Copeman's
Textbook of the Rheumatic Diseases

To all patients with rheumatic diseases, who hopefully await the progress of medical research, together with the generation of young clinicians and scientists throughout the world whose efforts are bent to their relief, this book is respectfully dedicated.

Copeman's Textbook of the Rheumatic Diseases

EDITED BY

J. T. Scott MD FRCP
Consultant Physician, Charing Cross Hospital, London; Honorary Physician, Kennedy Institute of Rheumatology, London

SIXTH EDITION

VOLUME ONE

CHURCHILL LIVINGSTONE
EDINBURGH LONDON MELBOURNE AND NEW YORK 1986

CHURCHILL LIVINGSTONE
Medical Division of Longman Group UK Limited

Distributed in the United States of America by Churchill Livingstone Inc., 1560 Broadway, New York, N.Y. 10036, and by associated companies, branches and representatives throughout the world.

First Edition 1948
Second Edition 1955
Third Edition 1964
Fourth Edition 1969
Reprinted 1970
Fifth Edition 1978
Sixth Edition 1986

ISBN 0 443 02689 0 (2 vols)

British Library Cataloguing in Publication Data
Copeman, William Sydney Charles
Copeman's textbook of the rheumatic diseases. — 6th ed.
1. Rheumatism
I. Title II. Scott, J. T.
616.7'23 RC927

Library of Congress Cataloging in Publication Data
Copeman, W. S. C. (William Sydney Charles), 1900–
Copeman's Textbook of the rheumatic diseases.
Includes bibliographies and index.
I. Rheumatism. I. Scott, J. T. (James Thomas)
II. Title. III. Title: Textbook of the rheumatic diseases. [DNLM: 1. Arthritis. 2. Collagen Diseases. 3. Rheumatism. WE 140 C782te]
RC927.C65 1986 616.7'23 85-19449

Printed and bound in Hong Kong
by Mandarin Offset Marketing (HK) Ltd.

Preface to the Sixth Edition

The continuing growth of rheumatology as a scientific clinical discipline within the framework of general internal medicine has now led to its recognition as such by clinicians in other fields, and to an increasing number of rheumatological textbooks and journals. We are now living in an age when basic science — especially molecular biology — is elucidating the mechanisms of health and disease to an extent undreamt of a decade or two ago. It has been generally felt that 'Copeman' — the authoritative British reference work on the rheumatic diseases — should keep pace with such progress in the form of yet a further edition.

Readers of previous editions will see that many of the sections and chapters — some of them classical contributions to rheumatological literature — have been updated but are essentially unchanged. There has again, however, been renewal and expansion: 46 chapters in the Fifth Edition, 69 in the Sixth Edition.

Two entirely new sections have been incorporated. Rapid developments in drug treatment have justified a section on clinical pharmacology as related to the rheumatic diseases; and a section on topographical rheumatology (regional disorders) allows a discussion of localised problems more conveniently than in previous editions.

Apart from the chapters in these sections, other new chapters have been written on a diversity of topics which seem to require more individual consideration than given previously: differential diagnosis of arthritis, biochemistry of connective tissue, examination of synovial fluid, immunogenetics in relation to the rheumatic diseases, metabolic bone disease, arthritis and blood disease, osteonecrosis, overlap syndromes, Sjögren's syndrome and imaging techniques.

A chapter on this last rapidly developing field is certainly justified; but I have continued to withhold a chapter on conventional radiology, since radiographic examples are amply provided in the various clinical chapters.

These changes have meant corresponding changes in the team of contributors, rather too numerous to mention individually. Two or three have retired to the touchline, some have changed their positions in the field, and there has been an influx of new young players of great potential.

Much as I hope and believe that this further edition will maintain and even enhance the reputation of the book, I have nevertheless come, during my editorship of the Fifth and Sixth Editions, to recognise two serious constraints in textbooks of this kind, with their ever-increasing authorship.

In the first place, writers on topics which are to some extent interrelated are bound to cover ground of common interest. I have tried to eliminate redundancies, discrepancies and contradictions as far as possible, but I hesitate to destroy the balance of a carefully written essay. And such essays, rather than mere reference chapters, have come to be a feature of the book. It therefore transpires that 'overlap syndromes' are something of a problem not only in the practice of clinical rheumatology but in the very books in which they are described.

A more serious difficulty is that of time. So much happens, so quickly. Dr Samuel Johnson wrote in his preface to his *Dictionary of the English Language* (1755), '. . . no dictionary of a living tongue can ever be perfect, since while it is hastening to publication, some words are budding, some falling away . . .'. If Johnson felt this about relatively static things like words, how much more do his comments apply to mobile scientific thoughts? The elucidation of immunogenetic mechanisms is no doubt 'budding'. Focal sepsis, at any rate in its conventional sense, has 'fallen away', but the concept has come alive again in discussions of reactive arthritis and seronegative spondarthritis. A lot can happen while the collective wisdom of 68 contributors hastens to publication.

I must again thank all my distinguished friends who have contributed to the book, to the staff of Churchill Livingstone for their efficient collaboration, and to my secretary Mrs Sheila Webber Spry, whose prodigious efforts have successfully seen the work to fruition.

London, 1986

J. T. Scott

Contributors

Barbara M. Ansell CBE MD FRCS FRCP
Consultant Rheumatologist, Wexham Park Hospital, Slough; Head, Division of Rheumatology, and Consultant Rheumatologist, Clinical Research Centre, Northwick Park Hospital, Harrow

Elizabeth M. Badley DPhil MSc
Deputy Director of the Arthritis and Rheumatism Council Epidemiology Research Unit, University of Manchester Medical School

J. Ball BSc MD FRCPath
Emeritus Professor of Osteo-articular Pathology, Department of Rheumatology, University of Manchester

Marilyn L. Baltz PhD
Senior Research Officer, MRC Acute Phase Protein Research Group, Immunological Medicine Unit, Royal Postgraduate Medical School, Hammersmith Hospital, London

Colin G. Barnes BSc FRCP
Consultant Physician, Department of Rheumatology, The London Hospital

H. Berry MA MRCP
Consultant in Rheumatology Rehabilitation, King's College Hospital, London

David Blake MRCP
Consultant Senior Lecturer, Department of Rheumatology, University of Birmingham

A. C. Boyle MD FRCP
Formerly Director, Rheumatology Department, The Middlesex Hospital, London

K. Alun Brown BSc PhD
Research Fellow, Department of Immunology, The Rayne Institute, St Thomas' Hospital, London

W. Watson Buchanan MD FRCP(Glas) FRCP(Ed) FRCP(C) FACP
Professor of Medicine and Regional Coordinator of Rheumatology, Department of Medicine (Rheumatology), McMaster University Health Sciences Centre, Chedoke-McMaster Hospitals, Hamilton, Ontario

E. G. L. Bywaters CBE MD(Liege) FRCP FRCP(C) FACP FRCS(C)
Emeritus Professor of Rheumatology, Royal Postgraduate Medical School, Hammersmith Hospital, London

E. D. R. Campbell FRCP
Consultant Rheumatologist, Royal Free Hospital, London

M. Anne Chamberlain BSc FRCP
Consultant Physician in Rehabilitation Medicine and Honorary Senior Lecturer, School of Medicine, University of Leeds

N. Christophidis PhD FRACP
Honorary Senior Registrar, St Bartholomew's Hospital, London

Mary Corbett FRCP
Consultant Rheumatologist, The Middlesex and Royal National Orthopaedic Hospitals, London

Charles F. Corke BSc MRCP
Research Registrar, St Bartholomew's Hospital, London

H. L. F. Currey MMed(Cape Town) FRCP
Professor of Rheumatology and Director of the Bone and Joint Research Unit, The London Hospital Medical College; Physician, Department of Rheumatology, The London Hospital

A. M. Denman FRCP
Head, MRC Connective Tissue Diseases Research Group, Clinical Research Centre, and Consultant Physician, Northwick Park Hospital, Harrow

W. C. Dick MD FRCP
Reader in Rheumatology and Honorary Consultant Physician, Royal Victoria Infirmary, Newcastle upon Tyne

Paul Dieppe BSc FRCP
Senior Lecturer (Rheumatology), University of Bristol; Consultant Rheumatologist, Bristol Royal Infirmary

Allan St J. Dixon MD FRCP
Consultant Physician, Royal National Hospital for Rheumatic Diseases, Bath; Visiting Professor, University of Bath

David V. Doyle MD FRCP(I)
Consultant Physician and Rheumatologist, Whipps Cross Hospital, London; Honorary Consultant Rheumatologist, St Bartholomew's Hospital, London

D. C. Dumonde MA PhD MD(Cantab) FRCPath CChem FRSC
Professor of Immunology, St Thomas' Hospital and Medical School, University of London

D. L. Gardner MD PhD(Ed) FRCP FRCPath
Professor of Histopathology, University of Manchester

T. Gibson MD FRCP
Consultant Physician, Department of Rheumatology, Guy's Hospital, London

Rodney Grahame MD FRCP
Consultant Rheumatologist, Guy's Hospital, London

Ian Griffiths BSc FRCP
Consultant Rheumatologist, Royal Victoria Infirmary and Freeman Hospital, Newcastle upon Tyne

Michael Gumpel FRCP
Consultant Physician (Rheumatology), Northwick Park Hospital, Harrow

E. B. D. Hamilton FRCP
Consultant Physician, Department of Rheumatology, King's College Hospital, London

Timothy E. Hardingham PhD DSc
Deputy Head, Biochemistry Division, Kennedy Institute of Rheumatology, London

Ian Haslock MD
Consultant Rheumatologist, South Tees District, Middlesbrough

Brian Hazleman MA FRCP
Associate Lecturer, Department of Medicine, University of Cambridge; Fellow of Corpus Christi College, Cambridge; Consultant Rheumatologist, Addenbrooke's Hospital, Cambridge, and Newmarket Hospital, Suffolk

E. J. Holborow MD(Cantab) FRCP FRCPath
Emeritus Professor of Immunopathology, The London Hospital Medical College

Peter John Lennox Holt FRCP(Ed) FRCP(Lond) DCH
Reader in Rheumatology and Physician in Charge, Rheumatism Research Centre, Manchester Royal Infirmary; Physician, Booth Hall Children's Hospital, Manchester

Graham R. V. Hughes MD(Lond) FRCP
Consultant Physician and Head of Rheumatology Unit, Hammersmith Hospital, London

E. C. Huskisson BSc MD FRCP
Consultant Physician and Senior Lecturer, St Bartholomew's Hospital, London

David B. Jack BSc PhD
Senior Lecturer, Department of Therapeutics and Clinical Pharmacology, The Medical School, University of Birmingham

Malcolm I. V. Jayson MD FRCP
Professor of Rheumatology, University of Manchester

David Katz BSc FRCR
Consultant Radiologist, Northwick Park Hospital and Clinical Research Centre, Harrow

Walter F. Kean MD FRCP(C) FACP
Associate Professor of Medicine, McMaster University Health Sciences Centre, Chedoke-McMaster Hospitals, Hamilton, Ontario

J. H. Kellgren MSc FRCS FRCP
Emeritus Professor of Rheumatology, University of Manchester

M. J. Kendall MD FRCP
Senior Lecturer in Therapeutics and Clinical Pharmacology, University of Birmingham; Honorary Consultant, Queen Elizabeth Hospital, Birmingham

J. K. Lloyd Jones MA FRCP
Consultant Rheumatologist, Harlow Wood Orthopaedic Hospital and Mansfield District General Hospital; Clinical Teacher, Nottingham University Medical School

Bruce Lynn PhD
Senior Lecturer in Physiology, University College London

R. N. Maini BA FRCP
Head, Division of Clinical Immunology, Kennedy Institute of Rheumatology, London; Professor and Head of Department of Immunology of Rheumatic Diseases, Charing Cross and Westminster Medical School; Honorary Consultant Physician, Charing Cross Hospital

J. A. Mathews MD FRCP
Consultant Physician, Department of Rheumatology, St Thomas' Hospital, London

R. Mitchell FRCR
Consultant Radiologist, Northwick Park Hospital

J. M. H. Moll BSc PhD FRCP
Consultant Physician in Rheumatology, and Head, Sheffield Centre for Rheumatic Diseases, Nether Edge Hospital, Sheffield; Honorary Clinical Lecturer in Rheumatic Diseases, University of Sheffield

Alastair G. Mowat FRCP(Ed)
Clinical Lecturer in Rheumatology, University of Oxford; Consultant Rheumatologist, Nuffield Orthopaedic Centre, Oxford

Helen Muir CBE MA DPhil DSc FRS
Head of Biochemistry Division and Director, Kennedy Institute of Rheumatology, London

A. B. Myles BA FRCP
Consultant Physician, Department of Rheumatology, St Peter's District General Hospital, Chertsey, Surrey

G. S. Panayi MD FRCP
Professor of Rheumatology, United Medical Schools, Guy's Hospital, London

M. B. Pepys MA MD PhD FRCP MRCPath
Professor of Immunological Medicine and Honorary Consultant Physician, Immunological Medicine Unit, Royal Postgraduate Medical School, Hammersmith Hospital, London; Head, MRC Acute Phase Protein Research Group

Philip N. Platt MRCP
Consultant Rheumatologist and Honorary Clinical Lecturer, Royal Victoria Infirmary, Newcastle upon Tyne

David G. I. Scott MD MRCP
Lecturer in Rheumatology, University of Birmingham

J. T. Scott MD FRCP
Consultant Physician, Charing Cross Hospital, London; Honorary Physician, Kennedy Institute of Rheumatology, London

M. H. Seifert FRCP
Consultant Physician, Department of Rheumatology, St Mary's Hospital, London

Michael L. Snaith MD FRCP
Consultant Rheumatologist, University College Hospital, London; Honorary Senior Lecturer, Faculty of Clinical Sciences, University College London

Trevor C. B. Stamp MD FRCP
Consultant Physician and Senior Lecturer, Royal National Orthopaedic Hospital and Institute of Orthopaedics, Brockley Hill, Stanmore, Middlesex

Michael W. Steward BSc PhD DSc FRCPath
Professor of Immunology, London University School of Hygiene and Tropical Medicine

Anthony K. Thould MD FRCP
Consultant Rheumatologist, Royal Cornwall Hospital (City), Truro, Cornwall

Patrick J. W. Venables MA MRCP
Lecturer in Immunology of the Rheumatic Diseases, Kennedy Institute of Rheumatology, and Charing Cross Hospital, London

Barrie Vernon-Roberts PhD MD MRCPath FRCPA FRCPath
Professor of Pathology, University of Adelaide; Head of Division of Tissue Pathology, Institute of Medical and Veterinary Science, Adelaide

Philip H. N. Wood FRCP FFCM
Director of the Arthritis and Rheumatism Council Epidemiology Research Unit, and Honorary Professor in Community Medicine, University of Manchester Medical School; Honorary Regional Specialist in Community Medicine, North Western Regional Health Authority, England

J. C. Woodrow MD FRCP
Consultant Rheumatologist, Royal Liverpool Hospital

V. Wright
Professor of Rheumatology, University of Leeds; Consultant Physician in Rheumatology, Leeds Western Health Authority, and Regional Rheumatology Centre, Royal Bath Hospital, Harrogate

D. A. H. Yates MD FRCP
Consultant Physician, Department of Rheumatology, St Thomas' Hospital, London; Consultant Rheumatologist, King Edward VII Hospital for Officers, London

D. B. Yates FRCP
Consultant Physician and Rheumatologist, Taunton and Somerset Hospitals, Taunton

Contents

Volume One

SECTION I: The Rheumatic Diseases

1. Historical 3
J. T. Scott
2. The basis of rheumatological practice, including nomenclature and classification 19
P. H. N. Wood
3. Epidemiology of individual rheumatic disorders 59
P. H. N. Wood E. M. Badley
4. Pain 143
B. Lynn J. H. Kellgren
5. The differential diagnosis of arthritis 161
A. St J. Dixon

SECTION II: Connective Tissue

6. Biochemistry of connective tissue 177
H. Muir T. E. Hardingham
7. Structure and function of connective tissue and joints 199
D. L. Gardner
8. Synovial fluid and its examination 251
B. Vernon-Roberts

SECTION III: Inflammation and Immunology in the Rheumatic Diseases

9. Inflammation 281
P. Dieppe D. Blake
10. Immunogenetics and rheumatic diseases 309
J. C. Woodrow
11. Immunological mechanisms and the rheumatic diseases 331
A. M. Denman
12. Autoantibodies in the rheumatic diseases 355
E. J. Holborow
13. Immune complexes and complement 376
R. N. Maini
14. The role of microbial infection in rheumatic disease 411
D. C. Dumonde M. W. Steward, K. A. Brown
15. Animal models of arthritis 468
H. L. F. Currey

SECTION IV: Clinical Pharmacology

16. The clinical pharmacokinetics of antirheumatic drugs 489
M. J. Kendall D. B. Jack
17. Salicylates 500
M. H. Seifert
18. Non-steroidal anti-inflammatory drugs 514
P. N. Platt W. C. Dick
19. Penicillamine, gold and antimalarials 525
H. Berry
20. Corticosteroids 535
A. B. Myles
21. Cytotoxic and immunomodulating drugs in the treatment of rheumatic diseases 547
C. F. Corke E. C. Huskisson N. Christophidis
22. Hypouricaemic drugs 569
T. Gibson
23. Intra-articular therapy 584
J. M. Gumpel

SECTION V: Rheumatoid Arthritis

24. The aetiopathogenesis of rheumatoid arthritis 595
G. S. Panayi
25. Pathology of rheumatoid arthritis 604
D. L. Gardner
26. Articular and systemic manifestations of rheumatoid arthritis 653
W. W. Buchanan W. F. Kean
27. The management of rheumatoid disease 706
M. Corbett

SECTION VI: Seronegative spondarthritis

28. Seronegative spondarthritides 723
J. M. H. Moll I. Haslock V. Wright
29. Ankylosing spondylitis 745
J. M. H. Moll
30. Psoriatic arthritis 775
V. Wright
31. Reiter's disease 787
V. Wright
32. Enteropathic arthritis 806
I. Haslock

Volume Two

SECTION VII: Osteoarthrosis

33. Aetiology and pathology of osteoarthrosis 821
J. Ball
34. Clinical aspects of osteoarthrosis 846
D. Doyle
35. Management of osteoarthrosis 874
D. Doyle

SECTION VIII: Metabolic Disease

36. Gout 883
J. T. Scott
37. Pyrophosphate arthropathy 938
E. B. D. Hamilton
38. Arthritis in ochronosis, haemochromatosis and Wilson's disease 950
E. B. D. Hamilton
39. Endocrine disorders 959
P. J. L. Holt
40. Metabolic bone disease 992
T. C. B. Stamp
41. Amyloidosis 1024
M. B. Pepys M. L. Baltz

SECTION IX: Arthritis in Children

42. Rheumatic fever 1057
E. G. L. Bywaters
43. Juvenile chronic arthritis 1100
B. M. Ansell E. G. L. Bywaters
44. Other forms of arthritis in childhood 1125
B. M. Ansell

SECTION X: Other forms of Arthritis

45. Infective arthritis 1137
B. M. Ansell
46. Heritable disorders 1162
R. Grahame
47. Arthritis and blood disease 1177
P. J. L. Holt
48. Osteonecrosis 1207
I. D. Griffiths
49. Miscellaneous 1229
C. G. Barnes

SECTION XI: Inflammatory Disorders of Connective Tissue

50. Overlap syndromes and mixed connective tissue disease 1269
P. J. W. Venables
51. Polymyalgia rheumatica and giant cell arteritis 1278
B. Hazleman
52. Vasculitis 1292
D. G. I. Scott
53. Systemic lupus erythematosus 1325
G. R. V. Hughes
54. Polymyositis and dermatomyositis 1350
B. M. Ansell
55. Systemic sclerosis 1364
M. I. V. Jayson
56. Sjögren's syndrome 1386
M. L. Snaith

SECTION XII: Topographical Rheumatology (Regional Disorders)

57. Back pain, spondylosis and disc disorders 1407
M. I. V. Jayson
58. The neck and shoulder 1435
D. A. H. Yates
59. The upper limb 1448
H. L. F. Currey
60. Lesions of the lower limb 1455
J. K. Lloyd Jones

SECTION XIII: Physical Treatment, Rehabilitation and Surgical Treatment

61. Physical treatment of the rheumatic diseases 1483
J. A. Mathews
62. Rehabilitation in the rheumatic diseases 1497
M. A. Chamberlain
63. Surgical treatment of arthritis 1518
A. G. Mowat

SECTION XIV: Clinical and Laboratory Techniques

64. History taking and physical examination 1569
A. K. Thould
65. Clinical trials and therapeutic evaluation 1581
E. C. Huskisson
66. Arthroscopy, arthrography and synovial biopsy 1597
D. B. Yates
67. Injection techniques 1612
A. C. Boyle
68. Electrodiagnosis in the rheumatic diseases 1621
E. D. R. Campbell
69. Modern imaging techniques 1627
D. Katz R. Mitchell

Index **I1**

SECTION I

The Rheumatic Diseases

1

J.T. Scott

Historical

It may be true, as Edmund Bourke wrote, that you can never plan the future by the past, but most doctors take a lively interest in the history of their art, gleaning what they can about the patterns of disease in former times, their impact on society and methods of treatment once used, knowing that their own efforts will in due course also come under the scrutiny of posterity.

Traditional sources of medical history, derived from texts dating back to classical times, occasionally shine with the clarity of a Sydenham or Harvey, but their interpretation is often made difficult by the confused ideas of the writers (which is not, however, a prerogative of our ancestors), together with problems of retrieval, transcription and translation from original languages. Palaeopathology, which examines diseases in antiquity from evidence provided by skeletons and other ancient remains, is a more recent and objective method of study. Diseases of bones and joints in particular leave their traces upon skeletons from which information can be obtained about the antiquity of some of the rheumatic diseases and changes in pattern and severity over the centuries (Steinbock, 1976).

Some of the rheumatic diseases have been recognised since the 5th century BC. The term 'rheumatism', derived from the Greek 'ρευμα' meaning a stream or flow, appears to have been introduced in medieval times to designate pain caused by a deranged flow from one of the four cardinal 'humours' — blood, phlegm, bile (choler) and black bile (melancholy) — which had been postulated by Galen in the 2nd century AD. Faulty humour from the blood was eliminated or discharged into one of the many cavities of the body including those of the joints. In this sense, of a humour dripping into a joint cavity, arose the word 'gout', by way of (Latin) 'gutta' — a drop.

'Rheumatism' no longer has any place in medical terminology, except that the term 'palindromic rheumatism' is used to designate a form of transient synovitis, of unknown cause, sometimes constituting the onset of rheumatoid arthritis. The term 'acute rheumatism', synonymous with 'rheumatic fever', has now passed out of usage. 'Arthritis' is an acceptable term, meaning simply inflammation of a joint, but unless qualified (rubella arthritis, tuberculous arthritis, etc.) tells nothing of the cause or type of joint inflammation.

Any physician, seeking honest and frank communication with his patient, has problems when confronted with the question, 'Do I have rheumatism, doctor?' I used to reply, 'I don't know what 'rheumatism' is', until a long-suffering lady retorted, 'Well, you certainly would if you had it'. A patient who is told by his doctor that he has 'rheumatism' is quite justified in asking for a more precise definition of his problem.

Out of this confusion we can still talk of the 'rheumatic diseases', expert knowledge of which is required by the rheumatologist. Rheumatology has been broadly defined by the International League against Rheumatism as follows: 'Rheumatology is a branch of medicine concerned with a heterogeneous group of diseases and disorders commonly affecting the locomotor system. They may arise from primary pathological processes in connective tissue structures, from disorders of their function, or as a manifestation of systemic disease. Their common denominator appears to be involvement of connective tissue. Although joints appear to be the main site of symptoms, the arthritis is only one component of a constitutional illness of considerable complexity.'

INFECTIVE ARTHRITIS

Various types of infective arthritis must have been common over the ages. A Saxon tibia has been described (Bourke, 1967), the shaft of which showed a sinus and changes typical of osteomyelitis, with evidence of suppurative arthritis proximally. Bourke quotes other examples, with comments on the difficulty of distinguishing with certainty infective from neuropathic joints in skeletal remains. In the Hippocratic Collection one Kriton is described as having pain in the great toe, which became red and swollen (Patrick, 1967); his death two days later indicates that infective arthritis with septicaemia was a more likely diagnosis than gout, an early exercise in the differential diagnosis of monarticular arthritis.

Signs of tuberculous arthritis in dried specimens of bones may be indistinguishable from those of other infectious or destructive diseases, but Morse (1967) reviews the extensive palaeopathological evidence for vertebral tuberculosis from prehistoric times onwards in the Old and New Worlds, and there are numerous descriptions of consumption in its various forms in the early literature. Copeman (1964) attributes the first sophisticated description of tuberculous arthritis to sergeant–surgeon Richard Wiseman (1622–1676) of Exeter, who recognised its scrofulous (tuberculous) association from the fact that lung disease often coexisted, together with enlarged lymph glands. Historical aspects of gonococcal arthritis and its differentiation from Reiter's syndrome are discussed by Benedek & Rodnan (1982).

The concept of bacterial infection which was developed in the 19th century has been followed — to a considerable extent — by its conquest during the 20th. Infective lesions can still be a difficult problem in the rheumatic diseases — when complicating rheumatoid arthritis, for example, or following the use of immunosuppressive drugs. Much remains to be learnt about various types of viral and fungal infection, and of course the possibility of some arcane type of infective process, in association with immunogenetic susceptibility, underlying the inflammatory disorders of connective tissue, constitutes today's central hypothesis in rheumatology.

RHEUMATIC FEVER

The Hippocratic writings (4th and 5th centuries BC) appear to describe rheumatic fever as an entity separate from gout, which may have been the form of arthritis most familiar to the Greeks: 'The joints become swollen and painful. The disease assumes an acute form and the pains, varyingly sharp, wander first from one articulation and later to another . . . the disease is short and acute, but not fatal. It usually attacks young people rather than the aged'.

Such a distinction, however, appears to have been largely ignored until the 17th century, the term 'arthritis' being used to designate any joint abnormality associated with pain (Copeman, 1964).

Guillaume de Baillou, of Paris, was the first modern medical writer to differentiate between gout and rheumatic fever, his posthumous work, *Liber de Rheumatismo*, being published in 1642 by his nephew. It was he who first used the term

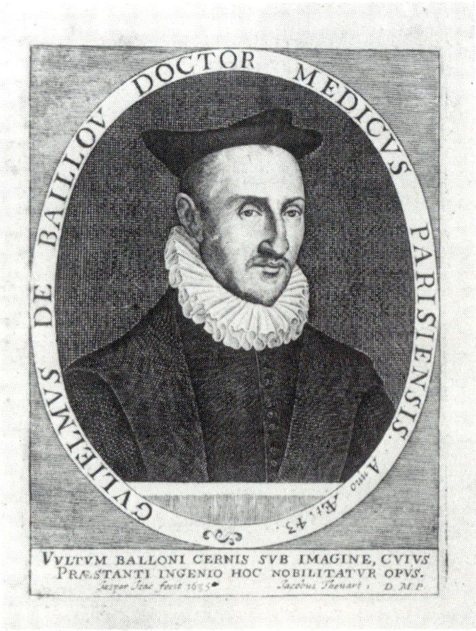

Fig. 1.1 Guillaume de Baillou (1538–1616). From an engraving by Jacques Thevart, after Jasper Isaac, dated 1635, in the Wellcome Institute of the History of Medicine, by courtesy of the Trustees.

'rheumatism' in the sense of an acute polyarthritis which has no connection with gout, and he is therefore often referred to as the 'Father of Rheumatism' (Fig. 1.1). In 1676 Thomas Sydenham (see Sydenham, 1848), the greatest English physician of his century, gave the first full description of acute rheumatism, from which an extract may be quoted. 'It is commonest . . . during the autumn, chiefly attacking the young and vigorous — those in the flower of their age'. After a few days 'the patient is attacked by severe pains in the joints — this pain changes its place from time to time, takes the joints in turn, and affects the one that it attacks last with redness and swelling'. Sydenham was also the first to describe chorea, and his name is still frequently attached to it although he did not connect it with the rheumatic diseases. His treatment of rheumatic fever was 'moderate' bleeding, ten ounces three or four times during the first week, combined with purgatives, rest in bed, and dieting.

William Heberden the Elder (1802) was one of the first to point out that rheumatic fever is largely a disease of childhood (Fig. 1.2). In his *Commentaries* he wrote; 'The rheumatism has appeared so early as in a child only four years old. I have seen several afflicted with it at the age of nine years; in which it differs from the gout, which I have never observed before the years of puberty'.

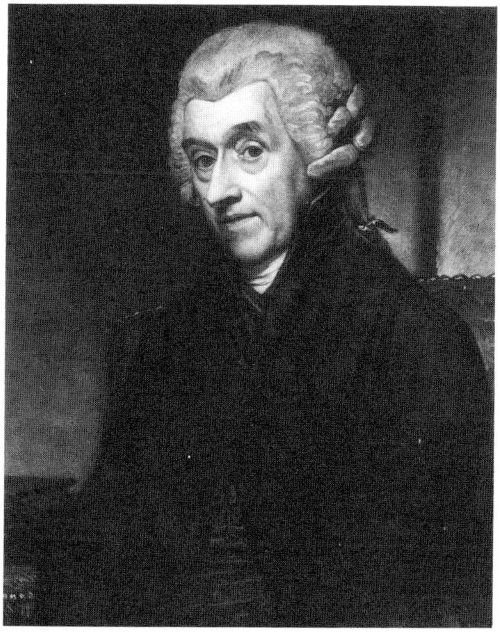

Fig. 1.2 William Heberden (1710–1801). From the mezzotint by James Ward after Sir William Beechey, in the Wellcome Institute of the History of Medicine, by courtesy of the Trustees.

William Cullen, who had been a pupil of Hermann Boerhaave of Leyden, in his Edinburgh lectures (1785) divided polyarthritis into 'two species, the one named the acute, the other the chronic rheumatism . . . although the limits between the acute and chronic rheumatism are not always exactly marked'. One can well understand the difficulty in distinguishing rheumatic fever from rheumatoid arthritis, at that time undescribed: rheumatic fever in those days was common and severe, and physicians may have seen the chronic subluxing arthropathy first described by Jaccoud (1869), which follows repeated attacks of rheumatic fever and which bears some clinical resemblance to rheumatoid arthritis, much more commonly than during recent years.

It was David Pitcairn, of St Bartholomew's Hospital, London, who first (in 1788) associated rheumatic fever with disease of the heart, a fact recorded by Mathew Baillie (1797) — a nephew of John Hunter — in his great work on morbid anatomy. This new knowledge resulted from the increasing practice of post-mortem examination. The following year Edward Jenner, the discoverer of vaccination, gave an address entitled 'Remarks on a disease of the heart following acute rheumatism, illustrated by dissection' although his manuscript was unfortunately lost. W.C. Wells (1812), an American by birth but later physician to St Thomas's Hospital and F.R.S. was the first to note the nodules of acute rheumatism. Sir Thomas Barlow and Dr Francis Warner (1881) emphasised their serious prognostic importance because of their association with progressive heart disease.

The French physician Bouillaud (1840), first described endocarditis, as distinct from pericarditis. He enunciated the view that heart disease is an intrinsic aspect of acute rheumatism, and not, as had previously been thought, an occasional complication. 'Rheumatism', he wrote, 'licks the joints but bites the heart'. In France rheumatic fever is still known as 'Bouillaud's disease'.

Subsequent to this a good deal of work was

carried out on the subject of rheumatic fever, chiefly in this country, culminating in the work of Dr Cheadle (1889) who was physician to St Mary's Hospital. He placed the wider view of this disease on a firm basis, saying that, 'in the rheumatism of early life arthritis is at its minimum: endocarditis, pericarditis, chorea and subcutaneous nodules at their maximum'. It was his pupil, F J Poynton, who instigated the modern approach to the problem of aetiology through the medium of bacteriology and immunology, although he failed to gain recognition for his 'diplococcus rheumaticus', which he believed to be causative of the disease. Aschoff (1904) described the specific miliary nodule of the myocardium which occurs in this disease and bears his name. Later work from the USA and elsewhere established that rheumatic fever is a sequel of Group A beta-haemolytic streptococcal infection.

Salicylate treatment for rheumatic fever was introduced by the Scottish physician Thomas MacLagan (1881), although unknown to him willow-bark had been used for rheumatic fever over a hundred years previously by the Reverend Edmund Stone who noted that, 'as this tree delights in a moist and wet soil where agues abound, the general maxim that natural maladies carry their cures with them . . . was so very appropriate that I could not help applying it'. More recent years have seen the introduction of corticosteroid hormones to supplement the use of salicylates, the treatment of streptococcal infection with penicillin, the prevention of recurrences by means of long-term antibiotic prophylaxis and surgical treatment of the late results of cardiac damage, in which the work of Blalock in the USA and Brock in England was pre-eminent. The dramatic decline in rheumatic fever in Western Europe and America has been associated with improved socioeconomic conditions, but in other parts of the world it remains one of the most important rheumatic diseases.

GOUT

Although, as we have seen, a certain amount of confusion has surrounded ancient descriptions of disease, particularly various forms of arthritis, there is no doubt that the lineage of gout extends down to us from antiquity and that the disorder was well recognised by writers of classical times.

Urate was identified in tophaceous deposits related to the feet of a skeleton in upper Egypt (Fig. 1.3) and an Egyptian mummy was found to contain a renal calculus with a nucleus of uric acid (Elliott-Smith & Dawson, 1924). Excavation of Roman and Saxon inhumations have shown, on direct inspection and radiography, lesions which were almost certainly gouty.

Gout is clearly described in Hippocratic writings (460–370 BC) as, 'the most violent, tenacious and painful of joint affections', non-fatal, often hereditary and frequently affecting the great toe. The Aphorisms (Adams, 1849) also refer to the rarity of gout in premenopausal women and boys, and to the immunity enjoyed by eunuchs, observations consistent, as far as they are applicable, with present-day experience. Gout also appears to have been common among the Romans, from the emperors downwards: the hands and feet of the emperor Galba (68–69 AD), for example, are said by the historian Suetonius to be so distorted that he could not endure a shoe for long, unroll a manuscript or even hold one. Cicero, Horace, Juvenal and Martial mention the disease and Galen (131–200 AD), physician to the emperor Marcus Aurelius, described gouty 'tophi' (Latin 'tophus' = 'porous stone').

The apparent frequency of gout in Romans is of interest. It has generally been ascribed to rich living and there is no doubt that immoderate eating and drinking were commonplace among the wealthy classes. Celsus (25 BC–50 AD) recognised this and stressed the importance of a regulated manner of living, the avoidance of corpulence and the need for moderate regular exercise. There may have been other factors, however. For example, Waldron (1982) reports a very high lead content in Romano-British bones from the excavations at Cirencester: 5% of samples contained an excess of 500μg/g, compared with a maximum modern concentration of 50μg/g, indicating exposure on a massive scale, presumably by ingestion, although excavations have given no clues as to how this occurred. Nriagu (1983) gives a detailed account of Roman enthusiasm for wine-drinking, pointing out how grape-syrup ('sapa'), boiled down slowly in lead pots, was used to

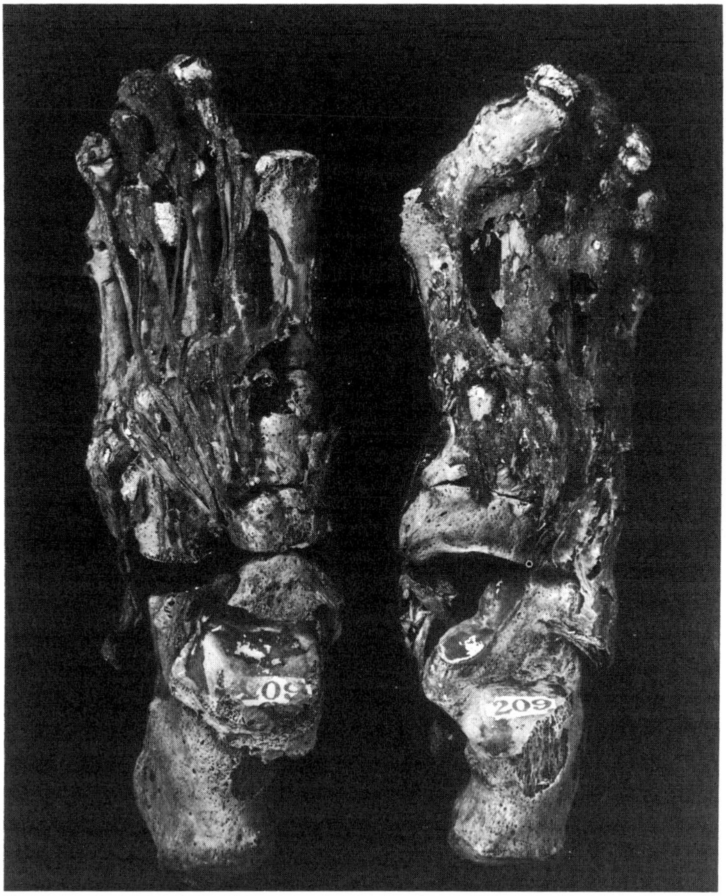

Fig. 1.3 Gouty feet from Upper Egypt. The white concretions were found to be composed of urate (Smith & Jones, 1910). Courtesy of Miss T I Molleson, Department of Palaeontology, British Museum (Natural History).

enhance the colour, sweetness and preservation of wine. Attempts to prepare sapa according to ancient recipes have produced lead concentrations of up to 1 g/l: one teaspoonful of such syrup would have been more than enough to cause chronic lead poisoning.

Early writings refer to podagra (Greek 'πους' 'foot', 'αγρα' = 'seizure') and cheiragra (Greek 'χειρ' = 'hand'). The word 'gout' itself, derived, as mentioned above, from the Latin gutta meaning a drop, was first used in its modern sense by Ralph Bocking, domestic chaplain to Saint Richard, Bishop of Chichester (1197–1258), who recounted that he was a great sufferer with 'gutta quam podagram vel arteticam vocant', cured by wearing a pair of the Bishop's boots (Copeman, 1964). Like other disorders, gout was considered to be caused by a disturbance in body fluids or humours, excess of which caused a gravitational flux particularly to the great toe: the word was also applied to a number of other affections which were remittent in character and so were considered to be of similar aetiology. Expressions such as 'a gouty stomach' or 'a gouty eczema' were in use until well into the present century, part of an underlying condition of the body (or 'diathesis') of which the joint trouble was only one manifestation.

Thomas Sydenham, himself a sufferer, gave such a detailed and accurate description of gout that it became possible to distinguish it from other types of arthritis. He subscribed to the humoral theory and referred to the 'impaired concoction of matters, both in the parts and the juices of the body', to which inactivity, gluttony and heavy drinking predisposed. The therapy advocated by sydenham was dietetic and cooling ('expectant'). The latter included moderate blood-letting, but not purging, a traditional form of treatment. Sydenham was not acquainted with colchicine, which had been extracted from the corm of a species of colchicum called 'hermodactyl' (finger of Hermes) by the Byzantine physician Alexander of Tralles (525–605 AD), and used to good effect in gout. Over the centuries the drug gradually passed into oblivion until its reintroduction by Storck of Vienna in 1763 and its popularisation as 'L'Eau d'Husson'.

Gout appears to have been very common in England during the 17th and 18th centuries and there is a formidable list of eminent victims — monarchs, politicians, scientists, physicians, clerics and men of letters. Satirical writers and caricaturists of these times did not fail to draw on such a rich source of material. The combinations of genetic and environmental factors which can contribute to gouty arthritis were well known at that time. Dr Samuel Johnson who described the pain of gout as 'the most diabolic to which man may be subjected' commented in 1773 that Dr William Cadogan's contemporary essay on the gout was foolish in maintaining that gout was not hereditary; the genetic basis of gout had been recognised by Galen. The parts played by food and drink were equally well appreciated. In 1840 the Reverend Sydney Smith wrote, 'What a singular disease gout it; it seems as if the stomach fell down into the foot. The smallest deviation from the right diet is immediately punished by limping and lameness, and the innocent ankle and blameless instep are tortured for the vices of the nobler organs.' And Sir Alfred Garrod (1859) (Fig. 1.4) in his classic review on gout: 'There is no truth in medicine better established than the fact that the use of fermented liquours is the most powerful of all the predisposing causes of gout.'

The same period, however, had seen the beginnings of the scientific study of purine metabolism and crystal synovitis. The appearance of urate crystals from a tophus were described by the Dutch microscopist Antonj van Leeuwenhoek in 1684 (McCarty, 1970). Scheele's discovery in Stockholm in 1776 of uric acid in a urinary calculus (lithic acid', Greek 'λιθος' = 'a stone'), was followed closely in 1797 by Wollaston's detection in London of the same substance from a gouty tophus. During the 19th century Sir Alfred Garrod demonstrated, by his famous thread test, that the blood of gouty subjects contained an excess of sodium urate which became deposited in crystalline form in the joints: such an excess could result from either increased formation or abnormal retention in the blood. The later work of Emil Fischer in 1889, establishing that uric acid was a purine compound and thus potentially related to the nucleic acid constituents adenine and guanine, and the improved methodology of uric acid determination in the blood described by Folin and Dennis in 1913 completed this part of the story.

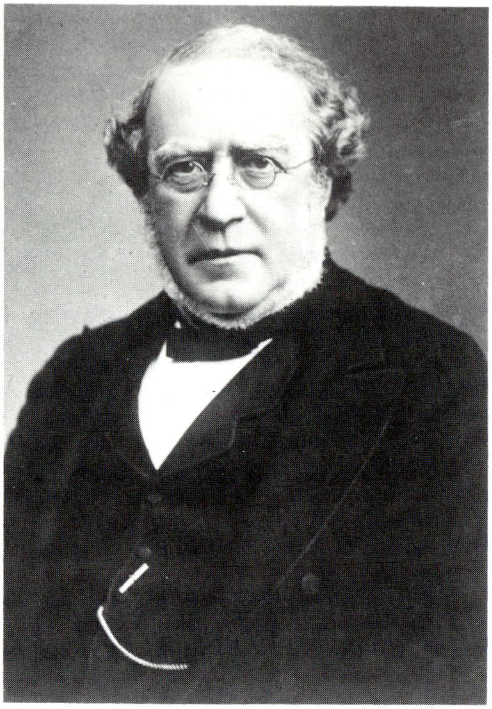

Fig. 1.4 Sir Alfred Garrod (1819–1907). From an original photograph in the Wellcome Institute of the History of Medicine, by courtesy of the Trustees.

Developments in recent years have included the realisation that hyperuricaemia and gout have many different causes; a swift advance, gained by biochemical, isotope and cell-culture techniques, in our knowledge of purine metabolism, including the discovery by Seegmiller and his colleagues in 1967 of the first specific enzymatic defect responsible for one special type of gout; the examination of joint fluid for crystals of urate as a routine diagnostic procedure (McCarty & Hollander, 1961); and, from the therapeutic aspect, a facility to control both the acute gouty attack and the level of uric acid in the blood, thus transforming this painful and crippling scourge of centuries into the most easily treatable of the rheumatic diseases.

Numerous articles on the history of gout, to which the reader is referred for further details, include those by Hartung (1957), Bywaters (1962), Copeman (1964), Rodnan (1965) and Talbott and Yü (1976).

OSTEOARTHROSIS

Osteoarthrosis (osteoarthritis) appears to be the commonest and best documented form of joint diseases to be encountered in palaeopathology (Fig. 1.5), a high frequency being described in numerous studies from different parts of the world (Bourke, 1967; Harman et al, 1981), although the pattern of disease has sometimes differed between series, e.g. the distribution of apophyseal osteoarthrosis in various parts of the vertebral column. There are also some differences observable between ancient forms and those of today: for example, the incidence of osteoarthrosis of the shoulder in relation to the hip in Saxon (Rogers

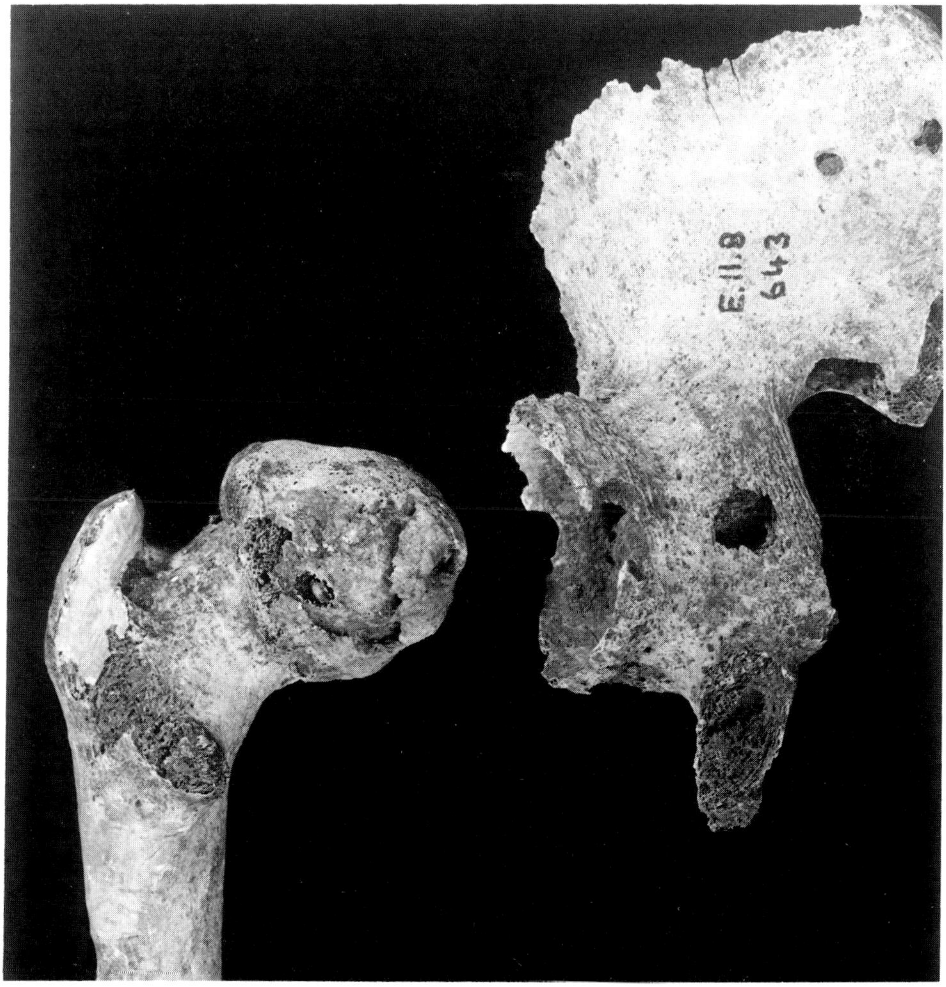

Fig. 1.5 Osteoarthritic hip from Romano-British cemetery at Cassington, Oxfordshire. Courtesy of Miss T I Molleson, Department of Palaeontology, British Museum (Natural History).

et al, 1981) and Romano-British (Wells, 1982) skeletons is far greater than is found in the UK today.

This type of joint disorder must therefore have been common throughout the ages, but lacking to some extent the striking clinical features of rheumatic fever and gout, its identification has been comparatively recent. The Hippocratic writings refer to 'an arthritis which seizes the great joints, which are able to contain it, but which does not usually go beyond there', but later writers such as Celsus do not appear to recognise the condition. In Sauvage's *Nosologia Methodica* (1763) there is a foretaste of the confusion in classification which, until lately, obscured the subject of arthritis. He divided 'gout' into fourteen varieties, and 'rheumatism' into ten. Osteoarthrosis would seem largely to correspond with his division 'rheumatismus arthriticus' — a form of 'gouty rheumatism' affecting chiefly large joints and showing no concretions.

William Heberden gave an account of osteoarthrosis in his *Commentaries*, calling particular attention to the fact that it has no connection with gout. He also described the small nodes which are usually called after him. His original description may be quoted:

'Digitorum Nodi. What are these little hard knobs, about the size of a small pea, which are frequently seen upon the fingers, particularly a little below the top near the joint? They have no connexion with the gout, being found in persons who never had it; they continue for life; and being hardly ever attended by pain, or disposed to become sores, are rather unsightly than inconvenient, though they must be of some little hindrance to the use of the fingers.'

Robert Adams of Dublin (1857) described two forms of chronic arthritis, one perhaps rheumatoid arthritis, involving the small joints of the extremities, the other, the larger joints 'either singly or in conjunction', a fair description of osteoarthrosis. He used the term 'malum coxae senilis' for osteoarthrosis of the hip, emphasising, however, that the disorder was confined to the aged. Nevertheless, Charcot (1881) failed to distinguish rheumatoid arthritis from osteoarthrosis and for many years the two conditions remained included in the overall term '*arthritis deformans*'. Charcot did, of course, recognise that special neuropathic form of osteoarthrosis which bears his name, correctly attributing it to the effects of syphilis.*

The designation 'osteoarthritis' appears first to have been used by Spender (1889) although he used the word synonomously with rheumatoid arthritis. However, Goldthwait (1904) pointed out that the findings are different in rheumatoid arthritis and osteoarthrosis, and proposed the names 'atrophic' and 'hypertrophic' arthritis. The distinction between the two diseases was made final by Sir Archibald Garrod's article in the 1907 issue of Allbutt and Rolleston's *System of Medicine*, in which he describes them separately, each with its own special pathology. Treatment throughout the 18th century was confined largely to guaiacum internally, and flannel worn externally, with Dover's powder for the relief of pain. Spa treatment was added during the 19th century as was aspirin. Later manipulation, intra-articular injection and physiotherapy were used with varying degrees of success, but the major development here has been the use of prosthetic hip replacement surgery, by Judet, Smith-Peterson, Charnley and other distinguished surgeons.

Current research into the biochemistry and biomechanics of cartilage will no doubt elucidate further the various forms of osteoarthrosis, but knowledge about aetiology — beyond 'unfair wear and tear', the importance of which has been known for many years — remains rudimentary.

RHEUMATOID ARTHRITIS

As Stockman (1920) and others have pointed out, from the earliest times until comparatively recently medical writers drew little or no distinction between the different types of 'chronic rheumatic arthritis', and today it is practically impossible to disentangle their descriptions. Nowhere in the writings of Hippocrates or Celsus, for example, do we find a description of rheumatoid arthritis comparable in clarity to that of gout. Caughey (1974), discussing the matter, makes a case for

* Not so well known is the fact that Charcot wrote two papers on *Joint Disease Secondary to Cerebral Disorders*. One described the neuropathic joint: the other is an excellent clinical and pathological description of the shoulder-hand syndrome (Charcot, 1868).

the Byzantine Emperor Constantine IX (980–1055 AD) being a victim: much earlier, the 'articularis morbus' which deformed the limbs of the Emperor Galba, and which is usually translated as 'gout', could equally well refer to rheumatoid arthritis.

Clues from palaeopathology are also scanty, recorded cases from ancient Egypt and elsewhere being few and of indeterminate authenticity (Bourke, 1967; Short, 1974; Steinbock, 1976; Buchanan & Murdoch, 1979; Rogers et al, 1981). As archaeologists point out, little attention had been paid in the past to detailed examination of small joints and future studies may produce more convincing evidence. Meanwhile, however, the case described by May (1897) dating from 5500 years ago, is highly suggestive of rheumatoid arthritis.

The paucity of archaeological findings, together with the absence of convincing early descriptions, either in literature or in medical writings, has raised the intriguing possibility that the disease is one of comparatively recent times, perhaps appearing from outer space as Hoyle (1983) has suggested in the case of smallpox and other virus diseases. Wood (1976), however, deals severely with such armchair speculation.

The first differentiation of the disease is usually attributed to Landré-Beauvais (1800), physician to the Salpêtrière Hospital in Paris, who published his observations as a thesis. He noticed that it mostly affected women, and described its most striking clinical features under the name of 'goutte asthénique primitive'. Sauvages (1763) had previously written of a secondary type of arthritis, which might follow acute rheumatism, forming swellings about the size of a nut on the fingers, but never forming concretions on the joints like gout. 'It is not', he pointed out, 'periodic in its attacks, but frequently has increasing light paroxysms which involve the hands, the feet and the knees. The fingers and hands become deformed and twisted and it lasts till death'. Heberden, in describing this type of arthritis, had commented upon the deterioration in the general health of the patient, as well as the local effects of contracture of the joints and muscles.

Garrod (1859) proposed the name 'rheumatoid arthritis' to replace the many aliases under which it was then spoken of, such as 'rheumatic gout', 'rheumatisme noueux', and 'chronic rheumatic arthritis'; and that name became widely adopted both in this and other countries. It is perhaps of interest to quote his reasons for doing so. He states that, 'the term rheumatic gout is given to a disease having a peculiar pathology in no way related to gout, and not necessarily to rheumatism — and which is sometimes termed chronic rheumatic arthritis'. He then says, '. . . Although unwilling to add to the number of names, I cannot help expressing a desire that one might be found for this disease . . . perhaps 'Rheumatoid Arthritis' would answer the object, by which term I should wish to imply an inflammatory affection of the joints not unlike rheumatism . . . but differing materially from it'. Bannantyne (1896) published a treatise on the pathological changes found in this disease, although he only finally differentiated it from osteoarthrosis in the fourth edition of his book in 1906. Strangeways (1907), under the auspices of the Cambridge Committee for the Study of Special Diseases, increased our knowledge of the pathology of rheumatoid arthritis and resuscitated the theory that the changes might be due to infection, a theory propounded by Bouchard (1891) who had pointed out that polyarthritis might be a sequel to a number of infections as diverse as gonorrhoea, dysentery and scarlet fever. The theory of focal sepsis was introduced by William Hunter (1901), and further popularised by Sir William Willcox (1935).

In 1896, G. F. Still, of Great Ormond Street children's Hospital, London, read a paper, *On a form of chronic joint disease in children*, basing his observations on 22 cases. Shortly afterwards this syndrome was described independently by Chauffard in France, where this form of juvenile rheumatoid arthritis is known as Chauffard–Still's disease. In 1924 A. R. Felty described five adult cases of rheumatoid arthritis in whom the spleen and lymphatic glands were enlarged, together with reduction in the white cell count, seen by him at Johns Hopkins Hospital — 'Felty's syndrome'.

The era of intensive investigation into the immunological aspects of rheumatoid arthritis and some related diseases may be said to have commenced with the independent discovery of rheumatoid factor by Waaler (1940) and by Rose and his colleagues (1948), the latter simultaneous with that of the L. E. cell test (Hargraves et al, 1948). The subsequent identification of various antinuclear antibodies shed further light on pathogenetic mechanisms and encouraged an integrated approach to rheumatoid arthritis and other inflammatory disorders of connective tissue — such as systemic lupus erythematosus — a concept which had been previously advanced by Klemperer et al (1942) who had used the term 'collagen disease' applied to lupus and scleroderma. More recent work on complement, immune complexes and cell-mediated immunity has had a direct bearing on rheumatoid arthritis, but underlying causes remain obscure and the possibility of infection is by no means discarded. For brief accounts of historical aspects of the inflammatory disorders of connective tissue, see Benedek & Rodnan (1982).

With regard to the treatment of chronic inflammatory arthritis, Sauvages recommended sulphur and other baths, whilst Haygarth (1805) added warm douching, and guaiacum internally, although he stated that no treatment is of much value. Heberden advised mild tonic treatment, with opium for pain. Rest, aspirin and physiotherapy were introduced early in this century.

Jacques Forestier (1935) published his favourable impression of treatment with gold salts which he had introduced in the belief that rheumatoid arthritis and tuberculosis shared a common aetiology, gold at that time being a fashionable remedy for tuberculosis and other infectious diseases, though it was a number of years before the value of gold in rheumatoid disease was demonstrated by controlled trials (Empire Rheumatism Council, 1961). The discovery that disease activity could be controlled by the use of cortisone was made by Hench & Kendall in 1948 (see Polley & Slocumb, 1976). Since then a variety of synthetically prepared non-steroidal anti-inflammatory drugs have been introduced. Further active therapeutic agents include antimalarials, penicillamine and immunoreactive compounds, but their toxicity makes extremely careful supervision mandatory. A major development in recent years has been the application of surgical procedures.

SPONDARTHRITIDES

In contrast to rheumatoid arthritis, many cases of ankylosing spondylitis have been reported from Egyptian skeletal material and from remains in many other parts of the world (Steinbock, 1976). It is true that there may have been some confusion about the different entities of ankylosing spondylitis and hyperostosis, but radiographs of Egyptian vertebral columns (Bourke, 1967) leave little doubt about the existence of ankylosing spondylitis in ancient times. This may not however reflect a higher prevalence of ankylosing spondylitis compared with rheumatoid arthritis: appearances of the disease are more easily recognisable in skeletons than those of rheumatoid disease. The age of onset is generally lower than that of rheumatoid arthritis, which would favour its relative predominance in short-lived populations.

The historical aspects of ankylosing spondylitis are set out in detail by Copeman (1964) and Bywaters (1980), while Francois (1976) gives a list of twenty-two synonyms with their respective authors, writing between 1897 and 1964. The anglicised form of the term recommended by Humphrey Rolleston in 1933 — 'spondylitis ankylopoietica' — is that which is now universally accepted.

Hippocratic writings, the 5th century Byzantine physician Caelius Aurelianus, the 16th century anatomist Realdo Colombo and Thomas Sydenham all described conditions corresponding to some extent with the clinical picture of the disease, but the present profuse literature on the subject starts with the description by the Irishman Bernard Connor in 1691 of a skeleton which he found in a graveyard while he was demonstrating anatomy in France, and which showed advanced stages of spondylitis. During the 19th century a number of cases were described, the best known being of Strümpell (Berlin) in 1884, Bechterew (St Petersburg) in 1897 and Marie (Paris) in 1898, who described nearly every feature of ankylosing spondylitis, which he called 'la spondylose rhizomélique'.

Because of the frequent involvement of peripheral joints, with clinical, radiological and pathological similarities to rheumatoid arthritis, ankylosing spondylitis came for a time, particularly in the USA, to be regarded as a 'variant' of rheumatoid disease, the term 'rheumatoid spondylitis' being a particular source of confusion. With the realisation that patients with ankylosing spondylitis were seronegative — that is, they did not have IgM rheumatoid factor — together with the appreciation of many obvious clinical and pathological differences, the separate identities of the two diseases were finally confirmed.

Rather has the overlap been with Reiter's disease, psoriatic arthritis and enteropathic arthritis, which may share features such as sacroiliitis and the various non-articular manifestations. Post-venereal urethritis, arthritis and conjunctivitis were described together by Sir Benjamin Brodie (1818). During the First World War, Reiter (1916) on the Balkan front and Fiessinger & Leroy (1916) on the Western front described the triad following dysentery. References to psoriasis associated with arthritis also appeared during the 19th century.

The remarkably close association between the presence of the histocompatibility antigen HLA B27 with ankylosing spondylitis, Reiter's disease and anterior uveitis, together with the concept of 'reactive arthritis' has been the latest chapter in the story.

NON-ARTICULAR RHEUMATISM

Hippocrates refers to; 'Those lighter pains which have no evident association with podagra and do not cause swellings', but little more is heard of non-articular pain until the 17th century.

The distinction between gout and acute rheumatism was made by Sydenham, and he mentions in connection with the latter a chronic form of 'scorbutical rheumatism' which will last for months and years, 'Nay, it will torment a patient throughout his miserable lifetime'. He also described lumbago as a third variety of rheumatism.

Frederick Hoffman (1729) initiated the tendency to refer to any kind of shifting pain as rheumatic; a tendency which has not yet died out entirely. He refers to 'scorbutic, dental, venereal, and other rheumatisms', evidently losing sight of rheumatism as a disease entity and using it as a synonym for pain. Sauvages de la Croix, in his great work on medical classification published in 1763, defined the word 'rheumatism' as a generic term for many diseases affecting the muscles and accompanied by pain and disability. He recognised that in these conditions the joints might become involved also, but thought that this was a secondary effect from affection of the muscle tendons inserted into or near them.

William Cullen (1785) divided the rheumatic diseases into acute and chronic rheumatism of joints and of muscles, whilst he dismissed all other forms of so-called 'rheumatic' pains as being symptomatic of other disease processes. He considered the primary causation to be cold, and not 'that peculiar acrimony' of the humours which has been mentioned as being the medieval idea of the aetiology of rheumatism.

Sciatica was generally considered by such authorities as Andrew Boorde (1575), physician to King Henry VIII, to be a manifestation of implication of the joints of the lumbar vertebrae or hip joint in gout or acute rheumatism. In Naples, Dominicus Cotunnius, or Cotugno (1764), published a booklet distinguishing for the first time two varieties: one due to swelling or irritation of the sciatic nerve — 'ischias nervosa' — and the other arising from inflammation of the hip joint. The role of the intervertebral disc in the causation of sciatica was described in Glasgow and Boston USA independently, in the early years of the present century.

The first systematic treatise on chronic rheumatism was published by Scudamore (1816). He asserted definitely that its true morbid anatomy was an inflammation affecting the white fibrous tissues of the body. He held that the fleshy parts of the muscles were not affected, but that the pain arose from their inflamed tendinous and fibrous parts being dragged upon. He defined chronic muscular rheumatism as 'pains affecting the ligamentous and tendinous textures, synovial membranes and nerves, without external signs of inflammation, and unaccompanied by fever but aggravated by motion'.

It was William Balfour (1816) of Edinburgh who first seems to have mentioned the occurrence of indurated 'nodules'. He pointed out that these were tender on pressure and that pains shot from them to neighbouring parts. His method of treatment was to apply to these nodules 'friction, percussion and compression'. Scudamore was also familiar with these nodules and pointed out that it is often 'impossible to effect a cure without the aid of friction and shampooing'. Throughout the military campaigns of the 18th century we find it recorded that 'muscular rheumatisms without fever' were a great waster of manpower.

Sir William Gowers (1904) proposed the name 'fibrositis' for this condition, since he believed the aetiology always to be an inflammation of the white fibrous tissues. This hypothesis was supported by Stockman (1904) of Glasgow with an account of the histology and structure of fibrous indurations which he had removed from sufferers. Such descriptions, however, were few in number and 'fibrositis' never achieved a place in scientific medical terminology. In recent years attempts have been made to revive the idea (Campbell et al, 1983).

Aetiologically chronic rheumatism was in earliest times attributed to an 'acrimony' between the 'humours' of the body. Later it was thought to be due to cold, and by some to a rigidity or atony of the muscular and fibrous tissues. Irritation and spasm of the muscles was also advanced as a cause, whilst Fuller (1854) argued that the real factor must be a general blood toxaemia, determined possibly by the action of cold, damp, and dietic factors. A little later Haig (1903) launched his theory, which enjoyed a short-lived popularity, that the cause was an excess of lactic or uric acid in the blood and tissues.

Treatment for chronic rheumatism remained the same as that for rheumatic fever and gout until these entities were separated finally in the 19th century. Bleeding, purging, dieting, and rest remained the keynotes. Some authors recommended sweating, whilst others recommended cold baths. Spa treatment was used by the Romans, and probably also by the Greeks before them; and physical methods of treatment in these centres may have approximated to modern practice so far as hydrotherapy, counter-irritation, soothing local applications, and massage are concerned. The drugs in use in the 18th and 19th centuries included sulphur, guaiacum, colchicum, quinine and others, whilst the beneficial effects of a dry climate and a cheerful nature are mentioned by Andrew Boorde.

Recent years have seen some progress in our understanding of the problem. It is recognised that a multiplicity of factors may precipitate pains of this nature, from minor trauma and nerve irritation to connective tissue disorders such as polymyositis and systemic lupus erythematosus. The syndrome known as 'polymyalgia rheumatica', often accompanied by temporal arteritis, has been defined as a common cause for musculoskeletal pain in the elderly, and current investigations will doubtless soon throw light on its aetiology. Our concept of many other forms of non-articular rheumatism, however, remains extremely unsatisfactory.

THE DEVELOPMENT OF RHEUMATOLOGY

Because many of the rheumatic diseases manifest themselves as chronic, painful disorders of the musculoskeletal system, lacking, at least until recently, adequate methods of prevention and treatment, their victims, not unnaturally, have concerned themselves with such palliative and symptomatic forms of physical therapy as are to be found at spas and similar centres. Nor is this in itself necessarily to be condemned: whatever the shortcomings of old-type cures and watering-places, properly applied physical treatment, with its modern tendency towards self-reliance often in a group environment, engenders a more positive reaction to illness and disability than does the consumption of pills, and the morbidity and mortality of balneotherapy (accidental or suicidal) is surely less than that of salicylates and other drugs which we prescribe so readily.

Such forms of treatment undoubtedly had a considerable influence on the early development of rheumatology. In 1931, for example, the Section of Balneology and Climatology of the Royal Society of Medicine joined with the Section of Electrotherapeutics to form the Section of Physical Medicine, which in 1973 became that of Rheumatology and Rehabilitation.

There have however been other influences, which can now be seen to have exerted a much more profound effect, such as the founding of academic departments (the first Chair in Rheumatology was established at Manchester in 1953), or similar units, which have contributed to the training of large numbers of rheumatologists throughout the world, besides stimulating research and setting exemplary standards of clinical practice. Within the framework of modern rheumatology have evolved many of the advances in clinical immunology and epidemiology, together with concepts of scientific clinical techniques such as the design of therapeutic trials and establishment of diagnostic criteria. Arguments about the historically-determined association of rheumatology with the important but separate problem of general medical rehabilitation are becoming resolved, although they may for some time be settled by local or individual circumstances. Certainly rheumatologists, who tend to concern themselves with the whole care of their patients, thereby set an example to their colleagues in other specialities. What is beyond dispute is the necessity for the discipline to advance as an integral part of internal medicine: as such it is now gaining momentum and attracting able recruits.

Along with these developments in the clinical field, national and international organisations have been established to initiate and co-ordinate the fight against the rheumatic diseases. The modern renaissance in these diseases and their prevention can be dated to papers such as Glover's (1927) Report on Chronic Rheumatism to the British Ministry of Health, and to the formation of the Committee on Chronic Rheumatic Diseases by the Royal College of Physicians in 1935. This formed the nucleus of the Arthritis and Rheumatism Council, which today supports much of the research and education in rheumatic diseases in this country, and to which the credit should be given of having made the Government aware of the great social and industrial importance of this group of diseases in Great Britain. The British League against Rheumatism consists of scientific and community sections, representing the medical and other health professions, patients and voluntary bodies. Affiliated organisations include the Arthritis and Rheumatism Council, the British Rheumatism and Arthritis Association (primarily concerned with patient welfare) and the British Council for Rehabilitation of the Disabled.

The International League against Rheumatism (ILAR) was formed in 1927, with Jan van Breemen of the Netherlands as one of its principal founders and first Secretary-General (Fig. 1.6). This was well before the present constitutent regional leagues EULAR (European League against Rheumatism), PANLAR (Pan American League against Rheumatism) and SEAPAL (South-East Asia and Pacific Area League against Rheumatism). The original function of ILAR and the regional leagues was to organise international scientific congresses every four years, but as part of the new constitution of 1974, six co-ordinated standing committees were set up:

1. *International and National Agencies*, co-ordinating ILAR's work with that of other international agencies and WHO.
2. *Education*, collecting data on education of rheumatologists and ancillary personnel and ident-

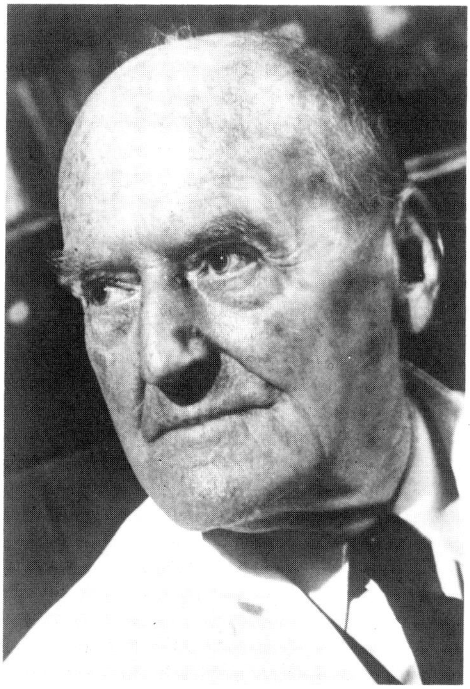

Fig. 1.6 Dr Jan van Breemen (1874–1961).

ifying areas where improvements can be made.
3. *Publications*, dealing with the ILAR *Handbook of Rheumatology* and any other publications issued with the authority of ILAR.
4. *Epidemiology*, studying rheumatic diseases in communities, nomenclature and diagnostic criteria.
5. *International Clinical Studies*, co-ordinating clinical trials to avoid reduplication and setting up reference centres on diagnostic criteria and laboratory tests, in collaboration with WHO.
6. *Social and Community Agencies*, developing parallel national, social and community agencies responsible for fund-raising, research, patient welfare, education and pressure on governmental departments to produce resources.

Coinciding with the fiftieth anniversary of its foundation, ILAR, together with its regional leagues, and with the support of WHO, designated 1977 as World Rheumatism Year, during which widespread activities were undertaken by all sections of the community aimed at increasing our knowledge of the rheumatic diseases, improving availability and quality of care in all its aspects and developing research policies.

Rheumatologists in most developed nations have also organised national scientific societies. Largest among these is the American Rheumatism Association, but equally virile, though smaller, associations have been formed in many other countries, In the UK, the Heberden Society was founded in 1936 and has played a leading part in advancing rheumatology in this country and overseas. However, a British Association of Physical Medicine was formed in 1942, becoming the British Association for Rheumatology and Rehabilitation (BARR) in 1970. The two bodies at first represented different interests and viewpoints, but in recent years the content of the meetings of BARR came to resemble more closely that of the larger Heberden Society. BARR also assumed the role of a professional association, a field of activity never really attempted by the Heberden Society. There has been increasing common membership between the two societies, and a good deal of pressure, particularly among younger members, for their replacement by a single society. In this way the British Society for Rheumatology has been formed in 1984 although the honoured name of William Heberden will be perpetuated in the Heberden Oration, the Heberden Round and the Heberden Library at the Royal College of Physicians, London.

REFERENCES

Adams F (translator) 1849 The genuine works of Hippocrates. Sydenham Society, London

Adams R 1857 Treatise on rheumatic gout, or chronic rheumatic arthritis, of all the joints. Churchill, London

Aschoff L 1904 Zur Myocarditisfrage. Verhandlungen der Deutschen Pathologischen Gesellschaft 8: 46–53

Baillie M 1797 The morbid anatomy of some of the most important parts of the human body, 3rd Edn. London

Baillou Guillaume de 1642 Liber de rhumatismo. J Quesnel, Paris. Translated into English by C C Barnard 1940 British Journal of Rheumatism 2: 141–162

Balfour W 1816 Observations with cases illustrative of a new, simple and expeditious mode of curing rheumatism and strains. Edinburgh

Bannantyne G A 1896 Rheumatoid arthritis: its pathology, morbid anatomy and treatment. Wright, Bristol

Barlow Sir Thomas, Francis Warner. On subcutaneous nodules connected with the fibrous structures occurring in children, the subjects of rheumatism and chorea. Transactions of the International Medical Congress, London, 2–9 August 1881. Session 7, 4:46H

Bechterew V M 1897 Deutsche Zeitschrift für Nervenheilkunde 11: 327–337

Benedek T G, Rodnan G P 1982 A brief history of the rheumatic diseases. Bulletin on the Rheumatic Diseases 32: 59–68

Boorde A 1575 The breviary of healthe. Thomas East, London

Bouchard C 1891 Semaine Medicale (Paris) 11:387

Bouillaud J B 1840 Traite clinique due rheumatisme articulare et de la loi de coincidence des inflammations due coeur avec cette maladie. Bailliere, Paris

Bourke J B 1967 A review of the paleopathology of arthritic diseases. In: Brothwell D, Sandison A T (eds) Diseases in antiquity Charles C Thomas, Springfield, Illinois, pp 352–370

Brodie B C 1818 Pathologic and surgical observations on diseases and joints. Longman, London

Buchanan W W, Murdoch R M 1979 That rheumatoid arthritis will disappear. Journal of Rheumatology 6: 324–329

Bywaters E G L 1962 Gout in the times and person of George IV: a case history. Annals of the Rheumatic Diseases 21: 325–338

Bywaters E G L 1980 In: Moll J M H (ed) Ankylosing spondylitis. Churchill livingstone, Edinburgh

Caughey D E 1974 The arthritis of Constantine IX. Annals of the Rheumatic Diseases 33: 77–80

Campbell S M, Clark S, Tindall E A, Forehand M E, Bennett R M 1983 Clinical characteristics of fibrositis. I. A 'blinded', controlled study of symptoms and tender points. Arthritis and Rheumatism 26: 817–824

Charcot J M 1868 Sur quelques arthropathies qui paraissent dependre d'une lesion du cerveau ou de la moelle epiniere: deuxieme article. Archives de Physiologie Normal et Pathologique 1: 399–400

Charcot J M 1881 Clinical lectures on senile and chronic diseases. Translated by Tuke W S. New Sydenham Society, London

Cheadle W B 1889 The various manifestations of the rheumatic state as exemplified in childhood and early life. Smith, Elder, London

Connor B 1691 Sur la continuite de plusieurs os, a l'occasion d'une fabrique suprenante d'un tronc de squelette humain, ou les vertebres, les cotes, l'os sacrum, let les os des iles, qui naturellements sont distincts et separes, ne font qu'un seul os continu et inseperable. Rheims

Copeman W S C 1964 A short history of the gout and the rheumatic diseases. University of California Press, Berkeley & Los Angeles

Cotugno D (Contunnius) 1764 De ischiade nervosa commentarius. Frat Simonios, Naples

Cullen W 1785 Synopsis nosologiae methodicae. Creech, Edinburgh

Elliott-Smith G, Dawson W R 1924 Egyptian mummies. Allen & Unwin, London

Empire Rheumatism Council 1961 Gold therapy in rheumatoid arthritis: final report of a multicentre controlled trial. Annals of the Rheumatic Diseases 20:315

Fiessinger N, LeRoy E 1916 Bulletin et memoires Societë Medicale des Hopitaux, Paris 40: 2030–2069

Felty A R 1924 Chronic arthritis in the adult, associated with splenomegaly and leucopenia. Bulletin of Johns Hopkins Hospital 35: 16–20

Forestier J 1935 Rheumatoid arthritis and its treatment by gold salts. Journal of Laboratory and Clinical Medicine 20: 827–840

Francois R J 1976 Le rachis dans la spondylarthrite ankylosante. Editions Arscia SA, Bruxelles

Fuller H W 1854 On rheumatism, rheumatic gout and sciatica, their pathology, symptoms and treatment. Wood, New York

Garrod A B 1859 Nature and treatment of gout and rheumatic gout. Walton & Maberly, London

Goldthwait J E 1904 Bostom Medical and Surgical Journal 151: 529–534

Glover J A 1927 Ministry of Health Reports on Public Health and Medical Subjects, No. 44. HMSO, London

Gowers W R 1904 British Medical Journal 1: 117–121

Haig A 1903 Uric acid as a factor in the causation of disease. Churchill, London

Hargraves M M, Richmond H, Morton R 1948 Presentation of two bone marrow elements: the 'Tart' cell and the 'L.E.' cell. Proceedings of the Staff Meeting of the Mayo Clinic 23: 25–28

Harman M, Molleson T I, Price J L 1981 Burials, bodies and beheadings in Romano-British and Anglo-Saxon cemeteries. Bulletin of the British Museum of Natural History (Geol) 35: 145–188

Hartung E F 1957 Symposium on gout. Historical considerations. Metabolism 6: 196–208

Haygarth J 1805 A clinical history of acute rheumatism. Cadell & Davies, London

Heberden W 1802 Commentaries on the history and cure of disease. Payne, London

Hoffman F 1729 Opera omnia physico-medica. Fratres de Tournes, Genevae

Hoyle F 1983 From virus to cosmology. Journal of the Royal Society of Medicine 76: 99–111

Hunter W 1901 Oral sepsis as a cause of septic conditions. Cassell, London

Jaccoud F S 1869 Lecons de clinique medicale faites a l'Hopital de la Charite, 2nd, Edn. Delahave, Paris

Klemperer P, Pollack A D, Baehr G 1942 Diffuse collagen disease: acute disseminated lupus erythematosus and diffuse scleroderma. Journal of the American Medical Association 119: 331–332

Landré-Beauvais A J 1800 Doit-on admettre une nouvelle espece du goutte sous la demoniation de goutte asthenique primitive? Paris

Maclagan T J 1881 Rheumatism: its nature, its pathology and its successful treatment. Pickering, London

McCarty D J 1970 A historical note: Leeuwenhoek's description of crystals from a gouty tophus. Arthritis and Rheumatism 13: 414–418

McCarty D J, Hollander J L 1961 Identification of urate crystals in gouty synovial fluid. Annals of Internal Medicine 54: 452–460

Marie P 1898 Sur la spondylose rhizomëlique. Revue de Medicine, Paris 28: 285–315

May W P 1897 Rheumatoid arthritis (osteitis deformans) affecting bones 5,500 years old. British Medical Journal ii: 1631–1632

Morse D 1967 Tuberculosis. In: Brothwell D, Sandison A T (eds) Diseases in antiquity. Charles C Thomas, Springfield, Illinois, USA

Nriagu J O 1983 Saturnine gout among Roman aristocrats. New England Journal of Medicine 308: 660–663

Patrick A 1967 Diseases in antiquity: ancient Greece and Rome. In: Brothwell D, Sandison A T (eds) Diseases in antiquity. Charles C Thomas, Springfield, Illinois

Pitcairn D 1788 Cited by Baillie M 1797

Polley H F, Slocumb C H 1976 Behind the scenes with cortisone and ACTH. Mayo Clinic Proceedings 51: 471–477

Poynton F J, Paine A 1913 Researches on rheumatism. Churchill, London

Reiter H 1916 Ueber eine bisher unerkanate Spirochaeteninfektion (Spirochaetosis arthritica). Deutsche Medizinsche Wochenschrift 42: 1435–1536

Rodnan G P 1965 Early theories concerning etiology and pathogenesis of the gout. Arthritis and Rheumatism 8: 599–609

Rogers J, Watt I, Dieppe P 1981 Arthritis in Saxon and medieval skeletons. British Medical Journal 283: 1668–1670

Rose H M, Ragan C, Pearce E, Lipman M O 1948 Differential agglutination of normal and sensitized sheep erythrocytes by sera of patients with rheumatoid arthritis. Proceedings of the Society of Experimental Biology (New York) 68: 1–6

Sauvages de la Croix 1763 Nosologia methodica sistens morborum classes, genera et species juxta Sydenhami mentem et botanicorum ordinem. Amsterdam

Scudamore C 1816 A treatise on the nature and cure of rheumatism. Longmans, London

Short C L 1974 The antiquity of rheumatoid arthritis. Arthritis and Rheumatism 17: 193–205
Smith G E, Jones F W 1910 Report on the human remains. Archaeological Survey of Nubia Report 1907–1908. Egyptian Survey Department, Cairo
Spender J K 1889 The early symptoms and the early treatment of osteoarthritis (commonly called rheumatoid arthritis). H K Lewis, London
Steinbock R T 1976 Paleopathological diagnosis and interpretation. Charles C Thomas, Springfield, Illinois
Still G F 1896–1897 On a form of chronic joint disease in children. Medica-Chirurgical Transactions 80:47
Stockman R 1904 Edinburgh Medical Journal N.S. 15: 107–223
Stockman R 1920 Rheumatism and arthritis. Green, Edinburgh
Strangeways T S P 1905–1907 Bulletins of the Committee for the Study of Special Diseases. 1: 55–78
Strúmpell E A G G 1884 Deutsche Zeitschrift fúr Nervenheilkunde. 11: 338–342
Sydenham R 1848 The works of Thomas Sydenham MD. Translated by R G Latham. Sydenham Society, London
Talbott J H, Yú T F 1976 History (of gout). In: Gout and uric acid metabolism. Stratton Intercontinental Medical Book Corporation, New York, pp 1–25
Waaler E 1940 On the occurrence of a factor in human sera activating specific agglutination of sheep blood corpuscles. Acta Pathologica et Microbiologica Scandinavica 17: 172–188
Waldron T 1982 Human bone lead concentrations. In: McWhirr A, Viner L, Wells C (eds) Cirencester Excavation II: Romano-British cemeteries at Cirencester. Cirencester Excavation Committee, Cirencester, p 203
Wells C 1982 The human burials. In: McWhirr A, Viner L, Wells C (eds) Romano-British cemeteries at Cirencester. Cirencester Excavation Committee, Cirencester, pp 135–201
Wells W C 1812 On rheumatism of the heart. Transactions of the Society for the Improvement of Medical and Chirurgical Knowledge 3: 373–424
Willcox W H 1935 Reports on chronic rheumatic diseases 1:72 Lewis, London
Wood P H N 1976 Is rheumatoid arthritis a recent disease? In: Dumonde D C (ed) Infection and immunology in the rheumatic diseases. Blackwell, Oxford, ch 76, pp 619–622

The basis of rheumatological practice, including nomenclature and classification

The purpose of this chapter is to set rheumatological practice in a broader context, both scientifically and socially. The foundation for specialist expertise mirrors the phases of scientific enquiry — how observations are made (criteria), how phenomena are referred to (nomenclature), how ideas are arranged (diagnosis and classification), and how conclusions are drawn (interpretation). Each of these will be discussed so as to establish the basis for the final phase, controlled study and experiment (such as a therapeutic trial). But these activities cannot be divorced from what makes them possible, the existence of problems that have both individual and social dimensions. Consideration of the two latter is important because it is by this means that resources are made available for the pursuit of rheumatological excellence. Finally, the background is ever changing and so thought also needs to be given to the direction for future endeavours.

Before embarking on this review there are two points to be made. The first is that the term 'rheumatology' is used in two different senses. On the one hand it connotes a body of knowledge, the branch of medical science that is concerned with advancing understanding of rheumatic disorders. Many disciplines contribute to this endeavour, the yield from which is described elsewhere in this book. The other sense is more concrete, denoting internists who specialise in the application of that knowledge to the identification and treatment of rheumatic conditions. It is with this latter, clinical, sense that this chapter is concerned, and with the resources that a practitioner of the specialty calls upon.

The second point is that it may be felt that definition of the specialty is sufficient to establish its identity. However, recognition has to be accorded by others as well as by practitioners of the craft, and this requires that the basis for such acknowledgement be made explicit. The autonomy of a profession is legitimated by society in recognition of the profession's ability to perceive the needs of that society, to equip itself to meet them, and to adapt itself to changes in those needs. In this context society may be interpreted both as the community at large and, for a specialty, as fellow members of the profession in other specialties. The points of practical relevance that command further examination, therefore, are how rheumatologists equip themselves to meet needs, what the burden of those needs is, and what changes can be anticipated.

RHEUMATOLOGICAL EXPERTISE

A common misconception is to attribute the scientific foundation of a branch of medicine to the less mission-oriented disciplines on which it draws for enlightenment (Kelley et al, 1981). Undoubtedly we have learned a great deal from medically-related enquiries in fields such as immunology and biochemistry. However, to imagine that invocation of T cells or disulphide bonds confers an aura of science on the practice of rheumatology is as wishful as the Bellman's confidence that what he asserted three times must be true. The danger of this misapprehension is that it may distract attention from various features of scientific endeavour as applied to clinical practice. These features include the language or terminology of rheumatology, the types of concept that are employed, the means by which conditions can be identified, and the use that is made of evidence. Each plays its part in establishing a foundation for specialist expertise.

Nomenclature

Like any domain of activity, rheumatology has its own language. However, equally as in other domains, vagaries of terminology and variations in usage create obstacles to communication. Perhaps more important, inappropriate nomenclature can distort our thinking in unhelpful ways. Some order in the use of technical language is therefore desirable, and this section is concerned with the general principles that should guide such endeavours.

Desiderata for terminology

Nomenclature deals with the selection of names for defined objects or concepts. It is thus a branch of terminology, which deals with all the special terms used in an art or science. A nomenclature is usually presented as a systematic list of terms relating to the members of a clearly defined conceptual or linguistic family, such as the names of all the different rheumatic disorders.

Terms tend to fall into one of three types. These are:

1. Defining identifiers, where the name in effect defines the entity (e.g. 'tuberculosis'). In many ways ideal, such names can be developed only if the entity has a uniquely defining attribute or hallmark.
2. Descriptive identifiers, which are more common though generally less satisfactory. Not only is a descriptive identifier not defining but, because ideal nomenclature is brief, a degree of arbitrariness in the feature selected for emphasis is inescapable (e.g. ankylosis is not a universal feature in people with ankylosing spondylitis).
3. Arbitrary identifiers, where the components of the name have no linguistic significance in relation to the condition being identified (e.g. eponymous designations, and terms such as 'fifth disease').

Ideally any one concept, such as a disease or syndrome, should be designated by only a single term in any one language. Unfortunately we are usually confronted with an array of choice which, however, can be simplified by designation of the preferred term, permitted synonyms, and rejected synonyms. The latter should be avoided, and every effort should be made to restrict formal usage to the preferred term. Although at times the discipline of following ideal nomenclature may appear to be irksome and even pedantic, it is worth recalling that 'pedantry' is the careless person's term for 'accuracy'.

Preferred terms should be selected by international or national organisations with authority in the particular field or, in the absence of such decisions, by usage. When usage has not crystallised, and especially if an individual is tempted to construct a new term, it is wise to consult *Medical Terminology and Lexicography* (CIOMS, 1966). This work includes guidelines, which are reproduced here in Table 2.1.

Underlying these desiderata is the implication that the criterion of utility is the overriding consider-

Table 2.1 Attributes of preferred terms for use in nomenclature (tabulated in descending order of importance).

A preferred term should be:

1. Specific and unambiguous; the term rheumatism is thus unacceptable in informed usage unless supported by a qualifying adjective, as it could indicate either rheumatic fever or non-specific pains experienced in soft tissue.
2. Reasonably short, easy to pronounce, and sufficiently flexible to permit formation of derivatives and combinations; whenever possible it should consist of a single word, one reason why (osteo)arthrosis is preferable to degenerative joint disease.
3. Self-explanatory, and certainly it should be sufficiently expressive, both in morphology and phonetics, to evoke instantly the concept it describes; this indicates why eponymous designations are generally undesirable, chauvinism apart, even though they are often difficult to avoid.
4. Generically similar for closely related concepts; 'lupus' is a generic term for skin tuberculosis so that, although it is too late to start afresh, lupus erythematosus is an undesirable designation because the condition bears no relation to tuberculosis.
5. Preferably at least similar if not identical in as many as possible of the five major languages of communication; note here the difficulty with colloquialisms because, whereas '*gicht*' is the German derivative of the latin '*gutta*', as is the English 'gout', in Bavarian usage it is non-specific and crudely equivalent to 'rheumatism'.
6. As far as is possible without infringing on the foregoing, euphonious and in keeping with the spirit of the language, as well as not being a hybrid with roots from two or more different languages; hence pauciarticular is preferable to oligoarticular.

ation — unambiguous and effective communication is more important than anything else. The importance of etymology in medical linguistics has been exaggerated considerably. Its main contribution is to shed light on the historical development of the word, rather than on its meaning; the latter is determined by context.

An important property of language, and especially of technical jargon, is the way in which it can imprison us (Bross, 1964). Our usage can condition our thinking so that we become in danger of being confined by ideas originating not so much from observation as from the biasing influence of the terminology we use. Hence the desirability of avoiding descriptive identifiers that predetermine issues needlessly, inappropriately, or inaccurately. For example, inclusion of the word 'idiopathic' in disease terms means that as soon as a cause is discovered the condition must be renamed, a futile additional burden; 'systemic sclerosis' is not necessarily inexorably progressive; and 'osteoarthritis' is thought by many not to involve articular inflammation.

The form of words also influences their meaning. For example, nouns generally have more specific meanings than their derivative adjectives. With the exception of hallowed usage, dignified classically in a word such as 'rheumatoid', it is preferable to avoid describing pathological processes by adjectives derived from other disease terms. Such usage is interpretative, and it is generally preferable to be more simply descriptive.

Perhaps the most important source of confusion in everyday dialogue arises from another property of language. We all recognise that the same word may have more than one meaning, but the context of its use usually indicates which meaning is intended; only rarely will we be uncertain whether 'the President's address' refers to an oration or where he lives. Nevertheless this is not always the case, and problems arise when writers use existing terms but attach to them personal idiosyncrasies of new meaning; this has occurred recently with 'fibrositis' (Reynolds, 1982).

More bewildering is the fact that the same word can be used in different senses, at times implying inclusion and at others the opposite (Fig. 2.1), and the context is frequently not enlightening. For example, if someone speaks of the community, and especially if this word is used as an adjective (e.g. community care), one is often uncertain whether the whole population is being referred to or only those not in institutions. Figure 2.1 displays the basis for the insufficiently appreciated distinctions. The problem arises because medical terminology has tended to concentrate on specific disease labels, neglecting the need for generic descriptors or collectives (Wood, 1980a).

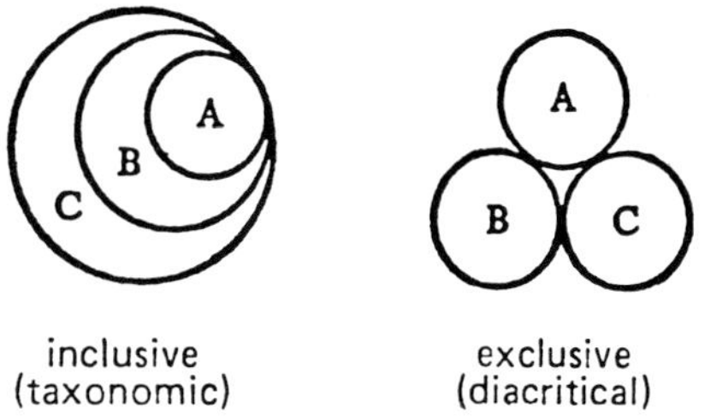

Fig. 2.1 Diagram to illustrate the two different senses in which a term may be used. In the example discussed in the text, C might represent juvenile rheumatoid arthritis. The inclusive North American sense includes a residue of less differentiated disorders, B, which itself includes, say, enteropathic arthropathies, A. Exclusive usage in Britain regards these three as distinct, and would refer to C in the left-hand diagram as juvenile chronic arthritis.

Rheumatology is beset by such difficulties, as perennial transatlantic differences over the signification of the term 'juvenile rheumatoid arthritis' (JRA) illustrate. In North America this label is used inclusively, as a collective referring to a range of conditions that could be designated less ambiguously (see *juvenile chronic arthritis*, Table 2.2). British rheumatologists, on the other hand, tend to use the term distinctively, confining 'JRA' to the occurrence in juveniles of the same disease that is encountered more commonly in adults. Both senses, the connotative and the denotative, represent real and legitimate needs which should be met. However, to confuse the two and, what is worse, to use the identifier for a specific entity as a generic descriptor is surely unhelpful.

Rheumatological nomenclature

A fairly exhaustive guide to preferred nomenclature was published as a thesaurus for the American Rheumatism Association (Ruhl & Sokoloff, 1965). I would refer the interested reader to this work, because I would differ from it in only a few and relatively unimportant instances. As far as was

Table 2.2 Selected examples of preferred usage in rheumatological nomenclature (for a more exhaustive listing see Ruhl & Sokoloff, 1965)

Algoneurodystrophy. Preferable as the generic term for conditions variously described as reflex or sympathetic dystrophy, the shoulder–hand syndrome, or Sudeck's atrophy.

Arthropathy. Preferable as the generic descriptor for articular disorders; these are indicated in colloquial usage by the term 'arthritis', but this has specific pathological connotations. Arthropathies can be qualified as inflammatory, whereas the occasionally encountered 'inflammatory arthritides' is both tautological and less euphonious.

Crystal arthropathy. A generic term to identify gouty arthritis and other articular disorders associated with the presence of crystals, and preferable to 'crystal deposition disease' because it is at once more specific and briefer. Although the term 'pseudo-gout' aptly conveys the clinical resemblance to urate gout, '(articular) chondrocalcinosis' is generally preferred.

Dorsopathy. This term has been suggested as a generic descriptor for the diversity of problems associated with or arising from the back. It is a linguistic hybrid, in contrast to 'notopathy', but is preferable because its origins are less unfamiliar. The term is more inclusive than 'spondylopathy', the latter referring only to the vertebral column.

Enthesopathy. Useful as a generic descriptor for disorders of ligamentous or muscular attachments. It is a valuable unifying concept that brings together a wide variety of otherwise disparate conditions such as particular forms of bursitis, epicondylitis, peri-arthritis, and tendinitis, as well as iliac crest and calcaneal spurs and the Pellegrini–Stieda syndrome. Also included is the 'frozen shoulder', but this terms tends to be used imprecisely; properly it is a synonym for 'adhesive capsulitis', in contradistinction to the rotator cuff syndrome.

Enteropathic arthropathy. Preferable as the term to designate arthropathies associated with inflammatory bowel disorders; not only is it more economical in words than the latter phrase but semantic difficulties are also avoided — infections such as shigellosis give rise to inflammation of the bowel, and yet it is usually only ulcerative colitis and regional enteritis that are being referred to.

Juvenile chronic arthritis. Preferable as the generic descriptor for arthritis in children. Previously this has been designated 'Still's disease' in Great Britain and 'juvenile rheumatoid arthritis' in the USA, but the heterogeneity of these conditions has now been established (Ansell & Wood, 1976). The subject of concern is arthritis with onset before the 16th birthday, regardless of the age at which a patient is first seen, and which lasts for three months or more — the latter to avoid confusion with more evanescent states. Agreement on nomenclature and classification are not sufficient to promote comparability in reported clinical experience unless a variety of specific disorders is excluded; for this purpose an exhaustive enumeration of conditions to be considered in differential diagnosis is less instructive than a structured presentation that takes account of the likelihood and degree of clinical resemblance (Wood, 1977). Having followed this procedure, the conditions remaining under consideration constitute juvenile chronic arthritis (JCA). Included under this heading it is possible to identify adult-type (IgM rheumatoid factor positive) rheumatoid arthritis occurring in juveniles, juvenile ankylosing spondylitis, psoriatic arthropathy, enteropathic arthropathies, and a residue of disorders that at present cannot be differentiated further other than by describing differences in the pattern of onset. Interpretation of laboratory and other findings has been confused by failure to make these distinctions, especially when confounded by different methods of patient selection. For example, reported frequencies of HLA B27 in JCA have ranged from 1 to 45%, a variation that appears to have been determined by whether or not consecutive new referrals were considered, and whether adolescents were included or excluded. The pattern of onset may be differentiated into systemic, polyarticular, and pauciarticular — 4 joints or less; monoarticular onset is a subset of pauciarticular, although it is noteworthy because the child may be referred to an orthopaedic surgeon rather than to a paediatric rheumatologist. Obviously the different onset subtypes may be observed equally in the various other specific diseases just listed; as the nature of these conditions may be revealed only after varying intervals extending up to some years from onset, it is unsatisfactory to arbitrarily exclude those patients who have been ascertained as suffering from these conditions at a particular point in time when many more may reveal themselves later. Nevertheless in reporting experience with JCA the numbers in the group studied that have been recognised as falling into the different categories should be mentioned.

Osteoarthrosis. Some of the problems associated with the use of this term have been reviewed (Wood, 1983a). Although etymologically confusing, the French '*arthrose*' being more rational, usage in English languages has hallowed the osteo- prefix. Designation as 'degenerative joint disease' is not only a mouthful, but is undesirable because it goes further than identifying an observable state; the gratuitous specification of aetiology gives rise to semantic difficulties when the changes are shown to result from, for example, particular metabolic derangements. Usage is confused by employing the same term in different contexts, when the meaning varies considerably (Wood, 1976a). For instance, 'clinical osteoarthrosis' (OA) connotes a patient with a complaint for whom some attempt at amelioration is called; 'radiographic OA' refers to characteristically abnormal shadows, but without telling anything of the influence these may have on the patient; and 'OA' in morbid anatomical terms describes pathological changes, but again out of relation to the patient's suffering. Further chaos is introduced by contentious partisans of the suffixes -osis and -itis; why cannot rheumatologists emulate their colleagues in gastroenterology, who use diverticulosis to describe the underlying structural abnormalities and diverticulitis to identify the patient who is suffering from these changes? The situation is additionally confused when 'OA' is used to subsume the specific but not necessarily related state of osteophytosis (Wood, 1971); the latter condition should not be equated automatically with the presence of OA. Another source of difficulty is generalised OA (GOA). Since this condition was first described (Kellgren & Moore, 1952) there has been a lax tendency to refer to any polyarticular OA as 'GOA'. However, the latter is a distinct disorder and it is preferable to speak of 'multiple OA' in those instances where the characteristic picture (Kellgren & Lawrence, 1958),

Table 2.2 — *continued*

including associated Heberden's nodes, is not observed. There is much to commend European usage in adding to the information value of identifiers by incorporating anatomical specification, as in the term 'coxarthrosis'.

Rheumatic disorders. Preferable as the generic descriptor for rheumatological conditions. It avoids the predicament with symptomatic diagnosis, whether a disease is present, and it also allows consideration of the consequences of soft-tissue trauma, whereas 'rheumatic diseases' customarily would not include conditions arising as a result of injury or developmental abnormality (the term 'disorder' is more inclusive than 'disease'). The term 'rheumatic complaints' is a permitted synonym, emphasising the subjective distress that characterises these conditions.

Rheumatoid factor. Although satisfactory as a generic, it is normally preferable to be more precise and specify which class of antigammaglobulin is present, IgM or IgG, or the method by which it is detected (such as by latex fixation or sheep-cell agglutination tests).

Spondylarthropathy. A useful generic descriptor for a number of different disorders that nevertheless exhibit various features in common, including peripheral arthropathy. These conditions include ankylosing spondylitis, Reiter's disease, psoriatic arthropathy, and arthropathies associated with ulcerative colitis, regional enteritis, and Whipple's disease, as well as with Behçet's disease and infection with *Yersinia enterocolitica*. Two terms have come into vogue in recent years, 'reactive arthritis' and 'seronegative polyarthritis' (or 'spondarthritis'), and yet both are undesirable. The former is intended to convey the remote and often indirect effects of an aetiological agent, in much the same way as rheumatic fever might have been designated as a 'reactive carditis'. However, to the extent that medicine operates on the assumption that every malady has an aetiology, and that the manifestations of the condition represent a reaction to the underlying process, the notion is unhelpfully non-specific. The other concept will be discussed further, under the heading of classification. As regards its nomenclature, the term 'spondylarthropathies' is more euphonoius than 'spondarthritides'; there is no justification for dropping the 'yl' component of the root (its omission suggests to me a different derivation, akin to that of a disyllabic metrical foot); and once attention has been directed from polyarthritis to spondylarthropathy specification as seronegative becomes redundant (what are the seropostive spondarthritides, anyway?).

Spondylosis. The many difficulties attending use of the term 'osteoarthrosis' have already been noted. Confusion is heightened when the same term is used indiscriminately to refer to abnormalities both in peripheral joints and in the spine, particularly when changes at the latter site differ in a number of important regards — notably because they are not exclusively related to synovial joints. The difficulties could be largely overcome by using an existing term, 'spondylosis', to identify spinal changes, restricting 'OA' to peripheral joints.

---

possible, the English version of the 9th revision of the *International Classification of Diseases* incorporated preferred nomenclature into the tabular listing of Chapter XIII, covering diseases of the musculoskeletal system and connective tissue. Because problems are exaggerated when trying to read papers in a language other than one's own, the European League against Rheumatism took initiative in developing an international nomenclature of rheumatology (Wood, 1974, 1980b); unfortunately financial constraints precluded publication of an exhaustive dictionary of equivalent terms. These sources acknowledged, there are certain terms about which a little more needs to be said (Table 2.2), mainly because of subsequent developments in our appreciation; most of these are inclusion terms or collectives, the need for which has already been noted.

A more general point is that an almost mystical significance is sometimes attached to the distinction between diseases and syndromes. Some idealists claim that disease status should be withheld in various instances, without specifying what the prerequisites for such designation are. I suspect aspirations for a uniquely defining hallmark, or for an established aetiology. As most rheumatic disorders cannot qualify in this sense, it is worth clarifying the distinctions. A disease is 'the sum of the abnormal phenomena displayed . . . in association with a specified common characteristic or set of characteristics . . . in such a way as to place (organisms) at a biological disadvantage' (Scadding, 1967; Campbell et al, 1979).

Most generally a syndrome represents an observed concurrence of various features, usually at more than one site, without the significance of such associations at first being known; for example, the Plummer–Vinson (or Paterson–Kelly–Ross) syndrome. The basis of the association may then become apparent as a particular manifestation or presentation of a specific disease, in other words a subset, such as Caplan's or Felty's syndromes. In some circumstances a new entity is recognised in this way, as when the sicca syndrome graduated into Sjögren's disease. What really matters is the nature of what is being identified, and there seems to be little justification for still referring to the syndromes of Reiter and Behçet — both appear to be specific entities and therefore to quality as diseases; to continue to downgrade them as syndromes perpetuates an unnecessary degree of uncertainty, as well as posing needless difficulties about whether the condition is present if, for example, all the features of Reiter's triad are not observed.

The situation is confounded by two other patterns of usage. One is that 'syndrome' has a wider applicability, being appropriate to non-disease phenomena such as congenital anomalies as well. For example, whilst it is correct to refer to Hansen's disease (leprosy) one can only speak of Down's syndrome; these, incidentally, are examples of the euphemistic use of eponyms as a means of reducing stigma. The other is the unacknowledged distinction between inclusive and exclusive senses, already noted, such as when some consider osteoarthrosis to be a specific disease entity whereas others, usually surgeons, regard it as only a syndrome and therefore include under the same heading the end results of ochronosis and other conditions that damage joints. Finally, it is worth noting that Raynaud's phenomenon is correctly so described because it refers to abnormalities confined to one location, the fingers.

In presuming to comment about rheumatological nomenclature, as I have done in Table 2.2, it has certainly not been my intention to prescribe, because only the vocabulary of our progeny will reveal what usage has established as correct or acceptable. I am not even optimistic about the power of enlightenment; as Gibbon remarked in his analysis of the Roman empire, 'the power of instruction is seldom of much efficacy except in those happy dispositions where it is almost superfluous'. Nevertheless it would have been remiss not to assume a component of rationality in the development of rheumatology, and it is to discourse on this plane that my observations are directed.

In concluding this brief discussion of nomenclature it may be helpful to identify another important contributory cause of difficulty. Vagaries of terminology are encouraged by the widespread misconception in medicine that a textbook type of description, one which amounts to an enumeration of characteristic features, constitutes a definition. This unhelpful notion arises from confusion over what it is that is being defined, and how this problem should be tackled. Although the broad endeavour may be to describe diseases, a label is in fact used to identify an idea or concept — in this instance the concept of a particular disease. The role of definition and the part it plays in the recognition of disease manifestations is indicated in Table 2.3 (stage 3).

Table 2.3 Stages in the recognition and differentiation of distinct disease manifestations.

1. In the beginning is perception of a concept, such as by identification of a syndrome, and this is rapidly followed by description of its features.
2. Once recognised one needs a means of referring to the concept, so that a name or label needs to be attached to it — which is what the remarks about nomenclature in Table 2.2 are intended to clarify.
3. The concept then needs to be defined, which is accomplished parsimoniously by specifying the broad class to which the concept belongs and sufficient of its characteristics to distinguish it from any other concept. Thus to define arthrodesis it suffices to say 'surgical fixation of a joint', where fixation identifies the broad class.
4. Formulation of a definition requires that interrelationships with other concepts be examined — this is the process of taxonomy or classification.
5. Finally, the means of recognising further examples of the concept have to be established — this requires consideration of necessary and sufficient conditions for assignment to the particular class, diagnosis being one example of the assignment process, and specification of identification criteria to facilitate this endeavour.

Classification

It has to be acknowledged that physicians are often as opinionated about how to classify diseases as they are about how to refer to them. In both instances a somewhat absolutist stance tends to be adopted, one which, reduced to its essentials, amounts to little more than assertion that others should do as they do. Yet there is no ultimate arbiter, no single approach which is correct and compared with which all others are in error. In the last analysis all that matters is usefulness — does one's terminology facilitate effective communication, and does one's taxonomy fulfil a practical need? Failure to appreciate this utilitarian foundation makes for a potent source of controversy even though the parties think they agree the facts of the situation, the different disease states. What happens is that non-factual arguments unwittingly develop because the participants fail to identify that their purposes and the contexts in which they are viewing phenomena are different (Crawshay-Williams, 1974); confusion over inclusive and exclusive senses illustrates this point. The difficulties are exacerbated because the empirical tradition in science tends to assume that there can be only one correct context, and it is not realized that taxonomy is a philosophical rather than a 'scientific' pursuit. These are the uncertainties I have to try to resolve.

Arranging ideas

As physicians we register phenomena in the natural world around us, and perceive resemblances and differences between them. We then organise these percepts and relate them together into concepts by a process of classification, a fundamental step in the development of understanding (Wood, 1982). However, it all depends on what is perceived. This can be illustrated by an old Hindu story about blind men encountering an elephant. One thought it was like a snake, another like tree-trunks, and a third like leather. Each perceived elements of the whole, but perception is selective. We are similarly selective in developing concepts and in integrating these into classification schemes. Simplifying assumptions allow us to reduce a complex problem to components that can be handled. Inevitably there are losses, because we are describing not the whole but only some of the parts. With different assumptions the losses, those similarities that are not taken into account, would almost certainly be different.

Development of a classification scheme thus involves making choices, balancing the gains and losses of those features that are highlighted and those which are neglected. The corollary of this state of affairs is that it is axiomatic that classification is subordinate to a purpose. As a result it is necessary to consider only a single criterion when evaluating a classification, that of utility — does the taxonomy do what you want it to do? It is noteworthy that most disputes about the relative merits of different classification schemes arise from failure to identify their specific purposes and the contexts in which they are to be applied. The reality is revealed by the following passage (Midgley, 1979):

> 'What counts as a fact depends on the concepts you use, on the questions you ask. . . . There is no neutral terminology. So there are no wholly neutral facts. All describing is classifying according to some conceptual scheme or other. We need concepts in order to pick out what matters for our present purpose from the jumble of experience, and to relate it to the other things that matter in the world. There is no single set of all-purpose 'scientific' concepts which can be used for every job. Different inquiries make different selections from the world. So they need different concepts.'

To make the sources of conflict explicit, 'Every scientific discourse is based on a set of culture and ideology-bound *metaphors*, and has therefore to be read as metaphor, and not as an 'objective' transparent language that would stand in a one-to-one relationship with an immutable, absolute reality' (Joris, 1980). The real caution then comes from Palmerston (Jenkins et al, 1972): 'Half the wrong conclusions at which mankind arrive are reached by the abuse of metaphors and mistaking general resemblance or imaginary similarity for real identity.'

Conceptual taxonomies

Having acknowledged that there is no one correct scheme, it must be recognised that 'superficial generalizations of wide validity and precise ones of limited scope are complementary to each other, and both are necessary' (Hinde, 1966). The most far-reaching schemes are related to an underlying paradigm, such as the concept of phylogeny on which 'standard' botanical and zoological taxonomies are based. Knowledge in medicine has not yet reached a stage that would permit development of so comprehensive a theoretical framework, and so our goals are usually more limited.

Three broad categories of purpose can be identified. The first is essentially practical, what might almost be regarded as administrative, and will be discussed later in this section. The second is concerned with clinical decision making, such as a system for displaying options as one proceeds to make a diagnosis, and will be considered under the latter heading. The third, what perhaps comes most readily to mind when thinking of classification, is directed at a deeper level — biomedical schemes that offer a framework for orienting understanding and research about disease phenomena.

Biomedical schemes. In the light of what has been said, it should be clear that one cannot argue that a taxonomy based on aetiology is necessarily superior to other approaches. Only some purposes would be better served by such a scheme, notably those concerned with prevention. In any case the aetiology of most rheumatic disorders is still ill-understood, so that is scarcely a serious option.

The same can certainly not be said of observable phenomena that characterise different pathological processes. This allows one to make a start, such as by grouping together the inflammatory polyarthropathies in contradistinction to other disorders. Proceeding on this sort of foundation, taxonomies were developed by the International League against Rheumatism (1960) and the American Rheumatism Association (Blumberg et al, 1964) and were included in early editions of this book (Copeman, 1969). However, in the immediately previous edition (Wood, 1978a) I declined to commend a particular scheme and endeavoured to indicate the basis for my reluctance. Being now under pressure to remedy this omission I have chosen to do two things — to reproduce one of the more recent rheumatological classification schemes (Mathies et al, 1979), which can be seen in simplified form in Table 2.4, and to discuss some of the difficulties that have to be confronted when undertaking such an exercise.

Any system of classification imposes an arbitrary basis for interrelating biomedical phenomena. The attempt to be comprehensive by incorporating more than one taxonomic principle gives rise to conflicts in priority. For example, logical inconsistency is unavoidable if a system founded on morbid anatomical features is extended to take account of causal influences; to which should more importance be attached, the fact that infections have an established aetiology or their manifestation, in common with other processes, of an inflammatory reaction? When inflammatory polyarthropathies are regarded as a class it is often not clear whether the primary emphasis is being placed on the pathological, synovitis as opposed to cartilage destruction, or on the anatomical, a single joint versus a polyarthritis and, at the same time, peripheral as opposed to axial joints. At a very different level is the blithe way we refer to inflammation, as if this can be regarded as a uniform whole. Yet unacknowledged differences between acute and chronic processes may well underlie confused debates about whether OA is inflammatory; certainly whatever may be observed in this condition is not the same as occurs in RA. Equally we speak of anti-inflammatory drugs, without distinguishing between different phases of the very complex process we designate as inflammation, individual drugs appearing to act at different stages of this process (Wood, 1966).

These difficulties bring one back to the fundamental concern with purpose and utility. Grouping the inflammatory arthropathies together at first appears to be meaningful not only pathologically, but also in terms of therapeutics. However, this depends on how far resemblances are pursued because there are important differences, both in the pathogenesis of the various forms of arthritis and in the therapies that are appropriate for them. As far as research endeavours are concerned I suspect that the level of generality in any comprehensive classification scheme renders the latter of limited value, as hypotheses need to be framed with greater precision if they are to be amenable to testing. This leads me to proceed to examination of a more restricted conceptual scheme, which brings out other difficulties.

Seronegative polyarthritis. The concept of seronegative polyarthritis (Wright & Moll, 1976) made important contributions to our understanding. Critical analysis of the underlying ideas and their implications is nevertheless rewarding, and I am indebted to the authors for permitting me to use this example as an illuminating case study. Three aspects call for examination: What does the concept signify? For whom might the concept have value? Is the designation satisfactory?

I will not belabour a literal interpretation of the term 'seronegative', other than to note that it would appear to imply that for a condition to be identified as rheumatoid arthritis (RA — which I imagine is what the opposite, seropositive polyarthritis, is taken to be) tests for rheumatoid factor should be positive. As regards the idea itself, a clinician would derive benefit from a concept that indicated differential diagnosis, one which conveyed diagnostic possibilities and at the same time emphasised these according to their relative frequency. It is for this quite sophisticated model that we are indebted to Wright and Moll. What it amounts to is that, when confronted by a patient with inflammatory polyarthropathy, two main possibilities should be borne in mind — first a specific, rheumatoid arthritis, and second a collective, indicating various other polyarthropathies. In referring to the latter, 'seronegative' is really being used as a shorthand term, to indicate that one should first make sure it isn't RA.

In a later development of their thesis (Moll et al, 1978) the nomenclature was modified. I have already noted some of the terminological difficulties (Table 2.2). What the term 'spondylarthropathy' helps to bring out is other features, without the need for further specification — i.e. that these conditions tend to affect fewer and more often the larger limb joints, especially those of the lower limb; they tend to be asymmetrical; they are often associated with sacroiliac and spinal involvement; and generally they carry a less unfavourable prognosis. However we may choose to refer to the notion, a means has been developed for acknowledging that various diseases may resemble or even mimic each other in their modes of presentation. It is now necessary to consider whether it is helpful to group these conditions together in biological as opposed to diagnostic contexts because, although any one individual may function as both clinician and research investigator, the purpose of these activities is quite different.

On one plane the concept of overlap phenomena certainly appears to be helpful; not only does it display similarities that call for explanation, but the means for accomplishing at least a part of this is now available since markers for susceptibility, the HLA antigens, have been identified. For other purposes the emphasis on resemblances is not so advantageous. After all, much though they may have in common, these diseases are still likely to be separate entities — each with particularities in susceptibility, and also in extraneous precipitants. The problems can be illustrated by a parable. Consider horses and donkeys. Compared with other four-footed creatures the similarities are overwhelming, and biologically it is helpful to stress these in order to depict evolution. But only the donkey was ridden in to Jerusalem, and we know of many other ways in which they differ. Moreover, if we concentrate too much on what they have in common we may be tempted to interbreed them — and the resultant mule is sterile. This highlights a general property of any conceptual taxonomy; although it may be very useful for some purposes it cannot help but violate other aspects of reality and, in the process, inhibit or retard awareness of the whole that is to be comprehended. Hence my reluctance to recommend any particular scheme for universal application.

Practical classifications

There are two situations in which practically oriented schemes are of interest. The first occurs when dealing with data relating to individual experiences, such as may be required for certain types of epidemiological enquiry and for health service planning. The raw material consists of terms that doctors of varying levels of sophistication have written down on pieces of paper, be these case records or certificates of sickness incapacity or death. The *International Classification of Diseases* (ICD) was developed for this purpose, originally as a means of facilitating comparability in mortality studies.

It is necessary to appreciate why it is not possible for the ICD to be structured in conformity with idealised classification schemes, even though every effort has been made to assimilate current clinical insights. In the first place conceptual taxonomies are usually the product of individual specialty groups, whereas the ICD has to span all body systems so as to embrace the entire range of morbid phenomena. Moreover, this exercise has to be accomplished on the basis of agreement not only between specialties, but also between statistical agencies in countries where health information systems vary considerably in their level of development. Compromises are therefore unavoidable; the interests of rheumatologists have to be reconciled with those of orthopaedic surgeons in regard to Chapter XIII of the ICD, diseases of the musculoskeletal system, and overall due weight has to be accorded to the principle of the greatest reliability of information, which tends to be related

Table 2.4 Outline classification of diseases of the locomotor apparatus, with selected examples of details (simplified from Mathies et al, 1979).

No.	Category of rheumatic disorder	ICD code	Approximately equivalent category of the ICD (9th revision)
1.	DISEASES OF THE JOINTS	710–719	Arthropathies and related disorders
11.	Inflammatory joint disease	711–714	(inflammatory arthropathies)
111	rheumatoid arthritis	714	rheumatoid arthritis and other inflammatory polyarthropathies
115	arthritis in disease not primarily in the locomotor apparatus (including psoriatic and enteropathic arthropathies)	713	arthropathy associated with other disorders classified elsewhere
116	reactive (allergic and toxic) arthritis	711	arthritis associated with infections (part)
119	joint infections	711	arthritis associated with infections
12.	Joint disease with various inflammatory and non-inflammatory components (including gout)	713 712	arthropathy associated with other disorders classified elswhere, and crystal arthropathies
13.	Degenerative joint disease	715	osteoarthrosis and allied disorders
14.	Changes in joints and synchondroses due to physical causes and surgery	840–848	Sprains and strains of joints and adjacent muscles (part)
15.	Disorders of joint development	736 754–756	acquired deformities of limbs (part), and congenital musculoskeletal anomalies (part)
16.	Joint tumors and hamartomas	var.	(neoplasm of bone, classified according to whether benign or malignant, and other categories)
2.	DISEASES OF THE SPINAL COLUMN AND NEIGHBOURING JOINTS	720–724	Dorsopathies
21.	Inflammatory diseases of the spinal column	720 730	ankylosing spondylitis and other inflammatory spondylopathies, and osteomyelitis, periostitis, and other infections involving bone (part)
22.	Static and functional disorders of the spinal column	737	curvature of spine (and other categories)
23.	Degenerative changes in the spine	721 722	spondylosis and allied disorders, and intervertebral disc disorders
24.	Diseases of the spine in internal and neurological disorders	713	arthropathy associated with other disorders classified elsewhere (part)
25.	Changes in the spine and neighbouring joints due to physical injury or surgery	846–847	sprains and strains of back
26.	Disorders of spinal development	737	curvature of spine (and other categories)
27.	Tumors of the spine	var.	(neoplasm of vertebral column, classified according to whether benign or malignant)
3.	DISEASES OF THE SOFT TISSUES OF THE LOCOMOTOR AND CONNECTIVE TISSUE SYSTEMS	725–729	Rheumatism, excluding the back
31.	Diseases of the muscles (including polymyalgia rheumatica)	725	polymyalgia rheumatica (and other categories)
32.	Diseases of the tendons, tendon sheaths, ligaments and fasciae	726–728	(see below)
33.	Disease of the bursae	727	other disorders of synovium, tendon, and bursa (part)
34.	Compound soft-tissue diseases	726	peripheral enthesopathies and allied syndromes (and other categories)
35.	Congenital contractures	754	congenital musculoskeletal deformities (part)
36.	Acquired contractures	735	acquired deformities of toe (and other categories)
37.	Neuropathy	357	other diseases of peripheral nerves
4.	ANGIOPATHY WITH MANIFESTATIONS IN THE LOCOMOTOR APPARATUS (including polyarteritis nodosa)	446	polyarteritis nodosa and allied conditions

5.		DISEASES OF THE SUBCUTANEOUS CONNECTIVE TISSUE	—	
6.		DISEASES OF CARTILAGE AND BONE	730–733	Osteopathies and chondropathies (and other categories)
7.		DISORDERS OF SKELETAL FORMATION, DEVELOPMENT AND GROWTH	754–756	Congenital musculoskeletal anomalies (and other categories)
8.		SYSTEMIC DISEASES WITH FACULTATIVE MANIFESTATIONS IN THE LOCOMOTOR APPARATUS	—	
	811	rheumatic fever	390–392	Acute rheumatic fever
	812	Reiter's disease	711.1	arthropathy in Reiter's disease
	813	systemic diseases of connective tissue	710	diffuse diseases of connective tissue
	815	Behçet's syndrome	711.2	arthropathy in Behçet's syndrome
	821	chondrocalcinosis	712	crystal arthropathies
9.		SYSTEMIC DISEASES NOT INVOLVING THE LOCOMOTIVE APPARATUS ASSOCIATED WITH DISEASES OF THE LATTER	—	

more to anatomical localisation than to aetiological or pathological considerations.

Two other specific features have to be recognised. First, disease terms in the ICD are used to identify people's illnesses and, because these are not mutually exclusive and an individual may suffer from more than one simultaneously, some system for arbitration on priority in assignment is necessary. For many years the concept of an underlying cause has been used for this purpose, being particularly appropriate to mortality studies. Secondly, specialists may find it difficult to accept that they cannot prescribe a vocabulary for their confreres (Mathies, 1980). However, doctors cannot be compelled to use only a preferred nomenclature, and so provision has to be made with a range of categories in order to cope with different levels of terminological specificity.

Clinicians are becoming more interested in information retrieval according to ICD categories, both as their activities are increasingly subjected to scrutiny and audit and as microcomputers facilitate such enquiries. Components of the ninth revision of the ICD (WHO, 1978) can be seen in Table 2.4. In contrast to earlier revisions, it is now possible to identify the rheumatic or articular manifestations of any disease through code numbers in Chapter XIII, so that the frustration of seeking conditions such as Reiter's disease and gout in other chapters, under infections and metabolic disorders respectively, can be avoided. This has come about because new demands, particularly in relation to studies of health care utilisation, have led to introduction of a means for ascertaining manifestations as an alternative to aetiologies based on the underlying cause concept.

The retrieval of case dossiers is also relevant. A system for filing medical records is analogous to a telephone directory. My telephone number tells you nothing about me, only how to get hold of me; all that is required is a unique place for each person or record, and no other assumptions are involved. It should be evident that as detail is added to a classification scheme, as has been done in the ninth revision of the ICD, so the difference from a nomenclature, a systematic list of terms, becomes progressively less. The merit of using ICD numbers for record retrieval is largely due to the fact that it is the most exhaustive widely available listing of disease terms, and one which at the same time can cope with variations in usage. Furthermore, as the production of routine statistics is usually linked with the processing of medical records, the economy of using ICD numbers for both purposes is evident.

The other practical situation to be considered is the setting up of a personal index of clinical experience. Again one is concerned with classification for purposes of retrieval, though this time the material is clinical information oriented to the interests of a particular doctor or group. The structure will be influenced by the characteristics in which the originators are interested, and by the form in which the index will be maintained, be it file cards, floppy disc, or a computer tape. Experience (Hewitt et al, 1979) indicates three guiding principles. For a specific project an index may represent a system of data abstraction on which analyses may be carried out. However, any general and continuing index that is not limited to defined purposes is unlikely to anticipate all one's requirements, so that the ultimate need to return to the source data, the case records, must be accepted. Indexes should therefore be selective, serving only as a pointer to other sources. Secondly, the more ambitious an index, the greater the detail it encompasses, then the less likely it is to be maintained, not least because few will share or maintain the dedication of the originator. Finally, by adopting diagnostic classes that are comparable with or convertible to ICD categories one gains the asset of wider comparability with others, without losing any options for alternative methods of manipulating the index.

Diagnosis

Although the word is often used in both senses it is helpful to make a distinction between classification proper, the exercise of constructing classes, and assignment, the allocation of entities to given classes. Many assignment schemes resemble a classification but, as the classes are predetermined, they must be regarded as secondary taxonomies. For example, the simple aetiological check-list, whether a condition is congenital, traumatic, neoplastic, inflammatory, or degenerative, is a secondary classification concerned with assignment, in this instance differential diagnosis.

However, before discussing such schemes there are more general aspects of diagnosis that demand consideration.

Diagnosis is the process whereby specific diseases are identified, where a patient's problems are assigned to a particular disease class. Much has been written about the so-called 'diagnostic process', but it would appear that pattern recognition is probably the cornerstone of individual diagnostic skill (Elstein, 1982); in other words, the ability to identify an elephant through having seen one before (Cohen, 1943). Nevertheless such a largely intuitive exercise is scarcely amenable to analysis, and so some attempt must be made to tease out components of the activity.

The ultimate goal is inference of morbid changes, and often internal anatomical abnormalities at that, and the process calls for extraordinary intellectual virtuosity. The evidence elicited from a patient is subjected to what amounts to a sequence of orders of assignment. The complexity of these exercises has been reviewed by Feinstein (1967), and has been illustrated for rheumatoid arthritis (Wood, 1970a). The process is confounded by the manner in which data from different sources and of varying qualities are integrated. Wood (1968) has shown how this can be a source of variation in assignment. For instance, diagnosis of rheumatoid arthritis can be represented symbolically by the equation

$$RA = IP + EA + RF$$

where IP represents the clinical features, inflammatory polyarthropathy; EA the radiographic changes, erosive arthritis; and RF the serological characteristics, usually rheumatoid factor; and with different weights being attached to each. This is but a different method of expressing the situation that Kellgren (1968) represented by a Venn diagram.

The diagnostic process can be regarded as a sequence of decisions, although the pathway may well vary between one clinician and another. Each step consists of assessment of the probabilities (Schoolman, 1982) according to the state of a particular discriminatory attribute, the presence or absence of a given sign. This decision tree approach has been applied successfully to the much simpler judgements made in selecting therapy (Emerson et al, 1974) and in attempts to reduce the risk of fatal thromboembolism after hip joint replacement (Kelsey et al, 1976). The diagnostic challenge is more complex, but a similar approach has been rewarding (Feldman et al, 1972). The contribution of the order imposed by such numerical methods has been shown clearly by work on abdominal pain (de Dombal et al, 1974).

Assignment schedules

With the exception of conditions submitted to computer diagnosis and discriminant function analyses, it is not possible to document sequential pathways for most clinical disorders. The effort could be rewarding as it should encourage transmission of the fruits of experience more explicitly in teaching. There is also a potential to economise in the amount of information required to reach a decision, or at least for these data to be elicited in a more coherent sequence than is the case with a standard data base. However, some progress can be made at a simpler level.

In botany the analogue of diagnosis is identification of the species to which a specimen belongs. This is accomplished by a means of a flora or key. Problems in medicine are at once more changeable and immediate, and they relate to processes rather than to objects like a plant. Nevertheless the reasoning is instructive, and an attempt to pursue this method with inflammatory arthropathies is presented in Figure 2.2. Although only a preliminary and intuitive analysis, this does indicate the essentials of the approach. It also highlights that diagnostic decision making may be explored more fruitfully by applying a series of discriminators in sequence than by matching a patient to a modal profile, which is the method implicit in the use of diagnostic criteria.

A flora used in botanical field studies attempts to be comprehensive, allowing you to start from any of a number of features — the number of petals or stamens, for instance, or the form of the leaves. Problems in medicine are usually narrowed in focus by the patient's presenting complaint, which permits a more selective approach. This has been exploited in diagnostic flow charts prepared for use by primary health workers in developing countries (Essex, 1977), an example of which is reproduced in Figure 2.3.

PATIENT'S COMPLAINT

- Pain and stiffness in limbs *localise to* .... A. Bones
  - B. Muscles
  - C. Nerves
  - D. Blood vessels
  - E. Joints (q.v.)
  - F. Psychosocial factors
- Other complaints (not considered further)

E. JOINTS

determine characteristics

- Signs of inflammation (red, hot, painful, swelling etc.) .....Inflammatory arthropathies (q.v.)
- Signs of mechanical derangement ....Deformities
  - Occupation
  - Osteoarthrosis
  - Connective tissue dystrophy
- Other complaints ....Osteoarthropathy
  - Osteochondritis
  - Algoneurodystrophy

INFLAMMATORY ARTHROPATHIES

observe distribution of joint involvement

- Monoarticular ....
  - *acute* ....Blood
    - Crystals
    - Pus
  - *subacute*
    - Monoarticular Still's disease (juvenile chronic polyarthritis)
    - Ankylosing spondylitis
    - Rheumatoid arthritis
    - Tuberculosis
- Pauciarticular ....
  - Chronic iridocyclitic Still's disease (juvenile chronic polyarthritis)
  - Ankylosing spondylitis
  - Arthropathy of regional enteritis and ulcerative colitis
  - Reiter's disease
- Polyarticular ....
  - *flitting* ....Rheumatic fever
    - Rheumatoid arthritis
  - *subacute* ...Systemic lupus erythematosus
    - Ankylosing spondylitis
    - Benign (viral) polyarthritis
    - Rheumatoid arthritis
    - Systemic Still's disease (juvenile chronic polyarthritis)
    - Other

Fig. 2.2 A suggested outline assignment key for inflammatory arthropathies.

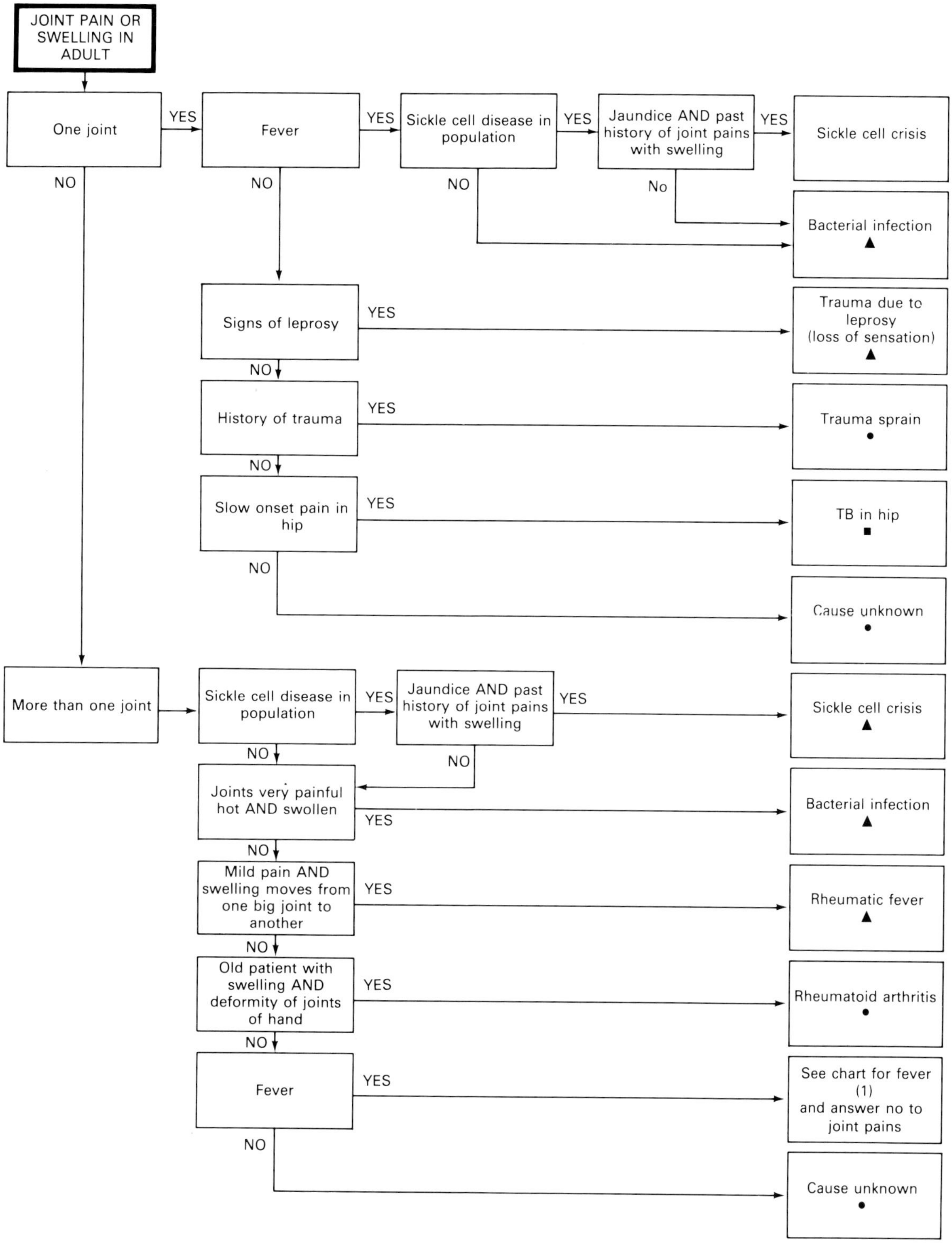

Fig. 2.3 Diagnostic flow chart for joint pain or swelling in an adult, for primary health workers (from Essex, 1977). Key to symbols: ● treat in outpatient clinic; ▲ admit to nearest health centre or hospital; ■ refer to hospital.

Analogous principles have been followed in developing material for distance learning (Wilkinson, 1982). In this approach diagnosis is reduced to a two-stage process, based on the assumption that most rheumatic problems present as one of only six clinical syndromes. These can be determined from the history and examination, and consist of acute or chronic monoarthritis, acute or chronic polyarthritis, low backache, and a myalgia syndrome. The diagnostic possibilities related to any particular syndrome are then reviewed and, when considered alongside the age and sex of the patient, the probable diagnosis is often sufficiently obvious that only a few confirmatory tests should be required.

So far I have considered assignment from the point of view of diagnosis. Certainly an ideal diagnosis should convey a lot of information — the aetiology, the nature of morbid changes, the most appropriate treatment, and the outlook or prognosis — with the subsequent course of the illness serving as a test of the validity of these inferences. Sadly, diagnosis of most rheumatic disorders cannot aspire to such heights of attainment, and it is therefore perhaps surprising that more has not been done to develop therapeutic assignments, a means of determining that this is an aspirin patient, this a radiotherapy patient, this a gold patient, and so on. Uncertainty in assessing the extent of benefit offered by specific therapies undoubtedly contributes to the difficulties, but further work is needed on the prediction of individual susceptibilities to both beneficial and adverse effects.

Criteria

The discussion on assignment focused largely on the discipline of practical problem-solving for an individual patient. However, as soon as one wishes to collect experience together and draw conclusions from what has been observed in a group of patients one enters a different domain. Deductive reasoning has to be based on the homogeneity and representativeness of the sample studied. Sampling strategies are concerned with the latter problem (Wood, 1983b) whereas, in the absence of a hallmark, the former has to be secured by methods of identification based on a cluster concept for clinical and related features (Wood, 1971). It is as a means of overcoming the cluster problem that diagnostic criteria have been developed.

Great credit must be paid to the American Rheumatism Association (ARA) both for pioneering efforts on uniform identification of RA (Ropes et al, 1956) and for work in the last decade on most of the major rheumatic disorders (Hunder, 1982). The initial approach was pragmatic, and it certainly encouraged a greater homogeneity in case material reported in clinical studies and drug trials. Epidemiological application of the criteria revealed difficulties (Wood, 1970b), and these were reviewed at international symposia (Bennett & Wood, 1968). Whilst the New York criteria for RA seem to have largely survived the test of time, those for ankylosing spondylitis have been more problematic (Moll, 1980).

Without question it is valuable to continue reporting criteria status in descriptive and research reports. On the other hand it is also helpful to appreciate their limitations. The fundamental approach to developing criteria is still empirical, although more systematic analytical techniques have helped to improve reliability. The question of validity has been tackled less satisfactorily, and necessary and sufficient discrimination still tends to be oversimplified by a summation of evidence of different qualities. Criteria tend to depict a modal profile, to which conformity is then sought. Logically, though, the need is to establish when an array of clinical features exceeds a threshold — which features, and with what severity, are sufficient to allow the boundary for decision to be crossed. Related to this, undue weighting of features (such as the triad of one joint, a second joint, and symmetry in the original ARA criteria for RA) has usually not been eliminated, and yet testing for the independence of attributes is not difficult (Bird et al, 1979).

What has also been appreciated insufficiently is that purposes vary and, although core components may be preserved, differences in both emphasis and tolerance are to be expected (Wood, 1983b). For example, population surveys are concerned primarily with the separation of disease from non-disease, and exclusions are almost impossible to apply systematically; clinical studies, on the other hand, are more exercised by discrimination between similar disorders, when exclusions come to play a critical role. The consequence is that criteria need to be adapted to the purpose in hand, and those for immunogenetic studies (Dawkins et al, 1983), for instance, probably need to be more stringent than for descriptive reviews of clinical experience. Moreover, such adaptations require reassessment of the reproducibility and validity of individual and combined criteria in the new context.

A witty review (Bywaters, 1982) highlighted that criteria are no more than standards for judgement. They thus represent a preliminary approach to the problem of measurement and quantification. But homogeneity is as necessary at the end as it is at the beginning. So there is a need for criteria of disease remission (Pinals et al, 1981), and criteria for the assessment of outcome (Kirwan et al, 1983), though work in these areas is still in its infancy. Similarly, there is a need for standardisation of approach in other activities, such as the interpretation of radiographs (Atlas, 1963; Larsen, 1974; Larsen et al, 1975) and the conduct of clinical trials of therapy (Lequesne & Mery, 1980).

Interpreting evidence

Having discussed various aspects of the process of assembling evidence, some thought should be given to the use that is made of this material. Medicine is commonly regarded as being born of a marriage between the scientific and an element of indefinable artistry. Unfortunately people frequently get the roles of bride and groom confused because, as Medawar (1969) remarks, 'it is the unbiased observation, the apparatus, the ritual of fact-finding and the inductive mumbo-jumbo that the clinician thinks of as 'scientific', and the other element, intuitive and logically unscripted, which he thinks of as a creative art'. So deep-rooted are these misconceptions that they need to be exposed, because they are obstacles to sound practice.

As Medawar goes on to say, 'the purpose of scientific enquiry is not to compile an inventory of factual information. . . . We should think of it rather as a logically articulated structure of justifiable beliefs about nature.' So the process of diagnosis is concerned with justifiable beliefs, and that of differential diagnosis with hypothesis testing. For these purposes knowledge of how to assess the function of every joint in the body is essential. However, rheumatologists tend to be more scientific than non-specialists not because they carry out an exhaustive examination of all these structures, but because they know when it is necessary to look at particular joints with special care in order to expose tentative ideas to falsification.

How disease arises

If scientific reasoning 'is a kind of dialogue between the possible and the actual' (Medawar, 1969) it is necessary to take account of what may be possible, in other words the role of theory and hypothesis. This may be accomplished by reviewing the manner in which disease arises and how various influences observed to be associated with it may be implicated in causation.

The search for causality is far from straightforward, and Murphy (1972) has reviewed some of the obstacles that have to be circumvented. One of the first questions to consider is the appropriateness of the idea of single-factor aetiology. Simple Mendelian inheritance of a trait is a prime example of this possibility. The implication is that a single factor is both necessary and sufficient to account for the occurrence of a condition. But in reality life is rarely so simple (Fig. 2.4). There is the complication of pleiotropy, that a single cause can lead to multiple effects. Think of the myriad manifestations of tuberculous infection; until Robert Koch isolated *Mycobacterium tuberculosis* who could have realised that Jane Austen's Addison's disease developed from essentially the same cause as Charlotte Brontë's consumption?

The distinction between single factor and multifactorial aetiology is usually more artificial than real. In practice what we find it useful to think of as a single factor condition is in fact only quasi-unifactorial (Bury & Wood, 1978). This means that the factor is a necessary cause, and that it accounts for a large proportion of the variance in the occurrence of the condition — but that nevertheless it fails to account for the whole of the circumstances. The dramatic successes of medicine have stemmed from situations like this, the infections, nutritional deficiencies, and industrial intoxications being obvious examples. However, we must be cautious about generalising too far from

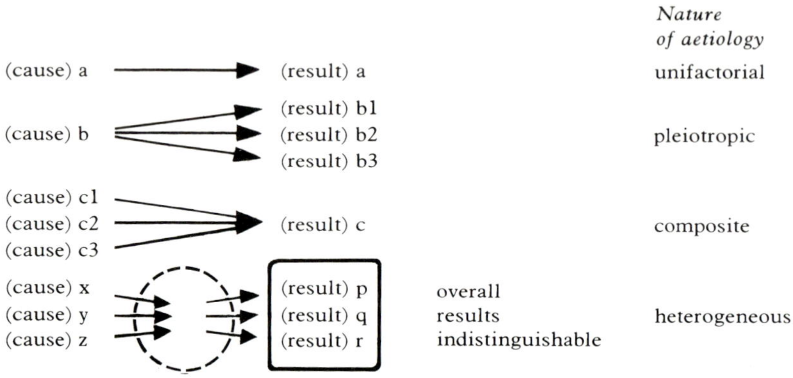

Fig. 2.4 Some of the relationships between causes and results (diseases). (Derived from Murphy, 1972; for description see text.)

this experience. There is no reason other than optimism to suppose that such simplistic models are necessarily appropriate to diseases of which the aetiology remains obscure.

It is more common for us to become aware of influences that appear to contribute to the development of a condition, without these being sufficient to provide a complete or even an adequate explanation. Present knowledge of ischaemic heart disease typifies this situation. We are often driven to further confuse our limited understanding by speaking of diverse aetiologies, but what does this concept signify? A distinction has to be made between heterogeneous and composite aetiologies (Fig. 2.4), and unfortunately one of the dangers with techniques of multivariate analysis is that the difference may be neglected.

Heterogeneity describes the situation where the causes are distinct but the results are indistinguishable. This can represent a big obstacle to understanding. For example, until a clinician realised that a cretin was different from other mentally retarded dwarfs, little progress could be made; the biochemistry of iodine, the geography of this element in relation to goitre, the epidemiology and other aspects, all were impossible until the clinician had posed a circumscribed problem. Equally, much that may be observed in the laboratory and which appears relatively non-specific, because it is detected in only a proportion of patients, may in fact have much greater import if it correlates with an entity we have so far failed to differentiate.

Heterogeneity can always be a problem when the late stages of disease are observed in a tissue with a limited range of responses, considerations that are probably relevant to osteoarthrosis. It is also a clinical challenge, the potential failure to recognise different disease entities, such as has now been shown with juvenile chronic arthritis (Ansell & Bywaters, 1959; Ansell & Wood, 1976) and as has been suggested may be the case for rheumatoid arthritis (Wood, 1968).

Composite aetiology refers to a given result occurring from the conjunction of multiple causes, what in loose usage is often referred to as being multifactorial. The interaction of a number of causal circumstances or factors is presumed to be necessary for a condition to develop. The concept is particularly apposite to the chronic diseases of later life, amongst which many rheumatic disorders loom large. One must suspect from their chronic nature that environmental components of aetiology are more complex; certainly the difficulties posed by induction and latency over long periods make them more difficult to elucidate. Furthermore, one is also tempted to suppose that genetic components are perhaps more important, if only because the age at which these diseases develop has rendered them less subject to selection pressures (Wood & Badley, 1984)

Nature and nurture. There are two main classes of explanation for the particularity of disease experience. First, that only a part of the population is susceptible, and secondly, that only a part is exposed to determining or precipitating circumstances. These two possibilities have often been treated as if they were mutually exclusive, leading to unenlightening questions of the type,

'Is this condition inherited?' Certainly with some of the inherited structural defects the contribution of environmental factors may be so small as to be indeterminate, but the situation can be very different with genetically determined metabolic abnormalities. Favism is undoubtedly an inherited disease, but if the fava bean does not feature in your environment you do not suffer from the condition.

The underlying web of causality is in fact very complex, involving what Knox (1968) has referred to as the combinatorial properties of a series of causal or contributory circumstances. Such circumstances include both individual and social factors, personality and biological variates such as age and sex on the one hand and the influence of culture and various aspects of social structure on life style and behaviour on the other (Wood & Badley, 1984). For the purposes of this discussion the realistic question can be reduced to pondering the relative magnitudes of the separate contributions of nature and nurture. The conclusions will describe persons and the time and place at which they are affected, information that will also be of some relevance to diagnosis and management.

What is known of environmental factors contributing to the development of rheumatic disorders has been reviewed recently (Wood, 1985). Our concrete knowledge of extraneous influences is generally rudimentary, and this despite much imaginative speculation about the role of factors such as infectious agents and immunological phenomena (Dumonde, 1976). Difficulty stems from loose usage of the term 'infection'. One immediately thinks of situations where Koch's postulates are satisfied, but the paradigm of the germ theory is being modified as more subtle interrelationships between microbe and man are discovered. The complexity of disease associations with Epstein–Barr virus illustrates this state of affairs. It is unfortunate that so far immunologists and virologists have been unable to specify the nature of the relations with greater precision, rendering it impossible for other disciplines to expose the ideas to falsification — such as by testing for space–time interaction (Wood, 1978b).

As far as the genetical background is concerned it is likely that there is an inherited component of virtually every disease, and that this probably determines susceptibility. Consider how, in the one species *Canis familiaris*, alsatians (German shepherds) are prone to dislocation of the hips, dachsunds to prolapse of the intervertebral discs, and dalmatians to hyperuricaemia. It seems that susceptibility or diathesis is the result of a number of factors, more than one of which may be genetically determined. Moreover, by being multifactorial it is likely that susceptibility is not an all-or-none state, but that it may exist to varying degrees in different individuals. If the disease is associated with an identifiable characteristic, such as blood groups with peptic ulcer, or HLA-B27 with ankylosing spondylitis, marker genes can yield a partial indication of susceptibility. Unfortunately it is not usually possible to get any absolute indication of susceptibility in the individual, even B27 being only a mark of increased risk for spondylitis (Grahame et al, 1975), but the concept is nevertheless valuable.

One of the theoretical attractions of the multifactorial determination of susceptibility is that it does provide a means of explaining disease associations. The increased likelihood of a patient with rheumatoid arthritis suffering from tuberculosis or peptic ulcer (Cobb & Hall, 1965) could be due to the fact that, of the genes determining susceptibility to these diseases, one could be common to all three conditions. A similar explanation could account for the association of psoriasis with various forms of arthropathy (Wright & Moll, 1971), and also for the occurrence of overlap of different collagen diseases, both in the kindreds of those suffering from one of these maladies and in the concept of mixed connective tissue disease.

Drawing inferences

One of the more creative acts in medicine can be the detection of associations. In a sophisticated form this is typified by the first description of a syndrome (Cochrane, 1965). Having observed an association, such as has been suggested between rheumatoid arthritis and hypogammaglobulinaemia (Good & Rotstein, 1960), we are likely then to ponder its significance and particularly to consider whether the relationship is causal. Unfortunately there are no simple answers to the difficulties, as the persisting uncertainty about hypogammaglobulinaemia indicates.

Many of the problems are highlighted by consideration of the challenge of interpreting changes associated with age, such as in relation to osteoarthrosis. Is an observed characteristic an integral part of ageing per se? If this were the case we should surely expect it to be consistent and universal. Or is it something that is not a feature of the ageing process but which nevertheless increases in frequency with age? If the latter, is the association the result of some relatively non-specific concomitant of age, such as greater exposure to wear, or is it the consequence of some specific pathological process which is itself commoner in those of greater age? Osteophytosis is probably an example of a non-specific concomitant (Wood, 1971) whereas osteoarthrosis is likely to be a disease; wear may be common to both, but with the latter it could be accelerated and abnormal. A corollary of this analysis is that any universal characteristic or process is of questionable relevance to elucidation of morbid changes, the concept of disease implying a less than universal experience.

Part of the difficulty arises from what has been referred to as the cross-sterilisation of disciplines, 'the bolstering up of arguments in one field with doubtful and imperfectly understood inferences made from another' (Frankfurter, 1948). As Murphy (1966) goes on to remark, 'if there is one piece of folly more remarkable than the belief that the tools of one's own specialty are suited to the solving of all problems, it is the naive belief that those from another are'. The proliferation of statistical props for clinical arguments is an obvious example of this, and the hazards get neglected (Altman, 1980; Gore, 1981). In this particular area the possibilities for bias are legion; Sackett (1979) has succeeded in identifying only one less than Heinz's celebrated varieties.

Central to the endeavour are the three causal fallacies: *post hoc ergo propter hoc*, the confusion of cause and effect, and the deception of common cause. One of the more celebrated examples of the latter was the train of intermediate conclusions on the aetiology of homologous serum jaundice (Paul, 1966); in one instance it was attributed first to diabetes, then to something about people attending diabetic clinics, and then to diabetics who were being injected. Obesity is vulnerable in this regard; we know it is associated with reduced life expectancy but no one has yet shown that losing weight lengthens life, prudent though advice to this effect would appear to be. The only really satisfactory proof of a causal relationship is to show that modification of the presumed aetiological factor leads to anticipated differences in the end result. Such evidence is usually not easy to contrive, but short of that the guide should be Bradford Hill's nine criteria — strength, consistency, specificity, temporality, biological gradient, plausibility, coherence, experiment, and analogy (Hill, 1965).

The need for caution in interpreting associations is illustrated by the relationship between brucellosis and rheumatic complaints (Cliff, 1981). Brucellosis is known to produce arthritis, and it has been assumed that much of that identified in agricultural workers is brucella-associated. However, work by Henderson (1967) suggests that the association shouldn't be taken at face value. Recurrent injury of the same anatomical site over a period of years may give rise to a clinical picture resembling chronic arthritis. The importance of the distinction is obvious because recurrent injury might be avoided by means different from those for the control of brucella infection.

In his description of the scientific approach Medawar (1969) specified a logically articulated structure, but he also noted that a defect of the hypothetico-deductive scheme is that it sets no upper limit to the number of hypotheses that might be propounded to account for observations. Part of the difficulty is that data tend to be 'submitted as objective because of the nature of the measurement and not because of the objectivety of the . . . method of applying the data to evaluation' (Preston, 1977).

Underlying this, though, the logic is vulnerable — we are often compelled to rely on what are called 'non-conclusive arguments' (Alexander, 1969) and an element of circularity is difficult to avoid, the latter being evident in the justification for many statistical procedures (Murphy, 1972). It is because logic alone does not usually allow us to reject other explanations consistent with available evidence that emphasis has been placed on attempts to expose ideas to falsification (Popper,

1959). The simplest, but often neglected, way of observing this caution is to look at inconsistencies in evidence — following Hamilton's (1974) advice to always concentrate on failures.

This strategy may be facilitated by seeking what amounts to methods of triangulation — other sources of data, and other means of acquiring information that has a bearing on the question. For example, Lawrence (1961) developed a measure of the frequency of RA from his studies of population samples. We attempted to estimate prevalence by a different route. Long-term follow-up studies of patients with RA (Reah et al, 1971) provided an indication both of the frequency of mention of the disease on the death certificates of decedent individuals and of the average duration of disease from the time of diagnosis in a representative group of affected persons. Applying this information in the fundamental theorem of epidemiology (prevalence = incidence × duration), together with reported mortality from RA for the whole of Great Britain, we were able to compute an independent prevalence estimate. This was of the same order of magnitude as Lawrence's measure.

RHEUMATIC SUFFERING

Medical practice exists because people wish to seek help when they develop problems that they relate to their state of health. The physician's insight on the problem is the concept of disease. Paradoxically, though, the very strength which has promoted biomedical understanding carries with it the danger of obscuring problems. This hazard arises from the dialectic between percepts and concepts, between subject and object relationships. Feinstein (1967) put his finger on the difficulty when he said that 'what is archaic in clinical medicine today is . . . the idea that the complex natural phenomena occurring in diseased people can be adequately classified by a taxonomy devoted only to disease'.

Illness and disease

Health in the individual relates to levels of physiological function, an equilibrium that is threatened or disturbed by disease. Such an appreciation encourages the view that health and disease are mutually exclusive states. This perspective of discontinuity is reinforced by clinical practice which, being a sphere of action, also imposes a dichotomy — whether or not to treat. The underlying reality, however, is that health and disease represent the poles of a continuum. The overwhelming majority of individuals lie at intermediate points on the spectrum, and there is a variable threshold of expression at which disease processes become manifest. Thus as a phenomenon disease must be seen as being graded rather than discontinuous, which has important implications for the types of explanation to be sought.

The concept of disease (Black, 1968) has been the foundation for most of our comprehension of biomedical derangements. This encourages us to regard the notion as having substance. In fact, though, disease has no existence outside the bodies of those that suffer from it (Wood, 1970a). It is no more than a simplifying assumption that enables us to perceive the similarities between the health problems or illnesses of different individuals. The contrast is between the abstract and the concrete and the latter, illness, is a reflection of the interaction between disease and the individual's body (Fig. 2.5). Seen in this light the attempt to combat disease can be recognised as one of the means of ameliorating a patient's illness; obviously it tends to be the most effective means because it is directed at eliminating the underlying cause of the problem.

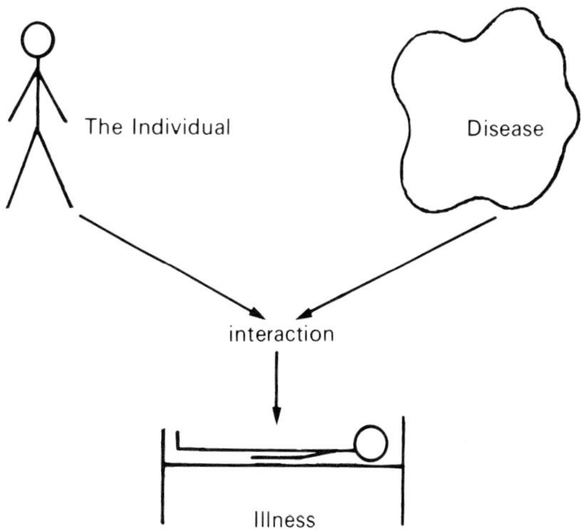

Fig. 2.5 The relationship between the individual, his disease, and his illness.

Illness status	Disease status	Clinical interpretation
Ill	Symptoms correlated with pathology	Clinical disease
Not ill	Pathology without symptoms (e.g. isolated 'abnormal' test)	(a) Subclinical disease (b) Misinterpretation of findings
Ill	Symptoms without discernible pathology	Symptomatic diagnosis (pejorative)

Fig. 2.6 The relation between symptoms, signs, and illness.

The possible interrelationships between disease and illness are quite complex, as may be seen in Figure 2.6. The usual situation is a correlation between symptoms and evidence of pathology, so-called 'clinical disease'. Increasingly, however, and especially with the introduction of biochemical profiles and multiphasic screening, we are confronted by abnormalities identified in the absence of related illness. The pathological significance of an isolated finding of hyperuricaemia is often difficult to determine. We may even create the difficulty for ourselves, because the notion of hyperuricaemia derives from exaggerated application of the concept of a 'normal range' (Murphy, 1966). The observation may in fact reflect little more than an extreme of 'normal' variation.

Even more problematic are symptoms that develop without a discernible pathological process to account for them. Symptomatic diagnosis is usually regarded pejoratively, though as much as anything it represents no more than failure of our powers of detection and understanding. If a syndrome can be recognised reproducibly, albeit solely on the basis of a number of characteristic symptoms, our disquiet is partially assuaged. However, many forms of soft-tissue or non-articular rheumatism fail to satisfy even this criterion (Wood et al, 1979).

The limitations of our medical knowledge cannot deny the existence of these problems, nor can they gainsay the suffering and the morbidity burden that result; a few of these states are fairly intractable, as some forms of back pain exemplify (Wood & Badley, 1980). The relatively mild nature of many of these conditions creates ethical problems in pursuing many lines of investigation by direct invasion, such as tissue biopsy. Clinicopathological facts are thus likely to remain beyond our grasp for some time, but a degree of progress could be anticipated if we restored merit to simple clinical observation or nosography.

These points may be summarised by definitions. Disease is a condition of the body in which its structure or function is disturbed or deranged. Illness is the state that is perceived by the individual when he or she is suffering from disease. Sickness, with which I have not dealt, is the state that develops as a reaction to illness, where the individual manifests behaviours in response to the expectations others have of him when he is ill.

Recognition of problems

Although disease is properly conceived of as a process, with an unfolding natural history, it is often unconsciously reduced to being thought of as a state. This then makes it too easy for it to be considered in isolation from the sequence of interactions that occur with the host body. Our disease nomenclature compounds the problem by being based largely on morbid or pathological anatomy. Pathological terminology inevitably relates mainly to form, to what can be observed visually, whereas most of the patient's symptoms derive from disturbances of function. By the very use of this nomenclature we automatically remove ourselves one stage, and a very important one, from the patient's problems.

Pathological features form the kernel of what is referred to as the medical model of illness which, in essentials, may be represented as:

$$\text{aetiology} \rightarrow \text{pathology} \rightarrow \text{manifestations.}$$

To respond to Feinstein's (1967) criticism (noted at the beginning of this section on suffering), what is needed is a conceptual framework for appreciation of the consequences of disease (Wood, 1975). In order to accomplish this it is necessary to extend the medical model along the following lines (Wood & Badley, 1978):

disease → impairment → disability → handicap.

To use a rheumatological example, limitation of motion of individual joints of the lower limb (impairments) may or may not interfere with the ability to walk, and it is the composite activity of walking that is considered in the context of disability — i.e. restriction of the ability to perform activities that are generally accepted as essential components of everyday life. Handicap is concerned with what disadvantage may ensue. Because an individual may have problems in walking one cannot necessarily infer that he or she is at a disadvantage; that will depend not only on the particular type of problem, but also on such factors as where they live (e.g. on the flat or with a need to climb) and what they expect of life (such as the more circumscribed aspirations of older people).

Perhaps the best-known attempt to draw attention to problems, as distinct from diagnosis, is that of Weed (1969) with his problem-oriented medical record. The practical remedies suggested are valuable, though difficulties are encountered with the display of a series of problems over time. However, Weed's work lacks an overall theoretical framework to take account of the hierarchical interrelationships between different dimensions of problem experience, along the lines just indicated. To meet this difficulty, the extended model of illness has been assimilated as the foundation for the World Health Organization's *International Classification of Impairments, Disabilities, and Handicaps* (WHO, 1980), and further guidance on the application of this scheme is available in a companion monograph (Wood & Badley, 1981a).

To a large degree individual problems are reflected by disabilities and handicaps much more than they are by diagnoses or impairments, though for operational purposes in relation to medical care the latter are naturally the major focus of concern. Nevertheless the more behavioural aspects are important, and their neglect gives rise to incongruence between the problem the physician identifies and the trouble that really concerns the patient. This can lead to difficulties in communication between the two parties (Bury & Wood, 1979). Some of the dangers can be mitigated by more explicit formulation of the aims of clinical intervention (de Blécourt et al, 1981). The different dimensions of disablement are also relevant to assessment of outcome and evaluation of therapy. If these considerations are neglected there can be a hazard of subsuming a problem in one of its expressions, such as by concentrating on a surrogate property such as grip strength when the relevant difficulty is a more general one of manual function (Wood, 1983c).

Consequences of rheumatic disorders

It is possible to derive some indication of the extent of more personal individual consequences from a consideration of those persons who are impaired to some degree by their rheumatic problem. One of the most representative sources for such information is the report on a study carried out by the Government Social Survey in Great Britain (Harris, 1971). In these data rheumatic disorders emerge as the biggest single class of impairments due to any cause. These conditions are responsible for 36% of the total burden, a proportion that approaches 50% in the over 65s. A measure of the impact of these disorders on everyday life style is shown in Table 2.5. Further details of the rates of impairment and severe disability from selected rheumatic disorders will be shown later (Table 2.9). In terms of impact the arthropathies are the dominant problem. Of all those more seriously affected, the severely and very severely disabled, rheumatoid arthritis is the underlying problem in 10% and other arthropathies account for a further 25%. Other noteworthy features of those impaired to any degree by rheumatic conditions are shown in Table 2.6. Difficulties in walking, already noted (Table 2.5), are to some extent compounded by other aspects. Thus a large proportion are elderly, many live alone, and the frequency of contact with many services is less than the average for chronically sick and disabled persons as a whole. Greater detail of the situation for disabled arthritics has been studied by Thompson et al (1974) and is shown in Table 2.7. Perhaps the most interesting conclusion of this work was that there appeared to be

Table 2.5 Impact of rheumatic disorders on everyday life style (expressed as ratios per thousand population at risk; source — Harris, 1971)

Rheumatic disorder	ICD rubric (8th revision)	Impaired persons (adults, > 16 yr of age)		Disadvantaged in major dimensions of activity (proportions of impaired rheumatic sufferers, as %)							
		all degrees	severe and very severe	Physical independence		Mobility				Occupation	
				confined to chair or bed	unable to bath themselves	wheelchair confined	wheelchair use	house-bound*	use sticks or crutches	have had to give up work	have had to change job
Arthropathies — rheumatoid arthritis	712	3.4	1.3	7.8	25.0	3.3	10.8	17.4	32.2	31.3	2.4
— osteoarthrosis**	713	18.7	3.0	1.8	17.9	0.4	3.4	13.9	36.4	18.9	1.7
Dorsopathies	353, 717.0 725, and 728	2.0	0.2	0.4	6.4	0.3	0.9	1.2	12.7	17.3	1.7
Other rheumatic disorders	274, 390–398 rem. 710–738 787, and N840–N848	8.1	0.9	2.1	12.1	0.3	2.2	6.4	25.6	16.8	2.1
All rheumatic disorders		27.8†	4.9	2.6	17.1	0.8	4.0	12.5	32.7	20.0	1.8

* Includes those who are confined to chair or bed.

** Arthritis unspecified has been included under osteoarthrosis because it resembles this later category in most associated characteristics.

† The total of impaired persons with all rheumatic disorders is less than the sum of the individual rates because more than one disorder was present in a proportion of people.

Table 2.6 Features of individuals impaired by rheumatic disorders (after Harris, 1971)

Feature	Proportion of impaired rheumatic sufferers mainfesting the feature (%)	Comparison of feature in rheumatic sufferers with all impaired persons*
Female sex	73.5	++
Age (years):		
16–49	10.6	–
65–74	33.6	+
Single or widowed	47.1	+
Private consultation:		
orthodox	10.7	+
heterodox	12.5	++
On local authority 'handicapped' register	2.1	=
Visited by:		
home helps	8.7	–
meals on wheels	2.4	=
district nurse or health visitor	8.6	–
social worker	3.4	–
remedial therapist	2.4	+
chiropodist	12.4	+
voluntary agencies	0.6	+

* Comparisons are indicated as greater or lesser proportions by + or – respectively, = denoting close similarity; differences greater than 5% are shown ++.

Table 2.7 Problems in self-care experienced by disabled arthritics (expressed as proportions of a sample of chronically sick and disabled persons with rheumatological problems; source — Thompson et al, 1974)

Activity	Does with difficulty (%)	Someone's help needed (%)	Totally dependent (%)	All degrees of impairment (%)
Personal hygiene:				
— shaving (by males)	0	0	0	0
— combing and brushing hair (by females)	3	1	2	6
— washing hands and face	4	1	1	6
— getting to and using toilet	10	1	2	14
— having a bath or all-over wash	29	16	4	49
— cutting toenails	21	19	14	54
Dressing:				
— getting dressed	6	2	2	10
— doing up buttons and zips	9	3	2	15
— putting on shoes and stockings	12	3	3	19
Within the home:				
— feeding	1	0	0	1
— preparing meals	11	6	5	21
— getting in and out of bed	21	2	1	24
— other housework	37	18	6	62
Mobility:				
— getting around the house	22	1	1	24
— using stairs in the house (where has to)	35	1	6	41
— getting out of the house	30	8	8	46
— coping with stairs outside the home	28	12	10	49
In the community:				
— local shopping	12	9	16	37
— using buses	25	10	15	49
— town shopping	12	17	24	53

considerable underutilisation of services. When compared with the potential for benefit this was true at all levels; there was underutilisation of the general practitioner, of all the hospital services, of remedial assistance, of aids to daily living, and of adaptations to the home.

The limitation of all this information is that it is cross-sectional, whereas for prognosis one wants longitudinal data. Unfortunately the latter have to be based on the experience of yesterday's patients, and few meticulous follow-up studies have been carried out. This means that it is not possible to estimate with any precision the probabilities for different outcomes, such as that an arthritic will become bed-ridden. Figure 2.7 shows the best indication we were able to derive from published experience; it almost certainly exaggerates the less favourable outcomes, as has happened in the past with systemic lupus erythematosus and multiple sclerosis (largely because of stringent criteria for inclusion of patients in such studies). Although this offers a feeling for what is likely to happen,

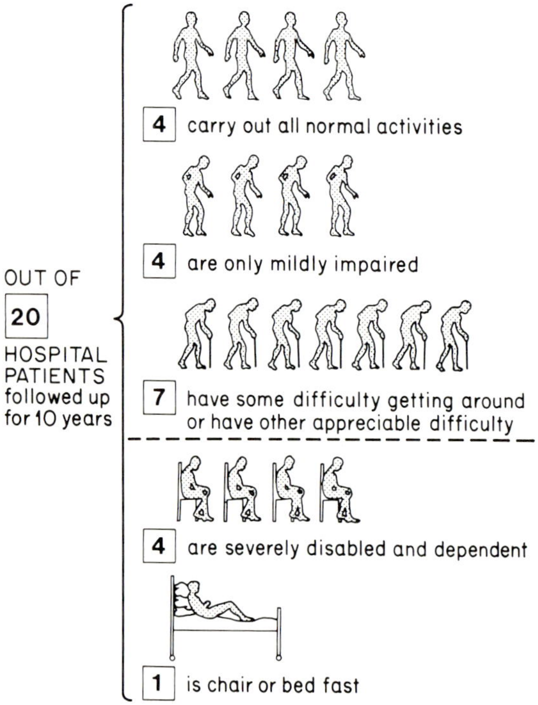

Fig. 2.7 A crude indication of prognosis in rheumatoid arthritis. (Derived from a teaching slide prepared for the Arthritis and Rheumatism Council, largely based on Duthie et al, 1964)

lack of rigorous documentation of long-term outlook denies us the opportunity of measuring changes in the effectiveness of treatment. It also implies that decisions about the benefit/risk ratio of various therapies have to be entirely intuitive.

Mortality experience. Reported death rates for various rheumatic disorders have been included in Table 2.9. Of the individual causes named, the most important has been rheumatic heart disease, which in very recent times was still responsible for 5500 deaths a year in England and Wales. The only other rheumatological cause reaching a four figure total has been rheumatoid arthritis, to which approximately 1000 fatalities were attributed in a recent year; these represent only one in eight of deaths occurring in persons in whom RA had been diagnosed earlier in hospital (Benn & Wood, 1972a).

One detail that may call for explanation is the attribution of death to conditions that are not generally regarded as leading to a fatal outcome; bursitis and synovitis, for example. If a person dies while undergoing treatment, such as a surgical operation, then the underlying cause rule will lead to the death being assigned to the condition which led to the operation. This is not an unreasonable assumption; if the individual had not suffered from the condition he or she would not have been submitted to surgery and so in all probability would not have died.

A practical aspect of mortality experience is worth noting. Studies documenting the course of any disease tend to be based on more severely affected patients. It is on such material that assurance companies have to establish their calculations on life expectancy for persons suffering from specific diseases. To some degree these computations of risks may therefore tend to exaggerate hazards — a point clinical investigators might bear in mind when deciding how to present their results. What is worse is that, if rejected for insurance by a company, a patient may be placed on what is known as the Association Register, jeopardising chances for obtaining cover from a competitor. The whole problem of insurance in chronic disease has been reviewed recently (Tomenson et al, 1984). It would be wise for physicians to advise patients that, rather than contacting companies direct, they should consult a broker or a voluntary organisation concerned with the interests of persons afflicted similarly.

The community burden

Studies of specific diseases are valuable for what they contribute to our overall understanding, as may be seen in the next chapter. However, the diverse nature of rheumatic suffering and the relatively non-specific character of many complaints inevitably determines that the burden of these conditions is greater than can be revealed just by summing experience of the individual diseases. This is evident when the array of subcategories in the *International Classification of Diseases* is contrasted with a more clinically oriented scheme such as, for example, that implicit in the chapter headings in this book. The lack of diagnostic specificity in much of the available information about the consequences of rheumatic disorders also contributes to the differences.

Unfortunately the discordance in these measures of community suffering tends to get reinforced. As professionals we are involved at a particular level of a health care system. Part of the difficulty in comprehending the scope of the problems is that patients are seen only in highly stylised situations, at a consultation, and the patients that are seen are only those individuals who have made contact with that particular level of the system — be it on their own initiative or by a process of selective referral. The physician is thus aware of only a part of illness phenomena, other than to the degree that knowledge is extended by personal experience of suffering. This section is intended as an antidote to these limitations.

The spectrum of rheumatic suffering has some value in providing a crude indication of the probabilities of different diagnoses. At the same time such data can influence the organisation of services to combat arthritis and rheumatism. In what follows the advantage of simplicity in presenting overall experience outweighs the fact that appreciable and important differences between the sexes are concealed. These differences are largely what would be expected when account is taken of age and the characteristics of the various rheumatological conditions. The information generally relates only to manifest disease and is therefore of very limited use for aetiological studies, although it is of some biological interest because it sets health-related problems in overall perspective. The information is ordered according to source, which gives a rough indication of the calls made on various levels of the service and hence of the states ascertained.

Rheumatic disorders in hospital

The medical student gains first awareness in hospital, and the specialist tends to pursue knowledge of rheumatological conditions in the same context. This, then, is probably the most appropriate level at which to start.

Some information on hospital admissions is available annually and has revealed patterns of change in recent years. Undoubtedly some of the latter reflect increasing use of surgical joint replacement, of which the associated influences have been reviewed elsewhere (Wood, 1976b). Taken together the various rheumatic disorders account for over 4% of all non-maternity admissions to hospital. Table 2.8 shows the principal characteristics related to these admissions, and a number of points call for comment. Perhaps most important, these data reflect the overall situation in England and Wales, and conceal fairly considerable variations between one region of the country and another.

We noted earlier (Benn & Wood, 1972b) that median waiting times for a bed had been increasing, probably partly due to greater use of waiting lists in preference to immediate admissions. The trend has continued more recently, but different factors have been at play. Whereas formerly there had been an increase in the admission rate and also in per capita bed usage, at least for rheumatoid arthritis and osteoarthrosis, the longer wait more recently has been experienced in the face of a fairly stable per capita admission rate. This has resulted from a reduction in available beds (i.e. the average number occupied daily), other than for OA, and for which shorter median durations of stay have not been entirely able to compensate. Overall the proportion of beds occupied by women has increased, due presumably at least in part to the predominance of this sex among the growing number of elderly people. It seems that hospital planners may not have appreciated the situation; the nature of rheumatic disorders,

Table 2.8 Characteristics of hospital utilisation for rheumatological disorders in England and Wales (derived mainly from Hospital In-Patient Enquiry (HIPE) for 1978 — DHSS, 1981)

Hospital utilisation characteristic	Rheumatoid arthritis	Osteoarthrosis	Other arthritis	Displacement of intervertebral disc	Other musculoskeletal and connective tissue disorders	All diseases of musculoskeletal system
ICD rubrics (9th revision):	714	715	remainder 711–716	722	remainder 710–739 excl. 717 and 730	710–739
Median waiting time for admission (weeks)	7.2	19.0	7.7	4.5	10.9	11.0
Admission rate (per thousand population)	0.3	0.8	0.1	0.3	1.8	3.9
Median duration of stay (days)	18	19	16	14	7	11
Average number of beds used daily (per million population)	46	73	9	14	60	211
Proportion of beds used for women (%)	82	79	77	43	58	69
Hospital death rate (% of admissions)	4.8	3.0	3.4	0.0	0.7	1.4
Operation rate (all procedures) as proportion of all admissions (%)*	26	53	27	48	35	54
Operative mortality (% of persons operated on)	0.3	0.9	2.8	0.0	0.3	0.4
Proportion of discharges and deaths treated in selected hospital departments (%):						
— rheumatology	31	3	7	3	—	—
— physical medicine	10	2	—	7	1	—
— orthopaedic surgery	30	58	44	67	67	—
— general medicine	15	4	—	3	—	—
— geriatric	11	16	13	—	1	

* Derived from HIPE 1976; operations include a diversity of procedures extending to biopsy, endoscopy, and even isotope scanning, as well as a variety of non-operative procedures of which the commonest is normal delivery in childbirth.

and the associated need for rehabilitation, do not allow rheumatology departments to reduce inpatient facilities to such a great extent as other medical units — particularly because there are limits to how much the durations of rheumatological stays can be shortened.

One other aspect of the national situation attracts comment. Much the greatest proportion of the case load is carried by orthopaedic departments. Rheumatology units deal with only a part of the whole, even if consideration is restricted to rheumatoid arthritis. This is due to the fact that their existence and size is so variable, though the increase in their numbers in recent years has been reflected by the diminishing proportion of patients with RA treated in internal medicine beds. Despite this trend, though, at the time of the 1982 reorganisation of the National Health Service a quarter of health authorities in the United Kingdom were without specialist advice in the currently linked fields of rheumatology and rehabilitation.

Unfortunately, routine statistics on outpatient attendances are available only by specialty and not by diagnostic categories. In a recent year, outpatient attendances in Great Britain, in thousands, were over 200 new and 700 reattendances at rheumatology clinics, and almost 1400 and 4000 respectively at orthopaedic clinics (Wood & Badley, 1981b). Arden (1972) has estimated that 35% of new attendances at the latter were related to pain arising from the spine. To this should be added an allowance for orthopaedic attendances for other rheumatic conditions, say 15% on a conservative basis. This would indicate that new attendances for rheumatological problems occur at the rate of approximately 23 per thousand adults every year. The individuals referred to hospital were generally likely to attend outpatients on an average of four occasions during the year.

Rheumatism outside hospital

The patients seen at hospital are referred there by their general practitioner. The GP sees a different cross-section of rheumatic suffering. This has been reviewed recently (Wood & Badley, 1983), and is depicted diagrammatically in Figure 2.8. For every 1000 persons of all ages on a general practitioner's list, 152 will consult with a rheumatic problem during the course of a year (OPCS, 1974).

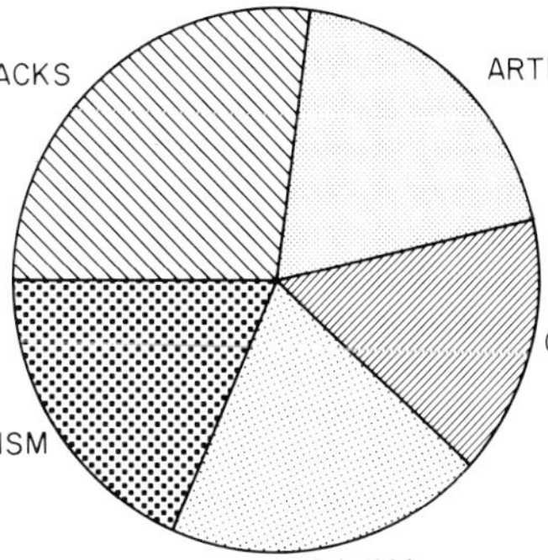

Fig. 2.8 Crude case mix in patients with rheumatic problems presenting to a general practitioner. (Derived from Second National Morbidity Study — OPCS, 1974.)

That is 15% of the individuals registered with the doctor, those at risk, but it accounts for 23% of all diseases and conditions presenting for consultation.

An attempt to rank conditions by their order of magnitude is open to manipulation unless comparably broad classes are used. Comparative rankings are therefore not usually instructive. However, it is noteworthy that the major classes of medical condition presenting to a GP are respiratory diseases, rheumatic conditions, and mental disorders.

Taking account of average list sizes, a GP is likely to see at least one new patient with some sort of rheumatic condition for every working day. It is important to realise that, although one is speaking of persons, these figures are in fact reflecting events, presentations to doctors, and so they should not be used as prevalence estimates for comparison with experience elsewhere. Nevertheless they do provide a measure of the calls being made on GPs, and they indicate that in excess of eight million people in Great Britain consult their doctors with one form or other of rheumatism every year.

A diagnostic breakdown of these conditions is given in Table 2.9, which shows the rates for consultations and for episodes as well as measures from other levels of the health service. Approximate estimates for the number of persons affected in Great Britain as a whole may be derived from the rates in Table 2.9 by multiplying them by the total population in thousands. The importance of complaints associated with trauma has been shown

Table 2.9 Measures of the frequency of experiences with rheumatic disorders (expressed as ratios per thousand population at risk for the year 1978 — Sources: OPCS, 1974,1981; DHSS, 1981; Harris, 1971.

Rheumatic disorder	ICD rubric (8th revision)	GP consultations (home population)		Sickness incapacity certifications (insured population)		Admissions to hospital (home population)	Impaired persons (adults, > 16 yr of age)		Deaths (home population)
		Consultations	Episodes	Spells	Days lost		All degrees	Severe and very severe	
Arthropathies		**79.9**	**35.6**	**7.64**	**964**	**1.47**	**22.10**	**4.30**	**0.05**
Gout	274	3.8	1.8	0.83	21	0.01	—	—	0.0007
Rheumatoid arthritis (incl. AS)	712	18.9	5.9	—	—	0.5	3.44	1.29	0.02
Spondylosis	713.1	13.7	7.6	—	—	—	—	—	0.002
other osteoarthrosis	rem. 713	43.5	20.3	3.12	421	0.8	3.56	0.52	0.015
Other arthritis	rem. 710–715	—	—	3.70	522	0.1	15.10	2.49	0.002
Connective tissue diseases	716 and 734	—	—	—	—	0.04	—	—	0.01
Back troubles		**68.0**	**36.1**	**20.69**	**738**	**0.88**	**2.00**	**0.20**	**0.0005**
Sciatica	353	3.3	1.7	2.79	115	0.06	0.34	0.01	0.00002
Lumbago	717.0	15.3	9.1	3.56	72	—	—	—	—
Displacement of intervertebral disc	725	17.5	6.4	3.79	277	0.3	1.66	0.19	0.0002
Vertebrogenic pain	728 excl. 728.9	10.9	5.4	3.54	120	0.5	—	—	0.0003
Other back pain	728.9	21.0	13.5	7.00	154	—	—	—	—
Non-articular rheumatism		**60.3**	**40.3**	**13.49**	**301**	**0.63**	—	—	**0.0004**
Frozen shoulder	717.1	3.2	1.8	—	—	—	—	—	—
Other rheumatism	rem. 717–718	14.3	9.9	—	—	—	—	—	0.0004
Other arthritis and rheumatism	rem. 710–718	9.2	5.9	7.01	165	0.07	—	—	0
Bursitis and synovitis	731	12.0	7.6	1.87	41	0.2	—	—	0.00002
Symptoms referred to limbs	787	21.6	15.1	4.61	95	0.4	—	—	0.00002
Other rheumatic disorders		**78.4**	**51.3**	**23.04**	**608**	**1.7**	**4.04**	**0.45**	**0.15**
Rheumatic fever and rheumatic heart disease	390–398	4.5	1.4	0.12	62	0.3	0.19	0.02	0.11
Internal derangement of joint	724	6.4	3.3	0.65	32	0.2	—	—	0.00002
Hallux valgus and varus	737	1.3	0.9	—	—	0.2	—	—	0
Other musculoskeletal disorders	rem. 720–738	19.5	13.2	1.82	139	0.9	3.04	0.34	0.04
Sprains and strains	N840–N848	46.6	32.5	20.45	375	0.1	0.81	0.09	0.0001
All rheumatic disorders		**286.5**	**163.3**	**64.85**	**2611**	**4.66**	**27.77**[b]	**4.91**	**0.2**
All diseases and conditions*		**3009.6**	**1808.6**[d] (671.7)	**429.41**	**15191**	**89.7**[c]	**77.99**	**12.66**	**11.93**[d]

a Sizes of populations for computation of national experience in England and Wales — multiply rate shown by home population, 49.1×10^3; insured population, 23.3×10^3; or adult population, 36.1×10^3; as appropriate. Population < 15 yr 13.0×10^3. (All population figures are quoted in thousands.)
b The total of impaired persons with all rheumatic disorders in less than the sum of the individual rates because more than one disorder was present in a proportion of people.
c Hospital admissions for all diseases and conditions exclude maternity admissions and those to psychiatric hospitals.
d The rate for episodes for all diseases and conditions is inflated by persons experiencing more than one episode, due to different causes; the rate in parentheses is that for patients consulting and is more useful for comparison with the rates shown.
* Includes all medical and surgical conditions, and are shown here for purposes of comparison.

by Weston & Wood (1971), and so strains and sprains have been included in addition to non-traumatic conditions; the former account for almost one-fifth of the totals derived from primary care. That noted, the great bulk of calls on the service are for relatively non-specific and ill-defined complaints referred to the musculoskeletal system, including the back.

Certain aspects of consultation patterns in primary care are of interest. The relative burden of rheumatic disorders is greater in older people. For instance, among individuals aged 45 years and older these complaints account for 31% of all diseases and conditions presenting. The average number of consultations per rheumatic patient is about two, so that a GP is likely to see at least two such individuals every working day. However, when return visits are considered further there is an impression that patients with rheumatic problems in general are seen slightly less frequently than those with other conditions.

Features of the GP's response to rheumatic disorders have been reviewed elsewhere (Wood & Badley, 1983). Whereas more than one-third of all patients seen are referred for outside help, only about one-fifth of rheumatic patients are so referred; for each type of referral the proportion of rheumatological patients is smaller than that for all diseases and conditions. Particularly noteworthy is the infrequency of referral for a local authority service. Hospital and specialist referral patterns are instructive because they offer some guidance to areas of need in postgraduate and continuing education.

Burden on society. The detailed experience just reviewed was derived from an ad hoc enquiry undertaken under the aegis of the Royal College of General Practitioners (OPCS, 1974). Generally it was not that different from an earlier study (Logan & Cushion, 1958, reviewed by Wood & McLeish, 1974). A cruder outline is available every year in statistics on sickness incapacity for work, and these have also been included in Table 2.9. However, the value of these data will be reduced in future as a consequence of changes in sickness insurance legislation, because they will be much less representative of the burden of suffering.

Incapacity data are derived from the working or insured population so that the denominator is smaller, the elderly not being covered and women being underrepresented. As can be seen in Table 2.9 the rates tend to be rather lower than those observed in the consultation studies covering all patients. However, by being based on employment statistics these data do allow one to estimate the productivity losses suffered by the community as a whole, an approximate method for this calculation being given by Benn & Wood (1972b). Such figures are vulnerable to the rapidity of change in values with inflation but, for what it is worth, the loss of productivity in a recent year had a cash value in excess of £1000 million (Wood & Badley, 1981b). This loss arose from over 1.5 million spells of certified rheumatic sickness incapacity, which caused more than 61 million days to be lost from work.

So far only contacts with different levels of health care arrangements have been discussed. By no means everyone goes to see their doctor when they develop a rheumatic complaint. Some thought therefore needs to be given to symptom experience in society at large. In a period of two weeks 29% of adults have experienced acheing in their limbs and joints, 21% have had backache, and 19% have had trouble with their feet (Dunnell & Cartwright, 1972). These categories are not exclusive and should be assessed in the context that adults experience an average of just under four symptoms during a 14-day period.

These figures indicate that some degree of rheumatic experience is almost universal, and it is likely that of the order of 20 million people in Great Britain suffer in this way during a year. This serves to reinforce McKeown & Lowe's (1974) comment that, if we accept the World Health Organization's euphoric definition of health as 'a state of complete physical, mental, and social well-being, and not merely the absence of disease or infirmity', then we are all sick.

ANTICIPATING THE FUTURE

In his letter of 22nd November 1757 to the Bishop of Waterford, Lord Chesterfield wrote 'physical ills are the taxes laid upon this wretched life; some are taxed higher, and some lower, but all pay something'. More than two centuries later the situation does not seem to have altered appreciably because, as I have tried to demonstrate, rheumatic complaints are a heavy tax that few escape. Moreover, and particularly as the proportion of elderly people in the population increases, the challenge is, if anything, growing (Wood et al, 1980). Some thought therefore needs to be given to the means for improving matters.

Control of rheumatic disorders

As with any class of health problem, the ultimate goal is to develop adequate measures for community control of rheumatic disorders. Three areas of great importance (WHO, 1976) are the identification of priorities and the development of strategies directed at improving rheumatic disease control; the promotion and co-ordination of collaborative research activities in rheumatology; and the development of educational opportunities to meet the needs of these programmes, as regards both research and clinical practice. It is with the first of these that this section is concerned.

The development of strategies for control has been considered elsewhere (Wood, 1983d). However, three prerequisites can be identified. Successful control results from increases in scientific knowledge, such as are described in this book. Appropriate technologies then need to be developed, to exploit understanding and translate it into practical expression. Finally, such technologies then need to be applied in response to the will of the people to overcome the problem (WHO, 1976). The will of the community is shaped by awareness of the nature and importance of the problem (Badley & Wood, 1979). It is a framework for orienting thoughts about strategic options that therefore merits more explicit consideration.

Levels of control

It is perhaps understandable that a physician's thoughts usually turn to treatment potential. However, a more global appreciation is necessary if the burden of suffering throughout the community is to be contained. For this purpose it is helpful to draw on the model developed by Leavell & Clark (1979).

Primary control. Prevention is customarily considered to be the best option, but present knowledge does not allow of many specific initiatives related to rheumatic disorders. Two levels of action should be considered — in regard to health promotion, and the containment of specific hazards. Both are amenable to influence largely through social policy initiatives, to the development of which physicians have important contributions to make insofar as health consequences are concerned.

Specific hazards have been reviewed elsewhere (Wood & Badley, 1984; Wood, 1985). As regards health promotion two aspects are relevant. The first is disease oriented, and there are three specific factors — exercise, diet, and beds — on which opinions are often held strongly but conflictingly. The evidence on all three is unsatisfactory, and so one can do no more than state common-sense views without endeavouring to bolster these with supposedly scientific justification.

To the extent that the integrity of the musculoskeletal system is preserved by the separate contributions of its individual parts, the protection of articular structures by their surrounding soft tissues is important. A general attribute such as muscle tone can therefore be critical, and hence thc value of adequate physical exercise — particularly in reducing liability to suffer from 'degenerative' changes in structures like the spine. Physical activity is influenced not only by individual preference but also by more general arrangements in society (e.g. the availability of sporting facilities, and particularly the decay in urban public transport — which fosters increasing reliance on private automobiles), so that there are health implications in many areas of social policy.

The determination of what happens within by what is taken in is firmly fixed in the minds of many, but the role of diet remains uncertain. Apart from the influence of specific foods on the uric acid pool, the only acceptable generality is that excess weight is liable to increase the stress transmitted across structures such as joints and so is best reduced if symptoms develop. There is thus a rheumatological component to be considered in relation to nutrition, and hence to agricultural, policies.

In regard to sleep the important observations are that a number of people with back pain find relief by sleeping on the floor, whereas the suffering of other individuals appears to be less dependent on physical support. There is therefore no pressing reason for medical considerations to feature in the choice of a bed, though having made it the lying is likely to be more comfortable for someone with back pain if the bed is not too soft.

The other aspect of health promotion is handicap oriented, and concerns implementation of a policy of enablement in anticipation of the problems likely to be experienced by persons disabled by arthritis. Relevant to this are urban design (in regard to isolation), educational and employment opportunities, transport policies, and social attitudes.

Secondary and tertiary control. As far as secondary control is concerned, the arrest of problems, there are again two levels to be considered — reaction to damage, and stabilisation to counter harm. The latter involves cure and amelioration, including the avoidance of impairment and disability by arrest of disease progression, and will be considered further in the next section. Reaction to damage calls for prompt response, mainly of relevance to injury, and for early detection and screening.

The most obvious rheumatological example of early detection concerns rheumatic fever, in order to minimise cardiac damage. There are few other instances where, in the light of current knowledge, a determined campaign for early detection would be justified. Screening is a problematic proposition, and before committing resources to such endeavours a number of desiderata should be borne in mind. These are (Smith, 1974):

Importance. In general the importance of a disorder is dependent on its frequency and severity, and under this head the major forms of arthritis would qualify. However, even a rare and localised condition may be deemed to be important if its progression can be modified by early intervention (e.g. congenital dislocation of the hip).

Safety and reliability of the test used in the process, considerations which are also relevant to its acceptability.

Discrimination. Determination of HLA status has a high sensitivity for ankylosing spondylitis (AS), but it is not very efficient in discrimination because it identifies those who have an innate susceptibility or predisposition rather than those who are going to develop the disease. Even if the claim that 20% of those positive for B27 are at risk of developing AS (Calin & Fries, 1975) were generally applicable, this would mean that at least 80% of those detected would not be at risk.

Specificity. Clinical reliance on specificity in pattern recognition encourages the attachment of too much importance to this criterion. When applied on a population basis, tests with high specificity still yield large numbers of false positives just because 'normals' considerably outnumber of the affected (Wood, 1972).

False positives. Although obviously not in the same class as cancer screening, there remains a possibility of generating anxiety in those 'falsely' detected.

Natural history. The full natural history needs to be known. In this context it is relevant to recall the prerequisites for prevention and cure. Prevention is a realisable goal only when circumstances extraneous to the potentially affected individual are responsible, so that the circumstances can be susceptible to manipulation in such a way as to eliminate their operation. Cure is feasible when the changes induced in the individual by the disease process are not, for a time at least, irreversible.

Benefit. The most critical aspect is that there is little point in early intervention unless this makes a marked difference to prognosis — screening for lung cancer is currently not worthwhile for this reason.

Take-up. Effective screening demands that you reach those whom you consider to be at risk. Ethical considerations are also relevant — for instance, would the likely benefits justify a venepuncture?

Costs. These are not limited to financial aspects, and have to be measured in terms of personpower and other scarce resources.

Against this background, perhaps the best candidate for a screening approach in regard to rheumatology is anticipatory care of the elderly — monitoring their health status so that rheumatic complaints are detected early, before they interfere seriously with mobility.

Tertiary control is concerned with repair and this, too, can be considered at two levels. The first is directed at the control of disability by restoration, either by reconstruction (such as a total hip replacement) or by rehabilitation. The other level is concerned with the control of handicap and involves continuing care (including monitoring for deterioration), support (such as welfare provision, assistance, and aid to the family), and enablement by means such as extension of opportunities and vocational resettlement.

Arrangements for care

Coming back to strategies for stabilisation, the processes of cure and amelioration, it is helpful to note that the critical distinction between medicine and science relates to the aims that are pursued (Platt, 1967). Whereas the latter aspires to discovery and generalisation, the former is concerned to particularise and plan action judged to be of best value to the individual. In pursuing these aims different decision strategies are adopted, epitomised in Sherrington's words: 'Science nobly declines as proof anything but complete proof; but common sense, pressed for time, accepts and acts on acceptance' (Cohen, 1943). The concepts that are utilised or invoked in such acceptance reflect the frames of reference in which the physician operates, and they determine the more immediate objectives.

The major considerations for planned care (Wood & Badley, 1976) help to illuminate aspects of clinical decision-making and the contribution to be expected from others involved in health care. These considerations are:

1. The nature of the disease process, which is considered in the other chapters of this book.

2 The activity of this process, be it acute exacerbation, a chronic course, remission, or exhaustion of active disease. Assessment may be aided by study of phenomena such as acute phase reactants, which will also be mentioned elsewhere in this book.

3. Particularities of the localisation of this process. In other words, problems which are associated with the specific sites affected, the joints and other structures and organs, and which manifest themselves as impairments. Rheumatology is confounded by an almost infinite potential of patterns with multilocus involvement, a difficulty that does not confront most other specialties. It is probably for this reason that a concept of locomotor failure has not emerged, valuable though this approach has been for other branches of medicine.

4. Complications of the disease process, including those affecting other systems of the body. These may be exemplified by the concept of rheumatoid disease, a designation which emphasises that involvement may not be restricted to the joints.

5. Complications of treatment. It is salutary that antirheumatic drugs are responsible for almost a quarter of all fatal therapeutic misadventures. The numbers of such deaths every year are in fact small, about 0.5% of all deaths attributed to rheumatic disorders. However, the additional occurrence of a diversity of other adverse effects highlights the need for a deliberate balancing of possible benefits against risks. Hence the concept that a patient must earn his treatment.

6. Comorbidity, the presence of other diseases. For instance, therapeutic choices for medication are often constrained by the simultaneous existence of a peptic ulcer or of renal failure.

7. The obligations the individual is expected to discharge, according to his life style. The person making contact with a health care system is likely to do so because of interference with the ability to discharge those functions that are expected of him or which he expects of himself. In other words, the individual is unable to sustain his accustomed social role and cannot maintain his customary relations with others. This view is sufficiently broad to take account of the vast majority of calls that are likely to be made on a health care system. At one extreme it embraces life-threatening illness, and at the other it includes less medical experiences such as anxiety or the wish for advice and counselling.

8. The environment, both at home and at work. The tragedy is that all too often heroic remedies have to be resorted to in order to compensate for inability to modify the environment suitably.

9. The role of the immediate family, both in giving support and in reinforcing advice, such as by ensuring that necessary exercises are carried out.

10. The response of the community. Awareness of the impact of rheumatic disorders on the life style of the individual and his family is generally limited, and the burden imposed on society is also

underestimated. Insufficient knowledge of these dimensions influences general attitudes to the problems, and may encourage the persistence of inappropriate attitudes. In turn the latter shape the expectations for the individual with a disability, and they also condone the perpetuation of physical barriers such as flights of stairs. The expressions of greatest general interest to physicians are the influences of constraints on resources and personpower.

11. Other psychological and social factors. One of the important challenges is advent of a chronic illness. Consider an individual developing rheumatoid arthritis. As soon as it is realised that the complaints are not a passing phenomenon some sort of reconciliation with the uncertainty in outlook has to be effected (Wiener, 1975). Performance becomes impaired, ways of life have to change, and relationships with others have to be modified. In these altered circumstances things that were done without thought call for deliberation, things that were easy become difficult or impossible. One has to search for latent qualities and strive to elaborate some new role, a compromise different from that to which one was accustomed. All of these developments affect one's body image, which in any case may be vulnerable to the stigma of visible deformity and reduced competence (Goffman, 1968). One's own sense of identity is also under assault, and has to undergo metamorphosis. Against this background it is evident that over time the individual is likely to be concerned much more with the consequences of his illness experience than with the actual illness itself. It is also clear that, unless a dramatic cure can be effected, contacts with a health care system are likely to play only a minor part in the adaptations the individual makes in the face of his problem. Moreover, as the individual strives to develop a stable view of his situation he is likely to be considerably influenced by his experiences with other sufferers.

It can be seen that in the first six of these considerations medical assessment is paramount. As far as rheumatic disorders are concerned, particular expertise in the medical aspects of these conditions is possessed by the rheumatologist. His special contribution still rests in examination of the articular system, which is the key to correct medical assessment. However, expensive investment in the first six areas can be largely wasted unless there is integration both of the means of assessing the last five and of meeting any needs identified by this process.

All professionals involved in care need a basic appreciation of the contribution of all these different factors. To confine activities to the last five, without regard to medical aspects, is as shortsighted and as counter-productive as for physicians and surgeons to neglect consideration of the individual who is harbouring the disease and the environment in which he lives (Wood et al, 1980).

Unfortunately medical efforts are often able to accomplish little more than amelioration, necessary and good though this is. In this connection it is instructive to recall the words of Dubos (1965): 'In their present state, the exact sciences fail to account for the phenomena which are of most direct relevance to the human condition. . . . In most cases, (man's) responses are determined less by the direct effects of the stimulus on his body fabric than by the symbolic interpretation he attaches to the stimulus.'

Education

The point not brought out in the immediately preceding discussion is the importance of devolution in arrangements for care (Wood & Badley, 1976), with general practitioners being encouraged to take more initiative. This has been inhibited by deficiencies in the educational background available to them in the past (Wood & Benn, 1972). Although there are welcome signs that the situation is improving, it may be helpful to recapitulate here what have been agreed nationally as the objectives for basic rheumatological education (Wood & Badley, 1981c). These are as follows.

Knowledge

1. The range of rheumatic disorders, as exemplified by:
   a. The diversity of different conditions — extending to some 200 in number, although they may more conveniently be grouped into articular disorders ('arthritis'), back problems, soft-tissue lesions, and certain

other diseases affecting the musculoskeletal system.
   b. The differential influence of age — extending from arthritis in children to the frequent degenerative disorders encountered in the elderly, a scope which calls for liaison with many other specialties.
   c. The array of disease manifestations — whereby rheumatology provides a model for a large part of medicine (cf. the former value of syphilis).
2. The effects of rheumatic disorders, including:
   a. The impact on the individual — especially the unfolding natural history of chronic conditions, and the influence exerted on life style and expectations.
   b. The burden imposed on the community — in terms of economic losses, etc., and the demands placed on others, including family members.
   c. The calls made on health services — both as regards the balance between community and specialist services, and the conflicts that may develop between the needs of the individual and those of the community.
3. The pathogenesis of rheumatic disorders, which may provide the key for the most cost-effective methods of control of rheumatic disorders, by prevention.
4. The experience of rheumatic suffering — including pain and the challenge to identity resulting from deformity and reduced functional capacity, which serve as models for the complexity of mind–body relationships.

Skills

1. Establishing a rheumatological data base, by means of:
   a. Eliciting the relevant features in the history.
   b. Examining the musculoskeletal system, particularly the most frequently affected joints.
   c. Recording the findings in appropriate form.
2. Assessing disablement status.
3. The approach to differential diagnosis, especially in regard to differentiation between acute and less urgent problems.
4. Rheumatological therapeutics.
5. Rehabilitation procedures for rheumatic disorders.
6. Counselling, particularly in regard to the limitations the patient has to learn to accept.

Attitudes

1. A holistic approach to the management of chronic illness — for which rheumatic diseases provide a paradigmatic model for problem-solving.
2. Enthusiasm and confidence in regard to rheumatic disorders — notably in relation to the results that can be achieved with appropriate treatment.
3. Co-operation in regard to the contributions that can be made by various health professionals and other members of the team.
4. Realism in regard to the limitations of current medical efforts to control rheumatic suffering.

By way of conclusion, it is worth recalling that Rosenheim (1968) remarked that if all research stopped tomorrow, the potential of medical care would continue to grow for another 20 years — just because this is the lag period before knowledge is applied. That is a measure of the challenge for improved educational efforts. However, the burden of rheumatic suffering documented earlier in this chapter indicates how sustained commitment to further research is also necessary if the problems are to be overcome.

REFERENCES

Alexander P 1969 An introduction to logic: the criticism of arguments. Allen & Unwin, London, Ch 2, p 30

Altman D G 1980 Statistics and ethics in medical research. British Medical Journal 281: 1182–1184; 1267–1269; 1336–1338; 1399–1401; 1473–1475; 1542–1544; 1612–1614; 1981 282: 44–47. See also *Statistics in practice*. British Medical Association, 1982, p 1–24

Ansell B M, Bywaters E G L 1959 Prognosis in Still's disease. Bulletin on the Rheumatic Diseases 9: 189–192

Ansell B M, Wood P H N 1976 Prognosis in juvenile chronic polyarthritis. In: Ansell B M (ed) Rheumatic disorders in childhood. Clinics in Rheumatic Diseases 2: 397–412

Arden G P 1972 In: Advisory Services Colloquium Proceedings — Back pain and soft tissue rheumatism. Advisory Services (Clinical and General) Ltd., London, p 10

Atlas of Standard Radiographs of Arthritis 1963 The

ascertainment of the affected, such as among attenders at hospitals and other institutions, and these case are taken as the numerator. The denominator is then assumed to be the catchment population for the health care facilities included in the study, the characteristics of which can be derived from sources such as a census.

Testing hypotheses about the influence of putative aetiological or precipitating circumstances can often be accomplished without using the whole population as a reference set. Having identified the affected, a comparison group is selected so as to resemble the cases in as many respects as possible apart from the presence of the condition of concern. This is the classical case–control approach, and the relative frequency of the circumstances of interest in the two groups is established. Lewis-Faning's rheumatological report (1950) is a model of the use of this technique, as are various enquiries undertaken by the Boston Collaborative Drug Study. Needless to say, the economy of the design is not without its own hazards (Ibrahim, 1979).

With any of these approaches the important caution concerns the representativeness of the samples studied because it is on this property, more than any other, that the validity of inference rests. A simple measure of representativeness is the completion rate, the extent to which usable information has been obtained from the target population for study. Unfortunately one cannot safely make assumptions about resemblances between respondents and those who are not seen, because response rates may be determined by influences that differ systematically between the two groups. An epidemiological aphorism emphasises that non-responders are a highrisk group; even though the risks may not necessarily be life-threatening for the individuals to whom they apply, they certainly pose sore hazards for the investigator who neglects to pay them due accord.

Methods of sampling for rheumatological studies have been discussed elsewhere (Wood, 1982a), but the dangers of systematic bias are everpresent. For example, it has been common experience that the bulk of cases of tuberculosis have been identified only towards the end of a community survey, when effort was sustained to increase the completion rate to something in excess of 90%. Similarly, in strategies that start with case ascertainment the neglect of particular health care facilities for recruitment can distort results. This happened when Buerger's disease was thought to be a disease of Jews; account was not taken of the fact that the original report was based on experience in a Jewish hospital.

Frequency estimates

Estimates of disease frequency need to be related to the purposes for which they were derived because this influences how illness was ascertained and the context in which the measurements were made.

When frequency estimates are applied to form the basis of aetiological hypotheses they must relate to the complete picture of disease. Severe disease is relatively easy to define, as is shown by the general acceptance of classical rheumatoid arthritis identified by the American Rheumatism Association (ARA) criteria. In contrast the significance of milder disease and of isolated abnormalities is much more difficult to assess, as the continuing uncertainty over diagnostic criteria and the aetiological importance of findings based on these serves to indicate.

To illustrate the difficulties, how should relatives with various titres of rheumatoid factor be treated in the analysis of family studies of rheumatoid arthritis? The decision on whether to regard isolated abnormalities or incomplete manifestations as evidence that the individual is affected by the disease has to be made on other grounds before the analysis is undertaken. The criteria were not directed to this problem, yet neglect of the difficulties means that one can make the results show almost whatever one wants depending on the choices that are made.

The other important use to which frequency estimates are applied is as an indication of the demand for services for amelioration. By being concerned with relatively severe illness this involves only the tip of the iceberg, which is why it is so important to be clear for what purpose one wants an indication of frequency. As just noted diagnostic criteria usually perform fairly well for this purpose, even though they were not developed in relation to treatment potential. However, service needs indicators are likely to be subject to the influence of other sources of variation, particularly to existing patterns in the availability of such services, and note must also be taken of these factors.

Expression of illness

When an individual becomes ill it is possible to identify different aspects of the unfolding of this process. The more obvious milestones are represented by incidents or events. These include the onset of disease, perception of illness, consultation with a physician, admission to or discharge from hospital, initiation or discontinuance of particular therapies, development of specific disabilities, and the ending of disease by recovery, death, or inactivation of the pathological process.

Incidence

The critical characteristics of these events are that they may be conceived of as being instantaneous and that they mark the beginning or end of a given state — of being ill or in hospital or under treatment. Experiences of this type are measured by counting the number of events during a particular period of time and relating this count to the population exposed to these events.

This measure is known as the *incidence* of the event and is expressed as a rate per unit time. Essentially one is considering not persons but events that happen to persons. The distinction is important because, when enumerating such occurrences, it must be remembered that some types of event may happen more than once to the same person. One may thus be exposed to the hazard of double counting, which inhibits direct translation of experience of events into experience by people.

In understanding how disease arises the circumstances of its origin are obviously most instructive. Studies of incidence are therefore likely to be of greatest aetiological interest, and the method has been used successfully with well-defined events like the onset of acute infectious fevers. Well-defined outcomes such as sudden death from ischaemic heart disease also lend themselves to this approach, particularly when the outcome is almost universal, as with cancer mortality in the absence of treatment.

Of rheumatic disorders, gout and acute rheumatic fever can be studied usefully in this way. But although the presence of most other rheumatic conditions can be established satisfactorily the processes are rarely punctuated by well-defined natural events; their onset is usually not clear and a fatal outcome is rare. This compels us to resort to prevalence studies, which must therefore be set in perspective.

Prevalence

It has been noted that events mark the beginning or the end of a given state. The characteristic of a state is that it has a duration. Being ill or in hospital or under treatment are not instantaneous experiences but extend over some period of time. Experiences of this type are measured by counting the number of persons in the particular state at a given point in time and relating this count to the population at risk to the experience.

This measure is known as the *prevalence* of the state and is expressed as a proportion or rate at an actual or average point in time. Thus when a survey is carried out the results are usually expressed as a point prevalence estimate. Obviously there would be difficulties if the phenomena under study were evanescent. However, providing the average duration of the state is longer than the duration of the survey, the fact that the observations were not all made at precisely the same point in time will not give rise to significant error.

As both incidence and prevalence relate to individuals experiencing episodes of illness the two measures are obviously interrelated, and the link may be stated formally as the fundamental theorem of epidemiology. Providing incidence remains constant and both incidence and duration are expressed in identical time units (e.g. annual incidence and duration in years), the prevalence of a state is the product of its average duration and the incidence of the event that initiates or terminates it.

DISEASE EPIDEMIOLOGY

We have tried to marshal the relevant information on each condition in a systematic manner, noting in sequence, where the evidence allows, its frequency (prevalence and incidence) and characteristics (both for identification and as regards natural history), and the influences of external factors and individual attributes on its occurrence.

A clarification of the way in which frequency estimates are presented may be helpful. In the epidemiological literature it is common for occurrences to be related to large denominators selected so as to yield frequency estimates in whole numbers; prevalence and incidence ratios therefore tend to be variably expressed as per thousand, per 100 thousand, per million, etc. In order to facilitate direct comparisons we have adopted a standard denominator in this chapter and, because it is a more familiar base for clinicians, we have expressed estimates in percentage terms (i.e. as ratios in a population of 100 persons). However, in order to remind readers that this complicates the multiplication together of such estimates, we have also often cited absolute rates (i.e. ratios to a base of unity) on which the arithmetic can be carried out direct.

Our intention is to contribute to a broader understanding of the origin and occurrence of rheumatic disorders. As the details and difficulties of particular epidemiological enquiries are not of immediate concern to the reader of a rheumatological text, we have not dwelt on these at any length. Some of these aspects, however, are taken up later to illustrate how misinterpretation and over-simplification are ever-present hazards.

INFLAMMATORY ARTHROPATHIES

This section will deal in turn with rheumatoid arthritis, juvenile chronic arthritis, ankylosing spondylitis, other spondylarthropathies, the crystal arthropathies, and arthropathies associated with other disorders. The connective tissue diseases will be considered in the next section.

Rheumatoid arthritis

Of all rheumatic disorders, rheumatoid arthritis (RA) is the condition that has been studied most extensively and over the longest period of time in the laboratory. This is also true of epidemiological enquiries, and especially of population surveys. It is frustrating to have to acknowledge that all this effort has not led to commensurate enlightenment, and our appreciation of how and why this disease arises (if, indeed, it is a single condition) remains rudimentary. Of the variations in frequency that have been reported it is at least as likely that technical and methodological features have been responsible as that meaningful biological clues have been missed.

The main conclusion one can draw is that, if significant aetiological clues are to be detected, it will be necessary to study very much larger samples of the population at risk than has been the case so far, and to follow them over a period of some years antedating onset of the disease; this is probably equally true of most other rheumatic disorders. The efficiency of such studies would be considerably enhanced could attention be confined to susceptible subpopulations. Unfortunately appropriately typed communites (if we yet know enough of the markers), and of sufficient size, do not exist at present and the readiest substitute, panels of blood donors, is far from representative of the population at large.

Frequency

An indication of the range of variation in prevalence estimates for RA is given in Table 3.2, and a more recent and exhaustive enumeration has been provided by Hochberg (1981). Although there are difficulties in making direct comparisons because methods varied and the age structure of samples studied was different, the prevalence of definite disease appears to be remarkably constant in most Caucasian groups at approximately 1% (absolute rate 0.01); probable disease is much more variable in its occurrence. The most outlying result in reported Caucasian studies, from the Deutsches Bundesrepublik, appears to have been related to a high frequency of men with bilateral knee involvement who had had dysentery during the Second World War (Behrend et al, 1972a). Prevalence increases fairly markedly with age because of chronicity and surviving cases.

From the population experience one would anticipate that a realistic estimate of the incidence of new cases would be at least 0.02% (absolute rate 0.0002) per annum. This is a conservative estimate as most reports (Cobb & Lawrence, 1957; den Oudsten et al, 1968; Linos et at, 1980) are consistent with an incidence at least twice as great, but allowance has been made for the fact that RA can-

Table 3.2 Estimates of rheumatoid arthritis in different countries derived from surveys conducted at similar times (after Kellgren, 1966, and Wood & Benn, 1972).

Country	Prevalence (by ARA criteria)			Mortality*	
	Probable and definite cases (%)	Definite cases (%)	Ratio of rates for 'probable and definite' in the sexes (f : m)	Standardised death rate	Ratio of rates in the sexes (f : m)
Finland	7.5	3.0	2.5	46.9	3.2
Germany (Federal Republic)	5.7	5.0	0.5	33.2	2.4
UK (Leigh, and England and Wales)	4.0	1.1	2.1	27.5	2.8
USA (Tecumseh)	2.5	0.5	4.7	13.6	2.1
Czechoslovakia	1.3	0.5	1.5	20.1	3.8
Japan	0.5	0.3	13.0	41.4	2.8

* Derived from World Health Statistics Annual 1966 (WHO, 1969), category A122, arthritis and spondylitis.

not be detected at a 7-year follow-up in some persons originally thought to have definite disease (Kellgren, 1962). A rogue study in North America (O'Sullivan et at, 1968) suggested an annual incidence of 0.3% but there are difficulties with this estimate; these will be discussed in the section of this chapter on gout.

The prevalence of RA in the first-degree relatives of affected persons, both hospital propositi and cases identified in a population sample, is of the order of 4% (range 3–8%); conflicting assessments of the degree of familial aggregation have been attributable to the means of applying criteria for identification of probands (Lawrence & Wood, 1968).

Identification

Standard diagnostic criteria were formulated at conferences in Rome and New York (Bennett & Wood, 1968) and have largely stood the test of time. The criteria are based on three types of evidence. Radiographic and serological features are observed in roughly similar proportions in the two sexes and increase in frequency with age. Clinical findings, to which the original ARA criteria gave most emphasis, are usually encountered more commonly in females.

Different syndromes of presentation can be identified by the criteria (Mitchell & Fries, 1982), and it has been suggested that the underlying clinicopathological spectrum may resemble that of leprosy (Panayi, 1982). A uniquely problematical feature of the criteria is the built-in Guttman scale; if symmetrical swelling is observed then three of the five criteria necessary for 'definite' RA are automatically fulfilled, and yet the specificity of this triad leaves a lot to be desired. The distinctive phenomenon of symmetrical involvement is challenging, and yet it has been the subject of surprisingly little thought or research.

Despite uncertainty about whether RA may be heterogeneous, criteria have certainly been valuable in promoting the homogeneity of material reported in clinical reviews and drug trials. Concentration on seropositive erosive disease is likely to yield the most closely similar collection of patients. The performance of criteria in the survey type of study is less reassuring (Allander & Bjelle, 1981), because of both difficulties in applying exclusions consistently and variability in the accuracy of recalled histories; the role of radiographs in such contexts has been reviewed recently (Wood, 1983a). The custom of dichotomising the results of tests for rheumatoid factor into positive or negative responses can give rise to misleading conclusions when comparing different groups of results unless it is first established that the cumulative titre distributions of the groups do not intersect (Badley et al, 1975).

Natural history

The widespread impression that seropositive, as

opposed to seronegative, RA has a worse functional outcome (Jacoby et al, 1973) can now be extended because Fleming et al (1976a) have identified a variety of other characteristics that are predictive of a less favourable prognosis. Long-term follow-up studies (Bywaters & Dresner, 1952; Reah 1963; Duthie et al, 1964; Rasker & Cosh, 1978) have helped to provide a basis for appreciating the variability in disease course and outcome indicated in Figure 2.7, although such assessments tend to exaggerate the overall severity of the impact of RA. Such studies have also suggested that median life expectancy is reduced in patients with RA, particularly in those in whom the disease starts before the age of 45 years (Benn & Wood, 1972a), and survival is notably less in people with more severe disease at the time of first diagnosis (Cobb et al, 1953; van Dam et al, 1961).

The two or threefold excess mortality is attributable to a variety of different conditions (Zlosnik & Wood, 1979), including infection (Uddin et al, 1970), renal disorders (Isomaki et al, 1975) and possibly lymphoproliferative malignancies (Calabro, 1967; Isomaki et al, 1978). Despite Sharpey-Schafer's anticipation that the repeated use of salicylate might give rise to stomach cancer, there is no apparent excess of solid tumours and, despite the postulated value of aspirin as secondary prophylaxis for thrombotic vascular disorders, no deficit of coronary heart disease (Monson & Hall, 1976). The lack of an excess mortality in a report on the Mayo Clinic study (Linos et al, 1980) could well be due to an unstable denominator and other methodological limitations (i.e. person-years of exposure were not taken into account).

Mortality experience can provide a useful comparative measure for assessing the hazard of particular complications, such as cervical subluxation (Smith et al, 1972). Non-fatal consequences of RA were indicated in the previous chapter as far as functional capacity is concerned. The reader is directed especially to a paper by Wiener (1975) on the uncertainty associated with a chronic and generally progressive illness.

Protection

A most remarkable observation is that the oral contraceptive pill appears to halve the incidence of RA (Wingrave & Kay, 1978; Vandenbroucke et al, 1982). Whether this may be related to MacMahon's view (quoted by Vandenbroucke, 1983) 'that more than 50 million women worldwide take regularly for contraceptive purposes a combination of hormones that essentially cuts off the function of their own ovaries' has not been established. Nor can the observation be immediately reconciled with the well-known remission of RA that occurs during some pregnancies (Hence, 1938; Unger et al, 1983) because averting a hazard is not necessarily the same as abating it once one has come under its sway. Nevertheless this incidental finding, which is not unchallenged (Linos et al, 1983), could be one of the most interesting observations ever made about the disease, even though both the practical and theoretical implications remain obscured.

Other external influences

It may seem arbitrary to consider areas of low prevalence under environmental influences and to discuss excess frequencies on the basis of genetic predisposition, but the evidence appears to accord with such interpretations. Data on RA from Japan have tended to be both variable and somewhat perplexing. Some of the earlier studies mentioned by Shichikawa et al (1981) showed low prevalence and a remarkable female preponderance. The low frequence of occurrence was not easy to reconcile with the high mortality shown in Table 3.2, suggesting that the survey results may not have been truly representative. For example, it is possible that admitting to subjective distress and suffering had different cultural significance in the two sexes, perhaps leading to underdetection of affected males. However, recent work (Shichikawa et al, 1981) has been more compatible with other studies. Radiation following the atomic bombs dropped on Hiroshima and Nagasaki appears to have had no influence on the occurrence of RA (Wood et al, 1967; Kato et al, 1971). Migrant studies should be illuminating, such as have proved to be so rewarding in regard to Japanese experience of breast cancer and ischaemic heart disease.

Prevalence also appears to be low in Africa, both in the bush (Beighton et al, 1975) and under tribal living conditions (Greenwood, 1969; Muller et al, 1972; Meyers et al, 1977), in Polynesia (Rose & Isdale, 1963), in Puerto Rico (Mendez-Bryan et al, 1964), and, anecdotally, in much of Asia, where

RA also appears to be less severe and to be associated with nodules only infrequently. Some of the criteria give rise to difficulty in tropical countries where the frequencies of rheumatoid factor and erosive changes are raised by infections and trauma respectively.

An illuminating observation is that the prevalence of RA in members of the same tribe in Africa is increased when they migrate from a rural to an urban environment (Solomon et al, 1975). We will discuss the interpretation of this finding later, in the section of this chapter on time as an aetiological influence. Why the disease appears to occur more commonly in those of lower social class is unknown (Wolfe, 1968), although what people believe about their affliction is also related to social class (Elder, 1973).

Although symptoms may vary with the weather, indicators of inflammation such as CRP and the ESR do not show similar changes (Latmant & Levi, 1980) and dampness is also not associated (Behrend et al, 1972b; Lawrence, 1977). However, the season may have some influence (Valkenburg, 1968). Anecdotal evidence suggests that joints stressed at work may become more severely damaged by RA, but overall no link with occupation (such as coal mining — Miall, 1955) has been detected. An isolated case–control study reported that, in the 5 years prior to disease onset, people developing RA had had more exposure to domestic pets (Gottlieb et al, 1974), but this work does not seem to have been repeated.

There is controversy about the appearance of the disease in history, and we shall take this up later. Possible more recent variations are likely to have been distorted by significant demographic changes. Suggestions that RA may be declining in frequency (Linos et al, 1980) and that it may also be getting less severe (Silman & Davies, 1981) are based on unconvincing testimony and the findings can be accounted for in other ways. A review of clinical evidence concluded that there had been no apparent changes in the pattern of rheumatoid disease over the previous 20 years (Valkenburg, 1976). One would like to be able to report improvements in outcome related to the increase in therapeutic options, especially with the introduction of delayed action or disease-modifying drugs but, with the exception of developments in surgery, the evidence to permit such conclusions is unfortunately not available.

Individual attributes

Most clinical studies have revealed a fall-off in incident cases of RA at older ages together with changes in the relative frequency of affection between the sexes, both of which are shown in Figure 3.1. However, the few population-based studies that have reported age and sex-specific incidence rates have appeared to show a progressive increase in incidence with age and a fairly consistent sex differential throughout the age range (Cobb & Lawrence, 1957; Linos et al, 1980), although the samples at individual ages on which these were based were inevitably small. It is common to condense key features of persons affected into statements such as 'the peak age at onset is about 40 years' but inspection of Figure 3.1 shows how unhelpful this is, either for diagnostic discrimination or biological understanding (an imaginative example of which is provided by Burch, 1968). The two or threefold female preponderance is well known and fairly consistent, but so far unexplained.

Familial aggregation can be observed, and the heritability of liability is of the order of 50–60% (Lawrence & Wood, 1968). Rheumatoid factors also show familial aggregation (Lawrence et al, 1970). There is a link between RA and HLA DR4/Dw4, and this extends to rheumatoid factor. It is interesting that the Japanese sample with the

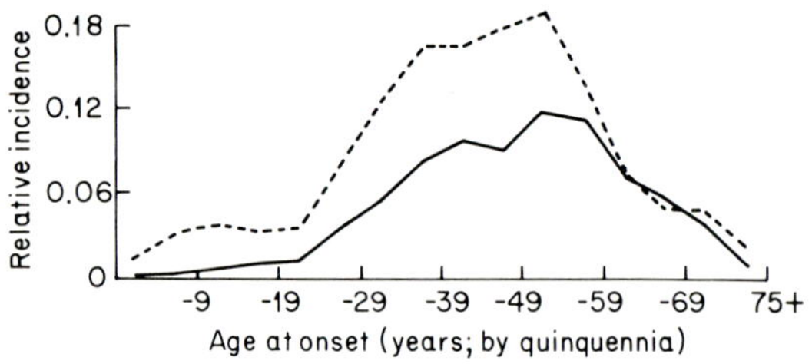

Fig. 3.1 Relative age-specific incidence rates for seropositive rheumatoid arthritis plotted against age at onset of symptoms (sample: 124 males and 175 females; from Wood, 1968). Moving averages of consecutive data pairs are plotted, based on patients attending the Manchester Royal Infirmary in 1964–1965. Relative incidence is derived by adjusting the samples to the mean number of cases seen per annum and relating these means to the population of the South-East Lancashire conurbation, from the 1961 Census. Females — interrupted line; males — continuous line.

lowest prevalence of RA had a high frequency of DR4 (Shichikawa et al, 1981). An unusually high frequency of RA has been reported in certain Amerind tribes, notably the Yakima (Beasley et al, 1973) and a Chippewa band (Harvey et al, 1981, 1983); in the latter this was associated with high frequencies of DR4 and of antinuclear antibodies, but the link with DR4 was not evident in the Yakima (Willkens et al, 1982).

Adverse reactions to drugs may be linked with genetic markers (e.g. DR3 and reactions to chrysotherapy — Gran et al, 1983), but available evidence is not consistent and cannot at present be used to predict hazard. Suppressed hostility and increased liability to divorce have been reported in persons afflicted with RA (Cobb et al, 1959). However, other studies have failed to find differences from 'controls' in those with early disease (Crown & Crown, 1973). Personality profiles are more likely to be a consequence of the malady rather than a contributory cause (Robinson et al, 1972), whilst the excess of divorces could be accounted for by lower rates of remarriage (Medsger & Robinson, 1972).

Clinical reports of disease associations, such as between RA and ankylosing spondylitis (Fallet et al, 1976), give rise to problems because the universe from which the patients under study were drawn is difficult to define; lacking this information the long odds for coincidental occurrence are not easy to evaluate. The lower prevalence of RA in persons who are mentally ill could be related to a possible negative association with schizophrenia (Pilkington, 1956). There appears to be a definite association with progressive massive fibrosis and pulmonary tuberculosis (Miall, 1955) and the link may extend to other infections and to peptic ulcer, with a reciprocal negative association with ischaemic heart disease, hypertension, and obesity (Cobb & Hall, 1965), and possibly arthrosis (other than that secondary to RA) and gout.

Juvenile chronic arthritis

The term 'juvenile chronic arthritis' (JCA) is a generic descriptor and therefore identifies a heterogeneous collection of conditions, as noted in Table 2.2. Failure to acknowledge this heterogeneity gives rise to problems of two types.

The first is concerned with hermeneutics or interpretation, and it is illustrated by the difficulty of attempting to understand the significance of elevated frequencies when the magnitude of increase is only intermediate. For example, early reports suggested that features such as rheumatoid factor, anti-nuclear antibodies (ANA), and the B27 antigen could each be observed in something like 20% of affected children, although the meaning of these observations was indeterminate. Such problems are of more general concern, and will be referred to again later.

Careful natural history studies should be able to overcome these difficulties. For instance, using the example already given, once various subtypes had been recognised on purely clinical grounds (Table 3.3 — Ansell & Wood, 1976) these biological attributes began to make sense — the seropositives suffered from juvenile RA and the B27-positives were spondylitics, reflecting the same types of associations seen in adults with these diseases, whilst the children with ANA had pauciarticular involvement and chronic iridocyclitis and were in hazard of blindness.

The second type of problem is more practical. Clinically it is obviously more difficult to offer a prognosis unless the distinctions between heterogeneous subsets are made, as the variations in outcome shown in Table 3.3 illustrate. Furthermore, in trying to organise clinical experience so as to learn from it the failure to differentiate subtypes leads to variation in sample composition (referred to in Table 2.2). Obviously our present task is made more difficult because reports vary in how clearly it is identified to which part of the disease spectrum any findings may apply.

Frequency

The estimated prevalence of JCA is of the order of 0.06% (absolute rate 0.0006) in children under the age of 15 years (Bywaters, 1968). Other estimates, based mainly on hospitalised patients, have been summarised by Hochberg (1981) and are of a similar order of magnitude. The prevalence of the JCA variants cannot be estimated satisfactorily, other than as proportions relative to other subtypes encountered in clinical experience. This is because sample sizes even from Taplow were rather small for this purpose, and other reports

Table 3.3 Heterogeneity of juvenile chronic arthritis revealed by follow-up for 15 years (after Ansell & Wood, 1976).

Variant	No. in sample	Mean age at onset (years)	Sex ratio (f : m)	Associated features	Outcome after 15 years† activity limitation none (%)	slight (%)	severe (%)	very severe* (%)	death (%)
Juvenile RA	26	11.0	1.9	Rheumatoid factor +ve	19	58	15	0	12
Juvenile AS	32	9.6	0.2	Sacroiliitis and B27 +ve	59	28	6	6	0
Onset subtypes (not included above)									
— monoarticular	42	6.2	2.2	Present to orthopaedics	50	31	12	2	2
— systemic	68	5.1	1.3	Splenomegaly, rash, etc.	35	19	26	3	15
— pauciarticular	13	3.2	1.6	ANA and chronic iridocyclitis	15	54	23	0	8
Residual forms	62	8.0	2.6	Bowel disease, psoriasis, etc.	48	24	15	5	5
All JCA	243	7.1	1.4		42	30	17	3	7

† Proportions may not sum to 100% because of missing information.
* Includes children who were helpless or restricted to a chair/bed existence.

are generally based on considerably less material.

Using the follow-up experience of children seen at Taplow (Ansell & Wood, 1976), an incidence estimate of the order of 0.006% (absolute rate 0.00006) per annum is obtained, which accords broadly with suggestions in the material reviewed by Hochberg (1981). The quoted prevalence figure will yield an overestimate in the population of all ages because it takes no account of the frequency of residual JCA in older persons. Lawrence (1969a) has reported a history of past JCA in 0.27% of adults. However, this exceeds the more direct estimate in the age-group at risk and, in the light of mortality experience in the Taplow children and the proportion that are left with no clinical residua, the overall prevalence of JCA in the population is probably more realistically regarded as being approximately 0.02% (absolute rate 0.0002).

Experience of the familial occurrence of JCA (Ansell et al, 1962, 1968, 1969) indicates a frequency in first-degree relatives of just over 1% for clinical AS, 9% for sacroiliitis, and 5% for polyarthritis. However, it is difficult to assess these findings in relation to the various subtypes of disease.

Characteristics

The WHO/EULAR criteria (Wood, 1977 — and see Table 2.2) draw heavily on the original Taplow proposals, and their main difference from those developed by the American Rheumatism Association (JRA Criteria Subcommittee, 1977) is that the latter require a minimum duration of disease of 6 rather than 3 months. The topic has been reviewed recently (Hanson, 1982; Kvien et al, 1982), but criteria have not yet been applied in population studies.

Some of the features predictive of a less favourable outcome can be inferred from Table 3.3. Overall, though, after the age of 15 years less than 10% of affected children are likely to be handicapped in regard to occupation and most marry and have children (a range of sources is reviewed by Hochberg, 1981, and Miller et al, 1982, have carried out a more recent study).

One case study reported a ten-fold excess mortality over the age period 5–30 years in children initially diagnosed as having JCA, which represents a case fatality rate of 7% (Ansell & Wood, 1976); the subtypes associated with higher mortality can be seen in Table 3.3. These figures almost certainly paint too gloomy a picture because they are based on experience at a national referral centre that would be likely to preferentially attract more severe cases with a less favourable outlook. Other studies (reviewed by Hochberg, 1981) present a more optimistic impression, but interpretation is confounded by transatlantic

sociology of this disorder (e.g. greater frequency in those following itinerant occupations) has not been more thoroughly documented.

A recurrence rate of 50% has been noted among individuals with non-specific urethritis who had previously developed Reiter's disease following this infection (Csonka, 1960). Arthritis or iritis led to some permanent disability in 42% of individuals 20 years after an initial postdysenteric attack; spondylitis was present in 7% but spinal symptoms were relatively mild (Sairanen et al, 1969). With venereally acquired Reiter's disease some 15% have one or more of permanently deformed feet, ankylosed peripheral joints, or recurrent iritis and its complications, though overall functional potential tends to be better than in RA and AS (Csonka, 1972).

Psoriatic arthropathy

Psoriasis has a population frequency of between 1 and 2% (0.01–0.02; Ingram, 1954; Baker, 1966), and Leczinsky (1948) has reported that inflammatory polyarthropathy may be observed in almost 7% of psoriatics. The product of these two estimates would indicate that psoriatic arthropathy probably has a frequency approaching 0.1% (0.001), although this figure does not take account of psoriatic spondylarthropathy and various other articular problems. Given some ambiguity in nosological distinctions, a population study of the relationship between arthritis and psoriasis appeared to yield broadly similar results (Hellgren, 1969). Much of the other available evidence is difficult to evaluate, although Wright &, Moll (1976) have undertaken an exhaustive review.

Criteria have been suggested by Moll & Wright (1973). Skin lesions usually precede the articular changes, occasionally they are synchronous, and in one-sixth they occur after the joint disorder (Roberts et al, 1976); the closest temporal relationship is between nail and distal interphalangeal joint changes (Wright, 1965). The basic characteristics of affected persons generally resemble those of individuals with the different forms of arthropathy with which psoriasis may be associated. Thus although onset may be observed in childhood, the rheumatoid type of seronegative polyarthritis has an age and sex distribution resembling RA and the same is true for spondylitis. The noteworthy features are that deforming arthritis tends to start in younger adults, and that distal joint arthropathy is commoner in men.

Psoriatic arthropathy occurs in 5.5% of the first-degree relatives of probands similarly affected, and the heritability of liability is of the order of 80% (Moll & Wright, 1973). Full details of this work, including familial frequencies of psoriasis, seronegative polyarthritis, sacroiliitis, and spondylitis, are summarised in Wright & Moll (1976). Overlap with other spondylarthropathies in families has already been noted. Discordance for psoriatic arthropathy in monozygotic twins has been reported (Gottlieb et al, 1979).

As might be anticipated, the HLA associations are complex and difficult to disentangle. The overall increase in B27 is most marked in those with spinal changes (Lambert et al, 1976), but this antigen may also indicate increased risk for developing peripheral arthropathy (Eastmond & Woodrow, 1977b). The latter has also been associated with Bw38 (Espinoza et al, 1978), but the most consistent links have been with B13 and B17 (Russell et al, 1972; White et al, 1972), and B17 appears to identify a subgroup characterised by a slightly earlier age at onset and a very strong familial tendency. The distribution of antigens is different in mixed Negro–Caucasoids (Green et al, 1981), in whom B27 is not so significant a marker for sacroiliitis whilst the haplotype A1/B8 is increased in psoriatics.

Little specific has been established about environmental determinants. Apart from the deforming arthritis, the overall impact of psoriatic arthropathy on the individual generally tends to be less than that related to other major rheumatic disorders (Roberts et al, 1976). Mortality data are meagre and earlier evidence is unrepresentative because of the use of corticosteroid therapy. It is interesting that syndesmophytes without accompanying sacroiliac changes have been observed in psoriatic spondylitis (Lambert & Wright, 1977), and that these patients are more likely to be B27-negative.

Crystal arthropathies

As a reflection of the considerable effort that has been invested in the study of gout and its associated characteristic, serum uric acid (SUA) levels, most of the discussion in this section will be devoted to urate arthropathy. Other crystal arthropathies will be dealt with briefly at the end.

Frequency of gout

Estimates of the frequency of gout must be approached with some caution because there are two significant sources of variation. The first concerns the means of diagnostic assignment. Surveys based on the experience of appropriate symptoms by respondents in a population sample seem to yield unduly high estimates (Badley et al, 1978a; Gardner et al, 1982b). It has been more common to rely on a clinical diagnosis made by a physician, from which lower measures are derived. The second problem relates to the episodic nature of gout, and what time span of occurrence is being considered. A few studies have used the McCarthy approach ('Are you now or have you ever been?'), and lifetime experience will obviously lead to high estimates. In other enquiries only attacks of gout in the recent past appear to have been considered.

Against this background the best estimate of prevalence is still probably the average value quoted by Kellgren (1964), less than 0.3% (0.003) in European and North American Caucasoids but rising to 6% in the first-degree relatives of gouty probands. A study in a 'representative general practice' (Currie, 1979) yielded a similar value, 0.26% in persons aged 15 years or more, and this was related to an incidence estimated as 0.025–0.035% (0.0003) per annum, which would appear to indicate a mean duration of the order of 10 years. One of the few North American studies of incidence (O'Sullivan, 1968) put this as high as 0.1% which, given a prevalence of 0.3%, a level similar to that found by O'Sullivan himself (1972), would suggest an average disease duration of only 3 years.

Some of these findings are incompatible with our knowledge of the natural history of gout, which is why we have emphasised inconsistencies in the evidence. Not only is prevalence likely to be underestimated, as we have already indicated, but it is also probable that incidence has been overestimated. Repeated examinations over relatively short periods of time would obviously be more sensitive in detecting what might have appeared to be new onsets of gout, and it was from studies like this that the high incidence estimates were derived. Barry (1968) has acknowledged that the estimates diminished when the Framingham study was extended over longer periods of time. The age composition of the groups examined relative to the modal age at onset of gout can also obviously influence the findings.

Characteristics

Ascertainment problems have already been indicated, and it is surprising that more emphasis has not been placed on these difficulties when criteria were formulated (see Bennett & Wood, 1968). The development of standardised means for identifying the affected has perhaps been too influenced by the model of criteria for RA, without taking sufficient account of the fact that gout is an episodic threshhold disorder. The latter qualities pose very different challenges for recognition in a survey, as the hallmark is a characteristic acute syndrome, typically affecting only a single joint, rather than a constellation of chronic features identifiable at a number of sites. To some degree this was acknowledged at New York, by eliminating SUA levels as a criterion. More recent work on behalf of the American Rheumatism Association (Wallace et al, 1977) has clearly been directed at diagnosis in clinical rather than population contexts.

Gout is almost certainly heterogeneous, being the common end-expression of a variety of metabolic and other defects including overproduction and underexcretion of uric acid. Direct complications can be detected in the kidney, and include calculus disease. Associations between gout and/or hyperuricaemia have been described with hypercholesterolaemia and other lipid abnormalities, hypertension, vascular disease, and diabetes. However, the evidence is not entirely consistent and in fact in the latter condition it has been suggested that the link is with prediabetes (Herman & Goldbourt, 1982). Representative mortality experience has not been adequately documented.

Much of the epidemiological literature has concentrated on the distribution of SUA levels in various circumstances. Certainly this attribute has to be regarded as a risk factor, but some caution should be exercised over how this is assimilated. The problem is not just analogous to whether one

Table 3.4 Proportions of males developing gout in the ensuing 12 years according to initial serum uric acid levels (Framingham data; after Hall et al, 1967).

Initial serum uric acid level (mg %)	Number of males examined	Proportion developing gout in 12 years (%)	Proportion of all men developing gout occurring in each SUA category (%)
< 6	1615	1.1	28.6
6–6.9	354	7.3	41.3
7–7.9	78	14.2	17.5
8–8.9	16	18.7	4.8
9 +	6	83.3	7.9

says a glass is half full or half empty, because different contexts may be implied. For example, in given circumstances risk may be increased seventy-fold and yet still only 6% of those with the characteristic may be affected. It is only in aetiological pursuits that the former expression, 'relative risk', is likely to be more helpful; for most clinical purposes the latter measure is generally better suited. The relevance of this point to SUA levels can be seen in Table 3.4 — two-thirds of new cases develop in those below the customary hyperuricaemia threshhold when first seen, and even of those at the very highest levels almost one-fifth don't manifest gouty arthritis.

External influences

An apparent increase in prevalence since the Second World War was indicated in our own study (Badley et al, 1978a), and has been documented by Mertz & Babucke (1971). There are problems in interpreting the likely significance of this change. Certainly awareness of the disease is greater than it used to be. However, interest tends to focus on the fact that today's diet is more abundant that the fare customary in wartime, conditions that are also relevant to changes in diabetes. Various other observations accord with this possibility. Gout occurs more frequently in those of high body bulk (Acheson & O'Brien, 1968), and both SUA levels and gout are increased by ingestion of a rich diet (Popert & Hewitt, 1962), especially one in which purines feature prominently, and by alcohol consumption; the most extreme example of these influences is seen in Rikishi (Sumo) wrestlers, who have not been shown to have any unusual genetic predisposition (Hayashi, 1971). The remedy, however, would appear to be moderation because unaccustomed deprivation, such as starvation, can also raise SUA levels and precipitate an acute attack.

Another factor has been the introduction of thiazide diuretics, which appear to have contributed to the increase in gout especially in postmenopausal women. Diuretic therapy was being taken by one-fifth of our gouty respondents, compared with 6.4% of the non-gouty, but again interpretation is not quite straightforward because virtually all of them were also taking other cardiac medication — and a likely link between gout and ischaemic heart disease has already been noted. Currie (1979) estimates that perhaps 10% of gout can be attributed to the thiazides, whilst in Finland 25% of cases show some association with diuretic therapy (Isomaki et al, 1977). There is a suggestion that the peak of the distribution of ages at onset may have shifted to some ten years older in both sexes (Grahame & Scott, 1970) when compared with older data (Lawrence, 1977), but whether this is connected with increased use of thiazides is indeterminate.

Another environmental factor is lead poisoning, and it has even been suggested that saturnine gout may have contributed to the fall of the Roman Empire (Nriagu, 1983). Lead also provides an illuminating example of pitfalls in hermeneutics. Emmerson (1960) described a kindred with familial hyperuricaemia and gout that he opined was due to an inherited metabolic disorder although, in contrast to the Lesch–Nyhan syndrome (Seegmiller et al, 1967), he did not identify the enzyme defect. Later (Emmerson, 1963) he discovered that the familial aggregation was due to chronic lead poisoning from an extraneous source.

There is certainly variation between different

localities (Badley et al, 1978a; Gardner et al, 1982b), and gout has been identified less frequently in densely populated parts of Scotland (Currie, 1979). Satisfactory explanations for these variations are lacking, although failure to find differences between mean SUA levels north and south of the Scottish border (Sturge et al, 1977) is not enlightening because, apart from the imperfect correlation between SUA and gout, similarity in means may conceal appreciable differences in extreme values; proximity of observed means cannot therefore be used to exclude differences in disease prevalence (Badley et al, 1978a). By the same token, gout probably occurs with a relatively high frequency in the United States.

Apart from exposure to lead, no links with occupation have been identified. We shall discuss the influence of social class in the section of this chapter on aetiological influences, but a high standard of living and postulated stress, which may act as recognised precipitators of gout, by no means tell the whole story — a proportion of attacks have no obvious immediate cause (Katz et al, 1975). The overall influence of culture and life style is indicated by the very low prevalence of gout under primitive conditions when compared with experience in urbanised Africans (Beighton et al, 1976).

Individual attributes

Underlying the three Hippocratic aphorisms on gout, concerned with boys, eunuchs, and the menopause, are the changes in SUA levels with age. Serum uric acid is found at low levels in both sexes in childhood and rises during puberty, attaining higher values in males than in females. From then on the pattern is fairly stable until, after the menopause, levels in women rise to approach those found in men. The incidence of gout shows an increase with age, so that this cannot simply be a function of SUA and other factors must be involved. Overall there is a six- or seven-fold male preponderance, although whether this holds throughout the age range does not seem to have been specifically examined (i.e. whether age-specific incidence rates might be similar in the later part of life). The other important feature of women who take the gout is their higher frequency of renal involvement (Grahame & Scott, 1970).

The strong familial tendency to gout is reflected by a heritability of liability of the order of 80% (Rondier & Wood, 1968). However, this observation is of limited significance considering the likely heterogeneity of the condition. The metabolic defects in gout have often been likened to inborn errors but there is difficulty with this analogy. Most major enzyme defects so far identified show a recessive or sex-linked pattern of inheritance and yet gout was once thought to show dominant transmission, so closely did the data on familial occurrence correspond to the pattern that would be expected in this situation; it is not easy to see how these impressions could be reconciled. It is also interesting that there is a 13% correlation in SUA levels between spouses.

Ethnic differences on the periphery of the Pacific Ocean have proved to be a rich field for study, and high frequencies have been reported in Polynesians, Micronesians, and Filipinos — what Kellgren (1964) referred to as 'one large gouty family'. Migrant studies have indicated that the key to this experience appears to be a blend of nature and nurture. Whether it be Pacific islanders moving to New Zealand (Prior et al, 1966) or Filipinos migrating to Hawaii and the west coast of the USA (Healey et al, 1967), acculturation appears to provoke higher frequencies of gout than are observed in neighbouring Caucasoids. It may be that there is an inborn inability to handle the higher purine loads imposed by 'European' diets (Healey et al, 1967), but hyperuricaemia and gout may be found in some of the Pacific groups even on their home grounds (Burch et al, 1966) and in fact a complex array of disease associations exists (Prior & Rose, 1966). This indicates that simplistic ethnic generalisations about 'Filipinos' or 'Polynesians' are inappropriate because a much more tangled skein is being concealed.

Behavioural aspects of gout have also been subjected to study. The vulnerability of SUA levels to stresses such as job loss (Kasl et al, 1968) and other events and elements of life style (Cobb, 1963; Lanese et al, 1969) has been documented, as has that of gout itself (Katz et al, 1975). A suggested link of SUA with intelligence (Brooks & Mueller, 1966) is interesting in view of the possibility that uric acid might function as an endogenous cortical stimulant but this finding, like the association with social status, is vulnerable to selection biases and the like. Perhaps understandably, effort seems to have directed at possible explanatory variables and other behavioural aspects, such as mood swings and the sufferer's advance awareness of an impending attack, appear to have been neglected.

Chondrocalcinosis

The sensitivity of detection of calcified shadows and their specificity in regard both to crystals in the synovial fluid and clinical attacks of pseudogout is uncertain, although calcium pyrophosphate deposition disease can occur without chondrocalcinosis (Utsinger et al, 1975). Differences in crystal composition suggest that the condition may be heterogeneous, and certainly there is a diversity of clinical presentations (McCarty 1975, 1976; Bjelle, 1979).

Only clinical reports are available on the occurrence of chondrocalcinosis in most joints (e.g. Dieppe et al, 1982), although an overall frequency of articular calcification of 0.6% has been observed in radiographs of the knees of respondents aged 35 years and over in Leigh, Wensleydale, and Watford (Mariakakis, 1969). The condition is commoner in the elderly (Ellman & Levin, 1975; Wilkins et al, 1981) and it has been estimated that 5% of the adult population have knee joint deposits at the time of death (McCarty, 1976), a frequency that may be increased by high resolution X-ray film (Ellman & Levin, 1975).

A recent report suggests marked differences between the sexes (Dieppe et al, 1982), women tending to have chronic polyarticular disease whilst men were usually 10 years younger, had a shorter history of disease, and suffered from recurrent acute episodes in the lower limb. There has been an assumption that chondrocalcinosis is a primary event, but later studies have suggested that it may be the result of pre-existing joint damage (Dieppe et al, 1982). Relevant evidence includes a relationship with hypermobility (Bird et al, 1978), previous joint surgery (Doherty et al, 1982 — radiographic chondrocalcinosis was detected in 20% of operated and only 4% of unoperated knees), and hyperparathyroidism (Pritchard & Jessop, 1977; Rynes & Merzig, 1978; Alexander et al, 1982); the finding of reduced joint space is also suggestive (Ellman et al, 1981).

The course of the condition has been admirably summarised by Zitnan & Sitaj (1976). No consistent link with the HLA system has been identified, but the influence of inherited factors is attested by kindreds showing apparent dominant transmission in Czechoslovakia, Chile, France, the Netherlands, and Spain (all reviewed by Rodriguez-Valverde et al, 1980) and in Quebec (Gaudreau et al, 1981) and Sweden (Bjelle et al, 1982). However, it seems likely that these relatively isolated occurrences probably represent a different form of the condition, and familial occurrence in representative communities has yet to be studied.

Other inflammatory arthropathies

A miscellany of other arthropathies associated with inflammatory processes has to be taken into account. Of greatest epidemiological interest are a variety of conditions in which micro-organisms have been implicated.

Micro-organisms

A complex set of responses to micro-organisms has become apparent as knowledge has been extended. Dumonde and Steward (Ch. 14) identify three definitive classes:

1. The classical situation of straighforward joint infection or septic arthritis, where organisms invade synovial tissue and microbial antigen is present in the joint.

2. Postinfective arthropathy, where microbial antigen is present but recovery of an organism is inconstant and there is no evidence of local multiplication. This class includes postmeningococcal arthritis, that associated with hepatitis B and with syphilis, and perhaps rubella and other viral arthropathies, and we shall not discuss these further.

3. A 'reactive' arthropathy, where microbial infection of the body is established but neither organisms nor antigens can be identified in the joint and the aetiological mechanism is still obscure although 'allergy' has often been invoked. The concept is useful, but difficulties with the designation 'reactive' were noted in Table 2.2; perhaps the term 'contingent' most closely conveys

these delayed and inconstant manifestations, although it seems unlikely to receive approbation. Certainly it is an oversimplification to identify resemblances in features such as a genetic element when the arthritis of rheumatic fever is included as well as sundry B27-associated spondylarthropathies. Whether Poncet's disease (articular or periarticular inflammation related to a distant tuberculous focus) should be included in this class as well, or in the preceding category, seems to be uncertain.

This is not the place to discuss speculation as to whether there may be a fourth class, one that could include rheumatoid arthritis and multisystem autoimmune disease.

This taxonomic scheme has an attractive theoretical coherence, but its application in clinical contexts is often far from straightforward. After commenting on this Olhagen (1980) proceeded to subdivide 'reactive' arthropathies following infection according to the primary locus or portal of entry of micro-organisms. Each of these sources merits some consideration.

The oronasopharynx. It is interesting that of streptococcal infections only those localised to the throat appear to give rise to an arthropathic reaction. Group A streptococci are responsible for rheumatic fever, but post-tonsillitic arthropathy has been observed following infection with other strains (i.e. non-Group A). A benign polyarthritis has also been associated with Group A strains of this organism (Abdin et al, 1977). Olhagen notes in addition that a rarity among respitory infections associated with arthropathy are those due to *Mycoplasma pneumoniae*.

The urinogenital tract. We have already discussed Reiter's disease, the venereal organism responsible for which has not yet been established with certainty — and Olhagen argues that what he refers to as chronic uroarthritis is a wider concept than Reiter's disease. He suggests criteria for establishing whether coexistent prostatitis and arthropathy should be regarded as uroarthritis, the B27 antigen being one of the features.

The intestine. Postdysenteric arthropathy complicates the issue because its clinical manifestations usually resemble those of sexually-acquired Reiter's disease. In postsalmonella arthropathy, on the other hand, both urethritis and conjunctivitis are rare. Other responsible organisms include the agent of non-specific enteritis and *Yersinia enterocolitica*, and the B27 antigen again plays some part in influencing susceptibility. Yersinial infections appear to be virtually endemic in Scandinavian countries, although an associated arthropathy has also been reported from the UK (Sheldon et al, 1982). The 'lag period' may be as short as a week after *Yersinia* infection, and erythema nodosum and a mild myocarditis are not uncommon. This organism has also been incriminated in polymyalgia rheumatica (Olhagen, 1980), although this appears to be an isolated claim. Clinical expression is influenced by the B27 antigen (Laitinen et al, 1977). Chronic brucellosis may give rise to a spondylarthropathy, and more commonly in those with B27 (Hodinka et al, 1978).

Septic arthritis

Difficulties are created if one tries to be too literal in nomenclature just because episodes of septic arthritis are not infectious in the common sense of being communicable, clinical signs of sepsis are not always manifest, and suppuration (i.e. a purulent synovial fluid) may not be evident in the earliest stages. The term 'infectious agent arthritis' has been put forward to cope with this predicament (Garcia-Kutzbach & Masi, 1974) but scarcely succeeds because it could apply equally well to the other classes of arthropathy associated with micro-organisms.

The apparent frequency with which septic arthritis affects those of a particular age and can be attributed to different microbial agents is very dependent on sampling, i.e. the range of clinical experience to which a particular investigator is exposed. Overall the occurrence of septic arthritis is not great, although there is insufficient evidence to justify a numerical estimate. The source of the infection may be a puncture wound, spread from adjacent infected tissues, or haematogenous dissemination from a distant focus.

Experience encourages subdivision into two types, gonococcal arthritis and infection due to other organisms (Manshady et al, 1980). The former is usually regarded as a benign condition, whereas outcome with the other infections may be more variable. Monoarticular involvement is considerably the more common and the knee is the most frequently affected site other than in infants, when it is more often the hip (Obletz, 1960).

There appear to be two broad patterns of non-gonococcal septic arthritis. What might be regarded as uncomplicated septic arthritis may occur at any age but is encountered more frequently in younger persons and is often associated with a history of some form of musculo-skeletal trauma. The other pattern is observed in those with what might be considered to be a predisposition, be it chronic debilitating illness such as rheumatoid arthritis, diabetes, alcoholism, or drug addiction (Argen et al, 1966) or treatment with corticosteroid or immunosuppressive drugs. An element of genetic determination can be identified from the predisposition that exists in individuals with RA, for example, for which condition an inherited contribution is more marked.

Although in absolute terms septic arthritis is rare in RA, when it does occur it is dangerous to limb and life (Editorial, 1976a). The patients most at risk are those with advanced seropositive nodular disease, especially if they have Felty's syndrome or are receiving full doses of corticosteroids.

Lyme disease

In the north-eastern part of the USA the syndrome of a bite by the tick, *Ixodes dammini*, followed 3–20 days later by erythema chronicum migrans and about 4 weeks after that by a pauciarticular arthropathy, often recurrent and occasionally sustained, is now well known (Harris, 1983). A proportion of those affected, especially if they carry HLA-DR2, are prone to develop meningoencephalitis with Bell's palsy or peripheral neuropathy, or myocarditis or transient heart block, at about the same time as the arthritis. The most recent finding has been isolation of a spirochaete from a small proportion of those with the disease. Suggestive cases have been reported from Europe (Gerster et al, 1981).

Behçet's disease

The protean manifestations of this rare condition introduce uncertainty over the comparability of estimates of both frequency and rates of affection in the two sexes, although criteria have been suggested by Mason & Barnes (1969). Chamberlain (1977) found a prevalence of about 10 cases per million population in Yorkshire, but the disease is some 13 times commoner in Japan and it is also encountered more frequently at the eastern end of the Mediterranean, especially in Turkey. Sparse data do not indicate any particular age predilection although onset appears to be commoner in the early half of life.

In the past it has been suggested that environmental pollutants such as organophosphates and organochloride pesticides might be implicated, but the emphasis in aetiology seems to have returned to the search for a viral agent; recent progress has been summarised by O'Duffy et al (1983). The risk of contracting the disease appears to be increased by previous respiratory infections, dental disease, peptic ulcer, and exposure to 'organic chemicals' and antibiotics. In areas of high prevalence Behçet's disease is an important cause of blindness from uveitis, and of neurological impairment from meningoencephalitis.

Most surveys have tended to rely on questionnaires rather than examination of respondents, so that much of the data on familial occurrence is of uncertain value. Chamberlain (1978) found that occasional first-degree relatives of affected persons had mouth, and less commonly genital, ulceration. A single anarthritic kindred in South Africa suggested dominant transmission (Berman et al, 1979). Sibs and other family members have been reported as affected in Japan, but in Turkey one or more suggestive symptoms have been found in spouses. The disease has not been reported in Japanese living on Okinawa or Hawaii, and in Israel it is commoner in immigrants than in the indigenous population. There have been a number of reports of a link with HLA-B5, and it has been postulated that HLA associations may be related to disease localisation.

Hypogammaglobulinaemia

On most of the other inflammatory arthropathies that might come to a clinician's mind in this context there are virtually no epidemiological data. However, a brief comment can be made about hypogammaglobulinaemia (HGG). An inflammatory polyarthropathy has been observed in 5% of patients with HGG, but the clinical features differed somewhat from those of rheumatoid arthritis (Lawrence & Bremner, 1976). First-degree relatives of such individuals did not differ appreciably from the populations with which they were compared.

CONNECTIVE TISSUE DISEASES

From an epidemiologist's point of view the connective tissue diseases have three important properties in common. First, they are relatively infrequent conditions when considered on a community scale. This means that, as an investigative approach, population surveys are likely to be inefficient — using the latter term in its strict sense, as the relationship between inputs and outputs. Obviously efficiency can be increased if one is able to gather useful data from every individual surveyed, such as by measurement of a universal characteristic. However, continuously distributed variates have not been meaningfully linked with any of the connective tissue diseases, although community studies do have some value in setting features such as autoantibodies in context (Greenbury & Wood, 1973). As a result, most of our understanding of the epidemiology of these disorders has been derived from studies that start by identifying cases, such as in those attending a clinic.

The other two properties are interrelated. One is concerned with the fact that our awareness of these conditions has increased markedly over the last 30 years, because of changes in the sensitivity of detection. This contributes to variability between different studies, and confounds interpretation of putative trends in frequency of occurrence over time. The other is derived from the way in which ascertainment has undergone change. Our perception of the spectrum of disease manifestations has been modified, leading to appreciation that earlier experience tended to be confined to the tip of the iceberg. We shall explore this further when discussing prognosis in SLE.

Systemic lupus erythematosus

The extensive literature on systemic lupus erythematosus (SLE) has excited comment on its discrepancy with the relative importance of this condition as a community health problem (Dixon, 1981). However, despite the criticism that much of the work has indubitably been little more than phenomenological philately, the disease does present many features that are of scientific interest. Perhaps more than with many other disorders, though, impressions about SLE have tended to be unduly influenced by experiences with series of patients, without the corrective of these cases being related to defined communities. This bias is likely to reflect the nature of medical care organisation in the USA, whence most of the work has come, but in fairness it must also be acknowledged that it is in this same country that many of the best and most ambitious population studies have been carried out. More recently a screening strategy for population studies has been put forward (Liang et al, 1980).

Frequency

Two population-related studies were carried out over much the same period on either side of the north Atlantic and yielded broadly similar results (Leonhardt, 1964; Siegel & Lee, 1968), the estimates for prevalence being 0.006% (0.00006) and for incidence between 0.001 and 0.002% per annum. The vulnerability of such measures to case-finding (i.e. methods of ascertainment) is illustrated by the apparently lower frequency observed in another part of the USA at a similar time (Siegel et al, 1970). Recognition of this problem led Masi (1968a) to suggest that increased sensitivity of screening for SLE probably accounted for the much higher frequency apparent in Rochester, Minnesota (Nobrega et al, 1968), where prevalence was seven times higher and incidence almost five times greater. On this basis he predicted that within 10–20 years New York City would be reporting rates comparable to Rochester, although the much smaller sample base in the latter (25 cases as opposed to 86, both relating to Caucasoids) may account for some of the variation. Current experience suggests that a similar frequency to Rochester, about 0.04% (0.0004), is observed in the United Kingdom.

A review of published family surveys revealed a prevalence of 1.5% in the first-degree relatives of probands with lupus (Masi, 1968b). This very high estimate is probably the result of selecting for study particularly those families in which more than one person was affected, a strategy adopted deliberately in a number of studies (e.g. Reinertsen et al, 1982). In contrast are the findings in three studies in which no definite SLE was identified in relatives (reviewed by Lawrence, 1977), and Lawrence concludes that a more realistic estimate of familial prevalence is probably of the order of 0.1%. Nevertheless associated features such as gammaglobulin and antinuclear factor are often encountered with increased frequency in relatives.

Characteristics

A multisystem disease obviously poses taxing challenges for reproducible identification and the scene has been transformed, first by description of the LE cell and then later by discovery of antinuclear antibodies (ANA). The British Medical Research Council offered a set of diagnostic criteria but these did not find wide acceptance and various individual workers used their own approaches; agreement was evident on the involvement of systems but not on the relative importance of specific features. The New York symposium (Bennett & Wood, 1968) felt unable to make a useful contribution, and a WHO project on the classification of diffuse connective tissue diseases, co-ordinated from Paris, shed little light on the difficulties. As has so often been the case with rheumatological criteria, it was left to the American Rheumatism Association to take more definitive initiatives. Preliminary suggestions from the ARA were not entirely satisfactory, but the most recent recommendations (Tan et al, 1982) take in a broader array of serological features.

Although there is some relationship between levels of antibodies to double-stranded DNA and disease activity, such estimations are not satisfactory as the sole criterion (Davis et al, 1977). Both evidence of active renal disease and the dose of corticosteroids are associated with an increased frequency of infection in persons with lupus (Ginzler et al, 1978). There is evidence of bimodality in the pattern of mortality, with early deaths being attributable to active disease and infection and late deaths occurring from vascular disease in those with inactive lupus (Urowitz et al, 1976); SLE vasculitis may predispose to endothelial damage, which could explain the vascular complications (Urowitz & Gladman, 1980). A similar pattern is found superimposed on a constant rate of death from renal failure in those with lupus nephritis (Karsh et al, 1979).

A multicentre study of outcome in the USA (Ginzler et al, 1982) found the highest mortality in those with initial serum creatinine levels greater than 3 mg/dl; survival was also correlated independently with entry haematocrit, degree of proteinuria, number of criteria fulfilled, and source of funding for medical care (a surrogate for socioeconomic status), but ethnic origin did not appear to be important. Variations in survival between centres appeared to be due mainly to differences in disease severity, and the latter did not appear to be related directly to disease duration prior to entry to the study. An apparent increase in the frequency of malignant disease has been reported (Canoso & Cohen, 1974); this could be related to therapy, and bladder cancer after cyclophosphamide has certainly been noted (Elliott et al, 1982).

Prognosis

The vexed question of whether the prognosis of SLE has really improved is sufficiently important for use to confront in some detail. A number of factors need to be considered. First, we have already noted an increase in ascertainment which will have led to growth in the pool of identified cases. This could lead to more deaths being linked to lupus even though extension of the disease spectrum, particularly by the inclusion of milder cases, would be expected to reduce the case fatality rate. At the same time we would still be left uncertain of how cases identified according to former and less sensitive criteria might have fared.

Secondly, and over and above the presumed expansion related to detection sensitivity, it has also been suggested that incidence is increasing. Here it is appropriate to sound a note of caution to clinicians; the population has grown, so the fact that more cases may be seen at a health care facility does not of itself necessarily indicate an increase in prevalence ratios. However, taking this postulated increase at face value one might still expect a growth in the actual number of attributed deaths even if mortality rates were unaltered. Thirdly, if treatment has become more effective then impressions will be distorted in another way — reduced case fatality rates will be associated with improved survival, which will increase prevalence without any need to postulate a rise in incidence.

How does the evidence allow one to choose between these possibilities? There are two main sources of data. The first is reported national mortality experience. This shows an overall decline in adjusted death rates in the early to middle part of life in the most recent period (Gordon et al, 1981). Without having a reliable estimate of prevalence this finding is difficult to interpret; for example, it might reflect a decline in prevalence, or a fall in mortality perhaps attributable to improvements in therapy (i.e. an improvement in prognosis).

The other source is direct observation of relatively unselected groups of patients over time. This evidence, too, appears to show an increase in survival when compared with earlier studies, despite some difficulties over comparability that were noted (Ginzler et al, 1982). As regards the latter point it would certainly help, when there isn't an event that is to be evaluated (such as X-ray therapy for AS), if everyone assessed durations from a point of biological significance, disease onset, rather than from one of administrative convenience, entry to a study. The relevance of this consideration is that variability is increased, the mean lag between appearance of multisystem disease and study entry being 37 ± 52 months in the most recent enquiry, with a median of 14 months; computation from study entry therefore also yields a less favourable outlook.

More important is that the evidence doesn't really warrant the conclusions, and could err in either direction. The authors were noticeably reticent about losses to follow-up, apart from recording that they formed a large proportion and thereafter euphemistically regarding them as censored data. Nor were we informed whether such losses occurred preferentially in some groups rather than others. Furthermore, whilst life table methods were used, the periods of observation were not acknowledged; from what is stated the minimum could have been 4 years, but with losses the duration of meaningful follow-up could have been very appreciably less. One is thus still left with what is only an intuitive impression that outcome is far from being as gloomy as was thought formerly. The same appears to apply when children contract the disease (Caeiro et al, 1981).

Individual attributes

Systemic lupus more frequently starts in adults before the age of 45 years, when a marked (about nine-fold) female preponderance is evident (Siegel & Lee, 1968). However, among incident cases where disease onset occurs either before puberty or at ages greater than 45, females outnumber males by only 2 to 1 (Masi & Kaslow, 1978). Later onset of disease is associated with less marked serological abnormalities, although rheumatoid factor may be identified more frequently (Wilson et al, 1981). Significant renal disease appears to be less common, whereas pleuropericarditis and arthritis are often more prominent. No satisfactory explanation for observed sex differences has emerged, despite speculation about a wide variety of influences including somatic mutation (Burch & Rowell, 1965, 1970).

Ethnic differences have been reported repeatedly, and in most of this work there has been an encouraging consistency between estimates of increased risk derived from different sources — prevalence, incidence, and mortality studies. Methodological shortcomings do not allow too much to be made of exact magnitudes, but it appears that races originating from eastern Asia and the Pacific region are at some four-fold greater risk than Caucasoids. This is true of the Sioux and related tribes of Amerinds (Morton et al, 1976), of Chinese and Japanese (Kaslow, 1982), and of Filipinos (Serdula & Rhoads, 1979) and Australian Aborigines (Bloor et al, 1982). In these groups the disease often appears earlier and to be more severe, but migrant effects have not been noted. The status of individuals of African origin is less consistent. In Africa itself SLE and autoimmune phenomena in general appear to be less common (Seedat & Pudifin, 1977), whereas American Negroes suffer from the disease at least three times as frequently as neighbouring Caucasoids (Siegel & Lee, 1968). West Indians of African origin appear to emulate their American cousins, whereas Puerto Ricans contract the disease with a frequency intermediate between these levels and those found in Caucasoids.

These crude and oversimplified generalisations

about the influence of race are likely to conceal more subtle differences, and this is reinforced by findings on the distribution of HLA antigens. In Caucasoids a number of HLA antigens have been associated with SLE, and in particular the haplotype A1, B8, DR3 appears to confer a two- to five-fold increase in relative risk for the disease (Black et al, 1982) and a liability to more severe illness (Rigby et al, 1978). Despite the greater frequency of SLE in other ethnic groups, associations with MHC products have been studied less extensively in them; the evidence is reviewed by Walport et al (1982).

Familial occurrence of a variety of abnormalities associated with SLE has been described. Some 5% of affected individuals offer a family history of the disease, and concordance rates up to 67% have been reported in monozygotic twins (Hughes & Batchelor, 1983). A number of rare inherited complement deficiencies have been found in association with SLE (Rynes, 1982), and genetic susceptibility appears to be related to complement polymorphisms (Fielder et al, 1983). Although subsets of the disease have been related to different autoantibody profiles (Bell & Maddison, 1980), these do not appear to be closely linked to different HLA antigens. Despite the strong evidence of inherited influences, though, familial aggregation of various phenomena is also seen in spouses and household contacts (Lowenstein & Rothfield, 1977), indicating that extraneous (environmental) factors are also important.

Drug-induced lupus

Drug-induced lupus is as difficult to assess as is thiazide-induced gout. More precise measures of the frequency of these relatively uncommon conditions are lacking and comparative estimates of the occurrence of the drug-induced state, particularly as one is unable to challenge all the population at risk with the drug, are even less accurate. It is therefore not always easy to resolve whether the drugs induce a distinct and specific entity in a susceptible subpopulation, or whether they alter the threshold at which preexistent occult disease expresses itself.

Recent work has helped to resolve these difficulties. The characteristic of drug-induced lupus is that there is a history of intake of a drug and that the signs and symptoms abate when the drug is withdrawn (Condemi et al, 1970). Prior to 1965 the most common source of trouble was hydralazine, and adverse effects are observed more readily in women and in slow acetylators who carry the DR4 antigen (Batchelor et al, 1980), persons with non-drug-induced lupus having acetylator phenotypes resembling those in comparison groups (Vansant et al, 1978).

Procainamide has been implicated more frequently in subsequent experience (Siegel et al, 1967), and it has been estimated that between 3 and 12% of all cases of SLE in New York City follow ingestion of a drug (Lee et al, 1966). Procainamide lupus shows a less marked female preponderance; Caucasoids appear to be more commonly affected than other ethnic groups; and, whilst renal involvement and antibodies to native DNA tend to be less common, disease affecting the pulmonary parenchyma is seen more frequently (DuBois, 1969).

In his review of the condition Lawrence (1977) noted that the risks of developing drug-induced lupus are 13% in hypertensives to whom large doses of hydralazine are given, and up to 30% in those on prolonged treatment with procainamide. Some two-thirds of patients exposed to the latter develop antinuclear antibodies. The disease may appear at any time from 2 weeks to 6 years after starting procainamide. Other agents that have been implicated occasionally include isoniazid, methyldopa, chlorthalidone, and the anticonvulsant ethosuximide.

Other external influences

Ultraviolet light is a well-established trigger factor, some 30% of patients with SLE exhibiting light sensitivity (DuBois & Tuffanelli, 1964) as opposed to only 5% in comparison groups. Although the ethnic groups at greater risk in the United States tend to live in deprived communities, their susceptibility to SLE does not appear to be directly related to poor housing, overcrowding, and migration (Siegel & Seelenfreund, 1965). Abortion rates are increased in women with SLE (Fraga et al, 1974), but the influence of pregnancy on the disease appears to give less cause for concern than was formerly thought to be the case (Zurier, 1980).

A viral aetiology for SLE has long been favoured, largely because of suggestive serological findings but also because of other indirect evidence, such as the implication of oncorna viruses in animal models. Family studies have often appeared to reinforce these views; for example, antinuclear antibodies have been found in similar proportions of consanguineous and nonconsanguineous relatives, which has been interpreted as encouraging the argument for a transmissible agent (Cleland et al, 1978). On the other hand inter-species exposure seems not to be important because the frequency of lupus-related phenomena was similar in all families with dogs even though only some of the latter had high titre antinuclear antibodies (Reinertsen et al, 1980). At the moment, therefore, all this infectious speculation remains in the field of possibility rather than that of probability.

Systemic sclerosis

As with SLE, there has been increasing ascertainment of systemic sclerosis (SS) over the last 25 years, presumably related at least in part to greater diagnostic awareness. This is particularly true of a variant known as the CREST (calcinosis, Raynaud's phenomenon, oesophageal dysfunction, sclerodactyly, and telangiectasia) syndrome, which has been recognised only within this period and about which little epidemiological information is available, although it generally appears to follow a milder course.

The other aspects to be borne in mind when assessing evidence are variability in identification and dermatological confounding, in which regard an analogy with lupus is strengthened — just as distinctions need to be made between systemic and discoid LE, so SS has characteristics that differ from those of localised morphoea. Although some workers made preliminary attempts to develop diagnostic criteria, a standardised collaborative approach under the aegis of the American Rheumatism Association has been adopted only recently (Masi et al, 1980).

Occurrence

Medsger & Masi (1971) observed an average incidence of 0.0002% (0.000002) per annum in Caucasoids, which accords with an observed annual death rate of 0.0002% per annum (Masi & D'Angelo, 1967) assuming that a fatal outcome occurred in the majority of diagnosed cases, as the title of the latter authors' paper would suggest. The Mayo Cinic estimates are higher, an annual incidence of 0.001% and a prevalence of 0.01% (Kurland et al, 1969), but this study was less satisfactory methodologically. The Tennessee study found a seven-fold increase in incidence over 20 years, from 0.00006 to 0.00045% per annum (Medsger & Masi, 1971), although the rise could be attributed in part to demographic change because incidence increases with age to a peak in those over 65 years.

It has been suggested that SS resembles RA in regard to age, sex, and race (Medsger & Masi, 1971), and this is certainly evident in the threefold female proponderance. However, the relationship to age is less straightforward. Differences in sampling may well account for the more favourable outlook reported from Great Britain (Bennett et al, 1971) when compared with American experience, where five-year survival was only 44% (Medsger et al, 1971a; Medsger & Masi, 1973). All of these studies indicated that the major force of mortality was in the early years after diagnosis, that survival was less when onset occurred at older ages, and that features suggestive of renal or trunk involvement were harbingers of a less favourable outcome. Age effects were taken into account, but it is opportune to stress another influence. The pattern of disease in the elderly is inevitably influenced by general properties associated with senescence, including changes in metabolism and other processes and reduced life expectancy. For example, the generally slow progress of a condition such as SS diagnosed for the first time in older persons can lead to an appearance of lesser severity, because they don't live long enough for the full ravages of the disease to become evident.

Epidemiological features

The importance of taking account of factors such as differential utilisation of medical care facilities is well illustrated in a report on US veterans (Medsger & Masi, 1978). After adjusting for such influences, it appears that there are no significant ethnic differences apart from the possible greater likelihood of an early unfavourable outcome in blacks suggested by the previous studies of these workers. Preliminary work on the HLA antigens failed to detect any differences in their distribution in SS (Birnbaum et al, 1977), although a recent report suggests that the frequency of DR5 may be increased (Gladman et al, 1981), a finding that others have not confirmed (Whiteside et al, 1983). Vertical transmission of SS and its variants in families has been described (Mund & Greenwald, 1978). Other family studies have been reviewed by Lawrence (1977).

It has been suggested that SS, like other connective tissue diseases, may be less common in New Zealand (Wigley & Borman, 1980), but significant geographical variation has not been detected in the USA (Medsger & Masi, 1978). In contrast to earlier statements by these workers the latter report did indicate predisposition to the disease in heavy consumers of alcohol and those engaged in less skilled occupations. It has been suggested that exposure to coal and other dusts may be important (Rodnan, 1963), a possibility encouraged by a report on fulminant disease in South African gold miners (Erasmus, 1957), and unfinished plastic polymers have also been implicated (Malloy, 1967). There has been nothing to suggest that an infectious agent may be involved, although antinuclear antibodies can be detected with increased frequency (Rothfield & Rodnan, 1968).

Polymyositis and dermatomyositis

Definition of these disorders is unsatisfactory (Dawkins, 1978) so that interpretation of available evidence cannot help but be speculative. The distorting influence of selection factors such as differential hospital utilisation and presentation to different medical specialties has encouraged a number of claims that polymyositis (PM) and dermatomyositis (DM) are seen with a frequency approaching that of gout and SLE. However, estimates related to populations at risk indicate that these conditions occur some ten times less commonly. More attention appears to have been devoted to PM than to DM, though the significance of this difference is uncertain and the two diseases will be treated together.

The average incidence of new cases in Caucasoids in a North American study, 0.0003% (0.000003) per annum (Medsger et al, 1970), was similar to an estimate for Britain, 0.0004% (Rose & Walton, 1966). Once again the Mayo Clinic estimates were somewhat higher, an annual incidence of 0.0006% per annum and a prevalence of 0.006% (Kurland et al, 1969) which at face value, as for SS, would suggest a mean duration of disease of 10 years. The latter is broadly in keeping with observed cumulative survival rates of 53% after seven years (Medsger et al, 1971b); an adverse outcome in this study was associated with being older at onset and with being black, and with dysphagia and muscle weakness, but no differences between PM and DM were noted. Somewhat similar results were obtained in another study (Carpenter et al, 1977), which also showed that high dosage of corticosteroids was not associated with increased likelihood of a fatal outcome.

The apparent increase in incidence over time in North American experience is largely attributable to an increase in the population of American blacks (Medsger et al, 1970). A four-fold female preponderance was reported, but the most important observation in this study was demonstration of bimodality in ages at onset, with peaks occurring at 10–14 and at ages over 45 years. Juvenile cases appear to escape the increased risk of malignant disease noted in older patients (some 13% in the latter — Barwick & Walton, 1963), and to be more likely to carry HLA B8 (Pachman et al, 1977). A case–control study of PM in childhood failed to identify significant factors apart from a suggestion of increased exposure to streptococcal infections (Koch et al, 1976). Various precipitant experiences have been suggested in adults, including photosensitivity and sulfonamide ingestion (Barwick & Walton, 1963), but no evidence to implicate an infectious agent or socioeconomic factors has been identified (Medsger et al, 1970). A point of particular relevance to rheumatologists is the increased risk of occurrence of PM and DM in persons treated with penicillamine (Carroll et al, 1982), a drug that is known to induce myasthenia gravis and other autoimmune phenomena. Familial occurrence has been discussed by Lawrence (1977).

Other connective tissue disorders

A notable feature of connective tissue disorders is the extent to which various characteristics may be common to more than one of these conditions. Examples include the female preponderance, involvement of a variety of tissues or organs, and the occurrence of serological abnormalities. Although in principle we favour the making of distinctions (i.e. we would encourage 'splitting') because important and distinct determinants may then be identified, we must confess to some uncertainty about the uniqueness of entities that are characterised by marked overlap in features.

Were significant differences in therapy necessary, other than those dictated by involvement of particular organs or systems, then we would be more confident in the value of nosological differentiation. As it is, though, we cannot help but wonder whether some, at least, of these disorders may represent no more than responses to similar external influences, the differences in response perhaps being attributable to intrinsic variation in tissue susceptibility determined by properties such as phenotype.

Mixed connective tissue disease

The ultimate in this nosological confusion is so-called 'mixed connective tissue disease' (MCTD), characterised as much as anything by the lack of predominant features associated with one of the others in this family of conditions. We have retained the term 'MCTD' because it is in common use, but the observations of Le Roy et al (1980) are relevant. The 'variant' is only ten years old, and most of the literature is devoted to clinical and laboratory studies. Familial occurrence has been described, both of MCTD itself (Horn et al, 1978) and of SLE in relatives (Ramos-Nienbro & Alarcon-Segovia, 1978).

Sjögren's disease

Some 50% of persons with keratoconjunctivitis sicca display other features of Sjögren's disease (Talal, 1966). The syndrome of keratoconjunctivitis sicca (xerophthalmia) and xerostomia may be encountered on its own, and when observed in the elderly without associated autoantibodies it has been suggested that it is more likely to result from acinar atrophy than an autoimmune process (Whaley et al, 1972). Somewhat more common is the classical triad of which musculoskeletal or connective tissue involvement is the third constituent; this was recognised in 58% of cases in one series, the conditions identified in these 100 patients being RA in 94, SLE in 4, SS in one, and psoriatic arthropathy in another (Whaley et al, 1973a, b). It has been estimated that 10–15% of sufferers from RA manifest the condition (Talal, 1966), and appreciable disability can result.

There was a nine-fold female preponderance in Whaley's series and the mean age was 57 years, although an earlier report indicated that half of those affected experience their first symptom before the age of 40 (Vanselow et al, 1963). Penicillin allergy is common, being reported by 40% of those with Sjögren's disease as compared with 16% in uncomplicated RA (Williams et al, 1969). Serological findings such as autoantibodies suggest that the disorder is likely to be an autoimmune phenomenon (Marcolongo et al, 1972). Both susceptibility and the severity of manifestations appear to be related to HLA-B8 and DR3 (Fye et al, 1978). An increased risk of reticuloendothelial malignancies has long been recognised (Talal & Bunim, 1964).

Polyarteritis nodosa

The only quantified estimates are from the Mayo Clinic, an incidence of 0.0007% (0.000007) per annum and a prevalence of 0.006% (Kurland et al, 1969). Other epidemiological evidence is scant, but Lawrence (1977) has discussed what is available.

ARTHROSIS AND DORSOPATHIES

Most people make a very basic taxonomic distinction by differentiating between two very broad classes of articular disorder. On the one hand are the inflammatory arthropathies that we have already discussed, and with which the connective tissue diseases are usually linked. On the other are so-called 'mechanical' or 'degenerative' disorders, and it is with these that we must now deal. It is helpful to begin by acknowledging some of the rather unsatisfactory characteristics that they have in common.

A very impressive feature is that these conditions form the most widespread type of rheumatic problem. Arthrosis and back troubles together account for at least a third of all rheumatic suffering (see Fig. 2.8), and they are much the commonest rheumatological causes of impairment and disability. In contrast to the inflammatory arthropathies, one cannot help but be struck by the fact that research endeavour has not been commensurate with the burden that has to be endured. Much of the explanation for this discrepancy lies with other characteristics of these conditions.

Obstacles to understanding

A series of interrelated features combine to retard appreciation of the nature of all these disorders. A large part of the difficulty can be attributed to how observations are regarded and how evidence is interpreted. One influence is really psychological, the notion of 'degeneration' and a wearing out of parts scarcely encouraging optimism about the possibilities for arrest or reversal of the underlying pathology. Such views derive largely from patterns of occurrence with age, a topic touched on in the previous chapter in the context of drawing inferences. At this stage it suffices to say that the case for regarding arthrosis as a degenerative or ageing process is open to serious question.

The most extensive parts of our knowledge are based on observations of structural changes, either directly, in morbid anatomical specimens, or indirectly through the medium of shadows on X-ray plates. Apart from levels of detail, such as that fibrillation of cartilage may be observed pathologically but cannot be identified radiographically, the two sources of evidence have yielded broadly compatible findings. The similarity of features observed at different sites of involvement has fostered the view that arthrosis is an almost universal phenomenon, to be explained by comparable mechanisms wherever it may be encountered. This in turn has also encouraged the notion of a degenerative process.

This line of reasoning glosses over a number of aspects. One is that the concatenation of features is often treated as a whole, neglecting the fact that some of those included are fundamental whereas others are only associated or confounding. As was noted in the previous chapter, osteophytes probably fall in the latter category. Another aspect is that what is observed to be similar structurally could nevertheless reflect just a common end-expression of a number of different processes.

Regularity at what can be regarded as the micro level tends to deflect attention away from important locus-specific differences. In turn this leads to rather sterile arguments about whether the chondrocyte or whatever is the originating source of trouble. Surely this is somewhat akin to considering pollination at the micro level and indulging in disputation about whether the male or female gamete is primordial — whilst neglecting that pollination failure is more likely to be explained by studying whether the process is dependent on self-fertilisation or the mediation of agents such as the wind or bees. Put another way, one is reminded of the chap searching under the streetlight, not because that was where he had dropped his belongings but because the chance of finding them should have been enhanced by the better illumination. This is not intended in derogation of pathologists, who deserve great credit for having taken most of the initiative in arthrosis research. However, it is difficult to avoid the impression that insufficient attention has been directed to what are likely to be more promising areas.

Another aspect, and clinically the most important, is that significant discontinuities in the evidence get neglected. Specific structural abnormalities are relatively easy to study, and they have been productive of useful biomedical concepts. These concepts tend to be linked to clinical problems on the basis of the observation that severe structural changes in a joint are often associated with symptoms. This leads to a common clinical syllogism (Wood, 1976a): osteoarthrotic changes cause symptoms; this patient has osteoarthrotic changes; therefore this patient's symptoms are due to the osteoarthrotic changes.

Although this is frequently a reasonable guide, the vulnerability of the conclusion is that the first premise does not state that all osteoarthrotic changes always cause symptoms. In other words, available biomedical concepts have a limited applicability in the elucidation of an individual's subjective problems. This is because there is an

Table 3.5 Discordance between symptom experience and evidence of structural change (derived from Lawrence, 1969c).

Complaint	Radiographic findings	Concordance* (complaint with X-ray changes)	Discordance† (X-ray changes without complaint)
Pain in hip	Arthrosis of hip	39	8
Pain in knee	Arthrosis of knee	68	12
Cervicobrachial pain	Cervical disc degeneration	50	35
Back-hip-sciatic pain	Lumbar disc degeneration	59	45

* Equivalent to sensitivity of radiographic changes as a criterion.
† Equivalent to complement of specificity, derived by subtracting latter from 100.

appreciable discordance between clinical problems and evidence of underlying abnormalities such as may be revealed by radiographs. This discordance is illustrated in Table 3.5. A major, but by no means exclusive, part of the discordance is attributable to the fact that most structural changes are irreversible whereas symptoms in any one individual tend to be inconstant. The latter is a feature that also makes clinical trials more difficult because non-therapeutic variation is greater.

We have illustrated these problems by reference to arthrosis, but the same difficulties obtrude on attempts to understand back pain. Similarly, the major implications apply equally to both types of condition. One is that terminology is undoubtedly unsatisfactory and confusing, as was indicated in Table 2.2. This is largely a reflection of the crudity of nosological distinctions, and appreciable heterogeneity is almost certainly being concealed at present. Underlying the problems with nomenclature has been poverty of clinical observation. For example, there has been a dearth of careful and detailed natural history studies, and this means that we are still uncertain about how uniformly progressive these disorders are, and at what rate. Basic biological changes have also not been adequately established, such as the possibility that symptom expression may alter with age (Acheson, 1982)

The other important implication concerns the use we make of concepts and how far we extend their application. On one plane it may be very helpful to regard arthrosis as being basically a disease of cartilage, or back pain as emanating from disturbance of the intervertebral disc. However, for many other purposes it is more profitable to examine form and alignment, such as the geometry of a joint or stenosis of the spinal canal, and for yet others to concentrate on patterns of use and overuse, including the influence of posture and habitual activities.

Peripheral joints

We would have preferred to discuss the occurrence of arthrosis at each individual joint in turn. Unfortunately the evidence is insufficiently comprehensive to justify pursuing such an approach, and it would also have been difficult to avoid a lot of repetition. To stay as close to our original aim as possible we shall begin by considering what is known of the localised occurrence of arthrosis, leaving remarks on polyarticular or generalised disease until the end.

Frequency

The tendency to quote frequency estimates based on structural changes is perhaps understandable in the absence of better alternatives. The work of Lawrence (1977) is extensive and has included all the most important individual joints. Moderate or severe arthrotic changes may be observed in radiographs of the hands and feet in 11% of persons (Lawrence, 1963), and radiographic abnormalities of at least mild degree occur somewhere in almost all individuals aged 65 years or more (Lawrence et al, 1966). Associated symptom rates generally increase with the severity of structural changes, although the discordance or 'false positive' rates indicate how incomplete an explanation for symptoms is provided by radiographs.

To treat these findings as if they related to an

entity, when in fact they represent an amalgam of changes at different anatomical sites, not only conceals important differences between the various locations but also may create misleading impressions of the size of the populations at risk of developing these changes (Wood, 1970a, 1971a). The more striking and useful observation is not that we shall all develop OA somewhere, but that most of us will not develop it in any one particular joint. This aspect has been considered further elsewhere (Wood, 1976a).

The knee is the most commonly involved major joint, but the most disabling site is undoubtedly the hip. The encouraging successes with total replacement of these joints has created a need for indications of the likely demand for such operations. Unfortunately we lack a satisfactory basis for deriving good estimates, but the subject has been considered in some detail by Laing & Taylor (1982).

Characteristics

Standards for interpretation of radiographic changes have been available for 20 years (Atlas, 1963) but a sustained approach to the construction of diagnostic criteria has been undertaken only recently (Altman et al, 1983), and that endeavour is confined to characterisation of arthrosis of the knee joint. A complementary approach is to concentrate on perceived health problems (Hunt et al, 1981).

The simplest method of subdividing OA is according to whether it is localised to a single site or multiple sites are involved. The former appears to be much commoner, particularly if the idea of a single site is extended so as to include similar joints in a group, such as both knees or the distal interphalangeal joints. The value of the distinction is that it directs attention to local factors in pathogenesis, but obviously it also provides a useful guide for clinical management. However, it emerges that in clinical, and perhaps especially in surgical practice, the search for involvement of sites other than the presenting joint is often cursory, so that relative frequencies of occurrence are difficult to establish with any confidence.

The discordance between symptoms and anatomical changes indicates a need for more detailed localisation of the source of complaints in structures surrounding the joints. Whilst it is possible that arthrotic changes may predispose to the development of various lesions in ligaments and other soft tissues, the outlook for such 'complications' is likely to be more optimistic than it would be for the underlying structural change, and certainly therapeutic options are extended. Moreover, it is in such lesions that the inflammatory basis for 'arthrotic' symptoms could be located.

We have remarked upon the poverty of longitudinal studies. However, progression of radiographic arthrosis in joints of the hand has been studied over time in a group of predominantly professional, technical, and managerial males. The maximum rate of change was observed in the distal interphalangeal joints, with an average increase of one standard X-ray grade per individual over a 12–16 year interval; rates of change were much less in the proximal interphalangeal joints (Plato & Norris, 1979).

Rheumatoid arthritis is commonly regarded as the most disabling form of arthropathy. Polyarticular involvement is encountered less frequently in OA and certainly a smaller proportion of sufferers from this disorder, only some 11%, are sufficiently disabled to need some help with everyday living activities. However, the very much higher prevalence of arthrosis puts this condition number one in the league table as being the most frequent physical cause of severe disablement in the community, and by a long lead (Badley et al, 1978b). Interference with sexual activity is also an important problem (Currey, 1970).

Heterogeneity of arthrosis

It has been common to make a distinction between primary and secondary OA, the former implying a condition that develops in the absence of any obvious predisposing factors and which therefore often gets attributed to some intrinsic defect of cartilage. The problems with this view have been considered before (Wood, 1976a) and Solomon (1976), following similar reasoning, has suggested that three patterns of pathogenesis should be recognised:

1. Failure of essentially normal cartilage subjected to abnormal or incongruous loading for long periods

2. Damaged or defective cartilage failing under normal conditions of loading
3. Break-up of articular cartilage due to defective subchondral bone.

These ideas are attractive, although what constitutes normal conditions of loading and how these may alter at different stages of life requires further clarification.

The prevalence of all forms of arthrosis increases with age, though the evidence is generally insufficient to allow one to determine whether rates of change with age differ between the various joints. The apparent lack of such differences is not helpful, because age patterns could indicate whether failure under normal or excessive loading was the more likely at any particular site. Some meaningful import must underlie not only the relative frequency with which different joints are affected, but also how these changes manifest themselves with age.

What is true of different sites may also apply to different areas within an individual joint. The knee is ideal to study with this possibility in mind because it is of sufficient size to allow of topographical discrimination between different regions on radiographs. Factor analysis of various observed features permits computation of scores for each individual as a means of describing how important different factors may be in any one person (Pole et al, 1974). Notable factors were those reflecting predominant involvement of either the medial or lateral compartments, the scores for which tended to be low in the majority of individuals but which were elevated in a small proportion of patients who were also more likely to be older. These patterns contrasted with the more uniform increase with age in scores for an osteophyte factor, which suggests that the latter may well represent a wear phenomenon, the reaction of a joint to prolonged use rather than being directly related to OA.

Overall the frequency of arthrosis appears to be fairly similar in the two sexes, but more detailed scrutiny of the evidence indicates a number of differences. First, though, it must be noted that men and women are more alike than different in their actual reporting of chronic joint symptoms (i.e. women are not more willing to complain and men are not more likely to under-report); sex differentials in complaints need to take account of treatment behaviour and disease state before conclusions can be drawn (Davis, 1981). The relationship between symptoms and changes in individual joints has been studied in some detail (Lawrence et al, 1966).

Men not only seem to develop arthrosis more frequently in the wrists and hips (Kellgren & Lawrence, 1958) but they also often appear to be affected at younger ages than do women, which has encouraged people to speculate about the role of trauma. On the other hand arthrosis in the hands is encountered more frequently and with greater severity in women (Acheson et al, 1970), which has led to a suggestion that 'systemic' factors underlie the development of 'degenerative' joint disease and that these are more important in females (Acheson & Collart, 1975). Women also exhibit arthrosis in the knees and sacroiliac joints more commonly than men (Kellgren & Lawrence, 1958).

Predisposing factors to arthrosis of the hip include deformations of the femoral head resulting from congenital dislocation of the hip, Legg–Calvé–Perthes disease, slipped epiphysis, trauma, and polyarthritis. It has been estimated that some 40% of cases can be attributed to these underlying causes, and that in such instances presentation occurs at younger ages (Kelsey, 1977). Although one may suspect that the hip is perhaps a special case, particularly by virtue of the variety of such predispositions, what appears to be peculiar to this joint could nevertheless be a more general phenomenon — so that we ought to be alert for heterogeneity in the factors predisposing to arthrosis in other joints.

Other individual attributes

Inherited factors obviously contribute to properties such as the geometry of joints as well as, potentially at least, to differences in cartilage composition and metabolism, but these have not been studied at all extensively. Most work on genetic aspects has focused on multiple OA, to be discussed shortly, although a familial coxarthrosis has been documented (Böni, 1959). Observed ethnic differences have been attributed more to patterns of use than to genetic influences. For example the greater frequency of arthrosis in the metacarpophalangeal and proximal interphalangeal joints of Tswana males has been related to trauma (Solomon et al, 1976), and the relative infrequency of arthrosis of the hip in Hong Kong Chinese (Hoaglund et al, 1973) and Malays and in Uganda, South Africa, and the West Indies (reviewed by Kelsey, 1977) has been linked to squatting, an activity that allows all areas of articular cartilage to be subject to pressure every day (Gunn, 1974).

Arthrosis of the hands is observed more frequently on the right side than the left, but this is apparently not related to dominance (Acheson et al, 1970). With unilateral hip disease the two sides seem to be affected at similar rates, although the hip on the side of the longer leg is affected more often in people with unequal leg lengths (reviewed by Kelsey, 1977). In lower limb amputees an increased frequency of arthrosis is observed in the contralateral limb (Burke et al, 1978). On the other hand the occurrence of arthrosis of the hip and knee is reduced in limbs affected by poliomyelitis, which suggests that neurological function may play some part in the development of or protection from the condition (Glyn et al, 1966).

Population studies have usually indicated an association between arthrosis and increased body mass but interpretation of this relationship is not straightforward; in some instances it may be a contributory factor whereas in others it may represent a consequence of arthrosis, being encouraged by reduced activity in response to pain. Much of the evidence is not easy to disentangle in regard to individual joints, but one of the more surprising links is that between obesity and arthrosis of the distal interphalangeal joints (Kellgren & Lawrence, 1958; Engel, 1968). Lawrence (1977) discusses some of the possible implications of these observations. It is in weight-bearing joints that the association might appear to be most plausible aetiologically, and certainly this view is commonly acted on clinically by endeavouring to persuade patients to lose weight. However, contrary opinions have been expressed (Goldin et al, 1976). For example, Watson (1976) implicated obesity in some cases of coxarthrosis whereas Saville & Dickson (1968) discounted this influence. Among the difficulties has been too great a reliance on clinical (i.e. selected) samples. Other problems have also been aired recently (Wood, 1983b).

Other constitutional influences, not of themselves of particular relevance to the common occurrence of arthrosis, are the presence of conditions such as ochronosis and acromegaly. Of greater interest is the possible role of joint laxity (Scott et al, 1979), and a relationship to bone density (Foss & Byers, 1972). The latter gives rise to what might appear to be a paradox in that essentially similar treatment is used at either extreme of a distribution, some form of hip replacement being used both when bone density is high (arthrosis) and when it is low (femoral neck fracture).

External influences

There are no clear patterns of occurrence of arthrosis with place, other than can be attributed to ethnic influences and factors mentioned elsewhere in this discussion. However, a distinctive form of arthrosis has been identified in eastern Siberia and is designated 'Kashin–Bek disease'; presumed to arise as a result of fungal spores from damp grain, the condition can therefore shed little light on more commonly occurring problems. One other geographical difference deserves comment. It is striking that OA appears to be recorded clinically with much greater frequency in Great Britain than it does in other countries, such as France, even though rigorous documentation of this impression from the literature is not possible. The difference is likely to be more apparent than real, and is probably due to variation in diagnostic practices. Although generalisation is hazardous it seems that most British physicians may more readily attribute symptoms to underlying structural changes, whereas French rheumatologists are perhaps more discriminating in the variety of conditions they identify in juxta-articular structures.

The influence of activity scarcely leads to any clear model of the role of use and stress. Among the interesting negative observations have been failure to find increased risk, such as in the hips and knees of physical education teachers (Eastmond et al, 1979), the hips of competitive runners (Puranen et al, 1975), the knees and ankles of parachutists (Murray-Leslie et al, 1977), and the ankles of professional footballers (Adams, 1979). The feature common to all these groups, of course, is that exposure to stress occurs after training, and the concomitant development of other musculoskeletal structures may offer protection from injury.

Occupation tends to impose hazards of a different type, and ones for which the individual has not been prepared by training. Trauma appears to be an important factor in distal interphalangeal arthrosis in cotton operatives (Lawrence, 1961), in arthrosis of the elbow in those carrying out heavy manual work, and especially in those using pneumatic drills (Lawrence, 1955), and in arthrosis of the knees in miners (Lawrence et al, 1963). Once again, though, the situation is not quite straightforward because wear and tear has been invoked to explain high rates of coxarthrosis in farmers and gardeners, yet the parts of the joint manifesting the earliest signs are not those most subjected to stress (Harrison et al, 1953). As a final antidote to thinking that may become too deterministic, it is also worth recalling that the joint space in a degenerated hip can show spontaneous recovery (Perry et al, 1972).

Polyarticular arthrosis

Polyarticular arthrosis was first described clinically, but full appreciation of multiple joint involvement really stemmed from radiographic studies. In a few instances the disorder is related to familial chondrodysplasia (Brown & Rose, 1966). More often multiple joints are affected without evidence of underlying developmental defects. We have already noted that a polyarticular pattern may often be missed if physical examination is only cursory. It also seems likely that multiple joint involvement, when it is recognised, may not always be appraised with sufficient discrimination. In fact two types of condition have been identified, and it is not helpful when both tend to be referred to by the same designation.

The situation is complicated further because distal interphalangeal arthrosis is encountered with each of the two conditions, and both also show aggregation of related features within families (Kellgren et al, 1963). However, in only one are there associated Heberden's nodes, and we will discuss this in a moment. The other, non-nodal, disorder presents with a different pattern of joint involvement in which arthrosis of the wrists and metacarpophalangeal joints are noteworthy. The distinctness of this condition is reinforced by observation of an increased frequency of inflammatory polyarthropathy, predominantly seronegative for rheumatoid factor, in affected kindreds. Other features, such as elevated erythrocyte sedimentation rates and serum uric acid levels and complaints of morning stiffness, also appear to be more common in this group.

The evidence is therefore suggestive that non-nodal polyarticular arthrosis often may be secondary to other joint disorders, notably rheumatoid-type polyarthritis and perhaps occasionally gout (Lawrence, 1969b). It is confusing to refer to this condition as 'generalised osteoarthrosis' (GOA). We suggest that multiple OA be designated as such when its nature has not been further elucidated, and even this term is probably best restricted to situations where at least five joints or groups are affected. We also suggest that the non-nodal disorder just delineated be identified by some other term, such as 'polyarticular arthrosis'.

Men tend to be affected by polyarticular arthrosis slightly more frequently than women, but more often than not the condition is asymptomatic at the time of an epidemiological survey (Lawrence, 1969b). In those aged 45 years and over the prevalence of radiographic changes at five or more sites approaches 9%.

Generalised osteoarthrosis

The other recognisable form of multiple OA is the primary nodal disorder described by Kellgren & Moore (1952), and for which the term 'GOA' is best reserved. Failure to observe this rigour probably accounted for the anomalously high frequency of non-typical GOA at some centres in our international diagnostic study (Kellgren et al, 1969). In population studies, and also in clinical practice, respondents may well complain of symptoms related to only a single joint or group of joints (Lawrence, 1969b), but radiographic investigation reveals the typical pattern.

Characteristically there is involvement of both distal and proximal interphalangeal joints, together with the first carpometacarpals and the metatarsophalangeals, especially the first. The appearance of hip involvement is different from when it occurs as an isolated or 'primary' lesion (Kellgren & Lawrence, 1961; Marks et al, 1979). These joints, together with the knees and the apophyseal joints of the spine, are somewhat less frequently affected than the smaller joints of the hands and feet.

The uniqueness of GOA appeared to be challenged when O'Brien et al (1968) were unable to detect bimodality in the distribution of the number of hand joints involved radiographically. However, the distinction between generalised and other forms of OA was substantiated when we found that the number of joints involved throughout the body was related to particular sites (Benn & Wood, 1975). Two broad patterns can be detected (Wood, 1976a) and the likelihood of arthrosis of phalangeal joints rises markedly as the number of sites affected increases.

Surveys of radiographs from the population indicate a prevalence of up to 15% in women aged 45 years and over, but only half of those affected complained of symptoms at the time and almost a third had never experienced pain (Lawrence, 1969b). What we now identify as GOA was described as menopausal arthritis by Cecil & Archer (1926) but the menopause does not seem to be a critical factor (Kellgren et al, 1963), even though the symptomatic condition presenting to hospital is observed overwhelmingly in females. Other endocrine aspects are discussed by Lawrence (1977). The disorder has been described in association with articular chondrocalcinosis, when a more destructive process that also involved the shoulders, elbows, and wrists was identified (Gerster et al, 1975a, b). However, the lower frequency of Heberden's and Bouchard's nodes in the chondrocalcinotic group suggests that some of these patients might have suffered from polyarticular arthrosis rather than GOA.

Spondylosis

In this section we shall consider the evidence on structural changes on its own, and then confront the more general problem of 'non-specific' back pain in the following section. We have used the term 'spondylosis' as a generic descriptor for 'degenerative' processes in the spine, be these in the apophyseal joints or related to intervertebral discs. For completeness we shall include remarks on other anatomical abnormalities at the end of the present discussion.

Characteristics

Epidemiological reports mirror the clinical literature in the poverty of information available on arthrosis of the diarthrodial interfacetal joints. Despite considerable detail in a report on the relationship between symptoms and radiographic changes (Lawrence et al, 1966), even in his meticulous monograph Lawrence (1977) makes little more than passing mention of the condition, other than to note that it can frequently be observed in women with GOA. The explanation probably lies with the fact that the commonly available lateral radiographs of the spine are less satisfactory for detecting apophyseal abnormalities than they are for revealing intervertebral disc degeneration.

Friberg & Hirsch (1948) described the triad of disc space narrowing, osteophytes on the vertebral bodies, and sclerosis of the vertebral end-plates that is characteristic of disc degeneration (DD), the disorder for which the term 'spondylosis' is often used as a synonym. Standards for radiographic gradings have been developed (Atlas, 1963), although Lawrence (1977) notes that intraobserver variation over time can still be an appreciable problem. Frykholm (1951) described osteophytes in two locations — ventral (anterior) spurs, especially in the thoracolumbar region, which do not seem to be related to DD; and lipping, either marginal or affecting the entire circumference, which could be observed throughout the spine and was presumed to be the consequence of DD with disc collapse. The latter can also result in subluxation of the corresponding interfacetal joints, leading to secondary osteophyte formation at these sites. However, it is difficult to pursue the epidemiology of these relationships with the limited radiographs available in population studies.

There is a paradox concerning the interpretation of X-ray findings related to DD. It is understandable that great weight should be attached to the most obvious features, osteophytes. On the other hand these changes are likely to indicate that the stable door has been secured after the occupant has

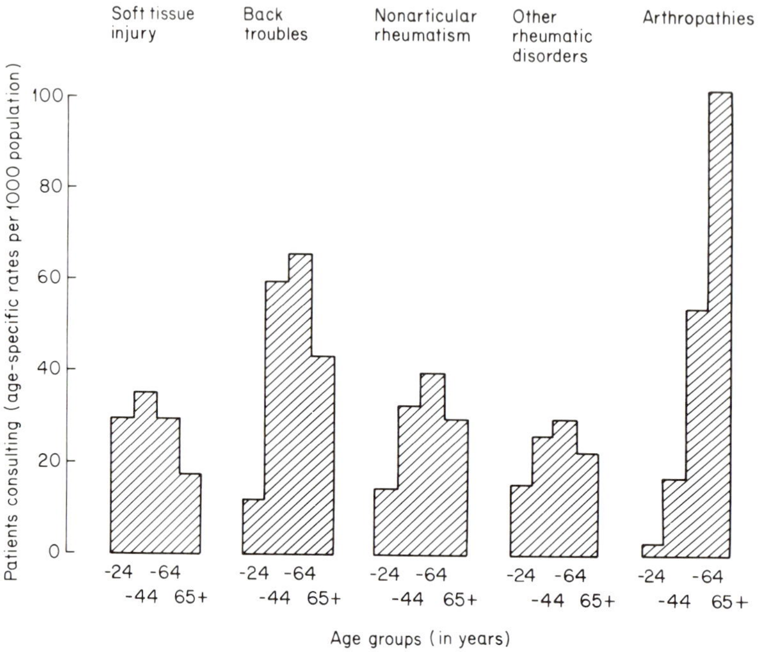

Fig. 3.3 Age-specific incidence rates for categories of rheumatic disorders in general practice (derived from OPCS, 1974).

bolted. Symptoms usually arise from an articular segment that is vulnerable to instability because of DD, and yet the presence of osteophytes generally indicates that stabilisation has probably begun to occur (Kellgren, 1977). This contrast offers a likely explanation for the fall-off in incidence of many back complaints with age (Fig. 3.3), despite the fact that radiographic abnormalities tend to show a sustained increase in extent and severity. More generally, it probably accounts for much of the discordance between symptoms and structural evidence of degeneration in the spine (Torgerson & Dotter, 1976; Table 3.5).

Epidemiology

The most extensive work on DD has been carried out by Lawrence (1969c), who has also (1977) reviewed the whole field, including the differential affection of individual segments of the spine; the reader is directed to these sources for further detail. In summary, the prevalence of DD increases with age, and after the age of 60 years it is rare to find a completely normal spine on radiographic investigation.

Frequency estimates obviously depend on the severity of changes to which attention is paid, although the patterns of progression with age are parallel for different grade thresholds. As Lawrence (1977) notes, lower values are generally obtained if the judgements of more than one observer are reconciled, as opposed to considering the results from individual observers working on their own. The age composition of samples studied also influences overall measures of frequency in the population. Taking all these factors into account the more recent work by Julkunen and his colleagues (1981a) appears to be broadly in accord with Lawrence's estimates, and an overall figure for the prevalence of DD in a population of adults is of the order of 45% (0.45).

Palaeopathological evidence from Eskimos, Pueblo Indians, and Caucasoids (Stewart, 1966) provides graphic examples of variation in the frequency of DD, both between different segments of the spine and as regards the upper and lower margins of the vertebral bodies. Such variation is most likely to represent not ethnic or geographical differences but differential stress related mainly to habitual patterns of use. Only infrequently are antecedent causes identifiable, such as adolescent kyphosis, scoliosis, tuberculous infection, spondylolysis or spondylolisthesis, and spinal osteochondrosis (Stoddard & Osborn, 1979).

The role of heavy manual work in encouraging multiple DD, especially as may be seen in the lumbar region in coalminers, appears to depend on both its nature (and particularly exposure to injury) and its duration. Sedentary workers exhibit frequencies of involvement of the cervical spine that are similar to those encountered in people engaged in physically more taxing pursuits, but in the former the severity of changes is only minimal. There is also evidence of variability in predisposition to DD. Ochronosis provides an obvious but uncommon example.

Familial aggregation has been described by Lawrence, and Bull and his colleagues (1969) observed both concordance in twins and relative freedom from cervical spondylosis in certain other families. However, until inherited influences on properties such as disc metabolism have been identified the results from genetic studies are not straightforward for interpretation. Families do differ in attributes such as habitual postures and mannerisms (i.e. patterns of use), but these could be related to cultural assimilation (unconscious mimicry, etc.) as much as to genetic factors. There is insufficient evidence to establish the characteristics of those in whom spondylosis is associated with the development of myelopathy, and so the role of constitutional factors in regard to this complication is indeterminate.

Ankylosing hyperostosis

Ankylosing hyperostosis (AH) is often referred to as Forestier's disease because of important reports by this author on the characteristic X-ray features (Forestier & Rotes-Querol, 1950) and on differentiation from AS (Forestier et al, 1956). Formerly qualified as being vertebral, the preferred term of 'AH' was put forward by Bywaters & Forestier (1967) in recognition of the fact that extraspinal features associated with peripheral complaints are not uncommon. More widespread involvement is also emphasised by the designation 'diffuse idiopathic skeletal hyperostosis' (DISH) (Resnick & Niwayama, 1976; Utsinger et al, 1976), which may attract some because it appears to form a new 'word'. However, this nomenclature is longer and yet no more informative than 'AH'; the latter had priority in usage; and 'DISH' has two features that are undesirable — there is gratuitous specification of an unknown aetiology, and needless problems of exclusion are created (i.e. if hyperostotic changes are not diffuse then the term 'DISH' would scarcely seem to be appropriate, even if the underlying pathology was the same).

Criteria for identification are discussed by Lawrence (1977) and Julkunen et al (1971). There has been controversy whether AH represents a unique 'degenerative' disorder (Forestier & Lagier, 1971) or just a particular variety of spondylosis (Ott et al, 1963). Most of the epidemiological work on the condition has been carried out by Julkunen and his colleagues (1971, 1975, 1979) and this has helped to clarify the status of AH. However, it is perplexing to find lack of apophyseal and peripheral involvement cited by these authors as a distinguishing feature of what they refer to as 'DISH'. Differences in distributional characteristics and linked features indicate that AH is distinct from spondylosis — the former occurs later in life, is unrelated to strenuous work, is associated with diabetes mellitus (Julkunen et al, 1981a), and has a lower risk in regard to future cardiovascular disease (Julkunen et al, 1981b). These sources also suggest that AH can be identified in association with acromegaly, hypoparathyroidism, essential hypocalcaemia, hypophosphataemia, and fluorosis, though the evidence leaves one uncertain whether spinal changes that might be specific to some of these disorders had been adequately discriminated.

The frequency of AH is 6–10 times less than that of spondylosis, although the ratio of the former relative to the latter increases with age (Julkunen et al, 1981a). Lawrence (1977) quotes prevalence ratios of 14% in men and 5% in women over the age of 34 but these estimates are much higher than those observed in the Finnish experience; the latter seem to be more specific and realistic, even though the units in which they were reported were not entirely clear. It is difficult to interpret the limited evidence on geographical differences. The occurrence of multiple cases in an unusual family has been reported (Beardwell, 1969); involvement was detected as young as 18 years, and there was an association with tylosis (punctate hyperkeratosis). No association could be detected with B27 (Brigode & Francois, 1977), nor with other HLA antigens in a study of Pima Indians (Spagnola et al, 1978) although skeletal fluorosis is common in this group.

Other anatomical abnormalities

Reviews of evidence on back pain usually identify specific abnormalities of structure that are assumed to be relevant. We have already mentioned some of these in passing. However, a general caution should be noted. Many of these conditions have been implicated on the basis of guilt by association, i.e. with back pain. This may be a productive starting point, but all too often the essential sequel has been neglected — to establish whether such conditions are necessary and sufficient causes of the complaints presented.

The challenge arises because we are not confronted by unique associations, such as that between exposure to asbestos particles and the development of pleural mesothelioma. Instead we observe what appear to be increases in risk, that given lesions seem to be more common in those with backache. It is the extent and nature of this risk that requires elucidation. As one of us noted some time ago (Wood, 1972), to resolve this problem it is necessary to study a group of people with a particular lesion, record their complaints, and then relate the findings to symptom experience in a comparable group of people without the lesion. With a few notable exceptions such testimony is largely lacking, although the work of Magora and his colleagues is exemplary.

What is particularly worrying is that not only does available evidence tend to be unsatisfactory, which retards research enquiry, but also that this does not deter people from prescriptive infringement of individual liberty. This is most evident in regard to pre-employment screening because anatomical abnormalities are the easiest features to detect radiographically. On the basis of currently inadequate knowledge, curtailing the individual's freedom of choice when seeking employment would appear to be scientifically and ethically unjustifiable in many instances. It is paradoxical that the operation of legal precedents supposed to protect the individual, such as in regard to liability and compensation, tend to neglect consequential intrusion on wider aspects of the preservation of rights.

Developmental anomalies. Conditions such as spina bifida occulta and transitional vertebra, especially sacralisation of L5, are probably commoner than has been realised (Magora & Schwartz, 1978, 1980). However, the evidence does not support the view that these anomalies have a meaningful relation to back complaints. A whole host of theories about the pathogenesis of associated pain therefore become suspect (Magora & Schwartz, 1978). The same also appears to be true of spondylolysis and spondylolisthesis, the epidemiology of which has been reviewed by Kelsey & White (1980). The situation is even less satisfactory in regard to scoliosis. Lateral spinal curvature can be identified in 15% of schoolchildren, but in two-fifths it is related to pelvic tilt due to inequality in leg lengths rather than to primary abnormality of the spine itself (Dickson, 1983). The greater the curvature the more likely the problem represented a true idiopathic scoliosis, which had an overall frequency of 0.2%. This condition occurs more frequently in girls, is associated with a median sagittal asymmetry, and tends to be progressive. The remaining children had spinal scoliosis, which probably represents irrelevant coronal asymmetry in normal healthy children. All one can conclude is that the extent of the contribution these different conditions make, both to DD and to back pain, has yet to be established.

Spinal stenosis. This condition is as much a functional as a structural abnormality. It represents disproportion between the sizes, and more specifically the cross-sectional areas, of the spinal canal and associated tunnels and foramina on the one hand and of the nervous structures disposed within them on the other. The result can be compression of the latter, and interference with the blood supply. A variety of lesions may give rise to the condition, and these and other clinical aspects have been reviewed recently (Critchley, 1982). Pulsed echo ultrasound offers an acceptable means for large-scale investigation and has been used in the study of patients and other selected groups, both of children and of adults in particular occupational groups (Porter et al, 1980). More evidence is required, especially on alterations over time, because observed trends in measurements such as oblique diameters could reflect cohort effects as much as changes associated with age. In the present state of knowledge it appears that the concept of spinal stenosis represents one factor of significance in certain clinical syndromes, though it appears to be less relevant in older patients and in those with root entrapment (Porter et al, 1980).

Other back troubles

Confronted by a subjective complaint, physicians are generally happier if they can find so-called 'objective' evidence to support a diagnostic conclusion. At the same time the tradition of medical practice encourages identification of an underlying pathological state, even if only by inference. Unfortunately back pain cannot easily be constrained in this manner. If associated physical signs can be detected they tend to be non-specific and are as likely to represent the consequence of the complaint, such as limitation of spinal mobility, as they are to provide an independent clue to the origin of the problem.

Such a state of affairs can encourage further investigation, especially by the use of radiographs. However, the discordance with symptoms already discussed (Table 3.5) indicates that all too often it is not possible to make very much of such findings. This would suggest that X-ray techniques have a limited role in clinical practice, and it has been argued that routine radiography should be reserved for those patients who have not recovered from their back complaints within three months (Currey et al, 1979).

A more general point to be acknowledged is that, although an array of different conditions may give rise to pain in the back, these are insufficiently differentiated to allow an epidemiologist to make any significant contribution. This is an example of the dependence of less specialised disciplines on being presented with clearly defined problems by clinical medicine (Himsworth, 1969). As a result one is limited to evidence of two types. The first is provided by frequency measures derived from health service utilisation and the uptake of benefits, such as were discussed in the previous chapter. The second is circumstantial evidence, what we referred to above as 'guilt by association', relating to the overall influence of various factors on the heterogeneity of conditions concealed by the term 'non-specific back pain'. Before considering this evidence, though, there is one other 'lesion' that has to be taken into account.

Disc prolapse

Much of the literature on back complaints is confused by references to prolapse of the intervertebral discs (PID). Although these structures undoubtedly may prolapse, herniate, or in other ways be displaced, the difficulty lies in establishing both when this may have happened and whether it is clinically significant. In severe cases there may be little doubt, especially when contrast radiography can be used to demonstrate the lesion. However, in most instances there are many sources of uncertainty — criteria for identification are notable for their vagaries and lack of uniformity in application; the source of pain is often not explored systematically, particularly as regards differentiation between articular, dural, and neurological origins; and confirmatory evidence cannot be derived from plain radiography. In particular, narrowing of the disc space on its own has never been established as having a relationship to symptoms (Troup, 1965).

The result is loose usage of the term 'disc prolapse' by both practitioners and the public. Whereas the former often mislead themselves, for reasons such as we have noted or perhaps to conceal ignorance, the latter may wish for more prestigious diagnostic status or may even seek secondary gain, such as through social security benefits or compensation. Serious and provocative challenges to the validity of the concept (Troup, 1961; Strange, 1966) have unfortunately not succeeded in stemming this tide.

Recognising this terminological carelessness, we are not satisfied that reports supposedly concerned with epidemiological aspects of disc prolapse in fact contribute any enlightenment on this condition. We prefer to acknowledge these uncertainties and to consider all that has been so ascribed in the more general context of non-specific back pain. However, readers wishing to pursue a specific focus on disc prolapse despite these caveats may consult a recent review (Kelsey & White, 1980).

Unfortunately the confusion extends to other areas of unspecialised research as well. For example, work on intradiscal pressures (Nachemson, 1975) is of interest in its own right in regard to the biology of discs. However, attempts to apply these insights to clinical problems suffer from the weaknesses we have discussed — i.e. to what extent can symptoms be ascribed or otherwise related to lesions that are only postulated, however plausible the inferences may appear to be? Underlying this is another difficulty, that the relationship between disc prolapse and DD has not been adequately elucidated so that one is often compelled to resort to generic designation of disc lesions. In fact much of the evidence, such as that on the mechanical properties of lumbar spine segments (Nachemson et al, 1979), would suggest that DD is of much more general importance than uncomplicated prolapse.

Occurrence of back pain

Estimates of prevalence for what is usually a relatively short-lived but nevertheless very common complaint are not particularly enlightening. More graphic is the appreciation Hult (1954a, b) developed in his pioneer work — that 60% of a sample of men up to age 69 years had at some time suffered from symptoms related to the lower back, and that the proportion increased to 80% when attention was focused on those involved in physically demanding occupations. Recent work employing the same concept of lifetime incidence has yielded similar results (Svensson & Andersson, 1982). The same report revealed that more than a quarter of those not admitting to such a history nevertheless had experienced time off work with low back pain, so that even these impressive figures represent an underestimate.

Confronted with such enormity one has to seek means of reducing the problem to comprehensible dimensions. At a crude level two aspects deserve more attention, relating to location and duration. Unfortunately it is not always clear from the literature to what extent these distinctions have been made. As a result there are often taxing difficulties over comparability between estimates from different sources. The first aspect is the more straightforward of the two. For some purposes it is useful to treat the spine or the back as a whole, perhaps especially when documenting the community burden. However, for aetiological or control-oriented enquiries it is essential to differentiate between the functional and anatomical regions of the spine.

This most important distinction requires separation of cervical from lumbar involvement, particularly as the former may be responsible for complaints that can be difficult to distinguish from parts of what we shall discuss later, soft-tissue syndromes. Lumbar disorders outnumber cervical by a factor of 2 : 1 (Fry, 1972), and so it is not surprising that the bulk of the literature is devoted to lumbosacral problems. However, even under the topic of low back pain there is generally insufficient differentiation between lumbago and sciatica, a distinction which the concept of disc prolapse has unhelpfully tended to blur. Both the thoracic region (Editorial, 1976b) and the sacroiliac joint also have to be considered; the latter is a not uncommon source of low backache (Davis & Lentle, 1978).

For the other aspect we have found it useful to employ a very simple taxonomy (Wood & Badley, 1980) that allows us to identify the broad areas to which published work appears to relate, so that constraints upon inference from one set of observations to another are made more evident. This scheme differentiates between three types of problem:

1. **Transient** back pain, the evanescent twinges that everyone probably experiences at some time in their lives. The hallmark is brevity, a passing awareness of discomfort or perhaps sharper sensations related to the back. By their very universality such symptoms make up much the biggest class of back pain. However, it is unlikely that this order of complaint is usually presented to a doctor, so that it tends to be outside our professional experience and to be neglected in consideration of the problem. Nevertheless the context has to be taken note of because enquiries about symptom experience may well tap an unknown part of this reservoir of discomfort, and this may be especially relevant to retrospective studies of lumbar symptomatology.

2. **Acute** back pain is probably what most readers are likely to think of in relation to this subject. The key distinction concerns duration, and this class consists of symptoms present for sufficient time to compel most sufferers to take

note of them; the range probably extends from some hours to a few weeks. A very considerable range of variation is embraced — the onset of complaints may be dramatic, as with the hexenschuss or witch's blow, or it may be gradual; the symptoms may be confined to the lumbar region (lumbago), or they may also radiate to other areas, or they may be present only in the lower limbs (sciatica); the severity of suffering may extend from the mild to the severe; and relief may be afforded differentially by support, warmth (Dixon et al, 1972), or other factors. Although reflected by measures such as consultations with general practitioners and certified incapacity for work, these sources are almost certainly not exhaustive because it is unlikely that all people with acute back pain seek medical advice. Problems in interpretation arise partly because of overlap between this category and more transient experiences when pursuing anamnestic enquiries, recall of durations being notoriously variable. However, a more particular difficulty stems from the fact that most research reports emanate from hospital-based doctors, and the selectivity of referral for specialist help will not be the same across the wide spectrum of back pain. Thus until clinical nosography has provided us with greater discriminatory power between different syndromes, and the criteria by which these may be identified have been applied rigorously, considerable caution is needed in determining how applicable the findings in one study may be in another context.

3. Chronic back pain is the minority class, including all those who suffer for periods in excess of a few weeks. Although the critical distinction between acute and chronic is largely a function of duration, there are other important differences in the nature of the difficulties encountered by this group. Of particular note are the influence on everyday life (Wood & Badley, 1980) and the tendency to be neglected because less people are affected by chronic back pain. Unfortunately what is perhaps the key question — whether chronic backs are such from the beginning or whether they progress from unfavourable response to an acute back — is difficult to answer because of the uncertain applicability of many clinical and research findings. Differentiation between acute and chronic backs is also complicated by uncertainty about the significance of episodic or recurrent complaints, particularly in aetiological terms.

Characteristics

In patients with back pain attending a referral clinic in a hospital for the first time it was not possible to identify information available to the clinician that had useful predictive value in regard to outcome (Currey et al, 1979), apart from a tendency for those who came to radiculography to have shorter histories and for those who became chronic attenders to have longer ones. However, when lifetime experience in the population was considered, where the cumulated incidence of lumbago, sciatica, and intermittent claudication of the cauda equina was 56, 24, and 6% respectively (Hasue & Fujiwara, 1979), the situation was a little more positive. The X-ray findings still had relatively little discriminatory value, and abnormalities revealed by contrast radiography were not necessarily associated with a poor prognosis. What did emerge was that a poor outlook was related more to the frequency of attacks than their duration, although in one group the recurrence rate was as high as 50%.

Experience in general practice is not dissimilar, the unfavourable omens being more than three previous episodes, gradual onset of symptoms, referral of pain distal to the femur, and delays in reporting complaints exceeding a month (Pedersen, 1981). These features appear to be relied upon quite frequently in primary care assessments (Hull, 1982), though how reliably the appraisals are carried out and then interpreted is another matter (Waddell et al, 1982).

Whilst the origin of most non-specific back pain remains uncertain, it is obviously possible that inflammatory processes such as those associated with AS may make some contribution to the overall burden. This contingency has been explored by Calin and his colleagues (1980), but unfortunately the results cannot be taken at face value. The approach started from a premise that now has to be discounted, as we shall note when discussing genotype later on. More important, though, is that very basic problems with sampling have been neglected by this group, especially in regard to the question 'Who got away?' (Wood, 1982a). There is always a hazard of preferential response by individuals with certain characteristics, of which latent AS could be an example in this instance, and results can then be seriously distorted if overall response rates are low.

A syndrome that appears to have attracted relatively little attention is the association of dull backache with skin hyperaesthesia, a tender spot, and limitation of spinal movement (Glover, 1960). Various other phenomena have been investigated for their association with back pain. These have included electromyographic recordings (Jayasinghe et al, 1978; Sweetman et al, 1980), muscle strength (Karvonen et al, 1980), capillary resistance (Sweetman & Anderson, 1975), nerve entrapment (Kirkaldy-Willis & Hill, 1979), pregnancy (Mantle et al, 1977), and how various biomechanical properties, already referred to, may influence clinical decision-making (Pope et al, 1979). The principal influence of comorbidity, such as chronic bronchitis, appears to be on symptom exacerbation with coughing rather than on developing back pain in the first place.

We shall discuss psychological factors shortly but, whatever part they may play, the affected individual is commonly regarded as being able to make personal contributions to recovery. Self-care initiatives depend on knowledge and understanding, so that patient education is important (Kvien et al, 1981); this is an important feature in 'back schools'. It is sometimes asserted that acute back complaints are more disabling than chronic problems (Hasue & Fujiwara, 1979) but we have tried to display the limitations in such a view (Wood & Badley, 1980). Certainly it is chronic backache that is often an important cause of premature retirement (Damlund et al, 1982) and of problematic medical assessments for purposes such as workmen's compensation (Lehmann & Brand, 1982). Hadler (1978) has exposed three moot issues that underlie the latter, and concludes that the law requires an inference of causality that is generally beyond medical determination. In regard to sickness absence, the longer the incapacity for work related to back complaints the less is the likelihood of a return to gainful employment (McGill, 1968).

Individual attributes

In his comprehensive review Andersson (1981) comments that data on individual factors are even more confusing to interpret than are those on occupational influences. Symptom experience seems to be similar in the two sexes, despite reports that disc prolapse appears to be observed more frequently in men. We have come to regard this field as one where male chauvinism is rather evident although Kelsey & Ostfield (1975) have offered a more charitable explanation, that women may be willing to wait for improvement from conservative therapy while men are more anxious to return to work quickly.

Relationships to age may require clarification. Figure 3.3 depicted the crude pattern observed in consultations with general practitioners, which reflects the maximal burden of complaints in the middle years of life. When this is translated into lifetime experience, symptoms are usually first experienced in the earlier part of adulthood. Surgical treatment is most commonly undertaken for those between the ages of 35 and 45 years, but durations of incapacity for work tend to increase progressively with age.

Although some studies have suggested that the risk of developing back pain is increased in those who are tall and those who are heavy (Hrubec & Nashold, 1975), no consistent relationship with anthropometric characteristics is evident in the bulk of reported work. Body disposition is influenced not only by structural abnormalities, already considered, but also by habitual postures. Standing height shows circadian fluctuations (Wood & Badley, 1983a), but longer term trends in the loss of height with age could bear some relationship to back pain. Such shrinkage is commonly attributed to reduction in intervertebral disc spaces, but the erectness required of long-serving military personnel is associated with less height loss (Lipscomb & Parnell, 1954) and whether such veterans experience less back pain does not seem to have been studied.

Physical fitness is related to activity and occupation, which we shall discuss shortly. However, one aspect that is more appropriately considered at this juncture is back mobility, which has been studied quite extensively and in different contexts. The latter have included development during adolescence (van Adrichem & van der Korst, 1973; Moran et al, 1979), cadaveric specimens (Hilton et al, 1979; Taylor & Twomey, 1980), screening for AS (Macrae & Wright, 1969; Moll & Wright, 1971; Hart el al, 1974), and more generally in regard to back pain (Loebl, 1967; Troup et al, 1968; Sweetman et al, 1974; Anderson & Sweetman, 1975; Kiernan, 1981; Lankhorst et al, 1982). There is little to suggest that spinal mobility has aetiological significance.

Crown (1978) has carried out a helpful systematic review of psychological aspects of back pain. There is some indication that significant life events in the preceding three months are experienced more frequently by those destined to develop backache than by those who do not (Rose, 1975), and the complaint is encountered with greater frequency in those with broken marriages (Westrin et al, 1972). It has been suggested that so-called 'non-organic' physical signs may be useful as a simple clinical screen to identify patients requiring more detailed psychological assessment (Waddell et al, 1980). Certainly psychological variables appear to influence the 'reliability' of proffered information (Westrin, 1974).

An interrelationship between spinal mobility and ability to cope with pain has been demonstrated, and this seems to influence recovery of normal motion (Pope et al, 1980). People suffering from backache are more likely to manifest features of anxiety (Gilchrist, 1976; Frymoyer et al, 1980). Earlier work was much concerned with low back pain as a possible expression of an underlying depressive state, loss of libido and appetite being useful discriminators for this condition (Forrest & Wolkind, 1974). The origins of such depression are uncertain, especially in regard to poor response to treatment, although Stevenson (1970) has argued that it may be a primary result of back injury rather than a reaction to treatment failure.

External influences

Data on incapacity for work show an increase in sickness absence from back troubles over time, but this is more likely to reflect secular changes in society rather than indicating a real increase in the occurrence of these complaints. Geographical comparisons have been few, and they are difficult to interpret because cultural influences on the expression of discomfort tend to vary pari passu. However, it is interesting that, as industrialisation increases in Africa, back pain appears to emerge as a problem on the same scale as in Western Europe and North America.

The topic investigated most abundantly has been the relationship between back pain and bodily activity, especially as determined at the workplace. Certainly there is much in the characteristics of occurrence of backache to suggest that mechanical factors are important. However, the mediation of such influences, and even their magnitude, remain to be elucidated. Many simplistic explanations have been offered, but most founder on neglected inconsistencies in the data.

The prima facie case rests on the generally greater frequency of back pain in blue as opposed to white collar workers (Hult, 1954b; Svensson, 1982) and the very striking differences in absences from work due to back disorders in heavy and light industry, the ratio between the two being 5 : 1 (Troup, 1968). However, similar sources yield data that are not easy to reconcile with a simple mechanical load hypothesis, such as the anomalous duration of intervertebral disc morbidity in insurance and banking (Wood & McLeish, 1974). Another example is that, although nurses claim their backache is precipitated by activities at work, the overall prevalence of the complaint is similar in teachers who customarily do not lift heavy people in bed (Cust et al, 1972). Only a part of the discrepancies is likely to be related to the fact that the severity of back pain tends to be greater when mechanical loading of the spine is increased.

Mechanical forces cannot be regarded as a uniform stress because the conditions of loading may vary. Two major types of situation have to be considered, but within these are also important subvarieties. Dynamic loading is the more obvious condition. A physiological example is afforded by pregnancy, multiparity being encountered more frequently among women with back pain than in those without (Frymoyer et al, 1980). The more common image is heavy physical work, and especially if this involves lifting — which itself tends to be associated with twisting and bending. This is the foundation for campaigns of instruction in manual handling and lifting, although satisfactory evidence on the protective effect of such educational initiatives is not available (Glover, 1971). More generally, physical work characterised by high energy demand is not consistently associated with back troubles.

We have already noted not only a relationship between dynamic loading and DD, but also how injury may play a part. The whole notion of injury to the back tends to be ill-defined, and inevitably it is also coloured by possibilities of fault and compensation. Slipping appears to be much more important than tripping as a cause of lumbosacral injury (Manning & Shannon, 1981), and falls are associated with longer absences from work and higher rates of recurrence of back pain (Troup et al, 1981). However, the importance of what can perhaps be regarded as cultural factors is highlighted by the influence of repetitive work. There is a greater frequency of backache among assembly-line workers than in their colleagues employed in offices at the same plant (Bergquist-Ullman & Larsson, 1977), although this only mirrors increases in sickness absence in general under such circumstances of work.

The other major class of condition is static loading, and this is influenced by posture. Backache appears to occur with increased frequency in those with sedentary occupations and in people in whom postures at work involve bending over. Prolonged sitting may be compounded by vibration, such as in vehicle driving (Kelsey & Hardy, 1975; Auquier et al, 1981; Buckle et al, 1980), but as with so much else the findings are not wholly consistent. Whereas insufficient physical exercise may increase the risk of developing back troubles so, too, does the other extreme in certain sporting activities (Kelsey, 1975; Billings et al, 1977).

A synthesis

How is one to seek enlightenment from this welter of information? A recurring theme is the notion that back pain is an epiphenomenon of cultural evolution of the human species. However, there is no agreement on what characteristic of this process might be implicated. It is likely that the complaint represents the resultant of a complex interplay of factors, such as has been reviewed by Wood (1980).

Within the heterogeneity of problems one can suggest at least two broad types of origin for common back pains, based on different patterns of occurrence with age (Wood & Badley, 1980). Some individuals are affected in early maturity; their complaints may often be labelled as the 'disc syndrome', and it is in these people that the search for precipitating circumstances, especially mechanical factors, may well be most profitable. The other type of back pain tends to become progressively more of a problem with increasing age, and is often rather loosely designated as being degenerative. It is difficult to assess the importance of these considerations until better delineation of syndromes is possible.

SOFT-TISSUE SYNDROMES

Dixon (1979) has described soft-tissue rheumatism as 'the great outback of rheumatology, a vast frontier land, ill-defined and little explored, its features poorly categorised and far from internationally agreed.' It is therefore scarcely surprising that we have only meagre fare to offer. In what follows we shall consider a generalised form of soft-tissue rheumatism, polymyalgia rheumatica, various occupational disorders, and sundry other non-articular problems.

Polymyalgia rheumatica

Being a disorder predominantly affecting older people, frequency estimates are especially vulnerable to the age structure of the population being considered; this applies particularly to what may be encountered in clinical series, and to most claims about how often polymyalgia is encountered in relation to other rheumatic diseases. Two other difficulties are that diagnostic criteria have only recently been submitted to rigorous testing (Bird et al, 1979) and that the relationship to temporal arteritis, close though this is, has nevertheless not been adequately quantified.

The best population estimate relates to temporal arteritis and indicates a prevalence of 0.04% (0.0004), with an incidence of 0.003% (0.00003) per annum (Hauser et al, 1971). The prevalence is markedly influenced by age, being 0.03% in the 60s age-group and rising to 0.8% in the over 80s. Hamrin's (1972) study of polymyalgia rheumatica (PMR) was not as large but suggested an incidence of a similar order of magnitude, 0.008% per annum. The condition is probably under-recorded, so that realistic estimates may well be somewhat higher. Ostberg (1973) has suggested that temporal arteritis occurs with a frequency of 0.012% per year, and Rhodes (1976) reported an annual incidence of 0.05% in a general practice.

Age-specific incidence rates are some three times higher in women which, because of the greater longevity of this sex, leads to an even more marked female preponderance in clinical practice. PMR is rare before the age of 50 years although it has been reported under 30 (Mowat & Hazleman, 1974). Familial aggregation has been described (Liang et al, 1974) but its interpretation remains open; some mother-daughter pairs have become affected within a year of each other and conjugal affection has been reported (Kvernebo & Brath, 1980; Nielsen, 1980), which might favour a common extraneous precipitant, but other relatives have developed PMR in the absence of evidence of space–time interaction. There have been conflicting reports of associations with HLA antigens, and a recent study (Malmvall et al, 1980) failed to find any consistent relationship with antigens at the A, B, and C loci.

Although described almost 100 years ago, PMR was not really thrust before people's notice until a number of papers were published in the early 1950s. In the absence of any durable morbid anatomical features, this means there can be no satisfactory evidence on whether the condition has changed over time. The geography of the disorder is indicated only indirectly by the origin of published papers, predominantly from Scandinavia, the UK, and northern cities in the USA, particularly when account is taken of the fact that life expectancy is less in most other parts of the world. In particular PMR has been reported in American blacks (Sanford & Berney, 1977), although the impression persists that the condition is rare in British immigrants originating from the Indian subcontinent.

Mowat (1979) has suggested that there may well be several different mechanisms responsible for a largely similar pattern of pain. An association with a prodromal illness resembling influenza or viral pneumonia has been noted (Mowat & Hazleman, 1974) but this appears to be coincidental as viral studies have been negative and bacterial causes, including chronic brucellosis, have been excluded (Bacon et al, 1975). A suggestion that sufferers were more likely to keep pet birds has now been discounted from aetiological consideration (White & Innes, 1972), but uncertainty about the role of previous exposure to hepatitis B persists (Bacon et al, 1975). No other external influences have been significantly implicated, although seasonality has been suggested.

The biggest hazard of both PMR and temporal arteritis is blindness, though the risk has not been adequately quantified. Life-table analysis does not show any reduction in survivorship (Hauser et al, 1971), and the occurrence of malignant disease resembles that in the general population (von Knorring & Somer, 1974).

Occupational disorders

These conditions have remained largely within the province of practitioners of occupational medicine, and rheumatologists have tended to ignore the problems. The same is generally true of musculoskeletal problems encountered in athletics and other forms of recreation.

The scope of occupational influences has been reviewed by Anderson (1971) and more recently by Lawrence (1977). Occupation plays a necessary part in certain industrial diseases affecting the musculoskeletal system, including Caplan's syndrome, aseptic necrosis of the femoral head in caisson disease, and what are known, in the context of industrial injury provisions, as prescribed diseases 32 — beat knee, 33 — beat elbow, and 34 — synovitis of the wrist. As we have already noted, the importance of occupation in regard to the occurrence of back pain is less certain. With most other rheumatic disorders one is confronted at most with an apparent increase in risk in certain industries, without being certain whether there is an absolute increase in risk or just that the rate of developing the disorder is accelerated. One may be tempted to introduce the concept of high risk groups, but our earlier remarks on pre-employment medical examinations are relevant in this context.

Lawrence (1977) has reviewed a series of specific

occupations in regard to the occurrence of various rheumatic diseases. Occupational disorders are of interest because, theoretically at least, it should be possible to devise methods of working that could prevent their development. Certainly sufferers are at present in considerable hazard of repeated attacks, as is indicated by recrudescence rates for the prescribed diseases — 12% for beat knee, 7% for beat elbow, and 6% for tenosynovitis of the wrist (Wood & McLeish, 1974).

Four aspects provoke comment (Wood et al, 1979):

1. The hatter's shakes may have faded into the past, as have weaver's bottom and housemaid's knee — if the latter persists today, it is in the housewife herself rather than her unobtainable maid. However, there is still a considerable array of work-induced bursitides, including Covent Garden hummy, Billingsgate or humper's hump, hodman's or dustman's shoulder, miner's elbow, and beat knee (evident in miners and nuns, among others), although changing patterns of work and increased mechanisation may be reducing the occurrence of many of these.
2. With tenosynovitis the old also gives way to the new, so that hopper's gout has been replaced by telegraphist's wrist.
3. Recreation adds to the range, with complaints such as baseball player's finger, the same sport's glass arm, and enthesopathies including golfer's shoulder and tennis elbow.
4. New technology produces its own problems, exemplified by diver's paralysis (caisson disease) and pneumatic-hammer disease (the white finger of Raynaud's phenomenon); however, pneumatic drillers do not appear to be particularly prone to osteoarthrosis (Burke et al, 1977) other than, as already noted, at the elbows.

These colloquialisms instruct by indicating aspects of aetiology. Thus the manner of use or overuse of parts of the body appears to play an important part in the pathogenesis of localised forms of soft-tissue rheumatism. This view encompasses soft-tissue injury, in the form of sprains and strains; the role of pressure in bursitis; and the contribution of repetitive movement to the development of tenosynovitis and perhaps to some enthesopathies and entrapment neuropathies. These aspects are reflected in ages at presentation to primary care, with a fall-off at older ages (Fig. 3.3). On the other hand it would also be of interest to learn why only a proportion of individuals exposed to particular methods of working in fact develop these conditions. Hadler (1977) has argued for development of industrial rheumatology as an investigative discipline to pursue these implications.

Other non-articular rheumatism

Development of the unifying concept of the enthesopathies marks some progress in this area, though the relative recency of the idea has precluded reappraisal of scattered evidence on a variety of clinical conditions. Lawrence's early work (summarised in Lawrence, 1977) reviews the occurrence of pain in various parts of the body. The only more recent population study that has included specific concern with certain forms of soft-tissue rheumatism is that by Allander (1974). Unfortunately age and sex-specific prevalence ratios were quoted only for four quinquennial groups between the ages of 30 and 75 years so that an overall population frequency cannot be derived. Nevertheless the data suggest surprisingly high rates, the unweighted mean prevalence in the groups being 16% for the painful shoulder, which by definition had to include restriction of movement, and 3% for tennis elbow. These findings cannot easily be reconciled with experience from health service utilisation (discussed in the previous chapter), nor even with a population survey by the Swedish National Central Bureau of Statistics and reported by the same author, which showed a prevalence of all forms of soft-tissue rheumatism of 1.6% in men and 3.6% in women (Bjelle et al, 1980).

Of localised problems the painful shoulder certainly ranks after the painful knee in frequency of presentation. Probably the best documented, though still ill-understood, problem is the so-called 'frozen shoulder' or 'adhesive capsulitis'. The peak incidence is between 50 and 70 years (Hazleman, 1972), and the condition is encountered slightly more commonly in women than in men. The left (non-dominant) shoulder is more frequently involved and, although rarely recur-

conditions. Moreover, in looking at the occurrence and distribution of rheumatic disorders in the population a number of both methodological and more theoretical considerations need to be borne in mind. The purpose of this section is to examine some of these issues, offering a necessary expansion of what was said about how disease arises in the previous chapter.

Our purpose, therefore, is two-fold; to alert investigators to considerations that ought to be borne in mind when carrying out and interpreting their studies, and to bring out implications for clinical practice and patient management. The topic has been explored in greater detail elsewhere (Wood & Badley, 1984), concentrating more on strategies for public health initiatives.

Given the complexity of determination of liability to disease from the interaction between susceptibility and exposure, a simplifying framework is necessary to bring the threads together. This has to start from appreciation that individuals of the human species, and their health, are in a dynamic and yet vulnerable state (Dubos, 1965). This ecological perspective indicates that the species is part of an ecosystem in which the balance of nature can be altered. One reflection of this is the manner in which disease experience has changed at different stages of evolution and history.

This broad view is so important in establishing context that it merits exemplification. The major problems for hunter–gatherer man appear to have been trauma and undernutrition. The latter was abated to some degree by improved food production following the neolithic revolution, but the resultant aggregation in villages promoted increased passage of epidemics so that infections became the dominant scourge. Both of these features were enhanced, respectively, by the much later agricultural and industrial revolutions. Following not long after, the sanitary revolution presaged reduction in the toll of infection so that so-called 'degenerative' conditions and mental ill-health emerged to the forefront. At the same time the nature of some infections altered, epitomized by the manner in which exposure to poliovirus became less universal and deferred to later in life so that a different pattern of illness was observed.

Against this background one can see that the sources of influence on health lie both within the individual and externally in the society in which he or she lives. Such influences may be health-promoting or deleterious, though few exhibit direct and immediate one-to-one relationships. A person's liability to illness is determined not only by genetic predisposition and exposure to environmental agents, but also by individual vulnerability. The latter is reflected by behaviour and life style and is the product, on the one hand, of personality and biological characteristics such as age, sex, and race, and on the other of cultural values and social arrangements.

EXTERNAL INFLUENCES

It is important to recognise that ethnicity reflects culture (including religious belief) at least as much as genetic similarity. Custom obviously influences the expression of illness, such as by how pain and distress are regarded (Zborowski, 1969), varying expectations in relation to gender and age, and whether recourse is made to folk remedies or heterodox practitioners (Hewitt & Wood, 1975). These aspects are obviously of relevance to diagnosis and, together with lay systems of belief (Fabrega, 1974; Badley & Wood, 1979; Bury & Wood, 1979), they also have to be taken into account in the approach to management. Their pertinence to aetiology has probably been underestimated, as should have been evident from the discussion of primary control of rheumatic disorders in the previous chapter.

Both social structure and social policy have implications for patient management. These can be detected in expressions such as social mobility, migration, and the availability of resources for health care initiatives. Occupation and social class are relevant to diagnosis and therefore influence items of the history to be elicited from a patient; exposure to hazards provides an obvious example (e.g. leptospirosis may not be considered unless the individual's work is taken into account). This emphasis serves to indicate the role of these experiences in aetiology.

Social class

We have already discussed occupational disorders,

and the strength and nature of the association between a variety of rheumatic phenomena and social status is equally problematical (Wood & McLeish, 1974), particularly when it is recalled that most morbid experience is recorded more commonly in those of lower social class. As with the apparaisal of occupational exposure the difficulty is the lack of a unique hypothesis. Less favourable social situations tend to be associated with a variety of other circumstances, such as a greater likelihood of engaging in manual labour or of working in heavy industry, as well as of living in less desirable housing that itself is often additionally exposed to environmental pollutants.

It is often thought that the notable exception to this gradient is gout, which is presumed to single out the more affluent. In fact the evidence for this is unsatisfactory and the notion is probably as much as anything an expression of past differences in both levels of nutrition and the availability of medical care, only the more wealthy being able to afford overindulgence and consultation with a doctor in order to have an elegant label applied. Experience since the Second World War has noted gout in those of lower social class, as well as higher serum uric acid levels at both extremes of the social class scale (Acheson, 1969). Gout, therefore, has almost come to resemble other so-called 'diseases of affluence', such as ischaemic heart disease, by being more notable for preferential occurrence in the least favoured in societies with material abundance.

Place

The influence of climatic factors is suggested by the extent to which they feature in folk mythology and has been pursued by Lawrence (1969d), but experimental appraisal has proved unrewarding (Hollander & Yeostros, 1963). It seems likely that the principal factor underlying the association between climate and rheumatism is the influence of ambient temperature on pain threshold. Interpretation of comparative studies in different parts of the world (Lawrence, 1968) is complicated by the profusion of variables. Apart from a variety of climatological factors there are differences in other experiences, such as the cyclicity of daylight, ethnicity, socioeconomic status, and predominant patterns of occupation. Perhaps even more fundamental is the variation in life expectancy, to which we shall refer later.

The confounding effects of multiple variables have been compounded by methodological shortcomings and these hampered earlier identification of significant variations in the occurrence of rheumatoid arthritis in different parts of the world (Wood & Benn, 1972). The most conservative interpretation of such data was that they failed to demonstrate any convincing geographical differences. The appearance of uniformity is biologically implausible. Not only are there no known instances of diseases that are distributed equally in all parts of the world but such a situation would defeat the primary aim of research endeavour, which is to seek differences. Even though age-specific inception rates for malignant disease appear to be universal (Brockington, 1975) this impression arises only when all tumours are considered together; the different distributions of cancers at various sites are very striking. This reinforces the suspicion that undetected heterogeneity may be frustrating our attempts to seek further enlightenment on RA.

Notwithstanding these problems, certain interesting and yet isolated differences have been reported. Some of these have not yet been adequately accounted for, such as localisation of the agent of epidemic polyarthritis, the Ross River virus, to parts of Australia. Others appear to depend on a suitable habitat for a vector, such as the black-legged tick that transmits Lyme arthritis or the mosquito indirectly responsible, in parts of Africa, for the polyarthritis associated with chikungunya and o'nyongnyong. Yet others are more likely to be genetic rather than environmental and include examples we have noted earlier.

Time

Crude changes with time have been quite marked, even in fairly recent experience, but they too are difficult to interpret because one cannot examine a unique hypothesis. As reflected by sickness incapacity in the period 1961–1967 (Wood, 1970b) rheumatic disorders have increased in frequency and in duration to a greater extent than have all causes of morbidity taken together. The components contributing most to these changes have

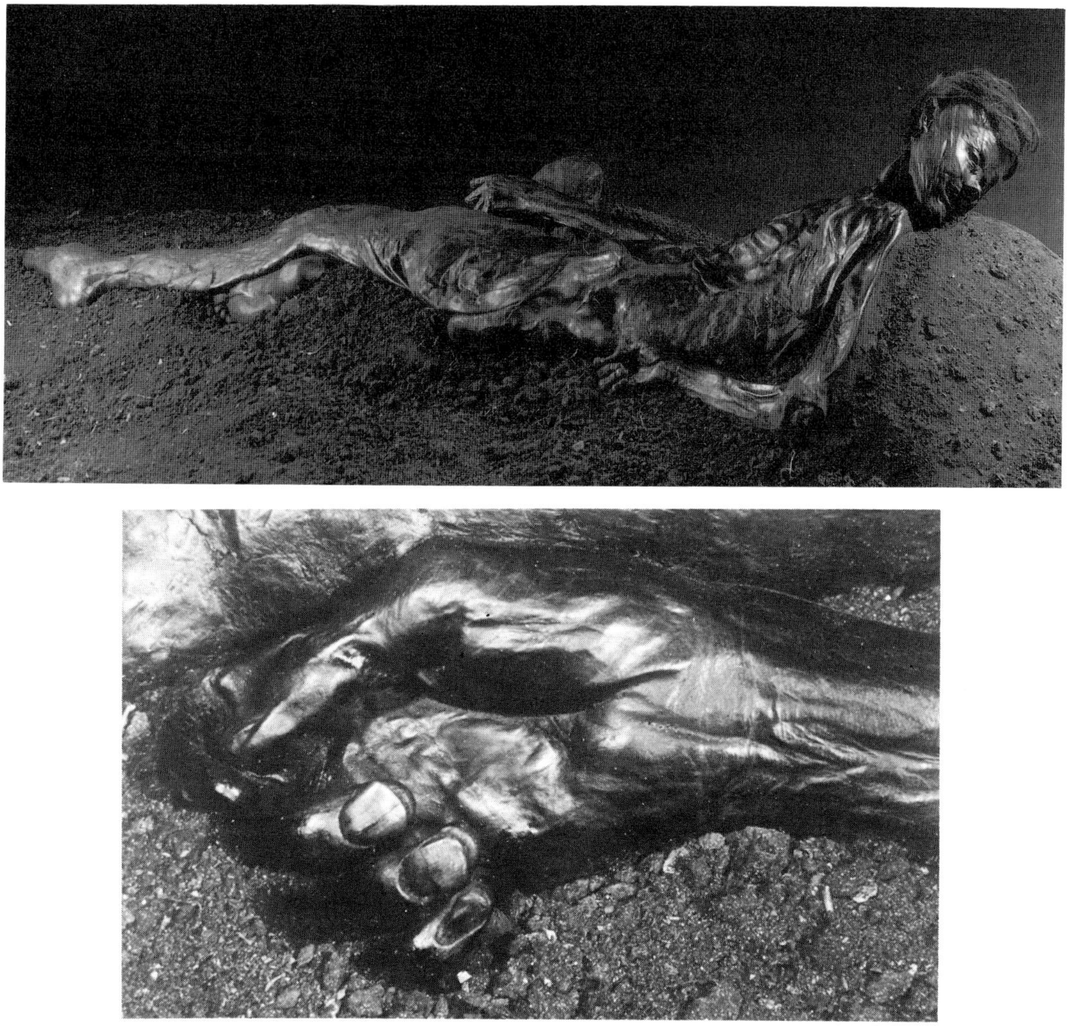

Fig. 3.4 Grauballe man (*c.* AD 400) who, it had been suggested, suffered from rheumatoid arthritis. (Reproduced by kind permission of Forhistorisk Museum, Moesgard, Denmark.)

been arthropathies and back troubles. Among the factors that could be influencing these patterns are changes in certification practices and in social mores in regard to attitudes to work.

Alterations in the occurrence of specific diseases over a longer time span are of interest because, by correlation with changes in cultural experience, it may be possible to uncover aetiological possibilities. Since an earlier paper on whether RA is a recent disease (Wood, 1976b) one of us has had the opportunity to visit Aarhus to examine Grauballe man (Fig. 3.4). He had his throat cut in ritual sacrifice before being cast into a peat bog in Jutland some 1600 years ago. Unfortunately it was not possible to endorse earlier suggestions (Glob, 1965) that his radiographs revealed evidence of RA. The question is left similarly open by the fascinating report on how the frequency of this disease increases in members of the same tribe as they migrate from the bush to urban environments (Solomon et al, 1975). The comparison encapsulates virtually the whole of human cultural evolution, and therefore fails to indicate at what stage in this process disease determinants, so far unknown, might have begun to operate.

More conventional studies of the health of

human populations attempt to display somewhat different lessons. We cannot compete on the scale of McKeown (1976), with his suggestion that tuberculosis has been the main factor influencing population expansion. The only way open for the study of longer term rheumatological time trends is with mortality statistics.

Most rheumatic disorders have been subject to fashions in diagnostic terminology, and they also appear on death certificates only infrequently. These considerations have led us to dismiss the change in sex ratios in standardised death rates from RA between 1881 and 1961, when the ratio of female to male deaths increased from unity to 3 : 1, as being without deep significance.

Changing patterns of disease can be studied more systematically in regard to rheumatic fever (RF). We were reassured that data quality was probably satisfactory on finding that mortality from other streptococcal diseases, such as scarlatina and erysipelas, showed roughly parallel trends over the 80 years studied, and again on finding consistent if delayed relationships between mortality from RF and rheumatic heart disease. We were also encouraged to note the emergence of a male preponderance in RF deaths about the time of the two World Wars, coinciding with the adolescent peak in incident cases to which we have already referred.

INDIVIDUAL CHARACTERISTICS

We have already indicated that it is a misconception to regard behaviour and life style as if they are intrinsic qualities of the individual. The problems arise partly because these attributes can be observed more directly than most of the influences that determine them (culture and social structure as well as personality), but also because of unacknowledged moral and political values that favour individualistic interpretations with their overtones of blame (Wood & Badley, 1984). More recent work has pursued influences outside the individual, such as life events, but the evidence so far is not very abundant.

A fairly extensive literature devoted to personality and other psychological aspects certainly alerts one to potential problems in patient management, especially in regard to rheumatoid arthritis. However, from an aetiological point of view the evidence remains unsatisfactory, and chicken-and-egg problems (whether one is observing no more than the consequences of affliction) have not been entirely overcome. What one may in the past have been justified in dismissing as woolly holism can no longer be so regarded. For example, empirical observations have shown that the psyche can influence immunological phenomena (Rogers et al, 1980). Other means of mediation for psychological influences have also begun to invoke biological mechanisms, and a review by McQueen & Siegrist (1982) sets this work in perspective.

Biological attributes

Whereas personality and genotype are unique to the individual, biological attributes identify features that tend to be more common to the species, or at least to definable subpopulations. We have already discussed various aspects of ethnicity but other characteristics deserve further consideration — both as regards diagnostic possibilities, and in relation to aetiological interpretation.

Age

Although it is unlikely that anyone escapes some form of rheumatic complaint during the course of his or her life, the chances do vary with age. Based on consultations with general practitioners (Wood & Badley, 1983b), approximately 5% of persons between the ages of 16 and 44 years present with a rheumatic disorder compared with 23% of persons between 45 and 64 and 41% of those 65 years and older.

The differences in regard to which type of complaint in the various age-groups most frequently leads to presentations in primary care were shown in Figure 3.3. Summarised briefly there are three contrasting patterns — soft-tissue trauma is notable in younger people, and less common in the elderly; back troubles, non-articular rheumatism, and (for what the observation is worth, as the category is very heterogeneous) other rheumatic disorders are less frequent in young adults but thereafter occur at roughly comparable rates; and the arthropathies show a very steep increase with age, reaching the highest peak in the elderly.

Attempts at interpretation should be related to

human biography, a precept of particular relevance when considering musculoskeletal disorders in the elderly (Wood & Badley, 1983a). In this context it is the characteristics of onset of a condition that are important. Four patterns can be identified:

1. **Reduced frequency with age,** when compared with earlier stages of adult life. Here one might include AS, sprains and strains of joints and adjacent muscles, and lesions of the menisci of the knee joint. Three classes of explanation are of special relevance when considering the tailing off of effects within a distribution. The one that comes most readily to mind is a difference in risk in relation to age; in other words, that older people are less exposed to some particular hazard — the converse of the situation that appears to apply to femoral neck fractures. The second type of explanation is that the susceptible subpopulation has been exhausted, either because all have been exposed at an earlier age or because vulnerability may be restricted to particular stages in the life cycle (circumstances that may be relevant to the occurrence of AS). The third type of explanation, and the one that is commonly neglected, is that survivors to old age are a selected subpopulation. This may operate in two ways. One is that the condition of interest may be strongly associated with some other disease which is itself lethal; this could have applied to the link between rheumatoid arthritis and tuberculosis (Cobb & Hall, 1965; Benn & Wood, 1977). In more general terms, the overall force of mortality experience earlier in life may have selectively removed persons who would otherwise have become susceptible to a particular condition. The other aspect of selection is that mortality associated with a specific disease obviously leads to attrition of those affected. Although most rheumatic disorders are generally regarded as having a low mortality (i.e. the case fatality rate is low), differential attrition could nevertheless distort impressions of relative frequencies at different ages.

2. **Increased frequency with age,** of which the most striking example is arthrosis. Such occurrences appear to conform to the criterion of sustained and progressive increase over a span of many years, but whether these phenomena should be equated with ageing or degeneration is another matter. It is undeniable that an arthrotic joint has degenerated from its formerly normal structure, but to generalize from this observation is tautologous and misleading — strictures that apply equally to cerebrovascular disease and many other supposedly degenerative disorders. The point that is being missed is that the term 'degenerative' suggests a universal process to which the tissues of the whole species are susceptible, whereas the phenomena of concern are non-universal, only a subpopulation being susceptible to such pathological changes at any given site.

3. **Concentration in the elderly.** Conditions such as polymyalgia rheumatica, Paget's disease, and ankylosing hyperostosis do not show a gradient of ages at onset corresponding to what would be anticipated with ageing or degenerative processes. Unfortunately the evidence is too scanty to permit much conjecture, but two comments are worth making. First, conventional possibilities, such as preferential exposure to particular agents, may have relevance to the incidence of fractures in the elderly but are difficult to conceive of in relation to microbial agents — although some old people may be congregated in residential accommodation, the majority are more notable for the solitariness of their existence. Secondly, a threshold concept has utility as a means of providing explanation for why progressive conditions such as osteoporosis tend to manifest themselves abruptly (e.g. vertebral collapse that suddenly impinges on nervous tissue). Progressive deterioration of the tissues may proceed to a qualitatively different state of swift collapse or vulnerability to some insult that formerly they were able to resist (a process perhaps in some way analogous to fatigue fracture in metal).

4. **Lack of age gradient,** conditions appearing to occur with similar frequency in middle and late life. Here one might consider rheumatoid arthritis, gout, and, despite what has been said about presentations to general practitioners, back troubles and various forms of soft-tissue (non-articular) rheumatism. This is the most unsatisfactory pattern from the point of view of seeking generic explanations, and there are a number of reasons for this. First, available data are rarely adequate to allow of certainty that any particular condition should not be assigned to one of the other three

categories of pattern in relation to age. Secondly, some of this uncertainty is coloured by failure to make an important distinction — that between incident cases (i.e. the frequency and characteristics of new onsets of particular disorders) and the case mix or prevalence encountered in everyday practice. The relative frequency of occurrence in the latter context is determined by general biomedical characteristics of the individual conditions, including influences such as the recruitment of incident cases, chronicity, and differential survival of sufferers. Thirdly, given such limitations in the data the influence of other distorting factors becomes potentially more important. For instance, there is evidence that older people make proportionately less use of health services in relation to their medically-defined 'needs', and lesser rates of consultation cannot help but influence ascertainment (this is why we have included backs and non-articular problems in this pattern category). Finally, there is the problem we have highlighted more than once, that of heterogeneity. This difficulty certainly poses a challenge when trying to unravel what may be at the root of back pain, the relative contributions of different causes being obscured as conditions such as osteoporosis and osteomalacia become superimposed on pre-existent spondylotic changes.

Sex and other attributes

Whereas few conditions are confined entirely to one or the other sex, many disorders exhibit differences in the frequency with which men and women are affected. If such is not observed it suggests a ubiquitous hazard for the species, of which many common infections provide examples. Given a difference, age patterns will usually prove to be illuminating.

Consistency in sex differentials over an age range could suggest that a behavioural characteristic may be important. For example, males have a greater likelihood of fracture both as children and in young adulthood, a difference that is commonly attributed to activity patterns. Secular change in such differences is now occurring with lung cancer, as the proportion of women that smoke tobacco has increased.

Perhaps more often the relationship between the patterns in the two sexes differs over the distribution of ages at onset, as may be seen in Figure 3.1. Only two classes of explanation can offered for such findings. One is the problem to which we have made recurring reference, heterogeneity — that the disease called rheumatoid arthritis (see Fig. 3.1) that is observed to develop in older people may in fact be different (i.e. distinct) from that affecting younger people. The other is that different factors may be influencing disease development and expression, factors which operate differently between the sexes when compared with younger groups. The two types of explanation are by no means mutually exclusive, but unfortunately there have been insufficient detailed clinical studies to provide evidence that might indicate which of the two might be more likely to apply. As a result the biological significance of such distributions remains obscured.

In attempting to seek explanations for sex differences two cautions should be borne in mind, both of which we have illustrated elsewhere (Wood & Badley, 1983a). First, excessive importance should not be attached to coincidence such as with phases in the life cycle, especially the menopause; falsification ought to be attempted by examining other possibilities. Secondly, and not unrelated to this, observations need to be set in an overall context. For example, so-called 'postmenopausal osteoporosis' is an inadequate explanation for the linear increase in femur fractures with age in women when men exhibit a parallel pattern, even though in them the rates are only half those observed in females.

Other biological attributes include characteristics such as birth order and family size. The latter may be of relevance to explanations for some experiences in the early part of life. Features such as earlier exposure to infections that may be carried home from school by older sibs (Monto & Ross, 1977) indicate some of the mechanisms that might be considered.

Genotype

In family studies one observes the results not only of individual susceptibility but also of environmental factors that may equally be operating within the family. This offers theoretical grounds for anticipating that a wide range of conditions will aggregate in families, and some of the common infectious fevers provide an example of this. The recognition of familial aggregation is therefore only a preliminary step, and isolated reports of twins or sibs affected with relatively common diseases can be of only limited interest.

The real challenge is to elucidate the nature and cause for aggregation, but this is a far from simple problem — even when markers are available, such as the HLA antigens. Not only are the individual's innate tendencies or susceptibilities likely to be a graded property but so, too, is the combination of external circumstances that makes him or her more or less likely to develop the disease (Wood & Badley, 1984).

Family studies

The resultant of these two influences is called liability (Falconer, 1965), and it is this attribute that is all one is usually able to consider in family studies. Moreover, although liability is a graded phenomenon, in most instances it has to be inferred from discontinuous occurrences because there is a threshold of expression of the presence of disease. Estimates of the heritability of liability can be derived (Falconer, 1965) which give an indication of the maximum extent to which genetic factors could account for the observed occurrence in families. One thus ends up with an estimate of where a given disease falls on the spectrum between nature and nurture, as has been done for a number of rheumatic conditions in Figure 3.5.

The genetic aspect is complicated further. A number of genes may determine whether one is susceptible to developing disease at all — perhaps of the order of three genes being involved in this process (Wood, 1982a). In addition, one's response, if the disease does develop, may be influenced by genetic factors. For instance, there may be familial tendencies affecting the severity of disease as well as the particular form it takes, such as which joints are most severely affected. However, our knowledge on these aspects is small at present although they are likely to contribute to observed aggregation.

Family studies of relatively common multifactorial conditions should be seen in their proper context. They represent observations in a regulated situation — by knowing the degree of relationship genetical similarity is controlled. Any differences from the anticipated degrees of genetical resemblance, therefore, must be due to non-genetic factors. There is some attraction in the idea of studying different degrees of relationship with their different proportions of shared genes. However, data on second as well as first-degree relatives by no means resolve the theoretical difficulties because environments are also usually more similar within families.

The principal clues likely to emerge from family studies will be to environmental rather than to inherited factors, which is the opposite of what so many people have in mind. Moreover, although this is not the place to deal with methodological problems, such as the representativeness of index cases selected for study, these aspects are very important because they can bias the results.

Immunogenetics

Medical journals are being assailed by reports of associations between immunogenetic markers and different diseases at what seems to be an ever-increasing rate. What is equally confusing, discussion of possible explanations for these observations continues unabashed even in the face of unresolved discrepancies in data. The ideas that have been stimulated by these findings are of great interest and their potential significance is considerable. However, the problems attendant on inconsistencies in the evidence must be examined seriously, even at the price of occasional repetition. The reader is referred to Dawkins (1982) for an up-to-date review of the field, which leaves us free to examine some of the neglected difficulties in hermeneutics or interpretation.

At the outset we must acknowledge the importance of purely technical factors, i.e. those influencing the reliability of test results. Account has to be taken not only of laboratory methods, but also of features such as bias introduced by the study of groups too small to embrace the range of variation; reported frequencies of HLA antigens in 'normal' people have often been vulnerable in this regard (Wood, 1982a). Of perhaps greater concern to us, though, are more profound problems related to validity.

The basic observations are of associations, such as the very strong link between B27 and AS. It should be well recognised that statistical relation-

Nature (genetic factors)										(environmental factors) Nurture
1. Diseases										
Marfan's syndrome										
Ehlers-Danlos syndrome	Congenital dislocation of hip	Ankylosing spondylitis	Psoriasis	Rheumatoid arthritis	Lupus erythematosus	Rheumatic fever	Osteoarthrosis of hip	Osteoarthrosis of other joints	(Back pain)	Septic arthritis
Hurler's syndrome		Gout	(Chondrocalci-nosis)			Serum sickness			(Entheso-pathies)	(Occupational synovitis of wrist)
2. Associated attributes										
		Sacroiliitis					Serum uric acid levels	Rheumatoid factor		

Fig. 3.5 Spectrum of various rheumatic disorders showing the approximate relative contributions of genetic and environmental factors. The scale of magnitude of inherited factors corresponds to estimates for the heritability of liability, the maximum extent to which genetic factors could account for the observed occurrence of disease in families. The figure is based on assessments of all available data, which were often poor, rather than on precise numerical estimates; conditions shown in parentheses are only guesstimates.

ships cannot of themselves logically imply causation; there are many celebrated examples of such fallacies. Ideas on causality have to be measured against the nine criteria identified in the previous chapter (Hill, 1965).

Measures of association. The strength and consistency of the association satisfy only the first two criteria. As regards the third, specificity, the evidence is not entirely satisfactory. Although most series have reported links that fall short of 100% association, some question remains about whether B27-negative AS actually exists — partly because interlaboratory comparisons have sometimes led to reassignment of antigen status, and false negatives seem more likely to be encountered than false positives. There is also evidence (reviewed by Woodrow, 1980) that B27-negative spondylitics may have a genetic predisposition to undeclared psoriatic or enteropathic arthropathy.

Four independent criteria. The fourth criterion, temporality (in Bradford Hill's delightful phrase, 'Which is the cart and which the horse?') might appear to be inapplicable because it is predetermined — i.e. a genetically programmed attribute must antedate later developments. However, more confirmatory prospective observations on disease experience in those of established antigen status would afford reassurance. Biological gradient, the fifth criterion, would in this instance be represented by findings in those homozygous at the relevant loci, on which the evidence is scant. The sixth, experimental, criterion is not easy to conceive of being satisfied without draconian intervention, such as by selective elimination of gametes carrying the responsible haplotype. On the other hand the seventh criterion, coherence, offers little difficulty because causal interpretations present no serious conflict with generally known biological facts.

Plausibility and analogy. It may seem a little contrived to examine with such care a phenomenon that most people take for granted. However, speculation has been rife, particularly in the area to which the last two criteria relate, and disciplined scrutiny does offer cautionary tales. There is a fairly widespread assumption that the presence of particular HL antigens has immunological significance in regard to disease pathogenesis. As the previous edition of this book went to press the preferred view was of linkage with postulated immune response genes that predispose to the development of specific diseases (Bodmer, 1975), certainly a mechanism that was biologically plausible. This idea was encouraged by analogy with the mouse, in which species histocompatibility genes appeared to be linked to those governing immune responses. However, at that time one of us stressed the limitations of analogy because other explanations could apply instead (Wood, 1978) and this seems to have come about, genetic influences now being thought to be mediated by the histocompatibility genes themselves (Adams, 1982).

The problems arise partly from invocation of unsubstantiated (and largely unsubstantiatable) explanatory concepts to account for discrepancies between data and a hypothetical model, an indulgence to which genetics seems to be especially prone. The relevant instance is the notion of linkage disequilibrium, an undoubted occurrence but scarcely to be bandied around so lightly. A more renowned example is the concept of incomplete penetrance which, as noted in the previous edition of this book (Wood, 1978), some medical geneticists once resorted to when they regarded the relatively infrequent development of AS in individuals with B27 as the lowest penetrance rate on record.

The reality is that such ideas can be little more than an attempt at post hoc rationalisation, an elegant obfuscation of the fact that observed data don't correspond to a pet hypothesis. The inescapable deduction has to be that the hypothesis is likely to be in error. In regard to incomplete penetrance the need to seek such exemption arises only from excessive devotion to the idea of unifactorial determination, and the Mendelian character of B27 was under threat only as long as its presence was erroneously interpreted as being a disease indicator rather than a marker for susceptibility.

Phenotypic expression of susceptibility certainly appears to be variable, but the likeliest explanation for this may well be a more complex inherited basis. How, for instance, is one to account for ethnic differences? The lower overall frequency of AS in American blacks has been estimated to correspond with the degree of their contamination with Caucasian genes. However, this cannot account for the observation that B27 appears to be less common in those blacks who do develop spondylarthropathy (Khan et al, 1976).

Equally problematical is that the marked male preponderance in AS can scarcely be accounted for by genes that are not sex-linked. This could indicate that susceptibility must have other determinants that have yet to be discovered. Alternatively B27 may indicate susceptibility to sacroiliitis rather than to clinically manifest AS; the radiographic changes tend to occur with a similar frequency in the two sexes, and perhaps clinical expression of a problem is the result of other influences that do differ between the sexes. The suggestion that AS can be detected in B27-positive individuals with a much greater frequency than had formerly been acknowledged (Cohen et al, 1976) and that this applied to women as much as men (Calin & Fries, 1975) should be largely discounted on the basis of unsatisfactory sampling procedures and variability in the interpretation of radiographs (Hollingsworth et al, 1983).

All that has been said so far relates to B27 in the context of AS. The situation is different when one turns to B27 in relation to other disorders; as we discussed in the section on spondylarthropathies associated with inflammatory bowel disease, psoriasis, and Reiter's disease, the contexts are different. Designation of 'B27-positive rheumatic disease' (Metzger et al, 1974) as if this were a homogeneous entity is confusing because it is analogous to the idea of cigarette-smoking disease; the concept may be valuable for some purposes but for serious nosology the confounding of lung cancer, chronic bronchitis, and ischaemic heart disease is unlikely to be helpful.

Clinical implications

The information available on the familial occurrence of the commoner rheumatic disorders, even when augmented by immunogenetic markers, is generally inadequate to serve as the basis for very positive action — other than to the extent that some markers appear to indicate idiosyncratic susceptibility to the actions of certain drugs (e.g. penicillamine — see reviews in Dawkins et al, 1982). How, then, should this generally imperfect knowledge influence clinical decisions? This topic is best considered under three headings:

1. **Diagnosis.** Recall of positive family histories tends to be greater by individuals who are similarly affected. Ascertainment is therefore a less serious problem than it might have been. However, the important question is the degree to which a positive family history influences the probability of a given diagnosis. An oversimplified example is provided by a patient with arthritis in whom one is considering the alternative diagnoses of rheumatoid arthritis (RA) and osteoarthrosis. To what extent does a positive family history for RA, for instance, help one to make this choice? The answer is dependent on the proportions of all arthritics who have RA, of patients with RA who give a positive family history, and of positive family histories given by arthritics without RA. When these relative frequencies are considered one realises that a family history can contribute very little to diagnosis, particularly when compared with the discriminatory value of other clinical information. There are, of course, certain important exceptions to this generality. The rare conditions that are probably due to single gene defects constitute a special case. Of the commoner rheumatic disorders, a family history of gout is important in awakening one to the possibility of this diagnosis. Somewhat similar is the record of sacroiliitis in the parents or sibs of a possible spondylitic. Despite the eclat and euphoria with which the HLA antigens have been received, their diagnostic value appears to be limited.

2. **Management.** The greatest clinical value of a positive family history for a rheumatic disease is in arousing one to the need for anticipation. The individual is likely to want to ask, 'Am I going to get like my mother?' This question in fact relates more to familial patterns of disease severity, about which less is known. However, recalling improvements in, and the increased availability of, treatment facilities during the period between the generations, one is usually justified in giving an encouraging and optimistic reply to the question. A more general point is that genetic aetiologies should be seen in perspective. We must learn more about inherited factors because they add to our knowledge of disease, and ultimately they may help us to identify susceptible subpopulations in whom some special preventive effort could be worthwhile. However, recognition that nature

plays a large part should not lead to pessimism. Even though with some conditions the environmental component is very small it may still be amenable to intervention — such as by withholding milk from the galactosaemic.

3. Counselling. There remains the more general problem of the risks of developing a rheumatic disease, given that a member of the individual's family is affected, and of the issue to be anticipated from union with a person similarly situated. The answer is fairly simple. The proportion of close relatives developing one of these diseases, given a case in the family, remains relatively small. Thus there are no grounds for attempting to deter prospective marriage partners. As far as the worried individual trying to anticipate his or her chances for the future is concerned, once again optimistic reassurance is justified — with the rider that the means of ameliorating rheumatic problems are improving all the time even if something did develop.

Procreation

It is also important not to lose sight of non-genetic aspects of procreation. There has been a suggestion that fertility may be reduced in women with RA (Kay & Bach, 1965), although a more recent study failed to find a deficit in children born but did detect some evidence of delay in conception (Al Azzawi & Wood, 1985). A quandary also arises over the unquantified possibility of a postpregnancy exacerbation. More important, though, is parental incapacity and the question of how a severe rheumatoid will cope with parenthood.

To be consulted about the wisdom of a known arthritic having another child gives rise to a dilemma. The response must be tempered by the individual situation but there is no simple answer. All one can do is to outline the possible consequences of the alternative courses and leave the individual couple to make their choice. The dilemma is in fact more serious and more general. Present knowledge does not allow us to exonerate antirheumatic medicaments from having teratogenic potential (Kay, 1982), and there is also concern that certain delayed-action drugs could be oncogenic for offspring; consumption of these products may be as important in the intending father as in the mother. Not only do rheumatologists appear to lack any consistent policy for the use of drugs in pregnancy but, if these potential hazards prove to be real, anticipatory modification of therapeutic regimens would be necessary in advance of conception. It is to be hoped that this problem will soon be studied further.

TYPES OF ENQUIRY

In the preceding sections readers will have been able to identify a variety of different techniques that have been used to shed light on the epidemiology of rheumatic disorders. As a contribution to promoting initiatives that might remedy the many deficiencies in the evidence, it may be helpful if we conclude with a brief review of approaches that may be followed.

One framework for considering the types of approach has been put forward by Morris (1975), and is shown in Table 3.6. Many of these approaches have perhaps not been exploited very fully. However, in trying to illustrate what may be expected of epidemiology it is wise to start with a caution. As Morris has indicated, and as applies with any discipline or technique, epidemiology may be a useful way of approaching many problems; it can also be the only way of seeking answers to some biomedical questions, but it is no way at all to answer many others. Expectations should therefore be realistic.

CLASSICAL APPROACHES

It should be clear that much of the work that has been described in both this and the previous

Table 3.6 Epidemiological approaches (after Morris, 1975).

Classical	
— Community diagnosis	— the health of the community
— History	— changing patterns of disease
— Aetiology	— seeking causes of health and disease
Recent	
— Syndromes	— identifying associations
— Natural history	— completing the clinical picture
— Risk factors	— estimating chances of disease
— Treatment	— effectiveness
	— controlled trials,
	— benefit *vs* risk, etc.
	— efficiency — working of health services

chapter falls into the class of community diagnosis, and no attempt will be made to say more about this. Of Morris's second approach, the historical perspective, we have already said enough when discussing time as an external influence on disease determination. However, this is perhaps an appropriate juncture to offer a summary of major points in our review, by bringing together the frequency estimates discussed under each individual rheumatic disorder into a single table (Table 3.7).

One general point is worth emphasising. Perhaps one of the major achievements of rheumatological epidemiology has been to pinpoint more accurately the nature of the burden of rheumatic suffering. Investigative effort in rheumatology needs to take account of the considerable morbidity burden from back pain and non-articular rheumatism, as well as of the problems with joint disease, and, within the latter, of arthrosis as least as much as of the inflammatory polyarthropathies. There are also important implications for what needs to be taught to students and doctors, and for the nature of specialist activities. As far as the health of the community as a whole is concerned, a rheumatologist who sees his or her function almost exclusively as an arthritologist is likely to be of limited value.

Aetiology

With many diseases, such as cancer, it is possible

Table 3.7 Summary of reported prevalence estimates for the various rheumatic disorders in Great Britain.

Disorder	Prevalence* (%)	
Inflammatory arthropathies	>2.2	
Rheumatoid arthritis	1.0	
Juvenile chronic arthritis	0.02	(0.06 in children < 15 yr)
Ankylosing spondylitis	0.15	
Enteropathic arthropathy	0.002	
Reiter's disease	0.001	
Psoriatic arthropathy	0.1	
Gout	<0.3	
Chondrocalcinosis	0.6	(on radiographic evidence)
Septic arthritis	—	(no satisfactory estimate)
Behçet's disease	<0.001	
Connective tissue diseases	>0.05	
Systemic lupus erythmatosus	0.04	
Systemic sclerosis	(0.004)	
Polymyositis and dermatomyositis	(0.003)	
Sjogren's disease	—	(no satisfactory estimate)
Polyarteritis nodosa	(0.006)	
Arthrosis and dorsopathies	?	(estimates for components not exclusive)
Peripheral joints	11.0	(on radiographic evidence)
Spondylosis	45.0	(on radiographic evidence)
Other back troubles	?	(lifetime incidence 60%)
Soft-tissue syndromes	?	(no satisfactory overall estimate)
Polymyalgia rheumatica	>0.04	
Occupational disorders	?	
Other nonarticular rheumatism	(2.5)	
Other rheumatic disorders	?	(no satisfactory overall estimate)
Inherited conditions	?	
Rheumatic fever	?	
Bone disorders (of rheumatological concern)	(>3.0)	
Dupuytren's contracture	(2.0)	
	contracture	

* In the adult population; the main value of the figures is to indicate relative frequencies of occurrence, as the precision of the estimates varies — less confidence can be placed in the accuracy of figures shown in parentheses.

to pursue various aetiological enquiries using routinely available data. This is largely a function of specificity in identification and completeness of ascertainment by these means. In sad contrast, the nosological characteristics of most rheumatic disorders relate to a cluster concept as a hallmark is lacking. The result is variability in ascertainment in research enquiries. This tends to vitiate comparisons, thus curtailing interpretation of the findings in family and twin studies (Wood, 1971a) as well as of population frequency estimates.

Despite these problems the undertaking of a survey is a fairly obvious way to study aetiology if other data are not available. Such was the case in the late forties, when Lawrence began his pioneer work; his prodigious activity has been summarised in a monograph (Lawrence, 1977). Seeking aetiological factors, Lawrence compared urban and rural environments, the influence of various occupations, exposure to fluoride in drinking water, and variation in prevalence in different parts of the world.

Disciplined enquiry is concerned with elucidating occurrences by determining their relation to other phenomena. The potential for any study to yield useful results is generally founded on the precision with which a hypothesis can be formulated, which itself is a synthesis of previous knowledge and imaginative speculation. Unfortunately, though, a community survey can not only appear to contrast unfavourably with a laboratory study, because of the scale of investment of human resources that the former will require, but it also has a greater likelihood of dashing wishful hopes, by exposing speculation that has too far outstripped what has been established. This arises not because of any inherent negative quality in epidemiology, but rather because such enquiries span additional dimensions in which postulated relationships may be observed not to hold — the dimensions being indicated in the quote from Lilienfeld at the beginning of this chapter.

Obviously the greater likelihood of negative findings can function as a disincentive to undertaking epidemiological studies. All is unlikely to be lost in the laboratory; the bench can usually accommodate more than one experiment at once, and each of these tends to require only fairly circumscribed commitments in time. A community study, on the other hand, usually demands the concentrated efforts of a team over quite lengthy periods, with trespass on unsociable hours as well if many respondents are to be reached. Personal impatience can then be reinforced by limited vision on the part of funding agencies, encouraging more economical approaches such as by use of a case–control design. Whilst not wishing to cast the latter in an unfavourable light, we would stress that such designs represent a very different 'experimental' situation because their purpose is different — economy results from the asking of a sharply focused question, but a corollary of this very restriction is that one is denied the opportunity of triangulation such as may be had when validity in the other dimensions to which we have referred can be examined at the same time.

By its very nature the community survey offers considerable potential to falsify poorly secured hunches. This is because clinical insights are put in a very different context. For example, although it is now assimilated as if it had never been regarded otherwise, it was epidemiological enquiry that revealed the non-specificity of cardinal features such as rheumatoid factor (Table 3.8). From Lawrence's work one was forced to conclude that atmospheric pollution probably played as large a part in determining the occurrence of positive tests as did the underlying presence of rheumatoid arthritis.

We have already mentioned the perplexing and often disappointing results from studies of the geography of rheumatic disorders. Earlier impressions that these conditions were uncommon in the tropics are likely to have been due to the

Table 3.8 Setting a diagnostic feature in context — the quantitative implications of specificity.

Rheumatoid factor is present in — 75% of patients with rheumatoid arthritis — 5% of 'normals' (hospital patients without RA)		
If these rates are applied to a sample of 1000 people from the general population:		
— 2% may have RA* =	20 people, 75% RF+ve =	15
— 98% do not have RA =	980 people, 5% RF+ve =	49
— Total with rheumatoid factor (RF)		64

* For purposes of illustration only, the prevalence of RA has been indicated as 2% so as to yield a whole number of seropositive individuals; actual estimates of the frequency of this disease are of the order of half this value.

generally lower life expectancy in such parts of the world (Wood, 1971a) — you have to live to the age at which a disease starts for it to become manifest. This exercise highlights one of the basic means for assessing validity, a technique that causes others to remark wryly that once an epidemiologist has finished with something it is broken down — by age and sex. Comparison of the patterns of age and sex-specific prevalence ratios is a powerful means for revealing inconsistencies or discordance in evidence, such as has been done for rheumatoid arthritis (Wood, 1968).

These remarks lead on to some more general considerations. The search for aetiological factors reflects a common misconception, one that is shared even by some epidemiologists. For reasons connected to what has just been said, epidemiological methods are generally better at tracing the operation of known or putative factors than they are at identifying such influences in the first place (Murphy, 1972). Experience with pellagra exemplifies this situation, as does that with the clustering of Hodgkin's disease in New York State (Vianna & Polan, 1973). Relevant to this is a point introduced in the previous chapter. Aetiological models developed by other disciplines need to specified with sufficient detail and precision. Moreover, the non-specificity postulated in regard to infectious agents gives rise to difficulty, threatening the concept of specific causation on which so much of the scientific approach has depended so far (Wood, 1982c).

RECENT APPLICATIONS

The average clinician may well be daunted by what has just been said about population-related projects. However, from our review of the various rheumatic disorders it should be evident that many of the gaps in knowledge could be filled by simple clinical description on a more systematic basis. Some of the problem areas to which such enquiries could be directed are therefore worth discussing.

We will begin with an uncertainty mentioned in relation to virtually every condition considered — potential failure to distinguish between things that are different, the problem of heterogeneity. It was not long ago (a few centuries, perhaps) that physicians could do little more than identify fever, failing to perceive that this might have different origins which themselves were associated with different constellations of clinical features — measles as opposed to quartan ague, for instance, for the distinction between which we are indebted to Sydenham (Wood, 1982c). In rheumatology we owe a great debt to people like Heberden and the Garrods, and to others already mentioned, for considerable progress in differentiating between different disorders. However, the race is far from won, and topics such as arthrosis, the dorsopathies, and soft-tissue syndromes present countless opportunities for improvements in clinical nosology.

The basic requirement is clinical acumen and an ability to detect differences where none have been perceived before. However, an epidemiologist can offer tools to help in such endeavours. One way in which these possibilities may be confronted is to study the regularity of age patterns. The pioneer of this approach was Rigoni Stern (1842) who published analyses of age-specific death rates in Verona from carcinoma of the breast and the same condition affecting the uterine cervix. By contrasting the continued increase in deaths from breast cancer with age with the peak of mortality from cervical cancer at about age 50 years, and by recognising the different distribution of the type of cancer according to marital status and parity, he laid the foundations for identifying hormone-dependent tumours. We have presented rheumatological applications of this approach in Figures 3.1 and 3.2. Admittedly such examples lack the profound implications of Stern's work, but nevertheless a means is indicated by which clinical inspiration may be complemented (Wood, 1968). At the moment a comparable ordering of data on most other rheumatic disorders is not available.

Why should an epidemiologist be concerned with these apparently clinical problems? In order to pursue clinically inspired questions an epidemiologist has to depend on the concepts and identification or assignment procedures transmitted to him even if, in the process, he modifies them. Heterogeneity may not only obscure associations, by diluting them with aetiologically unrelated conditions, but it may also encourage misleading conclusions. We have illustrated this in regard to the supposedly degenerative nature of arthrosis. One of the practical problems with conditions that are encountered infrequently is to collect together sufficient cases to establish the basic characteristics of the disease. It was to facilitate such enquiries that we became associated with establishment of the ARC National Case Register of Less Common Rheumatic Diseases.

Clinical picture

Once a syndrome has been recognised, it is then necessary to delineate its profile. In speaking of disease occurrence it is common to invoke the iceberg phenomenon, the idea that a considerable part of morbid experience is frequently not revealed — a situation evident in regard to the community burden, discussed in the previous chapter. Clinically perceived profiles tend to be unpresentative, being the product of selection processes influencing consultation and referral. The importance of recognising such limitations is because bioligical explanations are vulnerable to context; they can never be adequate as long as the complete picture is not taken into account.

There are two main ways in which the picture may be completed. One is to undertake natural history studies in known cases, following up series of patients over time so as to record the full spectrum of outcome. A comprehensive range of severity must be included in such studies so that a representative expression of course is obtained. If only the more marked and severe cases habitually seen in the clinic are included, an unduly gloomy view of prognosis may be obtained. An example of this has been referred to in regard to SLE. A particular value of follow-up studies is their potential to reveal unsuspected heterogeneity, as we have discussed in relation to JCA. Survival studies are more limited in their objectives, noted in the previous chapter, and yet they represent a more economical approach to some of the questions.

The other main means of completing the clinical picture is to follow-up community samples. As indicated in Table 3.1, the axis of enquiry contrasts with that in clinic-based studies and, as a result, the context in which phenomena should be comprehended is extended. Unfortunately the price of such revelation is too often the unwelcome demonstration of non-specificity — as we have already noted for rheumatoid factor (Badley et al, 1974; and see Table 3.8) but which applies equally to a 'normal' erythrocyte sedimentation rate as a criterion for arthrosis (Hargreaves et al, 1973). At the same time some care should be exercised over how phenomena are regarded. Like rheumatoid factor, serum uric acid levels are a continuously distributed variate (i.e. graded by concentration in the serum). To reduce such characteristics to dichotomous attributes, positive (i.e. hyperuricaemic) or negative, distorts reality and wastes data, the full range of responses. Such deformation can carry with it the danger of predetermining results, leading to erroneous conclusions about inherited influences (Wood, 1971a). An analogous example concerns the nature of hypermobility (Wood, 1971b).

Epidemiologists share with clinicians an interest in the identification of predictors, both of disease occurrence and of outcome. Among the more general class of characteristics with predictive value, those indicating increased likelihood of developing a particular disease in the first place are usually designated as risk factors. Of course this does not necessarily mean that such factors have causal significance, as continuing uncertainty about ischaemic heart disease illustrates. Nevertheless they can provide interesting clues to be pursued by other means. For example, at a crude level the identification of differential risks associated with attributes such as residence, such as we noted about Paget's disease, can provide the basis for stimulating further enquiry and the development of aetiological hypotheses. The source of such insights lies in community natural history surveys, and in case–control studies that set out to test the role of specific factors. Genetic markers obviously have some potential as risk factors as well.

Clinicians are perhaps more likely to be interested in attributes that can indicate the future outlook for those affected. Characteristics with predictive value for prognosis can be indentified by means of long-term follow-up studies of patients (Fleming et al, 1976a). A similar approach can also be exploited with uncertainties in patient management. To some extent one can predict the occurrence of thromboembolism following total replacement of the hip joint (Kelsey et al, 1976), which helps to provide the foundation for more rational choices about the prophylactic use of anticoagulant therapy. Many other therapeutic uncertainties could be resolved by analogous approaches.

The most crucial questions about therapy are concerned with efficacy and the balance between benefit and harm. Rheumatology deserves acknowledgement for its enlightened adoption of the technique of randomised controlled trials many years ago (Joint Committee, 1954). Outstanding difficulties have been mentioned in the previous chapter, notably the difficulty in evaluating benefit when chronic processes may perhaps be ameliorated and occasionally even aborted but scarcely ever reversed. Moreover, the valuation to be attached to these different outcomes is problematic. This was one of the considerations that stimulated us to develop an extended view of outcomes (Wood & Badley, 1981), making explicit the relationship between impairments, disabilities, and handicaps.

Therapeutic decisions are taken in a context, so that it is also necessary to be concerned with the working of health services, their efficiency and the equality of their distribution. Although rather humble by customary scientific standards, work in this area can nevertheless make potent contributions to social arithmetic. Our interest was aroused by awareness of the feelings of neglect that appeared to be widespread among rheumatism sufferers. Beginning with a study of the distribution of medical services (Wood, 1971c) we later extended this to ancillary staff and appliances (Benn & Wood, 1972c), the availability of surgical treatment (Wood, 1976c), and various other aspects. The fruits of most of these labours have been published as special reports for the Arthritis and Rheumatism Council, and were discussed in the previous chapter. However, much work remains to be done in many of these areas, not least in the context of improving access to specialist expertise. This could be to the benefit of both patients and general practitioners, and a variety of initiatives could be taken by clinicians.

REFERENCES

Abdin Z H, Ghanem M, Abdul-Fadl N, El-Ghobarey A F, Dick W C 1977 Benign polyarthritis in Egyptian children and adolescents: a new syndrome? Rheumatology 7: 69–74

Acheson R M 1969 Social class gradients and serum uric acid in males and females. British Medical Journal 4: 65–67

Acheson R M 1982 Heberden Oration 1981: Epidemiology and the arthritides. Annals of the Rheumatic Diseases 41: 325–334

Acheson R M, Collart A B 1975 New Haven survey of joint diseases — xvii relationship between some systemic characteristics and osteoarthrosis in a general population. Annals of the Rheumatic Diseases 34: 379–387

Acheson R M, O'Brien W M 1968 Some factors associated with serum uric acid in the New Haven survey of joint disease. In: Bennett P H, Wood P H N (eds) Population studies of the rheumatic diseases. International Congress Series No 148. Excerpta Medica Foundation, Amsterdam, Ch 49, p 365–370

Acheson R M, Chan Y-K, Clemett A R 1970 New Haven survey of joint diseases — xii: distribution and symptoms of osteoarthrosis in the hands with reference to handedness. Annals of the Rheumatic Diseases 29: 275–286

Adams D D 1982 Genetics of autoimmune disease in relationship to rheumatology. In: Dawkins R L, Christiansen F T, Zilko P J (eds) Immunogenetics in rheumatology — musculoskeletal disease and D-penicillamine. International Congress Series No 602. Excerpta Medica, Amsterdam, Ch 1.10, p 43–47

Adams I D 1979 Osteoarthrosis and sport. Journal of the Royal Society of Medicine 72: 185–187

Adams P, Davies G T, Sweetnam P 1970 Osteoporosis and the effects of ageing on bone mass in elderly men and women. Quarterly Journal of Medicine NS 39: 601–615

van Adrichem J A M, van der Korst J K 1973 Assessment of the flexibility of the lumbar spine, a pilot study in children and adolescents. Scandinavian Journal of Rheumatology 2: 87–91

Agarwal B L 1981 Rheumatic heart disease unabated in developing countries. Lancet 2: 910–911

Al Azzawi A J M, Wood P H N 1985 The relationship between fertility factors and the severity of rheumatoid arthritis in women. Annals of the Rheumatic Diseases (in press)

Alexander G M, Dieppe P A, Doherty M, Scott D G I 1982 Pyrophosphate arthropathy: a study of metabolic associations and laboratory data. Annals of the Rheumatic Diseases 41: 377–381

Allander E 1974 Prevalence, incidence, and remission rates of some common rheumatic diseases or syndromes. Scandinavian Journal of Rheumatology 3: 145–158

Allander E, Bjelle A 1981 Developments in epidemiological studies on rheumatoid arthritis. Scandinavian Journal of Rheumatology 10: 257–261

Allander E, Bjornsson O J, Olafasson O, Sigfusson N, Thorsteinsson J 1974 Normal range of joint movements in shoulder, hip, wrist and thumb with special reference to side: a comparison between two populations. International Journal of Epidemiology 3: 253–326

Altman R D, Meenan R F, Hochberg M C, Bole G G, Brandt K, Cooke T D V, et al 1983 An approach to developing criteria for the clinical diagnosis and classification of osteoarthritis: a status report of the American Rheumatism Association Diagnostic

Subcommittee on Osteoarthritis. Journal of Rheumatology 10: 180–183
Anderson J A D 1971 Rheumatism in industry: a review. British Journal of Industrial Medicine 28: 103–121
Anderson J A D, Sweetman B J 1975 A combined flexi-rule/hydrogoniometer for measurement of lumbar spine and its sagittal movement. Rheumatology and Rehabilitation 14: 173–179
Andersson G B J 1981 Epidemiologic aspects on low-back pain in industry. Spine 6: 53–60
Ansell B M, Wood P H N 1976 Prognosis in juvenile chronic polyarthritis. In: Ansell B M (ed) Rheumatic disorders in childhood. Clinics in Rheumatic Diseases 2: 397–412
Ansell B M, Bywaters E G L, Lawrence J S 1962 A family study in Still's disease. Annals of the Rheumatic Diseases 21: 243–2
Ansell B M, Bywaters E G L, Lawrence J S 1968 Family studies in Still's disease (juvenile R A). In: Bennett P H, Wood P H N (eds) Population studies of the rheumatic diseases. International Congress Series No 148. Excerpta Medica Foundation, Amsterdam, Ch 32, p 229–234
Ansell B M, Bywaters E G L, Lawrence J S 1969 Familial aggregation and twin studies in Still's disease. In: Rotstein J (ed) Population studies and genetics. Rheumatology 2: 37–61
Argen R J, Wilson C H Jnr, Wood P H N 1966 Suppurative arthritis: clinical features of 42 cases. Archives of Internal Medicine 117: 661–666
Atlas of Standard Radiographs of Arthritis 1963 The epidemiology of chronic rheumatism, Vol 2. Blackwell, Oxford
Auquier L, Henrard J C, Siaud J R 1981 Enquete controlée sur le rachis lombaire des tractoristes. In: Peyron J G (ed) Epidemiologie de L'arthrose, Symposium, Paris. Ciba Geigy, Paris, p 172–179
Bacon P A, Doherty S M, Zuckerman A J 1975 Hepatitis-B antibody in polymyalgia rheumatica. Lancet 2: 476–478
Badley E M, Wood P H N 1979 Attitudes of the public to arthritis. Annals of the Rheumatic Diseases 38: 97–100
Badley E M, Ball J, Wood P H N 1974 Rheumatoid factor, so-called — what does it portend for the population. Journal of Preventive and Social Medicine 20: 71–72
Badley E M, Ball J, Wood P H N 1975 Interpreting the biological significance of rheumatoid factor. Annals of the Rheumatic Diseases 34:463
Badley E M, Meyrick J S, Wood P H N 1978a Gout and serum uric acid levels in the Cotswolds. Rheumatology and Rehabilitation 17: 133–142
Badley E M, Thompson R P, Wood P H N 1978b The prevalence and severity of major disabling conditions — a reappraisal of the Government Social Survey on the handicapped and impaired in Great Britain. International Journal of Epidemiology 7: 145–151
Baker H 1966 Epidemiological aspects of psoriasis and arthritis. British Journal of Dermatology 78: 249–261
Ball J 1971 The Heberdern Oration 1970: Enthesopathy of rheumatoid and ankylosing spondylitis. Annals of the Rheumatic Diseases 30: 213–223
Barker D J P, Gardner M J 1974 Distribution of Paget's disease in England, Wales and Scotland and a possible relationship with vitamin D deficiency in childhood. British Journal of Preventive and Social Medicine 28: 226–232
Barker D J P, Clough P W L, Guyer P B, Gardner M J 1977 Paget's disease of bone in 14 British towns. British Medical Journal 1: 1181–1183
Barry H C 1969 Paget's Disease of Bone. Livingstone, Edinburgh
Barry P E 1968 In: Bennett P H, Wood P H N (eds) Population studies of the rheumatic diseases. International Congress Series No 148. Excerpta Medica Foundation, Amsterdam, p 376
Barwick D D, Walton J N 1963 Polymyositis. American Journal of Medicine 35: 646–660
Batchelor J R, Welsh K I, Tinoco R M, Dollery C T, Hughes G R V, Berstein R et al 1980 Hydralazine-induced systemic lupus erythematosus: influence of HLA-DR and sex on susceptibility. Lancet 1: 1107–1109
Baum J, Fink 1968 Juvenile rheumatoid arthritis in monozygotic twins: a case report and review of literature. Arthritis and Rheumatism 11: 33–36
Baum J, Ziff M 1971 The rarity of ankylosing spondylitis in the black race. Arthritis and Rheumatism 14: 12–18
Baum J, Alekseev L S, Brewer E J, Dolgopolova A V, Mudholkar G S, Patel K 1980 Juvenile rheumatoid arthritis, a comparison of patients from the USSR and USA. Arthritis and Rheumatism 23: 977–984
Beales J G, Keen J G, Holt P J L 1983 The child's perception of the disease and the experience of pain in juvenile chronic arthritis. Journal of Rheumatology 10: 61–65
Beardwell A 1969 Familial ankylosing vertebral hyperostosis with tylosis. Annals of the Rheumatic Diseases 28: 518–523
Beasley R P, Willkens R F, Bennett P H 1973 High prevalence of rheumatoid arthritis in Yakima Indians. Arthritis and Rheumatism 16: 743–748
Behrend T, Lawrence J S, Behrend H, Fischer K 1972a Prevalence of rheumatoid arthritis in rural Germany. International Journal of Epidemiology 1: 153–156
Behrend T, Lawrence J S, Behrend H, Koch R 1972b Eine longitudinale studie im Hinblick auf rheumatisch Erkrankungen in der Landlichen Bevolkerung von Oberhorlen in Hessen. Zeitschrift für Rheumaforschung 31: 153–167
Beighton P 1978 Inherited disorders of the skeleton. Churchill Livingstone, Edinburgh
Beighton P, Solomon L, Soskolne C L 1973 Articular mobility in an African population. Annals of the Rheumatic Diseases 32: 413–418
Beighton P, Solomon L, Valkenburg H A 1975 Rheumatoid arthritis in a rural South African negro population. Annals of the Rheumatic Diseases 34: 136–141
Beighton P, Daynes G, Soskolne C L 1976 Serum uric acid concentrations in a Xhosa community in the Transkei of Southern Africa. Annals of the Rheumatic Diseases 35: 77–80
Bell D A, Maddison P J 1980 Serologic subsets in systemic lupus erythematosus: an examination of autoantibodies in relationship to clinical features of disease and HLA antigens. Arthritis and Rheumatism 23: 1268–1273
Benn R T, Wood P H N 1972a Mortality in rheumatoid arthritis. British Journal of Preventive and Social Medicine 26:60
Benn R T, Wood P H N 1972b Mortality from Paget's disease of bone. Presented to Society for Social Medicine, Rennes, July
Benn R T, Wood P H N 1972c Services ancillary to physical medicine: regional variations in staff and appliances. Rheumatology and Physical Medicine 11: 403–412

Benn R T, Wood P H N 1975 Generalized osteoarthrosis, a problem of definition. Annals of the Rheumatic Diseases 34:466

Benn R T, Wood P H N 1977 Clustering of arthritis with other diseases on multiple-cause coded death certificates. Presented to Society for Social Medicine, Birmingham, September

Bennett P H, Wood P H N (eds) 1968 Population studies of the rheumatic diseases. International Congress Series No 148. Excerpta Medica Foundation, Amsterdam

Bennett R, Bluestone R, Holt P J L, Bywaters E G L 1971 Survival in scleroderma. Annals of the Rheumatic Diseases 30: 581–588

Bergquist-Ullmann M, Larsson V 1977 Acute low back pain in industry. Acta Orthopaedica Scandinavica (Suppl) 170

Berman L, Trappler B, Jenkins T 1979 Behçet's syndrome: a family study and the elucidation of a genetic role. Annals of the Rheumatic Diseases 38: 118–121

Billings R A, Burry H C, Jones R 1977 Low back injury and sport. Rheumatology and Rehabilitation 16: 236–240

Bird H A, Tribe C R, Bacon P A 1978 Joint hypermobility leading to osteoarthrosis and chondrocalcinosis. Annals of the Rheumatic Diseases, 37: 203–211

Bird H A, Esselinckx W, Dixon A St J, Mowat A G, Wood P H N 1979 An evaluation of criteria for polymalgia rheumatica. Annals of the Rheumatic Diseases 38: 434–439

Birnbaum N S, Rodnan G P, Rabin B S, Bassion S 1977 Histocompatibility antigens in progressive systemic sclerosis (scleroderma). Journal of Rheumatology 4: 425–428

Bjelle A 1979 Pyrophosphate arthropathy. Scandinavian Journal of Rheumatology 8: 145–153

Bjelle A, Allander E, Magi M 1980 Rheumatic disorders in the Swedish population and health care system. Journal of Rheumatology 7: 877–885

Bjelle A, Edvinsson U, Hagstam A 1982 Pyrophosphate arthropathy in two Swedish families. Arthritis and Rheumatism 25: 66–74

Black C M, Welsh K I, Fielder A, Hughes, G R V, Batchelor J R 1982 HLA antigens and Bf allotypes in SLE: evidence for the association being with specific haplotypes. Tissue Antigens 19: 115–120

Bloor G, Rigby R J, Richmond J M, Zilko P J, Dawkins R L 1982 Systemic lupus erythematosus in Australian Aborigines. Australian and New Zealand Journal of Medicine 12:553

Bodmer W F 1975 The HL-A system and its association with immune response and disease. Annals of the Rheumatic Diseases 34 (Suppl): 13–16

Böni A 1959 Familial coxarthrosis. Seminars International 8: 16–21

Bremner J M, Emery A E H, Kellgren J H, Lawrence J S, Roth H 1968 A family study in ankylosing spondylitis. In: Bennett P H, Wood P H N (eds) Population studies of the rheumatic diseases. International Congress Series No 148. Excerpta Medica Foundation, Amsterdam, Ch 40, p 299–304

Brigode M, Francois R J 1977 Histocompatibility antigens in vertebral ankylosing hyperostosis. Journal of Rheumatology 4: 429–433

Brockington F 1975 World health, 3rd Edn. Churchill Livingstone, Edinburgh, Ch 3, p 15–24

Brooks G W, Mueller E 1966 Serum urate concentrations among university professors — relation to drive, achievement, and leadership. Journal of the American Medical Association 195: 415–418

Brown A R, Rose B S 1966 Familial precocious polyarticular osteoarthrosis of chondrodysplastic type. New Zealand Medical Journal 65: 449–461

Bruckner F E, Nye C J S 1981 A prospective study of adhesive capsulitis of the shoulder ('frozen shoulder') in a high risk population. Quarterly Journal of Medicine 50: 191–204

Buckle P W, Kember P A, Wood A D, Wood S N 1980 Factors influencing occupational back pain in Bedfordshire. Spine 5: 254–258

Bulgen D Y, Hazleman B L, Voak D 1976 HLA-B27 and frozen shoulder. Lancet 1: 1042–1044

Bull J, El Gamnal T, Pophan M 1969 A possible genetic factor in cervical spondylosis. British Journal of Radiology 42: 9–16

Burch P R J 1966 Dupuytren's contracture: an auto-immune disease? Journal of Bone and Joint Surgery 48B: 312–319

Burch P R J 1968 An inquiry concerning growth, disease and ageing. Oliver & Boyd, Edinburgh

Burch P R J, Rowell N R 1965 Systemic lupus erythematosus: etiological aspects. American Journal of Medicine 38: 793–801

Burch P R J, Rowell N R 1970 Lupus erythematosus: analysis of the sex- and age-distributions of the discoid and systemic forms of the disease in different countries. Acta Dermato-venereologica 50: 293–301

Burch T A, O'Brien W M, Need R, Kurland L T 1966 Hyperuricaemia and gout in the Mariana Islands. Annals of the Rheumatic Diseases 25: 114–116

Burke M J, Fear E C, Wright V 1977 Bone and joint changes in pneumatic drillers. Annals of the Rheumatic Diseases 36: 276–279

Burke M J, Roman V, Wright V 1978 Bone and joint changes in lower limb amputees. Annals of the Rheumatic Diseases 37: 252–254

Bury M R, Wood P H N 1979 Problems of communication in chronic illness. International Rehabilitation Medicine 1: 130–134

Bywaters E G L 1968 Diagnostic criteria for Still's disease (juvenile R A). In: Bennett P H, Wood P H N (eds) Population studies of the rheumatic diseases. International Congress Series No 148. Excerpta Medica Foundation, Amsterdam, Ch 33, p 235–240

Bywaters E G L 1971 Still's disease in the adult. Annals of the Rheumatic Diseases 30: 121–133

Bywaters E G L, Dresner E 1952 The prognosis in rheumatoid arthritis. Proceedings of the 46th Annual General Meeting of the Association of Physicians of Great Britian and Ireland. Quarterly Journal of Medicine 21:463

Bywaters E G L, Forestier J 1967 Glossary of terminology of the spondylopathies. Reports and Abstracts, VI European Congress of Rheumatology, Lisbon, p 472–480

Caeiro F, Michielson F M C, Bernstein R, Hughes G R V, Ansell B M 1981 Systemic lupus erythematosus in childhood. Annals of the Rheumatic Diseases 40: 325–331

Calabro J J 1967 Cancer and arthritis. Arthritis and Rheumatism 10: 553–567

Calin A, Fries J F 1975 Striking prevalence of ankylosing spondylitis in 'healthy' W27 positive males and females: a controlled study. New England Journal of Medicine 293: 835–839

Calin A, Kaye B, Sternberg M, Antell B, Chan M 1980 The prevalence and nature of back pain in an industrial

complex; a questionnaire and radiographic and HLA analysis. Spine 5: 201–205
Canoso J J, Cohen A S 1974 Malignancy in a series of 70 patients with systemic lupus erythematosus. Arthritis and Rheumatism 17: 383–390
Carette S, Graham D, Little H, Rubenstein J, Rosen P 1983 The natural disease course of ankylosing spondylitis. Arthritis and Rheumatism 26: 186–190
Carpenter J R, Bunch T W, Engel A G, O'Brien P C 1977 Survival in polymyositis: corticosteroids and risk factors. Journal of Rheumatology 4: 207–214
Carroll G J, Peter J B, Garlepp M J 1982 D-pencillamine-induced dermatomyositis and polymyositis. In: Dawkins R L, Christiansen F T, Zilko P J (eds) Immunogenetics in rheumatology — musculoskeletal disease and D-penicillamine. International Congress Series no. 602. Excerpta Medica, Amsterdam, Ch 8.12, p 326–330
Carter C O, Fairbank T J 1974 The genetics of locomotor disorders. Oxford Monographs on Medical Genetics. Oxford University Press, London
Carter C, Wilkinson J 1964 Persistent joint laxity and congenital dislocation of the hip. Journal of Bone and Joint Surgery 46B: 40–45
Carter E T, McKenna C H, Brian D D, Kurland L T 1979 Epidemiology of ankylosing spondylitis in Rochester, Minnesota, 1935–1973. Arthritis and Rheumatism 22: 365–370
Catford J C, Bennet G C, Wilkinson J A 1982 Congenital hip dislocation: an increasing and still uncontrolled disability? British Medical Journal 285: 1527–1530
Cecil R L, Archer B H 1926 Classification and treatment of chronic arthritis. Journal of the American Medical Association 87: 741–746
Chalmers I M 1980 Ankylosing spondylitis in African blacks. Arthritis and Rheumatism 23: 1366–1370
Chamberlain M A 1977 Behçet's syndrome in 32 patients in Yorkshire. Annals of the Rheumatic Diseases 36: 491–499
Chamberlain M A 1978 A family study of Behçet's syndrome. Annals of the Rheumatic Diseases 37: 459–465
Chamberlain M A 1981 Socioeconomic effects of ankylosing spondylitis. International Rehabilitation Medicine 3: 94–99
Chief Medical Officer (CMO) 1974 Sexually transmitted diseases; extract from the Annual Report of the Chief Medical Officer of the Department of Health and Social Security for the year 1972. British Journal of Venereal Diseases 50: 73–79
Christiansen F T, Owen E T, Dawkins R L, Hanrahan P 1977 Symptoms and signs among relatives of patients with HLA B27 ankylosing spondylitis: correlation between back pain, spinal movement, sacroiliitis and HLA antigens. Journal of Rheumatology 3: 11–17
Cleland L G, Bell D A, Willans M, Saurino B C 1978 Familial lupus: family studies of HLA and serologic findings. Arthritis and Rheumatism 21: 183–191
Cobb S 1963 Hyperuricaemia in executives. In: Kellgren J H, Jeffrey M R, Ball J (eds) The epidemiology of chronic rheumatism. Blackwell, Oxford, Ch 21, p 182–186
Cobb S, Hall W 1965 Newly identified cluster of diseases — rheumatoid arthritis, peptic ulcer and tuberculosis. Journal of the American Medical Association 193: 1077–1079
Cobb S, Lawrence J S 1957 Towards a geography of rheumatoid arthritis. Bulletin on the Rheumatic Diseases 7: 133–134
Cobb S, Anderson F, Bauer W 1953 Length of life and cause of death in rheumatoid arthritis. New England Journal of Medicine 249: 553–556
Cobb S, Miller M, Wieland M 1959 On the relationship between divorce and rheumatoid arthritis. Arthritis and Rheumatism 2: 414–418
Cohen L M, Mittal K K, Schmid R F, Rogers L F, Cohen K L 1976 Increased risk for spondylitis stigmata in apparently health HL-A W27 men. Annals of Internal Medicine 84: 1–7
Collins D H 1956 Paget's disease of bone, incidence and subclinical forms. Lancet 2: 51–57
Condemi J J, Blomgren S E, Vaughan J H 1970 The procainamide-induced lupus syndrome. Bulletin on the Rheumatic Diseases 20: 604–608
Coventry M B 1953 Problem of painful shoulder. Journal of the American Medical Association 151: 177–185
Critchley E M R 1982 Lumbar spinal stenosis. British Medical Journal 284: 1588–1589
Crown S 1978 Psychological aspects of low back pain. Rheumatology and Rehabilitation 17: 114–124
Crown S, Crown J M 1973 Personality in early rheumatoid disease. Journal of Psychosomatic Research 17: 189–196
Csonka G W 1958 The course of Reiter's syndrome. British Medical Journal 1: 1088–1090
Csonka G W 1960 Recurrent attacks in Reiter's disease. Arthritis and Rheumatism 3: 164–169
Csonka G W 1972 Reiter's disease. British Journal of Hospital Medicine 7: 8–12
Currey H L F 1970 Osteoarthrosis of the hip and sexual activity. Annals of the Rheumatic Diseases 29: 488–493
Currey H L F, Greenwood R M, Lloyd G G, Murray R S 1979 A prospective study of low back pain. Rheumatology and Rehabilitation 18: 94–104
Currie W J C 1979 Prevalence and incidence of the diagnosis of gout in Great Britain. Annals of the Rheumatic Diseases 38: 101–106
Cust G, Pearson J C G, Mair A 1972 The prevalence of low back pain in nurses. International Nursing Review 19: 169–179
van Dam G, Lezwijn A, Bos J G 1961 Death-rate of patients with rheumatoid arthritis. Atti del X Congresso Lega Internazionale contro il Reumatismo. Minerva Medica, Torino 1: 161–164
Damlund M, Goth S, Hasle P, Munk K 1982 Low-back pain and early retirement among Danish semi-skilled constructive workers. Scandinavian Journal of Work and Environmental Health 8 (Suppl 1): 100–104
David T J, Burwood R L 1972 The nature and inheritance of Kirner's deformity. Journal of Medical Genetics 9: 430–433
Davis M A 1981 Sex differences in reporting osteoarthritic symptoms: a sociomedical approach. Journal of Health and Social Behaviour 22: 298–310
Davis P, Lentle B C 1978 Evidence for sacroiliac disease as a common cause of low backache in women. Lancet 2: 496–497
Davis P, Percy J S, Russell A S 1977 Correlation between levels of DNA antibodies and clinical disease activity in SLE — retrospective evaluation. Annals of the Rheumatic Diseases 36: 157–159
Dawkins R L 1978 Polymyositis and dermatomyositis: clinical problems. Australian and New Zealand Journal of Medicine 8 (Suppl 1): 139–142
Dawkins R L 1982 Concepts and models — introduction. In: Dawkins R L, Christiansen F T, Zilko P J (eds)

Immunogenetics in rheumatology — musculoskeletal disease and D-penicillamine. International Congress Series No 602. Excerpta Medica, Amsterdam, Ch 1.1, p 1–5
Dawkins R L, Christiansen F T, Zilko P J (eds) 1982 Immunogenetics in rheumatology — musculoskeletal disease and D-pencillamine. International Congress Series No 602. Excerpta Medica, Amsterdam
Detheridge F M, Guyer P B, Barker D J P 1982 European distribution of Paget's disease of bone. British Medical Journal 285: 1005–1008
Dickson R A 1983 Scoliosis in the community. British Medical Journal 286: 615–618
Dieppe P A, Alexander G J M, Jones H E, Doherty M, Scott D G I, Manhire A, Watt I 1982 Pyrophosphate arthropathy: a clinical and radiological study of 105 cases. Annals of the Rheumatic Diseases 41: 371–376
Dixon A St J 1979 Soft tissue rheumatism: concept and classification. In: Dixon A St J (ed) Soft tissue rheumatism. Clinics in Rheumatic Diseases 5: 739–742
Dixon A St J 1981 Editorial: Research is for now, too. Journal of Rheumatology 8: 361–363
Dixon A St J, Owen-Smith B D, Harrison R A 1972 Cold sensitive non-specific low back pain: a comparative trial of treatment. Clinical Trials Journal 9: 16–21
Doherty M, Watt I, Dieppe P A 1982 Localised chondrocalcinosis in post-meniscectomy knees. Lancet 1: 1207–1210
Donovan J, Adelstein A M 1974 Sequelae of virus infection in pregnancy. British Medical Journal 2:502
DuBois E L 1969 Procainamide induction of a systemic lupus erythematosus-like syndrome; presentation of six cases, review of literature, and analysis and follow-up reported cases. Medicine (Baltimore) 48: 217–228
DuBois E L, Tuffanelli D L 1964 Clinical manifestations of systemic lupus erythematosus. Journal of the American Medical Association 190: 104–111
Dubos R 1965 Man adapting. Yale University Press, New Haven, Ch 1, p 1
Duthie J J R, Brown P E, Truelove L H, Baragar F D, Lawrie A J 1964 Course and prognosis in rheumatoid arthritis: a further report. Annals of the Rheumatic Diseases 23: 193–202
Early P F 1962 Population studies in Dupuytren's contracture. Journal of Bone and Joint Surgery 44B: 602–613
Eastmond C J, Woodrow J C 1977a Discordance for ankylosing spondylitis in monozygotic twins. Annals of the Rheumatic Diseases 36: 360–364
Eastmond C J, Woodrow J C 1977b The HLA system and the arthropathies associated with psoriasis. Annals of the Rheumatic Diseases 36: 112–120
Eastmond C J, Hudson A, Wright V 1979 A radiological survey of the hips and knees in female specialist teachers of physical education. Scandinavian Journal of Rheumatology 8: 264–268
Ebringer R W, Cawdell D R, Cowling D, Ebringer A 1978 Sequential studies in ankylosing spondylitis: association of *Klebsiella pneumoniae* with active disease. Annals of the Rheumatic Diseases 37: 146–151
Editorial 1976a Septic arthritis in rheumatoid disease. British Medical Journal 2: 1089–1090
Editorial 1976b Thoracic discs are different. British Medical Journal 1:608
Editorial 1978 Enterobacteria, B27 and ankylosing spondylitis. Lancet 1:1242
Editorial 1981 Problems with the shoulder. Lancet 2: 564–565
Elder R G 1973 Social class and lay explanations of the etiology of arthritis. Journal of Health and Social Behaviour 14: 28–38
Elliot R W, Essenhigh D M, Morley A R 1982 Cyclophosphamide treatment of systemic lupus erythematosus: risk of bladder cancer exceeds benefits. British Medical Journal 284: 1160–1161
Ellman M H, Levin B 1975 Chondrocalcinosis in elderly persons. Arthritis and Rheumatism 18: 43–47
Ellman M H, Brown N L, Levin B 1981 Narrowing of knee joint space in patients with pseudogout. Annals of the Rheumatic Diseases 40: 34–36
Emery A E H, Lawrence J S 1967 Genetics of ankylosing spondylitis. Journal of Medical Genetics 4: 239–244
Emmerson B T 1960 Heredity in primary gout. Australasian Annals of Medicine 9: 168–175
Emmerson B T 1963 Chronic lead nephropathy: the diagnostic use of calcium edita and the association with gout. Australasian Annals of Medicine 12: 310–324
Engel A 1968 Osteoarthritis and body measurements as shown in data from the Health Examination Survey, 1960–1962. US Public Health Service Publication No. 1000, series 11, no. 29. Superintendent of Documents, Washington
Erasmus L D 1957 Scleroderma in gold miners on the Witwatersrand with particular reference to pulmonary manifestations. South African Journal of Laboratory and Clinical Medicine 3: 209–231
Espinoza L, Oh J H, Kinsella T D, Stacey C H, Osterland C K, Dove F B 1974 Ankylosing spondylitis: family studies and HL-A27 antigen distribution. Journal of Rheumatology 1: 254–259
Espinoza L R, Vasey F B, Oh J H, Wilkinson R, Osterland C K 1978 Association between HLA-BW38 and peripheral psoriatic arthritis. Arthritis and Rheumatism 21: 72–75
Evans J G, Acheson E D 1965 An epidemiological study of ulcerative colitis and regional enteritis in the Oxford area. Gut 6: 311–324
Fabrega H 1974 Disease and social behaviour: an interdisciplinary perspective. MIT Press, Cambridge, Massachusetts
Falconer D S 1965 The inheritance of liability to certain diseases estimated from the incidence among relatives. Annals of Human Genetics 29: 51–76. See also Falconer D S 1967 The inheritance of liability to diseases with variable age of onset with particular reference to diabetes mellitus. Annals of Human Genetics 31: 1–20
Fallet G H, Mason M, Berry H, Mowat A G, Boussina I, Gerster J-C 1976 Rheumatoid arthritis and ankylosing spondylitis occuring together. British Medical Journal 1: 804–807
Fielder A H L, Walport M J, Batchelor J R, Rynes R I, Black C M, Dodi I A, Hughes G R V 1983 Family study of the major histocompatibility complex in patients with systemic lupus erythematosus: importance of null alleles of C4A and C4B in determining disease susceptibility. British Medical Journal 286: 425–428
Filipowicz-Sosnowska A M, Roztropowicz-Denisiewicz K, Rosenthal C J, Baum J 1978 The amyloidosis of juvenile rheumatoid arthritis — comparative studies in Polish and American children. Arthritis and Rheumatism 21: 699–703
Fleming A, Crown J M, Corbett M 1976a Prognostic value of

Reiter's disease

Historical outline

As long ago as 1507 Pierre Van Forest described a patient who developed arthritis of the knee in association with urethritis, and Martiniere recognised arthritis as a complication of urethritis in 1664 (Sharp, 1972). Over 150 years ago Sir Benjamin Brodie (1818) described the syndrome which now carries the eponymous title of 'Reiter's disease'. This report appeared almost one hundred years before Hans Reiter (1916) described the case of a cavalry officer serving on the Balkan front who developed an acute dysenteric illness characterised by arthritis, urethritis and conjunctivitis. Since then over 97 synonyms have been used to describe this entity. It is generally accepted that 'Reiter's disease' is an unsatisfactory term for the syndrome; and, as Ford (1953a) has pointed out, Reiter's paper made only a negligible and somewhat misleading contribution to the subject: the illness of Reiter's patient followed dysentery, and the arthritis was attributed to syphilis — indeed, in the title, the phrase 'spirochaetosis arthritica' appeared.

The first description in the USA did not appear until 1942 (Bauer & Engelman, 1942), and the syndrome has become more widely recognised since the studies of Harkness (1950), Csonka (1958a, b, 1960), Ford (1953, 1958), and workers at the London Hospital (Murray et al 1958; Oates & Young, 1959; Hancock, 1960).

There seems little doubt that previous reviews have included patients with gonococcal disease. A study (Wright, 1963) of 214 patients with arthritis associated with venereal disease delineated gonococcal arthritis and Reiter's disease, and few today would doubt their existence as separate entities.

The classical triad of Reiter's disease comprises non-specific urethritis, arthritis and conjunctivitis. It is now appreciated that there is a spectrum of involvement and Hancock & Mason (1965) have summarised the disease as one of unknown cause, the most constant feature of which is a recurrent non-suppurative polyarthritis with a predilection for the joints of the lower limbs and sacroiliac joints, occurring in close association with non-specific inflammation of the lower urogenital tract. In an attempt to overcome the difficulties of definition, the American Rheumatism Association made a retrospective analysis of 66 different clinical features associated with 'typical' cases of Reiter's disease, and assessed the sensitivity and specificity of these features in delineating it from ankylosing spondylitis, psoriatic arthritis, gonococcal arthritis and seronegative rheumatoid arthritis (Wilkens et al, 1981). Their working definition was 'an episode of peripheral arthritis of more than one month's duration occurring in association with urethritis and/or cervicitis'. Cervicitis was not defined, and the preconceived ideas of the contributors would inevitably influence the outcome of this investigation, together with the fact that it was done in the USA, where a dysenteric form of Reiter's disease is less common than it is in Scandinavia.

Prevalence

In the United Kingdom and North America most cases follow extramarital sexual intercourse, whereas in other parts of Europe dysentery more frequently precedes the clinical symptoms. Csonka (1958a) commented that the disease seemed to be less severe in coloured patients. A paper from Papua showed that Reiter's disease accounted for the majority of cases of arthritis in young males, and epidemiological studies suggested a venereal transmission (Maddocks, 1967). It is difficult to arrive at a figure for the prevalence of Reiter's disease venereally acquired. Laird (1958) found a prevalence of 1.7% amongst 3500 cases of non-specific urethritis. The urethritis is usually assumed to be venereally acquired, although patients frequently deny sexual exposure. The time relationship with sexual intercourse, and the fact that the majority of patients acknowledge themselves to be sexually promiscuous (Csonka, 1958a) lends support to this. Indeed, 12–50% of patients do give a history or have signs of other diseases known to be venereal, usually gonorrhoea (King, 1957; & Levy, 1950; Csonka, 1958a, Steinmetz Green, 1959). However, there are cases which fall into this category in whom such a history cannot be obtained even by those most skilled in extracting such information, and, similarly, during a dysentery epidemic cases occur in patients who have no symptoms or signs of diarrhoea.

There are some who would still incriminate gonococcal infection in this disease, but the course of true gonococcal arthritis and its response to treatment distinguishes the diseases as groups (Wright, 1963). However, it is not necessarily true that the majority of so-called cases of 'gonococcal arthritis' were in fact examples of Reiter's disease (Harkness, 1950; Ford, 1953b; Kelly, 1958).

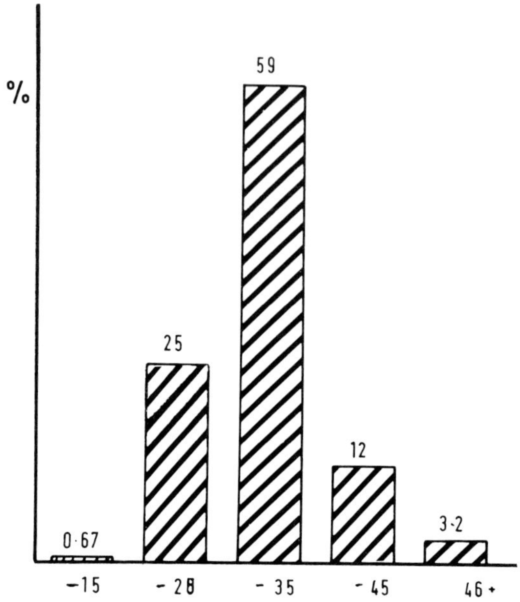

Fig. 31.1 Age of onset of Reiter's disease (739 cases).

Incidence

The majority of cases occur between the ages of 16 and 35 years (Fig. 31.1). Reiter's disease is the most common cause of peripheral inflammatory arthritis in young men (Arnett et al, 1976). The disease has been reported in children. The first published account of the syndrome in childhood did not appear until 1946 when Koster & Jansen reported a Dutch family in which three infants developed the triad. Since then, other cases have been published (Zewi, 1947; Paronen, 1948; Corner, 1950; Jacobs, 1961; Moss, 1964). Of particular interest is a case of Reiter's disease reported in a boy aged 32 months (Florman & Goldstein, 1948). Lockie & Hunder (1971) in an excellent review found in the literature only 20 adequately detailed cases of childhood Reiter's occurring under the age of 16. They found a higher frequency (75%) of diarrhoea in all childhood cases. Of the childhood cases so far reported only 7 have been from England (Corner, 1950; Jacobs, 1961; Gough, 1962; Moss, 1964; Iveson et al, 1975), and six from the United States (Florman & Goldstein, 1948; Margileth, 1962; Herman, 1966; Davies et al, 1969; Lockie & Hunder, 1971).

At the other end of the scale, older patients may be affected, and King (1957) found 25 of his 101 patients were between 41 and 60 years. A review of the literature suggests that 3.2% of patients develop the disease after the age of 45 years.

Reiter's disease is usually (some would say almost exclusively) confined to men. The ratio of 15 males to 1 female quoted by King & Nicol (1969) is similar to that of other authors. The only reports of childhood Reiter's disease occurring in girls have come from Europe (Zewi, 1947; Henckel, 1954). This gives a ratio of 1 girl to 4–5 boys which is similar to that found in Paronen's adult 'dysenteric' cases, of whom 10% were women; but higher than that of Oates & Csonka (1959) who found a ratio of approximately 1 female to 50 male patients seen in venereal disease clinics. This would seem to indicate that the childhood cases have more in common with the adult dysenteric than the venereal form.

Epidemiological studies

The source of any series influences the clinical pattern considerably, as is well shown by the sexually-acquired reactive arthritis described by Keat et al (1979), who looked at 57 patients with arthritis associated with non-gonococcal genital infection that presented at a venereal disease clinic.

A dysenteric form of Reiter's disease usually follows bacillary dysentery and the most extensive study has been undertaken by Paronen (1948) in a report of 344 cases in Finland following an outbreak of dysentery.

Aboard an American naval vessel 9 such cases followed an outbreak of bacillary dysentery affecting 602 personnel in whom there was no immediate venereal exposure (Noer, 1966). The disease, however, may also follow attacks of amoebic dysentery (Moorhead, 1916; Graby et al, 1949; Marche, 1955), and has been observed following seasonal toxic non-specific diarrhoea among French troops in Algeria (Roumagnac et al, 1958; Masbernard, 1959). The incidence and geographical distribution of these cases generally correspond with the behaviour of the preceding dysentery epidemic (Paronen, 1948), although this is not invariable (Manson-Bahr, 1943). The endemic sporadic form is related to the increase in the fly population (Marche, 1955), the seasonal incidence of diarrhoea, and lack of hygienic facilities. Newcomers to the area appear to be more susceptible (Roumagnac et al, 1958). Paronen found the frequency of Reiter's disease to be 0.24% amongst 150 000 cases of dysentery.

Reiter's syndrome follows *Shigella flexneri* 1b and 2a infections in about 1.5% of white adults with dysentery, women developing post-dysenteric Reiter's syndrome as often as men (Simon et al, 1981). In a Puerto Rican community *S. Sonnei* was not arthritogenic (Caslow et al, 1979).

Family studies

There are few data on familial aspects of the disease. A summary of the literature is shown in Table 31.1. Koster & Jansen (1946) reported attacks in three or four siblings; Paronen (1948) mentioned multiple cases in three families; Trier (1950) and Csonka (1958a) reported the occurrence in brothers, and Morton (1958) reported cousins who were affected. A hereditary predisposition to the arthritis of Reiter's disease was suggested by Csonka (1958a) on the basis that 13% of 109 patients gave a 'clear account of rheumatoid arthritis in their families', compared with only 2.2% of a control group of 400 patients with uncomplicated urethritis. However, little weight can be given to the recollection of patients, as rheumatologists concerned in family surveys will appreciate. A nationwide study of families of patients with Reiter's disease in the United Kingdom was attempted by Lawrence (1974). Results in 34 families showed an

Table 31.1 Reiter's disease affecting more than one member of family: summary of literature

		Index case				Secondary case(s)				
Author(s)	Year	Sex	Age	Diarrhoea	Triad	Relationship	Age	Diarrhoea	Triad	Interval[a]
Koster & Jansen	1946	M	15	+	+	Brother	11	0	0	14 days
						Brother	3	0	0	15 days
Glauner	1947	M	15	+	+	Brother	10	+	+	Not given
Schoeneich	1950	F	13	+	+	Brother	7	0	+	3 days
Fabregoule	1951	M	40+	+	+	Wife	40+	+	0	Simultaneous
						Son	16	+	0	Simultaneous
Davies et al	1969	M	39	+	0	Son	11	+	+	3 days
						Son	7	+	+	Few days
Trier	1950	M	Adult	0	0	Bro-in-law	—	0	+	1 month
						Brother	37	0	0	20 months
Morton	1958	M	36	0	+	1st cousin (male)	27	0	+	10 years
Gough	1962	M	Adult	0	0	Son	15	0	+	Not given
Mowat & Nicol	1968	M	29	0	+	Brother	21	0	+	26 months
Csonka	1969	M	31	0	+	Brother	34	0	+	9 months
		M	27	0	+	Brother	25	0	+	6 months
Good	1971	M	23	0	+	Brother	46	0	+	17 years

[a] Interval between onset index case to onset secondary case(s).

increased prevalence of sacroiliitis, spondylitis, and of psoriasis among relatives.

Aetiology

Reiter's disease usually follows an infection of the bowel or lower genitourinary tract. Enterocolitic agents which have been implicated as triggers are *Shigella flexneri* (serotypes 2a and 1b), *Salmonella typhimurium*, *Salmonella enteritidis*, *Salmonella heidelberg*, *Yersinia enterocolitica* (Marsal et al, 1981), *Yersinia pseudoberculosus*, and *Campylobacter fetus* (Weir et al, 1979; Urman et al, 1977). The nature of the agent responsible for the disease and its manner of operation are not clear. It has been suggested that the spinal changes might be due to an infective agent draining directly via the prostatic venous plexus to the sacroiliac joints (Grainger, 1959), or by the venous system described by Batson (1942) passing from the prostate and seminal vesicles to the sacroiliac joints (Oates & Young, 1959). This may also be the explanation of the sacroiliitis in women, occurring as a late sequel to acute salpingitis (Hagenfeldt & Szanto, 1980). A piece of evidence favouring this view is that sacroiliitis is said to occur in patients with paraplegia (Abel, 1950; Lodge, 1956). It was felt that genital inflammation causing sacroiliitis was 'a seductive hypothesis' (Mason et al, 1958), since nearly all the male paraplegic patients would be expected to have chronic prostatitis. A careful study of bone and joint changes in paraplegic men was unable to substantiate this (Wright et al, 1965). Sacroiliac changes occurred in 12 of 38 patients, but the changes differed from sacroiliitis. They appeared to be due to mechanical stresses operating on osteoporotic bones around the joints. There was no evidence to connect the sacroiliac joint changes with chronic genitourinary infection, but they were found more frequently in patients whose admission to a special unit had been delayed, in those who had been confined to bed for longer periods, and in those whose mobilisation had been delayed.

Much effort has been expended in trying to isolate an infective agent from patients with Reiter's disease (Levy et al, 1966), but so far without consistent success. Intermittently, the role of pleuropneumonia-like organisms (PPLO) has excited attention, and some have claimed to isolate them from patients with Reiter's disease (Bartholomew, 1965). Others have not been so successful (Ford & Rasmussen, 1964). PPLO cause arthritis in animals (Decker & Ward, 1966), but their role in Reiter's disease is far from clear. No virus has been implicated yet, despite strenuous efforts (Ford & Rasmussen, 1964).

More recently, attention has been directed to the *Bedsonia* genus of organisms (psittacocis-lymphogranuloma venereum-trachoma group). In sheep, *Bedsonia* cause arthritis, conjunctivitis and orchitis (Norton & Storz, 1967). They have been isolated from the synovium, urethra and conjunctiva of some patients with Reiter's disease (Engelman & Weber, 1967), and some of the patients also had complement-fixation titres of 1 : 16 or more against a Bedsonia group antigen (Schachter et al, 1966). *Chlamydia trachomatis* has been implicated as a probable causal agent (Vilppula et al, 1981), but other studies have not confirmed this, although there may be exaggerated antibody response to acute infection by *Chlamydia* (Keat et al, 1980).

It should be remembered that it is difficult to demonstrate an association between a disease and a virtually universal phenomenon, sexual intercourse. Furthermore, non-gonococcal urethritis is a feature of post-dysenteric Reiter's syndrome, occurring without sexual exposure. Urethritis is, therefore, an inherent feature of Reiter's syndrome, and need be considered only as another mucocutaneous lesion which is not necessarily a marker for the portal of entry of an infectious agent (Arnett, 1982).

It is possible that an infective agent initiates the disease and that many of its manifestations are immunologically produced. This may be the explanation for the prostatic antibodies found by a haemagglutination test in these patients (Grimble & Lessof, 1965). On the other hand, prostatititis from whatever cause could well produce such antiprostatic antibodies (Grimble, 1964). In rats, inoculation with complete Freund adjuvant produces a polyarthritis with an acute balanitis and urethritis, iritis or iridocyclitis and dermatitis (Pearson, 1963).

The most probable explanation of these features is that patients genetically predisposed to the disease develop it after exposure to an infective agent acquired either by venereal exposure or in a dysenteric attack. The high frequency of HLA-B27 antigen in patients with Reiter's disease (Brewerton et al, 1973; Morris et al, 1974; Brewerton et al, 1974; McCluskey et al, 1974) favours this suggestion, as discussed by Metzger et al (1974). However, it should be noted that only 20% of B27-positive persons develop arthritis after attacks of shigellosis, salmonellosis or yersinosis (Woodrow, 1979). This is a similar figure to the occurrence of sacroiliitis in B27 subjects from the population, and raises the possibility that these two diseases may be appearing independently in the same genetically predisposed host. The findings of immunoproteins in the synovium of the majority of patients with Reiter's syndrome, suggests that immunological mechanisms are involved in the pathogenesis of the disease (Baldassare et al, 1981). The findings of Ford and his colleagues (1980, 1981) would support this.

Clinical features

There is a wide spectrum of Reiter's disease. It is difficult to determine the frequency of various features, since some authors insist on the complete triad for the diagnosis of Reiter's disease, whereas others have less stringent criteria. This has been well shown by two published series of patients (Table 31.2).

In both the venereal and the diarrhoeal forms of Reiter's disease the arthritis begins between 1 and 3 weeks after the initial symptom. The average time is about 15 days.

Diarrhoea tends to be mild, short-lived and with absence of blood. The urethritis, likewise, is usually a mild disease with a mucoid urethral discharge, which is rarely bloodstained (Colby, 1944; Twiss & Douglas, 1946; Ford, 1953b; Reiter, 1957). There is usually some dysuria and occasionally the discharge may be purulent. Frequency of micturition is common and bladder involvement produces suprapubic discomfort.

Urogenital lesions

The non-specific urethritis associated with the beginning of the venereally-acquired disease may be asymptomatic and detected only by examination of the first urine specimen in the morning (the two-glass test) when shreds of mucoid material may be seen. Occasionally, however, it is severe. Acute haemorrhagic cystitis, confirmed cystoscopically, occurs (Berg et al, 1957; Berry & Berry, 1947) and prostatitis is an almost invariable accompaniment of the disease. This is diagnosed by examining the fluid obtained on prostatic massage and observing 10 or more leucocytes per half inch microscopic field. Interpretation of such findings must be cautious, however, and although prostatitis of this degree is an invariable accompaniment of Reiter's disease, the converse, that prostatitis is an evidence of genitourinary infection, should not be assumed. In men who are otherwise normal, 25% have evidence of 'chronic prostatitis' on these criteria (Oates, 1959; Catterall, 1960) and men with rheumatoid arthritis have a similar frequency (Mason et al, 1958).

Cystitis, which is said to occur in about 3% of patients (Paronen, 1948; Harkness, 1950; Csonka, 1958a), may produce serious shrinkage of the bladder (Piora, 1953) and cases of hydronephrosis arising from ureteric stenosis (Colby, 1944; Harkness, 1950) have been described.

Urethritis is frequent in the dysenteric form of Reiter's disease (Young & McEwen, 1947; Paronen, 1948; Noer, 1966). This raises the possibility that inflammation of the urogenital tract may be due to mechanisms other than direct infection, although there is no information on the incidence of prostatitis in these patients. Conversely, diarrhoea may occur in venereally-acquired Reiter's disease and has been reported in 32% of the patients described by Weinberger et al (1962) and 22% of those described by Hall & Finegold (1953).

Circinate balanitis is a characteristic feature of

Table 31.2 Frequency of complications in two series of cases with Reiter's disease

Authors	Series	No. of cases	% eye lesions	% mouth lesions	% penile lesions	% keratoderma
Montgomery et al (1959)	Triple	38	92	37+	80	30
Hancock (1960)	Unselected	76	44.7	10.5	26.3	7.8

the disease. It has the appearance of keratoderma elsewhere. The frequency of balanitis (26%) in the dysenteric form is similar to the figures of Hancock in the disease venereally acquired. Its appearance is influenced by whether the patient is circumcised. In uncircumcised subjects the initial lesion is a superficial ulcer of small diameter which may coalesce with others to form circinate patches. As these develop a clear centre is left and a scaly border appears. In the circumcised patient, however, the lesions may be discrete and the scaly border very hyperkeratotic (Montgomery et al, 1959; Weinberger et al, 1962). A classical example is shown in Figure 31.2. Circinate vulvitis has also been described (Thambar et al, 1977).

At the onset the patient may be pyrexial with a temperature reaching 103°F. Three-quarters of the patients in the literature are said to have had a raised temperature.

Arthritis

Joint symptoms are characteristically acute, short-lived and transient. A patient may have undoubted non-specific urethritis and then develop an acute monarticular arthritis which subsides within 3 or 4 days, regardless of the type of treatment.

Weight-bearing joints, particularly the knees and ankles, are most frequently involved initially (Fig. 31.3). The activity of arthritis may be extremely acute and attended by large tense

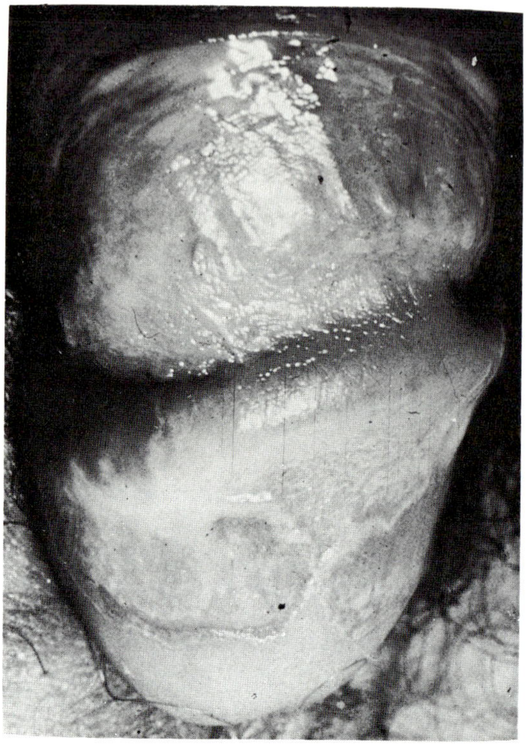

Fig. 31.2 Circinate balanitis.

effusions; this is particularly well seen at the knee which has been known to rupture early in the course of the disease (Weese & McCarthy, 1969; Garner & Mowat, 1972; Moll, 1973).

In nearly a quarter of patients the arthritis starts

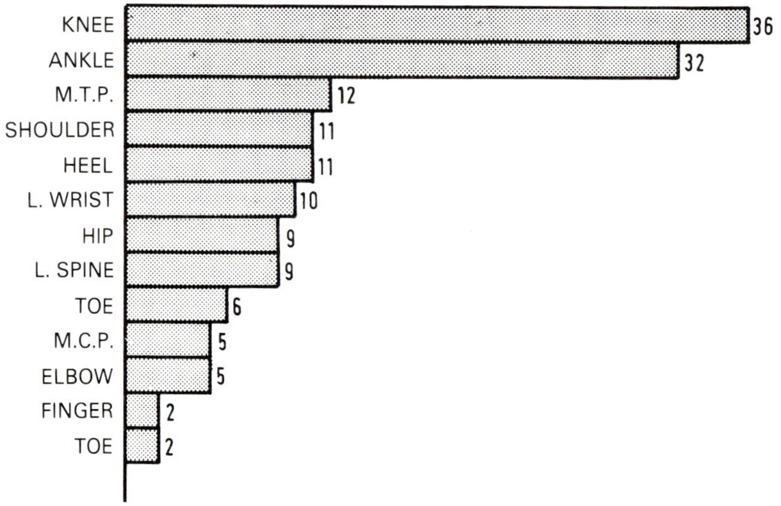

Fig. 31.3 Joints involved at onset of Reiter's disease.

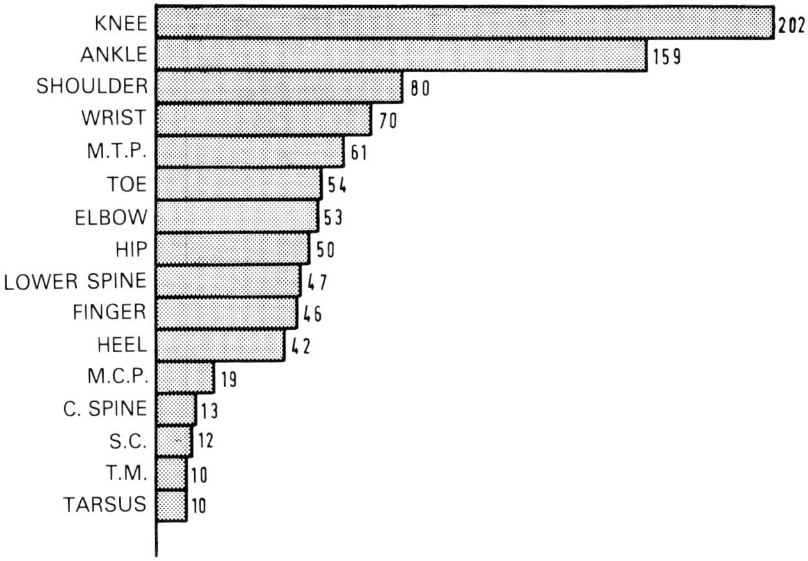

Fig. 31.4 Joints involved during the course of Reiter's disease.

in one joint. The arthritis may become widespread, and occasionally involves most joints of the body. More often it is confined to five or six joints, and the knees and ankles remain predominantly affected (Fig. 31.4). The arthritis is commonly asymmetrical.

A feature of the disease is the occurrence of fleeting pains in the back, the plantar fascia, the heels, the chest wall, and soft tissues of the lower limbs. The tendon sheaths may be involved, especially around the tendo Achilles, although tenosynovitis is not such a prominent feature as it is in gonococcal arthritis (Ford, 1953a; Wright, 1963). Csonka (1958a) found tendon involvement in 37 of 185 cases at the London Hospital.

Residual disability occurs in about 5% (Hancock & Mason, 1965). Permanent deformities of the feet (Fig. 31.5), pain at the insertion of the plantar fascia into the os calcis, metatarsophalangeal arthralgia, deformity of the fingers and spondylitis may

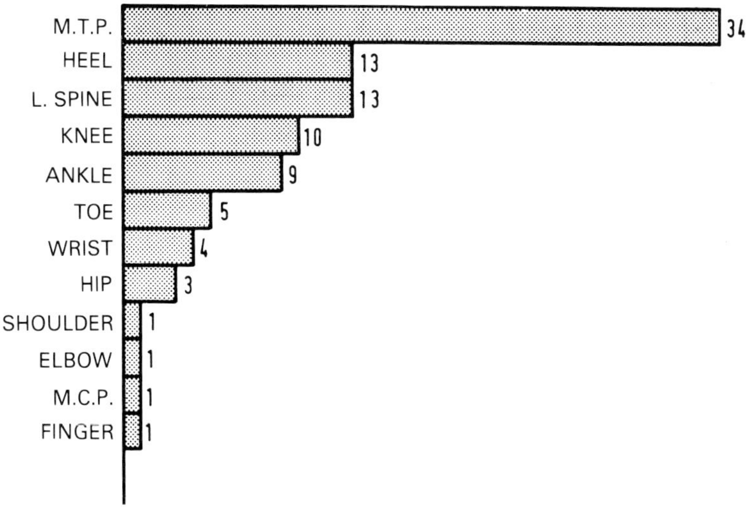

Fig. 31.5 Residual disability in Reiter's disease.

all occur. Precise data are not easily gleaned from the literature on this aspect, but in order of frequency the sites of residual symptoms appear to be metatarsophalangeal joints, heels, lumbar spine and knee.

Although Reiter's disease is self-limiting recurrences do occur. The more prolonged the follow-up of these patients the higher is the frequency of recurrence and Csonka (1960) in a 15-year experience of a single department found the likelihood of a second attack to be in the region of 62%. These recurrences may be associated with reinfection and more rarely with factors such as dilatation of urethral strictures, food poisoning, diarrhoea caused by antibiotics, tonsillitis (Csonka, 1958a), massage of the prostate (Olhagen, 1960), respiratory infections, and damage to the joints (Weinberger et al, 1962). It is interesting that a fresh infection producing non-specific urethritis does not necessarily provoke a recurrence of Reiter's disease (Csonka, 1960), and likewise a further attack of dysentery only preceded a second attack of arthritis in 4 of the 10 cases of recurrence reported by Paronen (1948). However, a longer follow-up study from 100 of the Finnish cases 20 years after the initial attack showed that only 20 patients had been free from symptoms since the original attack. In 32, symptoms and radiological findings of sacroiliitis or spondylitis were present, 18 had chronic active peripheral arthritis, and in 30 chronic arthritis had become inactive. A more or less severe disability was present in 42 patients (Sairanen et al, 1969).

The spinal involvement which is radiologically indistinguishable from ankylosing spondylitis (Ford, 1953b) is of particular interest.

Mason (1964) found sacroiliitis in 10% of patients with Reiter's disease of less than 5 years' duration and 54% of those of more than 5 years' duration. Comparable figures of Lawrence (1965) were 9% and 71%.

Ocular lesions

Conjunctivitis is part of the classical triad of Reiter's disease. Its reported incidence is higher in patients with dysentery, but these figure are of dubious significance since symptoms may be so mild as to escape the patient's notice (or at the most give the sensation of a little grittiness in the eye for a short time). The discharge is sterile and subsides in 1–4 weeks (Popert et al, 1964). The condition may progress, however, to produce episcleritis, keratitis, and corneal ulceration; uveitis may also occur. Uveitis affects less than 1 in 10 patients early in the course of the disease, but Ford (1953b) reported a frequency of 30% in patients with recurring chronic arthritis. Where sacroiliitis is present, half the patients may be affected (Csonka, 1959a). Looking at the problem from the opposite point of view Catterall (1961) examined 211 men with anterior uveitis in an opthalmological department and found Reiter's disease in 21.3% and ankylosing spondylitis in 12.3%.

Iritis may occur as an incident separate from arthritis in a protracted course of Reiter's disease. Less commonly intraocular haemorrhage or hypopyon (Paronen, 1948), optic neuritis (Zewi, 1947; Oates & Hancock, 1959), and retrobulbar neuritis (Lindsay-Rea, 1947) can also occur.

Integumentary lesions

Keratoderma blenorrhagica is the characteristic skin lesion of the disease (Fig. 31.6). In Hancock's series the rash occurred in 7.8%, whereas other authors quote figures as high as 30%. The lesions begin commonly on the soles of the feet, but may involve the palms and occasionally become extensive, spreading to the rest of the limbs, trunk, and scalp, and rarely involving the face. In such severe cases they may persist for as long as a year. Patients with the dysenteric form seem to have keratoderma less frequently and no more than 2% is the reported prevalence. Initially, the lesions occur as brown macules which progress to papulovesicles and pustules. Later, scales develop and the lesions come to resemble limpets.

The nails may be involved with a dystrophy affecting the whole nail, simulating the grosser changes of psoriasis (Fig. 31.7). Hyperkeratosis with heaping of cornified material under the nail can be severe enough to cause displacement or even shedding of the nail. Sometimes lakes of pus develop in the nailfold at the base and sides. Deep pits or even punched-out areas are also occasionally seen (Samman, 1972).

Histologically, the epidermis shows hyperkeratosis, parakeratosis and acanthosis, with irregular elongation of the rete ridges and frequent supra-

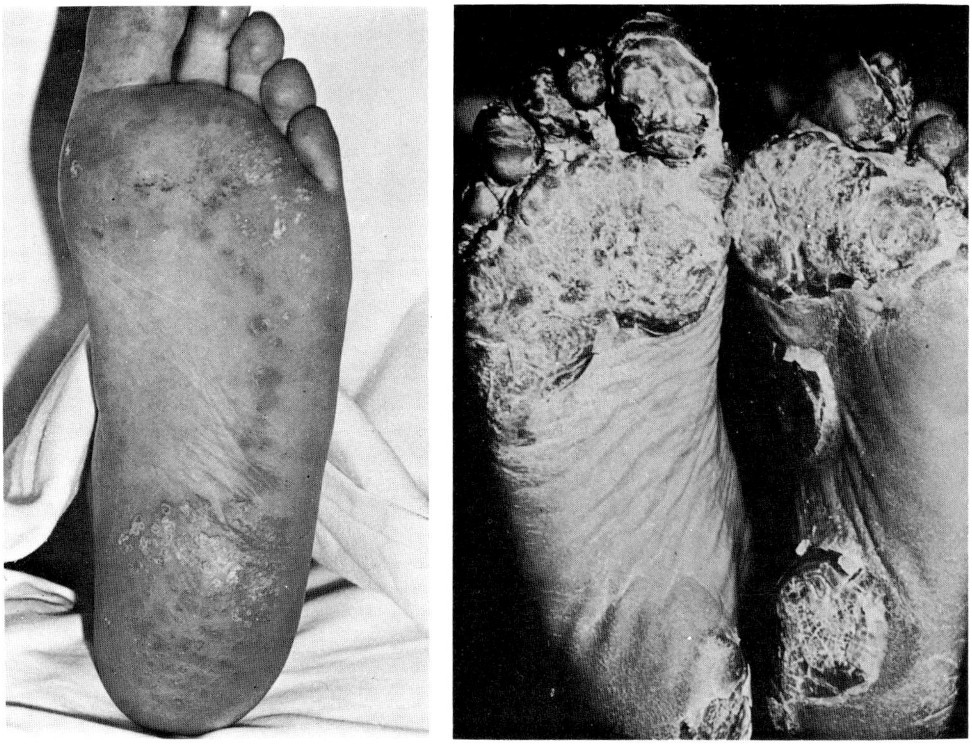

a b

Fig. 31.6 Keratoderma blenorrhagica. (a) Early lesions. (b) Advanced changes.

papillary thinning. There is a varying degree of vacuolisation and lysis of the superficial prickle cells, with focal neutrophil infiltration which may result in microabscesses. The papillary layer of the corium is infiltrated by lymphocytes and plasma cells with a few scattered neutrophils (Kulka, 1962; Weinberger et al, 1962; Wright & Reed, 1964: Maxwell et al, 1966). The appearances are indistinguishable from pustular psoriasis (Lever & Crawford, 1944), and 11 cases have been described in which the clinical appearance of the skin has progressed to frank psoriasis (Wright & Reed, 1964). This has since been confirmed by others (Khan & Hall, 1965; Maxwell et al, 1966; Perry & Mayne, 1965). It has been questioned whether this is not the coincidence of a fairly common disease, psoriasis, in these patients (Hancock, 1960), but careful observation lends support to the view that there is an association between Reiter's disease and psoriatic arthritis.

Oral lesions

Buccal erosions occur in about 8% of patients. They usually start as painless shiny red patches, and occur on the palate, tongue and mucosa of the cheeks or lips. Uncommonly, they proceed to confluent erythema of the soft palate, uvula and tonsillar regions, with purpura of the tongue (Montgomery et al, 1959; Hancock, 1960). Essentially, the histology of lesions affecting the skin,

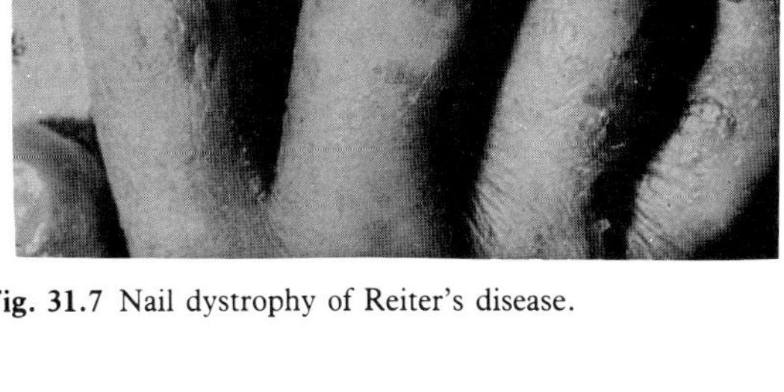

Fig. 31.7 Nail dystrophy of Reiter's disease.

glans penis and oral mucosa are the same. Epistaxis has occasionally been reported, and it may well have a similar basis.

Other lesions

Involvement of the heart is well recognised. Electrocardiographic changes include prolongation of the P-R interval (Feiring, 1945; Hall & Finegold, 1953; Csonka et al, 1961; Weinberger et al, 1962), complete heart block (Trier, 1950), and serial T-wave changes, elevation of the S-T segment or occasional abnormal Q-waves (Feiring, 1945; Vallee, 1946; Hall & Finegold, 1953; Weinberger et al, 1962). Clinically, the patient may complain of palpitations, and transient systolic murmurs may be heard (Paronen, 1948; Hall & Finegold, 1953; Masbernard, 1959). In the dysenteric form, cardiovascular complications occurred in 7% and a pericardial friction rub (or pericarditis) occurred in 2% (Paronen, 1948). This has also been noted in other series (Mayne, 1955; Csonka & Oates, 1957; Csonka et al, 1961).

Aortic incompetence has also been reported (Camp, 1956; Csonka et al, 1961; Cliff, 1971) in Reiter's disease. These lesions were indistinguishable from the aortic abnormality of ankylosing spondylitis. The prolonged follow-up of the Finnish series (Sairanen et al, 1969) showed serious heart disease in two patients (cardiac failure and total heart block).

Involvement of the central nervous system has been reported, but no consistent findings have emerged. The frequency of neurological complications is low, probably in the region of 1% (Hancock, 1964), and these include peripheral neuropathy (Walther, 1941; Wilke, 1943; Graby et al, 1949), neuritis of the shoulder girdle (Wilke, 1943; Oates & Hancock, 1959), transient hemiplegia (Lagon et al, 1955), and meningoencephalitis (Oates & Hancock, 1959). Cranial nerve lesions may also occur (Walther, 1941; Zewi, 1947; Csonka, 1958b).

In the respiratory system, pleurisy and pulmonary infiltrations have been reported in Reiter's disease (Thiers & Pinet, 1950; Lafon et al, 1955). Considering other similarities between Reiter's disease and ankylosing spondylitis it is interesting that recently lung lesions have also been reported in the latter. These consist of chronic infiltrative and fibrotic changes in the upper lobes (Hamilton, 1949; Campbell & MacDonald, 1965; Jessamine, 1968). This clinical and radiological picture appears to differ from the transient pulmonary infiltration reported in Reiter's disease.

Purpura (Makari, 1950), thrombophlebitis (Csonka, 1966), amyloidosis (Bleehen et al, 1966) and severe haemorrhage from gastrointestinal ulceration (Boyle & Buchanan, 1971) may all complicate Reiter's disease, but are rare.

Radiological features

In the early stages no abnormality is found radiologically. Later, however, particularly in patients with recurrent disease, juxta-articular osteoporosis, narrowing of the joint space, and erosive changes are all found (Guck & Wolf, 1952; Ford, 1953a; Mason et al, 1959; Reynolds & Csonka, 1958). The last authors described ankylosis of the small joints of the hands and feet as a rare finding, and this was also noted by Twiss & Douglas (1946) and Weldon & Scalettar (1961).

Periostitis may be a striking feature at times, occurring along the metatarsals, phalanges of the feet, tarsal bones, and around the pubis. Roughness at the insertion of the plantar fascia is also fairly characteristic of the disease (Fig. 31.8). Plantar spurs in Reiter's disease are typically large and fluffy although smooth spurs of smaller size and similar to those seen in rheumatoid arthritis

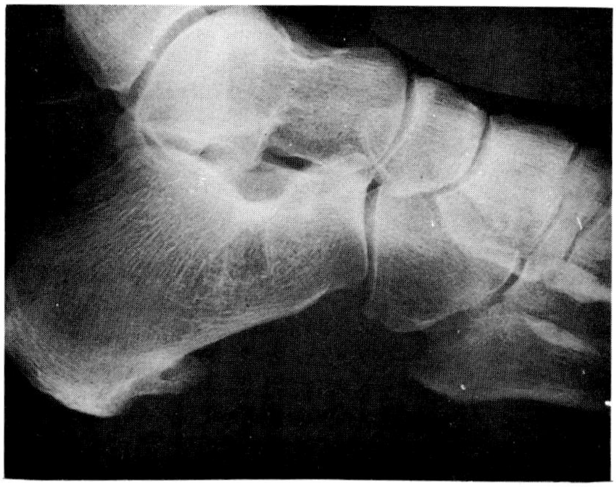

Fig. 31.8 Florid plantar spur in a man with Reiter's disease.

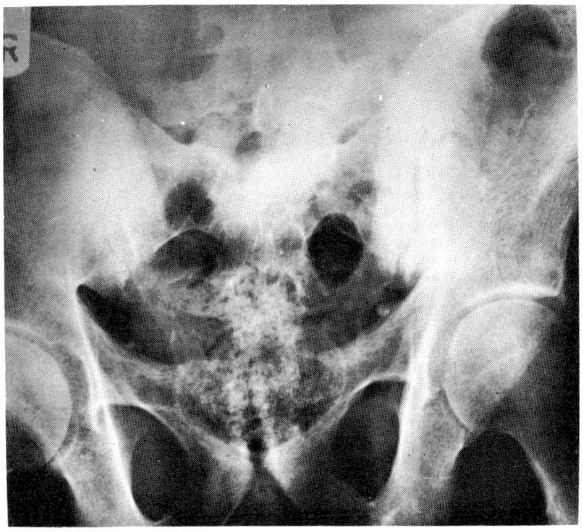

Fig. 31.9 Sacroiliitis in Reiter's disease.

and ankylosing spondylitis may also occur (Mason et al, 1959).

Changes of sacroiliitis are indistinguishable from those accompanying ankylosing spondylitis (Fig. 31.9). Sacroiliitis may be asymmetrical and in 17% of one series the changes were unilateral (Oates & Young, 1959). Sacroiliac involvement is found particularly in patients with longstanding, recurrent disease, and figures as high as 80% have been quoted (Marche, 1950). However, the usual frequency is nearer 30%. The longer the duration of the disease, the higher is the frequency (Mason, 1964; Lawrence, 1965). Patients who go on to develop psoriatic arthritis nearly all show some changes in the sacroiliac joints (Wright & Reed, 1964).

Some patients demonstrate apophyseal joint erosion and ankylosis, together with ligamentous calcification indistinguishable from that seen in uncomplicated ankylosing spondylitis (Ford, 1953a). It has been suggested that a characteristic finding in the early stage of spinal involvement in Reiter's disease is an isolated bony spur on a single vertebral body (Cliff, 1971). McEwen et al (1971) felt that the radiological picture of these patients was the same as in psoriatic arthritis, but different from that seen in uncomplicated ankylosing spondylitis.

Cliff (1971) reported three cases with unusual lateral bony bridging between the vertebral bodies of the dorsal spine and dorsolumbar junction. Two of these patients had a febrile illness erroneously attributed to subacute bacterial endocarditis, and all had aortic incompetence. This unusual type of spinal bony bridging (Fig. 31.10) was also noted by Weldon & Scolettar (1961), Montgomery et al, (1963), Good (1965) and Peterson & Silbiger (1967). The association with aortic value disease was described in one case by Rodnan et al (1964). These bony lesions must be distinguished from senile ankylosing hyperostosis of the spine (Forestier & Rotes-Querol, 1950) and the rare familial ankylosing vertebral hyperostosis (Beardwell, 1969). The skip lesions of the spine have certain similarities to the unusual progressive paraspinal calcification of psoriatic arthritis. Indeed, this may be another area where there is 'overlap', since some of the cases described by Bywaters & Dixon (1965) as examples of psoriatic arthritis also had features of Reiter's disease. Martel (1979) has described these as discontinuous spondylitis characterised by eccentric, laterally positioned vertebral hyperostoses which tend to bridge around the contiguous disc. He believes that these are characteristic, together with subtle periosteal bone

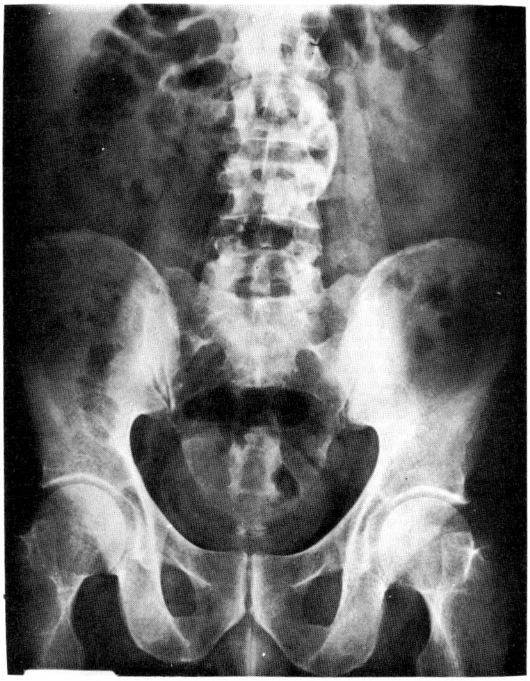

Fig. 31.10 Spinal bony bridging.

apposition of bony prominences, the increased frequency of regional panarthritis and hip and shoulder involvement, and the tendency for destructive arthritis to be confined to small joints, particularly in the feet.

Pathology

Where biopsy material is available, the unhelpful but accurate report of 'non-specific inflammation' is usually returned. Initially, there is oedema with vascular congestion and moderate infiltration of neutrophils, lymphocytes and occasional plasma cells, together with some proliferation of synoviocytes and fibroblasts. In specimens taken later in the disease, the changes are principally lymphocytic, and show perivenular infiltration of lymphocytes and plasma cells, and lymphocyte nodules which are indistinguishable from those of rheumatoid arthritis (Weinberger et al, 1962).

Biopsy of the skin lesions shows changes of keratoderma blenorrhagica or pustular psoriasis, and these have been discussed in Chapter 30. The mucous membrane lesions show similar changes.

Synovial Fluid

Examination of the synovial fluid reveals little that would not be expected with an inflammatory exudate. There is a protein content in the region of 50 g/litre and the mucin clot is poor (Weinberger et al, 1962); there is an elevated white count between 1000 and 50 000 cells/mm^3 of which 66% are polymorphonuclear leucocytes, although this proportion may be as high as 97% (Ellis & Bereston, 1959). Occasionally the joint fluid can contain so many polymorphs as to appear purulent, though sterile. This is important in the differential diagnosis from infective arthritis. In 20 joint aspirates reported in the literature, the mean white count was 18 000. The glucose was low in 3 of 11 patients in one series (Sharp et al, 1968), and in 13 of 23 in another (Weinberger et al, 1962), the mean being 16 mg/100 ml. It has been suggested that one feature distinguishing rheumatoid arthritis is the normal total haemolytic complement in Reiter's disease contrasted with low titres in rheumatoid arthritis (Fostiropoulos et al, 1965). However, synovial fluid : serum complement values appear to be reduced in Reiter's disease (Yates et al, 1975).

Blood tests

The ESR is often considerably raised and may be as high as 140 mm/h; this may persist for weeks after the acute attack and does not necessarily parallel joint activity. A mild hypo- or normochromic anaemia (Hall & Finegold, 1953; Sargent, 1945) may be present, together with leucocytosis, the white cell count occasionally rising to 32 000/mm^3 (Hamner & Grayowski, 1964). In these circumstances bacterial infection of a joint has to be excluded by diagnostic aspiration.

Serum proteins show little change apart from an occasional decrease in the albumen and an increase in the alpha 1 and alpha 2 globulin fractions. Serum uric acid is usually within the normal range (Young & McEwen, 1947; Csonka, 1959; Weinberger et al, 1962; Hancock, 1964; Noer, 1966).

There are few serological abnormalities. Rheumatoid factor, whether determined by the latex fixation test or the Rose–Waaler differential agglutination test, is usually absent from the sera in these patients (McEwen et al, 1958; Csonka, 1959; Kellgren et al, 1959; Oates & Csonka, 1959; Hancock, 1964). Anti-nuclear factor is negative and LE cells are absent (Noer, 1966). A haemaglutination test for prostatic antibodies (Grimble, 1964) is commonly positive, but is not specific. One-third of patients with ankylosing spondylitis have positive results, and the test has proved positive in 20% of women.

A striking laboratory development in Reiter's disease is the demonstration of a high proportion of HLA-B27-positive tests (75%) in Reiter's disease contrasted with only 9% in uncomplicated non-specific urethritis and 6% in controls (Brewerton et al, 1973).

In this study, HLA-B27 was particularly associated with patients with Reiter's disease complicated by ankylosing spondylitis, an observation confirmed by Bluestone et al (1973). The precise implications of these interesting results are still not clear, but it would seem that if a patient with non-specific urethritis is HLA-B27-positive he has a higher than expected chance of developing the full picture of Reiter's disease. Furthermore if a patient with Reiter's disease is HLA-B27-positive it might be expected that sacroiliitis or ankylosing spondylitis will be present, or if not present, it may be reasonable to keep the patient under close review in anticipation of its development in the future.

Differential diagnosis

The acute nature of the arthritis may raise the question of infective arthritis, systemic lupus erythematosus, osteomyelitis, brucellosis, rheumatic fever, gout and pseudogout. The multiple joint involvement, the distribution of joints involved, the relationship to non-specific urethritis or dysentery, and the course of the disease are all useful pointers. Where pyogenic arthritis is suspected, diagnostic aspiration is mandatory. Aspiration may also help to differentiate gout and pseudogout in that characteristic crystals of uric acid or calcium pyrophosphate may be seen with polarised microscopy. The presence of chondrocalcinosis radiologically may also alert the clinician to the possibility of pseudogout.

The differential diagnosis may be particularly difficult when the complete triad is not present. Yet few would doubt that 'incomplete' forms of the disease occur. The ocular lesions may be minimal, being experienced merely as a sense of grittiness in the eyes or indeed escaping the notice of the patients altogether. The urethral discharge may be barely perceptible (especially in women), or it may be denied even to those most skilful in extracting a history of venereal exposure. The course of the illness is similar in the incomplete forms, although the frequency of other features may be greater in patients with the complete triad (Table 31.2).

Although the chronic phase may mimic rheumatoid arthritis, the asymmetrical nature of the arthritis (particularly at its onset), the persistent absence of rheumatoid factor in the serum, and the involvement of the sacroiliac joints are all useful in differentiating the condition. A high ESR at the start of the illness may also point to the diagnosis of Reiter's disease rather than rheumatoid arthritis.

It has been suggested that the normal total haemolytic complement in the synovial fluid, compared with the low value in rheumatoid arthritis, may also be helpful in diagnosis. However, the synovial fluid : serum complement levels appear to be reduced in Reiter's disease (Yates et al, 1975).

In the venereally-acquired form of Reiter's disease gonococcal arthritis is the most important disease to differentiate. Gonococcal arthritis can only be diagnosed with certainty by culture of the organism from the synovial fluid. However, if it is cultured from the urethral discharge, the infection merits treatment in its own right, and the arthritis will subside dramatically and completely with penicillin or sulphonamides (Wright, 1963).

Psoriatic arthritis, Behçet's syndrome, and the Stevens–Johnson syndrome must also be considered. Genital ulceration is a common feature of true Behçet's syndrome, and the ocular involvement is usually more severe than in Reiter's disease, sometimes producing blindness. It has been suggested that in the Stevens–Johnson syndrome the skin lesions are less pustular than in Reiter's disease and not keratotic. The mucocutaneous lesions of these diseases have been well discussed by Robinson & McCrumb (1950). When psoriasis vulgaris and keratoderma blenorrhagica coexist it is impossible to make a distinction between psoriatic arthritis and Reiter's disease, since even the more florid lesions of the two conditions are indistinguishable clinically and histologically.

Management

There is no form of treatment that can consistently prevent attacks of Reiter's disease from progressing, can cause clear-cut and substantial reductions in the duration of established attacks, or can prevent the development of subsequent attacks. Treatment of all features is empirical and is aimed at reducing symptoms and the intensity of the inflammatory process until the disease undergoes a spontaneous remission. Specific treatment is, of course, available for antecedent dysentery or associated gonorrhoea.

The tetracyclines are usually preferred for the non-specific urethritis of Reiter's disease because they are most effective in the treatment of uncomplicated non-specific urethritis. (However, there is still no incontrovertible evidence to show that the two types of urethritis have the same cause.) A dose of 250 mg of tetracycline or oxytetracycline 6-hourly for 5 days is often sufficient. Continuing the treatment for longer appears to provide no further benefit unless *Chlamydia* have been isolated (Schofield, 1972). If there is a response, this is usually noted within 24–72 hours when dysuria, and the volume and purulence of the discharge diminish. Thereafter, the discharge may disappear altogether or remain as a scanty mucopurulent secretion detectable only by the early morning two-glass test. Even in patients without overt urethritis it is advisable to have an examination by a genito-urinary physician.

In patients with haemorrhagic cystitis tetracycline may be effective, and to relieve dysuria and strangury, potassium citrate and hyoscyamus mixture *BPC* is often beneficial.

When the activity of the urethritis, arthritis or ocular inflammation is controlled it is King's policy to examine the prostate, as chronic prostatitis (more accurately prostatovesiculitis) is almost invariably present (King, 1964). If prostatitis is present, twice-weekly prostatic massage and a 5-day course of tetracycline are given. During recovery serial examination of the prostate fluid may show diminution of the proportion of polymorphonuclear leucocytes and a decrease in their tendency to clump together. In other cases, despite subjective relief, the fluid remains the same.

While under treatment for the urogenital disorder, the patient should abstain from sexual activity and steps should be taken to examine the patient's sexual partner to exclude similar or other venereal disease, particularly gonorrhoea. Advice on the avoidance of promiscuous activity and the risk of recurrence should be given.

Schofield (1972) has suggested that the management of the urethritis is not complete without urethroscopy. This should be done after active urethritis has subsided in order to exclude urethral stricture, even if this complication is not suggested by clinical features. Outpatient review should be continued for a long time, preferably several years.

As far as the arthritis is concerned, preferably all but the mildest cases should be admitted to hospital and confined to strict rest in bed. Splinting should be minimal, but if necessary should be used for the shortest time in view of the risk of fibrous ankylosis. Muscle wasting, particularly of the quadriceps, may be marked in Reiter's disease and requires appropriate physical treatment. Severe cases will normally need indomethacin 100–150 mg daily individed doses. This produces substantial pain relief, often within a few days. When symptomatic relief has been obtained, the dose is reduced gradually. Other non-steroidal anti-inflammatory drugs may be equally effective, but have not been tried so extensively. A valuable guide to the activity of the disease is continuing fever. The ESR, which may be considerably elevated, is less reliable, sometimes remaining elevated long after improvement of other features has taken place. The patient's feeling of well-being and his response to exercise are better guides than the height of the sedimentation rate as to whether or not to discharge the patient from hospital.

Indomethacin should be continued for about the first month of outpatient supervision. If gastric intolerance arises other non-steroidal anti-inflammatory drugs may be used, but high doses will probably be required. Corticosteroids are indicated in patients with severe disease of acute onset attended by much pain, rapid wasting, continued fever, and high and increasing sedimentation rate which have failed to respond to indomethacin within a few days. Adequate control is likely to need large doses of corticosteroid (up to 60 mg of prednisolone or its equivalent). The symptoms of Reiter's disease tend to be more resistent to corticosteroids than those of rheumatoid arthritis.

The use of cytotoxic or immunosuppressive agents in severe or intractable Reiter's disease is not yet established. Methotrexate has been used successfully, according to uncontrolled studies (Mullins et al, 1966; Farber et al, 1967). Other antimitotic agents such as 6MP, azathioprine and cyclophosphamide also appear capable of suppressing Reiter's disease in tolerable doses (Sharp, 1972). However, all these preparations are potentially toxic drugs and are not recommended for general use, especially in those of reproductive age. On the other hand, there may be a place for their selective use, particularly in patients with severe or prolonged episodes of Reiter's disease with permanent residua which have been refractory to simpler forms of therapy. The management of acute recurrent attacks of Reiter's disease is similar to that of first attacks.

Pain in the region of the plantar fascia or Achilles tendon may be controlled by local corticosteroid injection. Effusions of the knees, which may be large, should be aspirated; they respond to intra-articular injections of corticosteroid.

Mild and transient conjunctivitis needs no local

treatment. When it is severe, however, the position is more difficult. It is generally felt by opthalmologists that corticosteroids alone are contraindicated in view of the possibility that Reiter's disease may be due to infection by a virus. This objection has not yet been tested by controlled study. Furthermore patients with conjunctivitis receiving systemic steroids for the arthritis have experienced no worsening of the conjunctivitis, and Jacobs (1961) has used topical steroid therapy without harm. However, until more evidence is available, it is probably judicious to withhold local steroids for conjunctivitis. Some clinicians use frequent instillations of chloramphenical drops until the conjunctivitis remits in order to reduce the chances of secondary infection.

All cases of anterior uveitis should have skilled opthalmological management. This usually includes dark glasses to relieve photophobia, atropine to dilate the pupil and to prevent adhesions of the iris, and topical corticosteroids to suppress inflammation. In severe cases systemic steroids may be necessary.

Keratoderma usually requires no treatment. Topical chlortetracycline (Cameron, 1956), penicillin, streptomycin and broad spectrum antibiotics (Levy, 1950; Ford, 1953b; Fowler & Knight, 1956; Albert & Crone, 1959; Montgomery et al, 1959), and corticosteroids (Myerson & Katzenstein, 1952; Schwartz & Kingma, 1952; Ford, 1953; Albert & Crone, 1959; Montgomery et al, 1959) have met with doubtful therapeutic success. Local triamcinolone, in view of its beneficial effect in psoriasis, is now being tried in Reiter's disease by some workers, but the results have not yet been formally evaluated. Aminopterin or methotrexate may afford complete or partial remission of keratoderma (Maxwell et al, 1966; Mullins et al, 1966), but in view of the frequency of serious side-effects these drugs are not recommended for routine use.

The moist lesions of circinate balanitis can usually be completely suppressed with applications of hydrocortisone or other corticosteroid cream. These preparations are best combined with an antibiotic in uncircumcised patients in order to deter secondary infection.

Mouth ulcers are usually pain-free and rarely require special treatment.

The infrequent but important occurrence of cardiac and neurological complications in Reiter's disease constitutes an indication for systemic corticosteroids (Schofield, 1972).

REFERENCES

Abel M S 1950 Sacroiliac joint changes in traumatic paraplegics. Radiology 55:235
Albert J, Crowe R 1959 Keratosis blennorrhagica (Reiter's disease?) and its treatment. Archives of Dermatology 79:581
Arnett F C 1982 Reiter's syndrome. Johns Hopkins Medical Journal 150: 39–44
Baldassare A R, Weiss T D, Tsai C C, Arthur R E, Moore T L, Zuckner J 1981 Immunoprotein deposition in synovial tissue in Reiter's syndrome. Annals of the Rheumatic Diseases 40: 281–285
Bartholomew L E 1965 Isolation and characterization of PPLO from patients with rheumatoid arthritis and Reiter's syndrome. Arthritis and Rheumatism 8:376
Batson O V 1942 Role of vertebral veins in metastatic processes. Annals of Internal Medicine 16:38
Bauer W, Engelman E P 1942 Syndrome of unknown aetiology characterized by urethritis, conjunctivitis, and arthritis (so-called Reiter's disease). Transactions of the Association of American Physicians 57:307
Beardwell A 1969 Familial ankylosing vertebral hyperostosis with tylosis. Annals of the Rheumatic Diseases 28:518
Berg R L, Weinberger H, Dienes L 1957 Acute haemorrhagic cystitis. American Journal of Medicine 22:848
Berry J V, Berry N E 1947 Acute exudative cystitis of undetermined aetiology. Journal of Urology 58:260
Bleehen S S, Everall J D, Tighe J R 1966 Amyloidosis complicating Reiter's syndrome. British Journal of Venereal Diseases 42:88
Bluestone R H, Schlosstein L H, Terasaki P, Pearson C M 1973 Paper presented at XIII International Congress of Rheumatology, Kyoto, Japan
Boyle J A, Buchanan W W 1971 Clinical rheumatology, 1st Edn. Blackwell, Oxford
Brewerton D, Caffrey M, Nicholls A, James D C O 1974 The histocompatility antigen (HL-A27) and its relation to disease. Journal of Rheumatology 1:249
Brewerton D A, Caffrey M, Nicholls A, Walters D, Oates J K, James D C O 1973 Reiter's disease and HL-A27. Lancet 2:996
Brodie B C 1818 Pathological and surgical obsercations on diseases of the joints. Longman, London, p 54
Bywaters E G, Dixon A St J 1965 Paravertebral ossifications in psoriatic arthritis. Annals of the Rheumatic Diseases 24:313
Cameron J M 1956 Keratodermia blennorhagica. British Journal of Veneral Diseases 32:7
Camp S 1956 Zur Klinik und Prognose der Reiter'schen Krankheit. Münchener medizinische Wochenschrift 98:334
Campbell A H, MacDonald C B 1965 Upper lobe fibrosis

associated with ankylosing spondylitis. British Journal of Diseases of the Chest 59:90
Catterall R D 1960 Uveitis, arthritis, and non-specific genital infection. British Journal of Veneral Diseases 36:27
Catterall R D 1961 Significance of non-specific genital infection in uveitis and arthritis. Lancet 2:739
Cliff J M 1971 Spinal bony bridging and carditis in Reiter's disease. Annals of the Rheumatic Diseases 30:171
Colby F 1944 Renal complications of Reiter's disease. Journal of Urology 52:415
Corner B D 1950 Reiter's syndrome in childhood. Archives of Disease in Childhood 25:398
Csonka G W 1958a The course of Reiter's syndrome. British Medical Journal 1:1088
Csonka G W 1958b Involvement of the nervous system in Reiter's syndrome. Annals of the Rheumatic Diseases 17:334
Csonka G W 1959 Bacteriological and biochemical investigation in Reiter's syndrome. British Journal of Venereal Diseases 35:84
Csonka G W 1960 Recurrent attacks in Reiter's disease. Arthritis and Rheumatism 3:164
Csonka G W 1966 Thrombophlebitis in Reiter's syndrome. British Journal of Venereal Diseases 42:93
Csonka G W 1969 Multiple cases in Reiter's syndrome. British Journal of Venereal Diseases 45:157
Csonka G W, Litchfield J W, Oates J K, Willcox R R 1961 Cardiac lesions in Reiter's disease. British Medical Journal 1:243
Csonka G W, Oates J K 1957 Pericarditis and electrocardiographic changes in Reiter's syndrome. British Medical Journal 1:866
Davies N E, Haverly J R, Boatwright M 1969 Reiter's disease associated with Shigellosis. Southern Medical Journal (Birmingham, Alabama) 62:1011
Decker J L, Ward J R 1966 The relationship of mycoplasma (PPLO) to RA and related diseases — working conference. Bulletin on Rheumatic Diseases 16:412
Ellis F A, Bereston E S 1959 Reiter's syndrome versus keratosis blenorrhagica sine blenorrhoea. Southern Medical Journal 52:828
Engleman E, Weber H M 1968 Reiter's syndrome. Clinical Orthopaedics 57:19
Fabregoule M 1951 Syndrome familial de Fiessinger–Leroy–Reiter syndrome. Algérie médicale 55:1054
Farber G A, Forshner J G, O'Quinn S E 1967 Reiter's syndrome: treatment with Methotrexate. Journal of the American Medical Association 200:171
Feiring W 1945 Reiter's disease with prolonged auricolo-ventricular conduction. Annals of Internal Medicine 25:498
Florman A L, Goldstein H M 1948 Arthritis, conjunctivities, and urethritis (so-called Reiter's syndrome) in a four-year old boy. Journal of Pediatrics 33:172
Ford D K 1953a Natural history of arthritis following venereal urethritis. Annals of the Rheumatic Diseases 12:177
Ford D K 1953b Arthritis and venereal disease. British Journal of Venereal Diseases 29:123
Ford D K 1958 Reiter's syndrome. Bulletin on Rheumatic Diseases 8:159
Ford D K, Rasmussen G 1964 Relationship between genitourinary infection and complicating arthritis. Arthritis and Rheumatism 7:220
Ford D K, Da Roza D M Shah P, Wenman W M 1980 Cell-mediated immune responses of synovial mononuclear cells in Reiter's syndrome against ureaplasmal and chlamydial antigens. Journal of Rheumatology 7: 751–755
Ford D K, Da Roza D M, Shah P 1981 Cell-mediated immune responses of synovial mononuclear cells to sexually transmitted, enteric and mumps antigens in patients with Reiter's syndrome, rheumatoid arthritis and ankylosing spondylitis. Journal of Rheumatology 8: 220–232
Forestier J, Roates-Querol J 1950 Senile ankylosing hyperostosis of the spine. Annals of the Rheumatic Diseases 9:321
Fostiropoulos G, Austen K F, Bloch K J 1965 Total haemolytic complement (CH 50) and second component of complement (C'2nd) activity in serum and synovial fluid (encl. Reiter's disease). Arthritis and Rheumatism 8:219
Fowler W, Knight G H 1956 Value of treatment in Reiter's disease. British Journal of Venereal Diseases 32:2
Garner R W, Mowat A G 1972 Joint rupture in Reiter's disease. British Journal of Surgery 59:657
Glauner W 1947 Ist die postinfektiöse Trias: Arthritis, Urethritis and Konjunktivitis eine Erkrankung sui generis? Deutsche medizinische Wochenschrift 72:522
Good A E 1965 Reiter's disease and ankylosing spondylitis. Acta Rheumatologica Scandinavica 11:305
Good A E 1971 Reiter's disease, ankylosing spondylitis and rheumatoid arthritis occurring within a single family Arthritis and Rheumatism 14:753
Gough K R 1962 Reiter's syndrome in father and son. Annals of the Rheumatic Diseases 21:292
Graby, Hosotte, Armand 1949 Cahiers médicaux de l'Union Francaise 4:93
Grainger R G 1959 Procto-colitis and other pelvic infections in relation to ankylosing spondylitis. Journal of the Faculty of Radiologists 10:138
Grimble A 1964 Auto-immunity in Reiter's syndrome. British Journal of Venereal Diseases 39:246
Grimble A, Lessof M H 1965 Anti-prostate antibodies in arthritis. British Medical Journal, 2:263
Guck J K, Wolf J 1952 Monarticular and destructive arthropathy in Reiter's syndrome. American Journal of the Medical Science 224:653
Hagenfeldt K, Szanto E 1980 Sacroiliitis in women: A late sequela to acute salpingitis. American Journal of Obstetrics and Gynecology 38: 1039–1041
Hall W H, Finegold S 1953 A study of 23 cases of Reiter's syndrome. Annals of Internal Medicine 38:533
Hamilton K A 1949 Pulmonary disease disease manifestation of ankylosing spondarthritis. Annals of Internal Medicine 31:216
Hamner J G, Gravowski E A 1964 Oral lesions compatible with Reiter's disease — a diagnostic problem Journal of the American Dental Association 69:560
Hancock J A H 1969 Surface manifestations of Reiter's disease in the male. British Journal of Venereal Diseases 36:36
Hancock J A H 1954 In: King A (ed) Recent advances in venereology, 1st Edn. Churchill, London, p 395
Hancock J A H, Mason R M 1965 In: Dixon A St J (ed) Progress in clinical rheumatology. Churchill, London, p 201
Harkness A H 1950 In: Non-gonococcal urethritis. Livingstone, Edinburgh, p 99–145
Henckel H 1954 Reitersche Krankheit bei Kinder. Zeitschrift für Kinderheilkunde 74:303
Herman M 1966 Reiter's syndrome in a 13-year-old boy. Wisconsin Medical Journal 65:195

The level at which pain enters consciousness is not clear but disturbances of both thalamic and cortical regions may give rise to abnormalities of pain sensibility and to 'central pain' syndromes. The individual's emotional and intellectual response to pain can be reduced by severing the connections to the frontal lobes of the cerebral cortex (prefrontal leucotomy).

Inhibitory controls

Activity within the posterior horns of the spinal cord is modulated in a complex manner by the small cells of the substantia gelatinosa. Powerful inhibitory effects are produced from the large mechanoreceptor afferent fibres as well as from descending tracts from the brainstem. These inhibitory interneurones form the 'gate control' mechanism proposed by Melzack & Wall (1965). According to this theory, continuous activity in the small pain afferents resulting from disease or injury tends to keep the gate open so enhancing pain sensations whilst activity in the large mechanoreceptor afferents, for example produced by rubbing the skin, by vibration or by electrical stimulation, tends to close the gate, so relieving pain. Such a mechanism can account for relief of pain by relatively innoccuous forms of counter-irritation, by transcutaneous peripheral nerve stimulators and possibly by acupuncture (Melzack & Wall 1982) (see also section on pain from nerve trunks and roots, below).

The spinal gate is also under control from a brainstem system that includes the periaqueductal grey matter (PAG) of the midbrain and the nucleus raphe magnus in the medulla (Fields & Basbaum, 1978). The PAG cells appear to be activated by endogenous narcotic-like agents (endorphins, enkephalins) and exogenous narcotics (e.g. morphine) probably act at least in part through this system (Snyder, 1977; Yaksh, 1981). In addition there are enkephalin-containing cells in the substantia gelatinosa of the spinal cord and so this is another site where morphine can exert an inhibitory action on nociceptive transmission.

Clearly the sensitivity of the transmission pathway for information about pain is subject to modulation at several levels. Recent studies have emphasised the importance of inhibitory 'gating' at the first synapses in the spinal cord or trigeminal nucleus. In addition similar inhibitory controls may be present at brainstem and thalamic levels. Finally, as mentioned above, the sensitivity of the receptors themselves can be greatly increased by local inflammatory processes.

LOCALISATION OF PAIN

The function of sensory localisation has two distinct components: the capacity to distinguish two spatially separate stimuli, often called two-point discrimination, and the capacity to place the origin of a given sensation in space. Two-point discrimination clearly requires (i) a certain density of innervation and (ii) that receptive fields are restricted in size. The placing of a sensation in space depends upon these factors and also on our awareness of space and of the position of our body within space.

The newborn infant is probably unaware of the existence of its limbs, but as a result of continuous tactile, proprioceptive and visual experiences body consciousness gradually develops until a full body image is acquired. In the adult's body image the skin and the more accessible and obvious deep structures are clearly represented, but structures lying buried in the trunk and limb girdles are poorly, if at all, represented. We are, for instance, quite unconscious of the existence of the body of a lumbar vertebra though we are aware of the tip of its spinous process. We think we know where our kidneys lie but a pelvic kidney is not recognised as such by its possessor. Obviously, we cannot place pain accurately in a structure when we are not aware of either its existence or location.

Skin pain

The normal skin is densely innervated and is well represented in our body image, and the source of cutaneous pain can be localised to within about 1 cm of the point stimulated, discrimination being equally accurate; but if the density of innervation is reduced, as when all forms of cutaneous sensibility are lost with the exception of delayed cutaneous pain, discrimination becomes very defective, although the source of pain is still correctly placed in the part stimulated.

In certain disorders of the pain pathways in the central nervous system pain from a single needle prick in the skin may spread widely over the body, so that it is possible for there to be a central breakdown of localisation; but under normal conditions cutaneous pain is always localised with considerable accuracy.

Deep pain

Unlike pain arising from the skin, deep pain is usually diffuse, poorly localised and often felt at some distance from the point stimulated, when it may be described as 'referred pain'. The degree of localisation varies greatly from one part of the body to another. Thus, structures at the periphery, such as fingers and toes, give pain which is fairly well localised, while structures lying deeply inside the body give very diffuse pain which may be widely referred over a segmental distribution.

The various deep structures have been systematically explored by passing needles through anaesthetic skin, and stimulating the muscle, ligament or joint in question by scratching or pricking. This stimulus gives a sudden flash of pain which is difficult to place, and the boundaries of which it is impossible to mark out, but if chemical solutions such as 1 mol/l NaCl are injected a steady pain is produced, lasting several minutes after the needle has been withdrawn and all mechanical stimulation ended. Pain produced in this way resembles most closely the pain of disease, and its distribution can be marked out with accuracy (Kellgren, 1938, 1939a). When the two forms of stimulus are compared it is found that the sudden flashes of pain produced by the needle point are placed somewhere within the area marked out for the continuous pain of saline. Figure 4.2 illustrates this point and also demonstrates the difference between pain from superficial and deep-lying structures. Thus, pain from the periosteum over the scapular spine, which is subcutaneous, is confined to the region stimulated; while the more deeply situated periosteum of the infraspinous fossa gives diffuse pain referred to the shoulder. The pain obtained from point stimulation of the subcutaneous deep fascia is confined to an area about 3 cm in diameter near the point stimulated, but usually somewhat distal to it. Focal pain of this type is obtained from all subcutaneous deep fascia, and from any periosteum, tendon, ligament or joint near the body surface.

The skeletal muscles give more diffuse pain with distant reference, and when situated deeply give pain of clear segmental distribution. Indeed the deep-lying structures in the trunk and limb girdles, whether joints, bones or muscles, all give very diffuse pain of full segmental distribution. Taking advantage of this fact, the deep-lying structures in the region of the laminae and articular processes of the spine were used to map out segmental pain areas. By injecting at the level of each vertebra, complete charts were obtained as shown in Figures 4.3 and 4.4. It will be noticed that these segmental areas for deep pain differ from the dermatomes and have been described as sclerotomes by Inman & Saunders (1944). In the trunk the dermatome forms a complete band

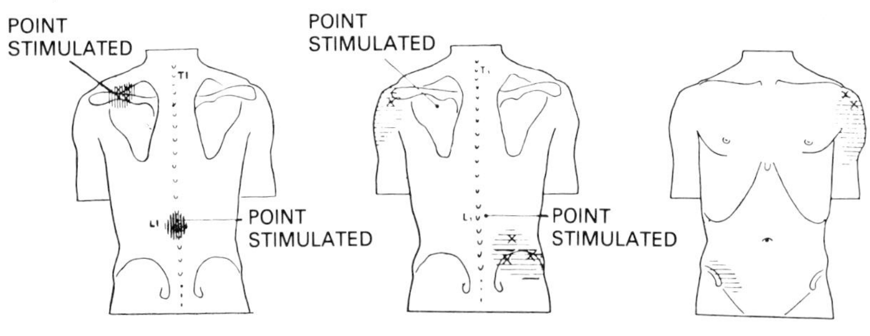

Fig. 4.2 The distribution of pain produced by saline from subcutaneous periosteum (vertical hatching) and deeply situated periosteum (horizontal hatching). Points stimulated are tip of spine and lamina of the first lumbar vertebra, and the spine and infraspinous fossa of the scapula. The crosses indicate where pain was placed when the periosteum at the site of injection was scratched with the needle point (three observations). (From Kellgren, 1939a.)

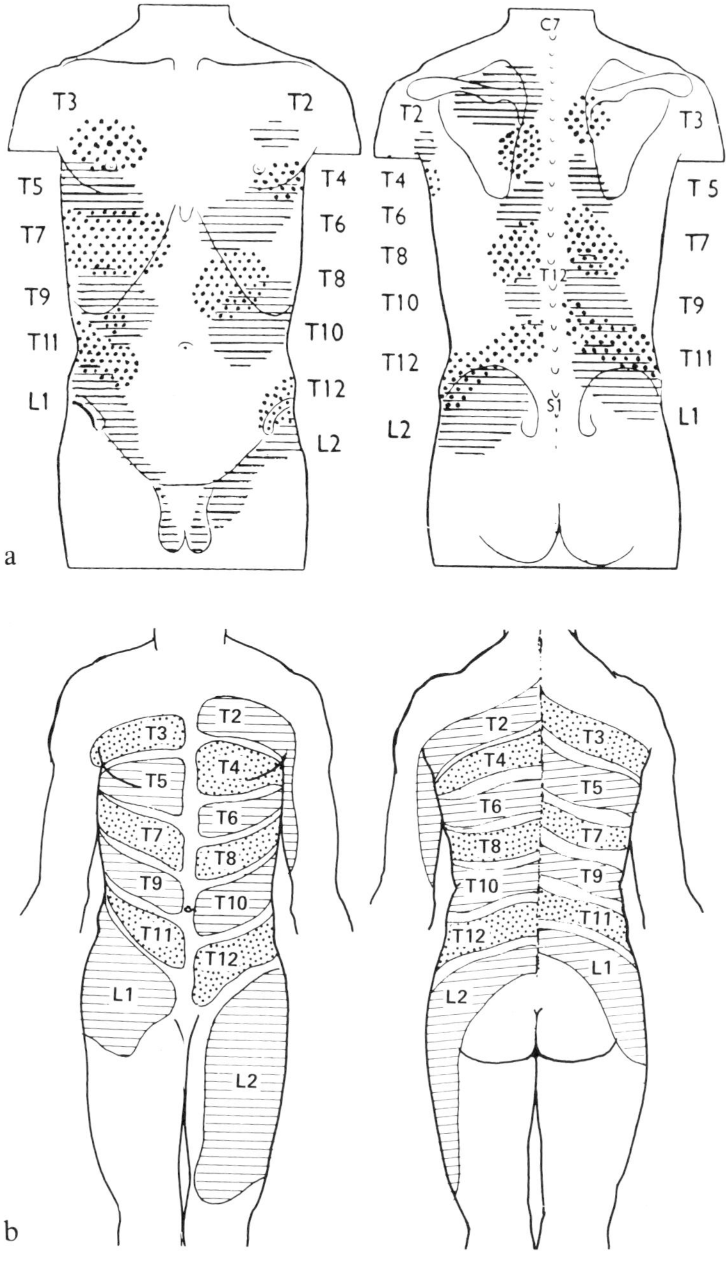

Fig. 4.3 (a) Distribution of pain from stimulating the region of the interspinous ligaments T2 to L2. Average of different subjects. For clarity, alternate areas have been hatched and stippled. (From Kellgren, 1939a.) (b) The dermatomes derived from Foerster (1933) and Carpenter (1976) are shown for comparison.

around the body while deep pain goes through from the back to front or vice versa, and in the limbs the dermatomes are more peripheral as shown in Figure 4.4.

The pain is not distributed evenly over these segmental areas as shown in Figures 4.2–4.5. On the contrary there are one or more areas of maximal pain within the full area. If pain is slight only the points of maximal pain will be appreciated, and it is only when pain is intense that the

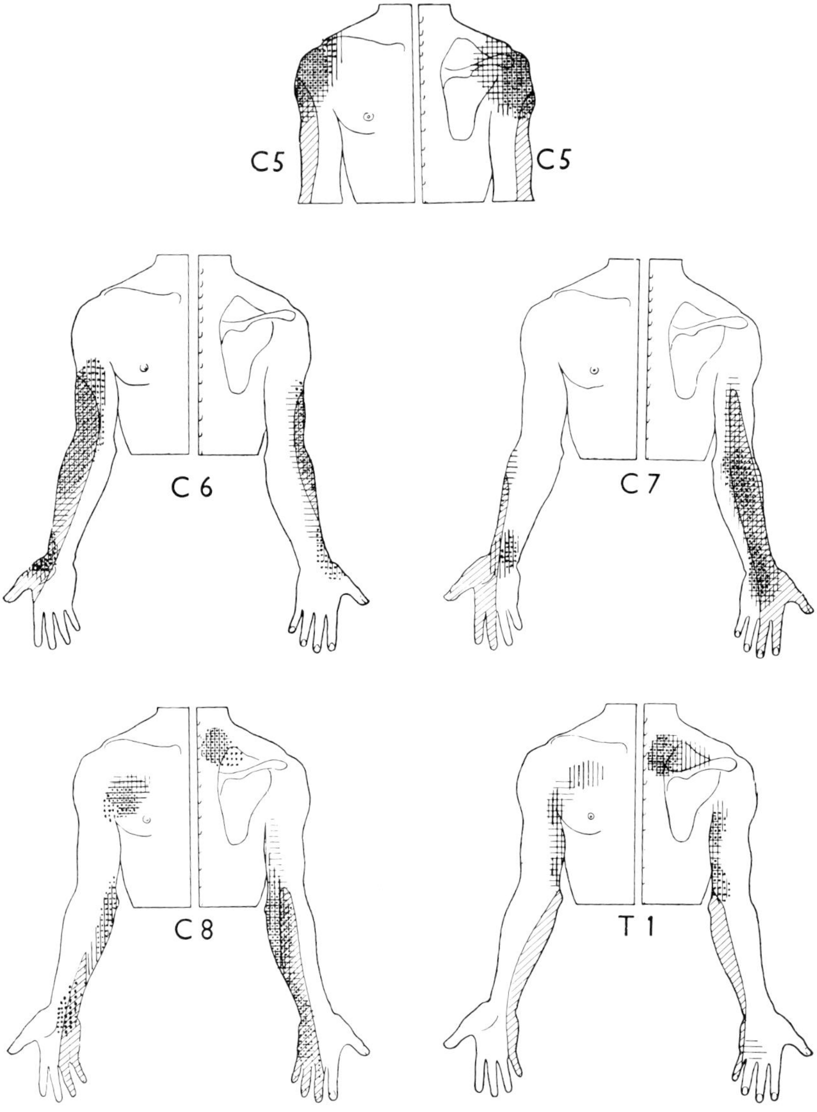

Fig. 4.4 Distribution of pain from stimulating the region of the interspinous ligaments C5 to T1 and L3 to S2. The results from different subjects — horizontal hatching, vertical hatching and stippling — have been superimposed to display individual variations. (From Kellgren, 1939a). The outline of the dermatomes derived from Foerster (1933) and Carpenter (1976) are shown for comparison (diagonal hatching).

full area can be mapped out. In the limbs these points of maximal pain are often located in the joints, and other prominent and sensitive structures, while in the trunk they correspond with the regions where the spinal nerves pierce the deep fascia and give it a rich nerve supply (Fig. 4.5). The reference of pain is quite striking when the pain comes from a muscle moving a particular joint. Thus pain from the tibialis anticus is felt in front of the ankle. The quadriceps gives pain in the knee, the long flexors of the fingers give pain in the knuckles, and so on. Conversely, pain from the joints of the spine and limb girdles is felt over the muscle masses of the trunk and limb girdles and this false localisation over muscles was responsible for the old concept of 'fibrositis'.

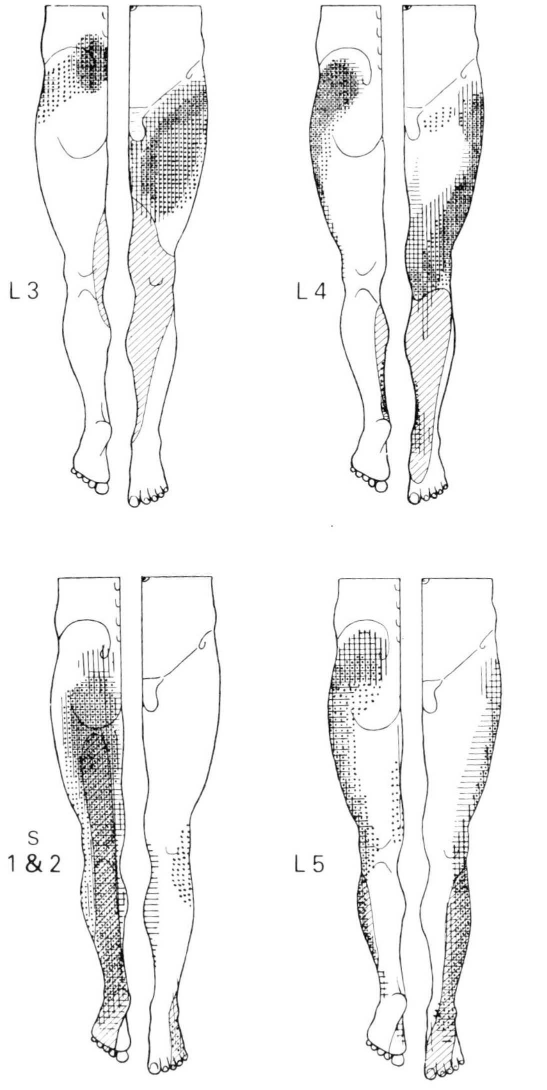

Fig. 4.4 (continued)

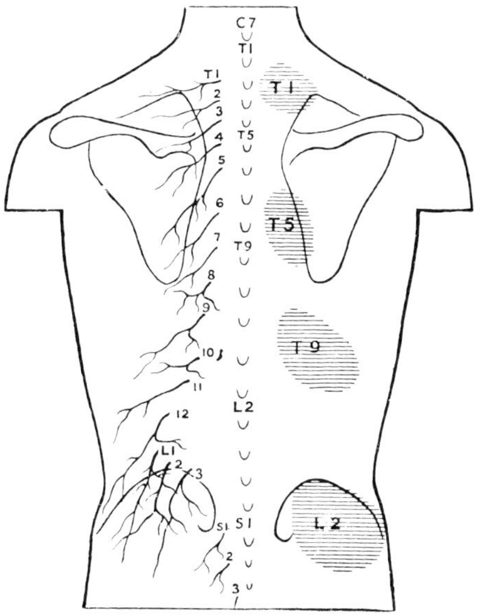

Fig. 4.5 On the left the posterior primary divisions of the spinal nerves are shown in their course after piercing the deep fascia. On the right the hatched areas represent some of the corresponding deep pain areas for comparison.

Pain from the joints follows the same lines as pain from the muscles, periosteum and fascia. Figure 4.6 illustrates the distribution of pain from different parts of the knee joint. It will be noticed that slight pain is felt in the knee region, but that, when severe, pain spreads up and down the limb within the appropriate segmental area.

The distribution of pain from the sacroiliac and hip joints is shown in Figure 4.7. The whole joint is not always involved in the genesis of pain so that hip disease can present with pain felt only in the knee, groin or buttock. Figure 4.8 shows the most frequent distribution of pain from the various joints of the shoulder and the subacromial bursa. All these examples represent the most common findings but there are individual variations deter-

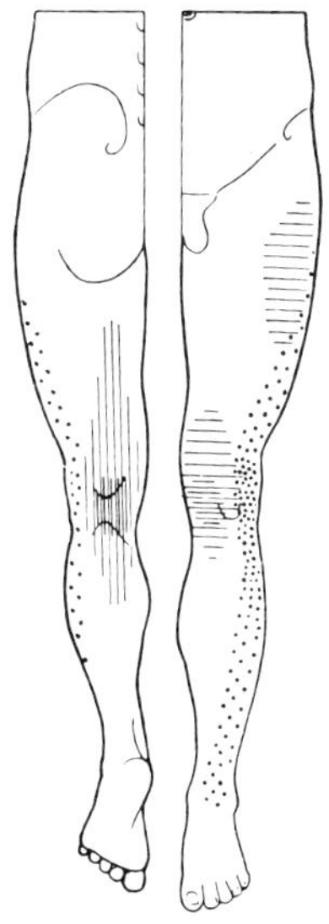

Fig. 4.6 The distribution of pain from structures around the knee. From medial ligament, horizontal hatching; from lateral ligament, stippling; from posterior part of capsule, vertical hatching. The pain extends over the wider areas only when severe, moderate pain being confined to the region of the knee. (From Lewis & Kellgren, 1939.)

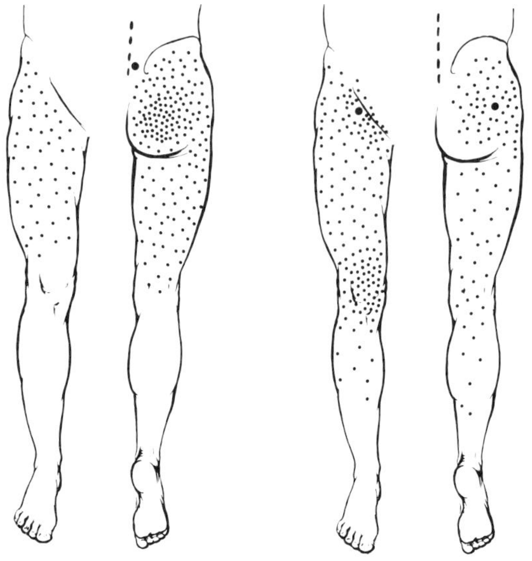

Fig. 4.7 Illustrates the distribution of pain arising from the sacroiliac and hip joints. Initially the pain is often only felt at one of the sites of election so that hip disease may present as pain felt only in the knee, groin or buttock.

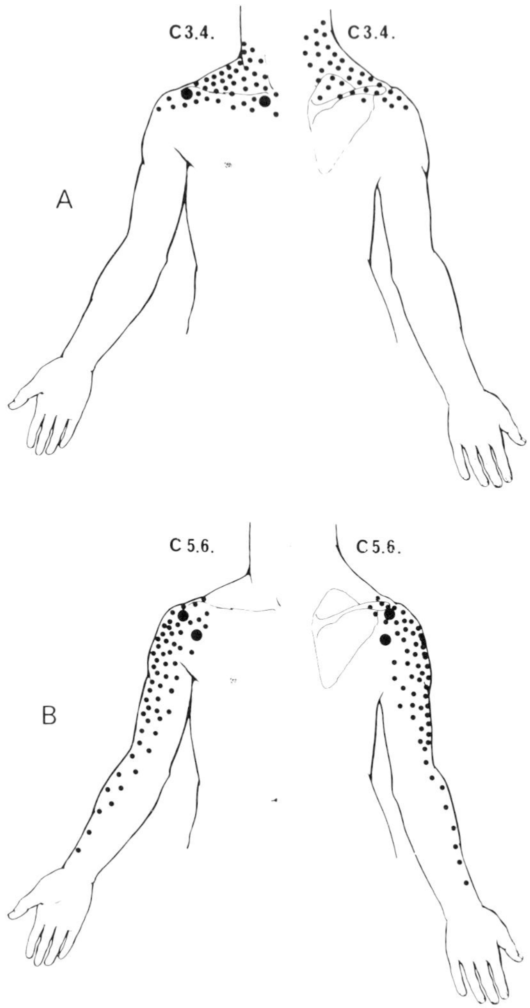

Fig. 4.8 Illustrates the most common distribution of pain arising from: A, the acromioclavicular or sternoclavicular joints; B, the scapulohumeral joint or subacromial bursa.

mined by variation in the segmental innervation of the joints concerned as well as the individual's past experience.

The site of greatest confusion is in the lower lumbar spine where the posterior divisions of the 4th and 5th lumbar nerves are small and innervate only the apophyseal joints and deeper muscles while the posterior longitudinal ligament, so often involved in disc disorders, is innervated from higher lumbar nerves by the descending nerve of Roofe (Roofe, 1940; Spurling & Grantham, 1940). The supraspinous ligaments are replaced by the strong tendon of the sacrospinalis which is also innervated by upper lumbar nerves. Disorders of the lower lumbar spine, therefore often give rise to back pain of upper lumbar distribution. This accounts for the exceptional difficulty of determining the anatomical source of low back pain in patients.

From these examples we can draw some general conclusions about the localisation of deep pain. Beneath the skin there is a second sensitive layer in which pain is localised with fair accuracy. This consists of the deep fascia encasing the limbs and trunk, together with any periosteum, ligament or joint that is subcutaneous. Deep to this layer all structures give diffuse pain which is poorly localised. With increasing depth from the surface the pain becomes more diffuse until from the deep-lying structures of the trunk and limb girdles we get pain which is very diffuse and referred over a segmental distribution. There is thus a gradual transition from focal to segmental pain.

The focal pain comes from structures of which we are normally conscious as a result of the everyday experience of palpation and movement, while diffuse pain comes from the deep-lying structures of which we are normally unconscious. Pain from these deep structures appears to be projected to the region of the structures of which

Chemical algogens

Alterations of pH, osmolarity and the concentration of various ions in the tissues all cause pain but it is unlikely that these are operative in disease. Keele & Armstrong (1964) found that in addition to histamine and acetylcholine there were many protein and polypeptide algogenic agents, the most interesting of which is bradykinin which is effective in very low concentrations producing both pain and hyperalgesia. The concentration of bradykinin in the tissues in vivo is controlled by the labile kallikrein kininase system and it may well be an important cause of the pain of acute inflammation.

The prostaglandins and lipoperoxides are also of special interest since they have been shown to produce prolonged sensitisation of cutaneous and joint pain receptors to algesic chemicals such as histamine (Ferreira, 1972) and bradykinin (Moncada et al, 1975). Since prostaglandins are produced locally during inflammatory changes, including those occurring in joints, they appear likely to contribute to the hyperalgesic state which is such a feature of the affected tissues in the rheumatic diseases. Furthermore many agents that reduce inflammatory pain, such as steroids (Blackwell et al, 1978) and aspirin (Vane, 1971) can block or reduce prostaglandin synthesis. For example, indomethacin reduces prostaglandin production in joint inflammation caused by carrageenin (Moncada et al, 1975). It has been proposed that this anti-prostaglandin synthesis action is the main mechanism behind the ability of such drugs to relieve inflammatory pains, like those occurring in rheumatic diseases (Vane, 1971).

The effects of alterations in blood flow on limb pains have been the subject of several studies. In acute inflammation caused by trauma, infection or gout, two to three minutes of arterial occlusion cause a dramatic increase in pain and hyperalgesia which is relieved at once by restoring the circulation (Addis et al, 1950). Similar findings have also been reported for pain and hyperalgesia from UV radiation (Lewis & Hess, 1933). These findings suggest that in such situations the pain producing substances are stable and freely diffusible and are therefore normally removed via the local blood vessels. Possible agents would be serotonin (5HT) or the more stable members of the prostaglandin family. In rheumatoid arthritis, the effect of arterial occlusion is much less pronounced and in ankylosing spondylitis, tuberculous arthritis and most cases of osteoarthritis, and also in acute heat-injured skin (Lynn, 1980), no effect of stopping the blood flow is observed. In these states, therefore, it appears that relatively unstable mediators that are locally destroyed may play a prominent part in producing pain and hyperalgesia.

Short periods of arterial occlusion also have no effect on the painful states observed in neuromata and digital nerve injuries, though ischaemia sufficiently prolonged to cause loss of all sensation except delayed pain has an enhancing effect on all painful states and this may be one factor causing the severe burning rest pain of impending gangrene. In most inflamed tissues, venous congestion only has slight effects on pain and so tissue tension is probably only a minor factor in such situations.

The ischaemic muscle pain of intermittent claudication (Lewis, 1942) is another example of a chemical algogenic agent produced by muscular contraction. Though its precise nature has not yet been established, it probably differs from the algogenic agents operating in inflammation.

A very puzzling condition is the hyperalgesic state in ligaments and periosteum that follows trauma or mechanical stress and which persists for months without any evidence of inflammation and which can be restored to normal by a single injection of local anaesthetic with or without corticosteroid, provided the hyperalgesic tissue is thoroughly and accurately infiltrated.

Temperature changes (cold pain)

If the normal deep tissues are cooled rapidly deep pain is experienced while the temperature of the tissues is falling from 30°C to 15°C but as cooling proceeds analgesia develops and becomes complete when the tissue temperature reaches about 10°C. If the tissues are cooled slowly analgesia develops without appreciable pain and this is what happens under normal conditions of exposure. If on the other hand the deep tissues are abnormally sensitive, as a result of trauma or disease, persistent pain may result from slow cooling and analgesia only develop slowly and partially (Kellgren et al, 1948).

Weather-sensitive patients often complain of pain during the cold front which precedes bad weather, as during this period rapid cooling gives rise to cold pain; similarly in cold damp weather an increased depth of cooling occurs in the limbs which will also aggravate cold pain. This mechanism of cold pain is found in most conditions in which there is hyperalgesia of the deep tissues, and since it is often accompanied by muscle spasm and vasospasm a thorough warming may give more than temporary relief and provides a valuable period of comfort, during which the function of the painful disused part may be restored. Alternatively profound cooling down to 10°C produces deep analgesia which allows painful joints to be exercised painlessly.

The effect of temperature changes on cutaneous pain is quite different. In normal skin, pain results from heating above 43°C or cooling below 10°C but in the erythralgic state and impending gangrene cutaneous pain may result from temperatures as low as 30°C or as high as 15°C. Thus, in these lesions warmth causes an increase of pain and cooling between 30°C and 15°C gives relief.

Abnormalities of pain pathways

Changes in pain pathways may result from tumours, vascular accidents, trauma or biochemical abnormalities. In these situations there may be spontaneous pain that can spread widely, involving a whole limb or half the body. These 'central' pains, such as 'thalamic syndrome' from damage to the thalamus, were well described by Head & Holmes (1911) and Head (1920). The pain threshold to peripheral stimuli may be either high or low, but the painful sensory response is characteristically explosive, exaggerated and prolonged. In lesions of the pain pathways there may be a curious paradoxical abnormality of pain sensibility; thus a point stimulus such as a pin-prick may give rise to no pain while a larger stimulus such as squeezing a fold of skin gives rise to a painful response which is both excessive and prolonged.

The mechanism by which abnormal pain responses are produced is but poorly understood and is likely to remain so until the anatomy and physiology of the parts of the brain involved are better understood. One new feature revealed by recent studies is the existence of powerful inhibitory influences on pain transmission. Clearly, some disorders of pain sensitivity may result not from direct influences on excitatory pain pathways, but rather from a lack of inhibition.

Psychogenic pain

True psychogenic pain is a rare condition in which the subject projects his emotional anguish into some convenient part of the body where he keeps it quite cheerfully as an 'agonising pain'. These pains are bizarre in distribution, constant in intensity, and completely unaffected by any form of therapy, and indeed we are probably doing the patient a disservice in attempting to undo his solution of his agonising problem. Then there are people in whom mental tension expresses itself as widespread muscular tension. These people move stiffly and awkwardly, contracting agonists and antagonists simultaneously. This muscular inefficiency leads to fatigue and painful muscle strains, the mechanism being of the psychosomatic type. Various psychoneuroses may also have pain as a presenting symptom. In such cases the pain is usually linked with organ, joint or limb, the part selected being determined by injury or a past or family history of disease or trauma, with a high dramatic and emotional content. In all these conditions the cause of pain lies wholly outside the part of which the subject complains, and extensive investigations or treatments directed at the 'painful' part are liable to confuse the physician and aggravate the patient's disability.

CONCLUDING REMARKS

A complaint of pain may result from disorders at many levels in the human organism, and different mechanisms may be involved at each level. Despite the considerable advances in recent years in our understanding of the basic anatomy and physiology of pain, its assessment in the clinic still presents many problems. Every patient must be considered as an individual problem, and only by careful assessment of the various components of his disorder and through a proper understanding of the mechanisms involved can we hope to relieve this most distressing symptom with more consistent success than is usual at the present time.

REFERENCES

Addis H St C C, Jepson R P, Kellgren J H 1950 On the effect of arterial occlusion and venous congestion upon limb pain. Clinical Science 9: 271–280

Beecher H K 1962 An inspection of our working hypotheses in the study of pain and other subjective responses. In: Keele C A, Smith R (ed) The assessment of pain in man and animals. UFAW, London, p 159–169

Bessou P, Perl E R 1969 Response of cutaneous sensory units with unmyelinated fibres to noxious stimuli. Journal of Neurophysiology 32: 1025–1043.

Blackwell G J, Flower R J, Nijkamp F P, Vane J R 1978 Phospholipase A_2 activity of guinea pig isolated perfused lungs: stimulation and inhibition by anti-inflammatory steroids. British Journal of Pharmacology 62: 79–89

Burgess P R, Perl E R 1967 Myelinated afferent fibres responding specifically to noxious stimulation of the skin. Journal of Physiology 190: 541–562

Carpenter M B 1976 Human neuroanatomy, 7th Edn. Williams & Wilkins, Baltimore

Coggeshall R E, Hong K A P, Langford L A, Schaible H-G, & Schmidt R F 1983 Discharge characteristics of fine medial articular afferents at rest and during passive movements of inflamed knee joints. Brain Research 272: 185–188

Cohen H 1947 Visceral pain. Lancet 2: 933–934

Ferreira S H 1972 Prostaglandins, aspirin-like drugs and analgesia. Nature New Biology 240: 200–203

Fields, H L, Basbaum A I 1978 Brainstem control of spinal pain transmission. Annual Review of Physiology 40: 217–248

Foerster O 1927 Die Leitungsbahnan des Schmerzgefuhls. Urban & Schwarzenburg, Berlin

Foerster O 1933 The dermatomes in man. Brain 56: 1–39

Gordon G 1977 Somatic and visceral sensory mechanisms. British Medical Bulletin 33: 89–182

Hardy J D, Wolff H G, Goodell H 1952 Pain sensations and reactions. Williams & Wilkins, Baltimore

Harpman J A 1948 Observations on cutaneous hyperalgesia. Brain 71: 34–47

Head H 1893 On disturbances of sensation, with especial reference to the pain of visceral disease. Brain 16: 1–133

Head H 1920 Studies in neurology. Oxford University Press, London

Head H, Holmes G 1911 Sensory disturbances from cerebral lesions. Brain: 34: 102–254

Head H, Rivers W H R, Sherren J 1905 The afferent nervous system from a new aspect. Brain 28: 99–115

Huskisson E C 1974a Measurement of pain. Lancet ii: 1127–1131

Huskisson E C 1974b Simple analgesics for arthritis. British Medical Journal 4: 196–200

Huskisson E C, Hart D F 1972 Pain thresholds and arthritis. British Medical Journal 4: 193–195

Inman V T, Saunders J B M 1944 Referred pain from skeletal structures. Journal of Nervous and Mental Disease 99: 660–667

Keele C A, Armstrong D 1964 Substances producing pain and itch. Edward Arnold, London

Kellgren J H 1938 Observations on referred pain arising from muscle. Clinical Science 3: 175–190

Kellgren J H 1939a On the distribution of pain arising from deep somatic structures with charts of segmental pain areas. Clinical Science 4: 35–46

Kellgren J H 1939b Somatic simulating visceral pain. Clinical Science 4: 303–309

Kellgren J H 1949 Deep pain sensibility. Lancet 1: 943–949

Kellgren J H, McGowan A J 1948 On the behaviour of deep and cutaneous sensibility during nerve blocks. Clinical Science 7: 1–11

Kellgren J H, McGowan A J, Hughes S R 1948 On deep hyperalgesia and cold pain. Clinical Science 7: 13–27

LeBars D, Dickinson A H, Besson J-M 1979a Diffuse noxious inhibitory controls (DNIC). I. Effects on dorsal horn convergent neurones in the rat. Pain 6: 283–304

LeBars D, Dickinson A H, Besson J-M 1979b Diffuse noxious inhibitory controls (DNIC). II. Lack of effect on non-convergent neurones, supra-spinal involvement and theoretical implications. Pain 6: 305–327

Leriche R 1939 The surgery of pain. Baillière, London

Lewis T 1936 Experiments relating to cutaneous hyperalgesia and its spread through somatic nerves. Clinical Science 2: 373–423

Lewis T 1942 Pain. Macmillan, New York

Lewis T, Hess W 1933 Pain derived from the skin and the mechanism of its production. Clinical Science 1: 39–61

Lewis T, Kellgren J 1939 Observations relating to referred pain, viscero-motor reflexes and other associated phenomena. Clinical Science 4: 47–71

Lewis T, Pochin E E 1937 The double pain response of the human skin to a single stimulus. Clinical Science 3: 67–76

Loh L, Nathan P W 1978 Painful peripheral states and sympathetic blocks. Journal of Neurology, Neurosurgery and Psychiatry 41: 664–671

Lynn B 1977 Cutaneous hyperalgesia. British Medical Bulletin 33: 103–108

Lynn B 1980 Heat pain sensitivity of human skin after mild heat injury and its lack of dependence on the local blood flow. Pain 8: 189–196

Lynn B 1983 Cutaneous sensation. In: Goldsmith L (ed) Biochemistry and physiology of the skin. OUP New York, p 654–684

Lynn B, Perl E R 1977 A comparison of four tests for assessing the pain sensitivity of different subjects and test areas. Pain 3: 353–365

Melzack R 1975a The McGill pain questionnaire: major properties and scoring methods. Pain 1: 277–299

Melzack R 1975b Prolonged relief of pain by brief, intense transcutaneous somatic stimulation. Pain 1: 357–373

Melzack R, Wall P D 1965 Pain mechanisms: a new theory. Science 150: 971–979

Melzack R, Wall P D 1982 The challenge of pain. Penguin Books, Harmondsworth, Middlesex

Merskey H 1978 Pain and personality. In: Sternbach R A (ed) The psychology of pain. Raven Press, New York, p 111–127

Moncada S, Ferreira S H, Vane J R 1975 Inhibition of prostaglandin biosynthesis as the mechanism of analgesia of aspirin-like drugs in the dog knee joint. European Journal of Pharmacology 31: 250–260

Mountcastle V B 1980 Pain and temperature sensibilities. In: Medical physiology, 13th Edn. Mosby, St Louis, Ch 13, p 391–427

O'Driscoll S L, Jayson M I V 1974 Pain threshold analysis in patients with osteo-arthritis of hip. British Medical Journal 3: 714–715

Roofe R G 1940 Innervation of annulus fibrosus and posterior longitudinal ligament. Archives of Neurology and Psychiatry 44: 100–103
Simons D J, May E, Goodell H, Wolff H G 1943 Experimental studies on headache: muscles of the scalp and neck as sources of pain. Proceedings of the Association for Research in Nervous and Mental Diseases 23: 228–244
Snyder S H 1977 Opiate receptors and internal opiates. Scientific American 236: 44–56
Spurling R G, Grantham E G 1940 Neurologic picture of herniations of the nucleus pulposus in the lower part of the lumbar region. Archives of Surgery 40: 375–388
Trotter W, Davies M 1909 Experimental studies in the innervation of the skin. Journal of Physiology 38: 134–246
Vane J R 1971 Inhibition of prostaglandin synthesis as a mechanism of action for aspirin-like drugs. Nature New Biology 231: 232–258
Wall P D 1984 Textbook of pain. Churchill Livingstone, London
Wall P D, Gutnick M 1974 Ongoing activity in peripheral nerves: the physiology of impulses originating from a neuroma. Experimental Neurology 43: 580–593
Webster K E 1977 Somesthetic pathways. British Medical Bulletin 33: 113–120
Weddell G, Sinclair D C, Feindel W H 1948 An anatomical basis for alterations in quality of pain sensibility. Journal of Neurophysiology 11: 99–109
Wolff B B 1978 Behavioural measurement of human pain. In: Sternbach R A (ed) The psychology of pain. Raven Press, New York, p 129–168
Yaksh T L 1981 Spinal opiate analgesia: characteristics and principles of action. Pain 11: 293–346
Yaksh T L, Hammond D L 1982 Peripheral and central substrates involved in the rostrad transmission of nociceptive information. Pain 13: 1–85

5

A. St J. Dixon

The differential diagnosis of arthritis

The differential diagnosis of arthritis is not concerned with late, chronic forms, the diagnosis of which will have been established years earlier. It is concerned first, with the differentiation of synovitis of joints from other painful conditions causing pain in, or deformity of, joints (Table 5.1). This is usually easy. Synovitis implies inflammation. Of the cardinal signs of inflammation redness and heat, but especially soft tissue joint swelling, distinguish synovitis from the painful bony enlargements and the mechanical displacements of non-inflammatory joint disease.

Table 5.1 Some painful conditions which resemble arthritis

Carpal tunnel syndrome (numerous causes, including tenosynovitis, hypothyroidism, acromegaly and myelomatosis, but many are idiopathic). 'Shoulder hand syndrome' (swelling of hand in association with painful stiff shoulder).
Osteomyelitis near joint. Sudeck's atrophy. Painful periostitis in syphilis, scurvy, leukaemia. Haemarthrosis (trauma after intra-articular fractures, intra-articular haemangioma, bleeding diseases).
Fractures near joints (e.g. stress fracture of the lower end of the fibula or 'March fracture' of the metatarsals). Acute and chronic scaphoid fracture at the wrist. Milkman's fractures in the pelvis or femora or scapulae in osteomalacia. Osteochondritis dissecans.

This done, it is concerned with distinguishing onsets of monarthritis, oligoarthritis or polyarthritis one from another with a view to establishing correct treatment and prognosis. Synovial membrane lines tendon sheaths and bursae as well as joints, thus tenosynovitis and bursitis often accompany and may precede acute arthritis.

THE LIMITATIONS OF CLINICAL FEATURES IN DIAGNOSIS

There is much overlap between different arthritic diseases in their physical manifestations. Synovial joints are moving structures. There may be more difference between two patients with rheumatoid arthritis (RA) because in one joint movements are restricted by pain and in the other they are not, than there is between different forms of arthritis where use and movement have remained much the same. Differential diagnosis often depends on such associated features as the presence or absence of nodules in RA, the rash in psoriatic arthritis and the urethral discharge in sexually acquired reactive arthritis (SARA). Because of this overlap, it is necessary to bear in mind all the common arthritic diagnoses in considering differential diagnosis.

Pathophysiology of arthritis

Except where inflammation in the joints follows disease in the underlying bone or periosteum (examples: osteomyelitis of the metaphysis, inflammatory periostitis behind the suprapatellar pouch in hypertrophic pulmonary osteoarthropathy), the inflammation of arthritis starts in the synovium, the first reaction of which is to increase the production of joint fluid. Excess joint fluid first distends the synovial space and any connecting bursae or tendon sheaths. There is much variation anatomically in this. Thus around the ankle, the synovial space of the talotibial joint may, or may not, connect with the posterior subtaloid joint and with the peroneal and posterior tibial groups of tendon sheaths at each side of the ankle. While the joint tissues are slack the intrasynovial pressure at first rises slowly but with increasing fluid the intrasynovial pressure climbs more steeply. The joint bulges in areas determined by the anatomy, and not by which kind of synovitis is present.

Inflammatory synovial effusions contain irritating mediators of inflammation which diffuse from the distended synovial cavity into the surrounding tissues, even to the overlying skin, causing the other cardinal signs of inflammation, namely heat, redness and pain with loss of function. Such signs do help a little in differentiating the type of synovitis. The heat and redness of crystal arthropathies (urate or pyrophosphate gout) or of septic arthritis are generally more severe than those of RA. Indeed this difference is most obvious in distinguishing gouty arthritis of the big toe from other forms of arthritis. In gout the skin is hot, dry and reddened, and the draining veins are distended. In rheumatoid or SARA of this joint, discolouration is more bluish, and the overlying skin is cool and sweating.

Synovial swellings of whatever cause may press on surrounding structures, causing 'non-synovial' symptoms, compression of the median nerve at the wrist being an example. A synovial effusion in a joint will lift the tendons running over the joint from their normal position. When these tendons are tensed by muscle contraction the forces acting through them will have vectors which compress the effusion within with the result that the intrasynovial pressure rises during use of the joint. (Pressures of over 1000 mmHg have been measured). Temporary, but repeated, elevations of intrasynovial fluid pressure have a number of consequences. One of these is rupture of the joint capsule with free escape of inflammatory joint fluid into the surrounding tissues (when the knee is involved this mimics deep crural vein thrombosis). This is most often seen in RA but can occur in any acute synovitis of the knee. Another is the formation of chronic synovial cysts which may in their turn cause symptoms and signs by compressing surrounding nerves or veins.

Normal synovial membrane, if in constant contact with the joint cartilage, will adhere to it and erode it and this is a tendency which is amplified when the synovial membrane is inflamed. Breaches of articular bone cortex caused by this erosion then expose the marrow cavity (which is at venous pressure) to the synovial fluid pressures and inflammatory synovial cavity contents. Not only is the synovial membrane, but also the synovial fluid with its cell content and debris, forced into the metaphysis producing the familiar X-ray erosions and cystic geodes.

Thus synovial swelling, redness and heat in overlying skin, pressure on neighbouring structures, the existence of synovial cysts, acute and chronic rupture of the joint, X-ray juxta-articular bone erosions with surface or cystic appearances, have relatively little force in differentiating one form of arthritis from another. Conversely the lack of these changes is seldom helpful. The physical changes of any form of arthritis are absent or diminished in the joints of paralysed limbs even though, on biopsy, disease is present (Thompson & Bywaters, 1962; Glick, 1966). In any form of polyarthritis changes are less severe or occur later in the non-dominant hand (Soila, 1963). The X-ray changes seen in the hands of manual labourers who continue to work despite RA differ from those seen in the hands of RA sufferers in non-manual occupations (Castillo et al, 1965). The X-ray erosions of joints seen in the hands of gout can mimic very closely those seen in the hands of manual workers with rheumatoid arthritis. Thus X-rays also have limitations in the differentiation of the forms of inflammatory joint disease.

SIGNS WHICH HAVE SOME DIAGNOSTIC FORCE

The differentiation of the individual rheumatic disease therefore depends on the presence of relatively few exclusive and essential features, for example, sodium biurate crystals in gout, and on the total clinical picture as arrived at by the summation of qualifying criteria and the absence of disqualifying criteria and by a knowledge of the probability of diagnoses derived from surveys of various age-groups or occupational groups. The earlier a patient is seen in the course of synovitis, the greater the likelihood that no firm diagnosis can be made. In many patients early synovitis recovers without sequelae. Observation over a prolonged period — especially in differentiating the subsets of juvenile chronic arthritis (JCA) —

may be needed. Accurate differential diagnosis of arthritis requires a full medical history and a full medical examination; important clues will otherwise be missed.

Differential diagnosis from non-inflammatory joint pain and swelling

A joint may be enlarged because of bony overgrowth, or apparently enlarged because of dislocations and subluxations. The most important sign of arthritis is soft tissue swelling of the joint. Without this the diagnosis of arthritis is suspect. Two important clues to joint swelling in the history are inability to wear rings on fingers which have swollen, or inability to wear previously comfortable shoes when the feet have swollen. Swelling of the wrists, elbows, ankles and knees is usually obvious on inspection. Swellings of the hip and shoulder joints are more difficult to detect.

The second most important sign is pain on movement coupled with limitation of movement. Beware the 'pons asinorum' of rheumalology, the patient with a painful hip in which the pain is referred to the anterior thigh and knee. Attempts to move the knee with the patient supine involve moving the hip and many such a patient has been diagnosed as having arthritis of the knee when the trouble is in the hip. The referred pains of brachialgia arising from the neck, or of sciatica arising from the lumbar spine are made worse by movements of the neck and spine respectively and not by movements of the limbs in which the pains are felt. This general principle, that pain arising in a joint is made worse by movement of the joint, whereas pain referred to a joint area when arising elsewhere is unaffected by joint movement, is the foundation for the differentiation of arthritis from other forms of rheumatic pain.

The next most important physical sign differentiating inflammatory arthritis from non-inflammatory arthrosis or joint deformity is warmth. The latter is felt with the back of the examiner's fingers. The presence of inflammation is confirmed by tests for acute phase reactants, of which the sedimentation rate, plasma viscosity and C-reactive protein estimations are the most helpful, and above all by the aspiration of inflammatory synovial fluid.

THE AGES OF ARTHRITIS

Infants and toddlers

Pains and difficulty in movement imitating arthritis can occur in scurvy and rickets because of subperiosteal and intra-articular haemorrhages or epiphyseal enlargement respectively. Rare conditions which mimic arthritis in an infant or in a young child are the painful periostitis of congenital syphilis or of leukaemic infiltration. True inflammatory synovitis is uncommon in babies and when it occurs infection must first be excluded. Tuberculous arthritis in infants is now rare in Western societies following the pasteurisation of milk but septic arthritis still occurs. Juvenile chronic arthritis of the Wistler–Fanconi type is possible. This condition, initially described by Still, is that variety of JCA characterised by remittant fever, rash, lymphadenopathy and splenomegaly with arthritis. The arthritis may be one of the later features to appear.

The 2–12 age-group

Thirty years ago arthritis in this age-group was automatically diagnosed as rheumatic fever until proved otherwise. Now rheumatic fever in affluent societies is so rare that it is often forgotten and should not be the first thought. But it still does occur in children, though much less frequently than do septic arthritis and the forms of JCA.

Rheumatic fever follows a proven Group A, β-haemolytic infection of the throat, and is confirmed by throat swab culture and rising titres of antistreptococcal antibodies, notably antistreptolysin-O and antihyaluronidase. The joint disease is transient, and the previous scourge of heart involvement (valvulitis, pericarditis, ECG changes and dysrhythmias) is nowadays virtually banished from the medical scene in affluent countries.

As in infants, osteomyelitis, painful periostitis from scurvy, syphilis or leukaemia, or bone tumours near joints need to be ruled out. Many patients in this age-group with painful limb joints are brought by their parents, the eventual diagnosis being 'growing pains'. It is doubtful if there is any such thing. Some are children who copy the complaints of their parents in order to gain sympathy. Others are experiencing the normal physiological cold-induced pain — as in the boy who spends 90 minutes standing on a cold ground watching a football match and comes home complaining that his feet ache. Juvenile chronic polyarthritis in this age-group may take several forms although the distinction of these forms may require time. The pauciarticular form affects one or two joints and may be associated with positive tests for anti-nuclear antigens and insidious development of chronic uveitis. The Wistler–Fanconi form occurs in the younger age-groups and there are rheumatoid factor positive juvenile forms of adult rheumatoid arthritis and (in boys) of HLA B27-associated adult ankylosing spondylitis. Juvenile systemic lupus erythematosus (SLE) (mainly in girls), juvenile psoriatic arthropathy and juvenile forms of reactive arthritis associated with inflammatory bowel disease are known but are rare. In the older children a transient or very rarely persistent arthritis can follow clinical rubella or immunisation against rubella (Grahame et al, 1983). Mumps, glandular fever, hepatitis B, Coxsackie B and chickenpox are other viral infections which have been observed on occasion to be followed by a synovitis which is usually transient and of little clinical consequence. Septic arthritis may be a diagnostic problem. Whenever a joint is inflamed and fluid is present it must be aspirated and cultured. Knees, hips and elbows are particularly liable to infection and the isolation of an infecting organism and its prompt treatment may save the function of the joint. In septicaemic illnesses, invasion of joints from the bloodstream is not uncommon. Staphylococci, streptococci, pneumococci, brucella abortus and brucella melitensis are some of the micro-organisms found. In meningococcal septicaemia (cerebrospinal fever, spotted fever), arthritis is usually of the reactive type, synovial fluid cultures being negative, and if the patient survives there is no residual damage to the joint. Rare immunodeficiency syndromes, including agammaglobulinaemia, may be associated with acute transient or persistent arthritis (Reviewed by Webster, 1983).

Adolescents and young adults

As the child becomes an adult, adult forms of RA and of psoriatic arthropathy and the various spondylarthropathies become more likely. For girls systemic lupus may present with arthritis, facial rash and systemic manifestations including pericarditis, pleurisy, fever, abortion, arthritis and loss of weight. The handsome young man with arthritis of a knee or ankle will probably have reactive arthritis, sexually acquired, but sometimes this is a prodromal manifestation of ankylosing spondylitis. Testing for the white cell group HLA-B27 is useful since if negative it makes ankylosing spondylitis or reactive arthritis, whether sexually acquired or postdysenteric, much less likely (a positive has to be evaluated in relation to the 7–10% of the population who possess this antigen, the majority of whom will never develop arthritis). Helpful clues include the development of the skin and nail changes of keratoderma blennorrhagica, balanitis, conjunctivitis, urethritis, cystitis, a history of diarrhoea, or the presence of psoriasis. Painful swelling of the Achilles tendon insertion at the heel, or pain in the plantar spur area are also strongly indicative of reactive arthritis. SARA also occurs in women — its incidence being generally underestimated (Neuwelt et al, 1982). Amongst sexually promiscuous females (Graber, 1965) and amongst practising male homosexuals, gonococcal arthritis is common. It is less common among heterosexual males, in whom gonorrhoea is discovered earlier and treated before arthritis occurs. The presentation is of a feverish illness with migratory oligoarthritis or tenosynovitis eventually settling in one or two joints, together with a scattered rash which may vary in appearance. It can be petechial or resemble the 'rose spot' macules of typhoid fever or the macules can be raised with a central pustule. The joint fluid is not always positive on culture for gonococci, partly because *Neisseria gonorrhoeae* is a fragile and fastidious micro-organism which easily dies out between bedside and laboratory, but often because the effusions are those of a reactive arthritis without direct infection. High vaginal swabs, urethral swabs and sometimes swabs after prostatic massage will be needed to establish the diagnosis in difficult cases. The gonococcal fixation test is unreliable. A positive serves only to alert suspicion. Urate gout is rare in this age-group. Hippocrates' third aphorism that 'a young man does not take the gout until he indulges in coitus' is more likely to refer to the involvement of joints of the feet by SARA in the light of modern knowledge.

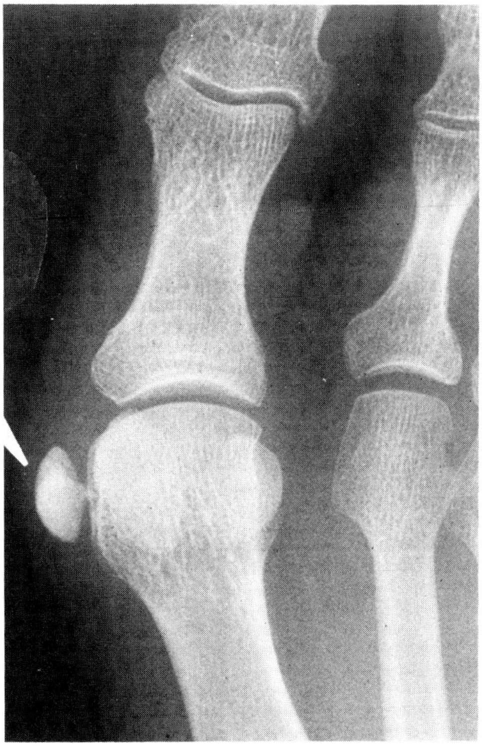

Fig. 5.1 Calcific tendinitis in capsule of hallux metatarsophalangeal joint (female aged 21).

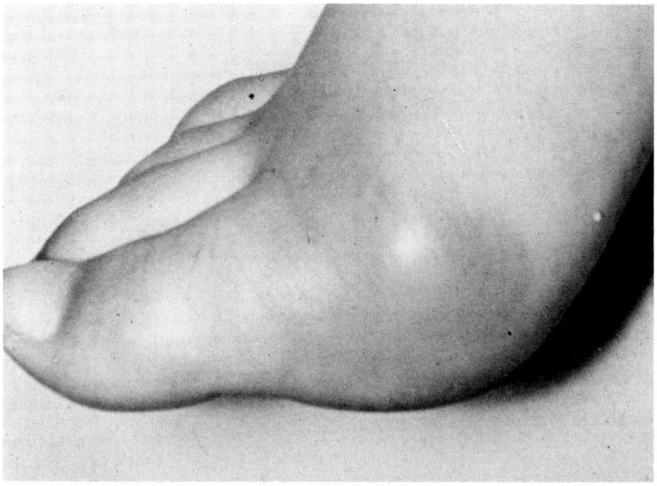

Fig. 5.2 Clinical appearance resembling gouty podagra.

But gout-like states have been observed in connection with the dispersal of deposits of hydroxyapatite in calcific tendonitis (see Figs. 5.1, 5.2) mostly in young women. 'Pseudo podagra' can occur at the first MTP as indeed it can in relationship to many joints or tendons, although acute subacromial bursitis due to deposits in the rotator cuff area, detectable by X-ray, are the most frequent.

The middle-aged and elderly

All too often synovitis in the 30–70 age-group is the onset of RA. In many such patients the blood titre for rheumatoid factor will already be positive when the patient is first seen. Kellgren & Ball (1959) were the first to show that the results of testing for rheumatoid factor can be predicted from the clinical and radiological features of the patients' polyarthritis with some confidence. Seropositive patients showed a typical distribution of joint involvement with symmetrical peripheral polyarthritis, which included involvement of both wrists, the index and middle metacarpophalangeal joints of both hands and the lateral metatarsophalangeal joints of the feet. (As the disease gets worse, other joints might become involved.) Seronegative patients could usually be predicted because they showed an atypical distribution of joint inflammation, affecting mainly the large, central joints, or with asymmetry of disease such that, for example, one knee might be severely damaged and the other normal. Dixon (1960) in a review of 61 seronegative patients from the same centre, found that 12 eventually developed positive tests for rheumatoid factor, and had typical distribution of joint disease. 23 others, otherwise similar, remained seronegative. However, 19 patients either developed other named polyarticular syndromes (11) or remained undiagnosable (8) by then current criteria. Thus persistent seronegativity, at the onset of polyarthritis, must give rise to the suspicion that diseases other than rheumatoid arthritis may eventually become apparent. Perhaps the most frequent of these is psoriatic arthropathy when the arthropathy antedates the rash. Onsets of urate gout become commoner in males of this age-group and 75% of such attacks start in the big toe. Onsets of the forms of reactive arthritis either sexually acquired or associated with dysenteric colitis or with *Yersinia* or *Campylobacter enterocolitis*, become less common. Forms of episodic recurrent or palindromic arthritis create a diagnostic puzzle (see below). From age 50 onwards and especially over the age of 60, polymyalgia rheumatica may occur. Classically it presents with severe, almost paralysing, morning stiffness affecting the shoulders and thighs in the *absence* of arthritis but in almost all reported series, transient, mild, non-deforming, non-erosive synovitis of peripheral joints or tendon sheaths has been observed in a few patients although usually not at the very onset of disease. In the older age-groups malignancy due to secondary deposits near joints, or leukaemic infiltration may mimic synovitis. Patients whose immune mechanisms are suppressed by disease or treatment are at risk from secondary septic arthritis caused by a variety of organisms, often with relatively mild signs. Acute arthritis in an old person admitted to hospital for another cause — a myocardial infarct, pneumonia, or a prostate operation, for example — is a common experience. In men it is often urate gout (especially when urate-retaining thiazide or loop diuretics have been taken) but in women it is more often chondrocalcinosis associated with calcium pyrophosphate deposition in joints which is causing the trouble.

In very old age

After the age of 70, first onsets of rheumatoid arthritis are increasingly rare. Gout, chondrocalcinosis, septic arthritis, are again the main causes of trouble. All too commonly non-inflammatory conditions which cause pain on movement are diagnosed as 'arthritis' in this group. Osteoarthrosis, fractures of femoral neck, osteomalacia, stress fractures of other bones, carcinomatous secondary deposits from the breast or prostate malignancies, Paget's disease near joints — these are often said to be 'arthritis' to the patient in the hope of softening the blow or covering up ignorance.

RARER CAUSES OF SYNOVITIS

Plant thorn synovitis in children is usually due to kneeling on a thorn, which eventually penetrates the synovium, while in adults it occurs in the finger joint, from gardening or similar activities. Synovectomy is curative.

Renal failure, renal transplantation, haemodialysis and peritoneal dialysis may all be followed by active synovitis associated with calcium pyrophosphate deposition within a joint, or hydroxyapatite around it. Mixed crystalline deposition occurs — urate and oxalate crystals have also been observed. Sickle cell disease and sickle-C haemoglobin disease present with fever and large joint arthritis, due to ischaemic infarction of the articular bone. Sickle-C trait should be suspected in those of Negro or mixed blood who develop acute pain from ischaemic joint disease after travelling in an aeroplane.

Villonodular synovitis occurs in children and young adults as a fixed, subacute joint swelling of one or two joints, hips and knees being most frequently affected. Synovial fluid is usually blood-stained and synovial biopsy is diagnostic.

Drugs are associated with synovitis. Drug-induced SLE complicates treatment with a variety of drugs. Hydrallazine, procainamide, and penicillamine are amongst those most often incriminated. A serum sickness-like reaction, with urticaria and arthritis, may follow penicillin or barbiturates. A polyarteritis nodosa-like syndrome may follow sensitivity to phenylbutazone and antithyroid drugs.

Huskisson & Hart (1978) have published a comprehensive list of most of the rare and not so rare associations of arthritis or joint pain.

SYMPTOMS AND SIGNS

Pain

This is the least reliable of the symptoms of arthritis in the differentiation of its various causes. The duration of pain and its accompaniments such as pain on movement, or pain on pressure, can be observed, but the intensity of pain cannot, since no-one can feel another's pain. The normal synovial membrane contains no pain nerve endings but the joint capsule and the ligamentous attachments around the joints have many. When a normal knee is experimentally distended with saline, there is at first little to feel. Then comes a feeling of stiffness in the joint but not until about 40 or 50 ml of fluid has been injected into the synovial cavity does it become painful at rest. Pain is therefore not a prominent symptom of the early mild arthritis. In RA severe pain felt in the arms at night is far more likely to be due to pressure on the median nerve in the carpal tunnel. Patients complain of weakness, tiredness and above all of frustration in the early stages of rheumatoid polyarthritis but relatively little of pain. However, when very inflammatory fluid fills the joint, the clinical picture is complicated by the presence in the fluid of chemical mediators of inflammation and pain. Pain at rest then becomes possible and it is a feature of gout and of septic arthritis.

Weakness

Inhibitory reflexes weaken the action of the muscles which move a distended joint. Painful weakness of grip is thus a feature of arthritis of the hands, particularly of the wrist.

Morning stiffness, rest stiffness

Careful measurements show circadial variation in normal joints. Thus, in the very early morning, the finger joints are one or two millimetres greater in circumference, the strength of grip is weaker and there is a feeling of stiffness in the joints, most pronounced before the normal waking increase in circulating cortisol levels. These changes in normal joints are exaggerated in all forms of arthritis and have little or no differential diagnostic force. The as yet unexplained severe morning stiffness of polymyalgia rheumatica, in the absence of joint swelling, is diagnostically helpful. Severe stiffness of movement may precede arthritis in the erythema nodosum syndrome.

Symmetrical distribution of joint involvement

When one joint is affected there can be no symmetry. With all joints affected there can be no asymmetry. In established RA, symmetry of involvement, particularly of the small joints of the hands and wrists, may be a striking feature — but symmetry or the lack of it is unhelpful in very early disease.

Monarticular synovitis

Synovitis of a single joint is not uncommon in rheumatology. Within the first month or so, this will often have declared itself by clinical course, X-ray, or laboratory investigation as gout, chondrocalcinosis, infection or the result of trauma such as the wrist swelling and pain which follows an ununited fracture of the scaphoid. But in a proportion of such patients, monarticular synovitis persists, most often in the knee, providing a problem in differential diagnosis. Fletcher & Scott (1975) analysed 151 such patients with single joint synovitis of at least 13 weeks duration followed-up to 350 weeks. At follow-up 32% still had 'synovitis of unknown cause' and were the largest group. In those to whom a firm diagnostic label could be attached, 29% had osteoarthritis, 9% (13 patients) developed rheumatoid arthritis (and in 12 of the 13, other joints became involved), 5% had traumatic synovitis, 5% osteochondritis dissecans, 14% had chondrocalcinosis and 4% a loose body in the joint. 18 patients had rarer conditions including psoriatic arthropathy, septic arthritis, Reiter's syndrome, ankylosing spondylitis, Crohn's disease, sarcoidosis, Freiberg's disease, neuropathic arthropathy, giant cell synovitis, malignant melanoma, osteoblastoma or hypermobility syndrome. Only one patient had tuberculosis, emphasising the near disappearance of bone and joint tuberculosis in Britain. Needle biopsy of the synovium was used to back up the diagnosis, but with few exceptions such as villonodular synovitis, or chondrocalcinosis, this does not often produce certainty.

Palindromic or intermittent forms of arthritis

Any chronic disease carries the implication of a dynamic equilibrium between the disease and the recovery process, otherwise the patient would be cured or dead. In the early stages of any form of chronic arthritis the cybernetics of the dynamic equilibrium may lead to 'hunting'. The clinical picture oscillates between bouts of disease and intervals of recovery before settling down to a steady state. 'Palindromic rheumatism' was the name coined by Hench to describe attacks of acute polyarthritis, sometimes with fever, which disappeared as mysteriously as they came leaving the patient well in-between bouts. 'Intermittent hydrarthrosis' is a descriptive term for recurrent swelling and effusion, usually in the knees. Rarely, cyclical forms of intermittent arthritis occur with a set sequence of involvement of, in turn, hips, knees, ankles and other joints. 'Palindromic' onsets of RA are seen and carry a poor prognosis, especially if associated ab initio with positive tests for IgM rheumatoid factor. In men, the picture may resemble the classical episodic onsets of urate gout with long periods of recovery between attacks. Palindromic or intermittent forms of polyarthritis have been observed evolving into RA, SARA, systemic lupus erythematosus and ankylosing spondylitis, as well as gout. In familial Mediterranean fever, episodes of fever, rash and arthritis are a common mode of onset. In a proportion of patients — perhaps around 50% — palindromic rheumatism eventually clears up without sequelae or just continues without ever evolving. The differential diagnosis depends heavily on the blood tests (RA factor, serum urate, DNA binding, HLA status) but eventually on the passage of time, and the unrolling of the full clinical picture.

Skin, hair, nail and mucous membrane changes

Psoriasis usually precedes psoriatic arthropathy and makes the diagnosis easy but occasionally the arthritis comes first or the psoriatic changes are cryptic and confined to changes in the nails, or to flexural psoriasis in the axillae, folds of the breasts, in the navel or natal cleft, which would be missed unless looked for. Any nail dystrophy should give rise to suspicion of psoriasis if associated with arthritis. Thimble pitting and nail-plate dystrophy are psoriatic changes which grow out with the nail. Subungual hyperkeratosis is a precocious separation of the free margin of the nail with accumulation of soft keratotic material under the nail plate. It increases in the direction contrary to nail growth. The association of subungual hyperkeratosis and terminal interphalangeal joint swelling in psoriatic arthropathy gives rise to one of the spot diagnoses of rheumatology (Fig. 5.3). Clubbing, if severe, is seldom related to joint disease but mild to moderate clubbing accompanies hypertrophic pulmonary osteoarthropathy (HPOA). The cigarette-tar-stained clubbed finger of the man coming into the rheumatology clinic for his painful limbs is another spot diagnosis, i.e. bronchial carcinoma with HPOA. Rashes are of diagnostic help in rheumatic fever (erythema marginatum),

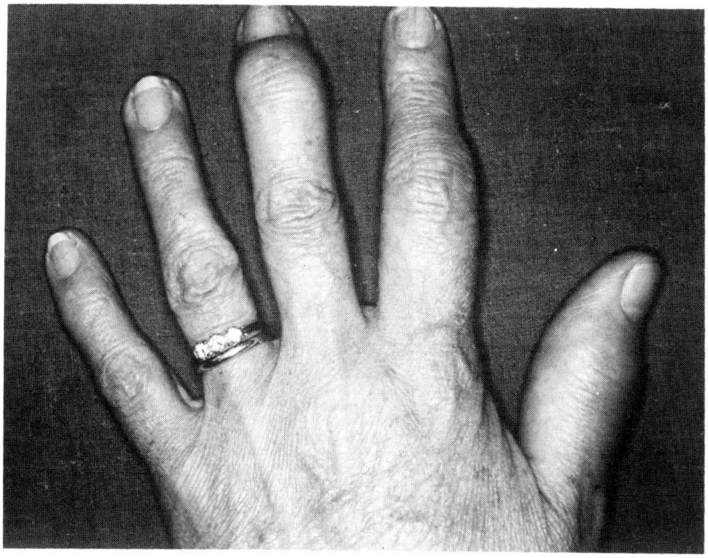

Fig. 5.3 Psoriatic arthropathy. Involvement of middle finger terminal interphalangeal and thumb interphalangeal joints. Early 'sausage finger' change in proximal and middle phalanges of index finger.

Henoch–Schönlein purpura, rubella arthritis and systemic lupus erythematosus. Erythema nodosum usually precedes, but sometimes follows, arthritis in a knee or ankle. Hair fall is quite common in young women suffering from systemic lupus erythematosus but is not sufficiently diagnostic to be included as one of the official criteria of that disease. Genital ulcers point to the diagnosis of Behçet's disease or sometimes of SARA (Reiter's disease), particularly if they are accompanied by mouth ulcers and arthritis. In practice orogenital herpes simplex is sufficiently common to be by chance associated with other forms of arthritis and viral studies should be done. The rash of keratoderma blennorrhagica is easy to overlook when mild. It occurs as fixed, deep patches of reddish-brown discolouration (varying in size from a few millimetres to a few centimetres across on the soles of the feet), which eventually develop into rupioid areas of heaped up keratotic material. The rash also occurs in the corona at the base of the glans penis. Failure to retract the foreskin in a young man with SARA will lead to missing a valuable clue. In multifocal reticulohistiocytosis there is a characteristic aggregation of tiny reddish nodules around the base of the nails which can be a spot diagnosis.

Pigmentation and scaling reflect the severity and duration of inflammation of the skin over a previously inflamed joint. Thus acute gout, if the attack is prolonged, will be followed by the development of sunburn-like pigmentation of the overlying skin which in turn is followed by scaling. However, the same changes can be seen over an area of cellulitis due to infection. Involvement of the interphalangeal joints in the toes in sexually acquired or other forms of reactive arthritis may lead to swollen sausage-like toes with a coppery pigmentation. In dark skinned peoples, arthritis — especially RA — is associated with greater intensity of pigmentation over involved joints. A brown skin may become black over the joint.

Fever

'When the body is sick, the joints weep'. A transient and usually trivial synovitis can occur in a wide variety of feverish illnesses. In those caused by infections, the synovitis may possibly reflect a bacteraemia without established joint infection. The clinical picture is usually dominated by the cause of the fever but fever with relatively mild or flitting synovitis is a feature of rheumatic fever, of systemic lupus, of Henoch–Schönlein purpura and certain forms of JCA, including the rare adult onset JCA, and gonococcal arthritis. Fever can be (rarely) an accompaniment of severe polyarticular gout but never of early gout. Septic arthritis with fever, with positive bacterial culture in joint fluid, is usually part of a septicaemia diagnosed by blood cultures but may occur paradoxically without fever in immunosuppressed patients.

Lymphadenitis, lymphangitis and splenic enlargement

Regional lymph node swelling is recognised but uncommon in early rheumatoid arthritis particularly in the younger subject but is to be expected in juvenile chronic arthritis and sexually acquired reactive arthritis. It is sometimes confused, even after biopsy, with Brill-Symmers' disease (follicular lymphoma). Lymphadenitis does not occur in gout. The writer has only once seen lymphangitis in gout and that not severe; lymphangitis does not occur with other non-infective causes of arthritis. The association of lymphangitis and lymphadenitis with a painful red foot indicates infection. Splenomegaly is not a helpful sign in early arthritis. It occurs in JCA, in lupus, and of course in lymphoproliferative conditions where arthritis and gout are minor manifestations. Marked or persistent splenomegaly associated with synovitis points to subacute bacterial endocarditis, leukaemia, or to polycythaemia rubra vera or myeloblastic anaemia with gout.

Subcutaneous nodules, tendon nodules

The presence of subcutaneous nodules considerably reduces the number of possible diagnoses (Table 5.2); although only rarely are nodules present at the onset of polyarthritis. Rheumatoid arthritis is the disease in which subcutaneous nodules are most often found. They may occur along the olecranon border of the forearm or in the walls of the olecranon bursae and occasionally over the prominences of the knuckles, knees, or malleoli. They also occur along the course of the digital extensor tendons and the Achilles tendon. Tophi of urate gout are late manifestations of that

Table 5.2 Subcutaneous nodules associated with arthritis

Common:	Rheumatoid arthritis
Less common:	Gouty tophi at elbow or behind the heel or subcutaneous nodules in systemic lupus and in rheumatic fever
Rare:	Calcific nodules in calcinosis circumscripta (idiopathic or accompanying dermatomyositis). Xanthomatous deposits near elbow or Achilles tendon. Intradermal nodules in multicentric reticulohistiocytosis
Unassociated:	Neurofibroma, lipoma, haemangioma, etc.

disease, though occasionally in older subjects with renal failure they may precede arthritis. Other nodules around the elbow include calcinosis circumscripta and xanthomatous deposits. Small nodules on the elbow, found better by inspection than palpation, occur in rheumatic fever and systemic lupus erythematosus and in multifocal reticulohistiocytosis. Coincidental elbow nodules include neurofibromata and lipomata diagnosable by the rest of the clinical picture and by biopsy. Garrod's pads (knuckle pads) sometimes cause confusion with the digital nodules of rheumatoid arthritis, particularly when accompanying osteoarthritis.

Rheumatoid subcutaneous nodules carry a high, almost 100%, association with positive tests for RA factor in the blood. Tendon nodules, particularly in the flexor tendons of the hands, are not so closely related to the presence of RA factor and may occur in various forms of seronegative polyarthritis and in multicentric reticulohistiocytosis. Heel nodules, felt by firm palpation in the cushion tissue under the heel have only a weak association with rheumatoid factor.

The patterns of joint involvement

There are characteristic patterns of involvement of the joints in the hand (Fig. 5.4; Kellgren, 1957).

The pattern in adults with early RA is wrists plus index and middle metacarpophalangeal joints affecting both sides symmetrically. The pattern in the early painful and slightly inflammatory stage of primary nodal osteoarthritis is in the terminal interphalangeal joints especially that of the index finger. The pattern of involvement in gouty hands is random. Psoriatic arthropathy gives terminal interphalangeal joint swelling, diagnostic if associated with subungual hyperkeratosis and accompanied by the 'sausage finger' sign, namely cylindrical swelling of the whole digit from a combination of proximal interphalangeal, distal interphalangeal and flexor tendon sheath swelling. Fusiform or spindle-shaped swelling of the proximal interphalangeal joints is more characteristic of JCA and younger subjects with RA.

In the feet it is the first metatarsophalangeal joints which are most often affected by urate gout, usually asymmetrically, and the lateral metatarsophalangeal joints by RA and SARA. However, other valuable clues occur in the feet. Nodules over the Achilles tendon need to be distinguished from the diffuse Achilles insertional tendinitis, a form of enthesopathy, which leads to a hard woody swelling of the Achilles tendon and its insertional area over the heel. If present, this is a strong pointer to reactive arthritis, usually sexually acquired, but also as an accompaniment of ankylosing spondylitis. Like the latter, it is highly correlated with the presence of HLA-B27 in the blood. In contrast, pain in the plantar spur area is often idiopathic, although occasionally associated with seronegative polyarthropathies.

Regional muscle wasting

This is not an early sign of arthritis but may come on with remarkable rapidity in tuberculous arthritis.

Involvement of the eyes

Conjunctivitis presents as a red, uncomfortable eye in SARA. The *painful* red eye with blurred vision of acute iritis points to ankylosing spondylitis. A more severe, but painless, chronic uveitis occurs in JCA and is often unnoticed until sight is threatened. It may precede the involvement of the joints. Conjunctivitis with arthritis occurs in Behçet's disease and may be associated with ophthalmoplegia or partial visual loss.

Other organ involvement

Pericarditis and occasionally pericardial tamponade are seen in JCA, RA and SARA but only in rheumatic fever or systemic lupus erythematosus are these presenting features. Myocarditis in rheumatic fever is shown by first or second degree heart block, or by T wave inversion. T wave

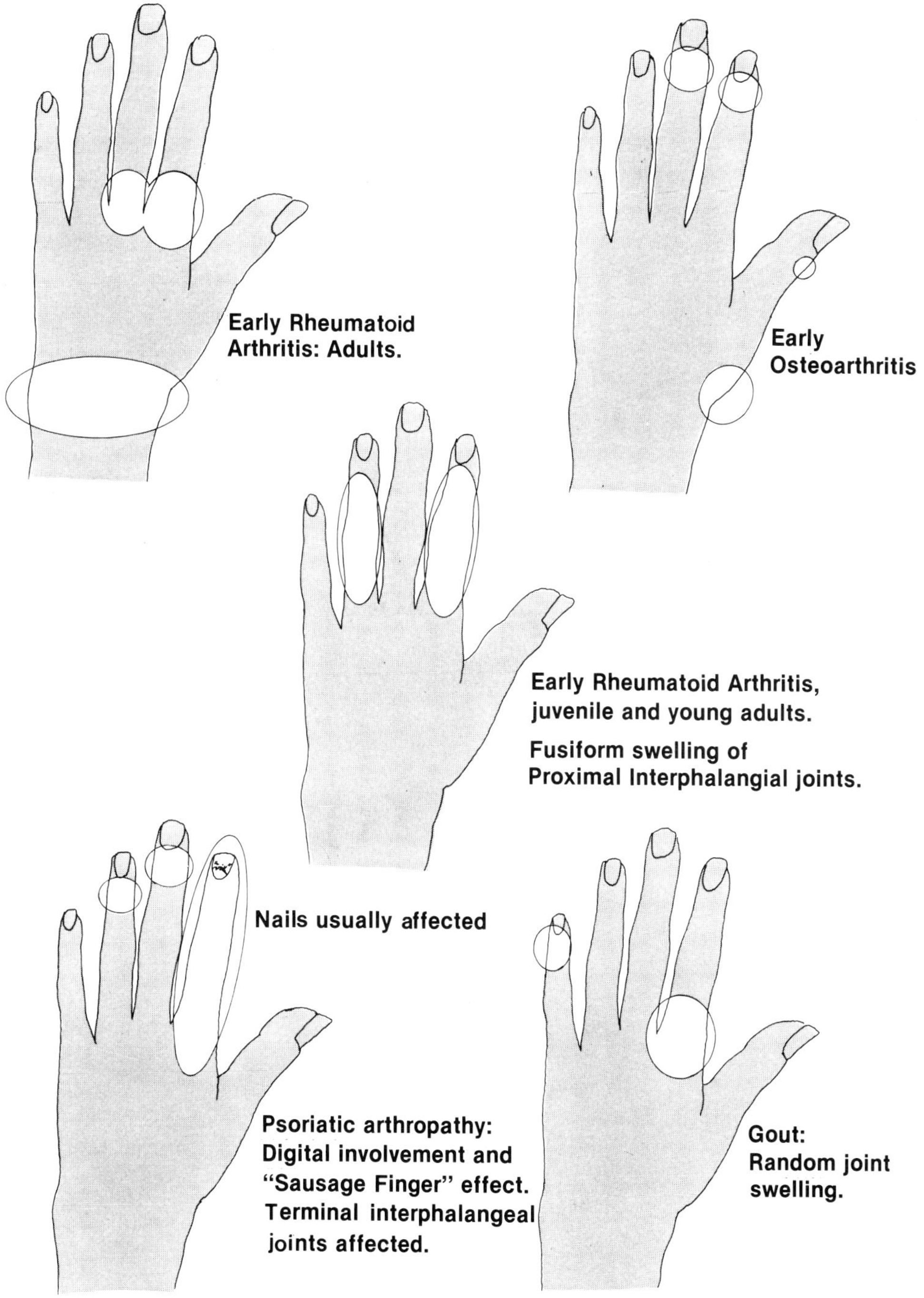

Fig. 5.4 Patterns of hand joint involvement in chronic joint diseases.

inversion in the anterior chest leads is also an occasional non-specific accompaniment of the erythema nodosum syndrome. Valvulitis in rheumatic fever or in the Libman–Sacks endocarditis of systemic lupus erythematosus may be helpful in diagnosis. Hilar node enlargement seen on chest X-rays is a common, predictable accompaniment of the erythema nodosum syndrome and is not specific. It does not imply that the lesions of visceral sarcoidosis will follow. Pulmonary involvement with segmental lung collapse and disproportionate dyspnoea accompany the early phase of systemic lupus erythematosus when the lung is involved. Curiously, it is in men destined to develop RA that pulmonary changes have been noted to antedate joint swelling. Pulmonary involvement takes one of several forms. Pulmonary nodules, either discrete or multiple and following exposure to coal dust (Caplan's syndrome) can precede the arthritis by months or years. So can pleurisy with effusion. Aspiration of pleural fluid may be helpful. A sterile, turbid fluid, with a low glucose concentration is predictive of subsequent RA.

Central nervous system involvement in association with arthritis points to systemic lupus erythematosus and sometimes to Behçet's disease. Proteinuria occurs in Henoch–Schönlein purpura with nephritis and in systemic lupus erythematosus. The most important genitourinary tract manifestation in the history and examination is non-specific urethritis or cystitis in sexually acquired reactive arthritis. Its presence may be difficult to detect. Urethritis in men varies from a slight gleet and nocturnal discharge with staining of the pyjamas to a painful urgency and frequency with haematuria. The two-glass test may show pus in the first few drops of urine. In young women almost any urinary symptoms, including urgency and frequency, pain and haematuria may be significant. Sexually acquired reactive arthritis occurs in women but its frequency is underestimated because of the greater difficulty in associating the genitourinary symptoms with the disease.

Carpal tunnel syndrome

Carpal tunnel syndrome, in varying degrees of severity, is a common early feature of synovitis of the wrist or of the digital flexor tendon sheaths in the carpal tunnel. The characteristic signs include pain in the arm, worse at night, often with a burning quality, for which the patient attempts to gain relief by hanging the hands outside the bedcloths or shaking them. Paraesthesiae are more accurately confined to the radial $3\frac{1}{2}$ digits, although the thumb is often spared. Abductor brevis weakness and electromyographic changes give late inconstant but if present supportive evidence but the best confirmation is the signal relief afforded by decompression of the carpal tunnel by a corticosteroid injection or by surgery. The carpal tunnel syndrome is present in about half of those affected by early RA. Differential diagnosis at this stage includes other causes of carpal tunnel syndrome, including hypothyroidism, acromegaly, myelomatosis and the fluid retention of pregnancy. It occurs as a late sequel of Colles' fracture and it is particularly confusing in patients with stiff, painful shoulders where the lack of elevation of the arm and of the pumping action of the forearm muscles lead to congestion in the hand.

Rheumatoid arthritis — unusual modes of onset

'Unusual manifestations of common diseases are commoner than usual manifestation of rare diseases' — is a good guide in differential diagnosis. Some of the rarer modes of onset of RA need to be remembered. Carpal tunnel syndrome has been mentioned. Other forms of tenosynovitis affect the extensor tendons on the back of the wrist and are often misdiagnosed as a ganglion. Tenosynovitis of the long thumb abductor tendon may mimick De Quervain's disease. To tenosynovitis around the ankle various names, including 'peroneal spasm' and 'acute flat foot', have been applied. Onsets in the lateral metatarsophalangeal joints are miscalled 'metatarsalgia' or 'dropped anterior arch'. Rheumatoid arthritis sometimes seems to start after a bunion operation suggesting that it was the arthritis rather than the bent toe which originally caused the patient to complain. Rarely RA starts in the neck, the temporomandibular joint or in the shoulder joint. From time to time patients, unaware of their arthritis, present for removal of large rheumatoid nodules. Palindromic onsets and rheumatoid lung changes anticipating the arthritis have already been mentioned.

X-RAYS IN DIFFERENTIAL DIAGNOSIS

Radiographs of joints do not often aid in the differential diagnosis of early arthritis but they help to eliminate bone disease in or near a joint, for example, a stress fracture or osteochondritis dissecans. However, they introduce additional sources of confusion. This is by no means confined to the unthinking radiologist who, investigating a painful back or neck, finds some harmless osteophyte or minor disc degeneration and informs the patient that she has "arthritis of the spine". Cystic erosions of subarticular bone (geodes), a feature of all forms of inflammatory arthritis including rheumatoid arthritis and gout, are very similar to the cysts seen in the metacarpal and styloid processes of the hands and wrists in osteoarthrosis, particularly in manual workers. However, such X-ray changes are relatively late. In early arthritis, when diagnostic difficulty may be experienced, cystic erosions are rare. Patterns of bone loss around the joint are largely determined by the pattern of vascular supply (Brower & Allman, 1982) and 'no one radiograph is specific for one disease'. The earliest X-ray changes (which are not seen until much later in the large joints) occur in the small joints of the hands and feet as extra-articular osteoporosis, a loss of joint 'space' and juxta-articular periosteal new bone growth. Soft tissue shadows are important. The subsynovial fatty layers can be visualised as a relatively translucent zone around a joint, a zone which is displaced or opacified when fluid accumulates in the joint, and when inflammatory oedema (with its higher calcium content) infiltrates the fat. Juxta-articular osteoporosis is particularly rapid in onset in pyarthrosis whether septic or tuberculous.

Other causes of articular osteoporosis includes Sudeck's atrophy and neighbourhood inflammation as in early osteomyelitis, not primarily in the joint. Loss of joint space occurs in osteoarthrosis but the bones themselves remain dense. Periosteal new bone formation in arthritis is either due to hypertrophic pulmonary osteoarthropathy (rare) or most commonly this is a reaction to intense inflammation in neighbouring tenosynovial sheaths and bursae. Periostitis along the shaft of a metacarpal or metatarsal bone is most often seen in children with JCA or in young adults with psoriatic arthropathy or reactive arthritis. It is rare in seropositive RA, but can occur in very acute aggressive disease.

It is in early ankylosing spondylitis and in SARA that X-rays of the sacroiliac joints are most helpful. The best view is obtained with an antero-posterior view of the whole pelvis, with the beam directed cephalward. Gonad shields interfere with the view in females but not in males. This view separates the anterior and posterior parts of the sacroiliac joints and allows comparison of one side with another and inspection of the pubic symphysis and entheses around the trochanters, iliac crests and ischial tuberosities. Early ossification in these areas may be seen. Postero-anterior or oblique views of the sacroiliac joints, theoretically carrying certain advantages, are in practice confusing. Sacroiliac X-rays should be done routinely in seronegative peripheral arthritis in young people, particularly when one or two large joints in the legs are affected. The early diagnostic changes are set out in Chapter 29. Spinal and peripheral joint symptoms in ankylosing spondylitis may on occasions precede sacroiliitis. Even earlier diagnosis using technetium scanning or computerised axial tomography scanning have not proved helpful in practice. One negative X-ray finding is sometimes of interest in differential diagnosis — namely that marginal osteophytes are never seen in inflammatory arthritis which shows continuing activity of the inflammatory process. They are also absent in the joint lysis which accompanies certain forms of chondrocalcinosis.

LABORATORY TESTS

Acute phase reactants are present in arthritis as in any inflammatory condition and their absence throws doubt on the diagnosis. The erythrocyte sedimentation rate, plasma viscosity and C-reactive protein tests are the most reliable but in some individuals one or more of these tests may be unexpectedly normal in the face of obvious arthritis. False negative tests are commonest in men with purely spinal ankylosing spondylitis but seldom occur if peripheral joints are also affected. Tests for IgM rheumatoid factor (Rose test, latex fixation test) help considerably. Positive results are to be expected in nodular RA (100%) and in about 80% of non-nodular RA of typical peripheral distribution. The frequency of positive tests is less in the first year of the disease. Positive tests for rheumatoid factor occur in about 30% of patients with systemic lupus erythematosus and polyarteritis nodosa when arthritis is also present. Tests for IgG rheumatoid factor are available but their diagnostic significance is not yet certain. Tests for recent infection by group A β-haemolytic streptococci (GpAβHS) include the anti-streptolysin O titre (ASO), anti-hyaluronidase and anti-desoxyribonuclease tests. These tests reflect mainly recent infection. Titres of 200 or more in the ASO are taken as significant but need careful interpretation. The average family with young children has at least two streptococcal infections of the throat every year, so a rising titre has more significance than isolated elevated titres as evidence of recent streptococcal infection in rheumatic fever. Only 80% of strains of GpAβHS produce streptolysin giving a possibility of 20% false negatives. The addition of the other tests improved the 'catch'. The ASO test is of most value when negative in ruling out rheumatic fever. Positive results in association with arthritis occur in some patients with erythema nodosum, Henoch–Schönlein purpura, or by chance in children with JCA.

Similar reservations apply to the serum urate level test for gout. Urate gout cannot occur in the absence of a raised serum urate (except in the course of treatment) but hyperuricaemia in population or hospital surveys is ten times more commonly unaccompanied then accompanied by gout, so much so that patients with other arthritic diseases may show false positive hyperuricaemia. Thiazide and loop diuretics which inhibit tubular secretion of urate and mild degrees of renal failure are the commonest sources of non-gouty hyperuricaemia but there are many others.

Tests for the white cell antigen HLA-B27 have proved helpful, especially in monarthritis or oligoarthritis and in reactive arthritis and in the peripheral arthritis associated with the back pain of ankylosing spondylitis. 95% of ankylosing spondylitis sufferers, about 85% of those with sexually acquired reactive arthritis (especially if the sacroiliac joints are affected) and 70–80% of rheumatoid factor negative monarthritis sufferers in this class are positive. However, in population surveys there are four or more people who are HLA-B27-positive without arthritis or spondylitis for every one who has or will develop these conditions.

Other laboratory methods in differential diagnosis

These include examination of joint fluid, biopsy of the synovial membrane and arthroscopy with biopsy. These are discussed in Chapters 8 and 66.

Biopsy of nodules is helpful in the uncommon patient whose gouty tophus at the elbow may resemble a rheumatoid nodule. In such instances the diagnosis is obvious to the naked eye as soon as the nodule is opened up. Biopsy will be needed to differentiate 'bogus' nodules such as a fibroma which are coincidental with early arthritis but not related to it. Biopsy of small nodules on the fingers and occasionally around the elbows may be needed in granuloma annulare, the histology of which somewhat resembles that of RA but this is a condition that is not associated with systemic arthritis.

Skin biopsy has been helpful in systemic lupus erythematosus with appropriate immunofluorescent staining.

REFERENCES

Brower A C, Allman R M 1982 Vascular influence on patterns of deossification. Arthritis and Rheumatism 25: 333–338

Castillo B A, El Sallab R A, Scott J T 1965 Physical activity, cystic erosions and osteoporosis in rheumatoid arthritis. Annals of Rheumatic Diseases 24: 522–527

Dixon A S 1960 'Rheumatoid arthritis' with a negative serological reaction. Annals of Rheumatic Diseases 19: 209–228

Fletcher M R, Scott J T 1975 Chronic monarticular synovitis: Diagnostic and prognostic features. Annals of Rheumatic Diseases 34: 171–176

Glick E N 1966 Asymmetrical rheumatoid arthritis after poliomyelitis. Lancet

Graber W J, Sanford J P, Ziff M 1960 Sex incidence of gonococcal arthritis. Arthritis and Rheumatism 3: 309–313

Grahame R, Armstrong R, Simmons N, Wilton J M A, Dyson M, Laurent R et al 1983 Chronic arthritis associated with the presence of intra synovial rubella virus. Annals of Rheumatic Diseases 42: 2–13

Huskisson E C, Hart F D 1978 Joint disease: all the arthropathies, 3rd Edn. John Wright, Bristol

Kellgren J H, Ball J 1959 Clinical significance of the Rheumatoid Serum Factor. British Medical Journal 1: 523–531

Neuwelt C M, Borenstein D G, Jacobs R P 1982 Reiter's syndrome: a male and female disease. Journal of Rheumatology 9: 268–272

Soila P 1963 A roentgenological study of asymmetry in rheumatoid arthritis. Acta Rheumatologica Scandinavica 9: 264–268

Thompson M, Bywaters E G L 1962 Unilateral rheumatoid arthritis following hemiplegia. Annals of Rheumatic Diseases 21: 370–377

Webster A D B 1983 Immunodeficiency and rheumatic diseases. Reports on Rheumatic Diseases, No. 84

SECTION II

Connective Tissue

6

H. Muir T.E. Hardingham

Biochemistry of connective tissue

The evolution of multicellular organisms made necessary the development of an extracellular matrix to protect cells and to bind them together in spatial arrangements needed for specialised anatomical and physiological functions.

All tissues are composed of cells that are surrounded by an extracellular matrix. The nature and extent of the matrix varies with the function of the tissue, but in connective tissues, where there is a mechanical function to perform, the extracellular matrix is particularly well developed. The broad range of physical properties encountered in different tissues is determined by variations in the relative proportion and molecular organisation of fibrous (collagen and elastin) and non-fibrous components. The fibrous elements provide the structural framework and tensile properties of the tissue, whereas the non-fibrous components (such as proteoglycan) influence the organisation of the fibrous components and control the water content and ionic composition of the tissue fluid (Muir, 1983). Connective tissues thus form the architecture of the body and this chapter reviews some of the properties of the extracellular macromolecules that are responsible for this role.

The articular joint is important in giving movement and mobility to an otherwise rigid bony skeleton. The function is essentially biomechanical, to transmit forces from one set of components to another. The loads applied to the different components are derived from body mass and muscle contractions.

The joint is composed of a number of tissues; bone, articular cartilage, synovium, soft connective tissue, ligaments and tendons and although of diverse physical properties they are all important for the biomechanical function of the joint. Connective tissue is relatively acellular and the specialised cells in each type of connective tissue synthesise and secrete the structural macromolecules of their extracellular matrix. They maintain it in its normal state and have some ability to repair any damage that may arise, but as the articular joint is dependent on the integrity of several kinds of connective tissue it is particularly vulnerable to changes in the physical properties of any one of its component parts.

The principal structural protein of animals is collagen, which is the most prevalent protein in

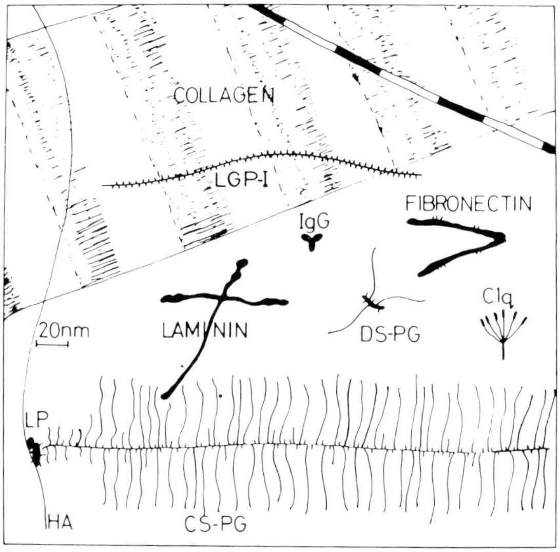

Fig. 6.1 Connective tissue macromolecules. A scale drawing of the molecular features of some major connective tissue macromolecules including hyaluronate (HA), cartilage proteoglycan (CS-PG), dermatan sulphate proteoglycan (DS-PG), lubricating glycoprotein (LPG-1), and also (for comparison) immunoglobulin (IgG) and the complement protein Clq. Details from: Engel et al, 1981; Perkins et al, 1981; Swann, 1978.

the body. It was first thought to be a single protein, but it is now known to consist of a family of similar but genetically distinct proteins which have specific distributions in the body and presumably, therefore, specific functions. The major collagens are fibrillar and endow the tissues with tensile strength (Fig. 6.1). However, the orientation of the fibres varies widely in different tissues: thus in skin, which is extensible, the fibres form a loose network, whereas in tendon, which is of high tensile strength and not extensible, the fibres are parallel and lie along the length of the tendon. In all connective tissues, interspersed throughout the collagen fibre network, are macromolecules which have properties that are complementary to those of collagen, such as proteoglycans (Fig. 6.1). These contain highly charged polysaccharides with many carboxylate and sulphate groups, which in consequence are extremely hydrophylic and thus retain water in the tissues. Most connective tissues contain about 70–80% water.

Elastin is also an important structural protein which is present in certain tissues requiring elasticity such as blood vessel walls and skin. It is structurally unrelated to collagen, but shares some biosynthetic features. It is now clear that a range of other proteins also participate in the molecular organisation of the extracellular matrix. Amongst these are fibronectin, which is widely distributed in many different tissues, and laminin which is also in many tissues, but with a restricted distribution as a component of basement membranes (Fig. 6.1). These proteins have the capacity to interact with collagen or other connective tissue macromolecules and may thus participate in further levels of molecular organisation amongst the fibrous and non-fibrous protein and carbohydrate components and with the cells of connective tissues. It has not yet been determined how these interactions contribute to the structural integrity of the matrix or what their role is in the biology of connective tissue cells. However, the selective distribution of the different components of connective tissue suggest they all make some distinct contribution to function and, far from being 'amorphous', the ground substance of each type of connective tissue is a highly organised assembly of selected components.

In this chapter, where cogent and clear reviews are available, reference to these will be given rather than to individual papers, as the latter can be obtained from the reviews.

COLLAGEN

Structure

(For reviews see Miller, 1978; Prockop et al, 1979; Burgeson, 1982; Nimni, 1983.) The molecular structure of fibrillar collagen is ideally designed to provide tensile strength to the tissue. The tensile strength of human knee cartilage is directly correlated with its collagen content and is greater when tested in a direction parallel to the predominant fibre orientation (Kempson et al, 1973). In tendon, a tissue particularly strong in tension, the fibres are arranged in parallel along the tendon. For an extensive review of the biomechanical properties of collagen, see Hukins (1982). Each molecule consists of three polypeptide chains (α chains) coiled in a left-handed helix with about three amino acids per turn. The three helical chains are then twisted round each other into a right-handed superhelix to form a structure like a segment of fine rope. Interchain and intermolecular cross-links further stabilise the molecular arrangement (see below). Each polypeptide chain contains about 1000 amino acid residues and with the exception of short non-helical regions at both ends of the chains (originally called 'telopeptides'), every third residue in each chain is glycine, the smallest amino acid. Its presence in every third position enables the three polypeptide chains when twisted together to approach closely at the glycine residues. Collagen therefore contains a high proportion of a repetitive amino acid sequence x-y-gly where about one-third of x is proline and y hydroxyproline. High contents of proline and hydroxyproline are characteristic of collagens, and hydroxyproline content is often used to measure the amount of collagen in tissues. However, hydroxyproline is not exclusive to collagen and occurs in small amounts in elastin and also in some non-connective tissue proteins, i.e. the complement component Clq which resembles a bunch of six tulips (Fig. 6.1), whose triple helical 'stalks' are composed of 'collagen-like' sequences (Reid, 1982) and acetylcholinesterase which has a collagen-like tail.

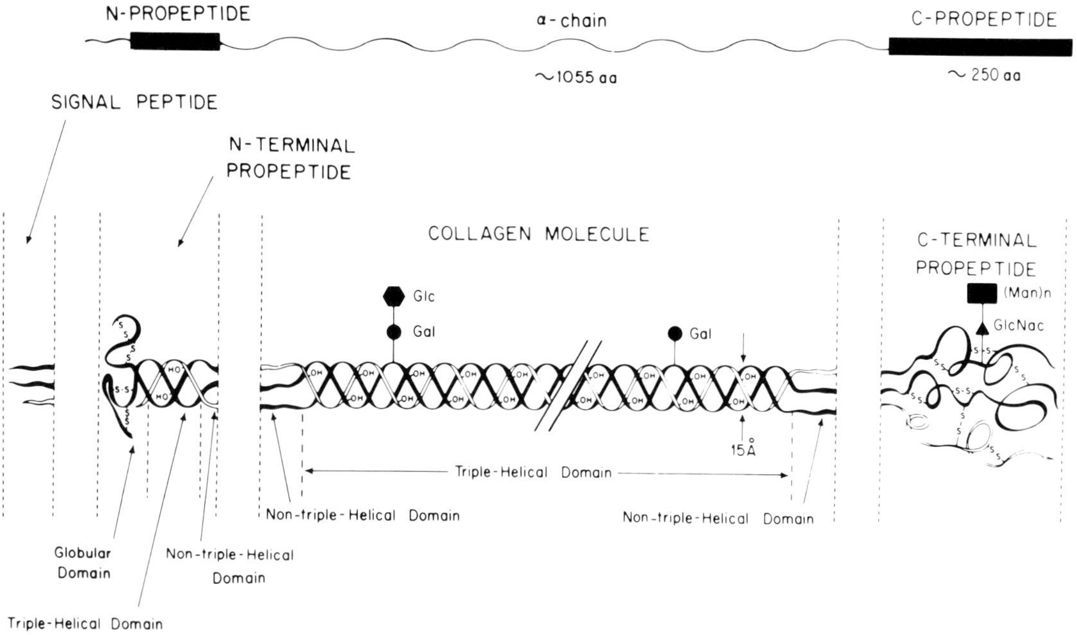

Fig. 6.6 Structure of type I pre-procollagen. Note the signal peptides at the N-termini are cleaved as nascent chains enter the endoplasmic reticulum, whereas N and C terminal propeptides are not removed until after secretion of procollagen from the cell. Oblique bars at the centre of the helical region denotes the collagenase cleavage site (from Olsen, 1981).

through the membranes into the cisternae of the rough endoplasmic reticulum (RER). A hydrophobic additional or signal sequence is first formed at the amino terminal ends of the polypeptide, which probably binds to the membrane of the rough endoplasmic reticulum and may direct the movement of the nascent polypeptide chain along the rough endoplasmic reticulum. The signal sequences are subsequently cleaved within the membrane during translation. The chains are initially formed as pro-α-chains with long extension peptides at both the carboxy- and amino-terminal ends which account for about a third of the weight of the pro-α-chain (Fig. 6.6). The extension peptides mainly are globular and markedly different in amino acid composition from the helical region of collagen, particularly in containing a number of cysteine residues which subsequently form disulphide bridges. The extension peptides also contain oligosaccharides linked to asparagine which are typical of glycoproteins and which do not occur in collagen itself. The pro-α-chains are progressively modified before secretion and also afterwards, and the complexity of the process, elucidated in the last few years, underlines the importance of ensuring the correct molecular structure to enable functional collagens fibres to be formed. Hydroxylation of proline to form hydroxyproline is an essential step, as otherwise the triple helix is not stable at body temperatures and a non-functional protein is produced. The hydroxylation of lysine is also essential for the formation of cross-links, which become converted to stable non-reducible forms (see above).

There are two enzymes which hydroxylate proline in the 4 and in the 3 position and a third enzyme which hydroxylates lysine. The 4-prolyl hydroxylase acts on proline residues in the y-position of the repeating triplets x-y-gly, and the 3-prolyl hydroxylase acts on proline residues in the x-position provided another proline in the y-position is already hydroxylated. Lysylhydroxylase acts on lysine residues in the triplet x-lys-gly (Prockop et al, 1979). All three enzymes require the same cofactors — ferrous ions, molecular oxygen, ascorbate and 2-oxoglutarate, which is decarboxylated in the process. The reaction is as follows:

$$\text{Substrate} + O_2 + CH_2 \begin{matrix} \nearrow CH_2\text{–}COOH \\ \searrow CO\text{–}COOH \end{matrix} \xrightarrow[\text{ascorbate}]{Fe^{++}} \text{substrate-OH} + \begin{matrix} CH_2\text{–}COOH \\ | \\ CH_2 \\ | \\ COOH \end{matrix} + CO_2$$

Neither ferrous ion nor ascorbate are consumed stoichiometrically in the reaction, but are essential. All three hydroxylases require the substrate to be non-helical and experimentally it has been shown that longer peptides are hydroxylated more efficiently than short ones. Once the peptides have formed triple helices, no further hydroxylation takes place, but since triple helices need about 90–100 hydroxyproline residues per chain to be stable at body temperatures, hydroxylation can proceed at least until this point is reached. As lysyl residues become hydroxylated, sugar residues are added by two specific enzymes; a galactosyl transferase attaches galactose residues to the lysyl hydroxyl group to form a β-glucoside and a glucosyltransferase then adds glucose to a proportion of the galactose residues already attached to hydroxylysine to form a disaccharide with an unusual α 1–2 O-glycoside bond. Like the hydroxylases, both enzymes require non-helical peptides as substrates, are more active on longer than shorter peptides and use sugars in the form of uridine diphosphate glycosides. A genetic defect in lysyl hydroxylase has been shown in some patients with type IV Ehlers–Danlos syndrome (Prockop et al, 1979).

As the procollagen peptides are formed and hydroxylated, they fold into secondary and tertiary structures. The assembly of three pro-α-chains to form the triple helix is aided by the formation of disulphide bonds between the chains in the carboxyterminal propeptides. If hydroxylation or the formation of interchain disulphide bonds is prevented experimentally, the molecules will not form triplehelices. They accumulate within the rough endoplasmic reticulum and are only slowly secreted as non-functional molecules. The absence of ascorbate prevents hydroxylation which explains why wound-healing is impaired in scurvy.

The normal triple helical procollagen molecule, i.e. the form secreted from the cell, is further modified outside the cell. The globular carboxy- and amino-terminal propeptides are each cleaved by different specific proteases which are most active on triple helical procollagen. These cleavages are necessary before collagen molecules can assemble into fibrils, which is a spontaneous but complicated multistep process. Genetic defects in cleavage of the amino-terminal propeptide results in impaired fibril formation as in type VII Ehlers–Danlos syndrome (Prockop et al, 1979).

The formation of intermolecular cross-links (Fig. 6.2) is the final stage in the production of functional collagen. As explained above, the cross-links arise from the interaction of lysine, hydroxylysine or glycosylated hydroxylysine with a lysine or hydroxylysine residue whose Σ-amino group has been oxidised by the enzyme lysyl oxidase. A deficiency of this enzyme is involved in type V Ehlers–Danlos syndrome and in some patients with cutis laxa and a congenital heart disease with a 'floppy valve syndrome' (Prockop et al, 1979). The enzyme is copper-dependent and hence copper deficiency reduces the number of cross-links and, therefore, the strength of the collagen. Penicillamine can interfere with cross-link formation not only by competing itself in forming Schiff bases (Robins, 1982) with the aldehyde groups of oxidised lysine residues, but since it complexes with copper, it reduces the copper available to lysyloxidase. Penicillamine is used in relatively high doses as a scavenger of copper in Wilson's disease but as it has no effect on ketoimine or mature cross-links: it impairs the strength only of newly formed collagen in soft tissues where aldimine rather than ketoimine cross-links predominate. At doses used to treat rheumatoid arthritis, no effects on skeletal or synovial collagen have been detected. In homocysteinuria, high circulating levels of homocysteine may interact with aldehydes produced by lysyloxidase and thus interfere with normal collagen cross-linking which accounts for the connective tissue changes seen in this disease (Prockop et al, 1979). Diseases associated with molecular abnormalities of collagen have been lately reviewed (Smith & Francis, 1982; Uitto & Bauer, 1982; Pope et al, 1983).

After the complex series of reactions discussed above have all taken place, mature collagen fibres are laid down in the extracellular matrix where they normally remain for a very long time. How collagen fibres are oriented in tissues in response to lines of stress and the control of fibre thickness and morphology in different tissues are not fully understood. The different distribution of each type of collagen implies that they have distinct properties appropriate to different morphological requirements. The fibres of type III collagen are thinner than those of other fibrillar collagens and type III collagen differs from type I and type II collagens in having interchain disulphide bridges at the amino-terminal end. There is a specific type III amino-terminal procollagen peptidase which does not remove the disulphide bridges when type III procollagen is converted to type III collagen. This is a relatively slow process and variable amounts of type III procollagen are present in many tissues where it may regulate the growth of fibres.

Degradation

(Reviews: Woolley & Evanson, 1980; Nimni, 1983; Barrett & Saklatvala, 1984.) Mature cross-linked collagens are very resistant to most proteolytic enzymes. Its very stability therefore poses problems for its removal during normal growth and remodelling of the body. The breakdown and dissolution of collagen fibres in vivo is an extracellular process that results from the stepwise concerted action of several proteolytic enzymes acting at neutral pH. Two of the most important steps are the cleavage of the helical region of the molecule which is otherwise resistant to proteolysis. Which of these steps comes first is disputed. There are specific collagenases which attack the helical region of all three chains in the molecule simultaneously at a particular position cleaving between glycine–isoleucine to give two products, three-quarters and one-quarter the length of the original molecule (Fig. 6.6). The helical cleavage products are no longer stable at temperatures above 33°C, when they are denatured and become susceptible to attack by many non-specific proteinases, which results in the complete dissolution of the collagen. There appear to be several specific collagenases derived from different kinds of cell which have a preference for native fibrillar collagen. These collagenases are metalloproteinases requiring calcium as a cofactor (Barrett & Saklatvala, 1984).

Collagenases are found in culture media of a variety of tissues including rheumatoid synovium (Woolley et al, 1975). The specificities of collagenases have been established from such cell and tissue culture studies. The rate of attack on a particular collagen type depends on the source of the collagenase. Human granulocyte enzyme attacks type I collagen faster than type III, type II collagen is more resistant and bone collagen is not degraded until demineralised, although bone is continuously remodelled throughout life. The rate of degradation of native type I and II collagen fibres by collagenase is increased four times by a rise of 2°C in the range 30–37°C, a factor which may be important when joints become inflamed as they are normally at temperatures of 30–33°C.

Because collagen is such an important structural protein, its degradation must be carefully regulated. Collagenases are normally present in a latent form, even that produced by translation of synovial cell mRNA in a cell-free system (Nagase et al, 1981). They can be activated by various proteinases such as trypsin, plasmin and other endogenous proteinases. The activation of plasminogen in the circulation, by plasminogen activator, a specific serine proteinase, provides one general mechanism, both direct and indirect, for localised dissolution of the extracellular matrix (Reich, 1978). The activator is cell-associated and once plasmin has been formed, it activates latent collagenase and also degrades proteoglycans exposing the collagen to enzymatic attack.

The site where collagenase is activated probably determines which proteinase participates in the activation. The mononuclear cell factor interleukin I stimulates collagenase production by synovial explants while the production of interleukin I is itself stimulated by the presence of aggregated immunoglobulin, a situation which could perpetuate the destructive process in rheumatoid joints.

Macrophages appear to play a pivotal role in tissue breakdown. They are themselves a source of proteinases including plasminogen activator, elastase and collagenase, and they also secrete factors which activate connective tissue cells, such as fibroblasts and chondrocytes to produce collagenase and other degradative enzymes themselves, thus recruiting connective tissue cells in the degradative process (Vaes, 1984). On the other hand, macrophages secrete factors which have a mitogenic effect on fibroblasts and which stimulate them to lay down collagen. Lymphocytes also produce factors which affect connective tissue cells directly and others which stimulate macrophages. The cellular interactions in inflammation are thus extremely complex and are only slowly being elucidated. The relative importance of these factors in vivo is not yet known (Vaes, 1984).

Joint fluids contain general proteinase inhibitors, such as α_2-macroglobulin, the principal proteinase inhibitor in plasma, which inactivates all types of proteinases by a trapping mechanism (Barrett & Starkey, 1973), and also α-anti-collagenase, which being of relatively low molecular weight could probably enter cartilage matrix (Barrett & Saklatvala, 1984). Moreover, a 30 000 MW inhibitor (known as 'tissue inhibitor of metalloproteinases' TIMP) has been isolated from various connective tissue cells and inhibits collagenase and other metalloproteinases (Cawston et al, 1981), while glucocorticoids inhibit the production of collagenase by synovial cells (Brinckerhoff &, Harris, 1981). Thus, the rate of turnover of collagen in normal and pathological tissues depends on the balance between activation and inhibition of collagenase.

The removal of the cross-linked portion of the collagen molecule (depolymerisation) is effected by elastase, a serine proteinase that degrades elastin which is resistant to other proteinases. Elastase is more restricted in distribution than collagenase but has a very wide specificity. Amongst other substrates, it degrades cartilage proteoglycans extensively and also type II collagen faster than type I collagen (Barrett & Saklatvala, 1984). It is found in pancreas and in azurophilic granules of polymorphonuclear leucocytes (Barrett, 1981). The activity of leucocyte elastase in tissues is likely to be controlled by α_1-proteinase inhibitor (α_1-anti-trypsin) and α_2-macroglobulin (Barrett & Saklatvala, 1984) and it is notable that the antirheumatic drug gold thiomallate inhibits leucocyte elastase. Macrophages also secrete an elastase which is distinct from the serine dependent elastase of leucocytes (Vaes, 1984).

ELASTIN

Elastin has a more restricted distribution than collagen and is found in tissues with elastic recoil properties such as aorta, lung, skin and ligaments. Elastin fibres consist of elastin surrounded by a microfibrillar glycoprotein which is rich in cysteine. Although seemingly amorphous in low resolution electron microscopy, under high resolution preparations of purified elastin have a filamentous structure (Gotte, 1977).

Much less is known about the structure and biosynthesis of elastin than of collagen. It has a unique amino acid composition with a preponderance of non-polar residues and glycine represents one-third of the amino acids as in collagen, but there is very little hydroxyproline. Analysis of peptides shows that there are repeating tetra-, penta- and hexapeptides, all of which contain proline and glycine (Franzblau & Faris, 1981). Soluble tropoelastin which is secreted from the cell has a molecular weight of about 70 000 (Mecham et al, 1977). The in vitro translation product of mRNA for tropoelastin has about the same molecular weight (Rosenbloom, 1982). Intermolecular cross-links are then formed as a result of the oxidative deamination of specific lysyl residues by lysyl oxidase to produce insoluble elastin.

The cross-links, which are polyfunctional amino acids with a pyridine nucleus are unique to elastin, although the intermediates are Schiff bases like those of collagen cross-links. The cross-links have been isolated as two geometric isomers desmosine and isodesmosine (Fig. 6.7) after strong acid hydrolysis of insoluble elastin. The desmosines are chemical markers of elastin in tissues, for which a radioimmunoassay is available (Skinner et al, 1983). Whether it is the same (Narayan et al, 1977), or a closely similar enzyme to that which oxidises lysyl residues in collagen, remains to be firmly established, as the primary sequences around the oxidised lysines in each protein are entirely different (Rosenbloom, 1982). Sequence analysis of peptides derived from tropoelastin (soluble elastin lacking cross-links) suggest that the

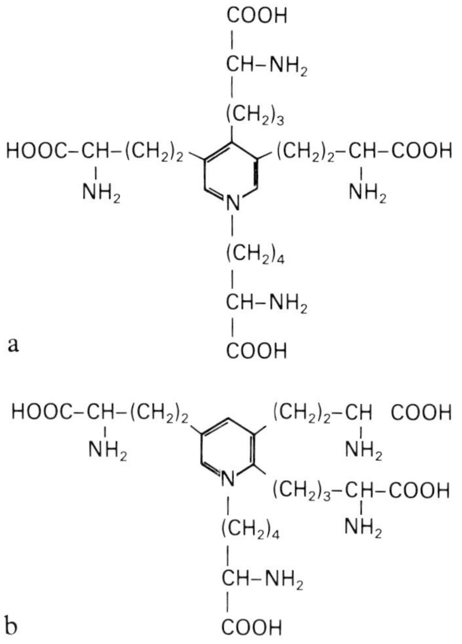

Fig. 6.7 Structure of (a) desmosine and (b) isodesmosine.

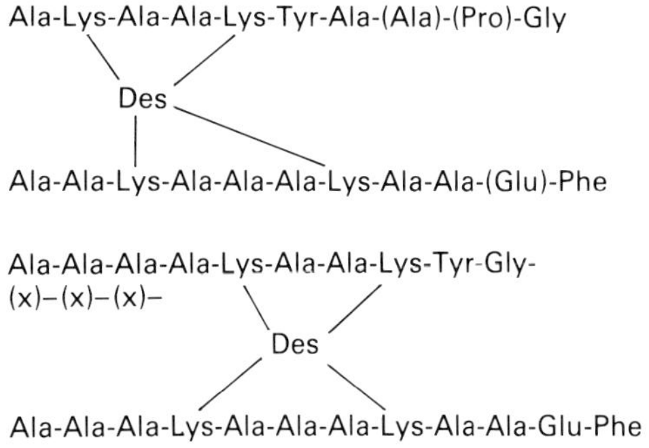

Fig. 6.8 Suggested sequence of amino acid residues flanking desmosine and isodesmosine cross-links. Note the clustering of alanine residues in the environment of the cross-links (Franzblau et al, 1977).

lysines occur in pairs separated by two or three amino acid residues and that these pairs are distributed all along the polypeptide chain. Several peptides containing desmosine cross-links have been partially sequenced and show that desmosine and isodesmosine occur in the same primary sequence (Franzblau et al, 1977).

Alanine residues are clustered near the lysines that become oxidised (Anwar, 1977) so that cross-linked peptides isolated from mature elastin are enriched in alanine (Franzblau & Faris, 1981). Thus, in the formation of desmosines three of the lysines that are oxidised are flanked by alanine residues and the fourth has alanine on one side and a hydrophobic residue on the other (Fig. 6.8).

The desmosines cross-link two polypeptide chains (Franzblau et al, 1977), which imposes a restriction on stretching so that the individual chains cannot slip past each other. On release of tension, the chains snap back into their original conformation which explains the rubber-like (elastomer) properties of elastin. During embryonic development, the rate of elastin synthesis in aorta and lung increases markedly, and lung distensibility is closely correlated with the elastin content of foetal lung, (Skinner et al, 1983), whereas in emphysema elastin content of lung is decreased (Mandl et al, 1977).

Elastin ligaments consist of elastin and collagen in a ratio of about 4 : 1 by weight. The central part of the ligament consists of elastin oriented longitudinally and in between are zones of collagen fibres apparently arranged in a spiral. Biphasic stretch/strain curves suggest that on stretching, the elastin is deformed first followed by the collagen, which is less extensible, and accounts for the steep part of the curve (Fig. 6.9) (Serafini-Fracassini & Field, 1977).

Elastin is resistant to most proteolytic enzymes, but is degraded by specific elastase enzymes which have been obtained from leucocytes, macrophages, aortic smooth muscle cells and pancreas. Interaction of elastin with fatty acids renders it more anionic and thence more susceptible to attack by elastase (Kagan et al, 1977), a factor which may be implicated in elastolysis in atherosclerosis. Elastases are neutral proteinases which have a wide specificity for other substrates, besides elastin, including proteoglycans and the part of the collagen molecule which bears cross-links (Barrett & Saklatvala, 1984; see above).

ATTACHMENT PROTEINS

Fibronectin

(Reviews: Yamada, 1981, 1983; Hynes, 1981; Aplin & Hughes, 1982.) Connective tissues apart from cartilage contain fibronectin (Fig. 6.1, Table

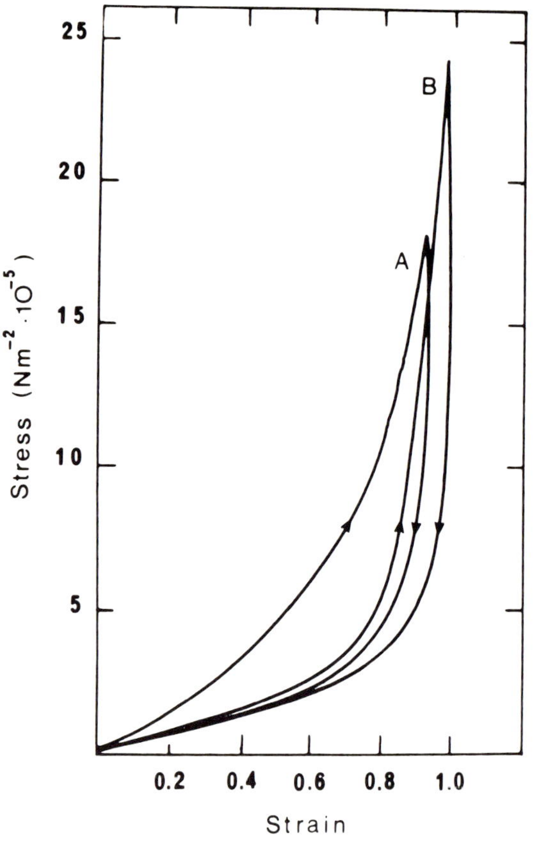

Fig. 6.9 Stress/strain curves of a strip of bovine ligamentum nuchae during the first two extensions — relaxation cycles (A & B) under high loads. Note the lower part of the curve represents extension of elastin and the steep part the much smaller extension of collagen fibres (from Serafini-Fracassini & Field, 1977).

6.3), an attachment protein that binds to collagen and forms a fibrillar matrix around cells.

Fibronectin is a dimeric glycoprotein consisting of two polypeptide chains held together by disulphide bonds, which has an elongated asymmetrical shape (Fig. 6.1). There are separate domains involved in binding to collagen, heparin and heparan sulphate and to fibrin and hyaluronic acid (Fig. 6.10). Fibronectin mediates in cell-substrate and cell — cell interactions in vitro and immunofluorescence studies show it to be widespread in extracellular matrices (Timpl & Martin, 1981). Changes in quantities of fibronectin are correlated with wound-healing inflammation and fibrosis. In granulation tissue fibronectin is synthesised before new collagen is laid down (Kurkinen et al, 1980). It is involved in cell attachment and spreading on substrates in vitro (Hynes, 1981). On the other hand, virally transformed cells which do not readily attach to substrates produce very little fibronectin. Fibronectin is also present in plasma (~ 300 μg/ml, previously identified as cold insoluble globulin), but plasma fibronectin is not identical with the fibronectin in the extracellular matrix and its function and relationship with the fibronectin of the matrix are not clear (Yamada et al, 1982; Hynes, 1981).

Mature cartilage differs from other types of connective tissue as it has very little fibronectin, but contains another attachment protein, chondronectin (see below). When chondrocytes differentiate in vitro and begin to form components of the matrix characteristic of cartilage, they cease to synthesise fibronectin. Similarly, when mesenchymal cells differentiate into muscle, fibronectin production decreases, whereas on differentiation into fibroblasts, fibronectin continues to be produced at a high level. Endothelial cells also synthesise large amounts of fibronectin in vivo and in vitro and fibronectin forms an integral part of the basement membrane below endothelial cells. The epithelial cells of most organs and glands are attached to basement membranes that contain fibronectin (and laminin, see below). Fibronectin is also present in loose stromal connective tissues throughout the body and like type IV collagen, it appears early in embryonic development at the late blastocyst stage (Adamson, 1982), and is involved in promoting and directing cellular migration (Hynes, 1981). Thus, the multiple functions of fibronectin make it an extremely important constituent of connective tissue.

There are other attachment proteins in the cell membrane which are exclusive to particular types of cell. An example is a 32 000 MW glycoprotein from the plasma membrane of differentiated chondrocytes termed 'anchorin'. It binds strongly to type II collagen and to chondronectin and would thus enable chondrocytes to be 'anchored' within the cartilage matrix (Mollenhauer & von der Mark, 1984). Other less well-characterised binding proteins have been described and as techniques improve for the isolation and characterisation of such hydrophobic membrane proteins, more are likely to be

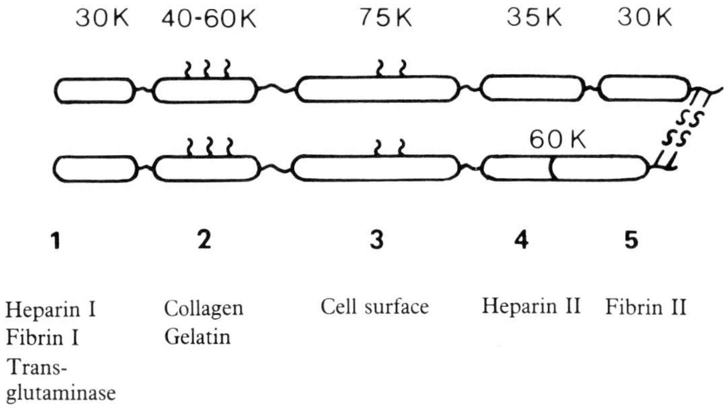

Fig. 6.10 The domain structure of plasma fibronectin. The molecule contains two disulphide bonded protein units (see Fig. 6.1), which contain similar domain structures, but one lacks an internal peptide sequence (shown as the lower unit) present on the other. The molecular weight and major interactions associated with five identified regions are illustrated. The short lateral projections show the general distribution of carbohydrate groups. After Yamada, 1983.

discovered in the future. Their existence underlines how exact and varied is the molecular organisation of connective tissues.

Laminin

(Reviews: Yamada, 1981; Aplin & Huges, 1982; Kleinman et al, 1984.) Laminin (Fig. 6.1 and Table 6.3) is a glycoprotein of 800 000 MW which is a major constituent of basement membranes (Timpl et al, 1979; Kleinman et al, 1982), including that of the vascular endothelium and it mediates the adhesion of several types of epithelial cell to type IV collagen. It appears early in the development of animals (Leivo et al, 1980). It has been isolated as a major component of a murine basement membrane tumour (EHS sarcoma) (Timple et al, 1979) and is composed of 2 B-chains (200 000 MW) and 1 A-chain (400 000 MW) held together by disulphide bonds and arranged in the shape of a cross (Fig. 6.1) as shown by electron microscopy (Engel et al, 1981). Within its structure, there are sites for interaction with type IV collagen, heparan sulphate (Rao et al, 1982) and cell surface components. Laminin is specific to basement membranes and is synthesised by epithelial cells. In culture, it promotes their growth and

Table 6.3 Attachment glycoproteins

	Molecular weight	Cell adhesion and interaction sites
Fibronectin a. Plasma b. Cellular (Yamada 1981, 1983; Hynes, 1981)	450K Dimer, 215–220K subunits 3–5% carbohydrate Dimer and multimer 220–240K subunits 3–5% carbohydrate	Promotes adhesion of many cell types. Interaction: type I and II collagen gelatin, heparin, hyaluronate, fibrin/fibrinogen, transglutaminase (see Fig. 6.10)
Laminin (Timpl & Martin 1981; Yamada, 1981)	800K 220K and 440K subunits 15% carbohydrate	Promotes epithelial cell adhesion. Component of basement membranes Interactions: type IV collagen and heparin/heparan sulphate
Chondronectin (Hewitt et al, 1982)	175K 60K subunits	Promotes chondrocyte adhesion. Interaction: type II collagen, chondroitin sulphate proteoglycan

influences their morphology. It is probably selective for epithelial cells as most mesenchymal cells do not utilise laminin for attachment and it actually inhibits attachment of fibroblast cells. Also found in association with laminin is a sulphated glycoprotein, entactin, of molecular weight 158 000 (Bender et al, 1982) which may also be involved in cell adhesion.

Chondronectin

An attachment glycoprotein, chondronectin (Table 6.3), which specifically promotes the adhesion of chondrocytes to type II collagen, has been identified in cartilage (Hewitt et al, 1982). Chondronectin is of 175 000 MW and contains disulphide bonded subunits of 60 000 MW and is resistant to trypsin digestion. It has some capacity to bind to cartilage proteoglycans and this appears to be necessary for its interaction with collagen (Hewitt et al, 1983). Proteoglycan may also play some part in the adhesion process. As well as occurring in cartilage, it is also present in vitreous humour and at low concentration in serum (~ 20 μg/ml).

Lubricating glycoprotein

A glycoprotein of particular interest to the physiology of the joint has been isolated from bovine synovial fluid. It has a molecular weight of 200 000 and was present in the fluid at a concentration of 20 μg/ml (Swann et al, 1981) and accounted for all the lubricating action of complete synovial fluid when compared by friction measurements between cartilage and glass. The molecule was shown by electron microscopy to be a partially extended flexible rod 220 nm long and analysis showed a carbohydrate content of about 50% (w/w), which consisted of many O-linked and a few N-linked oligosaccharides (Fig. 6.1). The present concept of boundary lubrication of articular cartilage by this glycoprotein is that it binds to the cartilage surface and is able to act as a lubricant by stabilising a layer of water at the surface.

PROTEOGLYCANS

(Reviews: Muir & Hardingham, 1975; Muir, 1980; Hascall & Hascall, 1981.) Proteoglycans form an important class of structural macromolecule amongst the non-fibrous components of connective tissues. They are a specialised family of glycoproteins in which a protein has attached to it from one to over 100 glycosaminoglycan chains. Few proteoglycans have been characterised in great detail, but sufficient is known to show that all glycosaminoglycans are synthesised on protein cores as proteoglycans and that each type of glycosaminoglycan may occur in several different proteoglycan structures. Their selective distribution suggests they have different roles to play in different tissues.

Glycosaminoglycans

The connective tissue glycosaminoglycans fall into four main types: hyaluronate, keratan sulphate, the chondroitin sulphate — dermatan sulphate group and the heparan sulphate — heparin group (Table 6.4). They are long chain polysaccharides with a repeating disaccharide structure and they are linked to protein via a characteristic short sequence of sugar residues. Although similar mechanisms for the biosynthesis of all the glycosamingolycans on proteoglycans have been proposed, hyaluronate is exceptional in that it is not synthesised on a protein core, but by the growth of a chain at the opposite end from that extended in normal glycosaminoglycan synthesis (Prehm, 1983). Hyaluronate thus has no linkage regions comparable with those of other glycosaminoglycans. The presence of sulphate and/or carboxylate groups on glycosaminoglycans makes the chains strong polyanions and this dominates their physical properties and to a large extent their interaction with other molecules. There is also considerable evidence of variation in the extent and sequence of sulphated or epimerised residues and this may be of importance in determining specific structures of interaction and self-association.

Structure of cartilage proteoglycan

Proteoglycans are particularly abundant in cartilage, where the major species present is of high molecular weight ($1–4 \times 10^6$) (Fig. 6.11) and forms aggregates by binding to hyaluronate (Fig. 6.1) (see Hardingham, 1981). Each proteoglycan contains up to 100 chondroitin sulphate chains and 50 keratan sulphate chains attached to a protein core of molecular weight $2–3 \times 10^5$. Structural investigations have identified three

Table 6.4 Glycosaminoglycans of mammalian tissues

Glycosaminoglycan	Molecular weight	Major disaccharide repeat structure		Linkage to protein	Major tissue distribution
HYALURONATE	0.5×10^6 to 5×10^6	GLUCURONATE β1–3	N-ACETYLGLUCOSAMINE β1–4	No covalent linkage to protein	Synovial fluid, vitreous humour, skin, blood vessel wall, cartilage, brain, embryonic tissues
CHONDROITIN 4 SULPHATE CHONDROITIN 6 SULPHATE	1×10^4 to 5×10^4	GLUCURONATE β1–3	N-ACETYLGALACTOSAMINE β1–4 4–0 sulphate or 6–0 sulphate	Gal β1–3 gal β1–4–xyl-o-serine	Cartilage, intervertebral disc, skin, bone, aorta, brain
DERMATAN SULPHATE	1×10^4 to 5×10^4	{ GLUCURONATE β1–3 or IDURONATE α1–3 some 2–0 sulphate }	N-ACETYLGALACTOSAMINE β1–4 4–0 sulphate or 6–0 sulphate	Gal β1–3 gal β1–4–xyl-o-serine	Tendon, skin, aorta, heart valve, lung parenchyma
HEPARAN SULPHATE	7×10^3 to 5×10^4	{ GLUCURONATE β1–4 or	(N-ACETYL)GLUCOSAMINE α1–4 some N-sulphate and 6–0 sulphate	Gal β1–3 gal β1–4–xyl-o-serine	Cell surface, basement membrane, lung parenchyma, aorta, heart valve
HEPARIN	1×10^4 to 1×10^5	IDURONATE α1–4 } some 2–0 sulphate Heparan sulphate: low in iduronate and all sulphate groups Heparin: high in iduronate and all sulphate groups			
KERATAN SULPHATE I-corneal II-skeletal	5×10^3 to 5×10^4	GALACTOSE β1–4 some 6–0 sulphate	N-ACETYLGLUCOSAMINE β1–3 6–0 sulphate	I corneal: β1–6 GlcNAc-N-asp | Sialic acid-Gal II skeletal: β1–6-GalNAc-o-serine (threonine)	I cornea, II cartilage, intervertebral disc

Abbreviations: GlcNAc, N-acetylglucosamine; GalNAc, N-acetylgalactosamine; gal, galactose, xyl, xylose; asp, asparagine

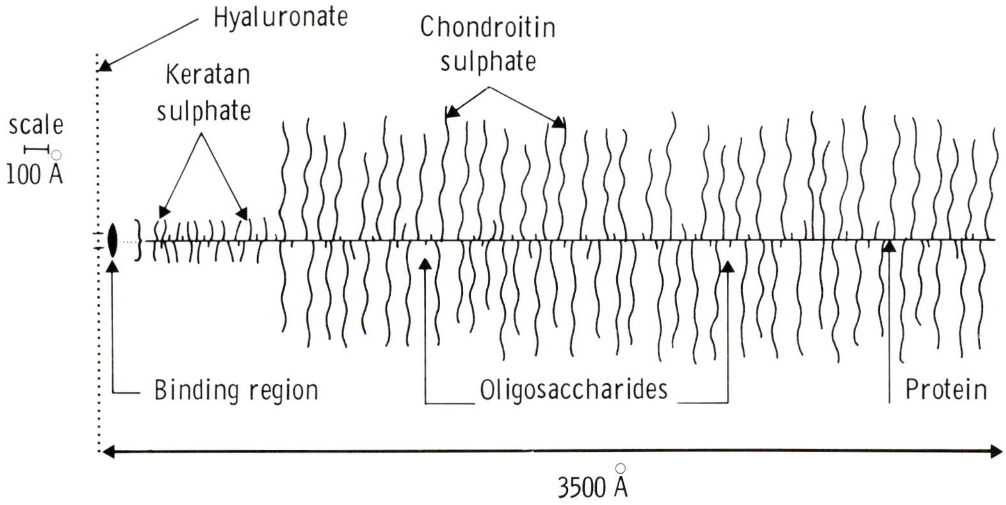

Fig. 6.11 Cartilage proteoglycan monomer. The protein core (MW 2×10^5 to 3×10^5) bears ~ 100 chondroitin sulphate and ~ 50 keratan sulphate chains, also ~ 50 O-linked oligosaccharides and a few N-linked oligosaccharides. Total MW 1×10^6 to 4×10^6 (note scale 1000 Å 0.1 μm) (from Perkins et al, 1981).

separate protein domains; a long extended region which bears most of the chondroitin sulphate chains, a shorter extended region rich in keratan sulphate and a globular terminal region which forms the specific sites involved in aggregation (Heinegård & Axelsson 1977; Hascall, 1977; Perkins et al, 1981). The protein core also has attached to it many O-linked oligosaccharides and a few N-linked oligosaccharides (Lohmander et al, 1981; Nilsson et al, 1982). The overall density of carbohydrate substitution of amino acid residues is thus extremely high, approaching one per 4 amino acids on the extended part of the molecule with only the binding region having a relatively low carbohydrate content.

Proteoglycan aggregates are formed by many proteoglycans binding to an extended hyaluronate chain via specific sites on the globular binding region of the protein core (Figs. 6.11, 6.12). A link protein of 40 000 MW also participates in aggregation by binding to proteoglycan and to hyaluronate such that it increase the stability of the proteoglycan — hyaluronate bond (Hardingham, 1979; Tang et al, 1979). Typically, to each hyaluronate chain of 1×10^6 MW, as many as 100 proteoglycans can bind, thereby forming large aggregates, which by electron microscopy are more than 2 μm long (Fig. 6.13; Buckwalter & Rosenberg, 1982).

Biosynthesis of proteoglycan by chondrocytes

Estimates of the turnover of proteoglycans in cartilage show fast turnover in young animals (5–10 days) but much slower turnover at maturity (100–300 days — Maroudas, 1979). All the components of proteoglycan aggregates are synthesised continuously by chondrocytes, within the tissue, and the controlled synthesis, secretion and assembly of proteoglycan aggregates are thus important in maintaining cartilage structure and

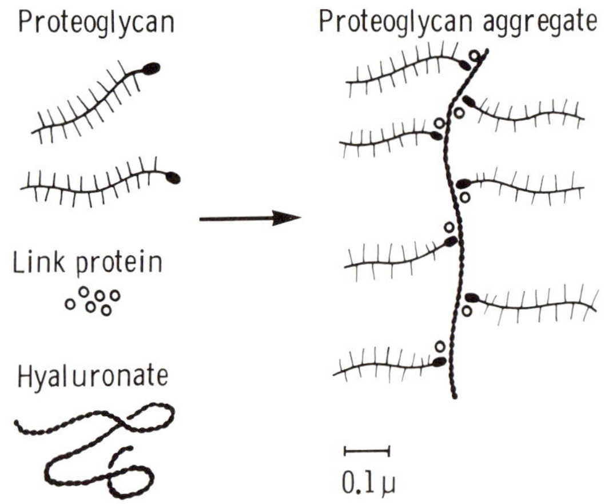

Fig. 6.12 Diagram of cartilage proteoglycan aggregation. Each hyaluronate chain in an aggregate is 1–4 μm long and binds up to 200 proteoglycan monomers to form an aggregate of MW 5×10^7 to 5×10^8 (from Hardingham, 1981).

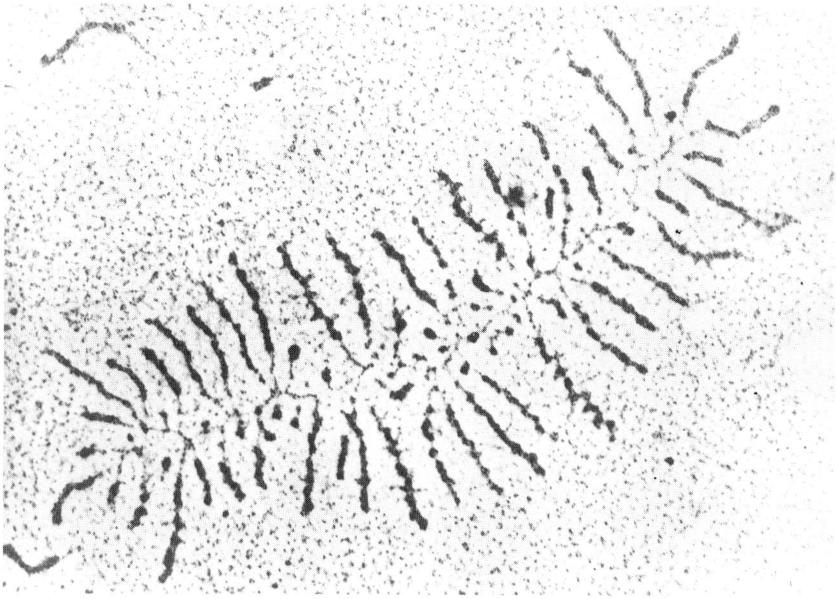

Fig. 6.13 Electron micrograph of cartilage proteoglycan aggregate (courtesy of Dr J. Buckwalter). Each arm represents a single proteoglycan monomer, as shown schematically in Figures 6.11, 6.12.

function. Proteoglycans are specialised glycoproteins which are synthesised along intracellular pathways like other secretory proteins. The protein core is first formed on membrane-bound polysomes and then migrates within the cisternae of the RER to the Golgi where chondroitin sulphate chain synthesis and sulphation occurs. It is likely that link protein also shares this route of synthesis as there is evidence that both are closely associated soon after secretion. The site of synthesis of hyaluronate within the chondrocyte has not been established, but in teratocarcinoma cells, it is synthesised by a mechanism entirely different from other glycosaminoglycans (Prehm, 1983), and there is evidence to suggest it is formed outside the compartments of protein synthesis and secretion (Mitchell & Hardingham, 1982). Thus, if proteoglycan and link protein are secreted separately from hyaluronate, it may explain why proteoglycan aggregation with hyaluronate and link protein occurs extracellularly.

Aggregating proteoglycans are particularly abundant in cartilage and are phenotypic of differentiated chondrocytes. In the development of cartilage, the differentiation of mesenchymal cells into chondrocytes is accompanied by a change in the type of proteoglycan synthesised from a small proteoglycan with long chondroitin sulphate chains to a large aggregating proteoglycan with many more, but shorter, chondroitin sulphate chains (Caplan & Hascall, 1980). There is also a greatly increased rate of synthesis. The deposition of a type II collagen network and the production of aggregating proteoglycans are two key factors in the expansion of the cartilage matrix. The role of proteoglycans is evident from studies on mutants with growth disorders such as those found in the brachymorphic mouse (Schwartz, 1983). This has a defect in which the proteoglycans are 50–65% undersulphated which results in a great reduction in the size of the epiphyseal growth plates and in growth of the long bones. This mutation is non-lethal but a more extensive deficiency of cartilage proteoglycan protein core synthesis has been described in the cmd/cmd mouse (Kimata et al, 1981), which stunts the development of long bones, trunk and head, such that the neonate is half normal length and rarely survives.

Function of proteoglycan in cartilage

Cartilage has been described in biomechanical

terms as a 'permeable fibre-reinforced composite solid matrix swollen with water' (Mow & Lai, 1980) and it is the presence of proteoglycan at high concentration that complements the role of collagen in making cartilage stiff, yet resilient (Kempson et al, 1970; Fig. 6.14). The large size of proteoglycans and their formation into supramolecular aggregates immobilises them within the collagen network and with a high concentration of anionic groups this creates a large osmotic swelling pressure. Water is drawn into the tissue and is balanced by tension developed in the collagen network. Cartilage is thus made stiff by being swollen with water, but on loading it shows slow compliance as proteoglycans oppose the redistribution of water within the tissue and it recovers elastically when the load is removed (Maroudas, 1979). The structural integrity of the collagen network and of the proteoglycans are thus both important in maintaining the biomechanical properties of cartilage. The erosion of cartilage in pathological conditions may be preceded by some damage to these components. This may be through direct action of invading pannus which releases enzymes to degrade the matrix in rheumatoid arthritis but may also be indirectly through the release of cytokines such as interleukin I (catabolin) which activate chondrocytes to degrade the matrix surrounding them (Dingle, 1979).

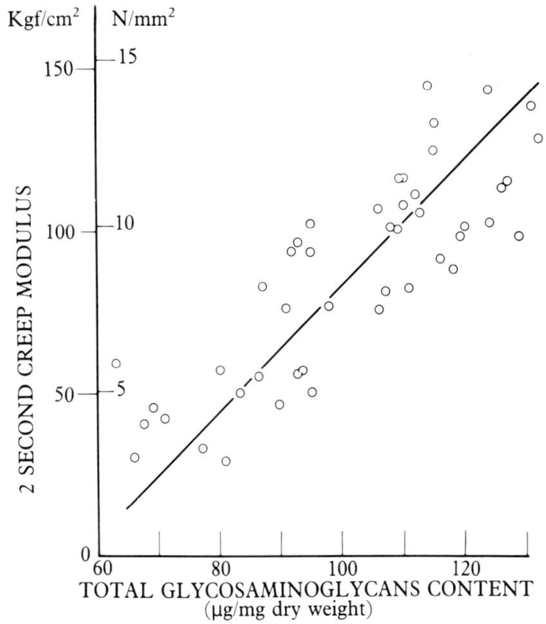

Fig. 6.14 Biomechanical properties of human articular cartilage. Variation of 2 second creep modulus with glycosaminoglycan (proteoglycan) content of human femoral head articular cartilage (Kempson et al, 1970) showing that a high proteoglycan content is responsible for cartilage stiffness in compression.

Dermatan sulphate proteoglycan

Dermatan sulphate is a structural isomer of chondroitin sulphate in which some sugar residues are epimerised from D-glucuronate to L-iduronate. This conversion only involves a switch in the carboxyl group at C_5 of the sugar ring from an equitorial to an axial position and it happens through enzyme action after the chain is synthesised. Dermatan sulphate is thus synthesised as chondroitin sulphate and is then epimerised to form dermatan sulphate. The conversion of all residues to L-iduronate is never complete and shows large variation from $<10\%$ to 90%. Few dermatan sulphate proteoglycans have been fully characterised, but one type found in ligament, aorta and skin has similar structural features suggesting a common protein core (Cöster & Fransson, 1981; Damle et al, 1982; Pearson et al, 1983). Analysis showed this to be of quite low MW 40 000 with 2–3 dermatan sulphate chains. This appeared comparable in structure to a small proteoglycan identified as comprising 80% of the proteoglycan in bovine flexor tendon. When purified, this proteoglycan was found to have a potent inhibitory effect on collagen fibrillogenesis in vitro (Vogel & Heinegård, 1983). Electron microscopy of tendon stained with an electron dense cationic dye (cuprolinic blue) showed regular binding of proteglycans to the outside of collagen fibrils at the 'd' band (Scott & Orford, 1981). Analysis of the tissue content showed that the amount of dermatan sulphate in tendon was directly related to the surface area of collagen fibrils over a wide range of growth and development. The specific binding of this small dermatan sulphate proteoglycan to type I collagen fibrils may thus play a role in fibril formation and stabilisation in tendon and other tissues.

A dermatan sulphate proteoglycan of this type was also shown to be synthesised by cultured skin fibroblasts (Carlsted et al, 1981), but they also synthesised a second dermatan sulphate proteoglycan of much higher molecular weight that was of lower iduronate content. The larger proteoglycan isolated from tendon was shown to have no inhibitory effect on collagen fibrillogenesis (Vogel & Heinegård, 1983) and may thus play a quite different role in the tissue.

Heparan sulphate proteoglycans

Heparan sulphate and heparin are glycosaminoglycans of closely related structure, but occur on different proteoglycans with quite separate morphological distribution and function. Although heparin is found in many connective tissues, it is present only as an intracellular component of mast cell granules, where it is stored in a partly degraded form (Stevens & Austen, 1981). It contains specific sequences that bind to antithrombin and on release into plasma this results in the accelerated inactivation of serine proteinases involved in clotting mechanisms (Lindahl & Höök, 1978). Heparan sulphate has the same disaccharide repeating structure as heparin, and undergoes the same polymer modifications that introduce N-sulphate, 2,O-sulphate and iduronate groups, but they are carried out incompletely leaving long sequences of unmodified N-acetylglucosamine and glucuronate residues. Heparan sulphate thus has a much lower charge density than heparin.

At least two heparan sulphate proteoglycans have been described. One of these is a cell surface component in which the protein core has a hydrophobic region that intercalates into the plasma membrane and contains only 1–3 heparan sulphate chains (Kjellén et al, 1981; Norling et al, 1981). This cell surface heparan sulphate is a common feature of many cell types (Kraemer, 1971). A further heparan sulphate proteoglycan isolated from aorta and skin is of much larger size and is an extracellular component that is a constituent of basement membranes (Hassell et al, 1980; Kleinman et al, 1982). Several studies have described the selective self-association of heparan sulphate chains (Fransson et al, 1982), which might provide some basis for a role in cell contact and recognition and, by interaction with other extracellular components, such as fibronectin and laminin, may form macromolecular networks.

Hyaluronate

Hyaluronate is a common component of all connective tissue matrices (Toole, 1981). It is an unbranched non-sulphated glycosaminoglycan of extremely long chain length (MW 10^6–10^7) and accounts for most of the viscosity of synovial fluid. It was at one time thought to provide the lubricating action of synovial fluid on the opposing articular surfaces, but this has since been shown to be the property of a specific lubricating glycoprotein (see above). It may, however, be important in soft tissue lubrication in the synovium and in helping to maintain the synovial fluid volume.

As well as occurring in synovial fluid, hyaluronate is present in all soft connective tissues such as skin, blood vessel walls, lung and the vitreous of the eye. It is also present in cartilage where it is an essential component of proteoglycan aggregates (see above). For this purpose, its content is only 1–5% of that of proteoglycan, but as the concentration of proteoglycan is very high (up to 100 mg/ml), the concentration of hyaluronate in cartilage (~1 mg/ml) is not very different from its concentration in synovial fluid (~2–3 mg/ml).

Hyaluronate occurs at higher concentration in embryonic and neonatal tissues than in the adult and this has been shown to be related to its abundance at times of cellular migration and its removal as cells differentiate and form new tissues and organs (Toole, 1981). It may thus play a role in tissue remodelling and repair when there is also much cell migration.

Concluding remarks

It is clear from this review that there is a great structural complexity in connective tissue and this will become increasingly evident as methods and techniques of investigation improve. Each tissue is well adapted for the particular function it has to perform by having a precise molecular organisation of its constituents. This organisation is acquired mostly during embryonic development with relatively minor changes thereafter. As organs increase in size and change in shape, carefully controlled remodelling has to take place by degradation and resynthesis of connective tissue constituents. Although turnover rates decline as maturity is reached, connective tissue continues to be turned over slowly throughout life while retaining its supermolecular organisation where the interplay of the constituents is crucial. The process of repair, on the other hand, produces scar tissue which is quite different from the surrounding highly organised connective tissue and, therefore, does not share its specific properties to the detriment of the overall function of the tissue. Understanding of how normal tissues are maintained is a prerequisite to understanding pathological processes.

REFERENCES

Adamson E D 1982 The effect of collagen on cell division, cellular differentiation and embryonic development. In: Weiss J B, Jayson M I V (eds) Collagen in health and disease. Churchill Livingstone, Edinburgh, Ch 13, p 218–243

Anwar R A 1977 Desmosine peptides: amino acid sequences and the role of these sequences in cross link formation. Advances in Experimental Biology and Medicine 79: 329–350

Aplin J D, Hughes R C 1982 Complex carbohydrates of the extracellular matrix. Structures, interactions and biological roles. Biochimica et Biophysica Acta 694: 375–418

Barrett A J 1981 Leucocyte elastase. Methods in Enzymology 80: 581–588

Barrett A J, Saklatvala J 1984 Proteinases in joint disease. In: Kelley W N, Harris E D, Ruddy S, Sledge C B (eds) Textbook of rheumatology. Saunders, Philadelphia, Ch 14 (in press)

Barrett A J, Starkey P M 1973 The interaction of α_2-macroglobulin with proteinases. Characteristics and specificity of the reaction and a hypothesis concerning its molecular mechanism. Biochemical Journal 133: 709–724

Bender B L, Carlin B, Jaffe R, Temple T, Chung A E 1982 Production and distribution of entactin and GP-2 in M1536-B3. Experimental Cell Research 137: 415–425

Brinckerhoff C E, Harris E D 1981 Modulation by retinoic acid and corticosteroids of collagenase production by rabbit synovial fibroblasts treated with phorbol myristate acetate or poly (ethylene glycol). Biochimica et Biophysica Acta 677: 424–432

Buckwalter J, Rosenberg L A 1982 Electron microscopic studies of cartilage proteoglycans. Journal of Biological Chemistry 257: 9830–9839

Burgeson R 1982 Articular cartilage intervertebral disc, synovia. In: Weiss J B, Jayson M I V (eds) Collagen in health and disease. Churchill Livingstone, Edinburgh, Ch 18, p 335–361

Caplan A I, Hascall V C 1980 Structure and developmental changes in proteoglycans. In: Naftolin F, Stubblefield J (eds) Dilation of the uterine cervix. Raven Press, New York, p 79–98

Carlstedt I, Cöster L, Malmström A 1981 Isolation and characterization of dermatan sulphate and heparan sulphate proteoglycans from fibroblast culture. Biochemical Journal 197: 217–225

Cawston T E, Galloway W A, Mercer E, Murphy G, Reynolds J J 1981 Purification of rabbit bone inhibitor of collagenase. Biochemical Journal 195: 159–170

Cöster L, Fransson L-Å 1981 Isolation and characterization of dermatan sulphate proteoglycans from bovine sclera. Biochemical Journal 198: 143–153

Damle S P, Cöster L, Gregory J D 1982 Proteodermatan sulfate isolated from pig skin. Journal of Biological Chemistry 257: 5523–5527

Dingle J T 1979 Recent studies on the control of joint damage: the contribution of the Strangeways Research Laboratory. Annals of Rheumatic Diseases 38: 201–214

Engel J, Odermatt E, Engel A, Madri J A, Furthmayr H, Rohde H, Timpl R 1981 Shapes, domain organisations and flexibility of laminin and fibronectin: two multifunctional proteins of the extracellular matrix. Journal of Molecular Biology 150: 97–120

Eyre D R 1981 Cross-link maturation in bone collagen. In: Veis A (ed) Chemistry and biology of mineralised connective tissues. Elsevier North Holland, New York, p 51–55

Eyre D R, Oguchi H 1980 The hydroxypyridinium cross-links of skeletal collagens. Their measurement, properties and proposed pathyway of formation. Biochemical and Biophysical Research Communications 92: 403–410

Eyre D R, Grynpas M D, Shapiro F D, Creasman C M 1981 Mature cross-link formation and molecular packing in articular cartilage collagen. Seminars in Arthritis and Rheumatism 11 (Suppl.1): 46–47

Fransson L Å, Carlstedt I, Cöster L, Malmström A 1982 The self-associating properties of fibroblast proteoheparan sulphate. Progress in Clinical and Biological Research 102A: 435–445

Franzblau C, Faris B 1981 Elastin. In: Hay E D (ed) Cell biology of the extracellular matrix. Plenum Press, New York, Ch 3, p 65–93

Franzblau C, Foster J A, Faris B 1977 Role of cross-linking in fiber formation. Advances in Experimental Biology and Medicine 79: 313–327

Fujimoto D, Moriguchi T, Ishida T, Hayashi H 1978 The nature of pyridinoline a collagen cross-link. Biochemical and Biophysical Research Communications 84: 52–57

Gotte L 1977 Recent observations on the structure and composition of elastin and elastic tissue. Advances in Experimental Medicine and Biology 79: 105–117

Grynpas M D, Eyre D R, Kirschner D A 1980 Collagen type II differs from type I in native molecular packing. Biochimic et Biophysica Acta 626: 346–355

Hardingham T 1979 The role of link protein in the structure of cartilage proteoglycan aggregates. Biochemical Journal 177: 237–247

Hardingham T 1981 Proteoglycans: their structure, interactions and molecular organization in cartilage. Biochemical Society Transactions 9: 489–497

Hascall V C 1977 Interactions of cartilage proteoglycans with hyaluronic acid. Journal of Supramolecular Structure 7: 101–120

Hascall V C, Hascall G K 1981 Proteoglycans. In: Hay E D (ed) Cell biology of the extracellular matrix. Plenum Press, New York, Ch 2, p 39–63
Hassell J R, Gehron Robey P, Barrach H J, Wilczek J, Rennard I, Martin G R 1980 Isolation of heparan sulphate containing proteoglycan from basement membrane. Proceedings of the National Academy of Science USA 77: 4494–4498
Heinegård D, Axelsson I 1977 Distribution of keratan sulphate in cartilage proteoglycans. Journal of Biological Chemistry 252: 1971–1979
Hewitt A T, Varner N H, Silver M H, Dessau W, Wilkes C M, Martin G R 1982 The isolation and partial characterization of chondronectin, an attachment factor for chondrocytes. Journal of Biological Chemistry 257: 2330–2334
Hewitt A T, Varner H H, Silver M H, Martin G R 1983 The role of chondronectin and cartilage proteoglycan in the attachment of chondrocytes to collagen. Progress in Clinical and Biological Research 110B 25–33
Hukins D W L 1982 Biomechanical properties of collagen. In: Weiss J B, Jayson M I V (eds) Collagen in health and disease. Churchill Livingstone, Edinburgh, Ch 4, p 49–72
Hynes R O 1981 Fibronectin and its relation to cellular structure and behaviour. In: Hay E D (ed) Cell biology of the extracellular matrix. Plenum Press, New York, Ch 10, p 295–334
Kagan H M, Jordan R E, Lerch R M, Mukherjee D P, Stone P, Franzblau C 1977 Factors affecting the proteolytic degradation of elastin. Advances in Experimental Medicine and Biology 79: 189–205
Kempson G E, Muir H, Pollard C, Tuke M 1973 The tensile properties of the cartilage of human femoral condyles related to the content of collagen and glycosaminoglycans. Biochimica et Biophysica Acta 297: 456–472
Kempson G E, Muir H, Swanson S A V, Freeman M A R 1970 Correlations between stiffness and the chemical constituents of cartilage of the human femoral head. Biochimica et Biophysica Acta 215: 70–77
Kimata K, Barrach H-J, Brown K S, Pennypacker J P 1981 Absence of proteoglycan core protein in cartilage from the cmd/cmd mouse. Journal of Biological Chemistry 256: 6961–6968
Kjéllen L, Pettersson I, Höök M 1981 Cell surface heparan sulfate: an intercalated membrane proteoglycan. Proceedings of the National Academy of science USA 78: 5371–5375
Kleinman H K, McGarvey M L, Liotta L A, Gehron Robey P, Tryggvason K, Martin G R 1982 Isolation and characterization of type IV pro-collagen, laminin and heparan sulfate proteoglycan from the EHS sarcoma. Biochemistry 21: 6188–6193
Kleinman H K, McGarvey M L, Hassell J R, Martin G R 1984 The role of laminin in basement membranes and in the growth, adhesion and differentiation of cells. In Trelstad R (ed) The role of Extracellular matrix in development. A. Liss, New York, p 123–143
Kraemer P M 1971 Heparan sulfates of cultured cells. Acid-soluble and precipitable species of different cell lines. Biochemistry 10: 1445–1451
Kühn K 1982 Relationship between amino acid sequence and higher structures of collagen. Connective Tissue Research 10: 5–10
Kurkinen M, Vaheri A, Roberts P J, Steinman S 1980 Sequential appearance of fibronectin and collagen in experimental granulation tissue. Laboratory Investigations 43: 47–51
Leivo I, Vaheri A, Timpl R, Wartiovaara J 1980 Appearance and distribution of collagens and laminin in the early mouse embryo. Developmental Biology 76: 100–114
Lindahl U, Höök M 1978 Glycosaminoglycans and their binding to biological macromolecules. Annual Review of Biochemistry 47: 385–417
Lohmander L S, De Luca S, Nilsson B, Hascall V C 1981 Oligosaccharides on proteoglycans from the Swarm rat chondrosarcoma. Journal of Biological Chemistry 255: 6084–6091
Mandl I, Darnule T V, Fiever J A, Keller S, Turino G M 1977 Elastin degradation in human and experimental emphysema. Advances in Experimental Biology and Medicine 79: 221–231
Maroudas A 1979 Physicochemical properties of articular cartilage. In: Freeman M A R (ed) Adult articular cartilage. Pitman Medical, Tunbridge Wells, Ch 4, p 215–290
Mecham R, Forster J, Franzblau C 1977 Proteolysis of soluble elastin. Advances in Experimental Biology and Medicine 79: 209–220
Miller E J 1978 The collagen of joints. In Sokoloff L (ed) The joints and synovial fluid, Vol I. Academic Press, New York, Ch 5, p 205–242
Mitchell D, Hardingham T 1982 Monensin inhibits synthesis of proteoglycan, but not of hyaluronate in chondrocytes. Biochemical Journal 202: 249–254
Mollenhauer J, Von der Mark K 1983 Isolation and characterization of collagen-binding glycoprotein from chondrocyte membranes. The EMBO Journal 2: 45–50
Mow V C, Lai W M 1980 Recent developments in synovial joint biomechanics SIAM Review 22: 275–317
Muir H 1980 The chemistry of the ground substance of joint cartilage. In: Sokoloff L (ed) The joints and synovial fluid, Vol II. Academic Press, New York, Ch 2, p 28–94
Muir H 1983 Proteoglycans are organizers of the intercellular matrix. Biochemical Society Transactions 11: 613–622
Muir H, Hardingham T E 1975 Structure of proteoglycans. In: Whelan W J (ed) MTP International Review of Science, Biochemistry, Series One, Vol 5. Butterworths, London, Ch 5, p 153–222
Nagase H, Jackson R C, Brinkerhoff C E, Vater C A V, Harris E D 1981 A precursor form of latent collagenase produced in a cell-free system with mRNA from rabbit synovial cells. Journal of Biological Chemistry 256: 11951–11954
Narayan A S, Page R G, Kazan F 1977 Studies on the action of lysyl oxidase on soluble elastin. Advances in Experimental Biology and Medicine 79: 329–350
Nilsson B, De Luca S, Lohmander L S, Hascall V C 1982 Structures of N-linked and O-linked oligosaccharides on proteoglycan monomer from the Swarm rat chondrosarcoma. Journal of Biological Chemistry 257: 10920–10927
Nimni M E 1983 Collagen: structure, function and metabolism in normal fibrotic tissues. Seminars in Arthritis and Rheumatism 13: 1–86
Norling B, Glimelius B, Wasteson A 1981 Heparan sulfate proteoglycan of cultured cells: demonstration of a lipid- and a matrix-associated form. Biochemical and Biophysical Research Communications 103: 1265–1272

Olsen B R 1981 Collagen biosynthesis. In: Hay E D (ed) Cell biology of the extracellular matrix. Plenum Press, New York, Ch 6, p 139–177

Pearson C H, Winterbottom N, Fackre D S, Scott P G, Carpenter M R 1983 The NH_2-terminal amino acid sequence of bovine skin proteodermatan sulfate. Journal of Biological Chemistry 258: 15101–15104

Perkins S J, Miller A, Hardingham T E, Muir H 1981 Physical properties of the hyaluronate binding region of proteoglycan from pig laryngeal cartilage. Journal of Molecular Biology 150: 69–95

Piez K A 1982 Structure and assembly of the native collagen fibril. Connective Tissue Research 10: 25–36

Pope F M, Nicholls A C, Dorling J, Webb J 1983 Molecular abnormalities of collagen: a review. Journal of the Royal Society of Medicine 76: 1050–1062

Prehm P 1983 Synthesis of hyaluronate in differentiated teratocarcinoma cells. Biochemical Journal 211: 181–198

Prockop D J, Kivirrikko K I, Tuderman L, Guzman N A 1979 The biosynthesis of collagen and its disorders. New England Journal of Medicine 301: 13–23

Rao C N, Margalies I M, Tralka T S, Terranova V P, Madri J A, Loitta L A 1982 Isolation of subunit of laminin and its role in molecular structure and tumour cell attachment. Journal of Biological Chemistry 257: 9740–9744

Reese C A, Widemann H, Kühn K, Mayne R 1982 Characterization of a highly soluble collagenous molecule isolated from chicken hyaline cartilage. Biochemistry 21: 826–830

Reich E 1978 Activation of plasminogen: A general mechanism for producing localised extracellular proteolysis. In: Berlin R D, Herrmann H, Lepow I H, Tanzer J M (eds) Molecular basis of biological degradative processes. Academic Press, New York, p 155–169

Reid K B M 1982 Proteins containing collagen sequences. In: Weiss J B, Jayson M I V (eds) Collagen in health and disease. Churchill Livingstone, Edinburgh, Ch 2, p 18–27

Robins S P 1982 Turnover and cross-linking of collagen. In: Weiss J B, Jayson M I V (eds) Collagen in health and disease. Churchill Livingstone, Edinburgh Ch 9, p 160–178

Rosenbloom J 1982 Elastin, biosynthesis, structure, degradation and role in disease processes. Connective Tissue Research 10: 73–91

Schwartz N B 1983 Defect in proteoglycan synthesis in brachymorphic mice. Progress in Clinical and Biological Research 110B: 97–103

Scott J E, Orford C R 1981 Dermatan sulphate-rich proteoglycan associates with rat tail-tendon collagen at the d band in the gap region. Biochemical Journal 197: 213–216

Serafini-Fracassini A, Field J M 1977 The ultrastructure and mechanics of elastic ligaments. Advances in Experimental Biology and Medicine 79: 97–101

Skinner S J M, Schellenberg J C, Liggins G C 1983 The estimation of elastin in fetal tissues by radioimmunoassay of isodesmosine. Connective Tissue Research 11: 113–121

Smith R, Francis M J O 1982 Disorders of collagen biosynthesis. Recent Advances in Endocrinology and Metabolism 2: 211–238

Stevens R L, Austen K F 1981 Proteoglycans of the mast cell. In: Becker E K, Simon A S, Austen K F (eds) Biochemistry of the acute allergic reactions. A. Liss, New York, Ch 6, p 69–98

Swann D A 1978 Macromolecules of synovial fluid. In: Sokoloff L (ed) The joints and synovial fluid, Vol 1. Academic Press, New York. Ch 9, p 407–435

Swann D A, Slayter H S, Silver F H 1981 The molecular structure of lubricating glycoprotein I, the boundary lubricant of cartilage. Journal of Biological Chemistry 256: 5921–5925

Tang L-H, Rosenberg L, Reiner A, Poole A R 1979 Proteoglycans from bovine nasal cartilage, properties of a soluble form of link protein. Journal of Biological Chemistry 254: 10523–10531

Timpl R, Martin G R 1981 Components of basement membranes. In: Furthmayr H (ed) Immunochemistry of the extracellular matrix, Vol II. CRC Press, Cleveland, Ch 5, p 119–150

Timpl R M, Rohde H, Geyron Robey P, Rennard S J, Foidart J M, Martin G R 1979 Laminin — a glycoprotein from basement membranes. Journal of Biological Chemistry 254: 9933–9937

Timpl R, Wiedemann H, Van Delder V, Furthmayr H, Kühn K 1981 A network model for the organization of type IV collagen molecules in basement membranes. European Journal of Biochemistry 120: 203–211

Toole B P 1981 Glycosaminoglycans in morphogenesis. In: Hay E D (ed) Cell biology of the extracellular matrix. Plenum Press, New York, Ch 9, p 259–294

Uitto J, Bauer E A 1982 Diseases associated with collagen abnormalities. In: Weiss J C, Jayson M I V (eds) Collagen in health and diseases. Churchill-Livingstone, Edinburgh, Ch 16, p 289–312

Vaes G 1984 Macrophage-secretory products and connective tissue remodelling: role of macrophage enzymes and of 'matrix regulatory monokines'. In: Dean R, Stahl P (eds) Developments in cell biology, Vol I. Butterworths, London (in press)

Veis A 1982 Collagen fibrillogenesis. Connective Tissue Research 10: 11–24

Vogel K, Heinegård D 1983 Proteoglycans in bovine fibrous tendon and their interactions with tendon collagen in vitro. Proceedings of the 7th International Symposium on Glycoconjugates, p 830–831

Woodhead-Galloway J 1982 Structure of the collagen fibril: an interpretation. In: Weiss J W, Jayson M I V (eds) Collagen in health and disease. Churchill Livingstone, Edinburgh, Ch 3, p 28–48

Woolley D E, Evanson J M (eds) 1980 Collagenase in normal and pathological connective tissue. John Wiley, New York

Woolley D E, Lindberg K A, Granville R W, Evanson J M 1975 Action of rheumatoid synovial collagenase on cartilage collagen. Different susceptibilities of cartilage and tendon collagen to collagenase attack. European Journal of Biochemistry 50: 437–444

Yamada K M 1981 Fibronectin and other structural proteins. In Hay E D (ed) Cell biology of the extracellular matrix. Plenum Press, New York, Ch 4, p 95–114

Yamada K M 1983 Cell surface interactions with extracellular materials. Annual Review of Biochemistry 52: 761–799

Yamada K M, Hayashi M, Akiyama S K 1982 Structure and function of fibronectin. In: Hawkes S, Wang J L (eds) Extracellular matrix. Academic Press, New York, p 25–34

7

D.L. Gardner

Structure and function of connective tissue and joints

With advancing age, stature diminishes, the back becomes curved, bone brittle, joints stiff, the skin wrinkled and eyesight impaired (Engel & Larsson, 1969; Gardner & O'Connor, 1985; Goldman & Rockstein, 1975; Vogel, 1973). These common results of altered connective tissue structure and function emphasise its ubiquity, its importance and its possible deficiencies.

Connective tissue changes throughout life: modifications in function determine alterations at molecular and at microscopic level that are expressions of senescence. The changes are strongly influenced, if not determined by, heredity and take place against a background of metabolic change in which every connective tissue, including bone, is continually lost and continually replaced. There is an habitual, normal turnover of the cells of connective tissue and of their products, a turnover that can be demonstrated by techniques such as radioisotopic labelling. For each material there is a normal half-life, that is, a time required for the loss and replacement of half the component molecules. The half-life of the chondrocytes of embryonic chick cartilage in culture is very brief, that of the cells of adult human femoral head articular cartilage exceedingly long. More is known of the half-lives of cartilage glycosaminoglycans than of the proteoglycans of which they are part (Ch. 6); the mean half-life for femoral head cartilage glycosaminoglycans may be as long as 800 days but there are other fractions with brief survival. The measurement of the half-life of cartilage collagen reveals the existence of at least two species of fibrils. Bone collagen survives for very long times but the life span of osteocalcin is not known.

This chapter reviews the anatomical structure, tissue organisation and microscopical detail of the components of the connective tissue system against a background in which their evolution, comparative anatomy and development are briefly considered. The chapter also discusses the function of those parts of the connective tissue system that are of importance in clinical rheumatology; particular attention is devoted to the articulations. The characteristics of the cells of connective tissue and their products are programmed genetically (Slavkin & Grenlich, 1976) and a word is said of this inheritance.

Like all body tissues, the connective tissues are composed of parent *cells* that synthesise and secrete a hydrated *extracellular matrix* that is formed of *proteoglycans* reinforced by a fibrous microskeleton of *collagen* and sometimes of *elastic material*. In special circumstances, the extracellular matrix is *mineralised*. During early embryonic growth, the structural varieties of connective tissue differentiate to assume *loose* or *compact* forms; some become *cartilage*, others *ligaments*, *tendons*, *menisci*, *labra*, *capsules* and *bone*. Where body movement is necessitated, adjacent skeletal units articulate at specialised zones that serve as *joints*.

Connective tissue is studied with continued vigour by physicians, physicists, chemists, immunologists, geneticists, pathologists and mechanical engineers (Wainwright et al, 1976). The flood of literature that is a product of this activity reflects the extraordinary diversity of the methods adopted for investigation. The function of the whole, intact joint of the living human is best analysed by a combination of radiological, engineering, rheological, telemetric and radioisotopic ('nuclear') techniques. Computerised axial tomography and nuclear magnetic resonance, non-invasive scanning methods, have special parts to play and exquisite detail can now be derived by these approaches and by microfocal radiography. The invasive procedures of the pathologist centre on fibreoptic arthroscopy. At the other end of the scale, the cytologist may choose to investigate individual cells in monolayer culture or parts of tissues in organ culture. The immunologist can now distinguish between the immunoglobulins and their components in cell preparations in serum and in sections and can identify the populations of cells by monoclonal antisera. The microscopist has at his command transmission and scanning electron microscopic techniques supplemented by X-ray diffraction analysis, electron probe X-ray microanalysis, low temperature techniques, backscattered electron imaging and replication. The variety of approaches is so large, the range of methods so great, that no short, comprehensible and comprehensive account is possible. In the present chapter, therefore, the connective tissues are considered only in the outline appropriate to a textbook of rheumatology. Access to the literature is facilitated by the provision of a heavy weighting of recent reviews.

EVOLUTION AND COMPARATIVE ANATOMY (Dillon, 1973)

Multicellular plants and animals form connective tissue to oppose gravity, to store water and minerals, and for protection (Alexander, 1978, 1979; Brown, 1975). Animals have developed cells and extracellular connective tissue around organs and between external and internal body surfaces (Mathews, 1975). Evolutionary trends cannot be defined in the many invertebrate phyla as succinctly as they can in the single subphylum that comprises the vertebrates (Torrey & Feduccia, 1971). The tetrapod limb is thought to have arisen from the pelvic or pectoral fins of members of the crossopterygian fish group (Currey, 1974). It is possible to identify precursors of the humerus/femur, ulna/fibula and radius/tibia. The remaining smaller bones have given rise to the carpals/tarsals. There are insufficient bones present to account for the metacarpals/metatarsals and digits and these bones are assumed to have evolved independently.

There is no complete record of the transition from the crossoptergian fin to the tetrapod limb (Webster & Webster, 1974). In the early tetrapods the limbs simply project at right angles to the sides of the body. The body is elevated by the presence of bends at the elbow and knee, an arrangement seen in salamanders, turtles and many lizards. This form of elevation is mechanically laborious; it is analogous to a man lying prone on the ground doing 'press-ups'.

A more efficient structure is found in the mammals. The hind limbs are rotated forwards so that the knees and feet point to the front. By contrast, the forelimbs are rotated backward and the elbows point to the rear. This process alone would leave the arms pointing backward. There has therefore been an evolutionary rotation of the wrist through 180°, about the vertical axis of the forearms. The forearm becomes twisted so that the radius and ulna cross. This arrangement permits free fore-and-aft movement and results in more efficient locomotion than the crawling movements that occur when the limbs are horizontal (Torrey & Feduccia, 1971). Further adaptations of the primitive structural arrangements are numerous. Thus, in birds the forelimb is modified to form a wing by specialisation of the first, second and third metacarpals and phalanges. In cattle and horses only the tips of the digits are used for walking; they are reduced in number.

The assumption by hominids of an erect posture led, in man, to the whole foot being placed on the ground. The upright position, and the consequent increase in weight borne by the leg bones, resulted in an increase in the circumference of the human femur that in primates is second only to that of the gorilla. Human legs are the longest among primates relative to trunk length (Badoux, 1974). To support the additional loads, there is an associated increase in the bearing surfaces of the joints. The femoral head and acetabulum become relatively large. Nevertheless, the condylar surface areas are smaller than those of the heaviest apes. This reduction stems from improved weight transmission down the leg, through the lateral condyle. The femoral neck is longer in hominidae than in monkeys and apes: the greater trochanter is farther from the femoral head, allowing abductor muscles greater purchase to support the trunk over the leg (Chiarelli, 1973).

In the mammalian embryo, a primitive, undifferentiated connective tissue, the mesenchyme, partly of mesodermal, partly of ectodermal origin, occupies embryonic sites where the axial skeleton and limb buds grow, filling in zones between organ rudiments into which vascular channels and nerve fibres extend. The proportion of intercellular material to cell numbers is high, the water content high but the relative quantity of fibrous proteins low. Mesenchymal differentiation proceeds in parallel with organogenesis. 'Differentiation' describes the organisation of specialised functions: the structural and enzymic proteins, and the nucleic acids necessary for the coded activity of individual cell populations, result from the phenotypic expression of genetic information. The whole range of postnatal connective tissue growth is therefore closely modulated by the genetic mechanism. From an early embryonic age, mutation or the actions of chemical agents, viruses and ionising radiations can impede this development and lead to skeletal malformation, the severity of which tends to be inversely proportional to the developmental age of the affected embryo. Individual organs such as the heart, eye and ear are particularly vulnerable during periods when they are assuming definitive forms.

In anatomical sites where differentiated connective tissue structures arise, such as axial and limb bones, intervertebral discs, fibrocartilaginous menisci and the lens for example, mesenchymal tissue progresses through a series of subtle and complex metamorphoses that are commonly described as 'condensations'. This term indicates the increasingly intense staining characteristics of these connective tissue structures viewed in microscopic section. Where a joint is to appear, liquefaction of the centre of an island of 'condensed' mesenchyme progresses to the formation of a fluid-filled connective tissue structure, an articulation equidistant between opposed skeletal elements. Prevention of movement by curarisation or by the administration of *Clostridium botulinum* neurotoxin can impair joint formation experimentally; but the coded information necessary for joint development is, of course, inherited and normal joints are not formed simply in response to the imposition of loads caused by movement.

Mesenchymal cells grow vigorously even under adverse conditions: they are robust and readily survive explantation or allografting. It is widely believed that varying numbers of cells, with the potential for growth and development of relatively primitive mesenchymal cells, persist into adult life in sites of loose and of fibrofatty connective tissue as well as within the skeleton and the viscera. From these mesenchymal cells there may emerge lines of daughter cells that lead in time to the formation of fibrous tissue, fat, cartilage, bone, synovial tissue and glial tissue. Glomerular mesangial cells and pulmonary alveolar septal cells may have comparable origins. So, too, may the dendritic cells of the mononuclear macrophage system.

UNITS OF STRUCTURE AND FUNCTION

Cells (Ross, 1975)

Fibroblasts (Abercrombie, 1978)

The fibroblast is the prototype of all differentiated connective tissue cells or mechanocytes (Willmer, 1970). Readily grown in monolayer culture and therefore capable of being harvested in large numbers, the shape, contractility, and multiplication of fibroblasts have been studied in detail and many investigations made of their response to ageing, their genetic characteristics and their synthetic and secretory properties. The fibroblast is the larger, more active, more versatile precursor of the mature fibrocyte that forms the cell population of all compact, non-mineralised connective tissue; it is the most common cell of the loose and areolar connective tissues. Connective tissue in which fibrocytes and secreted collagen predominate is said to be *fibrous*; the formation of such tissue under pathological circumstances is the process of *fibrosis*. Fibrous tissue formation is a necessary part of healing by replacement and is part of granulation tissue. The synthesis of abundant new collagen-rich fibrous tissue in scirrhous carcinomata is given the special name of 'desmoplastic response'.

Fibroblasts in cell culture are elongated, ~

50–100 μm long, 30 μm broad and 3 μm thick. Obviously, the plump shapes and attenuated or stellate forms seen in normal tissues are quite different but the shapes seen in monolayer culture have the merit of drawing attention to the capacity of fibroblasts to react to contact with their neighbours by the assumption of smoothly contoured outlines with projecting borders, and to tension by contraction. The normal cell has much endoplasmic reticulum; ribosomes and polyribosomes combine to yield a basophilic tinge with common dye combinations such as haematoxylin and eosin. In addition to the smooth reticulum, the tortuous spaces of which are related to the Golgi apparatus, there are bundles of contractile cytoplasmic microfilaments the actin–myosin nature of which is demonstrable by appropriate fluorescein-labelled antisera. The filaments respond to ATP by contraction and are found to be aligned in the direction of movement of a cultured cell. Mitochondria are numerous but lysosomes are rare and phagocytosis is not a property often expressed by fibroblasts. However, macromolecular species synthesised within the cell may accumulate under a wide variety of circumstances. Just as collagen and proteoglycan pass to the vesicular system associated with the Golgi apparatus before export, so defects of synthesis or impaired degradation result in the accumulation, within cytoplasmic vesicles, of the excess of abnormal products. The identification of accumulated glycosaminoglycan within cultured fibroblasts or in tissue excised from the conjunctiva by biopsy, is a preliminary guide to the recognition of the heritable disorders of glycosaminoglycan degradation.

The principal function of fibroblasts is the synthesis, secretion and modulation of the fibrous and non-fibrous proteins, particularly the proteoglycans and glycoproteins, that together give the connective tissues their distinctive physical properties and their unusual but essential biological characteristics.

All human somatic cells inherit the information necessary for the synthesis of the fibrous and non-fibrous structural proteins as well as the enzyme proteins, the non-genetic nuclear material and the other macromolecules of connective tissue. In differentiated cell lines much of this special information is repressed. Fibroblasts, however, are able to express a wide variety of synthetic abilities and in doing so become important sources of the collagens, proteoglycans, core proteins, some glycoproteins and other molecular species of which the most important are elastin and elastic microfibrillar glycoprotein (Jackson, 1978). In many instances it appears that the precise primary structure of the macromolecules formed by individual connective tissues is characteristic of, although not unique to, the individual tissue. Type II collagen (Ch. 6) is therefore the predominant collagen species of hyaline articular cartilage, type I of bone. In a growing number of examples two or more species of a particular macromolecule such as collagen are found in a single tissue; but the ratios of the different species are likely to be characteristic of individual tissues suggesting an extended, subtle range of differences in physical and mechanical properties consequent upon small but highly important variations in primary structure.

The fibroblast serves a central function in healing by replacement (Bourne, 1981). Following irreversible tissue injury or in the course of protracted inflammation, fibroblasts multiply and extend from the intact margins of injured zones in company with proliferating buds of young capillary endothelial cells. These cells and the new vascular channels derived from them, together with the fibroblasts and the fibrous and non-fibrous matrix materials that they export, comprise *granulation tissue*. In sustained inflammatory disorders such as rheumatoid arthritis or in chronic bacterial infections such as tuberculosis, vascular, cellular granulation tissue may persist for very long periods, its presence maintained by the persistence of foreign antigenic material or by the continuation of humoral or cell-mediated hypersensitivity responses to autoantigens. In circumstances in which healing progresses to completion or when inflammation subsides spontaneously or as a result of anti-inflammatory therapy, granulation tissue becomes gradually less vascular with fewer cells, less matrix material and a larger proportion of collagen, usually of type III. The collagen-rich connective tissue formed in this way comprises a *scar* (Glynn, 1981). When excessive scar tissue forms, the scar is said to be *hypertrophic*. When excess scar tissue recurs after excision or local irradiation, growing inexorably like an unsightly benign neoplasm, it is said to be a *keloid*, a process more common in Negroes than in Caucasians and particularly likely after burns and ear-piercing.

Chondrocytes

The complex and varied molecular components of hyaline, of fibro- and of elastic cartilage are synthesised and exported/secreted by chondrocytes (Stockwell, 1979). Chondrocytes in monolayer cell culutre may be indistinguishable by transmission electron microscopy techniques from fibroblasts. The most satisfactory definition of a chondrocyte is one that emphasises the large amount and characteristic form of the non-fibrous matrix macromolecules that the cell synthesises, not the morphology or size of the cell itself. A chondrocyte, by this reckoning, is a connective tissue cell that is programmed to form a relatively large amount of extracellular matrix rich in proteoglycan and that is especially likely to express this property in response to compressive, mechanical loading.

The mature, differentiated chondrocyte (Fig. 7.1) derives from less well-differentiated chondroblasts, the cytological characteristics of which are clearly recognisable in embryonic limb buds. There are analogous cell populations at the epiphyses. Here the vigorous growth of proliferating chondrocytes

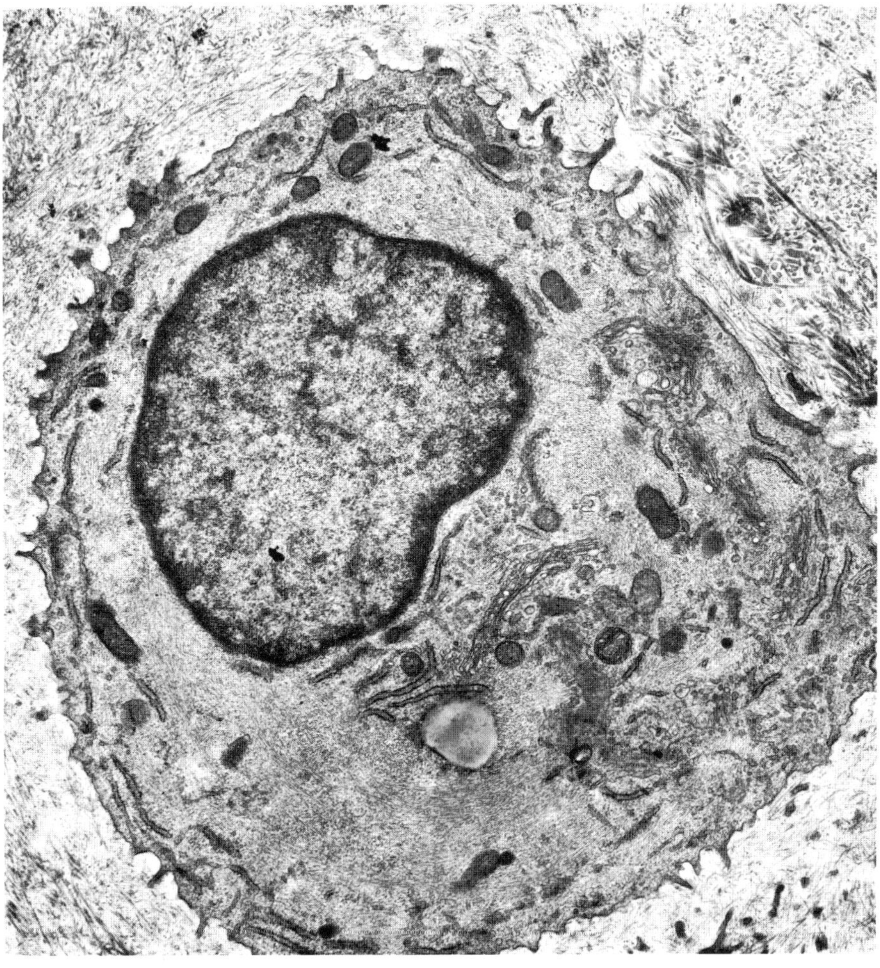

Fig. 7.1 Chondrocyte. A single cell lies within a pericellular matrix of delicate fibrils. At lower left, note larger, coarse collagen fibrils that indicate lacunar margin. External to this, much collagen and dispersed proteoglycan constitutes interlacunar (interterritorial) matrix. Transmission electron micrograph (TEM) ×4260.

is reflected in morphological features closer to those of the fibroblast than the chondroblast, an observation that emphasises the mutability of these connective tissue cells and the readiness with which environmental circumstances can derepress inherited capacities to assume distinctive functions and forms. When cartilage collagen synthesis is blocked, proteoglycan formation may still continue. Fibrocartilaginous cells are distinguished from hyaline cartilage chondrocytes by their tendency to synthesise and secrete relatively large amounts of collagen; elastic cartilage chondrocytes simultaneously synthesise and secrete elastin, elastic glycoprotein, collagen and proteoglycan.

Chondrocytes are ellipsoidal or discoid near the articular surface; ovoid, round or polygonal in the subsurface cartilage layers. They lie within 'lacunae' in which a protective buffer zone of matrix is bounded by a rim of condensed collagen (Poole et al, 1984). The proportion of cells to matrix decreases with age since the absolute quantity of matrix increases, an observation that apparently accounts for the increase of cartilage thickness with age.

The fine structure of chondrocytes is discussed in detail by Stockwell (1979) and reviewed by Ghadially (1983). The chondrocytes of superficial zone 1 hyaline articular cartilage are ellipsoidal or discoid; those of zones II and III are progressively more ovoid or spheroidal, and, depending on their site, paired rather than single. The transition from the ellipsoidal to the ovoid form is particularly well seen in the transitional zones of the synoviochondral margins. In the deeper layers of the hyaline articular cartilage, chondrocytes lie together in pairs, triplets or quadruplets. For reasons that are thought to be mechanical, each cell or cell group is protected within a distinctive island of specialised, pericellular matrix the margin of which, defined microscopically by a condensed lamina of circumferentially orientated collagen fibrils, is seen as the edge of a so-called '*lacuna*'.

Transmission electron microscopic evidence (Poole et al, 1984) suggests that the lacuna, disregarded in recent times because of an assumption that its appearance is artefactual, has a three dimensional form, with a finite fenestra in the fibrillar margin through which, it is supposed, electrolytes and water move quickly and reversibly. The matrix of the lacuna is distinguished from that of the perilacunar (territorial) and interlacunar (interterritorial) matrix by a rich content of sulphated, metachromatic and polyanionic proteoglycan. The proteoglycan of the chondrocyte lacuna is qualitatively distinct from that of the surrounding extralacunar matrix. Within the lacuna, collagen fibrils are rare; the numerous delicate microfibrils seen by electron microscopy are proteoglycan. External to the lacunar margin, collagenous material is more evident, the fibrils longer and wider (Fig. 7.2). Their orientation tends to be random except in the narrow, superficial surface region of articular cartilage. The histochemical definition of this matrix material is much influenced by the specificity of the staining techniques selected. The critical electrolyte concentration technique of Scott & Dorling (1965) is optimum. Modified for transmission electron microscopy (Scott, 1980), this method allows the locations of the glycosaminoglycans to be identified and their identity distinguished.

Chondrocytes contain lipid (Stockwell, 1979). The amount may be large and is markedly

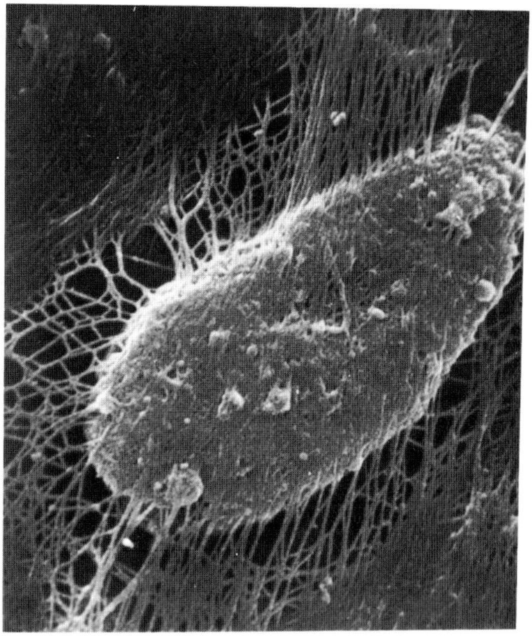

Fig. 7.2 Superficial chondrocyte suspended in collagen meshwork at the surface of rat femoral condylar cartilage after 30 min treatment with thiol proteinase, papain. Scanning electron micrograph (SEM) ×4743

increased in experiments in which lipid is injected into the synovial cavity (Ghadially et al, 1970; Mehta & Ghadially, 1973) when there may be a simultaneous loss of chondroitin sulphate, little change in keratan sulphate and no alteration in cellularity (Stockwell & Sprintz, 1981). There is also a variable content of glycogen both in mature articular and non-articular cartilage (Stockwell, 1967). Single cilia are often present (Wilsman, 1978).

Chondrocyte growth. Much insight into the behaviour of chondrocytes has come from cell culture studies (Sokoloff et al, 1973; Sokoloff, 1976). That the nature and amount of matrix material, such as glycosaminoglycans, synthesised and secreted by chondrocytes, is regulated by a feedback system, has long been suspected (Fitton Jackson, 1964). The proportion of hyaluronic acid in hyaline cartilage may determine proteoglycan production (Wiebkin et al, 1975; Wiebkin & Muir, 1973; 1975). Although some cell culture systems (Kuettner et al 1982; Kuettner et al 1982; Morales et al, 1983; Sanders & Prasad, 1983; Yang & Nandi, 1983) of bovine chondrocytes have proved more effective sources of new matrix material than others (Sokoloff et al, 1973), there is agreement that the physical conditions in which the cells are maintained, in particular whether they are grown as monolayers or free, in spinner culture, greatly influences the quantity and quality of the macromolecules formed (Sokoloff, 1980).

The *respiratory activity* of individual chondrocytes is thought to be comparable to that of other connective tissue cells. Nevertheless, in specialised connective tissues, where there is much extracellular matrix material and a low cell density, the integrated respiratory activity of the composite tissue is low. Whereas aerobic glycolysis is characteristic of the vascular synovium, of bone and of loose connective tissue, cartilage glycolysis is in part anaerobic. Cartilage is, indeed, remarkably resistant to prolonged periods of hypoxia that would be sufficient to cause irreversible injury to many tissues. These differentiated forms of connective tissue cell are metabolically active and vigorously synthesise new extracellular materials as well as structural and enzymic cell proteins. A simple test of chondrocyte metabolism is the demonstration of the incorporation of ^{35}S-sulphate into the chondroitin sulphates, one activity essential for the synthesis of the most common forms of proteoglycan side chain. Techniques such as the addition of actinomycin D or of puromycin, can be used to measure protein synthesis and amino acid incorporation by chondrocytes, respectively.

Enzyme activities. Chondrocytes from rat hyaline articular cartilage can be shown by histochemical techniques to possess lactate and glucose-6-phosphate dehydrogenase activities. There is high acid phosphatase and β-glucuronidase activity in the small cells of the superficial part of the marginal, tangential zone of cow cartilage (Scheinberg et al, 1982) and, in rats, high alkaline phosphatase activity limited to the deeper half of the weight-bearing cartilage. The presence of latent metalloproteinase is demonstrable in cultured bovine articular cartilage chondrocytes (Morales et al, 1983). The enzyme can be activated by incubation of the cells with agents like organomercurials, releasing an enzyme that degrades proteoglycan. Inhibitory activity against trypsin and collagenase is also present in bovine nasal cartilage. It is possible that these inhibitors are secreted into discrete tissue locations so that active enzymes that have diffused to these sites are prevented from disrupting matrix macromolecules (Morales et al, 1983). Whether a mechanism of this kind plays any part in cartilage degradation when synovium releases catabolin (p. 234) is not known.

Osteoblasts, osteocytes, osteoclasts

Understanding of the nature of these cells has advanced with recent progress in analysing the properties of bone marrow.

The supportive stromal tissue of the bone marrow is a network of fibroblast-like reticular cells and collagen fibres together with the endothelial cells of the marrow sinusoidal blood vessels (Owen, 1978). These *stromal connective tissue* elements are derived from lines of cells histogenetically distinct from the marrow *haemopoietic cells*. The marrow macrophages originating from the haemopoietic cells, intertwining with and wrapping round the stromal cells, appeared to be part of a composite *reticuloendothelial* system but it now seems clear that marrow macrophages, monocytes and their precursors comprise a distinct *mononuclear phago-*

cytic system, able to ingest foreign material at a very high rate. The components of the separate, supportive reticuloendothelial system ingest particles only slowly and by pinocytosis.

The stromal, supportive elements of the marrow gives rise to osteogenic, soft connective tissue; stromal cells merge into *preosteoblasts* and *osteoblasts* near bone surfaces. *Osteoclasts*, by contrast, also found with their precursors near bone surfaces, derive quite separately from mononuclear macrophages. The fibroblast-like stromal cells, capable of spontaneous bone formation, are said to be 'determined osteogenic precursor cells' other cells, including those of the undifferentiated mesenchyme, form bone only in the presence of an inducing agent and are said to be 'inducible osteogenic precursor cells'.

Osteoblasts. Osteoblasts line the external (periosteal) and internal (endosteal) surfaces of all young bone. In the adult, the resting, mature fibrocyte-like (preosteoblastic or osteoprogenitor) cells that comprise these surface layers retain a vigorous capacity to resume bone formation when provoked. Thus, comparatively slight periosteal trauma, the growth of a neoplasm or the more severe disturbance of a fracture, all lead very rapidly, in normal persons, to an abrupt resumption of differentiated synthetic and catalytic activities.

Osteoblasts are 15–80 μm in mean diameter, ovoid and elongated. There is much cytoplasmic RNA, prominent endoplasmic reticulum cisternae and free ribosomes and polyribosomes. The nucleus is large and ovoid with a single prominent nucleolus. Occasionally delicate intracellular fibrillar material can be recognised. Fine cytoplasmic processes extend into the openings of nearby superficial bone canaliculi where they make contact with other bone cells. When cytodifferentiation is provoked, the organisation of the cytoplasmic components and organelles of the preosteoblast is evident. Incorporation of ^{3}H-thymidine provides one guide to the synthesis of DNA and, in experimental studies, suggests that the life cycle of those young osteoblasts that divide is of the order of 2–3 days: at the end of this time the cell differentiates further to become an osteocyte that is incorporated in young, marginal bone. Osteoblasts inherit the capacity to synthesise and secrete the collagen and proteoglycan of bone matrix (osteoid) and the ability to catalyse mineralisation of this matrix by their highly active alkaline phosphatase.

Osteocytes (Jande & Belanger, 1971), the mature bone cells, lie within lacunae from which fine canaliculi communicate with the larger channels of the haversian vascular system (Ham, 1974; Vaughan, 1981, 1984). The cytoplasmic processes of osteocytes extend within these canaliculi and establish paths for metabolic and respiratory exchange. Although 'imprisoned', osteocytes near bone surfaces are still osteogenic and can incorporate radioactive isotopic precursors during osteogenesis. Osteocytes appear destined to die within their lacunae. A crude index of bone death histologically is loss of osteocyte nuclei from lacunae. There is no satisfactory evidence that osteocytes can revert to less mature osteoblasts during bone reabsorption.

Young osteocytes have much cytoplasm; cytoplasmic processes are short and few. With time, many longer processes appear: they contain no organelles but establish contact, through canaliculi, with adjacent cells. Tight junctions are recognisable. An exchange area of about 250 mm^{-2}/mm^{-3} permits easy metabolic relationships, within bone, between blood plasma and tissue fluid. The exchange surface area is greatly increased at fine structural level within bone matrix interfibrillar spaces.

An important property of surfaces laying down bone or dentine is a capacity to bind tetracycline. The deposited material, bound to bone or tooth matrix, is fluorescent in ultraviolet light. If tetracycline is given to a child, the teeth may remain permanently faint brown and fluorescent, to the individual's embarrassment. In adults, the deliberate in vivo labelling of skeletal tissue by this technique has allowed valuable measurements of the rate of bone growth to be made. Tetracycline may also be used to label osteoid in vitro (McClure, 1982). The characteristic metabolic disturbances of bone that may be encountered in the major connective tissue diseases have been analysed by Ellis (1981).

Much of the normal turnover of bone is

mediated by osteoclastic reabsorption. However, osteocytes contain an acid phosphatase, an aminopeptidase and a protease and appear capable of catalysing the insidious lysis of bone that some believe may complement the continual, more obvious activity of osteoclastic reabsorption. This process of osteocytic osteolysis may be exquisitely sensitive to parathyroid hormone and calcitonin concentration and may determine the minute-by-minute plasma calcium concentration. A view has been advanced that osteocytes act as pumps, transporting water from periosteal surfaces through canaliculi to the tissue fluid. Although this ingenious mechanism could convey dissolved calcium for exchange with bone mineral, it is equally possible that calcium exchange is by diffusion. Osteocytes may, in addition, play a part in facilitating the proven uptake of plasma proteins into bone matrix.

Osteoclasts (Hancox, 1972) are large, mobile multinucleated cells containing as few as two or as many as 200 nuclei. The usual location of the osteoclast is at a bone surface that is being absorbed. Here the giant cell often lies within a Howship's lacuna. The nuclei are close together. The cytoplasm contains a well-developed Golgi apparatus associated with specific granules, many vacuoles of lysosome-like structure, and small vesicles. The small number of ribosomes and scanty endoplasmic reticulum suggest limited synthetic activity but the numerous mitochondria are an index of high energy production. At the cell margin adjoining the bone surface is a characteristic brush (ruffled) border, a series of cytoplasmic processes and both channels and vacuoles with high enzyme activity. The vacuoles often contain crystals of bone mineral and fragmented collagen fibres.

Osteoclasts reabsorb normal calcified tissue by enzymes active at neutral or acid pH; among the most important is cathepsin B, a protease capable of degrading collagen by an unusual mechanism. Collagenolytic activity, possibly at neutral pH, has been confirmed by tissue culture techniques.

Among the control factors that regulate osteoclastic activity are parathormone, calcitonin, thyroid hormone, vitamin A, vitamin D and its derivatives, and the phosphonates. It remains possible that the plasma calcium level can affect the osteoclast directly.

Synovial cells

Synovial cells (synoviocytes) form the surface of the marginal, non-articulating vascular synovial connective tissue that is the source of synovial fluid and that provides the substances necessary for the survival of the chondrocytes of hyaline cartilage. It is widely accepted that the synovial lining cells are of two main types. Electron microscopic evidence established that one form of cell, with many villous cytoplasmic processes, phagocytic vacuoles and lysosomes was of a macrophage-like character: the cell was designated type A or M (macrophage). A second cell type contained much rough endoplasmic reticulum, few vacuoles, a conspicuous Golgi apparatus and occasional lysosomes. The cell resembled a fibroblast and was categorised as type B or F (fibroblast).

The *A(M), macrophage-like cells* (Fig. 7.3) are large, bear many pseudopod-like processes that extend into the synovial space and usually contain considerable numbers of phagocytic vacuoles and of lysosomes. Their principal function is believed to be the ingestion of autologous or foreign material that has gained access to the joint. This sequence is commonly observed when intra-articular bleeding has taken place or when foreign particles such as ^{198}Au or ^{90}Y are introduced into the joint for therapeutic reasons. The foreign material is enclosed within a phagocytic vacuole (phagosome) that merges with lysosomal particles. Phagocytosis is well-demonstrated by the injection of heavy metals such as gold or uranium (Ghadially et al, 1982; Ghadially, 1983). Single membrane-bounded, presumably lysosomal bodies ('aurosomes', 'uraniosomes') are formed in both type A and type B cells. Lysosomal enzymes, mainly acid hydrolases that include acid phosphatase, β-glucuronidase and proteinases, are activated within the phagocytic vacuoles. After degradation, the products of enzymatic action are extruded from the cell either into the synovial fluid or into the loose synovial connective tissue. Some, however, are held inert in an insoluble form within the phagocyte. Haemosiderin, for example, is retained for long periods within synovial cells, and so are

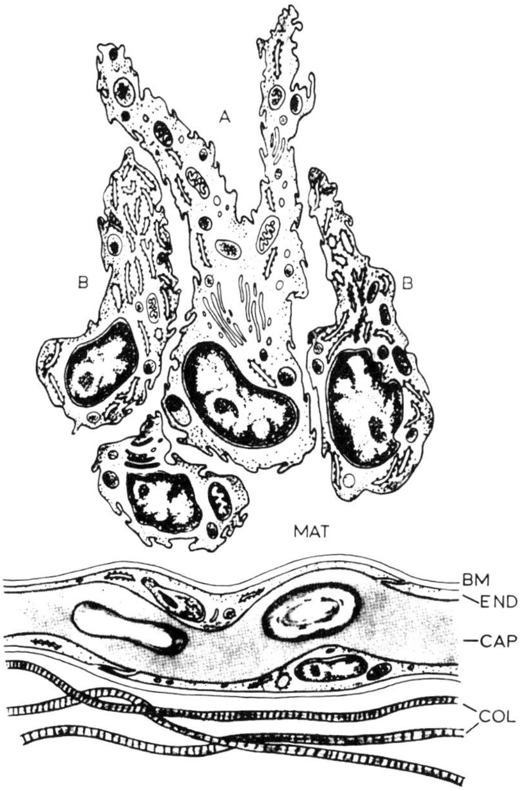

Fig. 7.3 Synovial cells. Type A and type B cells of normal synovial surface overlying synovial connective tissue matrix (MAT) and capillaries (CAP). BM: capillary basement membrane; END: capillary endothelial cells; COL: synovial collagen fibrils. (Redrawn from Barland P, Novikoff A B, Hamerman D (1962) Journal of Cell Biology 14: 207–220.)

lipids, gold and carbon. Immune complexes and other macromolecules can be quickly released from synovial cells to become conspicuous components of abnormal synovial fluid.

The *B(F), fibroblast-like cells.* The structure and function of these cells centre upon the synthesis and secretion of the hyaluronate-protein of synovial fluid (Ch. 8). There is much rough endoplasmic reticulum. Ribosomes and polyribosomes are numerous. A Golgi apparatus and smooth reticulum may be recognised and, as an index of oxidative enzyme activity and of oxidative phosphorylation, mitochondria are frequent and well formed. Synovial B cells are metabolically highly active and display many anabolic and catabolic processes that range from collagen, hyaluronic acid (Myers & Christine, 1983) and DNA synthesis to oxidative, lysosomal enzyme and collagenase activity (Henderson, 1981).

That synovial cells (Fig. 7.4) are of these two main forms is supported not only by conventional EM investigations but also by more sensitive analytical techniques. Thus, after the intra-articular injection of horseradish peroxidase, a first cell type, type A, absorbed the enzyme protein and contained many small cytoplasmic vesicles and large vacuoles. A second type, type S, did not absorb peroxidase but had a well-developed rough endoplasmic reticulum, a Golgi complex and many dense secretory granules. Serial, thin sections proved necessary to provide adequate information on different synoviocytic types (Graabek, 1982). Two distinct cell types are also found in monolayer and explant cultures (Krey et al, 1976); one form is macrophage-like, the other fibroblastic. Only the latter persists in culture; it displays no receptor sites for the Fc portion of IgG or for C3.

In spite of these and many other observations the distinction between the two main cell types is neither sharp nor absolute. Indeed, in a review of the articular territory of the reticulendothelial system, Ghadially (1980) stresses that the two main cell types, type A (macrophage-like) and type B (fibroblast-like) 'are not distinct and different races of cells with different functions but merely cells whose differences in morphology reflect the function they are performing at a given moment'.

The dual nature of synovial cells receives support from physiological studies in which mouse radiation chimeras are studied. The macrophage-like, type A cells, appear to be derived from the bone marrow like so many other cells of the mononuclear phagocyte system; the type B cells resemble bone marrow stromal cells and are fibroblast-like. Complementary functional studies with autoradiographic techniques support this view (Dreher, 1982) and show that synovial cell hyperplasia in experimental hypersensitivity arthritis does not occur after bone marrow irradiation. Even if functional and ultrastructural investigations show only two populations of synovial cells, the cells from patients with rheumatoid arthritis or with non-inflammatory joint disease can be divided into three populations on the basis of their expression of surface antigens as determined by

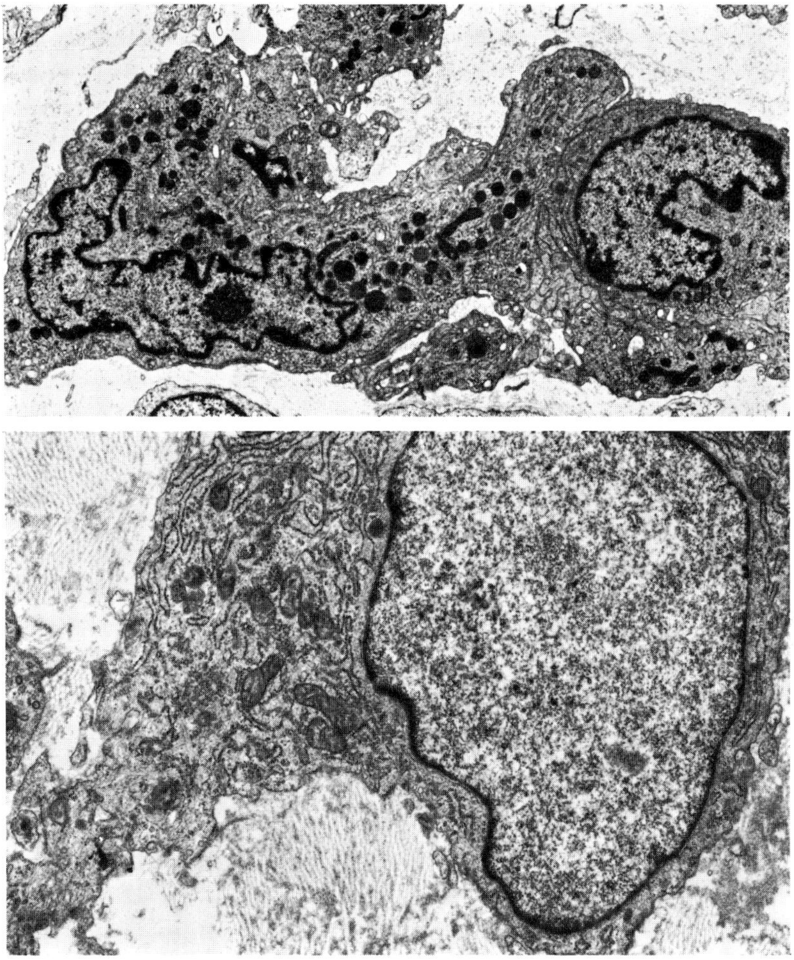

Fig. 7.4 Synovial cells. (Top) A(M) macrophage-like, phagocytic synovial cells: both have irregular shaped, indented nuclei and many dark-appearing cytoplasmic organelles that are lysosomes. EM ×4500.

(Bottom) B(F) fibroblast-like cell with prominent ovoid nucleus and cytoplasm containing much rough endoplasmic reticulum and many mitochondria. TEM ×6000.

monoclonal antisera against Ia and against antigens associated with mononuclear macrophages and fibroblasts (Burmester et al, 1983).

Mast cells

An important constituent of loose connective tissue is the *mast cell*. The metachromatic granules of these large versatile cells are readily lost during laboratory handling but the use of rapidly frozen, cryostat-cut material allows the cells to be viewed intact. The granules, well seen after reaction with acridine orange or after supravital staining, are electron dense, round or ovoid and membrane-bounded. Granular endoplasmic reticulum and ribosomes are scanty. Mast cells commonly lie near small blood vessels and, in this situation, are encountered in many of the viscera (Bromley et al, 1984).

The most important function of the mast cell is the synthesis and liberation of histamine. Mast cells bind IgE reaginic antibody through a surface receptor. On contact with the appropriate antigen, for example in the course of the local anaphylaxis that is one explanation for clinical asthma, mast cell granules are liberated. From the degranulated cell derive both histamine and other smooth muscle-reacting agents including 5-hydroxytryptamine. The granules store and release the polyanion heparin with which histamine and 5-hydroxytryptamine exist as counterions (Ch. 6) (Gardner & Dodds, 1976).

Histiocytes
The scavenging macrophages of normal loose connective tissue include blood neutrophil granulocytes and occasional monocytes. However, intrinsic large phagocytes, *histiocytes*, are also present. Histiocytes possess many lysosomes and have a marked capacity for the phagocytosis of degraded autologous cells and cell debris, including red blood cells, and for the elimination of foreign material such as dust. They engulf and retain crystals of intrinsic metabolic or of extrinsic origin. The capacity to phagocytose crystals is influenced by crystal size and displays species variability.

Fat cells
Lipoblasts give rise to two forms of mature fat cells, the cells of the brown fat sometimes seen in the retroperitoneal tissues, and the adipose tissue that supports and protects the viscera while acting as a store of energy. Mature *fat cells* display little oxidative enzyme activity. Although in the fetus and newborn several fat droplets lie within the individual fat cell, in the adult each cell usually contains a single large droplet that displaces the nucleus to one margin of the cell. When adipose tissue is injured, cell degradation liberates products that are irritant and vigorously chemotactic to plasma cells and histiocytes. The histological consequences of such injury are those of fat necrosis. The cells of *brown fat*, analogous with the brown fat cells of hibernating animals, are intensely active metabolically. They respond readily to catecholamines and convert chemical energy into heat, a reaction mediated by cyclic AMP.

Glial cells
The supporting *neuroglial* cells of the central nervous system are neuroectodermal in origin. They lay down glial fibres that provide the same support for nervous tissue as do collagen fibres for the remainder of the body. Precursor cells give rise to spongioblasts from which the mature astrocytes and oligodendrocytes arise. The third common form of neuroglial cell, the microglial cell, is widely regarded as an extrinsic derivative of the mononuclear macrophage system.

Fibres (Table 7.1)

Collagen
Collagen is a ubiquitous structural protein of the connective tissues and an essential part of the calcified and non-calcified skeleton. It may serve as a substitute biomaterial (Stenzel et al, 1974).

70% of the human body is water. The dry weight includes much collagen, forming about one-third of all body protein. Collagen comprises 75–85% of the dry weight of the dermis, 50% of the dry weight of cartilage and 30% of dry bone. Synthesised within all forms of connective tissue cell except specialised units that are essentially phagocytic in function such as the osteoclast, and within many other cells of mesodermal origin such as the arterial smooth muscle cell, mature collagen comes to be a wholly extracellular, largely insoluble structural material which becomes even less soluble and more rigid with advancing age.

The chemical composition of collagen, its synthesis, secretion and extracellular processing, are described in Chapter 6. There are excellent modern reviews (Gay & Miller, 1983; Minor, 1980; Prockop et al, 1979).

Collagen fibrils are unbranched, vary greatly in diameter and can aggregate to form bundles sufficiently large to be visible with the naked eye. Aggregated fibrils, fibres, can form 'ropes' in tendons and ligaments, 'sheets' in joint capsules and fascia or three-dimensional mesh-like supportive microskeletons in articular cartilage. Unique physical and chemical properties provide collagen fibres and fibre bundles with high tensile strength and a high elastic modulus that determines the most important properties of tendon and ligament; resistance to tensile stress in articular cartilage; and an orderly and optically translucent crystalline structure in the lens. In bone, it is probable that particular parts of the collagen fibril facilitate the calcium hydroxyapatite deposition in the process of mineralisation and ensure its orderly nature

Table 7.1

Fibre	Site of synthesis	Main properties	Staining characteristics
Collagen	Endoplasmic reticulum; transport within cells to Golgi apparatus; secretion across plasma membrane	High tensile strength, high elastic modulus; reinforcement of cartilage matrix; nucleation foci for bone mineralisation; crystalline translucent structure for lens and cornea	Red with picric acid fuchsin (van Gieson); blue with trichrome methods (e.g. MSB); purple/brown with silver impregnation. Doubly refractile (intensified by picro-Sirius red). Periodic axial structure revealed by anionic and cationic stains for electron microscopy, or by negative staining
Reticular	Presumably identical	Structural support for blood vessels, and skeleton of reticuloendothelial system	Blue with Mallory trichrome; black with silver impregnation. Not distinctive on electron microscopy
Basement membrane	Epithelial cells, mesangial cells, alveolar septal cells fibroblasts of epithelial lamina propria, and cells of vascular intima	The ultimate filter (pore size 70×70^4 daltons between plasma and extracellular fluid)	Brown-black to PAS-silver impregnation. Electron dense after uranyl nitrate staining
Elastic fibres	Chondrocytes of ear, nose, epiglottis, smooth muscle cells of arteries; septal cells of lung. Amino acids essential to polypeptides incorporated on endoplasmic reticulum	High extensibility. Resists large deformations without rupture. Support essential for blood vessels in face of pulsatile pressure changes	Dark blue/black with resorcein; faint brown with orcein; pink with Congo red; according to maturity, stains with potassium permanganate or phosphotungstic acid for electron microscopy

(Höhling et al, 1974). In non-osseous connective tissues such as tendon (Scott & Orford, 1981) and the cornea (Young, 1985) proteoglycan molecules are associated with collagen in a correspondingly orderly manner. In hyaline cartilage, proteoglycan is linked to collagen at the 'd' band (Orford & Gardner, 1984) and the intimacy and regularity of this association is likely to contribute to the structural integrity of articular structure.

Light microscopists stain collagen with the acid-fuchsin of the van Gieson reagents with which collagen is coloured red (Gardner & Dodds, 1976). The picro-Sirius red method gives a corresponding colouration and has the considerable advantage that the birefringence of collagen is enhanced so that recognition by colour and by double refractility are simultaneous. The commonly used trichrome methods such as Martius blue Scarlet (MSB) yield a blue colour, and silver impregnation techniques which bind to fibres and fibre bundles stain collagen black. Staining techniques appear capable of distinguishing between different collagens (Lillie et al, 1980) so that degraded and pathological forms can be identified by light microscopy.

For transmission electron microscopy (Fig. 7.5), it is convenient to contrast the results of positive and of negative staining. Positive staining with uranyl acetate and phosphotungstic acid reveals 5 major dark bands designated a–e. Negative staining, a technique in which phosphotungstic acid is used at neutral pH to define collagen fibrillar outlines, presumably by binding with carbohydrate, displays a darkly-stained 'gap zone' and a lightly-stained 'overlap zone' (Stockwell, 1979). The banding pattern of collagen fibrils stained for electron microscopy reflects the charge distribution that is determined by the primary amino acid sequence (Meek et al, 1979).

Much has been learnt of the significance of the cross-band pattern of collagen. When mammalian tissue is extracted at neutral pH, the subsequent transmission electron microscopic study of the extract reveals fibrils with a 'native' periodic structure of 67 nm. When the extract is prepared at acid pH, an entirely different, non-fibrillar structure is found composed only of segments of fibrils. The segments have many axial periods of 280 nm length, the same dimension as that of the tropocollagen molecule itself: they are said to be

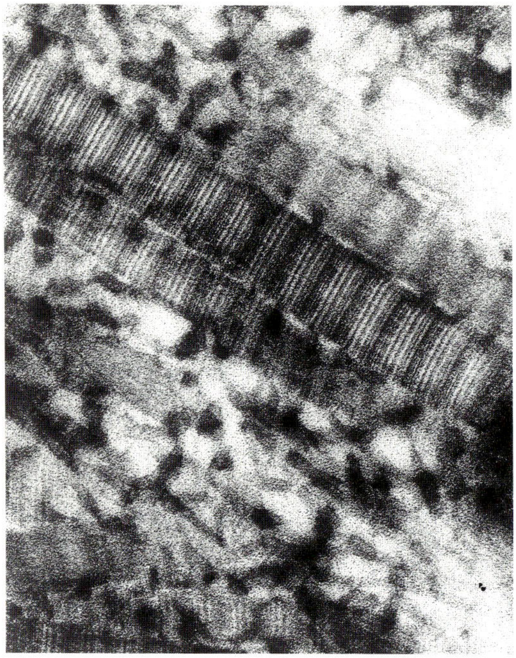

Fig. 7.5 Collagen fibril from Zone IV B of canine articular cartilage. Banding periodicity is ~ 60 nm in fixed, dehydrated tissue. Phosphotungstic acid/uranyl acetate. TEM ×96 625.

'segment long spacing' (SLS). There is evidence that the striated appearance of the SLS fibrils is the result of the laying down of laterally packed tropocollagen molecules in homoregister, that is, with all like molecular features in exact juxtaposition, an arrangement strongly suggested by transmission electron microscopic analyses. In vivo, however, the laying down of fibrils is 'staggered' so that each adjacent fibril is displaced by one period (D) in its relation to the adjacent fibril. The longitudinal displacement or 'stagger' with fibrils of 4.4 D each displaced 1 D in relation to its neighbour is a likely explanation for the ultrastructure of collagen in vivo as well as for that of 'native' fibrils artificially precipitated in the laboratory.

This widely accepted arrangement of tropocollagen molecules in collagen fibrils can only satisfactorily explain fibrillar structure if tropocollagen molecules are deposited in a monolayer. In a three-dimensional macromolecular structure of the kind that forms the 'native' collagen fibril, the monolayer can be considered to be wrapped into the form of a hollow cylinder. Each cylinder probably comprises five molecules, arranged as a filament. The filaments, retaining a 1D helical stagger, are aggregated into larger collagen fibrils, preserving a 1D periodicity (Serafini-Fracassini & Smith, 1974). In bone, the three-dimensional molecular arrangement is a quasi-hexagonal lattice (Miller, 1984).

Proteoglycans influence fibril formation in vitro and presumably in vivo. If proteoglycans are mixed with tropocollagen at neutral pH, fibrils with the 'native' 67 nm periodicity result; at acid pH, fibrils (not segments of fibrils) are found to form. They have a characteristically long periodic structure and are said to be 'fibril long spacing' (FLS). Their appearance is one indication of the important role of proteoglycans in determining collagen structure in the laboratory. It is reasonable to assume that proteoglycans play at least as significant a part in collagen fibrillogenesis 'in vivo'.

Human hyaline cartilage contains a number of collagens, perhaps as many as 10. In addition to the α 1(II) chain of type II collagen, the 1α and 2α chains have been extensively studied (Burgeson et al, 1982); they display similarities to the α1(V) and α2(V) chains of type V collagen. Interest in the antigenicity of the collagens has grown quickly. Monoclonal, anti-collagen antibodies can be employed to dissect the microscopic structure of the connective tissues at both light and electron microscopic levels (Evans et al, 1983; Foellmer et al, 1983) and type II collagen has been shown to be an effective and reproducible antigen for the production of a widely studied form of experimental arthritis (Trentham, 1982). Collagen has long been employed as a substrate for the culture of cells, either as a thin film or gel or to provide a three-dimensional environment (Kleinman et al, 1981; Yang & Nandi, 1983). The complex pathological processes of collagen degradation (Perez-Tamayo, 1978) and the role of collagenases in pathological states (Krane, 1982) are considered elsewhere (Ch. 6).

Elastic material (Kadar, 1979; Sandberg et al, 1981; Urry, 1983).

Ligaments; some articular cartilages; ear, nose and epiglottic cartilage; arteries; lungs, bronchi and many other tissues contain a lamellar and branched material, elastic, that has the reversible deformability of a rubber. Elastic* material in mammals is analogous to resilin in molluscs and to abductin in insect wings. In a number of the inflammatory connective tissue diseases of man, such as polyarteritis, polychondritis and polymyalgia rheumatica or giant cell arteritis, elastic material is actively and, to an extent, selectively destroyed. In other experimental disorders such as lathyrism in chicks and copper deficiency in pigs, elastic material formation and maturation are impaired; and in some non-inflammatory, neoplastic diseases such as the adenomatoid tumours and breast cancer, elastic material is formed in excess.

The lamellar and branched material of elastic is usually present in islands, *elastic aggregates*, that can be identified by electron but not by light microscopy. With the latter technique, elastic is seen, in arterial walls for example, as a discontinuous lamina or, in cartilage, as clusters of perichondrocytic fibres. Elastic material and elastic aggregates are formed of two principal components: a central, apparently amorphous substance that comprises the bulk of the mature lamina or fibre; and a microfibrillar component seen most clearly at the developing periphery of elastic aggregates. The islands or aggregates invariably lie within a broader, connective tissue extracellular matrix that comprises varying proportions of proteoglycan and of collagen which is usually of types I or III.

The *amorphous component* of the elastic aggregate is the unusual protein *elastin*, derived from a precursor, tropoelastin, and containing a unique proportion of the non-polar amino acids glycine, proline, alanine, valine, phenylalanine, isoleucine and leucine. There is debate concerning the orderliness of its structure (Urry, 1983) but it is increasingly likely that elastin, in spite of its limited double refractility in polarised light, is best described as isotropic and filamentous. Elastin has great resistance to chemical, physical and enzymatic digestion but characteristically aggregates with heat to form *coacervates*. Unlike rubber, with which there are similarities, elastin is hydrophobic: dry, it becomes hard and brittle. The structure of elastin determines the potential for cross-link formation throughout the polypeptide chain and, in turn, for the construction of a molecular meshwork of great size. The four-armed cross links contributed by desmosine and isodesmosine, heterocyclic nitrogen-containing molecules unique to elastin, contribute stability and insolubility. The cross-links exist in a part of the elastin molecule that is compact and rich in alanine; the extensible part of the molecule contains the hydrophobic amino acid residues.

The *microfibrillar component* of developing elastic aggregates is composed of beaded, glycoprotein filaments 10–12 nm in diameter. The microfibrils are formed before elastin can be identified and may serve as a framework upon which elastin accumulates during embryonic elastogenesis. The glycoprotein contains at least two constituents, MFPI, a collagenous glycoprotein with a molecular weight of 150 000 and MFP2, non-collagenous and with a molecular weight of only 35 000. Elastin is synthesised, inter alia, by the fibroblasts of ligaments, by the chondroblasts of elastic cartilage, by the smooth muscle cells of arteries and by pulmonary alveolar septal cells. It is of interest that, in the epiglottis, for example, each chondrocyte of this elastic cartilage is capable of the simultaneous synthesis and export of elastin, of the microfibrillar glycoproteins, of collagen and of proteoglycan as well as of its own structural and enzymic proteins and nucleoproteins. The interrelationship between the various extracellular macromolecules is extremely close and the formation and maturation of elastic material deposited outside chondrocytes or smooth muscle cells rests on the integrity of the remaining intercellular matrix materials.

During elastin synthesis, vesicles appear in those fibroblasts and smooth muscle cells that are producing this protein. The vesicles (Sandberg et al, 1981) are acanthosomes (spiny or coated vesicles): they have an inner, electron-dense core that may comprise proteoglycan, tropoelastin or elastin in an early phase of cross-linking. The vesicles pass to the plasma membrane and fuse with it. The

* Elasticity is the capacity of a material to recoil perfectly after stretching. The resistance of a material to deformation (stiffness) is expressed as Young's modulus which is an index therefore of the force required to cause a given deformation. Young's modulus for ox ligamentum nuchae is $10^4 N/m^{-2}$. Elastic tissue, in the biological sense, has a lower Young's modulus than collagen, i.e. 'elastic' tissue is more extensible than collagenous tissue.

core material is subsequently extruded into the zone of elastogenesis. Cross-link formation may begin within the acanthosomes.

The secretion and extracellular deposition of elastin and of the glycoprotein microfibrils are programmed genetically: each step begins at exactly defined times in the developing embryo. In the chick, for example, the onset of elastogenesis is at 5½ days and is first detected in the truncus arteriosus. Elastogenesis then extends peripherally until finally, after 12–14 days, elastic material is encountered in the smallest arteries (El-Maghraby & Gardner, 1969). Elastic formation extends from the periphery of arterial walls towards the lumen. Elastogenesis in rat epiglottic cartilage is not recognisable until 24 hours before birth. In the epiglottic cartilage of the human fetus elastogenesis begins at the 4th month. Little is known of the times of appearance of human arterial elastic and the cellular details of elastic synthesis in human elastic cartilage have been the subject of few recent investigations.

Elastic material (Fig. 7.6) is conveniently examined by light microscopy, after staining with dyes such as Weigert's resorcin-fuchsin or with orcein. Immature elastic material reacts positively with phosphotungstic acid-haematoxylin. The capacity for binding cationic dyes diminishes with developmental time; older material continues to be demonstrable with potassium permanganate. Just as the relative proportions of elastin and of the microfibrillar glycoproteins change with age, so, too, do the electron microscopic appearances. Phosphotungstic acid positivity is an index of the

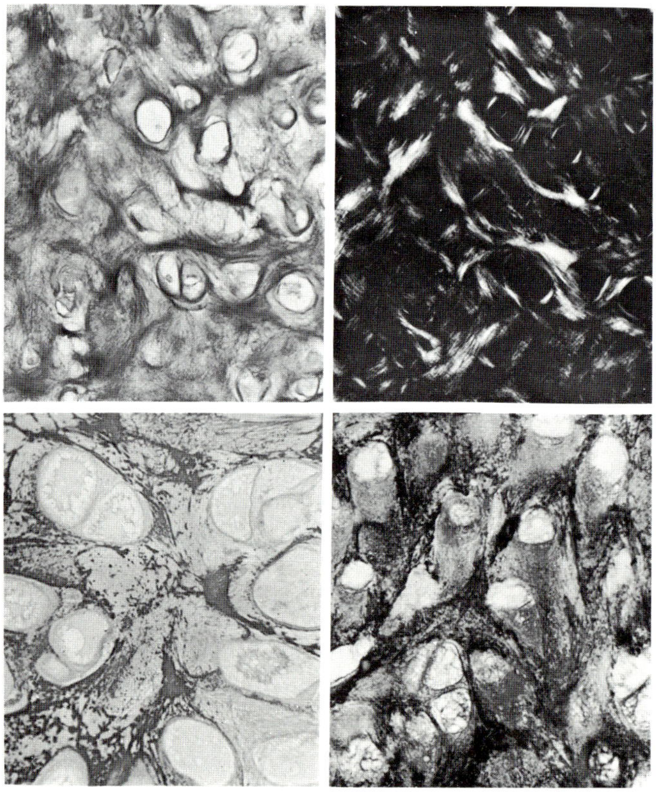

Fig. 7.6 Adult human epiglottic cartilage. Composite figure to show distribution of collagen and elastic material in relation to chondrocytes. Much alcian blue-positive glycosaminoglycan is also present but is not shown in this figure.

(Top) Collagen fibres, often condensed around chondrocyte lacunae, appear dark grey (left) and white (right). (Left) Picro-Sirius red × 150. (Right) Picro-Sirius red with polarised light ×150.

(Bottom) Compare with top fields. Elastic material is evident equidistant from and around chondrocytes where elastic aggregates form grey-appearing islands (left), dark grey islands (right). (Left) 1 μm section of Epon-embedded material. Aldehyde-fuchsin ×320. (Right) Conventional paraffin section of same material.Orcein ×240.

glycosaminoglycan content of the elastic material (Kadar, 1979); consequently young elastic material reacts strongly with phosphotungstic acid and this component resists the elastase digestion that degrades elastin. In the older individual, elastic material becomes increasingly calcified and the desirable biological properties are impaired.

Elastin can be examined with the transmission electron microscope after the application of heavy metal stains (Kadar, 1979); its presence can also be inferred by the demonstration of the vacuities remaining after tissue, embedded in a water soluble polymer, has been selectively digested with an elastase. Ultrasonication and negative staining demonstrate that elastin itself is formed of 30–40 nm diameter filaments arranged in the long axis of the gross elastic fibres. The filaments display an axial periodicity of approximately 4.0 nm.

Reticular fibres

Widely dispersed throughout the body, forming a delicate network around the walls of small arteries, and intimately related to the stromal framework of the lymphoreticular and reticuloendothelial systems, are fibres identified by light microscopy after the retention of silver by impregnation. This brown-grey argyrophilia suggests that these 'reticular' fibres are distinct from collagen fibres and fibre bundles which retain silver more completely to give a black appearance. 'Reticular' fibres are often closely associated with the deeper parts of basement membranes (see below) but they are not identical with the lamina densa. Differences in argyrophilia between mature collagen fibres and reticular fibres are thought to depend on subtle differences in the quantity of non-collagenous matrix macromolecules bound to each fibre. Thus, small bundles of thin collagen fibres invested with ruthenium red-staining material correspond to reticular fibres in number and distribution when judged by light microscopy.

Examination by transmission electron microscopy shows that reticular fibres, which appear extremely early in chick embryonic and yolk sac development and long before stainable collagen, are nevertheless identical with collagen in ultrastructural terms. The distinction between the collagen and reticular fibres is clearly therefore one of maturity, of quantity of associated material and, consequently, of stainability, rather than of primary structure. Reticular fibres and the fibrous long-spacing fibres (FLS) of collagen that result from collagenase incubation (Kajikawa et al, 1980) display the same spatial distribution, an observation suggesting that the substrate on which endogenous collagenase acts to produce FLS fibres is reticulin. This enzymatic process is likely to be influenced by carbohydrate.

Both reticular fibres and basement membranes contain appreciable amounts of glycoprotein; both react with the periodic acid-Schiff reagents; but they are distinct. Whereas basement membranes, often of epithelial cell origin, are laminar microfibrillar matrices, reticular fibres share many features with collagen.

Basement membranes (Martinez-Hernandez & Amenta, 1983)

Basement membranes are delicate, faintly eosinophilic, extracellular, composite matrices indentifiable by light microscopy close to the basal aspect of epithelial cells and between these cells and the connective tissue stroma. Basement membranes, found in all parts of the body and adjacent to endothelial, neurilemmal and skeletal muscle cells as well as to epithelia, play major roles in disease and are synthesised and secreted by the cells near which they lie: they are not usually connective tissue cell products although among their components (Table 7.2) are molecular species closely similar to those found in the connective tissue matrices elsewhere. Basement membranes have a characteristic microscopic appearance, a distinctive

Table 7.2 Components of basement membranes (after Leivo, 1983)

Component	All basement membranes	Restricted distribution
Collagen	Type IV	Type V
Non-collagenous	Laminin	Fibronectin
glycoproteins	Entactin	Antigens of bullous pemphigus and of Goodpasture's syndrome
Glycosaminoglycans	Heparan sulphate Chondroitin sulphate	

fine structure, a well-defined chemical composition and individual antigenic properties.

The appearances in thin paraffin sections is well shown by the periodic acid-Schiff stain but superior results are obtained when silver stains are used on these or on 0.5–1.0 μm sections embedded in polymers such as Epon; the silver reacts with the lamina densa. The thickness, integrity and arrangement of basement membranes can also be demonstrated with appropriate anti-basement membrane antibody, allowing them to be investigated in formalin-fixed, paraffin section by the PAP-immunoperoxidase method or in cryostat sections of unfixed, frozen material by immunofluorescence.

Electron microscopy (Fig. 7.7) reveals a continuous, uninterrupted structure comprising a 20–80 nm basal *lamina densa* representing the basement membrane material visible with the light microscope, and an electron lucent 10–30 nm *lamina rara* situated between the basal lamina densa and the plasma membrane of the parent cell. At high resolution, the lamina densa is found to comprise a thick meshwork of fine fibrils. When, as in the case of the pulmonary alveoli and renal glomeruli, basement membranes lie between adjoining epithelial cells or between epithelial and endothelial cells, a lamina rara is found on both aspects of the lamina densa.

Much can be learnt of the composition of basement membranes by histochemical and immunocytochemical analyses. Basement membranes possess antigens with antigenic determinants shared with those of nearby epithelial cells; some, at least, of these antigenic determinants are distinct from those of the other connective tissues. Cationic dyes reveal a component of glycosaminoglycan. Immunofluorescent studies with anticollagen antibodies confirm the presence of type IV and sometimes type V collagen. Laminin is found in both laminae; the lamina rara contains fibronectin.

Laminin is the principal, non-collagenous basement membrane glycoprotein; it is present in all basement membranes that have been investigated and is a large structure with a molecular weight of $0.8–1.0 \times 10^6$. Transmission electron microscopy reveals laminin as an asymmetrical cross with three short and one long arm. Many cultured cells synthesise laminin and fibroblasts secrete and deposit *entactin*, a similar sulphated polypeptide that is recognisable at glomerular epithelial and endothelial cell plasma membranes.

The *fibronectins* are a family of ubiquitous glyco-

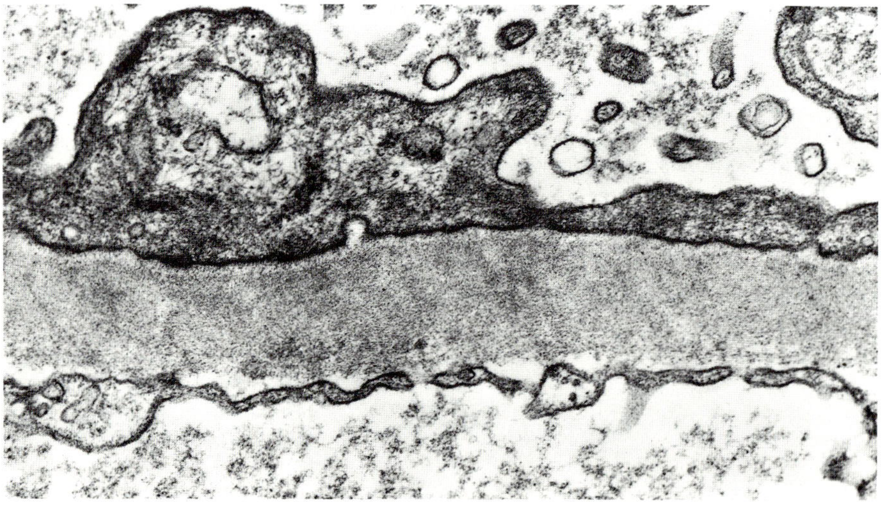

Fig. 7.7 Basement membrane (basal lamina) from human glomerular tuft. At top, endothelial cell adjoins relatively electronlucent zone of basement membrane. At bottom, epithelial cell cytoplasm is separated from membrane margin by artefactual space. Uranyl acetate/lead citrate TEM × 42 200

proteins. Fibronectin, secreted by many connective tissue cells, plays a part in cell adhesion and migration and is present in articular cartilage (Clemmensen et al, 1982) but not, apparently, in association with collagen 1α2α3α* or with collagen C–PS (Evans et al, 1983). In addition to the fibronectins and laminin, there is a suggestion that there may exist a further glycoprotein, *chondronectin*, which specifically mediates the attachment of chondrocytes to type II collagen Hewitt et al, 1982). Basement membranes contain ~ 1% glycosaminoglycan, the presence of which influences permeability. Heparan sulphate, with small amounts of chondroitin sulphate and hyaluronic acid, can be isolated.

The apparently compact structure of the tenuous but continuous basement membrane made it difficult for light microscopists to understand how small and large molecules, and, in some instances, cells and bacteria, could escape from channels lined by epithelia to enter the extracellular fluid spaces and lymphatics. Recent evidence shows that a basement membrane is not an inviolate, constant structure. Silver labelling has been used to demonstrate the habitual exchange of its structural molecules. There is a continual turnover of its components which are assembled as a molecular sieve of finite permeability. Transient discontinuities can appear and allow the passage of lymphocytes, cancer cells, bacteria or macromolecules. The most striking instance of this filter-like function is the renal glomerular capillary. Both the epithelial and endothelial cell layers of this unit are normally discontinuous, the basement membrane continuous. The basement membrane acts as a filter that allows the escape, to the urinary space, of water and of molecules that have molecular weights of not more than 7.0×10^4. Under physiological conditions, the basement membrane permits metabolites to reach and catabolites to leave glandular and other secretory cells although it is not certain whether the filtration is by molecular sieving or by ion exchange.

Injuries, such as those caused by some forms of diffuse glomerulonephritis, commonly provoke new basement membrane synthesis. The basement membrane can be lysed after local inflammation, presumably by lysosomal enzyme hydrolysis, and a physiological response appears to occur in mammary involution following lactation.

*Collagen type 1α2α3α is likely soon to be designated collagen type XI.

Non-fibrillar extracellular matrix (Meachim & Stockwell, 1979)

The connective tissue extracellular matrix is a fibre-reinforced gel in which highly hydrated, expanded proteoglycans (Ch. 6), arranged as aggregates about molecules of hyaluronic acid, are restrained within a three-dimensional meshwork of type II collagen fibrils. The matrix constitutes an amorphous, heterogeneous material that occupies the space between the connective tissue cells. The proteoglycans and, in particular, their glycosaminoglycan chains, give the matrix many of its distinctive physical and chemical properties.

Because ground substance not only forms the bulk of connective tissues such as hyaline cartilage but also occupies the interstices of all organs in all parts of the body, it has been described (Schubert & Hamerman, 1968) as 'the real internal medium' (*milieu interieur*) in which cells are immersed and across which anabolites and catabolites, water and gases pass constantly.

The connective tissues with the highest water content are those in which hyaluronic acid comprises the predominant matrix macromolecule. They include umbilical cord Wharton's jelly, the oestrogen-responsive skin of monkeys, the aqueous humour of the eye, the mesenchyme of the embryo, the young nucleus pulposus of the intervertebral disc, and the mucinous material synthesised by some cancer cells and by synovial 'ganglia'. When the water is removed, the dry residue comprises collagen, occasionally elastic material, proteoglycans, some glycoprotein, other unidentified proteins and small molecular species that range from glycosaminoglycans, oligo- and monosaccharides, amino acids and lipid, to electrolytes of which sodium chloride is the most abundant. Just as the proportion of collagen in different tissues varies from very high (ligaments, tendons, intervertebral annulus fibrosus, cornea, meniscus) to low (intervertebral nucleus pulposus, bursae, ganglia), so the quantity of the other principal non-aqueous component of the extracellular connective tissue, proteoglycan, tends to vary reciprocally. Where tensile strength, structural rigidity and elasticity are of overriding importance, collagen predominates. Where compressive strength and uniform stress distribution are prime requirements, proteoglycans form the principal fraction.

With many of the staining techniques used to prepare sections for the light microscope, the non-fibrous matrix cannot be recognised. Connective tissue components also tend to be lost during aqueous fixation: fixed, paraffin-embedded sections stained with haematoxylin and eosin therefore reveal a pale intercellular background. In unfixed material prepared at low temperature, the high proportion of polyanionic glycosaminoglycan gives ground substance a characteristic metachromasia with cationic dyes such as toluidine blue.

The properties of the dyes that stain glycosaminoglycans have been reviewed by Elliott (1976). The dyes comprise the *thiazins*, e.g. toluidine blue; the *azins*, e.g. safranin; the *acridines*, e.g. acridine orange; and the *phthalocyanins*, e.g. alcian blue 8GX. Valuable reactions are also evinced by dialysed ferric hydroxide and by colloidal iron or gold. Ruthenium red (Luft, 1965), and bismuth nitrate give electron-dense glycosaminoglycan complexes. In spite of their 1 : 2 diglycol links, most of the ground substance polysaccharides do not stain with the Schiff reagent after oxidation with periodic acid; this is because they react only slowly with periodate. The periodic acid — Schiff reaction is given, however, by epithelial 'mucins', secretions in which distinct oligosaccharides are attached to protein. A positive response can be recognised in ground substance where sufficient keratan sulphate is present.

The phthalocyanin dye alcian blue has attracted particular interest. Used in a critical electrolye concentration (CEC) technique (Scott & Dorling, 1965) with selected molar concentrations of magnesium chloride, the dye, which contains copper, can be employed to show the presence of the different glycosaminoglycans in filter paper, and, probably, in tissue preparations. Phthalocyanin derivatives with higher copper contents, in particular cuprolinic blue and cupromeronic blue (Scott et al, 1981) have been selected as electron-dense stains for transmission electron microscopy (Fig. 7.8)

Just as the CEC method has been used to show that the superficial zones of articular cartilage are rich in chondroitin sulphate, which increases with age, so the ultrastructural application of cuprolinic- and of cupromeronic blue has enabled the precise sites of proteoglycan–collagen relationships to be demonstrated in thin sections of cartilage, tendon and cornea. There is an apparently constant, periodic association between proteoglycan and the collagen 'd' band.

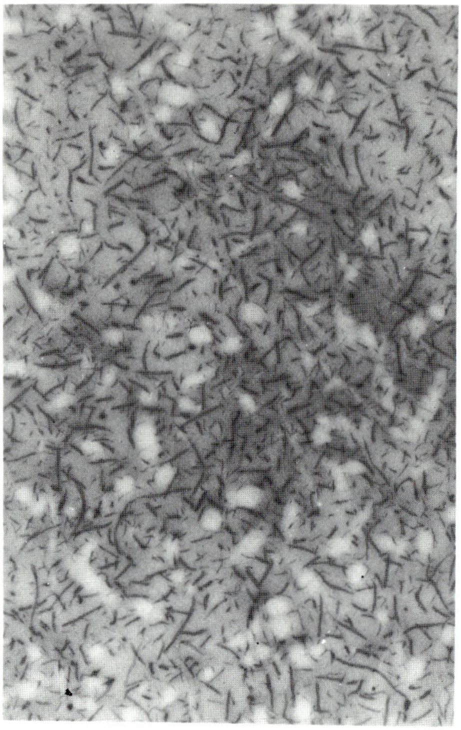

Fig. 7.8 Proteoglycans preserved in situ in Zone II of canine articular cartilage using a cationic dye, cupromeronic blue, in a critical electrolyte concentration technique to demonstrate sulphated glycosaminoglycans. Collagen fibrils are unstained and appear as pale outlines. Cupromeronic blue applied at 0.3M $MgCl_2$. TEM ×25 650

ORGANISED CONNECTIVE TISSUE

Loose, adipose, fibrofatty, compact, elastic

Loose connective tissue, widely distributed in almost all parts of the body, serves a supporting function; it is often arranged in thin, separating layers between viscera. There is much ground substance, many cells but relatively few fibres. Blood vessels and lymphatics are numerous, sensory nerve endings and specialised sensory receptors frequent. Much subcutaneous connective tissue is 'loose'; and loose connective tissue provides the flexible support for the synovial lining cells of the majority of the diarthrodial joints. The malleable texture of this form of connective tissue is an index of the high proportion of proteoglycan to fibres. Hyaluronate is abundant. The predominance of proteoglycan ensures a high water content. However, the absence of the kind of physical barriers provided by the dense fibrous laminae of fascia and aponeuroses explains why inflammatory reactions, and especially bacterial infections, extend so rapidly within loose connective tissue: there is direct continuity with the lymphatic system.

Adipose tissue is formed of fat cells grouped in lobules between which extend delicate collagenous septa bearing small blood vessels with associated mast cells, lymphatics and nerve fibres. The orderly lobular arrangement of adipose tissue is well seen at the surface of adipose synovial tissue such as that of the infrapatellar fat pad. Here scanning EM reveals a hexagonal packing of adjacent blunt adipose synovial processes.

Fibrofatty tissue is a common foundation for lining synovial cells. There is an intimate admixture of clusters of fat cells with interlacing bundles of collagen fibres in relation to which nerve fibres and blood and lymphatic vessels extend freely.

The term '**compact connective tissue**' is applicable to those forms where strength is a prime requirement rather than flexibility. Bone, tendons, ligaments, fascia, aponeuroses, menisci, labra, dura, lens, sclera and intervertebral discs fall within this broad category. Characteristically, there is much collagen, relatively little matrix material, and small numbers of differentiated cells. In bone, insoluble mineral increases strength still further.

Exceptionally, connective tissue is 'elastic'. The term is used in a descriptive, not in a precise mechanical sense. **Elastic connective tissue** has a characteristic yellow colour. It is clear that in elastic tissues such as the epiglottis and ear, the chondrocytes secrete elastin and the glycoproteins of elastic material as well as collagen, proteoglycan and other protein. The multiphase structure of elastic connective tissue is analogous with the complex composition of the extracellular matrix in 'elastic' arteries.

Joint capsule, fascia, aponeuroses, ligaments, tendons

Surrounding synovial joints and forming a mobile, protective tent, are *capsules* attached firmly to both opposing bone ends. At the bone ends, the capsule interlaces and is in continuity with the periosteum. Capsules are often discontinuous; the openings in their structure allow the synovial membrane to protrude to form bursae and permit the passage of tendons, the attachments for which lie inside the joint capsule.

In *fascia and aponeuroses* strength and flexibility are ensured by a sheet-like arrangement of randomly dispersed collagen bundles.

Ligaments are formed of dense parallel collagen bundles, incompletely attached one to the other and receiving a small arterial blood supply. The limited number of fibrocytes, and the ease with which blood flow is interrupted, explain why ligaments heal slowly after injury; their abundant sensory innervation determines the associated severe pain. Many ligaments are no more than localised thickenings of a joint capsule. Where this is so, the site of ligaments is determined by the form and direction of movement. In ball and socket joints, for example, ligaments lie to the side of maximum movement or, as in the hip joint, secure the opposing articulating surfaces by a central location (ligamentum teres). In hinge and many condylar joints the principal ligaments are lateral. Ligaments may be entirely intra-articular. There are also frequent anatomical associations of syndesmoses and synchondroses (p. 229). In all sites, ligament development and strength increase with normal intermittent use but decrease either with disuse or with constant, excess stress.

The attachment of a ligament to bone is an *enthesis* (Ball, 1971). Disorders of this junction, such as those encountered in ankylosing spondylitis, are said to be enthesopathies. Immediately before reaching the bone the ligamentous fibres become increasingly compact; they then become cartilaginous and finally calcified before attaching to bone by a cement line. There is substantial variation in the depth of the calcified zone. A significant vascular communication exists between the ligament and the Haversian system vessels or bone marrow. Ball (1971) stresses that the annulus fibrosus of the intervertebral disc is an important exception to this rule — all but the outer fibres are avascular. The available biochemical evidence shows that the enthesis is a site of active cell metabolism and molecular exchange.

Tendons are formed of numerous collagen fibrils clustered, as they are in ligaments, into parallel bundles and associated with very small numbers of fibrocytes. The collagen ensures strength, slight extensibility and a high modulus of elasticity. Within large tendons, groups of collagen bundles are arranged as fascicles that are separated by a small quantity of loose connective tissue in which are blood vessels and nerve fibres. At the myotendinous junction are sprays of non-myelinated nerve terminals, constituting the Golgi tendon organs. In the relaxed state, tendons assume a crimped pattern, a form that helps to explain the arrangement of the collagen fibres of which the tendon is formed (Gathercole & Keller, 1975).

Labra, intra-articular discs, menisci

Fibrocartilaginous rims in the shoulder and hip joints are known as **labra** (labrum glenoidale and labrum acetabulare respectively). Labra function to provide protection to the articular margins at extremes of movement. They may also give part origin to tendons (long head of the biceps) or ligaments (ligamentum teres of hip joint).

Intra-articular discs may be complete or incomplete. Complete fibrocartilaginous discs are present in the temporomandibular, inferior radioulnar and sternoclavicular joints; incomplete discs lie within the knee (menisci) and occasionally the acromioclavicular joints. The sternoclavicular and inferior radioulnar discs may become perforated with advancing age.

Menisci are crescent-shaped fibrocartilaginous discs that lie within synovial joints. It is interesting that their upper, free surfaces bear numerous microscopic tertiary features, comparable in size to those that cover hyaline articular cartilage. The menisci of the knee, the semilunar cartilages, are attached to the tibial condyles, increasing the congruence between femoral condyles and tibial plateaux, spreading load-bearing and acting as shock absorbers in walking and running. The medial knee meniscus is densely united with the tibial collateral ligaments. Particularly in extension, when the joints are close-packed, the medial collateral ligament and meniscus are vulnerable to rotational movements when the body weight pivots upon the knee.

Cartilage

In the human hip joint, forces approximating to 3–5 times the body weight are applied to the articulations twice in each walking cycle*. If it is assumed that an average adult takes 6000 steps each day, the hip joint is subjected to 2×10^6 episodes of loading each year or 10^8 loads in a lifetime. The bearing surfaces that withstand these loads are usually formed of hyaline (glass-like) cartilage supported by bone. Hyaline cartilage is therefore one of the most important connective tissue components of the mammalian body. The structure and properties of adult articular cartilage are reviewed in detail by Freeman (1979); by Kempson (1980) and by Myers & Mow (1983); those of embryonic, infantile and adolescent articular cartilage are described in appropriate anatomical texts (Warwick & Williams, 1980).

Whereas bone is a shell with an internal system of trabeculae that lie along the main stress trajectories, cartilage is a fibre reinforced gel (Maroudas, 1977; Maroudas et al, 1980). The fibres which entrap and restrain the gel are collagen. The gel is formed of macromolecules that are mutually repellent but which bind water within their domains. The osmotic forces generated in this way produce a swelling pressure which is equivalent to loading forces of approximately 0.35 MN/m^2 (50 lb/in^2). This swelling pressure affords hyaline cartilage its resistance to compression.

Hyaline cartilage (Fig. 7.9) (Kempson et al, 1973; Kempson et al, 1974; Stockwell, 1979) is not confined to diarthrodial joints. It is an integral part of the growth zone of bones formed by endochondral ossification; of the larynx, trachea and bronchi; and occasionally of other situations such

* Calculations show that in hip joint movement, loads of 0 to 3kN (647 lb) generate pressures of 0 to 3 MN/m^2 (435 lb/in^{-2}). A sliding speed of 0.025m/s is customary. The degree of surface roughness is indicated on p. 235. The viscosity of the lubricating synovial fluid is 10^{-2}–1 N/m^{-2}.

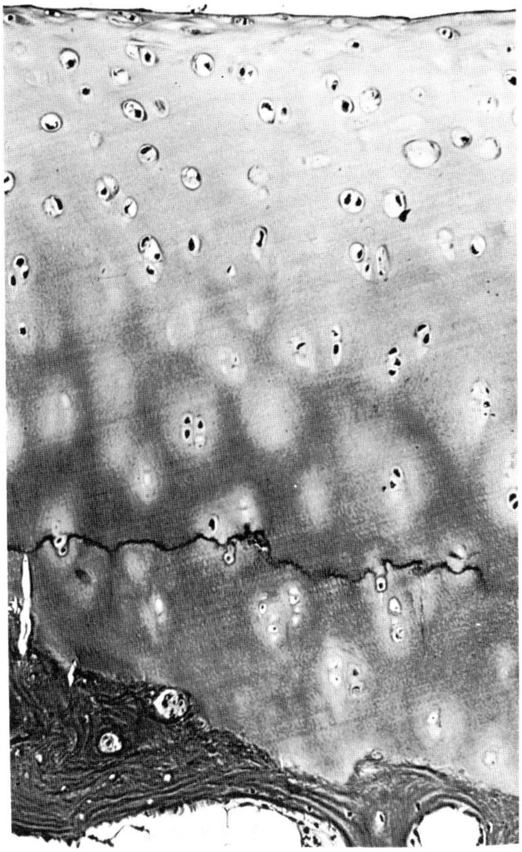

Fig. 7.9 Articular cartilage. Section perpendicular to surface of decalcified material from human interphalangeal joint. Note joint surface (top), chondrocytes within lacunae (centre), 'tide-line' separating non-calcified cartilage from calcified cartilage, and bone (bottom). Haematoxylin and eosin (H&E) × 130.

as the heart and aorta. Pig nasal cartilage has been a focus for biochemical study on the reasonable assumption that it shares many characteristics with the hyaline cartilage of other organs. The components of hyaline cartilage are cells; fibres that are predominantly collagen but occasionally elastic; and the abundant, intercellular matrix material (Scott, 1975).

Until recently, it had been accepted that the collagen fibres (Fig. 7.10) of hyaline cartilage were arranged in intermingling arcades: each fibre passed up from the underlying bony end plate to the articular surface and arched downwards to rejoin the bone with which it formed an extremely firm union. However, studies made with the scanning electron microscope have failed to confirm this arcade structure originally proposed by Benninghof. Detailed EM surveys show instead a meshwork or mat in which dense interlacing bundles of large collagen fibres lie parallel to the surface (Bozdech & Horn, 1975; Meachim et al, 1974; O'Connor et al, 1980). The surface meshwork of collagen is formed of many, predominantly unidirectional fibre laminae of approximately 20 nm diamter, interlacing mutually to provide a porous but stiff, strong and elastic protective surface mat. The surface disposition of the fibre bundles in this mat can be readily shown by making a series of pin-pricks in the surface and applying India ink (Fig. 7.11). Beneath the mat, other fibres are arranged at random,* not in arcades, and much more widely separated. The low proteoglycan/high collagen content of the surface lamina contrasts with the much larger relative proportion of proteoglycan in the matrix of the deeper cartilage. The deepest cartilage layer, adjoining the bone end, is to a varying degree calcified. When the more superficial, non-mineralised cartilage is removed by proteolytic digestion, the calcified layer of cartilage is found to display a form that simulates the dermal papillae of the skin, with narrow projections extending upwards and interdigitating with the corresponding, adjacent, downward-pointing islands of non-mineralised cartilage. Historically, it is interesting to note that this three-dimensional subcartilaginous structure was well known is the 19th century whereas the structure of the bearing surface itself was not defined until 1968.

Cartilage growth

The growth of cartilage has long been an object of intense interest. In man, there are easily recognisable, abnormal increases in heritable disorders such as the chondrodystrophies, in endocrine diseases such as acromegaly, and in the chondromata. Diminished growth is seen not only in hypopituitarism, the varieties of dwarfism and nutritional deficiency, but in limb joints remaining after partial amputation (Benichow & Wirotius, 1982).

* Nevertheless, the microscopic reconstruction of the orientation of the deeper collagen fibres has not yet been satisfactorily completed.

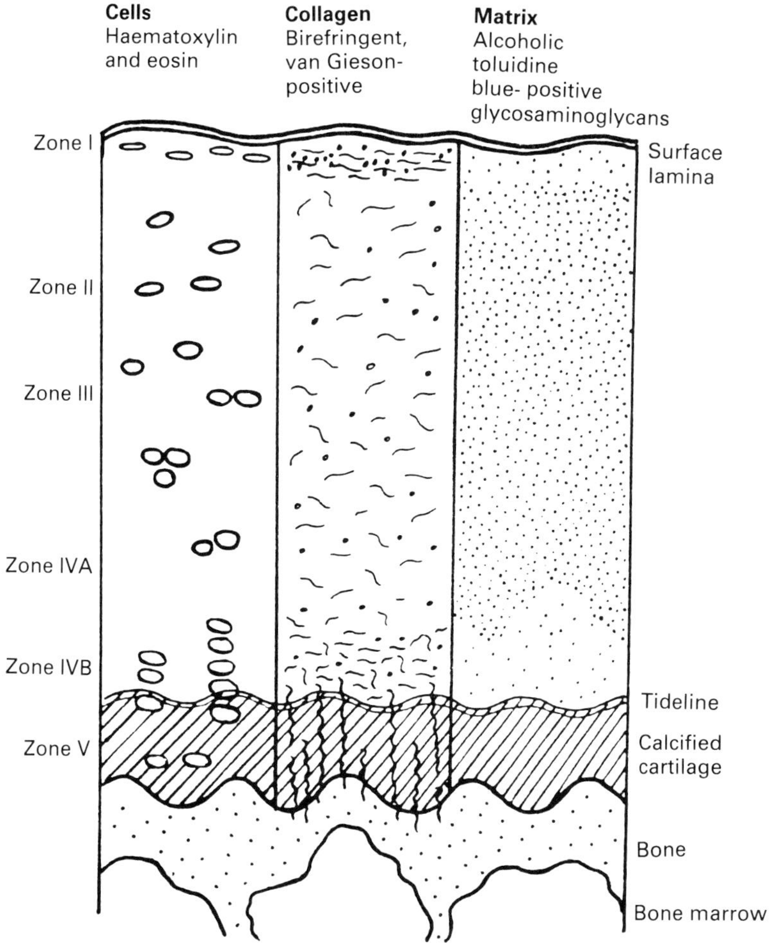

Fig. 7.10 Diagram of cartilage zones.

Experimentally, a chondrocyte growth factor is identifiable as a contaminant of the glycoprotein hormones of the anterior pituitary (Malemud & Sokoloff, 1978). Growth hormone promotes skeletal lengthening indirectly and the concept of the somatomedins envisages a role for growth hormone-dependent, circulating factors. Somatomedins, as well as analogues of cAMP, increase the number of rat chondrocytes synthesising DNA; their effects are synergistic (Hough et al, 1980). Fetal bovine cartilage contains analogous substances with somatomedin-like effects (Kato et al, 1982). Glucocorticoids diminish the proliferation of chondroprogenitor cells in neonatal mice (Silbermann et al, 1983) and it is of obvious relevance that somatostatin, which has extrahypothalamic sites of secretion and release, can locally inhibit the proliferation of cartilage precursor cells (Weiss et al, 1981). Many agents that exert purely local influences on cartilage survival and multiplication are recognised. Among the most interesting is prostaglandin A_1 (Kirkpatrick, 1980).

Neoplastic cartilage

The distinction between the hyaline cartilage of diarthrodial joints, the cartilage of fracture callus, the dysplastic cartilage of the chondrodystrophies and the neoplastic cartilage of benign neoplasms such as the chondromata is not well understood. The *quantity* of matrix material, and probably of the individual proteoglycan molecules present in these various forms of connective tissue, differs significantly, and the proportion and morphology

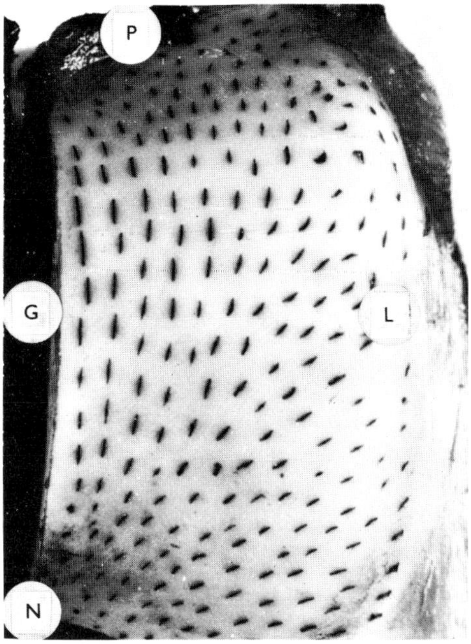

Fig. 7.11 Articular cartilage. Artificial splits made by pin-pricks display the orientation of the surface collagen fibre bundles on the lateral facet of this femoral patellar groove. From a male age 12 years. G: midline of groove; L: lateral edge; N: apex of intercondylar notch; P: proximal edge. ×2. (Reproduced by courtesy of Dr G. Meachim and the Editor, Journal of Anatomy. From Meachim G, et al (1974) Journal of Anatomy 118: 101–118.)

of the cells are distinctive. From the accumulating evidence that now exists to show variation in the species of collagen found in different tissues, it appears probable that hyaline cartilage collagen from synovial joints will prove to have a different molecular structure from the collagen of zones of endochondral ossification, of hamartomata and of the cartilaginous neoplasms.

Cartilage repair

In the absence of bone repair, hyaline articular cartilage undergoes repair with difficulty (Meachim & Roberts, 1971; Meachim, 1972). When holes are drilled experimentally into hyaline cartilage, a defect persists unless the hole extends through the underlying calcified cartilage into the vascular bone. Under these circumstances, the defect is repaired by a new formation of fibrocartilage (Salter et al, 1975); the main collagen in such defects is initially type I but becomes to a greater extent, but never completely, type II (Furukawa et al, 1980). Attempts have been made, without notable success, to introduce cultured chondrocytes into experimental partial thickness defects but there is difficulty in retaining the cells in the defects and little new hyaline cartilage forms.

Blood vessels and cartilage

Normally, hyaline cartilage, cornea, dentine, heart valves, the lens and epithelia do not undergo vascularisation. Their resistance to vascular invasion, studied in the chick chorioallantoic membrane (Eisenstein et al, 1973), appears to be due to the presence of diffusable substances that inhibit capillary endothelial cell growth. These anti-invasion factor(s) have been isolated and include at least 7 major protein bands (Kuettner & Pauli, 1983): the factors display activity against a variety of proteinases, including collagenases and proteoglycan-degrading enzymes. It appears likely that these factors play an important part in protecting articular cartilage from the adverse inflammatory responses that accompany minor and transient synovial disease.

Angiogenesis factors

By contrast with the anti-invasion factors, synovia in particular form, contain and liberate angiogenesis factors (Brown et al, 1980, 1983). The contact of articular cartilage with vascular tissue in the highly artificial circumstances of organ culture causes an extensive loss of proteoglycan and of collagen with fibroblastic transformation of the chondrocytes (Jubb, 1982). This effect is due partly to a direct action on the matrix, partly to activation of catabolic processes in the chondrocytes. The loss of matrix caused by vascular tissue appears to be precisely the same as that provoked by synovial tissue in the studies that led to the demonstration of catabolin (Fell & Jubb, 1977a, b) (p. 234) and it is reasonable to deduce that analogous responses in diseases such as rheumatoid arthritis can exert an important influence on the histological changes in affected joints.

Cartilage mechanics

Valuable information of the nature and behaviour of articular cartilage has come from mechanical experiments. If an external load is applied to cartilage, it will deform instantaneously due to the elasticity of the fibre-reinforced gel. With time, further deformation will occur as a result of fluid being squeezed out of the cartilage. The flow of fluid is resisted by entrapment within the collagen network. When the load is removed, there is an immediate recovery followed by the flow of fluid back into the loaded area. Under normal conditions of loading, there is very little, if any, fluid flow. Experiments on small, uniform blocks (Gore et al, 1983) and on thin slices of articular cartilage (Broom & Myers, 1980; Broom & Poole, 1983) suggest that deformation is not uniform through the whole thickness of articular cartilage.

These unusual features, together with the complex multiphase structure, have made it difficult for engineers to describe the material properties of cartilage. The complexity of theory required increases rapidly with the degree of precision with which cartilage is to be modelled. To assess the short-term behaviour of a large bulk of cartilage it is possible to visualise it as a simple elastic material. However, for more exact analysis, taking into account the different structure of cartilage at various depths, the flow of fluid through the matrix and other features, the concept of a fluid-filled porous, elastic material has recently gained favour.

Immobilisation results in degenerative changes in chondrocytes in the superficial (I) and mid (II and III) zones of articular cartilage, in parts that are not in contact during immobility. The changes advance with time. Chondrocyte necrosis, matrix loosening and the fragmentation of collagen in the superficial zones are found also in cartilage from areas that have been in contact with an opposing surface at the time of immobilisation. These changes, however, are much more severe, a result that suggests the importance for the survival of the superficial cartilage of diffusion of metabolites from the synovial fluid. A high, normal content of proteoglycan is necessary for the load-bearing requirements of joints: the consequent low hydraulic permeability and high swelling pressure limit the amount of fluid lost when cartilage is loaded normally in compression (Maroudas, 1976). Distortions of these relationships seem inevitable when immobilisation is combined with contact. Studies of proteoglycan change reveal little alteration in the quality or quantity of this molecular species when dog stifle joints are immobilised without compression, but a rapid deterioration and proteoglycan loss when the joint is used, and loaded, immediately after the period of immobility. If, by contrast, a period of 3–4 weeks recovery is permitted between the end of immobilisation and the beginning of use, no such deterioration is observed (Palmoski et al, 1979; Palmoski & Brandt, 1982).

Immunity to cartilage

In diseases such as rheumatoid arthritis and relapsing polychondritis in which cartilage is degraded there are humoral antibodies against components such as collagen (Greenbury & Skingle, 1979). The formation of anti-proteoglycan antibodies is not infrequent (Poole et al, 1981). It is uncertain whether this autoimmunity is associated with the pathogenesis of the disease. It is also unclear whether the articular lesions in rat anti-type II collagen arthritis (p. 478) are the result of immunity to autologous type II collagen or to cross-reactions between homologous or heterologous and autologous collagen.

Cartilage transplantation

Not only are the macromolecular components of cartilage matrix immunogenic but so also are the chondrocytes, an observation accounting for the rejection of a high proportion of allografts. Cells transplanted into athymic nu/nu (nude) mice are accepted however and form hyaline cartilaginous nodules (Lipman et al, 1983). Devitalized xenografts have been used to investigate graft reabsorption (Ksiazek & Thyberg, 1983). The role of living chondrocytes is not required and reabsorption is by macrophages. Because of the difficulties in enabling slices or blocks of cartilage to survive after grafting, half or whole joints have been transplanted with microvascular surgical anastomosis (Hurwitz, 1979). Whole joints survive well, are indistinguishable from normal joints, are demonstrably viable and display only slight limitation of movement.

Cartilage slices and blocks in organ culture have been used as explants to examine the beneficial influence on cartilage of agents such as hydrocortisone (Tyler et al, 1982). The maintenance of whole explanted chick embryo limb bones was the basis of similar earlier experiments (Fell, 1981) but it remained uncertain whether the results were applicable to adult tissues. Hydrocortisone prevents the breakdown of cartilage caused by synovial tissue in organ culture, by an inhibitory action on the production both of catabolin and of degradative enzymes, but not through an effect on chondrocytes.

Cartilage thickness.
Articular cartilage varies greatly in thickness in different species, in different joints and in different parts of the same joint (Fig. 7.12). Until recently, very few systematic measurements had been made of human cartilage thickness or volume. In canine and bovine joints cartilage thickness is inversely proportional to the congruence of the joints (Simon et al, 1973), i.e. the small areas, perhaps 1.5 cm^2 that are load-bearing at any

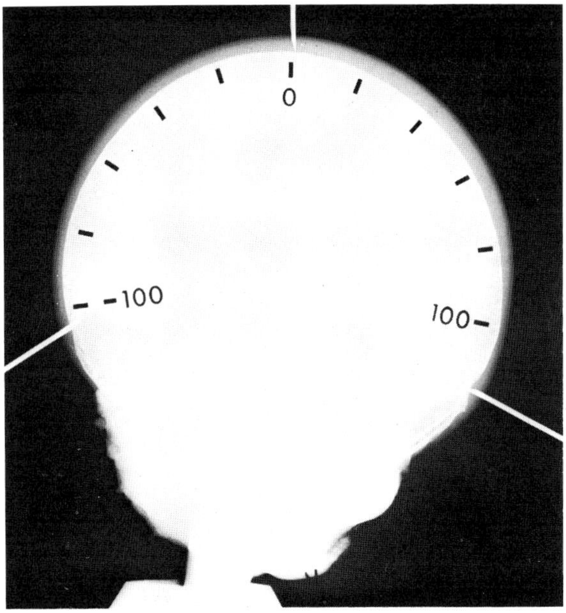

Fig. 7.12 Human femoral head cartilage. Radiograph, in lateromedial plane, of normal femoral head. The circumference of the head is marked in degrees (0 = zenith): the thickest zone of articular cartilage is anterior to the zenith. (From Armstrong & Gardner (1977) Annals of the Rheumatic Diseases 36: 407–412.)

time on the average adult human lateral femoral and tibial condyles, represent parts of very thick cartilage. The much larger cartilage area under load in the average adult human ankle joint corresponds to cartilage that is much thinner.

It has been suggested that the cartilage of large, load-bearing joints becomes thinner with age (Barnett et al, 1961). There is certainly considerable variability in the thickness of adult femoral condylar cartilage. Walker & Hajek (1972) recorded values ranging from 1.8–2.3 mm. However Meachim (1971) measured the mean thickness of human humeral cartilage in paraffin tissue sections and found no decrease with advancing age, a result that conformed with the observations made by Simon (1970, 1971) on patellar cartilage. More sophisticated methods of observation were adopted by Armstrong & Gardner (1977). Measurements made at 20° intervals around the circumference of defined planes of human femoral head cartilage showed clearly that the thickness of hyaline cartilage increased from minimum values at the synoviochondral junctions to a maximum value 20° anterior to the zenith (Fig. 7.12). Furthermore, the thickness of the thickest parts of the cartilage increased significantly within the age range 20–50 years. It appeared, therefore, that femoral head cartilage was distributed asymmetrically and that, with age, the thickness *increased* differentially.

Age changes (Gardner & O'Connor, 1985)
As age advances, articular cartilage displays a large range of alterations in colour, thickness, chemical composition and mechanical properties.

Young cartilage has a delicate blue translucence; aged cartilage becomes yellow and opaque. The yellow colour is asociated with a non-collagenous protein fraction but the chemical identity of the pigment, which is an acidic glycoprotein, is not wholly clear. Haemoglobin (M.W. 6.8 × 10^4 daltons) can penetrate cartilage but the pigment of ageing cartilage is unrelated to the iron-containing pigments of haemophilia and haemochromatosis which aggregate in cartilage matrix without significantly colouring it. There is no apparent relationship to ochronotic pigment. The possibility that the yellow pigment of ageing cartilage is a carotenoid has been raised (Meachim & Stockwell, 1979) only to be discounted.

With advancing age, there is a decrease in cartilage water (Venn & Maroudas, 1977; Venn, (1978). The quantity of proteoglycan changes little (Bayliss et al, 1983). The aggregatability of protein with hyaluronate is preserved but smaller proteoglycan monomers come to form a larger fraction of the total. In deep, zone IV cartilage there is an increasing proportion of keratan sulphate. Collagen cross-links increase in number and strength; with maturation, reducible cross-links gradually disappear and those that increase are of a stable, non-reducible kind (Schofield & Weightman, 1978).

Cartilage metabolic activity declines with age but this reflects a diminishing cellularity (Stockwell, 1979). The diminution in cell density selectively affects superficial zones, for example, of the humeral head and femoral condyle. There is a parallel increase in the total quantity of cartilage on a single bearing surface. Thickness increases on the femoral head between the ages of 20 and 50 years (Armstrong & Gardner, 1977) and humeral (Meachim, 1971) and patellar (Simon, 1971) cartilage thicknesses do not decline. These observations are not easy to reconcile with the observed falls in cell density unless it be supposed that there is an increase in the amount of matrix relative to the cell population. This supposition, in turn, is not easily related to observed decrements in water content.

There are corresponding alterations with age in cartilage mechanics. Tensile stiffness, fracture strength and fatigue resistance deteriorate (Kempson, 1979). Deformability in compression under peak loads increases greatly (Armstrong et al, 1979), an observation confirmed in tests on whole hip joints (Armstrong et al, 1979, 1980). The possibility arises that the large deformations caused in aged limb cartilage in response to normal loads establish a vicious circle predisposing to fibrillation (Ch. 33).

With advancing age, the frequency of the ~ 30 μm surface features of cartilage (p. 235) decreases. Since these features are now believed to be the superficial manifestation, at unloaded surfaces, of zone I chondrocytes (Middleton et al, 1984), this change is apparently a representation of the reduced cell density measured by Stockwell (1979). The ~ 30 μm features become wider and higher, a possible indication of the increased size of chondrocyte lacunae.

Particular attention has been directed to the marginal, *transitional zone* that comprises the circumferential boundary of the articular cartilage of diarthrodial joints (Thompson & Stockwell, 1983). At this site, cartilage, periosteum, synovial tissue and the fibrous capsule merge; inflammatory articular diseases begin here. The boundary is abrupt, the sudden transition attributable to the arrangement and amount of collagen and cells; the change in cell structure is gradual. There is an oblique edge-belt of collagen and here, the chondrocytes resemble those of the midzone (Zone III of Gardner, 1984). There are apparently no mast cells. The majority of the fibrils of the marginal synovium of the rabbit knee run around the perimeter of the cartilage and only a few bundles are radial. This is not necessarily true of human joints and in the synovial apophyseal joints, for example, the radial component is a large one.

The '*tidemark*' or 'tideline', delineating the non-mineralised hyaline articular cartilage of diarthrodial joints from the calcified cartilage, is a calcification front (Bullough & Jagannath, 1983). The line or lines stain with phloxine-tartrazine. Lipid in the form of calcium phospholipid complexes is present and there is both alkaline phosphatase and ATPase activity. A significant change occurs in the matrix proteoglycan at the tidemark. The nature of the regulating processes that take place in this site is still not wholly understood but specific cellular activity is proposed (Bullough & Jagannath, 1983) and transmission electron microscopy and scanning electron microscopy evidence suggests an active process (Redler et al, 1975), under cell control, related to the presence of extracellular membrane-bound matrix vesicles (p. 229).

Even less is known of the *osteochondral junction*. The cartilage and bone are bridged by the intermingling of unravelled collagen fibrils heavily laden with mineral crystallites (Hough et al, 1974). The loose texture and random arrangement of the collagen fibrils in the human osteochondral junction is believed by these authors to be responsible for the lack of birefringence. In young children and in animals where endochondral ossification is continuous, the junction contains little collagen.

Bone

By custom, bone has received less attention in texts on rheumatology than have the non-mineralised connective tissues. However, bone constitutes a large and important part of the supporting tissues and the literature attests to recent progress in understanding of skeletal structure and function (Vaughan, 1981). The mineralised skeleton provides support against gravity; protection for the viscera; the means by which muscular work is transmitted; and an important dynamic reservoir for water, electrolytes, calcium, phosphorus and protein.

Where tendons, muscles or periodontal membranes are attached to bone, thick collagen bundles, Sharpeys' fibres, extend into the bone to anchor these structures securely. Ligaments are attached at entheses. Bones conceal and accommodate the haemopoietic tissues and act as selective repositories for elements such as strontium but as less selective sites for lead, radium and plutonium.

The cells of bone, osteoblasts, osteocytes and osteoclasts, are considered on page 205. The matrix, osteoid, is formed of collagen, osteocalcin and proteoglycan. Bone collagen is often termed 'osteocollagen', a name that recalls the characteristic amino acid structure of bone collagen peptides. The ground substance of bone is similar but not identical to that of the other connective tissues (Engfeldlt & Hjerpe, 1976). The quantity and integrity of osteoid determine normal mineralisation, a process catalysed by the alkaline phosphatase of osteoblasts.

Mature bone is of two forms. The shaft of the femur, for example, is formed of *compact* bone which is analogous in engineering terms with the wall of a metal tube: it is of relatively low metabolic activity. By contrast, the interstices of the femur are occupied by delicate, ramifying struts of buttress-like bone processes constituting a honeycomb-like framework in which there is high metabolic activity. This open *cancellous* bone (Fig. 7.13) is arranged geometrically in a manner appropriate to the lines of stress that pass through each bone under load (Thompson, 1961).

The unit of structure of compact bone, the *osteon*, is formed by the laying down of 20–40 layers (lamellae) of type I (osteo) collagen around a vascular channel. The cylindrical unit formed in this way is a haversian system. These systems lie close together, the small spaces beween them filled by interstitial lamellae. The inner surfaces are lined by the osteoblasts of the endosteum, the outer surfaces by those of the periosteum. Both categories are osteogenic.

Cancellous bone does not have an osteonal configuration but is arranged as trabecular bone packets (Lips et al, 1978), units of structure and function that are *bone remodelling units* (*BRU*). The mean formation time of a unit is approximately 70 days. Because of the concentration of metabolic change at the surfaces of these units, cancellous bone is exquisitely susceptible to change in most metabolic bone diseases and provides early indications of such disorders.

Both compact and cancellous bone are often said to be *lamellar* because of the orderly laminae of mineralised matrix. This is in distinction to *woven bone* seen only in embryonic development, at sites of fracture repair and in disorders such as fibrous dysplasia.

Bone formation may be *direct*, as in the formation of the skull; or *indirect*, when as in the growth of long bones, a cartilaginous model is first produced only to be continuously and insidiously replaced by bone. Direct bone formation is said to be intramembranous, indirect to be endochondral. Both require critical amounts of calcium and of vitamin D; and both require the normal activity of the parathyroid gland and of the calcitonin-secreting C cells of the thyroid.

Bone is continually undergoing remodelling in a co-ordinated sequence in which osteoclasts are activated, bone matrix and mineral resorbed, osteoblasts activated and new matrix formed and subsequently mineralised (Ellis, 1981). Bone turnover rate depends on the birth rate of BRUs; resorption and formation are finely balanced so that a constant total skeletal mass is maintained. The normal rate of appositional laying down of osteoid is about 1 μm per day (Ellis, 1981).

It is commonly claimed that the mineral of bone (Table 7.3) is calcium hydroxyapatite

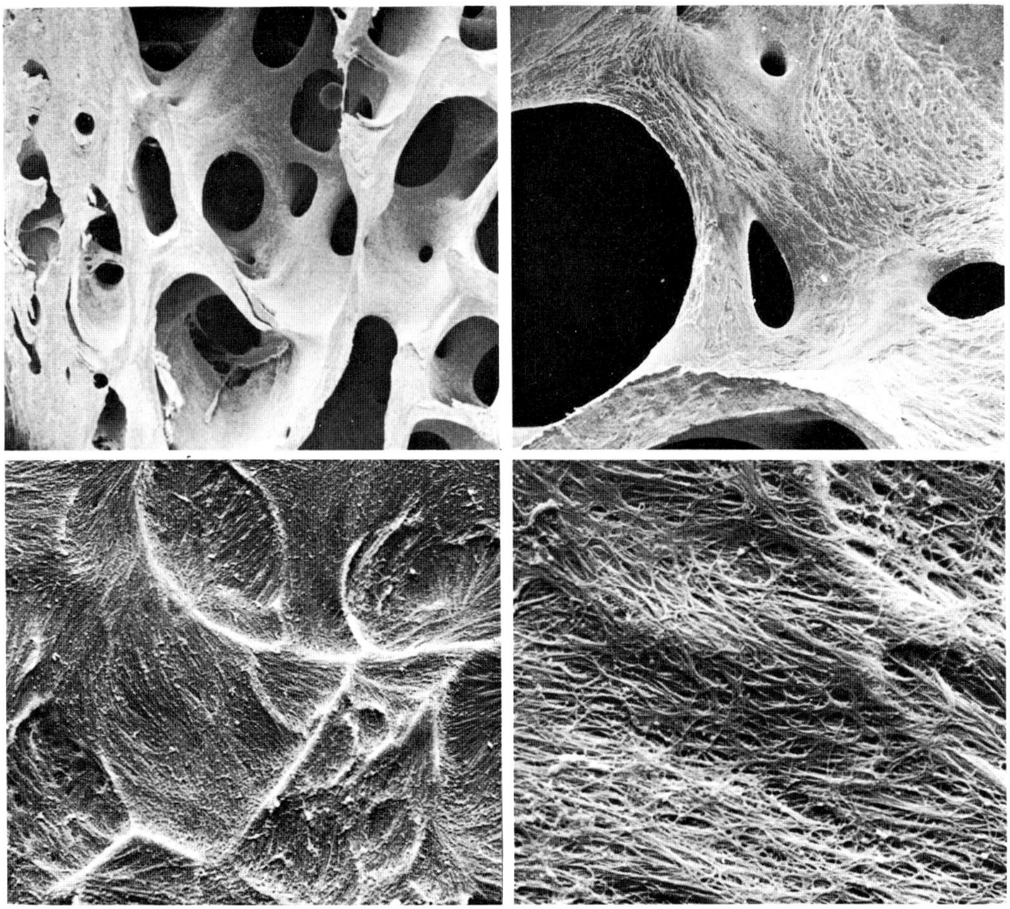

Fig. 7.13 Human iliac crest bone. (Top left) dense cortical bone at left margin, with cancellous medullary bone. Note (top right) higher power view of bone trabeculae from which haemopoietic tissue has been removed. Broad crescent-shaped zones of trabecular margin shown (bottom left) with collagen fibre bundles of same zone at higher magnification (bottom right). Scanning EM (Top left) ×20. (Top right) ×60. (Bottom left) ×600. (Bottom right) ×3000.

Table 7.3 Crystals deposited in human articular cartilage (from Dieppe et al, 1976)

Crystal	Phosphorus/calcium ratio
Calcium hydroxyapatite $CA_5\ OH(PO_4)_3.\ H_2O$	0.46
Calcium pyrophosphate $CA_2P_2O_7.\ 2H_2O$	0.77
Calcium orthophosphate $Ca\ HPO_4.\ 2H_2O$	0.77

Strictly, hydroxyapatite is $Ca_{10}\ (PO_4)_6(OH)_2$. However, there is lack of precision in bone terminology due to incomplete understanding of bone structure. $Ca_2OH(PO_4)_3H_2O$ is correctly termed 'calcium hydroxyapatite'.

$$(Ca_{10}\ (PO_4)_6\ (OH)_2)$$

However, it is probable that the crystalline deposit laid down through the action of chondrocytes in endochondral ossification, or of osteoblasts in direct ossification, is calcium hydroxylapatite ($Ca_5\ OH(PO_4)_3H_2O$).

The mechanisms of mineralisation and the fine structure of the matrix during this process are disputed. One view suggests that apatite crystals are deposited first in relation to a part of the orderly periodic structure of the bone collagen fibril, perhaps that part where proteoglycan is commonly bound (Boskey, 1981). Another view stresses the importance of randomly scattered, minute vesicle-like structures in the 'matrix': these vesicles can be recognised by electron microscopy (Anderson, 1980).

Vitamin D is essential for the absorption and use of calcium in bone mineralisation, and for the regulation of renal tubular phosphate loss. Vitamin D_3, cholecalciferol, is synthesised in the skin from 7-dehydrocholesterol under the influence of ultraviolet light; alternatively, it can be provided in the diet. It is now clear that many of the most important actions of vitamin D_3 are exercised not by cholecalciferol itself but by a metabolic product 1, 25-dihydrocholecalciferol (1, 25-DHCC) that is formed in the kidney from an intermediary 25-hydroxycholecaliciferol (25-HCC). 25-HCC is synthesised from cholecalciferol by the liver. 1, 25-DHCC has many of the properties of a hormone; in the gut, it leads to the production of a calcium-binding protein. Both 25-HCC and 1, 25-DHCC can directly influence calcium absorption and bone utilisation.

Parathormone is a polypeptide containing approximately 80 amino acids in a single chain. It can be assayed by immunological and bioassay techniques to facilitate the diagnosis of hypercalcaemia and of parathyroid adenoma. The hormone, like 1, 25-DHCC, acts on gut, kidney and bone. In addition to increasing intestinal phosphate absorption and reducing urinary excretion, parathormone increases osteoclastic bone reabsorption and the liberation of mineral. The relationship of the actions of parathormone to those of 1, 25-DHCC is by no means clear. However, parathormone can lead to a movement of calcium into cells: calcium may act as a 'second messenger' of parathormone.

The C- (parafollicular) cell of the thyroid, a member of the APUD series, secretes a 32- amino acid polypeptide, *calcitonin*, that acts on bone directly to inhibit osteoclastic reabsorption. When bone turnover is rapid, as in young persons, hypocalcaemia results: a lowering of blood calcium is not seen in the adult in spite of the direct effect on bone. Two main actions appear likely therefore: first, to oppose the influence of parathormone on bone so that when calcium is deficient, parathormone-induced bone loss is minimised while the other actions of parathormone continue; and second, and most important, the control of variations in blood calcium level that are likely when there is active bony reabsorption.

JOINTS

The review of the biology of joints by Davies (1969) is of lasting value. The upright posture and bipedal gait of man present unique problems in biomechanical terms. *Homo sapiens* and his ancestors, including *Australopithecus*, display skeletal and articular differences that distinguish them sharply from the apes and monkeys. For example, the human femoral neck is unusually long. This, it is suggested, helps to ensure stability for the very wide pelvic girdle that is the evolutionary corollary of the large human brain and cranium.

Muscular contractions, transmitted through ligaments and tendons, act upon bone to effect movements that are facilitated by the joints. Two fundamental joint types are recognised; those where there is both a cavity and free movement, the *synovial joints* (diarthroses) — and those without a cavity, the *synarthroses*. Synarthroses may be fibrous (syndesmoses), cartilaginous (synchondroses), or bony (synostoses). Where the bones are capped by hyaline cartilage and united by fibrocartilage and fibrous tissue, the term '*symphysis*' is applied to describe the unusually strong joint.

Synovial joints

Structure and classification

It is convenient to classify the synovial joints (Figs. 7.14 & 7.15) according to the shape of the articular surface(s) (Table 7.4).

Joints that permit movement in one plane only (*uniaxial*) include hinge (transverse axis) and trochoid (pivot) joints (longitudinal axis). In condylar joints movement is mainly around one axis but limited movement around a second axis is possible. Thus, a pair of convex knuckle-shaped condyles articulate with a pair of correspondingly concave condyles. When movement is allowed in two mutually perpendicular axes the joint is said to be *biaxial*. In ellipsoid joints, surfaces are oval, the opposite surfaces convex and concave. Flexion/extension and abduction/adduction move-

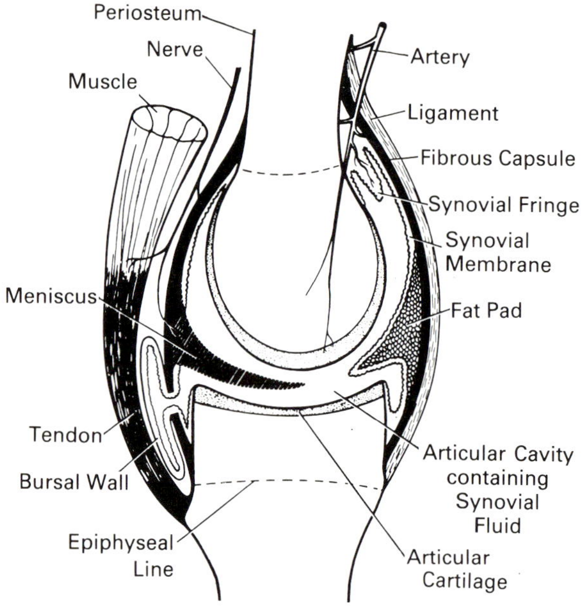

Fig. 7.14 Synovial joint. Diagram of knee joint structure. (Redrawn from Barnett et al (1961) Synovial joints: their structure and mechanics.

ments are possible, as at the wrist, but not rotation. In sellar (saddle) joints, such as the carpometacarpal joint of the thumb, rotary movement is permitted but only when flexion/extension or abduction/adduction occur. The rotary movement is said to be 'conjoint'.

The size of the diarthrodial joints varies greatly between different mammalian species and within a single species. There are analogous differences between the loads sustained by a particular joint so that, in one series, loads were greatest in the largest animal, the cow, smallest in the mouse (Simon, 1970). The proportion of a human articular cartilage surface in contact with the mating surface varies widely between joints, being greatest in the congruent ankle, least in the ball-and-socket hip. Nevertheless, the *proportion* is approximately the same among species that vary greatly in size.

The thickness of a lower limb articular cartilage is directly related to body weight, area of the tibial plateau and hip-to-shoulder length. The 'law of simple allometry' relates the growth of part of an organism to that of the whole, and the thickness and surface area of articular cartilages are 'scaled'

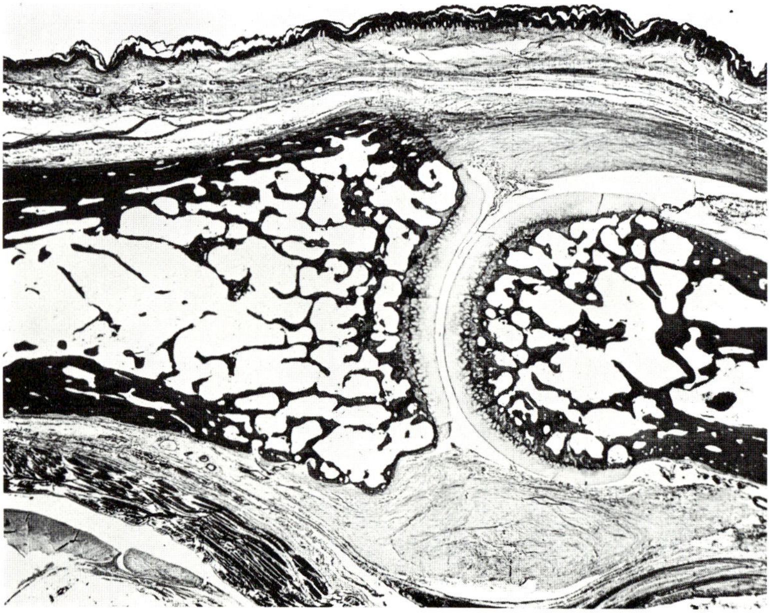

Fig. 7.15 Synovial joint. Compare with Figure 7.14. Human interphalangeal joint cut in longitudinal section after decalcification. Space separating hyaline articular cartilage surfaces is artefactually large due to separation of material during, or after, sectioning. H&E ×10.

Table 7.4 Classification of synovial joints

Shape	Anatomical description	Degrees of freedom to rotate	Example
Planar	Articular surfaces flat or only slightly curved	2	Carpometacarpal
Spherical	Ball-and-socket	3	Hip
Ellipsoidal (cotylic)	Modified spheroidal: articulating surface longer in one direction	2	Metacarpophalangeal
Hinge (ginglymus)	Hinge shape permits flexion and extension	1	Humeroulnar
Condylar (bicondylar)	Complex hinge, articulating on two distinct surfaces (condyles)	2	Knee
Trochoid	A pivot within a ring	1	Radioulnar
Sellar	Saddle-shaped: one surface convex in longest articulating distance, the other concave	2	Trapezium — first metacarpal

from small to large animals in accordance with this principle (Simon, 1970). By contrast, the compressive stresses on the cartilage of a particular joint are within one order of magnitude when small and large species are compared: the stresses are not related to the thickness of the cartilage. The limb structures, Simon believes, are 'optimally designed' to maintain low static pressures on the articular surfaces.

The most mobile synovial joints are *multiaxial*; the hip and the shoulder exemplify this structure. Both are ball-and-socket (spheroidal) joints: they permit flexion/extension, abduction/adduction, and rotation.

In a further category of *plane* joints, only limited gliding without angular movement is possible. There are groups of plane joints in the carpus and tarsus and between the vertebral arches. In such groups, the integrated influence of all the plane joints may permit arching and some twisting in the long axis in spite of the limited movement at individual articulations.

Joint movements are of four main varieties which may combine to give infinitely variable movements. The varieties are: gliding; angular movement; circumduction; and rotation. Angular movements are of two kinds: flexion/extension; and abduction/adduction. Circumduction is said to occur when a long bone circumscribes a conical space. The apex is the articulation, the base of the cone the course followed by the distal end of the bone (Harris, 1974; Warwick & Williams, 1980).

The science of kinesiology, a branch of biomechanics, has led to geometric studies of articular movement (MacConaill & Basmajian, 1969). One advantage of this work has been the adoption of a concept of the mechanical axis, a hypothetical line passing through the bone ends perpendicular to the centre of the articular surface. The relationship of this axis to movement at the articular surface is self-evident when a symmetrical long bone is considered. When, however, the head of the bone is offset, as in the case of the femur, complex limb movements can be predicted and analysed when they result from quite simple axial movements such as rotation.

When joint positions are analysed it is evident that any given pair of opposing ovoid articular surfaces only fit perfectly in one position of the joint. Full congruence is reached when the joint achieves the extreme of one of the most habitual movements. In the knee, this state is achieved at full extension. In this position, the tensions within capsule and ligaments are greatest; a final, spiral twist through conjunct rotation imposes a maximum congruence and maximum compression in a 'screwed home', *close-packed* position. In all other positions of the joint, the surfaces are not congruent and the joint is said to be *loose-packed*. In these latter positions, externally applied distractive forces can achieve separation of the articular surfaces: this is not possible when the joint is close-packed. Close-packed, the opposing bones are locked together as though there was no joint between them. In this position the articular structures are especially susceptible to traumatic injury.

Davies (1969) commends the view, advanced by Barnett et al (1961) that there are only two fundamental types of synovial joint, the ovoid and the saddle-shaped. All parts of both 'male' and 'female' surfaces are respectively convex and concave; in the saddle-shaped joints some parts of both surfaces are concave, others convex. In no human joint is there absolute geometrical regularity; *nor are there any true plane articular surfaces.* All are to some extent curved and in all gliding is inevitably accompanied by some rotation. Davies (1969) draws an interesting analogy between the human ankle joint where abduction/adduction are prevented by the malleolar projections, and the temporomandibular joints, where a comparable limitation is effected by the united movement of the two joints.

Synovial tissue

Synovial tissue (Figs. 7.16, 7.17) may be fatty, fibrofatty (areolar) or fibrous. The collagens are of type I and III (Eyre & Muir, 1975). The dual layer of synovial cells forms the surface of fatty and areolar synovia where they cover adipose and loose connective tissue respectively. Over fibrous and periosteal tissues, the synoviocytes are attenuated, forming a single layer of squamous character. At articular margins, where the synovial and cartilaginous tissues merge in the transitional zone, the synovial cells become flattened over the periarticular vascular fringe, ultimately disappearing in a circumferential rim where vessels loop back towards the periphery and where cartilage first becomes hyaline. Synovial tissue is often thrown into folds that provide a large absorptive and secretory surface. Villous processes are encountered particularly in articular recesses. Synovia cover tendon sheaths and constitute the lining of many bursae.

The large synovial surface (Fig. 7.18), where fibronectin is demonstrable (Linck et al, 1983), is seen *en face* as a series of packed hexagonal arrays; it is partly formed of type A(M) macrophage-like phagocytic cells and partly of type B(F) fibroblast-like synovial cells.

Most synovial tissues have a rich capillary bed, located superficially and well-placed to facilitate exchange processes (Knight & Levick, 1983). The capillary density is uneven however, ranging from 67–83 × 10^3 capillaries/cm^2 section over alveolar or adipose tissue to 2 × 10^2 capillaries/cm^2 section over tendon.

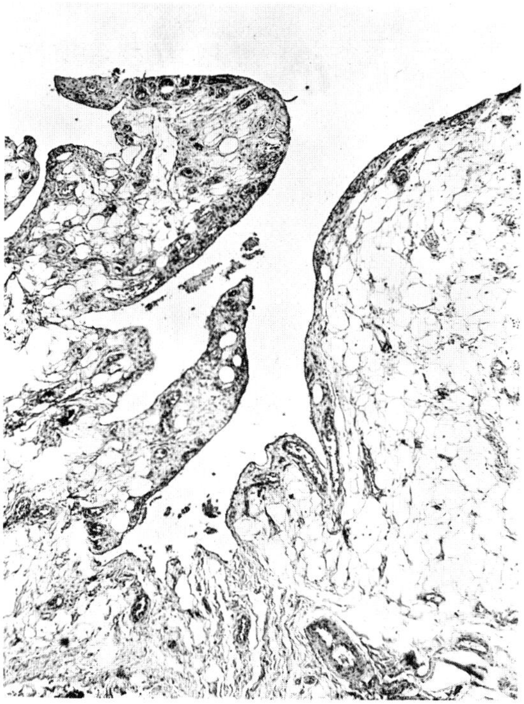

Fig. 7.16 Synovial villi. Margins of areolar (fibrofatty) synovial tissue seen at low magnification. Note numerous blood vessels some of which are well displayed lower right. H&E ×44. (From Gardner D L (1965) Pathology of the connective tissue diseases. Edward Arnold, London, Longmans Green.)

There is no basement membrane material beneath the 2–3 cell layer of synovial cells that comprises the synovial surface (Fig. 7.19). This structural feature demonstrates that synovial surfaces are not precisely analogous with epithelial membranes and suggests that the passage of fluid, metabolites and other molecules may not be regulated in the same way as they are, for example, in the glomerular tuft. It can be misleading, in connective tissue disease, to look for synovial disturbances therefore that precisely replicate those seen at epithelial surfaces. Synovial villi do not form simply by outgrowth (Edwards, 1982; Edwards et al, 1983): splitting and fusion are also observed.

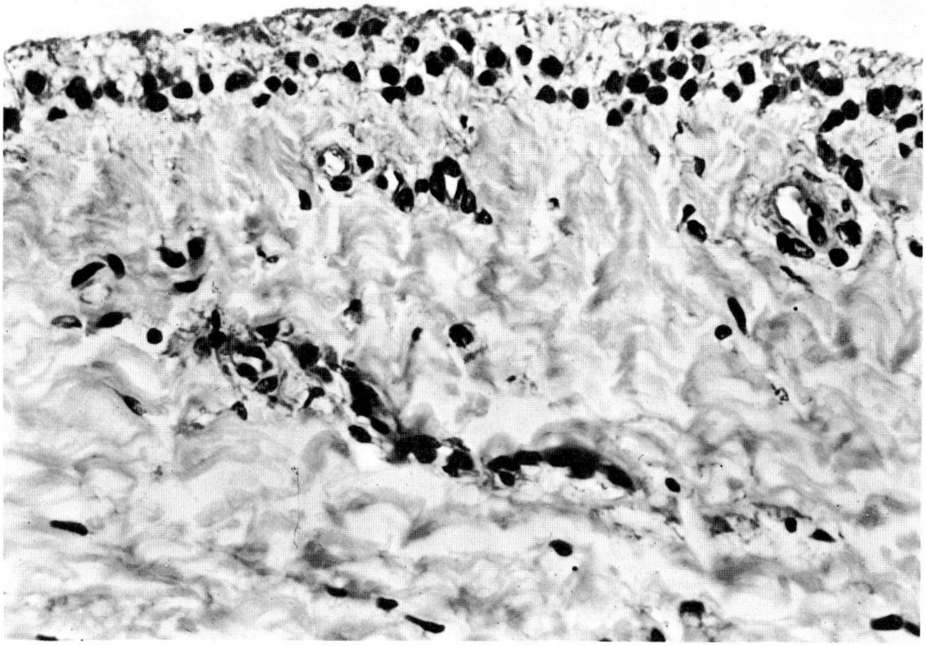

Fig. 7.17 Synovial surface. Two-three cell layer of synovial cells (top) forms surface communicating with joint cavity. Among the extensive collagen bundles (grey) beneath surface, note transected and diagonally dispersed small blood vessels. H&E × 80. (From Gardner D L (1965) Pathology of the connective tissue diseases. Edward Arnold, London, Longmans Green.)

The effects of synovium on cartilage-catabolin (Fell, 1981)

When synovial tissue particles in culture are placed *in contact with* either living or frozen-thawed, dead cartilage, the synovium causes severe breakdown of proteoglycan in both living and dead cartilage explants but much more breakdown of collagen in the living cartilage. When living and dead cartilage are placed in the same culture chamber as living synovial tissue, *but not in contact with it*, there is

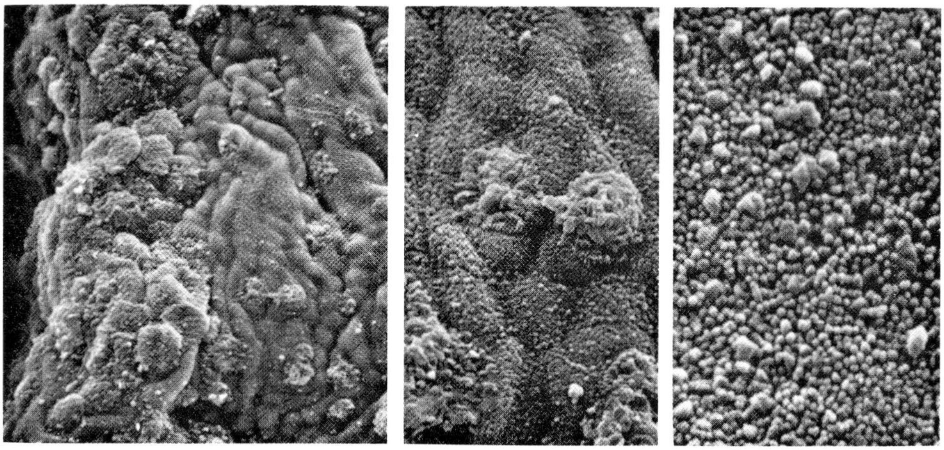

Fig. 7.18 Synovial surface. 3-D structure of synovial surface. SEM (left) ×40. (Centre) ×100. (Right) ×250. (From Gardner & Dodds (1976) Human histology. Churchill Livingstone, Edinburgh.

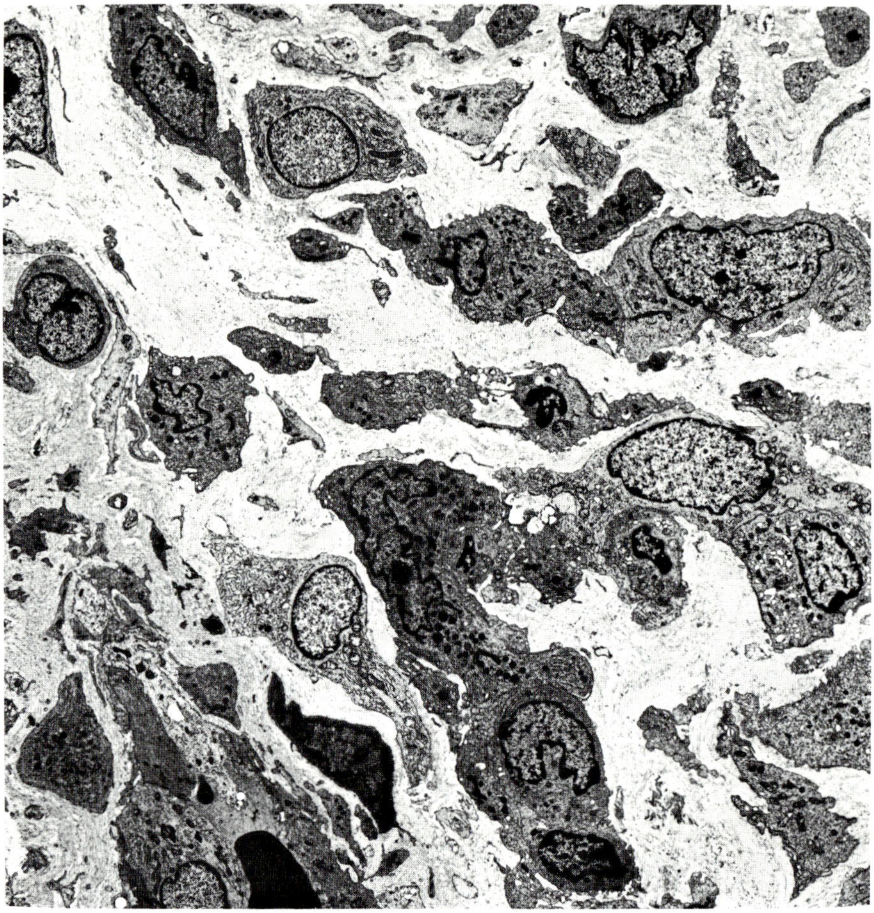

Fig. 7.19 Synovial tissue. Beneath the synovial surface, fibroblasts and macrophages lie among intercellular collagen bundles and nonfibrillar, pale-appearing ground substance. EM ×1720.

severe depletion of both proteoglycan and collagen from the living cartilage but not from the dead material. Fell & Jubb (1977a, b) deduced that living synovial tissue could exert two effects on cartilage, both of the greatest possible interest in attempts to understand the mechanisms of cartilage disease. First, there is a direct, enzymatic action on the matrix of either living or dead cartilage with which the synovium is in contact; second, there is an indirect action, mediated via living chondrocytes, for which contact is not necessary and which is without effect on cartilage in which chondrocytes are dead (Jubb & Fell, 1980). It is now evident that mononuclear macrophages stimulated with lectins also cause cartilage reabsorption in the same way.

The active agent from pig synovium was shown to be a small acidic protein of approximately 20 000 M.W. termed 'catabolin' (Saklatvala, 1981; Saklatvala & Sarsfield, 1982; Saklatvala et al, 1983). More recently, a similar protein capable of inducing cartilage resorption, has been demonstrated in human synovium and human mononuclear leucocytes (Saklatavala et al, 1983). The catabolin from pig leucocytes has been purified (Sakatvala et al, 1983) and can cause proteoglycan release from cultured bovine nasal cartilage at 20 pM. The protein is now thought to be identical with interleukin 1; however, there are similarities of action and present evidence suggests that the synovial cells responsible for the synthesis of catabolin/interleukin include the fibroblast-like B(F) cells (Pilsworth & Saklatvala, 1983).

Articular surfaces

Load-bearing and movement at synovial joints are facilitated by the juxtaposition of two or more surfaces covered, sometimes incompletely, by hyaline (glass-like) cartilage (Fig. 7.9). At arthrotomy or arthroscopy, living cartilage appears remarkably smooth and shining, appearances noted by William Hunter (1742–1743). When the thin, tenuous 30 nm film of viscous synovial fluid is washed from a disarticulated normal cartilage surface, the smoothness of the non-loaded cartilage is immediately seen to be artefactual: coarse 0.4–0.5 mm irregularities can be detected with a hand lens or dissecting microscope, finer orders of irregularity with an incident light compound microscope, with an interference microscope or by replication.

The delicate blue-white colour of normal young hyaline articular cartilage is modified near the margins of thin cartilage surfaces by the dark red-purple colour of the underlying blood vessels of the bone. When the objective of an incident light microscope is immersed in a drop of fluid placed on the surface of the cartilage, the vessels of the metaphysis can be visualised with ease if the fluid has a refractive index similar to that of the cartilage itself (i.e. 1.4). 1% polyvinylpyrrolidone is suitable for this purpose: its viscous nature recalls the physical properties of synovial fluid.

Hunter (1742–1743) believed that the articular cartilage of diarthrodial joints was vascular but it was quickly shown that hyaline articular cartilages have neither blood vascular nor nerve supplies and that there are no lymphatic communications. He also believed that hyaline articular cartilage was normally covered by a synovial membrane but this was satisfactorily disproved by Leidy (1849). Hunter described the surface of cartilage as strikingly smooth as indeed it appears when a freshly opened joint, with a thin, tenacious layer of viscous synovial fluid, is viewed *postmortem* or at biopsy. The apparent and conspicuous smoothness was emphasised by Davies (1969) although, by 1968, the reality of this appearance had been questioned (Dowson et al, 1968; Gardner & Woodward, 1968, 1969; McCall, 1968; Inoue et al, 1969). Incident light studies of fresh, unfixed and of living cartilage in a joint with an intact, normal vascular circulation then showed that the whole articular surface was covered by numerous, shallow, randomly dispersed 20–40 μm tertiary features ('undulations') (Fig. 7.20) interpreted variously as hollows when dry or as prominences when hy-

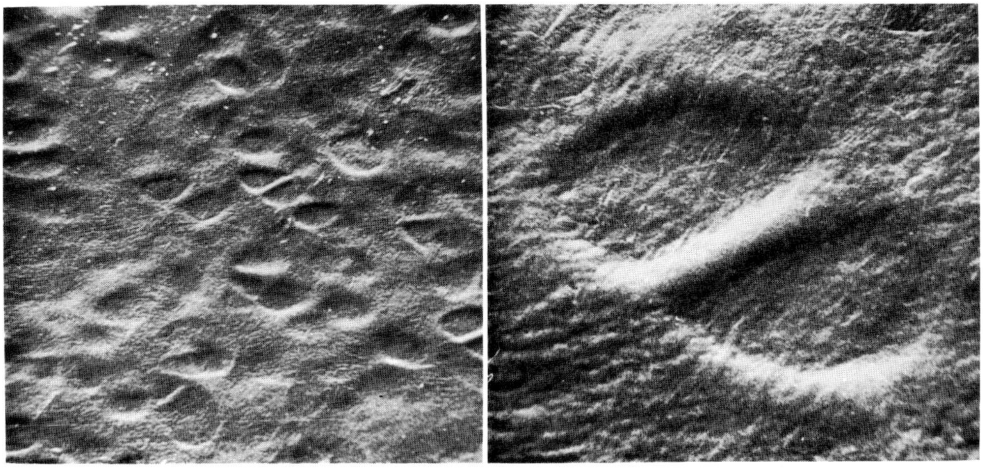

Fig. 7.20 Articular cartilage surface. (Left) part of the lateral femoral condyle of abnormal 25-year-old male. Observe clusters of surface hollows that correspond to superficial chondrocyte lacunae. (Right) higher power of surface above one 'figure-of-eight' lacuna that probably contains two chondrocytes. Glutaraldehyde, ethanol dehydration, propylene oxide, vacuum dried. SEM (left) ×160. (Right) ×1050.

drated. The presence of these hollows was confirmed by the scanning electron microscopy of fixed, dehydrated cartilage material whether or not the cartilage blocks remained on or were detached from underlying bone although they could not be recognised by transmission electron microscopy (Fig. 7.21). The hollows were superimposed on the 0.4–0.5 mm diameter features seen with a hand lens and were thought to correspond to the situation of the most superficial chondrocytes (Clarke, 1972, 1973) (Tables 7.5, 7.6). This view was later confirmed by X-ray micro-analytical studies in which comparisons were made between the elemental composition of the tissue immediately deep to the surface features and that of midzone chondrocytes prepared in perpendicular section of frozen (−190°) material (Middleton et al, 1984).

That these so called 'tertiary' features, whether identified as hollows or prominences, were not artefactual was strongly supported by the finding that they persisted on the non-loaded surface of exposed living human and animal cartilage (Gardner & McGillivray, 1971a, b; Gardner, 1972). It appeared possible that the hollows trapped and retained synovial fluid, boosting the lubrication mechanism at the articular surfaces (Walker et al 1968, 1969, 1970) but this view is now disputed.

The introduction of low temperature scanning electron microscopic techniques made it possible to compare the surface structure of unfixed, hydrated cartilage with that of blocks fixed and dehydrated before conventional scanning electron microscopy (Gardner et al, 1979; Gardner et al, 1981). Where hollows had been seen in dry material, gentle convex elevations were displayed (Fig. 7.22). The presence of these arrays of 20–40 m diameter surface features was not influenced by the separation of cartilage from bone during tissue preparation; the technique of preparing tissue on residual bone, rather than of detaching cartilage from bone during preparation, was repeatedly shown to avoid the introduction of the very fine, so-called 'quaternary irregularities' that Ghadially et al (1976) had

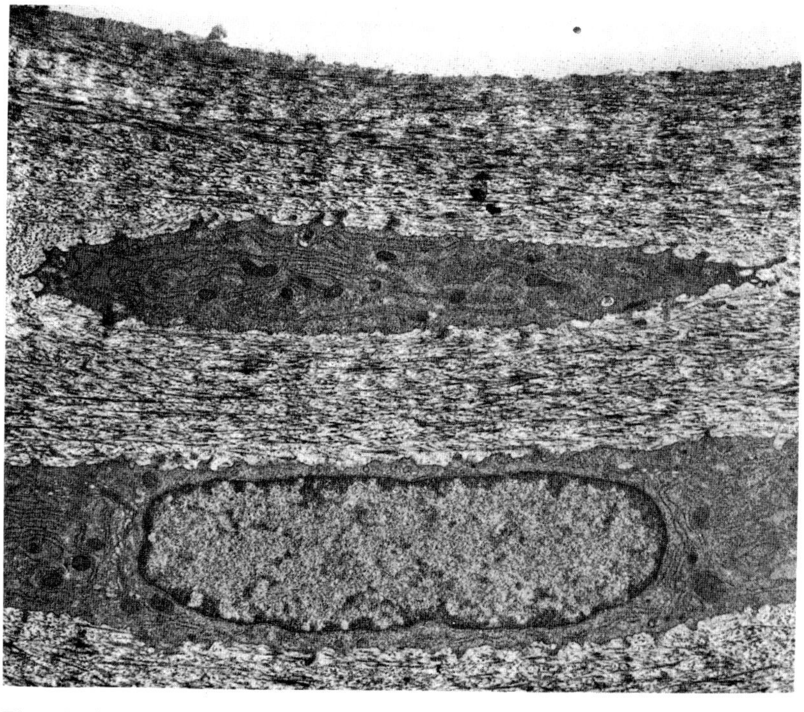

Fig. 7.21 Articular cartilage surface. Note fasicles of collagen at surface where they can be defected in longitudinal and in transverse section; and less orderly arrangement of collagen fibres below surface layer. Parts of two chondrocytes are seen. The more superficial cell is cut tangentially and the nucleus is not shown. TEM ×6300.

Table 7.5 Magnitude and frequency of *surface depressions* and *chondrocyte lacunae* on articular cartilage surfaces, measured by light- and by scanning electron microscopy (after Clarke, 1972)

Study	Subject	Area studied	Number of areas	Depression or lacunar diameter (μm)	Depression or lacunar frequencies (mm^{-2})	
					Range	Average
Reflected light microscopy	Adult human	Sectioned surface	11	13–60	191–366	287
Transmitted light microscopy	Adult human	Tangential section	22	10–71	295–725	427
	Immature human	Tangential section	5	7–25	647–1190	920
Scanning electron microscopy	Adult human	Sectioned surface	24	10–53	186–1007	611
		Articular surface	31	10–68	189–1070	588
			20–42 (*mean*)		488 (*mean*)	

Data from immature subjects excluded from mean values

Table 7.6 Comparison of *lacunar* frequencies obtained from tangential surface sections, with published data of *nuclear* frequency in radial sections from the superficial zone (after Clarke, 1972)

Report	Age range (years)	Site of specimen	Section	Cell or lacunar frequency (mm^{-3})
Meachim & Collins (1962)[a]	25–84	Upper end of humerus	Radial 0.22 mm deep	43 500–61 800
Stockwell (1967)	0–26 31–89	Lower end of humerus Lower end of humerus	Radial 0.22 mm deep Radial 0.22 mm deep	17 000–157 000 28 900–97 000 (*mean 62 000*)
Stockwell (1970)		Lower end of humerus	Radial 0.12 mm deep	(*mean 67 000*)
Clarke (1972)	0–2 32–76	Upper end of femur Upper end of femur	Tangential 10 m deep Tangential 10 mm deep	64–700–119 000 29 500–72 000

[a] Meachim G, Collins D H (1962) Annals of the Rheumatic Diseases 21: 45–50
[b] Stockwell R A (1967) Journal of Anatomy 101: 753–763
[c] Stockwell R A (1970) Personal communication to Clarke (1972)

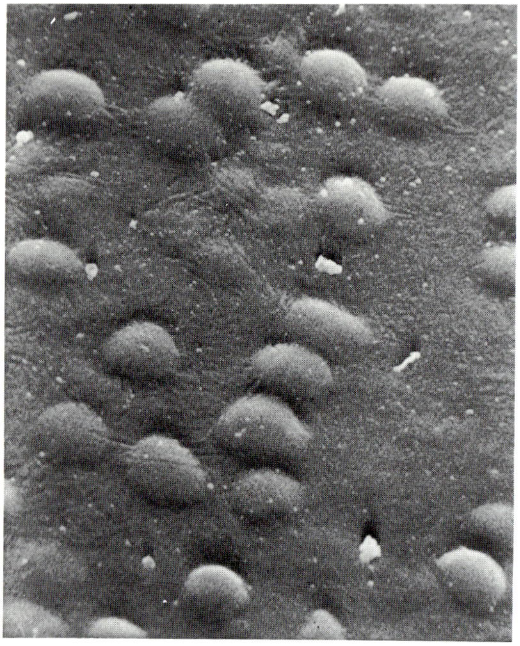

Fig. 7.22 Surface of frozen, fully hydrated dog femoral condylar cartilage covered by random array of tertiary elevations. Low temperature SEM at – 191°. ×1350.

long suspected might be artefactual. In further recent investigations of frozen, hydrated, non-fixed mammalian cartilage surfaces, the technique of low temperature replication was adopted to demonstrate, by transmission electron microscopy, an even smaller 'quinary' order of surface features that included superficial collagen fibres and expanded proteoglycans (Gardner et al, 1983) (Fig. 7.23).

As a result of these investigations, and to assist understanding of the scale of these various surface features, a hierarchy of surface structure was proposed (Fig. 7.24). The surfaces features, which had been analysed by Talysurf traces (Sayles et al, 1979), were measured. It became evident that in normal, unloaded articular hyaline cartilage, the height/depth of the tertiary features and their individual diameters tended to increase with age whereas the frequency decreased (Longmore, 1976; Longmore & Gardner, 1975, 1978).

It is of importance to note that the rough but orderly surface structure of articular cartilage becomes increasingly less orderly with age (Fig. 7.25). By the age of 40–45 years, severe cartilage surface disorganisation progresses to the structural, zonal, loss of cartilage. The changes of advancing age fuse with those of disease and fibrillation and this is one complication of these normal ageing processes.

At the articular surface (Fig. 7.21), the fibre

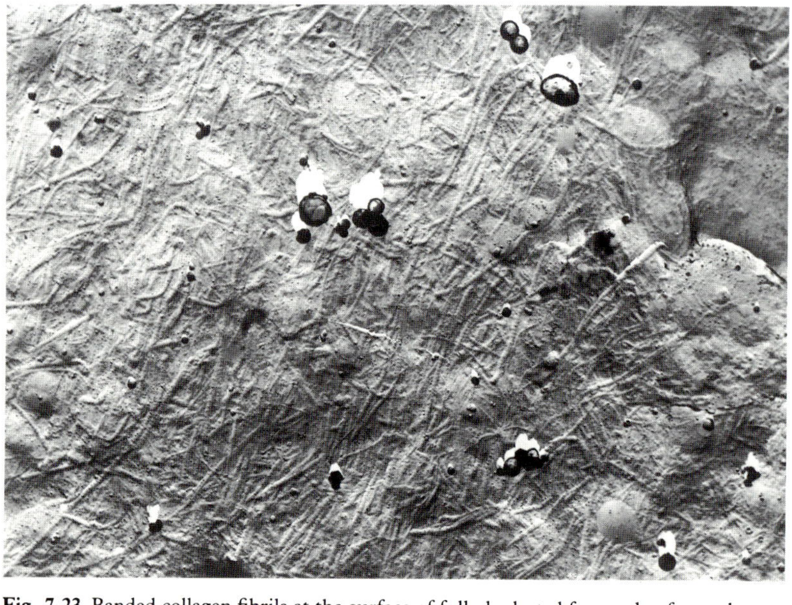

Fig. 7.23 Banded collagen fibrils at the surface of fully hydrated frozen dog femoral condylar cartilage. Transmission electron macrograph of replica taken at – 195°. ×7395.

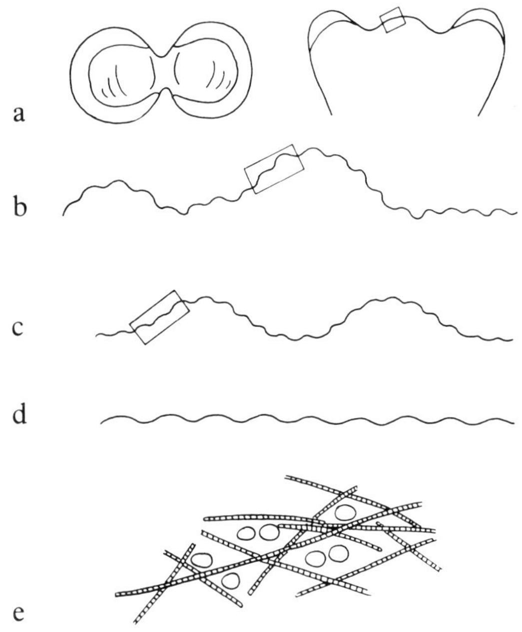

Fig. 7.24 Hierarchy of anatomical structure of human articular cartilage surfaces. (a) (Primary) Anatomical contours seen 'naked eye'. (b) (Secondary) Irregularities, 0.2–0.5 mm diameter, detected with hand-lens. (c) (Tertiary) Features, 20–40 μm diameter, seen on dry preparations as hollows, hydrated specimens as prominences. (d) (Quarternary) Striations, 1–4 μm diameter, 130–275 nm deep, seen by interference and by scanning electron microscopy when specimens have been detached from bone. (e) Quinary) Structures, including collagen fibrils of 68 nm periodicity and parts of expanded proteoglycans, 150 nm diameter, demonstrable in low temperature replicas by transmission electron microscopy.

bundles of type II collagen are arranged as an orderly, multilayered mat. The collagen bundles are arranged tangentially to the load-bearing surface and approximately at right angles to each other. Electron microscopic evidence shows that the most superficial collagen fibrils extend into an ultramicroscopic '*lamina obscurans*' (Balazs et al, 1966), a non-fibrillar chondroitin sulphate rich layer, ~ 400 nm thick, which is itself covered by a thinner, ~ 60 nm glycoprotein stratum in continuity with the hyaluronate-protein of the synovial fluid (Orford & Gardner, 1984). The ultramicroscopic lamina obscurans should be distinguished from the brightly illuminated surface seen by phase contrast light microscopy, the (lamina splendens) (MacConaill, 1951) which has now been shown to be an optical artefact (Aspden & Hukins, 1979).

Lubrication (Dowson & Wright, 1981; Kempson, 1975, 1979; McCutcheon, 1966–1967, 1978; Radin et al, 1976; Radin & Paul, 1972; Swanson, 1976, 1979)

No biological problem has exercised tribologists and engineers more severely than the unexplained excellence of the lubrication mechanism of synovial joints. For 70 or more years, tens of millions of movements, under widely varying loads (Day et al, 1975) are facilitated by a system in which low friction is the corollary of slow wear. Low wear is a function of the efficiency of load transmission and of lubrication. It is therefore a product of the physical properties of the opposing cartilage surfaces, the loads (forces) applied across these surfaces and the characteristics of the lubricant, synovial fluid (Paul, 1976; Radin et al, 1976) (Table 7.7). When cartilage is deformed by loading, it becomes electrically polarised (Andrew et al, 1973), a change that can facilitate lubrication. Whereas it was generally accepted that the hyaluronic acid of synovial fluid, in the form of a hyaluronate–protein complex, provided the unique lubricant (Table 7.7); it has been shown (Radin et al, 1976) that lubrication in vitro is determined by a glycoprotein fraction and not by the hyaluronate. This controversial evidence indicates that the glycoprotein is the key to the lubricant properties of the fluid between opposing cartilage surfaces and suggests that hyaluronate acts only to lubricate the non-weight-bearing surfaces of the marginal synovial tissues. Theoretically, there are several possible ways to ensure effective lubrication of human synovial joints. The limiting value of the tangential force required to move one flat surface across another is expressed as a fraction of the normal force holding the surfaces in contact: it is termed the 'coefficient of friction' (Table 7.7). In *boundary lubrication* the frictional force is a function of the properties of the opposing surfaces and of properties of the lubricant other than its viscosity. It depends on the adhesion of lubricant molecules to the surface so that these molecules slip over each other rather than over the dry surfaces. In *hydrodynamic lubrication*, lubrication under pressure, the shape and relative motion of the sliding surfaces cause the formation of a fluid film having sufficient pressure to separate the surfaces. The coefficient of friction is then a func-

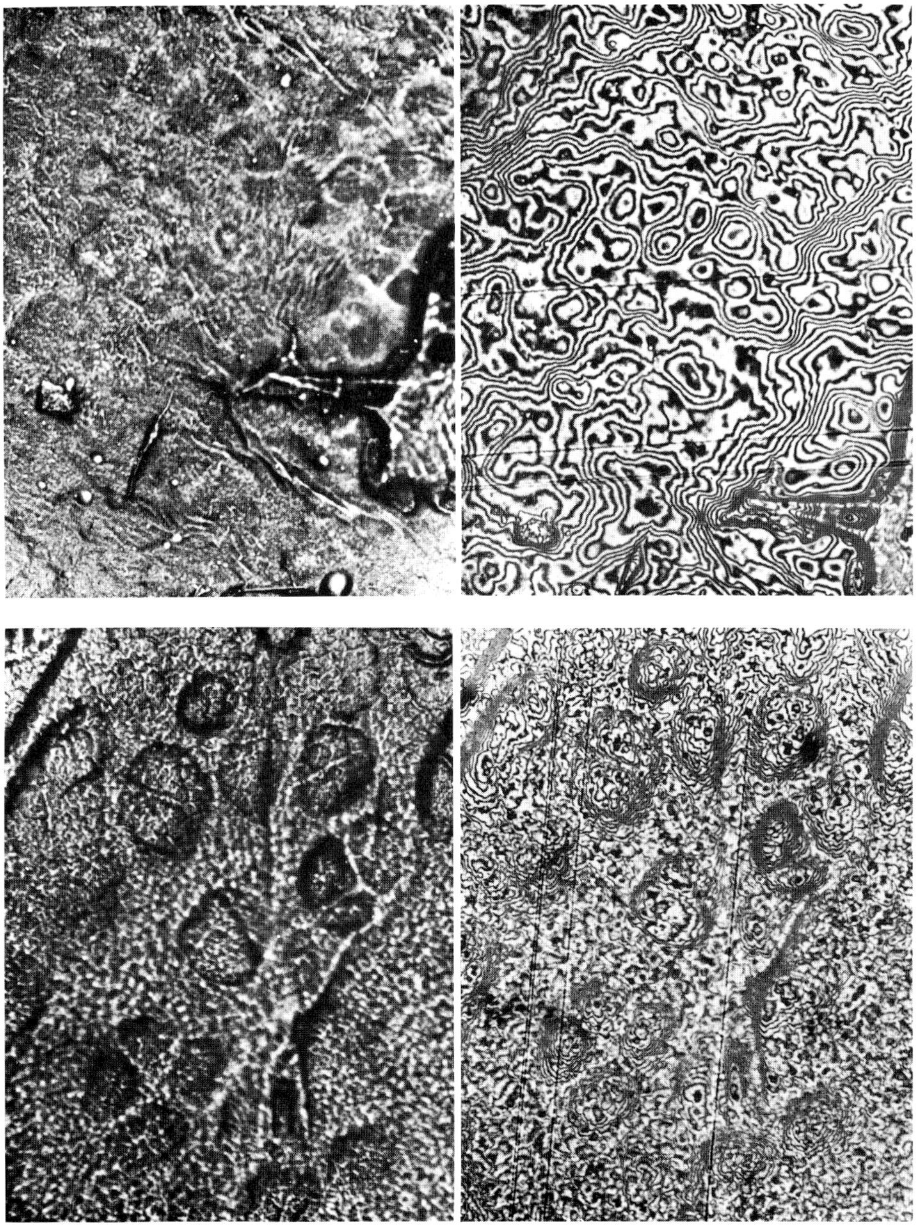

Fig. 7.25 Articular cartilage surfaces. (Top) Part of lateral femoral condylar surface from knee of normal 4-year-old female child viewed (left) by reflected white light, (right) by reflected green light (λ 550 nm). Contour distances exactly represent elevations and depressions on surface: fine, parallel reference lines (100 μm apart) allow diameter of undulations to be measured.

(Bottom) Under exactly similar viewing conditions, wider and steeper irregularities of surface of lateral femoral condylar cartilage of normal 23-year-old male are shown. Note vertical 100 μm reference lines. Reflected light interference microscopy. All fields. ×270.

tion of load, sliding speed and fluid viscosity. However, calculations of the thickness of the fluid film likely to be generated by hydrodynamic action in typical joints reveal that this is very much smaller than the irregularities of the surfaces. Extensions of the simple hydrodynamic theory have since been employed to model the behaviour of joints. For example, theoretical studies by Mow

Table 7.7 Coefficients of friction (from Swanson, 1973)

	Coefficient
Non-biological systems	
Clean, degassed smooth metal surfaces	100.00
Rubber tyre on dry road	1.0
Nylon against steel	0.3
Ball bearing	0.001
Entire synovial joints	
Human ankle	0.014–0.024
Human hip	0.003–0.015
Small pieces of cartilage (with synovial fluid as lubricant)	
Articular cartilage (on bone), against glass	0.008–0.1
Articular cartilage (on bone), against glass, rubber or plastic	0.15–0.8
Articular cartilage (on bone), against glass	0.0014–0.07

et al (1974a, b) examine the effect of a load moving across the cartilage and indicate that it may be possible for cartilage to produce a fluid film from the fluid squeezed out in front of, and in the leading half of, the contact area.

The concept of *squeeze-film lubrication* exploits the fact that if two surfaces are initially separated by a fluid film a finite time is required for this fluid to be squeezed out, particularly if the surfaces are congruous. This mechanism is useful when loads are of short duration. If opposing articular surfaces are relatively soft then the pressures which develop in a fluid film could deform the surfaces so that the load is distributed evenly and thicker fluid films made possible. This consequence might establish *elastohydrodynamic lubrication*, a possibility that is widely discounted. Other suggested modes of lubrication allow the operation of more than one mechanism. Thus there may be contact of the opposing solid surfaces *and* the possibility of fluid flow in the permeable cartilage. In *weeping lubrication* (McCutcheon, 1962), fluid could be squeezed out of the opposing cartilages into the loaded area, providing the hydrodynamic pressure to support most of the load. However, the rapid escape of fluid in this way is not possible. In *boosted lubrication* (Walker et al, 1968) fluid might escape from the contact area into cartilage and between the surfaces. As the surfaces closed, the large molecules of the synovial fluid could be trapped by the approaching surface irregularities, eventually forming a stable 'gel' approximately 30 nm thick between the surfaces. The possibility of 'boosted' lubrication is not agreed.

A Newtonian fluid displays a viscosity that is independent of the shear rate. Synovial fluid is non-Newtonian: its viscosity varies with the rate at which layers of fluid move (shear) relative to each other. The differences between boundary and viscous friction are consequently not clear-cut. Different forms of lubrication are almost certainly of critical importance under different operating conditions. For example, Unsworth et al (1975), using human femoral heads as fulcra, in a pendulum machine, show that when loading is sudden, squeeze-fluid film lubrication is present. At low loads, a self-generated fluid film process is recognised; at higher loads, boundary lubrication is important. Evidently in the walking cycle (Fig. 7.26) each of these modes of lubrication may be employed.

Friction in synovial joints is low by engineering standards (Table 7.7). Attempts have been made to replicate the properties of synovial fluid by synthetic materials but the results have been unsatisfactory. In searching for a synthetic fluid that can be injected into human joints it is essential that the fluid be capable of long-term retention within the joint, that it be non-toxic, non-antigenic and non-carcinogenic. No known fluid fulfils all of these criteria.

Because of the elastic and viscous forces exerted by muscles, tendons and ligaments, 'joint stiffness' measured in the intact human subject is not a valid index of joint friction. It is however a useful procedure in assessing the objective response to therapeutic agents and has been used in clinical trials of anti-inflammatory and analgesic agents.

Symphyses

Specialised secondary cartilaginous joints formed of hyaline and of fibrocartilage are called 'symphyses'. The opposing bones are separated by a fibrocartilaginous disc. Symphyses provide for growth by means of the layers of hyaline cartilage that lie between the fibrocartilage and the nearby bone. As age advances, the hyaline growth cartilage disappears. An additional feature of increasing age is the development of a cavity in the fibrocartilage of joints such as the manubriosternal and the pubic symphysis.

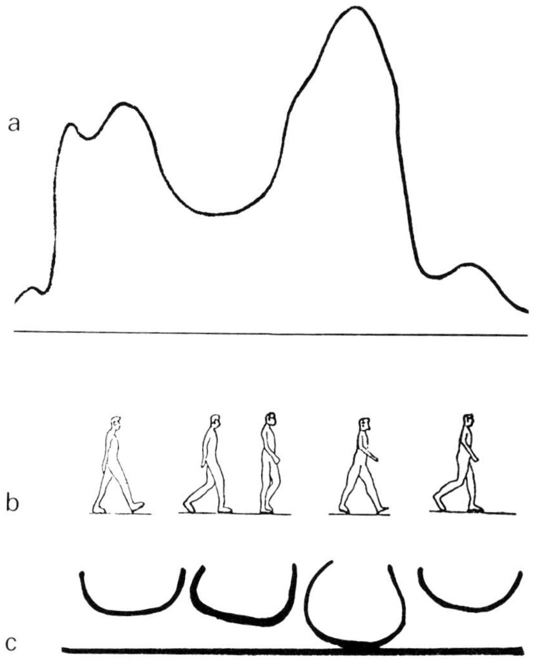

Fig. 7.26 Walking cycle, load and lubrication of hip joint. Relationship, expressed diagrammatically, between (a) contact stress on hip joint cartilage measured by experimental pendulum technique; (b) phases of cycle during walking movement; and (c) proposed lubrication mechanisms.

At heel strike, load on hip is 3–4 times body weight but there is no sliding motion. Lubrication is squeeze film. As walking continues, sliding motion, under lighter load, draws fluid into load-bearing zone, establishing fluid film lubrication. At extreme posterior position, fluid film is much reduced by high load and lubrication becomes boundary. (From Clarke (1972) PhD thesis, University of Strathclyde, Unsworth et al (1975) Annals of the Rheumatic Diseases 34: 277–285.)

Intervertebral joints. The most important secondary cartilaginous joints are those between the vertebral bodies. These articulations are entirely distinct from the paired intervertebral synovial joints comprising the opposed articular facets on the superior and inferior articular processes of adjacent vertebrae. The main joints between the vertebral bodies are formed by intervertebral discs that have a unique connective tissue structure, an unusual developmental origin and a most important supportive function (Golub et al, 1971). In the cervical region, it is occasionally possible to identify a third form of small marginal synovial (Luschka) joint that may influence the genesis of disorders of the cervical articulation. The Luschka joints lie at the intervertebral disc margins.

The 23 intervertebral discs are fibrocartilaginous plates that unite adjacent vertebrae. Each plate is formed of dense concentric bundles of collagen fibres displayed as an *annulus fibrosus* (Fig. 7.27). The collagen bundles are arranged around the geometric axis of the vertebral column. However, many bundles combine to provide an extremely strong junction between the vertebrae by extending upwards in an arc from one vertebral body to the next. At the same time, other bundles intermingle with them while running from the superior to the inferior body. The entire effect is the provision of a series of helical and concentric collagenous fascicles. The orientation of the collagenous bundles is less well-defined posteriorly. Here, the collagen is in random array; the strength of the union is correspondingly less. The posterior margins of the intervertebral discs are bound to a posterior longitudinal ligament which widens over the disc surface and which lies anterior to the vertebral foramen, spinal cord and corda equina. The ligament is deficient posterolaterally where there is a zone of relative weakness.

The *nucleus pulposus*, the residue of the embryonic notochord, is an ellipsoidal island of highly

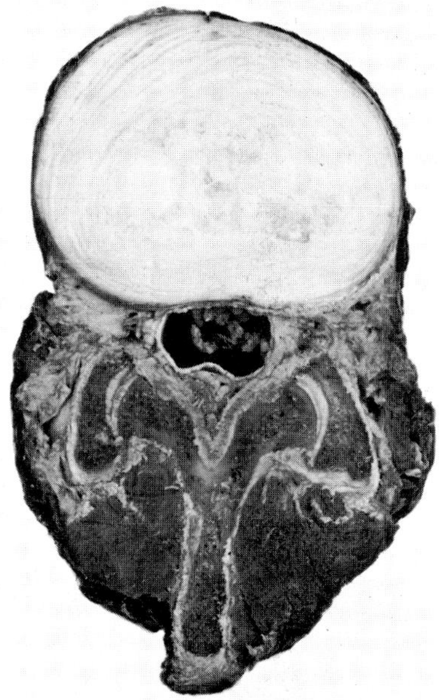

Fig. 7.27 Human adult intervertebral disc. The spine has been divided in a plane at right angles to the axis of the vertebral column. The concentric, marginal collagen bundles of the disc are seen.

hydrated connective tissue entirely distinct in structure from the dense surrounding annular collagen bundles. The nucleus is rarely at the centre of the disc: it is retained by the collagen fibres of the annulus, an arrangement which constitutes a hydrostatic pressure vessel, resisting compression vertically but allowing flexion and rotation about the vertical axis. The nucleus is analogous in structure and function to the fluid core of a classic golf ball; it gives elasticity and flexibility to the otherwise rigid union.

Much is now known of the histological structure and chemical composition of the intervertebral disc. The dense collagen of the annulus is of very low cellularity. There is relatively little non-collagenous matrix. Thicker and thinner collagen fibrils alternate (Inoue & Takeda, 1975). By contrast, the young nucleus contains little collagen and relatively large amounts of proteoglycan.

Sensory nerves supply the anterior and posterior longitudinal ligaments but are confined to the periphery of the annulus fibrosus. The discs are collectively the largest avascular structures in the mammalian body. The viability of the cells of the nucleus pulposus is dependent on diffusion. Anatomically, diffusion of metabolites may be *peripheral*, through the annulus fibrosus from marginal blood vessels; or *central*, from the bony plates that are the end products of the epiphyses of nearby vertebral bodies. Maroudas et al (1975) used ^{14}C glucose to compare the diffusion coefficients of the human *postmortem* annulus fibrosus and the hyaline cartilage end-plate. The results, 2.5 cm^2/sec and 2.4 cm^2/sec respectively, at 37°, were comparable to those obtained for articular cartilage elsewhere. Assuming a low rate of glycolysis, the whole annulus fibrosus appeared to be adequately nourished by peripheral blood vessels whereas part of the nucleus pulposus was sustained by the vasculature of the bony end-plates of the vertebrae. When a high rate of glycolysis was assumed, one-third of the annulus was provided with nutrients from the bony end-plate only, a source that was demonstrably inadequate. Thus, the nutritional state of the intervertebral disc appears precarious by comparison with that of other avascular structures such as hyaline articular cartilage, which is believed to have a 50% excess of supply over normal demand.

In other investigations it was possible to measure fluid expression under load and to suggest that the hydraulic permeability of the disc depends largely on the degree of disc hydration. Normally, the nucleus pulposus, a turgid island of gelatinous consistence, is hyperhydrated with a water content of almost 80%. The water content of the annulus is a great deal lower.

Age changes

There are pronounced changes with age in the histological structure, chemical composition, physical properties and mechanical behaviour of the intervertebral discs and of the adjacent bone. There is progressively less water and an increasing cross-linking of ageing collagen. Inevitably, reduced hydration influences the structure and function of the nucleus pulposus more than that of the annulus.

Estimates of glycosaminoglycan in intervertebral disc tissue from children and from old people show that there is a qualitative change in proteoglycan with age. The molecular weight of the proteoglycan decreases and the keratan sulphate content increases. A proportion of the proteoglycans have an enhanced association with disc collagen; and the remaining extractable molecules are of decreased hydrodynamic size (Adams & Muir, 1976). The amount of hyaluronate increases from the outer to the inner zone of the disc in parallel with a change in uronic acid. This gradient obtains in young and old discs. The aged discs contain no less hyaluronate than the young, and the nucleus, indeed, comes to have an increased hyaluronate fraction. The evidence suggests that any loss of proteoglycan from old discs is not due to hyaluronate deficiency.

The annulus fibrosus is unique because it contains both type I and type II collagen (Eyre & Muir, 1974). It is possible that the high type II collagen content is related to a response to high loading. The collagen of the disc periphery is entirely type I; at the central, nuclear zone, collagen is entirely type II. The interesting hypothesis has been proposed that each of these molecular types of collagen is restricted to one of the morphological types of fibre. Less is known of the age changes in collagen that are strongly suggested by alterations, such as those of tensile stiffness, observed up to the age of 26 years but not beyond (Galante, 1967). Hydroxyproline, an index of collagen content, does not change with age. Studies of collagen fibril diameter, measured in human fetal annulus fibrosus, show that this parameter does not increase in utero suggesting the possibility that diametric change may also not occur at later ages (Hickey & Hukins, 1980). Scanning electron microscopic studies suggest the converse (Takeda, 1975) and an increase in fibril diameter, at least to the end of maturation (~ 25 years) has been demonstrated. It remains of importance to note that those changes in intervertebral disc composition that occur with age, are anatomically selective so that at the age of 44 years the collagen content of the annulus fibrosus increases distally, a regional distinction not found at the age of 16 years. There is an analogous alteration in glycosaminoglycan composition of both annulus fibrosus and nucleus pulposus (Adams & Muir, 1976).

There are parallel age-related changes in the mechanical properties of the intervertebral discs. The compressive breaking of lumbar vertebrae at physiological strain rates varies greatly across the population (Hutton et al, 1979) although the difference in compressive strength between the upper and lower lumbar vertebrae is not significant.

Loads of more than 640 kg are required to significantly deform isolated segments of young vertebral column segments; but deformation of older specimens may occur with loads of no more than 160 kg. Pressures within discs range from 7 kg/cm^2 in the recumbent position, to 10 kg/cm^2 in the sitting position and to 15 kg/cm^2 standing. The structure of an individual vertebral column is influenced by diurnal variations in the water content of the nucleus pulposus so that the height of a person may be as much as 2 cm greater in the morning than in the later part of a day spent sitting or standing.

It is important to observe that severe alterations in the structure and function of the intervertebral discs with age invariably alter the forces imposed on the posterior intervertebral (apophyseal) joints which are therefore necessarily affected adversely by any form of age-related intervertebral disc degeneration. Cumulatively, ageing variations in water content and alterations in disc glycosaminoglycan concentration may combine with the exertion of severe, inappropriately directed forces to cause protrusion of part of an eccentrically located nucleus pulposus through the relatively weak posterolateral parts of the annulus and of the posterior intervertebral ligaments.

ACKNOWLEDGEMENTS
The completion of this chapter would not have been possible without the constant advice and constructive criticism of my colleagues, Dr C.G. Armstrong, Dr C.H.S. Cameron, Dr C.J. Kirkpatrick, Dr J. McClure, Dr K. Oates, Dr P. O'Connor and Dr C.R. Orford, each of whom has helped in the provision of material and illustrations from his/her own field of research. The laboratory is supported by the Arthritis and Rheumatism Council for Research, by the Medical Research Council, and by Ciba-Geigy (Pharmaceuticals).

REFERENCES

Abercrombie M 1978 Fibroblasts. Journal of Clinical Pathology 31; (Suppl 12): 1–6
Adams P, Muir H 1976 Qualitative changes with age of proteoglycans of human lumbar discs. Annals of the Rheumatic Diseases 35: 289–296
Alexander R McN 1978 The chordates. Cambridge, University Press
Alexander R McN 1979 The invertebrates. Cambridge, University Press
Anderson H C 1980 Calcification processes. Pathology Annual 15: 45–75
Andrew C, Bassett L, Pawluk R J 1972 Electrical behaviour of cartilage during loading. Science 178: 982–983
Armstrong C G, Gardner D L 1977 Thickness and distribution of human femoral head articular cartilage. Changes with age. Annals of the Rheumatic Diseases 36: 407–412
Armstrong C G, Bahrani A S, Gardner D L 1979 In vitro measurements of articular cartilage deformations in the intact human hip joint under load. Journal of Bone and Joint Surgery 61–A: 744–755.
Armstrong C G, Bahrani A S, Gardner D L 1980 Changes in the deformational behaviour of human hip cartilage with age. Journal of Biochemical Engineering 102: 214–220
Aspden R M, Hukins D W L 1979 The lamina splendens of articular cartilage is an artefact of phase contrast microscopy. Proceedings of the Royal Society B 206: 109–113
Badoux D M 1974 An introduction to biomechanical principles in primate locomotion and structure. In: Jenkins

F A (ed) Primate locomotion. New York, Academic Press
Balazs E A, Bloom G D, Swann D A 1966 Fine structure and glycosaminoglycan content of the surface layer of articular cartilage. Federation Proceedings 25: 1813–1816
Ball J 1971 Enthesopathy of rheumatoid and ankylosing spondylitis (Heberden oration 1970). Annals of the Rheumatic Diseases 30: 213–223
Barnett C H, Davies DV, MacConnaill M A 1961 Synovial joints: their structure and mechanics. London, Longmans Green
Bayliss M T, Ridgway G D, Ali S Y 1983 Differences in the rates of aggregation of proteoglycans from human articular cartilage and chondrosarcoma. Biochemical Journal 215: 705–708
Benichow C, Wirotius J M 1982 Articular cartilage atrophy in lower limb amputees. Arthritis and Rheumatism 25: 80–82
Boskey A L 1981 Current concepts of the physiology and bio-chemistry of calcification. Clinical Orthopaedics and Related Research 157: 225–257
Bourne G H 1981 Nutrition and wound healing. In: Glynn L E (ed) Tissue repair and regeneration: Handbook of inflammation, Vol 3. Amsterdam, Elsevier/North Holland Biomedical, p. 211–242
Bozdech Z, Horn V 1975 The morphology of growth cartilage using the scanning electron miscroscope. Acta Orthopaedica Scandinavica 46: 561–568
Bromley M, Fisher W D, Woolley D E 1984 Mast cells at sites of cartilage erosion in the rheumatoid joint. Annals of the Rheumatic Diseases 43: 76–79
Broom N D, Myers D B 1980 A study of the structural response of wet hyaline cartilage to various loading situations. Connective Tissue Research 7: 227–238
Broom N D, Poole C A 1983 Articular cartilage collagen and proteoglycans — their functional interdependency. Arthritis and Rheumatism 26: 1111–1119
Brown C H 1975 Vertebrata: internal skeletal structures. In: Structural materials in animals. London, Pitman, p 305–336
Brown R A, Weiss J, Tomlinson I W, Phillips P, Kumar S 1980 Angiogenic factor from synovial fluid resembling that from tumours. Lancet I: 682–685
Brown R A, Tomlinson I W, Hill C R, Weiss J B, Phillips P, Kumar S 1983 Relationship of angiogenesis factor in synovial fluid to various joint diseases. Annals of the Rheumatic Diseases 42: 301–307
Bullough P G, Jagannath A 1983 The morphology of the calcification front in articular cartilage — its significance in joint function. Journal of Bone and Joint Surgery 65–B: 72–78
Burgeson R E, Hebda P A, Morris N P, Hollister D W 1982 Human cartilage collagens. Comparison of cartilage collagen with human type V collagen. Journal of Biological Chemistry 257: 7852–7856
Burmester G R, Dimitriu-Bona A, Waters S J, Winchester R J 1983. Identification of three major synovial lining cell populations by monoclonal antibodies directed to Ia antigens and antigens associated with monocytes/macrophages and fibroblasts. Scandinavian Journal of Immunology 17: 69–82
Chiarelli A B 1973 Posture of the primates and the aquisition of an upright posture by man. In: Evolution of the primates. London, Academic Press, p. 269–283
Clarke I C 1972 A study of the structure and wear response of hip joint cartilage. PhD thesis, University of Strathclyde
Clarke I C 1973 Quantitative measurement of human articular surface topography in vitro by profile recorder and stereomicroscopy techniques. Journal of Microscopy 97: 309–314
Clemmensen I, Holund B, Johansen N, Andersen R B 1982 Demonstration of fibronectin in human articular cartilage by an indirect immunoperoxidase technique. Histochemistry 76: 51–56
Currey J D 1974 Animal skeletons. London, Edward Arnold
Davies D V 1969 The biology of joints. In: Copeman W S C (ed) Textbook of the rheumatic diseases, 4th Edn. London, E & S Livingstone, p. 40–86
Day W H, Swanson S A V, Freeman M A R 1975 Contact pressures in the loaded human cadaver hip. Journal of Bone and Joint Surgery 57–B: 302–313
Dieppe P A, Huskisson E C, Crocker P, Willoughby D A 1976 Apatite deposition disease. Lancet 1: 266–268
Dillon L S 1973 Evolution: Concepts and consequences. St Louis, C V Mosby
Dowson D, Wright V (ed) 1981 An introduction to the Biomechanics of joints and joint replacement. London, Mechanical Engineering Publications Ltd
Dowson D, Longfield M D, Walker P S, Wright V 1968 An investigation of the friction and lubrication in human joints. Proceedings of the Institution of Mechanical Engineers 182: 3–68
Dreher R 1982 Origin of synovial type-A cells during inflammation: an experimental approach. Immunobiology 161: 232–245
Edwards J C W 1982 The origin of type-A synovial lining cells. Immunobiology 161: 227–231
Edwards J C W, Mackay A R, Sedgwick A D, Willoughby D A 1983 Mode of formation of synovial villi. Annals of the Rheumatic Diseases 42: 585–590
Eisenstein R, Sorgente N, Soble L W, Miller A, Kuttner K E 1973 The resistance of certain tissues to invasion: penetrability of explanted tissue by vascularised mesenchyme. American Journal of Pathology 73: 765–774
Elliott R J 1976 Biochemical studies of age-associated changes in human articular cartilage. PhD thesis. The Queen's University of Belfast.
Ellis H A 1981 Metabolic bone disease. In: Anthony P, MacSween R N M (eds) Recent advances in histopathology, Vol. II. Edinburgh, Churchill Livingstone, p 185–202
El-Maghraby MAHA, Gardner D L 1969 Development of connective tissue components of small arteries in the chick embryo. Journal of Pathology 108: 281–291
Engel A, Larsson T 1969 Ageing of connective tissue and skeletal tissue. Thule International Symposia Proceedings: Nordiska Bokhandelns Forlag
Engfeldt B, Hjerpe A 1976 Glycosaminoglycans and proteoglycans of human bone tissue at different stages of mineralisation. Acta pathologica et microbiologica Scandinavica (A) 84: 95–106
Evans H B, Ayad S, Abedin M Z, Hopkins S, Morgan K, Walton K W, et al 1983 Localisation of collagen types and fibronectin in cartilage by immunofluorescence. Annals of the Rheumatic Diseases 42: 575–581
Eyre D R, Muir H 1974 Collagen polymorphism: two molecular species in pig intervertebral disc. FEBS Letters 42:192
Eyre D R, Muir H 1975 Type-III collagen: a major constituent of rheumatoid and normal human synovial membrane. Connective Tissue Research 4: 11–16

Fell H B 1981 The Strangeways Research Laboratory and cellular interactions. In: Dingle J T, Gordan J L (eds) Cellular Interactions. Amsterdam, Elsevier/North Holland Biomedical, p. 1–14

Fell H B, Jubb R W 1977a The effect of synovial tissue on the breakdown of articular cartilage in organ culture. Arthritis and Rheumatism 20: 1359–1371

Fell H B, Jubb R W 1977b The destructive action of synovial tissue on articular cartilage in organ culture. In: Gordon J I, Hasteman B I (eds) Rheumatoid arthritis. Amsterdam: Elsevier/North Holland Biomedical, p. 193–197

Fitton Jackson S 1964 Connective tissue cells. In: Brachet J, Mirsky A E (eds) The cell. New York, Academic Press, p. 387–520

Foellmer H G, Madri J A, Furthmayr H 1983 Methods in laboratory investigation. Monoclonal antibodies to Type IV collagen: probes for the study of structure and function of basement membranes. Laboratory Investigation 48: 639–649

Freeman M A R (ed) 1979 Adult articular cartilage, 2nd Edn. London, Pitman Medical

Furukawa T, Eyre D R, Koide S, Glimcher M J 1980 Biochemical studies on repair cartilage resurfacing experimental defects in the rabbit knee. Journal of Bone and Joint Surgery 62: 79–89

Galante J O 1967 Tensile properties of the human annulus fibrosus. Acta Orthopaedica Scandinavica (Suppl) 100: 8–91

Gardner D L 1972 The influence of microscopic technology on knowledge of cartilage surface structure. (Heberden Oration 1971). Annals of the Rheumatic Diseases 31: 235–258

Gardner D L 1978 Diseases of connective tissue: a consensus. Journal of Clinical Pathology 31 (Suppl 12): 223–238

Gardner Dl 1984 Anatomical Changes and pathogenesis of osteoarthrosis in man, with particular reference to the hip and knee joints. In: Birdwood G, Jasani C (eds) Studies in osteoarthrosis: Pathogenesis, intervention, assessment, New York, Academic Press (in press)

Gardner D L, Dodds T C 1976 Human histology, 3rd Edn. Edinburgh, Churchill Livingstone

Gardner D L, McGillivray D C 1971a Living articular cartilage is not smooth. Annals of the Rheumatic Diseases 30: 3–9

Gardner D L, McGillivray D C 1971b Surface structure of articular cartilage. Historical review. Annals of the Rheumatic Diseases 30: 10–14

Gardner D L, O'Connor P 1985 The musculoskeletal system — aging of articular cartilage. In Brocklehurst J C (ed) Textbook of geriatric medicine and gerontology, 3rd Edn. Edinburgh, Churchill Livingstone, p. 776–794

Gardner D L, Woodward D H 1968 Scanning electron microscopy of articular surfaces. Lancet II:1246

Gardner D L, Woodward D H 1969 Scanning electron microscopy and replica studies of articular surfaces of guinea-pig synovial joints. Annals of the Rheumatic Diseases 28: 379–391

Gardner D L, O'Connor P, Oates K 1979 Surface structure of mammalian articular cartilage viewed at low temperature. Lancet II:538

Gardner D L, O'Connor P, Oates K 1981 Low temperature scanning electron microscopy of dog and guinea-pig hyaline articular cartilage. Journal of Anatomy 132: 267–282

Gardner D L, O'Connor P, Middleton J F S, Oates K, Orford C R 1983 An investigation by transmission electron microscopy of freeze replicas of dog articular cartilage surfaces: the fibre-rich surface structure. Journal of Anatomy 137: 573–582

Gathercole L J, Keller A 1975 Light microscopic waveforms in collagenous tissues and their structural implications. In: Atkins EDT, Keller A (eds) Structure of fibrous biopolymers London, Butterworths, p. 153–187

Gay S, Miller E J. 1983 What is collagen, what is not? Ultrastructural Pathology 4: 365–377

Ghadially F N 1980 Overview article: The articular territory of the reticuloendothelial system. Ultrastructural Pathology 1: 249–264

Ghadially F N 1983 Fine structure of synovial joints. London, Butterworths

Ghadially F N, Mehta P N, Kirkaldy-Willis W H 1970 Utrastructure of articular cartilage in experimentally produced lipoarthrosis. Journal of Bone and Joint Surgery 52–A: 1147–1158

Ghadially F N, Ghadially J A, Oryschak A F, Yong N K 1976 Experimental production of ridges on rabbit articular cartilage: a scanning electron microscope study. Journal of Anatomy 121: 119–132

Ghadially F N, Lalonde J-M A, Yong N K 1982 Uraniosomes produced in the synovial membrane by uranyl acetate. Pathology 14: 121–128

Glynn L E 1981 The pathology of scar tissue formation. In: Glynn L E (ed) Tissue repair and regeneration: Handbook of inflammation, Vol 3. Amsterdam, Elsevier/North Holland Biomedical, p. 211–242

Goldman R, Rockstein M 1975 The physiology and pathology of human aging. New York, Academic Press

Golub B S, Rovit R L, Mankin H J 1971 Cervical and lumbar disc disease: a review. Bulletin of the Rheumatic Diseases 21: 635–642

Gore D M, Higginson G R, Minns R J 1983 Compliance of articular cartilage and its variation through the thickness. Physics in Medicine and Biology 28: 233–247

Graabaek P M 1982 Ultrastructural evidence for two distinct types of synoviocytes in rat synovial membrane. Journal of Ultrastructural Research 78: 321–339

Greenbury C L, Skingle J 1979 Anti-cartilage antibody. Journal of Clinical Pathology 32: 826–831

Ham A W 1974 Histology. Philadelphia, Lippincott, p. 410–413

Hancox N H 1972 The osteoclast. In: Bourne G H (ed) The biochemistry and physiology of bone, Vol I, 2nd Edn. New York, Academic Press, p. 45–67

Harris W H 1974 The hip. Proceedings of the 2nd Open Scientific Meeting of the Hip Society. St Louis, C V Mosby

Henderson B 1981 The biochemistry of the human synovial lining with special reference to alterations in metabolism in rheumatoid arthritis. Pathology, Research and Practice 172: 1–24

Hewitt A T, Varner M M, Silver M H, Dessau W, Wilkes C M, Marfin G R 1982 The isolation and partial characterization of chondronectin, an attachment factor for chondrocytes. Journal of Biological Chemistry 257: 2330–2334

Hickey D S, Hukins S W L 1980 X-ray diffraction studies of the arrangement of collagenous fibres in human foetal inervertebral disc. Journal of Anatomy 131: 81–90

Höhling H J, Steffens H, Ashton B A, Nicholson W A P 1974 Molekular biologie der Hartewebsbildung.

Verhandlung der Deutsche Gesellschaft fur Pathologie 58: 54–71
Hough A J, Banfield W G, Moltram F C, Sokoloff L 1974 The osteochondral junction of mammalian joints: an ultrastructural and microanalytic study. Laboratory Investigation 31: 685–695
Hough A J, Bomboy J D, Salmon W D 1980 Somatomedin and analogues of cyclic AMP increase the number of cells synthesizing DNA in cartilage from hypophysectomized rats. Acta Endocrinologica 93: 294–299
Hunter W 1742–1743 Of the structure and diseases of articulating cartilage. Philosophical Transactions of the Royal Society of London 42: 514–521
Hurwitz P J 1979 Experimental transplantation of small joints by microvascular anastomoses. Plastic and Reconstructive Surgery 64: 221–231
Hutton W C, Cyron B M, Stott J R R 1979 The compressive strength of lumbar vertebrae. Journal of Anatomy 129: 753–758
Inoue H, Takeda T 1975 Three-dimensional observation of the collagen framework of lumbar intervertebral discs. Acta Orthopaedica Scandinavica 46: 949–956
Inoue H, Kodama T, Fujita T 1969 Scanning electron microscopy of normal and rheumatoid articular cartilages. Archivum Histologicum Japonicum 30: 425–435
Jackson D S 1978 Collagens. Journal of Clinical Pathology 31: (Suppl 12): 44–48
Jande S S, Belanger L F 1971 Electron microscopy of osteocytes and the pericellular matrix in rat trabecular bone. Calcified Tissue Research 6: 280–289
Jubb R W 1982 Breakdown of articular cartilage by vascular tissue. Journal of Pathology 136: 333–343
Jubb R W, Fell H B 1980 The breakdown of collagen by chondrocytes. Journal of Pathology 130: 159–168
Kadar A 1979 The elastic fiber. Normal and pathological conditions in the arteries. Experimental Pathology Suppl 5: 7–130
Kajikawa K, Nakanishi I, Yamamura T 1980 The effect of collagenase on the formation of fibrous long spacing fibres. Laboratory Investigation 43: 410–417
Kato Y, Watanabe R, Hiraki Y, Suzuki F, Canalis E, Raisz L G, et al 1982 Selective stimulation of sulfated glycosaminoglycan synthesis by multiplication — stimulating activity, cartilage-derived factor and bone-derived growth factor. Comparison of their acttions on cultured chondrocytes with those of fibroblast growth factor and rhodamine fibrosarcoma-derived growth factor (BBA 21108). Biochimica et Biophysica Acta 704: 232–239
Kempson G E 1975 Mechanical properties of articular cartilage and their relationship to matrix degradation and age. Annals of the Rheumatic Diseases 34 (Suppl 2): 111–113
Kempson G E 1979 Mechanical properties of articular cartilage. In: Freeman M A R (ed) Adult articular cartilage, 2nd Edn. Tunbridge Wells, Pitman Medical, p 333–414
Kempson G E 1980 The mechanical properties of articular cartilage. In: Sokoloff L (ed) The joints and synovial fluid, Vol II. New York, Academic Press, p 177–239
Kempson G E, Muir H, Pollard C, Tuke M 1973 The tensile properties of the cartilage of human femoral condyles related to the content of collagen and glycosaminoglycans. Biochimica et Biophysica Acta 297: 456–472
Kempson G E, Spivey C J, Swanson S A V, Freeman M A R 1974 Patterns of cartilage stiffness on normal and degenerative femoral heads. Journal of Biomechanics 4: 597–609
Kirkpatrick C J 1980 The effects of prostaglandin A_1 and prostaglandin B_1 on the differentiation of cartilage in the chick embryo. Cell and Tissue Research 210: 111–120
Kleinman H K, Klebe R J, Martin G R 1981 Role of collagenous matrices in the adhesion and growth of cells. Journal of Cell Biology 88: 473–486
Knight A D, Levick J R 1983 The density and distribution of capillaries around a synovial cavity. Quarterly Journal of Experimental Physiology 68: 629–644
Krane S M 1982 Collagenases and collagen degradation. Journal of Investigative Dermatology 79 (Suppl I): 835–865
Krey P R, Scheinberg M A, Cohen A S 1976 Fine structural analysis of rabbit synovial cells. Arthritis and Rheumatism 19: 581–592
Ksiazek T, Thyberg J 1983 Electron microscopic studies on resorption of xenogeneic cartilage inplants. Virchows Archives A 399: 79–88
Kuettner K E, Pauli B U 1983 Inhibition of neovascularization by a cartilage factor. In: Nujent J, O'Connor M (eds) Development of the vascular system. Ciba Foundation Symposia 100: Tunbridge Wells, Pitman Medical, p 163–173
Kuettner K E, Pauli B U, Gall G, Memoli V A, Schenk R K 1982 Synthesis of cartilage matrix by mammalian chondrocytes in vitro. I. Isolation, culture characteritics and morphology. Journal of Cell Biology 93: 743–750
Kuettner K E, Memoli V A, Pauli B U, Wrobel N C, Thonar E J M A, Daniel J C 1982 Synthesis of cartilage matrix by mammalian chondrocytes in vitro. 2. Maintenance of collagen and proteoglycan phenotype. Journal of Cell Biology 93: 751–757
Leidy J 1849 On the intimate structure and history of the articular cartilages. American Journal of Medical Science 17: 277–294
Leivo I 1983 Structure and composition of early basement membranes: studies with early embryos and teratocarcinoma cells. Medical Biology 61: 1–30
Lillie Rd, Tracy R E, Pizzolato P, Donaldson P T, Reynolds C 1980 Differential staining of collagen types in paraffin sections — a color change in degraded forms. Virchows Archives A 386: 153–159
Linck G, Stocker S, Grimaud J-A, Porte A 1983 Distribution of immunoreactive fibronectin and collagen (Type I, III, IV) in mouse joints. Fibronectin, an essential component of the synovial cavity border. Histochemistry 77: 323–328
Lipman J M, McDevitt C A, Sokoloff L 1983 Xenografts of articular chondrocytes in the nude mouse. Calcified Tissue International 35: 767–772
Lips P, Courpron P, Meunier P J 1978 Mean wall thickness of trabecular bone packets in the human iliac crest: changes with age. Calcified Tissue Research 26: 13–17
Longmore R B 1976 Surface structure of ageing human cartilage: a reflected-light interference and scanning electron microscope study. PhD thesis, The Queen's University of Belfast
Longmore R B, Gardner D L 1975 Development with age of human articular cartilage surface structure. Annals of the Rheumatic Diseases 34: 26–37
Longmore R B, Gardner D L 1978 The surface structure of ageing human articular cartilage: a study by reflected light interference microscopy (RLIM). Journal of Anatomy 126: 353–365

Luft J H 1965 The fine structure of hyaline cartilage matrix following ruthenium red fixation and staining. Journal of Cell Biology 27:61A
McCall J G 1968 Scanning electron microscopy of articular surfaces. Lancet II:1194
MacConaill M A 1951 The movements of bone over joints. 4. The mechanical structure of articulating cartilage. Journal of Bone and Joint Surgery 33B: 251–257
MacConaill M A, Basmajian J V, 1969 Muscles and movements. Baltimore, Williams & Wilkins
McClure J 1982 The demonstration of calcification fronts by in vivo and in vitro tetracycline labelling. Journal of Clinical Pathology 35: 1278–1282
McCutcheon C W 1962 The frictional properties of animal joints. Wear 5: 1–17
McCutcheon C W 1966–1967 Physiological lubrication. Proceedings of the Institute of Mechanical Engineers 181 (3J): 55–62
McCutcheon C W 1978 Lubrication of joints. In: Sokoloff L (ed) The joints and synovial fluid, Vol I. New York, Academic Press, p 438–483
Malemud C J, Sokoloff L 1978 The effect of chondrocyte growth factor on membrane transport by articular chondrocytes in monolayer culture. Connective Tissue Research 6: 1–9
Maroudas A 1976 Transport of solutes through cartilage: permeability to large molecules. Journal of Anatomy 122: 335–347
Maroudas A 1976 Balance between swelling pressure and collagen tension in normal and degenerate articular cartilage. Nature (Lond) 260: 808–809
Maroudas A, Bayliss M T, Venn M F 1980 Further studies on the composition of human femoral head cartilage. Annals of the Rheumatic Diseases 39: 514–523
Maroudas A, Stockwell R A, Nachemson A, Urban J 1975 Factors involved in the nutrition of the human lumbar intervertebral disc: cellularity and diffusion of glucose in vitro. Journal of Anatomy 120: 113–130
Martinez-Hernandez A, Amenta P S 1983 The basement membrane in pathology. Laboratory Investigation 48: 656–677
Mathews M B 1975 Connective tissue, macromolecular structure and evolution. Berlin, Springer-Verlag
Meachim G 1971 Effect of age on the thickness of adult articular cartilage at the shoulder joint. Annals of the Rheumatic Diseases 30: 43–46
Meachim G 1972 Repair of the para-articular bone plate in the rabbit knee. Journal of Anatomy 113: 359–371
Meachim G, Roberts C 1971 Repair of the joint surface from subarticular tissue in the rabbit knee. Journal of Anatomy 109: 317–327
Meachim G, Stockwell R A 1979 The matrix. In: Freeman M A R (ed) Adult articular cartilage 2nd Edn. Tunbridge Wells, Pitman Medical, p. 1–67
Meachim G, Denham D, Emery I H, Williamson P H 1974 Collagen alignments and artificial splits at the surface of human articular cartilage. Journal of Anatomy 118: 101–118
Meek K M, Chapman J A, Hardcastle R A 1979 The staining pattern of collagen fibrils. Journal of Biological Chemistry 254: 10710–10714
Mehta P N, Ghadially F N 1973 Articular cartilage in corn-oil induced lipoarthrosis. Annals of the Rheumatic Diseases 32: 75–82
Middleton J F S, Oates K, O'Connor P, Orford C R, Gardner D L 1984 Demonstration by X-ray microprobe analysis of relationship between chondrocytes and tertiary surface structure of hyaline articular cartilage. Connective Tissue Research 13: 1–8
Miller A 1984 Collagen: the organic matrix of bone. Philosophical Transactions of the Royal Society of London B 304: 455–477
Minor R R 1980 Collagen metabolism: A comparison of diseases of collagen and diseases affecting collagen. American Journal of Pathology 98: 225–280
Morales T I, Kuettner K E, Howell D S, Woessner J F 1983 Characterization of the metalloproteinase inhibitor produced by bovine articular chondrocyte cultures. Biochimica et Biophysica Acta 760: 221–229
Mow van C, Lai W M, Redler I 1974a Some surface characteristics of articular cartilage. I. A scanning electron microscopy study and a theoretical model for the dynamic interaction of synovial fluid and articular cartilage. Journal of Biomechanics 7: 449–456
Mow van C, Lai W M, Eisenfeld, Redler I 1974b Some surface characteristics of articular cartilage. II. On the stability of articular surface and a possible biomechanical factor in etiology of chondrodegeneration. Journal of Biomechanics 7: 457–468
Myers E R, Mow Van C 1983 Biomechanics of cartilage and its response to biomechanical stimuli. In: Hall B K (ed) Cartilage, Vol I. Structure, function and biochemistry. New York, p 313–341
Myers S L, Christine T A 1983 Hyaluronate synthesis by synovial villi in organ culture. Arthritis and Rheumatism 26: 764–770
O'Connor P, Bland C, Gardner D L 1980 Fine structure of artificial splits in femoral condylar cartilage of the rat: a scanning electron microscope study. Journal of Pathology 132: 169–179
Orford C R, Gardner D L 1984 Proteoglycan association with collagen d-band in hyaline articular cartilage. Connective Tissue Research 12: 345–348
Orford C R, Gardner D L 1985 Ultrastructural histochemistry of the surface lamina of normal articular cartilage. Histochemical Journal (in press)
Owen M 1978 Histogenesis of bone cells. Calcified Tissue Research 25: 205–207
Palmoski M J, Brandt K D 1982 Proteoglycan aggregation in injured articular cartilage. A comparison of healing lacerated cartilage with OA cartilage. Journal of Rheumatology 9: 189–197
Palmoski M J, Perricone E, Brandt K D 1979 Development and reversal of a proteoglycan aggregation defect in normal canine knee cartilage after immobilisation. Arthritis and Rheumatism 22: 508–517
Paul J P 1976 Approaches to design. Force actions transmitted by joints in the human body. Proceedings of the Royal Society of London B 192: 163–172
Perez-Tamayo R 1978 Pathology of collagen degradation. American Journal of Pathology 92: 507–566
Pilsworth L M C, Saklatvala J 1983 The cartilage-resorbing protein catabolin is made by synovial fibroblasts and its production is increased by phorbol myristate acetate. Biochemical Journal 216: 481–489
Poole A R, Golds E E, Champion B R 1981 The immunopathology of inflammatory arthritis. Some new insights. Surgical Clinics of North America 61: 353–368
Poole C A, Flint M H, Beaumont B W 1984 Morphological and functional relationships of articular cartilage matrices. Journal of Anatomy 138: 113–138

Prockop D J, Kivirikko K I, Tuderman L, Guzman A 1979 The biosynthesis of collagen and its disorders. New England Journal of Medicine 301: 13–25; 77–85
Radin E L, Paul I L 1972 A consolidated concept of joint lubrications. Journal of Bone and Joint Surgery 54-A: 607–616
Radin E L, Ehrlich M M, Weiss C A, Parker H G 1976 Osteoarthrosis as a state of altered physiology. In: Buchanan W W, Dick W C (eds) Recent Advances in Rheumatology. Edinburgh, Churchill Livingstone p 1–18
Redler I, Mow van C, Zimny M L, Marilyn L, Mansell J 1975 The ultrastructure and biomechanical significance of the tidemark of articular cartilage. Clinical Orthopaedics and Related Research 112: 357–362
Ross R 1975 Connective tissue cells, cell proliferation and synthesis of extracelluiar matrix — a review. Philosophical Transactions of the Royal Society of London B 271: 247–259
Saklatvala J 1981 Characterization of catabolin, the major product of pig synovial tissue that induces resportion of cartilage proteoglycan in vitro. Biochemical Journal 199: 705–714
Saklatvala J, Sarsfield S J 1982 Lymphocytes induce resorption of cartilage by producing catabolin. Biochemical Journal 202: 275–278
Saklatvala J, Curry V A, Sarsfield S J 1983 Purification to homogeneity of pig leucocyte catabolin, a protein that causes cartilage resorption in vitro. Biochemical Journal 215: 385–392
Salter R B, Simmonds D F, Malcolm B W, Rumble E J, MacMichael D 1975 The effects of continuous passive motion on the healing of articular cartilage defects — an experimental investigation in rabbits. In: Proceedings of the Orthopaedic Research Society. Journal of Bone and Joint Surgery 57-A: 570–571
Sandberg L B, Soskel N T, Leslie J G 1981 Elastin structure, biosynthesis and relation to disease states. New England Journal of Medicine 304: 566–579
Sanders E J, Prasad S 1983 The culture of chick embryo mesoderm cells in hydrated collagen gels. Journal of Experimental Zoology 226: 81–92
Sayles R S, Thomas T R, Anderson J, Haslock I, Unsworth A 1979 Measurement of the surface microgeometry of articular cartilage. Journal of Biomechanics 12: 257–267
Scheinberg R D, Ehrlich M G, Lippiello L, Mankin H J 1982 Degradative enzyme activity in isolated chondrocyte populations. Clinical Orthopaedics and Related Research 164: 279–286
Schofield J D, Weightman B 1978 New knowledge of connective tissue ageing. Journal of Clinical Pathology 31 (Suppl 12): 174–180
Schubert M, Hamerman D 1968 A primer on connective tissue biochemistry. Philadelphia, Lea & Febiger, p 5–52
Scott J E 1975 Composition and structure of the pericellular environment. Philosphical Transactions of the Royal Society of London B 271: 235–242
Scott J E 1980 Collagen-proteoglycan interactions. Localization of proteoglycans in tendon by electron microscopy. Biochemical Journal 187: 887–891
Scott J E, Dorling J 1965 Differential staining of acid glycosaminoglycans (mucopolysaccharides) by alcian blue in salt solutions. Histochemie 5: 221–233
Scott J E, Orford C R 1981 Dermatan sulphate-rich proteoglycan associates with rat tail-tendon collagen at the d band in the gap region. Biochemical Journal 197: 213–216
Scott J E, Orford C R, Hughes E W 1981 Proteoglycan-collagen arrangements in developing rat tail tendon. Biochemical Journal 195: 573–581
Serafini-Fracassini A, Smith J W 1974 The structure and biochemistry of cartilage. Edinburgh, Churchill Livingstone
Silbermann M, Livne E, Lizarbe M A, von der Mark K 1983 Glucocorticoid hormone adversely affects the growth and differentiation of cartilage cells in neonatal mice. Growth 47: 77–96
Simon W H 1970 Scale effects in animal joints. I. Articular cartilage thickness and compressive stress. Arthritis and Rheumatism 13: 244–255
Simon W H 1971 Scale effects in animal joints. 2. Thickness and elasticity in the deformability of articular cartilage. Arthritis and Rheumatism 14: 493–502
Simon W H, Friedenberg S, Richardson S 1973 Joint congruence. A correlation of joint congruence and thickness of articular cartilage in dogs. Journal of Bone and Joint Surgery 55-A: 1614–1620
Slavkin H C, Grenlich R C 1976 Extracellular matrix influence on gene expression. New York, Academic Press
Sokoloff L 1976 Articular chondrocytes in culture. Arthritis and Rheumatism 19: 426–429
Sokoloff L 1980 In vitro culture of joints and articular tissues. In: Sokoloff L (ed) The joints and synovial fluid, Vol II. New York, Academic Press, p 1–26
Sokoloff L, Malemud C J, Srivastava V M L, Morgan W D 1973 In vitro culture of articular chondrocytes. Federation Proceedings 4: 1499–1502
Stenzel K H, Miyata T, Rudin A L 1974 Collagen as a biomaterial. Annual Review of Biophysics and Bioengineering 3: 231–253
Stockwell R A 1967 The lipid and glycogen content of rabbit articular hyaline and non-articular hyaline cartilage. Journal of Anatomy 102: 87–94
Stockwell R A 1979 Biology of cartilage cells. London, Cambridge University Press, p 245–247
Stockwell R A, Sprinz R 1981 Glycosaminoglycan content and cell density of rabbit articular cartilage in experimental lipoarthrosis. Journal of Anatomy 133: 309–315
Swanson S A V 1973 Lubrication. In: Freeman M A R (ed) Adult articular cartilage, 1st Edn. London, Pitman Medical, p 247–276
Swanson S A V 1976 Design and testing of replacement prostheses. Proceedings of the Royal Society of London B 192: 173–189
Swanson S A V 1979 Friction, wear and lubrication. In: Freeman M A R (ed) Adult articular cartilage, 2nd Edn. Tunbridge Wells, Pitman Medical, p 415–460
Takeda T 1975 Three-dimensional observation of collagen framework of human lumbar discs. Japanese Journal of Orthopaedics 49: 45–57
Thompson A M, Stockwell R A 1983 An ultrastructural study of the marginal transitional zone in the rabbit knee joint. Journal of Anatomy 136: 701–713
Thompson D A W 1961 On growth and form. Bonnar J T (ed). Cambridge, University Press
Torrey T W, Feduccia A 1971 Morphogenesis of the Vertebrates. New York, Wiley
Trentham D E 1982 Collagen arthritis as a relevant model for rheumatoid arthritis — evidence pro and con. Arthritis and Rheumatism 25: 911–916

Tyler J A, Fell H B, Lawrence C E 1982 The effect of cortisol on porcine articular tissues in organ culture. Journal of Pathology 137: 335–351

Unsworth A, Dowson D, Wright V 1975 Some new evidence on human joint lubrication. Annals of the Rheumatic Diseases 34: 277–285

Urry D W 1983 What is elastin; What is not. Ultrastructural Pathology 4: 227–251

Vaughan J 1981 The physiology of bone, 3rd Edn. Oxford, Clarendon Press

Vaughan J 1984 The influence of bone cells on the formation, and mineralization, of bone matrix. Philosophical Transactions of the Royal Society of London B 304: 453–454

Venn M F 1978 Variation of chemical composition with age in human femoral head cartilage. Annals of the Rheumatic Diseases 37: 168–174

Venn M F, Maroudas A 1977 Chemical composition and swelling of normal and osteoarthrotic femoral head cartilage. I. Chemical composition. Annals of the Rheumatic Diseases 36: 121–129

Vogel H. 1973 Connective tissue and ageing. Amsterdam, Excerpta Medica

Wainwright S A, Biggs W D, Currey J D, Gosline J M 1976 Mechanical design in organisms. London, Edward Arnold

Walker P S, Hajek V J 1972 The load-bearing area in the knee joint. Journal of Biomechanics 5: 581–589

Walker P S, Dowson D, Longfield M D, Wright V 1968 'Boosted lubrication' in synovial joints by fluid entrapment and enrichment. Annals of the Rheumatic Diseases 27: 512–520

Walker P S, Sikorski J, Dowson D, Longfield M D, Wright V, Buckley T 1969 Behaviour of synovial fluid on surfaces of articular cartilage. A scanning electron microscope study. Annals of the Rheumatic Diseases 28: 1–14

Walker P S, Unsworth A, Dowson A, Sikorski J, Wright V 1970 Mode of aggregation of hyaluronic acid protein complex on the surface of articular cartilage. Annals of the Rheumatic Diseases 29: 591–602

Warwick R, Williams P L 1980 Gray's anatomy, 36th Edn. Edinburgh, Churchill Livingstone

Webster D, Webster M 1974 Comparative vertebrate morphology. New York, Academic Press

Weibkin O W, Muir H 1973 The inhibition of sulphate incorporation in isolated adult chondrocytes by hyaluronic acid. FEBS Letters 37: 42–46

Weibkin O W, Muir H 1975 Influence of the cells on the pericellular environment. The effect of hyaluronic acid on proteoglycan synthesis and secretion by chondrocytes of adult cartilage. Philosophical Transactions of the Royal Society of London B 271: 283–291

Weibkin O W, Hardingham T E, Muir H 1975 The interaction of proteoglycans and hyaluronic acid and the effect of hyaluronic acid on proteoglycan synthesis by chondrocytes of adult cartilage. In: Burleigh P M C, Poole A R (eds) Dynamics of connective tissue macromolecules. Amsterdam, North-Holland p 81–98

Weiss R E, Reddi A H, Nimni M E 1981 Somatostatin can locally inhibit proliferation and differentiation of cartilage and bone precursor cells. Calcified Tissue International 33: 425–430

Willmer E N 1970 Cells in tissue culture: mechanocytes. In: Cytology and evolution, 2nd Edn. New York, Academic Press, p 20–63

Wilsman N J 1978 Cilia of adult canine articular chondrocytes. Journal of Ultrastructure Research 64: 270–281

Yang J, Nandi S 1983 Growth of cultured cells using collagen as substrate. In: Bourne G H, Danielli J F, Jeon K W (eds) International review of cytology, Vol 81. New York, Academic Press, p 249–286

Young R D 1984 Journal of Cell Science (in press)

Young R D 1985 The ultrastructural organisation of protoeglycans and collagen in human and rabbit scleral matrix. Journal of Cell Science 74 (in press)

8

B. Vernon-Roberts

Synovial fluid and its examination

Since almost all types of articular disease tend to increase the volume of synovial fluid and since the synovial fluid is actually in contact with diseased articular tissues, it would not be unreasonable to hope that changes in the character of a synovial effusion often might reflect accurately the pathological process in the affected joint. Taking into account the full spectrum of joint disease, disappointingly, analysis of the fluid gives a precise diagnosis only in a limited number of conditions and usually provides but a dim reflection of events taking place in the joint. The clinician and pathologist need, therefore, to have a clear picture of what useful information may be obtained by examining the synovial fluid and of the limitations of this investigation.

In crystal induced arthritis and infective arthritis (particularly acute suppurative arthritis) synovial fluid examination utilising appropriate techniques allows a precise and positive diagnosis to be made. The suspicion that either of these conditions may be the cause of an undiagnosed arthritis remains much the most important indication for diagnostic arthrocentesis. Moreover, even in patients in whom a precise diagnosis appears to have been established, examination of the synovial fluid can play an important role in the diagnosis of complicating factors, such as a superimposed bacterial infection in rheumatoid arthritis, calcium pyrophosphate dihydrate crystals in osteoarthritis, or crystals of corticosteroid inducing synovitis following intra-articular injection. In other circumstances the examination of synovial fluid provides important, but not pathognomonic, evidence supporting other clinical and laboratory findings by indicating, for example, the presence within the aspirated joint of an 'inflammatory' or 'non-inflammatory' effusion. The synovial fluid may be used also as a source of cells, proteins, enzymes, immunoglobulins, complement, electrolytes, and other substances which can be measured and stuied in a variety of clinical and experimental settings.

While this chapter briefly reviews the formation and function of synovial fluid and outlines techniques for joint aspiration, its main purpose is to consider the constituents of the fluid with a particular emphasis on useful information which may be gained to assist in the diagnosis of joint disease.

COMPOSITION OF SYNOVIAL FLUID

Proteins

Normal synovial fluid has been characterised as a dialysate of plasma to which the protein component of the hyaluronate proteoglycan is added by local synthesis by the joint tissues. Proteins which diffuse into the fluid are present in lower (approximately one-third) concentrations than in plasma, and appear to be allowed to pass into the fluid selectively from plasma circulating in the small vessels of the synovial tissue. The present data indicate that the concentration of a given synovial fluid protein relative to its serum concentration depends upon its molecular size and the degree of inflammation present, in the absence of local production or consumption.

Most of the protein (60–75%) in synovial fluid is albumin, and the larger globulin molecules are present in relatively lower concentrations. Plasma proteins of high molecular weight or asymmetrical shape are present in small amounts or are absent from normal fluid. The cause of this selective retardation of large molecule flux into the synovial fluid may be due, in part, to hyaluronic acid in the interstitial tissue of the synovium acting as a molecular filter (Nettelbladt et al, 1963). Whatever the exact mechanism of exclusion of large molecules, because of their size, molecules such as α_2-macroglobulin, lipoproteins, fibrinogen and IgM are present only in small amounts in normal and 'non-inflammatory' synovial fluids. The low concentration of fibrinogen in such fluid explains the absence of clot formation. By contrast, when the synovium becomes inflamed, the protein content of the 'inflammatory' synovial fluid increases and the quantity of large molecular weight proteins is greater than in normal fluid (Kushner & Somerville, 1971) with fibrin clot formation resulting from the presence of significant amounts of fibrinogen.

In 'inflammatory' synovial fluids, the distribution and concentration of protein approaches that of serum, and all factors present in serum are present in the fluid (Schur & Sandson, 1963). In classic rheumatoid arthritis, IgM and IgG concentrations are higher than would be predicted purely on the basis of augmented vascular permeability (Kushner & Somerville, 1971), and this observation is consistent with local immunoglobulin synthesis in synovial tissue in rheumatoid arthritis (Smiley et al, 1968).

The ratio of concentration of non-immunoglobulin proteins, such as α_1-acid-glycoprotein, transferrin, caeruloplasmin and α_2-macroglobulin in synovial fluid to that of serum (SF/S) is directly related to the molecular weight (Kushner & Somerville, 1971). In rheumatoid synovial fluid a threefold increase in the concentration of α_1-acid-glycoprotein, transferrin and caeruloplasmin compares with a tenfold increase in α_2-macroglobulin (Kushner & Somerville, 1971). The SF/S ratios of these constituents in rheumatoid arthritis, osteoarthritis and gout have been reported to correlate well with the clinical findings and serum C-reactive protein concentration. The data of Kushner & Somerville (1971) are consistent with the conclusion that the transfer of plasma proteins to synovial fluid is related quantitatively to the size and shape of the particular molecule and the degree of inflammation. While this conclusion is justified for higher molecular weight proteins, it would appear that the mechanisms regulating the transfer of plasma proteins are insensitive to molecular weight changes below about 100 000.

The type and quantities of plasma proteins present in the synovial fluid may be influenced also by the modification or catabolism of proteins during transit from the circulation to the fluid via the synovial membrane. This mechanism could, for example, provide an explanation for reports of unexpectedly low concentrations of haptoglobin in synovial fluid (Niedermeier et al, 1965; Nettlebladt & Sunblad, 1965) and the variability in the concentration of other plasma glycoproteins (Sunblad, 1965).

While serum levels of total haemolytic complement are normal or elevated in patients with rheumatoid arthritis in the absence of systemic vasculitis, synovial fluid levels are relatively depressed when compared with those from patients with osteoarthritis or other forms of arthritis (Perkin & Zvaifler, 1964; Hedberg, 1967). Early studies claimed that synovial fluid complement levels correlate closely with the concentration of total protein in the fluid, and that low synovial fluid complement or rheumatoid factor, or both, is associated with more severe disease and probable worse prognosis in rheumatoid arthritis (Bunch et al, 1974b). However, while subsequent studies have found that low levels of complement activity are found more frequently in the synovial fluid of patients with rheumatoid arthritis, low levels also may occur in patients with systemic lupus erythematosus, psoriatic arthritis and septic arthritis (Bunch et al, 1974b; Fostiropoulos et al, 1965, Pekin & Zvaifler, 1970; Sheppheard et al, 1981). Low complement levels have been found also in some patients with gout and pseudogout (Townes & Sowa, 1970). The relationship between synovial fluid complement activity and clinical joint activity, synovial fluid leucocyte counts, and synovial fluid protein concentration claimed in a number of publications has been challenged recently in studies showing that the measurement of total haemolytic complement in synovial fluid is of limited value in determining the diagnosis or prognosis in joint disease (Sheppheard et al, 1981). Moreover, while there is evidence that various forms of drug therapy in rheumatoid arthritis do not affect the level of synovial fluid complement (Pekin & Zvaifler, 1970; Shepphеard et al, 1981), there are conflicting reports as to the influence of gold salts on synovial fluid complement (Hedberg, 1967; Pritchard & Nuki, 1978).

The early reports that complement levels were lowered in the synovial fluid in rheumatoid arthritis, and the finding that rheumatoid synovial fluid complement levels (CH50, Clq and β1A) were inversely related to the amount of IgG immune complex-like material in the joint (Winchester et al, 1969), were consistent with the view that the lowered complement level in the fluid was due to local consumption by immune complexes formed by interaction between IgG and rheumatoid factor of IgG type within the joint. There is evidence also that alternative pathways in addition to the classic pathway may be activated intra-articularly in rheumatoid arthritis (Ruddy et al, 1975). Whether the activation of different pathways in seropositive rheumatoid arthritis reflects a separate initiating event, mediated by immune complexes of a particular immunoglobulin chain or by tissue products released at the height of the inflammatory response, or whether it is somehow linked directly to the intense activation of the classic pathway, is unknown.

The interpretation of complement levels in synovial fluid is made more complex by the knowledge that rheumatoid synovial tissue also synthesises certain of the components (C2, C3, C4 and C5) of the complement system (Ruddy & Colten, 1974).

In systemic lupus erythematosus, lowered synovial fluid complement levels may be a reflection of lowered serum levels; but the synovial fluid levels may also be lowered when serum levels are normal (Bunch et al, 1974), in which case local consumption by immune complexes presumably is the explanation. A number of factors, some of them non-immunological, may contribute to the lowered synovial fluid complement levels which may be observed in septic arthritis.

Synovial fluids contain DNA and DNA–protein complexes as well as immunoglobulins, antiglobulins, and antinuclear antibodies (Cracchiolo et al, 1971; Robitaille et al, 1973). The highest levels of DNA in synovial fluids have been found in seropositive rheumatoid arthritis, gout and pseudogout, with very low levels present in osteoarthritis and post-traumatic arthritis (Leon et al, 1981). Serial determinations of DNA and other criteria of disease activity (leucocytes and protein levels in synovial fluid, blood sedimentation rate) in individual patients have suggested a strong correlation of elevated levels of synovial fluid DNA with active episodes of arthritis (Leon et al, 1981), indicating that these parameters reflect tissue damage.

Hyaluronic acid

The characteristic sticky and viscous nature of synovial fluid is due largely to the presence of hyaluronate, a glycosaminoglycan, synthesised by the type-B synoviocytes. Hyaluronate consists of long chains of repeating disaccharide units. About 2500 of these units are linked covalently with a protein (probably also synthesised by the type-B synoviocytes) to form very large proteoglycan molecules with molecular weights exceeding one million. Kinked and coiled, these long molecules take up an overall globular shape about 4000 Å in diameter. When the proteoglycan is coagulated in the mucin test, the remaining fluid has a viscosity similar to that of water.

The viscosity of synovial fluid is known to be non-Newtonian, that is, it decreases with increasing shear rates. Viscosity measurements on synovial fluid give values in the range 4000–8000 ml/g for normal fluids and 3000–6000 ml/g for rheumatoid fluids (Balazs et al, 1967). It is assumed usually that the decrease in viscosity observed during the purification of hyaluronic acid and the lower values in rheumatoid synovial fluid is due to a depolymerisation (i.e. a decrease in the length of the chain), but there is little evidence to indicate that the viscosity drop is caused solely by a decrease in length (Swann, 1978). There are, on the other hand, considerable data to indicate that the polysaccharide chains can interact with other matrix constituents and occur in solution in ordered arrangements. On this basis, it appears entirely possible that the macromolecular hyaluronic acid present in synovial fluid with an apparent molecular weight of about 10^7 is not composed of linear polysaccharide chains but instead contains linear structures organised via specific interactions to form macromolecular complexes (Swann, 1978).

According to Swann (1978), an additional factor that probably contributes to the viscosity of synovial fluid in vivo is dispersed collagen fibres. Electron microscopic studies have detected the presence of collagen fibres in hyaluronic acid from synovial fluid (Swann et al, 1975). The fibres were too few to be detected by chemical means and were incompletely removed by filtration and centrifugation. It was found that treatment of the hyaluronic acid preparations with collagenase caused a decrease in the intrinsic viscosity.

The results of frictional measurements in entire joints point to the operation of boundary lubrication by adsorbed hyaluronate-protein, perhaps combined with fluid film lubrication by a fluid having a viscosity orders of magnitude higher than that of synovial fluid (Swann, 1978). Hyaluronate-protein can be adsorbed by articular cartilage, and, independent of the adsorption process, filtration of synovial fluid by cartilage can produce very rapidly a concentrate on the cartilage surface in the loaded region. While the work of Radin et al (1970) indicated that protein alone is responsible for the lubricating ability of synovial fluid, this does not invalidate completely the role of hyaluronate-protein since this is capable of lubricating to the same degree as protein alone (Swann, 1978). In this respect, it is possible that the principal lubricating function of the hyaluronate-protein in synovial fluid is that of protecting the cartilage surfaces against wear, and not the reduction of friction.

Glycoproteins

The specificity of the boundary-lubricating effect of synovial fluid, the failure of plasma proteins to inhibit lubrication, and the data available concerning the structure of hyaluronic acid, suggest that other constituent proteins endow synovial fluid with its boundary-lubricating properties. Supporting evidence for the latter arises from studies indicating that high molecular weight glycoprotein constituents are responsible largely for the lubricating activity of synovial fluid, and that the lubricating properties are associated with two distinct glycoproteins (LGP-1 and LGP-2) and a small amount of protein similar to γ-globulin (Swann & Radin, 1972; Swann, 1978). In particular, the LGP-1 constituent appears to possess characteristics which are well suited to a postulated unique role as an articular lubricant.

Fibronectins are a class of high molecular weight glycoproteins having affinity for both native and denatured forms of collagen, fibrinogen or fibrin, glycosaminoglycans, and collagen. It has been found that fibronectin levels are significantly higher in synovial fluids from patients with rheumatoid arthritis than with other forms of arthritis, and exceed those of plasma (Carsons et al, 1981; Scott et al, 1981; Clemmensen & Andersen, 1982). Synovial fluid fibronectin concentration may correlate directly with synovial leucocyte counts (Carsons et al, 1981), and the presence of degraded fibronectin in rheumatoid fluids suggests degradation of fibrin-fibronectin complexes or the destruction of matrix fibronectin from the synovial tissue (Clemmensen & Andersen, 1982). While the exact function of fibronectins is unknown, it has been suggested that they have an important structural and functional role in the organisation and repair of inflamed intra-articular structures (Scott et al, 1981), and it has been postulated that they may be concerned also as opsonising factors in the disposal of fibrin and collagen, and their degradation products, by the mononuclear phagocyte (reticuloendothelial) system.

Glucose, lactate, P_{O_2}, P_{CO_2} and pH

Electrolytes are distributed in concentrations according to Donnan's equilibrium theory with substances such as urea, amino acids and uric acid, diffusing freely from plasma into the synovial fluid (Simkin &Pizzorno, 1974). However, those cations which are bound significantly to protein are present in lower concentrations consistent with the lower concentrations of proteins in synovial fluid relative to plasma.

In normal synovial fluid, glucose is present in approximately the same concentration as in plasma. However, glucose enters the joint more rapidly than predicted from its diffusion coefficient (Simkin & Pizzorno, 1974) indicating facilitated diffusion or active transport into the joint cavity. The concentration of glucose in non-inflammatory joint diseases such as osteoarthrosis, post-traumatic arthritis and neuropathic joints is essentially normal, averaging less than 10 mg below that of the serum. In rheumatoid arthritis, septic arthritis and Reiter's disease the average glucose concentration is not uncommonly reduced by more than 10 mg below the serum level. There is frequently a very marked reduction below serum levels in cases of established septic arthritis and in rheumatoid effusions which have been present for more than one year (Ropes & Bauer, 1953). Thus, while a low or zero glucose level is not necessarily evidence of bacterial invasion, this should be excluded even in known cases of rheumatoid arthritis. In rheumatoid arthritis without infection, persistently low glucose levels are an indication of severe or long-continued disease. To explain low levels of glucose in inflammation or sepsis, it is necessary to postulate impaired delivery to the joint and increased utilisation by synovial components.

It has been reported that there is an inverse relationship between synovial fluid glucose and lactate levels (Ropes & Bauer, 1953). This may be explained by the knowledge that glucose diffuses into cells and is phosphorylated, which prevents it from diffusing out again until it is metabolised to pyruvate. Pyruvate is converted into lactate which diffuses out of the cells. In this connection, the very low synovial fluid P_{O_2} (below 30 mmHg) which has been observed in patients with rheumatoid arthritis and other forms of inflammatory arthritis is accompanied by a sharp rise in P_{CO_2} and lactate and a fall in pH (Lund-Olesen, 1970; Falchuk et al, 1970; Treuhaft & McCarty, 1971). The good correlation between lactate and both pH and P_{O_2} suggests that anaerobic glycolysis by an anaerobic synovium may be the most important underlying factor (Richman et al, 1981). These synovial fluid changes signify that the local tissue metabolism switches from predominantly aerobic to largely anaerobic (glycolytic) processes during inflammatory joint disease. Since the hypoxic changes in the synovial fluid occur in the absence of evidence of concomitant hypoxia or acidosis in the blood (Richman et al, 1981), intra-articular hypoxia most likely represents some form of circulatory imbalance at the level of the synovial membrane with the volume of synovial effusion and the compliance of the joint capsule probably being important determinants of the articular blood supply (Richman et al, 1981).

While correlation between P_{O_2} and synovial leucocyte counts has been reported to be poor in a study not including patients with septic arthritis (Richman et al, 1981), recent studies have suggested that lactic acid measurement is a useful and rapid test for differentiating between septic and non-septic arthritis, being markedly raised in septic joints (Brook et al, 1978; Riordan et al, 1982).

Studies of normal synovial fluid pH have shown slight variations in mean values in various studies resulting in an overall mean of about 7.4 (all studies) and a range (all studies) between 6.5 and 8.9 (Ropes et al, 1940; Jebens & Monk-Jones, 1959; Cummings & Nordby, 1966; Goldie & Nachemson, 1969). Under normal conditions synovial fluid and blood pH are only slightly different, whereas with systemic acidosis there is an associated synovial fluid acidosis (Joseph et al, 1946). The synovial fluid acidosis which has been observed in rheumatoid arthritis and other inflammatory conditions is not associated normally with clinical or electrolytic evidence of systemic acidosis, and more acid synovial fluid pH is associated with other evidence (cell count, acute phase proteins) or a greater degree of inflammatory activity in rheumatoid joints (Ward & Steigbigel, 1978; Farr et al, 1981).

Lipids

Normal human synovial fluid contains small amounts of phospholipids and cholesterol (Bole, 1962). Substantial amounts of cholesterol, phospholipids and triglyceride may be found in the synovial fluid of rheumatoid and osteoarthritic patients to the extent that total lipids equal 40–60% of serum concentration (Bole, 1962; Chung et al, 1962; Small et al, 1964). While findings in a rheumatoid patient having a chylous effusion have provided evidence for local cholesterol biosynthesis within the joint (Newcombe & Cohen, 1965), it is probable that the increased lipid levels in most effusions are derived chiefly from plasma. The cells in synovial effusions contain less than 10% of the total lipid (Bole, 1962) and no correlation has been shown to exist between lipid concentration and total cell count in synovial fluid.

Enzymes and enzyme inhibitors

Enzymes of lysosomal origin are present in very low concentrations in the cell-free supernatants of synovial fluids from normal joints or non-inflammatory joint diseases, such as osteoarthritis and traumatic arthritis. With increasing degrees of articular inflammation, there is a corresponding increase in the various enzymes. The effusions of rheumatoid arthritis and septic arthritis have the highest concentrations of lysosomal enzymes, and consistently smaller amounts are found in other inflammatory, non-rheumatoid joint diseases such as gout, psoriatic arthritis, and the arthritis of ankylosing spondylitis.

The majority of lysosomal enzymes are derived from neutrophil polymorphs by virtue of the dominant numbers and short lifespan of these cells in inflammatory effusions. The half-life of neutrophils in synovial fluid is only a few hours, and it has been estimated that in an average 30 ml rheumatoid effusion containing 25 × 10 neutrophils/mm^3, the daily breakdown in the synovial cavity may exceed one billion cells (Hollingsworth et al, 1967). This is associated with the release of great quantities of granule enzyme activities. Among enzymes of lysosomal origin which have been identified in synovial fluid are acid phosphatases, β-glucuronidase, muramidase (lysozyme), β-acetylglucasaminase, β-galactosidase, lactoferrin, myeloperoxidase, elastase, cathepsin C_T (cationic protein), arylsulphatase and collagenase. Of interest is the fact that collagenase has been shown to be located in specific granules of neutrophils (together with muramidase) and not in the azurophil granules which contain lysosomal hydrolases and neutral proteinases (Murphy et al, 1977).

Nonlysosomal (cytoplasmic) enzymes may be present in large amounts in synovial fluid. Thus lactic dehydrogenase has been studied extensively, and catalase activity has been shown to be roughly proportional to the total white cell count in various joint diseases.

Alkaline phosphatase occurs free in the synovial fluid and its concentration and isozyme pattern parallels serum levels (Lemperg et al, 1971).

While hyaluronidase is present in synovial fluid, and presumably plays a role in the initial cleaving of hyaluronic acid, current evidence indicates that synovial fluid hyaluronidase is produced extra-articularly and, like alkaline phosphatase, diffuses freely into the joint from the blood (Stephens et al, 1975).

While there is an abundant literature proposing important roles for synovial fluid enzymes in cartilage matrix degradation, it is unlikely that lysosomal enzymes in solution in the synovial fluid in vivo are primarily involved in cartilage destruction despite in vitro studies supporting such concepts. Thus, a recent study has shown that the amounts of various neutrophil lysosomal enzymes have a negative correlation with the degree of radiographic destruction of the joint from which the fluid was obtained (Hadler et al, 1979). The explanation for this important observation comes from a subsequent study (Hadler et al, 1981) which showed that protease inhibitors (α_1-antitrypsin, α_1-antichymotrypsin, α_2-macroglobulin, inter-α-trypsin inhibitor and C1 esterase inhibitor) correlate positively with the total protein in synovial fluid as well as the number of granulocytes and the concentration of granulocyte lysosomal enzymes in the fluid. As did the lysosomal enzymes, the protease inhibitors correlated negatively with radiographic destruction. While the findings in those studies indicate that the lysosomal enzymes in solution in inflammatory synovial fluid are rendered effete by the presence of protease inhibitors (Hadler et al, 1981), it is the case that some enzyme–inhibitor complexes can still hydrolyse low molecular weight substrates. However, in order to function to bind and inhibit a protease, most inhibitors are first substrates of the protease which they inhibit (James & Cohen, 1978), and the possibility exists also that other inactivators of enzymes inhibitors exist in inflammatory joint disease. Nevertheless, the weight of current evidence tells against synovial fluid enzymes playing a significant role in cartilage degradation.

An enzyme present in synovial fluid which has assumed major importance in recent years is superoxide dismutase. Superoxide dismutase, and catalase, appear to be capable of scavenging superoxide free radicals (O_2^-) produced by phagocytic leucocytes during the respiratory burst which follows exposure to soluble stimuli (including immune complexes and/or complement components) or during injection of particulate matter (including bacteria or crystals) (Dormandy, 1979; McCord & Wong, 1979; Greenwald, 1981). There is evidence that the free radicals play a role in initiating inflammation, damaging tissue and in degrading hyaluronic acid, and that superoxide dismutase plays a protective role by scavenging phagocyte-produced superoxide and preventing the production of neutrophil chemotactic factor (Petrone et al, 1980). A recent study has reported that superoxide dismutase activity in the synovial fluid of patients with rheumatoid arthritis was raised markedly when compared with osteoarthritis and was correlated significantly with C-reactive protein (Igari et al, 1982). These findings call into question, therefore, the pathological significance of superoxide production in inflammatory synovial fluids.

Kinins have been demonstrated in the synovial fluids of the knee joints of patients regardless of the aetiology of their arthritis (Melmon et al, 1967). Their importance relates to the ability of kinins to produce vasodilatation, increased capillary permeability, contraction of smooth muscle and pain. The possible role of kinins and related factors in relation to the activity of immune complexes was reviewed by Zvaifler (1973) who considered that discrepancies in various reports precluded definite conclusions being made at that time.

Trace metals

It has been reported, from a study of synovial fluids from 33 subjects without evidence of arthritis (post-mortem) and 13 patients with rheumatoid arthritis, that copper, iron, aluminium, rubidium, lithium and strontium were present in all fluids; barium, silver, manganese and caesium were present inconstantly in both groups; and nickel was not detected in any sample (Niedermeier et al, 1962). The study showed also that the synovial fluid of patients with rheumatoid arthritis contained increased concentrations of copper, iron and aluminium. The elevation of synovial fluid copper accompanied by a rise in caeruloplasmin has been stated to be characteristic of rheumatoid effusions (Scudder et al, 1978), and supports the concept of an abnormal copper and caeruloplasmin metabolism in rheumatoid arthritis.

Zinc, which is present in both normal and rheumatoid synovial fluids, is increased in the effusions of patients with rheumatoid arthritis despite normal serum zinc concentrations and increased urinary zinc excretion (Bonebrake et al, 1972). The increased synovial fluid zinc concentration appeared to correlate with increasing total leucocyte counts in the synovial fluid, but not with disease duration, rheumatoid factor titre, or synovial fluid mucin clot test (Bonebrake et al, 1972).

Cells

Normal synovial fluid contains very few cells, but the numbers are increased markedly in various diseases (see section below on synovial fluid analysis). Apart from occasional cells which are derived locally (synovial lining cells and chondrocytes), the cells which form the major solid constituents of synovial fluid under normal and pathological circumstances (lymphocytes, mononuclear phagocytes and neutrophil polymorphs) appear to be derived from the blood stream. There is an absence of significant information concerning the kinetics of cells in synovial fluid in normal and pathological circumstances.

FORMATION AND REMOVAL

The wide variation in the normal concentration of constituents probably is due to a number of factors such as the natural variability of biological systems, location of the joint, activity of movement of the joint, and factors which influence the composition of the blood and vascular permeability. Additional factors which may contribute to the variability in constituents of synovial fluid derived from plasma are the structure of the synovial vasculature and the surrounding connective tissue matrix. The synovial tissues have a rich blood supply. The capillaries have a fenestrated structure (Suter & Majno, 1964), and, while the cells lining the synovium have desmosome-like intercellular junctions (Groth, 1975) they do not form a continuous barrier and a basement membrane is absent. Thus, in places the ground substance of the synovial tissues is in contact with the articular cavity containing the synovial fluid. This structural arrangement suggests that the extravascular extracellular matrix of synovial tissue may play a regulating role in the transfer of substances between the blood and synovial fluid. Evidence supporting this concept was obtained by Nettelbladt et al (1963) who showed that sedimentation of plasma through hyaluronic acid produced an ultrafiltrate having a composition similar to that of normal synovial fluid.

The composition of synovial fluid probably is influenced to some extent by the outflow of constituents via the lymphatics. Early studies of the passage of intra-articularly injected plasma proteins have shown that albumin is detectable rapidly in lymph but globulins are not detectable (Bauer et 1933). Moreover, removal to local lymph nodes of colloids and fine particulate matter with particle sizes larger than that of serum globulin (Adkins & Davies, 1940), demonstrated that the differences in lymphatic removal of proteins is not related to molecular size.

The differential removal of plasma proteins via lymphatics differs from the transfer of intra-articularly injected albumin and globulin to the peripheral blood since they are absorbed from the joint space with little difference in rate (Rodnan & McLachlan, 1960). However, when IgG is reduced and heat aggregated its removal from both rheumatoid and osteoarthritic joints is enhanced (Sliwinsky & Zvaifler, 1969).

In summary, therefore, current evidence suggests that most large molecules appear to leave the joints at equivalent rates, unlike the rate at which they enter the joint cavity which is inversely proportional to molecular weight. There is evidence, however, which indicates that the clearance mechanism may be inadequate in inflamed joints. Synovial blood flow, which must have an important role in the rate of exchange of molecules, has been reported to be increased in inflamed joints in studies utilising the clearance of ^{133}Xe (Dick et al, 1970; Porter et al, 1970; Goetzl et al, 1971). The interpretation of those studies has been questioned in a critical analysis of the ^{133}Xe clearance technique (Phelps et al, 1972) in a study which suggested also that the increased intra-articular pressure associated with effusion (Jayson & Dixon, 1970a, b) can reduce synovial blood flow by a tampon effect on synovial microvasculature.

The cells lining the synovium, particularly the macrophage-like type A cells, ingest debris presented at the cell–synovial fluid interface. Normal synovial fluid contains small amounts of soluble and particulate constituents derived from the cells present in the fluid, but the amounts of cell debris arising from the death of neutrophil polymorphs may be very large in inflammatory fluids of rheumatoid arthritis, crystal-induced arthritis and septic arthritis. In normal and diseased joints the lining cells may play a minor role in removing non-cellular proteins from the synovial fluid, but the type A synoviocytes of rheumatoid joints can contain appreciable amounts of immune complexes and complement components due to the possession by these cells of specific receptors for IgG Fc and C3 (Theofilopoulos et al, 1980; Dayer et al, 1980).

INTRA-ARTICULAR PRESSURE

The intra-articular pressure of the normal knee is a negative one when compared with ambient atmospheric pressure, and becomes markedly negative with quadriceps contraction (Levick, 1979). In the presence of an effusion, the normal fall in intra-articular pressure is absent, or with larger effusions, reversed, so that a positive pressure results (Jayson & Dixon, 1970c). In the presence of effusion, the intra-articular pressure is least at about 30° of flexion (Jayson & Dixon, 1970c; Eyring & Murray, 1964). Further flexion or quadriceps contraction produces very high pressures which can lead to the rupture of the joint capsule, and may be associated with the presence of unusual bone cysts ('geodes') around the rheumatoid knee (Jayson & Dixon, 1970d; Jayson & Dixon, 1972). The extravasation of synovial fluid into the calf following rupture of the joint capsule can produce a condition resembling thrombophlebitis but can be distinguished from the latter condition by arthrography (Hall & Scott, 1966). There is some evidence that a one-way valve system operates between the knee joint cavity and popliteal or calf cysts (Genovese et al, 1972).

SYNOVIAL FLUID ANALYSIS

Technique of joint aspiration (arthrocentesis)

While the risk of introducing infection is low, aspiration of a joint should be carried out only when adequate precautions to ensure sterility are taken. Using disposable sterile equipment and a strict 'no touch' technique, it is permissible to carry out joint aspiration as an 'office' procedure in the case of an operator experienced in the technique of arthrocentesis and performing a straightforward aspiration with appropriate equipment.

After removal of sufficient clothing to provide adequate access to the joint, the joint in question is examined to confirm the presence of the effusion and to determine the point of entry of the needle. The planned point of entry can be marked with firm pressure from the end of a ball-point pen with the top retarded. The area to be aspirated should be examined carefully to exclude cellulitis or periarticular infection which could allow infection to be introduced into the joint during insertion of the needle. The points of entry into various joints can be selected as described by Miller (1956, 1957) and Owen (1981) (see also Chapter 67).

Much the most common source of synovial fluid for examination is the knee, and a detailed description of the technique for aspiration of this joint has been given by Currey & Vernon-Roberts (1976). Small articulations, such as the finger joints, are more difficult and require very careful technique if discomfort for the patient is to be avoided. However, any joint in which an effusion is clinically detectable usually is relatively easy to aspirate. The length to which the operator should go in attempting to obtain a sample of synovial fluid depends on the indications for arthrocentesis. Thus, if a diagnosis of septic arthritis is entertained, it is obligatory to obtain a specimen of synovial fluid for microbiological examination. Similarly, in order to be able to confirm or refute a diagnosis of crystal-induced arthritis, the obtaining of a sample is strongly indicated. In such circumstances, a firm diagnosis may be obtained from the examination of a very small sample. Thus, even in the case of an apparently unsuccessful 'dry tap', the contents of the needle may be sufficient to provide useful information if taken straight to the laboratory since one drop can be used for the examination for crystals, Gram stain, or culture.

Having ensured that the appropriate syringes, needles, specimen containers, microscope slides, culture media, injection material, and other items which may be required during the procedure, are available, the operator 'scrubs'. Gloves and drapes are not required providing the needle or the area to be aspirated is not touched. A wide area of skin is cleaned thoroughly (chlorhexidine 1% in 70% ethanol, pHisoHex, or iodine). When aspiration is likely to be a straightforward procedure undertaken by an experienced operator, there is little need for anaesthesia since deft penetration into a greatly distended knee joint cavity is relatively painless. Some operators prefer to spray the skin with ethyl chloride at the point of entry. In other circumstances it may be necessary to infiltrate the skin to the synovial lining with a small quantity of 1 or 2% local anaesthetic solution without adrenalin. A fine (25 gauge) needle is used. In children, it may be necessary to use general anaesthesia. The fluid present in almost all synovial effusion will pass readily through a 21 or a 20 gauge needle, and the use of a wide bore needle or high negative pressure seldom yields more fluid. Obstruction to the outflow of fluid, either by fronds of synovium, clumps of fibrin, or rice bodies, is overcome by gentle rotation and manipulation of the needle during aspiration.

It is usually the case that as much synovial fluid as can be obtained readily is aspirated regardless of the amount needed for diagostic purposes. However, perseverance in attempting to empty a joint can be traumatic and produce bleeding. After aspiration is completed, any substance to be injected into the joint is instilled by attaching a separate syringe to the aspiration needle. No special precautions are required following aspiration, and haemarthrosis is very rare.

SAMPLES REQUIRED FOR LABORATORY EXAMINATION

The type of laboratory investigation to be carried out depends on the indications for arthrocentesis and the diagnostic information sought. However, in general, three types of sample are useful (Currey & Vernon-Roberts, 1976):

1. A small sample (4 ml) into a sequestrin (EDTA, Versenate) tube as used for routine peripheral blood counts. This can be used for a total and differential cell count. Because of the viscosity of synovial fluid, care has to be taken in order to obtain dissolution of the anticoagulant before clotting starts.

2. Specimens placed in standard (20 ml) sterile, screw-top containers are suitable for microbiological investigation and for crystal examination. In the absence of a sterile container the fluid can be sent to the laboratory in the aspirating syringe. It goes without saying that specimens for microbiology should be sent to the laboratory immediately. By contrast, examination for crystals is usually perfectly satisfactory when performed on specimens even a few days old (provided the fluid remains sterile). Sending such specimens through the mail is thus feasible.

3. Specimens placed in standard (10 ml) heparin tubes and mixed immediately and thoroughly with the anticoagulant are suitable for all investigations in which it is necessary to separate cells and fluid. This applies to all biochemical and immunological tests, including complement determinations. In addition, the cells in these specimens can be used in investigations requiring live cells such as the LE cell test and more elaborate cell function tests.

Cells in the synovial fluid alter the chemical composition of the fluid both by their continuing active metabolism and also by breaking down to release their contents. Centrifugation should therefore not be delayed. In the case of complement determinations the timing is absolutely critical; such specimens require immediate centrifugation, after which the cell-free fluid is stored at –20° C (or colder) until examined.

As has been mentioned above, even in the case of an apparently 'dry tap', a drop of fluid in the lumen of the needle may be sufficient to identify an infecting organism or microcrystals of urate or pyrophosphate.

Volume

There is little correlation between the volume of an effusion and the aetiology, severity or duration of joint disease. Low volume does not imply the absence of an important intra-articular process. However, in inflammatory conditions, the amount of fluid present in the affected joints is generally at a maximum when signs of inflammation are at their height, and decreases as inflammation wanes. The normal knee joint contains 0.1–4.0 ml of fluid (Currey & Vernon-Roberts, 1976). The maximum amount which may be obtained from a diseased knee joint during any one aspiration varies markedly up to a maximum of about 250 ml.

Gross appearances

The gross appearances (summarised in Table 8.1.) can supply important diagnostic information.

Normal fluid is clear, pale yellow, highly viscous, and does not clot on standing.

In *osteoarthritis*, the fluid usually is increased in amount but retains its normal colour, clarity and high viscosity. Occasionally, the viscosity is reduced markedly in the absence of an increase in cellularity.

In *rheumatoid arthritis and other inflammatory arthropathies* the volume of fluid is increased, is cloudy due to its increased cellularity and may

Table 8.1 Gross appearance of synovial fluid (data from various sources)

	Opacity	Colour	Viscosity	Spontaneous clot
Normal	Clear	Pale yellow	High	Absent
Osteoarthritis	Clear	Pale yellow	High–low	Absent
Rheumatoid arthritis	Cloudy	Yellow–greenish	Low	Present
Systemic lupus erythematosus	Clear–cloudy	Yellow	Medium–High	Possible
Reiter's disease	Clear–cloudy	Yellow–greenish	Low	Present
Gout	Cloudy–purulent	Greenish–white	Low–turbid	Present
Pseudogout	Clear–cloudy	Yellow–greenish	High–low	Possible
Apatite arthropathy	Clear–cloudy	Yellow–white	High–low	Possible
Septic arthritis	Cloudy–purulent	Greenish–white	Low–turbid	Possible
Viral arthritis	Clear–purulent	Yellow–greenish	Low–turbid	Possible
Post-traumatic	Clear–bloody	Amber–bloody	High–low	Possible

have a greenish hue, the viscosity is reduced so that often it is watery in consistency, and may clot spontaneously on standing due to a high fibrinogen content.

In *acute episodes of gout and pseudogout* the fluid may be purulent in appearance due to its high cell content, it may be quite turbid, it may have a greenish hue or may be milky white if many urate crystals are present, and spontaneous clot formation is common. In the intervals between acute episodes, the fluid may be clear or cloudy depending upon its cellularity, the viscosity usually is reduced, and clot formation is variable.

In *septic arthritis* the fluid usually is frankly purulent in the established condition, but can be difficult to distinguish from an inflammatory arthropathy or crystal arthritis in the early stage when the cell count may be moderately increased and the viscosity is reduced.

In *post-traumatic* effusions, the fluid varies in appearance according to the amount and duration of haemorrhage, and the interval between bleeding and aspiration. Thus, the fluid may vary between faint pink to frank blood during or after recent bleeding, or may be yellow to amber according to the degree of xanthochromia if some period of time has elapsed since bleeding occurred.

In *ochronosis* the fluid may be speckled with dark patches like ground pepper (Hunter et al, 1974).

Following *arthroplasty*, the presence of metal or plastic wear material may discolour the fluid black or grey (Kitridou et al, 1969).

Slight or marked bleeding into the fluid occasionally may result from trauma during the aspiration procedure. It is important for the operator to record whether the blood-staining was mixed homogenously with the fluid throughout the aspiration, or occurred after non-blood-stained fluid initially had been aspirated.

Rice bodies

Rice bodies, so named because of their resemblance to polished white rice, may be seen in synovial fluid from various types of inflammatory arthritis including both juvenile and adult forms of rheumatoid arthritis (Berg et al, 1977; Wynne-Roberts & Cassidy, 1979), septic arthritis, and tuberculosis (Riese, 1895). They may be present in up to approximately one-quarter of inflamed joints (Berg et al, 1977). They consist primarily of fibrin and collagen, and their morphological and biochemical characteristics indicate a former connection and origin from the synovial membrane (Berg et al, 1977; Cheung et al, 1980).

The mucin clot test

Extensive studies were carried out on the concentration of 'mucin' in the synovial fluid by Ropes and Bauer (1953) who classified the types of mucin precipitate after the additon of acetic acid to the fluid. These authors described the following four types of precipitate seen in this 'mucin test':

1. A tight ropy clump of precipitate in an otherwise clear solution was seen in normals, oedema, post-traumatic arthritis of some duration, osteoarthrosis, rheumatic fever and intermittent hydrarthrosis.
2. A soft mass in a very slightly cloudy solution was seen in rheumatoid arthritis, ulcerative colitis, traumatic arthritis with haemorrhage and villonodular synovitis.
3. Small friable masses in a cloudy solution were seen in rheumatoid arthritis, gout, haemophilia, Reiter's disease, and septic arthritis.
4. Few or no flecks in a cloudy solution were seen in all types of inflammatory joint disease.

In individual diseases, Ropes & Bauer (1953) found wide variations in the precipitating characteristics of fluids and the chemical basis and significance of the phenomenon is uncertain.

It is generally known that the mucin test gives only rough clues and does not have significant advantages over a visual assessment of the relative viscosity of synovial fluid as the aspirated fluid is expressed from the syringe. The mucin test and viscosity are not a reliable basis for the classification of the pathogenesis of effusions.

Total cell counts

Freshly aspirated fluid should be placed in a suitable container having heparin or potassium EDTA as anticoagulant and mixed thoroughly. In the case of potassium EDTA it is essential that the appropriate volume of synovial fluid be added to the anticoagulant since, if too little fluid is added, intracellular crystal formation may occur (Currey & Vernon-Roberts, 1976). While it is desirable that total and differential cell counts be carried out within 24 hours of aspiration, it has been found that storage of anticoagulated fluid at 4°C ensures that there is no marked reduction in the total cell count for up to 3 days and differential cell counts are not rendered difficult. After 3 days of storage at 4°C or 24 hours at room temperature, there is rapid degeneration and breakdown of neutrophil polymorphs.

Assessment of the total leucocyte count is an important part of synovial fluid analysis. While it frequently is used as the basis of the classification of effusions into 'inflammatory' or 'non-inflammatory' types, there is a wide overlap in the ranges of total leucocyte counts in different disease categories (Table 8.2). Thus, the total cell count alone cannot be relied upon to exclude or confirm a diagnosis of septic arthritis. In sequential samples aspirated from the same joint, the total cell count may be taken to reflect the changing intensity of inflammation.

Total cell counts are made by examining a sample of anticoagulated fluid in a haemocytometer counting chamber; unless the cell count is very high (over 50 000 cells/mm^3) it is not necessary to dilute the fluid before counting, and even the most viscous fluids will spread evenly in the chamber. The rate at which the cells settle on the lower (grid) surface of the chamber is largely determined by the viscosity of the fluid, and highly viscous fluids may require to stand for over 30 minutes before the cells can be easily counted. Since the cells do settle on standing, even in highly viscous fluids, it is essential that the fluid should be very thoroughly agitated before being added to the counting chamber; this is simply and rapidly achieved using a bench vibratory mixer. Tilting or shaking the specimen tube by hand does not achieve satisfactory mixing.

When the total number of nucleated leucocytes is being assessed, it is important that they should be distinguishable from the non-nucleated erythrocytes which usually are present in appreciable numbers even in the absence of a history of trauma at the time of, or before, aspiration. The distinction between nucleated leucocytes and non-nucleated erythrocytes is easily achieved using phase-contrast examination of unstained cells, but large errors may arise if phase-contrast is not used. Alternatively, 0.3% saline may be used to lyse the erythrocytes (Hollander et al, 1961). For standard light microscopy, the addition of methylene blue can aid the recognition of nucleated cells.

When dilution of fluid is necessary, normal saline is used since the routine diluents (e.g. acetic acid) cause precipitation of mucin.

The average total cell count, together with minima and maxima, encountered in various conditions are listed in Table 8.2.

Normal fluid contains less than 750 leucocytes/mm^3 with an average count of about 150 leucocytes/mm^3. In *osteoarthritis* the total cell count seldom differs from the normal but may rise to 2000 leucocytes/mm^3 with an average of 500 leucocytes/mm^3. In *rheumatoid arthritis* the total cell count commonly is raised above 3000 leucocytes/mm^3 and may exceed 50 000 leucocytes/mm^3, with the average about 10 000 leucocytes/mm^3; the total cell count may be taken as a guide to the inflammatory disease activity within the joint. Thus the clinically 'inactive' or 'mildly inflamed' joint usually has a total cell count below 5000 leucocytes/mm^3, while the 'actively inflamed' joint commonly has a cell count in excess of 15 000/mm^3 (Currey & Vernon-Roberts, 1976). In *systemic lupus erythematosus* the total cell count rarely exceeds 3000 leucocytes/mm^3 (Pekin & Zvaifler, 1970; Labowitz & Schumacher, 1971). In the inflammatory arthropathies accompanying *Crohn's disease*, *ulcerative colitis*, *Reiter's disease*, *psoriasis* and *ankylosing spondylitis* the total cell count does not usually exceed 10 000 leucocytes/mm^3, although it may occasionally reach 50 000 leuco-

Table 8.2 Total leucocyte counts of synovial fluid (data combined from various sources)

	Leucocyte/mm^3	
	Average	Range
Normal	150	30–750
Osteoarthritis	500	30–2 000
Rheumatoid arthritis	10 000	1 000–100 000
Systemic lupus erythematosus	2 000	10–25 000
Reiter's disease	20 000	1 000–50 000
Gout	15 000	1 000–300 000
Pseudogout	5 000	500–50 000
Apatite arthropathy	2 000	250–50 000
Septic arthritis	50 000	5 000–500 000
Viral arthritis	5 000	30–100 000
Post-traumatic	500	10–5 000

cytes/mm^3 in active Reiter's disease (Weinberger et al, 1961). In *gout* the total cell count is dependent upon the number of crystals present; in active gout there may be up to 300 000 leucocytes/mm^3, but in quiescent intervals the cell count may only be slightly elevated above 1000 leucocytes/mm^3. In *pyrophosphate arthropathy* (*pseudogout*), although the cells may exceed 30 000 leucocytes/mm^2 in an acute episode, the count rarely exceeds 10 000 leucocytes/mm^3 and is frequently less than 1000 leucocytes/mm^3. It has been reported that acute pseudogout may take place without an increase in the number of synovial fluid leucocytes (Matthay et al, 1977). In arthritis associated with *apatite crystals* the total cell count rarely exceeds 5000 leucocytes/mm^3 (Dieppe et al, 1979; Halverson & McCarty, 1979) but occasionally exceeds 30 000 leucocytes/mm^3 (Schumacher et al, 1977). In *septic arthritis* the total cell count may be quite low in the early stages and may thus be easily confused with a non-infective inflammatory arthropathy; in the established condition the total count is generally greater than 100 000 leucocytes/mm^3 and frequently exceeds this figure. The cell count does not assist in differentiating infections by organisms such as staphylococci and streptococci from those caused by tubercle bacilli, meningococci, gonococci or fungi. In *virus-induced arthritis* the total cell count usually is below 15 000 leucocytes/mm^3 and may be only slightly elevated above 1000 leucocytes/mm^3. In *post-traumatic* effusions red blood cells may be numerous only for a short time after the traumatic episode has occurred, but they may also be numerous due to previous attempts at aspiration, to acute synovitis of any cause, to haemophilia, or to villonodular synovitis. Whatever the cause of bleeding into a joint, it may be accompanied by a rise in the leucocyte count but this rarely exceeds 5000 leucocytes/mm^3 and is generally much lower.

Microscopy of stained smears

While it is conventional to examine cell morphology and carry out differential cell counts by the microscopic examination of stained smears of synovial fluid, the various cell types can be differentiated easily using phase-contrast microscopy of fresh or stored (4°C) wet smears which allows also the easy visualisation of intracellular materials (Currey & Vernon-Roberts, 1976).

Thin smears of synovial fluid may be prepared on microscopic slides in the same manner as with peripheral blood smears or with the aid of a cytocentrifuge. Smears may be stained using one of the Romanowsky stains (e.g. Leishman, Wright, Giemsa), haematoxylin and eosin, or neutral red. When using the Romanowsky stains it is essential that the smears be thin since staining of proteoglycans and mucoprotein present in the fluid may obscure the cellular detail.

The three principal types of cell (Fig. 8.1) present in the synovial fluid are:

1. *Neutrophil polymorphonuclear leucocytes* (neutrophils), which have a morphology identical with the same cell in the blood but sometimes additionally contain intracytoplasmic inclusions in the form of vacuoles, crystals, fat droplets or micro-organisms.
2. *Lymphocytes*, which have a morphology identical with that of the small lymphocyte of the blood.
3. *Mononuclear phagocytes* (monocytes, macrophages, histiocytes), which may be similar to the blood monocyte, but frequently exhibit wide variations in morphology and may contain a variety of intracytoplasmic inclusion in the form of crystals, fat droplets, erythrocytes, neutrophil fragments, DNA, or micro-organisms.

The neutrophil polymorphs in rheumatoid arthritis may show a number of changes which, although not diagnostically specific, are suggestive of the disease. Many of the polymorphs show a loss of lysosomal granules, are markedly vacuolated, and have hypersegmented or pyknotic nuclear chromatin; but these changes are common in any inflammatory condition. Somewhat more specific for rheumatoid arthritis are intracytoplasmic globules of DNA which can be identified using the Feulgen stain, and which almost certainly represent ingested nuclear debris from degenerate leucocytes (Zvaifler, 1973). A cell which has been claimed to be quite unique for rheumatoid effusions is a neutrophil polymorph with the nuclear chromatin peripherally displaced by either a Feulgen-staining globule or a protein-

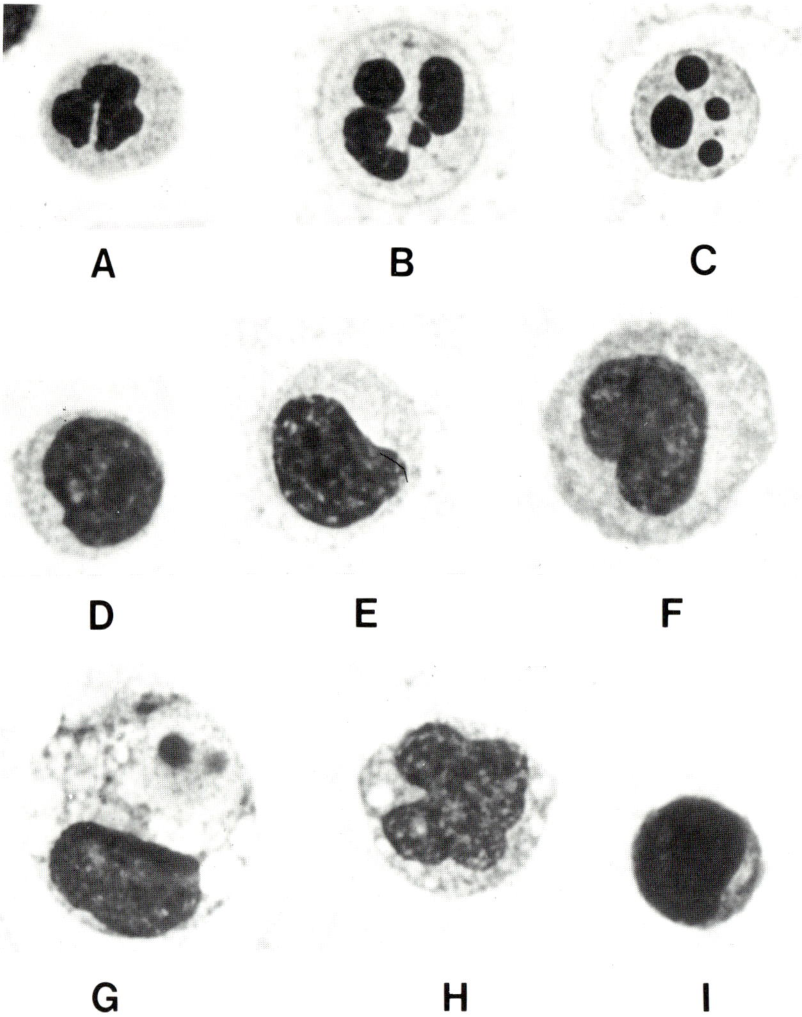

Fig. 8.1 Microscopic appearances of cells in synovial fluid after staining by Giemsa technique. A. Neutrophil polymorph. B. Neutrophil polymorph with markedly segmented nucleus: seen commonly in rheumatoid arthritis but not exclusive to that condition. C. Effete neutrophil polymorph with pyknotic nucleus. D–F. Mononuclear phagocytes showing variation in size and nuclear morphology. G. Mononuclear phagocyte containing intracytoplasmic effete neutrophil polymorph: seen commonly in Reiter's syndrome but not exclusive to that condition. H. Mononuclear phagocyte with numerous intracytoplasmic lipid droplets. I. Lymphocyte. (×1000)

aceous mass in about one percent of the cells present (Zvaifler, 1973).

Large mononuclear cells include mononuclear phagocytes, transformed lymphocytes, synovial lining cells (synoviocytes) and, rarely, chondrocytes. The distinction between these cell types is difficult. It has been suggested that transformed lymphocytes are present in rheumatoid arthritis but not in gout or pseudogout (Traycoff et al, 1976). While Sudan-negative type B synoviocytes have been reported to be distinguishable from Sudan-positive type A synoviocytes and mononuclear phagocytes by the use of Sudan black stain (Sheehan & Storey, 1947), it is not considered that the presence of synoviocytes has a particular diagnostic significance.

The characteristic LE cells frequently are present in systemic lupus erythematosus (Hollander et al, 1966), but also may be seen occasionally in rheumatoid arthritis. Haematoxylin bodies may also support a diagnosis of lupus erythematosus.

Mononuclear phagocytes and neutrophils may

contain a variety of diagnostically important intracellular inclusions, and appropriate special staining procedures should be employed to aid the specific recognition of intracytoplasma. *Crystals* of urate or calcium pyrophosphate should be identified positively using polarising microscopy (see below), but are often visible in smears stained by the Romanowsky technique despite the tendency for urates to dissolve in aqueous solution. The Von Kossa stain will demonstrate calcium pyrophosphate crystals and renders visible clumps of apatite crystals. *Bacteria* may be visible in smears routinely stained by the Romanowsky or haematoxylin techniques in septic arthritis, but, using Gram's stain, their presence should be sought routinely in the presence of a high neutrophil count even when the patient is known already to have rheumatoid arthritis or other inflammatory joint disease. The absence of bacteria in smears stained with Gram's stain is common during infection and does not exclude septic arthritis. If tuberculosis is suspected, the Ziehl-Neelsen stain should be applied although cultures and synovial biopsy usually are needed to establish the diagnosis. *Erythrocytes* commonly are present within mononuclear phagocytes following bleeding into the joint prior to aspiration and, like xanthochromia, are a useful guide to blood-staining being due to bleeding into the joint as distinct from fluid into which haemorrhage has occurred at the time of aspiration. Intracellular *fat droplets*, demonstrable with fat stains (Fig. 8.2), may be numerous following uptake of marrow fat following the breaching of the articular surface after trauma or 'aseptic necrosis' (Currey & Vernon-Roberts, 1976), but also may be present in some cases of acute arthritis associated with minor trauma (Graham & Goldman, 1978). *Amyloid* may be present within synovial fluid leucocytes in rare cases of amyloid arthropathy associated with multiple myeloma (Hickling et al, 1981), but is present extracellularly in the synovial fluid in up to 5% of multiple myeloma (Schumacher, 1972; Hickling et al, 1981). Aspirates of synovial fluid in patients with amyloidosis associated with multiple myeloma have been reported to contain small sequestered fragments of synovial villi containing amyloid (Gordon et al, 1973). Intracellular *metal or plastic wear particles*, best detected by polarised light microscopy of wet preparations, may be present in synovial fluid aspirated from joints having endoprostheses, and may be numerous when loosening has occurred.

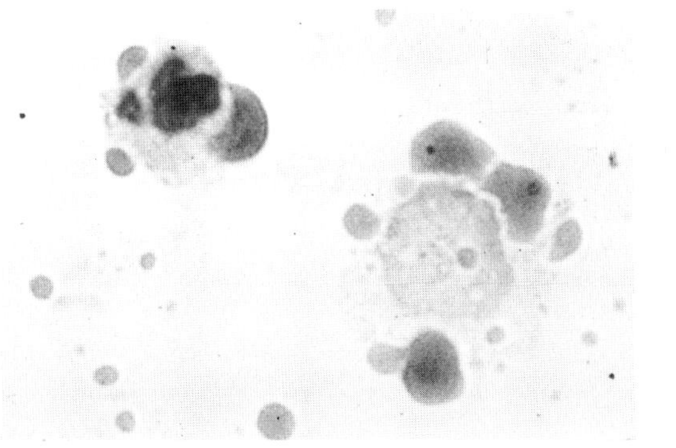

Fig. 8.2 Neutrophil polymorph (left) and mononuclear phagocyte (right) containing numerous intracellular globules of lipid which the cells have taken up due to fatty marrow being liberated into the joint cavity following collapse of the femoral head. Numerous free extracellular lipid globules also are present. Sudan III (×1000)

Eosinophils are present rarely (Ropes & Bauer, 1953) and do not reflect changes in the peripheral blood eosinophil count. However, significant numbers of eosinophils in the synovial aspirate have been recorded in some patients with rheumatoid arthritis (Collins, 1936; Panush et al, 1971), rheumatic fever (McEwen, 1935), Guinea worm infestation (Reddy et al, 1969), metastatic adenocarcinoma (Goldenberg et al 1975), radiation-associated arthritis (Hasselbacher & Schumacher, 1977), and following arthrography in gout (Hasselbacher & Schumacher, 1978).

While synovial effusions may arise from a synovial reaction or infiltration by carcinoma, sarcoma or leukaemia without malignant cells being detected in the synovial fluid (Spilberg & Meyer, 1972; Lagier, 1977), cases have been reported in which leukaemic cells (Dresner, 1950; Emkey et al, 1973) or metastatic carcinoma cells (Benedek, 1965; Goldenberg et al, 1975) have been present in the fluid.

Large vacuolated macrophages have been observed in the synovial fluid from a patient with *Whipple's disease*, but the periodic acid-Schiff (PAS) positive granules and ultrastructural presence of rod-like bodies were recorded in the synovial tissues alone (Rubinow et al, 1976). Large vacuolated foamy cells also have been recorded in the synovial fluid and synovial membrane of a patient with multicentric reticulohistiocytosis (Krey et al, 1974).

While electron microscopy currently appears to have a minor role in the routine diagnostic examination of synovial fluids, it is an essential procedure for the specific recognition of apatite crystals which usually are too small to be seen by light microscopy and are not birefringent (Dieppe et al, 1976). Transmission and scanning electron microscopy, with the availability of elemental analysis, already has played a significant role in the better understanding of the interactions of crystals and cells and no doubt will come to be used more widely to study the cells of synovial fluid in various forms of arthritis.

Differential cell counts

The differentiation of lymphocytes from mononuclear phagocytes is not absolutely essential for diagnostic purposes, and it is the relative proportion of polymorphonuclear cells to mononuclear cells which gives the best indication of the degree of inflammatory activity — particularly when this is correlated with the total number of leucocytes present (Currey & Vernon-Roberts, 1976). There is wide variation in the proportion of neutrophil polymorphs, lymphocytes and mononuclear phagocytes in normal and pathological fluids. When the total cell count is elevated, a differential count of over 90% neutrophil polymorphs indicates very active acute inflammation and suggests that sepsis should be excluded; over 80% indicates active inflammation; and below 80% indicates moderate inflammatory activity, low-grade inflammation, resolving or quiescent disease, depending on the percentage of neutrophils recorded and the total number of cells present. A *high percentage of neutrophils* may be the clue to septic arthritis, even when the total cell count is only modestly elevated. A predominance of mononuclear cells, in the presence of an elevated leucocyte count, has been described in some forms of arthritis associated with viral infections including rubella (Chambers & Bywaters, 1963), hepatitis B (Onion et al, 1971; Duffy et al, 1976), adenovirus (Utsinger, 1977), infectious mononucleosis (Adebonojo, 1972), chicken pox (Ward & Bishop, 1970; Friedman & Naveh, 1971; Priest et al, 1978); echovirus (Blotzer & Myers, 1978) and the epidemic polyarthritis associated with Ross River virus (Fraser et al, 1981). An acute monocytic arthritis, possibly of viral aetiology, also has been described (Brawer & Cathcart, 1979). Other forms of viral arthritis show a variable distribution of cell types, with a dominance of neutrophils being common (Sauter & Utsinger, 1978).

It has been reported also that the joint fluid of patients with late onset hypogammaglobulinaemia contains predominantly mononuclear cells (Asherson & Webster, 1980).

Microscopic examination of wet preparations

It is most important that a wet preparation of synovial fluid is examined. Ideally, this should be carried out using freshly aspirated fluid without anticoagulant. However, heparinised fluids also are suitable for examination. Crystals and cells become enmeshed in any clot which forms, so that a fragment of clot must be included with the drop of fluid which is transferred to a glass slide and on which a coverslip is placed. If desired, or if there is to be any delay before examination, the coverslip can be sealed around the edges with nail-varnish or petroleum jelly (e.g. Vaseline). Slides and coverslips must be very clean to minimise birefringent dirt which may be confused with crystals. For the optimum examination of cell morphology and crystals it is desirable for the cells to be given time to settle on the surface of the slides so that movement ceases and the cells are in the same plane. The greater the degree of viscosity of the fluid, the longer this process takes. It is aided if the wet preparation, with coverslip in place, is placed in an oven or incubator at 37°C for a minimum of 15 minutes.

Ordinary transmitted light microscopy of unstained wet preparations is capable of providing limited information only and does not allow the definite distinction of different types of cells, crystals or intracellular inclusions. Some limited assistance may be given by lowering the condenser or closing the diaphragm. While the principal cell types may be distinguished by ordinary transmitted light microscopy after supravital staining with neutral red and Janus green, or by the addition of methylene blue, this is not necessary when phase-contrast equipment is available. In

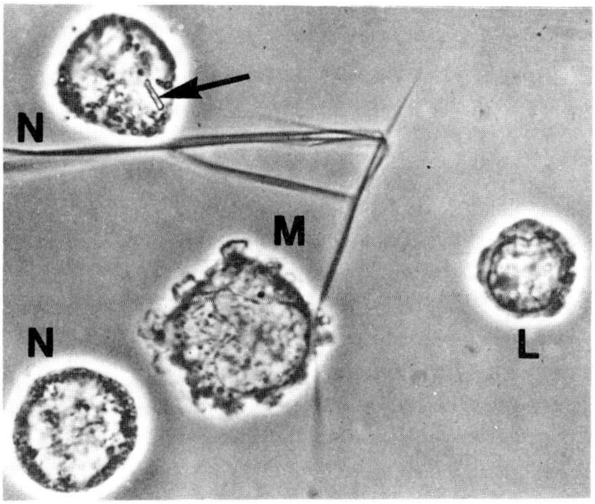

Fig. 8.3 Appearances of cells in wet smear preparation viewed by phase-contrast microscopy. Shows neutrophil polymorphs (N) with an intracellular crystal of calcium pyrophosphate dihydrate (arrow), mononuclear phagocyte (M), small lymphocyte (L), and strands of fibrin. (×850)

practice, phase-contrast examination of fresh or stored (4°C) unstained smears constitutes a very easy way of differentiating between the different types of cell present while allowing also the visualisation of crystals (Fig. 8.3), bacteria, fibrin, fat droplets, intracellular erythrocytes, cartilage fragments, chondrocytes, fragments of villi, 'ragocytes' (Fig. 8.4), prosthetic wear particles, or other solids. The specific identification of intracellular and extracellular materials may require compensated polarised light microscopy (see below) or the use of appropriate special staining techniques for the identification of bacteria, mycobacteria, fungi, and amyloid as stated earlier. The use of transmission or scanning electron microscopy is indicated in special circumstances, such as the identification of apatite crystals (Dieppe et al, 1979), or when crystals of urate or pyrophosphate are too small to be revealed or unambiguously identified by light microscopy (Honig et al, 1977; Gaucher et al, 1977). Phase-contrast is capable also of higher resolution than ordinary transmitted light microscopy, and allows the detection of fine fibrils (e.g. glass fibre), or small crystals (e.g. apatite), which are not demonstrable by polarised light microscopy.

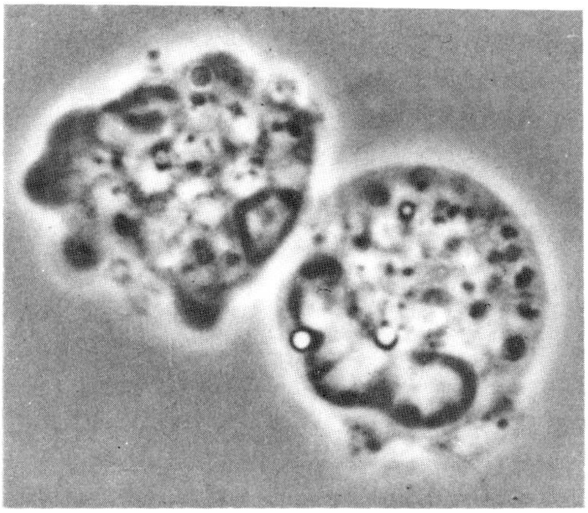

Fig. 8.4 Neutrophil polymorphs ('ragocytes' or 'RA cells') in rheumatoid synovial fluid showing many small dark intracytoplasmic inclusions when viewed by phase-contrast microscopy of a wet preparation. (×1750)

Wet unstained preparations of neutrophil polymorphs from freshly aspirated rheumatoid synovial fluid contain numerous dark intracytoplasmic granules (Fig. 8.4) from 0.5–1.5 μm in diameter: these granules were thought initially to be quite specific for rheumatoid arthritis (Hollander et al, 1965), but it is now generally agreed that these 'ragocytes', 'inclusion body cells' or 'RA cells' are not specific for rheumatoid arthritis although they are more numerous in this disease. Immunofluorescent and other techniques have shown the intracellular inclusions to be the result of neutrophils taking up immune complexes from the fluid, and the conclusions from these studies have been summarised by Zvaifler (1973) as follows:

1. IgG, IgM, complement components and rheumatoid factor are present in varying combinations in the cells from rheumatoid effusions.
2. IgG and complement components are frequently found in the cells from non-rheumatoid inflammatory effusion.
3. Anti-γ-globulin inclusions are correlated with rheumatoid factor in the serum or synovial fluid and a low level of joint complement.
4. The quantity of complement component within the cells is inversely proportional to the concentration of the same component in the accompanying fluid.
5. The first (Clq) and fourth (C4) components of complement are detected in most of the cells from patients with seropositive rheumatoid arthritis, but they are also found frequently in

the cells from patients with seronegative rheumatoid arthritis.
6. Immunofluorescent staining for IgM or C3 correlates closely with seropositive rheumatoid arthritis.

Polarised light microscopy for crystal identification

Providing that an appropriate microscope is available, the identification of crystals of urate or pyrophosphate may be carried out simply and readily on wet preparations of synovial fluid in the clinic, office or laboratory. Since these crystals and others often may be present when the diagnosis of crystal synovitis has not been suspected clinically as the cause of an effusion, it is sound practice to examine all aspirated fluids for the presence of crystals even in circumstances when the diagnosis of rheumatoid arthritis, for example, has been made on the basis of other clinical and laboratory findings.

A thorough understanding of the optical properties of crystals and polarised light microscopy is not necessary for the identification of urate and pyrophosphate crystals in synovial fluid. Nevertheless, a superficial account of the optical principles involved makes the procedure more logical and comprehensible.

While an ordinary basic biological microscope may be equipped for use as a polarising microscope, a special polarised light microscope is recommended for the rapid and accurate differentiation of urate and pyrophosphate crystals. The essential feature of a suitable polarising microscope is that the light emitted from the light source is oriented in a single plane by a polarising filter (the polariser) placed between the light source and the microscope stage. A second polarising filter (the analyser) is placed in the light path between the microscope stage and the eyepiece of the microscope. By rotating the polariser and analyser independently, the plane of polarisation of the light can be varied. Thus, when the planes are parallel the light travels uninterrupted through the analyser and the field viewed by the observer is bright; and, when the planes are at 90° to each other (i.e. 'crossed polars') the polarised light is blocked by the analyser so that the field appears to be dark to the observer. When a crystal is placed on the microscope stage, interposed between the crossed polars, the structural lattice of the crystal allows light from the polariser to travel through different planes of the crystal at different speeds. Such crystals are designated as *anisotropic* and this is recognised by the optical properties of *birefringence*. The deflection of some of the polarised light passing through the crystal now allows some light to pass through the analyser and is viewed by the observer as brightly visible against a dark background (Fig. 8.5). This brightness (birefringence) can be modified by rotating the crystal, using the rotating stage of the polarising microscope, through 360° so that the optical axes of the crystal change with respect to the plane of the polariser. When rotated, under these conditions, the crystal will pass through four bright positions and four dark positions (Fig. 8.6) and the relationship of the dark positions of the planes of the polars determines the 'angle of extinction'. This angle of extinction varies from crystal to crystal, and is *parallel in the case of urate* and *oblique in the case of calcium pyrophosphate dihydrate* (CPPD) (Currey, 1968; Currey & Vernon-Roberts, 1976). Colour changes also occur as the birefringent crystal is

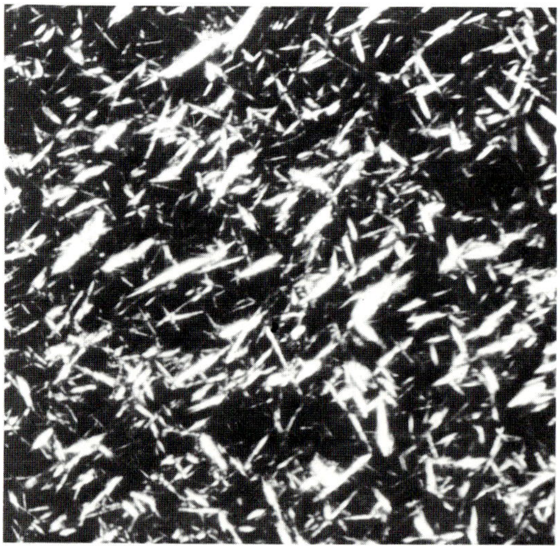

Fig. 8.5 Wet preparation of fluid from a case of active gout showing numerous needle-shaped crystals of monosodium urate when viewed by polarised light microscopy. The crystals are brightly birefringent when lying oblique to the planes of the polariser and analyser plates but are dark and invisible when lying parallel to those planes (parallel extinction). (×1000)

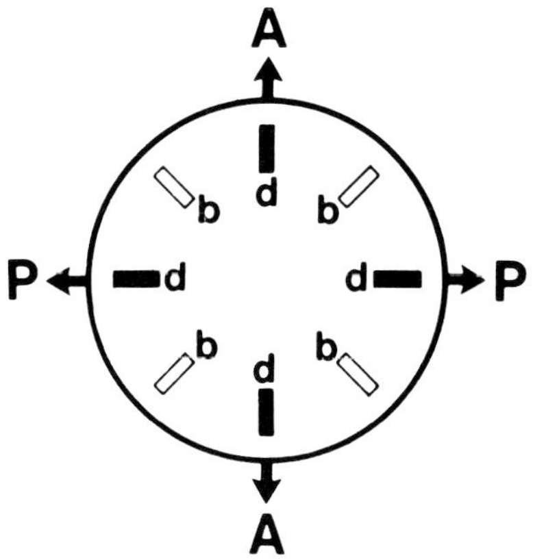

Fig. 8.6 Appearances of a birefringent crystal during rotation between crossed polars. P–P. Plane of polariser. A–A. Plane of analyser. b. Positions in which crystal appears bright. d. Positions in which crystal appears dark. The crystal illustrated has an angle of extinction (position 'd') which is parallel (with P–P and A–A), as in the case of urate. By contrast, crystals of calcium pyrophosphate dihydrate exhibit oblique extinction. (Reproduced with permission from Hughes & Currey, 1980.)

rotated since the combining of light of different speeds after passage through the crystal produces interference and changes of frequency (colour). The type and extent of the colour change is characteristic for different types of crystal.

While the use of polarised light microscopy and the determination of the angle of extinction of crystals present in synovial fluid samples plays a role in rapid screening for the presence of crystals, it is necessary to undertake *compensated* polarised light microscopy for the definitive separation of urate from CPPD crystals. This takes advantage of the fact that crystals can be characterised further by placing a birefringent flat quartz plate (the compensator) in the light path between the crossed polars. The compensator commonly used is a 'first order red plate' which is placed obliquely in the light path so that its slow component direction is at an angle of 45° to the plane of the polars. This produces a change in the observed background from black to rose-red.

Against this red background the presence of a birefringent crystal will produce a colour change by adding to or substracting from the birefringent effect of the quartz plate. The intensity of the colour change depends on the strength (*weak* to *strong*) of the birefringence, while the actual colour depends on the sign (*negative* or *positive*) of the birefringence. Thus, a urate crystal shows a marked colour change, turning yellow when the long axis of the crystal is parallel with the slow component of the first order red plate, and blue at right angles to this position (strong negative birefringence) (Fig. 8.7). CPPD crystals exhibit less marked changes with the colours reversed (weak positive birefringence). Rotated through 360° a urate crystal can be seen to take on these colours when it lies at 45° to the planes of the polars (Plate 8.1). When the long axis of the crystal is parallel with the axis of the polariser or analyser the crystal takes on the red colour of the background.

Formal identification of crystals employing optical methods (including the determination of refractive indices), is a highly precise technique. However, the examination of synovial fluids is greatly simplified because, in practice, there are only two types of crystal which need to be identified frequently, urate and CPPD. Practical procedures to be followed in examining synovial fluids for the presence of urate and pyrophosphate crystals are detailed elsewhere (Phelps et al, 1968; Currey, 1968; Fagin & Lidsky, 1974; Currey &

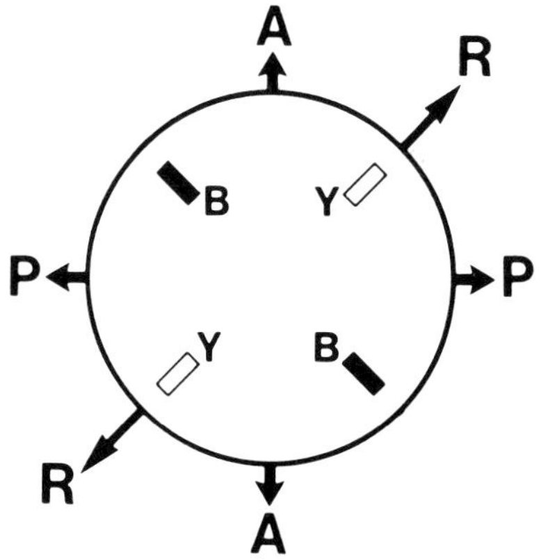

Fig. 8.7 Appearance of birefringent crystal during rotation between crossed polars and with the first order red compensator in position. P–P. Plane of polariser. A–A. Plane of analyser. R–R. Orientation of slow component of first order red compensator. B. Positions in which crystal appears blue. Y. Positions in which crystal appears yellow. In the intermediate positions (i.e. in the planes A–A and P–P) the crystal takes on the colour of the red background. The crystal illustrated is negatively birefringent as in the case of urate. By contrast, crystals of calcium pyrophosphate dihydrate exhibit opposite and less marked colour changes (weak positive birefringence). (Reproduced with permission from Hughes & Currey, 1980.)

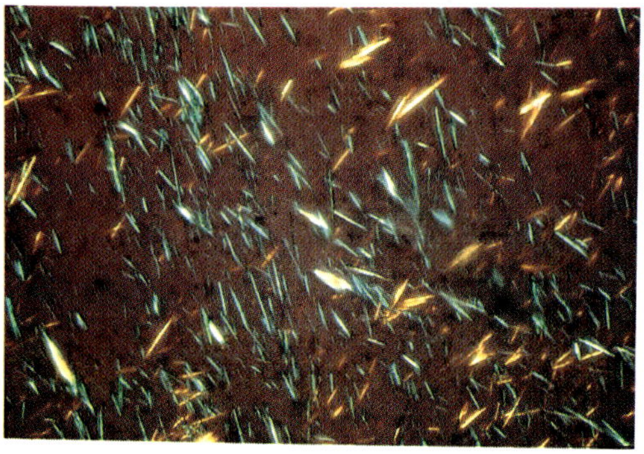

Plate 8.1 Crystals of monosodium urate in joint fluid from case of active gout viewed by compensated polarised light microscopy. The crystals appear yellow when their long axes are parallel with the slow component of the first order red plate, and appear blue at right angles to that position (strong negative birefringence). (×1000)

	Urate	Pyrophosphate
Size	2-10 μ	1-10 μ
Shapes	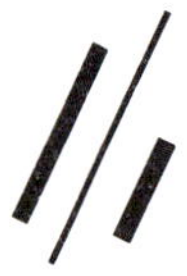	
Angle of extinction	Parallel	Oblique
Birefringence	Strong Negative	Weak Positive

Fig. 8.8 Comparison of the optical properties of the two types of crystal found in synovial fluid. (Reproduced with permission from Hughes & Currey, 1980.)

Vernon-Roberts, 1976; Gatter, 1977), but the characteristics of these crystals are summarised below, and in Figure 8.8.

Monosodium urate crystals of gout (Fig. 8.9) tend to be 2–10 μm long (but may reach 20 μm), are needle- or rod-shaped, exhibit parallel extinction and yellow colour changes when viewed by non-compensated polarised microscopy, and are brightly negatively birefringent. By contrast, CPPD crystals (Fig. 8.9) tend to be 1–10 μm long, are rod- or tablet-shaped, exhibit oblique extinction, and are weakly positively birefringent.

The finding of numerous crystals of urate or pyrophosphate, many present intracellularly within leucocytes, in the fluid from an inflamed joint is characteristic of acute crystal synovitis (Fig. 8.5). Similarly, fluids obtained from subacute or chronic gouty or pyrophosphate arthritis usually will contain enough crystals for a definite diagnosis. However, fluids from joints affected by a variety of other arthropathies occasionally may reveal small numbers of either urate or CPPD, or both, and the significance of this remains unclear.

Cholesterol crystals may be seen in acute or chronic joint effusions, including rheumatoid arthritis (Zuckner et al, 1964; Newcombe & Cohen, 1965; Griffin & Bole, 1969; Ettlinger & Hunder, 1979) and osteoarthritis (Fam et al, 1981). Cholesterol crystals form thin plates, each plate being equilateral and regular. The crystals

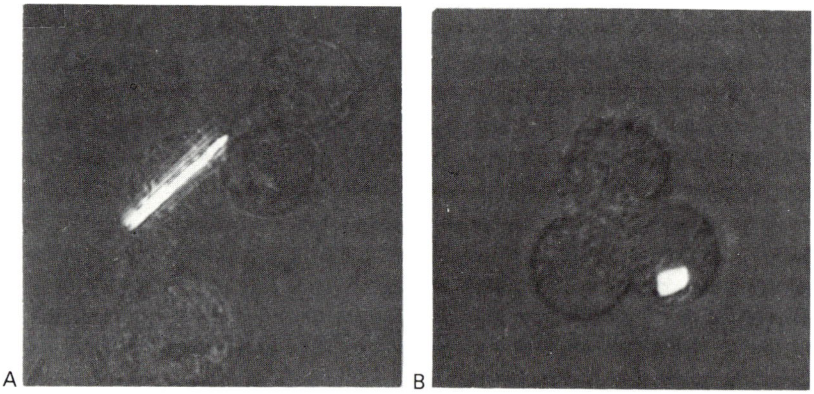

Fig. 8.9 Polarised light microscopy of crystal-containing neutrophil polymorphs in a wet preparation of synovial fluid. A. Birefringent (white) needle-shaped urate crystal at 45° to the planes of the polariser and analyser. B. Birefringent (white) rhomboid cyrstal of calcium pyrophosphate dihydrate lying parallel to the plane of the analyser. (×1300)

adhere to one another and, when viewed in stacks, there is an illusion that one or more crystal corners are indented or notched due to irregular overlap (Gatter, 1977). Occasionally they are needle-like in form.

Artefactual birefringent material is important. Lithium heparin (but not sodium heparin) anticoagulant will produce small crystals similar to CPPD (Tanphaichitr et et al, 1976). Calcium oxalate crystals may form also when the fluid is erroneously placed in an oxalated container, and form cubes similar to the oxalate crystals seen in urine (Schumacher, 1966). Crystals may also form if too little fluid is added to bottles containing potassium EDTA (Currey & Vernon-Roberts, 1976). All such crystals may be taken up by phagocytic leucocytes in vitro and may be seen intracellularly.

Corticosteroid crystals may be present in the synovial fluid up to many weeks after the injection of depot microcrystalline corticosteroid esters (Kahn et al, 1970). They appear as positively or negatively birefringent rods similar in size to crystals of urate or CPPD, or as granular or irregular debris.

Dicalcium phosphate dihydrate crystals are strongly positively birefringent and may be present admixed with weakly positively birefringent crystals of CPPD (Moskowitz et al, 1971).

Prosthetic wear particles in the form of metallic fragments of orthopaedic alloy (Kitridou et al, 1969) may be present in fluid aspirated from joints having endoprostheses in place. It has been established that ultra high molecular weight polyethylene debris is also shed into the fluid surrounding low-friction endoprostheses (Vernon-Roberts & Freeman, 1977). Metallic particles are distinguished from polyethylene particles with ease using polarised light microscopy (Vernon-Roberts & Freeman, 1977).

Birefringent congo red-positive amyloid fragments have been identified in synovial fluid (Gordon et al, 1973), and brightly birefringent large rectangular crystals composed of immunoglobulin have been observed in a tendon sheath effusion in a patient with unusual symptoms associated with a monoclonal cryoglobulinaemia (P. Goatcher, personal communication, 1976).

Cartilage and fibrin are not truly birefringent, but transmit and reflect light irregularly; they do not possess the regular profiles of crystals.

Glove powder is brightly birefringent and shows a Maltese cross appearance.

The absolute definitive identification of crystals requires X-ray diffraction. It is through previous basic work examining the same crystals by both compensated polarised light and by X-ray diffraction that confidence in the compensated polarising microscope has been established. Crystals which are observed under the microscope which do not fulfill the characteristics classically described may be definitively investigated therefore by X-ray diffraction.

Crystals also may be so small or few in number that it is necessary to use electron microscopy, possibly combined with electron diffraction and elemental analysis, to specifically identify the material present (Schumacher et al, 1975; Crocker et al, 1976; Honig et al, 1977; Gaucher et al, 1977). Electron microscopy plays an essential role in the detection of hydroxyapatite crystals in synovial fluid.

Detection of hydroxyapatite crystals

Crystals of hydroxyapatite (HA) have been identified by transmission and scanning electron microscopy in synovial fluids from patients usually with acute undiagnosed arthritis or exacerbations of osteoarthritis, and rarely in some miscellaneous conditions including renal dialysis patients, mixed collagen–vascular diseases, rheumatoid arthritis, and chondrocalcinosis (Dieppe et al, 1976; Schumacher et al, 1977; Dieppe et al, 1979). They also may be shed into the fluid from heavy deposits in the synovial tissues in progressive systemic sclerosis (Brandt & Krey, 1977). Crystals are rods or needles, 7.5–25 nm in diameter and up to 10 times as long, which can be seen individually only by electron microscopy. They may form clumps which can be observed by light microscopy as shiny globules in the wet smear, intracellular inclusions which stain purple with Romanowsky stains, or occasionally atypical positively or negatively birefringent crystals (Schumacher, 1977). Crystal clumps appear to contain hydroxyapatite as the only mineral on the basis of electron probe studies, but crystals of CPPD and other calcium salts may also be present in the synovial fluid in some cases (Dieppe et al, 1979). A binding technique employing [^{14}C] diphosphonate has been described for the identification and semiquantitation estimation of HA crystals in synovial fluids (Halverson & McCarty, 1979).

The relevance of HA crystals remains unknown. They have been demonstrated to have phlogistic properties (Schumacher et al, 1975; Dieppe et al, 1976), and must be suspected to be the explanation for some episodes of acute arthritis, exacerbations of osteoarthritis, and synovitis associated with calcific periarthritis.

Micro-organisms

Examination of synovial fluids for infecting organisms follows the conventional microbiological principles of staining and culture applicable to biological fluids generally. When a joint infection is suspected, every effort must be made to obtain an adequate sample of synovial fluid before any antimicrobial therapy is started. In the case of suppurative arthritis the Gram-stained smear may give an immediate guide to starting antibiotic therapy. Useful information can be obtained also by examination of synovial fluid obtained during therapy: the ability or otherwise to culture the organism subsequently provides some check on the success of treatment, while comparison of the antimicrobial activity of the blood and synovial fluid (against the organism cultured originally) provides evidence of the penetration of the antibiotics into the joint and the effective concentrations achieved there. The drug regimen should aim at producing bacterial concentrations within the synovial fluid.

Joint infection occasionally may be due to viruses, *Brucella*, *M. tuberculosis*, to non-tuberculous *Mycobacteria*, or to any of the pathogenic fungi. For these reasons it is important to consider at the outset all the tests that need to be instituted. When bacteriological examination of synovial fluid is negative in a patient in whom the suspicion of infection is high, synovial material should usually be obtained by biopsy for histology and further microbiological studies. It must be pointed out, however, that the gross appearance of synovial fluid is often a poor guide to the presence or absence of infection; apparently purulent fluids are occasionally found in (uninfected) joints affected by crystal synovitis or rheumatoid arthritis, while thin, serous synovial fluids may be seen in the early stages of severe pyogenic infections. Partial antibiotic treatment also can produce grossly misleading results.

Chemical tests applied to the synovial fluid cannot establish with certainty a diagnosis of septic arthritis although a very much reduced glucose level is suggestive and infection should be excluded even in known cases of rheumatoid arthritis and Reiter's disease in which the glucose concentration normally is low. It has been reported that the detection of an increase in lactic acid levels in the synovial fluid is a useful screening test for indicating the presence of joint infection (Brook et al, 1978; Riordan et al, 1982).

Immunology

Application of immunological tests to synovial fluids is of considerable theoretical interest, but at present the results seldom contribute decisively to establishing a diagnosis. It needs to be remembered that most proteins and other substances found in the synovial fluid have been derived from the plasma. Thus, in seeking evidence that the concentration of a particular substance in the synovial fluid reflects a local phenomenon such as synthesis, consumption or binding, it is necessary to consider also the concentration of the same substance in the plasma and the concentration of total protein in the synovial fluid. Other factors influencing the concentration of synovial fluid components are molecular size and the concentration and state of hyaluronate, with its 'volume excluding' effect.

Synovial fluid complement determination is of value predominantly when compared with serum levels and with serum and synovial fluid determinations. Cells must be removed promptly by immediate centrifugation of the fluid, and the supernatant should then be examined within two hours or stored at below −20°C until tested. The information concerning synovial fluid complement in disease, cited earlier, is mainly of theoretical interest, but the lowered levels in rheumatoid effusions (in the presence of normal serum levels) may be helpful in diagnosis.

Rheumatoid factors of IgM type usually are present in synovial effusions when detected in the serum of rheumatoid patients. Titres in the synovial fluid tend to be equal to or lower than those found in the serum (Bland & Clark, 1963). However, there is evidence that the synovial fluid titres sometimes may be higher than that in the serum due to local synthesis, or lower due to local consumption (Hannestad & Mellbye, 1967). In practice it is worth testing synovial fluid for rheumatoid factors when it becomes available in a case of seronegative polyarthritis. Very occasionally a positive result may contribute to the diagnosis.

Antinuclear factor (ANF) tests performed on synovial fluids also are of mainly theoretical interest, but ANF may occasionally be detected in the synovial fluid in many conditions in which it is not identifiable in serum. Generally, however, titres of ANF in synovial effusions are equal to or lower than those in serum (MacSween et al, 1968).

A variety of techniques exist for identifying subpopulations of lymphocytes as bone marrow-derived (B) cells or thymus-derived (T) cells, and a number of workers have applied these techniques to the study of subpopulations of these cells in synovial effusions in rheumatoid arthritis and systemic lupus erythematosus. The synovial fluids in these diseases show wide variations in the results obtained in various studies, particularly with regard to the percentage of B cells present and the immunoglobulin classes to which they belong. In the current state of knowledge, information useful for diagnosis is unlikely to be obtained by attempting to classify the lymphocyte-like cells in synovial fluids.

REFERENCES

Adebonojo F O 1972 Monoarticular arthritis: an unusual manifestation of infectious mononucleosis. Clinical Pediatrics 11: 549–550

Adkins E W O, Davies D V 1940 Absorption from joint cavity. Quarterly Journal of Experimental Physiology 30: 147–154

Asherson G L, Webster A D B 1980 Late onset hypogammaglobulinaemia. In: Diagnosis and treatment of immunodeficiency diseases. Blackwell, Oxford, p 44

Balazs E A, Watson D, Duff I F, Roseman S 1967 Hyaluronic acid in synovial fluid. I. Molecular parameters of hyaluronic acid in normal and arthrititic human fluids. Arthritis and Rheumatism 10: 357–375

Bauer W, Short C L, Bennett G A 1933 Manner of removal of proteins from normal joints. Journal of Experimental Medicine 57: 419–433

Benedek T G 1965 Lysis of the patella due to metastatic carcinoma. Arthritis and Rheumatism 8: 560–567

Berg E, Wainwright R, Barton B, Puchtler H, McDonald T 1977 On the nature of rheumatoid rice bodies: an immunologic, histochemical and electron microscope study. Arthritis and Rheumatism 20: 1343–1349

Bland J H, Clark L 1963 Rheumatoid factor in serum and joint fluid. Annals of Internal Medicine 58: 829–836

Blotzer J W, Myers A R 1978 Echovirus associated polyarthritis. Arthritis and Rheumatism 21: 978–981

Bole G G 1962 Synovial fluid lipids in normal individuals and patients with rheumatoid arthritis. Arthritis and Rheumatism 5: 589–601

Bonebrake R A, McCall J T, Hunder G G, Polley H F 1972 Zinc accumulation in synovial fluid. Mayo Clinic Proceedings 47: 746–750

Brandt T K D, Krey P R 1977 Chalky joint effusion. The result of massive synovial deposition of calcium apatite in progressive systemic sclerosis. Arthritis and Rheumatism 20: 792–796

Brawer A E, Cathcart E S 1979 Acute monocytic arthritis. Arthritis and Rheumatism 22: 294–301

Brook I, Reza M J, Bricknell K S, Bluestone R, Finegold S M 1978 Synovial fluid lactic acid: a diagnostic aid in septic arthritis. Arthritis and Rheumatism 21: 774–779

Bunch T W, Hunder G G, McDuffie F C, O'Brien P C, Markowitz H 1974a Synovial fluid complement determination as a diagnostic aid in inflammatory joint disease. Mayo Clinic Proceedings 49: 715–720

Bunch T W, Hunder G G, Offord K, McDuffie F C 1974b Synovial fluid complement: usefulness in diagnosis and classification of rheumatoid arthritis. Annals of Internal Medicine 81: 32–35

Carsons S, Mosesson M W, Diamond H S 1981 Detection and quantitation of fibronectin in synovial fluid from patients with rheumatic disease. Arthritis and Rheumatism 24: 1261–1267

Chambers R J, Bywaters E G L 1963 Rubella synovitis. Annals of the Rheumatic Diseases 22: 263–268

Cheung H S, Ryan L M, Kozin F, McCarty D J 1980 Synovial origins of rice bodies in joint fluid. Arthritis and Rheumatism 23: 72–76

Chung A C, Shanahan J R, Brown E M 1962 Synovial fluid lipids in rheumatoid and osteoarthritis. Arthritis and Rheumatism 5: 176–183

Clemmensen I, Andersen R B 1982 Different molecular forms of fibronectin in rheumatoid synovial fluid. Arthritis and Rheumatism 25: 25–31

Collins D H 1936 The pathology of synovial effusions. Journal of Pathology and Bacteriology 42: 113–140

Cracchiolo A, Goldberg L S, Barnett E V, Bluestone R 1971 Studies of cryoprecipitates from synovial fluid of rheumatoid patients. Immunology 20: 1067–1077

Crocker P R, Dieppe P A, Tylor G, Chapman S K, Willoughby D A 1976 The identification of particulate matter in biological tissues and fluids. Journal of Pathology 121: 37–40

Cummings N A, Nordby G L 1966 Measurement of synovial fluid pH in normal and arthritic knees. Arthritis and Rheumatism 9: 47–56

Currey H L F 1968 Examination of joint fluids for cystals. Proceedings of the Royal Society of Medicine 61: 969–971
Currey H L F, Vernon-Roberts B 1976 Examination of synovial fluid. Clinics in Rheumatic Diseases 2: 149–177
Dayer J M, Passwell J H, Schneeberger E E, Krane S M 1980 Interactions among rheumatoid synovial cells and monocyte-macrophages: production of collagenase stimulating factor by human monocytes exposed to Concanavalin A or immunoglobulin Fc fragments. Journal of Immunology 124: 1712–1720
Dick W C, Whaley K, St Onge R A, Downie W W, Boyle J A, Nuki G, Gillespie F C, Buchanan W W 1970 Clinical studies on inflammation in human knee joints: Xenon (133Xe) clearances correlated with clinical assessment in various arthritides and studies on the effect of intra-articularly administered hydrocortisone in rheumatoid arthritis. Clinical Science 38: 123–133
Dieppe P A, Crocker P, Huskisson E C, Willoughby D A 1976 Apatite deposition disease. A new arthropathy. Lancet 1: 266–269
Dieppe P A, Crocker P R, Corke C F, Doyle D V, Huskisson E C, Willoughby D A 1979 Synovial fluid crystals. Quarterly Journal of Medicine 48: 533–553
Dormandy, T L 1979 Free radical reactions in biological systems. Annals of the Royal College of Surgeons 80: 188–194
Dresner E 1950 The bone and joint lesions in acute leukaemia and their response to folic acid antagonists. Quarterly Journal of Medicine 19: 339–360
Duffy J, Lidsky M D, Sharp J T, Davis J S, Person D A, Hollinger F B, Min K W 1976 Polyarthritis, polyarteritis and hepatitis B. Medicine 55: 19–37
Emkey R D, Ragsdale B D, Ropes M W, Miller W 1973 A case of lymphoproliferative disease presenting as juvenile rheumatoid arthritis. American Journal of Medicine 54: 825–828
Ettlinger R E, Hunder G G 1979 Synovial effusions containing cholesterol crystals. Mayo Clinic Proceedings 54: 366–374
Eyring E J, Murray W R 1964 The effect of joint position on the pressure of intra-articular effusion. Journal of Bone and Joint Surgery 46A: 1235–1241
Fagin T J, Lidsky M D 1974 Compensated polarized light microscopy using cellophane adhesive tape. Arthritis and Rheumatism 17: 256–262
Falchuk K H, Goetzl E J, Kulka J P 1970 Respiratory gases of synovial fluids. An approach to synovial tissue circulatory-metabolic imbalance in rheumatoid arthritis. American Journal of Medicine 49: 223–231
Fam A G, Pritzker K P H, Cheng P T, Little A H 1981 Cholesterol crystals in osteoarthritic joint effusions. Journal of Rheumatology 8: 273–280
Farr M, Kendall M J, Bold A M, Hawkins C F 1981 Significance of pH in synovial fluid. Annals of the Rheumatic Diseases 40: 621
Fostiropoulos G, Austen K F, Bloch K J 1965 Total hemolytic complement and second component of complement activity in serum and synovial fluid. Arthritis and Rheumatism 8: 219–232
Fraser J R E, Cunningham A L, Clarris B J, Aaskov J G, Leach R 1981 Cytology of synovial effusions in epidemic polyarthritis. Australian and New Zealand Journal of Medicine 11: 168–173
Friedman A, Naveh Y 1971 Polyarthritis associated with chicken pox. American Journal of Diseases of Children 122: 179–180
Gatter R A 1977 Use of the compensated polarizing microscope. Clinics in Rheumatic Diseases 3: 91–103
Gaucher A, Faure G, Netter P, Malaman B, Steinmetz J 1977 Identification of microcrystals in synovial fluids by combined scanning electron microscopy and X-ray diffraction: application to triclinic calcium pyrophosphate dihydrate. Biomedicine 27: 242–244
Genovese J R, Jayson M I V, Dixon A St J 1972 Protective value of synovial cysts in rheumatoid knees. Annals of the Rheumatic Diseases 31: 179–182
Goetzl E J, Falchuk K H, Zieger L S, Sullivan A L, Hebert C L, Adams J P, Decker J L 1971 A physiologic approach to the assessment of disease activity in rheumatoid arthritis. Journal of Clinical Investigation 50: 1167–1180
Goldenberg D L, Kelley W, Gibbons R B 1975 Metastatic adenocarcinoma of synovium presenting as an acute arthritis. Arthritis and Rheumatism 18: 107–110
Goldie I, Nachemson A 1969 Synovial pH in rheumatoid knee joints. Acta Orthopedica Scandinavica 40: 634–641
Gordon D A, Pruzanski W, Ogryzlo M A 1973 Synovial fluid examination for the diagnosis of amyloidosis. Annals of the Rheumatic Diseases 32: 428–430
Graham J, Goldman J A 1978 Fat droplets and synovial fluid leucocytosis in traumatic arthritis. Arthritis and Rheumatism 21: 76–80
Greenwald R A 1981 Editorial. Oxy radicals and connective tissue. Journal of Rheumatology 8: 185–187
Griffin P E, Bole G G 1969 Cholesterol containing synovial effusions and cholesterosis of the synovial membrane. University of Michigan Medical Centre Journal 35: 170–176
Groth H P 1975 Cellular contacts in the synovial membrane of the cat and the rabbit: an ultrastructural study. Cell and Tissue Research 164: 525–541
Hadler N M, Spitznagel J K, Quinet R J 1979 Lysosomal enzymes in inflammatory synovial effusions. Journal of Immunology 123: 572–577
Hadler N M, Johnson A M, Spitznagel J K, Quinet R J 1981 Protease inhibitors in inflammatory synovial effusions. Annals of the Rheumatic Diseases 40: 55–59
Hall A P, Scott J T 1966 Synovial cysts and rupture of the knee joint in rheumatoid arthritis. An arthrographic study. Annals of the Rheumatic Diseases 25: 32–41
Halverson P B, McCarty D J 1979 Identification of hydroxyapatite crystals in synovial fluid. Arthritis and Rheumatism 22: 389–395
Hannestad K, Mellbye O J 1967 Rheumatoid factor in synovial effusions; local production and consumption. Clinical and Experimental Immunology 2: 501–509
Hasselbacher P, Schumacher H R 1977 Bilateral protrusio acetabuli following pelvic irradiation. Journal of Rheumatology 4: 189–196
Hasselbacher P, Schumacher H R 1978 Synovial fluid eosinophilia following arthrography. Journal of Rheumatology 5: 173–176
Hedberg H 1967 Studies on synovial fluid in arthritis. I. The total complement activity. Acta Medica Scandinavica (Suppl) 479: 1–37
Hickling P, Wilkins M, Newman G R, Pritchard M H, Jessop J, Whittaker J, Nuki G 1981 A study of amyloid arthropathy in multiple myeloma. Quarterly Journal of Medicine 50: 417–433

Hollander J L, Jessar R A, McCarty D J 1961 Synovianalysis: an aid in arthritis diagnosis. Bulletin of the Rheumatic Diseases 12: 263–264

Hollander J L, McCarty D J, Astorga G, Castro-Murillo E 1965 Studies on the pathogenesis of rheumatoid joint inflammation. I. The RA cell and a working hypothesis. Annals of Internal Medicine 62: 271–280

Hollander J L, Reginato A, Torralba T P 1966 Examination of synovial fluid as a diagnostic aid in arthritis. Medical Clinics of North America 50: 1281–1294

Hollingsworth J W, Siegel E R, Creasey W A 1967 Granulocyte survival in synovial exudate of patients with rheumatoid arthritis and other inflammatory joint diseases. Yale Journal of Biology and Medicine 39: 289–296

Honig S, Gorevic P, Hoffstein S, Weissmann G 1977 Crystal deposition disease. Diagnosis by electron microscopy. The American Journal of Medicine 63: 161–164

Hughes G R V, Currey H L F 1980 Laboratory investigations. In: Currey H L F (ed) Mason and Currey's clinical rheumatology. Pitman, Tunbridge Wells, p 340–354

Hunter T, Gordon B A, Ogryzlo M A 1974 The ground pepper sign of synovial fluid: a new diagnostic feature of ochronosis. Journal of Rheumatology 1: 45–53

Igari T, Kaneda H, Horiuchi S, Ono S 1982 A remarkable increase of superoxide dismutase activity in synovial fluid of patients with rheumatoid arthritis. Clinical Orthopaedics and Related Research 162: 282–287

James H L, Cohen A B 1978 Mechanism of inhibition of porcine elastase by human α_1-antitrypsin. Journal of Clinical Investigation 62: 1344–1353

Jayson M I V, Dixon A St J 1970a Intra-articular pressure in rheumatoid arthritis of the knee. I. Pressure changes during passive joint distension. Annals of the Rheumatic Diseases 29: 261–265

Jayson M I V, Dixon A St J 1970b Intra-articular pressure in rheumatoid arthritis of the knee. II. Effect of intra-articular pressure on blood circulation to the synovium. Annals of the Rheumatic Diseases 29: 266–268

Jayson M I V, Dixon A St J 1970c Intra-articular pressure in rheumatoid arthritis of the knee. III. Pressure changes during joint use. Annals of the Rheumatic Diseases 29: 401–408

Jayson M I V, Dixon A St J 1970d Valvular mechanisms in juxta-articular cysts. Annals of the Rheumatic Diseases 29: 415–420

Jayson M I V, Dixon A St J 1972 Unusual geodes ('bone cysts') in rheumatoid arthritis. Annals of the Rheumatic Diseases 31: 174–178

Jebens E H, Monk-Jones M E 1959 On the viscosity and pH of synovial fluid and the pH of blood. Journal of Bone and Joint Surgery 41-B: 388–400

Joseph N R, Need C I, Honberger E 1946 An in vivo study of pH of synovial fluid in dogs. American Journal of Physiology 146: 1–11

Kahn C B, Hollander J L, Schumacher H R 1970 Corticosteroid crystals in synovial fluid. Journal of the American Medical Association 211: 807–809

Kitridou R, Schumacher H R, Sbarbaro J L, Hollander J L 1969 Recurrent hemarthrosis after prosthetic knee arthroplasty: identification of metal particles in the synovial fluid. Arthritis and Rheumatism 12: 520–528

Krey P R, Comerford F R, Cohen A S 1974 Multicentric reticulohistiocytosis. Fine structural analysis of the synovium and synovial fluid cells. Arthritis and Rheumatism 17: 615–633

Kushner I, Somerville J A 1971 Permeability of human synovial membrane to plasma proteins. Arthritis and Rheumatism 14: 560–570

Labowitz R, Schumacher H R 1971 Articular manifestations of systemic lupus erythematosus. Annals of Internal Medicine 74: 911–921

Lagier R 1977 Synovial reaction caused by adjacent malignant tumours: anatomicopathological study of three cases. Journal of Rheumatology 4: 65–72

Lemperg R K, Beckman G M M, Beckman L E A 1971 Effect of intra-articular corticosteroid administration on acid and alkaline phosphatase activity in synovial fluid of patients with rheumatoid arthritis. Acta Rheumatologica Scandinavica 17: 195–202

Leon S A, Revach M, Ehrlich G E, Adler R, Petersen V, Shapiro B 1981 DNA in synovial fluid and the circulation of patients with arthritis. Arthritis and Rheumatism 24: 1142–1150

Levick J R 1979 An investigation into the validity of subatmospheric pressure recordings from synovial fluid and their dependence on joint angle. Journal of Physiology 289: 55–67

Lund-Olesen K 1970 Oxygen tension in synovial fluids. Arthritis and Rheumatism 13: 769–776

McCord J, Wong K 1979 Phagocyte produced free radicals: roles in cytotoxicity and inflammation. In: Oxygen free radicals and tissue damage, Ciba Foundation Symposium 65. Excerpta Medica, Amsterdam

McEwen C 1935 Cytologic studies on rheumatic fever. Journal of Clinical Investigation 14: 190–201

MacSween R N M, Dalakos T G, Jasani M K, Boyle J A, Buchanan W W, Goudie R R 1968 A clinico-immunological study of serum and synovial fluid antinuclear factors in rheumatoid arthritis and other arthritides. Clinical and Experimental Immunology 3: 17–24

Matthay M, Lindamood M, Steigerwald J C, Solomons C 1977 Acute pseudogout in the absence of synovial fluid leukocytes. Journal of Rheumatology 4: 303–306

Melmon K L, Webster M E, Goldfinger S E, Seegmiller J E 1967 The presence of a kinin in inflammatory synovial effusion from arthritides of varying etiologies. Arthritis and Rheumatism 10: 13–20

Miller J A 1956 Joint paracentesis from an anatomic point of view. I. Shoulder, elbow, wrist and hand. Surgery 40: 993–1006

Miller J A 1957 Joint paracentesis from an anatomic point of view. II. Hip, knee, ankle and foot. Surgery 41: 999–1011

Moskowitz R W, Harris B K, Schwartz A, Marshall G 1971 Chronic synovitis as a manifestation of calcium crystal deposition disease. Arthritis and Rheumatism 14: 109–116

Murphy G, Reynolds J J, Bretz U, Baggiolini M 1977 Collagenase is a component of the specific granules of human neutrophil leucocytes. Biochemical Journal 162: 195–197

Nettlebladt E, Sunblad L 1965 Haptoglobin in serum and synovial fluid. Acta Rheumatologica Scandinavica 11: 11–14

Nettlebladt E, Sunblad L, Jonsson E 1963 Permeability of the synovial membrane to proteins. Acta Rheumatologica Scandinavica 9: 28–32

Newcombe D S, Cohen A S 1965 Chylous synovial effusion

in rheumatoid arthritis. American Journal of Medicine 38: 156–164

Niedermeier W, Creitz E E, Holley H L 1962 Trace metal composition of synovial fluid from patients with rheumatoid arthritis. Arthritis and Rheumatism 5: 439–444

Niedermeier W, Cross R, Beetham W P 1965 The concentration of haptoglobin in synovial fluid of patients with rheumatoid arthritis. Arthritis and Rheumatism 8: 355–360

Onion D K, Crumpacker C S, Gilliland B C 1971 Arthritis of hepatitis associated with Australia antigen. Annals of Internal Medicine 75: 29–33

Owen D S 1981 Aspiration and injection of joints and soft tissues. In: Kelley W N, Harris E D, Ruddy S, Sledge C B (eds) Textbook of rheumatology. Saunders, Philadelphia, p 553–567

Panush R S, Franco A E, Schur P H 1971 Rheumatoid arthritis associated with eosinophilia. Annals of Internal Medicine 75: 199–205

Pekin T J, Zvaifler N J 1964 Hemolytic complement in synovial fluid. Journal of Clinical Investigation 43: 1372–1382

Pekin T J, Zvaifler N J 1970 Synovial fluid findings in systemic lupus erythematosus. Arthritis and Rheumatism 13: 777–785

Petrone W F, English D K, Wong K, McCord J M 1980 Free radicals and inflammation: superoxide dependent activation of a neutrophil chemotactic factor in plasma. Proceedings of the National Academy of Science, USA 77: 1159–1163

Phelps P, Steele A D, McCarty D J 1968 Compensated polarized light microscopy. Identification of crystals in synovial fluids from gout and pseudogout. Journal of the American Medical Association 203: 508–512

Phelps P, Steele A D, McCarty D J 1972 Significance of Xenon 133 clearance rate from canine and human joints. Arthritis and Rheumatism 15: 360–370

Porter B B, Nuki G, Buchanan W W, Dick W C 1970 Synovial perfusion of clinically normal knee joints in patients with rheumatoid arthritis. Annals of the Rheumatic Diseases 29: 649–652

Priest J R, Urick J J, Groth K E, Balfour H H 1978 Varicella arthritis documented by isolation of virus from joint fluid. Journal of Pediatrics 93: 990–992

Pritchard M H, Nuki G 1978 Gold and penicillamine: a proposed mode of action in rheumatoid arthritis based on synovial fluid analysis. Annals of the Rheumatic Diseases 37: 493–503

Radin E L, Swann D A, Weisser P A 1970 Separation of a hyaluronate-free lubricating fraction from synovial fluid. Nature 228: 377–378

Reddy C R R M, Parvathi G, Swaramappa M 1969 Adhesion of white blood cells to Guinea worm larvae. American Journal of Tropical Medicine and Hygiene 18: 379–381

Richman A I, Su E Y, Ho G 1981 Reciprocal relationship of synovial fluid volume and oxygen tension. Arthritis and Rheumatism 24: 701–705

Riese H 1895 Die Reiskörperchen in tuberculös erkrankten Synovalsäcken. Deutsch Zeitschrift für Chirurgie 42: 1–99

Riordan T, Doyle D, Tabaqchali S 1982 Synovial fluid lactic acid measurement in the diagnosis and management of septic arthritis. Journal of Clinical Pathology 35: 390–394

Robitaille P, Zvaifler N J, Tan E M 1973 Antinuclear antibodies and nuclear antigens in rheumatoid synovial fluids. Clinical Immunology and Immunopathology 1: 385–397

Rodnan G P, McLachlan M J 1960 The absorption of serum albumin and gamma globulin from the knee joint of man and rabbit. Arthritis and Rheumatism 3: 152–157

Ropes M W, Bauer W 1953 Synovial fluid changes in joint disease. Harvard University Press, Cambridge, Massachusetts

Ropes M W, Rossmeisl E C, Bauer W 1940 The origin and nature of normal synovial fluid. Journal of Clinical Investigation 19: 795–799

Rubinow A, Canoso J J, Goldenberg D L, Cohen A S 1976 Synovial fluid (SF) and synovial membrane (SM) pathology in Whipple's disease (WD).Arthritis and Rheumatism 19: 820

Ruddy S, Colten H R 1974 Rheumatoid arthritis biosynthesis of complement proteins by synovial tissues. The New England Journal of Medicine 290: 1284–1288

Ruddy S, Fearon D T, Austen K F 1975 Depressed synovial fluid levels of properdin and properdin factor B in patients with rheumatoid arthritis. Arthritis and Rheumatism 18: 289–295

Sauter S van H, Utsinger P D 1978 Viral arthritis. Clinics in Rheumatic Diseases 4: 225–240

Schumacher H R 1966 Intracellular crystals in synovial fluid anticoagulated with oxylate. New England Journal of Medicine 274: 1372

Schumacher H R 1972 Multiple myeloma with synovial amyloid deposition. Rheumatology and Physical Medicine 11: 349–353

Schumacher H R 1977 Pathogenesis of crystal induced synovitis. Clinics in Rheumatic Diseases 3: 105–131

Schumacher H R, Jimenez S A, Gibson T, Pascual E, Traycoff R B, Dorwart B B, Reginaton A M 1975 Acute gouty arthritis without urate crystals identified on initial examination of synovial fluid. Arthritis and Rheumatism 18: 603–612

Schumacher H R, Smolyo A P, Tse R L, Maurer K 1977 Arthritis associated with apatite crystals. Annals of Internal Medicine 87: 411–416

Schur P H, Sandson J 1963 Immunologic studies of the proteins of human synovial fluid. Arthritis and Rheumatism 6: 115–129

Scott D L, Wainwright A C, Walton K W, Williamson N 1981 Significance of fibronectin in rheumatoid arthritis and osteoarthrosis. Annals of the Rheumatic Diseases 40: 142–153

Scudder P R, McMurray W, White A G, Dormandy T L 1978 Synovial fluid copper and related variables in rheumatoid and degenerative arthritis. Annals of the Rheumatic Diseases 37: 71–72

Sheehan H, Storey G 1947 An improved method of staining leucocyte granules with Sudan Black B. Journal of Pathology and Bacteriology 59: 336–337

Sheppheard H, Lea D J, Ward D J 1981 Synovial fluid total hemolytic complement activity in rheumatic diseases — a reappraisal. Journal of Rheumatology 8: 390–397

Simkin P A, Pizzorno J E 1974 Transynovial exchange of small molecules in normal human subjects. Journal of Applied Physiology 36: 581–587

Sliwinsky A J, Zvaifler N J 1969 The removal of aggregated and nonaggregated autologous gamma globulin from rheumatoid joints. Arthritis and Rheumatism 12: 504–514

Small D M, Cohen A S, Schmid K 1964 Lipoproteins of

synovial fluid as studied by analytical ultracentrifugation. Journal of Clinical Investigation 43: 2070–2079

Smiley J D, Sachs C, Ziff M 1968 Synthesis of immunoglobulin by rheumatoid synovial membrane. Journal of Clinical Investigation 47: 624–632

Spilberg I, Meyer G J 1972 The arthritis of leukaemia. Arthritis and Rheumatism 15: 630–635

Stephens R W, Ghosh T, Taylor T K F, Gale C A, Swann J C, Robinson R G, Webb J 1975 The origins and relative distribution of poly-saccharidases in rheumatoid and osteoarthritic fluids. Journal of Rheumatology 2: 393–400

Sunblad L 1965 Glycosaminoglycans and glycoproteins in synovial fluid. In: Balazs E A, Jeanloz R W (eds) The amino sugars. Academic Press, New York, p 229–250

Suter E R, Majno G 1964 Ultrastructure of the joint capsule in the rat: presence of two kinds of capillaries. Science 202: 920–921

Swann D A 1978 Macromolecules of synovial fluid. In: Sokoloff L (ed) The joints and synovial fluid, Vol 1. Academic Press, New York, p 407–435

Swann D A, Radin E L 1972 The molecular basis of articular lubrication. I. Purification and properties of a lubricating fraction from bovine synovial fluid. Journal of Biological Chemistry 274: 8069–8073

Swann D A, Caulfield J B, Ceselski A 1975 Proteins associated with hyaluronic acid. Annals of the Rheumatic Diseases 34: Supplement 98–100

Swanson S A V 1973 Lubrication. In: Freeman M A R (ed) Adult articular cartilage. Pitman, London, p 247

Tanphaichitr K, Spilberg I, Hahn B 1976 Letter to the Editor. Lithium heparin crystals simulating calcium pyrophosphate dihydrate crystals in synovial fluid. Arthritis and Rheumatism 19: 966–968

Theofilopoulos A G, Carson D A, Tavassoli M, Slovin S F, Speers W C, Jensen F B, Vaughan J H 1980 Evidence for the presence of receptors for C3 and IgG Fc on human synovial cells. Arthritis and Rheumatism 23: 1–9

Townes A S, Sowa J M 1970 Complement in synovial fluid. Johns Hopkins Medical Journal 127: 23–37

Traycoff R B, Pascual E, Schumacher H R 1976 Mononuclear cells in human synovial fluid. Identification of lymphoblasts in rheumatoid arthritis. Arthritis and Rheumatism 19: 743–748

Treuhaft P S, McCarty D J 1971 Synovial fluid pH, lactate, oxygen, and carbon dioxide partial pressure in various joint diseases. Arthritis and Rheumatism 14: 475–484

Utsinger P D 1977 Adenovirus 7 Arthritis: Clinical and immunological studies. Arthritis and Rheumatism 20: 138

Vernon-Roberts B, Freeman M A R 1977 The tissue response to total joint replacement prostheses. In: Swanson S A V, Freeman M A R (eds) The scientific basis of joint replacement. Pitman, London, p 86–129

Ward J R, Bishop B 1970 Varicella arthritis. Journal of the American Medical Association 211: 1954–1956

Ward T T, Steigbigel R T 1978 Acidosis of synovial fluid correlates with synovial fluid leukocytosis. American Journal of Medicine 64: 933–936

Weinberger H W, Ropes M W, Kulka J P, Bauer W 1961 Reiter's syndrome clinical and pathologic observations. Medicine 40: 35–91

Winchester R J, Agnello V, Kunkel H G 1969 The joint fluid γG-globulin complexes and complement diminution. Annals of the New York Academy of Sciences 168: 195–203

Wynne-Roberts C R, Cassidy J T 1979 Juvenile rheumatoid arthritis with rice bodies: light and electron microscopic studies. Annals of the Rheumatic Diseases 38: 8–13

Zuckner J, Uddin J, Gantner G E, Dorner R W 1964 Cholesterol crystals in synovial fluid. Annals of Internal Medicine 60: 436–446

Zvaifler N J 1973 The immunopathology of joint inflammation in rheumatoid arthritis. Advances in Immunology 16: 265–336

SECTION III

Inflammation and Immunology in the Rheumatic Diseases

9

P. Dieppe   D. Blake

Inflammation

Inflammation can be defined as the response of living tissues to a sublethal injury. At its simplest level it is characterised by changes in small blood vessels and the accumulation of fluid and cells at the site of damage. This local reaction usually triggers a more systemic response including fever, leucocytosis, protein catabolism and altered hepatic synthesis of plasma protein, which may then influence the injured area. This fundamental biological reaction is a dynamic process, not a state. It is often perceived as harmful, but is designed to minimise local damage and inhibit its progression. Most inflammatory responses are short-lived (acute), illustrating the efficiency of the protective, reparative system. Indolent (chronic) inflammation often results in medical interference on the assumption that the response is doing more harm than good. Because of the enormous complexity of the inflammatory reaction, and the large number of interrelated mechanisms which influence it, such 'anti-inflammatory' therapy is often relatively ineffective, and its use remains controversial.

This chapter outlines the inflammatory process, and the complexity of its control. A historical approach has been adopted (Table 9.1); the resulting emphasis on one mechanism in preference to another reflects the nature of recent research rather than their respective importance.

HISTORICAL INTRODUCTION

Prehistoric man must have been familiar with inflammation and wound healing in the skin, which are mentioned in some of the earliest medical texts. The Smith Papyrus (*c*. 1650 BC) includes a word implying a 'hot thing' to describe suppurating wounds, and the Ebers Papyrus (*c*. 1600 BC) describes erysipelas and suggests that wounds should be allowed to heal by granulation (i.e. without interference).

Greek and Roman physicians wrote extensively about the inflammatory process. They apparently regarded it as undesirable, and evidence of imbalance of 'humours'; they also interfered with it, describing cleaning and suturing of wounds in an attempt to aid resolution. Celsus (*c*. 30 BC–30 AD) is noteworthy for his classical description of the four cardinal signs of inflammation: *Tumor* (swelling), *Rubor* (redness), *Calor* (heat) and *Dolor* (pain). A fifth sign, *Functio Laesa* (loss of function) was added by Virchow (1821–1902). This sign is often wrongly attributed to Galen (130–200 AD), the Greek physician whose writings dominated medicine for centuries (Majno, 1975).

Table 9.1 Selected landmarks in the history of inflammation

Early descriptions
Egyptian papyri, Greek and Roman tests.
Celsus (*c*. 30BC–30AD): The cardinal signs of inflammation.
Pathophysiology
Cohnheim (1839–1884): Vascular events.
Metchnikoff (1845–1916): Cellular events.
Starling (1896): Control of fluid exudation.
Lewis (1927): The 'triple response'.
Systemic response
Mankin and Beeson (1940s): Endogenous pyrogen isolated.
Selye (1950s): The 'general adaptation syndrome'.
1970s: Descriptions of the 'cytokines' — mediating local, systemic and immunological events.
Chemical mediators
Dale (1910): Histamine.
Von Eular (1935): Vasoactive prostaglandins.
Miles (1964): The kinin system.
Spector and Willoughby (1960s): Sequential release of chemical mediators.
Vane (1971): Inhibition of prostaglandin synthetase.

John Hunter (1728–1793) was one of the first to record the benefits of inflammation, describing it as a 'salutary reaction', and one whose purpose is 'to restore the parts to their natural functions'. Virchow's cellular concept of disease then led to the idea that inflammation is a physiological response to trauma that can take various forms in different tissues.

Cohnheim (1839–1884) provided the classical description of the vascular events in inflammation, and was able to relate them to the five cardinal signs. He concluded that the whole process was due to blood vessel injury. The Russian zoologist Metchnikoff (1845–1916) discovered phagocytosis, and described the protective role of cellular digestion of foreign material in many animal species. Metchnikoff showed that the influx of phagocytes to an area of injury was an active process, and declared that the whole purpose of the inflammatory process was 'mobilisation of the phagocyte'. He distinguished the early role of the 'microphage' (polymorphonuclear cell) from the later influx of the 'macrophage' (mononuclear cells). He also demonstrated increased phagocytosis on second exposure to an infective stimulus; an early illustration of the humoral (immunological) aspects of inflammation.

The humoral, as opposed to the cellular, aspects were also appreciated by Edward Jenner (1749–1839), who described the lasting protection against smallpox provided by vaccination with cowpox, and noted that vaccinated people reacted with a stronger inflammatory response. Louis Pasteur (1822–1895) extended Jenner's work, and described the value of humoral factors in providing protection in immunised patients. The concept that inflammation allows 'antitoxins' to get to a bacterial invader and neutralise its effects then developed.

Wound healing was also studied extensively by surgeons and physicians treating those injured in numerous wars. Thus both the protective and reparative role of the inflammatory response were delineated.

Hunter, who described the benefits of inflammation, was also quick to appreciate that it can be harmful. He wrote: 'when it cannot accomplish that salutory purpose ... it does mischief'. It is now appreciated that inflammation is a complex process controlled by numerous mediator and suppressor systems, and that an inappropriate stimulus, or loss of control of the effectors, can lead to unwanted tissue damage.

That inflammation is a process and not a state was emphasised by Burden-Sanderson (1828–1905): 'inflammation is the succession of changes which occurs in living tissue when it is injured'. He realised that the balance of the vascular, cellular and healing phases varies, as does the importance of the humoral and systemic responses. Changes in either the stimulus or the host can result in a shift of emphasis in the inflammatory reaction.

Early research therefore described the vascular, cellular, humoral and reparative events of inflammation. Recent work has concentrated on the mechanisms controlling it and the interrelationships between them (Florey, 1970; Majno, 1975; Ryan & Majno, 1977).

THE LOCAL INFLAMMATORY PROCESS

The inflammatory response at a site of injury can be divided into several parts, which overlap but dominate the response in a sequential way (Table 9.2). Full descriptions of the events can be found in the work of Cohnheim (1889), Metchnikoff (1905), Florey (1970), Hurley (1983), and Ryan & Majno (1977).

Table 9.2 Local events in the inflammatory process

Induction
Vasodilation
Increased vascular permeability
Formation of an exudate
Cellular infiltration:
Polymorphonuclear cells (early)
Macrophages (late)
Other cells
Phagocytosis of invaders and damaged tissue
Repair
Fibrogenesis
Neovascularisation
Tissue regeneration

These events occur in sequential, but overlapping, phases following acute injury. In prolonged inflammation different events may dominate the reaction according to the nature of the stimulus, and time from onset. In this chapter the local inflammatory response is described under these headings.

Changes in vascular calibre, blood flow and lymphatic drainage

Introduction

The early sequential changes of vasodilation, followed by slowing of blood flow, fluid exudation, cellular infiltration, the formation of new blood vessels and repair were beautifully described by Cohnheim, who examined the living frog mesentery. Thc initial vascular response to injury was also documented by Sir Thomas Lewis (1927), who analysed the changes following a firm stroke of the skin. They include the sequential development of a red line, swelling, and a flare (the 'triple response'). Lewis showed that the same response could be induced by several different stimuli, including histamine injection, and that denervation of the tissue reduce the flare and wheal.

Cohnheim, Lewis and others concentrated on the initial reactive changes occurring within hours of a single transient stimulus. Analysis of subsequent events is more recent, and has been dependent on the use of different models of inflammation, such as implantation of subcutaneous foreign bodies in rodents (Ryan & Spector, 1970). These studies have emphasised the evolution from the acute phase dominated by vasodilation, and exudation of fluid and polymorphonuclear cells, to a chronic phase dominated by exudation of mononuclear cells, the generation of new blood vessels (granulation tissue), tissue regeneration and fibroblast repair (Spector & Lykke, 1966). Chronic inflammation is therefore not synonymous with persistent inflammation.

Blood flow and lymphatic drainage

Direct trauma to blood vessels can cause a fleeting constriction of arteriolar smooth muscle. However, the dominant reaction of the arterioles is a persistent *vasodilation* lasting for the duration of the inflammatory response. This is the basis of the red flare in the triple response. Arteriolar dilation is mediated by local chemical and neuronal factors which cause relaxation of the muscular wall.

Vasodilation can result in a transient increase in the rate of blood flow through the capillary bed. But within minutes of injury there is *slowing of flow*, and in some capillarics complete stasis. Reduced flow may be accompanied by clumping of the erythrocytes (rouleaux formation, or 'sludging'), and intravascular thrombosis. The early reduction in blood flow appears to be caused by exudation of plasma raising the viscosity of the blood. As the response develops, increasing extravascular pressure, and chemical mediation of local thrombosis, may contribute further to vascular stasis (Hay & Movat, 1979).

Blood flow is normally laminar, the cells occupying the central fast stream, and plasma the outer, slower stream adjacent to the endothelial cell wall. The reduced flow in inflammation is accompanied by loss of these zones, increasing turbulence, and mixing of cells and plasma. This *loss of laminar flow* results in some cells coming into contact with the endothelium.

In a normal vessel, cells do not stick to the surface. In inflamed tissue, leucocytes which come in contact with the vessel wall are seen to roll along it, and then become adherent. Cellular *margination*, and *pavementing* of the endothelium with leucocytes is observed principally in the venules. It appears to be caused by increased 'stickiness' of the vessel wall, although the mechanism for this remains obscure (Wilkinson & Lackie, 1979).

Lymphatic drainage increases dramatically in inflamed tissue (Hay, 1979). Pressure and flow can both increase 100 fold or more, and debris, particles and cells are all carried swiftly by the lymphatic vessels to the draining lymph nodes. The sinuses of the regional nodes become engorged, and the macrophages respond. Follicular hyperplasia with the appearance of new germinal centres may occur — a picture described as a 'reactive' lymph node or 'reactive hyperplasia'. Increased lymph flow is caused by exudation of fluid from blood vessels and increased extravascular pressure. Unlike the capillaries, the lymphatics are kept open, and flow increases rather than decreases. This is facilitated by the anatomy of the vessel, which has tethering lines which become taut in engorged tissues, and keep the lymph channel open (Pullinger & Florey, 1935).

The formation of an exudate

(*a*) *Physiology of the terminal vascular bed.* The arterioles, capillaries and venules which form the terminal vascular bed are the 'business end' of the vascular tree (Fig. 9.1). They form the site for transport between the intra-vascular and extravascular spaces, and the site of control of the microcirculation. Transport back and forth across the vessel wall depends on physical forces, and on the vascular endothelium. Heidenheim (1891) suggested that transport depended on active secretion by endothelial cells, whereas Starling (1896) considered that the principles of diffusion controlled flow, and that the vessel wall acted as a passive filter. This controversy is still not fully resolved.

The Starling hypothesis (1896, 1909) proposes that fluid passage is a product of filtration pressure (the hydrostatic pressure is the capillary minus the hydrostatic pressure in the interstitial fluid) and the osmotic pressure across the capillary wall. Landis (1934) examining this hypothesis demonstrated that at the arterial end of the terminal vascular bed the filtration pressure exceeds the

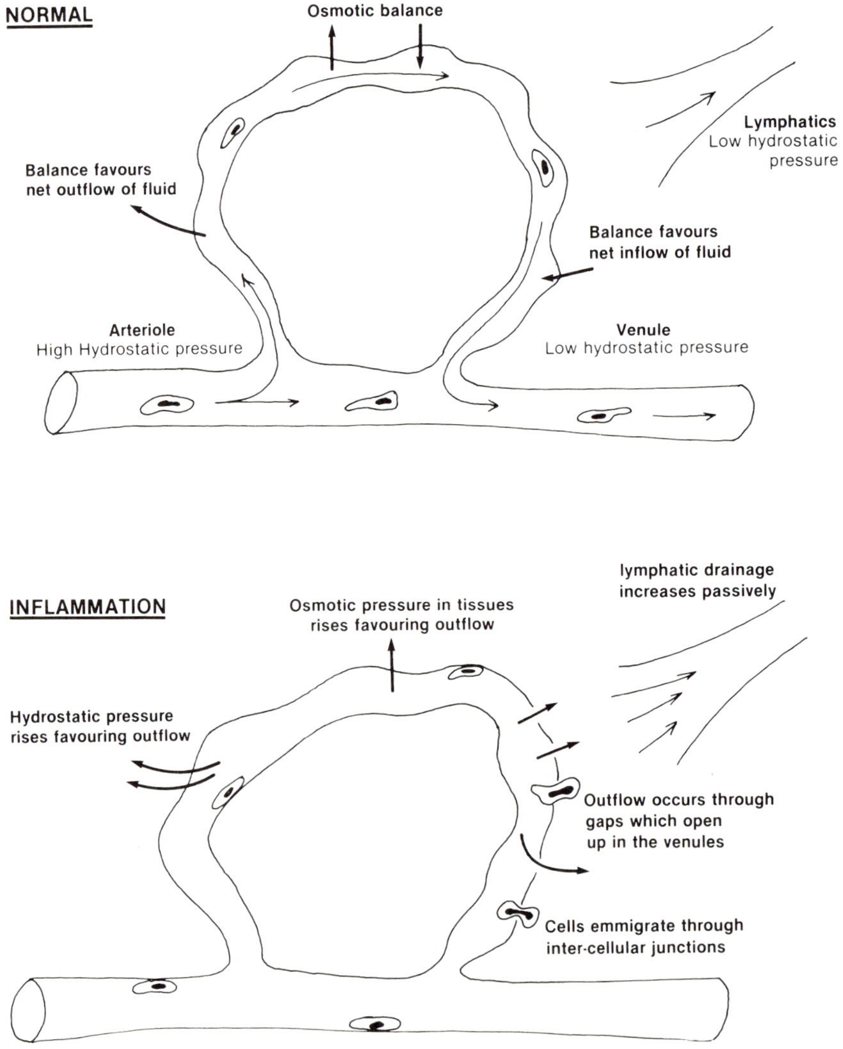

Fig. 9.1 The terminal vascular bed and the formation of an exudate. According to the hypothesis of Starling, there is bidirectional flow of fluid across the terminal vascular tree, dependent on the balance of hydrostatic and osmotic pressures in the vessels and tissue. In inflammation, various factors, including increased intravascular pressure, alterations in the vessel wall and increased osmotic pressure in the tissues, all tend to increase fluid movement into the extravascular space.

osmotic pressure, whereas the converse is true on the venous side (Fig. 9.1). Bidirectional flow may therefore occur at different locations, and the endothelium of the venule might be most sensitive to extravascular influences whereas the arteriole endothelium would be more sensitive to intravascular changes.

Vessel walls consist of endothelial cells and a basement membrane of collagen fibres. Normally the intercellular junctions are about 20 nm wide, but they vary in size and complexity. Cellular and fluid transport must occur either through the cells and basement membrane, or via gaps between cells and holes in the membrane. Pappenheimer (1953) predicted that a system of cylindrical pores, about 90Å in diameter, must exist to allow passage of large molecular weight proteins across capillary walls. Electron microscopy has not shown any evidence for such pores, but conspicuous intracellular vesicles aligned on the luminar and external margins of endothelial cells are seen. Palade and colleagues therefore suggested that they represent small pinocytic vesicles which ferry substances across vessel walls (Simonescu et al, 1975). The intercellular junction has been studied by Luft (1966). Using ruthenium red (a cationic stain) he demonstrated the presence of mucopolysaccharides in the junction as well as along the basement membrane, suggesting that an intercellular cement exists. Karnovsky (1967) introduced horseradish peroxidase (molecular weight 40 000) into the circulation and subsequently found it in both the intercellular vesicles and in the intracellular junctions. Clementi & Palade (1969) using ferritin particles (molecular weight 500 000) showed their presence in the vesicles only, with subsequent accumulation along the external basement membrane 10 minutes after injection.

In the normal vascular bed it therefore appears that the physical forces elucidated by Starling control the passage of water, electrolytes and other low molecular weight substance. However, the intercellular junctions and active transport by vesicles have an important role in transport of particles and high molecular weight substances. The relative importance of these different mechanisms probably varies in different organs according to the anatomy of the terminal vascular bed. Some have a continuous endothelium (e.g. skin, muscle, lungs); some are fenestrated, with areas in which the wall thins down to a narrow membrane (e.g. glomerulus and glandular tissue); others are discontinuous, with conspicuous gaps between endothelial cells (e.g. spleen and bone marrow).

The vascular bed of the synovial membrane has been studied both in health and disease (Rothschild & Masi, 1982; Ghadially, 1983). It is generally thought to have a deep population of capillaries with a continuous endothelium, but there is also a superficial capillary bed which is fenestrated (Mitnick et al, 1978; Ghadially, 1983). Electron microscopy shows that it changes dramatically in early synovitis (Schumacher & Kitridou, 1972).

(*b*) *Pathophysiology of the microcirculation in inflammation: exudation.* The 'tumor' described by Celsus and the 'wheal' of Lewis's triple response represent the fluid exudate of inflammation. Three main mechanisms cause fluid to leave the circulation in inflammation (Simon, 1979; Fig. 9.1).

1. Alteration in the balance of hydrostatic and osmotic pressures. Vasodilation of arterioles causes increased hydrostatic pressure. This 'pushes' fluid and electrolytes across the endothelium of arterioles, capillaries and venules. As the reaction develops the osmotic pressure also changes in favour of fluid passage from the intra- to the extravascular space because of the increasing concentration of protein in the inflammatory exudate. Much of the fluid swelling can therefore be accounted for by changing diffusion forces, favouring a transudate. This is opposed by a small increase in the hydrostatic pressure in the extracellular space, but this is often minimal due to the facility of the lymphatic vessels to respond by rapidly draining fluid from the extracellular space. This mechanism of fluid formation is mediated by chemical messengers and by neuronal influences causing dilation of arterioles (Ryan & Majno, 1977).

2. Formation of gaps in the venules. The second mechanism aiding formation of the exudate principally affects the venules. Gaps, about 1 μm wide, appear between the endothelial cells, and plasma pours out. These holes in the endothelium act as sinks, and can be observed holding back

cells, platelets, chylomicrons etc., which sometimes plug the gap, while plasma and its proteins pour into the traumatised area. The gaps appear to be produced by chemical mediators which cause active contraction of microfilaments in the endothelial cells, rounding up the cell, and pulling it away from its neighbour. Venules are affected partly because of their susceptibility to extravascular mediators (mentioned above), and partly because their endothelial cells seem to be richest in the contractile filaments (Ryan & Majno, 1977).

3. Trauma. A third, and rather obvious, mechanism of exudate formation is via direct vascular injury, allowing all elements of the blood to leak into the tissues. This is prominent at the centre of the injury, and persists until vessels are sealed by platelets and fibrin.

An exudate is, by definition, richer in protein than a transudate formed by simple diffusion forces. But not all inflammatory exudates are the same.

The protein content as well as the cell counts vary. This results in different visual appearances, and to descriptions of serous (low cell count), purulent (high cell count), fibrinous or haemorrhagic exudates. These variations may depend on the stimulus, the site of inflammation, and variation in host responses. Serous surfaces (e.g. pleura and pericardium) tend to form fibrinous exudates with a surface layer of polymerised fibrin. Synovial joints can behave similarly, and exudates rich in fibrin and fibronectin, with surface deposits on the membrane and cartilage, are common.

Cellular infiltration

The characteristic histological feature of an inflammatory lesion is the presence of a cellular infiltrate in the perivascular region and interstitial spaces.

Cell types

Most lesions are dominated by polymorphonuclear leucocytes ('microphages'), or mononuclear phagocytic cells ('macrophages'). The predominant type depends on the stimulus and the time course of the reaction (Van Furth & Willemze, 1979).

A short-lived, traumatic stimulus produces a triphasic response. There is an initial transient phase in which hardly any cells can be found (the 'disappearance' reaction). After about 30 minutes neutrophils start to enter the lesion, and within 4–6 hours the reaction peaks. The neutrophils then slowly disappear over the next 48 hours. The third phase is the appearance of the macrophages. Although a few are found within about 6 hours of the stimulus, their concentration in the exudate takes about 36 hours to reach a peak, and then subsides over 3–5 days (Van Furth, 1975).

Bacterial stimuli produce varying cellular reactions. 'Pyogenic' organisms get their name from their ability to attract masses of polymorphs, resulting in 'pus'. In contrast, the tubercle bacillus induces a reaction dominated by slow recruitment of mononuclear cells. Parasites excite the generation of an eosinophil chemoattractant, as does IgE-mediated mast cell degranulation; this results in an exudate dominated by the eosinophil species of polymorph. Basophils frequently appear in macrophage-dominated lesions. Lymphocytes and plasma cells are usually numerous in chronic immune-mediated inflammation, and multinucleate cells appear in chronic foreign body reactions.

Other cells found in the inflammatory exudate include erythrocytes and platelets. The platelet may have a major role in many types of inflammation, but has proved difficult to study and quantify (Gordon, 1976).

The origin of cells in the exudate

It is now generally accepted that both polymorphonuclear cells and macrophages are derived from the bone marrow. The influx of numerous neutrophils within a few hours of the stimulus is facilitated by their presence in large numbers in the blood (the marginated pool). Pyogenic stimuli induce release of more neutrophils from the bone marrow as part of the systemic response to inflammation (see below). The neutrophils are short-lived cells which subsequently degenerate and disappear.

The origin of the macrophages has been the subject of much debate. Metchnikoff (1905) believed that macrophages were derived from lymphocytes, but Volkman & Gowans (1965), in an elegant set of experiments, showed that they came from the bone marrow. They labelled bone marrow promonocytes with tritiated thymidine, and followed the labelled cells into the inflammatory lesions; they proved the point by abolishing the macrophage response through prior irradiation of the bone marrow. Spector and his colleagues have gone further and shown that macrophages also proliferate locally at the site of inflammation, and can transform into the epithelioid and multinucleate giant cells found in some chronic inflammatory lesions (Spector, 1979; Ryan & Spector, 1970).

The persistent macrophage response found in chronic inflammation is therefore facilitated by three factors:

1. The long life of the macrophage
2. The persistent emigration of cells derived from the bone marrow
3. Local proliferation and cellular transformation.

Lymphocytes are continually moving from the blood to the extracellular space, and thus to the lymphatics, the thoracic duct, and back to the blood. It has been presumed that lymphocytic cells found in inflammatory lesions originate from this pool, via attraction of cells during their passage from the terminal vascular bed to the lymphatics (Dumonde, 1978).

Leucocyte emigration

The pavementing of venules by leucocytes, and their subsequent emigration across the vessel wall has been described by numerous light microscopists. Marchesi & Florey (1960), using the electron microscope, confirmed the previous observations of passage of leucocytes through intercellular spaces of the venular endothelium. The chemical attraction of leucocytes was first investigated by Leber (1888) who observed movement of leucocytes to the site of an injected mold in the guinea-pig cornea. Subsequently Harris (1950) and Boyden (1962) developed more elegant in vitro systems for studying chemotaxis.

Pavementing. Endothelial cells and leucocytes are both negatively charged, inhibiting sticking. There is also a layer of glycoprotein on vessel walls which may alter in inflammation and could influence leucocyte pavementing on the endothelium. Experimental data suggests that changes in the leucocyte as well as the vessel wall may affect stickiness; the former tend to clump more easily in areas of inflammation, and the latter can be damaged by oxygen radicals perhaps reducing the normal charge property, or by degrading a natural anti-inflammatory protein which is perpetually synthesised in vivo to regulate endothelial cell contraction. Leucocyte sticking is dependent on both calcium and magnesium ions, suggesting that they may form 'ionic bridges' between cells (Wilkinson & Lackie, 1979; Oyanagui, 1981).

Diapedesis. Cells escape by amoeboid movement through the vessel wall. The process takes between 2 and 12 minutes. It would seem logical that the route chosen would be through the intracellular gaps opened up by mediators of increased vascular permeability, but this is not the case. The leucocytes appear to force their way through a normal intercellular bridge, which closes after the passage of the cell.

Chemotaxis. The diapedesis of cells, and their movement to the stimulus, depends on the generation of chemoattractants. Some of the mediators involved are discussed later.

Various experimental systems have been used to study the mechanism of chemotaxis (Boyden, 1962; Hurley, 1963; Wilkinson, 1982). The use of synthetic oligopeptides (e.g. fomyl Met-Leu-Phe) which produce analogous effects to bacterial derived chemotoxins has aided research (Schiffmann et al, 1975; Pike & Synderman 1982). In response to a stimulus the cells change shape and rapidly polarise, and the flat leading edge travels towards the source. Cell movement is achieved by changes in the internal microfilaments and microtubules; it is mediated through specific cell surface receptors, and can be blocked by calcium ionophores (Synderman, 1982).

Lymphocytic accumulation. Whereas red cells, platelets and phagocytic cells have the proven ability to migrate towards a stimulus, the passage of lymphocytes is less well characterised. De Sousa (1981) has reviewed the lack of understanding of the how and why of lymphocyte movement, and suggested that iron may play an important role in dictating sites of lymphocyte accumulation. Direct evidence to support this is lacking, but local iron has also been implicated in other recent studies (Blake et al, 1981). Dumonde (1978) has suggested that a disorder in the normal regulation of lymphocyte traffic may be caused by changes in blood vessels, resulting in the transformation of some inflammatory foci to aberrant lymph nodes.

Phagocytosis

The process of phagocytosis involves recognition of the particle, attachment to the cell surface, ingestion, degranulation and release of substances capable of destroying the invader. The main cells involved are the polymorphonuclear neutrophil and the macrophage.

Recognition and attachment. The fascinating ability of the phagocyte to recognise damaged self (e.g. dead cell fragments) and foreign particles has been documented by Stossel (1975) and others, but the mechanism is not fully understood.

The value of serum factors which enhance phagocytosis (opsonins) is well recognised. Opsonins are of two types — non-specific factors which probably include acute phase proteins (e.g. C-reactive protein), and the more specific antibodies which are programmed to recognise an individual foreign protein. The opsonins coat the foreign particles, and can then aid recognition by attaching to cell surface receptors. Receptors for C3 and the Fc component of immunoglobulins were described on phagocytic cells many years ago; recently receptors for glycoproteins and other substances have also been discovered (Weinbaum et al, 1982).

Opsonisation and attachment to receptors is not, however, the whole story. Washed cells, incubated in a protein-free medium, can recognise, attach to, and ingest a variety of particles, including inert diamond crystals, and show different responses to the different stimuli (Dieppe et al, 1983). The mechanisms involved are not clear.

Ingestion and degranulation. After attachment, the particle is internalised. The cell extends projections (pseudopods) which seem to flow around the foreign body, and then fuse together to produce a phagosome which is drawn back into the main body of the cell.

During this process, three other phenomena can be observed:

1. A respiratory burst from the cell
2. Release of lysosomal hydrolases and other cell-derived factors into the surrounding medium
3. Granules converging on the phagosome and discharging their contents into it (Fig. 9.2).

The respiratory burst provides energy, and generates toxic radicals (see 'free radicals and inflammation' below). Enzymes are released during ingestion, phagocytes being 'messy eaters' (Weissmann et al, 1979). The process of degranulation occurs as lysosomal granules fuse with the wall of the phagosome to form phagolysosomes. Neutrophils degranulate rapidly, often killing themselves in the process ('suicide cells'). Macrophages are phylogenetically younger, more discriminating, and less suicidal in their response; they secrete a variety of enzyme products and intercellular communicators according to the response (see 'enzyme products' and 'cytokines' below).

These products of the phagocyte are designed to destroy the foreign invader. They can also cause damage to surrounding tissues.

The healing process

Inflammation is a healing process, designed to repair tissue damage both quickly and efficiently.

At the simplest visual level there are four main elements to healing, involving four cell types (Table 9.3).

1. The phagocyte destroys damage tissue and removes debris
2. Fibroblasts help wound contraction, and put down a new connective tissue stroma of collagen
3. Endothelial cells proliferate to produce a new vascular bed, providing nutrition and a passage for the other cells
4. The cells of the damaged tissue show a variable degree of regeneration, or metaplasia, repairing the involved organ (Peacock & Van Winkle, 1976).

   The role of the phagocyte has already been described.

Fibroblasts

Proliferation of fibroblasts begins soon after injury, and reaches a peak between day 2 and day 10, when the cells are actively secreting collagen. After about 2 weeks, activity lessens, but cross-

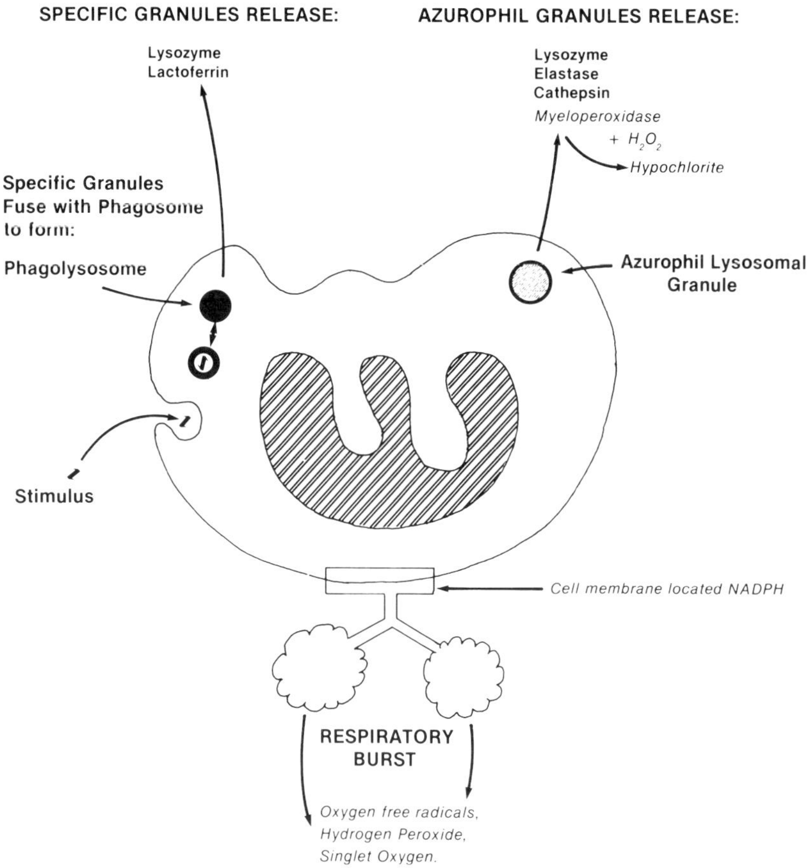

Fig. 9.2 Phagocytosis. The foreign invader (bacteria, crystal, immune complex, etc.), activates the cell membrane and causes release of enzymes from lysosomal granules. The respiratory burst generates oxygen radicals which have an important role in degrading the foreign stimulus. (Oxygen-dependent reactions shown in italics.)

linking continues, increasing the strength of the collagen, which becomes maximal some 3 weeks after induction of a wound. The precise stimuli which control and regulate fibroblast activity are unknown, although the macrophage is known to produce factors which affect fibroblast replication (Leibovich & Ross, 1976), including interleukin 1 (Schmidt et al, 1982).

Table 9.3 Cells involved in the repair phase of inflammation

The macrophage
Removal of damaged tissue
Activation of other cells
The fibroblast
Formation of a new connective tissue matrix
Wound contraction
Endothelial cells
Formation of new vessels: 'granulation tissue'
Tissue cells
Regeneration

The macrophage also secretes collagenase (Werb & Gordon, 1975) and new collagen may itself be chemotactic for macrophages (Postlethwaite & Kang, 1976). One can therefore envisage a system in which the fibroblast and the macrophage work hand-in-hand in the remodelling and repair of damaged and disorganised connective tissue. (Krane et al, 1982).

Majno's group recently showed that the fibroblast was also responsible for wound contraction (Gabbiani & Majno, 1972; Ryan & Majno, 1977). The cells apparently contain myofibrils, which allow contraction and pull together the edges of a resolving inflammatory lesion.

Vascular proliferation and granulation tissue

Neovascularisation is an essential feature of healing, as macrophages, fibroblasts and regenerating tissue must have a blood supply.

Growth of new blood vessels has been studied by Schoefl (1963) and others using trauma to induce inflammation and healing. The endothelial cells can be observed forming pseudopodia which stretch out into the lesion. The cells then migrate and proliferate to form a new tube budding off from an existing vessel. Capillary buds increase at an average rate of about 0.2 mm per day, and eventually meet up to form a new vascular bed. The lymphatics also regenerate, and manage to link up with their own vessels and not the capillaries.

Factors which might control this process were first discovered by Brem et al (1972), who described a factor in tumours responsible for angiogenesis. Since then factors derived from lymphocytes (Sidkey & Auerbach, 1975) and macrophages (Polverini et al, 1977) have also been implicated (see 'cytokines' below). Avascular tissues such as cartilage may contain specific inhibitors (angiogenesis inhibiting factor) which prevent neovascularisation (Brem & Folkman, 1975).

'Granulation tissue' is a term used to describe the advancing mass of new blood vessels and immature connective tissue stroma which fills up the gap in an open wound, and grows into areas of tissue damage. The vessels provide nutrition and channels for the scavenging macrophages and reparative fibroblasts which pull the wound together and repair it with collagen. The vascular element of granulation tissue then slowly reorganises itself into a new capillary network for the healed tissue.

Granulation tissue must be distinguished from a 'granuloma' which is a concentric aggregation of cells around an indolent inflammatory focus. The pattern and morphology of the cells varies with the chronicity of the reaction and the stimulus, allowing histological recognition of some granulomas.

Tissue regeneration

The ability of tissues to regenerate varies considerably. This, combined with variation in the other elements of healing, means that repair is quite different in the various organs of the body.

Skin healing is excellent. After an attack of erysipelas, for example, regeneration and repair are quick and return the tissue entirely to normal. In contrast, cells of the central nervous system cannot regenerate, and only scarring (collagen), can replace lost tissue. The liver has the ability to regenerate rapidly, but also scars easily; patchy areas of fibrosis and nodular regeneration are responsible for the cirrhotic liver. The synovial lining cells regeneate and proliferate rapidly in response to trauma, and the amount of new tissue formation often appears inappropriate (e.g. villous hypertrophy). The synovium sometimes demonstrates the other main element of tissue repair — metaplasia. Thus the cells may form a different type of tissue, as in synovial chondromatosis or osteochondromatosis.

THE SYSTEMIC RESPONSE TO INFLAMMATION

Local inflammatory responses are accompanied by a systemic response to injury. This is clinically apparent from signs such as fever, weight loss and general malaise, and has been recognised for centuries.

Selye (1950) studied this systemic response, describing it as a 'general adaptation syndrome'. He observed alterations in local vascular permeability and cell movement if the systemic reaction was large, and stressed the role of corticosteroid release to mobilise the whole of the body's defences to fight a local insult. It was clear to Selye that local and systemic responses were closely interrelated.

The alterations in endocrine function and electrolyte balance described by Selye have received less attention recently. Febrile responses continue to be monitored, and fever charts remain at the end of all hospital beds, but attention has now been shifted towards two other manifestations of the systemic response to injury:

1. Alteration in the number of cellular elements circulating in the blood
2. The hepatic synthesis of a variety of proteins (acute phase proteins).

It is also recognised that this systemic response can cause major changes in T and B lymphocyte function, altering, for example, the synthesis of immunoglobulins, and can result in muscle breakdown.

Until recently, both the mediation and biological significance of these reactions remained obscure. However, one exciting recent development in inflammation is the appreciation that many aspects of the systemic response are probably mediated by the same macrophage-derived factors (Bornstein, 1982; Dinarello, 1984).

Thus 'leucocyte-derived pyrogen', 'leucocytic endogenous mediator' and 'lymphocyte activating factor' are probably similar mediators, they are all now known as 'interleukin 1' (IL1) (Aarden et al, 1979). The present evidence suggests that macrophages, activated by the inflammatory process, produce these 15 000 dalton proteins which then activate the hepatocyte, altering its synthetic activity, and disturb hypothalamic function, to produce fever. IL1 has local effects on muscles and on lymphocyte function, and may have other local and distant effects (Table 9.4) (Bornstein, 1982; Dinarello, 1984).

The role of the systemic response is becoming clearer, and mechanisms to explain Selye's observation that general stress alters local inflammation are now being described.

Table 9.4 Interleukin 1

1 A family of cell-derived polypeptide mediators with similar (possibly identical) characteristics, including:
   Endogenous pyrogen
   Leukocytic endogenous mediator
   Lymphocyte activating factor
   B-cell activating factor
   Mononuclear cell factor

2. Main source: mononuclear phagocytic cells

3. Some factors inducing release of interleukin 1:
   Micro-organisms and microbial products
   Particulate inflammatory stimuli, e.g. urate crystals
   Antigens and lymphokines

4. A wide range of probable actions includes:
   Induction of fever
   Neutrophilia
   Altered synthesis of acute phase proteins
   Skeletal muscle proteolysis
   Immunoregulation
   Increased activity of fibroblasts and chondrocytes.

Fever

The febrile response is produced by an alteration in the hypothalamic regulatory system resulting in inappropriate vasoconstriction. This raises body temperature, and is followed by a phase of compensatory vasodilation and sweating.

The classical studies of Bennett & Beeson (1953) established that chemical mediators produced locally in inflamed tissue were responsible for fever. Using -pyrogen free conditions they extracted fluid from inflammatory exudates and showed that it induced hyperthermia. Subsequent work by Wood (1970), Atkins & Bodel (1972) and others established that the macrophage was the main source of the pyrogen. These workers have also documented the different pattern of the febrile response in different diseases.

A high temperature is recognised by everyone as a sign of inflammatory disease, but it is one aspect of the response whose purpose has yet to be fully defined.

Phagocytic cell activity increases at higher temperatures, and various immunological responses are facilitated by raising body temperature (Jampel et al, 1983). It is therefore likely that the systemic febrile response benefits the local inflammatory reaction in its attempts to eliminate invaders and repair tissue damage (Bernheim et al, 1979). The mediation of fever by interleukin 1, like muscle proteolysis, probably involves activation of arachidonic acid metabolism in cell membranes (Dinarello, 1984).

Changes in blood cells

A neutrophil leucocytosis with a 'shift to the left' (more immature cells in the circulation) is the classical feature of inflammation, especially if the stimulus is bacterial. Other changes may include a lymphocytosis, eosinophilia, and thrombocytosis.

Polymorphonuclear leucocytes are 'pooled' in the marrow reserve, and in the marginated pool within the circulation (cells stuck to vessel walls). Exercise and steroids will induce mobilisation of leucocytes, but in inflammation there is evidence that specific chemical mediators are also responsible. A leucocytosis-inducing factor (LIF) has been isolated from inflammatory lesions (Gordon, 1970). Some products of complement activation are chemotactic and a marrow colony-stimulating factor which may mobilise cells from the marrow has also been isolated (Golde & Cline, 1974). It remains unclear whether these observations are demonstrating the presence of one, or of several, different factors. Macrophage-derived IL1 may be the main cytokine responsible for neutrophilia (Dinarello, 1984).

Other blood cell changes, such as thrombocytosis, are often prominent in rheumatic diseases, and it appears that mechanisms exist to turn on, as well as turn off, the production of various cells from the marrow in response to injury. Lactoferrin may play a part in these inhibitory changes (Bagby et al, 1981).

As with the febrile response, the variability of the reaction in response to different inflammatory stimuli is striking.

Hepatic synthesis of proteins — the 'acute phase' response

The elevated ESR, so often used to measure inflammation, is largely caused by increased production of fibrinogen and globulin (Holdstock & Mitchell, 1977). It is now clear that there is a massive change in hepatic synthesis of many proteins in response to inflammation (Table 9.5). Some proteins are increased, others decrease (Whicher, 1981; Kushner, 1982).

'Negative' acute phase proteins

A few proteins fall in concentration in the plasma; examples are albumin, pre-albumin and transferin. This may be due to switching of aminoacids to other pathways, to a specific 'switch-off' mechanism, or to increased catabolism.

'Positive' acute phase proteins

There are some 20 known proteins whose synthesis is increased during inflammation. The response is quick, occurring within hours or days of the stimulus, but varies in degree. Some proteins, such as C3 and caeruloplasmin, only increase a little, others such as fibrinogen, and the enzyme inhibitors α_1 antitrypsin and α_1 antichymotrypsin increase in concentration 2–4 fold, and C-reactive protein (CRP) and serum amyloid A protein (SAA) increase several hundred fold.

All the proteins involved are synthesised by the hepatocyte, and they can be classified into several different classes (Table 9.5). Some are natural mediators of inflammation (e.g. kinins and complement components); others are natural inhibitors (e.g. C1 inactivator and α_1 antitrypsin). Caeruloplasmin has been described as 'beautiful but purposeless' by chemists and clinicians. It is a carriage protein for copper, but recent work suggests that it has an important role in inflammation, by acting as an antioxidant (Gutteridge & Stocks, 1981).

Several enzyme inhibitors are produced (e.g. α_2 macroglobulin and α_1 antitrypsin), and they may help inhibit damage. The final group is a miscellaneous collection of proteins which include CRP and SAA. Their function is not yet clear, although they may act as primitive scavengers and opsonins, or 'non-specific antibodies' (Kushner, 1982; Volanakis, 1982).

CRP responses and other protein changes are used widely in the assessment of chronic inflammatory disorders (Whicher, 1981). In common with other aspects of inflammation, the acute phase response differs according to the stimulus or

Table 9.5 Some of the acute phase proteins and their possible role in inflammation

'Negative' acute phase proteins (levels fall during inflammation)	
Albumin Pre-albumin Transferin	Carriage proteins
'Positive' acute phase proteins (levels rise during inflammation)	
Complement components Plasminogen Fibrinogen Prothrombin Factor VIII	Effector molecules involved in complement, coagulation and kinin cascades
C1 INH C3 b INA α_1 antitrypsin α_1 antichymotrypsin βIH	Inhibitors of complement cascade and enzyme inhibitors
Haptoglobin Haemopexin Ferritin	Iron retrieval from haemoglobin release
Caeruloplasmin	? Free radical elimination
C-reactive protein (CRP)	? Non-specific opsonisation ('primitive antibody')
α_1 acid glycoprotein (orosomucoid) Serum amyloid A-related protein (SAA) Gc globulin	Function unknown

disease present. Moreover, disease-specific defects in the response have recently been described; systemic lupus erythematosus rarely increases CRP levels (Pepys, 1981), and patients with scleroderma show a defective response when challenged with prostaglandins (Whicher et al, 1980). Although absolute deficiencies of response have not been described, if the role of these proteins is as extensive as is now suggested, these defects may have great significance in the pathogenesis of rheumatic disorders. Several studies indicate defective IL1 production from macrophages of patients with rheumatic diseases (Dinarello, 1984).

Other components

There are several other components to the systemic response to inflammation, which includes widespread metabolic and endocrinological changes. Weight loss is often striking in patients with inflammatory disorders, and muscle wasting and weakness are prominent. It has recently become clear that muscle proteolysis is induced as another part of the IL1-mediated response to local inflammation (Baracos et al, 1983). Immunoregulation is another vital function of IL1 (Dinarello, 1984), so it is clear that the local response, altered immune function, and widespread systemic changes are inextricably linked in inflammation.

THE CONTROL OF THE INFLAMMATORY RESPONSE

Extrinsic injury was regarded as the major factor in inflammation for centuries, but after the work of Metchnikoff, Cohnheim, Pasteur and others, there was a dispute in which the traumatic, cellular and humoral theorists competed with each other to explain the cause of inflammation. That local chemicals such as histamine could mediate the vascular changes was demonstrated by Lewis, who also observed the influence of the axonal reflex on vasodilation. It was subsequently shown that nerves were unnecessary for local inflammation, and neural mediators have been given surprisingly little further attention. Other systemic factors were stressed by Selye. In the 1940s Valey suggested that a large array of chemical mediators, each specific to a different aspect of the inflammatory process, much exist. They were conveniently named — leukotoxins, exudin and leukocytosis-promoting factors. Spector & Willoughby (1963) then summarised the features of the permeability response that strongly suggested a role for chemical mediators rather than direct physical effects. They are

1. The reversible nature of the inflammatory process
2. The consistent pattern of the response for a wide range of effective stimuli
3. Suppression by drugs
4. The existence of a latent period between the initial and delayed phase of increased permeability.

The chemical systems controlling inflammation remain poorly understood. There are many interrelated factors which are artificially divided into separate chemical systems, but clearly interact with each other in a complex fashion. For convenience these factors are often divided into:

1. Systems which recognise tissue injury, invasion or insult, and respond by initiating the inflammatory cascade
2. The main mediator and modulator systems controlling inflammation
3. The effector mechanisms which induce destruction of the insult, initiate repair, and also cause tissue damage.

This division is artificial, as many stimuli to inflammation trigger the main mediator and modulator systems, and they in turn activate repair and can damage host tissues.

The term chemical 'mediator' was first introduced to describe substances which transmitted nerve impulses across the neuromuscular junction (e.g. acetylcholine). Mediators involved in inflammation, as in other biological processes, are of two basic types:

1. Those produced at a distant site and carried by the blood to the effector system (e.g. oxytocin)
2. Those produced locally at their main site of action (e.g. histamine and bradykinin).

Inflammation is also influenced by *modulators*, which can be defined as compounds released locally or systemically which change the magnitude or quality of an event which has already been started. A mediator will therefore initiate or participate in the process of inflammation and a modulator will change it.

Mediators of inflammation can be classified in several different ways. Some are breakdown products of components of the plasma, others are derived from cells, and these may be stored, or synthesised in response to an insult. Chemically they range from the low molecular weight factors like histamine (involved in the early phase) to higher molecular weight peptides, like the cytokines (involved later in the reaction). They can be divided functionally into those which primarily affect the microcirculation, those which influence the cellular aspects of inflammation, and those that mediate the systemic effects (Table 9.6).

Each chemical system is controlled by positive and negative feedback systems, and by interaction with other mediators. The principles of physiological control, outlined by Claude Bernard, are exemplified by inflammatory mediators (Fig. 9.3). For example, histamine release results in negative feedback inhibition of further release, limiting mast cell degranulation, and the alternate complement pathway is under constant control from interacting inhibitors, and a positive accelerator loop.

The dual themes of interconnected systems, feedback inhibition, and/or amplification loops in inflammation are discussed further in the next sections.

Table 9.6 The origin of some of the mediators of vascular changes and cellular infiltration in inflammation

Mediator	Origin
Vasoactive	
Histamine	Stored in mast cells,
Serotonin	basophils, platelets.
Bradykinin	Formed by enzymatic cleavage
Complement components	of serum factors.
Prostaglandins (especially PGE_2 and $PGF_{2\alpha}$)	Synthesised from cell membrane arachidonic acid.
Neutrophil products	Cellular products
Chemotactic	
Complement products (especially C3a and C5b)	Formed by enzymatic cleavage of serum factors.
Neutrophil chemotactic factor	Cellular products
Other cellular chemotoxins	
Leukotriens (especially LTB_4)	Synthesised from cell membrane arachidonic acid.
Bacterial chemotactic factor	Derived from the inflammatory stimulus.

Recognition systems and the initiation of inflammation

The ability of the body to respond quickly to trauma, to recognise foreign invaders, and to discriminate damaged and dead tissues is central in the initiation of inflammation.

The recognition systems consist of

1. Mediators stored in cells in a 'pre-packaged' form released by trauma or other stimuli
2. Proteins and other chemicals in the serum which can be cleaved to release active mediators
3. Cell surface receptors which recognise and respond to a specific signal.

There is often a sequential development of mediator systems controlling vasodilation, as outlined by Di Rosa et al (1971). This is due to

a. Interactions between the systems
b. Feedback inhibition
c. A different time lag between systems which are prepackaged (e.g. histamine) and those which have to be synthesised in response to the stimulus (e.g. prostaglandin).

Several different stimuli are capable of inducing an inflammatory response. They include the following:

Trauma

Direct physical or chemical trauma causes damage to cells and connective tissues. Mast cells and platelets are particularly vulnerable, and if ruptured may spill stored low molecular weight vasodilators such as histamine and serotonin into the tissues. Exposed collagen can activate intravascular coagulation and inflammation by activating plasmin and Hagemann factor. More extensive trauma, breaking blood vessels and rupturing many cells, will cause the release of many more of the mediators and modulators described below, including proteases, which cleave protein systems such as complement components.

Charged surfaces

A variety of particles and organic materials with a charged surface initiate inflammation. Zymosan, products of bacterial cell walls and crystals are examples. The properties which dictate whether or not a crystal will induce inflammation have been studied in depth (Mandel & Mandel, 1982), and illustrate the discriminative powers of these systems. Critical features include the surface roughness and zeta potential of the particle. Similar factors probably determine the ability of bacterial lipopolysaccharides to trigger inflammation. Hagemann factor, the complement cascade and release of proteases from phagocytes are all activated by such particles.

Products of inflammation

Nearly all known mediators and modulators of inflammation also have the ability to activate other proinflammatory pathways (see below). Thus lysosomal proteases activate complement; the respiratory burst of phagocytosis produces radicals that can induce the formation of a chemoattractant; prostaglandins can activate immunological systems; and complement, Hagemann factor, kinin generation, and clotting are inextricably linked. Those interactions help explain the essential similarity of the response irrespective of its cause. They also illustrate the need for modulators and inhibitor systems to prevent all inflammatory reactions growing exponentially.

Damaged tissues, including cartilage, also induce inflammation

Chrismann et al (1965) showed that chemical extracts of rabbit cartilage could induce synovial inflammation in the same species in vivo. Kinin generation has been identified in response to such products (Moskowitz et al, 1970), and the inflammatory and antigenic potential of exposed and altered collagen has recently been recognised (Trentham et al, 1978). These pathways could perpetuate inflammation of joints and other connective tissues if not checked by other systems.

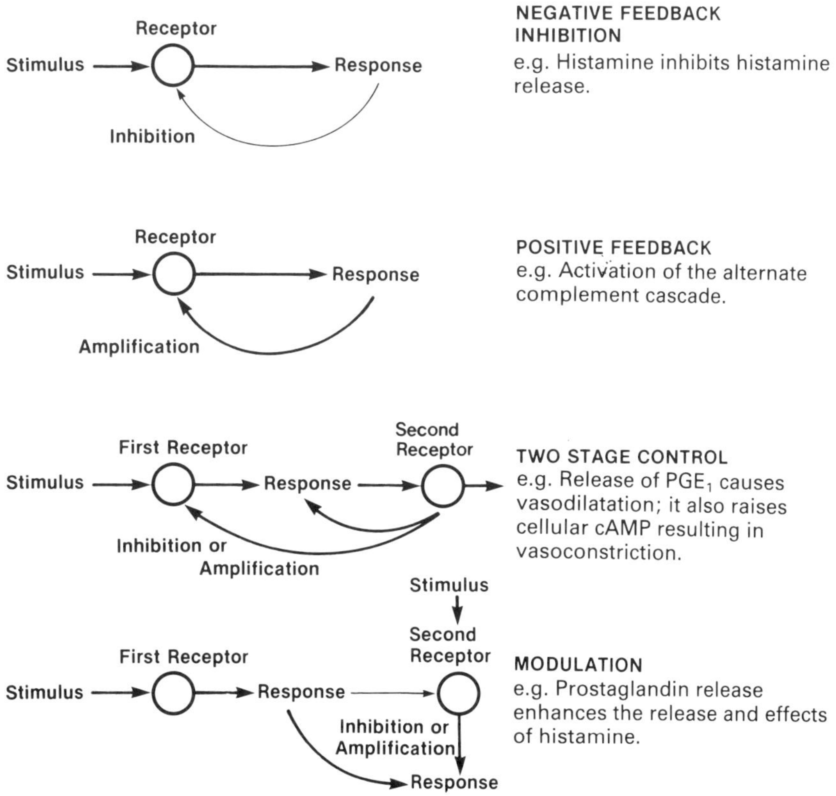

Fig. 9.3 Control mechanisms in inflammation. The figure shows in diagrammatic form some of the loops which operate to maintain control and to modulate the inflammatory process. The complex interaction of all the main mediator systems allows for the construction of many much more complicated pathways.

Immunological stimuli

The generation of antibody and reactive lymphocytes produces a system primed to activate an inflammatory response in tissues containing the antigen. The basic types of 'hypersensitivity' are covered elsewhere. The recognition systems include cell surface receptors for C3 and the Fc component of immunoglobulin on phagocytes, the first component of complement, and cellular responses to lymphokines released by activated lymphocytes.

Mediators and modulators of inflammation

For the sake of simplicity the main mediator systems will now be discussed as separate chemical entities, in accordance with their historical development. This approach minimises the enormous importance of the interaction of the different systems, and overemphasises the individual importance of each mediator or modulator.

Histamine

Histamine was first synthesised in 1907 and then found as an endogenous substance in the intestinal mucosa and elsewhere. It is widely distributed in mammalian tissues and is found in many different species (e.g. bee venom). Its concentration in tissues is directly related to the number of mast cells present, although it may exist elsewhere, and in blood it is limited to basophilic leukocytes. It is synthesised from histidine by the cytoplasmic enzyme histidine decarboxylase. It is stored within intracellular granules through firm ionic linkage to carboxyl groups on granular proteins. The vascular effects of histamine occur after it has been released from its storage sites and are short-lived because it is rapidly methylated or oxidised by enzymes such as histamine-N-methyl-transferase which is plentiful in most tissues.

The major pharmacological properties of histamines are contraction of smooth muscle, dilation of small blood vessels and stimulation of secretion from endocrine glands. One of the most striking effects of histamine is on the microvascular circulation. Shortly after injury, mast cells, which are particularly abundant around small blood vessels, degranulate and the histamine content of tissue fluid rises. This dilates the arterioles and increases the permeability of the postcapillary venules by causing the endothelial cells to contract. It is thought that increased permeability is mainly a function of the H_1 receptor, whilst vasodilation is mediated by both H_1 and H_2 receptors (Kozlowski et al, 1981; Beaven, 1976).

For a long time it was considered that the effect of histamine was transient, because in vitro studies show that histamine depletion and antihistamines only ameliorate the early vascular response. However, histamine has recently been found to have many other actions relevant to inflammation. In vivo work suggests that histamine may inhibit its own release as well as reducing basophil, eosinophil and neutrophil chemotaxis (Lett-Brown & Leonard, 1977). Chemokinesis (random motility) appears to be enhanced. These findings are associated with increased intracellular cyclic AMP, but cyclic GMP levels are unaffected (Anderson et al, 1977). The effects of histamine are also potentiated by various prostaglandins, and a complex interrelationship clearly exists between histamine and the products of arachidonic acid metabolism.

Vasoactive amines may also modulate immune responses (Askenase, 1977; Rocklin & Beer, 1983). Histamine can inhibit the expression of delayed cutaneous hypersensitivity, and inhibits T cell-mediated cytotoxicity, lymphocyte proliferation and lymphokine production in vitro. It has been suggested that histamine might serve as a negative feedback regulator of cellular immune reactions, a concept supported by Schwartz et al (1981) who have shown that histamine inhibits the generation of suppressor T lymphocytes induced by the mitogen Con A.

Bradykinin and the kallikrein–bradykinin system

The discovery of a permeability factor of plasma (PF/Dil) by Miles (1964) brought the kinin system to the attention of pathologists.

The peptide bradykinin is cleaved from the α_2 globulin bradykininogen by the protease kallikrein which is generated from prekallikrein by activated factor XII (Hagemann factor) (Fig. 9.4). This factor may be activated by a variety of mechanisms — acidification, dilution, treatment with organic solvents or by contact with charged surfaces such as crystals, or aggregates of immune complexes. The complexities of the system are compounded by the ability of Hagemann factor to influence the

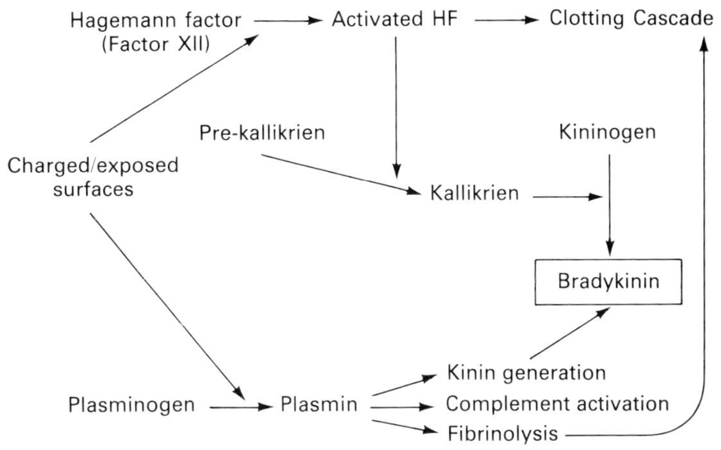

Fig. 9.4 Some of the pathways involved in activation of bradykinin and the clotting cascade in inflammation. Hagemann factor and plasminogen are both activated by charged surfaces. Activated Hagemann Factor (HF) precipitates the clotting cascade, it also activates prekallikrein, leading to the generation of the vasodilator bradykinin. Activated plasminogen can also lead to the generation of bradykinin, as well as complement activation and fibrinolysis. Different parts of these interrelated pathways are more or less dominant in different inflammatory reactions.

complement system, the intrinsic coagulation pathway, and the fibrinolytic system, and of bradykinin to induce histamine release, and suppress cellular immune responses (Kimura, 1983).

The exact role of the kinin system in inflammation still requires clarification. Its concentration depends upon the balance of formation and inactivation. A variety of inactivating tissue peptidases ensure that its effect is local, and make isolation difficult. However, at acid pH the inactivity enzymes are inhibited whereas the forming enzyme is little affected, so in inflammation its concentration may rise. Its effects depend entirely on the amount present; in concentrations as low as 10^{-8} M bradykinin will cause vasodilation and increased vascular permeability; at 10^{-7}–10^{-6} M it will cause pain, and at 10^{-5}–10^{-4} M it will induce leucocyte chemotaxis (Lewis, 1962; Elliott et al, 1960).

Should bradykinin escape into the circulation it is inactivated in the lungs by the same enzyme that converts the inactive decapeptide angiotensin I to the active octapeptide angiotensin II. The latter will cause generalised vasoconstriction (cf. bradykinin-induced local vasodilation), and release of aldosterone (Erdös, 1977). This provides an example of a local mediator inducing a systemic balancing reaction, and highlights the difficulty in assessing the importance of any individual mediator of the inflammatory reaction in isolation. Histamine has a similar effect on the endocrine system, inducing adrenaline release from the adrenal medulla, and thus opposing its own local vasodilatory actions.

The complement system

The complexities of the complement cascade are dealt with elsewhere (Ch. 13) and will only be discussed here to illustrate its interrelationship with other systems, and the modulating influence of complement on the inflammatory process. Examples of these specialised mediating and modulating influences of activated complement components include the release of histamine from mast cells, enhancement of vascular permeability, contraction of smooth muscle, chemotactic attraction of phagocytic cells, immune adherence, enhancement of phagocytes, degranulation and release of lysosomal enzymes from neutrophils, and stimulating prostaglandin E synthesis (Minta & Movat, 1979).

As with the kinin-generating pathway, the phenomenon of limited proteolysis is central to the functioning of the complement system. Specific but limited proteolytic reactions catalyse the cleavage of complement proteins, the development of active enzymes from their precursors, and the formation of protein–protein complexes. As with other effector systems, duplication of effects exists, e.g. factors derived from both the classical and alternate pathway both induce chemotaxis.

Control mechanisms also exist so that activation of either pathway does not inexorably lead to a cytotoxic conclusion. The necessity for precise control relates to the fact that the complement system is a physiological plasma constituent and as such is constantly available.

The many interrelated mediator and modulator functions of the complement cascade are probably involved in all types and phases of the inflammatory/immune reaction, and complement depletion reduces inflammation in response to traumatic, immunological and other stimuli (Di Rosa et al, 1971; Egwang & Befus, 1984).

Prostaglandins — enzyme catalysed lipid peroxidation

Virtually all mammalian cells have the capacity to synthesise prostaglandins, named by Von Eular in 1935, following the discovery that the polar fatty acids derived from seminal fluid were capable of causing vasodepression and contraction of the uterus. The precursors of prostaglandins are the polyunsaturated fatty acids in cell membranes derived from dietary essential fatty acids, and are susceptible to dietary maniuplation. The autacoids are synthesised (de novo) from three specific fatty acid precursors

1. Dihomo-γ-linolenic acid
2. Arachidonic acid
3. Eicosapentaenoic acid

with the formation of prostaglandins of the 1, 2, and 3 series respectively.

Arachidonic acid is the most abundant precursor in mammals. Acylhydrolases (e.g. phospholipase A_2) result in the polyenoic fatty acids being liberated from their membrane stores and once in free form they become substrates for cyclo-oxygenases and lipoxygenases. The subsequent pathway of enzymatic degradation are shown in Figure 9.5. Lipoxygenase inserts one oxygen molecule into the fatty acid acid resulting in a hydroperoxy intermediate (HPETE); cyclo-oxygenase inserts two oxygen molecules into one substrate molecule resulting in the formation of the prostaglandin endoperoxide PGG_2. Depending on the type of catalase present in different tissues formation of the classical prostaglandins (PGE_2, PGF_2 and PGD_2) and thromboxanes (TXA_2 and TXB_2) follows. Prostacyclin PGI_2 and its stable metabolite 6-Keto $PGF_{2\alpha}$ are also formed (Vane, 1976; Robinson et al, 1982).

Recently it has been shown that the formation of the 'slow releasing substances of anaphylaxis' (SRS-A), the lipid autacoid released from lungs following immunological challenge, is dependent on a lipoxygenase with a specificity for the 5 position of the arachidonate molecule. Samuellson et al (1979) discovered a new group of arachidonic acid metabolites which are formed in leucocytes via this 5-HPETE. Because of their origin, and presence of 3 conjugated double bends in their molecules, these new members of the AA family were named 'leukotrienes'. Leukotriene C is probably identical with SRS-A (Orning et al, 1980).

Virtually all of the products of arachidonic acid metabolism have been implicated in inflammation, although research is made difficult by the instability of some (e.g. TXA_2 and PGI_2) and problems in assaying others (e.g. leukotrienes).

In general cyclo-oxygenase derivatives affect the vascular phase of inflammation, whereas the lipoxygenase pathway produces cellular chemoattractants. Thus PGE_2 is a potent and important vasodilator, and LTB_4 is one of the most active polymorphonuclear cell chemotoxins known (Table 9.4).

Elevated levels of arachidonic acid and prostaglandins of the E and F series have been found in many inflammatory tissues, including synovial fluid. In addition to causing vasodilation, prostaglandins have other potentially important inflammatory properties, including the ability to enhance the effect of other mediators, and sensitisation of pain receptors (modulation). Inhibition of prostaglandin synthesis has been widely held to be an important 'anti-inflammatory' property since Vane (1971) discovered that aspirin and other non-steroidal drugs inhibited cyclo-oxygenase (for review see Robinson, 1983).

However, the actions of arachidonic acid derivatives are far from simple, and not all are proinflammatory. Thus many of the actions of PGF_2 are the opposite of those of PGE_2 and PGE_2 alters cyclic nucleotide levels, resulting in inhibition of

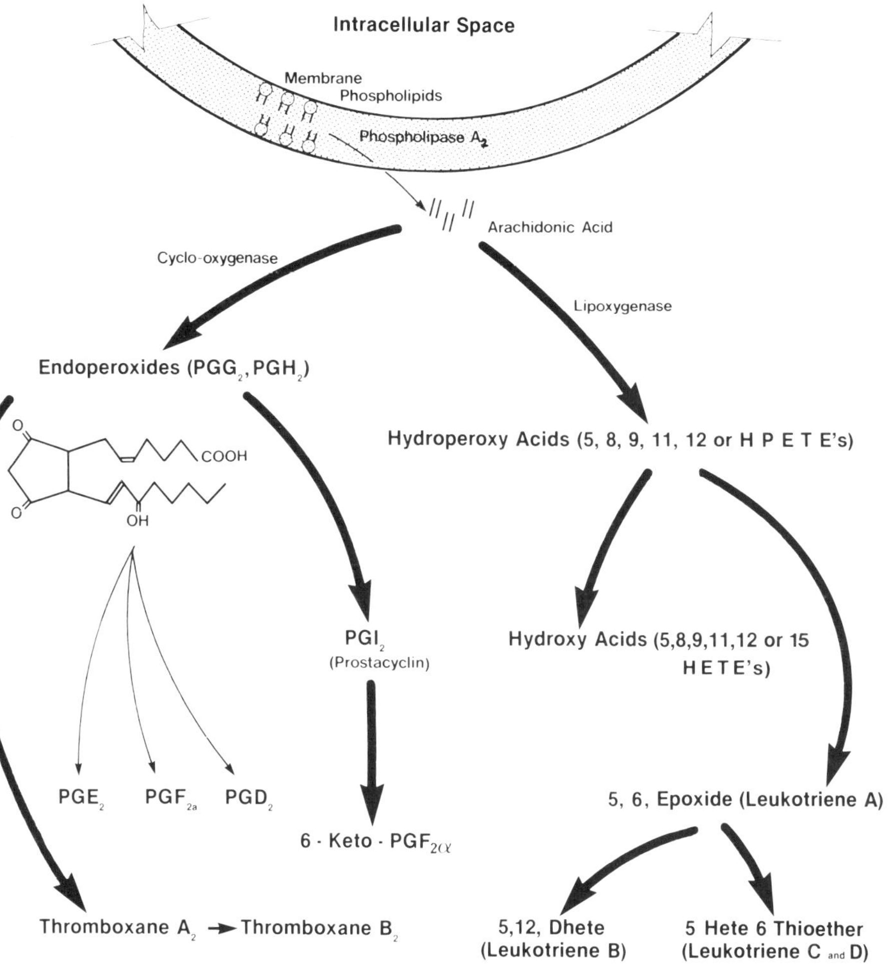

Fig. 9.5 Some pathways of arachidonic acid metabolism. The most important product of membrane phospholipid is arachidonic acid. This can be metabolised to the endoperoxides by cyclo-oxygenase, or to the hydroperoxy acids by lipoxygenase. The former pathway leads to a number of potent, short-lived vasoactive compounds including prostaglandins, prostacyclin and thromboxane; the lipoxygenase pathway leads to the formation of chemotactic agents such as leukotriene B.

its own actions (see below). Furthermore, enzymatic production of these derivatives is accompanied by the formation of free radicals that may cause futher tissue damage and more degradation of polyunsaturated fatty acids (Freeman & Crapo, 1982).

The role of arachidonic acid derivatives in inflammation is therefore still unclear; it is obviously complex, is interrelated with other mediators, and controlled by feedback inhibition and amplification loops. Prostaglandins have modulator as well as mediator actions, as may the leukotrienes. The importance of the other derivatives of membrane fatty acids such as platelet activating factor (PAF) also remains to be elucidated (Samuelsson, 1983).

Cyclic nucleotides

The cyclic nucleotides, like the prostaglandins, are present in nearly all human tissues and act as cellular mediators to a wide variety of agents including prostaglandin. Two cyclic nucleotides are important in the biology of inflammation (Goldberg & Haddox, 1977):

1. Adenosine 3′5′ — cyclic monophosphate (cAMP)
2. Guanosine 3′5′ — cyclic monophosphate (cGMP).

cAMP is synthesised from adenosine triphosphate (ATP) by the plasma membrane enzyme adenylate cyclase. This enzyme has both a receptor/regulator subunit and a catalytic subunit. The former allows interaction with hormones (including PGE, E_2, D_2 and I_2 and PG endoperoxides) which modulate the activity of the catalytic subunit located nearer the interior of the membrane. The less well documented cGMP has effects that are often antagonistic to cAMP, e.g. cholinergic agents decrease cardiac contraction and elevate cGMP, whilst β adrenergic agents increase cardiac contraction and stimulate cAMP. These opposing effects have been referred to as the 'yin–yang' phenomenon and have great potential relevance to the inflammatory cascade and its acute and chronic phases (Fig. 9.6; Weissmann et al, 1975).

A variety of in vitro immune reactions are suppressed by cAMP or by agents which stimulate adenylate cyclase and raise tissue cAMP levels (PGE_1 and E_2). These include immediate hypersensitivity reactions (histamine and SRSA release), and cellular immune reactions including antibody-dependent lymphocyte-mediated cytotoxicity. B cell mitogens and antibody production are enhanced by stimulation of cGMP and suppression of cAMP.

Lysosomal enzyme release appears to be similarly modified, with cAMP decreasing release

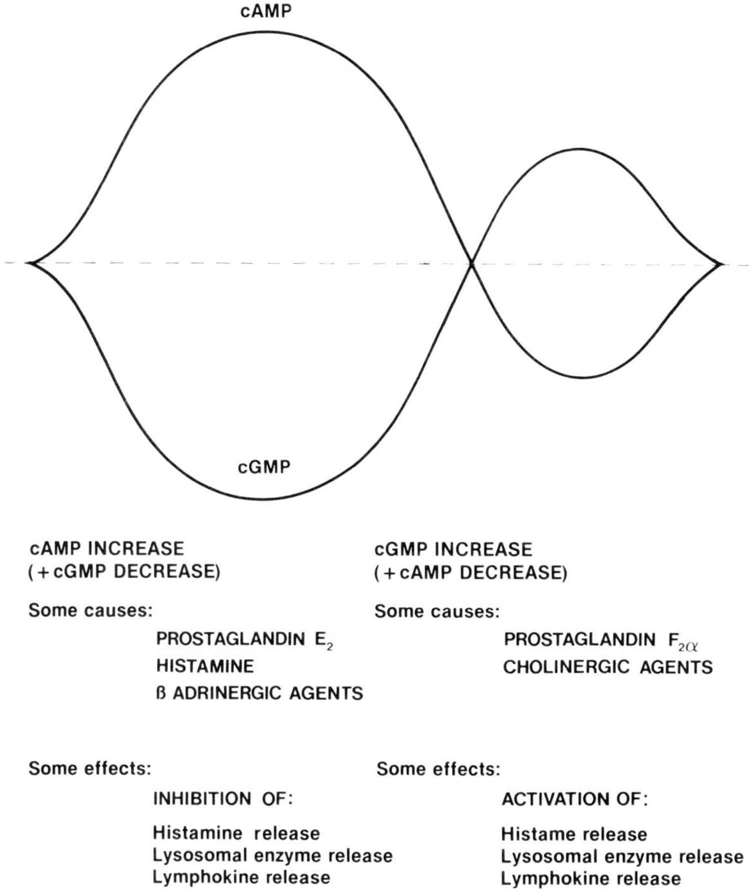

Fig. 9.6 The Yin–Yang hypothesis of mediator release in inflammation. The levels of the cyclic nucleotides cAMP and cGMP fluctuate in an acute inflammatory reaction precipitated by sudden exposure to an injurious stimulus. Initially cAMP levels rise and cGMP levels fall; later the situation is reversed. The two mediators tend to have opposing actions in inflammation, as listed. This finding led to the concept of fluctuating pro and anti-inflammatory factors controlling inflammatory reactions — the 'yin–yang' hypothesis.

whilst cGMP has the opposite effect. Neutrophil chemotaxis is enhanced by cGMP and inhibited by cAMP whilst the converse is true for monocytes (Genta & Hill, 1976). The subtle balance between acute and chronic inflammation could therefore be influenced by agents that altered cyclic neucleotide production. Cyclic AMP will inhibit several types of experimental inflammation, both acute and chronic. Such effects can be augmented by theophylline, an inhibitor of phosphodiesterase, and isoprenaline which will activate adenyl cyclase (Lewis & Mohd-Hidir, 1983). Polyamines (e.g. putricine, spermidine and spermine), which are simple aliphatic amines found in all living cells, also have anti-inflammatory properties and their production is controlled by cyclic AMP. However, the long-term clinical sequelae of prescribing these agents has yet to be discovered.

Enzyme products released by the neutrophil

The discovery of the fundamental role of the neutrophil in inflammation can be attributed to Metchnikoff (1882) who proposed that such cells may be involved in the liberation of substances capable of damaging adjacent tissues. The first direct evidence that the cytoplasmic granules of lysosomes were responsible for such lesions was provided by Thomas (1964) who injected lysosome intradermally followed by endotoxin intravenously and produced a localised Schwartzman reaction. Polymorphonuclear leucocytes contain both azurophil (primary) and specific (secondary) granules. Primary granules contain lysosomal hydrolases and peroxidase, whereas the smaller less dense secondary granules contain other enzymes including alkaline phosphatase, lysozyme and lactoferin. Macrophages contain large numbers of heterogenous granules which secrete a wide variety of different substances including acid hydrolases and many intercellular communicators (cytokines; see below).

The full identification of the products of lysosomes has revealed two main classes of compounds, the enzymatic proteinases and a variety of non-enzymatic cationic proteins (Wasi & Movat, 1979).

There are four major polymorphonuclear (PMN) proteinases that account for the bulk of lysosomal enzyme attack on extracellular structures.

1. Granulocyte collagenases. This metalloproteinase is present in specific granules. It preferentially attacks type I collagen present in some tendons and cartilage. Both macrophages and fibroblasts produce other collagenases which act both on type I and type III collagen.

2. Granulocyte elastase. This serine proteinase will attack proteoglycans within cartilage and the elastic fraction of ligaments, cartilage and blood vessels. The enzyme will also degrade type IV collagen of basement membrane.

3. Cathepsin G is another serine proteinase (along with trypsin, plasmin, thrombin and elastase) which will attack the chondroitin sulphate-rich segment of proteoglycan and thereby augment elastase which attacks the hyaluronic acid binding region.

4. Cathepsin D is a carboxyl proteinase sharing similarities with pepsin as an acid-acting proteinase within cells. It is active at an acid pH which may be below that present in many inflammatory lesions.

The activity of these neutrophil proteinases is regulated by the globulin inhibitors α_1 antitrypsin and α_2 macroglobulin. The predominance of the former in the serum suggests it is the major inhibitor. Their increase as part of the acute phase response to local inflammation suggests a modulation role.

Lysosome enzymes may also *modulate* other inflammation mediator systems. A neutral proteinase obtained from rabbit PMNs is capable of cleaving C5 into a chemotactically active fragment and a similar enzyme is present in human lysosomes (Ward & Hill, 1976). Human PMN granules also possess factors which contribute to both coagulation and fibronolysis (Niemetz, 1972). Neutral proteases from granulocytes have also been shown to be polyclonal B cell activators.

The non-enzymatic cationic proteins isolated from phagocytic cells include interleukin 1 and other cytokines mentioned below.

Oxygen free radicals and inflammation

The release of enzymes from phagocytic cells results from attempted phagocytosis or cell death. Stimuli which activate these cells also cause an increase in oxygen consumption, triggered by adhesion of the particles to the cell surface

(Fig. 9.2). The significance of this respiratory burst remained unknown until it was demonstrated that the increased oxygen uptake was associated with the production of hydrogen peroxide, and the superoxide radical ($O_2^{\cdot -}$), which are involved in the bacteriocidal activity of the phagocytic cell (Babior et al, 1973; Babior, 1978). The superoxide radical is the first univalent reduction product of oxygen and is termed a radical because of its unpaired electron. Its toxicity is also dependent on this inherently unstable situation, as it is obliged to seek electron pairing with any molecule in its environment. There is now a considerable literature to support the view that such species are important in damaging bacteria, though much less satisfactory data to support the view that they promote inflammation (Babior, 1978). However, the hydrogen peroxide and superoxide may react together in the presence of a trace metal catalyst such as iron to produce the hydroxyl radical, ($OH^{\cdot}$), a species that has been shown to degrade hyaluronic acid and promote the degradation of polyunsaturated fatty acids in vitro — lipid peroxidation. In this process the generation of organic oxygen radicals is followed by the formation of lipid peroxidases which can fragment further to produce gaseous hydrocarbons and reactive aldehydes potentially able to damage structural membranes and enzymes (Reily et al, 1974; Halliwell, 1981).

A complicated inhibitor system protects against such a process. The intracellular enzymes superoxide dismutase and catalase scavenge the superoxide radical and hydrogen peroxide, but have little effect within the extracellular environment, where caeruloplasmin is considered the important extracellular antioxidant. The ferroxidase activity of caeruloplasmin probably accounts for this property, as the oxidation of ferrous iron prevents it from catalysing hydroxyl radical formation (Gutteridge & Stocks, 1981). Free radicals inhibit the action of antiproteases thereby promoting the damaging effects of proteases liberated from lysosomes (Carp & Janoff, 1980). The superoxide radical also reacts with a component of normal human plasma to form a product chemotactic for neutrophils, so attracting more of them to the area (Weissman et al, 1979). There have been reports that $O_2^{\cdot -}$, H_2O_2 and $OH^{\cdot}$ are involved in prostaglandin metabolism, and that lipid peroxides stimulate prostaglandin synthesis, whilst the endoperoxides formed in such systems look like products of free radical attack. Superoxide generating systems also promote aggregation of platelets and release of serotonin from them (Handin et al, 1977) (for review see Blake et al, 1984).

Cytokines

Most of the mediators and modulators mentioned above influence vascular permeability or phagocytic cellular infiltration in an inflammatory lesion. Recently a group of poorly characterised soluble factors have been described which have a wide spectrum of other effects on the metabolism and function of many cells involved in inflammation (Fig. 9.7).

An extract of activated lymphocytes has the ability to transfer type IV hypersensitivity ('transfer factor'). Following this discovery, it was found that lymphocytes produce soluble factors with a wide spectrum of biological effects on other cells. One of the first to be delineated was a substance which inhibits the movement of macrophages ('migration inhibition factor' — MIF), and it was suggested that this facilitated inflammation by keeping macrophages at the site of the lesion (Yamamoto, 1975). Since then an enormous number of cellular changes have been observed in vitro in response to lymphocyte-derived factors, and the terms 'lymphokine' and 'IL2' were introduced to describe the substance or group of substances involved. Chemotactic, mitogenic and osteoclast activating factors have been described, which may have a crucial role in local lesions, and may or may not be the same chemical. Lymphokines can also stimulate fibroblasts (fibroblast stimulation factor') and affect endothelial cell proliferation ('angiogenesis inhibiting factor') (Baum, 1982).

Use of cell culture techniques has led to the discovery of a different set of cytokines. Castor & Lewis (1975) showed that factors derived from leucocytes had a profound effect on synovial cells in culture. He termed the process 'connective tissue activation', and has delineated a wide variety of connective tissue activating peptides (CTAPs),

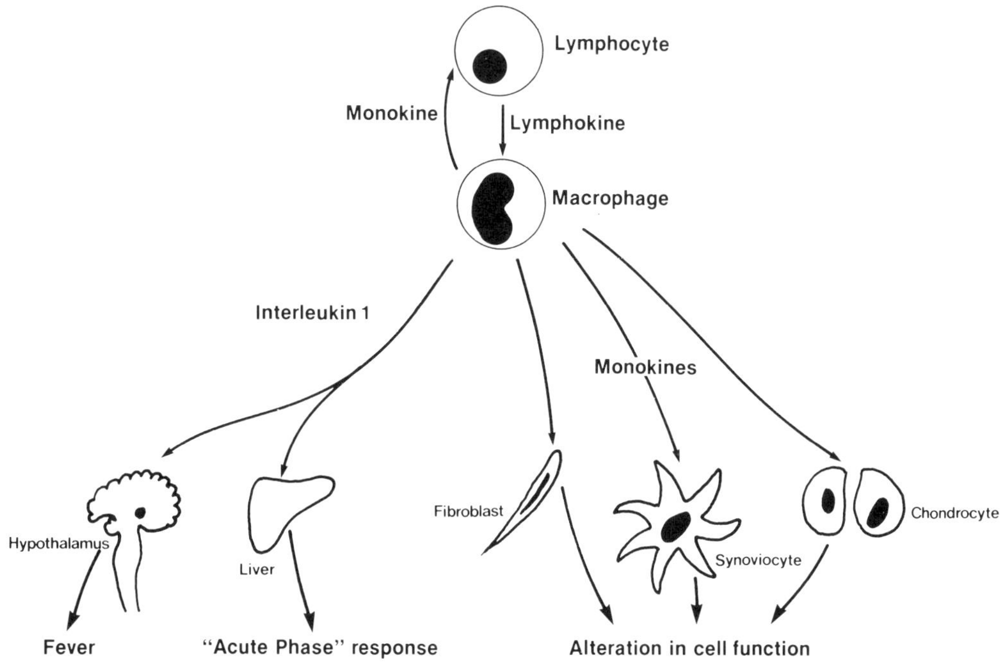

Fig. 9.7 Outline of some 'cytokines' involved in inflammation. Macrophages and lymphocytes 'talk' to each other through the production of factors called monokines and lymphokines respectively. The macrophage produces a factor which stimulates RNA synthesis in the hepatocyte and the production of acute phase proteins; it also mediates the hypothalamic production of fever (interleukin 1). Other cellular functions can be altered by products from the macrophage (monokines), and changes in fibroblasts, synoviocytes and chondrocytes are probably important in inflammation. It is not yet clear how many of these actions are mediated by the same factor, or whether a range of chemically different cytokines is produced by each cell type.

some of which are derived from monocytes, others from platelets (Castor et al, 1979). Fell (1978) used co-culture experiments to show that the synovium produced a factor which affects cartilage metabolism, inducing chondrocytes to autodigest the cartilage. This factor, called 'catabolin' by Dingle (1981), may be similar to the monocyte-derived factors which affect fibroblasts (MCF), delineated by Dayer and colleagues (1981), which is similar to macrophage-derived interleukin 1 (Dinarello, 1984; Table 9.4). An increasing number of in vitro biological effects produced by monocyte-derived factors ('monokines', 'IL1') are therefore being described, and IL1-like activity has been found in synovial fluids (Wood et al, 1983). As with 'lymphokine', it is difficult to know whether one or several chemicals are involved.

These factors re-emphasise the complex interrelationship between all cellular functions, and all aspects of the control of the inflammatory process. This may help to explain why attempts to inhibit the response with limited pharmacological agents are incomplete, relatively ineffective in preventing chronic changes, and unsatisfactory in the long-term (Otterness et al, 1984).

SUMMARY AND CONCLUSIONS

The inflammatory process

Inflammation is a dynamic response to injury with local and systemic aspects. It used to be divided into 'acute', short-lived inflammation dominated by vascular changes and PMN infiltration, and 'chronic', though not necessarily persistent, inflammation dominated by mononuclear cells and the reparative process. This distinction is artificial, as the response can shift to-and-fro, with one or other aspect of the local reaction dominating the overall picture at different times. It is clear that all components of this complex, reparative process are interrelated, and continually influencing each other.

Inflammation in the rheumatic diseases

Inflammation has been defined as the response of living tissue to sublethal injury. All rheumatic diseases cause tissue damage, and therefore have an inflammatory component. In some diseases this response dominates the picture, and is regarded as 'primary', in others it is less prominent and considered 'secondary' to some other pathological process. The highly vascularised synovium, with its fenestrated capillary bed, phagocytic cells, and synthetic functions, often shows the most prominent changes, and a marked vascular and cellular response is usually apparent. Periarticular sites such as the enthesis are also commonly affected. Articular cartilage, being a tight avascular matrix, does not react to injury with blood vessel changes or cellular infiltration, although alteration in cellular function with attempted repair or metaplasia of chondrocytes does occur. Products of the cartilage can also activate inflammation of the synovium, and synovial cytokines can affect cartilage metabolism. Just as all aspects of inflammation are interrelated, it is clear that all components of the joint interact in an inflammatory response.

Both local and systemic aspects of inflammation differ in the various rheumatic diseases. Gout, for example, has a short-lived, self-limiting, acute inflammatory component dominated by vascular changes and PMN infiltration; fever and a leucocytosis can also occur. Osteoarthritis is associated with a less obvious chronic inflammatory reaction, characterised by a mononuclear cell exudate and a prominent reparative phase resulting in extensive capsular fibrosis and new bone formation; there is little or no systemic response. Rheumatoid inflammation combines features of both 'acute' and 'chronic' reactions, and also has prominent immunological and systemic components. The rheumatoid response changes in severity and in character with time during the various exacerbations and remissions of the disease. In the connective tissue diseases inflammation occurs in many organs, and is very variable; the local component may be atypical, and there may be a deficit in the acute phase response in SLE and scleroderma. The fine balance of the various local and systemic mediator and modulator systems may be altered in favour of maintenance of inflammation in some of these conditions.

Although these differences occur, there are also striking similarities in all synovial responses. Thus it is often impossible to tell the difference between rheumatoid and osteoarthritic joints at post-mortem; crystals are the only distinctive feature of gouty inflammation; and the synovitis of connective tissue diseases is usually described as 'non-specific' by histopathologists. These similarities arise from the limited type of response a joint can show to injury, and the interrelationships of the various mediator, modulator and cellular systems (Vernon Roberts, 1983; Ghadially, 1983).

Inflammation is designed to limit and repair tissue damage. In joint disease it is usually thought to be doing more harm than good, although there is little hard evidence to support this belief. Our present attempts to reduce the response are crude and inadequate (Otterness et al, 1984). Although they reduce symptoms they may not be helping the joint in the long-term.

REFERENCES

Aarden L A, Brunner T K, Cerottini J C et al 1979 Revised nomenclature for antigen-non-specific T cell proliferation and helper factors. Journal of Immunology 123: 2928–2929

Anderson R, Glover A, Rabson A R 1977 The in vitro effects of histamine and metiamide on neutrophil mobility and their relationship to intracellular cyclic nucleotide levels. Journal of Immunology 118: 1690–6

Askenase P W 1977 Role of basophils, mast cells and vasoamines in hypersensitivity reactions with a delayed time course. Progress in Allergy 23: 119–320

Atkins E, Bodel P 1972 Fever. New England Journal of Medicine 286: 27–34

Babior B M, Kipnes R S, Curnutte J T 1973 Biological defense mechanisms. The production by leukocytes of superoxide, a potential bactericidal agent. Journal of Clinical Investigation 52: 741–744

Babior B M 1978 Oxygen dependent microbial killing by phagocytes. New England Journal of Medicine 298: 659, 721

Bagby G C, Rigas V D, Bennett R M, Vandenbark A A, Garewal H S 1981 Interaction of lactoferrin, monocytes and T lymphocyte subsets in the regulation of steady-state granuloporesis in vitro. Journal of Clinical Investigation 68: 56–63

Baracos V, Rodemann H P, Dinarello C A, Goldberg A L 1983 Stimulation of muscle protein degradation and prostaglandin E2 release by leukocyte pyrogen (IL–I). A mechanism for the increased degradation of muscle

proteins during fever. New England Journal of Medicine 308: 553–558
Baum J 1982 Mediators of inflammation. In: Panayi G S (ed) Scientific basis of rheumatology. Churchill Livingstone, Edinburgh, p 260–271
Beaven M A 1976 Histamine. New England Journal of Medicine 294: 30–36, 320–325
Bennett I L, Beeson P B 1953 Studies on the pathogenesis of fever. II. Characterisation of fever-producing substance from polymorphonuclear leukocytes and from the fluid of sterile exudates. Journal of Experimental Medicine 98: 493–508
Bernheim H A, Block L H, Atkins E 1979 Fever: Pathogenesis, pathophysiology and purpose. Annals of Internal Medicine 91: 261–270
Blake D R, Hall N D, Bacon P A, Dieppe P A, Halliwell B, Gutteridge J M C 1981 The importance of iron in rheumatoid disease. Lancet 2: 1142–1144
Blake D R, Lunec J, Winyard P, Brailsford S, Bacon P A 1984 Oxygen free radicals and inflammatory joint disease. Current Medical Literature. Scott J T, Decker J (eds) (in press)
Bornstein D L 1982 Leukocytic pyrogen: A major mediator of the acute phase reaction. Annals of the New York Academy of Science 389: 323–337
Boyden S 1962 The chemotactic effect of mixtures of antibody and antigen on polymorphonuclear leucocytes. Journal of Experimental Medicine 115: 453–466
Brem H, Folkman J 1975 Inhibition of tumor angiogenesis mediated by cartilage. Journal of Experimental Medicine 141: 427–439
Brem S, Cotran R S, Folkman J 1972 Tumor angiogenesis: a quantitative method for histologic grading. Journal of The National Cancer Institute 48: 347–356
Carp H, Janoff A 1980 Potential mediator of inflammation — phagocyte-derived oxidants suppress the elastase-inhibitory capacity of $alpha_1$ proteinase inhibitor in vitro. Journal of Clinical Investigation 66: 987–995
Castor C W, Lewis R B 1975 Connective tissue activation. X. Current studies of the process and its mediators. Scandanavian Journal of Rheumatology (Suppl 12): 41–54
Castor C W, Ritchie J C, Williams C H, Scott E M, Whitney S L, Myers S L, Sloan T B, Anderson B E 1979 Connective tissue activation. XIV. Composition and actions of human platelet autacoid mediator. Arthritis and Rheumatism 22: 260–272
Chrisman O D, Fessel J M, Southwick W O. 1965. Experimental production of synovitis and marginal articular exostoses in the knee joints of dogs. Yale Journal of Biological Medicine 37: 409–412
Clementi F, Palade G E 1969 Intestinal capillaries. I. Permeability to peroxidase and ferritin. Journal of Cell Biology 41: 33–58
Cohnheim J 1889 Lectures in general pathology, 2nd Edn. The New Sydenham Society, London, 1: 21–36
Dayer J M, Krane S M, Goldring S R 1981 Cellular and humoral factors modulate connective tissue destruction and repair in arthritic diseases. Seminars in Arthritis and Rheumatism XI (Suppl 1): 77–81
de Sousa M 1981 A circulation of lymphocytes: Reflections on the questions of how and why. In: Lymphocyte circulation, experimental and clinical aspects. Wiley, Chichester, p 197–217
Dieppe P A, Hornby J, Swan A 1983 The different effects of crystals on release of inflammatory mediators from human peripheral blood phagocytic cells. Annals of Rheumatic Diseases (Suppl) 42:112
Dinarello C A 1984 Interleukin-I. Reviews of Infectious Diseases 6: 51–95
Dingle J T 1981 The role of catabolin in arthritie damage. Seminars in Arthritis and Rheumatism XI (Suppl 1): 82–83
Dumonde D C 1978 The rheumatological significance of lymphokines. In: Dumond D C, Jasani M K (eds) Recognition of anti-rheumatic drugs. MTP, London, p 167–192
Egwang T G, Befus A D 1984 The role of complement in the induction and regulation of immune responses. Immunology 51: 207–224
Elliott D F, Horton E W, Lewis G P 1960 Actions of pure bradykinin. Journal of Physiology (Lond) 153: 473–480
Erdös E G 1977 The angiotensin 1 converting enzyme. Federal Proceedings 36: 1760–1765
Eular U S von 1935 Über die spezifische blutdrucksenkende. Substanz des menschlichen Prostata — und Samenblasensekretes. Klinische Wochenschrift 14: 1182–1183
Fell H B 1978 Synoviocytes. Journal of Clinical Pathology 31 (Suppl): 14–24
Florey H W (ed) 1970 General pathology, 4th Edn. Saunders, Philadelphia
Freeman B A, Crapo J D 1982 Biology of disease: Free radicals and tissue injury. Laboratory Investigation 47: 412–426
Gabbiani G, Majno G 1972 Dupuytren's contracture: Fibroblast contraction? American Journal of Pathology 66: 131–138
Genta G E, Hill H R 1976 Paradoxical influence of cyclic AMP on human monocyte chemotactic responses. Clinical Research 24:180A
Ghadially F N 1983 Fine structure of synovial joints. Butterworths, London
Goldberg N D, Haddox M K 1977 Cyclic GMP metabolism and involvement in biological regulation. Annal Review of Biochemistry 46: 823–896
Golde D W, Cline M J 1974 Regulation of granulopoiesis. New England Journal of Medicine 291: 1388–1395
Gordon 1976 Platelets in biology and pathology. Elsevier, Amsterdam
Gordon J L 1981 Platelets and inflammation. In: Kelley W N, Harris E D, Ruddy S, Sledge C B (eds) Textbook of rheumatology. Saunders, Philadelphia, p 163–178
Gordon J L, Milner A J 1976 Blood platelets as multifunctional cells. In: Gordon J L (ed) Platelets in biology and pathology. Elsevier, Amsterdam
Gutteridge J M C, Stocks J 1981 Caeruloplasmin: Physiological and pathological perspectives. CRC Critical Reviews in Clinical Laboratory Sciences 14: 257–329
Halliwell B 1981 Free radical oxygen toxicity and ageing. In: Sohal R S (ed) Age pigments. Elsevier, Amsterdam p 1–62
Handin R I, Karabin R, Boxer G J 1977 Enhancement of platelet function by superoxide anion. Journal of Clinical Investigation 59: 959–965
Hay J B 1979 Kinetics of the inflammatory response in regional lymph. Current Topics in Pathology 68: 89–109
Hay J B, Movat H Z 1979 Hyperemia, stasis and increase in vascular permeability: New methods for their quantitation. Current Topics in Pathology 68: 33–45
Harris H 1954 Role of chemotaxis in inflammation. Physiology Review 34: 529–562
Holdstock G, Mitchell J R A 1977 Erythrocyte sedimentation

rate before and after in vitro defibrination. Lancet 2: 1314–1316
Hurley J V 1963 Incubation of serum with tissue extracts as a cause of chemotaxis of granulocytes. Nature 198: 1212–1213
Hurley J V 1983 Acute inflammation, 2nd Edn. Churchill Livingstone, Edinburgh
Jampel H D, Duff G W, Gershan R K, Atkins E, Durum S K 1983 Fever and immunoregulation. Journal of Experimental Medicine 157: 1229–1238
Karnovsky M J 1967 The ultrastructural basis of capillary permeability studied with peroxidase as a tracer. Journal of Cell Biology 35: 213–236
Kimura Y 1983 Suppressive effect of bradykinin to cellular immune responses in vivo and in vitro. Advances in Experimental Medical Biology 156: 755–766
Kozlowski T, Raymond R M, Korthuis R J, Wang C Y, Grega G J, Robinson N E, Scott J B 1981 Microvascular protein efflux: Interaction of histamine and HI receptors. Proceedings of the Society of Experimental Biological Medicine 166: 263–270
Krane S M, Dayer J M, Goldring S R 1982 Consideration of possible cellular events in the destructive synovial lesion of rheumatoid arthritis. In: Gorini S (ed) Advances in inflammation research, Vol 3. Rheumatoid arthritis. Raven, New York, p 1–15
Kushner I 1982 The phenomenon of the acute phase response. Annals of the New York Academy of Science 389: 39–48
Landis E M 1934 Capillary pressure and capillary permeability. Physiology Review 14: 404–481
Leibovich S J, Ross R 1976 A macrophage-dependent factor that stimulates the proliferation of fibroblasts in vitro. American Journal of Pathology 84: 501–514
Lett-Brown M A, Leonard E J 1977 Histamine-induced inhibition of normal human basophil chemotaxis to C5a. Journal of Immunology 118: 815–818
Lewis D A, Mohd-Hidir S 1983 The anti-inflammatory action of drugs that raise adenosine 3′ 5′ cyclic monophosphate and putrescine levels in vivo (abstract). British Journal of Pharmacology 79: 348
Lewis G P 1962 Bradykinin — biochemistry, pharmacology and its physiological role in controlling local blood flow. The Scientific Basis of Medicine Annual Reviews 10: 242–258
Lewis T 1927 The blood vessels of the human skin and their responses. Shaw, London
Luft H J 1966 Fine structure of capillary and endocapillary layer as revealed by ruthinium red. Federal Proceedings 25: 1773–1783
Majno G 1975 The healing hand. Man and wound in the ancient world. Harvard University Press, Cambridge
Mandel N S and Mandel G S 1982 Structure of Crystals that Provoke Inflammation. In: Weissman G (ed) Advances in Inflammation Research. Raven Press, New York 4: 73–94
Marchesi V T, Florey H W 1960 Electron micrographic observations on the emigration of leucocytes. Quarterly Journal of Experimental Physiology 45: 343–348
Metchnikoff E 1905 Immunity in infective diseases. Cambridge University Press, London
Miles A A 1964 Large molecular weight substances as mediators of the inflammatory reaction. Annals of the New York Academy of Science 116: 855–865
Minta J O, Movat H Z 1979 The complement system and inflammation. In: Morat H Z (ed) Current topics in pathology, Vol 68 Inflammatory reaction. Springer-Verlag, Berlin. p 135–178
Mitnick H, Hoffstein S, Weissmann G 1978 Fate of antigen after intravenous and intra-articular injection into rabbits. Arthritis and Rhenumatism 21: 918–929
Moskowitz R W, Schwartz H J, Michel B, Ratnoff O D, Astrup T 1970 Generation of kinin-like agents by chondroitin sulphate, heparin, chitin sulphate, and human articular cartilage. Possible pathophysiologic implications. Journal of Laboratory Clinical Medicine 76: 790–798
Niemetz J 1972 Coagulant activity of leukocytes. Tissue factor activity. Journal of Clinical Investigation 51: 307–313
Orning L, Hammerström S, Samuelsson B 1980 Leukotriene D: A slow reading substance from rat basophilic leukaemia cells. Proceedings of the National Academy of Science USA 77: 2014–2017
Otterness I G, Capetola R J, Wong S (eds) 1984 Therapeutic control of inflammatory disease. (Advances in inflammation research, Vol 4.) Raven, New York
Oyanagui Y 1981 Steroid like anti-inflammatory effect of superoxide dismutase in serotonin, histamine and kinin induced edemata of mice. Biochemical Pharmacology 30: 1791–1798
Pappenheimer J R 1953 Passage of molecules through capillary walls. Physiology Review 33: 387–423
Peacock E, Van Winkle W V 1976 Wound repair, 2nd Edn. Saunders, Philadelphia
Pepys M B 1981 Serum C-reactive protein, serum amyloid P-component and serum amyloid A protein in autoimmune disease. Clinics in Immunology and Allergy 1:77
Pike M C, Synderman R 1982 Chemoattractant-receptor interactions in leucocytes In: Weissmann G (ed) Advances in inflammation research, Vol 4. Raven, New York, p 109–130
Polverini P J, Cotran R S, Gimbrone M A- Unanue E R 1977 Activated macrophages induce vascular proliferation. Nature 269: 804–806
Postlethwaite A E, Kang A H 1976 Collagen and collagen peptide-induced chemotaxis of human blood monocytes. Journal of Experimental Medicine 143: 1299–1307
Pullinger B D, Florey H W 1935 Some observations on the structure and function of lymphatics: their behaviour in local oedema. British Journal of Experimental Pathology 16: 49–61
Riely C A, Cohen G, Liebermann M 1974 Ethane evolution: a new index of lipid peroxidation. Science 183: 208–210
Robinson D R 1983 Prostagladins and the mechanism of action of anti-inflammatory drugs. American Journal of Medicine 75: 26–31
Robinson D R, Curran D P, Hamer P J 1982 Prostagladins and related compounds in inflammatory rheumatic diseases. In: Ziff M, Velo G P, Gorini S (eds) Advances in inflammation research, Vol 3. Rheumatoid arthritis. Raven, New York, p 17–28
Rocklin R E, Beer D S 1983 Histamine and immune modulation. Advances in International Medicine 28: 225–251
Di Rosa M, Giroud J P, Willoughby D A 1971 Studies of the mediators of the acute inflammatory response induced in rats in different sites by carrageenan and turpentine. Journal of Pathology 104: 15–29
Rothschild B M, Masi A T 1982 Pathogenesis of rheumatoid arthritis: A vascular hypothesis. Seminars in Arthritis and Rheumatism 12: 11–31

Ryan G B, Majno G 1977 Acute inflammation. A review. American Journal of Pathology 86: 185–276
Ryan G B, Spector W G 1970 Macrophage turnover in inflamed connective tissue. Proceedings of the Royal Society of London (B) 175: 269–292
Samuelsson B 1983 From studies of biochemical mechanism to novel biological mediators: prostagladin endoperoxides, thromboxanes, and leukotrienes. Nobel Lecture, 8 Dec 1982. Bioscience Reports 3: 799–813
Samuelsson B, Borgeat P, Hammarström S, Murphy R C 1979 Introduction of a nomenclature: Leukotrienes. Prostaglandins 17: 785–787
Schiffmann E, Corcoran B A, Wahl S M 1975 N-formyl methionyl peptides as chemoattractants for leucocytes. Proceedings of the National Academy of Science 72: 1059–1062
Schmidt J A, Mizel S B, Cohen D, Green I 1982 Interleukin-I: a potential regulator of fibroblast proliferation. Journal of Immunology 128: 2177–2182
Schoefl G I 1963 Growing capillaries: their structure and permeability. Archives of Pathology, Anatamy and Physiology 337: 97–111
Schumacher H R, Kitridou R C 1972 Synovitis of recent onset. A clinicopathologic study during the first month of disease. Arthritis and Rheumatism 15: 465–485
Schwartz A, Sutton S L, Askenase P W, Gershon R K 1981 Histamine inhibition of concanavalin A-induced supressor T-cell activation. Cell Immunology 60: 426–439
Selye H 1950 The physiology and pathology of exposure to stress: a treatise based on concepts of the general adaptation syndrome and the diseases of adaptation. Acta Medica, Montreal
Selye H, Somogye A, Vegh P 1968 Inflammation topical stress and the concept of pleuricasual diseases. In: Houck J C, Forsher B K (eds) Chemical Biology of Inflammation. Pergamon
Sidky Y A, Auerbach R 1975 Lymphocyte-induced angiogenesis. Journal of Experimental Medicine 141: 1084–1100
Simionescu N, Simionescu M, Palade G E 1975 Permeability of muscle capillaries to small heme-peptides. Evidence for the existence of patent transendothelial channels. Journal of Cell Biology 64: 586–607
Simon G T 1979 Ultrastructure of acute inflammation. Current Topics in Pathology 68: 1–32
Spector W G 1979 The macrophages and their role in inflammation. European Journal of Rhumatological Inflammation 2: 104–106
Spector W G, Lykke A W J 1966 The cellular evolution of inflammatory granulomata. Journal of Pathology and Bacteriology 92: 163–177
Spector W G, Willoughby D A 1963 The inflammatory response. Bacteriological Reviews 27: 117–154
Starling E H 1896 On the absorption of fluids from the connective tissue spaces. Journal of Physiology 19: 312–236
Stossel T P 1974 Phagocytosis. New England Journal of Medicine 290: 717–723, 774–780, 833–839
Synderman R 1980 Inflammation and autodestructive reactions initiated by antibody. In: Joklik E K, Willett H P, Amos D B (eds) Zinsser microbiology, 17th Edn. Appleton-Century-Crofts, New York, p 342–353
Thomas L 1964 Possible role of leukocyte granules in the Schwartzman and Arthus reactions. Proceedings of the Society of Experimental Biological Medicine 115: 235–240
Trentham D E, Dynesius R A, Rocklin R E, David J R 1978 Cellular sensitivity to collagen in rheumatoid arthritis. New England Journal of Medicine 299: 327–332
Vane J R 1971 Inhibition of prostaglandin synthesis as a mechanism of action for aspirin like drugs. Nature New Biology 231: 232–235
Vane J R 1976 Prostaglandins as mediators of inflammation. In: Samuelsson B, Paoletti R (eds) Advances in prostaglandin and thromboxane research, Vol 2. Raven, New York, p 791–801
Van Furth R 1975 An approach to the characterization of mononuclear phagocytes involved in pathological processes. In: Giroud J P, Willoughby D A, Velo G P (eds) Future trends in inflammation II. Birkhäuser Verlag, Basel, p 91–98
Van Furth R, Willenze R 1979 Phagocytic cells during an acute inflammatory reaction. Current Topics in Pathology 68: 179–212
Vernon Roberts B 1983 Rheumatoid joint pathology revisited. In: Carson Dick W, Moll J M H (eds) Recent advances in rheumatology, Vol 3. Churchill Livingstone, Edinburgh
Volanakis J E 1982 Complement activation by C-reactive protein complexes. Annals of the New York Academy of Science 389: 235–350
Volkman A, Gowans J L 1965 The origin of macrophages from bone marrow in the rat. British Journal of Experimental Pathology 46: 62–70
Ward P A, Hill H J 1970 C_5 chemotactic fragments produced by an enzyme in lysosomal granules of neutrophils. Journal of Immunology 104: 535–543
Wasi S, Movat H Z 1979 Phlogistic substances in neutrophil leukocyte lysosomes: their possible role in vivo and their in vitro properties. Current Tropics in Pathology 68: 213–237
Weinbaum D L, Sullivan J A, Mandell G L 1982 Orientation of membrance receptors on the neutrophil. In: Weissmann G (ed) Advances in inflammation research, Vol 4. Raven, New York, p 95–108
Weissmann G, Goldstein I, Hoffstein S, Chauvet G, Robinaux R 1975 Yin/Yang modulation of lysosomal enzyme release from polymorphonuclear leukocytes by cyclic nucleotides. Annals of the New York Academy of Science 256: 222–232
Weissmann G, Korchak H M, Perez H D, Smolen J E, Goldstein I M, Hoffstein S T 1979 Leukocytes as secretory organs of inflammation. In: Weissmann G, Samuelsson B, Paoletti R (eds) Advances in inflammation research, Vol 1. Raven, New York, p 95–112
Weissmann G, Serhan C, Korchak H M, Smolen J E 1982 Neutrophils: Release of mediators of inflammation with special reference to rheumatoid arthritis. Annals of the New York Academy of Science 389: 11–24
Werb Z, Gordon S 1975 Secretion of a specific collagenase by stimulated macrophages. Journal of Experimental Medicine 142: 346–360
Whicher J T 1981 Inflammation: The role of acute phase proteins. Diagnostic Medicine 52–69
Whicher J T, Martin M F R, Dieppe P A 1980 Absence of prostaglandin stimulated increase in acute phase proteins in systemic sclerosis. Lancet 2: 1187–1188
Wilkinson P C 1982 Chemotaxis and inflammation, 2nd Edn. Churchill Livingstone, Edinburgh
Wilkinson P C, Lackie J M 1979 The adhesion, migration and chemotaxis of leucocytes in inflammation. Current Topics in Pathology 68: 47–88
Wood D D, Ihrie E J, Dinarello C A, Cohen D L 1983

Isolation of an Interleukin-I-like factor from human joint effusions. Arthritis and Rheumatism 26: 975–983
Wood W B 1970 The pathogenesis of fever. In: Mudd S (ed) Infectious agents and host reactions. Saunders, Philadelphia, p 146–162
Yamamoto S 1975 Studies on mechanisms of immobilization of mononuclear cells in the delayed hypersensitivity reaction. In: Giroud J P, Willoughby D A, Velo G P (eds) Future trends in inflammation II. Birkhäuser Verlag, Basel, p 16–27

J.C. Woodrow

Immunogenetics and rheumatic diseases

It is likely that many of the major rheumatic disorders develop as a consequence of the effects of environmental agents in genetically predisposed individuals. In some instances, e.g. generalised osteoarthritis and the crystal-induced disorders, the processes involved are largely of a biochemical nature. There is good evidence, as documented in other sections in this volume, that in the case of several disorders of the musculoskeletal system immunologically mediated processes play a leading role in the development of an inflammatory process and in the destructive effects that result from this. In considering the possible pathogenesis of these disorders two main bodies of evidence are worth considering. Firstly, there is evidence in many instances that the condition aggregates in families to a greater or lesser degree, e.g. ankylosing spondylitis, psoriatic arthritis, reactive arthritis, rheumatoid arthritis and systemic lupus erythematosus. Secondly, there is the evidence that the various stages of the immune response are under genetic control. A convergence of these two lines of inquiry is proving to be of great value in our attempts to understand the aetiology of these disorders.

CLINICAL GENETICS

In studying disorders which are found to aggregate in families the first step is to analyse the pattern of segregation of the disorder within involved families. This may reveal a regular mode of inheritance indicating the presence of a gene of major effect such that it is, in the simplest case, necessary and sufficient of itself to give rise to the disorder. In this way Mendelian dominant or recessive traits or disorders are defined. Although there are rare abnormalities of the immune system of this type, there are none which predominantly affect the joints. For example, X-linked hypogammaglobulinaemia, in which there is a block in the development of immunoglobulin-producing B lymphocytes, may be associated with the development of a polyarthritis or of a condition resembling dermatomyositis but the main clinical effect is the occurrence of repeated pyogenic infection.

When it comes to the more common disorders, familial aggregation is shown by the observation that close relatives of patients have a greater incidence of the disorder than a suitable control population but no clear pattern of familial segregation emerges. Well studied examples are ankylosing spondylitis and rheumatoid arthritis. Sophisticated segregation analysis can be applied but may fail to reveal a clear-cut genetic structure and certainly little that can be directly applied in the field of clinical research. It is commonly concluded that the basis for such disorders is that they depend on the effects of an environmental agent or agents on individuals who are rendered susceptible by the action of several genes whose effects are either additive or interactive. It is here that knowledge gained from a study of immunogenetics, i.e. of the genetically-determined variability that exists between different individuals, becomes important. The discovery of associations between certain immunogenetic variables and these disorders suggests that susceptibility to them is dependent on quite subtle differences which can exert their effects at different points in the immune system.

GENETICS OF THE IMMUNE RESPONSE

The immune response to most foreign antigens is initiated by the processing of antigen by specialised macrophages. Antigenic determinants at the surface of these cells are recognised by T helper cells which then co-operate with B lymphocytes or with effector T lymphocytes, the latter cells having also recognised part of the foreign antigen. As a result, specific antibody or delayed hypersensitivity and cytotoxic T cells are induced. This immune response may be inhibited or suppressed by the appearance of T suppressor cells or by feedback inhibition by specific antibody or by anti-idiotype antibody (i.e. antibody to the antibody-combining site of specific antibody). Under normal circumstances the quality and degree of the immune response is thus carefully regulated.

There are two main genetic systems which determine the normal range of these specific immune responses. The first comprises those clusters of genetic loci which code for the specific antibody-binding sites of antibodies. These sites are constituted by the hypervariable (V) regions of light and heavy immunoglobulin chains so that the particular arrangement of amino acid sequences in these regions largely determines the antibody specificity. There is evidence that the great diversity of antibody specificities generated by each individual can be accounted for in large degree by the considerable number of available germ line V-genes. In the mouse it has been estimated that the number of V-region genes for heavy and light chains provides the possibility of something of the order of 10^6 different antibody specificities. There is also the likelihood that during clonal expansion of B lymphocytes, somatic mutation of V-genes adds to the diversity of the antibody repertoire. Experimental evidence suggests that variation in the ability to produce a specific antibody response can be due to V-region differences, but there is no good evidence that this plays an important role in the genetic control of the immune response.

The second major genetic system which determines the specific immune response is the major histocompatibility complex (MHC). The discovery of this system of genetic loci had its origins in pioneer investigations into genetic control of tissue graft rejection and, although it is now evident that the genetic systems thereby revealed have a much wider significance, the original terminology has been retained.

Before describing the MHC in man and the evidence pointing to its relevance to our understanding of the genetics of certain rheumatic disorders, it is necessary to summarise the present knowledge with regard to the homologous system in the mouse, the H-2 complex. The reason for this is that our present understanding of the physiological role of the MHC has come and could only have come from experimental animal studies. The availability of inbred strains, some differing only by virtue of differences in the MHC region (congenic) and the ability to use a variety of immunogenic stimuli and to measure various types of response, has provided insights of fundamental importance in our attempts to understand the genetic control of the immune response. This knowledge can be applied to human studies and provides a rich fund of ideas which can act as a potent stimulus to clinical research. For example, when the structure of a molecule determined by a human MHC gene is found to be homologous to one found in the H-2 region of the mouse, this immediately implies a similar function and valuable insights into this may already have been gained by experimental studies.

The H-2 complex of the mouse

The MHC of the mouse consists of a series of closely linked genetic loci as shown in Figure 10.1. The K and D/L loci were originally defined by their control over graft rejection and the generation of cytotoxic T cells, i.e, they determine the classical transplantation antigens. The products of the genes of these loci, class I molecules, are glycoproteins with a molecular weight of 45 000 and constitute integral membrane proteins of all nucleated cells, being associated at the cell surface with the small polypeptide, β_2-microglobulin (Fig. 10.2) (Coligan et al, 1981). Serological specificity is determined by the amino acid sequence at localised areas of the heavy chain but β_2-microglobulin is essential for its expression.

Class II molecules result from the combination of four types of polypeptide chains $A\alpha$, $A\beta$, $E\alpha$, $E\beta$. The α chains have a molecular weight of approximately 32 000 and the β chains of 28 000.

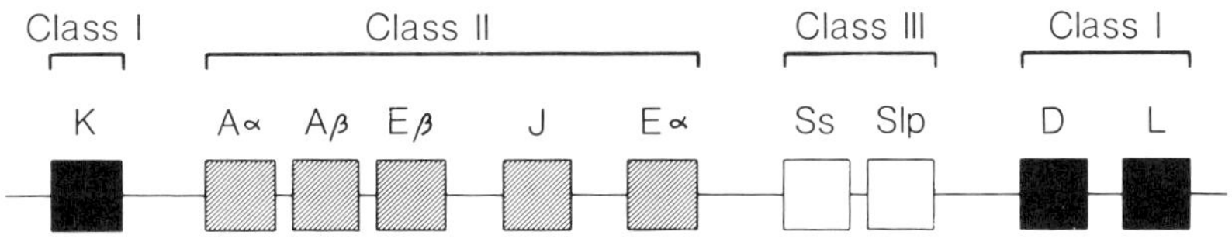

Fig. 10.1 Genetic loci in the H-2 chromosomal region of the mouse.

It is thought that these chains are synthesised separately but combine to form dimers which are then integrated into the plasma membranes particularly of B lymphocytes and macrophages. Thus Aα and Aβ form an I-A molecule and Eα and Eβ an I-E molecule. The I-J locus determines specificities present on T suppressor cells.

The class III products, Ss and Slp, are C4, a component of the classical complement pathway.

A notable feature is that several of these loci are highly polymorphic, i.e. K, D, Aβ, Eβ, whilst Aα appears constant and Eα shows little variation and

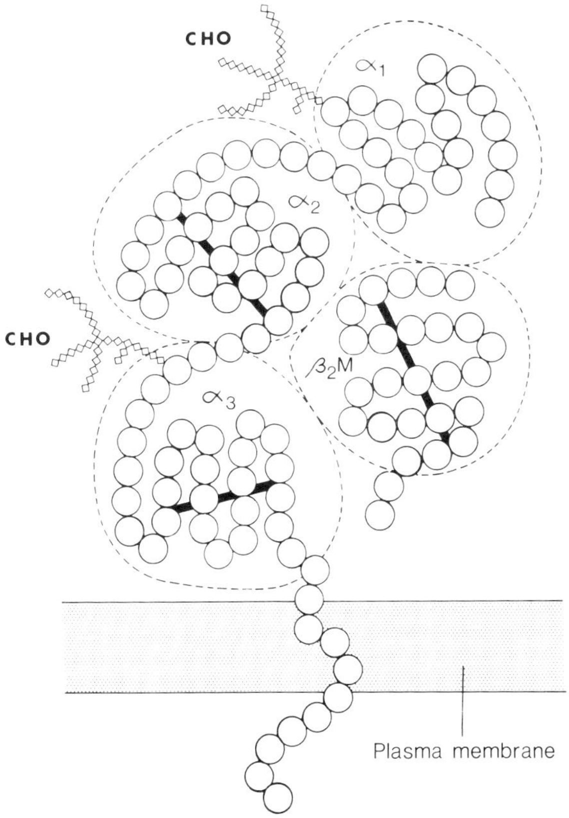

Fig. 10.2 General structure of class I glycoprotein molecules (after Coligan et al, 1981). Disulphide linkages are present in the α_2, α_3 and β_2M chains.

β_2-microglobulin is invariant (Klein & Figueroa, 1981). Thus each final product appears to consist of a highly variant chain and a smaller chain, which is either invariant or shows little variability. Serological specificity is associated largely with the variable chain.

We are concerned here with the physiological role of these genetic loci in the control of the immune response. Several related observations have thrown important light on this:

a. It was shown that optimal co-operation between T helper and B lymphocytes in the immune response only occurs when these cells share a common I-A gene product (Katz et al, 1973).

b. Cytotoxic T cells from mice infected with the virus of lymphocytic choriomeningitis could induce lysis in virus-infected target cells only when the latter cells carried the same K or D region antigens as the cytotoxic cells (Zinkernagel & Doherty, 1974). This phenomenon is so sensitive that single amino acid substitutions in the K and D protein chains, resulting from mutation, change the susceptibility of of target cells to lysis (Klein, 1978).

c. It has been shown that the proliferative response of T cells, previously primed to antigen and challenged by antigen-carrying macrophages, only occurred when the two types of cell carried the same I-A specificity (Schwarz et al, 1978). I-E molecules play a similar role and this restriction also applies to the response by unprimed T cells. In the induction of delayed hypersensitivity there is again evidence that the appearance of T cells mediating this function also depends on sharing of I-A specificities between antigen-presenting macrophage and T helper cell.

d. It has been established in several mammalian species that the specific antibody and delayed hypersensitivity responses to thymus-dependent antigens are controlled as dominant traits by genes (Ir) located in the MHC (Benaceraff & Katz, 1975).

Although the experimental studies involved antigens of restricted specificity, it is likely that the response to more complex natural antigens is also dependent on Ir genes. These genes do not operate by influencing the structure of antibody molecules. There is evidence that in some instances where an antibody response does not occur after antigenic challenge, T suppressor cells are generated and that this also is under the control of I-region genes — Is genes. The products of the Ir genes are referred to as 'immune-associated', hence 'Ia molecules'.

The above phenomena are all examples of MHC restriction and it is clear that this occupies a central role in the functions of the MHC. There are several possible mechanisms which might account for the observations:

a. T cells have two distinct receptors, one recognising foreign antigen and the other MHC-coded membrane antigen, e.g. K or D in the case of cytotoxicity, I-A or I-E in the cases of antigen presentation by macrophages and co-operation with B cells (dual recognition).

b. The T cell receptor is single and recognises the compound antigen provided by foreign antigen and MHC molecule (associative recognition).

c. The foreign antigen produces conformational changes in the MHC molecule which is recognised by T cell receptors (altered self).

d. There is cross-reactivity between foreign antigen and the MHC molecule such that the T cell receptor for the former will also interact with the latter (cross-reactivity).

It is still uncertain which of these explanations is physiologically the most likely. Whatever the mechanism of MHC restriction there remains the related question of how Ir-genes produce their effects. There is considerable evidence that the I-A and I-E molecules are themselves the product of the Ir genes (Nagy et al, 1981). Why does an immune response to an antigen occur in individuals with particular I-A or I-E specificities and not in others with other specificities?

There is firstly the possibility that in the non-responders, macrophages fail to present the antigen together with I-A or I-E molecules in a way which is recognised by the T helper cell receptors. Secondly, a concomitant induction of T suppressor activity could lead to lack of response (Nagy et al, 1981). Thirdly, there is the important possibility that the T cell repertoire does not include cells that have receptors for the combination of the particular antigen and I-A or I-E molecule. The development of precytotoxic T cells into cytotoxic cells has been shown to depend on recognition of K and D/L antigens as well as foreign antigens and thus class I antigens also act as immune response genes, for example in relation to viruses (Finberg & Benacerraf, 1981).

Experimental autoimmune disease

It has been shown that the development of autoimmune thyroiditis resulting from immunisation with thyroglobulin in Freund's adjuvant is under genetic control by a gene in the MHC region (Rose et al, 1973). Similarly susceptibility to experimental allergic encephalomyelitis in the rat is determined by genes in the MHC (Williams & Moore, 1973).

Although one cannot necessarily translate these observations into the context of human autoimmune disorders, it is nonetheless of interest that MHC-linked genes can have an important role in the development of autoimmune processes.

THE HUMAN MHC (HLA) SYSTEM

The possibility that human nucleated cells might possess inherited membrane antigenic specificities was first investigated by methods which were an extension of those traditionally applied to red cell blood group systems. Sera from repeatedly transfused individuals were examined for their ability to agglutinate peripheral blood leucocytes. Two major advances led to rapid progress. Firstly, it was found that pregnancy was often associated with the appearance of leukoagglutinins and because the source of the stimulating white cells was much more restricted, the possibility of defining discrete specificities was greatly increased. Secondly, the development of complement-dependent cytotoxicity assays proved to be greatly superior as a tool for detecting and analysing antisera (Terasaki & McClelland, 1964).

It became possible to define a number of antigenic specificities carried on lymphocytes and family studies show that these were inherited as codominant traits controlled by genes at three closely linked loci, i.e. HLA-A, B and C.

The application of cellular techniques, measuring the degree of proliferative response of lymphocytes from one individual stimulated in culture by those of another individual (the mixed lymphocyte culture — MLC response) led to the definition of the HLA-D locus. Findings in relation to the H-2 system in the mouse led to a search for antibody specificities which would define antigens of more restricted distribution, e.g. occurring on B lymphocytes rather than on all peripheral blood lymphocytes. As a result, the HLA-DR locus was defined, so named because of its close relationship to the HLA-D locus.

The observation that some of the components of the classical and alternative complement pathways showed genetically determined variants, allowed for linkage studies which mapped three of these components within the HLA chromosomal region (C2, C4 and factor B).

Linkage studies further showed that the HLA loci are situated on the short arm of chromosome 6.

Methods Used

Appropriate antisera for HLA typing are obtained for the most part from parous women. The antibodies appear as a result of stimulation by paternal antigens carried on fetal white cells which cross into the maternal circulation during pregnancy. Lymphocytes for typing are separated from peripheral blood by gradient sedimentation in ficoll-hypaque and are incubated with the test antisera in the presence of appropriate rabbit complement. Dead cells are identified by their uptake of dye, e.g. trypan blue or eosin, and the degree of cytotoxicity is assessed by counting the percentage of dead cells. Antisera are often multispecific and suitable test sera can only be obtained by testing against a large panel of previously typed lymphocytes. Problems in typing arise because of cross-reactivity between HLA antigens of different specificity. Thus the serum obtained from an individual, immunised with a cell thought to contain one HLA specificity, may react not only with that cell but with cells from other individuals lacking that specificity. For example, HLA-B7, B27, B22 and B40 constitute a cross-reactive group and mistakes in typing for B27 can be made unless an adequate panel of sera is available.

A basically similar method is commonly used for DR typing but the problem is that the B lymphocytes which carry these antigens constitute only 10–20% of the peripheral lymphocytes. One approach is to remove the T lymphocytes by adding sheep red cells with which the T lymphocytes form rosettes which sediment, leaving a B cell enriched supernate. Alternatively, the T lymphocytes may be separated out by using nylon wool columns. The separated B cells can then be tested in the cytotoxin assay described above.

A second approach is to avoid the need to separate the B cell population by adding fluorescein-labelled anti-Ig which reacts with surface immunoglobulin on B cells. The cytotoxic assay is carried out in the usual way using suitable DR antisera, dead cells being identified by their staining with ethidium bromide. Using a fluorescent microscope with suitable filters the B cells can be identified by the green rim of staining and dead cells by their red staining. The percentage of dead B cells is thus determined.

D-locus typing is dependent on carrying out a one-way mixed lymphocyte reaction (MLR). The test cell is ideally one homozygous for a known D specificity which has been inactivated, e.g. by mitomycin C, before incubating with the unknown cell. The proliferative response of the latter is measured by [^{3}H] thymidine uptake and a lack of response suggests that the unknown cell carries the specificity of the test cell.

The HLA specificities

Table 10.1 lists the specificities at the A, B, C, D and DR loci as agreed by the WHO committee on HLA nomenclature in 1980. A designation including 'w' denotes that there is some uncertainty as to whether the specificity is adequately defined.

Figure 10.3 shows the relative position of the loci in the HLA region on the short arm of chromosome number 6. There is still uncertainty as to the exact relationship between the D and DR specificities. Because of the close linkage, recombination between the loci is relatively uncommon. However, studies of recombinants gives infor-

Table 10.1 Recognised specificities at the HLA loci (WHO Nomenclature Committee, 1980)

HLA-A	HLA-B	HLA-C	HLA-D	HLA-DR
HLA-A1	HLA-B5	HLA-Cw1	HLA-Dw1	HLA-DR1
HLA-A2	HLA-B7	HLA-Cw2	HLA-Dw2	HLA-DR2
HLA-A3	HLA-B8	HLA-Cw3	HLA-Dw3	HLA-DR3
HLA-A9	HLA-B12	HLA-Cw4	HLA-Dw4	HLA-DR4
HLA-A10	HLA-B13	HLA-Cw5	HLA-Dw5	HLA-DR5
HLA-A11	HLA-B14	HLA-Cw6	HLA-Dw6	HLA-DRw6
HLA-Aw19	HLA-B15	HLA-Cw7	HLA-Dw7	HLA-DR7
HLA-Aw23(9)	HLA-Bw16	HLA-Cw8	HLA-Dw8	HLA-DRw8
HLA-Aw24(9)	HLA-B17		HLA-Dw9	HLA-DRw9
HLA-A25(10)	HLA-B18		HLA-Dw10	HLA-DRw10
HLA-A26(10)	HLA-Bw21		HLA-Dw11	
HLA-A28	HLA-Bw22		HLA-Dw12	
HLA-A29	HLA-B27			
HLA-Aw30	HLA-Bw35			
HLA-Aw31	HLA-B37			
HLA-Aw32	HLA-Bw38(w16)			
HLA-Aw33	HLA-Bw39(w16)			
HLA-Aw34	HLA-B40			
HLA-Aw36	HLA-Bw41			
HLA-Aw43	HLA-Bw42			
	HLA-Bw44(12)			
	HLA-Bw45(12)			
	HLA-Bw46			
	HLA-Bw47			
	HLA-Bw48			
	HLA-Bw49(w21)			
	HLA-Bw50(w21)			
	HLA-Bw51(5)			
	HLA-Bw52(5)			
	HLA-Bw53			
	HLA-Bw54(w22)			
	HLA-Bw55(w22)			
	HLA-Bw56(w22)			
	HLA-Bw57(17)			
	HLA-Bw58(17)			
	HLA-Bw59			
	HLA-Bw60(40)			
	HLA-Bw61(40)			
	HLA-Bw62(15)			
	HLA-Bw63(15)			
	HLA-Bw4[a]			
	HLA-Bw6			

mation on the relative position of the loci and on the genetic distance between them. The exact locations of the structural genes for C4, C2 and factor B are still somewhat uncertain but they are thought to be between B and D/DR.

The alleles present at the various loci on one chromosome are inherited in the great majority of cases as a unit and the genetic information thus provided is the haplotype. Individuals may be homozygous or heterozygous at any one locus. The HLA phenotype describes all the specificities found at the various loci, e.g. an individual's pheno-

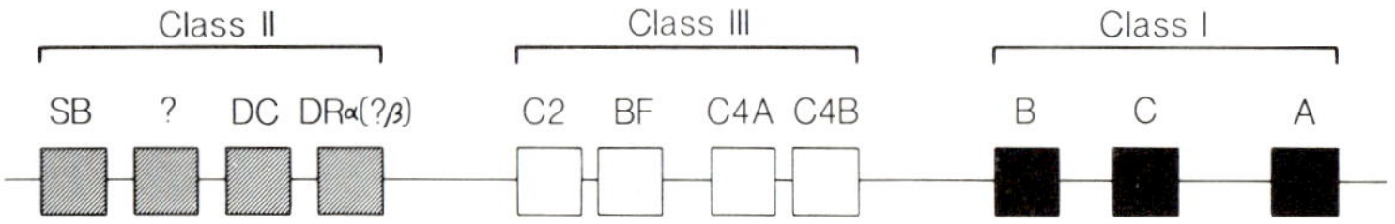

Fig. 10.3 Genetic loci in the HLA region. ? denotes likelihood for presence of at least one further locus for class II molecules.

type might be A1, A3, B7, B22, Cw1, Cw6, DR1, DR4. Family studies are required to determine the genotype, i.e. the specificities arranged in haplotypes e.g. A1, B7, Cw1, DR4 on one chromosome and A3, B22, Cw6, DR1 on the other. Figure 10.4 gives an example of the way in which HLA haplotypes are inherited.

The frequency with which a particular antigen occurs in the general population, as estimated from an appropriate sample, can be used to derive the gene frequency for that antigen. If f is the population frequency of the antigen, the gene frequency $(p) = 1 - \sqrt{(1-f)}$. Estimation of the frequency of particular haplotypes in a population is a more complex matter. The direct way is to carry out family studies on a suitably large sample of individuals and thus derive the genotypes of the probands, each of whom supplies two haplotypes. The different haplotypes can then be counted. There are other more indirect and more complex methods for deriving haplotype frequencies from phenotype frequencies. However derived, the estimation of haplotype frequencies reveals a striking tendency for certain specificities at the different loci to associate together in the same haplotype. General principles of population genetics suggest that the frequency with which two particular genes occur together on the same chromosome should, under equilibrium conditions and in the absence of selection, be the product of the two individual population gene frequencies. For example, if p (a) and p(b) are the gene frequencies for two genes, a and b, at two loci on the same chromosome, the frequency of the haplotype ab would be expected to be $p(a) \times p(b)$. In the HLA system frequent examples are observed where in fact the haplotype frequency is significantly greater than expected. The difference from expected is a measure of linkage disequilibrium, i.e. $p(ab) - [p(a) \times p(p)]$. In Caucasian population one of the earliest observed and most striking examples of this is the association between HLA-A1 and B8, e.g. typical population frequencies for A1 and B8 are 29% and 20% giving gene frequencies of 0.16 and 0.11 respectively. The expected frequency of the A1, B8 haplotype is thus 0.0176. In fact the observed frequency of the haplotype is 0.09 which is approximately five times the expected. The measure of linkage disequilibrium (D) is $0.09 - 0.0176 = 0.0724$ and this accounts for approximately four-fifths of the actual haplotype frequency. As more polymorphic loci are defined in the HLA region it becomes apparent that they are all involved to a greater or lesser degree in linkage disequilibria, so that particular haplotypes which involve all the known loci are characteristic of each population.

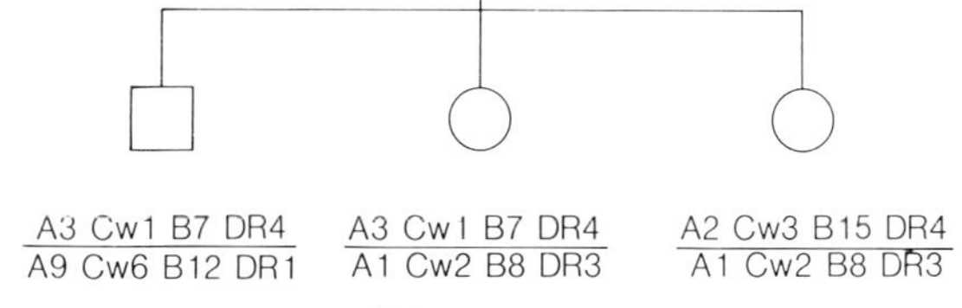

Fig. 10.4 Inheritance of HLA haplotypes in a family.

The existence of linkage disequilibrium has considerable importance when it comes to the interpretation of HLA and disease associations. It is postulated that the degree of linkage disequilibrium observed is in large part the result of selection. If a mutant gene results in increased fitness, then not only may the mutant gene increase in the population but the genes at loci closely linked to it will also tend to increase as a haplotype, a phenomenon called 'hitchhiking' (Thomson, 1977). Similarly, if a gene promoting increased susceptibility to a disease appears in the same chromosomal region, it also will tend to increase in frequency in the population and will become associated with the particular haplotype for many generations before repeated recombination gradually lessens the linkage disequilibrium.

Molecular structure

The products of the HLA-A, B, C and DR loci are glycoproteins integral to the cell membrane structure and float in the lipid bilayer. The molecules are transmembrane, the N-terminus being associated with the part of the polypeptide chain presenting on the external surface and the hydrophilic C-terminal end projecting into the cytoplasm (Orr et al, 1979).

Class I molecules (A, B and C) have a heavy polypeptide chain of 45 000 dalton molecular weight, the antigenic specificity of the molecule residing in the amino acid sequence at discrete lengths along the chain. This is associated at the surface with β_2-microglobulin, a 12 000 dalton molecular weight polypeptide chain which is not integral to the membrane and which is invariant. This molecule is coded for on chromosome 15. The heavy chain is made up of three domains (Fig. 10.5) and there is very considerable sequence homology between the three domains and β_2-microglobulin and the constant region domains of the heavy chain of immunoglobulin. These molecules are present on the surface of all nucleated cells and on platelets, and occur free in tissue fluids.

Class II molecules (DR) are constituted by two glycoprotein chains, a heavy (α) chain of 34 000 daltons and a lighter (β) chain of 28 000 daltons (Shackelford et al, 1982). The β chain appears to be the more polymorphic and the serologically defined antigens certainly occur on this chain. Both chains include two domains which show considerable sequence homology with those of class I molecules and with β-microglobulin and in some degree with constant region immunoglobulin domains. The molecules are present on B lymphocytes, T cells, macrophages (especially when activated), Langerhans cells in the skin and glomerular capillary endothelium.

Considerable progress has been made since the DR specificities listed in Table 10.1 were published. The application of more sophisticated techniques involving use of monoclonal antibodies and radio-immunoassay for typing has produced evidence of three closely linked loci in the DR region (Tanigaki & Tosi, 1982). The evidence points to the previously recognised DR molecules being the homologue of the I-E molecule in the H-2 system (Allison et al, 1978; Silver, et al, 1979). Another locus (DC) determines a series of molecules which are probably the equivalent of murine I-A molecules (Bono & Strominger, 1982).

Further complexity is evident in the definition of a series of specificities (SB) which are probably separate from those just described and which are defined by a cellular technique — the primed lymphocyte test (Shaw et al, 1981). It will be some time before a complete picture of this HLA region is obtained but it seems evident that there exists a series of closely linked polymorphic loci whose products are the homologues of class II molecules of the H-2 system, i.e. I-A and I-E.

CLASS III LOCI (C4, C2, FACTOR B)

C4 polymorphism

It appears most likely that there are two closely linked loci for C4 — C4A and C4B. Codominantly inherited allotypes are identified by preincubation of plasma with neuraminidase followed by electrophoresis in agarose gel. Each glycoprotein gene product is thus separated into three bands, those for C4A moving faster than the C4B bands. These are subjected to immunofixation by anti-human C4 serum and stained. At present, 12 C4A and 18

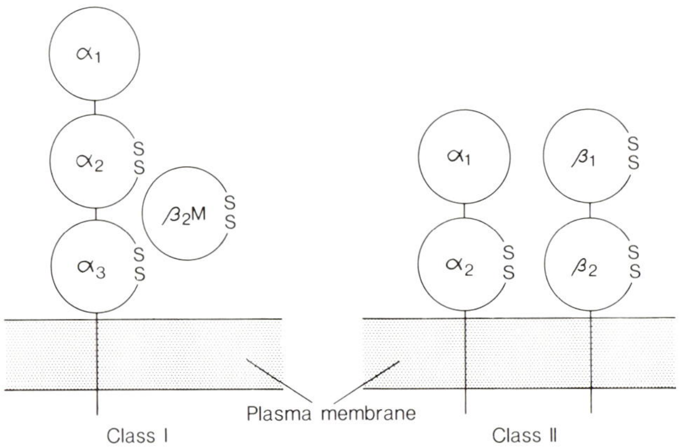

Fig. 10.5 General structure of HLA class I and class II molecules, showing arrangements in domains.

C4B allotypes are recognised and family studies allow haplotypes to be identified, e.g. a very common haplotype is C4A*3, C4B*1. There may be no expression of the gene present at these loci, the corresponding alleles being designated C4A*Q0 and C4B*Q0 and these are of quite appreciable frequency, e.g. 0.16 for the former and 0.09 for the latter. The technique may be supplemented by a haemolytic overlay assay, i.e. by overlaying the gel with sensitised sheep red cells and C4-deficient serum and observing the bands of haemolysis. This has shown that C4B allotypes regularly show little or no haemolytic activity.

C4 products occur in plasma and on the surface of red cells and the antisera which define the Rodgers (Rg) and Chido (Ch) blood group systems are directed at determinants on the C4d components of C4A and C4B molecules respectively. Thus sera showing no fast bands (C4A) are Rg (a−) and those showing no slow bands (C4B) are Ch (a−). Evidence of linkage disequilibria with the other complement and HLA polymorphisms includes C4A*4 with C4B*2, C4A*Q0 with HLA-B8, DR3 and C4B*Q0 with HLA Bw44, DR4.

C2 polymorphism

Allotypes are defined by isoelectric focussing followed by a haemolytic overlay assay. For each gene product several haemolytic bands are seen, one predominating. The commonest allotype is C2C, variants C2B and C2A being uncommon. Linkage disequilibrium is observed, e.g. C2*B with HLA-B15, Bw22, Cw3, BF*S, DR4.

C2 deficiency has allowed for the definition of a null allele, C2*Q0, which has a gene frequency of the order of 0.006 suggesting that 1:28 000 of the population are homozygous C2 deficient (Rynes, 1982). This allele is in marked linkage disequilibrium with A25(10), B18, C4A*4, C4B* 2, BF*S, Dw2/DR2.

Factor B polymorphism

By use of agarose gel electrophoresis and immunofixation by anti-factor B serum, two common gene products are observed, BFS and BFF, with two rarer variants, BFF1 and BFS 0.7. BFF1 is associated with HLA-B18 and DR3.

HLA ASSOCIATIONS WITH DISEASE

The purpose of looking for possible associations between the HLA polymorphisms and disease is to detect the presence of genes in the HLA chromosomal region which increase susceptibility to the particular disorders. Two main approaches are used involving:

a. Groups of patients and controls
b. Family studies.

Population studies

The frequency of the antigens at each locus is determined for a sample of patients with a particular disorder and compared with the frequencies in a suitable control sample. Because of the variability in these frequencies between different ethnic groups and between different regions within the same ethnic group, it is important that the control subjects are selected from the same ethnic group and preferably from the same geographical region. Moreover, it is important to define clearly the criteria by which the patient group has been selected.

For each antigen tested for, there is derived a 2 × 2 table as in Figure 10.6. The null hypothesis is that there is no significant difference between the two frequencies and the probability that this is not true is tested for by the goodness of fit test (χ^2 test) or by Fisher's exact probability test.

In starting such an investigation it must be remembered that one is looking for differences not in relation to any one particular antigen but involving *any* of the many antigens tested for. There are bound to be some differences in respect of some of the antigen frequencies and the problem to decide is whether these differences are worthy of note. The standard criterion for accepting a difference as being significant for a single comparison is the finding of a probability (p) value

	Patients	Controls
Number with antigen present	a	c
Number with antigen absent	b	d

Fig. 10.6 2 × 2 table used to measure the association between an HLA antigen and a disease.

of 0.05 or less. With multiple comparisons a probability less than this is required, e.g. if 20 antigens are being tested for, the required probability is 0.05/20, i.e. 0.0025. The usual practice is to multiply the p value derived from the 2 × 2 table by the number of antigens tested for and to regard a value of <0.05 as significant.

It is important to appreciate that these studies, of necessity, involve relatively small groups of patients and controls. If the association between the disorder and particular HLA antigen is real but not strong, a single study is unlikely to allow a firm conclusion to be drawn. One study may show no difference in frequency whilst one from another centre may show an apparent association and yet there may actually be no significant difference between the two sets of findings. It is often, therefore, necessary for several studies to be carried out in different centres before a firm conclusion can be drawn.

In relation to this, a useful measure of association is the relative risk which is equivalent to the odds ratio, i.e. the risk of developing the disorder for those in the population who possess the antigen, relative to the risk for those who do not. It is estimated from data in 2 × 2 tables (Fig. 10.6) as (a + 0.5) (d + 0.5)/(b + 0.5) (c + 0.5) (Haldane, 1955). It will equal 1 if there is no association. Data from several studies can be combined to give a combined relative risk and the corresponding probability estimated (Woolf, 1955). A test for heterogeneity is performed at the same time. If an association is real, a combination of the data in a series of studies, provided they involve homogenous groups of patients and ethnically comparable populations, should reinforce each other and give increasingly significant results, without heterogeneity. It is often of interest to subdivide a group of patients according to clinical or laboratory criteria. This can be useful in demonstrating heterogeneity within a particular disorder but there is a danger that, as the subgroups become smaller, difficulties may arise in drawing conclusions from small numbers.

Interest has been shown in the possibility of 'protective' genes in the HLA region which would lead to a negative association between a particular HLA antigen and a disease. The finding that only one antigen determined by a gene at a polymorphic locus is, relative to all other antigens, negatively associated with the disorder, would be evidence of such a protective gene. Where one or more antigens are positively associated with the disorder, it is to be expected that, relative to this, other antigens will be negatively associated. So far no clear evidence has been put forward for the existence of such genes.

Although the relative risk is a useful measure of the degree of association, its quantitative interpretation is not simple. It is used to give a measure of the degree of association between an HLA antigen and a disease but also to compare the degrees of association of different antigens with a disease, e.g. the relative risk for coeliac disease increases progressively from HLA-A1 to B8 to DR3. Theoretically the size of the relative risk is a function firstly of the degree of linkage disequilibrium between the HLA antigen and the disease susceptibility gene and secondly of the importance of this gene in the total variability underlying the disease. It is to be expected that, other things being equal, the closer the antigen locus is to the disease susceptibility gene locus, the greater will be the linkage disequilibrium and the higher the relative risk. However, the size of the relative risk does depend on the particular gene frequencies involved and although in general it is probably true that, as the relative risk for antigens at different HLA loci increases, one is approaching nearer to the disease susceptibility gene locus, some caution is necessary in this interpretation.

One way of examining the respective degrees of association of antigens of different HLA loci and the disease is to partition the data, e.g. if antigen A at the HLA-A locus and antigen B at the HLA-B locus are both associated with the disease, the frequency of B may be compared in A-positive patients and controls and conversely the frequency of antigen A, may be compared in B-positive patients and controls. Although there are some reservations, this will usually show which of the two antigens is primarily associated with the disease.

Haplotype associations

It is common to find that a disease is associated not just with one HLA antigen at one particular locus but with a series of antigens at different loci along the chromosome, i.e. the disease is associated with an HLA haplotype. This is not surprising in view of the marked degree of linkage disequilibrium between the various loci. The basis for the occurrence of linkage disequilibrium between a disease susceptibility gene and HLA haplotype may be closely related to the development of linkage disequilibrium between the various genes within that haplotype, i.e. both susceptibility gene and HLA haplotype may 'hitchhike' with a closely linked mutant gene which spreads in the population.

A particular antigen, e.g. DR, may be associated with a disorder but may itself be involved in two or more haplotypes in the population. When the frequencies of these haplotypes are studied in the patients it may be found that the frequency of one is increased but not so that of another, e.g. the disorder may be associated with DR3 and it may be found that DR3 is itself part of two separate haplotypes, one or both of which is associated with the disease. It may also be found that one particular haplotype is associated with two or more disorders and this raises interesting possibilities in regard to common pathogenetic factors, e.g. a haplotype involving DR4 may be common to insulin-dependent diabetes and rheumatoid arthritis.

Family studies

These can supplement information obtained from the study of groups of patients and can aid in the further analysis of the genetics of the disorder.

One can confirm the importance of the HLA association by carrying out a linkage analysis, i.e. measuring the degree to which the disease and the HLA antigen or haplotype segregate together with families. One approach is to compare the haplotypes of two or more siblings with the same disorder to determine whether there is a departure from random zygotic assortment of parental HLA haplotypes. If siblings share these haplotypes to a degree greater than expected by chance this is good evidence of an HLA-linked susceptibility gene (Green & Woodrow, 1977). Modifications of the classical methods of analysis of linkage are now being applied (Morton & Lalouel, 1981).

When a positive association is established, the most likely interpretation is that there are one or more disease susceptibility genes for the disorder in the HLA region. This can be interpreted in two ways:

1. The HLA antigen which is positively associated is itself the product of the susceptibility gene.
2. The susceptibility gene is at a locus closely linked to the HLA locus in question and is in linkage disequilibrium with the HLA antigen associated with the disorder, i.e. it is relatively more frequent on chromosomes carrying the gene for the HLA antigen than on those that do not.

There is no certain way of distinguishing these two possibilities but evidence may be sought along the following lines.

a. If an association is found between a particular antigen and a disease in different ethnic groups, this supports the possibility that the HLA antigen is itself the product of the susceptibility gene (see B27-associated disorders, below). On the other hand, if what appears to be the same disorder is associated with different HLA antigens in different populations, the second possibility is more likely. An example of this is that primary thyrotoxicosis is associated with quite different B and DR locus antigens in Caucasian, Chinese and Japanese populations.
b. Clinical heterogeneity may provide useful information. If one finds significant differences in clinical features between patients with a disease who are positive for an antigen and those who are negative, this suggests that the antigen itself is the susceptibility gene and that there is genetic heterogeneity. If all patients, positive for the HLA antigen or not, carried the same linked susceptibility gene, such clinical differences would not be expected.
c. There may be evidence of genetic heterogeneity. If the pattern of familial aggregation is different in the families of those patients positive for the particular antigen as compared with those negative, this supports the likelihood that the HLA antigen is directly involved in increasing susceptibility. If all patients, regardless of whether they were positive for the HLA antigen or not, carried the same linked susceptibility gene there should be no such genetic heterogeneity.
d. Precise information would be afforded that the HLA antigen is not the susceptibility gene if,

within a family, disassociation between the particular HLA antigen and the disease were shown to be due to genetic recombination. However, just finding that of two first degree relatives with the disease, one possessed the antigen and one did not, is not sufficient proof. One must show by following the segregation of other genetic markers along the chromosome that a recombination has occurred.

e. Study of haplotype associations may be informative. For example, if an HLA antigen, e.g. DR-X is associated with a disease, and is also part of more than one haplotype in the population, it is important to ask whether all these haplotypes are increased in frequency in individuals with the disease. If this is not found, it provides evidence against DR-X being the susceptibility gene.

Once the HLA association is established one can ask:

1. Are there one or more genes for susceptibility in the HLA region?
2. Is there genetic heterogeneity, e.g. some fraction of the cases not dependent on an HLA-linked gene?
3. Is the gene or genes involved acting in dominant, recessive or intermediate fashion?

Information in regard to the last question may provide evidence as to the possible mechanisms of action of the susceptibility gene.

The degree of sharing of HLA haplotypes between affected siblings can be analysed to give evidence on the genetic behaviour of an HLA-linked susceptibility gene (Thomson & Bodmer, 1977). Useful information also comes from the determination by family studies of the genotype of a series of patients, e.g. whether an individual is homozygous, heterozygous or negative for the associated HLA antigen (Thomson, 1983). The ratio between these is affected by the genetic behaviour of the susceptibility gene, e.g. if it results in a recessive phenotype there will be a relative excess of affected patients who are homozygous for the associated HLA antigen.

Further methods of analysis are currently being developed, using complex segregation and linkage analysis. What is usually done is to produce a genetic model and to see whether the actual family or genotype data fit this. There are, however, usually several unknowns in the equation, i.e. the gene frequency of the susceptibility gene in the population, its penetrance, the degree of genetic recombination between the proposed HLA-linked gene and the locus for the HLA antigen and the degree of genetic heterogeneity. These parameters have to be estimated during the analysis, using maximum likelihood methods.

HLA ASSOCIATIONS WITH RHEUMATIC DISEASES

HLA-B27 associated disorders

The group of clinical disorders which is associated with the inheritance of HLA-B27 constitutes one of the most striking examples of HLA and disease association. Previously there had been evidence that these disorders were associated clinically and genetically (Wright & Moll, 1976) and the finding of a common association with B27 has contributed greatly to our understanding of these observations. The first association found was with ankylosing spondylitis (Brewerton et al, 1973a; Schlosstein et al, 1973) followed by sexually-acquired reactive arthritis (Brewerton et al, 1973b; Woodrow et al, 1974), arthritis reactive to gastrointestinal infections (Aho et al, 1974; Friis & Svejgaard, 1974), anterior uveitis (Brewerton et al, 1973c; Woodrow et al, 1975) and peripheral psoriatic arthritis (Zachariae et al, 1974; Brewerton et al, 1974). A detailed documentation and analysis of these associations has been presented (Woodrow, 1977). Table 10.2 gives details of typical findings in a Caucasian population.

Table 10.2 Association between various disorders and HLA-B27

	Number	B27-positive No.	B27-positive %	Relative risk
Controls	*550*	*50*	*9.1*	
Ankylosing spondylitis	230	212	92.2	118
Reactive arthritis				
Sexually acquired	103	73	70.9	24.3
Gastrointestinal infection	10	10	100.00	4.0
Psoriatic arthritis	94	27	28.7	13.1
Acute anterior uveitis	90	51	55.7	

Ankylosing spondylitis

The odds ratio (relative risk) for ankylosing spondylitis suggests that the B27-positive individual is at least a hundred times as likely to develop spondylitis as one who is negative. One can ask the question whether the B27-negative patients are genetically different. Evidence of relevance in this regard comes from two main sources. Firstly, where sacroiliitis or spondylitis and inflammatory bowel disease coexist, the frequency of B27 is of the order of 54% (Woodrow, 1977). Thus in the presence of bowel disease, sacroiliitis or spondylitis not uncommonly occurs in the absence of B27. Similarly, when sacroiliitis is found in individuals with psoriasis the frequency of B27 is of the order of 75%. This suggests the possibility that genetic factors implicated in bowel disease and psoriasis may also be involved in the development of susceptibility to spondylitis in some individuals and this raises the possibility that, in some instances at least, B27-negative spondylitis is a result of genetic factors other than B27 (Woodrow & Eastmond, 1978). The second line of evidence relates to the question whether the major gene for spondylitis is that for B27 or whether it is situated at a locus very close to the HLA-B locus and in very strong linkage disequilibrium with B27. There can be no certainty on the basis of the present evidence, but it tends to favour the former possibility.

a. Ankylosing spondylitis is associated with B27 in all ethnic populations so far studied. This is so in populations where the B27 frequency is very high, e.g. in the Haida Indians (Gofton et al, 1975) and in those where it is low, e.g. in the Japanese (Sonozaki et al, 1975). In all the populations studied the relative risk for developing spondylitis is high for B27-positive individuals.

b. Although no clear cut clinical differences have been observed between B27-positive and negative patients, the age of onset appears to be somewhat higher in the latter group.

c. Families have been reported in which both B27-positive and negative first degree relatives have had spondylitis and this has suggested the possibility of genetic recombination between a spondylitis gene and the B27 gene. In some of the families inflammatory bowel disease has been present and this raises the possibility that other genes might be giving rise to the spondylitis in the B27-negative individual (Woodrow & Eastmond, 1977). No case has been recorded in which such disassociation has coincided with a proven chromosomal recombination.

d. If all cases of spondylitis were genetically the same one would expect the same pattern of familial aggregation in those B27-negative as in those positive. Studies so far have tended to show less familial aggregation in the case of B27-negative probands and this favours genetic heterogeneity, i.e. other, less penetrant genes are the basis for disease in these individuals.

If the gene for B27 is itself the spondylitis gene then the genetics is relatively simple in that the vast majority of patients with spondylitis are heterozygous B27 and this suggests a dominant trait. Even if this assumption is not made, analysis of the ratio of patients homozygous for B27 to those heterozygous, favours a dominant expression of the gene (Thomson & Bodmer, 1977). However, there is a suggestion in the available data that individuals homozygous for B27 are at a somewhat greater risk than heterozygotes (Woodrow, 1977; Kahn et al, 1978). Only a proportion of the first degree B27-positive relatives of B27-positive patients show evidence of sacroiliitis or spondylitis. One study suggested that approximately 50% of B27-positive brothers and fathers of probands had radiological sacroiliitis compared with approximately 20% of control B27-positive males (Woodrow et al, 1983). Several other family studies have been reported and although the methodology involved and the particular frequencies found varied considerably, they agree in finding a greater prevalence of evidence of disease in B27-positive relatives of affected probands than in controls (Kidd et al, 1977; Lochead et al, 1983; Calin et al, 1983; van der Linden et al, 1984). The finding is capable of several possible genetic interpretations. If there was variability in the B27 antigen and one variant was especially associated with increased susceptibility to spondylitis, the finding would be explained. Recently heterogeneity of B27 has been demonstrated by the use of monoclonal antibodies (Grumet, 1983) and by cellular techniques (Breuning et al, 1982). It has, however, not so far been demonstrated that one particular variant leads to greater susceptibility than another. Another explanation would be that there is another gene (or genes), possibly HLA-linked, which is segregating in the families of patients with spondylitis and interacts with B27 to increase susceptibility. HLA-A2 is positively associated with spondylitis although with a rather low relative risk and there is the possibility of a gene in the HLA-A region contributing to susceptibility.

Reactive arthritis

The relative risk associated with B27 of developing a peripheral arthritis and possibly mucocutaneous lesions following sexually-acquired non-specific urethritis is of the order of 24. A very similar risk is seen in respect of Yersinia arthritis (Leirisalo et al, 1982). It appears that an even stronger association is present in relation to the peripheral arthritis and enthesopathy following gastrointestinal infection with *Salmonella*, *Shigella* and *Campylobacter* organisms where it is rare to find the patient to be B27-negative. This is perhaps the most striking of all HLA and disease associations.

Uveitis

Approximately 50% of individuals experiencing one or more episodes of non-granulomatous anterior uveitis are B27-positive, giving a relative risk of 13. It is likely that this largely accounts for the association of ankylosing spondylitis and reactive arthritis with anterior uveitis and the great majority of patients with uveitis who develop either of these rheumatic disorders are B27-positive.

Peripheral arthritis and B27

B27-positive individuals, both male and female, during both the childhood and adult years, are liable to develop a predominantly lower limb arthropathy which is sometimes associated with calcaneal and metatarsal periostitis and tendo-Achilles bursitis. Although often self-limited and episodic, persistent synovitis especially involving the knees may occur. Sacroiliitis may be asymptomatic and only discovered on radiography. The arthropathy may precede or follow the onset of ankylosing spondylitis.

Psoriatic arthritis

Psoriasis itself is positively associated with HLA B13, B17, Cw6 and DR7 which are in linkage disequilibrium with each other in the population. Individuals with psoriasis who are B27-positive appear to be approximately four times more liable to get peripheral psoriatic arthritis than those who are negative. Evidence has been put forward to suggest an increased risk of developing peripheral arthritis for patients with psoriasis who are positive for a split of Bw16 and in particular for Bw39, but the evidence is far from clear on this, in part because of relatively small sample sizes and probably because of considerable heterogeneity in the cases included under the heading of psoriatic arthritis (Armstrong et al, 1983a; Beaulieu et al, 1983; McKendry et al, 1984).

Rheumatoid arthritis

Following the observations of Stastny et al (1978) and Panayi et al (1978) an association between DR4 and rheumatoid arthritis has been found in several populations of widely differing ethnic origins. Combination of data from different centres give relative risks for developing rheumatoid arthritis in DR4-positive individuals of 3.9 in Caucasians, 2.3 in Japanese, 5.0 in American blacks, 10.5 in Indians from New Delhi and 1.6 in Thais. There is significant heterogeneity between the populations but the common association is striking. Two studies, one from Israel (Schiff et al, 1982) and one involving Asian Indian immigrants in England (Woodrow et al, 1981) have found an apparent association with DR1 rather than DR4.

Childhood onset seropositive rheumatoid arthritis is also associated with DR4 (Clemens et al, 1983).

Evidence has been reported supporting an association with a particular haplotype which includes, in addition to DR4, Bw62(15), BfS, C4A3, C4B2.9 (McCluskey et al, 1984). This finding requires confirmation and the interpretation must remain uncertain until the degree of association of C4B2.9 with DR4 in the population is clarified.

Family studies have investigated the segregation of disease with HLA haplotypes. Analysis of sibships which include two or more individuals with rheumatoid arthritis has not so far shown a significant increase in the sharing of inherited haplotypes by affected siblings (Zilko & Dawkins, 1982; Khan et al, 1983; Grennan et al, 1983; Nunez et al, 1984). This could be the result of a high population frequency for the HLA-linked susceptibility gene(s) and major contributions from non-HLA-linked genes and environmental agents.

The evidence on the question as to whether DR4 is positively associated with seronegative as well as seropositive disease is contradictory, probably in part due to heterogeneity within the seronegative group. A recent study showed a significant difference in frequencies between the two groups (Alarçon et al, 1982). When this point is resolved, the evidence will be of great relevance when more is known of the role HLA-DR linked antigens play in the pathogenesis of rheumatoid arthritis. One study has shown that patients with Felty's syndrome are almost always DR4-positive (Dinant et al, 1980). Proteinuria resulting from gold therapy has been associated with DR3 (Panayi et al, 1978) and myasthenia gravis resulting from d-penicillamine therapy with DR1 (Garlepp et al, 1983).

Sicca syndrome

Where the sicca syndrome occurs in the absence of rheumatoid arthritis there is a positive association with Dw3 (Fye et al, 1978) and with DRw3 (Moutsopoulos et al, 1979). In the latter study the relative risk for DR3 in sicca syndrome without arthritis was 3.8 and in sicca syndrome with arthritis 0.3. It thus appears that there is heterogeneity in the genetic susceptibility to sicca syndrome.

Juvenile chronic arthritis

The investigation of HLA antigen frequencies within a heterogeneous group of clinical conditions may, in conjunction with clinical and laboratory features, help to establish more clearly defined entities within the group. HLA-B27 associated arthropathy may occur in children as well as in adults and it is not surprising, therefore, that there is an increase in frequency of B27 when juvenile arthritis as a whole is investigated. An increase in Dw5 and Dw8 and correspondingly in DR5 and DRw8 has been found (Fink & Stastny, 1980; Morling et al, 1981). Early onset pauciarticular arthritis appears to be associated with DR5 (Glass et al, 1980; Suciu-Foca et al, 1980), with relative risks of 6.0 and 7.4 respectively. Persistent pauciarthritis may be associated with DRw8 (Morling et al, 1981; Balogh et al, 1982).

Systemic lupus erythematosus

Evidence of familial aggregation and of a higher concordance rate in monozygotic twins than in dizygotic twins has suggested a genetic component in the pathogenesis of this disorder. Initial investigations of HLA antigen frequencies suggested an association with B8 with a relative risk of little over 2. Several studies have investigated the frequencies of DR antigens, and a combined analysis by Woolf's method of five such studies (Reinersten et al, 1978; Scherak et al, 1980; Celada et al, 1980; Black et al, 1982a; Ahearn et al, 1982), gives:

a. a combined relative risk for DR2 of 1.8, $p = 0.0006$, p for heterogeneity $= 0.04$
b. for DR3 a combined risk of 2.5, $p = 5.3 \times 10^{-8}$, p for heterogeneity $= 0.08$.

There appears to be a degree of agreement that DR2 and more consistently DR3 are positively associated with systemic lupus erythematosus. The possibility that a stronger association might appear when other polymorphisms closely linked to DR are studied is raised by the finding of a much stronger risk associated with positivity for a 'supertypic' antiserum MB1/MT1 (Reinersten et al, 1978) but this finding is not consistent (Schur et al, 1982).

The occurrence of systemic lupus erythematosus in patients with various types of complement deficiency has been repeatedly documented and the association is thought to be a real one (Rynes, 1982). The disorder is seen in approximately 30% of individuals homozygous for deficiency of C2, i.e. who are homozygous C2*QO. This gene is in linkage disequilibrium with A10(A25), B18, C4A*4, C4B*2, BF*S, DR2. Heterozygotes for C2 deficiency are also at risk of developing systemic lupus (Glass et al, 1976). A high frequency of C4A*QO and C4B*QO was reported by Fielder et al (1983) and family studies suggested that haplotypes including DR3 and C4 null alleles were particularly associated with a liability to SLE. It is possible to analyse these data to show that the association with C4 null alleles is primary to that with DR3 but direct involvement of the C4 gene products in susceptibility is not clearly established.

The appearance of a lupus-like syndrome in approximately 10% of individuals on prolonged treatment with hydralazine is more liable to occur in those who are DR4-positive (Batchelor et al, 1980). An association of procainamide-induced lupus with a different antigen, DR6Y, has also been documented (Whiteside et al, 1982).

Systemic sclerosis

The evidence for an association between systemic sclerosis and the HLA systems is far from clear. An association with DR5 has been claimed but combining the data from four studies (Gladman et al, 1981; Niks et al, 1982; Black et al, 1982a; Lynch et al, 1982) gives a combined relative risk of 1.7, $p = 5 \times 10^{-4}$, p for heterogeneity = 0.007. There is thus marked heterogeneity between the studies. This could be due to real differences between different populations or to different patient selection.

There is some evidence for a weak association with DR3 and combining data from five studies (Gladman et al, 1981; Kallenburg et al, 1981; Niks et al, 1982; Black et al, 1982b; Lynch et al, 1982) gives a combined risk of 1.6, $p = 1.4 \times 10^{-3}$, p for heterogeneity = 0.09.

Dermatomyositis

There is evidence of an increased risk of dermatomyositis in childhood in DR3-positive individuals with a relative risk of 3.1 (Pachman et al, 1980).

Behçet's syndrome

In most populations studied, Behçet's syndrome has been found to be positively associated with HLA-B5. The relative risks associated with B5 are 8.3 in Turkey (Muftuoglu et al, 1981), 6.7 in Japan (Ohno et al, 1977). Comparable values have been found in other countries but rather low relative risks have been documented in two studies in England, i.e. 1.7 and 2.1 (Lehner & Batchelor, 1979; Chamberlain, 1977) and 1.2 in the USA (O'Duffy et al, 1976). It has been suggested that different clinical manifestations may be associated with different HLA antigens, e.g. B5 with ocular involvement (Lehner & Batchelor, 1979) but findings are not consistent in this regard, e.g. Muftuoglu et al (1981) found no difference in the frequency of B5 in those with and those without ocular involvement.

It is likely that it is the Bw51 split of B5 that is associated with Behçet's syndrome (Yazici et al, 1980). No association with any DR antigen has been documented and it is possible that Bw51 (B5) is directly involved in increasing susceptibility. A high incidence of the condition appears to correlate with a high population frequency of B5.

Giant cell arteritis: polymyalgia rheumatica

Evidence for a positive association between these two disorders and DR4 has been reported by Barrier et al (1981) and Armstrong et al (1983b).

Possible mechanisms

We have no direct knowledge of the way in which HLA-linked genes predispose to disease. Increasing insight into the physiological role of MHC-linked genes has led to the formulation of various general hypotheses. It is likely that different mechanisms are operating in different disorders and in particular probably differ in those associated with class I antigens from those associated with class II antigens.

With regard to those disorders associated with class I antigens, e.g. B27 and B5, the available experimental evidence points to a role of cytotoxic T cells, although in the case of virus infection the same type of cells may also mediate delayed hypersensitivity (Lin & Askonas, 1981). Cytotoxic cells may be protective against viral infection by killing the relatively small number of virus-infected cells present early in the infection but may also be involved in the development of a pathological and damaging inflammatory reaction as in lymphocytic choriomeningitis in mice which is under the control of the MHC (Oldstone et al, 1973). Different class I antigens may differ in their ability to promote the generation of effector T cells against target cells carrying such viruses as influenza, herpes simplex and cytomegelovirus

(Biddison, 1982). Thus precytotoxic T cells may not be induced to proliferate even when they share the same class I antigen as the infected target cells. This could be because a particular class I antigen cannot interreact with the particular virus determinants to provide an appropriate stimulus. A T helper cell response is presumably also involved (Finberg & Benacerraf, 1981) and the appropriate cell, operating through a class II antigen, may be absent. The generation of T suppressor cells could also account for such non-response. In relation to the B27-associated disorders, one hypothesis that has been explored is that cross-reactivity between foreign proteins and the class I (e.g. B27) molecule could result in an impairment of the primary immune response to the foreign antigen, resulting in retention of antigen and finally in a response directed at self MHC (Young et al, 1978).In particular the possibility that certain strains of *Klebsiella* could play such a role has been investigated and evidence has been put forward for cross-reactivity (Ebringer et al, 1976; Avakian et al, 1980). Certain anti-*Klebsiella* sera raised in rabbits has been claimed to be cytotoxic to B27-positive lymphocytes from B27-positive spondylitics but not to those from healthy B27-positive individuals (Seager et al, 1979). These findings await confirmation.

The class II (DR)-related disorders are of particular interest because the antigens occur on molecules which appear to be homologous to those molecules in the mouse which, under experimental conditions, are the products of immune response genes. These are thought to play a key role in the generation of T helper (and T suppressor) response and in the interaction of these with effector T lymphocytes. Demonstration of HLA-linked genetic control of the immune response in man is constrained by experimental difficulties, but evidence for such control in respect of microbial antigens has been documented (Sasazuki et al, 1983).

With regard to the DR association found in rheumatoid arthritis, it is of interest that normal synovial lining cells contain a fraction of cells of the monocyte–macrophage type that express DR antigens (Klareskog et al, 1981).These increase greatly in number and in their expression of DR antigen in rheumatoid arthritis, when they become intimately associated with T helper lymphocytes (Janossy et al, 1981). Under appropriate conditions, synovial adherent cells could activate T cells in response to soluble antigens (Klareskog et al, 1982). The initiation and persistence of inflammatory changes may well depend on the presentation of foreign antigen by the dendritic-type macrophages in the synovium resulting in the local accumulation of T helper cells which are stimulated to co-operate with B and T cells in the production of antibody, lymphokines and cytotoxic cells. Different class II antigens may have differing potentialities to interact with antigen in this way. Further progress depends on a greater understanding of the immunogenic stimulus involved and on further clarification of the DR and closely related polymorphisms.

The association of DR3 with systemic lupus erythematosus and sicca syndrome may be related to a more general phenomenon in which disorders, where there is evidence that autoimmune processes are important, are associated with this DR antigen. A similar association with DR3 is seen in one group of patients with myasthenia gravis and in disorders of endocrine glands leading to atrophy or failure of function, especially where they occur as part of a polyglandular syndrome, i.e. insulin-dependent diabetes, primary thyrotoxicosis, atrophic thyroiditis, Addison's disease and gonadal failure. A common susceptibility gene in linkage disequilibrium with DR3 could account for this, but systemic lupus and the sicca syndrome are not clinically associated with these disorders and it seems likely that separate susceptibility genes are involved. It is possible that different genes leading to a failure of immunoregulation by quite different mechanisms may be associated with DR3. One non-specific mechanism has been suggested by Legrand et al (1982), who found that the variation in the ability of macrophages from different individuals to degrade sensitised erythrocytes was related to DR type, i.e. DR3-positive macrophages tended to have a reduced ability to degrade under the conditions of the experiment.

Conclusions

Apart from a limited clinical application, especially in relation to the B27-related disorders and perhaps susceptibility to drug toxicity, the discovery of evidence for HLA-linked disease susceptibility genes is only of value in so far as it leads to a greater understanding of the pathogenesis of the disorders involved. Progress over the next few years will depend on further clarification of the polymorphisms involved, and especially those involving class II molecules. Even more important will be a greater insight into their function. However, such increased knowledge will only achieve its application when it is studied in conjunction with information regarding other factors involved in pathogenesis and perhaps especially bacterial and viral agents. Some of the HLA associations are likely to turn out to be of greater importance than others but there can be no doubt that their discovery has provided a great stimulus for future research studies.

OTHER GENETIC POLYMORPHISMS

It is very likely that other genetic loci can influence susceptibility to HLA-associated disorders. Two genetically linked polymorphisms have been investigated from this point of view.

Immunoglobulin allotypes

The structural loci of the genes for heavy chains, κ light chains and λ light chains are on chromosomes 14, 2 and 22 respectively. Localised differences in amino acid structure of the heavy chains of IgG molecules can be detected serologically and are inherited codominantly (the Gm groups). Allotypes also exist for the IgA heavy chains (Am) and for κ light chains (Km).

The antibody response to certain bacterial antigens has been shown to be dependent in some degree on immunoglobulin allotypes, e.g. the response to salmonella monomeric flagellin (Whittingham et al, 1980) and meningococcal group B polysaccharide (Pandey et al, 1981).

No clear associations with any rheumatic disorder have yet been established.

α1-antitrypsin allotypes

The structural locus for this enzyme is situated on chromosome 14. Electrophoretically separable variants of this enzyme have been shown to be inherited and constitute the Pi system. Some variants, especially Z and S, determine decreased enzyme concentrations, e.g. the MZ phenotype is associated with just over half the normal level. Evidence for an increased frequency of Z heterozygotes in patients with rheumatoid arthritis has been documented (Buisseret et al, 1977; Arnaud et al, 1979; Cox & Huber, 1980). Combining the data from these three studies with those from three others (Geddes et al, 1977; Sjöblom & Wollheim 1977; Blundell et al, 1980), gives a combined relative risk for Z heterozygotes of 1.75, $p = 0.00049$, p for heterogeneity $= 0.024$. There is some evidence for a weak association between the deficient phenotype and rheumatoid arthritis, although the different studies do not agree on this.

Arnaud et al (1977) reported an increased frequency of the MZ phenotype in patients with juvenile chronic arthritis.

Combining the data from two studies of ankylosing spondylitis (Buisseret et al, 1977; Brewerton et al, 1978), the combined risk for the MZ phenotype is 2.8, $p = 0.04$, i.e. considering that several phenotypes are studied, the association is not proven.

Acute anterior uveitis was found to be associated with the MZ genotype by Brewerton et al (1978), the relative risk being 8.4.

The function of the enzyme involved suggested that control is not likely to act in the early stages of the initiation of these various disorders but rather on the effects of the inflammatory process, deficient phenotypes being associated with a lesser degree of inhibition of collagenases and neutral proteases.

REFERENCES

Ahearn J M, Provost T T, Dorsch C A, Stevens M B, Bias W B, Arnett F C 1982 Inter-relationships of HLA-DR, MB and MT phenotypes, autoantibody expression and clinical features in systemic lupus erythematosus. Arthritis and Rheumatism 25: 1031–1040

Aho K, Ahvonen P, Lassus A, Sievers K, Tiilikainen A 1974 HLA 27 in reactive arthritis: A study of Yersinia arthritis and Reiter's disease. Arthritis and Rheumatism 17: 521–526

Alarçon G S, Koopman W J, Acton R T, Barger B O 1982 Seronegative rheumatoid arthritis. Arthritis and Rheumatism 28: 502–507

Allison J P, Walker L E, Russell W A, Pellegrino M A, Ferrone S, Reisfeld R D 1978 Murine Ia and human DR

antigens: homology of amino-terminal sequences. Proceedings of the National Academy of Science USA 75: 3953–3956
Armstrong R D, Panayi G S, Welsh K I 1983a Histocompatibility antigens in psoriasis, psoriatic arthropathy, and ankylosing spondylitis. Annals of the Rheumatic Diseases 42: 142–148
Armstrong R D, Behn A, Myles A, Panayi G, Welsh K I 1983b Histocompatibility antigens in polymyalgia rheumatica and giant cell arteritis. Journal of Rheumatology 10: 659–661
Arnaud P R, Galbraith R, Faulk N P, Ansell B M 1977 Increased frequency of the MZ phenotype of alpha-l-protease inhibitor in juvenile chronic arthritis. Journal of Clinical Investigation 6: 1442–1444
Arnaud P, Galbraith R M, Faulk W P, Black C, Hughes G R V 1979 $Alpha_1$-antitrypsin in adult rheumatoid arthritis. Lancet i: 1236–1237
Avakian H, Welsh J, Ebringer A, Entwistle C C 1980 Ankylosing Spondylitis, HLA-B27 and Klebsiella II. Cross-reactivity studies with human tissue typing sera. British Journal of Experimental Pathology 61: 92–96
Balogh Z, Gyodi E, Petranyi G, Meretey K, Vozsok S 1982 HLA-DR antigens in juvenile chronic arthritis. Journal of Rheumatology 9: 448–450
Barrier J, Bignon J D, Soulillou J P, Grolleau J 1981 Increased prevalence of HLA-DR4 in giant cell arteritis. New England Journal of Medicine 305: 104–105
Batchelor J R, Welsh K I, Tinoco R M, et al 1980 Hydralazine-induced systemic lupus erythematosus: influence of HLA-DR and sex on susceptibility. Lancet i: 1107–1109
Beaulieu A D, Roy R, Mathon G, et al 1982 Reappraisal of HLA antigen frequencies in psoriasis and psoriatic arthritis. Arthritis and Rheumatism 25 (Suppl): 133 (Abstract)
Beaulieu A D, Roy R, Mathon G, Morissette J, Latulippe L, Lang J-V, et al 1983 Psoriatic arthritis: risk factors for patients with psoriasis — a study based on histocompatibility antigen frequencies. Journal of Rheumatology 10: 4, 633–636
Benacerraf B, Katz D H 1975 The histocompatibility-linked immune response genes. Advances in Cancer Research 21: 121–173
Biddison W E 1982 The role of the human major histocompatibility complex in cytotoxic T-cell responses to virus infected cells. Journal of Clinical Immunology 2: 1–9
Black C M, Welsh K I, Fielder A, Hughes G R V, Batchelor J R 1982a HLA antigens and Bf allotypes in SLE: evidence for the association being with specific haplotypes. Tissue Antigens 19: 115–120
Black C M, Batchelor J R, Welsh K I, Hughes G R V 1982b A comparison of the HLA antigens in SLE and systemic sclerosis. Annals of the Rheumatic Diseases 41: 195–196 (Abstract)
Blundell G, Lockhart M, Boyd M W J, Merrett D, Cole R B 1980 $Alpha_1$ antitrypsin phenotypes in patients with rheumatoid arthritis: a comparison of phenotyping techniques. Irish Journal of Medical Science 149: 148–151
Bono M R, Strominger J L 1982 Direct evidence of homology between human DC-1 antigen and murine I-A molecules. Nature 299: 836–838
Breuning M H, Lucas C J, Breur B S 1982 Subtypes of HLA-B27 detected by cytotoxic T lymphocytes and their role in self recognition. Human Immunology 5: 259–268
Brewerton D A, Hart F D, Nicholls A, Caffrey M, James D C O, Sturrock R D 1973a Ankylosing spondylitis and HL-A27. Lancet i: 904–907
Brewerton D A, Nicholls A, Oates J K, Caffrey M, Walters D, James D C O 1973b Reiter's disease and HL-A27. Lancet ii: 996–998
Brewerton D A, Caffrey M, Nicholls A, Walters D, James D C O 1973c Acute anterior uveitis and HL-A 27. Lancet ii: 994–998
Brewerton D A, Nicholls A, Caffrey M, Walters D, James D C O 1974 HL-A27 and arthropathies associated with ulcerative colitis and psoriasis. Lancet i: 956–957
Brewerton D A, Webley M, Murphy A H, Ward A M 1978 The alpha l-antitrypsin phenotype MZ in acute anterior uveitis. Lancet i:1103
Buisseret P D, Pembrey M E, Lessof M H 1977 αl-antitrypsin phenotypes in rheumatoid arthritis and ankylosing spondylitis. Lancet ii: 1358–1359
Calin A, Marder A, Becks E, Burns T 1983 Genetic differences between B27 positive patients with ankylosing spondylitis and B27 positive healthy controls. Arthritis and Rheumatism 12: 1460–1464
Celada A, Barras C, Benzonana G, Jeannet M 1980 Increased frequency of HLA-DRw3 in systemic lupus erythematosus. Tissue Antigens 15: 282–288
Chamberlain M A 1977 Behçet's syndrome in 32 patients in Yorkshire. Annals of the Rheumatic Diseases 36: 491–499
Clemens L E, Albert E, Ansell B M 1983 HLA studies in IgM rheumatoid-factor-positive arthritis of childhood. Annals of the Rheumatic Diseases 42: 431–434
Coligan J E, Kindt T J, Uehara H, Martinko J, Nathenson S G 1981 Primary structure of a murine transplantation antigen. Nature 291: 35–39
Cox D A, Huber O 1980 Association of severe rheumatoid arthritis with heterozygosity for αl-antitrypsin deficiency. Clinical Genetics 17: 153–160
Demaine A G, Vaughan R W, Behn A R, Myles A B, Panayi G S, Welsh K I 1983 Immunoglobulin (Gm) allotype frequencies in patients with giant cell arteritis and polymyalgia rheumatica. Journal of Immunogenetics 10: 343–348
Dinant H J, Muller W H, Berg-Loonen E M, Nijenhuis L E, Engelfriet C P 1980 HLA-DRw4 in Felty's syndrome. Arthritis and Rheumatism 23:1336
Ebringer A, Cowling P, Ngwa Suh N ,James D C O, Ebringer R W 1976 Crossreactivity between Klebsiella aerogenes and B27 lymphocyte antigens as an aetiological factor in ankylosing spondylitis. In: Dausset J, Svejgaard A (eds) HLA and Disease. INSERM, Paris 58:27
Fielder A H L, Walport M J, Batchelor J R, Rynes R I, Black C M, Dodi I A, Hughes G R V 1983 Family study of the major histocompatibility complex in patients with systemic lupus erythematosus: importance of null alleles of C4A and C4B in determining disease susceptibility. British Medical Journal 286: 425–428
Finberg R, Benacerraf B 1981 Induction, control and consequences of virus specific cytotoxic T-cells. Immunological Reviews 58: 157–180
Fink C W, Stastny P 1980 Results of serologic HLA-DR typing in juvenile arthritis and adult rheumatoid arthritis. Arthritis and Rheumatism 23:673
Friis J, Svejgaard A 1974 Salmonella arthritis and HLA-A27. Lancet i:1350
Fye K H, Terasaki P I, Michalski J P, Daniels T E, Opelz G, Talal N 1978 Relationship of HLA-DW3 and HLA-B8

to Sjögren's syndrome. Arthritis and Rheumatism 21: 337–342
Garlepp M J, Dawkins R L, Christiansen F T 1983 HLA antigens and acetylcholine receptor antibodies in penicillamine induced myasthenia gravis. British Medical Journal 286: 338–340
Geddes D M, Webley M, Brewerton D A 1977 α1-antitrypsin phenotypes in fibrosing alveolitis and rheumatoid arthritis. Lancet ii: 1049–1050
Gladman D D, Keystone E C, Baron M, Lee P, Cane D, Mervert H 1981 Increased frequency of HLA-DR5 in scleroderma. Arthritis and Rheumatism 24: 854–856
Glass D, Raum D, Gibson D, Stillman J S, Schur P 1976 Inherited deficiency of the second complement component. Journal of Clinical Investigation 58: 853–866
Glass D, Litvin D, Wallace K, et al 1980 Early-onset pauciarticular juvenile rheumatoid arthritis associated with human leucocyte antigen-DRW5, iritis and antinuclear antibody. Journal of Clinical Investigation 66: 426–429
Gofton J, Chalmers A, Price G E, Reeve C 1975 HL-A27 and ankylosing spondylitis in B.C. Indians. Journal of Rheumatology 2: 314–318
Green J R, Woodrow J C 1977 Sibling method for detecting HLA-linked genes in disease. Tissue Antigens 9: 31–35
Grennan D M, Dyer P A, Clague R, Dodds W, Smeaton I, Harris R 1983 Family studies in RA — the importance of HLA-DR4 and of genes for autoimmune thyroid disease. Journal of Rheumatology 10: 584–589
Grumet F C 1983 Monoclonal antibodies to HLA-B27. British Journal of Rheumatology 22 (Suppl 2): 110–118
Haldane J B S 1955 The estimation and significance of the logarithm of a ratio of frequencies. Annals of Human Genetics 20: 309–311
Janossy G, Duke O, Poulter L W, Panayi G, Bofill M, Goldstein G 1981 Rheumatoid arthritis: A disease of T-lymphocyte/macrophage immunoregulation. Lancet ii: 839–842
Kallenberg C G M, Voort-Beelen J M, D'Amaro J, The T H 1981 Increased frequency of B8/DR3 in scleroderma and association of the haplotype with impaired cellular immune response. Clinical and Experimental Immunology 43: 478–485
Katz D H, Hamoaka T, Dorf M E, Benacerraf B 1973 Failure of physiologic co-operative interactions between T and B lymphocytes from allogeneic donor strains in humoral responses to haptan protein conjugates. Journal of Experimental Medicine 137: 1405–1408
Khan M A, Kushner I, Braun W E, Zachary A A, Steinberg A G 1978 HLA-B27 homozygosity in ankylosing spondylitis: relationship to risk and severity. Tissue Antigens 11: 434–438
Khan M A, Kushner I, Weitkamp L R 1983 Genetics of HLA associated disease: rheumatoid arthritis. Tissue Antigens 22: 182–185
Kidd K K, Bernoco D, Carbonara A O, Daneo V, Steiger U, Ceppellini R 1977 Genetic analysis of HLA-associated diseases: 'The illness-susceptible' gene frequency and sex ratio in ankylosing spondylitis. In: Dausset J, Svejgaard A (eds) HLA and disease. Munksgaard, Copenhagen, p 72–79
Klareskog L, Forsum U, Malmnäs Tjernlund U, Kabelitz D, Wigren A 1981 Appearance of anti-HLA-DR-reactive cells in normal and rheumatoid synovial tissue. Scandinavian Journal of Immunology 14: 183–192
Klareskog L, Forsum U, Kabelitz D, et al 1982 Immune functions of human synovial cells. Phenotypic and T cell regulatory properties of macrophage-like cells that express HLA-DR. Arthritis and Rheumatism 25: 488–501
Klein J 1978 H-2 mutations: their genetics and effect on immune functions. Advances in Immunology 26: 56–146
Klein J, Figueroa F 1981 Polymorphism of the Mouse H-2 loci. Immunological Reviews 60: 23–57
Legrand L, Rivat-Perran L, Hutton C, Dausset J 1982 HLA and Gm-linked genes affecting the degredation rate of antigens (sheep red blood cells) endocytosed by macrophages. Human Immunology 4: 1–13
Lehner T, Batchelor J R 1979 Classification and immunogenic basis of Behçet's syndrome. In: Lehner T, Barnes C G (eds)Behçet's syndrome. Academic Press, London, p 13–32
Leirisalo M, Skylv G, Kousa M, et al 1982 Follow-up study on patients with Reiter's disease and reactive arthritis, with special reference to HLA-B27. Arthritis and Rheumatism 25: 249–259
Lin Y-L, Askonas B A 1981 Biological properties of an influenza A virus-specific killer T-cell clone. Inhibition of virus replication *in vivo* and induction of delayed type hypersensitivity reactions. Journal of Experimental Medicine 154: 225–234
van der Linden S M, Valkenburg H A, Dejongh B M, Cats A 1984 The risk of developing ankylosing spondylitis in HLA-B27 positive individuals. Arthritis and Rheumatism 27: 241–249
Lochead J A, Chalmers I M, Marshall W H, Larsen B, Skanes V M, Payne R H, Barnard J M 1983 HLA-B27 haplotypes in family studies of ankylosing spondylitis. Arthritis and Rheumatism 26: 1011–1016
Lynch C J, Singh G, Whiteside T L, Rodnan G P, Medsger T A, Rabin B S 1982 Histocompatibility antigens in progressive systemic sclerosis (PSS: Scleroderma). Journal of Clinical Immunology 2: 314–318
McCluskey J, Kay P H, Dawkins R L, Komory K, Christiansen F T,McCann V J 1984 Association of specific MHC supratypes with rheumatoid arthritis and insulin-dependent diabetes mellitus. Disease Markers 1: 197–212
McKendry R J R, Sengar D P S, DesGroseilliers J P, Dunne J V 1984 Frequency of HLA antigens in patients with psoriasis or psoriatic arthritis. Canadian Medical Association Journal 130: 411–415
Morling N, Hellesen C, Jakobsen B K, et al 1981 HLA-A, B, C, D, DR antigens and primed lymphocyte typing (PLT) defined DP-antigens in juvenile chronic arthritis. Tissue Antigens 17: 434–441
Morton N E, Lalouel J M 1981 Resolution of linkage for irregular phenotype systems. Human Heredity 31: 3–7
Moutsopoulos H M, Mann D L, Johnson A H, Chused T M 1979 The genetic differences between primary and secondary sicca syndrome. New England Journal of Medicine 301: 761–763
Muftuoglu A U, Yazici H, Yurdakul S, Pazarli H, Ozyazgan Y, Tuzun Y 1981 Behçet's disease: Lack of correlation of clinical manifestations with HLA antigens. Tissue Antigens 17: 226–230
Nagy Z A, Baxevanis C N, Ishii N, Klein J 1981 Ia antigens as restriction molecules in Ir-gene controlled T-cell proliferation. Immunological Reviews 60: 59–83
Niks M, Rovensky J, Nyulassy S, Buc M, Stefanovic J, Zitnan D 1982 Lack of association of HLA-DR antigens with progressive systemic sclerosis (scleroderma). Tissue Antigens 17: 238–239

Nunez G, Moore S E, Ball G V, Hurd E R, Stastny P 1984 Study of HLA antigens in ten multiple-case rheumatoid arthritis families. Journal of Rheumatology 11: 129–135

O'Duffy J D, Taswell H F, Elveback L R 1976 HL-A antigens in Behçet's disease. Journal of Rheumatology 3: 1–3

Oldstone M B A, Dixon F J, Mitchell G F, McDevitt H O 1973 Histocompatibility-linked genetic control of disease susceptibility. Murine lymphocytic choriomeningitis virus infection. The Journal of Experimental Medicine 137: 1201–1212

Ono S, Nakayama E, Suigiur S, Itakura K, Aoki K, Aizaw M 1975 Specific histocompatibility antigens associated with Behçet's disease. American Journal of Ophthalmology 80: 636–641

Orr H T, Lopez de Castro J A, Pavham P, Ploegh H L, Strominger H L 1979 Comparison of amino acid sequences of two human histocompatibility antigens HLA-A2 and HLA-B7. Biochemistry 18: 5711–5715

Pachman L M, Maryjouski M C, Friedman J M, et al 1980 Immunogenetic studies of juvenile dermatomyositis; increased occurrence of HLA-B8, DRW3 and their relation to PM-1 and other autoantibodies. Arthritis and Rheumatism 23:728 (abstract)

Panayi G S, Wooley P, Batchelor J R 1978 Genetic basis of rheumatoid disease: HLA antigens, disease manifestations and toxic reactions to drugs. British Medical Journal 2: 1326–1328

Pandey J P, Zollinger W D, Fudenberg H H 1981 Immunoglobulin allotypes and immune response to meningococcal group B polysaccharide. Journal of Clinical Investigation 68: 1378–1380

Reinertsen J L, Klippel J H, Johnson A J, Steinberg A D, Decker J L, Mann D L 1978 B-lymphocyte alloantigens associated with systemic lupus erythematosus. New England Journal of Medicine 299: 515–518

Rose N R, Vladutiu A O,David C S, Shreffler D C 1973 Autoimmune murine thyroiditis V Genetic influence on the disease in BSVS and BRVR mice. Clinical and Experimental Immunology 15: 281–287

Rynes R I 1982 Inherited complement deficiency states and SLE. In: Hughes G R V (ed) Clinics in rheumatic diseases, Vol 8, No. 1. Saunders, Philadelphia, Ch 3, p 29

Sasazuki T, Nishimura Y, Muto M, Ohta N 1983 HLA-linked genes controlling immune response and disease susceptibility. Immunological Reviews 70: 51–75

Scherak O, Smolen J S, Mayr W R 1980 HLA-DRw3 and systemic lupus erythematosus. Arthritis and Rheumatism 23: 954–957

Schiff B, Mizrachi Y, Orgad S, Yaron M, Gazit E 1982 Association of HLA-Aw31 and HLA-DR1 with adult rheumatoid arthritis. Annals of the Rheumatic Diseases 41: 403–404

Schlosstein L, Terasaki P I, Bluestone R, Pearson C M 1973 High association of an HL-A antigen, W27 with ankylosing spondylitis. New England Journal of Medicine 288: 704–706

Schur P H, Meger I, Garovoy M, Carpenter C B 1982 Associations between systemic lupus erythematosus and the major histocompatibility complex: clinical and immunological considerations. Clinical Immunology and Immunopathology 24: 263–275

Schwarz R H, Yano A, Paul W E 1978 Interaction between antigen-presenting cells and T lymphocytes: an assessment of Ir gene expression in the antigen-presenting cell. Immunological Reviews 40: 153–180

Seager K, Bashir H V, Geczy A F, Edmonds J, De Vere-Tyndall A 1979 Evidence for a specific B27-associated cell surface marker on lymphocytes of patients with ankylosing spondylitis. Nature 277: 68–70

Shackelford D A, Kaufman J F, Korman A J, Strominger J L 1982 HLA-DR antigens; structure, separation of subpopulations, gene cloning and function. Transplantation Reviews 66: 133–187

Shaw S, Kavathas P, Pollack M S, Charmot D, Mawas C 1981 Family studies define a new histocompatibility locus, SB, between HLA-DR and GLO. Nature 293: 745–747

Silver J, Walker L E, Reisfeld R A, Pellegrino M A, Ferrone S 1979 Structural studies of murine I-E and human DR antigens. Molecular Immunology 1979 17: 37–42

Sjöblom K G, Wollheim F A 1977 Alpha$_1$ antitrypsin phenotypes and rheumatic diseases. Lancet ii: 41–42

Sonazaki H, Seki H, Chang S, Okuyama M, Juji T 1975 Human lymphocyte antigen HL-A27 in Japanese patients with ankylosing spondylitis. Tissue Antigens 5: 131–138

Stastny P 1978 Association of the B-cell alloantigen DRw4 with rheumatoid arthritis. New England Journal of Medicine 298: 869–871

Sucui-Foca N, Godfrey M, Jacobs J, et al 1980 Increased frequency of DRw5 in pauciarticular JRA. In: Terasaki P I (ed) Histocompatibility testing 1980. UCLA Tissue Typing Laboratory, Los Angeles, California, p 953

Tanigaki N, Tosi R 1982 The genetic control of human Ia alloantigens: a three-loci model derived from the immunochemical analysis of 'supertypic' specificities. Transplantation Reviews 66: 5–37

Terasaki P I, McClelland J D 1964 Microdroplet assay of human serum cytotoxins. Nature 204: 998–1000

Thomson G 1977 Effect of a selected locus on linked neutral loci. Genetics 85: 753–788

Thomson G 1983 Investigation of the mode of inheritance of the HLA associated diseases by the method of antigen genotype frequencies among diseased individuals. Tissue Antigens 21: 81–104

Thomson G, Bodmer W F 1977 The genetic analysis of HLA and disease associations. In: Dausset J, Svejgaard A (eds) HLA and disease. Munksgaard, Copenhagen, p 84–93

Whiteside T, Mulhern L, Buckingham R, Luksick J 1982 Procainamide-induced lupus (PLE) is associated with an increased frequency of HLA-DR-6Y. Arthritis and Rheumatism 25 (Suppl): 233 (Abstract)

Whittingham S, Mathews J D, Schanfield M S, et al 1980 Interactive effect of Gm allotypes and HLA-B locus antigens on the human antibody response to a bacterial antigen. Clinical and Experimental Immunology 40: 8–15

Williams R M, Moore M J 1973 Linkage of susceptibility to experimental allergic encephalomyelitis to the major histocompatibility locus in the rat. Journal of Experimental Medicine 138: 775–783

Woodrow J C 1977 Histocompatibility antigens and rheumatic diseases. Seminars in Arthritis and Rheumatism 6: 257–276

Woodrow J C, Eastmond C J 1978 HLA-B27 and the genetics of ankylosing spondylitis. Annals of the Rheumatic Diseases 37: 504–509

Woodrow J C, Treanor B, Usher N 1974 The HLA system in Reiter's syndrome. Tissue Antigens 4: 533–540

Woodrow J C, Mapstone R, Anderson J, Usher N 1975 HLA 27 and anterior uveitis. Tissue Antigens 6: 116–120

Woodrow J C, Nichol F E, Zaphiropoulos G 1981 DR

antigens and rheumatoid arthritis: A study of two populations. British Medical Journal 283: 1287–1288

Woodrow J C, Nichol F E, Whitehouse G H 1983 Genetic studies in ankylosing spondylitis. British Journal of Rheumatology 22 (Suppl 2): 12–17

Woolf B 1955 On estimating the variation between blood groups and disease. Annals of Human Genetics 19: 251–253

World Health Organisation Nomenclature Committee on Leucocyte Antigens 1980 Nomenclature for factors of the HLA system, 1980. Bulletin of the World Health Organisation 58: 945–948

Wright V, Moll J M H 1976 Seronegative polyarthritis. North Holland, Amsterdam

Yazici H, Chamberlain M A, Schreuder I, D'amaro J, Muftuoglu M 1980 HLA antigens in Behçet's disease: a reappraisal by a comparative study of Turkish and British patients. Annals of the Rheumatic Diseases 39: 344–353

Young C R, Ebringer A, Archer J R 1978 Immune response inversion after hyperimmunisation. Possible mechanism in the pathogenesis of HLA-linked diseases. Annals of the Rheumatic Diseases 37: 152–158

Zachariae H, Hjortshøj A, Kissmeyer-Nielsen F, Svejgaard A, Svejgaard E, Zachariae E 1974 HLA antigens and psoriatic arthritis. Acta Dermatovener 54: 443–447

Zilko P J, Dawkins R L 1982 Rheumatoid arthritis: Family studies in immunogenetics in rheumatology. Exerpta Medica, Amsterdam, p 142

Zinkernagel R M, Doherty P C 1974 Restriction of in vitro T-cell mediated cytotoxicity in lymphocytic choriomeningitis within a syngeneic or allogeneic system. Nature 248: 701–702

11

A.M. Denman

Immunological mechanisms and the rheumatic diseases

This chapter reviews the mechanisms by which immune reactions contribute to the inflammatory and degenerative processes characteristic of the rheumatic disorders. It especially considers the factors which determine the susceptibility of joints to immunopathological damage. The main emphasis also is on immunological factors which may predispose to persistent inflammation in diseases of unknown aetiology. A systematic description of immunological principles is not included since these are described in numerous elementary guides to immunology (for example, Roitt, 1983) and in more detailed texts (for example, Lachmann & Peters 1982). Immune reactions are defined as those wholly or partly determined by the specific recognition of antigens by cellular or humoral mechanisms. There are three general ways in which immune reactions may lead to persistent inflammation in joints and other tissues characteristically involved in inflammatory disorders associated with arthritis (Table 11.1).

Table 11.1 Immunopathological features of the rheumatic disorders — general explanations

1.	Provoked by persistent antigen (e.g. microbial or chemical)
2.	Perpetuated by defective regulation of conventional immune responses (including autoimmune disease)
3.	Primary proliferative disorders of lymphocytes or their precursor cells

Antigen persistence

The most logical immunological explanation for chronic arthritis is the persistence of antigen which continues to provoke an immune response. Many potential sources of persistent antigen have been postulated. Indeed widely differing yet identifiable antigens reproduce many of the clinical and laboratory features of the rheumatic diseases both in human disease and in appropriate laboratory models. Unfortunately the non-specific nature of these abnormalities largely accounts for the failure of detailed analyses of the immunopathological features in the rheumatic diseases to produce decisive evidence about their aetiology.

Acute arthritis and vasculitic lesions are observed in a variety of bacterial infections (see Ch. 14) and the clinical manifestations are attributable to antibody responses to antigen directly deposited at sites of inflammation or else deposited in the form of antigen–antibody complexes. Meningococcal infection is a pertinent example (Greenwood & Whittle, 1976). However, bacterial infections rarely provoke chronic arthritis and its immunopathological features except in the special circumstances of reactive arthritis in individuals with a clear-cut genetic predisposition. Nevertheless bacterial cell wall products induce a variety of inflammatory reactions including arthritis in experimental animals whose distribution largely depends on the species in question (Hadler & Granovetter, 1978). Rats and guinea-pigs are particularly susceptible to chronic, often relapsing, arthritis with granulomatous inflammation in the synovial membrane. These observations indicate that bacteria can provoke chronic arthritis in special circumstances some of which may be immunologically determined. The constituents of bacterial cell walls responsible for those reactions have received particular attention. Peptidoglycans are effective stimulants of chronic inflammation, because of their resistance to proteolytic digestion and hence their persistence in sites of deposition. Bacterial cell wall components including peptidoglycans induce the entire range of classical immune responses. In addition they stimulate the synthesis and release of degredative enzymes by macrophages either directly or indirectly through immunological pathways. Moreover different bacterial cell wall constituents act selectively on immune reactions thereby disrupting the mechanisms which control the intensity and duration of such responses (Schwab, 1983). For example, under different experimental conditions, staphylococcal peptidoglycans may act as adjuvants to increase immune reactions in general, may be immunosuppressive, or may non-specifically activate lymphocytes (Dziarski, 1979). There are many difficulties in extending such experimental observations to man. For example, streptococcal antigens have been identified in circulating immune complexes in patients with infective endocarditis indicating that the well-known abnormalities in subacute bacterial endocarditis such as immune complex nephritis, hypergammaglobulinaemia, and autoantibody production may be at least partly attributable to the dissemination of bacterial products (Inman et al, 1982). However, it has proved difficult to pin-point the extent to which conventional immune responses account for tissue damage in other post-streptococcal disorders. Thus there is only indirect evidence implicating immune responses to streptococci in the pathogenesis of rheumatic carditis. Conventional tests for implicating specific micro-organisms in the pathogenesis of disease depend on demonstrating increased immune responses to microbial antigens. Paradoxically the abnormality in host responses which allows a continued inflammatory response to persistent streptococcal antigens may lie in a reduced cellular immune response to extracellular streptococcal products (Gray et al, 1981). Indeed the chronic arthritis induced by unusual infections with micro-organisms such as *Mycoplasma pneumoniae* and *Ureaplasma* in patients with unequivocal immunodeficiency disorders emphasises that impaired rather than exaggerated responses to ubiquitous agents may predispose to antigen persistence (Asherson & Webster, 1980). Furthermore bacterial products may produce inflammatory reactions which do not involve immunological mediation. For example Chetty et al (1983) have described a polysaccharide of group A streptococci which itself directly produces inflammatory oedema.

Persistent virus infections have often been proposed as the source of antigens perpetuating chronic arthritis (Denman, 1983). Whilst there is little evidence implicating any specific virus in the pathogenesis of diseases such as rheumatoid arthritis, virus infections provoke a wide range of immunopathological abnormalities encountered in the rheumatic diseases. Moreover, a variety of mechanisms have been identified by which virus infections can evade elimination by the host immune response (Table 11.2). In conventional virus infections, new infectious virus particles are produced which can be detected by standard techniques. However many viruses persist in forms which do not lead to the destruction of the infected cell, do not release infectious virus, and can only be detected by more sophisticated techniques.

Table 11.2 Mechanisms of viral persistence

1. **Viral peculiarities**
   Defective, latent or non-cytopathic infection (inadequate host response)
   Mutation (host responses directed at irrelevant antigens)
   Viral genome incorporated into host genes (risk of transformation)
2. **Host cell peculiarities**
   Certain cell types prone to persistent infection (e.g. lymphocytes, macrophages, oligodendrocytes)
3. **Viral immunosuppression**
   Specific suppression of antiviral immunity
   Non-specific suppression of host defences (e.g. neutrophils)
4. **Immune responses favour viral persistence**
   Congenital or acquired immunodeficiency
   Humoral immunity interferes with T cell responses
   Humoral immunity blocks (modulates) expression of viral antigens

Only principle mechanisms included; for detailed references see Denman, 1983.

However such infections may still induce changes in the membrane of the infected cells, which attract an immune response. These immune reactions are directed either at viral antigens on the cell membrane or at host antigens whose expression is altered by virus infection. This distinction is important because, in the latter instance, the immune response is directed against antigens which are not components of the infecting virus particles. Persistent infection by hepatitis B virus provides a cogent example of a human virus infection whose immunopathological manifestations are largely determined by the interaction between the surface antigens of persistently infected hepatocytes and different arms of the immune response (Zuckerman, 1982). Moreover virus expression is itself influenced by host immune responses in that antigen may be modulated, that is deleted from the cell membrane by exposure to antibody. Thus in many persistent virus infections the variable expression of viral antigens accounts for the fluctuations in inflammatory activity.

The notion that relatively simple chemical compounds might initiate rheumatic disorders has been strengthened by the realisation that immunopathological abnormalities regarded as characteristic of these diseases are also encountered in individuals exposed to chemicals. For example vinyl chloride toxicity may be accompanied by polyclonal hypergammaglobulinaemia, circulating immune complexes, increased complement consumption, and disturbances in the relative numbers of blood lymphocyte populations (Ward et al, 1976). It is also evident that drugs can induce syndromes resembling spontaneous connective tissue disorders. Whilst the drug-induced disorders may be clinically distinguishable, their immunopathological features are often similar to those encountered in the idiopathic diseases. For example, it is simplest to assume that in drug-induced systemic lupus erythematosus the offending drug acts as a simple immunogen and that the immunopathological picture is determined by the resulting immune response. However other mechanisms are involved which need not necessarily involve specific immunological recognition. Thus the drug practolol, formerly used as a β-adrenergic blocking agent, induced both inflammatory lesions and immunological aberrations in susceptible individuals (Behan et al, 1976). The distribution of the lesions in the skin, sclerae, and pleuroperitoneal membranes suggested that these were provoked by the local deposition of the drug or unidentified metabolites. However there is little evidence to suggest that a specific immune reaction to the drug contributed to the inflammation reaction. These immunological abnormalities, similar to those encountered in vinyl chloride toxicity, remain unexplained.

A wide range of environmental agents therefore could plausibly provide the continued antigen stimuli which would account for the general immunological features of the rheumatic diseases.

Antigen persistence and joints

Antigen persistence would most satisfactorily account for chronic arthritis if it could be shown that antigens from various sources persist in joints or related structures. In experimental models of arthritis there is little evidence that antigen is preferentially trapped in joints. Chronic arthritis usually ensues only when animals systemically immunised with a given antigen are challenged by intra-articular injection of the same or a closely related antigen. The frequency with which infectious diseases of man are associated with acute arthritis raises the suspicion that there are mechanisms by which infectious agents or their products specifically localise to joints. The possibility that there are specific receptors for bacterial polysaccharides on various synovial cells analogous to those found on some epithelial cells has not yet been explored. Similarly, arthritis commonly accompanies acute virus infections and, conceivably, joint cells could carry specific virus receptors. Rubella virus, for example, grows in the cartilage cells of experimental animals and can be transmitted to this site transplacentally in rabbits, thereby establishing persistent infections in rabbits (London et al, 1970). However, there is little evidence that other viruses associated with acute arthritis replicate in joints and, indeed, synovial membrane cells grown as micro-organ cultures replicate common viruses poorly (Bacon, 1983). Alternatively antigens may reach the joints in the form of antigen–antibody complexes. Transient arthritis is a prominent feature of acute immune complex disease and it is presumed although not formally proven, that the complexes localise to synovial cells with receptors for the Fc portion of the antibody molecule or complement components bound to the complexes.

Antigen persistence has not been demonstrated in chronic arthritis except in the special circumstances of infection produced by readily identifiable agents, for example in tuberculous synovitis or in immunodeficiency disorders. However, it is possible that unidentified antigens could continually reach the joints in circulating immune complexes. In addition such antigens could persist in immune complexes trapped in articular cartilage (Jasin & Cooke, 1978).

Immunodeficiency and arthritis

Arthritis is encountered in patients with both X-linked and acquired hypogammaglobulinaemia. The arthritis usually affects large joints, often unilaterally, and tenosynovitis is a prominent feature. Symmetrical involvement of small joints resembling rheumatoid arthritis is unusual and, when it does occur in patients with this disorder, is likely to be a complication of hypersensitivity reactions to gammaglobulin treatment. From the practical point of view, the most important responsibility of the clinician is to institute stringent microbiological attempts to characterise the causative organisms. *Mycoplasma pneumoniae* (Johnston et al, 1983), *Ureaplasma urealyticum* (Webster et al, 1978) and *Mycoplasma salivarium* (So et al, 1983) have all been recovered from infected joint fluids. Conventional microbiological techniques may be unsuccessful and the possibility of unusual opportunistic infections must be borne in mind. The arthritis usually responds to immunoglobulin treatment in hitherto undiagnosed patients (Webster et al, 1976) or to vigorous antibiotic treatment; prolonged courses of parenteral tetracyline may be necessary.

From the theoretical point of view, the association of immunodeficiency and specific mycoplasma infection is interesting in illustrating the arthrotropic properties of this group of organisms, although the clinical picture is entirely distinct from that of classical rheumatoid arthritis. In contrast, polymyositis accompanying echo-virus infections in patients with hypogammaglobulinaemia has some features in common with the idiopathic disorder, strengthening the notion that similar infections may be more difficult to detect in individuals with intact immune systems (Webster, 1983).

Incomplete immunodeficiency syndromes have also been mooted as predisposing to rheumatic disorders; IgA deficiency is commonly invoked. Whilst there is a suspicion that IgA deficiency may be more common in patients with juvenile chronic polyarthritis (Barkley et al, 1979), there is no conclusive evidence to this effect.

The synovial membrane and persistent immune responses

In most forms of chronic arthritis the immunopathological events noted in the synovial membrane are consistent with a persistent immune response to unknown stimuli despite the failure to identify the hypothetical antigens. The main events in the generation of immune responses must first be reviewed concentrating on those mechanisms which are relevant to the pathogenesis of joint inflammation. In general terms immune reactions involve a series of reactions (Fig. 11.1). Antigens are concentrated on the surface of dendritic (accessory) cells (Fig. 11.2), which are particularly concentrated in lymphoid organs such as the spleen and lymph nodes and are also widely distributed throughout other tissues such as the skin (Nussenzweig et al, 1981). Whilst dendritic

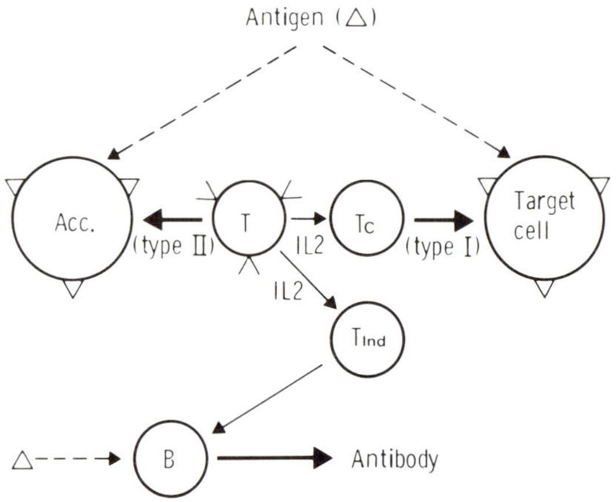

Fig. 11.1 Main events in the generation of specific immune responses. T = T lymphocyte (receptor for antigen); Tc = cytotoxic; TIND = inducer; B = B lymphocyte; IL2 = interleukin 2; Acc. = accessory cell; (Type I) = recognition controlled by class I HLA antigens; (Type II) = recognition controlled by class II HLA antigens.

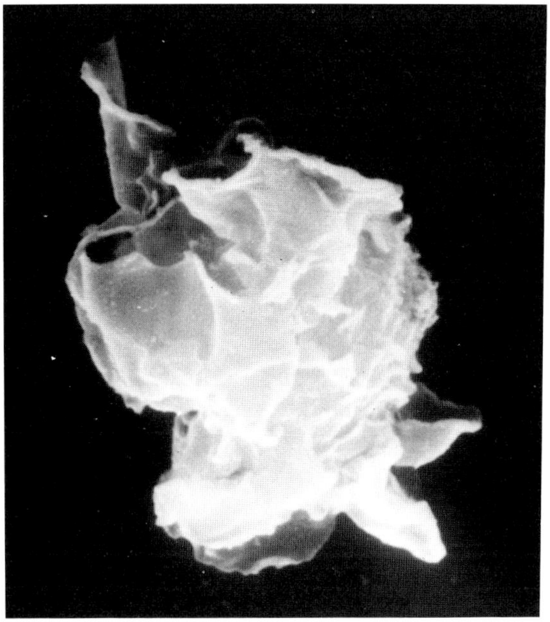

Fig. 11.2 Accessory cell seen by scanning electron microscopy showing the characteristic lacy cytoplasm ('veils'). Photograph by courtesy of Dr Brigid Balfour.

cells are for the most part specialised for this exclusive purpose it is important to note that other cells such as the endothelial cells lining blood vessels can also function in this manner (Ashida et al, 1981). The importance of antigen-presenting cells has been shown in a variety of immune reactions including the striking example of renal allograft rejection (Lechler & Batchelor, 1982). The accessory cells in the grafted organs are of critical importance in presenting alloantigens to the T lymphocytes of the recipient. Accessory cells are distinguished by the rich concentration of Ia antigens on their surface. These antigens synthesised under the direction of immune response (Ir) genes serve as recognition molecules which, in combination with antigen, provide signals for initiating specific immune responses. The extent to which accessory cells simply concentrate antigens on their surface or actively process antigens is unknown (Klinkert et al, 1982). The interaction between antigen and accessory cells generates soluble factors concerned in the generation of specific immune reactions, one of which has been characterised and identified as interleukin 1 (Rosenberg & Lipsky, 1981).

Antigens in combination with class 2 histocompatibility antigens induce several kinds of T lymphocyte response. Several experimental approaches suggest that T lymphocytes respond clonally to different antigens in a manner analogous to the clonal selection of antibody-synthesising cells. The most telling evidence for this view is the rapid development of techniques for selecting clones of T lymphocytes with specific patterns of antigen recognition and biological behaviour. The nature of the receptors on T cells has long been controversial (Matzinger, 1981). It is clear that T lymphocytes recognise foreign antigens in association with self-antigens but whether through a single receptor or different surface molecules is undecided. Until recently the chemical nature of the T cell receptors was also unknown and earlier views that these receptors are structurally analogous to immunoglobulin molecules have proved untenable (Jensenius & Williams, 1982). There is now strong evidence that T cell receptors consist of a novel disulphide — bridged dimer of 80–90 000 molecular weight linked to a glycoprotein of 20 000 molecular weight termed the 'T3 antigen' (Haskins et al, 1983). Once these molecules have been characterised, the genetic events conferring specificity on T cell clones should be analysable by the same methods that have helped to elucidate the generation of antibody diversity. There is good agreement that the interaction between antigens and T lymphocytes generate soluble factors which select the different functional populations of T cells involved in immune responses. These messengers are likely to contain sequences coded by Ir genes and are therefore also genetically controlled.

In vitro cloning techniques have confirmed the traditional view that three different populations of T lymphocytes are generated in response to antigenic challenge. These populations are not only functionally distinct but also release factors which mediate the same immune function as the cells producing them. Firstly, inducer T lymphocytes responding to a given antigen initiate the proliferation of other populations of T and B lymphocytes reactive with the same antigen. Human inducer T lymphocytes have been identified and characterised in a variety of in vitro experiments involving specific cell-mediated and antibody responses to antigens such as influenza virus and tetanus toxoid. T cells are also critical in determining the induction and suppression of immunoglobulin subclasses in response to antigens (Mongini et al, 1981).

Secondly, cytotoxic T lymphocytes destroy host cells bearing foreign antigens derived for example, from microbes, drugs or chemicals. Moreover cytotoxic T lymphocytes recognize antigens in association with class 1 histocompatibility antigens expressed on the surface of the target cells. The nature of this recognition is also controversial, although it appears most likely that separate surface receptors on cytotoxic T lymphocytes recognise self-antigen and foreign antigens independently. This dependence on recognising foreign antigens in association with self-antigens has been established in a variety of ways. For example, in vitro, cytotoxic T lymphocytes kill target cells infected with viruses such as influenza and Epstein–Barr (EB) efficiently if the effector and target cells carry the same class 1 HLA antigens; killing is less effective when these cells do not share HLA antigens. In vitro experiments of this kind have been confirmed by observations in human virus infections. Thus lymphocytes isolated from the blood and cerebrospinal fluid of children with mumps meningitis effectively killed autologous lymphocytes expressing mumps virus antigens but failed to destroy histoincompatible lymphocytes which were similarly infected (Kreth et al, 1982). The importance of this defence mechanism is attested by clinical situations in which defective killing of virus-infected cells by cytotoxic T lymphocytes predisposes to more severe or atypical infections in man. EB virus infects virtually all individuals and persists life-long in B lymphocytes but its reactivation is restricted by cytotoxic T lymphocytes (Wallace et al, 1982). Abnormal lymphoproliferative syndromes induced by EB virus are attributable to a variety of specific immune defects in handling the virus of which defective cytotoxic T cell killing is the most prominent (Harada et al, 1982). Indeed, it has been claimed that patients with rheumatoid arthritis have similar though less marked defects in controlling the proliferation of B lymphocytes induced by EB virus (Bardwick et al, 1980). Whilst cytotoxic T lymphocytes contribute to host defence by eliminating infected cells, this cytotoxicity may have immunopathological consequences if excessive numbers of host cells are destroyed. In animal models of virus infection the vigour of this response is genetically controlled. There are indication that these reactions are also genetically controlled in man raising the possibility that the immunopathological consequences of infections provoking cytotoxic T cell responses may vary in different individuals. The antigenic specificity of cytotoxic T cell responses also varies. Analysis of T cell clones shows that cytotoxic T cells often recognise a very restricted ranges of virus-coded antigens expressed on infected cells. However, there may also be extensive cross-reaction whereby, for example, cytotoxic T cells generated in response to earlier infection by one strain of influenza virus cross-react with group-specific antigens on target cells subsequently infected with a different strain of influenza virus (Reiss & Burakoff, 1981). Such considerations are important in predicting the pattern of cross-reactive cytotoxic responses induced by different antigens.

Finally, suppressor T lymphocytes inhibit the duration and magnitude of both humoral and cell-mediated immune responses. Their effects may be specific, exclusively inhibiting immune reactions to the provoking antigen or non-specific, affecting unrelated immune responses. Similarly the suppressor factors generated by suppressor cells may be specific or non-specific.

Suppressor T lymphocytes have been described and characterised in man following experimental in vitro immunisation with various antigens (Lehner, 1982). Supressor factors produced by human T cells are complex molecules with binding sites for the inducing antigen and determinannts coded by Ir genes (Lehner, 1983). However the precise composition of helper and suppressor factors produced in response to specific antigens awaits chemical and functional clarification (Zanders et al, 1983).

Humoral antibody is produced by B lymphocytes. These cells follow a series of differentiation steps which can be mapped in terms of their changing phenotype (Möller, 1981). This differentiation depends partly on exposure to antigen and partly on exposure to factors synthesised by inducer T lymphocytes. However, some antigens, referred to as T-independent antigens, stimulate B lymphocytes directly without the aid of antigen-specific inducer T lymphocytes. Whilst antigen induces the selective proliferation of B lymphocytes synthesising antibody reactive with that antigen, not all the immunoglobulin produced in response to antigen stimulation has this specificity. Indeed detailed studies of the antibody specificity of B lymphocytes responding to antigenic stimulation in experimental animals show that the immunoglobulin initially produced does not react with the stimulating antigen. Even in established antibody responses, the major part of the immunoglobulin synthesised by the responding B cells is polyclonal and does not react with the immunising antigen or has seemingly irrelevant specificities. Experimentally, antibodies of limited specificity are only produced after hyperimmunisation with highly purified antigens. The important mechanism governing this pattern of response may be that soluble factors produced by T lymphocytes in response to antigen stimulate not only the proliferation of B lymphocytes synthesising antibodies of the desired specificity but also other B cells. The most widely studied of these factors (formally termed 'lymphokines') is interleukin 2. This factor is produced by activated lymphocytes and promotes the proliferation of both T and B lymphocytes. It has been partly purified as a 16 000 molecular weight substance (Welte et al, 1982) and is produced by several different populations of lymphocytes (Luger et al, 1982). However its production is primarly stimulated by antigens presented in association with Ia antigens (Lattime et al, 1982).

B lymphocytes can also be non-specifically and directly stimulated by substances which do not function as conventional antigens but bypass the usual sequence of events for inducing B cell proliferation. Since the antibodies generally in this way combine with a wide range of antigens unrelated to the stimulating materials the latter are termed 'polyclonal activators'. Several substances possess this property including EB virus, many common human pathogenic bacteria, and bacterial lipopolysaccharides and proteins (Primi et al, 1977; Lipsky, 1980). Moreover, soluble bacterial antigens also trigger inducer T lymphocytes thereby providing additional pathways for the activation of B lymphocytes (Hank & Sondel, 1982). Factors generated during a variety of immune responses such as mixed lymphocyte reactions also stimulate B cells polyclonally (Chiorazzi et al, 1979). It is noteworthy that the active principle of bacterial peptidoglycans which induces adjuvant arthritis, namely N-acetylmuramyl-L-alanyl-D-isoglutamine, also stimulates B cells polyclonally during the induction of this disorder (Chang et al, 1981).

Non-specific host immunity

Host immunity also utilises many mechanisms which are non-specific in their actions and do not appear to depend on initial sensitization to specific antigens. Many of these mechanisms have been implicated in inflammatory arthritis. In particular natural killer (NK) cells destroy many tumour cells and cell lines in vitro without evidence of previous immunological sensitisation to the antigens carried by these cells. It is more likely that several different populations of effector cells possess this property rather than that NK cells are a separate category of mononuclear cells. For example, one cloned cell line with the cytotoxic properties of NK cells has been shown to possess the ultrastructure of basophils and to express IgE surface receptors, thereby indicating that basophilic granulocytes may function as NK cells (Galli et al, 1982). Mouse strains which are genetically deficient in NK cell activity show a low natural in vivo resistance to transplanted tumours or syngeneic leukaemias provoked by retroviruses or chemicals (Kärre et al, 1980). Cloned NK cells confer resistance to tumour induction and the ability to reject foreign bone marrow grafts on strains of mice which lack NK cells (Warner & Dennert, 1982). Observations of this kind demonstrate the in vivo relevance of NK cells whose cytotoxic properties were originally demonstrated entirely by in vitro systems. It is probable that NK cells detect minor changes in the pattern of membrane glycoproteins expressed by target cells and that they complement other cytotoxic mechanisms mediated by immunologically specific effector cells.

K cells are also a heterogenous population which react non-specifically with target cells sensitised by antibody bound to surface antigens.

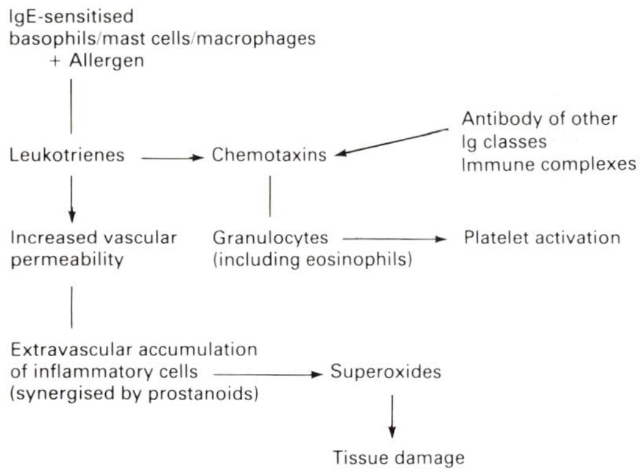

Fig. 11.3 Principal inflammatory pathways activated by immune responses.

Immune reactions generate several inflammatory reactions which may have pathological consequences (Fig. 11.3), further discussed in Chapter 9. Immediate hypersensitivity (type 1) reactions are generated by allergens combining with IgE antibody bound to mast cells and basophils. These cells release a family of peptidolipids termed 'leukotrienes', formally referred to as 'slow reacting substances'. Leukotrienes induce a variety of inflammatory reactions including vasoactive responses followed by increased vascular permeability and a change in the microenvironment of the extravascular space. These reactions generate chemotactic factors so that basophils and granulocytes accumulate in the extravascular space. The accumulating cells release proteolytic enzymes which damage tissues. In addition different oxidative products of arachidonic acid metabolism act synergistically to increase the local inflammatory response (Lewis & Austen, 1981). There is also evidence that leukotrienes are released from alveolar macrophages sensitised with IgE antibody and exposed to the relevant allergen (Rankin et al, 1982).

Immediate hypersensitivity reactions also stimulate granulocytes, notably eosinophils, to produce a potent factor which activates platelets thereby generating procoagulant activity. Antibody responses involving other immunoglobulin classes generate the same activity (Becker et al, 1981). Inflammatory cells attracted by any form of immune response may damage tissues through other mechanisms. Oxygen metabolites, termed 'superoxides', are generated by both granulocytes and monocytes after the phagocytosis of particulate material including that of microbial origin. These cells also generate superoxides during immediate hypersensitivity reactions, after ingesting immune complexes (Weiss & Ward, 1982), and after exposure to interleukins stimulated by antigens or non-specific mitogens (Nakagawara et al, 1982). Tissue damage results when superoxides are generated in excessive quantities or are inadequately neutralised by the appropriate enzyme systems.

In essence several forms of host defence operate in the extravascular space to degrade and eliminate foreign antigens. These may be activated non-specifically and therefore act as a rapid means of host defence in advance of those mechanisms which depend on immunologically specific reactions. These mechanisms are accompanied by intense local inflammation which is usually self-limited and therefore produces no life-lasting pathological consequences. Excessive tissue destruction results from the inappropriately prolonged activation of these mechanisms under circumstances which, for the most part, remain undefined. Whereas many major defects in complement inactivation have been precisely defined, few inhibitory pathways relating to other inflammatory mediators have yet been identified.

Several lines of evidence indicate that the synovial membrane is a site of intense immunological activity in chronic inflammatory disorders such as rheumatoid arthritis (Table 11.3). Detailed analysis of the rheumatoid synovial membrane has identified virtually all the main components of conventional immune reactions and their non-specific inflammatory consequences. The introduction of monoclonal antibodies has enabled investigators to classify the infiltrating mononuclear cells in terms of their phenotype and to reach some conclusions about their likely functional significance. Both cellular and humoral events have been analysed. T lymphocytes predominate among the mononuclear cells isolated from synovial effusions or eluted from the inflammatory membrane. This conclusion is based on methods for identifying surface receptors and reactivity with monoclonal antibodies specific for different cell populations. The function of the infiltrating cells has been partly deduced from studies comparing the characteristics of cells isolated from the joints with those obtained from the blood of the same patients. For

Table 11.3 Methods for characterising immunopathological events in persistent synovitis

Synovial effusion

Cells:
(i) Determine phenotype in terms of membrane antigens.
(ii) Predict function from above and assess this non-specifically (e.g. response to mitogens) or specifically (e.g. antigen presentation by accessory cells, autoantibody production by B cells).

Fluid
Assay for known inflammatory mediators (e.g. leukotrienes) *or* immunological mediators (e.g. immune complexes, interleukins).

Synovial membrane

Intact membrane
(i) Characterise cells and their products by electron microscopy, immunofluorescence–microscopy and immunochemical techniques in order to deduce the nature of the immunopathological response from the distribution and interrelationships of the infiltrating cells.
(ii) Measure specific function of micro-organ cultures (e.g. production of immunoglobulins).

Isolated cells
As for synovial effusion cells.

example, in one study, Fox et al (1982) compared the blood and effusion lymphocytes of patients with rheumatoid arthritis using a variety of monoclonal antibodies and concluded that the fluid contained a higher percentage of cells with the surface markers characteristic of inducer lymphocytes than the blood and that a significantly higher proportion of the effusion cells carried markers typical of activated T lymphocytes. These observations are in keeping with earlier morphological studies indicating that the perivascular infiltrates in rheumatoid synovial membranes are infiltrated with activated T cells (Ishikawa & Ziff, 1976). Accessory cells with readily detectable surface Ia antigen have also been identified in rheumatoid synovial effusions (Tyndall et al, 1983).

Histochemical techniques for characterising cells in tissue sections have enabled investigators to analyse the distribution of different mononuclear cells within the synovial membrane. Using the approach, Janossy et al (1981) and Konttinen et al (1981) have observed that the arterioles in rheumatoid synovial membranes are surrounded by a rich network of cells with the morphology and phenotype of accessory cells bearing a high surface concentration of Ia antigen. These cells are infiltrated with lymphocytes predominantly bearing the surface markers peculiar to inducer T lymphocytes. These features resemble those of the paracortical area of lymph nodes engaged in active immune responses but with an unusual predominance of lymphocytes with an inducer phenotype. Conversely, lymphocytes with the phenotype of suppressor cells are poorly represented. These observations are consistent with the notion that antigens concentrated on the surface of accessory cells in the synovial membrane attract an inducer cell population from the peripheral blood which in chronic synovitis is either continually recruited from this source or else is self-sustaining as the result of local proliferation.

However, current analyses largely depend on monoclonal antibodies for classifying the infiltration cells and it is commonly assumed that there is a constant relationship between phenotype and function. In reality there is often a poor correlation between the phenotype of freshly isolated lymphocytes or cloned T cell lines in vitro and their functional properties. Furthermore, immunological reactions themselves influence the pattern of antigens expressed by the target cells. Thus the epidermal cells and gut epithelial cells in animals with graft-versus-host disease express Ia antigens as a result of the immunological assault (Barclay & Mason, 1982). The possible contribution of non-specific cellular mechanisms is raised by the detection of NK cells in rheumatoid synovial fluid and in the inflamed membrane (Silver et al, 1982).

Lymphocytes and mature plasma cells contribute to the cellular infiltration in chronic arthritis. This is attested by morphological investigations using conventional light microscopic and ultrastructural techniques. Moreover the rheumatoid synovial membrane synthesises immunoglobulin of all the major classes in quantities comparable with those produced by conventional lymph nodes (Smiley et al, 1968). This immunoglobulin is polyclonal in terms of conventional immunochemical markers. The only specificity of locally synthesised antibody which has been convincingly shown is rheumatoid factor. No other specificities have been detected in terms of antibody eluted from synovial membranes or synthesised in vitro by tissues fragments or isolated cells from inflammatory synovial membranes. The juxtaposition of activated T cells and immunoglobulin-synthesising cells has encouraged speculation that immunoglobulin is synthesised by foci of intermingled inducer T cells and B cells. Another important consideration concerns the distinction between inflammatory events in the synovial membrane in general and those confined to the invading pannus responsible for cartilage erosion. Whilst inflammatory cells surrounding proliferating small blood vessels are prominent in areas of cartilage lysis (Kobayashi & Ziff, 1975), immunoglobulin is not detectable at these sites (Shiozawa et al, 1980). Indeed the cells in the pannus have the ultrastructural features of macrophages and fibroblasts rather than lymphocytes (Kobayashi & Ziff, 1975), emphasising the importance of correlating immunological studies with the histological organisation of the inflammatory lesions. The infiltration of cartilage by cells of this kind may however be provoked by the deposition of immune complexes in cartilage whether synthesised in the synovial membrane or filtered from the vascular compartment.

In keeping with the infiltration of the rheumatoid synovial membrane by cells engaged in immune responses, soluble factors concerned with mediating various forms of immune and inflammatory response have been detected in the synovial fluid and membrane. In terms of immediate hypersensitivity responses, prostaglandins, and particularly prostaglandin PGE 2, have been detected in rheumatoid synovial membrane, and immunoelectronmicroscopic observations suggest that the latter is synthesised by local macrophages (Shiozawa et al, 1982). A systematic search for other leukotrienes has not yet been reported but such mediators are being increasingly found in other pathological situations in which the sparse infiltration with basophils or eosinophils at first sight made it unlikely that such mediators would be detected. Indeed there are already indications that leukotrienes may contribute to inflammatory events in chronic arthritis (Klickstein et al, 1980). Complement activation by both the classical and alternative pathways is an accepted feature of chronic synovitis, but immune complex formation is tacitly assumed to be mainly responsible. In relation to cellular infiltration, both interleukin 1 (Fontana et al, 1982) and interleukin 2 activity (Wilkins et al, 1983) have been reportedly detected in rheumatoid synovial effusion fluid. Interferons are also produced by the infiltrating cells. Such activity is scarcely surprising in sites of intense cellular reactions. The extent to which soluble factors are responsible for perpetuating these reactions has not been elucidated and awaits the application of the more precise assays which are now becoming available.

There are several immunopathological mechanisms which could account for the characteristic erosive changes of persistent inflammatory arthritis. Prostaglandins synthesised in response to acute inflammatory mediators or interleukins are one obvious pathway to bone reabsorption (Bockman & Repo, 1981). Similarly prostaglandins in inflammatory synovial fluids could initiate the breakdown of proteoglycans in articular cartilage (Jones et al, 1982). There is both biochemical and ultrastructural evidence to suggest that proteolytic enzymes secreted by granulocytes and macrophages contribute to the degradation of collagen and proteoglycans in the cartilage matrix (Kimura et al, 1977). Cartilage breakdown has also been attributed to the activation of chondrocytes in response to a low molecular weight material, termed 'catabolin', synthesised by the synovial membrane (Dingle, 1980). Recent evidence suggests that catabolin may be synthesised by monocytes in the synovial membrane in response to interleukins (Jasin & Dingle, 1981). There are also extensive observations indicating that interleukins stimulate monocytes to release collagenase which also contributes to cartilage degradation (Krane et al, 1982). Fibroblasts derived from human synovial membrane have also been shown to synthesise plasminogen activator (Hamilton et al, 1981) indicating a pathway which could account for the prominent fibrin deposition on the surface of the articular cartilage noted in inflammatory arthritis. In addition both the normal and rheumatoid synovial membrane produce factors which stimulate the production of plasminogen activator by chondrocytes (Meats et al, 1980).

These observations are compatible with the idea that the synovial membrane is the site of a persistent immune response to an unknown antigen. However there are more reservations about the notion that in chronic arthritis, the synovial membrane functions as ectopic lymphoid tissue. In particular there is no evidence that exogenous antigens regularly localise to joints whether by the blood stream or via lymphatics. Indeed such evidence that has been adduced suggests that the synovial membrane does not respond to systemic antigenic challenge (Herman et al, 1971). In addition, whilst it is assumed that the relative enrichment of the synovial membrane for a given lymphocyte subpopulation at the expense of the blood implies that this population has homed selectively to the synovial membrane, there is a dearth of reliable information concerning the traffic patterns of lymphocytes between the blood and joints. Such data as are available are largely invalidated by reliance on isotopes which elute from the surface of the labelled cells after infusion.

Table 11.4 Regulation of immune responses — main mechanisms

Cell-mediated
a. Antigen-specific suppressor T lymphocytes
b. T cell suppressor factors — Antigen-specific — antigen non-specific
c. T cell control of antibody class expression (e.g. IgM→IgG 'switch')
d. Monocyte macrophages
Humoral
a. Anti-idiotype antibody
b. Antibodies recognising immunoglobulin allotypes or class determinants

Immunoregulation and chronic arthritis

Exogenous antigens have not been identified in the majority of chronic rheumatic disorders characterised by persistent immunopathological responses in the joints or other affected tissues. This failure has prompted speculation that the persisting inflammation arises from a defect in the control of conventional immune responses. Such defects would allow immune reactions which are normally ephemeral to be potentiated after the initiating antigen had been eliminated. Alternatively, conventional immune responses against exogenous antigens could be potentiated as autoimmune reactions.

Several important control mechanisms have been identified which limit the magnitude and duration of immune responses against the entire range of specific cell-mediated and humoral immune responses (Table 11.4). Indeed, even non-specific immune mechanisms are subject to feedback inhibition; thus lymphocyte subpopulations have been described which limit the activity of NK cells (DeBoer et al, 1981). An important mechanism involved in the control of humoral immunity is the production of antibodies reactive with the novel sequences or idiotypes displayed by antibodies synthesised in response to antigenic challenge. The idiotypes in the V region of both the heavy and light chains of antibody molecules not only determine the specificity of those antibodies but also serve as new antigenic determinants which in turn stimulate a fresh antibody response to those determinants (Cazenave, 1981) (Fig. 11.4). Different anti-idiotypic antibodies stimulate or inhibit the further secretion of antibodies of the appropriate specificity. Inhibitory anti-idiotypic antibodies react with surface receptors on B lymphocytes which inactivate the genes coding for specific antibody synthesis. These conclusions are based partly on animal experiments but also on observations in man. For example, anti-idiotypic antibody has been demonstrated during the normal human immune response to tetanus toxoid antigen (Geha, 1982). This regulatory mechanism has received close attention in the context of the rheumatic diseases.

Suppressor cell function in man has been most commonly assessed by counting the number of cells in blood and inflammatory lesions with the phenotype considered characteristic of suppressor cells. Judged by this criterion defects in suppressor T cell activity have been linked to the pathogenesis of such disorders as the hyperimmunoglobulin E syndrome (Geha et al, 1981) and insulin-dependent diabetes mellitus (Horita et al, 1982). Conversely, in patients with multiple sclerosis

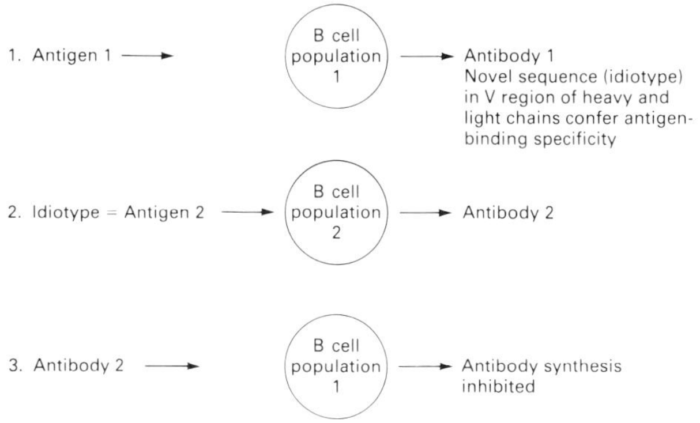

Fig. 11.4 Regulation of antibody production by anti-idiotype antibody.

suppressor lymphocytes with the phenotype of activated suppressor cells circulate in increased numbers during periods of remission prompting the speculation that phases of active diseases are associated with impaired suppressor cell function (Huddlestone & Oldstone, 1982). Cells with the phenotype of putative suppressor cells can also be detected in lymphocytic infiltrations by histochemical techniques employing monoclonal antibodies. Caveats about attributing functions to mononuclear cells on the basis of surface markers must again be stressed. Functional tests for suppressor activity have also been devised using systems in which blood lymphocytes stimulated with concanavalin A or soluble factors secreted by these cells are tested for their ability to suppress indicator immune reactions mediated by blood lymphocytes from the same donors in response to stimuli such as allogeneic lymphocytes (mixed lymphocyte reactions). However the results of these assays are unreliable because they do not take into account the likelihood that assays based upon the interactions of different lymphocyte populations proliferating in vitro may show mutual inhibition because of the constraints of in vitro culture rather than reflecting true in vivo suppressor functions (Farrant & Newton, 1981). Thus claims that such assays can detect abnormalities of T cell regulation in such diseases as SLE must be regarded with suspicion. Furthermore, abnormalities of the kind detected in SLE have also been observed in patients with the inflammatory disorder Henoch–Schönlein purpura, a disease in which the idea of suppressor T cell defects has not been seriously advocated (Beale et al, 1982). There is no convincing evidence for defects of suppressor T cell function in diseases such as rheumatoid arthritis judged by assays of blood lymphocytes. The increasing sophistication of techniques for inducing in vitro antibody responses to both exogenous and autoantigens offers the opportunity of testing suppressor T cell function more rigidly than has been possible with non-specific mitogens.

The apparent excess of inducer over suppressor lymphocytes in the rheumatoid synovial membrane has prompted speculation that persistent synovitis may result from a self-perpetuating inflammatory reaction which escapes feedback inhibition by suppressor T cells (Janossy et al, 1981; Klareskog et al, 1982). Nevertheless there are still reservations about accepting this interpretation. There have been few systematic reports of immunological events in a wide range of acute and chronic joint disorders of the kind carried out with classical histological techniques by Goldenberg & Cohen (1978). Thus it is still possible that the changes regarded as characteristic of rheumatoid arthritis are induced in any reaction in the joint regardless of its cause or natural history. In addition, inflammatory reactions may non-specifically influence the behaviour of lymphocytes in the lesions; for example, activated complement component C5a induces interleukin 1 by binding to macrophage receptors (Goodman et al, 1982) and could thereby be expected to provoke lymphoproliferative activity. Thus the grounds for attributing persistent synovitis to defects in the regulation of immune responses are still potentially tautological; the events described in this reaction may represent effects rather than causes.

Autoimmune reactions

Immune recognition of self-antigens and even reactions against such antigens are an integral part of the immune response to foreign antigens. This concept contrasts sharply with the classical view that autoimmune reactions are suppressed by climinating lymphocytes with this propensity. Several steps in the induction and execution of immune responses involve obligatory self-recognition (Fig. 11.5). Thus, since T lymphocytes recognise foreign antigens in association with self-antigens it is not surprising that T cell immunity to self-antigens arises transiently in the course of many common virus infections (Denman, 1981). There are three main problems in attempting to relate autoimmunity to the pathogenesis of the rheumatic diseases. The first is to identify the autoantigens which may be targets for persistent immune reactions. The second is to explain the circumstances under which such reactions acquire immunopathological significance and do not merely represent transient serological abnormalities. Finally the extent to which autoimmune reactions might account for the disease features of chronic rheumatic disorders must be elucidated.

Exogenous antigens provoke a wide range of autoimmune reactions to cross-reacting self-antigens. It is apparent, for example, that T lymphocytes sensitised to viral antigens commonly express a much wider range of antigen reactivity. Thus cloned cytotoxic T lymphocytes reactive with target cells infected with influenza virus also kill target cells bearing foreign histocompatibility antigens (Braciale et al, 1981). Moreover the introduction of monoclonal antibodies has increased the number of such reactions which have been recognised. Indeed this approach has revealed antigenic similarities in different cells and tissues whose existence had not hitherto been appreciated. For example, monoclonal antibodies against human T lymphocytes react with Purkinje cells in the central nervous system (Garson et al, 1982). Similarly common antigenic determinants have been detected in suppressor T lymphocytes and oligodendrocytes (Oger et al, 1982). Certainly there is the possibility that hitherto unsuspected autoantibodies may explain otherwise inexplicable disease features associated with autoimune diseases. For example, the exopthalmos of autoimmune thyroiditis has been linked to the presence of a circulating autoantibody reactive with a soluble antigen isolated from the muscles which control eye movements (Kodama et al, 1982). Some cross-reactions observed in experimental models give illuminating

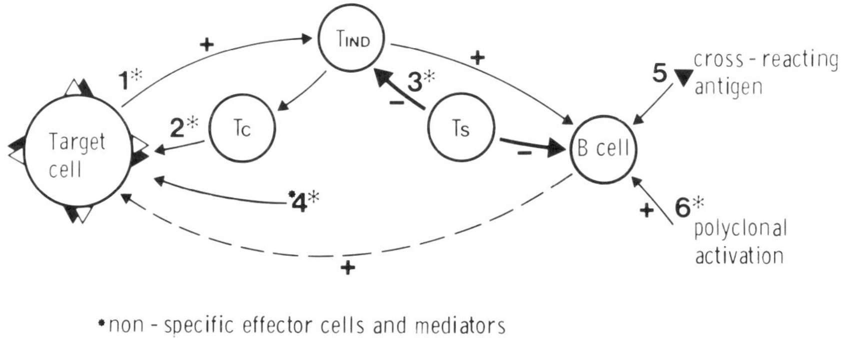

Fig. 11.5 This simplified diagram illustrates that autoimmune reactivity is inescapable in generating conventional immune responses. The numbers indicate the stages at which there is a risk of potentiating autoimmune diseases and the asterisks indicate which of these stages are genetically controlled:

1. Recognition of foreign antigens (▲) thereby priming autoreactive inducer T cells (T_{IND}).
2. Cytotoxic T cell (Tc) reactions against foreign antigens in association with self-antigens.
3. Feedback inhibition mediated by, for example, suppressor T cells (Ts) normally limits the proliferation of autoreactive T and B cells.
4. Cell-mediated immune responses are only in part mediated by specifically sensitised cells. Non-specific populations (e.g. monocyte-macrophages) and mediators (e.g. interferons) also contribute to such reactions.
5. Foreign antigens cross-reactive with self-antigens may elicit autoimmune responses.
6. The repertoire of antibodies elicited by polyclonal B cell stimuli may include self-antigens.

Genetic factors control the initiation, the briskness and the regulation of immune responses at the points indicated.*

insights into the manner in which the autoantibodies encountered in human connective tissue diseases may be generated. Mice immunised with various strains of cocci produce autoantibodies reactive with immunoglobulin determinants and also with a membrane glycoprotein common to lymphocytes and the immunising micro-organisms (Grooten et al, 1980). This model illustrates how such cross-reactions could account for the appearance of autoantibodies reactive with immunoglobulins and specific lymphocyte subpopulations in human disease. Furthermore there is evidence that the seemingly vast range of autoantigens to which patients with rheumatic diseases produce antibodies may in reality reflect autoimmunity against a limited range of antigenic determinants. This change in emphasis follows the introduction of techniques for analysing the specificity of autoantibodies produced by single clones of B lymphocytes immortalised by fusion with myeloma cell lines. Experiments in mice with genetically determined autoimmune diseases resembling human SLE have shown that the autoantibodies characteristic of these strains react with a common phosphodiester bond present in phospholipids in a variety of tissues (Lafer et al, 1981). Applying the same technique to human disease, Shoenfeld et al (1982) have shown that hybridomas derived from the B lymphocytes of patients with SLE produce antibody against the same phosphodiester bond found in a variety of tissues including nucleic acids. Thus the apparently diverse range of autoantibodies judged by conventional techniques which are encountered in this disorder may also be directed against a range of tissue antigens (Shoenfeld et al, 1983). Such observations make it more plausible that the autoantibodies found in the rheumatic diseases could arise as the result of cross-reaction between exogenous antigens, whether microbial or otherwise, and a relatively limited number of autoantigens.

B cells normally have the capacity to react with a wide repertoire of self-antigens and it is arguable that these cells can potentially respond as well to determinants on self-antigens as to those carried by foreign antigens. Indeed a small number of cells synthesising autoantibodies are detectable in normal individuals. Autoantibody production is sustained in a number of circumstances which abrogate the usual restrictions on this process (Allison, 1977). For example, whilst T lymphocytes normally recognise viral antigens and simple haptens in association with self-antigens expressed on cell surfaces, infections may increase the immunogenicity of membrane antigens which would otherwise elicit a weak immune response. This has been shown experimentally using target cells infected with viruses such as herpes simplex, Newcastle disease, or vaccinia virus (Bromberg et al, 1982). The important observation that T lymphocytes from patients with rheumatoid arthritis are sensitised to determinants on the light chains and Fab fragments of the heavy chains of IgG (Radoiu et al, 1982), encourages the view that the production of rheumatoid factors by B cells could be initated by unusual patterns of T cell recognition.

Polyclonal activation of B cells also accounts for many autoimmune disorders. For example, many bacterial infections produce polyclonal hypergammaglobulinaemia in which the gammaglobulin lacks any obvious antigen specificities. Nevertheless, the range of antibodies induced by polyclonal activators of B lymphocytes may include autoantibodies of varying specificities. For example, spleen cells cultured from normal strains of mice as well as those predisposed to autoimmune disease synthesise antibodies to double-stranded DNA after stimulation with the polyclonal stimulant *E. coli* lipopolysaccharide (Fish & Ziff, 1982).

In a clinical context some septicaemic illnesses provoke polyclonal hypergammaglobulinaemia which appears to be mainly non-specific but some of the IgG reacts specifically with platelet antigens resulting in thrombocytopenia (Kelton et al, 1979). The most telling clinical example of autoantibodies provoked by a polyclonal stimulating agent is EB virus infection; infectious mononucleosis is commonly associated with short-lived autoantibody production to a wide range of autoantigens and occasionally with overt autoimmune disease.

The transition from ephemeral to persistent autoimmune disorders needs further explanation and it is reasonable to invoke errors in immunoregulation and particularly those which may be genetically determined. The well-known influence of genetic factors in the induction of autoimmune disorders is also evident in this context. Thus the experimental arthritis induced by immunisation with collagen is dependent on B cell sensitisation (Klareskog et al, 1983) suggesting that B cell proliferation in response to this antigen is induced by the same general mechanisms that underlie many other forms of organ-specific autoimmune disease. Susceptibility to this disease is controlled by antigens linked to the major histocompatibility complex in a manner reminiscent of other autoimmune diseases induced experimentally by immunisation with organ-specific antigen and an appropriate adjuvant (Wooley et al, 1981). Conversely, genetic resistance to the induction of autoimmune disease by this kind of manoeuvre has been observed in other forms of experimentally induced autoimmune disease, notably experimental allergic encephalomyelitis (Waxman et al, 1981).

In some experimental models there is defective suppression of immune responses in general. Thus, whereas the conventional immune responses of normal mouse strains can be suppressed by passively administering antibody of the necessary specificity, similar reactions in mouse strains predisposed to autoimmune disease are not suppressible (Cowdery & Steinberg, 1982). Again crippling the suppressor mechanisms of normal mice by neonatal thymectomy enhances the induction of precipitating anti-DNA antibodies by the adjuvant Poly I Poly C (Smith et al, 1982). More specifically the lack of anti-idiotypic antibodies specifically reactive with autoantibodies may allow autoimmune reactions to persist. Whereas autoantibodies to red cells are common in NZB mice, anti-idiotypic antibodies to these autoantibodies prevent this complication in F1 hybrid of the same strain (Cohen & Eisenberg, 1982). In man there are indications that patients with diseases associated with autoantibody formation are defective in producing anti-idiotypic antibodies to those autoantibodies. Thus patients with active SLE lack anti-idiotypic antibody to antinuclear autoantibodies, whereas both patients with inactive disease and their unaffected family members possess these regulatory antibodies (Abdou et al, 1981). Similarly, it has been claimed that inflammatory uveitis associated with autoimmune reactions to retinal antigens is more severe in those patients who lack anti-idiotype antibodies to antiretinal antibodies (Dumonde et al, 1982); these authors propose that the circulating immune complexes in such patients consist of antiretinal antibodies and anti-idiotypic antibodies. However, anti-idiotypic antibodies may enhance as well as suppress antibody responses, particularly when the interacting antibodies are highly heteregeneous (Pollok et al, 1982). Furthermore patients with myasthenia gravis who carry autoantibodies reactive with the receptor for acetylcholine also possess naturally occurring anti-idiotypic antibodies to the anti-receptor antibodies without any obvious evidence that these modify the natural history of the disorder (Dwyer et al, 1983). These interactions need further analysis.

The regulation of immune responses by soluble factors may also be disordered in autoimmune disease. Since the proliferation of lymphocytes in response to specific antigens is partly regulated by soluble factors, theoretically either the defective production of such factors or inadequate responses could lead to autoimmune disorders. Spontaneous autoimmune diseases of mice have provided the opportunity for exploring this idea and there are indications that both the production of interleukin 2 and the responsiveness of lymphocytes to this mediator are defective in these murine models (Altman et al, 1981). Interestingly, the synthesis of interleukin 2 may be defective in ageing mice, raising the possibility that the propensity for autoimmune diseases to develop with age even in normal strains may result from similar defects (Thoman & Weigle, 1982). If soluble suppressor factors are important in limiting the extent of B cell activation (Fleisher et al, 1981) it is reasonable to suggest that deficiency of such mediators could account for the polyclonal B cell activation noted systemically in diseases such as SLE and locally in rheumatoid arthritis (Fauci & Moutsopoulos, 1981). Moreover, the observation that patients with SLE develop autoantibodies to the immunoregulatory molecule gamma-interferon (Panem et al, 1982) poses additional problems, since such autoantibodies could themselves interrupt normal regulatory pathways of this kind (Fleisher et al, 1982). Data of this kind are still fragmentary, but emphasise the need to take the products of several different lymphocyte subpopulations into account when analysing immune regulation in the rheumatic diseases. Given the increase in polyclonal B cell proliferation characteristic of many inflammatory rheumatic diseases, it is particularly difficult to determine when autoimmune reactions against a given tissue antigen are clinically or pathogenetically important. In clinical situations, the relationship between autoantibody production and disease manifestations is reasonably clear; for example platelets coated with autoantibody are readily removed by the Fc moiety of immunoglobulin binding to receptors on monocytes and macrophages. However, the association of autoantibodies with the rheumatic diseases need not necessarily have any pathogenetic significance. For example, autoimmunity to collagen has been advocated as an important immunopathological mechanism in rheumatoid arthritis and inflamatory arthritis can be induced in experimental animals by immunisation with type 2 collagen. It is attractive, therefore, to postulate that autoimmunity to collagen accounts for the persistence of inflammatory synovitis in man not only in rheumatoid arthritis, but also in other forms of inflammatory arthritis (Trentham et al, 1981). Nevertheless, there is no direct evidence that this form of autoimmunity directly contributes to the inflammatory process.

Difficulties in accepting the immunopathological significance of autoantibodies often arise from the poor correlation between disease manifestations and autoantibodies judged by standard assays. However, autoantibodies may only assume pathological significance under certain circumstances. For example, there is a generally poor correlation between the presence of rheumatoid factor as generally determined and the severity of rheumatoid arthritis in terms of its articular and extra-articular manifestations. However, high serum concentrations of rheumatoid factor in the form of low molecular weight IgM are associated with severe or active disease and also with rheumatoid vasculitis (Roberts-Thomas et al, 1981). It has been proposed that complexes between IgG and this form of IgM produces small circulating immune complexes which circulate for prolonged periods and are deposited in the tissues over a long timespan. The nature of the immune complexes formed between autoantigens and autoantibodies determine the pattern of inflammatory reactions and the sites of deposition. The ease with which immune complexes can be solubilised and removed by monocyte-macrophages also has a bearing on the pathological consequences of their circulation; thus the immune complexes formed in infectious mononucleosis are readily solubilised by autologous serum and cause only transient clinical features whereas those formed in SLE resist solubilisation (Charlesworth et al, 1982).

Immunoproliferative disorders and the rheumatic diseases

There has long been a hypothesis that unequivocally autoimmune diseases such as pernicious anaemia and disorders of unknown aetiology such as rheumatoid arthritis are primary immunoproliferative diseases in which the abnormal lymphocytes are autoreactive. Historically this process has been considered to arise from mutations in lymphocytes or their progenitor stem cells. The subsequent proliferation of these autoreactive clones has been attribute to the failure of the thymus or other selective processes to eliminate them (Burnet, 1959).

Recent advances in understanding the molecular basis of antibody synthesis (Nisonoff, 1982; Tonegawa, 1983) have confirmed that there are numerous possibilities for error in this process. However, the original theory must be modified by the realisation that mutation is an essential part of generating antibody diversity; it is the abnormal recombination of transforming genes and immunoglobulin genes which predisposes to uncontrolled lymphocyte proliferation.

The stages in antibody synthesis are outlined in Figure 11.6. The antibody molecule consists of a variable (V) region responsible for specific antigen binding and a constant (C) region which contributes to the general biological properties of the molecule. Given the diversity of antigens encountered in life the repertoire of antibodies has to be very large and probably exceeds one million. This figure is achieved by using combinations of several different genes to code for separate portions of the antibody molecule. The V region of the molecule consists of several regions termed 'complementarity-determining regions', interspersed with less variable framework regions. The former mainly deterimine the specificity of antigen binding.

Immunoglobulins are transcribed from genes situated on different chromosomes. The chromo-

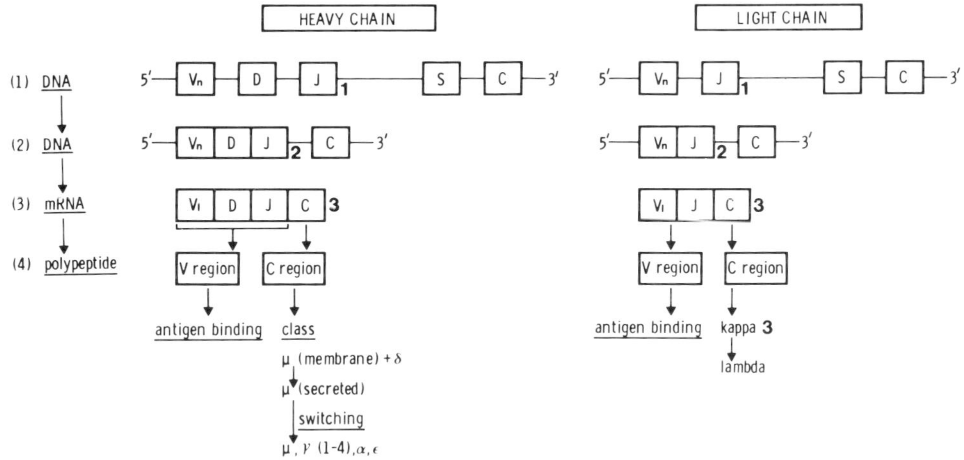

Fig. 11.6 This schematic representation outlines the main events in immunoglobulin synthesis. The chromosome segments are shown as if they were single genes; in reality they consist of several genes, e.g. 300 in the VH segment alone. However the transition from multiple unexpressed genes ('n' for VH) to one transcribed gene (V_1 in mRNA transcript) illustrates that the precursor B cell becomes irreversibly committed to synthesising antibody that combines with a single antigenic determinant. In particular there are multiple human C genes, some silent, others reduplicated. Their sequential activation is controlled by the S ('switch') gene and determines the heavy chain class or subclass of the Ig molecule eventually secreted by the fully differentiated B cell. Similarly there is sequential expression of kappa and lambda chains possibly only if the kappa genes are defective and spliced out. (1) Indicates the stage of extensive somatic mutation (estimated frequency 10^{-3}/base pair/generation), (2) the stage of gene recombination, and (3) the stage of RNA splicing when errors and arrested differentiation are most frequent. See text for full references.

somes coding for heavy chains are situated on chromosome 14, for kappa light chains on chromosome 2 and for lambda light chains on chromosome 22.

Immunoglobulin polypeptide chains are encoded by multiple gene segments which have to be brought together for the immunoglobulin to be synthesised. These genes (exons) are separated by silent genes (introns). Immunoglobulin heavy chain genes consist of four different families of genes, the variable genes (VH), diversity (D), joining genes (JH) and constant (CH). Light chains are the products of similar gene combinations with the exception of D genes which are only involved in the synthesis of H chains. There are several hundred different gene elements in the VH and V kappa or lambda segments with a smaller number in the DH gene segment. Coding for immunoglobulin synthesis is initiated by a signal peptide, transcribed from a separate L segment of the DNA. The V gene codes for most of the V region of the light chain molecule, namely the complementarity-determining regions and the framework regions with the exception of part of the framework regions which are encoded by the J segment. The C genes code for the entire C region of the molecule. An additional D gene codes for part of the complementarity-determining region in heavy chain molecules. Multiple genes code for the heavy chain C region. The mechanism of V-J and V-D-J joining is uncertain but it is likely that DNA binding proteins and enzymes remove the intervening introns probably by looping out and excision. RNA transcripts of the C region genes of heavy and light chains are joined to the products of the other genes by RNA splicing. This series of events largely explains the extraordinary diversity of antibodies which can be synthesised in response to different antigens. Because the V regions of heavy chains are encoded by 3 different genes as compared with 2 genes for light chains, more diversity can be generated in heavy chains than in light chains. In addition considerable recombination between different gene products takes place during B cell maturation independently of antigen stimulation. Indeed recombination between immunoglobulin-coding genes occurs at a higher level than does recombination in any other mammalian chromosome. Thus the genes coding for the V regions of heavy and light chains must be regarded as hot-spots of gene recombination abetted by promoter genes which have also been recently described (Boss, 1983). The assembly of the joining portions of the immunoglobulin genes is imprecise, thereby contributing further to antibody diversity. Further nucleotides may be also inserted at the junction between gene segments, again increasing the generation of diversity. This joining may be imprecise and be eventually non-productive so that diversity is achieved at the cost of considerable wastage in terms of generating functional antibodies. In summary, therefore, there are four methods for generating antibody diversity, namely somatic mutation within genes, recombinational events between genes, variation in the fusion of gene products and the insertion of additional nucleotides at the site of junction.

It has been shown that somatic mutation, defined as alterations in nucleotide sequence within genes, occurs in the genes coding for both heavy and light chains. It is likely that somatic mutations occur in V, J, and D gene segments. Moreover, these somatic changes usually involve a single base substitution. Whether the high background incidence of mutations within immunoglobulin genes is entirely spontaneous or governed by antigen stimulation is unknown.

Thus, it is not sufficient to talk about 'somatic mutation' as the basis for autoantibody production unless the circumstances which might lead to the inappropriate synthesis of antibody with specificity for autoantigens are more clearly defined.

Once the grouping of V-J-C genes has been established thereby allowing the cell to produce a particular immunoglobulin, all other possibilities for producing immunoglobulin of different specificity are removed (Coleclough, 1983). This irreversible selection allows plasma cells to secrete potent antibody of high affinity. Since the spontaneous recombinations of genes controlling immunoglobulin synthesis occurs at random, there is likely to be much fruitless rearrangement of genes in precursor cells which are destined never to differentiate into cells producing specific antibody. Moreover, maturing B cells become progressively and irreversibly differentiated with respect to the heavy and light chain classes they produce. Initially both kappa and lambda light chains are used in roughly equal proportions in order to synthesise specific antibody. Subsequently cells producing lambda light chains eliminate the majority of the genes involved in kappa chain production thereby providing a means of editing out aberrant transcripts and light chain fragments that might interfere with the final synthesis and assembly of the complete antibody molecule (Korsmeyer et al, 1982). The gene segments which determine heavy chain class are also sequentially expressed; the u gene is first expressed whilst subsequent switches involve the operation of switch or S regions which have structural similarity with similar gene complexes found in other species (Flanagan & Rabbitts, 1982). Whether or not these switches also depend on somatic mutation is unknown.

In a seminal paper Klein (1981) raised the possibility that genes responsible for malignant transformation might be translocated to chromosomes coding for immunoglobulin synthesis thereby inducing the excessive and unregulated synthesis of these molecules. The frequent recombination of these genes would encourage the integration of DNA sequences translocated from other chromosomes. This prediction has been largely borne out by observations in human lymphomas and leukaemias. Burkitt's lymphomas are monoclonal proliferations of malignant B lymphocytes and the tumour cells consistently show chromosome translocations between chromosome 8 and chromosomes containing immunoglobulin coding segments. The immunoglobulin chains produced by these lymphomas are correlated with the site of translocation; Burkitt's lymphomas cells with an 8–22 translocation express lambda type light chains whereas those with 8–2 translocation express kappa light chains; 8–14 translocation is associated with heavy chain synthesis (Lenoir et al, 1982). These observations suggest that the transforming genes (oncogenes) responsible for inducing malignancy in B cells induce the production of immunoglobulin by contiguous genes.

The nature of the oncogenes is currently of great interest. There is speculation that DNA derived from retroviruses may directly transform cells or activate oncogenes. Retroviruses are RNA viruses which replicate through the formation of a DNA copy which becomes integrated in the DNA of the host chromosome (Varmus, 1982; Weiss, 1982). Retroviruses can be transmitted either horizontally or vertically. The infection does not kill the cell and the integrated viral DNA becomes a stable component of host chromosomes. Recombination between retroviruses and oncogenes may provide the stimulus for immunoglobulin synthesis induced in neighbouring genes on chromosomes to which the oncogene becomes translocated. Retroviruses have frequently been discussed in the context of human lupus; furthermore caprine retrovirus induces arthritis in goats with many of the histopathological features of rheumatoid arthritis (Brassfield et al, 1982). Moreover, experimental studies show that the expression of retroviruses in mammalian cells is extremely variable depending upon the site of integration during embryogenesis and the extent to which methylation restricts its expression (Jähner et al, 1982). It is noteworthy that a human gene homologous with the murine retrovirus Abelson murine leukaemia virus has been located on chromosome 9 and that chronic myelocytic leukaemia is associated with the specific translocation of this oncogene to chromosome 22, the Philadelphia translocation associated with this form of leukaemia (De Klein et al, 1982). Similarly a human cellular homologue of an avian retrovirus has been discovered on chromosome 8 and termed the 'c-myc' gene. The nucleotide sequence of this gene and the proteins for which it codes have been fully determined (Watt et al, 1983). This sequence may initiate the transforming events following the translocation of segments of chromosome 8 in Burkitt's lymphoma.

There is as yet no evidence that human autoimmune diseases arise from unregulated immunoproliferative events in B cells or other lymphocytes in a manner analogous with that observed in overt malignant diseases. However, there are indications that the disturbances of immune function in both murine and human lupus are extensive involving the regulation of pleuripotential stem cells (Kumagai et al, 1982) and T cells (Taurog et al, 1981). Also of interest are observations in mice with genetically determined autoimmune diseases indicating that many of these disorders can be abrogated by preparing congenic mice with the genetic background of NZB mice and the immune deficiency gene xid linked to the X chromosome (Steinberg et al, 1982). Such mice with B cell immunodeficiency fail to develop the naturally occurring autoimmune disease characteristic of NZB F1 hybrid mice. The same authors also claim that these mice fail to develop autoantibodies to DNA after polyclonal B cell activation, although these may be induced be powerful activators such as bacterial polysaccharides (Smathers et al, 1982). Partial suppression of autoimmune disease in NZB mice and its hybrid strains can be achieved in crosses between NZB mice and CBA/n mice which also have X-linked immunodeficiency disorder (Romain et al, 1980). These observations strongly suggest that the polyclonal hypergammaglobulinaemia and autoantibody production characteristic of many chronic rheumatic disorders could arise from inherited defects in the maturation of stem cells and their lymphocyte progeny. These abnormalities could result from mutations secondary to the normal background of gene recombination in immunoglobulin synthesising cells. However, the links between retroviruses, oncogenes, and immunoproliferative diseases are still tenuous in murine models of autoimmune disease and are completely lacking in human disorders. Nevertheless the observation that lymphoblastoid cell lines infected with EB virus can produce monoclonal rheumatoid factor (Steinitz & Tamir, 1982) at least demonstrates that transformed cell lines can synthesise an autoantibody commonly encountered in human disorders.

CONCLUSIONS

Immune reactions similar to those produced in response to antigens are readily detectable in the synovial membrane and other tissues involved in acute and chronic rheumatic disorders. Moreover several immunopathological pathways have been identified which could account for the tissue damage encountered in these disorders including the degradation of articular cartilage and underlying bone. However, whilst such observations have done much to elucidate the mechanisms of tissue damage, they have not produced any specific guide to the aetiology of these disorders. The main problem is the similarity of the immunopathological picture produced by a wide range of differing stimuli including many of the serological abnormalities and disturbances in blood lymphocyte populations often considered characteristic of the rheumatic diseases. The chronic synovitis in rheumatic diseases is consistent with a persistent immune reaction to an unidentified antigen.

However, there is an alternative explanation which would account for the repeated failure to identify the postulated antigen, namely that defective immune regulation allows these responses to persist even after antigen has been eliminated. Evidence to this effect is still fragmentary and is largely based upon in vitro assays of lymphocyte functions and immunochemical analyses of biopsy material whose specificity is still in doubt. Similarly, autoimmune reactions accompany rheumatic disorders but there is no decisive evidence that these are of primary pathogenetic importance. The antigens and autoantibodies involved in the rheumatic disorders need to be better characterised, as do the factors which normally restrict the proliferation of autoreactive lymphocytes.

A growing appreciation of the genetic events which characterise normal immunoglobulin synthesis prompts a re-examination of the classical view that many rheumatic disorders may be primary immunoproliferative diseases originating in mutations of lymphocytes or their precursor cells. Transformations of this kind have been shown to contribute to malignant lymphoproliferative disorders. Their possible role in autoimmune disorders has not yet been evaluated. However, the introduction of techniques for identifying and sequencing genes coding for immunoglobulin synthesis and T cell recognition should allow these ideas to be tested.

REFERENCES

Abdou N I, Wall H, Lindsley H B, Halsey J F, Suzuki T 1981 Network theory in autoimmunity. In vitro suppression of serum anti-DNA antibody binding to DNA by anti-idiotypic antibody in systemic lypus erythematosus. Journal of Clinical Investigation 67: 1297–1304

Allison A C 1977 Autoimmune diseases: concepts of pathogenesis and control. In: Talal N (Ed) Autoimmunity: genetic, immunologic, virologic, and clinical aspects. Academic Press, London, p 91–139

Altman A, Theofilopoulos A N, Weiner R, Katz D A, Dixon F J 1981 Analysis of T cell function in autoimmune murine strains. Defects in production of and responsiveness to interleukin 2. Journal of Experimental Medicine 154: 791–808

Asherson G L, Webster A D B 1980 Diagnosis and treatment of immunodeficiency diseases. Blackwell, Oxford

Ashida E R, Johnson A R, Lipsky P E 1981 Human endothelial cell–lymphocyte interaction. Endothelial cells function as accessory cells necessary for mitogen-induced human T lymphocyte activation in vitro. Journal of Clinical Investigation 67: 1490–1499

Bacon T H 1983 Unpublished observations

Barclay A N, Mason D W 1982 Induction of Ia antigen in rat epidermal cells and gut epithelium by immunological stimuli. Journal of Experimental Medicine 156: 1665–1676

Bardwick P A, Bluestein H G, Zvaifler N J, Depper J M, Seegmiller J E 1980 Altered regulation of Epstein–Barr virus induced lymphoblast proliferation in rheumatoid arthritis lymphoid cells. Arthritis and Rheumatism 23: 626–632

Barkley D O, Hohermuth H J, Howard A, Webster D B, Ansell B M 1979 IgA deficiency in juvenile chronic polyarthritis. Journal of Rheumatology 6: 219–224

Beale M G, Nash G S, Bertovich J, MacDermott R P 1982 Similar disturbances in B cell activity and regulatory T cell function in Henoch–Schönlein erythematosus. Journal of Immunology 128: 486–491

Becker D, Ossowski L, Reich E 1981 Induction of plasminogen activator synthesis by antibodies. Journal of Experimental Medicine 154: 385–396

Behan P O, Behan W M, Zacharias F T, Nicholls J T 1976 Immunological abnormalities in patients who had the oculomucocutaneous syndrome associated with practolol therapy. Lancet ii: 984–987

Bockman R S, Repo M A 1981 Lymphokine-mediated bone resorption requires endogenous prostaglandin synthesis. Journal of Experimental Medicine 154: 529–534

Boss M A 1983 Enhancer elements in immunoglobulin genes. Nature 303: 281–282

Braciale T J, Andrew M E, Braciale V L 1981 Simultaneous expression of H-2 restricted and alloreactive recognition by a cloned line of influenza virus-specific cytotoxic T lymphocytes. Journal of Experimental Medicine 153: 1371–1376

Brassfield A L, Adams D S, Crawford T D, McGuire T C 1982 Ultrastructure of arthritis induced by a caprine retrovirus. Arthritis and Rheumatism 25: 930–936

Bromberg J S, Lake P, Brunswick M 1982 Viral antigens act as helper determinants for antibody responses to cell surface antigens. Journal of Immunology 129: 683–688

Burnet F M 1959 The clonal selection theory of acquired immunity. Cambridge University Press, London

Cazenave P-A 1981 Idiotypy of antibodies. In: Bona C, Cazenave P-A (eds) Lymphocytic regulation by antibodies. Wiley, New York, p 171–185

Chang Y, Pearson C M, Chedid L 1981 Adjuvant polyarthritis. V. Induction by N-acetylmuramyl-L-alanyl-D-isoglutamine, the smallest peptide subunit of bacterial peptidoglycan. Journal of Experimental Medicine 153: 1021–1026

Charlesworth J A, Endre Z H, Pussell B A, Yasmeen D, Peake P W 1982 Complement behavior in infectious mononucleosis: possible mechanisms for the prevention of immune complex injury. Journal of Infectious

Diseases 145: 505–513
Chetty C, Brown R G, Schwab J H 1983 Edema-producing activity of group A streptococcal polysaccharide and its possible role in the pathogenesis of cell wall-induced polyarthritis. Journal of Experimental Medicine 157: 1089–1100
Chiorazzi N, Fu S M, Kunkel H G 1979 Introduction of polyclonal antibody synthesis by human allogeneic and autologous helper factors. Journal of Experimental Medicine 149: 1543–1548
Cohen P L, Eisenberg R A 1982 Anti-idiotypic antibodies to the Coombs antibody in NZB Fl mice. Journal of Experimental Medicine 156: 173–180
Coleclough C 1983 Chance, necessity and antibody gene dynamics. Nature 303: 23–26
Cowdery J S, Steinberg A D 1982 Regulation of primary, thymus-independent, anti-hapten responses of normal and autoimmune mice by syngeneic antibody. Journal of Immunology 129: 1250–1255
DeBoer K P, Kleinman R, Teodorescu M 1981 Identification and separation by bacterial adherence of human lymphocytes that suppress natural cytotoxicity. Journal of Immunology 126: 276–281
deKlein A, van Kessel A G, Grosveld G, Bartram G R, Hagemeijer A, Bootsman D, et al 1982 A cellular oncogene is translocated to the Philadelphia chromosome in chronic myelocytic leukaemia. Nature 300: 765–767
Denman A M 1981 Viruses and autoimmune diseases. In: Halborow E J (ed) Autoimmunity. Clinics in Immunology and Allergy 1: 17–39
Denman A M 1983 Viruses and immunopathology. In: Holborow E J, Reeves W J (eds) Medical immunology, 2nd Edn. Grune & Stratton, New York, p 179–202
Dingle J T 1979 Recent studies on the control of joint damage: the contribution of the Strangeways Research Laboratory. Annals of the Rheumatic Diseases 38: 201–214
Dumonde D C, Kasp-Grochowska E, Graham E, Sanders M D, Faure J-P, deKozak Y, van Tuyen V 1982 Antiretinal autoimmunity and circulating immune complexes in patients with retinal vasculitis. Lancet ii: 787–792
Dwyer D S, Bradley R J, Urquhart C K, Kearney J F 1983 Naturally occurring anti-idiotypic antibodies in myasthenia gravis patients. Nature 301: 611–614
Dziarski R 1979 Relationships between adjuvant, immunosuppressive and mitogenic activities of staphylococal peptidoglycan. Infection and Immunity 26: 508–514
Farrant J, Newton C 1981 Relative ability to provide help: an explanation for Con A-induced suppression Clinical and Experimental Immunology 45: 504–513
Fauci A S, Moutsopoulos H M 1981 Polyclonally triggered B cells in the peripheral blood and bone marrow of normal individuals and in patients with systemic lupus erythematosus and primary Sjögren's syndrome. Arthritis and Rheumatism 24: 577–584
Fish F, Ziff M 1982 The in vitro and in vivo induction of anti-double-stranded DNA antibodies in normal and autoimmune mice. Journal of Immunology 128: 409–414
Flanagan J G, Rabbitts T H 1982 Arrangement of human immunoglobulin heavy chain constant region genes implies evolutionary duplication of a segment containing γ, ε and α genes. Nature 300: 709–713
Fleisher T A, Greene W C, Uchiyama T, Goldman C K, Nelson D L, Blaese R M, Waldmann T A 1981 Characterisation of a soluble suppressor of human B cell immunoglobulin biosynthesis produced by a continuous human suppressor T cell line. Journal of Experimental Medicine 154: 156–167
Fleisher T A, Attallah A M, Tosato G, Blaese R M, Greene W C 1982 Interferon-mediated inhibition of human polyclonal immunoglobulin synthesis. Journal of Immunology 129: 1099–1103
Fontana A, Hengartner H, Weber F, Fehr K, Grob P J, Cohen G 1982 Interleukin 1 activity in the synovial fluid of patients with rheumatoid arthritis. Rheumatology International 2: 49–53
Fox R I, Fong S, Sabharwal N, Carstens S A, Kung P C, Vaughan J H 1982 Synovial fluid lymphocytes differ from peripheral blood lymphocytes in patients with rheumatoid arthritis. Journal of Immunology 128: 351–354
Galli S J, Dvorak A M, Ishizaka T, Nabel G, Der Simonian H, Cantor H, Dvorak H F 1982 A cloned cell with NK function resembles basophils by ultrastructure and expresses IgE receptors. Nature 298: 288–290
Garson J A, Beverley P C L, Coakham H B, Harper E I 1982 Monoclonal antibodies against human T lymphocytes label Purkinje neurones of many species. Nature 298: 375–377
Geha R 1982 Presence of auto-anti-idiotypic antibody during the normal human immune response to tetanus toxoid antigen. Journal of Immunology 129: 139–144
Geha R S, Reinherz E, Leung D, McKee K T, Schlossman S, Rosen F S 1981 Deficiency of suppressor T cells in the hyperimmunoglobulin E syndrome. Journal of Clinical Investigation 68: 783–791
Goldenberg D L, Cohen A S 1978 Synovial membrane histopathology in the differential diagnosis of rheumatoid arthritis, gout, pseudogout, systemic lupus erythematosus, infectious arthritis and degenerative joint disease. Medicine 57: 239–252
Goodman M G, Chenoweth D E, Weigle W O 1982 Induction of interleukin 1 secretion and enhancement of humoral immunity by binding of human C5a to macrophage surface C5a receptor. Journal of Experimental Medicine 1156: 912–917
Gray E D, Wannamaker L W, Ayoub E M, Elkholy A, Abdin Z H 1981 Cellular immune responses to extracellular streptococcal products in rheumatic heart disease. Journal of Clinical Investigation 68: 665–671
Greenwood B M, Whittle H C 1976 The pathogenesis of meningococcal arthritis. In: Dumonde D C (ed) Infection and immunology in the rheumatic diseases. Blackwell, Oxford, p 119–127
Grooten J, De Baetselier P, Vercauteren E, Hamers R 1980 Anti-micrococcus antibodies recognise an antigenic marker of confluent mouse lymphoid cell lines. Nature 285: 401–403
Hadler N, Granovetter D A 1978 Phlogistic properties of bacterial debris. Seminars in Arthritis and Rheumatism 8: 1–16
Hamilton J A, Bootes A, Philips P E, Slywka J 1981 Human synovial fibroblast plasminogen activator. Arthritis and Rheumatism 24: 1296–1303
Hank J A, Sondel P M Soluble bacterial antigen induces specific helper and cytotoxic responses by human lymphocytes in vitro. Journal of Immunology 128: 2734–2738
Harada S, Sakamoto K, Seeley J K, Lindsten T, Bechtold T, Yetz J, Rogers G, Pearson G, Purtilo D T 1982 Immune

deficiency in the X-linked lymphoproliferative syndrome I Epstein-Barr virus-specific defects. Journal of Immunology 129: 2532–2535

Haskins K, Kuno R, White J, Pigeon M, Kappler J, Marrack P 1983 The major histocompatibility complex-restricted antigen receptor on T cells. I isolation with a monoclonal antibody. Journal of Experimental Medicine 157: 1149–1169

Herman J H, Bradley J, Ziff M, Smiley J D 1971 Response of the rheumatoid synovial membrane to exogenous immunization. Journal of Clinical Investigation 50: 266–273

Horita M, Suzuki H, Onodera T, Ginsberg-Fellner F, Fauci A C, Notkins A L 1982 Abnormalities of immunoregulatory T cell subsets in patients with insulin-dependent diabetes mellitus. Journal of Immunology 129: 1426–1429

Huddlestone J R, Oldstone M B A 1982 Suppressor T cells are activated in vivo in patients with multiple sclerosis coinciding with remission from acute attack. Journal of Immunology 129: 915–917

Inman R D, Redecha P B, Knechtle S J, Schned E S, van de Rijn I, Christian C L 1982 Identification of bacterial antigens in circulating immune complexes of infective endocarditis. Journal of Clinical Investigation 70: 271–280

Ishikawa.H, Ziff M 1976 Electron microscopic observations of immunoreactive cells in the rheumatoid synovial membrane. Arthritis and Rheumatism 19: 1–14

Jähner D, Stuhlmann H, Stewart C L, Harbers K, Löhler J, Simon I, Jaenisch R 1982 De novo methylation and expression of retroviral genomes during mouse embryogenesis. Nature 298: 623–628

Janossy G, Duke O, Poulter L W, Panayi G, Bofill M, Goldstein G 1981 Rheumatoid arthritis: a disease of T-lymphocyte/macrophage immuno-regulation. Lancet 2: 839NNC842

Jasin H E, Cooke T D 1978 The inflammatory role of immune complexes trapped in joint collagenous tissues. Clinical and Experimental Immunology 33: 416–424

Jasin H E, Dingle J T 1981 Human mononuclear cell factors mediate cartilage matrix degradation through chondrocyte activation. Journal of Clinical Investigation 68: 571–581

Jensenius J C, Williams A F 1982 The T lymphocyte antigen receptor-paradigm lost. Nature 300: 583–588

Johnston C L W, Webster A D B, Taylor-Robinson D, Rapaport G, Hughes G R V 1983 Primary late-onset hypogammaglobulinaemia associated with inflammatory polyarthritis and septic arthritis due to mycoplasma pneumoniae. Annals of the Rheumatic Diseases 42: 108–110

Jones I L, McGuire M B, Klämfeldt A 1982 Enhanced breakdown of bovine articular cartilage proteoglycans by conditioned synovial medium in vitro: a possible role for prostaglandins. Scandinavian Journal of Rheumatology 11: 177–183

Kärre K, Klein G O, Kiessling R, Klein G, Roder J C 1980 Low natural in vivo resistance to syngeneic leukaemias in natural killer-deficient mice. Nature 284: 624–626

Kelton J G, Neame P B, Gauldie J, Hirsch J 1979 Elevated platelet-associated IgG in the thrombocytopenia of septicemia. New England Journal of Medicine 300: 760–764

Kimura H, Tateishi H, Ziff M 1977 Surface ultrastructure of rheumatoid articular cartilage. *Arthritis and Rheumatism 20*: 1085–1098

Klareskog L, Forsum U, Scheynius A, Kabelitz D, Wigzell H 1982 Evidence in support of a self-perpetuating HLA-DR dependent delayed type cell reaction in rheumatoid arthritis. Proceedings of the National Academy of Science, USA 79: 3632–3636

Klareskog L, Holmdahl R, Larsson E, Wigzell H 1983 Role of T lymphocytes in collagen II induced arthritis in rats. Clinical and Experimental Immunology 51: 117–125

Klein G 1981 The role of gene dosage and genetic transpositions in carcinogenesis. Nature 294: 313–318

Klickstein L B, Shapleigh C, Goetzl E J 1980 Lipoxygenation of arachidonic acid as a source of polymorphonuclear chemotactic factors in synovial fluid and tissue in rheumatoid arthritis and spondyloarthritis. Journal of Clinical Investigation 66: 1166–1170

Klinkert W E F, LaBadie J H, Bowers W E 1982 Accessory and stimulating properties of dendritic cells and macrophages isolated from various rat tissues. Journal of Experimental Medicine 156: 1–19

Kobayashi I, Ziff M 1975 Electron microscopic studies of the cartilage-pannus junction in rheumatoid arthritis. Arthritis and Rheumatism 18: 475–485

Kodama K, Sikorska H, Bandy-Dafoe P, Bayly R, Wall J R 1982 Demonstration of a circulating autoantibody against a soluble eye-muscle antigen in Graves' ophthalmopathy. Lancet ii: 1353–1355

Konttinen Y T, Reitamo S, Ranki A, Häyry P, Kankaanapää U, Wegelius O 1981 Characterization of the immunocompetent cells of rheumatoid synovium from tissue sections and eluates. Arthritis and Rheumatism 24: 71–9

Korsmeyer S J, Hieter P A, Sharrow S O, Goldman C K, Leder P, Waldmann T A 1982 Normal human B cells display ordered light chain gene rearrangements and deletions. Journal of Experimental Medicine 156: 975–985

Krane S M, Goldring S V, Dayer J M 1982 Interactions among lymphocytes ,monocytes, and other synovial cells in the rheumatoid synovium. In: Pick E (ed) Lymphokines. Vol 7. Academic Press, London, p 75–736

Kreth H W, Kress L, Kress H G, Ott H F, Eckert G 1982 Demonstration of primary cytotoxic T cells in venous blood and cerebrospinal fluid of children with mumps meningitis. Journal of Immunology 128: 2411–2415

Kumagai S, Sredni B, House S, Steinberg A D, Green I 1982 Defective regulation of B lymphocyte colony formation in patients with systemic lupus erythematosus. Journal of Immunology 128: 258–262

Lachmann P J, Peters D K (eds) 1982 Clinical aspects of immunology, 4th Edn. Blackwell, Oxford

Lafer E M, Rauch J, Andrzejewski C, Mudd D, Furie B C, Furie B et al 1981 Polyspecific monoclonal lupus autoantibodies reactive with both polynucleotides and phospholipids. Journal of Experimental Medicine 153: 897–909

Lattime E C, Gillis S, Pecoraro G, Stutman O 1982 Ia-dependent interleukin 2 production in syngeneic cellular interactions. Journal of Immunology 128: 480–485

Lechler R I, Batchelor J R 1982 Immunogenicity of retransplanted rat kidney allografts. Journal of Experimental Medicine 156: 1835–1841

Lehner T 1982 The relationship between human helper and suppressor factors to a streptococcal protein antigen. Journal of Immunology 129: 1936–1940

Lehner T 1983 Characterization of human helper and suppressor factors with special reference to HLA-DR

determinants. Immunology 48: 695–702
Lenoir G M, Preud' Homme J L, Bernheim A, Berger R 1982 Correlation between immunoglobulin light chain expression and variant translocation in Burkitt's lymphoma. Nature 298: 474–476
Lewis R A, Austen K F 1981 Mediation of local homeostasis and inflammation by leukotrienes and other mast cell-dependent compounds. Nature 293: 103–108
Lipsky P E 1980 Staphylococcal protein A, a T cell-regulated polyclonal activator of human B cells. Journal of Immunology 125: 155–162
London W T, Fuccillo D A, Anderson B, Sever J L 1970 Concentration of rubella virus antigen in chondrocytes of congenitally injected rabbits. Nature 226: 172–173
Luger T A, Smolen J S, Chused T M, Steinberg A D, Oppenheim J J 1982 Human lymphocytes with either the OKT 4 or OKT 8 phenotype produce interleukin 2 in culture. Journal of Clinical Investigation 70: 470–473
Matzinger P 1981 A one-receptor view of T-cell behaviour. Nature 292: 497–501
Meats J E, McGuire M B, Russell R G G 1980 Human synovium releases a factor which stimulates chondrocyte production of PGE and Plasminogen activator. Nature 286: 891–892
Möller G (ed) 1981 Ontogeny of human lymphocyte function. Immunological Reviews 57
Mongini P K A, Stein K E, Paul W E 1981 T cell regulation of IgG subclass antibody production in response to T-independent antigens. Journal of Experimental Medicine 153: 1–12
Nakagawara A, DeSantis N M, Nogueira N, Nathan C F 1981 Lymphokines enhance the capacity of human monocytes to secrete reactive oxygen intermediates. Journal of Clinical Investigation 70: 1042–1048
Nisonoff A 1982 Introduction to molecular immunology. Sinauer Associates Inc, Sunderland, Mass
Nussenzweig M C, Steinman R M, Unkeless J C, Wimer M D, Gutchinov B, Cohn Z A 1981 Studies of the cell surface of mouse dendritic cells and other leukocytes. Journal of Experimental Medicine 154: 168–187
Oger J, Szuchet S, Antel J, Arnason B G W 1982 A monoclonal antibody against human T suppressor lymphocytes binds specifically to the surface of cultured oligodendrocytes. Nature 295: 66–68
Panem S, Check I J, Henriksen D, Vilcek J 1982 Antibodies to α-interferon in a patient with systemic lupus erythematosus. Journal of Immunology 129: 1–3
Pollok B A, Bhown A S, Kearney J F 1982 Structural and biological properties of a monoclonal auto-anti-(anti-idiotype) antibody. Nature 299: 447–449
Primi D, Hammarström L, Smith C I E, Möller G 1977 Characterization of self-reactive B cells by polyclonal B-cell activators. Journal of Experimental Medicine 145: 21–30
Radoiu N, Cleveland R P, Leon M A 1982 Peripheral T lymphocytes from rheumatoid arthritis patients recognise determinants on light chains and/or Fab fragments of immunoglobulin G. Journal of Clinical Investigation 70: 329–334
Rankin J A, Hitchcock M, Merrill W, Bach M K, Brachler J R, Askenase P H 1982 IgE-dependent release of leukotriene C_4 from alveolar macrophages. Nature 297: 329–331
Reiss C S, Burakoff S J 1981 Specificity of the helper T cell for the cytolytic T lymphocyte response to influenza viruses. Journal of Experimental Medicine 154: 541–551
Roberts-Thomson P J, Wernick R M, Ziff M 1981 Low molecular weight IgM in rheumatoid arthritis and other rheumatic disorders. Arthritis and Rheumatism 24: 795–802
Roitt I M 1978 Essential immunology, 3rd Edn. Blackwell, Oxford
Romain P L, Cohen P L, Fish F, Ziff M, Vitetta E S 1980 The specific B cell subset lacking in the CBA/N mouse is not required for the production of autoantibody in (CBA/N × NZB)F_1 male mice. Journal of Immunology 125: 246–251
Rosenberg S A, Lipsky P E 1981 The role of monocytes in pokeweed mitogen-stimulated human B cell activation. Separate requirements for intact monocytes and a soluble monocyte factor. Journal of Immunology 126: 1341–1345
Scwab J 1983 Bacterial interference with immunospecific defences. In: Smith H, Arbuthnott J P, Mims C A (eds) The determinants of bacterial and viral pathogenesis. Royal Society, London, p 59–71
Shiozawa S, Jasin H E, Ziff M 1980 Absence of immunoglobulins in rheumatoid cartilage-pannus junctions 1980. Arthritis and Rheumatism 23: 816–821
Shiozawa S, Williams R C, Ziff M 1982 Immunoelectron microscopic demonstration of prostaglandin E in rheumatoid synovium. Arthritis and Rheumatism 25: 685–693
Shoenfeld Y, Hsu-lin S C, Gabriels J E, Silberstein L E, Furie B C, Furie B, et al, 1982 Production of autoantibodies by human–human hybridomas. Journal of Clinical Investigation 70: 205–208
Shoenfeld Y, Raugh J, Massicotte H, Datta S K, Andre-Schwartz J, Stollar B D, Schwartz R S 1983 Polyspecificity of monoclonal lupus autoantibodies produced by human–human hybridomas. New England Journal of Medicine 308: 414–420
Silver R M, Redelman D, Zvaifler N J, Naides S 1982 Studies of rheumatoid synovial fluid lymphocytes. 1. Evidence for activated natural killer (NK)-like cells. Journal of Immunology 128: 1758–1763
Smathers P A, Steinberg B J, Reeves J P, Steinberg A D 1982 Effects of polyclonal immune stimulators upon NZB xid congenic mice. Journal of Immunology 128: 1414–1419
Smiley J D, Sachs C, Ziff M 1968 In vitro synthesis of immunoglobulin by rheumatoid synovial membrane. Journal of Clinical Investigation 47: 624–632
Smith H R, Green D R, Raveche E S, Smathers P A, Gershon R K, Steinberg A D 1982 Studies of the induction of anti-DNA in normal mice. Journal of Immunology 129: 2332–2334
So A K L, Furr P M, Taylor-Robinson D, Webster A D B 1983 Arthritis caused by mycoplasma salivarium in hypogammaglobulinaemia. British Medical Journal 286: 762–763
Steinberg B J, Smathers P A, Frederiksen K, Steinberg A D 1982 Ability of the xid gene to prevent autoimmunity in (NZB × NZW) F_1 mice during the course of their natural history, after polyclonal stimulation or following immunisation with DNA. Journal of Clinical Investigation 70: 587–597
Steinitz M, Tamir S 1982 Human monoclonal autoimmune antibody produced in vitro: rheumatoid factor generated by Epstein–Barr virus-transformed cell line. European Journal of Immunology 12: 126–133
Taurog J D, Raveche E S, Smathers P A, Glimcher L H, Huston D P, Hansen C T, Steinberg A D 1981 T cell

abnormalities in NZB mice occur independently of autoantibody production. Journal of Experimental Medicine 153: 221–234

Thoman M L, Weigle W O 1982 Cell-mediated immunity in aged mice: an underlying lesion in IL 2 synthesis. Journal of Immunology 128: 2358–2361

Tonegawa S 1983 Somatic generation of antibody diversity. Nature 302: 575–581

Trentham D E, Kammer G M, McCune W J, David J R 1981 Autoimmunity to collagen. A shared feature of psoriatic and rheumatoid arthritis. Arthritis and Rheumatism 24: 1363–1369

Tyndall A de V, Knight S C, Edwards A J, Clarke J B 1983 Veiled (dendritic) cells in synovial fluid. Lancet ii: 472–473

Varmus H E 1982 Form and function of retroviral proviruses. Science 216: 816–820

Wallace L E, Rickinson A B, Rowe M, Moss D J, Allen D J, Epstein M A 1982 Stimulation of human lymphocytes with irradiated cells of the autologous Epstein–Barr virus-transformed cell line. I. Virus-specific and non-specific components of the cytotoxic response. Cellular Immunology 67: 129–140

Ward A M, Udnoon S, Watkins J, Walker A E, Darke C S 1976 Immunological mechanisms in the pathogenesis of vinyl chloride disease. British Medical Journal 1: 936–938

Warner J F, Dennert G 1982 Effects of a cloned cell line with NK activity on bone marrow transplants, tumour development and metastasis in vivo. Nature 300: 31–34

Watt R, Stanton L W, Marcu K B, Gallo R C, Croce C M, Robera G 1983 Nucleotide sequence of cloned cDNA of human c-myc oncogene. Nature 303: 725–728

Waxman F J, Perryman L E, Hinrichs D J, Coe J E 1981 Genetic resistance to the induction of experimental allergic encephalomyelitis in rats. I. Genetic analysis of an apparent mutant strain with phenotypic resistance to experimental allergic encephalomyelitis. Journal of Experimental Medicine 153: 61–76

Webster A D B 1983 Echovirus myosits in hypogammaglobulinaemic patients. Clinics in Rheumatic Diseases (in press)

Webster A D B, Loewi G, Dourmashkin R D, Golding D N, Ward D J, Asherson G L 1976 Polyarthritis in adults with hypogammaglobulinaemia and its rapid response to immunoglobulin treatment. British Medical Journal 1: 1314–1316

Webster A D B, Taylor-Robinson D, Furr P M, Asherson G L 1978 Mycoplasmal (ureaplasma) septic arthritis in hypogammaglobulinaemia. British Medical Journal 1: 478–479

Weiss R A 1982 The persistence of retroviruses. In: Mahy B W J, Minson A C, Darby G K (eds) Virus persistence. Cambridge University Press, Cambridge, p 267–288

Weiss S J, Ward P A 1982 Immune complex induced generation of oxygen metabolites by human neutrophils. Journal of Immunology 129: 309–313

Welte K, Wang C Y, Mertelsmann R, Venuta S, Feldman S P, Moore M A S 1982 Purification of human interleukin 2 to apparent homogeneity and its molecular heterogeneity. Journal of Experimental Medicine 156: 454–464

Wilkins J A, Warrington R J, Sigurdson S L, Rutherford W J 1983 The demonstration of an interleukin 2-like activity in the synovial fluids of rheumatoid arthritis patients. Journal of Rheumatology 10: 109–113

Wooley P H, Luthra H S, Stuart J M, David C S 1981 Type II collagen-induced arthritis in mice I major histocompatibility complex, (I region) linkage and antibody correlates. Journal of Experimental Medicine 154: 688–700

Zanders E D, Fischer A, Smith S, Beverley P C L 1983 Antigen-specific and non-specific helper activities derived from supernatants of human influenza virus-specific T-cell lines. Immunology 48: 361–366

Zuckerman A J 1982 Persistence of hepatitis B virus in the population. In: Mahy B W J, Minson A C, Darby G K (eds) Virus persistence. Cambridge University Press, Cambridge, p 39–56

E.J. Holborow

Autoantibodies in the rheumatic diseases

Autoimmune phenomena are increasingly recognisable in human disease, and as the list of autoantibodies of defined specificity lengthens, it becomes a challenging task to identify which of them are most relevant to diagnosis or to the elucidation of pathogenesis. An aim of equal importance is to determine what irregularities of immune function account for their appearance, and, especially in the context of chronic inflammatory rheumatic disease, for their persistence.

The autoantibodies that feature most characteristically in rheumatic disease differ in character from those familiar in, for example, the autoimmune endocrinopathies, which are clearly directed at antigens localised in and peculiar to the affected organ. Instead, we are concerned here with non-organ-specific antibodies comprising, in the main, two different constellations reactive with antigenic determinants (epitopes) on IgG molecules, or with a wide variety of different molecular constituents of cell nuclei, and respectively designated rheumatoid factors (RFs) and anti-nuclear antibodies (ANAs). Non-organ-specific autoantibodies of these sorts cluster in patients with connective tissue disorders of systemic type, where the lesions, as well as affecting the musculoskeletal system, also appear extra-articularly in the form of scattered areas of vasculitis or endothelial cell injury affecting many possible sites.

Systemic lupus erythematosus (SLE) with its multisystem lesions and multiple autoantibody production has long been the paradigm of such autoimmune connective tissue disease. Non-organ-specific autoantibodies apparently generically similar are also more or less prominent immunological features of rheumatoid arthritis (RA) and its variants, of overlap syndromes between RA and SLE, of systemic sclerosis, of mixed connective tissue disease and of some forms of juvenile chronic polyarthritis. In other systemic rheumatic conditions, for example polymyositis, dermatomyositis and ankylosing spondylitis, detectable autoantibodies are usually more conspicuous by their absence, although in these conditions, as in systemic inflammatory rheumatic disorders in general, the presence of cell-mediated autoimmune reactions is by no means ruled out.

In both SLE and RA, the range of autoantibodies which may be present includes some which, while non-organ-specific, are distinctly cell-specific or organelle-specific. In SLE, for example, autoantibodies reactive with membrane antigens of red cells, platelets and lymphocytes may be present, and associated to varying extents in different patients with clinical evidence of their effects such as anaemia, thrombocytopenia or lymphopenia. Such anti-cell membrane autoantibodies also appear to be associated with a variety of other clinical manifestations of the disease, supposedly through cross-reactivity with membrane antigens on other cell types such as neurones and trophoblast cells. In rheumatoid arthritis, on the other hand, the range of autoantibody specificities seen includes those against intracellular cytoskeletal elements and related structures which seem to have no apparent associations with clinical features.

The diagnostic usefulness of RFs and ANAs has been recognised since the early 1950s, when serological test systems for their detection were first developed. The results of such tests have acquired added significance with the recognition that both of these groups of autoantibodies have important roles in pathogenesis, and the expectation that more precise tests capable of distinguishing and measuring specific reactions within each group should provide information useful in management and treatment as well as in diagnosis.

The explanation of the striking frequency, serum levels and distribution of antinuclear and antiglobulin antibodies in systemic connective tissue diseases is still uncertain. A recently discovered feature of several of these conditions which promises to throw light on the nature of the underlying immunological causes is their preferential occurrence in individuals who have inherited certain factors controlled by the major histocompatibility gene complex (MHC) on chromosome 6 which exerts a central directing role on most forms of the immune response. The incidence of autoimmune connective tissue diseases shows significant associations with certain cell membrane antigens coded at the HLA, HLA-DR and related loci in the MHC which are also associated with some other autoimmune or otherwise immune mediated diseases. HLA molecules at the cell surface are thought to guide the functions of T lymphocyte subsets in such a way that the immune system delivers appropriate responses to diverse forms of infection. It therefore seems likely that whatever the precise underlying causes of this group of systemic rheumatic conditions, they work through specific features of the genetic constitution of the individual which predispose to autoimmunity.

ANTIGLOBULINS AND RHEUMATOID FACTORS

Basis of methods of detection

A factor in human serum which agglutinates sheep erythrocytes sparingly coated with rabbit anti-sheep erythrocyte antibody was reported by Waaler in 1940, who found it in 35% of rheumatoid and 9% of non-rheumatoid patients and noted that his findings were a rediscovery of an initial observation by Meyer (1922).

The independent rediscovery of the reaction by Rose et al in 1948 was a stimulus to more extensive investigation of its diagnostic possibilities, and at the same time sowed the seed of immunological interpretation of pathogenesis in systemic connective tissue disease. The rheumatoid serum factor responsible for the Rose–Waaler reaction had the properties of a high molecular weight (IgM) gammaglobulin, and numerous modifications of the test, mostly depending on agglutination or flocculation of coated erythrocytes or other particles, were rapidly developed in attempts to improve its diagnostic efficiency.

Results with the latex particle agglutination test of Singer & Plotz (1956) and the F2 (tanned sheep cell) test of Jacobson et al (1956) clearly showed that whether antibody or not, the essential feature of the reactant coating the particles of red cells used in such tests is that it is gammaglobulin. They also showed that the gammaglobulin need not necessarily be from another species (e.g. rabbit in the Rose–Waaler test), but can be of human origin. Human group O, D-positive red cells coated with incomplete anti-D antibody from a rhesus-immunised subject were found to be equally agglutinable by many rheumatoid sera (Waller & Vaughan, 1956). It was Grubb's (1956) observation that some human sera inhibit agglutination when added to such a system that first revealed the existence of human gammaglobulin (or Gm) groups or allotypes, analogous to blood groups. This led to the realisation that there are alleles of the gene codings for the polypeptide chains of antibody molecules, and initiated the genetic analysis of allotypic markers. Grubb's discovery, together with emergence of evidence that in fact rheumatoid sera contain at least three types of factor, reactive with human, with rabbit, or with both human and rabbit IgG (Milgrom et al, 1962; Williams & Kunkel, 1963), emphasised the resemblance of the heterogeneity of rheumatoid factor activity to the cross-reactivity long recognised as typical of the behaviour of antibodies against protein antigens. The concept of rheumatoid factors as antiglobulin antibodies directed at human IgG thereafter assumed the central position in hypotheses of the autoimmune basis of rheumatoid arthritis from which it has yet to be dislodged.

Specificity of rheumatoid factors

The IgG molecule consists of two pairs of linked light and heavy polypeptide chains, composed of sequences of some 200 and 400 amino acids respectively. The enzyme papain splits it into large fragments, two of which (Fab fragments) retain the antigen binding property of intact antibody. The third, the Fc fragment, carries amino acid sequences whose conformation determines the various biological activities of IgG and also distinguishes the immunoglobulin classes and most allotypes. These sequences, like the idiotypic sequences which determine epitope binding specificity in the Fab portions, are genetically coded. Rheumatoid factor binds readily and selectively to Fc fragments, but it was for long a matter of doubt whether the binding sites on the free fragments are physically accessible in the intact native IgG molecule. It was known that another series of antiglobulin antibodies, the pepsin agglutinators, which are present in high titres in some chronic suppurative infections, but not in rheumatoid arthritis, react with sites on Fab fragments which are only revealed after proteolytic digestion (Waller et al, 1969).

The ability of human sera with high titres of classical rheumatoid factor to precipitate some gammaglobulin preparations (Epstein et al, 1956) and the fact that it needs heat-aggregated IgG to effect such precipitation (Edelman et al, 1958) gave rise to the notion that rheumatoid factor reactivity must be directed towards sites unmasked on conformationally altered IgG, such as might be exposed by configurational change brought about by the antibody molecule combining with its complementary antigen (Glynn et al, 1957). Alternatively, the aggregation process might merely be linking together 'univalent' IgG molecules to form a 'multivalent' antigen capable of forming a precipitation lattice with rheumatoid factor (Henney & Stanworth, 1965).

Large protein complexes (22s) identified in the sera of some rheumatoid patients proved to be dissociable into IgM with rheumatoid factor activity, and a monomeric IgG moiety (Franklin et al, 1957); and subsequently similar large complexes were artifically assembled in vitro by reacting purified IgM rheumatoid factor in the ultracentrifuge with aggregate-free monomeric preparations of normal IgG (Schur & Kunkel, 1965). These findings seemed to point to rheumatoid factors being autoantibodies against native autologous IgG. Against this interpretation, however, there was still a consistent failure to demonstrate reactivity between rheumatoid factor and autologous gammaglobulin, either in tanned cell haemagglutination systems (Fudenburg & Franklin, 1965) or in haemagglutination tests using human red cells coated with incomplete antibodies from the same patient (Milgrom & Witebsky, 1961). Again, only aggregated gammaglobulin effectively inhibited agglutination of sheep erythrocytes coated with human anti-sheep antibody (Aho et al, 1964). Furthermore, rather than autospecificity, the allotype reactivity of rheumatoid factors often appeared to display isospecificity, i.e. a preference for Gm or other allotypic determinants absent in each patient's own gammaglobulin. These paradoxes were largely resolved when it was shown that separation of the IgM fraction from rheumatoid sera by gel filtration at pH 4.0 dissociates bound IgG and releases the missing autoreactivity, which becomes demonstrable by, for example, agglutination of anti-D coated human cells, and totally inhibitable by addition of the patient's own serum, her isolated IgG, or serum from all normal subjects tested (Allen & Kunkel, 1966).

Further evidence that rheumatoid factor has a major autospecific reactivity with native IgG came from rheumatoid patients who had been immunised with sheep red cell stromata. Serum IgM from these patients, separated from inhibiting IgG by fractionation at acid pH, proved capable of agglutinating sheep erythrocytes coated with autologous IgG antibody, although their whole sera did not (Bandilla & McDuffie, 1969). In both investigations effects due to allotype, denaturation and immune complex formation could be excluded.

Dissociation and inhibition experiments by Allen & Kunkel (1966) and Gaarder & Natvig (1970) showed that the autospecificity of rheumatoid factors is well defined, being directed at determinants on the Fc part of IgG heavy chains, at least some of which are independent of Gm allotype. Williams & Kunkel (1965) and Glynn (1963) separately reached the conclusion that the factors in rheumatoid arthritis sera which exhibit certain Gm-specificities are not directed against the Gm sites at all, but against a neighbouring epitope influenced only in degree of exposure by the Gm sites.

This, the 'general' rheumatoid factor reactive determinant (Aho et al, 1965; Natvig & Turner, 1970), is thus structurally distinct from nearby Fc allotype markers of the Gm series, and is sited, probably as a complex dependent upon the configuration of the molecule as a whole (Stewart et al, 1973), in the C-terminal half of the Cγ2 'domain' (Hunneyball & Stanworth, 1976). Such a site probably corresponds with the isotypic Ga epitope present on IgG1, IgG2 and IgG4 subclasses, and on rabbit IgG (Johnson & Faulk, 1976). At least one other site of reactivity with rheumatoid factor seems to be present on an adjacent part (the Cγ3 domain) of the Fc fragment of any given IgG molecule (Steward et al, 1973).

Measurement of the binding constants of rheumatoid factor subunits for native and for aggregated human gammaglobulin, and for rabbit gammaglobulin, have shown that all three reactants yield values which, while low in comparison with other antigen antibody systems ($3–5 \times 10^5$ L/M), are virtually identical (Normansell, 1971, 1972).

Thus, despite the bewildering array of reactions with native, altered, autologous, homologous and heterologous gammaglobulins that has been used to demonstrate rheumatoid factor activity, there is a good measure of agreement that 'rheumatoid factor' consists of a set of separate antibody specificities each specific for part of a complex determinant, and that unique parts of the determinant are masked in each species tested (Normansell, 1972). That these specificities arise as autoimmune responses in rheumatoid arthritis is not seriously disputed. What imparts so striking an immunogenic property to autologous gammaglobulin in these patients is a question under intensive renewed study.

Non-rheumatoid antiglobulins

Only 25% of seropositive individuals in random population samples present clinical evidence of rheumatoid arthritis (Ball & Lawrence, 1961; Cathcard & O'Sullivan, 1969). In several population sample studies, there has been a tendency for the proportion of positive tests to be greater in older age-groups (Valkenburg, 1963), the incidence even of Rose–Waaler positives exceeding 5% by the age of 60 in some reports (Bartfield, 1969; Ball & Lawrence, 1961). At any age, the subsequent incidence of rheumatoid arthritis in positive reactors without previous histories of polyarthritis is low (Cathcart & O'Sullivan, 1969), even when titres are persistently high (Waller & Toone, 1968).

Among non-rheumatoid conditions in which RFs have been found, sometimes at high titres, are some bacterial and viral infections (especially viral hepatitis and infectious mononucleosis), some chronic infections and parasitic conditions (tuberculosis, leprosy, schistosomiasis, trypanosomiasis, and visceral larvae migrans) paraproteinaemias (when the RF activity is monoclonal) (Bartfield, 1969) and some chronic fibrosing lung diseases (Turner-Warwick & Haslam, 1971). In subacute bacterial endocarditis about half the patients studied have had positive latex tests, correlating with raised serum IgG levels and duration of disease (Messner et al, 1968) and disappearing after successful treatment (Williams & Kunkel, 1962). In seropositive non-rheumatoid conditions reactions with human IgG are more frequent than with rabbit IgG, but there are many instances where both are present.

Although RF reactive with rabbit IgG is aggregated in families, families of hospital patients with seropositive arthritis do not have significantly more RF than expected, nor than the families of patients with seronegative arthritis (Lawrence, 1970). This seems to point to disease processes rather than genetic disposition being the most usual causes of RF production.

Sensitivity and clinical specificity of RF tests

Table 12.1 illustrates the relationship between sensitivity and clinical specificity in testing for RFs, as exemplified by results by three methods, the DAT, a latex tube agglutination test, and the FII test, the two latter measuring anti-human IgG activity, the former anti-rabbit. It will be seen that, at the level of sensitization with rabbit amboceptor used in this series, the DAT results show good specificity, but less sensitivity for a diagnosis of rheumatoid arthritis. Greenbury (1960) showed that increasing the level of sensitisation of the sheep red cells increases the number of positives obtained with rheumatoid arthritis sera, but this imposes a requirement for greater technical expertise to maintain reproducibility, and the effect produced may not be consistent (Anderson & Cooper, 1970). The Rose–Waaler and DAT tests require sensitised sheep cells

Table 12.1 Antiglobulin antibodies (rheumatoid factors) in health and rheumatic disease (modified from Zutshi et al, 1969).

	Number	Age (range) (years)	DAT+ (%)	Latex +/++ (%)	FII titre 1/200 or more (%)	FII titre Mean tube titre[a]
1. Control subjects						
Healthy	70	39 (17–80)	0	0	11	1.4
Sick adults	71	40 (16–82)	0	4	16	1.2
Chest disease (adults)	65	53 (16–76)	1.5	11	26	1.8
2. Degenerative joint disease	84	57 (33–76)	1.2	1.2	20	1.7
3. Rheumatoid arthritis						
Classical/definite	435	53 (18–84)	42	75	87	7.4
Probable/possible	69	50 (20–79)	5	30	50	3.8
4. Ankylosing spondylitis	65	38 (15–65)	0	1	31	2.1
5. Gout	52	56 (31–80)	2	6	21	1.8

[a]Tube 1 = 1/25; tube 2 = 1/50; tube 3 = 1/100 . . . tube 10 = 1/12 800

freshly prepared for each batch of sera to be tested. Formalin-treated sheep red cells precoated with denatured rabbit IgG and lyophilised have been shown to reconstitute satisfactorily with distilled water to provide a reagent giving reproducible results comparable with those by other sheep cell methods (Finnie et al, 1974). A sheep cell reagent in this form (the RAHA test) is commercially available. The latex test in Table 12.1 was performed by a simple tube method at 1 : 20 serum dilution. It gave a higher percentage of positive results than the DAT in rheumatoid disease, but also a significant number of positives in non-rheumatoid conditions. If the latex test is titrated, the end-point taken as positive may be selected to give results more closely correlated with those by the DAT or other sheep cell agglutination tests (Ball et al, 1962), but nevertheless, some sera are positive in one but not both tests, and some remain negative. Table 12.1 shows that a sensitive test such as the FII test further increases the level of positivity among RA sera, but at the expense of a significant increase in the incidence of positives in non-rheumatoid patients and healthy people. This loss of diagnostic specificity of positive reactions is to some extent offset, however, by the much higher mean titre of rheumatoid sera in this type of test.

An alternative method of determining rheumatoid factor levels which is in increasing laboratory use is nephelometric measurement of increased light scattering by serum following the addition of soluble heat aggregated IgG. Comparison of the merits of agglutination methods and nephelometry has shown that the latter is both technically simple and more reliable than traditional sheep cell agglutination techniques, which may lack precision (Knight & Pritchard, 1982).

Cross-reactivity of RFs

Antibody specificities have also been ascribed to RF for antigenic determinants other than those of IgG. Reactivity of IgM RF with dinitrophenyl and trinitrophenyl groups was observed by Hannestad (1967). Several more recent reports have described cross-reactivity of a majority of isolated IgM RF preparations with epitopes present in normal cell nuclei (Johnson, 1981). In whole seropositive sera this reactivity is masked by the presence of excess IgG, so it is evidently a true cross-reaction. The epitopes in question appear to require the presence of both intact DNA and core histone protein for their expression, and thus are probably (like the Ga site with which rheumatoid factors normally react) strongly dependent on molecular conformation.

Molecular restriction of RFs

Although polyclonal, a marked kappa light chain predominance in the RF of rheumatoid patients compared with normal serum $\kappa : \lambda$ ratios has been noted, which is echoed in the antiglobulins of subacute bacterial endocarditis and in monoclonal macroglobulinaemic proteins with antiglobulin activity (Carson & Lawrence, 1978; Kunkel et al, 1974).

Isolated IgM RFs from rheumatoid patients also show restriction to one of the three possible kappa chain variable regions subgroups, often the V_H3 subgroup (Førre et al, 1977). Furthermore, cross-idiotypic specificities have been identified in polyclonal IgM RFs from different patients (Førre et al 1979) which may be inheritable (Pasquali et al, 1980). There is thus evidence that production of RFs in rheumatoid patients is clonally restricted, and of sharing of clones between patients.

IgG rheumatoid factor

Since it has subsequently appeared that IgG RFs contribute to the formation of pathogenic immune complexes in rheumatoid joints and probably extra-articularly as well, much attention has been given to developing methods of measuring IgG RF levels in serum and joint fluids separately from IgM RF. IgG RF is a poor agglutinator of IgG-coated particles, and hence indirect solid phase assays have had to be used for its detection. These have mostly taken the form of radioimmunoassay (Hay et al, 1979; Allen et al, 1981) or lately of enzyme-linked immunosorbent assay (ELISA) (March et al, 1982; Faith et al, 1982).

These methods use labelled antisera specific for human IgG or its specific Fab (Fd) determinants, and have the advantage that, by extending the range of anti-isotype specificities separately used, the laboratory performing them can measure IgM, IgG and IgA antiglobulin levels in parallel.

Incidence of raised RF levels in rheumatoid disease

IgM rheumatoid factors. As with many serum antibodies, the distribution of titres of RF is a continuous variable within any given population (Lawrence, 1965) so that any level chosen to separate the 'seropositive' from the 'seronegative' is arbitrary. In practice it is chosen to include as many patients clinically acceptable as rheumatoid, and to exclude as many non-rheumatoid subjects as possible. The latex slide test is usually performed at a serum dilution of 1 : 20, while in tube tests a titre of 1 : 40 (sometimes 1 : 80) or more in the latex test, and 1 : 16 or more in the sheep cell differential agglutination test (DAT) are usually taken as positive. The frequency of latex seropositivity in patients with clinical features of rheumatoid disease (American Rheumatism Association criteria) is 70–80%. As noted above, however, antiglobulin activity of IgM class cannot be equated simply with a diagnosis of rheumatoid arthritis.

Hidden and low molecular weight IgM RF. In some rheumatoid arthritis patients the reactivity of IgM RF in the serum is masked by its complexing with circulating IgG. This has been noted in certain cases of apparently seronegative nodular rheumatoid disease and of juvenile chronic polyarthritis (Moore et al, 1978).

Low molecular weight IgM (LMW IgM) is the monomeric subunit of pentameric IgM. LMW IgM is not present in normal serum, but levels are often high in rheumatoid sera, especially in rheumatoid vasculitis and Felty's syndrome (Roberts-Thompson et al, 1981). LMW IgM is also commonly found in systemic lupus erythematosus, primary biliary cirrhosis, Sjögren's syndrome, and in other conditions in which RF levels are raised. In RA sera a proportion (up to 40%) of LMW IgM is LMW IgM RF, levels of which correlate with those of the more usual pentameric IgM RF.

IgG rheumatoid factors. The measurement of IgG RFs is complicated by normal IgG being identified as IgG antiglobulin owing to complexing with IgM antiglobulin, and by self-association of IgG antiglobulin molecules modifying their reactivity.

Raised levels of IgG antiglobulins are usually found in patients with raised IgM RF levels (Carson et al, 1977; March et al, 1982). In seropositive adult RA, Wernick et al (1981) found levels (μg/ml) of IgG RF 100 times that of normals and 2.5 times that of IgM RF in the same patients, although IgM has long been regarded as the predominant class of RF in rheumatoid sera. Levels of IgG RFs are reported to be significantly higher in rheumatoid patients with nodules (Hay et al, 1979) or vasculitis (Allen et al, 1981) than in those without. There is lack of agreement about levels of IgG antiglobulins in normal subjects and in seronegative rheumatoid patients (Carson et al, 1977; Allen et al, 1981) which probably reflects methodological differences. The use of tests for IgG RF in a clinical context has so far added little to improve diagnosis or management of rheumatoid disease. The diagnosis of seronegative rheumatoid arthritis is in practice arrived at cautiously by exclusion, since it is well recognised that in joint disease provisionally so labelled, psoriasis, ankylosing spondylitis, inflammatory bowel disease and urethritis are all features more commonly present than in seropositive RA.

The biological role of rheumatoid factors

The physiological role of non-rheumatoid antiglobulins is not clear, but they may contribute both to defence mechanisms against infection, and to immunoregulation. The demonstration that the anti-IgG specificity of non-rheumatoid RFs may be against Fab rather than Fc fragments (March, 1983) is consistent with the concept of the latter function.

In experimental conditions, human rheumatoid RF can play a part in neutralising virus complexes with antibody, perhaps by assisting complement to cover the virion, and there is evidence also that RF can compete with complement for sites on the IgG molecule (Heimer & Levin, 1965; Tesar & Schmidt, 1970).

Rheumatoid factors and complement activation

The ability of RF to fix complement is of central relevance to the question of its immunopathogenetic potential. In vitro studies of the complement-fixing property of IgM RF did not prosper until the reactant, IgG antibody or aggregated IgG, was used in a reduced and alkylated form in which its own anti-complementary activity was blocked. Reacting with this material at 37°C IgM RF fixed human, though not guinea-pig complement through its own complement attachment sites (Zvaifler & Schur, 1968). Non-rheumatoid RF, whether monoclonal IgM RF or polyclonal (Bianco et al, 1974) was reported to be non-complement fixing, but whether this is a valid differentiating property between rheumatoid and non-rheumatoid RFs remains unsettled (March, 1983).

In the rheumatoid joint where they are synthesised, rheumatoid factors, both in their self-associative IgG form and in their IgM form reactive with the latter, activate complement (also locally synthesised by macrophages) through their complement attachment sites via the classical pathway (Zvaifler & Schur, 1968). The immunopathogenic role of RFs in rheumatoid synovitis is discussed fully in the next chapter, but it may be mentioned here that although binding of serum RFs to the reactive 'general rheumatoid' determinants on IgG molecules is inhibited better by rabbit than human IgG, the reactivity of RFs synthesised by lymphoid cells in the rheumatoid synovial membrane itself is more readily inhibited by human than by rabbit IgG, and is of considerably higher affinity (Robbins et al, 1978). The monomeric IgG molecule behaves as a univalent antigen in its reaction with RF (Normansell, 1970), but the predominance of self-associating IgG RF in the rheumatoid joint favours the spontaneous formation of intra-articular complexes of IgG composition. These two features of locally produced IgG RFs in rheumatoid joints — the linking of univalent IgG RF molecules to form multivalent aggregates, and the higher affinity of articular RFs — combine to promote formation of polymeric complexes composed of IgG and IgM which have an augmented complement fixing property, as the low levels of the early complement components C, C4 and C2, and of C3, in rheumatoid synovial fluids attest.

The immunopathogenic role of rheumatoid factors in rheumatoid synovitis and extra-articular rheumatoid disease

This aspect is also discussed in other chapters (Chs. 13, 24). The ability of rheumatoid RF to fix complement is a crucial factor is production of rheumatoid synovitis, for a striking difference between non-rheumatoid seropositive individuals and rheumatoid patients is that in the latter a principal site of production of RF is in the affected joints themselves. Immunofluorescence shows that the IgG or IgM synthesised by many of the plasma cells in the rheumatoid synovial membrane has RF activity. In cryostat sections, this cytoplasmic immunoglobulin binds labelled IgG aggregates specifically. In many of the IgG plasma cells, the IgG RF synthesised has already undergone intracellular self-association through its binding affinity for its own Fc determinants (Pope et al, 1974), so that its anti-IgG reactivity is demonstrable only on pretreatment of sections with pepsin in order to digest and remove Fc fragments and thus free its Fab antigen combining sites (Natvig & Munthe, 1975). Conditions in the rheumatoid joint thus favour the formation of RF immune complexes of complement-activating composition.

In the circulation, self-association of IgG RF molecules is less favoured. What determines the sites of extra-articular rheumatoid lesions is ill-understood, but it is reported that the presence of circulating immune complexes containing RF, IgG and complement correlates better with the clinical manifestations of vasculitis than with synovitis (Elson et al, 1983).

ANTIBODIES AGAINST NUCLEAR ANTIGENS

Antibodies reactive with nuclear antigens have a wide distribution and a high frequency in systemic connective tissue disease, and may be directed at a wide range of nuclear antigens.

Methods of detection

The LE cell test. Incubation of fresh clotted blood from a patient with systemic lupus erythematosus leads to the formation of 'LE cells', which result from the opsonisation of exposed dead cell nuclei by antinuclear antibody ('LE cell factor') in the patients' serum and their uptake as inclusions in surviving phagocytic cells. The LE cell factor was identified as a complement-fixing IgG antibody with specificity for insoluble nucleoprotein. The presence of typical LE cells in smears from such preparations was historically the first evidence of an autoimmune reaction in SLE, and provided a uniquely useful diagnostic laboratory sign hitherto lacking (Hargraves et al, 1948).

The immunofluorescence test. Searching a stained smear for LE cells is a time consuming process, and the prolonged microscopy necessary to exclude their even scanty presence in smears has led to replacement of the LE cell test by the much more routinely applicable immunofluorescence antinuclear antibody (ANA) test (Johnson & Holborow, 1983). In the ANA test patients' sera are incubated with rat liver sections (or other sources of cell nuclei) on slides, and after washing to remove non-specifically attached protein the uptake of ANA is detected by staining with fluorescent antiglobulin conjugate. This renders the reaction visible as nuclear fluorescence in the fluorescence microscope. Positive ANA tests, unlike positive LE cell tests, are found in a wide range of conditions with autoimmune features. The immunofluorescence ANA method gives no accurate information about the nuclear antigens responsible for a positive test. Where these are soluble nuclear constituents ('extractable nuclear antigens'), haemagglutination (Sharp et al, 1972), immunodiffusion (Mattioli & Reichlin, 1971), and counter-immunoelectrophoresis (Kurata & Tan, 1976) have been successfully used to determine the specificity of the anti-nuclear reactivity. In the case of anti-DNA antibodies, radioimmunoassay with isotope labelled DNA (Farr test) has become a routine method. An entirely different method of detecting anti-DNA antibodies is based on the ability of sera to give indirect immunofluorescent staining of the kinetoplasts in smears of the haemoflagellate *Crithidia luciliae*. In this protozoan, double-stranded mitochondrial DNA is concentrated in the single cytoplasmic kinetoplast, which stains characteristically with a serum containing anti-dsDNA antibody (Aarden & Smeenk, 1981). Recently, enzyme linked immunosorbent assay methods (ELISA) have been increasingly used to measure anti-nuclear antibodies specific for several different nuclear antigens (Smeenk, 1982; Venables et al, 1983).

ANA staining patterns on immunofluorescence

Homogeneous ANA. The pattern of ANA staining given by SLE sera is often homogeneous, that is to say the nuclei in the substrate tissue or cells are seen to fluoresce evenly. Homogeneous ANA staining is usually due to antibodies against deoxyribonucleoprotein or against histones (Tan et al, 1976). Homogeneous ANA is the pattern typical of SLE (both idiopathic and drug-induced) and is present in almost all cases with active disease, usually, though not invariably, at high titre. ANA is also found with variable but less frequency in a wide range of other conditions associated with autoimmune features (Table 12.2). These include rheumatoid arthritis. The highest levels of ANA in RA are seen in patients with vasculitis, nodules or infection and in Sjögren's and Felty's syndromes, where the incidence may reach 50–60%. In patients with established RA, the incidence of ANA

Table 12.2 Some conditions in which ANA has been reported.

Systemic lupus erythematosus
Progressive systemic sclerosis
Rheumatoid arthritis
Juvenile chronic polyarthritis
Polymyositis and dermatomyositis
Sjogren's syndrome
Polyarteritis nodosa
Chronic discoid lupus erythematosus
'Lupoid' hepatitis and other autoimmune liver diseases
Hyperglobulinaemic purpura
Myasthenia gravis
Thymoma
Hashimoto's thyroiditis
Pernicious anaemia
Ulcerative colitis
Chronic membranous glomerulonephritis
Chronic bronchitis
Cryptogenic fibrosing alveolitis
Asbestosis
Infectious mononucleosis
Dermatitis herpetiformis

at serum levels at or above 25 iu/ml is, in my laboratory, 14% for males and 25% for females. These incidence figures are based on an immunofluorescence method with cryostat sections of rat liver and sheep anti-whole human Ig conjugate, calibrated against a WHO/IUIS reference standard (Holborow et al, 1982).

Speckled ANA. This is the second commonest pattern, and appears as a finely granular or powdery staining. Speckled staining is usually due to antibodies against extractable nuclear antigens soluble in physiological saline. Such antigens are readily leached from nuclei during the washing steps of immunofluorescence staining, so that sera countaining only antibodies reactive with them may appear ANA-negative. Speckled ANA is a feature of mixed connective tissue disease (MCTD) (Sharp et al, 1972), the concept of which as a disease entity is discussed in Chapter 50. In MCTD patients, and some with SLE or scleroderma only, the high titres of speckled ANA are due to autoantibody against ribonucleoprotein (nRNP). Another antibody which gives a speckled ANA pattern is directed at a different determinant, Sm, and is found only in about 30% of SLE patients. Both Sm and nRNP are in the cell nucleus. The Sm determinant is present on a series of five small nuclear RNAs complexed with protein (snRNPs), while the anti-nRNP antibody reacts with a determinant present on only one (known as U1) of the the five small nuclear RNAs complexed with protein. U1 SnRNA appears to be involved functionally in the splicing of nuclear RNA to form mature messenger RNA. These two sites of antibody binding, which are both manifest as speckled ANA, are spatially separate (Lerner et al, 1982).

Another antibody giving a speckled ANA pattern, which is found in patients with the primary sicca syndrome and some patients with SLE, is directed at yet another nuclear antigen, known as SS-B or La. This is a protein (Venables et al, 1983) associated with another class of snRNPs (Lerner et al, 1982) in cell nuclei. A third class of RNP particles, this time apparently cytoplasmic rather than nuclear, is associated with another antigen, SS-A, or Ro, antibodies against which are again found in some patients with SLE and some with sicca syndrome. In accordance with the supposed cytoplasmic location of the SS-A antigen in cells, sera containing anti-SS-A do not give ANA patterns on immunofluorescence. That antibodies to nRNP, Sm, SS-B(La) and SS-A (Ro) recognise distinct epitopes is established by immunodiffusion, radio-immunoassay and ELISA analyses of their respective reactivities (Venables et al, 1983). In addition to these RNP-related antigens, ANA-positive sera have been shown to include some that react with ribosomal RNA and transfer RNA (Lerner et al, 1982).

Other varieties of non-homogeneous ANA may be recognised. These include coarse granular staining, the granules being sparse and tending to show a peripheral distribution within the nucleus. This is often seen at low titre in sera from patients with malaria (Greenwood, 1970).

Nucleolar ANA. This is the least common pattern seen alone (often in cases of systemic sclerosis) but is a frequent constituent of mixed staining patterns. It is attributed to reaction with nuclear RNA specific to the nucleolus. The major antigen involved appears to be slowly sedimenting (4s–7s) RNA localised in the nucleus (Miyawaki

& Ritchie, 1973) and distinct from the RNA antigens which react with antiribosomal antibodies (Sturgill & Carpenter, 1965) and from the Sm and RNP antigens described above.

Granulocyte-specific ANA. A different antinuclear antibody with specificity only for granulocyte nuclei (GS-ANA) is frequently present in Felty's syndrome, and although rare in other conditions, is also present in about 75% of rheumatoid patients, and 30% of SLE patients (Faber & Elling, 1966; Elling et al, 1968), independently of the presence or absence of ANAs which are not cell-type-specific.

Reproduction of the staining patterns described above demands strict adherence to the letter of the methods which have been used to display them. Artifacts due to diffusion of nuclear materials during the staining procedure can confuse the picture (Johnson et al, 1973), and varying the dilution of the serum under test can alter the pattern of fluorescence seen. In practice, immunofluorescence is best used as a screening procedure, and antinuclear antibody specificities deduced from the appearances of the nuclear staining are best regarded as approximations requiring confirmation by more specific tests.

The clinical incidence of positive antinuclear antibody tests

The immunofluorescence ANA test

The immunofluorescence ANA test is not diagnostic for SLE (Table 12.2) and when this diagnosis is considered possible, a positive ANA test is best interpreted as indicating the need for a DNA-binding (Farr) test. It has considerable value as a screening test to exclude a diagnosis of SLE, since a patient with a negative ANA test is unlikely to have lupus.

In a given serum, ANA activity may be present in one or more of the immunoglobulin classes IgG, IgA and IgM (Barnett et al, 1964). In SLE, antinuclear staining is predominantly due to IgG, while in rheumatoid arthritis there is a preponderance of IgM-ANA (Weir & Holborow, 1962; Baum & Ziff, 1962). When IgM rheumatoid factor is also present in the serum it may interact with IgG-ANA, so that nuclei binding the latter nevertheless appear to stain exclusively for IgM (Holborow & Johnson, 1965).

Most patients with SLE, systemic sclerosis or MCTD have IgG-ANA titres significantly higher than occur in other connective tissue diseases. Notwithstanding the clinical associations claimed for different ANA staining patterns, it appears to hold that, at any rate when routine immunofluorescence methods are used, the diagnostic implications of particular staining patterns should be cautiously interpreted. A detailed discussion of this subject is given by Tan (1982).

As noted above, the highest levels and incidence of ANA in rheumatoid arthritis are seen in patients with extra-articular disease, and in Felty's syndrome. The usual pattern of ANA staining given by RA sera is homogeneous. No single nuclear antigenic specificity appears to account for the positive ANAs in RA (Table 12.3), but a preference for histone has been demonstrated by immunofluorescence monitoring of the effects of acid extraction and histone reconstitution of the tissue sections used as substrate in the test (Tan et al, 1976; Aitchison et al, 1980).

A provocative observation confirmed from several sources (Johnson, 1981) is that rheumatoid factor isolated from rheumatoid sera not infrequently shows what appears to be true cross-reactivity with core histone protein complexes in association with DNA. This reactivity is masked in whole serum by the presence of IgG, so it appears not to be due to the anti-histone antibody activity separately demonstrable in many rheu-

Table 12.3 Specificities of antinuclear antibodies in rheumatoid sera (Aitchison et al, 1980).

Nuclear antigen	Frequency of antibodies No*	%
dsDNA	2	3.5
ssDNA	4	6.8
sNP	1	1.7
Sm	1	1.7
n-RNP	1	1.7
SS-A	4	6.8
SS-B	1	1.7
Histones	14	23.7

*Total number of sera tested = 59

matoid sera. Anti-histone antibodies are also present in sera from both idiopathic and drug-induced SLE following procainamide or hydralazine therapy (Rubin et al, 1982), but differ in isotype and in their reactivity with defined histone fractions and complexes (Tan, 1982).

Antibodies against soluble cellular antigens

The *anti-Sm antibody* described above is, when present, diagnostic of SLE. Although it produces a speckled ANA pattern on immunofluorescence, this is often obscured by concomitant homogeneous nuclear staining due to other anti-nuclear antibodies. The unequivocal demonstration of anti-Sm activity depends upon immunodiffusion analysis of the patient's serum against saline extract of rabbit thymus, the appearance of a precipitation line showing identity with that given by a reference serum confirming the specificity. In view of this, and the fact that it is present only in about 30% of SLE patients, the diagnostic usefulness of anti-Sm is limited.

Anti-nRNP antibody, although associated with certain clinical features (Raynaud's phenomenon, myositis, pulmonary fibrosis) lacks specificity as a diagnostic marker. This is fully discussed in Chapter 50.

Anti-SS-A and *anti-SS-B antibodies*, as we have already seen, are both associated clinically with the sicca syndrome alone and with Sjögren's syndrome in association with SLE. In Sjögren's syndrome associated with rheumatoid arthritis, however, anti-SS-B is not present, and anti-SS-A only infrequently (Alspaugh et al, 1976). Antibodies to extractable nuclear antigen, possibly anti-SS-A, were found in a majority of rheumatoid patients with extra-articular disease, digital vasculitis and circulating immune complexes with low serum complement levels being common features (Venables et al, 1980).

It has been reported (Wasicek & Reichlin, 1982) that in SLE patients with both anti-SS-A and anti-SS-B in their sera lupus nephritis is unusual, while a majority of SLE patients with anti-SS-A alone develop nephritis. This difference is reflected in a lower frequency of anti-DNA antibodies in patients with both anti-SS-A and anti-SS-B in their sera (Reichlin, 1982).

ANA-negative SLE. Patients with clinical features consistent with a diagnosis of SLE but nevertheless with sera negative on routine ANA testing have in some cases proved positive for anti-SS-A and/or anti-SS-B antibodies. Although negative for ANA on liver tissue sections, such sera may prove ANA-positive on cultured epithelial cell lines, at any rate if they contain anti-SS-B.

Anti-SS-A has also been found in neonatal lupus, both in the infant and the mother. The mother may be symptomless or have features of Sjögren's syndrome or SLE (Tan, 1982). There is also evidence that pregnant women with anti-SS-A are at risk of delivering an infant with congenital heart block (Maddison et al, 1983).

ANA in systemic sclerosis

Antinuclear antibodies are demonstrable by immunofluorescence in most patients with systemic sclerosis, especially when sera are tested on monolayers of tissue culture cells such as HEp-2. Patterns of staining seen are nucleolar and speckled, the antibody responsible for the latter also giving a pattern showing the characteristic clustering of chromatids during telophase in cells undergoing mitosis. This antibody has specificity for centromeres. Anti-centromere antibody is highly specific for the variant of systemic sclerosis characterised by 4 or all 5 of the features calcinosis, Raynaud's phenomenon, oesophageal dysmotility, sclerodactyly or acrosclerosis without diffuse scleroderma, and telangiectasia. More than 50% of patients with this so-called 'CREST' syndrome have this antibody. In interphase HEp-2 cells anti-centromere antibody gives a fluorescence pattern of large round granules. Another antibody reactive on immunodiffusion with a cell nuclear protein (Scl-70) has been found only in scleroderma, and on immunofluorescence gives a diffuse grainy pattern of nucleoplasmic staining (Douvas et al, 1979).

Antinuclear antibodies in juvenile chronic polyarthritis

The commonest mode of presentation among the seronegative childhood arthritides is with few (1–4) affected joints and little evidence of systemic disease. Within this category of pauciarticular juvenile chronic polyarthritis there is an important subgroup of young children particularly liable to develop a chronic insidious iridocyclitis with band opacities of the cornea, cataract and glaucoma as complications (see Ch. 43). An important marker identifying patients at risk is a positive immunofluorescent ANA test, which is found in at least 80% of such children with chronic iridocyclitis, usually preceding its development (Schaller, 1977).

Intracellular nuclear Ig deposits. Immunofluorescence studies of skin biopsies from patients with clinical features of MCTD, SLE or polymyositis and with serum antibodies to extractable nuclear antigens (usually nRNP) have shown speckled staining due to in vivo IgG deposits in the nuclei of epidermal cells of apparently normal skin (Andersen et al, 1983). Evidence of the ability of certain anti-nuclear antibodies to penetrate into living cells has been provided by Alarçon-Segovia (1981) who found that IgG anti-RNP antibody purified from the serum of an MCTD patient can penetrate living blood mononuclear cells in vitro, via Fcγ receptors on these cells. Further, intranuclear immunoglobulins have been observed by the same worker in a proportion of the circulating mononuclear cells in patients with MCTD, and in some patients with SLE, but in none with rheumatoid arthritis or scleroderma. Evidence was also adduced suggesting that this process of in vivo penetration of cells by IgG antinuclear antibody could lead to loss of T cells of suppressor type. More studies are needed to substantiate these findings.

Anti-RANA antibody. A third antibody reactive with a soluble cellular antigen was described by Alspaugh et al (1976). At first designated 'anti-SS-C', it was renamed 'rheumatoid arthritis precipitin' (RAP), since it was found in a majority of rheumatoid patients. RAP-positive sera were found to give a fine speckled staining pattern on unfixed cells of certain lymphoblastoid cell lines, which was attributed to the presence in these cells of a 'rheumatoid arthritis nuclear antigen' (RANA). RANA is apparently present only in human B lymphocytes transformed by Epstein–Barr virus. While Ferrell & Tan (1981) confirm the presence of anti-RANA antibody in a majority of seropositive RA subjects, with a less than 10% incidence in normal subjects, Venables et al (1981) have found a considerably higher incidence in normals. Studies of levels of Epstein–Barr virus antibodies in RA have produced somewhat conflicting results, but agree that there is a lack of complete concordance between their presence and the presence of anti-RANA. At the same time, evidence has been forthcoming that the in vitro response of rheumatoid lymphocytes to Epstein–Barr virus (EBV) infection is abnormal. When blood lymphocytes are exposed to EBV and cultured, the B cells infected undergo polyclonal activation, producing and secreting immunoglobulins. Virus-induced transformation of the B cells may then lead to emergence of permanent cell lines. With normal lymphocytes, such outgrowth is influenced and controlled by the regulatory activity of T cells present in the culture, but this T cell function is reported to be defective in RA, while rheumatoid B cells appear to transform more readily than normal cells on exposure to EBV (Stierle et al, 1983). Thus, although there is little evidence to implicate EBV in the causation of rheumatoid arthritis, EBV is a useful tool to reveal the immunoregulatory defect in RA which may prove to explain the autoantibody production typical of the disease and its variants.

Anti-DNA antibodies

In patients with active SLE, anti-nuclear factors are almost invariably, and antibodies to nucleoprotein and DNA are usually present, while serum haemolytic complement is low, especially in patients with renal disease. The finding of bound immunoglobulin and complement components in deposits in the glomeruli of lupus kidneys, together with experimental evidence that immune complexes formed under appropriate conditions of immunisation produce chronic glomerulonephritis through their deposition in the kidney (Dixon et al, 1961), led to investigation of the role of immune complexes involving nuclear antigens in the pathogenesis of lupus nephritis. Eluates from glomeruli of lupus kidney proved to contain not only a remarkably high concentration of elutable anti-nuclear antibodies, especially anti-DNA antibody, but also DNA itself. After dissociation of bound immunoglobulin from combination with the glomeruli, DNA was specifically and distinctly stainable with fluorescein-labelled anti-DNA antibody which had been isolated from SLE serum, the stained material showing the same coarsely granular distribution on the basement membrane as the immunoglobulin and complement deposits (Koffler et al, 1967). High titre serum anti-DNA antibodies, low serum complement levels and active renal disease (Schur & Sandson, 1968) thus appeared largely explicable as the correlates of immune complex formation, with DNA and anti-DNA as major protagonists. It seems probable that, at any rate with regard to lupus nephritis, complexes are for the most part formed in situ at the glomerular basement membranes affected, since the latter have a particular affinity for DNA (Izui et al, 1976). There is conflicting evidence as to whether or not the circulating complexes in SLE patients contain DNA (Izui et al, 1977; Bruneau & Benveniste, 1979). Another question is whether subpopulations of antibodies to DNA are especially nephritogenic (Hahn, 1982). For these reasons, and for their diagnostic implications, anti-DNA antibodies in SLE are the subject of unremitting clinical and laboratory investigation.

Initial studies that showed the presence of anti-DNA antibodies in patients with lupus led to the conclusion that three main groups of anti-DNA specificity could be identified. These are:

1. Antibodies reactive exclusively with single stranded DNA (ssDNA) and combining primarily with various combinations of single purine or pyrimidine bases, the analogous nucleosides and nucleotides, and with oligonucleotides containing mixed purine–pyrimidine sequences. All these distinct antibody specificities are related to co-existing reactivity with ssDNA molecules.
2. Antibodies combining with epitopes on the deoxyribose phosphate backbone of the DNA molecule which are common to both ds and ssDNA.
3. A rare type of antibody reacting preferentially with dsDNA.

The so-called 'anti-double-stranded DNA' antibodies which are characteristic of SLE have for the most part the second (ss and ds) specificity noted above.

Methods of detecting anti-DNA antibodies

The most widely used technique for measuring anti-DNA antibodies is the Farr radio-immunoassay, which has the advantage of being a primary binding method. It depends upon the precipitation of antibody-bound labelled DNA by half-saturated ammonium sulphate.

The precision and accuracy of the Farr assay are much influenced by the reaction conditions. It has for long been asserted that a prime requirement is the purity of the dsDNA used as antigen, and the standardisation of its molecular weight. The latter is clearly important, since binding of even a single IgG antibody molecule to a DNA molecule leads to its precipitation in the Farr assay (Aarden et al, 1976a). Avoidance of single stranded regions in the dsDNA molecule has been sought by the use of circular dsDNA from the bacteriophage PM2 (Aarden, 1976b). The Farr test does not detect immunoglobulin directly, and binding of non-immunoglobulin components may occur during the test owing to the strong negative charge on DNA molecules. The greater flexibility of ssDNA leads to serum components binding to it with higher avidity than to dsDNA, according to Aarden &Smeenk (1981). It might thus be argued that provided the immunoglobulin nature of the serum component binding to DNA in an assay is established, the strandedness of the DNA is immaterial. This question remain open.

The Farr assay method is limited by the dissociating effect of the high salt concentration at the precipitation stage, and also by the rise in pH due to loss of carbonic acid during incubation, both of which favour detection of high avidity antibody. A modification of the assay method in which 3.5% polyethylene glycol (PEG) (MW 6000) is used to precipitate the antibody-bound DNA has been introduced by Smeenk & Aarden (1980). This requires dextran sulphate to be incorporated in the test mixture to prevent high DNA binding with normal sera as a result of interaction with low-density lipoproteins. This PEG assay detects a population of anti-DNA antibody molecules missed by the Farr method because their low avidity makes them salt-labile.

The *Crithidia* test differs in kind from the other tests described above, since it provides direct evidence of the Ig nature of the DNA binding protein in the test serum. It can in fact be used to determine the isotype of the antibody. The *Crith-*

idia test is relatively simple and reliable and avoids the use of isotopes; it is thus suitable for routine screening of sera for DNA antibodies. Unlike the Farr test it is not dependent on avidity, but as an immunofluorescence test involving titration it is only semiquantitative. For accurate measurement of anti-DNA antibody levels without recourse to isotypes, ELISA tests with dsDNA or ssDNA bound to the wells of plastic plates by an intervening layer of protamine sulphate have been developed (Klotz et al, 1979). These have the same advantage of directly assaying Ig molecules with anti-DNA activity.

The clinical incidence of anti-dsDNA antibodies

The different assay methods described above each appear to detect a different fraction of the total spectrum of anti-DNA antibodies which may be present in patients' sera (Table 12.4). The Farr assay with its selectivity for high avidity antibody is the most useful diagnostic test at present. Definitely raised binding values are rarely found in diseases other than SLE, and then only in occasional cases of Sjögren's syndrome, rheumatoid arthritis, chronic active hepatitis and discoid lupus. The *Crithidia* test is a useful and relatively easily performed screening test positive in many SLE patients, but may miss some patients with low or moderate levels of antibody in the Farr test, presumably for reasons unconnected with avidity. The PEG test, used routinely, is reported to give positive results not only in patients fulfilling the disgnostic criteria for SLE (Tan et al, 1982), but also some in whom the diagnosis remains uncertain (Swaak et al, 1982a). Among the latter, signs of renal involvement were found to be present more often in those with positive Farr tests, and signs of central nervous system involvement more often in those with negative Farr tests.

Table 12.4 Comparison of PEG assay, ELISA, *Crithidia* and Farr assay on 289 sera (Smeenk, 1982)

PEG assay	ELISA	Crithidia	Farr assay	Number of sera
+	+	+	+	22
+	+	+	−	22
−	+	+	+	7
+	+	−	−	15
+	−	+	−	2
−	+	+	−	3
−	+	−	+	1
+	−	−	−	33
−	+	−	−	23
−	−	+	−	3
−	−	−	−	158
94	93	59	30	289

A high level of anti-dsDNA antibodies in the serum, while of diagnostic value, does not necessarily imply or predict disease activity (Hughes, 1979a). Changes in antibody levels have been studied by Swaak et al (1982b), who find that exacerbations as judged by major signs (Lightfoot & Hughes, 1976) are preceded by a continuous increase in anti-dsDNA levels with a doubling time of 6–10 weeks. The onset of clinical activity in the patients studied was immediately preceded by a sharp fall in antibody levels. In contrast (as noted above) patients with a constant high level of antibody may show no major signs of active disease. These observations indicate the value of serial antibody determinations.

Antinuclear antibodies in drug-induced SLE

The incidence of ANA and other autoantibodies during administration of hydralazine, procainamide and some other drugs is shown in Table 12.5. A small proportion of patients producing ANA may develop arthralgia, pleurisy and other features of SLE, but not nephritis (Ch. 53). The presence of ANA is detected by immunofluorescence, but a follow-up Farr test is negative, and antibodies against ssDNA are but rarely found. The ANA reactivity is mainly directed at nuclear histones (Fritzler & Tan, 1978). ANAs induced by procainamide and hydralazine react with histones of different classes (Tan & Portanona, 1981). In hydralazine-induced disease three genetic features act in concert to determine which patients develop this form of lupus — female sex, slow acetylator phenotype and HLA-DR4 tissue type (Batchelor et al, 1980).

Lymphocytotoxic antibodies

Antibodies reactive with lymphocyte surface antigens are present in most SLE patients. These are complement-dependent IgM antibodies, maxi-

Table 12.5 Approximate prevalence of autoimmune phenomena associated with the use of selected drugs. (Reproduced with permission from A S Russell. Clinics in Immunology and Allergy 1: 59.)

Drug	% developing the 'marker' autoantibody	% with 'autoimmune' disease
Procainamide	75	20
Hydralazine	50	10
Methyldopa	15[a]	0.1[b]
Practolol	20	<0.1
Chlorpromazine	20	exceedingly rare
Isoniazid	20	<0.5
Anti-epileptics	20	<0.5
Venocuran	90[c]	10
Penicillamine	0.5[d]	0.5[e]
	25[f]	

[a] Positive direct Coombs' test and ANA (similar frequency)
[b] Haemolytic anaemia, never lupus
[c] Antibodies to mitochondria
[d] Antibodies to acetylcholine receptor
[f] Antibodies to striated muscle
[e] Myasthenia gravis. Other diseases, pemphigus, immune complex glomerulonephritis, and even a lupus syndrome, are also seen but the prevalence is uncertain.

mally cytotoxic at 15°C and unable to kill cells at 37°C; and IgG antibodies reactive at 37°C but not cytotoxic (Charlesworth et al, 1983). The temperature-dependent cytotoxic activity of sera from SLE patients against autologous and allogeneic lymphocytes has, at least in part, specificity for common structures in the HLA-A and HLA-B antigenic molecular complex, and is directed also against HLA-DR antigens, and in the same study lymphocytoxins of similar anti-HLA specificities were found in the relatives of SLE patients (Messner et al, 1980). IgG antibodies preferentially cytotoxic for mitogen activated lymphocytes have also been found in a majority of SLE patients tested (Winfield et al, 1982).

The lymphopenia in SLE correlates to some extent with increasing activity of anti-lymphocyte antibodies, but direct evidence of a causal relationship is lacking.

There is some experimental evidence that anti-lymphocyte antibodies in SLE react directly with T cells involved in the generation of suppressor cells, and might thus favour hyperactivity of B cells and autoantibody production (Morimoto et al, 1979). Defective T suppressor cell generation in vitro has not been substantiated however Tsokos & Balow, 1982).

Anti-lymphocyte antibodies in SLE have been shown to cross-react with placental trophoblast antigens, and it has been suggested that this may explain the high incidence of spontaneous abortion in SLE patients. Antibodies against lymphocytes are reported to the absent during pregnancy in SLE patients, except in pregnancies ending in abortion (Hughes, 1979b).

Circulating lymphocytotoxic antibodies also appear to be associated with central nervous system involvement in SLE, since anti-lymphocyte antibodies in patients with CNS disease are absorbed from serum with brain tissue, whereas those in patients without CNS disease are not. An anti-neuronal antibody, the titre of which correlates with CNS disease activity is also described in SLE (Bresnihan et al, 1979). IgG anti-neuronal activity was similarly much higher in cerebrospinal fluid from lupus patients with active CNS disease than without (Bluestein & Woods, 1982).

Anti-collagen and anti-cartilage antibodies

Antibodies against cartilage detected by immunofluorescence have been found in patients with the rare condition relapsing polychondritis (Ebringer et al, 1981). In sera from 3% of a large group of rheumatoid subjects, Greenbury & Skingle (1979) found similar anti-cartilage antibody, which could be absorbed out with type 2 collagen. Using a fluoremetric assay, Beard et al (1979) also found only 3% of RA sera contained antibody to native type 2 collagen.

Three different antigenic sites on the triple helical conformation of the native collagen molecule or its constituent polypeptide chains are recognised by antibodies produced by immunising animals with soluble native collagen, and type-specific antibodies for the five most studied collagen types, differing in primary stucture, have been produced. Many investigators using a variety of test systems and forms of collagen have reported the presence of anti-collagen antibodies in a proportion (often a majority) of rheumatoid patients, but only rarely in normal subjects

(Steffen, 1980). These antibodies reacted with several different collagen types, and usually more frequently with denatured than with native collagen.

The results of Greenbury & Skingle (1979) and of Beard et al (1979) have called into question the validity of the conclusions from earlier work about the frequency and specificity of anti-collagen antibodies in rheumatoid arthritis, and the reader is referred to a useful discussion by Beard (1983).

Anti-perinuclear factor

Antibodies to perinuclear cytoplasmic inclusions in human buccal mucosal cells and detected by indirect immunofluorescence were initially described by Nienhuis & Mandema (1964) who found them in the sera of about 50% of the rheumatoid patients they tested. The cytoplasmic components in question are structures known as 'keratohyaline granules', and the presence of anti-perinuclear factor (APF) in RA sera has been confirmed with a positivity rate of 80%, as against 5–7% in other conditions and healthy subjects (Sondag-Tschroots et al, 1979; Johnson et al, 1981).

Anti-keratin antibodies

Another tissue-reactive antibody present in rheumatoid arthritis which is directed against an epithelial cell component has anti-keratin specificity (AKA). This was described by Young et al (1979) and is well demonstrated by indirect immunofluorescence on cryostat sections of rat oesophagus, the keratiniseal cell layer of the lining epithelium giving a characteristic laminar staining pattern. 30–50% of RA sera are reported to give this pattern of staining, which is rarely seen with normal sera (Johnson et al, 1981). AKA antibodies have also been reported in systemic sclerosis (Scott et al, 1981).

Anti-salivary duct antibody

A third distinct antibody against epithelial cells was described by Bertram & Halberg (1964). This stains salivary duct epithelium by immunofluorescence on cryostat sections of normal human parotid, submaxillary or sublingual glands. Anti-salivary duct antibody occurs with low incidence in the sicca syndrome, but in 65% of patients with Sjögren's syndrome with RA, and in about 25% of patients with RA alone (Whaley & Buchanan, 1980). It is thus associated with lacrimal and salivary gland involvement in rheumatoid disease. The mechanism of its production, like that of APF and AKA, is unknown.

Anti-intermediate filament antibodies

Antibodies against intermediate (10 nm) filaments of the cytoskeleton are present in a majority of patients with RA. These antibodies are usually of IgM class, and are found at low titre in less than 15% of normal subjects (Holborow, 1981). Anti-intermediate filament antibodies in RA have specificities for two of the intermediate filament constituent proteins, vimentin and prekeratin, but recognise different keratin determinants from those reacting with AKA above. The presence of anti-intermediate filament antibodies is not confined to RA. They are also frequently present in infectious mononucleosis, and in some other viral diseases (Milani et al, 1981; Pedersen et al, 1982).

Is there a link?

With the exception of rheumatoid factors and some of the antinuclear antibodies, the discovery of the collection of autoantibodies described above, and the differentiation of their specificities, has, at any rate so far, had little impact upon the diagnosis and management of the inflammatory arthropathies and related conditions. This chapter began by posing another material question; what irregularities of immune function, or other causes, lead to the appearance and persistence of the spectrum of autoantibodies of such different specificities that is found in these diseases? Are they linked by a common thread of causality?

That the arthropathies and other systemic rheumatic diseases in question so frequently express autoimmune features implies disturbances of immunoregulatory mechanisms in these patients. HLA cell membrane antigens coded for by the major histocompatibility gene complex (MHC) are thought to govern the activities of lymphocytes and macrophages in such a way as to promote immune responses appropriate to diverse forms of infection, while avoiding autoimmune responses. Although associations between different inflammatory arthropathies or related disease and HLA antigens have been increasingly established and elaborated for a decade, proof of the explanations advanced to account for them (immune response genes, molecular mimicry, virus or hormone receptors, as discussed in Chapter 10) remains inconclusive and fragmentary, and verifiable alternatives have hitherto been lacking. Nevertheless, new evidence of immunoregulatory lymphocyte defects in both RA (Stierle et al, 1983) and SLE (Green et al, 1982) is accumulating. Furthermore, the possibility that virus may after all play an aetiological role has regained relevance since the autoimmune sequelae of persistent viral infections of lymphocytes themselves have been more fully appreciated (Denman, 1983). An acceptable working hypothesis for the causation of autoimmunity in systemic rheumatic diseases might postulate disease susceptibility genes that lower resistance of lymphocytes to virus infection. As a result, the MHC products expressed at the cell surface are modified, with resulting restricted disturbance of immunoregulatory function. Hypotheses of this type may now to put to experimental test.

REFERENCES

Aarden L A, Smeenk R 1981 Measurement of antibodies specific for DNA. In: Lefkovits I, Pernis B. Immunological Methods, Vol II. Academic Press, London, p 75–82

Aarden L A, Lakmaker F, de Groot E R 1976a Immunology of DNA. IV. Quantitative aspects of the Farr test. Journal of Immunological Methods 11: 153–163

Aarden L A, Lakmaker F, Feltkamp T E W 1976b Immunology of DNA. II. The effect of size and structure of the antigen or the Farr assay. Journal of Immunological Methods 10: 39–48

Aho K, Harboe M, Leikola J 1964 Studies of the antibody nature of the rheumatoid factor. Immunology 7: 403–418

Aitchison C T, Peebles C, Joshin F, Tan E M 1980 Characteristics of antinuclear antibodies in rheumatoid arthritis. Arthritis and Rheumatism 23: 528–538

Alarçon-Segovia D 1981 Penetration of antinuclear antibodies into immunoregulatory T cells: Pathogenetic role in the connective tissue diseases. Clinics In Immunology and Allergy 1: 117–126

Allen C, Elson C J, Scott D G I, Bacon P A, Bucknall R C 1981 IgG antiglobulins in rheumatoid arthritis and other arthritides: Relationship with clinical features and other parameters. Annals of the Rheumatic Diseases 40: 127–131

Allen J C, Kunkel H G 1966 Hidden rheumatoid factors with specificity for native γ-globulins. Arthritis and Rheumatism 9: 758–768

Alspaugh M A, Talal N, Tan E M 1976 Differentiation and characterization of antibodies and their antigens in Sjögren's syndrome. Arthritis and Rheumatism 19: 216–222

Andersen I, Andersen P, Elling P, Graudal H 1983 Epidermal nuclear immunoglobulin depositis in some connective tissue diseases: Correlation with ENA antibodies. Annals of the Rheumatic Diseases 42: 163–167

Anderson S G, Cooper S 1970 Effects of two factors, source of sheep cells and concentration of amboceptor, on the estimated titre of rheumatoid factor. Bulletin of the World Health Organization 43: 681–685

Ball J, Lawrence J S 1961 Epidemiology of the sheep cell agglutination test. Annals of the Rheumatic Diseases 20: 235–243

Ball J, Graaff R, de Valkenburg H A, Boerma F W 1962 Comparative studies of serotopic tests for rheumatoid diseases. I. A comparison of a latex test and two erythrocyte agglutination tests in a random population sample. Arthritis and Rheumatism 5: 55–60

Bandilla K K, McDuffie F C 1969 Reactivity of rheumatoid factor with autologous IgG antibodies. Arthritis and Rheumatism 12: 74–81

Barnett, E V, Condemi J J, Leddy J P, Vaughan J H 1964 γ_2, γ_1A and γ_1M antinuclear factors in human sera. Journal of Clinical Investigation 43: 1104–1115

Bartfeld H 1969 Distribution of rheumatoid factor activity in non-rheumatoid states. Annals of the New York Academy of Sciences 168: 30–40

Batchelor J R, Welsh K I, Mansilla-Tinoco R, Hughes G R V, Bernstein R, Ryan P, et al 1980 Hydralazine-induced systemic lupus erythematosus: Influence of HLA-DR and sex on susceptibility. Lancet i: 1107–1109

Baum J, Ziff M 1962 7S and macroglobulin antinuclear fluorescence factors in systemic lupus erythematosus and rheumatoid arthritis. Arthritis and Rheumatism 5: 636–637

Beard H K 1983 The role of autoimmunity to collagen in rheumatoid arthritis. In: Maroudas A, Holborow E J (eds) Studies in joint disease II. Pitman, London, Ch 3, p 88–105

Beard H K, Lea D J, Ryvan R 1979 Anomalous reactions in the haemagglutination assay for anti-collagen antibodies: Studies on patients with rheumatoid arthritis or chronic low back pain. Journal of Immunological Methods, 31, 119–128

Bertram V, Halberg P 1964 A specific antibody against the epithelium of the salivary ducts in sera from patients with Sjögren's syndrome. Acta Allergologica (Kbh) 19:458

Bianco N E, Dobkin L W, Schur P H 1974 Immunological properties of isolated IgG and IgM anti-gamma globulins (rheumatoid factors). Clinical and Experimental Immunology, 17, 91–101

Bluestein H G, Woods V L 1982 Antineuronal antibodies in systemic lupus erythematosus. Arthritis and Rheumatism, 25, 773–777

Bresnihan B, Oliver M, Williams B, Hughes G R V 1979. An anti-neuronal antibody cross-reactive with erythrocytes and lymphocytes in systemic lupus erythematosus. Arthritis and Rheumatism, 23, 313–318

Bruneau C, Benveniste J 1979 Circulating DNA-anti DNA complexes in systemic lupus erythematosus. Journal of Clinical Investigation 64: 191–198

Carson D A, Lawrance S 1978 Light chain heterogeneity of

19S and 7S anti-γ-globulins in rheumatoid arthritis and subacute bacterial endocarditis. Arthritis and Rheumatism 21: 438–440

Carson D A, Lawrance S, Catalano M A, Vaughan J A, Abraham G 1977 Radioimmunoassay of IgG and IgM rheumatoid factors reacting with human IgG. Journal of Immunology 119: 295–299

Cathcart E S, O'Sullivan J B 1969 A longitudinal study of rheumatoid factors in a New England town. Annals of the New York Academy of Sciences 168: 41–51

Charlesworth J A, Quin J W, Yasmeen D 1983 Lymphocytotoxic antibodies in rheumatic diseases. In: Maroudas A, Holborow E J (ed) Studies in joint disease II. Pitman Medical, London, p 56–87

Denman A M 1983 Viruses and immunopathology. In: Holborow E J, Reeves W G (eds) Immunology in medicine, 2nd Ed. Academic Press, London, p 179–202

Dixon F J, Feldman J D, Vazquez J J 1961 Experimental glomerulonephritis. The pathogenesis of a laboratory model resembling the spectrum of human glomerulonephritis. Journal of Experimental Medicine 113: 899–920

Douvas A, Achten A, Tan E M 1979 Identification of a nuclear protein (Scl-70) as a unique target of human antinuclear antibodies in scleroderma. Journal of Biological Chemistry 254: 10514–22

Ebringer R, Rook G, Swana G T, Bottazzo G F, Doniach D 1981 Autoantibodies to cartilage and type II collagen in relapsing polychondritis and other rheumatic diseases. Annals of the Rheumatic Diseases 40: 473–479

Edelman G M, Kunkel H G, Franklin E C 1958 Interaction of the rheumatoid factor with antigen–antibody complexes and aggregated γ-globulin. Journal of Experimental Medicine 108: 105–120

Elling P, Graudal H, Faber V 1968 Granulocyte-specific antinuclear factors in serum and synovial fluid in rheumatoid arthritis. Annals of the Rheumatic Diseases 27: 225–233

Elson C J, Scott D G I, Blake D R, Bacon P A, Holt P D J 1983 Complement activating rheumatoid-factor-containing complexes in patients with rheumatoid vasculitis. Annals of the Rheumatic Diseases 42: 147–150

Epstein W, Johnson A M, Ragan C 1956 Observations of a precipitin reaction between serum of patient with rheumatoid arthritis and a preparation (Cohn Fraction II) of human gammaglobulin. Proceedings of the Society for Experimental Biology and Medicine 90: 235–237

Faber V, Elling P 1966 Leucocyte-specific antinuclear factors in patients with Felty's syndrome, rheumatoid arthritis, systemic lupus erythematosus and other diseases. Acta Medica Scandinavica 179: 257–267

Faith A, Pontesilli O, Ungar A, Panayi G S, Johns P 1982 ELISA assays for IgM and IgG rheumatoid factors. Journal of Immunological Methods 55: 169–178

Ferrell P B, Tan E M 1981 Epstein–Barr (EB) virus antibodies in rheumatoid arthritis. Springer Seminars in Immunopathology 4: 181–192

Finnie A, Mason M, Minn C 1974 Evaluation of the RAHA test for rheumatoid factor. Medical Laboratory Technology 31: 323–326

Førre Ø, Johnson P M, Natvig J B 1977 A study of the variable heavy chain (V_H) regions in human polyclonal IgM rheumatoid factors. Scandinavian Journal of Rheumatism 6: 113–117

Førre Ø, Dobloug J H, Michaelsen T E, Natvig J B 1979 Evidence of similar idiotypic determinants on different rheumatoid factor populations. Scandinavian Journal of Immunology 9: 281–289

Franklin E C, Holman H R, Muller-Eberhard H J, Kunkel H G 1957 An unusual protein component of high molecular weight in the serum of certain patients with rheumatoid arthritis. Journal of Experimental Medicine 105: 425–438

Fritzler M J, Tan E M 1978 Antibodies to histones in drug induced and idiopathic lupus erythematosus. Journal of Clinical Investigation 62: 560–567

Fudenberg H H, Franklin E C 1965 Rheumatoid factors and the aetiology of rheumatoid arthritis. Annals of the New York Academy of Sciences 124: 884–895

Gaarder P I, Natvig J B 1970 Hidden rheumatoid factors reacting with 'non a' and other antigens of native autologous IgG. Journal of Immunology 105: 928–937

Glynn L E 1963 Rheumatoid arthritis. In: Gell P G H, Coombs R R A (eds) Clinical aspects of immunology. Blackwell, Oxford, p 848–870

Glynn L E, Holborow E J, Johnson G D 1957 The nature of the Rose–Waaler factor. Proceedings of the Royal Society of Medicine 50: 469–471

Green I, Kumagai S, Steinberg A D 1982 Immune responses to hapten-modified self and their regulation in normal individuals and patients with systemic lupus erythematosus. Arthritis and Rheumatism 25: 824–827

Greenbury C L 1960 A comparison of the Rose–Waaler, latex fixation, 'RA test' and bentonite flocculation tests. Journal of Clinical Pathology 13: 325–330

Greenbury C L, Skingle J 1979 Anti-cartilage antibody. Journal of Clinical Pathology 32: 826–831

Greenwood B M 1970 Heterophile antibodies in Nigerian sera. Clinical and Experimental Immunology 6: 197–206

Grubb R 1956 Agglutination of erythrocytes coated with 'incomplete' anti-Rh by certain rheumatoid arthritic sera and some other sera. The existence of human serum groups. Acta Pathologica et Microbiologica Scandinavica 39:195

Hahn B H 1982 Characteristics of pathogenic subpopulations of antibodies of DNA. Arthritis and Rheumatism 25: 747–752

Hannestad K 1967 Monoclonal and polyclonal rheumatoid factors with anti-di and anti-tri nitrophenyl activity. Clinical and Experimental Immunology 4: 555–578

Hargraves M M, Richmond H, Morton R 1948 Presentation of two bone marrow elements: the 'tart' cell and the 'LE' cell. Proceedings of the Staff Meetings of the Mayo Clinic 23: 25–28

Hay F C, Nineham L J, Perumal R, Roitt I M 1979 Intra-articular and circulating immune complexes and antiglobulins (IgG and IgM) in rheumatoid arthritis. Correlation with clinical features. Annals of the Rheumatic Diseases 38: 1–7

Heimer R, Levin F 1965 Inhibition of complement fixation by rheumatoid sera. Annals of the New York Academy of Sciences 124: 879–883

Henney C S, Stanworth D R 1965 The reactivity of rheumatoid factor with human gamma G globulin. Immunology 9: 139–150

Holborow E J 1981 Autoantibodies in rheumatoid arthritis. Some new facts. Clinics in Immunology and Allergy 1: 127–138

Holborow E J, Johnson G D 1965 The nature of antinuclear immunoglobulins. Annals of the New York Academy of Sciences 124: 833–837

Holborow E J, Johnson G D, Chantler S 1982 Use of international reference preparations for immunofluorescence. In: Schauenstein K, Wick G (eds) Selected practical topics of immunofluorescent techniques. Elsevier, Amsterdam, Ch 2, p 1–10
Hughes G R V 1979a Antinuclear antibodies and lymphocytotoxic antibodies; how useful in the diagnosis and management of clinical subsets of SLE? In: Harper P S, Minn J R (eds) Advanced Medicine 15. Pitman, London, p 119–129
Hughes G R V 1979b The treatment of systemic lupus erythematosus: The case for conservative management. Clinics in Rheumatic Diseases Aug 1979: 641–655
Hunneyball I M, Stanworth D R 1976 The effects of chemical modification on the antigenicity of human and rabbit IgG. Immunology 30: 881–894
Izui S, Lambert P H, Miescher P 1976 In vitro demonstration of a particular affinity of glomerular basement membrane and collagen for DNA. Journal of Experimental Medicine 144: 428–443
Izui S, Lambert P H, Miescher P A 1977 Failure to detect circulating DNA-anti DNA complexes by four radioimmunological methods in patients with systemic lupus erhthematosus. Clinical and Experimental Immunology 30: 384–392
Jacobson A S, Kammerer W A, Wolf J, Epstein W V, Heller G 1956 The haemagglutination test for rheumatoid arthritis III. Clinical evaluation of the sheep erythrocyte agglutination (SEA) test and the gammaglobulin (FII) tests. American Journal of Medicine 20: 490–499
Johnson G D, Holborow E J 1983 The routine immunofluorescent test for serum antinuclear antibodies. Association of Clinical Pathologists Broadsheet No. 10. British Medical Association, London
Johnson G D, Smith M E, Holborow E J 1973 Precipitating antibody to DNA detected by two-stage electroimmunodiffusion. Lancet ii: 883–885
Johnson G D, Carvalho A, Holborow E J, Goddard D H, Russell G 1981 Antiperinuclear factor and keratin antibodies in rheumatoid arthritis. Annals of the Rheumatic Diseases 40: 263–266
Johnson P M 1981 Molecular nature and cross-reactions of rheumatoid factor. In: Holborow E J (ed) Clinics in immunology and allergy. Saunders, London, Ch 6, p 103–115
Johnson P M, Faulk W P 1976 Rheumatoid factor: its nature, specificity and production in rheumatoid arthritis. Clinical Immunology and Immunopathology 6: 414–430
Klotz J L, Minima R M, Teplitz R L 1979 An enzyme linked immunosorbent assay for antibodies to native and denatured DNA. Journal of Immunological Methods 29: 155–165
Knight R K, Pritchard M H 1982 Nephelometry compared with differential antibody titre in routine rheumatoid factor measurements. Annals of the Rheumatic Diseases 41: 428–429
Koffler D, Schur P H, Kunkel H G 1967 Immunological studies concerning the nephritis of systemic lupus erythematosus. Journal of Experimental Medicine 126: 607–624
Kunkel H G, Winchester R J, Joslin F G, Capra J D 1974 Similarities in the light chains of anti-γ-globulins showing cross-idiotypic specificities. Journal of Experimental Medicine 139: 128–136
Kurata N, Tan E M 1976 Identification of antibodies to nuclear acidic antigens by counter immunoelectrophoresis. Arthritis and Rheumatism 19: 574–579
Lawrence J S 1965 Surveys of rheumatic complaints in the population. In: Dixon A S J (ed) Progress in clinical rheumatology. Churchill, London
Lawrence J S 1970 Rheumatoid arthritis — nature or nurture? Annals of the Rheumatic Diseases 29: 357–379
Lerner E A, Lerner M R, Hardin J A, Janeway C A, Steitz J A 1982 Deciphering the mysteries of RNA containing lupus antigens. Arthritis and Rheumatism 25: 761–766
Lightfoot R W, Hughes G R V 1976 Significance of persisting serologic abnormalities in SLE. Arthritis and Rheumatism 19: 837–843
Maddison P J, Skinner R P, Hall N D, Esscher E, Taylor P V, Scott O, Scott J S 1983 Antibody to Ro(SS-A) and congenital heart block. Clinical Rheumatology 2:104
March R E 1983 Properties of normal and rheumatoid antiglobulins: Implications for the pathogenesis of rheumatoid arthritis. PhD Thesis, University of London
March R E, Reeback J S, Holborow E J, Jones V E, Jacoby R K 1982 The complement fixing properties and class distribution of rheumatoid factors (antiglobulins) in rheumatoid arthritis and other diseases. Clinical and Experimental Immunology 48: 555–560
Mattioli M, Reichlin M 1971 Characterization of a soluble nuclear ribonucleoprotein antigen reactive with SLE sera. Journal of Immunology 107: 1281–1290
Messner R P, Laxdal T, Quie P G, Williams R C 1968 Rheumatoid factors in subacute bacterial endocarditis — bacterium, duration of disease or genetic predisposition? Annals of Internal Medicine 68: 746–756
Messner R P, de Horatius R, Ferrone S 1980 Lymphocytotoxic antibodies in systemic lupus erythematosus patients and their relatives. Arthritis and Rheumatism 23: 265–272
Meyer K 1922 Uber Hämmagglutinin mehrung und Hämagglutination fordende Wirkung bei menschlichen seren. Immunotätsforschung Exp Ther 34:229
Milani M M, Osung O A, Badakere S S, Chandra M, March R E, Holborow E J 1981 Antibodies to cytoskeletal intermediate filaments in rheumatoid arthritis, osteoarthrosis and infectious mononucleosis. Abstract 0043, XV International Congress of Rheumatology, Paris
Milgrom E, Witebsky E 1961 The rheumatoid factor and its possible pathogenetic role. In: Grabar P, Meischer P (eds) Mechanism of cell and tissue damage produced by immune reactions. Immunopathology, Karger, Basel, 2nd International Symposium, p 337
Milgrom F, Witebsky E, Goldstein R, Loza V 1962 Studies on the rheumatoid and related serum factors. Journal of the American Medical Association 181: 476–484
Miyawaki S, Ritchie R J 1973 Nucleolar antigen specific for antinucleolar antibody in the sera of patients with systemic rheumatic disease. Arthritis and Rheumatism 16: 726–736
Moore T L, Zuckner J, Baldassare A R, Weiss T D, Dorner R W 1978 Complement fixing hidden rheumatoid factors in juvenile rheumatoid arthritis. Arthritis and Rheumatism 21: 935–941
Morimoto C, Abe T, Toguchi T, Kiyotaki M, Homma M 1979 Studies of anti-lymphocyte antibody in patients with systemic lupus erythematosus. I. Cause of loss of suppressor function. Scandinavian Journal of Immunology 10: 213–221
Natvig J B, Munthe E 1975 Self-associating IgG rheumatoid factor represents a major response of plasma cells in

rheumatoid inflammatory tissue. Annals of the New York Academy of Sciences 256: 88–95

Natvig J B, Turner M W 1970 Rheumatoid anti-Gm factors with specificity for the pFc subfragment of human immunoglobulin G. Nature 225: 855–857

Nienhuis R L F, Mandema E 1964 A new serum factor in patients with rheumatoid arthritis. The anti-perinuclear factor. Annals of the Rheumatic Diseases 23: 302–305

Normansell D E 1970 Anti-gammaglobulin in rheumatoid arthritis sera. I. Studies on the 22S complex. Immunochemistry 7: 787–797

Normansell D E 1971 Anti-gammaglobulin in rheumatoid arthritis sera. II. The reactivity of anti-γ-globulin rheumatoid factors with altered γ-globulin. Immunochemistry 8: 593–602

Normansell D E 1972 Anti-gammaglobulin in rheumatoid arthritis sera. III. The reactivity of anti-γ-globulin rheumatoid factors with heterologous γ-globulin. Immunochemistry 9: 725–736

Pasquali J L, Fong S, Tsoukas C, Vaughan J H, Carson D A 1980 Inheritance of immunoglobulin M rheumatoid factor idiotypes. Journal of Clinical Investigation 66: 863–866

Pedersen J S, Toh B H, Mackay I R, Tait B D, Gust I D, Kastelan A, Hadzic N 1982 Segregation of autoantibody to cytoskeletal filaments, actin and intermediate filaments with two types of chronic active hepatitis. Clinical and Experimental Immunology 48: 527–532

Pope R M, Teller D C, Mannik M 1974 The molecular basis of self-association of antibodies to IgG (rheumatoid factors) in rheumatoid arthritis. Proceedings of the National Academy of Science 71: 517–521

Reichlin M 1982 Clinical and immunological significance of antibodies to Ro and La in systemic lupus erythematosus. Arthritis and Rheumatism 25: 767–772

Robbins D L, Moore T L, Carson D A, Vaughan J H 1978 Relative reactivities of rheumatoid factors in serum and cells. Arthritis and Rheumatism 21: 820–826

Roberts-Thomson P J, Wernick R M, Ziff M 1981 Low molecular weight IgM in rheumatoid arthritis and other rheumatic diseases. Arthritis and Rheumatism 24: 795–802

Rose H M, Ragan C, Pearce E, Lipman M O 1948 Differential agglutination of normal and sensitized sheep erythrocytes by sera of patients with rheumatoid arthritis. Proceedings of the Society for Experimental Biology and Medicine 68:1

Rubin R L, Joslin F G, Tan E M 1982 Specificity of antihistone antibodies in systemic lupus erythematosus. Arthritis and Rheumatism 25: 779–782

Schaller J 1977 Iridocyclitis. Arthritis and Rheumatism 20: 227–228

Schur P H, Kunkel H G 1965 The reactivity of 19S anti-gamma globulins with native 7S gamma globulins. Arthritis and Rheumatism 8: 468 (Abstract)

Schur P H, Sandson J 1968 Immunologic factors and clinical activity in systemic lupus erythematosus. New England Journal of Medicine 278: 533–538

Scott D L, Delamere J P, Jones L J, Walton K W 1981 Significance of laminar anti-keratin antibodies to rat oesophagus in rheumatoid arthritis. Annals of the Rheumatic Diseases 40: 267–271

Sharp G C, Irvin W S, Tan E M, Gould R G, Holman A H 1972 Mixed connective tissue disease — an apparently distinct rheumatic disease syndrome associated with a specific antibody to an extractable nuclear antigen (ENA). American Journal of Medicine 52: 148–159

Singer J M, Plotz C M 1956 The latex fixation test. I. Application to the serologic diagnosis of rheumatoid arthritis. American Journal of Medicine 21:888

Smeenk R 1982 In: Low avidity antibodies to DNA. Thesis: Rodopi, Amsterdam, Ch 12

Smeenk R, Aarden L 1980 The use of polyethylene glycol precipitation to detect low avidity anti-DNA antibodies in systemic lupus erythematosus. Journal of Immunological Methods 39: 165–180

Sondag-Tschroots I R J M, Aaij C, Smit J W, Feltkamp T E W 1979 The anti-perinuclear factor. I. The diagnostic significance of the anti-perinuclear factor for rheumatoid arthritis. Annals of the Rheumatic Diseases 38: 248–251

Steffen C 1980 Collagen as an autoantigen in rheumatoid arthritis. In: Maroudas A, Holborow E J (eds) Studies in joint disease I. Pitman, London Ch 6, p 201–226

Steward M W, Turner M W, Natvig J B, Gaarder P I 1973 The binding affinities of the rheumatoid factors interacting with the Cγ3 homology region of human IgG. Clinical and Experimental Immunology, 15, 145–152

Stewart G A, Smith A K, Stanworth D R 1973 Biological activities associated with the Facb fragment of rabbit IgG. Immunochemistry 10: 755–760

Stierle H E, Brown K A, Perry J D, Holborow E J 1983 Increased responsiveness of rheumatoid B lymphocytes to stimulation by Epstein Barr virus. Rheumatology International 3: 7–11

Sturgill B C, Carpenter R R 1965 Antibodies to ribosomes in systemic lupus erythematosus. Arthritis and Rheumatism 8: 213–218

Swaak T, Smeenk R, Groenwald J, Aarden L 1982a Clinical differences between SLE patients in relation to the avidity of their anti-ds DNA. In: Low avidity antibodies to DNA. Thesis, Rodopi, Amsterdam, Ch XI

Swaak A J G, Groenwold J, Aarden L A, van Eps S L W, Feltkamp T E W 1982b Prognostic value of anti-ds DNA in SLE. Annals of the Rheumatic Diseases 41: 388–395

Tan E M 1982 Autoantibodies to nuclear antigens (ANA): Their immunobiology and medicine. In: Kunkel H G, Dixon F J (eds) Advances in immunology 33: 167–241

Tan E M, Portanova J P 1981 The role of histones as nuclear autoantigens in drug-related lupus erythematosus. Arthritis and Rheumatism 24: 1064–1069

Tan E M, Robinson J, Robitaille P 1976 Studies on antibodies to histones by immunofluorescence. Scandinavian Journal of Immunology 5: 811–818

Tan E M, Cohen A S, Fries J F, et al 1982 The 1982 revised criteria for the classification of systemic lupus erythematosus. Arthritis and Rheumatism 25: 1271–1277

Tesar J T, Schmid F R 1970 Conversion of soluble immune complexes into complement fixing aggregated by IgM rheumatoid factor. Journal of Immunology 105: 1206–1214

Tsokos G C, Balow J E 1982 Suppressor T cells in systemic lupus erythematosus: Lack of defective in vitro suppressor cell generation in patients with active disease. Journal of Clinical and Laboratory Immunology, 8: 83–90

Turner-Warwick M, Haslam P 1971 Antibodies in some chronic fibrosing lung diseases. I. Non-organ-specific antibodies. Clinical Allergy 1:83

Valkenburg H A 1963 Rheumatoid factor in populations. In: Kellgren J H, Jeffrey M R, Ball J (eds) Epidemiology of chronic rheumatism. Blackwell, Oxford, p 74

Venables P J W, Erhardt C C, Maini R N 1980 Antibodies to extractable nuclear antigens in rheumatoid arthritis: Relationship to vasculities and circulating immune

complexes. Clinical and Experimental Immunology 39: 146–153
Venables P W J, Roffe L M, Erhardt C C, Maini R N, Edwards J M B, Porter A D 1981 Titres of antibodies to RANA in rheumatoid arthritis and normal sera: Relationship to Epstein–Barr infection. Arthritis and Rheumatism 24: 1459–1461
Venables P J W, Charles P J, Buchanan R R C, Rung Yi, Mumford P A, Schreiber L, et al 1983 Quantitation and detection of isotypes of anti-SS-B antibodies by Farr and ELISA assays using affinity purified antigens: an approach to the investigation of Sjögren's syndrome and systemic lupus erythematosus. Arthritis and Rheumatism 26: 146–155
Waaler E 1940 On the occurrence of a factor in human serum activating the specific agglutination of sheep blood corpuscles. Acta Pathological Microbiologica Scandinaica 17:172
Waller M, Toone E C 1968 Normal individuals with positive tests for rheumatoid factor. Arthritis and Rheumatism 11:50
Waller M V, Vaughan J H 1956 The use of anti-Rh sera for demonstrating agglutination activating factor in rheumatoid arthritis. Proceedings of the Society for Experimental Biology and Medicine 92:198
Waller M, Richard A J, Mallory J 1969 Immunochemical and serological studies of enzymatically fragmented human IgG globulins. II. Hydrolysis with subtilisin elastase, trypsin and chymotrysin. Immunochemistry 6:207
Wasicek C A, Reichlin M 1982 Clinical and serological differences between SLE patients with antibodies to Ro versus patients with antibodies to Ro and La. Journal of Clinical Investigation 69: 835–843
Weir D M, Holborow E J 1962 Serum antinuclear factor: laboratory studies. Annals of the Rheumatic Diseases 21: 40–44
Wernick R, Lospalluto J J, Fink C W, Ziff M 1981 Serum IgG and IgM rheumatoid factors by solid phase radioimmunoassay. Arthritis and Rheumatism 24: 1501–1511
Whaley K, Buchanan W W 1980 Sjögren's syndrome and associated diseases. In: Parker C W (ed) Clinical immunology, Vol I. Saunders, Philadelphia, Ch 20
Williams R C, Kunkel H G 1962 Rheumatoid factor, complement and conglutinin aberrations in patients with subacute bacterial endocarditis. Journal of Clinical Investigation 41: 666–675
Williams R C, Kunkel H G 1963 Separation of rheumatoid factors of different specificities using columns conjugated with gammaglobulin. Arthritis and Rheumatism 6: 665–675
Williams R C, Kunkel H G 1965 Observations on anti-gamma globulin factors in human sera and antibodies against autologous gamma globulins produced in rabbits. Annals of the New York Academy of Sciences 124: 860–864
Winfield J B, Cohen P L, Litvin D A 1982 Antibodies to activated T cells and their soluble products in systemic lupus erythematosus. Arthritis and Rheumatism 25: 814–819
Young B J J, Mallya R K, Leslie R D G, Clark C J M, Hamblin T J 1979 Antikeratin antibodies in rheumatoid arthritis. British Medical Journal ii: 97–99
Zutshi D W, Reading C A, Epstein W V, Ansell B M, Holborow E J 1969 FII haeagglutination test for serum antigamma-globulin factors in arthritides seropositive and seronegative by other tests. Annals of the Rheumatic Diseases 28: 289–299
Zvaifler N J, Schur P 1968 Reactions of aggregated mercaptoethanol treated gammaglobulin with rheumatoid factor — precipitin and complement fixation studies. Arthritis and Rheumatism 11: 523–536

R.N. Maini

Immune complexes and complement

IMMUNE COMPLEXES

HISTORICAL BACKGROUND

The current interest in immune complexes in rheumatic diseases springs largely from their suspected role as mediators of tissue damage. The observation that originally contributed to this concept was made at the beginning of the century by Arthus (1903) when he found that subcutaneous injections of small quantities of horse serum into previously immunised rabbits resulted, within a few hours, in the production of erythema, oedema, petechial haemorrhages and tissue necrosis at the site of the injection. This reaction (the 'Arthus phenomenon') was subsequently analysed and shown to be dependent upon a process resulting from the union of the injected antigen with circulating specific antibody in the walls of blood vessels. In this example of tissue injury, the immune complexes were formed in situ by sequential deposition of antigen and antibody. The localised nature of the Arthus reaction contrasts with the systemic effects observed in serum sickness. This clinical syndrome was also first noted in the earlier part of this century when repeated injections of hyperimmune serum were employed in the therapy and prophylaxis of diphtheria, tetanus and other infections. Within 7–10 days following administration of the serum, a proportion of patients developed fever, lymphadenopathy, splenomegaly, rashes, arthritis, albuminuria and haematuria, which subsequently spontaneously subsided over a matter of one or two weeks. Von Pirquet (1911) recognised that the condition was a result of immunological reactions to the foreign protein injection and that its manifestations coincided with disappearance of the protein and appearance of circulating antibody. The role of circulating immune complexes in the pathogenesis of serum sickness awaited studies on experimental models and methodological developments in the detection and quantitation of antigens and antibodies in blood and tissues.

From the teleological point of view, the development of antibodies in response to antigens may be regarded as one part of the host defence mechanism. It results in benefit which is dependent on interaction of antigen with antibody, the formation of an immune complex, and its successful elimination by the phagocytic scavenging system. The formation of immune complexes does not always achieve a protective biological function, and may instead result in tissue damage and disease processes. This outcome is particularly likely to occur when an antibody response is perpetuated simultaneously with the chronic release of an antigen, as for example, could occur in autoimmune and neoplastic diseases and chronic infections.

The cellular basis of the immune response, the importance of environmental and genetic factors, the conditions favouring formation, persistence and tissue localisation of immune complexes , and the mechanisms of tissue damage are all subjects of intensive current investigation. Methods of detection of complexes and their application to studies of diseases in animals and man encourage the view that they are indeed involved in the pathogenesis of tissue damage, especially that observed in major vessels, visceral and cutaneous vessels, the glomerular wall, joint tissue and choroid plexus of the brain.

The techniques used for assessing immune complex mediated pathogenesis of diseases are very often indirect, as only in a few instances is the nature of the antigen known. Much of the current information in the rheumatic diseases, for example, is based on the demonstration of the coexistence of immunoglobulin and complement components in suitably prepared tissue sections, or by documenting changes in the individual components of complement in blood or tissue fluids of the type that suggest immune complex activation or consumption. Other tests rely on the physical characterisation of the complexes or studying their affinity for complement or rheumatoid factors or interactions with cell membrane receptors for complement or Fc part of heavy chain of immunoglobulin. Characterisation of the antigen component of putative immune complexes in diseases has only proved possible to a limited extent.

ANTIGEN–ANTIBODY INTERACTIONS

Composition of immune complexes

An immune complex is the macromolecule formed by the union of antigen to its specific antibody. A large number of antigens are soluble or freely dispersible in a fluid phase, and are therefore able to form immune complexes which can circulate in the blood or gain access to extravascular fluid compartments and interstitial fluid. Substances which are antigenic include biological molecules such as proteins, polypeptides, glycoproteins, lipoproteins, nucleic acids, polysaccharides as well as simpler organic and inorganic chemicals (usually bound as haptens to a carrier protein). Whole microbes (such as bacteria, viruses and fungi), mammalian cells and macromolecular or particulate constituents of cell membranes, cytoplasm and nuclei, also possess a number of potential antigenic sites which may form immune complexes which can circulate in blood or disperse in tissue fluids. Thus immune complexes may exist in an enormous range of sizes and physical forms. At one end of the spectrum exist 'soluble' macromolecules barely larger than a single IgG molecule, whilst at the other end are 'insoluble' immune precipitates visible to the naked eye. 'Particulate' immune complexes are typified by sensitised erythrocytes, leukocytes and platelets. A most convincing visual demonstration of circulating immune complexes of viral material and immunoglobulin (of hepatitis B antigen bound to its antibody) has been provided by electron microscopy in patients with serum hepatitis (Almeida & Waterson, 1969). In tissues antigenic determinants on the surface of cells, basement membrane and matrix components of tissues may specifically bind antibody, but this type of combination has to be distinguished from physical trapping of immune complexes and from binding of immunoglobulin or activated complement (as part of an immune complex) to heavy chain or complement receptors present on surfaces of certain cells.

Immune complexes, particularly those containing immunoglobulins of IgG_1, IgG_2, IgG_3 and IgM class, bind the first component of serum complement (Clq) and activate the complement sequence. Complement components bound to complexes in the circulation or tissues are therefore often part of the immune complex macromolecule. Since complement proteins and products of their breakdown possess distinct antigen specificities, it is possible to demonstrate them by the use of suitable antisera, for example, using immunofluorescent methods in tissue sections, or precipitation and agglutination reactions on serum speciments.

Structure of immunoglobulins

All immunoglobulin molecules consist basically of units of four polypeptide chains comprising two light (L) and two heavy (H) chains. The chains are arranged in two parts of H–L, joined to each other by disulphide (S–S) and non-covalent bonds. The antigenic valency of the basic unit of the molecule is two since each H–L pair provides one site for binding of antigen. In humans, IgG, IgD and TgE classes of immunoglobulin are usually found in this basic monomeric form, whereas IgM usually exists as a pentamer (i.e. five basic units of four chains each) and IgA as a monomer or dimer. It can be concluded that the maximum number of sites available for binding to antigen in the naturally occurring form of the IgG, IgD and IgE is two, whereas the number of sites available on IgA and IgM are four and ten respectively.

In 1959 Porter demonstrated that the four chain immunoglobulin unit could be split into three large fragments by the action of the enzyme papain which cleaves the H chain at a site immediately adjacent to the disulphide bond which binds the two H chains to each other. This results in the production of two fragments of Fab (ab for antigen-binding) and one of Fc (c for crystallisable). Whereas Fab fragments possess antigen-binding sites, the Fc fragment is responsible for mediating several of the biological properties relevant to understanding the role of immune complexes.

H and L chains themselves consist of regions (also termed 'domains') of approximately 100–120 amino acid sequences, each of which contains a characteristic 'intrachain' disulphide (S–S) bond. L chains consist of two such regions, the *N*-terminal half of which is known as the 'variable' (V_L) region (because of the wide variations in the sequence of amino acids) and the *C*-terminal region is known as the 'constant' (C_L) region (because its sequence does not vary apart from the differences noted in different classes of Ig and in different animal species). H chains also possess a variable domain in their *N*-terminal portion which is termed V_H and three domains of similar length in the constant portion, termed C_H1, C_H2 and C_H3. The V regions of the H and L chains provide for antigen binding specificity, and the C regions determine the class (or subclass) of the immunoglobulin molecule.

The site at which the immuneglobulin molecule is split by papain has been termed the 'hinge' region because the Fab portions of the molecule are flexible around this point in a manner which allows the angle formed by them to vary widely. This flexiblity allows the Fab portions on a single monomeric immunoglobulin molecule the ability to combine either with two antigenic determinant on the same molecule or alternatively with a single antigenic determinant on two separate molecules. Although polymeric forms of immunoglobulins can theoretically bind the number of antigenic molecules equivalent to the number of Fab portions available, in practice it has been found that the number of antigen molecules bound depends mainly on the size of antigen (Edberg et al, 1972), smaller antigens binding to more, and larger antigens to fewer antibody combining sites (probably as a result of physical steric hindrance).

Some physicochemical properties of immune complexes

The physicochemical and biological properties of immune complexes are governed to a certain extent by the properties of the constituent antigens and the antibodies involved. Important characteristics of antigens include their chemical structure, size, number of antibody combining sites per molecule ('valency') and their ability to induce an immune response ('immunogenicity'). The important features of the antibody molecule also include size (largely determined by their existence as monomers or polymers), valency and class or sub-class of the immunoglobulin (*see* above), as well as the energy of association exhibited on combination with antigen (termed 'avidity').

Size and lattice structure

The size of the immune complex is partly determined by its constituent antigen and antibody. Thus, antigens may vary from simple chemicals (haptens), to large particles of heterogeneous structure; and immunoglobulins from monomers to polymers containing up to 10 or more units bound together. In addition, the size of the complex is determined by the degree of lattice formation that takes place following combination of antigen and antibody (Marrack, 1938). For lattice formation to occur, the Fab combining sites of immunoglobulin molecules require to link together a large number of multivalent antigenic molecules or particles. Mono- or divalent antigens are unable to form a lattice-work with IgG because of the restriction imposed by the divalent monomeric structure of immunoglobulin, whereas multivalent antigens permit linkage between several molecules provided the relative proportions of antigen and antibody are appropriate. The effective valency of an 'antigen' might be theoretically increased by the presence of more than one antigen on the same carrier molecule reacting with their corresponding antibodies (of different specificities) in the same serum.

Solubility

The solubility of an immune complex is determined partly by the nature of the antigen; some antigens may themselves be insoluble. Combination of soluble antigens and antibodies may result in the formation of precipitates provided the conditions favour lattice formation. Precipitation is encouraged by combination of antigen and antibody in optimal proportions, which are achieved at equimolar concentrations ('equivalence'), whereas solubility is maintained in antigen excess (Fig. 13.1). Antibody excess usually leads to increased solubility but this varies according to the source and specificity of antibody; for example, antibodies raised in rabbits tend to remain insoluble even in great antibody excess (Nisonoff & Winkler, 1958). Other factors leading to precipitation are reviewed by Haurowitz (1968) and include the class of antibody (IgM precipitates more readily than IgG), avidity (high avidity may be expected to precipitate more readily than low avidity antibody) and the physical conditions in which the reaction takes place (e.g. precipitation being encouraged in semi-solid media, at neutral or alkaline pH and increased salt concentrations).

Structural alterations in immunoglobulin molecules following binding to antigens

The use of electron microscopy, measurement of optical rotation and X-ray diffraction techniques have revealed changes in the structure of the immunoglobulin molecule following combination with antigen (for reviews *see*: Nisonoff et al, 1975; Metzger, 1974). The interaction has been regarded as providing the stimulus for activation of sites responsible for the biological properties normally associated with CH2 and CH3 regions of the immunoglobulin molecule, such as complement activation, adherence to cell receptors and availability of sites for reaction with rheumatoid factors. However, the evidence is controversial since it has been claimed that structural alteration in immunoglobulin molecules occurs as a result of swivelling of Fab fragments at the hinge, without significant changes occurring in the Fc region, and that the active sites on CH2 and CH3 are too remote from the hinge region to be directly influenced by this mechanism. The alternative suggestion has been put forward that the mechanism of activation of the sites on Fc region depends on physical approximation and alignment of heavy chains which increases their binding affinity for Clq component of complement, rheumatoid factors and Fc cell surface receptors. The appropriate alignment of immunoglobulin molecules is achieved by combination with multivalent antigens and lattice formation or by the configurational changes secondary to heat aggregation of alkali denaturation.

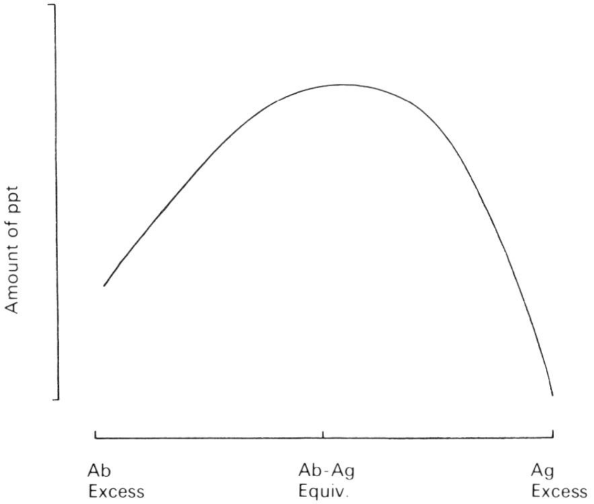

Fig. 13.1 Solubility of immune complexes in antibody and antigen excess. When certain antigens combine with antibody the maximum precipitate forms in the presence of equimolar concentrations of antigen and antibody (Ab–Ag equivalence). Increasing amounts of antigen and antibody lead to solubilisation of the precipitate.

Biological properties of immune complexes

Complement binding and activation

The site for binding of Clq, the first component of the classical complement pathway is believed to reside in the CH2 domain of IgG and in the case of human immunoglobulins it has been found that three of the four subclasses of IgG, i.e. IgG_3, IgG_1 and IgG_2, bind complement in decreasing order or efficacy (IgG_4 does not); and that pentameric IgM in equimolar concentrations is more effective than IgG (Augener et al, 1971). The binding of antigen–antibody complexes and aggregated IgG to Clq is more avid than to IgG or IgM alone. Complement binding is greatly increased by lattice formation (see p. 382) and by aggregation of the immunoglobulin molecule. Complement binding by immune complexes leads to activation of the complement sequence and is believed to be of central importance in mediating type III hypersensitivity reactions (Coombs & Gell classification, 1975) of the type seen in Arthus reactions, serum sickness and other forms of immune complex disease. The full details of the complement pathway and the biological and pathogenic role of complement is discussed in the section on complement (p. 397).

Interactions with cells

Immune complexes interact with cells bearing receptors for heavy chains of immunoglobulins (Fc) or complement (C) such as monocytes, macrophages and polymorphs capable of phagocytosis and release of inflammatory mediators. Of the four IgG subclasses in man, IgG_1, and IgG_3 have the highest avidity for human monocytes or macrophages (Abramson et al, 1970), an avidity which is influenced by the degree of lattice formation of immune complexes. Receptors of all subclasses of IgG and IgA have been demonstrated on polymorphonuclear neutrophils (Henson, 1971). Complexes bound to activated complement components attach themselves to C3 receptors on polymorphs (Lay & Nussenzweig, 1968) and human monocytes (Huber et al, 1968).

The phagocytosis of immune complexes which directly adhere to polymorphs by Fc or C3 receptors results in the release of lysosomal enzymes by mechanisms which either lead to loss of cell viability, or release of stored material and/or stimulation, synthesis and release of newly formed enzymes (Henson, 1971; Weismann, 1972). The phagocytosis of immune complexes by polymorphs has been regarded as the event responsible for lysosomal release and tissue damage in Arthus lesions, arteritis, certain forms of glomerulonephritis and within the joint cavity of rheumatoid arthritis (Henson & Cochrane, 1975). Lysosomal enzymes are also released by polymorphs adhering to complexes on non-phagocytosable surfaces, a process of possible importance in the damage to solid structures such as cartilage or glomerular basement membrane (Henson, 1971).

Immune complexes greatly enhance the production and release of lysosomal enzymes by mononuclear cells (Cardella et al, 1974). This mechanism has been considered to be of importance in the erosion of cartilage by pannus in rheumatoid arthritis (Allison et al, 1975).

Fc and C3b receptors are also present on platelets, although human platelets are apparently devoid of the C3b receptor. Interaction of immune complexes with platelets leads to aggregation and release of vasoactive constituents such as serotonin and other factors (Becker & Henson, 1973). C3b receptors on erythrocytes may provide an additional means of carriage and disposal of immune complexes to the RES (see section on complement).

Effect on the immune response

Antigen-presenting cells, such as macrophages, as well as B and some T lymphocytes possess Fc and C receptors. These receptors allow immune complexes to bind to these cells, and it has been shown in experimental systems that such interactions may have profound effects on the regulation of the immune response. Depending on the circumstances, both augmentory and suppressive effects on humoral and cellular immunity have been observed. The implications of such observations on the quantitative and qualitative aspects of immunological responses in health and in disease remain to be resolved. The following effects of immune complexes appear relevant:

Enhanced antibody production Immune complexes, especially in antigen excess, appear to be more efficient than antigen alone in the generation of primary and secondary antibody responses in vitro and in vivo (reviewed by Theofilopoulous & Dixon, 1979). The possible mechanisms for such augmentation could be mediated by an effect on macrophages (e.g. more effective antigen presentation and production of interleukin 1 which stimulates T cells), localisation in germinal centres allowing effective cellular cooperation, and the non-specific proliferation of lymphocytes induced by antigen–antibody complexes.

Regulation of antibody production. Immune complex formation provides a means of accelerating the elimination of the stimulating antigen. In addition, immune complexes have been shown to suppress antibody production by direct effects on antigen-binding sites and Fc receptors, B lymphocytes (Oberbarnscheidt & Koisch, 1978) and by their effects on the network of cellular interactions. Cellular interactions are now known to be important in suppression of B cell activity, the two main mechanisms proposed envisaging the participation of suppressor T cells and the anti-idiotype network. Of special interest is the possibility that immune complexes induce antigen-specific suppressor T cells (Taylor & Basten, 1976) which inhibit T helper cells or B cells directly. In addition, immune complexes can induce idiotypic specific suppressor T cells which inhibit production of antibodies bearing the corresponding idiotype (Caulfield et al, 1983).

Blocking of immune reactions Under certain experimental conditions in vitro, cells coated with low amounts of specific antibody (the 'target' cells) are 'killed' by a population of mononuclear cells resembling lymphocytes (sometimes referred to as 'K-cells' or the 'third' population). The mechanism of such antibody-dependent cell-mediated cytotoxicity (ADCC) (reviewed by Cerrottini & Brunner, 1974) appears to involve the binding of the effector cells to the free Fc portion of the antibody coating the target cell. This reaction occurs in the absence of complement, and should be distinguished from cytotoxicity induced by antibody in the presence of complement (Type II reaction as classified by Coombs & Gell). Antibody-dependent cell-mediated cytotoxicity (K-cell activity) is inhibited by the concurrent presence in tissue culture of soluble immune complexes or aggregated immunoglobulin, as a result of competition between the target cell and the free complexes or aggregates for Fc receptors on the 'killer' cells (MacLennan, 1972), a finding which indicates that soluble complexes protect against K-cell damage. The in vivo significance of these findings is largely unknown at present, although it has been proposed that ADCC may be involved in allograft rejection, tumour and viral immunity and in autoimmune disease. Depending on the circumstances, immune complexes could lead to beneficial or deleterious effects in such situations.

Monocytes and macrophages to which antibody or immune complexes have become bound by the Fc receptors also appear to acquire cytotoxic potential for tumour cells. The cytotoxicity of these so-called 'armed macrophages' may either be specific (i.e. dicated by antibody specificity for tumour cells) or 'non-specific' (i.e. directed against any tumour cells). The mechanism and possible significance of this type of experiment to inflammation in rheumatoid arthritis is discussed by Evans (1975). Experimental evidence has also implicated immune complexes in the 'blocking' of immune responses to tumours (Hellstrom et al, 1971). The concept of immunological unresponsiveness (or tolerance) can be broadened to include mechanisms involving the participation of immune complexes (Brent et al, 1976).

Reactions with rheumatoid-factors

A large number of antigenic sites on CH2 and CH3 domains of heavy chains react with a heterogeneous group of antibodies termed 'rheumatoid factors' (Natvig & Kunkel, 1973). The interaction of IgM rheumatoid factor with these Fc determinants is the basis of the precipitation and agglutination reactions widely employed for diagnostic purposes (e.g. latex fixation or sensitised sheep cell agglutination). It has been found that for precipitation or agglutination reactions to occur it is necessary to heat aggregate IgG or use sensitised particulate antigens (e.g. sheep erythrocytes) or use IgG passively adsorbed on latex or other particles. Soluble immune complexes are also precipitated by IgM rheumatoid factors (Edelman et al, 1958). The possibility has been considered that interaction between complexed or aggregated (altered) IgG and rheumatoid factor occur because conformational changes in the IgG molecule reveals previously hidden antigenic determinants. This is an unsatisfactory explanation since monomeric IgG does interact with rheumatoid factor (Normansell, 1971). A more plausible explanation is that whereas monomeric IgG is a monovalent antigen, altered IgG, being polyvalent, interacts with rheumatoid factor in a manner favouring lattice formation which is associated with precipitation or agglutination (see p. 378).

It has been suggested that interaction of IgM rheumatoid factor with soluble complexes converts them to larger complexes which are more readily phagocytosed and cleared by the reticuloendothelial system. This finding is compatible with an essentially beneficial role for rheumatoid factor in vivo, a view further elaborated by Goldberg & Fudenberg (1971). On the other hand the efficient phagocytosis of immune complexes leads to the release of lysosomal enzymes with attendant tissue damage. Furthermore, IgM rheumatoid factor converts complexes that bind little complement into those that bind complement efficiently (Tesar & Schmid, 1970) and the resulting complement activation should encourage a whole sequence of reactions, e.g. chemotaxis, phagocytosis and release of inflammatory mediators, which also contribute to tissue damage. Soluble immune complexes in the synovial fluid of patients lacking IgM rheumatoid factor are only phagocytosed by normal neutrophils when IgM rheumatoid factor is added (Hurd et al, 1970), a finding which has generally been interpreted as indicating its role in inducing joint damage. However it has been found that rheumatoid factor diminishes the generation of chemotactic activity by the action of immune complexes on fresh serum (Horowitz et al, 1971). Thus the role of rheumatoid factor in rheumatoid arthritis remains unresolved, although it is mostly regarded as contributing to tissue damage (reviewed by Zvaifler, 1973), a view in accord with the clinical association of the presence of rheumatoid factor with severe joint disease and the development of extra-articular manifestations.

The role of rheumatoid factor in microbial infections is equally controversial. The neutralisation of infectious herpes virus–antibody complexes in the presence of complement is assisted by rheumatoid factors (Ashe et al, 1971) and this type of mechanism should provide the host with antiviral protection. In contrast, it has been suggested that IgM rheumatoid factors impair protective immunity by inhibiting the opsonisation of bacteria by IgG (Messner et al, 1968).

FATE OF CIRCULATING IMMUNE COMPLEXES

The amount of immune complexes circulating in blood at any time is a function of the balance between their production and clearance by the reticuloendothelial system, degree of deposition in tissues, and the natural catabolic rates of the constituent immunoglobulin and antigen. If the complexes of the appropriate type persist in the circulation for a long enough period, deposition in tissues could occur and thereafter initiate the process of tissue damage.

Clearance

Certain types of circulating complexes are apparently actively cleared by phagocytic cells of the reticuloendothelial system in the lungs, liver and spleen (reviewed by Cochrane & Koffler, 1973). Insight into the mechanisms involved has been largely gathered from studies on the fate of artificially prepared complexes and of aggregated IgG (which behaves as an immune complex in many respects). Two main approaches have been employed:

a. The study of the clearance of complexes from the circulation and their uptake by the liver and spleen in vivo.
b. Interactions between cells and complexes in vitro.

Initial studies failed to recognise the fact that soluble and particulate complexes behave differently and that Fc and C receptors may function independently or synergistically. Moreover, particles (such as heat-damaged erythrocytes) may be cleared by non-immunological mechanisms. In assessing clearance in vivo, confusion has also arisen from failure to distinguish between passive pooling of blood in organs, as distinct from specific uptake by cells. Many of the previous conclusions need to be re-evaluated, and at the present time there is an incomplete picture of the precise site of clearance of different types of complexes, and of the role of C3 and Fc receptors in the eventual fate of complexes. The broad conclusions which have been drawn are that soluble complexes are predominantly cleared by Kupffer cells in the liver. Fc receptors are involved in clearing complexes containing IgG whereas C3b receptors are probably involved in the clearance of IgM and possibly particulate complexes (Van Es, 1981; Nussensweig, 1980). Some complexes and especially non-opsonised particulate material may also be removed bŷ the spleen, and IgA containing circulating complexes may be taken up by the hepatocyte and excreted into bile.

The clearance of immune complexes from the circulation is dependent on the following factors:

Size and lattice structure of the complex

As previously discussed (p. 378) this is determined by the nature of the antigen and antibody and by the relative amounts present. Injected antigen–antibody complexes formed near equivalence are cleared more rapidly than those formed in antigen excess (Weigle, 1958). Very large soluble complexes (greater than 19s on ultracentrifugation) are cleared within a few seconds compared to smaller complexes which persist for many hours (Cochrane & Hawkins, 1968; Lightfoot et al, 1970). Such complexes also have a well-defined lattice structure (Mannik et al, 1971).

Uptake by reticuloendothelial system and role of complement

Experiments suggest that large complexes with a well-developed lattice structure are cleared quickly because of efficient binding to surface receptors on phagocytic cells. Chemical alkylation and reduction of immunoglobulin abolishes the ability of immune complexes to bind to the cell receptors (without altering their size) and leads to impairment of their clearance from the circulation, and of binding to macrophages in vitro (Mannik et al, 1974). In the experiments of Mannik et al, 1971, depletion of circulating complement did not appreciably influence the rate of clearance of complexes containing IgG. However in other experiments complement has been shown to facilitate clearance of bacteria and erythrocytes coated with antibody (Spiegelberg et al, 1963). It seems that complement is required to clear complexes containing IgM antibody (Brown et al, 1970). This finding is in keeping with the observation that mononuclear phagocytes possess receptors for certain subclasses of IgG and complement but not IgM (Abramson et al, 1970). The role of complement in the clearance of complexes remains to be elucidated but there is compelling evidence of its importance (Nussensweig, 1980).

The possibility that the capacity of the reticuloendothelial system could be overwhelmed by the sheer load of immune complexes in large quantities is suggested by their prolonged persistence in the circulation of animals previously injected with increasing amounts of complexes (Mannik et al, 1974). Impaired clearance of complexes has also been documented in chronic serum sickness in rabbits (Wilson & Dixon, 1971) and NZB/NZW mice with evidence of renal disease (Mannik et al, 1974). A genetically determined variation in macrophage function has been found in different strains of mice (Morgan & Soothill, 1975). Using measurement of clearance of radiolabelled polyvinyl pyrolidine as an index of the phagocytic activity of the reticuloendothelial system in these investigations, it was found that strains of mice with low clearance rates also produced antibodies of low affinity. These strains of mice are known to be the most susceptible to immune complex disease. It is possible to suggest that production of low affinity antibody and impaired macrophage function (individually or together) lead to persistence of circulating immune complexes which are of pathogenetic importance. It is uncertain, at present, to what extent the observations on macrophage function in experimental animals have a parallel in diseases characterised by deposition of immune complexes in man. For example, in one recent investigation on patients with nephritis associated with immune complex deposition, in contrast with the results in animals, it was found that phagocytic activity (as measured by clearance of radiolabelled albumin) was increased (Drivas et al, 1976).

The nature of the antigen

Particular emphasis has been placed on the importance of the immunoglobulin and complement components of immune complexes in clearance studies. However, it is self-evident that the antigen moiety may be the rate-determining factor in some cases. This may be of particular importance for autoantigens (Schreiber et al, 1983).

The permeability of vessels

Immune complexes are normally unable to escape, either passively or during ultrafiltration across the vessel wall. This situation is altered in inflammatory diseases following damage to vessels (e.g. the glomerulus) and associated with rapid clearance from the circulation.

Tissue deposition

Circulating soluble complexes deposited in the walls of blood vessels of tissues show certain repeating patterns of preferential sites of localisation in both experimental and clinical situations. For example, in the acute serum sickness model the kidneys and blood vessels are mainly involved; in chronic serum sickness, and in the spontaneous

SLE-like syndrome in New Zealand mice, the kidneys; in Aleutian mink disease, the blood vessels, and to a lesser extent, the kidneys; in polyarteritis a patchy involvement of the medium-sized arteries; in SLE, varying combinations of the skin, kidney, joint, central nervous system or cardiorespiratory system; in Henoch–Schönlein purpura, the skin, joints, kidneys and gastrointestinal tract; and in serum hepatitis, the liver.

Several factors are involved in the process of deposition and localisation of complexes. An active process is implicated rather than a mere diffusion of the complex across vessel walls from the intravascular compartment (reviewed by Cochrane, 1971). An alteration in the permeability of vessel walls brought about by chemical mediators appears to be an important prerequisite. Intravenous colloidal carbon is deposited in the subendothelial region of the vessel walls of mice if vasoactive amines are simultaneously administered (Benacerraf et al, 1959). Preformed immune complexes are deposited in vessels only if administered with agents such as anaphylotoxin which liberate histamine. In acute and chronic serum sickness in rabbits the renal and vascular lesions can be prevented by administration of antagonists of histamine and serotonin (Kniker & Cochrane, 1968). The mechanism controlling release of vasoactive amines in acute serum sickness in rabbits has been defined and is dependent on interaction of antigen with circulating basophils sensitised with IgE antibody. This leads to the release of a mediator termed 'platelet aggregating factor' which in turn liberates vasoactive amines from platelets (Benveniste et al, 1972). It is uncertain the extent to which this mechanism can be regarded as a general phenomenon with wide applicability to all forms of immune complex disease.

Hawn & Janeway (1947) found that rabbits with an experimentally induced serum sickness-like disease tended to develop predominantly arteritic lesions involving large vessels if albumin was used as the challenging antigen, whereas glomerular lesions predominated if gammaglobulins were used. Although there are several possible explanations for this phenomenon, it should be considered that localisation of the complexes is determined by their size or a special affinity of antigen, antibody or complement for particular tissue components.

'Large' soluble immune complexes (which on ultracentrifugation sediment in the range equal or greater than 19s) are preferentially trapped in vessel walls (Cochrane, 1971). Such complexes are most efficient at binding complement and are also most efficiently eliminated by the reticuloendothelial system. The fate of such complexes is therefore a critical factor in determining whether tissue injury will occur as a result of deposition in tissues or whether their clearance will lead to sparing from damage. Complexes formed in considerable antigen excess (much smaller than 19s) do not appear to localise very much in tissues and apparently persist in the circulation (Cochrane & Hawkins, 1968), and have therefore been regarded as being relatively 'benign' in nature. To a certain extent these findings are supported by the observation that in the kidney, 'large' molecules localise in the subendothelial position (corresponding to molecular weight in excess of 500 000 daltons) and smaller molecules (80 000 to 250 000 daltons) penetrate the glomerular basement membrane and lodge within it or in the subepithelial layer (Oliver & Essner, 1972). The former position of complex deposition is best seen in the most severe forms of SLE nephritis, whereas the latter is seen with membranous nephropathies in which proteinuria (without severe impairment of glomerular filtration rate) is the predominant feature. In a study of SLE patients it was found that renal involvement occurred when the size of circulating complexes was in the region of 1 000 000 daltons, whilst extrarenal manifestations were present when the size of complexes was 2 500 000 to 4 000 000 (Levinsky et al, 1977).

Tissue receptors could be important in determining the site of localization of soluble circulating immune complexes. For example, Fc receptors have been described with an affinity for aggregated and complexed immunoglobulin on vascular endothelial cells of placenta (Johnson et al, 1973). C3b receptors which bind to erythrocytes coated with antibody and activated complement (forming EAC rosettes) have been found in the kidney glomerulus, and these receptors are blocked in diseases associated with immune complex deposits in the glomerulus (Gelfand et al, 1976).

In recent experiments it has been shown that DNA has considerable binding affinity for glomerular basement membrane and collagen, and it has been suggested that this affinity may be the basis of the observed sequential localisation of DNA followed by anti-DNA antibody on the glomerular basement membrane of an experimentally induced nephritis in mice (Izui et al, 1976). These experiments suggest the possibility that DNA-anti-DNA (antigen–antibody) complexes in the kidneys in SLE could arise as a result of a similar mechanism, and are therefore more akin to an Arthus-type reaction sequence (i.e. deposition of antigen followed by antibody) rather than an example of a disease entirely arising as a result of the deposition of circulating soluble complexes. Since anti-DNA antibodies are usually found in a non-complexed state in the circulation (Zubler & Lambert, 1977), the identity of the constituents of the readily demonstrable 'soluble complexes' in SLE remains to be elucidated.

The assumption that all forms of glomerulonephritis are a consequence of deposition of circulating complexes has been challenged, especially in view of the observation that only a minority of patients show the presence of immune complexes in blood. The view that in such diseases immune complex formation occurs in situ is gaining ground.

Tissues that are favoured sites of immune complex deposition share certain features. The glomerulus, synovial membrane, choroid plexus skin and uveal tract all have a fenestrated endothelium, a high blood flow rate and a filtering mechanism (Andrews & Penny, 1976). In the joint, periarticular tissues and cartilage have a special tendency to retain immune complexes (Cooke et al, 1975).

Mechanical and haemodynamic factors have also been regarded as being of some importance in the selection of the site of deposition. The glomerular basement membrane in kidneys and the internal elastic lamina of arteries provide examples of filtrating membranes which limit and trap circulating complexes by virtue of the high pressure forces across them. The turbulence of blood flow at points of origin and bifurcation of vessels may explain the involvement of coronary ostia and branches of the aorta (Germuth, 1953) and the increased intensity of vasculitic lesions in the presence of hypertension in serum sickness (Fisher & Bark, 1961). The widely appreciated clinical observation that rheumatoid nodules localise to sites of repeated trauma may have a similar explanation.

Pathogenicity of immune complexes

Immune complexes have been implicated as initiators of tissue damage. It has been considered that one important mechanism of tissue injury is dependent on immune complex induced release of lysosomal enzymes from polymorphs and macrophages present at the site of inflammation, which in turn leads to damage to connective tissue. Enzymes have been described with specificity for individual components such as proteoglycan-rich amorphous material, collagen and elastin found, for example, in cartilage, vessel walls and the supporting tissue of various organs. Although a large number of enzymes from various cell sources have been studied, it has become apparent that only a few are likely to be active at a physiological pH, and that their action is in any case counter-balanced by naturally occurring enzyme inhibitors. Nevertheless, since the observed tissue degradation is compatible with damage due to enzymatic attack, it could be suggested that a relative deficiency of enzyme inhibitors or selective access of the enzymes to the site of tissue degradation must exist (e.g. by close application of polymorphs or macrophages to connective tissue structures).

The mechanism of enzyme release by polymorphs and macrophages induced by immune complexes has been largely investigated in tissue culture. Release of enzymes consequent upon phagocytosis of particulate and large immune complexes occurs during the process of formation of the phagosome, a process termed 'regurgitation during feeding' (Weissmann et al, 1971). In addition, polymorphs adherent to complexes on non-phagocytosable surfaces release enzymes to the exterior by a process involving merger of lysosomal granules with the cell membrane and discharge of the enzyme (Henson, 1971), a process which has been termed 'reverse endocytosis' or 'frustrated phagocytosis'. This mechanism could be particularly important in mediating injury in lesions in which polymorphs are regularly found, for example, in the glomerular lesions in certain forms of glomerulonephritis and in Arthus-type vasculitic lesions. Immune complexes frequently found on the surface of cartilage and collagenous structures in the joints of patients with rheumatoid arthritis (Cooke et al, 1975) could provide a potential site for a similar reaction, although polymorph adherence to these structures is not a regular feature of the joint pathology. Indeed, in rheumatoid arthritis, only the synovial fluid is rich in polymorphs (some of which contain intracytoplasmic immune complexes, discussed below), and loss of cartilage and bone is most pronounced in the pannus contiguous with the hypertrophic synovial tissue in the region of the joint margin. It is possible that enzymes found in the joint fluid, and probably mainly derived from polymorphs, may contribute to joint damage (reviewed by Zvaifler, 1973) although enzyme inhibitors, also present in the fluid, should prevent enzymatic attack.

The interaction of complexes with polymorphs is facilitated by binding to specific membrane receptors. Experiments have indicated the presence of receptors for Fc and C3b, which allows interaction with immune complexes irrespective of whether they are bound to activated complement components (Henson, 1971). However, complement has been shown to enhance immune complex-dependent enzyme release, and, in addition, activated complement component C5 (C5a) itself leads to enzyme release without direct participation of complexes (Goldstein & Weissmann, 1974). Since C5 activation can be initiated by proteases (Lepow, 1971) additional mechanisms of complement-dependent injury may be perpetuated at sites of tissue damage following initiation by either the classical pathway (involving immune complexes) or other alternative pathways. Polymorphs are prominently involved in the Arthus reaction and their role in mediating tissue damage in such experimental models is supported by the observation that polymorph depletion reduces the severity of cutaneous Arthus reactions, as well as significantly reducing the lesions of arteritis in acute serum sickness (Cochrane & Koffler, 1973).

The exposure of mononuclear phagocytes to immune complexes in cultures is also accompanied by selective release of intracellular enzymes (Cardella et al, 1974). The most vigorous release of enzymes occurred with immune complexes prepared at equivalence and it was suggested that enzyme release was accompanied by increased synthesis upon prolonged exposure in culture. The presence of mononuclear cells at sites of inflammation enlarges our understanding of tissue damage in the absence of polymorphs. For example, the interaction of immune complexes with mononuclear phagocytic cells in the synovial membrane of patients with rheumatoid arthritis could explain the degradation of connective tissue of cartilage in the joint (Allison et al, 1975). The ability of the rheumatoid synovium to produce collagenase and to destroy cartilage in tissue culture has been documented (Evanson et al, 1967), but it is not yet clear whether the enzyme is produced by phagocytic cells or fibroblasts and to what extent immunological stimuli are important, or indeed whether such experiments bear any relationship to the situation in vivo.

THE CONCEPT OF IMMUNE COMPLEX DISEASE

The concept that vasculitis, arthritis and nephritis may be mediated by immune complexes is largely derived from an assumed causal relationship between the demonstration of immune complexes in tissues and in blood with disease features in man and in experimental models of disease. Experience over the last few years has shown that this may be a simplified view since immune complexes may be found in blood and tissues without evident pathology. In other patients with features assumed to be mediated by immune complexes, existing techniques do not confirm the presence of immune complexes. Certainly immune complexes are not pathogenic in themselves — they become pathogenic following interaction with cells and complement (as discussed above). They may also alter the rheology of blood, and by accumulating in tissues, they may exert physical effects on the function of tissues. Thus the pathogenic pathway is multifactorial and may exert its effect over a period of time. These factors make assessment of the importance of immune complexes in disease difficult and single measurements of little clinical value.

Nevertheless, the evidence that inflammatory rheumatic diseases can be regarded as examples of immune complex disease, although conjectural, is strong and is based on the following criteria:

a. Components of immune complexes can be identified in diseased tissues.
b. In many instances definable autoantigen–antibody complexes are found in blood and in tissues.
c. Evidence of hypercatabolism of complement is demonstrable.
d. Variation in circulating levels of immune complexes and hypercatabolism of complement correlates with disease.
e. Most, if not all, of these diseases occur in individuals with particular HLA phenotypes and complement allotypes, thus pointing to a susceptible genetic profile.

The current theory of immune complex rheumatic disease envisages that immune complexes are involved in the mediation of tissue lesions and clinical features, and in the main consist of autoantigen–antibody complexes with a particular liability to fix complement. The autoimmunity that is manifest in these patients is a result of disordered regulation of the immune response, which is itself influenced by various factors such as genes, gender, hormones and the environment (Fig. 13.2)

EXPERIMENTAL MODELS

Arthus reaction

In classical experiments, antigen injected into the skin of a pre-immunised animal is believed to form immune complexes in the walls of the small blood vessels and in the extravascular tissue space. For this reaction to occur, the vessel wall has to be permeable enough to allow antigen to diffuse inwards and for the circulating antibody to escape outwards, an event which may itself be initiated by the antigen first reacting with reagins (usually IgE antibody) present on tissue mast cells, thereby leading to the release of histamine and other vasoactive amines. The formation of immune complexes in optimal proportions leads to fixation and activation of serum complement and the generation of chemotactic factors which provide the means whereby the migration and attraction of polymorphs to the site of the immune complex is controlled. Phagocytosis of the complexes by polymorphs is believed to lead to release of lysosomal enzymes, which, together with other inflammatory mediators, damage blood vessel walls and result in enzymatic degradation of connective tissue and lead to necrosis, haemorrhage or infarction. The role of complement and polymorphs in the Arthus reaction is discussed by Henson & Cochrane (1975).

By means of immunofluorescent studies it is possible to follow the fate of injected antigen during the course of an Arthus reaction. At first it lies free or complexed with antibody in extracellular tissue spaces, and shortly afterwards in the walls of the vessels, especially between the endothelial cells and the basement membrane. Thereafter the complexes are phagocytosed and cleared by polymorphs (Humphrey & White, 1970). Once formed, the complexes are apparently rapidly cleared and do not persist at the site of injection for more than 48 hours (Cream et al, 1971).

Genes Gender Hormones Environmental factors	→ Disordered immune regulation	→ Autoimmunity and immune complex disease

Fig. 13.2 The aetiology of immune complex disease.

Serum sickness in rabbits; acute and chronic immune complex disease

Heterologous serum proteins have been commonly employed to produce acute and chronic serum sickness in experimental animals and these models serve as prototypes of immune complex disease in man (reviewed by Cochrane & Koffler, 1973). In the two models studied by Dixon and his associates (1958, 1961) rabbits were injected with a single large dose of bovine serum albumin (BSA) to produce acute immune complex disease, whereas repeated injection of smaller amounts of BSA over about 5–10 weeks were necessary before lesions of chronic immune complex disease became apparent. Since these models have contributed

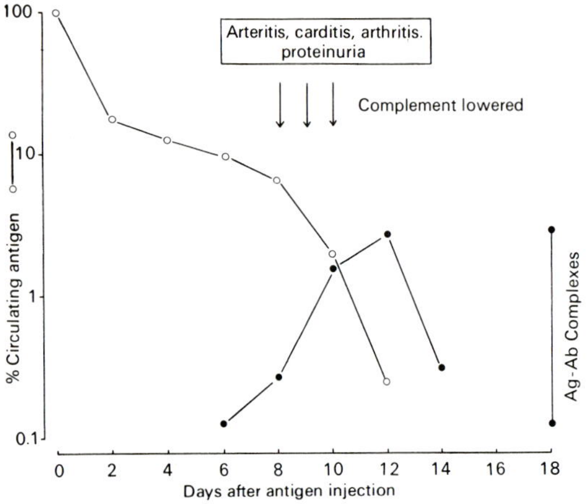

Fig. 13.3 Immune complex disease in acute serum sickness. Following injection of serum antigens (day 0) there is an initial phase of equilibration, followed by a slow rate of elimination due to catabolic processes. From the 6th day onwards circulating antibody levels begin to rise and are accompanied by accelerated removal of antigen. The appearance of circulating immune complexes coincides with hypocomplementaemia and a self-limiting disease characterised by arteritis, carditis, arthritis and glomerulonephritis. (Based on Dixon et al., 1958.)

significantly to current views on pathogenetic mechanisms, some of the features of the models are described below.

Acute immune complex disease occurs about eight days after antigen injection, when circulating BSA-anti-BSA complexes can be detected in the blood, and is characterised by a variety of multi-system lesions (Fig. 13.3). These include endocarditis, arteritis, glomerulonephritis and polyarthritis. The arteritis involves the origins of the coronary vessels and branching points of the aorta and pulmonary arteries and is of the necrotising type with intimal hyperplasia, disruption of the internal elastic lamina, and fibrinoid necrosis of the media with polymorph and mononuclear cell infiltration and inflammatory changes in the adventitia. Glomerulonephritis is characterised by proteinuria and haematuria; histological examination of the kidneys shows marked swelling of the endothelial cells of glomerular capillaries resembling changes observed in poststreptococcal acute nephritis. Using suitable techniques, antigen and antibody are demonstrable on the glomerular basement membrane (GBM). In simultaneous studies on kidney and blood, disappearance of circulating antigen corresponds with its deposition in kidneys, although the amount deposited represents only about 1/10 000 of the original injected dose (Wilson & Dixon, 1971). Immunofluorescent techniques at this stage demonstrate granular deposits of IgG and C3 component of complement as fine granules on the GBM. Spontaneous recovery is usual, and it is worthy of note that the healing phase of the glomerulonephritis is marked by a further increase in size of deposits of both IgG and C3, an important reminder that immune deposits in the tissues do not always indicate concurrent damaging processes, but in some situations are associated with healing.

Repeated injections of BSA in rabbits lead to the evolution of a disease predominantly involving kidneys; arthritis has been noted to occur but has not received detailed study until very recently. In the small proportion of animals that develop chronic arthritis, a synovitis (with a predominantly mononuclear cell infiltrate) and the formation of a pannus eroding cartilage resembling rheumatoid arthritis has been recently documented (Poole & Coombs, 1977). Histological studies of kidney at the onset of albuminuria and haematuria show a membranous type of glomerulonephritis. If antigen injections are continued, renal disease becomes more severe and is accompanied by hypoproteinemia and azotaemia, and eventually results in death. The histological lesions themselves vary in morphology from thickening of the GBM due to deposition of complexes only, or accompanied by endothelial cellular proliferation, polymorph accumulation, necrosis of cells and epithelial cell crescent formation in Bowman's capsule. Immunofluorescent studies on the kidney, before the onset of proteinuria, show fine granular immune deposits of BSA, IgG and C3 in the mesangial region; but when proteinuria is manifest, globular deposits of BSA, IgG and C3 are evident on the GBM, appearing as electron dense deposits within the basement membrane or in the subepithelial region (Wilson & Dixon, 1971).

In the acute serum sickness model an antibody response to the antigen begins to occur on about the eighth day, in the presence of a large excess of injected antigen (Fig. 13.3). The multisystem pathology occurs in this period of soluble immune complex formation and complement consumption (Dixon et al, 1958). The severity of the lesions is related to the amount of antigen deposited in the tissues (Wilson & Dixon, 1971). The most severe changes are seen in the kidneys of rabbits forming large amounts of antibody, and in these animals antigen is cleared most rapidly (by the twelfth day). It appears that the expression and severity of immune complex disease in this model is dependent on the production of an antibody response which results in the formation of immune complexes which possess maximal inflammatory potential.

In the chronic immune complex model the quantity of antibody and its quality are both important in establishing renal damage. If a fixed dose of BSA is injected daily, some rabbits (a minority) develop chronic glomerulonephritis. The amount of antibody in repeatedly immunised animals varies enormously, and if the antibody response is poor, no renal lesion is induced (Pincus et al, 1968). Provided the antigen dose is monitored so that the amount injected exceeds the amount of circulating antibody on each occasion, damage to kidneys is invariable in animals in whom antibodies are detectable (Dixon et al, 1961). Indeed, in this situation, rabbits which produce the largest antibody response detected as precipitating antibodies develop the most severe lesions and exhibit the greatest amounts of immune complex deposition. In experiments carried out by Pincus and his colleagues (1968) the rabbits with immune complex disease formed non-precipitating antibody, and in the presence of such antibody, elimination of antigen may be impaired and accompanied by prolonged circulation of soluble immune complexes (Christian, 1970). The finding that soluble immune complexes circulate in the blood for periods long enough to permit deposition in kidneys and other tissues in these and other similar studies has provided the basis of much current thought on the pathogenesis of disease processes, especially in relation to the kidneys.

'Allergic' arthritis in rabbits and adjuvant disease in rats

Injection of human fibrin into the knee or ankle joint of a rabbit that has been previously sensitised with this antigen in Freund's adjuvant (an oily emulsion containing mycobacteria) produces a chronic inflammatory arthritis which shows many features of the rheumatoid joint (Dumonde & Glynn, 1962). Subsequent experiments have shown that a similar arthritis can be induced with other foreign protein antigens (e.g. albumin) in a number of species of animals, and that the presence of mycobacteria in the adjuvant appears to be necessary (Glynn, 1975), possibly as a means of inducing cellular hypersensitivity, although their precise pathogenetic role remains undefined. The role of mycobacterial adjuvants and cellular immunity is better understood in the polyarthritis observed in rats injected with Freund's adjuvant (Pearson & Wood, 1963). The initial inflammatory reaction in the joint of rabbits with the Dumonde and Glynn type of model appears to be an Arthus response (Cooke et al, 1975). For several subsequent weeks a significant proportion of the antibody synthesised by plasma cells in the synovial membrane is directed against the inducing antigen (Cooke & Jasin, 1972). Experiments have also shown that antigen is retained in the joint for prolonged periods in the collagenous tissues of the cartilage and intra-articular ligaments in the form of immune complexes (Cooke et al, 1972). These experiments suggest that immune complexes provide a mechanism for sequestration of antigen in joints and that the subsequent availability of antigen could be responsible for perpetuating a local immune response which results in chronic synovitis. The induction of an allergic arthritis in the ankle joint of agammaglobulinaemic (bursectomised) chickens (Oates et al, 1972) however, implies that cell-mediated reactions are important in inducing inflammation and that the chronicity of the arthritis may be dependent on additional factors. Injection of bovine serum albumin (BSA) into the joints of rabbits previously immunised with BSA and Freund's incomplete adjuvant (containing oil but no mycobacteria) does not induce chronic arthritis, but is accompanied by the presence of immune complexes (IgG and C3) in cartilage (Fox & Glynn, 1975), further emphasising the possibility that immune complexes alone are not responsible for allergic inflammation in this model.

Spontaneous lupus in mice and dogs

The possible genetic basis of susceptibility to immune complex disease has been emphasised by studies on New Zealand mice in which spontaneous immune complex renal disease is believed to be induced by a virus and mediated by nuclear antigen–antibody complexes. It finds its most severe expression in the F1 hybrid offspring of mating between the black and white strains (Talal, 1970). Oldstone & Dixon (1969) have shown that mice infected in utero (or at birth) with lymphocytic choriomeningitis virus develop immune complex disease. In these animals tissue lesions are associated with deposits of viral–immunoglobulin–complement complexes. Further, it has been shown that infection of murine strains with the Scripps leukaemia virus (an example of a pathogenic oncorna virus) leads to the production of antinuclear antibodies in the majority of strains, but only certain genetic strains develop glomerulonephritis, the renal lesion being caused by immune complexes containing virus and nuclear antigens (Dixon et al, 1974). Soothill & Steward (1971) have shown that murine strains most susceptible to immune complex disease produce low avidity antibodies when challenged with antigens, whereas strains resistant to immune complex disease form high avidity antibody. A genetically determined abnormal immune response to common viruses, resulting in a low avidity antibody response and failure to eliminate virus, may favour formation of complexes and emergence of autoimmunity which may prove to be of aetiological importance in human diseases such as systemic lupus erythematosus.

A spontaneous lupus syndrome, predominantly occurring in female dogs with the serological abnormalities closely parelling disease in man, is of special interest because cell-free filtrates prepared from spleen of affected dogs injected into mice and beagle dogs induced anti-nuclear antibodies (Lewis & Schwartz, 1971). This finding suggests that a transmissable agent may be of aetiological importance in this disease.

An inbred strain of mice MRL-Lpr/Lpr has proved to be of great interest since the development of spontaneous lupus in these mice is not only genetically associated with the lpr 'gene', but is also characterised by immune complex mediated nephritis, and an erosive arthritis (Hang et al, 1982). These mice have circulating immune complexes with defects in clearance mechanisms. Antibodies to dsDNA and Sm as well as rheumatoid factors are present. Cellular interactions have been studied and show abnormalities in the generation of interleukin 2, and suppressor cell function. It promises to be a model which should allow the unravelling of the immune network abnormalities which lead to autoimmunity.

IMMUNE COMPLEXES IN RHEUMATIC DISEASES

The interest in the possible clinical significance of immune complexes has stimulated a proliferation of laboratory techniques for the detection and quantitation (for reviews see: Maini & Holborow, 1977; Theofilopoulous & Dixon, 1979; Jones & Orlans, 1981). The sensitivity, reproducibility, precision and specificity have been investigated up to a degree (Lambert et al, 1978). A lack of concordance has been observed in different assays and may reflect the varying principles which govern the basis of the assay as well as the fact that complexes vary in their size, concentration and relative ratios of antigen and antibody, each of which may affect aspects of quantitation and interpretation. The expression of results in equivalents of aggregated IgG may be of spurious value in this respect (McCarthy et al, 1981). The possibility that false-positive results may be obtained due to biologically reactive non-immune complex material raises a further problem in the use of the assays (Horsfall et al, 1981; Jones & Orlans, 1981). False-negatives are especially liable to occur if the pathogenic complexes contain IgA since the commonly used tests rely on interactions with complement (or its receptors) and rheumatoid factors. Moreover, the majority of assays are not antigen-specific.

In this section some of the approaches for the detection of immune complexes are examined with special reference to rheumatic diseases.

Microscopy

The availability of fluorescein-conjugated antisera to immunoglobulin and complement has permitted the wide application of immunofluorescent techniques for localisation of immune complexes within tissues and cells. Antisera with the appropriate specificity are employed as reagents, for example, directed against all classes of immunoglobulin ('polyvalent' antisera) a particular class or subclass ('monovalent' antisera), and a number of complement proteins, or their breakdown or activation products. Cryopreserved fresh tissues are cut into thin sections, placed on a glass slide and treated with fluoresceinated antisera and examined by the use of an ultraviolet light source, which causes fluorescence of the tissue-fixed reagent. The presence of immunoglobulin and complement in the same location in serial sections is taken as indirect evidence for the presence of a complement-fixing immune complex. Another method of demonstrating the coexistence of immunoglobulin and complement relies on the use of 'double-staining' of the same tissue section, for example, utilising fluorescein-conjugated antiserum for one of the proteins (which fluoresces green) and rhodamine-conjugated antiserum for the other protein (which fluoresces red); the coexistence of the two proteins is indicated by synthesis of the two colours, seen as yellow fluorescence (Plate 13.1).

a

b

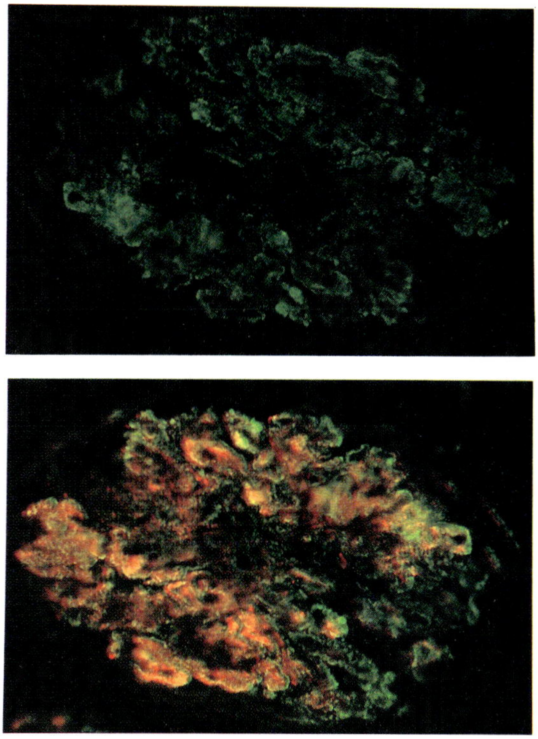

Plate 13.1 Adjacent cryostat sections of renal biopsy tissue obtained from a patient with systemic lupus erythematosus showing: (a) IgG deposits in the glomerular walls by using fluorescein-conjugated anti-IgG anti-serum (green); (b) 'Double-staining' for IgG and C3 (green for IgG, red for C3 and yellow where IgG and C3 are deposited together). (By courtesy of Dr Robin Butler and Dr David Woodrow.)

Frozen tissue sections may also be used for the demonstration of antigen provided a suitable antiserum is available and the appropriate controls are performed. The presence of antigen and immunoglobulin (with complement) in the same location in these circumstances provides direct evidence for the presence of immune complexes. In practice this is only rarely possible, either because the antigen implicated is not known or because no suitable antiserum is available, or because the antigen is 'hidden' in its complexed form or only present in minute amounts.

Using immunofluorescence, all classes of immunoglobulin, rheumatoid factor and C3 deposits have been demonstrated in the synovial membrane of patients with rheumatoid arthritis (Mellors et al, 1961; Fish et al, 1966; Rodman et al, 1967; Bononomo et al, 1970). The nature of the antigen and the specificity of immunoglobulin in the deposits is unresolved, although it has been claimed that the plasma cells in the membrane mainly synthesise rheumatoid factor (an anti-IgG antibody) which gives rise to the formation of complexes consisting of rheumatoid factor bound to autologous IgG (Natvig & Munthe, 1975). The possibility that infective agents could provide antigens against which the immune response is directed is attractive, but thus far no convincing evidence of such antigens (or isolation of infectious agents) is forthcoming. The lining layer cells of the synovial membrane obtained by trypsinisation have also been shown to contain IgG, IgM and C3 within their cytoplasm, presumably as a result of phagocytosis of immune complexes by the type A lining layer cell (Kinsella et al, 1970). Synovial fluid polymorphonuclear neutrophils obtained from patients with rheumatoid arthritis similarly contain intracellular phagocytosed complexes, a finding originally reported by Rawson and his colleagues (and cited by Hollander in support of the hypothesis that these cells were involved in mediating tissue injury (Hollander et al, 1965). Intracytoplasmic neutrophil inclusions contain rheumatoid factor, other immunoglobulins and C3, and their presence is inversely related to complement consumption as measured by levels of joint fluid C4 (Vaughan et al, 1968). Exposure of normal circulating polymorphs to synovial fluid from rheumatoid arthritis patients could be shown to lead to the development of intracytoplasmic inclusions of IgG, IgM and C3 only if the fluid was IgM rheumatoid factor-positive (Hurd et al, 1970). Addition of rheumatoid factor to IgM factor-negative fluids also led to the development of such inclusions, suggesting that complexes already present were rendered phagocytosable by rheumatoid factor. Whilst the immune complexes within the synovial membrane and synovial fluid are regarded as directly contributing to tissue damage, the discovery of immune complexes in the cartilage, menisci and ligaments of rheumatoid joints (Cooke et al, 1975) could be regarded as being of importance in retention of antigen in the joint, and an important factor in the perpetuation of the disease process. Immune complexes of IgG and IgM with antiglobulin activity have also been demonstrated in lymph nodes (McCormick, 1963) and rheumatoid nodules (Nowoslawski, 1971) and IgG, IgM and complement were found in the vasa nervosum in patients with rheumatoid vasculitis (Conn et al, 1972). These findings are regarded as implicating immune complexes in the pathogenesis of extra-articular manifestations of rheumatoid arthritis.

Systemic lupus erythematosus is widely regarded as a prototype of circulating immune complex disease with multisystem involvement explicable on the basis of deposition of complexes in vessel walls. Complexes of immunoglobulin and complement components are demonstrable by immunofluorescence in the glomeruli and consist, in part, of polynucleotide antigents and antibodies, particularly DNA and anti-DNA antibody (Koffler et al, 1967). Immunoglobulin and C3 have also been demonstrated in the choroid plexus (Atkins et al, 1972) and at the epidermodermal junction of skin (Tan & Kunkel, 1966). The deposition at the epidermodermal junction of skin could suggest that extravasated circulating anti-nuclear antibody may be combining with nuclear antigens released by degenerating epidermal cells. Although deposits of complement have been generally regarded as implying binding to immune complexes, studies indicate that alternative pathway complement components are also deposited in the skin (Schrager & Rothfield, 1976) and in kidneys et al, 1971), a finding implying that immune complexes are not necessarily the sole initiators of complement-mediated inflammation in systemic lupus erythematosus.

The finding of immune complexes (by immunofluorescent methods), containing Australia antigen, immunoglobulin and complement in the vessels of patients with polyarteritis nodosa (Gocke et al, 1971) has provided an important clue to the pathogenesis of the inflammatory multisystem vascular lesions in this disease. Studies undertaken on the synovial membrane in arthritis occurring in the prodromal phase of serum hepatitis and during the course of meningococcal septicaemia indicate that the arthritis in these infective conditions is mediated by immune complexes (Alpert et al, 1971; Greenwood et al, 1973). The findings of immune deposits in the vessels in skin and kidneys has also been observed in various other forms of vasculitis, including Henoch–Schönlein purpura (Urizar et al, 1968) and Wegener's granulomatosis (Fauci & Wolff, 1973). The childhood form of dermatomyositis is distinguished from the adult form by the presence, in the former, of complexes within vessel walls (Whitaker & Engel, 1972). The finding of complexes in the epimembranous part of the glomerular basement membrane has led to the concept that D-penicillamine-induced nephropathy is mediated by immune complexes. There are many other examples of demonstration of immune complexes in disease by immunofluorescence.

Electron microscopy

The examination of tissues by electron microscopy has greatly facilitated the demonstration and localisation of immune deposits. In the kidney, for example, the technique augments the results obtained by immunofluorescence and allows more precise characterisation of the sites of immune deposits and the structural changes that are observed (Fig. 13.4); such observations have contributed greatly to an understanding of the pathophysiology of immune complex disease.

The electron microscope has also provided important visual evidence of circulating immune complexes, for example, of Australia antigen and

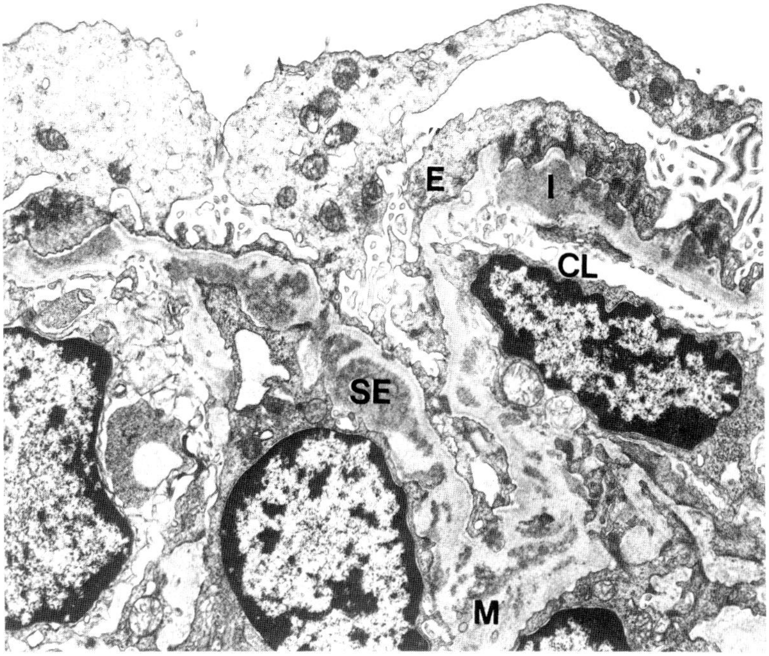

Fig. 13.4 Electron micrograph of a glomerulus from a patient with diffuse proliterative lupus nephritis. The electrondense deposits are present within the basement membrane, in the subendothelial space and within the mesangium. Foot process of epithelial cells are fused. (× 7600) E: Epithelial cell; CL: Capillary lumen; M: Mesangium; I: Intramembranous deposit within the capillary basement membrane; SE: Subendothelial deposit. (By courtesy of Dr David Woodrow and Professor J C Sloper.)

antibody in serum hepatitis (Almeida & Waterson, 1969), and of virus particles resembling Australia antigen in a third of the patients with polyarteritis nodosa (Gocke et al, 1971).

Ultracentrifugation

The technique of analytical ultracentrifugation provides a means of separating and visualising various components of circulating proteins. Under suitable conditions, the profile of normal serum shows the presence of a major peak in the 7s fraction (corresponding to IgG) and a minor peak in the 19s fraction (corresponding to IgM). Sera from patients with rheumatoid arthritis containing IgM rheumatoid factor have been shown to contain a peak which sediments more rapidly than IgM and is contained in the 22s fraction (Franklin et al, 1957) but which readily dissociates at acid pH to sediment in the 7 and 19s fractions. This phenomenon has been shown to depend on immune complex formation between autologous IgG and IgM rheumatoid factor. Immune complexes of 'intermediate' size (between 7 and 19s) have also been demonstrated in the sera of some patients with rheumatoid arthritis and are believed to occur as a result of association between IgG and rheumatoid factor of the IgG class (Kunkel et al, 1961). Similar complexes have been described in patients with hypergammaglobulinaemic purpura (Capra et al, 1971). The main disadvantage of this technique arises from its relative insensitivity in detecting complexes, and being purely analytical in nature, providing no opportunity of access to the protein fractions for analysis.

The use of the ultracentrifuge with density gradient sedimentation permits the separation of various fractions containing immune complexes. Using sucrose gradients, for example, the distribution of radiolabelled antigen bound to antibody in the various fractions (7–30s) was utilised to monitor the clearance of immune complexes of defined size (Cochrane & Koffler, 1973). The presence of IgG in the heavy fractions obtained as a pellet in a sucrose gradient indicated the presence of IgG aggregates or immune complexes in systemic lupus erythematosus (Bombardieri et al, 1973). Studies on intermediate size complexes in rheumatoid sera have indicated that the continuum of different sizes of protein obtained is a result of self-association of IgG rheumatoid factors as dimers, trimers, tetramers, etc. (Pope et al, 1974). In some patients with polyarteritis nodosa, typical electronmicroscopic appearance of Australia antigen were demonstrable in serum fractions separated by ultracentrifugation (Gocke et al, 1971).

Gel filtration

The separation of proteins by the use of gels may be used for detecting the presence of immune complexes. An example of the application of this procedure is the demonstration of complement component C3 in a macromolecular fraction larger than the molecular weight of free C3 (185 000 daltons), indicating that it is bound to an immune complex. Immune complexes were detected by this method in a majority of patients with active SLE and a few patients with rheumatoid arthritis (ten Bensel et al, 1968); the use of a more sensitive assay for C3 showed the occurrence of complexes in the majority of rheumatoid sera (Williams & Slaney, 1977).

Antigen and antibody complexes in blood, tissue eluates and other body fluids

In patients with SLE, circulating DNA was noted during phases of activity, and was found to alternate with the raised level of anti-DNA antibody in some patients (Koffler et al, 1974). The elution of antigen–antibody complexes containing polynucleotides and specific antibodies from the glomeruli of the same patients has contributed further to the view that the circulating complexes were deposited in the tissues in which injury occurred. Anti-nuclear antibodies have also been eluted from spleen (Svec & Allen, 1970). Sera of patients with SLE containing anti-DNA antibody were found to show greater amounts of antibody following DNAase digestion, indicating that some of the antibody was complexed to DNA (Harbeck et al, 1973). Using a similar technique complexes of DNA-anti-DNA antibodies were also found in the cerebrospinal fluid of patients with cerebral lupus (Keefe et al, 1974). Other workers have failed to confirm the presence of circulating DNA-anti-DNA antibodies, even though the sera were shown to contain immune complexes by other techniques (Zubler & Lambert, 1977).

About 30–40% of patients with polyarteritis nodosa have been reported to have persistent hepatitis B antigenaemia as well as evidence of circulating immune complexes, hypocomplementaemia and deposits of immune complexes at sites of vascular injury (reviewed by Gocke, 1974). The circulating immune complexes of the same antigen and antibody have been reported in the prodromal phase of hepatitis B infection of the liver and are a transitory phenomenon, not associated with the development of polyarteritis nodosa (Alpert et al, 1971). In experimental animals, persistent virus–antibody complexes have been demonstrated by a variety of techniques such as the depletion of infectious virus following precipitation by anti-immunoglobulin and anti-complement sera, and have been linked with the tissue injury process (Oldstone & Dixon, 1969).

Cryoprecipitation

Serum separated at 37°C and stored at 4°C may develop an immunoglobulin-rich precipitate which is resoluble on warming to 37°C, and in which immune complexes are concentrated. In connective tissue diseases such cryoprecipitates contain more than one class of polyclonal immunoglobulin and may contain complement components. In rheumatoid arthritis cryoglobulinaemia was originally described in patients with vasculitis (Weisman & Zvaifler, 1975) although in a subsequent study it was also found in patients with other extra-articular disease such as nodules, scleritis, ulcers, neuropathy and pulmonary disease (Erhardt et al, 1979). In the latter study a correlation with the Clq-binding test was noted, although the latter test did not descriminate between patients with extra-articular and articular disease. There was a negative correlation with haemolytic complement and a positive correlation with IgM-rheumatoid factor. Cryoglobulinaemia correlated with, but probably did not antedate, extra-articular disease, and was a marker of morbidity and mortality in the group of 52 patients studied. Cryoprecipitates are also found in patients with other connective tissue diseases such as SLE and Sjögren's syndrome (Cream, 1977).

Patients with cryoglobulins tend to exhibit clinical features of a syndrome characterised by Raynaud's phenomenon (or digital vasculitis) and purpura. The composition of the cryoglobulins in connective tissues diseases is of the so-called 'mixed' variety (i.e. the precipitate contains immunoglobulins of more than a single class). The composition of the cryoglobulins has been shown to include IgG and anti-IgG antibodies (rheumatoid factors) of different classes (Meltzer et al, 1966). In rheumatoid and SLE sera the cryoglobulins may also contain Clq (Hanauer & Christian, 1967; Agnello et al, 1970). SLE sera have been shown to contain DNA, anti-DNA antibodies, and IgM lymphocytotoxic antibodies (Winfield et al, 1975a,b). Cryoprecipitates of synovial fluids in rheumatoid arthritis are found to be rich in immune complexes containing IgG-anti-IgG and nuclear antigen and antibodies (Cracchiolo et al, 1971).

Polyethylene glycol (PEG) precipitation

PEG, a polymer, has been used to fractionate plasma proteins, and is useful in separating monomeric IgG and IgM from complexed material at concentrations of PEG between 2.5 and 4% (Chia et al, 1979; Digeon et al, 1977). As well as offering a simple test which can be used in most clinical laboratories, it offers a preliminary step for concentration of immune complexes which can subsequently be separated by other techniques such as complement affinity columns (Kilgallon et al, 1982).

Interactions with complement

Immune complex-initiated complement consumption may lead to depletion in the total activity of complement as measured by a haemolytic assay or to depletion of the individual complement component; a fall in the early components of the classical pathway (C1, C4 and C2) together with diminution in C3 is particularly indicative of immune complex activation (reviewed by Schur & Austen, 1972). This subject is fully discussed under the next section.

Anti-complementary activity of sera can be a function of the presence of immune complexes, and may be assessed by the addition of known quantities of fresh guinea pig complement and measuring its consumption by titrating the residual complement activity. Using this technique, with suitable precautions to avoid the generation of artefactual activity in vitro, complexes have been discovered in the majority of sera from SLE and polyarteritis patients (Johnson et al, 1975).

Precipitation of Clq (a subunit of the first component of complement) by immune complexes was described by Agnello et al (1970). Using this technique complexes were detectable in the sera of patients with systemic lupus erythematosus and in the joint fluid of patients with rheumatoid arthritis; but no reaction was obtained with sera from rheumatoid patients. In a test using radiolabelled Clq, serum is reacted with this reagent and precipitated with polyethylene glycol (Nydegger et al, 1974). Clq binding complexes have been demonstrated not only in patients with SLE but also in a significant number of patients with rheumatoid arthritis by this method (Lambert et al, 1975).

In another Clq binding assay, binding of immune complexes to Clq on a solid phase is assessed by radiolabelled anti-immunoglobulin (Hay et al, 1976). Binding of immune complexes containing C3bi to conglutinin has also been employed (Casali et al, 1977). Using these assays immune complexes are found in patients with rheumatoid arthritis and SLE. In a study comparing Clq-PEG and solid phase assays, a similar frequency of positive results were observed in rheumatoid arthritis, although discordant results were not infrequent (Mumford et al, 1982). Patients with extra-articular disease features tended to have a much higher frequency, as well as higher binding values of positive Clq binding, and showed evidence of hypercatabolism of C3 (Bourke et al, 1982). These findings strongly suggested that high levels of complement fixing complexes were associated with extra-articular disease.

Raji cells, a lymphoblastoid cell line with surface receptors for C3b and C3d, bind to immune complexes and aggregated IgG containing C3b or C3d (Theofilopoulous et al, 1976). Recent evidence has shown that the C3b receptor on Raji cells may in fact differ from the conventional receptor. Using the Raji cell binding assay a positive result was obtained in a smaller proportion of rheumatoid patients to that observed with the Clq binding assays (Mumford et al, 1982). The majority of sera with positive results were also positive in the Clq binding assays, suggesting that the Raji cell assay (which is more tedious to perform than Clq binding assays) offered no special advantages.

In SLE the proportion of patients who show a positive result in Clq binding PEG assay has been surprisingly low in most laboratories (e.g. 17% in the study by Mumford et al, 1982). In the same study, the solid phase assay was more frequently positive (51%) and the majority of patients were positive in the Raji cell assay (83%). However, the high frequency of positive results has to be interpreted with caution since antinuclear antibodies and other auto-alloantibodies which occur in SLE may also bind the surface membrane of Raji cells (Horsfall et al, 1981).

Immune complexes containing C3b may also bind to the C3b receptor of lymphocytes. Using antibody and complement coated erythrocytes, inhibition of rosette formation has been used to detect immune complexes in sera of patients with nephrotic syndrome and other renal diseases (Ezer & Hayward, 1974; Smith et al, 1975).

Immune complexes containing IgA may activate the alternative complement pathway and this leads to incorporation of C3b or C3bi into the complex. Hence the conglutinin and Raji cell assays with anti-IgA serum may be used to detect IgA complexes. Using a conglutinin-based assay IgA complexes have been found in certain forms of cutaneous vasculitis, Berger's disease with renal disease (Kaufmann et al, 1980).

Interactions with rheumatoid factors

Polyclonal and monoclonal rheumatoid factors bind to immune complexes containing IgG. Using monoclonal rheumatoid factor Winchester et al (1971) found precipitating immune complexes in rheumatoid sera. Using radioassays, and agglutination techniques, a number of assays have been devised (e.g. Cowdrey et al, 1975; Gabriel & Agnello, 1977; Cambiaso et al, 1977). Although these assays detect non-complement fixing IgG immune complexes and therefore extend the range of immune complexes detectable in the laboratory, they suffer from interference by high levels of IgG or intrinsic rheumatoid factors, coincidentally present in the sera, which reduce the binding activity of rheumatoid factor.

Low affinity IgM anti-human IgG is reported to bind to immune complexes and agglutinates IgG-coated latex particles. Inhibition of agglutination has been used to detect IgG complexes (Levinsky & Soothill, 1977), and can by modified to detect IgA containing complexes (Levinsky & Barrat, 1979).

Using these rheumatoid factor based assays, immune complexes have been found in rheumatoid arthritis, SLE and Henoch–Schönlein disease, although it is necessary to deplete intrinsic rheumatoid factor prior to the procedure, and this makes the assays cumbersome.

Other assays

In the test developed by Onyewotu et al (1974) the Fc receptors on guinea pig peritoneal exudate macrophages were used for detection of immune complexes. Immune complexes in sera were measured by their ability to inhibit (or enhance) the binding of radiolabelled aggregated IgG to this receptor. Using this technique, complexes which inhibited uptake of aggregated IgG were found in SLE patients, but, possibly as a result of the concurrent presence of rheumatoid factors, sera from some patients with rheumatoid arthritis contained circulating complexes which enhanced the uptake of aggregates.

In the platelet aggregation test, Fc receptors are also believed to be involved in the process whereby immune complexes bind to their surface and activate the process. Using this technique immune complexes have been detected in sera of patients with rheumatoid arthritis, systemic lupus erythematosus and other disorders (Penttinen, 1977).

Inhibition of antibody-dependent mononuclear cell-mediated cytotoxicity (K cell activity) has been utilised as a means of detecting immune complexes (MacLennan, 1972). Using this technique it is claimed that patients with certain inflammatory bowel disorders and ankylosing spondylitis possess circulating immune complexes (Jewell & MacLennan, 1973; Corrigaletal, 1978). The migration of guinea pig peritoneal macrophages from capillary tubes is inhibited by immune complexes (Spitler et al, 1969) but this technique has yet to be evaluated in diseases. Sera containing immune complexes lead to histamine release from lung preparation in vitro, a finding which has been utilised for detecting such biologically active factors in rheumatoid arthritis (Baumal & Broder, 1968).

USE OF IMMUNE COMPLEX ASSAYS IN CLINICAL PRACTICE

Although it has been argued from the previous section that immune complexes in the blood are implicated in the pathogenesis of rheumatic diseases, the complexity of aspects of measurement and the large number of assays that would be required to cover the range of species of complexes that may be pathogenic, makes it impractical for a routine laboratory to measure them. Evaluation of their use and cost-effectiveness in monitoring therapy, disease activity and prognosis is still in progress, but results of investigations suggest that carefully selected and appropriate assays offer an additional useful tool for the management of patients with systemic rheumatic disease (Schrieber & Maini, 1984). The main value of detection and analysis is in research into the identity of antigens which may be implicated in the pathogenesis of disease.

COMPLEMENT

The complement system consists of 14 circulating proteins which, under certain conditions, are activated in a sequential manner. The sequential activation is triggered by interaction between initiating factors and a complement component. The acquisition of specific enzymatic activity then exerts its action on another complement protein, thereby setting in motion a cascade of further interactions, modulated by inhibitors and amplification pathways. Four proteins are recognised which modulate and inhibit activate complement. Activation products and combinations of the components (soluble or tissue-fixed) are biologically active and are implicated in inflammatory and immunological reactions in certain rheumatic diseases.

COMPLEMENT SEQUENCE

Activation of complement is initiated along two principal pathways which result in the production of enzymes termed 'C3 convertases' with specificity for the C3 component (Fig. 13.5). The activation of complement is a complicated cascade of sequential generation of cell-associated and 'fluid phase' products with biochemical and biological activity. The reactions are modulated by the controlling proteins Cl-esterase inhibitor (Cl-INH), C4-binding protein, factor H and factor I (Fig. 13.5). Further details may be obtained by reference to a review of the subject by Lachmann & Peters (1982).

1. The classical pathway is activated by antigen-antibody complexes or aggregated IgG following combination with the Clq subunit of the first component of C1. Clq then combines with and activates Clr which enzymatically cleaves off a fragment from Cls and results in the formation of activated C1. Activated C1 splits C4 and C2 and generates a bimolecular complex C4b2b termed 'classical pathway C3 convertase' with enzymatic activity for C3, and simultaneously liberates fragments C4a and C2a into the fluid phase. C4 binding protein dissociates and increases susceptibility of C4b to cleavage by I.

Activation of C1 may also be initiated by complexes of polyanions and cations (e.g. heparin and protamine), C-reactive protein and certain viruses. Proteolytic enzymes such as plasmin, kallikrein and trypsin also cleave Cl and generate C4b2b. Thus a variety of initiating factors can be involved in activating the classical pathway in addition to immune complexes.

The initiating step of activation is inhibited by Cl-INH. Deficiency of Cl-INH is known to be associated with hereditary angioedema and leads to uninhibited activation of Cl, the generation of a C2-kinin and hypercatabolism of complement.

2. C3 convertase activity is also generated by the involvement of the alternative pathway proteins, factors B, D and P independent of Cl, C4 and C2. The understanding of initiation and am-

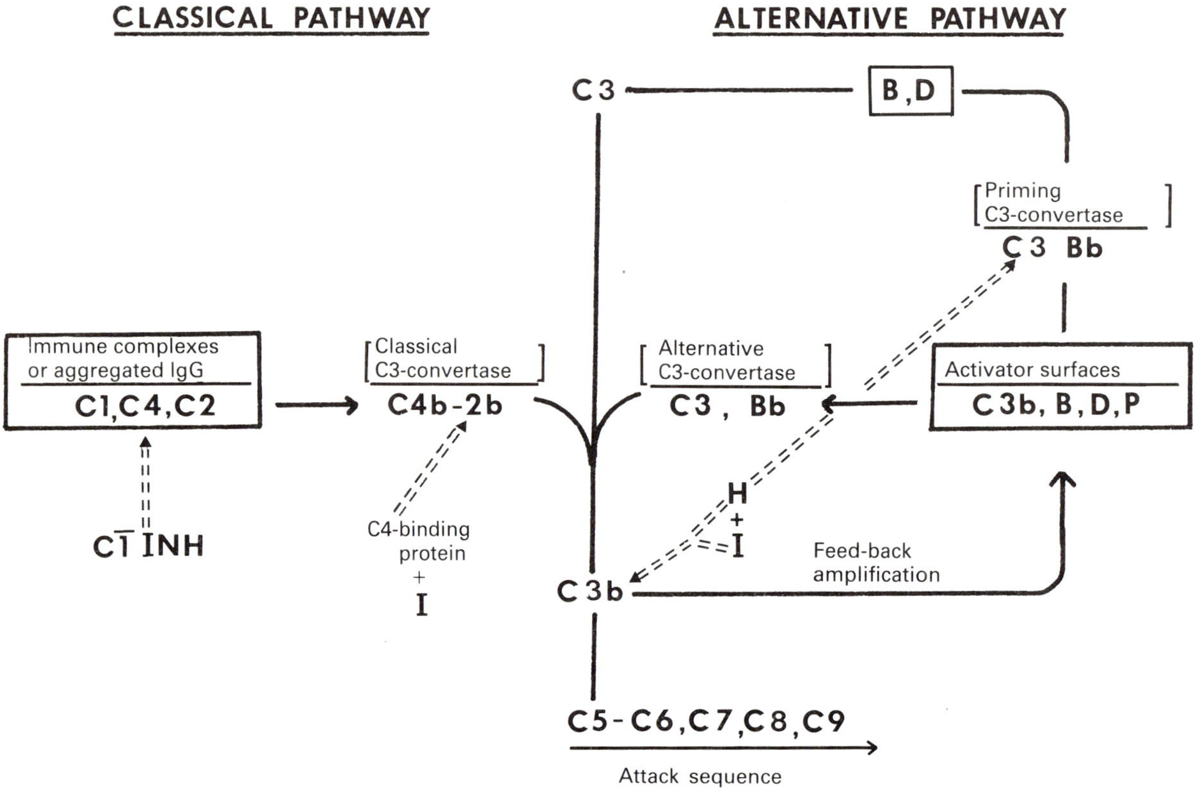

Fig. 13.5 Complement activation pathways. In the classical pathway, immune complexes or aggregated IgG combine with subunits of C1 and sequentially activate C4, C2 and generate $\overline{C42}$ (C4b 2b), the classical C3-convertase. Alternative pathway activation may occur by: (a) the generation of the priming C3-convertase (C3 Bb) by the action of spontaneously derived D on C3 complexed to factor B and lead to generation of C3b; (b) the generation of the alternative C3-convertase $\overline{C3B}$ (C3b Bb) which is initiated by the protection of small amounts of C3b spontaneously generated on activator surfaces (Zymosan, endotoxin, insulin and aggregated IgA) and allows the interaction of C3b and factor B enhanced by $\bar{D}$ and stabilised by properdin (p); (c) by feedback amplification induced by C3b generated by the classical pathway reaction and consequent interaction with factor B. The controlling effects and points of action of C1-INH, C4-binding protein and proteins H and I are shown by dotted lines. Synonyms: Factor B = C3 proactivator or glycine-rich beta globulin (GBG); Factor D = C3 proactivator convertase (C3PAse); H = beta 1H; I = KAF or C3b inactivator.

plification of this pathway has undergone major revision in the last decade (Fearon, 1981). The alternative pathway may become activated by three principal mechanisms:

a. De novo generation of a circulating convertase C3Bb (the priming C3 convertase)

b. The generation of the convertase C3bBb on activator (protected) particulate surfaces

c. The generation of C3bBb as an obligatory 'feedback' amplification system following cleavage of C3 by the classical pathway convertase C4b2b (Fig. 13.5).

Under normal circumstances, the circulating protein D is partially found in its activated form $\overline{D}$ and continuously activates altered (but undigested) circulating C3 complexed to factor B (C3B) to form the 'priming C3 convertase' C3Bb. C3Bb cleaves C3 into C3b which has a binding site for suitable surfaces. If a binding surface is not encountered in its immediate vicinity, the binding site of C3b rapidly decays and C3b itself complexes with H and is inactivated by I.

C3b attached to a 'non-activator' surface has a high affinity for H and is inactivated by I. On the other hand when attached to an 'activator' surface, C3b is protected from H and I, and instead, binds to B, to form C3bB which is cleaved by D to C3bBb, the alternative pathway convertase. C3bBb cleaves C3, forming more surface-associated C3b, which in turn leads to formation of further C3bBb. The molecule C3bBb is inherently subject to rapid and irreversible dissociation, but in the presence of properdin (P), the complex is stabilised. H controls the formation of further C3bBb and dissociates this molecule and Bb to Bbi, and thus allows I to split C3b to the inactivated form, C3bi.

Activator surfaces include zymosan, rabbit erythrocytes, particulate inulin and endotoxin. These activate the alternative pathway by protecting the enzymatic activity of the convertase C3bBb. C3 nephritic factor (C3-Nef) found in the Blood of patients with lipodystrophy and mesangiocapillary nephritis, is also known to activate complement.

C3-Nef is now known to be an IgG autoantibody directed against the alternative pathway convertase (Thompson, 1972) and stabilises the convertase by making it resistant to H and I (Daha et al, 1978). C3b generated by the action of the classical C3 convertase C4b2b (Fig. 13.5) may also lead to formation of C3bBb via the alternative pathway and provides a feedback amplification of breakdown of C3 during activation by the classical pathway.

It may be appreciated from the description of these reactions that the alternative pathway may be activated independently of the classical pathway, in which situation the proteins of the alternative pathway (properdin, factor D and factor B and C3) are consumed and their levels founds to be lowered, whilst C1, C4 and C2 levels remain normal. If the classical pathway is activated, C1, C4, C2 and C3 are consumed and their levels lowered but under these circumstances an obligatory feedback activation of the alternative pathway may lead to a certain degree of consumption of factor B.

C3 convertase activity produced by either of the two pathways leads to cleavage of C3 and the product of C3b is involved in enzymatic attack on C5. C5 to C9 sequential activation is necessary for membrane lysis and is termed the 'attack sequence'. Cleavage products of C3 and C5, namely C3a, C3b and C5a as well as the trimolecular complex formed by association of C5, C6 and C7 ($\overline{C567}$), all have important biological activities (see below).

BIOLOGICAL ACTIVITIES OF COMPLEMENT

These are summarised in Table 13.1.

Complement and interactions with receptors

There are at least three complement receptors:

Table 13.1 Biological activities of complement

Biological activity	Complement product	Mode of action	Result
Anaphylatoxin	C3a C5a	Histamine release from mast cells direct effect on vessels and smooth muscle	Increased vascular permeability; smooth muscle contraction
Chemotaxis	C3a C5a C567	Attraction of circulating leucocytes	Leucocyte accumulation
Immune adherence	C3b	C3b bound to antigen–antibody attaches to specific receptors on polymorphs and macrophages (monocytes)	Enhanced phagocytosis and release of lysosomal enzymes with tissue degradative properties
Exocytosis and activation	C5a	Acts on adherent polymorphs	Lysosomal enzyme release and generation of superoxide radicals
B-cell stimulation	C3b	Binding to complement receptor by antigen and activation	Antibody synthesis
Virus neutralisation	C14	Augmentation of specific antibody	Loss of virus infectivity
Membrane lysis	C1–9	Antibody and complement membrane attack	Lysis of cell membranes, bacteria and viruses

a. Receptors for C3b (termed CR1)
b. Receptors for C3d (termed CR2)
c. Receptors for C3bi (termed CR3).

C3b receptors have been well characterised and are distributed on erythrocytes, monocytes, macrophages, polymorphs and dendritic cells. C3b receptors also bind C4b. Isolated C3b receptor inhibits the alternative and classical pathway convertases (Fearon, 1979; Iida & Nussenzweig, 1981). The inhibitory activity may provide an essential protective mechanism from the membrane-damaging effects of the full assembly of the attack sequence (C5–9) for cells that bind C3b.

Recent investigations suggest that the density of C3b receptors may be genetically controlled and that there is a deficiency of these receptors in patients with SLE and rheumatoid arthritis (Wilson et al, 1982; Iida et al, 1982). It has been postulated that C3b receptor deficiency may lead to impaired clearance of C3b-bound immune complexes and perpetuate immune complex-mediated reactions.

C3b-receptors are involved in mediating adherence of C3b coated material such as immune complexes and microbes to phagocytic cells. However, Fc receptor interaction is required for phagocytosis (Czop et al, 1978). Such interactions are beneficial to the host and may be of special importance in the clearance of particulate and IgM-containing immune complexes. However, release of enzymes and superoxide anions during phagocytosis may cause tissue damage.

The receptors for C3b and C3d on lymphocytes may be involved in the activation of B cells (Dukor & Hartmann, 1973), generation of lymphokines and regulation of the immune response (Fearon, 1981).

C3b and C3bi receptors have been found on glomerular epithelial cells and may lead to retention of immune complexes (Gelfand et al, 1975).

Solubilisation of immune precipitates

Nussenzweig and his colleagues have shown that immune precipitates can be solubilised by an excess of complement, and although the classical pathway is implicated, the reaction is predominently dependent on the alternative pathway (Miller & Nussenzweig, 1978). This reaction appears to require intercalation of C3b into the antigen–antibody lattice and its fragmentation into soluble products. The solubilised material does not appear to be capable of binding to C3b receptors on phagocytes. Thus the effect may be important in mobilising complexes deposited in tissues, but once solubilised, the complexes become biologically inert and are presumably catabolised gradually. Complement also effectively prevents formation of immune precipitates (Schifferli et al, 1980) by a similar mechanism. It has been suggested that complement-modified complexes may be involved in generation of B cell memory in the spleen.

Generation of C3a and C5a

The biologically active peptides C3a and C5a are generated by activation of complement by the classical or alternative pathways. The effects of C3a and C5a have been reviewed by Lepow (1971) and Hugli & Muller-Eberhard (1978).

a. C3a and C5a are anaphylotoxins, and lead to exocytosis of histamine by mast cells and are spasmogenic for smooth muscle. The former is involved in leading to increased vascular permeability in inflammation.

b. C5a and $C\overline{567}$ are chemotactic for leukocytes, including polymorphs and mononuclear cells.

c. C5a is implicated in release of lysosomal enzymes from leukocytes and the generation of superoxide radicals, both of importance in protective microbial immunity and in inflammation.

Membrane lysis

Assembly of C5–9 leads to lysis of membranes of erythrocytes (e.g. paroxysmal nocturnal haemoglobulinuria), of viruses and of bacteria (especially of the genus *Neisseria*). Deficiency of the 'late' complement components is associated with gonococcal and meningococcal infections (Lachmann & Peters, 1982). Virus neutralisation is also described with the assembly of C1–4 on antibody coated viruses (Daniels et al, 1969).

DEFICIENCY OF COMPLEMENT SYNTHESIS AS AN ACQUIRED ABNORMALITY

It has been found that in some patients with diseases associated with hypocomplementaemia the low levels of complement result from decreased synthesis of C3, possibly due to a negative feedback inhibition induced by activated or split products of C3 (Alper & Rosen, 1967). This set of circumstances has been documented in patients with various disorders, particularly in a group with mesangiocapillary nephritis. Decreased synthesis of C3 has been documented in SLE (Sliwinski & Zvaifler, 1972), although the majority of patients with hypercatabolism of complement in SLE have an increased or normal synthetic rate (Ruddy et al, 1975).

GENETICALLY DETERMINED COMPLEMENT DEFICIENCIES AND PREDISPOSITION TO DISEASE

There are well recognised associations between genetically determined deficiencies of complement and a tendency to the development of infections and connective tissue diseases (Lachmann & Peters, 1982). The latter include SLE, juvenile chronic arthritis, glomerulonephritis and vasculitis. SLE has been observed in association with deficiency of C1, C4, C2 and C1 esterase inhibitor, although it should be noted that many individuals with such deficiencies are healthy. Early component deficiency in lupus syndromes should be suspected in all patients in whom the levels of C3 are normal whilst levels of CH_{50} remain persistently lower. The role of early components of the classical pathway in viral neutralisation, phagocytosis and immune clearance of microbial agents has prompted the hypothesis that early component deficiencies lead to disease as a result of failure of elimination of immunogenic viruses; a situation which also encourages emergence of autoimmunity. Some evidence of persistent infections has been found in a patient with Henoch–Schönlein purpura whose blood was found to harbour particles resembling mycoplasma, and in a patient with glomerulonephritis with viral particles in the renal biopsy, both patients being deficient of C2 (Lachmann & Peters, 1982). Although the association of lupus syndromes with C2 deficiency were originally observed in individuals with total deficiency of complement components (genetically homozygous for the deficiency) a partial deficiency of C2 (with 50% levels) has been described in association with an increased incidence of juvenile rheumatoid arthritis and systemic lupus erythematosus (Glass & Schur, 1977) suggesting that heterozygote individuals may also show increased disease susceptibility. A high degree of association of C2 deficiencies with HLA antigens A10 and/or B18 has led to the belief that genes controlling C2 synthesis are located in major histocompatibility complex on the 6th chromosome (for review see Schur, 1975). Since genes controlling immune responses are also thought to be located in the same region on the chromosome (see Maini et al, 1976) the occurrence of an immune complex disorder such as SLE in C2 deficiency presents novel opportunities for investigating the aetiology and pathogenesis of these diseases.

Deficiency of C3 is rate and may be associated with infections and nephritis. Patients with late component (C5–8) deficiencies are especially likely to develop gonococcal and meningococcal infections.

MEASUREMENT OF COMPLEMENT AND APPLICATION IN RHEUMATIC DISEASES

Methods

The observation that red cells coated with antibody (immune complexes) are lysed in the presence of complement is utilised to measure the total functional capacity of fresh serum complement. The results are usually evaluated by the procedures of Mayer (1961) or Kent & Fife (1963) and expressed in units of complement required to achieve 50% lysis. Lowered activity indicated diminution in the level of one or several components of the pathway and provides a valuable guide to increased consumption in vivo (e.g. by immune complexes or other activators) or decreased synthesis (e.g. as an acquired or congenital abnormality) without of course providing any indication of the specific mechanisms involved. Individual components may also be measured by haemolytic techniques.

Immunochemical measurements of individual complement proteins of both the classical and alternative pathways are now possible as a result of availability of antisera to C1, C4, C2, C3, C5, C6, C7, C9, properdin and factor B. For the purposes of quantitation, the radial immunodiffusion technique or the two-dimensional electrophoresis technique are employed, the latter having the advantage that the procedure may be completed in a short period thereby preventing the degradation of the proteins which otherwise interferes with quantitation. Antigenically intact complement components may not be functionally active, and conversely, functional activity may be inhibited by serum factors. For this reason it may necessary to measure complement components by both techniques in sophisticated investigative studies.

The findings of lowered levels of CH_{50} and C3 in the presence of simultaneous lowering of C1, C4 and C2 indicated utilisation of complement by the classical pathway, whereas lowered or absent CH_{50} with normal levels of C3 provides a clue to the existence of the isolated deficiency of C1, C4 or C2, usually on a congenital basis. Lowered CH_{50} and C3 with normal C1, C4 and C2 indicates a primary alternative pathway activation; more direct evidence of activation of this mechanism requires measurement of properdin and factor B, although it has to be noted that feedback activation of the alternative pathway by C3b may be associated with consumption of factor B.

Split products of C3, C4 and factor B may be measured as an indication of complement activation in vivo. Such products may be antigenically similar to their parent compounds in which case they are reactive with antisera to native C3, C4 and factor B, but because they have an altered electrophoretic charge may be detected by using the technique of two-dimensional immunoelectrophoresis (Versey et al, 1973). Changes in antigenic constitution of split products also allow the use of specific antisera for their detection, and the application by Perrin et al (1975a, b) and Bourke et al (1982) of the use of polyethylene glycol for fractionating and concentrating split products on the basis of their molecular size and then detecting them by two-dimensional immunoelectrophoresis has greatly increased accuracy and sensitivity. Tests for measuring components and their split products require great care in collection and storage and specimens to avoid spontaneous activation of complement components.

Since the levels of complement in blood reflect the balance between synthesis and metabolism, their measurement does not accurately reflect complement consumption. In several inflammatory diseases increased complement synthesis may well mask the degree of consumption. In addition it has recently become apparent that in some patients, decreased synthesis of complement components is the main factor in inducing hypocomplementaemia (Alper & Rosen, 1967). Differentiation between different mechanisms contributing to hypocomplementaemia requires documentation of the catabolic rates of radiolabelled components; however, such techniques are limited to experimental studies.

Deposition of complement components in fresh tissue sections may be detected by immunofluorescent microscopy by the use of appropriate antisera or to individual components of the classical and alternative pathway. Such studies have usually been undertaken in conjunction with localisation of immunoglobulin.

TISSUE FIXATION AND HYPERCATABOLISM OF COMPLEMENT IN RHEUMATIC DISEASES

The interest in the role of complement in rheumatic diseases has thus far focused on documenting its detection in tissues, or seeking evidence of hypercatabolism. The results have been compatible with the view that complement is an important mediator of allergic inflammation possibly usually initiated by immune complexes.

Systemic lupus erythematosus

Studies by immunofluorescence microscopy have been considered under the section on immune complexes, and it is noted that complement deposition in systemic lupus erythematosus has been documented in various tissues, e.g. kidneys, skin and choroid plexus. The component most frequently sought is C3, although in some studies early components of the classical pathway have also been documented. These studies indicate that complement is deposited together with immune complexes, including those formed by polynucleotide or protein antigens and antinuclear antibodies (Koffler et al, 1967). It has been suggested that the severity of renal lesions is related to the presence of complement-fixing immunoglobulins, although a high prevalence of classes of immunoglobulin that poorly fix complement raises the possibility that complement-independent injury may also occur (Lewis et al, 1970). Other studies have shown the deposition of properdin and factor B especially in the kidneys and skin, indicating alternative pathway participation (Schrager & Rothfield, 1976). It remains uncertain at present whether the alternative pathway activation demonstrated in such studies occur as a result of obligatory action of the C3b feedback pathway secondary to classical pathway activation, or as a result of independent initiating factors.

Hypocomplementaemia is regarded as a very useful guide of disease activity, especially when found in conjunction with elevated levels of anti-DNA antibody (Schur & Sandson, 1968). Hypocomplementaemia not only correlates with renal involvement, but is also seen when other manifestations of the disease are apparent, and provides a useful index for monitoring disease activity and therapy (Schur, 1975). For example, low CH_{50}, Clq, C4 and C3 levels (together or singly) may precede exacerbations of disease activity, very low levels of C3 are seen in patients with active and severe nephritis, very low levels of Clq tend to have a high morbidity and mortality. The finding of depressed levels of CH_{50} with normal C3 levels should lead to the suspicion of pre-existing complement component deficiency which is known to occur in a group of patients with SLE as a genetically acquired abnormality. Inverse correlations between hypocomplementaemia and the presence of immune complexes (detected by various techniques, e.g. cryoglobulins, Clq-binding or binding activity by the Raji cell assay) and between hypocomplementaemia and the presence of inactivation products of C4 and C3 have all indicated participation of activation and complement by immune complexes in this disease.

Examination of the cerebrospinal fluid has been reported to show diminished levels of C4 in certain patients with cerebral disease, although Hadler et al (1973) found that the absolute levels of C4 were not an accurate or reliable guide to cerebral involvement. In serial studies a fall in C4 levels correlated with disease activity, indicating complement fixation.

Measurement of complement levels in synovial fluid in patients with lupus have been undertaken simultaneously with measurement of the total haemolytic activity in serum (Pekin & Zvaifler, 1970). These studies have suggested that there are two groups of patients, one group in whom there is considerable local consumption of complement, and a second group in whom the hypocomplementaemia is already present as a systemic feature with little further increased consumption in the joint. This finding probably reflects the two types of synovitis which are seen in clinical practice, a chronic arthritis, resembling rheumatoid disease and a flitting synovitis or arthralgia more in keeping with the joint manifestation observed in acute serum sickness.

Rheumatoid arthritis

Complement components (usually C3) have been detected by immunofluorescent microscopy together with immunoglobulin of all classes in the interstitium, and within cells of the lining and deeper layers of synovial membrane, as well as inclusions in phagocytic cells in the synovial fluid, as previously noted. It has also been noted that complement may be found in conjunction with immunoglobulin in extra-articular sites such as rheumatoid nodules and lymph nodes. Measurement of synovial fluid total complement activity has suggested that local consumption of complement occurs in the majority of patients (Hedberg, 1963; Pekin & Zvaifler, 1964). The pattern of individual component depletion shows lowering of the early components suggestive of immune complex-induced activation of the classical pathway (Ruddy & Austen, 1970) and of the properdin pathway (Ruddy et al, 1975). The finding of intermediate size IgG–anti-IgG complexes which fix complement suggest that these complexes may be the main factor involved in complement utilisation in joints (Winchester et al, 1970). Other studies have shown split products of C3 (Zvaifler, 1969) and C4 (Perrin et al, 1975b) as well as factor B (Lambert et al, 1975) in the joint fluid indicating complement activation by both the major activating pathways. The finding of C5-related chemotactic activity in synovial fluid (Ward & Zvaifler, 1971) is also indicative of complement activation by either of the two pathways, although it should be noted that certain lysosomal proteases of the type found in rheumatoid synovial fluid can directly split C3 and C5 (Lepow, 1971).

In rheumatoid vasculitis, complement deposits have been described together with immunoglobulin in the blood vessels associated with nerves (Conn et al, 1972). Although total levels of circulating complement are normal or high in uncomplicated rheumatoid arthritis, low levels have been noted in patients with vasculitis (Bourke et al, 1982). Catabolic studies of radiolabelled C3 have shown an increased consumption in rheumatoid vasculitis (Weinstein et al, 1972).

Polyarteritis nodosa and vasculitis

Complement components and immunoglobulin have been noted in the vessel walls in polyarteritis nodosa, and in such patients, hypocomplementaemia as measured by CH_{50} levels was usual (Gocke et al, 1971). In the phase of the development of arthritis, cutaneous vasculitis and systemic complications in meningococcal septicaemia (Greenwood et al, 1973) and in a similar prodromal phase of hepatitis B (Alpert et al, 1971), complement has been noted to be lowered coincidentally with a disappearance of antigen circulating in blood. In some patients with dermatomyositis, especially children, C3 deposits in blood vessels of muscles have been noted and indicate that immune complex-mediated pathology may occur (Whitaker & Engel, 1972).

Other diseases

Low serum complement levels are found in some patients with Sjögren's syndrome, poststreptococcal and mesangiocapillary nephritis, subacute bacterial endocarditis, liver diseases and conditions associated with cryoglobulinaemia.

COMPLEMENT DEPOSITS IN TISSUES IN ABSENCE OF IMMUNOGLOBULIN

Deposits of complement in tissues occasionally occur in the absence of immunoglobulin. For example, in hypogammaglobulinaemic patients with an inflammatory polyarthritis, C3 deposits (without immunoglobulin) have been documented in the synovial membrane (Munthe et al, 1975). Barnett et al (1970) found evidence of depressed levels of C3 in the synovial fluid of a patient with arthritis and hypogammaglobulinaemia compared with serum, and C3-positive staining in the synovial membrane. In the study by Munthe et al (1975), the presence of properdin in the tissue lead to the speculation that complement activation was mediated via the alternative pathway.

It has been noted by Wilson & Dixon (1971) that complement persists at the site of immune complex deposition for periods longer than the Ig itself, for example as seen in nephritis of acute serum sickness in rabbits. The deposition of complement in the tubular basement membrane of kidneys in the absence of Ig has also been noted in various forms of nephritis and has been interpreted as residual C3 of immune complexes, technical artefact or as indicating an ill-defined role for complement in tissue damage (Lehman et al, 1975).

REFERENCES

Abramson N, Gelfand E W, Jandl J H, Rosen F S 1970 The interaction between human monocytes and red cells. Specificity for IgG subclasses and IgG fragments. Journal of Experimental Medicine, 132:1207

Agnello V, Winchester R J, Kunkel H S 1970 Precipitin reactions of the C1q component of complement with aggregated globulin and immune complexes in gel diffusion. Immunology 19:909

Allison A C, Cardella C, Davies P 1975 Immune complexes and induced release of lysosomal enzymes from mononuclear phagocytes in the pathogenesis of rheumatoid arthritis. Rheumatology 6:251

Almeida J, Waterson A P 1969 Immune complexes in hepatitis. Lancet, ii, 983

Alper C A , Rosen F S 1967 Studies of the in vivo behaviour of human C3 in normal subjects and patients. Journal of Clinical Investigation, 46:2021

Alpert E, Isselbacher K J, Schur P H 1971 The pathogenesis of arthritis with viral hepatitis. New England Journal of Medicine, 285:185

Andrewes B S, Penny R 1976 The role of immune complexes in the pathogenesis of disease. Australian and New Zealand Journal of Medicine 6: 591–602

Arthus M, Breton M 1903 Lésion cutanées produits par les injections de sérum de cheval chez le lapin anaphylactisé part et pour ce sérum. Comptes Rendus de la Société de Biologie 1478

Ashe W K, Daniels C A, Scott G S, Notkins A L 1971 Interaction of rheumatoid factor with infectious herpes simplex virus-antibody complexes. Science, 172:176

Atkins C J, Kondon J J, Quismorio F P, Friou G J 1972 The choroid plexus in systemic lupus erythematosus.

Annals of Internal Medicine, 76:65
Augener W, Grey H M, Cooper N R, Muller-Eberhard H J 1971 The reaction of monomeric and aggregated immunoglobulins with C1. Immunochemistry 8: 1011–1020
Barnett E V, Winkelstein A, Weinberger H J 1970 Agammaglobulinaemia with polyarthritis and subcutaneous nodules. American Journal of Medicine 48: 40–47
Baumal R, Broder L 1968 Studies into the occurrence of soluble antigen–antibody complexes in diseases. Clinical Experimental Immunology, 3:555
Becker E L, Henson P M 1973 In vitro studies of immunologically induced secretion of mediators from cells and related phenomena. Advances in Immunology 17: 93–193
Benacerraf B, McCluskey R T, Patras D 1959 Localisation of colloidal substances in vascular endothelium A mechanism of tissue damage I Factors causing the pathologic deposition of colloidal carbon. American Journal of Pathology, 35:75
Benveniste J, ll Henson P M, Cochrane C G 1972 Leukocyte-dependent mechanism of histamine release from rabbit platelets: the role of IgE, basophils and platelet-activating factor. Journal of Experimental Medicine, 136: 1356–1377
Bombardieri S, Lightfoot R W, Christian C L 1973 Serum IgG aggregates in systemic lupus erythematosus. Proceeding of the Society of Experimental Biology and Medicine, 144:148
Bonomo L, Tursi A, Trizio D, Gillardi U, Cammacco F 1970 Immune complexes in rheumatoid synovitis: a mixed staining immunofluorescence study. Immunology, 18:557
Bourke B E, Moss I K, Maini R N 1982. Measurement of the complement C3 breakdown product C3d by rocket immunoelectrophoresis. Journal of Immunological Method 48: 97–108
Bourke B E, Moss I K, Mumford P A, Horsfall A, Maini R N 1982 The complement fixing ability of putative circulating immune complexes in rheumatoid arthritis and its relationship to extra-articuar disease. Clinical and Experimental Immunology. 48: 726–732
Brent L, Brooks C G, Medawar P B, Simpson E 1976 'Transplantation tolerance' British Medical Bulletin, 32: 101–107
Brown D L, Lachmann P J, Dacie J V 1970 The in vivo behaviour of complement-coated red cells; studies in C5 deficient, C3-depleted and normal rabbits. Clinical Experimental Immunology, 7: 401–422
Cambiaso C L, Riccomi H, Masson P L 1977 Automated determination of immune complex by their inhibitors effect on the agglutination of IgG-coated particles by rheumatoid factor of C1q Annals of the Rheumatic Diseases, 36:(suppl 1):40
Capra J D, Winchester R J, Kunkel H R 1971 Hypergammaglobulinaemic purpura Medicine, 59:125
Cardella C J, Davies P, Allison A C 1974 Immune complexes induce lysosomal hydrolases from macrophages Nature, 247: 46–48
Casali P, Bossus A, Carpentier N A, Lambert P H 1977 Solid-phase enzyme immunoassay or radioimmunoassay for the detection of immune complexes based on their recognition by conglutinin: conglutinin binding test. Clinical and Experimental Immunology 29: 342–354
Caulfield M J, Luce K L, Proffitt M R, Cerny J 1983 Induction of idiotype-specific suppressor T cells with antigen/antibody complexes. Journal of Experimental Medicine, 157: 1713–1725
Cerottini J C, Brunner T 1974 Cell-mediated cytotoxicity, allographed rejection and tumour immunity. Advances in Immunology 18:67 Academic Press, London
Chia D, Barnett E V, Yamagata J, Knutson D, Restivo C, Furst D 1979 Quantitation and characterisation of soluble immune complexes precipitated from sera by polyethylene glyco (PEG). Clinical and Experimental Immunology, 37: 399–407
Christian C L 1970 Properties of immune complexes. In: Bonomo L, Turk J L (eds) Proceedings of the international symposium on immune complex diseases. Carlo Erba Foundation, Milan
Cochrane C G 1971 Mechanisms involved in the deposition of immune complexes in tissues. Journal of Experimental Medicine, 134:75 (s)
Cochrane C G, Hawkins D 1968 Studies on circulating immune complexes III Factors governing the ability of circulating complexes to localise in blood vessels. Journal of Experimental Medicine, 127:137
Cochrane C G, Koffler D 1973 Immune complex disease in experimental animals and man. Advances in Immunology, 16: 185–253
Conn D L, McDuffie F C, Dyck P J 1972 Immunopathologic study of sural nerves in rheumatoid arthritis. Arthritis and Rheumatism, 15:135
Cooke T D, Jasin H E 1972 The pathogenesis of chronic inflammation in experimental antigen-induced arthritis. I The role of antigen on the local immune response. Arthritis and Rheumatism, 15: 327–337
Cooke T D, Hurd E R, Ziff M, Jasin H E 1972 The pathogenesis of chronic inflammation in experimental antigen-induced arthritis. II. Preferential localisation of antigen–antibody complexes to collagenous tissues. Journal of Experimental Medicine, 135: 328–338
Cooke T D, Richer S, Hurd E, Jasin H E 1975 Localisation of antigen–antibody complexes in intra-articular collagenous tissues. Annals of the New York Academy of Science, 256: 10–15
Coombs R R A, Gell P G H 1975 In: Gell P G H, Coombs R R A, Lachmann P J (eds) Clinical aspects of immunology, Blackwell, Oxford
Cerottini J C, Brunner T 1974 Cell-mediated cytotoxicity, allographed rejection and tumour immunity. Advances in Immunology 18: 67. Academic Press, London
Chia D, Barnett E V, Yamagata J, Knutson D, Restivo C, Furst D 1979 Quantitation and characterisation of soluble immune complexes precipitated from sera by polyethylene glyco (PEG). Clinical and Experimental Immunology 37: 399–407
Christian C L 1970 Properties of immune complexes. In: Bonomo L, Turk J L (eds) Proceedings of the international symposium on immune complex disease. Carlo Erba Foundation, Milan
Cochrane C G 1971 Mechanisms involved in the deposition of immune complexes in tissues. Journal of Experimental Medicine 134:75 (s)
Cochrane C G, Hawkins D 1968 Studies on circulating immune complexes. III. Factors governing the ability of circulating complexes to localise in blood vessels. Journal of Experimental Medicine 127:137
Cochrane C G, Koffler D 1973 Immune complex disease in experimental animals and man. Advances in Immunology 16: 185–253
Conn D L, McDuffie F C, Dyck P J 1972 Immunopathologic study of sural nerves in rheumatoid

arthritis. Arthritis and Rheumatism 15:135
Cooke T D, Jasin H E 1972 The pathogenesis of chronic inflammation in experimental antigen-induced arthritis. I. The role of antigen on the local immune response. Arthritis and Rheumatism 15: 327–337
Cooke T D, Hurd E R, Ziff M, Jasin H E 1972 The pathogenesis of chronic inflammation in experimental antigen-induced arthritis. II. Preferential localisation of antigen–antibody complexes to collagenous tissues. Journal of Experimental Medicine 135: 328–338
Cooke T D, Richer S, Hurd E, Jasin H E 1975 Localisation of antigen–antibody complexes in intra-articular collagenous tissues. Annals of the New York Academy of Sciences 256: 10–15
Coombs R R A, Gell P G H 1975 In: Clinical aspects of immunology. Gell P G H, Coombs R R A, Lachmann P J (eds) Blackwell, Oxford
Corrigal V, Panayi G S, Unger A, Poston R N, Williams B D 1978 Detection of immune complexes in serum of patients with ankylosing spondylitis. Annals of Rheumatic Diseases 37: 159–163
Cowdrey J S, Treadwell P E, Fritz R B 1975 A radioimmunoassay for human antigen–antibody complexes in clinical material. Journal of Immunology 114:5
Cracchiolo A, Goldberg L S, Barnett E V, Bluestone R 1971 Studies of cryoprecipitates from synovial fluid of rheumatoid patients. Immunology 20:1067
Cream J J 1977 Immune complexes in cryoprecipitates. Annals of Rheumatic Diseases 36 (Suppl): 21–24
Cream J J, Bryceson A D M, Ryder G 1971 Disappearance of immunoglobulin and complement from the Arthus reaction and its relevance to studies of vasculitis in man. British Journal of Dermatology 84:106
Czop J K, Fearon D T, Austen K F 1978 Membrane sialic acid on target particles modulates their phagocytosis by a trypsin-sensitive mechanism on human monocytes. Proceedings of the National Academy of Sciences (USA) 75: 3831–3835
Daha M R, Austen K F, Fearon D T 1978 Heterogeneity, polypeptide chain composition and antigenic reactivity of C3 nephritic factor. Journal of Immunology 120: 1389–1394
Daniels C A, Borgos T, Rapp H J, Snyderman R, Notkins A L 1969 Neutralization of sensitised virus by purified components of complement. Proceedings of National Academy of Sciences 65:528
Digeon M, Laver M, Riza J, Bach J F 1977 Detection of circulating immune complexes in human sera by simplified assays with polyethylene glycol. Journal of Immunological Methods 16: 165–183
Dixon F J, Vazquez J J, Weigle W D, Cochrane C G 1958 Pathogenesis of serum sickness. Archives of Pathology 65:18
Dixon F J, Feldman J D, Vazquez J J 1961 Experimental glomerulonephritis. The pathogenesis of a laboratory model resembling the spectrum of human glomerulonephritis. Journal of Experimental Medicine 113:899
Dixon F, Croker B, Delvillano B, Jensen F, Lerner R 1974 Oncornavirus infection and 'auto' immune complex disease of mice. In: Brent L, Holborow J (eds) Progress in immunology, Vol 5. North Holland, Amsterdam, p 49
Drivas G, Kerr D N S, Wardle C N 1976 Reticule-endothelial phagocytosis in patients with nephritis. British Medical Journal i:321
Dukor P, Hartmann K V 1973 Bound C3 as the second signal for B-cell activation. Cellular Immunology 7:349
Dumonde D C, Glynn L E 1962 The production of arthritis in rabbits by an immunological reaction to fibrin. British Journal of Experimental Pathology 43: 373–383
Edberg S C, Bronson P M, Van Oss C J 1972 The valency of IgM and IgG rabbit anti-dextran antibody as a function of the size of the dextran molecule. Immunochemistry 9:273
Edelman G M, Kunkel H G , Franklin E C 1958 Interaction of the rheumatoid factor with antigen–antibody complexes and aggregated gammaglobulin. Journal of Experimental Medicine 108:105
Erhardt C C, Mumford P A, Maini R N 1979 The association of cryoglobulinaemia with nodules, vasculitis and fibrosing alveolitis in rheumatoid arthritis and their relationship to serum clq binding activity and rheumatoid factor. Clinical and Experimental Immunology 38: 405–413
Evans R 1975 Macrophage-mediated cytotoxicity: its possible role in rheumatoid arthritis. Annals of the New York Academy of Sciences 256: 275–287
Evanson J M, Jeffrey J J, Krane S M 1967 Human collagenase identification and characterisation of enzymes from rheumatoid synovium in culture. Science 158: 499–502
Ezer G, Hayward A R 1974 Inhibition of complement dependant rosette formation, a possible test for immune complexes. European Journal of Immunology 14:148
Fauci A S, Wolff S M 1973 Wegener's granulomatosis; studies in 18 patients and a review of the literature. Medicine 52:535
Fearon D T 1979 Regulation of the amplification C3 convertase of human complement by an inhibitory protein isolated from human erythrocyte membranes. Proceedings of the National Academy of Sciences USA 76: 5867–5871
Fearon D T 1981 Complement as a mediator of inflammation. In: Fauci A S (ed) Clinics in immunology and allergy. Saunders, Philadelphia, p 225–245
Fish A J, Michael A F, Gewurz H, Good R A 1966 Immunopathologic changes in rheumatoid arthritis synovium. Arthritis and Rheumatism 9:267
Fisher E R, Bark J 1961 Effect of hypertension on vascular and other lesions of serum sickness. American Journal of Pathology 39: 665–679
Fox A, Glynn L E 1975 Persistence of antigen in nonarthritic joints. Annals of the Rheumatic Diseases 34:431
Franklin E C, Holman H R,Muller-Eberhard H J, Kunkel H G 1957 An unusual protein component of high molecular weight in the serum of certain patients with rheumatoid arthritis. Journal of Experimental Medicine 105:425
Gabriel A, Agnello V 1977 Detection of immune complexes. Journal of Clinical Investigation 59: 990–1001
Gelfand M C, Shin M L, Nagle R B, Green I, Frank M 1976 The glomerular complement receptor in immunologically mediated renal glomerular injury. New England Journal of Medicine 295:10
Germuth F G Jr 1953 Comparative histologic and immunologic study in rabbits of induced hypersensitivity of serum sickness type. Journal of Experimental Medicine 97: 257–282
Glass D G, Schur P H 1977 Autoimmunity, genetic, immunologic, virologic and clinical aspects. In: Talal N (ed) Academic Press, London, Ch 18
Glynn L E 1975 The role of bacterial adjuvant in

experimental arthritis. In: Clot J, Samy J (eds) Rheumatology, Vol 6. Karger, Basel, p 283–288
Gocke D J 1974 Extrahepatic manifestations of viral hepatitis. American Journal of the Medical Sciences 270:49
Gocke D J, Hsu K, Morgan C, Bombardieri S, Lockshin M, Christian C L 1971 Vasculitis in association with Australia antigen. Journal of Experimental Medicine 134:330
Goldberg L S, Fudenberg H H 1971 Antiglobulins and human disease. Vox Sang 20:1
Goldstein I M, Weissmann G 1974 Cellular and humoral mechanisms in immune complex injury. In: Brent L, Holborow J (eds) Progress in immunology, Vol 5. North-Holland, Amsterdam, p 18
Greenwood B M, Whittle H C ,Bryceson A D M 1973 Allergic complications of meningococcal disease. II. Immunological investigations. British Medical Journal ii:2, 737
Hadler N M, Gerwin R D, Frank M M,Whitaker J N, Baker M, Decker J L 1973 The fourth component of complement in the cerebrospinal fluid in systemic lupus erythematosus. Arthritis and Rheumatism 16:507
Hanauer L B, Christian C L 1967 Studies of cryoproteins in systemic lupus erythematosus. Journal of Clinical Investigation 46:400
Hang L, Theofilopoulous A N, Dixon F J 1982 A spontaneous rheumatoid arthritis-like disease in MRL/1 mice. Journal of Experimental Medicine 155: 1690–1701
Harbeck R J, Bardana E J, Kohler P F, Carr R I 1973 DNA: anti-DNA complexes: their detection in systemic lupus erythematosus sera. Journal of Clinical Investigation 52:789
Haurowitz F 1968 Antigen–antibody interactions. In: Immunochemistry and biosynthesis of antibodies. Interscience Publishers USA
Hawn C V, Janeway C A 1947 Histological and serological sequences in experimental hypersensitivity. Journal of Experimental Medicine 85:571
Hay F C, Nineham L J, Roitt I M 1976 Routine assay for the detection of immune complexes of known immunoglobulin class using solid phase Clq. Clinical and Experimental Immunology 24: 396–400
Hedberg H 1963 Studies on the depressed haemolytic complement activity of synovial fluid in adult rheumatoid arthritis. Acta rheumatologica Scandinavica 9:165
Hellstrom I, Hellstrom K E, Allison A C 1971 Neonatally induced allographed tolerance may be mediated by serum born factors. Nature 230:49
Henson P M 1971 Interaction of cells with immune complexes: adherence, release of constituents, and tissue injury. Journal of Experimental Medicine 134:114 (s)
Henson P M, Cochrane C G 1975 The effect of complement depletion on experimental tissue injury. Annals of the New York Academy of Science 256: 426–440
Hollander J L, McCarty D J, Astorga G, Castro-Murillo E 1965 Studies on the pathogenesis of rheumatoid joint inflammation. I. The 'R.A. cell' and a working hypothesis. Annals of Internal Medicine 62:271
Horsfall A C, Venables P J W, Mumford P A, Maini R N 1981 Interpretation of the Raji cell assay in sera containing antinuclear antibodies and immune complexes. Clinical and Experimental Immunology 44: 405–415
Horwitz D A, Garrett M A T, Davis J S 1971 Modification of leukocyte chemotaxis by rheumatoid factor. Arthritis and Rheumatism 14:388
Huber H, Polley M J, Linscott W D, Fudenberg H H, Muller-Eberhard H J 1968 Human monocytes: distinct receptor sites for the third component of complement and for immunoglobulin G. Science 162:1281
Hugli T E, Muller-Eberhard H J 1978 Anaphylotoxins C3a and C5a. Advances in Immunology. Vol 26 pp 1–53. Academic Press
Humphrey J H, White R G 1970 Hypersensitivity mediated by antibodies. In: Immunology for students of medicine. Blackwell, Oxford, Ch 11, p 451
Hurd E R, LoSpalluto J, Ziff M 1970 Formation of leukocyte inclusions in normal polymorphonuclear cells incubated with synovial fluid. Arthritis and Rheumatism 13: 724–733
Iida K, Nussenzweig V 1981 Complement receptor as an inhibitor of the complement cascade. Journal of Experimental Medicine 153: 1138–1150
Iida K, Mornaghi R, Nussenzweig V 1982 Complement receptor (CRI) deficiency in erythrocytes from patients with systemic lupus erythematosus. Journal of Experimental Medicine 155: 1427–1438
Izui S, Lambert P H, Miescher P A 1976 In vitro demonstration of a particular affinity of glomerular basement membrane and collagen for DNA. Journal of Experimental Medicine 144:428
Jewell D P, MacLennan I C M 1973 Circulating immune complexes in inflammatory bowel disease. Clinical Experimental Immunology 14:219
Johnson A H, Mowbray J F, Porter K A 1975 Detection of circulating immune com lexes in pathological human sera. Lancet i:762
Johnson P M, Trenchev P, Page Faulk W 1973 Immunological studies of human placentae. Binding of complex immunoglobulin by stromal endothelial cells. Clinical Experimental Immunology 22: 133–138
Jones V E, Orlans E 1981 Isolation of immune complexes and characterisation of their constituent antigens and antibodies in some human diseases: a review. Journal of Immunological Methods 44: 249–270
Kauffmann R H, Hermann W A, Meijer C J L M ,Daha M R, Van Es L A 1980 Circulating and tissue-bound complexes in allergic vasculitis; relationship between immunoglobulin class and clinical features. Clinical and Experimental Immunology 41: 459–470
Keefe E B, Bardana E J, Harbeck R J, Pirofsky B, Carr R I 1974 Antibody to deoxyribonucleic acid (DNA) and DNA: anti-DNA complexes in cerebrospinal fluid. Annals of Internal Medicine 80:58
Kent I F, Fife E H 1963 Precise standardisation of reagent for complement fixation. American Journal of Tropical Medicine 12:103
Kilgallon W, Amlot P L, Williams B D 1982 Anti-Clq column: Ligand specific purification of immune complexes from human serum or plasma: Analysis of the interaction between Clq and immune complexes. Clinical and Experimental Immunology 78: 705–714
Kinsella T D, Baum J, Ziff M 1970 Studies of isolated synovial lining cells of rheumatoid and non-rheumatoid synovial membranes. Arthritis and Rheumatism 13:734
Kniker W T, Cochrane C G 1968 The localisation of circulating immune complexes in experimental serum sickness. The role of vasoactive amines and hydrodynamic forces. Journal of Experimental Medicine 127:119
Koffler D, Schur P, Kunkel H S 1967 Immunological studies concerning the nephritis of systemic lupus erythematosus. Journal of Experimental Medicine 126:607

Koffler D, Agnello V, Kunkel H S 1974 Polynucleotide immune complexes in serum and glomeruli of patients with systemic lupus erythematosus. American Journal of Pathology 74:109
Kunkel H G, Muller-Eberhard H J, Fudenberg H H, Tomasi T B 1961 Gammaglobulin complexes in rheumatoid arthritis and certain other conditions. Journal of Clinical Investigation 40:117
Lachmann P J, Peters D K 1982 Complement. In: Lachmann P J, Peters D K (eds) Clinical aspects of immunology, 4th Edn. Blackwell, Oxford, p 18–49
Lambert P H, Nyedeggar V E, Perrin L H et al 1975 Complement activation in seropositive and seronegative rheumatoid arthritis. In: Clot J, Sany J (eds) Rheumatology, Vol 6. Karger, Basel, p 52
Lambert P H, Dixon F J, Zubler R H et al 1978 A WHO collaborative study for the evaluation of eighteen methods for detecting immune complexes in serum. Journal of Clinical and Laboratory Immunology 1: 1–15
Lay W H, Nussenzweig V 1968 Receptors for complement on leukocytes. Journal of Experimental Medicine 128:991
Lehman D H, Wilson C B, Dixon F J 1975 Extraglomerular immunoglobulin deposits in human nephritis. American Journal of Medicine 58:765
Lepow I H 1971 Biologically active fragments of complement. In: Amos B (ed)Progress in immunology. Academic Press, New York, p 579
Levinsky R J, Soothill J F 1977 A test for antigen–antibody complexes in human sera using IgM of rabbit antisera to human immunoglobulins. Clinical and Experimental Immunology 29: 428–435
Levinsky R J ,Barrat T M 1979 IgA immune complexes in Henoch-Schoenlein purpura. Lancet ii: 1100–1103
Levinsky R J, Cameron J S, Soothill J F 1977 Serum immune complexes and disease activity in lupus nephritis. Lancet i:564
Lewis E J, Busch G J, Schur P H 1970 Gamma G globulin subgroup composition of the glomerular deposits in human renal disease. Journal of Clinical Investigation 49:1103
Lewis R M, Scwartz R S 1971 Canine systemic lupus erythematosus; genetic analysis of an established breeding colony. Journal of Experimental Medicine 134: 417–438
Lightfoot R W, Dursin R E, Christian C L 1970 Properties of soluble immune complexes. Journal of Immunology 105:1493
McCarthy D, Goddard D H, Holborow E J, Horsfall E J, Mumford P A, Maini R N 1981 The effect of IgG aggregate size and concentration on reactivity in immune complex assays. Journal of Immunological Methods 47: 349–358
McCormick J N 1963 An immunofluorescent study of rheumatoid factor. Annals of the Rheumatic Diseases 22:1
MacLennan I C M 1972 Competitions for receptors for immunoglobulin on cytotoxic lymphocytes. Clinical and Experimental Immunology 10:275
Maini R N, Glass D N, Scott J T 1976 Genetic factors, immune response, complement deficiency and susceptibility to inflammatory rheumatic diseases. In: Immunology of rheumatic diseases. Edward Arnold, London, Ch 13
Maini R N, Holborow E J 1977 Detection and measurement of circulating soluble antigen–antibody complexes and anti-DNA antibodies. Annals of Rheumatic Diseases (Suppl 1) 36: 1–142
Mannik M, Arend W P, Hall A P, Gilliland B D 1971 Studies on antigen–antibody complexes. I. Elimination of soluble complexes from rabbit circulation. Journal of Experimental Medicine 133:713
Mannik M, Haakenstad A O, Arend W P 1974 The fate and detection of circulating immune complexes. In: Brent L, Holborow J (eds) Progress in Immunology, Vol 5. North Holland, Amsterdam
Marrack J R 1938 The chemistry of antigens and antibodies. Special Report Series of the Medical Research Council No. 194. HMSO, London
Mayer M M 1961 Complement and complement fixation. In: Kabat E A, Mayer M M (eds) Experimental immunochemistry. Thomas, Springfield, p 135
Mellors R C, Nowoslawski A, Korngold L, Sengson B D 1961 Rheumatoid factor and the pathogenesis of rheumatoid arthritis. Journal of Experimental Medicine 113:475
Meltzer M, Franklin E C, Elias K, McCluskey R T, Cooper N 1966 Cryoglobulinaemia — A clinical and laboratory study. II. Cryoglobulins with rheumatoid factor activity. American Journal of Medicine 40:837
Messner R P, Laxdal T, Quie P G, Williams R C Jr 1968 Serum opsonin, bacteria and polymorphonuclear leukocyte interactions in subacute bacterial endocarditis. Anti-γ-globulin factors and their interaction with specific opsonins. Journal of Clinical Investigation 47:1109
Metzger H 1974 Effect of antigen binding on the properties of antibody. Advanced Immunology 18:169
Miller G W, Nussenzweig V 1978 A new complement function: solubilisation of antigen–antibody aggregates. Proceedings of the National Academy of Sciences USA 72: 418–422
Morgan A G, Soothill J F 1975 Relationship between macrophage clearance of PVP and affinity of anti-protein antibody response in inbred mouse strains. Nature 254:711
Mumford P A, Horsfall A C ,Maini R N 1982 The frequency of circulating immune complexes in rheumatoid arthritis and systemic lupus erythematosus: A comparative study using three immunoassays. Rheumatology International 1: 181–186
Munthe E, Hoyerall H M, Froland S S, Mellbye O J, Kass E, Natvig J B. Evidence for complement activation by the alternate pathway in the arthritis of hypogammaglobulinaemic patients. In: Clot J, Samy J (eds) Rheumatology, Vol 6. Karger, Basel, p 43–51
Natvig J B, Kunkel H G 1973 Human immunoglobulins: classes sub-classes genetic variance and idiotypes. In: Dixon F J, Kunkel H G (eds) Advanced immunology, Vol 16. Academic Press, London, p 1
Natvig J B, Munthe E 1975 Self associating IgG rheumatoid factor represents a major response of plasma cells in rheumatoid inflammatory tissues. Annals of the New York Academy of Sciences 256: 88–95
Nisonoff A, Winkler M H 1958 The reaction of chicken ovalbumin with homologous antibody in region of antibody excess. Journal of Immunology 81:65
Nisonoff A, Hopper J E, Spring S B 1975 In: Dixon F J, Kunkel H G (eds) The antibody molecule. Academic Press, London
Normansell D E 1971 Anti-γ-globulins in rheumatoid arthritis sera. II. The reactivity of anti-γ-globulin rheumatoid factors with altered γ-G-globulin. Immunochemistry 8: 593–603
Normansell D E, Stamworth D R 1968 Interactions between rheumatoid factor and native γ-G-Globulins studied in the ultracentrifuge. Immunology 15:549
Nowoslawski A 1971 Immunopathological features of

rheumatoid arthritis. In: Muller W, Harwerth H G, Fehr K (eds) Rheumatoid arthritis. Academic Press, London, p 325
Nussensweig V 1980 Interaction between complement and immune complexes: role of complement in containing immune complex damage. In: Fougereau M, Dausset J (eds) Progress in immunology IV. Academic Press, New York, p 1044–1056
Nydegger V E, Lambert P H, Gerber H, Miescher P A 1974 Circulating immune complexes in the serum in systemic lupus erythematosus and in carriers of hepatitis B antigen. Journal of Clinical Investigation 54:297
Oates C M, Payne L N, Maini R N, Dumonde D C 1972 In: Proceeding of the IV International Conference on Lymphatic Tissue, Dubrovnik. Plenum Press, New York
Oberbarensheidt J, Kolsch E 1978 Direct blockade of antigen-reactive B lymphocytes by immune complexes. Immunology 35: 151–157
Oldstone M B A, Dixon F J 1969 Pathogenesis of chronic disease associated with persistent lymphocytic choriomeningitis virus. Journal of Experimental Medicine 129:483
Oliver C, Essner E 1972 Protein transport in mouse kidney utilizing tyrosinase as an ultrastructural tracer. Journal of Experimental Medicine 136:291
Onyewotu I I, Holborow E J, Johnson G D 1974 Detection and radioassay of soluble circulating immune complexes using guinea pig peritoneal exudate cells. Nature New Biology 248:156
Pearson C M, Wood F D 1963 Studies of arthritis and other lesions induced in rats by the injection of mycobacterial adjuvant. VII. Pathologic details of the arthritis and spondylitis. American Journal of Pathology 42: 73–96
Pekin T J ,Zvaifler N J 1964 Haemolytic complement in synovial fluid. Journal of Clinical Investigation 43:1372
Pekin T J, Zvaifler N J 1970 Synovial fluid findings in systemic lupus erythematosus. Arthritis and Rheumatism 13:777
Penttinen K 1977 Platelet aggregation test. Annals of the Rheumatic Diseases 36, suppl. 1, 55
Perrin L H, Lambert P H, Miescher P A 1975a Complement breakdown products in plasma from patients with systemic lupus erythematosus and patients with membranoproliferative or other glomerulonephritis. Journal of Clinical Investigation 56:165
Perrin L H, Shiraishi S, Stroud R M, Lambert P H 1975b Detection and quantitation in plasma and synovial fluid of a fragment of human C4 with mobility generating during the activation of the complement system. Journal of Immunology 115:32
Pincus T, Haberkern R, Christian L 1968 Experimental chronic glomerulonephritis. Journal of Experimental Medicine 127:819
Poole A R, Coombs R R A 1977 Rheumatoid-like joint lesions in rabbits injected with bovine serum. International Archives of Allergy and Applied Immunology (in press)
Pope R M, Teller D C, Mannik M 1974 The molecular basis of self-association of antibodies to IgG (rheumatoid factors) in rheumatoid arthritis. Proceedings of the National Academy of Sciences of the United States of America 71:517
Porter R R 1959 The hydrolysis of rabbit γ-globulins and antibodies with crystalline papain. Biochemical Journal 73:119
Rodman W S, Williams R C, Bilka P J, Muller-Eberhard H J 1967 Immunofluorescent localisation of the third and fourth component of complement in synovial tissue from patients with rheumatoid arthritis. Journal of Laboratory and Clinical Medicine 69:141
Ruddy S, Austen F K 1970 The complement system in rheumatoid synovitis. Arthritis and Rheumatism 13:713
Ruddy S, Fearon D T, Austen F K 1975 Depressed synovial fluid levels of properdin and properdin factor B in patients with rheumatoid arthritis. Arthritis and Rheumatism 18:289
Ruddy S, Carpenter C B, Chin K W, Knostman J N, Soter N A, Gotzie O, Muller-Eberhard H J, Austen K F 1975 Human complement metabolism: analysis of 144 studies. Medicine 2:165
Schifferli J A, Bartolotti S R, Peters D K 1980 Inhibition of immune precipitation by complement. Clinical and Experimental Immunology 42:394
Schrager M A, Rothfield N F 1976 Clinical significance of serum properdin levels and properdin deposition in the dermal-epidermal junction in systemic lupus erythematosus. Journal of Clinical Investigation 57:212
Schrieber L, Maini R N 1984 Circulating immune complexes (CIC) in connective tissue diseases (CTD). Netherlands Journal of Medicine 27: 327–339
Schrieber L, Erhardt C C, Melsom R D, Venables P J W, McCarthy P A, Mumford P A, Maini R N 1983 In vivo fate of 125-I-SS-B (La) injected into mice. Immunology 48: 771–778
Schur P H 1975 Complement in lupus. Clinics in Rheumatic Diseases 3:519
Schur P H, Austen K F 1972 Complement in rheumatic diseases. Bulletin on Rheumatic Diseases 22:666
Schur P H, Sandson J 1968 Immunologic factors and clinical activity of systemic lupus erythematosus. New England Journal of Medicine 278:533
Sliwinski A J, Zvaifler N J 1972 Decreased synthesis of the third component in hypocomplementaemic systemic lupus erythematosus. Clinical Experimental Immunology 11:21
Smith M D, Barratt T M, Hayward A R, Soothill J F 1975 The inhibition of complement-dependant lymphocyte rosette formation by the sera of children with steroid-sensitive nephrotic syndrome and other renal diseases. Clinical and Experimental Immunology 21:236
Soothill J F, Steward M W 1971 The immunopathological significance of the heterogeneity of antibody affinity. Clinical Experimental Immunology 9: 193–199
Spiegelberg H L, Miescher P A, Benacerraf B 1963 Studies on the role of complement in the immune clearance of Escherichia coli and rat erythrocytes by the reticulo-endothelial system in mice. Journal of Immunology 90:751
Spitler L, Hubert H, Fudenberg H H 1969 Inhibition of capillary migration by antigen–antibody complexes. Journal of Immunology 102:404
Svec K, Allen S T 1970 Antibody to nuclear material eluted from isolated spleen vessels in systemic lupus erythematosus. Science 170:550
Talal N 1970 Immunologic and viral factors in the pathogenesis of systemic lupus erythematosus. Arthritis and Rheumatism 13:887
Tan E M, Kunkel H G 1966 An Immunofluorescent study of the skin lesions in systemic lupus erythematosus. Arthritis and Rheumatism 9:37
Taylor R B, Basten A 1976 Suppressor T cells in humoral immunity and tolerance. British Medical Bulletin 32:152
ten Bensel R, Cochrane C G, Williams R C 1968

Demonstration of complexes of gammaglobulin and complement in patients with SLE. Arthritis and Rheumatism 11:515 (abs)

Tesar J T, Schmid F R 1970 Conversion of soluble immune complexes into complement-fixing aggregates by IgM-rheumatoid factor. Journal of Immunology 105:1206

Theofilopoulous A N, Dixon F J 1979 The biology and detection of immune complexes. Advances in Immunology 28: 89–220

Theofilopoulos A N, Wilson C B, Dixon F J 1976 The Raji cell radioimmune assay for detecting immune complexes in human sera. Journal of Clinical Investigation 57:169

Van Es L A 1981 Factors affecting the deposition of immune complexes. In: Fauci A S (ed) Immune complexes in clinical medicine, Vol 1. Saunders, Philadelphia, p 281–304

Versey J M B, Hobbs J R, Holt P J L 1973 Complement metabolism in rheumatoid arthritis. Annals of the Rheumatic Diseases 32:557

Von Pirquet C E 1911 Allergy. Allergy Archives Internal Medicine 7:259 and 383

Ward P A, Zvaifler N J 1971 Complement-derived leukotactic factors in inflammatory synovial fluids of humans. Journal of Clinical Investigation 50:606

Weigle W O 1958 The elimination of antigen–antibody complexes from sera of rabbits. Journal of Immunology 81:204

Weinstein A, Peters K, Brown D, Bluestone R 1972 Metabolism of the third component of complement (C3) in patients with rheumatoid arthritis. Arthritis and Rheumatism 15:49

Weisman M, Zvaifler N 1975 Cryoglobulinaemia in rheumatoid arthritis. Journal of Clinical Investigations 56:725

Weissmann G, Zurier R B, Spieler P J, Goldstein I M 1971 Mechanisms of lysosomal release from leukocytes exposed to immune complexes and other particles. Journal of Experimental Medicine 134:149 (s)

Weissmann G S 1972 Lysosomal mechanisms of tissue injury in arthritis. New England Journal of Medicine 286:141

Westberg N G, Naff G B, Boyer J T, Michael A F 1971 Glomerular deposition of properdin in acute and chronic glomerulonephritis and hypocomplementaemia. Journal of Clinical Investigation 50:642

Whitaker J N ,Engel W K 1972 Vascular deposits of immunoglobulin and complement in idiopathic inflammatory myopathy. New England Journal of Medicine 286:333

Williams B D, Slaney J M 1977 Marcomolecular C3 — an indirect marker of circulating immune complexes. Annals of the Rheumatic Diseases 36 (Suppl 1):37

Wilson C B, Dixon F J 1971 Quantitation of acute and chronic serum sickness in the rabbit. Journal of Experimental Medicine 134:7 (s)

Wilson J G, Wong W W, Schur P H, Fearon D T 1982 Mode of inheritance of decreased C3b receptors on erythrocytes of patients with systemic lupus erythematosus. New England Journal of Medicine 307: 981–986

Winchester R J, Agnello V, Kunkel H G 1970 Gammaglobulin complexes in synovial fluids of patients with rheumatoid arthritis. Partial characterization and relationship to lowered complement levels. Clinical Experimental Immunology 6:689

Winchester R J, Kunkel H G, Agnello V 1971 Occurrence of globulin complexes in serum and joint fluids of rheumatoid arthritis patients: use of monoclonal rheumatoid factors in reagents for their demonstration. Journal of Experimental Medicine 134:286 (s)

Zubler R H, Lambert P H 1977 ^{125}I-Clq binding test for the detection of soluble immune complexes. Annals of the Rheumatic Diseases, supplement on, 'Detection and measurement of circulating soluble antigen–antibody complexes and anti-DNA antibodies'

Zvaifler N J 1969 Breakdown products of C3 in human synovial fluids. Journal of Clinical Investigation 48:1532

Zvaifler N 1973 The immunopathology of joint inflammation in rheumatoid arthritis. Advanced Immunology 16:265

14 *D.C. Dumonde M.W. Steward K.A. Brown*

The role of microbial infection in rheumatic disease

THE PARADOX OF INFECTION AND IMMUNITY

Rheumatoid arthritis and allied inflammatory rheumatic diseases have been thought to be due to infective processes almost since the time of Pasteur; yet intensive investigation has failed to reveal classical microbiological evidence for defined infective agents at sites of rheumatic inflammation. In the last few decades increasing laboratory evidence has highlighted immunological abnormalities in these disorders and attention has been drawn frequently to clinicopathological similarities with known infectious or hypersensitivity diseases in man and animals. Since the early 1970s the view has grown that these different inflammatory rheumatic syndromes arise through genetically-based immunopathological responses to microbial infection although it was continually conceded that much of the evidence supporting this view was circumstantial (see Dumonde, 1976).

Two principal kinds of derangement have been suggested by which such pathogenetic mechanisms may operate:

1. An inability to eradicate certain microbes or their products from the host and thus from potential sites of rheumatic inflammation.
2. A failure to stop a reaction produced to what would normally be regarded as an ephemeral stimulus to the host's immune system.

Herein lies the paradox of infection and immunity in the rheumatic diseases: for whereas the local tissue lesions look like hypersensitivity responses to persisting antigens, the microbiological and immunological evidence which would support this inference is, at best, indirect.

In this chapter we summarise the present state of this field from two points of view: first, the principal evidence which has sought to associate rheumatic diseases with specific microbial infections; and second, the principal immunopathological mechanisms which have been considered as linking rheumatic diseases with microbial infection. In discussing the first area we classify associations between microbial infection and arthritis syndromes and we derive the proposition that rheumatoid and allied diseases may be viewed as 'adverse' reactions precipitated by a potentially wide range of microbial agents. In discussing the second area we look 'outside' pathogenetic explanations of classical immunology by considering how disorders of the inflammatory process might give rise to aberrant or adverse reactions of a 'rheumatic' nature during the host response to certain kinds of microbial stimuli.

We consider that progress in this field in the last decade has been hampered by continued preoccupation with the need to reveal *specific* microbes as causative agents of inflammatory rheumatic disease. On the one hand we concur that it is socioeconomically justifiable to continue an enlightened and selective quest for evidence of persistent prokaryotic or viral agents (or their genomic fragments) in patients with these distressing diseases (Marmion, 1978). On the other hand, we present in this chapter a more optimistic note by viewing microbial stimulation as simply one of the events which may precipitate inflammatory rheumatic disease on the basis of a multifactorial aetiology and pathogenesis. We conclude that a less restrictive approach to the role of microbial infection may lead to scientific explanations of the rheumatic diathesis that will have special bearing upon disease control.

INVESTIGATIVE APPROACHES AND PRINCIPAL HYPOTHESES

Table 14.1 summarises the eight principal approaches which have sought to implicate specific micro-organisms in inflammatory rheumatic disease; and Tables 14.2–14.4 illustrate the kinds of detailed information that have been obtained by these approaches. Examination of Tables 14.1–14.4 reveals that the problem has been far more sophisticated and difficult than could be implied by the simple application of Koch's postulates. Thus for any one rheumatic syndrome (e.g. reactive arthritis) a multiplicity of micro-organisms has been implicated; and, moreover, any one given microbial species (e.g. *Salmonella*) seems capable of producing more than one rheumatic syndrome.

Certain general conclusions, however, seem justified:

a. Much clinical experience reveals that polyarthritis, vasculitis and other forms of 'rheumatic' inflammation can certainly develop in relation to defined infective and allergic states in man (see Table 14.2).

b. Much experimental knowledge in animals has been gained of the circumstances in which polyarthritis and other connective tissue pathology follow naturally-occurring or induced reactions to microbiological and immunological stimuli (see Table 14.3). These are discussed in Chapter 15.

c. Both direct and indirect evidence indicates that a *wide* (rather than a restricted) range of microbial agents are implicated in human inflammatory rheumatic disease (Table 14.4).

On the basis of these investigations and results there would seem to be three general ways by which microbial infection could initiate a generalised inflammatory rheumatic disease:

1. Dissemination of a specific microbe or its products throughout the host with local hypersensitivity reactions developing at 'risk sites' of rheumatic inflammation where the microbe or its antigens are deposited.

2. The induction or unmasking of autoimmune or immune complex disease by the precipitating effect of one or more microbial infections upon the susceptible host.

3. The development of reactive pathology at a distance from portals of microbial entry or colonisation, without needing to postulate the presence or retention of the microbe or its products at sites of disseminated ('rheumatic') inflammation.

Table 14.1 Principal approaches which have sought to implicate specific micro-organisms as aetiological agents in inflammatory rheumatic diseases

1. Attempts to isolate specific microbes from rheumatic lesions by techniques of microbial culture
2. Attempts to visualise microbes in rheumatic lesions by electron microscopy
3. Attempts to detect microbial products in rheumatic lesions by immunological or biochemical methods
4. Epidemiological or genetic evidence associating known infective and rheumatic disease
5. Immunological evidence associating rheumatic diseases with persistent host responses towards specific microbes or their antigens
6. Evidence derived from the study of arthritis and other connective tissue pathology temporally related to known infectious or hypersensitivity episodes in man
7. Evidence derived from the study of animal 'models' of inflammatory rheumatic disease occurring naturally or experimentally following known infectious episodes or hypersensitivity reactions
8. Evidence ascribing cell or tissue abnormalities in rheumatic disease to the sequelae of microbial infection

These considerations lead to hypotheses which implicate one or more of the following pathogenetic mechanisms:

a. That disseminated rheumatic lesions are the result of a persistent intense response by the immune system to an agent or 'target' outside its effector cells with the implication that for various reasons (e.g. molecular mimicry) the host is unable to eliminate the offending 'target' by immunological means (Marmion, 1978).

b. That the microbe or its genetic information persists inside or in association with cells of the immune system itself (i.e. macrophages or lymphocytes) resulting in a loss of normal immunoregulatory control ('immunological subversion'; see also Marmion, 1978) and which is revealed by exaggerated autoimmunity or by defective immune elimination of 'target' macromolecules.

Table 14.2 Examples of non-suppurative arthritis causally related to human infective or hypersensitivity states

	Nature and occurrence of 'rheumatic' syndrome		
Infective or hypersensitivity state	Principal features of arthritis	Associated clinicopathological features	Rheumatological interpretation (see also Tables 14.4, 14.5)
Vaccinia virus (? also variola, varicella, some rubella)	Acute, may be monoarticular; ascribed to local viral multiplication with synovial cell necrosis	Evidence suggests that arthritis resolves when virus eliminated as host develops immune response	Examples of 'infective' (class 1) arthritis with viral cytopathology as principal mechanism (Phillips, 1976a)
Rubella virus, rubella vaccine strains, mumps, hepatitis B, ? EB virus, ? arboviruses	Often subacute or migratory; some evidence of virus Ag or immune complexes in joint; no residual arthritis	Associations with hypersensitivity phenomena occurring during the infection (rashes; circulating immune complexes; depressed C′)	Examples of 'postinfective' (class 2) viral arthritis where hypersensitivity a principal mechanism (Phillips, 1976a; Hamerman, 1975; Sauter & Utsinger, 1978)
Arthritis of serum sickness and drug (e.g. antibiotic hypersensitivity)	Self-limiting migratory polyarthritis (with polymorphs in synovial fluid) after latent period	Associated with vasculitis, lymphadenopathy and renal involvement; latent period decreases on re-exposure to same agent (Lansbury & Joseph, 1966)	Example of joint involvement during systemic immune complex disease clinically different from postinfective arthritides
Meningococcal infection	Migratory, self-limiting polyarthritis in 2–10% subjects on antibiotic treatment with variable 'latent' period of onset	Other evidence of immune complex disease includes vasculitis and episcleritis but not glomerulonephritis; synovial exudate cells contain Ig and meningococcal Ag	Example of class 2 (postinfective) arthritis (Greenwood & Whittle, 1976)
Lepromatous leprosy	Migratory transient polyarthritis; sterile synovial fluid	Associated with cutaneous vasculitis, mucocutaneous lesions, proteinuria and high serum antibody titres	Immune complex pathogenesis (Turk & Belehu, 1974) of arthritis (? class 2)
Secondary syphilis	Rare examples of transient polyarthritis; sterile synovial fluid	Associated with cutaneous vasculitis, mucocutaneous lesions, proteinuria and high serum antibody titres	Immune complex pathogenesis of (class 2) postinfective arthritis (see also Turk & Belehu, 1974)
Tuberculosis	Migratory polyarthritis associated with erythema nodosum	? Doubtful entity of 'tuberculous rheumatism' (Brav & Hench, 1934)	? Class 2 (postinfective) or ? class 3 (reactive) arthritis
Group A streptococcal pharyngitis	Migratory polyarthritis in some 3% subjects during strep. epidemic but no evidence of streptococcal Ag in joint	No renal involvement; no fall in serum C′; arthritis dissociable from skin rashes and lymphadenopathy (Taranta, 1966)	Example of class 3 ('reactive') arthritis syndromes
Salmonella, shigella enteritis	Limited polyarthritis with sterile synovial fluid in some 3% subjects with antecedent diarrhoea	May develop spondylitic or Reiter's syndromes; HLA-B27 in 90%; tendency for recurrent arthritis with different precipitating factors (Aho et al, 1975)	Examples of class 3 (reactive) arthritis

Table 14.2 Examples of non-suppurative arthritis causally related to human infective or hypersensitivity states — *continued*

	Nature and occurrence of 'rheumatic' syndrome		
Infective or hypersensitivity state	Principal features of arthritis	Associated clinicopathological features	Rheumatological interpretation (see also Tables 14.4, 14.5)
Yersinosis	Up to 50% subjects may develop limited sterile polyarthritis	In 10% subjects, associations with erythema nodosum/multiforme and myocarditis raise differential diagnosis of RhF; HLA-B27 in 90%; tendency for recurrent peripheral or spondarthritis (in 10%) (Aho et al, 1975; Leino & Kalliomaki, 1974)	Class 3 (reactive) arthritis
Chlamydial infection (lymphogranuloma venereum)	Relapsing polyarthritis with sterile synovial fluid (Dawson & Boots, 1939)	Associated with DH (Frei-positive); and preceding erythema nodosum in some cases; not associated with HLA-B27 (Aho et al, 1975)	? Class 3 (reactive) arthritis
Non-gonococcal (non-specific) urethritis; ? chlamydial infection	Relapsing spondarthritis or peripheral arthritis; sterile synovial fluid	Assumed incidence of Reiter's syndrome in 1–2%; HLA-B27 positive in 80–90% of these (Aho et al, 1975)	? Class 3 (reactive) arthritis

Key: Ag, antigen; Ig, immunoglobulin; C′, complement; RhF, rheumatic fever; DH, delayed hypersensitivity.

Table 14.3 Illustrative animal models of inflammatory rheumatic disease: occurrence of arthritis and other connective tissue pathology associated with microbial agents or hypersensitivity reactions

Form of infective or hypersensitive animal disease	Principal pathological features of animal model	Rheumatological interest in special feature of animal models
Experimental serum sickness in rabbits produced by intravenous protein or immune complexes (Rich, 1947; Dixon, 1963)	Various patterns of vasculitis, glomerulonephritis and self-limiting polyarthritis associated with circulating immune complexes	Points to hypersensitivity mechanisms in polyarteritis: supports immune complex pathogenesis for lupus nephritis and for migratory polyarthritis following acute infections
Induction of experimental organ-specific autoimmune disease in normal rodents (Dumonde, 1966)	Immunization with corresponding tissue extracts in adjuvants leads to lymphocytic infiltration in brain, testis, liver, adrenal, thyroid; but prolonged immunisation or superimposed damage needed to obtain tissue specific autoimmune disease in other organs	Suggests requirement for non-immunological precipitating factors in relating tissue specific autoimmunity to disease
Response of normal rabbits to bacterial hyperimmunisation and of normal mice to bacterial endotoxin	Antiglobulin production by hyperimmunised rabbits; anti-DNA production by endotoxin-treated mice (Abruzzo & Christian, 1961; Fournié et al, 1974)	Antiglobulin and antinuclear antibodies viewed as potential responses to certain forms of microbial stimuli including endotoxins
'Adjuvant' disease in rats injected with killed mycobacteria or other 'arthritogenic' bacteria/extracts (Pearson, 1966; Pearson & Kohashi, 1977)	Acute and chronic peripheral and spondarthritis associated with nodular vasculitis, urethritis and anterior uveitis; different strains of inbred rats differ in susceptibility and disease pattern; marked periosteal new bone formation	Although hypersensitivity pathogenesis unclear (? types III & IV) may provide a model for reactive (spond-) arthritis following certain (bacterial) infections (e.g. 'class 3' arthritis; see Table 14.5)
Allergic monoarthritis in rabbits, rats, mice, guinea-pigs, chickens by intra-articular injection of sensitizing allergen (Dumonde et al, 1976, 1977)	Close histopathological resemblance to the rheumatoid joint includes lymphocyte and macrophage activation, cartilage/bone erosion, fibrosis and ectopic lymphoid foci (Dumonde & Glynn, 1962)	Points to involvement of both T cell and B cell activation in rheumatoid synovitis; to the joint as an immunising site; and permits immunopharmacological and genetic analysis of experimental model
Allergic subcutaneous granuloma to non-diffusible allergen in rabbits and guinea-pigs	Persistence of mixed cell granuloma comprising lymphocytes and macrophages with central fibrinoid mass and peripheral vasculitis and fibrosis (Dumonde & Glynn, 1965)	Experimental model of the rheumatoid nodule supports a role for allergic vasculitis in its pathogenesis
Follicular hyperplasia in guinea-pig or mouse lymph nodes by intralymphatic injection of lymphokine or regional injection of toxic Ag	Patterns of follicular hyperplasia associated with paracortical lymphocyte accumulation or with plasma cell differentiation in cortex in absence of specific Ab synthesis (Kelly & Wolstencroft, 1974; Dumonde et al, 1976)	Experimental model of rheumatoid lymph node suggests immunopharmacological control defect may underly characteristic follicular hyperplasia
Homologous disease in tolerant rats injected with allogeneic lymphocytes	Systemic 'graft-v-host' reaction with widespread cellular infiltration in viscera, joints and skin (Stastny et al, 1965)	Provides a model whereby systemic connective tissue disease can result from lymphocyte-mediated aggression

Table 14.3 Illustrative animal models of inflammatory rheumatic disease: occurrence of arthritis and other connective tissue pathology associated with microbial agents or hypersensitivity reactions — *continued*

Form of infective or hypersensitive animal disease	Principal pathological features of animal model	Rheumatological interest in special feature of animal models
Carditis in rabbits following group A streptococcal infection (Murphy, 1960)	Animals develop immunity to single infections but myocarditis and endocarditis only follow multiple infections with different M-types	Suggests host susceptibility to post-streptococcal rheumatic fever induced by multiple exposure to different streptococcal antigens and/or toxins
Chronic arthritis in pigs developing after systemic infection with *Erysipelothrix rhusiopathiae*	Acute followed by chronic polyarthritis associated with antiglobulins in serum and synovial fluid; enhanced severity of arthritis in animals previously vaccinated against erysipelas (see Drew, 1972)	Considerable variation in response of pigs to infection and in persistence of organisms/antigens in the joint provides investigative approach to role of infection and hypersensitivity in an animal model of rheumatoid arthritis
Chronic arthritis and subcutaneous nodules in pigs following change to excessive protein-rich diet (Mansson et al, 1971)	Rheumatoid-like synovitis with IgG-bearing lymphoid cells, pannus formation, cartilage and bone erosions; associated with change in bowel flora dominated by atypical clostridria	As a model of intestinal arthropathy it suggests that subclinical change in bacterial gut flora might act as precipitating event for reactive arthritis; pathogenesis is as yet unknown.
Mycoplasma arthritis in mammals and domestic fowl (see Taylor-Robinson & Taylor, 1976; Cole et al, 1976)	Chronic polyarthritis resembling rheumatoid histopathology; organisms not usually recovered from joints after acute phase; local antibody production can occur in synovia	Experimental models raise question of how chronic arthritis persists when organism is no longer recoverable from joints; animal strain differences may permit genetic studies
Polyarthritis in rabbits induced by single intra-articular injection of chlamydia (Smith et al, 1973)	Chronic lymphocytic synovitis with pannus and erosions runs parallel with ability to recover chlamydia from joint; tetracyclines fail to suppress established arthritis	Illustrates joint as a site for supporting immune and infective responses to chlamydia of human origin
Chronic herpes simplex arthritis in rabbits by single intra-articular injection of virus	Chronic erosive synovitis in infected (knee) joint with transient synovitis in contralateral joint (Webb et al, 1973)	Illustrates joint as a site for supporting immune and infective responses; offers approach to studying virus latency in synovial cells in vivo
Spontaneous polyarthritis in chickens and dogs attributed to viral infection	Electron microscopy of synovia suggests reovirus in chickens and paramyxovirus in dogs (Brandly & Jungherr, 1960)	Naturally occurring animal polyarthritides may offer investigative approach to viral aetiology/pathogenesis of RA
Aleutian virus disease in genetically susceptible mink (Nardo & Norton, 1971)	Systemic plasmacytosis, hypergammaglobulaemia, anti-globulins, anti-nuclear AB's, cryoprecipitates, immune complex nephritis and diffuse vasculitis. Disease worse in vaccinated animals; virus circulates as infective complexes; some animals develop monoclonal gammopathy	Example of immune complex disease accompanied by hyperglobulinaemia and antiglobulin production resulting from infection of genetically susceptible host with persistent virus
Lymphocytic choriomeningitis (LCM) and lactic dehydrogenase (LDH) virus infections of mice (Oldstone & Dixon, 1975)	Immune complex nephritis and circulating infective virus: antibody complexes following infection of thymectomised (LCM), neonatal (LCM) or adult (LDH) mice; genetic differences but no hyperglobulinaemia	Example of genetically-based immune complex disease without hypergammaglobulinaemia where virus circulates as infectious complexes

New Zealand (NZB/W) murine 'lupus' syndrome associated with expression of endogenous C-type leukovirus (MuLV) (Talal, 1975; Levy, 1974)	Glomerulonephritis associated with deposition of immune complexes containing DNA, RNA and C-type virus protein; generalized lymphocytic infiltration of viscera; antilymphocyte antibodies; monoclonal macroglobulinaemia; lymphomas	Severe renal disease in female B/W mice viewed as model for lupus nephritis, but spectrum of disease implicates genetic, immunoregulatory and viral factors in aetiology of SLE
Neonatal infection of various mouse strains with C-type MuLV (Lerner et al, 1974)	Spectrum of incidence of lymphomas, lymphosarcoma, visceral lymphomatosis. ANA-positive immune complex glomerulonephritis and circulating C-type virus protein	Demonstrates heterogeneity of expression of C-type viral genome in relation to animal models of systemic connective tissue disease
Canine lupus syndrome associated with evidence of C-type leukovirus (Lewis et al, 1973)	LE cells, anti-nuclear antibodies, autoimmune haemolytic anaemia, glomerulonephritis, polyarthritis, thyroiditis, thrombocytopenic purpura, lymphocytic follicles in thymus. LE cells and thymic follicles occur in asymptomatic animal relatives but no obvious genetic factor	Ability to confer antinuclear antibody production upon healthy dogs by spleen filtrates suggested horizontal transmission of canine lupus agent and relevance to human lupus epidemiology
Review of experimental models of rheheumatoid, lupoid, vasculitis syndromes: their comparison with human rheumatic disease (Glynn & Schlumberger, 1977)	Nature and form of 'rheumatic' lesions following experimental infection or hypersensitivity reactions implies dysregulation of inflammatory responses in human rheumatic disease	Selective study of experimental models should assist understanding of *cellular* mechanisms in rheumatic inflammation (Glynn & Schlumberger, 1977)
Review of experimental arthritis and vasculitis syndromes developing durin during hypersensitivity reactions and following exposure to bacterial products and bacterial, mycoplasma and viral infection (Deicher & Schultz, 1981)	Spectrum of cellular, vascular and haematological mechanisms implicated in pathogenesis of experimental models	Selective study of experimental models should assist understanding of *vascular* mechanisms in rheumatic inflammation (Deicher & Schultz, 1981)

Table 14.4 Illustrative evidence relating to involvement of specific microbial agents in inflammatory rheumatic diseases

Disease or syndrome; and microbe implicated	Nature of evidence relating disease and microbe: 'Direct' (evidence relating to microbes or antigens in cells or tissues)	'Indirect' (evidence from genetics, epidemiology, cell biology, or abnormal immune status)	Possible interpretation
RHEUMATIC FEVER (RhF)			
β-haemolytic streptococci (group A)	No evidence of streptococci or streptococcal Ag in RhF heart or RhF joints (Taranta, 1966);	Association of primary RhF with repeated infection by different group A types (Taranta, 1966)	
	Heart-muscle, vascular endothelium and basement membrane share antigens with group A streptococci (Kaplan & Svec, 1964; Kingston & Glynn, 1971)	Increased susceptibility of RhF subjects to reinfection with group A streps., or to RhF relapse, runs parallel with high or rising ASO titres and heart-reactive Ab but delay in onset of bactericidal Ab (Zabriskie, 1976)	Susceptibility of RhF is perhaps genetically linked to hyper-reactivity to group A streptococci on basis of 'immune restriction' permitting autoimmune pathogenesis of 'reactive' rheumatic disease on basis of type III or type IV hypersensitivity (Zabriskie, 1976)
		RhF subjects show persistently heightened cellular hypersensitivity to cross-reactive Ags of group A streptococcal membranes	
		Increased tendency for HLA sharing by parents of RhF children	
		Decreased complement (Cl, C4, C3) levels in synovial fluid	
RHEUMATOID ARTHRITIS (RA)			
Diphtheroids	Inconstant or unconfirmed isolations from lymph nodes, synovial membrane, synovial fluid; ? due to environmental contamination of cultures or ? opportunistic infection (Marmion, 1976)	Higher agglutinating Ab titres of RA sera for diphtheroid Ag but no elevation of CFT-Ab or cellular hypersensitivity (Maini et al, 1970; Duthie et al, 1976)	Present evidence suggests consequential, not causal role (Hamerman, 1975)
Atypical clostridia	High frequency of faecal group A *Clostridium perfringens* in RA and other inflammatory rheumatic diseases (Mansson & Olhagen, 1974)	Raised serum Ab titres to clostridial α-toxin and delayed hypersensitivity tests (Olhagen, 1976)	? Changes in gastrointestinal flora as a precipitating event (e.g. in 'class 3' syndromes (Table 14.5)
Mycoplasmas	Inconstant and unconfirmed isolations from SM/SF; no biochemical evidence for metabolising mycoplasma in SM; technical criticisms of direct and indirect isolation procedures (Hamerman, 1975; Marmion, 1976)	No differences in circulating Ab titres between RA and non-RA groups; heightened cellular hypersensitivity to *M. fermentans* ascribed to non-specific binding of γ-globulin by mycoplasmal Ag (Maini et al, 1975)	Present evidence suggests consequential not causal role (Hamerman, 1975; Marmion, 1976)

Bacterial L-forms	Unconfirmed isolations from RA blood and SF (Marmion, 1976)	Ill-defined concept of bacterial subphases as mediators of autoimmunity (Pease, 1969)	Role unsubstantiated (Marmion, 1976)
Group A streptococci	No evidence of group A streptococcal Ag in rheumatoid lesions	Reports of higher ASO titres and precipitating Ab to cell wall Ag in seronegative and seropositive RA (Braun & Holm, 1970)	? Slower elimination of pathogenic streptococci in RA
Group B streptococci	? More prevalent in RA nasopharynx; occasional isolation from RA-SF (Svartz, 1975)	No evidence concerning immunological status in RA	Role unsubstantiated
Any 'latent' virus	Unconfirmed reports of (heat-stable) active agent in RA synovial homogenates inducing articular disease in mice and chickens by embryonic or neonatal inoculation (Warren et al, 1969, 1971)	Cell biological properties of long-term rheumatoid synovial cells suggestive of latent virus infection; some RA synovial cell abnormalities 'transferable' to rabbit synovia (Hamerman, 1975; Smith & Hamerman, 1976)	Unsubstantiated role of 'scrapie-like' agent.
Rubella virus	Resistance of rheumatoid synovial cells to viral challenge in culture, including rubella (Smith & Hamerman, 1976)	Elevated titres of antirubella Ab in JRA; rise in rubella-related acute phase protein in RA sera (rho); unconfirmed susceptibility of rheumatoid synovial cells to lysis by antirubella serum and C′ (Hamerman, 1975)	? Rubella infection as precipitating event in some rheumatoids
	Unconfirmed reports of virus identification or isolation in a few RA patients (Grahame et al, 1981; Grahame et al, 1983)	Some evidence of altered lymphocyte reactivity in RA to rubella antigens (Ford et al, 1982)	Illustrates problems of implicating an arthritogenic virus in RA (Marmion, 1978)
Epstein–Barr virus (EBV)	Special nuclear antigen on B cell lines ('RANA') is identified preferentially by RA sera (Alspaugh & Tan, 1976)	Raised anti-EBV titres in RA (Alspaugh et al, 1981); EBV transforms RA lymphocytes more readily than normal lymphocytes (Slaughter et al, 1978); increased B cell susceptibility to EBV (Stierle et al, 1982) or lack of T cell control (Depper et al, 1981)	Persistent or active EBV infection (? secondary) could offer tenable explanation of increased auto-Ab production in RA
Oncogenic virus (e.g. C-type)	Suppression of lymphocyte mitogenic activation by co-culture with rheumatoid synovial explants (Denman et al, 1975)	RA sera contain Ab mediating K cell cytotoxicity of human neoplastic liver cells (Chang) in culture (Panayi, 1976)	
	Cytoplasmic particles resembling C-type viruses found in 'lymphoreticular' cells of rheumatoid synovia (Neumark & Farkas, 1976);	Increased incidence of lymphoreticular malignancy in RA and Sjögren's syndrome (Mason et al, 1973; Gutowska-Plachecka et al, 1975)	? Possibility of viral-induced neoantigen in association with lymphoid abnormalities and immunological response in some RA

Table 14.4 Illustrative evidence relating to involvement of specific microbial agents in inflammatory rheumatic diseases — *continued*

Disease or syndrome; and microbe implicated	Nature of evidence relating disease and microbe		
	'Direct' (evidence relating to microbes or antigens in cells or tissues)	'Indirect' (evidence from genetics, epidemiology, cell biology, or abnormal immune status)	Possible interpretation
	RNAse-sensitive DNA polymerase activity in rheumatoid synovia not a true (viral) reverse transcriptase (Norval et al, 1975)	Cellular hypersensitivity of RA leucocytes to 'lipoprotein' extracts of RA synovia (Bacon et al, 1973)	
Paramyxovirus	Several reports of paramyxovirus-like tubular structures and cytoplasmic buds in vascular endothelial cells of RA synovia (Neumark & Farkas, 1973; Schumacher, 1975)	Elevated serum Ab titres to measles virus in more than one RA series (Kalliomaki et al, 1975) Slight suppression of CMI reactivity in RA suggestive of viral infection or antigenic competition (Lockshin, 1976; Kantor, 1976)	? Paramyxovirus infection precipitates microvascular or lymphoid pathology
POLYMYOSITIS (P/M) AND DERMATOMYOSITIS (D/M)			
Paramyxovirus	Intranuclear and intracytoplasmic inclusions in vascular endothelial cells of paramyxovirus type (Sato et al, 1970)	Association of adult D/M and P/M with malignancy (carcinomata) (Pearson, 1966a); lymphocyte cytotoxicity for human fetal muscle cells but not evidence of specific antiviral immune response (Dawkins &Mastaglia, 1973)	? Tissue-specific autoimmunity and malignancy secondary to infection with different viruses
Picornavirus	Intracellular 'crystals' in muscle cells resembling Coxsackie virus (Chou, 1970)		
REITER'S SYNDROME			
Chlamydia	10–20% 'isolations' from joint, urethra, conjunctiva; 80% have urethral inclusions; yolk-sac inclusions from egg-inoculation of joint material (Catterall, 1976; Delbarre & Amor, 1976; Schachter, 1976)	Polyarthritis in 1–2% of subjects with urethritis; up to 80% Reiter's are HLA-B27-positive; 75% have elevated lymphocyte transformation to chlamydial Ag (Delbarre & Amor, 1976); Elevated CFT-Ab to chlamydia of same order as those with simple urethritis (Schachter, 1976)	? Genetically based immunopathological response to chlamydial infection
Mycoplasma	No predilection of T-strains for genitourinary tract of Reiter's subjects compared with non-specific urethritis (Catterall, 1976)	No evidence of abnormal host response to mycoplasma in Reiter's syndrome	No significant role for mycoplasma infection

Shigella	Precise bacteriological studies on Finnish epidemic (Paronen, 1948) not available (Aho et al, 1975)	No evidence of abnormal host response to shigella though up to 3% of exposed subjects developed syndrome (Aho et al, 1975)	? Reactive arthritis (class 3) following shigella infection
ANKYLOSING SPONDYLITIS (AS)			
Klebsiella spp.	Increased faecal carriage of klebsiella in AS (Ebringer et al, 1978); antigenic cross-reactivity between klebsiella and B27-positive (AS) lymphocytes (Seager et al, 1979)	Peripheral blood lymphocyte stimulation by klebsiella is defective in AS (Edmonds et al, 1981)	Disputed nature of all 'klebsiella' evidence (Kinsella et al, 1983) illustrates current difficulties
SYSTEMIC LUPUS ERYTHEMATOSUS			
C-type retrovirus	Minority (0.1%) of peripheral lymphocytes bear C-type virus-related antigen (Schwartz, 1975)	Reduced CMI responses by peripheral lymphocytes; subnormal DH responses (Horwitz, 1973)	
	SLE spleen, placenta, kidney contain substantial levels of C-type interspecies Ag (Strand & August, 1974; Mellors & Mellors, 1976)	High incidence of lymphocytotoxic Ab's (64%) in healthy relatives and household contacts (DeHoratius & Messner, 1975) Antibodies in both normal and SLE sera react with C-type interspecies Ags (Snyder et al, 1976)	? Enhanced expression of C-type viral Ags in SLE may provide stimulus for auto-Ab production against lymphocytes; ? Cause or effect of defective CMI responses
	IgG from immune complexes deposited in SLE kidneys reacts with major internal core protein of primate C-type virus (Reynolds & Panem, 1981)	Increased incidence of lymphoreticular malignancy in SLE (Dubois, 1974a) Epidemiological, cluster, family and twin studies suggest both genetic and environmental factors in SLE (Lee & Siegel, 1976)	
Paramyxovirus	Several confirmed reports of cytoplasmic tubuloreticular structures (TRS) in vascular endothelial cells (skin, kidney, synovium) and in peripheral lymphocytes (Fresco, 1970; Gyorker et al, 1973)	Elevated serum AB to measles, parainfluenza, and mumps viruses in different series (Phillips, 1975); selective decrease in cellular hypersensitivity to measles virus (Utermohlen et al, 1974)	? Special susceptibility of some SLE subjects to paramyxovirus which may have an immunogenetic basis
	Occasional reports of measles virus antigens in lupus leucocytes (Zhdanov, 1975)	Raised prevalence of certain HLA antigens in some SLE series (blacks: A1, B5; whites: B8, B15) (Svejgaard et al, 1975, 1983)	
	Measles virus RNA hybridises with DNA from leucocytes, lymph node and kidney (Zhdanov, 1975)		? Co-operation between paramyxovirus and C-type leukovirus in development of lupus syndromes

Table 14.4 Illustrative evidence relating to involvement of specific microbial agents in inflammatory rheumatic diseases — *continued*

	Nature of evidence relating disease and microbe		
Disease or syndrome; and microbe implicated	'Direct' (evidence relating to microbes or antigens in cells or tissues)	'Indirect' (evidence from genetics, epidemiology, cell biology, or abnormal immune status)	Possible interpretation
Other viruses, bacteria	Unconfirmed early reports of bacterial and viral isolation (Dubois & Arterberry, 1974)	Elevated serum Ab to rubella, reovirus, coronavirus, EB virus in different studies (Phillips, 1976b); antibodies to RNA have greater specificity for viral RNA (Talal et al, 1971)	? Secondarily raised Ab-levels; or SLE involves multiple (viral) infections (Phillips, 1975)
		Confirmation of raised anti-viral AB in SLE (Pincus et al, 1978); raised interferon levels in SLE sera (Strannegard et al, 1982); impaired antiviral Ab production in lymphocyte culture (Nies et al, 1980; Pelton & Denman, 1982)	Persistent or active infection with one or more viruses (? secondary) could offer tenable explanation of increased auto-Ab production in SLE
POLYARTERITIS NODOSA (PAN)			
Hepatitis B (HB) virus	Hepatitis B antigenaemia, or immunofluorescence detection of HBAg/Ab complexes and C′ in vessel walls or electronmicroscopic evidence of HBAg in circulating immune complexes in up to 30% patients with necrotising vasculitis (Sergent et al, 1976)	Minority of subjects with chronic HB antigenaemia develop PAN (Duffy et al, 1976); suggests that PAN might arise from hypersensitivity to a range of viral or non-viral agents (Rich, 1947)	? Role of genetic factors governing immune response to (HBAg) rather than susceptibility to virus infection itself
POLYMYALGIA RHEUMATICA			
Hepatitis B (HB) virus		Increased prevalence of serum antibody to HBAg in small series (Bacon et al, 1975)	? Vasculitis due to local deposition of immune complexes containing viral Ag

Key: SM, synovial membrane; SF, synovial fluid; CFT-Ab, antibody detected by complement fixation; CMI, cell-mediated immunity; DH, delayed hypersensitivity; Ab, antibody (other abbreviations as in Table 14.2)

c. That host genetic factors determine whether mechanism a, mechanism b, or both, are likely to be operating, and that the responsible genes are associated with those of the major histocompatibility complex, which control the specificity and extent of immunological responses.

d. That there is nothing immunologically specific about the aberrant host response to microbial infection which leads to disseminated rheumatic disease and that host susceptibility is viewed simply in terms of disorders of the *inflammatory* process at 'risk' sites of rheumatic inflammation.

In the next two sections we highlight the principal problems which have arisen in considering the association of different classes of microorganisms with rheumatic disease syndromes and we point to how the different pathogenetic hypotheses have been implicated to explain these associations.

ASSOCIATIONS BETWEEN RHEUMATIC DISEASE AND INFECTION BY BACTERIA OR OTHER PROKARYOTES

Recent progress

Since the last edition of this work (Dumonde & Steward, 1978) certain new information in this area has emerged which we wish to emphasise briefly.

First, the range of organisms capable of causing septic arthritis (especially in immunocompromised hosts) has been extended recently to include the fungi *Fusarum* (Jackle et al, 1983) and *Saccharomyces* (Feld et al, 1982), the Gram-negative bacilli *Moraxella* (Vincent et al, 1981), *Pasteurella* (Nitsche et al, 1982), *Arizona hinshawii* (Quismorio et al, 1983) and *Salmonella dublin* (Brodie & Ehresmann, 1983). In this context, two illustrative reports of septic arthritis in rheumatoid patients receiving extensive drug therapy are noteworthy. The first patient (with seropositive rheumatoid and psoriasis) developed septic arthritis due to *Listeria monocytogenes* whilst on long-term methotrexate (Newman et al, 1979); whilst the second patient developed septic arthritis due to *Streptococcus milleri* whilst on gold, prednisone and aspirin (Housten et al, 1980). The increased range of such organisms together with the evident susceptibility of known rheumatoids to such infections emphasises the general problem of attributing aetiological significance to specific microbes isolated from the joints of rheumatoid subjects.

Secondly, there has been much interest in describing cases of reactive arthritis outside Scandinavia and in distinguishing sexually-acquired reactive arthritis syndromes from those apparently triggered by intestinal infection. Illustrative reports are of *Brucella*-induced reactive arthritis in Peru without a raised frequency of HLA-B27 (Alarcon et al, 1981); of the recognition of *Shigella flexneri*-induced Reiter's syndrome in B27-positive American women (Simon et al, 1981); of the occurrence of *Yersinia*-related arthritis in Canadian Indians (Ford et al, 1977) and in the United Kingdom (Sheldon et al, 1982); and of B27-positive *Salmonella*-reactive arthritis in British Columbia (Stein et al, 1980). The increased recognition outside Scandinavia of reactive arthritis syndromes will be expected to throw light on genetic factors other than HLA-B27 as well as upon environmental factors which might affect patient susceptibility. The syndrome of polyarthritis triggered by *Chlamydia trachomatis* has been termed 'sexually acquired reactive arthritis' (SARA) by Keat et al (1978) to emphasise the importance of this route of infection. In this context a noteworthy publication on rheumatic fever (Taranta & Markowitz, 1981) emphasises its prevalence in tropical and subtropical developing countries and implies that reactive arthritis following pharyngeal infection with group A streptococci is in fact widely available for study.

Thirdly, an appreciation of the bacterial antigen load in the gastrointestinal tract (see below) has led to two hypotheses by which such bacterial products could trigger rheumatic disease:

1. Antigenic cross-reactivity between bacteria and HLA-determinants
2. Immunomodulation by bacterial constituents.

On the one hand, considerable research has been generated by reports that *Klebsiella* spp. have antigenic determinants in common with HLA-B27 (Ebringer et al, 1976; Seager et al, 1979); although controversial, these findings have highlighted immunogenetic interests in associations between secondary spondylitic syndromes and Gram-negative bacteria (Kinsella et al, 1983). On the other hand, an appreciation of the potent immunostimulatory and immunsuppressive effects of bacterial products (Friedman et al, 1982) is providing new explanations of how absorption of small quantities of such products might precipitate syndromes of reactive pathology (see Bennett, 1978.)

Although there has been little progress in defining the somewhat elusive state of 'post-infective' arthritis (Fain et al, 1979; Reginato et al, 1979; Goldman, 1981; Manicourt & Orloff, 1981; Brodie & Ehresmann, 1983), investigation of the role of prokaryotic micro-organisms in human arthritis syndromes is now poised for a renewed activity. It is hoped that the following comments on six of these areas will illustrate the wealth of potential research activity in this sphere.

Streptococci and rheumatic fever

Although haemolytic streptococci causing human pharyngitis may belong to Lancefield's groups A, C and G, it seems that only group A organisms 'cause' rheumatic fever. This association, supported by a large body of epidemiological and clinical evidence, is taken as being substantiated by long-term prospective studies which have shown that rheumatic fever does not recur without immunological evidence of intercurrent group A streptococcal infection (Taranta et al, 1964). It is of interest that most streptococcal infections which provoke recurrences of rheumatic fever are viewed as asymptomatic in being detected only by measurement of streptococcal antibody titres (Bisno & Stollerman, 1975); in fact, the repeated reactivation of rheumatic fever without clinical streptococcal disease led to an earlier suggestion that a variety of infectious agents or even physical trauma might also precipitate the syndrome (Taranta, 1966). In view of the known adjuvant or anamnestic effects of a variety of microbial infections upon antibacterial antibody titres, and the complete absence of evidence to implicate the localisation of group A streptococci or their antigens in rheumatic fever lesions, the possibility that other micro-organisms may play a contributory role cannot yet be discarded. In this context it is of interest to recall the New York studies which showed that the frequency of rheumatic fever relapse in patients receiving prophylactic penicillin and sulphonamides was related to the extent of rise in antistreptococcal antibody titres rather than to clinical or microbiological evidence of streptococcal reinfection (Taranta, 1966).

It is still not yet clear whether the rheumatic fever subject is more susceptible to group A streptococcal infection per se, or whether susceptibility lies in unusual features of the immunological response to 'normal' streptococcal infection. Several suggestions have been made: (1) that such subjects show a heightened cellular or humoral responsiveness to group A streptococcal antigens, including an aggressive response of cross-reactive autoimmunity to various cardiac and vascular tissue antigens (Zabriskie, 1976); or (2) that sharing of streptococcal and tissue antigens implies partial immunological tolerance of both and an opportunity for the development of genetically-based immunopathological responses to streptococcal infection (see Zabriskie, 1976). Family studies by Zabriskie and colleagues indicated a tendency to homozygosity and restricted representation of some leucocyte antigen types as a potential basis for histocompatibility-linked 'restricted' immune responses to certain extrinsic antigens (Zabriskie, 1976). If susceptibility to poststreptococcal rheumatic fever were determined by homozygosity for two unrelated recessive genes, then $\frac{1}{4} \times \frac{1}{4}$ (i.e. 6%) of a population would be susceptible, given the appropriate penetrance and stimulus; in fact, the overall attack rate is quoted as about 3% in closed epidemics of group A streptococcal infection. There is certainly no evidence that rheumatic fever subjects have abnormal immune responses to non-streptococcal antigens; but there is a tendency for most individuals to develop increased cell-mediated hypersensitivity to streptococcal antigens with increasing age. However, one of the principal difficulties concerning a simple 'allergic' hypothesis of rheumatic fever is that the latent period is not any shorter in recurrences than in first attacks (Taranta, 1966). Whether this feature can be accommodated by the pathogenetic capabilities of a cell-mediated anti-heart immune response, if it exists, presumably awaits further investigation of streptococcal infections in experimental animal models. At present, the arthritis of rheumatic fever must be viewed as a classic example of a 'reactive' arthritis (Aho et al, 1976), where the infecting microbial species is (presumably) known, but where the infecting organisms or their products have not yet been found at the sites of rheumatic pathology.

With the decline of acute rheumatic fever in developed countries there has been a fall-off in scientific reports which might have been expected to clarify ideas concerning its pathogenesis. Williams (1981) and Dumonde & Richards (1981) have reviewed evidence of abnormalities of white cell function, of the prevalence of circulating immune complexes, of the possible persistence of streptococcal cell wall components, and of limited HLA studies in rheumatic fever and rheumatic carditis. Taranta & Markowitz (1981) point out that it is the developing countries that now provide opportunities to study the disease in depth. We await renewed interest in the genetics and immunopathogenesis of rheumatic fever in geographical areas where it is still an important cause of mortality and morbidity in paediatric and adult medical practice (Taranta & Markowitz, 1981).

Streptococci and rheumatoid arthritis

Consideration of the association of rheumatic fever with antecedent group A streptococcal infection led predictably to the hypothesis that streptococci might also precipitate rheumatoid disease. At one time this was reinforced by the detection of high titres of streptococcal agglutinins in rheumatoid arthritis sera; but this serological reaction was later ascribed to enhancement of bacterial agglutination by circulating antiglobulins. Raised serum ASO titres are occasionally observed in individual rheumatoid subjects; but no evidence has been accumulated that serum titres against streptococcal products are unduly elevated in groups of rheumatoid subjects. Early reports of the isolation of group A streptococci from rheumatoid joints are now regarded as being due to contamination of the specimens in their handling; however, students of rheumatoid arthritis continue to be intrigued by anecdotal clinical information that tonsilitis and pharyngitis may be followed by a polyarthritis which at first appears to be rheumatic fever, but which evolves into classical rheumatoid disease. Svartz and her colleagues assembled evidence that certain group B streptococci could be isolated from the nasopharynx of 80–85% rheumatoid subjects, whereas the same organisms were only present in 15–20% of healthy subjects (Svartz et al, 1969). Serotaxonomy suggested that these group B organisms might be classified as *S. agalactiae*, possibly of bovine origin, present in human intestine and in some samples of milk; a few isolations were claimed from rheumatoid joints; and there was evidence that injection of these isolates into rats would produce a seropositive chronic progressive polyarthritis (Svartz, 1975).

Although there is continued interest in the possible role of persistent streptococcal cell wall components in provoking inflammatory disease in the host (Ginsburg et al, 1977; Cromartie, 1981) there is no real advance in further understanding of the possible role of streptococci in rheumatoid arthritis. Houba and colleagues (1964) found an enhanced rise in serum anti-streptokinase titres following the demonstration of diminished delayed skin reactions of rheumatoid subjects to streptococcal antigens; Braun & Holm (1970) reported raised serum antibody titres to an uncharacterised cellular antigen of group A type 12 streptococci; and there has been disputed evidence that synovial fluids from seronegative and seropositive rheumatoids contain precipitating antibodies for polysaccharide extracts of streptococci. In 1949 the *American Rheumatism Association Primer on Rheumatic Diseases* rejected the belief in 'focal infection' as an aetiological factor in rheumatoid arthritis (see Vaughan, 1966); and this view was supported by the Empire Rheumatism Council's report the following year (Lewis-Faning, 1950). However, it is conceded that controlled prospective studies of focal streptococcal infection in precipitating first attacks of rheumatoid disease are subject to the greatest difficulty. In summary, it seems that the possibility of streptococcal infection playing an aetiological role in the disease has still not yet been eliminated.

Diphtheroids, bacterial L-forms and mycoplasmas in rheumatoid arthritis

The bacteriology of rheumatoid arthritis is traditionally regarded as a 'slippery field' (Clasener, 1972); and the history of attempts to implicate diphtheroids, bacterial L-forms and mycoplasma provides ample illustration of this maxim. Several reviews have been published to which reference is recommended (e.g. Hamerman, 1975; Marmion,

1976); and the following comments are meant to serve the purpose of simplification.

The diphtheroid group, as yet taxonomically obscure, is a large heterogeneous collection of bacteria which is 'held together' by morphological and superficial cultural similarities to *Corynebacterium diphtheriae* and generally considered as harmless commensals. Over many years there have been occasional reports of the isolation of aerobic and anaerobic coryneforms from rheumatoid synovial fluids, membranes or lymph nodes; with much argument as to whether these arose by environmental contamination of specimens (Clasener & Biersteker, 1969). Interest in these organisms might have been lost but for the fact that they are powerful adjuvants in both animals and man; thus they will produce polyarthritis in rats, enhance both humoral and cell-mediated responses and stimulate mononuclear phagocyte ('reticuloendothelial') function. There is no evidence that they are especially arthrotropic, although certain serotypes of *C. acnes* have been implicated in postoperative infections. There seems to be only one report of elevated antibody titres to corynebacterial antigens in both seronegative and seropositive rheumatoids (Duthie et al, 1976); although by the leucocyte migration test, no evidence of cell-mediated immunity to one such corynebacterial isolate was obtained (Maini et al, 1970). In view of the particular taxonomic difficulties it is impossible to say whether rheumatoid subjects are unusually susceptible to infection or immunisation with this group of micro-organisms.

Microbiologists recognise many biochemical differences between L-phase bacteria and mycoplasmas, and emphasise the danger of attempting to identify these microbes by microscopy or morphology alone, whether of fresh specimens or of apparent 'colonies' on solid culture media. By electron microscopy, structures that resemble L-phase bacteria (Pease, 1969) or mycoplasma (Williams, 1968) have been reported in rheumatoid specimens; and Pease (1974) has described the visual identification of a bacterial L-form (*B. licheniformis*). There is much taxonomic uncertainty concerning the classification of bacterial L-forms in relation to their parent organisms, in particular concerning circumstances in which the L-phase might appear in vivo; accordingly it is of academic interest to consider that the failure to find bacteria in rheumatoid lesions is due to their regression to a subcellular or cryptogenic phase. On the other hand, a wide range of natural mycoplasma infection of animals is associated with arthritis; and the experimental production of mycoplasma polyarthritis in mice, rats, swine and chickens (Taylor-Robinson & Taylor, 1976) has focused attention on mycoplasma as possible aetiological agents in rheumatoid disease. Although there is increasing knowledge of the immunopathology of experimental mycoplasma infection, there is no confirmed evidence for the presence of mycoplasma components in rheumatoid synovia or for the prevalence of abnormal humoral or cellular immune status towards mycoplasma antigens in rheumatoid subjects. Much technical and microbiological controversy was directed towards the reported isolation of 'fastidious' mycoplasma from synovial fluid; and leucocyte migration reactivity to mycoplasma antigens (Williams et al, 1970) has been ascribed to their content of adsorbed immunoglobulin (Maini et al, 1975). The taxonomy of mycoplasma colonising man is still uncertain, and the immunosuppressive properties of these micro-organisms might suggest an 'escape clause' for a failure to detect heightened specific immune status towards the organisms themselves.

Despite these reservations there has been continued interest in the study of experimental animal models of mycoplasma infection (Washburn et al, 1982) which might yield clues concerning the immunopathology of mycoplasma infection in man (Taylor-Robinson, 1981). Having accepted the 'arthritogenicity' of most mycoplasmas it is admitted that the reason for mycoplasma localisation and persistence in the joints of experimental animals has never been elucidated satisfactorily. Mycoplasma have the ability to attach to lymphocyte surfaces and induce suppression or stimulation of lymphocyte function (Cole & Cassell, 1979) but it is not yet known whether these organisms can interact with particular HLA determinants on human lymphocytes. There is some evidence that *Mycoplasma pneumoniae* infection in man can induce a state of reactive arthritis (Ponka, 1979); mycoplasma infection is known to be associated with a variety of autoantibodies (Cole & Cassell, 1979) and mycoplasmas in culture can incorporate surface constituents of mammalian lymphocytes (Wise et al, 1978). However, at the present time, it must be conceded that diphtheroids, mycoplasmas or bacterial L-forms have not yet yielded the 'missing' exogeneous antigens in rheumatoid disease.

Genitourinary infection and inflammatory polyarthritis

It is salutary to recall that in 1818 Brodie expressed the view that the syndrome of arthritis, conjunctivitis and urethritis was caused by a sexually transmitted infectious agent; and subsequent clinical and microbiological problems associated with attempts to link seronegative arthritis syndromes with genitourinary infection by gonococci, mycoplasmas, viruses or chalmydia are well illustrated by several reviews (Ford, 1966; Csonka, 1972; Catterall, 1976). From the clinical point of view, the onset of polyarthritis within a few weeks of an episode of cystitis, prostatitis or urethritis is taken as suggestive evidence of Reiter's syndrome; and in a patient with typical ankylosing spondylitis, the development of peripheral arthritis or the exacerbation of spondylitic symptoms in association with urethritis or prostatitis suggests a role of genitourinary infection as a precipitating agent. Whereas the prevalence of HLA-B27 in these syndromes (Brewerton, 1979) should assist their recognition, pathogenetic considerations are made more complicated, if not more interesting, by the many vascular and other features comprising these overlapping disorders (Good, 1974) and by the heterogeneity of clinical patterns associated with the characteristic tendency to recurrence of disease (Ford, 1966). No satisfactory aetiological hypothesis for Reiter's syndrome, other than an infective one, has been presented; but it is assumed that any such microbiological relationships would be indirect and analogous to the relationship of streptococci to rheumatic fever. The clinical manifestations of Reiter's syndrome and to some extent, seronegative 'reactive' spondarthritis, are simulated by those of adjuvant arthritis in rats (Pearson, 1966). The initial claim of Reiter that a spirochaete was responsible has not been confirmed; in fact, it has been impossible to implicate any specific genitourinary bacterial infection, including gonococci, in the disease. Likewise, extensive and sophisticated virological studies have been uniformly negative; and sera from such patients have not shown significantly raised antibody levels to any known virus. Current microbiological attention is focused upon the apparent increase in the incidence of non-specific urethritis, upon the estimate that up to 2% of such patients develop Reiter's syndrome, and upon considerable attempts to implicate chlamydia and mycoplasma in these situations.

It is well established that chlamydia cause arthritis in sheep and cattle as part of naturally occurring systemic infectious diseases with recovery of the agents from blood, joints, conjunctivae and semen. In addition to the occasional occurrence of arthritis complicating human psittacosis and lymphogranuloma venereum, rheumatological interest in the trachoma-inclusion conjunctivitis (TRIC) agents arose from reports of typical TRIC agent inclusions in urethral epithelium of men with Reiter's syndrome and non-gonococcal urethritis. In California between 1964 and 1968, Schachter isolated chlamydia from synovia, urethra or conjunctiva in 10–15% of 89 patients with Reiter's syndrome together with negative results in 12 patients with ankylosing spondylitis (Schachter, 1976); subsequently in Paris, Amor and colleagues claimed an isolation rate of 66% exclusively in Reiter's syndrome, with evidence of urethral epithelial cell inclusions in 73% of Reiter's and 14% of ankylosing spondylitis patients (Delbarre & Amor, 1976). Both groups reported the ability of their chlamydial isolates to cause chronic arthritis on intra-articular injection in monkeys; and in the rabbit, chlamydial infection in the joint has been followed by recovery of organisms from ocular and visceral sites. However, conflicting results were obtained from other laboratories; reports of elevated serum antibodies to chlamydia in Reiter's syndrome ranged from 30–80%; and the Paris group reported positive lymphocyte transformation tests to chlamydial antigen in 76% of Reiter's and 40% of ankylosing spondylitis patients in whom the clinical picture was accompanied by peripheral arthropathy (Amor et al, 1972).

The term 'sexually acquired reactive arthritis' (SARA) has been introduced by Keat et al (1978) to emphasise the clinical similarity between polyarthritis complicating non-gonococcal urethritis

(NGU) and enterocolitic arthritis, whilst clearly separating the circumstances under which these reactive arthritides are triggered. The nosological value of the term SARA lies in the simplicity of principal criteria for its recognition (sterile synovitis following sexually acquired NGU) without the restrictions imposed by a need for the patients to develop a complete Reiter's triad; in fact many such patients have mild, self-limiting joint involvement without sacroiliitis or spondylitis (Keat et al, 1979). The prevalence of *Chlamydia trachomatis* in urethral exudates, or of raised IgM antibody to the organism was no different than in NGU patients (40–50%) who did not develop the SARA syndrome; however, titres of IgG anti-chlamydial antibody were much higher in SARA than in uncomplicated NGU or in other inflammatory rheumatic diseases (Keat et al, 1980). By analogy with syphilitic infection this feature suggests a longer history of sexual transmission than the apparent incubation period of SARA; and there seems to be continued interest in whether chlamydial and other sexually acquired infections trigger reactive arthritis syndromes (Vilppula et al, 1981; Kousa, 1982). At present we await clarification of whether HLA-B27 predisposes to SARA or to the full Reiter's triad by virtue of a special and selective pattern of immune response to chlamydia (Ford et al, 1982); and it seems likely that advances in the immunobiology of *Chlamydia* will also be required.

Intestinal bacteria and reactive arthritis syndromes

In the context of this chapter, the gastrointestinal tract must be regarded as an important source of micro-organisms and their products which could have the potential of precipitating onset or relapse of inflammatory rheumatic disease in appropriately susceptible subjects. The multiplicity of gastrointestinal micro-organisms that could be investigated is daunting; and perhaps it is hardly surprising that associations between inflammatory rheumatic disease and gastrointestinal infection have emerged from the 'dramatic' enteritic syndromes rather than from the recognition of more subtle changes in bowel flora. It is considered that Reiter's (1916) notable case was a postdysenteric arthritis; and among the intestinal pathogens, *Salmonella*, *Shigella* and *Yersinia* are currently regarded as including species of micro-organisms which can precipitate inflammatory rheumatic disease, though the pathogenetic mechanisms are completely unknown. Consideration of these syndromes gave rise to the term 'reactive arthritis', where the identity of the infection is generally known but in which the causative microbe cannot be isolated from synoval fluid (Aho et al, 1975, 1976). The classical clinical picture of these reactive syndromes, particularly in Scandinavia, comprises a seronegative sterile polyarthritis of limited duration and distribution which may include sacroiliitis, and which is unresponsive to antibiotics; however, the arthritis has a tendency to recur following an apparent variety of precipitating factors and some patients may eventually develop a chronic spondarthritis syndrome. Current evidence implicates the prevalence of HLA-B27 in 90% of subjects with postenteritic reactive arthritis though it is admitted that there may be other associations where the symptomatology is so mild as to escape clinical notice (Aho et al, 1975).

Yersinosis is considered of endemic prevalence in Finland, Sweden and possibly Denmark. The designations *Yersinia enterocolitica* and *Yersinia pseudotuberculosis* have been produced only in the last decade to delineate these Gram-negative bacteria, which also contain antigens giving serological cross-reactions with a variety of other micro-organisms. Elevated serum antibody titres to *Y. enterocolitica* serotype 3 are regarded as indicative of past or present infection, though the effect of anamnestic responses in not yet clear. In Finland, arthritis is one of the commonest symptoms of yersinosis, occurring in nearly 50% in one series, where it was considered that some patients previously diagnosed as having rheumatic fever actually may have had yersinosis (Leino & Kalliomaki, 1974). In Denmark, Larsen's serological analysis of 13 000 hospital patients indicated that some 3% had recent yersinia infection; that yersinia antibodies were elevated in 50–90% of cases of 'acute arthritis' and in 20% of chronic inflammatory rheumatic disease (Larsen, 1972). Although the syndrome of reactive arthritis following *Yersinia enterocolitica* infection was first defined in Scandinavia, it is premature to conclude that the organism is an important cause of chronic inflammatory rheumatic disease. A preliminary report from the United Kingdom suggested an impaired lymphocyte transformation response to yersinia antigen in HLA-B27-positive patients with ankylosing spondylitis as compared to those who lacked the B27 marker (Nikbin et al, 1975). There is no recent evidence which suggests that immunity to gastrointestinal organisms is defective in reactive arthritis syndromes.

In conclusion it is tempting to consider that an immune-response gene, linked to HLA-B27 (Brewerton, 1979), controls host reactions to a class of antigens represented on a variety of bacteria including those found in the gastrointestinal tract. However, much remains to be learnt about the immunotaxonomic relationships of organisms such as *Salmonella*, *Shigella* and *Yersinia*, particularly concerning their relative immunogenicity in man; and at present, there are no animal models of reactive arthritis syndromes following defined infections with these micro-organisms.

Ankylosing spondylitis and *Klebsiella* infection

In 1973 ankylosing spondylitis (AS) emerged from the 'backwash of scientific disinterest' (Kinsella et al, 1983) when its association with HLA-B27 was simultaneously described by two groups of investigators (Brewerton et al, 1973; Schlosstein et al, 1973). That B27-positive individuals have a 100-fold relative risk of developing AS, reinforced the view that inflammatory rheumatic diseases arise through genetically-based immunopathological responses to infection. 'Male dominance' in both AS and B27-positive Reiter's disease led to the suggestion that the local immunopathology of AS might arise from dissemination of microbial antigen to the spine via Batson's veins (Ziff, 1979). However, there was no explanation of why the B-locus (thought to be associated with lymphocyte effector mechanisms) rather than the D-locus (associated with immune induction) should be incriminated in susceptibility to AS; nor was there any evidence as to what kind of micro-organism could be implicated.

During the last seven years two different groups of investigators have claimed that *Klebsiella pneumoniae* could act as the disease trigger. In England the Ebringers reasoned that if there were antigenic similarities between the surfaces of B27-positive lymphocytes and certain enterobacteria, a host might give a defective antibacterial immune response resulting in increased bacterial carriage and reactive immunopathology. They found that sera from rabbits immunised with B27-positive lymphocytes contained agglutinating antibodies for *Yersinia enterocolitica* and *Klebsiella pneumoniae* (Ebringer et al, 1976) and that faecal carriage of klebsiella (in particular) was higher in AS patients with active disease, and those entering relapse, than in non-spondylitic controls, or in quiescent AS patients (Ebringer et al, 1978). The same group further reported that antigenic cross-reactivity between *Klebsiella pneumoniae* antigens and B27-positive lymphocytes was a general phenomenon displayed by rabbit antisera (Welsh et al, 1980) and by human tissue-typing sera (Avakian et al, 1980).

In Australia this conclusion was modified by a claim that selected antisera to certain klebsiella serotypes are cytotoxic preferentially for B27-positive lymphocytes of AS patients only (rather than controls) and that peripheral blood lymphocyte transformation to corresponding klebsiella serotypes is selectively diminished in AS (Seager et al, 1979; Edmonds et al, 1981). Accordingly the 'defective' immune response of AS patients to klebsiella was ascribed to interference by cross-reactive antibody with the effector phase of lymphocyte function rather than to an afferent defect in immune induction ascribable to 'cross-tolerance' or molecular mimicry (Marmion, 1978). The Australian group have reported three addition recent findings:

a. That the cross-reactive (heterogenetic) antigen is present on B cells, T cells, platelets and fibroblasts of B27-positive AS subjects as well as on Epstein–Barr virus-induced lymphoblastoid cell lines and skin fibroblasts cultured for up to 20 generations (Alexander et al, 1981)
b. That involved strains of klebsiella shed in culture a membrane glycoprotein which renders normal B27-positive lymphocytes of non-AS subjects temporarily susceptible to lysis by corresponding anti-klebsiella serum (Geczy et al, 1983)
c. That such klebsiella contained a plasmid which

could transfer to an *E. Coli* strain the ability to generate this lymphocyte-modifying factor (Cameron et al, 1983).

The authors suggest that immunomodulatory effects of bacterial products may include alterations of HLA-associated gene products which may then predispose to immunopathological responses to infection (Geczy et al, 1983); and they speculate that klebsiella plasmids might be able to induce permanent relevant modification of HLA-B27-positive lymphocytes thus increasing a host's tendency to develop ankylosing spondylitis (Cameron et al, 1983).

Almost every aspect of the 'klebsiella' connection has been disputed (Kinsella et al, 1983). Thus Archer (1981) and Beaulieu et al (1983) could not confirm the cytotoxicity of anti-klebsiella sera for B27-positive normal or AS lymphocytes; Warren & Brewerton (1980) could not confirm the association of disease activity with selectively increased faecal carriage of klebsiella; and Enlow et al (1982) failed to confirm the deficient lymphocyte reactivity to klebsiella. However, there have been no other explanations as to how the inflammatory disease we know as ankylosing spondylitis might be triggered or maintained by infective agents; and the application of gene mapping techniques to recognition structures of lymphocytes, to plasmids of Gram-negative bacteria and to their possible interactions might well provide unexpected insight into this field.

Conclusions concerning prokaryotic infection

At first sight there seems to be an atmosphere of despair pervading theories of the pathogenesis of prokaryotic arthritides. However it is now clear that the joint can support a wide variety of intra-articular infections and that a wide variety of microbial infections can induce syndromes of sterile polyarthritis ranging from transient, self-limiting joint involvement to severe clinical states of chronic, relapsing arthritis with mucosal inflammation distant from the primary infection. In all these situations, whether infective, post-infective or reactive (see Tables 14.5, 14.6) the role of local specific immunity (i.e. in the joint or at mucosal surfaces) awaits systematic investigation; and it is tempting to speculate that a pathophysiology of the mucosal-associated lymphoid system is involved in the pathogenesis of reactive arthritides. There is no real evidence of a prior genetic predisposition or systemic immune-deficiency of a specific nature to the primary infections themselves (whether in joint or mucosa) and it seems that a given bacterium can induce infective, post-infective or reactive arthritides in different individuals or even in the same individual. For these reasons Koch's postulates appear to be as gratuitous as does the search for experimental animal models (e.g. in the rabbit) of reactive arthritis syndromes. With the currently disputed exception of ankylosing spondylitis, the quest for associations between *specific* prokaryotic species and *idiopathic* inflammatory rheumatic disease seems as elusive as it did in the mid-1970s (Dumonde, 1976; Dumonde & Steward, 1978): one wonders whether it is in fact the 'right' approach.

A second feature apparently limiting progress may be inherent in the field of microbial taxonomy itself, where the laboratory rabbit or the bacteriophage are frequently asked to detect relevant differences between related organisms of different pathogenicity for man. On this basis it is not surprising that different klebsiella strains implicated in cross-reactions with HLA-B27 associated determinants do not share capsular serotypes or phage types with one another (Geczy et al, 1981). In general terms it would seem more appropriate to use reagents derived from components of the immune response of the 'naturally susceptible' or 'relevant' host species (i.e. man) in classifying differences between the pathogenetic potential of apparently related micro-organisms. The field of microbial immunotaxonomy is further complicated by the ability of microbes to transfer genetic information to one another: thus plasmid transfer from klebsiella to *E. Coli* also 'transfers' the ability to code for the B27-modifying agent (Cameron et al, 1983). One might ask, 'When is a klebsiella not a klebsiella?' — the answer being, 'When it's an *E. Coli*'. If such scenarios add anything to the understanding of infection and arthritis syndromes they point to the need to accommodate advances in bacterial genetics (Williamson, 1980–1982) alongside advances in human genetic methodology (Weatherall, 1982).

We close this section by recalling briefly the

thesis that infectious agents such as bacteria or mycoplasma might produce 'arthritogenic toxins' (Bennett, 1978). As yet there is no evidence that bacterial products such as exotoxins or endotoxins are selectively conveyed from a site of localised mucosal infection to joints and exert directly deleterious effects upon the local microvasculature or upon leucocyte–endothelial interactions implicated in the mechanics of inflammation. There is however growing evidence that bacterial and other prokaryotic products exert modulatory effects upon the immune system over and above their specific effects as antigens or immunogens or their ability to exert polyclonal B cell activation (Yamamura et al, 1982). Current activity in this aspect of immunopharmacology arises from the hope that it will yield therapeutic strategies in infectious, parasitic and neoplastic disease; however it cannot be long before its implications for reactive arthritis and the idiopathic inflammatory rheumatic diseases receive vigorous consideration (Friedman et al, 1982). We offer the optimistic prediction that interdisciplinary thinking inherent in research into bacterial-induced reactive arthritis syndromes will yield new incisive approaches to inflammatory rheumatic diseases in general.

VIRUSES IN THE AETIOLOGY OF INFLAMMATORY RHEUMATIC DISEASE

General considerations

It is considered impossible to define the term 'virus' succinctly, in view of the heterogeneity of their biological characteristics. Unlike prokaryotes, viruses contain no functional ribosomes or other cellular organelles; some viruses can be generated intracellularly from a single molecule of nucleic acid; and in certain viruses, all the genetic information is encoded in RNA, a situation unique in biology. On the one hand, the simplest 'viruses' may be transmitted between hosts and cells as naked molecules of nucleic acid, sometimes associated with host cell components. On the other hand, the large animal viruses can be relatively complex, consisting of DNA or RNA genomes enclosed within a protective coat incorporating carbohydrate or lipid of cellular origin. The description and nomenclature of viruses that cause classical infective disease in man and his domestic animals is relatively well advanced in comparison with those recoverable from invertebrates, plants, bacteria, fungi, algae, mycoplasmas and protozoa (Fenner et al, 1974). Some invertebrate and plant viruses show taxonomic similarities to those primarily infecting vertebrates, many of which are capable of multiplication in arthropods or other insects. The identification of natural hosts, reservoirs of infection and modes of transmission of many viruses presents problems of the greatest difficulty; and microbiologists value a viral classification based upon chemistry, morphology and strategy of multiplication (Fenner, 1976). In considering viruses as aetiological agents in human inflammatory rheumatic disease it must be appreciated that viruses may permanently alter host cell function without there being chemical, morphological or simple cultural evidence of viral persistence.

A viral aetiology for rheumatoid arthritis and related diseases gleans some support from the knowledge that syndromes of self-limiting polyarthritis, skin rashes, lymphadenopathy and fever accompany infections by a range of known viruses. Mosquitoes, sandflies and ticks transmit arboviruses to man from various animal reservoirs and can induce epidemics of polyarthritis which can involve the majority of a local population (Sauter & Utsinger, 1978), whilst arthritis is also associated with infection by rubella, hepatitis B, adenovirus, mumps and the pox viruses. The clinical features of these syndromes suggest that they are examples of infective (class 1) and post-infective (class 2) arthritides (Tables 14.5, 14.6) and there is evidence that both anti-viral immune complexes (Sauter & Utsinger, 1978) and specific cell-mediated immunity (Clarris et al, 1975; Fraser et al, 1981) contribute to the pathogenesis of joint involvement. The possibility that reactive arthritis syndromes may also occur is suggested by the association of an epidemic of Ross River polyarthritis with HLA-DR7 (Fraser et al, 1980). More detailed study of the pathogenesis of specific viral arthritides can be expected to throw considerable light upon the general role of virus infection in idiopathic inflammatory rheumatic disease (Hyer & Gottleib, 1978).

This optimistic note should temper the cumulative disappointment associated with years of research into the viral aetiology of diseases such as rheumatoid arthritis in which direct evidence of viral involvement has not been forthcoming (Christian et al, 1971). The current decade is witnessing great advances in the molecular and cell biology of viruses, including their ability to act as vectors for the insertion of other microbial genes into eukaryotic cells (Rigby, 1982). Current studies of viral oncogenesis, of slow virus infections and of experimental viral immunopathology are also providing concepts and techniques for application to investigative rheumatology. Over the years there have been many reviews which document the evolution of thought concerning viral involvement in rheumatic disease (Nardo & Norton, 1971; Hamerman, 1975; Kalliomaki & Halonen, 1975; Marmion, 1976; 1978; Phillips, 1975, 1976a, b; Denman, 1978, 1981). The following six topics are selected to illustrate the major approaches to this potentially unlimited field of enquiry.

Rubella virus and rheumatoid disease

Among the viral candidates considered as potential causes of rheumatoid arthritis, rubella virus has aroused recurrent interest. The arthritis associated with adult rubella can be regarded as a 'minority' complication (10–30% incidence) of a mild infection whose manifestations (e.g. rash) are easily missed, affecting young women more than men, occurring also in children, and frequently presenting as a symmetrical migratory polyarthritis whose appearance may be strikingly similar to acute rheumatoid disease. Rubella arthritis is often diagnosed retrospectively 'because of the paradox of apparent classic rheumatoid disease which completely disappears within days of its onset' (Kantor & Tanner, 1962). Vaccine strains of rubella virus also cause transient arthritis, particularly in the adult (female); the incidence of arthritis seems to depend on the strain of attenuated virus; and as with rubella arthritis itself, the virus has been recovered from synovial effusions (Lerman et al, 1971; Sauter & Utsinger, 1978). To this extent, rubella virus is regarded as 'arthrotropic', though the cellular basis of arthrotropism itself is shrouded in mystery. Further rheumatological interest in rubella virus derives from elevated serum antibody titres to the virus in juvenile chronic polyarthritis (Ogra & Hurd, 1972), occasional reports of raised serum antiglobulin in clinical rubella (Kacaki et al, 1970), and the occurrence of an acute phase protein ('rho') in rheumatoid sera which also occurs during clinical rubella (and pregnancy), but which can be produced by rubella virus-infected fibroblasts (Capell et al, 1974). Also, the rubella virus is classified within the *Togaviridiae* family of vertebrate arboviruses (Fenner, 1976) which is of interest in view of the occurrence of self-limiting polyarthritis as a manifestation of infection by this group (Bland & Phillips, 1972).

Despite these considerations, little is known of the pathology and immunopathology of joint involvement in rubella or in rubella-vaccination arthritis, particularly with respect to compartmentation of the virus. Congenitally-infected rabbits can harbour virus in articular chondrocytes; and both acute or chronic arthritis can be produced by intra-articular injection of rubella virus in the rabbit (Hamerman, 1975). A recent report describes Clq-binding immune complexes in the sera of three rubella vaccinated subjects with joint symptoms, and normal levels of Clq binding in all but one of seven symptomless vaccinated subjects (Vergani et al, 1980). It is not known whether rubella virus can enter the joint simply by infecting or traversing microvascular endothelium and then stimulate the release of inflammatory mediators by a direct action on certain cell types within the synovium. It is of course possible that such arthropathies arise by synovial deposition of systemically formed immune complexes or by the combination of virus with locally synthesised antibody; but it is not yet clear whether the virus selectively localises in any particular human synovial cell type. The possibility that rubella virus may be carried into the joint by recirculatory lymphocytes arises from the work of Chantler et al (1982) who reported its isolation from peripheral blood lymphocytes of six women with persistent rubella arthritis. In this study the virus was not isolated from the lymphocytes of a limited number of non-arthritic patients who had circulating anti-rubella antibodies or who had congenital rubella infection; and an essential step in virus isolation was the co-culturing of mitogen-stimulated lymphocytes with subconfluent monolayers of RK 13 cells (Chantler et al, 1982). To date, elucidation of the pathogenetic mechanisms of rubella arthritis still remains one of conjecture because of the lack of comprehensive immunopathological studies in this field. It is not known whether rubella virus can cause a reactive arthritis analagous to the bacterially-induced syndromes; and recurrent arthropathy following rubella vaccination does not seem to be associated with any particular HLA type (Griffiths et al, 1977). However, in the congenital rubella syndrome the virus displays its potential for establishing persistent infection and abnormalities of lymphocyte function (Dent, 1971), and the role of virus–lymphocyte interactions (Denman, 1979) in the various rubella syndromes is worthy of continued investigation.

Optimism concerning a possible implication of this virus in the aetiology of RA came from the demonstration of persistent arthropathy, in a minority of naturally-infected and rubella-vaccinated patients (Martenis et al, 1968; Spruance et al, 1977; Tingle et al, 1978) and the progression of one such patient to a chronic arthritis (Martenis et al, 1968). Serological studies have generally failed to demonstrate an increase in the frequency or titre of anti-rubella antibodies in sera and synovial fluid from rheumatoid patients when compared with controls (Smiley et al, 1969; Kacaki et al, 1970; Christian & Phillips, 1973; Wilkes et al, 1973; Deinard et al, 1974; Stanford, 1974). One report of high titres of rubella antibody in the sera of certain juvenile rheumatoid patients (Ogra et al, 1975) was not later confirmed (Schnitzer et al, 1977). Several attempts have been made to implicate rubella virus infection in synovial fibroblasts from rheumatoid subjects: initial reports (Ford & Oh, 1965; Smith & Hamerman, 1969; Grayzel & Beck, 1970) that cultured rheumatoid synovial fibroblasts were resistant to rubella virus infection (inferring intrinsic viral interference) were not confirmed by several other laboratories (Hamerman, 1975). Subsequently it was found that treatment of RA synovial fibroblasts with hyaluronidase before viral inoculation rendered them as susceptible to rubella virus infection as fibroblasts from non-RA synovia (Marmion, 1976). This resistance to rubella infection by RA fibroblasts appears to result from their excessive production of hyaluronate which acts as a simple barrier to penetration of rubella and other viruses (e.g. Newcastle disease and vesicular stomatitis viruses) (Clarris et al, 1974; Patterson et al, 1975). Interest in the possible expression of rubella virus antigens by rheumatoid synovial 'fibroblasts' emerged from the report (Patterson et al, 1973) that seven of nine such rheumatoid fibroblast lines were lysed by a monkey antirubella serum and complement in a similar fashion to cells from an infant with congenital rubella syndrome (Marmion, 1976). The inference that rubella-related antigens were present on rheumatoid fibroblasts was not supported by a study in which antigen identification was by immunofluorescence and radioimmunoassay (Hart & Marmion, 1977). Earlier attempts to isolate rubella virus from the synovial fluid of patients with polyarthritis, who had no evidence of rubella infection, failed (Wilkes et al, 1973) until Ford et al (1982) reported the isolation of the virus from one patient with RA and another with unexplained persistent knee arthritis. Grahame et al (1981) reported its isolation from five patients with seronegative arthritis and a sixth patient was included in a more detailed recent presentation (Grahame et al, 1983). In this study clinical features of typical rubella infection were absent in all six patients though most of them had high serum rubella haemagglutination inhibition titres. Rubella virus was implicated by resistance of cell cultures (when treated with patients' synovial fluid) to ECHO 11 virus, by immunofluorescent staining of synovial fluid leucocytes with anti-rubella antiserum, and by detection of the viral antigen in culture fluids using complement fixation tests. Furthermore, electron microscopy identified rubella-like inclusions in one of four synovial membrane biopsies examined. More recently, however, this group has been unable to confirm or extend these observations (C A Mims, personal communication, 1983): re-analysis of the clinical material has shown the immunofluorescence tests to be negative whilst inhibition of ECHO 11 multiplication by the synovial fluids is now thought to have been due to their content of interferon.

In summary there would seem to be insufficient evidence to implicate rubella virus as 'the' infective agent which 'causes' rheumatoid arthritis. Advocates of rubella virus involvement receive little support from clinical or cell biological studies; and it is equally plausible that cultural differences between RA and non-RA 'fibroblasts' were due to differences in exposure to autopharmacological mediators in vivo rather than to the possibility of latent rubella virus 'genetic' material in the cells, for rubella is a simple RNA virus with no mechanism of its own for incorporating itself into the host genome. The selection of rubella virus for continued inclusion in this chapter illustrates the problems inherent in clarifying the concept of viral arthrotropism (if indeed it exists as a cellular phenomenon) and of the remarkable lack of immunopathological information concerning an arthritis syndrome which can be ascribed to a known virus. On a more optimistic note, arthritis induced by this virus would seem to offer an excellent opportunity for studying mechanisms of viral arthropathy and how they may relate to rheumatoid and other arthritides in which viral aetiology is being considered. There will undoubtedly be continued interest in the possible role of subclinical rubella infection in precipitating the development of chronic rheumatoid disease in certain subjects without leaving behind any microbiological or even immunological evidence which would implicate its involvement (Marmion, 1978).

Paramyxoviruses and inflammatory rheumatic disease

Until designation of the family *Paramyxoviridae* (Fenner, 1976), viruses of three genera (*Paramyxovirus; Morbillivirus; Pneumovirus*) were grouped together under the term *Paramyxovirus*. This term is used (in the vernacular) to encompass those viruses whose genome consists of linear single-stranded RNA within a simple tubular nucleocapsid; whose pleomorphic lipoprotein envelope (100–300 nm diameter) carries specific haemagglutinin and sometimes a neuraminidase; and whose virion contains a conventional transcriptase. Such viruses (e.g. mumps, Newcastle disease, parainfluenza, measles/distemper) multiply in the cytoplasm and mature by budding from cytoplasmic or intracytoplasmic membrances; in addition to having a common morphology, they share the property of fusing cells because they have a biologically active envelope consisting of the converted membrane of the cell in which the virus multiplies. Paramyxovirus nucleocapsids may accumulate in huge cytoplasmic inclusions, clearly demonstrable by electron microscopy; and budding of virions from the plasma membrane is easily recognised in both spherical and filamentous forms. By immunofluorescence, large aggregations of viral protein are seen to accumulate in the cytoplasm of infected cells; and with some paramyxoviruses (notably the measles subgroup), nuclear inclusions are detectable by both electron microscopy and immunofluorescence (Fenner et al, 1974). In the case of measles virus, the normally long duration of immunity, even in the absence of reinfection for sixty or more years, has led to the speculation that these viruses may persist in a latent form and reappear perhaps due to a failure of cell-mediated immunity. Such a reappearance (e.g. in brain macrophages) is thought to be responsible for subacute sclerosing panencephalitis; and there has been much speculation as to the involvement of paramyxoviruses in multiple sclerosis (Norrby et al, 1974). Recent advances in viral immunopathology have clarified the paradoxical situation of developing an allergic response without protective immunity and of how quantitative or qualitative abnormalities in cellular and humoral responses may permit the establishment of chronic immune complex disease without viral elimination (Soothill & Steward, 1971; Notkins, 1975). Experimental studies suggest that paramyxoviruses can infect vascular endothelial cells, macrophages, lymphocytes and fibroblasts; hence their possible role in inflammatory connective tissue disease seems worthy of serious consideration.

Against this background it is of particular interest to view the numerous reports of paramyxovirus-like tubuloreticular structures in vascular endothelial cells, especially in renal tissue, skin and synovium, and in circulating lymphocytes, of patients with systemic or discoid lupus erythematosus (Dubois, 1974; Kalliomaki & Halonen, 1975). Secondly, in rheumatoid arthritis there are less frequent reports of similar intracytoplasmic or intranuclear inclusions in lymphocytes, macrophages and perivascular connective tissue cells (Kalliomaki & Halonen, 1975), with the most striking resemblance to membrane-associated paramyxoviruses being provided by Schumacher's (1975) electron micrographs of synovial vascular endothelial cells in early rheumatoid disease. Thirdly, in polymyositis and dermatomyositis there are confirmed reports of paramyxovirus-like nuclear and cytoplasmic inclusions in skeletal muscle (Chou, 1970) and vascular endothelial cells (Norton et al, 1970) with emphasis on involvement of the microvasculature. Definite identification of particles as viruses by electron microscopy of thin sections is recognised as being difficult. Sources of possible confusion include secretion granules, pinocytic vesicles, hyperplastic Golgi apparatus or endoplasmic reticulum; and most often, non-viral material resembles C-type viral particles (see below). Unfortunately, there is no immunological or microbiological confirmation of the presence of paramyxovirus (e.g. measles) antigens within rheumatic lesions (Phillips, 1975); and attempts to 'transmit' rheumatic diseases to mice (Warren et al, 1969) or to 'transfer' abnormal human synovial cell behaviour in culture to rabbit synovia (Hamerman, 1975) have not stood up to the test of confirmation. Increased serum levels of viral antibodies have been frequently reported in systemic lupus, though less frequently in rheumatoid arthritis; and although it has been suggested that this reflects 'hyper-reactivity' of the immune system (an unclarified concept: Phillips, 1975), the most constant finding has been increased serum antibody levels to measles virus with appearance of similarly raised titres in synovial fluid (Kalliomaki et al, 1975).

In multiple sclerosis and systemic lupus the possibility of a state of immune deviation towards measles virus antigen was suggested by a selectively suppressed inhibition of antiviral leucocyte migration in these diseases (Utermohlen et al, 1974); but these observations remain unconfirmed (Dumonde, 1978b) and were criticised on technical grounds (Nordal et al, 1975). A collaborative inter-Scandinavian study showed local production, in the central nervous system, of antibodies to paramyxoviruses in up to 60% of patients with multiple sclerosis (Norrby et al, 1974), which like RA, is accompanied by oligoclonal IgG production within the affected tissue (CSF; synovial fluid) and some linkage to HLA (Svejgaard et al, 1983). It is still not clear whether oligoclonal bands in rheumatoid synovial fluid have any consistent reactivity with paramyxoviruses of the type implicated in multiple sclerosis.

In summary, much circumstantial evidence in the 1970s implicated paramyxoviruses in inflammatory rheumatic syndromes; but, as with C-type retroviruses (see below) very little emerged in support of these agents (Marmion, 1978). Perhaps the last reported exhaustive virological study is that of Norval & Smith (1979) who extracted DNA and RNA from synovial membranes and cultured synovial fibroblasts and peripheral blood lymphocytes in order to determine whether these extracts would hybridise with a range of viral nucleic acids including measles virus RNA. The results were uniformly negative (Norval & Smith, 1979) and leave little room for further speculation other than to recall the hypothesis of Zhdanov (1975) who suggested that interaction between C-type retrovirus and other RNA viruses might result in genomic integration of the latter (see below).

Hepatitis B virus and chronic rheumatic disease

Although there are reports which show no significant prevalence of hepatitis B (HB) antigenaemia in rheumatoid disease (Burrell et al, 1972; Burssens et al, 1972), the occurrence of a serum-sickness-like syndrome during the prodromal phase of HB infection, with varying degrees of polyathralgia, diffuse vasculitis and glomerulonephritis (Gocke, 1975) has been viewed as a 'model' for a possible viral pathogenesis of chronic rheumatic disease (Phillips, 1976a). Like many other infectious agents, HB virus can give rise to the appearance of serum antiglobulins; and there is clear evidence that HB antigen can enter the joint space (Alpert et al, 1971), supporting an earlier concept (Marner, 1952) that there are 'arthritogenic' strains of HB virus. Furthermore, HB antigen-excess immune complexes have been demonstrated in serum by electron microscopy (Almeida & Waterson, 1969) and at various extrahepatic sites by immunofluorescence (Krawczynski et al, 1974). In the arthritides accompanying both acute and chronic hepatitis Schumacher & Gall (1974) showed by immunofluorescence and electron microscopy evidence for HB antigen in the synovia of two patients: particles of size 200–250 A° and 400–600 A° were seen in vascular endothelial cells and in both superficial and deep synovial cells. Several observers have noted depressed serum complement levels during the active stage of HB-arthritis (Sauter & Utsinger, 1978); however, like other viral arthritides the rheumatic symptoms are typically of short duration, resolving with the appearance of clinical hepatitis and free HB antibody in the serum, with the disappearance of serum HB antigen, and with the normalisation of serum complement. At the present time it is widely held that acute polyarthritis or transient diffuse vasculitis associated with acute HB infection is due simply to the deposition of circulating immune complexes; and that assembly of immune complexes locally may be of contributory importance (London, 1977).

The critical question is not whether HB antigen or immune complexes can be demonstrated in various parts of the microvasculature during acute hepatitis, but whether the virus does give rise to chronic rheumatic disease. Some reports have indicated that as many as 30% of patients with necrotising vasculitis may have HB_s-antigenaemia without a clinical history of liver disease (Gocke et al, 1970). All combinations of vasculitis and liver disease have been reported, including vasculitis as the initial clinical illness, vasculitis superimposed upon chronic active hepatitis, and vasculitis and acute hepatitis occurring at approximately the same time. The occurrence of HB_s antigen-positivity in one group of patients with vasculitis of more than a few weeks duration (e.g. 3–12 months: Sergent et al, 1976), and in another group, of persistent peripheral polyarthritis of up to several years duration (Duffy et al, 1976), was claimed as evidence that a known viral infection could cause chronic 'rheumatic' disease. In retrospect it is clear that the continued symptomatology of some of these patients differed from that of classical rheumatoid arthritis or systemic lupus. However, two such patients had been diagnosed earlier as rheumatoid arthritis; and only the presence of liver disease, which is often subclinical, separates HB_s antigen-positive patients with diffuse vasculitis from those who lack the antigen. Where HLA studies have been done, no special segregation has been observed. The finding of HB antibody in the serum of nine of a group of 12 patients with polymyalgia rheumatica (Bacon et al, 1975), added additional weight to these reports in view of the known association of this rheumatic syndrome with vasculitis. Additional studies by Levo et al (1977) claimed that one-third of a group of RA patients were seropositive for HB virus antibody and that HB viral antigen and its antibody were both present in cryoprecipitates of patients with mixed cryoglobulinaemia; however, cryoprecipitates from rheumatoid subjects were not examined for these constituents (Levo et al, 1980).

Recent considerations of the role of hepatitis B virus (HBV) in the acquired immunodeficiency syndrome (AIDS) may be relevant to the possible role of HBV in some patients with inflammatory rheumatic disease. It is appreciated that HBV can be transmitted horizontally via mucosal infection (as well as by blood), that vertical transmission of the virus may also occur, and that a significant proportion of HBV infections are asymptomatic (Ravenholt, 1983). It appears that HBV can replicate in cells other than hepatocytes, in particular, lymphoblastoid cells derived from bone marrow (Romet-Lemonne et al, 1983) and endothelial cells of the Kaposi sarcoma (Siddiqui, 1983). It further appears that a defective RNA retrovirus (the 'delta agent') can become physically associated with HB_s antigen and can depress HB-antigenaemia during infection (Rizzetto, 1981).

Accordingly, association of the delta agent with HB_s antigen is viewed as providing one model for the pathogenesis of AIDS in that there would seem to be no reason why other defective (retro) virus particles should not also be associated with HB_s antigen (McDonald et al, 1983). On this basis the physical association of a defective retrovirus with a double-stranded DNA virus product might not be unique to either HBV infection itself or to the dramatic phenomenon of AIDS; and it may be worth considering whether viral associations of this kind may underly those more subtle defects of the immune system that appear characteristic of the spectrum of rheumatic disease.

At present, it seems clear that diffuse inflammatory vascular disease, at times involving the synovial microvasculature, may result from the host response to HB infection and that certain such individuals may present with syndromes clinically indistinguishable from chronic inflammatory 'rheumatic' disease. There is little support for the hypothesis of a genetic predisposition to HB infection itself (Zuckerman et al, 1976) and no evidence yet that patients with rheumatic syndromes associated with hepatitis B are less capable of overcoming the virus infection than those without these apparent complications. In the field of demyelinating diseases there was much interest in the demonstration of a biologically active agent, in the serum of patients with multiple sclerosis (Henle et al, 1975), which exhibits certain of the features of an immune complex; in fact, extrahepatic syndromes associated with HB infection have been likened to slow-virus infection an animals (Gocke et al, 1970). The selection of HB for 'recitation' in the context of rheumatic disease illustrates current approaches to the identification of infectious agents and their genomes which resist recognition by conventional virological techniques.

Recent evidence implicating parvoviruses

During the 1960s a considerable number of vertebrate viruses were isolated from animals, animal tumours and from tumour cell lines, which shared the common characteristic of being small spherical non-enveloped DNA viruses of 20–25 nm diameter (Siegl, 1976). As these viruses were amongst the smallest DNA viruses known, they were given the family name *Parvoviridiae* (or by common usage, 'parvovirus'). The viruses are classified into two subgroups according to whether they replicate productively without the aid of a helper virus ('autonomous parvovirus') or whether they are 'defective' in the sense of being dependent upon adenovirus coinfection for their own replication in culture ('adeno-associated parvovirus'). In domestic and laboratory animals the parvoviruses are thought to be responsible for a variety of infectious diseases including panleukopenia (in cats), hepatitis (in dogs and geese) and the Aleutian mink disease of generalised lymphoid proliferation, hyperglobulinaemia, glomerulonephritis and arteritis (Ingram & Cho, 1974; Ward & Tattersall, 1978). Parvoviruses share a tendency to grow well in replicating cells including vascular endothelium, and the relatively high mitotic activity of tumours provides an explanation for their association with neoplasia. A number of these viruses induce dwarfism, bone deformities and haemorrhagic encephalopathy when injected into newborn or suckling laboratory rodents. Evidence of parvovirus-like particles in human sera was first described by Cossart et al (1975) during the screening of symptom-free blood donors for hepatitis B surface antigen: this 'serum parvovirus-like virus' (SPLV) was found to cause febrile illness in haematologically normal people (Shneerson et al, 1980) and aplastic crises in patients with haemolytic anaemia (Sergeant et al, 1981; Kelleher et al, 1983). In the present context it is relevant that the SPLV agent is adeno-independent, that it can be transmitted to haemophiliacs in clotting-factor concentrates, that the virus will suppress the growth of haemopoietic stem cells in vitro, and that it is implicated in transient bone marrow aplasia and forms of acquired immunodeficiency (Mortimer et al, 1983).

Recent work by Godzeski, Smith and their colleagues in the USA is now implicating the presence of a parvovirus-like agent in rheumatoid synovium (Godzeski et al, 1978; Simpson et al, 1983; C. Godzeski & C. A. Smith, personal communications, 1983). By long-term co-culture of rheumatoid synovial cells with human lung fibroblasts (Godzeski) or fetal rabbit synovial cells (Smith) these workers have isolated an agent by serial intracerebral passage in Swiss-Webster mice, which induced fatal encephalopathy if injected neonatally, and runting, limb deformities and kyphoscoliosis if injected later in the suckling period. The agent (termed 'RA-1' virus) appears as 24–25 nm particles by electron microscopy and resembles parvoviruses in other respects, such as resistance to chemical and physical treatment. One such isolate was obtained by the direct injection of cultured RA synovial cells into mice without the need for prior co-cultivation with accessory cells. In continued work (C A Smith, personal communication, 1983) it has been possible to develop an antiserum in rabbits reacting in ELISA with this ('RA-1') isolate and to show that six such additional isolates ('RA2–7') share antigenic similarities with the first isolate, but not with the SPLV agent (see above) or to any other known animal parvoviruses.

In collaboration with Dr Carol Smith we have recently prepared caesium chloride gradient fractions at the expected parvovirus buoyant density (about 1.4 g/l) of extracts of homogenised synovia from patients with rheumatoid arthritis and osteoarthritis with the aim of testing their reactivity with the antiserum to 'RA-1' and to the SPLV agent (also termed 'B19') as well as for ultrastructural study (G Stierle, K A Brown, S G Rainsford, I Chrystie, J Banatvala, C A Smith and D C Dumonde, 1983, unpublished work). Of eleven such RA synovial fractions, five reacted by ELISA with anti-RA-1 whilst none of the six OA fractions did so. Electron microscopy of the immunoreactive RA fractions showed abundant particles of 10 nm size although a similar isolate from very long-term RA synovial cultures showed a small number of 23 nm particles closely resembling the SPLV agent. None of the isolates reacted in ELISA or in counter-immunoelectrophoresis with antibodies to the 'B19' SPLV agent (kindly given by Dr Bernard Cohen, Colindale, London); thus, if parvovirus is present, it is more likely to be in a 'defective' form (e.g. dependent upon adenovirus co-infection).

This kind of work illustrates the recurrent problems experienced in attempting to incriminate possibly ubiquitous viruses as specific agents in rheumatoid synovitis. There are immense operational difficulties in the unwieldy approach of trying to isolate from rheumatoid tissues an agent pathogenic for immature or 'normal' animals. Warren's group claimed to have induced skeletal abnormalities in mice born after injection of the mother with an agent from homogenised RA synovial membranes (Warren et al, 1969, 1972) and also in chicks after similar injection of embryonated eggs (Warren et al, 1971); these investigators claimed that their agent was compatible with a small DNA virus of a buoyant density of 1.45 g/l (Warren et al, 1975, 1979) but other investigators failed to reproduce their findings (Cole et al, 1973). Using C5-deficient mice, Crocker et al (1974) claimed to have induced arthritis, deformities and runting by intraperitoneal injection of RA synovial extracts but no confirmatory reports of this work have appeared. In a recent report, Mackay et al (1983) injected mature and immature baboons intravenously and intra-articularly with cells from RA synovial fluids and synovial cultures: no arthritis or other pathology developed over a three year period of observation. One cannot hope to test the specificity of putative neutralising antisera to such agents using crude homogenates of synovia, scores of non-human primates, hundreds of suckling mice or thousands of embryonated eggs for each serum to be examined on a statistically satisfactory basis (Smith, 1979). If a parvovirus dissimilar to the 'B19' SPLV is incriminated in RA it must be identified by growth in cell culture, possibly with the help of adenoviruses, and techniques of cell hybridisation including monoclonal antibody production will be needed to detect its distinctive properties. However, the well-known ability of parvoviruses to replicate in vascular endothelium, to attach to erythrocytes, to grow in replicating cells, to be transported by circulating monocytes and to pass placental and other endothelial barriers (Margolis & Kilham, 1970) makes them attractive candidates for further investigation.

Epstein–Barr virus and rheumatoid arthritis

Epstein–Barr virus (EBV) is a ubiquitous DNA virus of the herpes group which was identified originally in cultured tumour cells derived from Burkitt's lymphoma and subsequently in nasopharyngeal carcinoma cells; accordingly it has been implicated as the causative agent in these conditions (Epstein & Achong, 1979). EBV is transmitted horizontally to the oral cavity where it replicates in epithelial cells of the nasopharnyx or salivary glands and is shed into the saliva. EBV infects all human populations. Ubiquitous primary infection in childhood or adolescence is either asymptomatic or induces a mild febrile illness with circulating antiviral antibodies; the virus is thought to be transferred to a receptor on a minority of B lymphocytes which then carry the viral genome and express nuclear (EBNA) and membrane (EMA, LYDMA) antigens thus providing immunogenic stimuli for long-lasting T cell immunity with persistent seropositivity (Rickinson et al, 1981). In a minority of individuals, primary EBV infection induces B cell proliferation in blood and lymphoid tissues with the appearance of heterophile antibodies, a varity of autoantibodies in addition to anti-viral antibodies, and (sometimes) polyclonal hyperglobulinanaemia; the resulting illness ('glandular fever') — infectious mononucleosis (IMN), which may include a transient polyarthritis, is accompanied by enhanced virus secretion in saliva and is thought to be terminated only when infected B lymphocytes are destroyed by cytotoxic T cells and other mechanisms. At all events, the majority of healthy adults (80% or more) retain the anti-viral antibodies and about 20% of these seropositive individuals shed EBV in the saliva (Gerber et al, 1972) thus providing a large human reservoir for horizontal virus transmission. In lymphocyte culture the addition of EBV induces B cells to secrete large amounts of polyclonal immunoglobulins including autoantibodies, and to proliferate ('transform') into permanent lymphoblastoid cell lines; B cells from a minority of seropositive healthy subjects will transform 'spontaneously' in culture, due to in vitro activation of the few cells carrying EBV genome. Permanent cell lines established in this way (e.g. RAJI, WIL2 or Daudi cells) carry antigens related to the EB virus within their cell nuclei (e.g. 'EBNA') as evidence of viral genomic persistence. In essence, the EB virus and its human host have come to terms with each other: for only a small minority of individuals will become irreversibly ill following primary infection; and yet man may have taken over from subhuman primates in becoming the virus's principal reservoir.

Until 1976 the only association between EBV and rheumatic disease was that of a self-limiting polyarthritis in some patients with 'glandular fever' (IMN). In 1976 Alspaugh & Tan reported that two-thirds of rheumatoid sera reacted with a special nuclear antigen present in human B lymphoblastoid cell lines carrying the EBV genome which was apparently distinct from the already known nuclear antigen EBNA (Alspaugh & Tan, 1976): accordingly the antibody was termed 'RAP' (rheumatoid arthritis precipitin) when detected by precipitation and 'anti-RANA' (rheumatoid arthritis nuclear antigen) when detected by immunofluorescence. Although anti-EBNA and anti-RANA titres are similar during the convalescent phase of IMN (Catalano et al, 1980), the antigens RANA and EBNA differ from each other in chemical sensitivity and in morphology by immunofluorescence (Ferrell et al, 1981), in patterns of expression during the cyclic phases of B-cell transformation, and by their independent segregation in B cell–fibroblast hybrids (Slovin et al, 1980, 1981), as well as by the independent occurrence of anti-RANA and anti-EBNA antibodies in occasional rheumatoid sera (Ng et al, 1980). Of eight such serological surveys between 1976 and 1982 the incidence of anti-RANA in RA sera has varied from 64–84% (Venables et al, 1980; Ng et al, 1980) and from 6–60% in normal subjects (Venables et al, 1981; Ferrell et al, 1981), most reports agreeing that anti-RANA titres in RA are significantly elevated above normal (Alspaugh et al, 1981).

Additional evidence then emerged to support an association between EBV infection and rheumatoid arthritis. Several investigators reported that both spontaneous and EBV-induced B-lymphocyte transformation to permanent cell lines was more successful with rheumatoid than normal lymphocytes and that EBV-transformed rheumatoid B lymphocytes secrete larger amounts of rheumatoid factor (RF) than non-rheumatoid B cell lines (Slaughter et al, 1978; Koopman & Schrohenloher, 1980). One explanation has been that in RA there may be an increased number of circulating immature B cells responding by RF production and proliferation following EBV infection or mitogen stimulation, 'intrinsic' B cell hyperreactivity being independent of T cell control (Stierle et al, 1983). This view is supported by the increased numbers of rheumatoid B lymphocytes which rosette with mouse erythrocytes (Room et al, 1982), a recognised feature of immature B cells capable of EBV-induced RF production (Fong et al, 1983). A second general explanation is that in RA there is impaired T cell control of B cell proliferation to EBV or other polyclonal activators and there is some evidence in vitro for this (Bardwick et al, 1980; Tosato et al, 1981; Depper et al, 1981; Stierle et al, 1983), including a decreased representation of OKT8-positive suppressor/cytotoxic T cells in RA peripheral blood (Stierle et al, 1983), A supplementary view ascribes this T cell surveillance to the production of interferon (Thorley-Lawson, 1981), which is claimed to be defective in RA (Hasler et al, 1983). Thus, in addition to the possibility that RA patients may have expanded numbers of immature B cells receptive to EBV stimulation (and then prone to RF production) there may also be a defective T cell control of B cell proliferation. This postulated 'immaturity' of lymphocyte function (Pasquali et al, 1981) then recalls that of cord blood, where B lymphocytes which respond poorly to mitogen (PWM) stimulation are very susceptible to EBV infection.

Enthusiasm for EBV in rheumatoid disease has, however, been tempered by a number of investigations. First, there is no evidence to suggest an increase of oropharyngeal EBV infection in rheumatoid subjects (Depper et al, 1982) unless they are on immunosuppressive drugs (Aitcheson et al, 1983). Secondly, the hallmark of 'normal' infection by EBV is the appearance of anti-capsid antibodies (anti-VCA: Henle et al, 1974) and the prevalence of these in RA is not elevated (Elson et al, 1979), whilst higher anti-VCA titres in RA (Henle et al, 1979) imply no disease specificity, for they also occur in patients with SLE or systemic sclerosis and in cancer patients receiving immunosuppressive drugs (Strauch et al, 1974). Thirdly, the choice of cell line may well influence the proportion of sera reported as 'positive' for anti-RANA; and the specificity and sensitivity of anti-RANA in RA remains a contentious issue. Fourth, reports that antibodies to intermediate filaments of the cytoskeleton occur in RA (Toh et al, 1979) as in IMN (Linder et al, 1979) are tempered by the fact that they also occur in a variety of other virus infections and human diseases. Fifth, the arthralgia of IMN, like other viral arthralgias, is typically mild and self-limiting (Urman & Bohrane, 1983).

Whereas the weight of evidence in this 'preliminary hearing of EBV versus RA' seems finely balanced, the verdict at present appears to be guilt by suspicion only. Epidemiological evidence associating the prevalence of IMN and RA in different populations is circumstantial and the suggestion that EBV can cause a reactive arthritis (Aho & Raunio, 1982) is speculative. RA lymphocytes differ from 'normal' lymphocytes in many features (Brown, 1983) other than their susceptibility to activation in vitro by EBV; and immunological explanations ascribing to RA a special defect in idiotypic network homeostasis or other mechanisms of T cell control are probably not specific for EBV itself. The most compelling evidence is that of EBV-induced polyclonal B cell stimulation and B cell immortalisation, but possessing the 'motive' does not implicate one as the instigator of the 'crime'. In summary, our verdict is that the virus may well contribute to the pathogenesis of RA but that a unique role in its induction seems unlikely unless there are other accomplices which have still to be detected. We await the outcome of 'trial by jury'.

Retroviruses, systemic lupus and rheumatoid arthritis

During the mid 1970s there was a surge of interest in searching for ultrastructural or immunological evidence of retrovirus infection in systemic lupus and rheumatoid arthritis, which followed the implication that C-type viruses are involved in the pathogenesis of lupus syndromes in New Zealand mice (Yoshiki et al, 1974; Lerner et al, 1974; Phillips, 1975). The family *Retroviridae*, originally called oncornaviruses (to which type-C viruses belong), possesses the unique enzyme RNA-dependent DNA polymerase (reverse transcriptase), which enables the virus to synthesise a DNA copy of its RNA genome. By insertion of this transcribed DNA into the host cell genome the virus can be transmitted vertically during mitotic division. Viruses which are transmitted in this manner are termed 'endogenous' in contrast to exogenous infection which is by horizontal transmission. Endogenous C-type viruses, which are found in a number of animal species including subhuman primates, and may be oncogenic, are generally 'ecotropic' (reinfecting cells of the same species of original isolation), whilst exogenous C-type viruses are 'xenotropic' (i.e. will only reinfect cells of a different species). A search for evidence of C-type virus infection in human rheumatic disease was further stimulated by a report implicating their presence in canine lupus (Lewis et al, 1973) and by repeated attempts to try to identify their presence in human leukaemia. It was reasoned that inappropriate expression of retrovirus genomes in lymphoid cells might alter cell behaviour in such a way as to promote autoimmunity, lymphoid neoplasia or both (Levy, 1974).

Between 1974 and 1977 there appeared several reports which indicated that this approach might be promising. Strand & August (1974) claimed to have detected by radioimmunoassay C-type virus interspecies antigens in human lupus kidney, and antigenic determinants related to the C-type virus of canine lupus were found by immunofluorescence on a small percentage of lymphocytes from lupus patients (Lewis et al, 1974; Schwartz, 1975). In 1976 Mellors & Mellors claimed that both C-type viral antigens and antibodies to them were deposited in the kidney of a lupus patient. Furthermore, Zhdanov (1975) reported the occurrence of reverse transcriptase in leucocytes and tissues of patients with systemic lupus, together with the presence of DNA sequences complementary to RNA of measles virus: this suggested that a retrovirus might induce reverse transcription of other RNA virus genomes into host cell DNA (e.g. of the lymphocyte) with appropriate pathophysiological consequences ascribable to 'phenotypic mixing' (Zhdanov, 1975).

As with so many related endeavours, enthusiasm for C-type retroviruses was tempered by inability to confirm or extend these observations. Because of the failure of electron microscopy to identify C-type virus particles exclusively in SLE tissue, many laboratories concentrated on demonstrating virus expression by identification of reverse transcriptase. Many of these studies have proved to be fruitless (Phillips & Christian, 1979), though this assay identified a putative retrovirus isolated from prolonged culture of cells which were derived from fusion of placental cells from an SLE patient with two animal cell lines. Isopycnic sedimentation for ^{3}H-uridine-labelled virus has failed to isolate the virus from SLE tissue (Phillips et al, 1976). Serological evidence indicated that all human sera, including SLE, contained antibodies reactive with oncogenic simian, feline and murine C-type virus proteins (Aaronson & Stevenson, 1974; Snyder et al, 1976); further serological study (by lactoperoxidase labelling) of the canine C-type viral-related antigen on SLE lymphocytes revealed that it was equally well 'represented' on T lymphocytes of healthy individuals (Markenson et al, 1977); and doubt has been cast on the specificity of antisera to putative C-type viruses that were available in the 1970s (Snyder et al, 1976; Reynolds & Panem, 1981). Exhaustive studies were undertaken by Marmion's group to test the supposition that C-type virus genomes were present in RA synoviocytes and in RA and SLE lymphocytes, using techniques including DNA hybridisation (Norval & Smith 1979). In these investigations lymphoblastoid cell lines from SLE patients were generated in culture by spontaneous activation of latent EBV genome; and infection with exogenous EBV was also used in the hope of activating or inducing expression of putative viruses. Analysis of these lines by electron microscopy, co-cultivation experiments, DNA hybridisation, reverse transcriptase assay and complement fixation for the presence of C-type virus were all negative (Hicks et al, 1979). An exhaustive study by Hart (1978) failed to detect any evidence of C-type interespecies antigens in extracts of rheumatoid synovial membrane or rheumatoid lymphocytes; and likewise failed to detect antibodies in rheumatoid sera reactive with primate C-type virus-infected cells. It appears that initial claims of selective expression of C-type virus antigens and antibodies in SLE (and rheumatoid arthritis) have foundered due to lack of confirmatory evidence, uncertain specificity of antiserum reagents, and the possibility of introducing cross-reacting retroviruses by laboratory contamination with animal material or cell cultures (Phillips & Hargrave-Grands, 1978; Norval et al, 1979; Hart et al, 1979).

No such mention of retroviruses in the mid-1980s can omit some reference to the human T cell leukaemia virus (HTLV) which, although not an endogenous virus, nevertheless (like murine retroviruses) has an envelope glycoprotein serologically related to cellular structures of thymus and of lymphocytes themselves (Weiss et al, 1983). Because this retrovirus (HTLV) has a particular tropism for helper T cells, and because its horizontal transmission has been implicated in states of T cell suppression (the acquired immunodeficiency syndrome 'AIDS', the AIDS-related lymphadenopathy syndrome, and some haemophiliacs), serological surveys of antibodies to HTLV cell-associated membrane antigen in SLE and other inflammatory rheumatic diseases may be expected. Although the retrovirus HTLV was first isolated as recently as 1980 there is evidence for seropositivity in healthy individuals (Evatt et al, 1983) and for the existence of more than one retrovirus variant (Groopman & Gottleib, 1983). Such viruses may use HLA antigens as receptors to enter helper T cells, so altering HLA expression on the cell surface and evading attack by cytotoxic T cells (Man et al, 1983). In view of the associations between HLA and rheumatic disease it is tempting to speculate that T cell retrovirus infection in susceptible individuals results in perturbation of T cell interactions of rheumatological significance. Accordingly, there is likely to be a revival of interest in lymphotropic retroviruses as aetiological and pathogenetic agents in those inflammatory rheumatic diseases associated with impaired T cell function or lymphoproliferative disorders (e.g. systemic lupus and Sjögren's syndrome). However, in AIDS there is insufficient evidence to judge whether only one given virus (e.g. EBV, cytomegalovirus, HBV, or HTLV itself) might be 'the' precipitating agent, or whether a variety of agents induce states of T cell depression which then predispose to those virus infections which can be identified. In the inflammatory rheumatic diseases where more subtle states of lymphocyte dysfunction are present, the problem of deciding whether any such virus is 'causative' or 'opportunist' will be at least as difficult as was experienced in AIDS by 1984 (Hamerman et al, 1982; McDonald et al, 1983).

Conclusions: viruses in inflammatory rheumatic disease

It is testimony to sheer determination that despite admittedly disappointing results, the search still continues for specific viruses or their genomes in cells, tissues or body fluids of rheumatic patients (Norval & Marmion, 1976; Norval & Smith, 1979; Hart & Norval, 1980). It is argued that because viruses can induce autoantibodies by a variety of mechanisms, and because rheumatoid factor production (in the mouse) is governed by genes linked to immunoglobulin (C_H) and major histocompatibility complex (MHC) genes, the association of rheumatoid factors with rheumatoid arthritis is itself evidence of prior or persistent viral infection (Editorial, 1984). Although there are no clear syndromes of known viral aetiology comparable to the bacterially-induced reactive arthritides, a wide range of virus diseases are complicated by arthritis of an infective or postinfective nature (Hyer & Gottlein, 1979). Opponents of the 'target' hypothesis (Marmion, 1978) of viruses in rheumatoid arthritis point out that the infective viral arthritides are commonly mild, non-erosive and self-limiting; that slow virus infections are characterised by a lack of inflammatory response; that there are no clear associations of viral arthritides with HLA types; that predisposing immune deficiency in viral arthritis (e.g. of complement components) is not a feature of rheumatoid disease; or that morphological and ultrastructural evidence of persistent or productive viral infection in the rheumatoid joint simply lacks credibility. Persistent advocates of the 'target' theory point to the important advances in molecular virology and viral oncology that should provide new probes and techniques, to mechanisms by which viruses or their products can evade the immune response, to the role of MHC gene products in presenting viral antigens for immune induction and elimination, and to occasional clinical reports suggesting that virus infections of medium duration can 'turn on' the rheumatic state (De Vere Tyndall et al, 1984). With the possible exception of work on parvovirus it seems likely that attempts to transmit virus-like pathology with human tissue extracts to experimental animals, ranging from mouse (Warren et al, 1969) to non-human primates (Mackay et al, 1983) will, for the moment, be a 'Cinderella' activity in the field of human autoimmune disease, in potential contrast to the more dramatic syndromes of acquired immunological dysfunction (London et al, 1983).

On the other hand it is conceded that there is at least a theoretical framework for pursuing the idea that unusual host responses to viruses subverting the immune system could lead to autoimmune and inflammatory rheumatic disease (Notkins, 1975). Advocates of the 'immune subversion' hypothesis point to the variety of autoimmune phenomena that accompany viral infections of lymphocytes, that a wide range of viruses are capable of infecting cells of the immune system, that virtually any immunoregulatory defect could arise (including disordered traffic of lymphocytes), and that the theoretical framework readily accommodates advances in understanding the role of MHC gene products in immune induction and expression (Denman, 1981). An interesting speculation would be to consider how a virus infection might perturb the idiotypic network of the immune system without leaving any conventional evidence of its prior existence in the host. A growing wave of interest may be anticipated in the potential of retroviruses to alter lymphocyte function (Pincus, 1982) and in their potential to become physically, genomically or phenotypically associated with other viruses. The ability of cell-derived transforming genes of retroviruses to alter growth regulation of connective tissue cells (Robbins et al, 1983) provides an illustration of how ubiquitous viruses might also perturb the function of nonlymphoid cells involved in the inflammatory process. In summary, there is no shortage of ideas in this area: there are plenty of animal models of autoimmune, immune complex, lymphoid and inflammatory disease following virus infection; and we share the opinion that susceptibility to certain forms of virally-induced subversion of lymphoid and inflammatory cell function contributes to the diatheses of the inflammatory rheumatic diseases in *Homo sapiens*.

CLASSIFICATION OF ASSOCIATIONS BETWEEN MICROBIAL INFECTION AND RHEUMATIC DISEASE

One purpose of devising disease classifications is to identify common characteristics between syndromes of diverse aetiology. For this reason we present such a classification and consider its aetiological and pathogenetic implications.

A four-fold classification of infection and arthritis

Tables 14.5 and 14.6 delineate the four principal ways in which microbial infection may be associated with arthritis syndromes. When the identity of the microbial species is known (i.e. the precipitating aetiology) the arthritis syndromes are classified as 'infective' (class 1), 'postinfective' (class 2) and 'reactive' (class 3) according to (i) whether the micro-organism is characteristically present in the lesion (i.e. the joint); and (ii) whether antigens of the micro-organism are known to be present at some stage at the site of inflammation during the disease process. In this classification the term 'inflammatory' is used to refer to the idiopathic inflammatory rheumatic diseases where microbial aetiology is considered plausible but where evidence is circumstantial (see above). This classification was first presented in Helsinki in 1975 at the Eighth European Rheumatology Congress (Dumonde, 1976). Its general form (Table 14.5) and immunological implications (Table 14.6) have been found applicable to other system-based disorders in which microbial infection is considered, e.g. encephalomyelitis syndromes (Dumonde, 1978b), carditis and vasculitis syndromes (Dumonde & Richards, 1981) and uveitis syndromes (Dumonde, 1985).

Associations of classes 1–3

In class 1 associations the responsible organism enters the joint (synovium) by extension of a local infective process or by haematogeneous spread from a distant site. Such organisms multiply in synovium and other articular tissue, and joint pathology arises from the ill-effects of local microbial multiplication, with superimposed pathogenetic mechanisms of type III and type IV hypersensitivity (Table 14.6). Predisposing factors are: being ill (e.g. with metabolic, neoplastic, immunodeficiency or inflammatory disease), being traumatised or neuropathic, or just being 'young'. There is however no evidence of a consistent immunoregulatory defect or of a genetic diathesis (Table 14.6). Despite the wide range of microbial species that can induce class 1 arthritis (see Ch. 45) we remain ignorant about many of its pathogenetic features: in the first instance, of how haematogeneous spread actually takes place — whether certain microbes are transported to the joint within or associated with effector cells of the immune system itself (e.g. macrophages or lymphocytes) or with other formed elements of the blood, or as infective immune complexes, or simply as 'free' microbes floating in the fluid phase. Secondly, we do not understand the role of local immunity: thus experimental studies reveal that the joint is an excellent site for immune induction, but little is known of the role of local antibody production, T cell sensitisation or accessory cell function in the pathology of class 1 arthritis. Thirdly, we do not know what determines whether a distant infection elsewhere will metastasise to the joint: thus we remain ignorant of the cellular basis of 'arthrotropism', and of the microvascular factors which may determine localisation of infec-

Table 14.5 A suggested classification of principal associations between infection and arthritis

Class of association	Microbial infection known	Presence or multiplication of organism at site of inflammation	Presence of microbial antigen at inflammatory site	Designation of rheumatic state	Illustrative examples
Class 1	Yes	Yes	Yes	'Infective'	Septic (suppurative) arthritis; infective viral arthritides
Class 2	Yes	Presence inconstant but probably no local multiplication	Yes	'Postinfective'	Postmeningococcal arthritis; PAN following HBV-infection; ? rubella arthritis
Class 3	Yes	No	No	'Reactive'	Arthritis of rheumatic fever; enterocolitic and sexually-acquired reactive arthritides
Class 4	No (? perhaps any of a number of infections)	—	—	'Inflammatory'	Rheumatoid, lupus syndromes, etc.

Table 14.6 Immunity and allergy in relation to microbial infection and rheumatic disease

Class of association (see Table 14.3)	Host immunity (resistance) to microbe	Allergic status of host	Immunoregulatory defect known	Genetic element
Class 1 (infective)	Impaired	Type III + Type IV hypersensitivity	No	No
Class 2 (post-infective)	Resistance develops with onset of rheumatic syndrome	Transient (? Type III + Type IV)	No	No
Class 3 (reactive)	Presumably normal	Not known	(? Cross-reactive autoimmunity)	Yes (HLA-B27)
Class 4 (inflammatory)	Presumably normal	Not known	Yes (antinuclear, antiglobulin, antilymphocyte responses)	Yes (DR4; A1-B8-DR3)

tive metastases. Many other examples could be given to display our ignorance of the pathogenesis of class 1 arthritides, yet acquisition of such knowledge would seem to be a vital importance in interpreting the pathogenesis of the other arthritis classes (Table 14.6).

In class 2 associations there is evidence that microbial antigen appears at the site of disease for some period of time during the postinfective process and that part of this localisation may be due to deposition of primary immune complexes from blood into the synovial microvasculature (Tables 14.5, 14.6). As with class 1 arthritis, there is no known immunoregulatory defect or genetic diathesis; but unlike class 1 arthritis, there is no evidence of local microbial multiplication. Accordingly the latent interval, self-limiting course, and some joint studies (see references to Table 14.2) suggest a self-limiting type III/IV hypersensitivity reaction in the synovium as host resistance develops to the primary infection. However, we remain ignorant of many aspects of pathogenesis, for example, whether the microbe was ever in the joint in an intact form, and whether the concept of 'primary' immune complex deposition is too simplistic. An unanswered question is whether the amount of antigen which localises in the synovium or other articular structures is sufficient by itself to explain the extent of joint pathology on the usual basis of hypersensitivity, or whether the pathology is greater than would have been expected from a knowledge of the allergic status of the host and of the amount of antigen in the joint. If one then adds the pathogenetic questions raised about class 1 arthritis (see above) our ignorance begins to appear 'cumulative'.

In class 3 associations, as in sexually-acquired arthritis, enterocolitic arthritis or rheumatic fever, there is no evidence that the microbe or its antigens actually enter the joint, there is no confirmed evidence of a *specific* allergy or anergy to the inciting microbe, and we remain clinically ignorant of what might determine chronicity or relapse. Despite increasing knowledge of HLA associations or speculation as to the role of cross-reactive autoimmunity (i.e. in rheumatic fever and spondarthritis syndromes), the pathogenesis of these reactive arthritides remains a 'cumulative mystery'. Moreover, Koch's postulates are unhelpful: a large range of microbial infections could well induce reactive arthritis syndromes; different microbes might precipitate different relapses in an individual patient; and there are no satisfactory animal models of reactive arthritis.

In view of the mucosal nature of the precipitating infection it could be proposed that sensitised lymphocytes of the mucosal-associated lymphoid system migrate to and sequester in the joint, awaiting host stimulation by reinfection at a distant site, as suggested for uveitis syndromes (Kaplan, 1983). There has been no other immunological explanation of why a focal infection, apparently localised to the pharynx, intestine or lower genitourinary tract, should in some 0.5–3% of subjects precipitate a reactive pathology, comprising vasculitic, arthritic, mucosal or other manifestations which are designated as a 'rheumatic' process.

'Class 4' associations

Let us now postulate a fourth class of association (Tables 14.5, 14.6) in which the rheumatic syndromes included share the following features:

1. Histological appearances of tissue lesions resemble hypersensitivity responses to persistent antigens
2. Clinical patterns of disease are chronic, progressive or relapsing
3. Investigation yields strong evidence of genetic associations and of non-organ-specific immunological abnormalities
4. Examination of skin, mucosa, blood, urine, lymphoid tissue, joints or serous cavities yields no specific extrinsic antigen
5. No single precipitating microbial infection can be identified.

For two principal reasons we use the term 'inflammatory' to designate this category of syndromes which of course comprises rheumatoid arthritis, ankylosing spondylitis, systemic lupus and their syndromic variants. First, the term seems taxonomically useful in communicating the common characteristics of idiopathic inflammation within connective tissue. Secondly, it implies that pathogenetic components in this group may include regulatory disorders of the inflammatory response, revealed by certain kinds of environmental stimuli.

Class 3 and class 4 syndromes viewed as 'adverse reactions' to microbial infection

In principle there seems to be every reason why microbes or their products should be able to induce 'adverse reactions' in a way similar to drugs. On this basis class 3 syndromes could be viewed as adverse reactions to a certain limited range of microbes colonising certain mucosal surfaces, whilst class 4 syndromes could be viewed as adverse reactions to a wide, possibly unlimited range of micro-organisms, entering the host by any known route. This view is compatible with a remarkable epidemiological feature: the prevalence of rheumatoid disease in the community (say 2%) is of the same order as the average incidence of class 3 (reactive) arthritis following focal infection with defined micro-organisms (0.5–3%).

Table 14.7 takes this discussion one stage further by drawing parallels between circumstances in which pseudoallergic reactions to drugs take place and circumstances in which adverse reactions to microbial infection might (also) give rise to syndromes of disseminated rheumatic

Table 14.7 Adverse reactions to microbes: features apparently shared with pseudoallergic reactions to drugs

Feature	Recognised adverse reactions to drugs	Postulated adverse reactions to microbes
Definition	Unexpected, unintended effect occurring at doses normally used for prophylaxis, diagnosis or treatment	Unexpected occurrence following 'normal' circumstances of exposure to the microbial agent
Clinical observation	Syndromes often 'pseudoallergic' (arthritis, vasculitis, lymphadenopathy, fever, haematological reactions)	Postulated 'pseudoallergic' reactions include those of inflammatory rheumatic disease
Inference	Effects not predictable from knowledge of the intended activity of the drug	Effects (e.g. inflammatory rheumatic syndrome) not predicted from knowledge of microbial taxonomy or acquired resistance mechanisms
Exclusions	Drug supersensitivity excluded (i.e. due to specific enzymatic deficiency)	Defined states of immunodeficiency excluded (i.e. hypogammaglobulinaemia)
Specificity	Intolerance may be present in the same individual to unrelated drugs	Intolerance (e.g. relapse) may be produced by taxonomically unrelated microbes
	A given drug may produce different syndromes of adverse reactions	A given microbe may produce different 'adverse reactions' in different individuals
Exposure factors	Adverse reactions more prevalent after prolonged administration of certain drugs	Class 3 arthritis syndromes (see Tables 14.5, 14.6) more prevalent after (repeated) infections with certain microbes (at mucosal surfaces)
	Other drugs show no dose-dependency (e.g. inducing SLE); range may be 'unlimited' (Alarcon-Segovia, 1969)	Perhaps the true range of microbes which *may* induce class 4 syndromes is 'unlimited'
Illustrative genetic (host) factors	HLA-DR4 in hydrallazine-induced SLE	HLA-B27 in some bacterially induced reactive arthritis syndromes
Suggested mechanisms	'*Allergenic*':drug acts as hapten or immunogen and host reacts allergically to subsequent doses	'*Allergenic*': exaggerated anti-microbial sensitisation, followed by host reactions of hypersensitivity to subsequent exposure
	'*Autoimmune*': drug induces autoimmunity and host reacts by developing autoimmune disease	'*Autoimmune*': infection induces autoimmunity and host reacts by developing autoimmune disease
	'*Autopharmacological*': drug perturbs cell/mediator systems normally controlling inflammatory and other homeostatic processes	'*Autopharmacological*': infection or microbial products perturb cell/mediator systems normally controlling inflammatory and other homeostatic processes
Rheumatological implications	Drug-induced inflammatory rheumatic disease involves a multifactorial aetiology and pathogenesis, much of which awaits clarification (Russell, 1981)	New approaches to the role of microbial infection in class 3 and class 4 rheumatic disease may well derive from improved knowledge of mechanisms involved in pseudoallergic drug reactions

disease. The first relevant feature of adverse reactions to microbes would seem to be their unexpected nature which could not be predicted from knowledge of their expected interactions with the host (i.e. immunotaxonomic status of the microbe or mechanisms involved in specific acquired immunity). Inspection of Table 14.7 reveals the wealth of research potential inherent in taking these comparisons further.

In this section we have presented a classification of associations between microbial infection and rheumatic disease (Table 14.5) and we have enlarged upon some immunological (Table 14.6) and pathogenetic (Table 14.7) implications. Amongst the many approaches which may be inferred from this discussion we suggest optimistically that identification of common factors that predispose to, or mediate, microbe-induced reactive arthritis syndromes (on the one hand) and drug-induced disseminated inflammatory disease (on the other hand) will make a major contribution to the understanding and control of the rheumatic diseases.

IMMUNOPATHOLOGICAL MECHANISMS IN RELATION TO INFECTION AND THE RHEUMATIC DISEASES

In this section we consider three interpretations of how rheumatic disease might arise through genetically-based immunopathological responses to specific microbial infection:

a. That disease arises through an inability to eradicate certain 'target' microbes or their interaction products from the host
b. That microbes induce 'classical' autoimmune or immune complex disease in the susceptible host
c. That a genetically-based or acquired defect in idiotypic network regulation of the immunological response allows the development of autoimmunity and immune complex disease in which the host has 'lost sight' of the inciting stimulus.

It is germane to recall that for some ten years there has been well-founded knowledge of five principal features of the immunological response to defined infection (see Moller, 1974):

1. Those allergic responses which accompany processes of immune elimination and which provide cellular and vascular mechanisms for initiating or completing the elimination process
2. 'Feed-back' cellular control mechanisms which are continually exercised to optimise elimination of microbes and their products, whilst normally minimising the extent and duration of allergic responses
3. How pathological responses may differ from physiological responses to infection by an undue intensity or duration of allergic reactions accompanying impaired immune elimination
4. The application of newer immunological, biochemical and microbiological techniques to analyse how cellular and humoral mechanisms involved in immune elimination become the actual mediators of tissue damage in allergic inflammation
5. The recognition that processes of cellular co-operation and feedback regulation are under genetic control.

It is against this background that the following three 'growth areas' are selected for discussion.

The 'target' theory

In its simplest form this proposes that syndromes of reactive (class 3) or inflammatory (class 4) disease arise through persistent hypersensitivity responses by a normally-functioning immune system reacting to specific microbial antigens deposited as 'targets' outside of the immune effector cells themselves (Marmion, 1978). Persistence of microbes or their products in such hosts has been viewed for a decade in terms of intracellular sequestration of the microbe, states of partial immunological tolerance due to antigenic sharing between host and microbe, production of non-metabolisable products at sites of inflammation, or immunosuppressive effects of the microbial infection itself (Porter & Knight, 1974; Moller, 1974). There is really hardly any evidence for the operation of any of these mechanisms and Ziff's aphorism that rheumatoid arthritis is an 'immaculate infection' (Ziff, 1976) still holds in this context. Persistent advocates of the 'target' theory postulate that the infective agents are immunosuppressive or evade rejection by antigen shedding or immunological enhancement, or that host-coded neoantigens (e.g. in synoviocytes) are derepressed (e.g. oncofetal antigens), or that a genetic minority (e.g. 2%) of individuals handle specific infections in a special way (Marmion, 1978). Let us accept that in this form, the 'target' view is at present unsupported by sufficient evidence (Table 14.5).

Induction of systemic autoimmune/immune complex disease

In any discussion of the role of infection in the rheumatic diseases, due consideration must be given to the heterogeneity of the normal immune response. Structural heterogeneity of the normal antibody response is recognised by the presence of isotypic, allotypic and idiotypic antigens on immunoglobulin molecules (Kindt & Sogn, 1977); functional heterogeneity is particularly evident in respect of the binding energy ('affinity') of antibody–antigen interaction (Steward, 1977); physiological differences in the effector functions of antibodies (e.g. immune elimination, fixation to macrophage surfaces) can now be partly ascribed to structural differences in the chemistry of immunoglobulin molecules. In view of the association of abnormally persistent immune complexes with inflammatory rheumatic disease it might be suggested that these disorders share an important defect in regulation of the normal heterogeneity of the immune response — in particular, of that aspect which controls the ability of antibodies to bind to their corresponding antigens.

In experimentally immunised animals it has long been known that immune complex deposition in the tissues particularly occurs following the development and persistence of soluble 'antigen-excess' immune complexes in the cirulation (Weigle, 1961). In mice this has been shown to be genetically associated with strains that produce circulating antibodies of unusually low affinity which fail to eliminate antigens from the circulation (Alpers et al, 1972), thus favouring deposition of antigen-excess immune complexes in the tissues (Soothill & Steward, 1971). Such mice may also have associated defects in macrophage and lymphocyte function which may be viewed as of primary or secondary pathogenetic significance (Passwell et al, 1974; Talal, 1975; Morgan and Steward, 1976); but all events, infection with a specific micro-organism (e.g. LCM virus) results in persistent viraemia, wide-spread vasculitis and tissue deposition of immune complexes containing specific viral antigen. In man it is likely that similar mechanisms underlie postinfective rheumatic syndromes (e.g. hepatitis — see above) where the responsible agent is shown to persist in both the circulation and tissue lesions in an immune-complexed form. In rheumatoid and lupus syndromes, where the identity of the precipitating (microbial) agent is not clear, it is necessary to modify this simplistic 'immune complex' interpretation of the significance of heterogeneity of the immune response.

Accordingly, the 'immune complex' view of chronic inflammatory rheumatic disease has been illustrated as follows (Fig. 14.1). The susceptible host is viewed as deviating on the side of a low affinity antibody production in response to a potentially wide range of microbial antigens, which at an early stage in the host's immune response are not eliminated quickly enough from the circulation to prevent immune complex deposition in the tissues (Petty et al, 1972). By analogy with experimental animals it may be further suggested that this displacement in heterogeneity of the immune response (Fig. 14.1) is itself genetically determined (Katz & Steward, 1975) and that in the syndromes of rheumatoid disease and systemic lupus there is an additional (genetically determined) propensity to develop antiglobulin and antinuclear antibody responses in which the 'rheumatic' host 'loses sight' of the original antigenic stimulus.

Support for this approach emerges from the demonstration that antiglobulins in rheumatoid disease and antinucleic acid antibodies in systemic lupus are indeed of low affinity (Steward et al, 1973, 1975). The rheumatoid subject may then be regarded simply as one who produces low affinity antiglobulin responses following certain precipitating (microbial) stimuli; and the lupoid diathesis may be similarly interpreted in respect of antinuclear responses. At present there is no real evidence for the existence of autoantibodies directed towards tissue-specific antigens of the

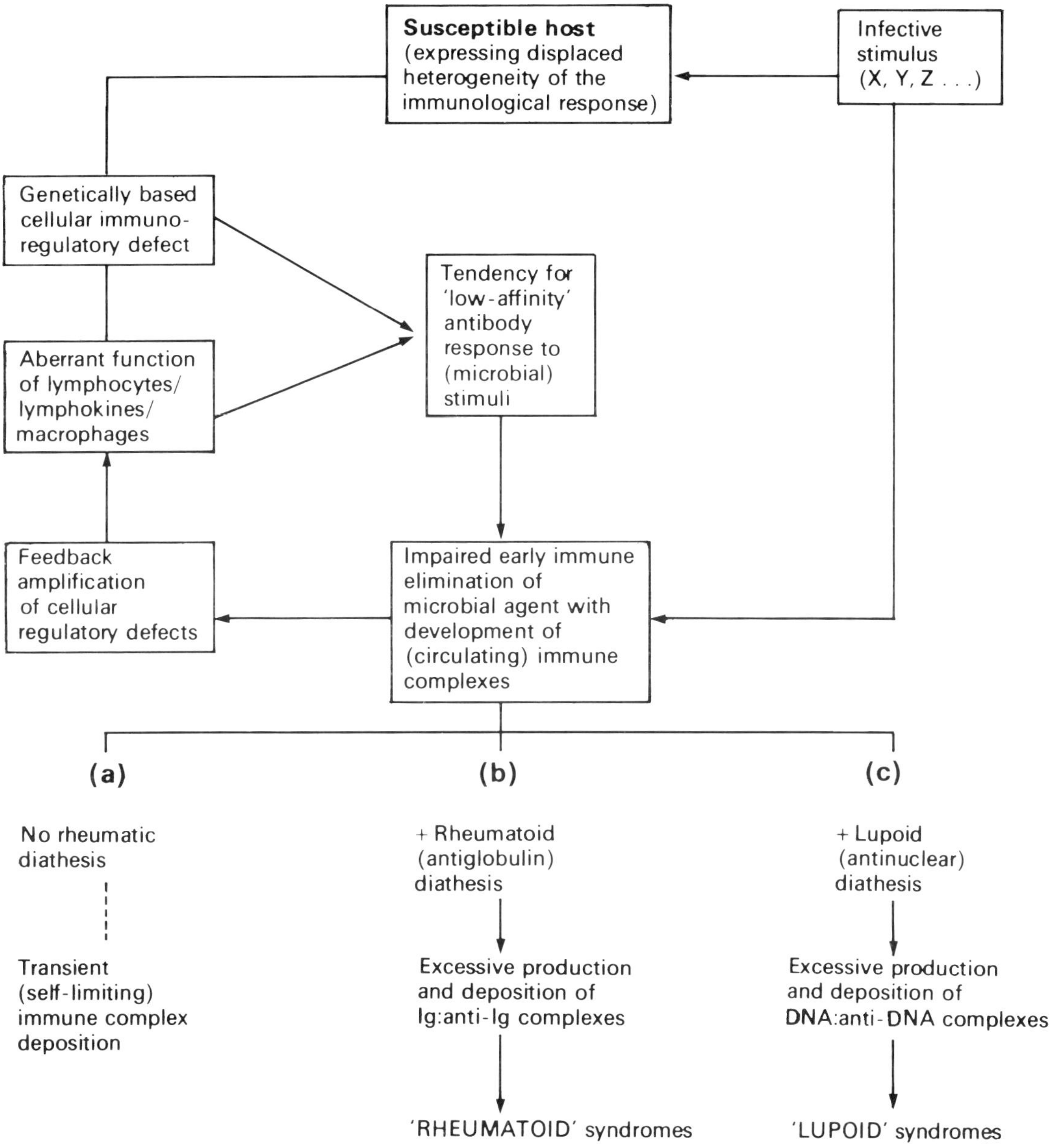

Fig. 14.1 Diagrammatic representation of 'immune complex' view of chronic inflammatory rheumatic disease. The diagram depicts the essential differences proposed in the course of immune complex responses to microbial infection where there is displaced heterogeneity of the immune response towards low affinity antibody production. (a) In the absence of additional 'rheumatic' diatheses the host develops transient immune complex disease following specific microbial infection. (b) A superimposed tendency to develop excessive anti-globulin responses is viewed as underlying chronic immune complex production and deposition in rheumatoid disease. (c) A superimposed tendency to develop excessive anti-nuclear responses is viewed as underlying chronic immune complex production and deposition in lupus syndromes. In both (b) and (c) the chronic or relapsing host response is viewed as being maintained by subclinical infectious episodes.

joint, which could develop by cross-reactive sensitisation to specific bacteria or viruses.

Rheumatological implications of the idiotypic network theory

Much contemporary immunology has developed against the background of the clonal selection theory of Burnet (1959) which proposes that individual lymphocytes are genetically programmed to produce antibodies of a particular specificity and that molecules of this antibody are incorporated into the lymphocyte membrane as cell surface receptors. Furthermore, it has been demonstrated that the hypervariable regions which constitute the antigen-combining sites of antibody molecules can behave as antigens themselves (idiotypes) and can elicit antibodies to them (anti-idiotypes). Jerne (1974) has proposed that the coexistence within an individual of both idiotypic and anti-idiotypic cellular receptors within the immune system could provide a new approach to the understanding of clonal interactions. Thus, lymphocytes have been viewed as being able to recognise both foreign antigenic determinants and the idiotypes on the immunoglobulin receptors of other lymphocytes. In this way, the immune system has been envisaged as a web of network of V-region domains in which the connections between the various T and B cells clones are idiotype–anti-idiotype linkages. The delicate balance between the clones and the cells regulating their expression can be perturbed by an external antigenic stimulus and by further idiotypes or anti-idiotypes. This 'network' concept has by no means received universal acceptance (Cohn, 1981) but its protagonists have accumulated a body of experimental evidence for its support (Urbain et al, 1981). This includes the demonstration that anti-idiotypes can be used to specifically suppress the expression of a dominant idiotype in an induced response and that auto-anti-idiotypic antibodies appear during the course of normal, antigen-induced immune responses. Furthermore, evidence has been obtained for the existence of idiotypes on both T and B cells; and anti-idiotypes have been associated with T helper and T suppressor cells. Thus during a response to a complex antigen such as a virus, T helper cells specific for one of the many epitopes on the virus collaborate with B cells specific for another epitope and a network of idiotype interactions is built up (of course accessory cells are also involved). Since an anti-idiotype is also antigenic, anti-anti-idiotypes may be produced which can act as 'internal images' of the original antigen. It is therefore possible that anti-idiotypic antibodies which regulate expression of idiotypes on the surface of lymphocytes may be important in the induction of tolerance to self antigens and to the avoidance of autoimmune reactions. Thus, immunoregulatory defects in the idiotype–anti-idiotype network could result in undue expression of autoreactive clones and exaggerated autoimmunity.

However, whilst these networks seem to be operative in experimental animals (Schechter et al, 1982), evidence for the existence in man is, not unexpectedly, far more difficult to acquire. Nevertheless, autoimmune disease in which antibodies to *immunoglobulins* can be demonstrated may be examples of situations in which there is a failure of such immunoregulatory networks. These autoantibodies are classically directed to antigens in the Fc of the host's immunoglobulin but can also react with allotypic structures on immunoglobulins. Antibodies to hidden determinants in the F $(ab')_2$ region (Osterland et al, 1963) and other anti-antibodies (Milgrom et al, 1966) have long been known; and there is evidence that autoimmunity to Fc-IgG gives rise to self-associated immune complexes of IgG antiglobulins of pathogenic potential in rheumatoid synovitis (Mannik, 1982). A report (Geltner et al, 1980) has shown the presence of anti-idiotypic anti-Ig antibodies in the cryoglobulins of patients with mixed cryoglobulinaemia, which could suggest that there is an immune network in man, but the role of anti-idiotypes in this disorder remains unknown. The suggestion has also been made, following studies of the role of anti-idiotype antibodies in human systemic lupus erythematosus (Abdou et al, 1981), that serum anti-DNA antibody levels are regulated both by suppressor cells and by anti-anti-DNA antibodies (anti-idiotypes). Thus (it was proposed) the regulation of anti-DNA antibodies by anti-idiotypic antibody might prevent disease expression in healthy individuals and induce disease remission in subjects with lupus (Abdou et al, 1981).

If it is accepted that idiotypic network interactions do occur in humans as in experimental animals then the possibility exists that abnormalities in this regulatory system may underlie autoimmune reactions and chronic antigen–antibody complex disease. One of the most perplexing aspects arising from analysis of circulating immune complexes in man is the failure, except in a few instances, to identify a specific exogenous antigen, whereas immunoglobulin and complement are readily demonstrated. Thus it is quite possible that circulating and tissue-localised complexes in a number of diseases including rheumatoid arthritis, in which a specific antigen cannot be demonstrated, may arise from idiotype–anti-idiotype interactions in a situation where the host has 'lost sight' of the initiating antigen; and against the background of a deficient immunoregulatory network, excessive production of anti–idiotypic-idiotype complexes continues.

Experimental evidence in support of this concept has been produced in Balb/c mice in which 95% of the anti-phosphoryl choline antibodies bear the same idiotype ('T15'): for following immunisation with the phosphoryl choline, antibodies to the antigen bearing the T15 idiotype are first produced and then clones are activated which produce antibody to the T15 idiotype (Cosenza, 1976). Circulating immune complexes have been demonstrated in phosphoryl choline-immunised Balb/c mice which consist of T15–anti-T15 idiotype (Rose & Lambert, 1980). In subsequent studies, these authors showed that polyclonal activation of Balb/c mice by bacterial lipopolysaccharide results in the production of anti-phosphorylcholine antibodies with T15 idiotype and also these mice produced anti-T15 idiotype antibodies. Furthermore, the LPS-treated mice produced circulating T15–anti-T15 complexes which could be demonstrated in glomerular lesions, and eluates of the kidneys contained immunoglobulins bearing the T15 idiotype and also anti-T15 antibody activity (Rose et al, 1982a; Goldman et al, 1982). Thus in this experimental situation where B cells were artificially made hyperactive, the production of idiotype–anti-idiotype reactions gave rise to glomerular deposits of immune complexes. In experimental African trypanosomiasis of mice (and in the human disease) there is an intense polyclonal proliferation of B cells with circulating immune complexes. When Balb/c mice were infected with trypanosomes, they produced T15–anti-T15 idiotype immune complexes (Rose et al, 1982b). It is thus theoretically possible that similar interactions could be involved in human immune complex-mediated immunopathology. Polyclonal antibody synthesis, a feature of a number of infections and autoimmune diseases, may result in the pertubations of the idiotypic network and give rise to the production of circulating complexes involving idiotype–anti-idiotype interactions.

Thus it is attractive to speculate that since the immunoglobulin-producing clonal repertoire of any individual represents an extensive source of antigens (idiotypes) and antibodies (anti-idiotypes), the search for putative antigens as initiating agents for immune complex-mediated pathology should be directed towards the identification of idiotypic reactants and of mechanisms which might disturb idiotypic network regulation. It seems plausible that the local or systemic formation of immune complexes comprised of an autoantibody linked to its anti-idiotype may be a compensatory host reponse to the development of autoimmunity itself and that some individuals may under-compensate or even over-compensate in this way. On this basis a host with a tendency to develop anti-globulin, anti-nuclear or other autoimmune responses (see Fig. 14.1 above) may have to balance the risk of immune complex disease against the risk of failing to modulate the initial state of autoimmunity. The clinical picture will reflect the balance between immune complex formation and autoimmunity and it is likely that different patients will respond to such diseases and their treatment in different ways (Dumonde et al, 1982). At the present time the question remains open of whether such regulatory defects in the idiotypic network might be ascribed to the presence of viruses or their genomic products inside the cells of the immune system itself (Marmion, 1978; Denman, 1979; Depper et al, 1981) or whether viruses can stimulate anti-idiotypic autoimmunity by interacting with cell membrane structures outside of the immune system (Plotz, 1983).

The problem of immunological specificity

The foregoing discussions present very little

encouragement that classical immunological techniques will reveal aetiological associations between *specific* micro-organisms and the 'idiopathic' (i.e. class 4) inflammatory rheumatic diseases. It seems that there is no evidence for the persistence of microbial antigens at sites of inflammation, or for persistence of unique viral or other foreign nucleic acid sequences within the host genome, or for the persistence of specific autoantibodies that cross-react with microbial constituents, or for the occurrence of specific microbial antigens in circulating immune complexes. There would seem to be two routes of 'escape' from this problem of immunological specificity. The first is to postulate that a disease like rheumatoid arthritis is initiated by certain specific infectious agents but that by the time the disease is manifest clinically, the host's immune system has lost sight of the inciting stimulus. The second is to postulate that the very idea of anti-microbial specificity is incorrect and that we should seek other explanations of how micro-organisms may be involved in disease diathesis and pathogenesis. In the remainder of this chapter we explore briefly some implications of this second line of enquiry.

PATHOPHYSIOLOGICAL, GENETIC AND CLINICAL CONSIDERATIONS

The nature of rheumatic inflammation

In this section we shall consider how microbial infections might affect certain pathophysiological mechanisms concerned with regulation of the inflammatory response that could underly features of the systemic rheumatic diseases. It is germane to recall controversy in the 19th century between the 'vascular' and 'cellular' theories of inflammation: Cohnheim envisaged a primary change in vascular endothelium followed by passive leucocyte adherence and diapedesis, whilst Metchnikoff viewed the microvasculature as passively supporting the active diapedesis of leucocytes towards the (extravascular) inflammatory stimulus (Rather, 1972). By the 1950s it was accepted that both vascular endothelium and intravascular white cells were actively involved in the inflammatory process (Ebert, 1974) and three theories of rheumatic inflammation had emerged: the 'vascular' (Gross, 1940), the 'collagen' (Klemperer et al, 1942), and the 'lymphoid' (Burnet, 1959). There being no subsequent evidence to ascribe rheumatic inflammation to a primary disorder of collagen, the 'vascular' view survived mainly in discussions of the pathogenesis of systemic sclerosis whilst the 'lymphoid' view has given rise to the wealth of immunohaematological investigations across the spectrum of rheumatic disease. This discussion envisages that in these syndromes there may be something 'wrong' with the control of inflammatory responses at risk sites of rheumatic inflammation, particularly concerning those processes that govern interactions between blood-borne leucocytes and vascular endothelium: and which take place in response to potentially injurious stimuli, microbial or otherwise, delivered to either compartment, intra-vascular or extravascular.

The concept of lymphoendothelial dysfunction

Although the term 'rheumatism' is said to lack a specific histopathological basis, a characteristic feature of early rheumatic inflammation is the accumulation of lymphocytes outside hypertrophic postcapillary venules in synovium, dermis and other tissues. 'Superimposed' upon this 'basic' lymphoendothelial pattern are other features of inflammation (e.g. macrophage accumulation and activation, granuloma formation, fibrosis, cartilage erosion) which by virtue of their striking nature, have attracted so much description and pathogenetic speculation. Experimental immunological models of rheumatoid inflammation are brought about simply by intense and persistent immunopharmacological stimulation to local lymphocytic emigration and activation in otherwise genetically normal animals (Dumonde et al, 1976). Against this background the basic pathology of rheumatoid disease can be viewed as a pathological triad of hyperplastic lymphadenitis, widespread subclinical vasculitis and lymphocytic polysynovitis (Dumonde, 1978a). The concept of lymphoendothelial dysfunction in inflammatory rheumatic diseases can be illustrated by considering the rheumatoid process as involving regulatory defects affecting the meeting points of the lymphoid and microvascular systems; and as manifest by a failure to control the activation of recirculatory lymphocytes during transmural passage within lymphoid tissue and at certain extralymphoid sites of lymphocyte

Table 14.8 Microvascular and lymphoid dysfunction in inflammatory rheumatic disease. (For references see Dumonde et al, 1976; Dumonde, 1978a.)

Evidence illustrating microvascular dysfunction	Evidence illustrating lymphoid dysfunction
Widespread subclinical vasculitis	Persistent autoantibody status.
Functional capillary abnormalities	Peripheral blood immunoblasts
Photosensitivity; vasomotor instability	Histopathology of lymphoid tissue
Circulating endothelial cells	Associations with lymphoid neoplasia
Fibrin/fibrinoid deposition and polyarthritis in haemophilia	Beneficial effects of thoracic duct drainage
Virus-like inclusions in endothelial cells	Virus-like inclusions in lymphoid cells
Endothelial hypertrophy and proliferation	Lymphokines in synovial fluid
Primary 'endothelial' hypotheses (Gross; Le Roy)	Primary 'lymphoid' hypotheses (Burnet)

recirculation (Dumonde et at, 1977; Dumonde, 1978a).

There are many indications that inflammatory rheumatic diseases are associated with regulatory disturbances of both lymphoid and microvascular function (Table 14.8; Dumonde & Steward, 1978). The lesions of rheumatoid disease appear to involve the selective accumulation and local activation of lymphocytes as in sustained local reactions of type IV hypersensitivity; however, there is no evidence for the persistence of extrinsic antigen at sites of chronic inflammation and the most reasonable hypothesis is that pathophysiological alterations in the migratory behaviour of lymphocytes and in lymphocyte–endothelial interactions may play an important part in the persistence and distribution of inflammatory rheumatic lesions.

This hypothesis of lymphoendothelial dysfunction is illustrated in Figure 14.2 which proposes the existence of a body system concerned with regulating the traffic and activation of recirculatory lymphocytes in connection with their passage through microvascular endothelium (Dumonde, 1978a, b). This 'lymphoendothelial system' (Dumonde et al, 1983) will clearly involve close physiological interactions between lymphocytes and endothelial cells, a situation which could so easily be disturbed by abnormalities of the lymphocyte, abnormalities of the endothelial cell, or abnormalities affecting the plasma milieu in which these interactions take place (Fig. 14.2). Virus infections present themselves as obvious candidates for inducing lymphoendothelial dysfunction in predisposed individuals. Thus many viruses are known to replicate within both lymphocytes and endothelial cells and to integrate themselves into the lymphocyte genome; virus infections can thereby alter lymphocyte function (Denman, 1979) and may also induce alterations in receptors for immunological reactants on endothelial cells (Cines et al, 1982). It is of particular interest that where virus-like inclusions have been observed in rheumatic tissues, it is the vascular endothelial cells which figure prominently in these descriptions. In health, microvascular endothelium is subject to continued onslaught by infective, toxic as well as haemodynamic factors; and normal endothelial repair mechanisms are known to involve increased mitosis following injury (Payling Wright, 1971). In bacterial infections, endotoxins released into the circulation may cause both lymphocyte activation and vascular endothelial damage; in endotoxic shock, vascular endothelial cells appear in the circulation (Payling Wright & Giacometti, 1972); vascular endothelial cells have even been detected in the circulation of rheumatoid subjects (H. Payling Wright, personal communication, 1976). The 'rheumatoid' response is compatible with a failure of feedback control of the activation of recirculatory lymphocytes to stimuli which would otherwise elicit only a self-limiting or subclinical lymphocyte activation episode, at or shortly after the transmural passage of cells through postcapillary venule endothelium, particularly in subcutis, subsynovium and lymphoid tissue. This concept of lymphoendothelial dysfunction may be said to bring together the vascular and lymphoid theories of pathogenesis against a background of experimental and clinicopathological evidence for dysfunction of both lymphoid and microvascular systems. On this basis a variety of infectious episodes, many of which could be subclinical, might well precipitate reactive clinical lymphoendothelial dysfunction at a distance from portals of entry of micro-organisms, without needing to postulate the retention of

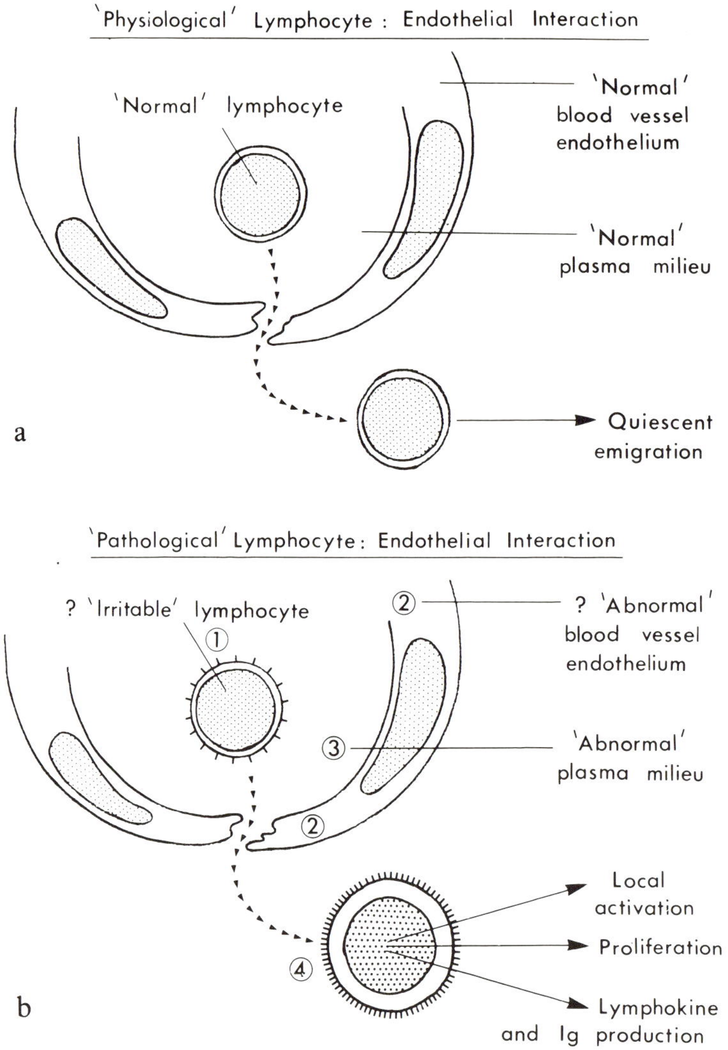

Fig. 14.2 The hypothesis of lymphoendothelial dysfunction in rheumatic disease. Diagrammatic representation of a proposed body system (the 'lymphoendothelial system') which is envisaged as regulating the traffic and activation of recirculatory lymphocytes through microvascular endothelium within lymphoid tissue and at widely distributed sites outside the lymphoid itself (e.g. subcutis: synovium). The 'system' is viewed as ensuring that when lymphocytes are entering extravascular connective tissue they will normally remain quiescent and migrate away from the site of transmural passage (a).

The diagrams depict the essential differences envisaged between lymphocyte behaviour when the lymphoendothelial system is 'normal' and when it is 'disturbed' by regulatory defects.

Regulatory disturbances in lymphocyte: endothelial interaction (b) could arise by virtue of:

(1) primary 'disease' of the lymphocyte (e.g. aberrant C-type virus expression; hormonal disturbance)

or (2) primary 'disease' of vascular endothelial cells (e.g. paramyxovirus or other infections; bacterial toxins; vasomotor or pharmacological abnormalities)

or (3) primary 'disease' of the milieu or environment in which these cellular interactions take place (e.g. presence of vasoactive mediators, immune complexes, etc. in the plasma)

— leading to:

(4) failure to keep lymphocytes 'quiet' during emigration (b).

Rheumatoid arthritis and allied rheumatic diseases are then viewed, not as 'primary' diseases of the connective tissue, but as disorders of the lymphocyte traffic which connective tissue carries. For example, the multiple actions of lymphokines on all major cell types in connective tissue could offer many opportunities for abnormally activated lymphocytes to set in motion the mechanisms which could lead to chronic inflammation at certain 'risk' sites of reactive pathology.

specific microbial antigens at widely distributed reactive sites of rheumatic pathology.

Pathophysiology of leucocyte interactions: the 'interleukin' hypothesis

'Superimposed' upon a 'basic' dysregulation of lymphocyte–endothelial interactions could well be additional defects in leucocytic interactions, which are implicated in the extravascular control of the inflammatory process. In the rheumatic diseases, various features of leucocyte dysfunction have long been sought, including abnormalities of chemotactic and phagocytic capacity (Wilkinson, 1982; Hurst et al, 1983), of arachidonic acid oxygenation pathways and other features of oxidative metabolism (Youssef & Baron, 1983), and of the representation of difference classes of white cells in blood and inflammatory exudates (Dumonde & Jasani, 1978). More recent approaches are illustrated by the 'interleukin' hypothesis which ascribes rheumatoid inflammation to defects in T lymphocyte–macrophage interaction, including the over-production of interleukin 1 (IL1) by macrophages together with an HLA-DR-linked propensity of antigen-presenting cells to overstimulate the production of interleukin 2 (IL2) by helper T cells (Janossy et al, 1981). The end result of failure of feedback mechanisms normally regulating extravascular white cell interactions is then viewed in terms of uncontrolled or imbalanced lymphokine production at sites of articular inflammation, leading to the known phenomena of macrophage accumulation and activation, granuloma formation, fibrosis and cartilage erosion (Krane et al, 1982).

Whether one views lymphocyte–endothelial or interleucocytic interactions as inherent, induced or linked features of rheumatic disease, these considerations illustrate growing interest in devising pathophysiological theories of rheumatic inflammation which allow an 'escape' from the restrictive concept of anti-microbial specificity. At this stage it is sufficient to point out the many current advances in molecular and cellular immunopharmacology, which may be expected to illustrate how a wide range of environmental stimuli may well trigger the onset of rheumatic inflammation in the susceptible subject (Hadden et al, 1983).

New genetic approaches

In this section we refer briefly to certain advances in human and microbial genetics which may bear upon the question of whether *specific* host–microbe interactions are involved in the genesis of 'class 4' inflammatory rheumatic diseases.

Over the past decade many idiopathic rheumatic diseases have been associated with one or other gene product of the major histocompatibility complex, and for the possession of any single HLA gene product, susceptibility to a rheumatic disease has been expressed as a relative risk which varies from about 100-fold for ankylosing spondylitis and HLA-B27, to about four-fold for rheumatoid arthritis and HLA-DR4 (Svejgaard et al, 1983). Prior to 1982 the favoured immunological interpretation was that a true susceptibility-gene for a given disease was more or less 'linked' to a single MHC gene which itself was expected to control induction, regulation or expression of an antigen-specific immunological response (Bodmer, 1980). It now appears that disease susceptibility may be more specifically related to combinations of alleles at different MHC loci ('supratypes') than to single MHC gene products, and that some of these combinations may include genes involved in the expression of complement components (Dawkins et al, 1983). Moreover there is a growing view that HLA-B and even HLA-A region gene products may contribute to general immunological reactivity and that the human immune response or immune suppression genes may not be associated exclusively with the HLA-D region (Moller, 1983). On this basis the concept of multiple genetic determinants of susceptibility to disease is more compatible with the operation of a variety of triggering factors than with a specific immunological stimulus initiating each disease syndrome (Brewerton, 1979).

Advances in microbial genetics and recombinant DNA research now indicate that transfer of genetic information between different species of prokaryotic organisms and from prokaryotes to eukaryotic cells may occur more frequently than thought hitherto (Williamson, 1980–1982). In the present context this carries two implications. First, if under normal epidemiological circumstances one kind of prokaryote (e.g. a bacterium) might acquire characteristics of another, the search for specific microbial agents as triggering factors in rheumatic disease could become almost a semantic problem. Second, if eukaryotic cells can acquire and express prokaryotic genomes (e.g. by transfection with viral vectors), then genetic factors determining disease susceptibility may be quite different from those determining the immune response to a single exogeneous antigen. As Weatherall has pointed out recently, the scope of the 'new genetics' is immense (Weatherall, 1982) and it is likely that nucleic acid probe techniques, currently applicable to the antenatal diagnosis of single-gene disorders, will be applied to the analysis of conditions where multiple genes determine disease susceptibility or expression. On this basis we may anticipate that parallel advances in human genetics and microbial genetics will provide the field of infection and rheumatic disease with a further route of 'escape' from the constraints applied by theories of antigen-specific immunopathology.

Identification of precipitating factors

This discussion leads to the question of whether it may be possible to identify those factors which initiate or precipitate the onset or relapse of inflammatory rheumatic disease in individual subjects or groups or subjects sharing some common (genetic or environmental) character.

Many lines of evidence imply that these diseases are the consequence of a multifactorial sequence, where the identity of the terminal or precipitating factor may be established for certain individuals or for lesions at certain sites (e.g. relapse of rheumatoid disease or ankylosing spondylitis following infections or immunisations; and the occurence of rheumatoid nodules at sites of persistent trauma). It seems likely that systemic infections may act as important precipitating agents by their two-fold action on both lymphoid and vascular systems; and careful clinical enquiry may reveal whether relapse of inflammatory rheumatic disease, such as rheumatoid arthritis or ankylosing spondylitis, in an individual subject, is regularly preceded by an identifiable infection through one or other major portals of entry. By such judicious clinical and laboratory study of relapsing rheumatic disease, it may be possible to determine whether certain patients show concordance or discordance between form of precipitating event and form of relapse. It is likely that certain types of infection will prove to be rare as precipitating factors but that others could be highlighted: such information might lead to the design of a selective microbiological and immunological screening programme for the assessment of patients who relapse without yielding clinical clues as to the nature of the precipitating event. On this basis the identification of certain microbial agents in precipitating relapses of ('class 4') inflammatory rheumatic disease may then be viewed as having the sort of implications for the clinical management, and perhaps prevention, of clinical relapse as did the identification of the aetiological role of group A streptococci in rheumatic fever (a 'class 3' association; see Table 14.5).

It is thus to relapse (De Vere Tyndall et al, 1984) rather than to onset (Lewis-Faning, 1950) of inflammatory rheumatic disease that such enquiries would seem to be particularly appropriate. It might be anticipated that precipitating events could act by neuroendocrine, vasomotor, autopharmacological, as well as immunological mechanisms; and that in any one patient the identity of the precipitating factor might vary from one relapse to another. Thus it would seem relevant to determine whether there are regulatory defects of both lymphoid and microvascular function in response to the action of different classes of autopharmacological mediators. Characterisation of the individual rheumatic subject in terms of the pathophysiology of both lymphoid and microvascular system may have important implications in terms of health care; for example, these approaches might facilitate the recognition of 'antirheumatic' drugs with selective value in correcting the homeostatic defects implied by this discussion.

Microbial infection in the multifactorial aetiology and pathogenesis of rheumatic disease

It therefore seems logical to view the role of microbial infection as part of the multifactorial aetiology of inflammatory rheumatic disease (Table 14.9) and to view the investigation of this field as a multidisciplinary exercise. To the immunologist, the part played by potential predisposing factors

Table 14.9 The multifactorial aetiology of inflammatory rheumatic disease

PREDISPOSING FACTORS	
Genes on the 6th chromosome	Genes on other chromosomes
Low affinity antibody diathesis	Diathesis for low threshold of autoimmune responses (rheumatoid factor, ANA, etc.)
Disturbed 'intrinsic' regulation of idiotypic networks	Disturbed 'intrinsic' regulation of T-cell activation
Lymphoendothelial disorder	Dysregulation of leucocyte interactions
Disturbed autopharmacological, neuroendocrine or metabolic responses to (microbial) stimuli	Homeostatic disorders of haematological responses to intravascular stimuli
Pathophysiological disorder affecting autonomic (neurovascular) control mechanisms	Abnormal reactivity of vascular endothelium to toxins and to inflammatory mediators
PRECIPITATING EVENT	
Subclinical microbial infection viewed as terminal event in a 'catastrophe' theory of the onset or relapse of inflammatory rheumatic disease	

such as a tendency to exhibit anti-globulin, antinuclear or other autoimmune responses to microbial stimuli, still needs clarification; this is true also of the role played by regulatory defects of the idiotype network system, of the control of antibody affinity, and of the control of specific cell-mediated immunity. To the microbiologist and microbial geneticist the challenge of inflammatory rheumatic disease presents an opportunity to apply recent advances in microbial taxonomy and in techniques of molecular microbiology to define the nature and phenotypic stability of those infective agents which may circumvene or evade the immune response or which may induce adverse reactions in the host. For the experimental pathologist or pharmacologist the study of these diseases has stimulated new ideas on how the inflammatory response may be controlled, and how it may be perturbed by environmental stimuli, microbial or otherwise; the parallel concept of adverse reactions to drugs and to microbial products may well have a pharmacological interpretation and these investigations should contribute to an understanding of the rheumatoid and lupus diatheses. The epidemiologist will naturally wish to consider whether the parallel study of infectious and rheumatic diseases will throw light upon differences in the severity or prevalence of rheumatic disease patterns in different communities; and the nosologist will wish to design more closely the clinical, diagnostic and therapeutic criteria which separate one rheumatic syndrome from another. The human geneticist will be expected to simplify the relationships between defined disease syndromes (or their stages of severity) and the prevalence of combinations of HLA types; at the same time the molecular biologist will be designing DNA or RNA probes with which to explore the host genome and the cell biologist will be seeking further molecular explanations of how prokaryotic or viral agents may permanently alter eukaryotic host-cell behaviour. A principal clinical challenge may lie in the investigation of factors which precipitate relapse of chronic inflammatory rheumatic disease as well as in the investigation of vascular and lymphoid responses to known infections. The multifactorial aetiology of inflammatory rheumatic diseases merits multidisciplinary approaches in which the role of microbial infection must still be regarded as one of the most important growing points in investigative rheumatology.

REFERENCES

Aaronson S A, Stephenson J R 1974 Widespread natural occurrence of high titres of neutralizing antibodies to a specific class of endogenous mouse Type-C virus. Proceedings of the National Academy of Sciences USA 71:1957

Abdou N I, Wall H, Lindsley H B, Halsey J F, Suzuki T 1981 Network theory in autoimmunity. In vitro suppression of serum anti-DNA antibody binding to DNA by anti-idiotypic antibody in systemic lupus erythematosus. Journal of Clinical Investigation 67:1297

Abruzzo J L, Christian C L, 1961 The induction of a rheumatoid factor-like substance in rabbits. Journal of Experimental Medicine 114:791

Aho K, Raunio V 1982 EB virus and rheumatoid arthritis: new insights into their interrelation. Medical Biology 60:49

Aho K, Ahvonen P, Alkio P, Lassus A, Sairanen E, Sievers K, Tiilikainen A 1975 HLA 27 in reactive arthritis

following infection. Annals of the Rheumatic Diseases 34 (Suppl:) 29
Aho K, Ahvonen P, Lasus A, Sievers K, Tiilikainen A 1976 Yersinia arthritis and related diseases: clinical and immunogenetic implications. In Dumonde D C (ed) Infection and immunology in the rheumatic diseases. Blackwell, London, Ch 44, p 341
Aitcheson C T, Wilson G L, Ferell P B, Tan E M 1983 Frequency of transforming Epstein–Barr virus in oropharyngeal secretions of rheumatoid arthritis patients. Intervirology 19:135
Alarcon G S, Bocanegra T S, Gotuzza E, Hinostroza S, Carrillo C, Vasey F B, et al 1981 Reactive arthritis associated with Brucellosis: HLA studies. Journal of Rheumatology 8:621
Alarcon-Segovia D 1969 Drug-induced lupus syndromes. Mayo Clinic Proceedings 44:664
Alexander K, Edwards C, Misko I S, Geczy A F, Bashir M V, Edmonds J P, 1981 The distribution of a specific HLA-B27-associated cell surface component on the tissues of patients with ankylosing spondylitis. Clinical and Experimental Immunology 45:158
Almeida J D, Waterson A P 1969 Immune complexes in hepatitis. Lancet ii:983
Alpers J H, Steward M W, Soothill J F 1972 Differences in immune elimination in inbred mice. The role of low affinity antibody. Clinical and Experimental Immunology 12:121
Alpert E, Isselbacher K J, Schur P H 1971 The pathogensis of arthritis associated with viral hepatitis. Complement component studies. New England Journal of Medicine 285:185
Alspaugh M A, Tan E M 1976 Serum antibody in rheumatoid arthritis reactive with a cell-associated antigen. Arthritis and Rheumatism 19:711
Alspaugh M A, Henle G, Lennett E T, Henle W 1981 Elevated levels of antibodies to Epstein-Barr virus antigens in sera and synovial fluid of patients with rheumatoid arthritis. Journal of Clinical Investigation 67:1134
Amor B, Kahan A, Lecoq F, Delbarre F 1972 Le test de transformation lymphoblastiques par les antigenes bedsoniens (TTL). Son interet nosologique et diagnostique dans le syndrome de Fiessenger-Leroy-Reiter. Revue de Rheumatologie 39:671
Archer J R 1981 Search for cross-reactivity between HLA-B27 and Klebsiella pneumoniae. Annals of the Rheumatic Diseases 40:400
Avakian H, Welsh K, Ebringer A, Entwistle C C 1980 Ankylosing spondylitis, HLA-B27 and Klebsiella. II. Cross-reactivity studies with human tissue typing sera. British Journal of Experimental Pathology 61:92
Bacon P A, Cracchoilo A, Bluestone R, Goldberg L S 1973 Cell mediated immunity to synovial antigens in rheumatoid arthritis. Lancet ii:699
Bacon P A, Doherty S M, Zuckerman A J 1975 Hepatitis-B antibody in polymyalgia rheumatica. Lancet ii:476
Bradwick P A, Bluestein H G, Zvaifler N J, Depper J M, Seegmiller J E 1980 Altered regulation of Epstein-Barr virus induced lymphoblast proliferation in rheumatoid arthritis lymphoid cells. Arthritis and Rheumatism 23:626
Beaulieu A D, Rousseau F, Israel-Assayag E, Roy R 1983 Klebsiella related antigens in ankylosing spondylitis. Journal of Rheumatology 10:102
Bennet J C 1978 The infectious aetiology of rheumatoid arthritis. Arthritis and Rheumatism 21:531
Bisno A L, Stollerman G H 1975 Streptococcal antibodies in the diagnosis of rheumatic fever. In: Cohen A S (ed) Laboratory diagnostic procedures in the rheumatic diseases, 2nd Edn. Little Brown & Co, Boston, Ch 7, p 207
Bland J H, Phillips C A 1972 Etiology and pathogenesis of rheumatoid arthritis and related multisystem diseases. Seminars in Arthritis and Rheumatism 1 (4):339
Bodmer W F 1980 The HLA system and disease. The Oliver Sharpey Lecture, 1979. Journal of the Royal College of Physicians of London 14:43
Brandly C A, Jungherr E L (eds) 1960 Advances in Veterinary Science, 6. Academic Press, New York
Braun D G, Holm S E 1970 Streptococcal anti-group A precipitins in sera from patients with rheumatoid arthritis and acute glomerulonephritis. International Archives of Allergy and Applied Immunology, 37:216
Brav E A, Hench P S 1934 Tuberculous rheumatism. Journal of Bone and Joint Surgery 16:839
Brewerton D A (Ed.) 1975 Symposium on histocompatibility and rheumatic disease. Annals of the Rheumatic Diseases 34 (Suppl): 1
Brewerton D A 1979 Inherited susceptibility to rheumatic disease. Journal of the Royal Society of Medicine 71:331
Brewerton D A, James D C O 1975 The histocompatibility antigen (HLA-27) and disease. Seminars in Arthritis and Rheumatism 4 (3):191
Brewerton D A, Hart F D, Nicholls A L 1973 Ankylosing spondylitis and HLA-B27. Lancet i:904
Brodie B C 1818 Pathological and surgical observations on diseases of the joints. Longman, London
Brodie T D, Ehresmann G R 1983 Salmonella Dublin arthritis: An initial case presentation. Journal of Rheumatology 10:144
Brown K A 1983 Electrophoretic analysis of lymphocytes and polymorphonuclear cells in rheumatoid arthritis. In: Maroudas A, Holborow E J (eds) Studies in joint disease, Vol 2. London, p 1
Burnet F M 1959 The clonal selection theory of acquired immunity. Cambridge University Press, London
Burrell C J, Dickson J D, Gerber H, McCormick J N, Marmion B P 1972 Rheumatoid arthritis, rheumatoid factor and tests for Australia or hepatitis-associated antigen. British Medical Journal iv:23
Burssens A, Dequeker J, Odeurs W 1972 Australian antigen in rheumatoid arthritis. British Medical Journal iv:549
Cameron F H, Russell P J, Sullivan J, Geczy A F 1983 Is a Klebsiella plasmid involved in the aetiology of ankylosing spondylitis in HLA-B27 positive individuals? Molecular Immunology 20:563
Capell R, Schleuderberg A, Gifford R H, Horstmann D M 1974 Characterization of a human acute phase protein in association with rubella virus infection. Journal of Experimental Medicine 139:497
Catalano M A, Carson D A, Niederman J C, Feorino P, Vaughan J M 1980 Antibody to the rheumatoid arthritis nuclear antigen: its relationship to in vivo Epstein–Barr virus infection. Journal of Clinical Investigation 65:1238
Catterall R D 1976 The role of microbial infection in Reiter's syndrome. In: Dumonde D C (ed) Infection and immunology in the rheumatic diseases. Blackwell, London, Ch 19, p 147
Chantler J K, Ford D K, Tingle A J 1982 Persistent rubella infection and rubella-associated arthritis. Lancet i:1323
Chou S M 1970 Picornavirus-like crystals in subacute

polymyositis. Neurology 20:205
Christian C L, Phillips P E 1973 Viruses and autoimmunity. American Journal of Medicine 54:616
Christian C L, Phillips P E, Williams R C (eds) 1971 Atypical virus infections: Possible relevance to animal models and rheumatic disease. Arthritis Foundation Conference Series No. 15. Arthritis Foundation, New York
Cines D B, Lyss A P, Bina M, Corkey R, Kelfalides N A, Friedman H M 1982 Fc and C3 receptors induced by Herpes simplex virus on cultured human endothelial cells. Journal of Clinical Investigation 69:123
Clarris B J, Fraser J R E, Rodda S J 1974 Effect of cell-bound hyalonic acid on the infectivity of Newcastle disease virus for human syncvial cells in vitro. Annals of the Rheumatic Diseases 33:240
Clarris B J, Doherty R L, Fraser J R E, French E L, Muirden K D 1975 Epidemic polyarthritis: a cytological, virological and immunochemical study. Australia and New Zealand Journal of Medicine 5:450
Clasener H 1972 Pathogenicity of the L-phase of bacteria. Annual Reviews of Microbiology 26:55
Clasener H A L, Biersteker P J 1969 Significance of diphtheroids isolated from synovial membranes of patients with rheumatoid arthritis. Lancet ii:1031
Cohn M 1981 (Commentary) Conversations with Niels Kaj Jerne on immune regulation: associations versus network regulation. Cellular Immunology 61:425
Cole B C, Cassell G H 1979 Mycoplasma infections as models of chronic joint inflammation. Arthritis and Rheumatism 22:1375
Cole B C, Ward J R, Smith C B 1973 Studies on the infectious aetiology of rheumatoid arthritis. Arthritis and Rheumatism, 16, 191
Cole B C, Golightly-Rowland L, Ward J R 1976 Arthritis of mice induced by Mycoplasma arthritidis. Humoral antibody and lymphocyte responses of CBA mice. Annals of the Rheumatic Diseases 35 (1):14
Cosenza A 1976 Detection of anti-idiotype reactive cells in the response to phosphoryl choline. European Journal of Immunology 6:114
Cossart Y E, Field A M, Cant W, Widdows D 1975 Parvovirus-like particles in human sera. Lancet i:72
Crocker J F S, Ghose T, Rozee K, Woodbury J, Stevenson B 1974 Arthritis, deformities and runting in C5-deficient mice injected with human rheumatoid arthritis synovium. Journal of Clinical Pathology 27:122
Cromartie W J 1981 Arthropathic properties of peptidoglycan-polysaccharide complexes of microbial origin. In: Deicher H, Schulz L C L (eds) Arthritis: Models and mechanisms. Springer Verlag, Berlin, p 24
Csonka G W 1972 Reiter's disease. British Journal of Hospital Medicine 7:8
Dawkins R L, Mastaglia F L 1973 Cell-mediated cytotoxicity to muscle in polymyositis. New England Journal of Medicine 268:434
Dawkins R L, Christiansen F T, Kay P H, Garlepp M, McCluskey J, Hollingsworth P N, Zilko P J 1983 Disease associations with complotypes, supratypes and haplotypes. Immunological Reviews 70:5
Dawson M H, Boots R L 1939 Arthritis associated with lymphogranuloma venereum. Journal of the American Medical Association 113:1162
Dehoratius R J, Messner R P 1975 Lymphocytotoxic antibodies in relatives of patients with systemic lupus erythematosus. Journal of Clinical Investigation 5:1254
Deicher H, Schulz L Cl (Eds.) 1981 Arthritis: Models and Mechanisms. Springer-Verlag, Berlin
Deinard A S, Venters M D, Bilka P J, Herrmann K L, Page A R 1974 Rubella antibody titres in rheumatoid arthritis. Lancet i:526
Delbarre F, Amor B 1976 Ankylosing spondylitis and Reiter's syndrome: genetic and microbiological studies. In: Dumonde D C (ed) Infection and immunology in the rheumatic diseases. Blackwell, London, Ch 21, p 159
Denman A M 1978 Rheumatoid arthritis — a virus disease? Journal of Clinical Pathology 31 (Suppl 12):132
Denman A M 1979 Lymphocyte function and virus infection. Journal of Clinical Pathology 32 (Suppl 13):39
Denman A M 1981 Viruses and autoimmune diseases. In: Holborow E J (ed) Clinics in immunology and allergy: Autoimmunity, Vol 1. Saunders, London, p 17
Denman A M, Pinder M, Pelton B K, Kinsley M 1975 Virus-lymphocyte interactions and the aetiology of connective tissue disease. In: Silvestri L G (ed) The immunological basis of connective tissue disorders. North-Holland, Amsterdam, p 3
Dent P 1971 The pathogenesis of chronic and congenital virus infections. In: Christian C L, Phillips P E, Williams R C (eds) Atypical virus infections: Possible relevance to animal models and rheumatic disease. Arthritis Foundation Conference Series No 15. Arthritis Foundation, New York
Depper J M, Bluestein H G, Zvaifler N 1981 Impaired regulation of EBV-induced lymphocyte proliferation in rheumatoid arthritis is due to a T cell defect. Journal of Immunology 127:1899
Depper J M, Zvaifler N J, Bluestein H G 1982 Oropharyngeal Epstein-Barr virus excretion in rheumatoid arthritis. Arthritis and Rheumatism 25:427
De Vere Tyndall A, Bacon T, Perry R, Tyrell D A J, Denman A M, Ansell B M 1984. Infection and interferon production in systemic juvenile chronic arthritis: a prospective study. Annals of the Rheumatic Diseases, 43:1
Dixon F J 1963 The role of antigen-antibody complexes in disease. Harvey Lectures Series, 1962–3. Academic Press, New York
Drew R A 1972 Erysipelothrix arthritis in pigs as a comparative model for rheumatoid arthritis. Proceedings of the Royal Society of Medicine 65:994
Dubois E L (Ed) 1974 Lupus erythematosus, 2nd edn. University of Southern California Press, Los Angeles
Dubois E L 1974a Malignancies in SLE. In: Dubois E L (ed) Systemic lupus erythematosus, 2nd Edn. University of Southern California Press, Los Angeles, p 639
Dubois E L, Arterberry J D 1974 Infection as a possible cause of systemic lupus erythematosus. In: Dubois E L (ed) Systemic lupus erythematosus, 2nd Edn. University of Southern California Press, Los Angeles, p 109
Duffy J, Lidsky M D, Sharp J T, Davis J S, Person D A, Hollinger F B, Min K-W 1976 Polyarthritis, polyarteritis and hepatitis B. Medicine 55:19
Dumonde D C 1966 Tissue-specific antigens. Advances in Immunology 5:266
Dumonde D C (ed) 1976 Infection and immunology in the rheumatic diseases. Blackwell, London
Dumonde D C 1978a The rheumatological significance of lymphokines. In: Dumonde D C, Jasani M K (eds) Recognition of anti-rheumatic drugs. MTP Press, Lancaster, p 167
Dumonde D C 1978b The paradox of infection and immunology in multiple sclerosis. In: Rose F C (ed)

Clinical neuroimmunology. Blackwell, Oxford, p 275
Dumonde D C 1985 Microbial agents in the pathogenesis of uveitis syndromes. In preparation
Dumonde D C, Glynn L E 1962 The production of arthritis in rabbits by an immunological reaction to fibrin. British Journal of Experimental Pathology 42:373
Dumonde D C, Glynn L E 1965 The reaction of guinea pigs to autologous and heterologous fibrin implants. Journal of Pathology and Bacteriology 90:649
Dumonde D C, Jasani M K (eds) 1978 Recognition of anti-rheumatic drugs. MTP Press, Lancaster
Dumonde D C, Richards T J 1981 The significance of immunological investigations in cardiovascular disease. In: Lessof M H (ed) Immunology of cardiovascular disease. Marcel Dekker, New York, p 75
Dumonde D C, Steward M W 1978 The role of microbial infection in rheumatic disease. In: Scott J T (ed) Copeman's textbook of the rheumatic diseases, 5th Edn. Churchill Livingstone, Edinburgh, p 222
Dumonde D C, Kelly R H, Morley J 1976 Lymphoid and microvascular dysfunction in experimental models of rheumatoid inflammation. In: Dumonde D C (ed) Infection and immunology in the rheumatic diseases. Blackwell, London, Ch 47, p 375
Dumonde D C, Jones E H, Kelly R H, Oates C M 1977 Experimental models of rheumatoid inflammation. In: Experimental models of chronic inflammatory diseases. Bayer Symposium VI. Springer-Verlag, Heidelberg
Dumonde D C, Hamblin A S, Kasp-Grochowska E, Pulley M S, Wolstencroft R A 1983 Lymphokines and the lymphoendothelial system: an illustration of immuno-regulatory integration. In: Fabris N, Garaci E, Hadden J, Mitchison N A (eds) Immunoregulation. Plenum Press, New York, p 177
Dumonde D C, Kasp-Grochowska E, Graham E, Sanders M D, Faure J-P, De Kozak Y et al 1982 Anti-retinal autoimmunity and circulating immune complexes in patients with retinal vasculitis. Lancet ii: 787
Duthie J J R, Stewart S M, McBride W H 1976 Do diphtheroids cause rheumatoid arthritis? In: Dumonde D C (ed) Infection and immunology in the rheumatic diseases. Blackwell, London, Ch 22, p 171
Ebert J 1974 The experimental approach to inflammation. In: Zweifach B W, Grant L, McClusky R T (eds) The inflammatory process. Academic Press, New York, p 3
Ebringer A, Cowling P, Ngwa Suh N, James D C O, Ebringer R W 1976 Cross-reactivity between Klebsiella Aerogenes and B27 lymphocyte antigens as an aetiological factor in ankylosing spondylitis. In: Daussett J, Svejgaard A (eds) HLA and disease INSERM, Paris, p 27
Ebringer R W, Cowdell D R, Cowling P, Ebringer A 1978 Sequential studies in ankylosing spondylitis: association of Klebsiella pneumoniae with active disease. Annals of the Rheumatic Diseases 27:146
Editorial 1984. The viral aetiology of rheumatoid arthritis. Lancet i:772
Edmonds J, Macauley D, Tydall A, Liew M, Alexander K, Geczy A, Bashir H 1981 Lymphocytotoxicity of anti-Klebsiella antisera in ankylosing spondylitis and related arthropathies. Arthritis and Rheumatism 24:1
Elson C J, Crawford D M, Bucknell R A, Allen C, Thompson J D, Epstein M A et al 1979 Infection with EB virus and rheumatoid arthritis. Lancet i:105
Enlow R W, Bias W B, Bluestone R 1982 Human lymphocyte response to selected infectious agents in Reiter's syndrome and ankylosing spondylitis. Rheumatology International 1:171
Epstein M A, Achong B G 1979 (eds) The Epstein–Barr virus. Springer-Verlag, Berlin
Evatt B L et al 1983 Antibodies to human T cell leukaemia virus-associated membrane antigens in haemophiliacs: evidence for infection before 1980. Lancet ii:698
Fain A G, Tenenbaum J, Stein J L 1979 Clinical forms of meningococcal arthritis: A study of five cases. Journal of Rheumatology 6:567
Feld R, Fornasier V L, Bombardier C, Hastings D E 1982 Septic arthritis due to Saccharomyces species in a patient with chronic rheumatoid arthritis. Journal of Rheumatology 9:637
Fenner F 1976 The classification and nomenclature of viruses. Journal of General Virology 31:463
Fenner F, McAuslan B R, Mims C A, Sambrook J, White D O 1974 The biology of animal viruses, 2nd Edn. Academic Press, London
Ferrell P, Aitcheson C, Pearson G, Tan E 1981 Sero-epidemiological study of relationships between Epstein–Barr virus and rheumatoid arthritis. Journal of Clinical Investigation 67:681
Fong S, Vaughan J H, Carson D A 1983 Two different rheumatoid factor-producing cell populations distinguished by the mouse erythrocyte receptor and responsiveness to polyclonal B cell activators. Journal of Immunology 130:162
Ford D K 1966 Reiter's syndrome. In: Hollander J L (ed) Arthritis and allied conditions, 7th Edn. Henry Kimpton, London, Ch 60, p 1001
Ford D K, Oh J O 1965 Use of 'synovial' cell cultures in the search for virus in rheumatoid arthritis. Arthritis and Rheumatism 8:1047
Ford D K, Henderson, Elizabeth, Price G E, Stein H B 1977 Yersinia-related arthritis in the Pacific Northwest. Arthritis and Rheumatism 20:1226
Ford D K, da Roza D M, Schulzer M 1982 The specificity of synovial mononuclear cell responses to microbiological antigens in Reiter's syndrome. Journal of Rheumatology 9:561
Ford D K, da Roza D M, Reid G D, Chantler J K, Tingle A J 1982 Synovial mononuclear cell responses to rubella antigen in rheumatoid arthritis and unexplained persistent knee arthritis. Journal of Rheumatology 9 (3):420
Fournie G J, Lambert P H, Miescher P A 1974 Release of DNA in circulating blood and induction of anti-DNA antibodies after injection of bacterial lipo-polysaccharides. Journal of Experimental Medicine 140:1189
Fraser J R, Tait B, Aaskov J G, Cunningham A L 1980 Possible genetic determinants in epidemic polyarthritis caused by Ross River virus infection. Australian and New Zealand Journal of Medicine 10:597
Fraser J R, Cunningham A L, Clarris B J, Asskov J G, Leach R 1981 Cytology of synovial effusions in epidemic polyarthritis. Australian and New Zealand Journal of Medicine 11:168
Fresco R 1970 Virus-like particles in systemic lupus erythematosus. New England Journal of Medicine 282:1231
Friedman H, Klein T W, Szentivanyi A 1982 Immunomodulation by bacteria and their products. Plenum Press, New York
Geczy A F, Bashir H V, Edmonds J P 1981 Klebsiella isolates which cross-react with an HLA-B27 associated determinant do not share capsular serotypes or

bacteriophage types. Journal of Rheumatology 8:1023
Geczy A F, Alexander K, Bashir H V, Edmonds J P, Upfold L, Sullivan J 1983 HLA-B27, Klebsiella and ankylosing spondylitis: biological and chemical studies. Immunological Reviews 70:23
Gellner D, Franklin E C, Frangione B 1980 Anti-idiotypic activity in the IgM fractions of mixed cryoglobulins. Journal of Immunology 125:1530
Gerber P, Lucus S, Wonoyama M, Perlin E, Goldstein L 1972 Oral excretion of Epstein-Barr virus by healthy subjects of patients with infectious mononucleosis. Lancet: 988
Ginsburg I, Zor U, Floman Y 1977 Experimental models of streptococcal arthritis: pathogenetic role of streptococcal products and prostaglandins and their modification by anti-inflammatory agents. In: Glynn L E, Schlumberger H D (eds) Experimental models of chronic inflammatory diseases. Bayer Symposium VI. Springer-Verlag, Berlin, p 256
Glynn L E, Schlumberger H D (eds) 1977 Experimental models of chronic inflammatory diseases. Springer-Verlag, Berlin
Gocke D J 1975 Extrahepatic manifestations of viral hepatitis. American Journal of the Medical Sciences 270:49
Gocke D J, Hsu K, Morgan C, Bombarieri S, Lockshin M, Christian C L 1970 Association between polyarteritis and Australia antigen. Lancet ii:1149
Godzeski C, Boyd R, Smith, Carol & Hamerman D 1978 Viral-like particles in co-cultivated rheumatoid synovial cells. Abstract III. 42nd Annual Meeting of the American Rheumatism Association
Goldman J A 1981 Patterns of gonococcal arthritis. Journal of Rheumatology 8 (5):707
Goldman M, Rose L M, Hochmann A, Lambert P H 1982 Deposition of idiotype-anti-idiotype immune complexes in renal glomeruli after polyclonal B-cell activation. Journal of experimental Medicine 155:1385
Good A E 1974 Reiter's disease: a review with special attention to cardiovascular and neurologic sequellae. Seminars in Arthritis and Rheumatism 3 (3):253
Grahame R, Armstrong R, Simmons N A, Mims C A, Wilton J M A, Laurent R 1981 Isolation of rubella virus from synovial fluid in five cases of seronegative arthritis. Lancet ii:649
Grahame R, Armstrong R, Simmons N, Wilton J M A, Dyson M, Laurent R, et al 1983 Chronic arthritis associated with the presence of intrasynovial rubella virus. Annals of the Rheumatic Diseases 42:2
Grayzel A I, Beck C 1970 Rubella infection of synovial cells and the resistance of cells derived from patients with rheumatoid arthritis. Journal of Experimental Medicine 131:367
Greenwood B M, Whittle H L 1976 The pathogenesis of meningococcal arthritis. In: Dumonde D C (ed) Infection and immunology in the rheumatic diseases. Blackwell, London, Ch 15, p 118
Griffiths M M, Spruance S L, Ogra P L, Thomson G R, DeWitt C W 1977 HLA and recurrent episodic arthropathy associated with rubella vaccination. Arthritis and Rheumatism 20:1192
Groopman J E, Gottleib M S 1983 AIDS: the widening gyre. Nature 303:575
Gross L 1940 The cardiac lesions in Libman–Sacks disease. With a consideration of its relationship to acute diffuse lupus erythematosus. American Journal of Pathology 16:375
Gutowska-Plachecka M, Polowiec Z, Abgarowicz T, Orlowska G, Luft S, Pazdur J, et al 1975 Syndromes of lymphoreticular proliferation in rheumatoid arthritis. VII European Rheumatism Congress. Scandinavian Journal of Rheumatology (Suppl 8): Abstract 14–01
Gyorkey F, Sinkovics J G, Min K W, Gyorkey P 1972 A morphologic study on the occurrence and distribution of structures resembling viral nucleocapsids in collagen diseases. American Journal of Medicine 53:148
Hadden J W, Chedid L, Dukor P, Spreafico F, Willoughby D (eds) 1983 Advances in immunopharmacology, Vol 2. Pergamon Press, Oxford
Hamerman D 1975 Evidence for an infectious etiology of rheumatoid arthritis. In: Perper E J (ed) Mechanism of tissue injury with reference to rheumatoid arthritis. Annals of the New York Academy of Sciences 256:25
Hamerman D, Gresser I & Smith C 1982 Isolation of cytomegalovirus from synovial cells of a patient with rheumatological arthritis. Journal of Rheumatology 9 (5):658
Hart 1978 Viruses in the aetiology of rheumatoid arthritis. PhD thesis, University of Edinburgh
Hart H, Marmion B P 1977 Rubella virus and rheumatoid arthritis. Annals of the Rheumatic Diseases 36:3
Hart H and Norval M 1980 Search for viruses in rheumatoid macrophage-rich synovial cell populations. Annals of the Rheumatic Diseases 39:159
Hart H, McCormick J N, Marmion B P 1979 Viruses and lymphocytes in rheumatoid arthritis. II. Examination of lymphocytes and sera from patients with rheumatoid arthritis for evidence of retrovirus infection. Annals of the Rheumatic Diseases 38:514
Hasler F, Bluestein H G, Zvaifler N J, Epstein L B 1983 Analysis of the defects responsible for the impaired regulation of Epstein–Barr virus-induced B cell proliferation by rheumatoid arthritis lymphocytes. I. Diminished gamma interferon production in response to autologous stimulation. Journal of Experimental Medicine 157:173
Henle W, Henle G E, Horwitz C A 1974 Epstein–Barr virus specific diagnostic tests in infectious mononucleosis. Human Pathology 5:551
Henle G, Koldovsky U, Koldovsky P, Henle W, Ackermann R, Haase G 1975 Multiple sclerosis-associated agent: neutralization of the agent by human sera. Infection and Immunity 12:1357
Henle G, Lennette E T, Alspaugh M A, Henle W 1979 Rheumatoid factor as a cause of positive reactions in tests for Epstein–Barr virus specific IgM antibodies. Clinical Experimental Immunology 36:415
Hicks J T, Aulakh G S, McGrath P P, Washington G C, Kim E, Alepa F P 1979 Search for Epstein–Barr and Type C oncornaviruses in systemic lupus erythematosus. Arthritis and Rheumatism 22:845
Horwitz D 1973 Impaired delayed hypersensitivity in systemic lupus erythematosus. Arthritis and Rheumatism 15:353
Houba V, Adam M, Malecek J, Teasserk B 1964 Delayed hypersensitivity and antibody response in rheumatoid arthritis. Experientia 20:522
Houston B D, Crouch M E, Finch R G 1980 Streptococcus MG-intermedius (Streptococcus milleri) septic arthritis in a patient with rheumatoid arthritis. Journal of Rheumatology 7:89
Hurst N P, Nuki G, Wallington T 1983 Functional defects

of monocyte C3b receptor-mediated phagocytosis in rheumatoid arthritis: evidence for an association with the appearance of a circulating population of non-specific esterase negative mononuclear phagocytes. Annals of the Rheumatic Diseases 42:487

Hyer F H, Gottleib N L 1978 Rheumatic disorders associated with viral infection. Seminars in Arthritis and Rheumatism 8 (1):17

Ingram D G, Cho H J 1974 Aleutian disease in mink: Virology, immunology and pathogenesis. Journal of Rheumatology 1:74

Jackle C, Leek J C, Olson D A, Robbins D L 1983 Septic arthritis due to Fusarium Solari. Journal of Rheumatology 10:151

Janossy G, Panayi G, Duke O, Bofill M, Poulter L W, Goldstein G 1981 Rheumatoid arthritis: a disease of T-lymphocyte/macrophage interaction. Lancet ii:839

Jerne N K 1974 Towards a network theory of the immune system. Annals of Immunology of the Pasteur Institute 125c:373

Kacaki J H, Balduzzi P C, Vaughan J H 1970 A study of rubella haemagglutination inhibition antibodies in rheumatoid arthritis. Clinical and Experimental Immunology 6:885

Kalliomaki J L, Halonen P 1975 The role of viruses in the aetiology of connective tissue diseases. Annals of Clinical Research 7:129

Kalliomaki J L, Halonen P, Salmi A 1975 Virus antibodies in serum and synovial fluid of patients with rheumatoid arthritis and other connective tissue disease. Annals of Rheumatic Diseases 34:43

Kantor F S 1976 Cellular immunity in microbial infections. In: Dumonde D C (ed) Infection and immunology in the rheumatic diseases Blackwell, London, Ch 3, p 13

Kantor T G, Tanner M 1962 Rubella arthritis and rheumatoid arthritis. Arthritis and Rheumatism 5:378

Kaplan H J 1983 Immunologic insights into the eye and uveitis. In: Kraus Mackin E, O'Connor G R (ed) Uveitis: pathophysiology and therapy. Thieme-Stratton, New York, p 231

Kaplan M H, Svec K H 1964 Immunological relation of streptococcal and tissue antigens. III. Presence in human sera of streptococcal antibody cross-reaction with heart tissue. Association with streptococcal infection, rheumatic fever and glomerulonephritis. Journal of Experimental Medicine 119:651

Katz F E, Steward M W 1975 The genetic control of antibody affinity in mice. Immunology 29:543

Keat A C, Maini R N, Nkwazi G C, Pegrum G D, Ridgeway G L, Scott J T 1978 Role of Chlamydia trachomatis and HLA-B27 in sexually acquired reactive arthritis. British Medical Journal 1:605

Keat A C, Scott J T, Ridgway G, Maini R N, Pegrum G D 1979. Sexually-acquired reactive arthritis. Annals of the Rheumatic Diseases 38:52

Keat A C, Thoma B J, Taylor-Robinson D, Pegrum G D, Maini R N, Scott J T 1980 Evidence of Chlamydia trachomatis infection in sexually-acquired reactive arthritis. Annals of the Rheumatic Diseases 39:431

Kelleher J F, Cuban N L C, Mortimer P D, Kamimura T 1983 The human serum 'parvovirus': a specific cause of aplastic crisis in hereditary spherocytosis. Journal of Paediatrics 102:720

Kelly R M, Wolstencroft R A 1974 Germinal centre proliferation in response to mitogenic lymphokines. Clinical and Experimental Immunology 18:321

Kindt T J, Sogan J 1977 The genetics of immunoglobulins. In: Glynn L E, Steward M W (eds) Textbook of immunochemistry. Wiley, London

Kingston D, Glynn L E 1971 A cross-reaction between Str. pyogenes and human fibroblasts, endothelial cells and astrocytes. Immunology 21:1003

Kinsella T D, Fritzler M J, McNeil D J 1983 Ankylosing spondylitis, a disease in search of microbes. Journal of Rheumatology 10:2

Klemperer P, Pollack A D, Baehr G 1942 Diffuse collagen disease: acute disseminated lupus erythematosus and diffuse scleroderma. Journal of the American Medical Association 119:331

Koopman W J, Schrohenloher R E 1980 Enhanced in vitro synthesis of IgM rheumatoid factor in rheumatoid arthritis. Arthritis and Rheumatism 23:988

Kousa M 1982 Evidence of chlamydial involvement in the development of arthritis. Scandinavian Journal of Infectious Diseases (Suppl) 32:116

Krane S M, Goldring S R, Dayer J-M 1982 Interactions among lymphocytes, monocytes and other synovial cells in the rheumatoid synovium. Lymphokines 7:75

Krawczynski K, Slusarczyk J, Brzosko W J, Nowoslawski A 1974 Viral-antigen: antibody complexes and the pathogenesis of degenerative vascular lesions. Advances in the Biosciences 12:435

Lansbury J, Joseph R R 1966 Serum sickness. In: Hollander J L (ed) Arthritis and allied conditions, 7th Edn. Kimpton, London, p 838

Larsen J H 1972 Human yersiniosis in Denmark. Scandinavian Journal of Immunology 1:412

Lee S L, Siegel M 1976 Systemic lupus erythematosus: epidemiological clues to pathogenesis. In: Dumonde D C (ed) Infection and immunology in the rheumatic diseases. Blackwell, London, Ch 40, p 307

Leino R, Kalliomaki J L 1974 Yersiniosis as an internal disease. Annals of Internal Medicine 81:458

Lerman S J, Nankervis G A, Heggie A D, Gold E 1971 A study of adolescent girls and young women given live attenuated virus vaccine (HPV-77: DE-5). Annals of Internal Medicine 74:67

Lerner R A, Dixon F J, Croker B P, Del Villano B C, Jenson F C, Kennel S J, McConahey P J 1974 The possible role of oncornaviruses in the etiology and pathogenesis of murine lupus. Advances in the Biosciences 12:356

Levo Y 1980 Nature of cryoglobulinaemia. Lancet i 285

Levo Y, Gorevic P D, Kassab H J. Zucher-Franklin D, Gigli I, Franklin E C 1977 Mixed cryoglobulinaemia — an immune complex disease often associated with hepatitis B virus infection. Transactions of the Association of American Pysicians 90:167

Levy J A 1974 Autoimmunity and neoplasia: the possible role of C-type viruses. American Journal of Clinical Pathology 62:258

Lewis R M, Tannebury W, Smith C, Schwartz R S 1974 C-type viruses in systemic lupus erythematosus. Nature 252:78

Lewis R M, Andre-Schwartz J, Harris G S, Hirsch M S, Black P H 1973 Canine systemic lupus erythematosus. Journal of Clincial Investigation 52:1893

Lewis-Faning E 1950 Report of a scientific advisory committee of the Empire Rheumatism Council into aetiological factors associated with rheumatoid arthritis.

Annals of the Rheumatic Diseases 9 (Suppl): 1
Linder E, Kivki P, Anderson L C 1979 Autoantibody to intermediate filaments in infectious mononucleosis. Clinical Immunology and Immunopathology 14:411
Lockshin M D 1976 Immunological status of patients with rheumatic disease. In: Dumonde D C (ed) Infection and immunology in the rheumatic diseases. Blackwell, London, Ch 70, p 541
London W T 1977 Hepatitis B virus and antigen-antibody complex diseases. New England Journal of Medicine 296:1528
London W T et al 1983 Experimental transmission of Simian acquired immunodeficiency syndrome (SIADS) and Kaposi-like skin lesions. Lancet ii:869
McAllister R M 1974 Viruses in human carcinogenesis. Progress in Medical Virology 16:48
McDonald M I, Hamilton J D, Durack D T 1983 Hepatitis B surface antigen could harbour the infective agent of AIDS. Lancet ii:882
Mackay J M K, Sim A K, McCormick J N, Marmion B P, McCraw A P, Duthie J R, et al 1983 Aetiology of rheumatoid arthritis: an attempt to transmit an infective agent from patients with rheumatoid arthritis to baboons. Annals of the Rheumatic Diseases 42:443
Maini R N, Stewart S M, Dumonde D C 1970 Peripheral leucocyte migration inhibited by diphtheroid organisms isolated from patients with rheumatoid arthritis. Annals of the Rheumatic Diseases 29:541
Maini R N, Lemcke R M, Windsor G D, Roffe L M, Magrath I T, Dumonde D C 1975 The significance of leucocyte migration inhibition by M. fermentans. Rheumatology 5:118
Man D L, Popovic M, Sarin P 1983 Cell lines producing human T-cell lymphoma virus show altered HLA expression. Nature 305:58
Manicourt D M, Orloff S 1981 Immune complexes in polyarthritis after Salmonella Gastroenteritis. Journal of Rheumatology 8:613
Mannik M 1982 Pathophysiology of circulating immune complexes. Arthritis and Rheumatism 25:783
Mansson I, Olhagen B 1974 Faecal Clostridium perfringens and rheumatoid arthritis. Journal of Infectious Diseases 130:44
Mansson I, Norberg R, Olhagen B, Bjorklund N E 1971 Arthritis in pigs induced by dietary factors. Clinical and Experimental Immunology 9:677
Margolis G, Kilham L 1970 Parvovirus infections, vascular endothelium and haemorrhagic encephalopathy. Laboratory Investigation 22 (5):478
Markenson J A, Phillips P E, Brinkman J P, Snyder H W, Christon C L 1977 Proteins on T-cell membranes from normals and patients with systemic lupus erythematosus (SLE) reactive with antisera to type-C viruses. Clinical Research 25:485
Marmion B P 1976 A microbiologist's view of investigative rheumatology. In: Dumonde D C (ed) Infection and immunology in the rheumatic diseases. Blackwell, London, Ch 32, p 245
Marmion B P 1978 Infection, autoimmunity and rheumatoid arthritis. In: Zvaifler N J (ed) Clinics in rheumatic diseases. Vol 4. Saunders, London, p 565
Marner I L 1952 The relation between hepatitis and polyarthritis. In: Slocumb C H (ed) Rheumatic diseases. Saunders, Philadelphia, p 237
Martenis T W, Bland J H, Phillips C A 1968 Rheumatoid arthritis after rubella. Arthritis and Rheumatism 11:683
Mason A M S, Gumpel J M, Golding P L 1973 Sjögren's syndrome: a clinical review. Seminars in Arthritis and Rheumatism 2:301
Mellors R C, Mellors J W 1976 Antigen related to mammalian Type-C RNA viral p30 proteins is located in renal glomeruli in human systemic lupus erythematosus. Proceedings of the National Academy of Sciences USA 73:233
Milgrom F, Dubiski S, Wozmezko G 1956 Human sera with anti-autobodies. Vox Sanguinis 1:172
Moller G (ed) 1974 The immune response to infectious diseases. Transplantation Review: 19
Moller G (ed) 1983 HLA and disease susceptibility. Immunological Reviews, 70, 1
Morgan A G, Steward M W 1976 Macrophage clearance function and immune complex disease in New Zealand black/white F_1 hybrid mice. Clinical and Experimental Immunology 26:133
Mortimer P P, Luban N L C, Kelleher J F, Cohen B J 1983 Transmission of serum parvovirus-like virus by clotting-factor concentrates. Lancet ii:482
Murphy G E 1960 Nature of rheumatic heart disease. Williams & Wilkins, Baltimore
Nardo J M, Norton W L 1971 Evidence for infectious etiologies in connective tissue disorders. Seminars in Arthritis and Rheumatism 1 (2):116
Neumark T, Farkas K 1973 Virus-like particles in rheumatoid synovium. Scandinavian Journal of Rheumatology 2:21
Neumark T, Farkas K 1976 Virus-like particles and some ultrastructural aspects of lymphoreticular cells in rheumatoid synovial membrane. In: Dumonde D C (ed) Infection and immunology in the rheumatic diseases. Blackwell, London, Ch 31, p 225
Newman J M, Waycott S, Cooney L M 1979 Arthritis due to Listeria monocytogenes. Arthritis and Rheumatism 10:1139
Ng K C, Brown K A, Perry J D, Holborow E J 1980 Anti-RANA antibody: A marker for seronegative and seropositive rheumatoid arthritis, Lancet i:447
Nies K M, Boyer R, Stevens R H, Louie J F 1980 Anti-tetanus toxoid antibody synthesis after booster immunization in systemic lupus erythematosus. Arthritis and Rheumatism 23:1343
Nikbin B, Brewerton D A, Byrom N, James D C O, Malka S, McLeod L et al 1975 Lymphocyte function in ankylosing spondylitis. Annals of the Rheumatic Diseases, 34 (Suppl): 49
Nitsche J F, Vaughan J H, Williams G, Curd J G 1982 Septic sternoclavicular arthritis with Pasteurella Multocida and Streptococcus Sanguis. Arthritis and Rheumatism 25:467
Nordal H J, Froland S S, Vandvik B, Norrby E 1975 Measles-virus-induced migration inhibition of human leucocytes: an immunologically unspecific phenomenon? Lancet ii:1266
Norrby E, Link H, Olsson J E, Panelius M, Salmi A, Vandvik B 1974 Comparison of antibodies against different viruses in cerebro-spinal fluid and serum samples from patients with multiple sclerosis. Infection and Immunity 10:688
Norton W L, Velayos E, Robinson L 1970 Endothelial inclusions in dermatomyositis. Annals of the Rheumatic Diseases 29:67
Norval M, Marmion B P 1976 Attempts to identify viruses in

rheumatoid synovial cells. Annals of the Rheumatic Diseases 35:106
Norval M, Smith C A 1979 Search for viral nucleic sequences in rheumatoid cells. Annals of the Rheumatic Diseases 38:456
Norval M, Ogilvie M, Marmion B P 1975 DNA polymerase in rheumatoid synovial membrane. Annals of the Rheumatic Diseases 34:205
Norval M, Hart M, Marmion B P 1979 Viruses and lymphocytes in rheumatoid arthritis. I. Studies on cultured rheumatoid lymphocytes. Annals of the Rheumatic Diseases 38:507
Notkins A L (ed) 1975 Viral immunology and immunopathology. Academic Press, New York
Obata Y, Ikeda H, Stockert E, Boyse E A 1974 Relation of G IX antigen of thymocytes to envelope glycoprotein of murine leukaemia virus. Journal of Experimental Medicine 141:188
Ogra P L, Herd J K 1972 Serological association of rubella virus infection and juvenile rheumatoid arthritis (JRA). Arthritis and Rheumatism 14:121
Ogra P L, Chiba Y, Ogra S S, Dzierba J L, Herd J K 1975 Rubella virus infection in juvenile rheumatoid arthritis. Lancet i:1157
Oldstone M B A, Dixon F J 1975 Immune complex disease associated with viral infections. In: Notkins A L (ed) Viral immunology and immunopathology. Academic Press, New York, p 341
Olhagen B 1976 Intestinal Clostridium perfringens in arthritis and allied conditions. In: Dumonde D C (ed) Infection and immunology in the rheumatic diseases. Blackwell, London, Ch 18, p 141
Panayi G S 1976 Antibody-mediated leucocyte cytotoxicity to Chang human liver cells in rheumatoid arthritis and other diseases. Annals of the Rheumatic Diseases 35:27
Paronen I 1948 Reiter's disease. A study of 344 cases observed in Finland. Acta Medica Scandanavica 131 (Suppl 212): 1
Pasquali J-L, Fong S, Tsoukas C D, Slovin S F, Vaughan J H, Carson D A 1981 Different populations of rheumatoid factor idiotypes induced by two polycloncal B cell activators, pokeweed mitogen and Epstein–Barr virus. Clinical Immunology and Immunopathology 21:184
Passwell J H, Steward M W, Soothill J F 1974 Inter-mouse strain differences in macrophage function and its relationship to antibody responses. Clinical and Experimental Immunology 17:159
Patterson R, Howard F, Deinhardt F 1973 Rubella virus and rheumatoid arthritis. Clinical Research 21:878
Patterson R L, Peterson D A, Deinhardt F, Howard F 1975 Rubella and rheumatoid arthritis: hyaluronic acid and susceptibility of cultured rheumatoid synovial cells to viruses. Proceedings of the Society of Experimental Biology and Medicine 149:594
Payling Wright H 1971 Endothelium and blood flow. Scientific Basis of Medicine Annual Reviews 1971:320
Payling Wright H, Giacometti N J 1972 Circulating endothelial cells and arterial endothelial mitosis in anaphylactic shock. British Journal of Experimental Pathology 52:1
Pearson C M 1966 Arthritis in animals. In: Hollander J L (ed) Arthritis and allied conditions, 7th Edn. Henry Kimpton, London, Ch 9, p 119
Pearson C M 1966a Polymyositis. Annual Reviews of Medicine 17:63
Pearson C M, Kohashi O 1977 Mechanisms of adjuvant-induced arthritis in the rat. In: Experimental models of chronic inflammatory diseases. VI Bayer Symposium, Springer, Heidelberg, p 36
Pease P 1969 Bacterial L-forms in blood and joint fluids of arthritis subjects. Annals of the Rheumatic Diseases 28:270
Pease P 1974 Identification of bacteria from blood and joint fluids of human subjects as Bacillus licheniformis. Annals of the Rheumatic Diseases 33:67
Pelton B R, Denman A M 1982 Defective B cell function in systemic lupus erythematosus. Clinical and experimental Immunology 48:513
Petty R E, Steward M W, Soothill J E 1972 The heterogeneity of antibody affinity and its possible immunopathologic significance. Clinical and Experimental Immunology 12:231
Phillips P E 1975 The role of viruses in systemic lupus erythematosus. Clinics in Rheumatic Diseases 1:505
Phillips P E 1976a Rheumatic disease during the course of known viral infections: models for the possible pathogenesis of rheumatoid arthritis. In: Dumonde D (ed) Infection and immunology in the rheumatic diseases. Blackwell, London, Ch 28
Phillips P E 1976b Recent attempts at implicating viruses in systemic lupus erythematosus. In: Dumonde D C (ed) Infection and immunology in the rheumatic diseases. Blackwell, London, Ch 34, p 265
Phillips P E, Hargrave-Granda 1978 Type C oncornavirus isolation studies in systemic lupus erythematosus. II. Attempted detection by viral RNA-dependent DNA polymerase assay. Annals of the Rheumatic Diseases 37:225
Phillips P E, Christian C L 1979 Infectious agents in chronic rheumatic diseases. In: McCarty D J (ed) Arthritis and allied conditions, 9th Edn. Lea & Febiger, Philadelphia, p 320
Phillips P E, Hargreave R, Stewart E 1976 Type C virus studies in SLE. II. Attempted detection of viral RNA-directed DNA polymerase (RDDP). Arthritis and Rheumatism 19:816 (abstr)
Phillips P E, Hargrave R, Stewart E, Sarkar N H 1976 Type C oncornavirus isolation studies in SLE. I. Attempted detection by isopycnic sedimentation of 3H uridine-labelled virions. Annals of the Rheumatic Diseases 35:422
Pincus T 1982 Studies regarding a possible function for viruses in the pathogenesis of systemic lupus erythematosus. Arthritis and Rheumatism 25:847
Pincus T, Steinberg A D, Blacklow N R, Decker J L 1978 Reactivities of systemic lupus erythematosus sera with cellular and virus antigen preparations. Arthritis and Rheumatism 21:873
Plotz P H 1983 Autoantibodies are anti-idiotype antibodies to anti-viral antibodies. Lancet ii:824
Ponka A 1979 Arthritis associated with Mycoplasma pneumoniae infection. Scandinavian Journal of Rheumatology 8:27
Porter R, Knight J (Eds) 1974 Parasites in the immunized host: Mechanisms of survival. Ciba Foundation Symposium 25 (new series). North-Holland, London
Quismorio F P, Jokes J T, Zarnow A J, Barber D, Kitridou R C 1983 Septic arthritis due to Arizona Hinshawie. Journal of Rheumatology 10:147
Rather L J 1972 Addison and the white corpuscles: an aspect of nineteenth century biology. Wellcome Institute of the History of Medicine, London

Ravenholt R T 1983 Role of hepatitis B virus in acquired immunodeficiency syndrome. Lancet ii:885
Reginato A J, Schumacher H R, Jimenez S, Maurer K 1979 Synovitis in secondary syphilis. Arthritis and Rheumatism, 22:170
Reiter H 1916 Uber eimer bisher unerkannte Spirochateninfektion (Spirochaetosis arthritica). Deutsche Medicinische Woschenschrift 42:1535
Reynolds J T, Panem S 1981 Characterization of antibody to C-type virus antigens isolated from immune complexes in kidneys of patients with systemic lupus erythematosus. Laboratory Investigations 40:410
Rich A R 1947 Hypersensitivity in disease with especial reference to periarteritis nodosa, rheumatic fever, disseminated lupus erythematosus and rheumatoid arthritis. Harvey Lectures Series 42:106
Rickinson A B, Moss D J, Wallace L E, Rowe M, Misko I S, Epstein M A, Pope J H 1981 Long-term T cell mediated immunity to Epstein–Barr virus. Cancer Research 41:4216
Rigby P W J 1982 Expression of cloned genes in eukaryotic cells using vector systems derived from viral replicons. In: Williamson R (ed) Genetic engineering, Vol 3. Academic Press, New York, p 84
Rizzetto M 1981 Biology and characterisation of the delta agent. In: Szmuness W, Alter H J, Maynard J E (eds) Viral hepatitis: 1981. Franklin Institute Press, Philadelphia, p 355
Robbins K C, Antoniades H N, Devare S G, Hunkapiller M W Aaronson S A 1983 Structural and immunological similarities between Simian sarcoma virus gene product and human platelet-derived growth factor. Nature 305:605
Romet-Lemonne, J-L, McLane M F, Elfassi E, Hazeltine W A, Azocar J, Essex M 1983 Hepatitis B virus infection in cultured human lymphoblastoid cells. Science 221:667
Room G R, Plater-Zyberk C, Clarke M F, Maini R N 1982 B-lymphocyte subpopulation which forms rosettes with mouse erythrocytes increased in rheumatoid arthritis. Rheumatology International 2: 175
Rose L M, Lambert P H 1980 The natural occurrence of idiotype-antiidiotype immune complexes during a secondary response to phosphoryl choline. Clinical Immunology and Immunopathology 15:481
Rose L M, Goldman M, Lambert P H 1982a The production of fanti-idiotype antibodies and of idiotype-anti-idiotype immune complexes following polyclonal B cell activation by bacterial LPS. Journal of Immunology 128:1126
Rose L M, Goldman M, Lambert P H 1982b Simultaneous induction of an idiotype, corresponding anti-idiotype antibodies and immune complexes during African trypanosomiasis in mice. Journal of Immunology 128:79
Russell A S 1981 Drug-induced autoimmune disease. In: Holborow E J (ed) Clinics in immunology and allergy: Autoimmunity. Saunders, London, p 57
Sato T, Walker D C, Peters H A, Reese H H, Chou S M 1970 Chronic polymyositis and myxovirus-like inclusions. Archives of Neurology 24:409
Sauter S V H, Utsinger P D 1978 Viral arthritis. In: Schmid F F (ed) Clinics in rheumatic diseases: Infectious arthritis, Vol 4. Saunders, London
Schachter J 1976 Can chlamydial infections cause rheumatic disease? In: Dumonde D C (ed) Infection and immunology in the rheumatic diseases. Blackwell, London, Ch 20, p 151
Schechter Y, Maron R, Elias D, Cohen I R 1982 Autoantibodies to insulin receptors spontaneously develop as anti-idiotypes in mice immunised with insulin. Science 216:542
Schlosstein L, Terasaki P I, Bluestone R, Pearson C M 1973 High association of an HLA antigen, W27, with ankylosing spondylitis. New England Journal of Medicine 288:704
Schnitzer T J, Ansel B M, Hawkins G T, Marshall W C 1977 Signifiance of rubella virus in juvenile chronic polyarthritis. Annals of the Rheumatic Diseases 36:468
Schumacher H R 1975 Synovial membrane and fluid morphologic alterations in early rheumatoid arthritis: microvascular injury and virus-like particles. Annals of the New York Academy of Sciences 256:39
Schumacher H R, Gall E P 1974 Arthritis in acute hepatitis and chronic active hepatitis. Pathology of the synovial membrane with evidence for the presence of Australia antigen in synovial membranes. American Journal of Medicine 57:655
Schwartz R S 1975 Viruses and systemic lupus erythematous. New England Journal of Medicine 293:132
Seagar K, Bashir H V, Geczy A F, Edmonds J de Vere, Tyndall A 1979 Evidence for a specific B27-associated cell surface marker on lymphocytes of patients with ankylosing spondylitis. Nature 277:68
Sergent J S, Lockshin M D, Christian C L, Gocke D J 1976 Vasculitis with hepatitis B antigenemia. Medicine 55:1
Serjeant G R, Topley J M, Mason K, Serjeant B E, Pattison J R, Jones S E et al 1981 Outbreak of aplastic crisis in sickle-cell anaemia associated with parvovirus-like agent. Lancet ii:595
Sheldon P J H S, Mair N S, Fox E 1982 Yersinia arthritis: a clinical, immunological and family study of two cases. Annals of the Rheumatic Diseases 41:153
Shneerson J M, Mortimer P P, Vandervelde E M 1980 Febrile illness due to a parvovirus. British Medical Journal ii:1580
Siddiqui A 1983 Hepatitis B virus in Kaposi's sarcoma. Proceedings of the National Academy of Sciences, USA 80:4861
Siegl G 1976 The parvoviruses. Virology monographs 15:1
Simon D G, Kaslow R A, Rosenbaum J, Kaye R L, Calin A 1981 Reiter's syndrome following epidemic Shigellosis. Journal of Rheumatology 8:969
Simpson R W, Smith C A, Godzeski C W, Boyd R, McGinty L, Simon L, Hamerman D 1983 Human rheumatoid arthritis synovium as a source of pathogens. Proceedings of the American Rheumatism Association, Boston, October 1982 (abstr) Clinical Research 1983
Slaughter L, Carson D A, Jensen F C, Holbrook T, Vaughan J H 1978 In vitro effects of Epstein–Barr virus on peripheral blood mononuclear cells from patients with rheumatoid arthritis and normal subjects. Journal of Experimental Medicine 148:1429
Slovin S F, Vaughan J M, Carson D A 1980 Expression of EBNA and RANA during different phases of the cell growth cycle. International Journal of Cancer 26:9
Slovin S F, Glassy M C, Dambaugh T, Catalano M A, Curry R A, Ferrone S, et al 1981 Discordant expression of two Epstein–Barr virus-associated antigens, EBNA and RANA, in man–rodent somatic cell hybrids. Journal of Immunology 127:585
Smith C A 1979 On a possible viral etiology of rheumatoid arthritis. Journal of Rheumatology 6:113
Smith C A, Hamerman D 1969 Significance of persistent differences between normal and rheumatoid synovial

membrane cells in culture. Arthritis and Rheumatism 12:629

Smith C, Hamerman D 1976 Evidence for a viral aetiology of rhematoid synovitis. In: Dumonde D C (ed) Infection and immunology in the rheumatic diseases. Blackwell, London, Ch 30, p 213

Smith D E, James P G, Schachter J, Engleman E P, Meyer K F 1973 Experimental bedsonial arthritis. Arthritis and Rheumatism 16:21

Snyder H W, Pincus T, Fleissner E 1976 Specificites of human immunoglobulin reactive with antigens in preparations of several mammalian type-C viruses. Virology 75:60

Soothill J F, Steward M W 1971 The immunopathological significance of the heterogeneity of antibody affinity. Clinical and Experimental Immunology 9:193

Spruance S L, Metcalf R, Smith C B, Griffiths M M, Ward J R 1977 Chronic arthropathy associated with rubella vaccination. Arthritis and Rheumatism 20:741

Stanford F 1974 Rubella-antibody titres in rheumatoid arthritis. Lancet i:1000

Stastny P, Stembridge V, Vischer T, Ziff M 1965 Homologous disease in the adult rat as a model for autoimmune disease. II. Findings in the joints, heart and other tissues. Journal of Experimental Medicine 122:681

Stein H B, Abdullah A, Robinson H S, Ford D K 1980 Salmonella reactive arthritis in British Columbia. Arthritis and Rheumatism 23:206

Steward M W 1977 The affinity of the antibody:antigen reaction and its biological signifance. In: Textbook of immunochemistry. Wiley, London

Steward M W, Katz F E, West N J 1975 The role of low affinity antibody in immune complex disease; the quality of anti-DNA antibodies in NZB/W F_1 hybrid mice. Clinical and Experimental Immunology 21:121

Steward M W, Turner M W, Natvig J B, Baarder P I 1973 The binding affinities of rheumatoid factors interacting with the Cγ3 homology region of human IgG. Clinical and Experimental Immunology 15:145

Stierle H E, Brown K A, Perry J D, Holborow E J 1983 Increased responsiveness of rheumatoid B lymphocytes to stimulation by Epstein–Barr virus. Rheumatology International 3:7

Strand M, August J T 1974 Evidence for type-C RNA virus expression in human tissue. Journal of Virology 14:1584

Strannegard O, Bjorkander J, Hermodsson S, Lundgren E, Strannegard I-L, Westberg G 1980 Production of interferon in lymphocyte cultures from patients with abnormal immune function. Annals of the New York Academy of Sciences 350:589

Strauch B, Siegal N, Andrews L, Miller G 1974 Oropharyngeal excretion of Epstein — Barr virus by renal transplant recipients and other patients treated with immunosuppressive drugs. Lancet i:234

Svartz N 1975 The origin of rheumatoid arthritis. Rheumatology 6:322

Svartz N, Hedman S, Soderberg O 1969 Two methods for producing in animals a macroglobulin similar to the rheumatoid factor. Acta Medica Scandanavica 186:135

Svejgaard A, Platz P, Ryder L P 1983 HLA and disease 1982 — a survey. Immunological Reviews 70:193

Svejgaard A, Nerup J, Platz P, Ryder L P, Nielsen L S, Thomsen M 1975 Human HLA histocompatibility antigens and disease. In: Silvestri L G (ed) The immunological basis of connective tissue disorders. V Lepetit Colloqium. North-Holland, Oxford, p 53

Talal N 1975 Animal models for systemic lupus erythematosis. Clinics in Rheumatic Diseases 1:485

Talal N, Steinberg A D, Daley G F 1971 Inhibition of polycytidylic acid in human and mouse sera by viral and synthetic ribonucleic acids. Journal of Clinical Investigation 50:1248

Taranta A 1966 Rheumatic fever: pathology, etiology, epiodemiology and pathogenesis. In: Hollander J L (ed) Arthritis and allied conditions, 7th Edn. Kimpton, London, Ch 41, p 667

Taranta A, Markowitz M 1981 Rheumatic fever: A guide to its recognition, prevention and cure — with special reference to developing countries. MTP Press, Boston

Taranta A, Kleinberg E, Feinstein A R, Wood H F, Tursky E, Simpson R 1964 Relation of rheumatic fever recurrence rate per streptococcal infection to pre-existing clinical features of patients. Annals of Internal Medicine 60 (Suppl 5):58

Taylor-Robinson D 1981 Mycoplasmal arthritis in man. Israel Journal of Medical Science 17:616

Taylor-Robinson D, Taylor G 1976 Do mycoplasmas cause rheumatic disease? In: Dumonde D C (ed) Infection and immunology in the rheumatic diseases. Blackwell, London, Ch 23, p 177

Thorley-Lawson D A 1981 The transformation of adult but not newborn human lymphocytes by Epstein–Barr virus and phytohaemoagglutinin is inhibited by interferon: the early suppression by T cells of Epstein–Barr infection is mediated by interferon. Journal of Immunology 126:829

Tingle A J, Ford D K, Price G E, Kettyls D W G 1978 Prolonged arthritis in identical twins after rubella immunisation. Annals of Internal Medicine 90:203

Toh B H, Yildiz A, Sotelo J, Osung O, Holborow E J, Kanakondi F, Small J V 1979 Viral infections and IgM autoantibodies to cytoplasmic intermediate filaments. Clinical and Experimental Immunology 37:76

Tosato G, Steinberg A D, Blaese R M 1981 Defective EBV-specific suppressor T cell function in rheumatoid arthritis. New England Journal of Medicine 305:1238

Turk J L, Belehu A 1974 Immunological spectra in infectious diseases. In: Porter R, Knight J (eds) Parasites in the immunised host. Ciba Foundation Symposium 25:101

Urbain J, Wuilmart C, Cazenave P A 1981 Idiotypic regulation in immune networks. Contemporary Topics in Molecular Immunology 8:113

Urman J D, Bohrone A M 1982 Acute polyarthritis and infectious mononucleosis. Western Journal of Medicine 136:151

Utermohlen V, Winfield J B, Zabriskie J B, Kunkel H G 1974 A depression of cell mediated immunity to measles antigen in patients with SLE. Journal of Experimental Medicine 139:1019

Vaughan J H 1966 Infectious and immunological considerations in rheumatic diseases. In: Hollander J L (ed) Arthritis and allied conditions, 7th Edn. Kimpton, London, Ch 33, p 577

Venables P J W, Edwards J M B, Maini R N 1980 Antibodies to RANA and other nuclear antigens in infectious mononucleosis and rheumatoid arthritis. Annals of the Rheumatic Diseases 39:191

Venables P J W, Roffe L M, Erhardt C C, Maini R N, Edwards J M B, Porter A D 1981 Titres of antibodies to RANA in rheumatoid arthritis and normal sera.

Relationship to Epstein–Barr virus infection. Arthritis and Rheumatism 24:1459
Vergani D, Morgan-Capner P, Davies E T, Anderson A W, Tee D E H, Pattison J R 1980 Joint symptoms, immune complexes and rubella. Lancet i:321
Vilppula A H, Yli-Kerttula U I, Ahlroos A K, Terho P E 1981 Chlamydial isolations and serology in Reiter's syndrome. Scandianavian Journal of Rheumatology 10:181
Vincent J, Podewell C, Franklin G W, Korn J H 1981 Septic arthritis due to *Kingella (Moraxella) kingii*. Journal of Rheumatology 8:501
Ward D C, Tattersall P (eds) 1978 Replication of mammalian parvoviruses. Cold Spring Harbor Laboratory, New York
Warren R E, Brewerton D A 1980 Faecal carriage of Klebsiella by patients with ankylosing spondylitis and rheumatoid arthritis. Annals of the Rheumatic Diseases 39:37
Warren S L, Marmor L, Leibes D M, Hollins R 1969 An active agent from human rheumatoid arthritis which is transmissible in mice. Archives of Internal Medicine 124:629
Warren S L, Marmor L, Boak R, Liebes D M 1971 Transmission of an active agent from rheumatoid arthritis synovial tissue to chicks. Archives of Internal Medicine 128:619
Warren S L, Mamor L, Liebes D M, Rosenblatt H M 1972 An active agent from rheumatoid synovial tissue. Archives of Internal Medicine. 130:899
Warren S L, Marmor L, Stamm M E, Lewis H, Horner H, Liebes D, et al 1975 Thermal inactivation and gradient studies of the active agent in rheumatoid arthritis. Rheumatology 6:361
Warren S L, Marmur L, Horner H E, Stanley W D, Stoeckel T A, Gerken S C et al 1979 Further studies on the specific infectious agent isolated in rheumatoid arthritis. Journal of Rheumatology, 6 (2):135
Washburn L R, Cole B C, Ward J R 1982 Chronic arthritis of rabbits induced by mycoplasmas. Arthritis and Rheumatism 25:937
Weatherall D J 1982 The new genetics and clinical practice. Nuffield Provincial Hospitals Trust, London
Webb F W, Bluestone R, Goldberg L S, Douglas S D, Pearson C M 1973 Experimental viral arthritis induced with herpes simplex. Arthritis and Rheumatism 16:241
Weigle W O 1961 Fate and biological action of antigen–antibody complexes. Advances in Immunology 1:283
Weiss R A 1983 Human leukaemia virus mimics cellular antigens. Nature 305:12
Welsh J, Avakian M, Cowling P, Ebringer A, Wooley P, Panayi G, Ebringer R 1980 Ankylosing spondylitis HLA-B27 and Klebsiella, I. Cross-reactivity studies with rabbit antisera. British Journal of Experimental Pathology 61:85
Wilkes R M, Simsarian J P, Hopps H E, Roth H, Decker J L, Aptekar R G, Mey H M 1973 Virological studies on rheumatoid arthritis. Arthritis and Rheumatism 16:447
Wilkinson P C 1982 Chemotaxis and inflammation. Churchill Livingstone, Edinburgh
Williams M H 1968 Recovery of mycoplasma from rheumatoid synovial fluid. In: Duthie J J R, Alexander W R M (eds) Rheumatic diseases. Williams & Wilkins, Baltimore, p 172
Williams M H, Brostoff J, Roitt I M 1970 Possible role of *Mycoplasma fermentans* in pathogenesis of rheumatoid arthritis. Lancet ii:277
Williams R C Jr 1981 Infective and post-infective disorders. In: Lessof M H (ed) Immunology of cardiovascular disease. Marcel Dekker, New York, p 105
Williamson R (ed) 1980–1982 Genetic engineering, Vols 1–4. Academic Press, New York
Wise K S, Cassell G H, Acton R T 1978 Selective association of murine T lymphoblastoid cell surface alloantigens with *Mycoplasma hyorhinis*. Proceedings of the National Academy of Science 75:4479
Yamamura Y, Kotani S, Azuma I, Koda A, Shibay T (eds) 1982 Immunoregulation by microbial products and related synthetic compounds. Excerpta Medica, Amsterdam
Yoshiki T, Mellors R C, Strand M, August J T 1974 The viral envelope glycoprotein of murine leukaemia virus and the pathogenesis of immune complex glomerulonephritis of New Zealand mice. Journal of Experimental Medicine 140:1011
Youssef A A R, Baron D N 1983 Leucocyte superoxide dismutase in rheumatoid arthritis. Annals of the Rheumatic Diseases 42:558
Zabriskie J B 1976 Rheumatic fever: a streptococcal-induced autoimmune disease? In: Dumonde D C (ed) Infection and immunology in the rheumatic diseases. Blackwell, London, Ch 13, p 97
Zhdanov V M 1975 Integration of viral genomes. Nature 256:471
Ziff M 1976 How far can rheumatic diseases be viewed as immunopathological responses to microbial infection? In: Dumonde D C (ed) Infection and immunology in the rheumatic diseases. Blackwell, London, Ch 79, p 627
Ziff M, 1979 Introduction to symposium on Reiter's syndrome. Annals of the Rheumatic Diseases 38 (Suppl):1
Zuckerman A J, Darnell R, Scalise G 1976 Hepatitis B infection illustrating problems of genetic susceptibility to infectious and rheumatic disease. In: Dumonde D C (ed) Infection and immunology in the rheumatic diseases. Blackwell, London, Ch 38, p 295

15

H.L.F. Currey

Animal models of arthritis

A variety of spontaneous and induced joint diseases in animals has been studied with the object of throwing light on the problems of human arthritis. In the main these have tended to provide intriguing parallels with human diseases rather than revealing the answers that were sought. Nevertheless, there are now available models which provide an approach to studying various growing points in current rheumatology research (Table 15.1).

Strategy in the selection of appropriate species to study has been determined by the availability of spontaneous disease models, by susceptibility to induced diseases, by the size of animals and their individual joints, cost and — more recently — the availability of inbred strains. Size is often critical. For the induction of mechanical damage by tendon section, dogs or pigs have generally been employed. However, surgical procedures such as synovectomy can readily be performed in the rabbit knee joint. The smaller guinea-pig knee joint has also been used for operative procedures, but this greatly increases the technical difficulty. The use of inbred rat and mouse strains, besides allowing cell transfer experiments, offers the opportunity of studying genetic influences on animal arthritis.

Table 15.1 Some animal models of arthritis used in the study of human joint disease. Page references are given in brackets.

Model	Species
Infective arthritis	
Erysipelothrix (469)	Pig, rabbit, guinea-pig, rat
Mycoplasma (470)	Pig, rat, mouse, turkey, rabbit
Virus (471)	Sheep, goat, rabbit
Injection of bacterial products	
Adjuvant disease (471	Rat
Streptococcal cell wall components (475)	Rat
Protein immunisation	
Antigen-induced arthritis (476)	Rabbit, guinea-pig, chicken, goat
'Serum sickness' (478)	Rabbit
Autoimmunisation	
Collagen type II arthritis (478)	Rat, mouse
Oral sulphonamide	
6-Sulphanilamidoindazole feeding (480)	Rat
Osteoarthritis	
Spontaneous osteoarthritis (480)	Mouse
Cruciate ligament section (481)	Dog, pig
Physical cartilage damage (481)	Rabbit
Papain injection (481)	Rabbit
Crystal-induced synovitis	
Intra-articular injection of crystals (482)	Dog, etc.
Dietary factors	
High protein diet (482)	Pig
Spontaneous autoimmune disease	
Rheumatoid-like disease (483)	Mouse

Considerations of cost and availability have greatly limited the use of primates. However, in his review of experimental arthritis in 1960, Gardner drew attention to the misleadingly similar appearances of the non-specific histological changes in various forms of small animal synovitis and those in human rheumatoid arthritis. His conclusion that the experimental approach to rheumatoid disease should concentrate on human — or possibly other primate — studies remains highly relevant. Sporadic reports have indeed appeared from time to time of spontaneous rheumatoid-like arthritis in monkeys, baboons, chimpanzees and gorillas (Bywaters, 1981). However, the experimental transfer of human rheumatoid material to baboons failed to induce disease (Mackay et al, 1983). By contrast there are available now animal models which provide a useful experimental approach to the study of osteoarthritis, crystal synovitis and infective arthritis.

In the descriptions which follow, the various models are discussed in the order in which they appear in Table 15.1.

INFECTIVE ARTHRITIS

Spontaneous joint infections are not uncommon in domesticated animals. So far none has proved to be a close model of human disease. However, there are parallels, particularly in the interplay of direct microbial and indirect immunological joint damage, which may be relevant to some human joint infections.

Erysipelothrix arthritis (Drew, 1972)

Erysipelothrix rhusiopathiae (*E. insidiosa*) is a small Gram-positive coccobacillus. In man it is the cause of erysipeloid. In a wide range of domestic and wild animals *E. rhusiopathiae* and closely related organisms can cause a variety of illnesses, including fatal septicaemia. In the laboratory, intravenous injection of live organisms will produce arthritis in rats, guinea-pigs rabbits and pigs. The interest of this organism to the rheumatologist lies in its predilection for articular tissues and in its ability to initiate an arthritis which later develops into a chronic proliferative synovitis and which persists, apparently sometimes without viable organisms being present in the joint.

Erysipelothrix arthritis ('rheumatoid arthritis') in pigs

Erysipelothrix arthritis ('rheumatoid arthritis') in pigs has been studied as a possible model for human arthritis. The natural disease takes one of three forms. The most acute is a septicaemia which is rapidly fatal in about 80% of cases. A somewhat less acute form occurs in which the main features are erythematous and urticarial skin lesions. In either of these two forms joint localisation may occur from the blood stream. However, the resulting acute synovitis is generally overshadowed by the systemic disease. The chronic form is characterised by polyarthritis with or without endocarditis. It may follow recovery from an acute systemic infection or may be the initial manifestation. Apparently healthy pigs can carry the organism in the tonsils, gut, spleen or bone marrow. When such pigs are stressed, clinical infection may appear.

Larger limb joints are mainly affected. The initial synovitis consists of vascular congestion and oedema, with a turbid or serosanguinous effusion. The animal is severely lame, and initially large numbers of organisms can be cultured from the joint. As the disease progresses proliferative changes appear and the organism becomes increasingly more difficult to recover. A majority of chronic joints are apparently sterile, and the response to antibiotics at this stage is disappointing. The persistence of organisms within joints is apparently not influenced by specific humoral immunity (Ajmal, 1970).

The chronic synovial changes are not unlike those of human rheumatoid arthritis. There is villous hypertrophy with lining cell hyperplasia, and a dense infiltrate of lymphocytes and plasma cells. Lymphoid follicles are common, sometimes with germinal centres. In advanced cases pannus formation is prominent and cartilage becomes eroded. Rheumatoid factor-like substances have been identified by some authors — not by others — both in the synovial fluid and the serum of affected animals. In infected rabbits, Astorga (1968) has described the appearance of anti-γ-

globulin factors in synovial fluid earlier than in the serum.

Mycoplasma arthritis

Mycoplasmas are the smallest and simplest self-replicating procaryotes (Razin, 1981). Equipped with a minimum set of organelles and having no cell wall, they are parasites of man, animals, anthropods and plants. In animals their primary habitat is moist mucosal surfaces such as the respiratory and genitourinary tracts. They also have a predilection for synovial linings of joints and tendon sheaths.

In farm animals such as pigs, cattle, goats and poultry, respiratory and other mycoplasmal infections are a significant cause of economic loss, and in all these animals arthritis may occur. In man *Mycoplasma pneumoniae* is now one of the most common causes of pneumonia in children and young adults. Another mycoplasma, *Ureaplasma urealyticum*, is one of the organisms which has been isolated from cases of non-gonococcal urethritis, but an aetiological role for this organism has not yet been proven (Taylor-Robinson et al, 1981). In the laboratory mycoplasmas are most familiar as a troublesome infection of rodents (murine respiratory mycoplasmosis) and as an equally troublesome contaminant of cell cultures. Experimental mycoplasma arthritis has been studied particularly in pigs, rabbits and rodents. It has also been induced in poultry.

Mycoplasma arthritis in pigs

Intravenous inoculation of certain strains of *Mycoplasma hyopneumoniae* into pigs produced arthritis in several limb joints (Lloyd & Etheridge, 1981). Clinical signs of polyarthritis appeared 8–15 days after inoculation. Post-mortem examination showed one or more proximal limb joints to be involved. There was a serofibrinous, sometimes blood-stained, effusion containing about 80% polymorphonuclear cells. The synovial membrane was thickened, congested and oedematous, with an intense infiltration predominantly of lymphocytes, plasma cells and macrophages. The propensity of different strains to produce arthritis was paralleled by mycoplasmaemia and serum complement-fixing antibody response.

Mycoplasma arthritis in rabbits

Washburn and his colleagues (1980) injected rabbits intra-articularly with *Mycoplasma arthritidis*, or *Mycoplasma pulmonis*. Joint swelling appeared within 2 days, and persisted in some animals for up to 1 year. In the early stages there were turbid synovial effusions. The synovial lining showed villous hypertrophy during the early weeks, and by 12 weeks pannus had begun to form. By 20 weeks the synovial effusion contained mainly mononuclear cells and spreading pannus was producing cartilage erosions. At 31 weeks there were bony erosions. By the 2nd week the synovial membrane was infiltrated with lymphocytes (some forming follicles) and plasma cells, together with smaller numbers of polymorphonuclear cells. The interesting feature of this study was that, despite the persistence of active arthritis, neither mycoplasmas nor mycoplasma antigens could be identified in joint tissues after seven weeks. Peak antibody titres coincided with this disappearance of the mycoplasmas. Despite these findings, persisting non-viable mycoplasmal antigen appears to be the most likely explanation for chronicity (Washburn et al, 1982).

Mycoplasma arthritis in rodents (Cassell et al, 1981)

Arthritis can be induced in both rats and mice by intravenous inoculation of *Mycoplasma pulmonis* or *Mycoplasma arthritidis*. Different strains of animal show marked differences in the pattern and severity of arthritis induced by the same organism. The evidence points to the presence of viable organisms in the joints usually being necessary for persistent arthritis and the condition responds to antibiotic treatment. Histologically the early acute phase gives way to a chronic picture of lymphocyte and plasma cell infiltration, pannus formation, and erosion of both cartilage and bone. Severe involvement may lead to bony ankylosis. F344 strain rats develop only tenosynovitis.

Mycoplasma host interactions (Bennett, 1978; Davis et al, 1981)

A number of features of the interplay between the host tissues and infecting mycoplasmas suggest that these models of experimental arthritis could have relevance to the study of rheumatic diseases in man. Failure to identify either living organisms or mycoplasma antigen in actively inflamed joints in rabbits is intriguing but needs to be interpreted with caution, as mycoplasmas can be difficult to recover. They are able to exchange antigenic material with host cells and this may account, on the one hand, for their propensity to provoke the production of various autoantibodies by the mammalian host. On the other hand, the transfer of host histocompatibility antigens to the organisms may provide them with protective 'immunological camouflage' and allow them to persist in immunocompetent hosts. Another form of antigenic disguise of which mycoplasmas may be capable is rapid mutation and selection. Mycoplasmas also interact with host lymphocyte populations, behaving as multivalent ligands and producing polyclonal B cell activation.

Viral arthritis

Speculation that viral infections may play a role in the causation of human arthritis lends interest to the occurrence of viral arthritis in animals. Two natural diseases of domestic animals have been studied, and herpes simplex virus arthritis has been induced in laboratory animals.

Natural viral arthritis in sheep (Norton & Storz, 1967)

Spontaneous arthritis in sheep is widespread in the western USA. The responsible agent belongs to the psittacosis-lymphogranuloma venereum-trachoma (PLT) group. Norton & Storz (1967) cultured the organism from synovial fluid obtained from a lamb with the natural disease, and innoculated 6-month-old sheep intramuscularly. Within 3 days the animals became febrile and toxic with a systemic disease. By 5 days the animals were lame, with obvious polyarthritis, particularly of larger limb joints. Maximum severity was reached by 2 weeks with gradual recovery thereafter. By the 5th week there was only some residual stiffness. The organism could be recovered from the synovial fluid of affected joints for about 4 weeks, but not thereafter. Microscopically there was a dense acute inflammatory cell infiltration at 2 weeks which then gave way to chronic synovitis with focal collections of plasma cells. Other lesions included tendinitis, conjunctivitis, orchitis and epididymitis.

Goat arthritis-encephalitis syndrome (Crawford et al, 1980; Cork & Narayan, 1980)

Caprine arthritis-encephalitis is a disease of domestic goats caused by a retrovirus (CAEV). It is a multisystem disease, affecting particularly synovial structures (joints, tendon sheaths, bursae), the brain, kidneys, and blood vessels. Secondary amyloidosis occurs in some animals. The central nervous system component affects particularly young animals as an acute demyelinating encephalomyelitis. The connective tissue component takes the form of chronic polyarthritis which progresses gradually over a period of years.

The joints develop a proliferative synovitis with infiltration by chronic inflammatory cells. Surface fibrin deposition and fibrinoid necrosis are both prominent. Later these changes give way to necrosis and secondary calcification. A detailed study of the synovial ultrastructure has recently been reported (Brassfield et al, 1982). The virus can be isolated from the synovial membrane. Natural infections are transmitted horizontally from mother to kid at an early age. Experimental transfer of the disease can be achieved by inoculation of virus by the intracerebral, intra-articular or intraperitoneal route.

Experimental herpes simplex arthritis in rabbits (Webb et al, 1973)

A single intra-articular injection of herpes simplex virus into the knee joint of rabbits induced a chronic erosive arthritis (Webb et al, 1973). After 3 months the injected knee in all of ten animals showed an active chronic synovitis with round cell infiltration. In some, marginal bony erosions and periostitis were appearing. In addition the opposite (non-injected) knees also developed some synovitis, indicating inflammatory changes in joints remote from the inoculation site.

INJECTION OF BACTERIAL PRODUCTS

Adjuvant arthritis in the rat

Following its description by Pearson in 1956, adjuvant disease in the rat has probably been studied more extensively than any other animal model of arthritis. The mechanism by which a single intradermal injection of dead tubercle bacilli in oil leads to polyarthritis remains uncertain, and no clear parallel with any human disease has yet been established. Nevertheless, this model is still studied extensively and used in screening drugs for anti-inflammatory activity.

Induction of arthritis

Adjuvant disease is generally induced by a single intracutaneous injection of dead tubercle bacilli suspended in mineral oil (Freund's complete adjuvant) into a footpad or the tailbase. The ear pinna and a lymph node are alterative sites. The volume injected (10–100 μl) is less critical than the concentration of tubercle, about 6 mg/ml being optimal. Thorough grinding of the tubercle aggregates is essential, arthritis depending on the presence of material which will pass through a sieve of pore size 90 μm (Liyanage et al, 1975).

The precise requirement for the sensitising 'antigen' has never been fully defined. Protein-free wax fractions of mycobacteria can readily induce the disease, as can several smaller protein molecules prepared from the cell walls of other bacteria, including *Nocardia, Streptomyces, Streptococcus* and *Lactobacillus.* Both bacterial and synthetic peptidoglycans, and peptidoglycan (dimer) fragments, in oil may induce arthritis. The requirement for conventional adjuvant properties appears to be more important than immunogenicity (Chang et al, 1980). This has been interpreted as suggesting a role for some endogenous antigen. However, it is notable that rats rendered tolerant to mycobacterial antigens are protected from adjuvant disease. Also, intraperitoneal injections of PPD during the incubation period increase the severity of arthritis, while similar injections of whole mycobacteria protect from arthritis (Currey, 1970). Competing antigens added to the adjuvant are also protective (Grey & Waksman, 1967).

Clinical course of adjuvant disease

Following the challenge with adjuvant there is some local inflammatory swelling at the site of the injection. This reaches a maximum after 24 hours and begins to subside after 48 hours. Polyarthritis appears from about the 9th to the 14th day. However, in those animals that received the initial challenge into a footpad, the injected foot may begin to swell again from about the 6th day. There are differences in susceptibility between different strains of rat. However, the incidence and severity of arthritis varies also from time to time — even within one laboratory and using an inbred rat strain — and the factors determining this have not been identified. With a good yield 100% of animals develop arthritis in all four limbs. The ankles and tarsus are usually most severely affected, but the wrists and digital joints are commonly involved too (Fig. 15.1). Affected joints are generally markedly swollen and tender, the overlying skin is bright red and the animal may walk with obvious difficulty. Changes in body weight and serum markers of inflammation point to the inflammatory activity reaching a maximum about day 15, then subsiding. In mildly affected rats this appearance and resolution of arthritis may be delayed for a week or more. Clinically joint swelling persists after body weight gain and serum changes indicate that the inflammatory disease has subsided. In the more severely affected joints irritability gives way to signs of bony thickening and ankylosis. Tail joint involvement, which may have been inconspicuous during the acute stage, can leave a rigid flexed tail which interferes with walking. Milder recurrences of inflammation may occasionally appear after about 60 or 100 days.

Extra-articular lesions appear about day 12 in severely affected animals. Most common are erythematous and nodular lesions on the pinna of the ear and along the tail. Balanitis may be obvious in male rats, sometimes conjunctivitis and rhinitis. Death attributable to adjuvant disease is rare.

Morbid anatomy (Fig. 15.2)

The early changes consist of oedema and round cell infiltration. This soon gives way to an intense infiltrate of mixed polymorphonuclear leucocytes and lymphocytes. There is marked vascular congestion, synovial effusion and fibrin deposition. Synovial proliferation then leads to pannus formation, with destruction of joint cartilage and underlying bone. There is a marked periosteal reaction which produces striking periarticular new bone formation. In the later stages bony overgrowth, fibrosis and ankylosis are the most obvious features. These latter changes are most readily seen on X-rays (Fig. 15.3). They persist after the inflammatory phase has settled. The nodular ear lesions show oedema and perivascular cuffing with

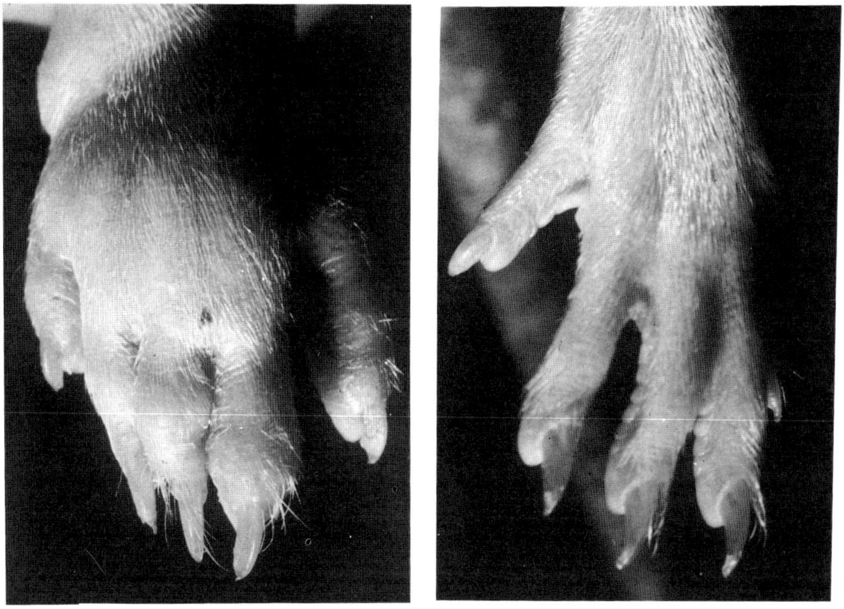

a b

Fig. 15.1 Adjuvant arthritis in the rat (a) Non-injected hind paw of an animal with severe arthritis on day 16. (b) Hind paw of a normal animal for comparison.

round cells. Scattered granulomata are found in internal organs.

Pathogenesis of adjuvant arthritis

There is no evidence that the joint lesions are the result of an infection. The role of the intracutaneous depot of tubercle in oil has been explored by Ward & Jones (1962) who found that polyarthritis occurred even when the depot was removed (by distal tail amputation) within two hours of injection. Newbould (1964) showed that the lymph nodes draining the injection site increased rapidly

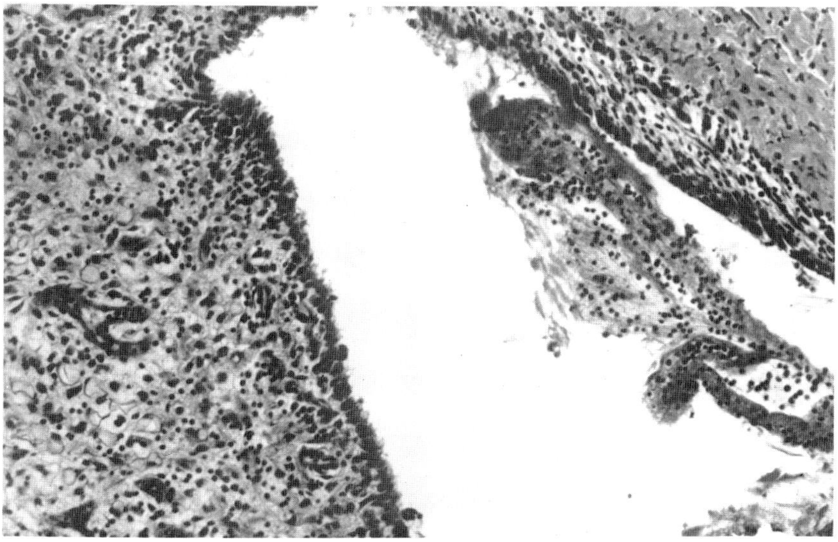

Fig. 15.2 Adjuvant arthritis in the rat. Synovium from non-injected hind paw joint of an animal with severe arthritis on day 16.

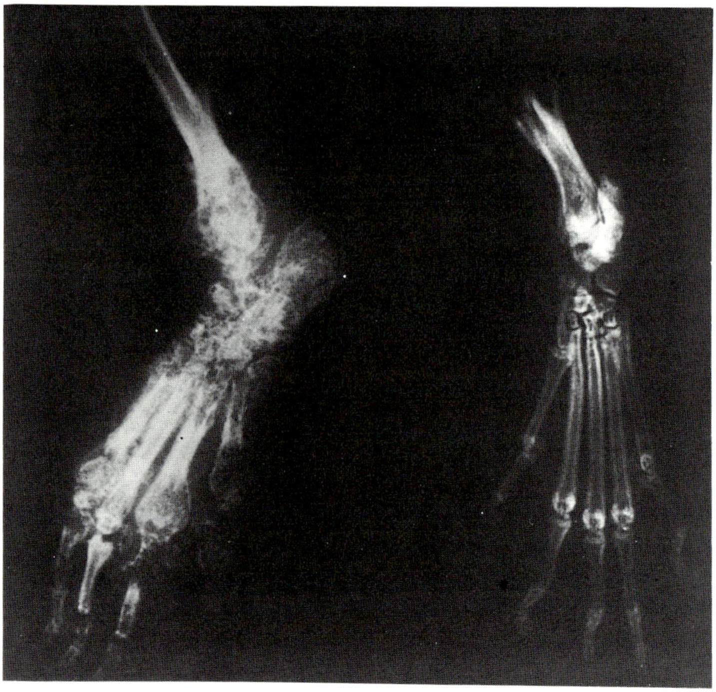

Fig. 15.3 Adjuvant arthritis in the rat. X-ray of non-injected hind paw of an animal with severe arthritis on day 23 (left). On right: X-ray of normal paw for comparison.

in weight during the first 5–7 days following injection. If these lymph nodes were excised before day 5, polyarthritis did not develop. Removal from day 7 onwards did not affect the appearance of arthritis. Vernon-Roberts and his colleagues (1976) showed by fluorescence techniques that the injected tubercle bacilli become distributed widely throughout many organs, and can be identified in the synovial lining of joints in non-injected limbs. Adjuvant arthritis can be transferred to syngeneic animals by lymph node and spleen cells from injected donors (Quagliata & Phillips-Quagliata, 1972). However, washed thoracic duct cells (capable of transferring delayed hypersensitivity to PPD) failed to transfer arthritis unless mycobacteria were added. Since the addition of mycobacterial components (probably already present in lymph node and spleen cell preparations) was necessary to transfer disease, together with sensitised thoracic duct cells, this appeared to point to adjuvant disease resulting from a cell-mediated reaction directed against mycobacterial components distributed to distal sites from the original injection depot. A recent study by Battisto et al (1982) employing inbred strains of rat suggests that susceptibility to adjuvant arthritis is inherited as a dominant trait controlled by an autosomal gene locus linked to the major histocompatability complex.

Quantitation of adjuvant disease activity

Adjuvant arthritis is so clinically obvious that it is a simple matter to use a subjective visual scoring system. Objective methods include displacement of mercury by immersion of the foot to a predetermined depth, or measurement of paw thickness by a light spring calliper. Glenn and his colleagues (1965) have described a variety of biochemical changes in the serum of arthritic rats. Nephelometrically-determined serum 'inflammation units' provide an objective, if non-specific, index of inflammatory activity.

Pharmacological studies using adjuvant arthritis

Adjuvant arthritis is suppressed to a measurable extent by all the anti-inflammatory drugs used in the treatment of rheumatoid arthritis (Ward & Cloud, 1965) and is widely used in the testing of such drugs. It is not influenced by 'slow acting' drugs such as gold, penicillamine and antimalarials, but it can be inhibited by immunosuppressive drugs such as azathioprine and antilymphocyte globulin. By varying the time of dosage, and following inflammation in the injected as well as non-injected limbs, and skin responses to tuberculin, it is possible to compare both the immunosuppressive and the anti-inflammatory activities of such drugs (Currey, 1971).

Streptococcal cell wall-induced arthritis in rats
(Cromartie et al, 1977)
Streptococcal cell wall preparations have been shown to produce a variety of inflammatory lesions in experimental animals. In mice the striking lesion is a pancarditis which has been regarded as a model of rheumatic fever in man; in rabbits the main feature is nodular inflammation of connective tissue. Direct injection of streptococcal material into rabbit joints produces a chronic and progressive monarthritis. Of greater interest, however, is a dramatic polyarthritis which appears in rats within hours of an intraperitoneal injection of a streptococcal sonicate.

Clinical features
Arthritis is produced by a single intraperitoneal injection of a whole cell sonicate of group A streptococci (total dose equivalent to 60 μg rhamnose per gram body weight). Amongst 35 Sprague-Dawley rats so injected, 100% developed polyarthritis (Cromatie et al, 1977). A few animals exhibited oligoarthritis lasting only days; the majority developed prolonged, either intermittent or remittent polyarthritis which was still present after four months. The pattern of arthritis was peripheral rather than proximal, and affected joints were hot, red, swollen and painful (Fig. 15.4). In striking contrast to adjuvant disease the arthritis appeared as early as 15 hours after injection. Rat strains differ in susceptibility and, as with adjuvant disease, the Buffalo strain is relatively resistant.

Histological changes
Microscopic changes appear before arthritis is clinically obvious, and evidence of inflammation

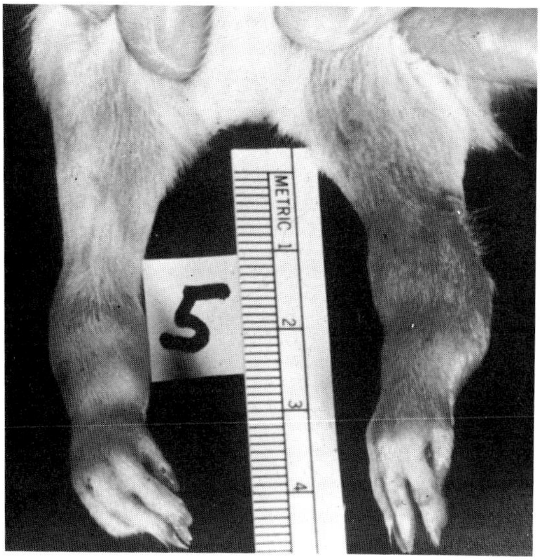

Fig. 15.4 Streptococcal cell wall arthritis. Front legs of a rat 79 days after injection of whole cell sonicate of group A streptococci. (Photograph kindly provided by Dr William J. Cromartie MD.)

is present within 5 hours of injection. Affected joints show acute exudative inflammation with infiltration by neutrophils, macrophages and lymphocytes. Fibrin deposition is prominent. These changes evolve into a chronic proliferative synovitis with pannus formation and erosion of cartilage and bone (Fig. 15.5). In severe cases there is joint destruction, sometimes with late bony ankylosis. Both the liver and the spleen become infiltrated with macrophages which have foamy cytoplasm. Fluorescent tracing studies have shown that streptococcal cell wall material is widely distributed and can be identified in synovial lining tissues. Significantly, such material has been shown to persist for months within macrophages at the sites of recurrent inflammatory episodes (Dalldorf et al, 1980).

Pathogenesis
Different species of streptococci vary in their ability to produce arthritis, and sonicates are more arthritogenic than heat-killed whole cell suspensions. The toxic moiety is a peptidoglycan-polysaccharide fragment of the cell wall. The ability of this material to induce arthritis may relate to the fact that it is highly resistant to degradation and it persists in the tissues for

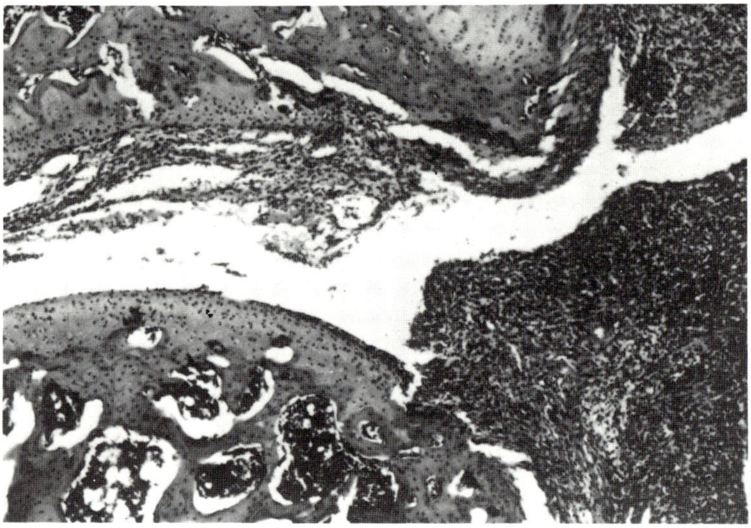

Fig. 15.5 Streptococcal cell wall arthritis. Erosive synovitis of a rat ankle joint 5 weeks after injection of whole cell sonicate of group A streptococci × 36. (Photograph kindly provided by Dr William J. Cromartie MD.)

long periods, particularly within macrophages.

How the peptidoglycan-polysaccharide complex induces synovitis is unknown. It could be a direct toxic effect. Alternatively it might act through an immume mechanism. However, the very short and variable incubation period is against this. Also, arthritis can be induced in neonatally thymectomised rats which do not mount a delayed hypersensitivity response to cell wall peptidoglycan (Hunter et al, 1980), and there is little correlation between disease and serum levels of antibodies against cell wall polysaccharides and peptidoglycans (Greenblatt et al, 1980). The studies of Schwab & Smialowicz (1975) suggest that the arthritogenicity of the cell walls of different streptococcal species depends on their resistance to degradation, and that the susceptibility of different rat strains may depend on the extent to which ingestion of such material induces their macrophages to become cytotoxic. Peptidoglycan-polysaccharide cell wall material can also activate the alternative complement pathway (Greenblatt et al, 1978). Predictably these observations have led to much speculation that this model provides a pointer to mechanisms involved in some types of human arthritis (Hadler, 1976).

Fox and his colleagues (1982) recently injected graded sizes of covalently bound polymers of peptidoglycan and group-specific polysaccharide isolated from the cell walls of group A streptococci. The resulting joint lesions followed a bimodal pattern, with a first peak at 5 days, followed by a chronic remittent, erosive arthritis lasting several months. The relative severity of the acute and chronic phases appeared to depend on the size of the polymers injected. Larger fragments (500×10^6 daltons) induced chronic lesions, smaller fragments (5.3×10^6 daltons) produced the most severe acute inflammation.

PROTEIN IMMUNISATION

Antigen-induced arthritis (Dumonde & Glynn, 1962; Glynn, 1968)

One of the best studied models of arthritis in animals is that in which an antigen is introduced directly into the joint of an animal previously sensitised to that substance. Early studies employed fibrin or products of inflammation as antigen and were interpreted as pointing to autosensitisation as a mechanism for the chronicity of inflammatory arthritis. However, subsequent studies have indicated that this is a more general phenomenon, and a wide variety of protein antigens are equally effective in inducing arthritis, provided that the animal is appropriately sensitised.

The close similarity between the morbid anatomical changes in this model and those in rheumatoid joints, the simplicity of the method of induction, its reproducibility and the convenience of working with the rabbit knee joint (and having the contralateral joint as a control) have tended to make this a standard experimental model of immune synovitis in animals. It has been used to study both pathogenic mechanisms and various therapeutic methods.

Method of inducing immune synovitis

A typical inducing regimen is to sensitise the rabbit with an emulsion containing equal volumes of (for example) ovalbumin 5 mg/ml in saline and Freund's complete adjuvant (2 mg tubercle/ml). 2 ml of this emulsion are injected intracutaneously, distributed between various sites. About 17 days later (at which stage skin testing should confirm delayed hypersensitivity to ovalbumin) a knee joint is injected with a sterile solution of 2.5 mg ovalbumin in 0.5 ml saline.

The rabbit is usually employed for production of this immune synovitis, but the guinea-pig, chicken and goat (with doses adjusted for size) are equally susceptible.

A notable point about the method of sensitisation is the requirement for the Freund's adjuvant to be 'complete' (i.e. to contain tubercle bacilli) in order for the subsequent intra-articular injection to induce a chronic synovitis. The experimental evidence points to this requirement reflecting the need for the animal to develop cell-mediated immunity to the sensitising antigen. It is perhaps relevant that there is a similar requirement for complete adjuvant in the induction of organ-specific autoimmune diseases such as thyroiditis and orchitis.

Morbid anatomical changes

Caged animals show little clinical evidence of disability. However, swelling of the injected knee can be detected within 24 hours. Histological changes are striking and may persist for 30 weeks or more (Fig. 15.6). These changes are very similar to those of human rheumatoid synovitis. There is both hyperplasia and hypertrophy of the lining cell layer, together with increased folding which may progress to villous transformation. Lymphocytic infiltration produces perivascular cuffing and follicle formation, sometimes with germinal centres. In addition there is an extensive, diffuse cellular infiltration in which plasma cells predominate. Continuing synovitis leads to

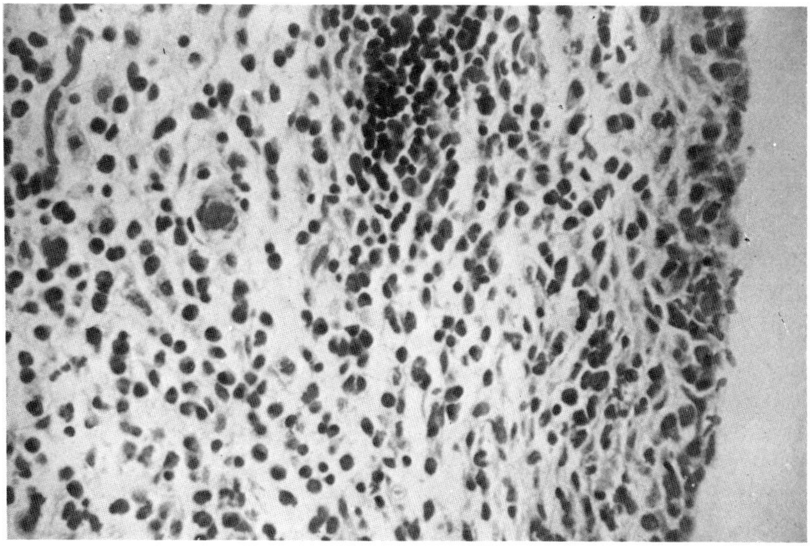

Fig. 15.6 Glynn model of immune synovitis. Rabbit knee joint synovium 3 weeks after antigen challenge. Lining cell hyperplasia and round cell infiltration.

outgrowth of a cellular pannus which spreads across the articular cartilage. In due course this invades first cartilage, then bone, to produce erosions which are entirely comparable to the destructive changes in rheumatoid disease. An impressive feature of this arthritis is that it may persist and progress for 6 months or more.

Studies using the immune synovitis model

Immune synovitis in the rabbit has been used extensively to study different aspects of inflammatory joint disease. Phillips & Page-Thomas (1979) have described techniques for quantitating the synovitis, and numerous studies have tested the influence on it of both systemic and local therapeutic measures including operative surgical procedures (Currey et al, 1970). Steffen et al (1982) showed that local X-ray treatment had an anti-inflammatory effect on the synovitis. This model has proved useful also for studying the biochemical changes in cartilage that occur in inflammatory arthritis, as well as the cellular and biochemical changes involved in invasion of connective tissues by pannus.

However, the main interest in this model lies in the opportunity it provides for studying factors which determine chronicity in the inflammatory synovitis. Cooke & Jasin (1972) and Cooke et al (1972) have shown that there is active local production of antibody to the injected antigen and that this is associated with selective retention of the antigen, in the form of immune complexes, within the collagenous joint structures. This has led to speculation that in rheumatoid arthritis also immune complexes trapped within, or bound to, collagen fibres may play a role in chronicity.

'Serum sickness' arthritis in rabbits (Poole & Coombs, 1977; Poole et al, 1978)

Inducing immune synovitis by the injection of antigen into animal joints introduces a highly artificial element into the model. In an attempt to overcome this, Coombs and his colleagues have studied the joints of rabbits injected intravenously with foreign proteins. Serum sickness has of course been much studied in laboratory animals, including rabbits (Dixon et al, 1961), but in the past little if any attention has been directed towards joint lesions.

When rabbits were given a single intravenous injection of bovine serum (5 ml/kg body weight) about 25% developed synovitis of both knees, which persisted for some weeks. A variety of different immunising regimens did not produce more consistent arthritis than the single intravenous injection, and delayed type hypersensitivity was not a prerequisite for arthritis.

Affected joints showed histological features very similar to human rheumatoid synovitis (Fig. 15.7). There was lining cell enlargement and hyperplasia, focal and diffuse infiltration with lymphocytes and plasma cells, pannus formation and loss of proteoglycan from the underlying cartilage. There was also a synovial effusion containing mainly polymorphonuclear cells. Fluorescent studies showed the presence of complement and immunoglobulin in the joints, suggesting local deposition of immune complexes.

In an interesting extension of these studies, Coombs & Oldham (1981) have shown that similar joint lesions can be identified, not only in rabbits receiving intravenous injections of cows' milk, but also in rabbits offered whole milk to drink in place of water (and receiving no injections).

AUTOIMMUNISATION

Collagen type II arthritis (Trentham et al, 1977)

A variety of organ-specific autoimmune diseases in man, e.g. thyroiditis, can be mimicked experimentally in rodents by a single injection of the tissue in question emulsified in Freund's complete adjuvant. In a series of reports Trentham and his colleagues have described what appears to be a comparable model in which immunisation against type II collagen (the type found in cartilage) produces polyarthritis in rats.

Arthritis was induced by type II collagen extracted from a variety of different human and animal sources, but not by other types of collagen. Limited pepsin digestion did not abolish arthritogenicity, suggesting that type-specific determinants residing in the helical region of the molecule were responsible for inducing the disease.

The inducing injection consisted on 0.5 mg of collagen in 0.1 *M* acetic acid, emulsified with either complete or incomplete Freund's adjuvant and injected intradermally in multiple sites. Intra-

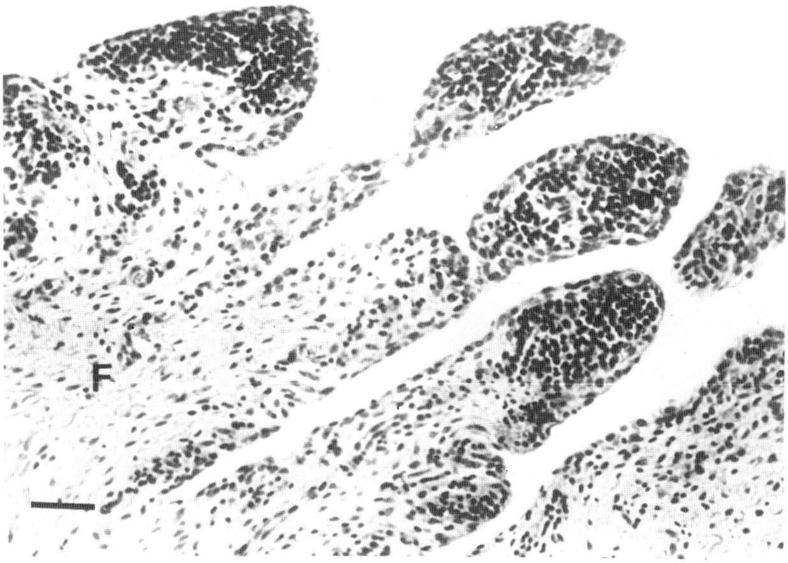

Fig. 15.7 Synovitis in the rabbit knee joint following intravenous injections of antigen. Villus formation, infiltration with lymphocytes and plasma cells, and fibroplasia (F). Scale = 50 μm. (Reproduced from Poole & Coombs, 1977, with kind permission of the authors and editor.)

peritoneal booster injections three weeks later (used in the early experiments) were subsequently found not to be necessary. Clinically the arthritis very closely resembles that of adjuvant disease (p. 471) except that only about 40% of injected rats develop arthritis, the onset is later (13–60 days postimmunisation), and the inflammation generally milder. Systemic manifestations and extra-articular features were less prominent than in adjuvant disease. However, this group subsequently described polychondritis affecting the ears of some animals (McCune et al, 1982). Cell transfer between inbred rats can induce arthritis in recipient animals.

An important question is whether collagen type II arthritis is a separate disease model, or whether it is no more than a modified form of adjuvant arthritis. On the present evidence — particularly the fact that it can be induced using Freund's *incomplete* adjuvant — it appears to have a separate pathogenesis, with a specific role for type II collagen.

Histological changes include early generalised lymphoid hypertrophy. Affected synovial joints show chronic proliferative synovitis with pannus formation and secondary destruction of cartilage and bone. The synovial inflammatory cell infiltrate consists mainly of mononuclear cells with fewer neutrophils. The observed changes are non-specific, and do not reveal significant differences (except in degree) from those found in adjuvant disease. As in the latter condition, periosteal new bone formation and late ankylosis are prominent.

Immunised rats develop humoral and cellular immunity to type II collagen. This response tends to be stronger in those rats which develop arthritis, but the correlation between immunity and arthritis is not close. Using seven inbred strains of rat, Griffiths and her colleagues (1981) conclude that both arthritis and immune responsiveness to type II collagen are controlled in part by genes within or closely linked to the rat major histocompatibility complex. As well as rats, certain strains of mouse are susceptible to collagen type II arthritis. Wooley and his colleagues (1981) found that only mice bearing the H-2*a* haplotype were susceptible to the disease, and all susceptible strains were high antibody responders to type II collagen.

Recent studies by Stuart et al (1982a) point strongly towards antibody directed specifically against type II collagen being responsible for the arthritis in mice, and serum transfer experiments in rats reported by this group (Stuart et al, 1982b) appear to confirm this.

Like adjuvant disease, this model of arthritis can be suppressed by anti-inflammatory and immunosuppresive drugs. However, current interest centres mainly round exploiting the model to learn more about the role of immunogenetics in arthritis susceptibility, and as a possible means of determining the significance of autoantibodies to collagen in the serum of rheumatoid patients.

ARTHRITIS INDUCED IN RATS BY ORAL 6-SULPHANILAMIDOINDAZOLE (Mielens & Rozitis, 1964; Miller et al, 1970, 1978)

Routine toxicity studies of the antibacterial agent 6-sulphanilamidoindazole (6-SAI) unexpectedly revealed that oral feeding of the drug induced arthritis in rats. This arthritis generally appeared about a week after the first oral feed, rapidly reached a peak of severity, remained acute for 2–3 days, then subsided over 2–3 weeks to leave non-inflamed joints which were stiff, with fibrosis and bony overgrowth. The ankles and hind paws were the joints usually involved, and the arthritis did not migrate. In some animals arthritis appeared as early as 2 days after the first dose. Affected paws were markedly swollen, erythematous and sometimes exuded a serous discharge. Steroidal and non-steroidal drugs suppressed the inflammation.

The incidence and severity of arthritis was related to both the dose of 6-SAI and the age of the rats. Two daily feeds of 250 mg/kg induced arthritis in some older rats (450 g). In general, higher dosages and older age of the rats yielded more arthritis. Parenteral administration of 6-SAI also produced arthritis. Later rechallenge produced somewhat milder arthritis in most animals. Different rat strains varied in susceptibility, while other species (monkeys and mice) did not develop arthritis following 6-SAI feeding, and related sulphonamides did not induce arthritis in rats. Histological studies showed, in the early stages, very gross periarticular oedema with round cell and polymorphonuclear infiltration. As the lesions evolved there developed striking proliferative changes, with overgrowth of fibrous connective tissue and new bone formation. The synovial membrane showed some cellular infiltration and proliferation, but the articular surfaces were generally well preserved. No significant systemic lesions were found.

Laboratory studies have failed to reveal the pathogenesis of this arthritis (or more correctly, periarthritis). An early report that mycoplasmas could be recovered from the joints and blood of affected animals has not been confirmed, and the features of the inflammation do not suggest a microbial cause. Likewise there is little to suggest an immunological basis. The incubation period (sometimes as short as 2 days) and spontaneous resolution despite continued administration of SAI, are difficult to reconcile with an immunological mechanism. Acute phase reactants, particularly fibrinogen, become raised early, but the available evidence does not point to a causative role for these.

EXPERIMENTAL MODELS OF OSTEOARTHRITIS

Models of osteoarthritis in laboratory animals are available which resemble the human disease much more closely than do animal models of inflammatory synovitis. In the first place most animal species develop osteoarthritis spontaneously. Using inbred strains of mice this has made it possible to study genetic influences in degenerative joint disease. However, in order to follow the sequential morbid anatomical and biochemical changes it has proved more convenient to induce secondary osteoarthritis in single joints in larger animals. Both operative procedures for inducing instability and biochemical insults to the articular cartilage have been employed for this (Troyer, 1982). The following are some of the models which have proved useful in studying osteoarthritis.

Spontaneous degenerative arthritis in mice

(Spilberg & Spilberg, 1971; Sokoloff et al, 1962)

All strains of mice so far studied develop osteoarthritis spontaneously, but there is a striking difference in incidence and severity between different strains. The course of the disease is conveniently followed in the knee joint. By 6 months of age the cartilage may show localised lose of nuclear staining, followed by surface fibrillation, increased cellularity and hypertrophy at the joint margins. In some animals this progresses to cartilage destruction and bony overgrowth. Sokoloff et al (1962) studying STR/IN hybrids found evidence of a polygenic pattern of inheritance with a non-sex-linked component. The Spilbergs (1971) have shown castration to have a protective effect in males and suggest a significant role for sex hormones in this species.

Experimentally-induced osteoarthritis in the dog (Pond & Nuki, 1973; McDevitt et al, 1977)

In a number of larger animals, surgical procedures which produce instability in the knee joint have been shown to lead to progressive osteoarthritis in the operated joint. The best studied model is the arthritis which follows closed section of the anterior cruciate ligament in the knee (stifle) joint in dogs. Spontaneous rupture of this ligament is a well known cause of hind limb lameness in dogs, and leads to secondary osteoarthritis. When this spontaneous rupture is mimicked by a surgical stab incision, the resulting arthritis appears to be entirely comparable. This induced arthritis allows the sequential morphological and biochemical changes to be followed. All the evidence points to the observed lesions resulting from joint instability, not from inflammatory changes induced by the incision, nor from lack of weight-bearing after the procedure.

The morphological changes tend to be most marked over the medial tibial condyle. Indian ink staining shows early fibrillation of this area after 2 weeks and overt fibrillation at 4 weeks. Early microscopic cartilage changes are seen after 1 week and these progress with time thereafter. By 16 weeks there is gross osteophyte formation and cartilage changes which are indistinguishable from those of secondary osteoarthritis following spontaneous anterior cruciate rupture.

McDevitt and his colleagues (1977) point out that this model is closely analogous to natural osteoarthritis in both man and dog. The size of the canine joints allows topographical biochemical as well as morphological changes to be studied. Since the time of onset is known, and the site at which changes occur is predictable, the disease can be followed in its early stages before overt lesions develop. Thus, increased cartilage hydration and changes in proteoglycans were apparent before the articular surface was damaged.

Surgically induced osteoarthritis in the rabbit knee

A variety of procedures in the rabbit knee joint may lead to progressive degenerative changes in a manner similar to cruciate ligament section in the dog (see above). However, most studies in the rabbit have employed more drastic procedures than have been used in the canine joint. These include cartilage freezing, scarification (which does not lead to progressive osteoarthritis — Mankin, 1982), compression and menisectomy. The Telhag procedure (Telhag & Lindberg, 1972) involves open operation with division of the medial collateral ligament, both cruciates and the flexor digitorum longus, combined with excision of the medial meniscus. Erlich and his colleagues (1975) have confirmed that rabbit knees so treated show histological and biochemical changes over the ensuing 6 months that are similar to those in human osteoarthritis.

Arthritis induced in rabbits by intra-articular papain

Murray (1964) has described a method of inducing degenerative changes in the rabbit knee joint by intra-articular injection of the enzyme preparation papain. The mechanism of the damage is presumed to be depletion of cartilage matrix. The injections consisted of 0.5 ml of a 1% solution of crude papain injected daily for 7 days.

Injected animals showed drooping of the tips of the ears, indicating that the effect of the enzyme is not limited to the injected knee. 10 days after injection the joint cartilage was roughened and friable, with some oedema of the synovium. By 3 weeks there was progressive erosion of cartilage. The role of mechanical factors even in this model of degenerative arthritis is shown by the observation that subcutaneous tenotomy of the patellar ligament significantly retards the development of papain arthritis.

CRYSTAL-INDUCED SYNOVITIS

In a series of classic experiments McCarty and his colleagues showed that injection of microcrystals of urate into the knee joints of both man and dog provokes an acute gouty attack (Faires & McCarty, 1962). Injection into the stifle joint of mongrel dogs of 6.5–20 mg sterile urate crystals suspended in 0.5 ml saline provoked acute arthritis within 2 hours. Aspiration of the tense effusion at 4 hours revealed highly cellular fluid containing intraleucocytic urate crystals.

This model has been used to establish the phlogistic properties of other types of crystals (McCarty & Hogan, 1964) and to test various theories about the mechanism of inflammation in acute crystal synovitis (Phelps et al, 1966). The same technique can be applied also to smaller laboratory animals.

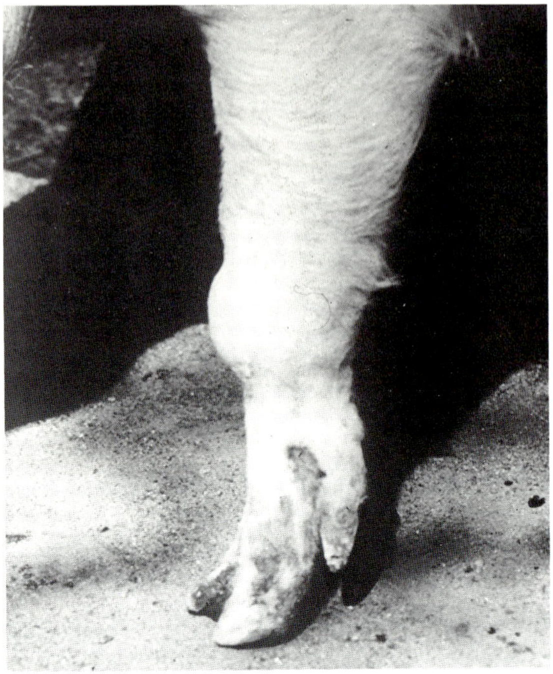

Fig. 15.8 Arthritis in the pig induced by a high protein diet. Swollen fetlock. (Photograph kindly provided by Professor B. Olhagen.)

ARTHRITIS INDUCED IN PIGS BY DIETARY FACTORS (Månsson et al, 1971)

The addition of 20% fish meal to the diets of 8-week-old pigs was shown by Månsson and his colleagues to induce polyarthritis which became clinically obvious after about 5 days. Joints in all four limbs were affected, sometimes with marked swelling (Fig. 15.8). The joint lesions consisted of synovitis with a cell-rich exudate. There was proliferation of synovial lining cells, with villous

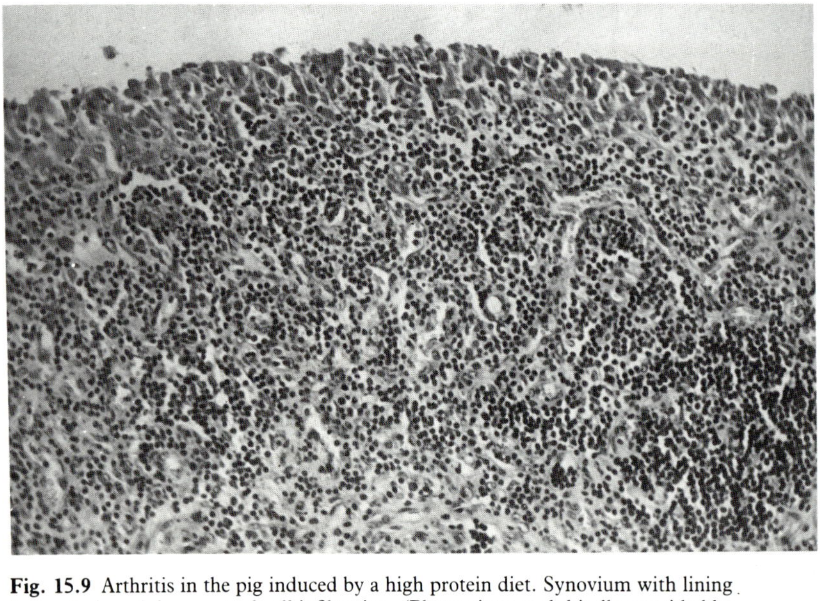

Fig. 15.9 Arthritis in the pig induced by a high protein diet. Synovium with lining hyperplasia and dense round cell infiltration. (Photomicrograph kindly provided by Professor B. Olhagen.)

hypertrophy and vascularised granulation tissue containing accumulations of lymphoid cells (Fig. 15.9). In some joints there was pannus formation and cartilage erosion. Subcutaneous nodules appeared in a proportion of animals, and these had many of the features of rheumatoid nodules. Most animals showed evidence also of some degree of proliferative glomerulonephritis. Culture of synovial material for microbial agents was completely negative.

Within 1 week of starting the high protein diet the animals developed abnormal intestinal microbial flora, the main feature of which was a significant increase in the number of atypical *Clostridium perfringens* type A. There was concomitant hypergammaglobulinaemia, with increased antibodies to *Cl. perfrigens* antigens. Administration of zinc preparations had a protective effect against the arthritis. The mechanism of this arthritis is unknown. Månsson and his colleagues suggest that the overgrowth of *Cl. perfringens* and the resulting immune response to this is the central causative event, operating through the formation of circulating immune complexes or some other mechanism.

SPONTANEOUS RHEUMATOID ARTHRITIS-LIKE DISEASE IN MICE

New Zealand B/W mice have long been studied as a model of SLE in man. Recent interest centres on two newer mouse models, the MRL/1 and the BXSB strains (Dixon, 1981). Hang et al (1982) describe how the disease in MRL/1 animals resembles rheumatoid polyarthritis, with circulating rheumatoid factors, polyarteritis, and enhanced helper T lymphocyte activity. Rordorf et al (1982) have shown that the acute phase plasma protein responses differ in the NZB/W and MRL/1 animals. In the former the levels remain normal, while in the latter they become markedly elevated. This represents an interesting parallel with C-reactive protein responses in human SLE and rheumatoid arthritis.

REFERENCES

Ajmal M 1970 Chronic proliferative arthritis in swine in relation to human rheumatoid arthritis. Veterinary Bulletin 40: 1–8

Astorga G P 1968 Immunological studies of a chronic experimental arthritis clinically resembling rheumatoid arthritis (Abstract). Arthritis and Rheumatism 11:813

Battisto J R, Smith R N, Beckman K, Sternlight M, Welles W L 1982 Susceptibility to adjuvant arthritis in DA and F_{344} rats. Arthritis and Rheumatism 25: 1194–1200

Bennett J C 1978 The infectious etiology of rheumatoid arthritis. New considerations. Arthritis and Rheumatism 21: 531–538

Brassfield A L, Adams D S, Crawford T B, McGuire T C 1982 Ultrastructure of arthritis induced by a caprine retrovirus. Arthritis and Rheumatism 25: 930–936

Bywaters E G L 1981 Observations on chronic polyarthritis in monkeys. Journal of the Royal Society of Medicine 74: 794–799

Cassell G H, Davis J K, Lindsey J R, Cole B C and Hartley M W 1981 Arthritis of rats and mice: implications for man. Israel Journal of Medical Sciences 17: 608–615

Chang Y-H, Pearson C M, Abe C 1980 Adjuvant polyarthritis. IV. Induction by a synthetic adjuvant: immunologic, histopathologic and other studies. Arthritis and Rheumatism 23: 62–71

Cooke T D, Jasin H E 1972 The pathogenesis of chronic inflammation in experimental antigen-induced arthritis. I. The role of antigen in the local immune response. Arthritis and Rheumatism 15: 327–337

Cooke T D, Hurd E R, Ziff M, Jasin H E 1972 The pathogenesis of chronic inflammation in experimental antigen-induced arthritis. II. Preferential localization of antigen-antibody complexes to collagenous tissues. Journal of Experimental Medicine 135: 323–338

Coombs R R A, Oldham G 1981 Rheumatoid-like joint lesions in rabbits drinking cows' milk. International Archives of Allergy and Applied Immunology 64: 287–292

Cork L C, Narayan O 1980 The pathogenesis of viral leukoencephalomyelitis-arthritis of goats. I. Persistant viral infection with progressive pathologic changes. Laboratory Investigation 42: 596–602

Crawford T B, Adams D S, Sande R D, Gorham J R, Henson J B 1980 The connective tissue component of the caprine arthritis-encephalitis syndrome. American Journal of Pathology 100: 443–454

Cromartie W J, Craddock J G, Schwab J H, Anderle S K, Yang C-H 1977 Arthritis in rats after systemic injection of streptococcal cells or cell walls. Journal of Experimental Medicine 146: 1585–1602

Currey H L F 1970 Adjuvant arthritis in the rat. Effect of intraperitoneal injections of either whole dead mycobacteria or tuberculin. Annals of the Rheumatic Diseases 29: 314–320

Currey H L F 1971 A comparison of immunosuppressive and anti-inflammatory agents in the rat. Clinical and Experimental Immunology 9: 879–887

Currey H L F, Moore C J, Prentice A I D 1970 Surgical synovectomy and experimental immune synovitis in the rabbit knee joint. Annals of the Rheumatic Diseases 29: 503–508

Dalldorf F G, Cromartie W J, Anderle S K, Clark R L, Schwab J H 1980 The relation of experimental arthritis to the distribution of streptococcal cell wall fragments. American Journal of Pathology 100: 383–402

Davis J K, Cassell G H, Minion F C, Wise K S 1981 Mycoplasma host-cell interactions resulting in chronic inflammation: acquisition of host antigens and other mechanisms. Israel Journal of Medical Sciences 17: 633–636

Dixon F J, 1982 Murine lupus — an overview. Arthritis and Rheumatism 25: 721–725

Dixon F J, Feldman J D, Vasquez J J 1961 Experimental glomerulonephritis. The pathogenesis of a laboratory model resembling the spectrum of human glomerulonephritis. Journal of Experimental Medicine 113: 899–920

Drew R A 1972 Erysipelothrix arthritis in pigs as a comparative model for rheumatoid arthritis. Proceedings of the Royal Society of Medicine 65: 42–46

Dumonde D C, Glynn L E 1962 The production of arthritis in rabbits by an immunological reaction to fibrin. British Journal of Experimental Pathology 43: 373–383

Erlich M G, Mankin H J, Jones H, Grossman A, Crispen C, Ancona D 1975 Biochemical confirmation of an experimental osteoarthritis model. Journal of Bone and Joint Surgery 57A: 392–396

Faires J S, McCarty D J 1962 Acute arthritis in man and dog after intrasynovial injection of sodium urate crystals. Lancet 2: 682–685

Fox A, Brown R R, Anderle S K, Chetty C, Cromartie W J, Gooder H, Schwab J H 1982 Arthropathic properties related to the molecular weight of peptidoglycan — polysaccharide polymers of streptococcal cell walls. Infection and Immunity 35: 1003–1010

Gardner D L 1960 The experimental production of arthritis: a review. Annals of the Rheumatic Diseases 19: 297–317

Gery I, Waksman B H 1967 Competition of antigens in adjuvant disease of rats. Arthritis and Rheumatism 10: 240–244

Glenn E M, Gray J, Kooyers W 1965 Chemical changes in adjuvant-induced polyarthritis of rats. American Journal of Veterinary Research 26: 1195–1203

Glynn L E 1968 The chronicity of inflammation and its significance in rheumatoid arthritis. Annals of the Rheumatic Diseases 27: 105–121

Greenblatt J J, Boackle R, Schwab J H 1978 Activation of the alternate complement pathway by peptidoglycan from streptococcal cell wall. Infection and Immunity 19: 296–303

Greenblatt J J, Hunter N, Schwab J H 1980 Antibody response to streptococcal cell wall antigens associated with experimental arthritis in rats. Clinical and Experimental Immunology 42: 450–457

Griffiths M M, Eichwald E J, Martin J H, Smith C B, De Witt C 1981 Immunogenetic control of experimental type II collagen-induced arthritis. I. Susceptibility and resistance among inbred strains of rats. Arthritis and Rheumatism 24: 781–789

Hadler N M 1976 A pathogenetic model for erosive synovitis. Lessons from animal arthritides. Arthritis and Rheumatism 19: 256–266

Hang L, Theofilopoulos A N, Dixon F J 1982 A spontaneous rheumatoid arthritis-like disease in MRL/1 mice. Journal of Experimental Medicine 155: 1690–1701

Hunter N, Anderle S K, Brown R R, Dalldorf F G, Clark R L, Cromartie W J, Schwab J H 1980 Cell-mediated immune response during experimental arthritis induced in rats with streptococcal cell walls. Clinical and Experimental Immunology 42: 441–449

Liyanage S P, Currey H L F, Vernon-Roberts B 1975 Influence of tubercle aggregate size on severity of adjuvant arthritis in the rat. Annals of the Rheumatic Diseases 34: 49–53

Lloyd L C, Etheridge 1981 Production of arthritis by intravenous inoculation of *Mycoplasma hyopneumoniae*: tests of five strains. Research in Veterinary Science 30: 124–126

McCarty D J, Hogan J M 1964 Inflammatory reaction after intrasynovial injection of microcrystalline adrenocorticosteroid esters. Arthritis and Rheumatism 7: 359–367

McCune W J, Schiller A L, Dynesius-Trentham R A, Trentham D E 1982 Type II collagen-induced auricular chondritis. Arthritis and Rheumatism 25: 266–273

McDevitt C, Gilbertson E, Muir H 1977 An experimental model of osteoarthritis; early morphological and biochemical changes. Journal of Bone and Joint Surgery 59B: 24–35

Mankin H J 1982 The response of articular cartilage to mechanical injury. The Journal of Bone and Joint Surgery 64A: 460–466

Månsson R, Norberg B, Olhagen B, Björklund N-E 1971 Arthritis in pigs induced by dietary factors. Microbiological, clinical and histological studies. Clinical and Experimental Immunology 9: 677–693

Mielens Z E, Rozitis J 1964 Acute peri-articular inflammation induced in rats by oral 6-sulfanilylindazole. Proceedings of the Society for Experimental Biology and Medicine 117: 751–754

Miller M L, Ward J R, Cole B C, Swinyard E A 1970 6-sulphanilamidoindazole induced arthritis and periarthritis in rats. A new model of experimental inflammation. Arthritis and Rheumatism 13: 222–235

Miller M L, Samuelson C O, Ward J R 1978 Hematologic and serologic studies in 6-sulphanilamidoindazole arthritis. Arthritis and Rheumatism 21: 681–689

Murray D G 1964 Experimentally induced arthritis using intra-articular papain. Arthritis and Rheumatism 7: 211–219

Newbould B B 1964 Role of lymph nodes in adjuvant-induced arthritis in rats. Annals of the Rheumatic Diseases 23: 392–396

Norton W L, Storz J 1967 Observations on sheep with polyarthritis produced by an agent of the psittacosis-lymphogranuloma venereum-trachoma group. Arthritis and Rheumatism 10: 1–12

Pearson C M 1956 Development of arthritis, periarthritis and periostitis in rats given adjuvants. Proceedings of the Society for Experimental Biology and Medicine 91: 95–101

Phelps P, Prockop D J, McCarty D K 1966 Crystal induced inflammation in canine joints. III. Evidence against bradykinin as a mediator of inflammation. Journal of Laboratory and Clinical Medicine 68: 433–444

Phillips N C, Page-Thomas D P 1979 Monitoring of experimental arthritis in rabbits. Annals of the Rheumatic Diseases 38: 89–93

Poole A R, Coombs R R A 1977 Rheumatoid-like joint lesions in rabbits injected intravenously with bovine serum. International Archives of Allergy and Applied Immunology 54: 97–113

Poole A R, Oldham G, Coombs R R A 1978 Early rheumatoid-like lesions in rabbits injected with foreign serum: relationship to localization of immune complexes in the lining tissues of joints and cellular content of synovial fluid. International Archives of Allergy and Applied Immunology 57: 135–145

Pond M J, Nuki G 1973 Experimentally-induced osteoarthritis in the dog. Annals of the Rheumatic Diseases 32: 387–388

Quagliata F, Phillips-Quagliata J M 1972 Competence of thoracic duct cells in the transfer of adjuvant disease and delayed hypersensitivity. Evidence that mycobacterial components are required for the successful transfer of the disease. Cellular Immunology 3: 78–87

Razin S 1981 Mycoplasmas: the smallest pathogenic procaryotes. Israel Journal of Medical Sciences 17: 510–515

Rordorf C, Schnebli H P, Baltz M L, Tennent G A, Pepys M B 1982 The acute-phase response in (NZB × NZW) F_1 and MRL/1 mice. Journal of Experimental Medicine 156: 1268–1273

Schwab J H, Smialowicz R 1975 Interaction of bacterial cell wall polymers and rat macrophages. Zeitschrift fur Immunitatsforschung 149: 283–288

Silberg R, Silberg M 1971 Skeletal growth and aging. Documents Geigy, Acta Rheumatologica. Ciba-Geigy, Basel, p 12–50

Sokoloff L, Crittenden L B, Yamamoto R S, Jay G E 1962 The genetics of degenerative joint disease in mice. Arthritis and Rheumatism 5: 531–546

Steffen C, Muller Ch, Stellamor K, Zeitlhofer J 1982 Influence of X-ray treatment on antigen-induced experimental arthritis. Annals of the Rheumatic Diseases 41: 532–537

Stuart J M, Townes A S, Kang A H 1982a Nature and specificity of the immune response to collagen in type II collagen-induced arthritis in mice. Journal of Clinical Investigations 69: 673–683

Stuart J M, Cremer M A, Townes A S, Karg A H (1982b) Type II collagen-induced arthritis in rats. Passive transfer with serum and evidence that IgG anticollagen antibodies can cause arthritis. Journal of Experimental Medicine 155: 1–16

Taylor-Robinson D, Tully J G, Furr P M, Cole R M, Rose D L, Hanna N F 1981 Urogenital mycoplasma infections of man: a review with observations on a recently discovered mycoplasma. Israel Journal of Medical Sciences 17: 524–530

Telhag H, Lindberg L 1972 A method for inducing osteoarthritic changes in rabbits' knees. Clinical Orthopaedics and Related Research 86: 214–223

Trentham D E, Townes A D, Kang A H 1977 Autoimmunity to type II collagen: an experimental model of arthritis. The Journal of Experimental Medicine 146: 857–868

Troyer H 1982 Experimental models of osteoarthritis: A review. Seminars in Arthritis and Rheumatism 11: 362–374

Vernon-Roberts B, Liyanage S P, Currey H L F 1976 Distribution of fluorescent material after footpad injection of rhodamine-labelled tubercle bacilli. Annals of the Rheumatic Diseases 35: 389–397

Ward J R, Cloud R S 1965 Comparative effect of antirheumatic drugs on adjuvant-induced polyarthritis in rats. The Journal of Pharmacology and Experimental Therapeutics 152: 116–121

Ward J R, Jones R S 1962 Studies on adjuvant-induced polyarthritis in rats. I. Adjuvant composition, route of injection and removal of depot site. Arthritis and Rheumatism 5: 557–564

Washburn L R, Cole B C, Gelman M I, Ward J R 1980 Chronic arthritis of rabbits induced by mycoplasmas. I. Clinical microbiologic and histological features. Arthritis and Rheumatism 23: 825–836

Washburn L R, Cole B C, Ward J R 1982 Chronic arthritis of rabbits induced by mycoplasmas. III. Induction with non-viable Mycoplasma arthritidis antigens. Arthritis and Rheumatism 25: 937–945

Webb F W, Bluestone R, Goldberg L S, Douglas S D, Pearson C M 1973 Experimental viral arthritis induced with herpes simplex. Arthritis and Rheumatism 16: 241–250

Wooley P H, Luthra H S, Stuart J M, David C S 1981 Type II collagen-induced arthritis in mice. I. Major histocompatibility complex (I region) linkage and antibody correlates. Journal of Experimental Medicine 154: 688–700

SECTION IV

Clinical Pharmacology

The clinical pharmacokinetics of antirheumatic drugs

The management of a patient with rheumatoid disease or one of the other rheumatic diseases usually requires a combined approach which may involve drugs, physiotherapy, physical, psychological and social support and, at times, other measures including surgery. In many cases drugs are the major part of treatment, and satisfactory control of symptoms, though undoubtedly related to the severity of the disease process, will depend on making the best use of those available.

There is a considerable choice of drugs to treat most rheumatic disorders and doctors need to be able to choose the best of those currently in use and also to assess the data presented on new agents, whose place in the therapeutic armamentarium is still to be determined. Data on the mode of action, evidence for efficacy, dose, and side-effects of the important antirheumatic drugs are presented in later chapters and the clinical relevance of this information is easy to understand. The pharmacokinetic data, indicating how these drugs are handled in the body and how they should be used to best advantage, are often less easy to comprehend. The meaning and relevance of such data are therefore presented in a non-mathematical way in this chapter.

Since pharmacokinetic data are derived from the plasma concentration of the drugs, which is the major but by no means only factor which determines the tissue concentrations, the relevance of plasma concentrations must be the starting point. It should be said at the outset that there is no simple, direct relationship between the circulating blood levels of anti-inflammatory drugs and their effects. Indeed, it would be remarkable if there were, since the clinical monitoring of the severity of inflammatory disease is not easily quantifiable. There is, consequently, no case to be made for routine therapeutic drug monitoring except perhaps to check compliance, although this is rarely a serious problem. A convincing case can, however, be made for the need for a proper understanding of the pharmacokinetics of anti-inflammatory agents in order to make the best use of them , to appreciate the factors which can affect their fate in the body and to be able to identify in advance potential drug interactions. Orme has published an interesting review of the plasma concentration and therapeutic effect of anti-inflammatory drugs (1982).

To exert an effect a drug must be able to reach its site of action in sufficiently high concentration. In inflammatory disease one of the main sites of action is probably the synovium and, to reach this, a drug must be able to cross a number of membranes within the body. There are several physicochemical factors which influence the extent and rate at which a drug is able to be transported across membranes, e.g. ionisation constant, partition coefficient and degree of protein binding. Although our understanding o f these factors is by no means complete, a great deal of information has been gathered and some important conclusions have been reached. These will be discussed below and areas where our knowledge is still scanty will be indicated.

PHARMACOKINETIC PRINCIPLES

Pharmacokinetics is simply a means of expressing, in quantitative terms, what happens to a drug in the body. What follows is a brief description of pharmacokinetic principles without the use of mathematics. This may irritate as many as it pleases. Readers seeking a simple and clear mathematical treatment are referred to the books by Smith & Rawlins (1976) and Ritschel (1977). More mathematical works by Shargel & Yu (1980) and Rowland & Tozer (1980) are also recommended. These latter works also contain references to the original literature.

An orally administered tablet or capsule will pass into the small intestine, which is the main site of absorption. The absorbed drug then passes through the liver to the systemic circulation and thereafter distributes itself throughout the body, some passing to the site of action which, in the case of rheumatological drugs, will include the synovial membrane. At the same time the active substance is being eliminated either directly through the kidney, indirectly through the biliary system or after biotransformation in the liver. As the concentration in plasma falls, more drug from the tissues will flow into the systemic circulation to be removed. These processes, the rate at which they occur and the factors which influence them are beginning to be understood. They are important because they determine the magnitude and duration of the effect which the active substance can have at its site of action.

Absorption and distribution

Many drugs are supplied in tablet form and may contain a dozen or more substances in addition to the therapeutically active compound. The additional substances are present for a variety of reasons: to prevent the drug decomposing due to the action of air, moisture or light, to bind the ingredients together to make tabletting easier, to make the tablet disintegrate rapidly once swallowed and to add bulk. Until the late 1960s these additional substances were assumed to be inert and have no effect on the action of the drug. However, several reports including one of an outbreak of phenytoin toxicity in Australia changed that (Tyrer et al, 1970). Today it is well recognised that small changes in the formulation, the recipe of the ingredients making up a tablet, can have a marked effect on the amount and rate of drug reaching the bloodstream. New formulations must now be compared with established ones using healthy volunteers to prove that the resulting blood drug profiles are closely similar with respect to the area under the plasma concentration/time curve, maximum drug concentration attained, time taken to reach this concentration and subsequent rate of elimination. If the formulations are comparable in all these respects they are judged to be 'bioequivalent' or to have the same 'bioavailability'.

The particle size of a drug substance can affect its rate of absorption: a study of benoxaprofen showed that a reduction in particle size (i.e. an increase in surface area) led to an increased rate of absorption (Smith et al, 1977). Many anti-inflammatory drugs are both acidic and prostaglandin synthetase inhibitors and may produce local irritation in the stomach. In an attempt to reduce this, many of the drugs are formulated as enteric preparations having a coating which is intended to delay release of the drug until it has passed into the small intestine. Once there, most anti-inflammatory drugs, particularly the non-steroidal organic acids, are very well absorbed.

The factors governing drug absorption are many and still not completely understood. However, the relative importance of a number of physicochemical properties of the drugs themselves is well recognised.

Ionisation or dissociation constant

This is important because it is now accepted that a molecule will pass more easily across a membrane when in its unionised form. Thus the pH on different sides of a biological membrane will help determine the passage of a drug. This will be of importance not only in determining absorption from the gastrointestinal tract into the bloodstream but also penetration into synovial fluid. Most drugs are capable of some degree of ionisation in an aqueous medium and the proportion of unionised to ionised molecules depends upon both the hydrogen ion concentration of the medium and the ionisation constant of the drug. These are most conveniently expressed in their logarithmic form as pH and pKa respectively. Acidic drugs will be almost completely unionised in strongly acidic media and almost completely ionised in alkaline media. Almost twenty years ago Cummings & Nordby (1966) demonstrated that the synovial fluid pH of subjects with rheumatoid arthritis was more acidic than that of osteoarthritic patients or normal controls. In the absence of any other factors, this would mean that the amount of drug passing into the synovial fluid of rheumatoid patients would be less than in a control group. This topic is discussed in some detail by Farr et al (1982). Absorption, however, is by no means simple and there are factors other than pH and pKa which may markedly influence transfer across membranes. These include the partition coefficient.

Partition coefficient

This is a measure of a drug's lipophilicity and is determined in the laboratory by observing how the drug partitions between an aqueous phase, usually buffered at pH 7.4, and a lipid phase, usually n-octanol. Lipophilic drugs concentrate in the octanol and have, therefore, a large partition coefficient, while hydrophilic drugs concentrate in the aqueous phase and have a small partition coefficient. A number of publications report partition coefficients for a few anti-inflammatory drugs, but direct comparison is impossible, unless they are measured under very similar conditions of temperature, buffer and lipid phase. Studies have been carried out to measure the partition coefficients of the most common non-steroidal anti-inflammatory drugs under a single set of conditions (Jack & Patel, 1982) and a simple ranking as high, intermediate and low lipophilicity is given in Table 16.1.

Generally the higher the partition coefficient the more easily will a drug cross a membrane. The fact that many drugs in Table 16.1 have high partition coefficients at pH 7.4, when they are almost completely ionised, means that even the *ionised* form of the drug is very lipid-soluble. However, lest one be lulled into a false sense of security, there are compounds which break all the rules: para-aminobenzoic acid, for example, has a low partition coefficient and is highly ionised at pH 7.4 yet it is extremely well absorbed (Yasuhara et al, 1978). Obviously our knowledge is still far from complete.

Protein binding

Plasma albumin binds many acidic drugs or drugs with strongly electronegative centres and at least four different binding sites have been identified, some with high affinity and others low (Sjöholm, 1978). One study has demonstrated that ibuprofen, flurbiprofen and naproxen are all bound to the 'diazepam' binding site, while azapropazone is bound to the 'warfarin' site (Kober & Sjöholm, 1980). Current thinking on protein-binding asserts that only the free (i.e. unbound) fraction of a drug is available for membrane transport and this is highly significant since almost all non-steroidal anti-inflammatory drugs are very highly bound (Table 16.1). A small change in binding can result in a much larger change in the free fraction. For example if a drug is 95% protein-bound the bound fraction is 0.95 and the free is 0.05. If a decrease of only 10% takes place in protein-binding, the bound fraction becomes 0.86 and the free 0.14. Thus a decrease of 10% in the bound produces an almost threefold increase in the free and this phenomenon becomes more pronounced the greater the degree of protein-binding. The increased amount of free drug then becomes available for transport across membranes including those of the liver and kidney, which may lead to an increased rate of elimination.

Changes in the degree of protein-binding can be brought about by alteration in the amount of circulating albumin (e.g. in renal disease) or by competition between drugs for the same binding site. Salicylates, which are frequently co-administered with other anti-inflammatory agents, are capable of displacing these from their binding sites. This will result in an immediate increase in the free fraction of drug, which is then redistributed to other tissues; the net result is a fall in total drug in the circulating bloodstream. This type of drug interaction is now well documented and is discussed later. It might be possible to use this interaction to advantage by co-administering salicylate with the drug to boost the tissue concentration of the latter. However, it should be remembered that the increased free drug is also available for hepatic or renal elimination.

Tissue-binding almost certainly takes place but the literature contains little information on this topic. There are, however, numerous examples of single dose studies of anti-inflammatory drugs where plasma and synovial fluid specimens have been withdrawn at intervals. Such profiles are of limited use and serve only to demonstrate that synovial fluid concentrations of drug lag behind those in the plasma. To obtain more meaningful data it would first be necessary to produce a steady-state concentration in plasma and synovial fluid and studies of this type are rare. Whitlam et al (1981) studied the distribution of ibuprofen between synovial fluid and serum in arthritic patients and found that the synovial concentration of total ibuprofen was about half that in serum. In addition the ratio of total drug in synovial fluid to that in serum correlated well with the albumin concentration ratio in the two fluids confirming that binding to this protein may be an important factor in determining tissue distribution. Farr et al (1982) have examined phenylbutazone concentrations under steady-state conditions and found that the synovial concentrations were lower than those in plasma, but related. Interestingly the synovial fluid concentrations of phenylbutazone were higher in patients with rheumatoid arthritis than in those suffering from osteoarthritis. This type of finding leads one to ask whether the nature of the synovial membrane in rheumatoid arthritis is different. Simkin & Pizzorno (1979) have shown that proteins enter the knee joint more rapidly in rheumatoid patients than normal subjects yet, paradoxically, the synovium appears less permeable to small molecules such as glucose. The authors account for these findings by suggesting microvascular changes that increase protein passage while interstitial changes decrease the passage of small molecules. It may be that anti-inflammatory drugs, highly bound as they are to albumin, may be capable to some extent of passage across the membrane in the bound state. In the study cited above, Farr et al demonstrated much higher total levels of phenylbutazone in the synovial fluid than would be predicted on the assumption that only the free fraction was capable of passage. The factors which determine the efficiency of drug transfer across synovial membranes into joint fluid obviously require further study.

A brief but clear discussion of other aspects of protein binding has been given by Lindup & Orme (1981) and an excellent critical review is contained in a book by Curry (1980). Wallis & Simkin (1983) have published an important review on synovial fluid and tissue concentrations of antirheumatic drugs.

Apparent volume of distribution

This is the hypothetical volume that would contain the drug dose were it present throughout the body in the same concentration as that observed in the blood. It can be most simply and reliably calculated from data obtained following intravenous drug administration and depends on the particular mathematical model used to describe the body. Although it does not always have a direct physiological significance (hence the word 'apparent'), a volume of distribution of around 7 l indicates that the drug is almost entirely confined to the plasma. Since many anti-inflammatory drugs are more than 95% bound to plasma albumin they often have apparent volumes of distribution of this magnitude. Larger volumes of distribution indicate that the drug is more widely distributed, e.g. 20 l (extracellular fluid), 30 l (intracellular fluid), 40 l (total body water). Very large volumes, 100–200 l, obviously have no direct physiological significance and indicate that the drug concentrates in some tissue such as fat or a particular organ.

Elimination

Once absorbed and distributed throughout the body a drug can be eliminated via the kidneys unchanged or as a polar, water-soluble conjugate. Alternatively a drug may be first metabolised in the liver with subsequent renal elimination of the metabolites. Although there are many cases where the metabolites possess some of the pharmacological activity of the parent drug, only rarely do they approach or surpass it. Elimination via the bile of drug and/or metabolites is also possible and this can prolong the time a drug spends in the body, since it may be reabsorbed from the intestine. Anti-inflammatory drugs provide examples of all these types of elimination as is indicated briefly in Table 16.1.

Elimination thus covers both renal and non-renal routes. If a drug is removed principally by the renal route then the dose may have to be reduced in renal disease and correspondingly the dose of a hepatically cleared drug may have to be reduced in liver failure. The concept of clearance is a useful one and is, in some respects, more helpful than the much quoted half-life. The latter is, however, firmly entrenched in the literature issued by drug companies and is certainly useful

Table 16.1 Some pharmacokinetic data on anti-inflammatory drugs. (Much of this material is presented as mean data and slightly different values may be found in individual studies.)

Drug type	Name	Dose	Half-life (hours)	Protein binding (%)	Lipophilicity at pH 7.4	Principal route of elimination	% Dose eliminated in urine
CARBOXYLIC ACIDS							
(a) Acetic acids	Diclofenac (Voltarol)	50 mg b.d. or t.d.s.	2	99.7	Intermediate	Metabolism and conjugation	60
	Fenclofenac (Flenac)	600 mg b.d.	21	96.0	Low	Conjugation, a little metabolism	60
	Indomethacin (Indocid)	75–150 mg daily	3	90.0	High	Metabolism and conjugation with a little unchanged	50
	Sulindac (Clinoril)	200 mg b.d.	7 (sulindac) 18 (sulphide)	93.0 98.0	Low –	Metabolism to active metabolites	50
	Tolmetin (Tolectin)	400 mg q.d.s.	5	99.0	Low	Metabolism and conjugation	100
(b) Salicylic acids	Aspirin	600–900 mg 6 times daily	15 min (aspirin) Salicylate dose-related	49.0 (aspirin) 80.0–90.0 (salicylate)	Low	Metabolism and conjugation	85
	Benorylate (Benoral)	10 ml b.d.	1	80.0–90.0 (salicylate)	Low	Metabolism to salicylic acid and paracetamol	–
	Diflunisal (Dolobid)	500 mg b.d.	11	98.0	High	Conjugation	95
(c) Propionic acids	Benoxaprofen (Opren)	600 mg o.d.	33	99.8	High	Conjugation	50
	Fenbufen (Lederfen)	600 mg o.d.	10	99.0	Intermediate	Metabolism to active metabolites	66
	Fenoprofen (Fenopron)	600 mg q.d.s.	3	99.0	Low	Metabolism and conjugation	85
	Flurbiprofen (Froben)	100 mg t.d.s.	4	99.0	Low	Metabolism and conjugation	100

Table 16.1 Some pharmacokinetic data on anti-inflammatory drugs — *continued*

Drug type	Name	Dose	Half-life (hours)	Protein binding (%)	Lipophilicity at pH 7.4	Principal route of elimination	% Dose eliminated in urine
	Ibuprofen (Brufen)	400–800 mg q.d.s.	2	99.0	Intermediate	Metabolism	60
	Ketoprofen (Orudis)	100 mg b.d. or t.d.s.	2	60.0–94.0	Low	Conjugation	70
	Naproxen (Naprosyn)	500 mg b.d.	14	99.0	Low	Conjugation	95
	Tiaprofenic acid (Surgam)	200 mg t.d.s.	2	97.9	–	Some unchanged & conjugation	96
(d) Fenamic acids	Flufenamic acid (Meralen)	200 mg q.d.s.	9	99.0	High	Metabolism	25
	Mefenamic acid (Ponstan)	500 mg q.d.s.	4	99.0	High	Metabolism	50
ENOLIC ACIDS							
(a) Pyrazolones	Azapropazone (Rheumox)	600 mg b.d.	12	99.5	–	Renal, unchanged	95
	Phenylbutazone (Butazolidin)	100 mg q.d.s.	75	98.0	Intermediate	Metabolism to active metabolite	60
(b) Oxicams	Piroxicam (Feldene)	20 mg daily	38	99.3	–	Metabolism	10
OTHERS	Gold (sodium aurothiomalate)	10 mg weekly i.m.	Not first order	91.0	–	–	40
	Penicillamine	125–250 mg daily	8 days	80	–	Metabolism	50
	Chloroquine	75–300 mg daily	54	55	–	Some metabolism	5

in the calculation of dosage schedules. To this end the half-lives of many of the frequently used anti-inflammatory drugs are given in Table 16.1.

If a drug is completely absorbed its total clearance can be obtained by simply dividing the dose by the area under the plasma drug concentration/time curve. Renal clearance can be calculated by collecting urine until the drug ceases to be excreted, measuring the total amount of unchanged drug present and dividing this by the area under the plasma drug concentration/time curve. The non-renal contribution to clearance is then obtained by subtracting the renal from the total clearance.

The phenomenon of *first pass effect* is now well recognised in clinical pharmacology. On oral dosing a drug is absorbed from the upper part of the gastrointestinal tract and passes via the portal circulation to the liver; if it is extensively metabolised there, very little will reach the systemic circulation. A large first pass loss is recognised by comparing the areas under the plasma drug concentration/time curves after an oral and after an intravenous dose. If the same dose is given the areas may be compared directly: if a different dose is given, an arithmetical correction must be made. First pass losses undoubtedly occur with anti-inflammatory drugs but little information is available since there are few intravenous preparations. Studies involving intravenous administration of fenoprofen (Rubin et al, 1972) and indomethacin (Kwan et al, 1976) have been published but it is not possible to calculate the extent of the first pass effect from these. The first pass loss of diclofenac has, however, been measured and found to be about 40%, assuming complete absorption of the oral dose (Willis et al, 1980).

If an extensive first pass effect is identified it can be compensated for by an adjustment of the dosage regimen. The effect is known to vary from individual to individual and to be influenced by food (McLean et al, 1981) and other drugs (Jack et al, 1982).

Finally, because the majority of anti-inflammatory drugs are acidic their renal excretion will be enhanced in alkaline urine since at a pH of 7.0 or more the drugs will be highly ionised and reabsorption through the renal tubules will be greatly reduced.

DRUG HANDLING BY THE PATIENT

Pharmacokinetic studies of drugs are usually performed on volunteers, initially within the particular drug company developing the preparation, and then sometimes by professional contract units or departments of clinical pharmacology. These studies yield valuable information about how the drug is handled in the body, what dose will be required and how often it needs to be given. The next question is, to what extent do these results apply to the patient with, for example, rheumatoid arthritis? In this section, the differences between the volunteer study and the clinical management of a rheumatoid patient will be considered. The relevance of each difference to a particular drug will depend on its pharmacokinetic characteristics. These may be found either in the previous section or in later chapters of this book.

The major differences which may be found between volunteer studies and clinical practice include the following:

	Volunteer study	Clinical practice
Administration	Single dose	Chronic dosing
Administration	Fasting	After food
Type of subject	Young	Old
Type of subject	Well	Ill
Interacting factors	On no other drugs	On other drugs

Chronic administration

The plasma concentrations after several weeks of administration may differ markedly from those obtained after the first dose given on day 1. The differences may arise because the drug (a) tends to accumulate (b) reduces or (c) increases its own rate of elimination.

(a) If further doses are given before all the drug from the last dose has been eliminated, the plasma levels will increase as the drug accumulates until a steady state is reached when absorption is balanced by elimination. Thus, unless a drug has a short half-life and is given infrequently, the plasma concentration on, say, day 10 will be greater than those attained after the initial dose.

Drugs with short half-lives such as ibuprofen and flurbiprofen (Adams & Warwick, 1979) and ketoprofen (Lewellen & Templeton, 1976) do not accumulate, while indomethacin does (Helleberg, 1981).

(b) Drugs may reduce their own rate of elimination, at least theoretically, by reducing hepatic or renal blood flow or by impairing hepatic (enzyme inhibition) or renal function. The beta adrenoceptor blocking drugs propranolol (Wood et al, 1978) and metoprolol (Kendall et al, 1980) produce larger areas under their plasma concentration/time curves (a measure of the amount of drug present in the body) after several days treatment. This is not known to be important for most rheumatological preparations, though phenylbutazone may act as an enzyme inhibitor.

(c) Drugs may increase their own rate of elimination. Although this is true of some anticonvulsants it is probably not relevant to drugs used by rheumatologists.

Food

Whereas most pharmacokinetic studies are performed after a 12 hour fast, many patients prefer, or are advised, to take their drugs after food. The effects of food have been extensively studied (Welling, 1977; Melander, 1978) and it has been shown that the absorption of different drugs may be influenced in different ways. However, it is not easy to remember detailed lists and therefore 'rules of thumb' are perhaps appropriate. These would be as follows:

1. Food tends to delay the absorption of drugs, but usually does not reduce the total amount absorbed.

2. Food probably does not materially alter the plasma concentrations attained during chronic administration.

3. Enteric coated preparations, because they only liberate their contents in the small intestine, may show markedly delayed absorption when taken after food. This has been demonstrated for aspirin (Bogentoft et al, 1978) and diclofenac (Willis et al, 1981a) but does not seem to be true for some enteric coated prednisolone preparations (Lee et al, 1979). Whether or not drugs likely to be used to treat patients with rheumatic diseases are taken before or after food is therefore important only if they are being given acutely to treat symptoms such as pain or stiffness. Relief will be achieved more rapidly if, for example, indomethacin (Wallusch et al, 1978), piroxicam (Brogden et al, 1981) or even effervescent aspirin (Volans, 1974) are taken on an empty stomach. This would obviously be important if a drug were being taken in the morning to control the pain and stiffness of rheumatoid arthritis. It should be reiterated, however, that food effects observed in single dose studies may disappear on chronic dosing (Willis et al, 1981b).

Age

Many patients are middle-aged or elderly and this factor may need to be taken into consideration before applying data from volunteers to clinical practice. However, although early reviews suggested theoretical reasons why in old age the body functions may deteriorate or diminish, more recent work suggests that age per se has relatively little effect on drug absorption (Hall, 1973), protein-binding and volume of distribution (Crooks et al, 1976) or on the metabolism of drugs (Willis & Kendall, 1978; Quarterman et al, 1981). The facts that we should remember are that old people

1. May show poor compliance
2. Do have less efficient renal function
3. May respond differently due to end-organ sensitivity
4. Are more likely to be on other drugs
5. Are more likely to be suffering from other diseases.

Even this list may be simplified for rheumatological practice. First, almost all non-steroidal anti-inflammatory drugs (azapropazone being an exception) and most other drugs used by the rheumatologist are broken down in the liver, a process not seriously impaired in the old. The impairment of renal function which occurs with advancing age is therefore not a serious problem. Secondly the responses which tend to be different in the old are those related to the central nervous system; thus the effects of nitrazepam are more marked and more prolonged (Castleden et al, 1977). It is, however, important to remember that adverse effects of drugs tend to be more common in the old (Greenblatt et al, 1982) and the aplastic anaemia associated with long-term phenylbutazone therapy might be considered as an example (Fowler, 1967). Apart from this aspect, it is probably true to say that simply being old will not seriously influence the way that the patient handles his or her anti-rheumatic medication. It is more important to be aware that other coexisting diseases or concomitant medication may well alter the pharmacokinetics of the drug in question.

The effect of being ill

A patient with a rather indolent osteoarthritis of the knees may be relatively well, with a normal erythrocyte sedimentation rate and biochemical profile. An acute rheumatoid, on the other hand, may be ill with fever, leucocytosis, a markedly raised sedimentation rate and his serum proteins and other biochemical indices, particularly those measured by the so-called 'liver function tests', may be abnormal. Does this matter?

Good data showing whether plasma drug concentrations are different from 'normal' when drugs are given to patients with acute inflammatory disorders are relatively sparse. The studies which are available suggest that, for the non-steroidal agents at least, the processes of absorption and metabolism are not seriously adversely affected by active disease. However since the inflammatory response includes changes in serum proteins, to which most non-steroidal drugs are extensively bound, changes in total plasma concentration would be expected. Drugs like propranolol (Schneider et al, 1979) and oxprenolol (Kendall et al, 1979) for example bind to acute phase proteins, and total plasma concentrations, particularly of propranolol, rise dramatically in inflammatory disorders like rheumatoid arthritis (Schneider et al, 1979). On the other hand, since many anti-inflammatory agents bind to albumin, the low plasma concentrations of this protein in chronic active rheumatoid disease will be associated with reduced plasma drug concentrations. This has been demonstrated for diclofenac (Crook et al, 1982), aspirin (Bayles, 1962) and fenclozic (Chalmers et al, 1969), though indomethacin levels appeared to be somewhat higher in patients (Emori et al, 1973). The relevance of these observations to the volume of distribution and the penetration into synovial fluid remains to be determined.

Drugs

Drugs may modify the absorption, distribution, protein binding, metabolism and renal elimination of other drugs. There is now an extensive literature on this subject and information pharmacists devote their working lives to collecting such data and answering questions about drug interactions. Here only a few examples which may be relevant to the management of rheumatological patients will be presented.

a. Absorption. Delayed absorption, which is generally only a problem when analgesic or anti-inflammatory drugs are being used to control pain acutely, is usually caused by taking the drug with some antacids (Emori et al, 1973; Brogden et al, 1979) or with drugs which have anticholinergic properties and therefore delay gastric emptying. These latter include the tricyclic antidepressants and the anticholinergic group of antiparkinsonian drugs such as benzhexol.

b. Protein binding and apparent volume of distribution. Salicylate appears to compete for protein binding sites and thereby displaces other non-steroidal anti-inflammatory drugs. The end result is to reduce the total drug concentration and by increasing the free fraction it increases the rate of elimination. Lower levels of naproxen (Brogden et al, 1979), diclofenac (Willis et al, 1980) and indomethacin (Helleberg, 1981) for example have been well documented following salicylate.

Non-steroidal drugs may compete with other highly bound drugs such as warfarin and the oral hypoglycaemic agents for binding sites. However, the problem is not usually related to possible changes in plasma levels of the non-steroidal agent but rather to the risk of affecting the other drug and possibly causing clotting or haemorrhage or unwanted changes in blood sugar concentration.

c. Metabolism. Drugs may increase the rate of metabolism by enzyme induction or reduce it by enzyme inhibition. The most important enzyme inducers are anticonvulsants, barbiturates, rifampicin and alcohol. The drugs most likely to be affected in rheumatological practice would be the corticosteroids, whose concentration and therefore efficacy would be reduced by enzyme inducers (Brooks et al, 1976; Jubiz & Meikle, 1979). Enzyme inhibition, if it ever modifies the response to drugs used in rheumatology, must be uncommon though phenylbutazone may inhibit the breakdown of phenytoin (Andreasen et al, 1973) and tolbutamide (Pond et al, 1977), and allopurinol that of warfarin (Self et al, 1975).

d. Renal excretion. This is not an important route of elimination for most of the active compounds used in rheumatology. Probenecid which competes for renal tubular transport will delay the excretion of numerous other drugs. Thus higher plasma concentrations of naproxen (Brogden et al, 1979) and of indomethacin (Helleberg, 1981) have been described.

CONCLUSIONS

Although the rheumatoid patient may differ in many ways from the healthy volunteer, some of these differences do not materially affect the way their antirheumatic medication is handled in the body. However besides wishing to know some of the pharmacokinetic characteristics of a new drug, the rheumatologist should also want to know about some of the variables described above. He should certainly want to see data on chronic dosing and on the effects of food and antacids on the rate of absorption. There should also be information on plasma concentrations attained in the patient group likely to receive the drug, with particular reference to the effects that active disease may have on protein binding. In this context he should know about the possible hazards of drug interactions that will be caused by modifying protein binding. It is then up to the clinician to take note of the other drugs that the patient may be taking and other diseases that may afflict the patient. It is also the responsibility of the clinical research worker to determine the factors which influence the rate and extent of penetration of the drugs into synovial membrane and other tissues.

REFERENCES

Adams S S, Warwick B J 1979 Ibuprofen and flurbiprofen. Clinics in Rheumatic Diseases 5: 359–379

Andreasen P B, Froland A, Skovsted L, Andersen S A, Hauge M 1973 Diphenylhydantoin half-life in man and its inhibition by phenylbutazone: the role of genetic factors. Acta Medica Scandinavica 193: 561–564

Bayles T B 1962 Plasma salicylate levels in rheumatoid arthritis. In: Dixon A, Martin B K, Smith M J H, Wood P H N (eds) Salicylates. An international symposium. Churchill, London, p 43–46

Bogentoft C, Carlsson I, Ekenved G, Magnusson A 1978 Influence of food on the absorption of acetylsalicylic acid from enteric coated dosage forms. European Journal of Clinical Pharmacology 14: 351–355

Brogden R N, Heel R C, Speight T M, Avery G S 1979 Naproxen up to date. Drugs 18: 241–277

Brogden R N, Heel R C, Speight T M, Avery G S 1981 Piroxicam: A review of its pharmacological properties and therapeutic efficacy. Drugs 22: 165–187

Brooks P M, Buchanan W W, Grove M, Downie W W 1976 Effects of enzyme induction on metabolism of prednisolone. Annals of the Rheumatic Diseases 35: 339–343

Castleden C M, George C F, Marcer D, Hallett C 1977 Increased sensitivity to nitrazepam in old age. British Medical Journal 1: 10–12

Chalmers I M, Pohl J E F, Platt D S 1969 The evaluation in man of fenclozic acid (ICI 54 450: Myalex) a new anti-inflammatory agent. Annals of the Rheumatic Diseases 28: 590–594

Crook P R, Willis J V, Kendall M J, Jack D B, Fowler P D 1982 The pharmacokinetics of diclofenac sodium in patients with active rheumatoid disease. European Journal of Clinical Pharmacology 21: 331–334

Crooks J, O'Malley K, Stevenson I H 1976 Pharmacokinetics in the elderly. Clinical Pharmacokinetics 1: 280–296

Cummings N A, Nordby G L 1966 Measurement of synovial fluid pH in normal and arthritic knees. Arthritis and Rheumatism 9: 47–56

Curry S H 1980 Drug disposition and pharmacokinetics, 3rd Edn. Blackwell, Oxford, p 88–100

Emori H W, Champion G D, Bluestone R, Paulus H E 1973 Simultaneous pharmacokinetics of indomethacin in serum and synovial fluid. Annals of the Rheumatic Diseases 32: 433–435

Farr M, Hawkins C F, Kendall M J, Willis J V 1982 Some observations and speculations on the factors influencing the concentration of phenylbutazone in synovial fluid. International Journal of Clinical Pharmacology Therapy and Toxicology 20: 589–594

Fowler P D 1967 Marrow toxicity of the pyrazoles. Annals of the Rheumatic Diseases 26: 344–345

Greenblatt D J, Sellers E M, Shader R I 1982 Drug disposition in old age. New England Journal of Medicine 306: 1081–1088

Hall M R P 1973 Drug therapy in the elderly. British Medical Journal 3:582

Helleberg L 1981 Clinical pharmacokinetics of Indomethacin. Clinical Pharmacokinetics 6: 245–258

Jack D B, Patel P D 1982 Prediction of the properties of non-steroidal anti-inflammatory drugs by chromatography. Unpublished work

Jack D B, Kendall M J, Dean S, Laugher S J, Zaman R, Tenneson M E 1982 The effect of hydralazine on the pharmacokinetics of three different beta adrenoceptor antagonists: metoprolol, nadolol and acebutolol. Biopharmaceutics and Drug Disposition 3: 47–54

Jubiz W, Meikle A W 1979 Alterations of glucocorticoid

actions by other drugs and disease states. Drugs 18: 113–121

Kendall M J, Quarterman C P, Bishop M, Schneider R E 1979 Effects of inflammatory disease on plasma oxprenolol concentrations. British Medical Journal 2: 465–468

Kendall M J, John V A, Quarterman C P, Welling P G 1980 A single and multiple dose pharmacokinetic and pharmacodynamic comparison of conventional and slow release metoprolol. European Journal of Clinical Pharmacology 17: 87–92

Kober A, Sjöholm I 1980 The binding sites on human serum albumin for some non-steroidal anti-inflammatory drugs. Molecular Pharmacology 18: 421–426

Kwan K C, Breault G O, Umbenhauer E R, McMahon F G, Duggan D E 1976 Kinetics of indomethacin absorption, elimination and entero-hepatic circulation in man. Journal of Pharmacokinetics and Biopharmaceutics 4: 255–280

Lee D A H, Taylor G M, Walker J G, James V H T 1979 The effect of food and tablet formulation on plasma prednisolone levels following administration of enteric coated tablets. British Journal of Clinical Pharmacology 7: 523–528

Lewellen O R V, Templeton R 1976 The pharmacokinetics of ketoprofen in man during and after repeated oral dosing (50 mg qid) with 'Orudis'. Scandinavian Journal of Rheumatology (Suppl) 14: 53–62

Lindup W E, Orme M C L'E 1981 Clinical pharmacology: Plasma protein binding of drugs. British Medical Journal 282: 212–214

McLean A J, Isbister C, Bobik A, Dudley F J 1981 Reduction of first-pass hepatic clearance of propranolol by food. Clinical Pharmacology and Therapeutics 30: 31–34

Melander A 1978 Influence of food on the bioavailability of drugs. Clinical Pharmacokinetics 3: 337–351

Orme M C L'E 1982 Plasma concentrations and therapeutic effect of anti-inflammatory and anti-rheumatic drugs. Pharmacology and Therapeutics 16: 167–180

Pond S M, Birkett D J, Wade D N 1977 Mechanisms of inhibition of tolbutamide metabolism: Phenylbutazone, oxyphenbutazone, sulfaphenazole. Clinical Pharmacology and Therapeutics 22: 573–579

Quarterman C P, Kendall M J, Jack D B 1981 The effects of age on the pharmacokinetics of metoprolol and its metabolites. British Journal of Clinical Pharmacology 11: 287–294

Ritschel W A 1980 Handbook of basic pharmacokinetics, 2nd Edn. Drug Intelligence Publications, Hamilton, USA

Rowland M, Tozer T N 1980 Clinical pharmacokinetics: Concepts and applications. Lea & Febiger, Philadelphia

Rubin A, Warrick P, Wolen R L, Chernish S M, Ridolfo A S, Gruber C M Jr 1972 Physiological disposition of fenoprofen in man. III. Metabolism and protein binding of fenoprofen. Journal of Pharmacology and Experimental Therapeutics 183: 449–457

Schneider R E, Bishop M, Hawkins C F 1979 Plasma propranolol concentrations and the erythrocyte sedimentation rate. British Journal of Clinical Pharmacology 8: 43–47

Self T H, Evans W E, Ferguson T 1975 Drug enhancement of warfarin activity. Lancet 2: 557–558

Shargel L, Yu A B C 1980 Applied biopharmaceutics and pharmacokinetics. Appleton-Century-Crofts, New York

Simkin P A, Pizzorno J E 1979 Synovial permeability in rheumatoid arthritis. Arthritis and Rheumatism 22: 689–696

Sjöholm I 1978 Binding of drugs to human serum albumin. Proceedings 11th FEBS Meeting, Copenhagen 50: 71–78

Smith G L, Goulbourn R A, Burt R A P, Chatfield D H 1977 Preliminary studies of absorption and excretion of benoxaprofen in man. British Journal of Clinical Pharmacology 4: 585–590

Smith S E, Rawlins M D 1976 Variability in human drug response. Butterworths, London

Tyrer J H, Eadie M J, Sutherland J M, Hooper W D 1970 Outbreak of anticonvulsant intoxication in an Australian city. British Medical Journal 4: 271–273

Volans G N 1974 Effects of food and exercise on the absorption of effervescent aspirin. British Journal of Clinical Pharmacology 1: 137–141

Wallis W J, Simkin P A 1983 Antirheumatic drug concentrations in human synovial fluid and synovial tissue: observations on extravascular pharmacokinetics. Clinical Pharmacokinetics 8: 496–522

Wallusch W W, Nowak H, Leopold G, Netter K J 1978 Comparative bioavailability: Influence of various diets on the bioavailability of indomethacin, International Journal of Clinical Pharmacology and Biopharmacy 16: 40–44

Welling P G 1977 Influence of food and diet on gastrointestinal drug absorption: a review. Journal of Pharmacokinetics and Biopharmaceutics 5: 291–334

Whitlam J B, Brown K F, Crooks M J, Room G F W 1981 Transsynovial distribution of ibuprofen in arthritic patients. Clinical Pharmacology and Therapeutics 29: 487–492

Willis J V, Kendall M J 1978 Pharmacokinetic studies on diclofenac sodium in young and old volunteers. Scandinavian Journal of Rheumatology (Suppl) 22: 36–41

Willis J V, Kendall M J, Jack D B 1980 A study of the effect of aspirin on the pharmacokinetics of oral and intravenous diclofenac sodium. European Journal of Clinical Pharmacology 18: 415–418

Willis J V, Kendall M J, Jack D B 1981a The influence of food on the absorption of diclofenac after single and multiple oral doses. European Journal of Clinical Pharmacology 19: 33–37

Willis J V, Jack D B, Kendall M J, John V A 1981b The influence of food on the absorption of diclofenac as determined by the urinary excretion of the unchanged drug and its major metabolites during chronic administration. European Journal of Clinical Pharmacology 19: 39–44

Wood A J J, Carr J, Vestal R E, Belcher S, Wilkinson G R, Shand D G 1978 Direct measurement of propranolol bioavailability during accumulation to steady state. British Journal of Clinical Pharmacology 6: 345–350

Yasuhara M, Kobayashi H, Kimura T, Muranishi S, Sezaki H 1978 Absorption and metabolism of p-aminobenzoic acid by rat small intestine in situ. Journal of Pharmacobio-Dynamics 1: 122–131

17

M.H. Seifert

Salicylates

HISTORICAL BACKGROUND

Salicylates have been used to treat disease for over two thousand years since Hippocrates recommended the leaves of the willow tree to relieve the pains of childbirth. In 1633, Calancha, an Augustinian monk living in Peru, discovered that when the bark of a certain 'fever tree' was powdered into a beverage it was able to reduce fever. This bark was used to treat the Countess of Chinchon, the wife of the Viceroy of Peru, and was therefore called cinchona bark gaining a wide reputation in Europe as an analgesic and antipyretic. Many years later the active ingredient and cause of its bitter taste was found to be quinine.

In 1763, the Reverend Edward Stone described a preparation of willow bark which he used as an antipyretic. It was whilst walking through a damp meadow in Chipping Norton that he tasted the bark of the common white willow (*Salix alba*) and was struck by its bitterness, reminding him of cinchona bark. He made an extract of the willow bark and on finding that it reduced the fevers of about fifty of his parishioners reported this to the Royal Society (Stone, 1763). As cinchona bark became more scarce and therefore expensive, willow bark became popular and from it salicin was isolated by Leroux in 1830.

Salicylic acid was prepared from salicin in 1838 and aspirin, the acetic ester of salicylic acid, in 1853. Felix Hoffman whilst working for the Bayer Pharmaceutical Company became interested in the salicylic acid, as his father who suffered from arthritis was intolerant of sodium salicylate. Together with his colleague Heinrich Dreser he developed a commercial method for synthesising aspirin in 1893, introducing it into medical practice in 1899. Aspirin is now widely prescribed and freely available in hundreds of preparations throughout the world (Leist & Banwell, 1974). Its ability to inhibit prostaglandin synthetase (Vane, 1971) and the discovery of its new-found therapeutic advantages are sure to guarantee its continued place in the therapeutic armamentarium.

CHEMISTRY

Because they are mild and therefore well tolerated when taken orally, the synthetic derivatives of salicylic acid are those that are used clinically. By a substitution in the hydroxy radical of salicylic acid a salicylate ester of acetic acid is formed: it is this that is called 'acetyl salicylic acid' or 'aspirin'. The sodium salt likewise is formed by substitution in the carboxyl radical (Fig. 17.1). Acetyl salicylic acid is a weak organic acid (pKa 3.5) which although stable in dry air hydrolyses to acetic and salicylic acids in the presence of water vapour. Considerable amounts of degraded drug may therefore be contained in tablets that have crumbled before use and this may account for differences in the bioavailability among aspirin preparations (Koch-Weser, 1974). Because aspirin and other salicylate derivates rapidly hydrolyse to salicylate in the plasma, the terms 'salicylate' and 'salicylic acid' will be interchangeable in this chapter.

PHARMACOLOGICAL PROPERTIES

Absorption

When ingested, salicylates are absorbed from the stomach and the upper small intestine by passive

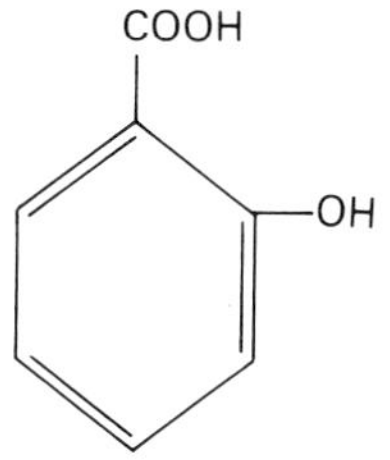

Salicylic acid

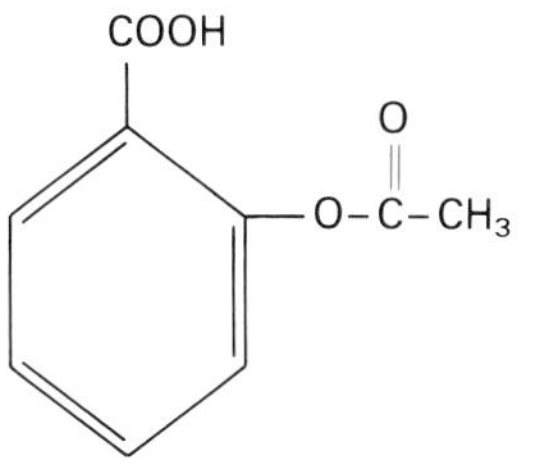

Acetyl salicylic acid (aspirin)

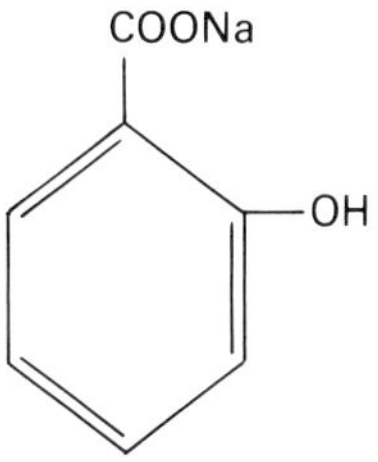

Sodium salicylate

Fig. 17.1 The structural formulae of the principal salicylates.

diffusion in the non-ionised lipid-soluble state (Rowland et al, 1972). Absorption is usually complete within 2–4 hours and significant plasma levels are obtained within 30 minutes. The amount and rate of absorption depends on the dissolution characteristics of the preparation used, the pH at the mucosal surface, and the gastric emptying time. Salicylates when taken in solution, such as effervescent buffered aspirin or easily soluble sodium aspirin, are more rapidly absorbed than a standard aspirin preparation (Leonards, 1963). Solid preparations must disintegrate and deaggregate before dissolution.

Aspirin is a weak organic acid and at low pH is in a non-dissociated form. In man the optimal gastric absorption occurs at pH 2.5–4 (Cohen, 1976). If the pH in the stomach is raised by the administration of buffers it might be expected that the rate of absorption of salicylate is decreased because more of it is ionised. However, a rise in pH also causes the salicylate to become more soluble and therefore enhances its absorption. Absorption in the small intestine is more rapid than in the stomach and as the pH is nearer neutrality the salicylates become ionised and solubility is enhanced.

The non-ionised molecules rapidly become ionised at the intracellular pH (7.0) of the mucosal cells after they pass through the lipid membrane, and concentrations of salicylate anion are 15–20 times higher in gastric mucosal cells than in the lumen of the stomach (Goodman & Gilman, 1970). Because of the smaller pH gradient however, much lower amounts accumulate in the intestinal cells.

Rectal absorption of salicylate is slow and incomplete and is therefore unreliable and certainly not a recommended route of administration if high plasma levels are required (Superstine et al, 1978). Gastric emptying time if delayed by disease such as migraine reduces absorption of aspirin as will the presence of food and fluid in the stomach (Koch et al, 1978).

Distribution

For the first 10–20 minutes after ingestion acetyl salicylic acid is the most dominant form of the drug detected in plasma (Mandel et al, 1954) and it may even be found in synovial fluid before salicylic acid (Soren, 1977). However, it can only be detected for a short time and 30 minutes after taking an oral dose of 650 mg of aspirin only 27% of the plasma salicylate remains in the acetylated form. Plasma concentrations of acetyl salicylic acid are therefore always low at usual therapeutic doses — approximately 2 mg%. The major portion of the resulting salicylic acid, in some instances up to 90%, is rapidly bound to plasma proteins, especially albumin (Levy et al, 1975), and competes for binding sites with such endogenous substrates as thyroid hormone, bilirubin and urates.

Competition also occurs between salicylates and other drugs such as steroids, penicillins, thiopentol, phenytoin and sulphinpyrazone. Whilst at one stage combination with non-steroidal anti-inflammatory agents was thought to produce an additive effect with naproxen (Willkens & Segre, 1976) and an increased toxicity with indomethacin (Brooks et al, 1975), it now seems that there is no advantage or disadvantage in using salicylates with these drugs (Kwan et al, 1978). The free hydroxy group is required for protein-binding. With increasing dose the proportion of non-protein-bound drug in plasma increases and when plasma albumin is low, for example in severe rheumatoid arthritis (Ballantyne et al, 1971) or elderly patients (Wallace & Whiting, 1976), less drug is protein-bound. This of course is important as it is the free drug that most probably mediates therapeutic activity and toxicity.

Acetyl salicylic acid is bound to protein to a much more limited extent (Tainter & Ferris, 1969). When it does bind to serum albumin it acetylates this protein. It can also acetylate hormones, DNA, platelets, haemoglobin and other proteins of which prostaglandin synthetase is the most notable example (Roth & Majerus, 1975).

The distribution of salicylate throughout the body is uneven. A two compartmental effect has been described (Rowland & Riegelman, 1968) in which a central compartment (blood, renal cortex and liver) contains high levels of salicylate and a peripheral compartment made up of various other organs contains lower levels of salicylate.

Aspirin and salicylates diffuse rapidly into cells and across membranes into the transcellular fluids such as synovial (Soren, 1977), spinal (Reed & Palmisano, 1975), and peritoneal fluids, saliva (Pohto, 1976), tears (Valentic et al, 1980) and milk, and across the placental barrier (Levy et al, 1975). Trace quantities of salicylate are found in sweat, bile and faeces, but aspirin has not been demonstrated in exudates.

When a constantly ingested dose of aspirin is prescribed a plateau is reached in a week (Gibson et al, 1975) but after this the concentration of serum salicylate decreases; this may explain why aspirin is thought to be less potent in some patients after being in continual use for months.

Metabolism

Salicylic acid is eliminated from the body by renal excretion and by conjugation in the endoplasmic reticulum and mitochondria of the liver. The metabolic products formed consist of salicyluric acid (the glycine conjugate), salicyl phenolic glucuronide, salicylacyl glucuronide, gentisic acid and gentisuric acid (the glycine conjugate of gentic acid) (Levy & Tsuchiya, 1972; Wilson et al, 1978). These metabolites and salicylic acid itself are excreted in the urine.

The studies of Levy & Tsuchiya (1972) have demonstrated that there is a limited capacity for glycine conjugation and phenolic glucuronidation. These processes proceed by capacity-limited (Michaelis — Menton) type kinetics. This is because those enzymes catalysing their formation become saturated and no matter how much the serum concentration of salicylic acid is increased, the rate of production of salicylurate and salicylphenylglucuronide remains the same. Gentisic acid, salicylic acid and salicylacyl glucoronide however are eliminated by first order kinetics so that as the plasma concentration of salicylic acid increases there is a proportional increase in their rates of excretion (Dromgoole et al, 1981).

Excretion

The metabolites are all excreted into the urine and never reach significant plasma levels so that their detection in plasma is only by very sensitive chemical techniques (Schachter & Manis, 1958). At physiologic pH the non-protein-bound salicylate is slowly filtered across the renal glomerulus. Salicylic acid and other metabolites are actively secreted by the proximal tubules and then passively reabsorbed across the distal tubule cell. Distal tubule reabsorption is dependent on urinary pH. If the urine in the distal tubule is acidic, a significant amount of non-ionised salicylate back-diffuses into the peritubular blood. Plasma salicylate levels can be more than doubled by changing urine pH from 6.5 to 5.5, and conversely salicylate clearance can be enhanced by alkalinisation of urine (Gibaldi et al, 1974). Salicylate excretion therefore changes from hour to hour depending on food, exercise and the general state of acid — base hydration and normal diurnal fluctuations of urinary pH (Ayres et al, 1977). Variations in renal function will also affect salicylate excretion.

If glomerular filtration rate is decreased or there is interference with the transport mechanisms of the proximal tubules by competition with drugs such as probenecid or acetazolamide then concentration of plasma salicylate increases (MacPherson et al, 1955).

THERAPEUTIC PROPERTIES

Analgesic actions

Salicylates are classified as mild but effective analgesics (Houde et al, 1960). They are suitable for the treatment of pain of slight to moderate intensity such as headache, myalgia and arthralgia and are more widely used and available for pain relief than any other class of drugs. Chronic use does not lead to tolerance or addiction. Relief of pain is by virtue of a peripheral and central nervous system effect.

A classical series of experiments on dogs (Guzman et al, 1964; Lim et al, 1964) has shown by cross-circulation studies that the induction of chemically induced peripheral pain can be suppressed by salicylates but the transmission or perception of painful stimuli are not blocked.

Direct effects of salicylates on the central nervous system have been described and a hypothalamic site of action for analgesic as well as antipyretic effect suggested.

Antipyretic action

One of the first and most troublesome clinical manifestations of connective tissue disease may be fever. The mechanism of this is unknown but it may be dependent on the release of leucocyte pyrogens from sites of inflammation. When released into the general circulation, they pass across the blood–brain barrier. This stimulates the release of prostaglandins from discrete sites within the brain and this has led to the detection of prostaglandin E within the third ventricle (Feldberg & Gupta, 1973). Salicylates and other antipyretics of the prostaglandin synthetase-inhibiting class have been shown to block this action (Feldberg & Gupta, 1973). It appears that the principal site for the antipyretic action of salicylates is the anterior hypothalamus (Wit & Wang, 1968; Avery & Penn, 1974).

Anti-inflammatory effects

The anti-inflammatory effects of salicylate are not dramatic (Deodhar et al, 1973) and methods of assessing them in the human subject are insensitive (Lee et al, 1973). The work of Boardman & Hart (1967) demonstrated that aspirin in a dose of 5.3 g/day reduced the pain and swelling of rheumatoid arthritis in the proximal interphalangeal joints of patients as measured by jewelers' rings, but at a dose of 2.6 g/day, only pain was affected.

Pain, swelling and erythema are only three of the features of the inflammatory process; other characteristics include leakage of blood cells, protein, electrolytes and fluid to the extracellular space and the migration of leucocytes into the inflamed tissues. There is also local liberation of histamine, 5-hydroxy-tryptamine, slow-reacting substance of anaphylaxis, various chemotactic factors, bradykinin and prostaglandins. Phagocytic cells migrate into the area and cellular lysosomal membranes are ruptured. The main effect of salicylates is upon prostaglandin and its interaction with bradykinin, and not on the other mediators of inflammation.

Immunological effects

A variety of antigen–antibody interactions can be demonstrated by in vitro experiments on human or animal lymphocytes. These include transformation in response to antigenic and mitogenic stimulation (Opelz et al, 1973; Panush & Anthony, 1976) and the production of migration inhibitory factor (Brown & Collins, 1977). These effects on normal lymphocytes are not cytotoxic and when the salicylates are withdrawn are reversible. Effects such as protection against the Schwartzman phenomenon in the rabbit are likely to be due to other actions of salicylates or to occur at extremely high salicylate doses beyond the clinical range.

Therapeutic doses of salicylate have been reported to depress lymphocyte transformation (Crout et al, 1975) or to have no effect (Smith et al, 1975).

Uricosuric effect

High doses of salicylate (over 5 mg/day) increase the urinary excretion of urates and this led at one stage to its use in the treatment of acute and chronic gout (Pollak & Mattenheimer, 1965). Salicylate affects both reabsorption and secretion of uric acid in the tubules. Low doses (1–2 g/day) may decrease urate excretion and elevate plasma urate concentration. If salicylate is used with other uricosuric drugs such as probenecid or sulphinpyrazone it blocks their uricosuric action (Kelley, 1975).

ADVERSE AND TOXIC REACTIONS

Gastrointestinal toxicity

The adverse effects of salicylates on the stomach are amongst the most common causes for discontinuation of the drug (Capell et al, 1979), and the process by which the gastric mucosa is damaged is complex (Fromm, 1978). Salicylates produce three major gastrointestinal side-effects; dyspepsia, occult bleeding and erosions with frank haemorrhage.

Dyspepsia

Although nausea, dyspepsia and heartburn are individually unpredictable, they are tolerated by most patients with chronic disease such as rheumatoid arthritis. These symptoms from high dose salicylate frequently disappear after a few days if the drug is continued (Alvarez & Summerskill, 1958) and they do not correlate with gastric bleeding (Vandam, 1972).

The type of aspirin preparation used does not appear to affect the incidence of gastrointestinal intolerance: both the buffered and unbuffered preparations can cause dyspepsia (Batterman, 1958; Cronk, 1958). Substituting enteric coated or liquid preparations can often overcome the discomfort, although if the intolerance persists an alternative non-steroidal anti-inflammatory drug will be required.

Gastrointestinal bleeding

Perhaps commoner than dyspepsia is microbleeding in the gastric mucosa; this occurs whether dyspepsia has been present or not (Scott et al, 1961). The small blood losses that range from 2.5–6 ml/day return to normal a few days after discontinuing the drug. It has been estimated that more than 70% of people taking high dose aspirin will have minor blood loss in this way (Leonards et al, 1973). However, it has been shown by epidemiological studies that only those persons taking aspirin regularly, on 4 or more days per week — 'heavy aspirin users' — are likely to suffer acute gastrointestinal bleeding (Levy, 1974). These serious consequences are rare, occurring in only 15 per 100 000 habitual aspirin users and there is therefore some justification for the belief that the adverse effects of aspirin on the gastric mucosa have been overemphasised (Rees & Turnberg, 1980).

The pathophysiology of the effects leading to gastric haemorrhage have been extensively studied (Weiss et al, 1961; Duggan, 1981). Local intracellular accumulation of salicylate anions in gastric mucosal cells leads to increased permeability of the mucosal barrier with a resultant back diffusion of hydrogen ions. This causes an erosive gastritis with desquamation of the gastric mucosa and haemorrhage from the subepithelial capillary plexus. The pH gradient favouring intracellular deposition of the salicylate crystals is greatest at the level of the stomach. These effects are facilitated by alcohol and bile. Although the ingestion of large doses of antacids with aspirin reduces blood loss compared with controls (Leonards & Levy, 1969), such buffering will also reduce salicylate levels. Reduction in salicylate-induced gastrointestinal bleeding as measured by [^{51}Cr] blood loss may also be produced by adding cimetidine, an H_2 receptor antagonist which reduces basal and stimulated acid secretion (Welch et al, 1978).

Peptic ulceration

That aspirin is a regular cause of peptic ulceration is still disputed although surveys do indicate that a proportion of patients with gastric ulceration had recently ingested aspirin (Levy, 1974).

Other epidemiological studies show the markedly increased incidence of chronic gastric ulcers associated with the introduction and popular use of headache powders in young Australian women (Duggan, 1976).

In endoscopic studies enteric-coated aspirin has been shown to produce much less gastric injury than standard or buffered aspirin at comparable concentrations of salicylate in the serum (Hoftiezer et al, 1980; Lanza et al, 1980). In patients prescribed aspirin for rheumatic diseases for at least 3 months, gastric ulcers have been found in about one-quarter of those taking conventional aspirin but in less than one in ten of those on the enteric-coated variety (Silvoso et al, 1979). Present knowledge therefore would advocate the use of enteric-coated aspirin if high dose salicylate is required to treat the rheumatic diseases.

There is no evidence that there is an association between aspirin use and duodenal ulceration (Levy, 1974), but aspirin consumption has been shown to be associated with benign oesophageal stricture (Heller et al, 1982).

Effects on the liver

Salicylates are metabolised in the liver and serum

transaminase levels have been reported to be elevated in a number of diseases in which salicylates are used. Juvenile rheumatoid arthritis (Athreya et al, 1975), rheumatoid arthritis and systemic lupus erythematosus (Seaman & Plotz, 1976) have all been shown to be diseases in which abnormal liver enzymes can follow aspirin ingestion. These abnormalities occur in the second week of therapy or if there is increase in dose. There does not appear to be any specific histological abnormality and the 'aspirin hepatitis' clears within a week of lowering the dose or stopping the drug. In juvenile rheumatoid arthritis transaminase levels return to normal despite continuation of aspirin (Miller & Weismann, 1976).

Effects on the kidney

When aspirin or salicylates are first ingested by normal subjects in therapeutic doses there is shedding of renal tubular cells and they are detected in the urine (Scott et al, 1963). The effect lasts several days and then disappears. It is not demonstrable again if the drug is stopped and then restarted. The mechanism is obscure, and like the effect aspirin has on decreasing renal blood flow (Beeley & Kendall, 1971), may be mediated by inhibition of prostaglandin synthesis (Flower, 1974). All this could contribute to the papillary and tubular necrosis reported in some patients taking aspirin-containing analgesics (Murray & Goldberg, 1975; Cove-Smith & Knapp, 1978). Aspirin as a cause of analgesic nephropathy, however, must be extremely uncommon in view of the vast amounts of the drug consumed annually and the normal renal function found after prolonged consumption of aspirin as a single drug (Akyol et al, 1982).

Berg (1977) noted that changes in renal function with rise of creatinine and decrease in creatinine clearance occurred in a series of patients with systemic lupus erythematosus and rheumatoid arthritis treated with aspirin; renal function being most affected in those with active disease. In another study, only on patients with systemic lupus erythematosus (Kimberley et al, 1978), a rise in prostaglandin could be demonstrated just before the fall in renal function. When the drug is stopped all these renal function changes rapidly improve; they must therefore be taken into account when assessing renal damage in such patients.

Central nervous system effects

Permanent neurological lesions never result from administration of salicylates in therapeutic doses. Temporary loss of hearing and tinnitus however is often noted and occasionally vertigo and loss of balance are recorded. Ototoxicity causes a change in the auditory threshold for pure tones and speech (Jardini et al, 1978). In patients with normal hearing tinnitus occurs universally if sufficient salicylates are taken, and as it occurs when the serum level of salicylates are within the anti-inflammatory range (200–300 μg/ml) it has been suggested as a guide to dosage (Mongan et al, 1973). Effects are reversible within 24–48 hours of discontinuing the drug (Miller, 1978). In advanced stages of intoxication with salicylates, blurred vision, confusion, hallucinations, delirium, convulsions and stupor or coma develop, but disappear often with withdrawal of the drug and restoration of fluid and electrolyte balance (Brown & Wilson, 1971).

Endocrine effects

It is not clear how aspirin acts as a hypoglycaemic agent but it is believed to increase the uptake of glucose in peripheral tissues of diabetic subjects (Gilgore & Rupp, 1961). Although this effect is not apparent in normal adults it can be an important cause of hypoglycaemia in the young (Limbeck et al, 1965).

With very large doses of salicylate, stimulation of the adrenals via the hypothalamus results in a rise of plasma cortisol; there is however abundant evidence that the anti-inflammatory effect of salicylates is independent of this rise in adrenocorticosteroids (Done et al, 1958).

Chronic administration of salicylate causes the competitive displacement by salicylate of thyroxine and tri-iodothyronine from prealbumin and thyroxine-binding globulin in plasma. The result of this is a decrease in plasma protein-bound iodine concentration, thyroidal uptake and clearance of iodine (Wolff & Austen, 1958).

Pulmonary and cardiovascular effects

Pulmonary oedema is a rare complication of salicylate consumption but its possibility must be kept in mind in the elderly (Andersen et al, 1976) especially if serum salicylate levels are elevated above 40 mg/%. Underlying heart disease is not a prerequisite (Tashima & Rose, 1974) but if carditis is present as in acute rheumatic fever there may be precipitation of congestive cardiac failure and pulmonary oedema, due to increase in circulating plasma volume and a fall in haematocrit and a resulting increase in cardiac output (Alexander & Smith, 1962).

Effects on the blood and coagulation

Aspirin has no effect on the total white cell count when taken in therapeutic doses although lymphocytes from subjects taking aspirin have been found to behave subnormally (Crout et al, 1975).

In patients with glucose-6-phosphate dehydrogenase deficiency haemolysis can be demonstrated after aspirin ingestion (Glader, 1976). Aspirin has an antithrombotic effect, the mechanism of action of which is complex. By inhibition of cyclo-oxygenase, which is the first enzyme in the arachidonic acid cascade, the formation of thromboxane A_2 and prostacyclin is unequally reduced. Thromboxane A_2 is a potent platelet aggregator found within platelets, and the platelet cyclo-oxygenase which forms it is more sensitive to aspirin than the cyclo-oxygenase which is responsible for the formation of prostacyclin, a potent vasodilator and inhibitor of platelet aggregation (Moncada & Vane, 1979).

Because of this unequal interaction the overall effect is an inhibition of platelet aggregation.

Vitamin K-dependent coagulation factors (II, VII, IX, X) may be reduced after ingestion of 2–8 g of aspirin per day in man. This effect is inconsistent and rarely a problem with aspirin toxicity (Loew & Vinazzer, 1976).

Because of the above mechanisms the protective effects of salicylates on the arteriovenous system have been exploited and will be discussed later.

Effects on pregnancy

Salicylates rapidly cross the placental barrier and fears are frequently expressed about the advisability of continuing salicylate therapy during pregnancy. There is no evidence that therapeutic doses of salicylate cause fetal damage in humans (Slone et al, 1976). If aspirin is taken daily through pregnancy, studies have shown a significant reduction in birth weight (Turner & Collins, 1975) and an increase in ante- and post-partum haemorrhage with a prolonged gestation and more complicated deliveries (Collins & Turner 1975; Stuart et al, 1982).

Salicylate intoxication

Because aspirin is one of the most commonly used and readily available analgesics it is not surprising that its abuse is a frequent cause for admission to hospital.

In children intoxication with aspirin occurs because of acute accidental ingestion or during the course of chronic use as used to be seen in the treatment of acute rheumatic fever. Small doses of acetyl salicylic acid can also be toxic in dehydrated children with fever. Accidental ingestion in children has fortunately been reduced following legislation to introduce 'child-proof' containers.

The problem with adults, however, persists and results in approximately 200 deaths from salicylate overdose in England and Wales every year.

Mild intoxication

Mild toxicity or salicylism occurs when plasma salicylate levels are greater than 35–50 mg/%. Among the symptoms the should alert the clinician are tinnitus, dizziness and headaches, confusion, sweating and thirst, nausea and hyperpnoea.

On withdrawal of the drug and with monitoring of plasma salicylate levels patients quickly recover (Anderson et al, 1976).

Major intoxication

When excessive plasma salicylate levels are reached a more florid picture develops. The most characteristic sign is an increase in the rate and depth of respiration. Although this results in metabolic acidosis in young children (Snodgrass & Rumack, 1981), in adults hyperventilation occurs producing a reduction in serum carbon dioxide and a resulting elevation in pH. The respiratory alkalosis thus produced is accompanied by fluid and electrolyte disturbances, high fevers, sweating and dehydration (Smith, 1968). At a later stage the accumulation of organic acids and the uncoupling of oxidative phosphorylation results in a metabolic acidosis. Patients die from complete circulatory collapse and respiratory failure, at times accompanied by pulmonary oedema, uraemia or massive gastrointestinal haemorrhage.

Treatment of major intoxication is aimed at correcting dehydration and metabolic disturbances. Urinary pH is usually alkaline in the early stages and then subsequently becomes acid. Measurement of the arterial blood gasses, pH and standard bicarbonate will show a respiratory alkalosis followed by a metabolic acidosis although usually a mixed acid — base disturbance is found. Hypokalaemia is usual but plasma sodium may be either high or low depending on the source of fluid loss and the type of replacement therapy. Prothrombin time is prolonged, forced alkaline diuresis to enhance salicylate elimination is well established (Lawson et al, 1969), but if renal failure is present, may be accompanied by pulmonary and cerebral oedema. In this situation urinary alkalinisation may be more effective in enhancing salicylate elimination (Prescott et al, 1982). Finally haemodialysis may be necessary; other more direct methods such as gastric lavage or the administration of activated charcoal are sometimes also indicated. Vitamin K administration or whole blood transfusion may also be required.

Monitoring of plasma salicylate levels is important but if slow-release or enteric-coated preparations have been taken then measurement of salicylate levels must be maintained for at least 70 hours after the overdose (Todd et al, 1981).

Hypersensitivity reactions

Small amounts of salicylate can precipitate a hypersensitivity reaction in some individuals, usually those with a known history of allergic reactions. This is related to the prostaglandin synthetase inhibitory effect of aspirin and other anti-inflammatory analgesics (Szczeklik et al, 1975). These reactions are not present with those analgesics that do not inhibit prostaglandins (Szczeklik et al, 1977).

The clinical effects can be divided into three categories: a reaction to aspirin demonstrated by bronchospasm (of which half have nasal polyps), an urticaria-angioedema reaction, and anaphylactic shock (Speer, 1975).

Patients with a history of such reactions should not only avoid salicylates and proprietary mixtures containing acetylsalicylic acid but also indomethacin, ibuprofen, fenoprofen, naproxen, tolectin and phenylbutazone. Mild reactions can be treated with antihistamines whilst epinephrine and corticosteroids will be needed in more severe anaphylactic reactions.

PROTECTIVE SIDE-EFFECTS OF SALICYLATES

The anti-platelet action of salicylates (see above) enables them to be used in clinical situations in which thrombus formation is a problem. A number of prospective clinical trials have been or are in the process of being conducted to establish the role salicylates play in preventing thrombus formation and at what dose they are most effective. Although the Medical Research Council Study (1972) failed to show a difference between 1.2 g aspirin daily and placebo in the prevention of post-operative venous thrombosis, there is good evidence that 1 g daily of aspirin, especially in men, prevents thrombus formation after hip surgery (Harris et al, 1982). The Canadian Co-operative Study (1978) showed that in aspirin-treated men there was a significant decrease in transient ischaemic attacks, stroke or death and suggested the use of aspirin in threatened strokes. Prospective studies on the effect of aspirin in preventing myocardial infarction or reinfarction are still under way but so far the data are inconclusive (Jick.&, Miettinen, 1976; Coronary Drug Project, 1976; EPSIM Research Group, 1982).

Finally there is non-conclusive evidence from uncontrolled trials that the development of cataract may be delayed in those patients taking aspirin for rheumatoid arthritis (Cotlier &, Sharma, 1981) and that aspirin may exert a protective effect on articular cartilage (Forney et al, 1973).

THERAPEUTIC USES OF SALICYLATES IN THE RHEUMATIC DISEASES

Salicylates are used to reduce fever, pain and inflammation in the rheumatic diseases, and because in most of their formulations they are completely absorbed, the particular type of salicylate preparation used is not critical. The generally accepted plasma salicylate level at which maximum anti-inflammatory effect is achieved is 200–300 μg/ml and only some enteric-coated salicylates or suppositories, being incompletely or erratically absorbed, do not achieve these levels. Because at anti-inflammatory serum levels salicylates have a long serum half-life, doses can be spaced out to twice or three times daily. Monitoring of plasma salicylate levels is important to achieve optimum anti-inflammatory effect. Tinnitus has been suggested as an indicator of this (Mongan et al, 1973) but if pre-existing hearing loss is present and patients are elderly this may be found unreliable. Steady-state serum salicylate levels are only reached in 5–7 days and if no toxicity is present measurement of serum salicylates should only be performed one week after each change in dosage.

In rheumatoid arthritis, aspirin must be given in full anti-inflammatory doses but just below those that produce tinnitus (5–6 g daily); some patients however will respond well to 3.6 g daily.

Children tolerate high serum levels of salicylate better than adults and for juvenile arthritis doses of 80–100 mg/kg/day or higher are acceptable. In rheumatic fever similar high levels are required and within 24–48 hours of adequate doses of salicylate there is considerable relief of pain, swelling and immobility.

In systemic lupus erythematosus aspirin has a useful role in combatting fever, arthritis, pleurisy and pericarditis and can be used prior to steroid therapy. Some patients with seronegative spondarthropathies respond to anti-inflammatory doses of aspirin and it has also been used for its analgesic effects in osteoarthrosis and non-articular rheumatism.

DRUG INTERACTIONS WITH ASPIRIN

Despite the large quantities of aspirin consumed and the likelihood of many potential drug interactions, very few of these are of clinical significance. The best documented is the displacement of drugs from protein binding sites by the more strongly bound salicylates. This results in pharmacological actions that may enhance or inhibit the effects of the displaced drug. The pharmacological effects of penicillin analogs, thyroid hormone, sulphonamide, methotrexate tolbutamide and coumarin anticoagulants are thus enhanced (Raisfeld, 1973).

In the neonate a dangerous situation may occur when bilirubin is displaced from its binding sites on albumin with a resulting kernicterus and hyperbilirubinaemia (Maisels, 1972).

The effects of aspirin on blood coagulation are twofold. By its effects on prothrombin time it can reduce the amount of anticoagulation needed (Loew & Vinazzer, 1976), and by interfering in the steps along the pathway to clotting, it disrupts this in heparinised patients (Yett et al, 1978).

Corticosteroids increase the renal excretion of salicylates so that when they are reduced or withdrawn salicylate levels rise sometimes into a toxic range (Klinenberg & Miller, 1965). There seems to be no evidence that the additive effect of aspirin and corticosteroids on the gastric mucosa causes any increase in dyspepsia or gastrointestinal haemorrhage.

There is no clinical significance in the interactions between aspirin and the non-steroidal anti-inflammatory drugs. For example there is no effect on plasma concentrations of indomethacin after aspirin ingestion and no clinical benefit if the two drugs are taken together (Brooks et al, 1975). Any dose of salicylate can inhibit the uricosuric activity of probenecid and sulphinpyrazone and the combination should be avoided (Kelley, 1975).

In addition to the above, other less important interactions have been reported (Buckingham, 1978).

FORMULATIONS OF SALICYLATE

There are more than 200 products containing aspirin in some form, the majority of which are available without a prescription (Leist & Banwell, 1974). Dosage forms include liquids, tablets, suppositories, creams and powders. Tablets and capsules are the most frequent preparations used by rheumatologists and differ only in their rates of disintegration, dissolution and site of absorption (Dromgoole et al, 1981).

Acetylated salicylate preparations (aspirin and benorylate) differ from non-acetylated preparations because their effect on platelet function lasts as long as 72 hours after each single dose of aspirin (Zucker & Rothwell, 1978). This effect is due to acetylation of platelet membrane which is irreversible and enables aspirin and benorylate to be given once or twice daily for an anti-platelet effect. The non-acetylated salicylates only affect platelets reversibly and for as long as they remain in the blood stream. Prostaglandin synthetase inhibition is produced equally by both preparations although the disadvantage of aspirin is that it produces bronchospasm in some asthmatics (Weinberger, 1978).

Acetylsalicylic acid (aspirin) preparations

Most aspirin is available in the form of tablets and capsules, some being combined with other drugs such as codeine, paracetamol or caffeine. Combinations of drugs should be avoided as the toxic effects of the added drug may become evident when attempting to achieve anti-inflammatory salicylate levels.

Fine particle size (microfined aspirin) has been shown experimentally to be more rapidly absorbed than coarser preparations (Leonards & Levy, 1967) and would therefore appear preferable.

As aspirin is more rapidly soluble at high pH, 'buffered' tablets have been developed to increase pH around the disintegrating tablet. Insoluble calcium and magnesium antacids and sodium bicarbonate have been used as buffers.

Enteric-coated tablets resist gastric fluids and are rapidly dissolved in the small intestine. Ideally the coating on the tablets should be soluble at pH values above 5 but frequently the stomach and small intestine do not conform to this and the result is an erratic and sometimes incomplete absorption of the drug. For chronic administration, however, when a steady-state is reached this formulation is well tolerated although periodic serum salicylate levels should be measured (Benson et al, 1976).

Sustained or time-release preparations of aspirin are available in which aspirin particles are microencapsulated in wax resins or plastics and have differing rates of disintegration. The effect of this is to flatten the plasma salicylate level time curve. They do not have any practical advantage over other formulations and may be, like enteric-coated preparations, extremely hazardous when taken as an overdose, because plasma salicylate levels frequently do not reach their highest values until 60 or 70 hours later (Todd et al, 1981).

The bioavailability of salicylates from suppositories is less than that of oral salicylate preparations but increases with retention time (first defaecation) so that the control of the amount of drug available needs careful monitoring with plasma salicylate levels (Connolly et al, 1979).

Newer salicylates

In the search for an acceptable formulation of salicylate with least side-effects, especially gastrointestinal, and maximum anti-inflammatory effect, a number of newer forms of salicylate have been introduced.

Benorylate

This is a condensation of aspirin and paracetamol which hydrolyses to release both drugs after absorption (Robertson, 1973). Salicylate levels equivalent to 1.2 g of aspirin have been shown to be produced by 2 g of benorylate. It is a potent anti-inflammatory compound with fewer gastrointestinal side-effects than aspirin (Croft et al, 1972) and readily enters synovial fluid in patients with rheumatoid arthritis (Aylward et al, 1975).

Salsalate

This is practically insoluble in the acid pH of the stomach and therefore causes less gastric irritation as it dissolves in the near neutral pH of the small intestine. 500 mg of salsalate are equivalent to 698 mg of acetyl salicylic acid in salicylic acid content.

It has a significant anti-inflammatory effect in rheumatic diseases and causes less occult gastrointestinal bleeding than aspirin alone (Cohen, 1979).

Diflunisal

By deliberate chemical alteration of the aspirin molecule the salicylate structure is modified with a diflurophenyl group and lacks an acetyl function. It is not metabolised to salicylic acid but is excreted unchanged in the urine. It is anti-inflammatory, analgesic and anti-pyretic and is useful in osteoarthritis, with few instances of gastric irritation and less gastrointestinal blood loss than equivalent doses of aspirin (Andrew et al, 1977).

Choline magnesium trisalicylate

Choline salicylate is an active, well-tolerated drug, but cannot be formulated as a tablet. Magnesium disalicylate is less hygroscopic and when combined they exhibit the properties of aspirin with reduced local irritant effects (Cohen & Garber, 1978). Each 500 mg tablet contains 293 mg of choline salicylate and 362 mg of magnesium salicylate, providing 500 mg of salicylate. This preparation is found to be particularly useful in the treatment of rheumatoid arthritis (Binus et al, 1982).

REFERENCES

Akyol S M, Thompson M, Kerr D N S 1982 Renal function after prolonged consumption of aspirin. British Medical Journal 1: 631–632

Alexander W D, Smith G 1962 Disadvantageous circulatory effects of salicylate in rheumatic fever. Lancet 1: 768–771

Alvarez A S, Summerskill W H J, 1958 Gastrointestinal haemorrhage and salicylate. Lancet 274: 920–925

Anderson R J, Potts D E, Gabow P A, Rumack B H, Schrier R W 1976 Unrecognized adult salicylate intoxication. Annals of Internal Medicine 85: 745–748

Athreya B H, Moser G, Cecil H S, Myers A R 1975 Aspirin induced hepatoxicity in juvenile rheumatoid arthritis: A prospective study. Arthritis and Rheumatism 18: 347–352

Avery D D, Penn P E 1974 Blockade of pyrogen induced fever by intrahypothalamic injections of salicyate in the rat. Neuropharmacology 13: 1179–1185

Aylward M, Maddock J, Rees, Thomas G M, Wheeldon R, Holly F 1975 Simultaneous pharmacokinetics of benorylate in plasma and synovial fluid of patients with rheumatoid arthritis. Scandinavian Journal of Rheumatology (Suppl) 13:9.12

Ayres J W, Weidler D J, MacKichan J, Wagner J G 1977 Circadian rhythm of urinary pH in man with and without chronic antacid administration. European Journal of Clinical Pharmacology 12: 415–420

Ballantyne F C, Fleck A, Dick W C 1971 Albumin metabolism in rheumatoid arthritis. Annals of the Rheumatic Diseases 30: 256–270

Batterman R C 1958 Comparison of buffered and unbuffered acetylsalicylic acid. New England Journal of Medicine 258: 213–219

Beeley L, Kendall M J 1971 Effect of aspirin on renal clearance of ^{125}I-diatrizoate. British Medical Journal 1: 707–708

Benson W G, Laskin C A, Paton T W, Little H A, Fam A G 1976 Twice daily dosing of enteric-coated aspirin in patients with rheumatic diseases. Journal of Rheumatology 6: 351–356

Berg K J 1977 Acute effects of acetylsalicylic acid in patients with chronic renal insufficiency. European Journal of Clinical Pharmacology 11: 111–116

Binus M A, Lyon J A, Nicolas J L 1982 Comparable serum salicylate concentrations from choline magnesium trisalicylate, aspirin and buffered aspirin in rheumatoid arthritis. Arthritis and Rheumatism 25: 464–466

Boardman P L, Hart F D 1967 Clinical measurement of the anti-inflammatory effects of salicylates in rheumatoid arthirtis. British Medical Journal 4: 264–268

Brooks P M, Walker J J, Bell M A, Buchanan W W, Rhymer A R 1975 Indomethacin-aspirin interaction. A clinical appraisal. British Medical Journal 3: 69–71

Brown G L, Wilson W P 1971 Salicylate intoxication and the CNS with special reference to EEG findings. Diseases of the Nervous System 32: 135–140

Brown K A, Collins A J 1977 Action of non-steroidal anti-inflammatory drugs on human and rat peripheral leucocyte migration in vitro. Annals of Rheumatic Diseases 36: 239–243

Buckingham R B 1978 Interactions involving anti-rheumatic drugs I and II. Bulletin on the Rheumatic Diseases 28: 960–971

Canadian Co-operative Study Group. 1978 A randomised trial of aspirin and sulfinpyrazone in threatened stroke. New England Journal of Medicine 299: 53–59

Capell H A, Rennie, J A N, Rooney P J, Murdoch R M, Hole D J, Dick W C, et al 1979 Patient compliance: a novel method of testing non-steroidal anti-inflammatory analgesics in rheumatoid arthritis. Journal of Rheumatology 6: 584–593

Cohen A 1979 Fecal blood loss and plasma salicylate study of salicyl-salicylic acid and aspirin. Journal of Clinical Pharmacology 19: 242–247

Cohen A, Garber H E, 1978 Comparison of choline magnesium trisalicylate and acetylsalicylic acid in relation to fecal blood loss. Current Therapeutic Research 23: 187–193

Cohen L S 1976 Clinical pharmacology of acetylsalicylic acid. Seminars in Thrombosis and Haemostasis 2: 146–175

Collins E, Turner G 1975 Maternal effects of regular salicylate ingestion in pregnancy. Lancet ii: 335–339

Connolly K, Lam L, Ward O C 1979 Rectal aspirin-absorption and antipyretic effect. Archives of Diseases of Childhood 54: 713–715

Coronary Drug Project Research Group 1976 Aspirin and coronary heart disease. Journal of Chronic Disease 29: 625–642

Cotlier E, Sharma Y R 1981 Aspirin and senile cataracts in rheumatoid arthritis. Lancet i: 338–339

Cove-Smith J R, Knapp M S 1978 Analgesic nephropathy, an important cause of chronic renal failure. Quarterly Journal of Medicine 47: 49–69

Croft D N, Cuddingham J H P, Sweetland C 1972 Gastric bleeding and benorylate, a new aspirin. British Medical Journal iii: 545–547

Cronk G A 1958 Laboratory and clinical studies with buffered and non-buffered acetylsalicylic acid. New England Journal of Medicine 258: 219–222

Crout J E, Hepburn B N, Ritts R E 1975 Suppression of lymphocyte transformation after aspirin ingestion. New England Journal of Medicine 292: 221–223

Deodhar S D, Dick W C, Hodgkinson R, Buchanan W W 1973 Measurement of clinical response of anti-inflammatory drug therapy in rheumatoid arthritis. Quarterly Journal of Medicine (New Series) 42: 387–401

Done A K, Ely R S, Kelley V C 1958 Symposium on adrenal

corticoid therapy: salicylates and the pituitary-adrenal system. Metabolism 7: 52–69
Dromgoole S H, Furst D E, Paulus H E 1981 Rational approaches to the use of salicylates in the treatment of rheumatoid arthritis. Seminars in Arthritis and Rheumatism 11: 257–283
Duggan J M 1976 Progress report. Aspirin in chronic gastric ulcer: an Australian experience. Gut 17: 378–384
Duggan J M 1981 The pathogenesis of the aspirin-related gastric lesion. Journal of the Royal College of Physicians of London 15: 117–118
E P S I M Research Group 1982 A controlled comparison of aspirin and oral anti-coagulants in prevention of death after myocardial infarction. New England Journal of Medicine 307: 701–708
Feldberg W, Gupta K P 1973 Pyrogen fever and prostaglandin-like activity in cerebrospinal fluid. Journal of Physiology 228: 41–53
Flower R J 1974 Drugs which inhibit prostaglandin biosynthesis. Pharmacological Reviews 26: 33–66
Forney H J Bentley G, Mathews R S 1973 Salicylates and repair in adult articular cartilage. Orthopaedics (Oxford) 6: 19–31
Fromm D 1978 Salicylates and gastric mucosal damage. Paediatrics 62: 938–942
Gibaldi M, Gundhofer B, Levy G 1974 Effects of antacids on pH of urine. Clinical Pharmacology and Therapeutics 16: 520–525
Gibson T, Zaphiropoulos G, Grove J, Widdop B, Berry D 1975 Kinetics of salicylate metabolism. British Journal of Clinical Pharmacology 2: 233–238
Gilgore S G, Rupp J J 1961 Response of blood glucose to intravenous salicylate. Metabolism 10: 419–421
Glader B E 1976 Evaluation of the haemolytic role of aspirin in glucose 6 phosphate dehydrogenase deficiency. Journal of Paediatrics 89: 1027–1030
Goodman L, Gilman A 1970 The pharmacological basis of therapeutics. Macmillan, New York
Guzman F, Braun C, Lim R K S, Potter G D, Rodgers D W 1964 Narcotic and non-narcotic analgesics which block visceral pain evoked by intra-arterial injection of bradykinin and other algesic agents. Archives Internationales de Pharmacodynamie et de Therapie 149: 571–588
Harris W H, Athanasoulis C A, Waltman A C, Salzman E W 1982 High and low dose aspirin prophylaxis against venous thromboembolic disease in total hip replacement. Journal of Bone and Joint Surgery 64A: 63–66
Heller S R, Fellows I W, Ogilvie A L, Atkinson M 1982 Non-steroidal anti-inflammatory drugs and benign oesophageal stricture. British Medical Journal 285: 167–168
Hoftiezer J W, Silvoso G R, Burks M, Ivery K J 1980 Comparison of the effects of regular and enteric coated aspirin on gastroduodenal mucosa of man. Lancet ii: 609–612
Houde R W, Wallenstein S L, Rogers M 1960 Clinical pharmacology of analgesics. I A method of assaying analgesic effect. Clinical Pharmacology and Therapeutics 1: 163–174
Jardini L, Findlay R, Burgi E 1978 Auditory changes associated with moderate blood salicylate levels. Rheumatology and Rehabilitation 17: 233–236
Jick, H, Miettinen O S 1976 Regular aspirin use and myocardial infarction. British Medical Journal 1: 1057
Kelley W N 1975 Effects of Drugs on uric acid in man. Annual Review of Pharmacology 15: 327–350
Kimberley R P, Gill J R, Bourden R E, Keiser H R, Plotz P H 1978 Elevated urinary prostaglandins and the effects of aspirin on renal function in lupus erythematosus. Annals of Internal Medicine 89: 336–341
Klinenberg J R, Miller F 1965 Effect of corticosteroids on blood salicylate concentration. Journal of the American Medical Association 194: 601–604
Koch P H, Schultz C A, Willis R J, Hallquist S L, Welling P G 1978 Influence of food and fluid ingestion on aspirin bioavailability. Journal of Pharmacological Science 67: 1533–1535
Koch-Weser J 1974 Bioavailability of drugs. New England Journal of Medicine 291: 503–506
Kwan K C, Breault G O, Davis R L, Lei B W, Czerwinski A W, Besselaar G H Duggan D E 1978 Effects of concomitant aspirin administration on the pharmacokinetics of indomethacin in man. Journal of Pharmacokinetics and Biopharmaceutics 6: 451–476
Lanza F L, Roger G L, Nelson R S 1980 Endoscopic evaluation of the effects of aspirin, buffered aspirin and enteric coated aspirin on gastric and duodenal mucosa. New England Journal of Medicine 303: 136–138
Lawson A A H, Proudfoot A T, Brown S S, MacDonald R H, Fraser A G, Cameron J C, et al 1969 Forced diuresis in the treatment of acute salicylate poisoning in adults. Quarterly Journal of Medicine 38: 31–48
Lee P, Sturrock D, Kennedy A, Dick W C 1973 The evaluation of anti-rheumatic drugs. Current Medical Research and Opinion 1: 427–443
Leist E R, Banwell J G 1974 Products containing aspirin. New England Journal of Medicine 291: 710–712
Leonards J R 1963 The influence of solubility on the rate of gastrointestinal absorption of aspirin. Clinical Pharmacology and Therapeutics 4: 476–479
Leonards J R, Levy G 1967 The role of dosage form in aspirin-induced gastrointestinal bleeding. Clinical Pharmacology and Therapeutics 8: 400–408
Leonards J R, Levy G 1969 Reduction or prevention of aspirin induced occult gastrointestinal blood loss in man. Clinical Pharmacology and Therapeutics 10: 571–575
Leonards J R, Levy G, Niemczura R 1973 Gastrointestinal blood loss during prolonged aspirin administration. New England Journal of Medicine 289: 1020–1022
Levy G, Tsuchiya T 1972 Salicylate accumulation kinetics in man. New England Journal of Medicine 287: 430–432
Levy G, Procknal J A, Garrettson L K 1975 Distribution of salicylate between neonatal and maternal serum at diffusion equilibrium. Clinical Pharmacology and Therapeutics 18: 210–214
Levy M 1974 Aspirin use in patients with major upper gastrointestinal bleeding and peptic ulcer disease. New England Journal of Medicine 290: 1158–1162
Lim R K S, Guzman F, Rogers D W, Goto K, Braun C, Dickerson G D, et al 1964 Site of action of narcotic and non-narcotic analgesics determined by blocking bradykinin-evoked visceral pain. Archives Internationales de Pharacodynamie et de Therapie 153: 25–58
Limbeck G A, Ruvalcaba R H A, Samols E, Kelley V C 1965 Salicylates and hypoglycemia. Americal Journal of Diseases of Children 109: 165–167
Loew D, Vinazzer H 1976 Dose dependent influence of acetylsalicylic acid on platelet functions and plasmatic coagulation factors. Haemostasis 5: 239–249

MacPherson C R, Milne M D, Evans B M 1955 The excretion of salicylate. British Journal of Pharmacology 10: 484–489
Maisels M J 1972 Bilirubin: Our understanding and influencing its metabolism in the New-born infant. Pediatric Clinics of North America 19: 447–501
Mandel H G, Cambosos N M, Smith P K 1954 The pressure of aspirin in human plasma after oral administration. Journal of Pharmacology and Experimental Therapeutics 112: 495–500
Medical Research Council 1972 Effect of aspirin on postoperative; venous thrombosis. Lancet ii: 441–445
Miller J J, Weismann B B, 1976 Correlations between transaminase concentrations and semi salicylate concentration in juvenile rheumatoid arthritis. Arthritis and Rheumatism 19: 115–118
Miller R R 1978 Deafness due to plain and long-acting aspirin tablets. Journal of Clinical Pharmacology 18: 468–471
Moncada S, Vane J R 1979 Arachidonic acid metabolites and the interactions between platelets and blood-vessel walls. New England Journal of Medicine 300: 1142–1147
Mongan E, Kelly P, Nies K, Porter W W, Paulus H E 1973 Tinnitus as an indication of therapeutic serum salicylate levels.
Journal of the American Medical Association 226: 142–145
Murray T, Goldberg M M 1975 Analgesic abuse and renal disease. Annual Review of Medicine 26: 527–550
Opelz G, Terasaki P I, Hirata A A 1973 Suppression of lymphocyte transformation by aspirin. Lancet ii: 478–480
Panush R S, Anthony C R 1976 Effects of acetylsalicylic acid on normal human peripheral blood lymphocytes. Inhibition of mitogenous antigen-stimulated incorporation of tritiated thymidine. Clinical and Experimental Immunology 23: 114–125
Pohto P 1976 Salicylates in saliva. Acta Odontologica Scandinavica 34: 155–161
Pollak V E, Mattenheimer H 1965 Glutaminase activity in the kidney in gout. Journal of Laboratory and Clinical Medicine 66: 564–570
Prescott L F, Balali-Mood M, Critchley J A J H, Johnstone A F, Proudfoot A T 1982 Diuresis or urinary alkalinisation for salicylate poisoning? British Medical Journal ii: 1383–1386
Raisfeld I 1973 Clinical pharmacology of drug interactions. Annual Review of Medicine 24: 385–418
Reed J R, Palmisano P A 1975 Central nervous system salicylate. Clinical Toxicology 8: 623–631
Rees W D W, Turnberg 1980 Reappraisal of the effects of aspirin on the stomach. Lancet ii: 410–413
Robertson A 1973 Benorylate — the rationale: A symposium on benorylate. Rheumatology and Rehabilitation 12: 7–16
Roth G J, Majerus P W, 1975 The mechanism of the effect of aspirin on human platelets. 1. Acetylation of a particulate fraction protein. Journal of Clinical Investigation 56: 624–632
Rowland M, Riegelman S 1968 Pharmacokinetics of acetylsalicylic acid and salicylic acid after intravenous administration in man. Journal of Pharmaceutical Sciences 57: 1313–1319
Rowland M, Riegelman S, Harris P A, Sholkoff S D 1972 Absorption kinetics of aspirin in man following oral administration of an aqueous solution. Journal of Pharmaceutical Sciences 61: 379–385
Schachter D, Manis J G 1958 Salicylate and salicyl conjugates: Fluorimetric estimation, biosynthesis and renal excretion in man. Journal of Clinical Investigation 37: 800–807
Scott J T, Denman A M, Dorling J 1963 Renal irritation caused by salicylates. Lancet: 344–348
Scott J T, Porter I H, Lewis S M, Dixon A St J 1961 Studies of gastrointestinal bleeding caused by corticosteroids, salicylates and other analgesics. Quarterly Journal of Medicine 30: 167–188
Seaman W E, Plotz P H 1976 Effect of aspirin on liver tests in patients with rheumatoid arthritis or systemic lupus erythematosis and in normal volunteers. Arthritis and Rheumatism 19: 155–160
Silvoso G R, Ivery K J, Butt J H 1979 Incidence of gastric lesions in patients with rheumatic disease on chronic aspirin therapy. Annals of Internal Medicine 91: 517–520
Slone D, Siskind V, Heinonen O P, Monson R R, Kaufman D W, Shapiro S 1976 Aspirin and congenital malformations. Lancet i: 1373–1375
Smith M J H 1968 The metabolic basis of major symptoms in acute salicylate intoxication. Clinical Toxicology 1: 387–407
Smith M J H, Hoth M, Davis K 1975 Aspirin and lymphocyte transformation. Annals of Internal Medicine 83: 509–571
Snodgrass W, Rumack B H 1981 Salicylate toxicity following therapeutic doses in young children. Clinical Toxicology 18: 247–259
Soren A 1977 Dissociation of acetyl salicylic acid in blood and joint fluid. Scandinavian Journal of Rheumatology 6: 17–22
Speer F 1975 Aspirin allergy: a clinical study. Southern Medical Journal 68: 314–318
Stone E 1763 An account of the success of the bark of the willow in the cure of agues. Philisophical Society Transactions 53: 195–200
Stuart M J, Gross S J, Elrod H, Groeber J E 1982 Effects of acetyl salicylic acid ingestion on maternal and neonatal hemostasis. New England Journal of Medicine 307: 909–912
Superstine S Y, Superstine E, Penchas S 1978 Comparison of the bioavailability of aspirin tablets and suppositories. Israel Journal of Medical Science 14: 292–294
Szczeklik A, Gryglewski R J, Czerniawska-Mysik G 1975 Relationship of inhibition of prostaglandin biosynthesis by analgesics to asthma attacks in aspirin sensitive patients. British Medical Journal 1: 67–69
Szczeklik K A, Gryglewski R J, Czerniawska-Mysik G 1977 Clinical patterns of hypersensitivity to nonsteroidal anti-inflammatory drugs and their pathogenesis. Journal of Allergy and Clinical Immunology 60: 276–284
Tainter M L, Ferris A J 1969 Aspirin in modern therapy. A review. Bayer Company Division of Sterling Drug, New York
Tashima C K, Rose M 1974 Pulmonary oedema and salicylates. Annals of Internal Medicine 81:274
Todd P J, Sills J A, Harris F, Cowen J M 1981 Problems with overdoses of sustained-release aspirin. Lancet i:777
Turner G. Collins E 1975 Fetal effects of regular salicylate ingestion in pregnancy. Lancet ii: 338–339
Valentic J P, Leopold I H, Dea F J 1980 Excretion of salicylic acid into tears following oral administration of aspirin. Ophthalmology 87: 815–820
Vandam L D 1972 Analgetic drugs — the mild analgetics. New England Journal of Medicine 286: 20–23

Vane J R 1971 Inhibition of prostaglandin synthesis as a mechanism of action for aspirin-like drugs. Nature New Biology 231: 232–235

Wallace S, Whiting B 1976 Factors affecting drug binding in plasma of elderly patients. British Journal of Clinical Pharmacology 3: 327–330

Weinberger M 1978 Analgesic sensitivity in children with asthma. Paediatrics 62: 910–915

Weiss A, Pitman E R, Graham E C 1961 Aspirin and gastric bleeding Gastroscopic observations with review of the literature. American Journal of Medicine 31: 266–278

Welch R W, Bentch H L, Harris S C 1978 Reduction of aspirin-induced gastrointestinal bleeding with cimetidine. Gastroenterology 74: 459–463

Willkens R F, Segre E J 1976 Combination therapy with naproxen and aspirin in rheumatoid arthritis. Arthritis and Rheumatism 19: 677–682

Wilson J T, Howell R L, Holladay N W, Brillis G M, Chrastil J, Watson J T, et al 1978 Gentisuric acid: Metabolic formation in animals and identification as a metabolite of aspirin in man. Clinical Pharmacology and Therapeutics 23: 635–643

Wit A, Wang S C 1968 Temperature-sensitive neurons in preoptic anterior hypothalamic region: Actions of pyrogens and acetylsalicylate. American Journal of Pysiology 215: 1160–1169

Wolff J, Austen F K 1958 Salicylates and thyroid function. 2. The effect on the thyroid-pituitary inter-relation. Journal of Clinical Investigation 37: 1144–1152

Yett H S, Skillman J J, Salzman E W 1978 The hazards of aspirin plus heparin. New England Journal of Medicine 298:1092

Zucker M B, Rothwell K J 1978 Differential influences of salicylate compounds on platelet aggregation and serotonin release. Current Therapeutic Research 23: 194–199

P.N. Platt W.C. Dick

Non-steroidal anti-inflammatory drugs

The intervening years since the previous edition of this textbook have seen the introduction of several new drugs to the already substantial list of non-steroidal anti-inflammatory drugs (NSAIDs) available to the clinician. Regrettably there have been few if any significant advances in efficacy. There has also been the unfortunate experience of having drugs suspended or withdrawn because of side-effects. This emphasises that NSAIDs produce significant morbidity and mortality (Girdwood, 1974) in patients suffering from predominantly non-fatal conditions, whilst at the same time they provide only symptomatic relief with no convincing evidence of disease modification. These drugs are being widely abused today.

MECHANISMS OF ACTION

The exact mechanisms of action of the NSAIDs are unknown. The past decade has been dominated by the prostaglandin synthetase inhibition theory following the description by Vane and his colleagues (Vane, 1971; Ferreira et al, 1971). Despite a decade of intensive research we are unsure whether prostaglandin synthesis is associated causally with inflammatory events or whether it occurs as an epiphenomenon (Metz, 1981).

The past ten years have seen a much greater understanding of the pathways of peroxidation of arachidonic acid, both by the classical cyclo-oxygenase pathway and by the more recently described lipoxygenase pathway (Hamberg & Samuelson, 1974; Borgeat et al, 1976) which gives rise to compounds containing a conjugated triene structure, the leukotrienes. The potent chemotactic activity of these products suggests that leukotrienes may have a role in the local accumulation of inflammatory cells.

All the presently available NSAIDs operate as selective cyclo-oxygenase inhibitors to variable degrees. With the withdrawal of benoxaprofen from the market there are no drugs available which inhibit lipoxygenase significantly at therapeutic concentrations. It has been suggested (Higgs et al, 1980) that the symptomatic relief produced by NSAIDs results from inhibition of formation of cyclo-oxygenase-derived products, but that the failure to produce a significant disease-modifying effect is related to the failure of these drugs to inhibit the lipoxygenase pathway at clinically relevant concentrations, allowing the more chronic leucocyte-mediated components of inflammation to proceed. The introduction of drugs capable of inhibiting both the known pathways may be a next step in the development of the NSAIDs.

The NSAIDs as a group have a wide range of pharmacological actions independent of prostaglandin synthetase inhibition. These include the scavenging of oxygen radicals (Kuehl et al, 1977) although some doubt has been cast on the significance of this as an anti-inflammatory property (Payne et al, 1982). The inhibition of production of superoxide radicals and lysosomal enzyme release (Smollen & Weissmann, 1980) has been reported, although the concentrations required to produce these actions may be supratherapeutic. However a role for toxic oxygen radicals as inflammatory agents cannot be ruled out, as the rate-limiting step in prostaglandin synthesis requires peroxidation of arachidonic acid and oxidation–reduction reactions involving oxygen radicals. Therefore the inflammatory changes associated with prostaglandin synthesis may be mediated to an unknown extent by these products (Metz,

1981) rather than the prostaglandins themselves.

Within the range of concentrations at which indomethacin inhibits cyclo-oxygenase it also inhibits cyclic nucleotide phosphodiesterase (Metz, 1981) leading to an increase in cAMP levels with potential anti-inflammatory actions. Widespread effects of NSAIDs can be demonstrated on flux of ions including calcium and potassium ions, transport of anions, and alteration of heterologous receptors. The significance of these findings in terms of anti-inflammatory actions is unclear.

In considering the biological effects of these drugs (Famaey et al, 1975) it is important to think in terms of those effects that are demonstrable at clinically realistic concentrations. It is also important to look for dose response relationships: dose response curves are often bimodal, displaying stimulation at low and inhibition at higher concentrations. This is demonstrated by the ability of indomethacin to enhance accumulation of cells in inflammatory exudates at low concentrations but to inhibit cell accumulation at high concentrations (Eakins et al, 1980). The differential effects at low and high concentrations may be due to the effect of inhibiting cyclo-oxygenase at low concentrations enhancing production of the highly chemotactic leukotrienes. At high concentrations the drug inhibits lipoxygenases in addition to the cyclo-oxygenases, thereby reducing production of leukotrienes.

Effects of NSAIDs have also been reported on control of lymphocyte function (Webb et al, 1979), including T and B cell activation and cell-mediated cytolysis. Inhibition of synthesis of IgM rheumatoid factor by several NSAIDs has been reported (Ceuppens et al, 1982), and this appears to be dependent on the presence of radiosensitive T cells; synthesis can be restored by addition of low dose PGE_2. This suggests that some of the 'disease modifying' properties attributed to NSAIDs on the basis of changes in rheumatoid factor and acute phase proteins may be purely prostaglandin inhibition-related phenomena.

SELECTION AND USE OF NON-STEROIDAL ANTI-INFLAMMATORY DRUGS

NSAIDs are symptomatic remedies that have no significant effect on the underlying disease process. The therapeutic goal is therefore to reduce symptoms to a level with which the patient can cope and can lead a full life. It is unrealistic for the patient, or physician for that matter, to expect abolition of symptoms. If there is doubt concerning the efficacy of a drug it should be withheld for the effect to be judged, and restarted if the effect is worthwhile. On occasions improvement may be noted when the drug is withdrawn.

A single drug should be used (Huskisson, 1977), and in the minimum dose required to produce relief. There is no evidence that any enhancement of effect is produced by the use of combination of NSAIDs (Buckingham, 1977). However there is evidence of increased toxicity when more than one anti-inflammatory agent is used, particularly in the case of gastro-intestinal lesions (Caruso & Bianchi Porro, 1980).

In view of the considerable variation in patient response to this group of drugs, the provision of a sequence of NSAIDs, each for a short period of time to allow patient assessment of efficacy, is a reasonable approach. A period of one week is normally adequate for assessment of each drug, and a sequence of not more than four or six drugs should suffice. The exact sequence of drugs will depend on the individual physician and the drugs with which he is familiar, and should include drugs from a variety of groups. This is no way is an abrogation of responsibility by the physician as patient participation is important in what is essentially a symptomatic treatment. The variations between patient responses often are greater than the variations between the different NSAIDs. If one drug proved to be significantly more effective than another in a population, there would still be individuals who would select the overall 'less effective' drug as their first choice.

ADVERSE EFFECTS AND INTERACTIONS

The NSAIDs as well as sharing common therapeutic actions appear to share a common pattern of adverse effects and interactions. It appears that many of these are related to prostaglandin synthesis inhibition. These include gastrointestinal irritation and ulceration, inhibition of platelet aggregation and prolonged bleeding time, central nervous system effects including headache, tinnitus, nervousness and confusion, impairment of renal function, oedema, and allergic manifestations.

The propensity for NSAIDs to produce ulceration appears to correlate with cyclo-oxygenase inhibition (Whittle et al, 1980), and the loss of cytoprotective effect, gastric acid inhibition and regulatory effects on blood flow. The prevention of these effects by administration of prostaglandins has been demonstrated in animals (Miller & Jacobsen, 1979) but extrapolation of this to man is tenuous.

The effects of NSAIDs on renal function probably reflect the disturbance of vasomotor control by prostaglandin inhibition (Walshe & Venuto, 1979) and loss of direct naturetic effect, and are generally reversible. The fluid-retaining effects of NSAIDs are most relevant in patients with limited cardiovascular reserve, and this is particularly important in the context of the demonstrated mutual antagonism between NSAIDs and a variety of diuretics (Brooks et al, 1974; Rawles, 1982) leading to considerably reduced diuresis.

In addition to these interactions the highly protein bound state of the majority of NSAIDs leads to potential interactions with other highly protein bound drugs including anticoagulants, oral hypoglycaemic agents and anticonvulsants.

INDOLE ACETIC ACIDS

Indomethacin

Indomethacin, 1-p-chlorobenzoyl-5-methoxy-2-methylindole-3-yl-acetic acid, is an indole acetic acid derivative (Fig. 18.1), with almost 20 years of use in the treatment of rheumatic conditions. It has become widely accepted as a reference compound against which other drugs are compared both for clinical effect, and also in the field of prostaglandin synthetase inhibition. It is well absorbed after oral administration producing peak plasma concentrations within 1–2 hours, with a very variable half-life of between 2 and 10 hours (Kwan et al, 1976). Attempts to prolong the effect of the drug have been made by the use of controlled release preparations. Rectal administration leads to earlier but lower plasma concentrations and appears to have no significant advantages over oral administration (Helleberg, 1981). Synovial fluid concentrations are initially lower than plasma levels after an oral dose. After approximately 5 hours the levels are equivalent and thereafter synovial fluid concentrations exceed plasma concentrations. The half-life of indomethacin is considerably prolonged in patients with obstructive jaundice, but is not affected by a moderate degree of renal insufficiency (Kunze et al, 1974). The rate and extent of absorption of indomethacin are reduced by concurrent administration of antacids (Emori et al, 1976).

Indomethacin is available as 25 or 50 mg capsules and in a slow release form in a 75 mg capsule. Many of the side-effects can be avoided if the drug is started in low dose, for example 25 mg three times daily, and gradually increased as required to a total of 200 mg daily. Acute gout is a exception to this where a large dose, for example 100 mg, should be given immediately and a further 200 mg over the next 24 hours, thereafter reducing the dose depending on the response. It is wise to use lower doses or avoid indomethacin completely in elderly patients. Indomethacin is particularly useful in patients with night pain and/or morning stiffness. An extra 50–75 mg at night is frequently effective in alleviating these symptoms and is a better approach than prescribing hypnotics.

Reviews of the numerous clinical trials of indomethacin in a variety of conditions including rheumatoid arthritis (Haslock, 1976), osteoarthritis, ankylosing spondylitis, gout, and acute musculoskeletal disorders (Rhymer & Gengos, 1979), confirm its superiority to placebo, and its equivalence to the other NSAIDs. Very few clinical trials are conducted in such a way (for example with respect to numbers of patients included and duration of treatment) to demonstrate any significant and consistent difference between NSAIDs. Therefore, all that can be said of any NSAID is that it is normally superior to placebo and equivalent in efficacy to aspirin and other NSAIDs.

Indomethacin is an effective antirheumatic drug, judicious clinical use being associated with an acceptable level of side-effects. About one-third of patients on conventional doses of indomethacin will experience side-effects. This represents the typical profile of NSAID side-effects probably related to prostaglandin synthetase inhibition, including dyspepsia and, less commonly, upper gastrointestinal tract ulceration and bleeding, central nervous system effects of headaches, confusion, tremor and rarely depression and psychosis, oedema, and increased bleeding time. Blood dyscrasias including agranulocytosis, thrombocytopenia and aplastic anaemias have been reported rarely, but additional drugs were usually being prescribed (Fowler, 1975).

Sulindac

Sulindac, (Z)-5-fluoro-2-methyl-1[p-(methylsulphinyl) phenyl]methylene-1H-indene-3-acetic acid, is an indene derivitive of indomethacin. It is a pro-drug with its activity residing in the sulphide metabolite which has a mean effective half-life of approximately 16 hours (Kwan et al, 1978). Sulindac is rapidly absorbed with peak serum concentrations occuring 1 hour after ingestion. Conversion to the active sulphide takes place predominantly in the liver, producing peak concentrations after 2 hours. The recommended dosage lies between 200 and 400 mg per day in a twice daily dose regime.

Clinical studies have shown sulindac to be of equivalent effect to other NSAIDs in a range of rheumatic conditions (Brogden et al, 1978; Rhymer, 1979). Sulindac appears to be well tolerated, the side-effects reported often being mild and associated predictably with conventional NSAIDs.

Tolmetin

This is a pyrrole derivative a (1-methyl-5-p-toluoyl) pyrrole-2-acetic acid, in which a pyrrole ring has been substituted for the indole nucleus of indomethacin. Tolmetin is rapidly absorbed when given orally, peak plasma and tissue concentrations being reached within 1 hour (Ayres et al, 1977). Plasma half-life has been reported variably as 1 hour (Cressman et al, 1976) and 4–6 hours (Ayres et al, 1977). It is highly protein bound (99%) but does not appear to interfere significantly with anticoagulants or antidiabetic drugs. Renal excretion of tolmetin is virtually complete within 24 hours, predominantly as the dicarboxylic acid metabolite.

Tolmetin is generally well tolerated, with an overall incidence of side-effects of 25–40%, withdrawal of treatment being required in some 5–8% of patients (Brogden et al, 1978). The incidence of gastrointestinal symptoms was similar with tolmetin and indomethacin in short-term trials (Ehrlich et al, 1975) but tolmetin was better tolerated in the long-term (Ehrlich & Roth, 1976). Adverse effects related to the central nervous system appeared to be less of a problem with tolmetin than indomethacin. In its normal dose range of 1200–1800 mg daily in divided doses, tolmetin has proved to be of equivalent effect to other non-steroidal anti-inflammatory drugs in a range of rheumatic diseases (Brogden et al, 1978).

PHENYLACETIC ACIDS

Diclofenac

Diclofenac, 2,6-dichlorophenyl-amino-phenylacetate, is an anti-inflammatory, analgesic and antipyretic agent with a potent inhibitory action on the cyclo-oxygenase pathway of prostaglandin synthesis. Maximum plasma concentrations are reached $1\frac{1}{2}$–2 hours after oral administration; elimination is also rapid, being 90% complete $1\frac{1}{2}$–$2\frac{1}{2}$ hours after the peak concentrations. With these kinetics significant steady-state concentrations are not achieved even with three times daily administration. Concentrations equivalent to those in the blood appear rapidly in the synovial fluid and persist much longer.

Pharmacokinetic studies in the elderly (Willis & Kendal, 1978) and in patients with renal failure (Stierlin et al, 1978) showed no evidence of accumulation, suggesting that no reduction of the normal dose was required. Diclofenac has proved to be an effective anti-inflammatory analgesic agent in a range of rheumatological conditions (Haslock et al, 1979) in a dose of 75–150 mg daily in two or three divided doses.

Fenclofenac

Fenclofenac, 2-(2,4-dichlorophenoxy) phenylacetic acid, is a relatively weak prostaglandin synthetase inhibitor. It is extensively bound to albumin and interferes with competitive binding assays for thyroid hormones by binding to thyroid binding globulin (Humphrey et al, 1980). Although the overall concentrations of thyroxine and triiodothyronine are reduced, the concentrations of free hormones are unchanged as is the level of thyroid stimulating hormone.

In the recommended dose range of 600–1200 mg daily in two divided doses, fenclofenac appears well tolerated, although there is a significant incidence of rashes — most commonly a maculopapular rash associated with pruritis. These were reported in up to 20% of patients and required withdrawal of the drug in 10% of patients (Goldberg & Godfrey, 1980).

PROPIONIC ACIDS

Ibuprofen

Ibuprofen, 2-(4-isobutylphenyl) propionic acid, was the first of the currently used propionic acid derivatives (Fig. 18.1) to be introduced for clinical use. It is a prostaglandin synthetase inhibitor, inhibiting the cyclo-oxygenase pathway. It is rapidly absorbed after oral administration, producing peak serum concentrations at 1–2 hours, with a half-life of 2 hours and synovial fluid concentrations above those of serum after 2–3 hours (Glass & Swannell, 1978). It is bound to albumin, but does not significantly displace warfarin or other heavily protein-bound drugs significantly.

Although initially introduced at suboptimal dose, it has proved to be well tolerated in its present recommended dosage range of 1600–2400 mg daily in three or four divided doses (Godfrey & de al Cruz, 1975; Brooks et al, 1973) and of comparable effect to other NSAIDs. Although dyspepsia is encountered with ibuprofen, there is evidence (Cardoe, 1970) that ibuprofen can be given safely to many patients who have experienced dyspepsia with other drugs or who have even had previous peptic ulceration. The main

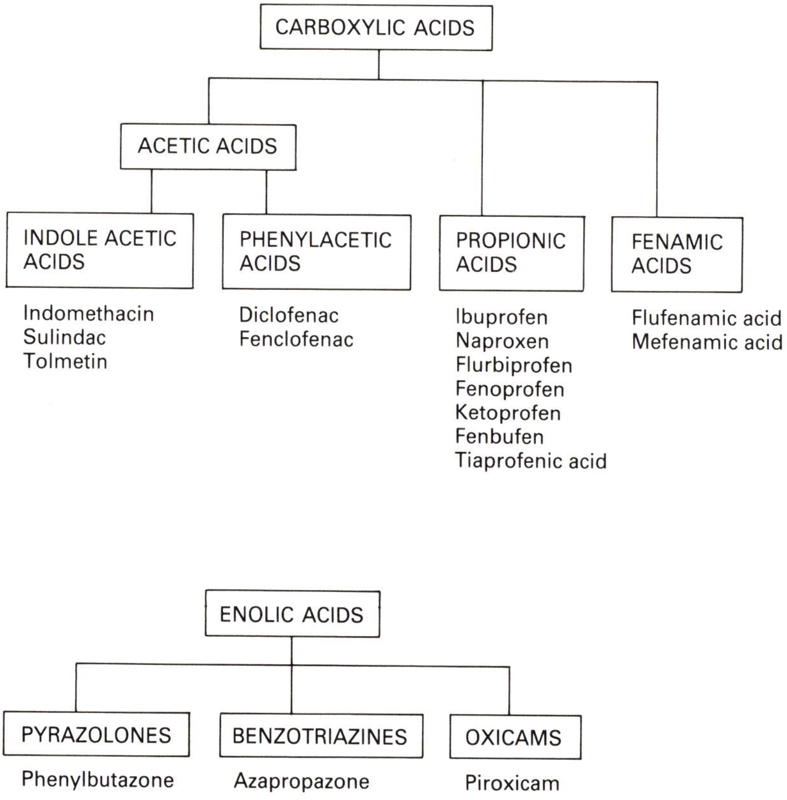

Fig. 18.1 Families of non-steroidal anti-inflammatory drugs.

advantage appears to be its low incidence of adverse reactions, rather than any particular potency of effect.

Flurbiprofen

Flurbiprofen, 2-(2-fluoro-4-biphenylyl) propionic acid, is a powerful anti-inflammatory agent with peripheral analgesic and antipyretic properties (Glenn et al, 1973). It is one of the most potent prostaglandin synthesis inhibitors (cyclo-oxygenase pathway), also exerting inhibitory effects on leucocyte migration and platelet aggregation.

Peak serum levels are obtained 1–2 hours after an oral dose, the half-life being 4 hours. It is bound to albumin but occupies less than 10% of the binding capacity and therefore is unlikely to displace other protein-bound drugs. The drug is metabolised in the liver and excreted predominantly in the urine.

Within its normal dose range of 100–300 mg daily in three or four divided doses, flurbiprofen appears to be well tolerated (Lee et al, 1976), gastrointestinal side-effects being less frequent than may be expected by its powerful prostaglandin synthetase inibition activity. The anti-inflammatory effect of this molecule resides in the parent compound and not in its metabolites, which may be of value in clinical or laboratory research.

Naproxen

Naproxen, d-2-(6-methoxy-2-naphthyl) propionic acid, is well absorbed when given orally and has a relatively long half-life of 13 hours allowing twice daily administration (Runkel et al, 1972). It takes some time for a steady-state to be reached because the drug is extensively protein bound and the steady-state depends on prior saturation of the binding sites and the equilibration of the free : bound drug ratio. Naproxen clearance is accelerated as the dose administered increases (Runkel et al, 1976). As the serum concentration rises, the capacity of protein binding sites is exceeded and the level of free drug rises sharply, the free drug being cleared much more rapidly by the kidney. Over 90% of a dose of naproxen is excreted in the urine within five days, the faecal excretion being minimal.

With a drug as extensively protein bound as naproxen the possibility of substantial effects on the free drug concentrations of other heavily bound drugs arises. Although a small increase in the free fraction of warfarin can be demonstrated, this is not accompanied by a clinically significant change in anticoagulation (Jain et al, 1979). Other drugs are unlikely to make a clinically significant impact on the pharmokinetics of naproxen with its high therapeutic index and shallow dose response curve.

The normal daily dose range of naproxen is 500–1000 mg divided into morning and evening doses. Doses of 1.5–2 g daily appear reasonably tolerated, although evidence of a dose response above 1 g daily is doubtful. The adverse reactions are relatively infrequent — 6% of patients with rheumatoid arthritis in a one year study requiring treatment to be withdrawn. Huskisson et al (1976) concluded that naproxen was as effective as any NSAID in controlling the symptoms of rheumatoid arthritis, with as low an incidence of side-effects as any other. The combination of efficacy and low level of side-effects make it one of the first choices among the NSAIDs.

Fenoprofen

Fenoprofen, DL-2-(3-phenoxyphenyl) propionic acid, is an effective anti-inflammatory, analgesic and antipyretic agent with a similar range of effects in vitro and in animal models to the other propionic acids. Following oral administration, peak plasma concentrations are obtained after 1 hour, with a plasma half-life of 1–2 hours. Absorption of the calcium salt is slightly delayed compared with the sodium salt although the bioavailability of these two forms is the same. It is metabolised predominantly to the glucuronide form which is then excreted by the kidney. Excretion is by the renal route and care should be taken in administration of fenoprofen to patients with impaired renal function.

Fenoprofen is extensively and strongly bound to plasma albumin. Of the drugs commonly interacting at this binding site only phenylbutazone will displace it (Rubin et al, 1974). Conversely fenoprofen will displace other protein-bound drugs including warfarin, hydantoins, sulphonylureas, etc. The addition of fenoprofen to a treatment regime including these drugs may require their dose being adjusted (Ridolfo et al, 1979) depending on changes in laboratory and clinical parameters. It is better clinical practice to avoid coprescription.

The dose range lies between 600 mg and 2.4 g taken in divided doses. In this dose schedule fenoprofen has proved to be of equivalent effect to other NSAIDs (Ridolfo et al, 1979) in a range of conditions including rheumatoid arthritis, osteoarthritis, ankylosing spondylitis and acute gout. The reported adverse reactions to fenoprofen are relatively infrequent and typical of the propionic acid group of drugs, dyspepsia being the most common.

Ketoprofen

Ketoprofen, 2-(3-benzoylphenyl) propionic acid, is very rapidly absorbed giving peak serum levels 45–60 minutes after rectal administration and 60–120 minutes after oral administration. With regular doses a plateau concentration is reached after 48 hours, with no evidence of accumulation in the body (Lewellen & Templeton, 1976). Following glucuronidation in the liver ketoprofen is excreted mainly in the urine, 50% of the dose being excreted in the first 6 hours. Synovial fluid concentrations of ketoprofen in patients with rheumatoid arthritis rise some time after blood levels and then remain elevated for longer, suggesting there is slow diffusion and retention of the ketoprofen in peripheral tissues (Mitchell et al, 1975).

The usual dose range is 100–300 mg daily in divided doses and it can also be given as suppositories in a dose of 100 mg. Clinical studies have shown anti-inflammatory analgesic effects comparable with aspirin and other NSAIDs (Tamisier, 1979) in a range of conditions, with significant side-effects outside the upper gastrointestinal tract being rare.

Fenbufen

Fenbufen, oxo(1,1′-biphenyl)-4-butanoic acid, is a biphenylpropionic acid, which acts as a prodrug. The anti-inflammatory, analgesic, prostaglandin synthetase inhibitor actions are properties of its p-biphenyl acetic acid derivative, one of the two main metabolites, which is chemically similar to diclofenac. The drug is rapidly absorbed, peak serum concentrations of total drug-related compounds being reached after 2 hours at which time only a small proportion is present as fenbufen. However the levels of the active metabolite, p-biphenyl acetic acid, peak after 8 hours and significant concentrations persist for a relatively long period (Mawdsley, 1980). Although fenbufen is highly protein bound there do not appear to be clinically significant interactions with other drugs such as warfarin.

The recommended dose is 600 mg daily in a single dose increasing to 900 mg in divided doses. In the light of experience with other drugs of this class this may be modified upwards in the future. Fenbufen appears to have effects similar to the other members of the propionic acid group both in therapeutic effects and adverse reactions. The drug was found to be well tolerated in patients with a previous history of gastric intolerance to other NSAIDs (Paice et al, 1982). Its use has also been studied in patients with impaired renal function in whom there appeared to be no significant evidence of accumulation despite renal excretion (Armstrong et al, 1982). There is a low overall incidence of side-effects, particularly gastrointestinal; however, rashes seem to occur more frequently with fenbufen than with other members of the propionic acids.

Tiaprofenic acid

Tiaprofenic acid, (benzoyl-2-thienyl) propionic acid, is the first of a new series of propionic acid derivitives containing a thiophene ring. It has typical anti-inflammatory analgesic antipyretic properties associated with the propionic acids and is a potent inhibitor of the cyclo-oxygenase pathway. The profile of prostaglandin inhibition by tiaprofenic acid is of interest. It displays some of the properties of tissue selectivity suggested by Whittle et al (1980) as a method of reducing gastrointestinal problems. Tiaprofenic acid is ten times as active as indomethacin in inhibiting the in vivo production of PGE_2 and PGF_2, but only half as active in inhibiting the formation of the mucosally protective PGI_2 (Deraedt et al, 1980). It is at present unclear whether this will convey any clinical advantages. Although tiaprofenic acid is well tolerated so are the other members of the propionic acid group.

Tiaprofenic acid is well absorbed, peak serum concentrations occurrring 90 minutes after oral administration. About 60% of an oral dose is eliminated in the urine in the form of tiaprofenic acid and its two main metabolites, mainly as acylglucuronide conjugates, the remainder being eliminated in the bile (Pottier et al, 1977). Although tiaprofenic acid is highly protein bound there does not appear to be clinically significant displacement of other drugs.

In a dose of 600 mg daily in divided doses, tiaprofenic acid appears to have effects comparable with other NSAIDs with the typically low incidence of side-effects associated with the propionic acid derivitives.

FENAMATES

Mefenamic acid and flufenamic acid

Mefenamic acid, N-2,3-xylylanthranilic acid, and flufenamic acid, N-(trifluoro-m-tolyl) anthranilic acid, are both active in animal models of inflammatory disease. Mefenamic acid is rapidly absorbed following ingestion; flufenamic acid produces more delayed peak blood levels 6 hours after administration. The half-life of flufenamic acid is also longer but both drugs are similarly metabolised by oxidation, with some 50% of the metabolites being excreted in the urine. There is also considerable biliary excretion and enterohepatic circulation.

Recommended doses are for mefenamic acid 1.5–2 g/day in three or four divided doses, for flufenamic acid 400–600 mg/day in divided doses. Both drugs are effective (Lee et al, 1976) but carry a higher incidence of side-effects than the propionic acids. These include dyspepsia, diarrhoea, skin rashes, leucopenia, thrombocytopenia, potentiation of anticoagulants and other protein-bound drugs, and a Coombs-positive haemolytic anaemia (Holmes, 1967).

THE PYRAZOLONES

Phenylbutazone

Phenylbutazone, 1,2 diphenyl 3,5 dioxo-4-N-butylpyrazolidine, possesses anti-inflammatory analgesic properties of the same order as aspirin and indomethacin (Fowler, 1975). Absorption is slow, peak levels occur after 72 hours, days being required for a steady-state to be reached on regular administration. Elimination of the drug is also slow, the drug being detectable in the urine up to two weeks after withdrawal. It circulates tightly bound to plasma proteins, predominantly albumin, and will displace other protein bound drugs.

Phenylbutazone is capable of inducing a wide range of side-effects of which gastrointestinal intolerance is the most common. The most alarming adverse reactions are its effects on the bone marrow. Aplastic anaemia tends to occur in the elderly, usually after a prolonged period of treatment. However, agranulocytosis may be seen in young people soon after treatment commences (Fowler, 1975).

Skin rashes of a very wide variety of type and severity up to and including Stevens–Johnson syndrome may be produced. The potent fluid-retaining properties of the drug may precipitate cardiac failure in those with limited cardiac reserve. Jaundice of both hepatocellular and obstructive type may be induced, together with the production of goitre, lymphadenopathy, hepatosplenomegaly and salivary gland swelling.

The frequency and potential severity of side-effects associated with the use of phenylbutazone have led to the imposition of restrictions on its use. In the UK phenylbutazone is now available only for the treatment of patients with ankylosing spondylitis by consultant physicians and oxyphenbutazone has been completely withdrawn.

BENZOTRIAZINES

Azapropazone

Azapropazone, 3-dimethylamino-7-methyl-1,2-(n-propyl-malonyl) 1,2-dihydro-1,2,4-benzotriazine, is a condensation product of a pyrazolidine ring with a benzotriazine ring (see Fig. 18.1). It has analgesic, anti-inflammatory and antipyretic actions in animal models of inflammatory arthritis. It inhibits prostaglandin synthesis and is uricosuric, its uricosuric action being blocked by pyrazinamide, suggesting increased tubular secretion as the mechanism (Sondervorst, 1979).

Azapropazone is well absorbed from the small intestine; plasma half-life is 12 hours but biological half-life is prolonged to 20 hours. The vast majority of azapropazone is excreted in the urine, predominantly unchanged with the rest as a hydroxylated metabolite. In view of this, care must be taken in patients with impaired renal function as so much of the active material depends on intact renal function for its excretion. Azapropazone significantly displaces warfarin from protein binding. Warfarin dose reductions of up to 50% may be required, so it would be wise not to coprescribe.

Azapropazone has proved to be an effective analgesic anti-inflammatory compound in a range of different clinical situations (Brooks & Buchanan, 1976; Grennan et al, 1976). Its successful use in both acute gout and as a long-term preventative treatment, by virtue of its uricosuric effect, have been reported recently (Dieppe et al, 1981; Higgens & Scott, 1984).

Adverse reactions reported to date have been predominantly gastrointestinal, skin rashes, central nervous system effects including headache confusion and depression, and fluid retention. The possibility of serious haematological side-effects suggested by the structural similarity to phenylbutazone has in practice proved not to be the case.

OXICAMS

Piroxicam

Piroxicam, 4-hydroxy-2-methyl-N-(2-pyridyl)-2H-1,2-benzothiazine1,1-dioxide, is the first and presently the only available member the oxicam group of NSAIDs (Fig. 18.1). It behaves as a conventional analgesic, anti-inflammatory agent in animal models, showing potent inhibition of the cyclooxygenase pathway of prostaglandin synthesis. In contrast to indomethacin the kinetic interaction with the enzyme is reversible (Carty et al, 1980).

The drug is well absorbed following oral administration, the absorption being almost complete after 2 hours. However peak plasma concentrations occur at 4 hours after administration. Its half-life is prolonged at 38 hours allowing the use of a single daily dose. It has been suggested that this improvement in convenience for the patient leads to an improvement in compliance (Blackwell, 1979). However compliance is excellent in symptomatic treatment for any chronic painful disease provided that the drug selected by the patient relieves pain and is not producing adverse reactions (Rooney et al, 1978).

In a recommended dose of 20–30 mg daily, piroxicam is as effective as conventional NSAIDs (Wiseman & Boyle, 1980), but also retains the side-effects of conventional NSAIDs. However it is a well tolerated drug, being better tolerated than aspirin, indomethacin and phenylbutazone (Pitts, 1980).

COLCHICINE

The use of colchicine, as an extract of the autumn crocus, in the treatment of acute gout has a history dating back to the 6th century AD and possibly before. The side-effects, particularly the purgative effects, led to it falling into disuse until its reintroduction in the late 18th century. It is now more of historical interest and of use as a laboratory reagent rather than in clinical practice.

Colchicine appears to have a multiplicity of actions on cells although many only occur at concentrations higher than those seen therapeutically. Colchicine appears to act in acute gout by suppressing the synthesis and secretion of a chemotactic factor produced in urate crystal-induced inflammation (Spilberg et al, 1979). This chemotactic factor does not appear to be a major mediator in other types of inflammation. Many of the effects of colchicine, including arrest in metaphase, may be related to its action in binding to tubulin (Borisy & Taylor, 1967), the microtubular subunit protein, interfering with its aggregation into microtubules.

Indications for colchicine include acute gout and short-term prophylaxis. Its use in calcium pyrophosphate arthropathy has also been suggested (Spilberg & Berney, 1979). Colchicine is contraindicated in patients with renal, liver, cardiac or gastrointestinal diseases. The recommended dose is 1 mg initially, followed by 0.5 mg every two or three hours until relief is obtained or until side-effects occur. A single course should not exceed 10 mg in total dose; gastrointestinal side-effects are frequent after a total dose of 6 mg. When used as a prophylactic agent the dose is 0.5 mg two or three times daily.

The most common side-effects are nausea, vomiting, abdominal pain, diarrhoea and gastrointestinal haemorrhage. Less frequently rashes or renal damage may occur; neuropathies and blood dyscrasias are occasional side-effects of long-term use.

REFERENCES

Armstrong R, Bradbrook I, Gibson T J, Morrison P, Rogers H J, Spector R G 1982 A study of repeated administration of fenbufen in patients with chronic rheumatic disorders and renal impairment. European Journal of Rheumatology and Inflammation 5: 294–300

Ayres J W, Weidler D J, MacKichan J, Sakmar E, Hallmark M R, Lemanowicz E F, Wagner J G 1977 Pharmacokinetics of tolmetin with and without concomitant administration of antacid in man. European Journal of Clinical Pharmacology 12: 21–28

Blackwell B 1979 Drug regimen and compliance. In: Haynes R B, Taylor D W, Sackett D C (eds) Compliance in health care. John Hopkins University Press, Baltimore

Borgeat P, Hamberg M, Samuelsson B 1976 Transformation of arachidonic acid and dihomo-gamma-linolenic acid by polymorphonuclear leucocytes. Journal of Biological Chemistry 251: 7816nnx7820

Borisy G G, Taylor E W 1967 The mechanism of action of colchicine. Binding of colchicine-3H to cellular protein. Journal of Cell Biology 34: 525–533

Brogden R N, Heel R C, Speight T M, Avery G S 1978a Sulindac: a review of its pharmacological properties and therapeutic efficacy in rheumatic diseases. Drugs 16: 97–114

Brogden R N, Heel R C, Speight T M, Avery G S 1978b Tolmetin: a review of pharmacological properties and therapeutic efficacy in rheumatic diseases. Drugs 15: 429–450

Brooks P M, Buchanan W W 1976 Azapropazone; its place in the management of rheumatic conditions. Current Medical Research and Opinion 4: 94–100

Brooks C D, Schagel C A, Sekhar N C, Sobota J T 1973 Tolerance and pharmacology of ibuprofen. Current Therapeutic Research 15: 180–190

Brooks P M, Bell M A, Lee P, Rooney P J, Dick W C 1974 The effect of frusemide on indomethacin plasma levels. British Journal of Clinical Pharmacology 1: 485–487

Buckingham R B 1977 Interactions involving antirheumatic drugs (part 1). Bulletins on the Rheumatic Diseases 28: 960–965

Cardoe N 1970 A review of the long term experience with ibuprofen with special reference to gastric intolerance. Rheumatology and Physical Medicine (Suppl 10): 28–31

Carty T J, Eskra J D, Lombardino J G, Hoffman W W 1980 Piroxicam: a potent inhibitor of prostaglandin production in cell culture. Structure activity study. Prostaglandins 19: 51–9

Caruso I, Bianchi Porro G 1980 Gastroscopic evaluation of anti-inflammatory agents. British Medical Journal 1: 75–7

Ceuppens J L, Rodriguez M A, Goodwin J S 1982 Non-steroidal anti-inflammatory agents inhibit the synthesis of IgM rheumatoid factor in vitro. Lancet 1: 528–530

Deraedt R, Jouquey S, Delevallee F, Flauhaut M 1980 release of prostaglandins E and F in an algogenic reaction and its inhibition. European Journal of Pharmacology 61: 17–24

Dieppe P A, Doherty M, Whicher J T, Walters G 1981 The treatment of gout with azapropazone: clinical and experimental studies. European Journal Of Rheumatology and Inflammation 4: 392–400

Eakins K E, Higgs G A, Moncada S, Mugridge K G, Vane J R 1980 The effects of indomethacin and BW755C on leukocyte migration and prostaglandin production in carregeenin-induced inflammation. British Journal of Pharmacology 69: 270–271

Ehrlich G E 1979 Tolmetin sodium: meeting the clinical challenge. Clinics in the Rheumatic Diseases 5: 481–497

Emori H W, Paulus H C, Bluestone R, Champion G D, Pearson C 1976 Indomethacin serum concentrations in man: effect of dosage, food, and antacids. Annals of Rheumatic Diseases 35: 333–337

Famaey J P, Brooks P M, Carson D W 1975 Biological effects of nonsteroidal anti-inflammatory drugs. Seminars in Arthritis and Rheumatism 5: 63–81

Ferreira S H, Moncada S, Vane J R 1971 Indomethacin and aspirin abolish prostaglandin release from the spleen. Nature 231: 237–239

Fowler P D 1975 Indomethacin and phenylbutazone. Clinics in the rheumatic diseases 1(2)

Girdwood R H 1974 Death after taking medicaments. British Medical Journal 1: 501–504

Glass R C, Swannel A J 1978 Concentrations of ibuprofen in serum and synovial fluid from patients with arthritis. British Journal of Clinical Pharmacology 6: 453–454

Glenn E M, Rohloff N, Bowman B J, Lyster S C 1973 The pharmacology of 2-(2-fluoro-4-biphenylyl) propionic acid (flurbiprofen). A potent non-steroidal anti-inflammatory drug. Agents and Actions 3: 210–216

Godfrey R, de la Cruz S 1975 Effect of ibuprofen dosage on patient response in rheumatoid arthritis. Arthritis and Rheumatism 18: 135–137

Goldberg A A J, Godfrey K E 1980 Fenclofenac. Clinics in the rheumatic diseases 6

Grennan D M, McLeod M, Watkins C, Dick W C 1976 Clinical assessment of azapropazone in rheumatoid arthritis. Current Medical Research and Opinion 4: 44–49

Hamberg M, Samuelsson B 1974 Prostaglandin endoperoxides. Novel transformation of arachidonic acid in platelets. Proceedings of the National Academy of Sciences of the USA 71: 3400–3404

Haslock I 1976 Indomethacin in rheumatoid arthritis: a review. In: Huskisson E C, Velo G P (eds) Inflammatory arthropathies. Excerpta Medica, Amsterdam, p 197–205

Haslock I, Eade A, Woolf D 1979 Diclofenac (Voltarol) in the treatment of rheumatic diseases: a conspectus of international experience. Rheumatology and Rehabilitation (Suppl 2)

Helleberg L 1981 Clinical pharmacokinetics of indomethacin. Clinical Pharmacokinetics 6: 245–258

Higgens C S, Scott J T 1984 The uricosuric action of azapropazone: dose-response and comparison with probenecid. British Journal of Clinical Pharmacology 18: 439–443
Holmes 1967 Fenamates in medicine. Annals of Physical Medicine (supplement) 36–42
Humphrey M J, Capper S J, Kurtz A B 1980 Fenclofenac and thyroid hormone concentrations. Lancet 1: 487–488
Huskisson E C 1977 Anti-inflammatory drugs. Seminars in Arthritis and Rheumatism 7: 1–20
Huskisson E C, Woolf D L, Balme H W M, Scott J, Franklyn S 1976 Four new anti-inflammatory drugs: responses and variations. British Medical Journal 1: 1048–9
Jain A, McMahon F G, Slattery J T, Levy G 1979 Effect of naproxen on steady state serum concentration and anticoagulant activity of warfarin. Clinical Pharmacology and Therapeutics 25: 61–66
Kuehl F A, Humes J L, Egan R W, Ham E A, Beveridge G C, Van Arman C G 1977 The role of prostaglandin endoperoxide PGG_2 in inflammatory processes. Nature 265: 170–172
Kunze M, Stein G, Kunze E, Traeger A 1974 The pharmacokinetics of indomethacin in relation to age, in patients with occlusion of the bile ducts, with reduced renal function and with signs of intolerance. Deutsche Gesundkeitswesen 29: 351–3
Kwan K C, Breault G O, Umbenhauer E R, McMahon F G, Duggan D E 1976 Kinetics of indomethacin absorption, elimination, and enterohepatic circulation in man. Journal of Pharmokinetics and Biopharmaceutics 4: 255–280
Kwan K C, Duggan D E, Van Arman E G, Shen T Y 1978 Sulindac: chemistry, pharmacology and pharmacokinetics. European Journal of Rheumatology and Inflammation 1: 9–11
Lee P, Anderson J A, Miller J, Webb J, Watson Buchanan W 1976 Evaluations of analgesic actions and efficacy of anti-rheumatic drugs. Journal of Rheumatology 3: 283–294
Lewellen O R V, Templeton R 1976 The pharmacokinetics of ketoprofen in man during and after repeated oral dosing (50 mg q.i.d.) with 'Orudis'. Scandinavian Journal of Rheumatology (Supplement) 14: 53–62
Mawdsley P 1980 Fenbufen. In: Huskisson E C (ed) Clinics in the rheumatic diseases 6(3) Anti-rheumatic drugs. Saunders, London, p 615–32
Metz S A 1981 Anti-inflammatory agents as inhibitors of prostaglandin synthesis in man. Medical Clinics of North America 65: 713–757
Miller T A, Jacobsen E D 1979 Gastro-intestinal cytoprotection by prostaglandins. Gut 20: 75–87
Mitchell W S, Scott P, Kennedy A C, Brooks P, Templeton R, Jeffries M 1975 Clinico-pharmacological studies on ketoprofen (Orudis). Current Medical Research and Opinion 3: 423–30
Paice E W, Tookman A J, White A G 1982 Fenbufen in patients with gastric intolerance. European Journal of Rheumatology and Inflammation 5: 301–3
Payne T G, Dewald B, Siegl H, Gubler H U, Ott H, Baggiolini M 1982 Radical scavenging and stimulation of prostaglandin synthesis not inflammatory? Nature 296: 160–2
Pitts N E 1980 Review of clinical experience with piroxicam. In: Piroxicam, a new non-steroidal anti-inflammatory agent. Proceedings of the Ninth European Congress of Rheumatology. Academy Professional Information Services, New York, p 48–66
Pottier J, Berlin D, Raynaud J P 1977 Pharmacokinetics of the anti-inflammatory tiaprofenic acid in humans, mice, rats, rabbits and dogs. Journal of Pharmaceutical Science 66: 1030–1036
Rawles J M 1982 Antagonism between non-steroidal anti-inflammatory drugs and diuretics. Scottish Medical Journal 27: 37–40
Rhymer A R 1979 Sulindac. Clinics in the Rheumatic Diseases 5: 553–568
Ridolfo A S, Nikander R, Mikulaschek W M 1979 Fenoprofen and Benoxaprofen. Clinics in the Rheumatic Diseases 5: 393–410
Rooney P J, Capell H, Paterson S, Buchanan W W, Dick W C 1978 Continued use of non-steroidal anti-inflammatory drugs — an index of clinical efficacy. British Journal of Clinical Pharmacology 5: 377–382
Rubin A, Chernish S M, Crabtree R, Gruber C M Jr, Helleberg L, Rodda B E, et al 1974 A profile of the physiological disposition and gastro intestinal effects of fenoprofen in man. Current Medical Research and Opinion 2: 529–544
Runkel R A, Chaplin M, Boost G 1972 Absorption distribution metabolism and excretion of naproxen in various laboratory animals and human subjects. Journal of Pharmaceutical Sciences 61: 703–8
Runkel R A, Chaplin M D, Sevelius H, Ortega E, Segre E 1976 Pharmacokinetics of naproxen overdoses. Clinical Pharmacology and Therapeutics 20: 269–277
Smolen J E, Weissmann G 1980 Effects of indomethacin, 5,8,11,14-eicosatetraynoic acid, and p-bromophenacyl bromide on lysosomal enzyme release and superoxide generation by human polymorphonuclear leucocytes. Biochemical Pharmacology 29: 533–538
Sondervorst M 1979 Azapropazone. Clinics in the Rheumatic Diseases 5: 465–480
Spilberg I, Mandell B, Simchowitz L, Rosenberg D 1979 The mechanism of action of colchicine in acute urate crystal-induced arthritis. Journal of Clinical Investigation 64: 775–380
Stierlin H, Faigle J W, Columbi A 1978 Pharmacokinetics of diclofenac sodium (Voltaren) and metabolites in patients with impaired renal function. Scandinavian Journal of Rheumatology (Suppl) 22: 30–35
Tamisier J N 1979 Ketoprofen. Clinics in the Rheumatic Diseases 5: 381–391
Vane J R 1971 Inhibition of prostaglandin synthesis as a mechanism of action of the aspirin like drugs. Nature 231: 232–5
Webb D R, Rogers T J, Nowowiejski I 1979 Endogenous prostaglandin synthesis and control of lymphocyte functions. Annals of the New York Academy of Science 332: 262–270
Whittle B J R, Higgs G A, Eakins K E, Moncada S, Vane J R 1980 Selective inhibition of prostaglandin production in inflammatory exudates and gastric mucosa. Nature 284: 271–273
Willis J V, Kendal M J 1978 Pharmacokinetic studies diclofenac sodium in young and old volunteers. Scandinavian Journal of Rheumatology (supplement) 22: 36–41
Wiseman E H, Boyle J A 1980 Piroxicam (Feldene). Clinics in the Rheumatic Diseases 6: 585–613

Penicillamine, gold and antimalarials

PENICILLAMINE

Abraham and his colleagues discovered penicillamine in 1942 when they found that acid hydrolysates of penicillin gave a strong blue-violet colouration with the ninhydrin reagent. It was also found that 59% of total nitrogen of the pure penicillin preparation could be estimated as amino-nitrogen after one hour's hydrolysis with n/10 sulphuric acid using the van Slyke method. This observation indicated that the substance responsible for the results of these reactions was an integral part of the penicillin molecule and they were able to report its isolation as a crystaline hydrochloride. To this amino acid degradation product of penicillin they gave the name 'penicillamine'. The chemical structure was determined later by Sir Ernest Chain in 1949. Subsequent animal experiments showed that the L-enantiomorph is the most toxic and therefore only D-penicillamine is now used therapeutically in man either as the hydrochloride or free amino acid.

ANIMAL TOXICITY

Acute toxicity

Experiments carried out at Dista laboratories under the auspices of Hugh Lyle confirm that D-penicillamine is not lethal to most rats although some died following a dose of 10 000 mg/kg body weight. The drug appears to exhibit anti-piridoxine activity in rats which can be corrected with vitamin B6. It also appears to have lathyrogenic properties in the same animal.

CLINICAL APPLICATION IN MAN

Walshe (1953) identified penicillamine in the urine of patients with advanced liver disease receiving parenteral penicillin therapy. Since the compound is excreted in the reduced -SH state, he deduced that the thiol group might prove active in chelation of copper. Further investigations confirmed that penicillamine prompted the urinary excretion of copper both in healthy people and patients with Wilson's disease. Penicillamine forms chelates with other divalent cations such as lead.

Disulphide exchange with cysteine

Tabachnick et al (1954) showed that penicillamine reacted readily with cysteine with formation of a mixed disulphide. It was not until ten years later that this observation was used in the treatment of patients with cystinuria. The excessive urinary excretion of cystine was shown to be reduced or abolished according to the dose of penicillamine administered. Penicillamine is capable of producing dissolution of cystine calculi in patients with cystinuria when added to other conventional techniques of treatment.

Pharmacological properties

All administered D-penicillamine is largely absorbed from the gastrointestinal tract but about half the effective dose is rapidly excreted in the urine mostly as a mixed D-penicillamine cysteine disulphide leading to cysteine depletion. Only a relatively small proportion of D-penicillamine taken up by the body is turned into s-methyl-D-penicillamine. It is partly excreted and partly catabolised by way of D-amino-acid oxydase in the liver. Roughly 20% of the administered dose is stored in the tissue, from which the serum pool is slowly refilled. This results in a steady rise in serum penicillamine level during continuous treatment and leads to an increase in storage of penicillamine in the tissues.

These observations are based on the comments of Perret and co-workers (1981) who themselves swallowed [^{14}C] D-penicillamine following which they recovered 35% of the radioactivity in the faeces, indicating incomplete resorption from the intestines or metabolic breakdown in the liver followed by biliary excretion. They recovered almost 50% of the administered dose from the urine. Van der Korst et al (1982) carried out similar studies. One of their group took a single intravenous dose of 50 mg of D-penicillamine and results were compared to the effect of an oral dose of 100 mg. In both instances a serum peak level of about 8 mg/ml was reached. However after intravenous administration, 75% of the dose administered was recovered from the urine, but from the oral dose only 28% was recovered. In summary, it appears that from an oral dose administered, two-thirds is resorbed from the gut; one-third or more is circulating as free D-penicillamine in the body, partly excreted as disulphide with itself or with cysteine and as a copper complex. Part of the free D-penicillamine becomes tissue-bound, from which the serum pool is constantly refilled presenting as the slow pool. The remainder, about 20%, is converted to s-methyl-D-penicillamine which is partly oxidised in the liver followed by a further breakdown whilst another part of the s-methyl-D-penicillamine is excreted in the urine.

Effects in rheumatoid disease

Jaffe (1962) demonstrated the dissociation of rheumatoid factor in synovial fluid when penicillamine was injected into the knee joint of a patient with rheumatoid arthritis. In 1963 he proved that oral administration in such a patient produced a consistent reduction of circulating rheumatoid factor accompanied by clinical improvement, but only after a latent period of a month or so on the treatment. He also reported beneficial response in a case of rheumatoid arthritis and a return to normal values of laboratory measurement of disease activity. Jaffe observed a drug-induced fall in IgG and IgM. Other workers have subsequently confirmed the drug's ability to lower all major immunoglobulin classes to normal. This does not necessarily correlate with clinical improvement. Jaffe also showed that penicillamine was capable of causing the level of immune complexes to decline on treatment.

Effects on lymphocyte function

If human lymphocytes stimulated with phytohaemagglutinin are studied there is a dose-related inhibition of lymphocyte transformation in the presence of D-L penicillamine. Schumaker et al (1975) showed that pre-exposure of mouse spleen T cells to D-penicillamine in vitro resulted in striking inhibition of cellular immune responses measured by the sheep erythrocyte rosette technique. This PHA-induced lymphocyte transformation inhibition has subsequently been confirmed by Maini & Roff (1977) but only after using high D-penicillamine concentrations. This led them to speculation that the therapeutic action of the drug might be through modulation of T cell function in vivo. Kendall and Hutchins (1978), experimenting on mouse spleen cells stimulated in culture by concanavalin A, observed that the true effect of penicillamine was enhancement of the lymphocyte transformation. This was observed when it was in the medium long enough to deplete cysteine supply, the rate of the depletion being dependent on penicillamine concentration. These apparently conflicting views are compatable in a truly biological system where enhancement and suppression represent evidence of effectiveness.

CLINICAL APPLICATIONS

Progressive systemic sclerosis (PSS)

Penicillamine seems to be of use for patients with morphoea, particularly in children (Moynahan, 1973). However its use in PSS is somewhat more controversial. Jayson et al (1977) concluded that it was of limited value for cutaneous features of PSS and of no value for the vascular or visceral manifestations of the disease.

Liver disease

There have been three trials in the use of penicillamine in primary biliary cirrhosis. The most significant finding appears to be a reduction in serum aspartate transaminase after three months, which is maintained at least to nine months. Liver copper concentrations fell in the pencillamine-treated patients (Jain et al, 1977). In chronic active hepatitis D-penicillamine appears to be a useful alternative therapy to corticosteroids in some patients (Stern et al, 1977)

Rheumatoid arthritis

Dosage

First studies in rheumatoid arthritis were originally carried out at somewhere around 1500 mg of penicillamine a day. The Multicentre Trial Group (1973) first confirmed efficacy in a placebo-controlled double blind study. Dixon et al (1975) reported that 600 mg/a day was a effective as 1200 mg/a day with a significant reduction in withdrawals for adverse effects. Response has been observed in some patients with as low a dose as 125 mg although the response is slow. The probability is that the right dose to start with is 250 mg daily. If there are beginnings of improvement around 6 weeks to 2 months, then this may be sufficient. Some patients however will need 500 or even 750 mg daily. However, the tendency these days is to increase the dose very slowly, possibly allowing a further 2–3 months again before the final increment to 750 mg. Only rarely will patients require 1 g/day.

Evidence for disease-modifying effect

There are now many papers showing that D-penicillamine is capable of improving all clinical measurements, including remission in some patients, certainly inducing disease modification in most other patients and causing some reversion towards normal of immunological changes (Jaffe, 1965); comparable trials against azathioprine (Berry et al, 1976), gold (Huskisson et al, 1974). pyrithioxine (Camus et al, 1981), fenclofenac (Berry et al, 1981) and levamisol (Mowat et al, 1981) have all confirmed the ability of penicillamine to induce remission of rheumatoid arthritis.

Unwanted effects

Unfortunately penicillamine does lead to a large number of unwanted drug effects.

1. Haematological — neutropenia, thrombocytopenia, pancytopenia and anaemia have all been described (Multicentre Trial Group, 1973).

2. Renal — proteinuria, early and frequently transient, or later a nephrotic syndrome, frequently occur (10% of patients) (Dische et al, 1976). The pathology shows immune complex glomerulonephritis very similar to the early changes of idiopathic membranous glomerular nephritis. IgG and C3 are found along the glomerular capillary loops. A rare renal complication is frank haematuria with renal failure developing with associated Goodpasture's syndrome (Gibson et al, 1976).

3. Skin complications — classically an early rash occurs which may well disappear even if the treatment is continued. Certainly on stopping treatment the rash will disappear and on reintroducing treatment the rash will not necessarily reappear.

A later and more troublesome complication is that of pemphigus or pemphigoid-like rashes. These consist of bullous lesions on the mucous membranes and surroundings that necessitate treatment with corticosteroids.

4. Alimentary tract — taste loss is described in early treatment with 10–15% of patients afflicted. This may last for up to two years, but all cases so far have been reversible (Jaffe, 1965). Nausea is another problem sometimes encountered which may lead to 5–10% of patients being withdrawn from treatment. A thorough search has failed to confirm peptic ulceration as being a problem with penicillamine therapy. In patients in whom this does occur it is much more likely to be due to a non-steroidal anti-inflammatory drug which the patient is taking in addition to the penicillamine. Diarrhoea and constipation appear to be described in equal numbers in most trials. In all probability the drug is not the cause of either.

5. Muscular side-effects — there have been case reports of polymyositis which appear to be drug-related (Fernandes et al, 1977).

6. Lung complications — an obliterative bronchiolitis and pulmonary fibrosis have been described as conceivably drug-induced. It is hard to be sure that these are necessarily drug-induced, as both these complications can occur as a complication of disease rather than of the drug (Turner Warwick, 1981).

7. Immunological disease — myasthenia gravis with antimotor end-plate antibodies appears to now be reasonably well substantiated as being caused by penicillamine (Bucknall et al, 1974). Lupus-like reactions with anti-nuclear antibodies are also well described (Camus et al, 1977; Walshe, 1981; Chalmers et al, 1982). If the drug is stopped soon after the onset of symptoms these will abate. On the other hand there are case reports of patients in whom the drug has been continued and in whom the disease has become fixed.

Effects in pregnancy
The only death described in an infant whose mother was taking penicillamine was not related to the drug, the child dying of small bowel atresia. However, the skin did exhibit features of the Ehlers–Danlos syndrome. Subsequently, in a series described by Lýle (1978), 27 patients taking D-penicillamine at some stage of pregnancy delivered children all of whom were normal except for one with a ventricular septal defect. It is probably wise to withhold administration of the drug during pregnancy, but it is not an indication for termination.

Continuation of therapy
Penicillamine, like all disease remitting agents, will take 3–6 months before it will have its maximum effect. At the end of that period the dosage should be reduced to the lowest level at which the patient still obtains a clinical remission. There is a certain amount of evidence suggesting that the lower doses will produce fewer side-effects although this is by no means universally agreed. It may well be necessary to continue the medication along with non-steroidal anti-inflammatory drugs. There are now many patients who have been treated successfully with penicillamine for at least 10 years.

There seems no reason for stopping the drug if it is holding the patient in clinical remission. It is however important to emphasise that continuing vigilence should be exercised by carrying out monthly full blood and platelet counts, also checking the urine and skin, because side-effects can occur at any point during the therapeutic use of the drug; patients have been known to develop proteinuria or neutropenia as late as 8 years after the commencement of treatment.

CHLOROQUINE

Chloroquine, a synthetic antimalarial drug, was introduced in 1943 at the same time as hydroxychloroquine. Early reports suggested benefit in systemic lupus and discoid lupus erythematosus. The first reports of success in rheumatoid synovitis were published in 1951. Very early on, the dose that was being considered was twenty times greater than that used for the treatment of malaria. It seemed to be toxic to the retina.

Pharmacological properties

There is little modern available information in terms of absorption, distribution, metabolism or excretion of this drug and there have been very few dose response studies. In part, this relates to the long history associated with this compound and the fact that it became available long before the Committee of Safety of Medicine was established. What is known is that it is absorbed from the upper intestinal tract rapidly and almost completely. It is then selectively localised in the liver, spleen and heart. It has an affinity for melanin and high concentrations are found in the iris, choroid and skin. Urinary excretion is slow and discontinuous. When the drug is withdrawn urinary output falls by 50% per week over a 4 week period, following which the excretion rate becomes stable at around 7.5 mg/24 h remaining at this level for months. It continues to be excreted for many months or even years after discontinuation of therapy. Metabolic breakdown in man proceeds by the formation of a secondary amine, the primary amine, the four aldehyde and the four carboxy derivative. Excretion is as follows: 60% drug unchanged, 37% secondary amine and 3% primary amine.

Clinical experience

In 1953 Haydu described 28 patients with active rheumatoid arthritis studied at dosages of 900 mg weekly for 6 months. Further open studies by Bagnell (1957) on 108 patients treated for more than 8 months showed 70% having a complete remission after one year of therapy with parallel improvement in haemoglobin levels and fall in sedimentation rate. Part of this study was double blind, 12 out of 19 cases showing improvement though with none out of 12 in the control group. Young (1959) showed that a variable dose gave better results, top dose utilised being up to 1800 mg weekly. Freedman & Steinberg (1960) carried out a double blind study, 53 patients being given chloroquine and 54 placebo. The patients also continued with aspirin and physiotherapy. One year's treatment was completed in 40 control patients and 42 in the chloroquine group. 80% of the 42 patients on chloroquine improved compared to 30% of the controls — 300 mg/day was the dose used in the study. By 1965 Lansbury had stated that chloroquine is probably less harmful in its side-effects than corticosteroids, phenylbutazone or gold salts in the treatment of rheumatoid arthritis. He used chloroquine for 10 years in a dosage of 125–250 mg daily and considered it safe. Chloroquine has been extensively used in discoid lupus and has even been tried in such unrelated conditions as basal cell epithelioma or squamous cell carcinoma of the skin, resistant asthma, rosacea, scleroderma, polyarteritis nodosa, granuloma annulare, dermatitis herpetiformis and chronic acrodermatitis atrophicans.

Therapeutic usage

It is not clear whether it is wiser to use a dosage of 300 mg of chloroquine or 400 mg of hydrochloroquine as a starting dose and then reducing to half that dose at the end of 3 months, or to start at the lower dose. Like all long-acting drugs the dose does not have an immediate action, taking up to 3 months before the drug has its main therapeutic effect. It should be given with a combination of non-steroidal anti-inflammatory drugs at least until remission is achieved. It should be reserved for those patients who are seropositive and/or erosive early in the course of the disease and in whom non-steroidal anti-inflammatory drugs alone are ineffective.

Side-effects

a. Rash — occurs in 1% of patients; it subsides on stopping the drug.

b. Digestive tract — increased flatus and bloating; there is audible peristalsis in many patients on this drug and irritable bowel syndrome occurs.

c. Pigment change — reversible greying or bleaching of the hair frequently occurs in patients who receive excessive doses of the drug.

d. The eye — fear of eye damage has constrained the use of chloroquine in the treatment of rheumatoid arthritis. It would appear that the original doses used were too high: there is a school of thought which believes that lower doses are associated with an almost negligible incidence of ophthalmic complications. Bernstein's review (1967) indicated that a dose of 250 mg daily was associated with an incidence of retinopathy of 0.4–0.6% in 1906 patients studied. He also describes corneal opacities. At 500 mg a day, the incidence of retinopathy becomes 3–6% in a series of 515 patients and at 750 mg a day the incidence is greater than 15% in 596 patients. Retinal effects include premaculopathy, which is defined as reversible change without permanent anatomical or functional injury (reversible scotoma to red characterises this phase and correlates with exceeding the toxic threshold of dosage). A maculopathy is the next lesion, showing a bulls-eye pattern of pigment: both the scotoma and reduced vision are reversible. Finally, there is a fully-fledged retinopathy in which permanent functional injury to vision occurs with a visible anatomical counterpart in the form of a bulls-eye pigment ring. There is both a scotoma and diminished visual activity. This is a preventable tragedy occuring sooner at high doses than at low doses. The question is really how to prevent this tragedy occuring. One test recommended by Percival & Berhman (1969) is to check visual field defects to red targets. This has been successfully used by these authors as a way of detecting premaculopathy but has subsequently been challenged. In the light of the work of Marks & Power (1979), the argument against using chloroquine on the grounds of retinopathy has probably been overstated and at low dosage the patient is probably safe. It is nevertheless advisable to continue three-monthly slit lamp examinations to check for corneal opacities (including preliminary base-line examination).

The usefulness of available tests to detect premaculopathy is controversial. Marks & Power (1979) recommended the use of recording visual activity, slit lamp corneal microscopy and fundal examination under mydriasis. Further tests include visual field testing to a red target fluorescein fundal angiography, colour vision and electroretinography.

GOLD

Gold was first used in rheumatoid arthritis by Jacques Forestier in 1929 on an empirical basis, as it appeared to have some effect on tuberculosis (then considered to be a possible aetiological factor in the disease). Since that time the popularity of gold has waxed and waned; it was really the Empire Rheumatism Council Report in 1961 that finally established clinical benefit from gold in a long-term controlled trial. It remains the last heavy metal in common clinical use although our knowledge of how it works has not progressed in the fifty years that it has been available.

Perhaps, however, we now understand better the diseases for which gold in appropriate and non-appropriate. In systemic lupus erythematosus, for example, gold treatment is at worst harmful and is at best usually unhelpful.

When gold is used early in the course of the disease, remissions appear to occur sooner, and in these circumstances frequency of injections can be reduced at the time of clinical remission.

Gold formulation

Until recently the only formulations of gold which have been available have been injectable. The two commonest have been sodium aurothiomalate in a 5% solution (Myocrisin) and 5% aurothioglucose (Solganal). Sodium aurothiomalate is in an aqueous solution and aurothioglucose is in oil suspension. This means that the sodium aurothiomalate is quickly absorbed, and the latter is more slowly absorbed. More recently an alternative means of administration of gold has been through an oral preparation (Auranofin).

Pharmacokinetics of gold

Pharmacokinetics of gold in blood and urine have been compared during intramuscular and oral therapy. Blood gold levels are 3–10 times higher with injectable thioglucose and thiomalate than with Auranofin but the serum half-life of the injectable compound is significantly shorter: 5.5 days compared to oral agent 14–21 days with a mean of 19 days. The gold content of the urine is 10 times higher with the intramuscular compounds than with the oral drug. Excretory pathways and tissue distribution of gold during conventional intramuscular therapy would suggest that 40% of the 50 mg injection of thiomalate is excreted in 7 days, of which 70% is recovered in the urine. Highest gold concentrations are found in the reticuloendothelial system, adrenal glands and kidneys, whilst the bone marrow, liver, skin and bone contain the greatest overall quantities of gold.

Using slowly increasing injectable gold, levels rise to around 3 μg/ml after 4 weeks. Elimination from serum occurs with a half-life of 3–5 days. During maintenance treatment with 50 mg monthly, serum gold concentration is held at around 1 μg/ml, maximum values being around 6 μg/ml with an elimination half-life of 11 days. 50% of the blood gold content is found associated with cellular components. Monitoring faeces and urine Gottlieb (1979) showed that 95% of Auranofin gold is recovered in the faeces and 5% in the urine. This contrasts with thiomalate where 40% of an injected dose is recovered, 70% in the urine. Less tissue gold is recovered than with parenteral therapy.

Comparing 20 weeks of Auranofin 6 mg a day with 20 weeks of Myocrisin 50 mg weekly, 66 mg of gold was retained in the Auranofin group compared with 300 mg of gold from the Myocrisin group.

Effect of gold on the immune response

Administration of gold is frequently followed by a decline in serum immunoglobuin levels and rheumatoid factor titres in rheumatoid arthritis. Gold inhibits stimulation of immunoglobulin cells. It also inhibits activation of classical and alternate complement pathways. Lorber et al (1979) showed that gold compounds inhibit the cell-mediated immune response to various mitogens and antigens such as concanvalin A and pokeweed. The inhibition may be due to the effects of gold on macrophages acting as helper cells in these reactions. Both Auranofin and Myocrisin seem to be effective in this way.

How to decide who should receive gold

Because the side-effects of gold can be so hazardous it would be useful to identify patients who would be likely to respond to gold therapy. Studies have been made of responders and non-responders and it has been shown that gold concentrations are similar in blood, urine, faeces, skin, hair and nails in both groups and also in patients with or without toxicity. There is however a suggestion that gold toxicity is related to dosage. Higher than conventional doses increase prevelance and severity of adverse responses. There is some suggestion that certain of the commoner side-effects of Myocrsin such as dermatitis, stomatitis and proteinuria may be fewer with the oral preparation, although diarrhoea may be commoner (Gottleib, 1979).

Dosage regimens

The first properly designed controlled trial that showed Myocrisin to be active was the Empire Rheumatism Council Trial in which 50 mg weekly was compared with 0.05 mg weekly; the response to the higher dose was significantly superior on all measurements. Subsequent studies have set out to assess whether such dosages are necessary or whether even higher doses should be employed. Furst et al (1977) compared 50 mg weekly with 150 mg weekly. Conventional doses were found to be as efficacious as high dosage with respect to rapidity and degree of response but the side-effects were much more frequent and severe in the high dose group. Sharp et al (1977) compared one group treated with 25 mg of gold weekly up to 30 weeks, then biweekly or monthly for up to 2 years of treatment, with another group who received double the dose at the same intervals. No difference was observed in therapeutic response of the two groups and the conclusion was that 25 mg or less per week may be the correct dose. Again in both these studies there appeared to be little correlation between either plasma levels or the rate at which gold disappeared from the serum and therapeutic response.

McKenzie (1981) compared a lower dose of 10 mg weekly with 50 mg weekly. There was no difference either in terms of efficacy or toxicity between these two dosages.

Cats (1976) evaluated the effect of different initial dosages followed by maintenance dosage. In the treatment of rheumatoid arthritis a high dosage of gold compound offered no advantage over the low dose. After a high dose a significantly higher number of side-effects occurred. The development of toxicity did not influence the ultimate results.

A second course of gold hardly appears to have any beneficial effect. Prolonged administration of gold is usually well tolerated although in the author's opinion its substantial therapeutic value is dubious. Progression of radiological abnormality can be observed at the same time that signs and other symptoms of the disease show improvement.

Therapeutic recommendation

Myocrisin

On the basis of all these studies the main aim of crysotherapy is to induce a remission. 50 mg weekly until remission is obtained is a reasonable therapeutic approach. After this maintenance therapy 50 mg monthly or six-weekly according to patient requirement should be continued. Regular monitoring (2–4-weekly) for unwanted effects remains essential, especially full blood count, differential white cell count, platelet count, urinalysis and the check of the skin for rash.

Auranofin

This relatively new agent has been submitted to a variety of clinical trials. 9 mg has been compared with 1 mg and 6 mg with 9 mg dosages. It would appear that 6 mg will be the recommended starting dose for most patients. It may be necessary for patients to continue on this oral medication indefinitely. Long-term studies suggest this may be its main problem: that patient compliance, whilst it can be regularised by injections, may be more difficult when patients are having to swallow daily tablets once the disease remits. Certainly Meyers (personal communication, 1982) suggests breakthrough of activity occurring after 3–4 years of the therapy because of poor compliance rather than lack of efficacy. Again a full haematological, dermatological and urinary monitoring programme remains essential.

Side-effects

Side-effects from gold have been well documented over the fifty years that the drug has been available. Most important are renal lesions (particularly proteinuria), skin rashes and bone marrow problems (particularly pancytopenia).

Renal lesions

The predominant renal complication is a minimal change lesion leading to persistent proteinuria or the nephrotic syndrome. Skrifvars (1979) described patients with microhaematuria, which appears rarely to lead to progressive renal failure. In these cases renal biopsy has disclosed granulomatous glomerulonephritis. Rovenska et al (1979) described a similar case of gold in juvenile chronic polyarthritis where membranous glomerulonephritis was seen and immunofluorescent examination revealed that the deposits contained IgG suggestive of an immune complex mechanism. Nelson & Birchmore (1979) described renal vain thrombosis associated with nephrotic syndrome and gold therapy.

Dermatological effects

The rash consists of an eczematous lesion often in the form of round plaques which can occur over any part of the body, particularly over the trunk. If gold therapy is continued the rash can become confluent and ultimately can exfoliate. A maculopapular rash occurs which can also become confluent. It is often difficult to decide whether a rash appearing during gold treatment is due to the drug or to some unrelated and coincidental cause. In all probability a large number of patients have had their gold therapy terminated as the result of a rash that may well not have been gold-induced.

Bone marrow suppression

The commonest form of bone marrow suppression is thrombocytopenia but neutropenia is also a frequent finding. For these reasons it is recommended that patients have weekly full blood counts, including differential white counts and platelet counts, for the first 8 weeks after starting therapy, followed by two-weekly counts up to the 1 g dosage, followed by four-weekly blood counts thereafter.

Other side-effects

1. Terho et al (1979) encountered 'gold lung'.
2. Mouth ulceration is not uncommon and can be quite difficult to overcome; hydrocortisone sodium succinate pellets ('Corlan pellets') are useful for the alleviation of this.
3. Griffin (1979) described cholestatic hepatitis.

Analysis of the incidence of side-effects

In an elegant study from Capetown, Majoos et al (1981), over the 8 year period from 1971–1979, studied 114 patients with rheumatoid arthritis who were treated with Myocrisin. 70 out of 104 patients benefitted from the drug, 40 going into complete remission. Therapy was discontinued in 58 patients, side-effects accounting for this in 33 cases. Adverse reactions included skin rashes in 41 patients (39%) renal complications in 16 patients (14%) and 7 (6%) developed haematological complications which resulted in death in two cases. Tissue typing in 37 patients with side-effects showed no increase in incidence of HLA-DW2 or 3 antigen. There was however a significant increase in HLA-DW4 antigen in both whites and blacks. Other studies have suggested that the drop-out rate on gold is anywhere between 50% and 75% by the end of the 18 months' treatment.

Side-effects on Auranofin

Side-effects on Auranofin appear to be fewer and less severe. The predominant side-effect is diarrhoea and this appears to be dose-related, a dose of 6 mg being associated with a lower incidence of diarrhoea than is 9 mg. Other side-effects such as rash, thrombocytopenia and proteinuria do occur but appear to be much less common. However further reports are necessary before drawing any firm conclusions about the toxcity of this compound.

Are there more side-effects to d-penicillamine after gold therapy?

This therapeutic problem has been extensively studied by Dodd et al (1981). In a study of 155 patients submitted to D-penicillamine, 125 took only D-penicillamine and 45 developed side-effects from the drug, whereas of the 27 patients with a history of gold toxicity 18 also reacted adversely to penicillamine. All patients who took penicillamine within 6 months after an adverse reaction to gold developed side-effects from penicillamine. 14 patients developed similar reactions to D-penicillamine and gold: the interval treatments in this group was significantly shorter than in those who developed either differing adverse reactions to both drugs or no reaction to D-penicillamine after treatment with gold. It would seem that if a gap of 6 months is left between the two treatments this reduces the risk of adverse reactions to D-penicillamine. Webley & Coombs (1979) considered 114 patients with rheumatoid arthritis who received treatment with penicillamine having previously received gold. Side-effects occurred in 50 patients; 60 were considered to have improved with the drug. Low and high maintenance regimes were compared and there was no significant difference in side-effects or clinical improvement. Previous gold therapy did not influence the therapeutic response or total incidence of side-effects observed with penicillamine. Rashes were perhaps more common in patients who received gold.

Tissue antigens and side-effects

Wooley et al (1980) attempted to relate HLA antigens and toxicity. 91 patients were studied; 71 had toxic reactions to either penicillamine or gold or both drugs. 19 out of 24 patients in which proteinuria developed were positive for HLA-B8 and HLA-DRW3. 14/15 episodes of aurothiomalate-induced proteinuria and 9/13 episodes of penicillamine-induced proteinuria occurred in patients with these antigens. All 13 episodes of proteinuria in which urinary protein exceeded 2 g/24 occurred in patients who were DRW3-positive. No significant association was found between any HLA antigens and the development of skin rashes and haematological receiving gold. Adverse reactions were found in increased frequency in patients who were B12 antigen-positive.

There have since been numerous studies published directed towards elucidating the important problem of histocompatability antigens and susceptibility to side-effects from gold and other drugs. Intensive current research leaves the present picture confused and controversial.

REFERENCES

Abraham D P, Baker W, Chain E, Florey H W, Holiday E R, Robinson R 1942 Penicillamine, characteristic degradation product of penicillamine. Nature 151: 107–9

Bagnell A W 1957 The value of chloroquine in rheumatoid disease A four year study of continuous therapy. Canadian Medical Association Journal 77: 182–94

Bernstein H N 1967 Chloroquine ocular toxicity. Survey of Opthalmology 12: 415–7

Berry H., Liyanage S P, Durance R A, Barnes C G, Berger L, Evans S 1976 Azathioprine and penicillamine in treatment of rheumatoid arthritis — a controlled trial. British Medical Journal 1:6017

Bucknall R C, Dixon A, St J. Glick E.N Woodland J, Zutshi D W, 1975 Myasthenia gravis associated with pencillamine treatment for rheumatoid disease. British Medical Journal 1 600–2

Camus J P, Crouzet J, Homberg J C, Bach J F 1977 Autoantibodies in rheumatoid arthritis treated with D-Penicillamine. In: Penicillamine research in rheumatoid disease. Fabritus & Sonner, Oslo, p 125–129

Camus J P, Crouzet J, Prier A, Bergerin H 1981. Pyrithioxine and thioprionine: new penicillamine-like drugs in rheumatoid arthritis. Journal of Rheumatology (Suppll) 7: 175–7

Cats A 1976 Multicentre controlled trial of the effects of different dosages of gold therapy followed by a maintenance dosage. Agents and Action 6: 355–63

Chalmers A, Thompson D, Stein H E, Reid G, Patterson A C, 1982 Systemic lupus erythematosus during penicillamine therapy for rheumatoid arthritis. Annals of internal medicine 97: 659–633

Dische F E, Swinson D R, Hamilton E B D, Parsons V 1976 Immunopathology of penicillamine-induced glomerular disease. Journal of Rheumatology 3: 145–54

Dixon A St J, Davis J, Dormandy T L et al 1975 Multicentre trial with synthetic D-penicillamine in rheumatoid arthritis: double blind controlled study of low and high dosage. Annals of Rheumatic Diseases 34: 416–21

Dodd M J, Griffith I D, Thompson M Adverse reactions to D-penicillamine after gold toxicity. British Medical Journal 280: 1498–500

Empire Rheumatism Council Report 1961 Gold therapy in rheumatoid arthritis. Final report of a multicentre controlled trial. Annals of Rheumatic Diseases 20:315

Fernandes L., Swinson D R, Hamilton E B D 1977 Dermatomyositis disease complicating penicillamine treatment. Annals of Rheumatic Diseases 36: 94–5

Forestier J M 1929 Bulletin et memoires de la Societé Médicale des Hopitaux de Paris, Vol 53. p 323

Furst D E, Levine S, Srinivasan R, Metzger A L, Bangst R, Paulus H E 1977 A double blind trial of high versus conventional dosages of gold salts for rheumatoid arthritis. Arthritis and Rheumatism 20: 1473–80

Gibson T, Burry H C, Ogg C, 1976 Goodpasture syndrome

and D-penicillamine Annals of Internal Medicine 84: 100
Gottlieb N L, 1979 Gold excretion and retention during Auranofin treatment — a preliminary report. Journal of Rheumatology (Suppl) 6: 61–7
Griffin A J 1979 Cholestatic hepatitis induced by gold. Rheumatology and Rehabilitation 18: 174–6
Haydu G C, 1953 Rheumatoid arthritis therapy — a rationale and the use of chloroquine diphosphate. American Journal of Medical Science 225:71
Huskisson E C et al 1974 Trial comparing gold and penicillamine — a preliminary report. Annals of Rheumatic Diseases 33: 532–5
Jaffe I A 1962 Intra-articular dissociation of the rheumatoid factor. Journal of Laboratory and Clinical Medicine 60: 409
Jaffe I A 1965 The effect of D-penicillamine on laboratory parameters in rheumatoid arthritis. Arthritis and Rheumatism 8: 1064–79
Jain S, Scheur P J, Samouriau S, McGee J O D 1977 A controlled trial of D-penicillamine therapy in primary biliary cirrhosis. Lancet 1: 831–4
Jayson M I V, Lovell C, Black C M, Wilson R S E, 1977 The effect of D-penicillamine in systemic sclerosis. Proceedings of Royal Society of Medicine 70 (Suppl 3):82
Kendall P A, Hutchins D, 1978 The effect of thiol compounds on lymphocytes stimulated in culture. Immunology 35: 189–201
Lansbury J 1965 Chloroquine in rheumatoid arthritis. Annals of Internal Medicine 62: 1065
Latts J R, Antel J P, Levinson D J, Amason B G, Medef M E, 1980 Histocompatability antigens and gold toxicity: a preliminary report. Journal of Clinical Pharmacology 20: 206–9
Lorber A, Simon T M, Leeb J, Peter A, Wilcox S A, 1979 Effects of crysotherapy on parameters of immune response. Journal of Rheumatology (suppl) 6: 82–90
Lyle W H, 1978 Penicillamine in pregnancy. Lancet 1: 606–7
McKenzie J M, 1981 Report on a double blind trial comparing small and large doses of gold in the treatment of rheumatoid disease. Rheumatology and Rehabilitation 20: 198–202
Maini R N Roff I 1977 D-Penicillamine and lymphocyte function in rheumatoid arthritis: the inhabitory and augmenting effects of D-penicillamine in vitro on phytohaemagglutin-induced lymphocyte transformation. In: Penicillamine research in rheumatoid disease. Fabritus & Sonner, Oslo, p 172
Majoos F L, Klemp P, Meyers O L, Briggs B 1981 Gold therapy in rheumatoid arthritis. South African Medical Journal 59: 971–4
Marks J S, Power B J, 1979 Is chloroquine obsolete in treatment of rheumatic disease? Lancet 1: 371–373
Mowat A G, Mowat A M 1982 D-Penicillamine versus levamisole in rheumatoid arthritis. Modulation of autoimmunity and disease. Praeger, Eastbourne, p 253–258
Moynahan E J 1973 D-Penicillamine in morphoea (localised scleroderma). Lancet 1: 428–9
Multicentre trial group 1973 Controlled trial of D-penicillamine in severe rheumatoid arthritis. Lancet I: 275–278
Nelson D C, Birchmore D A, 1979 Renal vein thrombosis associated with nephrotic syndrome and gold therapy in rheumatoid arthritis. South Medical Journal 72: 1616–1618
Percival S P B, Behrman J, 1969 Opthalmological safety of chloroquine. British Journal of Opthalmology 53:101
Perrett D 1981 The metabolism and pharmacology of D-penicillamine in man. Journal of Rheumatology (Suppl)7: 41–50
Rovenska E, Kappeller K, Rossman P 1979 Gold nephropathy in rheumatoid arthritis and in juvenile chronic arthritis. Czechoslovakian Medicine 2: 125–133
Schumaker K, Maeker-Alzar G, Preuss-R 1975 Effect of D-penicillamine on lymphocyte function. Arzneim Forsch 25(4) 600–3
Sharp J T, et al 1977 Comparison of two dosage schedules of gold salts in the treatment of rheumatoid arthritis. Relationhsip of serum gold levels to theraputic response, Arthritis and Rheumatism 20: 1179–1187
Skrifvars B 1979 Hypothesis for the pathogenesis of sodium aurothiomalate (myocrisin) induced immune complex nephritis. Scandinavian Journal of Rheumatology 8: 113–118
Stern R B, Wilkinson S P, Howarth P J N Williams R 1977 controlled trial synthetic D-penicillamine and prednisolone in maintenance therapy for chronic active hepatitis. Gut 18: 19–22
Tabachnick M., Eisen H N, Levine B, 1954 A new mixed disulphide Penicillamine-cysteine. Nature 174: 701–702
Terho E O, Torkka M, Valta R, 1979 Pulmonary damage associated with gold therapy. Scandinavian Journal of Respiratory Disease 60: 345–349
Turner-Warwick Margaret 1981 Adverse reactions affecting the lung: Possible association with D-penicillamine. Journal of Rheumatology (Suppl 7) 8: 166–168
Van der Korst J K, van de Stadt R J, Muijsers A O, Ament H J W, Henrichs A M A 1982 Pharmacokinetics of D-penicillamine in rheumatoid arthritis. Modulation of autoimmunity and disease. Praeger, Eastbourne, p 165–171
Walshe J M, 1953 Disturbances of aminoacid metabolism following liver injury: study by means of paper chromatography. Quarterly Journal of Medicine 22: 483–505
Walshe J M, 1981 Penicillamine and the SLE syndrome. Journal of Rheumatology (Suppl 7) 8: 155–161
Webley M, Coombs E N, 1979 An assessment of penicillamine therapy in rheumatoid arthritis and the influence of previous gold therapy. Journal of Rheumatology 6: 20–4
Wooley P H, Griffin A J, Panayi G S Batchelor S R, Welsh K L, Gibson T J, 1980 HLA-Dr Antigens and toxic reactions to sodium aurothiomalate and D-penicillamine in patients with rhuematoid arthritis. New England Jorunal of Medicine 303: 300–320
Young J P 1959 Chloroquine phophate in the long-term treatment of rheumatoid arthritis. Annals of Internal Medicine 51:1159

other forms of treatment: some initial improvement may be expected but postinflammatory degenerative joint changes will not be helped and it will be difficult to keep the dose to acceptable levels. The place for corticosteroid treatment is in those who have active disabling disease, who will presumably also receive some disease-modifying drug, but who require effective treatment while awaiting the possible results of such a drug. The precise indications depend upon the circumstances and age of the patient. Corticosteroids are avoided if possible in children because of the effect on growth and the fact that HPA suppression does seem to be more dangerous in the young. Corticosteroids, however, may be required for children with severe systemic involvement. There should be little hesitation in using corticosteroids when rheumatoid arthritis presents acutely in the elderly, rapidly leading otherwise to a bedbound patient. In the middle-aged majority the indication to use corticosteroids is the inability to carry on a normal life on account of active disease, whether this means running a family or being able to work.

Corticosteroid treatment for adults should normally be started in the form of 5 mg prednisolone daily in addition to other specific treatment and the use of analgesics. Corticosteroids are usually given as a single dose in the evening to alleviate morning stiffness although Kwanko et al (1982) have suggested that comparable relief can be provided by a single dose in the morning which may avoid HPA suppression. The aim should be to provide a reasonable degree of relief but not total suppression of the disease. If this is not achieved with 5 mg of prednisolone daily the dose should be increased by small increments of 1 mg at intervals of a few weeks up to a maximum of 10 mg daily; possibly 8 mg daily is maximal in women who are more prone to corticosteroid side-effects.

The patient must understand the principles of treatment, that there will be a maximum dose, and that dose reduction and withdrawal are anticipated if the arthritis goes into remission. Obviously this will not occur in all cases, and the patient, and indeed his doctor, may be tempted to think that benefit resulting from a dose of 10 mg daily would be proportionately greater if it were increased further. Experience has shown that this is not so. If the dose is confined to this level corticosteroid side-effects should not be severe but if the dose is increased even by a few milligrams they become inevitable and additional benefits are slight. There is a temptation, particularly when faced with an acute flare up of arthritis, to increase the dose of corticosteroid considerably as is done in the treatment of severe asthma, in the anticipation that the dose will be reduced to the previous level. This is very seldom possible in rheumatoid arthritis and should be avoided.

Complications of rheumatoid arthritis

Vasculitis. Relatively high corticosteroid doses are often advocated for those who develop vasculitis. The results are not impressive and it has been suggested these patients should receive pulsed corticosteroid therapy probably with the addition of cyclophosphamide (Scott et al, 1981).

Felty's syndrome. Corticosteroids have frequently been used to raise the neutrophil count in Felty's syndrome but relatively large doses — 20 mg a day or more — are required. Moreover, steroid treatment is not always effective and may itself increase the risk of infection. Furthermore, the increased blood neutrophilia may decrease the peripheral phagocytic effects of these cells. Other forms of treatment are usually preferable such as the use of disease-modifying drugs (Bennett, 1977; Fohrman et al, 1980).

Polyarteritis nodosa

Corticosteroids are the preferred treatment but unfortunately they are not remarkably effective. Temporary symptomatic relief may be expected but the long-term results are poor. It is probable that relatively high initial doses, 40–60 mg of prednisolone daily, should be used and that rapid control of the disease may improve the prognosis (Stack et al, 1975): immunosuppressive drugs are often used in association (Hollingworth et al, 1982).

Wegener's granulomatosis

This condition does not respond well to corticosteroid treatment and cyclophosphamide is considered to be the treatment of choice. Nevertheless corticosteroids may be required to produce rapid suppression of symptoms (Diaz-Jouanen & Alarcon-Segovia, 1980).

Polymyalgia rheumatica and giant cell arteritis

Corticosteroid treatment is mandatory in the treatment of giant cell arteritis to suppress ophthalmic involvement which may lead to blindness, usually permanent. Corticosteroids are also very much more effective than any other drugs in the relief of the unpleasant symptoms of polymyalgia rheumatica and protect against the complications of giant cell arteritis. There is little agreement about the dose or duration of treatment required, but in the UK most rheumatologists use relatively low doses such as 10 mg prednisolone daily for polymyalgia rheumatica, reducing the dose by 1 mg decrements provided that the symptoms are well controlled and the ESR has fallen. No precise dose or length of treatment can be recommended; each patient should be treated individually. The average duration of treatment is over three years and may be considerably longer.

Maintenance doses are usually relatively small and corticosteroid side-effects are infrequent, osteoporosis and vertebral collapse being the most common. Anti-inflammatory analgesic drugs such as phenylbutazone and indomethacin have been used with some symptomatic improvement but this is less than that provided by corticosteroids; moreover, these drugs do not suppress the development of giant cell arteritis. In those patients who have symptoms of giant cell arteritis there is less agreement about the dosage required (Jones & Hazelman, 1981). Many clinicians recommend high initial doses of 60 mg prednisolone daily (Graham et al, 1981) but there is no evidence that these higher doses provide greater protection than lower doses. A prospective study over 10 years of 191 patients (Behn et al, 1983) showed that a starting dose of 10 mg prednisolone daily for those with polymyalgia rheumatica alone, or 20 mg for those with clinical evidence of giant cell arteritis, produced adequate symptomatic relief and protection from any complications of giant cell arteritis. The incidence of corticosteroid side-effects was low, as would be expected.

Systemic lupus erythematosus

Corticosteroid treatment is not necessary in the majority of patients. In mild cases, with predominantly joint manifestations, small doses of corticosteroids may be helpful and can be given in very much the same way as in rheumatoid arthritis. Pleurisy and pericarditis are often suppressed rapidly by relatively small corticosteroid doses, such as 20 mg of prednisolone daily, which can usually be tapered off fairly rapidly. More serious complications such as autoimmune haemolytic anaemia and thrombocytopenic purpura usually require somewhat higher corticosteroid doses, such as 40–60 mg daily. Corticosteroids are usually required initially for the treatment of renal disease because the alternative forms of treatment — cytotoxic drugs — are not sufficiently rapid in effect. SLE affecting the central nervous system may be a serious and life-threatening problem. Corticosteroids are usually given in high doses but are often ineffective (Eyanson et al, 1980; Hollingsworth et al, 1982; Eisenberg et al, 1982).

Polymyositis and dermatomyositis

Corticosteroids are the mainstay of the treatment of these conditions. If there is a reasonable clinical suspicion of the disease, particularly if there is marked weakness, corticosteroid treatment should be started while investigations are performed, which include muscle biopsy, electromyography and muscle enzyme estimation. Delay in starting treatment, particularly if there is respiratory or pharyngeal involvement, may be fatal. High doses of prednisolone, 60 mg a day, should be used: polymyositis does seem to be a condition in which large initial doses ultimately produce a more satisfactory result. High doses may need to be continued for up to 6 months and it may take some years before treatment can be withdrawn altogether. Treatment is monitored mainly by clinical improvement but serial estimations of creatine kinase, and also of the urinary creatine/creatinine ratio may be helpful. If the response is inadequate a cytotoxic drug should be used in addition. The potassium-losing effect of prednisolone should be remembered and it is advisable to anticipate this by giving potassium supplements when treatment is started (Bradley, 1977).

CORTICOSTEROID TREATMENT OF OTHER CONDITIONS

Systemic corticosteroids are sometimes used in the treatment of frozen shoulder or severe adhesive capsulitis. They are also used in various forms of algodystrophy such as the shoulder–hand syndrome, Sudeck's atrophy and other forms of dystrophy. Relatively high doses of prednisolone, such as 30 mg daily, are given but they are rapidly reduced and the drug withdrawn over the course of about 6 weeks. Adequate trials are lacking but in the writer's experience this treatment is more effective than any other. Corticosteroids given for this short duration are almost free of significant side-effects.

SIDE-EFFECTS

Side-effects of corticosteroids result from sustained administration of a physiological substance in supraphysiological doses and are therefore to be expected in almost every case, although their nature and severity will obviously vary. There is little that can be done to prevent most of these effects, apart from using the smallest dose possible, withdrawing the drug as soon as it is no longer necessary and by intermittent administration, which certainly leads to fewer effects on the HPA axis and on growth (Myles & Daley, 1974a; David et al, 1970). The side-effects are summarised in Table 20.2. Some of these are discussed at greater length.

Gastrointestinal

One of the earliest and most feared complications of corticosteroid treatment was the reported high incidence of peptic ulceration leading to bleeding or perforation, and this continues to worry many clinicians. There is very little evidence, however, that corticosteroids increase the incidence of peptic ulceration. Conn & Blitzer (1976) reviewed the many publications on the subject and concluded that there was a marginal increase in peptic ulceration in those taking the equivalent of more than 20 mg of prednisolone a day, particularly in those taking these doses for long periods. It is difficult to estimate the incidence of ulceration which may be related to corticosteroids, since most chronic diseases including rheumatoid arthritis are associated with an increased incidence of peptic

Table 20.2 Side-effects of corticosteroid treatment

Alimentary	*Musculoskeletal*	*Neurological*
'Dyspepsia'	Myopathy	Euphoria
Peptic ulcer (high dose)	Osteoporosis	Insomnia
Pancreatitis	Osseous aseptic necrosis	Depression
		Benign intracranial hypertension
Endocrine	*Infection*	*Renal*
Growth impairment	Impaired resistance to infection including immunisation with live vaccines	Nocturia
HPA suppression		Sodium retention
Diabetes		Potassium loss
		Sterile pyuria
Ocular	*Cutaneous*	*Fat metabolism*
Posterior subcapsular cataract	Skin atrophy	Redistribution of fat
Glaucoma	Acne	Fatty infiltration of the liver
Deterioration of herpetic keratitis	Hirsutism	Hyperlipidaemia
Sub-conjunctival haemorrhage	Postprandial flushing	
Minor refractive changes		
Haematological		
Erythrocytosis		
Neutrophilia		
Lymphopenia		
Eosinopenia		
Thrombocytopenia		

ulceration. There are few theoretical reasons to account for possible ulcerogenic properties of corticosteroids, although there is some evidence of increased acid secretion. Some changes in the quantity and quality of gastric mucus have been described and corticosteroids do have some effect on prostaglandin release.

Corticosteroids are less likely to cause peptic ulceration than many anti-inflammatory analgesic drugs. The effect of corticosteroid treatment on patients already known to have peptic ulceration is uncertain but it is reasonable to assume that healing may be delayed and that corticosteroids should be avoided if possible. Corticosteroids, like almost any other drug given by mouth may lead to 'dyspeptic' effects which are unrelated to peptic ulceration. These symptoms may be modified by taking the corticosteroids with meals, by using soluble preparations or enteric-coated tablets.

Osteoporosis

Osteoporosis which occurs during corticosteroid treatment is similar to postmenopausal and senile osteoporosis. There is increased bone resorption and reduced new bone formation. Corticosteroids may impair the absorption of calcium from the intestine but there is little evidence that this is an important cause of osteoporosis in corticosteroid-treated patients. The incidence of osteoporosis is dose-related and is very much more common in women. No specific treatment has been shown to be helpful. There is no evidence that anabolic steroids are useful. Calcium supplements are usually given and it has been suggested that the use of microcystalline hydroxyapatite compound may provide some protection (Nilsen et al, 1978). Other more specific forms of treatment of osteoporosis, such as oestrogens or sodium fluoride, have not been evaluated in corticosteroid-induced osteoporosis.

Osseous aseptic necrosis (osteonecrosis)

Osseous aseptic necrosis is an important complication of corticosteroid treatment, particularly in high doses. It has seldom been reported with doses lower than 15 mg of prednisolone a day. Treatment is unsatisfactory. Corticosteroid withdrawal might halt the process but is seldom possible. Prolonged avoidance of weightbearing and osteotomy have been recommended but in most cases bone destruction continues. The most commonly involved bone is the femur, usually necessitating joint replacement in due course, but the head of any long bone may be involved.

The precise cause is uncertain. Surprisingly it does not appear to be related to osteoporosis. It is probable that fat microemboli are the cause. Corticosteroid treatment is known to cause fatty infiltration in the liver and an increase in blood lipids. Histological studies of involved bone have shown intravascular fat emboli in some cases. Osseous aseptic necrosis also occurs with alcoholism, chronic pancreatitis, sickle cell disease, decompression sickness and Gaucher's disease in all of which fat emboli have been described (Fischer & Bickel, 1971; see also Ch. 48).

Skin atrophy

Long-term corticosteroid therapy often leads to skin atrophy causing spontaneous bruising, or extensive bruising in response to minor trauma, which may lead to indolent ulceration, particularly of the legs. The appearance is similar to that of senile purpura, but unlike this condition, which occurs almost exclusively on the back of the hand and forearm, corticosteroid bruising may occur anywhere, especially on the legs. Fragile skin is an important source of disability and the patient may become housebound, knowing the results which minor trauma may produce, including examination by heavy-handed clinicians!

Corticosteroids and the hypothalamo–pituitary–adrenal axis

Decreased ability of the adrenal cortex to secrete hydrocortisone was one of the first recognised consequences of corticosteroid treatment. It is better understood than most and has been intensively investigated, in part because there are relatively simple tests available. Corticosteroids predictably suppress the release of ACTH from the pituitary, the circulating levels of ACTH and endogenous hydrocortisone being lowered by a single dose, the degree depending upon the amount and the time at which it is given. There is a circadian rhythm of ACTH and hydrocortisone secretion which is lowest at about midnight; corticosteroid administration at this time causes much greater and more prolonged suppression than in the morning when the plasma hydrocortisone is much higher. Longer intervals between doses allow a greater chance of HPA recovery. Intermittency rather than frequency should therefore be the aim.

The effect of a single dose is referred to as 'acute suppression' and has no clinical significance, HPA function returning to normal as soon as the administered corticosteroid has disappeared from the circulation. With continued administration, however, chronic suppression may occur; HPA function does not return to normal and may in due course become totally suppressed. It appears that chronic suppression of the pituitary occurs first, followed by suppression of the adrenal cortex. Chronic suppression depends on the dose, duration of treatment and the time of administration. Less than 7.5 mg of prednisolone daily causes little suppression, particularly if given in a single dose in the morning. With higher doses some degree of suppression is liable to occur, becoming inevitable when doses such as 15 mg of prednisolone daily are used. Chronic suppression appears very much more rapidly if the more potent corticosteroids are used, as a result of their longer action.

The short tetracosactrin test is a simple estimation of adrenal cortical function. The insulin hypoglycaemia test is less simple and has some dangers in the elderly but gives information about the integrity of the whole axis. It is the inability of the chronically suppressed HPA axis to respond to stress that causes concern to clinicians. The stress of an acute illness, an anaesthetic or an operation may lead to collapse if the secretion of hydrocortisone is not increased, although authenticated cases are few. It is a very infrequent complication of corticosteroid treatment considering the large numbers of people who receive it. Awareness of this danger led to the practice of corticosteroid cover for anaesthetics, operations and severe illnesses, though this has undoubtedly been overdone in the past. Unnecessarily high doses are still used and may themselves lead to postoperative complication.

A suggested cover is as follows:

1. For minor procedures, such as bronchoscopy, 100 mg of hydrocortisone hemisuccinate is given intramuscularly with the premedication.
2. For intermediate operations such as herniorrhaphy or synovectomy, 100 mg of hydrocortisone hemisuccinate is continued 8-hourly during the period of stress or heavy sedation, which will probably last until the following morning.
3. For major operations the injections need to be continued for as long as there is severe stress, but should be reduced as soon as possible to the maintenance dose.

Recovery form HPA suppression has also been studied extensively. During slow withdrawal recovery is normally full before reduction is complete and has nearly always occurred within a few days of withdrawal. The belief that corticosteroid cover is necessary for a year after receiving systemic steroids has no foundation in fact. HPA function recovers in all patients within 2 months and cover is not required after this period (Plumpton et al, 1969). Corticotrophin (ACTH) treatment has no clinically important effect on response to stress, and cover is not required except for those patients who have for some reason also received corticosteroids. Most of the supposition that the HPA axis takes many months to recover is anecdotal, but in part is derived from the compulsive study of Graber et al (1965), who studied 14 patients and concluded that recovery took up to 9 months in five elegantly defined stages. 8 of the patients however had Cushing's disease, which is very different from corticosteroid treatment and some patients had only one test performed. Those available at that time were imprecise, and in spite of the logical beauty of the study, its conclusions have not been confirmed. The facts concerning HPA suppression are now so well known that there is seldom any clinical need to perform HPA function tests in corticosteroid-treated patients.

Growth

It is well recognised that corticosteroid treatment leads to impairment of growth in children, although it must be remembered that chronic illness also impairs growth. If it is possible to withdraw corticosteroid treatment there is some catch-up but this is variable and clearly depends upon the time at which the corticosteroids are withdrawn. The precise mechanism of growth impairment is uncertain. The catabolic and anti-anabolic effects of corticosteroids probably play some part. Secretion of growth hormone is reduced by corticosteroid treatment and there is some correlation between HPA suppression and inhibition of growth hormone release during the insulin hypoglycaemia test. The use of human growth hormone however has not been shown to increase the rate of growth in these children. A possible effect of corticosteroids reducing the production of somatomedins from the liver remains uncertain.

Various methods are in use to reduce the degree of growth retardation. Corticotrophin (ACTH) certainly appears to cause less growth loss, but the reasons are uncertain. ACTH may lead to considerable impairment of growth hormone secretion in response to insulin hypoglycaemia and would be expected to produce as much growth suppression as corticosteroids if it were mainly due to a peripheral action. ACTH stimulates the release of sex hormones, which do play a part in growth.

The relative lack of growth suppression by ACTH may be merely due to intermittency of its dosage, since it is usually given in a single daily dose or sometimes less often. The use of corticosteroids in single morning doses on alternate days at present is the most effective way of reducing growth suppression although it is less effective in disease control, more anti-inflammatory analgesics being required for the corticosteroidfree days (Ansell & Bywaters, 1974; Byron et al, 1982).

CORTICOTROPHIN

The indications for ACTH are essentially similar to those for corticosteroid treatment. There is no evidence that it has any therapeutic advantages in the treatment of rheumatic diseases. It is the difference in the side-effects which may provide some advantage.

ACTH causes hypertrophy of the adrenal cortex but would be expected by increasing the plasma hydrocortisone to cause inhibition of the hypothalamus or pituitary. Some HPA function tests are abnormal, particularly the lysine vasopressin and the metyrapone tests; but the response to stress or to the insulin hypoglycaemia test are not impaired and there are no records of HPA failure leading to acute 'Addisonian' crises in ACTH-treated patients. The latter may be an important consideration in children, in whom HPA suppression appears to be more dangerous than in adults.

Dyspepsia does not occur and in the early days of treatment ACTH appeared to cause less peptic ulceration than cortisone or hydrocortisone, which were used at that time: however, peptic ulceration does not seem to be an important problem with synthetic corticosteroid treatment.

Withdrawal of ACTH therapy is considered to be easier than withdrawal of corticosteroid therapy for reasons that are uncertain, but are possibly due to the differing effects on the HPA axis. Skin atrophy and osteoporosis are possibly less marked with ACTH and this may in part be due to the stimulation of androgenic hormones from the adrenal cortex. There are, however, many disadvantages to ACTH treatment. It has to be given by injection, usually once a day, although sometimes alternate days or twice weekly administration is possible. Androgenic side-effects, particularly acne and hirsutes are more common than with oral corticosteroids and are particularly troublesome for women. ACTH has a melanocyte-stimulating action and pigmentation of the skin occurs with long-term therapy. Salt and water retention can be expected and considerable potassium loss may occur. Oedema, hypertension and cardiac failure may be precipitated. Since ACTH causes adrenal cortical hypertrophy, it has been used to overcome the adrenal atrophy that may arise from corticosteroid treatment. When the two are given together however, hypothalamopituitary response to stress is rapidly lost. ACTH and corticosteroid treatment should never therefore be combined.

Available preparations

The most commonly used ACTH is porcine in origin and marketed in the form of a gel. A synthetic ACTH, tetracosactrin, containing the 1–24 amino acids of ACTH has been made and has similar properties to ACTH. It was hoped that it would be more stable, more reliable and would not be immunogenic. It is complexed with zinc phosphate to increase the durarion of the action. The preparation available are very potent, are longer acting than the porcine gel and have now been shown to be immunogenic. There is no advantage in the use of these preparations and their longer action may be an actual disadvantage. It is possible that one of the advantages of ACTH is the relatively short action of the porcine gel over longer acting synthetic corticosteroids (Myles & Daly, 1974b).

ACTH dosage

ACTH is only useful in the treatment of conditions which would otherwise receive low dose prednisolone treatment as detailed previously. Since the response of the individual's adrenal cortex to ACTH stimulation cannot be accurately predicted, measurements of urinary metabolites of hydrocortisone were used to assess the response, the most usual being the 24 hour urinary excretion of 17-oxogenic steroids and the aim of the treatment was to double the pretreatment level. It is now realised that these measurements give little helpful information. The dose is judged by the clinical effects using the smallest amount that will provide reasonable control. The usual starting dose in adults is 30 units of porcine gel given in the evening with the anticipation that reduction will be possible and that alternative day treatment may be substituted when an adequate effect has been achieved: a starting dose of 20 units daily is usually adequate for children. If adequate control is not achieved with these doses, corticosteroid treatment is preferable, in view of the anticipated electrolyte disturbances of ACTH in large doses.

LOCAL CORTICOSTEROID TREATMENT

This subject is covered in detail elsewhere (Ch. 23). Intra-articular injection is a very valuable method of suppressing inflammation but all commonly used preparations are absorbed from the joint and exert a systemic effect. This can be demonstrated by the drop of plasma hydrocortisone levels after intra-articular injection of corticosteroids and in some cases by measuring the plasma levels of the injected corticosteroid (Reeback et al, 1980; Armstrong et al, 1981). The systemic absorption may be an advantage to the patient provided that excessively frequent injections are not given.

REFERENCES

Ansell B M, Bywaters E G L 1974 Alternate-day corticosteroid therapy in juvenile chronic polyarthritis. Journal of Rheumatology 1: 176–178

Armstrong R B, English J, Gibson T, Chakraborty J, Marks V 1981 Serum methylprednisolone levels following intra-articular injection of methylprednisolone acetate. Annals of the Rheumatic Diseases 40: 571–574

Bacon P A, Myles A B, Beardwell C G, Daly J R, Savage O 1966 Corticosteroid withdrawal in rheumatoid arthritis. Lancet 2: 935–937

Bayliss E M, Williams I A, English J 1982 High dose intravenous methylprednisolone 'pulse therapy' in patients with rheumatoid disease. Plasma methylprednisolone levels and adrenal function. European Journal of Clinical Pharmacology 21: 385–388

Behn A, Perera T, Myles A B 1983 Polymyalgia rheumatica and corticosteroids: How much and for how long? Annals of the Rheumatic Diseases (in press)

Bennett R M 1977 Extra-articular manifestations of rheumatoid arthritis. Clinics in Rheumatic Diseases 3: 433–467

Bernstein C A, Freiberg R H, 1961 Rheumatoid patients after five or more years of corticosteroid treatment: A comparative analysis of 183 cases. Annals of Internal Medicine 54: 938–953

Bradley G 1977 Polymyositis. British Journal of Hospital Medicine 17: 351–355

Brooks P M, Buchanan W W, Grove M, Downie W W 1976 Effects of enzyme induction on metabolism of prednisolone. Annals of the Rheumatic Diseases 35: 339–343

Brooks S M, Werk E E, Ackerman S J 1972 Adverse effects of phenobarbital on corticosteroid metabolism in asthmatics. New England Journal of Medicine 286: 1125–1128

Byron M A, Jackson J, Ansell B M 1982 The effect of different corticosteroid regimens on the hypothalmic–pituitary–adrenal (HPA) axis and linear growth in juvenile chronic arthritis. Annals of the Rheumatic Diseases 41:626

Conn H O, Blitzer B L 1976 Non-association of adrenocorticosteroid therapy and peptic ulcer. New England Journal of Medicine 294: 343–473

David D S, Grieco M H, Cushman P Jr 1970 Adrenal glucocorticoids after twenty years. Journal of Chronic Diseases 22: 637–711

Diaz-Jouanen E, Alarcon-Segovia 1980 Diagnostic and therapeutic approaches to the patient with vasculitis. Clinics in Rheumatic Diseases 6:453

Eisenberg D A, Morrow W J, Snaith M L 1982 Methylprednisolone 'pulse therapy' in the treatment of systemic lupus erythematosus. Annals of the Rheumatic Diseases 14: 347–351

Eyanson S, Passo M H, Aldo Benson M A, Benson M D

1980 Methylprednisolone 'pulse therapy' for non-renal lupus erythematosus. Annals of the Rheumatic Diseases 39: 377–380
Fischer D E, Bickel W H 1971 Corticosteroid induced avascular necrosis: A clinical study of seventy-seven patients. Journal of Bone and Joint Surgery 53A: 859–873
Fohrman D E, Mueller M N, Ward J R 1980 Felty's syndrome: Long term follow-up and response to medical therapy. Arthritis and Rheumatism 23:674
Forster P J G, Grindulis K A, Neumann V, Hubball S, McConkey B 1982 High-dose intravenous methylprednisolone in rheumatoid arthritis. Annals of the Rheumatic Diseases 41: 444–446
Graber A L, New R L, Nicholson W E, Island D P, Liddle G W 1965 Natural history of pituitary adrenal recovery following long term suppression with corticosteroids. Journal of Clinical Endocrinology 25: 11–16
Graber E K, Fan P T, Bluestone R, Wadsworth V A 1981 Realistic guidelines of corticosteroid therapy in rheumatic disease. Seminars in Arthritis and Rheumatism 1: 231–256
Graham C G, Champion G D, Day R O 1977 Patterns of plasma and urinary excretion of salicylates in rheumatoid arthritis. Clinical Pharmacology and Therapeutics 22: 410–420
Graham E, Holland A, Avery A, Ross-Russell R W 1981 Prognosis in giant cell arteritis. British Medical Journal 282: 269–271
Hahn B H, Pletscher L S, Munian M 1981 Immunosuppressive effects of deflazocort — a new glucosteroid with bone-sparing and carbohydrate-sparing properties: Comparison with prednisone. Journal of Rheumatology 8: 783–790
Hayes M, Alam A F M S, Bruckner F E, Doherty S M, Myles A, English J 1983 Plasma prednisolone studies in rheumatic patients. Annals of the Rheumatic Diseases 42: 151–154
Henderson R G, Wheatley T, English J 1979 Variation in plasma prednisolone concentrations in renal transplant recipients given enteric coated prednisolone. British Medical Journal 1: 1534–1536
Hollingworth P, et al 1982 Intensive immunosuppression versus prednisolone in the treatment of connective tissue diseases. Annals of the Rheumatic Diseases 41: 557–562
Joint Committee of the Medical Research Council and Nuffield Foundation on clinical trails of cortisone, ACTH and other therapeutic measures in chronic rheumatic diseases 1960. A comparison of prednisolone with aspirin or other analgesics in the treatment of rheumatoid arthritis. Annals of the Rheumatic Diseases 19: 331–337
Jones J G, Hazleman B L 1981 Prognosis and management of polymyalgia rheumatica. Annals of the Rheumatic Diseases 40: 1–5
Kwanko I C, Pownall R, Knapp M S, Swannell A J, Mahoney P G C 1982 Time of day of prednisolone administration in rheumatoid arthritis. Annals of the Rheumatic Diseases 41: 447–451
Lewis G P, Jusko W J, Burke C W, Graves L 1971 Prednisolone side effects and serum protein levels. Lancet 2: 778–780
Million R, Kellgren J H, Poole P H, Jayson M I V 1979 The long term management of early rheumatoid arthritis. Annals of the Rheumatic Diseases 38:573
Mills I H, Schendl H P, Chen P S, Bartter 1960 The effect of oestrogen administration on the metabolism and protein binding of hydrocortisone. Journal of Endocrinal Metabolism 20: 515–528
Myles A B, Daly J R 1974a Corticosteroid and ACTH treatment. Arnold, London, p 66–81
Myles A B, Daly J R 1974b Corticosteroid and ACTH treatment. Arnold, London, p 183–204
Nelson A M, Conn D 1980 Glucocorticosteroids in rheumatic disease. Mayo Clinic Proceedings 55: 758–769
Nilsen H N, Jayson M I V, Dixon A St J 1978 Microcrystalline calcium hydroxyapatite compound in corticosteroid-treated rheumatoid patients: A controlled study. British Medical Journal 2:1124
Pickup M E 1979 Clinical pharmacokinetics of prednisone and prednisolone. Clinical Pharmocokinetics 4: 111N–128
Plumpton F S, Besser C M, Cole P V 1969 Corticosteroid treatment and surgery 2. The management of steroid cover. Anaesthesia 24: 3–18
Reeback J S, Chakroborty J, Gibson T, Marks V 1980 Plasma steroid levels after intra-articular injection of prednisolone acetate in patients with rheumatoid arthritis. Annals of the Rheumatic Diseases 39: 22–24
Scott D G I, Bacon P A, Allen C, Elson C J 1981 IgG rheumatoid factor complement and immune complexes in rheumatoid synovitis and vasculitis: comparative and serial studies during cytotoxic therapy. Clinical Experimental Immunology 43: 54–64
Suchman A L, Condemi J J, Leddy J P 1983 Seizure after pulse therapy with methylprednisolone. Arthritis and Rheumatism 26:117
Thomas J P 1970 Nocturia in patients on long term steroid therapy. Clinical Science 38: 415–25
Williams I A, Bayliss E M, English J 1981 High dose intravenous methylprednisolone 'pulse therapy' in the treatment of rheumatoid disease. Scandinavian Journal of Rheumatology 10: 153–155

C.F. Corke E.C. Huskisson N. Christophidis

Cytotoxic and immunomodulating drugs in the treatment of rheumatic diseases

CYTOTOXIC DRUGS

RATIONALE FOR THE USE OF CYTOTOXIC DRUGS IN RHEUMATIC DISEASES

The basic premise upon which cytotoxic drugs were introduced into rheumatological practice has been continually challenged. This has resulted from an increasing understanding of the complexities of the immune response while the causes of most of the inflammatory connective tissue diseases remain unknown.

Cytotoxic drugs were introduced into the treatment of rheumatic diseases because the basic abnormality was thought to be a loss of tolerance to self-antigens allowing the proliferation of abnormal clones of lymphocytes with self-reactivity. Cytotoxic drugs, it was thought, might eliminate these clones and thereby control autoimmune diseases such as rheumatoid arthritis and systemic lupus erythematosus. The situation is now recognised to be far more complicated.

Both conventional and autoimmune reactions involve the interaction of several populations of lymphocytes and accessory cells, each with varying sensitivity to cytotoxic agents. There are populations of lymphocytes which control the nature and magnitude of all immune responses whether these are mediated by lymphocytes, antibodies or even by non-specific 'natural killer' cells. Thus cytotoxic drugs, which selectively effect these controlling cells may increase the vigour of immune responses if the cells which effect the responses are themselves resistant to the agent in question. In support of this concept there is evidence, from animal studies, that cytotoxic agents are capable of paradoxically enhancing or augmenting rather than suppressing an immune response (Chanmougan & Schwartz, 1966; Dixon & McConahey, 1963). Thus to call cytotoxic drugs immunosuppressive may be an oversimplification.

Although the basic mechanisms of both the rheumatic diseases and of cytotoxic drug therapy in these diseases remain unclear, certain basic concepts support the use of these agents. As outlined above cytotoxic agents might re-establish immune tolerance by antagonism of autoreactive clones. In support of this concept it has been shown that while the conventional secondary antibody response is resistant to cytotoxic agents, autoantibody production is more sensitive (Denman, 1982). Lymphoproliferation is associated with connective tissue disease and some features resemble those of lymphoma, justifying the application of cytotoxic agents. Finally the inflammatory reaction involves the interaction of various cell types some of which might be sensitive to cytotoxic agents and the reaction inhibited.

THE CLINICAL PHARMACOLOGY OF THE MORE COMMONLY USED CYTOTOXIC DRUGS IN RHEUMATIC DISEASES

Azathioprine is widely used as an 'immunosuppressive' drug in the UK whereas cyclophosphamide is more commonly used in North America (Hazleman & De Silva, 1982). Owing to the influence of de Seze and Kahn, chlorambucil has been the most commonly used immunosuppressive drug in France (Amor & Mery, 1980). The use of methotrexate is increasing and it is widely employed in psoriatic arthritis.

Mechanisms of action

Alkylating agents

Cyclophosphamide and chlorambucil (Fig. 21.1) are both alkylating nitrogen mustards. Alkylating agents covalently bond with various nucleophilic substances, including such biologically important moieties as phosphate, amino, sulphydryl, hydroxyl, carboxyl and imidazole groups (Price, 1975). The 7-nitrogen atom of guanine is particularly susceptible to the formation of a covalent bond with alkylating agents and may well represent the key target that determines the biological effects of these agents (Calabresi & Parks, 1980). Cross-linking of two nucleic acid chains, or the linking of a nucleic acid chain to a protein, by very strong covalent bonds results in major disruption of nucleic acid function (for further details see Price, 1975).

Azathioprine

Azathioprine is a derivative of 6-mercaptopurine. It was developed with the intention of blocking the rapid oxidation and methylation of 6-mercaptopurine (6MP) by attaching an imidazole ring to the sulphur atom at the 6-position in the molecule (see Fig. 21.1). There is evidence from experiments in rodents that azathioprine is more potent on a molar basis and in man it appears to have a better therapeutic index and can be used in effective doses for a longer period of time with less risk of thrombocytopenia or leucopenia than 6MP (Bertino, 1973).

Although purine analogues and their derivatives have been studied extensively, the mechanisms responsible for inhibiting cell replication are still not clear, but several sites of action have been elucidated (Calabresi & Parks, 1980; Hitchings & Elion, 1972).

Methotrexate

Methotrexate (4-amino-N-10 — methyl-folic acid) binds to the enzyme dihydrofolate reductase and thus inhibits the conversion of folic acid and dihydrofolic acid to the coenzyme tetrohydrofolic acid (Bertino, 1963). This coenzyme is the source of carbons 2 and 8 of the purine nucleus, the carbon of serine in the conversion of glycine to serine, the source for methylation of homocysteine

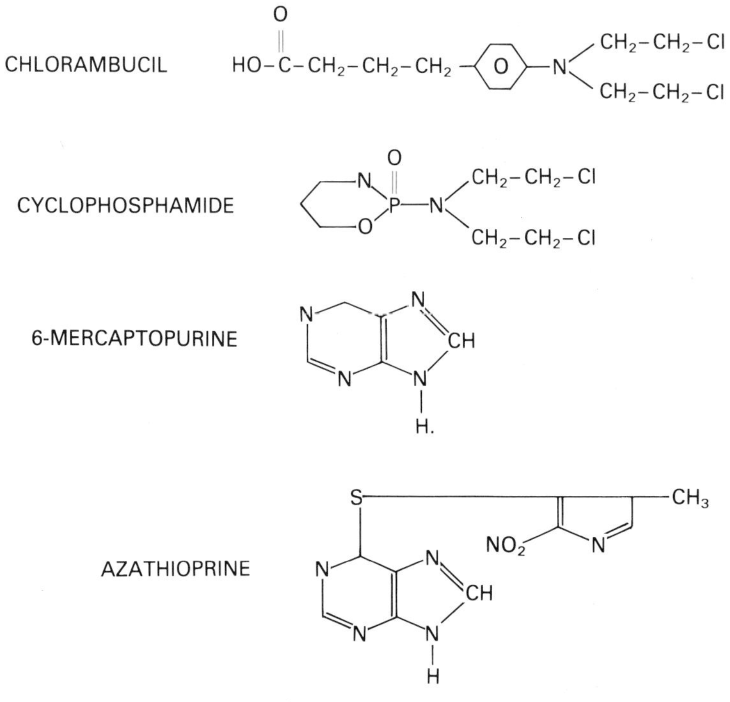

Fig. 21.1 Structural formulae of cytotoxic drugs.

to methionine and deoxyuridylate to thymidylate (Bertino, 1977). Vitamin B12 may also be required in these methylation reactions (Beck, 1973). Limitation of thymidylate synthesis by methotrexate results in impairment of DNA synthesis and is probably the most critical effect produced by methotrexate, resulting in cell death (Heynriuk & Bertino, 1971).

CYTOTOXIC DRUG THERAPY IN RHEUMATIC DISEASES

Rheumatoid arthritis

A significant number of patients, estimated at 5–20%, experience severe progression of disease despite adequate conventional treatment (Currey, 1971). As a result, a wide variety of cytotoxic drugs have been used including azathioprine, nitrogen mustard, cyclophosphamide, chlorambucil and methotrexate. Fosdick et al (1969) treated 108 rheumatoid patients with cyclophosphamide in an uncontrolled study. All the patients had severe active disease unresponsive to conventional therapy. Improvement occurred in 50 patients and of these 18 were able to discontinue corticosteroid therapy. These observations were confirmed in a randomised, controlled study conducted by the co-operating clinics of the American Rheumatism Association (1970); 48 patients were included in this study comparing 50–150 mg/day cyclophosphamide with 5–15 mg/day. The higher dose reduced disease activity as judged by grip strength, number of inflamed joints, duration of morning stiffness and walking speed. Sedimentation rate was a poor indication of improvement. Serial X-rays indicated minimal new erosions in patients receiving cyclophosphamide in a dose of 100 mg/day. However, the higher dose group had more toxic episodes than the lower dose group. Townes et al (1976) reported similar results in a double blind crossover study of 24 patients. 11 patients who completed 9 months of treatment, on a mean dose of 1.8 mg/kg. day^{-1} cyclophosphamide, demonstrated a significant decrease in painful or swollen joints, morning stiffness and increase in grip strength when compared to 11 patients on placebo. After crossover, significant improvement was observed in patients who switched to cyclophosphamide and deterioration was noted over several months in most patients who switched to the placebo.

Williams et al (1980) performed a 32 week, multicentre double blind trial comparing cyclophosphamide 150 mg/day with 75 mg/day in 88 patients. Both doses were equally effective. The incidence of alopecia and leucopaenia was significantly less in the lower dose group.

Several well-controlled studies have demonstrated significant improvement in patients with rheumatoid arthritis treated with azathioprine. In a double blind study to see if azathioprine could reduce the prednisolone requirement in severe rheumatoid arthritis, 49 patients who had been taking prednisolone 5–20 mg/day were randomised to receive either placebo or azathioprine for 12 months (Mason et al, 1969). The mean corticosteriod requirement was reduced by 36% without disease reactivation in the azathioprine-treated group, but no such reduction was possible in the placebo group. Levy et al (1972) found azathioprine to be significantly better than placebo in reducing the active joint count, improving grip strength and reducing morning stiffness. Urowitz et al (1971) showed azathioprine 2.0–2.5 mg/kg.day^{-1} to be significantly better than placebo, reducing the articular index and improving the grip strength. Woodland et al (1981) tested azathioprine at 2 dose levels, 2.5 and 1.25 mg/kg.day^{-1}, against placebo under double blind conditions over 24 weeks. Improvement on 2.5 mg/kg.day^{-1} was significantly better than on placebo while results in the 1.25 mg/kg.day^{-1} group tended to fall between the two other groups. It should be noted that significant improvement occurred in the placebo group in this study. Currey et al (1974) have compared azathioprine, cyclophosphamide and gold under double blind conditions in 121 patients with relatively early rheumatoid arthritis. Over a period of 18 months, azathioprine and cyclophosphamide produced clinical improvement comparable to that achieved with gold. Concomitant reduction of corticosteroid dosage was facilitated by the cytotoxic drugs but not by gold. Patients on azathioprine or cyclophosphamide showed less deterioration radiologically than the group treated with gold. Drug management was easiest with azathioprine, but cyclophosphamide was marginally more effective.

Most of the data on chlorambucil in rheumatoid arthritis are from studies carried out in France (Amor & Mery, 1980). A double blind placebo controlled study has been reported by Hatchuel (1972). 25 patients on chlorambucil were compared with 23 patients on placebo over a period of 3 months. The initial dose was 0.2 mg/kg.day^{-1}, but this was reduced with the appearance of leucopenia. Although the duration of treatment was comparatively short there was significant improvement on a global index which included pain, morning stiffness, functional ability and the number of joints affected. There were also significant falls in the ESR, rheumatoid factor and IgM. Using the grouped data from various authors' results, Kahn et al (1971) have estimated that 40–60% of patients improve on chlorambucil.

Michaels et al (1982) treated 14 patients with methotrexate. These patients had active classical rheumatoid arthritis and had failed to respond to gold. This was given intravenously each week increasing from 10–50 mg if tolerated. Once response had occurred the dosage interval was increased to 2–4 weeks. There was significant improvement in ESR, morning stiffness and articular index over a period of 7–20 weeks. Zeiders (1982) treated 183 out-patients with moderate/severe rheumatoid arthritis for up to 77 months. Most were steroid-dependent and unresponsive to remission-including drugs. The dose ranged from 2.5–25 mg/week, averaging 8.9 mg/week, usually given as a single tablet every other day. The incidence of side-effects with this regime was high at 36.1%. There is evidence that it is lower with weekly oral doses.

Systemic lupus erythematosus

There is controversy regarding the use of cytotoxic drugs in systemic lupus erythematosus (Pirofsky & Bardana, 1977; Hughes, 1979; Wagner, 1976). The majority of reports dealing with the use of the drug in SLE have been confined to renal, central nervous system and cardiopulmonary involvement.

Initial reports with azathioprine, cyclophosphamide or chlorambucil were uncontrolled but it was claimed that their combination with corticosteroids was more efficacious than either drug given alone, and a steroid-sparing effect has been claimed (Drinkard et al, 1970; Ginzler et al, 1975; Cameron et al, 1970; Feng et al, 1973; Gershwin et al, 1974; Hadidi, 1970; Epstein & Grausz, 1974; Snaith et al, 1973). Unfortunately, more recent randomised studies have failed to resolve the controversy which surrounds the use of these drugs in SLE. The studies have been mainly limited to cyclophosphamide and azathioprine although a controlled study of chlorambucil in active SLE, published in France, showed no benefit over placebo (Amor et al, 1972).

Fries et al (1973) in a controlled study involving 22 patients with active SLE, showed that cyclophosphamide alone, unlike prednisolone alone, did not induce remission in SLE with or without renal involvement. However the dose of cyclophosphamide was only 1 mg/kg.day^{-1}. 10 of 22 patients with similar forms of lupus nephritis were randomised into two groups of 5 patients. One group received cyclophosphamide alone and the other prednisolone alone. All those given cyclophosphamide were treatment failures. They were then given prednisolone to which 3 responded.

Steinberg et al (1971, 1972, 1974) randomised patients with biopsy proven lupus nephritis into groups to compare double blind the effects of azathioprine or cyclophosphamide with placebo. Nearly all had diffuse proliferative glomerulonephritis. Prednisolone up to 30 mg daily as needed was given to each group. The treatment period was 10 weeks. They noted that patients who received either azathioprine or cyclophosphamide showed improved immunological parameters, with less proteinuria. Extrarenal disease appeared to be controlled and smaller doses of corticosteroids were required. The net improvement in creatinine clearance was greatest in the cyclophosphamide group. Decker et al (1975) compared cyclophosphamide and azathioprine with corticosteroids in 38 patients with diffuse glomerulonephritis. The authors concluded that there was only marginal benefit obtained in patients treated with cytotoxic drugs. However, it was noted that no lupus-related deaths occurred in the 12 patients treated with cyclophosphamide. Renal failure was twice as common in the group treated with prednisolone alone compared to those treated with cyclophosphamide or azathioprine in addition.

Cade et al (1973) compared prednisolone,

azathioprine, azathioprine plus heparin and azathioprine plus prednisolone in a group of 50 patients of whom all but one had diffuse, proliferative lupus nephritis. Azathioprine was found to be remarkably efficacious. Only 2 of 15 patients on prednisolone alone survived, with a mean survival time of 19 months for the group. 9 of the 13 patients on azathioprine alone survived and the mean survival time for that group was 41 months. 7 of the 13 who received azathioprine and prednisolone survived; their average survival time was 29 months. 9 of the 13 who received azathioprine and heparin survived with a mean survival of 41 months.

These impressive results were not confirmed by Donadio et al (1972, 1974), who studied only 16 patients. These were randomly assigned to receive either azathioprine plus large doses of prednisolone or large doses of prednisolone alone for 6 months. The outcome for the two groups was similar. Biopsy 'activity' scores decreased markedly and equally; creatinine clearance, proteinuria and urine sediment findings were either stable or improved. After completion of 6 months therapy, patients were given the smallest dose of prednisolone that controlled extrarenal manifestations. The seven patients of the combined drug groups continued to receive azathioprine for another 12 months. The authors concluded that combined therapy was no more effective than prednisolone alone. More recently, Donadio et al (1978) have compared prednisolone alone with prednisolone plus cyclophosphamide given for 6 months followed by maintenance doses of prednisolone thereafter, in patients with diffuse proliferative lupus nephritis. 26 patients were in the prednisolone only group and 24 in the combined therapy group. During the 4 years follow-up the prednisolone only group had a higher recurrence of nephritis. Survival was the same.

Decker (1982) reported a 3-year follow-up on three groups of patients with lupus nephritis. One group of 12 received prednisolone alone, one group of 16 patients received cyclophosphamide and azathioprine daily by mouth and the third group of 11 received intermittent intravenous cyclophosphamide. There was no significant change in the serum creatinine in any of the groups and he concluded that neither cytotoxic drug was important in the management of SLE.

It is difficult from all these conflicting reports to reach any firm conclusion regarding the efficacy of these drugs in lupus nephritis, but overall, the therapeutic effect of azathioprine appears to be less than cyclophosphamide. Their role in central nervous system or cardiopulmonary involvement is even less clear.

Juvenile chronic arthritis

Amyloidosis is a serious complication of chronic juvenile arthritis. Despite a natural reluctance to treat young patients with cytotoxic drugs these have been employed in an attempt to improve the prognosis of this complication. In an open study of chlorambucil an improved prognosis has been reported (Schnitzer & Ansell, 1977).

Psoriatic arthritis

Cytotoxic agents have been shown to effectively relieve both skin and arthritic features in the minority of patients who have severe progressive psoriatic arthritis. In a double blind study of 21 patients intermittent parenteral methotrexate has been shown to effectively relieve both skin and arthritic manifestations (Black et al, 1964). The response was detectable within a few weeks of the initiation of therapy.

Azathioprine (2.5 mg/kg.day^{-1}) has been found to be effective in psoriatic arthritis and of comparable potency to oral methotrexate (10–25 mg/week) (Feldges & Barnes, 1974). In addition benefit has been reported with 6-mercaptopurine in 11 of 13 patients with psoriatic arthropathy, also with a rapid onset within 3 weeks of the start of therapy (Baum et al, 1973).

There is an impression that methotrexate is more effective for the dermatological features of psoriasis while azathioprine appears to be better for arthritis.

Polymyositis/dermatomyositis

Various cytotoxic drugs have been used in the treatment of polymyositis and dermatomyositis including 6-mercaptopurine, azathioprine, cyclophosphamide, methotrexate and chlormabucil (Haas, 1973; Benson & Aldo, 1973; Arnett et al, 1973; Metzger et al, 1974; El-Ghobarey et al,

1978; Christophidis & Huskisson, 1982; Bohan & Peter, 1975).

In steroid-resistant cases improvement has been observed in up to 75% of cases when steroid therapy was supplemented with weekly intravenous injections of 25–50 mg methotrexate (Metzger et al, 1974). The dose of prednisolone was able to be reduced and in some patients the frequency of methotrexate injections reduced to once a month. According to Pirofsky & Bardana (1977) azathioprine is equally effective in oral daily doses of 2–2.5 mg/kg.

In a recent controlled double blind trial Bunch et al (1980) compared 60 mg prednisolone/day plus either azathioprine (2 mg/kg.day^{-1}) or placebo over 3 months. There was no increased benefit with azathioprine; however this did not mean that azathioprine would not be effective in steroid-resistant cases or have a steroid-sparing effect. In fact in a later report giving their results of longer-term follow-up on these patients over a 3-year period, it was found that the patients on combined azathioprine and prednisolone therapy improved more with respect to functional ability and required lower doses of prednisolone than did the group on prednisolone alone (Bunch, 1981).

Polyarteritis nodosa

Patients who either fail to respond to steroids or required intolerably high doses to control their disease are now often treated with either cyclophosphamide or azathioprine (Lightfoot, 1979). The relative rarity of polyarteritis nodosa and the generally poor prognosis have precluded studies comparing treated patients with contemporary controls.

Garges et al (1973) have reported 15 biopsy-proven cases of polyarteritis nodosa treated with prednisolone and azathioprine (2–2.5 mg/kg.day^{-1}). 8 had hypertension and 9 had renal involvement. All but 2 required maintenance treatment with azathioprine. After a mean follow-up period of 26 months there were 14 survivors. Leib et al (1979) compared the outcome of 8 cases of polyarteritis nodosa treated supportively with 34 patients given corticosteroids and 22 treated with both cytotoxic agents and corticosteroids in combination. The median survival times were 3, 63 and 149 months respectively and the 5-year survival rates were 12%, 53% and 80% respectively. This suggests a better prognosis for treated patients and especially when a cytotoxic agent is given in addition to corticosteroid therapy.

UNWANTED EFFECTS OF CYTOTOXIC DRUGS

Organ-specific toxicity

By virtue of their rapid cell turnover, particularly susceptible are the reticuloendothelial system, the basal layer of the skin, the germinal epithelium and the gastrointestinal mucosa. Gastrointestinal intolerance is common with azathioprine and cyclophosphamide, less common with methotrexate and almost never seen with chlorambucil (Pirofsky & Bardana, 1977). Methotrexate can cause painful mouth ulcers which occasionally involve also the oesophagus and small bowel (Decker, 1973).

Alopecia reflects involvement of the basal layer of the skin. It is very common with cyclophosphamide, affecting 90% of patients. Alopecia is rare with azathioprine and methotrexate and not observed with chlorambucil.

Bone marrow depression is a major danger, but again should not be exaggerated. All cytotoxic agents can depress marrow function, and the concentrations of formed elements in the blood are usually used as guides to dosage since the degree of marrow suppression is dose related and can be modulated by dose changes (Decker, 1973; Steinberg & Decker, 1979). Treatment over months or years is often accompanied by progressive marrow depression so that the dosage tolerated after 2 years is lower than in the first 6 months. This type of depression is most common with the alkylating agents and is usually reversible. Prolonged marrow depression is very rare. The problem of increased susceptibility to infection is not as great as that seen in transplant patients (Decker, 1973). Most of the observed infections have occurred in patients made unduly leucopenic (Steinberg & Decker, 1979).

Fever and skin rashes are not uncommon with azathioprine, but resolve promptly when the drug is stopped. Acute and readily reversible hepatitis has been caused by both azathioprine and 6-mercaptopurine, often accompanied by fever and rash. Methotrexate may cause liver fibrosis, more commonly when given in daily oral doses and this complication is potentiated by alcoholism (Dahl et al, 1972; Metzger et al, 1974). Rarely hepatic fibrosis has been attributed to azathioprine and cyclophosphamide (Pirofsky & Bardana, 1977). Pulmonary toxicity may occur with methotrexate. The syndrome includes fever, cough, dyspnoea, diffuse pulmonary infiltration and variable eosinophilia. This is not dose related. It is usually non-recurring and sometimes clears despite continuing the drug, though clearing is more rapid after temporary drug withdrawal (Schein & Winokur, 1975).

Chemical cystitis occurs in at least 20% of patients maintained on cyclophosphamide for 1 year and fibrosis may occur (Steinberg & Decker, 1979; Johnson & Meadows, 1971). This is due to cyclophosphamide metabolites and can be reduced by maintaining a diuresis (with a high fluid intake). The risk of bladder complications increases with duration of treatment; they can appear without warning even after the drug has been stopped (Schein & Winokur, 1975). Transitional cell carcinoma of the bladder is also increased in patients on cyclophosphamide therapy (Steinberg & Decker, 1979). The alkylating agents, cyclophosphamide and chlorambucil, damage germinal epithelium. The effect on spermatogenesis, presumably because of rapid turnover, is most profound (Schein & Winokur, 1975). Cyclophosphamide causes azospermia or oligospermia within a few weeks of initiating therapy. Cessation of therapy is followed by a return of spermatogenesis within 3 years in about 50% of patients (Griffin & Wilson, 1980). However azospermia may be permanent after only six months treatment (Decker, 1973). Methotrexate has little effect on spermatogenesis and the purine analogues have none (Steinberg & Decker, 1979).

Ovulation is suppressed in about 30% of women on cyclophosphamide (Kumar et al, 1972). Only occasional patients recover ovarian function after 6–12 months of amenorrhoea (Uldall et al, 1972). Neither methotrexate nor the purine analogues alter ovarian function.

Teratogenesis

Teratogenic effects have been observed with each of the cytotoxic drugs used in rheumatology. However normal children have also been born even when therapy was continued throughout the pregnancy (Decker, 1973; Schein & Winokur, 1975).

Decker (1973) suggests that pregnancy in patients on these drugs should be proscribed and suggests a four month delay between stopping the drug and permitting conception. Development of the fetus in a treated patient should be followed closely with the aid of amniocentesis and ultrasound. If obvious gross anomalies are detected termination should be offered.

Tumour induction

Over the last decade considerable evidence has accumulated suggesting that cytotoxic drugs can cause an increased incidence of malignancy, particularly when used for long periods. Most of the evidence is derived from studies of patients receiving organ transplants and more anecdotal evidence comes from the use of these drugs in rheumatic diseases.

A recent propective study of 3823 patients who had received a renal transplant and 1349 other patients receiving cytotoxic drugs showed no clear increase in the incidence of most of the common cancers (Kinlen et al, 1979). However, follow-up of the renal transplant patients showed an almost 60-fold increase of non-Hodgkin's lymphoma together with an excess of squamous cell skin cancer and mesenchymal tumours. The patients without transplants showed an excess of the same tumours, though to a lesser extent. This increased incidence of lymphoma needs to be balanced against the increase associated with autoimmune diseases such as Sjögren's syndrome, rheumatoid arthritis and SLE, for which the cytotoxic therapy is given (Hazleman & De Silva, 1982).

Drug interactions

It is unwise to give cytotoxic drugs with other drugs which may suppress the bone marrow, such as gold, penicillamine or phenylbutazone (Huskisson, 1978).

Drug interactions resulting in reduced clearance of cytotoxic drugs may result in increased toxicity. Thus patients on allopurinol which prevents the breakdown of azathioprine and 6-mercaptopurine to 6-thiouric acid should have the dose of these purine analogues reduced by 75% (Coffcy et al, 1972; Decker, 1973). There is evidence that allopurinol prolongs the plasma half-life of cyclophosphamide (Bagley et al, 1973) and this may explain the increased toxicity observed with this combination (Boston Collaborative Drug Surveillance Program, 1974).

Probenecid and other organic acids may decrease the tubular secretion of methotrexate and thus result in toxic plasma levels (Leigler et al, 1969). Drug assays for methotrexate utilising bacterial dihydrofolate reductase may give spuriously high results in patients taking trimethoprim which antagonises this enzyme.

PHYSICAL IMMUNOSUPPRESSIVE THERAPIES

Thoracic duct drainage

Drainage of thoracic duct lymphocytes has been shown to beneficially reduce the clinical activity of rheumatoid arthritis (Paulus et al, 1977). Synovitis was relieved for a mean period of three months following drainage. However thoracic duct cannulation is impracticable as a routine procedure and the transient nature of the response has not encouraged further application of this technique.

Leucophaeresis

Two studies have indicated clinical benefit (Karsh et al, 1979; Tenenbaum et al, 1979) following leucophaeresis in patients with rheumatoid arthritis. In addition a double blind study by Karsh et al (1981) demonstrated a small but statistically significant clinical response. However in a recent double blind study of combined lymphoplasmaphaeresis no beneficial response was detected (Wallace et al, 1982).

Radiotherapy

Two recent studies of total nodal irradiation in patients with unresponsive rheumatoid arthritis have reported a beneficial response which persisted for some months (Kotzin et al, 1982; Trentham et al, 1982). A controlled study is indicated. However, anxiety about the carcinogenicity of this treatment together with the practical difficulties of performing the therapy in patients with advanced rheumatoid arthritis make it unlikely that such treatment could become widely applied.

DISCUSSION

There is evidence that cytotoxic agents effectively control features of rheumatoid arthritis and retard radiological progression. However, toxicity and apprehension concerning the association with neoplasia limits use of these agents, often until after a substantial degree of joint destruction has already occurred.

The situation with regard to SLE appears much less clear, though cytotoxic agents are frequently employed in patients with severe disease. There is however reasonable evidence that both methotrexate and azathioprine are useful agents in patients with severe psoriatic arthritis.

Over the last decade a number of novel agents have been introduced for use in oncology and in patients with tissue transplants. In general these new agents have been developed with a view to greater specificity without increased toxicity and may have value in rheumatological applications. Cyclosporin A is of particular interest in this regard, as it specifically inhibits T cells (particularly helper T cells) while exerting minimal toxic effects on the bone marrow. This and similiar agents may result in better clinical efficacy with less toxicity than current cytotoxic agents.

IMMUNOMODULATORS

Numerous abnormalities of immune function have been demonstrated in patients with rheumatoid arthritis and systemic lupus erythematosus. The appreciation of these abnormalities has fostered the impression that immunological imbalance might be of pathogenic importance in these conditions.

The immune system has been increasingly revealed as a complex interaction of regulatory pathways and it is evident that inhibition of the system at one point (for instance with a cytotoxic agent) might indirectly result in enhancement of other immune functions, from which control has been removed. There are, however, a small number of recently described agents, of which levamisole is the prototype, which have been demonstrated to stimulate various immune functions, apparently in a direct fashion (and not by inhibiting a controlling factor). Such agents with predominantly stimulatory actions on the immune system have been termed 'immunomodulatory', in recognition of the fact that their use may result in depression of other immune functions.

The concept of pharmacological regulation of the immune system, by stimulation of immune functions, presents an exciting therapeutic approach to diseases which may be associated with immunological imbalance.

Such an opportunity has been presented over the last decade since initial observations that the potent anti-heliminthic agent, levamisole, exerted various actions on the immune system (reviewed by Symoens & Rosenthal, 1977). Subsequently this drug has been extensively investigated, providing an increasingly detailed understanding of the possibilities and problems associated with immunomodulatory therapy.

Rational application of immunomodulatory therapy is dependent on the elucidation of relevant immunoregulatory abnormalities towards which therapy might be directed. Abnormalities which are currently thought to be of possible significance will be briefly reviewed, though this subject is more fully covered in Chapter 11. Such immunomodulatory therapy as has been clinically employed has almost entirely concerned rheumatoid arthritis, and immunological abnormalities in this condition will be the main area of consideration.

IMMUNOLOGICAL ABNORMALITIES IN RHEUMATOID ARTHRITIS

There is evidence of decreased T cell function in patients with rheumatoid arthritis as indicated by reduced response to those skin test antigens which induce a delayed hypersensitivity reaction (Toh et al, 1973). In addition the majority of authors have reported a decreased response by lymphocytes from rheumatoid patients to T cell mitogens (usually PHA), particularly when suboptimal mitogen concentrations are used (Lance & Knight, 1974; Lockshin et al, 1975; Silverman et al, 1976; Levy & Miller, 1976). Further evidence of abnormal T cell function is provided by the observation that T cells from rheumatoid patients are defective in their ability to inhibit the growth of Epstein-Barr virus-transformed B cells (Torsato et al, 1981).

In active rheumatoid arthritis an increased proportion of 'null' lymphocytes has been observed (Froland et al, 1973; Meijer et al, 1982) and recent analysis of T cell subsets, using monoclonal antibodies, has demonstrated a reduced proportion of OKT8 (suppressor/cytotoxic) cells in the peripheral blood (Veys et al, 1982).

In animal models, decreased T cell function is recognised to result in B cell hyperfunction, with increased immunoglobulin and autoantibody production (Yunis et al, 1967; Allison et al, 1971; Morse et al, 1974). A similar situation may pertain in rheumatoid arthritis where there is B cell hyperfunction; as evidenced by increased immunoglobulin turnover (Levy et al, 1970), high levels of serum IgG (though the rise is not uniform and values frequently fall within the normal range) (Barden et al, 1967; Marcolongo et al, 1967), rheumatoid factor production and plasma cell infiltration of the synovium.

Recognition of this immunological inbalance suggests two approaches to therapy. Firstly B cell activity may be inhibited by a cytotoxic agent such as cyclophosphamide, or alternatively an attempt may be made to enhance the depressed T cell function. It is this latter approach which has led to the introduction of immunomodulators as a therapeutic option in rheumatoid arthritis.

Levamisole

Levamisole, the levo-isomer of tetramisole (2,3,5,6-tetrahydro-6-phenylimidazo(2,1-b)thiazole hydrochloride), is a compound developed for its powerful antihelminthic properties (Thienpont et al, 1966). It is a selective inhibitor of mammalian alkaline phosphatases, with the exception of intestinal and human placental isoenzymes (Van Belle, 1976). Structurally levamisole is a heterocyclic, sulphur-containing compound which, on hydrolysis, possesses a free sulphydryl group.

Immunological activity

Levamisole has been shown to exert numerous effects on immune functions including: enhancement of delayed hypersensitivity (Szpilman et al, 1976; Dieppe et al, 1976); lymphocyte response to

T cell mitogens, both in vitro and in vivo (Levy & Miller, 1976; Hadden et al, 1975); macrophage phagocytosis and listericidal activity (Symoens & Rosenthal, 1977); neutrophil phagocytosis (De Cree et al, 1978; Verhaegen et al, 1973; Molin & Stendahl, 1977); clearance of colloidal particles by the reticuloendothelial system (Verhaegen et al, 1973; Hoebeke & Franchi, 1973).

In animal models of autoimmune disease levamisole has been shown to enhance the secondary lesions of adjuvant arthritis in rats (Dieppe et al, 1976; Trabert et al, 1976) and reduce the rate of progression of the 'systemic lupus erythematosus-like' disease which occurs spontaneously in NZB/W mice (Russell, 1976).

In man treatment with levamisole has been demonstrated to restore numbers of (T)lymphocytes forming rosettes with sheep red blood cells, in those patients initially found to have low numbers of such cells, in both Hodgkin's disease (Ramot et al, 1976) and rheumatoid arthritis (Basch et al, 1977; Di Perri et al, 1978). This restoration in the number of lymphocytes forming rosettes has been observed to persist for about 1 week, following a single dose of levamisole, in rheumatoid arthritis. Delayed hypersensitivity reactions to a variety of test substances have been restored by levamisole therapy when they have been depressed as a result of age (Symoens & Rosenthal, 1977), cancer (Brugmans et al, 1973) or rheumatoid arthritis (Basch et al, 1977; Rosenthal et al, 1976; Runge et al, 1977; Huskisson et al, 1976). The elevated numbers of 'null' lymphocytes associated with active rheumatoid arthritis have been seen to fall significantly in patients undergoing levamisole therapy (Rosenthal et al, 1976), and enhancement of the lymphocyte response to T cell mitogens has also been observed in such patients, particularly in the period shortly after the initiation of levamisole treatment (Scheinberg et al, 1978; Levy & Miller, 1976).

Mode of action

Review of the reported immunological effects of levamisole reveals a large number of conflicting results. Any real understanding of actions of levamisole must to some extent explain these conflicts.

In experiments employing an antigenic challenge great variation in the immune response is observed when levamisole is administered at various times in relation to the challenge; this variation ranges from marked potentiation to inhibition of the immune response (Renoux & Renoux, 1974). Similarly immune functions enhanced by a single dose of levamisole have been shown to become suppressed by repeated dosing (Verhaegen et al, 1973; Renoux & Renoux, 1974; Trabert et al, 1976; Dieppe et al, 1976).

The response to levamisole has been seen to vary between different strains of mice (Renoux et al, 1980) and similar variation might occur in other species, including man. This suggestion is supported by the observation that levamisole is extensively metabolised in the liver by various pathways, some of which include enzymes prone to genetic variation (Renoux, 1980).

In addition to the factors already considered, the pretreatment immunological status of the subject is another source of variation in the immune response. In this respect the age and sex are important factors, as is general debility, whether this is a result of a disease state or other factors such as starvation.

Further attempts to reconcile the rather conflicting findings of some studies have focused on the immunological activities of the various parts of the levamisole molecule. At least two groups within the levamisole molecule have been identified, each possessing distinctive actions on the immune system. The first group relates to the sulphur-containing moiety; this has been shown to induce the development of a serum factor which promotes the acquisition of T cell surface markers by thymocytes (indicating an enhancement of maturation). This effect is even apparent in athymic nu/nu mice and the factor generated in these mice by levamisole therapy is able, in vitro, to induce the development of T cell markers in human thymocytes (Renoux & Renoux, 1977). The factor is without action on B cells or their precursors and apparently affects the T cells by acting at a surface receptor. This action of levamisole on thymocytes has led to a comparison being made with thymopoietin, and to the suggestion that levamisole might act as a synthetic substitute for this factor (Goldstein, 1978).

The second active group of levamisole resides in

the imidazole ring. This structure has cholinergic activity and can be shown to alter intracellular cyclic nucleotide levels, seemingly in a direct fashion without the mediation of a surface receptor. Cyclic-GMP levels are increased while cyclic-AMP levels are decreased. This change in the cyclic nucleotide balance promotes cellular proliferative activity (Hadden, 1977), while inhibiting maturation (Scheid et al, 1978). Imidazole does not induce the development of T cell markers or enhance delayed hypersensitivity reactions in vivo (Renoux, 1980). These two immunologically active groups may have antagonistic effects and the overall result may represent a balance between these effects. Such a balance suggests a further source of variation in the response to levamisole.

In summary immunological actions of levamisole which might be of clinical significance in rheumatology include enhancement of T cell maturation and function and inhibition of B cell maturation may also be important. There is however a possibility that clinical efficacy of levamisole in rheumatoid arthritis might be unrelated to its actions on the immune system. In this context it is pertinent to recall that the rationales which supported the introduction of both gold (Forestier, 1935) and D-penicillamine (Ritzmann et al, 1960) to the treatment of rheumatoid arthritis have subsequently proved to be unfounded.

The sulphur-containing ring of the levamisole molecule may be cleaved to form OPMI (dl-2-oxo-3-(2-mercaptoethyl)-5-phenylimidazolidine). This compound has a free sulphydryl group, as occurs in D-penicillamine, which has been demonstrated to act as a scavenger of free radicals and to react with tubulin sulphydrals (DeBrabander et al, 1978). It has been suggested that this effect might be responsible for the effect of levamisole in rheumatoid arthritis.

Isoprinosine

Isoprinosine is a synthetic purine derivative which has been shown to potentiate the lymphocyte response to both T and B cell mitogens (Hadden et al, 1976; Morin et al, 1980) and also to promote T cell differentiation (as indicated by the generation of T cell surface markers) both in vivo and in vitro (Touraine et al, 1979). The mechanism of action of isoprinosine is unclear; the enhancement of the mitogenic response does not appear to be related to intracellular cyclic nucleotide changes (Hadden et al, 1976). nor the T cell maturing action to the generation of a mediating serum factor.

DTC

Diethyldithiocarbamate (DTC) is a simple sulphur-containing compound which also appears to possess a very low potential for toxicity. DTC enhances T cell mitogen reactions and promotes T cell surface marker generation in vivo, but is inactive in vitro. In vivo DTC appears to lack any direct action on cells of the B cell lineage. The T cell maturing action of DTC is mediated by a serum factor similar to that associated with levamisole therapy (Renoux & Renoux, 1980).

The putative mechanism of action of a number of immunostimulant agents is illustrated in Table 21.1.

D-Penicillamine

It has been suggested that D-penicillamine acts in rheumatoid arthritis by virtue of an immunosuppressive action (Mowat & Huskisson, 1975). However this agent has also been shown to have various stimulatory actions on immune functions. Enhancement of the delayed hypersensitivity reaction has been achieved by D-penicillamine administration to experimental animals (Bramm et al, 1979), though very high doses appeared inhibitory. Using *Bordetella pertussis* to induce delayed hypersensitivity, in rats both enhancement and inhibition of the reaction have been observed, depending on the timing of D-penicillamine administration (Arrigoni-Martelli & Bramm, 1976; Dieppe et al, 1976), a finding which closely parallels the behaviour of levamisole in this model (Arrigoni-Martelli et al, 1977). Enhancement of the response was observed when D-penicillamine was administered at the time of sensitisation or challenge, while inhibition was most consistently produced when therapy was commenced prior to sensitisation and continued up to the time of challenge. D-penicillamine has been shown to enhance the lymphocyte response to mitogens, when administered to rats with adjuvant arthritis (Binderup et al, 1980). In patients with rheuma-

Table 21.1 Actions of various immunomodulators on T cells

Agent	Mediator	Surface receptor	Intracellular cyclic nucleotide change	Result
Thymopoietin	–	T cell receptor (prothymocyte) T cell receptor (peripheral T cell)	cAMP cGMP	Induction of T cells Functional stimulation of T cells
Levamisole (sulphur group)	Serum factor	T cell receptor	cAMP	Induction of T cells
Diethyldithiocarbamate (DTC)	Serum factor	T cell receptor	cAMP	Induction of T cells
Levamisole (imidazole group)	–	–	cGMP	Functional stimulation of T cells Inhibition of maturation
Isoprinosine	–	–	No change shown	Induction of T cells Functional stimulation of T cells

toid arthritis restoration of the lymphocyte response to mitogens has been observed in patients treated with D-penicillamine (Maini & Roffe, 1976; Percy et al, 1978) and a similar effect has been observed during D-penicillamine treatment of Wilson's disease (Czlonowska, 1977). These responses occurred after long-term therapy (3 months or more) and the improvement may be, to some extent, associated with restoration of general health attributable to the treatment (rather than a primary effect of D-penicillamine on the lymphocytes).

Similarly delayed hypersensitivity reactions to skin test antigens have been seen to improve following D-penicillamine therapy (Huskisson, 1977; Zilko et al, 1977) and in Wilson's disease the delayed reaction to the sensitiser DNCB has improved following prolonged D-penicillamine therapy (Czlonkowska, 1977).

In contrast to immunosuppressive agents D-penicillamine has been shown to enhance the secondary lesions of adjuvant arthritis (Arrigoni-Martelli & Bramm, 1975; Willoughby & Dieppe, 1976). It may be concluded that D-penicillamine does exert stimulatory effects on some immunological functions particularly with reference to T cells, such effects are clearly demonstrated in animal models but in rheumatoid arthritis some of the demonstrated enhancement of depressed immune functions might be secondary to alleviation of the underlying disease state by the penicillamine therapy. The evidence supports the concept that penicillamine possesses significant immunostimulatory capability and might justifiably be classed an immunomodulator.

Thymic factors

The thymus has been shown to elaborate a number of polypeptides which exert various effects on the immune system (Goldstein et al, 1974; Low & Goldstein, 1979). Evidence that the major mechanism by which the thymus regulates immune function is humoral has been provided by Osoba & Miller (1964) who demonstrated maintenance of thymic-dependent immune function when thymectomised mice were grafted with thymic tissue contained within cell-impermeable chambers. Purification of thymic extracts has revealed numerous peptides (Table 21.2) and examination of some of these has revealed a lack of homology both with respect to structure and function. It appears that different thymic factors might regulate the various stages of lymphocyte maturation and examples of this specificity have been reported. Thymosin-α^1 has been shown (in mice) to be a potent inducer of T cells of the helper/inducer subset and to powerfully enhance E-rosette formation, while thymosin-α^7 appears to induce suppressor function (Low et al, 1979).

Partially purified thymic preparations act on the

Table 21.2 Thymus factors and thymus-derived serum factors

Factor	Prominent action	Reference
Thymosin (syn. fraction 5) more than 30 polypeptides including:		Low et al, 1979
Thymosin-α^1	Helper/inducer cell induction	
Thymosin-α^7	Suppressor/cytotoxic T cell induction	
Thymosin-β^1	No activity demonstrated	
Thymosin-β^3	?Induction of prothymocytes from stem cells	
Thymosin-β^4	?Induction of prothymocytes from skin cells	
Thymopoietin	Neuromuscular conduction inhibition	Goldstein, 1974
Factor thymique sérique (FTS)	Enhanced cell-mediated cytotoxicity	Bach et al, 1974
Various other factors as yet functionally ill-defined		

immune system in vitro and in vivo, both in animal models and in immunodeficient humans, but detailed analysis of these results is probably not of great value in view of the heterogeneity of the factors employed in each study. However a number of factors have now been sequenced and synthesised which will enable precise definition of the actions of the different factors on the immune system. Synthesis also promises to provide ample supplies of peptides with uniform biological activity for clinical application. Thymopoietin is an example of such a factor which has now been synthesised.

Thymopoietin has been highly purified (Goldstein, 1974), the constituent 49 amino acids sequenced (Schlesinger & Goldstein, 1975) and a pentapeptide (arginyl-lysyl-aspartyl-valyl-tyrosine) synthesised which corresponds to the 32–36 residues of thymopoietin and retains the activity of the whole factor on the immune system (Goldstein et al, 1979).

Thymopoietin has been shown to induce T cell maturation in vitro and in vivo and to enhance the response to peripheral T cells to allogenic stimulation (Sunshine et al, 1978). A cyclic-AMP second signal has been implicated in the transmission of the inductive signal in prothymocytes (promoting maturation) and cyclic-GMP as a second signal mediating functional enhancement in peripheral T cells. In contrast to the effect on T cell maturation, thymopoietin inhibits B cell maturation (Scheid et al, 1978).

Thymopoietin affects neuromuscular transmission — this led to the investigation of the relationship between this factor and the neuromuscular disease myasthenia gravis. The isolation of thymopoietin resulted from these studies. The neuromuscular effects of thymopoietin appear unique to this agent and have not been associated with the other thymic factors (Goldstein, 1974).

Thymopotein levels have been observed to decline with age (Lewis et al, 1978), which may be related to the deficiency of cell-mediated immune reactions in aged individuals.

In patients with rheumatoid arthritis the synthetic thymopoietin fragment (TP5) has been shown to restore the percentage of lymphocytes forming rosettes with sheep red blood cells (E-rosettes), both in vivo and in vitro.

In vivo the action of TP5 on rosetting was seen to persist up to 7 days after a single dose (DiPerri et al, 1978, 1980), though the half-life of TP5 after intravenous injection is extremely short (about 30 seconds) (Tischio et al, 1979).

Gold compounds

Despite the extended period over which gold compounds have been used in clinical medicine, the mode of action of these agents remains unclear. It has been suggested that these agents are immunosuppressive, an impression that is supported by the observation that gold thiomalate (GST) inhibits the development of the secondary lesions of adjuvant arthritis and inhibits the in vitro response of lymphocytes to mitogens by virtue of an action on monocyte-macrophages, which appear to serve an accessory function (Lipsky & Ziff, 1977).

Though there is some evidence of enhancement

of various immune functions both in experimental animals and patients treated with gold salts, the evidence suggests that the mechanism of action of these agents is predominantly suppressive.

CLINICAL PROPERTIES OF LEVAMISOLE AND THYMOPOIETIN IN RHEUMATOID ARTHRITIS

Levamisole

Levamisole has been very thoroughly investigated in rheumatoid arthritis. It was first used in a dose of 150 mg daily and shown to be an effective penicillamine-like drug. It soon became apparent that there were major differences in efficacy and toxicity of different dosage regimes and these are summarised in Table 21.3.

Efficacy

In the first reported controlled trial of levamisole, Huskisson et al (1976) showed that the drug was superior to placebo and comparable in efficacy to penicillamine. The time course of the action of the drug was similar to that of penicillamine with a plateau effect achieved after 4–6 months of treatment. These findings were confirmed in a large multicentre study carried out under the auspices of the European League against Rheumatism (Multi-Centre Study Group, 1978). In these studies levamisole relieved pain, reduced the duration of morning stiffness, articular index and other clinical criteria as well as reducing ESR and the titre of rheumatoid factor. There was also a demonstrable reduction in the need for symptomatic remedies including corticosteroids. The Multi-Centre Study Group (1982) compared single weekly doses of 50 and 150 mg using historical placebo data from the previous study. A single weekly dose of 150 mg was clearly superior to a single weekly dose of 50 mg in most clinical measures, though 50 mg weekly was superior to placebo in some of the measures. Combining the results of the two studies, carried out by the Multi-Centre Study Group using the same investigators and methods, it seems that the optimal dosage of levamisole is 150 mg weekly. 50 mg weekly is clearly less effective. The use of 150 mg on 3 or 7 days of each week produces little if any increase in efficacy.

Side-effects

While the different dosage regimens of levamisole may make little difference to its efficacy in rheumatoid arthritis, they profoundly influence the frequency and nature of adverse reactions. The toxicity of levamisole has been dominated by three side-effects — neutropenia, vasculitis and reactions which follow the administration of a single dose. Neutropenia has been reported in 5–10% of patients treated with levamisole in a dose of 150 mg daily on either 3 or 7 days of each week.

Williams et al (1978) reported 6 cases out of 60 treated for up to 2 years with levamisole. In these cases the neutrophil level fell to less than 1×10^9 cells/l after a period of 1–23 months of treatment. Smaller falls occurred in some patients and there was a trend towards falling white blood counts in the group as a whole. In some cases neutropenia

Table 21.3 Comparison of penicillamine and different dosage regimens of levamisole which have been used in rheumatoid arthritis

	Pencillamine	Levamisole, 150 mg per week × 7 days	Levamisole, 150 mg per week × 3 days	Levamisole, 150 mg in single weekly dose	Levamisole, 50 mg in single weekly dose
Effectiveness	+++	+++	+++	+++	+
Neutropenia	0	++	++	+	0
Vasculitis	0	++	+	0	0
'Reactions'	0	0	+	++	++
Proteinuria	++	0	0	0	0
Loss of taste, etc.	+	0	0	0	0
Withdrawals	+	+++	+++	+	+

was asymptomatic while in others it was associated with fever or mouth ulceration. There were no changes in haemoglobin or platelet levels. In one patient, the neutrophil count recovered while treatment was continued and in the remaining patients it recovered within 10 days of stopping treatment.

Bone marrow findings were variable, sometimes normal and sometimes showing promyelocyte arrest. None of these 6 patients were HLA-B27-positive, but in other studies neutropenia has been found to be more frequent in women with positive tests for rheumatoid factor and HLA-B27 (Veys & Mielants 1977).

Neutropenia is a serious complication and fatalities have occurred. The neutrophil count appears to reach a nadir 8–14 hours after levamisole administration, generally recovering over the next 24 hours. 'Flu-like' symptoms may be associated. Neutropenia appears less common with once weekly treatment (Veys & Mielants, 1977). Vasculitis is another serious reaction which has been described in patients receiving levamisole on 3 or 7 days each week for some months. Typical lesions appear on the lower limb and may be multiple. Very extensive lesions and ulceration may occur, requiring skin grafting. Rashes of other clinical types have been described in association with levamisole therapy including urticaria occurring early in the course of treatment, erythematous and lichenoid eruptions.

Reactions to intermittent dosage of levamisole were discovered only when the drug was given on 3 days of each week, and were found to be commoner when the drug was given weekly. The reactions were often associated with fever and flu-like symptoms, sometimes also of shivering, myalgia, arthralgia, malaise, headaches, chest pains, flushing and nausea. These reactions usually occur repeatedly with each exposure to the drug and if severe will demand withdrawal of treatment.

Various other side-effects have been reported in patients receiving levamisole. Some are apparently associated with cerebral stimulation and they include insomnia, sensory stimulation and a hyper-alert state. Gastrointestinal problems are unusual with the drug. As with other drugs of this class, side-effects are much more common in patients with rheumatoid arthritis than in those with other diseases. Neutropenia and rashes in particular are much commoner in patients treated for rheumatoid arthritis than those treated for cancer.

Indications and management

Levamisole is a useful alternative to drugs like penicillamine and gold in the treatment of rheumatoid arthritis which has either failed to respond to or progressed despite non-steroidal anti-inflammatory drugs. Levamisole has not been approved for use in rheumatoid arthritis, although it is already available in many countries for the treatment of worm infestation. Because of the optimal dosage regime of 150 mg in a single weekly dose, the drug is substantially cheaper than others of its class and may therefore have particular application in underdeveloped countries.

Patients selected for levamisole therapy should first be established on an optimal regime of analgesic anti-inflammatory drugs. Some assessment of the disease should be carried out before the start of treatment as a reference point for further assessments. Levamisole should then be introduced in a single weekly dose of 150 mg. A full blood count including differential should be carried out approximately 12 hours after each single weekly dose; the intervals between blood counts can be relaxed as treatment continues but should never exceed 4 weeks.

Perhaps the most important aspect of the monitoring of levamisole therapy is that the patient should be able to contact the physician in the event of some unusual occurrence. Disasters have been most likely to occur in patients given inappropriate treatment for complications of levamisole therapy by doctors who are not aware of the nature of the reaction. Patients who respond well to levamisole therapy should continue the drug indefinitely.

Thymopoietin

The clinical effects of the synthetic pentapeptide of thymopoietin closely resemble those of weekly levamisole.

Thrower et al (1982) reported 6 months experience with thymopoietin in a dose of 50 mg intravenously each week in rheumatoid arthritis. The drug was compared with levamisole and penicillamine. Efficacy was comparable to that of levamisole (150 mg weekly) and penicillamine, though reduction in ESR was small and there were no significant changes in rheumatoid factor. The time course of the response to thymopoietin was similar to that of penicillamine and levamisole. Two minor skin rashes occurred, but there were no serious reactions. Veys et al (1982) compared intravenous and intramuscular injection with placebo. Intramuscular thymopoietin in a single weekly dose of 1 mg was not superior to placebo while intravenous thymopoietin 50 mg weekly produced clinical effects comparable to those of gold or penicillamine. Side-effects were minor.

Though thymopoietin was introduced with the thought that it would reproduce the effects of levamisole, the effect in the individual patients did not support the view of a common mode of action. Thrower et al (1982) found that patients reacted very differently in terms of both efficacy and side-effects of thymopoietin and levamisole. Thymopoietin is a potentially useful approach to the treatment of rheumatoid arthritis. The major drawback at the present time is the need to give the drug by intravenous injection and further development should await the availability of a more convenient mode of administration.

Levamisole in the treatment of rheumatic diseases other than rheumatoid arthritis

In addition to rheumatoid arthritis levamisole has been used to treat other rheumatic diseases in which immunological functions have been shown to be abnormal or in which immunological factors have been thought to be important.

Systemic lupus erythematosus

Significant clinical improvement has been recorded in patients with systemic lupus erythematosus treated with levamisole in open studies (Gordon & Yanagihara, 1977; Rovensky et al, 1982). In the latter study levamisole was administered in a dose of 150 mg once weekly, while more frequent dosing was employed by Gordon & Yangihara. Laboratory parameters which have been noted to improve in patients on levamisole therapy include the responsiveness of lymphocytes to PHA (Smolen et al, 1977), numbers of E-rosette-forming cells (when numbers are initially low) and serum complement levels (Rovensky et al, 1982). However in a double blind study of levamisole (150 mg, once weekly) in active systemic lupus erythematosus no benefit was observed (Hadidi et al, 1981).

It must be concluded that the role of levamisole in the therapy of systemic lupus erythematosus remains unclear.

Ankylosing spondylitis

Significant improvement was reported in patients with ankylosing spondylarthritis treated with levamisole (three times weekly) in a double blind study (Goebel et al, 1977). In this study the majority of cases had classical ankylosing spondylitis; however, patients with chronic Reiter's disease or psoriatic arthritis were also included.

Behçet's disease

In two open studies of levamisole treatment of Behçet's disease, in which various dosage frequencies were used, benefit has been reported (de Merieux et al, 1981; Hamza et al, 1982).

Other diseases

Levamisole has been administered to small numbers of patients with other rheumatic diseases, including scleroderma, polymyositis and juvenile chronic arthritis. The results are generally conflicting and the numbers preclude any statistical evaluation of the results. Now that levamisole has dropped from favour it is unlikely that larger studies designed to determine the efficacy of this agent in conditions other than rheumatoid arthritis will be performed. It is to be hoped that should future immunomodulatory agents be evaluated, standard dosage frequencies will be administered to adequate numbers of patients with uniform diagnoses in order that meaningful conclusions can be reached.

DISCUSSION

Over the past decade numerous immunological abnormalities have been demonstrated in patients with rheumatoid arthritis, particularly during active phases. The possibility exists that some abnormalities of immune function might be of pathogenic significance. On the basis that the immune system embodies a complex network of regulatory circuits it has been thought preferable to restore immunological balance by stimulating natural control mechanisms rather than employing toxic agents which directly suppress a hyperactive immune system (e.g. cytotoxic agents).

To date only one synthetic agent with a clear ability to stimulate deficient immune functions has been widely employed clinically; this agent is levamisole. Levamisole has not proved a particularly satisfactory agent in rheumatological practice because of its side-effects. However levamisole is clinically effective and enhances various immune functions in treated rheumatoid patients. The clinical toxicity associated with levamisole therapy has to some extent been overestimated due to the high incidence of side-effects which were associated with the continuous therapy initially employed. Future developments should provide immunostimulant agents with low toxicity, and more potency than levamisole. Approaches towards this end include: attempted elucidation of the pathological significance of abnormalities of immune function in rheumatoid arthritis; clarification of those immunological actions of levamisole which might be of relevance to its clinical activity; attempts to relate the structural configurations of immunomodulatory agents with their actions on the immune system.

The dosage interval and optimal dose of levamisole has proved difficult to determine, particularly because it is unclear which immunological parameter should be monitored. However the recent introduction of monoclonal antibodies has permitted the observation of changes in populations of various subsets of immune cells; analysis of these changes may facilitate rational application of immunomodulatory therapy.

Levamisole has provided evidence that immunomodulation might offer a useful therapeutic approach to rheumatoid arthritis. As the prototype it is unlikely to be the optimal example of an agent of its type and it is reasonable to anticipate that the second generation of drugs of this type will be more effective in clinical use and will be associated with less toxicity.

REFERENCES

Allison A C, Denman A M, Barnes R D 1971 Co-operating and controlling functions of thymus derived lymphocytes in relation to autoimmunity. Lancet 2: 135–148

Amor B, Mery C 1980 Chlorambucil in Rheumatoid Arthritis. In: Huskisson E C (ed) Antirheumatic Drugs. II. Clinics in Rheumatic Diseases 6: 567–584

Amor B, Kahan A, Pompidou A, et al 1972 Efficacy of immunosuppression in systemic lupus erythematosus. Comparison of a series of 13 cases and 12 controls. Nouvelle Presse Medicale 1: 1699–1702

Arnett F C, Whelton C, Zizic T M, Stevens M B 1973 Methotrexate therapy in polymyositis. Annals of the Rheumatic Diseases 32: 536–546

Arrigoni-Martelli E, Bramm E 1975 Investigations on the influence of cyclophosphamide, gold sodium thiomalate and d-penicillamine on nyustalin oedema and adjuvant arthritis. Agents and Actions 5: 264–267

Arrigoni-Martelli E, Bramm E 1976 Development of models for penicillamine like drugs. Rheumatology and Rehabilitation 15: 207–210

Arrigoni-Martelli E, Bramm E, Binderup L 1977 Immunostimulant activity of d-penicillamine. Drugs Experimental and Clinical Research 2: 189–195

Bagley C M, Bostick F W, DeVita V T 1973 Clinical pharmacology of cyclophosphamide. Cancer Research 33: 226–233

Barden J, Franklin M, Waller M 1967 Immunoglobulin levels in rheumatoid arthritis: comparison with rheumatoid factor titres, clinical stage and disease. Arthritis and Rheumatism 10: 228–234

Bach R S, Goldstein G 1974 Induction of T-cell differentiation invitro by thymin, a purified polypeptide hormone of the thymus. Proceedings of the National Academy of Science USA 71: 1474–1478

Basch C M, Spitler L E, Engleman E G, Engleman E P 1977 Cellular immune reactivity in patients with rheumatoid arthritis and effects of levamisole. Journal of Rheumatology 4: 377–388

Baum J, Hurd E, Lewis D, Ferguson J L, Ziff M 1973 Treatment of psoriatic arthritis with 6-Mercaptopurine. Arthritis and Rheumatism 16: 139–147

Beck W S 1973 Haematology Harvard Pathophysiology Series, Volume 1. pp. 113–138 The Massachusetts Institute of Technology Press, USA

Benson M D, Aldo M A 1973 Azathioprine in polymyositis. Archives of Internal Medicine 132: 547–551

Bertino J R 1963 The mechanism of action of folate antagonists in man. Cancer Research 23: 1286–1306

Bertino J R 1973 Chemical Action and Pharmacology of methotrexate, azathioprine and cyclophosphamide in man. Arthritis and Rheumatism 16: 79–83

Bertino J R 1977 'Rescue' techniques in cancer chemotherapy: Use of leucovorin and other rescue agents after methotrexate treatment. Seminars in Oncology 4: 203–216

Binderup L, Bramm E, Arrigoni-Martelli E 1980 D-penicillamine in vivo enhances lymphocyte DNA synthesis: Role of macrophages. Scandinavian Journal of Immunology 11: 23–28

Black R L, O'Brien W M, Van Scott E J, Auerbach R, Eisen A Z, Bunim J J 1964 Methotrexate therapy in psoriatic arthritis; double blind study on 21 patients. Journal of the

American Medical Association 189: 743–747
Bohan A, Peter J B 1975 Polymyositis and dermatomyositis. The New England Journal of Medicine 292: 403–407
Boston Collaborative Drug Surveillance Program 1974 Allopurinol and cytotoxic drugs. Journal of the American Medical Association 227: 1036–1040
Bramm E, Binderup L, Arrigoni-Martelli E 1979 Delayed hypersensitivity to tuberculin in rats: Effects of antirheumatic drugs. Acta Pharmacology and Toxicology 44: 75–80
Brugmans J, Schuermans V, De Cock W, Thienpont D, Janssen P, Verhaegen H, Van Nimmen L, Louwagie A C, Stevens E 1973 Restoration of host defense mechanisms in man by levamisole. Life Sciences 13: 1499–1504
Bunch T W 1981 Prednisone and azathioprine for polymyositis. Long-term followup. Arthritis and Rheumatism 24: 45–48
Bunch T W, Worthington J W, Combs J J, Ilstrup D M, Engel A G 1980 Azathioprine with prednisone for polymyositis. Annals of Internal Medicine 92: 365–369
Cade R, Spooner G, Schlein E, et al 1973 Comparison of azathioprine, prednisone and heparin alone or combined in treating lupus nephitis. Nephron 10: 37–56
Calabresi P, Parks R E 1980 Antiproliferative agents and drugs used for immunosuppression. In: Gilman A G, Goodman L S, Gilman A (eds) The pharmacological basis of therapeutics, 6th edn. MacMillan, New York, p 1256
Cameron J S, Boulton-Jones M, Robinson R, Ogg C 1970 Treatment of lupus nephritis with cyclophosphamide. Lancet 2: 846–849
Chanmougan D, Schwartz R F S 1966 Enhancement of antibody synthesis by 6-mercaptopurine. Journal of Experimental Medicine 124: 363–378
Christophidis N, Huskisson E C 1982 Methotrexate therapy in steroid resistant polymyositis. A clinical and pharmacokinetic study (abstract). Annals of the Rheumatic Diseases 41:315
Coffey J J, White C A, Lesk A B, Rogers W I, Serpick A A 1972 Effect of allopurinol on the pharmacokinetics of 6-mercaptopurine (NSC 755) in cancer patients. Cancer Research 32: 1283–1289
Co-operating Clinics of the American Rheumatism Association 1970 A controlled trial of cyclophosphamide in rheumatoid arthritis. New England Journal of Medicine 283: 883–889
Currey H L F 1971 Immunosuppressive drugs in rheumatoid arthritis. In: Hill D F (ed) Modern trends in rheumatology, volume 2. Butterworths, London, pp. 174–198
Currey H L F, Harris J, Mason R M, Woodland J, Beveridge T, Roberts C J, Vere D W, St J Dixon A, Davies J, Owen-Smith B 1974 Comparison of azathioprine, cyclophosphamide and gold in treatment of rheumatoid arthritis. British Medical Journal 3: 763–766
Czlonkowska A 1977 The influence of prolonged treatment with d-penicillamine on the immunological response in Wilson's disease. European Journal of Clinical Pharmacology 12: 265–271
Dahl M G C, Gregory M M, Scheuer P J 1972 Methotrexate hepatotoxicity in psoriasis — Comparison of different dose regimens. British Medical Journal 1: 654–656
De Brabander M, Aerts F, Geuens G, Van Ginckel R, Van de Veire R, Van Belle H 1978 DL-2-oxo-3-(2-mercaptoethyl)-5-phenylimidazolidine. A sulphydryl metabolite of levamisole that reacts with microtubules. Chemical Biological Interactions 23: 45–63
de Merieux P, Spitler L E, Paulus H E 1981 Treatment of Behçet's syndrome with levamisole. Arthritis and Rheumatism 24: 64–70
Decker J L 1982 The management of systemic lupus erythematosus. Arthritis and Rheumatism 25: 891–894
Decker J L, Klippel J H, Plotz P H, Steinberg A D 1975 Cyclophosphamide or azathioprine in lupus glomerulonephritis. A controlled trial: Results at 28 months. Annals of Internal Medicine 83: 606–615
Decker J L 1973 Toxicity of immunosuppressive drugs in man. Arthritis and Rheumatism 16: 89–91
De Cree J, Emmery L, Timmermans J, Eeckels R, De Cock W, Verhaegen H 1978 Defective neutrophil chemotaxis and raised serum-IgE levels in a child with recurrent bacterial infections and eczema. The influence of levamisole. Archives of Disease in Childhood 53: 144–149
Denman A M 1982 Immunosuppression and the rheumatic diseases. Annals of the Rheumatic Diseases 41 (suppl): 3–8
Dieppe P A, Willoughby D A, Huskisson E C, Arrigoni-Martelli E 1976 Pertussis vaccine pleurisy: A model of delayed hypersensitivity. Agents and Actions 6: 618–621
Dieppe P A, Willoughby D A, Stevens C, Kirby J D, Huskisson E C 1976 Specific therapy in new and conventional animal models. Rheumatology and Rehabilitation 15: 201–206
DiPerri T, Auteri A, Pasini F L, Mattioli F 1978 A weekly oral dose of levamisole in the treatment of rheumatoid arthritis associated with E-rosette lymphocyte reduction. European Journal of Rheumatology 1: 155–164
DiPerri T, Pasini F L, Auteri A 1980 Immunokinetics of a single dose of thymopoietin pentapeptide. Journal of Immunopharmacology 2: 567–572
Dixon F J, McConahey P J 1963 Enhancement of antibody formation by whole body X-radiation. Journal of Experimental Medicine 117: 833–848
Donadio J V, Holley K E, Wagoner R D, Ferguson R H, McDuffie F C 1972 Treatment of patients with lupus nephritis with prednisone and combined prednisone-azathioprine. Annals of Internal Medicine 77: 829–835
Donadio J V, Holley K E, Wagoner R D, Ferguson R H, McDuffie F C 1974 Further observations on the treatment of lupus nephritis with prednisone and azathioprine. Arthritis and Rheumatism 17: 573–581
Donadio J V, Holley K E, Ferguson R H, Ilstrup D M 1978 Treatment of diffuse proliferative lupus nephritis with prednisone or combined prednisone and cyclophosphamide. The New England Journal of Medicine 299: 1151–1155
Drinkard J P, Stanley T M, Dornfield L, Austin R C, Barnett E V, Pearson C M, Vernier R L, Adams D A, Latta H, Gornick H C 1970 Azathioprine and prednisone in the treatment of adults with lupus nephritis. Medicine (Baltimore) 49: 411–432
El-Ghobarey A, Balint G, DeCeulaer K, Dick W C, Buchanan W W 1978 Dermatomyositis: observations on the use of immunosuppressive therapy and a review of the literature. Postgraduate Medical Journal 54: 516–527
Epstein W V, Grausz H 1974 Favourable outcome in diffuse proliferative glomerulonephritis of systemic lupus erythematosus. Arthritis and Rheumatism 17: 129–141
Feldges D H, Barnes C G 1974 Treatment of psoriatic arthropathy with either azathioprine or methotrexate. Rheumatology and Rehabilitation 13: 120–124
Feng P H, Jayartnam F J, Tock E P G, Seah C S 1973 Cyclophosphamide in the treatment of systemic lupus

erythematosus: 7 years experience. British Medical Journal 2: 450–452
Forestier J 1935 Rheumatoid arthritis and its treatment with gold salts: results of six years experiments. Journal of Laboratory and Clinical Medicine 20: 827–840
Fosdick W M, Parsons J L, Hill D F 1969 Long term cyclophosphamide therapy in rheumatoid arthritis: A progress report, 6 years experience. Arthritis and Rheumatism 11: 151–161
Fries J F, Sharp G C, McDevitt H O, Holman H R 1973 Cyclophosphamide therapy in systemic lupus erythematosus and polymyositis. Arthritis and Rheumatism 16: 154–162
Froland S S, Natvig J B, Husby G 1973 Immunological characteristics of lymphocytes in synovial fluid from patients with rheumatoid arthritis. Scandinavian Journal of Immunology 2: 67–73
Garges L, Beaulieu R, Bardana E J, Pirofsky B 1973 Combined azathioprine steroid therapy in polyarteritis nodosa (PAN) Clinical Research 21:268 (abstract)
Gershwin M, Goetzel E J, Steinberg A D 1974 Cyclophosphamide: Use in practice. Annals of Internal Medicine 80: 531–540
Ginzler E, Sharon E, Diamond H, Kaplan D 1975 Long-term maintenance therapy with azathioprine in systemic lupus erythematosus. Arthritis and Rheumatism 18: 27–34
Goebel K M, Goebel F D, Schubotz R, Hahn E, Neurath F 1977 Levamisole-induced immunostimulation in spondyloarthropathies. Lancet 2: 214–217
Goldstein G 1974 Isolation of bovine thymin: a polypeptide hormone of the thymus. Nature 247: 11–14
Goldstein G 1978 Mode of action of levamisole. Journal of Rheumatology 5 (suppl 4): 143–148
Goldstein G, Schied M P, Boyse E A, Schlesinger D H, Van Wauve J 1979 A synthetic pentapeptide with biological activity. Characteristic of the thymic hormone thymopoietin. Science 204: 1309–1310
Gordon B L, Yanagihara R 1977 Treatment of systemic lupus erythematosus with the T-cell immunopotentiator levamisole: a follow-up report of 16 patients under treatment for a minimum period of 4 months. Annals of Allergy 39: 227–236
Graziani G, DeMartin G L 1977 Pharmacokinetic studies on levamisole: On the pharmacokinetics and relative bioavailibility of levamisole in man. Drugs Experimental and Clinical Research 2: 235–239
Griffin J E, Wilson J D 1980 Diseases of the testes In: Harrison's principles of internal medicine, 9th Edn. McGraw-Hill Kogakinsha, p 1769
Haas D C 1973 Treatment of polymyositis with immunosuppressive drugs. Neurology 23: 55–62
Hadden J 1977 Levamisole, cyclic nucleotides and immunopharmacology. In: Chirigos M A (ed) Modulation of host immune resistance in the prevention or treatment of induced Neoplasias. Fogarty International Cancer Proceedings No. 28. US Government Printing Office Washington, pp 353–356
Hadden J W, Coffey R G, Hadden E M, Lopez-Corraes E, Sunshine G H 1975 Effects of levamisole and imidazole on lymphocyte proliferation and cyclic nucleotide levels. Cell Immunology 20: 98–103
Hadden J W, Hadden E M, Coffey R G 1976 Isoprinosine augmentation of phylohaemagglutinin induced lymphocyte proliferation. Infection and Immunity 13: 382–387
Hadidi T 1970 Cyclophosphamide in systemic lupus erythematosus. Annals of Rheumatic Diseases 29: 673–676
Hadidi T, Decker J L, El-Nagdy L, Samy M 1981 Ineffectiveness of levamisole in systemic lupus erythematosus. A controlled trial. Arthritis and Rheumatism 24: 60–63
Hamza M, Ayed K, Ben Ayed H 1982 Treatment of Behçet's disease with levamisole. Arthritis and Rheumatism 25: 714–715
Hatchuel R 1972 Efficate et mode d'action du chlorambucil dans la polyarthrite rhumatoide. Etude controlée en double insu. A propos de 47 obervations. Memoine pour L'obtention due certificat d'etudes Speciales en Rhumatologie. Paris (1972)
Hazleman B L, De Silva M 1982 The comparative incidence of malignant disease in rheumatoid arthritis exposed to different treatment regimens. Annals of the Rheumatic Diseases 41 (suppl): 12–17
Heyniuk W M, Bertino J R 1971 Growth rate and cell kill. Annals of the New York Academy of Sciences 186: 330–342
Hitchings G H, Elion G T 1972 Cancer chemotherapy II. The twenty-second Hahnemann symposium. Ed. Brodsky I, Kahn S B, Moyer J H (eds) Grune & Stratton, New York p 23–32
Hoebeke J, Franchi G 1973 Influence of tetramisole and its optical isomers on the mononuclear phagocytic system. Effect on carbon clearance in mice. Journal of the Reticuloendothelial Society 14: 317–323
Hughes G R V 1979 The treatment of systemic lupus erythematosus: The case for conservative management Clinics in Rheumatic Diseases 5: 641–655
Huskisson E C 1977 Is penicillamine an immunostimulant? Proceedings of the Royal Society of Medicine 70 (suppl 3): 142–143
Huskisson E C 1978 Drugs which apparently affect the rheumatoid disease process ('Long term or specific' agents). Hart F D (ed) Adis Press, p 44
Huskisson E C, Dieppe P A, Scott J, Trapnell J, Balme H W, Willoughby D A 1976 Immunostimulant therapy with levamisole in rheumatoid arthritis. Lancet 1: 393–395
Johnson W W, Meadows D C 1971 Urinary bladder fibrosis and telangiectasia associated with long term cyclophosphamide therapy. New England Journal of Medicine 284: 290–294
Kahn M F, Bedoiseau M, Six B, Le Goff P, De Seze S 1971 Le Chlorambucil dans la polyarthrite rhumatoide. Revue due Rhumatisme et des Maladies Osteo-Articulares 38:741
Karsh J, Wright D G, Klippel J H, Decker J L, Deisseroth A B, Flye M W 1979 Lymphocyte depletion by continuous flow cell centrifugation in rheumatoid arthritis: Clinical effects. Arthritis and Rheumatism 22: 1055–1059
Karsh J, Klippel J H, Plotz P H, Decker J L, Wright D G, Flye M W 1981 Lymphapheresis in rheumatoid arthritis: a randomised trial. Arthritis and Rheumatism 24: 867–873
Kinlen L J, Sheil A G R, Peto J, Doll R 1979 Collaborative United Kingdom — Australasian study of cancer in patients treated with immunosuppressive drugs. British Medical Journal 2: 1461–1466
Kotzin B L, Strober S, Engleman E G, Calin A, Hoppe R T, Kansas G S, Terrell C P, Kaplan H S 1982 Treatment of intractable rheumatoid arthritis with total lymphoid irradiation. New England Journal of Medicine 305: 969–976
Kumar R, Biggart J D, McEvoy J, McGeown R 1972

Cyclophosphamide and reproductive function. Lancet 1: 1212–1214
Lance E M, Knight S C 1974 Immunological reactivity in rheumatoid arthritis; response to mitogens. Arthritis and Rheumatism 17: 513–520
Lau C Y, Goldstein G 1980 Functional effects of thymopoietin 32–36 (TP5) on cytotoxic lymphocyte precursor units (CLP-U). 1. Enhancement of splenic CPL-U in vitro and in vivo after suboptimal antigenic stimulation. Journal of Immunology 124: 1861–1865
Leib E S, Restivo C, Paulus H E 1979 Immunosuppressive and corticosteroid therapy of polyarteritis nodosa. American Journal of Medicine 67: 941–947
Leigler D G, Henderson E S, Hahn M A, Oliverio V T 1969 The effect of organic acids on renal clearance of methotrexate in men. Clinical Pharmacology and Therapeutics 10: 849–857
Levy J, Barrett E V, MacDonald N S, Klineberg J B 1970 Altered immunoglobulin metabolism in systemic lupus erythematosus and rheumatoid arthritis. Journal of Clinical Investigation 49: 708–715
Levy J, Paulus H E, Barnett E V, Sokoloff M, Bangert R, Pearson C M 1972 A double blind controlled evaluation of azathioprine treatment in rheumatoid arthritis and psoriatic arthritis. Arthritis and Rheumatism 15:116 (abstract)
Levy J, Miller B 1976 Deficient cell mediated immune responses in rheumatoid arthritis and reversal with levamisole. Arthritis and Rheumatism 19:807
Lewis V M, Twomey J J, Bealmear P, Goldstein G, Good R A 1978 Age, thymic function and circulating thymic hormone activity. Journal of Clinical Endocrinology and Metabolism 47: 145–150
Lightfoot R W 1979 The vasculitis syndromes. In: McCarty D J (ed) Arthritis and allied conditions, 9th Edn. Lea & Febiger, p 723
Lipsky P E, Ziff M 1977 Inhibition of antigen and mitrogen induced human lymphocyte proliferation by gold compounds. Journal of Clinical Investigation 59: 455–466
Lockshin M D, Eisenhauer A C, Kohn R, Weksler M, Block S, Mushlin S B 1975 Cell mediated immunity in rheumatic diseases. Arthritis and Rheumatism 18: 245–250
Lorber A, Simon T M, Leeb J, Peter A, Wilcox S A 1979 Effect of chrysotherapy on parameters of immune response. Journal of Clinical Investigation 6 (suppl 5): 82–90
Low T L K, Thurman G B, Chincarimi C, McClure J E, Marshall G D, Hu S K, Goldstein A L 1979 Current status of thymosin research: evidence for the existence of a family of thymic factors that control T-cell maturation. Annals of the New York Academy of Science 332: 33–48
Maini R N, Roffe L 1976 D-Penicillamine and lymphocyte function in rheumatoid arthritis: The inhibitory and augmenting effects of d-penicillamine in vitro on phytohaemagglutinin-induced lymphocyte transformation. In: Munthe E (ed) Penicillamine research in rheumatoid arthritis. pp 172–184 Fabritus & Sons, Oslo
Marcolongo R Jr, Carcassi A, Frullini G, Bianco G, Bravi A 1967 Levels of immunoglobulins in patients with rheumatoid arthritis. Annals of the Rheumatic Diseases 26: 412–417
Mason M, Currey H L F, Barnes C G, Dunne J F, Hazleman B L, Strickland I D 1969 Azathioprine in rheumatoid arthritis. British Medical Journal 1: 420–421
Meijer C J L M, Lafeber G J M, Cnossen J, Damsteeg M G M, Cats A 1982 T-lymphocyte populations in rheumatoid arthritis. Journal of Rheumatology 9: 18–24
Metzger A L, Bohan A, Goldberg L S, Bluestone R, Pearson C M 1974 Dermatomyositis: Combined methotrexate and corticosteroid therapy. Annals of Internal Medicine 81: 182–189
Michaels R M, Nashel D J, Leonard A, Slivinski A J, Derbes S J 1982 Weekly intravenous methotrexate in the treatment of rheumatoid arthritis. Arthritis and Rheumatism 25: 339–342
Molin L, Stendahl D 1977 Enhancing effect of levamisole on the phagocytic activity of human neutrophil polymorphonuclear leucocytes in vitro. Scandinavian Journal of Haematology 19: 93–98
Morin A, Touraine J L, Renoux G, Hadden J W 1980 Isoprinosine as an immunomodulating agent. Symposium on new trends in human immunology and cancer immunotherapy. Montpellier, France, January 17–19, 1980
Morse H C, Steinberg A, Schur P H, Reed N D 1974 Spontaneous auto immune disease in nude mice. Journal of Immunology 113: 688–697
Mowat A G, Huskisson E C 1975 D-penicillamine in rheumatoid arthritis. Clinics in Rheumatic Diseases 1: 319–333
Osoba D, Miller J F A P 1964 The lymphoid tissues and immune responses of neonatally thymectomized mice bearing thymus tissue in millipore diffusion chambers. Journal of Experimental Medicine 119: 177–194
Paulus H E, Machleder H I, Levine S, Yu D T Y, MacDonald N S 1977 Lymphocyte involvement in rheumatoid arthritis: studies during thoracic duct drainage. Arthritis and Rheumatism 20: 1249–1262
Percy J S, Davis P, Russell A S, Brisson E 1978 A longitudinal study in vitro tests of lymphocyte function in rheumatoid arthritis. Annals of the Rheumatic Diseases 37: 416–420
Pirofsky B, Bardana E J 1977 Immunosuppressive Therapy in Rheumatic Disease Medical Clinics of North America 61: 419–437
Price C C 1975 Chemistry of Alkylation. In: Sartorelli A C, Johns D G (eds) Antineoplastic and immunosuppressive agents, Pt II. Handbuck der experimentellen parmakologie, Vol 3. Springer Verlag, Berlin, p 1–5
Ramot B, Biniaminov M, Shoham C, Rosenthal E 1976 Effect of levamisole on E-rosette forming cells in vivo and in vitro in Hodgkin's disease. New England Journal of Medicine 294: 809–811
Renoux G 1980 The general immunopharmacology of levamisole. Drugs 20: 89–99
Renoux G, Renoux M 1974 Modulation of immune reactivity by phenylimidothiazole salts in mice immunized by sheep red blood cells. Journal of Immunology 113: 779–790
Renoux G, Renoux M 1977 Thymus-like activities of sulphur derivatives on T-cell maturation. Journal of Experimental Medicine 145: 466–471
Renoux G, Renoux M 1977 Mechanismes d'action du levamisole, stimulant des reponses d'immunite cellulaire. Annales d'Immunologie 128c: 275–277
Ritzmann S E, Coleman S L, Levin W C 1960 The effect of some mercaptanes upon a macrocryogelglobulin; modifications induced by cysteamine, penicillamine and penicillin. Journal of Clinical Investigation 30: 1320–1329
Rosenthal M, Trabert U, Mueller W 1976 Immunotherapy with levamisole in rheumatic diseases. Scandinavian Journal of Rheumatology 5: 216–220
Rosenthal M, Trabert U, Mueller W 1976 The effect of levamisole on peripheral blood lymphocyte subpopulations

excretion and the magnitude of the increase of other urine oxypurines. Xanthine and hypoxanthine increase by only 25–30% of the reduction of uric acid (Wyngaarden et al, 1963). This phenomenon has been attributed to a suppressive effect of allopurinol on de novo purine synthesis. There are several possible explanations:

1. The effect is essentially dependent on the presence of hypoxanthine guanine phosphoribosyl tranferase (HGPRT) although not exclusively (Kelley et al, 1968). The conversion of allopurinol to its ribonucleotide requires HGPRT and could deplete cells of phosphoribosyl pyrophosphate (PRPP) thus influencing de novo synthesis (Fig. 22.2). This has been disputed (Elion & Nelson, 1974).

2. There may be enhanced purine salvage (Fig. 22.2) (Edwards et al, 1981).

3. Allopurinol may reduce absorption of dietary purines (Simmonds et al, 1974b).

There is good evidence of a close relationship between uric acid and ammonium excretion (Gibson et al, 1977). It is, therefore, of some interest that long-term allopurinol treatment may result in a reduction of ammonium as well as of uric acid excretion (Gibson et al, 1982). The significance of this in relation to the effect of allopurinol on purine metabolism is obscure.

In addition to these effects on purines, allopurinol may increase excretion of pyrimidines several fold (Simmonds et al, 1974a). Allopurinol appears to inhibit pyrimidine biosynthesis by interrupting orotidine-5-phosphate decarboxylase (ODC) activity. This is mediated by one or more ribonucleotide derivatives of allopurinol and oxipurinol or by xanthosine-5-monophosphate (Beardmore & Kelley, 1974). The resultant increase of pyrimidine excretion is manifest by orotidine and orotic aciduria which may theoretically induce depletion of the intracellular pool of pyrimidine. A clinical syndrome, with megaloblastic anaemia as the most consistent feature, is recognised amongst infants with congenital orotic aciduria (Fox et al, 1969). However, orotic acid excretion following allo-

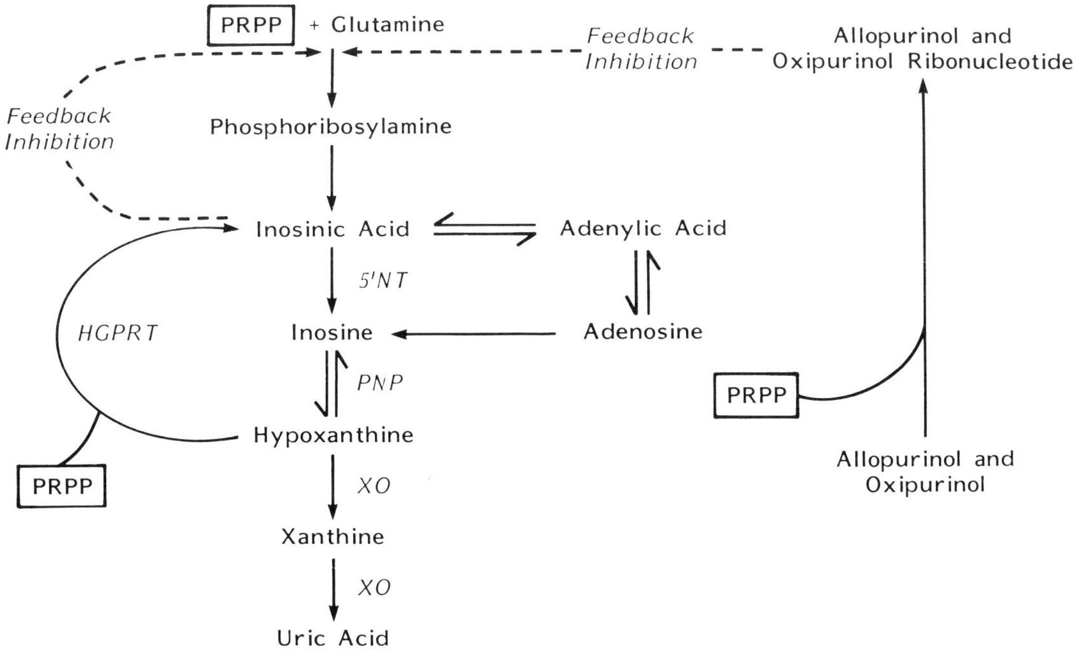

Fig. 22.2 A simplified representation of one.part of the purine pathway. During allopurinol treatment, de novo purine synthesis may be theoretically suppressed by: (a) consumption and depletion of PRPP during conversion of hypoxanthine, allopurinol and oxipurinol; (b) feedback inhibition of the first step by allopurinol and oxipurinol ribonucleotide; (c) increased salvage of hypoxanthine with subsequent feedback inhibition. 5′ NT = 5 nucleotidase; PNP = purine nucleoside phosphorylase; XO = xanthine oxidase; PRPP = phosphoribosylpyrophosphate; HGPRT = hypoxanthine guanine phosphoribosyl transferase.

purinol increases to only 1–5% of that seen in this disease and there have been no reports to suggest that a similar illness may be induced by allopurinol (Banholzer et al, 1980).

Therapeutic effect and dose

The efficacy of allopurinol as a hypouricaemic drug was quickly established (Yu & Gutman, 1964). It was found to be as effective as probenecid in this regard (Scott, 1966). Most patients require a daily dose of 300 mg to achieve normouricaemia but a minority may need up to 600 mg daily (Scott et al, 1966) and exceptionally 800–1000 mg (Rundles et al, 1966). At least one patient has been found to be totally resistant to doses of up to 600 mg daily. Whether this man simply failed to comply with treatment or represented an unusual variant of gout is uncertain (Simmonds et al, 1982). With increasing doses of allopurinol, there is a steady increase of allopurinol, oxipurinol and allopurinol riboside excretion. However, at a daily dose approaching 1500 mg, allopurinol riboside accounts for nearly 50% of metabolites and oxipurinol only 40% (Nelson & Elion, 1982). This implies that at a very high dose it is possible to saturate xanthine oxidase conversion of allopurinol to oxipurinol.

Initially, allopurinol was prescribed two or three times daily but it was subsequently shown that a single dose produced a sustained effect on blood uric acid levels (Brewis et al, 1975). An alternate day regime has been explored but unlike several uricosuric preparations, allopurinol is less likely to exert an adequate hypouricaemia effect when administered in this way. However, it has been claimed that alternate day therapy does not result in a higher incidence of gouty attacks (Nishizawa et al, 1978). Withdrawal of allopurinol after months or years of treatment is followed by a rapid rise of blood uric acid which attains pretreatment levels within two weeks (Loebl & Scott, 1974). Despite the abrupt return of hyperuricaemia, the majority of such patients who have received prolonged allopurinol before withdrawal will remain free of gout for long periods, often exceeding a year. A slow release preparation has been studied in Germany (Grobner et al, 1977). This is less effective than the conventional drug in reducing blood uric acid and it is associated with lower levels of plasma oxipurinol, suggesting incomplete absorption.

Patients who have severe tophaceous gout may be treated with a combination of allopurinol and a uricosuric drug. The effects of allopurinol and probenecid on blood uric acid are additive (Rundles et al, 1966). This may be surprising in view of the ability of probenecid to increase the excretion of oxipurinol because the latter makes an important contribution to xanthine oxidase inhibition (Elion et al, 1968). However, this is presumably compensated by the ability of allopurinol to increase the half-life of probenecid (Tjandramaga et al, 1972).

Effect on the kidneys

Three decades ago, before the availability of hypouricaemic drugs, it was commonly believed that hyperuricaemia posed a major threat to renal function. This was claimed to be a common cause of death amongst those with gout. Severe renal dysfunction is now uncommon and it is possible that this reflects the widespread use of available drugs. The evidence that allopurinol safeguards or improves kidney function is controversial. Levin & Abrahams (1966) found no improvement of kidney function in hyperuricaemic patients with renal impairment. Rundles et al (1966) and Wilson et al (1967) described improvements of kidney function in small numbers of patients with stones or renal impairment as did Chodorowski et al (1974) and Briney et al (1975). Allopurinol may prevent or retard the formation of calcific as well as uric acid calculi and is an effective treatment of recurrent stones, especially when these are accompanied by hyperuricosuria (Pak et al, 1978). There is no evidence at all that renal failure associated with hyperuricaemia in the absence of gout is influenced by allopurinol (Rosenfeld, 1974). In an attempt to determine whether allopurinol protects kidney function in primary gout, Gibson et al (1982) demonstrated subtle but significant slowing of the decline of GFR over two years. However, it is still uncertain whether such observations imply that allopurinol will prevent serious renal disease in those gouty subjects who are susceptible.

Adverse and toxic reactions

Early clinical experience with allopurinol indicated that it was a drug with a low incidence of toxicity. However, as with other hypouricaemic agents, almost half of gout patients may experience acute attacks of arthritis during the first few months of treatment (Yu & Gutman, 1964; Scott, 1966). In a large survey of hospital in-patients receiving allopurinol, 1–2% had unwanted effects (McInnes et al, 1981). These were not related to age, body weight or blood urea levels. A relationship between renal failure and toxicity, especially skin rashes, has been reported by others (Rundles et al, 1966). The most frequent side-effect is a rash. Diarrhoea, nausea, drug fever, bone marrow suppression and liver enlargement also occur, but none with an incidence of more than 0.2% (McInnes et al, 1981).

Severe reactions do occasionally arise, often associated with evidence of allergic hypersensitivity. Eosinophilia may be observed with rash, fever, renal failure and vasculitis (Kantor, 1970; Young et al, 1974). Severe toxic manifestations such as these are so unusual that their relationship to allopurinol may not be appreciated and they may be wrongly attributed to some other disease state.

Diarrhoea may rarely be associated with steatorrhoea and malabsorption (Chen et al, 1982). Liver dysfunction consistent with hepatocellular damage may accompany evidence of hypersensitivity and tends to be more common amongst those on diuretics or with renal dysfunction (Alkawas et al, 1981).

It is ironic that side-effects are more likely amongst patients with renal failure, the very group for whom the uricosuric alternatives are inappropriate. Although the situation rarely arises, there is a need for another xanthine oxidase inhibitor. Oxipurinol is one obvious substitute but this may exhibit cross reactivity with allopurinol in patients who have an allergic response (Lockard et al, 1976). Where the requirement for allopurinol is essential despite the presence of hypersensitivity, desensitisation may be attempted using small daily increments over a period of weeks (Meyrier, 1976).

Apart from the idiosyncratic adverse effects discussed above, the therapeutic properties of allopurinol may also have unwanted sequelae. Joint deformities may be accentuated by the resorption of tophi which have replaced bone (Gottlieb & Gray, 1977).

Successful treatment of hyperuricaemia is invariably accompanied by increased excretion of xanthine and hypoxanthine. Xanthine is less soluble than uric acid and it is surprising that renal xanthine stones do not occur more readily. At least one report has described xanthine calculi and crystalluria in a patient undergoing treatment with cytotoxic agents and allopurinol (Ablin et al, 1972). The authors recommended regular estimation of blood and urine oxypurines to avoid this complication but its occurrence is sufficiently rare to make this unjustifiable. In gout patients treated with allopurinol, crystals of hypoxanthine, xanthine and oxipurinol may be deposited regularly in muscles (Watts et al, 1971). This observation does not seem to be associated with any clinical evidence of myopathy.

Allopurinol is a poor substrate for HGPRT and allopurinol ribonucleotides are unlikely to account for any inhibition of de novo purine synthesis. However, a small concentration of nucleotide derivative could influence chromatid metabolism. There have been no reports to suggest that allopurinol is mutagenic and in vitro studies of tumour cells have failed to demonstrate any alteration of RNA patterns in response to allopurinol (Becher & Puschendorf, 1977). Examination of lymphocytes from treated patients have shown no chromosome aberrations and there is thus no evidence that either allopurinol or oxipurinol interfere with nucleoproteins at any stage of the cell cycle (Stevenson et al, 1976).

Drug interactions

Animal studies have suggested that allopurinol may reduce liver microsomal cytochrome content, impairing the metabolism of those drugs which are dependent on oxidation for their elimination. Two such preparations are phenylbutazone and warfarin but allopurinol has no effect on the blood concentration of phenylbutazone nor on the therapeutic effect of warfarin (Rawlins & Smith, 1973). On the other hand, probenecid biotransformation is also dependent to some extent on oxidation and an effect of allopurinol on liver microsomes may account for the increased half-life which is seen in some, but not all patients, when both drugs are given simultaneously (Tjandramaga et al, 1972).

Of interest is the report that rashes occur in 22% of those patients receiving ampicillin and allopurinol, whereas they appear in only 7 and 2% of those taking only ampicillin or allopurinol respectively (Boston Collaborative Drug Surveillance Program, 1972). The mechanism of rash potentiation and the drug which is primarily responsible are unknown. Ampicillin is the more likely culprit.

Interactions which may have serious or fatal consequences are those between allopurinol and cytotoxic drugs. The action of cyclophosphamide may be magnified, although the reason for this is not certain. Azathioprine and its active metabolite, 6-mercaptopurine, are dependent on xanthine oxidase for their eventual catabolism to thiouric acid. Allopurinol may, therefore, increase their cytotoxic action manyfold (Elion et al, 1963).

THIOPURINOL

The need for an alternative hypouricaemic drug which is not uricosuric has been discussed. In some countries of Europe, this requirement is met by the availability of thiopurinol (mercapto-4-pyrazolo-(3,4-d) pyrimidine). This drug is the 4-thio analogue of allopurinol and effectively reduces blood and urine uric acid. However, its mode of action is obscure, providing a puzzle which when unravelled may provide more information about the mechanism of allopurinol. It is readily absorbed and 50% is excreted as unchanged thiopurinol, and the remainder mainly as oxithiopurinol (Grahame et al, 1977). It does not inhibit xanthine oxidase and the subsequent lack of increased xanthine production could be of advantage in the exceptional instances where xanthine stones occur with allopurinol (Simmonds et al, 1974c). It does not reduce blood uric acid in the partial or complete absence of HGPRT (Grahame et al, 1974). Like allopurinol it does undergo conversion to its ribonucleotide (Auscher et al, 1974) and this may contribute to a direct suppression of de novo purine synthesis. In the absence of increased xanthine and hypoxanthine it is difficult to invoke any increase of the natural salvage pathway (Fig. 22.2). In the pig, thiopurinol appears to decrease absorption of dietary guanine and this provides another explanation for the effect of thiopurinol in man (Grahame et al, 1977).

URICOSURIC DRUGS

An appreciation of the renal handling of uric acid is fundamental to an understanding of uricosuric drugs (*see* Fig. 22.3).

Mode of action

In theory, uricosuric drugs may exert their effect by increasing the amount of uric acid filtered at A (Fig. 22.3), by inhibiting reabsorption at B and D or by enhancing urate secretion at C. It is probable that most drugs inhibit tubular reabsorption of uric acid and that they need to be within the lumen of the tubule to have this effect (Fanelli, 1975). The variable effect of drugs on uric acid excretion has provided the basis for an understanding of tubular handling. Small doses of aspirin impair urate clearance but large doses have a uricosuric effect. Aspirin inhibits both urate reabsorption and secretion, the net effect reflecting the size of dose (Fig. 22.3). The uricosuric response to large doses of aspirin is unaffected by pyrazinamide which reduces urate excretion by inhibiting its secretion. This implies that salicylates either block the action of pyrazinamide, or more likely, act at sites of pre- and postsecretory reabsorption (B and D, Fig. 22.3). By contrast, the uricosuric effects of both sulphinpyrazone and probenecid are abolished by pyrazinamide suggesting that they act at sites of postsecretory reabsorption (Diamond & Meisel, 1977a). Most uricosuric agents seem to affect the same sites as probenecid and sulphinpyrazone. Salicylates impair the uricosuric effect of sulphinpyrazone and probenecid probably by blocking their effect on tubular reabsorption (Yu et al, 1963; Fanelli & Weiner, 1979).

Many agents are known to be uricosuric and with few exceptions they are all weak organic acids like uric acid. It is likely that their inhibitory effect on uric acid reabsorption is competitive. Drugs which fall into this category but which are not employed in a therapeutic role as hypouricaemic compounds include acetoheximide, glyceryl guiacolate, dicoumarol, ethyl biscoumacetate and phenylindandione. Kelley (1975) has compiled a comprehensive catalogue of such agents. One addition to these is calcitonin which is used for the treatment of Paget's disease. It has a marked uricosuric effect and may reduce blood uric acid by 30% (Gattereau et al, 1979; RicoLenza et al, 1980).

One alternative mechanism of uricosuria has been postulated. In vitro studies of uric acid protein binding suggest that a range of drugs with uricosuric properties may displace urate from its binding site (Schlosstein et al, 1973), but this is unlikely to result in an increased clearance of uric acid (Holmes & Blondet, 1979). The first serious attempt to treat hyperuricaemia with a uricosuric drug involved the administration of 4.0–5.0 g/day of sodium salicylate (Yu & Gutman, 1951). By this means, normouricaemia was achieved and tophi disappeared. Comparisons of aspirin with probenecid and sulphinpyrazone subsequently showed that the dose of salicylate necessary to achieve an equivalent effect was unacceptable to patients (Gutman & Yu 1957; Emmerson, 1963). These early endeavours indicated that hypouricaemic therapy was feasible and worthwhile. They also provided the impetus for the evaluation and acceptance of probenecid and sulphinpyrazone.

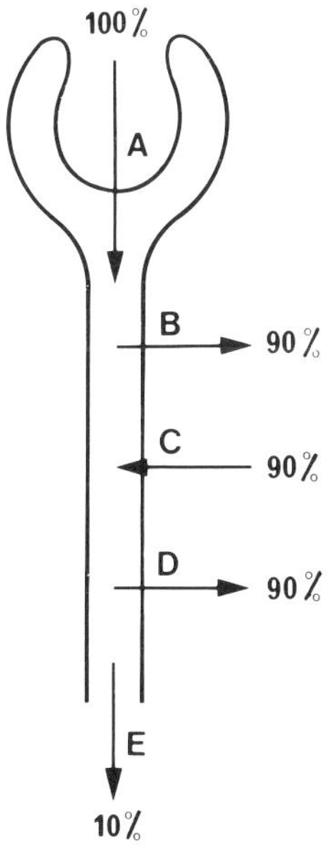

Fig. 22.3 Diagrammatic representation of renal handling of uric acid. This is completely filtered at the glomerulus then reabsorbed, secreted and reabsorbed again within the proximal tubule. The figures are not precise and merely reflect the net effect. Only 10% of uric acid filtered at the glomerulus is actually excreted. Uricosuric drugs may in theory increase filtration at A, inhibit reabsorption at B and D or increase secretion at C.

PROBENECID

Historical background

When penicillin was expensive and scarce, several drugs were synthesised in an attempt to find products which would delay its elimination and prolong its effect. Amongst these were carinamide and probenecid. It was found that such drugs altered the excretion of other weak organic acids, including uric acid. Probenecid was exceptional in its ability to accentuate uric acid excretion and this property was soon recognised as an important advance in the treatment of gout (Bishop et al, 1951).

Chemistry

Probenecid is a sulphonamide derivative — p-(dipropylsuphamoyl) benzoic acid. Its structure is illustrated in Figure 22.4.

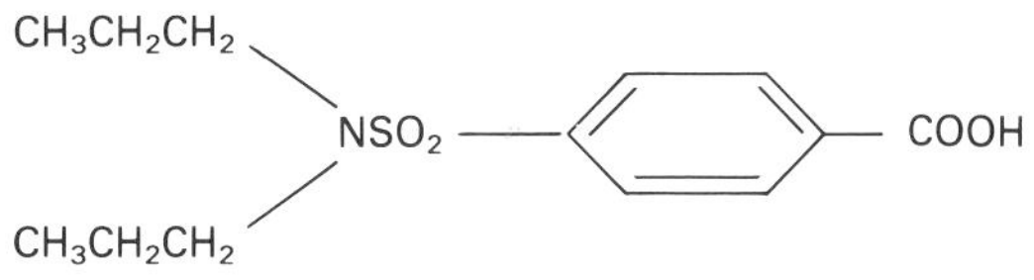

PROBENECID

Fig. 22.4 The structural formula of probenecid.

Pharmacological properties

Absorption

Probenecid is readily absorbed and peak plasma levels occur within 1–5 hours. Excretion of radiolabelled probenecid suggests that absorption is complete.

Metabolism

The drug is 80–90% bound to plasma albumin and its plasma half-life is 4–12 hours. Metabolism occurs principally by oxidation of its alkyl side-chains and glucuronide conjugation. These are less avidly bound to protein and less soluble in lipids than the parent compound. This accounts for their rapid clearance by the kidneys where they may have some uricosuric properties.

Excretion

After 48 hours, 5–11% of a single 2.0 g dose of probenecid is excreted unchanged, 16–30% as its monoacyl glucuronide, and the remainder as equal proportions of two monohydroxylated compounts, a carboxylated derivative and an N-depropylated metabolite (Dayton & Perel, 1971). The high degree of protein binding suggests that probenecid enters the urine by tubular secretion. Tubular reabsorption occurs and is nearly complete in acidic urine. It is known that excretion can be increased by alkalinisation. Pyrazinamide has no effect on probenecid excretion despite diminishing its uricosuric action. By contrast, the inhibitory effect of PAH on probenecid uricosuria is accompanied by a proportional decline of probenecid excretion (Diamond & Meisel, 1977b). Both PAH and probenecid are secreted by the tubules and when given together, compete for this function. These observations imply that probenecid must be secreted in order to exert its uricosuric effect.

Therapeutic effect and dose

Following an oral dose of probenecid, the uricosuric response is maximal within 30 minutes. At a daily dose of 1.0–2.0 g, urate clearance may be increased by 4–6 times. The limitations of probenecid are those of uricosuric agents in general. To avoid a rapid influx of uric acid into the tubules, probenecid is best administered twice daily. The conventional total daily dose of 1.0 g is adequate to achieve normal blood uric acid levels in the majority of patients with primary gout. Larger doses have been found necessary in some patients (Gutman & Yu, 1957). The efficacy is lessened by renal dysfunction and by the concurrent use of salicylates. The influence of probenecid on other drugs is due, in part, to inhibition of their excretion. This phenomenon has been exploited to effect higher circulating levels of several antibiotics of the penicillin and cephalosporin classes. However, the reduction of antibiotic excretion tends to be modest and may not account for the striking elevation of blood antibiotic levels. It has been suggested that probenecid induces a major alteration in the volume distribution of these drugs by blocking their uptake at tissue sites (Cunningham et al, 1981). This raises the question of whether increasing the circulating antibiotic level by this means is sometimes a self-defeating measure.

Effect on the central nervous system

Probenecid causes an accumulation of the major metabolites of noradrenaline, serotonin and dopamine in cerebrospinal fluid. This is due to inhibition of the active transport mechanism by which they are removed. There appear to be no harmful consequences and the effect has been extensively utilised in the investigation of psychiatric disorders (Tamarkin et al, 1970).

Adverse and toxic reactions

All uricosuric drugs entail the risk of uric acid crystallisation within the urine collecting system to produce small deposits or discrete stones. This is most apparent in the first few days of treatment and may be manifest by loin pain, dysuria or haematuria. Avoidance can be achieved by increasing fluid intake, at least during the first week of therapy. Alkalinisation of the urine will also help obviate this complication since uric acid cyrstallisation occurs more readily at a low urine pH.

The drug is in other respects remarkably free of side-effects. Gutman & Yu (1957) recorded rashes in 5% and some gastrointestinal disturbance in 8% of users. Serious toxicity is rare and a search of the literature reveals only isolated instances of nephrotic syndrome, hepatic failure and aplastic anaemia. Serious complications have been reported with less frequency than for allopurinol.

Drug interactions

The capacity of probenecid to alter the blood concentration of several drugs has been discussed. This effect may be mediated in part by reduced renal disposal. Other influences may be due to competition for plasma and tissue protein binding sites and an effect on the liver microsomal enzymes concerned with drug metabolism. Apart from increasing the circulating levels of penicillin and cephalosporin antibiotics, the concentration of rifampicin may also be accentuated, apparently by a decrease of hepatic uptake (Kenwright & Levi, 1973). Salicylates, naproxen and indomethacin are three anti-inflammatory drugs whose excretion is impaired and blood concentration increased by probenecid. Using 2.0–4.0 g probenecid daily, the plasma level of indomethacin may be raised by 50% (Skeith et al, 1968).

Other drugs whose action is increased by probenecid include heparin, methotrexate and perhaps chlorpropamide. The interaction of probenecid and allopurinol has been discussed in the section on allopurinol. Effects on barbiturates and sodium valproate have been reported in animals but not investigated in man (Cunningham et al, 1981).

SULPHINPYRAZONE

Historical background

Phenylbutazone was observed to have a uricosuric effect soon after its introduction. This was attributed to one of its metabolites and was a property that was shared by several phenylbutazone analogues. It was noted that a sulphoxide metabolite of one analogue was highly uricosuric (Burns et al, 1957). This was identified as sulphinpyrazone. It is of some interest that this new compound was initially attributed with weak anti-inflammatory activity.

Chemistry

The structure of sulphinpyrazone can be seen in Figure 22.5. Its formula is 4-(phenylthioethy)-1,2-diphenyl-3,5-pyrazolidinedione.

Pharmacological effects

Absorption

Sulphinpyrazone is very rapidly absorbed, reaching a peak plasma level within 1 hour. Absorption is virtually complete.

Metabolism

After absorption, sulphinpyrazone becomes extensively bound to plasma proteins. The half-life is only 1–3 hours and metabolism can be assumed to be rapid. The drug is converted to hydroxysulphinpyrazone in an analogous fashion to the

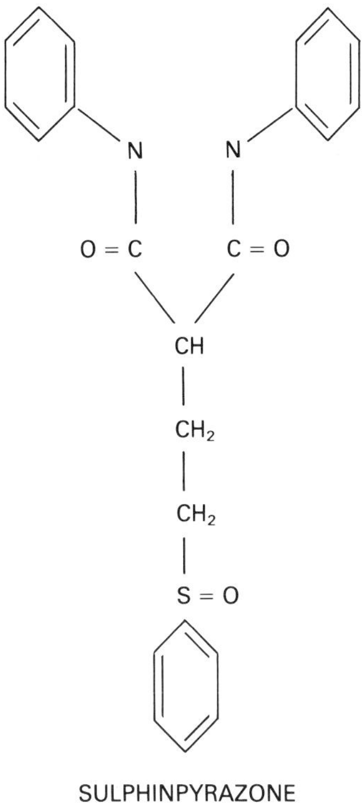

Fig. 22.5 The structure of sulphinpyrazone.

hydroxylation of phenylbutazone (Dayton et al, 1961).

Excretion

Most of the drug is excreted by the urine within 24 hours of a single oral dose. It is found mainly as the hydroxy metabolite but about 20% is excreted as unchanged sulphinpyrazone (Dayton et al, 1961). Surprisingly little is known about the tubular handling of sulphinpyrazone. It is probably secreted like probenecid and in a similar fashion competes successfully with salicylate at this level (Yu et al, 1963). However, there is evidence that its tubular secretion is inhibited by probenecid (Perel et al, 1969).

Therapeutic effect and dose

Sulphinpyrazone is one of the most uricosuric drugs known. Its rapid absorption and efficacy make it desirable that it should be given in divided doses throughout the day to avoid the hazards of uric acid precipitation in the renal tract. The precautions outlined for probenecid are equally applicable to sulphinpyrazone. The daily dose which is necessary to obtain normouricaemia is usually 300–400 mg. The effectiveness of this regime has been well documented (Persellin & Schmid, 1961) and the hypouricaemic response to 400 mg sulphinpyrazone is greater than that of 5.0 g aspirin and 1.5 g probenecid (Emmerson, 1963). Its uricosuric action is substantially greater than that of probenecid.

The drug shares with phenylbutazone and many other anti-inflammatory agents an ability to interfere with platelet aggregation (Packham et al, 1967) and thereby increase platelet survival (Smythe et al, 1965). This phenomenon provides a rationale for using sulphinpyrazone in ischaemic heart disease. Two double blind studies have demonstrated a reduction of death rates in the months following myocardial infarction (Anturane Reinfarction Trial Research Group, 1980; Anturane Reinfarction Italian Study Group, 1982). However, the design of these studies has been criticised and there remains some doubt about their interpretation. There is no evidence that sulphinpyrazone may act as a universal prophylactic against coronary thrombosis. There is some evidence that hyperuricaemia and coronary artery disease may be associated although not causally (Klein et al, 1973). In patients with gout and a history of myocardial ischaemia, there may be some merit in prescribing sulphinpyrazone for its dual effect. However, at present, the benefits must be viewed as theoretical. The use of sulphinpyrazone to prevent coronary occlusion is not devoid of risks and acute renal failure induced by uric urolithiasis has been described in just this setting (Kovalchik, 1981).

Adverse and toxic reactions

Sulphinpyrazone is associated with a range and incidence of side-effects which are similar to those of probenecid (Emmerson, 1963).

Drug interactions

Little is known about the effects of sulphinpyrazone on other drugs. There is an unfounded suspicion that it may alter their excretion and metabolism in the same way as probenecid.

The relationship between salicylates and sulphinpyrazone has been discussed. Aspirin lessens its uricosuric potential. Probenecid impairs its tubular secretion but surprisingly, their uricosuric effects tend to be additive (Perel et al, 1969).

BENZBROMARONE

Historical background

This drug was developed in France and is used extensively in many countries as an effective uricosuric alternative. It is not available in the UK. As a recently developed compound it has undergone intensive investigation and a lot more is known about its characteristics than is known about sulphinpyrazone.

Chemistry

Benzbromarone is structurally similar to another uricosuric agent, benziodarone, differing only in the substitution of two bromide radicles for iodine. Its formula is 2-ethyl-3 (4-hydroxy-3, 5-dibromobenzoyl)-benzofuran.

Pharmacological effects

Absorption

The drug is absorbed slowly with a peak plasma level which occurs 5–6 hours after an oral dose. Only about 50% is absorbed (Heel et al, 1977).

Metabolism

It is extensively dehalogenated in the liver to bromobenzarone and benzarone. A large proportion of these metabolites is conjugated with glucuronic acid.

Excretion

Half of a single dose is excreted in the faeces unchanged and about 8% in the urine. The metabolites are excreted in the gut via the biliary tract (Broekhuysen et al, 1972).

Therapeutic effect and dose

The hypouricaemic effect is due at least in part to increased renal clearance of uric acid. There is no increase of other urine oxypurines in man, suggesting that there is no inhibition of xanthine oxidase, although this does occur in the rat (Jain et al, 1974). The uricosuric effects of 80 mg of the

Annals of the Rheumatic Diseases 25: 623–626
Scott J T, Hall A P, Grahame R 1966 Allopurinol in treatment of gout. British Medical Journal 2: 321–327
Simkin P A 1979 Management of gout. Annals of Internal Medicine 90: 812–16
Simmonds H A 1969 Uricosuric excretion of purines, pyrimidines and pyrazolopyrimidines in patients treated with allopurinol or oxipurinol. Clinica Chimica Acta 23: 353–364
Simmonds H A, Levin B, Cameron J S 1974a Variations in allopurinol metabolism in xanthine subjects. Clinical Science and Molecular Medicine 47: 173–178
Simmonds H A, Cadenhead A, Jones A S, Hatfield P J, Cameron J S 1974 The effect of allopurinol on oral purine absorption and excretion in the pig. Advances in Experimental Medicine and Biology 41b: 653–655
Simmonds H A, Cadenhead A, Cameron J S, Rising T R, Grahame R, Dean B 1974c. Thiopurinol and purine metabolism. Metabolic and radioisotope studies. Annals of the Rheumatic Diseases 33: 548–553
Simmonds H A, Gibson T, Huston G J, Webster D R, Rodgers A V, Munro J 1982 Tophaceous gout resistant to allopurinol therapy: poor compliance or non-response. Journal of Clinical Chemistry and Clinical Biochemistry 20: 417–418
Sinclair D S, Fox I H 1975 The pharmacology of hypouricemic effect of benzbromarone. Journal of Rheumatology 2: 437–445
Skeith M D, Simkin P A, Healey L A 1968 Renal excretion of indomethacin and its inhibition by probenecid. Clinical Pharmacology and Therapeutics 9: 89–93
Smythe H A, Ogryzlo M A, Murphy E A, Mustard J F 1965 The effect of sulfinpyrazone (Anturan) on platelet economy and blood coagulation in man. Canadian Medical Association Journal 92: 818–821
Sorensen L B, Levinson D J 1976 Clinical evaluation of benzbromarone. A new uricosuric drug. Arthritis and Rheumatism 19: 183–190
Stevenson A C, Silcock S R, Scott J T 1976 Absence of chromosome damage in human lymphocytes exposed to allopurinol and oxipurinol. In vivo and in vitro studies. Annals of the Rheumatic Diseases 35: 143–147
Tamarkin N R, Goodwin F K, Axelrod J 1970 Rapid elevation of biogenic amine metabolites in human CSF following probenecid. Life Sciences 9: 1397–1408
Tjandramaga T B, Cucinell S A, Israeli Z H, Perel J M, Dayton P G, Yu T F, Gutman A B 1972 Observations on the disposition of probenecid on patients receiving allopurinol. Pharmacology 8: 259–272
Trevaks G, Lovell R 1965 Effect of Atromid and its components on uric acid excretion and on gout. Annals of the Rheumatic Diseases 24:572–575
Watts R W E, Scott J T, Chalmers R A, Bitensky L, Chayen J 1971 Microscopic studies on skeletal muscle in gout patients treated with allopurinol. Quarterly Journal of Medicine 40: 1–14
Wilson J D, Simmonds H A, North J D K 1967 Allopurinol in the treatment of uremic patients with gout. Annals of the Rheumatic Diseases 26: 136–142
Wyngaarden J B, Rundles R W, Silberman H R 1963 Control of hyperuricemia with hydroxypyrazolopyrimidine, a purine analogue which inhibits uric acid synthesis. Arthritis and Rheumatism 6: 306–307
Young J L, Boswell R B, Nies A S 1974 Severe allopurinil hypersensitivity. Association with thiazides and prior renal compromise. Archives of Internal Medicine 134: 553–558
Yu T S F, Gutman A B 1951 Mobilization of gouty tophi by protracted use of uricosuric agents. American Journal of Medicine 1: 765–769
Yu T S F, Gutman A B 1964 Effects of allopurinol (4-hydroxypyrazolo-(3,4-d) pyrimidine) on serum and urinary uric acid in primary and secondary gout. American Journal of Medicine 37: 885–898
Yu T S F, Dayton P G, Gutman A B 1963 Mutual suppression of the uricosuric effects of sulfinpyrazone and salicylate. Journal of Clinical Investigation 42: 1330–1339
Yu T S F, Berger L, Sarkozi L, Kaung C 1981 Effects of diuretics on urate and calcium excretion. Archives of Internal Medicine 141: 915–919

Intra-articular therapy

Intra-articular procedures date back to prehispanic Mexico, where thorny plants provide a ubiquitous needle to induce arthrocentensis (Alarcon-Segovia, 1980). The size of joint effusions has provided a lively correspondence in *Arthritis and Rheumatism* (1981–1982).

Corticosteroids undoubtedly play the major role in suppressing active synovitis, but most systemic medications have been injected into joints at one time or another — even cyclophosphamide, which has no direct local effect. The variety of diseases treated, the number of different substances used and varying indications make comparisons difficult. Even apparently well-controlled trials may be marred by the simultaneous injections of two different active substances, or an active and an inactive agent into different joints; and the use of a non-treated but involved joint may not be the perfect control. This chapter attempts to consider separately various intra-articular treatments for differing conditions without excessive overlap.

INTRA-ARTICULAR CORTICOSTEROID INJECTIONS

Rheumatoid arthritis and other forms of inflammatory polyarthritis

The whole subject of local corticosteroid treatment in rheumatic disorders has recently been comprehensively and excellently reviewed by Gray et al (1981), to whom the reader is referred for a detailed discussion and extensive bibliography.

Mechanisms by which local corticosteroids suppress synovial inflammation are not fully understood. Suggested processes have included stabilisation of lysozomal enzymes, decreased collagenase formation or prostaglandin synthesis in synovial cells, and a production of peptide factor which depresses polymorph migration. Steroids have also been shown to inhibit a variety of lymphocyte-mediated activities. Observed changes in rheumatoid arthritis include increased hyaluronate concentration and viscosity in synovial fluid with a reduction in polymorph count.

A number of corticosteroid preparations have been used. Those most commonly employed in the UK at present are hydrocortisone acetate (25 mg/ml), methylprednisolone acetate (40 mg/ml) and triamcinolone hexacetonide (20 mg/ml). The volume injected of each compound ranges from 0.2 ml of triamcinolone for a small joint (such as an interphalangeal joint) to 2.0 ml in a large joint such as the knee.

A recent controlled comparison of hydrocortisone acetate and saline (Bossingham et al, 1981) in rheumatoid arthritis showed prolonged improvement after hydrocortisone not only in walking time and pain but also in joint movement (as shown by electrogoniometry) which appeared only after the phase of maximum pain relief and persisted for 55 days. Numerous authors have compared the length of action of different corticosteroid esters both clinically and thermographically and have shown that triamcinolone hexacetonide appears to have the longest action (Bird et al, 1979). This does not necessarily displace the cheaper hydrocortisone acetate from the initial choice; the more potent and longer-acting esters may be reserved for subsequent use if the patient becomes refractory to hydrocortisone.

Local injection should be carried out using the strictest aseptic techniques, including scrupulous sterilisation of the skin, disposable syringes and needles, and no-touch technique; individual ampoules should be used for each injection rather than multidose containers. It is usual to anaesthetise the skin with a local anaesthetic, particularly when injecting small joints, but a controlled trial (Kirwan et al, 1984) did not show a patient preference for local anaesthetic.

Immediately following injection, dispersal of the injected fluid throughout the joint may be facilitated by a few passive movements. Thereafter, duration of effect may be prolonged by resting the joint for 24 hours after injection, as this may reduce extra-articular spread; some form of immediate splinting or rest may be necessary when injecting knees with large or leaking Baker's cysts. There is evidence that the volume of injection is important if the joint has been fully aspirated, in which case the addition of saline to produce a total volume of 5 ml or more (in the case of a knee or shoulder joint) may enhance the effect of the injection (Corbett et al, 1970).

Unsatisfactory results may be due to a true failure of response or undue reliance on corticosteroid alone. In certain situations corticosteroid combined with other remedial measures may give a longer and far greater response than corticosteroid alone: these include knee effusions with wasted quadriceps muscles or extensor lag, ankle swelling and/or tibialis posterior tenosynovitis with valgus feet, especially in seronegative arthropathies, and enthesiopathies at the lateral malleolus with flat feet. Corticosteroid injections may be relatively unsuccessful in weight-bearing joints with significant radiological evidence of damage, but in comparably damaged shoulders, elbows and wrists they can produce a long-lasting improvement. Particularly with the shoulder and soft tissue injections of enthesiopathies around the elbow, a very careful and prolonged examination to localise the exact site or cause of pain, and care in injecting that site (and recording it) may be more important than choice of injection substance.

The duration of effect is extremely variable, not just with different corticosteroids but with different patients, and the varying circumstances of clinical trials and the patients included make comparisons difficult. With individual patients seen personally, the duration of improvement following hydrocortisone acetate may vary from days to months.

Osteoarthritis

The literature reveals extensive variation in the apparent efficacy of injections in osteoarthritis. Most studies have involved the knee and detail regarding the condition of the joint prior to injection is rarely given. Personal experience suggests that there are marked differences in response between dry non-inflamed joints, those with effusion and those with effusion and synovial thickening, with increasing likelihood of response with increasing evidence of inflammation, and some limited support for this is given by Eymontt et al (1982) who studied synovial permeability before and after injection. In the knee, the state of the quadriceps muscle is an important factor in duration of response, and results in the first carpometacarpal joint are extremely variable.

Among the many report trials, that of Friedman & Moore (1980) is well presented: in knees the improvement noted with triamcinolone hexacetonide (20 mg) was transient and by four weeks was comparable to the control injected joint. Of interest is that the incidence of postinjection flare was comparable with active and non-active treatment.

Overall, local corticosteroids are generally regarded as being often useful in osteoarthritis, but their efficacy has not been established. They are specially indicated during acute flares of inflammation.

Non-invasive measures such as weight reduction, advice on careful use for carpometacarpal joints, muscle building exercises, correction of deformity — in particular leg length inequality — and physiotherapy may be more beneficial in the long-term than joint injection.

Gout and pseudogout

Although acute episodes of crystal synovitis improve rapidly following systemic treatment with non-steroidal anti-inflammatory drugs, they also respond immediately to local steroid injection. Diagnostic aspiration and a search for crystals is now a routine measure, and the opportunity can then be taken to give a local injection while the needle is in situ.

Non-articular soft-tissue lesions

Local corticosteroid injections are widely used in

the symptomatic treatment of digital flexor tenosynovitis, De Quervain's tenovaginitis, supraspinatus tendinitis, extensor humeral epicondylitis (tennis elbow), carpal tunnel syndrome and similar soft-tissue inflammatory lesions. Their effect is often dramatic, especially when combined with a local anaesthetic, but relapses often occur.

ADVERSE EFFECTS OF LOCAL STEROID TREATMENT

Postinjection flare

A transient acute synovitis occasionally follows injection. Though usually mild, it necessitates further aspiration to exclude infection. It is probably induced by the microcrystalline nature of the injected corticosteroid.

Infection

This is rare and indeed should never occur if proper aseptic precautions are taken, as outlined above. Thus experience from the Mayo Clinic, where 3000 injections are undertaken annually, reports a complete absence of this complication (Fitzgerald, 1976). However, infection is well documented, either directly introduced at the site of injection, or by a haematogenous route following local trauma. Rheumatoid joints are especially vulnerable, particularly if the patient is receiving systemic corticosteroids or other immunosuppressive agents. Naturally the possibility of infection demands immediate further arthrocentesis and antibiotic treatment.

Steroid arthropathy

Chandler et al (1959) drew attention to the production or acceleration of joint damage following repeated intra-articular injection of corticosteroid. It was suggested that articular damage was due to excessive joint mobility resulting from steroid-induced relief of pain, a situation analogous to a Charcot neuropathic joint. It is also possible that corticosteroids have a direct deleterious action on articular cartilage. Such an effect has been demonstrated in numerous experiments carried out on animals, fully reviewed by Gray et al (1981), who suggest that the potential danger may have been over-emphasised. It is certainly difficult to distinguish the effects of steroid arthropathy from those of the underlying disease. Nevertheless, it is generally felt to be unwise to inject the same joint frequently, and certainly not more often than once every two or three months.

Systemic effects

Extra-articular spread of corticosteroid is common. Bird et al (1979) noted clear differences in thermographic indices in the non-injected knee used as a control: triamcinolone hexacetonide produced the greatest effect in the non-injected knee, comparable to the decrease found in their study to the injection of methyl prednisolone acetate. Such extra-articular effect may be a factor in the differences between various studies, many using a saline-injected or non-injected joint as a control. Extra-articular effects are not confined to joints or to corticosteroids as it is possible to detect methotrexate by bioassay in the contralateral synovial cavity within half-an-hour of injection into a knee (Bird et al, 1977).

Depression of the hypothalamo–pituitary–adrenal axis has been demonstrated following injection of most corticosteroids. It may last a few days only but plasma cortisol levels may be depressed for 2–4 weeks following the longer-acting drugs (Bird et al, 1979). Armstrong et al (1981) found greater depression of serum cortisol levels when 80 mg of methylprednisolone acetate was injected as 40 mg into each of two knees than with 80 mg into one knee.

Systemic effects of intra-articular injection are not however a significant hazard and manifestations of chronic hypercorticism have not been reported.

Tissue atrophy

Rarely, dermal hypopigmentation and subcutaneous tissue atrophy can follow local injection, particularly if repeated at, say, a tennis elbow or similar local lesion. It is possible that hydrocortisone acetate may be safer in this respect than the more powerful and longer-acting corticosteroids.

Tendon rupture

Noyes et al (1977) demonstrated reduction of

tensile strength of ligaments in monkeys following local steroid injection and there are several clinical reports (reviewed by Gray et al, 1981) of spontaneous tendon and ligamentous rupture following topical injection. Frequent injections into tendon sheaths should probably be avoided, as should injection into tendon substance itself.

Joint capsule calcification

This is a very rare radiological finding of no clinical significance (McCarty, 1972).

ASPIRIN AND ORGOTEIN

Interest in other materials used intra-articularly has continued. Rylance et al (1980) used 20 and 100 mg acetylsalicylic acid in a controlled comparison with saline and 50 mg hydrocortisone acetate in patients with rheumatoid arthritis. All showed comparable effect. As aspirin is cleared rapidly from the joint (a one-way effect, as aspirin levels in joint fluid are low in subjects taking oral aspirin), their patients were maintained on high dose throughout the study periods.

Considerable interest remains in the action on joints of orgotein, a superoxide (0^{-2}) dismutase, which is believed to stimulate active biological defence mechanisms. Its disadvantage is that it is given by weekly intra-articular injections, but controlled trials in both osteoarthritis and rheumatoid arthritis have shown considerable improvement in the short-term compared with low dose (4 mg) aspirin (Goebel at al, 1981).

SILICONE OIL IN OSTEOARTHRITIS

The development of silicone oils and silicone implants inevitably led to the logical application of silicone into joints that had lost their natural lubrication, or had worn despite adequate lubrication. But a controlled comparison of silicone oil, hydrocortisone acetate and saline in osteoarthritis showed little benefit and a significant incidence of irritative synovitis (Corbett et al, 1970). In retrospect, this has saved rheumatologists from all the problems which have been posed by silicone breast implants.

GOLD IN RHEUMATOID ARTHRITIS

Sporadic interest has remained in intra-articular gold injections. Following Lewis & Ziff's (1966) observations on intra-articular gold, this has been used but rarely reported. Sloop (1982) studied the effect of 50 mg of sodium aurothiomalate in patients with rheumatoid arthritis on intramuscular gold in whom one or more joints were unresponsive, a situation normally treated by surgical synovectomy or radiocolloids. Patients were allocated either to one hydrocortisone injection or to serial intra-articular gold injections. The latter appeared to have some effect given in this way, with reduction in joint swelling, but hydrocortisone was more effective.

CHEMICAL AND RADIO-ISOTOPE SYNOVECTOMY ('SYNOVIORTHESIS')

Surgical synovectomy has long been a standard procedure of persistent chronic synovitis with effusion. In the hands of some orthopaedic surgeons, synovectomy is a relatively simple procedure from which patients make a rapid and trouble-free recovery. Unfortunately this is not universal and in one study (Gumpel & Roles, 1975) patients required an average of 64 hours individual physiotherapy following surgical synovectomy. Young adults appear to tolerate and recover well after synovectomy but children and older patients may have difficulty in regaining full mobility.

Compared with 2–6 weeks of incapacity following surgical synovectomy, an intra-articular injection with minimal hospitalisation becomes attractive. The past thirty years have therefore seen various attempts to suppress inflammation in diseased synovium by the intra-articular injection of chemical substances or radio-isotopes.

Osmic acid

Of several chemical agents used, osmic acid has been most widely reported. In the knee, osmic acid is administered as 10 ml of a 1% solution: the knee should be aspirated to dryness prior to the injection of 10 ml of 2% lignocaine, followed by osmic acid and then corticosteroid.

Unlike radio-isotopes, osmic acid reacts with cartilage as well as synovial membrane and there has been concern relating to the long-term effect of osmic acid on cartilage, especially in children. In long-term studies in adults, Nissila (1978) did not find any increased frequency of degenerative changes following osmic acid, and in a comparison of osmic acid with surgical synovectomy, Nissila et al (1978) found such changes in fact only after surgical synovectomy. A transient discolouration of urine is common soon after injection, but is without long-term effects. Considerable care is needed to avoid overdistension of the joint immediately following injection, as needle-tract fistulae have been reported (Sheppeard et al, 1981), and also to avoid application of osmic acid to tissues other than the joint itself.

A number of trials comparing osmic acid with other forms of synoviorthesis have been recently published. Sheppeard et al (1981), in a randomly allocated trial, compared the three year follow-up results in 91 knees treated with 10 ml of 1% osmic acid and methylprednisolone with those in 84 knees treated with 5 mCi of ^{90}Y silicate. Throughout the study, satisfactory results occurred more frequently following osmic acid treatment than after ^{90}Y but only after three years did the difference reach statistical significance, representing a greater deterioration in yttrium-treated knees after two years. At two years, 76% of osmic acid knees were satisfactory, compared to 68% of yttrium; at three years, 63% and 48%. In this respect, this early deterioration with yttrium is atypical.

Nissila et al (1978) compared the results of surgical synovectomy (21 knees) with osmic acid together with corticosteroid (22 knees) and ^{90}Y (23 knees) at one year. Surgical synovectomy was most successful in disposing of pain and effusion but was associated with a higher incidence of subsequent osteoarthritis radiological change and obviously presented greater rehabilitation problems as well as cost and hospital time. More yttrium-treated patients required corticosteroid injections in the following year and osmic acid-treated patients required fewest. Radiological progression of rheumatoid changes was least following surgical synovectomy and greatest following osmic acid. However, the only changes to reach statistical significance were those relating to radiological osteoarthritis following surgical synovectomy.

Menkes (1979), on a double blind basis, compared osmic acid (23 knees) with 4 mCi ^{90}Y citrate (25 knees). On reassessment, 6–12 months after injection, he found an excellent or good result in 72% of yttrium-treated patients, 52.2% with osmic acid and 38.1% with triamcinolone: the difference between yttrium and triamcinolone reached statistical significance.

However, because of painful inflammatory reactions (avoidable by concurrent anaesthetic and steroid) and the fear of long-term damage to cartilage, the use of osmic acid has not achieved general acceptance.

INTRA-ARTICULAR IRRADIATION

Radiocolloids in most countries are subject to central bureaucratic controls. Used intra-articularly, i.e. as localised irradiation, many of the theoretical hazards of whole-body irradiation are lessened but powerful β-emitters are recommended only in people over the age of 45 years. Many of the problems relating to extra-articular spread have been resolved and certainly in the UK radiocolloids are widely used, although their exact efficacy in comparison, for example, with long-acting local corticosteroid is difficult to assess.

A number of radioactive substances have been used, ^{198}Au, ^{90}Y citrate, ^{90}Y silicate, ^{90}Y ferric hydroxide, ^{186}Re, ^{169}Er. Some, such as ^{198}Au, are now rarely used: indications for others depend on their individual β-ray energy and various depths of penetration, making them suitable for joints of different sizes (Table 23.1). Care is needed to select a radio-isotope suitable for the joint to be treated. When injecting joints other than the knee, correct positioning of the needle within the joint should be ascertained by injecting a small amount of contrast medium as in arthrography.

^{90}Y in large joints

^{90}Y silicate is regularly used in the knee (usual dose 5 mCi), in the shoulder (3 mCi), in the elbow (2–3 mCi) and ankle (2 mCi). In France, ^{186}Re is used in the latter joints. As with osmic acid, the joint or joints to be treated should be the major site of active synovitis, reasonably stable and func-

Table 23.1 Some isotopes used for intra-articular therapy

Isotope	Half-life (days)	Emission	Max. energy of β(MeV)	Range in soft tissue (mm)		Range in cartilage (mm)	
				Mean	Maximum	Mean	Maximum
^{169}Er	9.5	β–	0.34	0.3	1.0	0.2	0.7
^{198}Au	2.7	β–γ	0.96	1.2	3.6	0.9	2.7
^{186}Re	3.7	β–(γ)	0.98	1.2	3.6	0.9	2.7
^{90}Y	2.7	β–	2.2	3.6	11.0	2.8	8.5

tional. Particularly in the knee, the absence of a major valgus, varus or flexion deformity is important.

Following injection, the joint should be immobilised for 48 hours to minimise extra-articular spread. We currently use bed-rest with a crepe bandage, or, if treated as an out-patient, the patient is fitted with a full length plaster of Paris cylinder with an aperture for injection purposes (Williams et al, 1981). Concurrent corticosteroids may be used, although there is no good scientific reason for so doing.

As with osmic acid, it is important to avoid needle-track reflux and subsequent radiation burns (Fig. 23.1), and the use of air or of corticosteroid to clear the needle is important, as well as full aspiration of the joint.

As mentioned above, comparable success rates with ^{90}Y to osmic acid have been obtained (Menkes, 1979; Szanto, 1977).

^{169}Er in small joints

The place of intra-articular radiotherapy in the joints of the hand remains controversial; results of clinical trials conflict. Much of the controversy arises from concurrent use of corticosteroid with ^{169}Er and it is likely that improvement is mainly due to corticosteroid. Ruotsi et al (1979) compared ^{169}Er in doses of 0.5 mCi for MCP joints and 0.25 mCi for PIP joints with 5 mg of triamcinolone hexacetonide. In the first 6 months after injection, triamcinolone-treated joints had a higher improvement rate than erbium-treated joints and the difference was striking and highly significant at 1 and 3 months. By 12 and 18 months after injection, no significant differences between the

a

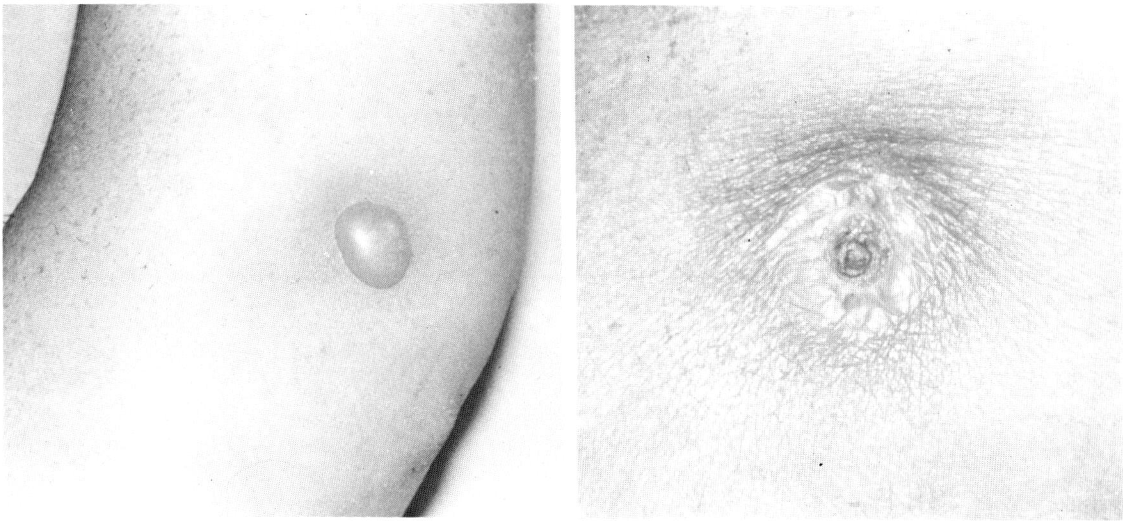

b

Fig. 23.1 (a) Needle-track radiation burn following intra-articular injection of ^{90}Y. The probable cause was injection of too great a volume of yttrium plus saline into a small (elbow) joint. (b) This later photograph shows healing after two months

two was noted, but improvements with both reached statistical significance compared with pretreatment assessments. Gumpel et al (1979) compared ^{169}Er with methylprednisolone acetate and found a similar rate of improvement with both preparations. These two reports contrast with previous studies (Menkes et al, 1977) who found greater improvement with ^{169}Er with prednisolone acetate than with prednisolone acetate and saline.

^{169}Er may well have a small place in the treatment of persistent and recurrent synovitis of joints of the hand that fail to show lasting improvement with corticosteroid injections. But the injections of radio-isotopes into small finger joints under radiographic control is a tedious process, commending itself only to the enthusiast.

SPECIAL INDICATIONS FOR INTRA-ARTICULAR RADIOTHERAPY

Pigmented villonodular synovitis

Recurrence rates following surgical synovectomy are of the order of 50%. We have arranged a referral from a number of orthopaedic surgeons of patients with this condition at the first sign of a recurrence following surgical synovectomy. We have now treated ten patients in this way, with successful results in a high proportion of these previously recurrent failures. It is necessary to use a large dose of ^{90}Y, say 8–10 mCi for a knee, and correspondingly for other joints.

Recurrent haemarthrosis in haemophilia

Successful reduction in frequency of haemarthrosis has been reported following osmic acid (Meaker et al, 1973) and radio-isotopes (Rivard et al, 1982). Haemophiliacs are usually young, and theoretical considerations suggest that osmic acid might be less hazardous in terms of possible late carcinogenesis. But radio-isotopes are first choice where factor VIII inhibitors are present, as the acute inflammatory reaction associated with osmic acid is thought to be likely to set off further bleeding. Other factors may be the prospective longevity of the patient.

Pyrophosphate arthropathy

In a controlled comparison of ^{90}Y silicate (5 mCi) with triamcinolone hexacetonide against saline with triamcinolone, Doherty & Dieppe (1981) demonstrated significant improvement following the irradiation.

REFERENCES

Alarcon-Segovia D 1980 Descriptions of therapeutic arthrocentesis and of synovial fluid in a Nahuatl text from prehispanic Mexico. Annals of the Rheumatic Diseases 39: 291–293

Armstrong R D, English J, Gibson T, Chakraborty J, Marks V 1981 Serum methylprednisolone levels following intra-articular injection of methylprednisolone acetate. Annals of the Rheumatic Diseases 40: 571–574

Bird H A, Ring E F J, Daniel R, Bacon P A 1977 Comparison of intra-articular methotrexate with triamcinolone hexacetonide by thermography. Current Medical Research and Opinion 5: 146–151

Bird H A, Ring E F J, Bacon P A 1979 A thermographic and clinical comparison of three intra-articular steroid preparations in rheumatoid arthritis. Annals of the Rheumatic Diseases 38: 36–39

Bossingham D H, McQueen A K, Mowat A G 1981 Knee function after intra-articular hydrocortisone. Rheumatology and Rehabilitation 20: 98–101

Chandler G N, Jones D T, Wright V, Hartfall S J 1959 Charcot's arthropathy following intra-articular hydrocortisone. British Medical Journal 1: 952–953

Corbett M, Seifert M H, Hacking C, Webb S 1970 Comparison between local injections of silicone oil and hydrocortisone acetate in chronic arthritis. British Medical Journal 1: 24–25

Doherty M, Dieppe P A 1981 Effect of intra-articular yttrium 90 on chronic pyrophosphate arthropathy of the knee. Lancet 2: 1243–1246

Eymontt M J, Gordon G V, Schumacher H R, Hansell J R 1982 The effects on synovial permeability and synovial fluid leucocyte counts in symptomatic osteoarthritis after intra-articular corticosteroid administration. Journal of Rheumatology 9: 198–203

Fitzgerald R H Jr 1976 Intrasynovial injection of steroids: uses and abuses. Mayo Clinic Proceedings 51: 655–659

Friedman D M, Moore M E 1980 The efficacy of intra-articular steroids in osteoarthritis: a double blind study. Journal of Rheumatology 7: 850–856

Goebel K-M, Storck U, Neurath F 1981 Intrasynovial orgotein therapy in rheumatoid arthritis. Lancet 1: 1015–1017

Gray R G, Tenenbaum J, Gottlieb N L 1981 Local corticosteroid injection treatment in rheumatic disorders. Seminars in Arthritis and Rheumatism 10: 231–254

Gumpel J M, Roles N C 1975 A controlled trial of intra-articular radio-colloids versus surgical synovectomy in persistent synovitis. Lancet 1: 488–489

Gumpel J M, Mathews S A, Fisher M 1979 Synoviorthesis with erbium 169: a double-blind controlled comparison of erbium 169 with corticosteroid. Annals of the Rheumatic Diseases 38: 341–343

Kirwan J R, Haskard D O, Higgens C 1984 Use of local anaesthetics. British Journal of Rheumatology 23: 210–213
Lewis D C, Ziff M 1966 Intra-articular administration of gold salts. Arthritis and Rheumatism 9: 682–692
McCarty D J 1972 Treatment of rheumatoid joint inflammation with triamcinolone hexacetonide. Arthritis and Rheumatism 15: 157–173
Menkes C J 1979 Is there a place for chemical and radiation synovectomy in rheumatic diseases? Rheumatology and Rehabilitation 18: 65–77
Menkes C J, Le Go A, Verrier P, Aignan M, Delbarre F 1977 Double-blind study of erbium 169 injection in rheumatoid digital joints. Annals of the Rheumatic Diseases 36: 254–256
Nissila M 1978 Absence of increased frequency of degenerative joint changes after osmic acid injections. Scandinavian Journal of Rheumatology 7: 81–84
Nissila M, Anttila P, Hamalainen M, Jalava S 1978 Comparison of chemical, radiation and surgical synovectomy for knee joint synovitis. Scandinavian Journal of Rheumatology 7: 225–228
Noyes F R, Grood E S, Nussbaum N S, Cooper S M 1977 Effect of intra-articular corticosteroids on ligament properties: a biomechanical and histologic study in rhesus knees. Clinical Orthopaedics 123: 197–209
Rivard G E, Girard M, Cliche C L, Guay J P, Belanger R, Besner R 1982 Synoviorthesis in patients with hemophilia and inhibitors. Canadian Medical Association Journal 127: 41–42
Ruotsi A, Hypen M, Rekonen A, Oka M 1979 Erbium 169 versus triamcinolone hexacetonide in the treatment of rheumatoid finger joints. Annals of the Rheumatic Diseases 38: 45–47
Rylance H J, Chalmers T M, Elton R A 1980 Clinical trials of intra-articular aspirin in rheumatoid arthritis. Lancet 1: 1099–1102
Sheppeard H, Aldin A, Ward D J 1981 Osmic acid versus yttrium 90 in rheumatoid synovitis of the knee. Scandinavian Journal of Rheumatology 10: 234–236
Sloop P R 1982 Intra-articular gold salts in rheumatoid arthritis. Arthritis and Rheumatism (letter) 9:1148
Szanto E 1977 Long term follow-up of yttrium 90 treated knee joint arthritis. Scandinavian Journal of Rheumatology 6: 209–212
Williams P L, Crawley J C, Freeman A M, Lloyd D C, Gumpel J M 1981 Feasibility of out-patient management after intra-articular yttrium 90: comparison of two regimens. British Medical Journal 282: 13–14

SECTION V

Rheumatoid Arthritis

The aetiopathogenesis of rheumatoid arthritis

DEFINITION OF RHEUMATOID ARTHRITIS

Diagnostic criteria

Rheumatoid arthritis (RA) is a chronic, symmetrical, inflammatory polyarthritis of unknown cause involving the diarthrodial joints and exhibiting, in a proportion of patients, a variety of extra-articular features such as vasculitis and nodules. Since there is no diagnostic test with high specificity and sensitivity, the diagnosis of RA is based on the recognition of certain clinical and laboratory features which have been set out as the American Rheumatism Association's diagnostic criteria (Ropes et al, 1958). These are:

1. Morning stiffness
2. Joint pain on motion or tenderness
3. Swelling of a joint
4. Second joint involvement
5. Symmetrical joint involvement
6. Subcutaneous nodules
7. Positive rheumatoid factor test
8. X-ray erosions
9. Poor synovial fluid mucin precipitate
10. Positive synovial biopsy
11. Positive nodule biopsy.

In addition to the features mentioned above there are others which need to be considered in any discussion of the aetiology and pathogenesis of the disease, and include: cutaneous vasculitis, lung involvement (effusions, nodules, fibrosis), cardiac involvement (effusion, involvement of the conducting tissues, constrictive pericarditis), eye involvement (episcleritis, scleritis, nodules), peripheral neuropathy, Felty's syndrome and amyloidosis. Thus RA is a multisystem disease but it is of considerable interest to note that these features of more severe disease are found in only a proportion of patients. These individuals tend to have high titres of rheumatoid factors (RF), both of the IgG and IgM subclasses, but this is not in itself a sufficient cause as there are patients with similar RF titres who do not have extra-articular manifestations. It is of additional interest to note that individuals have been described who have high RF titres and nodules (cutaneous and/or pulmonary) without arthritis (Eraut et al, 1978) and others with no RF but with erosive arthritis indistinguishable on X-ray from seropositive individuals (Dixon, 1960). Patients may remain 'true' to a particular type of disease or may swing from one type to another. Thus, one not uncommonly sees patients with intermittent bouts of vasculitis or crops of cutaneous nodules. Erosions, of course, once they have arisen are slow to heal so that recurrent episodes of erosive disease are more difficult to document since they will be noted as a progressive accumulation of erosive damage which becomes, over the years, more severe and involves more joints. This bewildering kaleidoscope requires a hypothesis by means of which one could attempt an understanding of the evolutionary history of RA in individual patients.

Clinicopathological spectrum

The concept that a disease may have a spectrum of clinical appearances based on a parallel immunopathological spectrum is well established in a variety of diseases including leprosy (Myrvang et al, 1973; Ridley & Jopling, 1966) and tuberculosis (Lenzini et al, 1977). The underlying immunopathological processes are the outcome of the host–parasite interaction which is determined by genetic factors regulating the immune response made by the host, as happens in leprosy (de Vries et al, 1981). This is, after all, the raw material of evolution. At one end or *pole* the parasite may gain the ascendancy with death of the host, whilst at the other pole the host may kill off the parasite. One can easily visualise gradations between these poles. The same situation can occur in human disease with severe and widespread infection at one pole (lepromatous leprosy, unreactive tuberculosis) and little or no pathogen found in tissues and organs at the other pole (tuberculoid leprosy, reactive tuberculosis). The descriptions of the intermediate forms of disease can be found in the references given. What is the relevance of such a spectrum should it be found in RA? By analogy with other diseases three compelling reasons can be given:

1. The aetiological agent is more likely to be found at one pole of the disease rather than at another.
2. Treatment and response to treatment may have to be different or modified depending on the phase of the disease.
3. Realisation that in a continuous spectrum there are indeed clinical syndromes to be recognised, but as part of a single disease, will help in diagnosis and classification of disease by removing the acrimonious disputes between so-called 'lumpers' and 'splitters'.

Let us therefore apply these concepts to RA but with the cautionary note that without knowing what the aetiological agent is it is not possible to perform the antigen-specific tests used in leprosy and tuberculosis (Panayi, 1982). Nevertheless, in clinical terms, one clinical pole of the spectrum should be characterised by little tissue destruction but much immune complex-mediated disease such as vasculitis, lymphadenopathy, splenomegaly, and peripheral neuropathy. Interestingly, all rheumatologists and many internists have experience of patients with widespread cutaneous or pulmonary RA nodules, no synovitis but with high titres of IgM RF in their serum. Some of these patients go on to develop the full picture of erosive arthritis. In addition to circulating immune complexes, the serum is characterised by the presence of very high titres of a variety of autoantibodies including antinuclear factors, antibodies to to Epstein–Barr virus-determined antigens (RANA, RAP), hypergammaglobulinaemia, cryoglobulins and increased turnover of complement in the circulation (Scott et al, 1981). This may be equivalent to lepromatous leprosy (characterised by hypergammaglobulinaemia, autoantibodies, circulating immune complexes) and to unreactive tuberculosis (characterised by hypergammaglobulinaemia and high titres of circulating antibodies to tuberculin PPD). A typical finding is the absence of delayed cutaneous hypersensitivity to the causative agent (lepromin or tuberculin respectively) at this pole of the spectrum. With no such test available in RA we have to rely on the indirect evidence that delayed cutaneous hypersensitivity to a variety of skin test antigens is often absent or depressed in RA in association with hyperactivity of the humoral immune response.

What is the rheumatoid disease equivalent of tuberculoid leprosy and of reactive tuberculosis? I would suggest that the erosive changes of articular cartilage and bone are the pathological consequences of activation of the cellular immune system in this disease. Hence, by analogy with the two prototypic diseases, erosive articular changes are evidence of a host immune response which is being partially successful in limiting the dissemination of the causative pathogen. It follows from this concept that patients with so-called 'seronegative rheumatoid disease' should cluster at this end of the spectrum. Although systematic analysis of the state of their cellular immune function either by the use of in vivo or in vitro tests has not yet been undertaken, it is already clear that they have little if any IgG or IgM rheumatoid factors in their serum, they do not possess other autoantibodies and have no clinical evidence of immune complex disease. Clinically these patients generally have a benign course with fewer joints eroded, good functional grade and without any of the extra-articular manifestations of lepromatous RA which adversely affect prognosis and functional outcome (Papadimitriou et al, 1982). The really intriguing questions, however, are the following: what does extreme tuberculoid RA look like and how does lepromatous RA present itself? As to the first, it should be remembered that Kellgren found from radiological surveys of large populations that healed erosive disease is probably as common as clinically apparent disease (Kellgren, 1968). Thus, it may be surmised that a large proportion of RA is a mild or asymptomatic disease leading to self-cure by efficient cellular immune processes just as happens in leprosy and in tuberculosis. As to the second question, a more critical look should be given to those vasculitides whose classification is difficult but in which there are very high titres of antiglobulins of the G, M and A immunoglobulin subclasses.

This hypothesis, therefore, leads to the description of two extreme or polar forms of rheumatoid disease with an undefined continuum between them. In the following sections we shall see how this concept helps us to understand other aspects of this disease.

THE AETIOLOGY OF RHEUMATOID ARTHRITIS

Since the aetiology of RA is unknown a variety of opinions jostle for our attention. There are two major hypotheses concerning its aetiology, the infective and the autoimmune, although as our knowledge of the genetic regulation of the immune response and of host–parasite interactions increases the distinction between these two possibilities becomes blurred. A variety of agents have been proposed in the past as aetiological agents of RA but none have stood the test of time. Amongst them may be included mycoplasma, diphtheroids, streptococci and a variety of viruses (Phillips, 1982). With so many 'autoimmune' features in RA it is not surprising that such a process should also be invoked in its causation. The autoimmune features include: hypergammaglobulinaemia, the presence of a variety of autoantibodies, especially RF, the presence of circulating and deposited immune complexes, cryoglobulins, plasma cells in the bone marrow, central lymphoid organs and synovial membrane making RF, and infiltration of the synovial membrane with mononuclear chronic inflammatory cells, especially lymphocytes. The central question concerns the mechanism whereby this autoimmunity is switched on. There are those who postulate that initiation of the disease is a genetically determined failure of tolerance to IgG while others maintain that external agents or factors activate autoimmunity to IgG by the breaking of tolerance through a variety of mechanisms such as excessive helper activity, loss of suppressor activity and activation of macrophages (Carson, 1982). Recent experimental work has demonstrated that the production of antiglobulins and anti-nuclear factors is a very prominent component of a normal immune response although the physiological function of such autoantibodies is not known (Dresser, 1978; Steele & Cunningham, 1978).

Environmental factors

Epidemiological studies have always played an important part in defining the role of environmental factors in the causation of disease. Needless to say similar efforts have been made in RA. Curiously one part of this investigation has been conducted in libraries and museums in which investigators have tried to ascertain the antiquity or otherwise of RA by studying ancient medical and religious texts, the remains of fossils, skeletons and mummies, and by the scrutiny of paintings and drawings. The consensus seems to be that RA is a 'new' disease, the first clear description having been given by Beauvais in 1801 (Short, 1974). One of the major demographic changes taking place in Europe from the 18th century onwards was increasing urbanisation and industrialisation which led to the spread of such diseases as rheumatic fever and tuberculosis. In the modern world such a demographic change with a change in the prevalence of RA seems to have been observed in South Africa. Because of the apartheid system operating in that country the movement of black people can be strictly controlled and documented and, as a consequence, it has been possible to observe changes in disease prevalence in a genetically homogeneous group of people as they migrated from their traditional rural environment to a modern urban way of life. This has indeed happened to the Xhosa as they moved from the countryside into the Soweto township. In rural villages, their original home, Beighton and his colleagues were able to find only one woman with an inflammatory joint disease which met the ARA criteria for possible RA while in Soweto the prevalence and clinical form of RA was similar to that found in whites living in nearby Johannesburg

(Beighton et al, 1975; Solomon et al, 1975). In the USA, RA seems to be as prevalent in blacks as in whites so that the reported paucity of the disease from tropical and subtropical Africa and other parts of the world may relate to these demographic changes. Indeed RA seems to have been reported from all African states with rheumatological services (Bagg et al, 1979).

What is the 'urban' factor? No one knows. The changes that take place in such migrations are legion and involve alterations in diet, sexual habits, living conditions and exposure to new environmental agents both microbial and chemical. The pattern of infant mortality and morbidity changes with urbanisation and this could have profound biological relevance in allowing the survival of individuals with aberrant host responses to a common environmental microorganism. As an example of this one need only compare the non-paralytic form of poliomyelitis found in overcrowded slums, where children are infected early in life, with the paralytic form of the disease in privileged middle class homes where infection occurs later in life.

Indirect evidence for such an environmental factor comes from the work of Wasmuth et al (1972) who showed that the probability of the non-consanguineous spouse of a proband with RA developing the disease was related to the length of time the two individuals had lived together. Similar conclusions have been arrived at by Lawrence & Wood (1968). However, studies of the distribution of RF in families with one member at least having RA have not shown the presence of an intrafamilial environmental agent as have the studies using ANF and lymphocytotoxic antibodies in lupus families. Whatever the environmental factor it would seem to behave differently from *Mycobacterium tuberculosis*, since tuberculosis has been declining in Europe for the last hundred years while RA seems to have appeared, and still to be appearing, in the last two hundred.

That environmental factors are of crucial importance in the manifestation of such a complex biological entity as a 'disease' can be illustrated by the dramatic impact of the oral contraceptive pill on the prevalence of RA. Three separate studies from three different parts of the world have shown that the prevalence of RA has declined during the time that the 'pill' has been used (Wingrave & Kay, 1979; Linos et al, 1980; Vandenbroucke et al, 1982) although a recent case-control study by Linos and her colleagues (1983) has failed to confirm the findings of their 1980 population study. The nature of the mechanism whereby this hormonal therapy has apparently prevented the development of RA is not known but may be related to that leading to improvement in disease activity seen in 75% of rheumatoids during pregnancy (Unger et al, 1983).

Genetic factors

Family and mono- and dizygotic twin studies have shown that there is a weak genetic factor in RA. There the matter rested until the importance of the major histocompatibility complex (MHC) in immune responses was realised in the 1970s (see Ch. 10). In RA the important observation was the finding that HLA-D4 and HLA-DR4 are significantly elevated in RA, being found in 60–80% of patients compared to 20% of control subjects (Panayi et al, 1978; Stastny, 1978). This is true for all populations studied except Israel where the association is with HLA-DRl (Schiff et al, 1982). This finding indicates that the disease susceptibility gene is in linkage disequilibrium with DR alleles. The conclusion from this must be that an individual MHC product may not of itself be necessary for initiation of disease. Family studies confirm the association of DR4 with RA in Caucasians but have shed no additional light on further genetic factors or on the exact location of the RA disease susceptibility gene within the MHC. Clearly genes at other loci and even on other chromosomes may be involved since some immunoglobulin Gm haplotypes are found more frequently in sibling pairs than would be expected by chance (Zilko et al, 1980).

The association of RA with HLA-DR4 raises some important questions: does DR4 predispose to the production of rheumatoid factors and is DR4 a marker for disease severity rather than disease susceptibility? The concensus of current research is that HLA-DR4 is not a marker for the propensity to develop rheumatoid factors (for review, see Panayi & David, 1983) either in normals or in patients with RA. Thus the scenario which envisages rheumatoid factors as being central to the aetiopathogenesis of RA through the formation of immune complexes cannot be related in a direct manner to DR4. It is more likely that once disease has been initiated, in ways related to DR4, rheumatoid factors are then made by mechanisms which are DR4-independent. This is in agreement with earlier family studies which showed that the inheritance of erosive joint disease and of rheumatoid factors behave as two independently segregating variables (Ziff et al, 1958; Lawrence, 1967)

There is evidence, however, that HLA-DR4 may be a marker for an immune response gene to denatured collagen in that DR4-positive individuals, whether healthy controls or patients with RA, are able to mount a T lymphocyte response to this antigen whereas DR4-negative individuals fail to do so (Smollen et al, 1980; Solinger et al; 1981). The unresponsiveness of DR4-negative individuals may be due to the presence of circulating suppressor T lymphocytes able to switch off this response (Solinger & Stobo, 1982). Nevertheless, despite these findings there must be other factors involved in the susceptibility to developing RA since only a small proportion of DR4-positive individuals in the community have the disease. It may be that following joint damage initiated by other means, cell-mediated immunity to collagen in DR4-positive patients would accentuate tissue destruction by secondary 'auto immune' reactivity.

This leads to the concept that DR4 is a marker for disease severity rather than disease susceptibility. This is a contentious area at present. The majority opinion is of the view that DR4 is *not* a marker for disease severity but the matter is bedevilled by differences in patient selection and clinical criteria of disease assessment between the different studies. There is evidence, however, that the possession of DR2 is associated with milder disease and with a better response to second-line drug treatment — especially sodium aurothiomalate (Panayi et al, 1978; Griffin et al, 1983). Indeed, many of the clinical/genetic studies of RA may be vitiated by as yet unknown relationships between drug therapy and genetic factors which could influence the selection of patients. Thus, it is already known that HLA-DR3 is linked to myocrisin-induced glomerulonephritis (Wooley et al, 1980) or thrombocytopenia (Coblyn et al, 1981) and that some toxic manifestations of D-penicillamine may be related to the slow sulphoxidiser status of the individual (Panayi et al, 1983). This is an area where many interesting and clinically important observations are still to be made. Unfortunately, the associations between these toxic manifestations and the corresponding genetic marker are not sufficiently strong for clinical application in patient management as yet. It is to be hoped that the techniques of molecular genetics, with their inherently greater power to detect polymorphism at the DNA level, may solve this problem.

THE PATHOGENESIS OF RHEUMATOID ARTHRITIS

Rheumatoid arthritis is a systemic disease with evidence of abnormal immune reactivity in the bone marrow, lymph nodes and spleen as well as in the synovial membrane itself. The simplest hypothesis to explain this phenomenon is that RA is a disease determined by genetic and environmental factors, namely an infectious agent (see above), which is systemically distributed in the patient, but has a particular predilection for synovial joints. The agent persists because of an exquisite inability, which is genetically determined, on the part of the patient to develop protective immunity against it; the patient's immune system, however, is capable of mounting an effective response against other antigens possessed by the agent so that immune hyperactivity develops. A variant of this hypothesis would be that the agent is 'defective' in that it fails to develop or to express the antigen(s) responsible for protective immunity but the outcome would, in operational terms, be the same. This situation is illustrated by the very high titres of anti-measles antibody in the cerebrospinal fluid of patients with subacute sclerosing panencephalitis in which measles virus is thought to persist in the central nervous system. Similarly in RA, as a consequence of the persistence of the postulated 'RA agent' and the consequent chronic stimulation of the immune response, a variety of autoantibodies are formed and in particular rheumatoid factor; such autoantibodies occur in many inflammatory and immunological states (burns, malaria, leprosy, etc.). It is these factors and their ability to form immune complexes which are thought to be responsible for some of the inflammatory lesions, especially the extra-articular features, seen during the course of the disease. Some of the immune complexes are formed locally in the joint while others may be formed in the circulation with subsequent deposition in tissues. Whether any of the immune complexes contain antigenic material related to the 'RA agent' is still a matter of dispute but if they do they must be in the minority. The inflammatory potential of immune complexes is determined by a variety of factors, including their ability to activate the complement cascade, and this has been reviewed elsewhere (see Ch. 13).

The synovial membrane

The hypertrophic and hyperplastic rheumatoid synovial membrane is infiltrated with chronic inflammatory cells such as macrophages, T and B lymphocytes and plasma cells. Some 70% of the latter are producing IgG and IgM rheumatoid factors but the nature of the immunoglobulin produced by the remainder is not known. Immune complexes are present in abundance both extracellularly and intracellularly either as phagocytosed material or as self-associated IgG rheumatoid factors within plasma cells (Munthe, 1978). The finding of phagocytosed immunoglobulins and complement is prominent in neutrophils of the synovial fluid but noticeable by its absence in the phagocytic type A cells of the synovial lining. This raises interesting questions about the phagocytic and degradative abilities of these cells — questions which have not been answered. The mechanism whereby the numbers of synovial lining cells are increased is also unknown and could be due to increased trafficking from the bone marrow, since they are bone marrow-derived cells, or to increased replication as a result of locally released growth factors. There is also an increase in the number of blood vessels in the inflamed synovial membrane and this could be due to the production of angiogenesis-promoting factors or to loss of angiogenesis-inhibiting factors normally made by articular chondrocytes. These findings are general to any inflammatory process in the synovium and specific markers allowing one to diagnose rheumatoid arthritis, ankylosing spondylistis or psoriatic arthritis, for example, are still not available.

How do these changes come about? The earliest lesion, at least in RA, involves the blood vessels running through the synovium, followed by the perivascular accumulation of lymphocytes, and, lastly, by changes in the synovial lining cell layer. Histological examination of tissue of necessity gives a rather static picture of a dynamic and active situation but we have no information on changes in lymphocyte and other cell traffic through the joints or central lymphoid tissues, and we know nothing of the molecular events involved in lymphocyte–endothelial interactions in the synovium although we know that such recognition structures are of major importance in lymphocyte migration through other tissues such as lymph node (Chin et al, 1982). The perivascular lymphoid aggregates in the rheumatoid synovium are predominantly localised around areas of high venular endothelium (HVE) where lymphocyte trafficking normally takes place as a consequence of specific lymphocyte-recognition-structures being present on HVE cells. Recent studies using histochemistry and immunohistology have shown that there are dendritic, interdigitating cells of a similar phenotype to antigen-presenting cells in the T dependent areas of lymph nodes (HLA-DR-positive, lysosomal enzyme-negative, adenosine triphosphatase-positive) scattered throughout the synovial membrane (both normal and inflamed) but particularly in a perivascular distribution. In the rheumatoid synovium these cells are intimately associated with T lymphocytes of a helper/inducer phenotype (OKT4-positive) (Fig. 24.1). These cells are the majority T cell population except at the periphery of the perivascular aggregates, where T lymphocytes of the suppressor/cytotoxic phenotype (OKT8-positive) may, on occasions, predominate and in small lymphocyte collections scattered in the synovium where the ratio of T4 to T8 lymphocytes is close to unity (Duke et al, 1982; Poulter et al, 1983). This arrangement is particularly suited for lymphocyte activation and the generation of a wide variety of interleukins, lymphokines and other inflammatory mediators. Thus the activation of T4 helper lymphocytes would lead to B cell activation

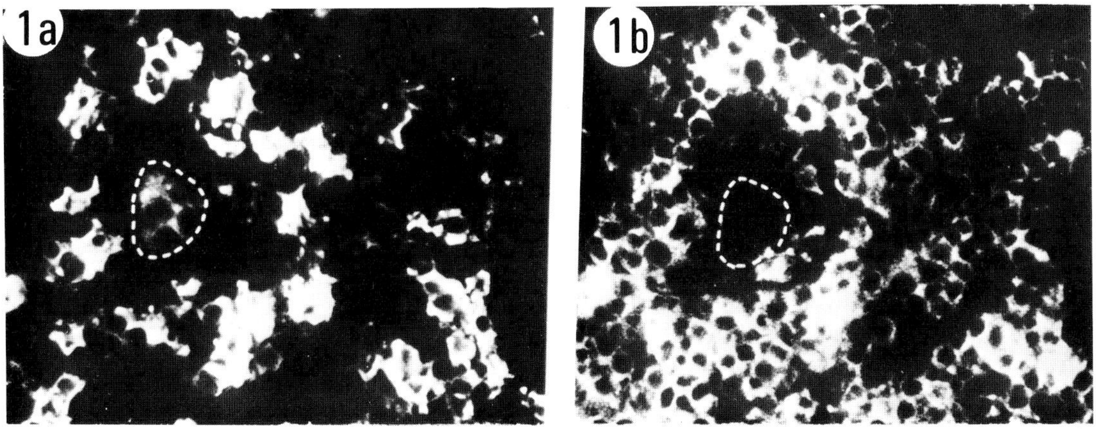

Fig. 24.1 Rheumatoid synovial membrane stained with anti-HLA-DR antiserum and monoclonal antibody OKT4 directed against T lymphocytes of the helper/inducer phenotype. (a) Large numbers of HLA-DR positive stellate cells thought to have antigen-presenting function (taken using a rhodamine-sensitive filter). (b) OKT4-positive T lymphocyte are prominent in the same area (taken using a fluorescein-sensitive filter). The dotted line identifies a blood vessel. (From: Poulter et al (1983) by kind permission of the editor of *Clinical and Experimental Immunology*.)

and differentiation into plasma cells producing RF and other immunoglobulins. It should be noted, however, that on this view the predominant immunopathological event in the RA synovium is a T-dependent one (Janossy et al, 1981) and that the previous emphasis on its B cell nature (the presence of germinal follicles, plasma cells and the production of immunoglobulin by synovial explants) may have been the result of an overenthusiastic interpretation of the findings. It is worth remarking here that most accounts of the lymph node architecture in RA still dwell on the hypertrophy and hyperplasia of the germinal follicles (B cell areas) to the unwarranted neglect of the T-dependent or paracortical areas.

Some of the factors released in the inflamed synovium could have a variety of effects. Thus activated macrophages could release interleukin 1 (ILI) which would have local as well as systemic effects. Systemic effects would, in particular, include the stimulation of the acute phase response including elevation of C-reactive protein. T4-positive helper/inducer lymphocytes produce interleukin 2 which would then activate other T cells to proliferate, others to make interleukin 3 capable of activating macrophages, and yet others to produce B cell activating and differentiating factors with the ultimate generation of immunoglobulin-producing plasma cells. The activation of macrophages or of large stellate synovial cells by ILI (mononuclear cell factor) leads to the production of collagenase and prostaglandins with obvious tissue degradative and inflammatory potential (Baum, 1982). What keeps this inflammed tissue active year after year? The arrangement of the helper/inducer lymphocytes around antigen-presenting cells with a paucity of T8 suppressor cells is eminently suitable for continued immunological activation. This could happen as a result of the arrival of foreign antigen, either alone or already bound to APC, in the synovium. This would then act as a trigger for the accumulation and subsequent stimulation of the T4 lymphocytes with the consequences which have been described above. Persistent disease would then be the result of the persistence of antigen ('RA agent') and/or inadequate T lymphocyte suppression so that a chronic, self-perpetuating inflammatory system could be set up (Fig. 24.2). There is even the possibility that after the initial trigger by exogenous antigen the whole process could become autostimulatory as in the autologous mixed lymphocyte reaction (Janossy et al, 1981). If so, rheumatoid arthritis would be the first of a new type of autoimmune disease whose persistence depends on the failure to switch off autoreactivity to the DR products of the major histocompatibility complex.

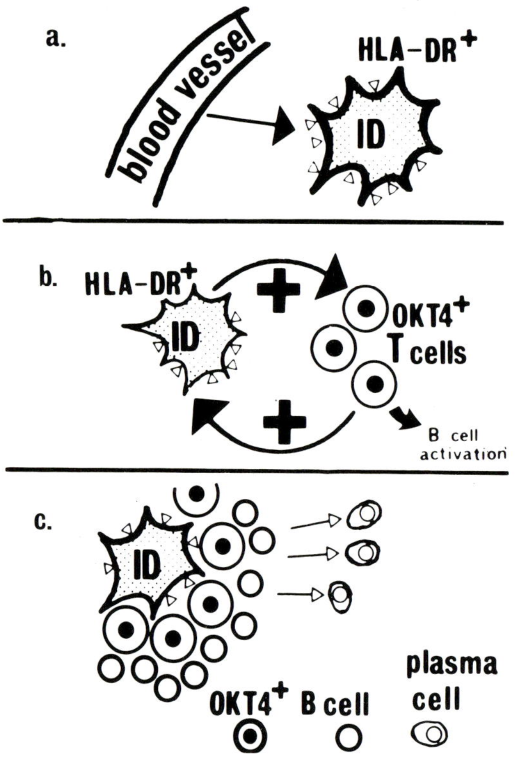

Fig. 24.2 The development of chronicity in rheumatoid arthritis. (a) Antigen (small triangles) arrives via the blood stream and is presented by HLA-DR-positive stellate interdigitating cells (ID). (b) OKT4-positive lymphocytes arrive and a vicious cycle of stimulation is set up due to failure of T lymphocyte suppression. (c) As a result of the release of soluble factors and cell/cell interactions, T cells are activated to participate in cell-mediated immunity and B cells to differentiate into immunoglobulin-producing plasma cells (including rheumatoid factor). (From: Janossy et al (1981) by kind permission of the editor of *The Lancet*.)

SUMMARY

In conclusion, RA may be thought of as:

1. A disease caused by an environmental agent, which evades the host immune system as a result of an exquisite and genetically-determined immunodeficiency on the part of the host
2. The entry of lymphocytes into the joint by means of specific recognition structures on lymphocytes and on high venular endothelium through which cells migration takes place
3. Persistence of the agent and/or failure of immune regulation leading to immune hyper-reactivity including the generation of RFs and immune complexes
4. The release of a variety of mediators with effects on lymphocytes, macrophages, osteoclasts, vascular endothelium and chondrocytes.

It is obvious that the potential for therapeutic intervention in RA is immense but, to date, this newly accumulated knowledge has not been used for the generation of new drug treatments. The future therefore promises not only to be exciting to the rheumatologist but full of hope to the patient.

REFERENCES

Bagg L R, Hansen D P, Lewis C, Houbra V 1979 Rheumatoid arthritis in Kenya. I. Clinical observations. Annals of the Rheumatic Diseases 38: 23–25

Baum J 1982 Mediators of inflammation. In: Panayi G S (ed) The scientific basis of rheumatology. Churchill Livingstone, Edinburgh, p. 260–271

Beighton P, Solomon L, Valkenberg H A 1975 Rheumatoid arthritis in a rural South African Negro population. Annals of the Rheumatic Diseases 34: 136–142

Carson D A 1982 Antiglobulin antibodies. In: Panayi G S (ed) The scientific basis of rheumatology. Churchill Livingstone, Edinburgh, p. 114–130

Chin Y–H, Carey G D, Woodruff J D 1982 Lymphocyte recognition of lymph node high endothelium. IV. Cell surface structures mediating entry into lymph nodes. Journal of Immunology 129: 1911–1915

Coblyn J S, Weinblatt M, Holdswoth D, Glass D 1981 Gold-induced thrombocytopenia. A clinical and immunogenetic study of twenty-three patients. Annals of Internal Medicine 95: 178–181

Dixon A St J 1960 'Rheumatoid arthritis' with negative serological reaction. Annals of the Rheumatic Diseases 19: 209–228

Dresser D W 1978 Most IgM-producing cells in the mouse secrete autoantibodies (rheumatoid factor). Nature 274: 480–483

Duke O, Panayi G S, Janossy G, Poulter L W 1982 An immunohistological analysis of lymphocyte subpopulations and their microenvironment in the synovial membranes of patients with rheumatoid arthritis using monoclonal antibodies. Clinical and Experimental Immunology 49: 22–30

Eraut D, Evans J, Caplan M 1978 Pulmonary necrobiotic nodules without rheumatoid arthritis. British Journal of Diseases of the Chest 72: 301–306

Griffin A J, Wooley P, Panayi G S, Batchelor J R 1983

HLA-DR antigens and disease expression in rheumatoid arthritis. Annals of the Rheumatic Diseases (in press)
Janossy G, Panayi G S, Duke O, et al 1981 Rheumatoid arthritis: a disease of T-lymphcoyte/macrophage immunoregulation. Lancet 2: 839–842
Kellgren J H 1968 Epidemiology of rheumatoid arthritis. In: Duthie J J R, Alexander W R M (eds) Rheumatic diseases. Edinburgh University Press, Edinburgh, p. 7–18
Lawrence J S 1967 Genetics of rheumatoid factor and rheumatoid arthritis. Clinical and Experimental Immunology 2: 769–783
Lawrence J S, Wood P H N 1968 Genetic influences in rheumatoid arthritis. In: Duthie J J R, Alexander W R M (eds) Rheumatic diseases. Edinburgh University Press, Edinburgh, p. 19–28
Lenzini L, Rottoli P, Rottoli L 1977 The spectrum of human tuberculosis. Clinical and Experimental Immunology 27: 230–237
Linos A, Worthington J W, O'Fallon W M, Kurland L T 1980 The epidemiology of rheumatoid arthritis in Rochester, Minnesota: a study of incidence, prevalence and mortality. American Journal of Epidemiology 11: 87–98
Linos A, Worthington J W, O'Fallon W M, Kurland L T 1983 Case-control study of rheumatoid arthritis and prior use of oral contraceptives. Lancet 1: 1299–1300
Munthe E 1978 Deposition of immune complexes in synovial membrane and fluid. In: Panayi G S, Johnson P M (eds) Immunopathogenesis of rheumatoid arthritis. Reed Books, Chertsey, p. 85–88
Myrvang B, Godal T, Ridley D S, Froland S S, Song Y K 1973 Immune responsiveness to *Mycobacterium leprae* and other mycobacterial antigens throughout the clinical and histopathological spectrum of leprosy. Clinical and Experimental Immunology 14: 541–543
Panayi G S 1982 Does rheumatoid arthritis have a clinicopathological spectrum similar to that of leprosy? Annals of the Rheumatic Diseases 41: 102–103
Panayi G S, David C (eds) 1983 Clinical immunology 1: Immunogenetics. Butterworths, London
Panayi G S, Huston G, Shah R R, et al 1983 Deficient sulphoxidation status and d-penicillamine toxicity. Lancet 1:414 (letter)
Panayi G S, Wooley P, Batchelor J R 1978 Genetic basis of rheumatoid disease: HLA antigens, disease manifestations, and toxic reactions to drugs. British Medical Journal 2: 1326–1328
Papadimitriou G M, Bacon P A, Hall N D 1982 Circulating activated lymphocytes in rheumatoid arthritis: a marker of synovial inflammation. Journal of Rheumatology 9: 217–223
Phillips P E 1982 Infection and the pathogenesis of connective tissue diseases. In: Panayi G S (ed) The scientific basis of rheumatology. Churchill Livingstone, Edinburgh, p. 1–21
Poulter L W, Duke O, Hobbs S, et al 1983 The involvement of interdigitating (antigen-presenting) cells in the pathogenesis of rheumatoid arthritis. Clinical and Experimental Immunology 51: 247–254
Ridley D S, Jopling W H 1966 Classification of leprosy according to immunity: a five group system. International Journal of Leprosy 34: 255–261
Ropes M W, Bennett G A, Cobb S, Jacox R, Jessar R A 1958. 1958 revision of diagnostic criteria for rheumatoid arthritis. Bulletin of the Rheumatic Diseases 9: 175–176
Schiff B, Mizrachi Y, Orgad S, et al 1982 Association of HLA-Aw31 and HLA-DR1 with adult rheumatoid arthritis. Annals of the Rheumatic Diseases 41: 403–404
Scott DGI, Bacon P A, Allen C, et al 1981 IgG rheumatoid factor, complement and immune complexes in rheumatoid synovitis and vasculitis: comparative and serial studies during cytotoxic therapy. Clinical and Experimental Immunology 43: 54–63
Short C L 1974 The antiquity of rheumatoid arthritis. Arthritis and Rheumatism 17: 193–205
Smolen J S, Menzel E J, Scherak O, et al 1980 Lymphocyte transformation to denatured type I collagen and B lymphocyte alloantigens in rheumatoid arthritis. Arthritis and Rheumatism 23: 424–431
Solinger A M, Bhatnagar R, Stobo J D 1981 Cellular molecular and genetic characteristics of T cell reactivity to collagen in man. Proceedings of the National Academy of Sciences (USA) 78: 3877–3881
Solinger A M, Stobo J D 1982 Immune response genes control reactivity in man: collagen unresponsiveness in HLA-DR4 negative unresponders is due to the presence of T-dependent suppressive influences. Journal of Immunology 129: 1916–1920
Solomon L, Robin G, Valkenberg H A 1975 Rheumatoid arthritis in an urban South African Negro population. Annals of the Rheumatic Diseases 34: 128–135
Stastny P 1978 Association of the B-cell alloantigen DRw4 with rheumatoid arthritis. New England Journal of Medicine 298: 869–871
Steele E J, Cunningham A J 1978 High proportion of Ig-producing cells making autoantibody in normal mice. Nature 274: 483–484
Unger A, Kay A, Griffin A J, Panayi G S 1983 Disease activity and pregnancy-associated 2-glycoprotein in rheumatoid arthritis during pregnancy. British Medical Journal 286: 750–752
Vandenbroucke J P, Valkenburg H A, Boersma J W, et al 1982 Oral contraceptives and rheumatoid arthritis: further evidence for a preventive effect. Lancet 2: 839–842
de Vries RRP, van Eden W, van Rood J J 1981 HLA-linked control of the course of *M. leprae* infections. Leprosy Review (Suppl. 1) 52: 109–119
Wasmuth A G, Veale A M O, Palmer D G, Highton T C 1972 Prevalence of rheumatoid arthritis in families. Annals of Rheumatic Diseases 31: 85–91
Wingrave J J, Kay C R 1979 Reduction in incidence of rheumatoid arthritis associated with oral contraceptives. Lancet 1: 569–571
Wooley P H, Griffin J, Panayi G S, et al 1980 HLA-DR antigens and toxic reaction to sodium aurothiomalate and d-penicillamine in patients with rheumatoid arthritis. New England Journal of Medicine 303: 300–302
Ziff M, Schmid F R, Lewis A J, Tanner M 1958 Familial occurrence of rheumatoid factor. Arthritis and Rheumatism 1: 392–399
Zilko P J, Feeney D, Christiansen F T, Hawkins B R, Dawkins R L 1980 HLA and Gm typing in families with rheumatoid arthritis. Arthritis and Rheumatism 23:767 (abstract)

25

D.L. Gardner

Pathology of rheumatoid arthritis

Rheumatoid arthritis (RA) is a common, symmetrical inflammatory but non-suppurative polyarticular disease unique to modern man. There is a genetic predisposition. Microbial agents are periodically associated with the disease but the cause remains uncertain. Psychological and physical agents have been invoked and there is a female preponderance. Rheumatoid disease attacks the 187 synovial joints but it is not confined to them and the many visceral manifestations have led to the classification of RA as a systemic disorder of the immunological mechanism. Of the visceral lesions, anaemia and a focal subcutaneous granuloma are the most characteristic. Some cases of RA, particularly those that are seropositive, are fulminating and rapidly progress to severe deformity. In others there is a remitting course (Fig. 25.1). The most characteristic pattern associates slowly advancing articular disease with progressive disability and systemic illness. There is no specific treatment but deformity can be minimised and disability reduced, by many new medical and surgical forms of prophylactic and remedial treatment. Some of these regimes are accompanied by their own pathological complications.

Rheumatoid arthritis has not been conclusively demonstrated in archeological remains and the morbid anatomical lesions were first described by Robert Adams (1857a, b) at almost the same moment that RA was given its contemporary name by Garrod (1859). Although there are hints that RA existed in Belgium in the late 17th century

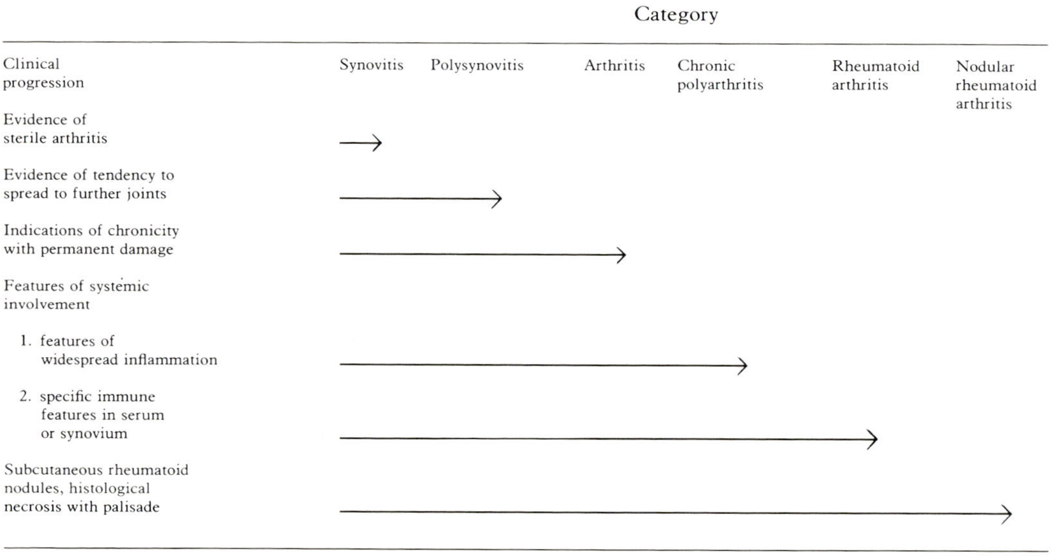

Fig. 25.1 A simple progressive system proposed by Schilling (1973) and advocated by Fassbender (1975), relating the clinical progression of rheumatoid disease and the pathological category in a stepwise fashion.

(Appelboom & Erhlich, 1981), it was only with the control of the great infectious diseases, and the prolongation of life in Western Society, that RA became a major health problem.

Articular disease

Any of the synovial joints may be the site of early inflammation. Very commonly, the disease first affects the peripheral joints of the limbs so that the interphalangeal, metacarpophalangeal and metatarsophalangeal articulations are the site for early morning pain, redness, swelling, heat and disability, the cardinal signs of inflammation. Several or many joints are simultaneously attacked and in decreasing order of frequency the wrists, ankles, knees, shoulders, elbows and hips are affected. The synovial (apophyseal) joints of the spine are involved and so are the inconstant neurocentral joints of the cervical region. To date, the evidence suggests sparing of the synovial component of the sacroiliac joints. RA of the small, intrinsic joints of the larynx is, however, common and characteristic.

The target for RA is the synoviochondral junction where delicate arcades of thin-walled capillaries define the symmetrical margins of the hyaline articular cartilage (Gardner, 1972). Because the inflammatory reaction is synovial and therefore circumferential (Fig. 25.2), the red, swollen synovial membrane attracted early attention and became known as a '*pannus*'. In addition, however, inflammation of the tendon sheath synovium, the joint recesses and the bursae, and of the vascular parts of the articular capsules, tendons, ligaments and menisci, is commonplace, and the non-cartilaginous lesions that result contribute materially to the natural history of the disease. It is interesting that the passive accumulation of immunoglobulin in superficial hyaline cartilage is much less than its accumulation in articular structures such as the knee menisci, capsule and ligaments (Cooke et al, 1975; Ohno & Cooke, 1978). Bone is affected. Secondary destruction of hyaline cartilage is inevitable but the synchondroses and symphyses are not sites of RA inflammation.

Synovial disease

Early changes

The cardinal, clinical signs of inflammation are evidence of an initial, microscopic synovitis (Soko-

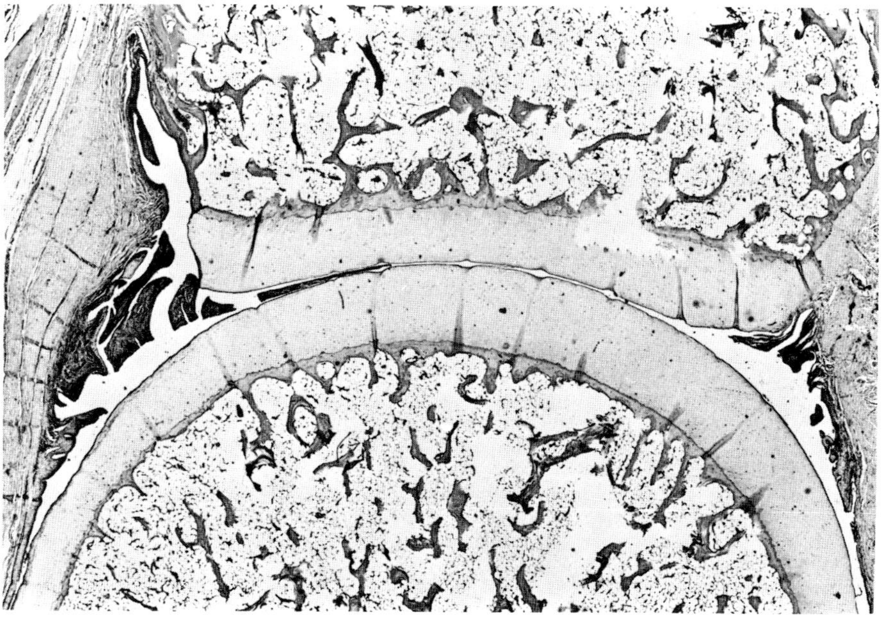

Fig. 25.2 Early rheumatoid synovitis. Enlarged, black-grey appearing synovial villi protrude into joint margin and extend over load-bearing articular cartilage surfaces. H & E ×4.

loff, 1966) (Fig. 25.3). Capillary and venular congestion reflect this initial reaction and oedema is seen. Endothial necrosis and venular thrombosis were described in one of the first studies of early RA synovitis (Kulka et al, 1955; Kulka, 1966) but most later biopsy specimens display intact endothelia. As blood flow slows, neutrophil polymorphs marginate and actively migrate through venous endothelial intercellular gaps, coming to lie in the extracellular tissue spaces of the subsynoviocytic layer. Here they are joined by increasing numbers of more slowly migrating macrophages. The absence of a true subsynoviocytic basement membrane accelerates the tendency for the rapidly moving polymorphs to pass among the synoviocytes themselves and escape into the synovial fluid where, in early RA synovitis, they are the predominant cell type. The constant presence, even in persistently active RA of longer duration, of significantly raised numbers of polymorphs, has been held to be an important factor in the marginal cartilage degradation of RA (Mohr & Wessinghage, 1978; Mohr, 1980; Menninger et al, 1980). The polymorphs release enzymes such as elastase that have collagenolytic activity. Their ability to produce superoxide and peroxide has also attracted much interest (Blake et al, 1981; Rowley & Halliwell, 1983).

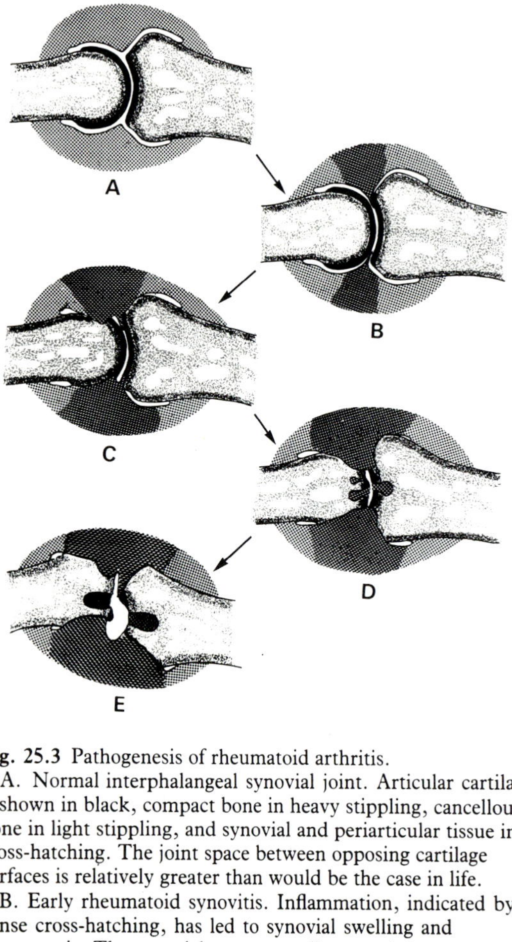

Fig. 25.3 Pathogenesis of rheumatoid arthritis.

A. Normal interphalangeal synovial joint. Articular cartilage is shown in black, compact bone in heavy stippling, cancellous bone in light stippling, and synovial and periarticular tissue in cross-hatching. The joint space between opposing cartilage surfaces is relatively greater than would be the case in life.

B. Early rheumatoid synovitis. Inflammation, indicated by dense cross-hatching, has led to synovial swelling and hyperaemia. The synovial processes adhere to the cartilage surfaces at the joint periphery.

C. The marginal destruction of cartilage, granulation tissue formation and the osteoclastic reabsorption of nearby bone, have caused the loss of tissue that can be detected radiologically as 'erosion'.

D. Granulation tissue, formed in continuity with the inflamed synovial membrane, has continued to replace bone and cartilage at the circumference of the articular surfaces and has extended through the surfaces to form the radiolucent zones that are called pseudocysts. The extent of the synovitis and of the fascitis, tendinitis and cellulitis is now much greater. Adhesions between the joint surfaces have formed.

E. Laxity of ligaments, and capsule, with muscle atrophy and tendinitis, have permitted subluxation to develop. Little or no normal articular cartilage remains. Secondary osteoarthrosis has developed and there is osteoporosis. Fibrous ankylosis is likely. Shortening of the finger or toe is observed.

Soon after the early phase of acute inflammation, the exogenous cell population of the synovial membrane changes (Schumacher & Kitridou, 1972). Plasma cells, at first scanty, become numerous (Fig. 25.4). Readily identified by their high content of pyroninophilic RNA, these cells

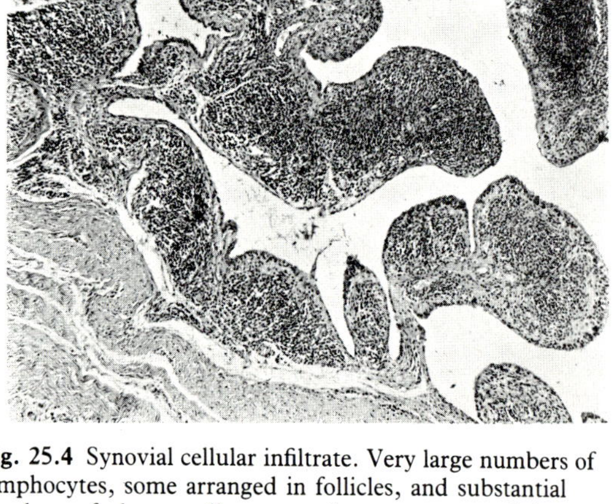

Fig. 25.4 Synovial cellular infiltrate. Very large numbers of lymphocytes, some arranged in follicles, and substantial numbers of plasma cells occupy the greater part of these enlarged synovial processes. H & E ×40.

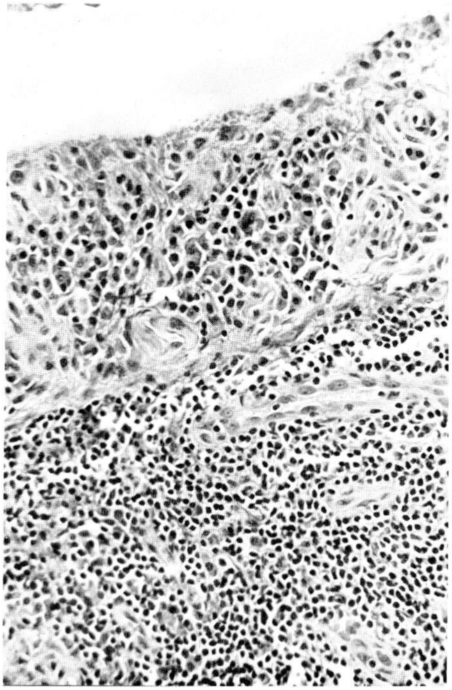

Fig. 25.5 Synovial surface. Synovial cell layer (top) merging with subsynoviocytic connective tissue extensively infiltrated by plasma cells. Lower half of field, with many small blood vessels, is almost wholly occupied by T lymphocytes. H & E ×200.

are known to be B lymphocytes. Their presence draws attention to the possibility that the synovial membrane is responding to exogenous or to autologous antigen. However, synovial cells may also be reacting to the products of mononuclear cells themselves (Baker et al, 1983). Subsequently, the B cell infiltrate is outnumbered by a diffuse infiltrate of T lymphocytes (Fig. 25.5).

From the earliest moment in RA synovitis, altered venular permeability allows plasma proteins to pass into the extravascular tissue spaces where they can be identified in the oedematous fluid. This proteinaceous exudate tends to be reabsorbed into synovial lymphatics but some is removed by phagocytes. The IgG, IgM and IgA immunoglobulins, together with complement, take part in local antigen–antibody reactions but remain localised, for example to the endothelium of small blood vessels. Fibronectin is present (Clemmensen et al, 1983). Fibrinogen represents only a small fraction of the total exudate but readily polymerises in the extracellular spaces. The resultant accumulation of insoluble fibrin (Figs. 25.6, 25.7) is a characteristic and almost invariable microscopic feature not only of persistent RA synovitis but also of other chronic arthritides such as tuberculosis and, to a much smaller extent, of systemic lupus erythematosus (SLE).

Although much fibrin remains within the subsynoviocytic tissue, a large part of the initial exudate escapes through the readily permeable synovial cell layer into the joint space (Holland et al, 1982) (Fig. 25.8). Here, the quantity of polymerised fibrin may be so large that it aggregates into melon-seed-shaped structures, often called 'rice bodies' (Popert et al, 1982). The fibrin is detected at synovial fluid examination. The rice bodies trap small numbers of free synovial fluid cells and gradually develop a thin, cellular covering; they also contain fibronectin. Persistence of polymerised fibrin has led to the suggestion that the long-standing presence of this protein itself can

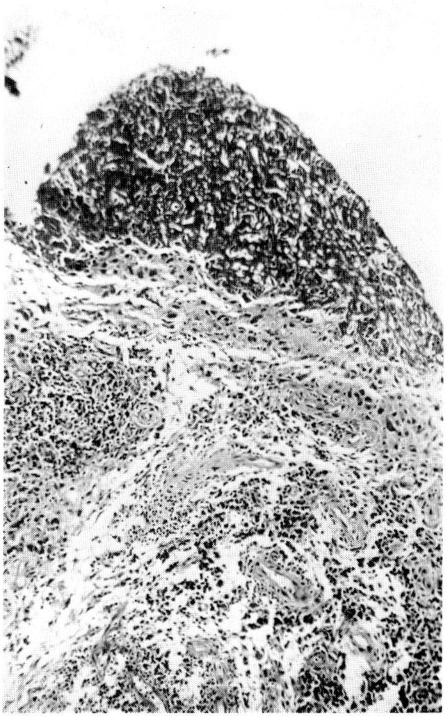

Fig. 25.6 Synovial fibrin. Fibroareolar synovial tissue widely infiltrated by mononuclear cells and capped (top) by aggregate of polymerised fibrin that is not yet covered by synovial cells, i.e. not yet incorporated in the synovium. H & E × 175.

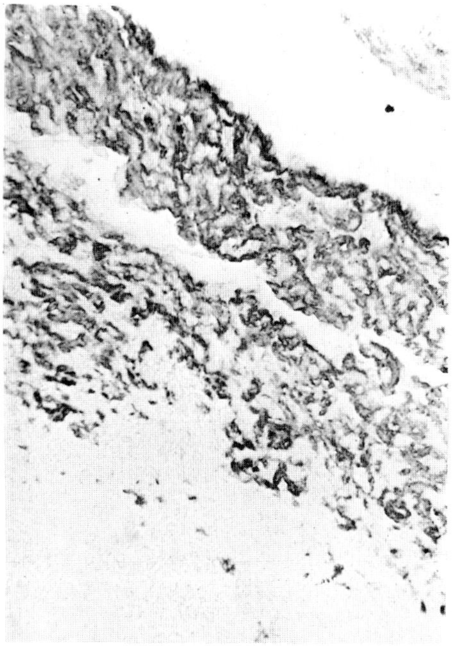

Fig. 25.7 Synovial fibrin. A loose meshwork of fibrin lies within the synovial surface layer, extending between the synoviocytes and between the deeper, subsynoviocytic vascular and connective tissue cells. Martius-scarlet-blue ×175.

contribute to or even account for the extraordinary chronicity of RA. A mechanism is postulated by which, after polymerisation, the fibrin undergoes a change in antigenic structure; it comes to assume an altered, foreign form, eliciting an autoimmune reaction that ensures perpetuation of the inflammation (Glynn, 1968, 1972). Some support is given to this view by experimental evidence. Although the eosinophilic exudate retained within the synovial membranes and on their surfaces is still occasionally termed 'fibrinoid', the main value of this description is in immediate, differential diagnosis and in reminding the observer of the aetiological analogies between RA, SLE and the other systemic connective tissue diseases. The use of the descriptive term 'fibrinoid' does not imply identity of composition or of cause.

Occasionally, and in a small proportion of cases, microscopy reveals foci of necrotic material within the subsynoviocytic connective tissue. True intra-articular granulomata (p. 625) have been described (Kampner & Kuzell, 1976). Exceptionally, the necrotic focus may communicate with the synovial cavity, constituting a hemigranuloma; there may be loss of part of the synovial, lining-cell layer with ulceration. The necrotic focus resembles the subcutaneous RA granuloma and the margin, of pallisaded A (M)-derived cells or of histiocytes, has a characteristic structure and serpiginous outline. The focus is sterile. Its recognition is one of the most valuable steps in histological diagnosis but its inconstancy renders this success improbable. One explanation for the development of focal RA synovial granuloma is the local accumulation of immune complexes. Another is the entrapment, between two hypertrophied, inflamed villi, of part of the inflammatory exudate.

Exploration of early cases has shown great variation in the extent and severity of the inflammatory reaction between different patients and within a single joint (Cruickshank, 1952). A diffuse proliferative synovitis, virtually confined at first to the synoviocytic and subsynoviocytic layers, is followed by hypertrophy and lymphocytic infiltration (Kulka et al, 1955). Lymphocytic foci appear but only rarely lymphoid follicles. There is a mononuclear cell infiltrate, oedema, the presence of poorly-differentiated mesenchymal cells, and disruption and hyalinisation of collagen fibre bundles. Geiler & Emmrich (1980) compared the synovial distribution, in the hands, fingers and knees in 13 early and 16 late cases, of 32 histological abnormalities. Five early changes were particularly significant: increased glycosaminoglycan, constituting a layer of mucoid change in the outer synovial tissue; vasculitis or perivasculitis; slight plasma- or lymphocytosis; little fibrin and few polymorphs; and an absence of fibrosis and hyaline change. Synovial cell hyperplasia was much less pronounced than in later cases but the presence of immunocompetent cells was characteristic. These observations are controversial. The inflammatory reaction is accompanied by altered redox potentials and other indices of changed metabolic activity (Butcher et al, 1973; Henderson, 1981). However, there is little direct evidence of altered synoviocytic metabolism; although DNA has been used as a guide to cellularity, rates of mitotic division have rarely been measured.

The transmission electron microscope (TEM) has clarified synovial ultrastructure (Davies & Pal-

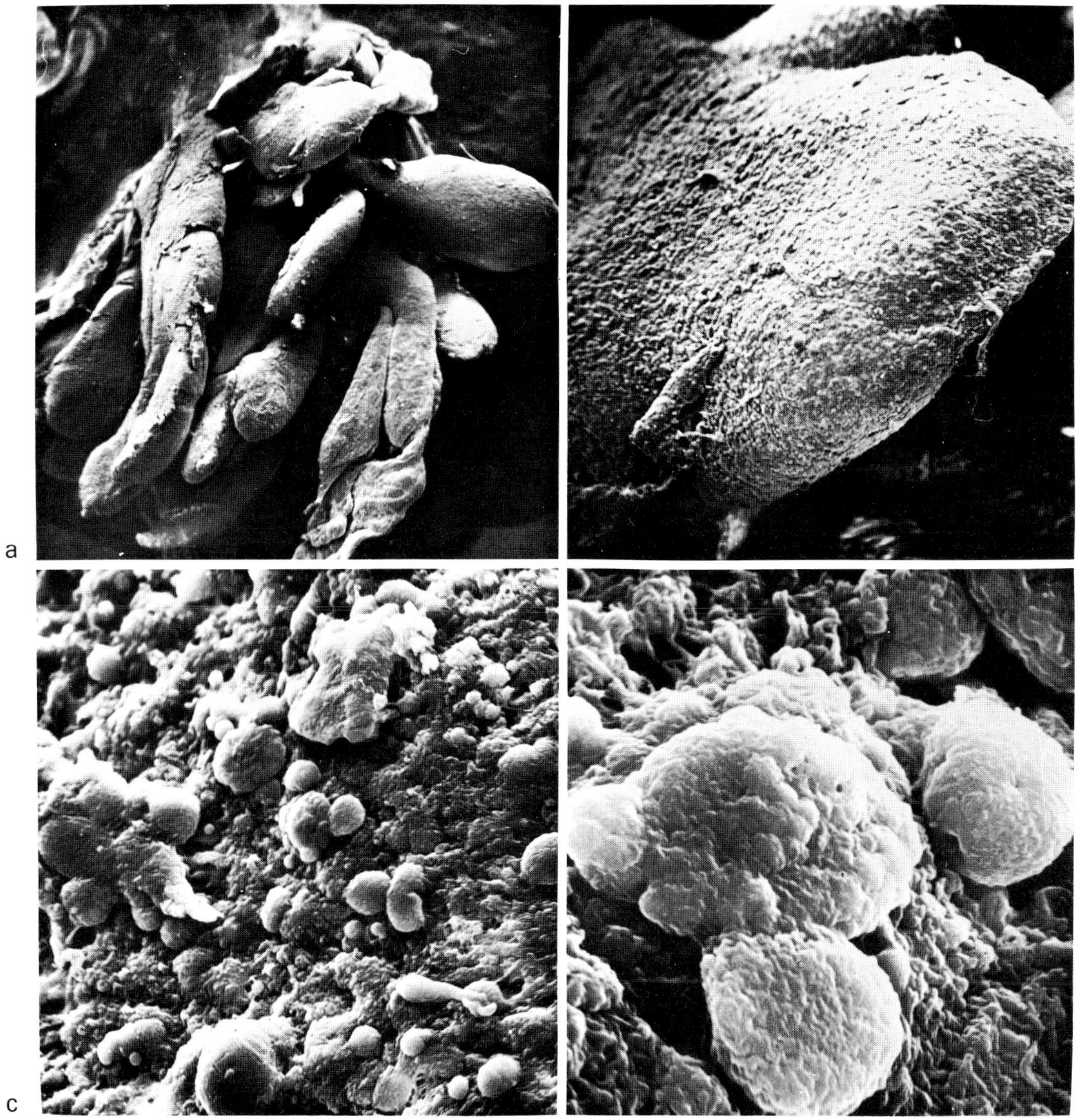

Fig. 25.8 Surface structure of synovial tissue.
(a) Synovial processes, enlarged and with a much increased surface area. SEM ×20.
(b) High power view of part of one synovial process. SEM ×90.
(c) Cells lying free upon surface of synovial process. The majority are polymorphs and lymphocytes. The normal delicate surface processes of the underlying synovial cells are obscured by fibrin and exudate. SEM ×830
(d) Detail of three inflammatory cells upon synovial process surface. SEM × 4425.

frey, 1967; Ghadially,1983; Ghadially & Roy, 1967, 1969). The covering strands of fibrin display a characteristic 10–25 nm periodicity. The synovial cells are of increased height and number. A (M) cells bear many filopodia and contain coated vesicles, cell debris and lysosomes (Fig. 25.9). The morphology of the lysosomes varies; some contain iron. The rough endoplasmic reticulum of the B(F) cells (Fig. 25.10) is accompanied by cisternal dilatation. Golgi complexes are few and small, large vacuoles scanty and lipid droplets frequent. Fine filaments may be abundant. Amyloid microfibrils have been identified. These observations largely confirm the early work of Barland et al

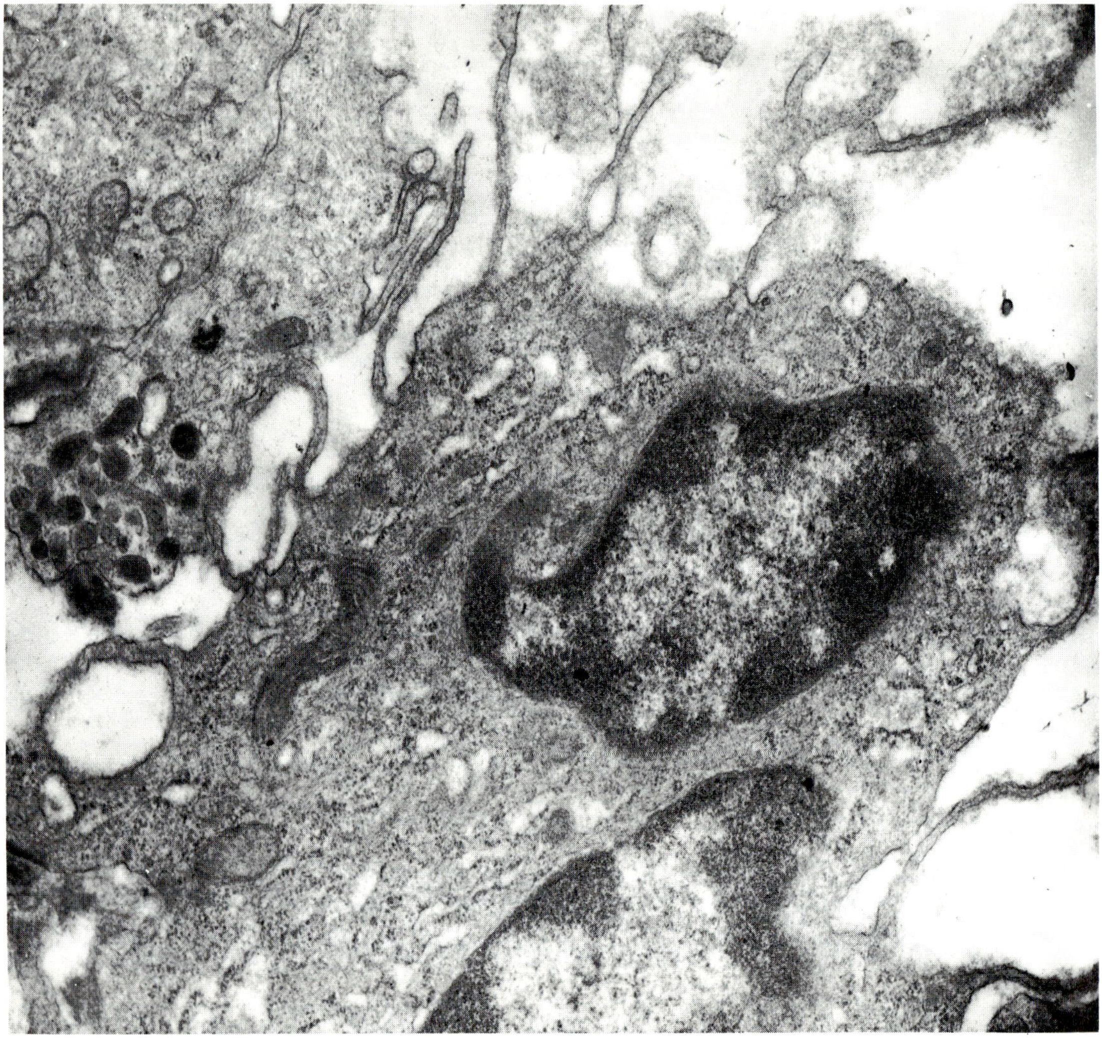

Fig. 25.9 Synovial A (M) cells. Part of two phagocytic A (M) cells, at a free synovial border. Filopodia extend from the cell surface. *At left*, a cluster of dense bodies lies within the cytoplasm of one cell. *At centre*, a nucleus is divided tangentially; the nearby cytoplasm contains many free ribosomes and some endoplasmic reticulum the cisternae of which are dilated. The formation of phagocytic vacuoles at the cell surface can be envisaged. Uranyl acetate and lead citrate (TEM) ×16 000.

(1963) and of Hirohata & Kobayashi (1964). Gold particles injected intra-articularly demonstrate continuity between the articular and extracellular tissue spaces (Norton & Ziff, 1964, 1966). TEM evidence supports the concept that synovial multinucleated giant cells originate from A(M) cells (Ghadially & Roy, 1967; 1969). Mesenchymal transformation (p. 612) of subsynoviocytic cells is suggested by the observations of Bierther & Wegner (1971) although the involvement of a cell type intermediate between the A(M) and B(F) cells remains possible (Huth et al, 1972). Pannus, analysed by TEM, resembles a 'secondary synovial membrane' rather than simple granulation tissue (Bierther & Wagner, 1974). However, there may be two patterns of transition between cellular pannus and cartilage:

1. Vascular invasion followed by cellular infiltration
2. Direct cellular invasion (Kobayashi & Ziff, 1973, 1975) with the secondary formation of a reparative, fibrous pannus.

These observations have been confirmed (Shiozawa et al, 1983) although it remains difficult to deter-

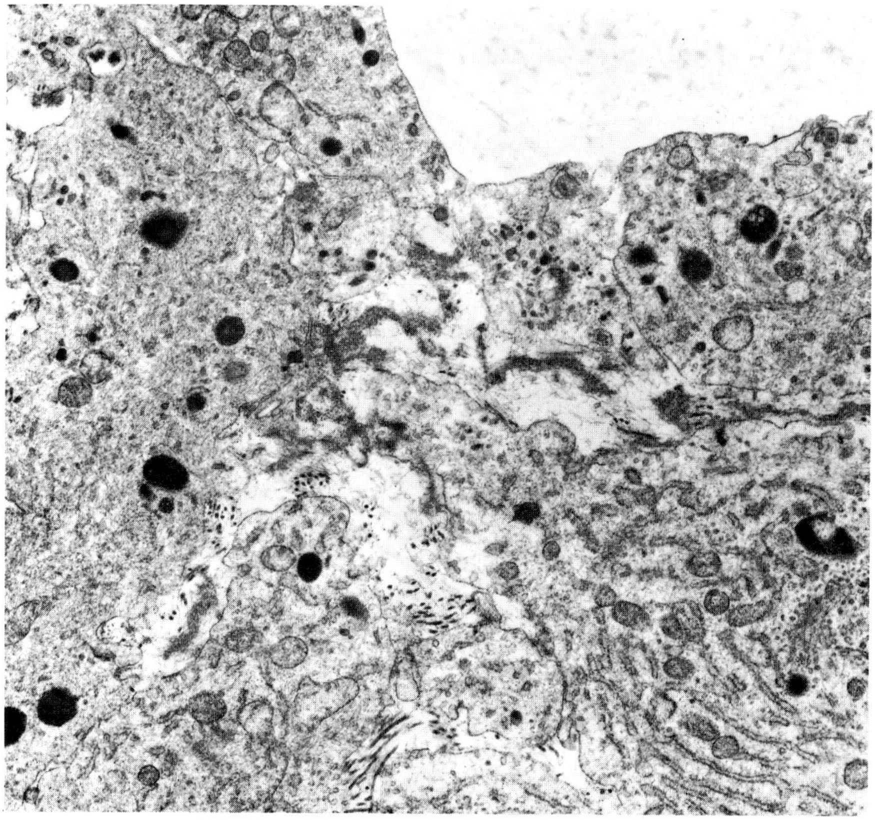

Fig. 25.10 Synovial B(F) cells. In centre of field delicate fibrils of collagen cut in longitudinal and transverse section, separate borders of two synovial cells. At right, type B cell cytoplasm contains numerous parallel arrays of endoplasmic reticulum. At surface, adjacent cells are linked at occasional tight junctions. Uranyl acetate and lead citrate (TEM) ×10 800.

mine the chronology of a single, individual case (Hollywell et al, 1983).

Proliferation

With time, the active RA inflammatory responses settle into a cycle of exudation, destruction (p. 615), proliferation and repair. A characteristic feature is the multiplication, by mitotic division, of the synovial cells. The normal single or double cell lamina is replaced by a proliferating, cellular array that may come to be 5, 7 or more cells in thickness.

Microdensitometry can be employed to measure the corresponding increase in DNA. A papillary structure is often assumed, the internal, lining surface layer displaying a greatly increased internal surface area. The synovial cell hyperplasia is characteristic of but not unique to RA and is encountered in response to almost any event, such as surgical trauma, that tends to provoke sterile synovitis. The multiplying cells retain a capacity for phagocytosis. Many contain ferritin (Muirden, 1966). During division, it is evident that some mitotic cycles are abnormal. Cell separation is incomplete and small numbers of multinucleated, large (giant) cells remain in and immediately deep to the synoviocytic layer (Fig. 25.11). These cells were first described by Collins (1949) and subsequently analysed in detail by Grimley & Sokoloff (1966). The giant cells, 40–50 μm in diameter, display acid phosphatase activity and periodically ingest red blood cells; these properties support the view that they arise by defective division of type A(M) synoviocytes. The 8–12 peripheral nuclei and the TEM appearances distinguish the RA cell from other multinucleated giant cells (Grimley, 1967; Muirden, 1970) found in the synovium, particularly those of pigmented villonodular

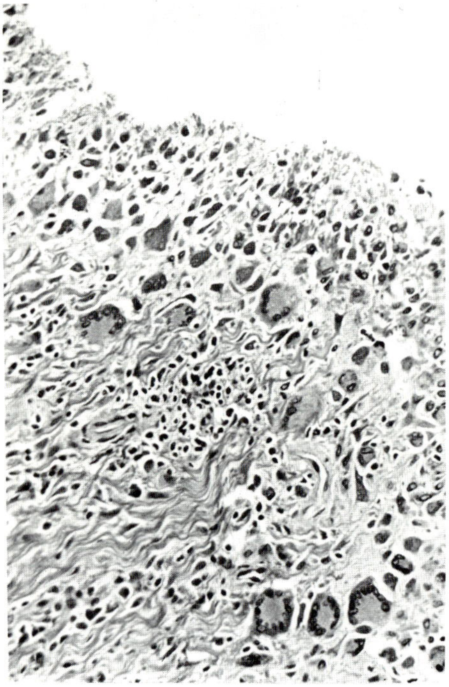

Fig. 25.11 Synovial giant cells. Numerous multinucleated giant cells are present. Those at top are smaller and display some similarity to the cells of the synoviocytic layer from which they may be derived. Those at bottom, distinct from foreign body and mulberry giant cells, recall the appearance of the Langhans' cell of tuberculosis. H & E ×200.

synovitis, of xanthogranuloma, of virus disease, of tuberculosis, of sarcoid and of reactions to foreign bodies and crystals. The ultrastructural features resemble those of the A(M) synoviocyte and include elaborate filopodia, granular endoplasmic reticulum, some smooth-surfaced vesicles and cytoplasmic micro-filaments, and sparse micro-tubules.

A proliferative response also characterises the mesenchymal cells of the subsynoviocytic tissue. Plump fibroblasts with open, vesicular nuclei dominate some areas and form islands of high cellular activity. The appearances have suggested a neoplastic-like behaviour and the phenomenon has been given the title 'mesenchymoid transformation' (Fassbender, 1980, 1983; Fassbender & Simmling-Annefeld, 1983). There is an analogy with the clonal characteristics of smooth muscle cells in atheroma. The further suggestion that the transformed cells derive from the endothelium of small synovial blood vessels, is less easy to accept (Simmling-Annefeld & Fassbender, 1979).

Immunopathology

Each clone of plasmacytes secretes a single immunoglobulin species. The synovial tissues in RA are infiltrated by these cells and it was not surprising that they could be shown to contain or bind anti-IgG rheumatoid factors (Figs 25.12–25.14). Immune complexes were demonstrated within free, synovial fluid phagocytes and the importance of humoral, immunological mechanisms for the destruction of tissue in RA was further underlined when C3 and C4 were shown in or on synovial cells positive for IgG. This coincidence, together with the demonstration of fibrin as a sign of active inflammation, indicated that humoral immunological mechanisms were implicated. That phagocytes containing

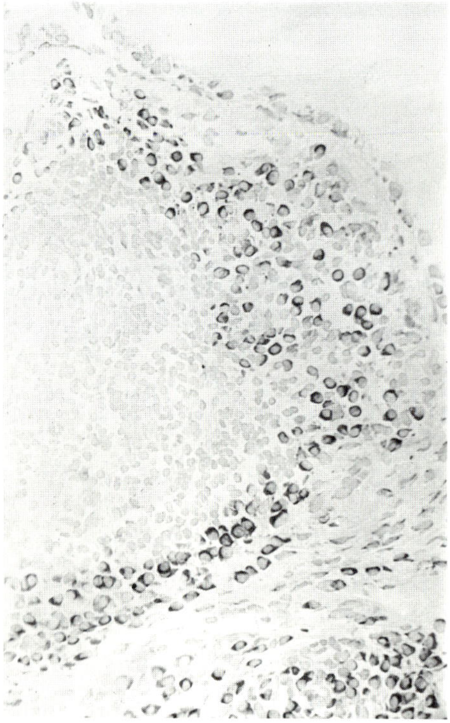

Fig. 25.12 Synovium: IgG. IgG-reacting plasma cells stain deeply. They form a marginal array around a synovial germinal centre. It is important to note that germinal centre formation in the lymphoid follicles of the synovium in rheumatoid arthritis is unusual. Unlabelled antibody peroxidase–antiperoxidase (PAP) without counterstain. PAP ×175.

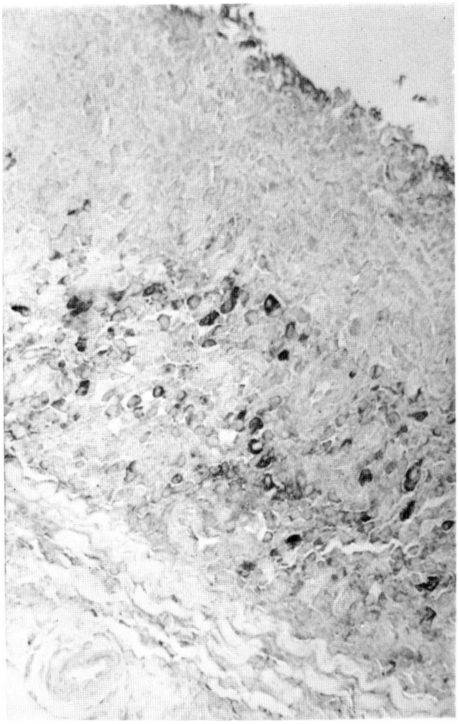

Fig. 25.13 Synovium: IgM. IgM-reacting plasma cells are observed constantly in modest number. They are usually much fewer than those reacting for IgG. PAP ×175.

immune complexes existed within the synovial fluid reflected the escape of these cells from the synovium. Although activated lysosomal hydrolases are released from the synovial cells, the attack zone for articular injury is the synoviochondral junction, not the principal, weight-bearing surface exposed to the hydrolases. The emphasis must remain on the significance of cell-derived enzymes at the joint circumference. It is reasonable to deduce that the synovial fluid changes are coincidental. The action of the immune complexes is not confined to the synovial tissue however and it has been established that they aggregate in and may injure associated fibrocartilaginous menisci and tendons (Cooke et al, 1975). Cartilage surface areas free from pannus contain easily detectable deposits of IgG whereas areas covered by pannus do not. It is suggested that the extension into cartilage of the mononuclear and polymorphonuclear cells of pannus liberates trapped immune complexes.

Cell-mediated immunological mechanisms play a critical part in determining the lesions of RA. Alterations in the proportion of circulating B and T cells have been demonstrated but the absolute number of circulating T cells is debated. The synovial mononuclear cell changes mirror those of the circulation. Monoclonal antisera, available for the identification of B and T cell subsets and for HLA characterisation, have been used, together with lymphocyte cytotoxicity, autoradiography,

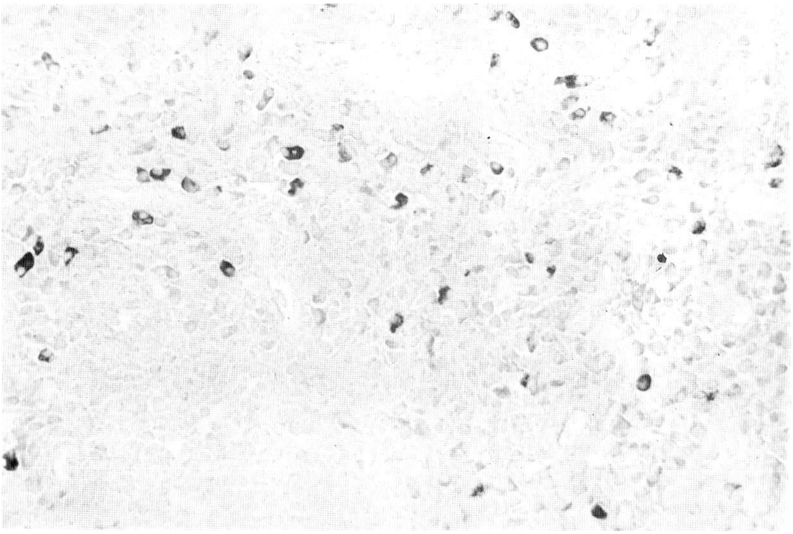

Fig. 25.14 Synovium: IgA. IgA is detected in relation to synovial plasma cells in approximately 25% of cases of rheumatoid arthritis. PAP ×250.

enzyme markers and nuclear birefringence, to analyse the synovial populations. Up to 85% of the mononuclear cells disaggregated from synovial tissue are T cells and up to 30% of the T lymphocytes in the perivascular, lymphoid tissues have the TEM characteristics of Sezary cells, suggesting first, that they may be inducer-type T cells and second, that there may be a local disturbance of T cell function such as that which is known to be expressed by altered reactions to EB virus. Many RA synovial T cells have microanatomical similarities to those of the paracortical regions of lymph nodes (Janossy et al, 1981). Also present are large, HLA-DR-positive, macrophage-like interdigitating cells with high lysosomal enzyme activity. These cells display characteristics identical to the interdigitating cells of the lymph node paracortex (Poulter et al, 1983), forming close contacts with inducer T cells. There are few suppressor/cytotoxic T cells between the clusters of macrophage-inducer cells. An abnormal stimulus to B lymphocyte (plasmacytic) activation is suggested due to the impaired suppression resulting from EB virus. The consequential immunoglobulin synthesis may be defective.

Fibrosis and repair

Within a few days of the onset of rheumatoid synovitis, reparative processes of granulation tissue formation and fibrosis are evident (Fig. 25.15). Because the opportunity for repeated biopsy at relatively short intervals is exceptional, there are few human records of serial studies. Nevertheless, indirect and circumstantial evidence shows that the cellularity, the glycosaminoglycan content of the synovia, the proportion of different glycosa-

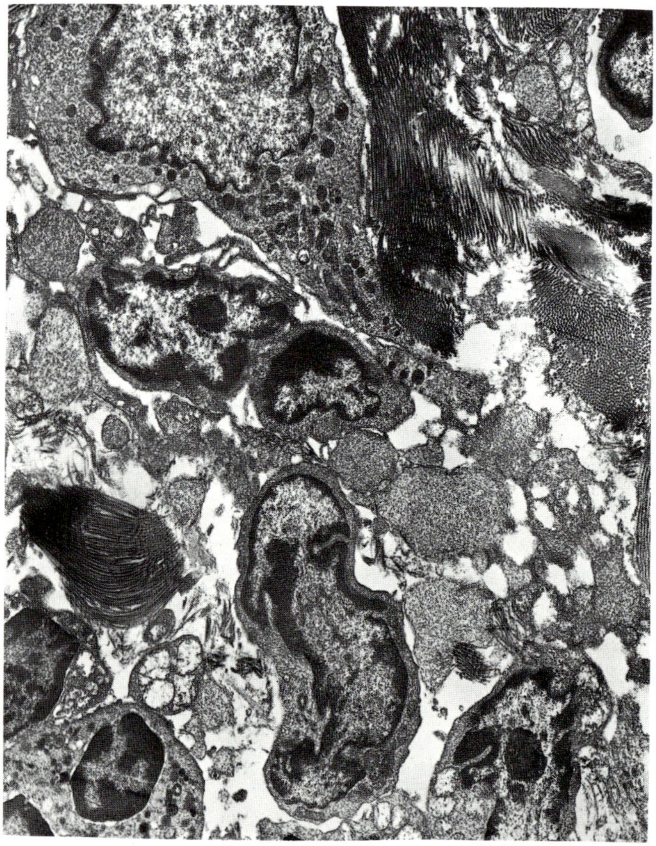

Fig. 25.15 Synovial connective tissue. Several mononuclear phagocytes are seen among bundles of synovial collagen. The appearances represent those that are common in vascular granulation tissue near the margin of eroded cartilage. Uranyl acetate and lead citrate (TEM) ×7200.

minoglycans and the collagen content, change and evolve with time and with the progress of the disease.

Active disease, assessed microscopically, often persists when the clinical state is quiescent (Gardner, 1972). The synovium becomes dull-red, granular and less swollen. Cartilage destruction and the extension of pannus are accompanied by the formation of new fibrous tissue which links and then binds together the peripheral margins and, later, the more central parts of the opposed, articulating surfaces. Synoviocytic hyperplasia, lymphocytic infiltration, mastocytosis, retained haemosiderosis (Fig. 25.16) and fibrin are features commonplace in chronic, active synovitis. Arteriolitis, is however, most exceptional, and necrotising granuloma unusual.

As a secondary consequence of tendinitis, tendinous and meniscal synovitis and of the local bone reabsorption, osteoporosis and remodelling that invariably accompany articular disease, temporary and then permanent deformities ensue.

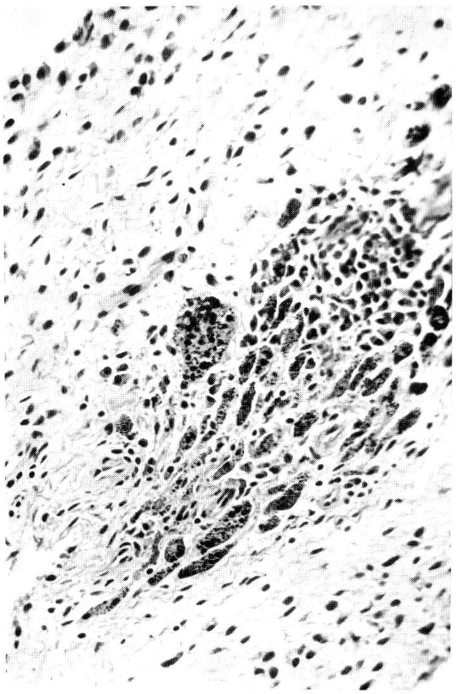

Fig. 25.16 *Synovial iron.* Dense, black-appearing granules of haemosiderin are seen (centre) within large mononuclear macrophages of subsynovial connective tissue. Granules of haemosiderin are frequently also extracellular.

Subluxation and ulnar deviation of the fingers are followed by dislocation, shortening, swan neck deformity, main-en-griffe and other characteristic disorders. Fibrous ankylosis eventually determines immobility. Bony ankylosis does not occur. Particular problems relate to neurocentral spinal synovitis and disease of the temporomandibular joints, but the deformities of increasing proportions of peripheral joints can be alleviated by surgery.

Cartilage destruction

The natural history of RA is dominated by the inexorable destruction of hyaline cartilage (Sheppeard, 1983). Cartilage destruction impairs movement and load-bearing and leads to inefficient lubrication. The replacement of the avascular cartilage by the vascular granulation tissue of the pannus further impedes movement and provokes fibrous ankylosis.

The first microscopic sign of cartilage degradation is thought to be the loss of metachromatic matrix material. Diminished metachromasia reflects decreased proteoglycan aggregation, increased proteoglycan breakdown, loss of glycosaminoglycan and, consequently, an altered water content. These matrix changes are first recognised at the periphery of the articular surfaces, in the junctional zone where synovium adjoins cartilage (Figs 25.17–25.19). At this site, there is diminished fibronectin (Shiozawa & Ziff, 1983). With matrix proteoglycan loss, there is an impairment of the capacity of the uninjured chondrocytes to effect repair by increased proteoglycan synthesis. The relationship between cartilage proteoglycan and collagen is extremely close: it it quickly disturbed and the subsequent, irreversible injury to the collagenous microskeleton prejudices cartilage recovery by new matrix synthesis.

The mechanism by which this centripetal breakdown of cartilage is effected is debated. Three patterns of enzymic release and activation, not mutually exclusive, appear possible: first, degradation may be primarily the result of collagenolysis; second, degradation may be the direct consequence of proteoglycan destruction; and third, both major populations of macromolecule may be attacked in sequence (Woessner & Howell, 1980). The enzymes that have been shown to be capable of degrading collagen include: the specific

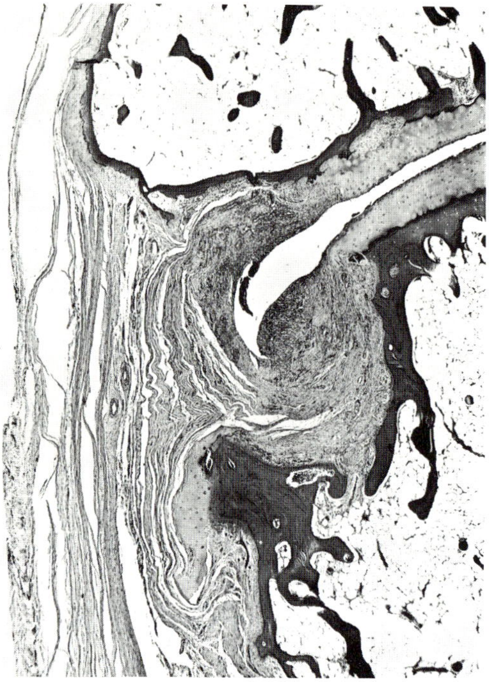

Fig. 25.17 Early pannus. Both the articular cartilages and the subjacent, osteoporotic bone are replaced by granulation tissue which constitutes an early pannus. H & E ×15.

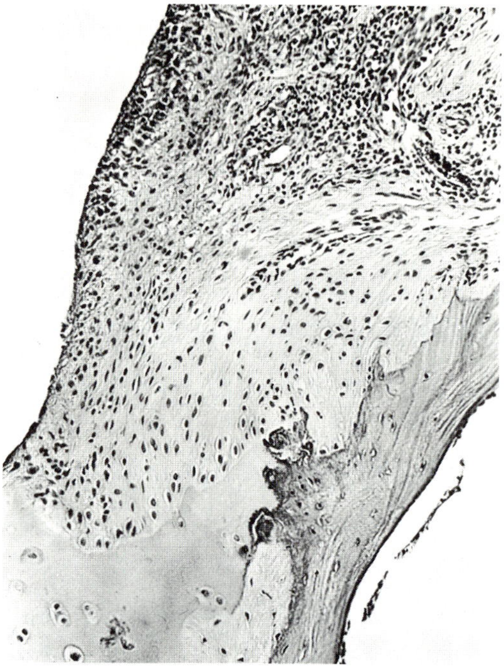

Fig. 25.18 Pannus formation. Vascular granulation tissue containing many lymphocytes, plasma cells and histiocytes (top) replaces hyaline articular cartilage (bottom left). Note the periosteal extension of granulation tissue into bone (at right) with lacunar reabsorption. H & E ×110.

collagenases, some effective at neutral pH; acid cathepsins; other neutral proteases; and enzymes that could further destroy collagen that had been partly degraded by catalysts of broader specificity. Enzymes capable of catalysing in vivo the breakdown of human proteoglycan include those capable of disorganising the multi-unit aggregate or the monomer; those degrading the glycosaminoglycan side-chains of the proteoglycan subunits; and those influencing the breakdown of the proteoglycan protein core. The enzymes may act extracellularly or within cells.

There is only a restricted variety of cell types from which these enzymes can be derived: the endothelial cells of small, synovial blood vessels at the synoviochondral fringe; blood-derived polymorphs (Menninger et al, 1980); macrophages; synoviocytes; chondrocytes; and bone cells, particularly osteoclasts. The intimate relationship between polymorphs and zones of cartilage degradation and erosion has already been remarked upon: polymorphs are sources not only of acid proteases derived from specific granules but also of: elastase (Menninger et al, 1980); cathepsins B, D and G associated with the azurophilic lysosomes; acid, collagenolytic cathepsin; and a neutral metalloproteinase (Saklatvala & Barrett, 1980), an enzyme which, with cathepsin D, has also been traced to the macrophage. Synoviocytes are sources of: neutral collagenase; a neutral metalloproteinase; a peptidase; and acid cathepsins. The chondrocyte itself secretes a collagenase, a metalloproteinase, acid cathepsins and a peptidase (Woessner & Howell, 1980); and the dendritic synovial macrophages secrete neutral collagenase (Woolley et al, 1979, 1980).

There are therefore at least three possible ways in which cartilage can be broken down in active RA.

1. Polymorphs and subsequently macrophages, escaping from the bloodstream at sites of synovitis, degrade cartilage by the extracellular release of enzymes, active at neutral pH, that destroy matrix proteoglycan, proteoglycan–collagen links, and,

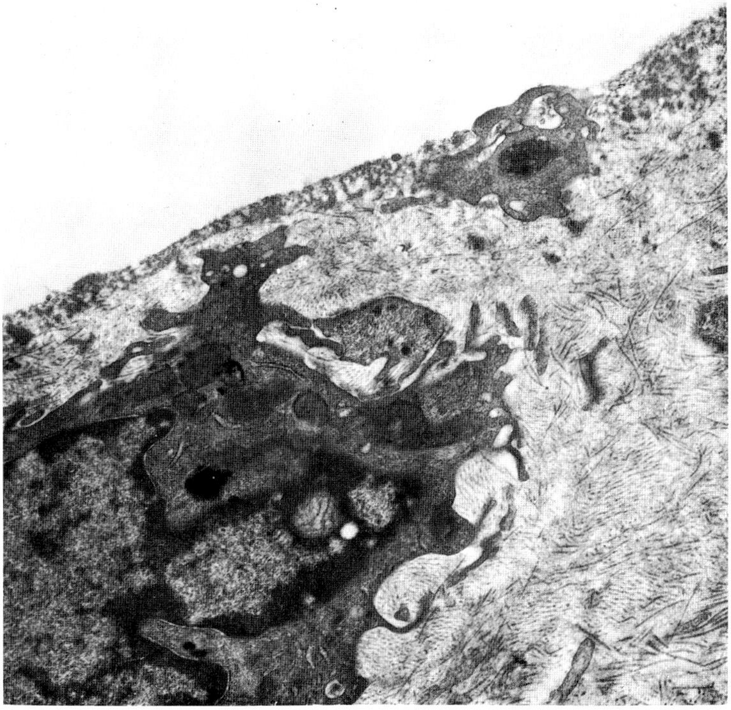

Fig. 25.19 Early pannus formation. Experimental allergic arthritis. Surface articular cartilage showing extension of process of cell (top right) that is occupying part of the load-bearing surface. Remainder of surface is formed of interlacing, transected bundles of collagen. Uranyl acetate and lead citrate (EM) ×10 500.

ultimately, collagen. Polymorph elastase and neutral collagenase have been implicated.

2. Synoviocytes themselves, at sites of inflammation, release neutral metalloproteases, especially collagenase (Evanson et al, 1967). The involvement of a small, 33 000 MW, Ca-dependent enzyme is suspected (Woolley & Evanson, 1977). Immunoreactive enzyme is present at the pannus–cartilage junction (Woolley et al, 1977). Enzyme activity, slight when the tissue is excised, becomes widespread after short-term culture (Woolley et al, 1980), a manifestation of released collagenase inhibitor. The balance between collagenase and inhibitor may hold the key to the extent and rapidity of cartilage destruction (McGuire et al, 1981, 1982).

3. Chondrocytes evince a capability in vitro to degrade their own perilacunar matrix (Fell & Jubb, 1977). This effect is elicited by a humoral agent, released from the cells of viable explanted synovium. The agent, catabolin (Saklatvala & Dingle, 1980; Dingle, 1981), is a small protein; it may be identical with interleukin 1. Catabolin is believed to act as a messenger, stimulating chondrocytes to synthesise and release proteolytic enzymes that break down proteoglycan around the cell. Although it is reasonable to postulate that this mechanism may be at work in RA, there is not yet substantive evidence that this is so.

Some help has been obtained about the process of cartilage erosion by electron microscopy. There is desquamation of collagen from the surface (Kimura et al, 1977), and excavation (Inoue et al, 1969). Chondrocytes may be surrounded by large moats; others accumulate lipid (Mitchell & Shepard, 1970). Dissolution of perichondrocytic proteoglycan can be shown but is inconstant (Mitchell & Shepard, 1978). Collagen fibrils, dissociated from proteoglycan, are phagocytosed. Since loss of proteoglycan may be remote from the margin of the cell exudate, the significance of catabolins (interleukins) should not on this evidence be discounted.

The role of the blood vessels and the influence

of blood flow on cartilage injury in RA is under close scrutiny. Normal cartilage inhibits vascularisation. Inflamed and non-inflamed synovial tissue can secrete angiogenesis factors (Brown et al, 1983), catalysing new vessel formation. There are analogies between the possible role of such factors in facilitating cartilage loss in RA and the vascularisation of experimental neoplasms (Sorgente et al, 1975). Neoplastic angiogenesis factors may derive from mast cells and their action can be blocked by heparin-inhibitors. Mast cells are numerous in, and correlate with, the activity of experimental arthritis (Gryfe et al, 1971). It is possible that mast cells play a hitherto unsuspected part in cartilage destruction in RA (Bromley et al, 1984).

A further local consequence of the increased regional blood flow that accompanies the synovitis of RA is bone reabsorption. The frequent coexistence of peripheral vascular diseases such as atherosclerosis does not impair this process. Osteoporosis in RA is not confined to the regions of active inflammation. Local osteoporosis is, however, one factor contributing to the formation of the frequent *peri-* and *subarticular pseudocysts*. These are small, radiolucent foci lying beneath or near cartilage at sites of severe RA synovitis. The pseudocyst is a solid structure histologically; it comprises loose, vascular granulation tissue and is usually in continuity with marginal pannus. Continuity may not be demonstrable, however, without serial section. Pseudocysts are likely to be simple extensions of RA granulation tissue (Collins, 1949). Alternatively, but less probably, a pseudocyst may represent an intraosseous RA granuloma (Magyar et al, 1974a, b). A third view of pseudocyst formation postulates that pseudocysts are formed when the very high hydrodynamic pressure generated by flexion of a limb, forces small amounts of synovial fluid through the bony end-plate. This is most probable when a large effusion is present and when subjacent bone is osteoporotic. Those parts of the cortical bone covered only by attenuated synovial tissue, the 'bare areas' of Schilling (1974), are susceptible. In support of this suggestion is the direct evidence obtained by Myers & Broom (1982). Using thin cartilage slices tested mechanically in a microscopic loading device, they demonstrated that, under stress, pannus tracks between cartilage lacunae or breaches in the subchondral bony endplate. The geological term 'geode', used to describe subarticular pseudocysts, is misleading. Geodes are rock cavities containing crystals and the analogy is confusing (Gardner, 1972).

Anatomical consequences

Anatomical studies are almost always at a late stage of the clinical disease. By the time reconstructive surgery or necropsy is performed, secondary phenomena such as amyloidosis, osteoarthrosis, osteoporosis and fracture complicate the initial polyarthritis; they are associated with the mechanical results of deformity and disease.

The key to the anatomical progression of RA is the marginal centripetal, erosive synovitis (Fig. 25.20). Peripheral cartilage destruction in any or all of the 187 diarthrodial joints with granulation tissue formation is recognised at arthroscopy or arthrotomy as a rim of pale-red, exuberant material linked by bands of young fibrous tissue establishing adhesions that become denser and more numerous with time (Fig. 25.21). Fibrous ankylosis is commonplace (Figs 25.22, 25.23). For reasons that invite comparison with the late consequences of suppurative arthritis and with anky-

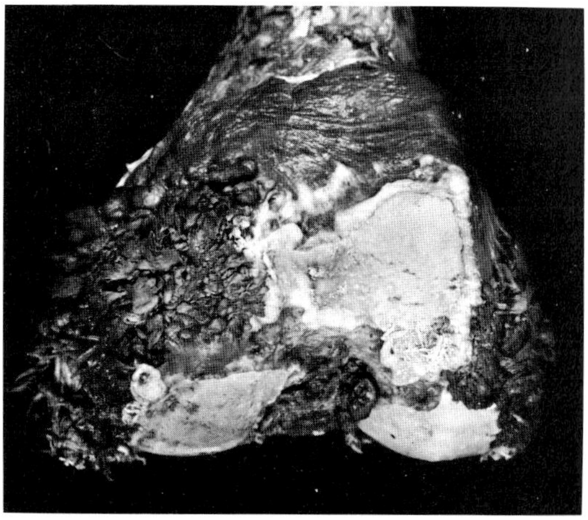

Fig. 25.20 Pannus. In this knee joint, bounded by hyperplastic, grey-black appearing synovial villi, granulation tissue, constituting a pannus, forms a sharply defined boundary for the remaining zones of load-bearing articular cartilage. Approximately one-half of the cartilage of the anterior surface of this knee joint has been destroyed. ½ natural size.

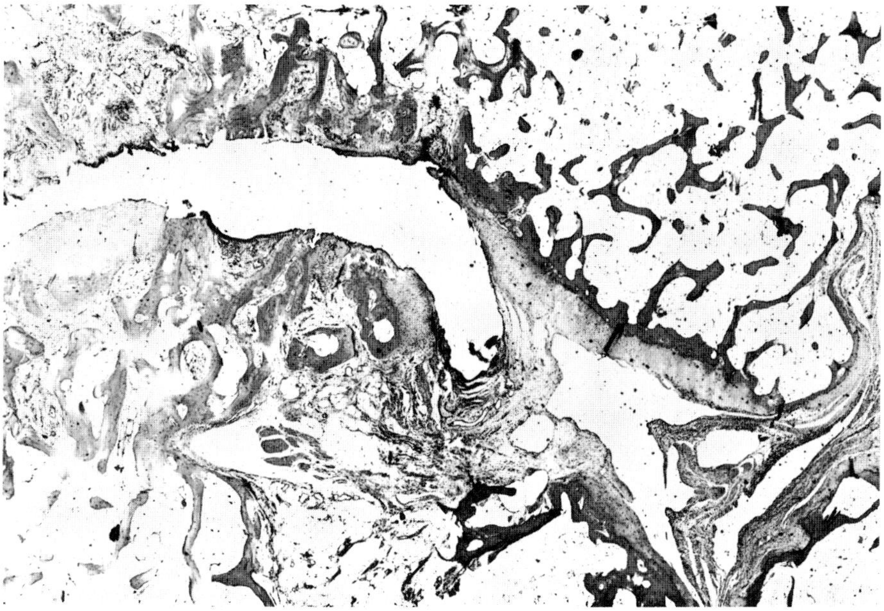

Fig. 25.21 Fibrous ankylosis. Metacarpophalangeal joint showing severe secondary osteoarthrosis (left) and fibrous adhesion binding opposing joint surfaces (centre). There is osteoporosis; and vascular connective tissue in continuity with the adhesion, extends into the osteoporotic bone (centre). H & E ×4.

losing spondylitis, bony ankylosis is most exceptional: its recognition suggests the coincidence of another disorder such as bacterial infection or trauma. Large synovial effusions are thought to delay ankylosis. Secondary osteoarthrosis (Gardner, 1983) is itself complicated by inflammation when fragments of bone are taken up by the synovium. As marginal osteoclastic bone

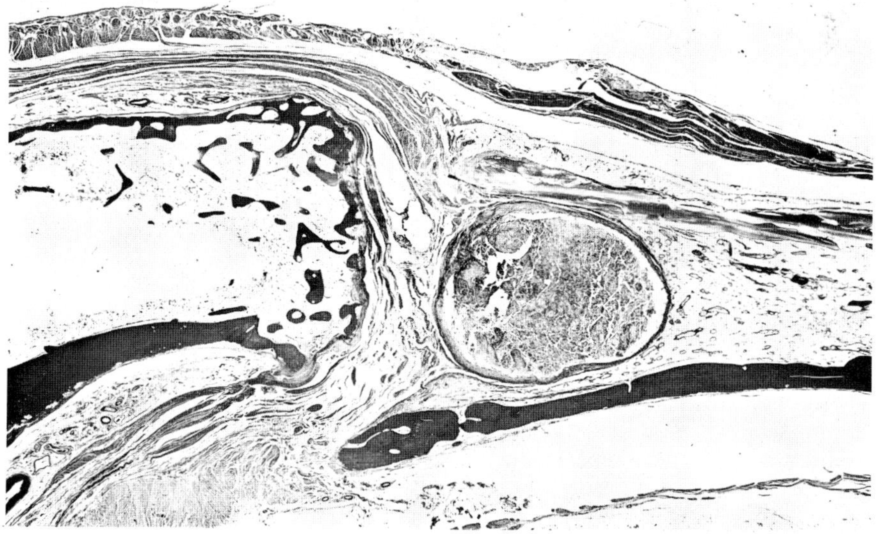

Fig. 25.22 Pseudocyst. Within osteoporotic bone (centre) adjoining metacarpophalangeal joint that has been entirely replaced by fibrous tissue, with resultant fibrous ankylosis, is a pseudocyst containing necrotic tissue and cell debris and bounded by a lamina of dense connective tissue. Note severe osteoporosis of bones. H & E ×6.

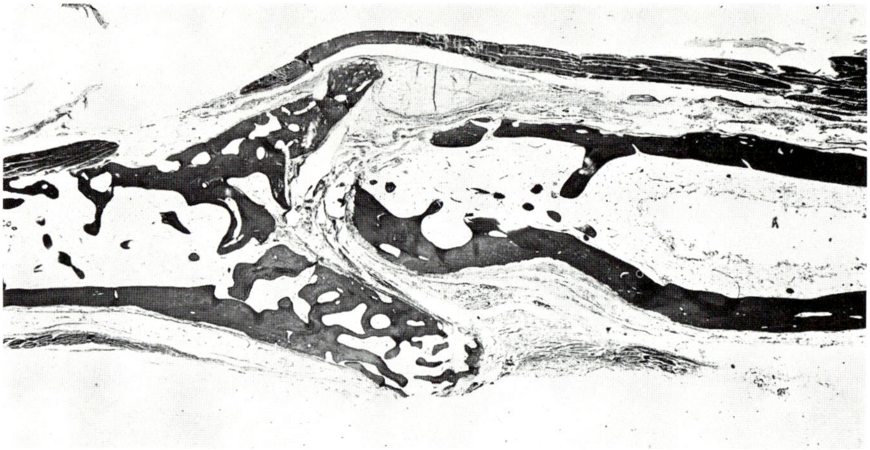

Fig. 25.23 Late fibrous ankylosis. The shaft of one osteoporotic phalanx, the cartilage covering of which has been entirely replaced by fibrous tissue, is impacted into the end of the adjacent bone. Observe remodelling of the bone structure. H & E ×6.

reabsorption advances, the erosions become recognisable radiographically: gross deformity accelerates and creates new, abnormal mechanical stresses that establish a vicious circle of destruction not amenable to medical treatment.

Juxta-articular connective tissues

Bursae and tendon sheaths are common sites of RA synovitis. The popliteal, and olecranon bursae are most often affected but the subacromial, subdeltoid and tendo achilles bursae are periodically inflamed. Chronic inflammation of the popliteal bursa, with distension and fibrosis of the wall, constitutes a 'Bakers' cyst' rupture of which may follow the pressure changes that occur when an inflamed knee joint containing a large exudate is flexed. The suprapatellar pouch may be involved. Occasionally, a valve-like mechanism permits the exudate to enter the popliteal bursa but not return. The signs of rupture simulate thrombophlebitis.

The wall of the inflamed bursa is formed of dense collagen. There is a chronically inflamed synovium-like lining, a variable lymphocytic and plasmacytic infiltrate, with few lymphoid follicles (Wagner & Abgarowicz, 1970) and a content of thin fluid and much cell debris. Villous hypertrophy is not evident but the presence of haemosiderin confirms that bleeding takes place into the bursa.

Among other less frequent complications of bursal disease are: urinary bladder compression from bilateral structures in continuity with the hip joint (Watson & Ochsner, 1967; Levy et al, 1982); venous obstruction due to iliopsoas bursa (Chilton & Darke, 1980); and peripheral neuropathy.

Tendons and tendon sheaths are often affected by RA (Scudamore, 1816; Stockman, 1904; Kellgren & Ball, 1950). The result is 'tendinous rheumatism'. The inflammatory exudate is recognised by light microscopy, by SEM (Inoue et al, 1970) and by TEM. Tissue degradation results from the activation of lysosomal hydrolases and other enzymes. Granulation tissue replaces the peritenon and mesotenon. A true tendinitis accompanies tendinous synovitis and the focal necrosis of tendon collagen that develops simulates the microscopic structure of RA granuloma. The rupture that follows may appear 'spontaneous' and is occasionally bilateral (Tarr, 1974). Support to nearby joints is diminished. The long flexor tendons of the fingers are particularly susceptible. However, involvement of the sheath of the carpal tunnel may trap both tendons and median nerve and the carpal tunnel syndrome which results (Page, 1961; Vaughan-Jackson, 1966) must be distinguished from the local effects of amyloidosis, tuberculosis and chondrocalcinosis. On rare occasions, rupture of an apparently intact tendon has followed the local injection of corticosteroids (Bedi & Ellis, 1970).

Bone disease

The skeleton in patients with RA displays changes in excess of those anticipated with age and sex. Stress fractures are frequent (Miller et al, 1967; Fam et al, 1983). There is decreased bone strength (Mueller & Jurist, 1973). Studies of the state of the skeleton demonstrate reduced bone mass (Reid et al, 1981) but increased bone turnover (Rajapakse et al, 1983) not explicable by immobilisation or associated metabolic disease.

The pathological evidence is limited. Locally, bone is destroyed at articular margins by osteoclastic reabsorption (Fig. 25.24). It is likely that this response is calcitonin-dependent: it may be susceptible to diphosphonates. The local bone change may coincide with coincidental hyperparathyroidism but there are no known and consistent changes in parathyroid gland structure. The absence of reactive, new bone formation is unexplained. Few investigations have been made by modern morphometric methods; meanwhile, there is little to demonstrate abnormal mineralisation or mineralisation fronts, altered osteoid or systemic change in osteoblastic or osteocytic activity. The osteoblasts retain a normal capacity for repair after fracture.

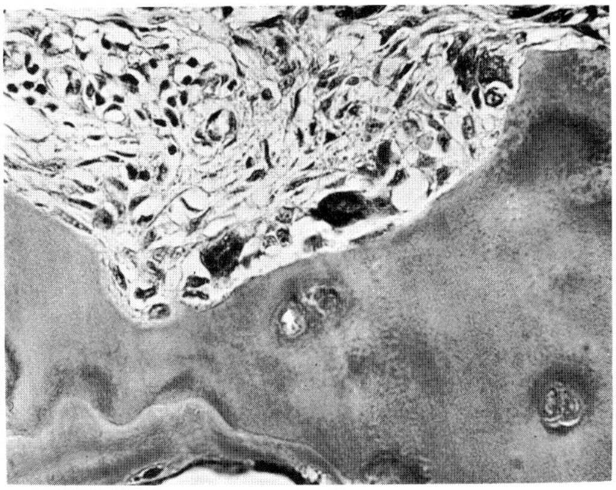

Fig. 25.24 Osteoclastic bone reabsorption. A common result of the formation and growth of granulation tissue (pannus) at synovial joint margins is the activation of osteoclasts. Note two of these cells (centre) within marginal bone lacunae. H & E ×210.

Since articular blood flow is dramatically increased in active synovitis, it is suspected that altered, increased blood flow may be an explana-

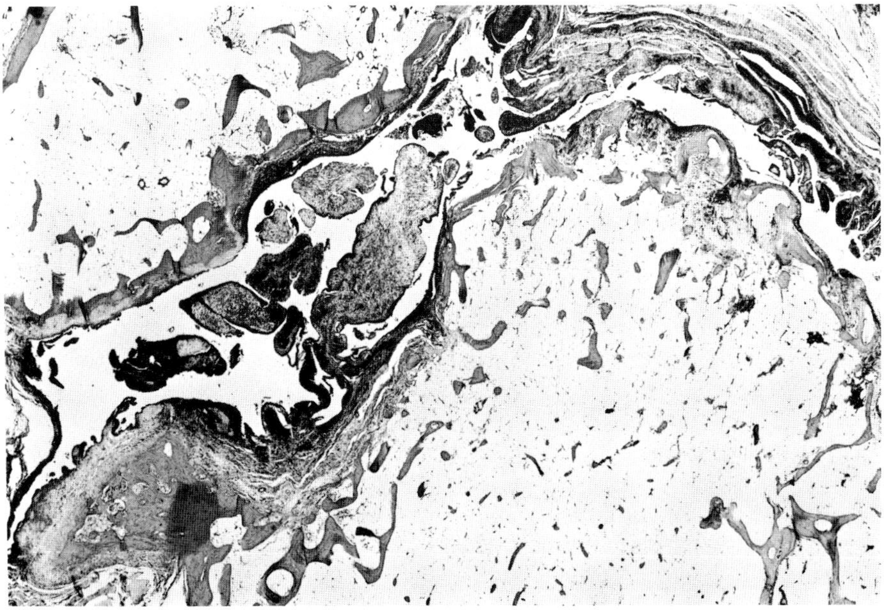

Fig. 25.25 Bone destruction. Severe active synovitis, indicated by fibrin aggregates (black) is accompanied by advanced osteoporosis. Little surface cartilage remains and granulation tissue extends, by lysis and by osteoclastic reabsorption, into the porotic bone. H & E ×15.

tion for local bone destruction. However, osteoporosis in RA (Fig. 25.25) is not simply a result of the administration of agents like corticosteroids that alter bone mass.

Regional disease

The pathological consequences of RA are concentrated upon the small joints of the hands and feet, upon the wrists and elbows, and upon the other large, limb joints. However, there is increasing recognition of the importance of involvement of articulations that are less often studied microscopically and the intrinsic joints of the ear and larynx, the temporomandibular joints and those of the spine merit special consideration. In many instances, RA affecting these structures can be severely disabling; in some, death may be a direct result.

The *incudostapedial* and *incudomalleal* joints are synovial. Aural RA (Gardner, 1972) can be obscured by the effects of salicylates or age but auricular ankylosis can cause mechanical impediment. There are very few histological descriptions of the affected joints. *Laryngeal* arthritis (Montgomery & Goodman, 1980) is a frequent and serious problem. Only in recent years has the frequency of cricoarytenoid arthritis been proved. As many as one patient in four may be affected by this form of regional arthritis. There is cartilage destruction and the lymphocytic and plasmacytic infiltrate may extend to adjacent muscle. The cricothyroid joint is affected with comparable frequency. The effects are distinguishable from rheumatoid laryngeal vasculitis.

Temporomandibular arthritis may be uni- or bilateral and may develop early in life as part of a juvenile polyarthritis (Carlsson et al, 1978). The lower compartment is first affected but the upper is soon involved. Pannus covers the degraded articular surfaces and disc. Fibrous adhesions form, resulting in ankylosis. Condylectomy may be necessitated. The hazards of this procedure and of laryngeal intubation in RA have been diminished by fibreoptic instruments but such severe deformity and impaired growth ('bird-face') may occur in juvenile polyarthritis that little can be done to alleviate the mandibular micrognathia.

There is widespread awareness of the prevalence and complications of spinal RA. Arthritis of the *atlanto-occipital, atlantoaxial, neurocentral* and *apophyseal* joints constitutes a crippling syndrome and destruction of the cervical articulations can be hazardous (Mantz et al, 1983). In one series, of 26 atlantoaxial joints, there was significant subaxial dislocation in 3, mobile atlantoaxial dislocation in 9 and fixed atlantoaxial luxation in 3 (Ball & Sharp, 1971). It has become clear that the problem of cervical RA stems from neurocentral synovitis; erosion of the margins of the annulus fibrosus of the principal intervertebral joints is followed by the extension of granulation tissue to replace the discs. Marginal osteophytes do not form and cervical dislocation is particularly likely (Weiner et al, 1982). Analogous RA changes have been described in the costovertebral joints (Bywaters, 1981).

Diagnostic biopsy

Although fibreoptic arthroscopy is commonplace, the older and unsatisfactory technique of blind needle biopsy is still widely practiced. The pathologist prefers to receive tissue in ample quantity from identified sites so that the larger blocks obtainable at open arthrotomy offer the best prospects of balanced interpretation and diagnostic accuracy. With advances in EM and immunopathological techniques, it is advantageous for fresh pieces of tissue to be snap-frozen and for small, representative samples to be placed in chilled, buffered glutaraldehyde. The availability of the results of synovial fluid analysis and culture is presumed (Ch. 8).

The specificity of the histological findings in RA is low. No single light microscopic feature or combination of features offers absolute diagnostic accuracy. The very uncommon microscopic synovial granuloma comes nearest to being a characteristic lesion. Its infrequency is diagnostically disadvantageous. Fibrinous exudates are encountered in many forms of arthritis and are usual in RA: fibrin incorporation into the synovium occurs. The mononuclear infiltrate of lymphocytes and plasmacytes is very frequent but is found not only in the seronegative spondyloarthropathies but in viral and postviral arthritis. Polymorphs are numerous in the early disease as they are in so many other forms of crystal, microbial, foreign body and immunological reaction. Synovial cell hyperplasia is characteristic of, but not unique to RA: it follows almost any mechanical, surgical or traumatic synovial disturbance. Multinucleate giant cell forms are recognised in a considerable variety of synovial diseases (Soren, 1978a). Mast cells appear in many forms of synovitis and increase in osteoarthrosis (OA) when inflammation supervenes. The proliferation of subsynoviocytic, mesenchymal cells is acknowledged: the change is not pathognomonic. Necrotising vasculitis in RA synovitis is rare; subacute arteritis is also uncommon and the fibromuscular intimal proliferation seen in large limb arteries may be difficult to identify in the small, thick-walled articular vessels. Accumulations of haemosiderin, common in RA, may succeed any traumatic or surgical episode. Equally, the particles of cartilage and bone, found in advanced disease, indicate secondary, hard connective tissue injury, not rheumatoid synovitis itself. The fibrosis of RA is a common sequel to virtually every form of non-lethal, sustained, joint injury, infection or irritation. The site and extent of fibrosis reflect duration and severity of disease, not specificity.

Two advances offer the hope of diminishing these diagnostic difficulties.

1. The increasingly wide availability of poly- and monoclonal antisera against autologous and foreign antigens means that there is continual improvement in the accuracy with which histological components can be exactly identified (Førre et al, 1982). The plasma cells of RA synovial tissue synthesise rheumatoid factors and approximately half of the IgG-synthesising cells of both seropositive and seronegative cases contain such factors. The majority of plasma cells in regions rich in IgM-synthesising cells also contain rheumatoid factor. No distinctive diagnostic synovial pattern of humoral IgG or IgM antibody or complement distribution is, however, demonstrable (Ghose et al, 1975) but IgA has been found with surprising frequency (Ghose et al, 1975; Alexander, 1983) as it has in seronegative arthritis (Revell & Mayston, 1982). Extravascular immunoglobulins are not confined to the synovium but are often detectable in the joint capsule (Cooke et al, 1975; Fritz et al, 1980).

These observations have done much to assist views on the pathogenesis of RA but have not yet resolved, for the diagnostic histopathologist, the intractable problem of accurate recognition of the disease. Immunoelectronmicroscopic analyses of synovial fluid cells have been made with the peroxidase–antiperoxidase (PAP) technique; both polymorphs and mononuclear phagocytes have been shown in this way to contain vacuolar inclusions of IgG, IgM and C3 and, less often, of IgA and fibrin (Cherian & Schumacher, 1983). Although these demonstrations, equally applicable to synovial tissue samples, are distinguishable from the negative results obtained in control tests, there is not yet any evidence that such methods will aid differential diagnosis to any greater extent than the PAP and fluorescein isothiocyanate (FITC) methods applied, in searches for Ig and C, to light microscopic preparations.

Comparable advances are now being made with antisera directed against lymphocytes and their subsets (Duke et al, 1983). Studies on blood samples suggest that RA patients may be deficient in the Epstein–Barr virus-specific cytotoxic T cell precursor population (Moss et al, 1983) and observations of this type have renewed interest in the identity of the lymphocytes present in the synovium (Ford & Daroza, 1983). Light and electron microscopic studies with the PAP technique have therefore been made using monoclonal antisera to identify cell subsets (Kurosaka & Ziff, 1983). Approximately 80% of lymphocytes in this study were T cells, staining with OKT 3. Lymphocytic accumulations varied in composition and size, even within a single sample. However, the percentage of OKT 4 (helper/inducer) cells correlated positively, and the percentage of OKT 8 (suppressor/cytotoxic) cells correlated negatively, with the percentage of lymphocytes in any given area. By contrast, the percentage of OKT 4 cells correlated negatively and the percentage of OKT 8 cells correlated positively with the percentage of macrophage-like cells in the same areas.

It is possible that OKT 8 cells proliferate in immunologically reactive areas, following local stimulation of a T cell-mediated immunological response and that, where there are numerous quiescent small lymphocytes, OKT 4 cells preponderate. The difficulty now remains, to develop diagnostic histopathological techniques based on this kind of information and to correlate synovial cell patterns with clinical severity and the response to treatment. There is little doubt that the answers to these challenging questions will have emerged by the time of publication of the next edition of this book.

2. There have been serious attempts to overcome the diagnostic limitations inherent in biopsy material, by the introduction of computer-based statistical analyses in which the significance of particular combinations of microscopic findings have been tested. Retrospective (Cooper et al, 1981; Goldenberg & Cohen, 1978; Rosenberger et al, 1981; Soren, 1978a, 1980) and a few prospective (Stiehl & Geiler, 1974) investigations have been made. *Prospectively*, the degree of inflammatory activity, judged by synovial fluid cytology, correlates with synovial tissue 'actual' activity; but 'basic' synovial cell proliferative activity does not correlate with the clinical disease state (Stiehl & Geiler, 1974). *Retrospectively*, only the presence of lymphoid follicles was specific for RA in one series taken by needle biopsy (Goldenberg & Cohen, 1978) although the degree and intensity of synoviocytic hyperplasia and the extent of macrophage infiltration were characteristic. These views were not accepted by Soren (1978a, 1980) who found lymphoid follicles almost as often in other forms of synovitis as in RA. Nor could he confirm the specificity of multinucleated, synovial giant cells. Soren (1978a) questioned the diagnostic value of vasculitis and agreed with Fassbender (1975) and Lindner (1968) that the significance of synovial granulomata or hemigranulomata was great, their frequency (~ 2%) low. The presence of large fibroblasts (Fassbender, 1975) was the most frequently observed and diagnostically most useful synovial change but this is a view that does not find wide acceptance. Only in psoriatic arthropathy was fibroblast proliferation more common.

Soren's (1978) work was elaborated upon. 127 specimens from cases of RA, seen over a 15-year period, were scored for 37 histological features. The proportion of cases showing each feature was derived. The significance of each feature in influencing the diagnosis in a future, unknown case was then calculated. As an example: 16 features argued against the diagnosis of OA in a biopsy from suspected RA; 4 features, capillary proliferation, hyperaemia, slight synovial cell proliferation, and severe oedema, argued in favour.

There are difficulties in the way of accepting some of the conclusions from Soren's (1978) work: they have been discussed by Gardner (1984). However, there is little doubt that any pathologist with sufficient time could establish a data-base, using, say, the previous 5 or 10 years accumulation of clinically validated cases, to prepare a record against which to quickly calculate the significance of each significant histological observation in any new case presenting for diagnosis. It is important to observe that these methods can offer a *measure* of the weight and importance of the discriminatory value of each observation.

Entirely distinct, quantitative approaches to diagnosis involve the application of measurements, by microdensitometry or image analysis, of tissue chemical components such as DNA, enzyme reaction products, antibody-labelled cells or morphology (Stiehl, 1982). There is a possibility that these techniques also will improve diagnostic accuracy when they are applied to biopsies.

EXTRA-ARTICULAR DISEASE

Rheumatoid arthritis is always a systemic and frequently a visceral disorder. Extra-articular disease, ranging from anaemia, lymphadenopathy and splenomegaly to skin, pulmonary and arterial abnormalities, is therefore seen with varying but considerable frequency (Williams, 1974). Subcutaneous granulomata have long been recognised. The development of extra-articular lesions in RA was noted by early students of the cardiovascular system (Baggenstoss & Rosenberg, 1943). Christie (1950) and Sinclair & Cruickshank (1956) described widespread organ involvement. The presence of significant titres of circulating rheumatoid factor was found to be characteristic of visceral rheumatoid disease. There is rapid progression and a poor prognosis. Inspite of this, the description 'malignant' is better reserved for cancer rather than applied as an index of severity to RA.

Coincidental disease

The age and sex pattern of RA determines that

many people with this common form of polyarthritis coincidentally develop cholecystitis, myocardial infarction, cerebrovascular disease and cancer although the prevalence of myocardial infarction and of cerebral vascular disease, it has been claimed (Ball, 1968), is less than would be expected. In one series of 142 cases (Gardner, 1972), 18% had malignant neoplasms. Moesman (1969) encountered malignant tumours in 14% and 43% of 85 and of 28 RA patients respectively, figures claimed to be 2.0–2.2 times those expected to occur randomly in a control, matched population. The mortality in the two series was 2.6 and 1.3 times the expected figures, observations precisely the converse to those of Ball (1968). Perhaps the true state of affairs is reflected in the studies of Owen et al (1970) who identified malignant neoplasms in 4% of rheumatoid arthritics and in 4% of controls. In the age range 50–74 years, malignancy was more closely associated with steroid treatment than with arthritis.

Rheumatoid arthritis predisposes to osteoporosis, pathological fracture and osteoarthrosis. There is an unexpectedly high frequency of chronic peptic ulcer (Ball, 1968). The coexistence of amyloidosis is discussed below (p. 638). Renal papillary necrosis is recognised as a common complication when phenacetin has been used in treatment but the claim that chronic pyelonephritis is more common in RA than would be expected (Ball, 1968) is not clearly understood. Septicaemia and other forms of secondary infection are recognised to be frequent; there is a diminished resistance to systemic microbial spread. Other drugs are responsible for a further category of iatrogenic disease and the widespread growth of reconstructive and plastic surgery has brought an attendant category of complications.

For many years, it has been apparent that a number of systemic disorders of the connective tissue system share common clinical and pathological characteristics. Currently, the term 'overlap syndrome' is used to describe this clinical phenomenon. Pathological 'overlap' was recognised by Klemperer and his colleagues (Klemperer et al, 1942) and lay at the heart of their original, classical description of the 'diffuse diseases of collagen'. The phrase 'viscerocutaneous collagenosis' was used by Pagel & Treip (1955) to denote the sharing of pathological features by diseases distinguishable on clinical grounds and it is relatively frequent to encounter vasculitis in RA and systemic lupus erythematosus (SLE), pulmonary fibrosis in RA and systemic sclerosis (SS) and renal disease in SLE and SS. Shared immunological characteristics are commonplace and have contributed to the introduction of obscure designations such as 'mixed connective tissue disease' (Ch. 50).

Granulomata

The most frequent tissue lesion in extra-articular rheumatoid disease is the subcutaneous granuloma; it is also histologically the most characteristic (Moore & Willkens, 1977). Subcutaneous granulomata are found in ~ 20% of cases, usually seropositive. However, granulomata may develop in seropositive individuals before the onset of arthritis: nodulosis is then said to be anarthritic (Ganda & Caplan, 1974; Frayha et al, 1976; Eraut et al, 1978; Bywaters, 1979; Wisnieski & Askari, 1981).

The granulomata of RA form in the subcutaneous tissues; they may, however, be small, transient and dermal (Figs 25.26–25.28). They are sterile. Parts exposed to repetitive, physiological, mechanical stress are particularly susceptible so that the occiput, the spinal processes, the scapulae, the extensor aspects of the forearms, the lateral margins of the phalanges and the ischial tuberosities are examples of bones over which subcutaneous granulomata arise. However, histologically closely similar lesions have been identified in the

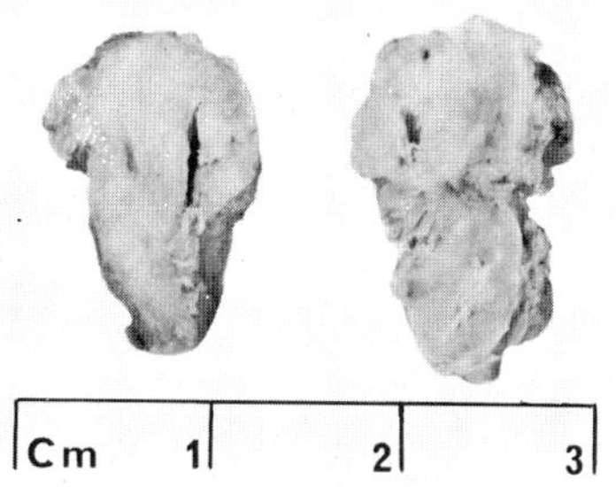

Fig. 25.26 Subcutaneous granuloma. This subcutaneous nodule, removed from the olecranon region, has a fluid filled centre and pale, grey/white surrounding zones where inflammatory cells and granulation tissue merge with nearby subcutaneous connective tissue.

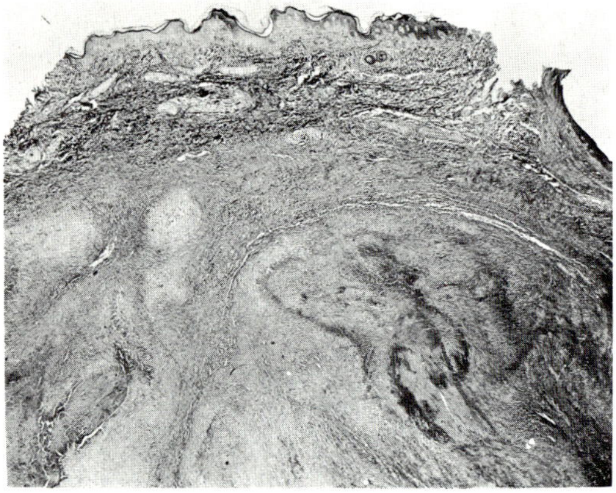

Fig. 25.27 Skin: subcutaneous nodule. The nodule is composed of several confluent areas of necrosis each bounded by pallisaded histiocytes and by a rim of marginal fibrous connective tissue. H & E ×8.

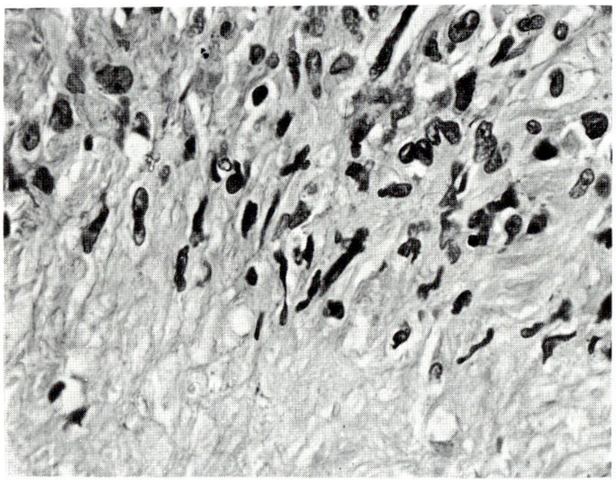

Fig. 25.28 Subcutaneous granuloma. The margin of the granuloma includes a layer of histiocytes that are orientated radially from a central zone of necrosis (top). H & E ×420.

choroid plexus (Kim et al, 1982), vertebral artery wall, retropharynx and base of heart valves and lung, so that physical factors are not the only agents responsible. Granulomata are rare in juvenile chronic polyarthritis but they are common features of severe forms of rheumatoid disease with visceral lesions.

The usual anatomical form of the established subcutaneous granuloma is that of a 2–3 cm diameter, circumscribed, smooth-surfaced loculated structure in which the presence of a soft, necrotic and often fluid centre is concealed, until dissection, by a concentric wall of firm, fibrous tissue. The nodules cause cosmetic difficulty rather than initial discomfort. Early lesions may be identified when of no more than 2–3 mm diameter; several may coalesce to form a multiloculated swelling. The yellow-white, lipochrome-containing margins become slowly but increasingly collagenous. Ulceration may occur and permits the introduction of pathogenic bacteria such as *Staphylococcus aureus*. Infection is indolent, antibiotic-resistance embarrassing and occasionally hazardous (Gardner et al, 1962).

Microscopically, RA granulomata bear a generic resemblance to those caused by mycobacterial infection or by crystal aggregates. However, no definitive foreign material, crystal or microorganism is present. The centre is an island of necrotic tissue debris containing fragments of collagen fibrils. Ultrastructural observations confirm the presence of cell and nuclear derivatives, a meshwork of fibrin, other plasma proteins, lipid and glycosaminoglycans (Cochrane et al, 1964). There is little calcium. Gieseking (1969) and Gieseking et al (1969) believe that the cells which comprise the cellular wall bounding the necrotic zone are proliferating, vascular parietal cells. The majority, however, favour the view that these bounding cells are histiocytes: they are elongated, radially disposed and form a pallisade-like zone arranged in a characteristic serpiginous form. The bounding cells do not take up neutral red but are potent sources of proteases that are presumably liberated into the ischaemic central zone. Multinucleate giant cells are occasionally seen among the histiocytes of the granuloma margins; their resemblance to Touton cells may indicate that they are a reaction to lipid.

RA granulomata can involute, but a persistent, indolent behaviour is usual.

The pathogenesis of the granulomata remains obscure. Anti-immunoglobulin (Ig) sera react with the central necrotic material but not with the marginal histiocytes. Nearby blood vessels, in which vasculitis has been demonstrated by meticulous serial section (Sokoloff, 1963), react for fibrin and for IgG. Vasculitis has therefore been held to be a causative factor but this is disputed (Rasker & Kuipers, 1983). The central Ig is both in free form and in the form of IgG/IgM complexes. Aggregated IgG exists as granules and as bumpy deposits between the residual collagen; labelled

IgM rheumatoid factor can be found, as can complement (C). Recent studies using FITC-labelled anti-IgG and anti-fibrinogen have led to the proposal that a series of evolutionary stages in the natural history of the subcutaneous granuloma can be recognised: acute, granulomatous, and fibrotic (Fukase et al, 1980).

Repeated attempts have been made to reproduce RA granulomata experimentally. Bentonite, polymerised fibrin, autologous blood, and autologous and heterologous synovial fluid have been tested in animal and in human tissues. None has replicated the RA lesion precisely. The implantation of insoluble fibrin into an animal sensitised to this material evokes a prolonged inflammatory reaction. Mechanisms of hypersensitivity can impair this local reaction and there is a strong suspicion that the human RA lesion may be perpetuated by a change in the antigenicity of the original, persistent protein. Such alterations can lead both to the local formation of immune complexes and to their capacity to activate a complement-mediated inflammatory response, sometimes with vasculitis. Once a nidus of antigenically distinct, necrotic tissue debris has formed in susceptible tissue of relatively low vascularity, the stimulus required to prolong its presence need not be strong.

Cardiac disease

As many as 5–10% of cases of RA have some form of cardiac disease (Lebowitz, 1966). Early descriptions included those of Bayles (1943), Rosenberg et al (1943), Levin et al (1955), Sokoloff (1953, 1964), and Cruickshank (1958).

Pericarditis is the most frequently recognised disorder (Prakash et al, 1973). In one series, there were 37 instances in 150 necropsy cases (Gardner, 1972); 15 were examples of acute, fibrinous pericarditis, 22 of chronic inflammation with fibrosis, fibrous adhesions or obliteration of the pericardial sac. Inflammation is localised or generalised. Effusion is seldom of functional significance but tamponade has been diagnosed (Thadani et al, 1975) and pericardiectomy is occasionally required because of constriction (Batley et al, 1969). The microscopic changes are characteristic, with low-grade, active inflammation, granulation tissue formation and fibrosis. They are only pathognomonic when necrotic foci resembling the subcutaneous granuloma are seen. Pericarditis has been found to precede synovitis but diagnosis by biopsy is seldom indicated.

Myocardial disease may be an integral part of the systemic inflammatory response. 10–20% of cases examined at necropsy in one series displayed focal, interstitial, non-specific myocarditis (Lebowitz, 1966) and it has long been acknowledged that the response is quite distinct from that of rheumatic myocarditis. In addition, however, there is increasingly common recognition of myocardial ischaemia, the result not only of coincidental coronary artery atheroma but also of coronary artery RA vasculitis, a condition now susceptible to surgical correction (Susmano et al, 1973). Occasionally myocardial granulomata are present and attempts can be made pathologically to distinguish this lesion, characteristically present in seropositive cases who also display vasculitis, from foci of hypersensitivity myocarditis caused by drugs used clinically.

Valvular, *endocarditic* disease is frequently (~ 30%) of an indeterminate nature. The valvulitis displays a lymphocytic, plasmacytic and increasingly histiocytic infiltrate. Vascularisation results. Fibrosis follows with focal or diffuse scarring; contracture with deformity leads to stenosis or incompetence. In a further 3% of cases there are aortic or mitral valve rheumatoid granulomata (Fig. 25.29). The granulomata are usually small

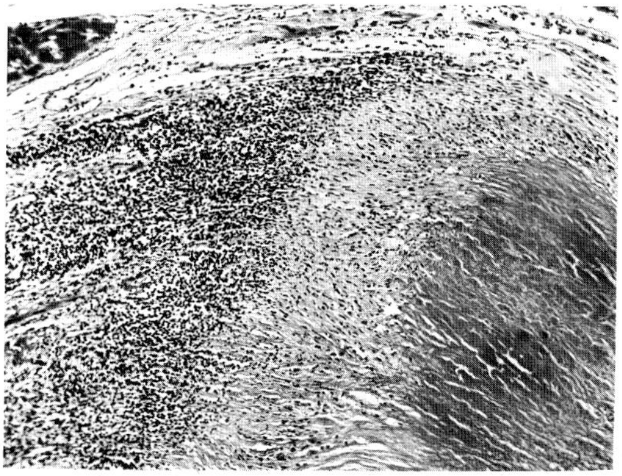

Fig. 25.29 Cardiac granuloma. At the base of a heart valve a granuloma is shown, having , at right, a zone of central necrosis, a margin of granulation tissue, and, at left, a fringe of lymphocytes and plasma cells. The resemblance to a subcutaneous granuloma is close. H & E ×54.

and do not cause mechanical defect. Occasionally, they are sufficiently large to occupy much of the base of the valve. All valves may be simultaneously affected (Roberts et al, 1968) but thrombosis and verrucous vegetations seldom form (Iveson & Pomerance, 1977). There may be a resemblance to and overlap with the aortic valvulitis of ankylosing spondylitis (Reimer et al, 1976). The scarred valve in RA can be replaced surgically (Yates & Scott, 1975) and valve prolapse is an occasional reason for emergency surgery (Linch et al, 1980).

The mitral valvular disease of RA is granulomatous as often as the aortic. Functionally, the mitral lesion is less important (Iveson & Pomerance, 1977) but aortic disease may coexist. It is general experience that there is a poor correlation between the frequency with which both mitral and aortic valve disease are diagnosed clinically and the (much higher) frequency with which they are found at necropsy. Although systemic bacterial infection is common in RA, bacterial endocarditis is very infrequent. Conduction defects develop from time to time, either because granulomata affect the conducting tissue or because of more diffuse inflammation. Complete heart block is regularly but rarely described (Harris, 1970; Ahern et al, 1983). Among other comparable cases are nodulosis of all four valves and left bundle branch block (Carpenter et al, 1967), heart block from secondary amyloidosis (Thery et al, 1974) and from coronary RA vasculitis (Lebowitz, 1966).

Vasculitis. Interest in arteritis derives from the early years of this century but has grown quickly in the present decade (Bannatyne, 1896; Ball, 1954; Cruickshank, 1954; Sokoloff & Bunim, 1957; Karten, 1969b; Glass et al, 1976; Koizumi et al, 1979; Scott et al, 1981). Arteritis is a feature of severe forms of RA and vascular involvement is an index of seropositivity, granuloma formation and neuropathy. There is a poor prognosis.

With the exception of coincidental atherosclerosis, medial sclerosis and aneurysm, 3 forms of *arterial disease* are recognised: a frequent, active, non-necrotising subacute arteritis (Cruickshank, 1954); a florid, necrotising arteritis which spares the synovium (Ball, 1954); and a bland, non-inflammatory fibromuscular obliterative lesion with thrombosis, occlusion and peripheral circulatory insufficiency (Bywaters, 1957; Gardner, 1972).

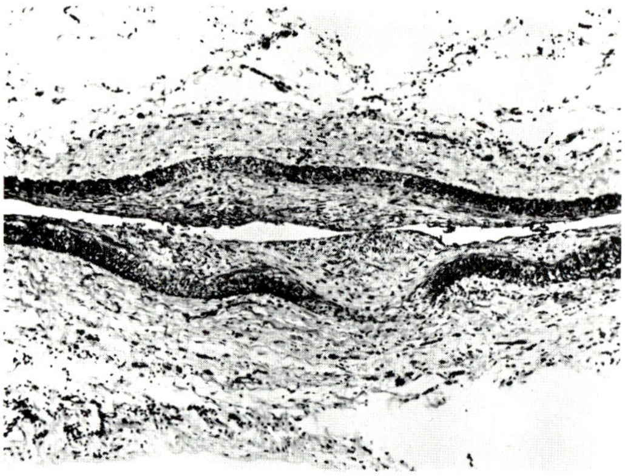

Fig. 25.30 Subacute arteritis. A low grade inflammatory response surrounds this small artery which lies in the connective tissue near the sciatic nerve. A zone of media is incompletely interrupted and the intima contains an excess of fibromuscular connective tissue and matrix covered internally by a continuous layer of endothelium. H & E ×40.

The *subacute arteritis* comprises a limited, often neglected intra- and periarterial infiltration by lymphocytes, histiocytes and occasional plasma cells (Fig. 25.30). The lesion has been detected not only in relation to the nerve sheaths of peripheral nerves and in skeletal muscle but also in the intrinsic vasculature and nerve fibre bundles of unexpected sites such as the larynx. The coexistence of myocardial disease with angina pectoris (Susmano et al, 1973) suggests that while this form of arterial lesion may by itself be insufficient to cause peripheral ischaemia or neuritis, it may complement the defect resulting from coincidental atherosclerosis.

The *necrotising vasculitis* of RA may be indistinguishable from microscopic polyarteritis nodosa (Fig. 25.31). There is an identical visceral distribution and the lesions of the medium-size, musculoelastic arteries are focal and segmental. However, much smaller vessels are also affected and this arteriolitis may dominate the pathological scene, affecting systemic and, exceptionally, pulmonary vessels. Aneurysm formation is much less frequently recognised than in polyarteritis nodosa. The cause of RA arteritis and arteriolitis must now be sought in the circulating, medium-size immune complexes that can be identified clinically in the serum.

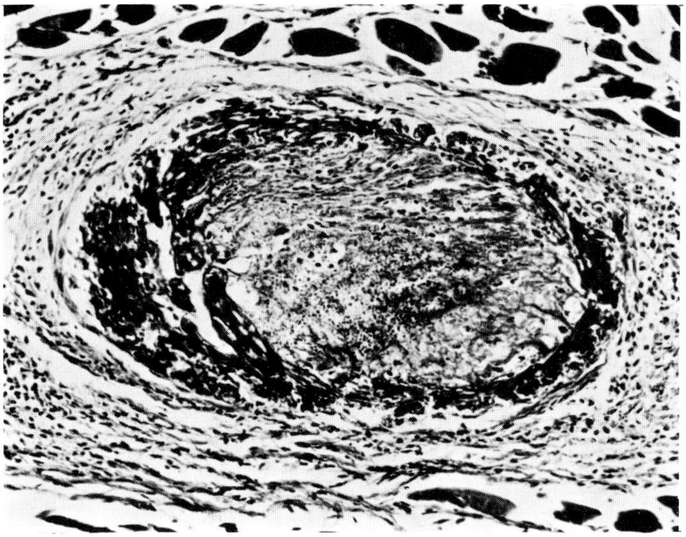

Fig. 25.31 Necrotising arteritis. Within skeletal muscle, a medium-sized musculoelastic artery, transected, is seen to be occupied by recent thrombus. The media is necrotic and occupied by fibrin and the vessel is surrounded by lymphocytes, polymorphs and histiocytes. The appearances are indistinguishable from those of some forms of polyarteritis. H & E ×150.

Intimal *fibromuscular hyperplasia* is a common disorder of the peripheral, limb vessels (Fig. 25.32). The digital arteries, for example, may be wholly or partly obstructed. Thrombosis supervenes but recanalisation may prevent early gangrene. Nevertheless, in older patients with associated medial

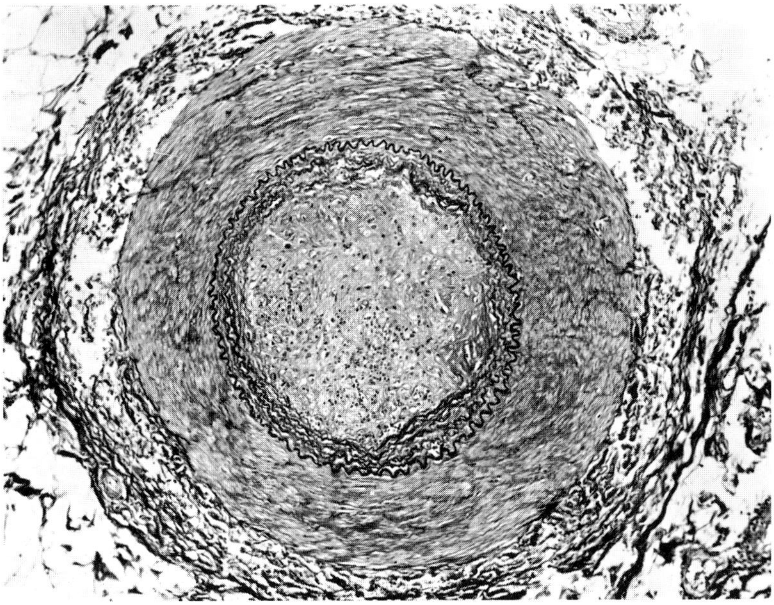

Fig. 25.32 Digital artery thrombosis. The well defined internal elastic lamina separates the intima from the hypertrophied muscular media. The lumen is occupied by recent organizing thrombus. The elastic lamina is reduplicated. H & E ×50.

arterial calcification and atherosclerosis, gangrene is a likely sequel to a period of claudication or Raynaud's phenomenon.

The skin circulation in RA has attracted attention. Nail-fold capillaries behave abnormally in response to altered environmental temperatures. Brown stains, nail-fold and nail-edge lesions and ischaemic ulceration draw attention to underlying obliterative, thrombotic or necrotising arterial disease. Analogous changes develop in the gastrointestinal tract.

Arteritis occurs focally in RA during the episodic formation of large immune complexes and their persistence in the circulation. Sites of complex deposition elicit complement-mediated inflammation. The cycle of complex formation is particularly likely in those with high circulating titres of IgM rheumatoid factor but high titres of anti-nuclear factor, IgG rheumatoid factor, cryoglobulinaemia, anti-complementary activity and other changes are common associations. Recently, immunoglobulins and complement have been found in the walls of affected vessels (Conn et al, 1976; Ullman et al, 1978). Rectal biopsy is of value in diagnosis (Scott et al, 1981) and the levels of IgG rheumatoid factor, anti-complementary activity and C4, which is diminished, are the best clinical markers for systemic vasculitis.

Table 25.1 Frequency of lung and bronchial disease at death, determined for 142 patients with rheumatoid arthritis dying in hospital. (From Gardner D L 1972 Pathology of rheumatoid arthritis. Edward Arnold, London.)

Pleural fibrosis	56	(41%)
Bronchopneumonia	54	(40%)
Emphysema	31	(23%)
Pulmonary embolism	14	(10%)
Tuberculosis	13	(10%)
Pulmonary hypertension	9	(7%)
Pulmonary infarction	8	
Acute pleuritis	8	
Pulmonary primary tumours	7	
Abscess	6	
Bronchiectasis	6	
Atelectasis	5	
Interstitial fibrosis	4	

Respiratory

A significant number of patients with RA develop disease of the larynx, bronchi, lungs or pleura (Table 25.1). Several of these disorders are characteristic of RA but, apart from the pulmonary granulomata, none is pathognomonic. In a survey of 516 patients, Walker & Wright (1969) found that 197 had had pleuritis, 16 bronchiectasis, 8 interstitial pulmonary fibrosis and 2 granulomata. These observations suggested the scale of the problem of respiratory disease in RA (Danieli et al, 1980). The evidence comes as no surprise to the pathologist since almost half of rheumatoid patients dying in hospital display evidence of pleural fibrosis.

One in four RA patients is thought to have arthritis of the intrinsic synovial joints of the *larynx* but anatomical studies suggest a much higher frequency of laryngeal disease (Bridger et al, 1980). Synovitis occurs (Montgomery & Goodman, 1980) and the laryngeal cartilages are eroded and destroyed, a process accompanied by inflammatory changes in nearby soft tissues. Granulomata develop. Laryngeal articular inflammation is succeeded by fibrous ankylosis. The difficulties that this offers to intubation for anaesthesia have been much reduced by the availability of fibreoptic instruments. Nevertheless, few pathologists in routine necropsy practice examine the larynx as closely as may be desirable so that the intrinsic joints and the perineuronal vasculitis that affect the recurrent laryngeal nerve are readily overlooked.

Bronchial disease is occasional, bronchiolar disease commonplace. Endobronchial granulomata have been recognised before the onset of sero-negative RA (Johnston et al, 1982) and in rare instances, bronchocentric granulomatosis has been diagnosed (Hellems et al, 1983). A considerable proportion of the cases studied in large series of RA in Western countries have had chronic bronchitis dating back to periods before the onset of arthritis and this may be a part explanation for the frequency of later episodes of bronchopneumonia.

Attention was drawn to the lungs in RA by Ellman & Ball's (1948) demonstration of a fibrosing pneumonic lesion. The most common forms of fibrosis, excluding those such as tuberculosis and scirrhous carcinoma that coexist by chance, are

1. Pulmonary granulomata, sometimes with pneumoconiosis (Fig. 25.33)
2. Diffuse interstitial fibrosis, the fibrosing alveolitis of Scadding (1969) (Figs 25.34, 25.35)

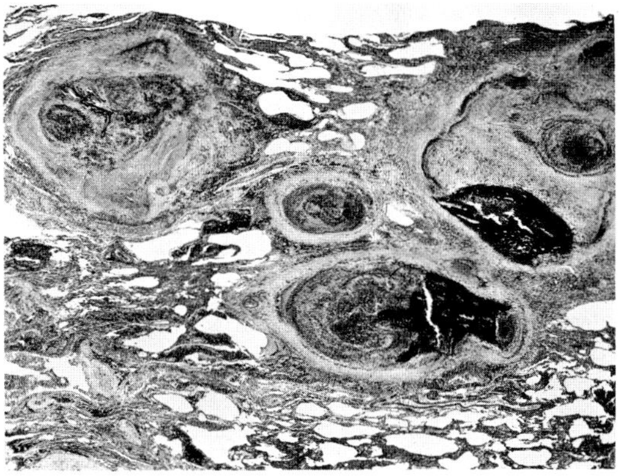

Fig. 25.33 Lung: granulomata. The appearances are those encountered in the Caplan syndrome. Within emphysematous and fibrotic lung tissue is a cluster of rheumatoid granulomata impregnated to a varying extent by dense, black carbon pigment, bounded by laminated collagen that becomes confluent. Each has a central zone of necrosis. H & E ×5.

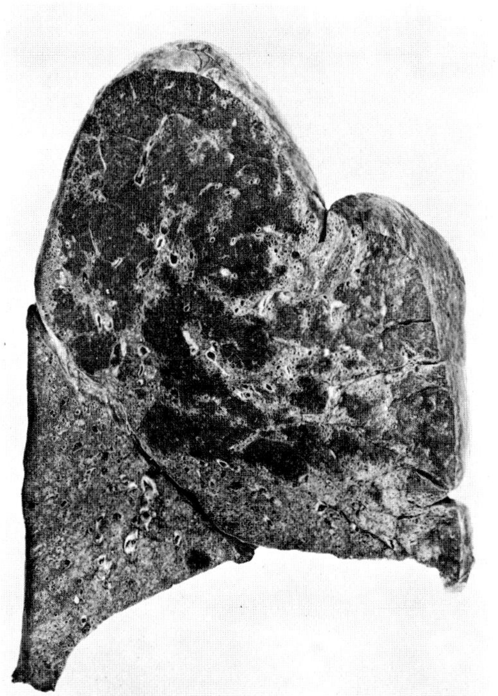

Fig. 25.34 Lung. In this long-standing case, there is widespread consolidation, necrosis and cyst formation of the lower lobe and of the lower part of the upper lobe. At age 55 this female patient had been treated with corticosteroids for systemic lupus erythematosus. Later the onset of peripheral vascular insufficiency was accompanied by pulmonary hypertension, cor pulmonale and congestive cardiac failure. $\frac{1}{4}$ natural size.

3. Obstructive bronchiolar disease
4. Pulmonary arteritis or arterial sclerosis.

Recently, obliterative bronchiolitis has gained notoriety (Geddes et al, 1977): it is rapidly progressive and intractable (Forman et al, 1982).

The granulomata form discrete, rounded, faintly radio-opaque shadows, lying close to a pleural surface or within the lung substance. They vary in diameter from 1–6 cm and may be single or multiple, related or not related to coexistent pneumoconiosis. In seropositive patients, the development of pulmonary granulomata may coincide with the formation of a subcutaneous lesion. Occasionally, the lung granulomata may be recognised in pneumoconiotic men who only subsequently manifest RA. Histologically, a central zone of eosinophilic necrosis is circumscribed by dust-laden, concentric cellular and increasingly fibrous margins. Cavitation has been described and ulceration into the pleural cavity can precipitate pyopneumothorax. Granulomata, effusion and empyema may coexist (Jones & Blodgett, 1971).

Fibrosing alveolitis is described clinically in 1–2% of cases. It is a rare finding pathologically. Diffuse interstitial fibrosis is the end-point. Numerous mononuclear phagocytes desquamate into the alveoli and alveolar ducts. The walls of these spaces thicken. Later, the air spaces are defined by fibrosis accompanied by inflammatory destruction of the normal connective tissue skeleton of the lung and the formation of a honeycomb-like meshwork in which pulmonary arterial branches display fibromuscular end arterial change and a pronounced reduction of their lumina. These later changes are irreversible and do not respond to agents such as the corticosteroids.

Obstructive bronchiolar disease can now be identified clinically in a group of patients who develop rapidly progressive breathlessness, and are not responsive to bronchodilators, antibiotics or corticosteroids (Geddes et al, 1977). The condition is analogous to the obliterating bronchiolitis of systemic sclerosis (Forman et al, 1982). Careful injection and serial section is necessary to prove the presence *postmortem* of bronchiolar constriction. There is neither excess mucus secretion nor mucosal gland hypertrophy. The subjects are non-smokers and small airways are destroyed in a

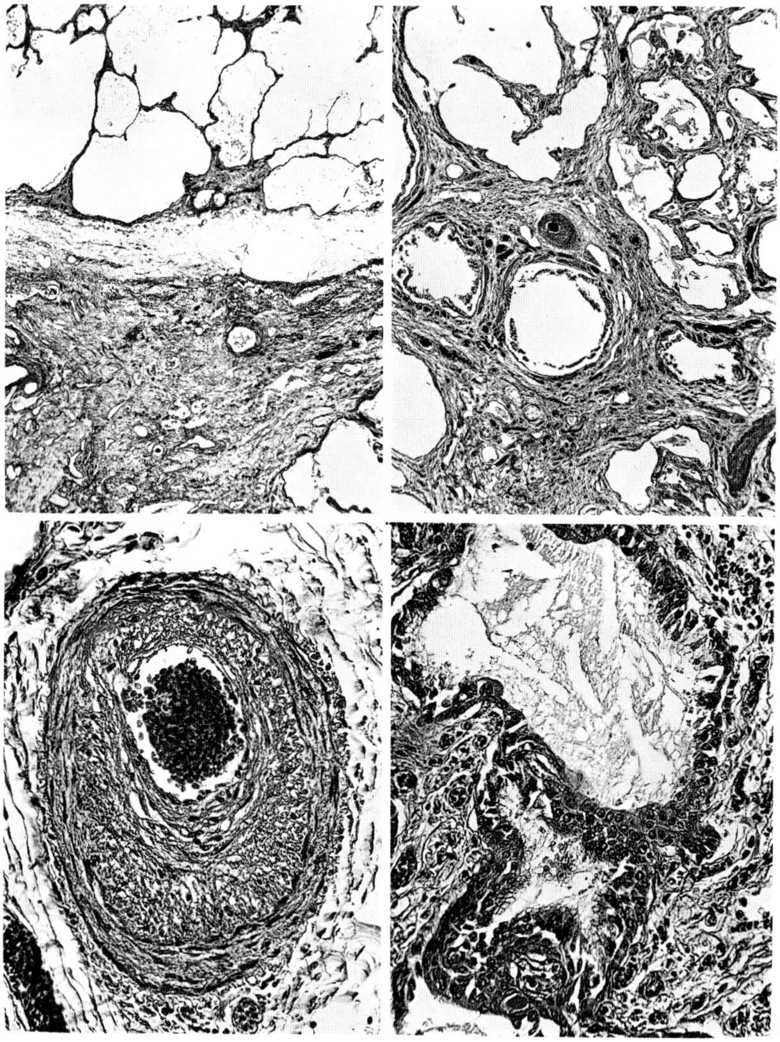

Fig. 25.35 Lung.

(a) Interlobar septum of lung shown in Fig. 25.34. Emphysema with slight interstitial fibrosis of upper lobe (top). Lower lobe (bottom) occupied by fibrous tissue with few residual alveolar spaces having a lining of low cuboidal epithelium. H & E ×18.

(b) Enlarged alveolar spaces, destruction of interalveolar septa and pulmonary arterial branch (centre) partly occupied by intimal fibromuscular hyperplasia. H & E × 18.

(c) High power view of field at top right to show structure of pulmonary artery. H & E ×190.

(d) In those parts of the cystic-appearing lung, residual air spaces are lined by hyperplastic cuboidal alveolar or low columnar bronchiolar epithelium. H & E ×140.

lymphoplasmacytic reaction that has much in common with the parotid gland lesion of Sjögren's syndrome (p. 641).

Excess eosinophils may indicate a particularly aggressive phase of RA but the reason for the occasional development of eosinophilic pneumonia (Cooney, 1981) is not known.

Pulmonary vascular disease in RA may assume a vasculitic form acutely, or as in Wegener's granulomatosis, with thrombosis and organisation. Pulmonary artery intimal fibromuscular hyperplasia is occasionally responsible for pulmonary hypertension and this condition has been recognised as one result of primary arteriolar disease (Gardner et al, 1957).

Pleural effusion is frequent in RA, empyema occasional. Empyema may be silent and bilateral. Chemical studies allow the effusions to be distinguished from those of SLE and in both disorders immune complexes can be found (Halla et al, 1980), an observation helping to exclude effusions due to non-rheumatoid disease. The pleural mesothelial cells phagocytose immune complexes and must be differentiated from the cells of carcinoma invading the pleura (Nosanchuk & Naylor, 1967; Boddington et al, 1971). Subsequent to effusion, fibrosis is commonplace: it is to be regarded as a measure of the high frequency of underlying lung infection, bronchiectasis, interstitial pneumonitis and bronchiolitis. Decortication may be required (Brunk et al, 1966).

Urinary disease

In one series, 72% of necropsy cases displayed significant renal lesions (Lawson & MacLean, 1966). In my own study, I found examples of hydronephrosis, polycystic kidney, calculus and pyonephrosis among the gross lesions in 142 cases (Gardner, 1972) (Table 25.2). Hypertensive vascular disease is common. Urinary infections complicate chronic disability and there is a high frequency of amyloidosis (p. 638). Rheumatoid nodules may cause ureteric obstruction (Adelson al, 1982). Although there is evidence, based on tests of excretory function, that glomerular filtration rates are often low, there is still debate on the question as to whether a specific rheumatoid glomerulitis occurs. The cellularity of the glomeruli is not increased above normal. Immune complex deposition has been implied (Skrifvars, 1979) but glomerulitis is not invariable. The possibility of a rheumatoid tubular disease has been raised; peritubular lymphocytic and plasmacytic infiltrates can clearly lead to tubular dysfunction, as in Sjögren's syndrome.

Antirheumatic and analgesic drug nephropathies remain of concern. Acute tubular necrosis in gold therapy is a rare, fatal complication but the membranous nephropathy that occurs in chrysotherapy responds to treatment (Samuels et al, 1978). Penicillamine directly injures glomeruli: immune complexes are deposited beneath the glomerular epithelium and a membranous glomerulonephritis leads to the nephrotic syndrome. Non-obstructive pyelonephritis and papillary necrosis were complications of phenacetin treatment. Papillary necrosis has been found, in isolated cases, during the administration of indomethacin and of phenylbutazone (Jackson & Lawrence, 1978). Salicylates may impair renal tubular function by causing epithelial cell desquamation (Burry et al, 1976).

Table 25.2 Frequency of renal disease in 142 hospital cases of rheumatoid arthritis examined at necropsy. (From Gardner D L 1972 Pathology of rheumatoid arthritis. Edward Arnold, London.)

Pyelonephritis	39	(20%)
Papillary necrosis	11	(8%)
Hydronephrosis	4	(3%)
Cystic kidney	3	—
Tubular necrosis	3	—
Calculus	2	—
Pyonephrosis	2	—

Alimentary disease

All chronic RA patients are liable to manifest disorders of the salivary glands. Salivary duct ectasia, duct strictures, the formation of calculi and gland atrophy are encountered. These lesions are particularly probable in patients with the 'sicca syndrome' (Ericson, 1968) and in these subjects local immunoglobulin synthesis and lymphocytosis are prominent.

Peptic ulcers, particularly of the stomach, are encountered in at least 38% of RA patients. Salicylates are thought to exacerbate erosion and thus ulceration. Intestinal function may be impaired and systematic investigations have revealed villous atrophy more often in seronegative than in seropositive individuals. Exceptionally, when total villous atrophy is found, clinical signs of arthritis may vanish when a gluten-free diet is given. A relationship to latent coeliac disease is suggested. The small intestinal arteries and arterioles are regular sites for vasculitis, sometimes necrotising, and amyloid deposits may coexist.

In spite of much study, debate continues on whether the liver is a primary target of RA. 10% of patients have hepatomegaly (Webb et al, 1975; Tiger et al, 1976). Conventional, older tests of liver function are often found to be abnormal. Even when the raised levels of hepatic alkaline phosphatase are considered, however, there is little correlation between their activity and the severity of liver parenchymal cell disease. A further difficulty in the interpretation of liver histology is the frequency with which potentially hepatotoxic drugs such as salicylates, phenylbutazone, gold and azathioprine are administered. Although, therefore, liver cell disease is frequently but not constantly identified (Mills et al, 1980), and although liver dysfunction may contribute to death, the relationship of liver disorder to RA usually remains equivocal.

In Sjögren's syndrome there is a raised frequency of liver disease (Whaley & Buchanan, 1971) so that when the syndrome coincides with primary biliary cirrhosis and RA (Ellman et al, 1974) it has been difficult to ascertain the sequence of cell disorder. Nodular, non-cirrhotic liver disease, regenerative hyperplasia, is a feature of Felty's syndrome (Thorne et al, 1982) but is not pathognomonic of RA. Finally, in a survey of the livers of 31 cases of classical or definite RA, only 4 were microscopically normal (Mills et al, 1980). Four cases revealed definitive lesions: primary biliary cirrhosis; chronic active hepatitis; amyloidosis; and alcoholic cirrhosis; or displayed non-specific changes. The difficulty remains to decide whether this pattern of liver abnormality differs from that found in a selected series of chronic *non-RA* inflammatory disease such as fibrocaseous pulmonary tuberculosis or schistosomiasis.

Haemopoietic disease

Although moderate, normocytic, hypochromic anaemia is characteristic of RA, the pathogenesis of the red cell disorder remains uncertain. Marrow lymphocytic foci are found. Plasma cells are frequent. Marrow amyloidosis and vasculitis are occasional.

The proportions of marrow red cell, white cell and platelet precursors may be disturbed with a reduced number of normoblasts. Iron, absorbed normally, is used inadequately for haemoglobin synthesis. Interest has been devoted to ineffective erythropoiesis (Samson et al, 1977) with a decreased haem turnover by approximately normal numbers of cells. There is a highly significant inverse correlation between the number of erythroid colonies formed when circulating erythrocyte progenitor cells are cultured in vitro, and the levels of serum IgM and rheumatoid factor (Harvey et al, 1983). Nevertheless, it remains unclear how these abnormalities relate to the tendency for iron to sequestrate in the cells of the mononuclear macrophage system, including the phagocytic A(M) cells of the synovium (Muirden, 1970). A slightly increased rate of peripheral red blood cell destruction is suspected. Normal red blood cells transfused to RA patients survive normally but the individuals' own cells have a diminished life span. When these disparate observations are summarised, it appears that the active, RA inflammatory process can influence haemopoiesis and the blood in a number of characteristic ways, one consequence of which is a particular form of anaemia. Leucopenia is more often the result of drug therapy than of Felty's syndrome (p. 640).

Lymphoreticular disease (Gardner, 1972; Dorfman & Warnke, 1974; Talal & Schnitzer, 1977).

Very many of those with active, adult RA have widespread lymph node enlargement at necropsy

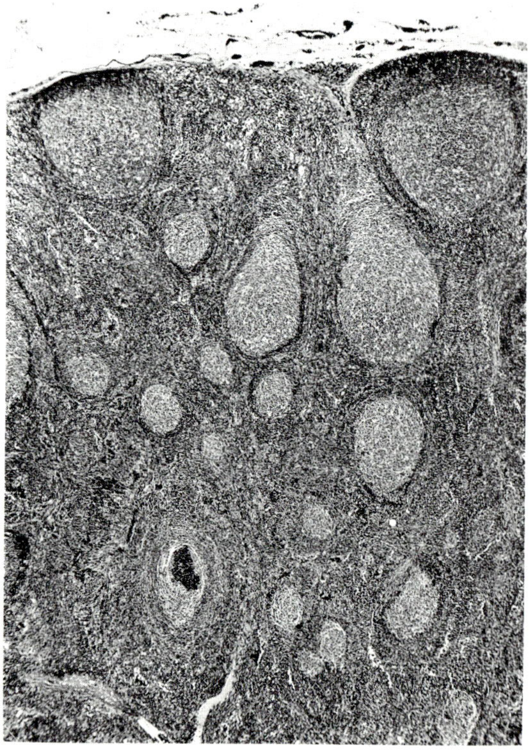

Fig. 25.36 Lymph node. Within the cortex are many prominent, large follides each having extremely large germinal centres. Occasionally, such follicles impinge upon each other, obliterating the intervening cortex. H & E ×25.

and groups of nodes may attract attention during life, sometimes leading to biopsy for suspected lymphoma. The anatomical distribution of the enlarged nodes does not closely mirror the pattern of articular disease. There is cortical hyperplasia. The interfollicular tissues may be obliterated to a degree that results in an appearance resembling follicular lymphoma (Fig. 25.36). Capsular fibrosis, with lymphocytic infiltration, interfollicular plasmacytosis of the thymic-dependent cortex and the sinus accumulation of raised numbers of histiocytes, are some of the features seen (Tables 25.3–25.5). When peripheral arthritis is active and progressive, lymph node oedema and the presence of neutrophil polymorphs reflect this activity and are particularly conspicuous when there is silent joint infection with opportunistic bacteria.

It is generally accepted that the involvement of the lymphoreticular system in RA reflects or is a manifestation of a generalised disturbance of the immunological mechanism. Apart from the abnormal lymph node structure referred to above, the frequent presence of serum rheumatoid factors, altered T cell function and the nature of the cellular synovial response, are all in accord with this view. The lymph nodes have been held to show many of the features of acute, high-antigen-dose stimulation (Dumonde et al, 1976).

Lymphoproliferative neoplasms may be more frequent in RA patients than would be anticipated by chance (Goldenberg et al, 1969). Although chronic lymphocytic leukaemia can be coincidental

Table 25.3 Cellular characteristics of lymph nodes in 51 fatal cases of rheumatoid arthritis. (From Gardner D L 1968 In: Duthie J J R, Alexander W R M (eds) Rheumatic diseases. Pfizer medical monograph No. 3. Edinburgh University Press.)

	Prominent germinal centres	Plasmacytosis	Sinus-cell hyperplasia
Lymph nodes (47)	15 (32%)	23 (49%)	33 (70%)
Spleen (51)	9 (18%)	18 (35%)	20 (40%)

Of the 18 spleens displaying plasmacytosis, 8 contained amyloid; amyloid, however, was identified in only 5 of the 23 lymph nodes with plasma cell excess.

Cytological assessments were made on a 5-point scale: 0 Nil; 1 Slight; 2 Moderate; 3 Marked; 4 Severe. Only those cases with moderate, marked or severe reactions are included in this table.

(Dmoszynska & Pytko, 1976), compounds occasionally used in treating RA, such as cyclophosphamide, are leukaemogenic. Both acquired and spontaneous immunological deficiency predispose to the development of malignant lymphomata; such deficiencies may also predispose to RA-like polyarthritis in which, therefore, the lymphomata are only expressions of the underlying disease.

Splenomegaly is characteristic of RA but the degree of splenic enlargement is not often sufficient to be detected by palpation (Table 25.6). Felty's syndrome is an exception. Histologically, the changes mirror those of the regional lymph nodes. Iron is present in abundance. Amyloidosis occasionally results in the appearance of 'sago' spleen but, more often, amyloid deposits are diffuse.

Neurological disease (Kim & Collins, 1981)
The lesions encountered from time to time in the brain, spinal cord and peripheral nerves may be primary or secondary. Some are iatrogenic.

Encephalopathy (Kim, 1980) may be the consequence of: vasculitis, intracranial granulomata and 'RA meningitis' (Spurlock & Richman, 1983); choroid plexus immune complex deposition; amyloidosis; microbial infection; or the action of a variety of drugs ranging from iron to corticosteroids. Active cerebral vasculitis is detected *post-mortem* more often than might be suspected clinically. Aneurysms develop and ischaemic infarcts result. RA granulomata are particularly likely within the dural reflections and falx cerebri but have been identified in the cerebral parenchyma, choroid plexus and vertebral arteries. The selective location of cerebral RA granulomata presumably indicates the susceptibility of certain vascular territories to immune complex deposition. Bacterial, mycotic and protozoal infections are features of long-term treatment with immunosuppressive drugs; they occasionally follow the development of bacterial resistance to antibiotics.

Myelopathy is likely to result from bone and articular disease of the spine. Rare instances of spinal vasculitis have been described (Watson, 1979; Watson et al, 1977). The synovial joints of the vertebral column are prone to destructive disease. The atlanto-occipital and apophyseal articulations are often found to be affected but

Table 25.4 Lymph nodes in rheumatoid arthritis (9 cases). (From Lennert K 1961 Cytologie und Lymphadenitis. In: Uehlinger E (ed) Handbuch der speziellen pathologischen Anatomie und Histologie. Springer, Berlin.)

Register No.	Age: Sex	Site	Size	Follicular lymphoid hyperplasia	Diffuse lymphoid hyperplasia	Sinus catarrh	Sinus leucocytosis	Mastocytosis[a]	Plasmacytosis	Clinical features
8687/52	61♀	Axilla	Plum-size	++++	0	0	o	(+)1455	0	Generalised lymph node enlargement
6084/54	69♀	Axilla	Cherry-size	+++++ plasma cells	0	+	+++	(+)1259	+	Tumour-like swellings in axilla and inguinal region
553/56	56♀	Axilla	Cherry-stone size	+	+	(+)	0	+5128	(+)	
554/56	48♀	Axilla	Cherry-size	++	+	+	(+)	(+)2319	+	
6071/56	49♂	Axilla	Cherry-size	++++	o	(+)	+	Diminished 100	0	
13 070/56	61♀	Groin	Cherry-stone size	++	0	(+)	+	(+)1120	(+)	
7682/53	39♂	Axilla	Cherry-size	++	0	+	0	++13 604	++	Felty's syndrome
4247/54	36♂	Axilla	Cherry-size	+	0	++RBC	++	(+)2278	++	Felty's syndrome
10 972/53	33♀	Hilum of spleen	Hazel-nut size	++++	0+	0	0	Diminished	0	Felty's syndrome

[a] Figures denote numbers of mast cells/cm^2

Table 25.5 Cell quantitation of three lymph nodes in rheumatoid arthritis. (From Lennert 1961 Cytologie und Lymphadenitis. In: Uehlinger E (ed) Handbuch der speziellen pathologischen Anatomie und Histologie. Springer, Berlin.)

No. of investigation	1	2	3
Lymphocytes	936	939	870
Basophil stem cells	—	1	—
Gerninoblasts: large	4	4	17
medium	—	7	19
small	—	2	12
Plasmablasts	—	—	1
Preplasma cells	1	—	1
Plasma cells	9	4	4
Stimulated reticulum cells: large	6	5	15
medium	22	12	27
small	—	3	5
Reticulum cells (large and medium)	7	4	4
Histiocytes (monocytes)	2	5	15
	5		
	15		
Phagocyte with nuclear fragment	—	—	—
Epithelioid cells	1	1	2
Tissue mast cells	1	1	—
Basophils	—	1	—
Eosinophils	—	2	—
Neutrophils	11	9	8

neurocentral synovitis is of particular importance since it may lead to disorganisation of the main cervical intervertebral joints; the associated disease of the spinal ligaments contributes to subluxation and even dislocation. The most common site for this potentially lethal form of RA synovitis is the atlantoaxial joint where the spinal canal is wide, but other levels may be affected and several vertebrae can be displaced simultaneously. Horizontal atlantoaxial dislocation is more common than vertical (Smith et al, 1980); the former leads to cervical cord injury, the latter to brain stem compression. If lower cervical segments are affected, the anterior surface of the cord may be indented (Davidson et al, 1977); anterior horn necrosis develops but other tracts may be implicated. The pattern of compression is distinct from that resulting from spondylosis (Kim & Collins, 1981).

Table 25.6 Organ weights in rheumatoid arthritis and in control cases matched for age and sex (necropsy records). (From Gardner D L 1972 Pathology of rheumatoid arthritis. Edward Arnold, London.)

	Mean weight (g)	
	Spleen	Liver
Rheumatoid arthritis	224	1490
Control cases	120	1435
Difference	104	55
SE	±26.1	±86

Peripheral neuropathy (Neumark et al, 1979) results from inflammation, ischaemia, compression or even amyloidosis. Histological evidence of perineuritis is much more frequent than signs of clinical disease. Endarterial fibrosis is recognised but necrotising vasculitis has been described. When the clinical evidence demonstrates involvement of the principal fascicles of the mid-upper arm and mid-thigh, it can be assumed that vasculitis is extensive (Kim & Collins, 1981). Entrapment neuropathy, encountered in 45% of cases of flexor tendon synovitis RA, is a consequence of disease of the carpal tunnel but amyloidosis can provoke the same complication. The posterior tibial nerve may be affected similarly.

Among the disorders that follow RA neuropathy of the autonomic nervous system are impairment of the thermoregulatory and heating responses (Bennett & Scott, 1965). Pre- and postganglionic lesions occur; postural hypotension and gustatory sweating are recorded (Edmonds et al, 1979).

Myopathy (Magyar et al, 1977). Muscle weakness is often disproportionate to the severity of RA. Occasionally, definitive muscle diseases such as myasthenia gravis coincide with RA but this is most exceptional. It has become convenient to divide the muscle disease of RA into six groups on the basis of new techniques such as selective biopsy, electromyography, and quantitative histochemistry (Reza & Veritz, 1977). The collaboration of specialised laboratories is desirable to enable full advantage to be taken of these sophisticated methods. In *a minimal lesion myopathy* muscle mass is not reduced but there are raised creatine phosphokinase levels. Microscopic changes are slight; for example there may be rare, angular, atrophic cells suggesting a role for single cell denervation. When there are significant lymphocytic foci (lymphorrhages) but little endomysial fibrosis and sparse atrophic angular cells, *inflammatory myopathy* is identified (Fig. 25.37). *Type II (dark, fast) muscle cell atrophy* discriminates against this cell; the normal type I/type II mosaicism is lost. In severe cases of seropositive RA with visceral disease and nodulosis, *neurogenic syndromes* develop. Microscopically, there is fascicular disruption, increased endomysial fibropla-

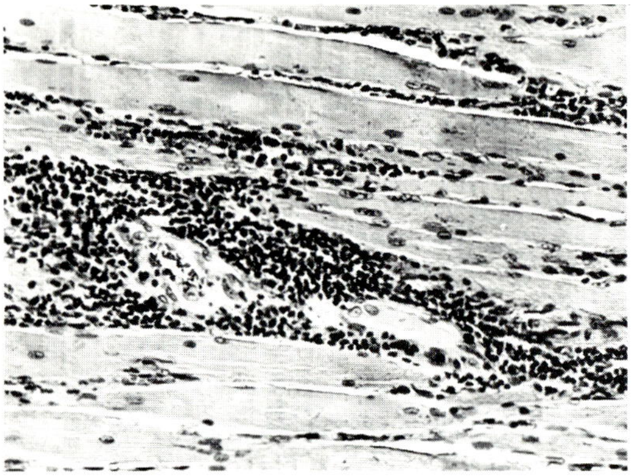

Fig. 25.37 Skeletal muscle. Lymphorrhage. Around a small intramuscular artery and within the intermuscular connective tissue is a substantial island of lymphocytes constituting a lymphorrhage. The presence of these structures is common to rheumatoid arthritis and myasthenia gravis and suggests the action locally of cell-mediated immune mechanisms. H & E × 150.

sia and vascular prominence, and inflammatory changes. The term 'cross-over syndrome' is suggested to designate a category in which myositis and synovitis coincide without the features of childhood polymyositis. There is variability of cell size, type II cell atrophy and rare, angular, atrophic cells. A final group of cases with *vasculitis* may simulate polyarteritis or polymyalgia.

Finally, it is necessary to recognise that the extended use of corticosteroids can create an important variety of myopathy (Haslock et al, 1970).

Ocular disease

The relationship between eye disease and RA remains debatable. Not only can important drugs such as chloroquine cause eye damage, but the interpretation of the lesions is disputed. Hazelman & Watson (1977) state that the ocular lesions are often the first evidence of the RA and run hand-in-hand with those of the joints, whereas Pisko et al (1982) could not relate the eye lesions in 97 cases treated with NSAID either to RA or to drug therapy.

In Sjögren's syndrome, biopsy conveniently confirms the minor salivary gland changes that accompany keratoconjunctivitis sicca. In these patients, it is suspected that antinuclear antibodies can damage the conjuctiva. Similar vascular and fibrotic lesions can be provoked by practolol and an analogy with the origin of retroperitoneal fibrosis is therefore suggested.

Endocrine disease

Many aspects of autoimmunity find expression in RA and its variants. Hashimoto's thyroiditis and RA is one association and anti-thyroid autoantibodies have been said to be demonstrable in unselected cases of RA more frequently than in control cases (Buchanan et al, 1961). However, confirmatory evidence of thyroiditis and of diabetes mellitus in RA was not recognised (Linos et al, 1980). No particular thyroid or pancreatic lesions have been found anatomically although the pituitary and adrenals are common sites for amyloidosis and every endocrine gland may be affected periodically by necrotising vasculitis.

Amyloidosis

Deposits of amyloid, containing protein AA, are widespread in some 13–17% of cases of RA examined *post-mortem* in hospital (Table 25.7).

Amyloid is described in detail elsewhere (Ch. 41). Almost every organ may be affected, but those of the lymphoreticular system, the liver and kidneys are especially vulnerable. Diagnosis by rectal biopsy has succeeded lingual biopsy as a safe, sensitive and reliable procedure. The amyloid deposits, which may be localised solely to the walls of mucosal arterioles, are identified by the alkaline Congo-red stain with which polarised light yields a characteristic apple-green dichroic response. Substantial glomerular deposits lead to amyloid nephrosclerosis so that renal excretory failure, with uraemia, is a relatively common cause of death in RA. Synovial and cartilage amyloid deposits are now identifiable but are very uncommon.

ASSOCIATED SYNDROMES

Juvenile chronic arthritis (Ansell, 1983)

In both poly- and pauciarticular forms there is an inflammatory reaction closely resembling that of adult RA but of lesser severity (Wynne-Roberts et al, 1978). There are many mast cells. The young cartilage is destroyed more slowly than the old: granulation tissue advances insidiously. Tenosynovitis is a frequent association. Biopsy is helpful

Table 25.7 Incidence of amyloidosis in reported *post-mortem* series of rheumatoid arthritis cases. (From Missen & Taylor, 1956.)

	No. of cases of RA	Amyloid found in	Percentage incidence of amyloid		Remarks
			Overall	Conservative	
Fingerman & Andrus (1942–43)	61	13	21.3	17.2	Active tuberculosis in 3 of the 13 amyloid cases
Baggenstoss & Rosenberg (1943)	30	2	6.7	3.4	Chronic suppurative prostatitis in 1 amyloid case
Bayles (1943)	23	3	13.0	9.1	1 of the 3 amyloid cases had AS (not RA)
Bennett (1943)	48	0	0	0	—
Solomon (1943)	7	1	14.3	14.3	Amyloid case treated for 3 years with coccal vaccine
Young & Schwedel (1944)	38	5	13.2	11.4	2 (without amyloid) were cases of AS Pulmonary tuberculosis in 1 amyloid case
Unger et al (1948)	58	4	6.9	6.9	—
Teilum & Lindahl (1954)	28	17	60.7	59.3	1 amyloid case AS, not RA. Histological examination in every case of methyl violet-stained sections
Gedda (1955)	45	11	24.4	24.4	9 of the 11 died of renal amyloidosis: 'amyloid-shrunken' kidneys in 7
Missen & Taylor (1956)	47	8	17.0	13.3	Alternative possible cause for amyloid in 2 cases
Gardner (1972)	148	17	11.8	11.8	Cases covering the years 1929–66
Total	533[a]	81[b]	Mean 17.2	Mean 15.5	

Key: AS = ankylosing spondylitis; RA = rheumatoid arthritis
[a] Includes 4 cases of ankylosing spondylitis.
[b] Includes 2 cases of ankylosing spondylitis.

in diagnosis (Bywaters & Edmonds, 1975) and the synovial fluid resembles that of the adult disease. disease.

Electron microscopy demonstrates poor preservation of the synovial cell layer (Wynne-Roberts et al, 1978). Remaining synovial A(M) cells contain many micropinocytotic vesicles, filopodia and long cytoplasmic processes. Lysosomes and phagolysosomes containing lipid lie within the cytoplasm; some giant forms retain cell debris. B(F) cells display much endoplasmic reticulum, cisternae that are more dilated than normal and nuclei devoid of inclusions. Within synovial macrophages are short, wavy 23 nm diameter tubules and similar structures are identified in the synoviocytes.

The visceral lesions of the seronegative juvenile disease are less common and less conspicuous than in those of the seropositive adult. The very uncommon subcutaneous nodule resembles the rheumatic fever lesion more closely than the adult granuloma (Sokoloff, 1966). Zones of necrosis and marginal histiocytic pallisading are unusual. Visceral granulomata are rare. An occuloarticular triad has been recorded (Hinzpeter et al, 1971). Vasculitis is most exceptional. A mild pericarditis occurs but does not advance to constriction; however, tamponade has been reported (Scharf et al, 1976). Amyloidosis accounted for 3 of the deaths (7.4%) is one series of 161 cases (Ansell, 1980), an outcome confined to those of insidious onset, among whom infection also led to 3 fatalities. Congenital heart disease, renal failure and aplastic anaemia are other occasional, fatal phenomena.

Psoriatic arthropathy

There are five categories of related disease (Kammer et al, 1979; Wright & Moll, 1976) but few pathological analyses. The older literature demonstrated articular destruction and bone reabsorption (Bauer et al, 1941). True pannus formation was not evident but the most severe lesions, distinct from RA, included replacement fibrosis, fibrous, and later bony, ankylosis (Sherman, 1952). These destructive lesions (Bollet & Turner, 1958) and those that segregate the joint changes from RA (Coste & Solnica, 1966) indicate less lymphocytosis, more fibrosis and the presence of small thick-walled blood vessels (Espinoza et al, 1982). Recent arthroscopic evidence supports Wright's (1981) view that in those with RA-like clinical disease, there are RA-like synovial changes. On histopathological, not clinical, evidence, Soren (1978b) postulated early and late progressive, and advanced stages. In early progression, there was slight synovial cell hypertrophy and hyperplasia: the widened intercellular spaces were filled with granular material. Surface fibrin lay in contiguity with the hypertrophic synoviocytes. Fibrosis ensued, with much superficial and deep plasmacytic infiltration; the fibrin accumulated and became organised. Occasional small, multinucleated 'giant cells' were related to the hypertrophic and hyperplastic synovial cells. Progressive collagen synthesis was the product of the numerous fibroblasts and fibrocytes. The relative quantity of subsynovial tissue increased.

The synovial lesions do not resemble those of the skin. Theoretically, local, synovial trauma could provoke synovitis in the same way that a pin-prick may promote a new psoriatic skin lesion at the site of pricking (the Koebner phenomenon). This hypothesis has not been tested. The very severe, destructive joint lesions seen in exceptional cases (arthritis mutilans) recall those of neurogenic arthropathy but, again, there is no published evidence regarding the histological state of the central, peripheral or autonomic nervous systems in psoriasis. One case in 10 develops amyloidosis and amyloid nephrosclerosis with renal failure is a cause of death. Anaemia is frequent and the features of Felty's syndrome may coexist. There is occasional hyperuricaemia but the coincident changes in uric acid metabolism or excretion have not been explained.

Felty's syndrome

The lymphoreticular disorders of RA may be exaggerated, constituting an unusual syndrome (Felty, 1924) in which splenomegaly and hypersplenism accompany granulocytopenia and increased susceptibility to infections such as bronchiectasis. In one series of 25 cases, from an original cohort of 34, 5 of the 9 fatalities were related to sepsis (Thorne & Urowitz, 1982). The pathological characteristics of Felty's syndrome centre upon the exaggerated function of the enlarged spleen the mean weight of which has been described as approximately 900 g (mean weight at age 60 ~ 120 g) (Barnes et al, 1971) (Table 25.8). There is increased elastic tissue in the follicular arteries and endothelial hyperplasia. The enlarged lymphoid tissue of the white pulp displays germinal centre hyperplasia: these centres are hyperactive but hyaline material is present. Extramedullary erythropoiesis and erythrophagocytosis in the red marrow distinguish the Felty spleen from the spleen of classical RA but amyloidosis is exceptional. In spite of the clinical and laboratory evidence of disordered splenic function, with shortened red cell survival, and the presence of leucocyte agglutinis and leucopenia, splenectomy does not protect against infection and may, on occasions, contribute to its occurrence (Thorne & Urowitz, 1982).

Table 25.8 Frequency of histological abnormalities in the spleen in Felty's syndrome. (From Barnes et al 1971 Annals of the rheumatic diseases 30: 359–374)

	Cases of Felty's syndrome (13)	Rheumatoid control cases (22)
White pulp		
Follicular arteries		
amyloid	0	2
hyaline	13	13
endothelial hyperplasia	13	6
increased elastic	11	0
perivascular fibrosis	0	0
Lymphoid tissue		
hyperplasia	7	0
germinal centre hyperplasia	7	0
'active' germinal centres	4	1
hyaline	10	5
amyloid	0	2
Red pulp		
Venous sinusoids		
congestion	10	17
sinus hyperplasia	13	8
erythrophagocytosis	13	10
excess iron	7	13
non-iron pigment	12	22
amyloid	0	1
Splenic cords		
reticulin increase	7	3
plasma cell hyperplasia	13	9
reticulum cell hyperplasia	6	1
excess iron	7	13
non-iron pigment	13	22
extramedullary haemopoiesis	13	3
amyloid	0	1

Secondary liver dysfunction develops (Blendis et al, 1969). Portal tract lymphocytic infiltrates are common. Nodular regenerative hyperplasia is characteristic (Blendis et al, 1974). The mortality is high, and the mean age at death is ~ 65 years (Thorne et al, 1982).

Sjögren's syndrome (see also Ch. 56)
The characteristic pathological changes are of the lacrimal and salivary glands; of the lymphoreticular system; and of epithelial structures. There is a close relationship to the other disorders such as SLE and SS, with which Sjögren's syndrome may be associated. Particular subsets of patients may display other systemic manifestations (Alexander et al, 1983), including vasculitis and haematological abnormalities; and links have been shown between the pathological features of Sjögren's syndrome, fibrosing alveolitis and renal tubular acidosis; and between Sjögren's syndrome, primary biliary cirrhosis and renal tubular acidosis. These associations, and the high frequency of shared immunological abnormalities, emphasise the importance of disorders of the immune mechanism, often of an autoimmune character, in promoting these varieties of systemic connective tissue disease.

The synovial joints display the changes characteristic of RA. However, the major and minor salivary glands are extensively affected by a focal or diffuse, low-grade inflammatory reaction that leads to acinar atrophy. The reaction is in excess of the lymphocytic and histiocytic reactions seen in the salivary glands of a proportion of non-RA persons of the same age. The glands enlarge but the lobular architecture is preserved. Lymphoid infiltration of individual glands may become extreme and benign lymphoepithelial lesions have been recognised. Germinal centre formation is occasionally accompanied by hyperplasia or metaplasia of duct epithelium and characteristic myoepithelial islets are seen in ~ 40% of biopsies (Bloch et al, 1965).

Labial salivary gland biopsy performed under local anaesthesia provides useful diagnostic information (Chisholm & Mason, 1968) but is a less sensitive test of gland behaviour than salivary flow determinations and lymphangiography. The nature of the salivary glandular lesions has not been clarified by periodic acid-Schiff, alcian blue or toluidine blue histochemistry (Fava-de-Moraes et al, 1978) although Gardner (1972) has suggested that the disorder, in part analogy with cystic fibrosis, might be based on a primary heritable disorder of protein-polysaccharide metabolism.

The syndrome may become part of a generalised lymphoproliferative disorder, affecting regional and peripheral lymph nodes, lung, kidney, spleen and bone marrow and simulating lymphoma or macroglobulinaemia. In the early stages of such a disorder, coincidental disease is difficult to exclude and the ambiguous term 'pseudolymphoma' has been used. There is evidence of an association with immunoblastic lymphadenopathy (Lukes & Tindle, 1975).

PATHOLOGICAL CONSEQUENCES OF TREATMENT

An increasingly diverse range of medical and surgical treatments may cause inconvenient, dangerous or even fatal complications.

Medical

The variety of drugs is too great to be considered in detail. Among the pathological processes that have attracted notoriety are: peptic ulcer and the perforation of stomal ulcer after corticosteroids (Gardner, 1972); gastric erosions and bleeding after salicylates; penicillamine nephropathy; renal papillary necrosis after phenacetin; bone marrow suppression after phenylbutazone; and the toxic reactions to gold.

The reactions to gold have been the object of detailed enquiry. Cells containing electron-dense gold bodies, aurosomes, have been detected by TEM in synoviocytes after the regressive and destructive changes caused by myocrysin (Ghadially et al, 1976, 1978; Ghadially, 1979). Similar bodies are found within chondrocytes up to 14 months after local administration (Ghadially & Lalonde, 1978). In a human case, black pigmentation of the synovium persisted for up to 12 years after injection, perhaps due to a high concentration of carrier ^{197}Au in the preparation containing the unstable isotope ^{198}Au (Pritzker et al, 1980). Blue-grey discoloration of the face, neck and hand skin has been found in longstanding cases (Beckett et al, 1982), a condition analogous with argyria, and TEM confirms the presence of gold-coated granules in the cells of both skin and synovium.

The uptake of ^{90}Y and ^{198}Au by regional lymph nodes following articular injection, and the possible relationship of this hazard to lymphoma, has been the subject of comment.

Consequences of surgery

A wide range of joints has been subjected to synovectomy (Clayton & Ferlic, 1975). Although there is a diversity of individual response (Patzakis et al, 1973; Myllala et al, 1983), a complete new synovial layer forms (Rosenthal et al, 1972) and after 3 years the synovium is indistinguishable from that of non-operated joints.

Arthroplasty has been employed with success to excise and replace RA joints. The complications include: deep vein thrombosis and thromboembolism (3%); bacterial infection; loosening of the bone/acrylic interface without infection; and adverse tissue reactions to bone cement (polymethylmethacrylate), polyethylene, and to metal, particularly cobalt–chrome steel. These reactions have been admirably reviewed by Revell (1982). Reactions can also be anticipated to silicone elastomer (silastic), and ceramics, now being tested, are not inert. The principal adverse reactions to metals, to polyethylene and to silicone, come from minute particles. Each variety provokes a characteristic, cellular response that can be distinguished from the barium sulphate that may have been used to enable bone cement to be traced radiographically. It is now appreciated that there are chondrogenic reactions to the plastic screws employed in the cementless fixation of prostheses.

Surgery in RA is complicated from time to time by aerobic infection with organisms such as *Staphylococcus aureus* and *Streptococcus haemolyticus*. Careful searches with appropriate techniques are now revealing an increasing proportion of anaerobic infections.

Coincidental infection

The possibility that RA is the direct or indirect result of bacterial, mycoplasmal, chlamydial or viral infection has been under close scrutiny for more than 50 years (Kellgren et al, 1958; Editorial, 1976). The search for causative micro-organisms has been plagued by the frequency with which rheumatoid joints and tissue are the focus for opportunistic infection, often clinically silent. The susceptibility of rheumatoid tissues to such infections is enhanced by the use of immunosuppressive and cytotoxic drugs that compromise the host defences. The frequency of infection among rheumatoid hospital patients is high (Parker, 1965). *Staphylococcus aureus* is the most commonly identified organism but streptococci, pneumococci, pasteurella, haemophilus, proteus and coliforms are among aerobes that infect the hip, wrist and knee (Karten, 1969a).

CAUSES OF DEATH; MORTALITY

(Abruzzo, 1982)

It has long been believed that there is a modest reduction in life expectation (Cobb et al, 1953; Duthie et al, 1964; Uddin et al, 1970) (Table 25.9). In spite of bias introduced by the selection for review of hospital patients, cardiovascular (Monson & Hall, 1976) and renal disease, and infection are the main immediate causes of death (Isomäki et al, 1975). When a survey was made over 11 years, the increased mortality in RA derived from the 75% of patients who had been in hospital during the 13 years before initial case selection (Allebeck et al, 1981). The apparent abbreviation of life may be a result of incorporating the records of a particular subset of patients likely to develop severe disease and likely therefore to receive aggressive treatment. This accords with the evidence of a further prospective study of 100 cases of definite or classical disease followed over 18 years (Rasker & Cosh, 1981). RA caused 9 of the 43 deaths and in a further 7 infection and drug treatment were important contributory factors. These 16 patients developed RA at an earlier age and died at an earlier age than the 27 in whom death was not attributable to RA.

Cervical vertebral subluxation or dislocation, necrotising renal papillitis, amyloidosis, vasculitis, cardiac granulomata and mesenteric arterial thrombosis are integral or associated disorders that kill. There is an increased susceptibility to infection (Parker, 1965; Gardner, 1972) (Table 25.10). Bacteraemia and bacterial endocarditis may follow surgery and disseminated intravascular coagulation is recognised when there has been visceral surgery, shock and fluid imbalance. Urinary tract infection and deep vein thrombosis complicate prolonged immobilisation.

For each sex at each year of follow-up, the cumulative survival rate in RA is lower than normal; the rate is lower in males than females. Chronic peptic ulcer is more common than usual (Ball, 1968) and there is a relatively high frequency of necrotising vasculitis, amyloidosis, septicaemia, pyelonephritis and necrotising papillitis. Conversely, cerebral haemorrhage, cerebral infarction, and cancer, with the exception of leukaemia and Hodgkin's disease, may be less prevalent than in a control population (Ball, 1968).

Table 25.9 Mean age at death of 142 hospital cases of rheumatoid arthritis examined at necropsy between 1929–66. (From Gardner D L 1972 Pathology of rheumatoid arthritis. Edward Arnold, London.)

	Number	Mean age
Of 142 cases[a] of rheumatoid arthritis examined *postmortem* 1929–1966		
Males	44	59.0
Mean age at death of whole male population		67.0[b]
Females	98	63.0
Mean age at death of whole female population		72.8[b]
Female/male sex ratio 2.2/1.0		
Of 106 cases examined *postmortem* 1950–66		
Males	31	58.7
Females	75	63.4

[a] Includes 4 cases of Still's disease, mean age at death 26 years.
[b] Registrar-General for Scotland, 1964.

Table 25.10 Pathological changes at death in 142 cases of rheumatoid arthritis. (From Gardner D L 1972 Pathology of rheumatoid arthritis. Edward Arnold, London.)

Amyloid	17
Arteries	
arteritis	7
arterial thrombosis	8
Bladder	
cystitis	7
Blood	
anaemia, megaloblastic	2
Bone	
fractures (2 cervical)	8
osteoporosis	41
Bone marrow	
hypoplasia	7
Brain	
meningitis	4
Drug toxicity	
colchicine	1
gold	12
iron	
phenylbutazone	2
steroids	17
Duodenum	
ulcer	7
Heart	
aortic valve disease	13
failure	12
endocarditis	9
infraction	9
mitral valve disease	24
myocardial fibrosis	12
pericarditis	
(subacute)	6
(chronic)	22
Infection	
generalised	8
Joints	
septic arthritis	3
Kidney	
calculus	2
cystic	3
hydronephrosis	4
papillary necrosis	11
pyelonephritis	39
pyonephrosis	2
tubular necrosis	3
Liver	
cirrhosis	2
extramedullary-haemopoiesis	1
haemangioma	1
hepatitis	2
necrosis	7
pylephlebitis	1
Lung	
abscess	6
atelectasis	5
bronchiectasis	6
bronchitis, purulent	30
bronchopneumonia	54
cystic disease	1
pulmonary embolism	14
emphysema	31
empyema	3
pulmonary hypertension	9
infarction	8
interstitial fibrosis	4
lobar pneumonia	2
nodules[a]	1
pleuritis	
(acute)	8
(fibrous)	56
pneumonoconiosis	3
tuberculosis	13
tumours	7
Lymph nodes	
enlargement	41
Muscle	
polymyositis	1
Nerve	
polyneuritis	1
Operations	
(recent)	9
Peritoneum	
adhesions	10
acute peritonitis	8
Psoriasis	3
Retroperitoneal abscess	3
Still's disease	4
Stomach	
ulcer	8
Thyroid	
adenoma or nodular	6
fibrous or thyroiditis	17
Tumours	
basal cell carcinoma	1
gall bladder	1
liver	1
malignant	24
breast	1
bronchus	7
colon	3
carcinoid	2
ovary	1
rectum	1
stomach	1
uterus	1
mesothelioma	1
oesophagus	1
sarcoma	1
Veins	
thrombosis	13

[a] Subcutaneous tissues unlikely to have been exhaustively searched.

REFERENCES

Abruzzo J L 1982 Rheumatoid arthritis and mortality. Arthritis and Rheumatism 25: 1020–1023

Adams R 1857a Illustrations of the effects of rheumatic gout or chronic rheumatic arthritis on all the articulations: with descriptive and explanatory statements. John Churchill, London

Adams R 1857b A treatise on rheumatic gout or chronic rheumatic arthritis of all the joints. John Churchill, London

Adelson G L, Saypol D C, Walker A N 1982 Ureteral stenosis secondary to retroperitoneal rheumatoid nodules. Journal of Urology 127: 124–125

Ahern M, Lever J V, Cosh J 1983 Complete heart block in rheumatoid arthritis. Annals of the Rheumatic Diseases 42: 389–397

Alexander E L, Arnett F C, Provost T T, Stevens M B 1983 Sjögren's syndrome: association of anti-Ro (SS-A)antibodies with vasculitis, hematologic abnormalities, and serologic hyper-reactivity. Annals of Internal Medicine 98: 155–159

Alexander I S 1983 An investigation of human and experimental arthritis by histological and immunocytochemical techniques. PhD thesis, University of Manchester

Allebeck P, Ahlbom A, Allander E 1981 Increased mortality among persons with rheumatoid arthritis but where RA does not appear on the death certificate. Scandinavian

Journal of Rheumatology 10: 301–306
Ansell B M 1980 Rheumatic disorders in childhood. Butterworths, London, p. 87–151
Ansell B M 1983 Arthritis in young children. British Medical Journal 286: 1917–1918
Appelboom T, Ehrlich G E 1981 Rubens and the question of antiquity of rheumatoid arthritis. Journal of the American Medical Association 245: 483–486
Baggenstoss A H, Rosenberg E F 1943 Visceral lesions associated with chronic infectious (rheumatoid) arthritis. Archives of Pathology 35: 503–516
Baker D G, Dayer J M, Roelke M, Schumacher H R, Krane S M 1983 Rheumatoid synovial cell morphologic changes induced by a mononuclear cell factor in culture. Arthritis and Rheumatism 26: 8–14
Ball J 1954 Rheumatoid arthritis and polyarteritis nodosa. Annals of the Rheumatic Diseases 13: 277–290
Ball J 1968 Postmortem findings and articular pathology in rheumatoid arthritis. In: Duthie J J R, Alexander W R M (eds) Rheumatic diseases: Pfizer Medical Monograph No 3. University Press, Edinburgh, p. 124–126
Ball J, Sharp J 1971 Rheumatoid arthritis of the cervical spine. In: Hill A G S (ed) Modern trends in rheumatology. Butterworths, London, p. 117–138
Bannatyne G A 1896 Rheumatoid arthritis: its pathology, morbid anatomy and treatment, 1st Edn. Wright, Bristol
Barland P, Novikoff A B, Hamerman D 1963 Fine structure and cytochemistry of the rheumatoid synovial membrane, with special reference to lysosomes. Journal of Cell Biology 44: 853–866
Barnes C G, Turnbull A L, Vernon-Roberts B 1971 Felty's syndrome, a clinical and pathological survey of 21 patients and their response to treatment. Annals of the Rheumatic Diseases 30: 359–374
Batley W J, Uddin J, Kelly H G 1969 Rheumatoid arthritis complicated by constrictive pericarditis; report of a case treated successfully by pericardiectomy. Canadian Medical Association Journal 100: 863–866
Bauer W, Bennett G A, Zeller J W 1941 Pathology of joint lesions in patients with psoriasis and arthritis. Transactions of the Association of American Physicians 56: 349–352
Bayles T B 1943 Rheumatoid arthritis and rheumatic heart disease in autopsy cases. American Journal of Medical Sciences 205: 42–48
Beckett V L, Doyle J A, Hadley G A, Spear K L 1982 Chrysiasis resulting from gold therapy in rheumatoid arthritis: identification of gold by X-ray microanalysis. Mayo Clinic Proceedings 57: 773–777
Bedi S S, Ellis W 1970 Spontaneous rupture of the calcaneal tendon in rheumatoid arthritis after local steroid injection. Annals of the Rheumatic Diseases 29: 494–495
Bennett G A 1943 Comparison of the pathology of rheumatic fever and rheumatoid arthritis. Annals of Internal Medicine 19: 111–113
Bennett P H, Scott J T 1965 Autonomic neuropathy in rheumatoid arthritis. Annals of the Rheumatic Diseases 24: 161–168
Bierther M F W, Wegner K W 1971 Elektronenmikroskopische Untersuchungen synovialer Gafässveranderungen bei chronischer Polyarthritis. Zeitschrift für Rheumaforschung 30: 214–222
Bierther M F W, Wagner R 1974 Electron microscope studies of the pannus in rheumatoid arthritis. Zeitschrift für Rheumatologie 33: 32–42
Blake D R, Hall N D, Bacon P A, Dieppe P A, Halliwell B, Gutteridge J M C 1981 The importance of iron in rheumatoid disease. Lancet ii: 1142–1144
Blendis L M, Ansell I D, Lloyd Jones K, Hamilton E, Williams R 1969 Liver in Felty's syndrome. British Medical Journal i: 131–134
Blendis L M, Parkinson M C, Shilkin K B, Williams R 1974 Nodular regenerative hyperplasia of the liver in Felty's syndrome. Quarterly Journal of Medicine 43: 25–32
Bloch K J, Buchanan W W, Wohl M J, Bunim J J 1965 Sjögren's syndrome A clinical, pathological, and serological study of sixty-two cases. Medicine 44: 187–231
Boddington M M Spriggs A I Morton J A, Mowat A G 1971 Cytodiagnosis of rheumatoid pleural effusions. Journal of Clinical Pathology 24: 95–106
Bollet A J, Turner R E 1958 Psoriatic arthritis. Annals of the New York Academy of Science 73: 1013–1019
Bridger M W M, Jahn A F, Vannostrand A W P 1980 Laryngeal rheumatoid arthritis. The Laryngoscope 90: 296–303
Bromley M, Fisher W D, Woolley D E 1984 Mast cells at sites of cartilage erosion in the rheumatoid joint. Annals of the Rheumatic Diseases 43: 76–79
Brown R A, Tomlinson I W, Hill C R, Weiss J B, Phillips P, Kumar S 1983 Relationship of angiogenesis factor in synovial fluid to various joint diseases. Annals of the Rheumatic Diseases 42: 301–307
Brunk J R, Brash E C, Swineford O 1966 Rheumatoid pleuritis successfully treated with decortication. Report of a case and review of the literature. American Journal of Medical Sciences 251: 546–551
Buchanan W W, Crooks J, Alexander W D, Kourtras D A, Wayne E J, Gray K G 1961 Association of Hashimoto's thyroiditis and rheumatoid arthritis. Lancet I: 245–248
Burry H C, Dieppe P A, Bresnihan F B, Brown C 1976 Salicylates and renal function in rheumatoid arthritis. British Medical Journal I: 613–615
Butcher R G, Bitensky L, Cashman B, Chayen J 1973 Differences in the redox balance in human rheumatoid and non-rheumatoid synovial lining cells. Beiträge zür Pathologischen Anatomie und Allgemeinne Pathologie 1148: 265–274
Bywaters E G L 1957 Peripheral vascular obstruction in rheumatoid arthritis and its relationship to other vascular lesions. Annals of the Rheumatic Diseases 16: 84–103
Bywaters E G L 1979 On two papers dealing with nodules. Journal of Rheumatology 6: 243–246
Bywaters E G L 1981 Thoracic intervertebral discitis in rheumatoid arthritis due to costovertebral joint involvement. Rheumatology International 1: 83–97
Bywaters E G L, Edmonds J P 1975 Biopsies and tissue diagnosis in the rheumatic diseases In: Jayson M I V (ed) Clinics in rheumatic diseases, Vol 2. 1. Diagnosis and assessment. Saunders, Philadelphia, p. 179–209
Carlsson G E, Kopp S, Öberg T 1978 Arthritis and allied diseases of the temporomandibular joint. In: Carlsson G E, Zarg G A (eds) The temporomandibular joints — function and dysfunction. Munksgaard, Copenhagen
Carpenter D F, Golden A, Roberts W C 1967 Quadrivalvular rheumatoid heart disease associated with left bundle branch block. American Journal of Medicine 43: 912–929
Cherian P V, Schumacher H R 1983 Immunoelectronmicroscopic characterization of intracellular inclusions in synovial fluid cells of patients with rheumatoid arthritis. Ultrastructural Pathology 5: 15–27
Chilton C P, Darke S G 1980 External iliac venous

compression by a giant iliopsoas rheumatoid bursa. British Journal of Surgery 67: 641

Chisholm D M, Mason K D 1968 Labial salivary gland biopsy in Sjögren's disease. Journal of Clinical Pathology 21: 656–660

Christie G S 1950 The general changes in rheumatoid arthritis. In: King E S J, Lowe T E, Cox L B (eds) Studies in pathology. Presented to Peter MacCallum, Melbourne University Press, Jubilee, Victoria, p. 133–144

Clayton M L, Ferlic D C 1975 The wrist in rheumatoid arthritis. Clinical Orthopaedics and Related Research 106: 192–197

Clemmensen I, Holund B, Andersen R B 1983 Fibrin and fibronectin in rheumatoid synovial membrane and rheumatoid synovial fluid. Arthritis and Rheumatism 26: 479–485

Cobb S, Anderson F, Bauer W 1953 Length of life and cause of death in rheumatoid arthritis. New England Journal of Medicine 249: 553–556

Cochrane W, Davies D V, Dorling J, Bywaters E G L 1964 Ultramicroscopic structure of the rheumatoid nodule. Annals of the Rheumatic Diseases 23: 345–363

Collins D H 1949 The pathology of articular and spinal diseases. Edward Arnold, London

Conn D L, Schroeter A L, McDuffie F C 1976 Cutaneous vessel immune deposits in rheumatoid arthritis. Arthritis and Rheumatism 19: 15–20

Cooke T D, Hurd E R, Jasin H E, Bienenstock J, Ziff M 1975 Identification of immunoglobulins and complement in rheumatoid articular collagenous tissues. Arthritis and Rheumatism 18: 541–551

Cooney T P 1981 Interrelationship of chronic eosinophilic pneumonia, bronchioloitis obliterans and rheumatoid disease: a hypothesis. Journal of Clinical Pathology 34: 129–137

Cooper N S, Soren A, McEwen C, Rosenberger J L 1981 Diagnostic specificity of synovial lesions. Human Pathology 12: 314–328

Coste F, Solnica J 1966 La polyarthrite psoriasique. Revue Francaise D'Études Cliniques et Biologiques 11: 578–599

Cruickshank B 1952 Interpretation of multiple biopsies of synovial tissue in rheumatic diseases. Annals of the Rheumatic Diseases 11: 137–145

Cruickshank B 1954 The arteritis of rheumatoid arthritis. Annals of the Rheumatic Diseases 13: 136–146

Cruickshank B 1958 Heart lesions in rheumatoid disease. Journal of Pathology and Bacteriology 76: 223–240

Danieli G, Corvetta A, Mariuzzi G M, Beltrami C A, Osculati F, Cinti S, et al 1980 Rheumatoid lung disease (a clinical physiological and histological study in 33 patients). La Ricerca in Clinica e in Laboratorio 10: 597–608

Davidson R C, Horn J R, Herndon J H. Grin O D 1977 Brain-stem compression in rheumatoid arthritis. Journal of the American Medical Association 238: 2633–2634

Davies D V, Palfrey A J 1967 The fine structure of normal and rheumatoid synovial membrane. In: Hill AGS (ed) Modern trends in rheumatology (2) Butterworths, London, p. 1–20

Dingle J T 1981 Catabolin — a cartilage catabolic factor from synovium. Clinical Orthopaedics and Related Research 156: 219–231

Dmoszynska A, Pytko H K 1976 Chronic lymphatic leukaemia in rheumatoid arthritis: a case. Polski Tygodnik Letarski T 31: 161–162

Dorfman R F, Warnke R 1974 Lymphadenopathy simulating the malignant lymphomas. Human Pathology 5: 519–550

Duke O, Panayi G S, Janossy G, Poulter L W, Tidman N 1983 Analysis of T-cell subsets in the peripheral blood and synovial fluid of patients with rheumatoid arthritis by means of monoclonal antibodies. Annals of the Rheumatic Diseases 42: 357–361

Dumonde D C, Kelley R H, Morley J 1976 Lymphoid and microvascular dysfunction in experimental models of rheumatoid inflammation. In: Dumonde D C (ed) Infection and immunology in the rheumatic diseases. Blackwell, Oxford, p. 375–403

Duthie J J R, Brown P E, Truelove L H, Baragar F D, Lawrie A J 1964 Course and prognosis in rheumatoid arthritis: a further report. Annals of the Rheumatic Diseases 23: 193–204

Editorial 1976 Septic arthritis in rheumatoid disease. British Medical Journal ii: 1089–1090

Edmonds M E, Jones T C, Saunders W A, Sturrock R D 1979 Autonomic neuropathy in rheumatoid arthritis. British Medical Journal 2: 173–175

Ellman M H, Weis M J, Spellberg M A 1974 Liver disease in rheumatoid arthritis. American Journal of Gastroenterology 62: 46–53

Ellman P, Ball R E 1948 'Rheumatoid disease' with joint and pulmonary manifestations. British Medical Journal ii: 816–820

Eraut D, Evans J, Caplin M 1978 Pulmonary necrobiotic nodules without rheumatoid arthritis. British Journal of Diseases of the Chest 72: 301–306

Ericson S 1968 The parotid gland in subjects with and without rheumatoid arthritis. Acta Radiologica (Stockh) 275: 7–167

Espinoza L R, Vasey F B, Espinoza C G, Bocanegra T S, Germain B F 1982 Vascular changes in psoriatic synovium. A light and electron microscopic study. Arthritis and Rheumatism 25: 677–684

Evanson J M, Jeffrey J J, Krane S M 1967 Human collagenase: identification and characterization of an enzyme from rheumatoid synovium in culture. Science 158: 499–502

Fam A G, Shuckett R, McGillivray D C, Little A H 1983 Stress fractures in rheumatoid arthritis. Journal of Rheumatology 10: 722–726

Fassbender H G 1975 The pathology of rheumatic diseases. Translated by G Loewi. Springer Verlag, Berlin, p. 79–220

Fassbender H G 1980 Structural basis and pathomechanisms of arthritis and arthrosis. Deutsche Medizinische Wochenschrift 105: 864–867

Fassbender H G 1983 Histomorphological basis of articular cartilage destruction in rheumatoid arthritis. Collagen and Related Research 3: 141–156

Fassbender H G, Simmling-Annefeld M 1983 The potential aggressiveness of synovial tissue in rheumatoid arthritis. Journal of Pathology 139: 399–406

Fava-de-Moraes F, Friedman H, Egami M I, Bevilacqua E M A F, Cossermelli W 1978 Histochemical study of labial salivary glands in Sjögren's syndrome. Journal of Oral Pathology 7: 135–142

Fell H B, Jubb R J 1977 The effect of synovial tissue on the breakdown of articular cartilage in organ culture. Arthritis and Rheumatism 20: 1359–1371

Felty A R 1924 Chronic arthritis in the adult, associated, with splenomegaly and leucopenia: a report of five cases of an unusual clinical syndrome. Bulletin of the Johns Hopkins Hospital 35: 16–20

Fingerman D L, Andrus F C 1943 Visceral lesions associated with rheumatoid arthritis. Annals of the Rheumatic Diseases 3: 168–181
Ford D K, Daroza D M 1983 Observations on the responses of synovial lymphocytes to viral antigens in rheumatoid arthritis and Reiters' syndrome. Journal of Rheumatology 10: 643–646
Forman M B, Zuri S, Gear A J, Kallenbach J, Wing J 1982 Severe airway obstruction associated with rheumatoid arthritis and Sjögrens syndrome. South African Medical Journal 61: 674–676
Førre O, Thoen J, Lea T, Doblong J H, Mellbye O J, Natvig J B, et al 1982 In situ characterization of mononuclear cells in rheumatoid tissues, using monoclonal antibodies. Scandinavian Journal of Immunology 16: 315–320
Frayha R, Ayyash R, Gehshan A, Gemayel N 1976 Rheumatoid disease without arthritis. Johns Hopkins Medical Journal (Suppl) 138: 69–72
Fritz P, Müller J, Wegner G, Assfalg P, Laschner W (1980) Beiträg zum enzymhistochemischen Nachweis von Immunoglobulin in Gelenkkapseln bei chronischer Polyarthritis und entzündlish aktivierter Arthrose. Zeitschrift für Rheumatologie 39: 331–342
Fukase M, Koizumi F, Wakaki K 1980 Histopathological analysis of sixteen subcutaneous rheumatoid nodules. Acta Pathologica Japonica 30: 871–882
Ganda O P, Caplan H I 1974 Rheumatoid disease without joint involvement. Journal of the American Medical Association 288: 338–339
Gardner D L 1972 The pathology of rheumatoid arthritis. Edward Arnold, London.
Gardner D L 1983 The nature and causes of osteoarthrosis. British Medical Journal 286: 418–424
Gardner D L 1984 Pathological basis of the connective tissue diseases. Edward Arnold, London (in preparation)
Gardner D L, Duthie J J R, Macleod J, Allan W S A 1957 Pulmonary hypertension in rheumatoid arthritis: report of a case with intimal sclerosis of the pulmonary and digital arteries. Scottish Medical Journal 2: 183–188
Gardner D L, Krieg A F, Chapnick R 1962 Fatal systemic fungus disease in rheumatoid arthritis with cardiac and pulmonary mycotic and rheumatoid granulomata. Interamerican Archives of Rheumatology 5: 561–586
Garrod A B 1859 The nature and treatment of gout and rheumatic gout. Walton & Maberly, London
Gedda P O 1955 On amyloidosis and other causes of death in rheumatoid arthritis. Acta Medica Scandinavica 150: 443–452
Geddes D M, Corrin B, Brewerton D A, Davies R J, Turner-Warwick M 1977 Progressive airway obliteration in adults and its association with rheumatoid disease. Quarterly Journal of Medicine 46: 427–444
Geiler G, Emmrich J 1980 Veränderungen an der Synovialmembran bei Frühfällen der rheumatoiden Arthritis. Zeitschrift für Rheumatologie 39: 33–45
Ghadially F N 1979 The aurosome. Journal of Rheumatology 6 (Suppl 5): 45–50
Ghadially F N 1983 Rheumatoid arthritis. In: Fine structure of synovial joints. Butterworths, London, p. 212–235
Ghadially F N, Lalonde J-M A 1978 Long-term effects of myochrysine in articular cartilage. Virchows Archives B Cell Pathology 28: 31–37
Ghadially F N, Roy S 1967 Ultrastructure of synovial membrane in rheumatoid arthritis. Annals of the Rheumatic Diseases 26: 426–443
Ghadially F N, Roy S 1969 Ultrastructure of synovial joints in health and disease. Butterworths, London, p. 151–175
Ghadially F N, Oryschak A F, Mitchell D M 1976 Ultrastructural changes produced in rheumatoid synovial membrane by chrysotherapy. Annals of the Rheumatic Diseases 35: 67–72
Ghadially F N, Lalonde J-M A, Thomas I, Massey K L 1978 Long-term effects of myochrysine on the synovial membrane and aurosomes. Journal of Pathology 125: 219–224
Ghose T, Woodbury J F L, Ahmad S, Stevenson B 1975 Immunopathological changes in rheumatoid arthritis and other joint diseases. Journal of Clinical Pathology 28: 109–117
Gieseking R. 1969 Das feinmikroskopische Bild des Rheumatismus nodosus. Beiträge zur Pathologischen Anatomie und Allgemeinen Pathologie 138: 292–320
Gieseking R, Bäumer A, Backmann L 1969 Electron microscopic studies on granulomas in nodular rheumatism. Zeitschrift für Rheumaforschung 28: 163–175
Glass D, Soter N A, Schur P H 1976 Rheumatoid vasculitis. Arthritis and Rheumatism 19: 950–952
Glynn L E 1968 The chronicity of inflammation and its significance in rheumatoid arthritis. Annals of the Rheumatic Diseases 27: 105–121
Glynn L E 1972 Pathology, pathogenesis and aetiology of rheumatoid arthritis. Annals of the Rheumatic Diseases, 31: 412–420
Goldenberg D L, Cohen A S 1978 Synovial membrane histopathology in the differential diagnosis of rheumatoid arthritis, gout, pseudogout, systemic lupus erythematosus, infectious arthritis and degenerative joint disease. Medicine 57: 239–252
Goldenberg G J, Paraskevas F, Israels L G 1969 The association of rheumatoid arthritis with plasma cell and lymphocytic neoplasms. Arthritis and Rheumatism 12: 569–579
Grimley P M 1967 Rheumatoid arthritis: ultrastructure of the synovium. Annals of Internal Medicine 66: 623–624
Grimley P M, Sokoloff L 1966 Synovial giant cells in rheumatoid arthritis. American Journal of Pathology 49: 931–954
Gryfe A, Sanders P M, Gardner D L 1971 The mast cell in early rat adjuvant arthritis. Annals of the Rheumatic Diseases 30: 24–30
Halla J T, Schrohenicher R E, Volanakis J E 1980 Immune complexes and other laboratory features of pleural effusions — a comparison of rheumatoid arthritis, systemic lupus erythematosus, and other diseases. Annals of Internal Medicine 92: 748–752
Harris M 1970 Rheumatoid heart disease with complete heart block. Journal of Clinical Pathology 23: 623–626
Harvey A R, Clarke B J, Chui D H K, Kean W F, Buchanan W W 1983 Anaemia associated with rheumatoid disease. Inverse correlation between erythropoiesis and both IgM and rheumatoid factor levels. Arthritis and Rheumatism 26: 28–34
Haslock D I, Wright V, Harriman D G F 1970 Neuromuscular disorders in rheumatoid arthritis: a motor-point muscle biopsy study. Quarterly Journal of Medicine 39: 335–358
Hazelman B L, Watson P G 1977 Ocular complications of rheumatoid arthritis. In: Bluestone R, Bacon P A (eds) Clinics in rheumatic diseases, Vol 3. 3. Extraarticular

manifestations of rheumatoid arthritis. Saunders, Philadelphia, p. 501–526
Hellems S O, Kanner R E, Renzetti A D Jr 1983 Bronchocentric granulomatosis associated with rheumatoid arthritis. Chest 83: 831–832
Henderson B 1981 The biochemistry of the human synovial lining with special reference to alterations in metabolism in rheumatoid arthritis. Pathology, Research and Practice 172: 1–24
Hinzpeter E N, Naumann G, Bartelheimer H K 1971 Ocular histopathology in Still's disease. Ophthalmic Research 2: 16–24
Hirohata K, Kobayashi I 1964 Fine structure of the synovial tissues in rheumatoid arthritis. Kobe Journal of Medical Sciences 10: 195–225
Holland C D, Rennie J A N, Hassan I F, Jasani M K, Jayson M I V 1982 Extravascular (e-v) fibrin in rheumatoid arthritis (R A):persistence and continuous turnover. Annals of the Rheumatic Diseases 41: 311
Hollywell C, Morris C J, Farr M, Walton K W 1983 Ultrastructure of synovial changes in rheumatoid disease and in seronegative inflammatory arthropathies. Virchows Archiv A: Pathological Anatomy and Histology 400: 345–355
Huth F, Soren A, Klein W 1972 Structure of synovial membrane in rheumatoid arthritis. Current Topics in Pathology 56: 55–78
Inoue H, Kodama T, Fujita T 1969 Scanning electron microscopy of normal and rheumatoid articular cartilages. Archivum Histologicum Japonicum 30: 425–435
Inoue H, Julkunen H, Oka M, Vainio K 1970 Scanning electron microscopic studies of extensor tendon degeneration in rheumatoid arthritis. Acta Rheumatologica Scandinavica 16: 311–318
Isomäki H A, Mutru O, Koota K 1975 Death rate and causes of death in patients with rheumatoid arthritis. Scandinavian Journal of Rheumatology 4: 205–208
Iveson J M I, Pomerance A 1977 Cardiac involvement in rheumatoid disease. In: Bluestone R, Bacon P A (eds) Clinics in rheumatic diseases, Vol 3. 3. Extraarticular manifestations of rheumatoid arthritis. Saunders, Philadelphia, p. A67–500
Jackson B, Lawrence J R 1978 Renal papillary necrosis associated with indomethacin and phenylbutazone treated rheumatoid arthritis. Australian and New Zealand Journal of Medicine 8: 165–167
Janossy G, Panayi G, Duke O, Bonfill M, Poulter L W, Goldstein G 1981 Rheumatoid arthritis: a disease of T-lymphocyte/macrophage immunoregulation. Lancet ii: 839–842
Johnston T S, White P, Weiss S T, Weiss W, Weinberger S E 1982 Endobronchial necrobiotic nodule antedating rheumatoid arthritis. Chest 2: 199–200
Jones F L Jr, Blodgett R C Jr 1971 Empyema in rheumatoid pleuropulmonary disease. Annals of Internal Medicine 74: 665–671
Kammer G M, Soter N A, Gibson D J, Schur P H 1979 Psoriatic arthritis: a clinical, immunologic and HLA study of 100 patients. Seminars in Arthritis and Rheumatism 9: 75–97
Kampner S L, Kuzell W 1976 Intra-articular rheumatoid nodule of the knee joint. Clinical Orthopaedics and Related Research 114: 243–247
Karten I 1969a Septic arthritis complicating rheumatoid arthritis. Annals of Internal Medicine 70: 1147–1158
Karten I 1969b Arteritis, myocardial infarction and rheumatoid arthritis. Journal of the American Medical Association 210: 1717–1720
Kellgren J H, Ball J 1950 Tendon lesions in rheumatoid arthritis. Annals of the Rheumatic Diseases 9: 48–65
Kellgren J H, Ball J, Fairbrother R W 1958 Suppurative arthritis complicating rheumatoid arthritis. British Medical Journal i: 1193–1200
Kim R C 1980 Rheumatoid disease with encephalopathy. Annals of Neurology 7: 86–91
Kim R C, Collins C H 1981 The neuropathology of rheumatoid disease. Human Pathology 12: 5–15
Kim R C, Collins C H, Parisi J E 1982 Rheumatoid nodule formation within the choroid plexus — report of a 2nd case. Archives of Pathology and Laboratory Medicine 106: 83–84
Kimura H, Tateishi H, Ziff M 1977 Surface ultrastructure of rheumatoid articular cartilage. Arthritis and Rheumatism 20: 1085–1098
Klemperer P, Pollack A D, Baehr R 1942 Diffuse collagen disease; acute disseminated lupus erythematosus and diffuse scleroderma. Journal of the American Medical Association 119: 331–332
Kobayashi I, Ziff M 1973 Electron microscope studies of lymphoid cells in the rheumatoid synovial membrane. Arthritis and Rheumatism 16: 471–486
Kobayashi I, Ziff M 1975 Electron microscopic studies of the cartilage-pannus junction in rheumatoid arthritis. Arthritis and Rheumatism 18: 475–483
Koizumi F, Fukase M, Wakaki K 1979 Rheumatoid arthritis with systemic necrotizing arteritis. Acta Pathologica Japonica 29: 825–836
Kulka J P 1966 Vascular derangement in rheumatoid arthritis. In: Hill A G S (ed) Modern trends in rheumatology, 1st Edn. Butterworth, London, p. 49–69
Kulka J P, Bocking D, Ropes M W, Bauer W 1955 Early joint lesions of rheumatoid arthritis: report of eight cases, with knee biopsies of lesions of less than one year's duration. Archives of Pathology 59: 129–150
Kurosaka M, Ziff M 1983 Immunoelectron microscopic study of the distribution of T cell subsets in rheumatoid synovium. Journal of Experimental Medicine 158: 1191–1210
Lawson A A H, MacLean N 1966 Renal disease and drug therapy in rheumatoid arthritis. Annals of the Rheumatic Diseases 25: 441–449
Lebowitz W B 1966 The heart in rheumatoid disease. Geriatrics 21: 194–198
Levin M H, Kaplan L, Marans S, Weinberger H J 1955 Heart in rheumatoid arthritis: clinical-pathologic correlation of 43 autopsied patients. Annals of the Rheumatic Diseases 14: 430–431
Levy R N, Hermann G, Haimov M, Sherry H S, Train J S, Davison S. 1982 Rheumatoid synovial cyst of the hip. Arthritis and Rheumatism 25: 1382–1384
Linch D C, Gilmer D J, Whimster W F, Keates J R W 1980 Rheumatoid aortic valve prolapse requiring emergency aortic valve replacement. British Heart Journal 43: 237–240
Lindner J 1968 Rheumatic connective tissue metabolism and pathological structure of the connective tissue in rheumatoid arthritis. Verhandlungen der Deutschen Gesellschäft für Innere Medizin 74: 1315–1349
Linos A, Worthington J W, Palumbo P J, O'Fallon W M, Kurland L T 1980 Occurence of Hashimoto's thyroiditis

and diabetes mellitus in patients with rheumatoid arthritis. Journal of Chronic Diseases 33: 73–77
Lukes R J, Tindle B H 1975 Immunoblastic lymphadenopathy. A hyperimmune entity resembling Hodgkin's disease. New England Journal of Medicine 292: 1–8
McGuire M K B, Murphy G, Reynolds J J, Russell R G G 1981 Production of collagenase and inhibitor (TIMP) by normal, rheumatoid and osteoarthritic synovium in vitro: effects of hydrocortisone and indomethacin. Clinical Science 61: 703–710
McGuire M K B, Meats J E, Ebsworth N M, Murphy G, Reynolds J J, Russell R G G 1982 Messenger function of prostaglandins in cell to cell interactions and control of proteinase activity in the rheumatoid joint. International Journal of Immunopharmacology 4: 91–102
Magyar É, Talerman A, Fehér M, Wouters H W 1974a Giant bone cysts in rheumatoid arthritis. Journal of Bone and Joint Surgery 56-B: 121–129
Magyar E, Talerman A, Fehér M, Wouters H W 1974b The pathogenesis of the subchondral pseudocysts in rheumatoid arthritis. Clinical Orthopaedics and Related Research 100: 341–344
Magyar É, Talerman A, Moháecy J, Wouters H W, de Bruijn W C 1977 Muscle changes in rheumatoid arthritis. A review of the literature with a study of 100 cases. Virchows Archiv A. Pathological Anatomy and Histology 373: 267–278
Mantz H J, Luessenhop A J, Robertson D M 1983 Cervical myelopathy due to atlantoaxial and subaxial subluxation in rheumatoid arthritis. Archives of Pathology and Laboratory Medicine 197: 94–98
Menninger H, Putzier R, Mohr W, Wessinghage D, Tillmann K 1980 Granulocyte elastase at the site of cartilage erosion by rheumatoid synovial tissue. Zeitschrift für Rheumatologie 39: 145–156
Miller B, Markheim H R, Towbin N 1967 Multiple stress fractures in rheumatoid arthritis. A case report. Journal of Bone and Joint Surgery 49A: 1408–1414
Mills P R, MacSween R N M, Dick W C, More I A, Watkinson G 1980 Liver disease in rheumatoid arthritis. Scottish Medical Journal 25: 18–22
Missen G A K, Taylor J D 1956 Amyloidosis in rheumatoid arthritis. Journal of Pathology and Bacteriology 71: 179–192
Mitchell N, Shepard N 1970 The ultrastructure of articular cartilage in rheumatoid arthritis. A preliminary report. Journal of Bone and Joint Surgery 52A: 1405–1423
Mitchell N S, Shepard N 1978 Changes in proteoglycan and collagen in cartilage in rheumatoid arthritis — study by light and electron microscopy. Journal of Bone and Joint Surgery 60A: 349–354
Moesmann G 1969 Malignancy and mortality in subacute rheumatoid arthritis in old age. Acta Rheumatologica Scandinavica 15: 193–199
Mohr W 1980 Pathogenesis of inflammatory cartilage destruction in chronic polyarthritis. Deutsche Medizinische Wochenschrift 105: 868–872
Mohr W, Wessinghage D 1978 The relationship between polymorphonuclear granulocytes and cartilage destruction in rheumatoid arthritis. Zeitschrift für Rheumatologie 37: 81–86
Monson R R, Hall A P 1976 Mortality among arthritics. Journal of Chronic Diseases 29: 459–467
Montgomery W W, Goodman M L 1980 Rheumatoid cricoarytenoid arthritis complicated by upper esophageal ulcerations. Annals of Otology, Rhinology and Laryngology 89: 6–8
Moore C P, Willkens R F 1977 The subcutaneous nodule: its significance in the diagnosis of rheumatic disease. Seminars in Arthritis and Rheumatism 7: 63–79
Moss D J, Klestov A, Burrows S, Kane R G 1983 A comparison of Epstein–Barr virus-specific T-cell immunity in rheumatoid arthritis and osteoarthritis patients. Australian Journal of Experimental Biology and Medical Science 61: 509–516
Mueller M N, Jurist J M 1973 Skeletal status in rheumatoid arthritis: a preliminary report. Arthritis and Rheumatism 16: 66–70
Muirden K D 1966 Ferritin in synovial cells in patients with rheumatoid arthritis. Annals of the Rheumatic Diseases 25: 387–401
Muirden K D 1970 Giant cells, cartilage and bone fragments within rheumatoid synovial membrane: clinico-pathological correlations. Australasian Annals of Medicine 19: 105–110
Myers D, Broom N D 1982 Morphological and biomechanical studies of rheumatoid pannus and cartilage. Journal of Rheumatology 9: 502–513
Myllala T, Peltonen L, Puranen J, Korhonen L K 1983 Consequences of synovectomy of the knee joint — clinical, histopathological and enzymatic changes and changes in 2 components of complement. Annals of the Rheumatic Diseases 42: 28–35
Neumark T, Dombay M, Gáspárdy G 1979 Ultrastructural studies in rheumatoid polyneuropathy. Acta Morphologica 27: 205–220
Norton W L, Ziff M 1964 The ultrastructure of rheumatoid synovium and subcutaneous nodules. Arthritis and Rheumatism 7:335
Norton W L, Ziff M 1966 Electron microscopic observations on the rheumatoid synovial membrane. Arthritis and Rheumatism 9: 589–610
Nosanchuk J S, Naylor B 1967 A unique cytologic picture in pleural fluid from patients with rheumatoid arthritis. American Journal of Clinical Pathology 50: 330–335
Ohno O, Cooke T D 1978 Electron microscopic morphology of immunoglobulin aggregates and their interactions in rheumatoid articular collagenous tissues. Arthritis and Rheumatism 21: 516–527
Owen D S, Waller M, Toone E C 1970 Rheumatoid arthritis and malignancy. Medical College of Virginia Quarterly 6: 8–10
Page J W 1961 Spontaneous tendon rupture and cervical vertebral subluxation in patients with rheumatoid arthritis. Journal of the Michegan Medical Society 60: 888–892
Pagel W, Treip C S 1955 Viscero-cutaneous collagenosis. A study of the intermediate forms of dermatomyositis, scleroderma and disseminated lupus erythematosus. Journal of Clinical Pathology 8: 1–18
Parker M T 1965 Infection acquired in medical wards (Public Health Laboratory Service Report). Journal of Hygiene, London 63: 457–477
Patzakis M J, Mills D M, Bartholomew B A, Clayton M L, Smyth J C 1973 A visual, histological and enzymatic study of regenerating rheumatoid synovium in the synovectomized knee. Journal of Bone and Joint Surgery 55A: 287–300
Pisko E J, Turner R A, Yeatts R P, Burch P G, McKinley P H, Collins R L 1982 Ocular pathology, tear production and tear lysozyme in rheumatoid arthritis. Journal of Rheumatology 9: 708–711

Popert A J, Scott D L, Wainwright A C, Walton K W, Williamson N, Chapman J H 1982 Frequency of occurrence, mode of development and significance of rice bodies in rheumatoid joints. Annals of the Rheumatic Diseases 41: 109–117

Poulter L W, Duke O, Hobbs S, Janossy G, Panayi G, Seymour G 1983 The involvement of interdigitating (antigen-presenting) cells in the pathogenesis of rheumatoid arthritis. Clinical and Experimental Immunology 51: 247–254

Prakash R, Atassi A, Poske R, Rosen K M 1973 Prevalence of pericardial and mitral-valve involvement in rheumatoid arthritis without cardiac symptoms. New England Journal of Medicine 289: 597–600

Pritzker K P H, Adams M E, Cheng P-T, Omar S A, Cruickshank B 1980 Black synovium: a consequence of intraarticular gold therapy. Arthritis and Rheumatism 23: 496–504

Rajapakse C, Thompson R, Grennan D M, Winston B M, Patel P, Nuttall P M, et al 1983 Increased bone metabolism in rheumatoid arthritis as measured by the whole-body retention of Tc-99m methylene diphosphonate. Annals of the Rheumatic Diseases 42: 138–141

Rasker J J, Cosh J A 1981 Cause and age at death in a prospective study of 100 patients with rheumatoid arthritis. Annals of the Rheumatic Diseases 40: 115–120

Rasker J J, Kuipers F C 1983 Are rheumatoid nodules caused by vasculitis — a study of 13 early cases. Annals of the Rheumatic Diseases 42: 384–388

Reid D M, Kennedy N S J, Tothill P, Eastall R, Smith M A, Nuki G 1981 The assessment of osteoporosis in rheumatoid arthritis using total body calcium and radiogrammetry. Clinical Science 62 (MRS Suppl):15

Reimer K A, Rodgers R F, Oyasu R 1976 Rheumatoid arthritis with rheumatoid heart disease and granulomatous aortitis. Journal of the American Medical Association 235: 2510–2512

Revell P A 1982 Tissue reactions to joint prostheses and the products of wear and corrosion. In: Berry C L (ed) Bone and joint disease. Current topics in pathology, Vol 7. Springer Verlag, Berlin, p. 73–101

Revell P A, Mayston U 1982 Histopathology of the synovial membrane of peripheral joints in ankylosing spondylitis. Annals of the Rheumatic Diseases 41: 579–586

Reza M J, Veritz M A 1977 Neuromuscular manifestations of rheumatoid arthritis: a clinical and histomorphological analysis. In: Bluestone R, Bacon P A (eds) Clinics in rheumatic diseases, Vol. 3. 3. Extraarticular manifestations of rheumatoid arthritis. Saunders, Philadelphia, p. 565–588

Roberts W C, Kehoe J A, Carpenter D F, Golden A 1968 Cardiac valvular lesions in rheumatoid arthritis. Archives of Internal Medicine 122: 141–146

Rosenberg E F, Baggenstoss A H, Hench P S 1943 The cause of death in 30 cases of rheumatoid arthritis. Annals of Internal Medicine 19: 114–115

Rosenberger J L, Cooper N S, Soren A, McEwen C 1981 A statistical approach to the histopathologic diagnosis of synovitis. Human Pathology 12: 329–337

Rosenthal R E, Oda J E, Lesker P A 1972 Experimental synovectomy in the rabbit knee: structural and functional considerations. Clinical Orthopaedics and Related Research 88: 241–246

Rowley D A, Halliwell B 1983 Formation of hydroxyl radicals from hydrogen peroxide and iron salts by superoxide — and ascorbate dependent mechanisms: relevance to the pathology of rheumatoid disease. Clinical Science 64: 649–653

Saklatvala J, Barrett A J 1980 Identification of proteinases in rheumatoid synovium. Detection of leukocyte elastase, cathepsin G and another serine proteinase. Biochimica et Biophysica Acta 615: 167–177

Saklatvala J, Dingle J T 1980 Identification of catabolin, a protein from synovium which induces degradation of cartilage in organ culture. Biochemical and Biophysical Research Communications 96: 1225–1231

Samson D, Halliday D, Gumpell J M 1977 Role of ineffective erythropoiesis in the anaemia of rheumatoid arthritis. Annals of the Rheumatic Diseases 36: 181–185

Samuels B, Lee J C, Engleman E P, Hopper J 1978 Membranous nephropathy in patients with rheumatoid arthritis: relationship to gold therapy. Medicine 57: 319–328

Scadding J G 1969 The lungs in rheumatoid arthritis. Proceedings of the Royal Society of Medicine 62: 227–238

Scharf J, Levy J, Benderly A, Nahir M 1976 Pericardial tamponade in juvenile rheumatoid arthritis. Arthritis and Rheumatism 19: 760–762

Schilling F 1973 Reflex dystrophien und dystrophische Pseudoarthritiden der unteren Extremitäten. Zeitschrift für Rheumaforschung 32: 375–384

Schilling F 1974 Knochenveränderungen bei entzundlich rheumatischen Erkrankungen vom klinisch-radiologischen Standpunkt. Verhandlungen der deutschen Gesellschaft für Rheumatologie 3: 142–157

Scott D G I, Bacon P A, Tribe C R 1981 Systemic rheumatoid vasculitis a clinical and laboratory study of 50 cases. Medicine 60: 288–297

Schumacher H R, Kitridou R C 1972 Synovitis of recent onset. A clinico-pathologic study during the first month of disease. Arthritis and Rheumatism 15: 465–485

Scudamore C 1816 A treatise on the nature and cure of gout. London

Sheppeard H 1983 An update on mechanisms of cartilage destruction in rheumatoid arthritis. Australian and New Zealand Journal of Medicine 13: 195–200

Sherman M S 1952 Psoriatic arthritis — observations on the clinical, roentgenographic and pathological changes. Journal of Bone and Joint Surgery 34A: 831–852

Shiozawa S, Ziff M 1983 Immunoelectron microscopic demonstration of fibronectin in rheumatoid pannus and at the cartilage–pannus junction. Annals of the Rheumatic Diseases 42: 254–263

Shiozawa S, Shiozawa K, Fujita T 1983 Morphologic observations in the early phase of the cartilage pannus junction — light and electron microscopic studies of active cellular pannus. Arthritis and Rheumatism 26: 472–478

Simmling-Annefeld M, Fassbender H G 1979 Transformation of the capillary wall elements in synovial tissue in rheumatoid arthritis. Zeitschrift für Rheumatologie 38: 153–162

Sinclair R J G, Cruickshank B 1956 A clinical and pathological study of sixteen cases of rheumatoid arthritis with extensive visceral involvement ('rheumatoid disease'). Quarterly Journal of Medicine (N.S.) 25: 313–332

Skrifvars B 1979 Immunofluorescence study of renal biopsies in chronic rheumatoid arthritis. Scandinavian Journal of Rheumatology 8: 241–247

Smith H P, Challa V R, Alexander E 1980 Odontoid compression of the brain stem in a patient with rheumatoid

arthritis — case report. Journal of Neurosurgery 53: 841–845
Sokoloff L 1953 The heart in rheumatoid arthritis. American Heart Journal 45: 635–643
Sokoloff L 1963 The pathophysiology of peripheral blood vessels in collagen diseases. In: Orbison J H, Smith D E (eds) The peripheral blood vessels. Williams & Wilkins, Baltimore, p. 297–325
Sokoloff L 1964 Cardiac involvement in rheumatoid arthritis and allied disorders: current concepts. Modern concepts of cardiovascular diseases 33: 847–850
Sokoloff L 1966 The pathology of rheumatoid arthritis and allied disorders. In: Hollander J L (ed) Arthritis and allied conditions, 7th Edn. Lea & Febiger, Philadelphia, p. 187–210
Sokoloff L, Bunim J J 1957 Vascular lesions in rheumatoid arthritis. Journal of Chronic Diseases 5: 668–685
Solomon W M 1943 Amyloidosis in chronic atrophic arthritis. Annals of Internal Medicine 18: 846–850
Soren A 1978a Histodiagnosis and clinical correlation of rheumatoid and other synovitis. Lippincott, Philadelphia, p. 116–122
Soren A 1978b Histodiagnosis and clinical correlation of rheumatoid and other synovitis. Lippincott, Philadelphia, p. 137–142
Soren A 1980 The diagnostic significance of certain histopathologic changes for rheumatoid arthritis. Zeitschrift für Rheumatologie 39: 74–78
Sorgente N, Kuettner K E, Soble L W, Eisenstein R 1975 The resistance of certain tissues to invasion II. Evidence for extractable factors in cartilage which inhibit invasion by vascularized mesenchyme. Laboratory Investigation 32: 217–222
Spurlock R G, Richman A V 1983 Rheumatoid meningitis: a case report and review of the literature. Archives of Pathology and Laboratory Medicine 107: 129–131
Stiehl P 1982 Correlational study on synovial membranes and joint effusions for the quantification of the activity diagnosis in cases of rheumatoid arthritis. Acta Histochemica (Suppl) 26: 437–442
Stiehl P, Geiler G 1974 Morphological activity estimation of rheumatoid arthritis: a comparative study of synovial fluid and synovial membrane. Zeitschrift für Rheumatologie 33: 54–62
Stockman R 1904 The causes, pathology and treatment of chronic rheumatism. Edinburgh Medical Journal 15(NS): 107–116, 223–235
Susmano A, Muenster J J, Javid H, Carleton R A 1973 Coronary arteritis in rheumatoid arthritis. Archives of Internal Medicine 132: 241–244
Talal N, Schnitzer B 1977 Lymphadenopathy and Sjögren's syndrome. In: Bluestone R, Bacon P A (eds) Clinics in rheumatic diseases, Vol. 3. 3. Extraarticular manifestations of rheumatoid arthritis. Saunders, Philadelphia p. 421–432
Tarr K H 1974 Spontaneous rupture of tendons in rheumatoid arthritis. New Zealand Medical Journal 79: 651–653
Teilum G, Lindahl A 1954 Frequency and significance of amyloid changes in rheumatoid arthritis. Acta Medica Scandinavica 149: 449–455
Thadani U, Iveson J M I, Wright V 1975 Cardiac tamponade, constrictive pericarditis and pericardial resection in rheumatoid arthritis. Medicine 54: 261–270
Thery C, Lekeiffre J, Gosselin B, Warembourg H 1974 Le bloc auriculo-ventriculaire de la polyarthrite rheumatoide. Etude histologique du systemé de Hi-Tawara. Archives des Maladies du Coeur, des Vaisseaux et du Sang 10: 1181–1191
Thorne C, Urowitz M B 1982 Long-term outcome in Felty's syndrome. Annals of the Rheumatic Diseases 41: 486–489
Thorne C, Urowitz M B, Wassless I 1982 Liver disease in Felty's syndrome. American Journal of Medicine 73: 35–40
Tiger L H, Gordon M H, Ehrlich G E, Shapiro B 1976 Liver enlargement demonstrated by scintigraphy in rheumatoid arthritis. Journal of Rheumatology 3: 15–20
Uddin J, Kraus A S, Kelly H G 1970 Survivorship and death in rheumatoid arthritis. Arthritis and Rheumatism 13: 125–130
Ullman S, Halberg P, Hentzer B, Sylvest J 1978 Deposits of complement and immunoglobulins in dermal and synovial vessels in psoriasis. Archives of Dermatology and Venereology (Stockholm) 58: 272–273
Unger P N, Zuckerbrod M, Beck G J, Steele J M 1948 Amyloidosis in rheumatoid arthritis: report of ten cases. American Journal of Medical Science 216: 51–56
Vaughan-Jackson O J 1966 The rheumatoid hand. In: Pulvertaft R G (ed) Clinical surgery, the hand. Butterworth, London, p. 173–196
Wagner T, Abgarowicz T 1970 Microscopic appearance of Baker's cyst in cases of rheumatoid arthritis. Reumatologia 8: 21–26
Walker W C, Wright V 1969 Diffuse interstitial pulmonary fibrosis and rheumatoid arthritis. Annals of the Rheumatic Diseases 28: 252–259
Watson J D, Ochsner S F 1967 Compression of bladder due to 'rheumatoid' cysts of hip joint. American Journal of Roentgenology 99: 695–696
Watson P 1979 Intracranial haemorrhage with vasculitis in rheumatoid arthritis. Archives of Neurology 36:58
Watson P, Fekete J, Deck J 1977 Central nervous system vasculitis in rheumatoid arthritis. Canadian Journal of Neurological Science 4: 269–272
Webb J, Whaley K, MacSween R N M, Nuki G, Dick W C, Buchanan W W 1975 Liver disease in rheumatoid arthritis and Sjögren's syndrome. Prospective study using biochemical and serological markers of hepatic dysfunction. Annals of the Rheumatic Diseases 34: 70–81
Weiner S, Bassett L, Spiegel T 1982 Superior, posterior and lateral displacement of C1 in rheumatoid arthritis. Arthritis and Rheumatism 25: 1378–1381
Whaley K, Buchanan W W 1971 Recent advances in Sjögren's syndrome. In: Hill AGS (ed) Modern trends in rheumatology: 2. Butterworths, London, p. 139–157
Williams R C Jr 1974 Rheumatoid arthritis as a systemic disease. Saunders, Philadelphia
Wisnieski J J, Askari A D 1981 Rheumatoid nodulosis — a relatively benign rheumatoid variant. Archives of Internal Medicine 141: 615–622
Woessner J F, Howell D S 1980 The enzymatic degradation of connective tissue matrices. In: Owen R, Goodfellow J, Bullough P (eds) Scientific foundations of orthopaedics and traumatology. Churchill Livingstone, Edinburgh, pp 232–241
Woolley D E, Evanson J M 1977 Collagenase and its natural inhibitors in relation to the rheumatoid joint. Connective Tissue Research 5: 31–35
Woolley D E, Crossley M J, Evanson J M 1977 Collagenase at sites of cartilage erosion in the rheumatoid joint. Arthritis and Rheumatism 20: 1231–1239
Woolley D E, Brinckerhoff C E, Mainardi C L, Vater C A,

Evanson J M, Harris E D 1979 Collagenase production by rheumatoid synovial cells: morphological and immunohistochemical studies of the dendritic cell. Annals of the Rheumatic Diseases 38: 262–270
Woolley D E, Tetlow L C, Evanson J M 1980 Collagenase immunolocalization studies of rheumatoid and malignant tissues. In: Woolley D E, Evanson J M (ed) Collagenase in normal and pathological connective tissues. Wiley & Sons, London, p. 105–125
Wright V 1981 Psoriatic arthritis. In: Kelley W N, Harris E D, Ruddy S, Sledge C B (eds) Textbook of rheumatology. Saunders, Philadelphia, p. 1047–1062
Wright V, Moll J M H 1976 Seronegative polyarthritis. North Holland, Amsterdam
Wynne-Roberts C R, Anderson C H, Turano A M, Baron M 1978 Light- and electron-microscopic findings of juvenile rheumatoid arthritis synovium: comparison with normal juvenile synovium. Seminars in Arthritis and Rheumatism 7: 287–302
Yates D B, Scott J T 1975 Cardiac valvular disease in chronic inflammatory disorders of connective tissue. Annals of the Rheumatic Diseases 34: 321–325
Young D, Schwedel J B 1944 The heart in rheumatoid arthritis. American Heart Journal 28: 1–33

Articular and systemic manifestations of rheumatoid arthritis

Doit-on admettre une nouvelle espèce de goutte sous la dénomination de goutte asthènique primitive?
A J Landré-Beauvais (1880)

Perhaps the most remarkable fact about rheumatoid arthritis, which today affects between 1 and 2% of the adult population in developed countries, is that it was first only clearly described in 1800 (Landré-Beauvais, 1800) and named in 1859 (Garrod, 1859). There is no unequivocal instance of the disease in ancient skeletal remains (Reymand, 1979), although there are good examples of osteoarthritis and ankylosing spondylitis (Spencer et al, 1980) and even a case of ochronotic arthropathy (Stenn et al, 1979). Hippocrates and other Greek and Roman writers gave possible descriptions of the disease (Short, 1974), and there are suggestive descriptions in the Sanskrit writings of Caraka Samhita of 100 AD (Sturrock et al, 1977) and by the 17th century English physician, Thomas Sydenham (Short, 1974). There is no description of the disease in either the Bible or in the works of Shakespeare (Ehrlich, 1967), and the 'flying gout' which Robert Burns suffered from in the last years of his life was probably due to subacute bacterial endocarditis (Buchanan & Kean, 1982). Dequeker (1977) examined the paintings of the Flemish school between 1400 and 1700, and found only five hand lesions suggestive of rheumatoid arthritis. The most impressive of these is illustrated in Figure 26.1. Appelboom et al (1981) have suggested that Rubens (1577–1640) may have suffered from rheumatoid arthritis, but the clinical description is also consistent with gout. Mary Queen of Scots has been thought by some to have suffered from rheumatoid arthritis

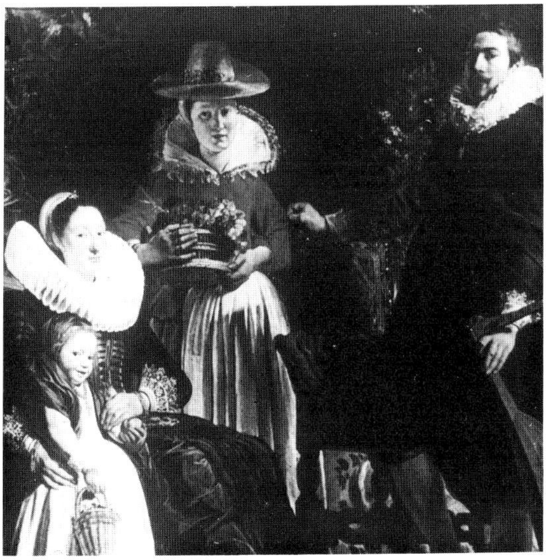

Fig. 26.1 The hands carrying the basket of fruit in the famous painting known as *The Printer's Family* are very suggestive of rheumatoid arthritis. This painting by the Flemish artist, Jacob Jordaens (1593–1678), now hangs in the Prado Museum, Madrid, Spain.

(Copeman 1964) but this could have resulted from Marfan's syndrome, since she was five feet eleven inches tall (Fraser, 1970). Christopher Columbus developed 'gout of all his joints accompanied by a low fever' on his third crossing of the Atlantic in 1498 (Copeman, 1964). However, he also suffered from 'severe and painful attacks of ophthalmia' (Copeman, 1964) which is suggestive of Reiter's syndrome. Caughey (1974) has provided better evidence that the Emperor Constantine IX developed rheumatoid arthritis when in his early sixties. The Emperor's biographer, Michael Psellus wrote, 'I myself saw his fingers, once so beautifully formed, completely altered from their natural shape, warped and twisted with hollows here and projections there, so that they were incapable of grasping anything at all. His feet were bent and his knees, crooked like the point of a man's elbow, were swollen, making it impossible for him to walk steadily or stand upright for any length of time. Mostly he lay on his bed and, whenever he wished to give audience, others tried to prop him up and make him comfortable'. There is no example of rheumatoid arthritis in the extensive pathological collection of William Hunter (1718–1783) in the Royal Infirmary, Glasgow, Scotland (Palmer et al, 1977).

Thus, from a historical perspective rheumatoid arthritis appears either to have been absent or relatively rare or present in a milder form before the 19th century (Buchanan & Murdoch, 1979). An outline of the articular and extra-articular manifestations of the disease as it is seen today in clinical practice follows.

Rheumatoid arthritis, like so many other autoimmune diseases, predominantly affects females, in a ratio of 2–3 females to 1 male. The disease varies considerably in its severity from the almost asymptomatic to an extremely severe crippling variety associated with vascular and granulomatous complications.

TYPE OF ONSET

The onset is usually insidious, occurring especially in the 4th and 5th decades. Occasionally the onset may be acute, as in Still's disease (see Ch. 43) with high and often spiking fever, evanescent rash, leucocytosis, lymphadenopathy, splenomegaly, pleuritis and pericarditis (Bywaters, 1971; Esdaile et al, 1980). The arthritis in this type of onset more commonly involves large rather than small joints of the hands and feet, and wrist involvement progressing to bony ankylosis has been described as highly suggestive of adult-onset Still's disease (Medsger & Christy, 1976). DeMulder & van de Putte (1982) have described a patient with adult-onset Still's disease with severe destructive arthritis of the distal interphalangeal joints of the hand, associated with transient capsular calcification. In the elderly the onset is usually insidious, but occasionally acute and surprisingly often associated with a favourable outcome (Corrigan et al, 1974). The nature of onset, whether acute, subacute, or gradual, has not been found in general in adults to be related to prognosis (Luukkainen et al, 1983).

PRODROMAL SYMPTOMS

Prodromal symptoms, including vague ill health, undue fatigue, weight loss, poor appetite, transient muscular pain and stiffness and numbness or tingling in the hands and feet, have been described preceding the onset of joint manifestations (Short et al, 1957) but are rare in the authors' experience. A single joint may be first affected, on occasion following a minor injury. Occasionally weeks or even months may elapse before other joints become involved (Jacoby et al, 1973). A diagnosis of traumatic synovitis may be considered at this stage, but the presence of a persistently raised erythrocyte sedimentation rate should alert the physician to the presence of inflammation. Frequently when the disease is monoarticular tests for rheumatoid factor are negative, and it is imperative in patients presenting with an inflammatory monoarthritis that further investigation including arthroscopy and/or synovial membrane biopsy be carried out to exclude tuberculous or other pathology.

More commonly the arthritis is polyarticular and symmetrical from the outset (Hernandez et al, 1980). The test for serum rheumatoid factor is usually positive at this state (Jacoby et al, 1973). The traditional view is that small peripheral joints are affected first, but in one large study large joints were affected first in 52% of patients (Short et al 1957).

Rarely patients may present with repeated afebrile attacks of acute arthritis and periarthritis. The attacks are usually of sudden onset and last from a few hours to several days, and then subside completely without residual disability. The intervals between attacks are irregular, unlike intermittent hydroarthrosis, and the diagnosis of rheumatoid arthritis may only become possible when the patient develops chronic polyarthritis and a positive test for rheumatoid factor. Although uncommon, this presentation of so-called 'palindromic rheumatism' is important, since at least one-third of patients with the syndrome subsequently develop classical rheumatoid arthritis. (Williams, et al 1971). The only difference between those patients who develop rheumatoid arthritis and those who continue to have attacks of palindromic rheumatism is that the former tend to have a persistently raised erythrocyte sedimentation rate and develop a positive test for rheumatoid factor.

COURSE AND PROGNOSIS

The clinical course of the disease is very variable. At least three main types can be distinguished. In the first the disease has an acute onset with widespread joint involvement and marked systemic upset. Surprisingly such patients often have a favourable prognosis. In the second type the disease starts insidiously with involvement of only a few joints, and progresses relentlessly with a steady deterioration in functional ability, but with little constitutional upset, although eventually the patient becomes severely crippled. The third category lies between these two extremes, the disease tending to run an irregular course of exacerbations and remissions. The eventual outcome of patients in this category is extremely varied.

In several large series of patients followed up over a period of years in the United Kingdom and in the United States up to one-quarter of the patients had inactive disease and good functional ability and another quarter had only mild to moderate activity with only slight functional impairment. The remaining patients, however, had persistent disease activity and were severely crippled, with many becoming chairbound or bedridden (Short & Bauer, 1948; Ragan, 1949; Short et al, 1957; Duthie et al, 1964). Thus, the prognosis on the whole is reasonably good in at least 50% of patients. It must be emphasised that all these studies were conducted on patients who had been referred to hospital. The prognosis, therefore, of rheumatoid arthritis among the general population must be very much better. It is also known that there is a surprising number of persons of both sexes in the general population with undoubted clinical, radiological and serological disease who never seek medical advice (Kellgren et al, 1953).

Temperature, atmospheric pressure and humidity all influence the symptoms of rheumatoid arthritis: a warm dry atmosphere produces a sense of well-being and less pain and stiffness in the joints, whereas cold damp weather produces discomfort (Latman, 1981). However, there is no evidence that climate influences the prognosis of the disease or tests such as the erythrocyte sedimentation rate and C-reactive protein (Latman, 1981).

Although certain factors such as acute onset of short duration, initial asymmetrical and limited joint involvement, absence of joint effusions and erosions, and a favourable response to treatment, appear to favour a better prognosis the most important single index is the titre of serum rheumatoid factor (Feigenbaum et al, 1979). Patients with persistently high titres of rheumatoid factor have in general a poor prognosis, whereas those with low titres or intermittently weakly positive rheumatoid factor tests run a favourable course (Duthie et al, 1964; Feigenbaum et al, 1979). In patients with persistently negative rheumatoid factor titres, which have not resulted from therapy with second line drugs such as injectable gold complexes or D-penicillamine, the diagnosis should be held in question. In a study by Burns & Calin (1983) the authors reported that patients labelled as having seronegative arthritis in whom other possible associated arthropathies have been excluded, have a radiological profile which is distinctly different from that of seropositive rheumatoid arthritis. They (Burns & Calin, 1983) suggested that at least one group of so-called 'seronegative' rheumatoids may be the adult equivalent of seronegative, HLA-DR4-negative juvenile polyarthritis. The antigen HLA-DR4 is related to seropositivity and is especially found in females with a positive family history of rheumatoid arthritis, but surprisingly not with prognosis (Gran et al, 1983). In the report by Lewis et al (1980), and their accompanying revision of the literature, it would appear that males have more severe disease than females.

ARTICULAR FEATURES

The term 'rheumatoid disease' was often used in the past to emphasise widespread involvement of many different organs and tissues (Ellman & Ball, 1948). However, the main brunt of the disease is borne by the diarthrodial joints, and most rheumatologists still prefer to use the term 'rheumatoid arthritis'. The pathological process in the joint is essentially a chronic synovitis, and it is the inflamed synovium which causes erosion of cartilage, with resulting loss of joint space on X-ray, and erosion of articular bone (Fig. 26.2). Bone cysts or 'géodes' (Fig. 26.3) often develop in the juxta-articular bone owing to the inflamed synovium being forced into the porous cancellous bone by increases in intra-articular pressure (Jayson et al, 1970). Large géodes appear to develop in patients who do hard manual work (Castillo et al, 1965; Gaunt & Rinker, 1970). However, patients who retain a good physique and muscular power do not necessarily develop géodes (De Haas et al, 1974). In the later stages of rheumatoid arthritis fibrous and/or bony ankylosis may supervene.

The juxta-articular decrease in bone density so classical of rheumatoid arthritis, does not occur in all patients. Indeed, those patients with coexistent diffuse idiopathic skeletal hyperostosis (DISH) have well preserved bone density and even osteophytosis. Forster et al (1981) have described two patients with rheumatoid arthritis with coexistent DISH in which the vertebral features of DISH were absent.

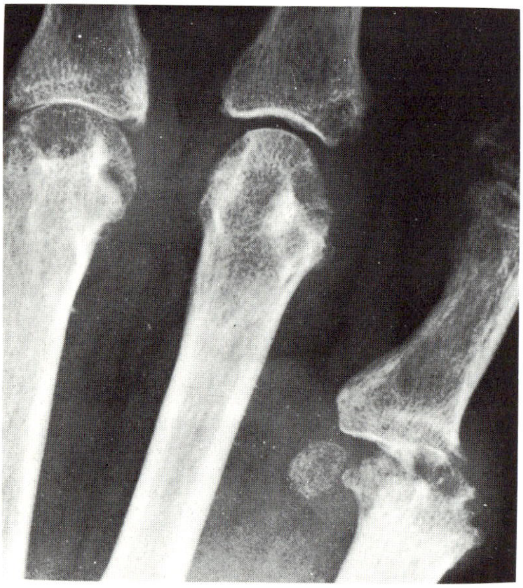

Fig. 26.2 Typical X-ray changes in the metacarpophalangeal joints in a patient with rheumatoid arthritis. Note the loss of joint space and very typical erosive changes.

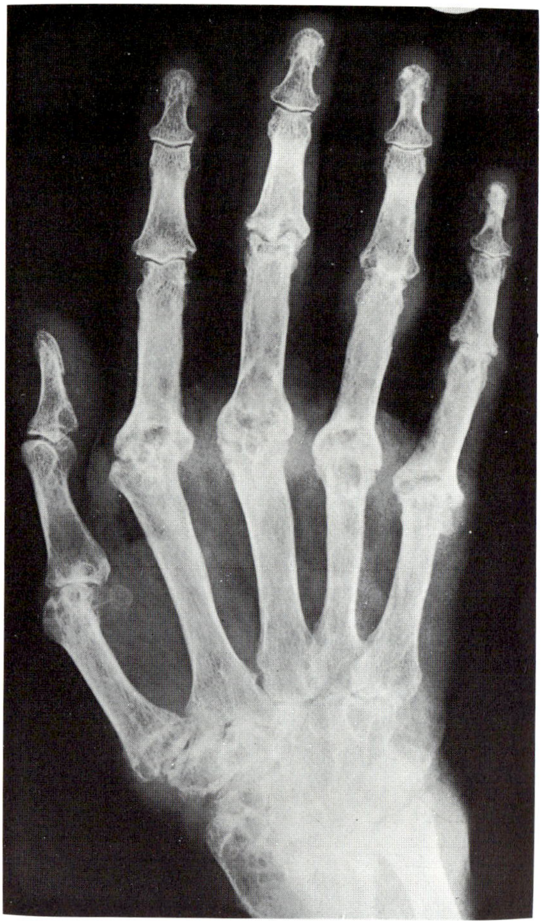

Fig. 26.3 Extensive changes in the joints of a hand of a patient with rheumatoid arthritis. The presence of juxta-articular bone cysts or géodes is particularly evident.

The clinical features of the arthritis conform to the cardinal features of inflammation with one exception — redness is never present. A 'red' rheumatoid joint must always be suspected as being infected, and demands immediate arthrocentesis. The joint in rheumatoid arthritis is liable to secondary infection, usually with *Staphylococcus aureus* (Kellgren et al, 1958; Rimoin & Wennberg; 1966, Karten, 1971; Baum, 1971; Huskisson & Hart, 1972).

Joint stiffness is especially troublesome in the morning, attributed to increased fluid content of the joint tissues (Scott, 1960). Stiffness of the joints after sitting for some time — so-called 'gelling' — is also very characteristic of rheumatoid arthritis, although also found in other forms of inflammatory joint disease. Efforts to explain stiffness in normal and diseased joints have not been particularly successful (Wright & Johns, 1960, 1961; Wright & Plunkett, 1966).

INDIVIDUAL JOINTS

Despite years of study in many different parts of the world there is no adequate description of the pattern of joint involvement. In general joints with a lot of synovium, e.g. the knee joint, are frequently affected, whereas joints with little synovium are less frequently affected. It is a remarkable fact that the pattern of joint involvement is so often symmetrical, but there are surprisingly no data on just how frequently this occurs. Most clinicians would agree, however, that the joints most frequently involved are the proximal interphalangeal joints of the fingers, the interphalangeal joints of the thumbs, the metacarpophalangeal joints, the wrist, elbow and shoulder joints, the knee joints and the metatarsophalangeal joints in the feet (Jacoby et al, 1973; Fleming et al, 1976a, b).

Involvement of the temperomandibular joint and the cervical spine are commonly present as early features in the disease presentation (Fleming et al, 1976a). Severe disease is generally associated with early wrist and metatarsophalangeal involvement (Fleming et al, 1976a), and also with a large joint distribution involving shoulders, elbows, wrists and knees (Fleming et al, 1976b).

Cervical spine

The prevalence of clinical and radiological involvement of the cervical spine in rheumatoid arthritis varies widely in different reports, owing presumably to differences in severity of disease studied (Bland, 1967, 1974). However, what is certain is that cervical spine involvement is by no means rare; it is a frequent cause of pain and disability and an occasional cause of spinal cord medulla oblongata injury. Lawrence (1961) found a surprisingly high prevalence of radiological changes in the cervical spine in otherwise healthy members of the population. A firm correlation between the severity of peripheral erosive joint destruction and cervical spine subluxation has been reported (Winfield et al, 1983) but it is also widely accepted that rheumatoid arthritis may involve the cervical spine with little or no clinical expression peripherally (Bland, 1967, 1974).

Involvement of the cervical spine is usually diagnosed by X-ray examination. Lateral X-rays in full flexion and extension are essential, and an anteroposterior view of the occipitoatlantoaxial region through the open mouth is often very useful. Tomography and cineradiography may be required in difficult cases, especially in patients in whom surgical treatment is contemplated. The absence of radiological signs in the cervical spine does not, of course, exclude involvement (Bland, 1967, 1974). Computerised axial tomography (CAT) in evaluation of atlantoaxial subluxation has

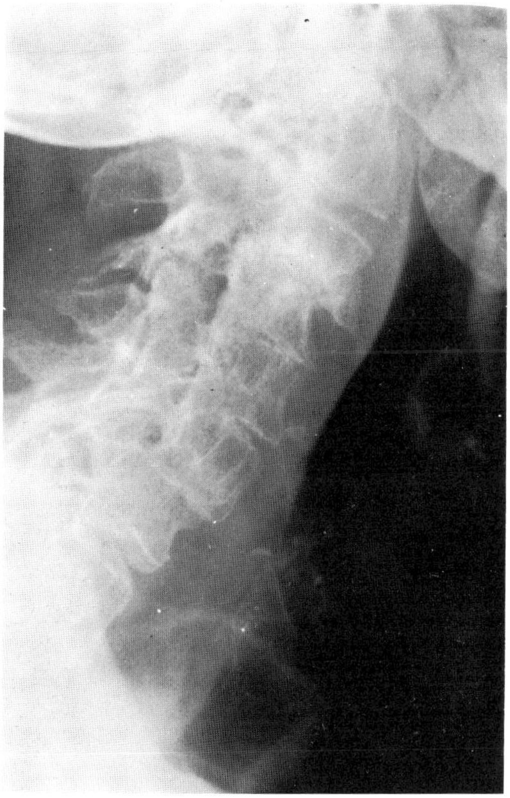

Fig. 26.4 Severe involvement of the cervical spine in a patient with rheumatoid arthritis. Note the severe anterior subluxations at C2, C3, C6 and C7.

been shown in one study to be better than plain X-ray in identifying the severity of cord compression and in correlating with clinical neurological findings (Raskin et al, 1983).

Atlantoaxial subluxation and multiple subluxations of C2–3, C3–4, C4–5, and C5–6 are very characteristic of involvement of the cervical spine by rheumatoid arthritis (Fig. 26.4). These subluxations occur more often in patients with severe, long-standing disease. Separation of the anterior surface of the odontoid peg from the posterior surface of the anterior arch of the atlas by more than 2.5 mm in females and 3 mm in males is pathological (Bland et al, 1965) (Fig. 26.5). Subluxation of the atlas on the axis is held in check by the alar ligaments. Subluxation may be either symmetrical or asymmetrical. The lateral masses of the atlas and the occipital condyles may become eroded and collapse, with resulting basilar impression (Rana & Taylor, 1971; Smith et al, 1972; Swinson et al, 1972). A useful measurement to determine the extent of basilar impression is to draw a line from the inferior margin of the occipital curve to the posterior edge of the hard palate. This line is known as McGregor's line (McGregor, 1948). Another useful measurement of basilar invagination of 'platybasia' is the angle between the foramen magnum plane and the clivus, which should not normally exceed 135° (Bland, 1967). The distance between the posterior arch of the atlas and the spinous process of the axis can be measured by subtracting the value in flexion from that in extension. Excess 'tipping' of atlas on the axis is indicated by a measurement of 7 mm or more (Bland et al, 1965). The lateral atlantoaxial joints frequently show 'pinching' when there is asymmetrical 'sliding' of the axis on the atlas, especially on the transbuccal view of the occipito–atlas–axis region. In addition, erosions of these joints are not uncommon (van Kerckhove, 1970) and unilateral erosive disease can result in lateral subluxation (Burry et al, 1978). Although extremely rare, posterior subluxation of the atlas on the axis has been reported in cases of odontoid erosion, fracture or congenital absence of the odontoid (Hart et al, 1981).

Changes in the odontoid peg include: loss of cortex, erosions, pointing, and diminution in size.

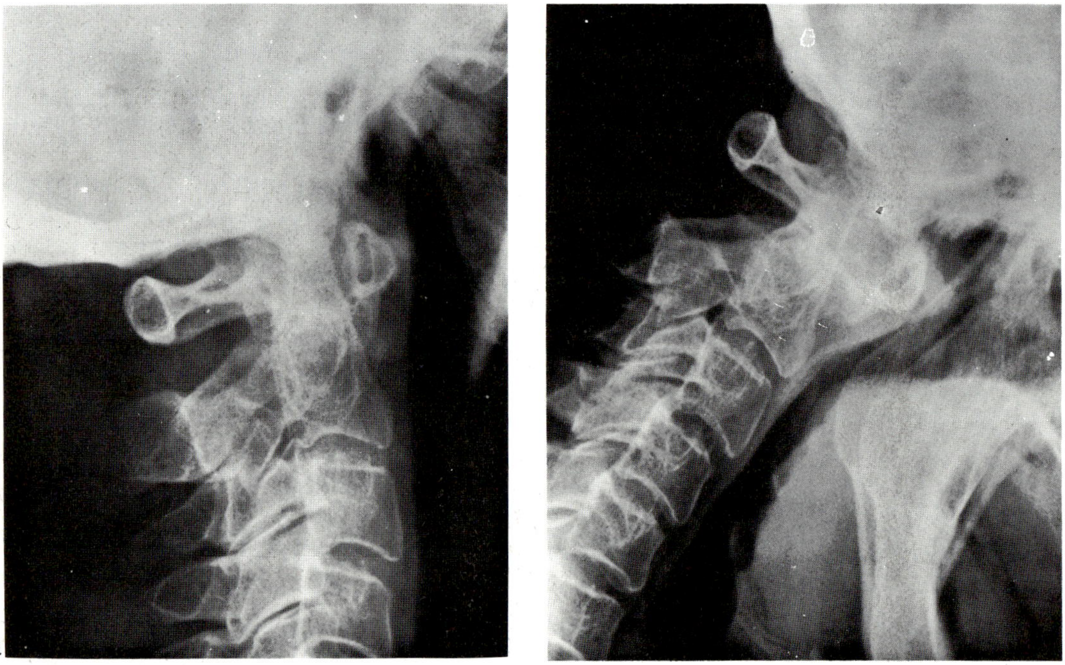

a b

Fig. 26.5 (a) Normal atlantoaxial articulation. (b) Marked separation of the anterior surface of the odontoid peg from the posterior aspect of the anterior arch of the atlas.

Occasionally the odontoid peg may be so reduced in size that it slips backwards under the transverse ligament so causing anterior subluxation of the atlas on the axis (Bland, 1967). Sclerosis of the odontoid peg is frequently present, and pathological fractures are not uncommon (Martel & Bole, 1968). Since the mastoid process lies close behind the odontoid peg on lateral films, it is necessary always to identify the mastoid process before interpreting the air cells of the mastoid as erosive changes in the odontoid (Bland, 1967).

Osteoporosis of the bones of the cervical spine parallels osteoporosis in other parts of the skeleton. In addition to anterior subluxations of C2–3 to C5–6, narrowing of the disc spaces with little or no osteophytosis is pathognomonic at C2–3 and C3–4 and highly suggestive at C4–5 and C5–6 of rheumatoid arthritis involving the cervical spine (Sharp et al, 1958; Bland et al, 1965). Erosions of the vertebrae, especially the vertebral plates, are very characteristic of rheumatoid arthritis involving the cervical spine (Sharp et al, 1958; Bland et al, 1965; Conlon et al, 1966). It appears that granulation tissue from the neurocentral joints erodes the disc annulus and disc bone border, especially laterally and posteriorly (Ball, 1971). That cervical disc erosion is secondary to an erosive process arising in the neurocentral joints is supported by the fact that these changes are only found in the cervical spine, and not in the thoracic or lumbar spine where there are no neurocentral joints. According to Ball (1971) thoracic and lumbar destructive disc lesions in patients with rheumatoid arthritis are due to other causes, such as disc degeneration, depressed fractures of the vertebral end plates, and infections. The rarity of erosive disc lesions in juvenile rheumatoid arthritis can be explained by the fact that the neurocentral joints are not fully developed until about 20 years of age (Ecklin, 1960). Apophyseal joint erosion and narrowing of the joint spaces are commonly seen in the cervical spine in rheumatoid arthritis, but are often difficult to interpret. Cortical erosions of the spinous process may be evident in severe disease.

The clinical features of cervical spine involvement in rheumatoid arthritis vary considerably from the completely asymptomatic to severe pain, quadriparesis and even death (Kornblum et al, 1952; Sharp et al, 1958; Martel & Page, 1960; Martel & Abell, 1963; Conlon et al, 1966; Robinson, 1966; Hopkins, 1967; Ahlgran & Fog, 1968; Martel, 1968; Reitan, 1968; Webb et al, 1968; Whaley & Dick, 1968; Mathews, 1969; Isdale & Corrigan, 1971; Meikle & Wilkinson, 1971; Ornilla et al, 1972; Sukoff et al, 1972; Swinson et al, 1972). Pain is the most frequent symptom of cervical spine involvement in rheumatoid arthritis. In some patients it is brief in duration, but in most it is persistent. With atlantoaxial subluxation pain is often experienced in the temporal and retro-orbital regions, and probably is referred from pain arising in the atlanto-occipital membrane and in the alar and transverse ligaments. Occipital pain is also common and may also be felt over the vertex and as a band-like tightness round the forehead. Occipital pain is considered to arise from C2–3 or below. Patients not infrequently have a sense of weakness in the neck and have to use their hands to support their heads. Abnormal movements of the head may occur and the patient may experience a frightening 'clunking' sensation on flexing the neck. Pain is often triggered by movements of the head, and gross subluxation of the atlas on the axis may produce pressure on the occipital nerve with occipital neuralgia. Bland (1967) maintains that cervical traction always makes the symptoms due to cervical spine involvement much worse, and is a useful diagnostic test.

Local examination of the cervical spine often reveals a bony prominence in the mid-suboccipital region due to prominence of the spinous process of the second cervical vertebra. This prominence is often tender on pressure. Sharp & Purser (1961) have described a test to elicit atlantoaxial instability, which consists of the physician placing one hand on the forehead and the index of the other hand on the spinous process of the axis. Normally pressure on the forehead when the patient is sitting erect produces no appreciable movement, but when atlantoaxial subluxation is present a backward gliding movement of the head can be felt as the subluxation is reduced. Clinical examination of the neck usually gives little information as the neck is often very painful and held rigid by the patient.

Neurological involvement may accompany gross

atlantoaxial subluxation, especially when there are subaxial subluxations. However it is surprising how often there may be no neurological sequelae and how good the prognosis is even when gross changes are present (Isdale & Corrigan, 1971; Mathews, 1974). Weakness of the arms and legs and difficulty in holding up the head, which feels 'heavy', are common complaints. Pyramidal signs may occur and wasting of the muscles of the hands may result as a consequence of neurological involvement. Paraesthesiae in both the upper and lower limbs may be brought on by movement of the head, and jolts to the body produce electric-shock-like sensations. Vertebral-basilar vascular insufficiency may cause transient blindness, nystagmus, vertigo and loss of consciousness. The anterior spinal arteries may be occluded with resulting anterior horn cell lesions. Spinal cord compression may result in limb weakness, spasticity and quadriplegia. Vertical subluxation of the atlas may lead to medullary compression and sudden death (Martel & Abell, 1963). Death has also been reported following quadriplegia due to subaxial subluxation (Whaley & Dick, 1968) or thrombosis of the vertebral arteries (Webb et al, 1968).

The importance of cervical spine involvement in rheumatoid arthritis cannot be overemphasised, especially since orthopaedic surgery is playing an ever-increasing role in management. Manipulation of the spine during induction of anaesthesia is potentially hazardous in a patient with severe neck involvement. Ornilla et al (1972) have suggested the very wise precaution of sending patients with neck involvement to the operating theatre wearing a cervical collar in order to alert the anaesthetist.

Shoulder joint

Involvement of the shoulder joint is one of the heaviest crosses the patient with rheumatoid arthritis has to bear. For not only can there be severe pain, but the patient may develop marked limitation of movement of the joint. The primary site of involvement is the glenohumeral joint. Tenderness can best be tested by applying firm pressure just below the coracoid process. Arthrograms of the shoulder joint often show irregular filling defects due to synovial hypertrophy, and on plain X-ray erosion of the capsular insertion above the greater tuberosity gives the best radiological indication of severity (Ennevaara, 1967). Limitation of shoulder joint movement is the clinical feature which correlates best with radiographic changes (McNair et al, 1969). Shoulder joint bursae may become inflamed and contribute to shoulder pain: these too can be visualised by arthrography (Weston, 1969), as can synovial rupture of the shoulder joint (Lane et al, 1972). Severe shoulder joint disease can also be associated with superior rib margin erosions. This feature of rib erosions was originally described in 1963 by Martel & Dixon and recently reviewed in detail by McKendry & Hogan (1981).

Elbow joint

Elbow joint involvement in rheumatoid arthritis is a common cause of disability. On examination the elbow joint is often found to be incapable of a full 180 degrees extension, and in severely involved elbow joints there is also limitation of flexion. Normally there is a sulcus below the radial head, but in rheumatoid arthritis this may become filled in with hypertrophied synovial tissue, which has a spongy or rubbery feel. Firm pressure over this area usually elicits tenderness. Visible swelling of the elbow joint usually becomes apparent over the lateral area between the radial head and the olecranon especially in full extension (Bilka, 1970).

Juxta-articular cysts in the forearm adjacent to the elbow joint have been described (Ehrlich, 1972; Ehrlich & Gutman, 1973). These cysts communicate with the elbow joint, and rice bodies and synovial proliferation may act as ball valves, allowing fluid to flow from the joint cavity into the cyst but not the reverse. Rupture of the elbow joint has also been described. Occasionally these cysts may lie posteriorly (Pirani et al, 1982). Rupture of the elbow joint may occur and cause forearm oedema. Leakage of synovial fluid from an olecranon bursa has also been described as a cause of the latter (MacFarlane & Van der Linden, 1981).

Synovial hypertrophy at the elbow joint may be evident on plain films and can be confirmed by arthrography (Jackman & Pugh, 1970; Weston, 1971).

Hand and wrist

The joints of the hand and wrist are seldom spared in rheumatoid arthritis. The following clinical features should be noted:

Dorsal surface

1. Synovial hypertrophy of the wrist joint
2. Extensor tendon and extensor pollicis longus involvement
3. Prominence of the ulnar styloid
4. Wasting of the dorsal interossei
5. Involvement of the metacarpophalangeal joints with ulnar deviation
6. Involvement of the proximal interphalangeal joints with 'buttonhole' and 'swan-neck' deformities
7. The typical Z-shaped deformity of the thumb.

Volar surface

1. Swellings along flexor sheaths and 'trigger finger'
2. Heaping up of the flexor retinaculum, with compression of median and ulnar nerves
3. Wasting of the intrinsic muscles due to median and/or ulnar nerve compression, or peripheral neuropathy.

Synovial swelling along the extensor tendons on the dorsum of the wrist joint may be difficult to distinguish from synovial hypertrophy arising from the wrist joint. Arthrography has shown that communications not only occur between the carpal joints, but also between the wrist joint and the extensor tendon sheaths (Harrison et al, 1971). Synovial hypertrophy in the wrist joint in arthrograms is shown by a corrugated pattern (Ranawat et al, 1969).

Dorsal subluxation of the ulnar styloid (Fig. 26.6) is a common deformity in the rheumatoid wrist. The ulnar collateral ligament is stretched by the hypertrophied synovium of the radioulnar joint until it is torn from its attachment to the ulnar styloid. This results in the distal end of the ulna springing upwards. The ulnar head often shows erosions early in the course of the disease. Rheumatoid involvement of the inferior radioulnar joint is often very troublesome for the patient, giving rise to pain, especially on wrist rotation. Bony spikes have been described (Vaughan-Jackson, 1948) against which the extensor tendons to the little finger chafe and rupture. Bäckdahl (1963) pointed to the caput ulnae as the cause of extensor tendon rupture due to the hypermobility of the ulnar head. However, Backhouse et al (1971) found neither of these causes important, the tendons having ruptured owing to necrosis as a result of granulomatous infiltration. Any of the extensor tendons to the fingers may rupture, as may the extensor pollicis longus.

Instability of the wrist may cause the carpus to sublux from the lower end of the radius towards the palm of the hand. This results in severe loss

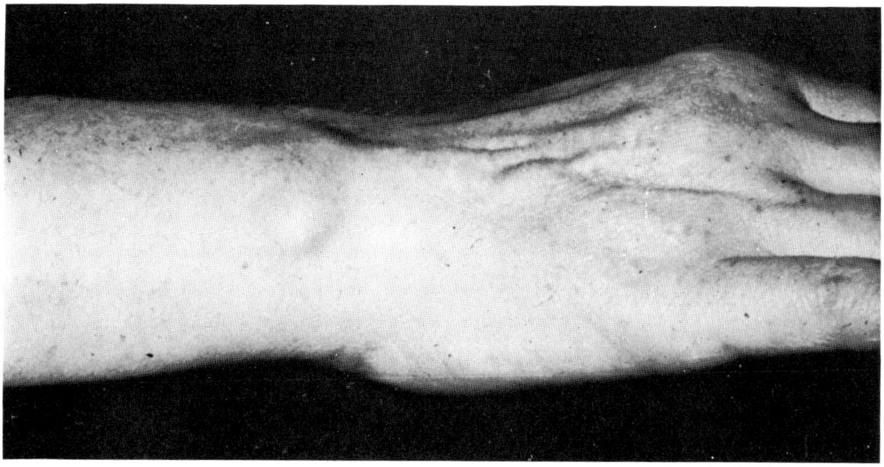

Fig. 26.6 Ulnar head prominence in a patient with rheumatoid arthritis.

of grip power, which may also be associated with a diminished ability to discriminate differences in weights placed in the hand (Korin & Tobis, 1971). There may also be radial or ulnar deviation of the wrist joint.

In addition to ulnar head erosion, X-ray of the wrist may show joint space widening in the radioulnar, navicular-capitate and navicular-lunate joints in early disease (Collins et al, 1972). Cyst formation and sclerosis of the radius has been attributed to impinging of the radius against the lunate during flexion and extension, or ulnar movement of the wrist, as shown by cineradiography (Arkless, 1967). A carpal notch or indentation is often seen on the radial aspect of the scaphoid: this must not be interpreted as a rheumatoid erosion as it is a normal anatomical finding in healthy subjects (Swezey & Alexander, 1969).

Flexor tendons may become involved at the wrist (Ranawat & Straub, 1970), and the median and (less commonly) the ulnar nerves may undergo compression under the flexor retinaculum (carpal tunnel syndrome) (Fig. 26.7).Compression of the median nerve produces weakness and wasting of the abductor pollicis brevis and opponens pollicis, with resulting hollowing of the lateral edge of the thenar eminence. Winding a watch becomes difficult due to weakness of abduction and opposition of the thumb. Sensory disturbance occurs in the thumb, index, middle and ring fingers. Diffuse pain in the hands is common, and may be more severe at night. Extension of the wrist, percussion over the median nerve (Tinel's sign), and ischaemia induced by inflation of a brachial arterial cuff provoke and exacerbate symptoms.

Ulnar nerve entrapment at the wrist produces wasting of the interossei and muscles of the hypothenar eminence. Sensory symptoms may occur in the ring and fifth finger. When ulnar nerve entrapment occurs as a result of elbow joint disease the flexor carpi ulnaris and flexor digitorum profundus are also weakened.

The late Dr Philip Hench used to refer to the arthritic patient's hand as his 'calling card'. Certainly in the patient with rheumatoid arthritis this is particularly relevant, and the feature which 'announces' the diagnosis is the ulnar deviation of the metacarpophalangeal joints (Fig. 26.8). The pathogenesis of ulnar deviation is complex, but there is a significant correlation between the position of the wrist and metacarpophalangeal angulation in rheumatoid disease that does not

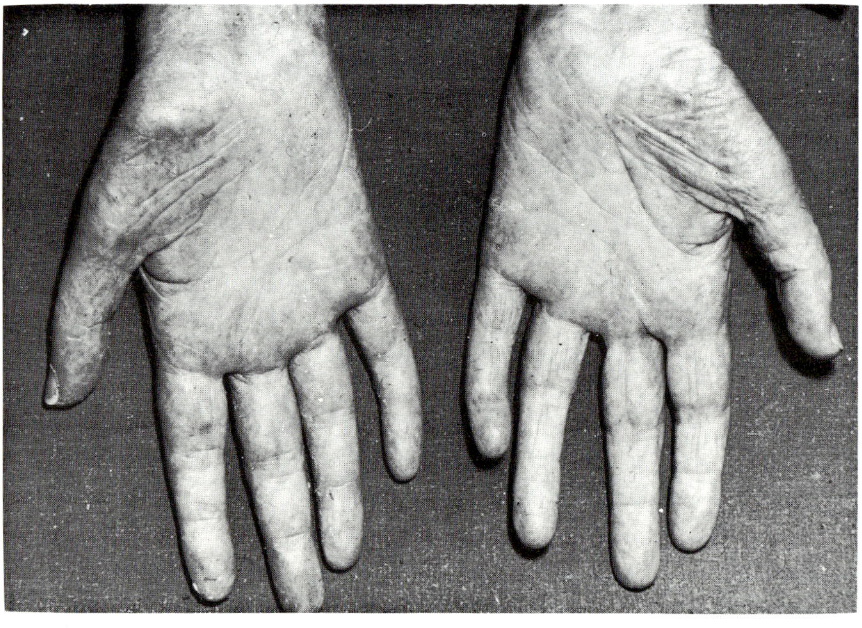

Fig. 26.7 Bilateral carpal tunnel syndrome in a patient with rheumatoid arthritis. Note the marked wasting of the hands.

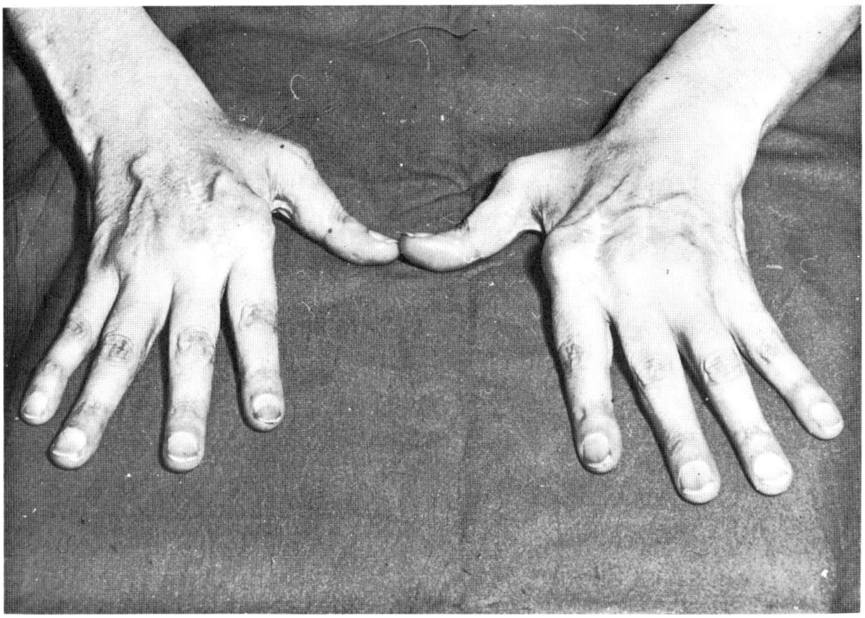

Fig. 26.8 Typical ulnar deviation of the fingers in a patient with rheumatoid arthritis.

appear to present in normals nor in other joint diseases (Read et al, 1983).

The events in order of importance according to Swezey (1971–1972) are:

1. Chronic inflammation of the synovial lining of the metacarpophalangeal joints (Fearnley, 1951).
2. Stretching of the volar supports of the flexor tendon sheaths, weakened by adjacent joint inflammation, by the long finger flexors of the three central digits during pinching activity (Snorrason, 1951; Smith et al, 1966; Hakstian & Tubiana, 1967; Backhouse, 1968).
3. Overstretching of the anatomically weaker radial collateral ligament (Vainio & Oka, 1953; Hakstian & Tubiana, 1967; Eaton, 1969; Backhouse, 1972).
4. Loss of the stabilising bulwark of the fifth digit because of the powerful ulnar pull of the abductor digiti quinti on the weakened radial collateral ligament (Fearnley, 1951; Brewerton, 1957; Straub, 1959–60).
5. Stretching of the horizontal fibres of the radial side of the extensor hood weakened by adjacent inflammation (Backhouse, 1968).
6. Weakening of the pull of the radial interosseous muscle by virtue of stretched hood attachment (Fearnley, 1951).
7. Further stretching of the extensor hood and ulnarward deviation of the extensor tendon by synovium bulging through the weak area between the central and horizontal slips of the extensor tendon over the metacarpophalangeal joint (Fearnley, 1951).
8. Ulnar drift of the long extensor tendon into the ulnar sulcus adjacent to the affected metacarpophalangeal joints allowing an ulnar bowstring force of the long extensor to further pull the digit into ulnar deviation (Fearnley, 1951; Snorrason, 1951; Brewerton, 1957, 1965). Disease in the carpi with ulnar displacement of the proximal row and associated radial rotation of the distal carpi and metacarpals due to the relatively unopposed force of the radial carpal extensors and flexor muscles is followed by 'compensatory' ulnar phalangeal drift enhanced by the greater ulnar angulation of the flexor tendons as they emerge from the wrist (Shapiro, 1968; Pahle & Raunio, 1969; Shapiro, 1970).

However, this last concept of a 'zig-zag' phenomenon occurring between the wrist and the metacarpophalangeal joints, although present in some patients, is by no means a constant finding (Swezey, 1971–1972).

Gravity and lateral pressure on the hand during everyday manoeuvres, such as pulling out a chair, have been discounted as causes of ulnar deviation (Lush, 1952). However, during grasping, pressure is transmitted against the index finger in a radial direction (Fearnley, 1951; Flatt, 1959; Hakstian & Tubiana, 1967). Radial deviation of the fingers occasionally occurs, especially in young patients (Brewerton, 1957).

Clinical examination of the metacarpophalangeal joints in early stages of the disease often reveals soft tissue swelling around the metacarpal heads (Fig. 26.9). Tenderness can be elicited by firm pressure exerted directly on the metacarpal heads or alternatively by lateral pressure on the second and fifth metacarpal head. Soft tissue swelling can be seen on X-rays of the metacarpophalangeal joints, and capsular distension may give rise to separation of the metacarpal heads. Very fine periosteal reaction proximal to the metacarpal head is often transient and may precede cortical erosion (Bywaters, 1960). Cortical erosions, if not seen on anteroposterior films, may become apparent on tomography (Kersley et al, 1964) or when X-rays are taken with the hands and wrists in a halfway supinate position (Nørgaard, 1965) or in a tangential projection (Brewerton, 1967). Early erosions have a 'soft' or fuzzy base: healed erosions, which often result in a hook-like appearance (Bywaters, 1960) have a 'hard' clear base.

In early disease the proximal interphalangeal joints may show marked soft-tissue swelling, giving rise to the characteristic spindle-shaped deformity. This, however, is not specific for rheumatoid arthritis, since any condition giving rise to swelling of the proximal interphalangeal joint, while sparing the distal interphalangeal joint, can give rise to spindling. Increase in pigmentation may be seen overlying the skin of the proximal interphalangeal joint in early disease in dark-skinned individuals. In more advanced disease a 'swan-neck' deformity (Fig. 26.10) may occur. This consists of a hyperextension of the proximal interphalangeal joint, associated with flexion of the terminal interphalangeal joint. The deformity is complex in its pathogenesis. Tightness of the intrinsic muscles may be primary, but more often is secondary to synovial hypertrophy or forward subluxation of the metacarpophalangeal joint

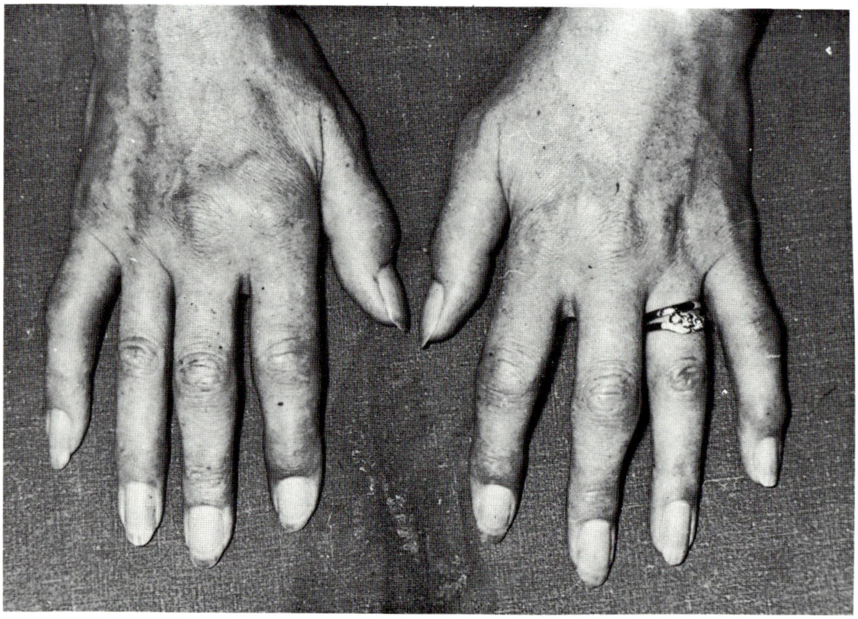

Fig. 26.9 Early rheumatoid arthritis of the hands. Note the swelling of the metacarpophalangeal and proximal interphalangeal joints and interphalangeal joints of the thumbs.

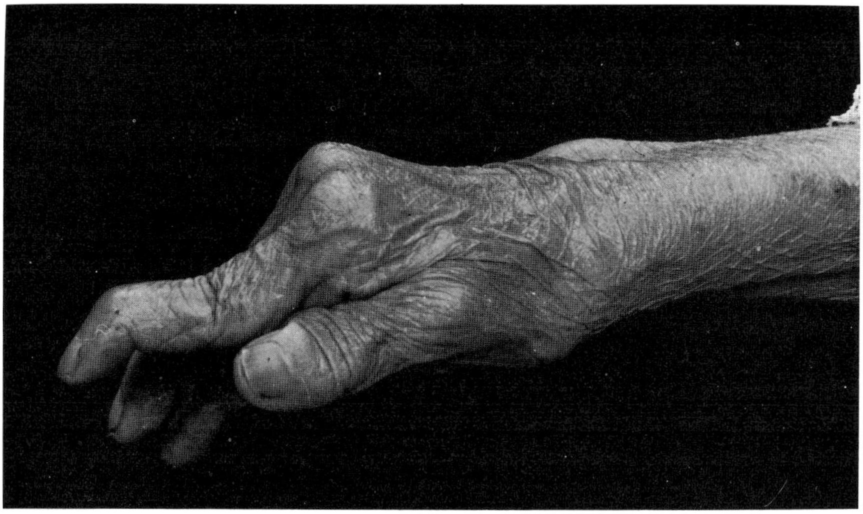

Fig. 26.10 Typical 'swan-neck' deformity.

which causes the intrinsic muscles and tendons to be stretched tight. This 'intrinsic plus' deformity, as it is often called, causes the metacarpophalangeal joints to flex as the fingers are extended. If there is laxity or destruction, however, of the volar plate of the proximal interphalangeal joint, then hyperextension of this joint will occur owing to the tight interossei (Brewerton, 1957). The interossei on histological examination usually show normal muscle fibres and no fibrosis (Vainio, 1967). Tightness of the intrinsic muscles can be tested clinically by extension of the metacarpophalangeal joints, which increases tension on the intrinsic muscles, thus resulting in increase in the deformity. Flexion of the metacarpophalangeal joints causes relaxation of the intrinsic muscles permitting flexion of the proximal interphalangeal joints. Section of the intrinsic tendons relieves the swan-neck deformity (Littler, 1949). In severe long-standing cases of swan-neck deformity, fibrous and bony ankylosis of the proximal interphalangeal joints may occur (Swezey, 1971–1972).

In the swan-neck deformity the distal interphalangeal joint becomes flexed, owing to the pull of the extended profundus tendon which exceeds the pull of the long extensor tendon which is bowstrung across the proximal interphalangeal joints (Straub, 1959–1960). Flexion of the distal interphalangeal joint may occur owing to avulsion of the distal phalangeal extensor tendon insertion with resulting mallet finger deformity (McCarty & Gatter, 1966). A mallet finger deformity may itself result in a swan-neck deformity (Littler & Eaton, 1967). Occasionally rupture of the sublimis tendon may result in a swan-neck deformity (Vaughan-Jackson, 1962).

As a consequence of chronic inflammation of the proximal interphalangeal joint the insertion of the central slip of the extensor tendon may become stretched or torn from its insertion into the base of the middle phalanx. This causes the proximal interphalangeal joint to protrude upwards through the lateral extensions of the extensor tendon like a button through a buttonhole, hence the term 'buttonhole' or 'boutonnière' deformity (Brewerton, 1957; Flatt, 1959; Littler & Eaton, 1967), (Fig. 26.11). The lateral fibres of the extensor tendons slip down on each side of the proximal interphalangeal joint and act as flexors to the joint (Littler & Eaton, 1967).

Casagrande (1965) has also made the interesting suggestion that the buttonhole deformity may result from tautness of the sublimis tendon, which is obstructed at the entrance to the flexor tendon sheath either by nodule formation or proliferative tenosynovitis. The sublimis tendon is inserted into the base of the middle phalanx and the proximal interphalangeal joint is consequently pulled into flexion.

The thumb is often very severely involved in

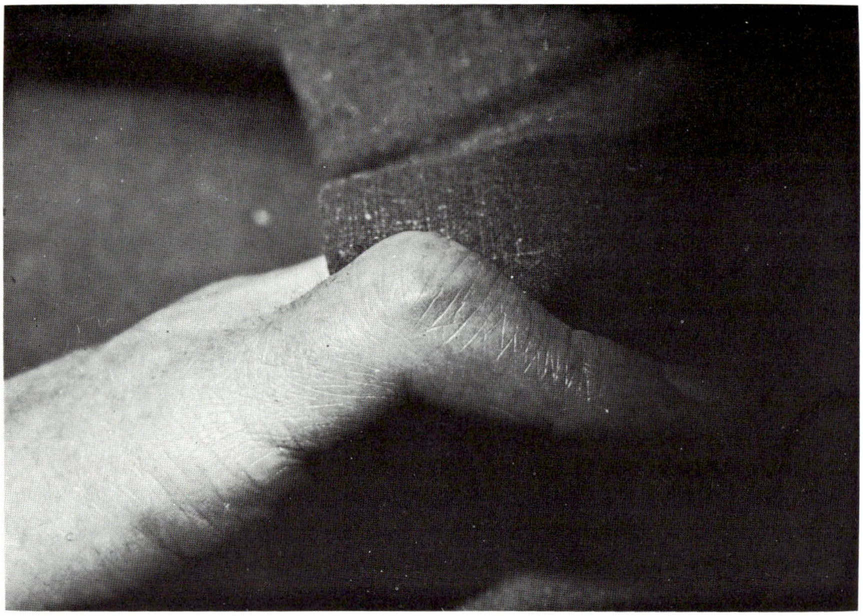

Fig. 26.11 Typical 'buttonhole' deformity.

rheumatoid arthritis. If the metacarpophalangeal joint is severely damaged the long and short thumb extensors are displaced volarwards on the ulnar side of the thumb. This causes loss of extension of the metacarpophalangeal joint (extrinsic minus). Hyperextension of the distal phalanx now occurs due to tension on the long thumb extensor. This deformity is often termed the 'Z-shaped' or 'hitch-hikers's' deformity (Fig. 26.12).

Other deformities of the thumb may be found when there is severe disease of the carpometacarpal joint. This causes volar subluxation of the first metacarpal, resulting in contracture of the adductor hallucis (intrinsic plus) and adduction of

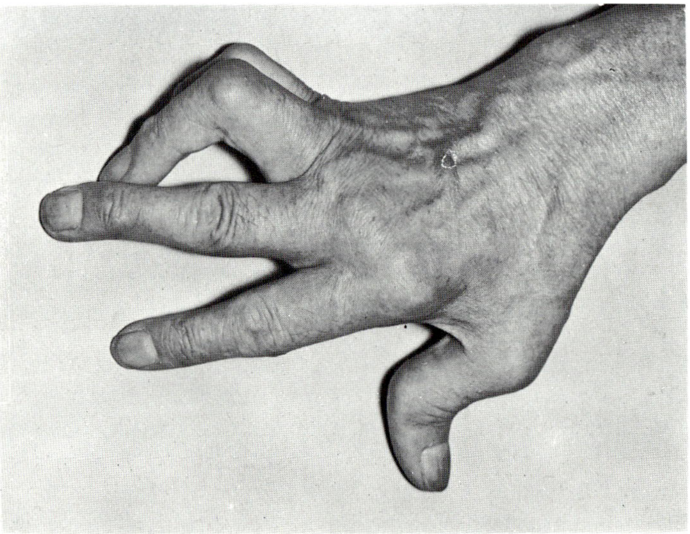

Fig. 26.12 Typical Z-shaped deformity of the thumb in a patient with rheumatoid arthritis.

the proximal thumb. Hyperextension of the metacarpophalangeal or interphalangeal joint may then occur, depending on which of the joints is more lax as a result of rheumatoid involvement (Swezey, 1971–1972).

It is extremely important to recognise synovitis of both flexor and extensor tendon sheaths in rheumatoid arthritis. Triggering of the flexor tendon at the level of the metacarpal head as it enters the flexor sheath is not uncommon. The profundus tendon may be entrapped at the level of the proximal interphalangeal joint just distal to the sublimis decussation, and cause limitation of passive flexion. The diagnosis of entrapment of the sublimis tendon can be confirmed clinically: when the proximal interphalangeal joint is put into maximum flexion there is loss of voluntary flexion at the distal interphalangeal joint. Rupture of flexor tendons is often unrecognised.

Extensor tendon synovitis is easily recognized as a mass just distal to the extensor retinaculum, but, as previously mentioned, it may occasionally be difficult to differentiate between synovitis of the extensor tendon sheaths and synovial hypertrophy arising from the wrist joint. Dropped fingers are caused by attrition or rupture of the extensor tendons as a result of tendon synovitis (Fig. 26.13). It must also be remembered that dropped fingers may be mimicked by lengthening and weakness of the extensor tendons due to dislocation (Helal, 1974). Another cause of dropped fingers is posterior nerve interosseus nerve palsy, due to involvement of the radial nerve at the elbow joint (Helal, 1974).

In longstanding cases of rheumatoid arthritis the joints may become ankylosed owing to fibrous or bony union. Alternatively severe erosive disease may produce 'egg and cup' radiological appearances which in severe cases results in the 'main-en-lorgnette' deformity or 'opera glass' hand (Silver & Steinbrocker, 1953) (Fig. 26.14). Palmar erythema is often seen in severe rheumatoid arthritis, but it no more common in patients with rheumatoid arthritis than in age and sex-matched controls (McAvoy et al, 1969). Longitudinal ridging of the nails appears to occur at an earlier age in patients with rheumatoid arthritis (Hamilton, 1960).

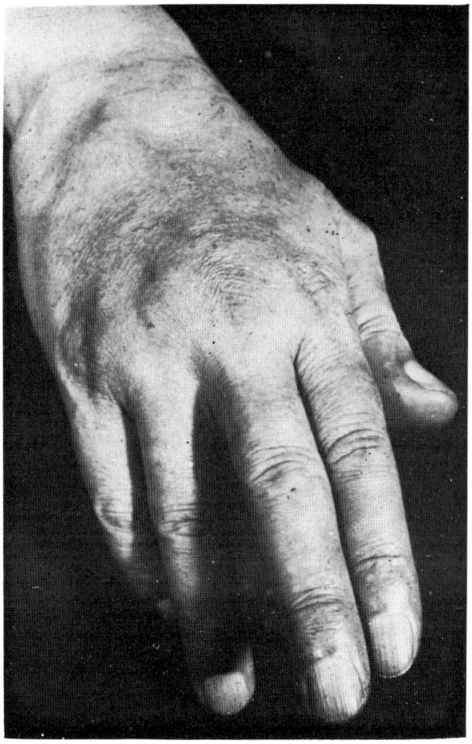

Fig. 26.13 Rupture of the extensor tendons to the 4th and 5th digits in a patient with rheumatoid arthritis.

Although it is universally taught that rheumatoid arthritis affects the proximal and not the distal interphalangeal joints McCarty & Gatter (1966) have clearly shown that clinical and radiological evidence of distal interphalangeal joint involvement occurs frequently. Moreover, Collins and his colleagues (Collins et al, 1971; Dick et al, 1972) have shown that the uptake of radioactive pertechnetate (^{99m}Tc) is as high in the distal as in the proximal interphalangeal joints.

Examination of the hands plays an important part in the overall assessment of a patient's progress. Measurement of grip strength by a sphygmomanometer cuff has proved useful (Lee et al, 1974). Recording the circumference of the proximal interphalangeal joints and interphalangeal joints of the thumbs by either jeweller's rings or a plastic spring gauge is the standard method for assessing anti-inflammatory effect of antirheumatic drugs (Webb et al, 1973). Uptake of radioisotopes by inflamed finger joints has also been shown to be of value in assessing anti-inflamma-

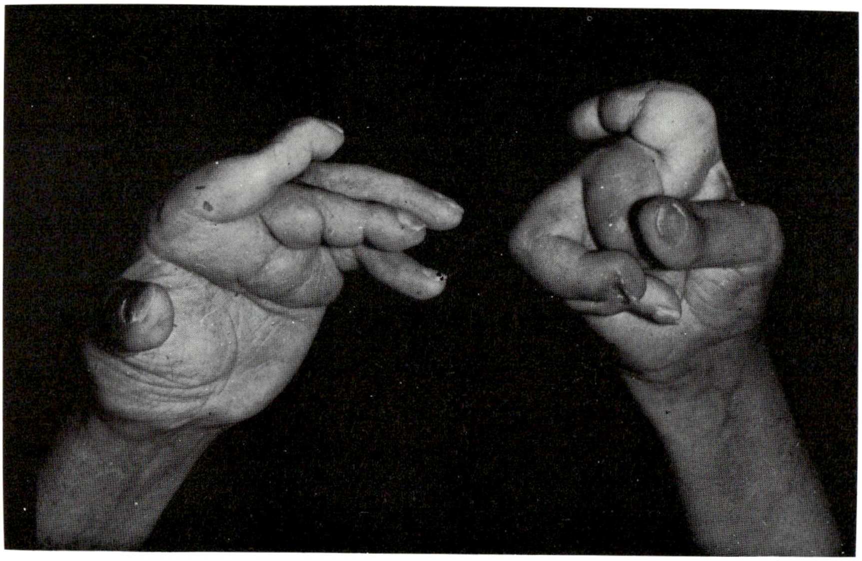

Fig. 26.14 Extremely severe deformity of the hands in rheumatoid arthritis. The joints of the left hand had completely been destroyed so that the joints could be pulled in and out like a concertina.

tory action of drugs (Collins et al, 1971; Dick et al, 1972). Sharp et al (1971) have evolved a quantitative method for recording radiographic abnormalities in the hands and wrists.

Hip joints

The hip joints are mercifully spared in most patients with adult rheumatoid arthritis; this is probably due to a relative paucity of synovial tissue, compared with joints such as the knee joint. By contrast, the hip joints are frequently involved in juvenile rheumatoid arthritis, where bony ankylosis is not an infrequent outcome in severe cases (Jacqueline et al, 1961). Even mild involvement of the hip joint can produce severe pain and disability.

It is important when examining hip joint movement to have the patient lying relaxed on his back and to use both hands! One hand should be placed on the iliac crest in order to detect pelvic movement and not mistake it for true hip movement, while the other hand is used to move the leg. According to Bilka (1968b) internal rotation, extension and abduction are lost earlier than flexion, adduction or external rotation. It is difficult to test for synovial tenderness, as most patients are 'sensitive' to palpation in the femoral area. Occasionally an anterior bulging may be present as a result of synovial hypertrophy. Patients with involvement of the hip joint invariably walk with a limp and have apparent shortening of the leg, which can be differentiated from real shortening, which is extremely rate, by measuring the distance between the anterior superior iliac spine to the medial malleolus. Tenderness over the greater trochanter may be present in rheumatoid arthritis, due to bursitis. Atrophy of muscles with flattening of the buttocks may be apparent with severe involvement of the hip joints, and rheumatoid nodules may be palpated over the sacrum and ischial tuberosities.

The earliest and most common radiological finding in the hips in rheumatoid arthritis is loss of joint space (Duthie & Harris, 1969). In patients with severe hip involvement resorption and destruction of the acetabular side of the joint may occur, giving rise to protrusio acetabuli. This radiological finding has often been said to occur only in rheumatoid arthritis and other inflammatory arthritides, but it may also occasionally be seen in patients with osteoarthritis. Osteophytosis is rarely seen in the hip joint severely affected by rheumatoid arthritis (Duthie & Harris, 1969). Avascular necrosis of femoral head is not uncommon in patients with rheumatoid arthritis, especially those being treated with corticotrophin or oral corticosteroid therapy. The pathogenesis of avascular necrosis in rheumatoid arthritis is unknown, but probably results from the collapse of the osteoporotic bone in the femoral head (Sweetnam et al, 1960). It has been claimed that capsular thickening may be seen on plain X-rays of the hip joint, but this has been doubted by Weston (1970).

Cysts occasionally arise from the hip joint, similar to Baker's cysts behind the knee. These have been found to contain fibrovascular tissue (Colton & Darby, 1970). Hip cysts have been reported to present as a 'psoas bursa' below the inguinal ligament displacing forward the femoral artery (Jeremy, 1969), and also to penetrate into the pelvis causing bladder compression (Watson & Ochsner, 1967).

Raman & Haslock (1982) have drawn attention to trochanteric bursitis as a frequent cause of 'hip' pain in rheumatoid arthritis.

Sacroiliac joint

Asymptomatic radiological changes in the sacroiliac joints in rheumatoid arthritis are not uncommon (Sharp, 1957; Dixon & Lience, 1961; Sievers & Laine, 1963; Wilkinson & Meikle, 1966). The changes include joint narrowing and fusion, and in a few patients para-articular sclerosis and erosions (Wilkinson & Meikle, 1966).

Symphysis pubis

Changes may be seen on plain X-rays of the symphysis pubis in patients with rheumatoid arthritis, especially in those with disease of long duration (Dilsen et al, 1962). These changes include small erosions, which are better visualised by tomography (Kormano, 1971). As with the sacroiliac joints, involvement of the symphysis pubis in rheumatoid arthritis is usually asymptomatic.

Knee joint

Knee joint involvement is particularly troublesome in rheumatoid arthritis, and patients often walk more stiffly than would be expected from clinical examination (Kettelkamp et al, 1972). The most frequently overlooked abnormality in the early stages of rheumatoid arthritis affecting the knee joint is loss of knee joint extension (Bilka, 1968b). Minimal knee joint flexion deformities can be corrected, if detected early enough, but if they have been present for several months only 50% will be completely corrected, and the relapse rate is high (Convery et al, 1971). It is important in testing knee movement that full extension to 180° be looked for, otherwise mild flexion contractures can easily be missed (Bilka, 1970). Goniometry is useful to chart progress in knee joint flexion, and has a remarkably low intra- and inter-observer error (Mitchell et al, 1975). In addition to lateral and medial ligament and anterior and posterior cruciate ligament laxity, mobility of the patella should also be tested. Synovial hypertrophy can be ascertained by careful palpation, and the presence of effusion can be detected by ballottement of the patella or radiologically (Weston, 1971). Very small effusions can be recognised clinically by stroking the medial aspect of the joint firmly from above downwards (to displace fluid laterally) and immediately thereafter stroking the lateral aspect of the joint in the same direction: this sends a fluid wave to the medial aspect of the joint, which can be seen as a sudden ballooning out of the skin just medial to the patella (Cary, 1966). Popliteal cysts or Baker's cysts (Fig. 26.15) as they are often termed (Baker, 1877), are best examined by

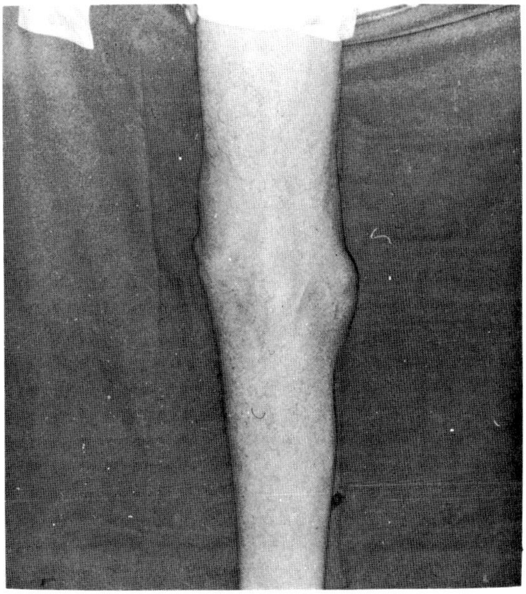

Fig. 26.15 Tense Baker's cyst in the knee joint of a patient with rheumatoid arthritis.

palpating the popliteal fossa with the patient lying prone as they can easily be missed (Genovese et al, 1972).Atrophy of the quadriceps should always be noted, because if not corrected by physiotherapy it may contribute to joint instability.

The bursae at the back of the knee joint, especially the gastrocnemius and semimembranosus bursae, may become enlarged and tender. These cysts may become huge and descend into the calf (Fig. 26.16) and reach as far as the ankle (Perri et al, 1968). Occasionally they may become infected (Hall & Healey, 1968). Pressure studies indicate that in the presence of effusion knee joint movement produces high intra-articular pressures, in contrast to the subatmospheric pressures in the normal joint (Caughey & Bywaters, 1963; De Andrade et al, 1965; Jayson & Dixon, 1970). This increased intra-articular pressure reduces synovial blood flow (Jayson & Dixon, 1970) and may give rise to popliteal cysts, or, if the increase in pressure is very acute, to rupture of the joint itself (Dixon, 1964; Hall & Scott, 1966; Tait et al, 1967; Myles, 1971). Popliteal cysts appear to have a valvular mechanism allowing synovial fluid to enter the cyst from the joint, but not to return (Jayson & Dixon, 1970; Taylor & Rana, 1973). The joint capsule in rheumatoid arthritis shows an increase in the numbers of inter- and intramolecular cross linkages of collagen, producing effective shortening of collagen fibre length (Steer et al, 1971); this presumably predisposes the joint to rupture with increased intra-articular pressure. Acute rupture of the knee joint or of a Baker's cyst presents as a sudden severe pain in the calf of the leg, which becomes swollen and tender. Oedema of the ankle, slight pyrexia, leucocytosis, and a positive Homan's sign may lead to an erroneous diagnosis of deep venous thrombosis. After the rupture swelling in the knee joint and Baker's cyst often subsides. Arthrography usually clinches the diagnosis of a ruptured cyst or joint (Palmer, 1969; Hughes & Pridie, 1970; Lapayowker et al, 1970). Ultrasound is useful in diagnosing popliteal cysts, but has the disadvantage of not being able to detect a cyst which is leaking, and is of no value when acute rupture of the joint or cyst is suspected (Meire et al, 1974). Nuclear magnetic resonance tomography has not only been shown to be a useful diagnostic tool for detecting popliteal cysts, but may also be useful in estimating and monitoring therapeutic response as demonstrated by changes in the proton skin-lattice relaxation time (T_1) (Hull et al, 1984). ^{125}I-fibrinogen uptake is used widely as a test of deep venous thrombosis, and will give a false positive test in acute rupture of the knee joint or popliteal cyst (Gibbons & Phillips, 1975).

The synovium may become markedly hypertrophied and aggressive causing severe joint destruction (Convey & Clawson, 1971) and even rarely fistula formation (Bennett et al, 1972). The synovium may 'punch' through cortical bone of the femur or tibia, giving rise to huge cysts or géodes in these bones (Jayson et al, 1970). Not all popliteal massess should be assumed to be popliteal cysts. Griffiths et al (1984) have described a popliteal swelling in a 50-year-old patient with seropositive rheumatoid arthritis and foot drop, to be a neural sheath fibrosarcoma and also a popliteal swelling in a 69-year-old non-rheumatoid female which on biopsy was revealed to be a multilocu-

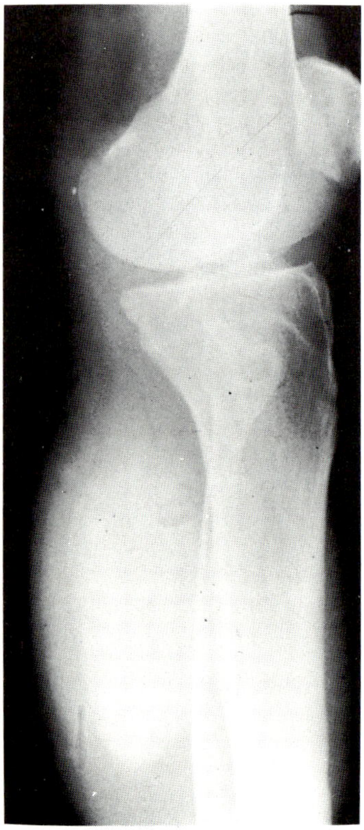

Fig. 26.16 Arthrogram of knee joint showing filling of a Baker's cyst which has tracked down into the calf.

lated spindle cell liposarcoma. We, ourselves, have recently seen two elderly patients with aneurysms of the popliteal artery, which had been diagnosed as Baker's cysts.

Ankle joint

Unlike the knee joint, the ankle joint has relatively little synovial tissue and rheumatoid arthritis is, therefore, uncommon in this site (Dixon, 1971). Pain in the region of the ankle joint is, however, common, being usually due to tendinitis of the posterior tibial and peroneal tendons. The normal ankle joint allows dorsiflexion of at least 15° and plantar flexion of 40° (Bilka, 1970). Synovial hypertrophy can occasionally be marked in the ankle joint and may be palpated or seen radiologically as bulging masses anterior and lateral to the joint margin (Saunders & Weston, 1971). Thickening and nodule formation of the tendon Achilles may be detected clinically and radiologically (Fig. 26.17) and the bursa deep to the tendon Achilles may become inflamed and enlarged (Weston, 1970). Erosions of the os calcis are found in a small proportion of patients: these occur at two sites — one immediately above the insertion of the tendon Achilles, and the other approximately 1 cm posterior to the insertion of the plantar aponeurosis (Fang, 1948; Soila, 1958; Bywaters, 1954; Calabro, 1962; Ennevaara et al, 1965). Periostitis may be seen over the posterior aspect of the os calcis (Fang, 1948). Calcaneal spurs are only slightly more common in patients with rheumatoid arthritis than in controls (Bassiouni, 1965). Achilles tendon rupture is rare in rheumatoid disease but has been reported in association with oral (Rask, 1978) and with local corticosteroid therapy (Bedi & Ellis, 1970; Unverforth & Olix, 1973). Bilateral Achilles tendon rupture has been reported in patients taking corticosteroids for other diseases, e.g. respiratory disorders and polymyalgia rheumatica (Haines, 1983). No doubt the normal use of the foot and ankle in the non-arthritic corticosteroid users contributed to the resultant rupture in Haines' patients.

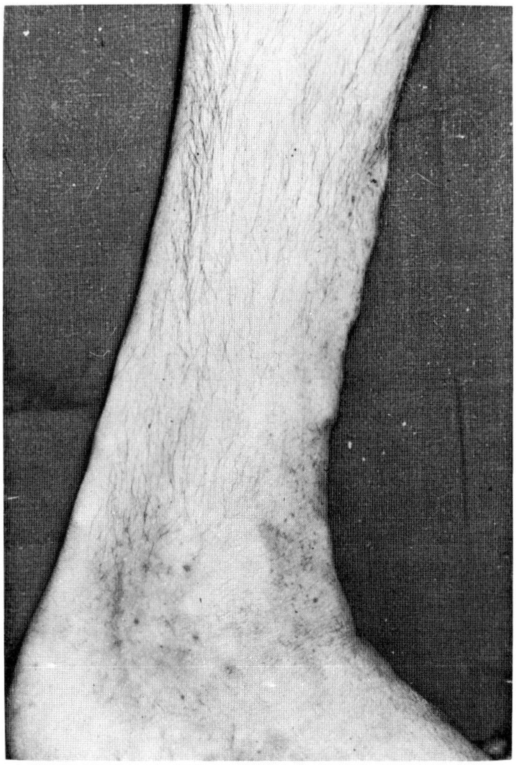

Fig. 26.17 Nodules on the anterior tibial tendons and on the tendo Achillis in a patient with rheumatoid arthritis.

The subtalar or talocalcaneal joint is largely responsible for inversion of the ankle of about 30° and eversion of 20–25° (Bilka, 1970). Unlike the ankle joint it is commonly involved in rheumatoid arthritis (Dixon, 1971). The joint changes are best visualised on a lateral X-ray of the hind foot. Severe involvement of the talonavicular joint leads to a painful valgus deformity of the foot. Subtalar joint disease results in malalignment of the true ankle joint and alters gait. There is a lack of plantar flexion at heel strike and there is a late heel rise. Mechanical compensation takes place at the thigh, knee and ankle to produce a characteristic gait pattern. In severe cases of subtalar disease, the gait of the rheumatoid patient is reduced to a shuffle (Marshall et al, 1980). As a consequence of subtalar disease and also disease in the first and second MTP joints, greater load is thrown on to the three lateral metatarsal heads.

Feet

The feet are frequently involved in rheumatoid arthritis, and pain in the feet is a not uncommon mode of presentation. The most common joints to be affected are the lateral metatarsophalangeal joints (Vidigal et al, 1975). On examination, soft tissue swelling over the metatarsophalangeal joints may be seen and the toes are often separated. Normally in an adult the toes are packed together with the wearing of shoes, but the oedema around the metatarsal heads pushes them apart, allowing 'daylight' to be seen between them (Dixon, 1971). Tenderness of the metatarsal heads can be elicited by lateral tarsal pressure, or by pressure between forefinger and thumb over each metatarsal head. Involvement of the proximal interphalangeal joints of the toes often gives rise to rather square-looking toes, and if oedema of the toes is present the 'sausage-shaped' toes of psoriatic arthritis, where both distal and proximal interphalangeal joints are involved, may be simulated.

Long-standing disease is characterised by marked deformities of the fore-feet, with hallux valgus and packing together of the lateral toes, which may override or underride the hallux or each other (Dixon, 1971) (Fig. 26.18).

With destruction of the metatarsophalangeal joints (Fig. 26.19) the toes become subluxed upwards on the metatarsal heads (Fig. 26.20). The fibro-fatty cushion which normally lies below the metatarsal head moves forward so that there is no longer any protection for the tender eroded metatarsal head, which now has to bear the patient's weight covered only by plantar skin. The toes become clawed and the fat pad under the

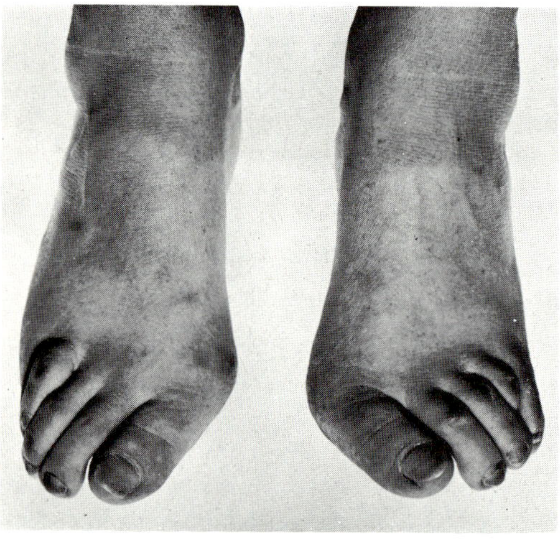

Fig. 26.18 Typical forefoot deformities in a patient with heumatoid arthritis.

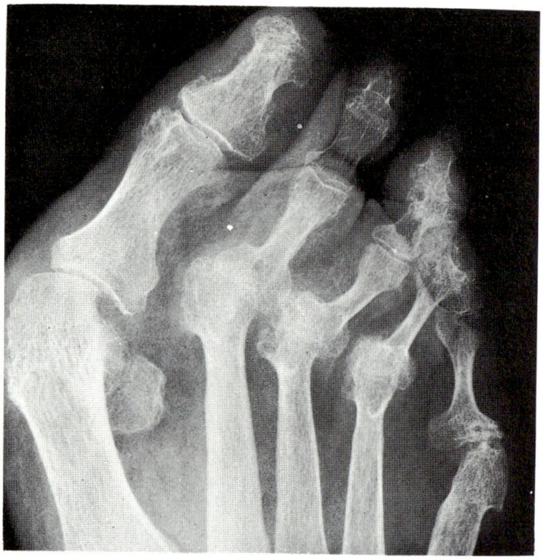

Fig. 26.19 Destruction of the metatarsophalangeal joints in rheumatoid arthritis.

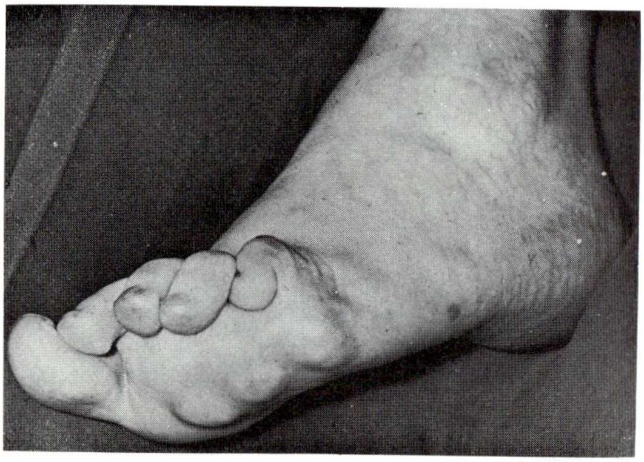

Fig. 26.20 Prominence of the metatarsal heads in the foot of a patient with rheumatoid arthritis. It can be appreciated why patients feel that they are walking on pebbles.

distal phalanx slips backwards so that painful callosities develop over the undersurface of the distal parts of the toes. The skin over the flexed proximal interphalangeal joints likewise becomes painful and inflamed due to the pressure of the shoes. Painful callosities develop under the second and third metatarsal heads in particular (Dixon, 1970), presumably as pressure on standing in the normal foot passes mostly through these two heads and least through the fifth metatarsal head (Collins & Jayson, 1972). The patient often describes the pain over the metatarsal heads as 'if they were walking on pebbles'. Fibrous septa attached to metatarsal bones which have not subluxed often pull on the plantar skin giving rise to clefts. Fluid-filled bursae may develop between the metatarsal heads (Bienenstock, 1975) and fistulae may rarely occur (Bywaters, 1953; Rosin & Toghill, 1963).

Osteoporosis of metatarsal bones sometimes causes March fractures (Dixon, 1971). The tarsal tunnel syndrome is extremely rare in rheumatoid arthritis (Lloyd & Agarwal, 1970) but should always be kept in mind when a patient is being investigated for peripheral neuropathy in the feet. Although tendon involvement is common in the foot actual rupure is rare.

Oedema of the feet and around the ankle joints is common in rheumatoid arthritis. Often it is due to extension of inflammation from acute synovitis, but it can also occur in patients with little or no clinical evidence of synovitis in the ankle or feet. Except in patients with amyloid disease it cannot usually be explained on a basis of hypoalbuminaemia; there is evidence that it is related to an abnormality of capillary function (Jayson & Barks, 1971) and to slowing of lymphatic drainage (Jayson et al, 1971). The oedema is often refractory to diuretic therapy and in long-standing cases may be associated with subcutaneous calcification. Calcification in blood vessels may be seen radiologically around the ankle and in the feet, especially in patients receiving long-term corticosteroid therapy (Kalbak, 1972).

Acromioclavicular, coracoclavicular, sternoclavicular and manubriosternal joints

The acromioclavicular, coracoclavicular, and sternoclavicular joints are frequently tender on pressure in patients with rheumatoid arthritis (de Haas et al, 1965; Nakata & Russell, 1970). Tomography of the manubriosternal joint has revealed erosions in approximately three-quarters of patients (Kormano, 1970; Laitenen et al, 1970). Subluxation or dislocation of the manubriosternal joint can occur (Wiseman, 1981). Although this is a cartilaginous joint, synovial lining can develop as a result of abnormal movement. Khong & Rooney (1982) have stated that manubriosternal dislocation in rheumatoid disease occurs as a consequence of severe cervical disease.

Temporomandibular joint

The frequency of involvement of the temporomandibular joint is emphasised in descriptions of the disease in the 19th century, yet it is only in the last three decades that interest has been taken again in this joint in rheumatoid arthritis (Russel & Bayles,

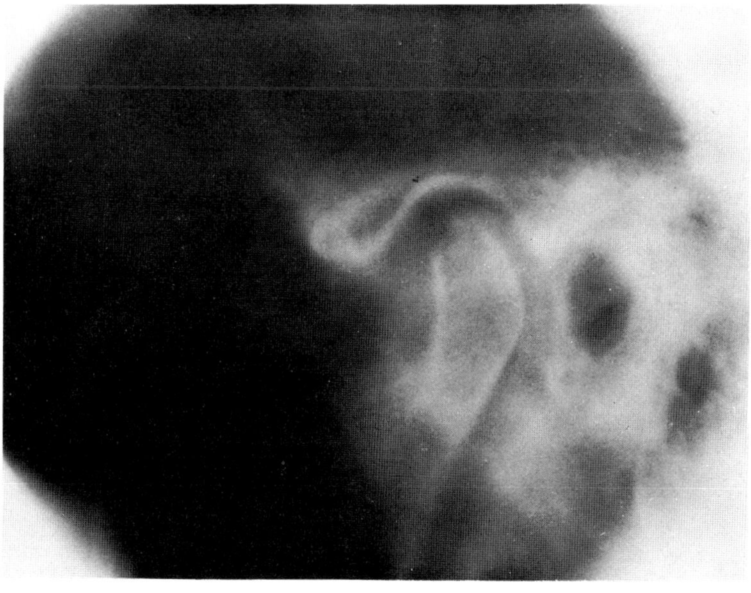

Fig. 26.21 Circular tomography of the temporomandibular joint showing surface erosions of condylar head.

1941; Uotila, 1964; Goodwill & Steggles, 1966; Ericson & Lundberg, 1967; Marbach & Spier, 1967; Chalmers & Blair, 1973). One or more clinical abnormalities were found in 71 of 100 patients with adult rheumatoid arthritis by Chalmers & Blair (1973). Radiological abnormalities were found in 79 of the patients and correlated well with clinical symptoms. Pocket and surface erosion (Fig. 26.21), flattening and marginal proliferations correlated well with limitation in opening the mouth, stiffness, referred pain, tenderness on biting and crepitus. Blair and his colleagues (Blair & Chalmers, 1972; Blair et al, 1973) found that circular tomography appeared to have advantages over other radiological techniques, such as orthopantomography and lateral transcranio-oblique radiography. Although more common in juvenile rheumatoid arthritis, foreshortening of the lower jaw and ankylosis of the temporomandibular joint may occur in the adult disease (Goodwill & Steggles, 1966).

Joints of the inner ear

The joints of the inner ear are diarthrodeal joints. As such they could be involved by rheumatoid arthritis, but this has, as yet, not been described (but see p. 622). There is no loss of hearing in the disease, apart from that produced by salicylates (Goodwill et al, 1972).

Cricoarytenoid joint

Involvement of the cricoarytenoid joints occurs more frequently in rheumatoid arthritis than is generally realised. Hoarseness, pain radiating to the ears, fullness of the throat on swallowing or speaking, and dyspnoea are prominent symptoms. Laryngoscopy often reveals inflammatory swelling of the arytenoid cartilage and vocal cords. In chronic arthritis of the cricoarytenoids one or both vocal cords may become paralysed, and if ankylosis of the joints supervenes, the vocal cords are held in adduction (Montgomery et al, 1955). Acute laryngeal distress may be precipitated by upper respiratory infections and tracheostomy may be required to relieve stridor. Typical changes of rheumatoid arthritis are present in the joints (Baker & Bywaters, 1957; Copeman, 1957; Bienenstock et al, 1963). Hoarseness may also be due to ischaemic recurrent laryngeal nerve paresis (Wolman et al, 1965) and to rheumatoid nodules of the vocal folds (Webb & Payne, 1972).

SYSTEMIC MANIFESTATIONS

Subcutaneous nodules

Perhaps the commonest non-articular manifestation of rheumatoid arthritis is the granulomatous nodule, which is characteristically found near the olecranon process in 20–30% of patients with 'definite' or 'classical' rheumatoid arthritis, as defined by the American Rheumatism Association (Ropes et al, 1959). Although most frequently situated at the elbow (Fig. 26.22), rheumatoid nodules occur in many different sites including tendons (Kellgren & Ball, 1950; McFarland & Hoffer, 1968), bones (Bywaters, 1949; Hunder et al, 1965, Lefkovits, 1969; Dorfman et al, 1970; Ginsberg et al, 1975), heart and pericardium (Baggenstoss & Rosenberg, 1944; Raven et al, 1948), lungs, pleura and larynx (Raven et al, 1948), vocal folds (Webb & Payne, 1972), peritoneum and abdominal wall (Raven et al, 1948), and scalp, sclera and skin (Baker et al, 1971). When present over the pinna of the ear they may be mistaken for gouty tophi, on the bridge of the nose as basal cell carcinomas (Healey et al, 1967), and when present in tendons as xanthomata (Watt & Baumann, 1967; Ginsberg et al, 1975). Occasionally subcutaneous nodules may present as multiple ulcerating papules on the skin (Baker et al, 1971), or as intraspinous masses causing nerve root compression (Friedman, 1970; Linquist & McDonnell, 1970). Not all nodules at the olecranon are necessarily rheumatoid: the wide differential diagnosis includes gouty trophi, rheumatic fever nodules, calcinosis, xanthomata, neurofibromata, non-specific bursal thickening and epidermoid cysts (Wilson & Sokoloff, 1970). If necessary, biopsy will settle the issue.

Sokoloff et al (1953) on the basis of careful dissection of early rheumatoid nodules came to the conclusion that they had a vasculitic basis. This has been refuted by Rasker & Kuipers (1983). However, nodules and clinical features of vasculitis frequently coexist, which supports Sokoloff's hypothesis (Harris, 1972).

Rheumatoid nodules may develop rapidly. Usually, however, they have an insidious onset and persist unchanged for many months or years. The

pleural effusions as in synovial fluid, but it is not certain to what extent this is the case in tuberculous or neoplastic effusions in patients with seropositive rheumatoid arthritis. Although pleural biopsy may reveal typical rheumatoid granulomatous infiltration, it more often shows non-specific changes only (Ward, 1961).

Caplan's syndrome (Caplan, 1953) consists of nodular opacities varying in size from 0.5–5 cm throughout both lungs in a patient with rheumatoid arthritis (Caplan, 1953, 1959) or in a subject with minimal or no rheumatoid arthritis but with positive tests for rheumatoid factor (Miall et al, 1953; Kantor & Morrow, 1958; Caplan et al, 1962). Other industrial dust diseases, such as asbestosis, have been implicated in the pathogenesis of Caplan's syndrome (Campbell, 1958; Richards & Barrett, 1958). The radiological appearance of Caplan's syndrome is of nodular opacities against a background of minimal pneumoconiosis.

Although extremely rare, chronic interstitial pulmonary fibrosis (Fig. 26.31), when it does occur, is sometimes a fatal complication of rheumatoid arthritis (Ellman & Ball, 1948; Cruickshank, 1957; Brannan et al, 1964; Patterson et al, 1965; Thompson, 1965; Walker & Wright, 1968). At least one case of restrictive lung defect has been described in adult-onset Still's disease (Corbett et al, 1983). Males are more commonly affected than females, although both idiopathic chronic interstitial pulmonary fibrosis and rheumatoid arthritis are more common in women (Walker & Wright, 1968). The clinical features of chronic interstitial pulmonary fibrosis in patients with rheumatoid arthritis are the same as those in patients with the idiopathic variety (Walker & Wright, 1968). Cough, dyspnoea, chest pain both pleuritic and non-pleuritic, and haemoptysis are common. Approximately 10% of patients are asymptomatic (Patterson et al, 1965). Cyanosis may be present and finger clubbing is common. Clinically no abnormality may be found on physical examination of the chest, but basal crepitations are often present (Patterson et al, 1965). On chest X-ray

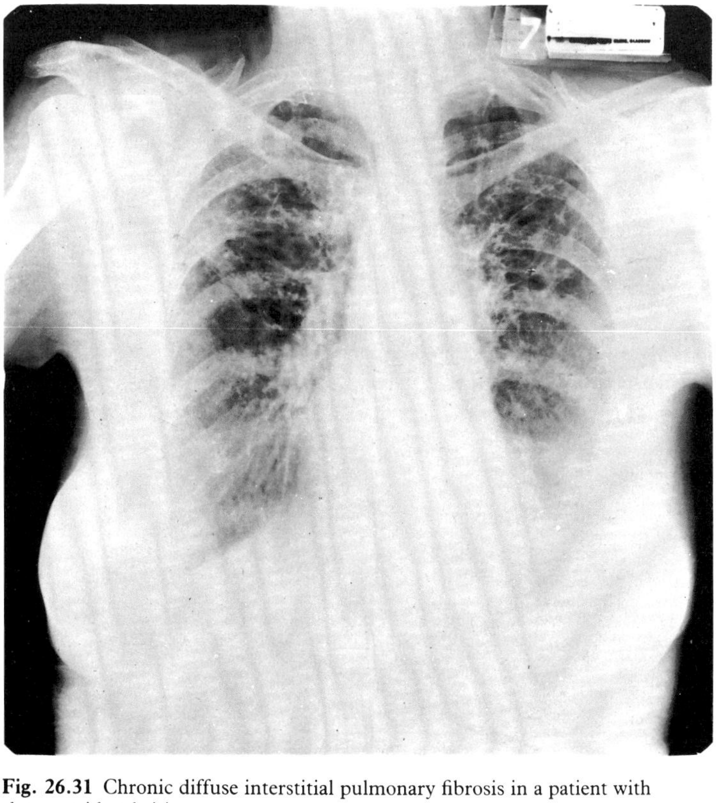

Fig. 26.31 Chronic diffuse interstitial pulmonary fibrosis in a patient with rheumatoid arthritis.

reticulation and mottling are most marked at the lung bases. Cystic changes with honeycombing may be seen in severe cases, and pneumothorax may occur owing to rupture of a cystic bulla (Rubin et al, 1967). Although upper lobe cavitation is a recognised feature of ankylosing spondylitis, there are at least two reports of upper lobe nodule formation and necrosis, cavitation, and fibrosis in rheumatoid arthritis (Petrie et al, 1980; MacFarlane et al, 1984).

Chronic interstitial pulmonary fibrosis may precede arthritis (Fig. 26.31) (Brannan et al, 1964; Walker & Wright, 1968). Surprisingly it may run a relatively benign course in patients with rheumatoid arthritis (Walker & Wright, 1968). Patients who develop chronic interstitial pulmonary fibrosis usually have subcutaneous nodules and positive tests for rheumatoid factor (Walker & Wright, 1968). De Horatius & Williams (1972) have shown in rabbits that human IgM rheumatoid factor accentuates the pulmonary lesions associated with experimental diffuse proliferative lung disease.

Microscopically there is proliferation of interstitial fibrous tissue around the small bronchioles and in the alveolar walls which become thickened with subsequent impairment of gas transfer. A lymphocytic and plasma cell infiltrate is found in the interstitial spaces. Fibrosis may be intense with distortion of bronchi. There appears to be an increased risk of development of alveolar-cell carcinoma (Stack & Grant, 1965).

Pulmonary rheumatoid nodules may occur at any time in the course of rheumatoid arthritis, and have even preceded the onset of arthritis (Portner & Gracie, 1966; Scadding, 1969; Eraut et al, 1978; Hull & Mathews 1982). The size of these nodules varies considerably, from the minute up to 7 cm in diameter (Walker & Wright, 1968). Occasionally cough and haemoptysis may occur (Spence, 1955; Locke, 1963). Cavitation of nodules may be followed by rupture into the pleural cavity and pyopneumothorax (Cudkowicz et al, 1961; Crisp et al, 1982). Finger clubbing has been reported in association with pulmonary rheumatoid nodules. Rheumatoid pulmonary nodules are almost always associated with subcutaneous nodules. If they are single, diagnosis from other causes of a 'coin' lesion, such as tuberculoma or neoplasm, cannot be made with certainly without histological examination.

The pulmonary arteries may be involved in rheumatoid arthritis (Price & Skelton, 1956, Gardner et al, 1957; Jordan & Snyder, 1964; Onodera & Hill, 1965). The pathology is similar to that seen in unexplained pulmonary hypertension and progressive systemic sclerosis. Patients with pulmonary hypertension secondary to pulmonary artery involvement may have digital arterial involvement and Raynaud's phenomenon.

Pneumonia occurs with increased frequency in patients with rheumatoid arthritis (Aronoff et al, 1955; Short et al, 1957; Talbott & Calkins, 1964; Kay, 1967; Walker & Wright, 1968). Aronoff et al (1955) and Kay (1967) found an increased incidence of chronic bronchitis in patients with rheumatoid arthritis compared to controls, but Walker & Wright (1968) found this only in male patients. Sutton et al (1982) demonstrated that lung mucociliary clearance is normal in rheumatoid patients compared to controls, therefore the explanation for the increased incidence of respiratory infection in rheumatoid patients must be related to some other aspect of host resistance. There is evidence that bronchiectasis is also slightly more frequent in patients with rheumatoid arthritis (Aronoff et al, 1955; Stack & Grant, 1965; Walker & Wright, 1968). Penny et al (1982) have recently described obliterative bronchiolitis as a complication of rheumatoid arthritis.

Cardiac involvement

Heart involvement in rheumatoid arthritis is not a particularly common clinical problem. Although approximately 40% of patients show evidence of chronic pericarditis at post-mortem examination (Sokoloff, 1953), only rarely does pericarditis manifest during life, usually at the onset of the disease in a young febrile patient. It is possible that the low incidence of pericarditis found clinically may, as suggested by Wilkinson (1962), be 'due to failure of recognition on the part of both patients and physicians'. Occasionally extensive pericardial fibrosis and constrictive pericarditis require pericardiectomy (Liss & Bachman, 1970). Granulomatous infiltration of the myocardium and conducting system may rarely occur and lead to conduction defects, cardiac arrhythmias and acute myocardial failure (Carpenter et al, 1967). Granulomatous involvement of the valves may lead to valvular insufficiency (Carpenter et al, 1967) when surgical replacement may become necessary (Iveson et al, 1975). Rheumatic heart disease is no more common in patients with rheumatoid arthritis than controls (Bonfiglo & Atwater, 1969). Although coronary arteritis may rarely cause myocardial infarction and death, it is true to say that cardiac deaths in rheumatoid arthritis are usually the result of non-rheumatoid disease, rather than a specific complication of rheumatoid arthritis itself.

Ocular manifestations

Episcleritis is relatively common, and results in mild, often intermittent, ocular pain and injection of the eye. It tends to occur in patients with other evidence of vasculitis and usually resolves leaving no permanent sequelae.

Scleritis (Fig. 26.32), however, is much more important than episcleritis, and may lead to visual impairment and even blindness. Scleritis usually has an insidious onset, but eventually leads to severe pain. The entire uveal tract is inflamed and anterior synechiae may form with the risk of subsequent closed-angle glaucoma. Thinning of the sclera may occur in severe scleritis, and may cause exophthalmos (Kennedy & McGavin, 1975). Blue discolouration of the sclera following severe scleritis does not necessarily indicate thinning of the sclera or the likelihood of immediate rupture.

Scleromalacia perforans results from necrosis and sloughing of a rheumatoid nodule situated in the sclera, leaving a punched-out hole through which the black uveal tract may be seen. Secondary infection may then necessitate enucleation of the eye, or the contents of the eye may pour out leaving the patient blind.

Keratoconjunctivitis sicca occurs in approximately 10% of patients with rheumatoid arthritis (Bloch et al, 1965). The condition may easily be overlooked, and patients may complain of dryness and grittiness of their eyes only on direct questioning. On physical examination the eye may appear normal, and a Schirmer tear test and Rose Bengal staining of the conjunctiva (Fig. 26.33) cornea may be necessary to detect the presence of keratoconjunctivitis sicca. Punctate and filamentary keratitis is best detected by biomicroscopy (Bloch et al, 1965; Whaley et al, 1973).

The diagnosis of keratoconjunctivitis sicca can be made on the basis of a statistical analysis of ocular symptoms and signs (Anderson et al, 1972). Dryness of the eyes may result in extensive symblephora due to shrinkage of the conjunctiva

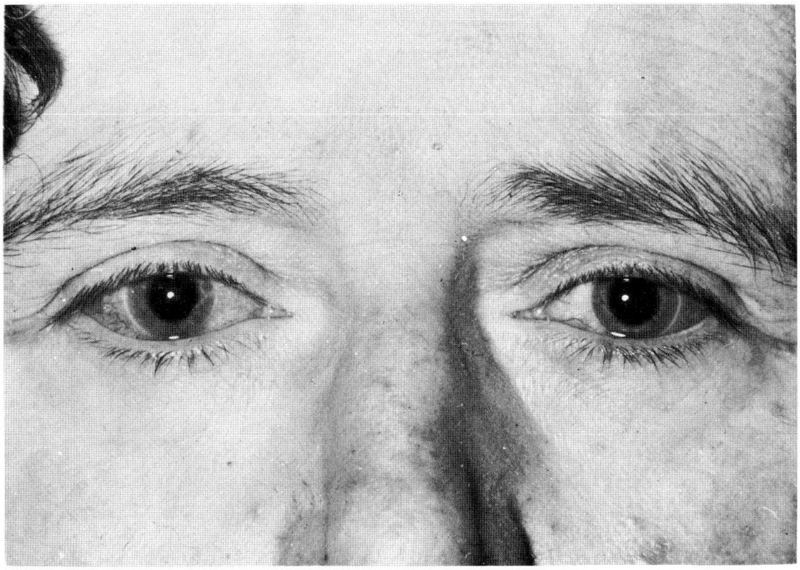

Fig. 26.32 Bilateral scleritis in a patient with rheumatoid arthritis. The eyes were painful and red.

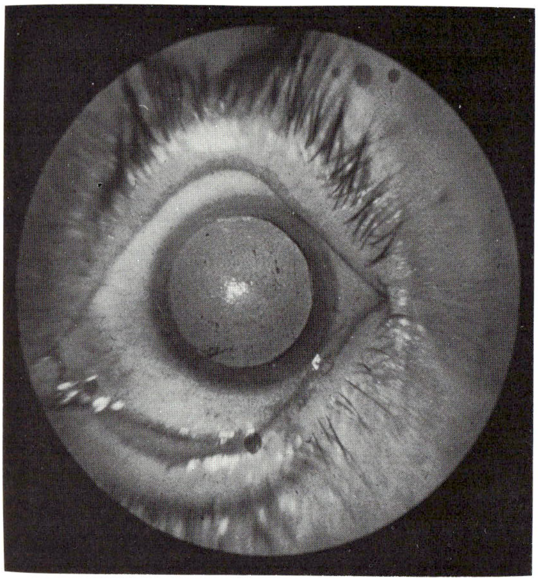

Fig. 26.33 Keratoconjunctivitis sicca. Rose bengal staining of the conjunctiva showing interpalpebral staining in the typical triangular areas.

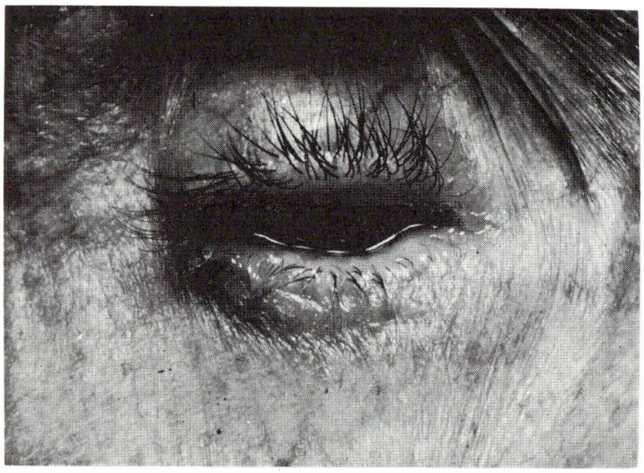

Fig. 26.34 Keratoconjunctivitis sicca. External symblephora due to shrinkage of the conjunctiva.

(Fig. 26.34) or perforation of the cornea with subsequent infection of the eye tissues (Table 26.1). Lacrimal gland enlargement occurs only rarely in rheumatoid arthritis.

Table 26.1 Ocular complications of keratoconjunctivitis sicca

Infection — bacterial and fungal
Corneal ulceration and perforation
Shrinkage of conjunctival fornices leading to exposure keratitis
Symblepharon leading to exposure keratitis

Sjögren's syndrome (see also Ch. 56)

Sjögren's syndrome, first clearly described by Henrik Sjögren in 1933, comprises the triad: dry eyes of keratoconjunctivitis sicca, xerostomia with or without salivary gland enlargement, and in one-half to two-thirds of patients a connective tissue disease, usually rheumatoid arthritis (Bloch et al, 1965; Whaley et al, 1973a, b). When only the first two features are present the term 'sicca syndrome' is often used.

In addition to the ocular and oral manifestations, previously described, patients with Sjögren's syndrome may develop clinical features from involvement of other organs and tissues. These are summarised in Table 26.2. The salient laboratory findings are recorded in Table 26.3. It should be noted that patients with the sicca syndrome appear peculiarly prone to develop lymphoid neoplasms, especially if they receive X-ray therapy for swollen lacrimal or salivary glands (Anderson & Talal, 1972). Patients with lymphomas often develop hypogammaglobulinaemia (Fig. 26.35) (Talal & Bunim, 1964).

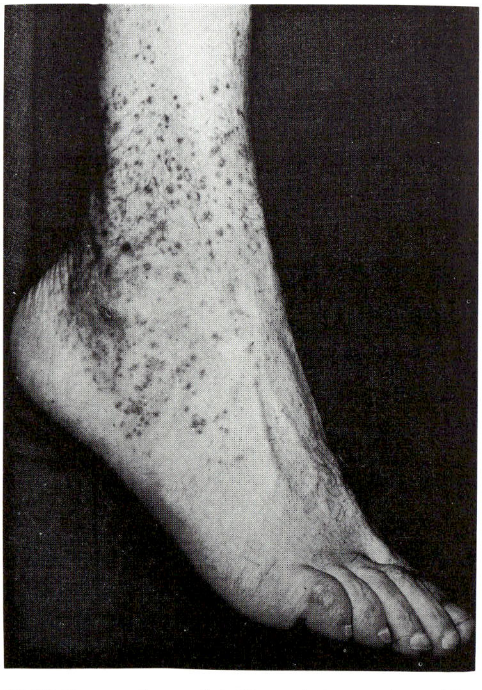

Fig. 26.35 Purpura hyperglobulinaemia in a patient with Sjögren's syndrome.

Table 26.2 Clinical features of Sjögren's syndrome other than ocular and oral symptoms

Respiratory tract	*Nose*	Nasal dryness, crusting, epistaxis, atrophy of nasal mucosa
	Nasopharynx:	Dryness
	Oropharynx:	Dryness, pain on deglutition, dysphagia, and postcricoid web (Paterson–Brown–Kelly or Plummer Vinson syndrome)
	Laryngopharynx:	Hoarseness of the voice
	Ear:	Dryness of skin of external auditory meatus, dry or absent cerumen, blockage of the Eustachian tube by crusts in nasopharynx causing conduction deafness
	Lungs:	Pneumonitis secondary to dryness of trachea and bronchi, chronic interstitial
Skin	Dryness, chronic inflammatory changes in sweat glands Purpura hyperglobulinaemia (Fig. 26.35) Raynaud's phenomenon	
Vagina	Dryness and dyspareunia	
Gastrointestinal system	Chronic atrophic gastritis and achlorhydria Focal biliary cirrhosis Diminution of exocrine/pancreatic excretion and chronic pancreatitis	
Thyroid	Hashimoto's thyroiditis and primary hypothyroidism	
Kidney	Renal tubular acidosis, aminoaciduria, and glycosuria	
Central nervous system	Cranial and peripheral neuropathy Myasthenia gravis	
Drug allergy	Penicillin especially	
Reticuloendothelial system	Lymphadenopathy and splenomegaly	
Connective tissue disease	Rheumatoid arthritis in 50–75% of patients. Rarely systemic lupus erythematosus, polymyositis, progressive systemic sclerosis, and polyarteritis nodosa	
Neoplasm	Extra- and intrasalivary lymphoreticular neoplasms especially in patients with sicca syndrome who have received X-irradiation. Other tumours have included malignant thymoma and Waldenström's macroglobulinaemia	

Table 26.3 Laboratory findings in Sjögren's syndrome

Haematological changes	Anaemia associated with rheumatoid arthritis. (Rarely Coombs positive haemolytic anaemia.) Leucopenia and lymphopenia, eosinophilia
Serum proteins	Diffuse elevation of all three immunoglobulins. Macroglobulinaemia and cryoglobulinaemia rare, as is hyperviscosity syndrome. Hypogammaglobulinaemia in patients with lymphoreticular neoplasm
Autoantibodies	Rheumatoid factors in very high percentage of patients with sicca syndrome, in addition to those with rheumatoid arthritis. High titres of antinuclear antibodies, especially with speckled and nucleolar patterns of staining. DNA antibodies and LE cells only rarely. Non-tissue-specific precipitins. Autoimmune complement fixation tests. Salivary duct autoantibodies, especially in patients with rheumatoid arthritis . Mitochondrial antibodies. Thyroglobulin and thyroid microsomal autoantibodies. Gastric parietal cell autoantibodies.

Involvement of the salivary glands can be detected by salivary flow determination, hydrostatic sialography (Fig. 26.36), radio-isotopic scanning and labial mucosal biopsy (Whaley et al, 1973).

Anaemia

Many patients with rheumatoid arthritis have an anaemia which responds poorly to standard haematinic therapy (Mowat, 1971). Fortunately, the degree of anaemia is rarely severe enough to be incapacitating per se, and there is a correlation between the severity of the disease and the degree of anaemia (Grennan et al, 1975). Morphologically the anaemia is normocytic and normochromic or slightly hypochromic. The bone marrow is normoblastic with an increase in plasma cells, stainable iron is usually present but there is poor haemoglobinisation of red cells. Serum iron levels are low, iron-binding capacity being normal or slightly reduced. Iron absorption is reduced

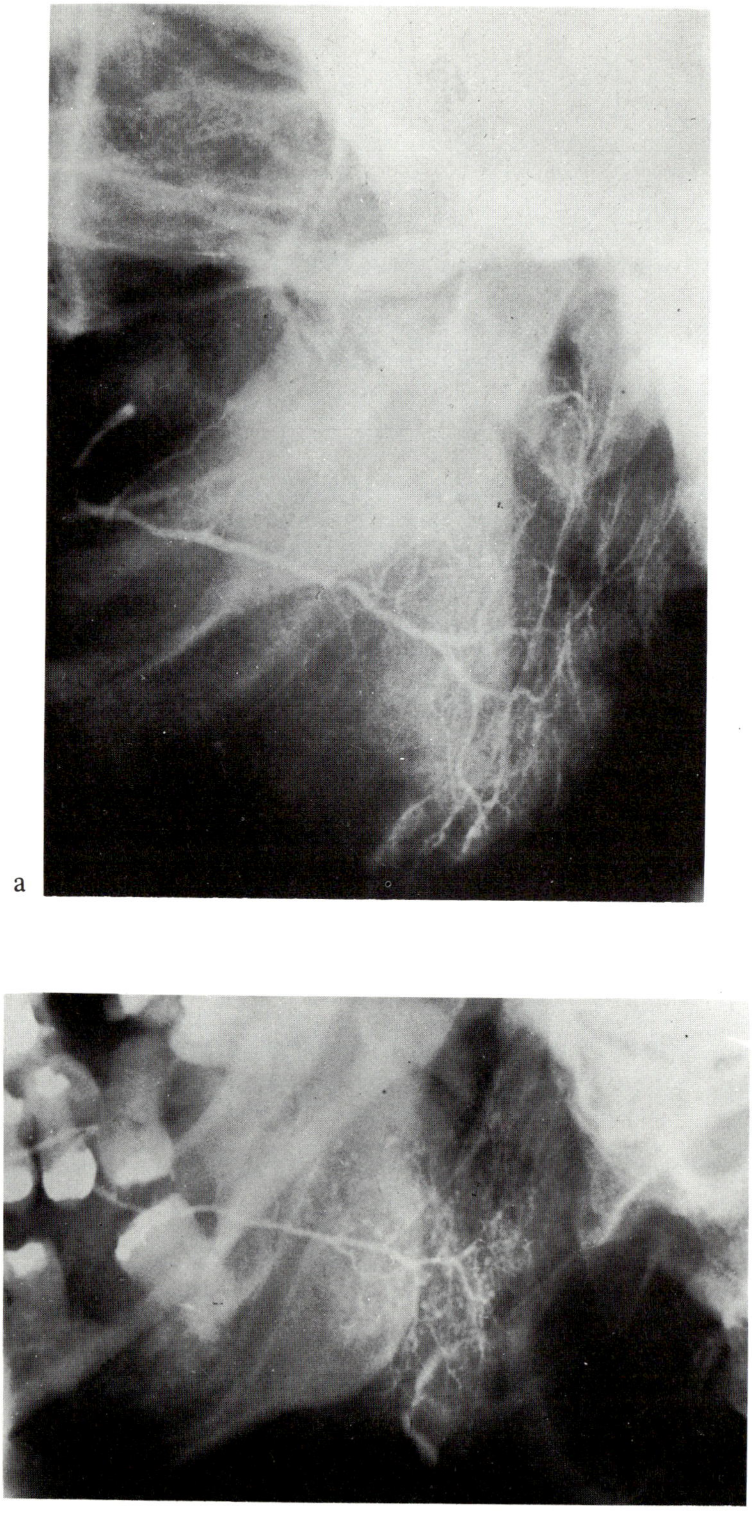

a

b

Fig. 26.36 Hydrostatic sialography: (a) normal parotid sialogram; (b) punctate sialectasis; (c) globular sialectasis; (d) cavitary or destructive sialectasis with irregular main duct dilatation; (e) atrophy of parotid gland.

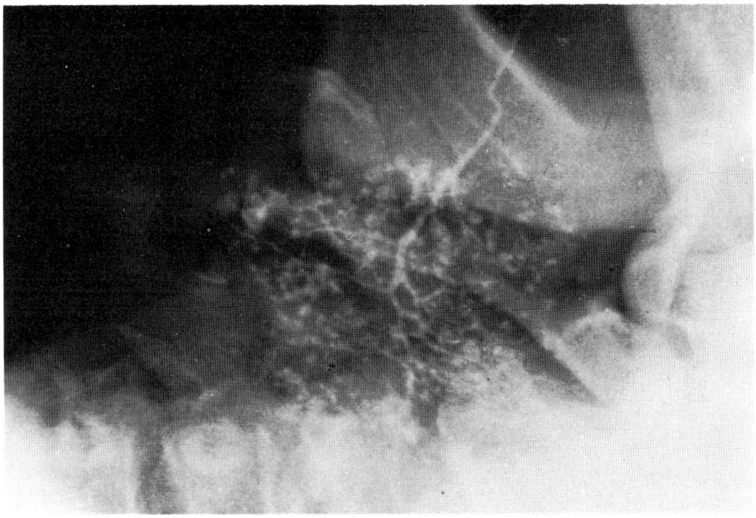

c

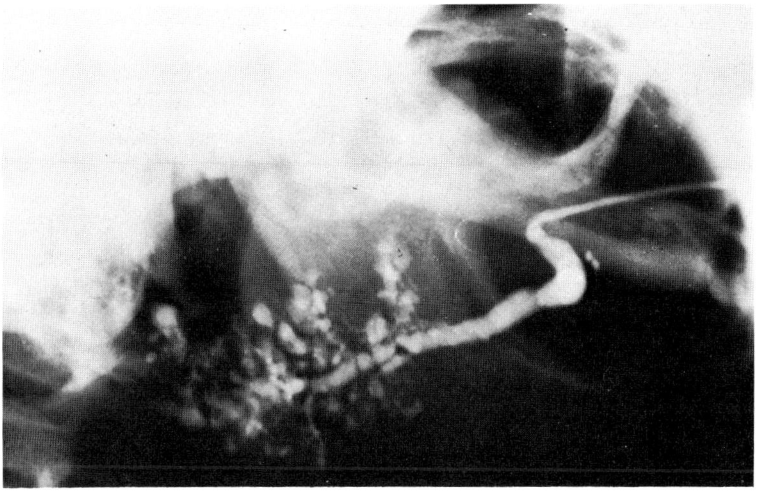

d

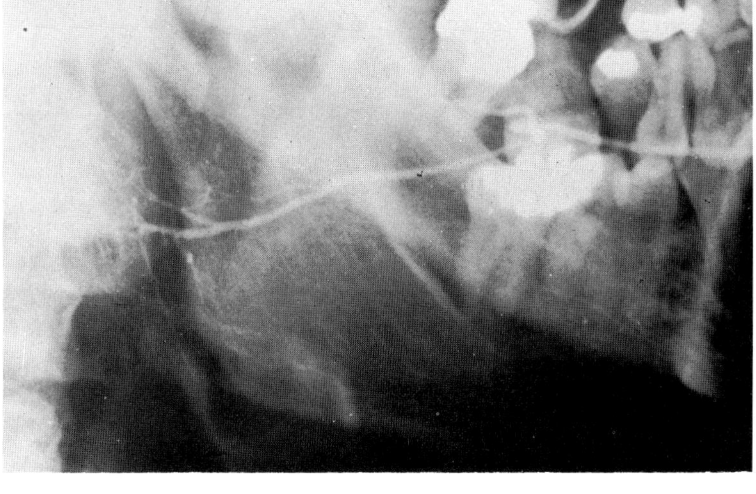

e

(Roberts et al, 1963; Raymond et al, 1965). Large numbers of ferritin molecules are present in synovial lining cells, but the iron is probably inaccessible for haemopoiesis in this site (Raymond et al, 1965; Muirden, 1966; Owen & Lawson, 1966; Lawson et al 1967; Mowat & Hothersall, 1968; Muirden, 1970). The pathogenesis of rheumatoid anaemia is complex (Mowat, 1971) and many abnormalities have been described including shortened red cell survival (Dinant, 1978; Richmond et al, 1978), reduced serum and red cell folate concentration (Omer, 1968), impairment of compensatory increase in iron absorption in response to anaemia (Boddy & Will, 1969), impaired erythropoietin release in response to anaemia (Ward et al, 1969), increased ineffective erythropoiesis (Dinant, 1978), synovial iron deposition (Muirden & Senator, 1967), and an abnormal pattern of iron handling characterised by rapid serum iron clearance and defective release of stored iron from the reticuloendothelial system (Friereich, et al 1957; Owen & Lawson, 1966, Bennett et al, 1974). The reticuloendothelial system probably acts as a reservoir which takes up iron (Freireich, et al 1957; Owen & Lawson, 1966) since rapid serum iron clearance correlates with disease activity (Roy et al, 1954; Mowat et al, 1969). Excessive reticuloendothelial iron is present in some patients with rheumatoid arthritis (Gardner & Roy, 1961; Muirden, 1970), but failure to use this iron as the primary course of rheumatoid anaemia should result in a microcytic hypochromic blood picture which is uncommon (Weinstein, 1959). Although failure to utilise available iron is an accepted factor in the pathogenesis of 'anaemia of chronic disease' it does not explain the mechanism nor aetiology. It is likely that alternative and additional factors cause suppression of the proliferative capacity of the erythroid marrow as has been demonstrated by bone marrow cytology (Richmond et al, 1956) and in ferrokinetic studies (Cavill & Bentley, 1982). Immune mechanisms to explain suppression of haemopoiesis have been demonstrated in many disease states (Cline & Golde, 1978) by both humoral (Dainiak et al, 1980; Goldberg et al, 1980) and cell-mediated mechanisms (Abodu et al, 1978). Recent work from our own laboratory by Harvey (Harvey et al, 1983) has shown that the mean colony counts of circulating erythroid burst forming units (BFU-E) from peripheral blood mononuclear cells of anaemic rheumatoid patients studied are lower than the mean counts for the non-anaemic rheumatoid patients and healthy control groups. This did not appear to be related to a T cell inhibition, but the BFU-E colony counts were universely related to the titre of rheumatoid factor and the serum IgM levels, suggesting that a humoral inhibition of erythropoiesis was a pathogenetic factor. Two general mechanisms for humoral immune suppression may be proposed:

a. Destruction of progenitor cells in vivo by specific cytotoxic antibodies, thus reducing the numbers of viable circulating colony forming cells, or
b. Immunoglobulin as immune complexes or as free protein may bind non-specifically to the progenitor cell surface in vivo.

Three cases of pure red cell aplasia in patients with rheumatoid disease have recently been reported. In one patient there was an IgG inhibitor of autologous erythroid colony forming and burst forming unit growth. The authors considered that the red cell aplasia was a manifestation of the rheumatoid disease and was related to drugs (Dessypris et al, 1984).

Chronic administration of antirheumatic drugs can lead to gastrointestinal blood loss (Scott et al, 1961), but this does not appear to be an important factor in the anaemia of rheumatoid arthritis (Gibberd, 1966). Although Lewis & Porter (1960) found no evidence of increased erythrocyte destruction this has been reported to be of mild degree by several workers (Alexander et al, 1956; Freireich et al, 1957; Weinstein, 1959).

There is evidence that the incidence of macrocytic anaemia is higher than expected in patients with rheumatoid arthritis (Partridge & Duthie, 1963) largely owing to folate deficiency (Gough et al, 1964; Omer & Mowat, 1968). Although there is no evidence that pernicious anaemia occurs with increased frequency in patients with rheumatoid arthritis, it is of interest that rheumatoid factor has an increased prevalence in patients with pernicious anaemia (Ghazi, 1972).

An inhibitor to factor VIII has been described

in patients with rheumatoid arthritis leading to extensive bleeding (Payne & Harris, 1972).

Eosinophilia occurs in patients with vasculitis, nodules and other visceral complications (Panush et al, 1971; Winchester et al 1971).

Platelet abnormalities

Thrombocytosis is a common finding in acute and severe rheumatoid disease. It correlates with most parameters of disease activity such as erythrocyte sedimentation rate, white blood cell count, plasma viscosity, liver enzymes, rheumatoid factor and acute phase reactants (Farr et al, 1983). Thrombocytopenia is not a feature of rheumatoid disease except in Felty's syndrome, or as a result of gold (Kean & Anastassiades, 1979) and D-penicillamine therapy (Kean et al, 1980). Shortened platelet survival is found in a minority of patients with rheumatoid disease but these patients usually have a normal or raised platelet count (Farr et al, 1980; Kelton et al, 1983). In patients with platelet counts greater than 1 000 000/mm^3, an alternative cause of the thrombocytosis should be considered.

Felty's syndrome

In 1924 Felty described the clinical association of leucopenia, splenomegaly and rheumatoid arthritis in five patients. Other features included lymphadenopathy, weight loss, anaemia, generalised skin pigmentation or chronic leg ulceration. Most rheumatologists have considered Felty's syndrome to be a variant of rheumatoid disease, but some challenge this unitarian concept, considering that Felty's syndrome indicates the presence of two diseases (Denko & Zumpft, 1962). Females predominate; the patients usually have severe arthritis complicated by systemic complications, including Sjögren's syndrome (deGruchy & Langley, 1961; Ruderman et al, 1968; Barnes et al, 1971; Goldberg & Pinals, 1980; Logue, 1979). A small proportion of patients with Felty's syndrome develop nodular regenerative hyperplasia of the liver, which may occasionally result in portal hypertension and bleeding oesophageal varices (Blendis et al, 1974; Thorne et al, 1982). The clinical importance of Felty's syndrome lies in the dangers to health and life from intercurrent infection due to leucopenia. The pathogenesis of the neutropenia is multifactorial: anti-neutrophil antibodies, antigen-antibody complexes, myelosuppression by a humoral inhibitor as well as a mononuclear suppressor cell, have all been described (Calabresi et al, 1959; Kimball et al, 1973; Rosenthal et al, 1974; Vincent et al, 1974; Wiik & Munthe, 1974; Gupta et al, 1975; Wiik, 1975; Goetzl, 1976; Logue, 1976; Turner et al, 1976; Joyce et al, 1980; Goldberg & Pinals 1980; Logue et al, 1981; Bucknall et al, 1982). Haemolysis contributes to the anaemia (Hume et al, 1964), which improves with corticosteroids (Pengelly, 1966) and splenectomy (Rackow, 1953, Gibberd et al, 1965; Green & Fromke, 1966; O'Neill et al, 1968; Ruderman et al, 1968; Sandusky et al, 1968; Barnes et al, 1971; Moore et al, 1971). The treatment of Felty's syndrome used to consist primarily of splenectomy especially in patients with recurrent life-threatening infections. Good short-term haematological responses occur in most patients after splenectomy, but recurrent infections remain a problem in 60% of patients so treated (Barnes et al, 1971; Moore et al, 1971; Goldberg & Pinals, 1980; Joyce et al, 1980; Blumfelder et al, 1981; Logue et al, 1981. Successful results have been reported with chrysotherapy, penicillamine, lithium and testosterone, but these therapies have not been subjected to controlled evaluation (Gupta et al, 1975; Goldberg & Pinals, 1980; Luthra et al, 1981.

Hyperviscosity syndrome

Patients with high titres of rheumatoid factor have slightly increased serum viscosity (Shearn et al, 1963). Occasionally this may be marked and give rise to the hyperviscosity syndrome (Jason et al, 1970; Pope et al, 1975; Cryer et al, 1981). The clinical features are protean and consist of: dyspnoea, dizziness, ataxia, visual blurring and diplopia, paraesthesiae, epistaxis, skin haemorrhages, menorrhagia and rectal bleeding. Examination of the fundi reveals venous engorgement, blot haemorrhages and soft exudates, and in severe cases papilloedema. Although intermediate complexes have been detected in patients with rheumatoid arthritis who have the hyperviscosity syndrome (Pope et al, 1975) and may have a bearing on the pathogenesis, the precise cause has not been established.

Lymph nodes

Local lymphadenopathy in the region of an inflamed joint is not uncommon in rheumatoid arthritis, but is sometimes impressive enough to raise the possibility of a lymphoma or secondary neoplasm. Lymph node biopsy shows the presence of germinal centres, and occasionally the appearances may resemble giant follicular lymphoma (Bumin et al, 1955). Generalised lymphadenopathy, although common in Still's disease, is rare in adults, and reticulosis should be borne in mind, especially since tumours of the reticuloendothelial system occur more commonly in patients with rheumatoid arthritis (Lea, 1964). Lymphangiography in patients with rheumatoid arthritis shows a picture of non-specific inflammatory change, which, although different from that seen in malignant reticulosis, is not sufficiently distinctive to be diagnostic in early cases (Robertson et al, 1968).

Renal manifestations

A proportion of patients with rheumatoid arthritis die in uraemia. This may be due to chronic pyelonephritis or other renal disease, amyloidosis, or analgesic nephropathy. There is still doubt whether rheumatoid disease may involve the kidneys per se. Arteritis may do so, but infrequently, and reduced glomerular function has been reported (Sørensen, 1960; Burry, 1972). Bacteriuria is no more common in patients with rheumatoid arthritis than in age and sex-matched controls (Burry, 1973).

Muscle

Muscle weakness and atrophy are not uncommon around inflamed joints in patients with rheumatoid arthritis. Histologically the changes in striated muscle include atrophy, degeneration, nodular myositis (Wegelius et al, 1969) and changes in the muscle spindles (Magyar et al, 1973). Lack of muscle necrosis serves to distinguish the condition from polymyositis. There are no specific features of muscle involvement (Riley & Harrison, 1968) and serum muscle enzymes are normal (Hendrich et al, 1966). Muscle atrophy may occur with remarkable rapidity in rheumatoid arthritis as a result of joint disease, and may be severe. Myopathy may occur following prolonged use of corticosteroid drugs, especially the 9α-fluorinated group (Golding & Begg, 1960).

Skin lesions

Atrophy and bruising of the skin on the dorsum of the forearms and the extensor surfaces of the legs are common in patients treated with corticosteroids. (Scarborough & Shuster, 1960). Leg ulcers are also common and may be due to friability of the skin due to corticosteroid therapy and/or arteritis of dermal vessels (Wilkinson & Kirk, 1965). Lesions of the skin may rarely occur as a result of vasculitis and multiple lesions of the skin may result from ulceration of cutaneous nodules. Longitudinal ridging of the nails such as occurs in elderly persons is found in patients with rheumatoid arthritis (Hamilton, 1960).

Bones

Periarticular and generalised osteoporosis is common in rheumatoid arthritis. The pathogenesis of generalised osteoporosis is multifactorial, involving duration of disease, age and sex of the patient, and use of corticosteroid drugs (McConkey et al, 1965; Bjelle & Nilsson, 1971; Mueller & Jurist, 1973; Kennedy et al, 1974). From these studies and others (Kennedy et al, 1979; Reid et al, 1982), the significance of high or low dose corticosteroid therapy in the development of decrease in bone density is still not clear. A radiological study by Hajirousou & Webley (1984) showed that rheumatoid patients treated with 5 mg/day of prednisolone for an average of 9.4 years had a decrease in radiological density by two standard techniques (Barnet & Nordin, 1960; Saville, 1967), when compared to control rheumatoid patients who had never received prednisolone. The differences, however, were not statistically significant. The increased metabolic activity of bone in rheumatoid disease is not only in the juxta-articular area but in the mid-shaft of non-articular bone (Rosenspire et al, 1980; Rajapakse et al, 1983). It should be noted that the increased turnover occurring in 'non-joint' bone of rheumatoid patients could compromise the results of investigation which used 'non-joint' bone as a reference standard joint imaging in rheumatoid arthritis patients (Rosenspire et al, 1980). Recent studies suggest that patients with rheumatoid arthritis may have hypercalcaemia and secondary hyperparathyroidism. Plasma zinc concentrations are depressed in patients with rheumatoid arthritis and may be related to the pathogenesis of osteoporosis (Kennedy et al, 1975).

Osteomalacia may also occur in patients with rheumatoid arthritis, due to vitamin D deficiency as a result of inadequate intake and lack of sunshine due to confinement indoors. As in non-rheumatoid patients osteomalacia may also be due to malabsorption.

Rarely massive osteolysis may occur in rheumatoid artiritis (Williams et al, 1966). Aseptic necrosis of the pubic ramus has been described in an elderly rheumatoid patient who had rheumatoid vasculitis. A large 6 × 8 cm encapsulated cystic mass adjacent to the pubic ramus, had histological features of acute necrotising vasculitis and fibrinoid necrosis (Shupak et al, 1983). Rarely osteomyelitis may occur as a septic complication in rheumatoid patients (Crook & Gray, 1982).

AMYLOIDOSIS

Although rheumatoid arthritis is now recognised as one of the commonest causes of amyloidosis in the Western world, it is still slightly less common than tuberculosis as a causative factor (Kennedy et al, 1974).

It is of interest that Ozdemir et al (1971) have suggested that the incidence of secondary amyloidosis in patients with rheumatoid arthritis is no higher than in age and sex-matched controls, and the 'increased' incidence in patients with rheumatoid arthritis can be explained on the basis of ageing, amyloidosis being common in the elderly. However, in Still's disease amyloidosis is relatively common, and certainly more so than among the childhood population in general. At least one case report in the literature has claimed the finding of amyloidosis in a patient with adult Still's disease (Harrington et al, 1981).

At post-mortem, amyloid deposits can be detected in as many as 60% of cases (Teilum & Lindahl, 1954). If carefully sought, approximately 5% of living patients with rheumatoid arthritis have amyloidosis detected by gingival or rectal biopsy, and approximately 12.5% have amyloid deposits on percutaneous renal biopsy (Brun et al, 1965). Microdeposition of amyloid may occur in the joints (Goffin et al, 1981). In spite of the high prevalence of amyloid disease in rheumatoid arthritis, it must be emphasised that such patients are not necessarily ill as a result of amyloidosis.

The clinical features of secondary amyloidosis are protean and are determined by the extent and site of amyloid deposition (Cohen, 1968). Amyloidosis occurs equally in both sexes, indicating an increased susceptibility of the male patient to develop the condition. Patients who develop secondary amyloidosis have usually had their disease for three years or more, often in a severe form. However, there are no specific features of rheumatoid arthritis which are related to the onset of amyloidosis, including the presence of rheumatoid factor, and amyloidosis has been reported in agammaglobulinaemia. Renal involvement is common and potentially the most serious complication (Fearnley & Lackner, 1955). The kidneys are characteristically enlarged, but may be of normal size or even reduced. Proteinuria, and occasionally haematuria, are frequently present and a typical nephrotic syndrome may occur. Patients who develop persistent proteinuria while receiving gold therapy or D-penicillamine should be investigated for possible amyloidosis (Bourke et al, 1981). Hypertension is frequent (Triger & Joekes, 1973). Hepatosplenomegaly is rarely found (Ennevaara & Oka, 1963). Malabsorption may result from extensive small bowel involvement (Babb et al, 1967). Amyloidosis involving the small bowel and causing ulceration has been reported in association with a refractory iron deficiency anaemia and intestinal haemosiderosis (Lee et al, 1978). Cardiac involvement is rare, but may result in undue sensitivity to digitalis (Cohen, 1968).

The diagnosis can be confirmed by gingival, rectal mucosal or abdominal fat biopsy (Stenvist et al, 1974). Abdominal fat biopsy by an ordinary needle and syringe is a useful diagnostic tool. There is little discomfort to the patient and the tissue sample can be stained at the bedside and read on a polarisation microscope (Westermark, 1984). Hepatic and kidney biopsies are extremely useful, but are not without risk of uncontrolled haemorrhage. The Congo red test is not without its limitations; anaphylactic reactions to the dye may occur if care is not taken in its preparation (Cohen,

1968). In the author's opinion it is a philosophical point whether efforts should be made to diagnose a condition for which there is no therapy. However, most rheumatologists believe that amyloidosis is an indication for treating disease activity as energetically as possible, e.g. with immunosuppressive drugs, but there is no evidence that this alters the prognosis. It should be noted that the prognosis in amyloidosis is much better than was previously thought (Brandt et al, 1968). Renal transplantation was successful in two patients with life-threatening disease (Cohen et al, 1971).

For a further discussion of amyloid see Chapter 41.

SEPTIC COMPLICATIONS

There seems little doubt that patients with rheumatoid arthritis are prone to infection, and that this may be a major cause of mortality (Cobb et al, 1953; Duthie et al, 1964). Pulmonary infection (Walker, 1967) and pyelonephritis at necropsy (Lawson & McLean, 1966) are common, but suprisingly urinary tract infection during life is no more common than among age and sex-matched controls (Mowat & Baum, 1971; Burry, 1973). Uddin and his colleagues (1970) have suggested that there is a ten-fold susceptibility to infection among patients with rheumatoid arthritis compared to healthy controls.

Septic arthritis is a well-recognised complication of rheumatoid arthritis (Kellgren et al, 1958; Cohen, 1965; Rimoin & Wennberg, 1966; Karten, 1969; Baum, 1971; Russell & Ansell, 1972). In approximately 75% of patients the offending organism is *Staphylococcus aureus* (Cohen, 1965; Rimoin & Wennberg, 1966; Myers et al, 1969; Russell & Ansell, 1972). However, many other organisms may infect the joints including streptococci, *Haemophilis influenzae*, pneumococci, coliforms and such rarities as *Pasteurella multocida* and *Candida quilliermondi*, and bacteroids (Dodd et al, 1982).

Septic arthritis occurs particularly in older patients with severe debilitating arthritis usually of long duration (Buchanan & Harvey, 1983). In patients with rheumatoid arthritis septic arthritis is a relatively uncommon occurrence when compared to all types of septic arthritis, but when it does occur, serious generalised infection such as pneumonia or meningitis may result (Manshady et al, 1980). Infection is usually haematogenous from a primary site elsewhere in the body, usually the skin, but occasionally the infection may be introduced by intra-articular injections (Gowans & Granieri, 1959; Kelly et al, 1970) or occur directly as a result of fistulous rheumatism. Septic arthritis is somewhat surprisingly no more common in patients treated with corticosteroid therapy (Kellgren et al, 1958; Rimoin & Wennberg, 1966). Patients with Felty's syndrome are especially susceptible to infections, including septic arthritis (De Gruchy, 1965; Ruderman et al, 1968; Barnes et al, 1971).

The onset of septic arthritis is protean in character. It may be fulminant with high fever, rigors and other classical symptoms and signs of septicaemia. Alternatively the onset may be ingravescent and fevers, rigors and leucocytosis may be absent (Kellgren et al, 1958; Cohen 1965; Rimoin & Wennberg, 1966; Karten, 1969; Russel & Ansell, 1972). It should be noted that a normal white cell count occurs in 50% of patients with staphylococcal septicaemia (Smith, 1975). Septic arthritis may complicate rheumatoid arthritis in one joint, but it is important for the physician to appreciate that it may involve two or more joints. The patient may, indeed, be suspected of having merely an exacerbation of arthritis, especially if there are no symptoms and signs of infection. A red, hot, swollen joint in a patient with rheumatoid arthritis should always be suspected as being septic, and demands immediate aspiration. The fluid in septic arthritis is purulent with a leucocytosis of 50 000 cells/mm^3 or more, the vast majority of the cells being polymorphonuclear leucocytes. The glucose concentration is depressed, and there is usually an abundance of microorganisms which can be seen on a film and grown on culture. This may not be so, however, if the patient has been given an antibiotic before aspiration, a situation which can lead to considerable diagnostic difficulty.

DIFFERENTIAL DIAGNOSIS

The diagnosis of classical rheumatoid arthritis presents no difficulty. In its early stages the disease may present a picture which invokes a differential diagnosis of such length that almost any disorder affecting joints and connective tissue may be mimicked. Diagnosis in general depends on the presence of observable phenomena and it is conceivable that rheumatoid arthritis is a syndrome and not a single disease entity. At present the diagnosis of rheumatoid arthritis rests on the coincidental presence of the triad of inflammatory polyarthritis, radiological evidence of juxta-articular erosions, and a positive test for rheumatoid factor by standard laboratory methods. When one of the triad is absent the diagnosis becomes less certain. For example, Dixon (1960) showed this very clearly in patients with severe active 'rheumatoid arthritis' with negative tests for rheumatoid factor: of 61 such patients followed over a period of 5 years, 11 had proven or probable disease other than rheumatoid arthritis, including gout, generalised osteoarthrosis, psoriatic arthropathy, reticulohistiocytosis, Takayashu's disease, Reiter's disease, and myelomatosis. The diagnostic criteria of the American Rheumatism Association (see Ch. 24) are of little practical clinical value to the physician dealing with individual patients, although they are invaluable to clinical research workers. The criteria are, however, useful in providing a list of exclusions. Other diseases, such as hypereosinophilic syndrome, may mimic classical rheumatoid arthritis, but are rare (Brogadir et al, 1980). The coexistence of other arthritides (such as Reiter's syndrome) with rheumatoid arthritis seems to be rarer than would be expected from the incidence of the two diseases, and needs to be explained (Fallahi et al, 1983).

REFERENCES

Abdou N I, Napombejara C, Balentine L, Abdou N L 1978 Suppressor cell-mediated neutropenia in Felty's syndrome.

Abel T, Andrews B S, Cunningham P H, Brunner C M, Davis J S, Horwitz D A 1980 Rheumatoid vasculitis: Effect of cyclophosphamide on the clinical course and levels of circulating immune complexes. Annals of Internal Medicine 93: 407–413

Adler R H, Norcross B M Lockie L M 1962 Arteritis and infarction of the intestine in rheumatoid arthritis. Journal of the American Medical Association 180:922

Ahlgren P, Fog J 1968 Atlanto epistrophical subluxation in rheumatoid arthritis. Acta Rheumatologica Scandinavica 14:210

Akers, W A, Miller D A 1966 Rheumatoid nodules in adults without rheumatoid arthritis. Archives of Dermatology 93:428

Alexander W R M, Richmond J, Roy L M H, Duthie J J R 1956 Nature of anaemia in rheumatoid arthritis. II. Survival of transfused erythrocytes in patients with rheumatoid arthritis. Annals of the Rheumatic Diseases 15:12

Anderson J A, Whaley K, Williamson J, Buchanan W W 1972 A statistical and to the diagnosis of keratoconjunctivitis sicca. Quarterly Journal of Medicine NS 41:175

Anderson L G, Talal N 1972 The spectrum of benign to malignant lymphoproliferation in Sjörgren's syndrome. Clinical and Experimental Immunology 10:199

Appelboom et al as in typescript.

Ansell B M, Loewl G 1977 Rheumatoid arthritis: general features. Clinics in Rheumatic Diseases 3: 385–401

Appelboom T, de Boelpaepe C, Ehrlich G E, Famaey J P 1981 Rubens and the question of antiquity of rheumatoid arthritis. Journal of the American Medical Association 245: 483–486

Arkless R 1967 Rheumatoid writs: cineradiography. Radiology 88:543

Aronoff A, Bywaters I G L, Fearnley G R 1955 Lung lesions in rheumatoid arthritis. British Medical Journal ii:228

Aronoff S, Johnson L, Dworkin S 1960 Arteritis in rheumatoid arthritis. Canadian Medical Association Journal 83: 355–364

Babb R R, Alarcon-Segovia D, Dressner G R, McPherson J R 1967 Malabsorption in rheumatoid arthritis: an unusual complication caused by amyloidosis. Arthritis and Rheumatism 10:63

Backdahl M 1963 The caput ulnae syndrome in rheumatoid arthritis. Acta Rheumatologica Scandinavica Suppl 5:5

Backhouse K M 1968 The mechanics of normal digital control in the hand and an analysis of the ulnar drift of rheumatoid arthritis. Annals of the Royal College of Surgeons 43:154

Backhouse K M 1972 Extensor expansion of the rheumatoid hand. Annals of the Rheumatic Diseases 31:112

Backhouse K M, Kay A G L, Coones E N, Kates A 1971 Tendon involvement in the rheumatoid hand. Annals of the Rheumatic Diseases 30:236

Baggenstoss A H, Rosenberg E F 1944 Unusual cardiac lesions associated with chronic multiple rheumatoid arthritis. Archives of Pathology 37:54

Baker W M 1877 On the formation of synovial cysts in the leg in connection with disease of the knee joint. Saint Bartholomew's Hospital Report 13:245

Baker O A, Bywaters E G L 1957 Laryngeal stridôr in rheumatoid arthritis due to cricoarytenoid joint involvement. British Medical Journal ii:1400

Baker R J, Johnson W C, Burgoon C F 1971 Unusual skin lesions of rheumatoid arthritis. Dermatologica 143:305

Ball J 1954 Rheumatoid arthritis and polyarteritis nodosa. Annals of the Rheumatic Diseases, 77:277

Ball J 1971 The Hebenden Oration. 1970 Enthesopathy of rheumatoid and ankylosing spondylilis. Annals of the Rheumatic Diseases 30:213

Barnes C G, Turnbull A L, Vernon-Roberts B 1971 Felty's syndrome. A clinical and pathological survey of 21 patients

and their response to treatment. Annals of the Rheumatic Diseases 30:359
Barnett E, Nordin B E C, 1960 The radiological diagnosis of osteoporosis: a new approach. Clinical Radiology, 11: 166–174
Bassiouni M 1965 Incidence of calcaneal spurs in osteoarthrosis and rheumatoid arthritis and in control patients. Annals of the Rheumatic Diseases 24:490
Baum J 1971 Infection in rheumatoid arthritis. Arthritis and Rheumatism 14:135
Beck E R, Hoffbrand B I 1966 Acute lung changes in rheumatoid arthritis. Annals of the Rheumatic Diseases, 25:459
Beckett V L, Dinn J J 1972 Segmental demyelination in rheumatoid arthritis. Quarterly Journal of Medicine, New Series 41:71
Bedi S S, Ellis W 1970 Spontaneous rupture of the calcaneal tendon in rheumatoid arthritis after local steroid injection. Annals of the Rheumatic Diseases 29:494
Belin D C, Abeles M, Weinstein A 1979 Rheumatoid markers in the absence of arthritis. Journal of Rheumatology 6: 293–299
Bennett P H, Scott J T 1965 Autonomic neuropathy in rheumatoid arthritis. Annals of the Rheumatic Diseases 24:168
Bennett R M, Hughes G R V, Bywaters E G L, Holt P J L 1972 Studies of a popliteal synovial fistula. Annals of the Rheumatic Diseases 31:482
Bennett R M, Holt P J L, Lewis S M 1974 Role of the reticuloendothelial system in the anaemia of rheumatoid arthritis: a study using the ^{59}Fe-labelled dextran model. Annals of the Rheumatic Diseases 33: 147–152
Berger H W, Seckler S G 1966 Pleural and pericardial effusions in rheumatoid disease. Annals of Internal Medicine 64:1291
Bienenstock H 1975 Rheumatoid plantar synovial cysts. Annals of the Rheumatic Diseases 34:98
Bienenstock H, Ehrlich G E, Freyberg R H 1963 Rheumatoid arthritis of the cricoarytenoid joint: a clinicopathologic study. Arthritis and Rheumatism 6:48
Bilka P J 1968a Rheumatoid arthritis — a systemic disease. Medical clinics of North America 52:493
Bilka P J 1968b Physical signs in rheumatoid arthritis. Medical Clinics of North America 52:493
Bilka P J 1970 Physical examination of the arthritic patient. Bulletin on the Rheumatic Diseases 20:596
Binder H J, O'Brien W M, Spiro H M, Hollingsworth J W 1966 Gluten and the small intestine in rheumatoid arthritis. Journal of the American Medical Association 195: 857
Bjelle A O, Nilsson B E 1971 The relationship between radiological changes and osteoporosis of the hand in rheumatoid arthritis. Arthritis and Rheumatism 14:646
Blair G S, Chalmers I M 1972 Radiology of the temporomandibular joint. A comparison of circular tomography with orthopantomography and lateral transcranio-oblique radiography. Journal of Dentistry 1:69
Blair, G S, Chalmers I M, Leggat T G, Buchanan W W 1973 Circular tomography of the temporomandibular joint. Oral Surgery, Oral Medical, Oral Pathology 35:416
Bland J H 1967 Rheumatoid arthritis of the cervical spine. Bulletin on the Rheumatic Diseases 18:471
Bland J H 1974 Rheumatoid arthritis of the cervical spine. The Journal of Rheumatology 2:319
Bland J H, Van Buskirk F W, Tampas J P, Brown E, Clayton E 1965 A study of roentgenologic criteria for rheumatoid arthritis of the cervical spine. The American Journal of Roentgenology, Radium Therapy and Nuclear Medicine 95:949
Blendis L M, Parkinson M C, Shilkin K B, Williams R 1974 Nodular regenerative hyperplasia of the liver in Felty's syndrome. Quarterly Journal of Medicine N.S. 43: 25–32
Bloch K J, Buchanan W W, Wohl M J, Bunim J J 1965 Sjögren's syndrome. A clinico-pathologic study of 63 cases. Medicine (Baltimore) 44:187
Blumfelder T M, Logue G L, Shimm D S 1981 Felty's syndrome: effects of splenectomy upon granulocyte count and granulocyte associated IgG. Annals of Internal Medicine 94: 623–628
Bonfiglo T, Atwater E D 1969 Heart disease in patients with seropositive rheumatoid arthritis. Archives of Internal Medicine 124:714
Bourke B E, Woodrow D F, Scott J T 1981 Proteinuria in rheumatoid arthritis — drug induced or amyloid. Annals of the Rheumatic Diseases, 40: 240–244
Brannan H M, Good C A, Divertie M B, Baggenstoss A H 1964 Pulmonary disease associated with rheumatoid arthritis. Journal of the American Medical Association 189:138
Brandt K, Cathcart E S, Cohen A S 1968 A clinical analysis of the course and prognosis of 42 patients with amyloidosis. American Journal of Medicine 44:955
Brewerton D A 1957 Hand deformities in rheumatoid disease. Annals of the Rheumatic Diseases, 16:183
Brewerton D A 1965 The rheumatoid hand. In: Dixon A St J (ed) Progress in clinical rheumatology Churchill, London, p 56
Brewerton D A 1967 A tangential radiographic projection for demonstrating involvement of metacarpal heads in rheumatoid arthritis. British Journal of Radiology 40:233
Brogadir S P, Goldwein M I, Schumacher H R 1980 A hypereosinophilic syndrome mimicking rheumatoid arthritis. American Journal of Medicine, 69: 799–802
Brown M M, Hadler W M, Sams W M, Wilson J, Snyderman R 1979 Rheumatoid nodulosis, Sporadic and familial diseases. Journal of Rheumatology 6: 286–292
Bu C Osn T S, Rasschou F, Sorensen A W S 1965 Renal biopsy in rheumatoid arthritis. Nephron 2:65
Buchanan W W, Harvey A R 1983 Pyoarthrosis complicating rheumatoid arthritis. The British Journal of Clinical Practice (Suppl 21): 11–12
Buchanan R C R, Kraag G 1980 Is there a lower incidence of deep venous thrombosis after joint replacement in rheumatoid arthritis? Journal of Rheumatology 7: 551–554
Buchanan W W, Kean W F 1982 Robert Burns' illness revisited. Scottish Medical Journal 27: 75–88
Buchanan W W, Murdoch R M 1979 Hypothesis: that rheumatoid arthritis will disappear. The Journal of Rheumatology 6: 324–329
Bucknall R C, Davis P, Bacon P A, Verrier-Jones J 1982 Neutropenia in rheumatoid arthiritis. Studies on possible contributing factors. Annals of the Rheumatic Diseases, 41: 242–247
Bunim J J, Sokoloff L, Williams R R, Black R L 1955 Rheumatoid arthritis: a review of recent advances in our knowledge concerning pathology, diagnosis and treatment. Journal of Chronic Diseases 1:168
Burns T M, Calin A 1983 The hand radiograph as a diagnostic discriminant between seropositive and seronegative

'rheumatoid arthritis': a controlled study. Annals of the Rheumatic Diseases 42: 605–612

Burry H C 1972 Reduced glomerular function in rheumatoid arthritis. Annals of the Rheumatic Diseases 31:65

Burry H C 1973 Bacteriuria in rheumatoid arthritis. Annals of the Rheumatic Diseases 32:208

Burry H C, Tweed J M, Robinson R G, Howes R 1978 Lateral subluxation of the atlanto-axial joint in rheumatoid arthritis. Annals of the Rheumatic Diseases 37: 525–528

Bywaters E G L 1949 A variant of rheumatoid arthritis characterised by recurrent digital pad nodules and palmar fasciitis, closely resembling palindromic rheumatism. Annals of Rheumatic Diseases 8:2

Bywaters E G L 1953 Fistulous rheumatism, a manifestation of rheumatoid arthritis. Annals of the Rheumatic Diseases 12:114

Bywaters E G L 1954 Heel leasions of rheumatoid arthritis. Annals of the Rheumatic Diseases 13:42

Bywaters E G L 1960 The early radiological signs of rheumatoid arthritis. Bulletin of the Rheumatic Diseases 11:231

Bywaters E G L 1971 Still's disease in the adult. Annals of the Rheumatic Diseases 30: 121–133

Bywaters E G L 1971 Skin manifestation of rheumatic diseases in dermatology and general medicine. Fitzpatrick T B (ed) McGraw-Hill, New York p 1535–1545

Bywaters E G L 1979 On two papers dealing with nodules (Editorial). The Journal of Rheumatology 6: 243–246

Calabresi P, Edwards E A, Schilling R F 1959 Fluorescent antiglobulin studies in leukopenic and related disorders. Journal of Clinical Investigation, 38: 2091–2100

Calabro J J 1962 A critical evaluation of the diagnostic features of the feet in rheumatoid arthritis. Arthritis and Rheumatism 5:19

Campbell J A 1958 A case of Caplan's syndrome in a boiler-scaler. Thorax 13:177

Caplan A 1953 Certain unusual radiological appearances in the chest in coalminers suffering from rheumatoid arthritis. Thorax 8:29

Caplan A 1959 Rheumatoid disease and pneumoconiosis (Caplan's syndrome). Proceedings of the Royal Society of Medicine 52:1111

Caplan A, Payne R B, Withey J L 1962 A broader concept of Caplan's syndrome related to rheumatoid factors. Thorax 17:205

Carmichael D S, Golding D N 1967 Rheumatoid pleural effusion with 'RA cells'. British Medical Journal, ii:814

Carpenter D F, Golden A, Roberts W C 1967 Quadrivalvular rheumatoid heart disease associated with left bundle branch block. American Journal of Medicine 43:922

Cary G R 1966 Methods for determining the presence of subtle knee joint effusion. The Journal of the Louisiana State Medical Society 118:147

Casagrande P 1965 Surgical rehabilitation of upper extremities. In: Dixon A St J (ed) Progress in clinical rheumatology. Little Brown & Co, Boston, p 74

Castillo B A, El Sallab R A, Scott J T 1965 Physical activity, cystic erosions and osteoporosis in rheumatoid arthritis. Annals of the Rheumatic Diseases, 24:522

Caughey D E, Bywaters E G L 1963 Joint fluid pressure in chronic knee effusions. Annals of the Rheumatic Diseases 22:106

Cavsey J Q 1972 Isolated subcutaneous rheumatic-like nodules in an adult. Southern Medical Journal 65:633

Caughey D E 1974 The arthritis of Constantine IX. Annals of the Rheumatic Diseases 33: 77–80

Cavill I, Bentley D P 1982 Erythropoiesis in the anemia of rheumatoid arthritis. British Journal of Haematology 50: 583–590

Chalmers I M, Blair G S 1973 Rheumatoid arthritis of the temporomandibular joint. A clinical and radiological study using circular tomography. Quarterly Journal of Medicine, New Series 42:369

Chamberlain M A, Bruckner F E 1970 Rheumatoid neuropathy. Annals of the Rheumatic Diseases 29:609

Chamberlain M A, Corbett M 1970 Carpal tunnel syndrome in early rheumatoid arthritis. Annals of the Rheumatic Diseases 29:149

Cline M J Golde D W 1978 Immune suppression of hematopoiesis. American Journal of Medicine 64: 301–310

Cobb S, Anderson F, Bauer W 1953 Length of life and cause of death in rheumatoid arthritis. New England Journal of Medicine 249:553

Cohen A S 1968 Amyloidosis associated with rheumatoid arthritis. Medical Clinics of North America 52:643

Cohen A S, Briccetti A B, Harrington J T, Mannick J A 1971 Renal transplantation in two cases of amyloidosis Lancet ii:513

Cohen C 1965 Staphylococcal septicaemia with multiple pyoarthrosis complicating rheumatoid disease. Gerontology Clinics 7:231

Collins K E, Deodhar S, Nuki G, Whaley K, Buchanan W W, Dick W C 1971 Radioisotope study of small joint inflammation in rheumatoid arthritis. Radioactive technetium (^{99m}Tc) uptake in the proximal interphalangeal joints and the effects of oral corticosteroids. Annals of the Rheumatic Diseases 30:401

Collins L C, Lidsky M D, Sharp J T 1972 Malposition of carpal bones in rheumatoid arthritis. Radiology 103:95

Collins W J M F, Jayson M I V 1972 Measurement of pedal pressures. An illustration of a method. Annals of the Rheumatic Diseases 31:215

Colton C, Darby A 1970 Giant granulomatous lesions of the femoral head and neck in rheumatoid arthiritis. Annals of the Rheumatic Disease 29:626

Conlon P W, Isdale I C, Rose B S 1966 Rheumatoid arthritis of the cervical spine. An analysis of 333 cases. Annals of the Rheumatic Diseases 25:120

Conn D L, McDuffie F C, Dyck P J 1972 Ummunopathologic study of sural nerves in rheumatoid arthritis. Arthritis and Rheumatism 15:135

Convery F R, Conaty J P, Nickel V L 1971 Flexion deformities of the knee in rheumatoid arthritis. Clinical Orthopaedics 74:90

Convey F R, Clawson D K 1971 The rheumatoid knee. American Family Physician 4:52

Copeman W S C 1957 Rheumatoid arthritis of the crico-arytenoid joints. British Medical Journal i:1398

Copeman W S C 1964 A short history of the gout and the rheumatic diseases. University of California Press, Los Angeles p 161–162

Corbett A J, Zizic T M, Stevens M B 1983 Adult-onset Still's disease with an associated severe restrictive pulmonary defect: a case report. Annals of the Rheumatic Diseases 42: 452–454

Corrigan A B, Robinson R G, Terenty T R, Dick-Smith J B, Walters D 1974 Benign rheumatoid arthritis of the aged. British Medical Journal i:444

Crisp A J, Armstrong R D, Grahame R, Dussek J E 1982 Rheumatoid lung disease, pneumothorax, and eosinophilia. Annals of the Rheumatic Diseases 41: 137–140
Crook P R, Gray J 1982 Bacteriodes causing osteomyelitis in rheumatoid arthritis. Annals of the Rheumatic Diseases 41: 645–646
Cruickshank B 1957 Rheumatoid arthritis and rheumatoid disease. Proceedings of the Royal Society of Medicine, 50:462
Cudkowicz L, Madoff I M, Abelmann W H 1961 Rheumatoid lung disease. A case report which includes respiratory function studies and a lung biopsy. British Journal of Disease of the Chest 55:35
Cummings J K, Taleisnik J 1971 Peripheral gangrene as a complication of rheumatoid arthritis. Report of a case and a review of the literature. Journal of Bone and Joint Surgery 53A:1001
Dainiak N, Hardin J, Floyd V, Callahan M, Hoffman R 1980 Humoral suppression of erythropoiesis in systemic lupus erythematosus (SLE) and rheumatoid arthritis. American Journal of Medicine, 69: 537–544
De Andrade J R, Grant C, Dixon A St J 1965 Joint distension and reflex muscle inhibition in the knee. Journal of Bone and Joint Surgery 47A:313
De Gruchy G C 1965 Diagnosis and treatment of Felty's syndrome. Geriatrics 20:219
De Gruchy G C, Langley G R 1961 Felty's syndrome. Australasian Annals of Medicine 10:292
De Haas WHD, Kingma M J, Drucker F 1965 The coracoclavicular joint and related pathological conditions. Annals of the Rheumatic Diseases 24:257
De Haas W H D, De Boer W, Griffioen F, Oosten-Elst P 1974 Rheumatoid arthritis of the robust reaction type. Annals of the Rheumatic Diseases 33:81
DeHoratius R J, Williams R C Jr 1972 Rheumatoid factor accentuation of pulmonary lesions associated with experimental diffuse proliferative lung disease. Arthritis and Rheumatism 15:293
Denko C W, Zumpft C W 1962 Chronic arthritis with splenomegaly and leukopenia. Arthritis and Rheumatism 5:478
DeQueker I 1977 Arthritis in Flemish paintings (1400–1700). British Medical Journal, 1, 1203–1205
Dequeker J, Rosberg G 1967 Digital capillaritis in rheumatoid arthritis. Acta Rheumatologica Scandinavica 13:299
Dessypris E N, Baer M R, Sergent J S, Krantz S B 1984 Rheumatoid arthritis and pure red cell aplasia. Annals of Internal Medicine 100: 202–206
Dick W C, Jasani M K, Boyle J A 1968 A study of capillary resistance in rheumatoid arthritis with special reference to the effects of long-term low-dosage oral corticosteroid therapy Acta Rheumatologica Scandinavica 14:265
Dick W C, Collins K E, Buchanan W W 1972 Clinical studies on inflammation in small diarthrodial joints, Technetium (^{99m}Tc) percentage uptakes in various arthritides and studies on the effect of aspirin in rheumatoid arthritis. Clinical Science 42:383
Dilsen N, McEwen C, Poppe M, Gersh W J, Didata D, Carmel P 1962 A comparative roentgenologic study of rheumatoid arthritis and rheumatoid (ankylosing) spondylitis. Arthritis and Rheumatism 5:341
Dinant H J 1978 Erythropoiesis and mean red cell lifespan in normal subjects and patients with the anemia of active rheumatoid arthritis. British Journal of Haematology 39: 437–444
Dixon A St J 1960 'Rheumatoid arthritis' with negative serological reaction. Annals of the Rheumatic Diseases 19:209
Dixon A St J 1963 Radiological aspects of rheumatoid arthritis. Proceedings of the International Symposium. International Congress Series. Excerpta Medica Foundation, Amsterdam, p 259
Dixon A St J 1964 Acute rupture of the knee in rheumatoid arthritis. Proceedings of the Royal Society of Medicine 57:1129
Dixon A St J 1970 Medical aspects of the rheumatoid foot. Proceedings of the Royal Society of Medicine 63:677
Dixon A St J 1971 The rheumatoid foot. In: Hill A G (ed) Modern trends in rheumatology 2. Butterworths, London Ch 11, p 158–173
Dixon A St J, Lience E 1961 Sacro-iliac joint in adult rheumatoid arthritis and psoriatic arthropathy. Annals of the Rheumatic Diseases 20:247
Doig J A, Whaley K, Dick W C, Nuki G, Williamson J, Buchanan W W 1971 Otolaryngological aspects of Sjögren's syndrome. British Medical Journal iv:460
Dorfman H, Norma A, Smith R 1970 Bone erosion in relation to subcutaneous rheumatoid nodules. Arthritis and Rheumatism 13:69
Douglas W 1965 The digital artery lesion of rheumatoid arthritis. An immunofluorescent study. Annals of the Rheumatic Diseases 24:40
Duthie J J R, Brown P E, Truelove L H, Baragar F D, Lawrie A J 1964 Course and prognosis in rheumatoid arthritis: a further report. Annals of the Rheumatic Diseases 23:193
Duthie R, Harris C 1969 Aradiographic and clinical survey of the hip joints in seropositive rheumatoid arthritis. Acta Orthopaedica Scandinavica 40:346
Eaton R G 1969 The extensor mechanism of the fingers. Bulletin of the Hospital for Joint Diseases 30:39
Ecklin U 1960 Die Altersveränderungen der Halswirbelsäule. Springer, Berlin, p 17, 28
Ehrlich G H 1967 Shakespeare's rheumatology. Annals of the Rheumatic Diseases 26: 562–563
Ehrlich G E 1972 Antecubital cysts in rheumatoid arthritis — a corollary to popliteal (Baker's) cysts. Journal of Bone and Joint Surgery 54A:165
Ehrlich G E, Guttman G G 1973 Valvular mechanisms in antecubital cysts of rheumatoid arthritis. Arthritis and Rheumatism 16:259
Ellman P, Ball R E 1948 'Rheumatoid disease' with joint and pulmonary manifestations. British Medical Journal ii:816
Ennevaara K 1967 Painful shoulder joint in rheumatoid arthritis. Acta Rheumatological Scandinavica (Supplement 11)
Ennevaara K, Oka M 1963 Amyloidosis in ankylosing spondylitis. Annals of the Rheumatic Diseases 22:336
Ennevaara K, Kajander A, Sillanpaa M, Laine V 1965 On radiological appearance of the calcaneus in rheumatoid arthritis and ankylosing spondylitis. Acta Rheumatologica Scandinavica 11:299
Epstein W V, Engleman E P 1959 The relation of the rheumatoid factor content of serum to clinical neurovascular manifestations of rheumatoid arthritis. Arthritis and Rheumatism 2:250
Eraut C D, Evans J A, Caplin M 1978 Pulmonary necrobiotic nodules without rheumatoid arthritis. British Journal of Diseases of the Chest 72: 301–306
Erhardt C C, Mamford P, Maini R N 1979 The association

of cryoglobulinaemia with nodules, vasculitis, and fibrosing alveolitis in rheumatoid arthritis and their relationship to serum Clq binding activity and rheumatoid factor. Clinical Experimental Immunology 38: 405–413

Ericson S, Lundberg M 1967 Alterations in the temporomandibular joint at various stages of rheumatoid arthritis. Acta Rheumatologica Scandinavica 13:257

Esdaile J M, Tannenbaum H, Hawkins D 1980 Adult Still's disease. American Journal of Medicine 68: 825–830

Fallahi S, Miller R K, Halla J T 1983 Coexistence of Reiter's syndrome and rheumatoid arthritis in a genetically susceptible individual. Annals of the Rheumatic Diseases 42: 210–212

Fang H C 1948 Periostitis of the os calcis; osteo-periosteal manifestations of rheumatoid arthritis. Chinese Medical Journal 66:57

Farr M, Scott D L, Constable T J, Hawkder R J, Hawkins C F, Stuart J 1983 Thrombocytosis of active rheumatoid disease. Annals of the Rheumatic Diseases 42: 545–549

Fearnley G R 1951 Ulnar deviation of the fingers. Annals of the Rheumatic Diseases 10:126

Fearnley G R, Lackner R 1955Amyloidosis in rheumatoid arthritis and significance of 'unexplained' albuminuria. A report of eight cases. British Medical Journal i:1129

Feigenbaum S L, Masi A T, Kaplan S B 1979 Prognosis in rheumatoid arthritis: a longitudinal study of newly diagnosed younger adult patients. American Journal of Medicine 66: 377–384

Felty A R 1924 Chronic arthritis in the adult, associated with splenomegaly and leucopenia. A report of five cases of an unusual clinical syndrome. Johns Hopkins Hospital Bulletin 35:16

Ferguson G C 1966 Cholesterol pleural effusion in rheumatoid lung disease. Thorax 21:577

Ferguson R H, Slocumb C H 1961 Peripheral neuropathy in rheumatoid arthritis. Bulletin on Rheumatic Diseases 11:251

Finkbiner R B, Decker J P 1963 Ulceration and perforation of the intestine due to necrotising arteriolitis. New England Journal of Medicine 268:14

Flatt A E 1959 Surgical rehabilitation of the arthritic hand. Arthritis and Rheumatism 11:278

Fleming A, Crown J M, Corbett M 1976a Incidence of joint involvement in early rheumatoid arthritis. Rheumatology and Rehibilitation 15: 92–96

Fleming A, Benn R T, Corbett M, Wood P H N 1976b Early rheumatoid disease. II Patterns of joint involvement. Annals of the Rheumatic Diseases 35: 361–364

Forster T J, Leek J C, Robbins D L 1981 Peripheral hyperostosis in rheumatoid arthritis in the absence of axial involvement. Journal of Rheumatology 8: 653–657

Franco A E, Schur P H 1971 Hypocomplementemia in rheumatoid arthritis. Arthritis and Rheumatism 14:231

Fraser A 1970 Mary Queen of Scots. Panther, London,

Freireich E J, Ross J F, Bayles T B, Emerson C P, Finch S C, MacDonald C 1957 Radioactive iron metabolism and erythrocyte survival studies of the mechanism of the anaemia associated with rheumatoid arthritis. Journal of Clinical Investigation 36:1043

Friedman H 1970 Intraspinal rheumatoid nodule causing nerve root compression. Case report. Neurosurgery 32:689

Gample W S, Abbruzzese A, Gray S J, Bayles T B 1969 Rheumatoid arthritis and xylose tolerance test. American Journal of Gastroenterology 52:445

Gardner D L, Roy L M H 1961 Tissue iron and the reti culoendothelial system in rheumatoid arthritis. Annals of the Rheumatic Diseases 20: 258–264

Gardner D L, Duthie J J R, MacLeod J, Allan WW S A 1957 Pulmonary hypertension in rheumatoid arthritis: report of a case with intimal sclerosis of the pulmonary and digital arteries. Scottish Medical Journal 2:183

Garrod, Sir Alfred B 1859 The nature and treatment of gout and rheumatic gout. Walton & Malberly, London

Gaunt W D, Rinker C T 1970 Gout-like X-rays in active men with rheumatoid arthritis. Missouri Medicine 67:225

Genovese G R, Jayson M I V, Dixon A St J 1972 Protective value of synovial cysts in rheumatoid knees. Annals of the Rheumatic Diseases 31:179

Ghazi H A 1972 Pernicious anaemia and rheumatoid arthritis. British Medical Journal i:144

Gibberd F B 1966 The haemoglobin level in patients with rheumatoid arthritis. Acta Rheumatologica Scandinavia 12:122

Gibberd F B, Gilbertson C, Jepson E M 1965 Felty's syndrome. Annals of the Rheumatic Diseases 24:46

Gibbons D, Phillips M 1975 Acute calf swelling. British Medical Journal (correspondence) i:335

Ginsberg M H, Genant H K, Yu T F, McCarty D J 1975 Rheumatoid nodulosis. An unusual variant of rheumatoid disease. Arthritis and Rheumatism 18:49

Goetzl E J 1976 Defective responsiveness to ascorbic acid of neutrophil random and chemotactic migration in Felty's syndrome and systemic lupus erythematosus. Annals of the Rheumatic Diseases 35: 510–515

Goffin Y A, Thoua Y, Potvliege P R 1981 Microdeposition of amyloid in the joints. Annals of the Rheumatic Diseases 40: 27–33

Goldberg J, Pinas R S 1980 Felty syndrome. Seminars in Arthritis and Rheumatism 10: 52–63

Goldberg L S, Bacon P A, Bucknall R C, Fitchen J, Cline M J 1980 Inhibition of human bone marrow-granulocyte precursors by serum from patients with Felty's syndrome. Journal of Rheumatology 7: 275–278

Golding D N, Begg T B 1960 Dexamethasone myopathy. British Medical Journal ii:1129

Good A, Lang K, Olson J, Frishette W 1970 Cardiac necrobiotic (rheumatoid) granulomas without arthritis. Arthritis and Rheumatism 13:166

Goodwill C J, Ford I J, Jones R P K 1972 Hearing in rheumatoid arthritis. A clinical and audiometric survey. Annals of the Rheumatic Diseases 31:170

Gough K R McCarthy C, Read A E, Mollin D L, Waters A H 1964 Folic-acid deficiency in rheumatoid arthritis. British medical Journal i:212

Gowans J D C, Grainieri P A 1959 Septic arthritis. Its relation to intra-articular injections of hydrocortisone acetate. New England Journal of Medicine 261:502

Gray R G, Poppo M J 1983 Necrotising vasculitis as the initial manifestation of rheumatoid artiritis. Journal of Rheumatology 10: 326–328

Green R A, Fromke V L 1966 Splenectomy in Felty's syndrome. Annals of Internal Medicine 64:1265

Grennan D, Anderson J A, Kennedy A C, Mitchell W, Dick W C, Buchanan W W 1975 Relationship between haemoglobin and the other clinical and laboratory parameters in rheumatoid arthritis. Current Medical Research and Opinion 3:104

Griffiths H T, Elston C W, Colton C L, Swannell A J 1984 Popliteal masses masquerading as popliteal cysts. Annals of the Rheumatic Diseases 43: 60–62

Gupta R C, Robinson W A, Smyth C J 1975 Efficacy of lithium in rheumatoid arthritis with granulocytopenia (Felty's syndrome). A preliminary report. Arthritis and Rheumatism 18: 179–184
Gupta R, Robinson W A, Albrecht D 1975 Granulopoietic activity in Felty's syndrome. Annals of the Rheumatic Diseases 34: 156–161
Hajiroussou V J, Webley M 1984 Prolonged low-dose corticosteroid therapy and osteoporosis in rheumatoid arthritis. Annals of the Rheumatic Diseases 43: 24–2
Hakstian R W, Tubiana R 1967 Ulnar deviation of the fingers. Journal of Bone and Joint Surgery 49A:299
Hall A P, Healey I A 1968 Infected synovial cysts arising as a complication of septic arthritis in a patient with rheumatoid arthritis. Arthritis and Rheumatism 11:579
Hall A P, Scott J T 1966 Synovial cysts and rupture of the knee joint in rheumatoid arthritis. An arthrographic study. Annals of the Rheumatic Diseases 25:32
Hall S, Ginsberg W W, Vollertsen R S, Hunder G G 1983 The coexistence of rheumatoid arthritis and giant cell arteritis. Journal of Rheumatology 10: 995–997
Halla J T, Koopman W J, Schrohenloner R E, Darby W L, Heck L W 1983 Local synthesis of IgM and IgM rheumatoid factor in rheumatoid pleuritis. Journal of Rheumatology 10: 204–209
Hamilton E B D 1960 Nail studies in rheumatoid arthritis. Annals of the Rheumatic Diseases 19:167
Harrington T M, Moran J T, Davis D E 1981 Amyloidosis in adult onset Still's disease. Journal of Rheumatology 8: 833–836
Harris E D Jr 1972 A collagenolytic system produced by primary culture of rheumatoid nodule tissue. Journal of Clinical Investigation 51: 2973–2976
Harrison M O, Freiberger R H, Ranawat C S 1971 Arthrography of the rheumatoid wrist joint American Journal of Roentgenology 112:480
Hart F D, Golding J R 1960 Rheumatoid neuropathy ii:1594
Hart L E, Bianchi F A, Banna M 1981 Posterior atlanto-axial subluxation in rheumatoid arthritis Journal of Association of Canadian Radiology 32: 240–241
Haskard D D, Higgens C S, Temple C N, Currey H L F 1983 Spontaneous rupture of the spleen in rheumatoid arthritis. Annals of the Rheumatic Diseases 42: 411–414
Hasock D I, Wright V, Harriman D G F 1970 Neuromuscular disorders in rheumatoid arthritis. Quarterly Journal of Medicine 39:335
Healey L A, Wilske K R, Sagebiel R W 1967 Rheumatoid nodules simulating basal-cell carcinoma. New England Journal of Medicine 277:7
Helal B 1974 The reconstruction of rheumatoid deformities of the hand. British Journal of Hospital Medicine 12:617
Hendrich F, Kuthan F, Tovarek J, Vitulova V 1966 The enzymatic pattern in serum of rheumatoid patients related to muscular wasting. Scripta Medica 39:63
Hernandez L A, Maurikakis M E, Balint G P, 1980 Early rheumatoid arthritis: a clinical, radiological, isotopic and immunological study. Rheumatology 10: 35–48
Hopkins J S 1967 Lower cervical rheumatoid subluxation with tetraplegia. Journal of Bone and Joint Surgery 49B:46
Horler A R, Thompson M 1959 The pleural and pulmonary complications of rheumatoid arthritis. Annals of Internal Medicine 51:1179
Hughes G R, Pridie R B 1970 Acute synovial rupture of the knee — a differential diagnosis from deep vein thrombosis. Proceedings of the Royal Society of Medicine 63:587
Hull R G, Rennie J A N, Eastmond C J, Hutchison J M S, Smith F W 1984 Nuclear magnetic resonance (NMR) tomographic imaging for popliteal cysts in rheumatoid arthritis. Annals of the Rheumatic Diseases 43: 56–59
Hull S, Mathews J A 1982 Pulmonary necrobiotic nodules as a presenting features of rheumatoid arthritis. Annals of the Rheumatic Diseases 41: 21–24
Hume R, Dagg J H, Fraser T N, Goldberg A 1964 Anaema of Felty's syndrome. Annals of the Rheumatic Diseases 23:267
Hunder G G, Ward L E, Ivins J C 1965 Rheumatoid granulomatous lesions simulating malignancy in the head and neck of the femur. Proceedings of the Mayo Clinic 40:766
Isdale I C, Corrigan A B 1971 Backward luxation of the atlas. Two cases of an uncommon condition. Annals of the Rheumatic Diseases 29:6
Iveson J M I, Thadani U, Ionescu M, Wright V 1975 Aortic valve incompetence and replacement in rheumatoid arthritis. Annals of the Rheumatic Diseases 34:312
Jackman J, Pugh D 1970 The positive elbow fat pad sign in rheumatoid arthritis. American Journal of Roentgenology, Radium, Thermo-Nuclear Medicine 108:812
Jacoby R F, Jayson M I V, Cosh J A 1973 Onset, Early Stages, and Prognosis of Rheumatoid Arthritis: A clinical study of 100 patients with 11-year follow-up. British Medical Journal 2: 96–100
Jacqueline F, Boujot A, Canet L 1961 Involvement of the hips in juvenile rheumatoid arthirits. Arthritis and Rheumatism 4:500
Jason H E, Lo Spalluto J, Ziff M 1963 Serum viscosity in rheumatic disease and macroglobulinaemia. Archives of Internal Medicine 112:684
Jayson M I V, Barks J S 1971 Oedema in rheumatoid arthritis: changes in the coefficient of capillary filtration. British medical Journal ii:555
Jayson M I V, Dixon A St J 1970 Valvular mechanisms in juxta-articular cysts. Annals of the Rheumatic Diseases 29:415
Jayson M I V, Cavill I, Barks J S 1971 Lymphatic clearance rates in rheumatoid arthritis. Annals of the Rheumatic Diseases 30:638
Jayson M I V, Ruberstein D, Dixon A St J 1970 intra-articular pressure and rheumatoid géodes (bone 'cysts'). Annals of the Rheumatic Diseases 29:496
Jeremy R 1969 Acute psoas bursitis and unusual joint cysts in rheumatoid arthritis. Medical Journal of Australia 2:1106
Jordan J D, Snyder C H 1964 Rheumatoid disease of the lung and cor pulmonale. American Journal of Diseases of Childhood 108:174
Joyce R A, Boggs D R, Chervenicj P A, Lalezari P 1980 Neutrophil kinetics in Felty's syndrome. The American Journal of Medicine 69: 695n702
Kalback K 1972 Incidence of arteriosclerosis in patients with rheumatoid arthritis receiving long-term cortisteroid therapy. Annals of the Rheumatic Diseases 31:196
Kantor M, Morrow C S 1958 Caplan's syndrome. American Review of Respiratory Diseases 78:274
Karten I 1969 Arteritis, myocardial infarction and rheumatoid arthritis. Journal of the American M dical Association 210:1717
Kay A 1967 Infection in rheumatoid arthritis. Lancet ii:152
Kean W F, Anastassiades T P 1979 Long term chrysotherapy. Incidence of toxicity and efficacy during

sequential time periods. Arthritis and Rheumatism 22: 495–501
Kean W F, Dwosh I L, Anastassiades T P, Ford P M, Kelly H G 1980 The toxicity pattern of D-penicillamine therapy: A guide to its use in rheumatoid arthritis. Arthritis and Rheumatism 23: 158–164
Kean W F, Kassam Y B, Lock C J L, Buchanan W W, Rischke J, Nablo L 1984a Antithrombin activity of gold sodium thiomalate. Clinical Pharmacology and Therapeutics 35: 627–632
Kean W F, Lock C J L, Kassam Y B, Rooney P J, Rischke J, Nablo L, Buchanan W W 1984b A biological effect on platelets by the minor component of gold sodium thiomalate. A by-product of heat sterilization and exposure to light. Clinical and Experimental Rheumatology 2: 321–328
Kellgren J H, Ball J 1950 Tendon lesion in rheumatoid arthritis: a clinicopathological study. Annals of the Rheumatic Diseases 9:48
Kellgren J H, Ball J 1959 Clinical significance of the rheumatoid serum factor. British Medical Journal i:523
Kellgren J H, Lawrence J S, Aitken-Swan J 1953 Rheumatic complaints in an urban population. Annals of the Rheumatic Diseases 12:5
Kellgren J H, Ball J, Fairbrother R W, Barnes K L 1958 Suppurative arthritis complicating rheumatoid arthritis. British Medical Journal 1:1193
Kelly P J, Martin W J, Coventry M B 1970 Bacterial (suppurative) arthritis in the adult. Journal of Bone and Joints Surgery 52A:2595
Kelton J G, Carter C J, Rodger C, Bebenek R T, Gauldie J, Rooney P J, et al 1983 The relationship between platelet-associated IgG, platelet life-span and retirculo-endothelial cell function. Blood (submitted for publication)
Kennedy A C, McGavin D D M 1975 Rheumatoid scleritis producing exophthalmos. The British Journal of Clinical Practice 29:73
Kennedy A C, Burton J A, Allison M E M 1974 Tuberculosis as a continuing cause of renal amyloidosis. British Medical Journal 3:795
Kennedy A C, Smith D A, Anderson J A, Buchanan W W 1974 Osteoporosis in rheumatoid arthritis: its natural history and statistical prediction. Rheumatology 4:441
Kennedy A C, Fell G S, Rooney P J, Stevens W, Dicks W C, Buchanan W W 1975 Zinc; its relationship to osteoporosis in rheumatoid arthritis. Scandinavian Journal of Rheumatology 4:243
Kennedy A C, Boddy K, Williams E D 1979 Whole body elemental composition during drug treatment of rheumatoid arthritis: a preliminary study. Annals of the Rheumatic Diseases 38: 137–140
Kersley G D, Ross F G M, Fowles S J, Johnson C 1964 Tomography in arthritis of the small joints. Annals of the Rheumatic Diseases 23:280
Kettelkamp D B, Leaverton P E, Misol S 1972 Gait characteristics of the rheumatoid knee. Archives of Surgery 104:30
Khong T K, Rooney P J 1982 Manubrio-sternal joint subluxation in rheumatoid arthritis. Journal of Rheumatology 9: 712–715
Kimball H R, Wolff S, Talal N, Plotz P H, Decker J L 1973 Marrow granulocyte reserves in the rheumatic diseases. Arthritis and Rheumatism 16:345
Korin H, Tobis J S 1971 Kinesthetic perceptical disturbance in musculoskeletal disease. Journal of Chronic Disease 24:209
Kormano M 1970 A microadiographic and histological study of the manubriosternal joint in rheumatoid arthritis. Acta Rheumatologica Scandinavica 16:47
Kormano M 1971 Radiographic appearance of the pubic symphysis in old age and in rheumatoid arthritis. Acta Rheumatological Scandinavica 17:286
Kornblum D, Clayton M L, Nash H H 1952 Nontraumatic cervical dislocations in rheumatoid spondylitis. Journal of the American Medical Association 149:431
Kosmin M, Vail J T Jr, Sturman M J 1964 Streptococcal infection and isolated rheumatic-like subcutaneous nodules. Method Bulletin of the United States Army Europe 21:28
Laitenen H, Saksanen S, Suoranta H 1970 Involvement of the manubrio-sternal articulation in rheumatoid arthritis. Acta Rheumatologica Scandinavica 16:40
Landré-Beauvais A J 1800 Doit-on admettre une nouvelle espece de goutte sous la demonstration de goutte asthenique primitive?
Thesis, University of Paris. Cited by Parish L C 1963 An historical approach to the nomenclature of rheumatoid arthritis. Arthritis and Rheumatism 6: 135–138
Lane P W F, Dyer N H, Hawkins C F 1972 Synovial rupture of shoulder joint. British Medical Journal i:356
Lapayowker M, Cliff M, Tourtellotte C 1970 Arthrography in the diagnosis of calf pain. Radiology 95:319
Latman N S 1981 Annual fluctuation in rheumatoid arthritis. Journal of Rheumatology 8: 725–729
Lawrence J S 1961 Prevalence of rheumatoid arthritis. Annals of the Rheumatic Diseases 20:11
Laws J W, El Sallab R A, Scott J T 1967 An arteriographic and histological study of digital arteries. British Journal of Radiology 40:740
Lawson A A H, McLean N 1966 Renal disease and drug therapy in rheumatoid arthritis. Annals of the Rheumatic Diseases 25:441
Lawson A A H, Owen E T, Mowat A G 1967 Nature of anaemia in rheumatoid arthritis. VII. Storage of iron in rheumatoid disease. Annals of Rheumatic Diseases 26:552
Lea A L 1964 An association between the rheumatic diseases and the reticulosis. Annals of the Rheumatic Diseases
Lee F D, El-Ghobarez A F, Buchanan W W, Browne M K 1978 Rheumatoid arthritis, amyloidosis, intestinal ulceration, refractory iron deficiency anaemia and intestinal haemosiderosis: a new clinical syndrome? Heamatology 7: 121–124
Lee P, Baxter A, Dick W C, Webb J 1974 An assessment of grip strength measurement in rheumatoid arthritis Scandinavian Journal of Rheumatology 3:17
Lefkovits A 1969 Synovial cyst of ischial tuberosity in Felty's syndrome. Journal of the American Medical Association 209:1089
Lewis S M, Porter I H 1960 Erythrocyte survival in rheumatoid arthritis. Annals of the Rheumatic Diseases 19:54
Lewis R B, Sanders L L, Lipsmeyer E. (1980). Characteristics of rheumatoid arthritis in a male population. Journal of Rheumatology. 7: 559–562
Lindsay M K, Tavadia H B, Whyte A S, Lee P, Webb J 1973 Acute abdomen in rheumatoid arthritis due to necrotising arteritis. British Medical Journal ii:592
Linquist P, McDonnell D 1970 Rheumatoid cyst causing extradural compression. A case report. Journal of Bone and Joint Surgery 52A:1235
Liss J P, Bachmann W T 1970 Rheumatoid constrictive

pericarditis, treated by pericardiectomy. Arthritis and Rheumatism 13:869
Littler J W 1949 Tendon transfers and arthrodeses in combined median and ulnar nerve paralysis. Journal of Bone and Joint Surgery 31A:225
Littler J W, Eaton R G 1967 Redistribution of forces in the correction of the boutonnière deformity. Journal of Bone and Joint Surgery 49A:1267
Lloyd K, Agarwal A 1970 Tarsal-tunnel syndrome, a presenting feature of rheumatoid arthritis. British Medical Journal iii:32
Locke G B 1963 Rheumatoid lung. Clinical Radiology 14:43
Logue G 1976 Felty's syndrome: granulocyte-bound immunoglobulin G and splenectomy. Annals of Internal Medicine 85: 437–442
Logue G L, Huang A T, Shimm D S 1981 Failure of splenectomy in Felty's syndrome. The role of antibodies supporting granulocyte lysis by lymphocytes. The New England Journal of Medicine 304: 580–583
Lowneg E D, Simons H M 1963 Rheumatoid nodules of the skin. Archives of Dermatology 88:221
Lush B 1952 Ulnar deviation of the fingers. Annals of the Rheumatic Diseases 11:219
Luthra H S, Conn D L, Ferguson R H 1981 Felty's syndrome: response to parenteral gold. Journal of Rheumatology 8: 902–909
Luukkainen R, Isomaki H, Kajander A 1983 Prognostic value of the type of onset of rheumatoid arthritis. Annals of the Rheumatic Diseases 42: 274–275
McAvoy B, Whaley K, Nuki G, Dick W C, Downie W W 1969 Liver in rheumatoid arthritis. Annals of the Rheumatic Diseases 28:606
McCarty D J, Gatter R A 1966 A study of distal interphalangeal joint tenderness in rheumatoid arthritis. Arthritis and Rheumatism 9:325
McConkey B, Frazer G, Bligh A 1965 Transparent skin and osteoporosis — a study in patients with rheumatoid arthritis. Annals of the Rheumatic Diseases 24:210
McFarland G B J, Hoffer M M 1968 Rheumatoid nodules in synovial membranes and tendons. Clinical Orhtopaedics 58:165
MacFarlane J D, Van der Linden S J 1981 Leaking rheumatoid olecranon bursitis as a cause of forearm swelling. Annals of the Rheumatic Diseases 40: 309–311
MacFarlane J D, Franken C K, Van Leeuwen AWFM 1984 Progressive cavitating pulmonary changes in rheumatoid arthritis: a case report. Annals of the Rheumatic Diseases 43: 98–101
McGregor M 1948 Singificance of certain measurements of skull in diagnosis of basilar impression. British Journal of Radiology 21:171
McKendry R J R, Hogan D B 1981 Superior margin rib defects in rheumatoid arthritis. Journal of Rheumatology 8: 673–678
McNair M M, Boyle J A, Buchanan W W, Davidson J K 1969 A clinical and radiological study of rheumatoid arthritis with a note on the findings in osteoarthrosis — 1. The shoulder joint. Clinical Radiology 20:269
Magyar E, Talerman A, Wouters H W 1973 Histological abnormalities in the muscle spindles in rheumatoid arthritis. Annals of the Rheumatic Diseases 32:143
Manshady B M, Thompson G R, Weiss J J 1980 Septic arthritis in a General Hospital 1966–77. Journal of Rheumatology 7: 523–530
Marbach J J, Spier H 1967 Rheumatoid arthritis of the temporomandibular joints. Annals of the Rheumatic Diseases 26:538
Marcolongo R, Bayeli P F, Montagnani M 1979 Gastrointestinal involvement in rheumatoid arthritis: a biopsy study. Journal of Rheumatology 6: 163–173
Marmor L, Lawrence J F, Dubois E L 1967 Posterior interosseous nerve palsy due to rheumatoid arthritis. Journal of Bone and Joint Surgery 49A:381
Marshall R N, Myers D B, Palmer D G 1980 Disturbance of gait due to rheumatoid disease. Journal of Rheumatology 7: 617–623
Marshall T R 1967 Digital arterial changes in rheumatoid arthritis. General Practitioner 35:143
Marshall T R 1968 Radiographic changes in rheumatoid arthritis in the digits. Radiology 90:121
Martel W 1963 Radiological aspects of rheumatoid arthritis. Proceedings of the International Symposium. International Congress Series. Excerpta Medica Foundation, Amsterdam, p 64
Martel W 1968 Cervical spondylitis in rheumatoid disease. American Journal of Medicine 44:441
Martel W, Abell M R 1963 Fatal atlanto-axial luxation in rheumatoid arthritis. Arthritis and Rheumatism 6:224
Martel W, Bole G G 1968 Pathologic fracture of the odontoid process in rheumatoid arthritis. Radiology 90:948
Martel W, Page J W 1960 Cervical vertebral erosions and subluxations in rheumatoid arthritis and ankylosing spondylitis. Arthritis and Rheumatism 3:546
Mathews J A 1969 Atlanto-axial subluxation in rheumatoid arthritis. Annals of the Rheumatic Diseases 28:260
Mathews J A 1974 Atlanto-axial subluxation in rheumatoid arthritis. A 5-year follow-up study. Annals of the Rheumatic Diseases 33:526
Medsger T A, Christy N C 1976 Carpal arthritis with ankylosis in late onset Still's disease. Arthritis and Rheumatism 19: 232–242
Meikle J A K, Wilkinson M 1971 Rheumatoid involvement of the cervical spine. Radiological assessment. Annals of the Rheumatic Diseases 30:154
Meire H B, Lindsay D J, Swinson D R, Hamilton E B D 1974 Comparison of ultrasound and positive contrast arthrography in the diagnosis of popliteal and calf swellings. Annals of the Rheumatic Diseases 33:221
Miall W F, Caplan A, Cochrane A L, Kilpatrick G S, Oldham P D 1953 An epidemiological study of rheumatoid arthritis associated with characteristic chest x-ray appearances in coal-workers. British Medical Journal iv:1231
Mitchell W S, Millar J, Sturrock R D 1975 An evaluation of goniometry as an objective parameter for measuring joint motion. Scottish Medical Journal 20:57
Mongan E, Cass R, Jacox R, Vaughan J H 1969 A study of the relation of sero-negative and sero-positive rheumatoid arthritis to each other and to necrotising vasculitis. American Journal of Medicine 47:23
Montgomery W W, Perone P M, Schall L A 1955 Arthritis of the crico-arytenoid joint. Annals of the Otalogy, Phenology and Laryngology 64:1025
Moore R A, Brunner C M, Sandusky W R, Leavell B S 1971 Felty's syndrome: Long-term follow-up after splenectomy. Annals of Internal Medicine 75:381
Mowat A G 1971 Haematological abnormalities in rheumatoid arthritis. Seminars in Arthritis and Rheumatism 1:195
Mowat A G, Baum J 1971 Chemotaxis of polymorphonuclear leukocytes from patients with rheumatoid arthritis. Journal of Clinical Investigations 50:2541

Mowat A G, Hothersall T E 1968 Nature of anaemia in rheumatoid arthritis. VIII. Iron content of synovial tissue in patients with rheumatoid arthritis and in normal individuals. Annals of the Rheumatic Diseases 27:34

Mowat A G, Hothersall T. . .E, Aitcheson W R C 1969 Nature of anaemia in rheumatoid arthritis, XI. Changes in iron metabolism induced by the administration of corticotrophin. Annals of the Rheumatic Diseases 28: 303–309

Mueller M N, Jurist J M 1973 Skeletal status in rheumatoid arthritis. Arthritis and Rheumatism 16:66

Muirden K D 1966 Ferritin in synovial cells in patients with rheumatoid arthritis. Annals of the rheumatic Diseases 25:387

Muirden K D 1970 Lymph node iron in rheumatoid arthritis. Histology, ultastructure and chemical concentration. Annals of the Rheumatic Diseases 29:81

Muirden K D Senator G B 1967 Iron in the synovial membrane in rheumatoid arthritis and other joint diseases. Annals of the Rheumatic Diseases 27: 38–47

Myer A R, Miller L M, Pinals R S 1969 Pyarthrosis complicating rheumatoid arthritis. Lancet 2: 714–716

Myles A B 1971 Posterior synovial leaks in arthritis of the knee. Proceeding of the Royal Society of Medicine 64:262

Nakata H, Russell W 1970 Chest roentgenograms in rheumatiod arthritis: Hiroshima-Nagasaki. American Journal of Roentgenology, Radium and Nuclear Medicine 108:819

Nørgaard F 1965 Earliest roentgenological changes in polyarthritis of the rheumatoid type: rheumatoid arthritis. Radiology 84:1

Omar A, Mowat A G 1968 Nature of anaemia in rheumatoid arthritis. IX. Folate metabolism in patients with rheumatoid arthritis. Annals of the Rheumatic Diseases 27:414

Onedera S, Hill J R 1965 Pulmonary hypertension. Report of case in association with heumatoid arthroid arthritis. Ohio Medical Journal 61:141

O'Neill J A Jr, Scott H W, Billings F T, Foster J H 1968 The role of splenectomy in Felty's syndrome. Annals of Surgery 167:81

Ornilla E, Ansell B M, Swannell A J 1972 Cervical spine involvement in patients with chronic arthritis undergoing orthopaedic surgery. Annals of the Rheumatic Diseases 31:364

Owen E T, Lawson A A H 1966 Nature of anaemia in rheumatoid arthritis. VI. Metabolism of endogenous iron. Annals of the Rheumatic Diseases 25:547

Ozdemir A I, Wright J R, Calkins E 1971 Influence of rheumatoid arthritis on amyloidosis of aging comparison of 47 rheumatoid patients with 47 controls matched for age and sex. New England Journal of Medicine 285:534

Pahle J A, Raunio P 1969 The influence of wrist position on finger deviation in the rheumatoid hand. Journal of Bone and Joint Surgery 51B:664

Pallis C A, Scott J T 1965 Peripheral neuropathy in rheumatoid arthritis. British medical Journal i:1141

Palmer D G 1969 Synovial cysts in rheumatoid disease. Annals of Internal Medicine 70:61

Palmer D G, Marshall A J, Buchanan W W 1977 Eighteenth century bone and joint disease: William Hunter's collection, Pathology Department, Royal Infirmary Glasgow. Rheumatology 7: 113–118

Panush R S, Franco A E, Schur P H 1971 Rheumatoid arthritis associated with eosinophilia. Annals Internal Medicine 75:199

Parker R A, Thomas P M 1959 Intestinal perforation and widespread arteritis in rheumatoid arthritis during treatment with cortisone. British Medical Journal i:540

Partridge R E H, Duthie J J R 1963 Incidence of macrocytic anaemia in rheumatoid arthritis. British Medical Journal 1:89

Patterson C D, Harville W E, Pierce J A 1965 Rheumatoid lung disease. Annals of Internal Medicine 62:685

Payne R W, Harris M C 1972 Factor VIII inhibitor: acquired haemostatic defect in a non-haemophiliac patient with rheumatoid arthritis. Scottish Medical Journal 17:310

Pengelly C D R 1966 Felty's syndrome. Good response to adrenocorticosteroids: possible mechanism of the anaemia. British Medical Journal iv:986

Penny W J, Knight R K, Rees A M, Thomas A L, Smith A P 1982 Obliterative bronchiolitis in rheumatoid arthritis. Annals of the Rheumatic Diseases 41: 469–472

Pernis B, Ballabio C B, Chiappino G 1963 Presence of the rheumatoid factor in vascular lesions of aggravated (malignant) rheumatoid arthritis: fluorescent antibody studies. Rheumatismo 15:187

Perri J A, Rodnan G P, Mankin H J 1968 Giant synovial cysts of the calf in patients with rheumatoid arthritis. Journal of Bone and Joint Surgery 50A:709

Petrie G R, Blomfield P, Grant I W B, Crompton G K 1980 Upper lobe fibrosis and cavitation in rheumatoid disease. British Journal of Diseases of the Chest. 74: 263–267

Pettersson T, Wegelius O, Skrifvars B 1970 Gastrointestinal disturbances in patients with severe rheumatoid arthritis. Acta Medica Scandinavica 188:139

Pirani M, Lange-Mechlen I, Cockshott W P 1982 Rupture of a posterior synovial cyst of the elbow. Journal of Rheumatology 9: 94–96

Pitcher C S, Lindsay D J, Hill A G S 1970 Absorption of vitamin B_{12} in rheumatoid arthritis. Annals of the Rheumatic Diseases 29:533

Pope R M, Mannik M, Gilliland B C, Teller D C 1975 The hyperviscosity syndrome in rheumatoid arthritis due to intermediate complexes formed by self-association of IgG-rheumatiod factors. Arthritis and Rheumatism 18:97

Portner M M, Gracie W A 1966 Rheumatoid lung disease with cavitary nodules, pneumothorax and eosinophilia. New England Journal of Medicine 275:697–700

Price T M L, Skelton M O 1956 Rheumatoid arthritis with lung lesions. Thorax 11:234

Rackow F 1953 Felty's syndrome treated by splenectomy. British Medical Journal 2:1415

Ragan C 1949 The general management of rheumatoid arthritis. Journal of the American Medical Association 141:124

Rajapakse C, Thompson R, Grennan D M, Winston B M, Patel P, Nuttall P M, et al 1983 Increased bone metabolism in rheumatoid arthritis measured by the whole-body retention of $^{99}Tc^{m}$ methylene diphosphonate. Annals of the Rheumatic Diseases 42:138–141

Raman D, Haslock I 1982 Trochanteric bursitis — a frequent cause of 'hip' pain in rheumatoid arthritis. Annals of the Rheumatic Diseases 41: 602–603

Rana N A, Taylor A R 1971 Upward migration of the odontoid peg in rheumatoid arthritis. Proceedings of the Royal Society of Medicine 64: 717–718

Ranawat C S, Straub L R 1970 Volar tenosynovitis of wrist in rheumatoid arthritis. Arthritis and Rheumatism 13:112

Ranawat C S, Freiberger R H, Jordan L R, Straub L R 1969

Arthrography in the rheumatoid wrist joint. A preliminary report. Journal of Bone and Joint Surgery 51A:1269
Rask M A 1978 Achilles tendon rupture owing to rheumatoid disease. Journal of the American Medical Association 239: 435–436
Rasker J J, Kuipers F C 1983 Are rheumatoid nodules caused by vasculitis? A study of 13 early cases. Annals of the Rheumatic Diseases 42: 384–388
Raskin R J, Schnapf D J, Wolf C R, Killian P J, Lawless O J 1983 Computerized tomography in evaluation of atlanto-axial subluxation in rheumatoid arthritis. Journal of Rheumatology 10: 33–41
Raven R W, Weber F P, Price L W 1948 The necrobiotic nodules of rheumatoid arthritis: case in which the scalp, abdominal wall involving striped muscle, larynx, pericardium (involving myocardium), pleurae (involving lungs) and peritoneum were affected. Annals of the Rheumatic Diseases 7:63
Raymond F D, Bowie M A, Dugan A 1965 Iron metabolism in rheumatoid arthritis. Arthritis and Rheumatism 8:233
Read G O, Solomon L, Biddulph 1983 Relationship between finger and wrist deformities in rheumatoid arthritis. Annals of the Rheumatic Diseases 42: 619–625
Redisch W, Messina E J, Hughes G 1970 Capillaroscopic observations in rheumatic diseases. Annals of the Rheumatic Disease 29:244
Reid D M, Kennedy N S J, Smith M A, Tothill P, Nuki G 1982 Total body calcium in rheumatoid arthritis: effects of disease activity and corticosteroid treatment. British Medical Journal 285: 330–332
Reitan H 1968 Anterior subluxation of the atlas in rheumatic disease. Acta Rheumatologica Scandinavica 11:24
Reymand T A 1979 The search for 'arthritis' in antiquity: paleo-arthritis workshop. Henry Ford Hospital Medical Journal 27: 32–37
Richards A G, Barrett G M 1958 Rheumatoid lung changes associated with asbestosis. Thorax 13:185
Richmond J, Gardner D L, Roy L M G, Duthie J J R 1956 Nature of anaemia in rheumatoid arthritis. III. Changes in the bone marrow and their relation to other features of the disease. Annals of the Rheumatic Diseases 15: 217–225
Riley M, Harrison S H 1968 Interossous muscle biopsy during hand surgery for rheumatoid arthritis. British Journal of Plastic Surgery 21:342
Rimoin D, Wennberg J 1966 Acute septic arthritis complicating rheumatoid arthritis. Journal of the American Medical Association 196:617
Roberts F D, Hagedorn A B, Slocumb C H, Owen C A 1963 Evaluation of the anaemia of rheumatoid arthritis. Blood 21:470
Robertson M D J, Hart F D, White W F, Nuki G, Boardman P L 1968 Rheumatoid lymphadenopathy. Annals of the Rheumatic Disease 27:253
Robinson H S 1966 Rheumatoid arthritis — atlanto-axial subluxation and its clinical presentation. Canadian Medical Association Journal 94:470
Ropes M W, Bennett G A, Cobb S, Jacox R, Jessar R A 1959 1958 Revision of diagnostic criteria in rheumatoid arthritis. Bulletin of the Rheumatic Diseases 9:175
Rosenspire K C, Kennedy A C, Steinback J, Blau M, Green F A 1980 Investigation of the metabolic activity of bone in rheumatoid arthritis. Journal of Rheumatology 7: 469–473
Rosenthal F D, Beeley J M, Gelsthorpe K, Doughty R W 1974 White-cell antibodies and the aetiology of Felty's syndrome. Quarterly Journal of Medicine NS 43:187
Rosin A J, Toghill P J 1963 Fistulous rheumatism. An unusual complication of rheumatoid arthritis. Postgraduate Medical Journal 39:96
Roy L M H, Alexander W R M, Duthie J J R 1954 Nature of anaemia in rheumatoid arthritis. I. Metabolism of iron. Annals of the Rheumatic Diseases 14: 63–71
Rubin E H, Gordon M, Thelmo W L 1967 Nodular pleuropulmonary rheumatoid disease. American Journal of Medicine 42:567
Ruderman M, Miller L M, Pinals R S 1968 Clinical and serologic observations on 27 patients with Felty's syndrome. Arthritis and Rheumatism 11:377
Russell A S, Ansell B M 1972 Septic arthritis. Annals of the Rheumatic Diseases 31:40
Russell L A, Bayles T B 1941 The temporomandibular joint in rheumatoid arthritis. Journal of the American Dental Association 140:659
Sandusky W R, Rudolf L E, Leavell B S 1968 Splenectomy for control of neutropenia in Felty's syndrome. Annals of Surgery 167:744
Saunders C G, Weston W J 1971 Synovial mass lesions in the anteroposterior projection of the ankle joint. Journal of the Canadian Association of Radiologists 22:275
Saville P D 1967 A quantitative approach to simple radiographic diagnosis of osteoporosis: its application to the osteoporosis of rheumatoid arthritis. Arthritis and Rheumatism 10: 416–422
Scadding J G 1969 The lungs in rheumatoid arthritis. Proceedings of the Royal Society of Medicine 62: 227–238
Scarborough H, Shuster S 1960 Corticosteroid purpura. Lancet i:93
Schmid F R, Cooper N S, Ziff M 1961 Arteritis in rheumatoid arthritis. American Journal of Medicine 30:56
Schneider R E, Dobbins W O 1968 Suction biopsy of the rectal mucosa for diagnosis of arteritis in rheumatoid arthritis and related diseases. Annals of Internal Medical 68:561
Schraibman I G, Goudie R B 1969 Limb gangrene associatev° with rheumatoid arthritis: clinico-pathological conference. Scottish Medical Journal 14:361
Schumacher H R Jr, Ligot P N, Barry P E 1968 Conjunctival and nailfold micro-circulation in patients with rheumatoid arthritis and normal subjects. Acta Rheumatologica Scandinavica 14:253
Scott J T 1960 Morning stiffness in rheumatoid arthritis. Annals of the Rheumatic Diseases 19:361
Scott J T, Porter I H, Lewis S M, Dixon A St J 1961 Studies of gastronintestinal bleeding caused by corticosteroids, salicylates, and other analgesics. Quarterly Journal of Medicine NS 30:167
Scott J T, Hourihane D O, Doyle F H, Steiner R E, Laws J W, Dixon A St J, Bywaters E G L 1961 Digital arteritis in rheumatoid arthritis. Annals of the Rheumatic Diseases 20:224
Scott J T, El Sallab R A, Laws J W 1967 The digital artery lesion in rheumatoid arthritis: further observations. British Journal of Radiology 40:748
Shapiro J S 1968 The wrist in relation to ulnar drift of the finger in rheumatoid arthritis. Presbyterian St. Lukes Hospital Medical Bulletin 7:69
Shapiro J 1970 A new factor in the etiology of ulnar drift. Clinical Orthopaedics 68:32
Sharp J 1957 The differential diagnosis of ankylosing spondylitis. British Medical Journal i:975
Sharp J, Purser D W 1961 Spontaneous atlanto-axial

dislocation in ankylosing spondylitis and rheumatoid arthritis. Annals of the Rheumatic Diseases 20:47
Sharp J, Purser D W, Lawrence J S 1958 Rheumatoid arthritis of the cervical spine in the adult. Annals of the Rheumatic Diseases 17:303
Sharp J T, Lidsky M D, Collins L C, Moreland J 1971 Methods of scoring the progression of radiologie changes in rheumatoid arthritis. Correlation of radiologic, clinical and laboratory abnormalities. Arthritis and Rheumatism 14:706
Shearn M A, Epstien W V, Engleman E P 1963 Serum viscosity in rheumatic disease and marcroglobulinaemia. Archives of Internal Medicine 112:684
Short C L The antiquity of rheumatoid arthritis. Arthritis and Rheumatism 17: 193–205
Short C L, Bauer W 1948 Course of rheumatoid arthritis in patients receiving simple medical and orthopaedic measures. New England Journal of Medicine 238:142
Short C L, Bauer W, Reynolds W E 1957 Rheumatoid arthritis. Harvard University Press, Cambridge
Shupak R, Bernier V, Rabinovich S, Gordon D A, Wright T 1983 Avascular necrosis of bone with rheumatoid vasculitis. Journal of Rheumatology 10: 261–266
Sievers K, Laine V 1963 The sacro-iliac joint in rheumatoid arthritis in adult females. Acta Rheumatologica Scandinavica 9:222
Silver M, Steinbrocker O 1953 Resorptive osteopathy in inflammatory arthritis ('absorptive arthritis' 'opera-glass hand'). Bulletin of the Hospital for Joint Diseases 14:211
Simons F E R, Schaller J G 1975 Benign rheumatoid nodules. Pediatrics 56:29
Sinclair R J G, Cruickshank B 1956 A clinical and pathological study of sixteen cases of rheumatoid arthritis with extensive visceral involvement. Quarterly Journal of Medicine 25:313
Smith E M, Juvinall R C, Bender L F, Pearson J R 1966 Flexor forces and rheumatoid metacarpophalangeal deformity. Journal of the American Medical Association 198:150
Smith H 1975 Infectious diseases Part 2. Medicine (CIBA) 2:61
Smith P H, Benn R T, Sharp J 1972 Natural history of rheumatoid cervical luxations. Annals of the Rheumatic Diseases 31:431
Snorrason E 1951 The problem of ulnar deviation of the fingers in rheumatoid arthritis. Acta Medica Scandinavica 140:359
Soila P 1958 Roentgen manifestations of adult rheumatoid arthritis, with special regard to the early changes. Acta Rheumatologica Scandinavica Suppl 1: 1–144
Soila P 1964 Some features of angiographic findings in rheumatoid arthritis and scleroderma. Acta Rheumatologica Scandinavica 10:189
Sokoloff L 1953 The heart in rheumatoid arthritis. American Heart Journal 45:635
Sokoloff L, Wilens S L, Bunim J J 1951 Arteritis of striated muscle in rheumatoid arthritis. American Journal of Pathology 27:157
Sokoloff L, McCluskey R T, Bumin J J 1953 Vasculatiry of the early subcutaneous nodule in rheumatoid arthritis. Archives of Pathology 55:475
Sørensen A W S 1960 Investigation of kidney function in rheumatoid arthritis. Acta Rheumatologica Scandinavica 6:115
Spence M P 1955 Rheumatoid disease of the lungs and pleura. Archives of the Middlesex Hospital 5:95
Spencer D G, Sturroch R D, Buchanan W W 1980 Ankylosing spondylitis yesterday and today. Medical History 24: 60–69
Stack B H R, Grant I W B 1965 Rheumatoid interstitial lung disease. British Journal of Diseases of Chest 59:202
Stage D E, Mannik M 1971 M-Globulin in rheumatoid arthritis. Evaluation of its clinical significance. Arthritis and Rheumatism 14:440
Steer G, Jayson M I V, Dixon A St J, Beighton P 1971 Joint capsule collagen. Analysis by the study of intra-articular pressure during joint distension. Measurements in the knees of control subjects and patients with rheumatoid arthritis and Ehlers-Danlos syndrome. Annals of the Rheumatic Diseases 30:481
Stenn F F, Milgram J W, Lee S L, Weigand R J, Veis A, Rogers F 1979 (Biochemical discovery of homogentisic acid pigment in an ochronotic Egyptian mummy. Henry Ford Medical Journal 27: 44–48
Stenvist B, Westermark P, Wibell L 1974 Simple method of diagnostic screening for amyloidosis. Annals of the Rheumatic Diseases 33:75
Straub L R 1959–1960 The etiology of finger deformities in the hand affected by rheumatoid arthritis. Bulletin of the Hospital for Joint Diseases 20–21:322
Sturgill B B, Allan J 1970 Rheumatoid-like nodules presenting as pump bumps in a patient without rheumatoid arthritis. Arthritis and Rheumatism 13:175
Sturroch R D, Sharma J J, Buchanan W W 1977 Evidence of rheumatoid arthritis in ancient India. Arthritis and Rheumatism 20: 42–44
Sturrock R D, Cowden E A, Howie E, Grennan D M, Buchanan W W 1975 The forgotten nodules: complications of sacral nodules in rheumatoid arthritis. British Medical Journal iv:92
Sukoff M H, Kadin M M, Moran T 1972 Transoral decompression for myelopathy caused by rheumatoid arthritis of the cervical spine. Case report. Journal of Neurosurgery 37:493
Sullivan S, Hamilton E B D, Williams R 1978 Rheumatoid arthritis and liver involvement. Journal of the Royal College of Physicians (London) 12: 416–422
Sutton P P, Kadir H, Pavia D, Sheahan N F, Clarke S W 1982 Lung mucociliary clearance in rheumatoid disease. Annals of the Rheumatic Diseases 41: 47–51
Sweetnam D R, Mason R M, Murray R O 1960 Steroid arthropathy of the hip. British Medical Journal i:1392
Swezey R L 1971–1972 Dynamic factors in deformity of the rheumatoid arthritis hand. Bulletin on the Rheumatic Diseases 22:649
Swezey R, Alexander S 1969 Notching of the carpal navicular. Annals of the Rheumatic Diseases 28:45
Swinson D R, Hamilton E B D, Mathews J A, Yates D A H 1972 Vertical subluxation of the axis in rheumatoid arthritis. Annals of the Rheumatic Diseases 31:359
Tait G B W, Bach F, Dixon A St J 1965 Acute synovial rupture. Annals of the Rheumatic Diseases 24:273
Talal N, Bunim J J 1964 The development of malignant lymphoma in the course of Sjögren's syndrome. American Journal of Medicine 36:529
Talbott J A, Calkins E 1964 Pulmonary involvement in rheumatoid arthritis. Journal of the American Medical Association 189:911
Taylor A R, Rana N A 1973 A valve. An explanation of the formation of popliteal cysts. Annals of the Rheumatic Diseases 32:419

Teilum G, Lindahl A 1954 Frequency and significance of amyloid changes in rheumatoid arthritis. Acta Medica Scandinavica 150:443

Theofilopoulos A N, Burtonboy G, Lospalluto J L, Ziff M 1974 IgG rheumatoid factor and low molecular weight IgM. An association with vasculitis. Arthritis and Rheumatism 17:272

Thompson M 1965 In: Dixon A St J (ed) Progress in clinical rheumatology. Churchill, London, p 10–26

Thomson D, Gardener D L 1969 Thrombotic microangiopathy in rheumatoid arthritis. Scottish Medical Journal 14:190

Thorne C, Urowitz M, Wanless I, Roberts E, Blendis L M 1982 Liver disease in Felty's syndrome. American Journal of Medicine 73: 35–40

Thurtle O A, Cawley I D 1983 The frequency of leg ulceration in rheumatoid arthritis: A survey. Journal of Rheumatology 10: 507–509

Topp J R, Hart G D 1967 Widespread necrotising arteritis in rheumatoid arthritis. Canadian Medical Association Journal 97:412

Triger D R, Joekes A M 1973 Renal amyloidosis — a fourteen-year follow up. Quarterly Journal of Medicine NS 42:15

Turner R, Collins R, Browner S, Kaufmann J, Schumacher H R, Parker M, deChatelet L 1976 Neutrophil and rheumatoid factor-immunoglobulin G insoluble complex interactions: phagocytosis and sequelae. Journal of Rheumatology 3: 109–117

Uddin J, Krus A S, Kelly H G 1970 Survivorship and death in rheumatoid arthritis. Arthiritis and Rheumatism 13:125

Unverforth L J, Olix M L 1973 The effect of local steroid injection on tendons. Journal of Bone and Joint Surgery 55A:1315

Votila E 1964 The temporomandibular joint in adult rheumatoid arthritis. A clinical and roentgenologic study. Acta Odontologica Scandinavica 22 (Suppl 39)

Vainio K 1967 Rheumatoid changes in the metacarpophalangeal region as a cause of Bunnell's sign. Annals of the Rheumatic Diseases 26:328

Vainio K, Oka M 1953 Ulnar deviation of the fingers. Annals of the Rheumatic Diseases 12:122

Van Kerckhove H 1970 Involvement of the lateral atlanto-axial joints as first and late symptom of rheumatoid arthritis. Acta Rheumatologica Scandinavica 16:197

Vaughan-Jackson O J 1948 Rupture of extensor tendons by attrition at inferior radio-ulnar joint; report of 2 cases. Journal of Bone and Joint Surgery 30B:528

Vaughan-Jackson O J 1962 Rheumatoid hand deformities considered in the light of tendon imbalance. Journal of Bone and Joint Surgery 44B:764

Vincent P C, Levi J A, MacQueen A 1974 The mechanism of neutropenia in Felty's syndrome. Journal of Haematology 27:463–475

Walker W C 1967 Pulmonary infections and rheumatoid arthritis. Quarterly Journal of Medicine NS 36:239

Walker W C, Wright V 1968 Pulmonary lesions and rheumatiod arthritis. Medicine (Baltimore) 47:501

Ward R 1961 Pleural effusion and rheumatoid disease. Lancet ii:1336

Watson D, Ochsner S F 1967 Compression of bladder due to 'rheumatoid' cysts of hip joint. American Journal of Roentgenology 99:695

Watt L, Baumann R R 1967 Pseudo-xanthomatous rheumatoid nodules. Archives of Dermatology (Chicago) 95:156

Webb F W S, Hickman J A, Brew D S 1968 Death from vertebral artery thrombosis in rheumatoid arthritis. British Medical Journal ii:537

Webb J, Payne W H 1970 Abdominal apoplexy in rheumatoid arthritis. Australasian Annals of Medicine 19:1

Webb J, Payne W H 1972 Rheumatoid nodules of the vocal folds. Annals of the Rheumatic Diseases 31:122

Webb J, Downie W W, Dick W C, Lee P 1973 Evaluation of digital joint circumference measurements in rheumatoid arthritis. Scandinavian Journal of Rheumatology 2:127

Webb J, Whaley K, MacSween R N M, Nuki G, Dick W C, Buchanan W W 1975 Liver disease in rheumatoid arthritis and Sjögren's syndrome. Propective study using biochemical and serological markers of hepatic dysfunction. Annals of the Rheumatic Diseases 34:70

Wegelius O, Pasternack A, Kuhlbäck B 1969 Muscular involvement in rheumatoid arthritis. Acta Rheumatologica Scandinavica 15:257

Weinstein I M 1959 A correlative study of the erythrokinetics and disturbances in iron metabolism associated with the anaemia of rheumatoid arthritis. Blood 14:950

Weller R, Bruckner F, Chamberlain M 1970 Rheumatoid neuropathy: a histological and electrophysiological study. Journal of Neurology, Neurosurgery and Psychiatry 33:593

Westermark P 1984 Diagnosis and characterisation of systemic amyloidosis by biopsy of subcutaneous abdominal fat tissue. Internal Medicine for the Specialist 5: 154–160

Weston W J 1969 The enlarged subdeltoid bursa in rheumatoid arthritis. British Journal of Radiology 42:481

Weston W J 1970 The bursa deep to tendo Achilles Australasian Radiology 14:327

Weston W J 1971 The synovial changes at the elbow in rheumatoid arthritis. Australasian Radiology 15:170

Weston W J 1971 The extrasynovial and capsular fat pads on the posterior aspect of the knee joint. British Journal of Radiology 44:277

Whaey K, Dick W C 1968 Fatal subaxial dislocation of cervical spine in rheumatoid arthritis. British Medical Journal ii:31

Whaley K, Williamson J, Chisholm D M, Webb J, Mason D K, Buchanan W W 1973 Sjögren's syndrome 1. Sicca components. Quarterly Journal of Medicine NS 42:279

Whaley K, Webb J, McAvoy, Huges G V R, Lee P, MacSween R N M, Buchanan W W 1973 Sjögren's syndrome 2 Clinical associations and immunological phenomena. Quarterly Journal of Medicine NS 42:513

Wiik A 1975 Circulating immune complexes involving granulocyte-specific antinuclear factors in Felty's syndrome and rheumatoid arthritis. Acta Pathologica Microbiologica Scandinavica 83: 354–365

Wiik A, Munthe E 1974 Complement-fixing granulocyte-specific antinuclear factors in neutropenic cases of rheumatoid arthritis. Immunology 26: 1127–1134

Wilkinson M 1962 Rheumatoid pericarditis. British Medical Journal ii:1723

Wilkinson M, Kirk J 1965 Leg ulcers complicating rheumatoid arthritis. Scottish Medical Journal 10:175

Wilkinson M, Meikle J A K 1966 Tomography of the sacro-iliac joints. Annals of the Rheumatic Diseases 25:433

Wilkinson M, Torrance W N 1967 Clinical background of rheumatoid vascular disease. Annals of the Rheumatic Diseases 26:475

Williams L E, Bland J H, Lipson R L 1966 Cervical spine subluxations and massive osteolysis in the upper extremities in rheumatoid arthritis. Arthritis and Rheumatism 9:348

Williams M H, Sheldon P J H S, Torrigiani G, Eisen V, Mattingly S 1971 Palindromic rheumatism. Clinical and immunological studies. Annals of the Rheumatic Diseases 30:375–380

Wilson J, Sokoloff L 1970 Epidermoid cysts simulating rheumatoid nodules. Journal of the American Medical Association 214:593

Winchester R J, Litwin S D, Koffler D, Kunkel H G 1971 Observations on the easinophilia of certain patients with rheumatoid arthritis. Arthritis and Rheumatism 14:650

Winfiled J, Young A, Williams P, Corbett M 1983 Prospective study of the radiological changes in hands, feet and cervical spine in adult rheumatoid disease. Annals of the Rheumatic Diseases 42: 613–618

Wiseman M J 1981 Dislocation of the manubriosternal Joint in rheumatoid arthritis. Annals of the Rheumatic Diseases 40: 307–308

Wolman L, Darke C S, Young A 1965 The larynx in rheumatoid arthritis. Journal of Laryngology 79:403

Wright V, Johns R J 1960 Physical factors concerned with the stiffness of normal and diseased joints. Bulletin of Johns Hopkins Hospital 106:215

Wright V, Johns R J 1961 Quantitative and qualitative analysis of joint stiffness in normal subjects and in patients with connective tissue diseases. Annals of the Rheumatic Diseases 20:36

Wright V, Plunkett T G 1966 Scientific assessment of the results of physical treatment — measurement of stiffness. Annals of Physical Medicine 8:280

The management of rheumatoid disease

'No two patients present the same combination of symptoms nor are their problems to be met in exactly the same manner' said Irons in 1935. Proper management of any potentially chronic disease such as rheumatoid arthritis deals not only with the physical impact of disease but also with the way it affects the patient's personality and everyday life, and in addition, anticipates what problems may lie ahead. Such an approach requires a team of professionals comprising the family doctor, rheumatologist, nurse, orthotist, remedial therapists, orthopaedic surgeon and perhaps a clinical psychologist as well.

HISTORY

The first meeting with the patient involves taking a history of joint symptoms and ascertaining what functional problems have been caused. Patients with hip problems will volunteer that they have difficulty climbing stairs or hills but gentle and sympathetic questioning is necessary if they are to admit to problems with going to the lavatory or having sexual intercourse. Similarly, patients with problem fingers will admit to having trouble with fastening buttons but not necessarily to problems like letting off the handbrake in the car or squeezing a tube of toothpaste. A patient with several hours of crippling early morning stiffness may well mention the difficulties of getting the children off to school but not necessarily complain about having to get out of bed hours earlier than usual in order to loosen up for the day's activities.

A family history may give clues to potential problems if it reveals that a relative was crippled with rheumatoid disease or had disastrous side-effects from drug treatment. Certain drugs and procedures may also be avoided if there is a family history say of diabetes mellitus or hypertension.

Of paramount importance is the social history. The physician must know about the patient's occupation, his ambitions and hopes for the future as well as his family commitments, how many stairs he has to climb at home, where the bathroom is and how far away he lives from relatives, friends and shops.

The economic and social impact of rheumatoid arthritis can be crippling. Yelin et al (1979) found that the resulting loss of income to American patients was 3 times as much as the cost of their medical care and that 75% of patients with severe rheumatoid disease had been obliged to change their place or hours or type of work. Meenan et al (1981) confirmed major losses in areas of work, finance and family structure; patients were earning only half their expected salary, 60% were unable to work at all after 9 years of disease and 16% had divorced or separated.

EXAMINATION

A thorough examination of all systems must be made and the range of movement of the joints recorded as a baseline. The physician has to decide whether disease is active and therefore potentially reversible or whether it is inactive with mechanical joint damage secondary to old and now quiescent inflammatory disease.

EXPLANATION

By now the physician has an idea of his patient's personality and this will help to guide him in explaining the disease to the patient in such a way that hope will be retained. Patients either never register or else forget about half of what is said at a consultation (Ley & Spelman, 1965; Joyce et al, 1969; Anderson et al, 1979) and is therefore important that the patient be invited to attend again for further discussion. Accurate prognosis at an early stage is difficult but it can be useful for the patient to know that mild, self-limiting and even single attacks of rheumatoid arthritis can occur (Hench, 1949; Short, 1968) and that the diagnosis does not necessarily mean a crippling disease. O'Sullivan & Cathcart (1972) were able to show that some 30% of patients diagnosed on the New York criteria (Lawrence, 1977) and some two-thirds classified as having 'definite' disease on the ARA criteria (Ropes et al, 1959) had no clinical evidence whatever of disease some 3–5 years later. Beall & Cobb (1961) make the point that there is a spectrum of disease: at one end a high proportion of patients briefly affected and at the other, patients whose disease is continuous. About 70% of patients follow a progressive course (Short et al, 1957) but even so, some 45% treated with only simple measures excluding gold between 1930 and 1936 had improved many years later (Short & Bauer, 1948). Linos et al (1980) judged that 13.5% of their 521 patients were in remission 10 years after diagnosis.

Patients can be told therefore that even if there is no 'cure' for rheumatoid disease, the prospects are good and even if the disease does not settle spontaneously, the likelihood is that modern treatment can bring it under control.

At this stage, a simple explanation of how untreated chronic inflammation leads to joint damage later is essential if the patient is to understand the value of protecting the joints from overuse and the rationale of treatment with drugs to modify inflammation. There are two aspects of joint disease to be understood by both patient and doctor. First is the inflammatory component which causes pain and stiffness and where the physical treatment is that of resting the joint. Second is the pain and disability caused by damage which is secondary to the inflammatory phase and where mobilisation and pain relief are required rather than disease-modifying drugs.

PATIENTS' PROBLEMS

The worst problem for the patient is fear. He is frightened of losing his independence and of becoming a burden to others. As Hawkins says (1980), talking has a powerful therapeutic effect. Plenty of time must be allowed for the physician to explain and for the patient to ask questions. Patients appreciate being given a booklet on rheumatoid arthritis such as that published by the Arthritis and Rheumatism Council; they and their relatives can read it at leisure and then return to ask further questions.

Patients commonly ask if rheumatoid arthritis runs in families and may be worried about the risk of their children developing the disease. They can be told that the number of families where this is so is relatively few, that in any case a triggering factor as yet unidentified is required as well as genetic factors and that the results of current research look promising. Another common question concerns climate. The fact that rheumatoid arthritis occurs in all world populations should be explained and also that joint symptoms often feel worse in a humid climate but are not in the long-term aggravated by it. It may be useful at this juncture to seek to dissuade the patient from moving to another climate far away from the help of his friends and relatives.

Patients often ask about diet. There is no good evidence that dietary factors are relevant in the vast majority of patients. Elimination of dairy products and wheat may help a few (Williams, 1981; Parke & Hughes, 1981; Panush et al, 1983) but Sundqvist et al (1982) found that patients improved after fasting only to relapse when allowed a diet containing no milk or protein. Special diets are fashionable, appealing to many who seek relief by methods other than drugs, but Pearson et al (1983) found a high incidence of psychological disorders in patients who attributed a wide variety of symptoms to ingestion of particular foodstuffs but in whom allergy could not objectively be shown on double blind provocation testing. Lessof (1983) says that food allergy is not proven unless symptoms remit on an elimination diet and recur after placebo-controlled challenge.

Excessive tiredness worries some patients. They should be told that it is an integral part of rheumatoid arthritis (Rogers et al, 1982) and understandable as they need to put more effort than do other people into everyday activities. They should also be told that rheumatoid arthritis affects both body and soul (Hart, 1966).

The question of work or return to work is an important one. If a patient with a manual job already has or is likely to develop severe joint damage, it is prudent to refer him early to the Disablement Resettlement Officer for advice about changing or adapting his job (Sheppeard et al, 1981). Robinson (1973) reports that return to work is more likely for the well-educated and well-motivated. Problems can include the attitudes of the employer, work-mates and trades unions, difficulties with pensions and insurance as well as the problem of general unemployment.

Whether suitable gainful employment is available or not, the physically disabled and potentially physically disabled need as much as anybody else to pursue activities other than those of merely existing. An occupied mind suffers less than an unoccupied one (Hart, 1979) and outside interests should be actively encouraged. Societies such as that of Arthritis Care can help in the UK with arranging group activities and organising holidays. Some groups publish journals with articles on rheumatoid disease and its management; they can also give specific advice on problems of daily living and how to overcome them.

Patients sometimes ask if they should marry. Wright & Owen (1976) found that some housewives had marital difficulties because of their arthritis with its consequent anxieties but that those who married after the onset of disease were much better adjusted. No doubt the same is true of husbands. Certainly both partners should be given the opportunity to discuss possible difficulties.

Problems with sexual intercourse are rarely fully discussed either because of mutual embarrassment or, on the clinician's side, lack of imagination (Ehrlich, 1973). The physical barriers of pain and limitation of movement as well as the psychological barrier of loss of self-esteem are nevertheless very real. Brattström et al (1982) showed that more than half the patients who had received a total hip replacement for inflammatory joint disease had experienced considerable sexual problems beforehand and would have been grateful for discussion or literature on the subject. If the clinician himself cannot advise, he can at least ascertain if the patient has problems and can suggest suitable reading such as the excellent booklet entitled *Marriage, sex and arthritis* written by Dr Wendy Greengross and published by the Arthritis and Rheumatism Council. He could consider too whether a chat with a Marriage Guidance Counsellor would help. Also he must bear in mind the fact that certain drugs can affect sexual performance (Swinburn, 1976).

Patients may also wish to discuss starting a family. This should generally be encouraged but the clinician should remember that women with (and indeed, even before the onset of disease) rheumatoid arthritis are less fertile than others (Empire Rheumatism Council, 1950; Kay & Bach, 1965). Rheumatoid arthritis is not a contraindication to pregnancy though due consideration must be given to the drugs being taken, if possible before conception. Couples should be advised however about spacing their families. As Chamberlain (1979) points out it is difficult to care for a small baby and a toddler at the same time; new mothers also need advice and as much practical help as possible in caring for the baby.

A frequent question is whether the patient should try to keep going rather than resting. An association between physical activity and more severe erosive joint damage was shown by Castillo et al in 1965, and patients who have active synovitis should be advised to rest their joints. The management of rheumatoid arthritis is aimed at minimising tissue damage and loss of function (Hunder & Bunch, 1982), hence the concept of 'joint protection' which aims to protect the joints from overuse and deformity. These principles are best demonstrated to the individual patient with his individual needs by the occupational therapist, the physiotherapist or the health visitor. A home visit to assess these needs can be invaluable. In this context, controlled studies (Katz et al, 1968; Vignos et al, 1972; Duff et al, 1974) demonstrate that fewer patients deteriorate in the activities of daily living, economic independence and even disease activity itself, if their care is undertaken by multidisciplinary clinics with regular home visits by trained paramedical staff.

All patients with joint disease should be encouraged to do exercises designed to retain or build up muscle bulk in an effort to stabilise and protect joints. Patients with actively inflamed joints can be encouraged to perform isometric muscle exercises which involved very little use of the joints themselves. Hench et al (1934) believed that the most potent single therapeutic measure was that of resting the joints. They are supported in this view by the controlled trial of Partridge & Duthie (1963) which showed that inflammatory synovitis could be rapidly controlled by rest in bed and local splintage. Contrary to what patients expect, limbs thus treated and stiff after immobilisation in plaster for 4 weeks regained movement within a fortnight. Local splintage relieves pain and also prevents deformity. A Futuro or Remploy-type working wrist splint allows finger function and may actually increase grip strength by holding the wrist in a slightly dorsiflexed position. Serial splintage of a fixed flexed knee may allow recovery of extension, and valgus insoles help to hold the valgus hind foot in a more neutral position thus protecting it and possibly the knee itself from irreversible valgus deformity.

Rest in bed improves widespread synovitis. Lee et al (1974) showed that active synovitis could be improved over a 4-week period with modified bed-rest in hospital but no improvement occurred in outpatients. The physical improvement is on its own often not sustained for long but allows the patient to see for himself the value of resting inflamed joints in the correct functional position and of building up muscle strength with isometric exercises. Admission also allows him to learn more about his disease from the medical and nursing staff as well as from his fellow patients. It may accustom him to the routine of regular medication and the precautions necessary with it.

Physical treatment and rehabilitation in the rheumatic diseases are discussed in Chapters 61 and 62.

MEDICATION

The rheumatoid robustus type (Haas et al, 1974) of patient has an unusual reaction to disease. These workers describe 9 nodular, seropositive and erosive men, all strong and athletic, 8 of whom were still engaged in heavy manual work even after 9 years of disease. Such patients seem neither to need nor to accept treatment. They are however unusual and almost all patients expect advice to take drugs to reduce inflammation. Always the balance between possible side-effects and the potential benefits must be weighed up. This equation:

$$\text{Amount of inflammation} \times \text{Time} = \text{Degree of joint damage}$$

was formulated by Bayles in 1966. In choosing drugs therefore, it is important to gauge how long the 'time' factor is likely to be; that is, to have some idea of the ultimate prognosis.

Some prognostic factors have been reported. Patients with an abrupt and acute onset often do well compared with those having an insidious onset of disease (Sharp et al, 1964; Fleming et al, 1976; Masi et al, 1976; Hart, 1977), though Luukkainen et al (1983) found no relationship between types of onset (acute, subacute or gradual) and the amount of radiological joint damage 7–8 years later. The prognosis is also better in patients with a short history of disease (Short & Bauer, 1948; Bywaters & Dresner, 1952; Duthie et al, 1957; Otten & Boerma, 1959; Ragan & Farrington, 1962; Feigenbaum et al, 1979) especially if they are male and seronegative. An episodic form of synovitis called 'palindromic rheumatism' (Hench & Rosenberg, 1941) may in about half the patients so affected develop into rheumatoid disease but it is usually not severe (Mattingly et al, 1981).

There is little evidence to suggest that the initial site of joint involvement correlates with outcome but Fleming et al (1976) showed that a combination of clinical wrist and metatarsophalangeal involvement in younger patients and that of shoulder, elbow, wrist and knee involvement in older patients seemed to suggest a worse prognosis.

Given that the clinical diagnosis of rheumatoid disease has been made, one of the best prognostic factors is seropositivity to rheumatoid factor, patients with highly seropositive disease faring worst (Otten & Boerma, 1959; Ragan & Farrington, 1962; Bland & Brown, 1964; Jacoby et al, 1973; Fleming et al, 1976a; Feigenbaum, et al, 1979). Seropositivity is however not a feature of very early disease (Schumacher & Kitridou, 1972), appearing if ever it does within the first year (Sharp et al, 1964; Short, 1968).

The finding of rheumatoid factor does not by itself denote the presence of rheumatoid disease (Waller & Toone, 1968; Mikkelson & Dodge, 1969). Waller et al (1964) found that rheumatoid factor occurs in healthy people, the incidence rising with age and approaching 30% in persons of over 64 years of age.

A normal ESR may be found in rheumatoid disease (Rotès-Quérol & Roig-Escofet, 1968). Whilst Jacoby et al (1973) did not find it valuable prognostically, Fleming et al (1976a) and Mäkisara & Mäkisara (1982) linked a high ESR with a bad prognosis, McConkey et al (1972) even going so far as to say that disease-modifying treatment should be begun if the ESR or C-reactive protein (CRP) are even moderately raised.

Many now believe that to wait for the appearance of radiological erosive damage before instituting disease-modifying treatment is to wait too long. Erosive damage correlates with a more severe clinical outcome (Brook et al, 1977) and the rate of radiological joint damage is most rapid when it occurs during the early phase of disease (Sjöblom et al, 1982).

The majority opinion at least in the UK (Haslock, 1983) is that active disease should be treated aggressively. Placebos can be effective in the disease if only for a short time (Traut & Passarelli, 1957) and thus any drug used for rheumatoid disease must be shown to be better than placebo. There is no drug treatment which is both effective and completely safe (British Medical Journal, 1977) and as an attack of the disease may be short-lived, it is wise to try the least toxic drugs first, for the study of Brooks et al (1975) probably underestimates the number of deaths resulting from side-effects. In their study of 143 deaths they found that 11 (7 on corticosteroids) had died from the actual side-effects of drugs and that drugs had contributed to the deaths of another 5 patients (3 on corticosteroids).

Drugs (see also Section IV)

The use of salicylate drugs in high dosage has largely gone out of fashion because of the high incidence of gastric upset and tinnitus but these drugs are effective and can be tolerated well by some patients. Newer and more expensive variations, such as benorylate and diflunisal, seem to cause less upset.

All the so-called 'non-steroidal anti-inflammatory drugs' (NSAIDS) may cause gastrointestinal upsets, many can cause skin rashes and exacerbate asthma and, particularly in elderly patients, cause problems with water retention. The tendency, because these drugs are highly protein-bound, to increase the effects of anticoagulant treatment can also be a problem. It may be necessary to try several of them in turn for 2 or 3 weeks at a time in a particular patient. Amongst the propionic acid derivates, ibuprofen is useful and even in the proper anti-inflammatory dose of about 2.4 g per day seems to cause less gastric upset than the others. Naproxen, though it has more side-effects, is also useful as it can be taken twice daily.

Indomethacin is very effective when tolerated but has a high incidence of side-effects, particularly those of peptic ulceration, water-retention, headaches and dizziness. The latter two can sometimes be avoided if the drug is given at night and in a low dose to begin with. The NSAIDS are contraindicated in peptic ulceration but drugs available in suppository form such as indomethacin (Lanza et al, 1982) and naproxen may be tolerated, while the drug fenbufen which is a 'pro drug' and not broken down till it reaches the liver, can be used as an alternative.

Care must be taken to use the lowest effective dose of these drugs, particularly in the elderly where side-effects are more common. The actual style of container may present a problem too to elderly patients who dislike blister packaging (Wright & Hopkins, 1972) and who find 'child-resistant' containers difficult (Lisberg et al, 1983).

Rheumatoid arthritis usually goes into remission during pregnancy (Persellin, 1976; Ungar et al, 1983; Østensen et al, 1983), improvement occurring within the first 3 months and exacerbation being the rule after delivery. Absolute safety for the foetus exposed to maternal ingestion of the antirheumatic drugs cannot be guaranteed and where at all possible, these drugs should be stopped during pregnancy. In particular, the prostaglandin inhibitors which may cause the premature closure of the ductus arteriosus should be withheld before and during the first trimester (Drug and Therapeutics Bulletin, 1981; Woodland, 1982). A small dose of aspirin is probably safe both for mother and child during pregnancy (Collins & Turner, 1975; Slone et al, 1976; Shapiro et al, 1976; Kay, 1982) and also in lactation. Through none of the pharmaceutical companies would claim entire safety in lactation, some of the NSAIDS such as ibuprofen, naproxen, ketoprofen and fenbufen are probably fairly safe (Drug and Therapeutics Bulletin, 1983) and can be useful if disease flares after delivery just at the time when the mother requires full mobility.

If the NSAIDS are not effective, disease-modifying drugs such as aurothiomalate (gold) or D-penicillamine are the next group to be considered. The order of so-called 'second line treatment' does not seem to matter (Steven et al, 1982), both gold and D-penicillamine being effective. Gold can alter the course of rheumatoid disease (Empire Rheumatism Council, 1960; Sigler et al, 1974) and can even halt radiological damage (Luukkainen et al, 1977; Sharp et al, 1982). Though a schedule of 50 mg intramuscularly per week for the first few months has traditionally been used, there is now a trend towards lower doses (Sharp et al, 1977; Griffin et al, 1983) and a lower incidence of side-effects has been noted by McKenzie (1981).

D-penicillamine can give results similar to those of gold (Gibson et al, 1976; Shiokawa et al, 1977) and now that it is used in low dosage (Hill et al, 1979), has a similar incidence of side-effects.

Both drugs may cause rashes although it is sometimes possible cautiously to reintroduce the drug once the rash has gone. Both drugs may cause proteinuria or even the nephrotic syndrome so regular urinalysis must be performed, though it should be remembered that a coincidental and often asymptomatic urinary infection is a much more common cause of proteinuria. The urine is tested before each gold injection and the result tabulated on a record card. If more than a trace of protein is present, gold must be stopped pending further investigation for a urinary infection and the 24-hour urinary protein must be measured if the urine culture is negative. Once the urine is clear, gold may be started again if the proteinuria was only moderate, such as 0.4–2 g/l (Newton et al, 1983). The patient on D-penicillamine is asked to test his own urine monthly for proteinuria and to record the result on a chart. D-penicillamine may safely be continued if the amount of proteinuria is not increasing and if the 24-hour specimen contains no more than 2 g/l. All types of gold reaction and the renal side-effects of D-penicillamine seem to be more common with the tissue type CW7, B8 and DR3 (Bardin et al, 1982).

A potentially more serious side-effect with these two drugs is that of bone marrow depression, even aplasia. Some advise a white cell and platelet count before each gold injection but as haematological side-effects usually occur suddenly and without warning, others are content to warn the patient to report immediately if there is spontaneous bruising or stomatitis and to have a blood count done every 4–6 weeks. A monthly blood count is mandatory with D-penicillamine and the results are entered on a chart. A trend towards a drop in the white cells or platelets is an indication to stop the drug or to lower the dose. Obviously other drugs known to cause bone marrow suppression should not be given concomitantly with gold or D-penicillamine but De Silva & Hazelman (1981) report that a combination of gold and azathioprine seemed to be of benefit to some patients and was not particularly toxic to the bone marrow.

There have been reports that patients who have had side-effects from gold are more likely to experience side-effects with D-penicillamine (Dodd et al, 1980; Smith et al, 1982; Stein et al, 1983) but Steven et al (1982) found that toxicity with one drug did not influence toxicity with the other and in a 5-year prospective study, Kean et al (1982) report no difference in the adverse effects of D-penicillamine between patients who had received gold without side-effects and those who had shown toxicity to gold.

If possible, all drugs should be stopped in pregnancy but it is said that gold is not necessarily contraindicated (Jessop, 1979) and D-penicillamine is said to be 'fairly safe' in pregnant women with rheumatoid disease (Lyle, 1979).

Other disease-modifying drugs include the antimalarials, sulphasalazine and dapsone. Amongst the cytotoxic drugs, azathioprine is used more frequently and is probably safer than chlorambucil, cyclophosphamide and methotrexate. Moens & Brocteur (1965) even suggest that the beneficial effect of azathioprine is due to an anti-inflammatory rather than an immunosuppressing action. Azathioprine decreases steroid requirements (Harris et al, 1971) and though in theory it might induce malignant change, Hunter et al (1975) found none in 40 patient-years at a dose of 1.5–2.5 mg/kg body weight, whilst Lewis et al (1980), studying patients given doses of up to 5 mg/kg body weight, report more neoplasia in the age-group 45–64.

So-called 'heroic' treatments used in rheumatoid disease when all else has failed include total lymphoid irradiation (Kotzin et al, 1981; Trentham et al, 1981) and 'combination treatment' with cyclophosphamide, azathioprine and hydroxychloroquine (McCarty & Carrera, 1982). Total lymphoid irradiation might induce neoplasia and an editorial in the Lancet (1982) pleads for controlled data. On the other hand, Ehrlich (1982) commenting on 'combination treatment' says that rheumatoid disease itself can be just as destructive as malignancy.

Systemic corticosteroid drugs are less often used for rheumatoid disease than formerly. Ehrlich (1982) makes the point that steroids fail to alter the course of the disease in a favourable way and what is more, create problems ultimately more threatening to both life and life-content than the disease for which they were prescribed. Some clinicians, however, do use steroids in severe disease whilst waiting for gold or D-penicillamine to work. The difficulty here is that of weaning the patient from the steroids once disease has been modified, not to mention the other difficulty which is that of recognising the occurrence of disease modification. A useful alternative could prove to be methylprednisolone pulse therapy which so far seems to be a reasonably safe and effective method of inducing short-term improvement (Liebling et al, 1981; Forster et al, 1982; Williams et al, 1982).

When life-threatening complications occur, steroid treatment is sometimes essential. Hart (1969) suggested that all patients with severe nodular disease had a diffuse vasculitis and that the increase in incidence of vasculitis seen at that time was running in parallel with corticosteroid overdosage. Certainly vasculitis seems to be less common now, but when it occurs it often does so in a patient with severe long-standing rheumatoid disease treated with long-term steroids. A short-term increase in steroid dosage for problems such as coronary arteritis may actually save life. Beck & Hoffbrand (1966) report a patient with pleuropericarditis and pneumonia in whom steroids were life-saving but in the case of fibrosing alveolitis, Walker & Wright (1968) doubt if steroids help except on a temporary basis.

In addition to the drugs which may influence inflammation, analgesics are often required to relieve pain, both that of inflammation and that caused by secondary degenerative change. Simple paracetamol or low-dose aspirin may be sufficient and if taken at night may result in sleep rather than a night disturbed by pain. Another cause of loss of sleep is depression and an antidepressant taken at night may help sleep as well as mood.

EXTRA-ARTICULAR COMPLICATIONS AND THEIR MANAGEMENT

A study undertaken between 1965 and 1966 of 127 consecutive inpatients with definite or classical rheumatoid disease and a mean disease duration of 11.5 years (Gordon et al, 1973), showed that 76% of patients had one or more extra-articular lesions. These included 53% with rheumatoid nodules, 20% with pulmonary fibrosis, 15% with digital vasculitis, 13% with skin ulceration, 12% with lymphadenopathy, 10% with non-compressive neuropathy, 9% with splenomegaly and 2% with pericarditis. The finding of extra-articular lesions denoted more severe disease both clinically and radiologically. Over a 5-year period, mortality in those with extra-articular lesions was twice as great as in those without and particularly striking in the group aged under 50. Infection contributed to death in at least 40% of the 23 who died.

Those patients who have highly seropositive nodular rheumatoid disease tend to have an unremittingly severe course (Sharp et al, 1964; Short, 1968) and also to have extra-articular lesions.

Cardiovascular system

The commonest lesion is pericarditis. This often goes unnoticed but is found at autopsy in some

30% of patients with long-standing, seropositive disease (Cosh, 1972). Pericarditis is sometimes followed by effusion which should be aspirated to prevent tamponade and to reduce the risk of later constrictive pericarditis.

Though myocardial infarction occurs in rheumatoid patients as frequently as in the normal population (Zaplicki et al, 1978), coronary arteritis is an uncommon cause (Karten, 1969; Voyles et al, 1980). If it is suspected. prompt treatment with corticosteroids and azathioprine should be instituted.

Heart block caused by rheumatoid granulomata in or near conducting tissue (Cosh, 1972) is treated symptomatically and if necessary, with a pacemaker. Granulomata can also involve the mitral or aortic cusps and the resulting haemodynamic abnormality may require valve replacement (Iveson et al, 1975).

Arteriosclerotic arteries as seen on X-ray of the ankles occur as frequently as in controls but are 3 times commoner in rheumatoid patients on steroid treatment (Kalbak, 1972).

Lungs

Ellman & Ball (1948) were the first to suggest that joint and lung lesions in rheumatoid disease were manifestations of the same pathological process.

There was no lung disease whatever in 180 of 253 consecutive patients presenting between 1938 and 1948 and followed for many years by Aronoff et al (1955) but 5 patients had pulmonary fibrosis and 2 had silicosis.

Walker & Wright (1968) compared 516 rheumatoid patients with 301 who had degenerative joint disease. Twice as many of the rheumatoid patients had had pleurisy and 6 times as many had had a pleural effusion. Two patients (both male) had pleural nodules, 3.1% of the rheumatoid patients had bronchiectasis and 0.3% of controls. Three-quarters of the 1.6% of patients with fibrosing alveolitis (Walker & Wright 1969) were male and of these, nearly all had nodules.

Lung involvement can precede joint involvement and vice versa (Brannan et al, 1964). In the former instance, difficulties in diagnosis arise. Pleural effusions and rheumatoid nodules either in pleura or lung require no specific treatment but such lesions may be due to malignancy or to infection and may have to be investigated further.

The management of pulmonary fibrosis is difficult; it is doubtful whether the corticosteroid drugs help except temporarily (Walker & Wright, 1968) but they are usually tried for worsening symptoms.

Neuropathy

Compression neuropathies such as the carpal tunnel syndrome and cervical myelopathy are mechanical in origin but peripheral neuropathy usually occurs only in severe systemic rheumatoid disease. Patients who have distal sensory signs only do quite well, but those who go on to develop distal sensorimotor signs do badly (Pallis & Scott, 1965). They are usually male and have malignant, erosive, nodular and highly seropositive rheumatoid disease (Chamberlain & Bruckner, 1970). The affected limb(s) must be supported in a functional position; cytotoxic treatment with or without steroid therapy can be life-saving, as the arteritis which in the case of peripheral nerves affects the vasa nervorum is likely to be already present in tissue throughout the body.

Ocular complications

Keratoconjunctivitis sicca is frequently found in rheumatoid disease. Symptomatic treatment with artificial tears often relieves the distressing symptoms and affords some protection to the dry eye but it may be necessary to block the lower punctum.

Scleritis which may damage visual acuity is present in 0.7% of rheumatoid patients and is associated with nodular disease, other extra-articular lesions and early mortality (McGavin et al, 1976). Indomethacin is sometimes helpful but high dose steriod drugs may be necessary if sight is to be preserved.

The corneal melting syndrome in rheumatoid arthritis seems to be associated with fewer systemic complications and even with inactive disease (Jayson & East, 1977). Nevertheless if sight is to be preserved, the use of azathioprine or D-penicillamine may be necessary, systemic corticosteroids seeming to make the condition worse.

Anaemia

The treatment of anaemia is difficult. It is an

integral part of active rheumatoid inflammation. Though true iron deficiency may occur from poor diet and drug-induced blood loss and is demonstrated by a response to oral iron and a value of serum ferritin below that of 55 μg/l in the rheumatoid patient (Blake et al, 1981), a more usual finding is that of the anaemia of chronic disease. This is shown by low haemoglobin, low serum iron, normal total iron-binding capacity, reduced transferrin and by red cells which are normochromic and normocytic.

Ferritin is the soluble intracellular storage form of iron. Blake et al (1981) postulate that inflammation directly stimulates the production of ferritin which may act itself as an anti-inflammatory protein (Blake et al, 1981). A high serum ferritin is associated with systemic disease (Blake & Bacon, 1981). Blake et al (1980) suggest that in active disease, the reticuloendothelial cells within the synovium may, when stimulated by inflammation, take up iron in direct competition with the bone marrow storing it within the synovium in the form of ferritin. Harvey et al (1983) have indirect evidence suggesting that a serum immunoglobulin M or rheumatoid factor itself may suppress erythropoiesis.

Whatever the mechanism of anaemia, it seems quite clear that only by correction of the underlying disease process will lasting improvement be obtained (Bentley & Williams, 1982). Furthermore, the administration of iron especially by the intravenous route may actually lead to disease exacerbation (Lloyd & Williams, 1970; Blake & Bacon, 1981; Blake et al, 1982). It seems reasonable therefore to treat true iron deficiency with iron (Rajapakse et al, 1980) and to treat the disease itself rather than the anaemia of chronic disease.

Infection

Death in rheumatoid arthritis occurs from the usual causes but often at an earlier than expected age (Cobb et al, 1953; Bywaters et al, 1960; Uddin et al, 1970; Benn & Wood, 1972; Isomäki et al, 1975; Allebeck, 1982) with infection frequently being the cause of death (Uddin et al, 1970; Isomäki et al, 1975; Mutru et al, 1976; Rasker & Cosh, 1981; Alleback et al, 1981). Any obvious bacterial infection occurring in rheumatoid disease must therefore be treated vigorously. Patients with rheumatoid damage to joints seem to be especially prone to bacterial invasion of their joints with or without an obvious nidus of infection such as a corn. Very often, fever and leucocytosis are absent so that worsening of any joint should alert the physician to consider infection. The suspected joint should be aspirated and if the fluid is obviously infected, antibiotic treatment should be begun before the results of cultures are available. The causative organism is most often a staphylococcus. Similarly, patients (especially those with severe disease and those who are on steroids) not infrequently develop a septicaemia (Huskisson & Hart, 1972). If the patients suddenly becomes ill, early and frequent blood cultures together with serial samples of the serum for bacterial antibody levels must be taken.

Though neoplasm is less common in rheumatoid patients than in controls (Mutru et al, 1976), lymphoma and leukaemia are more common (Isomäki et al, 1978) and though lymphadenopathy is a common feature of active rheumatoid disease, it does not occur above the clavicle (Robertson et al, 1968) so glands occurring in the neck should, unless clearly related to an infection, be biopsied. Whether cytotoxic treatment of rheumatoid disease predisposes to an increased risk of malignancy is not yet know; the results of the long-term prospective study under the auspices of EULAR are eagerly awaited.

SURGERY

The physical impact of destructive rheumatoid disease has been greatly lessened by recent major advances in orthopaedic surgery and by close cooperation between surgeons and physicians. The physician needs to know what is technically possible and also, given the general health of his patient and the level of motivation, to know what is possible for his individual patient. He advises the surgeon when surgery is required and if a number of procedures are to be embarked upon, the order in which they may best be done. Unless the indication were solely that of pain relief, it would not, for instance, help the patient to receive total hip replacement if his arms were so badly affected that he could not use crutches or if the state of his knees and feet were such that he would still be unable to walk. Also if a patient needs a joint replacement, any deformity such as dislocated toes or bunions which might in the future predispose to infection should be treated first. There is no place for cosmetic surgery in rheumatoid disease; the indications for surgery are those of intolerable pain and of loss of function which cannot be treated medically.

Close liaison with the anaesthetist is important. First the patient must be fit for surgery. If he is anaemic, preoperative blood transfusion may be required. If renal function, the lungs or the myocardium are impaired, as much corrective treatment as possible must be given even if that means admitting the patient some time before the operation.

There are mechanical problems too. The amount of mouth opening may, due to temporomandibular joint involvement, be too little to allow orthodox intubation and any cervical subluxation already present may be worsened during the manoeuvres required for intubation, so much so that some rheumatologists insist that a cervical collar be worn by any rheumatoid patient going to theatre.

Finally it must be remembered that any operation, however dramatic at the time and however splendid the outcome, is only one incident in the total management of the patient with rheumatoid disease. Surgical treatment of the rheumatic diseases is discussed in Chapter 63.

REFERENCES

Allebeck P 1982 Increased mortality in rheumatoid arthritis. Scandinavian Journal of Rheumatology 11: 81–86

Allebeck P, Ahlbohm A, Allender E 1981 Increased mortality amongst persons with rheumatoid arthritis but where RA does not appear on the death certificate. Scandinavian Journal of Rheumatology 10: 301–306

Amos R S, Crockson R A, Crockson A P, Walsh L, McConkey B 1978 Rheumatoid arthritis: C-reactive protein and erythrocyte sedimentation rate during initial treatment. British Medical Journal 1:1396

Anderson J L, Dodman S, Kopelman M, Fleming A 1979 Patient information recall in a rheumatology clinic. Rheumatology and Rehabilitation 18: 18–22

Aronoff A, Bywaters E G L, Fearnley G R 1955 Lung lesions in rheumatoid arthritis. British Medical Journal 2: 228–232

Bardin T, Dryll A, Debeyre N Ryckwaert A, Legrand L, Marcelli A, Dausset J 1982 HLA system and side-effects of gold salts and D-penicillamine treatment of rheumatoid arthritis. Annals of the Rheumatic Diseases 41: 599–601

Bayles T B (1966) Why treat rheumatoid arthritis? In: Ingelfinger F J, Relman A S, Finland M (eds) Controversy in internal medicine, 1st Edn. Saunders, Philadelphia, p 561

Beall G, Cobb S 1961 The frequency distribution of episodes of rheumatoid arthritis as shown by periodic examination. Journal of Chronic Diseases 14: 291–310

Beck E R Hoffbrand B I 1966 Acute lung changes in rheumatoid arthritis. Annals of the Rheumatic Diseases 25: 459–462

Benn R T, Wood P H N 1972 Mortality in rheumatoid arthritis. British Journal of Preventive and Social Medicine 26:60

Bentley D P, Williams P 1982 Parenteral iron therapy in the anaemia of rheumatoid arthritis. Rheumatology and Rehabilitation 21: 88–92

Blake D R, Bacon P A 1981 Serum ferritin and rheumatoid disease. British Medical Journal 282: 1273–1274

Blake D R, Bacon P A, Eastham E J, Brightham K 1980 Synovial fluid ferritin in rheumatoid arthritis. British Medical Journal 281: 715–716

Blake D R, Waterworth R F, Bacon P A 1981 Assessment of iron stores in inflammation by assay of serum ferritin concentrations. British Medical Journal 283: 1147–1148

Blake D R, Hall N D, Bacon P A, Dieppe P A, Halliwell B, Gutteridge J M C 1981 The importance of iron in rheumatoid disease. Lancet 2: 1142–1144

Blake D R, Ahern M, Ring F, Bradfield J, Bacon P A 1982 I.V. Iron therapy for rheumatoid arthritis — revisited. The Combined Meeting of British Association for Rheumatology and Rehabilitation, Heberden Society, RoyalSociety of Medicine Section of Rheumatology and Rehabilitation, Irish Society of Rheumatology and Rehabilitation. Abstract 29

Bland J H, Brown E W 1964 Seronegative and seropositive rheumatoid arthritis. Clinical, radiological and biochemical differences. Annals of Internal Medicine 60: 88–94

Brannan H M, Good A, Divertie M B, Baggenstoss A H 1964 Pulmonary disease associated with rheumatoid arthritis. Journal of the American Medical Association 189: 914–918

Brattström M, Alfe G, Brattström H 1982 Sexual problems in patients with inflammatory joint disease treated with total hip replacement. Scandinavian Journal of Rheumatology Supp 45:p 27

British Medical Journal Editorial 1977 Planning treatment for rheumatoid arthritis. 1:1120

Brook A, Fleming A, Corbett M 1977 Relationship of radiological change to clinical outcome in rheumatoid arthritis. Annals of the Rheumatic Diseases 36: 274–275

Brooks P M, Stephens W H, Stephens M E B, Buchanan W W 1975 How safe are anti-rheumatic drugs? A study of possible iatrogenic deaths in patients with rheumatoid arthritis. Health Bulletin (Edinburgh) 33: 108–111

Bywaters E G L, Dresner E 1952 Prognosis in rheumatoid arthritis. The Quarterly Journal of Medicine 12:463

Bywaters E G L, Curwen M, Dresner E, Dixon St J A 1960 Ten year follow-up of rheumatoid arthritis. Lancet 2: 1381

Castillo B A, El Sallab R A, Scott J T 1965 Physical activity,

cystic erosions and osteoporosis in rheumatoid arthritis. Annals of the Rheumatic Diseases 24: 522–527
Chamberlain M A 1979 Social implications of rheumatoid arthritis in young mothers. Rheumatology and Rehabilitation (Suppl 1): 70–73
Chamberlain M A, Bruckner F E 1970 Rheumatoid neuropathy: Clinical and electrophysiological features. Annals of the Rheumatic Diseases 29: 609–616
Cobb S, Anderson F, Bauer W 1953 Length of life and cause of death in rheumatoid arthritis. Annals of the Rheumatic Diseases 12:323
Collins E, Turner G 1975 Maternal effects of regular salicylate ingestion in pregnancy. Lancet 2: 335–337
Cosh J A 1972 The heart and the rheumatic diseases. Rheumatology and Physical Medicine 11: 267–280
Czaplicki S, Gietka J, Sulek K 1978 The frequency of coronary heart disease and myocardial infarction in rheumatoid arthritis patients. Cor et Vasa 20: 249–254
De Silva M, Hazelman B L 1981 Long-term azathioprine in rheumatoid arthritis: a double-blind study. Annals of the Rheumatic Diseases 40: 560–563
Dodd M J, Griffiths I D, Thompson M 1980 Adverse reactions to D-pencillamine after gold toxicity. British Medical Journal 280: 1498–1500
Drug and Therapeutics Bulletin 1981 Choosing a non-steroidal anti-inflammatory drug. Published by the Consumers Association 19: 53–56
Drug and Therapeutics Bulletin 1983 Drugs which can be given to nursing mothers. published by the Consumers Association 21: 5–8
Duff I F, Carpenter J O, Neukom J E 1974 Comprehensive management of patients with rheumatoid arthritis. Some results of the regional arthritis control programme in Michigan. Arthritis and Rheumatism 17: 635–645
Duthie J J R, Brown P E, Knox J D E, Thompson M 1957 Course and prognosis in rheumatoid arthritis. Annals of the Rheumatic Diseases 16: 411–424
Ehrlich G E 1973 Sexual problems of the arthritic patient. In: Ehrlich GE (ed) Total management of the arthritic patient. Lippincott, Philadelphia, p 193–208
Ehrlich G E 1982 Heroic treatment for non-malignant disease. Journal of the American Medical Association 248: 1743–1744
Ellman P, Ball R E 1948 'Rheumatoid Disease' with joint and pulmonary manifestations. British Medical Journal 2: 816–820
Empire Rheumatism Council Scientific Advisory Committee 1950 Report on an enquiry into the aetiological factors associated with rheumatoid arthritis. Annals of the Rheumatic Diseases 9 (Suppl)
Empire Rheumatism Council 1960 Gold therapy in rheumatoid arthritis. Annals of the Rheumatic Diseases 19: 95–120
Empire Rheumatism Council 1961 Gold therapy in rheumatoid arthritis. Final report of a multi-centre controlled trial. Annals of the Rheumatic Diseases 20: 315–334
Feigenbaum S L, Masi A T, Kaplan S B 1979 Prognosis in rheumatoid arthritis. A longitudinal study of newly diagnosed younger adult patients. American Journal of Medicine 66: 377–383
Fleming A, Benn R T, Corbett M, Wood P N H 1976 Early rheumatoid disease II. Patterns of joint involvement. Annals of the Rheumatic Diseases 35: 361–364
Fleming A, Crown J M, Corbett M 1976 Early rheumatoid disease. I. Onset. Annals of the Rheumatic Diseases 35: 357–360
Fleming A, Crown J M, Corbett M 1976a Prognostic value of early features in rheumatoid disease. British Medical Journal 1: 1243–1245
Forster P J G, Grindulis K A, Neumann V, HubballS, McConkey B 1982 High-dose intravenous methylprednisolone in rheumatoid arthritis. Annals of the Rheumatic Diseases 41: 444–446
Gibson T, Huskisson E C, Wojtewlewski J A, Scott P J, Balme H W, Burry H C, Gimborne R, Hart F D 1976 Evidence that D-penicillamine alters the course of rheumatoid arthritis. Rheumatology and Rehabilitation 15: 211–215
Gordon D A, Stein J L, Broder I 1973 The extra-articular features of rheumatoid arthritis. American Journal of Medicine 54: 445–452
Griffin A J, Gibson T, Huston G 1983 A comparison of conventional and low-dose sodium aurothiomalate treatment in rheumatoid arthritis. British Journal of Rheumatology 22: 82–88
Haas W H D, De Boer W, De Griffioen F, Oosten-Elst P 1974 Rheumatoid arthritis of the robust reaction type. Annals of the Rheumatic Diseases 33: 81–85
Harris J, Jessop J D, Chaput de Saintonge D M 1971 Further experience with azathioprine in rheumatoid arthritis. British Medical Journal 4: 463–464
Hart F D 1966 Complicated rheumatoid disease. British Medical Journal 2: 131–135
Hart F D 1969 Rheumatoid arthritis: extra-articular manifestations. British Medical Journal 3: 131–136
Hart F D 1977 Presentation of rheumatoid arthritis and its relation to prognosis. British Medical Journal 2: 621–624
Hart F D 1979 Pain as an old friend. British Medical Journal 1: 1405–1406
Harvey A R, Clarke B J, Chui D H K, Kean W F, Buchanan W W 1983 Anaemia associated with rheumatoid disease. Arthritis and Rheumatism 26: 28–34
Haslock I (1983) Report of the combined annual provincial meeting of the British Association for Rheumatology and Rehabilitation, the Herberden Society, the Royal Society of Medicine Section of Rheumatology and Rehabilitation and the Irish Society of Rheumatology and Rehabilitation. British Journal of Rheumatology 22: 57–58
Hawkins C 1980 Viewpoint. For every ill a pill. Annals of the Rheumatic Diseases 39: 198–199
Hench P S 1949 The potential reversibility of rheumatoid arthritis. Proceedings of the Staff Meetings at the Mayo Clinic 24: 167–178
Hench P S, Rosenberg E F 1941 Palindromic rheumatism. A 'new' oft-recurring disease of joints (arthritis, peri-arthritis, para-arthritis) apparently producing no articular residues: report of thirty-four cases. Proceedings of the Staff Meetings at the Mayo Clinic 16: 808–815
Hench P S, Bauer W, Fletcher A A, Ghrist D, Hall F, White P 1934–1935 The present status of the problem of 'rheumatism'. A review of recent American and English literature on 'rheumatism' and 'arthritis'. Annals of Internal Medicine 8: 1495–1555
Hill H F H, Hill A G S, Day A T, Brown R M, Golding J R, Lyle W H 1979 Maintenance dose of penicillamine in rheumatoid arthritis: a comparison between a standard and a response-related flexible regimen. Annals of the Rheumatic Diseases 38: 429–433
Hunder G H, Bunch T W 1982 Treatment of rheumatoid

arthritis. Bulletin on the Rheumatic Diseases 32: 1–7
Hunter T, Urowitz M B, Gordon D A, Smythe H A, Ogryzlo M A 1975 Azathioprine in rheumatoid arthritis. Arthritis and Rheumatism 18: 15–20
Huskisson E C, Hart F D, 1972 Severe, unusual and recurrent infections in rheumatoid arthritis. Annals of the Rheumatic Diseases 31: 118–121
Irons E E 1935–1936 Chronic arthritis, a general disease requiring individualized treatment. Archives of Internal Medicine 9: 1658–1663
Isomäki H A, Mutru O, Koota K 1975 Death rate and causes of death in patients with rheumatoid arthritis. Scandinavian Journal of Rheumatology 4: 205–208
Isomäki H A, Hakulinen T, Joutsenlahti U 1978 Excess risk of lymphomas, leukaemia and myeloma in patients with rheumatoid arthritis. Journal of Chronic Diseases 31: 691–696
Iveson J M I, Thadani U, Ionescu M, Wright V 1975 Aortic valve incompetence and replacement in rheumatoid arthritis. Annals of the Rheumatic Diseases 34: 312–320
Jacoby R K, Jayson M I V, Cosh J A 1973 Onset, early stages and prognosis of rheumatoid arthritis: a clinical study of 100 cases with 11-year follow-up. British Medical Journal 1: 96–100
Jayson M I V, East D L 1977 Ulceration of the cornea in rheumatoid arthritis. Annals of the Rheumatic Diseases 36: 428–432
Jessop J D 1979 Gold in the treatment of rheumatoid arthritis — why, when and how. Journal of Rheumatology Supp. No 5, 6: 12–17
Joyce C R B, Caple G, Mason R M, Reynolds E, Mathews J A 1969 Quantitative study of doctor–patient communication. Quarterly Journal of Medicine 38: 183–194
Kalbak K 1972 Incidence of arteriosclerosis in patients with rheumatoid arthritis receiving long-term corticosteroid therapy. Annals of the Rheumatic Diseases 31: 196–200
Karten I 1969 Arteritis, myocardial infarction and rheumatoid arthritis. Journal of the American Medical Association 210: 1717–1724
Katz S, Vignos P J, Moskowitz R W, Thompson H M, Svec K H 1968 Comprehensive out-patient care in rheumatoid arthritis: A controlled study. Journal of the American Medical Asssociation 206: 1249–1254
Kay A 1982 Anti-rheumatic drugs and pregnancy. Rheumatology in Practice (published by Medical News Group, London) No. 6: 6–8
Kay A, Bach F 1965 Subfertility before and after the onset of rheumatoid arthritis in women. Annals of the Rheumatic Diseases 24: 169–173
Kean W F, Lock C J L, Howard-Lock H E, Buchanan W W 1982 Prior gold therapy does not influence the adverse effects of D-penicillamine in rheumatoid arthritis. Arthritis and Rheumatism 25: 917–922
Koota K, Isomäki H, Mutru O 1977 Death rate and causes of death in rheumatoid arthritis patients during a period of 5 years. Scandinavian Journal of Rheumatology 6: 241–244
Kotzin B L, Strober S, Engelman E G, Calin A, Hoppe R T, Kansas G S, Terrell C P, Kaplan H S 1981 Treatment of intractable rheumatoid arthritis with total lymphoid irradiation. New England Journal of Medicine 305: 969–976
Lancet editorial 1982 Total lymphoid irradiation in rheumatoid arthritis. 1: 25–26
Lanza F L, Umbenhauer E R, Nelson R S, Rack M F, Daurio C P, White L A 1982 A double-blind randomised placebo controlled gastroscopic study to compare the effects of indomethacin capsules and indomethacin suppositories on the gastric mucosa of human volunteers. Journal of Rheumatology 9: 415–419
Lawrence J S 1977 Rheumatism in Populations. William Heinemann London p 519–520
Lee P, Kennedy A C, Anderson J, Buchanan W W 1974 Benefits of hospitalisation in rheumatoid arthritis. The Quarterly Journal of Medicine 63: 205–214
Lessof M H 1983 Food intolerance and allergy — a review. Quarterly Journal of Medicine 52: 111–119
Lewis P, Hazelman B L, Hanka R, Roberts S 1980 Cause of death in patients with rheumatoid arthritis with particular reference to azathioprine. Annals of the Rheumatic Diseases 39: 457–461
Ley P, Spelman M S 1965 Communications in an out-patient setting. British Journal of Social and Clinical Psychology 4: 114–116
Liebling M R Leib E, McLaughlin K, Blocka K, Furst D E, Nyman K, Paulus H E 1981 Pulse methylprednisolone in rheumatoid arthritis. Annals of Internal Medicine 94: 21–26
Linos A, Worthington J W, O'Fallon W M, Kurland L T 1980 The epidemiology of rheumatoid arthritis in Rochester, Minnesota. American Journal of Epidemiology 111: 87–98
Lisberg R B, Higham C, Jayson M I V 1983 Problems for rheumatic patients in opening dispensed drug containers. British Journal of Rheumatology 22: 95–98
Lloyd K N, Williams P 1970 Reactions to total dose infusion of iron dextran in rheumatoid arthritis. British Medical Journal 2: 323–325
Luukkainen R, Kajander A, Isomäki H 1977 Effect of gold on progression of erosions in rheumatoid arthritis. Scandinavian Journal of Rheumatology 6: 189–192
Luukkainen R, Isomäki H, Kajander A 1983 Prognostic value of the type of onset of rheumatoid arthritis. Annals of the Rheumatic Diseases 42: 274–275
Lyle W H 1979 Penicillamine in pregnancy. Letter to Lancet 1: 606–607
McCarty D J, Carrera G F 1982 Intractable rheumatoid arthritis. Treatment with combined cyclophosphamide, azathioprine and hydroxychloraquine. Journal of the American Medical Association 248: 1718–1723
McConkey B, Crockson R A, Crockson A P 1972 The assessment of rheumatoid arthritis. Quarterly Journal of Medicine 41: 115–125
McGavin D D M, Williamson J, Forrester J V, Foulds W S, Buchanan W W, Dick W C, Lee P, MacSween R N M, Whaley K 1976 Episcleritis and scleritis. A study of their clinical manifestations and association with rheumatoid arthritis. British Journal of Ophthalmology 60: 192–226
McKenzie J M M 1981 Report on a double-blind trial comparing small and large doses of gold in the treatment of rheumatoid arthritis. Rheumatology and Rehabilitation 20: 198–202
Mäkisara G–L, Mäkisara P 1982 Prognosis of functional capacity and work capacity in rheumatoid arthritis. Scandinavian Journal of Rheumatology Suppl 45:48
Masi A T, Maldonado-Cocco J A, Kaplan S B, Feigenbaum S L, Chandler R W 1976 Prospective study of the early course of rheumatoid arthritis in young adults: comparison of patients with and without rheumatoid factor positivity at entry and identification of variables correlating with

outcome. Seminars in Arthritis and Rheumatism 5: 299–326

Mattingly S, Jones D W, Robinson W M, Williams R A, Dunn E C 1981 Palindromic rheumatism. Journal of the Royal College of Physicians of London 15: 119–123

Meenan R F, Yelin E H, Nevitt M, Epstein W V 1981 The impact of chronic disease. A sociomedical profile of rheumatoid arthritis. Arthritis and Rheumatism 24: 544–549

Mikkelsen W M, Dodge H 1969 A four-year follow-up of suspected rheumatoid arthritis: the Tecumseh, Michigan, Community Health Study. Arthritis and Rheumatism 12: 87–91

Moens C, Brocteur J 1965 Treatment of rheumatoid arthritis with immunosuppressive drugs. Acta Rheumatologia Scandinavica 11: 212–220

Mutru O, Koota K, Isomäki H 1976 Causes of death in autopsied RA patients. Scandinavian Journal of Rheumatology 5: 239–240

Newton P, Swinburn W R, Swinson D R 1983 Proteinuria with gold therapy: when should gold be permanently stopped? British Journal of Rheumatology 22: 11–17

Østensen M, Aune B, Husby G 1983 Effect of pregnancy and hormonal changes on the activity of rheumatoid arthritis. Scandinavian Journal of Rheumatology 12: 69–72

O'Sullivan J B, Cathcart E S 1972 The prevalence of rheumatoid arthritis. Annals of Internal Medicine 76: 573–577

Otten H A, Boerma W B 1959 Significance of the Waaler–Rose test, streptococcal agglutination and antistreptolysin titre in the prognosis of rheumatoid arthritis. Annals of the Rheumatic Diseases 18: 24–28

Pallis C A, Scott J T 1965 Peripheral neuropathy in rheumatoid arthritis. British Medical Journal 1: 1141–1147

Panush R S, Carter R L, Katz P, Kowsari B, Longley S, Finnie S 1983 Diet therapy for rheumatoid arthritis. Arthritis and Rheumatism 26: 462–471

Parke A L, Hughes G R V 1981 Rheumatoid arthritis and food: a case study. British Medical Journal 282: 2027–2029

Partridge R E H, Duthie J J R 1963 Controlled trial of the effect of complete immobilisation of the joints in rheumatoid arthritis. Annals of the Rheumatic Diseases 22: 91–99

Pearson D J, Rix K J B, Bentley S J 1983 Food allergy: how much in the mind? Lancet 1: 1259–1261

Persellin R H, 1976–1977 The effect of pregnancy on rheumatoid arthritis. Bulletin on the Rheumatic Diseases. The Arthritis Foundation Atlanta Georgia 27: 922–926

Pinals R S, Baum J, Bland J, Fosdick W M, Kaplan S B, Masi A T, et al 1982 Preliminary criteria for clinical remission in rheumatoid arthritis. Bulletin on the Rheumatic Diseases 32: 7–10

Ragan C, Farrington E 1962 The clinical features of rheumatoid arthritis. Prognostic indices. Journal of the American Medical Association 181: 663–667

Rajapakse C N A, Holt P J L, Perera B S 1980 Diagnosis of true iron deficiency in rheumatoid arthritis. Abstract 2 The Heberden Round

Rasker J J, Cosh J A 1981 Cause and age at death in a prospective study of 100 patients with rheumatoid arthritis. Annals of the Rheumatic Diseases 40: 115–120

Robertson M D J, Hart F D, White W F, Nuki G, Boardman P L 1968 Rheumatoid lymphadenopathy. Annals of the Rheumatic Diseases 27: 253–260

Robinson H S 1973 Prognosis: return to work — arthritis. In: Ehrlich (ed) Total management of the arthritic patient. Lippincott, Philadelphia, p 183–192

Rogers M P, Liang M H, Partridge A J 1982 Psychological care of adults with rheumatoid arthritis. Annals of Internal Medicine 96: 344–348

Ropes M W, Bennett G A, Cobb S, Jacox R, Jessar R A 1959 Diagnostic criteria for rheumatoid arthritis. Annals of the Rheumatic Diseases 18: 49–51

Rotès-Quérol J, Roig-Escofet D 1968 Début de l'arthrite rheumatoide étude de 68 cas vus la première année d'évolution. Revue du Rheumatisme et des Maladies Osteoarticulaires 35: 21–30

Schumacher H R, Kitridou R C 1972 Synovitis of recent onset. Arthritis and Rheumatism 15: 465–485

Shapiro S, Siskind V, Monson R R, Heinonen O P, Kaufman D W, Slone D 1976 Perinatal mortality and birth weight in relation to aspirin taken during pregnancy. Lancet 1: 1375–1376

Sharp J T, Calkins E, Cohen A S, Schubart A F, Calabro J J 1964 Observations on the clinical, chemical and serological manifestations of rheumatoid arthritis based on the course of 154 cases. Medicine 43: 41–58

Sharp J T, Lidsky M D, Duffy J, Thompson H K, Person B D, Masri A F Andrianakos A A 1977 Comparison of two dosage schedules of gold salts in the treatment of rheumatoid arthritis. Arthritis and Rheumatism 20: 1179–1187

Sharp J T, Lidsky M D, Duffy J 1982 Clinical responses during gold therapy for rheumatoid arthritis: changes in synovitis, radiologically detectable erosive lesions, serum proteins and serological abnormalities. Arthritis and Rheumatism 25: 540–549

Sheppeard H, Bulgen D, Ward D J 1981 Rheumatoid arthritis: returning patients to work. Rheumatology and Rehabilitation 20: 160–163

Shiokawa Y, Horiuchi Y, Honma M, Kageyama T, Okada T, Azuma T 1977 Clinical evaluation of D-penicillamine by multi-centric double-blind study in chronic rheumatoid arthritis. Arthritis and Rheumatism 20: 1464–1472

Short C L 1968 Rheumatoid arthritis: types of course and prognosis. Medical Clinics of North America 52: 549–557

Short C L, Bauer W 1948 The course of rheumatoid arthritis in patients receiving simple medical and orthopaedic measures. New England Journal of Medicine 238: 142–148

Short C L, Bauer W, Reynolds W E 1957 Rheumatoid arthritis. Harvard University Press, Cambridge, Massachusetts, p 223

Sigler J W, Bluhm G M, Duncan H, Sharp J T, Ensign D C, McCrum W R 1974 Gold salts in the treatment of rheumatoid arthritis. Annals of Internal Medicine 80: 21–26

Sjöblom K G, Saxne T, Petterson H, Wollheim F 1982 Factors related to the progression of joint destruction in rheumatoid arthritis. Scandinavian Journal of Rheumatology Suppl 45:p 22

Slone D, Siskind V, Heinonen P H, Monson R R, Kaufman D W, Shapiro S 1976 Aspirin and congenital malformations. Lancet 1: 1373–1375

Smith P J, Swinburn W R, Swinson D R, Stewart I M 1982 Influence of previous gold toxicity on subsequent development of penicillamine toxicity. British Medical Journal 285: 595–596

Stein H B, Ruedy J, Atkins C J, Offer R C 1983 Penicillamine compared to previous chrysotherapy in

rheumatoid arthritis. Journal of Rheumatology Rheumatology 10: 319–322
Steven M M, Hunter J A, Murdoch R M, Capell H A 1982 Does the order of second-line treatment in rheumatoid arthritis matter? British Medical Journal 284: 79–81
Sundqvist T, Lindström F, Magnusson K–E, Sköldstam L, Stjernström I, Tagesson C 1982 Influence of fasting on intestinal permeability and disease activity in patients with rheumatoid arthritis. Scandinavian Journal of Rheumatology 11: 33–38
Swinburn W R 1976 Sexual counselling for the arthritic. In: Wright V (ed) Clinics in rheumatic diseases 2. Saunders, London, Ch 9, p 639–651
Traut E F, Passarelli E W 1957 Placebos in rheumatoid arthritis. Annals of the Rheumatic Diseases 16: 18–22
Trentham D E, Belli J A, Anderson R J, Buckley J A, Goetzi E J, David J R, Austen K F 1981 Clinical and immunologic effects of fractionated total lymphoid irradiation in refractory rheumatoid arthritis. New England Journal of Medicine 305: 976–982
Turner G, Collins E 1975 Foetal effects of regular salicylate ingestion in pregnancy. Lancet 2: 338–339
Uddin J, Kraus A S, Kelly H G 1970 Survivorship and death in rheumatoid arthritis. Arthritis and Rheumatism 13: 125–130
Ungar A, Kay A, Griffin A J, Panayi G S 1983 Disease activity and pregnancy associated α_2-glycoprotein in rheumatoid arthritis during pregnancy. British Medical Journal 286: 750–752
Vignos P J, Thompson H M, Katz S, Moskowitz R W, Fink S, Svec K H 1972 Comprehensive care and psycho-social factors in rehabilitation in chronic rheumatoid arthritis: a controlled study. Journal of Chronic Diseases 25: 457–467
Voyles W F, Searles R P, Bankhurst A D 1980 Myocardial infarction caused by rheumatoid arthritis. Arthritis and Rheumatism 23: 860–863
Waller M, Toone E C 1968 Normal individuals with positive tests for rheumatoid factor. Arthritis and Rheumatism 11: 50–55
Waller M, Toone E C, Vaughan E 1964 Study of rheumatoid factor in a normal population. Arthritis and Rheumatism 7: 513–520
Walker W C, Wright V 1968 Pulmonary lesions and rheumatoid arthritis. Medicine (Baltimore) 47: 501–520
Walker W C, Wright V 1969 Diffuse interstitial pulmonary fibrosis and rheumatoid arthritis. Annals of the Rheumatic Diseases 28: 252–259
White E G, Zaphiropoulos G C 1982 Haematuria occurring during anti-rheumatoid therapy. The combined annual provincial meeting of the British Association for Rheumatology and Rehabilitation, the Heberden Society, the Royal Society of Medicine Section of Rheumatology and Rehabilitation and the Irish Society of Rheumatology and Rehabilitation. Abstract 7
Williams I A, Bayliss E M, Shipley M E 1982 A double-blind placebo controlled trial of methylprednisolone in active rheumatoid disease. Lancet 2: 237–240
Williams R 1981 Rheumatoid arthritis and food: a case study. British Medical Journal 283:563
Woodland J 1982 Non-steroidal anti-inflammatory drugs. In: Hawkins C, Currey H L F (eds) Reports on rheumatic diseases. The Arthritis and Rheumatism Council, London, No. 81
Wright V, Hopkins R 1976 Administration of anti-rheumatic drugs. Annals of the Rheumatic Diseases 35: 174–180
Wright V, Owen S 1976 The effect of rheumatoid arthritis on the social situation of housewives. Rheumatology and Rehabilitation 15: 156–160
Yelin E H, Feshbach D M, Meenan R F, Epstein W V 1979 Social problems, services and policy for persons with chronic disease: the case of rheumatoid arthritis. Social Science and Meoicine 13C: 13–20

SECTION VI

Seronegative Spondarthritis

Seronegative spondarthritides

Some years ago it was fashionable to support the school of 'lumpers' which regarded rheumatoid arthritis as a non-specific syndrome that could be triggered by diverse aetiological factors such as psoriasis, urethritis, or ulcerative colitis. In most classifications at this time, psoriatic arthritis, Reiter's disease, and ankylosing spondylitis were considered 'atypical special forms of rheumatoid arthritis'. Later the trend changed in favour of the school of 'splitters' which regarded all so-called 'variants' of classical rheumatoid arthritis as discrete entities (McEwen et al, 1958; Leader, *BMJ*, 1956). This change in classification was mirrored by the system proposed by the American Rheumatism Association in 1963 (Copeman, 1969), in which rheumatoid arthritis, ankylosing spondylitis, psoriatic arthritis, and Reiter's disease were classified as separate entities. Another change in the 1963 classification was that the arthritides of ulcerative colitis, Crohn's disease, Whipple's disease, and Behçet's syndrome appeared for the first time.

Since the paper of Wright & Reed in 1964, attention has been drawn to possible interrelationships between certain seronegative 'variants of rheumatoid arthritis' and subsequently the concept has been further amplified (Moll et al, 1974; Wright & Moll, 1976; Wright, 1980; Moll, 1982). Despite suggestive evidence to uphold the idea of relationships between certain seronegative arthritides, it is still not clear which disease should be included in this network. A further problem concerns the choice of a suitable name for such a group. A term such as the 'seronegative *arthritides*', if left unqualified, might cause confusion with seronegative rheumatoid arthritis destined to become seropositive, or other inflammatory arthritides such as gout and the arthritis of haemochromatosis. The term 'seronegative *spond*arthritides' or simply the 'spondarthritides' has been used for the network under consideration — the prefix 'spond' emphasizing the strong association between each member of the group and ankylosing spondylitis. This term therefore identifies an interesting group of non-rheumatoid disorders in which striking clinical and familial interrelationships can be demonstrated. There is still imperfect agreement regarding the best term for this group of disorders, and the Americans, in particular, favour 'spondyloarthropathies'. Other terms include 'spondylarthropathies', 'spondylarthritides', 'spondyloarthritides', 'enthesopathies', and 'HLA-B27-positive disorders'. We favour 'spondarthritides' as it is shorter and more euphonic than the American term and its variants, and more accurate than the last two terms. The continued use of the term 'rheumatoid variants' (usually by non-rheumatologists) is not recommended and only serves to retard the spondarthritis idea and its central message stressing the non-rheumatoid nature of spondarthritic disorders.

CRITERIA FOR MEMBERS OF THE SPONDARTHRITIS GROUP

The following criteria should be satisfied when considering an arthropathy as one of the seronegative spondarthritides:

1. Absence of rheumatoid factors. (Tests for antinuclear factor are also negative.)
2. Absence of subcutaneous ('rheumatoid') nodules.
3. Inflammatory peripheral arthritis (often asymmetrical).

4. Radiological sacroiliitis with or without ankylosing spondylitis.
5. Evidence of clinical 'overlap' between members of the group. This should include two or more of the following features: psoriasiform skin or nail lesions; ocular inflammation, including conjunctivitis or anterior uveitis; buccal ulceration of small or large intestine; genital ulceration; genitourinary infection (particularly urethritis and/or prostatitis); erythema nodosum; pyoderma gangrenosum; thrombophlebitis.
6. Tendency to familial aggregation. Evidence for this may be obtained from individual pedigrees or from family surveys. In individual pedigree studies, familial aggregation has been defined as the presence of two or more examples of the same disease, or two or more different diseases within a single family. 'Disease' refers to members of the spondarthritis group (see 7). When there are different diseases within a family this type of aggregation has been termed a familial association (interrelationship). In the context of epidemiological studies, familial aggregation has been defined as a statistically significant increase in the familial prevalence of a disease compared with its prevalence in population or spouse controls. Clearly, an increased disease prevalence in blood relatives compared with the prevalence in the general population implies environmental and/or genetic factors as the cause, whereas an increased prevalence in relatives compared with the prevalence in spouse controls indicates the operation of genetic factors alone.
7. Significant association with the HLA-B27 antigen.

The clinical entities which appeared to justify inclusion in the seronegative spondarthritis group when the concept first evolved were as follows:

1. Uncomplicated ankylosing spondylitis
2. Psoriatic arthritis
3. Reiter's disease
4. Ulcerative colitis
5. Crohn's disease
6. Whipple's disease
7. Behçet's syndrome.

Subsequent evidence (see below) has led to a revision of this list to the following:

1. Uncomplicated ankylosing spondylitis
2. Psoriatic arthritis
3. Reiter's disease
4. Ulcerative colitis
5. Crohn's disease
6. Whipple's disease
7. Juvenile chronic arthritis
8. Reactive arthritis
9. Acute anterior uveitis
10. Behçet's syndrome.

EVIDENCE FOR SPONDARTHRITIS CRITERIA

Evidence that allows recruitment of the above disorders to the spondarthritis group and which also provides support for the concept of interrelationships between members of this group is derived from epidemiological surveys and from isolated observations. The supporting data have been divided into:

1. Evidence to support the 'basic' criteria 1–4 (summarised in Table 28.1)
2. Evidence to illustrate clinical overlap (criterion 5)
3. Evidence to illustrate familial aggregation (criterion 6).

Evidence for clinical overlap

One of the most striking clinical associations is that which exists between psoriatic arthritis and Reiter's disease (Fox & McLeod, 1901; Epstein, 1939; Hall & Finegold, 1953; Perkins, 1961; Wright & Reed, 1964; Maxwell et al, 1966; Dunlop et al, 1968; Dryll et al, 1969; Boxley, 1973). Thus, Wright & Reed reported a group of patients in whom it was impossible to make an unequivocal diagnosis of either disease; in some patients the disease appeared to be psoriatic arthritis with features of Reiter's disease; in others Reiter's disease with features of psoriatic arthritis. A particularly difficult diagnostic problem in these patients was the marked similarity, both clinical and histological, between pustular psoriasis and keratoderma blenorrhagica.

Table 28.1 Evidence to support basic seronegative spondarthritis criteria 1–4

Member of seronegative spondarthritis group	Seronegativity	Absence of subcutaneous nodules	Increased prevalence of polyarthritis	Increased prevalence of sacroiliitis
Psoriatic arthritis	Wright (1956); Reed et al (1961)	Baker et al (1963a); Reed & Wright (1966)	Leczinsky (1948)	Reed (1961); Wright (1961); Bywaters & Dixon (1965); Baker (1966); Jajić (1968); Moll (1971)
Reiter's disease	Ziff (1957); Reed et al (1961)	King (1964); King & Mason (1969)	King et al (1946); King & Mason (1969); Ford (1970)	Oates & Young (1959); King (1964)
Ulcerative colitis	Heller et al (1955); Dixon (1960)	Wilske & Decker (1965); Wright & Watkinson (1966)	Fernandez & Herlihy (1959); Wright & Watkinson (1966)	Bywaters & Ansell (1958); Acheson (1960); Wright & Watkinson (1965); Macrae & Wright (1973)
Crohn's disease	Bowen & Kirsner (1965); Soren (1966); Haslock & Wright (1973)	Ford & Vallis (1959); Wilske & Decker (1965)	Van Patter et al (1954); Daffner & Brown (1958)	McBride et al (1963); Stewart & Ansell (1963); Ansell & Wigley (1964); Haslock (1972)
Whipple's disease	Caughey & Bywaters (1963)	Wilske & Decker (1965)	Eyler & Doub (1956); Farnan (1959); Kelly & Weisiger (1963); Maizel (1970)	Puite & Tesluk (1955); Kelly & Weisiger (1963)
Behçet's syndrome	Strachan & Wigzell (1963); Mason & Barnes (1969)	Not yet reported	Dowling (1961); Oshima et al (1963); Mason & Barnes (1969)	Perkins (1961); Wright (1966); Dilsen (1967); Barnes (1969)
Ankylosing spondylitis	Heller et al (1955); McEwen et al (1958)	McEwen et al (1958); Sharp (1965)	Sharp & Easson (1954); Hart & Maclagan (1955); Sharp (1957); Kellgren & Ball (1959); Robinson (1963)	By definition 100%
Juvenile chronic arthritis	*See text for references*			
Reactive arthritis	*See text for references*			
Acute anterior uveitis	*See text for references*			

Strong similarities also exist between ulcerative colitis and Crohn's disease (Hammer et al, 1968). Not only do both disorders have in common a seronegative polyarthritis of similar pattern (asymmetrical, non-destructive, and tending to affect lower limb joints) and spondylitis, but in addition they share many other features such as ocular inflammation (conjunctivitis and uveitis), erythema nodosum, pyoderma gangrenosum, thrombophlebitis (Wilske & Decker, 1965), and buccal ulceration (Croft & Wilkinson, 1972).

Many of these clinical features — particularly ocular inflammation, buccal ulceration, erythema nodosum, and thrombophlebitis — are also seen in Behçet's syndrome, which may also be associated with colonic involvement indistinguishable from that seen in ulcerative colitis (Mason & Barnes, 1969). A further point of clinical overlap between Behçet's syndrome and the 'enteropathic' arthritides is the close similarity in the pattern of their peripheral arthritis (an asymmetrical, non-destructive lower limb joint synovitis). To extend the clinical spectrum further, Behçet's syndrome also has many points in common with Reiter's disease. These include ocular inflammation, genital and buccal ulceration, and bowel involvement (Bøe et al, 1958). However, although an increased frequency of sacroiliitis has been reported in

Behçet's syndrome by some workers (see Table 28.1), this has not been supported by recent studies (Chamberlain, 1977; Yazici et al, 1981). Reports on an increased prevalence of HLA-B27 in Behçet's syndrome have also been conflicting. For example, Chamberlain's study based only on X-rayed patients showed some increase (about 27%), despite the exclusion of premenopausal females, whereas the study of Ohno et al (1975) failed to show any increase. For these reasons, the place of Behçet's syndrome in the spondarthritis complex has lost some ground and must remain sub judice.

Further interrelationships have been reported between: Reiter's disease and ankylosing spondylitis (Oates & Young, 1959; Good, 1965); ankylosing spondylitis and Crohn's disease (Acheson, 1960); ulcerative colitis and Reiter's disease (Billson et al, 1967); ankylosing spondylitis and ulcerative colitis (Acheson, 1960; Jayson & Bouchier, 1968; Jayson et al, 1970); psoriatic arthritis and ulcerative colitis (Moll, 1971) and psoriasis and Crohn's disease (Haslock, 1972).

Dysentery has also been considered in relation to the seronegative spondarthritides. In this context, the study of Paronen (1948) is of particular interest. In a study of 344 patients with Reiter's disease, Paronen found that most cases originated from a widespread epidemic of Flexner dysentery on the Karelian isthmus, Finland, in the summer of 1944. In about 70% of patients the complete triad (articular, ocular and urethral manifestations) was present. Articular manifestations occurred in 97%, eye afflictions were observed in 89% and the urogenital organs were involved in 79% — urethritis being the most common manifestation. Two-thirds of patients developed Reiter's disease within 11–30 days of the onset of dysentery.

Some important clinical overlap phenomena are

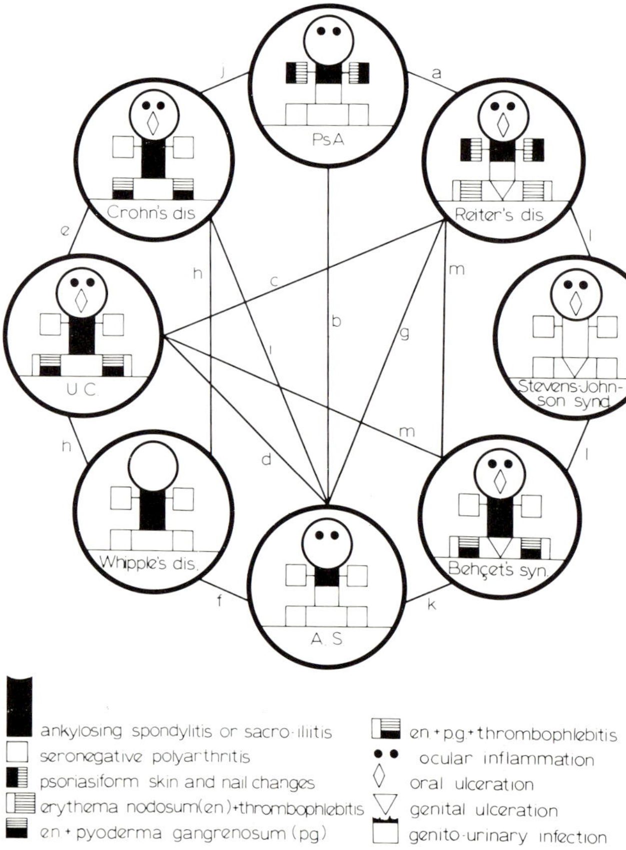

Fig. 28.1 Diagrammatic summary of clinical overlap phenomena. References to the relationships (denoted by letters a–m) are shown in Table 28.2.

summarised diagrammatically in Figure 28.1, and the references used to construct this diagram are shown separately in Table 28.2.

The inclusion of the Stevens–Johnson syndrome in the diagram does not imply its unequivocal acceptance as a member of the seronegative spondarthritis group. Although it satisfies many criteria, present evidence is not sufficient to justify its formal inclusion. However, the network of interrelationships would be incomplete without indicating the place of this syndrome in the mucocutaneous-ocular complex of Robinson & McCrumb (1950). These authors described a triad of disorders (Stevens–Johnson syndrome/Reiter's disease/Behçet's syndrome) each member exhibiting a number of similar clinical features, including ocular inflammation and orogenital ulceration.

The inclusion of juvenile chronic arthritis in the seronegative spondarthritis group has recently gained considerable support (Ansell, 1980; Rosenberg & Petty, 1982). At present it would appear that these patients represent a heterogeneous collection of diseases. Thus, some patients are undoubtedly suffering from ankylosing spondylitis (Ladd et al, 1971; Edmonds et al, 1974; Davidson et al, 1975; Ansell & Wood, 1976; Schaller, 1977), psoriatic arthritis (Lambert et al, 1976; Shore & Ansell, 1982), Reiter's disease (Iveson et al, 1975; Jacobs, 1977; Singson et al, 1977), or the arthritis of ulcerative colitis or Crohn's disease of juvenile onset (Schaller, 1976; Lindsley, 1977), and reactive arthritis (Rosenborg & Petty, 1982). Other patients have systemic, polyarticular, or pauciarticular Still's disease. Yet others have seropositive rheumatoid arthritis similar in pattern to that of the adult disease. It would seem reasonable to exclude the last group from the seronegative spondarthritides, but the other forms of juvenile chronic arthritis mentioned undoubtedly warrant inclusion, a claim strengthened by the finding of HLA-B27 is a significant proportion of the various subgroups mentioned (Edmonds et al, 1974; Hall et al, 1975; Jacobs et al, 1982).

Acute anterior uveitis

It is becoming clear that uveitis (particularly acute anterior uveitis) may represent not only a 'peripheral' co-disease in the spondarthritis network but also a primary member of the group in its own right. There is now abundant evidence that inflammation of the uveal tract (the portion of the eye that includes the iris, ciliary body, and choroid) is associated with a variety of systemic diseases including ankylosing spondylitis (Brewerton et al, 1973), Reiter's syndrome (Brewerton et al, 1973), psoriatic arthritis (Lambert and Wright, 1976), ulcerative colitis (Wright et al, 1965) and Crohn's disease (Greenstein et al, 1976), Behçet's syndrome (James, 1979), and juvenile chronic polyarthritis (Smiley, 1974; Glass et al, 1980). In many spondarthritic conditions the uveitis is of the acute anterior type but patterns of uveal inflammation vary (Rosenbaum & Cousins, 1982). For example, in ankylosing spondylitis and Reiter's disease the

Table 28.2 References to clinical associations shown in Figure 28.1

Diagram number	Author and date	Nature of clinical association
a	Wright & Reed (1964)	Psoriatic arthritis–Reiter's disease
b	Hill (1961)	Psoriatic arthritis–Ankylosing spondylitis
c	Billson et al (1967)	Reiter's disease–Ulcerative colitis
d	Acheson (1960)	Ulcerative colitis–Ankylosing spondylitis
e	Hammer et al (1968)	Ulcerative colitis–Crohn's disease
f	Puite & Tesluk (1955)	Ankylosing spondylitis–Whipple's disease
g	Oates & Young (1959)	Ankylosing spondylitis–Reiter's disease
h	Wilske & Decker (1965)	Whipple's disease–Ulcerative colitis
		Whipple's disease–Crohn's disease
i	Bowen & Kirsner (1965)	Crohn's disease–Ankylosing spondylitis
j	Ansell & Wigley (1964)	Crohn's disease–Psoriatic arthritis
k	Perkins (1961)	Behçet's syndrome–Ankylosing spondylitis
l	Robinson & McCrumb (1950)	Stevens-Johnson syndrome–Reiter's disease
		Stevens-Johnson syndrome–Behçet's syndrome
m	Bøe et al (1958)	Behçet's syndrome–Reiter's disease
		Behçet's syndrome–Ulcerative colitis

uveal tract disorder is an acute, unilateral, recurrent, non-granulomatous anterior uveitis associated with HLA-B27. In Behçet's syndrome it is a severe panuveitis often with hypopyon and HLA-B5. In pauciarticular juvenile chronic arthritis it is a low-grade chronic anterior uveitis with severe sequelae and associated with HLA-DRw5. These patients are usually seronegative for IgM rheumatoid factor but nearly 90% are positive for antinuclear antibodies (Schaller et al, 1974).

Further evidence for an association between anterior uveitis and rheumatic disorders of the seronegative type has recently been reported by Saari et al (1982). In a retrospective examination of 154 patients with acute anterior uveitis, associated rheumatic symptoms were observed in 64 (41.6%). 41 patients (26.6%) had ankylosing spondylitis and 39 (25.3%) manifestations of Reiter's disease. Radiographic sacroiliitis was seen in 35 (34%) of 103 patients and HLA-B27 occurred in 35 (87.5%) of 40 HLA-typed patients with acute anterior uveitis. Associated rheumatic diseases occurred in 18 (51.4%) of the 35 HLA-B27-positive patients, but in none of the HLA-B27-negative patients. These workers concluded that a pleiotropic HLA-B27-associated gene may determine the susceptibility to acute anterior uveitis, ankylosing spondylitis, and Reiter's disease.

Reactive arthritis

Although not included in the original delineation of the spondarthritis concept, reactive arthritis is now considered to belong to this group of disorders. The term 'reactive arthritis' is based on the model of rheumatic fever in which a microorganism precipitates arthritis by a purported immunological process rather than by direct infection (see also Chapter 14). Three enteric pathogens, *Shigella flexneri* (Schittenhelm & Schlecht, 1918; Paronen, 1948; Noer, 1966), *Salmonella* spp. (Warren, 1970; Frus & Svejgaard, 1974; Hakansson et al, 1976; Jones, 1977), and *Yersinia enterocolitica* (Aho et al, 1976; Schilling, 1976; Ford et al, 1977; Laitinen et al, 1977; Russell, 1977), can also induce a reactive arthritis, sometimes closely resembling that of rheumatic fever. However, the reactive arthritides of all three enteric pathogens differ from that of a group A streptococcus (true rheumatic fever) in that they are significantly associated with the HLA-B27 antigen. Moreover, certain *clinical* features characterising the reactive arthritides also differentiate these reactive syndromes from rheumatic fever and, indeed, were responsible for raising the question of their relationship to the spondarthritides. Prominent among these features were those of Reiter's phenomena (Leirisalo et al, 1982). These include urethritis, ocular inflammation (conjunctivitis or iritis), mucocutaneous lesions (palatal ulcers and balanitis), and erythema nodosum. The arthritis, too, has many features shared by certain spondarthritides, notably Reiter's disease and the enteropathic arthropathies of ulcerative colitis and Crohn's disease. Depending on the organism responsible, the joint disturbance (which may affect both peripheral and spinal joints) tends to appear one to several weeks after the onset of the bowel disturbance. For example, in shigellosis 85% of cases of arthritis begin within 4 weeks of the onset of diarrhoea, and in salmonellosis the interval is between 1 and 2 weeks. The knee and ankle joints are most often involved. The arthritis is non-migratory and usually clears completely within 3 months. A minority exhibit a monarthritis, or extend to a symmetrical rheumatoid-type pattern.

Evidence for familial aggregation

There is much evidence from the literature to suggest the presence of familial aggregation in each of the disorders of the seronegative spondarthritis group. However, with the possible exception of uncomplicated psoriasis and uncomplicated ankylosing spondylitis, it is still not established whether this aggregation represents a purely genetic effect, a purely environmental effect, or the effect of both these factors. Difficulties in drawing definite conclusions from many of the previous reports in the literature include: lack of spouse controls, lack of comparable population controls, small size of survey populations, and inadequacy and lack of uniformity of diagnostic criteria.

The most complete evidence for familial aggregation is that for uncomplicated ankylosing spondylitis. This has been fully reviewed by Kellgren (1964) who has drawn attention to the 40-fold increase in ankylosing spondylitis in relatives of probands with this disease. Although the importance

of genetic factors in ankylosing spondylitis is no longer challenged, the mode of inheritance is still not entirely clear. Stecher (1957) concluded that the disease is due to an autosomal dominant factor with 70% penetrance in males and 10% penetrance in females. Pedigree characteristics reported by Riecker, et al (1950), and Graham & Uchida (1957) support this hypothesis. However, a more recent interpretation of genetic data has favoured a multifactorial mechanism (Emery & Lawrence, 1967), and this mechanism would explain some features including:

1. The lack in most series of any obvious Mendelian pattern
2. The poor correlation between observed and expected rates of manifestation of the disease
3. The evidence that environmental factors such as genitourinary infecton may be important in aetiology.

In uncomplicated psoriasis the evidence for familial aggregation is also strong, and it has been proposed that this is due to genetic factors, Many genetic mechanisms have been proposed to explain the transmission of psoriasis. These have included a double recessive mechanism (Steinberg et al, 1951), and autosomal dominance with incomplete penetrance (Lomholt, 1963). More recently, simple Mendelian theories have given way to the idea of multifactorial inheritance in this disease (Watson et al, 1971). Evidence is also accumulating to support a similar mode of transmission in psoriatic arthritis (Baker, et al, 1963; Theiss et al, 1969).

Familial aggregation has been recorded in Reiter's disease by many workers and the subject has been well reviewed by Good (1971). Aggregation has been observed in both post-dysenteric Reiter's disease (Paronen, 1948), and in non-dysenteric Reiter's disease (Mowat & Nicol, 1968). Whether the concentration within families is due to genetic factors or infectious agents, or both, is still not understood.

Published data on familial aggregation in Behçet's syndrome are limited. Berlin (1960) has reported classical Behçet's syndrome in two siblings, and Sezer (1956) has observed the syndrome in three brothers. Behçet's syndrome with neurological manifestations has been reported in two sisters by Fowler et al (1968). In the experience of Mason & Barnes (1969), familial aggregation in Behçet's syndrome is not infrequent, and in four of their 33 patients another member of the family was affected.

Spriggs (1934) published the first report of familial aggregation in ulcerative colitis, and since this observation there have been several others (Sloan et al 1950; Houghton & Naish, 1958; Barker, 1962; Sherlock et al, 1963; Goligher et al, 1968). Kirsner & Spencer (1963) have provided further evidence for familial clustering in ulcerative colitis, and in a study of over 1000 colitic patients found 66 with a positive family history of the disease. McConnell (1966) thinks that familial aggregation in ulcerative colitis represents a genetic aetiology, and that this is probably multifactorial.

There is mounting evidence to suggest that Crohn's disease is in part genetically determined, and, in fact, Crohn (1934) himself suggested the term 'familial ileitis' for the disease. Crohn's disease in twins has been reported in a number of instances (Krisner & Spencer, 1963; Sherlock et al, 1963), but the fallacy of this type of evidence, unless based on unselected data, is well known. McConnell (1966) favours genetic rather than environmental factors in Crohn's disease in view of the fact that when the disease is observed in families it affects relatives in different generations. Another suggestive feature is the wide separation in time of onset of the bowel disease in relatives. However, it is probably that both factors are involved and, as with ulcerative colitis, a multifactorial mechanism seems most likely.

The aetiology of Whipple's disease remains unknown, but there is reasonable evidence for an infective agent (Chears & Ashworth, 1961; Yardley & Hendrix, 1961; Kurtz et al, 1962; Kent et al, 1963). It is possible that genetic factors may also be involved. The rarity of Whipple's disease has so far precluded even small family studies, and the only familial data available stem from individual pedigree reports. Thus, Puite & Tesluk (1955) described an interesting family in which two brothers had proven Whipple's disease and arthritis, and their mother and maternal grandmother had what was probably the same disease. Gross et al (1959) have also reported two brothers with Whipple's disease, and Scott & Hosie (1957) noted that a brother of their patient with Whipple's disease was thought to have had 'rheumatoid arthritis' and to have 'withered away'. McConnell (1966) suggests that heredity could be concerned in determining an unusual reaction to bacterial agents.

In many members of the spondarthritis group, with the exception of Behçet's syndrome and Whipple's disease, examples of familial association have been found. For example, relatives of patients with psoriatic arthritis have been found to exhibit not only psoriatic arthritis, but also ankylosing spondylitis (Moll, 1971), and Reiter's disease (Lawrence, 1965). Another example is provided by patients with Crohn's disease in whose families increased prevalences of uncomplicated psoriasis, ulcerative colitis, and ankylosing spondylitis have been demonstrated (Hammer et al, 1968). These workers have also observed Crohn's disease in the relatives of patients with ulcerative colitis. Kirsner & Spencer (1963) have reported additional evidence to support an association between ulcerative colitis and Crohn's disease. These workers have shown an increased frequency of ulcerative colitis and of Crohn's disease in families of probands with each disease. An interesting family has been reported by Sherlock et al (1963) in which there were two cases of ulcerative colitis, four of uncomplicated Crohn's disease, and one of Crohn's disease associated with ankylosing spondylitis. A pedigree has been reported by Good (1971) in which two siblings had Reiter's disease and a third, classical ankylosing spondylitis.

In order to examine the question of familial aggregation and the phenomenon of familial association within members of the seronegative spondarthritides, family studies of psoriatic arthritis (Moll, 1971; Mill & Wright, 1973), ulcerative colitis (Macrae & Wright, 1973), and Crohn's disease (Haslock, 1972) have been carried out at Leeds.

Studies of families of probands with psoriatic arthritis have revealed a highly significant increase in the prevalence of psoriasis ('complicated' and 'uncomplicated') in relatives (19.7%) compared with spouse and population controls. The prevalence of psoriatic arthritis (5.4%) was also significantly higher in relatives compared with spouse and population controls. Interesting, too, was the increased frequency of sacroiliitis (8%). Ulcerative colitis was found in two relatives (0.9%) and this was statistically significant when compared with the population prevalence of 0.6%.

Among the relatives of probands with ulcerative colitis, the most striking feature was the increased frequency of sacroiliitis (4.7%) and ankylosing spondylitis (3.2%) compared with the population figures for these conditions (1.10 and 0.19% respectively). Two relatives had ulcerative colitis (1.0%), which was statistically significant compared with the population frequency.

The study of relatives of probands with Crohn's disease revealed results comparable to those found in the colitis study, namely a significant increase in the prevalence of sacroiliitis (6.2%) compared with population data (0.01%). However, no examples of classical ankylosing spondylitis were found among these relatives, suggesting that spinal involvement in these families is relative mild. The prevalence of Crohn's disease in relatives (1.4%) was significantly higher than in population controls (0.01%)

An overall summary of data demonstrating familial aggregation and association within the seronegative spondarthritides is shown in Table 28.3.

The picture emerging from these data suggests a set of genes, some of which may provide predisposition to more than one clinical condition and which may interact to produce various patterns of disease susceptibility. For further details concerning genetic influences and interrelationships within the spondarthritides, the reader is referred to a recent review by Woodrow (1980).

SUPPORT FROM HLA STUDIES

General comment

Since 1960, the serological analysis and recognition of human leucocyte isoantigens (HLA antigens) has assumed increasing importance (see Ch. 10). The realisation that human cells carry isoantigens other than ABO antigens has, however, been slow to evolve. This is because of a failure to appreciate that the mature human red cell (in contrast to the white cell) does not carry these other isoantigenic determinants, as is the case with the mouse H systems.

Table 28.3 Summary of evidence supporting the concept of familial aggregation and association among the seronegative spondarthritides

Index disease (proband diagnosis)	Increased prevalence of associated disease in first-degree relatives	Reference
Uncomplicated ankylosing spondylitis	Ankylosing spondylitis	Kellgren (1964)
	Uncomplicated psoriasis	Lawrence (1965)
Uncomplicated psoriasis	Psoriasis	Lomholt (1963)
	Psoriatic arthritis	Lawrence (1967)
	Uncomplicated seronegative arthritis	Lawrence (1967)
	Ankylosing spondylitis	Lawrence (1967)
Psoriatic arthritis	Psoriatic arthritis	Baker et al (1963b); Moll (1971); Moll & Wright (1973)
	Uncomplicated psoriasis	Reed & Wright (1966)
	Ankylosing spondylitis	Lawrence (1967)
	Uncomplicated seronegative arthritis	Lawrence (1967)
	Reiter's disease	Lawrence (1967)
Reiter's disease	Reiter's disease	Paronen (1948)
	Uncomplicated psoriasis	Lawrence (1965)
	Ankylosing spondylitis	Lawrence (1965)
Ulcerative colitis	Ulcerative colitis	Kirsner & Spencer (1963); Macrae & Wright (1973)
	Ankylosing spondylitis	Macrae & Wright (1973)
	'Polyarthritis'	Hammer et al (1968)
	Crohn's disease	Hammer et al (1968)
Crohn's disease	Crohn's disease	Haslock (1972); Kirsner & Spencer (1963)
	Uncomplicated psoriasis	Hammer et al (1968)
	Ulcerative colitis	Kyle (1971)
	'Polyarthritis'	Hammer et al (1968)
	Ankylosing spondylitis	Hammer et al (1968)
Whipple's disease	Whipple's disease	Puite & Tesluk (1955)
Behçet's syndrome	Behçet's syndrome	Mason & Barnes (1969)

After an initial period of confusion in the naming of antigens (due to each laboratory necessarily adopting its own terminology), a series of joint workshops led to the development of an official World Health Organization Committee on Nomenclature.

It is now established that the inherited antigen HLA-B27 is present in a very high proportion of patients with ankylosing spondylitis. (This antigen was previously designated 'W27' when it was at the workshop stage; its current official status is reflected by the 'HLA' prefix.) The interesting association between HLA-B27 and ankylosing spondylitis was reported from the the United Kingdom (Caffrey & James, 1973; Brewerton et al, 1973) and from the United States (Schlosstein et al, 1973) almost simultaneously.

From the studies of Brewerton et al (1974) it has been calculated that only 5% of men and 0.6% of women born with HLA-B27 will develop clinical ankylosing spondylitis as currently defined. From this it follows that other factors must also be involved in determining disease susceptibility, including both genetic and environmental factors.

The HLA-B27 antigen has been found in 8% of Caucasians and in 4% of American Negroes. However, it has been shown to be absent in African Negroes (Albert et al, 1973). The low frequency in American Negroes suggests that the antigen may have come from a Caucasian admixture. The observation that the prevalence of ankylosing spondylitis in the Japanese is about 0.4% (which is comparable with the prevalence in the white Western population) is of interest in view of reports showing that the HLA-B27 antigen is present in only about 1% of normal Japanese (Albert et al, 1973).

HLA-B27 has been found in 8 of 10 black males with ankylosing spondylitis (Schlosstein et al,

1973) — a frequency similar to that found in Caucasian spondylitics. A recent report of the co-existence of HLA-B27 in only 3 of 7 black females with ankylosing spondylitis is of particular interest when compared with the higher prevalence in black males (Swezey et al, 1974). The comparatively low prevalence of HLA-B27 in black females suggests that factors in addition to the HLA-B27 antigen operate in the development of ankylosing spondylitis.

The association of HLA-B27 antigen with hip joint involvement and with aortic valvulitis suggests the possibility that this antigen may predispose patients to more severe spondylitic complications.

It is interesting to speculate how histocompatibility genes could predispose an individual to a disease such as ankylosing spondylitis, and in this context many research centres are now looking for specific immune responses in various members of the spondarthritis group. A particularly intensive study is being directed towards the 'reactive arthritides'. In these arthritides it is established that an organism is involved, but the precise way in which reactions to them are produced is not yet known.

It seems likely that from the gut (the site of initial infection) there is dissemination either of the organisms themselves (during a bacteraemic phase) to the joints, or alternatively dissemination of bacterial antigens. In either case, reaction to this event probably represents an immune response failure at the initial site of infection. Evidence for this has come from a demonstration of a relationship between cell-mediated immune responses to antigens of certain enterobacteria and specific major histocompatibility antigens (Glynn, cited by Allison, 1975.) Further evidence for this concept has emerged from Westminster Hospital (Nikbin et al, 1975). These workers have found that in HLA-B27-positive individuals there is a non-specific defect in cell mediated immunity manifested by diminished mixed lymphocyte reactions, and also a possible specific defect — namely in reactions to the Yersinia bacterium. The authors conclude that a poor T cell response to Yersinia may be inherited in associated with HLA-B27.

In Reiter's disease prevalences of over 90% have also been documented (Morris et al, 1974; Harris et al, 1975). When ankylosing spondylitis is found associated with inflammatory bowel disease, HLA-B27 has been noted in over 70% of patients (Morris et al, 1974; Brewerton et al, 1974). The arthropathy related to inflammatory bowel disease, however, is not directly associated with the HLA-B27 antigen. In patients with psoriatic arthritis, it seems that the antigen is highly correlated with spinal involvement (Brewerton et al, 1974; McClusky et al, 1974; Metzger et al, 1975), although less strongly than in uncomplicated ankylosing spondylitis. HLA-B27 is also increased in peripheral psoriatic arthritis without spinal involvement, but the statistical association is not striking (Brewerton et al, 1974). There is also a subpopulation of children with juvenile chronic arthritis that bear the HLA haplotype (Edmonds et al, 1974). It has been suggested that these patients may represent the juvenile counterpart of ankylosing spondylitis. Furthermore, there are reports describing the association of HLA-B27 with Yersinia arthritis (Aho et al, 1973) and idiopathic anterior uveitis (Brewerton et al, 1973).

This antigen is not present in increased frequency in the 'non-spondarthritic' rheumatic disease (rheumatoid arthritis, systemic lupus erythematosus, scleroderma, dermatomyositis, gout and osteoarthrosis), or in non-rheumatic disease states. In view of the striking relationship between the presence of antigen HLA-B27 and spondylitis-associated disorders, the new designation 'HLA-B27-positive rheumatic disease' has been proposed (Metzger et al, 1974) although this description has found less favour than the more clinically apposite term 'seronegative spondarthritides'.

As the association of HLA-B27 positivity with both ankylosing spondylitis and Reiter's disease is the strongest yet found for *any* human disease, this antigen must in some way be viewed as integral to their respective pathogeneses. Moreover, the strikingly high association between HLA-B27 positivity and the spondylitis of juvenile rheumatoid arthritis, psoriatic arthritis, and the arthritis of inflammatory bowel disease, strongly suggests that HLA-B27 identifies some genetic factor common to disorders of the seronegative spondarthritis spectrum. Precisely how this antigen links a susceptible patient and the eventual developments of these conditions remains unknown.

It has been suggested that tissue typing should make it possible to examine in more detail the nature of relationships between spondarthritides, their individual disease penetrance rates, and their preclinical and clinical evolution (Metzger et al, 1974). Moreover, now that so much of the clinical taxonometry has been completed, it will be up to the geneticist and the immunobiologist to discover the central links in the jigsaw connecting HLA-B27-positive subjects and their particular rheumatic disease syndrome.

For further details concerning HLA-B27 patterns in the various members of the spondarthritis network, the reader is referred to the individual chapters concerned with those disorders.

DISORDERS DISPLAYING SPONDARTHRITIS-LIKE FEATURES

Certain disorders manifest spondarthritic characteristics. However, whether some or all should be accepted as true members of the spondarthritis network remains to a greater or lesser extent undetermined.

Undifferentiated seronegative peripheral arthritis

Undifferentiated or unclassified seronegative peripheral arthritis continues to raise problems concerning nosological status within rheumatic disorders. Undoubtedly some of these patients have rheumatoid arthritis, and conversion to seropositivity for IgM rheumatoid factors attests to this. Some probably have true seronegative rheumatoid arthritis, although the cellular basis for non-expression of rheumatoid factor is still not understood (Alarcón et al, 1982a). It has been further suggested that although some patients with seronegative arthritis are in fact true rheumatoids, a further distinction can be made on the grounds of HLA-DR4 positivity — seropositive DR4-positive disease differing from seronegative DR4-positive disease in that the presence of DR4 in the latter provides an index of disease severity based on joint destruction (Alarcón et al, 1982b). These authors even go as far as to suggest that sero-negative DR4-positive rheumatoid is a distinct immunogenetic disease. Whether seropositive or seronegative for IgM rheumatoid factor or seropositive or seronegative for DR4, these patients are negative for HLA-B27.

There is little doubt, too, that some patients with undifferentiated seronegative peripheral arthritis represent lanthanic spondarthritis. These patients, often HLA-B27-positive, have been observed to develop spondarthritic features such as sacroiliitis, psoriasis, inflammatory bowel disease and features of Reiter's disease.

HLA-B27-positive patients who remain free from spondarthritic stigmata have revealed no special features with regard to joint pattern or sex distribution compared with HLA-B27-negative patients with unclassified seronegative peripheral arthritis (Amor et al, 1976; Esdaile et al, 1976).

Further study of undifferentiated HLA-B27-positive seronegative peripheral arthritis is needed to determine more precisely its relationship to the spondarthritides. The solution is unlikely to come from solely clinical or clinicoradiological studies, as this approach is too crude, and has doubtless been responsible for retarding progress in this field. More promising are studies of D locus antigens, in addition to the already established work on B locus antigens, and already such an approach is helping to discriminate between subcategories in rheumatoid arthritis, as has been indicated.

Pustulotic arthro-osteitis (see also Ch. 49).

Arthro-osteitis of the anterior chest wall has recently been reported in 12 of 128 consecutive patients with pustolosis palmaris et plantaris (a disorder variously debated among dermatologists as being either a variant of pustular psoriasis or a distinct entity). The authors (Sonozaki et al, 1981a) have proposed the term 'pustulotic arthro-osteitis' for this condition. In a further report (Sonozaki et al, 1981b) these workers suggested that the features of this condition warranted its inclusion in the seronegative spondarthritis group. Clinical features of 53 Japanese patients with pustulotic arthro-osteitis were described. Anterior chest wall symptoms such as intersternocostoclavicular or manubriosternal lesions were observed in all of the 53 patients. Spondylitis or spondylodiscitis was found in 18 patients. Sacroiliitis resembling that found in ankylosing spondylitis was seen in seven patients. Peripheral inflammatory arthritis (14 patients) was non-erosive and oligoarthritic, and disappeared within 1–2 months, leaving no residue. HLA-B27 was not found, and all patients were negative for rheumatoid factor. Histological examination revealed non-specific chronic inflammation of bone and soft tissue. Of further interest is a report describing overlap between pustolosis palmaris et plantaris and psoriasis (Ashurst, 1964). Although Sonozaki and colleagues did not study the familial aspects of pustolotic arthro-osteitis, one such report has been published (Kumagaya et al, 1973). This showed a pedigree in which 2 brothers and 2 sisters had pustulosis palmaris et plantaris and the brothers in addition had bilateral arthritis involving the clavicles.

Intestinal bypass arthritis–dermatitis syndrome

(see also Chapters 32, 49)

In 1956 Payne et al found that jejunocolic bypass was effective in treating morbid obesity but that it was associated with many complications, particularly vasculitic and rheumatic abnormalities. This observation, including the occurrence of postoperative arthritis in over 30% of patients, has since been confirmed by others (Shagrin et al, 1971; Mir-Madjlessi et al, 1974). Jejunoileal anastomosis is associated with a lower frequency of arthritis (Buchanan & Willkens, 1972; Campbell et al, 1977; Fernandez-Herlihy, 1977). The knees, ankles, fingers, wrists and shoulders are the areas most commonly involved. The arthritis tends to be non-destructive and transient. Two reports have drawn attention to axial skeleton involvement. One described sacroiliac sclerosis in 6 of 31 patients, although these were thought to be not typical of sacroiliitis (Stein et al, 1981). The other report (Rose et al, 1978) described two patients in whom spondylitis, associated with HLA-B27 and circulating immune complexes, was a prominent feature.

Further studies of this syndrome need to be done to determine more definitely whether or not it represents an 'experimental' model of other enteropathic spondarthritides, such as those associated with ulcerative coilitis, Crohn's disease, and Whipple's disease. At present, however, the place of this syndrome in the spondarthritis complex remains unconvincing.

Erosive spondylopathy

This disorder (alternatively termed 'spondylitis erosiva', 'chronic evolutive spondylodiscitis', 'isolated rheumatic spondylodiscitis'), has been reported with increasing frequency in recent years (Coste et al, 1963; Hicklin, 1968; Cawley et al, 1972; Little et al, 1974). The main argument is whether or not it should be regarded as an atypical presentation of ankylosing spondylitis, with vertebral erosions occurring earlier than usual. Courtois et al (1980) put forward reasons for regarding the condition as separate from ankylosing spondylitis. These include:

1. Female predominance
2. Normal chest mobility
3. Low frequency of sacroiliitis
4. Lower frequency of HLA-B27 than ankylosing spondylitis, but higher than control values
5. Absence of development of classical ossification of spinal ligaments.

Other workers, including Jajić et al (1982), view the condition as a feature of ankylosing spondylitis. Jajić and colleagues reported 9 patients, 7 of whom had ultimately developed sacroiliitis, and were HLA-B27-positive. One patient had a positive family history for ankylosing spondylitis.

Certainly, the localised erosive changes, usually of one or more lumbar vertebrae, often in the absence of sacroiliitis, with complete regression in some instances, are unlike the pattern seen in classicial ankylosing spondylitis. However, it is possible that the syndrome represents nothing more than an unusual manifestation of a disorder known to possess a wide spectrum of radiological expression. Whether to 'lump' erosive spondylitis with classical ankylosing spondylitis or whether to 'split' it from this disorder still leaves one with the conclusion that the condition belongs to the spondarthritides.

Diffuse idiopathic skeletal hyperostosis (DISH) (ankylosing hyperostosis, Forestier's disease)

The criteria proposed for this disorder are as follows:

1. The presence of flowing calcification and ossification along the anterolateral aspect of at least 4 contiguous vertebral bodies
2. Absence of extensive degenerative disc disease
3. Absence of both apophyseal ankylosis and sacroiliac erosion, sclerosis, or fusion.

The first criterion helps to distinguish DISH from typical spondylosis, the second from degenerative disc disease, and the third from ankylosing spondylitis (Resnick et al, 1978). Of interest in this respect is a recent study (Resnick et al, 1978) which revealed that 16 of 47 white patients (34%) had the HLA-B27 antigen. However, three subsequent studies of HLA typing in DISH have failed to confirm an increased prevalence of HLA-B27 (Brigode et al, 1977; Ercilla et al, 1977; Rosenthal et al, 1977). In conclusion, the bulk of clinical, radiological and serological evidence is very much against including this disorder as one of the spondarthritides.

Erosive osteoarthritis (Crain, 1961; Kidd & Peter, 1966; Peter et al, 1966; Swezey & Alexander, 1971)
This disorder, first reported in the 1960s, is confined to the distal and proximal interphalangeal joints. It closely resembles psoriatic arthritis sine psoriasis, although some workers claim to be able to differentiate between the disorders (Martel et al, 1980; Gold et al, 1982). Although some of these patients probably represent atypical rheumatoid arthritis — Ehrlich found that 15% develop rheumatoid features (Ehrlich, 1972) — it is likely that most of the patients have neither rheumatoid arthritis nor classic osteoarthritis. The probability that erosive osteoarthritis represents a distinct syndrome has been widely voiced, and it will be interesting to see if its clinicoradiological features of spondarthritis receive support from immunogenetic sources. However, at present we feel that this disorder reflects nothing more than a subset of the osteoarthritis/osteoarthrosis syndrome, one with inflammatory features predominating and one in which the suffix 'itis' as opposed to 'osis' might be particularly relevant. This comment is made despite certain resemblances between the distal interphalangeal joint changes of erosive osteoarthritis and psoriatic arthritis of distal joint variety.

COMMENTS ON AETIOPATHOGENESIS
(see also above and Chapter 29)

Despite the wealth of genetic, immunogenetic and immunological data that have emerged in recent years since the initial elaboration of the spondarthritis concept from largely clinical roots, the aetiopathogenesis of this group of disorders is still imperfectly understood.

It is possible, however, to express in general terms likely principles and pathways concerned. Any such hypothesis should take into account:
1. Certain fundamental characteristics displayed by these disorders regarded individually
2. The interrelationships that bind together the various spondarthritic entities.

It is now generally accepted that genetic factors provide a backcloth for diseases in this group, and that genetic expression in predisposed individuals requires the intervention of 'environmental triggering'. The multifactorial inheritance model for the spondarthritides therefore seems likely, but details regarding the balance between 'nature' and 'nurture' in individual disorders has yet to be elucidated.

The nature of genetic influences has been uncovered in part since the discovery of the cell surface antigens at the major histocompatibility complex. Notable among these is HLA-B27 in ankylosing spondylitis and in spondarthritic disorders associated with spondylitis such as psoriasis, ulcerative colitis, Crohn's disease, Reiter's disease, reactive arthritis, acute anterior uveitis and certain forms of juvenile chronic polyarthritis. Whether HLA-B27 is itself the 'spondylitis gene' (one gene theory) or whether it is in close linkage disequilibrium with a 'spondylitis-susceptibility' gene (two gene theory) has yet to be determined. The story is doubtless not as simple as this, and the presence of other HLA antigens at the B locus such as B13 and B17 in psoriasis, and B5 in Behçet's syndrome, raises the question of multiple genes operating to explain the myriad of phenotypic presentations. The relevance of genes at other HLA loci — A, C and D loci genes — has so far not thrown much further light on the genetic transmission of individual entities, nor on an association between them. However, the tentative evidence that A2 may be linked with spondylitis and Reiter's disease is interesting.

However encouraging these early findings, further immunogenetic work is required to unravel the nature and significance of, and interdependency between, the multiple loci and alleles involved in the spondarthritis network.

The place of the environment in generating clinically expressed syndromes from genetically predisposed states remains another poorly understood field. However, the likelihood of the existence of environmental triggers, and the fact that they exist in a wide spectrum is becoming well accepted. The association of certain micro-organisms with certain spondarthritic syndromes adds weight to the idea of environmental influences. In this context the phenomenon of reactive arthritis in yersinia infection, salmonellosis and shigellosis might be cited. Interesting, too, are recent reports that active ankylosing spondylitis is associated with positive faecal cultures for *Klebsiella aerogenes*. The relevance of infection either in a 'primary infective' or 'reactive' sense has of course been long realised in Reiter's disease, as has the triggering of psoriasis in children with certain streptococcal throat infections.

It would probably be naïve to believe that micro-organisms represent the only environmental triggers. The effect of trauma appears to be related to the onset of some spondarthritic disorders, and in others it appears to provide an aggravating effect out of proportion to the size of the injury. Conditions in which trauma appears to be influential are in the peripheral arthritis and skin lesions of psoriatic arthritis, and in certain spinal manifestations of ankylosing spondylitis such as 'spondylodiscitis'.

The mechanism through which trauma exerts long-term effects is not known but could arise from antigenic release from injured tissues.

The significance of other environmental threats such as pollutants, dietary factors, drugs and chemicals, might be worth examining.

Exactly how the individual blends of genetic and environmental factors combine to initiate pathogenetic pathways is not known. Also poorly understood is the nature of the pathogenetic mechanism or mechanisms. Currently fashionable is the pursuit of immunological abnormalities in spondarthritic disorders, and an attractive idea is that the core of pathogenesis is in fact immunopathogenesis. The plausibility of this concept is strengthened by findings in the mouse in which Ir (Immune response) and Ia (Immune associated) genes are known to be closely related to the loci of certain H-2 antigens (H-2k and H-2d). Unfortunately it is not yet clear whether it is possible to demonstrate the human equivalents of the mouse Ir/Ia system. However, further research to examine parallels between mice and men may prove useful in adding meaning to isolated immunological abnormalities (e.g. raised IgA levels, activation of the complement system, depressed lymphocyte responses) so far revealed in ankylosing spondylitis and allied disorders.

The exciting implications raised by immunological mechanisms rest on therapeutic possibilities through immunisation, or perhaps more optimistically in controlling environmental factors which may contribute in converting the genotype into the phenotype.

PRACTICAL IMPORTANCE OF THE CONCEPT

Associations between the seronegative spondarthritides have several practical implications:

1. As seronegative spondarthritides represent distinct clinical entities, and not variants of rheumatoid arthritis, this will enable the clinician to give a more optimistic prognosis.
2. Clinical associations existing between members of the spondarthritis group, by heightening the index of clinical suspicion, will allow earlier diagnosis in the case of seronegative arthritides presenting atypically.
3. The considerably increased prevalence of sacroiliitis, and even classical ankylosing spondylitis, in patients with psoriasis, Reiter's disease, the intestinal arthropathies, and Behçet's syndrome will more readily draw attention to the possibility of inflammatory arthritis of the spine in patients who might otherwise be erroneously diagnosed as having lumbar disc disease. The therapeutic and prognostic importance of differentiating true spondylitis from disorders

of the lumbar disc cannot be overemphasised.

4. Familial associations between the spondarthritides underline the importance of taking a detailed family history in patients with seronegative arthritis. Not only may this help to clarify the diagnosis of the proband, but, in addition, treatable and possibly otherwise unnoticed disease in relatives may be brought to light.
5. The concept also has profound aetiological implications. These stem particularly from accumulating evidence to suggest an infective cause in Reiter's disease and in Whipple's disease. Moreover, it is well known that psoriasis in children may be provoked by infection, especially with streptococci. In some diseases, infection perhaps represents the necessary environmental triggering agent to precipitate arthritis in the genetically predisposed. There is some evidence to suggest that trauma may be one environmental trigger.

CONCLUSIONS: WHERE NEXT?

Despite active interest in the spondarthritides in recent years there remain many unresolved issues. This is despite detailed clinical, serological, radiological, and family studies, and, not least, energetic study of HLA patterns, well summarised in a volume devoted to the subject (Brewerton, 1977).

The problem could relate to the absence of a generally agreed basis for the study of these disorders. For instance, should the ultimate criterion — 'the index of truth' — continue to be radiological sacroiliitis, or should it be the presence of the HLA-B27 antigen? Assumption of either will pose difficulties. For example, Behçet's syndrome conforms to the spondarthritis idea on clinical grounds, but is convincingly associated with neither sacroiliitis nor HLA-B27. The newly described disorder 'pustulotic arthro-osteitis' (although not yet an established member of the spondarthritides) is associated with sacroiliitis but not with HLA-B27. Frozen shoulder was found to be associated with HLA-B27 in 42% of one group of patients (Bulgen et al, 1976), though no other spondarthritic features, including sacroiliitis, have yet been reported to substantiate this. This HLA-B27 association raises the more general question of the relationship between 'systemic enthesopathies' and 'local enthesopathies' (Lawrence, 1977; Niepel & Sit'aj, 1979). A further problem concerns the difference between disorders characterised by HLA-B27-positive sacroiliitis and sacroiliitis in disorders not possessing the antigen. In this respect, Jayson (1977) has described sacroiliac lysis in addition to acro-osteolysis in patients with vinyl chloride disease, although the sacroiliac changes were described as not resembling ankylosing spondylitis. (Studies of HLA-B27 in this disease have not yet been reported.) Osteitis condensans ilii sometimes presents a sacroiliac appearance difficult to distinguish from sacroiliitis in which sclerosis is prominent. However, the non-spondarthritic nature of this disorder is supported by negative findings for HLA-B27 (de Bosset et al, 1975). Furthermore, within the realm of better established spondarthritic entities, how should one regard sacroiliitis-positive versus sacroiliitis-negative versions of, say, psoriasis, Reiter's disease, and chronic inflammatory bowel disorders? Are these merely variants of the same disease or are they subspecies with specific generic status?

The answer to these and other nosological conundrums could derive from a more global approach along the following lines?

1. Continued recognition of the importance of characteristic clinical features — both 'primary' and 'secondary'.
2. Continued recognition of the importance of radiological sacroiliitis.
3. Continued recognition of the importance of the HLA-B27 antigen.
4. A more flexible approach to allow for the wide spectrum involved in the spondarthritic network — particularly to include the idea of 'formes frustes'.
5. A wider approach to the possible relevance of other B locus antigens, already hinted at by the association of B5 with Behçet's syndrome and various B antigens (B13, Bw17) with psoriasis and psoriatic arthritis. Extension of such studies to other diseases in the spondarthritis matrix has so far led to conflicting results, such as variable reports in enteropathic arthritis.
6. A more precise differentiation between 'rheumatoid' and 'non-rheumatoid' by means of test-

ing for D locus antigens, particularly DR4.

7. The more widespread use of centres for the special study of the spondarthritides. This would have the advantage of allowing more realistic comparisons between the findings derived from different disorders. Much of the present inconsistency of results and variations in interpretation probably arise from differences in nomenclature, criteria and methodology.
8. The use of data banks to enable a more perspective view of clinical, radiological, and immunogenetic findings.

SUMMARY

The concept of seronegative spondarthritis has been discussed and updated in the light of new evidence.

Proposed criteria for spondarthritic conditions are as follows:

1. Absence of rheumatoid factors;
2. Absence of subcutaneous 'rheumatoid' nodules;
3. Inflammatory peripheral arthritis (often asymmetrical);
4. Radiological sacroiliitis with or without ankylosing spondylitis;
5. Evidence of clinical 'overlap';
6. Tendency to familial aggregation and familial 'overlap';
7. Significant association with the HLA-B27 antigen.

The original clinical entities included in the spondarthritis network were: uncomplicated ankylosing spondylitis, psoriatic arthritis, Reiter's disease, ulcerative colitis, Crohn's disease, Whipple's disease, and Behçet's syndrome. Latterly certain forms of juvenile chronic polyarthritis, reactive arthritis, and acute anterior uveitis have

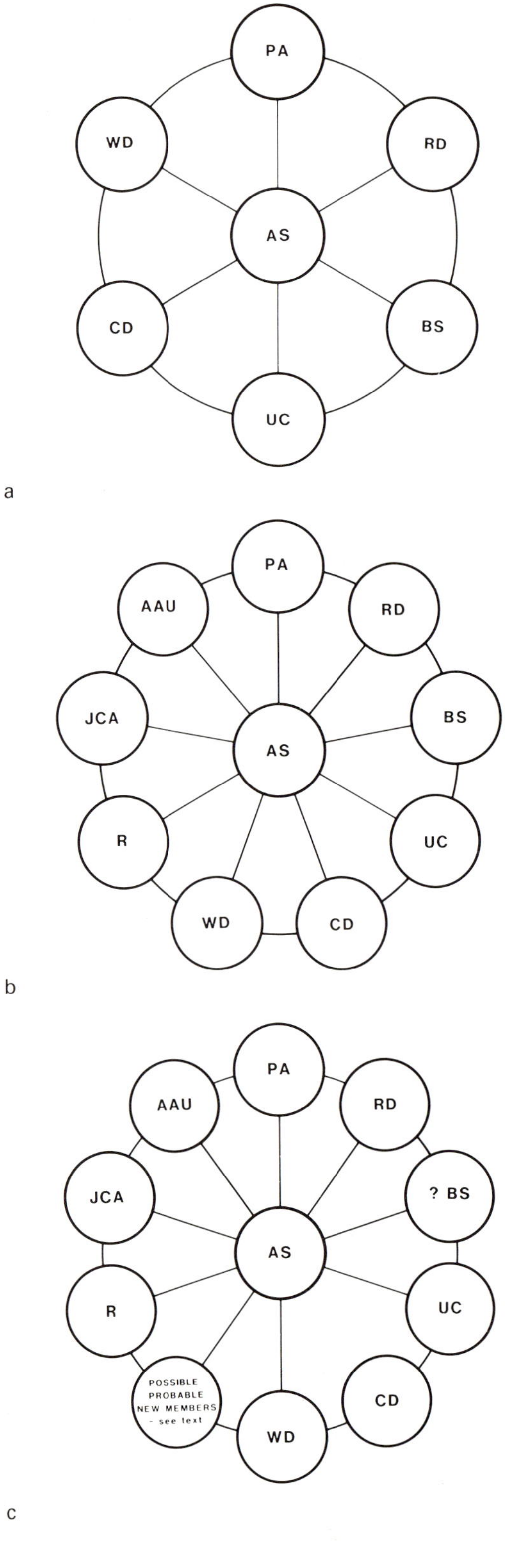

Fig. 28.2 Evolution of the spondarthritis concept (a, b, c) in terms of clinical entities fulfilling basic criteria. Key to symbols: AS = ankylosing spondylitis; PA = psoriatic arthritis; RD = Reiter's disease; BS = Behçet's syndrome; UC = ulcerative colitis; CD = Crohn's disease; WD = Whipple's disease; AAU = acute anterior uveitis; JCA = juvenile chronic arthritis; R = reactive arthritis. For further details see text.

been added to the group. The place of Behçet's syndrome, due to unconvincing confirmation of the association with sacroiliitis and HLA-B27, remains sub judice. Whether or not further entities should be included will require further evidence. Disorders falling within a spondarthritis-like category, though not yet fully established members of the group, include: undifferentiated seronegative arthritis; pustulotic arthro-osteitis; intestinal bypass arthritis–dermatitis syndrome; and erosive spondylopathy.

The place of diffuse idiopathic skeletal hyperostosis and erosive osteoarthritis remains very doubtful. Figure 28.2 summarises the evolution of the spondarthritis concept in terms of clinical entities fulfilling basic criteria. The practical importance of the spondarthritis concept, apart from its academic interest due to genetic and immunogenetic implications in clarifying rheumatological classification, lies in the realm of prognosis, differential diagnosis, and treatment.

Likely channels for elaborating the concept further are careful clinical observations, family studies, and the search for immunogenetic markers.

REFERENCES

Acheson E D 1960 An association between ulcerative colitis, regional enteritis and ankylosing spondylitis. Quarterly Journal of Medicine 29:489

Aho K, Ahvonen P, Lassus A, Sievers K & Tiilikainen, A 1973 HL-A 27 and reactive arthritis. Lancet 2: 157

Aho K, Ahvonen P, Lassus A, Sievers K, Tiilikainen A 1976 Yersinia arthritis and related diseases: clinical and immunogenetic implications. In: Dumond D C (ed) Infection and immunology in the rheumatic diseases. Blackwell, Oxford

Alarcón G S, Koopman W J, Acton R T, Barger B O 1982a Seronegative rheumatoid arthritis. A distinct immunogenetic disease? Arthritis and Rheumatism 25:502

Alarcón G S, Koopman W J, Schrohenloher R E 1982b Differential patterns of in vitro IgM rheumatoid factor synthesis in seronegative and seropositive rheumatoid arthritis. Arthritis and Rheumatism 25:150

Albert E D, Mickey M R, Terasaki, P I 1973 Genetics of the HL-A system in four populations: American Caucasians. Japanese Americans, American Negroes and Mexican Americans. In: Dausset J, Bolombani J (ed) Fifth International Histocompatibility Workshop, Histocompatibility Testing, 1972. Copenhagen, Munksgaard, p 233

Allison, A C 1975 Concluding remarks. In: Brewerton D A (ed) Symposium on histocompatibility and rheumatic disease. Annals of the Rheumatic Diseases, 34: 59

Amor B, Kahan A, Delbarre F 1976 HLA B27 in unclassified inflammatory rheumatic diseases. First International Symposium on HLA and Diseases, Paris, June 23–25

Ansell B M 1980 Juvenile spondylitis and related disorders. In: Moll J M H (ed) Ankylosing spondylitis. Churchill Livingstone, Edinburgh, Ch 11

Ansell B M, Wigley R A D 1964 Arthritic manifestations in regional enteritis. Annals of the Rheumatic Diseases, 23:64

Ansell B M, Wood P H N 1976 Prognosis in juvenile chronic arthritis. Clinics in Rheumatic Diseases 2:397

Ansell B M, Bywaters F G I, Lawrence J S 1968 Family studies in Still's disease (Juvenile RA). In: Bennett P H, Wood P H N (eds) Population studies of the rheumatic diseases. Proceedings of the 3rd International Symposium, New York, 1966. Excerpta Medica Foundation, Amsterdam, p 229

Ashurst P J C 1964 Relapsing pustular eruptions of the hands and feet. British Journal of Dermatology 76:169

Baker H, Golding D N, Thompson M 1963a Psoriasis and arthritis. Annals of Internal Medicine 58:909

Baker H, Golding D N, Thompson M 1963b Atypical polyarthritis in psoriatic families. British Medical Journal 2:348

Barker W F 1962 Familial history of patients with ulcerative colitis. American Journal of Surgery, 103:25

Barnes C G 1969 In: Mason R M, Barnes C G. Behçet's syndrome with arthritis. Annals of the Rheumatic Diseases, 28:95

Berlin C 1960 Behçet's disease as a multiple symptom-complex. Report of ten cases. Archives of Dermatology, 82:73

Billson F A, de Dombal F T, Watkinson G, Goligher J C 1967 Ocular complications of ulcerative colitis. Gut: Journal of the British Society of Gastroenterology, 8:102.

Bøe J, Dalgaard J B, Scott D 1958 Muco-cutaneous-ocular syndrome with intestinal involvement. American Journal of Medicine 25:857

Bowen G E, Kirsner J B 1965 The arthritis of ulcerative colitis and regional enteritis (intestinal arthritis). Medical Clinics of North America, 49:17

Boxley J D 1973 Reiter's disease and psoriasis. Proceedings of the Royal Society of Medicine, 66:440

Brewerton D (ed) 1977 Clinics in rheumatic diseases: Immunogenetics and rheumatic disease. Saunders, London

Brewerton D A, Caffrey M, Nicholls A, Walters D, James D C O 1973 Acute anterior uveitis and HL-A27. Lancet 2:996

Brewerton D A, Caffrey M F P, Hart F D, James D C O, Nicholls A, Sturrock R D 1973 Ankylosing spondylitis and HL-A27. Lancet 1:904

Brewerton D A, Caffrey M F P, James D C O 1974 The histocompatability antigen (HL-A 27) and its relation to disease. Journal of Rheumatology, 1:249

Brigode M, Francois R J 1977 Histocompatibility antigens in vertebral ankylosing hyperostosis. Journal of Rheumatology 4:429

Buchanan R F, Willkens R F 1972 Arthritis after jejeunoileostomy. Arthritis and Rheumatism 15:644

Bulgen D Y, Hazleman B L, Voak D 1976 HLA-B27 and frozen shoulder. Lancet 1:1042

Bywaters E G L, Ansell B M 1958 Arthritis associated with ulcerative colitis. Annals of the Rheumatic Diseases, 17:169

Bywaters E G L, Dixon A St J 1965 Paravertebral ossification in psoriatic arthritis. Annals of the Rheumatic Diseases, 24:313

Caffrey M F P, James D C O 1973 Human lymphocyte antigen association in ankylosing spondylitis. Nature, 242:121

Campbell J M, Hunt T K, Karam J H, Forsham P H 1977 Jejunoileal bypass as a treatment for mobid obesity. Archives of Internal Medicine 137:602

Caughey D E, Bywaters E G L 1963 The arthritis of Whipple's syndrome. Annals of the Rheumatic Diseases, 22:327

Cawley M I D, Chalmers T M, Kellgren J H, Ball J 1972 Destructive lesions of vertebral bodies in ankylosing spondylitis. Annals of the Rheumatic Diseases 31:345

Chamberlain M A 1977 Behçet's syndrome in 32 patients in Yorkshire. Annals of the Rheumatic Diseses 36:491

Chears W C, Ashworth C T 1961 Electron microscopic study of the intestinal mucosa in Whipple's disease. Demonstration of encapsulated bacilliform bodies in the lesion. Gastroenterology, 41:129

Copeman W S C 1969 Introductory note on the nomenclature and classification of the rheumatic diseases. In: Copeman W S C (ed) Textbook of the rheumatic diseases, 4th edn. Livingstone, Edinburgh, p 12

Coste F, Delbarre F, Cayla J, Massias P, Beasley E 1963 Spondylites destructives dan la spondylarthrite ankylosante. Presse Médical 71:1013

Courtois C, Fallet G H, Vischer T L, Wethstein P 1980 Erosive spondylopathy. Annals of the Rheumatic Diseases 39:462

Crain D C 1961 Interphalangeal osteoarthritis characterised by painful inflammatory episodes resulting in deformity of the proximal and distal articulations. Journal of the American Medical Association 175:1049

Croft C B, Wilkinson A R 1972 Ulceration of the mouth, pharynx and larynx in Crohn's disease of the intestine. British Journal of Surgery, 59:249

Daffner J E, Brown C H 1958 Regional enteritis. I: Clinical aspects and diagnosis in 100 patients. Annals of Internal Medicine, 49:580

Davidson C, Wojtulewski J A, Bacon P A, Winstock D 1975 Temporo-mandibular joint disease in ankylosing spondylitis. Annals of the Rheumatic Diseases 34:87

de Bosset P, Gordon D A, Singel D P, Smythe H A, Vrowitz M B 1975 Comparison of osteitis condensans ilii (OCI) and ankylosing spondylitis in female patients: clinical, radiological and HL-A typing characteristics. Annals of the Royal College of Physicians and Surgeons of Canada 8:78 (abstract)

Dilsen A N 1967 Sacro-iliitis and ankylosing spondylitis in Behçet's disease. In: 8th European Rheumatology Congress, Helsinki. Scandinavian Journal of Rheumatology (Suppl) 8: abstract 20

Dixon A St J 1960 Rheumatoid arthritis with negative serological reaction. Annals of the Rheumatic Diseases 19:209

Dowling G B 1961 Discussion on Behçet's disease. Proceedings of the Royal Society of Medicine, 54:101

Dryll A, Kahn M F, Solnica J, Mitrovic D, Sèze S de 1969 Les formes de passage entre Poculo-urèthro-synovite de Fiessinger-Leroy-Reiter et le rheumatisme psoriasique: à propos de 7 observations personnelles. Semaine des Hôpitaux de Paris 8:499

Dunlop E M C, Harper I A, Jones B R 1968 Sero-negative polyarthritis. The Bedsonia (chlamydia) group of agents and Reiter's disease. Annals of the Rheumatic Diseases 27:234

Edmonds J, Morris R I, Metzger A I 1974 Follow-up study of juvenile chronic polyarthritis with particular reference to histocompatibility antigen W 27. Annals of the Rheumatic Diseases 33:289

Edmonds J, Metzger A, Terasaki P, Bluestone R, Ansell B M, Bywaters E G L 1974 HL-A antigen W27 in juvenile chronic polyarthritis. Annals of the Rheumatic Diseases 33:576

Ehrlich G E 1972 Inflammatory osteoarthritis. I. The clinical syndrome. Journal of Chronic Diseases 25:317

Emery A E, Lawrence J S 1967 Genetics of ankylosing spondylitis. Journal of Medical Genetics 4:239

Epstein E 1939 Differential diagnosis of keratosis blenorrhagica and psoriatic arthropathy. Archives of Dermatology and Syphilology 40:547

Ercilla M G, Brancos M A, Breysse Y, Alonso G, Vives J, Castillo R, Rotes-Querol J 1977 HLA antigens in Forestier's disease, ankylosing spondylitis, and polyarthrosis of the hands. Journal of Rheumatology 4 (Suppl 3): 89

Esdaile J M, Stein H B, Dwosh I L, Urowitz M G, Falk J, Smythe H A, Ogryzlo M A 1976 HLA-B27 typing in seronegative arthritis. Arthritis and Rheumatism 19:795

Eyler W R, Doub H P 1956 Extra-intestinal Roentgen manifestations of intestinal lipodystrophy. Journal of the American Medical Association 160:534

Farnan P 1959 Whipple's disease. The clinical aspects. Quarterly Journal of Medicine 29:163

Fernandez-Herlihy L 1959 The articular manifestations of chronic ulcerative colitis; an analysis of 555 cases. New England Journal of Medicine 261:259

Fernandez-Herlihy L 1977 Arthritis after jejunoileostomy for intractable obesity. Journal of Rheumatology 4:135

Ford D K 1970 Reiter's syndrome. Bulletin of Rheumatic Diseases 20:588

Ford D K, Vallis D G 1959 The clinical course of arthritis associated with ulcerative colitis and regional ileitis. Arthritis and Rheumatism 2:526

Ford D K, Henderson E, Price G E, Stein H B 1977 Yersinia-related arthritis in the Pacific North West. Arthritis and Rheumatism 20:1226

Fowler J J, Humpston D J, Nussey A M, Small M 1968 Behçet's syndrome with neurological manifestations in two sisters. British Medical Journal ii:473

Fox T C, MacLeod J M H 1901 On a case of parakeratosis variegata. British Journal of Dermatology 13:319

Frus J, Svejgaard A 1974 Salmonella arthritis and HLA 27. Lancet 1:1350

Glass D, Litvin D, Wallace K, Chylack L, Garovoy M, Carpenter B B, Schur P H 1970 Early-onset pauciarticular juvenile rheumatoid arthritis associated with human leukocyte antigen-DRw5, iritis and antinuclear antibody. Journal of Clinical Investigation 66:426

Gold R H, Bassett L W, Theros E G 1982 Radiologic comparison of erosive polyarthritides with prominent interphalangeal involvement. Skeletal Radiology 8:89

Good A E 1965 Reiter's disease and ankylosing spondylitis. Acta rheumatica Scandinavica 11:305

Good A E 1971 Reiter's disease, ankylosing spondylitis and

rheumatoid arthritis occurring within a single family. Arthritis and Rheumatism 14:753
Goligher J C, de Dombal F T, Watts J McK, Watkinson G 1968 Ulcerative colitis. Baillière, Tindall & Cassel, London, p 59
Graham W, Uchida I A 1957 Heredity in ankylosing spondylitis. Annals of the Rheumatic Diseases 16:334
Greenstein A J, Janowitz J D, Sachar D B 1976 The extraintestinal complications of Crohn's disease and ulcerative colitis: a study of 700 patients. Medicine 55:401
Gross J B, Wollaeger E E, Sauer W G, Huizenga K A, Dahlin D C, Power M H 1959 Whipple's disease; a report of four cases, including two in brothers, with observations on pathologic physiology, diagnosis and treatment. Gastroenterology 36:65
Hakansson V, Eitrem M H, Low B, Winblad S 1976. HLA antigen B27 in cases with joint affections in an outbreak of salmonellosis. Scandinavian Journal of Infectious Diseases 8:245
Hall W H, Finegold S 1953 A study of 23 cases of Reiter's syndrome. Annals of Internal Medicine 38:533
Hall M A, Ansell B M, James D C O, Zylinski P 1975 HLA antigens in juvenile chronic polyarthritis (Still's disease). Annals of the Rheumatic Diseases 34:36
Hammer B, Ashurst P, Naish J 1968 Diseases associated with ulcerative colitis and Crohn's disease. Gut: Journal of the British Society of Gastroenterology 9:17
Harris J R W, Gelsthorpe K, Doughty R W, Lee D, Morton R S 1975 HL-A 27 and W 10 in Reiter's syndrome and non-specific urethritis. Acta Dermato-Venereologica (Stockholm) 55:127
Hart F D, Maclagan N F 1955 Ankylosing spondylitis: a review of 184 cases. Annals of the Rheumatic Diseases 14:77
Haslock I 1972 The arthritis associated with Crohn's disease: A family study. University of Edinburgh, MD Thesis
Haslock I, Wright V 1973 The musculo-skeletal complications of Crohn's disease. Medicine, Baltimore 53:217
Heller G, Kolodny M H, Lapow I H, Jacobson A S, Rivera M E, Marks G H 1955 The haemagglutination test for rheumatoid arthritis. Journal of Immunology 74:340
Hicklin J A 1968 Erosive vertebral disease in ankylosing spondylitis. Annals of Physical Medicine 9:206
Hill A G S 1961 In: Dixon A St J, Lience E. Sacro-iliac joint in adult rheumatoid arthritis and psoriatic arthropathy. Annals of the Rheumatic Diseases 20:247
Houghton E A W, Naish J M 1958 Familial ulcerative colitis and ileitis. Gastroenterologia (Basel) 89:65
Iveson J M, Nauda B S, Hancock J A 1975 Reiter's disease in three boys. Annals of the Rheumatic Diseases 34:364
Jacobs J C 1977 Incomplete Reiter's syndrome in young children. In: Proceedings of the XIV International Congress of Rheumatology, San Francisco, 1977. New York, Arthritis Foundation, abstract 170, p 57
Jacobs J C, Berdon W E, Johnston A D 1982 HLA-B27-associated spondyloarthritis and enthesopathy in childhood: clinical, pathologic, and radiographic observations in 58 patients. Journal of Pediatrics 100:521
Jajić I 1968 Radiological changes in the sacroiliac joints and spine of patients with psoriatic arthritis and psoriasis. Annals of the Rheumatic Diseases 27:1
Jajić I, Furst Z, Vuksic B 1982 Spondylitis erosiva: report on 9 patients. Annals of the Rheumatic Diseases 41:237
James D C 1979 Behçet's syndrome. New England Journal of Medicine 301:431
Jayson M I V 1977 Vinyl chloride diseases. Annals of the Rheumatic Diseases 36 (Suppl 2):39
Jayson M I V, Bouchier I A D 1968 Ulcerative colitis with ankylosing spondylitis. Annals of the Rheumatic Diseases 27:219
Jayson M I V, Salmon P R, Harrison W J 1970 Inflammatory bowel disease in ankylosing spondylitis. Gut 11:506
Jones R A K 1977 Reiter's disease after Salmonella typhimurium enteritis. British Medical Journal 1:1391
Kellgren J H 1964 The epidemiology of rheumatic diseases. Annals of Rheumatic Diseases 23:109
Kellgren J H, Ball J 1959 Clinical significance of rheumatoid serum factor. British Medical Journal 1:523
Kelly J J, Weisiger B B 1963 The arthritis of Whipple's disease. Arthritis and Rheumatism 6:615
Kent T H, Layton J M, Clifton J A, Schedl H P 1963 Whipple's disease: light and electron microscopic studies combined with clinical studies suggesting an infective nature. Laboratory Investigation 12:1163, reference to hyperthermia. British Journal of Venereal Diseases 22:1
Kidd K I, Peter J B 1966 Erosive osteoarthritis. Radiology 86:640
King A J 1964 Reiter's disease. In: Recent Advances in Venereology, Churchill, London, p 395
King A J, Mason R M 1969 Reiter's disease. In: Copeman W S C (ed) Textbook of the rheumatic diseases, 4th Edn. Livingstone, Edinburgh, p 336
King A J, Williams D I, Nichol C S, London J 1946 The treatment of infective arthritis with special reference to hyperthermia. British Journal of Venereal Diseases 22:1
Kirsner J B, Spencer J A 1963 Familial occurrences of ulcerative colitis, regional enteritis and ileocolitis. Annals of Internal Medicine 59:133
Kumagaya H, Tomishige M, Kagawa M, Yamada T, Okuda T, Naruto Y, Matsuo K, Kuwabara K 1973 Two brothers with pustulosis palmaris et plantaris associated with lesions of the bilateral clavicles. Orthopaedic Surgery and Traumatology 22:522 (abstract)
Kurtz S M, Davis T D, Ruffin J M 1962 Light and electron microscopic studies of Whipple's disease. Laboratory Investigation 11:653
Kyle J 1971 An epidemiological study of Crohn's disease in northeast Scotland. Gastroenterology 61:826
Ladd J R, Cassidy J T, Martel W 1971 Juvenile ankylosing spondylitis. Arthritis and Rheumatism 14:579
Laitinen O, Leiresalo M, Skylv G 1977 Relationship between HLA-B27 and clinical features in patients with Yersinia arthritis. Arthritis and Rheumatism 20:1121
Lambert J R, Wright V 1976 Eye inflammation in psoriatic arthritis. Annals of the Rheumatic Diseases 35:354
Lambert J R, Ansell B M, Stephenson E, Wright V 1976 Psoriatic arthritis in childhood. Clinics in Rheumatic Diseases 2:339
Lawrence J S 1965 A family study of Reiter's disease. Paper read to the Medical Society for the prevention of Venereal Disease
Lawrence J S 1967 In: Thompson M, Holt G. Microcirculatory studies of the skin in the investigation of seronegative polyarthritis. 6th European Congress of Rheumatology, Lisbon, p 29
Lawrence J S 1977 Rheumatism in populations. Heinemann, London, p 282

Leading Article 1956 Haemagglutination tests for rheumatoid arthritis. British Medical Journal 1:1157
Leczinsky C G 1948 The incidence of arthropathy in a ten-year series of psoriasis cases. Acta Dermato-Venereologica (Stockholm) 28:483
Leirisalo M, Skylv G, Kousa M, Voipio-Pulkki L-M, Suoranta H, Nissilä M et al 1982 Followup study on patients with Reiter's disease and reactive arthritis, with special reference to HLA-B27. Arthritis and Rheumatism 25:249
Lindsley C B 1977 Arthritis in inflammatory bowel disease in children. Arthritis and Rheumatism 20 (Suppl 2):411
Little H, Urowitz M B, Smythe H A, Rosen P H 1974 A symptomatic spondylodiscitis. An unusual feature of ankylosing spondylitis. Arthritis and Rheumatism 17:483
Lomholt G 1963 Psoriasis: Prevalence, spontaneous course and genetics. A census study on the prevalence of skin diseases on the Faroe Islands. Gad, Copenhagen, p 157
McBride J A, King M J, Baikie A G, Crean G P, Sircus W 1963 Ankylosing spondylitis and chronic diseases of the intestines. British Medical Journal 2:483
McClusky O E, Lordon R E, Arnett F C 1974 HL-A 27 in Reiter's syndrome and psoriatic arthritis: a genetic factor in disease susceptibility and expression. Journal of Rheumatology 1:263
McConnell R B 1966 The genetics of gastrointestinal disorders. Oxford University Press, London, p 135
McEwen C, Ziff M, Carmel P, Ditata D, Tanner M 1958 The relationship to rheumatoid arthritis of the so-called variants. Arthritis and Rheumatism 1:481
MacRae I, Wright V 1973 A family study of ulcerative colitis with particular reference to ankylosing spondylitis and sacroiliitis. Annals of Rheumatic Diseases 32:16
Maizel H, Ruffin J M, Dobbins W O 1970 Whipple's disease: a review of 19 patients from one hospital and a review of the literature since 1950. Medicine (Baltimore) 49:175
Martel W, Stuck K J, Dworin A M, Hylland R G 1980 Erosive osteoarthritis and psoriatic arthritis: a radiological comparison in the hand, wrist, and foot. American Journal of Radiology 134:125
Mason R M, Barnes C G 1969 Behçet's syndrome with arthritis. Annals of the Rheumatic Diseases 28:95
Maxwell J D, Greig W R, Boyle J A, Pasielzny T, Schofield C B S 1966 Reiter's syndrome and psoriasis. Scottish Medical Journal 11:14
Metzger A L, Morris R I, Bluestone R 1974 Biological significance of HL-A W 27 in rheumatic diseases (Editorial). Journal of Rheumatism 1:247
Metzger A L, Morris R I, Bluestone R, Terasaki P I 1975 HL-A W 27 in psoriatic arthropathy. Arthritis and Rheumatism 18:111
Mir-Madjlessi S H, Mackenzie A H, Wiukelman E I 1974 Articular complications in obesity patients after jejunocolic bypass. Cleveland Clinics Quarterly 41:119
Moll J M H 1971 A family study of psoriatic arthritis. University of Oxford, DM Thesis
Moll J M H 1982 Seronegative arthropathies. Journal of the Royal Society of Medicine 76:445
Moll J M H, Wright V 1973 Familial occurrence of psoriatic arthritis. Annals of the Rheumatic Diseases 32:181
Moll J M H, Haslock I, Macrae L, Wright V 1974 Associations between ankylosing spondylitis, psoriatic arthritis, Reiter's disease, the intestinal arthropathies, and Behçet's syndrome. Medicine, Baltimore 53:343
Morris R I, Metzger A I, Bluestone R T, Terasaki P I 1974 A useful discriminator in the arthropathies of inflammatory bowel disease. New England Journal of Medicine 290:1117
Mowat A G, Nicol C S 1968 Reiter's disease in two brothers. British Journal of Venereal Diseases 44:334
Niepel G A, Sit'aj S 1979 Enthesopathy. In: Dixon A St J (ed) Clinics in rheumatic diseases: Soft tissue rheumatism. Saunders, London, Ch 9
Nikbin B, Brewerton D A, Byrom N, James D C O, Malka S, McLeod L et al 1975 Lymphocyte function in ankylosing spondylitis. In: Brewerton D A (ed) Symposium on histocompatability and rheumatic disease. Annals of the Rheumatic Diseases 34 (Suppl 1):49
Noer H R 1966 An 'experimental' epidemic of Reiter's syndrome. Journal of the American Medical Association 198:693
Oates J K, Young A C 1959 Sacro-iliitis in Reiter's disease. British Medical Journal 1:1013
Ohno S, Makayama E, Sugiura S, Itakura K, Aoki K, Aizawa M 1975 Specific histocompatibility antigens associated with Behçet's disease. American Journal of Ophthalmology 80:636
Oshima Y, Shimizu T, Yokohari R, Matsumoto T, Kano K, Kagami T, Nagaya H 1963 Clinical studies on Behçet's syndrome. Annals of the Rheumatic Diseases 22:36
Paronen I 1948 Reiter's disease. A study of 344 cases observed in Finland. Acta Medica Scandinavica 131 (Suppl 212):1
Patter W N, Van Bargen J A, Dockerty M B, Feldman W H, Mayo C W, Waugh J M 1954 Regional enteritis. Gastroenterology 26:347
Payne J H, De Wind L T, Commons R R 1963 Metabolic observations in patients with jejunocolic shunts. American Journal of Surgery 106:272
Perkins E S 1961 Ophthalmological aspects of Behçet's disease. Proceedings of the Royal Society of Medicine 54:106
Peter J B, Pearson C M, Marmar L 1966 Erosive osteoarthritis of the hands. Arthritis and Rheumatism 9:365
Puite R H, Tesluk H 1955 Whipple's disease. American Journal of Medicine 19:383
Reed W B 1961 Psoriatic arthritis. A complete clinical study of 86 patients. Acta Dermato-Venereologica (Stockholm) 41:396
Reed W B, Wright V 1966 Psoriatic arthritis. In: Hill A G S (ed) Modern trends in rheumatology. Butterworth, London, Ch 26, p 375
Reed W B, Heiskell C L, Becker S W 1961 Negative latex fixation test in psoriatic arthritis. Archives of Dermatology 86:653
Resnick D, Shapiro R F, Wiesner K B, Niwayama G, Utsinger P D, Shaul S R 1978 Diffuse idiopathic skeletal hyperostosis (DISH) [ankylosing hyperostosis of Forestier and Rotes-Querol]. Seminars in Arthritis and Rheumatism 7:153
Riecker H H, Neel J V, Test A 1950 The inheritance of spondylitis rhizomélique (ankylosing spondylitis) in the K. family. Annals of Internal Medicine 33:1254
Robinson H M, McCrumb F R 1950 Comparative analysis of the mucocutaneous-ocular syndrome. Archives of Dermatology and Syphilology 61:539
Robinson W D 1963 Diseases of the Joints. In: Beeson P B, McDermott W (eds) Textbook of medicine, 11th Edn. Saunders, London, p 1485

Rose E, Espinoza I R, Osterland C K 1977 Intestinal bypass arthritis: association with circulating immune complexes and HLA B27. Journal of Rheumatology 4:129
Rosenbaum J T, Cousins S W 1982 Uveitis and arthritis: experimental models and clinical correlates. Seminars in Arthritis and Rheumatism 11:383
Rosenberg A M, Petty R E 1982 A syndrome of seronegative enthesopathy and arthropathy in children. Arthritis and Rheumatism 25:1041
Rosenthal M, Batious I, Muller W 1977 Increased frequency of HLA B8 in hyperostotic spondylosis. Journal of Rheumatology 4 (Suppl 3):94
Russell A S 1977 Reiter's syndrome in children following infection with Yersinia enterocolitica and shigella. Arthritis and Rheumatism 20 (Suppl):471
Saari R, Lahti R, Saari K M, Kangasniemi R, Starck J, Seppänin S, Laitinen O 1982 Frequency of rheumatic diseases in patients with acute anterior uveitis. Scandinavian Journal of Rheumatology 11:121
Schaller J 1976 The arthritis of inflammatory bowel disease in children. Archives of Rheumatic Diseases 2:353
Schaller J G 1977 Ankylosing spondylitis of childhood onset. Arthritis and Rheumatism 20 (Suppl 2):398
Schaller J G, Johnson G D, Holborrow E J, Ansell B M, Smiley W R 1974 The association of antinuclear antibodies with the chronic iridocyclitis of juvenile rheumatoid arthritis (Still's disease). Arthritis and Rheumatism 17:409
Schilling F 1976 Yersinia-arthritis. Deutsche Medizinische Wochenschrift 101:1515
Schittenhelm A, Schlecht A 1918 Uber Polyarthritis enterica. Deutsche Archiv Klinische Medizin 126:329
Schlosstein L, Terasaki P I, Bluestone R T, Pearson C M 1973 High association of an HL-A antigen, W 27, with ankylosing spondylitis New England Journal of Medicine 288:704
Scott P W, Hosie R T 1957 Whipple's disease. Archives of Internal Medicine 100:280
Sezer N 1956 Further investigations on the virus of Behçet's disease. American Journal of Ophthalmology 41:41
Shagrin J W, Frame B, Duncan H 1971 Polyarthritis in obese patients with intestinal bypass. Annals of Internal Medicine 75:377
Sharp J, Easson E C 1954 Deep X-ray therapy in spondylitis. British Medical Journal 1:619
Sharp J 1957 The differential diagnosis of ankylosing spondylitis. British Medical Journal 1:975
Sharp J 1965 Ankylosing spondylitis, a review. In: Dixon A St J (ed) Progress in clinical rheumatology. Churchill, London, p 180
Sherlock P, Bell B M, Steinberg H, Almy T P 1963 Familial occurrence of regional enteritis and ulcerative colitis. Gastroenterology 45:413
Shore A, Ansell B M 1982 Juvenile psoriatic arthritis — an analysis of 60 cases. Journal of Pediatrics 100:529
Singson B, Bernstein B H, Koster-King K, Glovsky M M, Hanson V 1977 Reiter's syndrome in childhood. Arthritis and Rheumatism 20 (Suppl 2):402
Sloan W P, Bargen J A, Gage R P 1950 Life histories of patients with chronic ulcerative colitis: a review of 2,000 cases. Gastroenterology 16:25
Smiley W K 1974 The eye in juvenile rheumatoid arthritis. Transactions of the Ophthalmalogical Societies of the United Kingdom 94:817
Sonozaki H, Kawashima M, Hongi O, Yaoita H, Ikeno M, Matsuura M et al 1981a Incidence of arthro-osteitis in patients with pustulosis palmaris et plantaris. Annals of the Rheumatic Diseases 40:554
Sonozaki H, Mitsui H, Miyanaga Y, Okitsu K, Igarashi M, Hayashi Y, Matsuura M, Azuma A, Okai K, Kawashima M (1981b) Clinical features of 53 cases with pustulotic arthro-osteitis. Annals of the Rheumatic Diseases 40:547
Spriggs E I 1934 Chronic ulceration of the colon. Quarterly Journal of Medicine 3:549
Stecher R M 1957 Heredity in joint diseases. Documenta Rheumatologica (Geigy, No. 12)
Stein H B, Otto L A, Schlappner A, Boyko W, Gourlay R H, Reeve C E 1981 The intestinal bypass arthritis-dermatitis syndrome. Arthritis and Rheumatism 24:684
Steinberg A G, Becher S W, Fitzpatrick T B, Kierland R R 1951 A genetic and statistical study of psoriasis. American Journal of Human Genetics 3:267
Stewart S S, Ansell B M 1951 Ankylosing spondylitis associated with regional enteritis. Gastroenterology 45:265
Strachan R W, Wigzell F W 1963 Polyarthritis in Behçet's multiple symptom complex. Annals of the Rheumatic Diseases 22:26
Swezey R L, Alexander S J 1971 Erosive osteoarthritis and the main en lorgnette deformity. Archives of Internal Medicine 128:269
Swezey R L, Zucker L M, Terasaki P I 1973 Reduced prevalence of HL-A antigen W 27 in black females with ankylosing spondylitis. Journal of Rheumatology, 1, No. 3, 260
Theiss von B, Schnyder U W, Böni A, Wagenhäuser F 1969a Intrafamiliäre Untersuchungen bei Psoriasis-Arthritis. Zeitschrift für Rheumaforschung 28:403
Warren C P W 1970 Arthritis associated with Salmonella infections. Annals of the Rheumatic Diseases 29:483
Watson W, Cann H M, Farber E M, Nall M L 1971 Genetics of psoriasis: family study. In: Farber E M, Cox A J (eds) Psoriasis: Proceedings of the international symposium. Stanford University Press, Stanford, p 16
Wilske K R, Decker J L 1965 The articular manifestations of intestinal disease. Bulletin of Rheumatic Diseases 15:362
Woodrow J C 1980 Genetics. In: Moll J M H (ed) Ankylosing spondylitis. Churchill Livingstone, Edinburgh, Ch 3
Wright V 1956 Psoriasis and arthritis. Annals of the Rheumatic Diseases 15:348
Wright V 1961 Psoriatic arthritis: a comparative study of rheumatoid arthritis and arthritis associated with psoriasis. Annals of the Rheumatic Diseases 20:123
Wright V 1966 Personal communication cited by Ansell B M, Rheumatism in childhood. In: Hill A G S (ed) Modern trends in rheumatology. Butterworth, London, p 27
Wright V 1980 Relationships between ankylosing spondylitis and other spondarthritides. In: Moll J M H (ed) Ankylosing spondylitis, Churchill Livingstone, Edinburgh, p 42
Wright V, Moll J M H 1976 Seronegative polyarthritis. North-Holland, Amsterdam
Wright V, Reed W B 1964 The link between Reiter's syndrome and psoriatic arthritis Annals of the Rheumatic Diseases 23:12
Wright V, Watkinson G 1965 Sacro-iliitis and ulcerative colitis. British Medical Journal 2:675
Wright V, Watkinson G 1966 Articular complications of ulcerative colitis. American Journal of Proctology 17:107
Wright R, Lumsden K, Luntz M H, Sevel D, Truelove S C

1965 Abnormalities of the sacro-iliac joints and uveitis in ulcerative colitis. Quarterly Journal of Medicine (New Series) 34:229
Yardley J H, Hendrix T R Combined electron and light microscopy in Whipple's disease demonstration of 'bacillary bodies' in the intestine. Bulletin of the Johns Hopkins Hospital 109:80
Yazici H, Tuzlaci M, Yurdakul S 1981 A controlled survey of sacroiliitis in Behçet's disease. Annals of the Rheumatic Diseases 40:558
Ziff M 1957 The agglutination reaction in rheumatoid arthritis. Journal of Chronic Diseases 5:644

29

J.M.H. Moll

Ankylosing spondylitis

NOMENCLATURE

'Ankylosing* spondylitis' is now the universally accepted term for this disease, although 'rheumatoid spondylitis' enjoyed some popularity in the mid-1950s, particularly in the United States.

It is now acknowledged that ankylosing spondylitis is not rheumatoid arthritis of the spine. Among many differentiating features is the fact that the sacroiliac joints are rarely involved in rheumatoid arthritis and also that the cervical region is the only part of the spine commonly affected in that disease.

Other terms for ankylosing spondylitis include 'bamboo spine', 'Bechterew's disease', 'Marie–Strümpell' disease, 'pelvospondylitis ossificans', 'rheumatismal ossifying pelvispondylitis', 'poker back', 'spondilarthritis ankylopoietica', 'atrophic spondylitis', 'atrophic ligamentous spondylitis', 'ossifying ligamentous spondylitis', 'spondylitis deformans' and 'rhizomelic spondylosis'.

DEFINITION AND DIAGNOSTIC CRITERIA

Ankylosing spondylitis is an inflammatory arthritis of the spine always involving the sacroiliac joints and less commonly the peripheral joints. It affects predominantly young men in the third decade. It is often self-limiting and the aetiology is unknown (Mason, 1969).

* *Ankylosis* (also spelt *anchylosis*) is derived from the Greek *ankylos* (αγκνλος) meaning 'stiffening of a joint'. The Oxford dictionary definition of *ankylosing* is 'the formation of a stiff joint by consolidation of the articulating surfaces; the coalescence of two bones originally distinct'. *Spondylitis* (*G. spondilos* (σπόνδυλος), vertebra) implies inflammation of one or more vertebrae.

In order to assist the diagnosis of other than well established examples of the disease, diagnostic criteria for ankylosing spondylitis have been laid down at conferences in Rome and New York. These are shown in Tables 29.1 and 29.2. The number of clinical criteria and associated radiological changes necessary for a diagnosis of ankylosing spondylitis are shown at the bottom of each table. Both sets of criteria require limitation of spinal mobility and limitation of chest expansion. A recent evaluation of the New York criteria for ankylosing spondylitis has shown these to be un-

Table 29.1 Rome clinical criteria for ankylosing spondylitis (Kellgren et al 1963)

1. Low back pain and stiffness for more than 3 months
2. Pain and stiffness in the thoracic region
3. Limited motion in the lumbar spine
4. Limited chest expansion
5. History or evidence of iritis or its sequelae.

Ankylosing spondylitis present if bilateral sacroiliitis associated with any *one* of the above clinical criteria.

Table 29.2 New York clinical criteria for ankylosing spondylitis (Bennett & Wood, 1968)

1. Limitation of motion of the lumbar spine in all three planes (anterior flexion, lateral flexion and extension)
2. A history of pain or the presence of pain at the dorsolumbar junction or in the lumbar spine
3. Limitation of chest expansion to 1 inch (2.5 cm) or less, measured at the level of the fourth intercostal space.

Definite ankylosing spondylitis present if:

1. Grade 3–4 bilateral sacroiliitis associated with at least one clinical criterion
2. Grade 3–4 unilateral or grade 2 bilateral sacroiliitis associated with clinical criterion 1 or with both clinical criteria 2 and 3

Probable ankylosing spondylitis present if:
Grade 3–4 bilateral sacroiliitis exists without any clinical criteria.

satisfactory in that back pain is too sensitive and too non-specific, whereas limitation of spinal movement and limitation of chest expansion are too specific and too insensitive (Moll & Wright, 1973a).

The value of these criteria would probably be considerably improved by weighting each clinical measurement as has been done in thyrotoxicosis (Crooks et al, 1959).

Another approach has involved the formulation of criteria from questionnaire data (Schurman et al, 1977). These workers have pointed out that in early ankylosing spondylitis the disease may be difficult to distinguish from non-specific back pain as laboratory aids are few and radiological changes uncertain. On a questionnaire basis good separation was achieved on clinical history alone. Ankylosing spondylitis differed from non-specific back pain in the following ways: age of onset under 40 years; insidious onset; duration of at least 3 months; morning stiffness; improvement with exercise.

As the author has pointed out elsewhere (Moll, 1980) perhaps future application of statistical methods developed in other fields of medicine (e.g. conditional probability, likelihood ratio, numerical taxonomy, multivariate analysis), combined with clinical material collected in data banks, will lead to further refinements in diagnostic criteria for ankylosing spondylitis.

HISTORY

There is evidence from Egyptian and Nubian skeletons that ankylosing spondylitis existed thousands of years before Christ. Hippocrates mentioned a painful spinal disease that extended to the ossacrum. Caelius Aurelianus in the fifth century referred to a patient who 'was afflicted with pain in the nates, moved slowly, and could only bend or stand erect with difficulty' (Mettler, 1947). Thomas Sydenham described what he termed 'rheumatic lumbago', and it is likely from his description that the disease was ankylosing spondylitis (O'Connell, 1956). The first pathological account of the disease was given by Bernard Connor (1691). Benjamin Brodie in 1818 was the first to note iritis as a feature of spondylitis, and it is probable that he was also the first to correlate the pathological appearance of the disease with the clinical picture (cited by Copeman, 1964).

However, little further prominence was given to the disease until later in the nineteenth century when Vladimir Bechterev (alternatively spelt 'Bechterew', 'Bechtereff' and 'Bekhterew') (1893), Adolf Strümpel (1897) and Pierre Marie (1898) carefully reported several cases. Of these physicians, there is little doubt that Marie deserves most of all to be linked eponymously with the disease. His paper entitled *La Spondylose Rhizomélique* contains a remarkably accurate description of ankylosing spondylitis, including such characteristic features as the typical gait, the flattened lumbar spine, the forward craning of the neck, the flexing of the hips and knees, and the Z-shaped posture. From post-mortem examinations he was aware of the fusion of the spine, chest and hips, and commented on the difficulty in breathing and walking that must have resulted from such extensive joint ankylosis.

PREVALENCE

The prevalence of ankylosing spondylitis varies according to the sex and age structure of the population studied. Boland & Shebesta (1946) found spondylitis in 18% of 6000 admissions to a United States Army Rheumatism Centre, and Savage (1942) found the disease in 5% of 270 service patients with rheumatic symptoms. Kellgren (1964), reviewing epidemiological literature up to 1963, quotes a mean prevalence of 0.1%. This figure corresponds closely with a recent estimate by de Blécourt (1972) who has found ankylosing spondylitis in 0.08% of a Dutch population.

A higher prevalence of ankylosing spondylitis and sacroiliitis has been found in Haida Indians (Gofton et al, 1966), and the same workers have found a lower than normal prevalence in Blackfeet Indians. Spondylitis is also less common in Negroes than in Caucasians (Baum & Ziff, 1971).

It is generally accepted that there is a male : female preponderance of the disease, but the sex ratio varies between surveys from 9 : 1 to 4 : 1 (Polley & Slocumb, 1947; West, 1949; Sharp & Easson, 1954; Wilkinson & Bywaters, 1958).

A disease very much like human ankylosing spondylitis has been described in prehistoric crocodiles, in monkeys (Zorab, 1961), in horses (Stecher & Goss, 1961), and in experimental rats (Francis et al, 1972).

CLINICAL FEATURES

Symptoms

The age of onset is most commonly in the 15–24 decade. 10% develop their first symptom before puberty (Hart, 1954; Mason et al, 1958).

The insidious onset of ankylosing spondylitis, which is observed in approximately 80% of patients, often delays diagnosis. In one study (Cheshire & Nichols, 1955) the average interval between onset of symptoms and diagnosis was one year seven months, and in another series (Hart et al, 1949) the delay in diagnosis was even longer (almost three years). The commonest first symptom, as well as the commonest presenting symptom, in ankylosing spondylitis is low backache (Cheshire & Nichols, 1955).

The initial aching and stiffness of the back are most prominent in the morning on rising, and are aggravated by physical inactivity and climatic changes. The back symptoms are often improved by mild exercise and by local heat. At first, pain and stiffness are episodic, each bout lasting for only a few days. Less often the first symptoms are even more short-lived and consist of fleeting sharp pains in the buttocks, hips and low back. These may be triggered by twisting, jolting, coughing or sneezing, but often occur spontaneously.

As the disease progresses the pain becomes more constant. Pain and stiffness often prompt the spondylitic to get up early in order to relieve the discomfort by moving around. In many patients spinal stiffness is more prominent than pain, but in many subjects there is difficulty in differentiating between these two symptoms.

In about 10% of patients the first symptom is sciatic pain, which must be differentiated from the sciatica associated with prolapse of a lumbar disc. In spondylitis there are no paraesthesiae or other indications of nerve root involvement, and furthermore the sciatica is usually relieved by activity and made worse by sitting for long periods. However, diagnostic difficulty may still arise from other points of similarity, particularly the aggravation of the sciatica in both disorders by coughing and sneezing.

Occasionally, chest pain can be the presenting feature in ankylosing spondylitis, and attention has been drawn to its importance in the differential diagnosis of heart pain (Good, 1963).

In about 15% of patients the first symptom is in one or more peripheral joints, usually the knee or ankle (Sharp, 1965). This presentation is particularly common in juvenile ankylosing spondylitis (Ladd et al, 1971).

In some patients, pain at sites of tendinous insertion may be a troublesome feature — particularly in the heel, the pelvic brim, and the ischial tuberosity. Other less usual modes of presentation include recurrent iritis (Birkbeck et al, 1951), fever of unknown origin and acute lumbago. Occasionally, patients may advance to the stage of severe spinal deformity without any spinal symptoms, the presenting feature in these patients usually being marked postural abnormality.

Physical signs

Before the 'formal examination' much can be gleaned by simply watching the patient walking into the clinic, sitting down, standing up, turning, undressing, and getting on and off the couch. The characteristic stiffness involved in these movements constitutes a most valuable sign in its own right.

Chest and spinal rigidity

Physical signs may be minimal or absent in early ankylosing spondylitis. However, sooner or later, the normal lumbar lordosis is effaced and movement of the lumbar spine becomes limited. At first the spinal stiffness is probably due to paravertebral muscle spasm associated with inflammatory arthritis of the apophyseal joints. Later, however, fibrous and eventually bony ankylosis supervene to produce the typical rigidity of the 'poker' back. Even without objective measurement of the limitation of spinal movement, it is usually easy to recognise the absence of the normal arching of the lumbar spine and also the absence of skin stretching over the lumbar spinal spaces as the patient attempts to bend forward. In established spondylitis the spine moves characteristically in one piece as a flat immobile segment. A useful method to assess semi-objectively movement of the lumbar spine is to place the thumb and middle finger on the lumbar spine and observe the degree of separation of the digits. Although this estimation will be affected by age and sex, a separation between finger and thumb of more than 3–4 cm is probably normal. Using the same principle, a more sophisticated tapemeasure method to record the distraction of skin marks on the lumbar spine has been described by Schober (1937), and has been further refined by Macrae & Wright (1969). A range of normal values for anterior flexion has been reported (Moll & Wright, 1971), and these data have emphasised the importance of correcting spinal mobility for the effects of age, sex, and wide scatter of normal values. There is also a wide scatter of spondylitic values for anterior flexion, and considerable overlap exists between the spondylitic range and the normal range (Fig. 29.1). This applies not only to other planes of spinal mobility but also to chest expansion (Moll & Wright, 1973). The traditional 'fingertips-to-floor' method for measuring anterior spinal flexion is no longer recommended. The unreliability of this technique stems from the fact that if the patient has a good range of hip movement he can often touch the floor with ease despite severe spinal rigidity.

In patients with suspected ankylosing spondylitis, measurement of lateral spinal flexion and extension should also be made, preferably using objective clinical methods (Loebl, 1967; Moll et al, 1972a, b). The value of measuring several directions of spinal movement is particularly important in differentiating between ankylosing spondylitis and prolapse of a lumbar disc. In the former, spinal mobility is usually limited both anteriorly and laterally, whereas in disc prolapse lateral flexion is often normal.

In advanced ankylosing spondylitis 'le signe de la corde de l'arc' is sometimes observed on lateral flexion. In normal individuals, the paravertebral muscles relax on the concave side during lateral flexion and those on the side of spinal convexity contract. In ankylosing spondylitis this pattern is reversed, the muscles on the concave side being tightly stretched like the taut string of a bow (Durrigl et al, 1965). Another feature associated with diminished lateral flexion is raising of the heel on the contralateral side as the patient forces himself to gain maximal lateral movement.

Chest expansion is diminished relatively early in ankylosing spondylitis. It is important to allow for the normal decrease in expansion with age, and

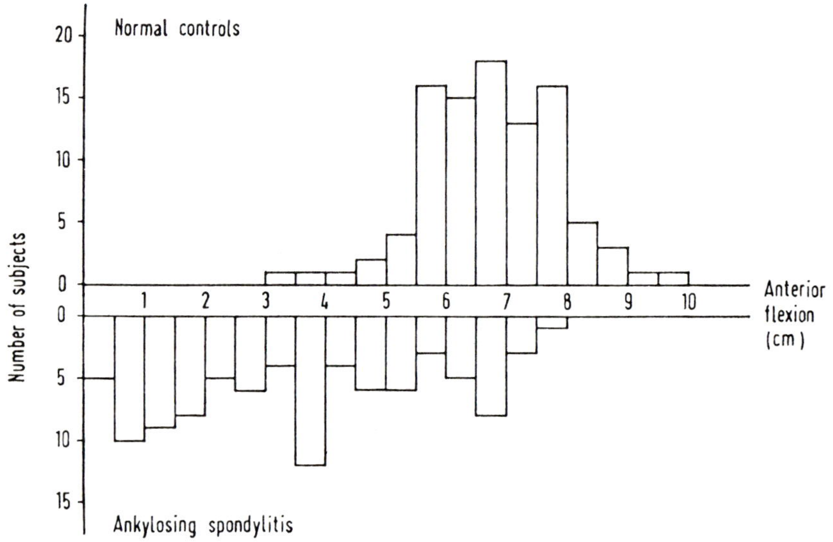

Fig. 29.1 Overlap between measurements of anterior spinal flexion in normal controls and patients with ankylosing spondylitis. (Moll & Wright, 1973; by courtesy of the Editor of *Rheumatology and Rehabilitation*.)

also the fact that male expansion exceeds that of females (Moll & Wright, 1972). Another relatively common but often unrecognised feature of spondylitic chest expansion is the jerky inspiratory phase compared with the smooth uninterrupted inspiratory movement in normal individuals. In view of this it is important when measuring chest expansion in spondylitics to allow plenty of time for the patient to reach his inspiratory maximum. Another source of diagnostic error arises from the often considerable reduction of chest mobility associated with chronic pulmonary disease and obesity. A useful adjunct for assessing the significance of chest immobility in a patient with suspected spondylitis is to measure the degree of diaphragm movement. In ankylosing spondylitis, even when complete chest rigidity is present, reasonable diaphragm mobility is retained (or even increased), in contrast to the pattern observed in chronic chest disease in which both chest and diaphragm movements are minimal.

A spondylitic index:

$$\frac{\text{chest expansion}}{\text{diaphragm excursion} + \text{abdominal 'ballooning'}}$$

has been reported (Moll, 1975). This makes use of the decrease in chest expansion and increase in diaphragm and abdominal movement in ankylosing spondylitis. It was found that 92% of spondylitics had an index less than 0.7 (the best dividing line between patients and controls), contrasted with controls in whom 80% had an index greater than 0.7.

Newton (1957) has emphasised the importance of pain on stressing the sacroiliac joints as an early sign of sacroiliitis. This may be carried out in various ways:

1. By placing the hands on the anterior superior iliac spine and applying pressure to force the pelvis backwards
2. Compressing the iliac bones towards each other
3. Pressing firmly downwards on the sacrum with the patient lying prone.

Another method to elicit sacroiliac pain is to fix one shoulder with the patient lying supine and flex the ipsilateral thigh (Latham, 1965). A similar method (Gaenslen's sign) is to hyperextend one hip while fully flexing the other (Romanus & Ydén, 1955). However, a recent study (Russell et al, 1981) has shown, contrary to common belief, that tests to stress the sacroiliac joints are of no value in distinguishing between ankylosing spondylitis and other causes of chronic low back pain.

Extra-articular bony tenderness

Tenderness over bony points constitutes another important physical finding in ankylosing spondylitis. Typical sites for such tenderness include the symphysis pubis, greater trochanter, iliac crest, ischial tuberosities, spinous processes, and heels. Tenderness may also be elicited over the manubrium sterni, and also on deep palpation over the costal cartilages.

Peripheral joint involvement

Peripheral arthritis occurs at some point during the course of ankylosing spondylitis in at least a half of patients (Polley, 1955; Sharp, 1957), and may in fact be the presenting feature in 15% (Sharp, 1965). The changes are often transient and relatively mild, and usually develop during the first 10 years of the disease (Wilkinson & Bywaters, 1958). In about a quarter of spondylitics with peripheral joint involvement, the arthritis becomes chronic. In patients with peripheral arthritis it is the proximal or root joints (hips and shoulders) which are most commonly affected. The most frequent root joint to be involved is the hip; in three-quarters of patients with hip arthritis this is bilateral. It is the tendency to develop arthritis of root joints which has given rise to the name 'spondylitis rhizomélique'. Joints other than root joints that are often affected include the knees, ankles, elbows and wrists. The small joints of the hands and feet may also be involved, but less commonly (Simpson & Stephenson 1949; Wilkinson & Bywaters, 1958; Adler & Carmon, 1961). Sternoclavicular joint involvement has been reported (Reuler et al, 1978), as has involvement of cricoarytenoid joints (Bienenstock & Lanyi, 1977). Peripheral joint involvement, excluding involvement of root joints, is often asymmetrical (Rosen & Graham, 1962).

From the practical standpoint, it is involvement

of the hips that is particularly important. In fact, hip disease in some patients may be far more incapacitating than spinal rigidity, and often makes continuing at work impossible (Hart et al, 1949). Not only does limitation of hip movement interfere with walking but, ultimately, because of flexion contractures of the hips, posture is also affected. Flexion contracture at the hip results in flexion at the knees to maintain an 'erect' posture, thus resulting in the typical Z-shaped posture first described by Marie (1898).

Posture

The characteristic posture of ankylosing spondylitis occurs earlier than has been previously realised. The posture is sometimes known as the 'Bechterew stoop' or the 'hang-dog appearance'. The essential features of the spondylitic posture are: forward craning of the neck, high dorsal kyphosis, rounding of the shoulders, obliteration of the normal lumbar lordosis, wasting of the buttocks, flattening of the chest and 'ballooning' of the abdomen. The stance is characteristically wide-based (Fig. 29.2). Inguinal herniae occur more commonly in spondylitic patients (Blumberg & Ragen, 1956), and this may stem from increased intra-abdominal pressure resulting from increased movements of the diaphragm. In the most advanced stage of the disease, the spinal deformity may resemble a question mark. The field of vision in these unfortunate patients is often restricted to an area just in front of the feet, and prismatic spectacles may be required in order to permit forward vision. One of the principal aims of modern treatment is to prevent this incapacitating development.

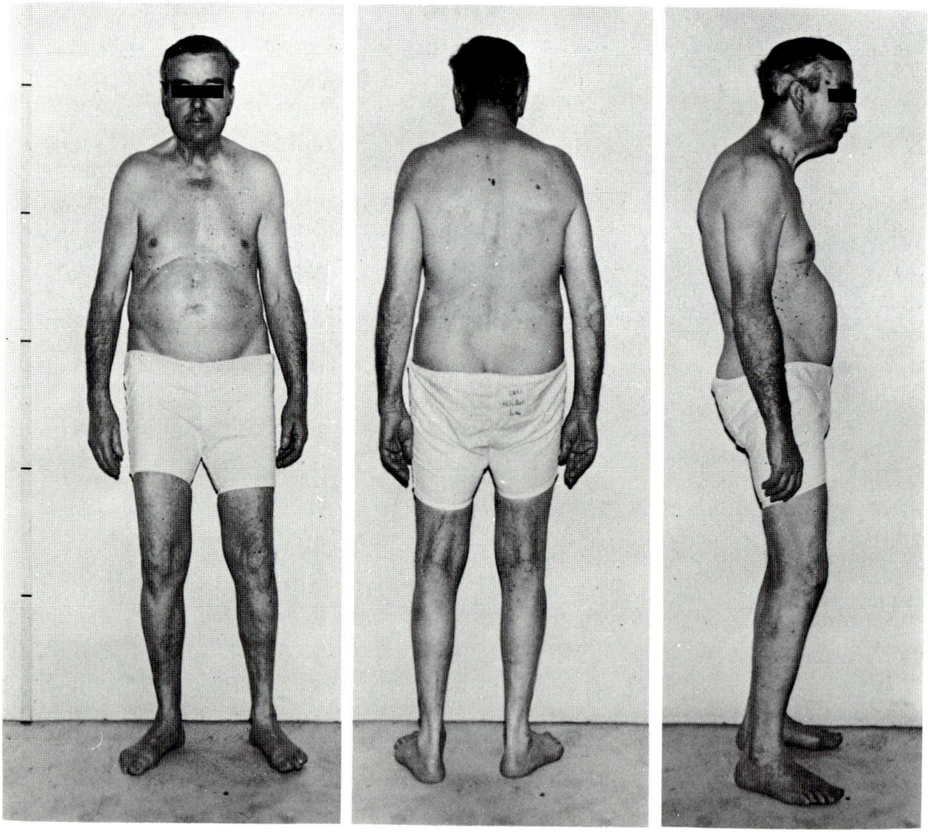

Fig. 29.2 Characteristic posture in ankylosing spondylitis. Note the dorsal kyphosis, forward craning of the neck, abdominal 'ballooning', and wide-based stance.

COMPLICATIONS

The familial and clinical associations between ankylosing spondylitis, psoriasis, ulcerative colitis, Crohn's disease, Whipple's disease, Reiter's disease and Behçet's syndrome are discussed fully in Chapter 28.

Iritis

Iritis (non-granulomatous anterior uveitis) occurs in about 20% of patients with ankylosing spondylitis (Blumberg & Ragan, 1956; Ogryzlo & Rosen, 1969), and is usually unilateral. It appears to be unrelated to the severity of the spondylitis, but occurs more frequently in patients with peripheral arthropathy (Wilkinson & Bywaters, 1958). Iritis may be the presenting feature of ankylosing spondylitis (Birbeck et al, 1951), and therefore in any young man with this eye disorder a careful search should be made to exclude spinal disease.

Heart disease

The most characteristic form of heart disease in sondylitis is lone aortic incompetence due to inflammatory changes in the aorta and aortic valve (Clark & Bauer, 1948; Schilder et al, 1956; Ansell et al, 1958; Sobin & Hagstrom, 1962). Heart disease is particularly common in long-standing spondylitis, and the frequency is higher in those with peripheral arthritis and prominent systemic manifestations such as fever, weight loss, and anaemia (Clark et al 1957). Graham & Smythe (1958) found heart disease in 3.5% of 519 patients with ankylosing spondylitis of at least 15 years' standing. Aortic incompetence, cardiomegaly and conduction defects are the commonest findings, although complete atrioventricular heart block complicated by Stokes-Adams attacks may occur (Julkunen & Luomanmäki, 1964; Hoffman & Leight, 1965). Acute fulminant aortic and mitral insufficiency have been reported recently (Stewart et al, 1978). Cardiomyopathy (Takkunen et al, 1970) and pericarditis (Graham & Smythe, 1958) have also been reported in ankylosing spondylitis.

Pathologically the aortic lesion resembles that seen in syphilitic aortitis (Mallory, 1936), and is quite unlike the nodular granulomata of rheumatoid arthritis (Clark et al, 1957; Graham & Smythe, 1958). Microscopically the aortic ring and ascending aorta are dilated (Davidson et al, 1963), and the valve cusps are fibrotic and thickened but not fused (Ansell et al 1958). In addition to aortic valve disease and involvement of the aortic root, involvement of the ascending aorta and part of the descending aorta with aneurysm formation has been described (Duvernay & Schatz, 1966).

Vascular lesions other than those observed in the aorta are rare in ankylosing spondylitis. A clinical picture resembling polyarteritis has been reported in a patient with spondylitis by Ball & Hathaway (1966), and a similar case has been observed by the author.

Central nervous system complications

Patients with ankylosing spondylitis may develop spontaneous atlantoaxial subluxation or dislocation (Kornblum et al, 1952; Martel, 1961; Sharp & Purser, 1961; Reid & Hill, 1978). Spinal cord damage may also result from fracture of the cervical spine after relatively mild trauma. There is a high risk of tetraplegia in these patients and the immediate mortality is about 50%. Cervical fracture most commonly occurs at the C5/6 interspace (Hollin et al, 1965). Good (1967) has reported a nontraumatic thoracic interspace fracture in a patient with spondylitis in whom displacement of adjacent vertebral bodies occurred. More recent reports have added support to the fracture-proneness of the spondylitic spine (Gelman & Umber, 1978; Hunter & Dubo, 1978; Martel, 1978). It has been suggested that the spondylitic patient may be particularly liable to fracture, not only because of the brittleness of his inelastic and demineralised spine, but also because of destructive changes.

Rarely a clinical picture simulating an expansive intraspinal process may be seen in ankylosing spondylitis (Hauge, 1961), and lesions of the cauda equina (Bowie & Glasgow, 1961; Russell et al, 1973; Milde et al, 1977) detectable by electromyography, and computerised tomography (Young et al, 1981), and a radiculopathy (Cumming & Saunders, 1978) may occur. Good et al (1982) have recently reported progressive paraparesis due to an epidural mass at D8–9 in a patient with ankylosing spondylitis. This was thought to be due to a combination of spinal meningeal disease and a fibroadipose mass associated with a non-infective destructive disc space lesion.

Amyloidosis

Secondary amyloidosis occurs in ankylosing spondylitis, and according to one necropsy series 6% of spondylitic patients died of uraemia from this complication (Cruickshank, 1960).

Pulmonary complications

Considering the thoracic fixity that occurs in ankylosing spondylitis, pulmonary function remains remarkably well preserved, probably owing to the substantial diaphragmatic contribution to ventilation (Zorab, 1962). However, lung disease does occur, and the change may simulate apical tuberculosis (Hamilton, 1949; Campbell & Macdonald, 1965; Jessamine, 1968; Cohen et al, 1971; Davies, 1972; Richards, 1974; Rosenow et al, 1977; Gupta & Johnston, 1978). Lung involvement in spondylitis typically appears several years after the onset of joint symptoms. Clinically, cough, sputum, dyspnoea, and later haemoptysis are present and serial radiographs show diffuse mottling in the upper half of each lung field. Cavities develop in most cases, and these are often colonised by *aspergilli*, with the formation of mycetomata. The fibrotic inflammatory appearance of the lung lesions is similar to that which has been observed in the aortae of patients with spondylitis (Leading article BMJ, 1971).

Complications of treatment

In an extensive necropsy series, Cruickshank (1960) has found that in a proportion of patients the cause of death in spondylitis was connected with its treatment. In 3% death followed operation on the spine or hips, in 10% death was from leukaemia, in 2% patients died from aplastic anaemia, and in 3% death was due to transverse myelitis possibly related to radiotherapy. Further evidence implicating radiotherapy as a cause of leukaemia and aplastic anemia in ankylosing spondylitis has been reported by Goodman (1956), Court Brown Doll (1957, 1965) and Spiers (1968).

RADIOLOGICAL FEATURES

Sacroiliitis

Sacroiliitis is the crucial feature in the diagnosis of ankylosing spondylitis, and definitive diagnosis of the disease is not possible in its absence. It is likely, however, that although sacroiliac involvement occurs early in the course of spondylitis (Forestier, 1931; Krebs, 1934; Scott, 1936), some patients will be seen with typical symptoms at a time when sacroiliitis has not yet reached the stage of radiological abnormality. Some workers refer to this stage of the disease as 'prespondylitis'.

The optimal radiographic technique to demonstrate early sacroiliitis is the postero/anterior projection with the patient in a prone position (Grainger, 1957). There is little evidence to support the alleged superiority of oblique projections or tomography, although the latter may be more useful to demonstrate joint narrowing and fusion (Wilkinson & Meikle, 1966).

Sacroiliitis appears initially as a patchy destructive process, later becoming replaced by complete ankylosis. One of the earliest changes is poor definition of the lower portion of the sacroiliac joint, probably due to localized decalcification. This is seen as blurring in the dense subchondral cortical streak on the iliac side of the joint, and the joint fissure may appear wider than usual ('pseudowidening'). Later, marginal erosions of varying size

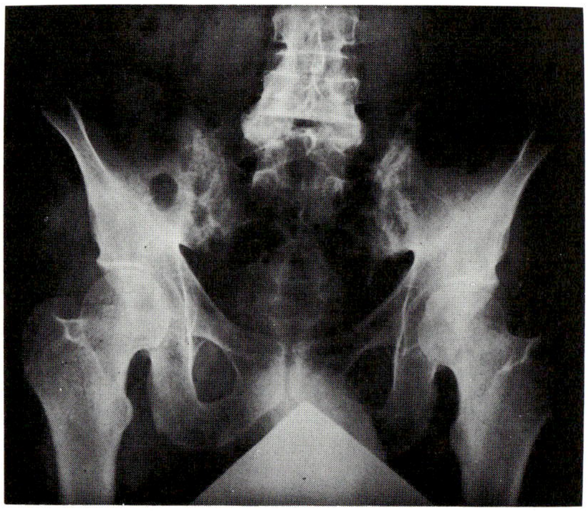

Fig. 29.3 Bilateral sacroiliac erosions in ankylosing spondylitis. The changes are particularly well shown in the right sacroiliac joint.

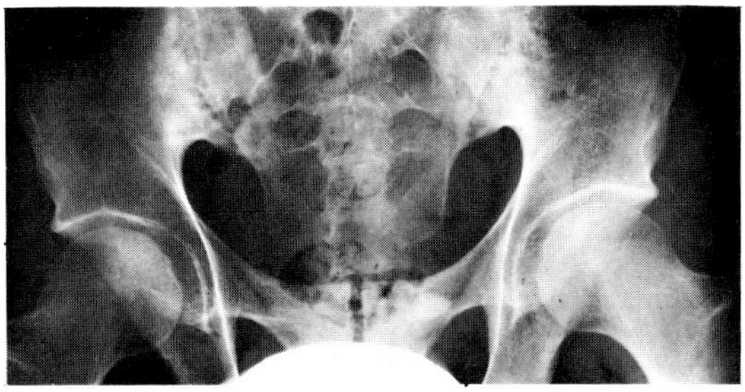

Fig. 29.4 Bilateral sacroiliac sclerosis in ankylosing spondylitis. Note that the sclerosis is present on both sides though more marked on the iliac side of the joint. Erosions are also evident.

and number appear (Fig. 29.3), and the edges of the articular surfaces become irregular and ragged. A parallel change is sclerosis (Fig. 29.4) seen at both sides of the joint, though more marked on the iliac side. At a relatively early stage of the sacroiliitis, new bone formation occurs in areas affected by destructive lesions; this process increases until complete ankylosis and obliteration of the joint occurs (Fig. 29.5). Later the sclerosis decreases and the bone structure gradually resumes its normal appearance, often leaving a star-shaped area of bony condensation in the upper third of each joint. In the final stages of sacroiliitis all that is left of the original joint is a fine faint line, sometimes referred to as the 'ghost joint'. If the presence of ankylosis is difficult to establish, the best indication is to follow the curved bony contour of the lower ilium and sacrum, and if this is continuous across the sacroiliac joint (Fig. 29.5) then ankylosis is likely to be present. However, even this

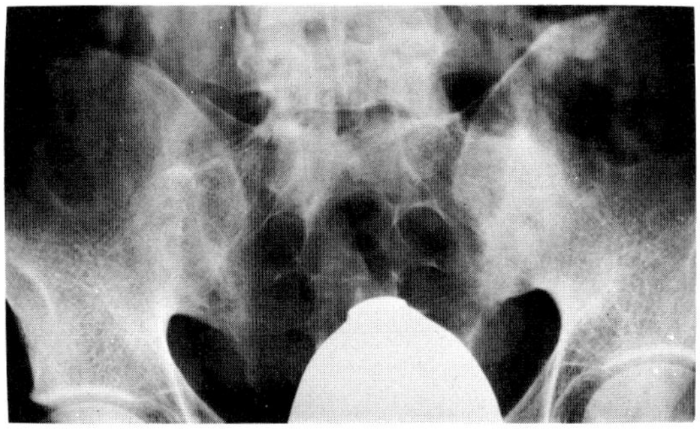

Fig. 29.5 Bilateral sacroiliac ankylosis in ankylosing spondylitis.

sign may be unreliable as positional changes may give rise to this effect in a normal joint.

Further diagnostic difficulty may be created by factors that obscure proper definition of the sacroiliac joint (Macrae et al, 1971; Moll, 1971):

1. Bowel shadow
2. Paget's disease
3. Osteosclerotic prostatic metastases
4. Calcified mesenteric glands
5. Osteitis condensans ilii
6. The 'adolescent sacroiliac joint syndrome' (Rogers & Cleaves, 1945)
7. Radiographic under- or overexposure
8. Osteoporosis resulting in 'pseudosclerosis'.

Interobserver variation is minimal for advanced bilateral disease but may be substantial when changes are mild and/or unilateral (Hollingsworth et al, 1983).

Many of these problems can be minimised by taking a full PA view of the pelvis, in constrast to a masked view including only the sacroiliac joints. Full pelvic views also have the advantage of allowing examination of the lower lumbar spine, hips, symphysis pubis and ischia for additional evidence of spondylitis. Furthermore, this view also provides a valuable opportunity to assess the degree of sacroiliac sclerosis against the normal 'control' sclerosis of the hip joint if this is not arthritic.

Spinal changes

From a diagnostic point of view spinal changes in ankylosing spondylitis are less important than changes in the sacroiliac joint because involvement of the spine usually occurs after the initial lesions of sacroiliitis. Romanus & Ydén (1955), in a detailed radiological study of 250 patients with spondylitis, have divided the spinal changes in spondylitis as follows:

1. *'Paravertebral' (intervertebral) ossification.* One of the most characteristic radiological features of spondylitis is the formation of bony bridges between adjacent vertebral bodies (Fig. 29.6). Forestier et al (1951) have shown by histological studies that this ossification occurs in the periphery of the intervertebral disc, rather than in the paravertebral ligaments as had been previously thought. These authors proposed the term 'syn-

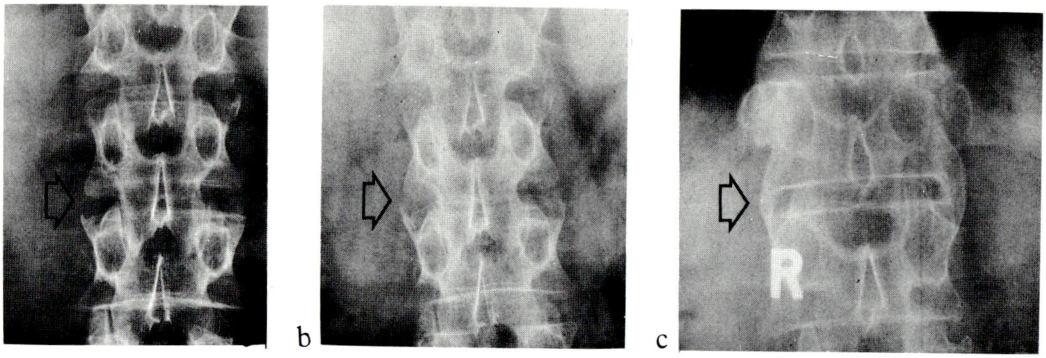

Fig. 29.6 Evolution of bony bridge between adjacent vertebral bodies in ankylosing spondylitis. (a) Early syndesmophyte. (b) Intermediate stage. (c) Complete bony bridge.

desmophyte' for the ossifying vertebral lesions. Syndesmophytes should be differentiated from osteophytes (Table 29.3). The most typical site for an early syndesmophyte is at or near the dorsolumbar junction, usually on the lateral aspect of the vertebral body. Syndesmophytes may also occur anteriorly (Fig. 29.7), and, much less frequently, posteriorly. The term 'bamboo-spine' is classically given to the undulating lateral contour of the spine when widespread bilateral intervertebral bridging has occurred (Fig. 29.8).

Table 29.3 Differentiation between the osteophyte and the syndesmophyte (Riley et al, 1971)

Osteophyte	Syndesmophyte
1. Associated with disc narrowing	1. No disc narrowing or protrusion
2. Marginal and HORIZONTAL bony plate built up at the base with subperiosteal bone	2. VERTICAL plate or wedge of bone in outer layer of annulus fibrosus
3. Base lies against protruded disc substance	3. Will ultimately form a bridge between one vertebral body and the next

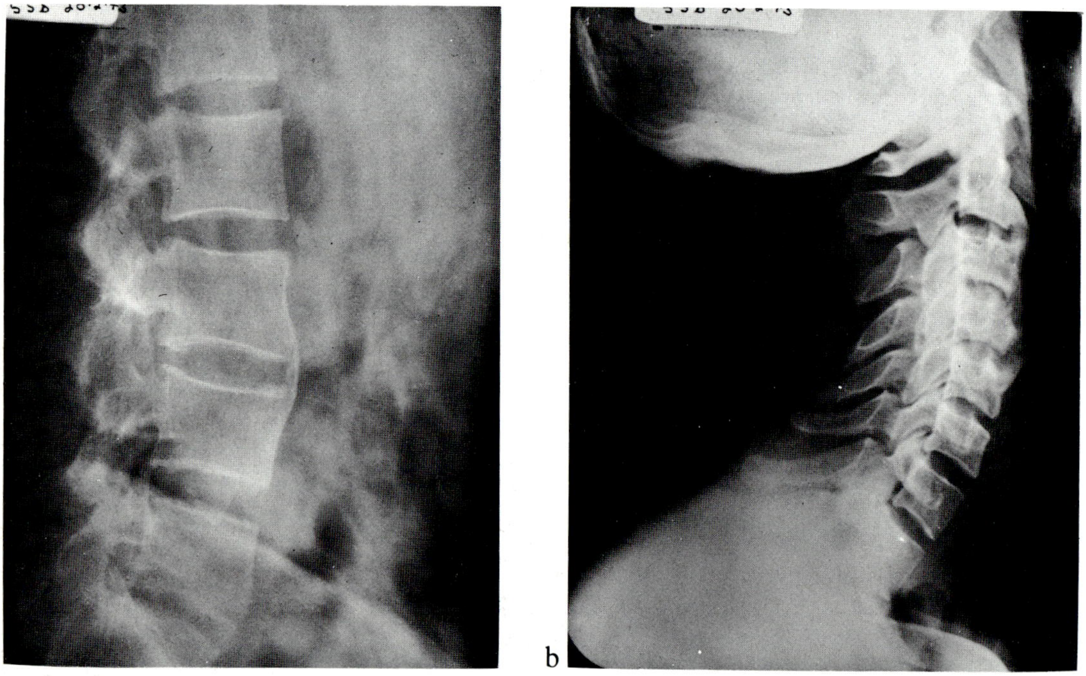

Fig. 29.7 Anterior syndesmophytic bridging in (a) lumbar spine and (b) cervical spine.

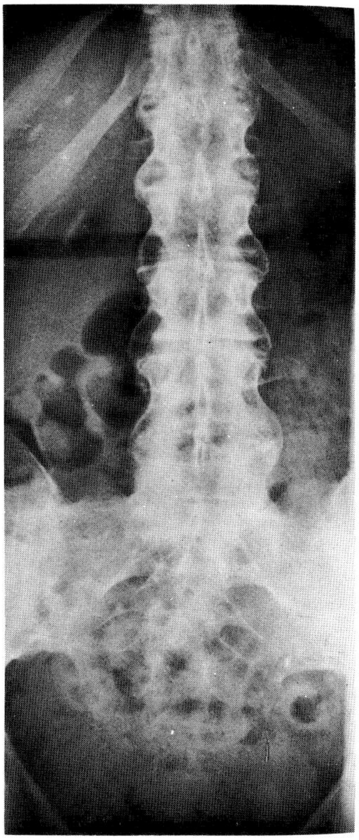

Fig. 29.8 Typical 'bamboo-spine' in ankylosing spondylitis. Note the undulating lateral contour of the spine due to widespread intervertebral bridging.

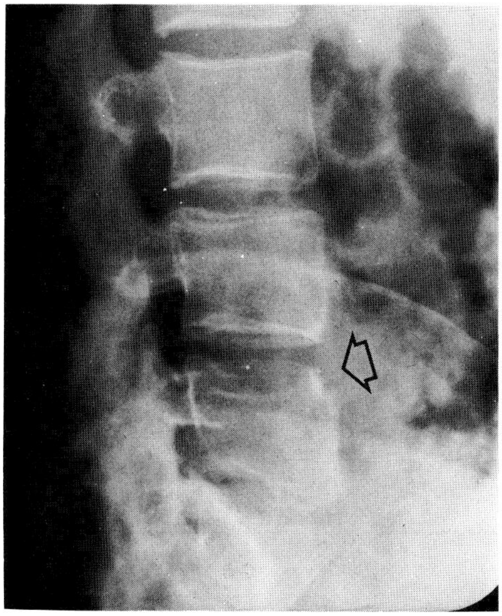

Fig. 29.9 'Romanus lesion' in ankylosing spondylitis. Note the area of erosion and sclerosis at the upper anterior corner of L5.

2. *Anterior spondylitis* ('Romanus lesions' and vertebral squaring). Romanus & Ydén (1955) have described destructive vertebral lesions confined to the upper and lower parts of the anterior vertebral surface (Fig. 29.9). These areas have since been termed 'Romanus lesions'. As these lesions heal, the anterior corners of the vertebral body lose their normal convexity and appear as if they had been planed down (Fig. 29.10). This is one explanation for the so-called 'square vertebra' in spondylitis. However, another theory to explain 'squaring' is based on the filling in with new bone of the convex anterior vertebral surface (Rolleston, 1947).

3. *Osteoporosis* (Fig. 29.10). This feature is usually considered to be a relatively late sign of spondylitis, but when it does occur early the outlook is usually poor (Forestier et al, 1951).

4. *Changes in the intervertebral disc* ('*spondylodiscitis*'). Evidence from discography and from disc biopsy has shown that disc space narrowing in spondylitis is probably due to involvement of the

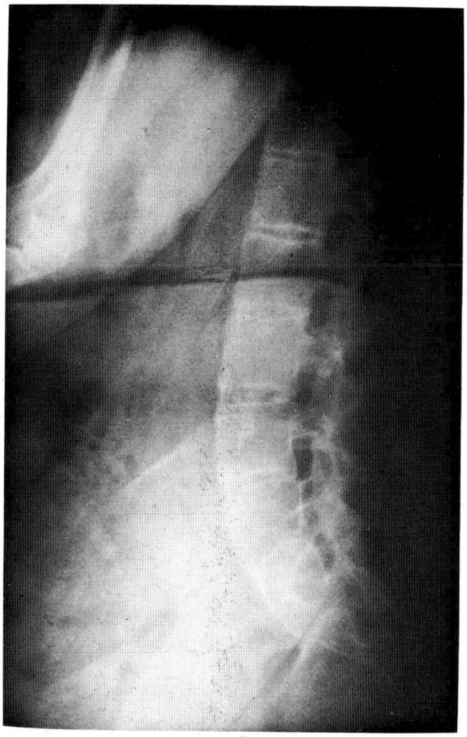

Fig. 29.10 Square vertebrae in ankylosing spondylitis. Note also vertebral osteoporosis and areas of ossification in the disc spaces (healed spondylodiscitis).

disc by the spondylitic process rather than by coexisting disc degeneration (Romanus & Ydén, 1955). Calcification of the disc may also occur, and in some instances the inflammatory changes in the disc may advance to massive destruction of adjacent vertebral bodies (Wholey et al, 1960; Seaman & Wells, 1961; Cawley et al, 1972). The healing of the lesions of spondylodiscitis may lead to bony ankylosis of adjacent vertebrae (Fig. 29.10).

5. *Apophyseal joint involvement.* This is seen in the lumbar spine and later in the thoracic and cervical areas (Fig. 29.11). It is difficult to see on routine lateral views, but may be clearly visualised on special oblique views. The latter, however, are probably not justified as routine radiographs in spondylitis in view of the late appearance of apophyseal joint involvement.

6. *Interspinous ossification.* This appears as a radio-opaque streak on a PA view, and is particularly well seen in the lumbosacral spine (Fig. 29.12). It is sometimes referred to as the 'dagger sign'.

7. *Peripheral arthritis.* Radiologically, the changes in the peripheral joints in ankylosing spondylitis are much the same as those seen in seropositive rheumatoid arthritis. However, in spondylitis there is less tendency to joint erosion, but a greater tendency to ankylosis, particularly in the hip joint which is the most commonly affected peripheral joint.

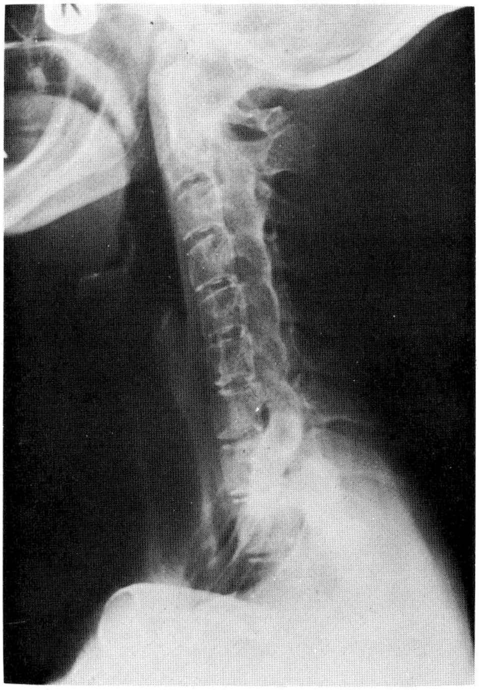

Fig. 29.11 Extensive apophyseal joint fusion in the cervical spine. Note also minimal fusion anteriorly.

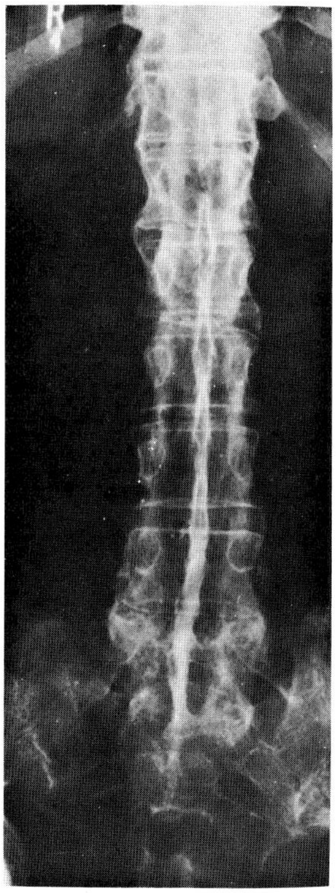

Fig. 29.12 Interspinous ossification in lumbosacral spine (dagger sign).

8. *Other bone and joint changes.* A number of radiological changes may be found in areas other than those in the spine and peripheral joints. These have been reviewed by Guest & Jacobson (1951), Wilkinson & Bywaters (1958), Graham (1960), and Dilsen et al (1962) and are as follows: erosion, sclerosis and ankylosis of cartilaginous joints (symphysis pubis, costosternal and manubriosternal joints); ossification of the sacrotuberous, sacrospinous, iliolumbar, coracoclavicular, and other ligaments; irregular periosteal new bone formation at various sites including the ischial tuberosities (Fig. 29.13), and iliac crests; erosion of the posterior cortex of the calcaneum, greater tubercles of the humeri and greater trochanters; spur formation at the external occipital protuberance and at the insertion of the plantar ligament. Spurs

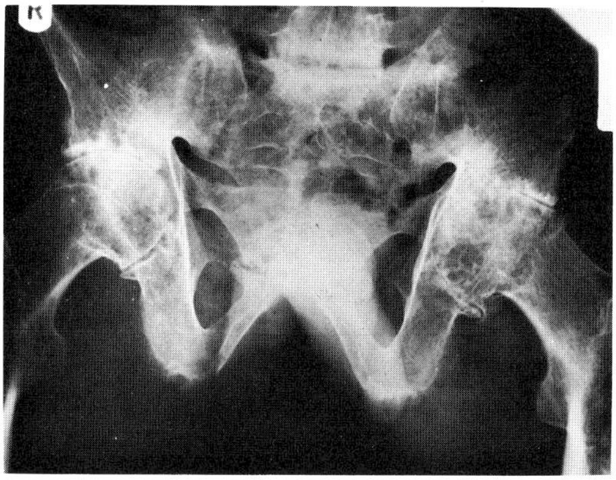

Fig. 29.13 Irregular periosteal new bone formation at the ischial tuberosities ('ischial whiskering'). Note also extensive involvement of the sacroiliac and hip joints.

in ankylosing spondylitis are usually less fluffy and less exuberant than those in Reiter's disease (Mason, 1964), and are less common than the spurs of rheumatoid arthritis (Dilsen et al, 1962).

SCINTIGRAPHY (see also Chapter 69)

Since the last edition of this book quantitative scanning techniques (scintigraphy) have been studied with much vigour in the hope that the method would enhance early diagnosis of ankylosing spondylitis (Lentle et al, 1977 a, b; Namey et al, 1977; Szanto et al, 1977; Berghs et al, 1978; Goldberg et al, 1978; Szanto & Lindvall, 1978; Chalmers et al, 1979; Domeij-Nyberg et al, 1980; Scott et al, 1980; Rothwell et al, 1981). It may be concluded that quantitative sacroiliac scintigraphy may be useful in detecting early ankylosing spondylitis before the development of radiological changes and that it can identify an organic basis for backache in patients with a spondylitis-like syndrome. However, it is important to take account of the individual clinical circumstances as scintigraphic abnormalities are not diagnostic of any specific disease entity. There is some evidence (Domeij et al, 1980) that [^{99m}Tc] EHDP gives more reliable results than [^{99m}Tc] pertechnetate.

AXIAL TOMOGRAPHY

A relatively new approach to studying the sacroiliac joint is axial tomography. By providing a craniocaudal axial view of the sacroiliac joints it enables ventral ankylosis to be demonstrated which is not visible or can only be suspected on AP films (Dory & Francois, 1978). Application of this technique to the spine may also help to delineate other spondylitic changes such as those of the cauda equina syndrome (Young et al, 1981).

PATHOLOGY

There is difficulty in studying the pathology of ankylosing spondylitis owing to its usually non-fatal outcome. Relative differences between rheumatoid and spondylitic synovitis include the following which are seen rarely in rheumatoid arthritis but frequently in ankylosing spondylitis:

1. Progression of fibrous ankylosis to bony ankylosis
2. Occurrence of synovial haemorrhage
3. Greater frequency (in non-irradiated patients) of endarterial fibrosis
4. Less active inflammatory reaction.

However, even the seemingly specific features of the spondylitic synovitis can be matched with similar lesions in rheumatoid arthritis (Cruickshank, 1951).

The differential points between rheumatoid arthritis and ankylosing spondylitis are more evident in the spine (van Swaay, 1950; Aufdermaur, 1957; Ball, 1971). The last author has produced convincing evidence to support a concept based on an abnormality of the 'enthesis' — a term first used by Niepel et al (1966) to describe a zone of ligamentous attachment to bone. Ball refers to the abnormal enthesis in ankylosing spondylitis as an 'enthesopathy'. The enthesopathy in spondylitis consists of a focal microscopic inflammatory lesion localised to ligamentous attachments and associated with an erosive defect in adjacent cortical bone (Figs 29.14–29.16). These lesions are particularly well seen in the iliac crest, greater trochanter, patella and intervertebral disc. In Ball's view, the syndesmophyte grows by apical new bone formation as part of a repair process in the inflammatory erosive lesion involving the edge of the annulus fibrosus. Furthermore, endochondral ossification of the vertebral endplate, excessive calcification of the disc, disc atrophy and osteoporosis of vertebral bodies are all secondary reactions

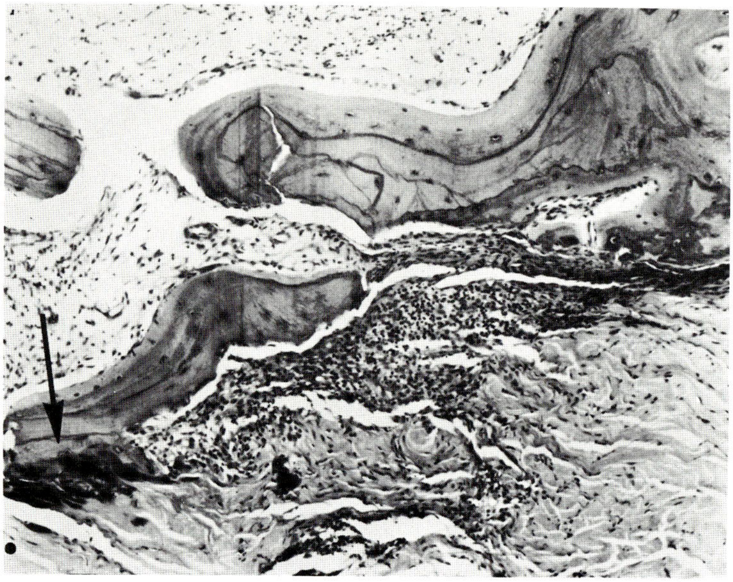

Fig. 29.14 Spondylitic enthesopathy. Iliac crest. An active inflammatory erosive lesion localised to the ligamentous attachment to bone (the enthesis). Arrow points to an unaffected part of the ligamentous attachment at the edge of the lesion. (H & E × 100) (By courtesy of Dr John Ball.)

to intervertebral bony ankylosis. Apophyseal ankylosis is thought to develop in the same way as the syndesmophyte, i.e. by capsular ossification starting as a capsuloligamentous attachment lesion. Again, Ball uses the same pathological principle to explain the findings in the sacroiliac joints — the initial lesion being peripheral bony ankylosis followed later by central endochondral ossification.

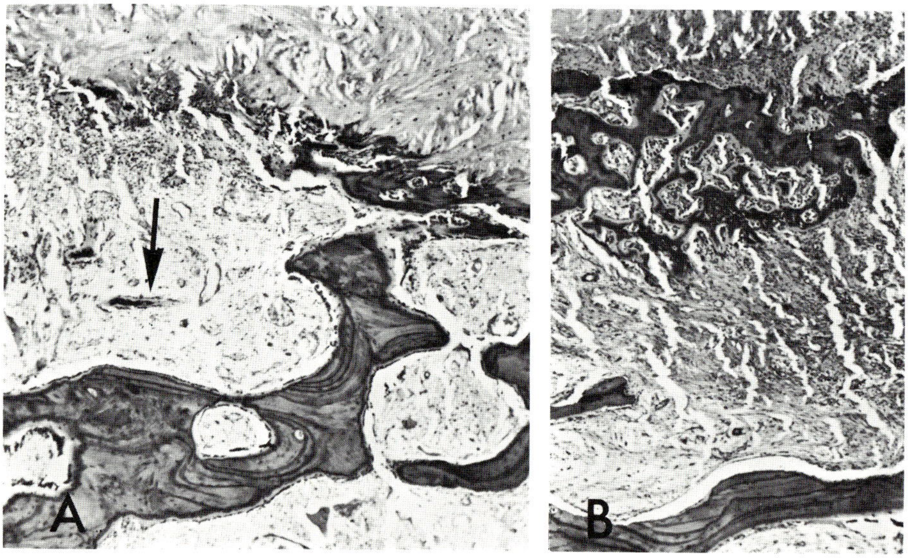

Fig. 29.15 Spondylitic enthesopathy. Greater trochanter. (A) Above left the ligamentous attachment has been destroyed. Arrow points to spicules of reactive bone indicating the onset of repair. (H & E ×40) (B) A later stage of repair. Reactive bone trabeculae (above) have filled in the defect and rejoined the ligament to the bone. (H & E ×100) (By courtesy of Dr John Ball.)

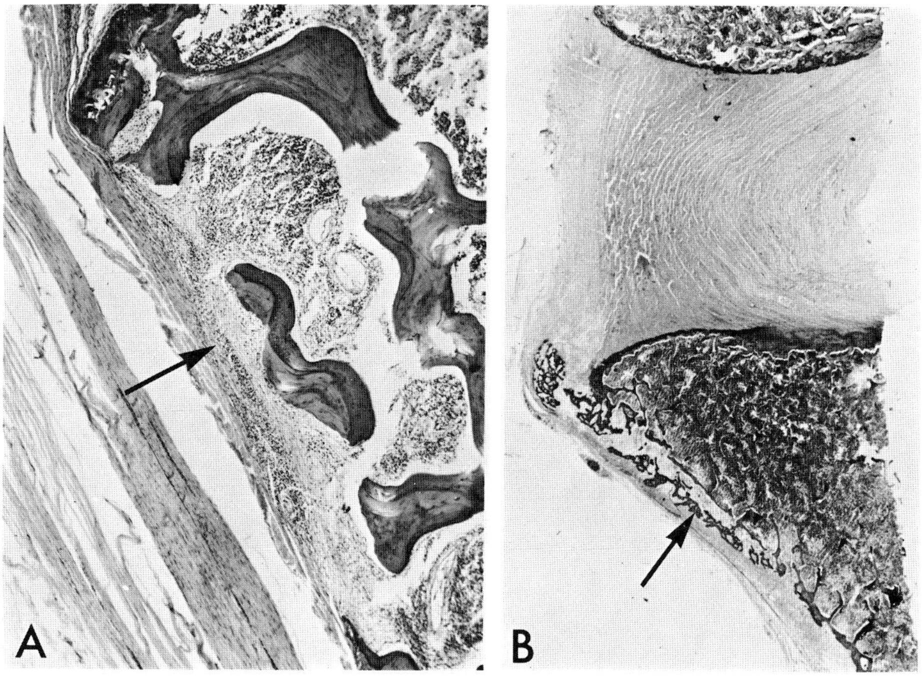

Fig. 29.16 Spondylitic enthesopathy. Lumbar vertebral body. (A) Arrow points to eroded attachment of the outer fibres of the annulus just below the vertebral rim (upper left) (H & E × 40) (B) Early repair in a vertebral enthesopathy. Arrow points to a layer of new reactive bone in the same position as the erosive lesion shown in (A). The new bone fills in the eroded attachment and begins to form a syndesmophyte (H & E 4.5) (By courtesy of Dr John Ball.)

So-called 'erosions' and 'apparent widening' of the sacroiliac joints are ascribed to irregular progression of endochondral ossification. Sacroiliac sclerosis is thought to represent appositional laying down of highly radio-opaque lamellar bone.

Cruickshank (1971) has pointed to a further characteristic though non-specific feature of spondylitis. This concerns the involvement of synchondroses such as the manubriosternal joint and the symphysis pubis. In these areas it is common to find a mild osteitis with infiltration by chronic inflammatory cells and proliferation of vascular fibrous tissue. Periosteum, cartilage, and bony trabeculae are invaded by granulation tissue, leading to bony erosion and destruction of joint tissue. Some sclerosis of adjacent bone accompanies the process, but eventually the joint is replaced by fibrous or bony ankylosis.

Rare occurrences of rheumatoid nodules in ankylosing spondylitis (London & Bland, 1963; Valkenburg et al, 1972) probably represent the fortuitous coexistence of two different diseases.

LABORATORY FINDINGS

The erythrocyte sedimentation rate is raised in approximately 80% of patients in the early phase of the disease, and a fall may occur in the later stages (Polley & Slocumb, 1947; Polley, 1955). However, the sedimentation rate is of little use as a guide to the activity of the disease, to its progression, or to its response to treatment (Hart et al, 1949).

Anaemia and leucocytosis may occur but are uncommon (Rosen & Graham, 1962). Non-specific changes in the plasma proteins include raised levels of α_2- and γ-globulin (Ogryzlo, 1972). The serum albumen may be decreased. Usually, however, the serum proteins are normal.

The sheep cell agglutination and latex tests for rheumatoid factor are negative in most patients. Occasionally spondylitic patients are seropositive, but the occurrence of positive tests does not exceed the frequency found in the general population (Kellgren & Ball, 1959). The seronegativity of patients with ankylosing spondylitis is a major factor in considering the disease as nosologically separate from rheumatoid arthritis.

Tests for LE factor have similarly been negative (Ogryzlo, 1972). Slight elevation of the cerebrospinal fluid protein (45–60 mg%) has been reported, particularly in patients with sciatica (Ludwig et al, 1943). Increased complement levels in spondylitic synovial fluid, such as have been seen in Reiter's disease, have been reported (Pekin et al, 1967). Increased complement levels have also been found in spondylitic plasma (Whaley et al, 1974).

Dixon et al (1981) have recently compared the serum biochemistry in ankylosing spondylitis with that of seronegative arthritis and seropositive rheumatoid arthritis. The following features were reported:

1. Total serum sulphydryl and haemoglobin discriminated well between ankylosing spondylitis and seropositive rheumatoid arthritis
2. IgG, IgA and acute-phase reactants discriminated between seropositive and seronegative arthritis
3. In active ankylosing spondylitis a normal ESR was often seen with abnormal C-reactive protein and plasma viscosity.

Many recent reports have suggested altered immunity in ankylosing spondylitis, although the significance of these laboratory data, where they have been consistent, is still uncertain. Features of altered immunity have included: the presence of immune complexes (Gabay et al, 1977; Corrigall et al, 1978); selective IgA deficiency (Good et al, 1977); raised serum IgA (Cowling et al, 1980); increased frequency of leucocyte-reactive antinuclear antibody (Vasey & Kinsella, 1977); diminished mixed lymphocyte response (Wee & Daymond, 1978). Zilko et al (1977) have also studied immune function in ankylosing spondylitis and have reported an apparent relationship between streptococcal responses and HLA-B27. T lymphocytes have also been studied in ankylosing spondylitis and the proportion of T_G cells (T lymphocytes with receptors for the Fc portion of IgG) was noted to be increased in half the population studied. T_m cells were found in normal distribution (Nilsson & Biberfeld, 1980). However, despite these findings, the role of T lymphocytes in ankylosing spondylitis is still debatable, the balance of evidence coming down against their being of immunopathogenetic significance in this disease.

The striking association between ankylosing spondylitis and HLA-B27(over 95%) has received substantial further confirmation since publication of the last edition of this book (Brautbar et al, 1977; Calin et al, 1977; Contu et al, 1977; Davatchi et al, 1977; Duquesnoy et al, 1978; Säfwenberg et al, 1978).

Typical ankylosing spondylitis has also been observed in HLA-B27-negative patients, especially in blacks (Khan et al, 1977; Van der Linden et al, 1977; Khan et al, 1977).

No differences in HLA-DR antigens have been observed in patients with ankylosing spondylitis (Dejeto et al, 1978), thus providing additional support for histocompatibility differences between spondylitis and seropositive rheumatoid arthritis.

The significance of HLA-B27 in aetiology and pathogenesis will be discussed below.

AETIOLOGY AND PATHOGENESIS

Genetic factors

Kellgren (1964) has estimated the degree of familial aggregation in ankylosing spondylitis to be 40. This figure was based on the mean prevalence of spondylitis in relatives (4%) compared with population controls (0.1%). The familial nature of spondylitis has been amply documented in other reports (Rogoff & Freyberg, 1949; Böni & Hauptmann, 1950; Hersh et al, 1950; Romanus, 1953; Stecher, 1957). The likelihood of genetic factors as the cause of familial aggregation in spondylitis is suggested by observations of concordance for the disease in monozygotic twins (Rae, 1932; Foxworthy et al, 1960; Kornstad & Kornstad, 1960; Moesmann, 1960). Eastmond & Woodrow (1977) however found discordance for spondylitis in two monozygotic twin pairs and a marked difference in disease severity in a third pair. This finding supports the concept that environmental factors are also important in the aetiology of the disease.

The mode of inheritance in spondylitis is still not entirely clear. Stecher (1957) has concluded that the disease is due to an autosomal dominant factor with 70% penetrance in males and 10% penetrance in females. Pedigree characteristics reported by Riecker et al (1950), and Graham & Uchida (1957) support this hypothesis. Other views, however, invoke a multifactiorial mechanism (Emery & Lawrence, 1967). Such a mechanism would explain some features including:

1. The lack in most series of any obvious Mendelian pattern
2. The poor correlation between observed and expected rates of manifestation of the disease
3. The evidence that environmental factors such as genitourinary infection may be important in aetiology.

The findings of Brewerton et al (1973) and Schlosstein et al (1973) have produced additional evidence for genetic factors in ankylosing spondylitis. Their tissue typing studies have demonstrated the presence of HLA-B27 in 31 of 60 (53%) first-degree relatives of spondylitic probands.

This early genetic work using HLA-B27 in family studies has been extended recently and has shown prevalences of ankylosing spondylitis or a related spondarthritis in 15–20% of first-degree relatives of spondylitis probands (Contu et al, 1977; Daneo et al, 1977; Hochberg et al, 1978; Migone et al, 1978).

Patients who are homozygous for HLA-B27 have been shown to be more susceptible to ankylosing spondylitis (Khan et al, 1978), to have more severe axial and/or peripheral arthritis (Arnett et al, 1977; Khan et al, 1978), and to exhibit more overlap with other HLA-B27-associated disorders (Sikora et al, 1978).

There is evidence to suggest that there are genes *controlling* antigens related to HLA-B27, such as Cw1 and Cw2 (Arnett et al, 1978; Duquesnoy et al, 1978; Kozin et al, 1978). There is also evidence for genes *cross-reacting* with HLA-B27, such as B7 (Khan et al, 1978) and Bw42 or A28 (Hochberg et al, 1978).

The role of HLA-B27 antigens remains in dispute but two concepts have been proposed:

1. *'Indirect' concept*. This suggests that the HLA-B27 antigen is unimportant but that its coding allele is in strong linkage disequilibrium with another gene that causes or permits the development of the disease and possibly acts by modifying immune responsiveness (Van der Berg-Loonen et al, 1977; Arnett et al, 1978; Dejelo et al, 1978; Khan et al, 1978; Kozin et al, 1978).

2. *'Direct' concept*. This suggests that the HLA-B27 antigen, a glycoprotein on the cell surface, contributes directly to the development of the disease. It is proposed that it does this either by acting as a receptor for a virus or other environmental agent, with the formation of a complex that initiates an immune response, or by resembling an environmental agent, thereby allowing continuing infection or an abnormal immune response. *K. pneumoniae* and other *Klebsiella* spp. have been implicated in this (Ebringer et al, 1977, 1978; Cowling et al, 1980; Eastmond et al, 1980, 1982). Furthermore, Calguneri et al (1981) have found raised values of salivary secretory IgA in patients with active spondylitis and have concluded that this suggests the presence of an antigenic stimulus from the gastrointestinal system in these patients whether or not this is due to *Klebsiella* spp. Despite the recent interest in the possible importance of Klebsiella as an inciting agent in ankylosing spondylitis, the evidence remains conflicting, and some workers in this field doubt its relevance.

Other factors

Romanus (1953) has stressed the importance of genitourinary infection as a cause of ankylosing spondylitis. He found evidence of genitourinary infection, usually prostatovesiculitis, in 89% of males with ankylosing spondylitis. Romanus suggested that pelvic infection may spread by way of lymph routes or the vertebral venous plexus of Batson (Batson, 1940, 1942a, b) to the sacroiliac joints, and thence to the spine and pelvis. He also suggested that infection may spread from the prostate and seminal vesicles to the general circulation, thus giving rise to systemic upsets and symptoms in the peripheral joints, tendons and uvea. However, it needs to be emphasised that the rates of prostatovesiculitis in men without spondylitis reported by urologists, although using less strict diagnostic criteria than those of Romanus, vary between 35% and as much as 50% (Pelouze, 1921; Hinman, 1935; Payr, 1947; Wilde, 1949).

Further evidence for an association between ankylosing spondylitis and genitourinary infection has been found by Ford (1953) who reported ankylosing spondylitis in four patients occurring after non-specific urethritis. Mason et al (1958) found 83% of patients with spondylitis to have definite evidence of chronic prostatitis, compared with 32% rheumatoid controls. Additional evidence for this relationship has been furnished by Catterall & Perkins (1961) who demonstrated an association between prostatitis, anterior uveitis, and sacroiliitis.

With regard to the possibility of pelvic infection as an inciting factor in the aetiology of ankylosing spondylitis, the now acknowledged associations between spondylitis and certain chronic bowel diseases (ulcerative colitis, Crohn's disease, and Whipple's disease) are of interest. It has been suggested that the common denominator in all these spondylitis-associated diseases is the spread of infection to the spine via the pelvic lymphatics. The main flaw in this hypothesis is the relatively common occurrence of ankylosing spondylitis appearing before manifest genitourinary infection or bowel disease. Nevertheless, it is possible that in these patients genitourinary infection or bowel disease was already established, but in latent form.

Other suggested aetiological factors, though now outdated, include trauma (Erhardt, 1905; Graber-Duvernay, 1951), parathyroid disease (Junghanns, 1939), and pulmonary tuberculosis (Scott, 1936). Schmorl & Junghanns (1971) cite further causal agents including: lead intoxication, upper respiratory infection, and other infections such as the common cold, gonorrhoea and focal sepsis. These and other outmoded theories, such as those invoking allergy or endocrine and metabolic defects, have little or no evidence to support them.

It is likely that ankylosing spondylitis is caused by a combination of genetic and environmental factors, and it is tempting to speculate that in many patients pelvic infection acts as the environmental trigger in genetically predisposed subjects.

COURSE AND PROGNOSIS

With appropriate management and treatment the outlook in ankylosing spondylitis is usually much better than has been traditionally thought. In only a minority (probably not more than 5% of patients) does the disease take an unfavourable course from the onset. In these subjects, permanent incapacity due to widespread ankylosis usually occurs within a few years. Normally, however, the progression of the disease is much more gradual, extending in a low-grade fashion over many years. The mechanical results of the disease on the spine and chest are sometimes so insidious in their development that they pass unnoticed by the patient until they are drawn to his attention. In some patients symptoms may completely subside at a relatively early stage, although there is always the chance of recurrence in later years.

The reasonable outlook in spondylitis is reflected in the fact that 85% of patients remain gainfully employed with little absenteeism (Ogryzlo, 1972). In another study, two-thirds or more were able to support themselves and their families after twenty years of symptoms (Blumberg & Ragan, 1956; Wilkinson & Bywaters, 1958).

Patients usually learn to adapt remarkably well to their disease, and often it is surprising how minimal is their disability considering the degree of spinal stiffness. As Sharp (1965) has stressed, the main limitations to working capacity are the severity of hip disease and the level of the patient's morale. Hip disease may also severely limit the patient's ability to perform sexual intercourse.

The course of ankylosing spondylitis is similar in females. Pregnancy does not seem to produce the remissions frequently seen in rheumatoid arthritis (Hart & Robinson, 1959). Considering the pelvic and spinal fixity imposed by the disease, pregnancy and childbirth usually proceed surprisingly well. Furthermore, in a recent study of 87 spondylitic pregnancies it was observed that the disease appeared to have no harmful effects on the fetus or the newborn. A short postpartum flare was observed in 45% of spondylitic mothers and postpartum uveitis occured in 20% (Østensen et al, 1982). (In this survey 12% of offspring who were 18 years old or more had developed definite ankylosing spondylitis.)

Originally it was thought that ankylosing spondylitis did not itself contribute to mortality. However, a recent study of 836 patients who had never received X-ray therapy has indicated that at least in men ankylosing spondylitis has life-threatening consequences related to multiple organ system involvement (Radford et al, 1977). The excess of mortality in these patients was thought to be contributed to by many factors — particularly ulcerative colitis, nephritis, tuberculosis and other respiratory diseases, gastrointestinal disorders, accidents, suicide, and cerebrovascular and circulatory diseases. A further study in Doll's unit (Smith et al, 1977) has shown that cancer deaths, and specifically leukaemia deaths, were no higher than expected rates among non-irradiated spondylitis patients. These workers concluded therefore that the excess of leukaemia and other malignancies in spondylitis can be attributed directly to X-ray therapy, and is unrelated to the disease process itself. Khan et al (1981) have also recently demonstrated lower-than-expected survival figures for a population of spondylitis in the USA (calculated from life tables, and matched for sex, age, race, geographic area and calendar year). Most of these patients had not had radiotherapy. This study therefore supports the claim that spondylitis itself contributes to mortality. However, the figures reported by Khan et al may have been biased in that all spondylitics were hospital-referred patients.

DIFFERENTIAL DIAGNOSIS

On the whole, the clinical and radiological features of uncomplicated ankylosing spondylitis are indistinguishable from those seen in the spondylitis of other seronegative disorders such as psoriatic arthritis, Reiter's disease, and the intestinal arthropathies. However, McEwen et al (1971) have divided their spondylitic patients into two groups according to clinical and radiological characteristics. In one group are placed uncomplicated ankylosing spondylitis and the spondylitis associated with ulcerative colitis and Crohn's disease, and in the other group the spondylitis associated with psoriasis and the spondylitis of Reiter's disease. The main difference between the two groups stems from the higher proportion of 'other-than-marginal' syndesmophytes in psoriatic and Reiter's spondylitis. However, as the authors themselves have pointed out, the differences between the groups are quantitative rather than qualitative.

Further points of differentiation have been made between the spondylitic features of members of the seronegative spondarthritides. Thus, Cliff (1971) described characteristic bony bridges in Reiter's spondylitis. These bridges or 'skip lesions' are often isolated and unilateral and usually join the mid portions of adjacent vertebral bodies rather than their corners, as in uncomplicated ankylosing spondylitis. The lesions may ultimately extend to form the characteristic bamboo spine of uncomplicated ankylosing spondylitis (Good, 1965).

Bywaters & Dixon (1965) have reported an unusual type of paravertebral ossification in patients with psoriasis. This appears as an interrupted wavy band of ossification running parallel to the lateral border of the spine and separated from it by a gap of 0.5–1.5 mm. However, this pattern of spinal ossification is rare.

Other causes of paravertebral ossification such as hyperparathyroidism and fluorosis may produce changes similar to those seen in uncomplicated ankylosing spondylitis, but in these diseases the sacroiliac joints are normal. The ankylosing arthropathy of vitamin D-resistant hypophosphataemic rickets may also be confused with ankylosing spondylitis (McKusick, 1972). Patients with this disorder develop spinal ankylosis as well as ankylosis of peripheral joints. Calcaneal spurs, roughening of the ischium, and capsular calcification of the hip may also occur. The sacroiliac joints of the patient reported by McKusick were not involved.

Radiographic lesions that may be confused with the syndesmophyte include the osteophyte and the bony spur of ankylosing hyperostosis. Essentially, however, the syndesmophyte is a vertically disposed structure, whereas the osteophyte and the hyperostotic spur tend to lie more horizontally. Bywaters et al (1971) have reported syndesmophyte-like lesions in spinal haemochromatosis, but these 'pseudosyndesmophytes' differ from those seen in ankylosing spondylitis.

The sacroiliac joint may be abnormal in gout (Malawista et al, 1965), and in tuberculosis (Wells, 1965), but in these conditions the destructive changes are usually unilateral.

Tuberculosis, brucellosis, and pyogenic abscess may enter into the differential diagnosis of inflammatory lesions of the intervertebral disc, and these may be sufficiently marked to produce destruction of adjacent vertebral bodies. However, this feature occurs late in ankylosing spondylitis, by which time the diagnosis is usually established.

Bony ankylosis of the sacroiliac joints has been described in dissection studies of normal pelves in elderly subjects (Sashin, 1930; Horwitz & Smith, 1940). However, radiography of these specimens has shown that bony fusion was confined to the upper part of the joint, and that complete ankylosis of the type associated with ankylosing spondylitis was rare.

Sacroiliac changes similar to those seen in ankylosing spondylitis have been observed in paraplegics (Abramson & Kamberg, 1949; Abel, 1950; Lodge, 1956). Wright et al (1965) have confirmed a sacroiliac abnormality in paraplegics, but disagree with previous workers about the similarity of these changes to those seen in true spondylitis. In the patients of Wright and colleagues, sacroiliac sclerosis was found in paraplegics, but there was no evidence of convincing joint erosion or ankylosis.

Observations from the United States (Dodson et al, 1971), and more recently from the United Kingdom (Darke, 1975), have revealed sacroiliac erosion and sclerosis, and also distal phalangeal osteolysis, in patients chronically exposed to polyvinylchloride (PVC).

The differentiating points between ankylosing spondylitis and ankylosing hyperostosis (diffuse idiopathic skeletal hyperostosis — see p. 734) are summarised in Table 29.4.

Bluestone et al (1971) have drawn attention to spinal hyperostosis in patients with acromegalic arthropathy. These changes are almost indistinguishable from ankylosing hyperostosis except that the disc space is often larger than normal in acromegaly, and these patients may also have erosion and sclerosis of the symphysis pubis. Another feature distinguishing acromegalic spinal involvement from both ankylosing hyperostosis and ankylosing spondylitis is that in acromegaly spinal mobility is often increased.

Differentiating between early spondylitis and acute lumbar disc prolapse may be a problem. This may be particularly so in youth and early adulthood when developmental changes in the sacroiliac joint often obscure proper assessment of sacroiliitis (Rogers & Cleaves, 1935). In both conditions there may be lumbago, sciatica, and spinal stiffness. However, in ankylosing spondylitis sciatica is not associated with paraesthesiae, and the restriction of spinal movement usually occurs in all directions (anterior flexion, lateral flexion, and extension), in contrast to disc prolapse in which lateral flexion is usually spared.

Few other conditions give rise to the spinal rig-

Table 29.4 Differential diagnosis between ankylosing hyperostosis and ankylosing spondylitis: summary of clinical and radiological findings. (After Forestier & Lagier, 1971.)

Feature	Ankylosing hyperostosis	Ankylosing spondylitis
Age	Elderly and aged	Adolescents and young adults
Pain	Mild dorsolumbar pain; root pain rare	Night pain at onset; frequent thoracic lumbar, and sciatic pain
Posture	Normal or slight kyphosis	Pronounced kyphosis in 60% of patients
Spinal rigidity	Slight stiffness in dorsal spine; lumbar and cervical spine mobility normal	Ascending lumbar rigidity leading to total spinal stiffness
Chest expansion	According to age	Progressive diminution
Incapacity	Moderate	Variable, sometimes considerable
ESR	Normal	Elevated in 75% of patients
Vertebral bodies	Continuous and thick outgrowth on lateral and oblique views which extends over the entire height of the vertebral bodies. No osteoporosis	Initial rarefying stage at the vertebral angles; squaring of vertebrae; syndesmophytes on PA view. Osteoporosis
Apophyseal joints	Normal	Joint space partially or completely obliterated
Sacroiliac joints	Normal	Bilateral erosive changes often leading to effacement of joint space

idity and postural abnormality observed in ankylosing spondylitis. However, in advanced Parkinsonism the clinical appearance may superficially resemble spondylitis. Rare and still poorly understood disorders of muscle such as the 'Stiff man syndrome' (Gordon et al 1967) and the 'Rigid spine syndrome' (Dubowitz, 1973), may also give rise to marked truncal rigidity, but in these syndromes there is an associated electromyographic abnormality.

MANAGEMENT AND TREATMENT

The management of ankylosing spondylitis may be considered under four headings:

1. Physical measures and appliances
2. Medication
3. Irradiation
4. Surgery.

In general, the management and treatment of uncomplicated spondylitis is the same as that of the spondylitis complicating psoriasis, Reiter's disease, and inflammatory bowel disease.

Physical measures and appliances

Patients should be encouraged to exercise in order to prevent postural abnormality and also to prevent limitation of movement of the spine, chest, and peripheral joints. The exercise régime is usually taught initially by the physiotherapist and later continued at home. Exercises should include the following:

a. Breathing exercises to encourage apical, costal and diaphragmatic breathing.
b. Static (isometric) muscle contraction to strengthen quadriceps, glutei, abdominal muscles, and rhomboids.
c. Lying prone on bed or floor to prevent hip flexion deformity.
d. Neck movements and shoulder shrugging exercises.
e. Arm exercises, particularly of the elbow-circling type.
f. Postural discipline while sitting, standing and walking.
g. Swimming. This is an excellent form of general exercise for all muscle groups. The breast-stroke is particularly good for the thorax and hips. The crawl is principally a chest exercise, and sculling provides exercise for all muscle groups. High diving should be prohibited in view of the increased danger of cervical injury.
h. The bed should have a firm, supported mattress, and preferably no pillow. However, if patients cannot tolerate this, one pillow should be allowed. The chair should have a firm, upright, high back.
i. Trunk exercises are not included in this scheme as most patients with early disease do these automatically as part of their normal daily routine.

In most patients with early postural deformities, these can be corrected by exercise alone. Spinal braces are usually reserved for patients with more severe disease and with deformities that cannot be corrected by exercise alone. Severe postural defects have been successfully reduced by means of the divided plaster bed (Rose, 1961), the halo splint (Perry & Nickel, 1959), and by methods of skull traction (Lee, 1963).

Further appliances that may help the severe spondylitic include:

a. Prismatic spectacles to extend the visual field in patients with gross kyphosis
b. Adjustable mirror for attachment to the bed in order to provide the patient with an improved view of his surroundings
c. A device consisting of two convex mirrors placed at right angles which may be fixed to the motor car bonnet to improve vision to left and right, particularly at road junctions (Derini, 1973).

In order to consolidate therapeutic advice to patients, and also to provide good general advice about the disease, the illustrated handbook produced by the Arthritis and Rheumatism Council (ARC, 1979) is recommended.

If the patient has problems with sexual intercourse because of hip or spinal rigidity, another handbook of value is *Marriage, Sex and Arthritis*, also produced by the Arthritis and Rheumatism Council (ARC, 1972).

Medication

The aim of medication is to reduce pain, stiffness and inflammation. Many different analgesic anti-inflammatory preparations are useful in ankylosing spondylitis; these include phenylbutazone,* indomethacin and aspirin. Some physicians consider aspirin the drug of first choice, particularly in mild cases, but others prefer phenylbutazone (100–300 mg daily), or indomethacin (100–150 mg daily). Both phenylbutazone and indomethacin are available in suppository form, and given at night this is a useful route of administration if nocturnal pain or morning stiffness are troublesome.

Phenylbutazone is particularly useful and has a remarkable specificity for symptomatic relief in ankylosing spondylitis. A small proportion of patients with ankylosing spondylitis seem to be completely refractory to the effect of phenylbutazone. The drug is contraindicated in patients with renal, cardiac or peptic disease. In a study of the side-effects of phenylbutazone (Wright, 1975) among 736 patients, 5.7% were found to have dyspepsia, 1.5% had oral ulceration and 1.5% had fluid retention. Skin eruptions, peptic ulceration, vertigo, insomnia and visual disturbances may also occur. Chromosomal abnormalities have also been found in patients taking phenylbutazone (Stevenson et al, 1971), but it is still too early to assess the importance of this observation.

In view of the possibility of dyspepsia, there may be a case for the routine use of the enteric form of phenylbutazone for long-term therapy.

Fowler (1967) has shown in a national survey that agranulocytosis may occur early in treatment, but that aplastic anaemia is related to the duration of treatment with phenylbutazone and also to the age of the patient (higher frequencies of aplastic anaemia having been found in elderly patients). Toxic effects also increase with the dose as well as with the duration of treatment with phenylbutazone, and in view of the fact that blood levels do not increase once the recommended dose has been reached, it is pointless and may be harmful to exceed conventional doses. (The higher prevalence of phenylbutazone-induced marrow suppression in past years was undoubtedly due to the much higher doses — often over 1 g/day — that were in popular use at this time.) Most patients can be adequately controlled on 300 mg daily, and usually a dose of 100 mg appears to be sufficient once control has been established.

Indomethacin has been found to give results comparable with phenylbutazone in ankylosing spondylitis (Godfrey et al, 1972). Treatment is usually started with capsules of 25 mg three times daily, and increased if necessary to 150 mg daily. A portion of the dose may usefully be given in suppository form (100 mg). If the suppositories are not retained or give rise to local irritation, two 50 mg capsules may be given instead. More recently a 75 mg sustained-release capsule has been marketed. This may be given at night instead of suppositories in patients with prominent night pain and morning stiffness. Some patients prefer capsules on aesthetic grounds. Side-effects include headache, dizziness, dyspepsia, drowsiness, faintness, feelings of drunkenness and rashes. Side-effects, including the commonest, headache and dizziness, often subside on persisting with treatment.

Hill & Hill (1973) have shown naproxen (500 mg daily) to be another effective agent in the treatment of ankylosing spondylitis. 22 of 30 patients found the drug equal or superior to previous therapy (including phenylbutazone and indomethacin).

Since the Hills' work on naproxen many other non-steroidal anti-inflammatory agents have been tested in spondylitic patients (e.g. ibuprofen, flurbiprofen, ketoprofen, diclofenac, fenclofenac, azapropazone, feprazone, flufenamic acid, sulindac), and the whole question of therapeutics in this disorder has been recently reviewed in detail (Hill, 1980). In summary, however, no 'new magic' has appeared since the last edition of this book was published.

Gold and antimalarials are not usually helpful in ankylosing spondylitis compared with their effect in rheumatoid arthritis. Systemic steroids or ACTH are not used routinely, but are sometimes useful in severe, progressive disease uncontrolled by other measures. Local corticosteroids may be the treatment of choice for the control of iritis. Their intra-articular injection is governed by the same principles as in rheumatoid arthritis.

* Now restricted in the UK to patients under hospital control.

Irradiation

Irradiation, although popular a few years ago, has now fallen into disrepute in view of the increased rates of aplastic anaemia, leukaemia, and other malignancies attributed to this form of therapy. Court Brown & Abbatt (1955) and Court Brown & Doll (1965) have estimated that the risk of developing leukaemia after radiotherapy is ten times that of non-irradiated patients or of the general population. Separate studies have shown that demonstrable marrow aplasia during the first 6 months after radiotherapy occurs in almost all patients, and that regeneration is incomplete for as long as 14 years (Steward & Dische, 1956). It has also been reported that such treatment induces extensive chromosomal damage in blood leucocytes, and that this may persist after exposure for 5 years or even longer (Buckton et al, 1962).

The transverse myelitis that has been observed after radiotherapy of the spine (Cruickshank, 1960) should not occur if the dose is kept within the range normally used for treatment of malignant disease (Brewin, 1973).

Nowadays radiotherapy to the spine is reserved only for special cases not responding to safer and more conventional treatment. In these patients the dose should not exceed 1500 r. Radiation may also have a place in the treatment of localised extraspinal areas such as painful hip involvement.

Surgery

Flexion deformity of the spine may be corrected by posterior spinal osteotomy in the middle or upper lumbar region. The technique was first described by Smith et al (1945). Several modifications of the original procedure have evolved over the years (Chapelle, 1946; Briggs, 1947; Herbert, 1948; Adams, 1952). In England, results of one of the most experienced workers in this field have revealed a 13% mortality from this operation (Law, 1952). Among the major complications in straightening the spine by this method are gastric dilatation (due to stretching of the superior mesenteric artery over the third part of the duodenum) and abdominal ileus. Principally because of neck rigidity, the danger of aspirating vomit in these patients is very real (Simmons, 1971). It is generally agreed that in its present form the operation should be restricted to skilful and experienced surgeons, and only used in clinical situations that are uncontrollable by other means.

Severe involvement of the hips, with flexion deformity unresponsive to traction and other physical measures, can often be improved by arthroplasty. The procedure of choice until recently has been the cup (mould) arthroplasty (Law, 1948; Bickel & Bryan, 1966; Calabro, 1968). However, in view of the problem of reankylosis of the hip joint which often occurs after cup arthroplasty (Law, 1948, 1952; Schwartzmann, 1959), total hip replacement has become more popular in patients with ankylosing spondylitis (Fig. 29.17). In the series of Welch & Charnley (1970) no postoperative reankylosis oc-

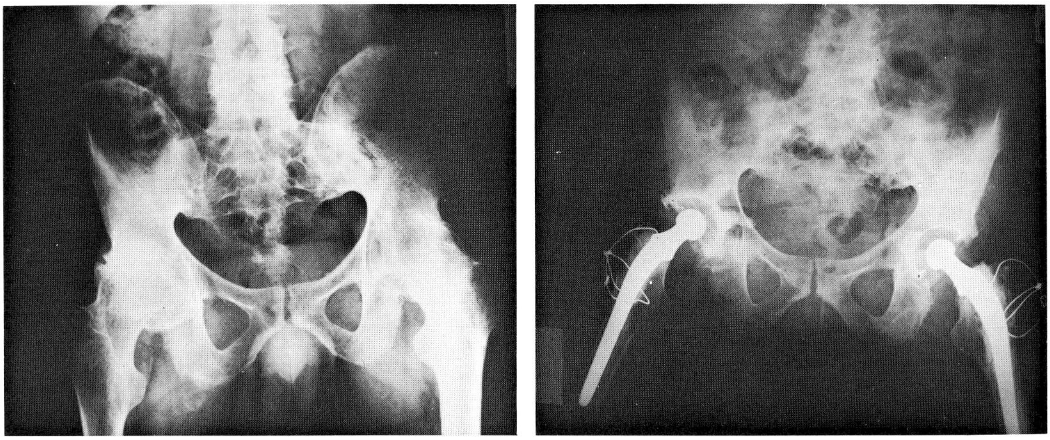

A B

Fig. 29.17 (A) Patient with advanced ankylosing spondylitis with bilateral hip involvement. (B) Same patient after Charnley arthroplasty.

curred in 33 total hip replacements in patients with ankylosing spondylitis, despite the fact that 23.5% of these patients had ankylosed hip joints preoperatively.

SUMMARY AND CONCLUSIONS

The classical epidemiological, clinical, radiological and laboratory features of ankylosing spondylitis have been described, and newer developements in the fields of aetiopathogenesis, diagnosis, and management have been reported. These last may be summarised as follows:

Aetiopathogenesis. In recent years the place of ankylosing spondylitis as the key disorder in the spondarthritis concept has continued to gain strength, not least through histocompatibility (HLA) studies. These have not only helped to clarify the immunogenetics of ankylosing spondylitis itself, but have also supported earlier epidemiological and clinicoradiological evidence pointing to associations between spondylitis and other members of the spondarthritis group (see Ch. 28). Furthermore, evidence is now emerging to indicate abnormalities of immune response in ankylosing spondylitis. However, the precise nature of the aetiopathogenesis remains unclear, although it is possible that the disease may be triggered by environmental factors such as certain microorganisms (e.g. *Klebsiella*) in patients with a genetic predisposition. Immunological factors may then contribute to perpetuation of the disease.

Diagnosis. Despite the availability of newer techniques such as scintigraphy, axial tomography, and histocompatibility typing for HLA-B27, the bedrock of diagnosis continues to be clinical observation coupled with conventional radiographical assessment for sacroiliitis. To offset the tendency by some clinicians to regard the HLA-B27 antigens as a useful index in clinical diagnosis (as opposed to its value as a research tool) it has been stressed that whereas most patients with ankylosing spondylitis carry the antigen, most people who carry it do not suffer from spondylitis.

Management. The principles of management have not changed in recent years, and remain firmly based on a vigorous approach to exercise, analgesic/anti-inflammatory drugs (when necessary), and surgery for patients with severe disability due to hip and/or spinal disease. Radiotherapy continues to be viewed with circumspection in view of the well-established long-term risks of malignant disease. However, its use may be justified in special circumstances to treat localised peripheral inflammatory events in areas unlikely to expose bone marrow to irradiation. Although several new non-steroidal analgesic/anti-inflammatory drugs have been shown to be helpful in controlling ankylosing spondylitis, none has been shown to be therapeutically superior to 'classical' drugs such as phenylbutazone or indomethacin, although some may be attended by fewer and less serious side-effects. Despite abortive thrusts in this direction, the need continues for a long-term suppressant (disease-modulating) drug for ankylosing spondylitis.

REFERENCES

Abel M S 1950 Sacroiliac joint changes in traumatic paraplegics. Radiology 55:235

Abramson D J, Kamberg S 1949 Spondylitis, pathological ossification and calcification associated with spinal-cord injury. Journal of Bone and Joint Surgery 31A:275

Adams J C 1952 Technique, dangers and safeguards in osteotomy of the spine. Journal of Bone and Joint Surgery 34B:226

Adler E, Carmon A 1961 Ankylosing spondylitis — a review of 115 cases. Acta Rheumatologica Scandinavica 7:219

Ansell B M, Bywaters E G L, Doniach I 1958 The aortic lesion of ankylosing spondylitis. British Heart Journal 20:507

Arnett F C, Schacter B Z, Hochberg M C, Hsu S H, Bias W B 1977 Homozygosity for HLA-B27: impact on rheumatic disease expression in two families. Arthritis and Rheumatism 20:797

Arnett F C, Hochberg M C, Bias W B 1978 HLA-C Locus antigens in HLA-B27 associated arthritis. Arthritis and Rheumatism 21:885

Arthritis and Rheumatism Council 1979 Ankylosing spondylitis: A handbook for patients. Rheumatism Council, London

Arthritis and Rheumatism Council 1972 Marriage, sex and arthritis. Prepared by the Arthritis and Rheumatism Council with the collaboration of W Greengross. Arthritis and Rheumatism Council, London

Aufdermaur M 1957 The morbid anatomy of ankylosing spondylitis. In: Documenta rheumatologica geigy, No 2. Geigy, Basle

Ball G V, Hathaway B 1966 Ankylosing spondylitis with widespread arteritis. Arthritis and Rheumatism 9:743

Ball J 1954 Rheumatoid arthritis and polyarteritis nodosa. Annals of the Rheumatic Diseases 13:277

Ball J 1971 Enthesopathy of rheumatoid and ankylosing spondylitis. Annals of the Rheumatic Diseases 30:213

Batson O V 1940 The function of the vertebral veins and their role in the spread of metastases. Annals of Surgery 112:138

Batson O V 1942a Role of the vertebral veins in metastatic processes. Annals of Internal Medicine 16:38

Batson O V 1942b Vertebral vein system as mechanism for spread of metastases. American Journal of Roentgenology 48:715

Baum J, Ziff M 1971 The rarity of ankylosing spondylitis in the black race. Arthritis and Rheumatism 14:12

Bechterev V M 1893 Steifigkeit der Wirbelsäule und ihre Verkrümmung als besondere Erkrankungsform. Neurologisches Centralblatt 12:426

Bennett P H, Wood P H N 1968 Population studies of the rheumatic diseases Proceedings of the 3rd International Symposium, New York, 1966 Excerpta Medica Foundation, Amsterdam, p 456

Berghs H, Remans J, DriesKens L, Kiebooms L, Polderman J 1978 Diagnostic value of sacroiliac joint scintigraphy with 99^m technetium pyrophosphate in sacroiliitis. Annals of the Rheumatic Diseases 37:190

Bickel W H, Bryan R S 1966 Results of cup arthroplasty of the hip in patients with rheumatoid arthritis and ankylosing spondylitis. Surgery, Gynecology and Obstetrics 123:243

Bienenstock H, Lanyi V F 1977 Cricoarytenoid arthritis in a patient with ankylosing spondylitis. Archives of Otolaryngology 103:738

Birkbeck M Q, Buckler W St J, Mason R M, Tegner W S 1951 Iritis as the presenting symptom in ankylosing spondylitis. Lancet 2:802

Blécourt J J de 1972 533 patients with ankylosing spondylitis, seen and followed in the period 1948–1971. Heberden Society, London

Bluestone R, Bywaters E G L, Hartog M, Holt P J I, Hyde S 1971 Acromegalic arthropathy. Annals of the Rheumatic Diseases 30:243

Blumberg B, Ragan C 1956 The natural history of rheumatoid spondylitis. Medicine 35:1

Boland E W, Shebesta E M 1946 Rheumatoid spondylitis: correlation of clinical and roentgenographic features. Radiology 47:551

Böni A, Hauptmann F 1950 Familiares Vorkommen von Morbus Bechterew in der Schweiz. Zeitsschrift für Rheumaforschung 9:273

Bowie E A, Glasgow G L 1961 Cauda equina lesions associated with ankylosing spondylitis. Report of three cases. British Medical Journal 2:24

Brautbar C, Porat S, Netken D, Gabriel K, Cohen R 1977 HLA B27 and ankylosing spondylitis in the Israeli population. Journal of Rheumatology 4 (Suppl 3):24

Brewerton D A, Caffrey M, Hart D F, James D C O, Nicholls A, Sturrock R D 1973 Ankylosing spondylitis and HL-A27. Lancet 1:904

Brewin T B 1973 Personal communication

Briggs H, Keats S, Schlesinger P T 1947 Wedge osteotomy of the spine. Journal of Bone and Joint Surgery 29:1074

Buckton K E, Jacobs P A, Court Brown W M, Doll R 1962 A study of the chromosome damage persisting after X-ray therapy for ankylosing spondylitis. Lancet 2:676

Bywaters E G L, Dixon A St J 1965 Paravertebral ossification in psoriatic arthritis. Annals of the Rheumatic Diseases 24:313

Bywaters E G L, Hamilton E B D, Williams R 1971 The spine in idiopathic haemochromatosis. Annals of the Rheumatic Diseases 30:453

Calabro J J 1968 An appraisal of the medical and surgical management of ankylosing spondylitis. Clinical Orthopaedics 60:125

Calguneri M, Swinburne L, Shinebaum R, Cooke E M, Wright V 1981 Secretory IgA: immune defence pattern in ankylosing spondylitis and Klebsiella. Annals of the Rheumatic Diseases 40:600

Calin A, Bennett P H, Jupiter J, Terasaki P I 1977 HLA B27 and sacroiliitis in Pima Indians — association in males only. Journal of Rheumatology 4 (Suppl 3):44

Campbell A H, Macdonald C B 1965 Upper lobe fibrosis associated with ankylosing spondylitis. British Journal of Diseases of the Chest 59:90

Cawley M I D, Chalmers T M, Kellgren J H, Ball J 1972 Destructive lesions of vertebral bodies in ankylosing spondylitis. Annals of the Rheumatic Diseases 31:345

Catterall R D 1960 Uveitis, arthritis and non-specific genital infection. British Journal of Venereal Diseases, 36:27

Catterall R D, Perkins E S 1961 Uveitis and urogenital disease in the male. British Journal of Ophthalmology, 45:109

Chalmers I M, Lentle B C, Percy J S, Russell A S 1979. Sacroiliitis detected by bone scintiscanning: a clinical, radiological, and scintigraphic follow-up study. Annals of the Rheumatic Diseases 38:112

Chapelle E H La 1946 Osteotomy of the lumbar spine for correction of kyphosis in a case of ankylosing spondylarthritis. Journal of Bone and Joint Surgery 28:851

Cheshire D J E, Nichols P J R 1955 The early stages of ankylosing spondylitis. Rheumatism 11:79

Clark W S, Bauer W 1948 Cardiac changes in rheumatoid arthritis. Annals of the Rheumatic Diseases 7:39

Clark W S, Kulka J P, Bauer W 1957 Rheumatoid aortitis with aortic regurgitation: unusual manifestation of rheumatoid arthritis (including spondylitis). American Journal of Medicine 22:580

Cliff J M 1971 Spinal bony bridging and carditis in Reiter's disease. Annals of the Rheumatic Diseases 30:171

Cohen A A, Natelson E A, Fechner R E 1971 Fibrosing interstitial pneumonitis in ankylosing spondylitis. Chest 59:369

Connor B 1691 Sur la continuité de plusieurs' os, a l'occasion d'un trone de squelette humain, òu les vertèbres, les côtes, l'os sacrum, et les os des iles, qui naturellements son distincts et separés, ne font qu'un seul os continu et inséperable. MD Thesis, Rheims

Contu L, Capelli P, Sale S 1977 HLA B27 and ankylosing spondylitis: population and family studies in Sardinia. Journal of Rheumatology 4 (Suppl 3):18

Copeman W S C 1964 A short history of the gout and the rheumatic diseases. University of California Press, Berkeley, p 174

Corrigall V, Panayi G S, Unger A, Poston R N, William B D 1978 Detection of immune complexes in serum of patients with ankylosing spondylitis. Annals of the Rheumatic Diseases 37:159

Court Brown W M, Abbatt J D 1955 The incidence of leukaemia in ankylosing spondylitis treated with X-rays. A preliminary report. Lancet 1:1283

Court Brown W M, Doll R 1957 Leukaemia and aplastic anaemia in patients irradiated for ankylosing spondylitis.

Special Report Series, No 295. Medical Research Council, London
Court Brown W M, Doll R 1965 Mortality from cancer and other causes after radiotherapy for ankylosing spondylitis. British Medical Journal 2:1327
Cowling P, Ebringer R, Cawdell D, Ishii M, Ebringer A 1980a C-reactive protein, ESR, and Klebsiella in ankylosing spondylitis. Annals of the Rheumatic Diseases 39:45
Cowling P, Ebringer R, Ebringer A 1980b Association of inflammation with raised serum IgA in ankylosing spondylitis. Annals of the Rheumatic Diseases 39:545
Crooks J, Murray I P C, Wayne E J 1959 Statistical methods applied to the clinical diagnosis of thyrotoxicosis. Quarterly Journal of Medicine 28:211
Cruickshank B 1951 Histopathology of diarthrodial joints in ankylosing spondylitis. Annals of the Rheumatic Diseases 10:393
Cruickshank B 1960 Pathology of ankylosing spondylitis. Bulletin on the Rheumatic Diseases 10:211
Cruickshank B 1971 Pathology of ankylosing spondylitis. Clinical Orthopaedics and Related Research 74:43
Cumming W J K, Saunders M 1978 Radiculopathy as a complication of ankylosing spondylitis. Journal of Neurology, Neurosurgery and Psychiatry 41:569
Daneo V, Migone N, Modena V, Bianchi S D, Alfieri G, Diotallevi P et al 1977 Family studies and HLA typing in ankylosing spondylitis and sacroiliitis. Journal of Rheumatology 4 (Suppl 3):5
Darke C S 1975 Personal communication
Davatchi F, Nikbin B, Ala F 1977 Histocompatibility antigens (HLA) in rheumatic diseases in Iran. Journal of Rheumatology 4 (Suppl 3):36
Davidson P, Bagenstoss A H, Slocum C H, Daugherty G W 1963 Cardiac and aortic lesions in rheumatoid spondylitis. Proceedings of Staff Meetings, Mayo Clinic 38:427
Davies D 1972 Ankylosing spondylitis and lung fibrosis. Quarterly Journal of Medicine 41:395
Dejelo C L, Braun W E, Khan M A, Clough J D 1978. HLA-DR antigens and ankylosing spondylitis. Transplant Proceedings 10:971
Derini M S 1975 Personal communication
Dilsen N, McEwen C, Poppel M, Gersh W J, Ditata D, Carmel P 1962 A comparative roentgenologic study of rheumatoid arthritis and rheumatoid (ankylosing) spondylitis. Arthritis and Rheumatism 5:341
Dixon J S, Bird H A, Wright V 1981 A comparison of serum biochemistry in ankylosing spondylitis, seronegative and seropositive rheumatoid arthritis. Annals of the Rheumatic Diseases 40:404
Dodson V N, Dinman B D, Whitehouse W M, Nast A N, Magnuson H J 1971 Occupational acro-osteolysis. 3. A clinical study. Archives of Environmental Health 22:83
Domeij-Nyberg B, Kjällman M, Nylén O, Pettersson N-O 1980 The reliability of quantitative bone scanning in sacro-iliitis. Scandinavian Journal of Rheumatology 9:77
Dory M A, Francois R J 1978 Craniocaudal axial view of sacroiliac joint. American Journal of Roentgenology 130:1125
Dubowitz V 1973 Rigid spine syndrome: muscle syndrome in search of a name. Proceedings of the Royal Society of Medicine 66:219
Duquesnoy R J, Kozin F, Rodney G E 1978 High prevalence of HLA-B27 Cw1 and Cw2 in patients with seronegative spondyloarthritis. Tissue Antigens 12:58
Durrigl T, Mezulic L, Androic A, Vitaus M 1965 Anylosing spondylitis — clinical examination. Rheumatism 21:79
Duvernoy W F C, Schatz I J 1966 Rheumatoid spondylitis associated with aneurysmal dilatation of the entire thoracic aorta. Henry Ford Hospital Medical Bulletin 14:309
Eastmond C J, Woodrow J C 1977 Discordance for ankylosing spondylitis in monozygotic twins. Annals of the Rheumatic Diseases 36:360
Eastmond C J, Willshaw H E, Burgess S E P, Shinebaum R, Cooke E M, Wright V 1980 Frequency of faecal Klebsiella aerogenes in patients with ankylosing spondylitis and controls with respect to individual features of the disease. Annals of the Rheumatic Diseases 39:118
Eastmond C J, Calguneri M, Shinebaum R, Cooke E M, Wright V 1982 A sequential study of the relationship between faecal Klebsiella aerogenes and the common clinical manifestations of ankylosing spondylitis. Annals of the Rheumatic Diseases 41:15
Ebringer R, Cooke D, Cawdell D R, Cowling P, Ebringer A 1977 Ankylosing spondylitis: Klebsiella and HLA B27. Rheumatology and Rehabilitation 16:190
Ebringer R, Cawdell D R, Cowling P, Ebringer A 1978 Sequential studies in ankylosing spondylitis: association of Klebsiella pneumoniae with active disease. Annals of the Rheumatic Diseases 37:146
Emery A E, Lawrence J S 1967 Genetics of ankylosing spondylitis. Journal of Medical Genetics 4:239
Erhardt O 1905 Uber chronische ankylosierende Wirbelsäulenversteifung. Mitteilungen aus den Grenzgebieten der medizin und chirurgie 14:726
Ford D K 1953 Natural history of arthritis following venereal urethritis. Annals of the Rheumatic Diseases 12:177
Forestier J 1931 Le diagnostic des rheumatismes vertebraux d'apres les methodes modernes d'examen. Presse thermale et climatique 72:268
Forestier J, Jacqueline F, Rotés-Querol J 1951 La spondylarthrite ankylosante. Masson & Cie, Paris
Fowler P D 1967 Marrow toxicity of the pyrazoles. Annals of the Rheumatic Diseases 26:344
Foxworthy D T, Montogomary M M, Barton E M 1960 Rheumatoid (ankylosing) spondylitis and osteochondritis of a lumbar vertebra in identical twins. Arthritis and Rheumatism 3:444
Francis M D, Flora L, King W R 1972 The effects of disodium ethane-1-hydorxy-1, 1-diphosphonate on adjuvant induced arthritis in rats. Calcified Tissue Research 9:109
Gabay R, Zubler R H, Nydegger U E, Lambert P H 1977 Immune complexes and complement catabolism in ankylosing spondylitis. Arthritis and Rheumatism 20:913
Gelman M I, Umber J S 1978 Fractures of thoracolumbar spine in ankylosing spondylitis. American Journal of Roentgenology 130:485
Godfrey R G, Calabro J J, Mills D, Maltz B A 1972 A double-blind crossover trial of aspirin, indomethacin and phenylbutazone in ankylosing spondylitis. Arthritis and Rheumatism 15:110
Gofton J P, Lawrence J S, Bennett P H, Burch T A 1966 Sacro-iliitis in eight populations. Annals of the Rheumatic Diseases 25:528
Goldberg R P, Genant H K, Shimshak R, Shames D 1978 Application and limitation of quantitative sacroiliac joint scintigraphy. Radiology 128:683
Good A E 1963 The chest pain of ankylosing spondylitis. Its place in the differential diagnosis of heart pain. Annals of Internal Medicine 58:926

Good A E 1967 Nontraumatic fracture of the thoracic spine in ankylosing spondylitis. Arthritis and Rheumatism 10:467
Good A E, Casidy J T, Mutchnik M G, Reed R E, Lederman H M 1977 Ankylosing spondylitis with selective IgA deficiency and a circulating anticoagulant. Journal of Rheumatology 4:297
Good A E, Keller T S, Weatherbee L, Braunstein E M 1982 Spinal cord block with a destructive lesion of the dorsal spine in ankylosing spondylitis. Arthritis and Rheumatism 25:218
Goodman G B 1956 Radiation leucopenia in ankylosing spondylitis. Journal of the Faculty of Radiology 7:167
Gordon E E, Januszko D M, Kaufman I 1967 A critical survey of the stiff man syndrome. American Journal of Medicine 42:582
Graber-Duvernay J 1951 Ankylosing spondylarthritis (rhizomelic spondylosis) of traumatic origin. Rheumatism 7:49
Graham D C 1960 Ankylosing spondylitis. Canadian Medical Association Journal 82:671
Graham D C, Smythe H A 1958 The carditis and aortitis of ankylosing spondylitis. Bulletin on the rheumatic Diseases 9:171
Graham W, Uchida I A 1957 Heredity in ankylosing spondylitis. Annals of the Rheumatic Diseases 16:334
Grainger R G 1957 Radiological aspects of sacro-iliac arthritis. Proceedings of the Royal Society of Medicine 50:854
Guest C M, Jacobson H G 1951 Pelvic and extrapelvic osteopathy in rheumatoid spondylitis. A Clinical and roentgenographic study of 90 cases. American Journal of Roentgenology 65:760
Gupta S M, Johnston W H 1978 Apical pulmonary disease in ankylosing spondylitis. New Zealand Medical Jouranl 88:186
Hamilton K A 1949 Pulmonary disease manifestations of ankylosing spondylarthritis. Annals of Internal Medicine 31:216
Hart F D 1954 Ankylosing spondylitis: A survey. Annals of the Rheumatic Diseases 13:186
Hart F D, Robinson K C 1959 Ankylosing spondylitis in women. Annals of the Rheumatic Diseases 18:15
Hart F D, Robinson K C, Allchin F M, Maclagan N F 1949 Ankylosing spondylitis. Quarterly Journal of Medicine 18:217
Hauge T 1961 Chronic rheumatoid polyarthritis and spondylarthritis associated with neurological symptoms and signs occasionally simulating an intraspinal expansive process. Acta Chirurgica Scandinavica 120:395
Herbert J J 1948 Vertebral osteostomy. Journal of Bone and Joint Surgery 30A:680
Hersch A H, Stecher R M, Solomon W M, Wolpaw R, Hauser H 1950 Heredity in ankylosing spondylitis; study of 50 families. American Journal of Human Genetics 2:391
Hill A G S 1980 Drug therapy. In: Moll J M H (ed) Ankylosing spondylitis. Churchill Livingstone, Edinburgh, Ch 14, p 163–175
Hill H F H, Hill A G S 1973 Naproxen in ankylosing spondylitis. Scandinavian Journal of Rheumatology 2:121
Hinman F 1935 The principles and practice of urology. Saunders, Philadelphia, p 111
Hochberg M C, Bias W B, Arnett F C 1978 Family studies in HLA-B27 associated arthritis. Medicine 57:463
Hoffman F G, Leight I 1965 Complete atrio-ventricular block associated with rheumatoid arthritis. American Journal of Cardiology 16:585
Hollin S A, Gross S W, Levin P 1965 Fracture of the cervical spine in paitents with rheumatoid spondylitis. American Surgeon 31:532
Hollingsworth P N, Cheah P S, Dawkins R L, Owen E T, Calin A, Wood P H 1983 Observer variation in grading sacroiliac radiographs in HLA-B27 positive individuals. Journal of Rheumatology 10:247
Horwitz M T, Smith R M 1940 Anatomical, pathological and roentgenological study of intervertebral joints of lumbar spine and of sacroiliac joints. American Journal of Roentgenology 43:173
Hunter T, Dubo 1978 Spinal fractures complicating ankylosing spondylitis. Annals of Internal Medicine 88:546
Jessamine A G 1968 Upper lung lobe fibrosis in ankylosing spondylitis. Canadian Medical Association Journal 98:25
Julkunen H, Luomanmäki M 1964 Complete heart-block in rheumatoid (ankylosing) spondylitis. Acta Medica Scandinavica 176:401
Junghanns H, Henke H, Lubarsch O (eds) 1939 Handbuch der speziellen pathologischen Anatomic and Histologie. Springer Berlin, Vol 9, Ch 4
Kellgren J H 1964 The epidemiology of rheumatic diseases. Annals of the Rheumatic Diseases 23:109
Kellgren J H, Ball J 1959 Clinical significance of the rheumatoid serum factor. British Medical Journal 1:523
Kellgren J H, Jeffrey M R, Ball J (eds) 1963 The Epidemiology of Chronic Rheumatism. Blackwell, Oxford, Vol 1, p 326
Khan M A, Kushner I, Braun W E 1977 Comparison of clinical features in HLA B27-positive and -negative patients with ankylosing spondylitis. Arthritis and Rheumatism 20:909
Khan M A, Braun W E, Kushner I, Grecek D E, Muir W A, Steinberg A G 1977 HLA B27 in ankylosing spondylitis: differences in frequency and relative risk in American Blacks and Caucasians. Journal of Rheumatology 4 (Suppl 3):39
Khan M A, Kushner I, Braun W E 1978 Subgroup of ankylosing spondylitis associated with HLA-B7 in American blacks. Arthritis and Rheumatism 21:528
Khan M A, Kushner I, Braun W E, Zachary A A, Steinberg A G 1978 HLA-B27 homozygosity in ankylosing spondylitis: relationships to risk and severity. Tissue Antigens 11:434
Khan M A, Khan M K, Kushner I 1981 Survival among patients with ankylosing spondylitis: a life-table analysis. The Journal of Rheumatology 8:86
Kornblum D, Clayton M L, Naish H H 1952 Non-traumatic cervical dislocations in rheumatoid spondylitis. Journal of the American Medical Association 149:431
Kornstad A M, Kornstad L 1960 Ankylosing spondylitis in two families showing involvement of female members only, with a search for linkage to genes determining blood group antigens. Acta Rheumatologica Scandinavia 6:59
Kozin F, Duquesnoy R, Rodey G E, lightfood R W, Ryan L M 1978 High prevalence of HLA-Cw1 and Cw2 antigens in spondylarthritis. Arthritis and Rheumatism 21:889
Krebs W 1934 Das Rötgenbild des Bechens bei der Bechterewschen Krankheit. Fortschritte auf dem Gebiete der Röntgenstrahlen 50:537
Ladd J R, Cassidy J T, Martel W 1971 Juvenile ankylosing spondylitis. Arthritis and Rheumatism 14:579
Latham B A 1965 Ankylosing spondylitis. Bulletin of the

Post-Graduate Committee in Medicine, University of Sydney 20:294
Law W A 1948 Post-operative study of the vitallium mold arthroplasty of the hip joint. Journal of Bone and Joint Surgery 30B:76
Law W A 1952 Surgical treatment of the rheumatic diseases. Journal of Bone and Joint Surgery 34B:215
Leading article 1971 The lungs in ankylosing spondylitis. British Medical Journal 3:492
Lee M I H 1963 Orthopaedic problems in ankylosing spondylitis. Rheumatism 19:79
Lentle B C, Russell A S, Percy J S, Jackson F E 1977a Scintigraphic findings in ankylosing spondylitis. Journal of Nuclear Medicine 18:524
Lentle B C, Russell A S, Percy J S, Jackson F E 1977b Scintigraphic investigation of sacroiliac disease. Journal of Nuclear Medicine 18:529
Lodge T 1956 Bone, joint and soft tissue changes following paraplegia. Acta Radiologica (Stockholm) 46:435
Loebl W Y 1967 Measurement of spinal posture and range of spinal movement. Annals of Physical Medicine 9:103
London M G, Bland J H 1963 Ankylosing spondylitis with subcutaneous nodules. New England Journal of Medicine 268:991
Ludwig A O, Short C L, Bauer W 1943 Rheumatoid arthritis as a cause of increased cerebrospinal-fluid protein — a study of one hundred and one patients. New England Journal of Medicine 228:306
Macrae I F, Wright V 1969 Measurement of back movement. Annals of the Rheumatic Diseases 28:584
Macrae I F, Haslock D I, Wright V 1971 Grading of films for sacro-iliitis in population studies. Annals of the Rheumatic Diseases 30:58
Malawista S E, Seegmiller J E, Hathaway B E, Sokoloff L 1965 Sacroiliac gout. Journal of the American Medical Association 194:954
Mallory T B 1936 Case records of the Massachusetts General Hospital. Case 22141 and 22142. New England Journal of Medicine 214:690
Marie P 1898 Sur la spondylose rhizomélique. Revue de Médicine 18:285
Martel W 1961 The occipito-atlanto-axial joints in rheumatoid arthritis and ankylosing spondylitis. American Journal of Roentgenology 86:223
Martel W 1978 Spinal pseudoarthrosis: a complication of ankylosing spondylitis. Arthritis and Rheumatism 21:485
Mason R M 1964 Spondylitis. Proceedings of the Royal Society of Medicine 57:533
Mason R M 1969 Ankylosing spondylitis. In: Copeman W S C (ed) 4th Edn. Textbook of the rheumatic diseases. Livingstone, Edinburgh, p 344
Mason R M, Murray R S, Oates J K, Young A C 1958 Prostatitis and ankylosing spondylitis. British Medical Journal 1:748
McEwen C, Di Tata D, Lingg C, Porini A, Good A, Rankin T 1971 Ankylosing spondylitis and spondylitis accompanying ulcerative colitis, regional enteritis, psoriasis and Reiter's disease. Arthritis and Rheumatism 14:291
McKusick V A 1972 Heritable and developmental disorders of connective tissues and bone. In: Hollander J L, McCarty D (eds) Arthritis and allied conditions. A textbook of rheumatology 8th Edn. Lea & Febiger, Philadelphia, p 1352
Mettler C C 1947 History of medicine. Blakiston, Philadelphia
Migone N, Modena V, Carbonara A O, Ceppellini R 1978 Sacroiliitis and HLA. A clinical and genetical study. Annals of the Rheumatic Diseases 37:513
Milde E J, Aarli J, Larsen J L 1977 Cauda equina lesions in ankylosing spondylitis. Scandinavian Journal of Rheumatology 6:118
Moesmann G 1960 Hereditary and exogenous etiological factors in ankylosing spondylitis in two sets of monozygotic twins. Acta Rheumatologica Scandinavica 6:144
Moll J M H 1971 A family study of psoriatic arthritis. DM Thesis, University of Oxford
Moll J M H 1975 A diagnostic feature of spondylitis. Scandinavian Journal of Rheumatology 4 (suppl 1): Abstract 20:17
Moll J M H 1980 Diagnostic criteria and their evaluation. In: Moll J M H (ed) Ankylosing spondylitis. Churchill Livingstone, Edinburgh, Ch 12, p 137–150
Moll J MH, Wright V 1971 Normal range of spinal mobility: an objective clinical study. Annals of the Rheumatic Diseases 30:381
Moll J M H, Wright V 1972 An objective clinical study of chest expansion. Annals of the Rheumatic Diseases 31:1
Moll J M H, Wright V 1973a New York clinical criteria for ankylosing spondylitis: statistical evaluation. Annals of the Rheumatic Diseases 32:354
Moll J M H, Liyanage S P, Wright V 1972a An objective clinical method to measure lateral spinal flexion. Rheumatology and Physical Medicine 11:225
Moll J M H, Liyanage S P, Wright V 1972b An objective clinical method to measure spinal extension. Rheumatology and Physical Medicine 11:293
Namey T C, McInture J, Buse M, LeRoy E C 1977 Nucleographic studies of axial spondarthritides. I. Quantitative sacroiliac scintigraphy in early HLA-B27-associated sacroiliitis. Arthritis and Rheumatism 20:1058
Newton D R I 1957 Discussion on the clinical and radiological aspects of sacro-iliac disease. Proceedings of the Royal Society of Medicine 50:850
Niepel G A, Kostka D, Kopecky S, Manca S 1966 Enthesopathy. Acta Rheumatologica et Balneologica Pistintana, No 1
Nilsson E, Biberfeld G 1980 Subpopulations of T lymphocytes in patients with ankylosing spondylitis. Annals of the Rheumatic Diseases 39:566
O'Connell D 1956 Ankylosing spondylitis. The literature up to the close of the nineteenth century. Annals of the Rheumatic Diseases 15:119
Ogryzlo M A, Rosen P S 1969 Ankylosing (Marie–Strümpell) spondylitis. Postgraduate Medicine 45:182
Ogryzlo M A 1972 Ankylosing spondylitis. In: Hollander J L, McCarty D J (eds) Arthritis and allied conditions, 8 Edn. Lea & Febiger, Philadelphia, p 699
Øtensen M, Romberg Ø, Husby G 1982 Ankylosing spondylitis and motherhood. Arthritis and Rheumatism 25:140
Payr E 1947 Warum ist die Bechterew–Strümpell–Mariesche Krankheit fast ausschliesslich auf das Männliche Geschlecht beschränkt? Zentralblatt für Chirurgie 72:241
Pekin T J, Malinin T I, Zvaifler N J 1967 Unusual synovial fluid findings in Reiter's syndrome. Annals of Internal Medicine 66:677
Pelouze P S 1921 The role of the prostate in focal infection. Medical Record (New York) 100:412
Perry J, Nickel V L 1959 Total cervical-spine fusion for neck paralysis. Journal of Bone and Joint Surgery 41A:37

Polley H F, Slocumb C H 1947 Rheumatoid spondylitis: a study of 1035 cases. Annals of Internal Medicine 26:240
Polley H F 1955 The diagnosis and treatment of rheumatoid spondylitis. Medical Clinics of North America 39:509
Radford E P, Doll R, Smith P G 1977 Mortality among patients with ankylosing spondylitis not given X-ray therapy. New England Journal of Medicine 297:572
Rae M B 1932 Spondylitis in twins. Proceedings of the Royal Society of Medicine 25:325
Reid G D, Hill R H 1978 Atlanto-axial subluxation in juvenile ankylosing spondylitis. Journal of Pediatrics 93:531
Reuler J B, Girard D E, Nardone D A 1978 Sternoclavicular joint involvement in ankylosing spondylitis. Southern Medical Journal 71:1480
Richards A J 1974 Ankylosing spondylitis and pulmonary apical fibrosis. Proceedings of the Royal Society of Medicine 67:45
Riecker H H, Neel J V, Test A 1950 The inheritance of spondylitis rhizomélique (ankylosing spondylitis) in the K. family. Annals of Internal Medicine 33:1254
Riley M J, Ansell B M, Bywaters E G L 1971 Radiological manifestations of ankylosing spondylitis according to age at onset. Annals of the Rheumatic Diseases 30:138
Rogers M H, Cleaves E N 1935 The adolescent sacro-iliac joint syndrome. Journal of Bone and Joint Surgery 17:759
Rogoff B, Freyberg R H 1949 The familial incidence of rheumatoid spondylitis. Annals of the Rheumatic Diseases 8:139
Rolleston G L 1947 The early radiological diagnosis of ankylosing spondylitis. British Journal of Radiology 20:288
Romanus R 1953 Pelvo-spondylitis ossificans in the male (ankylosing spondylitis, morbus Bechterew–Marie–Strümpell) and genito-urinary infection; the aetiological significance of the latter and the nature of disease based on a study of 117 male patients. Godvil, Stockholm
Romanus R, Ydén S 1955 Pelvo-spondylitis ossificans. Rheumatoid or ankylosing spondylitis. A roentgenological and clinical guide to its early diagnosis (especially anterior spondylitis). Munksgaard, Copenhagen, p 22
Rose G K 1961 The surgical management of ankylosing spondylitis. Rheumatism 17:63
Rosen P S, Graham D C 1962 Ankylosing (Strümpell–Marie) spondylitis — a clinical review of 128 cases. Archives of Interamerican Rheumatology 5:158
Rosenow E C, Strimlan C V, Muhm J R, Ferguson R H 1977 Pleuropulmonary manifestations of ankylosing spondylitis. Mayo Clinics Proceedings 52:641
Rothwell R S, Davis P, Lentle B C Radionuclide bone scanning in females with chronic low back pain. Annals of the Rheumatic Diseases 40:79
Russell A S, Maksymowych W, LeClercq S 1981 Clinical examination of the sacroiliac joints: a prospective study. Arthritis and Rheumatism 24:1575
Russell M L, Gordon D A, Ogryzlo M A, McPhedran R S 1973 The cauda equina syndrome of ankylosing spondylitis. Annals of Internal Medicine 78:551
Säfwenberg J, Domeij-Nyberg B, Kjällman M 1978 HLA antigens in females with ankylosing spondylitis and other forms of seronegative rheumatic diseases. Scandinavian Journal of Rheumatology 7:177
Sashin D A 1930 A critical analysis of the anatomy and the pathologic changes of the sacro-iliac joints. Journal of Bone and Joint Surgery 12:891
Savage O 1942 Management of rheumatic diseases in the forces. British Medical Journal 2:336
Schilder D P, Harvey W P, Hufnagel C A 1956 Rheumatoid spondylitis and aortic insufficiency. New England Journal of Medicine 255:11
Schlosstein L, Terasaki P I, Bluestone R, Pearson C M 1973 High association of an HL-A antigen, W27, with ankylosing spondylitis. New England Journal of Medicine 288:704
Schmorl G, & Junghanns H 1971 The human spine in health and disease, 5th Edn. Grunes Stratton, New York, p 398
Schober P 1937 Ledenwirbel säule und Kreuzschmerzen. Münchener medizinische Wochenschrift 84:336
Schurman D, Calin A, Fries J, Porta J 1977 The clinical history as a screening test for ankylosing spondylitis. In: Proceedings of the XIV International Congress of Rheumatology, San Francisco, 1977, Abstract 770. Arthritis Foundation, New York, p 181
Schwartzmann J R 1959 Arthroplasty of the hip in rheumatoid arthritis. A follow-up study of sixty-eight hips. Journal of Bone and Joint Surgery 41A:705
Scott S G 1936 Chronic infection of sacro-iliac joints as possible cause of spondylitis adolescens. British Journal of Radiology 9:126
Scott D L, Smith A H, Eastmond C J, Hayter C J, Wright V 1980. An evaluation of the techniques of sacro-iliac scintiscanning. Rheumatology and Rehabilitation 19:76
Seaman W B, Wells J 1961 Destructive lesions of the vertebral bodies in rheumatoid disease. American Journal of Roentgenology 86:241
Sharp J 1957 The differential diagnosis of ankylosing spondylitis. British Medical Journal 1:975
Sharp J 1965 Ankylosing spondylitis, a review. In: Dixon A St J (ed) Progress in clinical rheumatology. Churchill, London, p 180
Sharp J 1965 Ankylosing spondylitis, a review. In: Dixon A St J (ed) Progress in clinical rheumatology. Churchill, London, p 180
Sharp J, Easson E C E 1954 Deep X-ray therapy in spondylitis. British Medical Journal 1:619
Sharp J, Purser D W 1961 Spontaneous atlanto-axial subluxation in ankylosing spondylitis and rheumatoid arthritis. Annals of the Rheumatic Diseases 20:47
Sikora K, Webster S, Sachs J, Festenstein H 1978 Associated clinical syndromes in a patient homozygous for HLA B27. British Medical Journal 1:1184
Simmons E H 1971 Surgery of the spine in rheumatoid arthritis and ankylosing spondylitis. In: Cruess R L, Mitchell N S (eds) Surgery of rheumatoid arthritis. Lippincott, Philadelphia, p 101
Simpson N R W, Stephenson C J 1949 An analysis of 200 cases of ankylosing spondylitis. British Medical Journal 1:214
Smith Petersen N M, Larsen C B, Aufranc O E 1945 Osteotomy of the spine in rheumatoid arthritis. Journal of Bone and Joint Surgery 27:1
Smith P G, Doll R, Radford E P 1977. Cancer mortality among patients with ankylosing spondylitis not given X-ray therapy. British Journal of Radiology 50:728
Sobin I H, Hagstrom J W C 1962 Lesions of cardiac conduction tissue in rheumatoid aortitis. Journal of the American Medical Association 180:1
Spiers F W 1968 Radioisotopes in the human body: physical and biological aspects. Academic Press, New York, p 236

Stecher R M 1957 Heredity in joint diseases. Documenta Rheumatologica, No 12, Geigy, Basle, p 41

Stecher R M, Goss I J 1961 Ankylosing lesions of the spine of the horse. Journal of the American Veterinary Medical Association 138:248

Stevenson A C, Bedford J, Hill A G S, Hill H F H 1971 Chromosomal studies in patients taking phenylbutazone. Annals of the Rheumatic Diseases 30:487

Stewart J W, Dische S 1956 Effect of radiotherapy on bone marrow in ankylosing spondylitis. Lancet 2:1063

Stewart S R, Robbins D L, Castles J J 1978 Acute fulminant aortic and mitral insufficiency in ankylosing spondylitis. New England Journal of Medicine 299:1488

Strumpell A 1897 Bermerkungen uber die chronische ankylosirende Entzudung der Wirbelsäule und der Huftgelenke. Deutsche Zeitschrift für Nervenhetlkunde 11:338

Swaay H van 1950 Spondylosis Ankylopoëtica. Een Pathogentische Studie p 69. Leiden: Ijdo

Szanto E, Lindvall N 1978 Quantitative ^{99m}Tc pertechnetate scanning of the sacro-iliac joints: follow-up study of patients with suspected sacro-iliitis. Scandinavian Journal of Rheumatology 7:93

Szanto E, Axelsson B, Lindvall N 1977 Detection of sacroiliitis: a comparison between profile scanning with the use of ^{99m}Tc pertechnetate and scintigraphy with ^{99m}Tc disphosphonate. Scandinavian Journal of Rheumatology 6:129

Takkunen J, Vuopala U, Somaki H I 1970 Cardiomyopathy in ankylosing spondylitis. I. Medical history and results of clinical examination in a series of 55 patients. Annals of Clinical Research 2:106

Valkenburgh W G van, Georges I P, Irby R 1972 Aortic insufficiency and pelvo-spondylitis in a seropositive female with rheumatoid nodules. Arthritis and Rheumatism 15:544

Van den Berg-Loonen P M, Dekker-Saeys A J, Meuwissen S G M, Nijenhuis L E 1977 Histocompatibility antigens and other markers in ankylosing spondylitis and inflammatory bowel diseases. Journal of Rheumatology 4 (Suppl 3):57

Van der Linden J M J P, de Ceulaer K, van Romunde L K J, Cats A 1977 Ankylosing spondylitis without HLA B27. Journal of Rheumatology 4 (Suppl 3):54

Vasey F B, Kinsella T D 1977 Increased frequency of leukocyte-reactive anti-nuclear antibody in patients with ankylosing spondylitis. Journal of Rheumatology 4:158

Wee S L, Daymond T J 1978 Diminshed mixed lymphocyte response in ankylosing spondylitis. Tissue Antigens 11:409

Welch R B, Charnley J 1970 Low-friction arthroplasty of the hip in rheumatoid arthritis and ankylosing spondylitis. Clinical Orthopaedics 72:22

Wells J 1965 The sacro-iliac joint in ankylosing spondylitis. Rheumatism 21:100

West H F 1949 The aetiology of ankylosing spondylitis. Annals of the Rheumatic Diseases 8:143

Whaley K, Canesi B, Moseley A, Morrow W, Sturrock R, Mitchell W, Dick W C 1974 Complement metabolism in the seronegative arthritides. Annals of the Rheumatic Diseases 33:495

Wholey M H, Pugh D G, Bickel W H 1960 Localised destructive lesions in rheumatoid spondylitis. Radiology 74:54

Wilde H 1949 Diagnose and Behandlung der chronischen Prostatitis. Deutsche Gesundheitswesen 4:915

Wilkinson M, Bywaters E G L 1958 Clinical features and course of ankylosing spondylitis as seen in a follow up of 222 hospital referred cased. Annals of the Rheumatic Diseases 17:209

Wilkinson M, Meikle J A K 1966 Tomography of the sacro-iliac joints. Annals of the Rheumatic Diseases 25:433

Wright V, Catterall R D, Cook J B 1965 Bone and joint changes in paraplegic men. Annals of the Rheumatic Diseases 24:419

Wright V 1975 Personal communication

Young A, Dixon A, Getty J, Renton P, Vacher H 1981 Cauda equini syndrome complicating ankylosing spondylitis: use of electromyography and computerized tomography in diagnosis. Annals of the Rheumatic Diseases 40:317

Zilko P J, Thevathasan M, Dawkins R L 1977 Immuno function in ankylosing spondylitis: apparent relationship between streptococcal responses and HLA B27. Journal of Rheumatology 4 (Suppl 3):49

Zorab P A 1961 The historical and prehistorical background of ankylosing spondylitis. Proceedings of the Royal Society of Medicine 54:415

Zorab P A 1962 The lung in ankylosing spondylitis. Quarterly Journal of Medicine 31:267

Psoriatic arthritis

Since attention was drawn to the association of psoriasis and arthritis (Alibert, 1822; Bourdillon, 1888), there has been much discussion about the validity of 'psoriatic arthritis' as an entity separate from rheumatoid arthritis. Definitions of the condition have varied from a disease confined to the distal interphalangeal joints to severely destructive arthritis associated with psoriasis (Table 30.1).

There is increasing clinical, radiographic, serological and epidemiological evidence to support the classification of psoriatic arthritis as a true entity. Extensive series (Vilanova & Piñol, 1951; Coste et al, 1958; Wright, 1959a; Reed et al, 1961; Baker et al, 1963) suggest that most previous definitions are segments of a disease with a wide spectrum. Undue prominence has been given to the severely destructive form of arthritis, which rarely occurs. Few would subscribe to the view that psoriatic arthritis is a variant of rheumatoid arthritis, although it is recognised and that two diseases as common as psoriasis and rheumatoid arthritis may coincide.

Table 30.1 Definitions of psoriatic arthritis

1. Arthritis confined to the distal joints associated with psoriasis (Bauer et al, 1941; Meaney & Hays, 1957)
2. Atypical arthritis accompanying atypical psoriasis (Dawson & Tyson, 1938)
3. Atrophic arthritis associated with psoriasis, having synchronous remissions and relapses of skin and joint changes (Jeghers & Robinson, 1937; Epstein, 1939)
4. Arthritis following long-standing, uncontrolled psoriasis (Hench, 1927; Carrier, 1958)
5. Severely destructive arthritis associated with psoriasis (Fawcett, 1950; Sterne & Schneider, 1953)
6. Inflammatory polyarthritis associated with psoriasis, usually having a negative S.C.A.T. (Wright, 1956)
7. Coincidence of psoriasis and rheumatoid arthritis (Pillsbury et al, 1956; Short et al, 1957)

Prevalence

It is difficult to obtain accurate figures for the incidence of polyarthritis in patients with psoriasis, since hospital populations are highly selected and indeed the skin lesions may be so trivial that the patient is unaware of their presence or nature. Romanus (1945) found that the prevalence of inflammatory polyarthritis among the general population over 50 years of age in Sweden was 2.8% for males and 5.3% for females. Among patients with psoriasis of the same age he found arthritis in 1.4% of the males and 4.1% of the females. Church (1958) found arthritis in 2% of patients with psoriasis, and Hellgren (1969) found 5.4% of 534 psoriatic patients had rheumatoid arthritis by ARA criteria. Tiedeman (1951) found psoriatic arthritis in 2.2–3% of a group with psoriasis, males being affected 3 times as often as females.

Conversely, figures for the prevalence of psoriasis amongst patients with polyarthritis have been 3.1–4.5% (Wassmann, 1949; Gribble, 1955; Hellgren, 1969). Leczinsky (1948) found that 6.8% of 543 psoriatic inpatients had 'chronic (rheumatoid) polyarthritis' (5.8% in men; 7.9% in women). By contrast a control population of 543 non-psoriatic dematological patients has a prevalence of only 0.7%. It has been shown that taking into account the presence of rheumatoid factor makes a considerable difference (Baker, 1965). In seropositive rheumatoid arthritis Baker found a prevalence of psoriasis similar to that of a control hospital population, but the prevalence in seronegative 'rheumatoid arthritis' was over four times as great.

Psoriasis is found slightly more frequently among women than men. In contrast the male predominance in psoriatic arthritis has been stresed by some authors (Bollet & Turner, 1958; Reed, 1961). The sex ratio is determined to some extent by the type of patient the author sees. Arthritis predominantly affecting distal joints occurs more frequently in men, but in other patients there are more women (Wright, 1959a).

Aetiology

Heredity is a prominent factor in the occurrence of psoriasis, although the exact mode of inheritance is not clear. Hoede (1957) and Lomholt (1963) proposed dominant transmission with incomplete penetrance, but Steinberg et al (1951) supported a double recessive mechanism. It is now appreciated that psoriatic pedigrees have remarkable variability; pedigrees can be found which conform to the 'simple' (Mendelian) modes of inheritance, but there are a great many more which cannot be explained on a single gene basis. This realisation has led to the view that psoriasis is probably a multifactorial disorder (Watson et al, 1971; Farber & Nall, 1971).

There is an increased frequence of HLA-B13 and B37 among patients with psoriasis (Karvonen et al, 1974; McClusky et al, 1974; Metzger et al, 1975; White et al, 1972; Russell et al, 1972; Green et al, 1981; Tsuji et al, 1979). There is a strong association between Cw6 and psoriasis (Tsuji et al, 1979; Tillikainen et al, 1980; Batchelor & Morris, 1978; Hawkins et al, 1980). Marcusson (1979) in a careful family study showed that psoriasis often occurs in close relatives who share one disease-predisposing HLA haplotype with the proband. Some of the carriers of disease-associated HLA haplotypes have no signs of dermal involvement, but have subjective or objective signs of arthritic lesions. He, therefore, suggested that psoriasis and/or arthritic lesions may be different clinical manifestations of disease in individuals carrying psoriasis-predisposing haplotypes. On the basis of these findings he favoured a dominant inheritence pattern. Moreover, it was thought that at least two HLA-linked genes co-operated in the development of disease. These genes could occur in *cis*-position on the same haplotype, or in *trans*-position on different haplotypes. In the former case, disease inheritance would seem to be dominant, whereas in the latter case disease would occur mainly in HLA-identical siblings of the proband.

Russell et al (1972) found B17 to be a useful genetic marker for detecting a subgroup of psoriatic patients characterised by a high rate of affected relatives and a slightly earlier age at onset. HLA-B12, on the other hand, appeared to detect a subgroup with an infrequent family history of the disease.

Heredity appears to be a factor in the causation of the arthritis of psoriatic subjects judging from individual pedigree reports (Bauer & Vogl, 1931; Tiedmann, 1951; Ward & Stephens, 1961; Wright, 1969) and family surveys (Baker et al, 1963a; Theiss et al, 1969, 1970; Vilàghy & Krebs, 1970). An extensive controlled study of over 100 families of patients with psoriasis and arthritis has demonstrated psoriatic arthritis to be aggregated in first-degree relatives of psoriatic arthritis probands almost 50 times more often than has been reported in the general population (Moll, 1971; Moll & Wright, 1973a). A significant difference was also found between the prevalence of the disease in relatives and that in spouse controls, thus suggesting genetic rather than environmental factors as the cause of the familial aggregation. No definite Mendelian pattern of inheritance could be found in the Leeds pedigrees and it was concluded that genetic transmission was multifactorial.

There is a high concordance between HLA-B27 and sacroiliitis in patients with psoriatic arthritis (Bluestone et al, 1973; Amor et al, 1974; Brewerton et al, 1974; Karvonen et al, 1974; McClusky et al, 1974; Metzger et al, 1975; Lambert et al, 1976). The Guy's Hospital group (Armstrong et al, 1983) have confirmed the raised frequency of Cw6 in patients with psoriasis, and noted those with arthritis not only had an increased frequency of B27, but also of DR7. DR3 in their series was associated with erosions.

Environmental factors are probably of importance in the development of psoriatic arthritis as well as genetic ones. These suggested factors have included trauma (Buckley & Raleigh, 1959; Biernacki et al, 1968; Williams & Scott, 1967; Miller et al, 1971), neurotrophic effect (Brailsford, 1953;

Weddell et al, 1965), microvascular changes (Redisch et al, 1970; Monacelli, 1971; Espinoza et al, 1982), and infection (Mustakallio & Lassus, 1964).

Pathology

Bauer et al (1941) found the histological lesions in the terminal joints were similar to those occurring elsewhere, except in one patient with arthritis limited to these joints, in whom there was marked articular destruction and resorption of bone with pronounced shortening of the middle phalanges at the distal joints of the fingers and toes. The resorption was less marked at the proximal ends of the bones, but cup-like deformities were formed by pronounced marginal overgrowth of bones at the sites of insertion of tendons. Dense acellular fibrous tissue with little or no inflammatory change replaced the joint spaces in most of the digits. In early lesions found at surgery the synovial membrane was pale with oedematous granulation tissue extending out from the joint and a few millimetres along the shafts of the bone (Sherman, 1952). The membrane later became thickened and injected, often eroding articular margins, but without pannus formation. Finally, there was complete destruction with cancellous stubs embedded in fibrous tissue. Characteristic rheumatoid granulomata have not been found and the usual reports have been of chronic inflammatory changes with villous hypertrophy, fibrosis and destructive changes in cartilage and bone (Bollett & Turner, 1958). Certain differences from rheumatoid arthritis were reported in synovial biopsies (Coste & Solnica, 1966). These comprised fewer round cell aggregations, more fibrosis and many thick walled small vessels. In our experience, however, those with an arthritis indistinguishable from rheumatoid disease but with a persistently negative sheep cell agglutination test have histology similar to rheumatoid disease. In the case of one such patient, whom we have observed over many years, the late Professor D. N. Collins had set aside the histology of her synovium as typical of rheumatoid disease.

Arthroscopy has not demonstrated any macroscopic differences between the joint appearances of psoriatic arthritis and rheumatoid arthritis (Jayson & Henderson, 1973).

Clinical features

There is a wide spectrum of presentations of psoriatic arthritis and five broad clinical groups have been recognised (Moll & Wright, 1973b).

1. Patients with classical psoriatic arthritis in whom the distal interphalangeal joints are predominantly, although rarely exclusively, involved.
2. A severely deforming type of arthritis, usually characterised by widespread ankylosis. Very rarely *arthritis mutilans* occurs with 'opera glass' hands and a similar condition in the feet.
3. Many cases appear clinically indistinguishable from rheumatoid disease apart from the absence of rheumatoid factor in the serum. The arthritis tends to be less extensive and more benign in its course.
4. Patients with single or asymmetrical oligo- (or mono-) arthritis. This group has been emphasised on the continent (Serre et al, 1969; Schattenkirchner, 1970; Nazzaro & Gigante, 1971).
5. Patients in whom there is ankylosing spondylitis, accounting for about 5% of all types of psoriatic arthritis.

Arthritis was found 10 times more commonly in patients with severe involvement of the skin than in those with mild involvement (Leczinsky, 1948), but there is no other relation between the extent or type of skin lesions and joint changes, except that in the deforming type of arthritis the psoriasis tends to be long-standing, extensive and exfoliative. Pustular psoriasis may also occur on the palms and soles in these patients (Bollett & Turner, 1958; Wright, 1959b; Baker et al, 1963a). Skin lesions usually precede the arthritis, but the onset is sometimes synchronous, and in a small proportion of cases arthritis comes first. Some patients with seronegative 'rheumatoid arthritis' may later develop psoriasis (Dixon, 1958). Occasionally there are synchronous exacerbations and remissions of skin and joint lesions, but this is uncommon. The arthritis is more closely related to nail changes than to skin changes. 81% of patients with psoriatic arthritis have nail changes, compared with 18% of an unselected series of patients with psoriasis and 32% of patients with uncomplicated psoriasis matched by age and sex (Wright, 1957a).

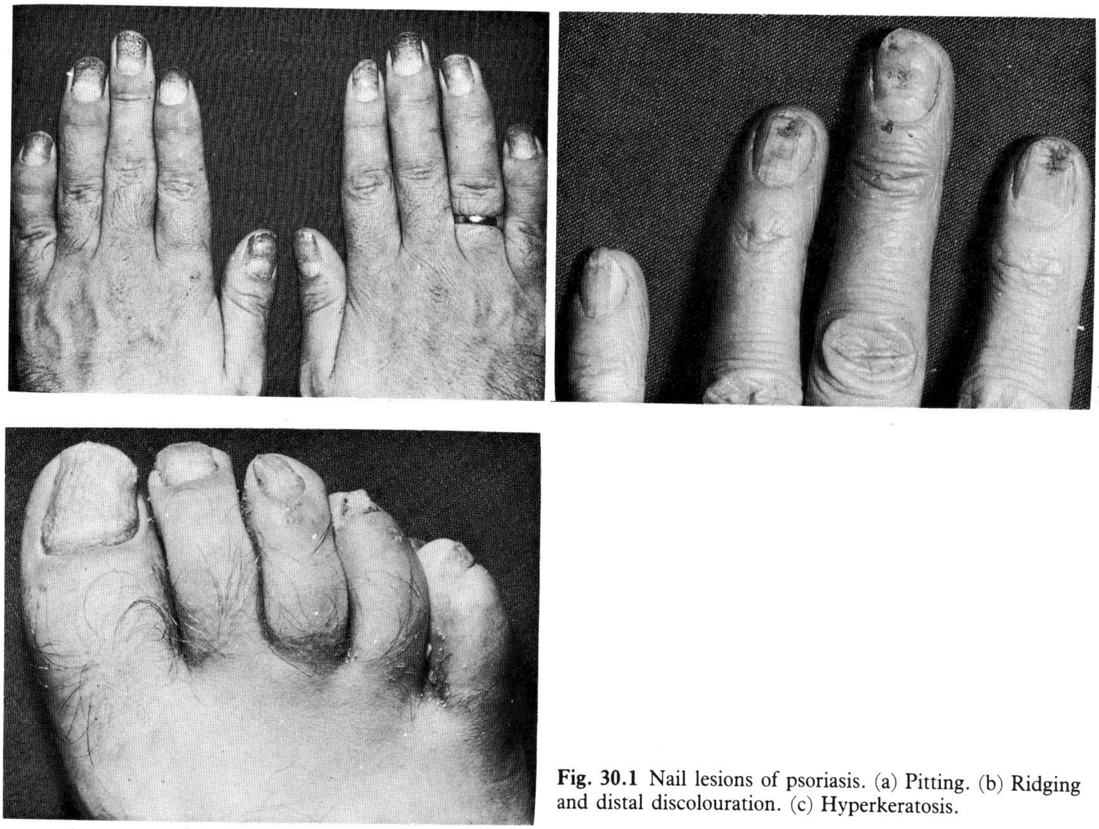

Fig. 30.1 Nail lesions of psoriasis. (a) Pitting. (b) Ridging and distal discolouration. (c) Hyperkeratosis.

Typical nail lesions include discolouration of the distal edge of the nail plate with undermining, pitting, hyperkeratosis (especially in the toes) and ridging (Fig. 30.1). Occasionally there is a topographical relationship between the involvement of distal joints and affected nails (Fig. 30.2). The nails are more frequently involved at the onset of arthritis than the skin.

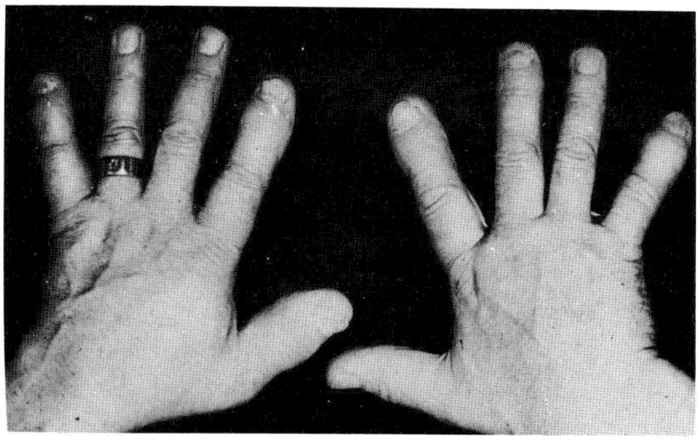

Fig. 30.2 Topographical association of nail and joint changes in psoriatic arthritis.

The age of onset of the deforming type of arthritis is earlier than in rheumatoid arthritis (Wright, 1956). Involvement of the distal and proximal interphalangeal joints, together with tendon sheath involvement, may give the digit a sausage shape. Asymmetry of joint involvement is seen more commonly than in rheumatoid disease. There may be a gout-like onset of the arthritis.

Juvenile psoriatic arthritis usually starts in the knee (Lambert et al, 1976; Shore & Ansell, 1982). Additional joints arc involved sporadically in an asymmetrical pattern, in both upper and lower limbs, so that 80% ultimately have polyarticular disease. Although in the series of Shore & Ansell 40% were asymptomatic at follow-up, 6 required bilateral hip replacement.

The association with spondylitis has been described over the years (Reiter & Norholm-Pederson, 1953; Graber-Duvernay, 1957; Coste et al, 1958; Reed, 1961; Baker et al, 1963a; Coste & Solnica, 1966). The familial evidence showing aggregation of sacroiliitis and spondylitis in blood relatives of patients with psoriatic arthritis lends support to the association (Moll, 1971).

Extra-articular features are much less frequent in psoriatic arthritis than in rheumatoid arthritis. Subcutaneous nodules are characteristically absent, and extensor tendon sheath effusions are less common. Ocular inflammation occurs in nearly one-third. Conjunctivitis was the most common (19.6%); iritis occurred in 7.1%, scleritis in 1.8% and keratoconjunctivitis sicea in 2.7% (Lambert & Wright, 1976). Spondylitic heart disease may be found, the skin lesions usually being pustular (Reed, 1961).

Prognosis

Apart from the rare destructive type of arthritis, to which undue attention has been paid in the literature because of its striking clinical and radiographic appearance, psoriatic arthritis tends to produce less pain and disability than rheumatoid arthritis. Death may occur from amyloidosis. Of 32 patients with psoriatic arthritis who died 3 had amyloidosis and 15 died from conditions in which corticosteroid therapy may have been a contributory factor (Reed & Wright, 1966). Most of these patients were from the USA, and the pattern of mortality may have been due to selection. In a 10-year study of patients in the United Kingdom, however, ischaemic heart disease was the commonest cause of death (as it is in the national mortality figures), occurring in 7 of 16 patients (Wright & Moll, 1976).

Ancillary investigations

The most striking feature in the blood tests is the absence of rheumatoid factor in the serum of the majority of patients with polyarthritis and psoriasis. In a 10-year follow-up study of 227 patients the SCAT was positive in 16% of the group indistinguishable from rheumatoid arthritis, fluctuating in a further 10% (Roberts et al, 1976).

Patients with psoriatic arthritis have raised levels of IgG antiglobulins, the results being similar to those in patients with rheumatoid arthritis (Howell et al, 1972). This is of little diagnostic significance since raised levels are also found in patients with uncomplicated psoriasis and with gout. It may be that the inflammatory process in these conditions is mediated by a common pathway. However, leucocytes in the synovial fluid are said to show the same 'RA cells', containing rheumatoid factor, as are present in rheumatoid arthritis (Hollander et al, 1965; Rawson et al, 1965). There may be some degree of anaemia, and the ESR is raised in the active phase of the disease, although this is said to be moderate compared with rheumatoid arthritis (Lodin et al, 1957).

Raised levels of circulating immune complexes have been found in the plasma of patients with psoriasis and of those with psoriatic arthritis (Laurent et al, 1981). Serum immunoglobulin G and A were equally raised in both patient groups. Levels of C-reactive protein, fibrinogen, alpha-l-antitrypsin and the 9th component of complement were raised in psoriatic arthritis but normal in patients with psoriasis alone. C-reactive protein and fibrinogen correlated best with clinical activity.

Hyperuricaemia has been frequently cited as a feature of psoriasis (Steinberg et al, 1951; Barmann & Jillson, 1961; Walton et al, 1961; Lawrence, 1966), although some authors have doubted this (Tickner & Mier, 1960). It is said to be commoner in patients with extensive involvement of the skin (Eisen & Weissman, 1962). There is an increased glycine incorporation into urinary uric acid in psoriatic patients, the degree of incorporation being proportional to the extent of skin involvement (Eisen & Seegmiller, 1961). Increased excretion of uric acid and pseudouridine has also been found (Weissman et al, 1962). A carefully controlled study of our patients, however, in which all drugs which might influence the level of serum uric acid were withdrawn, has not shown any difference from a group of matched patients with rheumatoid arthritis.

Other abnormalities have been reported: normal erythrocyte phosphoglucose isomerase activity (Gaedicke et al, 1970); absence of anti-nuclear factor (Macsween et al, 1968; Sonnichsen, 1969a, b); elevated gamma and alpha-2-globulin (Robillard, 1968); decreased IgM levels in mild psoriatic arthritis and elevated levels in severe psoriatic arthritis (Petres & Majert, 1968); elevated IgA levels (Danielsen, 1965). Heiskell et al (1962) found a consistent elevation of beta globulins in psoriatic arthritis but not in rheumatoid arthritis. Zachariae & Zachariae (1969) could not find any specific immunological pattern in psoriatic arthritis and

Baker et al (1963b) found no consistent correlation between clinical activity or severity in the degree of protein disturbance. Lysozyme activity has been found to be normal in the serum and synovial fluid (Prusanki & Orgyzlo, 1972). The increased frequency of histocompatibility antigens B13, B17, B27, Cw6, DR7 and DR3 have been discussed earlier under the heading of 'Aetiology'.

Radiographic findings

Many features are indistinguishable from rheumatoid arthritis. In some patients there are few joint changes apart from soft tissue swelling, while in others it is the pattern of asymmetrical oligoarthritis which is prominent. Some findings which have been regarded as characteristic, such as lack of porosis despite destructive changes (Fawcett, 1950; Clemmeson & Arsno, 1952), a relative sparing of the metacarpophalangeal joints even when the wrists are involved, and an involvement of the radioulnar rather than the radionavicular joint at the wrist (Sherman, 1952), have not been substantiated by controlled studies (Wright, 1957b). More characteristic features include involvement of the distal interphalangeal joints of the fingers and toes (Fig. 30.3) with marginal erosions at the very edge of the articular cartilage as one of the earliest signs (Plenk, 1950; Sherman, 1952), progressing to complete involvement of the joint with hypertrophic alterations around them (Wright, 1961; Baer & Witten, 1962) The tips of the terminal phalanges may be eroded (Fig. 30.4) and this is seen most clearly in the hallux (Wright, 1957b).

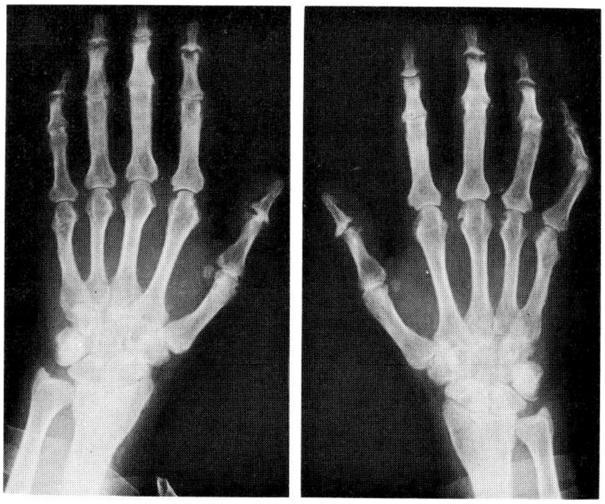

Fig. 30.3 Distal interphalangeal changes in psoriatic arthritis.

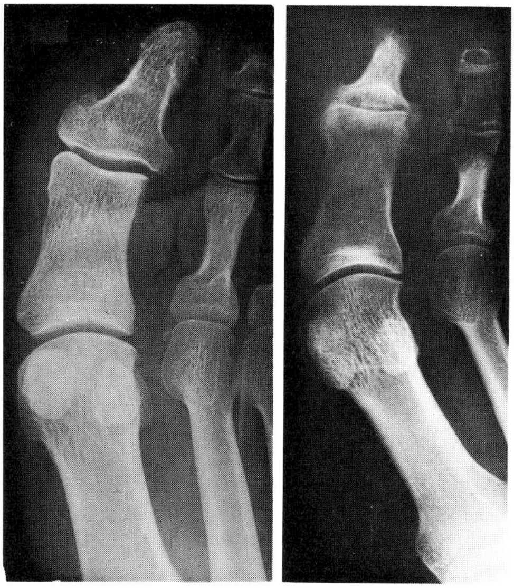

a b

Fig. 30.4 Terminal phalangeal tuft erosion (acro-osteolysis) in psoriatic arthritis. (a) Within 1 year of onset of arthritis. (b) 2 years later, showing progression.

It has been suggested that these changes are similar to those produced by vascular phenomena in Raynaud's disease and systemic sclerosis (Brailsford, 1953). Cheesebrough (1979) reported a patient with psoriasis showing tuft osteolysis with no evidence of arthropathy. He felt that psoriatic involvement of the nail-bed had stimulated bone absorption directly. Irregular destruction may extend along the shaft of the phalanges, metacarpals and matatarsals, sometimes with marked periosteal reaction (Sherman, 1952; Sterne & Schneider, 1953). This may progress to dissolution of the bones (Strom, 1921; Epstein, 1939; Clarke, 1950; Fawcett, 1950; Sherman, 1952; Brailsford, 1953; Gribble, 1955; Avila et al, 1960). The resulting telescoping of digits and tapering of metatarsal and metacarpal bones produce a picture similar to that seen in neuropathic joint disease (Fig. 30.5). These changes occurred in 3.4% of an unselected series of patients with psoriasis and polyarthritis (Wright, 1959a).

In most of the patients with deforming arthritis, ankylosis predominates, and fusion of the sacroiliac joints is the rule. Sacroiliitis has been reported in 10–30% of patients with psoriatic arthritis (Dixon & Lience, 1961; Hill, 1961; Reed et al, 1961; Wright, 1961; Baker et al, 1963a). Spinal involvement similar to that found in ankylosing

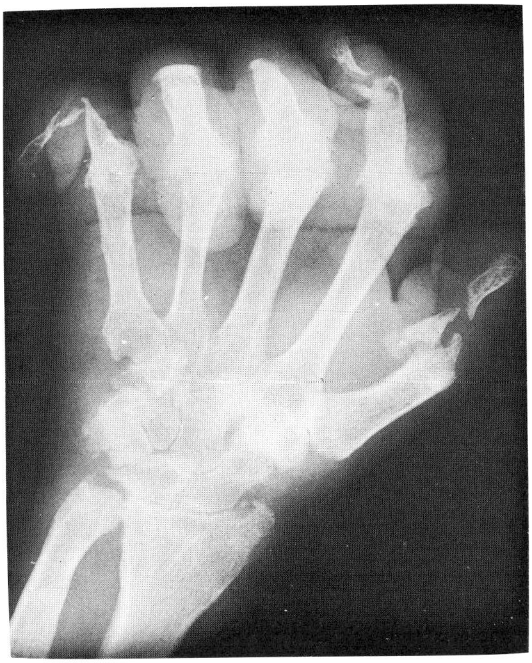

Fig. 30.5 Arthritis mutilans with psoriasis.

spondylitis may develop, and this may affect the cervical spine (Wright, 1957b; Porrini et al, 1964). It has been suggested that there is a specific cervical lesion associated with psoriasis (with or without arthritis) comprising apophyseal sclerosis, joint narrowing, and anterior ligamentous calcification (Kaplan et al, 1964). A rare type of paravertebral ossification in the lumbar and thoracic areas may occur at some distance from the vertebral body (Bywaters & Dixon, 1965; Coste & Solnica, 1966). On the basis of syndesmophyte morphology, McEwen et al (1971) placed the spondylitis associated with psoriasis in a group with Reiter's disease and distinguished it from another group of patients with idiopathic ankylosing spondylitis and the spondylitis associated with ulcerative colitis.

In a review of 130 patients with psoriatic arthritis, spondylitis was noted in 40% (Lambert & Wright, 1977). Syndesmophytes were noted in 25% of patients, and in 60% of these the sacroiliac joints were normal radiologically. Anterior syndesmophytes alone were found only in the cervical spine and were more common in patients without sacroiliitis. Lateral syndesmophytes were most commonly found in the lumbar and lower dorsal vertebrae and were slightly less common in patients without sacroiliitis.

Differential diagnosis

Problems in the diagnosis of psoriatic arthritis may conveniently be divided into the separate diagnostic difficulties posed by individual features of the disease — psoriasis, polyarthritis and spondylitis (Moll & Wright, 1973).

Psoriasis of the skin and scalp may be so minimal as to escape the attention of both patient and clinician. Particularly elusive are small lesions at the internatal cleft, perineum, umbilicus, submammary area, axilla, and groin. Scalp lesions may also be confined to a small plaque, often in the occipital region. As this may be the only manifestation of psoriasis, the scalp should always be examined meticulously in any patient with an arthritis of psoriatic pattern but without obvious psoriasis of skin or nails. Scalp psoriasis must be differentiated from seborrhoea capitis. The latter is characterised by poor demarcation between involved and normal scalp and also the fact that seborrhoeic lesions are not usually palpable. Other seborrhoeic features, such as scaly involvement of the eyebrows and otitis externa, may further simplify diagnosis.

Psoriatic nail involvement may be the only manifestation of psoriasis, and in these cases it is important to exclude other causes of nail dystrophy. If fungal infection is suspected, cuttings of the nail should be examined microscopically.

The differentiation of psoriatic arthritis from Reiter's disease may be particularly difficult in certain cases (Wright & Reed, 1964) and this is discussed in more detail in Chapter 31. The close similarities between nail involvement in these two conditions may be confusing and difficulty arises in distinguishing keratoderma blenorrhagica from pustular psoriasis of the palms and soles.

Other causes of asymmetrical distal interphalangeal and proximal interphalangeal joint arthritis in a patient with psoriasis may be mistaken for true psoriatic arthritis. Recently, erosive (Crain, 1961; Peter et al, 1966; Kidd, 1966; Swezey & Alexander, 1971) and ankylosing (Smukler et al, 1971) forms of osteoarthrosis have been described, and, because of their predilection for scattered distal interphalangeal and proximal interphalangeal joints, it may be impossible to distinguish these forms of arthritis from psoriatic arthritis. Osteoarthrosis may also cause diagnostic confusion when associated with Heberden's nodes: early active nodes may be red and swollen in the same way as in psoriatic arthritis of the distal interphalangeal joints. In osteoarthrosis, often it is only later that the single globular swelling of the distal interphalangeal joint settles to reveal the hard double node so typical of the disease. Advanced osteoarthrosis of the distal interphalangeal joint may be similar radiologically to psoriatic arthritis. This is due to gross irregularity of the joint margin and subchondral cysts, which, even to an experienced eye, may be mistaken for erosions.

At times an acute psoriatic joint may resemble gouty arthritis. Barber (1950) and Sherman (1952) have both commented that the clinical appearance of the joints in psoriatic arthritis may simulate gout. This is particularly true in the patients with distal joint arthritis (Wright, 1959b). It must be remembered also that coincidental gout and psoriasis will present occasionally at the rheumatology clinic. A considerably raised level of serum uric acid makes the diagnosis of psoriatic arthritis unlikely, the presence of serum uric acid crystals in the synovial fluid may provide the diagnosis, and the response of the disease to colchicine may be a useful diagnostic aid. In the series at Leeds there is only one patient that has caused sufficient confusion for diagnosis over a 12-year follow-up period to be changed from psoriatic arthritis to that of gout.

We have observed several psoriatic patients who have presented with post-traumatic pain and swelling of the knee. These patients were usually diagnosed as having a mechanical derangement until arthrotomy revealed synovial prolifcration and not a torn meniscus. There appears to be a susceptibility in patients with psoriatic arthritis to trauma and any 'traumatic' arthritis in a patient with psoriasis failing to settle in the usual way should be considered to be monarticular psoriatic arthritis until proved otherwise. Occasionally, patients with the classical clinicoradiological picture of psoriatic arthritis are found to be seropositive. Most of these patients are probably examples of true psoriatic arthritis associated coincidentally with the positive test for rheumatoid factor which is present in 5% of the general population (Walter & Toone, 1958).

The relationship to ankylosing spondylitis is dealt with in the preceding paragraphs on radiographic features and in other chapters in this section concerned with seronegative spondarthritis.

Treatment

Extensive skin lesions are best treated with the Goerkerman (Ingram) regime of dithranol, ultraviolet light and tar baths daily. Localised lesions may be treated at home with hydrarg.ammon.picis carb. or triacetoxyanthracene paste. Betamethasone ointment may be useful when lesions itch, although many dermatologists prefer to avoid this because of the likelihood of skin atrophy. For the treatment of the skin systemic steroids are rarely indicated, particularly as the condition usually relapses despite continued therapy. When they are used, triamcinolone has been advocated (Shelley et al, 1958; Hollander et al, 1959). Folic acid antagonists have been employed in the treatment of severe, uncontrolled psoriasis, and it has been claimed the skin and joints have improved (Black et aal, 1964). Effective doses produce marrow depression and it is doubtful whether such noxious remedies will ever be used generally in a non-lethal condition. Azathioprine has been given with benefit to 66% of a group of patients with psoriasis (du Vivier et al, 1974). The drug was used when patients required frequent inpatient treatment (or had failed to clear with this), when they had suffered toxic effects from methotrexate or failed to be controlled by it, when they were receiving corticosteroids, when they had exfoliative or pustular psoriasis, or when they were socially disabled by the disease. However, 8 of 29 developed some portal fibrosis in the liver. Fortunately, psoriasis is not usually resistant to treatment.

The nails are resistant to treatment, but clear temporarily with radiotherapy. It has been suggested that this treatment may improve the distal joints (Popp & Addington, 1941). Abell (1972) achieved marked improvement of nails in 21 of 27 patients with psoriasis using triamcinolone acetonide injected with a needle-less injector 3 times a week.

The arthritis does not usually subside with treatment of the psoriasis, contrary to previous claims (Jeghers & Robinson, 1937; Epstein, 1939;

O'Leary, 1943). Often it is sufficiently mild not to require treatment, but if needed it usually responds to a regimen similar to that for rheumatoid arthritis. Antimalarial drugs may provoke exfoliation (Cornbleet, 1956; Reed & Becker, 1960). The older literature gave a high incidence of exacerbation of psoriatic lesions by such therapy, but a recent review of 50 patients with psoriatic arthritis treated with hydroxychloroquine commented that there was no exacerbation of skin lesions (Kammer et al, 1979). In reviewing the situation Luzar (1982) reported an exacerbation in 1 of 3 psoriatic patients whom he had so treated but felt there was a low incidence of such exacerbations, probably in the realm of 1–2% on the basis of the work of MacKenzie & Scherbel (1980). Gold is not associated with any more skin reactions than in rheumatoid disease (Wright, 1961), but the risk of provoking a dermatitis makes some hesitant to use it. Uncontrolled studies have reported benefit for more resistant cases (Dorwart et al, 1978; Kammer et al, 1979; Richter et al, 1980). Baum et al (1973) have used 6-mercaptopurine in 13 patients with psoriatic arthritis, of whom 11 improved. Those with nail changes responded strikingly, and low doses (25–50 mg daily) sufficed, producing little toxicity. Cyclosporin A brought about an impressive improvement in the psoriatic lesions of 4 cases, but the effect on the arthropathy was variable (Muller & Graf, 1981). An enthusiastic report on the response of patients with psoriatic arthritis to the oral retinoid, tigason, was made on the basis of 24 patients treated, but the study was uncontolled (Stollenwer et al, 1981).

It has been said that patients with psoriatic arthritis are particularly prone to infection after prosthetic surgery (Kummerle et al, 1971; Lambert & Wright, 1979), but we have not been able to confirm this. Even incisions through psoriatic plaques do not increase the frequency of wound infection. However, it is not always appreciated that psoriatic scales are heavily infected and may produce cross-infection. Patients with psoriasis should therefore be kept in surgical wards for as short a time as possible. The more exuberant fibrotic reaction in psoriatic arthritis and the tendency to osteolysis and ankylosis do not appear to jeopardise results of surgery in these patients.

REFERENCES

Abell E 1972 The treatment of psoriatic nail dystrophy. British Journal of Dermatology 86:79

Alibert J L 1822 In: Precis theorerique et practique sur les maladies de la peau, 2nd Edn. Caille & Ravier, Paris

Amor B, Feldmann J, Delbarre F, Hors J, Beaujan M, Daussett J 1974 HL-A antigen W27-A genetic link between ankylosing spondylitis and Reiter's syndrome. New England Journal of Medicine 290:572

Armstrong R D, Panayi G S, Welsh K I 1983 Histocompatability antigens in psoriasis, psoriatic arthropathy and ankylosing spondylitis. Annals of the Rheumatic Diseases (in press)

Avila R, Pugh D G, Slocumb C H, Winkelman R K 1960 Psoriatic arthritis — A roentgenological study. Radiology 75:691

Baer R L, Witten V H 1962 In: Year book of dermatology. Year Book Publishers, p 9–39

Baker H 1965 M D Thesis, University of Leeds

Baker H, Golding D N, Thompson M 1963a Psoriasis and arthritis. Annals of Internal Medicine 58:909

Baker H, Golding D N, Thompson M 1963b Atypical polyarthritis in psoriatic families. British Medical Journal 2:348

Barber H W 1950 Psoriasis. British Medical Journal 1:219

Batechelor J R, Morris P J 1978 HLA and disease — joint report. In: Bodmer W F, Batchelor J R, Bodmer J G, Festenstein H, Morris P J (eds) Histocompatability testing, 1977. Munksgard, Copenhagen, p 205

Baumann R R, Jillson O F 1961 Hyperuricaemia and psoriasis. Journal of Investigative Dermatology 36:105

Bauer J, Vogl A 1931 Psoriasis und Gelenkleiden. Klinische Wochenschrift, 10:1700

Bauer W, Bennett G A, Zeller J W 1941 Pathology of joint lesions in patients with psoriasis and arthritis. Transactions of the Association of American Physicians 56:349

Baum J, Hurd E, Lewis D, Ferguson J L, Ziff M 1973 Treatment of psoriatic arthritis with 6-mercaptopurine. Arthritis and Rheumatism, 16:139

Biernacki R, Sadowska-Wroblewska M, Zabrokrycki J 1968 Acro-osteolysis in the course of ankylosing spondylitis. Reumatologia, 6:163

Black R L, O'Brien W M, Van Scott E J, Auerbach R, Eisen A Z, Bunim J J 1964 Methotrexate therapy in psoriatic arthritis. Journal of the American Medical Association 189:743

Bluestone R H, Schlosstein I H, Terasaki P, Pearson C M 1973 Paper persented at VIII International Congress of Rheumatology, Kyoto, Japan

Bollet A J, Turner R A 1958 Psoriatic arthritis. Annals of the New York Academy of Science 73:1013

Bourdillon C 1888 In: Psoriasis et arthropathies. Lecrosnier & Babe, Paris

Brailsford J F 1953 In: The radiology of bones and joints, 5th Edn. Churchill, London, pp 63, 77, 174

Brewerton D A, Caffrey M, Nicholls A, Walters D and James D C O 1974 HLA-B27 and arthropathies associated with ulcerative colitis and psoriasis. Lancet 1: 956–957

Buckley W R, Raleigh R L 1959 Psoriasis with acro-osteolysis. New England Journal of Medicine, 261:539

Bywaters E G L, Dixon A St J 1965 Paravertebral ossification in psoriatic arthritis. Annals of the Rheumatic Diseases 24:313

Carrier J W 1958 Psoriatic arthritis. American Journal of Roentgenology 75:612

Cheesbrough M J 1979 Osteolysis and psoriasis. Clinical and Experimental Dermatology 4: 341–344

Church R 1958 The prospect of psoriasis. British Journal of Dermatology 70:139

Clarke O 1950 Arthritis mutilans associated with psoriasis. Lancet 1:249

Clemmeson S, Arsno E 1952 In: Rheumatic disease. Based on the proceedings of the VII International Congress of Rheumatic Diseases. Saunders, Philadelphia, p 54–66

Cornbleet T 1956 Action of synthetic animalarial drugs on psoriasis. Journal of Investigative Dermatology 26:435

Coste F, Francon J, Touraine R, Loyau G 1958 Polyarthrite psoriasique. Revue du rhumatisme et des maladies ostéo-articularies 25:75

Coste F, Solnica J 1966 La polyarthrite psoriasique. Revue Francaise d'études cliniques et biblogipques, 11:58

Crain D C 1961 Interphalangeal osteoarthritis characterised by painful inflammatory episodes resulting in deformity of the proximal and distal articulations. Journal of the American Medical Association 175:1049

Danielsen L 1965 Immuno-electrophoretic analysis of serum proteins in psoriasis and psoriatic arthritis. Acta Rheumatologica Scandinavica 11:112

Dawson M H, Tyson T L 1938 Psoriasis arthropathia with observations on certain features common to psoriasis and rheumatoid arthritis. Transactions of the Association of American Physicians 53:303

Dixon A St J 1958 Rheumatoid polyarthritis associated with a negative sheep cell agglutination test. Annals of the Rheumatic Diseases 17:252

Dixon A St J, Lience E 1961 Sacro-iliac joints in adult rheumatoid arthritis and psoriatic arthropathy. Annals of the Rheumatic Diseases 20:247

Dorwat B B, Gall E P and Schumacher R H 1978 Chryrotherapy in psoriatic arthritis. Efficacy and toxicity compared to rheumatoid arthritis. Arthritis and Rheumatism *21*: 513–518

Du Vivier A, Munro D D, Verbov J 1974 Treatment of psoriasis with azathioprine. British Medical Journal 1:49

Eisen A Z, Seegmiller J E 1961 Uric acid metabolism in gout. Journal of Clinical Investigation 40:1486

Eisen A Z, Weissman S 1962 Pseudouridine (S-ribosyl uracil) excretion in psoriasis. Journal of Investigative Dermatology 37:35

Epstein E 1939 Differential diagnosis of keratosis blenorrhagica and psoriatic arthropathy. Archiv für Dermatologie und Syphilis 40:547

Espinoza L R, Vasey F B, Espinoza C G, Bocanegra T S, Germain B F 1982 Vascular changes in psoriatic synovium; a light and electron microscopic study. Arthritis and Rheumatism, 25:677

Farber E M, Nall M L 1971 In: Psoriasis. Proceedings of the International Symposium, Stanford University. University Press, Stanford, p 7–13

Fawcett J 1950 Bone and joint changes associated with psoriasis. British Journal of Radiology 23:440

Gaedicke H, Kaiser W, Mathies H 1970 Die Bestimmung der Phosphoglucose-Isomerase-Aktivitat in den Erythrocyten und ihre Bedeutung also diagnostisches Kriterium der Arthritis psoriatica. Kunische Wochenschrift, 48:1456

Graber-Duvernay J 1957 A propos de la spondylarthrite psoriasique. Revue du rhumatisme et des maladies osteo-articulaires, 24:288

Green L, Meyers O L, Gordon W, Briggs B 1981 Arthritis in psoriasis. Annals of the Rheumatic Diseases 40: 366–369

Gribble M de G 1955 Rheumatoid arthritis and psoriasis. Annals of the Rheumatic Diseases 14:198

Hawkins B R, Tiwari J L, Lowe N, Wolfish P, Pollock C A, Cho Y W, Terasaki P I 1981 HLA and psoriasis. In: Terasaki P I (ed) Histocompatability testing. UCLA Tissue Typing Laboratory, Los Angeles, p 711–714

Heiskell C L, Reed W B, Weimer H E, Becker S W, Carpenter C M 1962 Serum protein profiles in psoriasis and arthritis. Archives of Dermatology, 85:708

Hellgren L 1969 Association between rheumatoid arthritis and psoriasis in total populations. Acta rheumatologica Scandinavica 15:316

Hench P S 1927 Arthropathia psoriatica — presentation of a case. Proceedings, Mayo Clinic, 2:89

Hill A G S 1961 Sacro-iliac joint in adult RA. Annals of the Rheumatic Diseases 20:256

Hoede K 1957 Zur Frage der Erblichkeit der Psoriasis. Hautarzt Zeitscheift für Dermatologie, Vererologie und Verwändie Gebiete 8:433

Hollander J L, Brown E M, Jessar R A, Udell I, Cooperhard S, Smuckler B M 1959 The effect of triamcinolone on psoriatic arthritis. Arthritis and Rheumatism 2:513

Hollander J L, McCarty D J Astorga G, Castro-Murillo E 1965 Studies on the pathogenesis of rheumatoid joint inflammation. I. The 'RA cell' and a working hypothesis. Annals of Internal Medicine 62:271

Howell F A, Chamberlain M A, Perry R A, Torrigiani C, Roitt I M 1972 IgG antiglobulin levels in patients with psoriatic arthropathy, ankylosing spondylitis and gout. Annals of the Rheumatic Diseases 31:129

Jayson M I V, Henderson D R E 1973 Arthroscopy in the diagnosis of inflammatory joint disease. Rheumatology and Rehabilitation 12:195

Jeghers H, Robinson L J 1937 Arthropathia psoriatica — report of a case and discussion of the pathogenesis diagnosis and treatment. Journal of the American Medical Association 108:949

Kammer G M, Sotar N A, Gibson D J 1979 Psoriatic arthritis; a clinical, immunologic and HLA study of 100 patients. Seminars in Arthritis and Rheumatism 9: 513–518

Kaplan D, Plotz C M, Nathanson L, Frank L 1964 Cervical spine in psoriasis and in psoriatic arthritis. Annals of the Rheumatic Diseases 23:50

Karnoven J, Lassus A, Sievers V, Tiilikainen A 1974 HL-A antigens in psoriatic arthritis. Annals of Clinical Research 6: 304–307

Kidd K L, Peter J B 1966 Erosive osteoarthritis. Radiology 86:640

Kummerle F, Wessinghage D, Schweikert C H 1971 Risks of alloplastic replacements in degenerative and inflammatory diseases of joints. Acta Orthopaedica Belgica 37:541

Lambert J R, Wright V 1976 Eye inflammation in psoriatic arthritis. Annals of the Rheumatic Diseases 35:354

Lambert J R, Wright V 1977 Psoriatic spondylitis; a clinical and radiological description of the spine in psoriatic arthritis. Quarterly Journal of Medicine 46: 411–425

Lambert J R, Wright V 1979 Surgery in patients with psoriasis and arthritis. Rheumatology and Rehabilitation *18*: 35–37
Lambert J R, Ansell B M, Stephenson E, Wright V 1976 Psoriatic arthritis in childhood. In: Ansell B M (ed) Clinics in rheumatic disease, Vol 2. Saunders, London, p 339–352
Lambert J R, Wright V, Rajah S M, Moll J M H 1976 Histo-compatability antigen in psoriatic arthritis. Annals of the Rheumatic Diseases 35: 526–530
Laurent M R, Panayi G S, Shepherd P 1981 Circulating immune complexes, serum immunoglobulins, and acute phase proteins in psoriasis and psoriatic arthritis. Annals of the Rheumatic Diseases 40: 66–69
Lawrence J S 1966 Symposium on gout and other diseases of purine metabolism. Proceedings of the Royal Society of Medicine 59:325
Leczinsky C G 1948 The incidence of arthropathy in a ten-year series of psoriasis cases. Acta dermato-venereologica 28:483
Lodin A, Gentele H, Lagerholm B, Karltorp N 1957 Psoriatic arthritis and elevated E.S.R. Acta dermato-venereologica 37:459
Lomholt G 1963 In: Psoriasis, prevalence, spontaneous course and genetics. Gad, Copenhagen
Luzar M J 1982 Hydroxychloroquine in psoriatic arthropathy; exacerbations of psoriatic skin lesions. Journal of Rheumatology 9: 462–464
McClusky O E, Lordon R E, Arnett F C 1974 HLA27 in Reiter's syndrome and psoriatic arthritis; a genetic factor in disease susceptibility and expression. Journal of Rheumatology 1: 263–268
McEwen C D, Tata D, Lingg C, Porini A, Good A, Rankin T 1971 Ankylosing spondylitis accompanying ulcerative colitis, regional enteritis, psoriasis and Reiter's disease. Arthritis and Rheumatism 14:291
Mackenzie A H, Scherbel A L 1980 Chloroquine and hydroxychloroquine. In: Huskisson E C (ed) Clinics of rheumatic diseases. Saunders, London, p 545–566
MacSween R N M, Dalakos T G, Jasans M K, Boyle J A, Buchanan W W, Goudie R B 1968 A clinico-immunological study of serum and synovial fluid antinuclear factors in rheumatoid arthritis and other arthritides. Journal of Clinical and Experimental Immunology 3:17
Marcusson J 1979 Psoriasis and arthritic lesions in relation to the inheritance of HLA genotypes. Acta Dermato-Venereologica 59 Supplement 82
Meany T F, Hays R A 1957 Roentgen manifestations of psoriatic arthritis. Radiology 68:403
Metzger A L, Morris R I, Bluestone R, Terasaki R I 1975 HL-A W27 in psoriatic arthropathy. Arthritis and Rheumatism 18:11
Miller J L, Soltani K, Tourtellotte C D 1971 Psoriatic acro-osteolysis without arthritis. Journal of Bone and Joint Surgery 53A:371
Moll J M H 1971 D M Thesis, University of Oxford
Moll J M H, Wright V 1973a Psoriatic arthritis. Seminars in Arthritis and Rheumatism 3:55
Moll J M H, Wright V 1973b Familial occurrence of psoriatic arthritis. Annals of the Rheumatic Diseases 32:181
Monacelli M 1971 In: Psoriasis. Proceedings of International Symposium, Stanford University. Stanford University Press, Stanford, p 99–104
Mueller W, Graf U 1981 The use of cyclosporin A, a new immunosuppressant, in the treatment of psoriatic arthritis. Schwiz Med Wochenschr 111: 408–413
Mustakallio K K, Lassus A 1964 Staphylococcal alpha-antitoxin in psoriatic arthropathy. British Journal of Dermatology 76:544
Nazzaro P, Gigante D 1971 In: Psoriasis. Proceedings of International Symposium, Stanford University. Stanford University Press, Stanford, p 137–139
O'Leary P A 1943 A method of treating psoriasis. Canadian Medical Association Journal 48:34
Peter J B, Pearson C M, Marmor I 1966 Erosive osteoarthritis of the hands. Arthritis and Rheumatism 9:365
Petres J, Majert P 1968 Immunelekrophorese bei psoriatischer Arthropathie. Archiv für klinische und experimentelle Dermatologie 232:398
Pillsbury D M, Shelley W B, Kligman A M 1956 In: Dermatology. Saunders, Philadelphia, p 728–729
Plenk H D 1950 Psoriatic arthritis — report of a case. American Journal of Roentgenology 64:635
Popp W C, Addington E A 1941 Roentgen therapy for psoriasis of nails and psoriatic arthritis. Radiology 36:98
Porrini A, McEwan C, Ditata D, Poppel M, Lingg C 1964 Roentgenologic and clinical study of ankylosing spondylitis and spondylitis accompanying ulcerative colits, psoriasis and Reiter's disease. Arthritis and Rheumatism 7:338
Prusanski W, Orgyzlo M A 1972 Lysozyme in rheumatic diseases. Seminars in Arthritis and Rheumatism 1:361
Rawson A J, Abelson N M, Hollander J L 1965 Studies on the pathogenesis of rheumatoid joint inflammation. II. Intracytoplasmic particulate complexes in rheumatoid synovial fluids. Annals of Internal Medicine 62:281
Redisch W, Messina E J, Hughes G, McEwen C 1970 Capillaroscopic observations in rheumatic diseases. Annals of the Rheumatic Diseases 29:244
Reed W B 1961 Psoriatic arthritis — a complete clinical study of 86 patients. Acta dermato-veneralogica 41:396
Reed W B, Becker S W 1960 Psoriasis and arthritis. Archives of Dermatology 11:577
Reed W B, Wright V 1966 In: Hill A G S (ed) Modern trends in rheumatology. Butterworths, London, p 375–383
Reed W B, Heiskell C L, Becker S W 1961 Negative latex-fixation test in psoriatic arthritis. Archives of Dermatology 83:653
Reiter H F H, Norholm-Pederson H 1953 Relation between psoriasis and polyarthritis. Acta dermato-venereologica 33:372
Richter M B, Kinsella P, Corbett M 1980 Gold in psoriatic arthropathy. Annals of the Rheumatic Diseases 39: 279–280
Roberts M E T, Wright V, Hill A G S, Mehra A C 1976 Psoriatic arthritis; follow-up study. Annals of the Rheumatic Diseases 35:206
Robillard J 1968 Le rhumatisme psoriasique (a Propos de 53 Observations). Thése, Lyon
Romanus T 1945 Psoriasis from a prognostic and hereditary point of view. In: Psoriasis from a prognosis and hereditary point of view. Dissertation, Uppsala
Russell T J, Lorain M D, Schults M, Kuban D J 1972 Histocompatibility (HL-A) antigens associated with psoriasis. New England Journal of Medicine 287:738
Sany J, Seignalet J, Guilhou J J, Serre H 1975 HL-A et rhumatisme psoriasique. Revue du Rhumatologie 42:451

Schattenkirchner M 1970 Zur Symptomatologie der Arthritis psoriatica. Medizinische Klinik 65:1360

Serre H, Simon L, Sany J 1969 Le rhumatisme psoriasique. Journal de Medecine de Montpellier 4:3

Shelley W B, Harun J S, Pillsbury D M 1958 The treatment of psoriasis and other dermatoses with triamcinolone (Aristocort). Journal of the American Medical Association 167:959

Sherman M S 1952 Psoriatic arthritis — observations on the clinical, roentgenographic and pathological changes. Journal of Bone and Joint Surgery 34A:831

Shore A, Ansell B M 1982 Juvenile psoriatic arthritis — an analysis of 60 cases. Journal of Pediatrics 100: 529–535

Short L C, Bauer W, Reynolds W E 1957 In: Rheumatoid arthritis. Harvard University Press, Cambridge, Massachusetts, p 38–42

Smukler W M, Edeimen J, Giuliano V J 1971 Ankylosis in osteoarthritis of the finger joints. Radiology 100:525

Sönnichsen N 1969a Vergleichende immunologische Untersuchungen bei Lupus erythematodes, primär chronischer Polyarthritis und Psoriasis arthropathica. Allergie und Asthma 15:1

Sönnichsen N 1969b Immunologische Untersuchungen zur nosologischen Stellung der Psoriasis arthropathica. Allergie und Asthma 15:124

Steinberg A G, Becker S W, Fitzpatrick T B, Kierland R R 1951 A genetic and statistical study of psoriasis. American Journal of Human Genetics 3:267

Sterne E H, Schneider B 1953 Psoriatic arthritis. Annals of Internal Medicine 38:512

Stollenwerk E, Fischer-Hoinkes H, Komenda K, Schilling F 1981 Clinical observations on oral retinoid therapy of psoriatic arthropathy (RO10–9359). In: Orfanos C E (ed) Retinoids. Springer Verlag, Berlin, p 205–209

Strom S 1921 A case of arthropatia psoriatica. Acta radiologica 1:21

Swezey R L, Alexander S J 1971 Erosive osteoarthritis and the main en lorgnette deformity. Archives of Internal Medicine 128:269

Theiss B, Schnyder U W, Böni A, Wagenhauser F 1969 Intrafamiliäre Untersuchungen bei Psoriasis-Arthritis. Zeitscheift für Rheumaferschung 28:403

Theiss B, Schnyder U W, Böni A 1970 Intrafamiliäre immunochemische Untersuchungen bei Psoriasis-Arthritis und Psoriasis-Spondylarthritis. Archiv für klinische und experimentelle Dermatologie 239:248

Tickner A, Mier P D 1960 Serum cholesterol, uric acid and proteins in psoriasis. British Journal of Dermatology 72:132

Tiedemann G 1951 Symptomatologie und Aetiologie der Psoriasis arthropathica. Zeitschrift für menschliche Vererbungs-und Konstitutionsletre 30:248

Tillikainen A, Lassus A, Karvonen J, Vartainen P, Julin M, Psoriasis and HLA Cw6. British Journal of Dermatology 102: 179–184

Tsuji K, Inouye H, Nose Y, Sasazuki T, Ozawa A, Ohkido M 1979 Further studies in HLA A B C D DR and haptotype antigen frequencies in psoriasis vulgaris. Acta Dermatologica-venereologica 59 (Supplement 87): 107–108

Vilaghy I, Krebs A 1970 Untersuchungen uber die Vererblochkeit des Syndrome Psoriasis arthropathica. Dermatologica (Basel) 140:209

Vilanova X, Pinol J 1951 Psoriasis arthropathica. Rheumatism 7:197

Waller M, Toone E C 1968 Normal individuals with positive tests for rheumatoid factor. Arthritis and Rheumatism 11:50

Walton R, Black W D, Heyde J 1961 A comparative study of uric acid values of whole blood in patients with psoriasis and other dermatoses. Journal of Investigative Dermatology 36:125

Ward J H, Stephens F E 1961 Inheritance of psoriasis in a Utah kindred. Archives of Dermatology 84:589

Wassmann K 1949 Rheumatoid arthritis and psoriasis — statistical statement. Annals of the Rheumatic Diseases 8:70

Watson W, Cann H M, Farber E M, Nall M L 1971 In: Psoriasis. Proceedings of International Symposium, Stanford, University. Standford University Press

Weddel G, Cowan M A, Palmer E, Ramaswamy S 1965 Psoriatic skin. Archives of Dermatology 91:252

Weissman S, Eisen A Z, Karon M 1962 Pseudouridine metabolism, urinary excretion in gout, psoriasis, leukemia and heterozygous oroticaciduria. Journal of Laboratory and Clinical Medicine 59:852

White S, Newcomer V, Mickey M, Terasaki P 1972 Disturbance of HL-A antigen frequency in psoriasis. New England Journal of Medicine 287:740

Williams K A, Scott J T 1967 Influence of trauma on the development of chronic inflammatory polyarthritis. Annals of the Rheumatic Diseases 26:532

Wright V 1956 Psoriasis and arthritis. Annals of the Rheumatic Diseases, 15:348

Wright V 1957a Psoriasis and arthritis. British Journal of Dermatology 69:1

Wright V 1957b Psoriatic arthritis: a comparative study of rheumatoid arthritis and arthritis associated with psoriasis. British Journal of Radiology 30:113

Wright V 1959a Psoriatic arthritis: a comparative study of rheumatoid arthritis and arthritis associated with psoriasis. Archives of Dermatology 80:27

Wright V 1959b Rheumatism and psoriasis — a re-evaluation. American Journal of Medicine 27:454

Wright V 1961 Psoriatic arthritis — a comparative study of rheumatoid arthritis and arthritis associated with psoriasis. Annals of the Rheumatic Diseases 20:123

Wright V 1969 In: Copeman W S C (ed) Psoriatic arthritis. Livingstone, Edinburgh, p 632–633

Wright V, Reed W B 1904 The link between Reiter's syndrome and psoriatic arthritis. Annals of the Rheumatic Diseases 23:12

Wright V, Moll J M H 1976 Seronegative polyarthritis. North Holland, Amsterdam, p 169–235

Zachariae H, Zachariae E 1969 Antinuclear factors, the anti-human globulin consumption test, and Wassermann reaction in psoriatic arthritis. Acta Rheumatica Scandinavica 15:62

Reiter's disease

Historical outline

As long ago as 1507 Pierre Van Forest described a patient who developed arthritis of the knee in association with urethritis, and Martiniere recognised arthritis as a complication of urethritis in 1664 (Sharp, 1972). Over 150 years ago Sir Benjamin Brodie (1818) described the syndrome which now carries the eponymous title of 'Reiter's disease'. This report appeared almost one hundred years before Hans Reiter (1916) described the case of a cavalry officer serving on the Balkan front who developed an acute dysenteric illness characterised by arthritis, urethritis and conjunctivitis. Since then over 97 synonyms have been used to describe this entity. It is generally accepted that 'Reiter's disease' is an unsatisfactory term for the syndrome; and, as Ford (1953a) has pointed out, Reiter's paper made only a negligible and somewhat misleading contribution to the subject: the illness of Reiter's patient followed dysentery, and the arthritis was attributed to syphilis — indeed, in the title, the phrase 'spirochaetosis arthritica' appeared.

The first description in the USA did not appear until 1942 (Bauer & Engelman, 1942), and the syndrome has become more widely recognised since the studies of Harkness (1950), Csonka (1958a, b, 1960), Ford (1953, 1958), and workers at the London Hospital (Murray et al 1958; Oates & Young, 1959; Hancock, 1960).

There seems little doubt that previous reviews have included patients with gonococcal disease. A study (Wright, 1963) of 214 patients with arthritis associated with venereal disease delineated gonococcal arthritis and Reiter's disease, and few today would doubt their existence as separate entities.

The classical triad of Reiter's disease comprises non-specific urethritis, arthritis and conjunctivitis. It is now appreciated that there is a spectrum of involvement and Hancock & Mason (1965) have summarised the disease as one of unknown cause, the most constant feature of which is a recurrent non-suppurative polyarthritis with a predilection for the joints of the lower limbs and sacroiliac joints, occurring in close association with non-specific inflammation of the lower urogenital tract. In an attempt to overcome the difficulties of definition, the American Rheumatism Association made a retrospective analysis of 66 different clinical features associated with 'typical' cases of Reiter's disease, and assessed the sensitivity and specificity of these features in delineating it from ankylosing spondylitis, psoriatic arthritis, gonococcal arthritis and seronegative rheumatoid arthritis (Wilkens et al, 1981). Their working definition was 'an episode of peripheral arthritis of more than one month's duration occurring in association with urethritis and/or cervicitis'. Cervicitis was not defined, and the preconceived ideas of the contributors would inevitably influence the outcome of this investigation, together with the fact that it was done in the USA, where a dysenteric form of Reiter's disease is less common than it is in Scandinavia.

Prevalence

In the United Kingdom and North America most cases follow extramarital sexual intercourse, whereas in other parts of Europe dysentery more frequently precedes the clinical symptoms. Csonka (1958a) commented that the disease seemed to be less severe in coloured patients. A paper from Papua showed that Reiter's disease accounted for the majority of cases of arthritis in young males, and epidemiological studies suggested a venereal transmission (Maddocks, 1967). It is difficult to arrive at a figure for the prevalence of Reiter's disease venereally acquired. Laird (1958) found a prevalence of 1.7% amongst 3500 cases of non-specific urethritis. The urethritis is usually assumed to be venereally acquired, although patients frequently deny sexual exposure. The time relationship with sexual intercourse, and the fact that the majority of patients acknowledge themselves to be sexually promiscuous (Csonka, 1958a) lends support to this. Indeed, 12–50% of patients do give a history or have signs of other diseases known to be venereal, usually gonorrhoea (King, 1957; & Levy, 1950; Csonka, 1958a, Steinmetz Green, 1959). However, there are cases which fall into this category in whom such a history cannot be obtained even by those most skilled in extracting such information, and, similarly, during a dysentery epidemic cases occur in patients who have no symptoms or signs of diarrhoea.

There are some who would still incriminate gonococcal infection in this disease, but the course of true gonococcal arthritis and its response to treatment distinguishes the diseases as groups (Wright, 1963). However, it is not necessarily true that the majority of so-called cases of 'gonococcal arthritis' were in fact examples of Reiter's disease (Harkness, 1950; Ford, 1953b; Kelly, 1958).

Incidence

The majority of cases occur between the ages of 16 and 35 years (Fig. 31.1). Reiter's disease is the most common cause of peripheral inflammatory arthritis in young men (Arnett et al, 1976). The disease has been reported in children. The first published account of the syndrome in childhood did not appear until 1946 when Koster & Jansen reported a Dutch family in which three infants developed the triad. Since then, other cases have been published (Zewi, 1947; Paronen, 1948; Corner, 1950; Jacobs, 1961; Moss, 1964). Of particular interest is a case of Reiter's disease reported in a boy aged 32 months (Florman & Goldstein, 1948). Lockie & Hunder (1971) in an excellent review found in the literature only 20 adequately detailed cases of childhood Reiter's occurring under the age of 16. They found a higher frequency (75%) of diarrhoea in all childhood cases. Of the childhood cases so far reported only 7 have

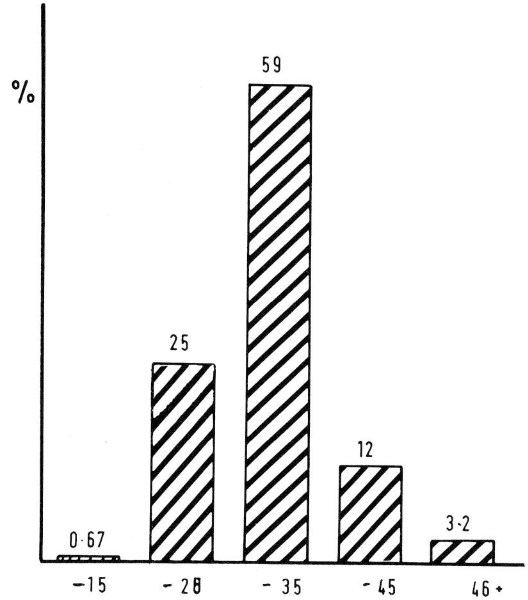

Fig. 31.1 Age of onset of Reiter's disease (739 cases).

been from England (Corner, 1950; Jacobs, 1961; Gough, 1962; Moss, 1964; Iveson et al, 1975), and six from the United States (Florman & Goldstein, 1948; Margileth, 1962; Herman, 1966; Davies et al, 1969; Lockie & Hunder, 1971).

At the other end of the scale, older patients may be affected, and King (1957) found 25 of his 101 patients were between 41 and 60 years. A review of the literature suggests that 3.2% of patients develop the disease after the age of 45 years.

Reiter's disease is usually (some would say almost exclusively) confined to men. The ratio of 15 males to 1 female quoted by King & Nicol (1969) is similar to that of other authors. The only reports of childhood Reiter's disease occurring in girls have come from Europe (Zewi, 1947; Henckel, 1954). This gives a ratio of 1 girl to 4–5 boys which is similar to that found in Paronen's adult 'dysenteric' cases, of whom 10% were women; but higher than that of Oates & Csonka (1959) who found a ratio of approximately 1 female to 50 male patients seen in venereal disease clinics. This would seem to indicate that the childhood cases have more in common with the adult dysenteric than the venereal form.

Epidemiological studies

The source of any series influences the clinical pattern considerably, as is well shown by the sexually-acquired reactive arthritis described by Keat et al (1979), who looked at 57 patients with arthritis associated with non-gonococcal genital infection that presented at a venereal disease clinic.

A dysenteric form of Reiter's disease usually follows bacillary dysentery and the most extensive study has been undertaken by Paronen (1948) in a report of 344 cases in Finland following an outbreak of dysentery.

Aboard an American naval vessel 9 such cases followed an outbreak of bacillary dysentery affecting 602 personnel in whom there was no immediate venereal exposure (Noer, 1966). The disease, however, may also follow attacks of amoebic dysentery (Moorhead, 1916; Graby et al, 1949; Marche, 1955), and has been observed following seasonal toxic non-specific diarrhoea among French troops in Algeria (Roumagnac et al, 1958; Masbernard, 1959). The incidence and geographical distribution of these cases generally correspond with the behaviour of the preceding dysentery epidemic (Paronen, 1948), although this is not invariable (Manson-Bahr, 1943). The endemic sporadic form is related to the increase in the fly population (Marche, 1955), the seasonal incidence of diarrhoea, and lack of hygienic facilities. Newcomers to the area appear to be more susceptible (Roumagnac et al, 1958). Paronen found the frequency of Reiter's disease to be 0.24% amongst 150 000 cases of dysentery.

Reiter's syndrome follows *Shigella flexneri* 1b and 2a infections in about 1.5% of white adults with dysentery, women developing post-dysenteric Reiter's syndrome as often as men (Simon et al, 1981). In a Puerto Rican community *S. Sonnei* was not arthritogenic (Caslow et al, 1979).

Family studies

There are few data on familial aspects of the disease. A summary of the literature is shown in Table 31.1. Koster & Jansen (1946) reported attacks in three or four siblings; Paronen (1948) mentioned multiple cases in three families; Trier (1950) and Csonka (1958a) reported the occurrence in brothers, and Morton (1958) reported cousins who were affected. A hereditary predisposition to the arthritis of Reiter's disease was suggested by Csonka (1958a) on the basis that 13% of 109 patients gave a 'clear account of rheumatoid arthritis in their families', compared with only 2.2% of a control group of 400 patients with uncomplicated urethritis. However, little weight can be given to the recollection of patients, as rheumatologists concerned in family surveys will appreciate. A nationwide study of families of patients with Reiter's disease in the United Kingdom was attempted by Lawrence (1974). Results in 34 families showed an

Table 31.1 Reiter's disease affecting more than one member of family: summary of literature

		Index case				Secondary case(s)				
Author(s)	Year	Sex	Age	Diarrhoea	Triad	Relationship	Age	Diarrhoea	Triad	Interval[a]
Koster & Jansen	1946	M	15	+	+	Brother	11	0	0	14 days
						Brother	3	0	0	15 days
Glauner	1947	M	15	+	+	Brother	10	+	+	Not given
Schoeneich	1950	F	13	+	+	Brother	7	0	+	3 days
Fabregoule	1951	M	40+	+	+	Wife	40+	+	0	Simultaneous
						Son	16	+	0	Simultaneous
Davies et al	1969	M	39	+	0	Son	11	+	+	3 days
						Son	7	+	+	Few days
Trier	1950	M	Adult	0	0	Bro-in-law	—	0	+	1 month
						Brother	37	0	0	20 months
Morton	1958	M	36	0	+	1st cousin (male)	27	0	+	10 years
Gough	1962	M	Adult	0	0	Son	15	0	+	Not given
Mowat & Nicol	1968	M	29	0	+	Brother	21	0	+	26 months
Csonka	1969	M	31	0	+	Brother	34	0	+	9 months
		M	27	0	+	Brother	25	0	+	6 months
Good	1971	M	23	0	+	Brother	46	0	+	17 years

[a] Interval between onset index case to onset secondary case(s).

increased prevalence of sacroiliitis, spondylitis, and of psoriasis among relatives.

Aetiology

Reiter's disease usually follows an infection of the bowel or lower genitourinary tract. Enterocolitic agents which have been implicated as triggers are *Shigella flexneri* (serotypes 2a and 1b), *Salmonella typhimurium*, *Salmonella enteritidis*, *Salmonella heidelberg*, *Yersinia enterocolitica* (Marsal et al, 1981), *Yersinia pseudoberculosus*, and *Campylobacter fetus* (Weir et al, 1979; Urman et al, 1977). The nature of the agent responsible for the disease and its manner of operation are not clear. It has been suggested that the spinal changes might be due to an infective agent draining directly via the prostatic venous plexus to the sacroiliac joints (Grainger, 1959), or by the venous system described by Batson (1942) passing from the prostate and seminal vesicles to the sacroiliac joints (Oates & Young, 1959). This may also be the explanation of the sacroiliitis in women, occurring as a late sequel to acute salpingitis (Hagenfeldt & Szanto, 1980). A piece of evidence favouring this view is that sacroiliitis is said to occur in patients with paraplegia (Abel, 1950; Lodge, 1956). It was felt that genital inflammation causing sacroiliitis was 'a seductive hypothesis' (Mason et al, 1958), since nearly all the male paraplegic patients would be expected to have chronic prostatitis. A careful study of bone and joint changes in paraplegic men was unable to substantiate this (Wright et al, 1965). Sacroiliac changes occurred in 12 of 38 patients, but the changes differed from sacroiliitis. They appeared to be due to mechanical stresses operating on osteoporotic bones around the joints. There was no evidence to connect the sacroiliac joint changes with chronic genitourinary infection, but they were found more frequently in patients whose admission to a special unit had been delayed, in those who had been confined to bed for longer periods, and in those whose mobilisation had been delayed.

Much effort has been expended in trying to isolate an infective agent from patients with Reiter's disease (Levy et al, 1966), but so far without consistent success. Intermittently, the role of pleuropneumonia-like organisms (PPLO) has excited attention, and some have claimed to isolate them from patients with Reiter's disease (Bartholomew, 1965). Others have not been so successful (Ford & Rasmussen, 1964). PPLO cause arthritis in animals (Decker & Ward, 1966), but their role in Reiter's disease is far from clear. No virus has been implicated yet, despite strenuous efforts (Ford & Rasmussen, 1964).

More recently, attention has been directed to the *Bedsonia* genus of organisms (psittacocis-lymphogranuloma venereum-trachoma group). In sheep, *Bedsonia* cause arthritis, conjunctivitis and orchitis (Norton & Storz, 1967). They have been isolated from the synovium, urethra and conjunctiva of some patients with Reiter's disease (Engelman & Weber, 1967), and some of the patients also had complement-fixation titres of 1 : 16 or more against a Bedsonia group antigen (Schachter et al, 1966). *Chlamydia trachomatis* has been implicated as a probable causal agent (Vilppula et al, 1981), but other studies have not confirmed this, although there may be exaggerated antibody response to acute infection by *Chlamydia* (Keat et al, 1980).

It should be remembered that it is difficult to demonstrate an association between a disease and a virtually universal phenomenon, sexual intercourse. Furthermore, non-gonococcal urethritis is a feature of post-dysenteric Reiter's syndrome, occurring without sexual exposure. Urethritis is, therefore, an inherent feature of Reiter's syndrome, and need be considered only as another mucocutaneous lesion which is not necessarily a marker for the portal of entry of an infectious agent (Arnett, 1982).

It is possible that an infective agent initiates the disease and that many of its manifestations are immunologically produced. This may be the explanation for the prostatic antibodies found by a haemagglutination test in these patients (Grimble & Lessof, 1965). On the other hand, prostatititis from whatever cause could well produce such antiprostatic antibodies (Grimble, 1964). In rats, inoculation with complete Freund adjuvant produces a polyarthritis with an acute balanitis and urethritis, iritis or iridocyclitis and dermatitis (Pearson, 1963).

The most probable explanation of these features is that patients genetically predisposed to the disease develop it after exposure to an infective agent acquired either by venereal exposure or in a dysenteric attack. The high frequency of HLA-B27 antigen in patients with Reiter's disease (Brewerton et al, 1973; Morris et al, 1974; Brewerton et al, 1974; McCluskey et al, 1974) favours this suggestion, as discussed by Metzger et al (1974). However, it should be noted that only 20% of B27-positive persons develop arthritis after attacks of shigellosis, salmonellosis or yersinosis (Woodrow, 1979). This is a similar figure to the occurrence of sacroiliitis in B27 subjects from the population, and raises the possibility that these two diseases may be appearing independently in the same genetically predisposed host. The findings of immunoproteins in the synovium of the majority of patients with Reiter's syndrome, suggests that immunological mechanisms are involved in the pathogenesis of the disease (Baldassare et al, 1981). The findings of Ford and his colleagues (1980, 1981) would support this.

Clinical features

There is a wide spectrum of Reiter's disease. It is difficult to determine the frequency of various features, since some authors insist on the complete triad for the diagnosis of Reiter's disease, whereas others have less stringent criteria. This has been well shown by two published series of patients (Table 31.2).

In both the venereal and the diarrhoeal forms of Reiter's disease the arthritis begins between 1 and 3 weeks after the initial symptom. The average time is about 15 days.

Diarrhoea tends to be mild, short-lived and with absence of blood. The urethritis, likewise, is usually a mild disease with a mucoid urethral discharge, which is rarely bloodstained (Colby, 1944; Twiss & Douglas, 1946; Ford, 1953b; Reiter, 1957). There is usually some dysuria and occasionally the discharge may be purulent. Frequency of micturition is common and bladder involvement produces suprapubic discomfort.

Urogenital lesions

The non-specific urethritis associated with the beginning of the venereally-acquired disease may be asymptomatic and detected only by examination of the first urine specimen in the morning (the two-glass test) when shreds of mucoid material may be seen. Occasionally, however, it is severe. Acute haemorrhagic cystitis, confirmed cystoscopically, occurs (Berg et al, 1957; Berry & Berry, 1947) and prostatitis is an almost invariable accompaniment of the disease. This is diagnosed by examining the fluid obtained on prostatic massage and observing 10 or more leucocytes per half inch microscopic field. Interpretation of such findings must be cautious, however, and although prostatitis of this degree is an invariable accompaniment of Reiter's disease, the converse, that prostatitis is an evidence of genitourinary infection, should not be assumed. In men who are otherwise normal, 25% have evidence of 'chronic prostatitis' on these criteria (Oates, 1959; Catterall, 1960) and men with rheumatoid arthritis have a similar frequency (Mason et al, 1958).

Cystitis, which is said to occur in about 3% of patients (Paronen, 1948; Harkness, 1950; Csonka, 1958a), may produce serious shrinkage of the bladder (Piora, 1953) and cases of hydronephrosis arising from ureteric stenosis (Colby, 1944; Harkness, 1950) have been described.

Urethritis is frequent in the dysenteric form of Reiter's disease (Young & McEwen, 1947; Paronen, 1948; Noer, 1966). This raises the possibility that inflammation of the urogenital tract may be due to mechanisms other than direct infection, although there is no information on the incidence of prostatitis in these patients. Conversely, diarrhoea may occur in venereally-acquired Reiter's disease and has been reported in 32% of the patients described by Weinberger et al (1962) and 22% of those described by Hall & Finegold (1953).

Circinate balanitis is a characteristic feature of

Table 31.2 Frequency of complications in two series of cases with Reiter's disease

Authors	Series	No. of cases	% eye lesions	% mouth lesions	% penile lesions	% keratoderma
Montgomery et al (1959)	Triple	38	92	37+	80	30
Hancock (1960)	Unselected	76	44.7	10.5	26.3	7.8

the disease. It has the appearance of keratoderma elsewhere. The frequency of balanitis (26%) in the dysenteric form is similar to the figures of Hancock in the disease venereally acquired. Its appearance is influenced by whether the patient is circumcised. In uncircumcised subjects the initial lesion is a superficial ulcer of small diameter which may coalesce with others to form circinate patches. As these develop a clear centre is left and a scaly border appears. In the circumcised patient, however, the lesions may be discrete and the scaly border very hyperkeratotic (Montgomery et al, 1959; Weinberger et al, 1962). A classical example is shown in Figure 31.2. Circinate vulvitis has also been described (Thambar et al, 1977).

At the onset the patient may be pyrexial with a temperature reaching 103°F. Three-quarters of the patients in the literature are said to have had a raised temperature.

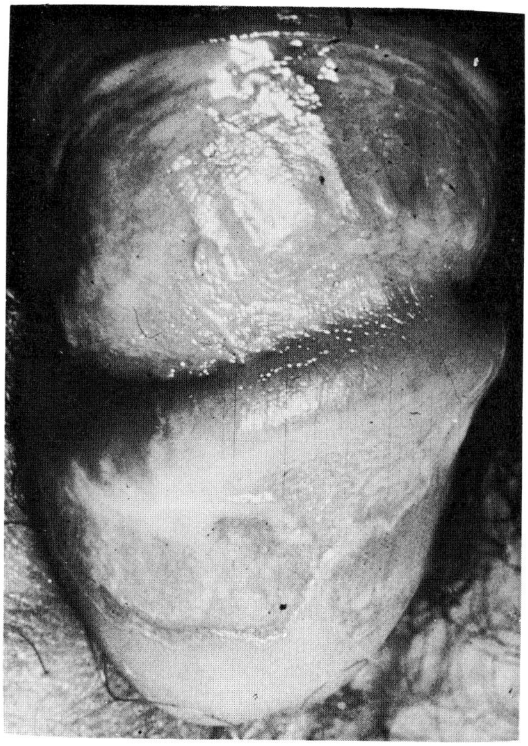

Fig. 31.2 Circinate balanitis.

Arthritis

Joint symptoms are characteristically acute, short-lived and transient. A patient may have undoubted non-specific urethritis and then develop an acute monarticular arthritis which subsides within 3 or 4 days, regardless of the type of treatment.

Weight-bearing joints, particularly the knees and ankles, are most frequently involved initially (Fig. 31.3). The activity of arthritis may be extremely acute and attended by large tense effusions; this is particularly well seen at the knee which has been known to rupture early in the course of the disease (Weese & McCarthy, 1969; Garner & Mowat, 1972; Moll, 1973).

In nearly a quarter of patients the arthritis starts

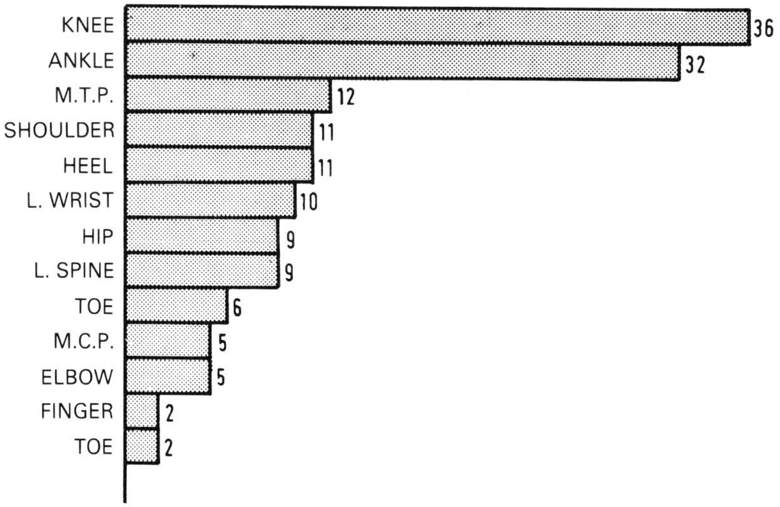

Fig. 31.3 Joints involved at onset of Reiter's disease.

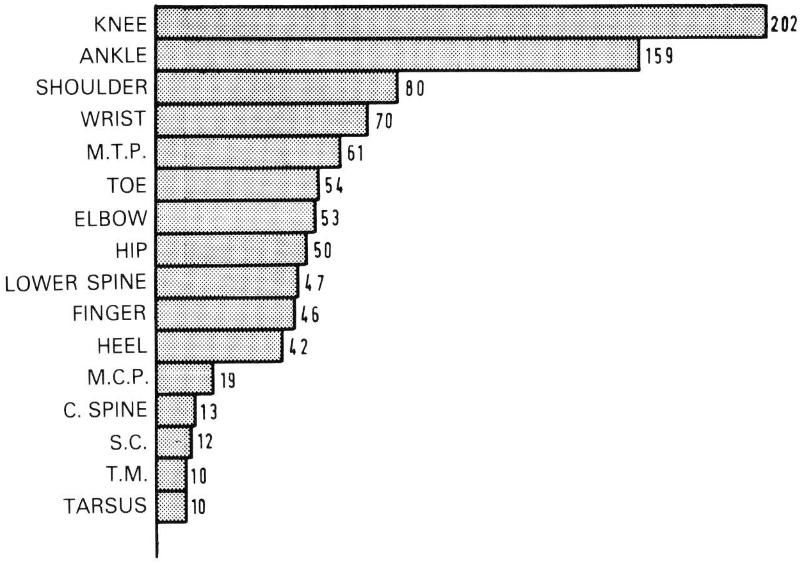

Fig. 31.4 Joints involved during the course of Reiter's disease.

in one joint. The arthritis may become widespread, and occasionally involves most joints of the body. More often it is confined to five or six joints, and the knees and ankles remain predominantly affected (Fig. 31.4). The arthritis is commonly asymmetrical.

A feature of the disease is the occurrence of fleeting pains in the back, the plantar fascia, the heels, the chest wall, and soft tissues of the lower limbs. The tendon sheaths may be involved, especially around the tendo Achilles, although tenosynovitis is not such a prominent feature as it is in gonococcal arthritis (Ford, 1953a; Wright, 1963). Csonka (1958a) found tendon involvement in 37 of 185 cases at the London Hospital.

Residual disability occurs in about 5% (Hancock & Mason, 1965). Permanent deformities of the feet (Fig. 31.5), pain at the insertion of the plantar fascia into the os calcis, metatarsophalangeal arthralgia, deformity of the fingers and spondylitis may

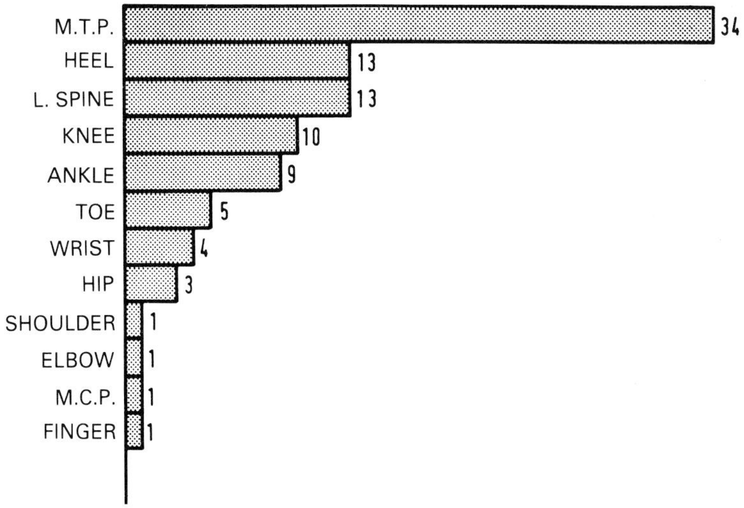

Fig. 31.5 Residual disability in Reiter's disease.

all occur. Precise data are not easily gleaned from the literature on this aspect, but in order of frequency the sites of residual symptoms appear to be metatarsophalangeal joints, heels, lumbar spine and knee.

Although Reiter's disease is self-limiting recurrences do occur. The more prolonged the follow-up of these patients the higher is the frequency of recurrence and Csonka (1960) in a 15-year experience of a single department found the likelihood of a second attack to be in the region of 62%. These recurrences may be associated with reinfection and more rarely with factors such as dilatation of urethral strictures, food poisoning, diarrhoea caused by antibiotics, tonsillitis (Csonka, 1958a), massage of the prostate (Olhagen, 1960), respiratory infections, and damage to the joints (Weinberger et al, 1962). It is interesting that a fresh infection producing non-specific urethritis does not necessarily provoke a recurrence of Reiter's disease (Csonka, 1960), and likewise a further attack of dysentery only preceded a second attack of arthritis in 4 of the 10 cases of recurrence reported by Paronen (1948). However, a longer follow-up study from 100 of the Finnish cases 20 years after the initial attack showed that only 20 patients had been free from symptoms since the original attack. In 32, symptoms and radiological findings of sacroiliitis or spondylitis were present, 18 had chronic active peripheral arthritis, and in 30 chronic arthritis had become inactive. A more or less severe disability was present in 42 patients (Sairanen et al, 1969).

The spinal involvement which is radiologically indistinguishable from ankylosing spondylitis (Ford, 1953b) is of particular interest.

Mason (1964) found sacroiliitis in 10% of patients with Reiter's disease of less than 5 years' duration and 54% of those of more than 5 years' duration. Comparable figures of Lawrence (1965) were 9% and 71%.

Ocular lesions

Conjunctivitis is part of the classical triad of Reiter's disease. Its reported incidence is higher in patients with dysentery, but these figure are of dubious significance since symptoms may be so mild as to escape the patient's notice (or at the most give the sensation of a little grittiness in the eye for a short time). The discharge is sterile and subsides in 1–4 weeks (Popert et al, 1964). The condition may progress, however, to produce episcleritis, keratitis, and corneal ulceration; uveitis may also occur. Uveitis affects less than 1 in 10 patients early in the course of the disease, but Ford (1953b) reported a frequency of 30% in patients with recurring chronic arthritis. Where sacroiliitis is present, half the patients may be affected (Csonka, 1959a). Looking at the problem from the opposite point of view Catterall (1961) examined 211 men with anterior uveitis in an opthalmological department and found Reiter's disease in 21.3% and ankylosing spondylitis in 12.3%.

Iritis may occur as an incident separate from arthritis in a protracted course of Reiter's disease. Less commonly intraocular haemorrhage or hypopyon (Paronen, 1948), optic neuritis (Zewi, 1947; Oates & Hancock, 1959), and retrobulbar neuritis (Lindsay-Rea, 1947) can also occur.

Integumentary lesions

Keratoderma blenorrhagica is the characteristic skin lesion of the disease (Fig. 31.6). In Hancock's series the rash occurred in 7.8%, whereas other authors quote figures as high as 30%. The lesions begin commonly on the soles of the feet, but may involve the palms and occasionally become extensive, spreading to the rest of the limbs, trunk, and scalp, and rarely involving the face. In such severe cases they may persist for as long as a year. Patients with the dysenteric form seem to have keratoderma less frequently and no more than 2% is the reported prevalence. Initially, the lesions occur as brown macules which progress to papulovesicles and pustules. Later, scales develop and the lesions come to resemble limpets.

The nails may be involved with a dystrophy affecting the whole nail, simulating the grosser changes of psoriasis (Fig. 31.7). Hyperkeratosis with heaping of cornified material under the nail can be severe enough to cause displacement or even shedding of the nail. Sometimes lakes of pus develop in the nailfold at the base and sides. Deep pits or even punched-out areas are also occasionally seen (Samman, 1972).

Histologically, the epidermis shows hyperkeratosis, parakeratosis and acanthosis, with irregular elongation of the rete ridges and frequent supra-

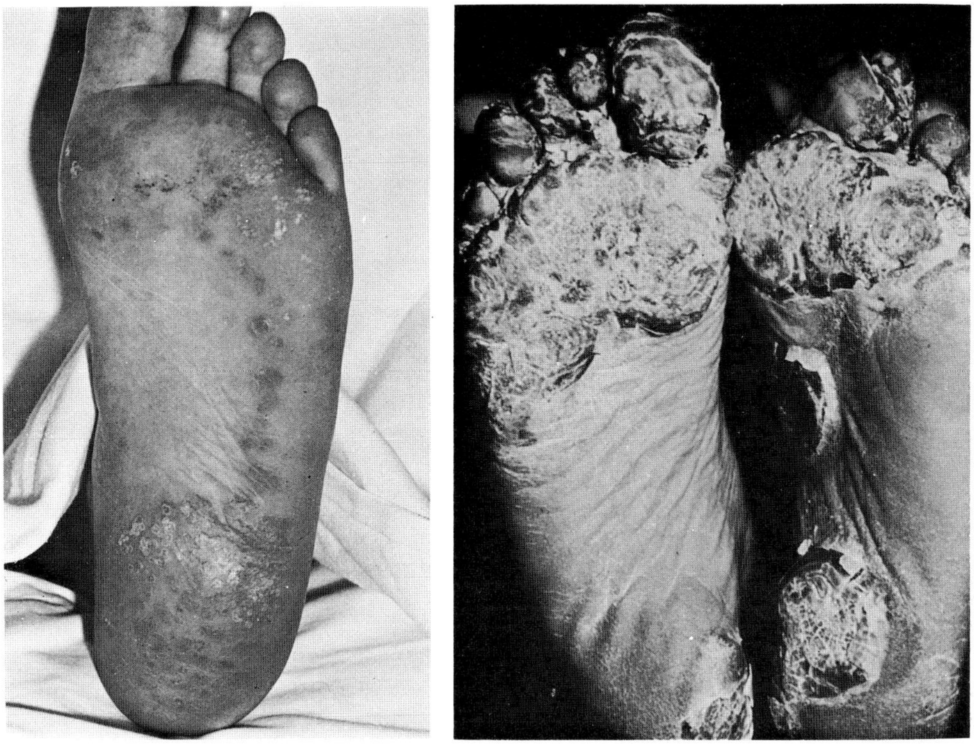
a b

Fig. 31.6 Keratoderma blenorrhagica. (a) Early lesions. (b) Advanced changes.

papillary thinning. There is a varying degree of vacuolisation and lysis of the superficial prickle cells, with focal neutrophil infiltration which may result in microabscesses. The papillary layer of the corium is infiltrated by lymphocytes and plasma cells with a few scattered neutrophils (Kulka, 1962; Weinberger et al, 1962; Wright & Reed, 1964: Maxwell et al, 1966). The appearances are indistinguishable from pustular psoriasis (Lever & Crawford, 1944), and 11 cases have been described in which the clinical appearance of the skin has progressed to frank psoriasis (Wright & Reed, 1964). This has since been confirmed by others (Khan & Hall, 1965; Maxwell et al, 1966; Perry & Mayne, 1965). It has been questioned whether this is not the coincidence of a fairly common disease, psoriasis, in these patients (Hancock, 1960), but careful observation lends support to the view that there is an association between Reiter's disease and psoriatic arthritis.

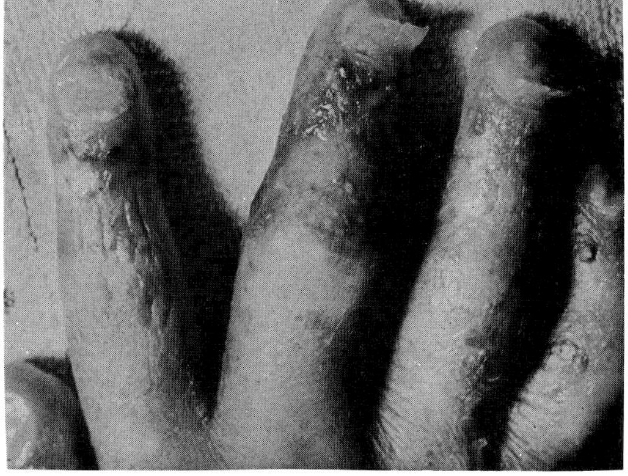

Fig. 31.7 Nail dystrophy of Reiter's disease.

Oral lesions

Buccal erosions occur in about 8% of patients. They usually start as painless shiny red patches, and occur on the palate, tongue and mucosa of the cheeks or lips. Uncommonly, they proceed to confluent erythema of the soft palate, uvula and tonsillar regions, with purpura of the tongue (Montgomery et al, 1959; Hancock, 1960). Essentially, the histology of lesions affecting the skin, glans penis and oral mucosa are the same. Epistaxis has occasionally been reported, and it may well have a similar basis.

Other lesions

Involvement of the heart is well recognised. Electrocardiographic changes include prolongation of the P-R interval (Feiring, 1945; Hall & Finegold, 1953; Csonka et al, 1961; Weinberger et al, 1962), complete heart block (Trier, 1950), and serial T-wave changes, elevation of the S-T segment or occasional abnormal Q-waves (Feiring, 1945; Vallee, 1946; Hall & Finegold, 1953; Weinberger et al, 1962). Clinically, the patient may complain of palpitations, and transient systolic murmurs may be heard (Paronen, 1948; Hall & Finegold, 1953; Masbernard, 1959). In the dysenteric form, cardiovascular complications occurred in 7% and a pericardial friction rub (or pericarditis) occurred in 2% (Paronen, 1948). This has also been noted in other series (Mayne, 1955; Csonka & Oates, 1957; Csonka et al, 1961).

Aortic incompetence has also been reported (Camp, 1956; Csonka et al, 1961; Cliff, 1971) in Reiter's disease. These lesions were indistinguishable from the aortic abnormality of ankylosing spondylitis. The prolonged follow-up of the Finnish series (Sairanen et al, 1969) showed serious heart disease in two patients (cardiac failure and total heart block).

Involvement of the central nervous system has been reported, but no consistent findings have emerged. The frequency of neurological complications is low, probably in the region of 1% (Hancock, 1964), and these include peripheral neuropathy (Walther, 1941; Wilke, 1943; Graby et al, 1949), neuritis of the shoulder girdle (Wilke, 1943; Oates & Hancock, 1959), transient hemiplegia (Lagon et al, 1955), and meningoencephalitis (Oates & Hancock, 1959). Cranial nerve lesions may also occur (Walther, 1941; Zewi, 1947; Csonka, 1958b).

In the respiratory system, pleurisy and pulmonary infiltrations have been reported in Reiter's disease (Thiers & Pinet, 1950; Lafon et al, 1955). Considering other similarities between Reiter's disease and ankylosing spondylitis it is interesting that recently lung lesions have also been reported in the latter. These consist of chronic infiltrative and fibrotic changes in the upper lobes (Hamilton, 1949; Campbell & MacDonald, 1965; Jessamine, 1968). This clinical and radiological picture appears to differ from the transient pulmonary infiltration reported in Reiter's disease.

Purpura (Makari, 1950), thrombophlebitis (Csonka, 1966), amyloidosis (Bleehen et al, 1966) and severe haemorrhage from gastrointestinal ulceration (Boyle & Buchanan, 1971) may all complicate Reiter's disease, but are rare.

Radiological features

In the early stages no abnormality is found radiologically. Later, however, particularly in patients with recurrent disease, juxta-articular osteoporosis, narrowing of the joint space, and erosive changes are all found (Guck & Wolf, 1952; Ford, 1953a; Mason et al, 1959; Reynolds & Csonka, 1958). The last authors described ankylosis of the small joints of the hands and feet as a rare finding, and this was also noted by Twiss & Douglas (1946) and Weldon & Scalettar (1961).

Periostitis may be a striking feature at times, occurring along the metatarsals, phalanges of the feet, tarsal bones, and around the pubis. Roughness at the insertion of the plantar fascia is also fairly characteristic of the disease (Fig. 31.8). Plantar spurs in Reiter's disease are typically large and fluffy although smooth spurs of smaller size and similar to those seen in rheumatoid arthritis

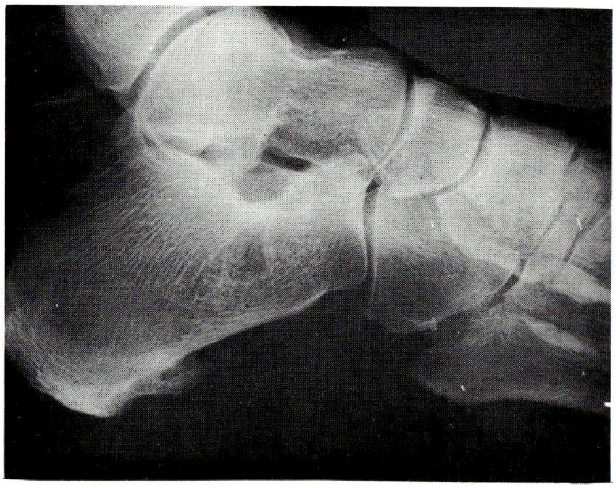

Fig. 31.8 Florid plantar spur in a man with Reiter's disease.

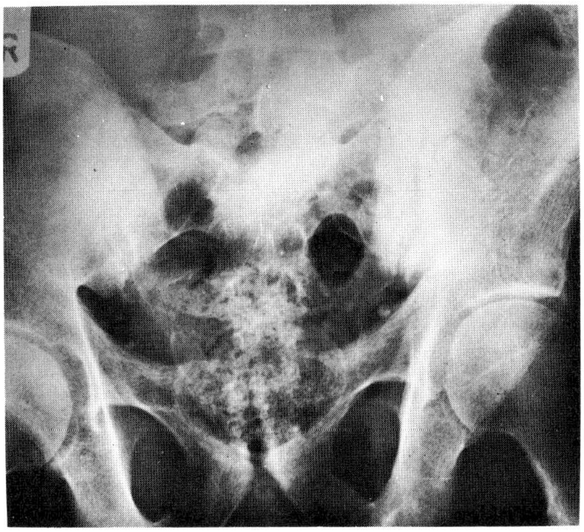

Fig. 31.9 Sacroiliitis in Reiter's disease.

and ankylosing spondylitis may also occur (Mason et al, 1959).

Changes of sacroiliitis are indistinguishable from those accompanying ankylosing spondylitis (Fig. 31.9). Sacroiliitis may be asymmetrical and in 17% of one series the changes were unilateral (Oates & Young, 1959). Sacroiliac involvement is found particularly in patients with longstanding, recurrent disease, and figures as high as 80% have been quoted (Marche, 1950). However, the usual frequency is nearer 30%. The longer the duration of the disease, the higher is the frequency (Mason, 1964; Lawrence, 1965). Patients who go on to develop psoriatic arthritis nearly all show some changes in the sacroiliac joints (Wright & Reed, 1964).

Some patients demonstrate apophyseal joint erosion and ankylosis, together with ligamentous calcification indistinguishable from that seen in uncomplicated ankylosing spondylitis (Ford, 1953a). It has been suggested that a characteristic finding in the early stage of spinal involvement in Reiter's disease is an isolated bony spur on a single vertebral body (Cliff, 1971). McEwen et al (1971) felt that the radiological picture of these patients was the same as in psoriatic arthritis, but different from that seen in uncomplicated ankylosing spondylitis.

Cliff (1971) reported three cases with unusual lateral bony bridging between the vertebral bodies of the dorsal spine and dorsolumbar junction. Two

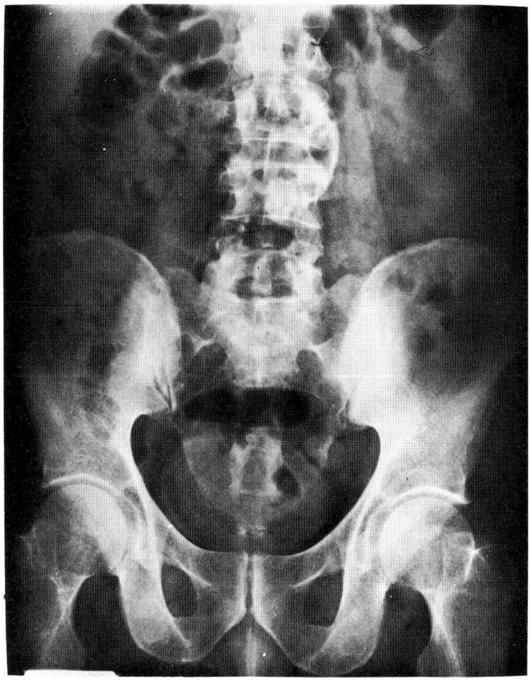

Fig. 31.10 Spinal bony bridging.

of these patients had a febrile illness erroneously attributed to subacute bacterial endocarditis, and all had aortic incompetence. This unusual type of spinal bony bridging (Fig. 31.10) was also noted by Weldon & Scolettar (1961), Montgomery et al, (1963), Good (1965) and Peterson & Silbiger (1967). The association with aortic value disease was described in one case by Rodnan et al (1964). These bony lesions must be distinguished from senile ankylosing hyperostosis of the spine (Forestier & Rotes-Querol, 1950) and the rare familial ankylosing vertebral hyperostosis (Beardwell, 1969). The skip lesions of the spine have certain similarities to the unusual progressive paraspinal calcification of psoriatic arthritis. Indeed, this may be another area where there is 'overlap', since some of the cases described by Bywaters & Dixon (1965) as examples of psoriatic arthritis also had features of Reiter's disease. Martel (1979) has described these as discontinuous spondylitis characterised by eccentric, laterally positioned vertebral hyperostoses which tend to bridge around the contiguous disc. He believes that these are characteristic, together with subtle periosteal bone apposition of bony prominences, the increased frequency of regional panarthritis and hip and shoulder involvement, and the tendency for destructive arthritis to be confined to small joints, particularly in the feet.

Pathology

Where biopsy material is available, the unhelpful but accurate report of 'non-specific inflammation' is usually returned. Initially, there is oedema with vascular congestion and moderate infiltration of neutrophils, lymphocytes and occasional plasma cells, together with some proliferation of synoviocytes and fibroblasts. In specimens taken later in the disease, the changes are principally lymphocytic, and show perivenular infiltration of lymphocytes and plasma cells, and lymphocyte nodules which are indistinguishable from those of rheumatoid arthritis (Weinberger et al, 1962).

Biopsy of the skin lesions shows changes of keratoderma blenorrhagica or pustular psoriasis, and these have been discussed in Chapter 30. The mucous membrane lesions show similar changes.

Synovial Fluid

Examination of the synovial fluid reveals little that would not be expected with an inflammatory exudate. There is a protein content in the region of 50 g/litre and the mucin clot is poor (Weinberger et al, 1962); there is an elevated white count between 1000 and 50 000 cells/mm^3 of which 66% are polymorphonuclear leucocytes, although this proportion may be as high as 97% (Ellis & Bereston, 1959). Occasionally the joint fluid can contain so many polymorphs as to appear purulent, though sterile. This is important in the differential diagnosis from infective arthritis. In 20 joint aspirates reported in the literature, the mean white count was 18 000. The glucose was low in 3 of 11 patients in one series (Sharp et al, 1968), and in 13 of 23 in another (Weinberger et al, 1962), the mean being 16 mg/100 ml. It has been suggested that one feature distinguishing rheumatoid arthritis is the normal total haemolytic complement in Reiter's disease contrasted with low titres in rheumatoid arthritis (Fostiropoulos et al, 1965). However, synovial fluid : serum complement values appear to be reduced in Reiter's disease (Yates et al, 1975).

Blood tests

The ESR is often considerably raised and may be as high as 140 mm/h; this may persist for weeks after the acute attack and does not necessarily parallel joint activity. A mild hypo- or normochromic anaemia (Hall & Finegold, 1953; Sargent, 1945) may be present, together with leucocytosis, the white cell count occasionally rising to 32 000/mm^3 (Hamner & Grayowski, 1964). In these circumstances bacterial infection of a joint has to be excluded by diagnostic aspiration.

Serum proteins show little change apart from an occasional decrease in the albumen and an increase in the alpha 1 and alpha 2 globulin fractions. Serum uric acid is usually within the normal range (Young & McEwen, 1947; Csonka, 1959; Weinberger et al, 1962; Hancock, 1964; Noer, 1966).

There are few serological abnormalities. Rheumatoid factor, whether determined by the latex fixation test or the Rose–Waaler differential agglutination test, is usually absent from the sera in these patients (McEwen et al, 1958; Csonka, 1959; Kellgren et al, 1959; Oates & Csonka, 1959; Hancock, 1964). Anti-nuclear factor is negative and LE cells are absent (Noer, 1966). A haemaglutination test for prostatic antibodies (Grimble, 1964) is commonly positive, but is not specific. One-third of patients with ankylosing spondylitis have positive results, and the test has proved positive in 20% of women.

A striking laboratory development in Reiter's disease is the demonstration of a high proportion of HLA-B27-positive tests (75%) in Reiter's disease contrasted with only 9% in uncomplicated non-specific urethritis and 6% in controls (Brewerton et al, 1973).

In this study, HLA-B27 was particularly associated with patients with Reiter's disease complicated by ankylosing spondylitis, an observation confirmed by Bluestone et al (1973). The precise implications of these interesting results are still not clear, but it would seem that if a patient with non-specific urethritis is HLA-B27-positive he has a higher than expected chance of developing the full picture of Reiter's disease. Furthermore if a patient with Reiter's disease is HLA-B27-positive it might be expected that sacroiliitis or ankylosing spondylitis will be present, or if not present, it may be reasonable to keep the patient under close review in anticipation of its development in the future.

Differential diagnosis

The acute nature of the arthritis may raise the question of infective arthritis, systemic lupus erythematosus, osteomyelitis, brucellosis, rheumatic fever, gout and pseudogout. The multiple joint involvement, the distribution of joints involved, the relationship to non-specific urethritis or dysentery, and the course of the disease are all useful pointers. Where pyogenic arthritis is suspected, diagnostic aspiration is mandatory. Aspiration may also help to differentiate gout and pseudogout in that characteristic crystals of uric acid or calcium pyrophosphate may be seen with polarised microscopy. The presence of chondrocalcinosis radiologically may also alert the clinician to the possibility of pseudogout.

The differential diagnosis may be particularly difficult when the complete triad is not present. Yet few would doubt that 'incomplete' forms of the disease occur. The ocular lesions may be minimal, being experienced merely as a sense of grittiness in the eyes or indeed escaping the notice of the patients altogether. The urethral discharge may be barely perceptible (especially in women), or it may be denied even to those most skilful in extracting a history of venereal exposure. The course of the illness is similar in the incomplete forms, although the frequency of other features may be greater in patients with the complete triad (Table 31.2).

Although the chronic phase may mimic rheumatoid arthritis, the asymmetrical nature of the arthritis (particularly at its onset), the persistent absence of rheumatoid factor in the serum, and the involvement of the sacroiliac joints are all useful in differentiating the condition. A high ESR at the start of the illness may also point to the diagnosis of Reiter's disease rather than rheumatoid arthritis.

It has been suggested that the normal total haemolytic complement in the synovial fluid, compared with the low value in rheumatoid arthritis, may also be helpful in diagnosis. However, the synovial fluid : serum complement levels appear to be reduced in Reiter's disease (Yates et al, 1975).

In the venereally-acquired form of Reiter's disease gonococcal arthritis is the most important disease to differentiate. Gonococcal arthritis can only be diagnosed with certainty by culture of the organism from the synovial fluid. However, if it is cultured from the urethral discharge, the infection merits treatment in its own right, and the arthritis will subside dramatically and completely with penicillin or sulphonamides (Wright, 1963).

Psoriatic arthritis, Behçet's syndrome, and the Stevens–Johnson syndrome must also be considered. Genital ulceration is a common feature of true Behçet's syndrome, and the ocular involvement is usually more severe than in Reiter's disease, sometimes producing blindness. It has been suggested that in the Stevens–Johnson syndrome the skin lesions are less pustular than in Reiter's disease and not keratotic. The mucocutaneous lesions of these diseases have been well discussed by Robinson & McCrumb (1950). When psoriasis vulgaris and keratoderma blenorrhagica coexist it is impossible to make a distinction between psoriatic arthritis and Reiter's disease, since even the more florid lesions of the two conditions are indistinguishable clinically and histologically.

Management

There is no form of treatment that can consistently prevent attacks of Reiter's disease from progressing, can cause clear-cut and substantial reductions in the duration of established attacks, or can prevent the development of subsequent attacks. Treatment of all features is empirical and is aimed at reducing symptoms and the intensity of the inflammatory process until the disease undergoes a spontaneous remission. Specific treatment is, of course, available for antecedent dysentery or associated gonorrhoea.

The tetracyclines are usually preferred for the non-specific urethritis of Reiter's disease because they are most effective in the treatment of uncomplicated non-specific urethritis. (However, there is still no incontrovertible evidence to show that the two types of urethritis have the same cause.) A dose of 250 mg of tetracycline or oxytetracycline 6-hourly for 5 days is often sufficient. Continuing the treatment for longer appears to provide no further benefit unless *Chlamydia* have been isolated (Schofield, 1972). If there is a response, this is usually noted within 24–72 hours when dysuria, and the volume and purulence of the discharge diminish. Thereafter, the discharge may disappear altogether or remain as a scanty mucopurulent secretion detectable only by the early morning two-glass test. Even in patients without overt urethritis it is advisable to have an examination by a genito-urinary physician.

In patients with haemorrhagic cystitis tetracycline may be effective, and to relieve dysuria and strangury, potassium citrate and hyoscyamus mixture *BPC* is often beneficial.

When the activity of the urethritis, arthritis or ocular inflammation is controlled it is King's policy to examine the prostate, as chronic prostatitis (more accurately prostatovesiculitis) is almost invariably present (King, 1964). If prostatitis is present, twice-weekly prostatic massage and a 5-day course of tetracycline are given. During recovery serial examination of the prostate fluid may show diminution of the proportion of polymorphonuclear leucocytes and a decrease in their tendency to clump together. In other cases, despite subjective relief, the fluid remains the same.

While under treatment for the urogenital disorder, the patient should abstain from sexual activity and steps should be taken to examine the patient's sexual partner to exclude similar or other venereal disease, particularly gonorrhoea. Advice on the avoidance of promiscuous activity and the risk of recurrence should be given.

Schofield (1972) has suggested that the management of the urethritis is not complete without urethroscopy. This should be done after active urethritis has subsided in order to exclude urethral stricture, even if this complication is not suggested by clinical features. Outpatient review should be continued for a long time, preferably several years.

As far as the arthritis is concerned, preferably all but the mildest cases should be admitted to hospital and confined to strict rest in bed. Splinting should be minimal, but if necessary should be used for the shortest time in view of the risk of fibrous ankylosis. Muscle wasting, particularly of the quadriceps, may be marked in Reiter's disease and requires appropriate physical treatment. Severe cases will normally need indomethacin 100–150 mg daily individed doses. This produces substantial pain relief, often within a few days. When symptomatic relief has been obtained, the dose is reduced gradually. Other non-steroidal anti-inflammatory drugs may be equally effective, but have not been tried so extensively. A valuable guide to the activity of the disease is continuing fever. The ESR, which may be considerably elevated, is less reliable, sometimes remaining elevated long after improvement of other features has taken place. The patient's feeling of well-being and his response to exercise are better guides than the height of the sedimentation rate as to whether or not to discharge the patient from hospital.

Indomethacin should be continued for about the first month of outpatient supervision. If gastric intolerance arises other non-steroidal anti-inflammatory drugs may be used, but high doses will probably be required. Corticosteroids are indicated in patients with severe disease of acute onset attended by much pain, rapid wasting, continued fever, and high and increasing sedimentation rate which have failed to respond to indomethacin within a few days. Adequate control is likely to need large doses of corticosteroid (up to 60 mg of prednisolone or its equivalent). The symptoms of Reiter's disease tend to be more resistent to corticosteroids than those of rheumatoid arthritis.

The use of cytotoxic or immunosuppressive agents in severe or intractable Reiter's disease is not yet established. Methotrexate has been used successfully, according to uncontrolled studies (Mullins et al, 1966; Farber et al, 1967). Other antimitotic agents such as 6MP, azathioprine and cyclophosphamide also appear capable of suppressing Reiter's disease in tolerable doses (Sharp, 1972). However, all these preparations are potentially toxic drugs and are not recommended for general use, especially in those of reproductive age. On the other hand, there may be a place for their selective use, particularly in patients with severe or prolonged episodes of Reiter's disease with permanent residua which have been refractory to simpler forms of therapy. The management of acute recurrent attacks of Reiter's disease is similar to that of first attacks.

Pain in the region of the plantar fascia or Achilles tendon may be controlled by local corticosteroid injection. Effusions of the knees, which may be large, should be aspirated; they respond to intra-articular injections of corticosteroid.

Mild and transient conjunctivitis needs no local

treatment. When it is severe, however, the position is more difficult. It is generally felt by opthalmologists that corticosteroids alone are contraindicated in view of the possibility that Reiter's disease may be due to infection by a virus. This objection has not yet been tested by controlled study. Furthermore patients with conjunctivitis receiving systemic steroids for the arthritis have experienced no worsening of the conjunctivitis, and Jacobs (1961) has used topical steroid therapy without harm. However, until more evidence is available, it is probably judicious to withhold local steroids for conjunctivitis. Some clinicians use frequent instillations of chloramphenical drops until the conjunctivitis remits in order to reduce the chances of secondary infection.

All cases of anterior uveitis should have skilled opthalmological management. This usually includes dark glasses to relieve photophobia, atropine to dilate the pupil and to prevent adhesions of the iris, and topical corticosteroids to suppress inflammation. In severe cases systemic steroids may be necessary.

Keratoderma usually requires no treatment. Topical chlortetracycline (Cameron, 1956), penicillin, streptomycin and broad spectrum antibiotics (Levy, 1950; Ford, 1953b; Fowler & Knight, 1956; Albert & Crone, 1959; Montgomery et al, 1959), and corticosteroids (Myerson & Katzenstein, 1952; Schwartz & Kingma, 1952; Ford, 1953; Albert & Crone, 1959; Montgomery et al, 1959) have met with doubtful therapeutic success. Local triamcinolone, in view of its beneficial effect in psoriasis, is now being tried in Reiter's disease by some workers, but the results have not yet been formally evaluated. Aminopterin or methotrexate may afford complete or partial remission of keratoderma (Maxwell et al, 1966; Mullins et al, 1966), but in view of the frequency of serious side-effects these drugs are not recommended for routine use.

The moist lesions of circinate balanitis can usually be completely suppressed with applications of hydrocortisone or other corticosteroid cream. These preparations are best combined with an antibiotic in uncircumcised patients in order to deter secondary infection.

Mouth ulcers are usually pain-free and rarely require special treatment.

The infrequent but important occurrence of cardiac and neurological complications in Reiter's disease constitutes an indication for systemic corticosteroids (Schofield, 1972).

REFERENCES

Abel M S 1950 Sacroiliac joint changes in traumatic paraplegics. Radiology 55:235

Albert J, Crowe R 1959 Keratosis blennorrhagica (Reiter's disease?) and its treatment. Archives of Dermatology 79:581

Arnett F C 1982 Reiter's syndrome. Johns Hopkins Medical Journal 150: 39–44

Baldassare A R, Weiss T D, Tsai C C, Arthur R E, Moore T L, Zuckner J 1981 Immunoprotein deposition in synovial tissue in Reiter's syndrome. Annals of the Rheumatic Diseases 40: 281–285

Bartholomew L E 1965 Isolation and characterization of PPLO from patients with rheumatoid arthritis and Reiter's syndrome. Arthritis and Rheumatism 8:376

Batson O V 1942 Role of vertebral veins in metastatic processes. Annals of Internal Medicine 16:38

Bauer W, Engelman E P 1942 Syndrome of unknown aetiology characterized by urethritis, conjunctivitis, and arthritis (so-called Reiter's disease). Transactions of the Association of American Physicians 57:307

Beardwell A 1969 Familial ankylosing vertebral hyperostosis with tylosis. Annals of the Rheumatic Diseases 28:518

Berg R L, Weinberger H, Dienes L 1957 Acute haemorrhagic cystitis. American Journal of Medicine 22:848

Berry J V, Berry N E 1947 Acute exudative cystitis of undetermined aetiology. Journal of Urology 58:260

Bleehen S S, Everall J D, Tighe J R 1966 Amyloidosis complicating Reiter's syndrome. British Journal of Venereal Diseases 42:88

Bluestone R H, Schlosstein L H, Terasaki P, Pearson C M 1973 Paper presented at XIII International Congress of Rheumatology, Kyoto, Japan

Boyle J A, Buchanan W W 1971 Clinical rheumatology, 1st Edn. Blackwell, Oxford

Brewerton D, Caffrey M, Nicholls A, James D C O 1974 The histocompatility antigen (HL-A27) and its relation to disease. Journal of Rheumatology 1:249

Brewerton D A, Caffrey M, Nicholls A, Walters D, Oates J K, James D C O 1973 Reiter's disease and HL-A27. Lancet 2:996

Brodie B C 1818 Pathological and surgical obsercations on diseases of the joints. Longman, London, p 54

Bywaters E G, Dixon A St J 1965 Paravertebral ossifications in psoriatic arthritis. Annals of the Rheumatic Diseases 24:313

Cameron J M 1956 Keratodermia blennorhagica. British Journal of Veneral Diseases 32:7

Camp S 1956 Zur Klinik und Prognose der Reiter'schen Krankheit. Münchener medizinische Wochenschrift 98:334

Campbell A H, MacDonald C B 1965 Upper lobe fibrosis

associated with ankylosing spondylitis. British Journal of Diseases of the Chest 59:90
Catterall R D 1960 Uveitis, arthritis, and non-specific genital infection. British Journal of Veneral Diseases 36:27
Catterall R D 1961 Significance of non-specific genital infection in uveitis and arthritis. Lancet 2:739
Cliff J M 1971 Spinal bony bridging and carditis in Reiter's disease. Annals of the Rheumatic Diseases 30:171
Colby F 1944 Renal complications of Reiter's disease. Journal of Urology 52:415
Corner B D 1950 Reiter's syndrome in childhood. Archives of Disease in Childhood 25:398
Csonka G W 1958a The course of Reiter's syndrome. British Medical Journal 1:1088
Csonka G W 1958b Involvement of the nervous system in Reiter's syndrome. Annals of the Rheumatic Diseases 17:334
Csonka G W 1959 Bacteriological and biochemical investigation in Reiter's syndrome. British Journal of Venereal Diseases 35:84
Csonka G W 1960 Recurrent attacks in Reiter's disease. Arthritis and Rheumatism 3:164
Csonka G W 1966 Thrombophlebitis in Reiter's syndrome. British Journal of Venereal Diseases 42:93
Csonka G W 1969 Multiple cases in Reiter's syndrome. British Journal of Venereal Diseases 45:157
Csonka G W, Litchfield J W, Oates J K, Willcox R R 1961 Cardiac lesions in Reiter's disease. British Medical Journal 1:243
Csonka G W, Oates J K 1957 Pericarditis and electrocardiographic changes in Reiter's syndrome. British Medical Journal 1:866
Davies N E, Haverly J R, Boatwright M 1969 Reiter's disease associated with Shigellosis. Southern Medical Journal (Birmingham, Alabama) 62:1011
Decker J L, Ward J R 1966 The relationship of mycoplasma (PPLO) to RA and related diseases — working conference. Bulletin on Rheumatic Diseases 16:412
Ellis F A, Bereston E S 1959 Reiter's syndrome versus keratosis blenorrhagica sine blenorrhoea. Southern Medical Journal 52:828
Engleman E, Weber H M 1968 Reiter's syndrome. Clinical Orthopaedics 57:19
Fabregoule M 1951 Syndrome familial de Fiessinger–Leroy–Reiter syndrome. Algérie médicale 55:1054
Farber G A, Forshner J G, O'Quinn S E 1967 Reiter's syndrome: treatment with Methotrexate. Journal of the American Medical Association 200:171
Feiring W 1945 Reiter's disease with prolonged auricolo-ventricular conduction. Annals of Internal Medicine 25:498
Florman A L, Goldstein H M 1948 Arthritis, conjunctivities, and urethritis (so-called Reiter's syndrome) in a four-year old boy. Journal of Pediatrics 33:172
Ford D K 1953a Natural history of arthritis following venereal urethritis. Annals of the Rheumatic Diseases 12:177
Ford D K 1953b Arthritis and venereal disease. British Journal of Venereal Diseases 29:123
Ford D K 1958 Reiter's syndrome. Bulletin on Rheumatic Diseases 8:159
Ford D K, Rasmussen G 1964 Relationship between genitourinary infection and complicating arthritis. Arthritis and Rheumatism 7:220
Ford D K, Da Roza D M Shah P, Wenman W M 1980 Cell-mediated immune responses of synovial mononuclear cells in Reiter's syndrome against ureaplasmal and chlamydial antigens. Journal of Rheumatology 7: 751–755
Ford D K, Da Roza D M, Shah P 1981 Cell-mediated immune responses of synovial mononuclear cells to sexually transmitted, enteric and mumps antigens in patients with Reiter's syndrome, rheumatoid arthritis and ankylosing spondylitis. Journal of Rheumatology 8: 220–232
Forestier J, Roates-Querol J 1950 Senile ankylosing hyperostosis of the spine. Annals of the Rheumatic Diseases 9:321
Fostiropoulos G, Austen K F, Bloch K J 1965 Total haemolytic complement (CH 50) and second component of complement (C'2nd) activity in serum and synovial fluid (encl. Reiter's disease). Arthritis and Rheumatism 8:219
Fowler W, Knight G H 1956 Value of treatment in Reiter's disease. British Journal of Venereal Diseases 32:2
Garner R W, Mowat A G 1972 Joint rupture in Reiter's disease. British Journal of Surgery 59:657
Glauner W 1947 Ist die postinfektiöse Trias: Arthritis, Urethritis and Konjunktivitis eine Erkrankung sui generis? Deutsche medizinische Wochenschrift 72:522
Good A E 1965 Reiter's disease and ankylosing spondylitis. Acta Rheumatologica Scandinavica 11:305
Good A E 1971 Reiter's disease, ankylosing spondylitis and rheumatoid arthritis occurring within a single family Arthritis and Rheumatism 14:753
Gough K R 1962 Reiter's syndrome in father and son. Annals of the Rheumatic Diseases 21:292
Graby, Hosotte, Armand 1949 Cahiers médicaux de l'Union Francaise 4:93
Grainger R G 1959 Procto-colitis and other pelvic infections in relation to ankylosing spondylitis. Journal of the Faculty of Radiologists 10:138
Grimble A 1964 Auto-immunity in Reiter's syndrome. British Journal of Venereal Diseases 39:246
Grimble A, Lessof M H 1965 Anti-prostate antibodies in arthritis. British Medical Journal, 2:263
Guck J K, Wolf J 1952 Monarticular and destructive arthropathy in Reiter's syndrome. American Journal of the Medical Science 224:653
Hagenfeldt K, Szanto E 1980 Sacroiliitis in women: A late sequela to acute salpingitis. American Journal of Obstetrics and Gynecology 38: 1039–1041
Hall W H, Finegold S 1953 A study of 23 cases of Reiter's syndrome. Annals of Internal Medicine 38:533
Hamilton K A 1949 Pulmonary disease disease manifestation of ankylosing spondarthritis. Annals of Internal Medicine 31:216
Hamner J G, Gravowski E A 1964 Oral lesions compatible with Reiter's disease — a diagnostic problem Journal of the American Dental Association 69:560
Hancock J A H 1969 Surface manifestations of Reiter's disease in the male. British Journal of Venereal Diseases 36:36
Hancock J A H 1954 In: King A (ed) Recent advances in venereology, 1st Edn. Churchill, London, p 395
Hancock J A H, Mason R M 1965 In: Dixon A St J (ed) Progress in clinical rheumatology. Churchill, London, p 201
Harkness A H 1950 In: Non-gonococcal urethritis. Livingstone, Edinburgh, p 99–145
Henckel H 1954 Reitersche Krankheit bei Kinder. Zeitschrift für Kinderheilkunde 74:303
Herman M 1966 Reiter's syndrome in a 13-year-old boy. Wisconsin Medical Journal 65:195

Iveson J M I, Nanda B S, Hancock J A H, Pownall P J, Wright V 1975 Reiter's disease in three boys. Annals of the Rheumatic Diseases 34:364
Jacobs A F 1961 A case of Reiter's syndrome in childhood. British Medical Journal 2:155
Jessamine A G 1968 Upper lung lobe fibrosis in ankylosing spondylitis. Canadian Medical Association Journal 91:25
Kaslow R A, Ryder R W, Calin A 1979 Search for Reiter's syndrome after an outbreak of Shigella sonnei dysentry. Journal of Rheumatology 6: 562–566
Keat A C, Maini R N, Pegrum G D, Scott J T 1979 The clinical features and HLA association of reactive arthritis associated with non-gonococcal urethritis. Quarterly Journal of Medicine 48: 323–342
Keat A C, Thomas B J, Taylor-Robinson D, Pegrum C D, Maini R N, Scott J T 1980 Evidence of Chlamydia trachomatis infection in sexually acquired reactive arthritis. Annals of the Rheumatic Diseases 39: 431–437
Kelly M 1958 Reiter's syndrome. British Medical Journal 2:449
Kellgren J H, Ball J, Bier F 1959 Clinical significance of the rheumatoid serum factor. British Medical Journal 1:523
Khan M Y, Hall W H 1965 Progression of Reiter's syndrome to psoriatic arthritis. Archives of Internal Medicine 116:911
King A J 1957 Arthritis and venereal urethritis. Excerpta Medica 11:125
King A 1964 In: Recent advances in venereology. Churchill, London, p 457
King A, Nicol C 1969 In: Venereal diseases, 2nd Edn. Balliere, Tindall & Cassell, London
Koster M S, Janson M T 1946 Reiter's disease. Nederlandsch tijdschreift voor Geneeskunde, 90:483
Kulka J P 1962 The lesions of Reiter's syndrome. Arthritis and Rheumatism 5:195
Lafon R, Pages P, Roux J, Temple J P, Minvlelle J 1955 Syndrome de Fiessinger-Leroy-Reiter, avec infiltrates pulmonaires lobaires et hemiplegie regressive — Organisons dans le secretions uretrales. Revue neurologique 92:611
Laird S M 1958 Figures and fancies. British Journal of Venereal Diseases 34:137
Lawrence J S 1965 Personal communication
Lawrence J S 1974 Family survey of Reiter's disease. British Journal of Venereal Diseases 50:140
Lever W F, Crawford G M 1944 Keratosis blennorrhagica without gonorrhoea (Reiter's disease?). Archives of Dermatology and Syphilology 49:389
Levy B 1950 Arthritis in venereal disease with particular reference to aetiology. Medical Journal of Malaya 5:42
Levy B 1951 Value of anti-histamine drugs in treatment of infective arthritis and Reiter's disease. Journal of the Royal Army Medical Corps 97:93
Levy J P, Ryckewaert D, Silvestre D, Kahn M F, Mitrovic D 1966 Etude par microscopie electronique des inclusions des cellules synoviales dans un cas de syndrome oculo-urethro-synovial. Pathologie et biologie 14:216
Lindsay-Rea A 1947 Un cas de maladie de Reiter. Congress of Ophthalmology SUK 67:241
Lockie G N, Hunder G G 1971 Reiter's syndrome in children. Arthritis and Rheumatism 14:767
Lodge T 1956 Bone joint and soft tissue changes following paraplegia. Acta Radiologica 46:435
McClusky O E, Lordon R E, Arnett F C Jr 1974 HL-A27 in Reiter's syndrome and psoriatic arthritis — a genetic factor in disease susceptibility and expression. Journal of Rheumatology 1:263
McEwen C D, Tata D, Lingg C, Porini A, Good A, Rankin T 1971 Ankylosing spondylitis and spondylitis accompanying ulcerative colitis, regional enteritis, psoriasis and Reiter's disease. Arthritis and Rheumatism 14:291
Maddock I 1967 Reiter's disease in Port Moreby, Papua. British Journal of Venereal Diseases 43:280
Makari J G 1950 Journal of Tropical Medicine 53:39
Manson-Bahr P 1943 In: The Dysenteric Disorders. Cassel, London
Marche J 1950 L'atteinte des articulations sacroiliaque dans le syndrome dit de Reiter. Revue du Rhumatisme et des maladies osteo-articulaires 17:449
Marche J 1955 Spondylarthritc ankylosantc ct syndrome de N. Fiessinger-Leroy-Reiter-Deux aspects de la meme maladie rhumatismale. France médicale 18:7
Margileth A M 1962 Reiter's syndrome in children. Clinical Paediatrics 1:143
Marsal L, Winblad S, Wollheim F A 1981 Yersinia enterocolitica arthritis in southern Sweden; a four-year follow-up study. British Medical Journal 283:101
Martel W. Radiologic features of Reiter's disease. Radiology 132: 1–10
Mashernard A 1959 Le syndrome de Fiessinger-Leroy-Reiter, l'etude de 80 cas observes en Tunisie. Revue du rhumatisme et des maladies osteo-articulaires 26:21
Mason R M 1964 Spondylitis. Proceedings of the Royal Society of Medicine 57:533
Mason R M, Murray R S, Oates J K, Young A C 1958 Prostatitis and ankylosing spondylitis. British Medical Journal 1:748
Mason R M, Murray R S, Oates J K, Young A C 1959 A comparative radiological study of Reiter's disease rheumatoid arthritis and ankylosing spondylitis. Journal of Bone and Joint Surgery 41B:137
Maxwell J D, Greig W R, Boyle J A, Pasieczny T, Schofield C B S 1966 Reiter's syndrome and psoriasis. Scottish Medical Journal 11:14
Mayne G O 1955 Electrocardiographic changes in Reiter's syndrome. British Journal of Venereal Diseases 31:238
Metzger A L, Morris R I, Bluestone R 1974 Biologic significance of HL-A W27 in rheumatic disease. Journal of Rheumatology 1:247
Moll J M H 1973 Unpublished data
Montgomery M M, Poske R M, Barton E M, Foxworthy D T, Baker L A 1959 The mucocutaneous lesions of Reiter's syndrome. Annals of Internal Medicine 51:99
Montgomery M M, Poske R M, Pilz C E, Barton E M, Foxworthy D T 1963 Reiter's syndrome, General Practice (Kansas City). General Practitioner 27:88
Moorhead T 1916 A note on dysenteric arthritis. British Medical Journal 1:483
Morris R, Metzger A L, Bluestone R, Terasaki P I 1974 HL-A W27 — a clue to the diagnosis and pathogenesis of Reiter's syndrome. New England Journal of Medicine 240:554
Morton R S 1958 Reiter's syndrome in first cousins. British Journal of Venereal Diseases 34:50
Moss I 1964 Reiter's disease in childhood. British Journal of Venereal Diseases 40:166
Mowat A G, Nicol C S 1968 Reiter's disease in two brothers. British Journal of Venereal Diseases 44:334
Mullins J F, Maberry J D, Stone O J 1966 Reiter's

syndrome treated with folic acid antagonists. Archives of Dermatology 94:335
Murray R S, Oates J K, Young A C 1958 Radiological changes in Reiter's syndrome and arthritis associated with urethritis. Journal of the Faculty of Radiologists (London) 9:37
Myerson R M, Katzenstein L 1952 Keratosis blennorrhagica successfully treated with corticotropin. Journal of the American Medical Association 149:838
Moer H R 1966 An 'experimental' epidemic of Reiter's syndrome. Journal of the American Medical Association 197:693
Norton W L, Storz L 1967 Observations on sheep with polyarthritis produced by an agent of the psittacosis-lymphogranuloma venereum-trachoma group. Arthritis and Rheumatism 10:1
Oates J K 1959 Reiter's disease and ankylosing spondylitis — is there common cause. British Journal of Venereal Diseases 35:81
Oates J K, Csonka G W 1959 Reiter's disease in the female. Annals of the Rheumatic Diseases 18:37
Oates J K, Hancock J A H 1959 Neurological symptoms and lesions occurring in the course of Reiter's disease. American Journal of the Medical Sciences 238:79
Oates J K, Young A C 1959 Sacro-iliitis in Reiter's disease. British Medical Journal 1:1013
Olhagen B 1960 Chronic uro-polyarthritis in the male. Acta medica Scandinavica 168
Paronen I 1948 Reiter's disease — a study of 344 cases observed in Finland. Acta medica Scandinavica, 131 (Suppl):212
Pearson C M 1963 Experimental joint disease. Observations on adjuvant-induced arthritis. Journal of Chronic Diseases 16:863
Perry H O, Mayne J G 1965 Psoriasis and Reiter's syndrome. Archives of Dermatology 92:129
Peterson C C, Silbiger M L 1967 Reiter's syndrome and psoriatic arthritis — Roentgen spectra and some interesting similarities. American Journal of Roentgenology 101:860
Piora J 1953 Cystitis and haematuria as the predominant symptoms of Reiter's disease. Acta medica Scandinavica 144:284
Popert A J, Gill A J, Laird S M 1964 A prospective study of Reiter's syndrome — an interim report on the first 82 cases. British Journal of Venereal Diseases 40:160
Reiter H 1916 Uber eine bisher unerkannte Spirochateninfektion (Spirochaetosis arthritica) Deutsche medizinische Wochenschrift 42:1535
Reiter H 1957 Reiter's disease. German Medical Monthly 2:346
Reynolds D F, Csonka G W 1958 Radiological aspects of Reiter's syndrome ('venereal' arthritis). Journal of the Faculty of Radiologists 9:44
Robinson H M, McCrumb F R 1950 Comparative analysis of the mucocutaneous-ocular syndrome. Archives of Dermatology and Syphilology 61:539
Rodnan G P, Benedek T G, Shaver J A, Fennell R H 1964 Reiter's syndrome and aortic insufficiency. Journal of the American Medical Association 189:889
Roumagnac H, Ferrand M, Pernod J, Memim Y, Eirhart Ch, Contant A 1958 Etude statistique sur le syndrome de Fiessinger-Leroy-Reiter. Revue du Corps de Santé Militaire 14:502
Sairanen B, Paronen I, Mahonen H 1969 Reiter's syndrome — a follow up study. Acta Médica Scandinavica 185:57
Samman P D 1972 In: The nails in disease, 2nd Edn. Heinemann, London, p 69–70
Sargent J C 1945 Reiter's syndrome. Journal of Urology 54:556
Schachter J, Barnes H G, Jones J P, Engleman E P, Meyer K F 1966 Isolation of bedsoniae from joints of patients with Reiter's syndrome. Proceedings of the Society for Experimental Biology and Medicine 122:283
Schoeneich P 1950 Zur Symptomatologie und Atiologie der Reiterschen Krankheit. Geschlechtskr 8:48
Schofield C B S 1972 Sexually Transmitted Diseases. Churchill Livingstone, Edinburgh, p 184
Schwartz H, Kingma H 1952 Keratodermia blennorrhagica treated with cortisone. British Journal of Dermatology 64:388
Sharp J T 1972 In: Hollander J L, McCarthy D J (eds) Arthritis and allied conditions, 8th Edn. Lea & Febiger, Philadelphia, p 1229–1241
Sharp J T, Lidsky M D, Riley W A 1968 Clinical studies on gonococcal arthritis and Reiter's syndrome and measurement of gonococcal and Bedsonia antibodies. Arthritis and Rheumatism 11:569
Simon D G, Kaslow R A, Rosenbaum J, Kaye R L, Calin A, Reiter's syndrome following epidemic Shigellosis. Journal of Rheumatology 1981, 8: 969–973
Steinmetz P R, Gren J P 1959 Reiter's syndrome. United States Armed Forces Medical Journal 10:1185
Thamdar I V, Dunlop R, Thin R N, Huskisson E C 1977 Circinate vulvitis in Reiter's syndrome. British Journal of Venereal Diseases 53: 260–262
Thiers H, Pinet A 1950 Syndrome de Reiter avec urétrite à inclusions, infiltrat pulmonaire labile et keratodermie. Lyon Médical 184:51
Trier M 1950 On Reiter's syndrome with special reference to cardiac complications and familial occurrence of the syndrome. Acta Medica Scandinavica (Suppl) 239:123
Twiss J R, Douglas A H R 1946 Reiter's disease — a report of two cases. American Internal Medicine 24:1043
Urman J D, Zurier R B, Rothfield N F 1977 Reiter's syndrome associated with campylobacter fetus infection. Annals of Internal Medicine 86: 444–445
Vallee B L 1946 Reiter's disease. Archives of Internal Medicine 77:295
Vilppula A H, Yli-Kerttula U, Ahlroos A K, Terho P E 1981 Chlamydial isolations and serology in Reiter's syndrome. Scandinavian Journal or Rheumatology 10: 181–185
Walther G 1941 Nachkrankheiten in der Ruhrrekonvalescens als ausdruck allergischer vorgänge. Münchener Medizinische Wochenschrift 88:381
Weese W C, McCarthy D J 1969 Spontaneous rupture of the knee joint in Reiter's syndrome. Journal of the American Medical Association 208:825
Weinberger H W, Ropes M W, Kulka J P, Bauer W 1962 Reiter's syndrome, clinical and pathological observations — a long term study of 16 cases. Medicine 41:35
Weir W, Keat A C, Welsby P D, Brear G 1979 Reactive arthritis associated with Campylobacter infection of the bowel. Journal of Infection 1: 281–284
Weldon M V, Scalettar P 1961 Roentgen changes in Reiter's syndrome. American Journal of Roentgenology 86:344
Wilke G 1943 Polyneuritiden chronischer enterocolitis insbesondere nach ruhr. Deutsche medizinische Wochenschrift 69:443
Wilkens R F, Arnett F C, Bitter T 1981 Reiter's syndrome. Arthritis and Rheumatism 24: 844–849

Woodrow J C 1979 Genetics of B27-associated diseases. Annals of the Rheumatic Diseases (Suppl 1) 38: 135–141
Wright V 1963 Arthritis associated with venereal disease. Annals of the Rheumatic Diseases 22:77
Wright V, Reed W B 1964 Reiter's syndrome and psoriatic arthritis. Annals of the Rheumatic Diseases 23:12
Wright V, Catterall R D, Cooke J B 1965 Bone and joint changes in paraplegic men. Annals of the Rheumatic Diseases 24:419
Yates D B, Maini R N, Scott J T, Sloper J C 1975 Complement activation in Reiter's syndrome. Annals of the Rheumatic Diseases 34:468
Young R H, McEwen E G 1947 Bacillary dysentery as the cause of Reiter's syndrome. Journal of the American Medical Association 134:1456
Zewi M 1947 Morbus Reiteri. Acta Ophthalmologica 25:47

Enteropathic arthritis

It has been recognised since the last century that inflammatory gut disease may be complicated by arthritis. This association has been generally termed 'enteropathic arthritis', a name which suggests that the cause of the joint disease lies in the intestine. This type of arthritis is a common complication of Crohn's disease, ulcerative colitis and Whipple's disease but is not the only rheumatic complaint found in patients suffering from these conditions. The musculoskeletal complications of each of these diseases are here considered separately, but it will be seen that there are marked similarities among them. These similarities and their significance are elaborated in Chapter 28.

CROHN'S DISEASE

The first systematic description of Crohn's disease was presented to the American Medical Association in 1932 and published in the same year (Crohn et al, 1932). The disease had, however, been described previously and in one early 19th century account, presentation of the disease with rheumatic symptoms was described (Abercrombie, 1830).

Enteropathic arthritis

Enteropathic arthritis was first recognised when large series of patients with Crohn's disease were studied (Van Patter et al, 1954; Crohn & Yarnis, 1958). It was described as 'rheumatoid polyarthritis' and diagnosed in 6% of patients in an early review of the extra intestinal manifestations of Crohn's disease (Daffner & Brown, 1958). The first systematic study of this arthritis was by Ansell & Wigley (1964), who examined 91 patients with Crohn's disease finding past or present inflammatory arthritis in 14. Patients with disease involving the large intestine were excluded from this study as the concept of 'Crohn's colitis' was not generally accepted at that time. It had already been suggested, however, that arthritis was more common in patients with large intestinal disease (Cornes & Stecher, 1961). This has been confirmed subsequently (Rankin et al, 1979) and is the most likely explanation for the higher incidence of arthritis, slightly more than 20%, found in studies of patients with gut disease at all levels (Haslock & Wright, 1973; Selby et al, 1979). As the commonest extraintestinal manifestation of Crohn's disease, arthritis has an important place in the Crohn's disease activity index (Best et al, 1979).

Great care must be taken in assessing the comparative incidence of enteropathic arthritis in ulcerative colitis and Crohn's disease from different series. The diagnostic criteria for both the gut and joint disease must be comparable and the studies should be temporally, methodologically and geographically as close as possible. Where comparative studies have taken place, enteropathic synovitis is found more commonly in Crohn's disease than ulcerative colitis. The 20.7% incidence in Crohn's disease and 12.1% in ulcerative colitis found in one carefully conducted survey probably reflects the true difference between the two conditions (Haslock et al, 1974).

Clinical features

Enteropathic arthritis is an acute synovitis, monarticular in most cases but occasionally polyarticular, involving large and lower limb more often than small and upper limb joints. The knee is most commonly affected, followed by the ankle, shoul-

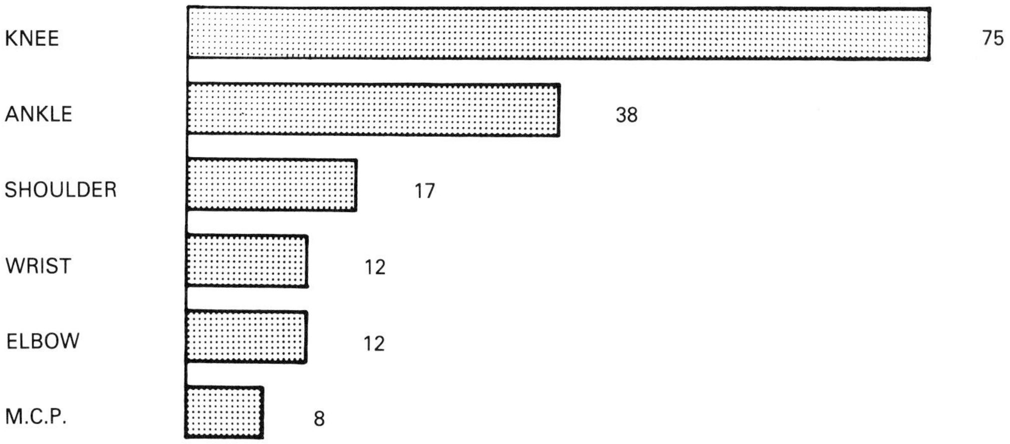

Fig. 32.1 Enteropathic arthritis in Crohn's disease. Joints involved (%). (After Haslock & Wright, 1973.)

der, wrist and elbow and the small joints of the hands and feet (Fig. 32.1). The attacks are self-limiting and resolve with subssquent clinical normality of the involved joints. The arthritis, which is occasionally associated with erythema nodosum, occurs either coincidentally with the onset of the gut disease or at any time during its course. There is a tendency for exacerbations of gut and joint disease to occur together, but surgery does not necessarily abolish the arthritis, which may indeed have a postoperative onset. This reflects the impracticality of a radical surgical cure for Crohn's disease. There is a tendency for arthritis to be more common in patients with other extraintestinal manifestations of their disease, especially perianal ulceration, as this too is more common where the colon is involved.

Investigations

Investigations are helpful to the diagnosis of enteropathic arthritis only by excluding other conditions. The sheep cell agglutination test is negative. Examination of synovial fluid and synovial tissue shows non-specific inflammatory changes (Soren, 1966; Austad et al, 1968). X-rays of affected joints remain normal irrespective of the number of attacks of synovitis.

Aetiology

The cause of enteropathic arthritis is unknown, but the strong temporal association between activity in the gut and the presence of synovitis suggests that some factor within the gut initiates the arthritis. A possible sequence of events in shown in Figure 32.2. Abnormalities of gut flora and gut wall abnormalities have been demonstrated as have antibodies to a variety of intestinal organisms. Circulating immune complexes have not been found in all studies but where they have been detected, high titres have been found in association with extraintestinal disease. The isolation of immune complexes from joints has not been achieved; therefore this pathogenetic mechanism remains hypothetical.

Two alternative pathogenetic mechanisms have been proposed. Biopsies were taken at arthroscopy from 10 patients with Crohn's disease and knee joint pain (Heuman et al, 1981). Crystalline deposits were observed in 7 patients and positively birefringent crystals were demonstrated histologically in 4, 8 of the 10 patients showing evidence of crystal formation. The crystals were considered to be pyrophosphate, and it was suggested that they may have aetiological significance in production of the synovitis. The influence of food on

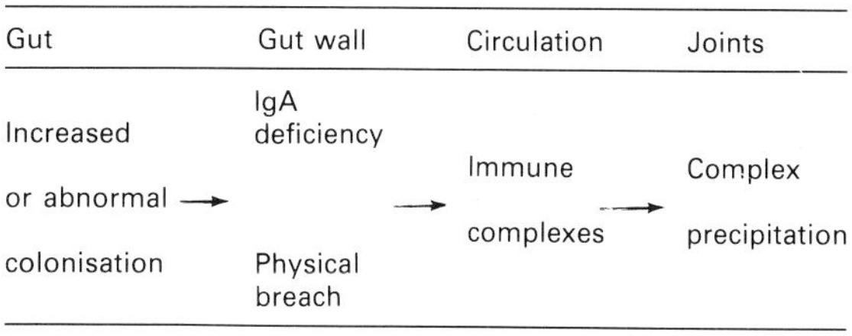

Fig. 32.2 Putative pathogenesis of enteropathic arthritis.

the course of the disease has also been studied. It has been suggested that some patients who experience flares of their arthritis following certain foods are, in fact, absorbing protein, which acts as an antigen initiating the formation of immune complexes and immune complex synovitis. There are too few data available to judge the relevance of this phenomenon, but it may be that a minority of patients will prove to have a 'food allergy' cause for their enteropathic synovitis.

Treatment
Analgesic/anti-inflammatory agents may be given in short courses to control the joint disease. Care must be taken in the selection of these drugs as all may, to some extent, cause gastrointestinal upset. Indomethacin suppositories may cause proctitis, the fenamates should be avoided because of their propensity to produce diarrhoea, and aloxiprin is too frequently costive to be recommended. The bleeding caused by phenylbutazone is not limited to the gastric mucosa but may involve both the small and large intestine and this drug should be avoided. The drugs of choice are now benorylate or one of the propionic acid derivatives such as naproxen. The absorption of fenbufen as a prodrug may decrease gut irritation, but oral indomethacin may be required if these fail. Aspiration of a swollen joint with instillation of hydrocortisone produces rapid pain relief. Surgical synovectomy has been reported, but even in this rare case the articular cartilage was found to be normal (Soren, 1966). Long-term therapy is unnecessary and the presence of enteropathic arthritis should not influence the introduction of drugs such as corticosteroids or azathioprine.

Ankylosing spondylitis
The coincidental development of ankylosing spondylitis and Crohn's disease has been studied from three viewpoints. Firstly, a statistical association has been found between the two diseases in hospital record surveys. These also yielded the information that the onset of spondylitis could antedate that of bowel disease by many years (Acheson, 1960). Secondly, Crohn's disease has been found in patients with 'idiopathic' ankylosing spondylitis with unexpected frequency (McBride et al, 1963). Finally both case reports and formal studies show an increased incidence of sacroiliitis and ankylosing spondylitis in patients with Crohn's disease. About 16% of Crohn's disease patients show radiological sacroiliitis. The proportion of these diagnosed as having true ankylosing spondylitis varies according to the criteria used, but approximately 6% of Crohn's patients will have unequivocal signs of this disease.

Clinical features
Sacroiliitis may be asymptomatic. Clinical cases occur with similar frequency in men and women. Spondylitic symptoms of pain and stiffness associated with reduced back movement and chest expansion may first present either in advance of the bowel symptoms or in patients with established gut disease. Patients with ankylosing spondylitis are a minority of the 56% of patients with Crohn's disease who complain of back pain (Haslock, 1972), but this diagnosis must be actively excluded by thorough clinical and radiological examination. Although gut distension may give rise to referred pain in many areas, including the back (Swarbrick et al, 1980), this diagnosis appears to be made too frequently without proper examination to exclude local lumbar pathology. The course of the arthritis is identical to that of idiopathic ankylosing spondylitis. There is no temporal relationship between exacerbations of the joint and gut disease, and treatment of the gut disease does not influence the progress of the arthritis. Spondylitis does not appear to be associated with disease in any specific part of the gut and in particular is not preferentially associated with colonic disease (Mueller et al, 1974).

Investigations
Radiology shows the presence of sacroiliitis, which may be seen unexpectedly on abdominal films taken for other purposes (Fig. 32.3). Where spinal disease occurs the appearances are identical to those of idiopathic ankylosing spondylitis. Some patients appear to show little or no progression of the disease radiologically beyond the pelvis. This may be interrelated with the relatively high number of female patients with Crohn's disease and spondylitis, as ankylosing spondylitis in women may follow a milder course than that in men (Hart, 1980). Quantitative sacroiliac scanning has been

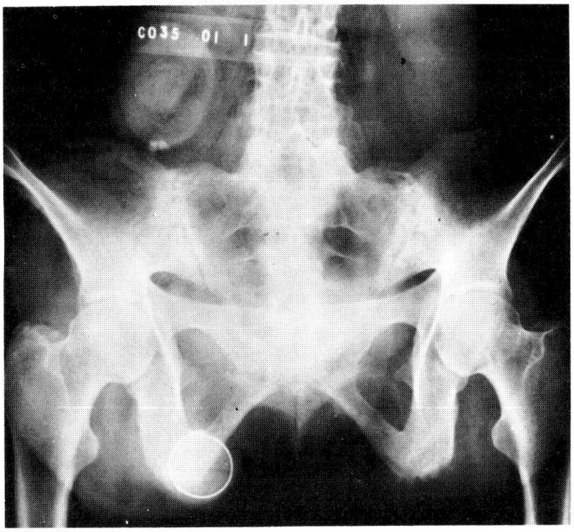

Fig. 32.3 Crohn's disease and ankylosing spondylitis. The ileostomy appliance does not obscure the appearance of sacroiliitis.

undertaken in patients with Crohn's disease and found to be positive in 52% (Davis et al, 1978). The significance of this observation is uncertain. Peripheral joint involvement occurs in two-thirds of the patients with spondylitis and may be distinguished from enteropathic arthritis by the presence of radiological change in the involved joints and by the associated sacroiliac and spinal disease.

Aetiology

When the families of 99 patients with Crohn's disease were studied, sacroiliitis was found in 8.3% of first-degree and 1.9% of second-degree relatives. No sacroiliitis was found in the patients' spouses (Haslock, 1973). This contrasts with a population incidence of 1.1%. From this finding, and the independent clinical progress of the two conditions, it was concluded that ankylosing spondylitis and Crohn's disease coexisted on a hereditary basis. Tissue typing of patients with Crohn's disease does not show an excess of HLA-B27, but studies of those with ankylosing spondylitis have shown between 14 and 91% to possess this antigen (Dekker-Saeys et al, 1978). However, if the relationship is studied in reverse, the proportion of patients with B27 and Crohn's disease who have ankylosing spondylitis appears to be very high indeed, all the patients with Crohn's and B27 having ankylosing spondylitis in some series (Huaux et al, 1977). There is evidence, therefore, of both hereditary and Crohn's disease-associated factors in the development of ankylosing spondylitis in these patients. While simple association of the arthritis with an intestinal antigen source produced by the disease, as is suggested for enteropathic arthritis, cannot be adduced as the aetiology of the spondylitis because the spondylitis may develop before the gut disease, there may be some as yet undetermined common factor present which predisposes to the development of both conditions.

Treatment

This does not differ from the treatment of idiopathic ankylosing spondylitis. The preservation of spinal mobility is achieved by an appropriate, regular exercise regime. Additional physiotherapy may be needed in the periods of relative immobility during exacerbations of the gut disease or pre- and postoperatively. The considerations governing the choice of an analgesic/anti-inflammatory agent in the treatment of enteropathic arthritis apply to an even greater extent where spondylitis is present, as therapy may be prolonged. Whichever drug is chosen, checks for occult bleeding must be undertaken throughout the time it is prescribed.

Other musculoskeletal disorders

Coincidental rheumatic diseases occur in conjunction with Crohn's disease with the expected frequency. Clubbing has been reported in up to 40% of patients. Its incidence is higher where the upper part of the small intestine is involved (Anderson et al, 1957). Its presence has also been shown to correlate with fibrosis in resected specimens, and it tended to regress after resection of macroscopic disease (Kitis et al, 1979). In contrast, hypertrophic pulmonary osteoarthropathy is extremely rare (Neale et al, 1971; Farman et al, 1971). One study reported an increased incidence of cervicobrachial pain in patients with Crohn's disease (Haslock and Wright, 1973) but this has yet to be confirmed.

Infective arthritis may occur and usually involves the hip (London & Fitten, 1970). It probably arises from psoas abscess formation, of which Crohn's disease is now the most common cause (Kyle, 1971). Rare reports of aseptic necrosis may reflect the therapeutic use of corticosteroids (Brom et al, 1971). There are rare reports that granulomas similar to those found in the gut have been demonstrated on synovial biopsy of patients with persistent monarthritis (Lindström et al, 1972; Frayha et al, 1975). X-rays may show erosive changes. Similar granulomas in bone have been incriminated as a cause of limb pain which was relieved by high dose prednisolone therapy (Nugent et al, 1976). Both granulomatous synovitis and granulomatous bone disease appear to be rarities, but should be considered in patients with persistent arthritis or radiological signs of cartilage loss. Granulomatous myositis has also been reported (Menard et al, 1976), and the demonstration of granulomas in biopsy specimens from patients not known to be suffering from Crohn's disease should lead to thorough gastrointestinal investigation.

ULCERATIVE COLITIS

Enteropathic arthritis

The association between colitis and arthritis was first described towards the end of the 19th century (White, 1895). There has been subsequent confusion regarding its nature, incidence and nomenclature. It was at first dismissed as coincident rheumatoid arthritis, but closer studies showed it to be a seronegative arthritis with distinctive features. The names 'colitic arthritis', 'intestinal arthritis' and 'enteropathic arthritis' have been successively and synonymously applied to the condition, the last term now finding general acceptance. Different series have shown incidences of arthritis varying from 0–22%. Selection plays an important part in determining such figures, but the incidence of 11.5% found in a large unselected series is typical (Wright & Watkinson, 1966).

Clinical features

As in the case of Crohn's disease, enteropathic arthritis is an acute synovitis, monarticular in most cases but occasionally polyarticular, which is sometimes accompanied by erythema nodosum. It occurs either coincident with the onset of ulcerative colitis or during the course of the disease. There is a close temporal association between exacerbations of the gut and joint disorders. A higher incidence of arthritis is found in patients with extensive and severe intestinal involvement and those with other complications such as oral ulceration, pyoderma gangrenosum, pseudopolyposis, perianal suppuration and massive haemorrhage. Enteropathic arthritis goes into remission after removal of the diseased bowel segment and is abolished by panproctocolectomy.

Arthritis has been described as the commonest extracolonic manifestation of ulcerative colitis in children, in whom it may become apparent before diarrhoea is noticed (Ament, 1975).

The knees are most commonly involved, closely followed by the ankles with synovitis of the elbows, wrists, small joints of the hands and feet and shoulders occuring less frequently (Fig. 32.4). Individual attacks are self-limited, 50% lasting less than 6 months and only 20% persisting longer than a year. Even when recurrent they do not lead to permanent joint damage or deformity.

Investigations

There are no characteristic laboratory features of enteropathic arthritis. Synovial fluid shows non-specific inflammatory changes with poor mucin clot formation. The cell count is in the range of 4–40 000/mm^3, up to 98% being polymorphs. Synovial tissue shows similarly non-specific inflammatory changes (Bywaters & Ansell, 1958). The sheep cell agglutination test is negative both in blood and synovial fluid. X-rays show no gross abnormality even after recurrent attacks of synovitis, though soft tissue swelling and mild osteoporosis may be seen during acute exacerbations.

Aetiology

The cause of enteropathic arthritis is unknown. There are a number of pointers to the concept that some factor within the intestine initiates the arthritis. These include absence of joint disease when the gut is unaffected, quiescent or removed, the temporal association of exacerbations of gut and joint disease and the increased incidence of arthritis where gut disease is widespread, severe or complicated. In all these situations the conditions are favourable for the release of large quantities of antigen into the circulation. Such periods of antigen excess predispose to the formation of soluble antigen–antibody complexes which can enter the

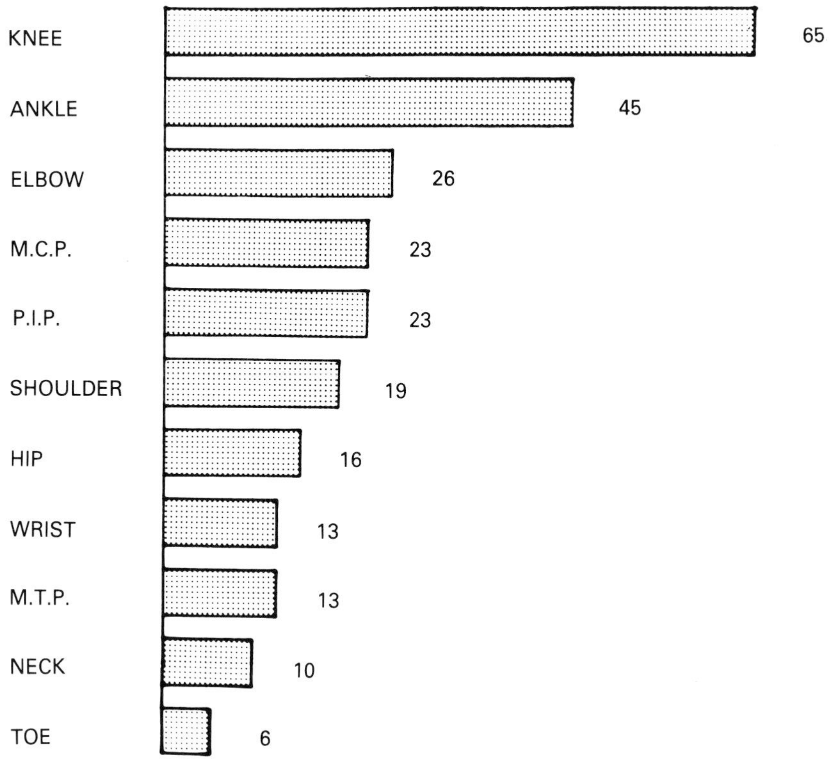

Fig. 32.4 Enteropathic arthritis in ulcerative colitis. Joints involved (%). (After Wright & Watkinson, 1965a.)

joint, producing a reactive synovitis. As with Crohn's disease, direct evidence for this hypothesis is lacking although there does seem to be an association between the presence of circulating immune complexes and abnormalities in the complement system with extraintestinal disease (Hodgson et al 1977; Lake et al, 1979).

Treatment

Enteropathic arthritis is self-limiting and non-deforming. The best therapy lies in control or cure of the underlying ulcerative colitis. Short courses of non-steroidal anti-inflammatory agents, chosen with due regard to the abnormality in the gut, may be required. Intra-articular hydrocortisone may give rapid relief, but systemic corticosteroids should not be used to control the joint disease although they may be required for treatment of the colitis. The fact that total proctocolectomy will abolish enteropathic arthritis should be explained to patients preoperatively, as some are worried about their joint disease limiting their ability to manipulate ileostomy appliances.

Ankylosing spondylitis

Studies of Veterans Administration Hospital records in the USA identified the coincidence of ankylosing spondylitis and ulcerative colitis, and also showed that the spondylitis frequently preceded the gut disease (Acheson, 1960). This was confirmed in the gastroenterology and radiotherapy departments at Edinburgh, where the incidence of spondylitis was studied in colitics and that of colitis in spondylitics. An unexpectedly high association of the two diseases was found under both circumstances (McBride et al, 1963). Subsequently, rheumatological assessment of an unselected group of 234 patients with ulcerative colitis showed 6.4% to have ankylosing spondylitis. In addition, 14% had asymptomatic sacroiliitis (Wright & Watkinson, 1965b). Investigation of 47 patients diagnosed as having idiopathic ankylosing spondylitis showed signs of inflammatory gut disease on barium enema, sigmoidoscopy or biopsy in 8, 3 of whom were asymptomatic (Jayson et al, 1970). Although a subsequent study failed to show an increase in bowel disease in spondylitics (Green et al, 1973), all the major series show that the bowel disease is as likely to precede as to succeed the spondylitis and it remains likely, therefore, that some patients with mild, unnoticed or absent symptoms from their gut disease will occur in groups of diagnosed spondylitics.

Clinical features

Spondylitis accompanying ulcerative colitis is identical to idiopathic ankylosing spondylitis. Low back pain and stiffness are the usual presenting complaints with restriction of chest and spinal movements detected clinically. 30% of patients with ulcerative colitis complain of back pain (Wright & Watkinson, 1965a) and each must be carefully examined clinically and radiologically to differentiate ankylosing spondylitis from other musculoskeletal causes of back pain and from referred pain arising from the gut. Peripheral joints are involved in two-thirds of cases, most commonly the hips and shoulders, less commonly the more distal joints. Such peripheral joint disease is distinguished from enteropathic arthritis by the presence of sacroiliac or spinal involvement, the independent nature of the gut and joint complaints and the appearance of clinical and radiological evidence of joint damage.

Investigations

The importance of the radiological signs of ankylosing spondylitis is the frequency with which they can be found on X-rays taken for gastrointestinal investigation (Fig. 32.5). These are frequently overlooked because attention is focused on the bowel. Sacroiliitis, which may be asymptomatic, spinal involvement with syndesmophyte formation or complete bony bridging, and narrowing progressing to fusion of the hips are all within the compass of films taken for barium studies. The general radiological features, and in particular those in the spine, are identical to those of idiopathic ankylosing spondylitis (McEwen et al, 1971).

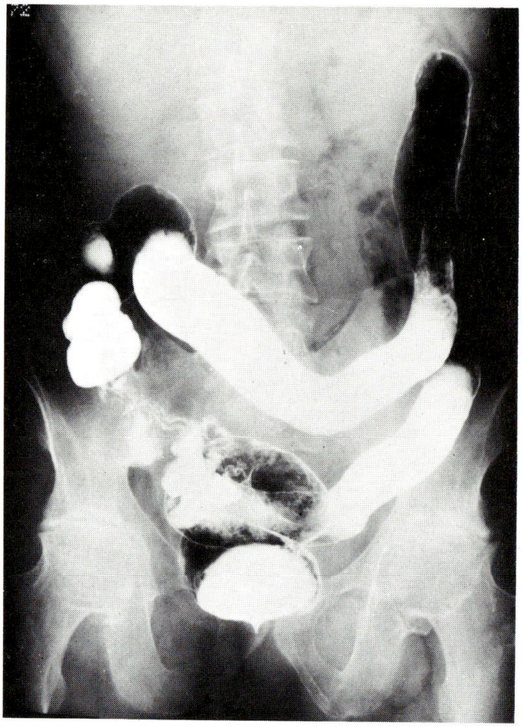

Fig. 32.5 Ulcerative colitis and ankylosing spondylitis in a 22-year-old man. Although the colon (which shows loss of normal haustration, typical of colitis) obscures the sacroiliac joints, spondylitic involvement of both hips can be seen.

Treatment

The most important aspect of treatment is maintenance of spinal and thoracic mobility by a regular exercise regime. This is of particular importance during acute exacerbations of gut disease and pre- and postoperatively. Care is needed in choosing analgesic/anti-inflammatory agents as all may cause gastrointestinal blood loss. The joint and gut diseases progress independently and treatment of the colitis, including cure by total proctocolectomy, does not influence the course of the spondylitis.

Aetiology

The clinical impression that ulcerative colitis and ankylosing spondylitis are two diseases which coexist rather than being causally related has been reinforced by the finding that relatives of patients with ulcerative colitis have an increased incidence of sacroiliitis and ankylosing spondylitis (Macrae

& Wright, 1973). This provides an example of the interrelationship of diseases encompassed in the concept of seronegative spondarthritis (Moll et al, 1974). The histocompatibility antigen HLA-B27, which is found in over 90% of patients with ankylosing spondylitis, was found in 13 of 18 patients with spondylitis and colitis (Brewerton et al, 1974), further reinforcing this concept. It has been suggested that the overall incidence of HLA-B27 is increased in ulcerative colitis (Woodrow et al, 1978) but this has not been reflected in an increased incidence of spondylitis compared with Crohn's disease patients.

Other musculoskeletal disorders

Clubbing is a well-recognised complication of ulcerative colitis, although hypertrophic pulmonary osteoarthropathy appears to be extremely rare (Farman et al, 1976). Young (1966) studied 156 patients with ulcerative colitis, 7 of whom showed finger clubbing. All these patients were in the group of 77 whose disease included areas of the colon supplied by the vagus, whereas no clubbing was seen in the 79 patients whose disease was confined to extravagal areas of the gut. This association with vagal innervation has more recently been demonstrated in both ulcerative colitis and Crohn's disease (Kitis et al, 1979).

Patients with ulcerative colitis are as commonly affected by other rheumatic diseases as other members of the population from which they are drawn. Wright & Watkinson (1965a) found musculoskeletal disorders in 45% of the patients they studied. Many suffered from coexistent rheumatic diseases, and this highlights the need for expert rheumatological appraisal of these patients if they are to be correctly diagnosed and managed.

WHIPPLE'S DISEASE

Whipple's disease is a chronic wasting disease which is more common in men than women. The four most common clinical features are weight loss, diarrhoea, arthritis and abdominal pain. Loss of weight is almost universal and may be severe. The diarrhoea is often continuous and may be watery or steatorrhoeic. It can be accompanied by gastrointestinal bleeding, either occult or frank. The abdominal pain is often poorly characterised and localised but is usually epigastric and may be exacerbated by food. The diagnosis is confirmed by the demonstration of PAS-positive macrophages in small intestinal biopsy specimens.

Several patients have been described in whom Whipple's disease followed a less typical clinical course. Although lung involvement has been recognised since the original report, it dominated the case described by Winberg et al (1978) causing a delay in diagnosis. Presentation with hypothalamic symptoms has also been described (Bayless & Knox, 1979) and overall Whipple's disease is emerging as a multisystem disorder with increasingly variable presentation.

Enteropathic arthritis

Arthritis or arthralgia has been noted as a symptom of Whipple's disease since the first case report (Whipple, 1907). It has subsequently been described in up to 90% of patients (Maizel et al, 1970).

Clinical features

The form of enteropathic arthritis associated with Whipple's disease is rather more variable than that accompanying ulcerative colitis and Crohn's disease. There may be arthralgia alone, or a synovitis affecting one or more joints with a tendency to symmetrical polyarticular involvement. This may be transient, lasting only hours, or can persist for several weeks. The arthritis is often described as migratory. Joint involvement is in the typical pattern with knees and ankles predominating and other joints involved less frequently.

Arthritis associated with Whipple's disease is of greatest importance as a harbinger of other symptoms of the disease such as abdominal pain, diarrhoea and weight loss. In about 60% of patients arthritis is the presenting symptom, often preceding other symptoms by many years.

Investigations

Studies of the synovial fluid and membrane are rare. Caughey & Bywaters (1963) found non-specific inflammatory changes in both. No excess of PAS-positive cells was seen and tests for rheumatoid factor were negative. Rod-shaped organisms identical to those found in the jejunum were demonstrated by electron microscopy in synovial biopsies taken from a patient with active joint disease (Hawkins et al, 1976). These were regarded as being responsible for the inflammatory arthropathy.

Radiologically the involved joints are normal. The importance of investigations in Whipple's disease lies in the recognition of enteropathic arthritis without apparent gut disease. This is most unusual in the inflammatory enteropathies, and should lead to a search for PAS-positive macrophages in small intestinal specimens obtained by peroral biopsy.

Aetiology

The aetiology of the arthritis is unknown. The presence of bacteria-like particles on electron microscopy and the response to antibiotic treatment suggests an infective cause for the underlying disease, but no specific organism has yet been identified. Investigation of the immune system of patients with Whipple's disease has suggested a persistent defect in T cells, more severe in those in whom the disease was active. The presence of HLA-B27 in 4 of 9 patients studied suggested that this immune deficiency, which could predispose the patient to infection, was primary rather than secondary (Feurle et al, 1979).

Treatment

Whipple's disease in uniformly responsive to prolonged antibiotic treatment, usually with tetracycline. The arthritis abates as the gut disease is controlled, and no specific therapy is needed (Maizell et al, 1970). The persistence of synovitis once adequate antibiotic therapy is established is a sign of non-responsiveness of the disease in general, and the antibiotic regime should be revised. Sulphamethoxazole-trimethoprim has been used successfully under these circumstances (Tauris & Moesner, 1978).

Ankylosing spondylitis

The frequency of the association between Whipple's disease and ankylosing spondylitis is a matter of controversy. Definite cases, with HLA-B27, do occur, and it has been estimated that the true incidence is at least 4 times that expected in the population and similar to that found in inflammatory bowel disease (Canoso et al, 1978). Pseudospondylitis, presumably due to synovitis in the spinal apophyseal joints, has been reported in association with Whipple's disease. It is distinguished from true spondylitis by the absence of radiological sacroiliitis and the response to antibiotic therapy (Bowman et al, 1983).

ARTHRITIS ASSOCIATED WITH INTESTINAL BYPASS SURGERY (see also Chs 28, 49)

The operations of jejunocolic and jejunoileal anastamosis have been used in the treatment of morbid obesity for more than 25 years. In one series of 31 patients, 7 (23%) developed a seronegative polyarthritis. All these patients were drawn from the 22 who had had jejunocolostomy, those with jejunoileostomy being arthritis free. The arthritis was usually transient, but lasted for more than 2 years in 2 patients. Because of the severity of the arthritis, one patient had her gut continuity restored, following which she had a prompt resolution of her articular symptoms (Shagrin et al, 1971). Since then a similar arthropathy has been reported from many centres including those using the jejunoileal procedure. Some studies suggest that locomotor symptoms are not found in excess in this group of patients when compared with similar patients (Danish Obesity Project, 1979) but a recent careful comparison of jejunoileal bypass with procedures such as jaw wiring and gastric reduction showed an arthralgia unique to this group in 38 of 107 patients, with active synovitis in 8. Again the symptoms resolved in all patients who had restoration of their gut continuity (Delamere et al, 1982). Osteomalacia and gout may also be found in these patients as a result of the metabolic changes induced by surgery.

Aetiology

The presence of cryoprotein complexes was demonstrated in 3 patients who had developed arthritis following a bypass operation, but not in 2 without arthritis (Wands et al, 1976). These complexes comprised IgG, IgM, IgA, complement components C3, C4, C5 and IgG antibody against *E. coli* and *B. fragilis*. It was suggested that intestinal bacterial antibodies were absorbed leading to the formation of circulating cryoprotein complexes. These complexes, which were shown to be capable of activating both the classical and alternative pathways, were considered to be of importance in the pathogenesis of the arthritis. Similar complexes were found in a further group of patients, and in this study it was shown that rheumatoid factor was selectively concentrated in the cryoglobulin (Ginsberg et al, 1979). The strong implication that this is an immune complex synovitis is not only of interest in this clinical situation, but may provide a model for enteropathic arthritis associated with other gut diseases.

Treatment

Short courses of non-steroidal anti-inflammatory agents are usually all that is required to treat this condition, but restoration of gut continuity may be needed in those patients in whom the symptoms are severe.

ARTHRITIS ASSOCIATED WITH GUT INFECTION

Arthritis following infectious diarrhoea has been recognised for several centuries (Bollet, 1981). The largest epidemic of Reiter's disease ever reported followed an epidemic of *Shigella* dysentry (Paronen, 1948) and a synovitis produced as a reaction to infection, rather than direct invasion of the joints, has been recognised increasingly since (Table 32.1). The term 'reactive arthritis' has been applied to this condition, which in its initial stages bears a strong resemblance to enteropathic arthritis, being short-lived, often monarticular and usually affecting large joints. It may also be associated with erythema nodosum (Aho, 1983). However, symptoms of acute sacroiliitis may also occur, and there may be considerable systemic upset associated with the arthritis, even when the enteritis has been cured, with a high plasma viscosity and deranged liver function tests. Some patients also show features of acute Reiter's syndrome, with urethritis and conjunctivitis, and it has been suggested that Reiter's syndrome would be better referred to as a 'reactive arthritis' or 'reactive spondarthritis', subdivided into 'sexually acquired reactive arthritis' (SARA; see p. 427) and 'enteropathic reactive arthritis' (ERA). This suggestion is strongly supported by

Table 32.1 The association between gut infection and arthritis

	Organism	GIT disease	Joint disease
Ch. 29, this volume	*Klebsiella pneumoniae*		?Ankylosing spondylitis
Paronen, 1948	*Shigella flexneri*	Acute diarrhoea	Reactive arthritis Reiter's syndrome
Ahvonen et al, 1969	*Yersinia enterocolitica*	Acute diarrhoea (occasionally mistaken for Crohn's disease)	Reactive arthritis Reiter's syndrome
Chalmers et al, 1978	*Yersinia pseudotuberculosis*	Acute diarrhoea	Reactive arthritis Reiter's syndrome
Vairtiainen & Hurri, 1964	*Salmonella tyhphimurium*	Acute diarrhoea	Reactive arthritis Reiter's syndrome
Jones et al, 1979	*Salmonella enteritidis*	Acute diarrhoea	Reiter's syndrome
Richardson et al, 1977	*Salmonella okatie*	None (positive stool culture: PUO)	Acute sacroiliitis
Gumpel et al, 1981	*Campylobacter*	Acute diarrhoea	Reactive arthritis
Bolton et al, 1981	*Clostridium difficile*	Pseudomembranous colitis	Reactive arthritis
Jaramillo et al, 1978	*Strongyloides stercolonis*	Diarrhoea, vomiting, abdominal distention	Reiter's syndrome
Hughes & Hind, 1983	*Staphylococcus epidermidis*	Peritonitis	Reactive arthritis
Ch. 45, this volume	*Brucella*	Non-specific	Chronic arthritis which may have sacroiliac and spinal components

a follow-up study of 160 patients with Reiter's disease, 144 with *Yersinia* arthritis and 9 with *Salmonella* arthritis (Leirisalo et al, 1982) which showed that all three groups were liable to develop a chronic arthritis, especially if they possessed B27, and that there was no significant difference in outcome in patients with differing initial diagnoses.

Investigations
Isolation of the initiating organism may be possible where active gut infection is still present at the time of presentation of the arthritis. The plasma viscosity and white cell count may reflect the infection, but the viscosity is likely to remain high while synovitis persists. True septic arthritis is unusual in these patients, occurring most frequently in response to *Salmonella* infections in children (David & Black, 1960). Aspiration and culture must be undertaken if infection is suspected. Liver function tests may remain deranged during the course of the synovitis, with the alkaline phosphatase and gamma glutamyl transferase both falling as the synovitis improves. The cause of this observation is yet to be determined.

Several studies have shown that the possession of HLA-B27 makes patients more likely to develop reactive arthritis and more likely to have severe and recurrent disease. Tissue typing, therefore, conveys some prognostic information.

Aetiology
Reactive arthritis is probably an immune complex synovitis, and complexes have been found both in blood and synovial fluid (Sheldon et al, 1982). The range of precipitating infections is wide, although it is of interest that *Shigella sonnei* does not appear to precipitate this condition (Lewis, 1982). The more unusual infections with *Strongyloides* and *Staph. epidermidis* were associated with immunosuppression chronic ambulatory peritoneal dialysis respectively.

It is possible that the arthritis reported in association with cimetidine therapy (Khong & Rooney, 1980) may be a reactive arthritis associated with bacterial colonisation of the stomach or alteration in the lower gut flora (Lancet, 1981).

Treatment
Although the initial attack is usually self-limiting, reactive arthritis may persist for many months. Treatment with non-steroidal anti-inflammatory agents, particularly indomethacin, supplemented if necessary by intra-articular corticosteroids, is usually adequate, but we have recently had to resort to pulsed methylprednisolone treatment in order to achieve disease control. This form of therapy has still to be fully evaluated. Treatment of the more chronic disease is the same as that of Reiter's syndrome (Ch. 31).

REFERENCES

Abercrombie J 1830 Pathological and practical researches on diseases of the stomach, the intestinal canal, the liver and other viscera of the abdomen, 2nd Edn. Waugh & Innes, Edinburgh

Acheson E D 1960 An association between ulcerative colitis, regional enteritis and ankylosing spondylitis. Quarterly Journal of Medicine (New Series) 29: 489–499

Aho K 1983 Yersinia reactive arthritis. British Journal of Rheumatology 22 (Suppl 2): 41–45

Ahvonen P, Sievers K, Aho K 1969 Arthritis associated with yersinia enterocolitica infection. Acta Rheumatologica Scandinavica 15: 232–253

Ament M E 1975 Inflammatory diseases of the colon: ulcerative colitis and Crohn's colitis. Journal of Pediatrics 86: 322–334

Anderson D O, Mullinger M A, Bagoch A 1957 Regional enteritis involving the duodenum, with clubbing of the fingers and steatorrhoea. Gastroenterology 32: 917–926

Ansell B M, Wigley R A D 1964 Arthritic manifestations in regional enteritis. Annals of the Rheumatic Diseases 23: 64–72

Austad W R, Thompson G R, Joseph R R 1968 Regional enteritis presenting as acute arthritis. Michigan Medicine 67:5: 324–329

Bayless T M, Knox D L 1979 Whipple's disease: a multisystem infection. New England Journal of Medicine 300: 920–921

Best W R, Becktel J M, Singleton J W 1979 Rederived values of the 8 coefficients of the Crohn's disease activity index (CDAI). Gastroenterology 77: 843–846

Bollet A J 1981 A report of reactive arthritis following dysentry in 1743. Arthritis and Rheumatism 24:860

Bolton R P, Wood G M, Losowsky M S 1981 Acute arthritis associated with *Clostridium difficile* colitis. British Medical Journal 283: 1023–1024

Bowman C, Dieppe P, Settas L 1983 Remission of pseudo-spondylitis with treatment of Whipple's disease. British Journal of Rheumatology 22: 181–182

Brewerton D A, Nicholls A, Caffrey M, Walters D, James D C O 1974 HL-A27 and arthropathies associated with ulcerative colitis and psoriasis Lancet 1: 956–958

Brom B, Bank S, Marske I N, Cobb J J 1971 Periostitis,

aseptic necrosis and arthritis occurring in a patient with Crohn's disease. Gastroenterology 60: 1106–1109
Bywaters E G L, Ansell B M 1958 Arthritis associated with ulcerative colitis. Annals of the Rheumatic Diseases 17: 169–183
Canoso J J, Saini M, Hermos J A 1978 Whipple's disease and ankylosing spondylitis. Simultaneous occurrence in HLA B27 positive male. Journal of Rheumatology 5: 79–84
Caughey D E, Bywaters E G L 1963 The arthritis of Whipple's syndrome. Annals of the Rheumatic Diseases 22: 327–335
Chalmers A, Kapgrove R E, Reynolds W J, Urowitz M B 1978 Postdiarrhoeal arthropathy of *Yersinia pseudotuberculosis*. Canadian Medical Association Journal 118: 515–516
Cornes J S, Stecher M 1961 Primary Crohn's disease of the colon and rectum. Gut 2: 189–201
Crohn B B, Yarnis H 1958 Regional ileitis, 2nd Edn. Grune & Stratton, New York
Crohn B B, Ginzburg L, Oppenheimer G D 1932 Regional ileitis: a pathological and clinical entity. Journal of the American Medical Association 156: 1323–1328
Daffner J E, Brown C H 1958 Regional enteritis: clinical aspects and diagnosis in 100 patients. Annals of Internal Medicine 49: 580–594
Danish Obesity Project 1979 Randomised trial of jejunoileal bypass versus medical treatment in morbid obesity. Lancet 2: 1255–1258
David J R, Black R L 1960 Salmonella arthritis. Medicine (Baltimore) 39: 385–403
Davis P, Thomson A, Lentle B 1978 Quantitative sacroiliac scintigraphy in patients with Crohn's disease. Arthritis and Rheumatism 21: 234–237
Dekker-Saeys B J, Meuwissen S G M, van den Berg-Loonen E M, de Haas W H D, Meijers K A F, Tytgat G N J 1978 Clinical characteristics and results of histocompatibility typing (HLA B27) in50 patients with both ankylosing spondylitis and inflammatory bowel disease. Annals of the Rheumatic Diseases 37: 36–41
Delamere J P, Baddeley R M, Walton K W 1982 Jejunoileal bypass arthropathy. Paper presented to the Combined Meeting of the British Association for Rheumatology and Rehabilitation and the Heberden Society, Cambridge
Farman J, Effman E L, Grnja V 1971 Crohn's disease and periosteal new bone formation. Gastroenterology 61: 513–522
Farman J, Twersky J, Fierst S 1976 Ulcerative colitis associated with hypertrophic osteoarthropathy. Digestive Diseases 21: 130–135
Feurle G E, Dorken B, Schopf E, Lenhard V 1979 HLA B27 and defects in the T-cell system in Whipple's disease. European Journal of Clinical Investigation 9: 385–389
Frayha R, Stevens M B, Bayless T M 1975 Destructive monarthritis and granulomatous synovitis as the presenting manifestations of Crohn's disease. Johns Hopkins Medical Journal 137: 151–155
Ginsberg J, Quismorio F P, De Wind L T, Mongan E S 1979 Musculoskeletal symptoms after jejunoileal shunt surgery for intractable obesity: clinical and immunologic studies. American Journal of Medicine 67: 443–448
Green F A, Alea J A, McCluskey R T 1973 The bowel in spondylitis — a controlled study. Arthritis and Rheumatism 16:549
Gumpel J M, Martin C, Sanderson P J 1981 Reactive arthritis associated with *Campylobacter* enteritis. Annals of the Rheumatic Diseases 40: 64–65
Hart F D 1980 Clinical features and complications. In: Moll J M H (ed) Ankylosing spondylitis. Churchill Livingstone, Edinburgh
Haslock I 1972 The arthritis associated with Crohn's disease: a family study. MD thesis, University of Edinburgh
Haslock I 1973 Arthritis and Crohn's disease: a family study. Annals of the Rheumatic Diseases 32: 479–486
Haslock I, Wright V 1973 The musculoskeletal complications of Crohn's disease. Medicine (Baltimore) 53: 217–225
Haslock I, Macrae I F, Wright V 1974 Arthritis and intestinal disease: a comparison of two family studies. Rheumatology and Rehabilitation 13: 135–140
Hawkins C F, Farr M, Morris C J, Hoare A M, Williamson N 1976 Detection by electron microscopy of rod-shaped organisms in synovial membrane from a patient with the arthritis of Whipple's disease. Annals of the Rheumatic Diseases 35: 502–509
Heuman R, Boeryd B, Gillquist J, Sjödahl R, Tagesson C 1981 Arthralgia and crystal deposits in Crohn's disease. Scandinavian Journal of Rheumatology 10: 313–317
Hodgson H J F, Potter B J, Jewell D P 1977 Immune complexes in ulcerative colitis and Crohn's disease. Clinical and Experimental Immunology 29: 187–196
Huaux J P, Fiasse R, de Bruyere M, de Deuxchaisnes C N 1977 HLA B27 in regional enteritis with and without ankylosing spondylitis or sacroilitis. Journal of Rheumatology Supplement 3: 60–63
Hughes B R, Hind C R K 1983 Reactive arthritis associated with *Staphylococcus epidermidis* peritonitis in patients undergoing continuous ambulatory peritoneal dialysis. British Medical Journal 286: 188–189
Jaramillo D, Leon W, Cardenas V, Cortes A 1978 Reiter's syndrome, immunosuppression and *Strongyloides*. Journal of Cutaneous Pathology 5: 200–208
Jayson M I V, Salmon P R, Harrison W J 1970 Inflammatory bowel disease in ankylosing spondylitis. Gut 11: 506–511
Jones M B, Smith P W, Olnhausen R W 1979 Reiter's syndrome after salmonella infection: occurrence in HLA B27 positive brothers. Arthritis and Rheumatism 22: 1141–1142
Khong T K, Rooney P J 1980 Arthritis associated with cimetidine. Lancet 2:1380
Kitis G, Thompson H, Allan R N 1979 Finger clubbing in inflammatory bowel disease: its prevelance and pathogenesis. British Medical Journal 2: 825–828
Kyle I 1971 Psoas abscess in Crohn's disease. Gastroenterology 61: 149–155
Lake A M, Stitzel A E, Urmson J R, Walker W A, Spitzer R E 1979 Complement alterations in inflammatory bowel disease. Gastroenterology 76: 1374–1379
Lancet Leading Article 1981 Bacteria in the stomach. Lancet 2: 906–907
Leirisalo M, Skylv G, Kousa M, Voipio-Pulkki L M, Souranta H, Nissilä M et al 1982 Follow up study on patients with Reiter's disease and reactive arthritis with special reference to HLA B27. Arthritis and Rheumatism 25: 249–259
Lewis R B 1982 The absence of reactive arthritis after *Shigella sonnei* infection. Arthritis and Rheumatism 25:1267
Lindström C, Wramsby H, Ostberg G 1972 Granulomatous arthritis in Crohn's disease. Gut 13: 257–259
London D, Fitton J M 1970 Acute septic arthritis

complicating Crohn's disease. British Journal of Surgery 57: 536–537

McBride J A, King M H, Baikie A G, Crean G P, Sircus W 1963 Ankylosing spondylitis and chronic inflammatory disease of the intestine. British Medical Journal 2: 483–486

McEwen C, Di Tata D, Lingg C, Porini A, Good A, Rankin T 1971 A comparative study of ankylosing spondylitis and spondylitis accompanying ulcerative colitis, regional enteritis, psoriasis and Reiter's disease. Arthritis and Rheumatism 14: 291–318

Macrae I F, Wright V 1973 A family study of ulcerative colitis with particular reference to ankylosing spondylitis and sacroiliitis. Annals of the Rheumatic Diseases 32: 16–20

Maizel H, Ruffin J M, Dobbins W O 1970 Whipple's disease — a review of 19 patients from one hospital and a review of the literature since 1950. Medicine (Baltimore) 49: 175–205

Menard D B, Haddad H, Blain J G, Beaudry R, Devroede G, Masse S 1976 Granulomatous myositis and myopathy associated with Crohn's colitis. New England Journal of Medicine 295: 818–819

Moll J M H, Haslock I, Macrae I F, Wright V 1974 Associations between ankylosing spondylitis, psoriatic arthritis, Reiter's disease, the intestinal arthropathies and Behçet's syndrome. Medicine (Baltimore) 53: 343–364

Mueller C E, Seeger J F, Martel W 1974 Ankylosing spondylitis and regional enteritis. Radiology 112: 579–581

Neale G, Kelsall A R, Doyle F H 1968 Crohn's disease and diffuse symmetrical periostitis. Gut 9: 383–387

Nugent F W, Glaser D, Fernandez-Herlihy L 1976 Crohn's colitis associated with granulomatous bone disease. New England Journal of Medicine 294: 262–263

Paronen I 1948 Reiter's disease: a study of 344 cases observed in Finland. Acta Medica Scandinavica 131 (Suppl 213): 1–114

Rankin G B, Watts H D, Melnyk C S, Kelley M L 1979 National cooperative Crohn's disease study: extraintestinal manifestations and perianal complications. Gastroenterology 77: 914–920

Richardson S B, Uttley A H C, Pettingale K W 1977 Acute sacroiliitis due to *Salmonella okatie*. British Medical Journal 1: 1449–1450

Selby W S, Kater R M H, Heap T R, Gallagher N D 1979 Crohn's disease: a review of 122 cases. Australia and New Zealand Journal of Medicine 9: 145–150

Shagrin J W, Frame B, Duncan H 1971 Polyarthritis in obese patients with intestinal bypass. Annals of Internal Medicine 75: 377–380

Sheldon P J H S, Mair N S, Fox E 1982 Yersinia arthritis: a clinical, immunological and family study of 2 cases. Annals of the Rheumatic Diseases 41: 153–158

Soren A 1966 Joint affections in regional iliitis. Archives of Internal Medicine 117: 78–83

Swarbrick E T, Bat L, Hegarty H E, Williams C B, Dawson A M 1980 Site of pain from the irritable bowel. Lancet 2. 443–446

Tauris P, Moesner J 1978 Whipple's disease. Acta Medica Scandinavica 204: 423–427

Van Patter W N, Bargen J A, Dockerty M B, Feldman D V M, Mayo C W, Waugh J M 1954 Regional enteritis. Gastroenterology 26: 347–450

Vairtiainen J, Hurri L 1964 Arthritis due to salmonella typhimurium. Acta Medica Scandinavica 175: 771–776

Wands J R, La Mont J T, Mann E, Isselbacher K J 1976 Arthritis associated with intestinal bypass procedure for morbid obesity. New England Journal of Medicine 294: 121–124

Whipple G H 1907 A hitherto undescribed disease characterised anatomically by deposits of fat and fatty acids in the intestinal and mesenteric lymphatic tissues. Johns Hopkins Hospital Bulletin 18: 382–391

White M H 1895 Colitis. Lancet 1: 538–539

Winberg C, Rose M, Rappaport H 1978 Whipple's disease of the lung. American Journal of Medicine 65: 873–880

Woodrow J, Leumonia R, McConnell R, Berg-Loonen E M, Meuvissen S G M, Dekker-Saeys B J et al 1978 HLA antigens in inflammatory bowel disease. Tissue Antigens 1: 47–52

Wright V, Watkinson G 1965a The arthritis of ulcerative colitis. British Medical Journal 2: 670–675

Wright V, Watkinson G 1965b Sacroiliitis and ulcerative colitis. British Medical Journal 2: 675–680

Wright V, Watkinson F 1966 Articular complications of ulcerative colitis. American Journal of Proctology 17: 107–115

Young J R 1966 Ulcerative colitis and finger clubbing. British Medical Journal i: 278–279

Index

Entries in italic type denote pages where illustrations appear; entries in bold type indicate a complete chapter on the subject.

Abdomen, physical examination 1574
Achilles tendon
  lesions 1474
  peritendinitis 1474
  rupture 1474
  tendinitis, injection technique 1619
Achondroplasia 1172–1173, *1173*
Acne arthritis 1239
Acquired immune deficiency syndrome (AIDS) 1199
Acromegalic arthropathy
  association with hypertrophic arthropathy 966
  backache 961
  clinical features 960
  compression neuropathies 962
  limb arthropathy 961–962
  neuromuscular manifestations 963
  pathology 963–965
  radiology 966–967
  treatment 966–967
Acromegaly 960
  association with osteoarthrosis 851–852
Acromioclavicular joint, osteoarthrosis 864
Acropachy, thyroid 1253, 1457
Acrosclerosis 1367
ACTH (Corticotrophin) 544–545
  see also Corticosteroids
  in acute gout 921
  in juvenile chronic arthritis 1114
  in rheumatic fever 1088
Acthar Gel, in juvenile chronic arthritis 1116, *1116*
Actinomyces bovis 1153
Acute anterior uveitis 727–728
Addresses, of organisations associated with rehabilitation 1517
Adductor origin, strain 1458
Adenine phosphoribosyltransferase (APRT) 904
Adenohypophysis 959–960
Adenoviral arthritis 1151
AIDS 1199
Aids, rehabilitation 1504–1514
Albers-Schoenberg disease (osteopetrosis) 999–1000
Alcohol, associations with
  gout and hyperuricaemia 915
  hypertriglyceridaemia 196
  osteonecrosis 1223
Alkaptonuria, and osteoarthrosis 853
Allopurinol 569–574
  in gout, long term management 922–924, *924*
Alopecia, in systemic lupus erythematosus 1327
American Rheumatism Association (ARA) 16, 34
Amoebic dysentery, arthritis 1146
Amyloid
  constituents 1024–1025
  definition 1024–1025
  fibril
    degradation 1040–1041
    deposition 1039–1041
    formation 1039–1040
    proteins and their precursors 1031
  importance 1025–1026
  pathogenesis of effects 1041
  P component 1036–1039
  senile 1030
Amyloidosis 691–692, **1024 – 1053**
  addendum (1985) 1044–1045
  in ankylosing spondylitis 752
  association with
    immunocyte dyscrasia, monoclonal protein amyloidosis 1028–1029
    causes 1028
    clinical features 1028–1029
    prevalence 1029
  clinical syndromes 1026–1030
  diagnosis 1041–1043
    biopsy 1041–1043
  familial Mediterranean fever 1029
  heredofamilial systemic 1029
  in juvenile chronic arthritis 1109
  leukaemia 1194–1195
  localised 1029–1030
  management 1043–1044
  in psoriatic arthritis 779
  in pyrophosphate arthropathy 944
  in rheumatoid arthritis 638
  systemic 1029
    associations 1027
    causes 1027
    clinical features 1027–1028
    reactive 1027
Anabolic steroids, in juvenile chronic arthritis 1116
ANA-negative lupus 1335
Anaphylactoid (Henoch-Schönlein) purpura 1235–1236
  abdominal pain 1235–1236
  association with familial Mediterranean fever 1235
  clinical features 1235
  joint involvement 1236
  pathology 1235
  sex incidence 1235
  treatment 1236
Angioimmunoblastic lymphadenopathy 1195–1196
  lymph node histology 1195
  rheumatic features 1195
  treatment 1196
Ankle
  see also Achilles tendon
  arthroscopy 1604–1605
  bursitis 1474
  calcaneal ephphysis 1474
  examination 1578–1579
  injection technique 1619–1620
  ligamentous injuries 1474
  osteoarthrosis 868
  surgery 1534–1535
  'weak ankle' 1474
Ankylosing hyperostosis (Forestier's disease) *764*
  epidemiology 97–98
  osteoarthrosis 859–860
Ankylosing spondylitis 321–322, 429–430, **745 – 774**
  aetiology 760–762
  association with Crohn's disease, ulcerative colitis, Whipple's disease 762
  see also Crohn's disease, ulcerative colitis, Whipple's disease
  axial tomography 757
  back pain 1429
  bone and joint changes, other than spine 756–757
  clinical features 747–750
  complications 751–752

Ankylosing spondylitis *cont*
amyloidosis 752
central nervous system 751–752
heart disease 751
iritis 751
pulmonary 752
treatment 752
course 762–763
Crohn's disease 808–810
definition 745
diagnostic criteria 745–746, *745*
differential diagnosis 764–765
from ankylosing hyperostosis *764*
enthesopathy of insertion of patellar tendon 1466, *1467*
epidemiology 70–72
genetic factors 760–761
genitourinary infection 761–762
hip replacement 1542
historical background 746
intubation 1524
irradiation 767
laboratory findings 759–760
HLA-B27 760
T-cells 760
levamisole therapy 562
management 765–768
appliances 765
patients' handbook 765
physical measures 765
medication 766
nomenclature 745
pathogenesis 760–762
pathology 757–759
apophyseal ankylosis 758
peripheral arthritis 756
physical signs 747–750
chest and spinal rigidity 747–749
extra-articular bony tenderness 749
peripheral joint involvement 749–750
posture 750, *750*
physical treatment 765
exercise 1495
prevalence 746–747
prognosis 762–763
scintigraphy 757
spine 1547
indications for osteotomy 1547
summary 768
surgery 767–768
therapeutic evaluation 1593
ulcerative colitis 811–813
Whipple's disease 814
Annulus fibrosus 1409, *1409*
Anterior tibial compartment 1471–1472
Antibodies 365–70, 394
see also Autoantibodies
Antigens
see also Immune complexes
Anti-malarial drugs **525 – 534**
chloroquine 528–530
in juvenile chronic arthritis 1117–1118
in SLE 1343
Antinuclear antibodies
see also Immune complexes
in SLE 1337, *1337*
Apatite arthritis 945–946
Aponeuroses 219
Apophyseal joint
involvement in ankylosing spondylitis 756, *756*
Apophyseal osteoarthrosis 1416–1418
Appliances
in ankylosing spondylitis 765
rehabilitation 1504–1514
Apprentice's foot 1476
Arachnoiditis 1423
Arborviruses 1151–1152
Arteritis
giant cell 1278–1291
granulomatous *1305*
large vessel 1316
polymyalgia rheumatica 1278–1291
Takayasu's 1316–1317
temporal **1278 – 1291**, 1316, 1440–1441
Arthralgia, menopausal 986
Arthritis
acne 1239
acute
clostridium difficile colitis 1146
suppurative 1137–1139
adenoviral 1151
in adolescents, advice 1515
apatite 945–946
associated microbial infections 443–447
classification *444*, *446*
carcinoma 1251
cervical 622
in childhood 1125–1133, *1125*
see also Juvenile Chronic Arthritis
connective tissue disorders, rarer 1131–1132
dermatomyositis 1131
familial Mediterranean fever 1132
mixed connective tissue disease 1131
Raynaud's phenomenon 1131–1132
sarcoidosis 1132
SLE 1131
juvenile psoriatic arthritis 1130–1131
HLA–B27 1130
incomplete Reiter's syndrome 1130
reactive arthritis 164, 166, 169–170, 322, 428–429, 728
juvenile spondylitis 1127–1130
complications 1129
course 1129
diagnosis 1129
drugs 1129
family history 1129
HLA–B27 1129
inflammatory bowel disease 1130
investigations 1129
iridocyclitis 1128
management 1129
onset 1127
radiology 1127–1129
sex ratio 1127
surgery 1129
seropositive juvenile arthritis 1125–1127
complications 1126
disease progression 1126
management 1126
onset 1125
pattern 1125
sex distribution 1125
spondyloarthropathies 1127–1130
complications, radionuclide imaging 1636
Crohn's disease 806–808
deformans *see* Osteoarthrosis
differential diagnosis 161–164
dysentery, bacillary 1146
enteric infections 1145–1146
enteropathic 808–818
experimental, animal models **468 – 485**, *468*
see also Experimental arthritis
gonococcal 1139–1140
gut infection 815–816
association with arthritis *815*
haemochromatosis 952–956
infective 1137–1161
inflammatory
intestinal bypass surgery 814–815, 1241
aetiology 814–815
treatment 815
shoulder 1444
lepromatous 1145
Lyme 1149–1150
lymphosarcomatous 1251
meningococcal 1140–1141
in mixed connective tissue disease 1271–1272
mumps 1151
in ochronosis 950–952
psoriatic 775–786
juvenile 1130–1131
reactive 164, 166, 169–170, 173, 322, 428–429, 728
campylobacter jejuni 1146
yersinia enterocolitica 1146
rubella 1150–1151
in single weight-bearing joint 1515–1516
in Sjögren's syndrome 1392–1393
smallpox 1152
surgical treatment 1518–1565
see also Surgery
tuberculous 1142–1144
Wilson's disease 956
Arthritis and blood disease **1177 – 1206**
complement 397–404, 1202
cryoglobulinaemia 1197–1198
deficiency 400–401, *1202*
haemoglobinopathies 1185–1191
haemophilia 1177–1185
hyperviscosity syndrome 1199
immune complex disease 1198
see also Immune complexes
immune deficiency 1199–1201
iron overload arthropathy 1191
leukaemia 1191–1196
lipid dermatoarthritis 1196–1197
multicentric reticulohistocytosis 1196–1197
clinical features 1196
course 1197

Arthritis and blood disease *cont*
purpura, hypogammaglobulinaemic 1199
thrombocytosis 1185
Arthritis and Rheumatism Council 15
Arthrocentesis 259
Arthrodesis 1531
elbow 1550
fingers 1559
hand/wrist 1559
in osteoarthrosis 879
Arthrography 1607–1608
double contrast 1607
single contrast 1607
ultrasonic examination 1607, 1608
xeroradiography 1607
Arthropathy
acromegalic 960–976
associated with non-articular neoplastic disease 1250–1251
chronic subluxing (Jaccoud's) 5
hypertrophic 1251–1253, 1475
in hypothyroidism 969–970
inflammatory 1229–1241
iron overload 1191
pyrophosphate 938–949
shoulder 1447
Arthroplasty
criteria 1530–1531
elbow 1550
fingers 1557–1559
hand/wrist 1557–1559
hinge replacement 1537–1538
complications *1538*
non-linked total knee replacement 1538–1539
replacement in osteoarthrosis 878
Arthroscopy 1597–1607
appearances
crystal synovitis 1606–1607
degenerative joint disease of knee internal derangement 1606–1607
inflammatory synovitis 1605–1606
physiological variations 1605
pigmented villonodular synovitis 1606
rheumatoid synovitis 1606
comparison with arthrotomy 1597–1598
examination technique
ankle 1604–1605
elbow 1604
hip 1605
knee joint 1599–1604
metacarpophalangeal joints 1605
fibreoptic arthroscope 1597, *1597, 1598*
historical background 1597
surgery 1535–1604
value and uses
assessment of extent of cartilage or synovial disease 1599
complications 1599
investigation of internal derangement of knee 1598–1599
non-arthritis 1598–1599
operative 1599
as research tool 1599
synovial biopsy 1598
therapeutic benefit 1599
Arthrotomy
comparison with arthroscopy 1597–1598
Articular indices 1591
Articular tumours 1241–1253
(or para-articular)
arising from bone/cartilage 1246
arthropathies associated with non-articular neoplastic disease 1250–1251
carcinoma arthritis 1251
lymphosarcomatous arthritis 1251
secondary neoplastic deposits 1251
benign 1244
developmental defects
diaphyseal aclasis 1246–1247, *1247*
enchondromatosis 1246, *1246*
differential diagnosis 1241
malignant neoplasms 1247–1250
chondrosarcoma 1247
fibrosarcoma 1247
giant cell tumours 1247
osteo-sarcoma 1247, *1248*
reticulum-cell sarcoma 1247
secondary neoplastic deposits 1244
synovioma 1244–1246
melanotic sarcoma 1246
myeloma 1247–1248, *1248*
osteoid osteoma 1248–1250, *1250*
pathological classification 1241
synovial chondromatosis 1241–1242
terminology *1242*
synovial chondrosarcoma 1246
Aschoff 6
Aschoff nodules 1066, *1066*
Aseptic necrosis
see also osteonecrosis 1207–1228
bone 837–838
leading to osteoarthritis 849, *850*
Legg-Perthes disease 851
radionuclide imaging 1636–1637
Aspergillosis 1153
Aspirin
see also Salicylates **500 – 513**
drug interactions 508
intra-articular injection 587
preparations 509
in SLE 1343
Asymptomatic hyperuricaemia 925–926
Atrial myxoma 1259
Attachment proteins 187–190
chondronectin 190
fibronectin 187–189
laminin 189–190
lubricating glycoprotein 190
Auranofin 530
side-effects 532
Auricular ankylosis 622
Autoantibodies 355–371
antibodies against nuclear antigens 362–366, *363*
clinical incidence of positive tests 364–366
specificities *364*
anti-cartilage antibodies 369
anti-collagen antibodies 369
anti-DNA antibodies 366–368
methods of detection 367–368
anti-dsDNA antibodies 368
clinical incidence 368
antiglobulins 356–362
anti-intermediate filament antibodies 370
anti-keratin antibodies 370
anti-perinuclear factor 370
anti-salivary duct antibody 370
assays, comparison *368*
lymphocytotoxic 368–369
rheumatoid factors 356–362
and complement activation 361–362
raised levels, incidence in rheumatoid disease 360–361
Autoimmune reactions 343
Avascular necrosis 1459
see also Osteonecrosis **1207 – 1228**
sickle cell disease 1188
Axial osteomalacia 1019
Azapropazone 521–522
in management of gout 921
Azathioprine 547–554

Bacillary dysentery arthritis 1146
Back pain
arachnoiditis 1423
classification 1411
causes *1411*
coccygeal pain 1427
disc degeneration
influence of geometric factors 1410
radiology 1407, *1407*
disc disorders 1407–1434
DISH 1428
early treatment 1427
epidemiology 99–104
exposure to cold and damp 1425
fibrositic nodules 1424
fibrositis 1424
fractures 1422–1423
frequency *1407*
inflammatory 1429
infection 1429
polymyalgia rheumatica 1429
rheumatoid arthritis 1429
seronegative spondylopathies 1429
local anaesthetic and steroid injection 1416
loose back syndrome 1424
lumbosacral pain 1411–1426
apophyseal osteoarthrosis 1416–1418
congenital abnormalities 1422
investigations 1414–1416
appearance 1416
CAT scanning 1416
conventional radiography 1414
discography 1415–1416
epidural myelography 1415
injection 1415
myelography 1414
nuclear magnetic resonance 1416

Back pain *cont*
pain production 1416
radiculography 1415
vertebral venography 1415
lumbar nerve roots, identification of sites, principal changes used *1413*
lumbar spondylosis 1416–1418
posture 1414
prolapsed intervertebral disc 1411
referred pain 1413–1414
Schmorl's nodes 1412, *1413*
lumbosacral strain 1424
magnitude of problem 1407
management 1425–1426
metabolic bone disease 1430–1431
neoplasms 1429–1430
nerves 1411, *1411*
non-specific low back pain 1423–1425
nucleus pulposus, variations of pressure 1410, *1410*
occupational factors 1408
Paget's disease 1430
posture 1424
pre-employment screening 1427
prevalence 1408
prevention 1426–1427
limitation of load bearing lift/strength rating 1426–1427
manual handling techniques 1427
posture 1427
radionuclide scanning 1637
referred pain 1431
sacroiliac strain 1424
Scheuermann's osteochondritis 1427–1428
Schmorl's nodes 1412, *1413*
sciatica 1413
sciatic scoliosis 1414, *1414*
spinal stenosis 1418–1420
causes *1419*
diagnosis 1420
management 1420
spine, structure and function 1408–1411
spondyolisthesis
association with lumbar spondylosis 1421
degenerative 1421–1422
spondyolysis 1420
spondylolytic spondylolisthesis 1422
spondylosis 1407–1434
'stuck' back 1424
treatment 1425–1426
Bacteria
see also infections, bacterial 1137–1145
Baillou, Guillaume de 4–5, *4*
Baker's cysts 669, 1465–1466, *669*
in hypermobile subjects 1168
Balanitis, of Reiter's disease 791–792, *792*
Bamboo spine 754, *754*
Basement membranes 215–217, *215*
chondronectin 217
fibronectin 216
laminin 216
B-cells 273, 310–313, 336–337
see also immune response, immunogenetics
autoimmune reactions 344
immune deficiency 1199
Sjögren's syndrome 1398–1399
synovial disease 607, 613
Behçet's disease 324, 1231–1235
arthritis 1233, 1234, *1234*
associations 1233
classification 1232–1233, *1232*
possible manifestations 1232–1233
diagnosis 1232
epidemiology 81
family history 1231
forms 1232
histology 1235
HLA 1233
immunological disturbance 1231
joints affected *1234*
levamisole therapy 562
prevalence 1233
treatment 1235
Benign intracranial hypertension 537
Benorylate 509
Biochemistry of conective tissue
see also Connective tissue **177 – 198**
Biomechanics 231
Blastomycosis, North American 1153–1154
Blood
see also Arthritis and blood disease **1177 – 1206**
abnormalities in SLE 1334
AIDS 1199
complement deficiency and rheumatic disease 1202, *1202*
cryoglobulinaemia 1197–1198
haemoglobinopathies 1185–1191
haemophilia 1177–1185, *1177*
hypergammaglobulinaemia purpura 1199
hyperviscosity syndrome 1199
hypogammaglobulinaemia 1199–1200
immune complex disease 1198
immune deficiency 1199–1201
iron overload arthropathy 1191
leukaemia 1191–1196
thrombocytosis 1185, *1186*
Bloodhound facies 1166
Blount's disease 1212
Bone
aseptic necrosis 837–838
Brittle Bones Society 1003
disease 612–622
dysplasias *998*
calcitonin 229
cancellous 227
collagen 227
compact 227
constitutional diseases, international nomenclature *998*
formation 227
hormonal control of metabolism 994–997
infarction, radio nuclide imaging 1636–1637
lamellar 227
metabolic bone disease **992 – 1023**
ageing 992–994
axial osteomalacia 1019
back pain 1130–1131
bone dysplasias 997, *998*
constitutional diseases, international nomenclature *998*
primary metabolic abnormalities *997*
endocrine disorders 987
fibrodysplasia ossificans progressiva 1019
fibrogenesis imperfecta ossium 1018
growth 992–994
heterotopic ossification 1019
hypophosphatasia 1001
infarction, radionuclide imaging 1636–1637
metabolism, hormonal control 994–997, *995*
multiple epiphyseal dysplasia 998–999, *999*
myositis ossificans progressiva 1019
osteogenesis imperfecta 1001–1003
proposed nomenclature *1002*
osteopetrosis 999–1000
osteoporosis 1004–1008, *1006*
oestrogren replacement therapy 1008
Paget's disease 1016–1018
parathyroid disorders 1014–1015
chondrocalcinosis 1015
diagnosis 1015
hypoparathyroidism 1015–1016
osteitis fibrosa 1014
primary hyperparathyroidism 1014–1015
rickets and osteomalacia 1008–1004, *1009*
biochemical changes 1012–1013, *1013*
vitamin D therapy 1013–1014
turnover 992–994
van der Hoeve's triad 1003
osteitis fibrosa 1014
osteocollagen 227
osteogenesis imperfecta 1001–1003
osteomalacia 1008–1014, *1009, 1013*
osteoporosis 1004–1008, *1006*
Paget's disease 1016–1018
parathormone 229
parathyroid disorders 1014–1015
primary metabolic abnormalities *997*
rickets 1008–1014, *1009, 1013*
vitamin D 229
woven bone 227
Bouchard's nodes 861, *863*
Boutonnière finger deformities, surgery 1559–1560, *1559*
British Association of Physical Medicine 16
British Association for Rheumatology and Rehabilitation (BARR) 16
British Council for Rehabilitation of the Disabled 15
British League Against Rheumatism 15
British Rheumatism and Arthritis Association 15
British Society for Rheumatology 16

Brittle Bones Society 1003
Brucellosis 1141–1142
Bunion 1477
Bursae
  injection techniques 1619
    infrapatellar 1619
    suprapatellar 1619
  surgical excision 1549
Bursitis
  acute calcific 1442, *1443*
  chronic 1442
  effusions 1450
  iliopsoas 1459
  infrapatellar 1465
  injection technique, supratrochanteric 1618
  olecranon 1450
  retrocalcaneal 1474
  semimembranous 1465
  student's elbow 1450
  treatment 1450
  trochanteric 1465
  water on the elbow 1450

Calcaneal epiphysitis 1474
Calcaneal spur 1475
Calcific tendonitis 165, *165*
Calcification,
  acute, in knee 1467
Calcitonin 229
Calcium pyrophosphate crystal deposition 857, 859, 938–949
Calcospherites 839–840, *840*
Calve's disease 1212
Campylobacter jejuni arthritis 1146
Candida infections 1155
Caplan's syndrome 681
Carcinoma arthritis 1251
Cardiac disease, in rheumatoid arthritis 627–630
Carpal tunnel syndrome 172, 1125, 1194
  in acromegalic arthropathy 967
  frequency in rheumatoid arthritis 1451
  in hypothyroidism 968
  injection technique 1615–1616, *1616*
    complications 1616
  management 1450–1451
  in myeloma 1248
  in rubella arthritis 1150
Cartilage
  age changes 225
  angiogenesis factors 223
  blood vessels 223
  destruction in rheumatoid arthritis 615–618
  fibrillation
    age factor 824–825
    nature 825–831
    pathology 831–833
  growth 221
  immunity 224
  mechanics 223–224
  neoplastic 222
  proteoglycans
    function 193–194
    structure 190–192
  thickness 225
  transplantation 224–225
CAT scanning in back pain 1416
Catabolin 223, 234, 617
Cat-scratch fever 1153
Cauda equina syndrome, axial tomography 757
Central nervous system disease in SLE 1333–1334
Cephalosporium 1155
Cervical spine 1435–1441
  anatomical relationships *1435*
  disease in rheumatoid arthritis 1545–1546
  examination 1575
  intubation 1524
  surgery 1545–1546
Charcot's joints 975, 1147, *1147*
  associated conditions 1253
  destructive arthropathy 1254
  in leprosy 1145
  radiology 1253–1254
  tabes dorsalis 1254
  treatment 1254
Cheiroarthropathy, diabetic 979–980, *979*
Chest, physical examination 1574
Chickenpox arthritis 1151
Chikungunya virus 1151–1152
Chilblains 1478
Children, therapeutic evaluation, 1593–1594
Chlorambucil 547–554
Chloroquine 528–530
  clinical experience 528–529
  pharmacological properties 528
  side-effects 529–530
  therapeutic usage 529
Choline magnesium trisalicylate 510
Chondrocalcinosis
  see also pyrophosphate arthropathy 938–949, *941*
  acromegalic arthropathy 966
  asymptomatic 942
  epidemiology 79
  gout 944
Chondrocytes 203, *203*
  acromegalic arthropathy 963, *964*
  enzyme activity 205
  growth 205
  respiratory activity 205
Chondromalacia patellae 1463–1464
Chondronectin 190, 217
Chondroprotective compounds, in treatment of osteoarthrosis 877
Chondrosarcoma 1247
Chorea 1078–1081, 1131
  see also rheumatic fever
  complications 1080–1081
  differential diagnosis 1079
  relapse 1080–1081, *1080*
  symptoms 1079
  treatment 1081
Christmas disease 1177, *1177*
Chronic subluxing arthropathy (Jaccoud's) 5
Chronopharmacology, in clinical trials 1583
Class III loci (C4, C2, Factor B) 316–317
Claw-foot 1476–1477
Clergyman's knee 1465
Clinical trials **1581 – 1596**
  analgesics, simple 1584–1585
    design of studies, three-way crossover *1584*
  anti-inflammatory drugs 1585–1586
    design of studies, short-term parallel group *1585*
  articular indices 1591
  chronopharmacology 1583
  design 1581–1584
    aims 1581
    anti-rheumatic drugs, classification *1581*
    programme *1582*
    protocol, how to write 1582
  dolorimeter 1591
  inflammation
    infra-red thermography 1591–1592
    objective measurements 1591
    technetium index 1592
  measurements
    Arthritis Impact Measurement Scale 1591
    articular index 1590–1591
    composite indices 1593
    disease severity 1590–1592
    functional 1591–1592
    grip strength 1590–1591
    indirect methods 1589–1590
    inflammation 1590–1591
    laboratory 1592
    McMaster Health Index Questionnaire 1591
    number 1593
    pain
      graphic rating 1589, *1589*
      other methods 1589
      relief, methods 1589
      simple descriptive scale 1588
      visual analogue scale 1588–1589
    range 1587–1594, *1587*
    side-effects 1594
    Standard Health Assessment Questionnaire 1591
    stiffness 1590
    swelling 1590
    tenderness 1590–1591
    toxicity 1594
  open trials 1584
  outcome 1584
  pharmacokinetics 1584
  pilot trials 1584
  post-marketing surveillance 1587
  progression, radiological 1592–1593
  slow acting drugs, design of studies 1586–1587, *1586*
  slowly appearing phenomena (e.g. toxicity) 1586–1587, *1586*
  statistics 1594
    interpretation 1595
  therapeutic evaluation

Clinical trials *cont*
ankylosing spondylitis 1593
children 1593–1594
gout 1593
osteoarthrosis 1593
treatment other than drugs 1594
uncontrolled trials 1584
Clostridium difficile colitis arthritis 1146
Clutton's joints, 1147, 1238–1239
Coalminer's 'beat knee' 1465
Coccidiomycosis 1154
Coccygeal pain 1427
Colchicine 522–523
in management of acute gout 921
Cold
physical treatment 1494
Colitis
clostridium difficile arthritis 1146
Collagen 178–186, 210–212, *211*
biosynthesis 182, *182*
degradation 185–186
structure 178–182
Complement 397–404
in absence of immunoglobulin 404
activation 397–398
in arthritis and blood disease 1202
binding, of immune complexes 379–380
biological activities 399–400, *399*
C3a, C5 generation 400
deficiency
as acquired abnormality 400–401
genetic determination; predisposition to disease 401
deficiency and rheumatic disease 1202, *1202*
arthritis symptoms 1202
investigations 1202
other diseases 404
polyarteritis nodosa 404
rheumatoid arthritis 403–404
serological findings 1202
SLE 402–403
treatment 1202
vasculitis 404
deposits in tissues in absence of immunoglobulin 404
immune precipitates, solubilisation 400
interaction with receptors 399–400
measurement
hypercatabolism 402
methods 401
in rheumatic diseases 401–402
tissue fixation 402
pathways 397–398, *398*
role in clearance of immune complexes 383
sequence 397–399
Computerised axial tomography (CAT scanning) in back pain 1416
Computerised tomography (CT) 1627–1632
disorders of spine
disc herniation 1627
facet joints 1628–1629
spinal stenosis 1629
femoral anteversion 1631–1632
quantitative bone mineral analysis 1632
sacroiliitis 1627
soft tissue lesions 1631
trauma 1630–1631
Connective tissue
adipose 219
biochemistry 177–197
attachment proteins 187–190
cartilage proteoglycan structure 190
chondronectin 190
collagen 178–186
biosynthesis 182–185, *182*
degradation 185–186
structure 178–182
elastin 186–187
fibronectin 187–189
glycosaminoglycans 190
laminin 189–190
lubricating glycoprotein 190
proteoglycans 190
biosynthesis by chondrocytes 192–193
dermatan sulphate 194–195
function in cartilage 193–194
heparan sulphate 195
hyaluronate 194
compact 219
elastic 219
fibrofatty 219
juxta-articular 620
loose 218–219
Connective tissue diseases in childhood 1131–1132
Connective tissue and joints
structure and function **199 – 250**
aponeuroses, ligaments, tendons 219–220
articular surfaces 235–239
basement membranes 215, *215*
bone 227–229
cartilage 220–227
cells 207–210
chondrocytes 203, *203*
enzyme activity 205
growth 205
osteo blasts 205
osteoclasts 206
osteocytes 207
collagen 210–212, *211*
comparative anatomy 200–201
elastic material 212–215
fibres 210
reticular 215
histiocytes 210
joint capsule fascia 218–219
labra intra-articular discs, menisci 220
lubrication 239–241
non-fibrillar extracellular matrix 217
organised connective tissue 218–219
symphyses 241–244
synovial joints 232
synovial tissue 232
synovium, effect on cartilage catabolin 233–235
units of structure and function 201
Contraceptive pill
rheumatic symptoms 986–987
Corticosteroids 535–545
acute gout, management 921
benign intracranial hypertension 537
corticotrophin (ACTH) 544–545
local treatment 545
drug interaction 537–538
in rheumatic diseases 538
intra-articular injections 584–586
in juvenile chronic arthritis 1114
metabolism 535
osteonecrosis, role in aetiology 1219–1220
physical treatment 1495
potency *536*
side-effects 537–544
gastrointestinal 541–542
growth, impairment 543–544
hypothalamo-pituitary adrenal axis 542–543
osteonecrosis 542
osteoporosis 542
skin atrophy 542
in SLE 1343–1344
synthetic 535–536
treatment
dermatomyositis 540
Felty's syndrome 539
giant cell arteritis 540
other conditions 521
polyarteritis nodosa 539
polymyalgia rheumatica 540
polymyositis 540
rheumatoid arthritis 538–539
SLE vasculitis 539
Wegener's granulomatosis 539–540
withdrawal 537
Corticotrophin (ACTH)
see also corticosteroids 544–545
Cortisol 980–982
anti-inflammatory 981
cardiovascular 981
immunological 981
metabolic 981
CPPD
(calcium pyrophosphate crystal deposition)
association with osteoarthrosis 857, 859
Cramp, occupational (writer's) 1453
C-reactive protein, in rheumatic fever 1081
CREST syndrome 1375
Crohn's disease
association with ankylosing spondylitis 762
enteropathic arthritis
aetiology 807
clinical features 806–807
food allergy 808
investigations 807
pathogenesis *807*
treatment 808
musculoskeletal disorders 809–810
Cryoglobulinaemia 1197–1199
essential 1197
essential mixed in vasculitis 1316
hyperviscosity 1197

Cryoglobulinaemia *cont*
mixed (polyclonal) 1197
unmixed (monoclonal) 1197
Cryoglobulins in SLE 1339
Cryptococcosis (torulosis) 1154
Crystal arthropathies
see also Epidemiology, Gout
epidemiology 75–79
Crystal synovitis
arthroscopic appearance 1607
Crystals in gout
identification by polarising microscope 895, *895*, *986*
Cutaneous vasculitis 1316
Cutis laxa 1166
Cysts, calf 1469–1471
Cytomegalic virus 1152
Cytotoxic drugs 547–554
azathioprine 547–554
chlorambucil 547–554
clinical pharmacology 547–549
cyclophosphamide 547–554
mechanisms 548–549
methotrexate 547–554
rationale 547
side-effects 552–554
structure *548*
treatment
dermatomyositis 551–552
juvenile chronic arthritis 551
polyarteritis nodosa 552
polymyositis 551–552
psoriatic arthritis 551
rheumatoid arthritis 549–550
SLE 550–551

Dagger sign 756, *756*
Debridement, in osteoarthrosis 879
Decompression sickness, acute
in aviators 1223
osteonecrosis, incidence 1223
radiology 1222, *1223*
Deformity, prevention 1515
De Quervain's syndrome 1452
Dermatoarthritis, lipid 1196–1197
Dermatomyositis 324, **1350 – 1363**
aetiology 1351–1352
in childhood 1132, 1354–1361
electromyographic triad 1358
laboratory aspects 1357–1358
prognosis 1357
classification 1350–1351
clinical manifestations 1352–1354
cytotoxic drug therapy 551–552
differential diagnosis 1355
epidemiology 87
hypogammaglobulinaemia, association 1200
incidence 1352
management 1358–1361
overlap with mixed connective tissue disease 1272–1273
precipitating factors 1352
Diabetes mellitus
associations
obesity 972
osteoarthrosis 852
carpal tunnel syndrome 978–979
Charcot joints 975
cheiroarthropathy 979–980, *980*
Dupuytren's contracture 978–979
gout 972
hyperuricaemia 917, 972
neuropathy 975–976
osteoarthritis 974–975
osteolysis (forefoot) 976
osteomyelitis 976
periarthritis of shoulder 980
peripheral neuropathy 975
soft tissue contracture 977
spinal neuropathy 976
trophic ulceration 976
vertebral ankylosing hyperostosis 973, 974
Diagnosis
see also Electrodiagnosis
acute phase reactants 1110
aids 1110–1111
blood count 1110
differential **161 – 174**, 1111–1112, *1111*
immunoglobulins 1111
laboratory tests 173–174
radiology 172–173, 1111
serology 1111
synovial membrane biopsy
Diaphyseal aclasis 1246–1247, *1247*
Diaphyseal dysplasia, progressive 1000
Diclofenac 517
Diffuse idiopathic skeletal hyperostosis (DISH) 656, 734–735, 1428
see also ankylosing hyperostosis, Forestier's disease
and osteoarthrosis 859–860
Diflunisal 509
Disc disorders 1407–1434
Discoid lupus 1335
Discs, intervertebral 1438
DISH
see also diffuse idiopathic skeletal hyperostosis, ankylosing hyperostosis, Forestier's disease
Dolorimeter 1591
D-penicillamine 557–558
see also penicillamine
comparison with levamisole *560*
side-effects
after gold therapy 532
in Sjögren's syndrome 1400
Drug-induced lupus 1335–1336, *1336*
Drugs
see also under individual drugs, pharmacokinetics
anti-malarials in SLE 1343
anti-rheumatic in clinical trials, classification 1594, *1581*, *1582*
(for details see Clinical Trials)
aspirin in SLE 1343
corticosteroids in SLE 1343
cytotoxic 547–554
hypouricaemic 569–583
immunosuppressive 547–554
immunosuppressive agents in SLE 1344
isotopes in drug studies 1635
NSAIDs in SLE 1343
in osteoarthrosis 875–876
side effects in Sjögren's syndrome 1400
in surgical treatment 1524–1526
uricosuric 574
in long-term management of gout 925
DTC (diethyldithiocarbamate) 557
Dupuytren's contracture 978–979, 1454
epidemiology 110
Dupuytren's contracture and diathesis 1254–1255
Dupuytren's diathesis 1444
Dysentery arthritis
amoebic 1146
bacillary 1146

Echovirus, type 6 1152
Ehlers-Danlos syndrome 1164–1166, *1165*, *1166*
articular complications 1165
clinical manifestations 1165
connective tissue disorders, types 1164
eye 1166
non-articular sequelae 1165
pregnancy 1166
skin
appearance 1164
trauma 1166
Elastin 186–187, 213–215
Elbow
arthrodesis 1550
arthroplasty 1550
arthroscopy 1605
effusions 1450
examination 1577
golfer's 1449–1450
humeral epicondylitis 1449–1450
injection techniques 1614–1615, *1615*
olecranon bursitis 1450
radial neuropathy 1452
student's elbow 1450
surgery 1549–1550
synovectomy 1549–1550
tennis 1449–1450
treatment 1449–1450
ulnar neuropathy 1452
water on the elbow 1450
Electrodiagnosis 1621–1626
clinical applications
myasthenia gravis 1625
myasthenic syndrome 1626
myopathic disorders 1624–1625
nerve compression 1623
nerve entrapment 1624
peripheral neuropathy 1624
electromyography 1623
latency measurements 1621
methods 1621
nerve conduction speed 1621–1623, *1622*
techniques 1621

Electromyography 1623
Enchondromatosis 1246, *1246*
Endocarditis 5
Endocrine disorders 959–991
  acromegalic arthropathy 960–967
  adenohypophysis 959–960
  hyperthyroidism 970–971
  hypothyroidism 968–970
  iatrogenic pituitary-adrenal insufficiency 982
  pregnancy 982–986
  in rheumatoid arthritis 638
  thyroid 967–968
  thyroid acropachy 971
Endocrine pancreas 972–980
Enteropathic arthritis 806–818
  ankylosing spondylitis 808–810, *809*
    aetiology 809
    clinical features 808
    HLA-B27 809
    investigations 808–809
    treatment 809
  Crohn's disease 806–808
    aetiology 807
    clinical features 806–807
    investigations 807
    pathogenesis *807*
    treatment 808
  gut infection 815–816, *815*
    aetiology 816
    investigations 816
    treatment 816
  intestinal bypass surgery 814–815
  ulcerative colitis 810–813
    aetiology 810–811
    ankylosing spondylitis 811–812
    clinical features 810
    investigations 810, *811*
    joints involved *811*
    musculoskeletal disorders 813
  Whipple's disease 813–814
    aetiology 814
    clinical features 813
    HLA-B27 814
    investigations 813–814
    treatment 814
Enteropathic reactive arthritis (ERA) 815–816
Enthesis 219
Enthesopathy 219, **723 – 744**, 1449
  see also Seronegative Spondarthritides
  ankylosing spondylitis 757–758, *758, 759*
  epidemiology 106–107
  insertion of patellar tendon 1467, *1467*
Enzymes, abnormalities in gout 904–906
Eosinophilic fasciitis 1257–1259, *1259*
Epidemiology 59–142
  acute back pain 100–101
  aetiological factors 110
  anatomical abnormalities 98
  ankylosing hyperostosis 97–98
  ankylosing spondylitis 70–72
  applications 124–126
  arthrosis 88–94
  back pain 99–104
  Behcet's disease 81
  biological attributes 114–116
  bone disorders 109–110
  chondrocalcinosis 79
  chronic back pain 101
  congenital dislocation of hip 108
  connective tissue diseases 82–88
  crystal arthropathies 75–79
  dermatomyositis 87
  developmental anomalies 98
  disc prolapse 99
  dorsopathies 88–94
  drug-induced lupus 85
  Dupuytren's contracture 110
  enteropathic arthropathy 73–74
  enthesopathies 106–107
  external influences 111–114
  generalised osteoarthrosis 94–95
  genotype 116–121
  gout 76–79
  HLA-B27 72–73
  hypermobility 107–108
  hypogammaglobulinaemia 81–82
  individual characteristics 114
  inflammatory arthropathies 79–82
  inherited conditions 107
  juvenile chronic arthritis 67–70
  Lyme disease 81
  micro-organisms 79–80
  non-articular rheumatism 106–107
  occupational disorders 105–106
  occurrence of back pain 100
  osteoporosis 110
  other spondylarthropathies 72–75
  Paget's disease 109–110
  peripheral joints, arthrosis 90–94
  polyarteritis nodosa 88
  polyarticular arthrosis 94
  polymyalgia rheumatica 104–105, 1279–1280
  psoriatic arthropathy 75
  reactive arthritis 72–80
  Reiter's disease 74–75, 788–789
  rheumatoid arthritis 63–67
  rheumatic disorders, individual 59–142
  rheumatic fever 108–109, 1066
  septic arthritis 79–80
  Sjögren's syndrome 88
  SLE 82–86, 1325–1326
  soft-tissue syndromes 104–107
  spinal stenosis 98–99
  spondylosis 95–99
  systemic sclerosis 86–87
  techniques 121–124
  transient back pain 100
Epiphyseal dysplasia
  in congenital hypothyroidism 970
  multiple 998–999, *999*
Epstein-Barr virus 438–440, 1152
Erbium (^{169}Er), intra-articular irradiation 589–590
Erosive osteoarthrosis 735, 856–857
Erosive spondylopathy 734
Erythema infectiosum, parvovirus cause 1153
Erythema nodosum 1229–1230, *1229*
  associations 1230
  histology 1229
  joint manifestations 1230
  treatment 1230
Erythrocyte sedimentation rate (ESR)
  in ankylosing spondylitis 799
  in juvenile chronic arthritis 1110
  in osteoarthrosis 869
  in Reiter's disease 798
  in rheumatic fever 1081
European League Against Rheumatism (EULAR) 15
Examination, physical 1573–1580
Exercise 1490–1492
  active
    assisted 1491
    hydrotherapy 1492
    resisted 1491–1492
  passive (movement) 1490
  in spondylitis 1495
Exocrine function, impaired in sicca syndrome 1388
Exocrine pancreas, failure 980
Experimental arthritis, animal models **468 – 485**
  autoimmunisation 478–480
  bacterial products, effect 471–476
  infective arthritis 469–471
  oral 6-sulphanilamidoindazole 480
  osteoarthrosis 480–481
  protein immunisation 476–478
  synovitis, crystal induced 482
Extractable nuclear antigen (ENA)
  see also Immunology
  in SLE 1338
Exudation 283–286
  formation 283–285, *285*
  origin of cells 286–287
Eyes, physical examination 1574

Familial juvenile gout 919–920
Familial Mediterranean fever 1029
  in childhood, mimicking juvenile chronic arthritis 1132
  familial recurrent polyserositis 1236
Fascia 219
Felty's syndrome 689
  association with rheumatoid arthritis 640–641, *641*
  corticosteroid therapy 539
Femoral anteversion, computerised tomography 1631–1632
Femur
  aseptic necrosis of proximal capital epiphysis 851
  slipped epiphysis leading to osteoarthrosis 850–851
Fenbufen 520
Fenclofenac 517–518
Fever
  cat-scratch 1153
  rheumatic 1057–1099
  Rocky Montain spotted 1150
Fibroblasts 201–203

Fibroblasts *cont*
in inflammation 288–290
Fibrodysplasia ossificans progressiva 1019
Fibrogenesis imperfecta ossium 1019
Fibronectin 187–189, 216–217
Fibrosarcoma 1247
Fibrosing alveolitis
in mixed connective tissue disease 1272
in systemic sclerosis 1374
Fibrosis 201
Fibrositic nodules 1424
Fibrositis 14, 20, 150, 1424
of shoulder 1446
Fibula, stress fractures 1472–1473
Fingers
clubbing in ulcerative colitis 813
in hypertrophic osteoarthropathy 1475
deformities
boutonnière 1559, *1559*
swan-neck 1560
injection techniques 1617, *1617*
stenosing tenovaginitis 1453, 1617, *1617*
surgery 1554–1560
trigger finger 1453, 1617, *1617*
Foot
examination 1579
flat 1476
forefoot
hallux rigidus 1533
hallux valgus 1533
osteoarthrosis 868
surgery 1531–1534
Freiberg's disease 1477
Freiberg's infraction 1477
hindfoot
osteoarthrosis 868
injection technique 1619–1620
Köhler's disease of metatarsal head 1477
march fracture 1477
metatarsal pain 1477
Morton's metatarsalgia 1477
painful foot, causes 1475–1478
pes cavus (claw-foot) 1476–1477
rheumatoid arthritis 1477
Foot drop
in rheumatoid vasculitis *1312*
Forestier's disease (ankylosing hyperostosis)
diabetes 973–974
epidemiology 97–98
osteoarthrosis 859–860
Fractures, vertebral
spinal pain 1422–1423
Freiberg's disease 1210, 1477, *1210*
Freiberg's infraction 1477
Frozen shoulder 1444
Fungal infection 1153–1155

Galen 3
Garrod, Sir Alfred 8, *8*
Gastrointestinal tract
in Sjögren's syndrome 1393
in systemic sclerosis 1372–1373
pathology 1372
Gaucher's disease 1219
and osteoarthrosis 853–854
Geigy gauge 1590
Genitourinary infection, causing ankylosing spondylitis 761–762
Geodes 258, 670
Giant cell arteritis 324
clinical features 1284–1285
corticosteroid therapy 540
and polymalgia rheumatica **1278 – 1291**
Giant cell tumours 1247
Gigantism 960
Glucose-6-phosphate, deficiency in gout 910
Glutathione reductase, increased activity in gout 910
Glycosaminoglycans 190
Goerkerman (Ingram) treatment of psoriatic arthritis 782
Gold 559
analysis 532
auranofin 531
comparison with D-penicillamine 532–533
dosage 531
effect on immune response 530–531
formation 530
in juvenile chronic arthritis 1117, *1117*
patient selection 531
rheumatoid arthritis, intra-articular injection 587
side-effects 532
in Sjögren's syndrome 1400
tissue antigens 533
therapeutic recommendation 531–533
Golfer's elbow 1449–1450
injection technique 1616, *1615*
Gonococcal arthritis 1139–1140
Gout **883 – 937**
see also Hyperuricaemia and Uric acid
acute
clinical features 884–886
differential diagnosis 898
long-term management 921–925
pathology 887–888
age of onset 884, *884*
alcohol 915
blood levels of uric acid 899–901
bodyweight, relation to uric acid 914–915, *915*
chronic
clinical features 884–887
differential diagnosis 898–899
pathology 890–891
chronic tophaceous
clinical features 886–887
corticosteroid injection 585
crystal identification 895, *895, 896*
diagnosis 894–899
differential diagnosis 164, 166, 897–899
epidemiology 76–79
familial juvenile 919–920
Heberden's nodes 898
historical background 6–9, 883
hyperlipoproteinaemia 1238
hyperuricaemia 906–917
age range 914
genetic factors 914
race 914
sex ratio 914
hypouricaemia 917–918, *917*
hypouricaemic drugs 569–583
intelligence 915
joints involved 885
lead poisoning 913
Lesch-Nyhan syndrome 906–909, *907*
leukaemia 1193
management 920–925
allopurinol 922–924, *924*
diet 925
hypertension 925
life-style 925
long-term management 921–925
uricosuric drugs 925
monosodium urate monohydrate, crystalline 890
histological demonstration 890
myeloid metaplasia 1196
pathology 887–891
crystal deposition 888–889
inflammatory response 889–890
prevalence 883–884
primary
association with hypertension, renal disease 892–894
hyperuricaemia, causes 918–919
uric acid calculi 892
prodromal symptoms 885
purines 902–905
pyrophosphate arthropathy 944
radiology 897
renal lesions 893–894
saturnine gout 913
secondary
accompanying myelomatosis 1248
serum uric acid 894–895
conversion scale *899*
levels 899, *899*
sex ratio 884, *884*
in sickle cell disease 1190
social class 915
synovial tissue, examination 895–896
therapeutic evaluation 1593
tophi 169
examination 895–86, *896*
urates, sites of deposition 891, *891*
uric acid
calculi 892
formation 892
hyperuricaemia 901
lithiasis 892
metabolism 901
Granulation tissue 202
Graunloma(s), Crohn's disease 810
Granulomatous arteritis
see also granulomatous vasculitis
Granulomatous vasculitis 1293–1294, 1304–1314, *1305*
overlap with polyarteritis nodosa 1293–1294
relationship to arteritis *1293*
Gut infection 815–816
association with arthritis *815*

Haemarthrosis, recurrent in haemophilia
  intra-articular radiotherapy 590
Haemochromatosis
  chondrocalcinosis 953–954
  clinical features 952–953
  differential diagnosis 953
  HLA 952
  osteoarthrosis 853
  pathogenesis 954–956
  pseudo-gout 953
  pyrophosphate arthropathy 943–944, 954
  radiology 953–954
  sex ratio 952
Haemoglobin
  rheumatic fever 1081
  uric acid levels 917
Haemoglobinopathies 1185–1191
  osteoarthrosis 854
  osteonecrosis 1218–1219
  sickle cell disease 1186–1190
  thalassaemia 1186, 1191
Haemophilia 1177–1185, *1177*
  aetiopathogenesis 1180–1181
  arthropathy, subacute 1179
  chronic arthropathy 1179
  clinical severity 1178
  corticosteroid therapy 1184
  definition 1178, *1177*
  factor VIII and IX replacement 1183
  haemarthrosis
    acute 1178
    recurrent, intra-articular radiotherapy 590
  management 1182–1185
  muscular contractures *1180*
  osteoarthrosis 854
  patient education 1185
  patient independence 1185
  physical adaptations 1184
  physiotherapy 1184
  prophylactic injections 1184
  radiology 1181—1185
  radiosynoviorthesis 1184
  soft-tissue bleeding 1179–1180
  splinting 1184
  surgery 1184–1185
Hagemann factor 296
Hairy cell leukaemia 1193
Hand
  arthroscopy 1605
  examination 1577–1578
  injection techniques 1616–1617, *1617, 1618*
  osteoarthritis, surgery, 1560
  success rating *1556*
  surgery 1554–1560
Hand-foot syndrome in sickle cell disease 1190
Hallux rigidus 1477
Hallux valgus 1477
Haverhill fever 1149
Headache
  giant cell arteritis 1284
  temporal arteritis 1440
Heart
  mitral valve prolapse associated with hypermobility 1169
  physical examination 1574
  rheumatic fever 1066
    clinical picture 1075–1076
    failure 1076–1077
    pericarditis 1076
    rhythm change 1076
    treatment 1089
  rheumatic pneumonia 1077–1078
    treatment 1089
  SLE 1328–1329
  subacute bacterial endocarditis
  complicating rheumatic fever 1082
    prevention *1090*
  systemic sclerosis 1374
Heat
  physical treatment 1493–1494, *1493*
Heberden, William 5, 16, *5*
Heberden Library 16
Heberden Oration 16
Heberden Round 16
Heberden Society 16
Heberden's nodes 861, *838*
  in gout 898
  heredity 856
  in primary osteoarthrosis 856
Heel, painful 1474–1475
Henoch-Schönlein purpura 1235–1236, 1315–1316
Hepatitis, acute
  arthritis 1151
Hepatitis B 435–437
Hereditary multiple aclasis 1246–1247, *1247*
Heritable disorders 1162–1176
  bloodhound facies 1166
  cutis laxa 1166
  Ehlers-Danlos syndrome 1164–1166, *1165, 1166*
  of fibrous proteins 1162
  homocystinuria 1163–1164
  hyperlysinaemia 1164
  hypermobility (in healthy subjects) 1166–1170, *1167*
  mucopolysaccharidoses 1170–1171, *1171*
  osteogenesis imperfecta 1001–1003, *1002*
  pseudo-xanthoma elasticum 1164
  skeletal
    achondroplasia 1172–1173, *1173*
    cleiodocranial dyostosis 1174
    diaphyseal aclasis 1175
    epiphyseal dysplasia 1173
    fibrodysplasia ossificans progressiva 1172
    microdactyly osteopoikilosis *1173*
    multiple epiphyseal dysplasia 1173
    myositis ossificans progressiva 1172
    osteopetrosis 1173–1174
    pycnodyostosis 1173
    spondyloepiphyseal dysplasia 1173
Herpes zoster 1461
Heterotopic ossification 1019
Hilton's law 1436
Hip
  arthography 1607–1608
  arthroscopy 1605
  congenital dislocation, epidemiology 108
  cysts 1459
  examination 1578
  injection techniques 1617–1618
    joint 1618, *1618*
    supratrochanteric bursitis 1618
  joint replacement surgery in osteoarthrosis 877–878
  osteoarthrosis 866–867
  pattern of pain referral from joint 1459
  and pelvis 1455–1456
  'snapping' 1456
  total replacement 1540–1545
  see also Surgery
Histiocytic lymphoma 1247
Histoplasma capsulatum, histoplasmosis 1154
Histoplasma duboisin 1154
Historical background of rheumatic diseases **3 – 18**
History-taking 1567–1573
HLA, associations with disease 317–320
  with rheumatic diseases 320–326, *320*
HLA-B27 730–733
  acne arthritis 1239
  ankylosing spondylitis 760
  associated disorders 320, *320*
  bacillary dysentery 1146
  Reiter's disease 791
  yersinia arthritis 322, 428–429, 1146
Hoffa's disease 1466
Homocystinuria 1163–1164
Host immunity 337
Housemaid's knee 1465
Housewife's shoulder 1446
HPOA (hypertrophic pulmonary osteoarthropathy) 1251–1253
Human MHC (HLA) system 312–316
Human thyroid stimulator (HTS) 972
Humeral epicondylitis 1449–1450
Hurler's syndrome 1171–1172, *1172*
Hyaluronate 195
Hydroxyapatite crystals
  deposition, association with osteoarthrosis 859
  detection in synovial fluid 271–272
Hypercalcaemia, in hyperuricaemia 914
Hypergammaglobulinaemic purpura 1199
Hyperlipidaemia, osteonecrosis 1223
Hyperlipoproteinaemia 1236–1238
  abnormality patterns 1237, *1237*
  eruptive 1237
  involving tendons, lytic lesions in bone 1237–1238
  hyperuricaemia 1238
  Type II (hypercholesterolaemic) arthritis 1238
  Type IV arthralgia, arthritis 1238
  xanthomata 1237–1238
Hyperlysinaemia 1164
Hypermobility
  associations
    chronic back pain 1168
    loose back syndrome 1168

Hypermobility *cont*
mitral valve prolapse 1169
clinical effects 1168
clinical stigmata *1167*
connective tissue disorder 1169
epidemiology 107–108
management 1170
premature osteoarthrosis 1168
race 1168
sex ratio 1168–1169
syndrome 1168
Hyperparathyroidism
association with acromegalic arthropathy 966
chondrocalcinosis 1015
diagnosis 1015
osteitis fibrosa 1014
primary, bone disease 1014–1015
pyrophosphate arthropathy 943
Hypersensitivity vasculitis 1314–1316
Hypertension 925
essential, in hyperuricaemia 193
Hyperthyroidism 970–971
Hypertriglyceridaemia
alcohol induced 916
in gout 916
Hypertrophic osteoarthropathy 1251–1253, 1475, *1251*
histology 1252
pachydermoperiostosis 1252–1253, *1253*
pathogenesis 1252
primary 1252
pulmonary 1475
pulmonary osteoarthropathy 1252
radiology 1251–1252
radionuclide scanning 1637
secondary, associations 1252
Hypertrophic pulmonary osteoarthropathy (HPOA) 1252
Hyperuricaemia
see also Gout, Uric acid
age range 914
alcohol 915
asymptomatic 925–926
bodyweight, relation to uric acid 914–915, **915**
cardiovascular disease 916–917
diabetes 917
familial juvenile gout 919–920
genetic factors 914
gout 906
causes in primary 918–919
haemoglobin and uric acid levels 917
hypercalcaemia 914
hyperlipoproteinaemia 1238
hyperparathyroidism 914
hypertriglyceridaemia 916
intelligence 915
lead poisoning 913
leukaemia 1193
myeloid metaplasia 1196
myxoedema 914
osteonecrosis 1223
plasma
lipids 916
proteins and uric acid levels 917
race 914
saturnine gout 913
sex ratio 914
in sickle cell disease 1190
social class 915
Hyperviscosity syndrome 689, 1189
Hypogammaglobulinaemia 1199–1200
epidemiology 81–82
Hypo-hyperparathyroidism 1016
Hypomagnesaemia, pyrophosphate arthropathy 944
Hypoparathyroidism 1015–1016
Hypophosphatasia 1001
calcinosis 944
pyrophosphate arthropathy 944
Hyposplenism 1028
Hypothyroidism 968–970
arthropathy 969–970
carpal tunnel syndrome 968
congenital 970
epiphyseal dysplasia 970
muscle 969
myopathy 969
osteonecrosis 1223–1224
pyrophosphate arthropathy 944
rheumatological manifestations 968
Hypouricaemia 917–918, *917*
Hypouricaemic drugs 569–583
allopurinol 569–574, *470*
chemistry 569
dose 572
drug interactions 573–574
historical background 569
kidneys 572
pharmacological properties 570–572
side-effects 573
therapeutic effect 573–574
anti-inflammatory drugs 579–580
benzbromarone 578–579
diuretics 579
lipid-lowering 580
probenecid 575–577
sulphinpyrazone 577–578
thiopurinol 574
uricosuric 574, 579, *575*
Hypoxanthine guanine phosphoribosyl transferase (HGPRT)
decreased activity in Lesch-Nyhan syndrome 906
purine metabolism 901

Iatrogenic pituitary-adrenal insufficiency 982
Ibuprofen 518–519
Iga, selective deficiency 1200–1201
Iliopsoas bursitis 1459
Imaging techniques **1627 – 1642**
computerised tomography 1627–1632
radionuclide scanning 1633–1642
Immune complex disease
concept 386–387
experimental
adjuvant disease 389
aetiology *387*
allergic arthritis 389
arthus reaction 387
prognosis 1198
purpura 1198
serum sickness 387–388, *387*
skin manifestations 1198
spontaneous lupus 389
treatment 1198
Immune complexes 376–397
antigen-antibody interactions 377
assays, use in clinical practice 396–397
biological properties 379
cell interaction 380
circulating immune complexes
clearance 382–383
fate 382–386
tissue deposition 383–385
complement binding 379
composition 377
detection, methods
cryoprecipitation 394–395
gel filtration 394
interaction with complement 395
interaction with rheumatoid factors 396
microscopy 390–392
electronmicroscopy 392–393
other assays 396–397
polyethylene glycol (PEG) precipitation 395
ultracentrifugation 393–394
effect on immune response 380
enhanced antibody production 380
historical background 376
immune reactions, blocking 381
immunoglobulins, structure 377
lattice structure 378, 382–383
nature of antigen 383
pathogenecity 385–386
permeability of vessels 383
physicochemical properties 378
reactions with rheumatoid factors 381–382
regulation of antibody production 380–381
role of complement 395–396
size 378, 382–383
solubility 378–379, *379*
tissue
damage 385–386
deposition 383–385
receptors 385
uptake by reticuloendothelial system 383
Immune deficiency 1199–1201
AIDS 1199
B-cell defects 1199
dermatomyositis associated with hypogammaglobulinaemia 1200
hypogammaglobulinaemia
acquired, late onset 1199
associations 1200
background 1200
bacterial infection 1200
clinical picture,
differences with arthritis of rheumatoid arthritis 1200
familial factor 1199
incidence 1199

Immune deficiency *cont*
non-infective arthritis 1200
onset, time 1199
pathological differences 1200
sex-linked (Bruton) 1199
selective Iga deficiency
diagnosis 1201
frequency in juvenile arthritis 1200
non-infective arthritis, pathogenesis 1201
treatment 1201
T-cell defects 1199
Immune response, autoimmune disease 345–346
Immunodeficiency and arthritis 334
Immunogenetics **309 – 330**
clinical genetics 309
experimental autoimmune disease 312
H-2 complex of mouse 310–312
HLA associations
disease 317–320
rheumatic disease 320–326, *320*
human MHC (HLA) system 312–316
immune response genetics 310–312
other genetic polymorphisms 326
Immunoglobulins
altered, following antigen-binding 379
in rheumatic fever 1081–1082
structure 377–378
Immunological mechanisms 331–354, *331, 332*
Immunology
in SLE 1336–1340
anti-DNA antibodies 1337–1338, *1338, 1339*
anti-ENA 1338
antinuclear antibodies 1337, *1337*
antiviral antibodies 1338
LE cells 1337
rheumatoid factor 1339
T-cell suppressor function 1336
Sjögren's syndrome 1396–1398
synovial fluid 272–273
Immunomodulators 554–563
clinical properties of *560*
D-penicillamine 554–558
DTC 554
gold 559
levamisole 560–561
thymopoietin 559, 561–562
effect on T-cells *558*
immunological abnormalities 555
isoprinosine 554
levamisole 555–557
levamisole therapy in
ankylosing spondylitis 562
Behçet's disease 562
other rheumatic diseases 562
SLE 562
rheumatoid arthritis 562
thymic factors 558–559, *559*
Immunoproliferative disorders 346–349
Immunoregulation, chronic arthritis 341–342, *341*
Immunosuppression, physical therapies 554
Immunosuppressive agents in SLE 1344
Immunosuppressive drugs 547–554
Immunosuppressive therapy in juvenile chronic arthritis 1188
Indomethacin 516–517
in acute gout 921
Infection
see also infective arthritis **1137 – 1161**
acute hepatitis 1151
adenoviral arthritis 1151
after total joint replacement 1155–1156
ankylosing spondylitis 429–430
arboviruses 1151–1152
association with arthritis 443–447
classification *444, 446*
back pain 1429
bacterial 423–430, 1137–1145
candida 1155
chickenpox 1151
clinical considerations 452–457
Coxsackie B 1153
cytomegalic virus mimicking Epstein-Barr viral infections 1152
enteric 1145–1146
fungal 1153–1155
genetic considerations 452–457
genitourinary 427–428
gonococcal 1139–1140
immunity 411–412
inflammatory polyarthritis 427–428
inflammatory rheumatic diseases, involvement 418, *422*
interleukin 455
intestinal, reactive arthritis 428–429
investigation 412–423, *423, 418, 422*
leptospirosis 1149
microbial 411–467
mumps 1151
paramyxoviruses 434–435
parvoviruses 437–438
pathological considerations 452–457
prokaryotic, conclusions 430–431
rat bite fever 1149
reactive immunopathology 447–452
recent progress 423–424
rheumatic diseases, involvement in aetiology and pathogenesis 456–457, *457*
rheumatic fever 424–425
rheumatoid arthritis 424–425
Rocky Mountain spotted fever 1150
in SLE 1334
smallpox 1152
spirochaetal 1146–1150
syphilis 1146–1148
viral 1150–1153
in vasculitis 1296
see also viruses
Infectious mononucleosis 1152
Infective arthritis **1137 – 1161**
actinomyces bovis 1153
acute hepatitis 1151
acute suppurative arthritis 1137–1139
adenoviral 1151
after total joint replacement 1155–1156
amoebic dysentery 1146
arthritis associated with microbial infection *1137*
aspergillosis 1153
atypical mycobacteria 1145
bacillary dysentery 1146
bacterial infections 1137–1145
blastomycosis 1153–1154
North American geography 1153
brucellosis 1141–1142
campylobacter jejuni enteritis 1146
candida infections 1155
cat-scratch fever 1153
complications 1153
cephalosporium 1155
chickenpox 1151
Chikungya virus 1151–1152
clostridium difficile colitis 1146
coccidiomycosis 1154
Coxsackie B infection 1153
Crohn's disease 809
cryptococcosis 1154
cytomegalic virus 1152
Echovirus type 6 1152
enteric infections 1145–1146
erythema infectiosum, parvovirus cause 1153
experimental models 469–471
fungal infections 1153–1155
gonococcal 1139–1140
Haverhill fever 1149
histoplasma capsulatum, histoplasmosis 1154
infectious mononucleosis 1152
leprosy 1145
leptospirosis 1149
Lyme arthritis 1149–1150
lymphogranuloma venereum 1155
madura foot (mycetoma pedis) 1154–1155
meningococcal 1140–1141
mumps 1151
mycoplasma 1142–1145
mycoplasma pneumoniae 1142
nocardia 1155
O'Nyong-Nyong virus 1151–1152
petrullidium boydis 1155
rat-bite fever 1149
Rocky Mountain spotted fever 1150
Ross River virus 1151–1152
rubella 1150–1151
salmonella 1145–1146
smallpox 1152
spirochaetal infections 1146–1150
sporotrichosis 1155
syphilis 1146–1148
tuberculosis 1142–1144
viral infections 1150–1153
yaws 1148–1149
yersinia enterocolitica 1146
Inflammation **281 – 308**
cell types 284
cellular infiltration 286–288
control of inflammatory response 293, *294, 295*
healing process 288–290, *289*
historical background 281, *281*

Inflammation *cont*
inflammatory process 282–290, 303–304
local events *282*
measurement 1590–1592
mediators 296–303
modulators 296–303
objective measurements 1591–1592
in rheumatic diseases 304
systemic response 290–293, *292*
Inflammatory arthritis of shoulder 1444
Inflammatory arthropathy 1229–1241
acne arthritis 1239
anaphylactoid purpura 1235–1236
Behçet's syndrome 1231–1235
Clutton's joints 1238–1239
erythema nodosum 1229–1230, *1229*
Henoch-Schönlein purpura 1235–1236
hyperlipoproteinaemia 1236–1238
intestinal bypass surgery arthritis 1241
pigmented villondular synovitis 1242–1244
pustolotic arthro-osteitis 1239–1240
pyoderma gangrenosum 1240–1241
sarcoidosis 1230–1231
traumatic synovitis 1239
tumours 1241–1253
Inflammatory back pain 1429
Inflammatory bowel disease in children 1130
Inflammatory polyarthritis, early, severe, rehabilitation 1515
Inflammatory synovitis, arthroscopy 1605–1606
Infrapatellar bursitis 1465
Injection techniques **1612 – 1626**
Achilles tendinitis 1619
ankle 1619–1620
elbow 1614–1615, *1615*
fingers 1617, *1617, 1618*
foot 1619–1620
hand 1616–1617
heel, painful 1619–1620
hip 1617–1618, *1618*
knee 1618–1619
miscellaneous 1620
shoulder 1613–1614, *1613*
steroid, local 1612–1620
wrist 1615–1616, *1616, 1617*
Interleukin 1, 234, 291–293, 617, *291*
infection 455
in rheumatoid synovial membrane 601
Intermittent claudication 1473
International Classification of Diseases (ICD) 23, 27, 28, 45
International League Against Rheumatism (ILAR) 15, 16
definition of rheumatology 3–4
Interspinous ossification 756
Intervertebral joints 242–244
age changes 243–244
annulus fibrosus 242
nucleus pulposus 242–244
Intestinal bypass surgery arthritis 814–815, 1241
dermatitis syndrome 734
Intra-articular discs 220
Intra-articular therapy **584 – 591**
aspirin 587
corticosteroid 584–585
gold in rheumatoid arthritis 587
irradiation 588–590
^{169}Er in small joints 589–590
special indications for use 590
^{90}Y in large joints 588–589
orgotein 587
osmic acid 587–588
in osteoarthrosis 876
side-effects 586–587
silicone oil in osteoarthrosis 587
soft-tissue lesions, non-articular 585–586
synoviorthesis 587
Iridocyclitis 1128
in juvenile chronic arthritis 1107–1108
Iron overload arthropathy 1191
Irritable hip syndrome 1192
Ischaemic pain 1457
Ischial tuberosity 1457
Ischial whiskering 757–758, *757*
Isoprinosine 557
Isotopes 1632–1639

Jaccoud's arthropathy 5
Joint capsule 219
Joints
acromioclavicular 1443–1444
antigen persistence 331–334
apophyseal 1410
arthrography 1607–1608
arthroscopic appearances 1605–1607, *1602, 1604*
arthroscopy 1603–1605
articular surfaces 235–239
aspiration 259
Charcot 975, 1147, 1253–1254, *1147*
Clutton 1147
elbow, surgery 1549–1550
examination 1574–1579
function 199–250
gout
acute 885
chronic 886
hip 1459
total replacement 1540–1545
imagine techniques 1627–1642
injection techniques 1612–1620
knee 1462–1467
cysts 1536
surgery 1535–1540
limited joint mobility syndrome 979–980, *979*
lubrication 239–241
neuropathic 975, 1253–1254
osteoarthrosis 861–869
prosthetic
infection 1527–1528
painful 1528–1529
replacement
in osteoarthrosis 877–878
radionuclide scanning 1639
shoulder 1441–1447
frozen 1444
surgery 1547–1549
structure 199–250
superior tibiofibular synovitis 1467
surgery 1534–1535
assessment 1520–1521
symphyses 241–242
synovial 229–232
cervical spine 1437–1438
in systemic sclerosis 1371
wrists, surgery 1550–1553
Jumper's knee 1464
Juvenile chronic arthritis (Still's disease) **1100 – 1124,** *22*
Acthar Gel 1116, *1116*
ACTH therapy 1114
aetiology 1101–1103
age distribution 1101, *1101*
amyloidosis 1109
anabolic steroids 1116
association with rheumatoid arthritis 638
clinical aspects 1103–1106
corticosteroid therapy 1114
growth impairment 1114
criteria 1100
cytotoxic drug therapy 551
death, causes 1109, 1110, *1110*
definition 1100
diagnosis 1111–1112, *1111*
drugs 1114–1118
anti-malarials 1117–1118
gold 1117, *1117*
treatment 1114–1118, *1117, 1118, 1119*
encephalitis 1106
epidemiology 67–70
fever 1104, *1104*
fractures 1109
growth defects 1108, 1114, *1108, 1115, 1116*
heredity 1103
historical background 1100
immunological basis 1101–1103
incidence 1100–1101
iridocyclitis 1107–1108
joint involvement, pattern 1106–1107
keratitis punctata *1108*
kidney involvement 1106
liver enlargement 1104
lone Iga deficiency 1200
lymphadenopathy 1104
management 1112–1114
myocarditis 1106
nodules 1107
NSAIDs 1114
onset
pauciarticular 1106
polyarticular 1106
pericarditis 1105
pleurisy 1106
prevalence 1100–1101
prognosis 1112, *1112, 1113*
pulmonary fibrosis 1106
serositis 1105

Juvenile chronic arthritis (Still's disease) *cont*
sex distribution 1101, *1101*
splenomegaly 1104
surgery 1118–1120
synovial membrane biopsy 1111
systemic features 1104
tenosynovitis 1107
Juvenile psoriatic arthritis 778, 1130–1131
Juvenile rheumatoid arthritis 21

Kashin-Beck disease 855
Keratitis punctata *1108*
Keratoconjunctivitis sicca 683–684, 1386–1390, *684*
diagnosis 1389–1390
fluorescein dilution 1390
osmolality 1390
Schirmer's test 1389
tear film break-up time 1389
tear protein profiles 1390
Ketoprofen 520
Ketosis, effect on uric acid excretion 912, *913*
Kidney, in systemic sclerosis 1374
Kienböck's disease 1217, *1217*
Kinesiology 231
Knee
acute calcification 1467
arthrography 1607–1608
arthroscopy 1598–1604
appearances 1607, *1602, 1603*
bursitis 1465
examination 1578
injection techniques 1618–1619
joint replacement in osteoarthrosis 878
lesions 1462–1467
differential diagnosis 1466
Hoffa's disease 1466
internal derangements 1463
Osgood-Schlatter disease 1466
Pellegrini-Stieda disease 1466–1467
superior tibiofibular joint, synovitis 1466
synovial shelf syndrome 1463
osteoarthrosis 867–868
patella 1463–1465
chondromalacia patellae 1463–1464
dislocation 1464
nail-patella syndrome 1464
popliteal cysts 1465–1466
differential diagnosis 1466
pre-patellar bursitis 1465
surgery 1535–1540
arthroplasty 1536–1539
arthroscopic 1535–1536
choice of procedures *1540*
joint cysts 1536
osteotomy 1539
synovectomy 1536
total knee replacement 1538–1539
synovial biopsy 1608–1611
tendinitis 1467
Kohler's disease 1210, 1476, *1210*

Laboratory tests, differential diagnosis 173–174
Labra 220
Lactic acidaemia 912
Laminin 189–190, 216
Laryngeal arthritis 622
Lateral popliteal nerve palsy 1461–1462
LE cells in SLE 1337
Lead poisoning 913
Leg
long-leg syndrome 1467–1468
Legg-Perthes disease in children, leading to adult osteoarthritis 851
Leprosy arthritis 1145
Leptospirosis 1149
Leriche's syndrome 1457
Lesch-Nyhan syndrome 906–909, *907*
xanthine stone formation 909
Leukaemia 1191–1196
amyloidosis 1194–1195
angioimmunoblastic lymphadenopathy 1195–1196
association with rheumatoid arthritis 1191
hairy cell leukaemia 1193
irritable hip syndrome 1192
leukaemic reticuloendotheliosis 1193
lymphoblastic 1191–1192
lymphoma 1193
myelogenous 1192
differentiation from juvenile arthritis 1192
myeloid 1193, *1192*
myeloid metaplasia 1196
myelomatosis 1193–1194
T-cells 1193
Waldenström's macroglobulinaemia 1195
Leukaemic reticuloendotheliosis 1193
Levamisole 555–557, 560–561
comparison with penicillamine in rheumatoid arthritis *560*
Ligaments 219–220
Limb, lower **1455 – 1480**
ankle, painful 1474–1475
anterior tibial compartment syndrome 1471–1472
bursitis 1465–1466
foot, painful 1475–1478
heel, painful 1474–1475
intermittent claudication 1473
knee joint, lesions 1462–1467
lesions 1455–1480
long leg syndrome 1467–1468
nerve entrapment syndrome 1461–1462
pain 1455–1460
stress fractures 1472–1473
synovial rupture 1468–1471
Limb, upper **1448 – 1454**
Lipid dermatoarthritis 1196–1197
Liver, involvement in Sjögren's syndrome 1393
Liver disease
penicillamine 526–527
Long leg syndrome 1467–1468
Loose back syndrome 1168, 1424
Looser's zone 1010, 1458, *1011*
Lumbar spine flexion check 1575, *1576*
Lumbar spondylosis 1414–1418
Lumbosacral pain 1411–1426
Lumbosacral strain 1424
Lubricating glycoprotein 190
Lungs
changes in rheumatic fever 1077
involvement in SLE 1330
radionuclide scanning in fibrosing diseases 1638–1639
'shrinking' 1330, *1330*
Lupus
ANA-negative 1335
discoid 1335
drug-induced 1335–1336, *1336*
Lyme arthritis 1149–1150
epidemiology 81
Lymphoma 1193
histiocytic 1247
Lymphogranuloma venereum 1155
Lymphosarcomatous arthritis 1251

Madura foot 1154–1155
Manubriosternal joint in osteoarthrosis 864
Marble bones disease 999–1000
March fracture 1477
Marfan's syndrome 1162–1163, *1162, 1163*
McCune-Albright syndrome 999
McGregor's line 658
Measurements 1591
Melanotic sarcoma 1246
Melorheostosis 1000
Menginococcal arthritis 1140–1141
Menisci 220
Menopausal arthralgia 986
Meralgia paraesthetica 1461
Metabolic bone disease **992 – 1023**
see also Bone
Metacarpophalangeal joints, osteoarthrosis 861–863
Methotrexate 547–554
Mexican hat 1541, *1541*
Microbial infection **411 – 467**
see also Infection
Microdactyly 1172
Microscopy
electron 266
stained smears 263–266
wet preparations 266–268
Milwaukee shoulder 863–864, 974, 1446, *946*
Miscellaneous conditions 1229–1266
Mixed connective tissue disease (MCTD) **1269 – 1277**, 1375
antibodies to nuclear ribonuclear protein, 1269–1270, *1270*
arthritis 1271–1272
clinical characteristics 1272, *1271*
clinical features 1270–1271
clinical findings 1272, *1272*
diagnosis 1274–1275
diagnostic criteria 1275

Mixed connective tissue disease (MCTD) *cont*
as 'distinct clinical entity' 1275–1276
epidemiology 88
fibrosing alveolitis 1272
overlap features 1272–1273
overlap with SLE 1336
prognosis 1274–1275
Raynaud's phenomenon 1272
treatment 1275
response 1274–1275
Morton's metatarsalgia 1477
Mouth, physical examination 1574
Mucin clot test 261
Mucopolysaccharidoses 1170–1171, *1171, 1172*
osteonecrosis 1219
Multicentric reticulohistocytosis 1196–1197
Multiple myeloma 1193–1194
Mumps arthritis 1151
Muscle, in systemic sclerosis 1371
Myalgia, pericapsular 1446
Myasthenia gravis, electrodiagnosis 1625–1626
Myasthenic syndrome, electrodiagnosis 1625–1626
Mycetoma pedis 1154–1155
Mycobacteria, atypical arthritis 1145
Mycoplasma pneumoniae arthritis 1142
Myeloid metaplasia 1196
Myeloma 1247–1248, *1248*
Myelomatosis 1193–1194
Myocarditis, overlap with MCTD 1272–1273
Myocrisin 530
Myopathic disorders, electrodiagnosis 1624–1625
Myopathy, in hypothyroidism 969
Myositis ossificans progressive 1019
Myxoedema, hyperuricaemia 914

Necrosis, avascular
see also osteonecrosis **1207 – 1228**
Nail-patella syndrome 1464
Naproxen 519
Natural killer (NK) cells, immune response 337
Neck and shoulder **1435 – 1447**
arteries 1440
cervical spine
examination 1436
functional anatomy 1435–1437
Hilton's law 1436
segmental innervation 1435–1436, *1436*
sites of origin of pain *1437*
torticollis 1436
cervical spondylosis 1437–1438
contra-indications for mobilising treatment 1440
intervertebral discs 1438
ligaments 1440
muscles 1440
nerve roots, spinal cord 1438–1439
polymyalgia rheumatica 1440
posture, poor cervical 1440
shoulder 1441–1447
synovial joints 1437–1438
temporal arteritis 1140–1141
thoracic outlet syndrome 1438–1439
thoracic viscera 1441
vertebrae
developmental abnormalities 1439–1440
disease 1440
Sprengel's shoulder 1439
whip-lash effect 1440
Necrosis, aseptic
see aseptic necrosis 837–838
Neoplasms, back pain 1429–1430
Nerves
back pain 1411, *1411*
carpal tunnel syndrome 1450–1451
central nervous system disease in SLE 1333–1334
compression syndromes 1461–1462
surgery 1553–1554
ulnar nerve 1554
electrodiagnosis 1621–1626
entrapment
neuropathy 1450–1451
syndromes 1461–1462
intermittent claudication 1473
neuralgic amyotrophy 1446–1447
neurologic conditions, primary, mimicking rheumatic disorders 1448
neuropathy 1452
peripheral neuritis causing foot pain 1477–1478
roots 1438–1439
damage 1413
lumbar 1413
pain pathways 155
trunks
pain pathways 155
in systemic sclerosis
Neuralgic amyotrophy 1446–1447
Neuropathic joints 975, 1253–1254
Neuropathy, in diabetes 975–976
Nocardia 1155
Nodules 1126
in juvenile chronic arthritis 759
rheumatoid, in ankylosing spondylitis 759
subcutaneous 169–170, 674–676, *170*
surgical excision, from elbow 1549
tendon 169–170
Nomenclature **19 – 58**
preferred terms 20, *20*
seronegative polyarthritis 26–27
Non-articular rheumatism 13–14
chronic 13–14
indurated nodules 13–14
polymyalgia rheumatica 14
sciatica 13
Non-steroidal anti-inflammatory drugs (NSAIDs) **514 – 524,** *518*
action, mechanisms 514–515
benzotriazines
azapropazone 521–522
colchicine 522–523
oxicams 522
piroxicam 522
indoleacetic acids
indomethacin 516–517
sulindac 517
tolmetin 517
phenylacetic acids
diclofenac 517
fenclofenac 517–518
proprionic acids
fenbufen 520
fenoprofen 519–520
ibuprofen 518–519
ketoprofen 520
naproxen 519
tienilic acid 520–521
pyrazolones
phenylbutazone 521
selection 515
in SLE 1343
use 515
NSAIDs *see above*
Nuclear magnetic resonance, in back pain 1416
Nucleoprotein, increased turnover in gout 910
Nucleus pulposus, pressure variations 1410, *1410*

Occupation, relation to osteoarthrosis 855–856
Occupational cramp 1453
Occupational disorders, epidemiology 105–106
Ochronosis 950–952
Ocular disease, relationship with rheumatoid arthritis 638
Oestrogen replacement therapy in osteoporosis 1008
Olecranon bursitis 1450
Ollier's disease 1246, *1246*
Onycho-osteodysplasia 1464
O'Nyong-Nyong virus 1151–1152
Organ transplantation, complicated by osteonecrosis 1220
Orgotein, intra-articular injection 587
Os calcis 1212
painful 1475
Osgood-Schlatter disease 1211–1212
Osmic acid, in synoviorthesis 587–588
Osteitis deformans 1460
Osteitis fibrosa 1014
Osteitis pubis 986, 1457
Osteoarthritis
see Osteoarthrosis
Osteoarthropathy
hypertrophic 1251–1253, 1475, *1253*
radionuclide scanning 1637
Osteoarthrosis **821 – 880**
aetiology 821–841
alkaptonuria 853
apophyseal 1416–1418

Osteoarthrosis *cont*
  articular index 1591
  clinical aspects 846–872
  clinical categories 847
  diabetes 974–975
  diarthrodial joints 821–824
  differential diagnosis 870
  experimental models 853–854
  Gaucher's disease 853–854
  haemachromatosis 853, 950–958
  haematological disorders 1177–1185
  haemoglobinopathies 854, 1177–1196
  haemophilia 854, 1177–1185
  historical background 9–10, 846
  individual sites 861–868
  intra-articular injection
    corticosteroid 585
    silicone oil 587
  investigations 869–870
  Kashin-Beck disease 855
  management, medical 874–880
  mixed crystal deposition 859
  mucopolysaccharidoses 853
  neurological disorders 854
  occupation, relationship 855–856
  ochronosis 950–958
  pathology 821–824
  premature, result of hypermobility 1168
  prevalence 846–847
  primary 856–860
  secondary 851–856
  sex hormones 852–853
  signs 860–861
  sport 855
  storage diseases
    see Heritable Disorders and Miscellaneous (Chs 46 & 49)
  surgery 877–879
    hand 1560
  symptoms 860–861
  synonyms 821
  synovial joints 229–241
    classification *231*
  therapeutic evaluation 1593
  thyroid disease 852
  Wilson's disease 853, 950–958
Osteoblasts 205–206
Osteochondritis
  dissecans 1211, *1211*
  Scheuermann's 1427–1428
Osteochondromatosis 1241–1242
Osteochondrosis 1207
  see also Osteonecrosis
Osteoclastoma 1257
Osteoclast grafts 1000
Osteoclasts 205, 207
Osteocytes 205–207
Osteogenic sarcomata 1247
Osteogenesis imperfecta 1001–1003, 1002
Osteoid osteoma 1248–1250, 1460, *1250, 1460*
Osteolysis, differential diagnosis from osteonecrosis 1225
Osteoma, post-traumatic, para-articular 1466–1477
Osteomalacia 1008–1014
  axial 1019
  hip pain 1456
Osteonecrosis **1207 – 1228**
  alcoholism 1223
  allied conditions 1225–1226
  classification 1207, *1215*
  in corticosteroid therapy 524
  diagnostic procedures 1224
  dysbaric, incidence in
    acute decompression sickness 1222
    aviators 1222
    radiology *1223*
  environmental *1215*
  experimental models 1216–1217
  genetically determined 1218–1219
  hyperlipidaemia 1223
  hyperuricaemia 1223
  hypothyroidism 1223–1224
  idiopathic 1217, *1217*
  miscellaneous conditions 1220–1222, *1221*
  multiple epiphyseal dysplasias 1212–1213
  non-articular 1207–1213
  osteochondroses 1209–1213
    disorders of articular epiphysis 1209–1211
    disorders of physeal epiphysis 1212
    spinal 1212
  pancreatitis 1224
  pathology 1214–1216
  pregnancy 1223
  radiological progression *1223*
  terminology 1207
  trauma 1217–1218
  treatment 1224–1225
    corticosteroid 1219–1220
    organ transplantation 1220
    related 1219–1220
    radiotherapy 1220
Osteopetrosis 999–1000, 1173–1174
Osteophytes 622, 833–834, 836–837
  in ankylosing hyperostosis 859, *859*
  in cervical spondylosis 1437
  differentiation from syndesmophytes in osteoarthrosis of spine 754, 865–866, *754, 865*
Osteoporosis
  ankylosing spondylitis 755, *755*
  corticosteroid therapy 542
  differential diagnosis from osteonecrosis 1226
    diffuse childhood 1226
    regional migratory 1226
  epidemiology 110
  oestrogen replacement therapy 1008
  in surgery 1527
  in Wilson's disease 956
Osteosarcomata 1247
Osteotomy 1531
  hip 878
  knee 879, 1539
  indications for in ankylosing spondylitis 1547
Oestrogen replacement therapy, in osteoporosis 1008
Ott's disease 851
Overlap syndromes 1269–1277
Oxford grading of muscle function 1499, *1499*

Pachydermoperiostosis 1252–1253, *1253*
Paget's disease 1016–1018, 1460
  back pain 1430
  epidemiology 109–110
  juvenile 1001
  osteosarcoma 1247
Pain **143 – 160**
  abnormalities 158
  assessment of severity 156
  chemical algogens 157
  deep 148–153
  definition 143–144
  distribution 151, *150, 152*
  inhibitory controls 147, *145*
  localisation 147
  measurement 1588–1589
    of relief 1589
    scales
      graphic rating 1588–1589, *1589*
      visual analogue 1588–1589, *1588*
  mechanisms 156–158
  nerve roots 156
  nerve trunks 155
  pathways 144–147
  protective role 143
  psychogenic 158
  receptors 144–147
  referred 148, 150, 153–154
  skin 147
    reflex tenderness 154
  source 143
  temperature changes 157–158
  threshold 156
  transition, focal to segmental 152–153
  types 144
  visceral 154–155
Paleopathology 3, 4, 11
Palindromic rheumatism 167–168
Pan American League Against Rheumatism (PANLAR) 15
Pancreas, endocrine 972–980
  failure 980
Pancreatitis, osteonecrosis 1224
Panner's disease 1210, *1211*
Para-articular tumours 1241–1253
Paramyxoviruses 434–435
Parathormone 229
Parathyroid bone disease 1014–1016
Parvoviruses 437–438
Patella 1463–1465
  see also Knee
  chondromalacia patellae 1463
  dislocations 1464
  lesions 1463
  nail-patella syndrome 1464
  tendinitis 1464
Pellegrini-Stieda disease 1466–1477
Pelvis
  see also Hip and pelvis 1455–1456

Pelvis *cont*
intra-pelvic lesions 1459
Penicillamine 525–528, 532–533
Penicillin therapy
gonococcal arthritis 1140
meningococcal arthritis 1141
rat-bite fever 1149
rheumatic fever 1088
side-effects in Sjögren's syndrome 1400
yaws 1149
Periarthritis of shoulder, in diabetes 980
Pericapsular myalgia 1446
Pericarditis in rheumatic fever 1076
Peripheral arthritis and B27 322
Peripheral neuritis causing foot pain 1477–1478
Peripheral neuropathy, electrodiagnosis 1624
Peripheral vascular disease in systemic sclerosis 1365–1366
Peritendinitis 1474
Perths disease 1209–1210
Pes cavus 1476–1477
Petrullidium boydis 1155
Pharmacokinetics **489 – 499,** *493, 494*
in clinical trials 1584
Phenylbutazone 521
in management of acute gout 921
5-phosphoribosyl-1-pyrophosphate (PRPP)
increased activity in gout 909
in purine biosynthesis 902
Physical examination 1573–1580
Physical treatment
see Treatment, physical **1483 – 1496**
Pigmented villonodular synovitis 1242–1244
arthroscopic appearance 1606
intra-articular radiotherapy 590
Piroxicam 522
Pituitary-adrenal insufficiency, iatrogenic 982
Plant-thorn synovitis 166
Plantar fasciitis 1475
Plasma proteins, uric acid levels 917
Polarised light microscopy, crystal identification 268–271
Polyarteritis nodosa **1293 – 1304**
association with hairy cell leukaemia 1193
clinical features 1299–1304
corticosteroid therapy 539
cytotoxic drug therapy 552
diagnosis 1298–1299
epidemiology 88
overlap with granulomatous vasculitis 1293–1294
Polyarthritis, rehabilitation
adult, chronic 1516–1517
early, severe inflammatory 1515
surgery, assessment 1521
Polychondritis, relapsing 1255–1257
Polymyalgia rheumatica 324, **1278 – 1291**
aetiology 1280–1281
back pain 1429
clinical features 1283–1284
corticosteroid therapy 540
diagnosis 1286–1287
differential diagnosis *1287*
epidemiology 104–105, 1279–1280
and giant cell arteritis **1278 – 1291**
historical background 1278–1279
neck involvement 1440
overlap with MCTD 1272–1273
pain in hips and pelvis 1455–1456
pathogenesis 1280–1281
pathology 1281–1283
shoulder involvement 1440
treatment 1287–1288
Polymalgia rheumatica and giant cell arteritis **1278 – 1291**
abnormalities of liver and thyroid function 1286
laboratory findings 1286
relationship 1285–1286
Polymyositis **1350 – 1363**
acute, differential diagnosis 1351
aetiology 1351–1352
classification 1350–1351, *1350*
clinical manifestations 1352–1354
cytotoxic drug therapy 551–552
differential diagnosis 1350
epidemiology 87
incidence 1352
laboratory aspects 1351
management 1358–1361
Polyostotic fibrous dysplasia 999, *1000*
Popliteal cysts 1465–1466
Posture 1424, 1427
in ankylosing spondylitis 750, *750*
in back pain 1410, 1414, *1414*
in bed rest 1484, *1484*
pericapsular myalgia 1446
poor, cervical 1440
physical examination 1573
Pregnancy
Ehlers-Danlos syndrome 1166
osteonecrosis 1223
rheumatic complications 982–986
rheumatic fever 1083–1084
SLE 1335
Prepatellar bursitis 1465
Probenecid 575–577
Progressive systemic sclerosis
penicillamine therapy 526
Proteins, attachment 187–190
chondronectin 190
fibronectin 187–189
laminin 189–190
lubricating glycoprotein 190
Proteoglycans 190–195
Protocol, in clinical trials
instructions on writing 1582, *1582*
Protrusio acetabuli 851
Pseudocysts 618, *619*
Pseudofracture 1010, *1011*
Pseudogout
see pyrophosphate arthropathy 938–949
corticosteroid injection 585
diabetes 973
Pseudohypoparathyroidism 1016, *1016*
Pseudopodagra 165, *165*
Pseudo-pseudohyperparathyroidism 1016
Pseudotumour cerebri 537
Pseudo-xanthoma elasticum 1164
Psoriatic arthritis 322, **775 – 786**
aetiology 776–777
age of onset 778
amyloidosis 779
ancillary investigations 779–780
associations
rheumatoid arthritis 640
spondylitis 778
clinical features 777
cytotoxic drug therapy 551
definition 775, *775*
differential diagnosis 781–782
environmental factors 776–777
epidemiology 75
familial aggregation 776–779
genetic background 776
HLA aetiology 776
juvenile 778, 1130–1131
laboratory findings 779–780
nail changes 777–778, *778*
ocular inflammation 779
pathology 777
prevalence 775–776
prognosis 779
radiology 780–781
sex ratio 776
spondylitic heart disease 779
treatment 782–783
Pubic rami, lesions 1458–1459
Public symphysis, stress lesions 1458
Pulmonary involvement in systemic sclerosis 1373–1374
Pulmonary hypertension in SLE 1329
Pulse steroid therapy in SLE 1344
Purines
biosynthesis 902, *903*
derivation 902
high-purine diet 910
influence of endogenous chemicals 905–911
Purpura
hypergammaglobulinaemic 1199
in immune complex disease 1198
Pustulotic arthro-osteitis 1239–1240
Pyoderma gangrenosum 1240–1241
Pyrophosphate arthropathy **938 – 949**
amyloidosis 944
apatite arthritis 945–946
associations with metabolic disease 943–944
in haemochromatosis 954
hereditary 938
hypomagnesaemia 944
hypophosphatasia 944
hypothyroidism 944
intra-articular therapy 590
Milwaukee shoulder 946, *946*
pathogenesis 944–945
radiology 940–941
sporadic 938–943

Radial neuropathy 1452

Radioisotopic imaging, osteonecrosis 1224
Radiological features 752–757
 sacroiliitis 752–753, *752*
 spinal changes 753–757
Radionuclide imaging 1632–1639
 aseptic necrosis 1636–1637
 back pain 1637
 bone infarction 1636–1637
 crush fractures 1637
 fibrosing diseases of lungs 1638–1639
 joint replacement 1639
 hypertrophic osteoarthropathy 1637
 radiopharmaceuticals 1632
 reflex dystrophy syndrome 1637–1638
 role in arthritis complications 1636
 sacroiliac joint quantification 1635–1636
 salivary scintigraphy 1638
 use of isotopes 1632
 use in joint disease 1533–1635
Radiopharmaceuticals 1632–1633
Radiotherapy, in osteoarthrosis 876
Raynaud's phenomenon 1153–1154
 in acromegaly 963
 atrial myxoma 1259
 childhood 1131
 MCTD 1272
 SJögren's syndrome
 systemic sclerosis 1365–1366
Reactive arthritis 164, 166, 169–170, 173, 322, 428–429, 728
 see also Sexually Acquired Reactive Arthritis
 campylobacter jejuni 1146
 in childhood 1130
 epidemiology 72, 80
 gut infection 815–816
 yersinia enterocolitica 1146
Referred pain 148, 150, 153–154
Reflex dystrophy syndrome, radionuclide scanning 1637–1638
Rehabilitation **1497 – 1517**
 addresses 1517
 adult chronic polyarthritis, management 1517
 aids and adaptations 1503–1514
 assessment of patient 1498–1502
 classification of handicap *1498*
 health visitor 1514
 key situations 1515–1517
 nursing 1514
 occupational therapy 1503
 patient education 1514–1515
 physiotherapy 1502
 resources 1503
 social work 1514–1515
 spa treatment 1497
 WHO definition 1497–1498
Reiter's disease **787 – 805**
 aetiology 790–791
 age of onset 788, *788*
 arthritis 792–794
 bacillary dysentery 1146
 balanitis 791–792
 blood tests 798
 clinical features 791
 complications
  frequency *791*
  neurological 796
 differential diagnosis 799
 epidemiology 74–75, 788–789
 family studies 789–790, *789*
 gut infection 815–816
 heart involvement 796
 historical background 787
 HLA-B27 791
 incidence 788
 incomplete forms 1130
 integumentary lesions 794–795
 joint involvement 792–793, *792, 793*
 management 799–801
 ocular lesions 794
 oral lesions 795–796
 other lesions 790
 pathology 798
 prevalence 787–788
 pulmonary involvement 796
 radiological features 796–798
 recurrence 794
 residual disability 793–794, *793*
 salmonella 1146
 sex ratio 788
 spinal involvement 794
 synovial fluid 798
 triad 787
 urogenital lesions 791–792
 venereal transmission 788
Relapsing polychondritis 1255–1257
Renal disease
 overlap in MCTD 1273
 in Sjögren's syndrome 1394
Respiratory disease 630–633
Rest
 see physical treatment of rheumatic diseases 1483–1496
Resticuloendothelial system in SLE 1330
Reticulohistocytosis, multicentric 1196–1197
Reticulum cell sarcoma 1247
Retrocalcaneal bursitis 1474
Retroviruses 440–442
Rheumatic complications in pregnancy 894–986
Rheumatic diseases
 see also Rheumatological practice
 arrangements for care 52–53
 attitudes 54
 burden on society 49
 classification 24–30, *28*
 community burden 45
 consequences of rheumatic disorders 41–44, *42*
 control of rheumatic disorders 50–52
 International Classification of Diseases 37–30
 knowledge 53–54
 mortality 44
 nomenclature 2–24, *20, 22, 23, 24*
 physical treatment **1483 – 1496**
 rheumatic disorders in hospital 45–46, *46*
 outside hospital 47–49
 rheumatic suffering 39–50
 skills 54
 WHO International Classification of Impairments, Disabilities and Handicaps 41
Rheumatic fever **1057 – 1099**
 acute attack, management 1086
 aetiology 1063–1065
 after-care 1089
 age incidence 1063
 arthritis 1070–1073
 chorea 1087–1081, *1080*
 see chorea for detail
 clinical aspects 1069
 complications 1082–1083
 course 1083
 criteria 1057
 definition 1057
 differential diagnosis
  Duckett-Jones criteria *1084*
  Hallidie-Smith and Bywaters criteria *1085*
  from rheumatoid arthritis 1086
 environmental factors 1064–1065
 epidemiology 108–109, 1066
 erythrocyte sedimentation rate 1081
 genetic factors 1065
 geographical factors 1063–1064
 heart involvement 1075–1076, 1079, 1089
  clinical aspects 1075–1076
  failure 1076
  pericarditis 1076
  rhythm change 1076
  subacute bacterial endocarditis 1082
 historical background 4–6
 hospital admission 1057
 infection 1059–1063
  and streptococci 1059–1063, *1065*
 laboratory aids 1081–1082
 lung changes 1077
 mortality 1064
 nodules 1068, 1074, *1068, 1075*
 pathology 1066
 pneumonia 1069, *1069*
 pregnancy 1083–1084
 prevalence 1057–1059
 prognosis 1083
 prophylaxis 1089–1091
  vaccination 1091
 pulse 1069–1070
 renal involvement 1078
 respiration 1069–1070
 rheumatic pneumonia 1077
  treatment 1078
 seasonal factors 1063–1064, *1058*
 serositis 1078
 sex incidence 1063
 skin manifestations 1073–1074
 streptococci 424–425, 1059–1063, *1065*
 symptomatology 1069
 temperature 1069–1070
 therapy 1086–1091
  ACTH 1088
  penicillin 1088

Rheumatic fever *cont*
salicylates 1087–1088
steroid 1088
Rheumatic heart disease 1057–1058, 1063
mortality 1064
prevalence 1057–1058, *1058*
Rheumatoid arthritis **515 – 719**
aetiology 597–599
aetiopathogenesis 595–602
amyloidosis 691–692
anaemia 685–688, 713–714
ankle 671
articular features 655–674
articular manifestations 653–705
back pain 1429
bacterial infection 425–427
Baker's cysts 669, *669*
bones 691–692
cardiac involvement 682–683
cardiovascular system 712–713
carpal tunnel syndrome 1451
cervical spine 657–660
disease, surgery 1545–1546
clinicopathological spectrum 595–597
corticosteroid therapy 539
course 655
cytotoxic drug therapy 549–550
death statistics 643–644, *643, 644*
definition 595–597
diagnostic criteria 595
differential diagnosis 692–693
drugs 710–712
ear 674
elbow 660
environmental factors 597–598
epidemiology 63–67
explanation 706–707
extra-articular complications 712–714
Felty's syndrome 11, 640–641, 689, *640*
foot 671–673
gastrointestinal tract 678–679
genetic factors 589–599
hand 661–668
historical background, 10–12, 653–654
history-taking 706
hyperviscosity syndrome 689
infection 714
intra-articular corticosteroid 584–585
intra-articular gold 587
juvenile chornic arthritis 638
knee 699–671
lungs 713
lymph nodes 690
management 706–719
medication 709–712
neuropathy 713
ocular complications 713
ocular manifestations 683–684
onset 654
pathology 604–652, *604*
anatomical consequences 618–620
articular diseases 605
associated syndromes 638, 640–642
bone disease 621–622
cartilage destruction 615–618
cell proliferation 611–612
coincidental disease 624–638
consequences of treatment 642–643
medical 642
surgical 642–643
diagnostic biopsy 622–624
fibrosis and repair 614–615, *615*
immunopathology 612, *612, 613*
juxta-articular connective tissues 620–621
synovial disease 605
patients' problems 707–709
penicillamine 527–528
peripheral neuropathy 678
prodromal symptoms 654–655
prognosis 655
psoriatic arthropathy 640
pulmonary involvement 680–682
retroviruses 440–442
septic complications 692
shoulder 660
Sjögren's syndrome 684–685, *685*
skin lesions 690
subcutaneous nodules 674–676
surgery 714–715
systemic manifestations 674–691
vasculitis 676–678, 1309–1314
wrist 661–668
Rheumatoid factor 355–362, *359*
in SLE 1339
Rheumatoid synovitis, arthroscopic appearance 1606
Rheumatoid vasculitis 676–678
clinical features 1310–1313, *1311*
diagnosis 1309–1310
laboratory tests 1313, *1313*
prognosis 1313
treatment 1314
Rheumatological practice **19 – 58**
see also Rheumatic diseases
Rice bodies 261, 1200
Rickets 1008–1014, *1009, 1013*
Rider's bone 1458
Rigid spine syndrome 765
Ritchie index (articular) *1571, 1591*
Rocky Mountain spotted fever 1150
Romanus lesion 755, *755*
Rose-Waaler test 356
Ross River virus 1151–1152
Rubella arthritis 1150–1151

Sacroiliac joint, radionuclide imaging, quantification 1653–1636
Sacroiliac strain 1424
Sacroiliitis
ankylosing spondylitis, radiology 752, *752, 753*
computerised tomography 1627
elicitation of pain 749
pain 1456–1457
Salicylates **500 – 513**
acute gout, management 921
aspirin 508–509, 587, 1343
benorylate 509
chemistry 500
choline magnesium trisalicylate 510
diflunisal 509
historical background 6, 500
pharmacological properties 500–502
in rheumatic fever 1087–1088
salsalate 509
side-effects 503–509
blood, coagulation 506
cardiovascular 505
central nervous system 505
dyspepsia 504
endocrine 505
gastrointestinal bleeding 504
gastrointestinal toxicity 503–504
hypersensitivity 507
kidney 504
liver 505
pregnancy 506
protective 507
pulmonary 506
salicylate intoxication 506–507
therapeutic properties 502–503
therapeutic use in rheumatic diseases 507–508
Salivary glands
in Sjögren's syndrome, investigations 1390–1392
in systemic sclerosis 1364
Salivary scintigraphy 1638
Salmonella
arthritis 1145–1146
infection predominantly causing osteomyelitis in sickle cell disease 1190
Salsalate 509
SARA
see Sexually Acquired Reactive Arthritis
Sarcoidosis 1230–1231
childhood 1132
diagnosis 1230
incidence 1230
joint disease, patterns 1230
in negroes 1230
prognosis 1230
radiology 1230
remission 1230
salivary scintigraphy 1638
sarcoid myopathy 1231
sex ratio 1230
Sarcoma
chondrosarcoma 1247
fibrosarcoma 1247
melanotic 1246
osteosarcoma 1247, *1248*
reticulum-cell 1247
synovial 1244–1246
Scheuermann's disease 1212
Scheuermann's osteochondritis 1427–1428
Schirmer's test 1389
Schmorl's nodes, 1212, 1412, *1413*
Sciatica 1413
Sciatic nerve compression 1461
Sciatic scoliosis 1414, *1414*
Sclerodactyly 1367
Scleroderma
see systemic sclerosis **1364 – 1385**

Scleroderma *cont*
–like features in MCTD 1273
Sclerosis, systemic **1364 – 1385**
Scoliosis, sciatic 1414, *1414*
Septic arthritis, epidemiology 80–81
Seronegative spondarthritides **723 – 744**
see also Ankylosing spondylitis, Enteropathic arthritis, Psoriatic arthritis, Reiter's disease
acute anterior uveitis 727–728
aetiopathogenesis 735–736
associations 736–737
clinical overlap 724–727, *724*
criteria 723–733, *725*
DISH 733–735
disorders showing spondarthritis-like features 733–735
erosive osteoarthritis 735
erosive spondyloarthropathy 734
familial aggregation 728–730
HLA–B27 730–733
intestinal bypass arthritis, dermatitis syndrome 734
irradiation 767
pustulotic arthro-osteitis 733–734
reactive arthritis 728
undifferentiated seronegative peripheral arthritis 733
Seronegative spondylopathies, back pain 1429
Seropositive (Igm rheumatoid factor) juvenile arthritis 1125–1127
Serositis 1078
Serum antistreptolysin O titre in rheumatic fever 1082
Serum complement levels in SLE 1339
Serum urate, indications for lowering in acute gout 922
Serum uric acid
alcohol, effect of 915
in gout 894–895
values 899
hypouricaemia 917–918, *917*
Sever's disease 1212
Sex hormones and osteoarthrosis 852–853
Sexually acquired reactive arthritis (SARA) 320, 423–424, 815–816
see also reactive arthritis
bacterial infection 427–428
Sharpey's fibres 227
Shober's method (lumbar spine flexion check) 1575, *1576*
Shoulder
acromioclavicular joint 1443–1444, 1614
acute calcific bursitis 1442–1443, *1443*
arthrography 1607–1608
arthropathies 1445–1446
aseptic necrosis 1445–1446
chronic bursitis 1442
examination 1442, 1576–1577
extra-capsular lesions 1442
fibrositis 1446
frozen 1444
history-taking 1442
housewife's 1446
inflammatory arthritis 1444
intra-capsular lesion 1444
mechanisms 1442–1442
Milwaukee shoulder 1446
muscle wasting 1442
and neck 1441–1447
see Neck and shoulder **1435 – 1477** for detail
neuralgic amyotraphy, mosaic form 1446–1447
osteoarthrosis 863–864
periarthritis in diabetes 980
pericapsular myalgia 1446
posture 1446
sepsis 1445–1446
shoulder-hand syndrome 1444–1445
subacromial bursa 1442–1443
surgery 1547–1549
syringomelia *1445*
tendinitis 1443
tendinitis, injection techniques
bicipital 1613–1614
supraspinatus 1613, *1613*
terminology 1442
trauma 1444
Shoulder-hand syndrome 1444–1445
Dupuytren's diathesis 1444
predisposition 1444
treatment 1444–1445
'Shrinking' lungs 1330, *1330*
Sicca syndrome 323
Sickle-cell disease 1186–1190
avascular necrosis 1188–1189
diagnosis 1190
gout 1190
hand-foot syndrome 1190
hyperuricaemia 1190
osteomyelitis predominantly caused by *Salmonella* infection 1190
racial factor 1186
radiology *1187, 1189*
synovial effusions 1190
Sindig-Larsen syndrome 1212
Sindig-Larsen-Johansson disease 1464
Sjögren's syndrome 684–685, **1386 – 1403,** *685*
aetiology 1400–1401
arthritis 1392–1393
associated conditions 1387
miscellaneous 1395–1396
other causes of sicca syndrome 1395–1396
rheumatoid arthritis 641–642
symptoms 1388
autoimmune exocrinopathy 1390–1391
clinical manifestations 1394
cutaneous manifestations 1394
definition 1386
differential diagnosis 1386
drug reactions 1400
epidemiology 88
exocrine function, impaired 1388
gastrointestinal disease 1393
genetics 1398
haematological disturbances 1395
historical background 1387
immunopathology 1396–1398
keratoconjunctivitis sicca, diagnosis 1389–1390
liver involvement 1393
lymphoproliferation 1398–1399
malignancy 1398–1399
neurological involvement 1394–1395
pathological manifestations 1387
primary 1386
pulmonary involvement 1395
Raynaud's phenomenon 1393
relationship between autoimmune diseases and sicca features *1386*
Schirmer's test 1389
secondary 1386
SLE 1331
systemic features 1392–1395
treatment 1399–1400
drugs, side effects 1400
general management 1399
problems of reduced secretions 1399–1400
systemic 1400
xeropthalmia 1387
xerostomia 1388
Skin
atrophy in corticosteroid therapy 542
changes in systemic sclerosis 1367–1371
in SLE 1327–1328
Small vessel vasculitis 1314–1316
Smallpox arthritis 1152
Snapping hip 1456
Soft tissue lesions
computerised tomography 1631
non-articular corticosteroid injection 585–586
Solganol 530
South-East Asia and Pacific Area League against Rheumatism (SEAPAL) 15
Spa treatment 10, 14, 1497
Spinal cord 1438–1439
Spinal stenosis 1418–1420
causes 1629, *1419*
computerised tomography 1629
criteria 1629–1630
diagnosis 1420
epidemiology 98–99
management 1420
Spine
cervical intubation 1524
computerised tomography 1628–1630
examination 1575–1576
function 1408–1411
osteoarthrosis 864–866
radionuclide scanning 1637
referred pain 1457, 1459
spinal cord 1438–1439
structure 1408–1411
surgery 1545–1547
in osteoarthrosis 897
Spondarthritides
historical background 12–13
seronegative **723 – 744**
Spondylitis
brucellar 1142
exercise 1495

Spondylitis *cont*
juvenile 1127–1129
physical treatment 1495
Spondyloarthropathies **723 – 744**
see also seronegative spondarthritides
in children 1127–1132, *1127*
Spondylodisciitis 755–756, *755*
Spondylolisthesis 1420–1422
spondylotic 1422
Spondylosis 1420–1422
Spondylosis
back pain **1407 – 1434**
cervical 1437–1438
disc disorders 1407–1434
epidemiology 95–99
lumbar 1416–1418
Spondylotic spondyolisthesis 1422
Sporotrichosis 1155
Sprengel's shoulder 1439
Starvation, predisposing factor in gout 912, *913*
Statistics 1594
Stenosis, spinal 1418–1420
causes 1629, *1419*
computerised tomography, criteria 1629–1630
diagnosis 1420
management 1420
Sternoclavicular joint, osteoarthrosis 864
Steroids in rheumatic fever 1088
Stevens-Johnson syndrome 726, 1142, *726*
Still's disease
see Juvenile chronic arthritis **1100 – 1124**
Stiff man syndrome 765
Stiffness, measurement 1590
'Stuck' back 1424
Student's elbow 1450
Sudek's atrophy 1478
Sulindac 517
Sulphinpyrazone 577–578
Superior tibiofibular joint synovitis 1466
Suppurative arthritis, acute 1137–1139
Sural nerve compression 1462
Surgery **1518 – 1565**
aims 1519
ankle 1534–1535
arthrodesis 1531, 1559
arthroplasty 1530–1531
arthroscopy 1535–1536
drug therapy 1524–1525
elbow 1549–1550
feet 1531–1534
fingers 1554–1559
deformities 1559–1560, *1559*
general considerations 1522
health, local disease
hand 1554–1559
in osteoarthrosis 1560
influencing factors 1523
intestinal bypass surgery arthritis 814–815, 1241
dermatitis syndrome 734
intubation 1524
knee 1535–1536, 1539–1540, *1540*
hip, total replacement 1540–1545
complications 1542–1545
nerve compression syndromes 1553–1554
osteotomy 1531
patient assessment 1519–1522
patient handling 1524
shoulder 1547–1549
spine 1545–1547
synovectomy 1529–1530
technical considerations 1526–1528
thromboembolism 1525–1526, *1526*
wrist 1550–1553, 1554–1559
wound healing 1522–1524
Swelling, measurement, Geigy gauge 1590
Sydenham Thomas 5, 7, 8
Syndesmophyte(s)
in ankylosing spondylitis 754, 757–758, *758, 759*
differentiation from osteophyte(s) 754, *754*
psoriasis 781
Syndrome de la loge de Guyon 1554
Synovectomy 1529–1530, 1536
hand and wrist 1556–1557
elbow joint 1549–1550
wrists and tendon sheaths 1550–1553
Synovial biopsy
arthroscopic methods 1597, 1608–1609
interpretation 1609
histopathology of synovitis 1609–1610
Synovial cells 207–209, 258, 264
Synovial chondromatosis 1241–1242
Synovial chondrosarcoma 1246
Synovial effusions in sickle cell disease 1190
Synovial fluid **251 – 277**, 824
analysis 259–273
arthrocentesis 259
cell counts
differential 266
total 261–263, *261*
composition 251–257
examination 251–277
formation 257–258
gross appearances 260–263, *260*
hydroxyapatite crystals, detection 271–272
immunology 272–273
intra-articular pressure 258
joint aspiration 259
micro-organisms 272
microscopy 263–266
mucin clot test 261
in osteoarthrosis 869–870
pathology 838–839
in Reiter's disease 798
removal 257–258
rice bodies 261
samples 259–260
volume 260
Synovial joints 229–232
classification 229–231, *231*
cervical spine 1437–1438
movement 231–232
structure 229–231
Synovial membrane 334–340, *339*
Synovial rupture 1469–1471
co-existing thrombosis 1471
investigation 1469
management 1470
Synovial sarcoma 1244–1246
Synovial shelf-syndrome 1463
Synovial tissue 232
in gout, examination 895–896
Synovioma 1244–1246
Synovitis
crystal, arthroscopic appearance 1607
histopathology 1610–1611
inflammatory, arthroscopic appearance 1605–1606
methods of quantitation 1634
pigmented villondular 1242–1244
arthroscopic appearance 1606
radionuclide imaging 1633–1634
relationship with osteoarthrosis 840–841
rheumatoid, arthroscopic appearance 1606
superior tibiofibular joint 1466
traumatic 1239
Synovium 824
cartilage-catabolin, effects on 233–235
osteoarthrosis, pathology 839–840
synovial chondromatosis 1241–1242
Syphilis
acquired 1147–1148
congenital 1146–1147
Syringomelia 1445, *1445*
Systemic lupus erythematosus (SLE) 323–324, **1325 – 1349**
aetiology 1330–1341
age of onset 1131
animal models 1341
ANA-negative lupus 1335
blood
abnormalities 1334
vessels 1329–1330
cardiovascular system 1328–1329
central nervous system
disease 1333–1334
involvement 1131
in childhood 1131
clinical features 1131, 1325–1334
clinical manifestations 1326, *1326, 1327*
congenital heart block 1329
corticosteroid therapy 540
cytotoxic drug therapy 550–551
differential diagnosis 1341–1342
additional features *1342*
ARA criteria *1342*
drug-induced lupus 1335–1336, *1336*
epidemiology 85
effect of UV light 1341
epidemiology 82–86, 1325–1326
gastrointestinal system 1331
genetic factors 1340
historical background 1325
hormonal factors 1340–1341
hypercatabolism, tissue fixation and 402–403
immunological features 1336–1340
infection 1334

Systemic lupus erythematosus (SLE) *cont*
levamisole therapy 562
–like features in MCTD 1273
management 1343–1345
anti-malarials 1343
aspirin 1343
corticosteroids 1343–1344
general 1342
immunosuppressive agents 1344
NSAIDs 1343
plasmapheresis 1345
pulse steroid therapy 1344
sex hormone therapy 1345
musculoskeletal system 1328
ocular lesions 1334
organ-specific antibodies 1340
osteonecrosis 1220–1222
radiological changes 1222, *1221*
overlap with MCTD 1336
pathology 1326
pregnancy 1335
prevalence 1325
prognosis 1131, 1345, *1344*
pulmonary hypertension 1329
pulmonary involvement, pleurisy 1330
racial incidence 1326
renal involvement 1331–1333, *1332*
reticuloendothelial system 1330–1331
retroviruses 440–442
sex ratio 1325
'shrinking' lungs 1330, *1330*
thrombophlebitis 1329–1330
tissue fixation and hypercatabolism 402–403
variants 1335–1336
abortion 1335
discoid lupus 1335
neurological disease 1335
thrombosis 1335
vasculitis 1329–1330
viral agents 1341
Systemic sclerosis 324, **1364 – 1385**
age incidence 1364
cardiac involvement 1374
changes
connective tissue 1376
immunological 1377–1379
inflammatory 1377–1379
microcirculatory 1376–1377
classification 1364–1365, *1364*
clinical features 1365–1376
CREST syndrome 1375
diagnostic criteria 1364, *1364*
disease sub-types 1375–1376
electromyographic abnormalities 1371
environmental factors 1365
eosinophilic fasciitis 1375–1376
epidemiology 86–87, 1364–1365
frequency of organ involvement *1365*
gastrointestinal involvement 1372–1373
pathology 1372
genetic factors 1365
incidence 1364
joints 1371
kidney involvement 1364
mixed connective tissue disease 1375
muscle involvement 1371
neurological involvement 1371
occupational factors 1364–1365
overlap syndromes 1375–1376
pathogenesis 1376–1379
pathology 1365–1376
peripheral vascular disease 1365–1366
presenting features 1365
prognosis 1379
pulmonary involvement 1373–1374
fibrosing alveolitis 1374
hyperplastic changes 1374
race factor 1364
Raynaud's phenomenon 1365
salivary glands 1373
sex ratio 1364
skin changes 1367–1371
acrosclerosis 1367
proximal scleroderma 1368
sclerodactyly 1367
typical findings 1368–1371
specific organ involvement, management 1380–1381
tendons 1371
treatment 1379–1381
anti-fibrotic drugs 1380
anti-inflammatory therapy 1380
general 1379
immunosuppressive therapy 1380
improvement of peripheral microcirculation 1379–1380
symptomatic 1379

Takayasu's arteritis 1316–1317
Tarsal tunnel syndrome 1462
T-cells 273
ankylosing spondylitis 760
effect of immunomodulators *558*
immune deficiency 1199
immunogenetics 310–313
leukaemia 1193
in rheumatoid synovial membrane 600–601
suppressor function in SLE 1336
in synovial disease 607, 613–614
Temporal arteritis **1278 – 1291**, 1316, 1440–1441
Temporomandibular arthritis 622, 864
Tendinitis 1443
Achilles 1619
bicipital 1448–1449
knee 1467
patellar 1464
surgery 1549
Tendons 220
repairs 1553
rupture *1553*
in systemic sclerosis 1371
Tennis elbow 1449–1450
injection technique 1614–1615, *1615*
Tenosynovitis, ankle 1474
injection technique 1616, *1616*
Tenovaginitis
of abductor pollicis longus 1452
stenosing 1453
Thalassaemia 1186, 1191
haemosiderosis 1191
pathogenesis of synovitis 1191
race factor 1186
radiology 1191
radiotherapy 1191
treatment 1191
Therapeutic evaluation **1581 – 1596**
see Clinical Trials for detail
Thiemann's disease 851, 1213, *851, 852, 1213*
Thiopurinol 574
Thoracic outlet syndrome 1438–1439
Thoracic pain 1427
Thrombocytosis 1185
correlation with complications and severity of rheumatoid disease *1186*
Thromboembolism, in surgery 1525–1526, *1526*
Thrombosis (deep vein) and synovial rupture 1471
Thymopoietin 559, 561–562
Thyroid 967–968
acropachy 971, 1263, 1475
and osteoarthrosis 852
Tiaprofenic acid 520–521
Tibia, stress fractures 1472–1473
Tienilic acid, in management of gout 925
Tolmetin 517
Tophi 886–887
in gout, examination 895–896, *866*
Torticollis 1436–1438, 1440–1441
Torulosis 1154
Touraine-Solente-Gole syndrome 1252–1253, *1253*
Trapezium excision in osteoarthrosis 878
Trauma
computerised tomography 1630–1631
inflammation 294
traumatic synovitis 1239
Treatment, physical
see Rheumatic diseases, physical treatment **1483 – 1496**
Treatment, surgical
see Surgery **1518 – 1565**
Trigger finger 1453
Trochanteric bursitis 1456
Tuberculosis
arthritis 1142–1143
diagnosis 1143
incidence 1142
management 1143–1144
pattern 1142
sites 1142–1143
Tumours
arising from bone/cartilage 1246–1250
articular 1241–1253
arthropathies associated with non-articular neoplastic disease 1250–1251
back pain 1429–1430
benign 1244
malignant 1244–1250

Ulcerative colitis
aetiology 810–813
association with ankylosing spondylitis 762, 810–812
clinical features 810–812, *811*
enteropathic arthritis 810–813
finger clubbing 813
HLA-B27 813
investigations 810–812
joints involved *811*
musculoskeletal disorders 813
spondylitis 812
treatment 811–812
Ulnar neuropathy 1451
Undifferentiated connective tissue disease (UCTD) 1276
Urate(s)
acute gout 887–890
chronic gout 891
crystals in gout 891, *891*
deposition, sites 891, *891*
identification 895, *895, 896*
histological demonstration 890
increased clearance causing hypouricaemia 917–918
monosodium urate monohydrate, crystalline 890
Uric acid
see also Hyperuricaemia
asymptomatic hyperuricaemia 925–926
calculi 892
formation 892
cardiovascular disease 916–917
decreased excretion
alterations in fluid volume, renal function 911
effects of drugs 911–912
effects of starvation and ketosis 912, *913*
essential hypertension 913
hypercalcaemia 914
hyperparathyroidism 914
lactic acidaemia 912
lead poisoning 913
myxoedema 914
saturnine gout 913
excretion 905–906
gout
see also Gout
serum levels 894–895, 899
conversion scale 899n, *899*
haemoglobin plasma protein 917
hyperuricaemia
age variations 901
from increased formation 906–909
genetic factors 901, 908
non-gouty conditions 899
sex ratio 900–901
increased formation 906–911
lithiasis 892
metabolism 901
formation 901
structural formulae *902*
molecular components 901
origins *902*
Uricosuric drugs in long-term management of gout 925
Uveitis 322

van Breemen, Jan 15, *15*
van der Hoeve's triad 1003
Vascular disease, peripheral in systemic sclerosis 1365–1366
Vasculitis **1292 – 1324**
associated with other connective tissue diseases 1314
classification 1292–1294, *1292, 1293*
clinical syndromes
lymphoid granulomatosis 1308
overlap syndrome with other necrotising arteritides 1308–1309
polyarteritis nodosa
classical 1297–1304
localised 1302
systemic necrotising arteritis 1297–1309
corticosteroid therapy 539
definition 1292
granulomatous 1293–1294, 1304–1306
allergic angiitis 1304–1306
clinical features *1305*
diagnosis 1304–1305
differential diagnosis from polyarteritis nodosa 1304
laboratory features 1305
overlap with polyarteritis nodosa 1293–1294
prognosis 1305
relationship to arteritis 1293
treatment 1305–1306
large vessel arteritis 1316–1317
Takayasu's 1316–1317
temporal 1316
pathogenetic mechanisms 1294–1297
rheumatoid 1309–1314, *1309*
in SLE 1329–1330
small vessel arteritis 1316
viral infection 1296
Vertebrae
cervical,
developmental abnormalities 1439–1440
disease 1440
fracture, spinal pain 1422–1423
intervertebral discs 1438
Vertebral ankylosing hyperostosis, diabetes 973–974
Viral infection in vasculitis 1296
Virus(es) 1152–1153
infection 1150–1153
Visual disturbances in giant cell arteritis 1284–1285
Vitamin D 229
in bone metabolism 995–997, *996*
von Gierke's disease 910
von Recklinghausen's disease 999
von Willebrand's disease 1177–1178, *1177*

Waldenström's macroglobulinaemia 1195
diagnosis 1195
management 1195
Wegener's granulomatosis 539–540, 1306–1308
clinical features 1306–1308
diagnosis 1306
laboratory tests 1308
prognosis 1308
treatment 1308
Whip-lash injury 1440
Whipple's disease 729–730
aetiology 814
association with ankylosing spondylitis 762, 814
clinical features 813–814
enteropathic arthritis 813
HLA-B27 814
investigations 813–814
treatment 814
White cell count in rheumatic fever 1081
WHO International Classification of Impairments, Disabilities and Handicaps 41
Wilson's disease 956
and osteoarthrosis 853
Wrist
arthrography 1607–1608
De Quervain's syndrome 1452
examination 1577
injection techniques 1615–1616, *1616, 1617*
median nerve compression 1450
osteoarthrosis 863
surgery 1550–1560
success rating *1556*
tenovaginitis of abductor pollicis longus 1452
writer's cramp 1453

Xanthine oxidase
inhibitors 905, 915, 922–924, *924*
principal action in man 905
Xanthomata in hyperlipoproteinaemia 1237–1238
Xeropthalmia 1387
Xerostomia 1388
X-rays in differential diagnosis 172–173

Yaws 1148–1149
Yersinia enterocolitica arthritis 322, 428–429, 1146
Yttrium (^{90}Y), intra-articular irradiation 588–589

Copeman's
Textbook of the Rheumatic Diseases

To all patients with rheumatic diseases, who hopefully await the progress of medical research, together with the generation of young clinicians and scientists throughout the world whose efforts are bent to their relief, this book is respectfully dedicated.

Copeman's Textbook of the Rheumatic Diseases

EDITED BY

J. T. Scott MD FRCP
Consultant Physician, Charing Cross Hospital, London; Honorary Physician, Kennedy Institute of Rheumatology, London

SIXTH EDITION

VOLUME TWO

CHURCHILL LIVINGSTONE
EDINBURGH LONDON MELBOURNE AND NEW YORK 1986

CHURCHILL LIVINGSTONE
Medical Division of Longman Group UK Limited

Distributed in the United States of America by Churchill Livingstone Inc., 1560 Broadway, New York, N.Y. 10036, and by associated companies, branches and representatives throughout the world.

First Edition 1948
Second Edition 1955
Third Edition 1964
Fourth Edition 1969
Reprinted 1970
Fifth Edition 1978
Sixth Edition 1986

ISBN 0 443 02689 0 (2 vols)

British Library Cataloguing in Publication Data
Copeman, William Sydney Charles
Copeman's textbook of the rheumatic diseases. — 6th ed.
1. Rheumatism
I. Title II. Scott, J. T.
616.7'23 RC927

Library of Congress Cataloging in Publication Data
Copeman, W. S. C. (William Sydney Charles), 1900–
Copeman's Textbook of the rheumatic diseases.
Includes bibliographies and index.
I. Rheumatism. I. Scott, J. T. (James Thomas)
II. Title. III. Title: Textbook of the rheumatic diseases. [DNLM: 1. Arthritis. 2. Collagen Diseases. 3. Rheumatism. WE 140 C782te]
RC927.C65 1986 616.7'23 85-19449

Printed and bound in Hong Kong
by Mandarin Offset Marketing (HK) Ltd.

Preface to the Sixth Edition

The continuing growth of rheumatology as a scientific clinical discipline within the framework of general internal medicine has now led to its recognition as such by clinicians in other fields, and to an increasing number of rheumatological textbooks and journals. We are now living in an age when basic science — especially molecular biology — is elucidating the mechanisms of health and disease to an extent undreamt of a decade or two ago. It has been generally felt that 'Copeman' — the authoritative British reference work on the rheumatic diseases — should keep pace with such progress in the form of yet a further edition.

Readers of previous editions will see that many of the sections and chapters — some of them classical contributions to rheumatological literature — have been updated but are essentially unchanged. There has again, however, been renewal and expansion: 46 chapters in the Fifth Edition, 69 in the Sixth Edition.

Two entirely new sections have been incorporated. Rapid developments in drug treatment have justified a section on clinical pharmacology as related to the rheumatic diseases; and a section on topographical rheumatology (regional disorders) allows a discussion of localised problems more conveniently than in previous editions.

Apart from the chapters in these sections, other new chapters have been written on a diversity of topics which seem to require more individual consideration than given previously: differential diagnosis of arthritis, biochemistry of connective tissue, examination of synovial fluid, immunogenetics in relation to the rheumatic diseases, metabolic bone disease, arthritis and blood disease, osteonecrosis, overlap syndromes, Sjögren's syndrome and imaging techniques.

A chapter on this last rapidly developing field is certainly justified; but I have continued to withhold a chapter on conventional radiology, since radiographic examples are amply provided in the various clinical chapters.

These changes have meant corresponding changes in the team of contributors, rather too numerous to mention individually. Two or three have retired to the touchline, some have changed their positions in the field, and there has been an influx of new young players of great potential.

Much as I hope and believe that this further edition will maintain and even enhance the reputation of the book, I have nevertheless come, during my editorship of the Fifth and Sixth Editions, to recognise two serious constraints in textbooks of this kind, with their ever-increasing authorship.

In the first place, writers on topics which are to some extent interrelated are bound to cover ground of common interest. I have tried to eliminate redundancies, discrepancies and contradictions as far as possible, but I hesitate to destroy the balance of a carefully written essay. And such essays, rather than mere reference chapters, have come to be a feature of the book. It therefore transpires that 'overlap syndromes' are something of a problem not only in the practice of clinical rheumatology but in the very books in which they are described.

A more serious difficulty is that of time. So much happens, so quickly. Dr Samuel Johnson wrote in his preface to his *Dictionary of the English Language* (1755), '. . . no dictionary of a living tongue can ever be perfect, since while it is hastening to publication, some words are budding, some falling away . . .'. If Johnson felt this about relatively static things like words, how much more do his comments apply to mobile scientific thoughts? The elucidation of immunogenetic mechanisms is no doubt 'budding'. Focal sepsis, at any rate in its conventional sense, has 'fallen away', but the concept has come alive again in discussions of reactive arthritis and seronegative spondarthritis. A lot can happen while the collective wisdom of 68 contributors hastens to publication.

I must again thank all my distinguished friends who have contributed to the book, to the staff of Churchill Livingstone for their efficient collaboration, and to my secretary Mrs Sheila Webber Spry, whose prodigious efforts have successfully seen the work to fruition.

London, 1986

J. T. Scott

Contributors

Barbara M. Ansell CBE MD FRCS FRCP
Consultant Rheumatologist, Wexham Park Hospital, Slough; Head, Division of Rheumatology, and Consultant Rheumatologist, Clinical Research Centre, Northwick Park Hospital, Harrow

Elizabeth M. Badley DPhil MSc
Deputy Director of the Arthritis and Rheumatism Council Epidemiology Research Unit, University of Manchester Medical School

J. Ball BSc MD FRCPath
Emeritus Professor of Osteo-articular Pathology, Department of Rheumatology, University of Manchester

Marilyn L. Baltz PhD
Senior Research Officer, MRC Acute Phase Protein Research Group, Immunological Medicine Unit, Royal Postgraduate Medical School, Hammersmith Hospital, London

Colin G. Barnes BSc FRCP
Consultant Physician, Department of Rheumatology, The London Hospital

H. Berry MA MRCP
Consultant in Rheumatology Rehabilitation, King's College Hospital, London

David Blake MRCP
Consultant Senior Lecturer, Department of Rheumatology, University of Birmingham

A. C. Boyle MD FRCP
Formerly Director, Rheumatology Department, The Middlesex Hospital, London

K. Alun Brown BSc PhD
Research Fellow, Department of Immunology, The Rayne Institute, St Thomas' Hospital, London

W. Watson Buchanan MD FRCP(Glas) FRCP(Ed) FRCP(C) FACP
Professor of Medicine and Regional Coordinator of Rheumatology, Department of Medicine (Rheumatology), McMaster University Health Sciences Centre, Chedoke-McMaster Hospitals, Hamilton, Ontario

E. G. L. Bywaters CBE MD(Liege) FRCP FRCP(C) FACP FRCS(C)
Emeritus Professor of Rheumatology, Royal Postgraduate Medical School, Hammersmith Hospital, London

E. D. R. Campbell FRCP
Consultant Rheumatologist, Royal Free Hospital, London

M. Anne Chamberlain BSc FRCP
Consultant Physician in Rehabilitation Medicine and Honorary Senior Lecturer, School of Medicine, University of Leeds

N. Christophidis PhD FRACP
Honorary Senior Registrar, St Bartholomew's Hospital, London

Mary Corbett FRCP
Consultant Rheumatologist, The Middlesex and Royal National Orthopaedic Hospitals, London

Charles F. Corke BSc MRCP
Research Registrar, St Bartholomew's Hospital, London

H. L. F. Currey MMed(Cape Town) FRCP
Professor of Rheumatology and Director of the Bone and Joint Research Unit, The London Hospital Medical College; Physician, Department of Rheumatology, The London Hospital

A. M. Denman FRCP
Head, MRC Connective Tissue Diseases Research Group, Clinical Research Centre, and Consultant Physician, Northwick Park Hospital, Harrow

W. C. Dick MD FRCP
Reader in Rheumatology and Honorary Consultant Physician, Royal Victoria Infirmary, Newcastle upon Tyne

Paul Dieppe BSc FRCP
Senior Lecturer (Rheumatology), University of Bristol; Consultant Rheumatologist, Bristol Royal Infirmary

Allan St J. Dixon MD FRCP
Consultant Physician, Royal National Hospital for Rheumatic Diseases, Bath; Visiting Professor, University of Bath

David V. Doyle MD FRCP(I)
Consultant Physician and Rheumatologist, Whipps Cross Hospital, London; Honorary Consultant Rheumatologist, St Bartholomew's Hospital, London

D. C. Dumonde MA PhD MD(Cantab) FRCPath CChem FRSC
Professor of Immunology, St Thomas' Hospital and Medical School, University of London

D. L. Gardner MD PhD(Ed) FRCP FRCPath
Professor of Histopathology, University of Manchester

T. Gibson MD FRCP
Consultant Physician, Department of Rheumatology, Guy's Hospital, London

Rodney Grahame MD FRCP
Consultant Rheumatologist, Guy's Hospital, London

Ian Griffiths BSc FRCP
Consultant Rheumatologist, Royal Victoria Infirmary and Freeman Hospital, Newcastle upon Tyne

Michael Gumpel FRCP
Consultant Physician (Rheumatology), Northwick Park Hospital, Harrow

E. B. D. Hamilton FRCP
Consultant Physician, Department of Rheumatology, King's College Hospital, London

Timothy E. Hardingham PhD DSc
Deputy Head, Biochemistry Division, Kennedy Institute of Rheumatology, London

Ian Haslock MD
Consultant Rheumatologist, South Tees District, Middlesbrough

Brian Hazleman MA FRCP
Associate Lecturer, Department of Medicine, University of Cambridge; Fellow of Corpus Christi College, Cambridge; Consultant Rheumatologist, Addenbrooke's Hospital, Cambridge, and Newmarket Hospital, Suffolk

E. J. Holborow MD(Cantab) FRCP FRCPath
Emeritus Professor of Immunopathology, The London Hospital Medical College

Peter John Lennox Holt FRCP(Ed) FRCP(Lond) DCH
Reader in Rheumatology and Physician in Charge, Rheumatism Research Centre, Manchester Royal Infirmary; Physician, Booth Hall Children's Hospital, Manchester

Graham R. V. Hughes MD(Lond) FRCP
Consultant Physician and Head of Rheumatology Unit, Hammersmith Hospital, London

E. C. Huskisson BSc MD FRCP
Consultant Physician and Senior Lecturer, St Bartholomew's Hospital, London

David B. Jack BSc PhD
Senior Lecturer, Department of Therapeutics and Clinical Pharmacology, The Medical School, University of Birmingham

Malcolm I. V. Jayson MD FRCP
Professor of Rheumatology, University of Manchester

David Katz BSc FRCR
Consultant Radiologist, Northwick Park Hospital and Clinical Research Centre, Harrow

Walter F. Kean MD FRCP(C) FACP
Associate Professor of Medicine, McMaster University Health Sciences Centre, Chedoke-McMaster Hospitals, Hamilton, Ontario

J. H. Kellgren MSc FRCS FRCP
Emeritus Professor of Rheumatology, University of Manchester

M. J. Kendall MD FRCP
Senior Lecturer in Therapeutics and Clinical Pharmacology, University of Birmingham; Honorary Consultant, Queen Elizabeth Hospital, Birmingham

J. K. Lloyd Jones MA FRCP
Consultant Rheumatologist, Harlow Wood Orthopaedic Hospital and Mansfield District General Hospital; Clinical Teacher, Nottingham University Medical School

Bruce Lynn PhD
Senior Lecturer in Physiology, University College London

R. N. Maini BA FRCP
Head, Division of Clinical Immunology, Kennedy Institute of Rheumatology, London; Professor and Head of Department of Immunology of Rheumatic Diseases, Charing Cross and Westminster Medical School; Honorary Consultant Physician, Charing Cross Hospital

J. A. Mathews MD FRCP
Consultant Physician, Department of Rheumatology, St Thomas' Hospital, London

R. Mitchell FRCR
Consultant Radiologist, Northwick Park Hospital

J. M. H. Moll BSc PhD FRCP
Consultant Physician in Rheumatology, and Head, Sheffield Centre for Rheumatic Diseases, Nether Edge Hospital, Sheffield; Honorary Clinical Lecturer in Rheumatic Diseases, University of Sheffield

Alastair G. Mowat FRCP(Ed)
Clinical Lecturer in Rheumatology, University of Oxford; Consultant Rheumatologist, Nuffield Orthopaedic Centre, Oxford

Helen Muir CBE MA DPhil DSc FRS
Head of Biochemistry Division and Director, Kennedy Institute of Rheumatology, London

A. B. Myles BA FRCP
Consultant Physician, Department of Rheumatology, St Peter's District General Hospital, Chertsey, Surrey

G. S. Panayi MD FRCP
Professor of Rheumatology, United Medical Schools, Guy's Hospital, London

M. B. Pepys MA MD PhD FRCP MRCPath
Professor of Immunological Medicine and Honorary Consultant Physician, Immunological Medicine Unit, Royal Postgraduate Medical School, Hammersmith Hospital, London; Head, MRC Acute Phase Protein Research Group

Philip N. Platt MRCP
Consultant Rheumatologist and Honorary Clinical Lecturer, Royal Victoria Infirmary, Newcastle upon Tyne

David G. I. Scott MD MRCP
Lecturer in Rheumatology, University of Birmingham

J. T. Scott MD FRCP
Consultant Physician, Charing Cross Hospital, London; Honorary Physician, Kennedy Institute of Rheumatology, London

M. H. Seifert FRCP
Consultant Physician, Department of Rheumatology, St Mary's Hospital, London

Michael L. Snaith MD FRCP
Consultant Rheumatologist, University College Hospital, London; Honorary Senior Lecturer, Faculty of Clinical Sciences, University College London

Trevor C. B. Stamp MD FRCP
Consultant Physician and Senior Lecturer, Royal National Orthopaedic Hospital and Institute of Orthopaedics, Brockley Hill, Stanmore, Middlesex

Michael W. Steward BSc PhD DSc FRCPath
Professor of Immunology, London University School of Hygiene and Tropical Medicine

Anthony K. Thould MD FRCP
Consultant Rheumatologist, Royal Cornwall Hospital (City), Truro, Cornwall

Patrick J. W. Venables MA MRCP
Lecturer in Immunology of the Rheumatic Diseases, Kennedy Institute of Rheumatology, and Charing Cross Hospital, London

Barrie Vernon-Roberts PhD MD MRCPath FRCPA FRCPath
Professor of Pathology, University of Adelaide; Head of Division of Tissue Pathology, Institute of Medical and Veterinary Science, Adelaide

Philip H. N. Wood FRCP FFCM
Director of the Arthritis and Rheumatism Council Epidemiology Research Unit, and Honorary Professor in Community Medicine, University of Manchester Medical School; Honorary Regional Specialist in Community Medicine, North Western Regional Health Authority, England

J. C. Woodrow MD FRCP
Consultant Rheumatologist, Royal Liverpool Hospital

V. Wright
Professor of Rheumatology, University of Leeds; Consultant Physician in Rheumatology, Leeds Western Health Authority, and Regional Rheumatology Centre, Royal Bath Hospital, Harrogate

D. A. H. Yates MD FRCP
Consultant Physician, Department of Rheumatology, St Thomas' Hospital, London; Consultant Rheumatologist, King Edward VII Hospital for Officers, London

D. B. Yates FRCP
Consultant Physician and Rheumatologist, Taunton and Somerset Hospitals, Taunton

Contents

Volume One

SECTION I: The Rheumatic Diseases

1. Historical 3
J. T. Scott
2. The basis of rheumatological practice, including nomenclature and classification 19
P. H. N. Wood
3. Epidemiology of individual rheumatic disorders 59
P. H. N. Wood E. M. Badley
4. Pain 143
B. Lynn J. H. Kellgren
5. The differential diagnosis of arthritis 161
A. St J. Dixon

SECTION II: Connective Tissue

6. Biochemistry of connective tissue 177
H. Muir T. E. Hardingham
7. Structure and function of connective tissue and joints 199
D. L. Gardner
8. Synovial fluid and its examination 251
B. Vernon-Roberts

SECTION III: Inflammation and Immunology in the Rheumatic Diseases

9. Inflammation 281
P. Dieppe D. Blake
10. Immunogenetics and rheumatic diseases 309
J. C. Woodrow
11. Immunological mechanisms and the rheumatic diseases 331
A. M. Denman
12. Autoantibodies in the rheumatic diseases 355
E. J. Holborow
13. Immune complexes and complement 376
R. N. Maini
14. The role of microbial infection in rheumatic disease 411
D. C. Dumonde M. W. Steward, K. A. Brown
15. Animal models of arthritis 468
H. L. F. Currey

SECTION IV: Clinical Pharmacology

16. The clinical pharmacokinetics of antirheumatic drugs 489
M. J. Kendall D. B. Jack
17. Salicylates 500
M. H. Seifert
18. Non-steroidal anti-inflammatory drugs 514
P. N. Platt W. C. Dick
19. Penicillamine, gold and antimalarials 525
H. Berry
20. Corticosteroids 535
A. B. Myles
21. Cytotoxic and immunomodulating drugs in the treatment of rheumatic diseases 547
C. F. Corke E. C. Huskisson N. Christophidis
22. Hypouricaemic drugs 569
T. Gibson
23. Intra-articular therapy 584
J. M. Gumpel

SECTION V: Rheumatoid Arthritis

24. The aetiopathogenesis of rheumatoid arthritis 595
G. S. Panayi
25. Pathology of rheumatoid arthritis 604
D. L. Gardner
26. Articular and systemic manifestations of rheumatoid arthritis 653
W. W. Buchanan W. F. Kean
27. The management of rheumatoid disease 706
M. Corbett

SECTION VI: Seronegative spondarthritis

28. Seronegative spondarthritides 723
J. M. H. Moll I. Haslock V. Wright
29. Ankylosing spondylitis 745
J. M. H. Moll
30. Psoriatic arthritis 775
V. Wright
31. Reiter's disease 787
V. Wright
32. Enteropathic arthritis 806
I. Haslock

Volume Two

SECTION VII: Osteoarthrosis

33. Aetiology and pathology of osteoarthrosis 821
J. Ball
34. Clinical aspects of osteoarthrosis 846
D. Doyle
35. Management of osteoarthrosis 874
D. Doyle

SECTION VIII: Metabolic Disease

36. Gout 883
J. T. Scott
37. Pyrophosphate arthropathy 938
E. B. D. Hamilton
38. Arthritis in ochronosis, haemochromatosis and Wilson's disease 950
E. B. D. Hamilton
39. Endocrine disorders 959
P. J. L. Holt
40. Metabolic bone disease 992
T. C. B. Stamp
41. Amyloidosis 1024
M. B. Pepys M. L. Baltz

SECTION IX: Arthritis in Children

42. Rheumatic fever 1057
E. G. L. Bywaters
43. Juvenile chronic arthritis 1100
B. M. Ansell E. G. L. Bywaters
44. Other forms of arthritis in childhood 1125
B. M. Ansell

SECTION X: Other forms of Arthritis

45. Infective arthritis 1137
B. M. Ansell
46. Heritable disorders 1162
R. Grahame
47. Arthritis and blood disease 1177
P. J. L. Holt
48. Osteonecrosis 1207
I. D. Griffiths
49. Miscellaneous 1229
C. G. Barnes

SECTION XI: Inflammatory Disorders of Connective Tissue

50. Overlap syndromes and mixed connective tissue disease 1269
P. J. W. Venables
51. Polymyalgia rheumatica and giant cell arteritis 1278
B. Hazleman
52. Vasculitis 1292
D. G. I. Scott
53. Systemic lupus erythematosus 1325
G. R. V. Hughes
54. Polymyositis and dermatomyositis 1350
B. M. Ansell
55. Systemic sclerosis 1364
M. I. V. Jayson
56. Sjögren's syndrome 1386
M. L. Snaith

SECTION XII: Topographical Rheumatology (Regional Disorders)

57. Back pain, spondylosis and disc disorders 1407
M. I. V. Jayson
58. The neck and shoulder 1435
D. A. H. Yates
59. The upper limb 1448
H. L. F. Currey
60. Lesions of the lower limb 1455
J. K. Lloyd Jones

SECTION XIII: Physical Treatment, Rehabilitation and Surgical Treatment

61. Physical treatment of the rheumatic diseases 1483
J. A. Mathews
62. Rehabilitation in the rheumatic diseases 1497
M. A. Chamberlain
63. Surgical treatment of arthritis 1518
A. G. Mowat

SECTION XIV: Clinical and Laboratory Techniques

64. History taking and physical examination 1569
A. K. Thould
65. Clinical trials and therapeutic evaluation 1581
E. C. Huskisson
66. Arthroscopy, arthrography and synovial biopsy 1597
D. B. Yates
67. Injection techniques 1612
A. C. Boyle
68. Electrodiagnosis in the rheumatic diseases 1621
E. D. R. Campbell
69. Modern imaging techniques 1627
D. Katz R. Mitchell

Index **I1**

SECTION VII

Osteoarthrosis

33

J. Ball

Aetiology and pathology of osteoarthrosis

SYNONYMS

Arthritis deformans is an old term, introduced by Virchow, which describes both osteoarthrosis and rheumatoid arthritis. It is no longer used.

Arthrosis deformans is occasionally used by continental European writers.

Osteoarthritis is often used, but many prefer the term **osteoarthrosis**. Neither is entirely satisfactory, but 'osteoarthrosis' serves to emphasise the distinction from primary inflammatory joint disease.

Degenerative joint disease describes both osteoarthrosis and intervertebral disc degeneration.

INTRODUCTION

Although man has probably always suffered from osteoarthrosis, it was not until recent times that it was delineated as an entity distinct from rheumatoid arthritis (Garrod, 1907; Hoffa & Wollenberg, 1908; Nichols & Richardson, 1909). Studying the pathology of non-tuberculous arthritis, Nichols & Richardson recognised two types of joint change — 'the proliferative type which tends to destroy joint cartilage and lead to ankylosis of adjacent joint surfaces, and the degenerative type which tends to destroy the joint cartilage and produce deformity without ankylosis'. The degenerative type is now known as 'osteoarthrosis' (OA).

OA is an abnormality of diarthrodial (synovial) joints characterised by focal splitting and fragmentation (fibrillation) of articular cartilage which is not attributable to direct contact with inflammatory tissue. Fibrillation is not discernible in a radiograph. It may or may not be accompanied by subchondral bone sclerosis, subchondral bone cysts, narrowing of the joint space and bony outgrowths at the joint margins (osteophytes) — all of which can be seen in radiographs, and which can be regarded as manifestations of abnormal articular remodelling. When these radiological changes are prominent, cartilage fibrillation will usually have progressed to full-thickness loss in some part of the articular surface. At present OA is best defined in these anatomical terms; and radiology is the main diagnostic tool.

Various conditions predispose to OA, and when an antecedent lesion can be identified the OA is said to be 'secondary.' Otherwise OA is said to be 'primary' (the term used in this chapter), 'idiopathic' or 'non-specific'.

Radiological evidence of OA is common and almost all elderly people are found to have it to some extent, though it is often symptomless (Lawrence et al, 1966; Gordon, 1968). Nevertheless, in an English industrial town it was found that among the rheumatic diseases OA was the commonest cause of loss of work in women and the third commonest cause in men (Kellgren et al, 1953) — and this was confirmed in studies of miners and dockworkers (Anderson et al, 1962; Anderson & Duthie, 1963). In Great Britain in 1969, 37 million days were lost from work due to rheumatic complaints, over 5 times more than the loss from industrial disputes (Statistical Appendix, 1972). This testifies that OA is more than just a geriatric problem.

BIOLOGY OF DIARTHRODIAL JOINTS

This subject is described in Chapter 7. Here it will suffice to recall briefly certain features of the healthy mature synovial joint before considering the changes that occur in OA.

Articular cartilage

This consists of cells (chondrocytes) and extracellular fibrous and non-fibrous components. The surface exhibits ovoid features about 10–35 μm in diameter and about 0.5–2.0 μm deep which appear as hollows in dried specimens and as circumscribed elevations in hydrated unloaded specimens. It is thought they may reflect different states of subsurface chondrocytes (Gardner et al, 1981). To what extent this apparently rough surface persists under load is not known and its relevance to joint function remains obscure (Swanson, 1979). The extracellular matrix is uncalcified except for a narrow zone which forms an impervious layer lying immediately above the supporting subchondral bone. The following remarks apply to uncalcified hyaline articular cartilage. Uncalcified cartilage does not contain blood vessels or lymphatics and, having no nerves, lacks all forms of sensibility. The extracellular matrix consists essentially of collagen fibrils embedded in a gel of proteoglycans, the water in which contains various solutes. The proportions of the main components vary somewhat from joint to joint and in different regions and levels from the surface in a given anatomic site such as the femoral head. Care is needed therefore to achieve strict comparability when studying articular cartilage in health and disease. In the upper region of the femoral head in young adults the mean water content is approximately 73%, the collagen 18% and the proteoglycans 7% of the wet weight (Maroudas et al, 1980).

Most if not all of the collagen is a genetically distinct type known as type II or by the formula $(\alpha\ 1(II))_3$ which describes its three polypeptide chains. Type II collagen is found only in cartilage, intervertebral disc and vitreous humour. (Recently, small amounts of four other types of collagen, namely type V, 1α2α3α, C-PS1 and C-PS2 have been detected in perichondrocytic zones in bovine nasal cartilage; and 1α2α3α has been found in immature human articular cartilage (Burgeson, 1982; Evans et al, 1983). Whether these occur in adult human articular cartilage is not known.) In the thin superficial zone of articular cartilage, which is about 5–10% of the total thickness, the collagen fibrils lie parallel to the articular surface in sheet formation and tend to be oriented in the direction of joint movement. This zone merges with a thicker, intermediate, zone where the fibrils are less closely packed and more or less randomly disposed in a three-dimensional meshwork. This layer merges with the deep zone where the fibrils tend to be aligned perpendicular to the surface and run into the calcified layer thus tethering the cartilage to the supporting bone (Hukins, 1982). The turnover of collagen in the adult is negligible (Maroudas, 1979).

A proteoglycan consists of a protein core along the length of which long-chain carbohydrate moieties (glycosaminoglycans) are attached. The glycosaminoglycans are mainly chondroitin sulphate with smaller amounts of keratan sulphate. Most of the proteoglycans in cartilage are uniquely capable of forming aggregates in which several proteoglycans are joined to a single long-chain molecule of hyaluronic acid, each junction being stabilised by a glycoprotein (link-protein). A minority of the proteoglycans are unable to react with hyaluronic acid to form aggregates and are relatively easily extracted by solutions of physiological ionic strength. Still other proteoglycans resist extraction even with strongly dissociating solvents, perhaps because of some as yet unidentified firm interaction with the collagen fibrils (Muir, 1979). The turnover time (defined as the time taken for all glycosaminoglycans to be replaced) in adults is of the order of 3 years (Maroudas, 1979). Turnover is greater in the mid-zone than in the superficial layers and greater in cartilage with a relatively low proteoglycan content (Brocklehurst & Maroudas, 1981). Different proteoglycan fractions probably have different turnover rates. Degradation is mediated by neutral proteinases (Sapolsky et al, 1976), cathepsins active at acid pH (Bayliss & Ali, 1978a) and possibly hyaluronidase (Stack & Brandt, 1982). Degradative activity may presumably be modified by enzyme inhibitors known to exist in the cartilage. Cartilage also normally contains compounds which inhibit vascular invasion (Kuettner et al, 1977).

Load carriage

Proteoglycans swell in the presence of water. The

internal swelling (osmotic) pressure generated in cartilage in this way is balanced by tensile forces in the mesh of collagen fibrils in which the proteoglycans are trapped. Unlike other connective tissues articular cartilage shows little tendency to swell when fragments are immersed in saline or even in water (Maroudas, 1980). Thus in unloaded cartilage the collagen mesh is probably normally stressed in tension. Cartilage is therefore a hydraulically self-pressurised prestressed rigid structure in which the collagen and proteoglycan gel are functionally interdependent. The greater the concentration of proteoglycans the greater the swelling pressure, the lower the hydraulic permeability and the greater the resistance to compressive forces, i.e. the stiffer the cartilage. In healthy joints, cartilage is stiffest in areas transmitting most of the load and softest at articular margins (Kempson, 1980).

When an area of cartilage is loaded perpendicular to its surface there is instantaneous deformation with compression of the loaded area, bulk movement of proteoglycans and water and a consequent increase in pressure in the surrounding more peripheral 'unloaded' cartilage. If the load is of brief duration there is instantaneous recovery. If the load is not quickly removed a progressive slow viscous deformation or 'creep' occurs due mainly to the movement of water (but not proteoglycans) out of the cartilage. On removing the load, water re-enters the cartilage from the synovial fluid and recovery takes place. But recovery probably requires a longer load-off period than the load-on period. Hence if there is abnormally rapid repetitive loading the cartilage may be unable to recover completely between loads (Weightman & Kempson, 1979; Maroudas, 1980).

The force across a joint including weight-bearing joints is due mainly to the contraction of muscles which span the joint. During walking, loads in the hip, knee and ankle reach several times body weight, albeit for only a fraction of a second in each step (Paul, 1980). Little is known of the peak pressures at specific sites within joints which may be more important than the overall load. According to Day et al (1975) these may differ appreciably between apparently healthy hip joints, perhaps because of minor anatomic variations. The strain induced in cartilage by a given load depends on the area over which the load is distributed. Any condition which reduces the area of load carriage and hence increases the force per unit area is potentially damaging. Articular cartilage with its large water content tends to increase contact areas and to improve stress distribution. According to Freeman et al (1975) cartilage can protect subchondral bone from fracture during repeated application of loads in the physiological range. However the subchondral bone is more effective than the thin layer of cartilage in attenuating rapidly applied loads causing high transient stresses because there is much more cancellous bone to attenuate the stress (Radin & Paul, 1970).

Nutrition

In the smaller adult human joints the cartilage is adequately nourished by diffusion of small solutes such as glucose and amino acids from the synovial fluid, provided that stagnant pools of fluid are avoided by joint movement (Maroudas, 1980). In larger joints such as the hip there may be an additional subchondral source of nutrition but the evidence (discussed by McKibbin & Maroudas, 1979) seems to the present writer to be unconvincing. The diffusion of solutes into and through cartilage is a function of the 'pore' size or permeability of the proteoglycan gel which diminishes as the concentration of the gel increases and vice versa. Solutes with a molecular weight above 70 000 are virtually excluded from healthy unloaded cartilage. However it should be noted that while the diffusion of small solutes is largely independent of proteoglycan concentration the diffusion of large molecules is very sensitive to proteoglycan concentration, small reductions in which may allow penetration of molecules as large as IgG (Maroudas, 1979). Furthermore, while the pumping action of cyclic loading is unnecessary for cartilage nutrition, recent studies show that it may be associated with reversible penetration of large molecules such as albumin (Maroudas, 1980).

Lubrication

The mechanisms involved in joint lubrication remain debatable. Evidence for fluid film, squeeze film and boundary lubrication mechanisms has been reported in human joints depending on the loading conditions (Unsworth et al, 1975). In test conditions favouring boundary lubrication Swann et al (1974, 1981) found that the friction-reducing property of synovial fluid depended not on its viscosity (which depends on its hyaluronic acid content) but on the presence of a glycoprotein. However using human hip joints in a system simulating walking Roberts et al (1982) report that at low loads friction is increased after hyaluronidase digestion of synovial fluid.

As hyaluronic acid is too large to pass into cartilage, Maroudas (1979) argues that when opposing cartilage surfaces come together the fluid between them looses water leaving a gel-like film about 0.02 μm thick which keeps the surfaces apart in physiological loading conditions. A renewable gel of this kind may reduce the wear on the bearing surfaces which are also essentially hydrophilic gels.

Articular stability

In some joints articular geometry obviously contributes to stability. Thus the deep acetabulum with its fibrous labrum will hold the femoral head in place (in vitro) when other constraints are severed. Joint movement is ultimately limited by articular ligaments together with the joint capsule. Within the normal range of movement, stability is maintained by musculo ligamentous tension. Neuromuscular control of joint movement is mediated on the afferent side by sensory receptors in ligaments, joint capsule and extra capsular structures (Wyke, 1967; Grigg et al, 1973).

Synovium and synovial fluid

The synovium consists essentially of a discontinuous intimal lining layer of cells, synoviocytes, and subjacent adipose or fibrous tissue. The synovium is supported by the fibroligamentous joint capsule. Synoviocytes have phagocytic and synthetic capability including the production of hyaluronic acid. Synovial capillaries are perforated and there is no basement membrane beneath the synoviocytes.

The synovial fluid consists of a plasma ultrafiltrate plus materials added by the synovial tissues. Normally the protein content does not exceed 2.5 g/dl and the cell count, mainly lymphocytes, does not exceed 2×10^8/l.

PATHOLOGY

Age and osteoarthrosis

During skeletal growth articular cartilage undergoes marked changes but here we are concerned only with mature cartilage. Elderly joints often contain cartilage which on inspection seems none the worse for wear, even when areas of fibrillated cartilage are present elsewhere in the joint. When apparently healthy cartilage is tested with an indentor its compressive stiffness remains constant in adult life (Sokoloff, 1966). This was confirmed by Armstrong et al (1980) in a study of femoral head cartilage, but when these workers applied large compressive loads in vitro to the intact hip joint, zones of increased deformation of the femoral head cartilage were found in older joints. However the duration of loading in this study was much greater than that which occurs in vivo. The tensile strength of thin discs of cartilage cut parallel to the surface of the femoral condyle (Kempson, 1982) and the fatigue resistance of femoral head cartilage in tension (Weightman et al, 1978), both of which depend on cartilage collagen, have been found to fall with age in adult life. It is difficult to reconcile this apparent weakening of the collagen meshwork with the observation (see below) that the water content of cartilage falls with age. Furthermore in most elderly people the articular cartilage of the zenith of the femoral head is remarkably healthy, degeneration occurring in only about 10% of the population of the UK.

Recent biochemical studies of cartilage the surface of which is macroscopically normal show that minor changes do occur as it ages during adult life. These include

a. A fall in the water content with no change in cartilage thickness
b. A rise in total glycosaminoglycan content due to an increase in keratan sulphate
c. A rise in the protein to uronic acid ratio and the keratan sulphate to chondroitin sulphate ratio (Rüttner et al, 1974; Venn, 1978; Maroudas et al, 1980).

These changes are the opposite of those found in the fibrillated cartilage of OA. Furthermore, unlike fibrillated cartilage, the proteoglycans of macroscopically healthy but ageing cartilage remain capable of aggregation (Bayliss & Ali, 1978b), exhibit no increase in extractability (Simunek & Muir, 1972) and show only slight change in the wet volume per unit weight of collagen which according to Maroudas et al (1980) is a measure of the integrity of the collagen meshwork, at least in unloaded cartilage. These biochemical findings seem to show that OA is not based on ageing.

Although cartilage fibrillation is clearly not an inevitable accompaniment of advancing years it is certainly age-related. This was first thoroughly documented by Heine (1926) who inspected the articular surfaces of several joints in 1002 necropsies. His data show that the prevalence and severity of cartilage degeneration increases with age. Minor degrees of fibrillation are seen in the 3rd decade but severe cartilage loss with bone exposure rarely occurs before the 5th decade, and there is much variation in susceptibility between joints. Radiological surveys of random population samples in the UK and USA are in accord with Heine's findings (Lawrence et al, 1966; Gordon, 1968).

Morbid anatomic studies show that fibrillation is often first seen in the so-called 'non-contact' areas such as the periphery of articular surfaces and the boundaries between articular territories (Fig. 33.1). Specific examples include the peripheral regions of the inferomedial zone of the femoral head, the medial part of the medial facet of the patella, the periphery of the glenoid and the rim of the radial head (except for the triangular facet which is in contact with the ulna) (Harrison et al, 1953; Goodfellow & Bullough, 1967; Byers et al, 1970; Meachim & Emery, 1973 and 1974; Bullough et al, 1973). Mild fibrillation in these sites is common in young adults and almost universal in the elderly, even in joints such as the hip which are infrequently affected by radiologically detectable OA. This type of fibrillation is sometimes referred to as 'age-related' or 'non-progressive' fibrillation (Meachim & Emery, 1973; Byers et al, 1970). Significantly, it was almost as prevalent in the hip joints of a Chinese population in which radiological OA was less common than in a comparable Caucasian population, thus emphasising the dissociation between the fibrillation in 'non-contact' areas and clinically significant OA, at least in the hip joint (Byers et al, 1974). The cause of non-progressive fibrillation remains speculative. Peripheral cartilage, being thinner and more compliant than other parts of the articular surface (Venn, 1979), is possibly less able to resist the internal stresses to which it may be subjected when the loaded part of a joint expands laterally (Weightman & Kempson, 1979). The existence of non-progressive fibrillation suggests that, whatever initiates the process, local mechanical factors may be needed to produce clinically significant damage.

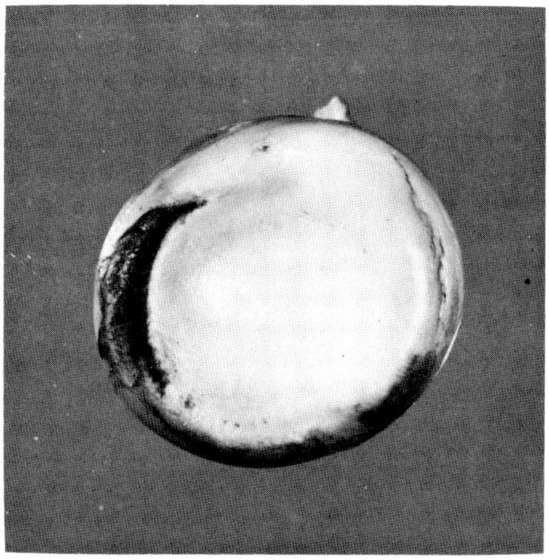

Fig. 33.1 Head of radius of a female aged 40. Areas of minimal cartilage degeneration (stained black by Meachim's (1972b) indian ink method) are limited to the peripheral (non-contact) part of the articular surface.

Severe fibrillation with exposure of calcified cartilage and bone usually has a different topographical distribution from fibrillation in 'non-contact' areas (Fig. 33.2). Thus, severe OA is more often found in the central part of the radial head, the zenith of the femoral head and in the central and lateral parts of the patella. However, according to Meachim & Emery (1974) peripheral fibrillation in the knee may sometimes spread to involve other areas; and 'medial OA' of the hip with severe involvement of the infero-medial zone of the femoral head is a well known subtype of coxarthrosis (see Fig. 33.15).

In old age amyloid is found in various tissues including articular cartilage and joint capsules, but this process is unrelated to OA (Goffin et al, 1981; Ladefoged, 1982).

The nature of cartilage fibrillation

If certain rare forms of secondary OA such as that

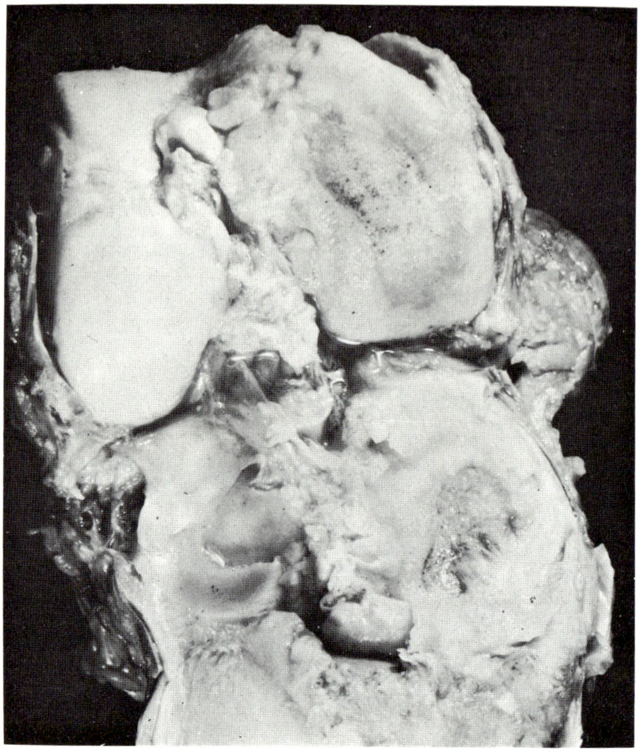

Fig. 33.2 The knee joint of a female aged 62 showing on the right complete loss of cartilage over the central area of the medial condyle of femur and tibia, and fraying of the medial meniscus. In contrast the lateral compartment is healthy.

associated with ochronosis are excluded, fibrillated cartilage is morphologically and metabolically the same in patients with OA as in subjects with radiologically normal joints provided the grade of fibrillation is the same (Maroudas, 1973). The softening, splitting and fragmentation which characterise fibrillation begin in a *focal* area of the articular *surface*. Cartilage which is apparently normal can exist in a joint in which there is an area of severe fibrillation (Brocklehurst & Maroudas, 1981). The vertical, oblique and horizontal clefts which occur in the surface layers of the cartilage impart a velvety or flaky appearance and produce fragments, usually of microscopic size, which are cast off into the synovial fluid (Figs 33.3, 33.6). The splitting and fragmentation may spread to involve a larger area of cartilage surface and/or progress vertically so that the cartilage gradually becomes thinner until calcified cartilage and, ultimately, bone are exposed (see Figs 33.14, 33.15). When a cleft reaches a calcified layer it tends to progress horizontally along the junction between the calcified and non-calcified layers, undermining healthy cartilage and sometimes creating small cartilage sequestra in the deep zones.

Occasionally deep clefts reaching down to the calcified layer are seen in cartilage of normal thickness (Fig. 33.4). In a case of this kind involving a patella removed at operation following a diagnosis of 'chondromalacia patellae' there was clinical evidence of trauma to the knee and histological evidence of trauma in the subchondral bone beneath the cleft, suggesting that deep clefts in cartilage of normal thickness may indicate a traumatic aetiology. Goodfellow et al (1976) suggest that deep clefts without surface loss may characterise the syndrome of 'chondromalacia patellae' in some patients.

In the tags of fibrillated cartilage, basophilia, metachromasia and the affinity for alcian blue and

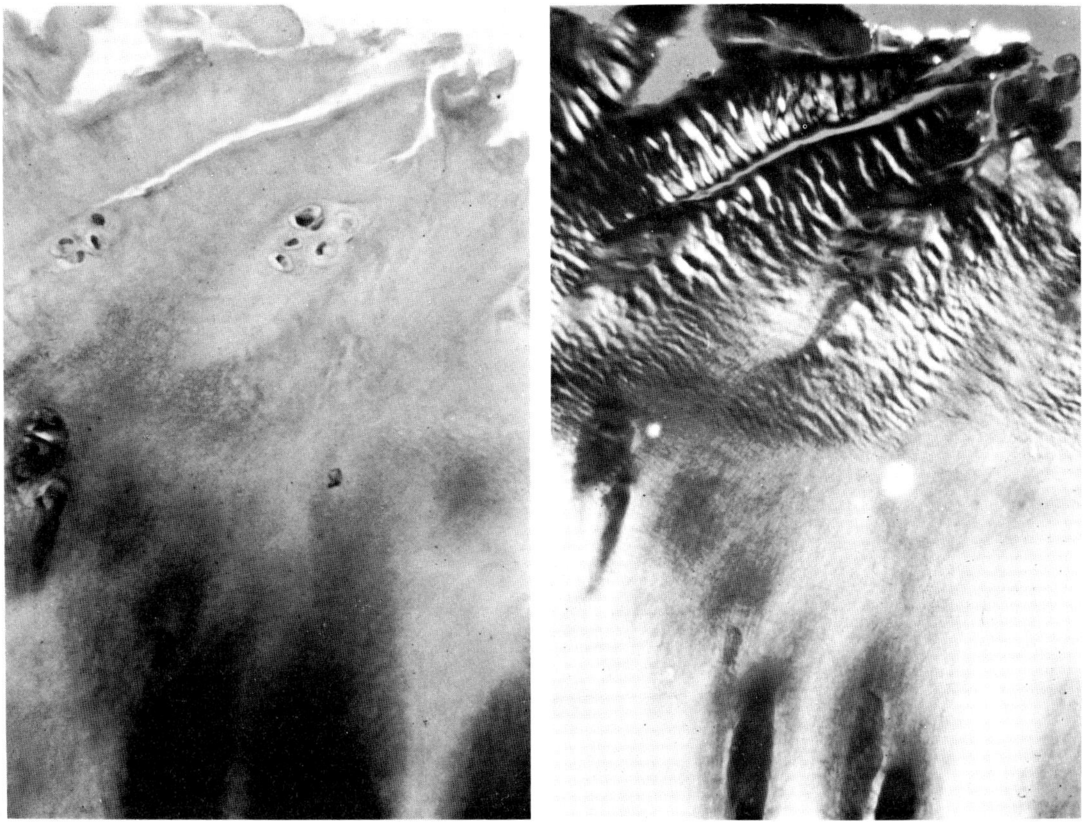

a b

Fig. 33.3 (a) Fibrillation of the surface of residual cartilage in an osteoarthrosic femoral head removed at arthroplasty. (H & E × 260) (b) Same field in polarised light showing the wavy or crimped appearance of the tags and the neighbouring cartilage in contrast to the featureless sheen of the healthy cartilage below.

safranin are all reduced indicating some loss of glycosaminoglycans (Meachim et al, 1965; Sokoloff, 1969; Mankin et al, 1971). This has been amply confirmed biochemically (see below). A reduction in glycosoaminoglycan staining may occur in histologically intact cartilage (Meachim et al, 1965) and occasionally the loss appears to be more pronounced in the perichondrocytic zones as might be expected if matrix depletion is chondrocyte-mediated (Fig. 33.5). In this connection it is relevant to recall that when cartilage was incubated in vitro at pH 5.0 proteoglycan depletion was first seen around chondrocytes, and only later in the interterritorial regions (Ali & Evans, 1973).

Chondrocyte loss occurs to a variable extent in the superficial parts (Figs. 33.3, 33.6) and may be seen at an early stage (Vignon & Arlot, 1981b). This is offset by the development of clusters (clones) of chondrocytes in the deeper parts (Figs 33.4, 33.6). These cells, which are known to show degrees of metabolic activity (Mitrovic et al, 1981), lie in matrix which may or may not be more basophilic than the nearby depleted matrix. These findings suggest that metabolic activity may vary widely in different parts of the affected area. As similar clusters of chondrocytes develop after experimental injury to the surface of articular cartilage they are probably a secondary reactive phenomenon (Carlson, 1957; Meachim, 1964; Mankin, 1974). Studies of DNA synthesis in fibrillated cartilage (Mankin et al, 1971) and in cultured chondrocytes (Sokoloff, 1974) indicate that the clusters result from cell division, possibly due to matrix depletion allowing access to growth factors normally excluded from cartilage. In both human and experimentally-produced fibrillation this chon-

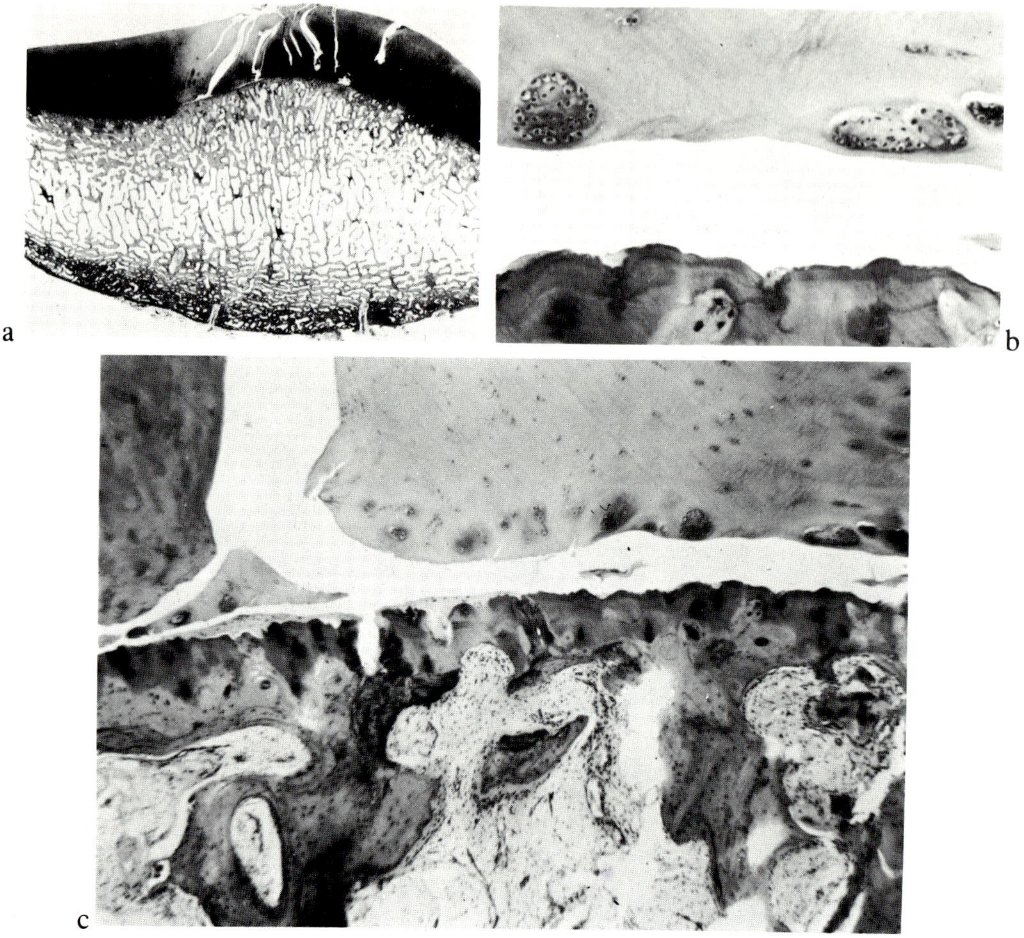

Fig. 33.4 (a) Section of patella removed at operation in a male aged 22. Clinical diagnosis 'chondromalacia patellae'. A localised group of deep clefts in cartilage of normal thickness near the ridge separating medial and lateral facets. (b) Lower end of a cleft showing splitting of cartilage along the junction of calcified and non-calcified zones, the formation of a triangular cartilaginous sequestrum, and bony repair of a crack in the subchondral plant. (H & E × 40) (c) Enlargement of part of the horizontal cleft shown to the right of (b). Calcified cartilage below; cell clusters (chondrones) in uncalcified cartilage at the edge of the cleft (above). (H & E × 100)

drocytic response is conspicuously ineffective in terms of tissue repair.

Microscopically the tags of fibrillated cartilage (and sometimes adjacent cartilage) have a wavy, striated or crimped appearance, best seen when viewed between crossed polars, whereas healthy cartilage has a featureless appearance in polarised light (Figs 33.3, 33.7). Crimped cartilage is also seen in 'buckled' surfaces which may be a prefibrillation stage in some cases (Fig. 33.7). A similar crimped pattern is characteristic of healthy fibrous structures in which the collagen fibres are not stressed in tension, normal cartilage and bone being notable exceptions to this rule (Viidik, 1973); Hukins, 1982). The significance of this change is uncertain but it suggests that fibrillation is associated with reorganisation of the collagen meshwork.

Electron microscopic studies have not as yet significantly advanced our understanding of the cartilage changes. In fibrillated specimens there are fewer matrix granules (which are thought to represent aggregated proteoglycans) and a greater variability in the diameter of collagen fibrils which tend to form tightly packed bundles (Ali & Bayliss, 1974). Weiss & Mirow (1972) draw atten-

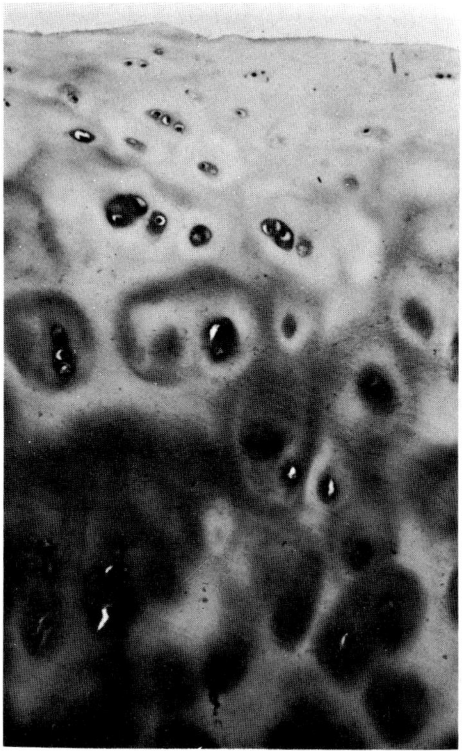

Fig. 33.5 Perichondrocyte loss of basophilia in the intact surface layers of the cartilage of a femoral head. This area adjoined a zone of overt fibrillation. (H & E × 130)

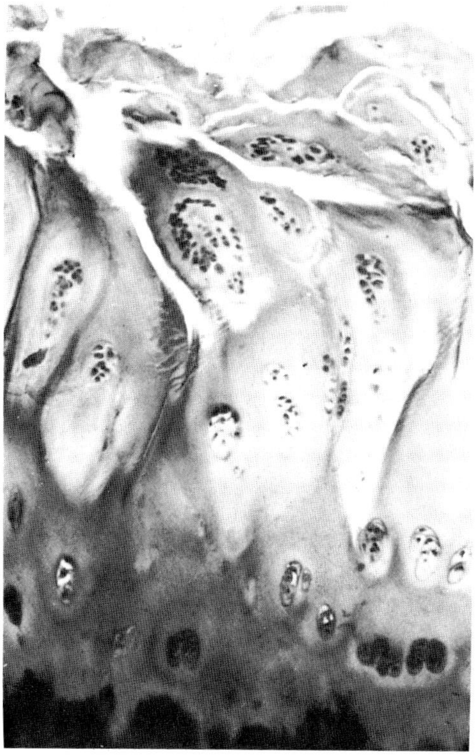

Fig. 33.6 The upper third of the cartilage is fragmented by horizontal and vertical clefts. Superficially there is a loss of chondrocytes, but cell clusters have developed in deeper layers near the clefts. (H & E × 100)

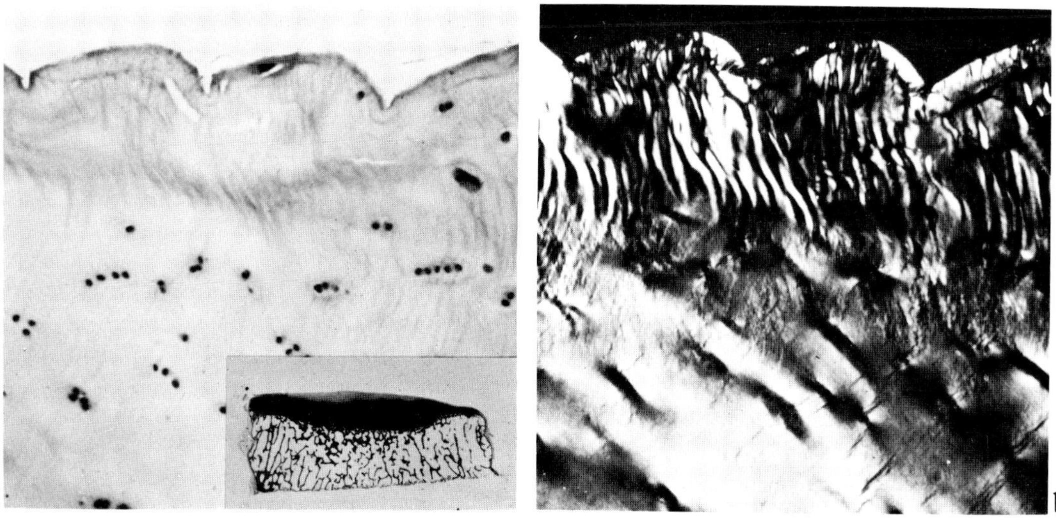

a b

Fig. 33.7 (a) The central part of a section of the medial facet of the patella (shown inset). The surface has a buckled or crimped appearance. (H & E × 130) (b) Same field in polarised light showing the wavy, crimped appearance in the superficial layers in contrast to the normal appearance below.

tion to the array of fine fibrils lying parallel to the surface of clefts and suggest that this indicates that cartilage clefts may in some cases be initiated by 'buckling or infolding' rather than splitting of the surface (Fig. 33.8).

Biochemically, fibrillated cartilage contains a reduced amount of proteoglycans and the ratio of keratan sulphate to chondroitin sulphate is reduced (Mankin et al, 1971; Maroudas et al, 1973; Sweet et al, 1977; Mankin et al, 1981; Brocklehurst & Maroudas, 1981). Furthermore the proteoglycans are more easily extracted, individual proteoglycans tend to be smaller and the proportion which are aggregated is reduced (Brandt, 1977; Sweet et al, 1977). The collagen content on the other hand remains unchanged (Mankin et al, 1971). The type of collagen is also normal (Lippiello et al, 1977) except for small amounts of type I collagen demonstrable immunohistochemically in and around the cells within the reactive cell clusters (Gay et al, 1976). The water content and the wet volume per unit weight of collagen are increased; and when slices of the cartilage are immersed in salt solutions there is excessive swelling, especially in the zones of cartilage deep to the fibrillated tags where there is little or no loss of proteoglycans (Maroudas & Venn, 1977; Sweet et al, 1977; Maroudas et al, 1980; Brocklehurst & Maroudas, 1981). Maroudas interprets these findings as indicative of weakness in the collagen meshwork at an early stage in the process of fibrillation. In the damaged cartilage, synthesis of DNA and matrix components, including collagen, continues (Mankin et al, 1971; Lippiello et al, 1977), but reports vary as regards the degree of metabolic activity and its relation to the severity of the disease (Thompson & Oegema, 1979; Mankin et al, 1981; Brocklehurst & Maroudas, 1981; Mitrovic et al, 1981). Degradation of matrix components also continues and raised levels of chondrocyte-derived cathepsins, neutral proteoglycanase and collagenase have been reported (Ali & Bayliss, 1974; Bayliss & Ali, 1978a; Ehrlich et al, 1978; Howell et al, 1979). Less is known about the enzyme inhibitors but there is some evidence they may be reduced (Kuettner et al, 1977).

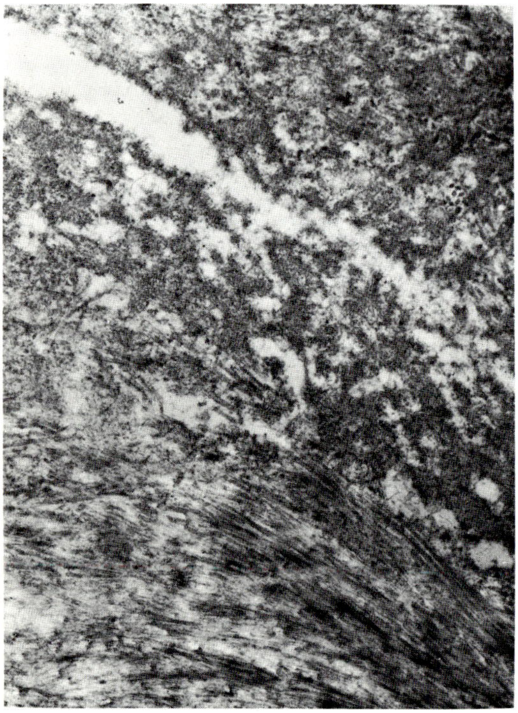

Fig. 33.8 Electron micrograph of a cleft in minimally fibrillated cartilage. The surface of the cleft is covered by an amorphous layer containing fine fibrils similar to that sometimes found over normal cartilage surfaces. Densely packed thin fibrils lie parallel to the surface of the cleft. (× 20 000)

Cartilage with an intact surface which is near to a fibrillated area may be normal (McKenzie et al, 1977; Brocklehurst & Maroudas, 1981) or have an increased water content (Sweet et al, 1977; Brocklehurst & Maroudas, 1981) and increased metabolic activity (Mitrovic et al, 1981). Similarly it may or may not be mechanically normal (Kempson, 1980). The reason for the inconsistent findings is not known; perhaps they reflect known differences in the rate of progression of OA.

In about a third of patients with severe OA undergoing surgery, deposits of immunoglobulins and complement have been demonstrated in the cartilage and other joint structures (Cooke et al, 1981). Their pathogenetic significance is obscure but according to Cooke et al they are probably a secondary phenomenon, not the initiator of fibrillation.

These various observations on human OA suggest that overt fibrillation may be preceded by a reduction in the stability of the collagen meshwork which allows increased hydration and swelling. The ability of the cartilage to resist deformation (and to recover from it) is further reduced by some loss of proteoglycans and their failure to aggregate normally. Chondrocyte malfunction (whether induced mechanically or in some other way) is conspicuous and could account for all these changes. Experimental studies (see below) confirm and extend these conclusions. It is also conceivable that in some cases the instability of the collagen meshwork is not enzymatically produced but results from fatigue failure — a purely mechanical process.

The essentially focal nature of cartilage fibrillation, and the fact that severe OA commonly occurs in the radiohumeral joint but rarely in the humeroulnar joint (Goodfellow & Bullough, 1967), which share the same joint cavity, suggests that OA is not due simply to a failure of lubrication. Some support for this comes from the observation that the coefficient of friction was much the same in human hip joints whether the cartilage was macroscopically normal or severely fibrillated (Swanson, 1979), and from the work of Davis et al (1978) who found that the boundary lubricating ability of synovial fluid obtained from human osteoarthrosic knees was not reduced, at least during the quiescent stages of the disease. It seems unlikely therefore that OA is initiated by a failure of lubrication.

Cartilage fibrillation could be initiated by an increase in subchondral bone density. This possibility has been explored experimentally and in human OA and is discussed below.

It should be noted that much of the data described above has been derived from studies of OA of the hip which may not be entirely representative of primary nodal generalised osteoarthrosis (PGOA), which is the commonest type.

Experimental pathology

Studies of experimental models have provided additional data and new insights into the nature of fibrillation. Attempts to produce OA by superficial scarification, laceration or tangential slices which do not penetrate the subchondral bone plate have signally failed (Carlson, 1957; Meachim, 1964; Ghadially et al, 1977; Mankin, 1982). These procedures lead to a prompt but transient increase in metabolic activity with increased turnover of proteoglycans and collagen (Repo & Mitchell, 1971; Mankin, 1982). The damaged cartilage neither heals nor gets worse. Thus factors other than discreet discontinuities in the collagen meshwork are needed to cause a significant degree of OA. Even local cartilage defects which breach the subchondral plate and which become filled by repair tissue originating in the bone do not necessarily promote progressive cartilage damage (Campbell, 1969; Mankin, 1982). Parenthetically, a lesion closely resembling this is occasionally seen in 'chondromalacia patellae', thus emphasising the possible role of trauma in some of these cases (Fig. 33.9).

Enzymic degradation of the cartilage matrix by intra-articular injections of papain into the hip joint of rabbits over a period of a few days leads during the course of the next few months to a severe form of OA (Murray, 1964; Bentley, 1972).

OA is also regularly induced in various models in which abnormal mechanical conditions have been created, as might be expected from observations in humans. In rabbits, extra-articular operations designed to produce a valgus deformity of the knee cause fibrillation on the excessively stressed side of the joint within 3 months (Reimann, 1973). Partial menisectomy in the rabbit also produces severe OA and has been shown to

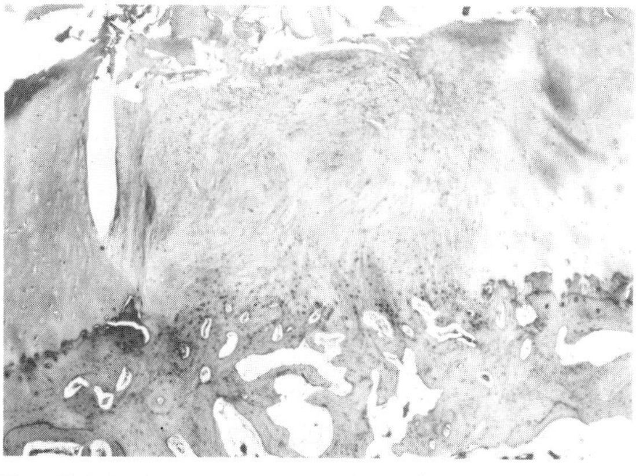

Fig. 33.9 Lesion at a transverse ridge of the patella. Centrally, all cartilage zones have been replaced by fibrous and fibrocartilaginous tissue. Clinical diagnosis — 'chondromalacia patellae'. (H & E × 20)

be associated with defective aggregation of proteoglycans even in apparently normal areas (Moskowitz et al, 1979).

Severance of the anterior cruciate ligament in the dog leads to OA which closely mimics natural canine gonarthrosis. The operation causes instability and postoperative immobilisation prevents the development of OA (Palmoski & Brandt, 1982). This model has been extensively investigated by Muir (1977) and McDevitt et al (1977). About a month after the operation when histological changes are minimal, the slightly swollen articular cartilage contains more water, there is defective aggregation of proteoglycans which are more easily extracted and the ratio of keratan sulphate to chondroitin sulphate is reduced; but the proteoglycan content is unaltered and there is no change in the type of collagen being synthesised. These findings indicate a weakened collagen meshwork or an increase in internal osmotic pressure but the latter seems unlikely for reasons discussed by Maroudas & Venn (1977). Studying the same model Altman et al (1980) reported that the swelling is mainly in the upper mid-zone and is associated with stress in the tangential fibres in the surface layer — findings which accord with Hukin's (1982) concept of articular cartilage as a pressure vessel and possibly explain why fibrillation in OA usually starts in the surface. Muir (1977) showed that the biochemical changes noted above occurred both in areas which later became fibrillated and areas (like the patella) which did not; and there was some evidence that in the areas which did not progress to overt fibrillation the changes were to an extent reversible — a feature noted in another model (see below). A fall in proteoglycan content was seen only in overtly fibrillated cartilage. Chondrocyte necrosis was not a feature of the early stages; and, as in the human, chondrocyte clusters were a relatively late manifestation (McDevitt et al, 1977). Thus this model supports several of the concepts emerging from the study of human OA. The model also points to the possibility that chondrocyte-mediated qualitative biochemical changes which appear to presage fibrillation can occur throughout the cartilage of a joint shortly after the onset of mechanical trauma but may be transient; for overt fibrillation and progressive OA to occur it seems that, in addition, localised excessive loading and a fall in proteoglycan content are required. The clinical implication would seem to be that when a joint suffers a traumatic episode (even a trivial one in a susceptible joint) it should be relieved of stress so that any reversible change in the cartilage may recover. By the same token the use of drugs which speed up the return to activity may in the long-term be harmful.

In the rabbit model studied by Radin et al (1978, 1982) it was shown that repetitive impulse loading can within a few days cause heightened chondrocyte activity (with increased incorporation of ^{3}H thymidine and $^{35}SO_4$), some loss of proteoglycans and an increase in stiffness of the subchondral bone — changes which under relatively modest loading conditions are to some extent reversible. In vitro studies of a similar model have also shown that artificially increasing subchondral bone stiffness, or extracting proteoglycans, can increase the rate of cartilage damage. The role of subchondral bone structure in the initiation or promotion of OA in humans is uncertain. OA of the hip and femoral neck fracture seem to be mutually exclusive. In patients with coxarthrosis cortical bone density in metacarpal or radial diaphysis has been reported to be normal (Solomon et al, 1982; Carlsson et al, 1979) or increased (Foss & Byers, 1972; Roh et al, 1974). On the other hand Roh et al (1974) and Carlsson et al (1979) agree that in women the cancellous bone density (which is more relevant) is increased in the lower end of the radius. Two more recent studies have compared patients with PGOA, which is the commonest clinical form of OA and is predominantly female, with controls. In one (Nuki, 1983) metacarpal cortical bone density and total body calcium (which mainly reflects cortical bone mass) were the same in patients and controls. In the other (Price et al, 1983) there was also no difference in cortical bone density between patient and controls but the cancellous bone density at the lower end of the radius (the site assayed) was statistically significantly increased in the patients with PGOA, all of whom were female. However the increased trabecular bone density (and hence presumably the subchondral bone stiffness) was not associated with an increase in OA at the radiocarpal joint which, as is well known, is not as a rule involved in PGOA.

Further studies will obviously be needed to clarify the situation. If, for instance, there is in PGOA a tendency to increased bone density from an early age, the cartilage and other structures might be able to adapt during the period of skeletal maturation. Thus the tendency to PGOA, in which there appears to be a genetic component, and increased bone mass might be genetically linked but pathogenetically independent.

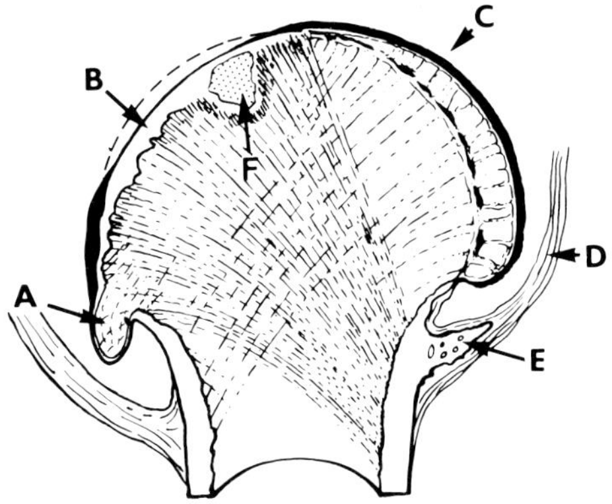

Fig. 33.10 Diagram of articular remodelling. A, Osteophyte at margin of articular cartilage. Residual cartilage shown in black. B, Sclerosed subchondral bone in area of regressive remodelling. The original joint contour is marked by an interrupted line. C, Area of progressive remodelling. Original joint contour marked by the interrupted black layer of residual calcified cartilage at the base of the bony outgrowth. D, Joint capsule with osteophytic bone growth (E) at its attachment. F, Subchondral bone cyst.

Articular remodelling

When fibrillation has progressed to the deep layers of the cartilage there is usually radiological evidence of remodelling of the end of the supporting bone. In its mildest form this consists of increased density in the region of the subchondral bone plate with little or no alteration in the general shape of the articular surface. In more severe cases local expansions and local recessions occur in the articular contour, sometimes referred to respectively as 'progressive' and 'regressive' remodelling (Fig. 33.10). Changes in contour are usually accompanied by alterations in the trabecular bone pattern within the end of the bone (Fig. 33.11a).

Progressive remodelling

Progressive remodelling (Figs 33.10–33.12) depends on enchondral ossification, that is, the vascular invasion and erosion of the subchondral bone plate and calcified cartilage and the subsequent deposition of bone on the eroded calcified cartilage surfaces. This process which is analogous to bone growth at an epiphyseal plate involves progressive calcification and in some cases growth of the hyaline cartilage (Johnson, 1962; Vignon & Arlot, 1981b). In the femoral head, progressive remodelling is commonly seen in the inferomedial part

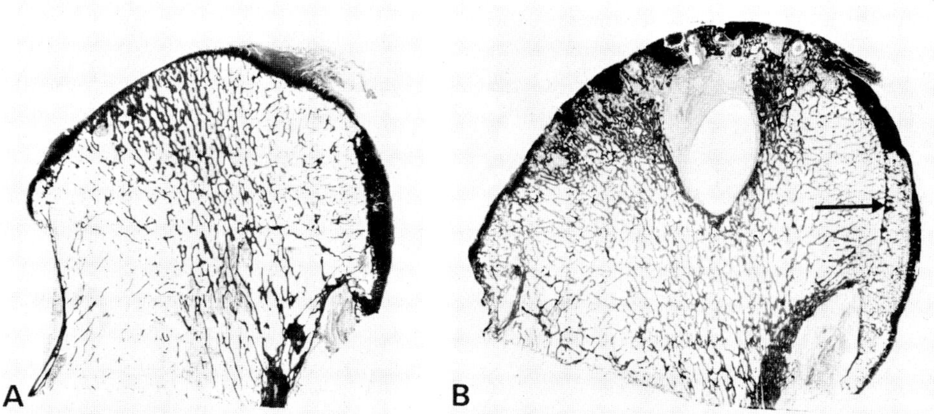

Fig. 33.11 Superolateral OA of the femoral head. (A) Early stage of remodelling with bone exposure (upper left) and beginning enchondral ossification of upper and lower parts of the medial cartilage. There is unusual prominence of trabeculae joining the superolateral surface to the medial cortex of the neck. (B) Later stage with gross flattening, sclerosis and cyst formation superolaterally (upper left). The lower two-thirds of the medial cartilage has been largely replaced by bone; arrow points to remnants of original calcified cartilage layer.

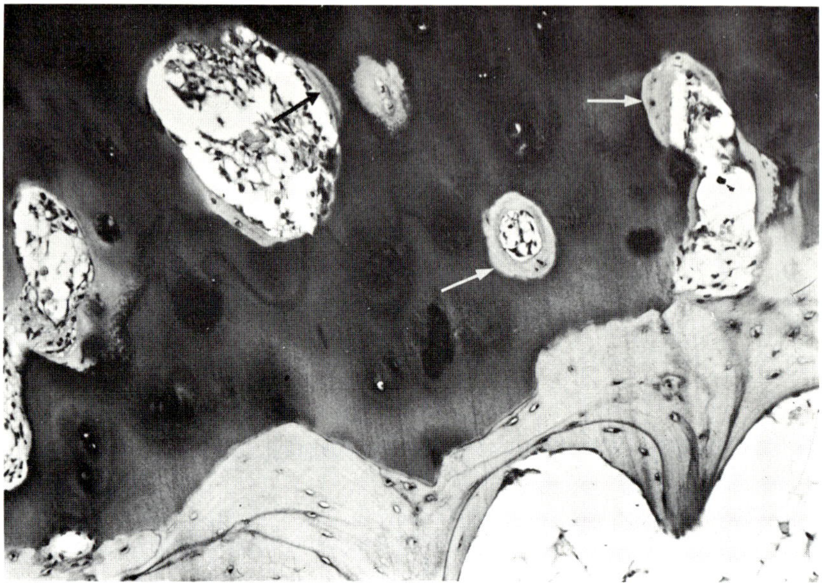

Fig. 33.12 Enchondral ossification in OA of the femoral head. Several cavities in the cartilage, formed by invasion of blood vessels from the marrow (below right), are partly or completely lined by bone (arrows). (H & E × 100)

and at the articular margins. All stages between microscopic replacement of cartilage and large bony outgrowths (osteophytes) can be seen. Unresorbed remnants of the original calcified cartilage zone enable the original joint contour to be identified, and may appear in radiographs as a 'double line' at the joint surface. As a rule the cartilage covering this type of osteophyte has a smooth surface but it should be distinguished from normal and early fibrillated cartilage because metabolic activity associated with enchondral ossification may be present and because it contains 'unmasked fibres' — features not seen in normal or early fibrillation (Vignon & Arlot, 1981a). Progressive remodelling usually occurs in those parts of the joint in which an abnormal reduction in stress has probably developed. This suggestion is supported by the following observations: firstly enchondral ossification is the mechanism by which the cartilage of joints immobilised by capsular ossification (Ball, 1970) or by myositis ossificans (Cocchi, 1951) and hence relieved of load-bearing is replaced by bone; secondly enchondral ossification can be induced in areas of joints experimentally relieved of compressive stress (Thompson & Bassett, 1970); and thirdly the bone produced by progressive remodelling is characteristically porotic but undamaged.

Synovial overgrowth of the joint margin may be seen but it does not cause radiological visible erosion. In most cases it can probably be regarded as part of the remodelling process (Meachim, 1972a).

Progressive remodelling is accompanied by regressive remodelling elsewhere in the joint.

Regressive remodelling (Figs 33.10, 33.11, 33.14)
Regressive remodelling occurs in the main load-bearing areas. It leads to an articular surface which lies deep to the plane of the original bone contour. It is associated with zones of bone sclerosis and cystic cavities in the bone at the joint surface. In the femoral head the articular surface in an area of regressive remodelling consists of eburnated (polished) bone studded with varying numbers of fibrous or fibrocartilaginous plugs each approximately 0.5–2 mm in diameter and about 1–2 mm in depth. In macerated specimens they are digested leaving pits in the surface (Fig. 33.13). Some of these plugs appear to be callus formed in response to the collapse of the thin roof of a subchondral cyst or to localised infractions of the bone surface (Fig. 33.14). The uncalcified cartilage at the periphery of an eburnated area is thin, and wedge-shaped in section (Fig. 33.15) and at the

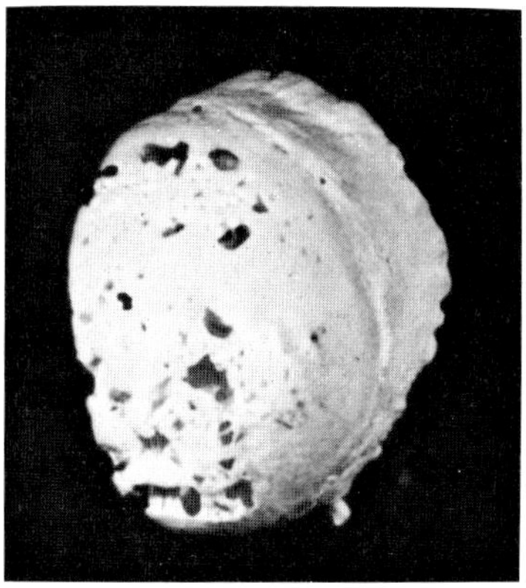

Fig. 33.13 The surface of a hemisected and macerated femoral head showing the pits in the eburnated surface which in the fresh state were occupied by fibrocartilaginous plugs. There is an osteophytic curtain (lower left).

junction with the eburnated surface the calcified layer is exposed. Some abrasion is probably inevitable at this site and may be assumed to cause further destruction of the hyaline cartilage and the shedding of calcific dust (calcospherites) from the calcified layer into the joint fluid.

In areas of regressive remodelling, foci of excessive active bone resorption and reactive bone deposition may be conspicuous especially in the vicinity of cysts and in relation to trabecular microfractures. In these activated foci the marrow spaces in the trabecular bone are oedematous and hyperaemic, but scanty inflammatory cells are only occasionally seen. On the other hand the trabecular bone surfaces may be smooth and inactive and the marrow spaces normal even when a joint articulates on eburnated bone. Thus the bone in late OA may be structurally stable or unstable and in the latter case the bone itself may be a source of pain (Fig. 33.16).

The hyperaemia of articular remodelling, which was documented by Harrison et al (1953), may be associated with increased intraosseous pressure and Arnoldi et al (1972) suggested that this may cause pain. However, Termanson et al (1981)

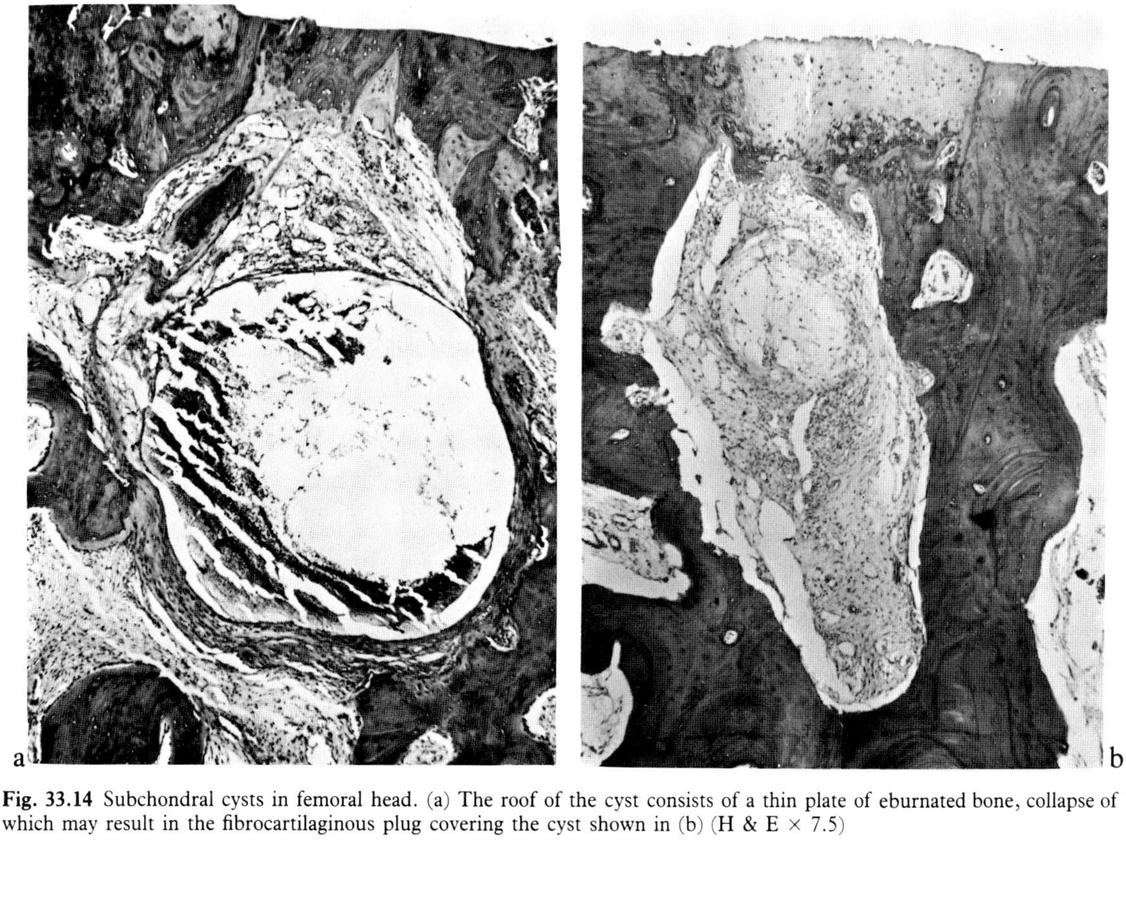

Fig. 33.14 Subchondral cysts in femoral head. (a) The roof of the cyst consists of a thin plate of eburnated bone, collapse of which may result in the fibrocartilaginous plug covering the cyst shown in (b) (H & E × 7.5)

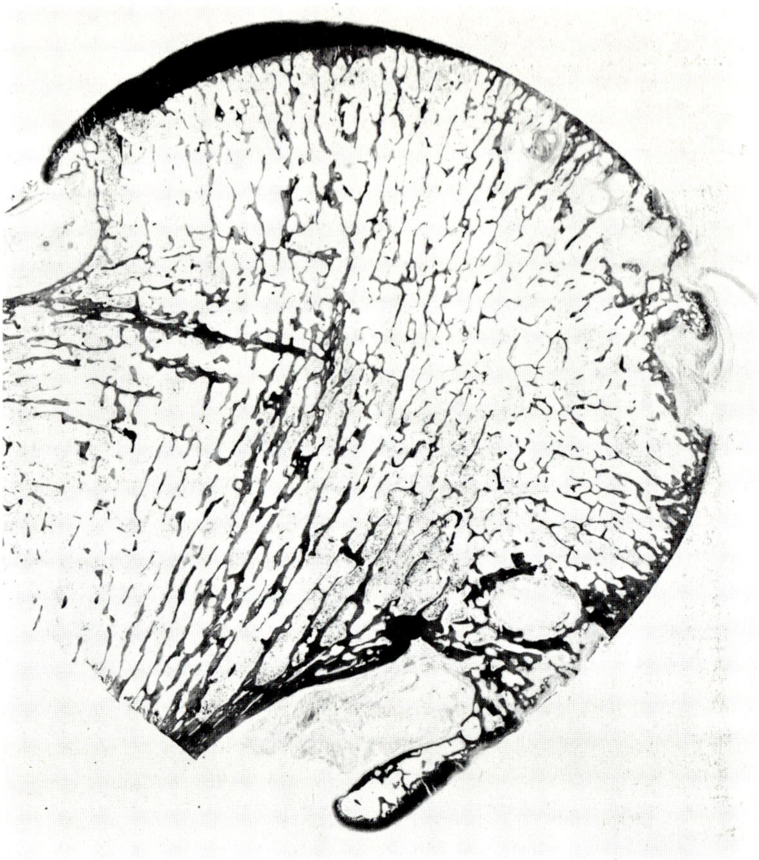

Fig. 33.15 Medial OA of the femoral head in a female aged 60 with GOA and bilateral coxarthrosis. There is bone exposure and cyst formation on the medial (right) side above and below the fovea, but the general shape of the head is largely maintained. Superolaterally the cartilage is well preserved. There is an osteophytic curtain at the joint margin.

found no relation between the intraosseous pressure in the femoral head in patients with primary coxarthrosis and the severity of rest-pain or walking-ability. This does not of course mean that active regressive remodelling is not a source of pain. In this connection it is noteworthy that occult stress fracture of the tibial plateau has been reported as a cause of pain of sudden onset in the early stages of OA in elderly patients (Lotke & Ecker, 1981).

Subchondral bone cysts (Figs 33.11, 33.14) are a characteristic but inconstant feature of OA. They lie singly or in groups just beneath the articular surface and vary from about 1.0 mm–2.0 cm in diameter. Centrally, they usually contain a variable amount of mucinous fluid surrounded by a fibrous layer, supported by a shell of reactive, sclerosed bone. Their pathogenesis remains obscure. In some instances a minute communication with the joint cavity can be demonstrated histologically, but whether this develops before or after the cyst has formed is not known. Another possibility is that they result from the focal transmission to the subchondral marrow of an excessive pulsatile force — a well-known stimulus to bone resorption. Subchondral bone cysts may be absent even in a joint with extensive bone exposure (Fig. 33.16).

Osteophytes are bony outgrowths which most commonly arise at the margin of the joint where perichondrium synovium and bone meet, and they may be restricted to this site (Figs 33.10, 33.15). But progressive remodelling can give rise to an

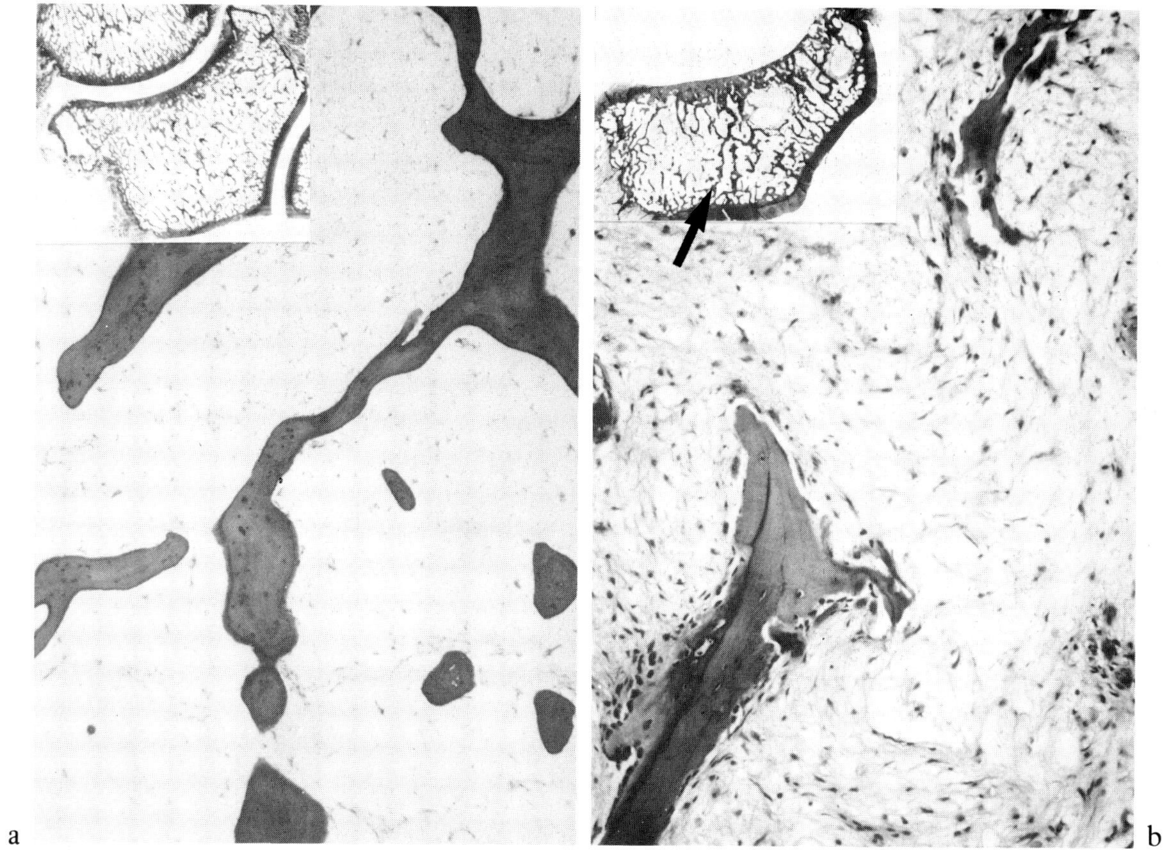

Fig. 33.16 PGOA, 1st CMC joint. (a) Necropsy specimen. The cancellous bone of the trapezium (inset) is healthy (H & E × 50). (b) Surgical specimen from female whose job involved pinch-grip lifting of heavy lead plates and whose pain was cured by excision of the trapezium. Oedema, excessive osteoclastic activity and a healing microfracture in part of the cancellous bone (arrow) of the trapezium (inset). (H & E × 100) In (a) and (b) the joint articulates on eburnated bone.

osteophyte which covers a larger area of the articular surface (see above and Fig. 33.11B). Osteophytes may also arise in the bony attachments of the joint capsule and articular ligaments (Figs 33.10, 33.17). This type of osteophyte may result from a single traumatic incident or reflect prolonged muscular activity (Burke et al, 1977). It is therefore hardly surprising that osteophytes are sometimes seen in the absence of other radiological signs of OA. According to Danielsson (1964) joints of this kind rarely develop unequivocal OA. For these reasons, some workers studying OA of the hip have excluded cases with minor osteophytosis but no other radiological sign of the disease (Hoaglund et al, 1973). In Meachim & Emery's (1974) study of the patellofemoral joints at necropsy, osteophytes were seen only in subjects aged over 50 years. In women there was a good correlation between osteophytosis and full thickness cartilage loss with bone exposure; in men however, the correlation was poor because of the more frequent occurrence of minor marginal osteophytes in the absence of full thickness cartilage loss, though some degree of cartilage fibrillation was present in every case.

Aseptic necrosis

Subchondral aseptic necrosis predisposes to OA, but in the literature it does not appear as a complication of OA due to other causes. This may be partly due to diagnostic difficulties. Plain radiography is insensitive and, histologically, considerable care is required to detect the smaller infarcts which may occupy only a small proportion of the articular surface (Fig. 33.18).

In most specimens of OA some empty osteocyte

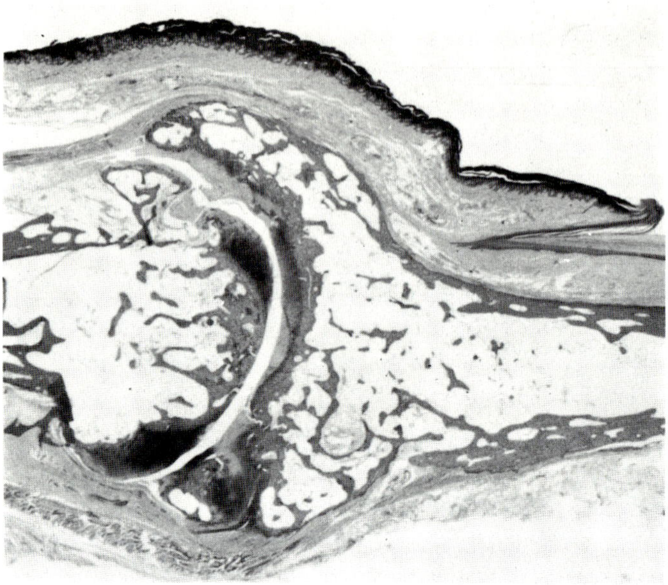

Fig. 33.17 Heberden's node. A bony spur occupies the dorsal capsular tissues. The proximal articular surface consists of eburnated bone centrally.

lacunae (the criterion of bone-cell death) are seen in the surface of eburnated bone and may be assumed to be the direct result of the rubbing of bone on bone. They are also sometimes seen in the thin wall of bone separating adjacent subchondral cysts. But otherwise osteocyte necrosis is inconspicuous and bone infarction as it is commonly understood is not seen in most cases. Nevertheless, it is probably commoner than has been assumed to be the case, at least in the hip where the present writer has occasionally encountered unequivocal evidence of a bone infarct unsuspected clinically or radiologically in patients with coxarthrosis. Recently, Habermann & Hartzband (1982) and Houpt et al (1982) have drawn attention to occult aseptic necrosis as a cause of pain of sudden onset in the knees of elderly patients with radiological signs of OA.

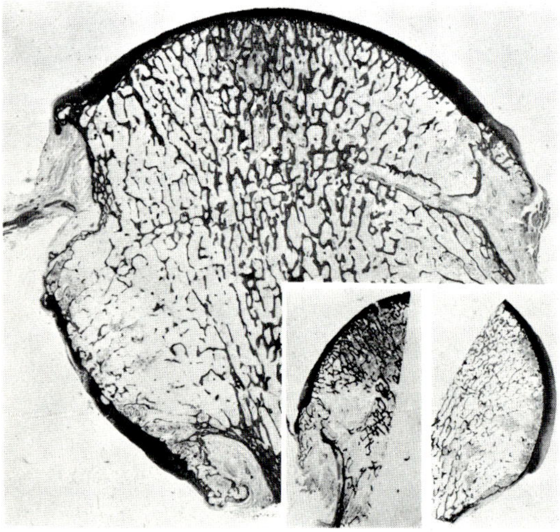

Fig. 33.18 OA and aseptic necrosis in a female aged 73 who suffered from GOA. Femoral head removed at arthroplasty. There is thinning of the cartilage superiorly, but elsewhere it is well preserved as is the general shape. There is a small dark area of dead bone at the zenith, but the bulk of the infarct is in the upper half of the sagittal section of the anterior part of the head (inset left). For comparison a similar section of the posterior part of the head is shown (inset right).

Synovial fluid

Synovial fluid may be normal but small effusions (sometimes misleadingly referred to as 'non-inflammatory') are not uncommon. In these effusions the fluid is usually viscous and forms a fair to good mucin clot. The white cell count is increased but rarely exceeds 5×10^9/l and in most cases is less than 1×10^9/l. Unlike gout, pseudogout and RA, lymphocytes predominate; and unlike RA, immunoblasts are absent (Eghtedari et al, 1980) and complement is not reduced (Bunch et al,

1974). Microscopic fragments of cartilage may be seen. Chemical analysis of the fluid shows the presence of type II but not type I or type III collagen (Cheung et al, 1980). Hydroxyapatite occurs in the form of ultramicroscopic (Dieppe et al, 1976) and microscopic (Gibilisco et al, 1982) clusters of crystals ('calcospherites') especially in severe cases. Surprisingly, they may be found in association with calcium pyrophosphate dihydrate (CPPD) — even in cases which by any other criteria would be diagnosed as OA (Halverson & McCarty, 1979). The significance of hydroxyapatite in OA is discussed below.

An effusion, especially if sudden in onset, may be found to be a haemarthrosis; and repeated haemorrhages are possibly the cause of the rare occurrence of cholesterol crystals (Fam et al, 1981). These crystals are only very weakly phlogistic and the fluids containing them have low cell counts.

Synovium

The inner layer of the joint capsule may be normal, inflamed or fibrosed (Lloyd-Roberts, 1953; Goldenberg et al, 1982). In a post-mortem study of the knee, synoviocyte hyperplasia or lymphocytic infiltration was found in about 16% of cases with minimal or no OA and in about a half of those with moderate or severe OA (Schumacher et al, 1981). In patients with coxarthrosis undergoing prosthetic surgery almost all have some degree of synovial inflammatory cell infiltration and occasionally this may be indistinguishable from that seen in rheumatoid arthritis (Pringle et al, 1978). When present, the synovitis is usually mild: hyperplasia of synoviocytes which show increased lysosomal enzyme activity (Reimann & Christensen, 1979), subintimal and perivascular oedema, hyperaemia and scattered small perivascular lymphocytic aggregates, sometimes admixed with plasma cells may be seen (Fig. 33.19). Unlike rheumatoid arthritis the synoviocytes do not contain inclusions of immunoglobulin and complement (Kinsella et al, 1970), and diffuse lymphocytic and plasma cell infiltration, and surface deposits of fibrin, are rarely seen (Cooper et al, 1981). The changes in OA closely resemble those found in patients with 'post-traumatic synovitis' (Soren et al, 1978), and a similar if less severe 'serous synovitis' occurs in young people with traumatic internal derangements such as a torn meniscus. Since the arthrosic joint may be mechanically defective and liable to recurrent ligamentous sprains (Kellgren, 1961) it is likely that trauma (the commonest cause of transient inflammation) is largely responsible for the synovitis, at least in some cases. Joint laxity

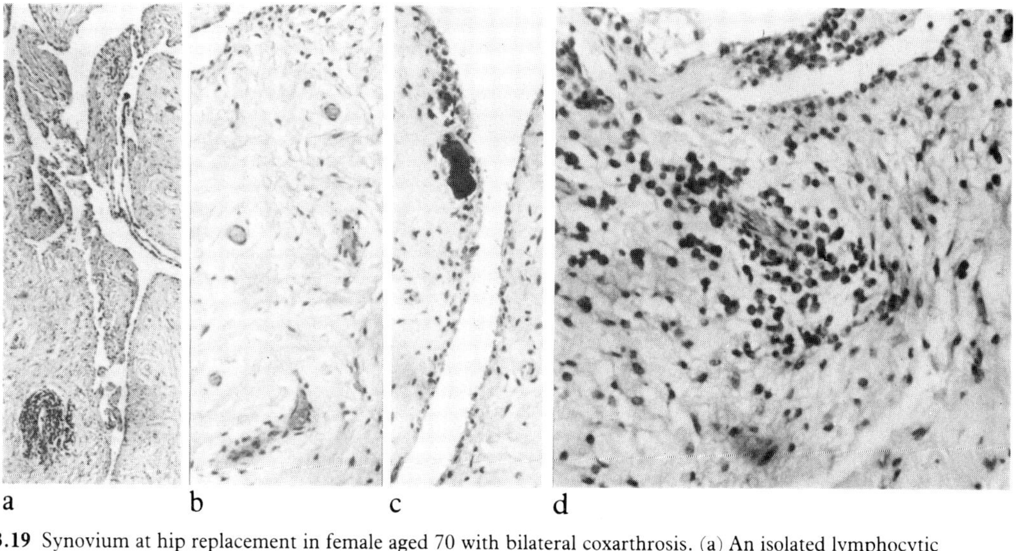

Fig. 33.19 Synovium at hip replacement in female aged 70 with bilateral coxarthrosis. (a) An isolated lymphocytic aggregate. (H & E × 30) (b) Perivascular oedema but no inflammatory cell infiltration. (H & E × 80) (c) A calcific fragment embedded in surface. (H & E × 80) (d) Focal plasma cell and lymphocytic infiltration. (H & E × 155)

may be more important than excessive use as a cause of synovitis in young adults (Bird & Wright, 1981).

In severely damaged joints small fragments of degenerate cartilage or bone are found here and there in the superficial layers of the synovium. They may be associated with a foreign body type reaction but not as a rule with other inflammatory cells; more often they are embedded in bland fibrous tissue. These findings and the report of Golds et al (1981) that peripheral blood mononuclear cells in OA are unresponsive to type II collagen and cartilage proteoglycans seem to indicate that the synovitis is not due to an immune response to cartilage matrix antigens. These relatively large fragments of joint detritus clearly act as a mild irritant, at least for a time, but as they probably accumulate slowly it is questionable whether they alone are ever a cause of the episodic effusions in OA — though this is often implied in the literature.

In patients with OA, particles of hydroxyapatite (calcospherites) similar to those sometimes found in the synovial fluid may be seen in the synovium but here they are usually inconspicuous (Doyle, 1982). Their provenance is uncertain but exposed calcified cartilage and areas of calcification in the fibrocartilaginous plugs are obvious potential sources; and in cases with aseptic necrosis calcified deposits in the dead marrow are another potential source. The attractive hypothesis (Dieppe et al, 1976) that the calcospherites in the fluid and/or synovium are a major cause of synovitis has now been abandoned on clinical (Dieppe, 1981) and pathological (Doyle, 1982) grounds. Rarely, prominent deposits of calcospherites occur in the superficial synovium especially in cases of aseptic necrosis (personal observations). In these cases there is marked hypertrophy and hyperplasia of synoviocytes and a deeper histiocytic reaction including giant cells but other inflammatory cells are conspicuously sparse (Fig. 33.20). It is clear from studies of the 'Milwaukee shoulder' (McCarty et al, 1981) that joint damage, massive deposits of calcospherites in synovium and synovial fluid and excessive production of neutral protease and active collagenase by synoviocytes (Cheung et al, 1981) may occur with no increase in inflammatory cells in the synovial fluid. Thus if calcospherites have a significant role in OA it might reside in their ability to stimulate the release from macrophages of degradative enzymes and possibly factors causing pain. However, active collagenase was not detected by Halverson et al (1981) in the OA fluids they tested. Perhaps as Halverson & McCarty (1979) suggest, the relatively small amount of calcospherites in fluid and/or synovium simply reflect severity in OA.

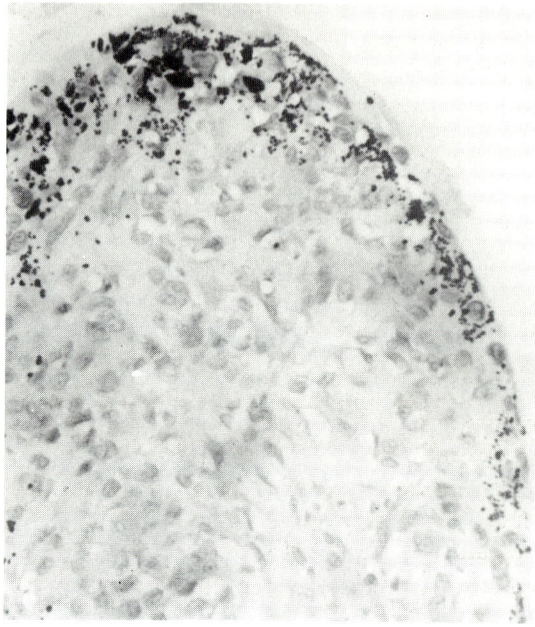

Fig. 33.20 Synovium at hip replacement in aseptic necrosis. Numerous calcospherites in superficial layers; synoviocyte hyperplasia and histiocytic infiltration but no other inflammatory cells. (Von Kossa and neutral red × 300)

In OA associated with pyrophosphate arthropathy crystals of CPPD are deposited in the synovium in which a cellular reaction, if present, is usually histiocytic. The relationship between CPPD and OA is discussed elsewhere (Ch. 37). Here it may be noted that the crystal size of CPPD and its propensity to form large deposits in the superficial layers of articular cartilage set it apart from apatite and accord with the concept (Dieppe et al, 1982) that whilst its deposition is favoured by primary cartilage disorders its presence promotes OA.

The relationship between synovitis and OA

Inflammatory joint diseases such as gout and rheumatoid arthritis, if not too severe, predispose to OA. The mechanisms have yet to be defined. Disuse, which can cause reversible chondrocyte-mediated loss and defective aggregation of proteoglycans (Palmoski et al, 1979), the increased metabolism in the joint as a whole, and 'mononuclear cell factor', which, in vitro, induces cartilage matrix degration by chondrocyte activation (Jasin & Dingle, 1981), may all be involved.

By definition the cause of primary OA is unknown. Nevertheless, Kellgren et al (1963) found an excess of seronegative polyarthritis in relatives of probands with primary non-nodal GOA suggesting that this relatively uncommon form of OA may be the late result of an occult synovitis. In primary nodal GOA (the commonest type of OA) some patients experience an initial painful phase, the nature of which is obscure but which, according to Kellgren (1961), differs in several ways from the pain due to trauma or inflammatory states such as rheumatoid arthritis. Recent in vitro studies have shown that, in culture, normal pig synovium (Jubb & Fell, 1980) and human synovium from joints with primary OA (Herman et al, 1981) contain and/or produce a factor which can induce a reversible chondrocyte-mediated reduction in glycosaminoglycan synthesis. Whether such a 'synovial factor' is involved in the *aetiology* of primary OA is unknown. The episodic secondary synovitis (see above) which commonly occurs in primary and secondary OA is obviously a potential source of 'synovial factor' and possibly of 'mononuclear cell factor' but to what extent, if any, these contribute to the *progression* of OA remains speculative.

'Erosive osteoarthritis' (EOA)

This term was introduced by Peter et al (1966) to describe a symmetrical seronegative arthropathy mainly affecting the hands, especially the distal and proximal interphalangeal joints in which articular erosions occur in addition to subchondral cysts and osteophytes. Ehrlich (1972) used the term 'inflammatory osteoarthritis' to describe these cases and showed that in a minority definite rheumatoid arthritis supervened. The synovium was histologically similar to active rheumatoid arthritis in 3 of the 6 patients studied by Peter et al but there was little or no inflammation in the others. In 10 of the 15 patients examined by Utsinger et al (1978) the synovial fluid white cell count was less than 2×10^9/l and synovial fluid immune complexes were detected by the Raji cell test in only two. However Utsinger & Fite (1982) reported that in EOA, unlike OA, there is an increase in the OKT8 subset of T lymphocytes in the synovial fluid (as there is in rheumatoid arthritis) indicating the presence in EOA of an immunologically determined inflammatory process. Perhaps EOA represents, at least in some patients, the coincidence of two common diseases, GOA and a mild variant of rheumatoid arthritis both of which commonly affect the hands of middle-aged and elderly females.

Comparative pathology

As in man, primary and secondary OA occur in wild and domesticated animals. For example, coxarthrosis in the German Shepherd dog is the result of acetabular dysplasia; but other breeds of dog suffer from a more generalised form of OA for which a cause has not been identified and in which the hip is rarely affected (Sokoloff, 1969, 1981). The hip is also spared and the knee always affected in the polyarticular OA to which some strains of mice are susceptible. In the STR/IN strain the OA has been shown to be genetically based but genetically dissociated from the obesity to which these mice are also prone (Sokoloff et al, 1962). In parenthesis it may be noted that the influences of obesity in OA in the human is mainly expressed in the knees, perhaps, as suggested by Radin et al (1972) because people with obese thighs tend to walk bow-legged thus excessively loading the medial compartment of the knee. The distribution of OA in STR/IN mice implies involvement of local factors. In STR/ORT mice (a substrain of STR/IN mice) it has indeed been shown that the OA in the knee is due to patellar dislocation and does not occur if this is surgically prevented (Walton, 1979). Thus it seems that in this joint the genetic influence is expressed as a local anatomic defect. In other joints it is not known how the genetic factor operates.

In most strains of mice males are more often affected than females whereas in human GOA the opposite is the case. In man and mouse the nature of the sex factor is unexplained.

REFERENCES

Ali S Y, Evans L 1973 Enzymic degradation of cartilage in osteoarthritis. Federation Proceedings 32: 1494–1498

Ali S Y, Bayliss M T 1974 Enzymic changes in human osteoarthrotic cartilage. In: Ali S Y, Elves M W, Leaback D H (Eds) Normal and osteoarthrotic articular cartilage. Institute of Orthopaedics, University of London, p 189–203

Altman R D, Pardo V, Tenenbaum J, Latta L L, Alzamora D, Howell D S 1980 Morphologic changes and swelling properties of osteoarthritis dog cartilage. Arthritis and Rheumatism 23: 648–649

Anderson J A D, Duthie J J R 1963 Rheumatic complaints in dockyard workers. Annals of the Rheumatic Diseases 22: 401–409

Anderson J A D, Duthie J J R, Moody B P 1962 Social and economic effects of rheumatic diseases in a mining population. Annals of the Rheumatic Diseases 21: 342–352

Armstrong C G, Bahrani A S, Gardner D L 1980 Changes in the deformational behaviour of human hip cartilage with age. Journal of Biomechanical Engineering 102: 214–220

Arnoldi C C, Linderholm H, Mussbichler H 1972 Venous engorgement and intraosseous hypertension in osteoarthritis of the hip. The Journal of Bone and Joint Surgery 54-B: 409–421

Ball J 1970 Enthesopathy of rheumatoid and ankylosing spondylitis. Annals of the Rheumatic Diseases 30: 213–223

Bayliss M T, Ali S Y 1978a Studies on cathepsin B in human articular cartilage. Biochemical Journal 171: 149–154

Bayliss M T, Ali S Y 1978b Age-related changes in the composition and structure of human articular-cartilage proteoglycans. Biochemical Journal 176: 683–693

Bentley G 1972 Papain-induced degenerative arthritis of the hip in rabbits. The Journal of Bone and Joint Surgery 53-B: 324–337

Bird H A, Wright V 1981 Traumatic synovitis in a classical guitarist: a study of joint laxity. Annals of the Rheumatic Diseases 40: 161–163

Brandt K D 1977 Proteoglycans: Structure and metabolism. Arthritis and Rheumatism 20 (Suppl): 109–114

Brocklehurst R, Maroudas A 1981 Comparative studies of composition and sulphate uptake in normal and osteoarthrotic cartilage from the knee, the hip and the ankle. In: Peyron J G (ed) Epidemiology of osteoarthritis. Ciba-Geigy, Paris, p 124

Bullough P G, Goodfellow J W, O'Connor J J 1973 The relationship between degenerative changes and load-bearing in the human hip. The Journal of Bone and Joint Surgery 55-B: 746–758

Bunch T W, Hunder G G, McDuffie F C, O'Brien P C, Markowitz H 1974 Synovial fluid compliment determination as a diagnostic aid in inflammatory joint disease. Mayo Clinic Proceedings 49: 715–720

Burgeson R 1982 Articular cartilage, intervertebral disc, synovia. In: Weiss J B, Jayson M I V (eds) Collagen in health and disease. Churchill Livingstone, London, Ch 18, p 335–361

Burke M J, Fear E C, Wright V 1977 Bone and joint changes in pneumatic drillers. Annals of the Rheumatic Diseases 36: 276–279

Byers P D, Contepomi C A, Farkas T A 1970 A post mortem study of the hip joint including the prevalence of features on the right side. Annals of the Rheumatic Diseases 29: 15–31

Byers P D, Hoaglund F T, Purewal G S, Yau A C M C 1974 A comparison between articular cartilage changes in Caucasian and Asian hip joints. Annals of the Rheumatic Diseases 33:157

Campbell C J 1969 The healing of cartilage defects.·Clinical Orthopaedics and Related Research 64: 45–63

Carlson H 1957 Reactions of rabbit patellary cartilage following operative defects. Acta Orthopaedica Scandinavica, Supplement 28

Carlsson A, Nilsson B E, Westlin N E 1979 Bone mass in primary coxarthrosis. Acta Orthopaedica Scandinavica 50: 187–189

Cheung H S, Ryan L M, Kozin F, McCarty D J 1980 Identification of collagen subtypes in synovial fluid sediments from arthritic patients. The American Journal of Medicine 68: 73–79

Cheung H S, Halverson P B, McCarty D J 1981 Release of collagenase neutral protease and prostaglandins from cultured mammalian synovial cells by hydroxyapatite and calcium pyrophosphate dihydrate crystals. Arthritis and Rheumatism 24: 1338–1344

Cocchi U 1951 Hereditary disease with bone changes. In: Schintz H R, Baensch W E, Friede E, Uelinger E (eds) Roentgen diagnosis, 5th Edn (English translation). Heinemann, London, p 644–868

Cooke T D, Bennett E, Wright L, Wyllie J 1981 Relationships of immune deposits in osteoarthritic (OA) cartilage to disease site, pattern and synovial reaction. In: Peyron J G (ed) Epidemiology of osteoarthritis. Ciba-Geigy, Paris, p 113–123

Cooper N S, Soren A, McEwen C, Rosenberger J L 1981 Diagnostic specificity of synovial lesions. Human Pathology 12: 314–328

Danielsson L G 1964 Incidence and prognosis of coxarthrosis. Acta Orthopaedica Scandinavica (Suppl 66)

Davis W H, Lee S L, Sokoloff L 1978 Boundary lubricating ability of synovial fluid in degenerative joint disease. Arthritis and Rheumatism 21: 754–760

Day W H, Swanson S A V, Freeman M A R 1975 Contact pressures in the loaded human cadaver hip. The Journal of Bone and Joint Surgery 57-B: 302–313

Dieppe P A 1981 Calcium phosphate crystal deposition and clinical subsets of osteoarthritis. In: Peyron J G (ed) Epidemiology of osteoarthritis. Ciba-Geigy, Paris, p 71–80

Dieppe et al 1982 Pyrophosphate arthropathy: a clinical and radiological study of 105 cases. Annals of the Rheumatic Diseases 41: 371–376

Dieppe P A, Crocker P R, Huskisson E C, Willoughby D A 1976 Apatite deposition disease: A new arthropathy. Lancet 2: 266–269

Doyle D V 1982 Tissue calcification and inflammation in osteoarthritis. The Journal of Pathology 136: 199–216

Eghtedari A A, Bacon P A, Collins A 1980 Immunoblasts in synovial fluid and blood in the rheumatic diseases. Annals of the Rheumatic Diseases 39: 318–322

Ehrlich G E 1972 Inflammatory osteoarthritis: II. The superimposition of rheumatoid arthritis. Journal of Chronic Diseases 25: 635–643

Ehrlich M G, Houle P A, Vigliani G, Mankin H J 1978 Correlation between articular cartilage collagenase activity and osteoarthritis. Arthritis and Rheumatism 21: 761–766

Evans H B et al 1983 Localisation of collagen types and

fibronectin in cartilage by immunofluorescence. Annals of the Rheumatic Diseases 42: 575–581
Fam A C, Pritzker K P H, Cheng P T, Little A H 1981 Cholesterol crystals in osteoarthritic joint effusions. The Journal of Rheumatology 8: 273–280
Foss M V L, Byers P D 1972 Bone density, osteoarthrosis of the hip, and fracture of the upper end of the femur. Annals of the Rheumatic Diseases 31: 259–264
Freeman M A R, Swanson S A V, Manley P T 1975 Stress-lowering function of articular cartilage. Medical Biological Engineering 13: 245–251
Gardner D L, O'Connor P, Oates K 1981 Low temperature scanning electron microscopy of dog and guinea-pig hyaline articular cartilage. Journal of Anatomy 132: 267–282
Garrod A E 1907 Rheumatoid arthritis, osteoarthritis and arthritis deformans. In: Allbutt T C, Rolleston H D (eds) A system of medicine. Macmillan, London, 3: 3–43
Gay S, Muller P K, Lemmen C, Remberger K, Matzen K, Kuhn K 1976 Immunohistological study on collagen in cartilage-bone metamorphosis and degenerative osteoarthrosis Klinike Wochenschrift 54: 969–976
Ghadially F N, Thomas I, Oryschak A F, La Ronde J M 1977 Long term results of superficial defects in articular cartilage. A scanning electron microscope study. The Journal of Pathology 121: 213–217
Gibilisko P A, Schumacher H R, Sieck M, Reginato A, Paul H 1982 Studies on the role of synovial fluid apatite and calcium pyrophosphate crystals in osteoarthritis. Arthritis and Rheumatism 25 (Suppl): 43
Goffin Y A, Thoua Y, Potvliege P R 1981 Microdeposition of amyloid in the joints. Annals of the Rheumatic Diseases 40: 27–33
Goldenberg D L, Egan M S, Cohen A S 1982 Inflammatory synovitis in degenerative joint disease. The Journal of Rheumatology 9: 204–209
Golds E E, Poole A R, Esdaile J, Strawcynzki H, Cooke T D V 1981 Stimulation of mononuclear cell factor synthesis in patients with connective tissue disease. Arthritis and Rheumatism 24 (Suppl): 93
Goodfellow J W, Bullough P G 1967 The pattern of ageing of the articular cartilage of the elbow joint. The Journal of Bone and Joint Surgery 49-B: 175–181
Goodfellow J, Hungerford D S, Woods C 1976 Patello-femoral joint mechanics and pathology. 2. Chondromalacia patellae. The Journal of Bone and Joint Surgery 58-B: 291–299
Gordon T 1968 Osteoarthrosis in U S adults. In: Bennett P H, Wood P H N (eds) Population studies of the rheumatic diseases. International Congress Series No 148. Excerpta Medica, Amsterdam
Grigg P, Finerman G A, Riley L H 1973 Joint position sense after total hip replacement. The Journal of Bone and Joint Surgery 55-A: 1016–1025
Habermann E T, Hartzband M A 1982 Osteonecrosis of the knee. Arthritis and Rheumatism 25 (Suppl): 9
Halverson P B, McCarty D J 1979 Identification of hydroxyapatite crystals in synovial fluid. Arthritis and Rheumatism 22: 389–395
Halverson P B, Cheung H S, McCarty D J, Garancis J, Mandel N 1981 'Milwaukee shoulder' — association of microspheroids containing hydroxyapatite crystals, active collagenase and neutral protease with rotator cuff defects. II. Synovial fluid studies. Arthritis and Rheumatism 24: 474–483
Harrison M H M, Schajowicz F, Trueta J 1953 Osteoarthritis of the hip: A study of the nature and evolution of the disease. The Journal of Bone and Joint Surgery 35-B: 598–626
Heine J 1926 Über die arthritis deformans. Virchows Archives für Pathologische Anatomie 260: 521–663
Herman J H, Appel A M, Pordy M G, Hopson C N 1981 Modulation of chondrocyte glycosaminoglycan synthesis and induction of cartilage proteoglycan degradation by primary osteoarthritic synovium. Arthritis and Rheumatism 24 (Suppl): 68
Hoaglund F T, Yau A C M C, Wong W L 1973 Osteoarthritis of the hip and other joints in southern chinese in Hong Kong. Incidence and related factors. The Journal of Bone and Joint Surgery 55-A: 545–557
Hoffa A, Wollenberg G A 1908 Arthritis deformans und sogenannter chronischer Gelenrheumatismus. Eine rontgenologische und anatomische studie. Enke, Stuttgart
Houpt J B et al 1982 Spontaneous osteonecrosis of the medial tibial plateau. The Journal of Rheumatology 9: 81–90
Howell D S, Woessner J F, Jimenez S, Seda H, Schumacher H R 1979 A view on the pathogenesis of osteoarthritis. Bulletin on the Rheumatic Diseases 29: 996–1001
Hukins D W L 1982 Biomechanical properties of collagen. In Weiss J B, Jayson M I V (eds) Collagen in health and disease. Churchill Livingstone, London, Ch 4, p 49–72
Jasin H E, Dingle J T 1981 Human mononuclear cell factors mediate cartilage matrix degradation through chondrocyte activation. Arthritis and Rheumatism 24 (Suppl): 106
Johnson L C 1962 Joint remodelling as the basis for osteoarthritis. Journal of the American Veterinary Medical Association 141: 1237–1241
Jubb R W, Fell H B 1980 The effect of synovial tissue on the synthesis of proteoglycan by the articular cartilage of young pigs. Arthritis and Rheumatism 23: 545–555
Kellgren J H 1961 Osteoarthrosis in patients and populations. British Medical Journal 2: 1–6
Kellgren J H, Lawrence J S, Aitken-Swan J 1953 Rheumatic complaints in an urban population. Annals of the Rheumatic Diseases 12: 5–15
Kellgren J H, Lawrence J S, Bier F 1963 Genetic factors in generalised osteoarthrosis. Annals of the Rheumatic Diseases 22: 237–255
Kempson G E 1980 The mechanical properties of articular cartilage. In: Sokoloff L (ed) The joints and synovial fluid. Academic Press, London, 11: Ch 5, p 177–238
Kempson G E 1982 Relationship between the tensile properties of articular cartilage from the human knee and age. Annals of the Rheumatic Diseases 41: 508–511
Kinsella T D, Baum J, Ziff M 1970 Studies of isolated synovial lining cells of rheumatoid and nonrheumatoid synovial membranes. Arthritis and Rheumatism 13. 734–753
Kuettner K E, Harper E, Eisenstein R 1977 Protease inhibitors in cartilage. Arthritis and Rheumatism 20 (Suppl): 124–132
Ladefoged C 1982 Amyloid in osteoarthritic hip joints: a pathological and histological investigation of femoral head cartilage. Acta Orthopaedica Scandinavica 41: 512–519
Lawrence J S, Bremner J M, Bier F 1966 Osteoarthrosis. Annals of the Rheumatic Diseases 25: 1–24
Lippiello L, Hall D, Mankin H J 1977 Collagen synthesis in normal and osteoarthritic human cartilage. Journal of Clinical Investigation 59: 593–600
Lloyd-Roberts G C 1953 The role of capsular changes in

osteoarthritis of the hip joint. The Journal of Bone and Joint Surgery 35-B: 627–642
Lotke P A, Ecker M L 1981 Painful knee in older patients — II. Possible stress fracture in tibial plateau. Arthritis and Rheumatism 24 (Suppl): 61
McCarty D J, Halverson P B, Carrera G F, Brewer B J, Kozin F 1981 'Milwaukee shoulder' — association of microspheroids containing hydroxyapatite crystals, active collagenase, and neutral protease with rotator cuff defects. I. Clinical aspects. Arthritis and Rheumatism 24: 464–473
McDevitt C A, Gilbertson E M M, Muir H 1977. An experimental model of osteoarthritis; early morphological and biochemical changes. The Journal of Bone and Joint Surgery 59-B: 24–35
McKenzie L S, Horsburgh B A, Ghosh P, Taylor T K F 1977 Sulphated glycosaminoglycan synthesis in normal and osteoarthrotic hip cartilage. Annals of the Rheumatic Diseases 36: 369–373
McKibbin B, Maroudas A 1979 Nutrition and metabolism. In: Freeman M A R (ed) Adult articular cartilage 2nd Edn. Pitman Medical, London, Ch 8, p 461–486
Mankin H J 1974 The reaction of articular cartilage to injury and osteoarthritis. The New England Journal of Medicine 291: 1285–1292
Mankin H J 1982 The response of articular cartilage to mechanical injury. The Journal of Bone and Joint Surgery 64-A: 460–466
Mankin H J, Dorfman H, Lippiello L, Zarins A 1971 Biochemical and metabolic abnormalities in articular cartilage from osteoarthritic human hips. The Journal of Bone and Joint Surgery 51-A: 1591–1600
Mankin H J, Johnson M E, Lippiello L 1981 Biochemical and Metabolic abnormalities in articular cartilage from osteoarthritic human hips. The Journal of Bone and Joint Surgery 63-A: 131–139
Maroudas A 1973 Physico-chemical properties of articular cartilage. In: Freeman M A R (ed) Adult articular cartilage. Pitman Medical, London, Ch 4, p 131–170
Maroudas A 1979 Physicochemical properties of articular cartilage. In: Freeman M A R (ed) Adult articular cartilage, 2nd Edn. Pitman Medical, London, Ch 4, p 215–290
Maroudas A 1980 Physical chemistry of articular cartilage and the intervertebral disc. In: Sokoloff L (ed) The joints and synovial fluid. Academic Press, London, 11: Ch 6, p 239–291
Maroudas A, Venn M F 1977 Chemical composition and swelling of normal and osteoarthrotic femoral head cartilage. Annals of the Rheumatic Diseases 36: 399–406
Maroudas A, Evans H, Almeida L 1973 Cartilage of the hip joint. Topographical variation of glycosaminoglycan content in normal and fibrillated tissue. Annals of the Rheumatic Diseases 32: 1–9
Maroudas A, Bayliss M T, Venn M F 1980 Further studies on the composition of human femoral head cartilage. Annals of the Rheumatic Diseases 39: 514–523
Meachim G 1964 Sulphate metabolism of articular cartilage after surgical interference with the joint. Annals of the Rheumatic Diseases 23: 372–380
Meachim G 1972a Articular cartilage lesions in osteoarthritis of the femoral head. The Journal of Pathology 107: 199–210
Meachim G 1972b Light microscopy of Indian ink preparations of fibrillated cartilage. Annals of the Rheumatic Diseases 31: 457–469
Meachim G, Emery I H 1973 Cartilage fibrillation in shoulder and hip joints in Liverpool necropsies. Journal of Anatomy 116: 161–179
Meachim G, Emery I H 1974 Quantitative aspects of patello-femoral cartilage fibrillation in Liverpool necropsies. Annals of the Rheumatic Diseases 33: 39–47
Meachim G, Ghadially F N, Collins D H 1965 Regressive changes in the superficial layer of human articular cartilage. Annals of the Rheumatic Diseases 24: 23–30
Mitrovic D, Gruson M, Demignon J, Mercier Ph, Aprile F, De Seze S 1981 Metabolism of human femoral head cartilage in osteoarthrosis and subcapital fracture. Annals of the Rheumatic Diseases 40: 18–26
Moskowitz R W, Howell D S, Goldberg V M, Muniz O, Pita J C 1979 Cartilage proteoglycan alterations in an experimentally induced model of rabbit osteoarthritis. Arthritis and Rheumatism 22: 155–163
Muir H 1977 Molecular approach to the understanding of osteoarthrosis. Annals of the Rheumatic Diseases 36: 199–208
Muir H 1979 Biochemistry. In: Freeman M A R (ed) Adult articular cartilage, 2nd Edn. Pitman Medical, London, Ch 3, p 145–214
Murray D G 1964 Experimentally induced arthritis using intra-articular papain. Arthritis and Rheumatism 7: 211–219
Nichols E H, Richardson F L 1909 Arthritis deformans. Journal of Medical Research 21: 149–222
Nuki G 1983 Personal communication
Palmoski M J, Brandt K D 1982 Immobilisation of the knee prevents osteoarthrosis after anterior cruciate ligament transection. Arthritis and Rheumatism 25: 1201–1208
Palmoski M J, Perricone E, Brandt K D 1979 Development and reversal of a proteoglycan aggregation defect in normal canine knee cartilage after immobilisation. Arthritis and Rheumatism 22: 508–517
Paul J P 1980 Joint Kinetics. In: Sokoloff L (ed) The joints and synovial fluid. Academic Press, London, 11: Ch 4, p 139–176
Peter J B, Pearson C M, Marmor L 1966 Erosive osteoarthritis of the hands. Arthritis and Rheumatism 9: 365–388
Price T, Reeve J, Mitchell R, Hesp R 1983 Bone density in generalised osteoarthritis. Annals of the Rheumatic Diseases 42: 227–228
Pringle J A, Byers P D, Brown M E A 1978 Immunofluorescence in osteoarthritis. Nature 274:94
Radin E L, Paul I L 1970 Does cartilage compliance reduce skeletal impact loads? Arthritis and Rheumatism 13: 139–144
Radin E L, Paul I L, Rose R M 1972 Role of mechanical factors in pathogenesis of primary osteoarthritis. Lancet i: 519–522
Radin E L, Ehrlich M G, Chernack R, Abernethy P, Paul I L, Rose R M 1978 Effect of repetitive impulse loading on the knee joints of rabbits. Clinical Orthopaedics and related research 131: 288–293
Radin E L, Swann D A, Paul I L, McGrath P J 1982 Factors influencing articular cartilage wear in vitro. Arthritis and Rheumatism 25: 974–980
Reimann I 1973 Experimental osteoarthritis of the knee in rabbits induced by alteration of the load-bearing. Acta Orthopaedica Scandinavica 44: 496–504
Reimann I, Christensen S B 1979 A histochemical study of alkaline and acid phosphatase activity in osteoarthritic

synovial membrane. Scandinavian Journal of Rheumatology 8: 39–42
Repo R U, Mitchell N 1971 Collagen synthesis in mature articular cartilage of the rabbit. The Journal of Bone and Joint Surgery 53-B: 541–548
Roberts B J, Unsworth A, Mian N 1982 Modes of lubrication in human hip joints. Annals of the Rheumatic Diseases 41: 217–224
Roh Y S, Dequeker J, Mulier J C 1974 Bone mass in osteoarthrosis, measured in vivo by photon absorption. The Journal of Bone and Joint Surgery 56-A: 587–591
Rüttner J R, Spycher A M, Werner G, Amado R 1974 Biochemical and morphological studies on the cartilage of the femoral head. Verhandlungen der Deutschen Gesellschaft für Pathologie 58: 392–394
Sapolsky A I , Keiser H, Howell D S, Woessner J F 1976 Metalloproteinases of human articular cartilage that digest cartilage proteoglycan at neutral and acid pH. Journal of Clinical Investigation 58: 1030–1041
Schumacher H R, Gordon G, Paul H 1981 Osteoarthritis, crystal deposition and inflammation. Seminars in Arthritis and Rheumatism (S1) 11: 116–119
Simunek Z, Muir H 1972 Changes in the protein-polysaccharides of pig articular cartilage during prenatal life, development and old age. Biochemical Journal 126: 515–523
Sokoloff L 1966 Elasticity of ageing cartilage. Federation Proceedings 25: 1089–1095
Sokoloff L 1969 The biology of degenerative joint disease. The University of Chicago Press, Chicago
Sokoloff L 1974 Cell biology and the repair of articular cartilage. The Journal of Rheumatology 1: 1–16
Sokoloff L 1981 Comparative pathology of degenerative joint disease. In: Peyron J G (ed) Epidemiology of osteoarthritis. Ciba-Geigy, Paris, p 81
Sokoloff L, Crittenden L B, Yamamoto R S, Jay G E 1962 The genetics of degenerative joint disease in mice. Arthritis and Rheumatism 5: 531–546
Solomon L, Schnitzler C M, Browett J P 1982 Osteoarthritis of the hip: the patient behind the disease. Annals of the Rheumatic Diseases 41: 118–125
Soren A, Klein W, Huth F 1978 The synovial changes in post-traumatic synovitis and osteoarthritis. Rheumatology and Rehabilitation 17: 38–45
Sorgente N, Kuettner K E, Soble L W, Eisenstein R 1975 The resistence of certain tissues to invasion. II. Evidence for extractable factors in cartilage which inhibit invasion by vascularised mesenchyme. Laboratory Investigation 32: 217–222
Stack M T, Brandt K D 1982 Identification and characterisation of articular cartilage hyaluronidase. Arthritis and Rheumatism 25 (Suppl): 100
Statistical Appendix 1972 Morbidity and mortality and hospital services for rheumatism sufferers. Annals of the Rheumatic Diseases 31: 522–529
Swann D A, Radin E L, Nazimiec M, Wrisser P A, Curran N, Lewinnek G 1974 Role of hyaluronic acid in joint lubrication. Annals of the Rheumatic Diseases 33: 318–326
Swann D A, Block K J, Sotman S, Shipner R, Swindell D 1981 Isolation of a purified glycoprotein lubricating fraction from human synovial fluid. Arthritis and Rheumatism 24 (Suppl): 88
Swanson S A V 1979 Friction, wear and lubrication. In: Freeman M A R (ed) Adult articular cartilage, 2nd Edn. Pitman Medical, London, Ch 7, p 415–460
Sweet M B E, Thonar E J M A, Immelman A R, Solomon L 1977 Biochemical changes in progressive osteoarthrosis. Annals of the Rheumatic Diseases 36: 387–398
Termansen N B, Jeglbjaerg P S, Sorensen K H 1981 Primary osteoarthritis of the hip. Interrelationship between intraosseous pressure, X-ray changes, clinical severity and bone density. Acta Orthopaedica Scandinavica 52: 215–222
Thompson R C, Bassett C A 1970 Histological observations on experimentally induced degeneration of articular cartilage. The Journal of Bone and Joint Surgery 52-A: 435–443
Thompson R C, Oegema T R 1979 Metabolic activity of articular cartilage in osteoarthritis. The Journal of Bone and Joint Surgery 61-A: 407–416
Unsworth A, Dowson D, Wright V 1975 Some new evidence on human joint lubrication. Annals of the Rheumatic Diseases 34: 277–285
Utsinger P D, Fite F L 1982 Immunologic evidence for inflammation in osteoarthritis: High percentage of Ia+ T lymphocytes in the synovial fluid and synovium of patients with erosive osteoarthritis. Arthritis and Rheumatism 25 (Suppl): 44
Utsinger P D, Resnick D, Shapiro R F, Wiesner K B 1978 Roentgenologic, immunologic and therapeutic study of erosive (inflammatory) osteoarthritis. Archives of Internal Medicine 138: 693–697
Venn M F 1978 Variation of chemical composition with age in human femoral head cartilage. Annals of the Rheumatic Diseases 37: 168–174
Venn M F 1979 Chemical composition of human femoral head cartilage: influence of topographical position and fibrillation. Annals of the Rheumatic Diseases 38: 57–62
Vignon E, Arlot M 1981a Macroscopically normal cartilage from the human osteoarthritic femoral head. The Journal of Rheumatology 8: 440–446
Vignon E, Arlot M 1981b Macroscopically normal cartilage from the human osteoarthritic femoral head. The Journal of Rheumatology 8: 447–450
Viidik A 1973 Functional properties of collagenous tissues. In: Hall D A, Jackson D S (eds) International review of connective tissue research. Academic Press, London, 6: Ch 3, p 127–215
Walton M 1979 Patella displacement and osteoarthrosis of the knee joint in mice. The Journal of Pathology 127: 165–172
Weightman B, Kempson G E 1979 Load carriage. In: Freeman M A R (ed) Adult articular cartilage, 2nd Edn. Pitman Medical, London, Ch 5, p 291
Weightman B, Chappell D J, Jenkins E A 1978 A second study of tensile fatigue properties of human articular cartilage. Annals of the Rheumatic Diseases 37: 58–63
Weiss C, Mirow S 1972 An ultrastructural study of osteoarthric changes in the articular cartilage of human knees. The Journal of Bone and Joint Surgery 54-A: 954–972
Wyke B D 1967 The neurology of joints. Annals of the Royal College of Surgeons of England 41: 25–50

Clinical aspects of osteoarthrosis

Osteoarthrosis is best regarded as the clinical manifestation of joint failure. It is not a single disease entity, but the final common pathway of many different pathological processes, which accounts for the fact that OA is the most common of the arthropathies by an overwhelming margin. Synonyms for the disease, such as 'osteoarthritis' and 'degenerative joint disease' reflect the varied aetiology. It may be defined in pathological terms as a degenerative condition affecting the axial skeleton and peripheral diarthrodial joints in which there is breakdown of the hyaline articular cartilage and remodelling of the subchondral bone with sclerosis and osteophyte formation. These changes lead to the characteristic radiological picture of joint space narrowing, bony sclerosis with subchondral cysts, and marginal osteophyte formation.

Clinically the condition is characterised by the gradual development of joint pain, stiffness, limitation of movement and swelling. It is slowly progressive. Traditionally, clinicians have subdivided OA into two main categories, primary OA in which the aetiology of the process is unclear, and secondary OA in which the joint degeneration is secondary to some known predisposing factor.

OA has afflicted man and other vertebrates from prehistoric times. Degenerative changes have been noted in the fossilised remains of *Pithecanthropus erectus* (Java man), an early ancestor of modern man. Similar changes have been reported in the bones of Nubian cave dwellers who lived about 10 000 BC (Brugsch, 1957) and in Anglo-Saxon skeletons (Rogers et al, 1981)

Hippocrates clearly recognised OA as a disease entity (Copeman, 1964). He described it as 'an arthritis which seizes great joints which are able to contain it but which does not actually go beyond these'. In subsequent centuries this clinical knowledge was forgotten and it was not until the late 18th century, some 2000 years later, that clinicians once again attempted to subdivide arthropathies. Though William Heberden's name is most widely associated with OA, he described only the nodes of the distal interphalangeal joints and did not link these nodes with OA at other sites (Heberden, 1806).

The first description of OA was in fact published at almost the same time by John Haygarth (1805). His description was detailed and clinically remarkably accurate but unfortunately went unrecognised. Indeed it was not until the paper of Cecil & Archer in 1926 that OA was widely accepted as a distinct rheumatic disease.

PREVALENCE OF OA

Though OA is an extremely common condition the exact prevalence has been difficult to establish. This has been due in part to difficulty in defining the condition under study. If radiological criteria alone are used to detect OA then a high prevalence figure will emerge. If clinical criteria are added then the prevalence figure is lower. The prevalence of OA is also influenced by age, sex, race and heredity. Much of our knowledge on prevalence in the United Kingdom has come from the epidemiological work of Kellgren & Lawrence (1958). In an X-ray study in 1958 of a random sample of the Leigh population aged 55–64 years, they found that 87% of females and 83% of males had osteoarthritic joint changes in one or more joint groups.

Lawrence et al (1966) later demonstrated that the prevalence of radiologically defined OA in the areas of Leigh and Wensleydale increased with age. The condition affected 67% of males and 61% of females in the 45–54 years age-group, but 97% of both sexes in the 65 years and over age-group.

However the radiological prevalence of OA far outstrips the prevalence of symptomatic OA. In Lawrence's study (1966), for example, the distal interphalangeal joints of the hands were affected radiologically in 56% of males, yet only 9% had any pain at this site. The figures for the female population were similar; 67% had degenerative changes on X-ray yet only 13% had symptoms. In weight-bearing joints the correlation between X-ray findings and symptoms is closer but never very strong, e.g. in the over 55 year age-group 27% of males had radiological OA and 43% of these had symptoms; 45% of females had radiological OA and 57% of these had symptoms. Studies in the USA have yielded comparable results. In a Pittsburg population survey Cobb et al (1957) found that only 30% of subjects with radiological OA had symptoms in the affected joint. Another problem in assessing the clinical prevalence of OA is that symptoms at a joint site may be due to a cause other than OA. Lawrence et al (1966) found that 27% of the population over 55 years had pain in the knee joint but did not have OA. It would seem prudent on this evidence to include both radiological and clinical criteria in any definition of OA.

The world prevalence of OA seems remarkably uniform though local factors do appear to modify the prevalence of OA of certain joints, e.g. OA of the hip is less common in the Southern Chinese (Hoaglund et al, 1973) than in Caucasian populations; OA of the lumbar spine is more prevalent amongst miners than it is in the general population (Kellgren & Lawrence, 1952).

The enormous economic consequences of this common disease are evident if one looks at the morbidity it causes in the community. It has been suggested that OA in the United Kingdom is responsible for the loss of 4.7 million days from work per year (Wood & McLeish, 1974). Together, peripheral joint and spinal OA constitute the most common rheumatic cause of loss of time from work in Britain (Wood 1971).

CLINICAL CATEGORIES

OA has been traditionally divided into two main categories — primary OA where the initiating event is unknown, and secondary OA where there is an apparent explanation for the development of the disease.

There is considerable dispute about what constitutes an acceptable predisposing factor in the development of secondary OA and so the percentage of patients who fall into each category is uncertain. In the case of the hip joint, for example, it has been suggested that congenital subluxation underlies the later development of OA in a significant number of cases. A predisposing abnormality of the hip joint was present in 26% of patients in the series reported by Wiberg (1939) and in 21% of those in the series of Lloyd-Roberts (1955). Murray (1965) has suggested that 65% of patients with primary OA of the hip can be shown to have a pre-existing anatomical abnormality of the joint. As these figures illustrate, there is no clear accepted dividing line between primary and secondary OA, but on our present knowledge the majority of cases of OA fall into the primary category.

SECONDARY OA

The recognised causes of secondary OA are numerous and the major categories are listed in Table 34.1. Suspicion that degenerative changes within a joint are secondary to some underlying cause should be raised wherever such changes are seen at an early age or in a single joint.

Table 34.1 Causes of secondary osteoarthrosis

Mechanical derangement
Trauma, e.g. fracture of joint surface, major injury to supportive ligaments, post-meniscectomy
Septic arthritis
Inflammatory joint diseases, e.g. rheumatoid arthritis, psoriatic arthritis, gout
Aseptic necrosis
Long leg arthropathy
Congenital and developmental abnormalities
Congenital hip dysplasia
Slipped femoral epiphysis
Legg–Perthes' disease
Chondrodysplastic conditions
Protrusio acetabuli

(cont.)

Table 34.1 *cont.*

Systemic diseases
Endocrine disorders
  Acromegaly
  Diabetes mellitus
  Hypothyroidism
  Sex hormone disorders
Metabolic disorders
  Haemochromatosis
  Wilson's disease
  Alkaptonuria (ochronosis)
  Storage disorders
    mucopolysaccharidoses
    Gaucher's disease
Haematological disorders
  Haemophilia
  Haemoglobinopathies — SS
  SC and S-thalassaemia
Neurological disorders
  Neuropathic arthropathy in association with tabes dorsalis, diabetes mellitus, peripheral nerve lesions
Kashin–Beck disease

Sport
  Doubtful predisposing factor

Occupation
  Chronic trauma may predispose to OA, e.g. lumbar spine in miners

OA secondary to structural deformity

Trauma, sepsis, inflammation

Structural deformity, whether the result of trauma to a joint or the consequence of abnormal development, may predispose to OA. For example, a fracture which involves the joint surface or a ligament injury which results in mechanical instability may lead to OA. The interval between injury and the ensuing OA varies widely: if a joint surface has

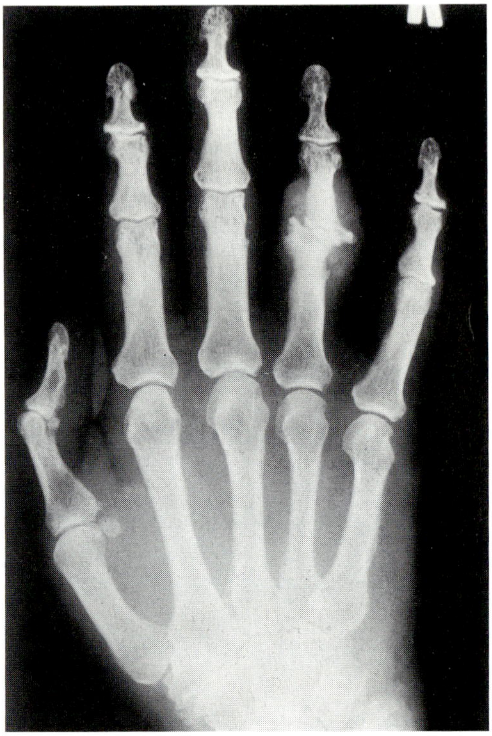

Fig. 34.2 Secondary degenerative changes in a gouty joint. A large tophus surrounds the proximal interphalangeal joint of the 4th finger. Destruction of the normal joint architecture by the gouty process has resulted in a secondary degenerative arthritis of the joint with obliteration of the joint space, bony sclerosis and marginal osteophyte formation.

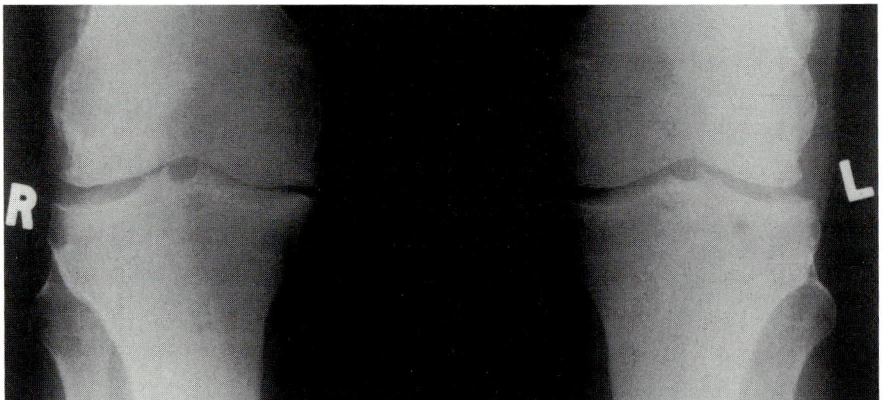

Fig. 34.1 Osteoarthrosis of the knee following meniscectomy. 15 years after removal of the medial meniscus, the right knee shows narrowing of the medial compartment of the joint together with marginal osteophyte formation. The left knee shows no degenerative changes.

been fractured, the degenerative changes may be evident within a matter of months of the injury, whereas in the case of a knee damaged by menisectomy there may be a delay of 10–15 years before the osteoarthritic changes become apparent (Fig. 34.1). Degenerative changes will also supervene in a joint which has been damaged by septic arthritis or inflammation, e.g. gout or rheumatoid arthritis (Fig. 34.2). Kashin–Beck disease may be another example of degenerative arthritis following infection.

OA secondary to aseptic necrosis
Degenerative changes rapidly supervene in a joint following aseptic necrosis (Fig. 34.3). The major causes of aseptic necrosis are listed in Table 34.2. The femoral head is most commonly affected, but the shoulders and femoral condyles can also be involved. As the joint surface collapses, the organised structure of the joint is destroyed and degenerative changes will develop as remodelling of the bony structure occurs (see Ch. 48).

Long-leg arthropathy
Inequality of leg length may lead to a degenerative arthritis of the knee joint in the longer leg (Dixon & Campbell-Smith, 1969). Backache may also be a symptom as the normal postural compensation

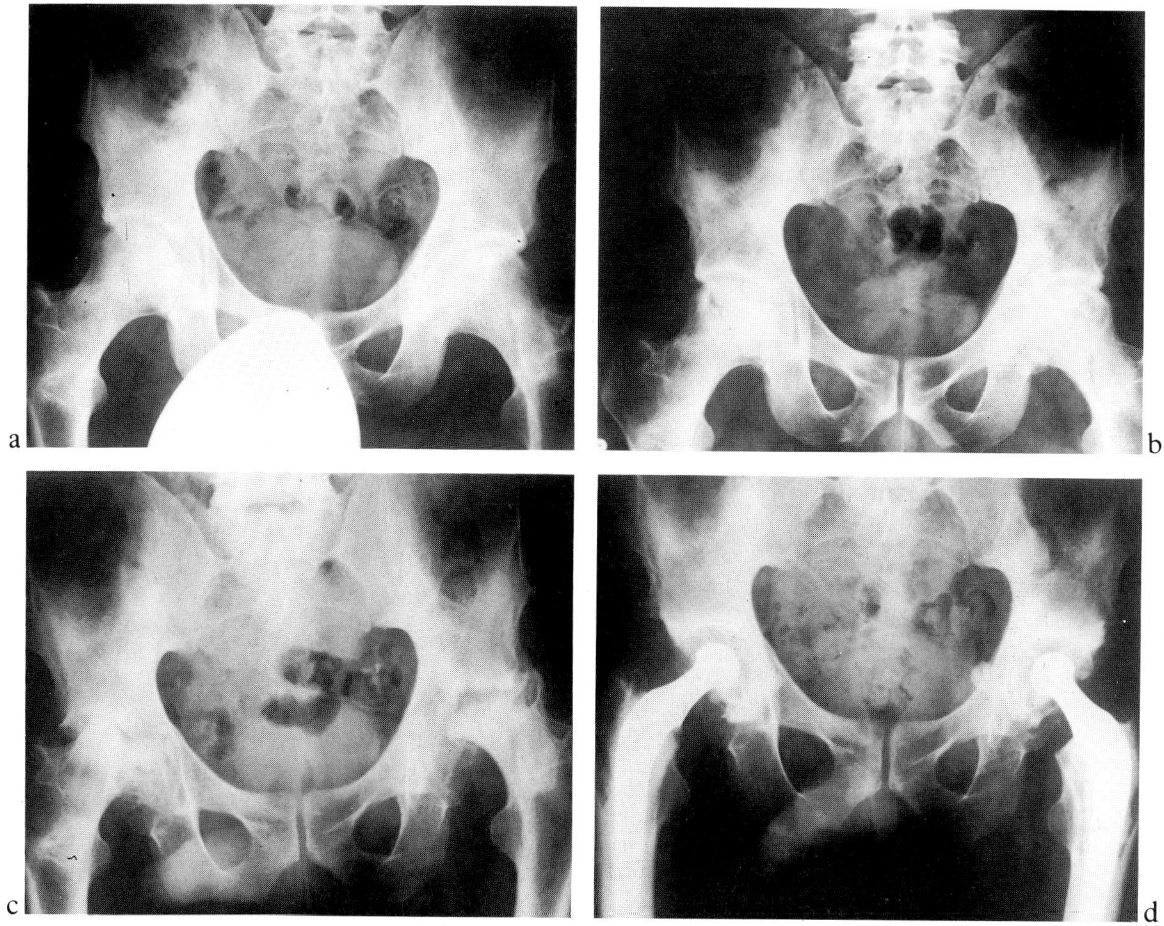

Fig. 34.3 Aseptic necrosis of the hip joint. The patient had received chemotherapy and radiotherapy treatment for acute leukaemia and shortly afterwards presented with pains in both hips. (a) Normal hip joints. (b) Several lucent areas are present in the femoral heads. There is flattening of the superior surfaces of both heads. (c) Collapse of the femoral heads has occurred. (d) Hip function has been restored by bilateral hip replacement operation. The interval between film (a) and film (c) was 18 months.

Table 34.2 Causes of aseptic necrosis

Trauma
e.g. Fracture of femoral neck, multiple injuries
Secondary to systemic disease
Rheumatoid arthritis
Psoriatic arthritis
Systemic lupus erythematosus
Haematological diseases, e.g. haemoglobinopathies, SS, SC, S-thalassaemia
Neoplastic disorders, e.g. lymphomas, leukaemias
Endocrine disorders, e.g. Cushing's syndrome, diabetes mellitus
Storage disorders, e.g. Gaucher's disease
Neuropathic disorders, e.g. syringomyelia
Extensive burns
Secondary to medical treatments
High dose steroid treatment
Cytotoxic drugs
Radiotherapy
Local steroid injection
Caisson's Disease
Alcoholism
Thiemann's Disease

for inequality of leg length is pelvic tilting which will result in a lumbar scoliosis.

OA secondary to congenital and developmental abnormalities

Developmental abnormalities of the hip joint such as congenital hip dysplasia, Legg–Perthes disease and slipped femoral epiphysis have been reported as being an underlying factor in 20–50% of cases of OA of the joint (Lloyd-Roberts, 1955; Adam & Spence, 1958; Nicoll & Holden, 1961; Solomon, 1976). Premature OA also characterises the chondrodysplastic diseases and Thiemann's disease (see below).

Congenital hip dysplasia

The underdevelopment of the acetabulum in this condition is accompanied by either subluxation or dislocation of the femoral head. If the condition passes unrecognised at birth, the acetabulum and femoral head may be malaligned, and premature degenerative changes may supervene (Fig. 34.4). Twin studies suggest that several genes with incomplete penetrance are involved in the development of congenital hip dysplasia (Carter & Wilkinson, 1964). Females are affected more often than males. It would also appear that environmental and social factors play a role since congenital hip dysplasia is more common after breech birth (Record & Edwards, 1958). It is also rare among the Chinese who carry their babies on their backs, ensuring that the child's hip is flexed and abducted, a position which will tend to reduce any subluxation (Hoaglund et al, 1973).

Slipped femoral epiphysis

This condition occurs in overweight children, particularly boys between the ages of 9 and 15. Clinically, the onset is insidious with pain and a limp. If the deformity is not corrected, OA may develop

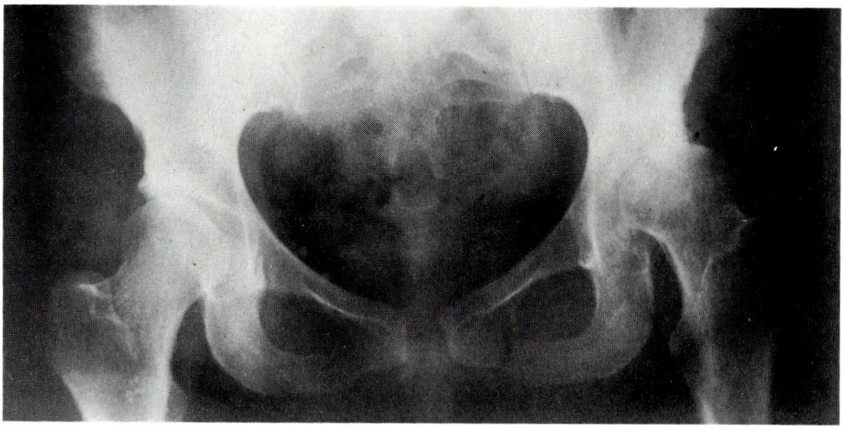

Fig. 34.4 Osteoarthrosis secondary to acetabular dysplasia. The acetabulum on the left side is shallow and there is a break in Shenton's line. Advanced degenerative changes are present in the left hip joint.

in early adult life. In about 50% of children both hips will be affected. Murray (1965) has suggested that slipped femoral epiphysis may be an underlying aetiological factor in as many as 40% of those with OA of the hip joint.

Legg–Perthes disease
Aseptic necrosis of the proximal capital femoral epiphysis is characteristically seen in boys of 4–8 years of age. This condition is unilateral in 90% of cases. The presenting symptom is usually hip and thigh pain with an associated limp. Though 75% resolve spontaneously within weeks or months, about 20% will be left with a structurally abnormal hip joint and will develop premature OA (Gower & Johnston, 1971).

Chondrodysplastic conditions
Premature joint degeneration is a characteristic late development in this rare group of diseases in which normal joint architecture is disrupted by the defective development of the epiphyses. Multiple epiphyseal dysplasia is one variant, inherited as an autosomal dominant trait, which involves many bones and usually presents in childhood. The presenting symptom is characteristically pain and limitation of the affected joints, most commonly the hips, hands, shoulders, knees and ankles. Spondyloepiphyseal dysplasia is clinically similar though the vertebral bodies are involved in addition. It may be transmitted as an autosomal dominant characteristic, in which case it presents in early childhood, or as a sex-linked recessive condition which presents in late childhood. Interestingly, these two examples of premature OA show an increased prevalence of pyrophosphate crystal deposition. Thiemann's disease is another rare familial condition predisposing to OA. It is characterised by avascular necrosis of the epiphyses of the small bones (particularly the phalanges) of the hands and the feet (Figs 34.5, 34.6). It is transmitted as an autosomal dominant and characteristically presents with premature Heberden and Bouchard nodal OA at about the age of puberty (Rubinstein, 1975).

Protrusio acetabuli (Otto's disease)
Otto's disease is probably determined by an autosomal dominant gene and presents in childhood with inward displacement of the hip joint and limited movement (Montagu, 1959).

OA secondary to systemic disease

OA and endocrine disease (see also Ch. 39)

OA in association with acromegaly. The arthritis of acromegaly is similar to idiopathic OA with cartilage degeneration and subchondral sclerosis with cyst formation. The hypertrophic changes induced by growth hormone in the soft tissues and bone of the spine may lead to cord compression. It has been suggested that increased levels of circulating growth hormone are a feature of idiopathic OA (Franchimont & Denis, 1968; Burssens et al, 1974), but this has been disputed. The perfusion of growth hormone through the liver produces somatomedins and it is thought that circulating somatomedins will enter the synovial fluid and modulate chondrocyte function (Ash & Francis, 1975). No increase in circulating or in synovial fluid somatomedin activity (measured through a cartilage bioassay) was detected by Coates et al (1978) in a study of patients with either OA or inflammatory joint diseases. Similarly, using a radio-immunoassay to measure circulating somatomedin, another group was unable

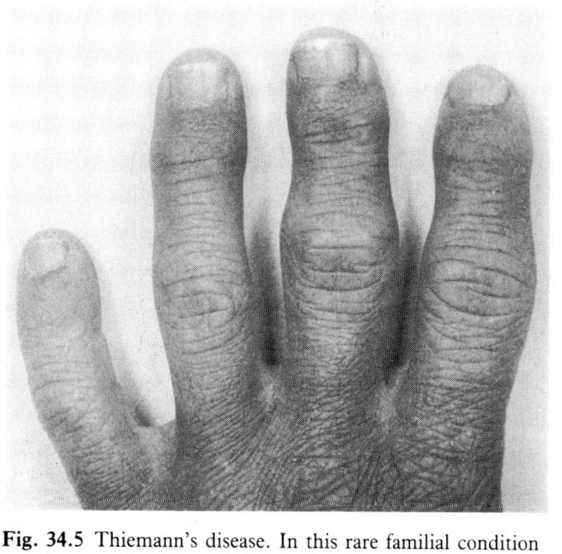

Fig. 34.5 Thiemann's disease. In this rare familial condition aseptic necrosis of the epiphyses of the small bones of the fingers results in short phalanges and in premature osteoarthrosis of the adjacent joints. This patient presented at the age of 16 years.

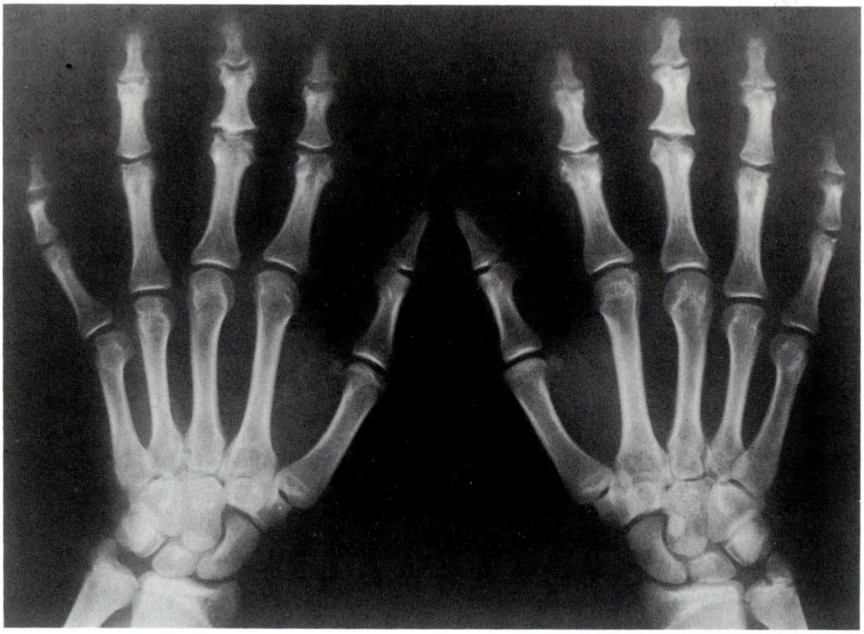

Fig. 34.6 Thiemann's disease. The X-ray shows flattening and irregularity of the epiphyses of the phalanges. The middle and distal phalanges are short and there is cupping of the articular surfaces of several of the interphalangeal joints. Premature degenerative changes can be seen in the distal interphalangeal joints.

to show any increase in levels amongst patients with OA when compared to matched rheumatoid controls (Doyle et al — unpublished observation).

OA in association with diabetes mellitus. The prevalence of OA in patients with diabetes mellitus is said to be increased (Silberberg R & Silberberg, M 1964), but the relationship is obscured by the increased prevalence in the diabetic population of other factors which may predispose to joint degeneration, e.g. obesity, neuropathy. Diabetes complicated by neuropathy may be accompanied by a severe degenerative arthritis of a neuropathic type, involving most commonly the metatarsophalangeal joint of the feet. The association between calcium pyrophosphate dihydrate crystal (CPPD) deposition, diabetes mellitus and OA is disputed. Though 4 of the 7 patients reported by McCarty et al (1962) in his original description of pseudogout had mild diabetes mellitus, subsequent investigations have failed to demonstrate a convincing association between pyrophosphate arthropathy and diabetes (McCarty, 1976).

Ankylosing hyperostosis (Forestier & Rotes-Querol, 1950; Forestier & Lagier, 1971), a florid degenerative spinal arthritis which may result in ankylosis, is one type of OA which is definitely associated with diabetes mellitus, particularly in the elderly patient (Julkenen et al, 1971, 1981).

OA and thyroid disease. An association between hypothyroidism and the deposition of CPPD crystals has been described (Dowort & Schumacher, 1975; Alexander et al, 1981). The joint disease in the other respects did not resemble OA.

OA and sex hormones. Cecil & Archer (1926) were the first to note that primary generalised OA often developed in middle-aged women about the time of the menopause. Despite this association, trials of oestrogen therapy have been unhelpful in relieving the symptoms and signs of OA (Kellgren & Moore, 1952). In experimental animals, however, some evidence has been presented to suggest that androgens precipitate and oestrogens retard the onset of degeneration of joints (Silberberg M & Silberberg, R 1964, 1970; Silberberg R & Silberberg, M 1965; Silberberg

& Hasler, 1971), but there is no evidence that the suppression of androgen production by orchidectomy will slow the progression of existing OA in mice.

OA and metabolic diseases (see also Ch. 38)

Haemochromatosis. The arthropathy which accompanies this disorder of iron metabolism can resemble primary OA, but the classical picture is one of degenerative arthritis accompanied by chondrocalcinosis, and pyrophosphate crystals can be found in the synovial fluid (Hamilton et al, 1967; Dymock et al, 1970). It is also of interest that a similar arthropathy has been reported in secondary haemosiderosis.

Wilson's disease. This inherited condition, which results in excessive retention of copper, may be accompanied in the later stages by OA and calcium pyrophosphate dihydrate crystal deposition (Feller & Schumacher, 1972; Golding & Walshe, 1977).

Alkaptonuria. Degenerative arthritis of the spine and large joints is a characteristic accompaniment of this inherited metabolic defect (O'Brien et al, 1963). The lack of homogentisic acid oxidase leads to deposition of homogentisic acid within the articular tissues. Characteristically, calcification of intervertebral discs is seen.

Gout. Joints affected by chronic tophaceous gout frequently show degenerative changes due to disruption of the normal joint architecture (see Fig. 34.2).

OA and storage diseases (see also Chs. 46, 49)

Mucopolysaccharidoses. This group of conditions is characterised by mucopolysacchariduria and by deposits of mucopolysaccharides in various tissues. There are eight recognised categories, all of which are recessively inherited (McKusick et al, 1978). The storage of the mucopolysaccharides may disrupt the articular soft tissues and the normal bony architecture, and a degenerative arthritis is seen in some of the subgroups.

Gaucher's disease. A recessive disorder of lysosomal sphingolipid storage, this condition may result in aseptic necrosis of bone and premature OA. The hip and shoulder joints are characteristically involved. X-rays show a patchy osteosclerosis (Figs 34.7–34.9). Avascular necrosis of the shoulder and hip joint may be evident and the

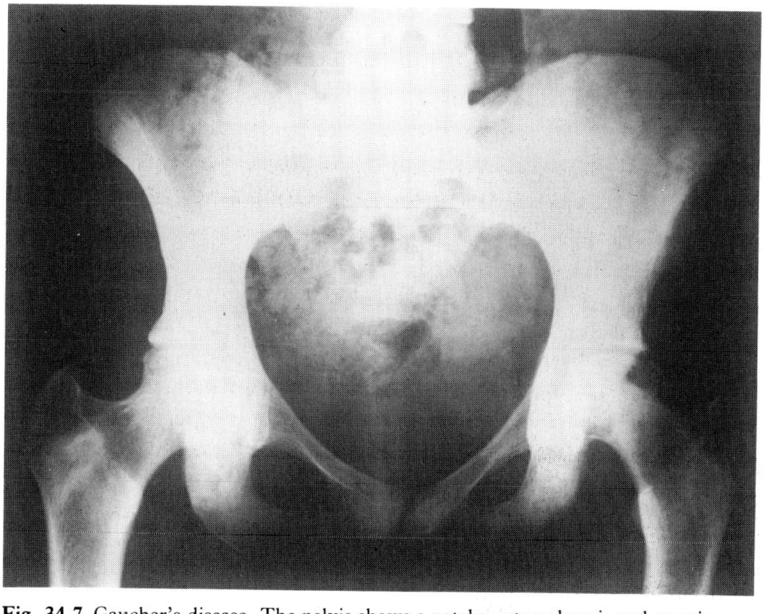

Fig. 34.7 Gaucher's disease. The pelvis shows a patchy osteosclerosis and aseptic necrosis of the heads of both femora.

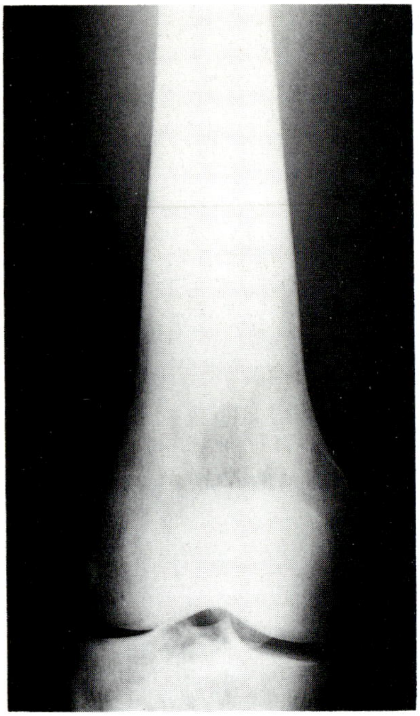

Fig. 34.8 Gaucher's disease. The femur is sclerotic and is expanded in its lower half to give the classical Ehrlenmeyer flask appearance.

lower end of the femur is characteristically expanded (Ehrlenmeyer flask appearance).

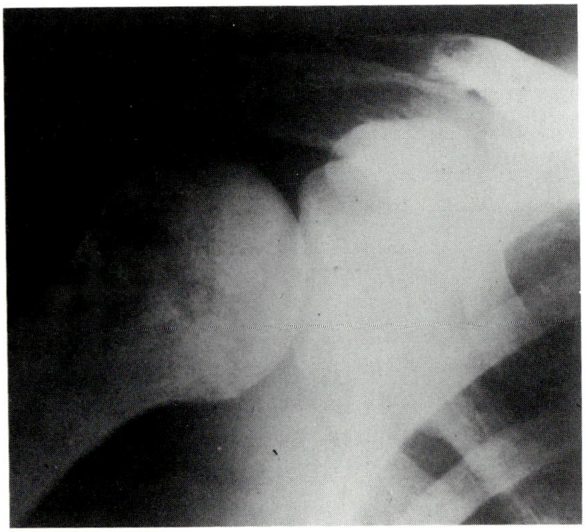

Fig. 34.9 Gaucher's disease. The shoulder joint shows a patchy sclerosis. A lucent line has developed 1 mm below the articular surface of the humeral head indicating early aseptic necrosis.

OA secondary to haematological disorders (see Ch. 47)

Haemophilia. Degenerative changes within joints are a late consequence of repeated intra-articular haemorrhage. The elbows and knees are most commonly affected.

Haemoglobinopathies. Avascular necrosis with consequent joint degeneration is a well recognised complication of sickle cell disease (both SS and SC disease) and has been reported with S-thalassaemia (Chung & Ralston, 1969).

OA and neurological disorders

A very destructive form of arthritis is seen in neuropathic disorders (Figs 34.10, 34.11). This was first described by Charcot (1868) and has been reviewed recently by Bruckner & Howell (1972). It is thought that impairment of the normal pathways for pain and proprioceptive sensation interferes with the physiologic mechanisms which protect a

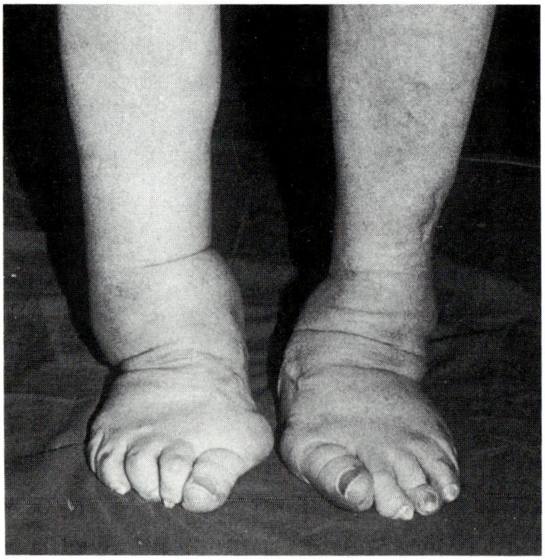

Fig. 34.10 Neuropathic joints. This 70-year-old woman had developed progressive deformity of both ankles over a 7-year period. Despite the gross deformity she was able to walk about without support and suffered only mild discomfort. No neurological abnormality which would explain her pain insensitivity was discovered, but it is of interest that she also suffered from florid generalised osteoarthritis with associated pyrophosphate crystal deposition. It is possible that her destructive ankle arthropathy was at least partly the result of crystal deposition disease.

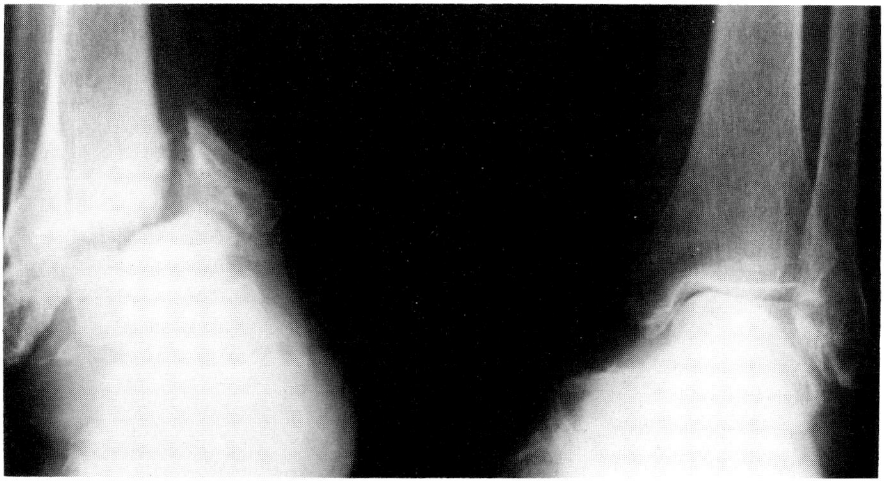

Fig. 34.11 Neuropathic joint. The X-rays of the patient shown in Figure 34.10 demonstrate the characteristic radiological features of a neuropathic joint. There is sclerosis of the bone ends, with a longstanding non-united fracture of the medial malleolus of the right ankle. The articular surfaces are disorganised, the joint space narrowed and there are calcified loose bodies and osteophytes in and around the joint margins.

joint when in motion and allows the articular structures to be damaged. This type of lesion may occur in tabes dorsalis, syringomyelia, sensory neuropathies such as in diabetes mellitus, peripheral nerve lesions and with malformations of the cord such as meningomyelocoele.

Kashin–Beck disease

Kashin–Beck disease, which is endemic in Eastern Siberia, Northern China and Northern Korea, is characterised by defective growth of bony epiphyses and metaphyses and results in a severe degenerative polyarthritis (Nesterov, 1964). It is thought to be due to an infection of the cereal grain with the fungus *Fusaria sporotrichiella*.

Sport and OA

There is little evidence to support the contention that OA is more common in sportsmen. Though there is a wealth of literature on the subject, many of the studies are poorly designed and without a control group for comparison. It may be of reassurance to the sportsman that in a well designed study of former Finnish distance runners, whose mean age was 55 years, Puranen et al (1975) were unable to show any increase in the prevalence of OA of the hip joint. Indeed, degenerative hip disease was present in 4% of the athletes and 8.7% of the controls. Solonen (1966), in a study of footballers, showed that there was no increase in the prevalence of radiological OA of the knee in the study group when compared with controls, but that degenerative changes in the ankle were more common among footballers.

Occupation and OA

The idea that chronic trauma might predispose to the development of OA has led to many investigations of the relationship between occupation and OA. Kellgren & Lawrence (1958) reported that OA of the lumbar spine was more common among miners. Similarly, OA of the shoulders, elbows and hands is increased in those who work with pneumatic drills (Hunter et al, 1945), and OA of the elbows is said to be more common amongst foundry workers (Mintz & Fraga, 1973). In these groups, the development of OA does appear to be related to chronic trauma. There is also some evidence that repetitive usage of joints in certain occupations will predispose to clinical and radiological OA (Hadler, 1977; Hadler et al, 1978; Hadler, 1981). In a study of female workers in a worsted mill, all of whom had completed at least 20 years at a sterotyped task, Hadler (1981) has shown that

OA was more common and more severe in those joints which were most used.

PRIMARY OA

The majority of patients with OA fall into this category, though there is argument in the case of OA of the hip (Murray, 1965). Despite the fact that the aetiology of the condition is unknown, patients with primary OA share many common characteristics, some of which are discussed below.

Sex

OA determined radiologically shows a similar pattern of distribution and severity in men and women up to the age of 54 but the condition is more severe and more generalised in women after this age (Kellgren et al, 1963). Over the age of 55 involvement of the distal interphalangeal, proximal interphalangeal, and the first carpometacarpal joints appears to be more common in women, whereas the hip joint is more frequently a problem in men. Overall, women are affected more often than men, the ratio being about 2 : 1 (Huskisson et al, 1979).

Race

There appears to be a striking uniformity in the geographic prevalence of OA but studies which highlight differences deserve mention. OA of the hip is less prevalent amongst Chinese (Hoaglund et al, 1973; Byers et al, 1974). In Greenland it is said that OA of the knee is more common amongst women on the west coast than amongst those on the east coast (Anderson & Winckler, 1979). The west coast women more commonly work outside the home and it is suggested that the difference in prevalence is related to occupational stresses. A low prevalence of OA of the metatarsophalangeal joints in black South Africans and Jamaicans has been attributed to the fact that they walk barefoot (Bremner et al, 1968; Soloman et al, 1975). The diagnostic criteria used in these studies were not uniform and the explanation for the differences in the prevalence of OA are speculative. This is a field which demands further investigation.

Heredity

A pattern of heredity for Heberden's nodes has been suggested (Stecher et al, 1953; Stecher, 1955). This involves an autosomal dominant gene in women and a recessive gene in men. Nodal generalised OA may have a similar pattern of inheritance, but non-nodal OA in contrast appears to have polygenic modes of inheritance.

Obesity

The relationship between obesity and OA is uncertain and disputed. A positive correlation between obesity and OA of weight-bearing joints such as the knee has been suggested by Lawrence et al (1966) on the basis of population surveys. On the other hand, an increased incidence in obese people of OA of non-weight-bearing joints such as the sternoclavicular and distal interphalangeal joints has also been reported (Silberberg et al, 1959; Silberberg M & Silberberg R, 1964; Silberberg R & Silberberg M, 1964). Other radiological studies have not shown any excess of OA in the hands, feet, knees or hips of an overweight study group (Danielsson, 1964; Engel, 1968). Animal work has also failed to provide conclusive evidence of a link between obesity and joint degeneration (Sokoloff et al, 1962; Walton, 1979).

Clinical subgroups of primary OA

Generalised OA and Heberden's nodes (Figs 34.12, 34.13)

This distinct subgroup of OA was delineated by Kellgren & Moore (1952). In a study of 391 cases of OA they found 120 patients, largely middle-aged women, who had a polyarthritis with a distinct pattern of joint involvement and a characteristic presentation and course. The joints involved were distal interphalangeal joints (86%), the carpometacarpal joints of the thumb (60%), proximal interphalangeal joints (41%), metatarsophalangeal joint of the big toe (33%), knee (53%, and nearly always with bilateral involvement), spine (48%) and hips (30%). The onset of symptoms was often acute and accompanied by signs of joint inflammation. The mean age at presentation was 52 years. 20% gave a family history of similar joint disease, suggesting an hereditary influence in its development.

Erosive OA (Fig. 34.14)

Occasionally, OA of the distal interphalangeal and

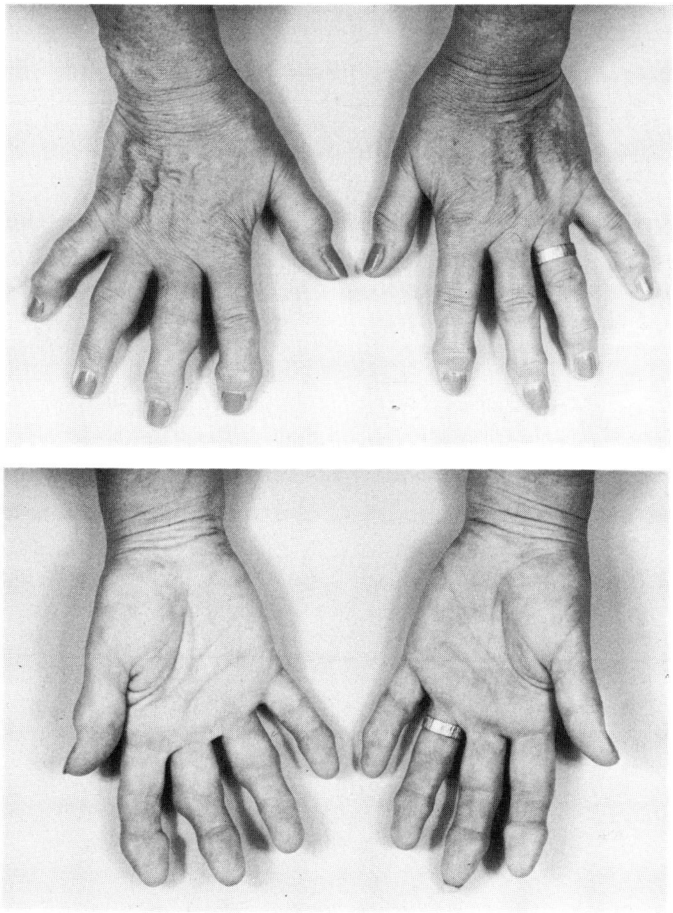

a

b

Fig. 34.12 Primary generalised osteoarthrosis with Heberden's nodes. The hands show bony enlargement of the distal interphalangeal joints. The pattern is symmetrical in both hands. There is also evidence of Bouchard node formation at the proximal interphalangeal joints of the 3rd and 4th fingers of the right hand.

proximal interphalangeal joints of the hand may present as an acute painful inflammatory arthritis (Kellgren & Moore, 1952; Crain 1961; Peter et al, 1966; Ehrlich, 1972, 1975). The term 'erosive arthritis' was coined by Peter et al (1966) but the disease entity they described would appear to share many of the characteristics of the acute form of generalised osteoarthrosis with Heberden's nodes described by Kellgren & Moore (1952), and inflammatory interphalangeal OA reported by Crain (1961).

Characteristically this acute presentation is seen in postmenopausal women. They suffer recurring acute flares and the affected joints may be red, warm and swollen. Gelatinous cysts develop around the affected joints. Eventually, joint deformity develops and X-rays will show loss of joint space, subchondral sclerosis, osteophyte formation and bony erosion. Bony ankylosis may occur. Histology of the synovial membrane shows non-specific inflammatory features (synoviocyte hyperplasia, lymphocytic aggregates and fibrin deposition)

OA with associated calcium phosphate crystal deposition (see Ch. 37)

OA associated with calcium pyrophosphate crystal deposition (Figs 34.15, 34.16). McCarty (1976) has suggested the term 'pseudo-osteoarthritis' to describe this group of patients. They are pre-

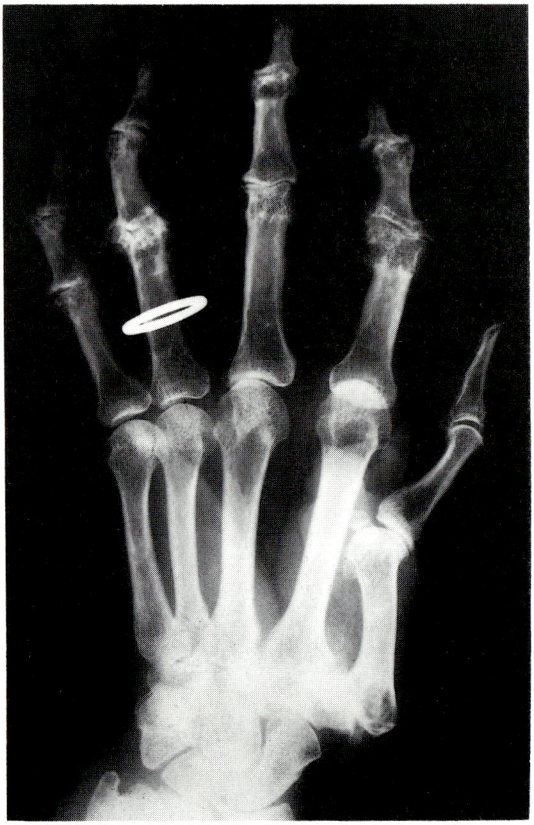

Fig. 34.13 Primary generalised osteoarthrosis of the hands. The characteristic radiological changes of juxta-articular sclerosis, joint space narrowing and marginal osteophyte formation can be seen at the distal and proximal interphalangeal joints and at the first carpometacarpal joint. There is also some soft tissue calcification around the first carpometacarpal joint. Such calcification is frequently seen in advanced osteoarthrosis.

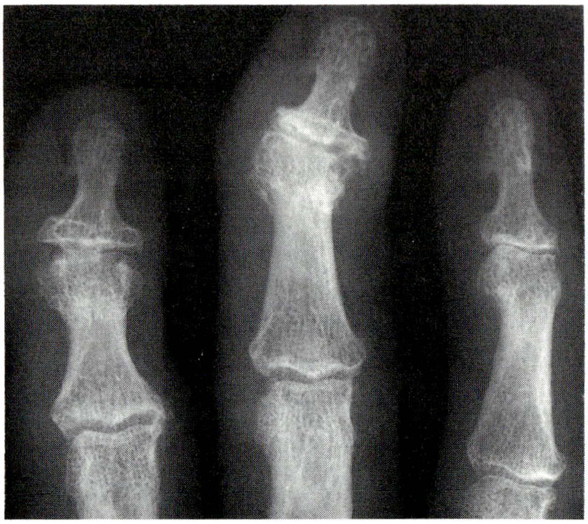

Fig. 34.14 Erosive osteoarthrosis. Degenerative arthritis of the distal interphalangeal joints may present acutely with signs of inflammation. This picture is usually seen in women of menopausal age. The X-ray will occasionally show evidence of marginal joint erosion as seen in the 3rd finger in this illustration.

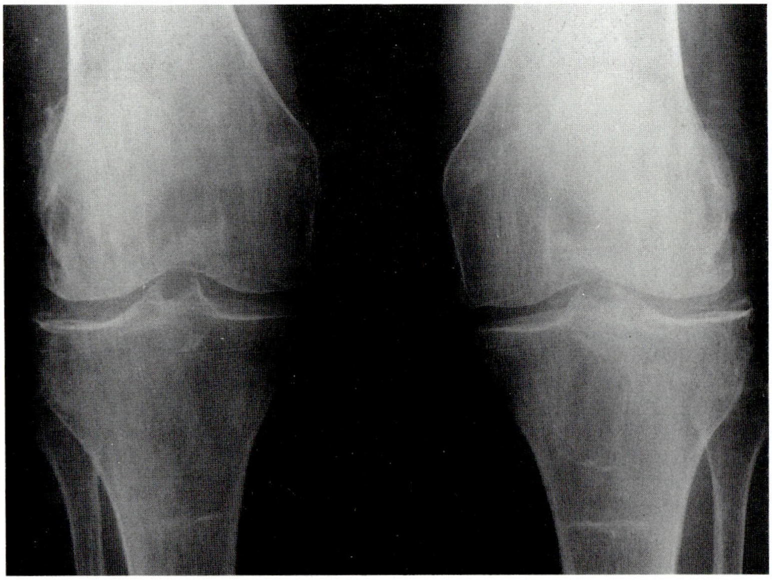

Fig. 34.15 Degenerative arthritis of the knee with associated chondrocalcinosis. Joint space narrowing is evident in the right knee. There is juxta-articular bony sclerosis, marginal osteophyte formation and linear calcification within the joint space. There are also some calcified bodies in the periarticular tissues of the lateral aspect of both knee joints.

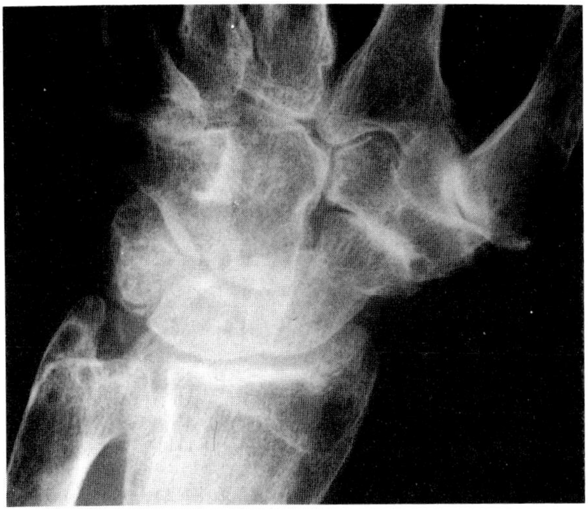

Fig. 34.16 Deposition of crystals of calcium pyrophosphate in the triangular ligament of the wrist.

dominantly women and have a degenerative arthritis affecting the knees, wrists, metacarpophalangeal joints, hips, shoulders, elbows and ankles. The course of the disease is punctuated in some by episodes of acute synovitis. Overall, about 50% of the total population of patients with calcium pyrophosphate crystal deposition disease fall into the subgroup with pseudo-osteoarthritis.

OA associated with hydroxyapatite crystal deposition. This association was first reported by Dieppe et al (1976). The hydroxyapatite crystals were found in the synovial fluids of 6 patients whose clinical pattern of disease resembled primary generalised OA. 3 of the patients had had episodes of acute synovitis reminiscent of those seen in OA accompanied by pyrophosphate arthropathy.

OA with mixed crystal deposition (hydroxyapatite and calcium pyrophosphate dihydrate crystals). The presence of both calcium phosphate crystals in the joint fluid of patients with OA has been reported (Doyle et al, 1977; Dieppe et al, 1978). The clinical pattern of disease in the patients with mixed crystal deposition was indistinguishable from that seen in patients with OA associated with deposition of either crystal alone, and from the pattern seen in patients with generalised OA without crystal deposition.

The significance of crystal deposition in the pathogenesis of OA is not fully understood, but since its presence does not appear to significantly modify the disease process it is more likely to be an epiphenomenon than a major factor in the pathogenesis.

Ankylosing hyperostosis (Forestier's disease; diffuse idiopathic skeletal hyperostosis)
(Fig. 34.17) (see above, and p. 973)

This florid form of OA of the spine was originally described by Forestier & Rotes-Querol (1950). The condition is characterised by large marginal osteophyte formation. Classically the new bone is laid down on the anterolateral aspect of the dorsal vertebrae across the front of the vertebral disc. The process forms a bony bridge immobilising the involved segment of the spine. Surprisingly, the

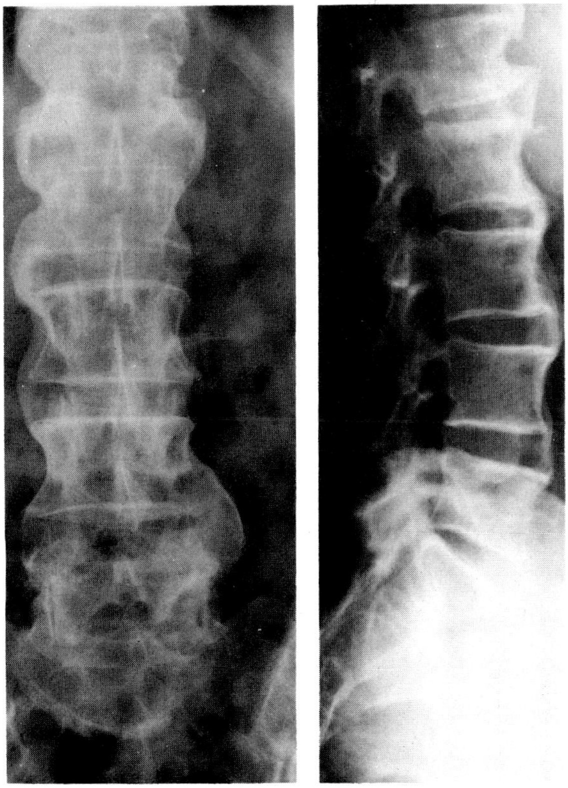

a b

Fig. 34.17 Ankylosing hyperostosis. This condition is characterised by the exuberant growth of osteophytes from the anterolateral aspects of the vertebral bodies. They extend both upwards and downwards and often join to form a bony bridge between the vertebrae. In contrast to ankylosing spondylitis, the normal concave appearance of the anterior aspect of the vertebral bodies is preserved and the sacroiliac joints are normal.

patient is often asymptomatic. In ankylosing hyperostosis the vertebral discs are usually well preserved in contrast to the more usual forms of spinal OA. The tendency to florid ossification is seen at other sites also, e.g. cervical and lumbar spine, calcaneum (spur formation). It has been suggested that the HLA-B27 antigen is more common in this condition than in the general population (Shapiro et al, 1976), and that the B27 gene may in some way stimulate bone production, but this has not been confirmed (see p. 735).

SYMPTOMS AND SIGNS OF OA

PAIN

Though OA is present radiologically in 85% of the population over the age of 55 (Kellgren & Lawrence, 1958), many will have no symptoms. For example, only 9% of men with involvement of the distal interphalangeal joint experienced any discomfort, and even in the case of large weight-bearing joints (hip or knee), only half of those with radiological OA have pain (Lawrence et al, 1966). If symptoms do develop, pain is the most common presentation. The discomfort, initially, is noted after exercise and relieved by rest. With more advanced disease, pain is often present at rest and nocturnal pain may become a major management problem. The pain is usually localised to the affected joint but it can be referred to another site, e.g. pain from an osteoarthritic hip may be felt in the thigh or knee; degenerative arthritis of the cervical or lumbar spine may cause radicular pain in the upper or lower limb respectively.

The site and mode of generation of pain sensation within a joint is poorly understood. Since it is devoid of sensory innervation, the articular cartilage does not appear to play a role, but the surrounding joint capsule and subchondral bone are well innervated and may be the source of pain sensation, though the mechanism is uncertain. It has been suggested that pain may arise as a result or periosteal elevation due to osteophyte formation, and that subchondral trabecular microfractures, venous distension and intracapsular ligament strains may also contribute. It is evident, too, in more advanced disease that chronic inflammatory changes develop within the joint and the resultant synovitis may contribute to the symptoms (Doyle, 1982).

STIFFNESS

Stiffness in the affected joint is usually a prominent symptom. This is characteristically noted on getting out of bed in the morning and when mobilising after sitting for a period. The duration of morning stiffness in OA is much shorter than in rheumatoid arthritis, lasting usually less than 30 minutes (Huskisson et al, 1979).

SWELLING, DEFORMITY AND RESTRICTION OF MOVEMENT

Swelling of an osteoarthritic joint is a common symptom. This may be due to synovitis with effusion, as frequently seen in a knee joint, or it may be the result of osteophyte formation as in the case of a Heberden's node. The chronic synovitis in OA is probably a consequence of many different processes. Occasionally calcium crystal formation may be responsible for acute flares, e.g. hydroxyapatite (Dieppe et al, 1976) or calcium pyrophosphate dihydrate (McCarty, 1976), but usually the synovial inflammatory changes are of a chronic type and appear to be a response to debris shed from the degenerating articular cartilage and subchondral bone (Doyle, 1982).

The bony enlargement which accompanies osteophyte formation leads to joint deformity. These changes are often most obvious in the distal interphalangeal joints of the fingers and in the knee joint. The osteophytes can be palpated at the joint margins and the swelling which they cause is bony in contrast to the fluctuant swelling of a joint effusion.

The swelling and deformity restrict the range of movement and crepitus may be felt by the patient and the examiner when the joint is moved. In advanced disease, gross deformity may occur. The articular cartilage is lost, the eburnated subchondral bone collapses and the secondary osteophyte formation fails to support the joint. The result is a deformed, poorly functioning, painful joint, which in some cases is unstable. The degree of disability depends, of course, on the site involved. In the case of a hip or knee joint advanced OA may immobilise the sufferer, whereas similar changes in a distal interphalangeal joint may cause few symptoms. It is not only OA of large joints which causes functional incapacity, however. OA of the first carpometacarpal joint in the hand may cause major disability, because it interferes with pinch grip and manual dexterity.

CHARACTERISTICS OF OA AT INDIVIDUAL SITES

DISTAL INTERPHALANGEAL JOINTS OF THE FINGERS (HEBERDEN'S NODES) (see Figs 34.12, 34.13)

Though William Heberden described these nodes (1806), he did not relate them to a generalised form of OA. This relationship was described by Haygarth (1805) and later revived by Kellgren (1952). The node is the result of the overgrowth of cartilage and bone along the medial, lateral and dorsal aspects of the distal interphalangeal joint. The changes often develop slowly and without symptoms over many years, and though movement of the affected joints is restricted, hand function remains satisfactory. Occasionally the onset is sudden, painful and associated with signs of inflammation such as redness, swelling and cyst formation. The latter presentation is seen in primary generalised OA as described by Kellgren & Moore (1952) and usually occurs in women of menopausal age. A similar acute presentation characterises the subgroup of patients who develop erosive OA (Crain, 1961; Peter et al, 1966; Ehrlich, 1972). The Heberden node is usually hard to touch, the joint is visibly deformed and occasionally there is some instability. Sometimes a soft cystic swelling may form around the joint and a clear viscous material consisting largely of hyaluronic acid may be aspirated (Begg & Scott, 1966). It does not contain calcium crystals. Similar swellings are seen on rare occasions along the flexor tendon sheaths. Unlike rheumatoid swellings they do not appear to be related to tissue inflammation and may persist for years causing little or no discomfort. It is thought that repetitive loading and excessive use may influence the development of Heberden's nodes. They are more common and more severe in the dominant hand, and paralysis of a limb seems to block their development (Acheson, 1970; Bland & Eddy 1968). The nodes are usually multiple and often symmetrically distributed in both hands, but a very similar node may develop in isolation following injury to a distal interphalangeal joint (Figs 34.18, 34.19). The polyarticular nodes are thought to be genetically determined, and Stecher (1955) has suggested that an autosomal dominant gene may be responsible in women and an autosomal recessive in men, and that penetrance is complete by the 8th decade.

PROXIMAL INTERPHALANGEAL NODES (BOUCHARD'S NODES) (Fig. 34.20)

The clinical onset is very similar to that of Heberden's nodes. Again, Bouchard's nodes are often painless, and though movement may be restricted, they have surprisingly little effect on hand function. Bouchard's nodes are usually part of the clinical pattern of generalised OA and the involvement is almost always symmetrical in both hands. However, trauma can produce similar degenerative changes (Figs 34.18, 34.19).

METACARPOPHALANGEAL JOINTS

These joints are rarely involved in OA unless there is associated deposition of crystals of calcium pyrophosphate dihydrate. This type of joint disease has been labelled 'pseudo-osteoarthritis' (McCarty, 1976). Secondary degenerative changes may occasionally develop following trauma (e.g. occupational) or preceding inflammatory joint disease such as rheumatoid arthritis.

THE FIRST METACARPOPHALANGEAL JOINT (Fig. 34.13)

After the distal interphalangeal joints, the first carpometacarpal point of the thumb is the joint most commonly involved in OA. Unlike the other small joints of the hand, OA at this site is usually painful, and hand function is often compromised. The patient will classically complain of clumsiness, a tendency to drop things and difficulty in gripping or manipulating objects. The joint may be tender to touch and there is usually crepitus on movement. With more advanced disease, 'squaring' of

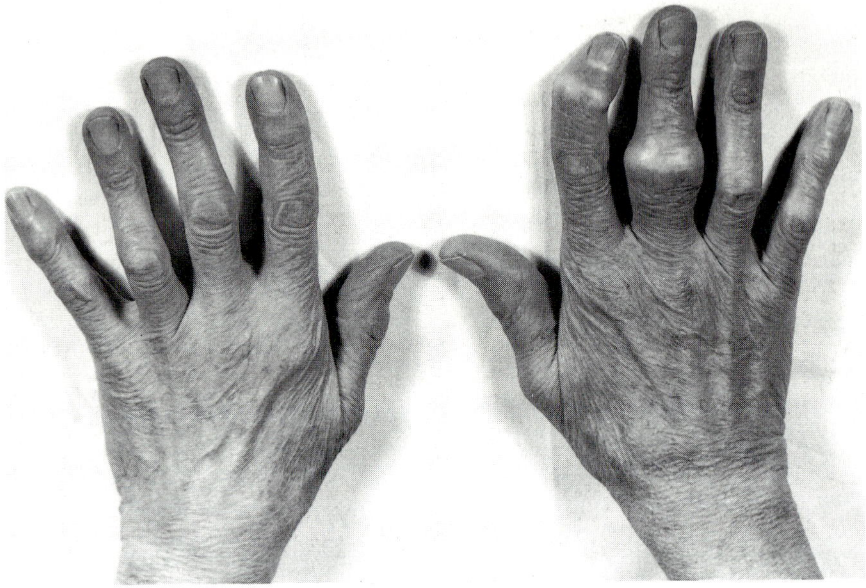

Fig. 34.18 Degenerative arthritis following trauma. Injury to an interphalangeal joint may produce clinical and radiological changes which are indistinguishable from idiopathic osteoarthrosis. This patient's index finger Heberden's node and middle finger Bouchard's node are the result of a hand injury. Note the lack of degenerative changes at other sites.

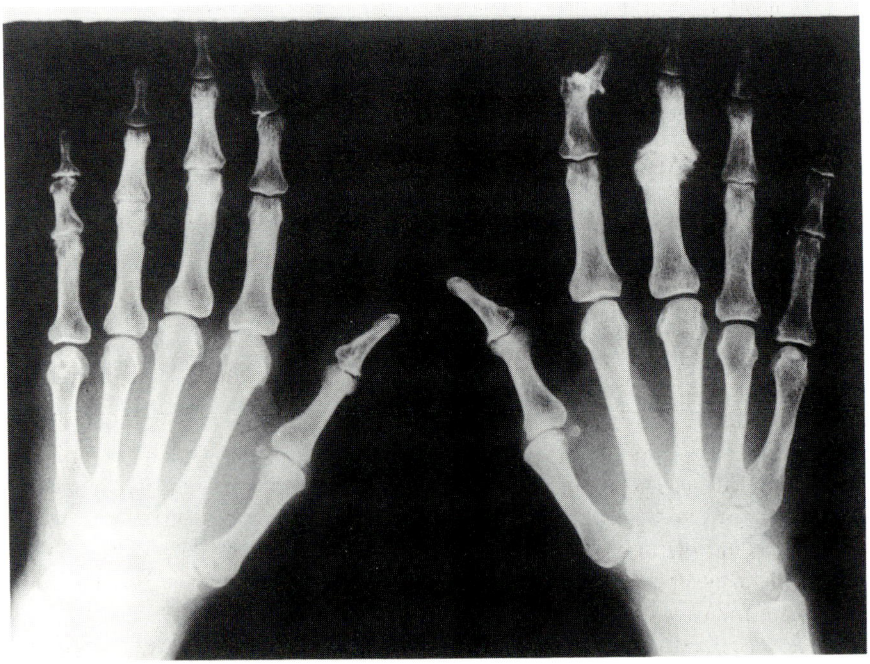

Fig. 34.19 Degenerative arthritis following trauma. X-rays of the patient shown in Fig. 34.18 exhibit changes of joint degeneration at sites of injury only.

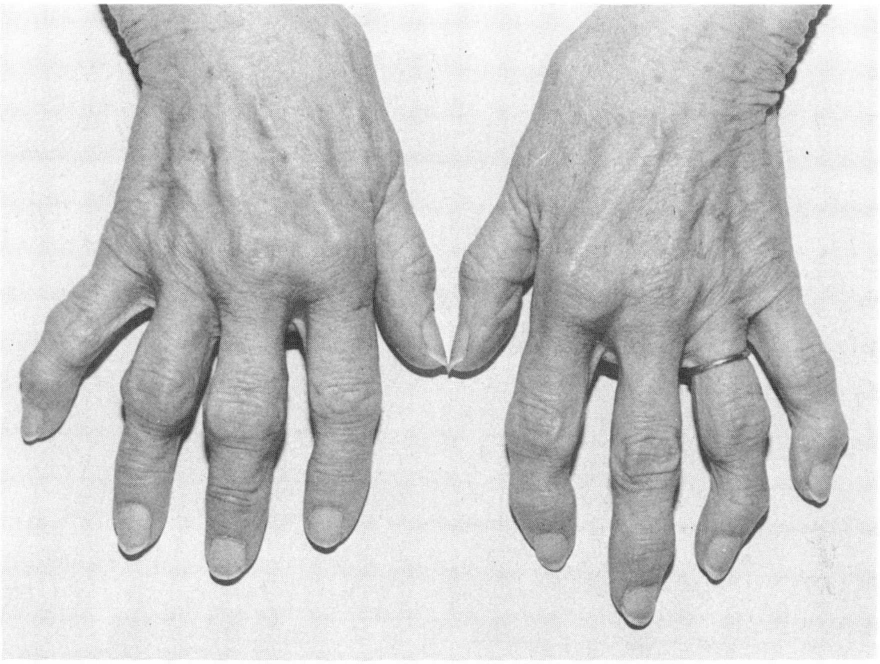

Fig. 34.20 Bouchard's nodes. Degenerative arthritis of the proximal interphalangeal joints of the hands produces a classical picture of bony enlargement of the joint. The pattern is usually symmetrical in both hands.

the base of the thumb will be evident. Restriction of movement of the first carpometacarpal joint results in disuse atrophy of the thenar muscles. The pain experienced by the sufferer may lessen as joint movement becomes grossly restricted.

The treatment of OA is discussed in Chapter 35, but it should be mentioned here that surgical arthrodesis of this joint is sometimes necessary to relieve pain. Excision of the trapezium or of the head of the first metacarpal is also effective in relieving pain but may lead to instability of the joint.

CARPUS AND WRIST JOINTS

The trapezioscaphoid joint is often involved in OA but usually it is seen in conjunction with OA of the first carpometacarpal joint and the symptoms from the latter joint tend to predominate. Primary OA rarely occurs at other sites in the carpus or wrist joint, though degenerative changes may develop at these sites following joint damage by trauma or inflammation.

ELBOW

The elbow is rarely involved by OA, but has been reported amongst certain groups of workers such as miners (Lawrence, 1955) and pneumatic drillers (Hunter et al, 1945). Though elbow OA is usually mild and not disabling, severe symptoms may occur in these groups. Florid OA of the elbow joint may lead to a compression neuropathy of the ulnar nerve.

SHOULDER JOINT (Fig. 34.21)

Involvement of the shoulder by OA is unusual, and if seen it is usually secondary to other pathology, most commonly trauma or inflammatory disease such as rheumatoid arthritis. It is also seen in association with pyrophosphate crystal deposition (McCarty, 1976). Primary OA of the shoulder is rare.

A painful degenerative condition of the shoulder has been described by McCarty et al (1981). This arthropathy, called 'Milwaukee shoulder' by the

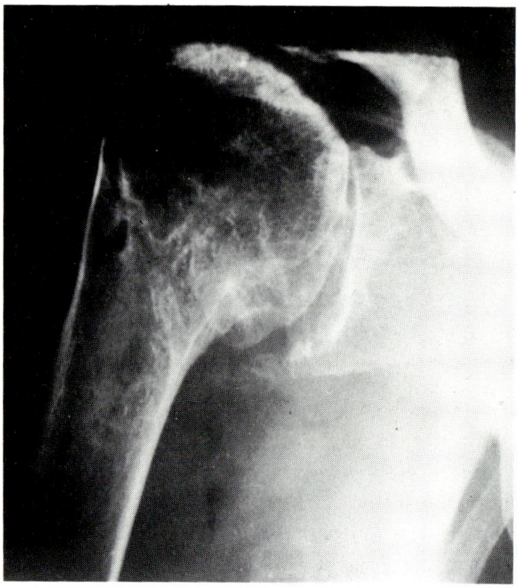

Fig. 34.21 Degenerative arthritis of the shoulders is not common. This X-ray shows narrowing of the joint space, some flattening of the articular surfaces and cystic change within the head of the humerus.

authors, presents with pain, swelling and limitation of the shoulder. A large effusion, rich in collagenase, neutral protease and microspheroids containing hydroxyapatite, is characteristic and there is usually evidence of rotator cuff disruption, soft tissue calcification and degenerative change within the humeral head. The Milwaukee shoulder does appear to be a distinct arthropathy and it is not part of the usual picture of generalised OA.

ACROMIOCLAVICULAR JOINT

OA in this joint causes a poorly localised pain in the region of the shoulder joint. The acromioclavicular joint may become enlarged and tender to touch. If passive movement of the glenohumeral joint is full, and neck movements do not exacerbate the discomfort, it should be suspected that the shoulder ache is due to involvement of the acromioclavicular joint.

STERNOCLAVICULAR AND MANUBRIOSTERNAL JOINTS

Tender enlargement of the sternocalvicular joint may occur in generalised OA. More rarely, similar changes occur at the manubriosternal joint. Local discomfort will be felt when pressure is put on these sites, e.g. when lying on one side, but persistent symptoms are unusual.

TEMPOROMANDIBULAR JOINT

Degenerative changes may develop in the temporomandibular joints. There is no satisfactory evidence to support the popular supposition that the changes result from malocclusion or abnormal mastication (Schwartz, 1959). The patient may complain of pain and stiffness in the joint, and the joint may be tender on palpation.

THE SPINE (Figs 34.22–34.24)

The spine is the site most frequently affected by OA. By the age of 70, it is virtually universally present (Schmorl & Junghanns, 1971). It is often accompanied by OA at other sites. It should be stated at once that the correlation between clinical and radiological OA of the spine is poor. Amongst a population without OA on spinal X-ray, Lawrence et al (1966) found that 50% complained of lumbar pain and 40% of cervical pain. Conversely,

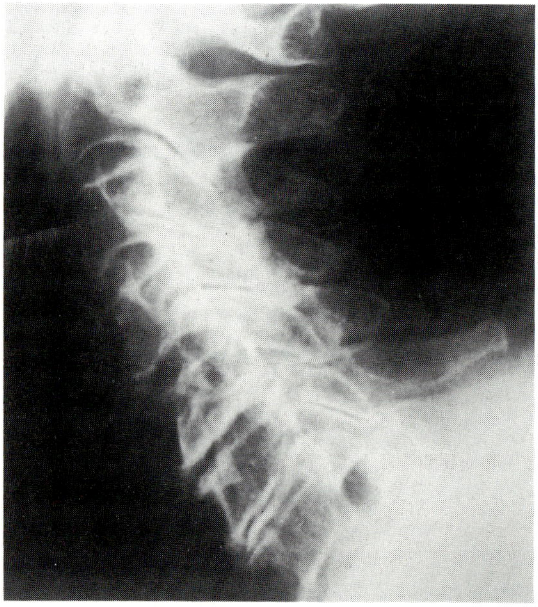

Fig. 34.22 Degenerative disease of the cervical spine. Proliferation of osteophytes around the disc margin may limit cervical movement. Posterior osteophytes may compress the spinal cord or trap existing nerve roots.

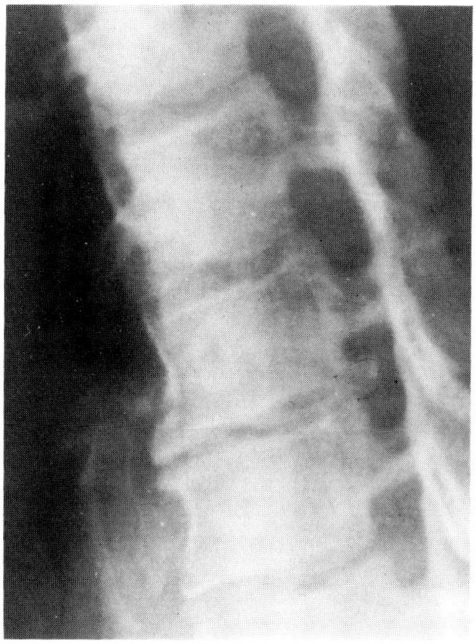

Fig. 34.23 Degenerative disease of the cervical spine. This oblique view shows an osteophyte encroaching on a neural foramen.

only 58% of those with lumbar OA radiologically and 44% of those with cervical OA complained of pain.

Though the term 'osteoarthrosis' is generally restricted to degenerative disease of the diarthrodial joints, in the spine the term is used (interchangeably with 'spondylosis') to encompass degeneration of both the fibrocartilaginous discs and the diarthrodial apophyseal joints. As the intervertebral disc degenerates and the disc space narrows, osteophytes develop along the margins of the vertebrae, particularly anteriorly. These appear to cause few symptoms. Concomitantly, however, degenerative changes occur in the apophyseal joints and posterolaterally around the neural foramina. Lesions at these sites frequently cause symptoms either through disruption of the normal anatomy or through pressure on nerve roots or on the spinal cord.

The osteoarthritic changes are usually most severe at the apices of the lordotic segments of the

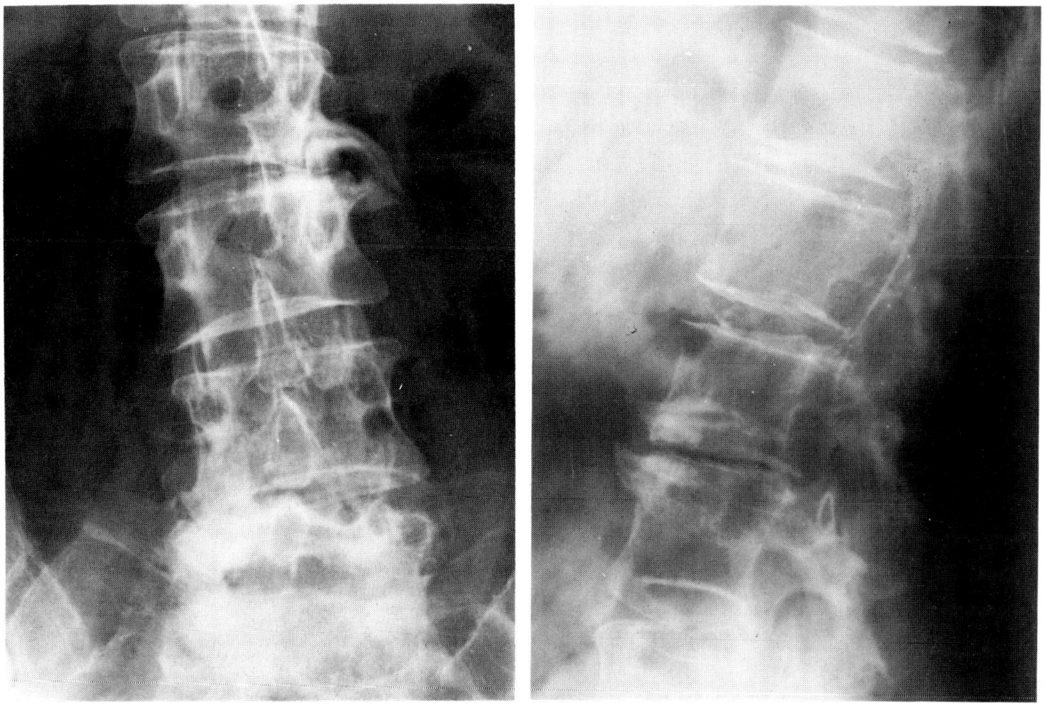

a b

Fig. 34.24 Degenerative disease of the lumbar spine. (a) Anteroposterior view. Large bridging osteophytes can be seen along the left lateral margins of the 3rd and 4th lumbar vertebrae. (b) Lateral view. The disc space between the 3rd and 4th lumbar vertebrae is narrowed and there is abundant anterior osteophyte formation. The disc space contains a small pocket of gas, the 'vacuum phenomenon' sometimes seen with degenerative disc disease. Linear calcification is seen within the disc space between the 1st and 2nd lumbar vertebrae.

spine, i.e. at C5–C6, T7–T8 and L3–L4 levels. With advancing age the changes may be seen throughout the spine, the most florid changes being seen in those with ankylosing hyperostosis. In this condition the osteophyte growth may ankylose whole segments of the spine. OA may develop prematurely in the spine in acromegaly and ochronosis.

Pain and stiffness are the characteristic symptoms of OA of the spine. As with OA at other sites, it is thought that symptoms may arise from the joint capsules, surrounding ligaments and periosteum and from the growth osteophytes. In addition, some discomfort may arise from paraspinal muscle spasm and from nerve root compression with referred radicular pain and paraesthesiae. Referred pain is most common in the C5, C6 and C7 dermatomes of the arms, and in the L4, L5 and S1 dermatomes in the legs, and may be associated with alteration of sensation, power and reflexes in the affected limbs. Occasionally entrapment of the lowest cervical and upper thoracic nerve roots may give rise to chest wall pain which can be mistaken for ischaemic cardiac pain.

Osteophytes may encroach on the spinal cord and cause cord compression. This is most commonly seen with OA of the lower cervical spine as at this point the canal is relatively narrow and the cord is relatively large. The signs of nerve root and cord compression may be detected in the absence of neck pain. Pallis et al (1954) in a study of 50 patients who were over the age of 50 and in hospital for investigation of complaints not related to the cervical spine or central nervous system, found signs of cord compression in 50% and of root compression in 40%.

Osteophyte formation within the spinal canal may also compress the blood supply to the spinal cord, causing a spinal claudication syndrome. Most common of these is claudication of the cauda equina in which the patient will complain of pain and paraesthesia in the legs which are related to exercise and the neurological deficit may be apparent only after exercise. Osteophyte growth may occasionally compress the vertebral arteries, as they course through the vascular foramina of the cervical vertebrae, and this will result in basilar artery insufficiency syndromes, presenting in a variety of ways, most commonly with headache, dizziness, nausea and ataxia. The neurological complications of spinal OA are frequently disabling and may be irreversible. Surgery to decompress the spinal cord or a nerve root may be undertaken in some circumstances, but the results of decompression are unpredictable, as often the neurological deficit has developed slowly and is irreversible by the time of presentation.

SACROILIAC JOINTS

These may be involved by the degenerative process, but as there have been no reported studies of this joint in OA, the frequency of symptoms and of radiological change are not known. The symptoms are of low back pain and stiffness, and local joint tenderness is a common finding. Secondary degenerative changes may occur in this joint after septic arthritis.

HIP JOINT (Fig. 34.25)

Particular forms of secondary degenerative arthritis of the hip joint have been discussed above. The estimates as to the percentage of cases which are secondary to some other pathology vary from 20–70% (Wiberg, 1939; Lloyd-Roberts, 1955; Murray, 1965). Primary OA of the hip is commonly unilateral, and men are affected more often than women.

The patient with degenerative hip disease complains of pain which may be felt in the groin region, the buttocks, the thigh or knee. The discomfort is exacerbated by movement of the joint and by weight-bearing. The referred pain in the thigh is thought to be due to the fact that both the hip joint and the skin of the medial thigh receive their innervation through the obturator nerve and its branches. Stiffness on rising and after inactivity are also characteristic symptoms, though they are usually overshadowed by the pain.

Restriction of movement may not be noticed by the patient initially, as flexion of the joint tends to be preserved. Extension and internal rotation movements are usually the first to be restricted and later flexion and abduction are compromised. With advanced disease flexion and abduction deformity of the joint may develop. The leg will be held in fixed flexion adduction and external rotation. This

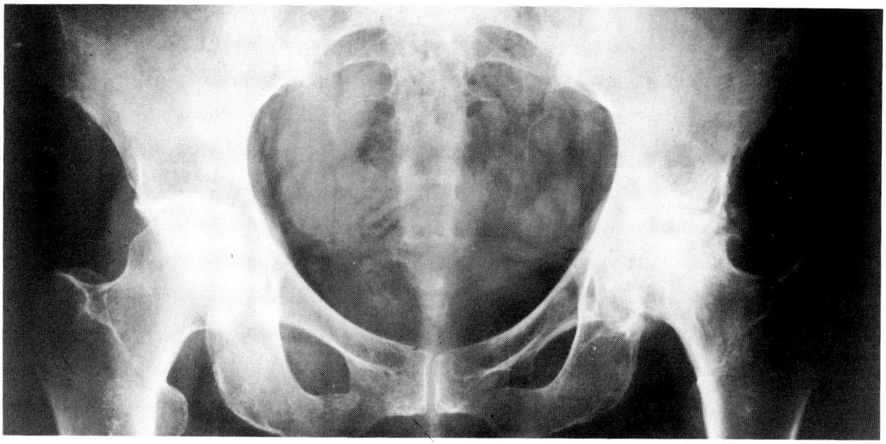

Fig. 34.25 Degenerative arthritis of the hip joint. The left hip shows marked narrowing of the joint space superiorly and medially and the femoral head is flattened superiorly. The joint margins are sclerotic and there is osteophytic buttressing of the acetabulum and the femoral head. Large lucent degenerative cysts are present in the acetabulum and in the head of the femur.

results is apparent shortening of the limb, but true shortening may also supervene if there is collapse of the substance of the femoral head. With painful restriction of hip movements, atrophy of the gluteal and quadriceps muscle occurs. The gait in patients with OA of the hip is usually antalgic (i.e. the stance phase is shortened on the affected side, and this results in a shorter period of weight-bearing on the affected limb). Frequently the patient will in addition lurch towards the involved side, in which case the gait may be described as coxalgic. The transfer of weight to the affected joint has the effect of reducing the amount of abductor muscle activity needed to maintain a level pelvis when walking. Some patients with longstanding hip disease develop a Trendelenberg gait because of their hip adduction deformity and associated abductor muscle weakness. The pelvis drops on the non-affected side when weight-bearing on the affected leg.

Two major patterns of OA of the hip joint have been described. The first is termed 'superolateral OA', as the maximum narrowing of joint space occurs in the superolateral segment of the joint. The head of the femur may sublux upwards and out of the acetabulum with progression of the disease. The second type is characterised by narrowing of the joint space medially with marginal osteophytic buttressing. This may be accompanied by a degree of protrusio acetabuli. The second type is thought to be more common amongst patients with generalised OA, and is said to have a better prognosis, less frequently requiring surgery than the first type.

Solomon et al (1982) have suggested an alternative subgrouping comprising a hypertrophic form of hip joint degeneration and an atrophic form. The hypertrophic group is characterised by abundant new bone formation and localised cartilage loss and there may be evidence of mechanical or anatomical abnormalities. The atrophic form on the other hand features extensive cartilage loss with little bone reaction and the patients frequently show evidence of polyarticular osteoarthrosis. Neither subgrouping however is entirely self-contained and it is likely that other subgroupings based on clinical, pathological and biochemical findings will be delineated in the future.

KNEE (Fig. 34.26)

OA of the knee joint is usually seen as part of the picture of primary generalised OA. In Kellgren & Moore's original series (1952) of patients with generalised OA, 50% had knee involvement and in the majority the condition was bilateral. As is the case with other weight-bearing joints, OA of the knee is likely to present with symptoms. Lawrence et al (1966) found that 43% of men and 57% of women who had radiological OA of the knee

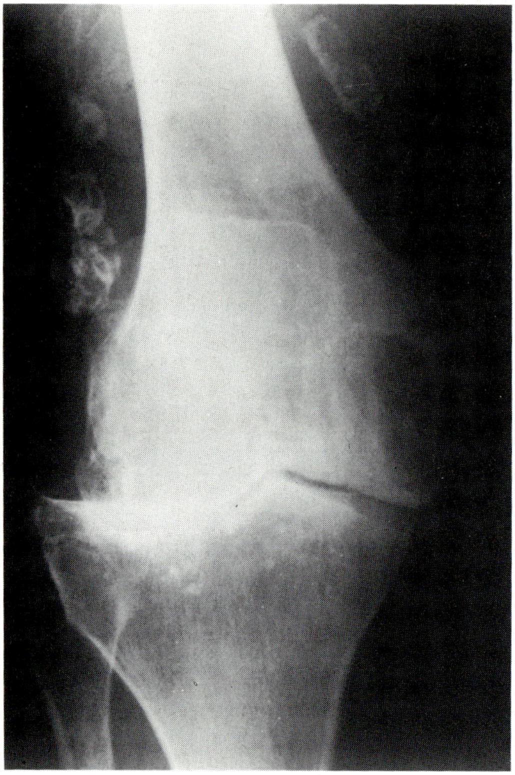

Fig. 34.26 Degenerative arthritis of the knee joint. Osteoarthritic changes are present in both knees but are most marked on the right side. There is loss of joint space, increased bone density, marginal osteophyte formation and some periarticular soft tissue calcification. There is also medial subluxation of the right femur on the tibia and a large degenerative cyst is present in the medial condyle of the right femur.

joint also had symptoms referable to that joint. This is in contrast to OA of the small joints of the hands, which causes discomfort much less frequently.

OA of the knee may involve the medial tibiofemoral, the lateral tibiofemoral and the patellofemoral compartments of the joint. Pain on movement and stiffness on waking and after inactivity are the major symptoms. Like OA of the hip joint, advanced disease may give rise to distressing pain while in bed at night.

On examination, the osteoarthritic knee may be obviously enlarged, either as a result of synovial effusion accompanying a low-grade synovitis, or as a consequence of bony overgrowth due to marginal osteophyte formation. The joint margins are frequently tender on palpation, and movement of the joint will often produce crepitus, most commonly in the patellofemoral joint. As joint degeneration progresses, a varus or valgus deformity may develop and occasionally this deformity will be accompanied by instability of the joint. Progressive wasting of the quadriceps usually develops hand in hand with the degenerative knee disease, and the lack of muscular support for the joint may further impair the patient's mobility, causing the knee to 'give way' in certain situations, e.g. when descending stairs or stepping off a pavement. The osteoarthritic knee is frequently the site of deposition of crystals of calcium pyrophosphate dihydrate. The prevalence of such deposition increases with age, and the knee joint is a characteristic site. In the 7th decade the prevalence is about 5% (McCarty, 1976) but by the 9th decade it may be as high as 28% (Ellman & Levin, 1975). The pyrophosphate crystals, if released into the joint space, will cause episòdes of acute synovitis which contrast with the usually chronic course of OA of the knee.

Chondromalacia patellae, a condition seen in young adults and characterised by patellofemoral discomfort on knee movements, is no longer thought to be a precursor of OA of the knee joint (Goodfellow et al, 1976; Abernethy et al, 1977).

ANKLE JOINTS AND HIND FOOT

Osteoarthritic involvement of the ankle joint is rare. It is occasionally seen following trauma to the joint, and is said to be more common among footballers (Brodelius, 1961) and lacrosse players (Thomas, 1971). OA at other sites in the hindfoot is rare.

FOREFOOT

OA of the metatarsophalangeal joint of the great toe is very common, and is often part of the clinical picture of primary generalised OA. The degenerative changes may develop without great toe deformity, or in association with hallux valgus. In those without deformity the patient will experience pain and stiffness in the affected joint as with OA at other sites. Symptoms may be hastened by the development of hallux rigidus, when extension of the toe is blocked by osteophyte formation and normal gait becomes painful. When hallux valgus is present, a bursa frequently develops over the medial aspect of the joint. Excessive valgus deformity of the great toe will result in subluxation of the 2nd and 3rd metatarsophalangeal joints, and in collapse of the transverse arch of the foot, with consequent pain on standing and walking.

INVESTIGATION OF OA

The diagnosis of OA is largely clinical. X-rays may provide useful confirmatory evidence of the condition, but laboratory investigations are usually of little help, except perhaps in detecting the underlying cause in certain rarer forms of secondary OA.

RADIOLOGICAL INVESTIGATIONS

The earliest change on X-ray in OA is joint space narrowing. This is usually accompanied by bony sclerosis around the joint margins, in contrast to rheumatoid disease which is characterised by juxta-articular osteoporosis. With advancement of disease, marginal osteophytes and subchondral bone cysts will develop (Fig. 34.25) and finally, in end-stage disease, the normal structures of the joint may be difficult to make out and gross bony deformity will be evident (see Figs 34.3, 34.10, 34.26).

Calcification within the articular soft tissues is an extremely common finding in OA. This may take the form of chondrocalcinosis in which the crystal deposited is calcium pyrophosphate dihydrate. The knee, wrist and symphysis pubis are the characteristic sites for such deposits. In the knee joint the crystals are laid down in linear fashion in the meniscus and in the hyaline articular cartilage (see Fig. 34.15); in the wrist the deposition tends to occur in the triangular ligament (see Fig. 34.16) and in the symphysis pubis in the fibrocartilage. OA of the metacarpophalangeal joints is said to be a characteristic of those patients with chronic pyrophosphate arthropathy (McCarty, 1976).

Non-linear deposits of calcium crystals are commonly seen in the periarticular soft tissues of patients with OA, especially in advanced disease (Fig. 34.26). Though these appear to be loose bodies on X-ray, they are usually within the synovial tissues. Some represent bone fragments which have broken away from the eburnated articular surface and have then been incorporated into the synovium, others may be growing deposits of crystals of calcium pyrophosphate dihydrate, and a further group may be the result of metaplastic change within the synovial tissues with cartilage formation and subsequent calcification of this cartilage. These calcified bodies can break free and form loose bodies which will severely hamper joint movement.

The term 'erosive arthritis' was coined by Crain (1961) and is used to describe OA with an acute inflammatory onset, typically involving the distal interphalangeal joints. X-rays of such joints shows erosions along the joint margins (see Fig. 34.14) in addition to the degenerative changes already described.

Joint ankylosis, though relatively rare in OA, characterises ankylosing hyperostosis, a florid degenerative condition of the spine (see Fig. 34.17). Bony spur formation, usually more marked on the right side of the spine, progresses until bony bridges have formed between vertebrae, and spinal ankylosis has occurred. The disc spaces are often well preserved and the sacroiliac joints are normal.

Bony ankylosis in OA may also occur in erosive OA (McEwan 1968) and in OA of the first metatarsophalangeal joint.

LABORATORY INVESTIGATIONS

Blood

The blood count, erythrocyte sedimentation rate (ESR) and bone biochemistry are normal in OA.

Synovial fluid

The synovial fluid is viscous, straw-coloured, and contains a small number of cells, predominantly mononuclear cells and macrophages. In advanced disease the fluid will contain fragments of the degenerating articular surface, e.g. cartilage fragments, bone fragments and hydroxyapatite or calcium pyrophosphate crystals. When calcium crystals are released into the joint space a vigorous inflammatory response is provoked and the synovial fluid will be less viscous and will contain numerous polymorphonuclear leucocytes. When viewed under polarised light the crystals may be seen free in the joint fluid and within the polymorphonuclear leucocytes.

Other investigations

Radionuclide joint imaging has been advocated in OA, but has yet to prove a useful investigative or therapeutic tool in this disease (Hoffer & Genant, 1976; Desaulniers et al, 1973). Thermography, arthroscopy and arthrography have also failed to achieve a useful diagnostic niche in the investigation of OA.

DIFFERENTIAL DIAGNOSIS OF OA

Since OA is the manifestation of joint failure and may result from many different pathological processes, the differential diagnosis must include the long list of potential causes of this condition. These have been discussed earlier. A clinical problem which is commonly encountered is whether a particular symptom can be accounted for by the finding of degenerative changes on X-ray of that site. Degenerative changes on X-ray examination are extremely common over the age of 55, but such changes are not always associated with symptoms. This is particularly true of small joints such as the distal interphalangeal joints, where only 10% of those with radiological OA will have pain in that joint. Even in the case of weight-bearing joints such as the hip or knee or spine, only 50% of those with radiological OA will experience pain (Lawrence et al, 1966). The converse is also true. Patients may experience pain at a particular site and show no radiological evidence of OA. This is particularly true of patients with low back pain, 50% of whom will show no degenerative changes on X-ray (Lawrence et al, 1966). The presence of OA on X-ray, therefore, does not necessarily explain a patient's symptoms. Supportive clinical findings must be used to substantiate a diagnosis of OA, and in the osteoarthritic age-group other causes of limb and joint pain and stiffness should be excluded. For example, pain in patients of this age-group may be due to malignant disease which has involved bone, or Paget's disease. Similarly, stiffness may be due to another condition such as polymyalgia rheumatica, Parkinson's disease or spasticity.

A particular diagnostic difficulty may be encountered in those elderly patients already suffering from OA who develop superimposed inflammatory rheumatic diseases such as rheumatoid arthritis and polymyalgia rheumatica. In this situation the marked increase in morning stiffness, the systemic symptoms and the sudden change in pattern of the illness should alert the physician to the presence of a second pathology. In the case of rheumatoid arthritis the classical pattern of joint involvement will usually point to the diagnosis, and an elevated ESR together with positive rheumatoid factor test may help confirm it. A high index of suspicion is necessary if polymyalgia rheumatica is to be detected early. It is, of course, characterised by shoulder and pelvic girdle myalgia, severe morning stiffness and systemic symptoms, but in an elderly patient these may be wrongly attributed to OA. A sudden change in the pattern of the patient's symptoms, together with the finding of a high ESR should point to the alternative diagnosis.

REFERENCES

Abernethy P J, Townsend P R, Rose R M 1977 Chondromalacis patellae as a separate entity. Arthritis and Rheumatism 20:105

Acheson R M, Chan Y, Clemett A R 1970 New Haven survey of joint diseases. XII. Distribution and symptoms of osteoarthrosis in the hands with reference to handedness. Annals of the Rheumatic Diseases 29: 275–286

Adam A, Spence A J 1958 Intertrochanteric osteotomy for osteoarthresis of the hip. A review of fifty eight operations. Journal of Bone and Joint Surgery 408: 219–226

Alexander G J M, Scott D G I, Dieppe P A 1981 Disease associations and laboratory investigations in pyrophosphate arthropathy. Annals of the Rheumatic Diseases 40:515

Andersen S, Winckler F 1979 The epidemiology of primary osteoarthritis of the knee in Greenland. Archives of Orthopaedic and Traumatic Surgery (Munchen) 93: 91–94

Ash P, Francis M J O 1975 Response of isolated rabbit articular and epiphyseal chondrocytes to rat liver somatomedin. Journal of Endocrinology 66: 71–78

Begg M W, Scott J E 1966 Hyaluronic acid and protein in simple ganglia and Heberden's nodes. Annals of the Rheumatic Diseases 25: 145–148

Bland J H, Eddy W M 1968 Hemiplegia and rheumatoid hemiarthritis. Arthritis and Rheumatism 11: 72–80

Bremner J M, Lawrence J S, Miall W E 1968 Degenerative

joint disease in a Jamaican rural population. Annals of the Rheumatic Diseases 27: 326–332

Brodelius A 1961 Osteoarthrosis of the talar joints in footballers and ballet dancers. Acta Orthopaedica Scandinavica 30: 309–314

Bruckner F E, Howell A 1972 Neuropathic joints. Seminars in arthritis and rheumatism 2: 47–49

Brugsch H G 1957 Rheumatic diseases, Rheumatism and arthritis. Philadelphia, p. 6

Burssens A, Dequeker J, Bouillon R, De Moor P, Mulier J C 1974 Growth hormone and osteoporosis. Israel Medical Journal 10: 1473–1474

Byers P D, Hoaglund F T, Purewal G S, Yau A C M C 1974 Articular cartilage changes in Caucasian and Asian hip joints. Annals of the Rheumatic Diseases 33: 157–161

Carter C O, Wilkinson J A 1964 Genetic and environmental factors in the etiology of congenital dislocation of the hip. Clinical Orthopaedics and Related Research 33: 119–128

Cecil R L, Archer B H 1926 Classification and treatment of chronic arthritis. Journal of the American Medical Association 87: 741–746

Charcot J M 1868 Sur quelques arthropathies qui paraissent dépendre d'une lesion du cerveau ou de la moelle épinière. Archives de Physiologie Normale et Pathologique 1: 161–178

Chung S M K, Ralston E L 1969 Necrosis of the femoral head associated with sickle cell anaemia and its genetic variants. A review of the literature and study of thirteen cases. Journal of Bone and Joint Surgery 51A: 33–58

Coates Claire, Geoffrey Buswell R, Lloyd-Jones K, Swannell A J, Walker G, Selby C 1978 Somatomedin activity in synovial fluid from patients with joint diseases. Annals of the Rheumatic Diseases 37: 303–314

Cobb S, Merchant W R, Rubin T 1957 The relation of symptoms to osteoarthritis. Journal of Chronic Diseases 5: 197–204

Copeman W S C 1964 A short history of the gout and the rheumatic diseases. University of California Press, p. 185

Crain D C 1961 Interphalangeal osteoarthritis characterised by painful, inflammatory episodes resulting in deformity of the proximal and distal articulations. Journal of the American Medical Association 175: 1049–1053

Danielsson L G 1964 Incidençe and prognosis of coxarthrosis. Acta Orthopaedica Scandinavica (Suppl) 66: 1–61

Desaulniers M, Fuks A, Hawkins D, Lacourciere Y, Rosenthall L 1973 Radiotechnetium polyphosphate joint imaging. Journal of Nuclear Medicine 15: 417–423

Dieppe P A, Huskisson E C, Crocker P, Willoughby D A 1976 Apetite deposition disease: a new arthropathy. Lancet 1: 266–269

Dieppe P A, Doyle D V, Huskisson E C, Willoughby D A, Crocker P R 1978 Mixed crystal deposition disease and osteoarthritis. British Medical Journal 1:150

Dixon A St J, Campbell-Smith S 1969 Long leg arthropathy. Annals of the Rheumatic Diseases 28: 359–365

Dorwort B B, Schumacher H R 1975 Joint effusions, chondrocalcinosis and rheumatic manifestations of hypothyroidism. American Journal of Medicine 59: 780–790

Doyle D V 1982 Tissue calcification and inflammation in osteoarthritis. Journal of Pathology 136: 199–216

Doyle D V, Dieppe P A, Crocker P R, Ibe K, Willoughby D A 1977 Mixed crystal deposition in an osteoarthritic joint. Journal of Pathology 123: 1–4

Dymock I W, Hamilton E B D, Laws J W, Williams R 1970 Arthropathy of haemochromatosis. Clinical and radiological analysis of 63 patients with iron overload. Annals of the Rheumatic Diseases 29: 469–476

Ehrlich G E 1972 Inflammatory osteoarthritis — 1. The clinical syndrome. Journal of Chronic Diseases 25: 317–328

Ehrlich G E 1975 Osteoarthritis beginning with inflammation. Definitions and correlations. Journal of the American Medical Association 232: 157–159

Ellman M H, Levin B 1975 Chondrocalcinosis in elderly persons. Arthritis and Rheumatism 18: 43–47

Engel A 1968 Osteoarthritis and body measurements: United States 1960–62. PHS Publication 1000, Series 11, No. 29, Washington, DC

Feller E R, Schumacher H R 1972 Osteoarticular changes in Wilson's diseases. Arthritis and Rheumatism 15: 259–266

Forestier J, Lagier R 1971 Ankylosing hyperostosis of the spine. Clinical Orthopaedics and Related Research 74: 65–83

Forestier J, Rotes-Querol J 1950 Senile ankylosing hyperostosis of the spine. Annals of the Rheumatic Diseases 9: 321–330

Franchimont P, Denis F 1968 Determination du taux de la somatotrophine et des gonadotrophines dans des cas d'arthrose apparaissant lors de la ménopause. Journal Belge de Rheumatologie et de Medicine Physique 23: 59–64

Golding D N, Walshe J M 1977 Arthropathy of Wilson's disease. Study of clinical and radiological features in 32 patients. Annals of the Rheumatic Diseases 36: 99–111

Goodfellow J, Hunergford D S, Wood C 1976 Patello-femoral joint mechanics and pathology. 1. Functional anatomy of the patello-femoral joint. Journal of Bone and Joint Surgery 588: 287–290

Gower W E, Johnston R C 1971 Legg-Perthes' disease. Longterm follow-up of 36 patients. Journal of Bone and Joint Surgery 53A: 759–768

Hadler N M 1977 Industrial rheumatology. Clinical investigations into the influence of pattern of usage on patterns of regional musculoskeletal disease. Arthritis and Rheumatism 20: 1019–1025

Hadler N M 1981 The variable of usage in the epidemiology of osteoarthrosis. In: Peyron J G (ed) Epidemiology of osteoarthritis. Ciba-Geigy, Rueil-Malmaison

Hadler N M, Gillings D B, Imbus H R, Levitin P M, Makuc D, Utsinger P D et al 1978 Hand structure and function in an industrial setting. Influence of three patterns of stereotyped repetitive usage. Arthritis and Rheumatism 21: 210–220

Hamilton E B D, Williams R, Barlow K A, Smith P M 1967 The arthropathy of idiopathic haemochromatosis. Quarterly Journal of Medicine 37: 171–182

Haygarth J 1805 A clinical history of disease. Gadell & Davies, London

Heberden W 1806 Commentaries on the history and cause of Diseases, 3rd Edn. Printed for T Payne of Pall Mall, p. 148

Hoaglund F T, Yau A C M C, Wong W L 1973 Osteoarthritis of the hip and other joints in Southern Chinese in Hong Kong. Journal of Bone and Joint Surgery 55A: 545–557

Hoffer P B, Genant H K 1976 Radionuclide joint imaging. Seminars in Nuclear Medicine 6: 121–137

Hunter D, McLaughlin A I G, Perry K M A 1945 Clinical effects of the use of pneumatic tools. British Journal of Industrial Medicine 2: 10–16

Huskisson E C, Dieppe P A, Tucker A K, Cannell B 1979 Another look at osteoarthritis. Annals of the Rheumatic Diseases 38: 423–428
Julkenen H, Heinonen D P, Pyorala K 1971 Hyperostosis of the spine in an adult population, its relationship to hyperglycaemia and obesity. Annals of Rheumatic Diseases 30: 605–612
Julkenen H, Knekt P, Aromaa A 1981 Diffuse idiopathic skeletal hyperostosis in relation to spondylosis deformans in Finnish population. Proceedings of XV International Congress of Rheumatology. Abstract 0984
Kellgren J H, Lawrence J S 1952 Rheumatism in miners. Part II. X-ray study. British Journal of Industrial Medicine 9: 197–207
Kellgren J H, Lawrence J S 1958 Osteoarthrosis and disk degeneration in an urban population. Annals of the Rheumatic Diseases 17: 388–397
Kellgren J H, Moore R 1952 Generalised osteoarthritis and Heberden's nodes. British Medical Journal 1: 181–187
Kellgren J H, Lawrence J S, Bier F 1963 Genetic factors in generalised osteoarthrosis. Annals of the Rheumatic Diseases 22: 237–255
Lawrence J S 1955 Rheumatism in miners. III. Occupational factors. British Journal of Industrial Medicine 12: 249–261
Lawrence J S, Bremner J M, Bier F 1966 Osteoarthrosis, prevalence in the population and relationship between symptoms and X-ray changes. Annals of the Rheumatic Diseases 25: 1–24
Lloyd-Roberts G C 1955 Osteoarthritis of the hip. A study of the clinical pathology. Journal of Bone and Joint Surgery 37B: 8–47
McCarty D J 1976 Calcium pyrophosphate dihydrate deposition disease — 1975. Arthritis and Rheumatism 19: 275–285
McCarty D J, Kohn N N, Faires J S 1962 The significance of calcium phosphate crystals in the synovial fluid of arthritis patients: the 'pseudogout syndrome'. I. Clinical aspects. Annals of Internal Medicine 56: 711–737
McCarty D J, Halverson P B, Carrera G F, Brewer B J, Kozin F 1981 'Milwaukee shoulder' — association of microspheroids containing hydroxyapatite crystals, active collagenase, and neutral protease with rotator cuff defects. 1. Clinical aspects. Arthritis and Rheumatism 24: 464–473
McEwan C 1968 Osteoarthritis of the fingers with ankylosis. Arthritis and Rheumatism 11: 734–744
McKusick V A, Neufeld E F, Kelly T E 1978 The mucopolysaccharide storage diseases. In: Stanbury J B, Wyngaarden J B, Fredrickson D S (eds) The metabolic basis of inherited disease, 4th Edn. McGraw-Hill, New York, p. 1282–1307
Mintz G, Fraga A 1973 Severe osteoarthritis of the elbow in foundary workers. Archives of Environmental Health 27: 78–84
Montagu A 1959 Human heredity World Publishing Co, Cleveland, p. 331
Murray R D 1965 The aetiology of primary osteoarthritis of the hip. British Journal of Radiology 38: 810–824
Nesterov A I 1964 The clinical course of Kashin–Beck disease. Arthritis and Rheumatism 7: 29–40
Nicoll E A, Holden N T 1961 Displacement osteotomy in the treatment of osteoarthritis of the hip. Journal of Bone and Joint Surgery 438: 50–60
O'Brien W M, La Du B N, Bunim J J 1963 Biochemical, pathological and clinical aspects of alkaptonuria, ochronosis and ochronotic arthropathy. Review of the world literature (1584–1962). American Journal of Medicine 34: 813–838
Pallis C, Jones A M, Spillane J D 1954 Cervical spondylosis. Brain 77: 274–289
Peter J B, Pearson C M, Marmor L 1966 Erosive osteoarthritis of the hands. Arthritis and Rheumatism 9: 365–388
Puranen J, Ala-Ketola L, Peltokallio P, Saarela J 1975 Running and primary osteoarthritis of the hip. British Medical Journal 2: 424–425
Record R G, Edwards J H 1958 Environmental influences related to the aetiology of congenital dislocation of the hip. British Journal of Preventive and Social Medicine 12: 8–22
Rogers J, Dieppe P, Watt I 1981 Arthritis in Saxon and mediaeval skeletons. Annals of the Rheumatic Diseases 40:206
Rubinstein H M 1975 Thiemann's disease. A brief reminder. Arthritis and Rheumatism 18: 357–360
Schmorl G, Junghanns H 1971 The human spine in health and disease. Grune & Stratton, New York
Schwartz L 1959 Disorders of the tempero-mandibular joints. Saunders, Philadelphia
Shapiro R F, Utsinger P D, Wiesner K B, Resnick D, Bryan B, Castles J 1976 The association of HLA B27 with Forestier's disease (vertebral ankylosing hyperostosis). Journal of Rheumatology 3: 4–8
Silberberg M, Silberberg R 1964 Dyschondrogenesis and osteoarthrosis in mice. Archives of Pathology 70: 385–390
Silberberg M, Silberberg R 1970 Age-linked modification of the effect of estrogen on joints and cortical bone of female mice. Gerontologia 16: 201–211
Silberberg R, Hasler M 1971 Submicroscopic effects of hormones on articular cartilage of adult mice. Archives of Pathology 91: 241–255
Silberberg R, Silberberg M 1964 Pathogenesis of osteoarthrosis. Pathologie Microbiologia 27: 447–457
Silberberg R, Silberberg M 1965 Ageing changes and osteoarthrosis in castrate mice receiving progesterone. Journal of Gerontology 20: 228–232
Silberberg M, Frank E L, Jarrett S R, Silberberg R 1959 Ageing and osteoarthritis of the human sternoclavicular joint. American Journal of Pathology 35: 851–865
Sokoloff L, Crittenden L B, Yamamoto R S, Jay G E Jr 1962 The genetics of degenerative joint disease in mice. Arthritis and Rheumatism 5: 531–546
Solomon L, Beighton P, Lawrence J S 1975 Rheumatic disorders in the South African negro. Part II. Osteoarthrosis. South African Medical Journal 49: 1737–1740
Solomon L 1976 Patterns of osteoarthritis of the hip. Journal of Bone and Joint Surgery 58B: 176–183
Solomon L, Schnitzler C M, Browett J P 1982 Osteoarthritis of the hip: the patient behind the disease. Annals of the Rheumatic Diseases 41: 118–125
Solonen K A 1966 The joints of the lower extremities of football players. Annales Chirurgiae Gynaecologiae Fenniae 55: 176–180
Stecher R M, Hersh A H, Hauser H 1953 Heberden's nodes. The family history and radiographic appearance of a large family. American Journal of Human Genetics 5: 46–60
Stecher R M 1955 Heberden's nodes; a clinical description of osteoarthritis of the finger joints. Annals of the Rheumatic Diseases 14: 1–10

Thomas R B 1971 Chronic injury — Lacrosse. In: Larson J A (ed) Encyclopaedia of sports, sciences and medicine. Macmillan, New York
Walton M 1979 Obesity as an aetiological factor in the development of osteoarthrosis. Gerontology 25: 36–41
Wiberg G 1939 Relation between congenital subluxation of the hip and arthritis deformans. (A Roentgenological study). Acta Orthopaedica Scandinavica 10: 351–371
Wood P N H 1971 Rheumatic complaints. British Medical Bulletin 27: 82–88
Wood P N H, McLeish C L 1974 Statistical appendix — digest of data on the rheumatic disease: 5 morbidity in industry, and rheumatism in general practice. Annals of the Rheumatic Diseases 33: 93–105

Management of osteoarthrosis

MEDICAL MANAGEMENT OF OA

Management of OA has two main aims: first to relieve symptoms; secondly to preserve the function of the failing joints.

Joint degeneration is usually fairly advanced by the time a patient presents with symptoms and, though in some cases there may be a correctable predisposing cause, the existing degeneration of the joint is not reversible. For this reason, the treatment of primary and secondary OA is generally similar.

The most important step in management is to explain the nature of the disease to the patient. The reassurance that the condition, though not reversible, is generally benign and only slowly progressive, will often allay the patient's anxiety about a diagnosis of arthritis.

The role of rest, exercise and diet

Excessive loading of an osteoarthritic joint will cause pain and disability, and may perhaps accelerate the degenerative process. A review of a patient's daily routine at home and at work may bring to light situations which unduly stress involved joints, and it may be possible to afford considerable pain relief by modifying this routine. For example, a rest period from weight-bearing may alleviate the symptoms of an osteoarthritic lower limb joint while still allowing the patient to complete the task in hand. It often helps to explain to a patient that overuse of an osteoarthritic joint will cause pain, but that he can safely exercise an affected joint within these limits. Complete rest of a joint is rarely useful, perhaps the only indication being acute crystal synovitis (e.g. pseudogout) in association with the osteoarthritic process. The load on an osteoarthritic joint can often be relieved by the correction of posture. For example, if shortening of a leg has developed as a result of OA of the hip joint, the correction of the shortening with a heel-raise may, by correcting posture, relieve symptoms. A walking stick or frame may similarly reduce the load on an arthritic hip or knee and increase the patient's ability to exercise.

Restriction of joint movement is usually accompanied by wasting of the muscles which support and move that joint. For example, wasting of the glutei occurs with OA of the hip, and quadriceps wasting with OA of the knee. A regular programme of controlled exercises may be the key to preserving the function of an osteoarthritic joint as it will restore the lost muscle bulk and provide some support for the degenerating joint. Though there is no firm evidence to suggest that excess weight will exacerbate a patient's symptoms, through overloading joints, weight reduction will frequently alleviate the symptoms of OA of weight-bearing joints, particularly in the case of the lumbar spine, hip and knee joints.

Role of remedial therapists in the treatment of OA

The importance of exercise in preserving function of the ostoearthritic joint has ensured a therapeutic role for the remedial therapist in the management of the patient with OA.The physiotherapist's skills should be used to devise and direct the patient's exercise programme, tailoring it to the individual's needs. Local measures such as heating (dry heat, ultrasound, short-wave diathermy, wax baths) or cooling (ice) may provide a useful analgesia prior to exercise, but offer no lasting relief as treatments. The aim of the physiotherapist should be to correct abnormal posture, to reduce joint deformity and to build up muscle power to support damaged joints. Exercise in a hydrotherapy pool or using suspension slings may be of help to the patient with advanced OA, as both measures eliminate the effects of gravity and facilitate joint mobilisation. In general, isometric exercises are used more often than isotonic because they build muscle as effectively, but impose less stress on a joint. The correction of a fixed flexion deformity of an osteoarthritic hip or knee may be difficult because joint movement is often restricted by marginal osteophytes. Serial splinting of the flexed joint by a physiotherapist and daily prone lying exercises may however produce some correction and are worth trying. The occupational therapist will contribute to the management of the patient with OA in several ways. Most practically she will assess the patient's disability in his home and work environment and report on any physical problems which may need correcting. For example, the patient with OA of the hips and lumbar spine may have great difficulty with bathing, climbing stairs or with reaching low-set power points, and minor alterations to correct such problems will often greatly improve a patient's ability to cope. Occupational therapy departments will usually have both light and heavy workshops and outdoor work facilities so that accurate work assessments can be made and advice given on employment. These facilities can also be used as part of a therapeutic exercise programme to improve joint function.

The orthotist may help the patient with osteoarthrosis. For example, corrective footwear may greatly relieve the symptoms of an osteoarthritic forefoot and the simple expedient of a heel raise to correct leg shortening may help to alleviate the symptoms of an osteoarthritic hip and lumbar spine.

The wide range of services which may be used to benefit the patient with OA must be coordinated by the physician, and the key to successful management hinges around a team approach by members of the different services.

Drug treatment of OA

By the time a diagnosis of OA has been made, joint degeneration is usually well established. Conventional drug treatment of OA aims to relieve pain but it will not halt or reverse the degenerative process. Because the main purpose of treatment is relief of discomfort, the evaluation of the efficacy of any remedy must allow for a placebo response which can be expected in at least 30% of patients treated (Evans, 1974). Such a response could clearly upset the assessment of any treatment of OA if a control group is omitted.

Analgesic and non-steroidal anti-inflammatory drugs

Since OA is primarily a degenerative condition, pure analgesic treatment has been advocated in preference to non-steroidal anti-inflammatory drugs. The latter group of compounds, however, is widely used in the treatment of OA and they have been shown in many studies to be effective treatment. In a study comparing an analgesic remedy (Distalgesic) with a non-steroidal anti-inflammatory drug in the treatment of OA, Doyle et al (1981) were able to show significant reduction in joint tenderness, and a definite patient preference for the non-steroidal compound, perhaps reflecting the fact that OA is frequently accompanied by low-grade joint inflammation. Virtually all of the large range of non-steroidal anti-inflammatory compounds now available can be shown to be as effective as aspirin in the field of pain relief, but the variation in the response of different individuals to any given compound does mean that if one agent fails to relieve symptoms it is still worth trying the other compounds (Huskisson et al, 1976). Most of the newer anti-inflammatory drugs cause fewer toxic effects than aspirin and are therefore better tolerated. This may be particularly important in the treatment of OA where the aims of therapy are limited to relief of pain and inflammation and where the treatment is not curative and will probably be continued for a long period. Long-term compliance with the treatment will be determined not only by the efficacy of a compound in relieving symptoms, but also by its side-effect profile and by the complexity of the dosage regimen. It is recognised that between 25 and 50% fail to take the treatment prescribed for them by their doctors and that non-compliance rises with the duration of the course of treatment (Blackwell, 1973). Simplicity of the dosing schedules has also been shown to influence the compliance with drug treatments. Gatley (1968) has shown that 67% of patients will adhere to a once daily treatment, whereas only 32% will manage to stick to a 4 times daily schedule. The relationship between compliance and the complexity of the drug regimen is not straightforward, however. It would appear that rheumatoid patients with severe disease appear to be more compliant than those with less active disease (Lee & Tan, 1979). Similarly patients with rheumatoid disease (mean compliance 73.3%) tend to be more compliant than those with OA (mean compliance 53.9%) (Deyo et al, 1981; Deyo, 1982). Perhaps the ideal treatment for OA, a chronic disease, should be effective in relieving symptoms, well tolerated and given once daily, and these characteristics should be used as a yardstick in selecting the anti-inflammatory or analgesic drug to be given to the patient with OA.

The most commonly used groups of analgesic and non-steroidal anti-inflammatory compounds used in the management of OA are listed in Table 35.1. Phenylbutazone and oxyphenbutazone have been excluded from this list because of the serious adverse reactions which may occur with their use. Aplastic anaemia is more common in patients over 55 years old and is more frequent in those who have taken these drugs for long periods. Clearly, the average patient with OA is over 55, and may require long-term treatment, and these two compounds should therefore be avoided.

Table 35.1 Drugs commonly used in the treatment of osteoarthrosis

Simple analgesics
Low dose aspirin
Paracetamol
Dextropropoxyphene
Codeine
Dihydrocodeine
Nefopam
Fixed-dose combinations, e.g. paracetamol and dextropropoxyphene (distalgesic)
Non-steroidal analgesic anti-inflammatory drugs
Aspirin and related compounds, e.g. benorylate, choline magnesium trisilicate, salsalate
Indomethacin
Propionic acid derivatives, e.g. ibuprofen, naproxen, ketoprofen, fenoprofen, flurbiprofen, fenbrufen, tiaprofenic acid
Drugs with clinical effects similar to those of the propionic acid derivatives, e.g. azapropazone, sulindac, diclofenac, diflunisal, piroxicam, mefanamic acid, flufenamic acid

Intra-articular steroid therapy

The value of intra-articular steroid treatment in OA has been disputed. Shah & Wright (1967) reported that such treatment was no more effective than the intra-articular injection of saline. Short-term improvement following intra-articular steroid was reported in a double-blind study by Friedman & Moore (1980), but by the end of 1 month this effect had disappeared. Similar results have been reported by Dieppe et al (1980) in another controlled study. Both of these studies involved the knee joint, however, and it is possible that intra-articular steroid may provide more prolonged relief at other sites. Mayer (1970) has reported a long-lasting benefit from intra-articular steroid injection of osteoarthritic carpometacarpal joints. It is also probable that acute synovitis due to crystals in an osteoarthritic joint will repond well to intra-articular injection of steroids (Dieppe et al, 1980).

Systemic steroid therapy has not been shown to be of any value in the treatment of OA.

Intra-articular radio-isotope therapy

The use of yttrium-90 (^{90}Y) to treat chronic pyrophosphate arthropathy has been advocated (Doherty & Dieppe, 1981). The hazards of exposure to radiation may be unacceptable in the younger patient where the long-term sequelae must always be considered, but since the patient with OA and associated pyrophosphate arthropathy is usually elderly the treatment may be considered reasonable. The knee is the most commonly affected joint and is ideally suited to the administration of treatment by the intra-articular route. Over a 6-month period ^{90}Y proved more effective than. intra-articular steroid in relieving symptoms, but it should be remembered that the long-term effectiveness of intra-articular steroid has not been established and that the consequences of cartilage irradiation on the progression of OA are unknown.

Radiotherapy

Gibson et al (1973) have shown that radiotherapy has a short-term advantage over conventional physiotherapy in the treatment of OA of the knee, but such treatment is not widely used, as the risks of ionising radiation outweigh the slight potential benefits of the treatment.

Intra-articular lubricants
Despite favourable reports in early uncontrolled studies, the treatment of OA by the local injection of a joint lubricant appears to be ineffective. Using silicone in a carefully controlled study, Wright et al (1971) showed a deterioration in the silicone-treated joints at one week when compared to the saline-injected control joints.

Alternative drug treatments for OA ('chondroprotective compounds')
The term 'chondroprotective' was coined to describe a group of compounds of high molecular weight that are said to protect and possibly restore the articular cartilage in OA. Examples of these compounds are glycosaminoglycan polysulphate (Arteparon), glycosaminoglycan sulphate peptide (Rumalon) and pentosan polysulphate. Pharmacokinetic studies suggest that glycosaminoglycan polysulphate has an affinity for the articular cartilage (Enislidis, 1972; Bach et al, 1977; Gallacchi et al, 1979) and it has been suggested that the protective action is the result of inhibition of cartilage degrading enzymes (Galacchi et al, 1979). Glycosaminoglycan sulphate peptide (Rumalon), which is a cartilage and bone extract, has been shown to have a marked stimulatory effect on proteoglycan synthesis in connective tissue, and Kalbhen (1981) has demonstrated a protective effect in biochemically induced OA in rat knee joints. A similar protective effect has been demonstrated in mechanically-induced OA in dogs (Newton et al, 1981). The value of these agents in treating human OA has yet to be established. In a prolonged open study using Rumalon in patients with OA of the hip Denko (1979) showed improvement of clinical measurements in the majority of the 20 patients treated, and regression of the X-ray changes in 4 of the 20 patients. A larger long-term study of Rumalon has been reported from Czechoslovakia (Rejholec & Kralova, 1979) in which 136 patients were randomly allocated to treatment with either Rumalon or B12 injections. Over a 14 year follow-up, the group treated with Rumalon appeared to lose less time from work and to have less disability. Similar success has been reported with Arteparon. In a double-blind study comprising 71 patients Wagenhauser (1982) compared the effects of intra-articular Arteparon and intra-articular saline. After 2 months, the end of the blind study period, both groups showed an equal improvement, but after a further 3 months of open follow-up the Arteparon-treated group was clearly superior. These studies illustrate the need for further controlled investigation of the effects of the 'chondroprotective' compounds on the progression of OA.

SURGICAL TREATMENT OF OA (see also Ch. 63)

The very fact that there is no preventative or curative treatment for OA ensures that surgery has a place in its management. The surgical treatment will be considered under 4 headings:

a. Joint replacement surgery
b. Surgical procedures to relieve pain e.g. osteotomy, arthrodesis
c. Debridement procedures
d. Surgery for OA of the spine.

Joint replacement surgery
Replacement of the hip joint, and to a lesser extent the knee joint, with a prosthesis is now established surgical practice. The high prevalence of OA in the community, the frequency of involvement of these two joints, and the lack of curative treatment has led to an enormous demand for joint replacement surgery.

Hip joint replacement
Hip joint replacement with Charnley prostheses (Charnley, 1961) is the most widely practised procedure, though the McKee & Watson-Farrar (1966) and the Ring (1968) prostheses have also proved satisfactory. The long-term results of hip replacement are extremely encouraging, Charnley & Cupic (1973) reporting a 92% success rate in 9 and 10 year follow-up. In a similar vein Beckenbaugh & Ilstrup (1978) in a 5 year follow-up of hip arthroplasties found that 97% of the patients had little or no pain. The rate of wear in a Charnley prosthesis has been calculated at 0.15 mm per year (Charnley & Halley, 1975) and is thought to be unrelated to body weight or degree of activity. The prosthesis should therefore remain satisfactory for

about 33 years, a functional life-span which exceeds the life expectancy of the average patient with OA undergoing hip replacement.

Infection is the most worrying complication of hip joint replacement. The infection rate in many centres is 0.5–1.5% and was thought to be similar whether a laminar airflow or a conventional theatre was used (Collis & Steinhaus, 1976; Mallory et al, 1978). However, a recent multicentre study has suggested that hip or knee joint replacement in an ultraclean air theatre may halve the deep infection rate (Lidwell et al, 1982). Infection once established produces devastating results. In one series of 135 patients with infected prostheses, all but 1 had pain at the site of the prosthesis, 23 died, and only 17 managed to retain their prostheses (Hunter & Dandy, 1977).

A more common but less serious complication is loosening of the prosthesis. In Charnley's 10 year follow-up series loosening of the femoral component occurred in 1%, and of the acetabular component in 2% of patients (Charnley & Cupic, 1973). The frequency of loosening increases with time and appears to be more common in overweight and active patients.

Knee joint replacement
The results of knee joint replacement are less predictable than those of the hip joint, a fact which is reflected by the very large numbers of different prostheses in use around the world. Generally, these fall into 3 main groups:

a. Non-constrained prostheses, e.g. unicondylar, polycentric, duocondylar prostheses
b. Semiconstrained prostheses, e.g. Imperial College London Hospital (ICLH), Sheehan, total condylar prostheses
c. Constrained prostheses, e.g. Stanmore and Guepar prostheses.

Knee replacement surgery produces a good result in 37–90% of patients (Insall et al, 1976; Insall et al, 1979). As with total hip replacement surgery infection is the most serious complication of knee joint replacement and the rate of infection varies with the type of replacement used (Freeman et al, 1978; 1981; Borden et al, 1982). A figure of 6.4% has been reported for Guepar prostheses in contrast with 0.5% with total condylar replacement (Insall et al, 1976). Freeman et al (1978, 1981) have recorded a 4% incidence of infection with the ICLH prosthesis despite the use of prophylactic antibiotics. It appears that the rate of infection may be lower in patients with OA than in those with rheumatoid arthritis.

Loosening of prosthetic knee joints has also been reported as a major problem (Cracchiolo, 1976) but this appears to have been due to defective prosthesis design since much lower figures have been reported with newer prostheses, e.g. 1 loose prothesis out of 923 total condylar replacement operations (Insall et al, 1979). The durability of knee replacement has yet to be reliably established, but as the majority of osteoarthritic patients undergoing such procedures will be elderly with a limited life expectancy, this may not be a problem in many cases.

Trapezium excision or replacement arthroplasty
These two procedures are occasionally used to treat OA of the carpometacarpal joint of the thumb. The excision arthroplasty, in which the trapezium is excised, results in good relief of pain, but at the cost of a reduction in pinch grip strength. Trapezium replacement arthroplasty produces a better functional result but is technically more difficult to perform.

Surgical procedures to relieve pain
Osteotomy and arthrodesis are both procedures used to relieve the symptoms of OA.

Osteotomy of the hip
The use of osteotomy in the treatment of OA was first advanced by McMurray (1935), and intertrochanteric osteotomy was widely performed before hip replacement procedures became commonplace. Though it produces good pain relief in 2/3 of patients in the early years, the results after 10 years of follow-up are disappointing, particularly in the elderly patient (Weisl, 1980). Intertrochanteric osteotomy may still have a place in the management of the young patient with OA of the hip, in whom hip replacement is considered undesirable. It does not preclude a later total jont replacement operation.

Osteotomy of the knee

Tibial osteotomy (Jackson, 1958; Jackson & Waugh, 1961; Wardle, 1964) and double (tibial and femoral) osteotomy (Benjamin, 1969) are widely used in the treatment of OA of the knee. The indication for operation is severe pain, unrelieved by other treatments. These operations produce good pain relief in knees which have 90° or more of flexion whether or not an angular deformity is present (Jackson, 1958; Benjamin, 1969; Huskisson & Phillips, 1973; Angel et al, 1974). Huskisson & Phillips (1973) have shown that double osteotomy produces greater relief of pain than immobilisation of the arthritic joint in a plaster splint. The mechanism of pain relief is not understood. Double osteotomy appears to be no more effective than tibial osteotomy and it may impair the postoperative range of joint movement (Philips & Cullen, 1968).

Insall et al (1973) has advocated low femoral osteotomy for correction of valgus deformity of the osteoarthritic knee as he has demonstrated that tibial osteotomy is a less successful procedure for correcting this particular deformity.

Arthrodesis

Pain relief at the expense of mobility is achieved by arthrodesis. A good functional result and relief of discomfort can be expected with arthrodesis of the carpometacarpal joint of the thumb or the first metatarsophalangeal joint, but with other joints the result is less predictable. Arthrodesis of the hip is occasionally advocated in young patients in whom the long-term risks of hip replacement are considered too great. The procedure should make standing and walking comfortable but it does transfer strain to the lumbar spine and opposite hip, and sitting in cramped surroundings, e.g. a car or a theatre, may be difficult. Arthrodesis does not preclude a later total hip replacement operation. Arthrodesis of the knee has declined in popularity in the surgical management of OA of the knee. The procedure is now reserved for the treatment of severe monoarticular OA in a young patient in whom total knee replacement is considered hazardous in the long-term, and as a salvage procedure for a failed knee arthroplasty.

Debridement procedures

Arthrotomy to remove loose fragments of bone or cartilage from an osteoarthritic joint may be of help if recurrent locking of a joint has been a symptom, but there is no evidence that debridement procedures to remove osteophytes have any place in the management of OA. The only exception is perhaps osteophyte formation in the spine which has produced pressure effects on the spinal cord or nerve roots. In this situation Symon (1971) has shown that laminectomy with decompression improves 60% of patients.

Surgical treatment of the osteoarthritic spine

The role of surgery in the management of OA of the spine is very limited, and is usually advocated only if there is evidence of spinal cord or nerve root entrapment. The operation performed will depend on the nature and site of the lesion and may include discectomy, laminectomy, removal of encroaching osteophytes, decompression of the vertebral artery and fusion procedures.

REFERENCES

Angel J C, Liyanage S P, Griffiths W E G 1974 Double osteotomy for relief of pain in arthritis of the knee. Rheumatology and Rehabilitation 13: 109–119

Bach G L, Panse P, Zeiller P 1977 Glycosaminoglycanpolysulfat (GAGPS, Arteparon R) Zur Basistherapie der arthrose. III: Biochemisch — diagnostische und klinische Untersuchungen zur intramusklaren Andwendung von GAGPS. Zeitschrift fur Rheumatologie 36: 269–274

Beckenbaugh R D, Iistrup D M 1978 Total hip arthroplasty. Journal of Bone and Joint Surgery 60A: 694–699

Benjamin A 1969 Double osteotomy for the painful knee in rheumatoid arthritis and osteoarthritis. The Journal of Bone and Joint Surgery 51B: 694–699

Blackwell B 1973 Drug therapy. Patient compliance. New England Journal of Medicine 289: 249–252

Borden L S, Heyne T, Belhobek G, Marks K E, Stulberg B N, Wilde A H 1982 Total condylar prosthesis. Orthopaedic Clinics of North America 13: 123–139

Charnley J 1961 Arthroplasty of the hip: a new operation. Lancet 1: 1129–1132

Charnley J, Cupic F 1973 The nine and ten year results of low function arthroplasty of the hip. Clinical Orthopaedics and Related Research 95: 9–25

Charnley J, Halley D K 1975 Rate of wear in total hip

replacement. Clinical Orthopaedics and Related Research 112:170

Collis D K, Steinhaus K 1976 Total hip replacement without deep infection in a standard operating room. Journal of Bone and Joint Surgery 58A: 446–450

Cracchiolo A 1976 Editorial comment. Statistics of total knee replacement. Clinical Orthopaedics and Related Research 120: 2–3

Denko C W 1979 Restorative chemotherapy in degenerative hip disease. Abstracts IX European Congress of Rheumatology, Wiesbaden 1043

Deyo R A 1982 Compliance with therapeutic regimens in arthritis: tissues, current status and a further agenda. Seminars in Arthritis and Rheumatism 12: 233–244

Deyo R A, Inui T S, Sullivan B 1981 Compliance with arthritis drugs: Magnitude, correlates and clinical implication. Journal of Rheumatology 8: 931–936

Dieppe P A, Sathapatayavongs B, Jones H E, Bacon P A, Ring E F J 1980 Intra-articular steroids in osteoarthritis. Rheumatology and Rehabilitation 19: 212–217

Doherty M, Dieppe P A 1981 Effect of intro-articular yttrium-90 (^{90}Y) on chronic pyrophosphate arthroplasty (CPA) of the knee. Annals of the Rheumatic Diseases 40:626

Doyle D V, Dieppe P A, Scott Jane, Huskisson E C 1981 An articular index for the assessment of osteoarthritis. Annals of the Rheumatic Diseases 40: 75–78

Enislidis A C 1972 Gewebsverteilung von Tritium — markiertem Glycosaminoglycanpolysulfat nach intraartikularer injektion. Medizinische Welt (Stuttgart) 23: 733–735

Evans F J 1974 The placebo response in pain reduction. In: Bonica J J (ed) Advances in neurology. Raven Press, New York

Freeman M A R, Todd R C, Bambert P, Day W H 1978 ICLH arthroplasty of the knee: 1968–1977. Journal of Bone and Joint Surgery 60B: 339–344

Freeman M A R, Blaha J D, Insler M 1981 Replacement of the knee in rheumatoid arthritis using the Imperial College London Hospital (ICLH) prosthesis. Reconstruction Surgery and Traumatology 18: 147–173

Friedman D M, Moore M E 1980 The efficacy of intra-articular steroids in osteoarthritis: a double-blind study. The Journal of Rheumatology 7: 850–856

Gallacchi G, Gächter A, Dick W, Miiller W 1979 Die Einlagerung intramuskulär applizierten Glykosaminoglykanpolysulfats im menschlichen Gelenkknorpel. Aktuelle Rheumatologie 4: 145–151

Gatley M S 1968 To be taken as directed. Journal of the Royal College of General Practitioners 16: 39–44

Gibson T, Winter P J, Grahame R 1973 Radiotherapy in the treatment of osteoarthrosis of the knee. Rheumatology and Rehabilitation 12: 42–46

Hunter G, Dandy D 1977 The natural history of the patient with an infected total hip replacement. Journal of Bone and Joint Surgery 59B: 293–297

Huskisson E C, Phillips H 1973 Controlled trial of double osteotomy for rheumatoid arthritis. Rheumatology and Rehabilitation 12: 214–218

Huskisson E C, Woolf D L, Balme H W, Jane Scott, Sue Franklin 1976 Four new anti-inflammatory drugs: responses and variation. British Medical Journal 1: 1048–1049

Insall J, Shoji H, Mayer V 1973 High tibial osteotomy for ostoearthritis of the knee with valgus deformity. Journal of Bone and Joint Surgery 55A: 963–973

Insall J, Ranawat C S, Aglietti P, Shine J 1976 A comparison of four models of total knee replacement prostheses. Journal of Bone and Joint Surgery 58B: 754–765

Insall J, Scott W N, Ranawat C S 1979 The total condylar knee prosthesis. A report of 220 cases. Journal of Bone and Joint Surgery 61A: 173–180

Jackson J P 1958 Osteotomy for osteoarthritis of the knee. Journal of Bone and Joint Surgery 40B:826

Jackson J P, Waugh M 1961 Tibial osteotomy for ostoearthritis of the knee. Journal of Bone and Joint Surgery 43B: 746–751

Kalbhen D A 1981 Experimentall-pharmakoloische Prufung der antiarthrotischen Wirkung des Knorpelknochenmarkextraktes Rumalon R. Therapiewoche 31: 4983–5001

Lee P, Tan L J P 1979 Drug compliance in outpatients with rheumatoid arthritis. Australian and New Zealand Journal of Medicine 9: 274–277

Lidwell D M, Lowbury E J L, Whyte W, Blowers R, Stanley S J, Lowe D 1982. Effect of ultraclean air in an operating room on deep sepsis in the joint after total hip or knee replacement: a randomised study. British Medical Journal 285: 10–14

Mayer J H 1970 Carpometacarpal osteoarthritis of the thumb. Lancet 2:270 (letter)

McKee G K, Watson-Farra J 1966 Replacement of arthritic hips by the McKee-Farrar prosthesis. Journal of Bone and Joint Surgery 48B: 245–259

McMurray T P 1935 Ostoearthritis of the hip. British Journal of Surgery 22: 716–727

Mallory T H, Meyer T L, Bombach J D 1978 Six hundred and ninety total hip replacements; a comparative study. Ohio State Medical Journal 74: 123–127

Mayer J H 1970 Carpometacarpal ostoearthritis of the thumb, Lancet 2:270 (letter)

Newton C D, Jimenez S A, Bashey R I, Fetter A W 1981 Abstracts of VX International Congress of Rheumatology 1515

Phillips R S, Cullen C H 1968 Surgical treatment of osteoarthritis. Geriatrics 23: 161–178

Rejholec V, Kralova M 1979 Can working ability and disablement of patients with coxarthrosis be influenced by longterm tissue extract treatment? (14 year controlled study with Rumalon). Abstracts IX European Congress of Rheumatology, Wiesbaden 967

Ring P A 1968 Complete replacement arthroplasty of the hip by the ring prosthesis. Journal of Bone and Joint Surgery 50B: 720–731

Shah K D, Wright V 1967 Intra-articular hydrocortisone in osteoarthritis. Annals of the Rheumatic Diseases 26: 316–318

Symon L 1971 Surgical Treatment. In: M Wilkinson (ed) Cervical spondylosis. Heinemann, London

Wagenhauser F J 1982 Basic drug treatment of arthrosis. In: Dettmer N, Greiling H (eds): International durg symposium: Arteparon. Eular Publishers, Basle, p 103–106

Wardle E N 1964 Osteotomy of the tibia and fibula in the treatment of chronic osteoarthritis of the knee. Postgraduate Medical Journal 40: 536–542

Weisl H 1980 Intertrochanteric osteotomy for osteoarthritis. The Journal of Bone and Joint Surgery 62B: 37–42

Wright V, Haslock I, Dowson D, Sellar P, Reeves B 1971 Evaluation of silicone as an artificial lubricant in osteoarthritis joints. British Medical Journal 2: 370–373

SECTION VIII

Metabolic Disease

J.T. Scott

Gout

I have jocosely called the GOUT an honour, because it is seriously affirmed by every physical writer, that it is the Inheritance only of the Acute and Sensible, tho' others possibly may acquire it. If the reader should chance not to be Gouty, and hath an inclination to indulge any Pleasantry upon this observation, though philosophical reasons for it are not wanting, I have no objection: but notwithstanding our advantages, and that our Order is very Honourable, (for the greatest men, even Kings and Emperors, have ranked in it) yet he may take my word, it is not worth his envy.

Ferdo Warner
A Full and Plain Account of the Gout
Cadell, London (1768)

'The gout, sir,' replied Mr Weller, 'The gout is a complaint as arises from too much ease and comfort. If ever you're attacked with the gout, sir, just you marry a widder as has got a good loud voice, with a decent notion of using' it and you'll never have the gout again. It's a capital prescription, sir. I takes it reg'lar, and I can warrant it to drive away any illness as is caused by too much jollity.' Having imparted this valuable secret, Mr Weller drained his glass once more, produced a laboured wink, sighed deeply and slowly retired.

Charles Dickens
The Pickwick Club

Gout is a disease with a strong familial tendency seen predominantly in adult men, characterised by episodes of acute arthritis, and later also by chronic damage to joints and other structures. It is caused essentially by *hyperuricaemia*, an excess of urate in the blood and tissues, which in some people (but not all) leads to the deposition of crystals of sodium urate in the joints and elsewhere. These crystalline deposits are now recognised to be the cause of the acute gouty attack, and further accumulations of crystalline and amorphous urate form the *tophi* (Latin *tophus* = porous stone) which are a feature of the advanced untreated disease.

With increasing knowledge of uric acid metabolism it has now become evident that there are many factors which can influence the development of hyperuricaemia and hence of gout. Gouty arthritis may therefore be regarded as the end result of a number of different biochemical processes (to be described later). The term *primary gout* is used when hyperuricaemia is due principally to an inherited metabolic abnormality and *secondary gout* when it is largely the result of an acquired disease or some environmental factor. In most patients with gout, however, a combination of inherited and environmental influences appears to be operating, as will be discussed below.

Some historical aspects of gout are mentioned in Chapter 1 and it only needs to be emphasised again, as well pointed out by the late Gerald Rodnan (1982), how gouty arthritis and attendant tophaceous disease respond so well to treatment nowadays that it is difficult for the young physician to appreciate the dread once inspired by this disorder. There is a vast literature on gout but three modern books to which the reader is referred for extensive discussion and bibliography are the works of Wyngaarden & Kelley (1976), Kelley & Weiner (1978) and Dieppe & Calvert (1983).

PREVALENCE

From analysis of a large series of outpatient records in Germany it was estimated that gout accounted for 6.3% of rheumatic diseases as seen at a hospital clinic (Mertz & Babucke, 1971), a figure close to that of 5% earlier proposed by Hench (1935) in the USA.

Results, such as they are, obtained from epidemiological surveys vary widely. For example, from the Framingham, USA, study came an estimated prevalence of gout of 28 per 1000 for males and 4 per 1000 for females (Hall et al, 1967). In this country Popert & Hewitt (1962) found no cases of gout among 891 individuals in Wensleydale, Yorkshire, and 2, or possibly 3, cases among 380 persons in the 55–64 age-group in Leigh. From an extensive study carried out in representative general practice samples in Great Britain, Currie (1979) found an overall prevalence of 2.6 per 1000. The prevalence in England was greater than in the rest of the United Kingdom and the prevalence in Wales was greater than that in Scotland. In 10% of the cases the gout was believed to be secondary, with induction by diuretics being the most frequent cause.

Prevalence figures can be taken as very general approximations only. Apart from usual problems of case selection, the diagnosis of an episodic disorder such as gout presents the epidemiologist with great difficulty. As will be discussed below, the prevalence of hyperuricaemia and gout is known to vary between different populations, and there appears little doubt that it can change, owing to environmental and particularly dietary factors, in the same population over quite a short period of time. For example, it is generally held that gout is much more common in Europe than it was during the Second World War; it is seen quite frequently today in Spain, where it was almost unknown during the Civil War (Barcello, 1976). It is also clear that the incidence of gout has been increasing in other countries during recent years, such as Japan (Nishioka & Mikanagi, 1981) and Finland (Isomäki et al, 1977). In a study of four South African populations gout was found among whites only (Beighton et al, 1977), but it is likely that the incidence is increasing among urban blacks (Lowenthal & Dymond, 1977: Mody & Naidoo, 1984).

Epidemiological aspects of gout and hyperuricaemia are discussed further in Chapter 3.

CLINICAL FEATURES

People who develop gout have usually lived for many years, unbeknown to themselves, with a raised plasma level of uric acid (*asymptomatic hyperuricaemia*), until eventually crystals of sodium urate, precipitated in a joint, provoke a sudden tissue reaction which leads to the first attack of *acute gouty arthritis*. Acute attacks each last for only short periods, being followed by intervals of widely varying duration during which there is again complete freedom from symptoms (*intercritical gout*), although hyperuricaemia persists. Some people may have only one or two episodes of acute gouty arthritis in the whole of their lives, while others suffer repeated attacks of increasing duration, severity and frequency, one running into another and involving joint after joint. In time some joints no longer return to their normal stage; deposits of urate (*tophi*) form around the joints and elsewhere: and the patient has entered the stage of *chronic tophaceous gouty arthritis*.

As will be discussed below, blood levels of uric acid are generally higher in men than in women, and this is reflected by the predominance of gouty arthritis among men. Onset is most often in the 4th, 5th and 6th decades. Distribution of age at onset and sex in a large British series of cases is shown in Figure 36.1. Of the 354 patients, 311 (88%) were men and 43 (12%) women.

Acute gout

Acute gouty arthritis starts, nearly always in a

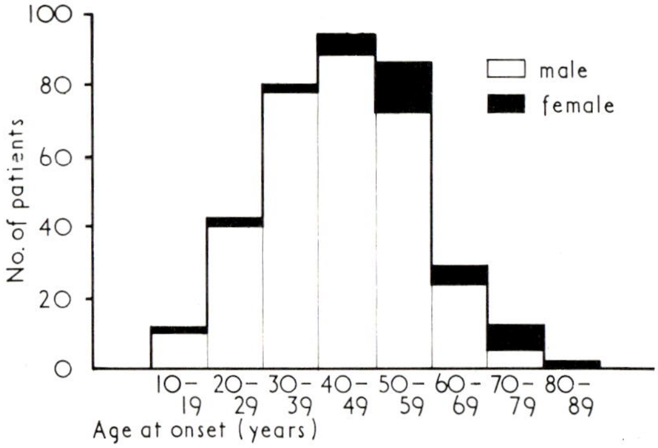

Fig. 36.1 Age of onset and sex incidence in 354 cases of gout. (Grahame & Scott, 1970. Reproduced by courtesy of the Editor of the *Annals of the Rheumatic Diseases*.)

single joint, as a sensation of discomfort developing over a period of hours and days into pain which can be extremely severe. Indeed, the pain which has to be endured during a fully developed attack of gout is one of the most excruciating torments to be encountered in medical practice, although less dramatic forms are not uncommon and with modern drugs the most violent paroxysms are seen less often than formerly. Attacks of gout often start at night, and may awaken the victim from his sleep. The affected joint becomes reddened, shiny, swollen and exquisitely tender with distension of superficial veins. The weight of a sheet on the foot may be intolerable and the apprehensive sufferer will often not allow an examining hand to approach the painful limb, let alone palpate it. Erythema is a prominent feature over the smaller joints: in the knee joint it may be less evident but an effusion is detectable, giving an opportunity for diagnostic aspiration and the detection of crystals. Unless terminated by colchicine or other drugs an attack of gout may last several days or weeks, but the condition of the joint eventually returns to normal. An irritating desquamation of the skin is sometimes seen as the attack subsides; this is a useful, thought not specific, diagnostic sign.

The metatarsophalangeal joint of the great toe is involved in over 70% of cases (Fig. 36.2), followed in frequency by the ankle or other joints in the foot, knee, fingers (Fig. 36.3), elbow and wrist (Grahame & Scott, 1970). Thus gout tends to affect distal rather than proximal joints and involvement of the axial skeleton is very rare indeed. Occasionally, more than one joint can be involved simultaneously, and indeed acute polyarticular gout may be more common than is generally appreciated (Hadler et al, 1974; Raddatz et al, 1983). Apart from joints, acute gout can occur in tendon-sheaths and in bursae (Canoso & Yood, 1979).

Attention is often drawn to so-called 'prodromal symptoms', such as changes in appetite or mood, nausea or flatulence, occurring before a gouty crisis. The authenticity of such symptoms is rather doubtful except of course for a certain degree of readily understandable irascibility or apprehension as the attack develops. Nor are constitutional features prominent, though during a very severe attack there may be pyrexia with leucocytosis and

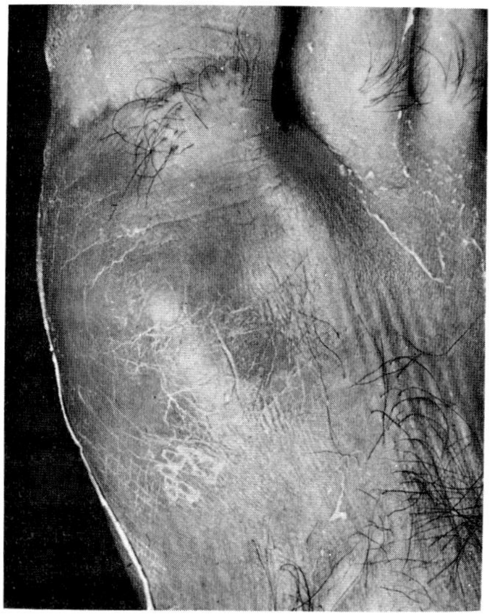

Fig. 36.2 Acute gouty arthritis in great toe, showing desquamation of the skin which sometimes accompanies a severe attack.

a raised sedimentation rate. Acute gout is not normally associated with changes in the plasma or urinary urate, which tend to be the same during the attack as during intervals of freedom, unless influenced by drug treatment.

Attacks of gout are often spontaneous, but are

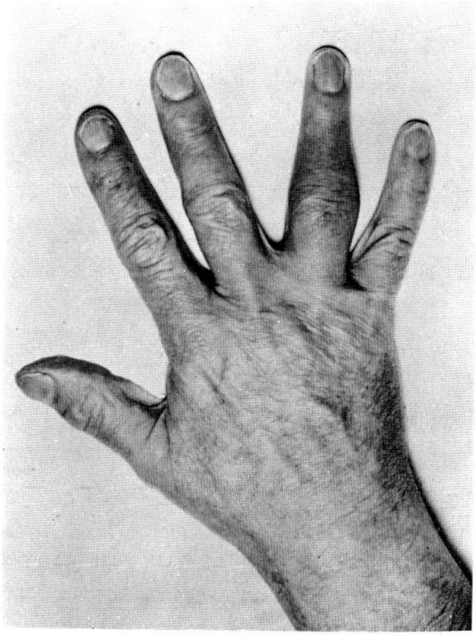

Fig. 36.3 Acute gouty arthritis in a proximal interphalangeal joint.

specially liable to occur in certain predisposing situations (Wallace et al, 1977; Wallace et al, 1979). Of these, trauma is not unusual, a blow on the knee or wrist, for example, being followed several hours later by an attack of gout in that joint. The special susceptibility of the great toe may be related to the repeated minor stresses sustained during walking. Gout also has a tendency to occur during systemic illnesses such as pneumonia or following myocardial infarction, and has been reported to follow emotional stress (Katz et al, 1975). It is well known that acute gout sometimes follows surgical operation, the mechanisms responsible being uncertain, although it has been shown that urinary excretion of uric acid is greatly increased in the postoperative period (Snaith & Scott, 1972). Acute gout is also seen early in the course of treatment aimed at lowering the serum uric acid. Other predisposing factors, such as dietary or alcoholic indiscretion, or starvation, probably exert at least part of their effect by a direct action on serum levels of uric acid, as discussed later, an acute attack being perhaps precipitated by a further transient elevation of uric acid superimposed on pre-existing hyperuricaemia.

Chronic tophaceous gout

Chronic gouty arthritis is due to depositions of solid urate (tophi) in relation to articular structures, leading to a destructive arthropathy with secondary degenerative changes. It usually follows repeated acute attacks but can develop insidiously in a previously unaffected joint. Acute attacks may continue to occur in the same joint, but tend to disappear late in the course of the disease. Such permanent changes are usually found in a number of different situations and are often prominent in the proximal and distal interphalangeal joints of the fingers, where periarticular tophi lead to bizarre asymmetrical swelling (Fig. 36.4). The skin overlying such tophi becomes thinned and shiny and through it can be seen the white mass of underlying sodium urate, which may later discharge itself as the skin breaks and ulcerates. Recurrent ulceration of this sort can be very troublesome but infection is rarely a problem.

The distribution of chronic joint involvement is similar to that of acute gouty arthritis although deformity in the hands is often more striking than in the feet. Gouty arthritis of the wrist joints occasionally causes a carpal tunnel syndrome (De Sèze & Phankim-Koupernik, 1964). Involvement of proximal joints is uncommon, but changes have been described in the sacroiliac joints (Malawista et al, 1965) and vertebrae, sometimes producing paraplegia (Kosoff et al, 1953; Hall & Selin, 1960). About one-fifth of patients with gout develop tophi and permanent joint damage (Grahame & Scott,

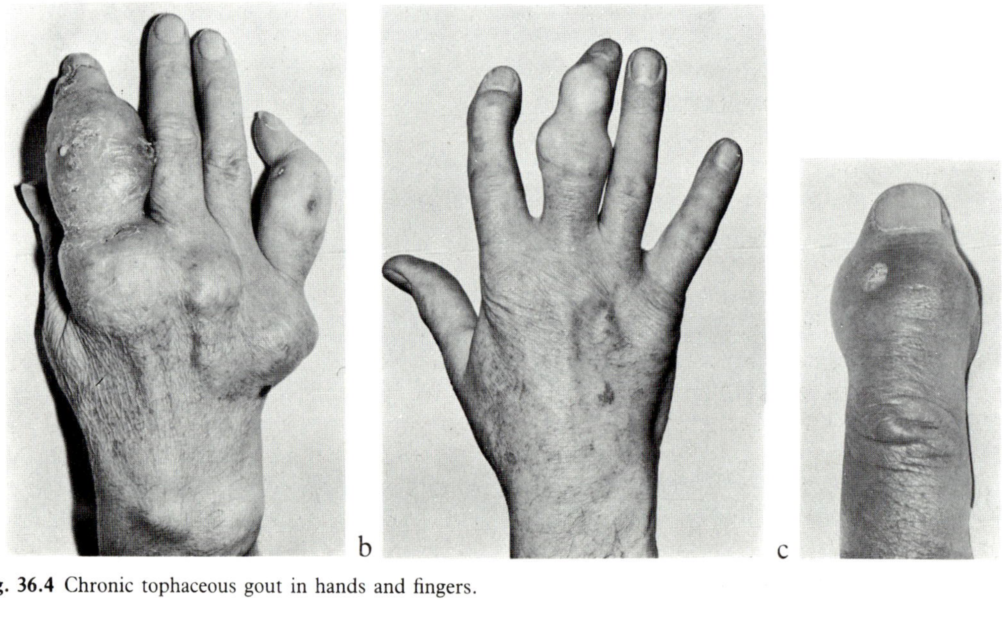

a b c

Fig. 36.4 Chronic tophaceous gout in hands and fingers.

a 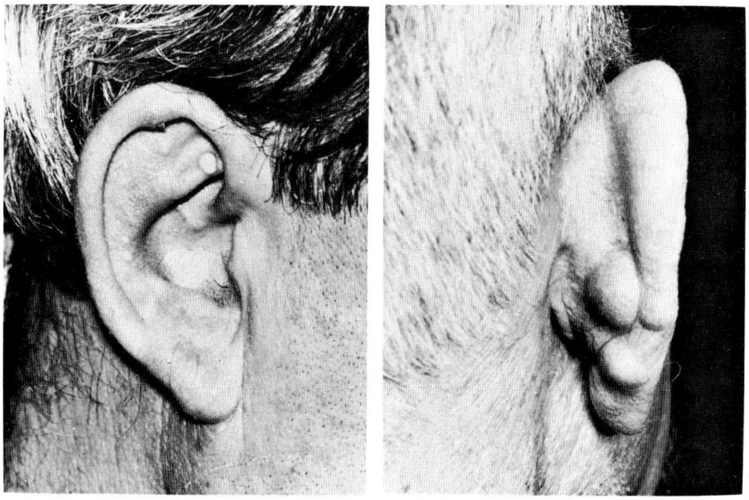 b

Fig. 36.5 Gouty tophi on the ear.

1970); the figure may have been higher in the past and is no doubt falling with modern methods of controlling uric acid levels.

Tophi are found in other situations beside periarticular subcutaneous tissue. They have a predilection for cartilage and are particularly common on the cartilage of the ear, where they form small white excrescences, usually about 1–4 mm in size (Fig. 36.5). Other sites include the olecranon and prepatellar bursae, tendons, and, less commonly, the eyelids. Rare patients have been described with extensive visceral deposition in intestine (Hawkins et al, 1965), larynx (Lefkovits, 1965), conducting tissue of the heart (Virtanen & Halonen, 1970), heart valves and myocardium (Pund et al, 1960),vertebrae and discs (Lagier & MacGee, 1983), also the eyes, penis, tongue, bronchi, pleura, pericardium and meninges (Talbott & Yü, 1976). Tophi in the extradural space have caused spinal compression (Sequeira et al, 1981; Magid et al, 1981). The special case of the kidneys is considered below. Tophi are characteristically absent from voluntary muscle, liver, spleen, lungs and nervous tissue. Amyloid has occasionally been reported secondary to gout, but this must be extremely rare (Rubinow & Sennenblick, 1981).

PATHOLOGY

Acute gouty arthritis

A level of uric acid in blood and tissue fluids sufficiently high to produce crystal deposition is a sine qua non in the pathogenesis of gout, all the features of the disease being associated with the presence of solid urate in one form or another. This has long been accepted with regard to the clinical manifestations of chronic gouty arthritis but the part played by urate in acute gout has until recently been more controversial, despite Garrod's (1876) early suggestion that precipitation of sodium urate crystals was a critical event. It was pointed out by earlier writers that levels of serum and urinary uric acid did not alter during acute attacks, that infusion or injection of urate solution into joints of gouty subjects did not precipitate an inflammatory episode, that it is possible to sustain a consistently elevated uric acid level without developing gout, that acute gout often ceases to occur in joints which are severely affected by chronic disease, and that some drugs, such as colchicine, are effective in terminating an acute attack without altering the serum uric acid level, while drugs which do lower the serum urate have no action in acute gout (indeed, their use may tend to precipitate attacks for a time).

The association of crystalline urate with acute gout is now however clearly established. Urate can be demonstrated within synovial tissue during an attack (Sokoloff, 1957), and examination of joint fluid for the presence of urate crystals (McCarty & Hollander, 1961) has now become a routine diagnostic measure, as will be discussed in more detail later. Using polarised light they can been seen as negatively birefringent needles, often lying within polymorphs, which form the principal type of cell in the synovial exudate. The synovial membrane itself is hyperplastic and infiltrated with polymorphs. It seems evident that urate crystals initiate the gouty attack, since injection of crystalline particles of appropriate size and shape — not only urate, but also oxalate and other substances — can produce an inflammatory response in skin, subcutaneous tissues and joints of man and animals (Faires & McCarty, 1962; Seegmiller et al, 1962). A similar mechanism no doubt operates in the other form of crystal-induced synovitis which is a feature of chondrocalcinosis, acute joint inflammation there being a response to crystals of calcium pyrophosphate dihydrate (see Ch. 37).

The exact mechanisms of crystal deposition and the subsequent inflammatory response, however, remain uncertain.

Crystal deposition

It is arguable whether crystals of urate are initially precipitated in synovial fluid or whether they are deposited first in synovial membrane or cartilage, as they are in other connective tissues, with subsequent release into the joint space. Perhaps both processes are involved, sometimes occurring almost simultaneously. Factors influencing crystal nucleation, growth and dissolution are certainly complex, particularly in biological systems, and have recently been reviewed in detail (Dieppe & Calvert, 1983).

Supersaturation of tissue fluids with monosodium urate appears to be a necessary but not sufficient precondition for crystal deposition. Concentration of urate is uniform through most body fluids: the solubility of monosodium urate under physiological conditions (pH 7.4, 37°C in the presence of 0.14M sodium ions) is also influenced by the presence of urate-binding proteins, though the magnitude of this remains uncertain. Saturation of urate in plasma probably occurs at a level of about 7.0 mg/100 ml (420 μmol/l), and it has been shown that the risk of developing gout increases with the degree of superstaturation above this level (Hall et al, 1967). Attacks of gout may occur at lower levels, particularly in patients recently commencing urate-lowering treatment, but such attacks represent an inflammatory response to crystals which were formed when the levels were higher.

However, although urate levels of gout patients are above saturation values, they are often well below those at which precipitation occurs spontaneously in vitro. This metastable situation — one between saturation and supersolubility leading to precipitation — probably obtains in the large number of hyperuricaemic subjects who never develop gout, or who do so only after long symptom-free periods. Other factors must be involved in actual nucleation and growth of urate crystals (Fiddis et al, 1983).

Urate deposition tends to occur in connective tissues rich in proteoglycans, particularly cartilage. Katz & Schubert (1970) proposed that destruction of proteoglycans following normal or accelerated tissue turnover could result in a reduction of binding capacity for urate, with consequent precipitation from saturated tissue fluids. Katz (1975) found increased serum uronic levels in patients with gout, reflecting enhanced turnover of connective tissue in such patients. However, the suggestion that proteoglycan aggregates of connective tissue are capable of initiating urate precipitation, losing this property on degradation (Katz & Schubert, 1970), has not been confirmed (Perricone & Brandt, 1978), and the whole field of urate deposition in cartilage awaits clarification.

The solubility of monosodium urate in the presence of physiological concentrations of sodium has been shown to fall sharply with decreasing temperature (Loeb, 1972), a point which may be relevant to the peripheral distribution of gouty arthritis. Cooling of extremity joints during rest may be contributory to the development of acute gout.

Urate solubility is increased by a number of other factors including the presence of albumin, lack of which in interstitial fluids may therefore predispose to its precipitation (Kippen et al, 1974). Simkin (1973) has demonstrated that urate concentration rises in resolving effusions and has suggested that the resolution of small traumatic effusions in the metatarsophalangeal joints and elsewhere predisposes to crystal deposition. Acute gouty arthritis may certainly follow trauma or exercise, particularly in the first metatarsophalangeal joint. Conceivably mechanical damage to cartilage predisposes to crystal deposition, or an attack is set off following desquamation of crystals from an articular crust. The severity of experimental urate arthritis in dogs in enhanced by exercise (Agudelo et al, 1972), a further experimental observation with clinical implications.

Inflammatory response

The capacity of a crystal to induce an inflammatory response depends on a number of things including size, shape, surface properties and protein coating (Dieppe & Calvert, 1983). Thus either very small amorphous deposits of urate or large crystals (> 20 μm long) are relatively ineffective, whereas crystals of about 5 μm in length are most reactive. It has been suggested (Mandel, 1976) that the key factor is the surface roughness in atomic terms, smooth crystals like cysteine being inactive in contrast to urate with many active charged groups sticking out from the surface. The relation of crystal structure to inflammatory properties has recently been discussed (Mandel & Mandel, 1982).

Urate and pyrophosphate crystals bind protein avidly, including IgG: this is likely to change surface characteristics and may enhance reactions with cell membranes, phagocytosis and activation of cell-free inflammatory mechanisms (Kozin & McCarty, 1976). Monosodium urate crystals precoated with IgG stimulated superoxide anion release by human polymorphs to a greater extent than did uncoated crystals, the effect not being observed when the crystals had been exposed to undiluted serum (Abrahamson et al, 1982). The complexity of the spectrum of crystal–plasma protein interaction has been demonstrated by Terkeltaub et al (1983), who have mapped numerous proteins from plasma and serum which bind to monosodium urate crystals, using 2-dimensional gel electrophoresis.

Experiments by Van Arman et al (1974) suggested the possibility that bacterial endotoxin adsorbed on to urate crystals might also induce inflammation.

Polymorph leucocytes appear to play an essential role in gouty arthritis. The inflammatory response to urate in dogs is dependent upon their presence (Phelps & McCarty, 1966; Chang & Gralla, 1968). Events following addition of urate crystals to phagocytic cells have been described (Rajan, 1975; Schumacher, 1977). Following rapid phagocytosis the crystal is surrounded by a phagosome with subsequent lysosomal fusion, membrane lysis, cell degranulation, rupture and death. Release of lysosomal enzymes after phagocytosis, together with release of lactic dehydrogenase following cell death, may both contribute to the inflammatory reaction. Colchicine appears to inhibit random motility and chemotaxis (Phelps, 1970). Gout can, however, occur in the absence of synovial fluid leucocytes (Ortel & Newcombe, 1974), suggesting that phagocytic cells in the synovial membrane can carry out a similar function. Platelet stimulation by urate crystals, mediated by membrane proteins, has been demonstrated by Jaques & Ginsberg (1982).

No clear picture of inflammatory mediators emerges from the considerable amount of experimental work undertaken (Spilberg, 1978; Platt & Dick, 1983). Kellermeyer (1968) and associates demonstrated that Hageman factor (clotting factor XII), which converts prekallikrein into kallikrein, and which is normally present in synovial fluid, was activated in vitro by urate crystals; and kinins are present in synovial fluid with spontaneous or crystal-induced gout in man (Melmon et al, 1967). However, it appears unlikely that the Hageman factor-kallikrein-kinin systems have a primary role in initiating the inflammatory response. For example, urate crystal synovitis can be induced in chickens, which lack Hageman factor, with no kinin activity being demonstrated in the synovial fluid (Spilberg, 1974). Activation of the complement sequence by monsodium urate crystals has been demonstrated (Naff & Byers, 1973; Terkeltaub et al, 1983; Russell et al, 1983; Boogaerts et al, 1983) and Doherty et al (1983) claim that inflammatory cystals can activate the alternate pathway of complement, but reductions of complement components in gouty effusions reported by Townes & Sowa (1970) have not been confirmed (Bunch et al, 1974). The part played by prostaglandins also remains uncertain: they have been implicated in urate synovitis (Rosenthale et al, 1972; Wigley et al, 1983) and many of the drugs effective in acute gout, such as indomethacin, are known to be potent inhibitors of prostaglandin synthetase, but aspirin, a strong inhibitor, has little therapeutic effect. The content of leucotriene B_4 in gouty joint effusions is higher than that found in rheumatoid arthritis and osteoarthrosis (Rae et al, 1982). Moreover, metabolism and biological deactivation of leucotriene B_4 by polymorphonuclear leucocytes are partly inhibited by crystals of monosodium urate. It is therefore possible that the crystals act not only as a stimulus for the production of this important chemotactic mediator, but also help towards its persistence.

Why are attacks of gout transient and why do crystals not always produce inflammation? They certainly do not invariably do so: urate crystals can be demonstrated in asymptomatic joints (Weinberger et al, 1979; Rouault et al, 1982; Gordon et al, 1982; Kennedy et al, 1984) and a particularly instructive case was that of a man with severe polyarticular gout who become asymptomatic immediately his hyperuricaemia was corrected with allopurinol, but whose knee joint, arthroscoped and biopsied before and again 6 months after the commencement of treatment, showed an apparently identical extent of urate deposition on the two occasions (Scott, 1978). Subtle undetected changes in crystal size or morphology may have occurred, and of possible relevance is the finding of Malawista et al (1979) that injury to cells exposed to silica crystals was related to the degree of dissolved urate in the system.

Also of possible relevance is the apparently rare association of acute gouty arthritis with certain other disorders, notably connective tissue diseases such as rheumatoid arthritis and systemic lupus erythematosus (Moidel & Good, 1981), and chronic renal failure, despite the presence of considerable hyperuricaemia. Various explanations have been offered: the occurrence of tophus formation without acute arthritis in such patients suggests that urate crystals are changed in some way, perhaps by the alteration of a protein coat, so that they do not stimulate an acute inflammatory response (Hollingworth et al, 1983). It has also been suggested, conversely, that hyperuricaemia can inhibit the activation of rheumatoid inflammation (Turner et al, 1983).

Reasons for the self-limiting nature of acute gout are thus unknown. It is clear that crystals can remain present after the attack ceases, although their nature may have been altered in some way. Perhaps some anti-inflammatory process is activated.

Chronic gouty arthritis

Deposition of crystalline monosodium urate monohydrate (Howell et al, 1963), as well as of granular and amorphous urates, leads to chronic inflammatory and degenerative reactions. The characteristic lesion of gout is the tophus, which consists of a multicentric deposit of crystals, often arranged radially, associated with an interstitial matrix and a foreign-body giant cell reaction (Fig. 36.6). The matrix may become partially calcified. With fresh deposition of urate the intervening inflammatory tissue tends to disappear leaving large chalky or stony concretions.

Demonstration of urates in histological sections requires special care because of their water-solubility. Fixation of tissue in absolute alcohol preserves crystals, which being birefringent can be seen under the polarising microscope; or they can be stained brown-black with silver nitrate (De Galantha, 1935), although this is not entirely specific for urate. Unless crystals are identified it may be difficult to distinguish with certainty the lesions of gout from other granulomatous foci.

Urates show a tendency to deposition in cartilage, periarticular soft tissue, bursae, epiphyseal

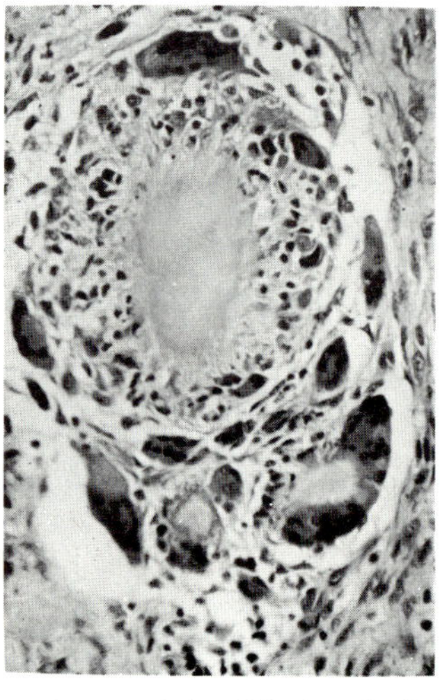

Fig. 36.6 Microphotograph (× 120) of periarticular gouty tophus showing oval area of matrix (from which crystals have been dissolved out) surrounded by foreign-body giant cells.

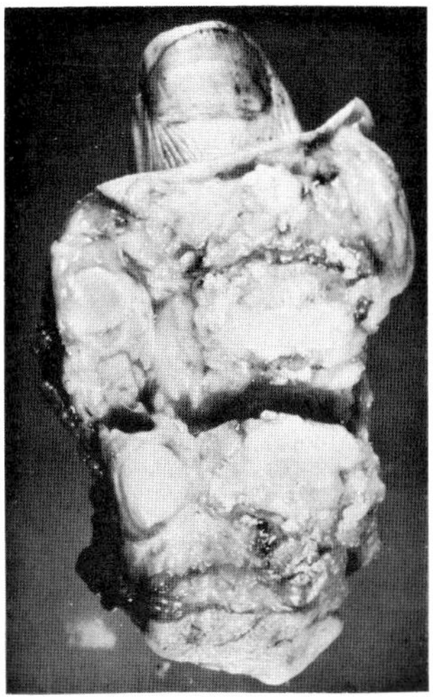

Fig. 36.7 Chronic gouty arthritis. Deposition of urate in 1st metatarsophalangeal joint. Note that the 2nd metatarsophalangeal joint, seen to the left, is normal.

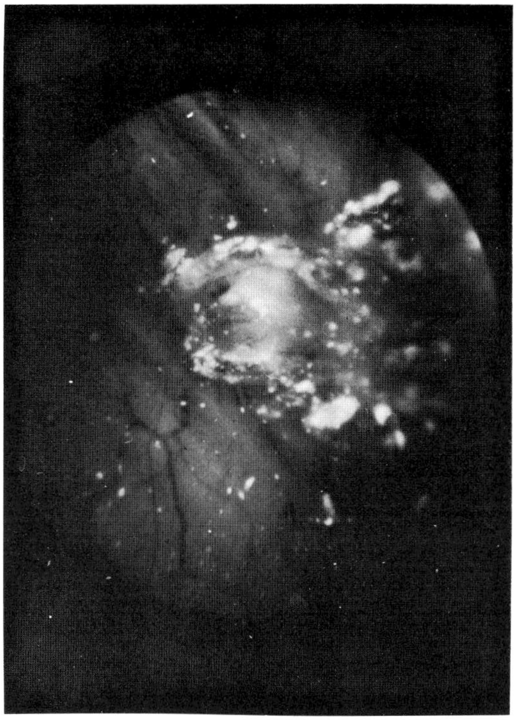

Fig. 36.8 Urate deposition on synovial membrane in the knee as seen through the arthroscope (Dr D. B. Yates).

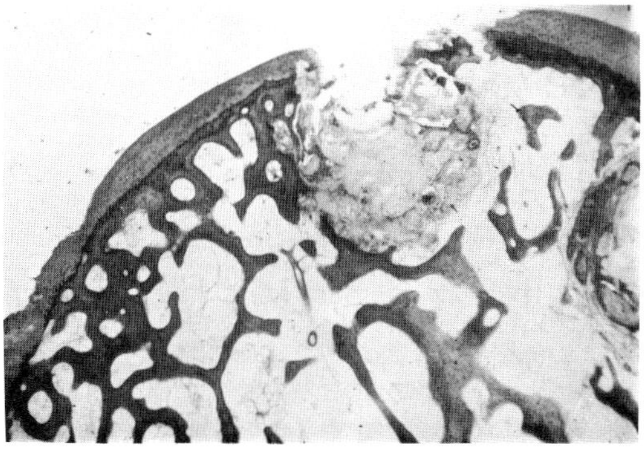

Fig. 36.9 Microphotograoh (× 6.5) of 1st metatarsophalangeal joint showing cartilage destruction over subchondral tophaceous deposit.

bone and kidneys. Tophi commonly occur on the pinna of the ear, in olecranon and patellar bursae, and tendon sheaths, also in the less common situations already described. In the joints themselves the articular cartilage becomes coated with white chalky urate (Fig. 36.7) and crystals are also formed within its superficial portions, as well as in synovial, capsular and periarticular tissues (Fig. 36.8). In the marrow of subchondral bone, tophus formation leads to collapse of articular cartilage and 'punched-out' lesions (Fig. 36.9) which give a characteristic radiological appearance. Further progressive changes include disintegration of cartilage with secondary osteoarthrosis and proliferation of marginal bone, obliteration of joint structure by urate deposition, proliferative tophaceous synovitis and occasionally fibrous or bony ankylosis.

The nature and significance of the tophaceous matrix are uncertain: it has been shown to contain lipids and glycosaminoglycans which are presumably formed between the crystals as part of a tissue response, but such tissue alterations may themselves help to precipitate or maintain the development of the tophus (Sokoloff, 1957). Favoured sites of urate deposition, such as articular and other cartilages, are rich in ground substance containing acid glycosaminoglycans. Proteoglycans from bovine nasal cartilage increase the solubility of urate, a feature not found with unbound chondroitin sulphate or trypsin-digested cartilage (Katz & Schubert, 1970), so that destruction of proteoglycans following normal or accelerated tissue turnover, as noted above, could possibly precipitate urate crystals from saturated tissue fluids.

PRIMARY GOUT, RENAL DISEASE AND HYPERTENSION

It is commonly held (Dieppe & Calvert, 1983; Emmerson, 1983) that in former times, when gout was severe, tophaceous, progressive and untreatable, kidney disease was common and serious, though data are hard to come by. It is less so today, at least in its grosser forms.

Uric acid calculi

Of the various forms of renal disease found in association with gout the first to be recognised was stone formation. Estimates of the frequency of stone formation among gout patients vary widely, ranging from 4% in an American series (Kuzell et al, 1955) to 73% in Israel (Atsmon et al, 1963). In another large series in the USA (Yü & Gutman, 1967) the incidence was 22% in primary gout and 42% in gout secondary to conditions such as polycythaemia or leukaemia where there are high degrees of hyperuricaemia and hyperuricosuria. A history of renal calculi was obtained from 11% of patients with gout in a British series (Grahame & Scott, 1970). Such variations may be due to racial differences and geographical factors — leading for example to relative dehydration and highly concentrated urine — as well as to differences in case selection, care of history-taking and diagnostic criteria. Evidence of urolithiasis may precede gouty arthritis, or the condition may be associated with hyperuricaemia but without gout.

Stones in patients with gout are usually composed of uric acid: the pKa_1 and pKa_2 of uric acid are 5.8 and 10.3, so that at a urinary pH of about 5 it is uric acid which is laid down, in contrast to the deposits of sodium urate which are found in the interstitial tissue of the kidney and elsewhere in the body (Howell et al, 1963). About one-quarter of stones contain additional calcium salts, and sometimes the calculi are composed entirely of calcium oxalate or phosphate, it being possible that hyperuricaemia and hyperuricosuria play a role in the formation of calcium stones (Smith et al, 1969; Coe, 1978; Pak et al, 1978). In most parts of the world stones composed wholly or mainly of uric acid constitute only a small proportion of all calculi, but again there is a wide variation, an incidence of 40% being found in Israel (Atsmon et al, 1963).

Uric acid lithiasis is classified by Gutman & Yü (1968) as

1. Idiopathic, i.e. without hyperuricaemia or hyperuricosuria
2. Associated with hyperuricaemia due to metabolic abnormalities (including primary gout, Lesch–Nyhan syndrome and glycogen storage disease, see below) or to myeloproliferative diseases
3. Associated with dehydration, and
4. Associated with hyperuricosuria without significant hyperuricaemia, due, for example, to uricosuric drugs, high purine intake, or defects in the tubular reabsorption of uric acid.

Factors leading to stone formation are incompletely understood, but important in their pathogenesis are hyperuricosuria and persistent undue acidity in the urine, the latter a feature said to be shown by gout patients in general and due to high titratable acidity; ammonium excretion in relation to pH is normal in stone-formers except in patients with impairment of renal function (Metcalfe-Gibson et al, 1965). Patients with chronic diarrhoea or ileostomies, who have low urinary pH values, are a special group showing a tendency to uric acid calculi (Clarke & McKenzie, 1969).

Uric acid stones, which are radiotranslucent unless they contain calcium, are usually small and are passed without difficulty although they may cause renal colic. They also predispose to pyelonephritis and renal functional impairment. Therapeutic measures consist of reduction in dietary purine content, adequate hydration, the reduction of urinary acidity by the administration of an alkalinising agent such as sodium bicarbonate and the use of allopurinol (see below). Uricosuric drugs predispose to uric acid calculi and are contraindicated in persons with a history of urinary calculi, or in whom the urinary uric acid is high (greater than 600 mg (3.6 mmol)/24 hours) on a low-purine diet.

Acute uric acid nephropathy, in which massive deposits of uric acid crystals form within the renal tubules, does not occur in primary gout, but is a consequence of excessive nucleoprotein degradation, occurring most commonly after chemotherapy for lymphoma or leukaemia (Bluestone et al, 1977).

Other renal lesions

Other renal lesions encountered in patients with gout and their relation to uric acid metabolism, renal function and hypertension, remain difficult to interpret. Uric acid stones can lead to renal functional impairment either directly or by secondary renal infection, and the same may be the case with interstitial deposition of urate (Fig. 36.10). Conversely, abnormalities of tubular function or gross failure of glomerular filtration will lead to hyperuricaemia. Evidence is sometimes available (from the clinical history or previous records) to indicate either that renal disease was present before gout occurred or that gouty arthritis developed before any indication of renal impairment, but it is often difficult, in an individual patient, to establish the sequence of events which has taken place.

Renal disease is undoubtedly frequent in gout and renal failure and has been said to be the commonest mode of death (Talbott & Terplan, 1960). However, most patients with primary gout appear to die from common and probably unrelated causes (Grahame & Scott, 1970) and life expectancy is not significantly reduced (Talbott & Lilienfeld, 1959). In fact, coronary artery disease, not renal disease, is the commonest cause of death (Yü & Talbott, 1980); this does not imply any specific association between gout and coronary artery disease, the incidence of which is now tending to fall as in the general population. The explanation for this apparent discrepancy almost certainly lies in the fact that, as discussed below, gouty patients do not represent a homogeneous disease process. Thus it seems that many show slight renal functional impairment, but that a small group, often young, have gout associated with hypertension and severe renal disease which lead to their early death. Examples of this are the oft-quoted family reported by Duncan & Dixon (1960) and the more recent study of Simmonds et al (1980a, b), but the concept of 'hyperuricaemic nephropathy' with its implication of cause and effect — a raised serum uric acid leading to renal disease — is probably an over-simplification. As Van Goor et al (1971) point out, reporting a similar family, such patients probably represent a hereditary disorder characterised by kidney damage, hypertension and hyperuricaemia, differing clinically and pathologically from classical gout. In the family studied by Hollingworth & Scott (1983), glomerular filtration rate was reduced in half of the subjects, with impaired urate clearance and hyperuricaemia in only a few of them. In such circumstances it is at least possible that the renal disease is not a direct consequence of hyperuricaemia (see Familial juvenile gout, p. 919).

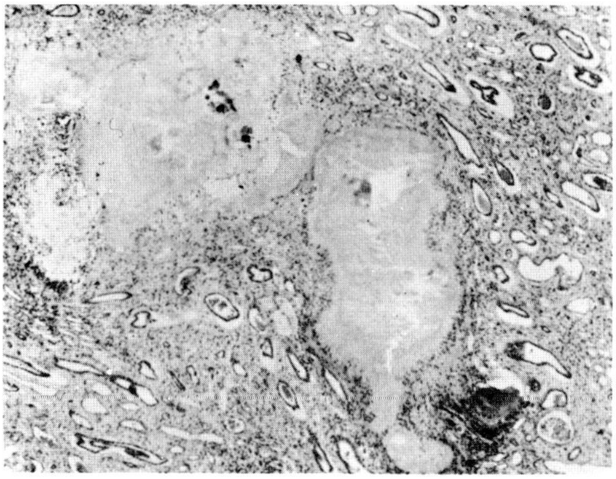

Fig. 36.10 Tophaceous deposit in kidney of a patient with gout and renal failure, showing tubular atrophy and fibrosis.

Indeed, the exact effect of hyperuricaemia per se, as contrasted with hyperuricosuria, on renal function is not at all clear. In a random-allocation controlled trial, Rosenfeld (1974) followed a group of hyperuricaemic subjects, some normotensive and some hypertensive, for over $2\frac{1}{2}$ years, and was unable to detect any difference in glomerular filtration rate between those whose serum urate had been lowered with allopurinol and the untreated subjects. An extensive investigation by Yü & Berger (1982a), in which glomerular and tubular function was measured in a large series of patients, indicated that hyperuricaemia, or uncomplicated gout alone, does not in itself cause renal insufficiency which, when seen in patients with gout, tends to correlate with the presence of hypertension, ischaemic heart disease or primary pre-existent renal insufficiency — views similar to those of Fessel (1979). The conclusion by Gibson et al

(1982) to the effect that allopurinol, by correcting hyperuricaemia, retards an apparent decline in renal function, must be viewed with caution in the light of initial differences in renal function between the groups studied. From a study of patients with HGPRT deficiency (see below), where urate overproduction is clearly primary and renal disease secondary, Emmerson & Row (1975) have put forward a working hypothesis concerning the evolution of the gouty kidney, taking into account the renal excretory capacity for urate, urinary uric acid levels, crystalluria and renal insufficiency.

Renal function in primary gout has been studied by a number of other workers, such as Barlow & Beilin (1968), who found evidence of renal insufficiency, nearly always mild and related to increasing age, in 41% of their patients. Impaired kidney function in gout has been confirmed by the controlled study of Gibson et al (1980), who showed a generally mild diminution of glomerular filtration rate and urine-concentrating ability in gouty subjects, whose urine showed a low pH and high excretion of titratable acid with a deficit of ammonium excretion. Proteinuria is found in about one-quarter of gout patients, usually small in amount and not progressive. The gouty kidney is characterised pathologically by urate crystals in the medulla and pyramids with a surrounding cellular reaction, vascular nephrosclerosis and chronic pyelonephritis (Brown & Mallory, 1950; Sokoloff, 1957; Talbott & Terplan, 1960), sometimes with early changes of tubular damage and focal interstitial cellular infiltration (Fig. 36.10).

Similar considerations apply to the association between gout and hypertension. Grahame & Scott (1970) found mild hypertension, defined as a diastolic blood pressure of between 91 and 130 mmHg, in 43% of cases and more severe hypertension in 9%. The incidence of hypertension was not related to disease duration, indicating that there is probably no added risk of developing hypertension with increasing duration of gout. The incidence of mild hypertension rose with increasing age of onset, but that of severe hypertension was highest in the decade 10–19. This again indicates the existence of a separate group of young subjects with gout, severe hypertension and renal failure. Conversely, about one-quarter of non-treated hypertensive patients are hyperuricaemic (Breckenridge, 1966). Filtered load of urate is higher than in normouricaemic hypertensive patients, but urate clearance is lower, indicating a tubular abnormality of uric acid excretion. An association between hypertension, hyperuricaemia and renal blood flow has been documented by Messerli et al (1980), who consider that hyperuricaemia in a hypertensive population is probably a reflection of hypertensive vascular disease.

The kidney in gout is reviewed by Diamond (1982) and by Yü & Berger (1982b).

DIAGNOSIS

The diagnosis of gout is primarily clinical, but it must be confirmed by the demonstration of a raised serum uric acid level. Other aids to diagnosis are the demonstration of crystals in joint fluid, histological examination of tophi or synovial tissue and radiological examination. As with other rheumatic diseases much consideration has been given to recommended diagnostic criteria (Bennett & Wood, 1966; Wallace et al, 1977). Although arbitrary criteria may be of some value in epidemiological surveys or other studies their value in ordinary clinical practice is very limited.

Serum uric acid

It is usually necessary to demonstrate a raised serum uric acid before the diagnosis of gout can be considered to be established. Some drugs, such as salicylate, can alter the plasma urate, so a careful drug history must be taken; if necessary the investigation is repeated after drugs have been withheld for a period of several days. Apart from the effect of drugs and other factors which can temporarily influence the serum uric acid, the level for any individual tends to remain fairly constant and it does not alter during an acute attack of gout.

It is true that there have been reports of acute gout occurring with normal serum urate levels in the absence of medication capable of altering them (Snaith & Coomes, 1977; Wallace et al, 1979), but such a situation is rare.

The most accurate measurement of uric acid is obtained by spectrophotometry, measuring the change in absorbency of serum or urine after treatment with purified uricase (Liddle et al, 1959). Though relatively expensive and time-consuming, this is preferable to older manual colorimetric methods, such as those based on a reaction with Folin's phosphotungstic acid reagent, which present difficulties due to coprecipitation of urate with plasma proteins, turbidity, non-linearity of colour yield, and interference by other reducing agents. However, automated colorimetric analysis has been shown to produce less variation in routine hospital laboratories than either manual colorimetric or uricase methods (Bywaters & Holloway, 1964; Whitehead et al, 1973); results for plasma agree reasonably closely with those of enzymatic spectrophotometric methods, but a much greater discrepancy is found with urine samples owing to the larger quantities or interfering reducing agents (Scott, 1983). Colorimetric autoanalysis, as widely used in hospitals in the United Kingdom, is a satisfactory method for routine clinical use as far as plasma is concerned, but is quite unreliable for the determination of urinary uric acid. For a detailed account of uric acid determination in blood and urine, see Watts (1974) and Scott (1983). Normal values and their variation are discussed below.

Identification of crystals in joint fluid by polarising microscopy

The presence of urate crystals in synovial fluids provides absolute confirmation of gouty arthritis. Fluid is easily examined when an effusion is present in a large joint such as the knee, but is less readily obtainable when small joints are involved. Nevertheless it is always worthwhile, using adequate local anaesthesia, to needle small joints in the fingers and toes: a few drops of often sanguinous fluid can usually be obtained in which crystals are readily detected. Synovial fluid is collected without anticoagulant and a drop examined on a slide under a coverslip. The search for crystals is facilitated by centrifugation; they may be seen lying freely in the fluid or within polymorphonuclear leucocytes, and are visible in large numbers when enmeshed in a fragment of fibrin. Crystals can be observed on ordinary light microscopy, but are detected more readily with the polarizing light microscope. A detailed account of the examination of synovial fluid for crystals is given in Chapter 8. See also Gatter (1977).

Crystals of sodium urate are needle-shaped, between 2 and 20 μ in length (Fig. 36.11) and show a strong negative sign of birefringence (Plate 36.1). They have to be distinguished from those of calcium pyrophosphate, which occur in chondrocalcinosis. Pyrophosphate crystals are much more pleomorphic than urate (Fig. 36.12) and show weakly positive birefringence.

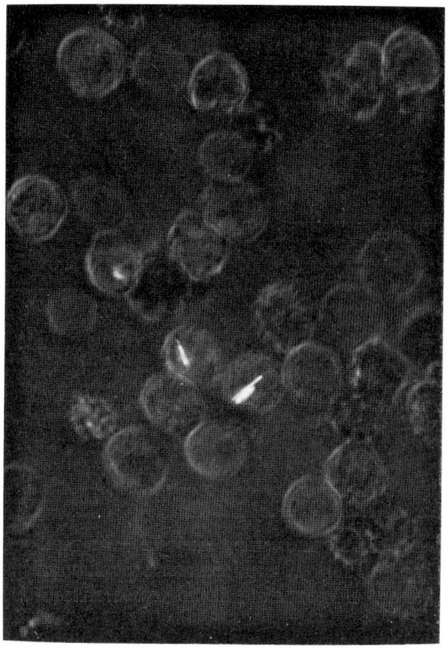

Fig. 36.11 Intracellular crystals of monosodium urate from joint fluid viewed under polarised light. (× 700)

Urate crystals are not invariably found in acute gouty joints, being undiscovered in 16% of patients in one study (Wallace et al, 1977). Moreover, as noted above, crystals can be recovered from asymptomatic joints. Very occasionally, both urate and pyrophosphate crystals can be recovered from the same joint, and there appears to be a tendency for an associated presence of urate gout and chondrocalcinosis (Stockman et al, 1980). Nevertheless, in ordinary clinical practice, the detection of urate crystals is quite specific for gouty arthritis and should always be attempted before urate-lowering treatment is commenced. A patient with a history suggestive of gout, but who is free of symptoms at the time of consultation, should be requested to present himself immediately his next attack occurs so that the affected joint can be needled.

Examination of tophi and synovial tissue

The contents of tophi may also be examined. For

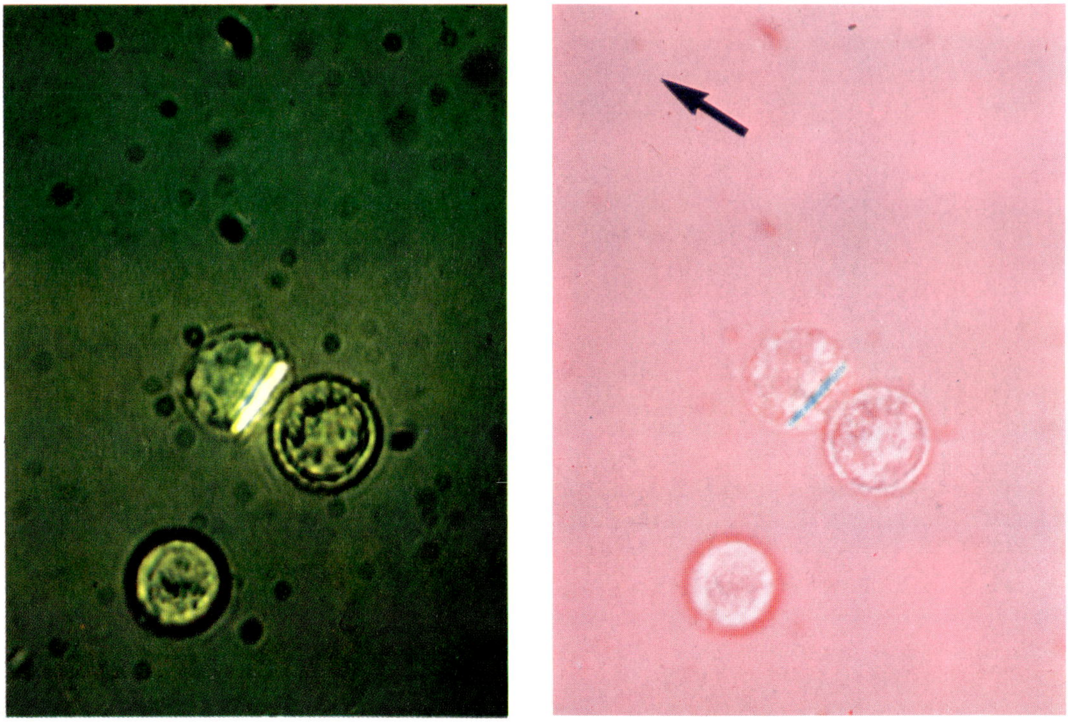

a b

Plate 36.1 Crystal of monosodium urate from joint fluid: (a) under polarised light; (b) with first order red quartz compensator, the slow axis lying in the direction arrowed. (× 1000)

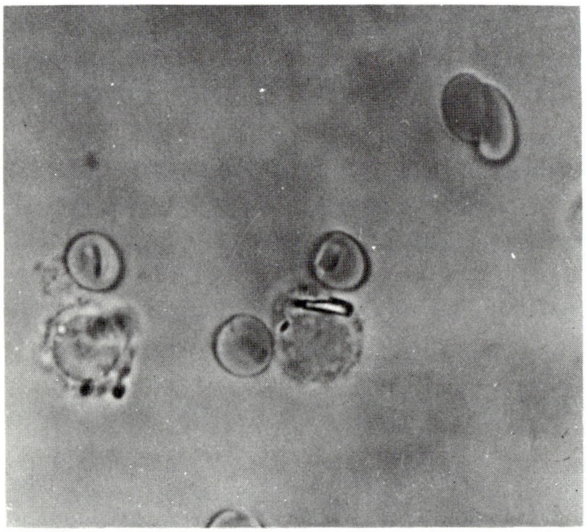

Fig. 36.12 Crystal of calcium pyrophosphate dihydrate from joint fluid viewed under polarised light. (× 1100)

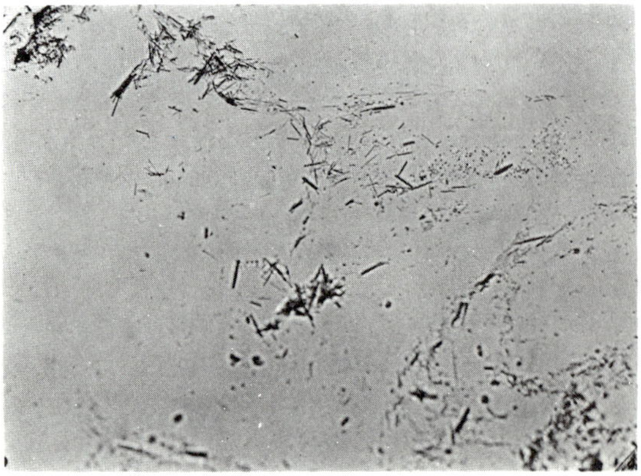

Fig. 36.13 Crystals of urate from a tophus. (× 325)

example, the contents of a small lesion of the ear or finger-pulp, suspected to be a tophus, can easily be extruded with a needle and examined under the microscopy, when the needle-shaped crystals of urate are clearly seen (Fig. 36.13). In the murexide test, rarely employed today, the contents of the tophus are heated with a few drops of dilute nitric acid in an evaporating dish until dry. When the residue (alloxan) is cool, ammonium hydroxide is added, giving a purple red colour (ammonium murexide). Arthroscopy and synovial biopsy are occasionally useful in the diagnosis of gout, but are rarely needed.

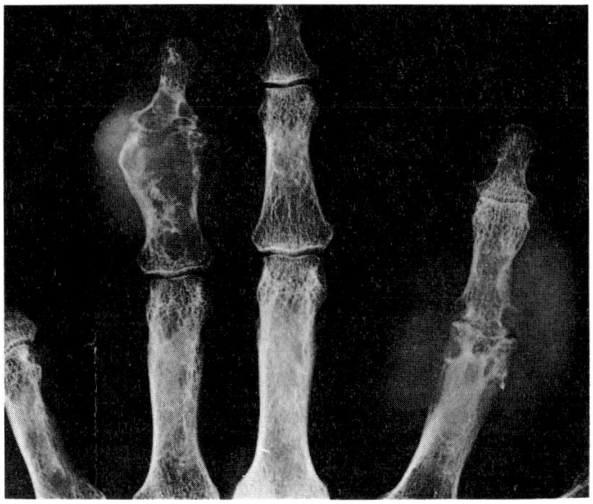

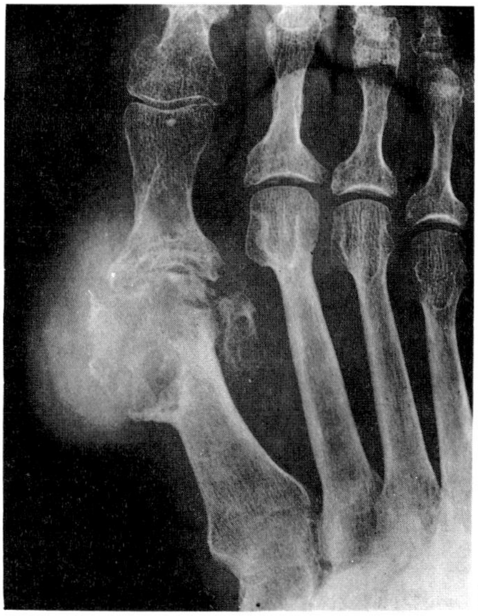

Fig. 36.14 Radiographs of (a) fingers and (b) great toe in advanced chronic tophaceous gout.

Radiology

Radiographs in the early stages of gout are normal but as time passes destruction of bone and cartilage by subchondral deposition of urate produces the characteristic radiological appearance of a bony defect, often with a rather sclerotic sharply defined circular margin (Fig. 36.14). Such a lesion, occurring asymmetrically in a site of predilection for gouty arthritis, is highly suggestive of the disease, but it is not specific; and it is impossible to distinguish it with certainty from, for example, an unusual form of rheumatoid erosion or from other diseases producing cystic changes in bone, such as tumours, sarcoidosis, myeloma and tuberculosis. Sometimes, especially in the 1st metatarsophalangeal joint, the lesion is situated centrally and such an appearance is extremely suggestive of gout (Fig. 36.15).

As chronic changes supervene, secondary osteoarthrosis develops with cartilage narrowing and osteophyte formation. Tophi are usually radiotranslucent but occasionally show calcium deposition (Fig. 36.16).

In general, radiological changes are relatively late, non-specific and therefore of only limited help in diagnosis.

The differential diagnosis of gout

A history of recurrent synovitis with intervening periods of complete remission, occurring usually in adult males (or post-menopausal women), often with a family history of the disease, and associated with hyperuricaemia, usually leads to a correct diagnosis without much difficulty. The appearances of acute and chronic gouty joints in their typical forms are highly characteristic, but there are a

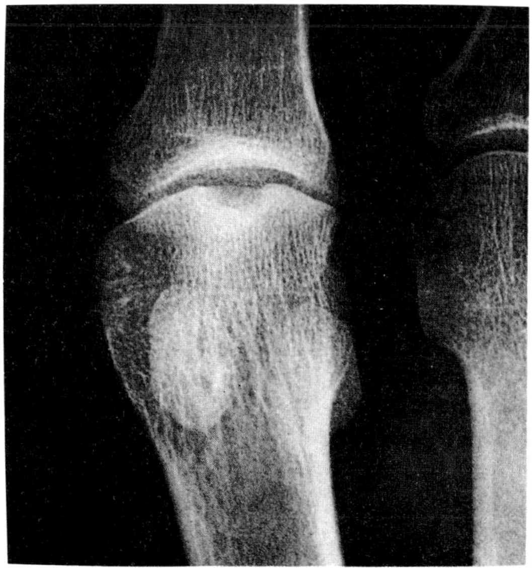

Fig. 36.15 Radiograph of great toe showing central erosion in metatarsophalangeal joint.

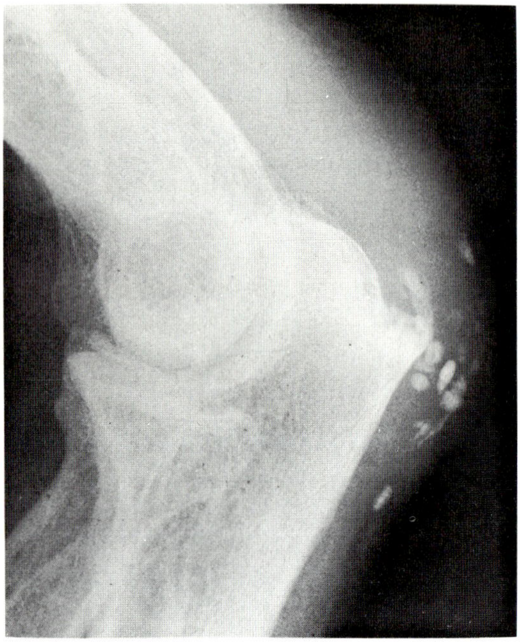

Fig. 36.16 Radiograph showing calcium deposition in a gouty tophus over the olecranon process.

number of conditions which have to be considered in the differential diagnosis.

The appearance of *acute gout* may be simulated by cellulitis of the foot, and the interdigital clefts of the toes should always be inspected for the presence of epidermophytosis, a possible portal of entry for streptococci. Although in both conditions local tenderness may be exquisite, the joints can often be moved painlessly with cellulitis (provided that the foot and toes are held away from the tender area); this is not the case with acute gout. Gout in the great toe must also be distinguished fron an inflamed bursa (bunion) on the medial side of the joint and from traumatic synovitis occurring in an osteoarthrotic metatarsophalangeal joint; the latter is occasionally difficult, especially since trauma may bring on an acute attack of gout. Haemarthrosis, either post-traumatic or secondary to haematological disorder, can also simulate gout. Acute gout and suppurative arthritis may resemble each other, and in doubtful cases joint aspiration must be carried out at once. The history of so-called 'palindromic rheumatism' — an episodic synovitis with periods of remission and often the precursor of chronic rheumatoid arthritis — is similar to that of recurrent gouty arthritis. As already noted, the patient should be asked to present himself during an acute attack, when the diagnosis may be clarified by further measures such as examination of joint fluid, needle biopsy of synovium and assessment of response to colchicine (though the diagnosis of gout by therapeutic tests is usually rather unsatisfactory). Gout, particularly when polyarticular, also has to be distinguished from various other forms of inflammatory synovitis such as rheumatoid disease itself, rheumatic fever, Reiter's disease and psoriatic arthritis, the latter two conditions, when presenting with relatively acute involvement of a single toe or finger, being especially deceptive mimics of gouty arthritis. Finally, attacks of urate gout may be clinically indistinguishable from pyrophosphate arthropathy occurring in association with chondrocalcinosis, formerly called 'pseudogout'. In both there is episodic synovitis, sometimes with a familial incidence, and chronic degenerative changes may occur in the joints. Urate gout, however, is more common in the great toe, whereas chondrocalcinosis occurs most frequently in the knee; gout predominates in men while in chondrocalcinosis the sex incidence is about equal; radiological appearances are distinctive, X-rays in chondrocalcinosis showing cartilage calcification without erosion; and crystals of sodium urate can be distinguished from those of calcium pyrophosphate as already described.

Chronic gouty arthritis is usually unmistakable but the bony swelling of Heberden's nodes (osteoarthrosis) at the distal interphalangeal joints of the fingers can be mistaken for gouty joints, as can osteoarthrosis of the metatarsophalangeal joints of the great toe. Indeed, the two conditions are not mutually exclusive: urate gout has been documented in Heberden's nodes (Simkin et al, 1983), a combination especially characteristic of diuretic-induced gout occurring in elderly ladies. Again, chronic inflammatory polyarthritis, particularly the asymmetrical finger involvement of psoriatic arthritis, has to be considered. *Tophi* are also easily recognisable, especially when they are ulcerating and discharging their chalky contents, but there are a number of conditions which may resemble them. These include small cartilagenous excrescences on the pinnae of the ears; olecranon bursae; sebaceous cysts; subcutaneous nodules of rheumatoid arthritis or rheumatic fever; tumours such as lipoma, neurofibroma or secondary carcinoma; xanthomata; and calcinosis, as seen in scleroderma and dermatomyositis. Diagnosis is usually reached by clinical assessment, but occasionally biopsy is necessary.

Finally, it is necessary to remember that many people have a raised serum urate without developing symptoms of gout, and that they may moreover have unrelated arthritic disorders. While, therefore, a raised uric acid level is necessary to establish a diagnosis of gout (unless the patient has been taking a urate-lowering drug), the presence of hyperuricaemia in itself does not necessarily mean that a particular symptom is due to gouty arthritis. Not infrequently a uric acid estimation is carried out on a patient who has an obviously non-gouty condition, such as pericapsulitis of the shoulder or osteoarthrosis of the hip. The serum uric acid, if elevated, may then be lowered with appropriate drugs, but of course such misdirected treatment is unsuccessful. This condition of 'non-gout' is very common today.

The old adage 'when in doubt, think of gout' remains sound enough, but its implication of easily missed diagnosis requires qualification. Gout is today an overdiagnosed disease. In fact, the less typical the presentation, the less likely — by far — the diagnosis of gout. Terms such as 'the lisping of the gout' and 'visceral gout' are seldom heard nowadays, but they represent an age-old mythology which has not yet been completely demolished and a confusion which modern methods of diagnosis and treatment have by no means dispelled.

BLOOD LEVELS OF URIC ACID

Despite the importance of local factors, as yet incompletely understood, which predispose towards the deposition of urate in solid form, and hence to the onset of symptoms, the development of gout must be regarded as primarily related to the degree and duration of hyperuricaemia. Concentration of urate in synovial fluid correlates closely with that in serum (Weinberger et al, 1981).

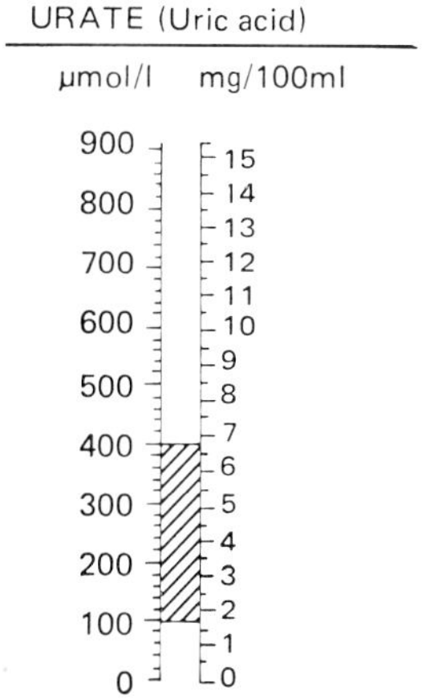

Fig. 36.17 Conversion scale uric acid.

Although there is an overlap between 6.0 and 7.5 mg/100 ml,* serum uric values for gouty and non-gouty subjects form two separate distribution curves (Fig. 36.18). The prevalence of gout is high in populations whose uric acid levels are above those found in Europe, and epidemiological surveys have shown a correlation between the height of the serum urate value and the prevalence of gout. Data from the Framingham, USA, study (Hall et al, 1967) indicated an incidence of 90% of gout among subjects with urate levels of about 9 mg/100 ml, and a 40% incidence of renal stones. However, only 10 men showed this degree of hyperuricaemia and other studies have not confirmed such a high incidence of gout and calculi. For example, Fessel (1972) found that only 3 out of 66 men with levels about 9 mg/100 ml (in whom pre-existing gout, cardiovascular and renal disease and diabetes had been excluded) developed gout after 4 years.

Plasma levels are relatively low in children — mean 3.6 mg/100 ml (Harkness & Nicol, 1969)

*Levels of uric acid are now generally expressed in SI units on the continent of Europe, but not in the USA. Conversion to SI units has taken place in the United Kingdom, but most readers throughout the world will be quite conversant with urate levels expressed in mg/100 ml, whereas the opposite does not apply. In this chapter, therefore, urate levels are expressed in mg/100 ml. To convert to SI units (μmol/l) the figure should be multiplied by 60 (more accurately 59.5). Thus a serum urate level of 5.0 mg/100 ml is approximately 300 μmol/l. A conversion scale is shown in Figure 36.17.

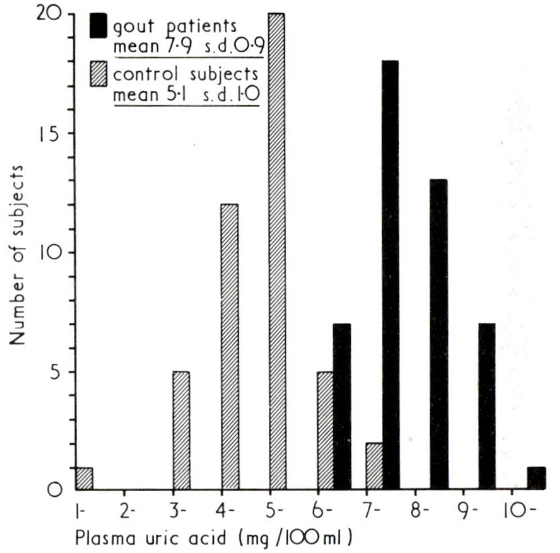

Fig. 36.18 Distribution curves of serum uric acid levels in 46 gout patients and 46 male control subjects (Snaith & Scott, 1971. Reproduced by courtesy of the Editor of the *Annals of the Rheumatic Diseases.*)

— with no difference between the sexes. Levels rise at puberty, more in boys than in girls, so that during young adult life the level for men is about 1 mg/100 ml higher than in women. After middle-age, values for women rise to approach those of men. There is little (Rubin et al, 1969) if any circadian variation in serum uric acid levels, although urinary uric acid excretion is reduced at night (Leathes, 1906). There is some evidence for a seasonal variation in serum levels, with highest values in July and August (Goldstein et al, 1972).

Mean urate values in two large American studies were 4.9 (s.d. 1.4) mg/100 ml for men and 4.2(s.d. 1.2) mg/100 ml for all adult women at Tecumseh, Michigan (Mikklesen et al, 1965); and 5.1 (s.d. 1.1) mg/100 ml for men and 4.0 (s.d. 0.9) mg/100 ml for women at Framingham, Massachusetts, (Hall et al, 1967). These figures are similar to those of an earlier English study (Popert & Hewitt, 1962) and a more recent investigation involving three populations in England and Scotland (Sturge et al, 1977b: Fig. 36.19).

It should be noted that in all these studies, and several others, the sex-specific distribution curve is broader for men than women and that both are skewed to the right. While hyperuricaemia may be defined as a serum urate concentration lying more than two standard deviations above the mean, this statistical concept presents difficulties in real bio-

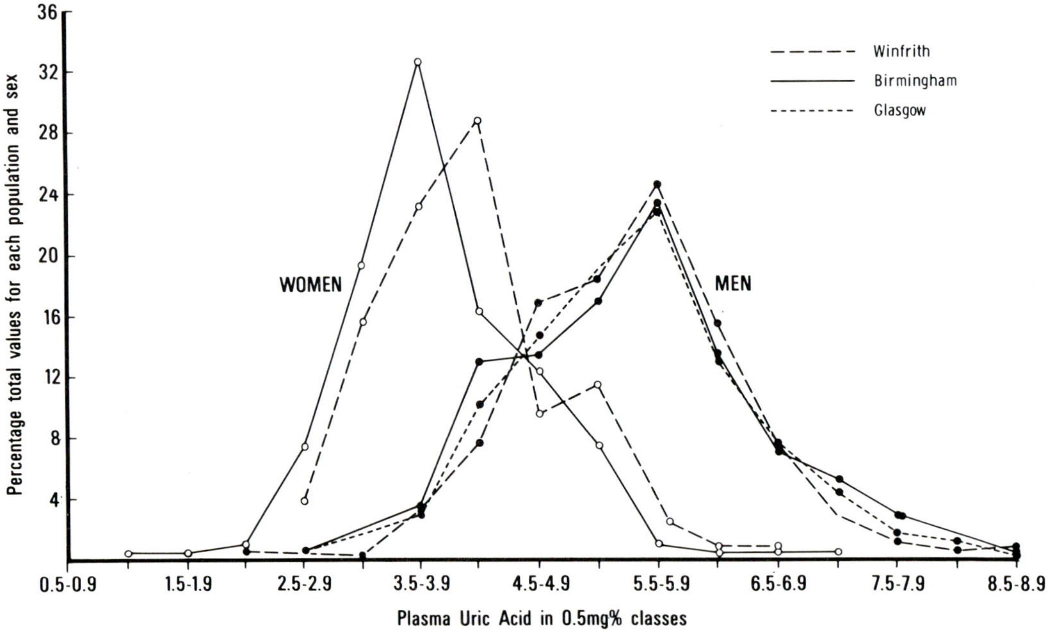

Fig. 36.19 Distribution curves of uric acid concentrations in three normal populations in the UK. (Sturge et al, 1977b. Reproduced by courtesy of the Editor of the *Annals of the Rheumatic Diseases.*)

logical terms when it is appreciated that we are dealing with a continuous variable and skewed distribution.

It is also possible to attempt a physicochemical definition of hyperuricaemia (Wyngarden & Kelley, 1976) based on the solubility of urate in plasma, which at 37°C is about 7.0 mg/100 ml. Factors such as protein-binding of urate have a bearing on such considerations.

Urate in the blood is mainly in the free form. Binding to plasma proteins was formerly considered to be negligible (Yü & Gutman, 1953) but an affinity has been demonstrated between the urate ion and both albumin and a specific α_1-α_2 globulin, and some patients with gout have been said to show a reduced urate binding capacity (Alvsaker, 1966; Klinenberg & Kippen, 1970). Campion et al (1975) found no significant difference in binding capacity between gout patients and controls. A number of drugs, including uricosuric agents, have been reported to reduce urate binding to plasma macromolecules in vitro (Bluestone et al, 1970). However, substantial urate binding at 4°C may be much less marked at body temperature (Sheikh & Møller, 1968), and the clinical significance of urate binding remains uncertain.

It will therefore be appreciated that a rigid definition of hyperuricaemia is not possible. In general terms and for practical purposes the upper limit of normal may be taken as 7.0 mg/100 ml for men and 6.0 mg/100 ml for women. Higher concentrations carry a proportionately increased risk of gout and renal stone formation.

In addition to variations with age and sex, there are significant ethnic differences in serum urate concentrations. For example, the Maoris of New Zealand (Brauer & Prior, 1978; Gibson et al, 1984) and the Polynesian peoples of the Western Pacific (Burch et al, 1966) have very high urate concentrations with a correspondingly increased prevalence of gout. Genetic factors must be important, but there are also environmental influences, such as purine, calorie and alcohol consumption. Thus Filipinos who have emigrated to the USA have higher urate concentrations than those in the Philipine Islands (Decker et al, 1968) and urban South African Negroes have higher concentrations than those in rural communities (Beighton et al, 1974). Japanese-American men living in Hawaii have higher levels than Japanese men living in Japan (Yano et al, 1977).

The epidemiological studies to which reference has so far been made have had a cross-sectional design, that is, single estimations of urate levels have been carried out at a certain point in time. Of particular interest is the study of Glynn et al (1983), in which serial urate measurements were repeated in a large population of adult male volunteers in the USA over a number of years. The levels were found to rise steadily between 1961 and 1978. Predictors of an increase were weight gain, alcohol consumption and triglyceride level, but these variables did not in themselves adequately account for the rise in urate which was observed. Also of interest was the fact that the trend appeared to halt after 1978, a situation inviting comparison with rates of heart disease.

METABOLISM OF URIC ACID

The three compounds by which nitrogen excretion is effected are urea, uric acid and ammonia, the first being predominant in mammals (ureotelic excretion) and the second in birds and reptiles (uricotelic excretion). Uric acid is 2,6,8-trioxypurine (Fig. 36.20). In man and the higher primates it is the end-product of purine metabolism, being excreted as such, whereas in other mammals it is further oxidised by the enzyme uricase (lost by primates in the course of evolution), with disruption of the purine ring, to allantoin. Uric acid is a weak acid owing to ionisation of hydrogen atoms at positions 9 (pKa 5.75) and 3 (pKa 10.3). In plasma and most body fluids at pH 7.4 nearly all is in the form of the monovalent sodium salt: at the lower pH of the urinary tract much is converted to free uric acid.

Uric acid formation

From the use of labelled substrates it has been possible to identify the atomic origins of the purine ring from various precursors (Fig. 36.21). A complex system of enzymatic interconversion controls the synthesis and catabolism of purines (adenine, guanine, hypoxanthine and xanthine), nucleosides (purine base + ribose), nucleotides (nucleoside

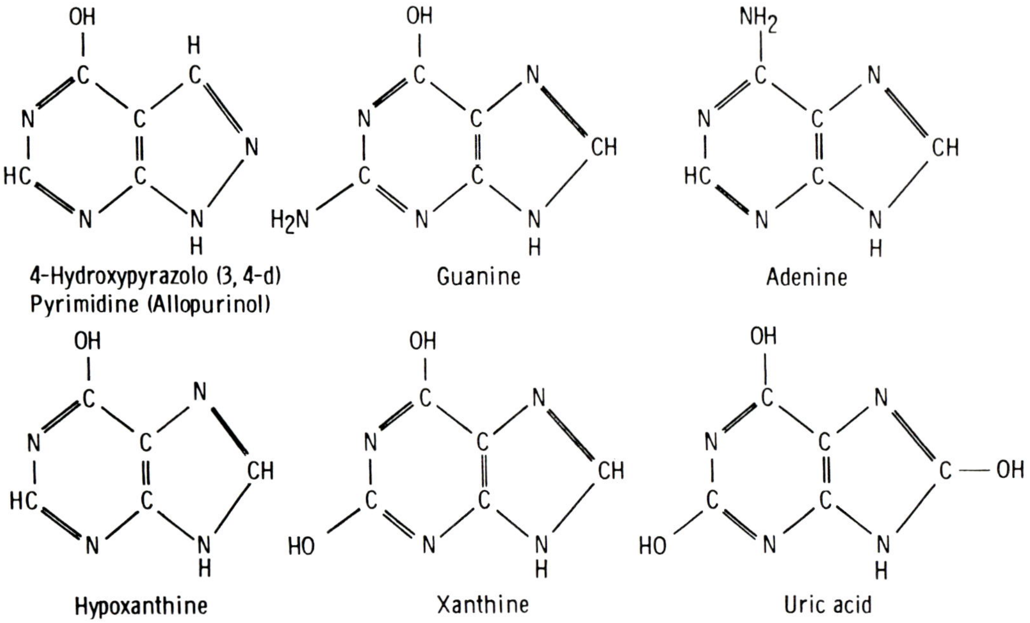

Fig. 36.20 Structural formulae of uric acid and some related molecules.

+ phosphate), nucleic acids (complexes of nucleotides) and nucleoprotein (combinations of protein and nucleic acids). Detailed accounts of purine metabolism include those by Seegmiller (1980), Wyngaarden & Kelley (1983) and Emmerson (1983), and the writer is grateful to Dr Anne Simmonds for comments on this section.

Purines are derived exogenously from the diet or endogenously either from the turnover of preformed nucleotide pools in cells and tissues (ATP, GTP, or the nucleic acids DNA and RNA, etc.) or by de novo biosynthesis. Careful studies have

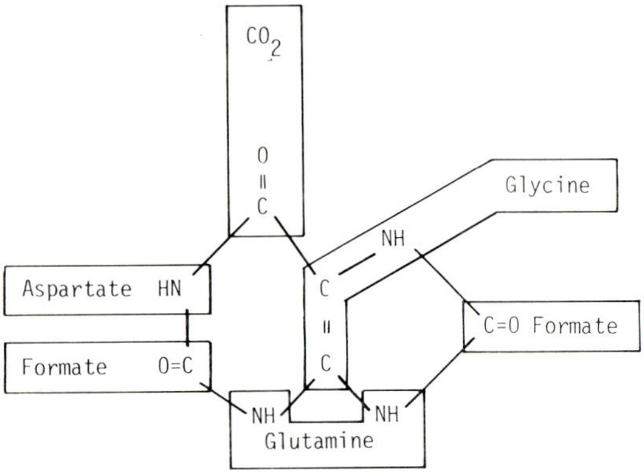

Fig. 36.21 Origins of uric acid molecular components.

shown that dietary purines are not incorporated into intracellular purine nucleotide pools but instead are rapidly degraded to uric acid (Loffler et al, 1982).

A key compound in purine biosynthesis is 5-phosphoribosyl-1-pyrophosphate (PRPP), synthesis of which from ribose-5-phosphate and ATP is catalysed by the enzyme PRPP-synthetase. The first specific step in purine biosynthesis, and one which appears to be rate-limiting for the whole subsequent sequence of reactions, consists of the conversion of PRPP to 5-phosphoribosylamine, the pyrophosphate group being replaced by the amide group of glutamine. The reaction is mediated by the enzyme glutamine PRPP-amidotransferase, possible factors in its regulation being the availability of PRPP and feedback control from the end-product purine nucleotides adenylic acid (adenosine monophosphate — AMP) and guanylic acid (guanosine monophosphate — GMP), so that variations in the concentrations of these nucleotides could regulate the rate of this initial reaction. PRPP-amidotransferase appears to exist in two molecular forms, a catalytically active form of low molecular weight and an inactive form of high molecular weight. Conversion of the former to the latter takes place in the presence of AMP and

GMP, the reverse reaction occurring in the presence of PRPP (Holmes et al, 1973). However evidence for feedback inhibition of the enzyme by nucleotides in intact as distinct from lysed mammalian cells is lacking (Bagnara et al, 1974) and PRPP availability appears to be the main regulator of de novo purine biosynthesis. Further steps are shown in Figure 36.22, culminating in the formation of the purine ring in the purine nucleotide inosinic acid (inosine 5′ monophosphate — IMP).

Inosinic acid is the first complete purine nucleotide formed by the ten-step de novo pathway (Fig. 36.23). IMP may be converted to adenosine monophosphate (AMP) or guanosine monophosphate (GMP) which are precursors of the corresponding triphosphates, the coenzymes and the nucleic acids. AMP, IMP and GMP may also be broken down by specific 5′-nucleotidases or non-specific phosphatases to ribonucleosides during the normal process of cell turnover. In most tissues, with the possible exception of the heart (Henderson & Paterson, 1973), the degradation of AMP normally occurs via prior deamination to IMP. By contrast dAMP arising from nucleic acid turnover is not a substrate for AMP deaminase and must be broken down to deoxyadenosine. The nucleosides inosine and guanosine, and their deoxyanalogues, are then cleaved by purine nucleoside phosphorylase (PNP) to hypoxanthine and guanine. Adenosine and deoxyadenosine are not substrates for PNP in mammalian cells and degradation occurs via prior deamination to inosine (or deoxyinosine) by adenosine deaminase (ADA). Consequently the only free purines formed from purine nucleotide

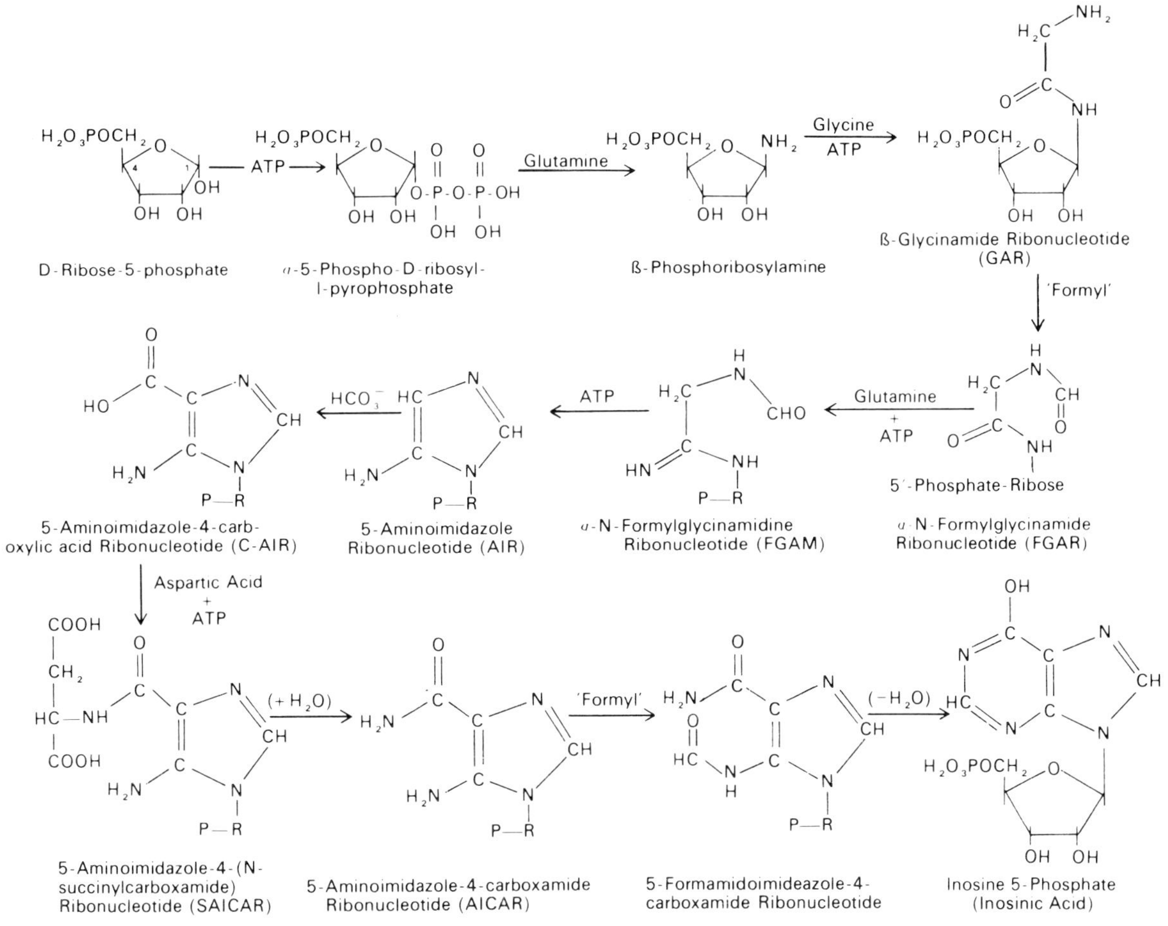

Fig. 36.22 Biosynthesis of the purine ring. (Wyngaarden & Kelley, 1972, used with permission of McGraw-Hill Book Company.)

degradation are hypoxanthine and guanine. There is normally extensive recycling of both bases by the so-called 'salvage pathway' resulting in minimal loss of endogenously derived purines form the body. The salvage pathway is a single step process involving condensation of either base with PRPP. This reaction, catalysed by the enzyme hypoxanthine guanine phosphoribosyltransferase (HGPRT) is energetically less expensive than the ten-step de novo pathway, the nucleotides so reformed acting as feedback inhibitors of de novo biosynthesis.

The finding of greatly accelerated rates of purine formation, hyperuricaemia and gout in patients with complete or partial deficiencies of HGPRT indicates the essential regulatory role of this enzyme in purine metabolism (Fig. 36.23). Inability to recycle hypoxanthine and guanine results in the removal of this important feedback inhibitory control mechanism. Cells deficient in HGPRT contain an excess of PRPP not utilised in the salvage reaction which further stimulates purine biosynthesis (Rosenbloom et al, 1968). This is underlined by the accelerated purine synthesis also found in patients deficient in the enzyme PNP where the precursors inosine and guanosine cannot be broken down to the corresponding base to provide the essential substrates for the HGPRT reaction. Consequently children completely deficient in PNP are also in effect HGPRT-deficient and demonstrate raised intracellular PRPP levels, gross purine overproduction and clinical symptoms relating to both defects, i.e. neurodevelopmental retardation, in addition to the severe T cell immunodeficiency (Watson et al, 1984).

A deficiency of the companion salvage enzyme adenine phosphoribosyltransferase (APRT) is not associated with purine overproduction or raised PRPP levels, indicating that adenine salvage via this route is not critically involved in the overall control of purine biosynthesis (Simmonds & Van Acker, 1983). The clinical consequence of APRT deficiency is kidney stones (frequently confused with uric acid) composed of the very insoluble 2,8-dihydroxyadenine (2,8-DHA). Studies in APRT-

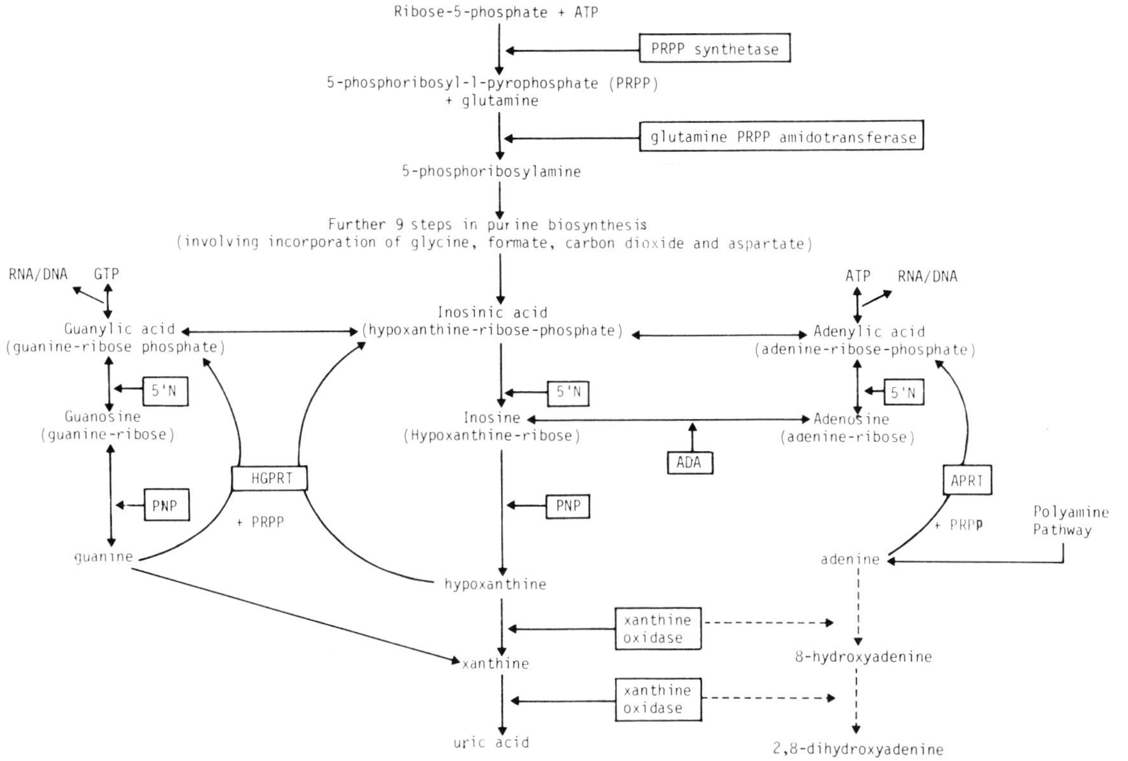

Fig. 36.23 Purine ribonucleotide interconversion reactions (HGPRT, hypoxanthine guanine phosphoribosyl transferase; APRT, adenine phosphoribosyl transferase; 5′N, 5′-nucleotidase; PNP, purine nucleoside phosphorylase; ADA, adenosine deaminase).

deficient subjects have established that a significant amount of adenine arises endogenously as a by-product of the polyamine pathway. In the absence of APRT it is converted by xanthine oxidase to 2,8-DHA via the 8-hydroxy intermediate (Fig. 36.23). However the principal action of xanthine oxidase in normal man is the conversion of hypoxanthine or xanthine (derived from guanine by the action of the enzyme guanase), not utilised in the salvage reaction, to uric acid. Activity of this enzyme is found almost exclusively in liver and intestinal mucosa (Watts et al, 1964). Plasma contains very little hypoxanthine (1–4 μmol/l) and xanthine (<1 μmol/l) under normal circumstances. Studies in patients with APRT- and PNP-deficiency have also shown that the alternative route of purine base recycling, a two step process via the nucleoside, is inoperative for adenine because of lack of reactivity with PNP and for inosine and guanosine because of the absence of an effective kinase in vivo for either (Simmonds et al, 1984a).

A wide variety of drugs and chemical compounds can influence purine biosynthesis. An inhibitory effect, for example, is found with compounds such as orotic acid, allopurinol and adenine, which compete for PRPP in phosphoribosyltransferase reactions. PRPP is utilised during the conversion of allopurinol to its ribonucleotide and erythrocyte concentration of PRPP is significantly reduced by allopurinol (Fox et al, 1970). The glutamine analogues azaserine and 6-diazo-5-oxo-1-norleucine (DON) inhibit steps of purine synthesis where glutamine is a substrate, and the ribonucleotides of 6-mercaptopurine, 6-azaguanine, 6-thioguanine and allopurinol inhibit the action of glutamine PRPP amidotransferase. The inhibitory effect of azathioprine is probably due to its hydrolysis to 6-mercaptopurine. Methotrexate inhibits purine synthesis by preventing absorption of single carbon fragments into the purine ring.

Xanthine oxidase is inhibited by many purine analogues and pyrimidines, allopurinol (4-hydroxypyrazolo-(3,4-d)pyrimidine) being a major drug in the treatment of gout. It is a competitive inhibitor of xanthine oxidase, by which it is rapidly metabolised to oxipurinol, itself an inhibitor but less effective therapeutically (Chalmers et al, 1968). Allopurinol has a short biological half-life of 3 hours; oxipurinol has a longer half-life of 28 hours and is excreted unchanged by the kidney.

Uric acid excretion

Lacking the enzyme uricase, man excretes uric acid as such, apart from a very small amount possibly broken down in the tissues; for example, human leucocytes have been shown to oxidise uric acid through a peroxidase reaction (Howell & Seegmiller, 1962). About one-third of the uric acid to be excreted passes into the gastrointestinal tract, where it is oxidised to allantoin, allantoic acid, urea and carbon dioxide by uricase and other enzymes present in intestinal bacteria: approximately 200 mg of uric acid is excreted this way daily (Sorensen, 1960).

Disposal of uric acid, however, is mainly through the kidney. The normal daily urinary excretion of uric acid on a purine-free diet averages 400 mg(2.4 mmol), and is usually less than 600 mg (3.6 mmol), though it can rise to as much as 1000 mg or more on an unrestricted diet. Mean estimates of renal clearance of urate in normal subjects range from 5.8 ml/min (Snaith & Scott, 1971) to 8.7 ml/min (Gutman & Yü, 1957), less than one-tenth of inulin clearance. Despite uncertainties concerning the significance of plasma urate binding, it is generally accepted that most uric acid in the plasma is freely filterable at the glomerulus, that a large part of the filtrate is reabsorbed in the proximal renal tubule, and that urinary urate is largely derived from further active tubular secretion (Milne, 1966; Steele, 1971). Evidence for active tubular secretion comes from various sources. Rare cases have been described of hypouricaemia associated with urate clearance which exceeded that of inulin, following the original report by Praetorius & Kirk in 1950; it is possible, under certain experimental conditions, to raise urate clearance above that of inulin in normal individuals (Gutman et al, 1959); while the paradoxical effect of salicylates and other uricosuric agents, which reduce urate excretion in low doses but enhance it when given in higher dosage, is most readily explained by postulating inhibition of secretion alone at low dose levels, and inhibition of both secretion and absorption at higher levels (Yü & Gutman, 1959).

Although bidirectional tubular transport of

urate is reasonably well established in different mammalian species (Roch-Ramel & Weiner, 1980), details of its components remain to be clarified. These include filtration followed by a bidirectional tubular transport system involving reabsorption, secretion and finally post-secretory reabsorption. The exact sites of these transport systems within the nephron are not known and they may coexist extensively throughout the proximal tubule (Weiner, 1979). Attempts have been made to identify the parts played by filtration, reabsorption and secretion by the pyrazinamide suppression test (Steele & Rieselbach, 1967a), on the assumption that the drug pyrazinamide, which drastically reduces uric acid excretion, blocks tubular secretion of urate without altering reabsorption. The decremental fall in uric acid excretion following the administration of pyrazinamide was thus supposed to provide a quantitative measure of active secretion. The assumption is no longer regarded as valid and studies employing this type of technique must be interpreted with caution (Holmes & Kelley, 1974). The interrelationship of reabsorption and excretion is extremely complex: there is, for example, some evidence that further reabsorption takes place in segments distal to or coextensive with the site for active secretion and that a proportion of secreted urate is itself reabsorbed (Diamond & Paolino, 1973).

In chronic renal disease, urate secretion is markedly decreased but with an increase in the fractional excretion of filtered urate. In severe renal disease 45% of filtered urate may escape reabsorption and be excreted. Thus while tubular secretion is the principal mechanism for urate excretion in normal and moderately diseased kidneys, glomerular filtration takes on this role in advanced disease (Steele & Rieselbach, 1967b).

Current concepts of renal excretion of uric acid are further reviewed by Steele (1978).

HYPERURICAEMIA

The serum uric acid can be raised by a number of factors, inborn or environmental, acting either alone or in combination. They involve basically:

1. An increased rate of formation or
2. A decreased rate of excretion. There are also
3. Other factors associated with hyperuricaemia and gout, the exact mechanism of which remains uncertain (Table 36.1).

Table 36.1 Hyperuricaemia

Increased formation of uric acid
1. Specific enzyme abnormalities
Decreased activity of HGPRT
Increased activity of PRPP synthetase
Deficiency of glucose-6-phosphatase
Increased activity of glutathione reductase
2. Increased turnover of nucleoprotein
3. Diet
4. Exogenous chemicals
Decreased excretion of uric acid
1. Alterations in renal function and contraction of extracellular fluid volume
2. Drugs
3. Lactic acidaemia
4. Starvation and ketosis
5. Essential hypertension
6. Lead poisoning
7. Hypercalcaemia
8. Myxoedema
Other factors
1. Race, sex and age
2. Genetic factors
3. Body weight
4. Social class and intelligence
5. Alcohol
6. Cardiovascular disease
7. Diabetes
8. Haemoglobin and plasma proteins

Increased formation of uric acid

Specific enzyme abnormalities

Decreased activity of HGPRT. The *Lesch–Nyhan syndrome* is a rare X-linked disorder of males; normal at birth, affected children develop choreoathetoic movements and spasticity during infancy and early childhood. Most patients appear to be mentally deficient although this may be party due to dysarthria and difficulty of communication. The most striking feature is compulsive self-destruction, so that restraint and sometimes dental extraction are necessary to prevent biting and severe mutilation of the lips and fingers (Fig. 36.24). Aggressive behaviour, such as spitting, may be directed at others, but this is combined with a friendly personality aware and regretful of its strange aberration. Urinary uric acid output is

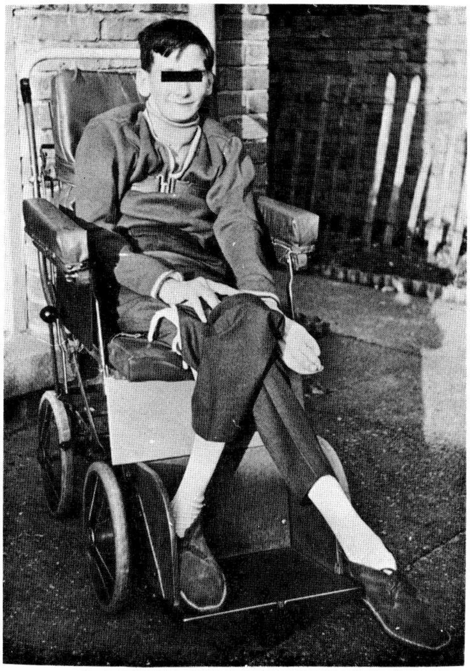

Fig. 36.24 Boy with Lesch–Nyhan syndrome. Spasticity, choreoathetotic movements: teeth have been extracted because of self-multilation.

greatly increased, detectable by measurement of 24-hour urinary urate, or, as a more simple screening procedure, by a raised uric acid : creatinine ratio in a random urine sample (Kaufman et al, 1968). However uric acid overproduction thus estimated may be masked in the presence of coexisting renal failure (Dillon et al, 1984). Urinary crystals may be the first indication of the disease and its course may be complicated by uric acid stone formation leading to death from renal failure, autopsy revealing shrunken kidneys with deposits of monosodium urate and uric acid. The serum uric acid is usually but not invariably raised and gouty arthritis may occur after about the age of 12 or so. Isotope studies show rapid incorporation of ^{14}C-glycine into uric acid, indicating an accelerated rate of de novo purine biosynthesis.

It was discovered by Seegmiller et al (1967) that erythrocytes from these children lacked the enzyme hypoxanthine-guanine phosphoribosyltransferase (HGPRT), which catalyses the conversion of hypoxanthine and guanine to their respective nucleotides, inosinic acid and guanylic acid, with the utilisation of PRPP (Fig. 36.23). The defect is also present in other tissues including liver, brain and cultured skin fibroblasts. Low levels of activity may be present, the enzyme showing other deviations from normal such as relative thermolability and variable lack of product inhibition by inosinic acid and guanylic acid, indicating considerable heterogeneity of mutation (Kelley & Meade, 1971; Becker & Seegmiller, 1975). Lesch–Nyhan erythrocytes, though usually showing no detectable activity, can cross-react with antibody prepared against normal HGPRT, indicating that essentially normal amounts of inactive enzyme are present and that the mutations involve structural gene coding for HGPRT (Kelly, 1972). However, most patients show no cross-reactive protein (Upchurch et al, 1975). Considerable advances have been made in the past decade. Single amino acid substitutions in variant forms of human HGPRT have been described (Wilson et al, 1984) and a nucleotide-binding domain in the first 120 amino acids of the human HGPRT protein has been proposed (Wilson et al, 1983). Cloned cDNA sequences of the human HGPRT gene have been isolated. A possible link between DNA methylation and X-chromosome inactivation has been proposed (Wolf et al, 1984) and molecular evidence for new mutations at the HGPRT locus demonstrated from DNA analysis in affected kindreds (Yang et al, 1984).

Possible mechanisms by which HGPRT deficiency produces overproduction of urate are:

1. Decreased synthesis of inosinic and guanylic acids, with consequent lack of inhibition of purine biosynthesis (Nuki et al, 1973). Consistent with this hypothesis severe GTP depletion has been noted in red cells of Lesch–Nyhan patients (but not partial HGPRT-deficient subjects) as well as in PNP-deficient red cells and those from a patient with uric acid overproduction due to an aberrant PRPP synthetase (Simmonds et al, 1984b).

2. Decreased utilisation, and therefore increased concentrations, of PRPP leading to accelerated purine biosynthesis (Rosenbloom et al, 1968), high intracellular levels of PRPP favouring dissociation of PRPP amidotransferase into its active subunits (Holmes et al, 1973). This appears to be a more important mechanism.

3. Break in so-called 'inosinate cycle' produced by a defect in HGPRT or PNP, not the level of

PRPP, can cause purine overproduction (Willis et al, 1984), the rate of purine synthesis increasing correspondingly to compensate for loss of purine nucleotides necessary for normal cellular functions.

The activities of several erythrocyte enzymes associated with purine and pyrimidine interconversions are secondarily altered in patients with a deficiency of HGPRT. Notably, activity of adenine phosphoribosyltransferase in erythrocytes is increased.

As well as hypoxanthine and guanine several purine analogues are substrates for HGPRT. For example, allopurinol, apart from its inhibitory effect on xanthine oxidase, is also converted to its ribonucleotide by HGPRT with utilisation of PRPP and may also exert a feedback effect upon purine biosynthesis as demonstrated by a significant reduction in total purine excretion. However, recent studies have questioned the extent to which allopurinol produces a substantial reduction in total endogenous purine production and excretion in vivo, claiming that this effect is relatively minor on a purine-free diet, and significant only on a purine-rich diet (Loffler et al, 1983). The original concept was based on the failure of HGPRT subjects to show any reduction in total oxypurine excretion on allopurinol (Fig. 36.25). Such patients have normally been studied on a restricted purine

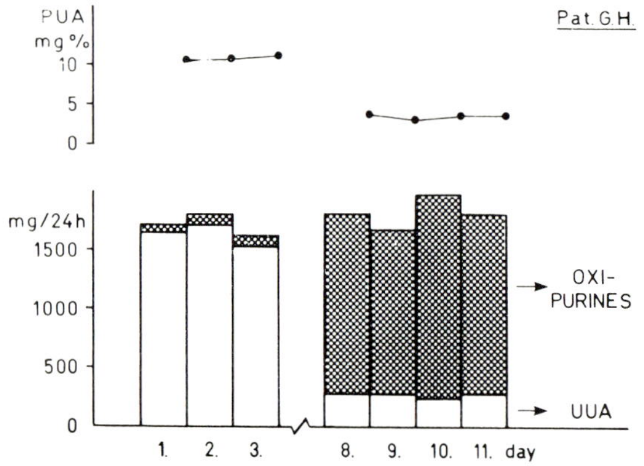

Fig. 36.25 Urinary purine excretion before (left) and during (right) treatment with allopurinol 400 mg daily in a patient with deficiency of HGPRT. The fall in urinary uric acid is equalled by a corresponding increase in oxipurine (xanthine and hypoxanthine) excretion, so that total urinary purine is unchanged. Allopurinol normally produces a fall in total urinary purine.

intake. A major effect of allopurinol may nevertheless be on dietary purine absorption. 8-Azaguanine, 6-mercaptopurine and azathioprine are all purine analogues which are also substrates of HGPRT. Their pharmacological use is dependent on intact HGPRT activity as demonstrated by their inability to inhibit de novo purine synthesis in vitro in HGPRT cells (Nyhan et al, 1968).

The pattern of inheritance is consistent with an X-linked mode of transmission, males being affected by transmission through carrier females. Heterozygotes are mosaics as far as enzyme activity is concerned, the presence of two cell populations — one normal, the other without activity — being demonstrable by fibroblast culture, cloning and chemical separation (Migeon, 1970).

Gene-mapping techniques, examining the expression of human HGPRT in human–rodent hybrids which retain the human X-chromosome, have demonstrated that the gene coding for HGPRT is located on the long arm of the X-chromosome, between the genes coding for PRPP synthetase and glucose-6-phosphate dehydrogenase (Goss & Harris, 1975; Becker et al, 1979).

Heterozygotes can also be detected by enzyme assay of hair follicles (Gartler et al, 1971), and prenatal diagnosis has been made by amniocentesis (DeMars et al, 1969), and more recently methods using recombinant DNA technology have been investigated. Prenatal diagnosis has now been carried out at an even earlier stage using chorionic biopsy material (Gibbs et al, 1984). Heterozygote female carriers can overproduce purines, but increased excretion usually keeps plasma levels of uric acid normal (Emmerson et al, 1976).

In contrast to these rapid developments in the understanding of purine metabolism in the Lesch–Nyhan syndrome, the pathogenesis of the neurological abnormalities, which constitute the most striking feature of the syndrome, is unknown, as is that of the megaloblastic anaemia which is often present. Uric acid itself can hardly be the cause of the neurological condition, since CSF levels are normal and antihyperuricaemic treatment has no effect on CNS function. The oxypurines xanthine and hypoxanthine are found in CSF in increased quantities, but they are also raised in patients with partial deficiency (see below), where neurological features are usually lacking. Patients with the syndrome are said to show elevated plasma dopamine-β-hydroxylase activity with an absent pressor response to acute sympathetic stimulation (Rockson et al, 1974). Recent data indicate that the concentration of free amino acids in the brain is lower in the Lesch–Nyhan syndrome and that this may restrict precursors essential for neurotransmitter or protein synthesis. Alteration in brain amino acid levels may also contribute to the decrease in catecholamine levels noted in basal ganglia (Rassin et al, 1982).

Management of these cases is difficult. Excessive urate production and its consequences are controlled by allopurinol but Lesch–Nyhan subjects are exquisitely sensitive to the drug, particularly in the presence of coexisting renal failure (Dillon et al, 1984), and the dose must be carefully controlled to prevent the development of either xanthine and/or oxipurinol calculi (Greene et al, 1969) or bone marrow depression which can result from excessive oxipurinol retention in renal failure (Shapiro, 1974). No effective treatment has been discovered for the neurological disorder (Watts et al, 1982): numerous drugs and chemical agents have been tried without success (Kelley & Wyngaarden, 1983). Future approaches envisage enzyme replacement with erythrocyte ghosts or liposome-trapped enzyme (Desnick et al, 1978), or chromosome- or DNA-mediated transfer of the HGPRT gene (Peterson & McBride, 1980; Lester et al, 1980; Jolly et al, 1983). Since mental retardation is often not as severe as it at first appears to be, these children should be educated and trained with as much care and expertise as possible.

Hyperuricaemia and overproduction of urate, but without the full neurological features of the Lesch–Nyhan syndrome, have been associated with partial deficiency of HGPRT, but the relation of clinical features to erythrocyte enzyme activity is not always close (Emmerson & Thompson, 1973; Bunn et al, 1975). Nevertheless, the degree of enzyme deficiency measured in intact fibroblasts correlates well with severity of clinical symptoms (Page et al, 1981). Such patients account for only a very small proportion — less than 1% — of gout cases (Yü et al, 1972).

Allison et al (1975) have reported subnormal percentages of B lymphocytes, IgG levels, serum isohaemagglutinin titres and lymphocyte responses to pokeweed mitogen in patients with the Lesch–Nyhan syndrome, contrasted with normal delayed hypersensitivity and T lymphocyte counts, suggesting that the salvage pathway catalysed by HGPRT may contribute to the proliferation and function of B lymphocytes. This observation is to date unconfirmed (Scott, 1977a). Its relation to the association of combined immunodeficiency disease with deficiency of adenosine deaminase (Giblett et al, 1972) or to that of T cell deficiency with lack of purine nucleoside phosphorylase activity (Ullman et al, 1976), is uncertain. The identification of these two inherited purine disorders associated with immunodeficiency has stimulated further interest in the role of purine metabolism in the immune response. However, despite more than a decade of research the basal mechanism remains undefined. (For review of purine disorders and immunodeficiency see appropriate chapters in Stanbury et al, 1983).

Increased activity of PRPP synthetase. Increased activity of PRPP synthetase with consequently elevated levels of PRPP was originally identified as the cause of uric acid overproduction and gout in two pairs of siblings (Sperling et al, 1972; Becker et al, 1973). Since then a total of 8 families have been described. Several different mutant forms of the enzyme have been identified which show either a reduced sensitivity to the nucleotide inhibitors ADP or GDP, increased specific activity per enzyme molecule, increased affinity for ribose-5-phosphate, or a combination of these (Becker, 1984). The normal enzyme comprises a single subunit which undergoes reversible aggregation to forms containing 2,4,8,16, and 32 subunits, only the latter being compatible with normal enzyme function. In 2 families a more severe form of the defect has been identified which is manifest in early infancy and in addition to the purine overproduction is associated with neurodevelopmental retardation and inherited nerve deafness. Whether as in HGPRT-deficiency this represents the complete syndrome whereas the late presenters escape the serious CNS involvement remains to be determined (Simmonds et al, 1984b). Like HGPRT-deficiency this is an X-linked disorder. Female heterozygotes show increased purine synthesis and uric acid excretion; in the families with the CNS involvement they also have sensorineural deafness.

Deficiency of glucose-6-phosphatase. Deficiency of glucose-6-phosphatase (type 1 glycogen storage disease, von Gierke's disease) is associated with hyperuricaemia and gouty arthritis develops in adult life. This is attributable in part to impaired excretion of uric acid due to competitive inhibition of renal tubular secretion of urate by lactate and ketones (see below). However, isotope studies have demonstrated excessive production of uric acid (Kelley et al, 1968). It is possible that deficiency of glucose-6-phosphatase leaves more glucose-6-phosphate available for conversion to ribose-5-phosphate, the substrate for PRPP synthetase, with consequent increased availability of PRPP.

Increased activity of glutathione reductase. Increased glutathione reductase activity is found as an autosomal recessive trait in Negroes and is associated with hyperuricaemia and gout. Pentose-phosphate shunt activity is increased with consequent generation of ribose-5-phosphate (Long, 1967).

Increased turnover of nucleoprotein

Hyperuricaemia due to overproduction of nucleoprotein accompanies proliferative disorders of the haemopoeietic system. In such patients the urinary urate level is high, Gutman & Yü (1962) finding a mean 24-hour excretion of 634 mg compared to 497 mg in a control group, and uric acid calculi are more common than in primary gout. Isotope studies showing an increase in the turnover rate of urate, and an excessive incorporation of radioisotopic precursors into uric acid (Wyngaarden, 1957), confirm that an exaggerated turnover of nucleic acid purines is the cause of hyperuricaemia in these patients. In myeloproliferative disorders maximum incorporation of isotope into urinary uric acid occurs after 7–14 days, whereas in primary overproducers peak incorporation takes place within 48 hours (Seegmiller et al, 1963a). It is, however worth noting that even in this indisputable form of overproduction hyperuricaemia, a combination of factors can operate. For example, Denman et al (1966) found that more marked degrees of urate elevation and gouty arthritis in a group of patients with polycythemia vera tended to be associated with renal failure rather than with the degree of platelet elevation, megakaryocyte proliferation or myelofibrosis. Hyperuricaemia, and sometimes gout, are also found in various types of leukaemia, myelomatosis, haemoglobinopathies, sickle-cell disease (Ball & Sorensen, 1969) and infectious mononucleosis (Cowdrey, 1966), as well as in secondary polycythaemia due to cardiac or respiratory disease (Lewis, 1961) or to renal tumour (Conley et al, 1957). Hyperuricaemia has been observed in a proportion of patients with psoriasis. It has been observed to correlate in degree with the extent of skin involvement, and to be associated with excessive ^{14}C-glycine incorporation into urinary uric acid, indicating that increased nucleic acid turnover in the skin lesions is responsible (Eisen & Seegmiller, 1961). However, the association may not be so quantitatively direct (Mariani et al, 1984) and indeed may not exist (Lambert & Wright, 1977; Scott & Stodell, 1984).

High-purine diet

A diet rich in purines is well known to raise the serum urate: as an extreme example it is possible to double the level by consuming 4 g of ribonucleic acid daily. Fractional turnover of uric acid pool is increased during dietary purine administration, suggesting an increased total body uric acid clearance as a result of the increased renal clearance which is observed: endogenous uric acid synthesis is not inhibited by dietary purines (Löffler et al, 1982). Conversely, a purine-free diet produces a mean fall in serum urate level of about 1.0 mg/100 ml (Seegmiller et al, 1961).

The hyperuricaemia of beer-drinking gout patients may be partly due to ingested purine nitrogen derived from the beer, augmenting the hyperuricaemic effect of alcohol itself (see below) (Gibson et al, 1983).

Indeed, relatively little is known about the precise identity and quantity of individual purines in most of the foods that we eat. Overall protein consumption is often invoked as a contributory cause of hyperuricaemia but it may have the opposite effect, high protein diets being associated with increased excretion of urate (Waslien et al, 1968; Matzkies et al, 1980).

Exogenous chemicals

The rate of purine biosynthesis is increased by 2-ethylamino-1,3,4-thiadiazole, one of a group of drugs which has been used in experimental cancer chemotherapy (Seegmiller et al, 1963b). The mechanism responsible for this effect appears to involve a marked increase in hepatic cell levels of PRPP (Lalanne & Henderson, 1975). Production of ribose-5-phosphate, hence of intracellular PRPP and purine biosynthesis, is enhanced by methylene blue in erythrocytes and other cells (Kelley et al, 1970).

Infusions of fructose also lead to hyperuricaemia and uricaciduria (Narins et al, 1974; Van den Berghe, 1978). This is a consequence of the consumption of ATP in phosphorylation of fructose with subsequent reactions resulting in a reduction of total adenyl nucleotides through conversion of AMP to IMP and further catabolic products. Urinary inosine, hypoxanthine, xanthine and uric acid all increase following fructose administration. Fructose infusion also results in stimulation of purine biosynthesis de novo, probably a secondary consequence of a reduced hepatic content of ADP, a nucleotide that is thought to be an important inhibitor of PRPP synthetase.

Decreased excretion of uric acid

Alterations in renal function and fluid volume

Urate clearance is related to changes in renal plasma flow, reduction of which may be associated with hyperuricaemia, as seen for example after administration of angiotensin or noradrenaline (Ferris & Gorden, 1968) or in patients with vasopressin-resistant diabetes insipidus (Gorden et al, 1971). Uric acid excretion varies directly with the rate of urine flow: the state of expansion or contraction of extracellular fluid volume influences tubular handling of urate, extracellular volume expansion being associated with decreased net reabsorption (Diamond et al, 1972), and extracellular volume contraction is an important factor in the hyperuricaemic effect of diuretics (see 'Drugs' below).

There is an overall relationship between uric acid clearance and inulin clearance (Davies & Shock, 1950). Urate clearance falls with the glomerular filtration rate, but with renal failure there is a relative increase in fractional urate excretion, i.e. as the number of functioning nephrons falls, there is an increase in the urate excretion per nephron (Steele & Reiselbach, 1967b). Nevertheless, the absolute value for the 24-hour urinary excretion of urate falls with the glomerular filtration rate, and it is likely that a larger percentage of produced urate is excreted by extrarenal routes. Hyperuricaemia due to renal insufficiency does not rise progressively as do serum concentrations of urea and creatinine and the serum urate seldom exceeds 10 mg/100 ml in stable chronic renal failure unless there are other factors operating such as drug therapy or uncontrolled hypertension. Lead nephropathy produces a disproportionate degree of hyperuricaemia (see below), and other varieties of chronic renal disease said to do the same include polycystic disease of the kidneys, renal amyloidosis, analgesic nephropathy, medullary cystic disease and obstructive uropathy due to bilateral hydronephrosis (Emmerson, 1980).

In these circumstances duration of disease is not usually long enough to produce sufficient tissue accumulation of urate for clinical gout, and secondary gout due to chronic renal disease is therefore rare. In any case, faced with a patient presenting with a combination of hyperuricaemia and renal failure, it is often difficult or impossible to ascertain the preceding sequence of events (Wallace & Bernstein, 1963). Patients with chronic renal failure probably do occasionally develop gout in the absence of any other contributory cause (Sorensen, 1960; Richet et al, 1965).

Episodes of acute synovitis are sometimes seen in patients undergoing haemodialysis for chronic renal failure, especially when biochemical control is not well maintained. They may sometimes represent true gout, but crystals of calcium phosphate rather than monosodium urate have been found in joint fluid, similar to deposits occurring in the muscles and elsewhere in these patients (Moskowitz et al, 1969).

Drugs

The antituberculous drug pyrazinamide (or in fact its metabolite pyrazinoic acid) is a potent inhibitor of uric acid excretion (Weiner & Tinker, 1972).

The limitations of the pyrazinamide suppression test have been mentioned above. Ethambutol and nicotinic acid also cause a renal hyperuricaemia.

The hyperuricaemic action of thiazides and other diuretics such as frusemide, ethacrynic acid and chlorthalidone represents a situation frequently encountered in clinical practice. Their mode of action is complex: whether due mainly to inhibition of tubular secretion or to more avid reabsorption, it appears to be dependent upon extracellular fluid volume contraction (Steele & Oppenheimer, 1969; Manuel & Steele, 1974).

In very high dosage, however, urate excretion is enhanced by chlorothiazide (Demartini et al, 1962), a biphasic reaction seen also with many other drugs including such commonly used uricosuric agents as probenecid, phenylbutazone and sulphinpyrazone, which increase urate excretion in normal therapeutic dosage but which can cause urate retention when administered in very small amounts. This paradoxical effect is most easily demonstrated with salicylate (Yü & Gutman, 1959), plasma levels of 10 mg/100 ml or less causing impairment of urate excretion and higher levels uricosuria (Fig. 36.26). The critical factor determining urate excretion by the kidney appears to be the concentration of free salicylate in the tubular urine. Low urinary concentrations probably suppress tubular secretion causing urate retention, while high concentrations produce greater suppression of tubular reabsorption with an overall uricosuric effect.

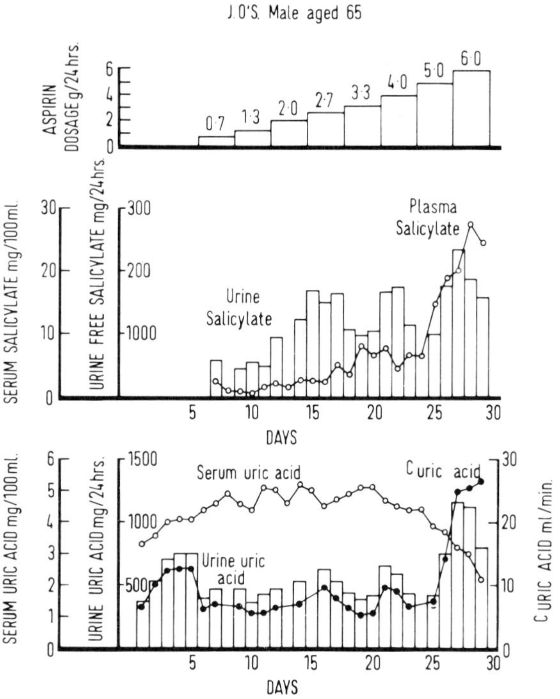

Fig. 36.26 Effect of increasing doses of salicylate upon serum and urinary uric acid. Low doses cause urate retention, but high doses (5–6 g daily) have a uricosuric effect.

Lactic acidaemia

Lactic acid causes hyperuricaemia by diminishing renal excretion of urate, probably as a result of suppressed tubular secretion (Yü et al, 1957). To this effect has been attributed the hyperuricaemia sometimes found in toxaemia of pregnancy (Handler, 1960), muscular exercise and parturition (Steenstrup, 1960). Lactic acidaemia may also be a contributory factor in the hyperuricaemia accompanying type 1 glycogen storage disease, acute alcoholic intoxication (Lieber et al, 1962), and chronic beryllium disease (Kelley et al, 1969).

Starvation and ketosis

Short periods of ketosis, occurring for example during complete starvation, high-fat diet intake, or diabetic coma, are accompanied by a fall in urate excretion and hyperuricaemia (Fig. 36.27). Uric acid clearance is impaired during infusion of betahydroxybutyric acid, which, like lactic acid, probably suppresses tubular secretion of urate by a direct competitive action (Scott et al, 1964b). Starvation can precipitate acute attacks of gout in predisposed subjects (MacLachlan & Rodnan, 1967).

The situation may therefore be regarded as reasonably well elucidated, but the picture changes during prolonged fasting, when the serum uric acid level falls coincident with a rise in urate clearance, despite continued ketonaemia; at this time an infusion of lactate produces a paradoxical uricosuric response (Fox et al, 1976). There are clearly ill-understood factors operating here, involving perhaps not only the renal tubule, but also urate production and enteral uricolysis, as indicated by the preliminary work on circadian variations of uric acid elimination by Owen-Smith (1983), extension and clarification of which is awaited.

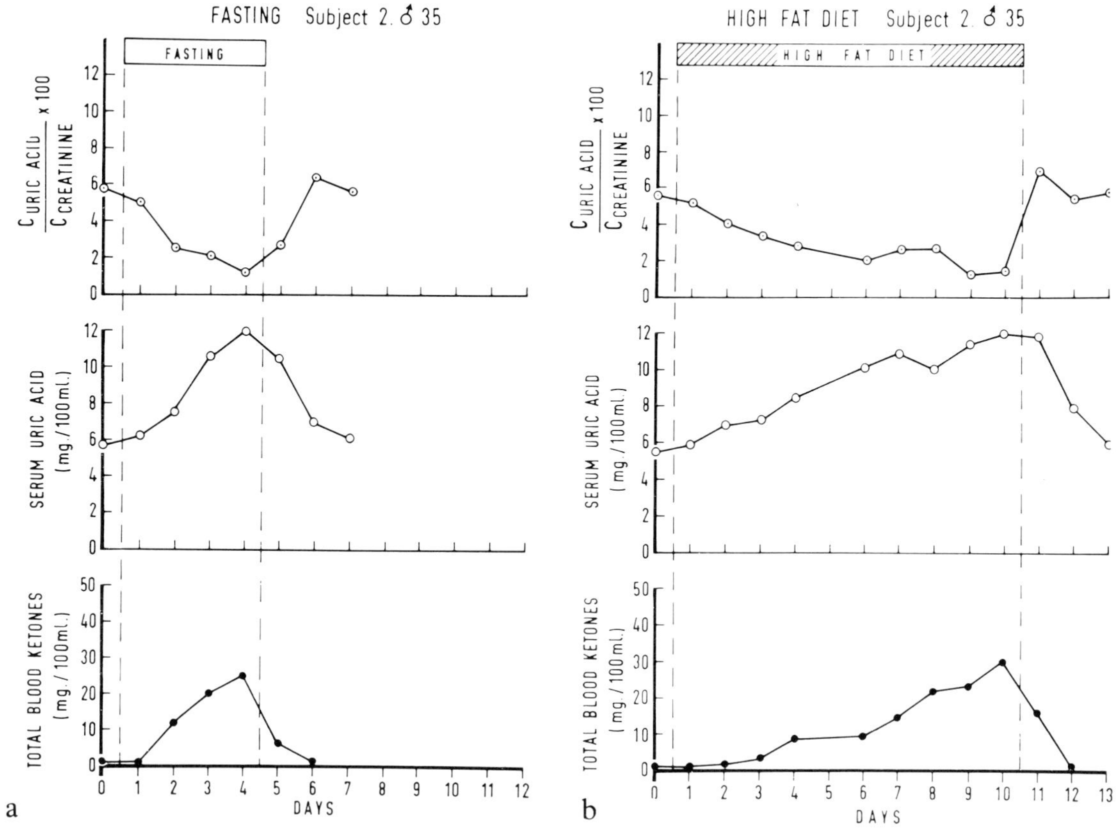

Fig. 36.27 Changes in blood ketones, serum uric acid and uric acid: creatinine clearance ratio produced by (a) fasting and (b) a high fat diet (Scott et al, 1964b).

Essential hypertension

As pointed out above (p. 894) there appears to be a defect in tubular secretion of urate in some patients with essential hypertension.

Lead poisoning ('saturnine gout')

The association of gout with lead poisoning was noted by Garrod over 100 years ago, but with the rarity of plumbism saturnine gout is now seldom seen in this country. Hyperuricaemia and gout associated with lead poisoning do however occur in certain special situations, such as in Australia following exposure to leaded paint in childhood, among American 'moonshiners', whose home-brewed liquor made from illicit stills contains an appreciable quantity of lead (Halla & Ball, 1982), and in Spain after prolonged contact with leaded petroleum (Rapado, 1969). Following the finding of greater quantities of lead mobilised by EDTA in patients with gout and renal disease compared with patients without renal disease, it has been suggested that the role of lead in gout nephropathy in the USA may be more significant than is generally supposed (Batumen et al, 1981), perhaps preventable by treatment with chelating agents (Wedeen, 1983).

However, Reynolds et al (1983) consider that while excessive lead stores in some gout patients are indicative of lead exposure the amount absorbed is usually insufficient to result in clinically recognisable toxicity, the abnormality in renal handling of urate being attributable to other genetic or acquired factors.

The available evidence indicates that exposure to lead can cause renal damage, a particular feature of which is a tubular defect leading to uric acid retention, perhaps associated with chronic plasma volume contraction resulting from abnormalities in the renin–angiotensin–aldosterone system (Emmerson et al, 1971).

Hypercalcaemia

In hyperparathyroidism, and occasionally in other hypercalcaemic conditions, hyperuricaemia is common and may be accompanied by clinical gout (Scott et al, 1964a). This may be partly attributable to renal failure, but it is possible that there is a certain type of renal lesion associated with calcium deposition in those parts of the tubule associated with uric acid secretion. Infusion of parathyroid hormone does not influence urate excretion (Shelp et al, 1969). Studies of uric acid levels following parathyroidectomy have given conflicting results (Castrillo et al, 1984). It is important to distinguish, on the basis of synovial fluid crystal examination if possible, attacks of urate gout from the calcium pyrophosphate arthropathy which can occur in hyperparathyroidism.

Myxoedema

Leeper et al (1960) found hyperuricaemia with a low excretion of uric acid to be common among patients with myxoedema, the values tending to be corrected after treatment; the association of gout and myxoedema has been noted by others (Kuzell et al, 1955; San Miguel, 1964; Scott, 1969). However, serum urate elevations were not found to be elevated in patients with hypothyroidism studied by Boyle et al (1966b) and by Golding (1970).

Other factors related to hyperuricaemia and gout

Race, sex and age

The variations of uric acid levels with race, sex and age have been outlined on pages 899–901. As pointed out, ethnic variations are probably due to a combination of genetic and environmental factors. The cause of sex variation is unknown, but a difference in renal excretory mechanisms appears probable, since renal clearance of urate is greater in women than in men (Wolfson et al, 1949). It is tempting to postulate a direct action of oestrogenic or androgenic hormones on the kidney, a concept supported by an apparent increase in urate excretion produced by administration of stilboestrol (Nicholls et al, 1973). On the other hand, Bengtsson & Tibblin (1974) found that the rise in serum urate shown by middle-aged women was unrelated to the menopause, pre- and post-menopausal levels in women of the same age showing no difference.

Genetic factors

A familial element to gout and hyperuricaemia has been emphasised by nearly all writers on the subject. There is a high incidence of gout in the relatives of patients, e.g. 36% in a recent British study (Grahame & Scott, 1970), and about 25% of asymptomatic relatives are hyperuricaemic (Talbott, 1940). It is evident from what has already been written, however, that apart from situations where a defined biochemical abnormality, such as HGPRT-deficiency, is being studied, family and epidemiological investigations can have only a limited value, since numerous causative mechanisms are operating. It is no longer possible to regard gout as a single entity following a 'Mendelian dominant pattern of inheritance with incomplete penetrance' (Stecher et al, 1949). A family study of some significance was that of Hauge & Harvald (1955), who compared serum urate values in the siblings of gouty patients with those of a control group. Values were significantly higher in the former. Moreover, serum urate values in the siblings could not be fitted to any Mendelian pattern of inheritance, but fell into a normal distribution curve, suggesting cumulative and multifactorial influences. Scott & Pollard (1970) found a graded correlation to exist between levels of urate clearance in gouty patients and those of first-degree relatives, which implies that the concept of multifactorial influences operating upon the level of uric acid in the blood may be extended to the handling of urate by the kidney. With regard to the relative importance of genetic as opposed to environmental influences we have little information but the study by Boyle et al (1967) of intrapair variances in monozygotic and dizygotic twins indicated a strong genetic component determining serum uric acid levels in females; this was not detected in males, and the significance of the sex difference remains uncertain.

Body-weight

It is generally accepted, and confirmed by Kahn (1976), that people with gout esteem their food highly, with eating and drinking being two of their greatest pleasures in life. Apart from the specific effects of a high-purine diet (p. 910) and alcohol (see below), the actual energy content of the diet probably influences the development of hyperuricaemia, the relation of which to body-weight has been shown in numerous epidemiological studies in Britain (Sturge et al, 1977b), the United States (Hall et al, 1967), and elsewhere. Notwithstanding many individual exceptions, the sufferer from gout tends to be a 'big, well developed and portly individual' (Williamson, 1920) and surveys of patients with gout have shown an increased incidence of obesity. For example, in a British study of 354 patients with gout, 38% were more than 15% over their ideal body-weights (Grahame & Scott, 1970), and comparable findings have been reported from other countries including Denmark (Brøchner-Mortensen, 1941), the United States (Wallace, 1975), and Australia (Emmerson & Knowles, 1971). The relation appears to be one of cause and effect since loss of weight lowers the serum urate concentration (Emmerson, 1973; Nicholls & Scott, 1972; Scott & Sturge, 1976). Data are shown in Table 36.2. How this comes about is not yet understood, but obesity is probably a more important factor in the pathogenesis of hyperuricaemia and gout than has been generally appreciated (Scott, 1977b).

Social class and intelligence

The social class of patients with gout is significantly higher than that of matched control hospital patients (Grahame & Scott, 1970) and an intriguing correlation exists between serum uric acid and intellectual level, particularly with regard to drive, achievement, range of activities and leadership (Brooks & Mueller, 1966; Dunn et al, 1960). These associations are reviewed by Wyngaarden & Kelley (1976). Their significance is unknown; it has been suggested (Orowan, 1955) that the development of intelligence in primates has been enhanced by evolutionary loss of uricase, urate perhaps bestowing a certain intellectual stimulation analogous to that conferred by methylated purines such as caffeine. There is no direct evidence for such a hypothesis. On the other hand, hyperuricaemia is associated with mental deficiency in the Lesch-Nyhan syndrome and in Down's syndrome (Kaufman & O'Brien, 1967; Pant et al, 1968).

Alcohol

The age-old belief that gout is often (but not always) associated with over-indulgence in alcohol has acquired some scientific corroboration by a number of observations which indicate some complex interrelationships:

1. Acute alcoholic intoxication can produce a transient state of lactic acidaemia and ketosis, leading to inhibition of renal tubular secretion and consequent hyperuricaemia (MacLachlan & Rodnan, 1967).
2. Because of its very high calorific value, long-term ingestion of alcohol predisposes towards obesity and therefore presumably to hyperuricaemia.
3. Prolonged consumption of alcohol may raise the serum uric acid independently of weight changes. Delbarre et al (1967) produced evidence that uric acid production is higher during periods of alcohol ingestion than during abstinence. In their study of Polynesian populations, Evans et al (1968) found that the mean serum uric acid level of those with a large habitual alcohol intake was higher than that of the others, and that this difference was independent of the association of uric acid levels with body bulk.

Faller & Fox (1982) examined the effects of long-term oral and short term intravenous administration of alcohol in patients with gout. During the long-term study, serum and urinary urate concentrations rose, as did urinary oxypurines and the daily turnover of uric acid. Short-term intravenous administration of alcohol produced no substantial

Table 36.2 Uric acid data before and after mean weight loss of 7 kg (Scott & Sturge, 1976).

	No. of subjects	Initial	Final	Mean fall	Significance
Serum uric acid (mg/100 ml)	35	7.0	6.3	0.7	$P = 0.000025$
Urinary uric acid (mg/24 hour)	35	603	516	87	$P = 0.0006$

changes in urate clearance but urinary oxypurines were increased and after administration of radioactive adenine, urinary radioactivity was also increased. The conclusion drawn was that alcohol increases urate synthesis by enhancing the turnover of adenine nucleotides.

4. Alcohol excess will produce moderate hypertriglyceridaemia (see 'Plasma lipids' below), which usually disappears on withdrawal of alcohol: after familial hypertriglyceridaemia and diabetes, alcohol is probably the commonest cause of hypertriglyceridaemia (Chait et al, 1972), possibly acting by decreasing hepatic oxidation of fatty acid and thereby increasing the availability of fatty acid for triglyceride synthesis. Gibson & Grahame (1974) found that alcohol-drinking gout patients had higher triglyceride levels than weight-matched controls or non-drinking gout patients.

5. As well as such more or less specific associations, alcohol is also a 'marker' of rich living. 'It seems that wine is guilty only by association. Its primary role was that of washing down these huge platters of meat . . .' (Healey, 1975).

6. Recent studies investigating the effect of beer on uric acid levels found an increased not decreased excretion and clearance of uric acid in control as well as gout patients despite an increase in serum lactate. The former was attributed to the high purine content of the beer rather than a direct effect on purine synthesis (Rodgers et al, 1984).

Despite the complexity of these relationships, the picture is emerging of chronic consumption of alcohol producing an increased synthesis of urate with acute intoxication providing an additional element of renal shutdown.

The high incidence of abnormal sulphobromophthalein retention found among gout patients (Grahame et al, 1968) may be at least partly due to alcohol-induced liver damage.

Plasma lipids

A number of studies claiming an association between hyperuricaemia and hypercholesterolaemia have been unconfirmed (Mielants et al, 1973). Patients with a raised triglyceride level in type IV hyperlipoproteinaemia often have a raised serum urate, and hypertriglyceridaemia is common in patients with gout, often associated with an excess of pre-β-lipoprotein which is usually ascribed to hypertriglyceridaemia of endogenous origin (Fredrickson et al, 1967; Darlington & Scott, 1972; Mielants et al, 1973). Obesity is to some extent a common factor (Gibson & Grahame, 1974) but the association does not appear to relate entirely to body-weight (Emmerson & Knowles, 1971; Wiedemann et al, 1972). Nevertheless, there is good evidence that the association between hyperuricaemia and hypertriglyceridaemia is due to the common factors of alcohol excess and obesity rather than to a direct causal mechanism (Gibson et al, 1979; Darlington, 1984). The hypertriglyceridaemia of gout patients is not found in their first-degree relatives (Darlington et al, 1982). Further investigation will require greater individual categorisation of patients and the use of modern techniques of lipid analysis and classification. Rheumatological aspects of hyperlipoproteinaemias are discussed further in Chapter 49.

Cardiovascular disease

The problem of uric acid and vascular disease also remains to be clarified. Associations with renal disease and hypertension have been considered above (p. 892). Reports of hyperuricaemia (Kohn & Prozan, 1959) and increased pool size and turnover rate (Dosman et al, 1974) associated with myocardial infarction must be interpreted with caution, because this situation does not readily lend itself to adequately controlled studies and the influences of such factors as changes in body fluid compartments are difficult to assess.

A relation between hyperuricaemia and atheroma has been suggested in the past (Dreyfuss, 1960; Eidlitz, 1961; Hansen, 1966), but this is not borne out by clinical experience (Grahame & Scott, 1970) or epidemiological studies (Hall, 1965; Myers et al, 1968). In the Framingham survey (Hall et al, 1967), a relationship was found between the occurrence of gouty arthritis and signs of coronary artery disease, but on removal of patients with gout from the analysis any association between coronary disease and hyperuricaemia was no longer apparent. Uric acid was not one of the variables found to be associated with the development of angina pectoris in the 5-year study of Medalie et al (1973). Neither male nor female gout patients after presentation to hospital, nor their male or female first-degree relatives, were found to have an increased risk of dying from coronary artery or cardiovascular disease (Darlington et al, 1983). A trend towards an increased prevalence of coronary heart disease in hyperuricaemic subjects (Klein et al, 1973) was found to lack significance when the factors of body-weight, hypertension and medication were taken into account. Hyperuricaemia in the absence of such associations does not appear to be a coronary risk factor.

Diabetes

Apart from the established fact that diabetic ketoacidosis, like any other form of ketosis, can produce transient hyperuricaemia because of impaired renal excretion of urate (Scott et al, 1964; Healey et al, 1966), the relationships between glucose, uric acid and lipid metabolism and body-weight are again by no means simple.

An association has been claimed between gout and diabetes but this is not the general clinical impression today (Denis & Launay, 1969) and the epidemiological survey in Framingham, USA, showed no such association (Hall et al, 1967). The Tecumseh survey showed no relationship between urate and blood sugar levels (Myers et al, 1968). Beckett & Lewis (1960) found serum uric acid levels to be lower in diabetics than in control subjects and only 8 cases of gout among 1000 diabetics.

Abnormal glucose tolerance and obesity tend to be a feature of type IV hyperlipidaemia (Fredrickson et al, 1967). Impaired glucose tolerance is found in many gout patients (Berkowitz, 1966), largely in those with hypertriglyceridaemia. Body-weight, however, again has an important bearing: there is no difference in oral or intravenous glucose tolerance, or in absolute plasma insulin responses, between gout subjects and weight-matched controls (Boyle et al, 1969; Wiedemann et al, 1972). Diamond et al (1974) found diabetic glucose tolerance curves in 9 of 21 gout patients, with a higher incidence in those who were obese, but mean glucose tolerance was similar in obese and non-obese subjects, indicating that impaired glucose tolerance in gout may not be entirely attributable to excess body-weight.

From a large prospective study, Herman & Goldbourt (1982) conclude that serum uric acid levels are higher in pre-diabetics than in non-diabetics, contrasting with a fall in uric acid with established diabetes. The study is difficult to interpret, not least because of a progressive rise in uric acid levels in a control population.

Other factors

Correlations have also been demonstrated between levels of uric acid and haemoglobin (Acheson & O'Brien, 1966) and plasma proteins (Acheson et al, 1969).

HYPOURICAEMIA (Table 36.3)

Problems of definition discussed earlier in the chapter with regard to hyperuricaemia apply also to hypouricaemia — an abnormally low level of serum uric acid — since one is dealing with a continuous but skewed distribution curve. Taking a normal range as the central 95% segment of the distribution, lower limits of normal distribution are about 2.1 mg/100 ml in women and 2.5 mg/100 ml in men.

Table 36.3 Hypouricaemia

Decreased formation of uric acid
1. Allopurinol; azathioprine
2. Xanthinuria
Increased excretion of uric acid
1. Uricosuric drugs
2. Expansion of extracellular fluid volume
3. Generalised defect in renal tubular transport (Fanconi syndrome), e.g. Wilson's disease, neoplasia
4. Isolated defect in renal tubular transport
5. Jaundice
Other factors
Pregnancy, pernicious anaemia, acute intermittent porphyria, inappropriate antidiuretic hormone secretion

Decreased production of uric acid follows the use of allopurinol and other xanthine oxidase inhibitors. Azathioprine reduces de novo purine biosynthesis. The rare condition of xanthinuria (Wyngaarden, 1972) is characterised by gross deficiency of xanthine oxidase and hence by a very low serum level of uric acid. An infant with hypouricaemia and mental retardation was found to have a low level of erythrocyte PRPP activity (Wada et al, 1974).

Increased excretion of uric acid is caused by a large number of uricosuric drugs which inhibit the overall tubular reabsorption of uric acid (Kippen et al, 1974; Kelley, 1975a). Some of these, such as probenecid, sulphinpyrazone and ethebenecid, are used in the treatment of gout, but the list of uricosuric compounds also includes salicylates (in high dosage), phenylbutazone, dicoumerol, ethyl triscoumacetate, phenylindandione, azauridine, the hypolipidaemic drug halofenate (Ravenscroft et al, 1973), some anticholinergic agents (Postlethwaite et al, 1974), chlorprothixine and radiographic contrast agents (Mudge, 1971). Benzofuran derivatives such as benzodiarone and benzbromarone (Jain et al, 1974) are powerful uricosuric agents, possibly with an additional inhibitory effect on xanthine oxidase activity (Marcolongo et al, 1972). Unawareness or oversight when any of these drugs are being used can lead to diagnostic error.

Uric acid excretion is increased by expansion of extracellular fluid volume (Steele, 1969) and is also found associated with rare defects in renal transport, either isolated, a situation analogous to that present in the Dalmatian coach-hound (Greene et al, 1972; Kuster et al, 1972; Healey et al, 1974) or generalised, sometimes associated with aminoaciduria. Examples of the latter include Fanconi syndrome (Bode et al, 1971), Wilson's disease (Bearn et al, 1957), in which treatment with penicillamine may lead to a decrease in uric acid clearance (Sorensen & Kappas, 1966), Hartnup disease (Baron et al, 1956), treatment with outdated tablets of tetracycline (Gross, 1963) and various types of neoplasm (Ramsdell & Kelley, 1973; Van Peenen, 1973), including acute myeloid leukaemia (Afzel Mir & Delamore, 1974) and Hodgkin's disease, where hypouricaemia has been related to disease activity (Bennett et al, 1972; Kay & Gottlieb, 1973). Hypouricaemia associated with increased clearance of urate is found in patients with liver disease and jaundice (Schlosstein et al, 1974; Michelis et al, 1974). Serum urate is also lowered during pregnancy (Boyle et al, 1966a), and hypouricaemia has been reported in association with pernicious anaemia and acute intermittent porphyria (Ramsdell & Kelley, 1973), also with inappropriate antidiuretic hormone secretion (Dorhout Mees et al, 1971).

PRIMARY AND SECONDARY GOUT; CAUSES OF HYPERURICAEMIA IN PRIMARY GOUT

The concept of primary and secondary gout was developed by Talbott (1959). The term 'primary gout' implies that the cause of hyperuricaemia is attributable to an inherent metabolic abnormality, occasionally identified (e.g. HGPRT-deficiency) but nearly always, as yet, unknown. 'Secondary gout' has signified a situation where an identifiable and usually acquired cause can be demonstrated; originally it was applied to proliferative haemopoietic disorders such as polycythaemia rubra vera where the excess of uric acid was caused by tissue breakdown of nucleic acids, and later it was extended to include circumstances where hyperuricaemia is due to a definable renal factor. These various mechanisms have been reviewed above.

There is no doubt that the increased body content of uric acid in primary gout, as shown by an elevated serum level, or by an increase in the miscible pool of urate, to which it tends to be related (Scott et al, 1969) can be due to a number of different mechanisms. Overproduction of uric acid is found in some of these patients: about 25% of a group studied by Gutman & Yü (1957) excreted uric acid in excess of 600 mg daily on a low-purine diet, and excessive incorporation of isotopic precursors into uric acid has been demonstrated in a higher proportion, e.g. 9 out of 14 patients studied by Seegmiller et al (1961). Wyngaarden & Kelley (1983) have summarised collected reports of 1-^{14}C-glycine incorporation. In gouty subjects with uric acid excretions of less than 590 mg/day, the cumulative incorporation of ^{14}C was excessive in about two-thirds of the patients. In subjects with higher rates of excretion incorporation was invariably increased. Even in subjects in whom total incorporation after administration of ^{15}N-glycine is normal there may be evidence of relatively increased enrichment of N-3 and N-9 in the uric acid molecule indicating accelerated kinetics of purine production (Sperling et al, 1973). Kelley (1975b) suggested that an accelerated rate of purine biosynthesis de novo contributes to the development of hyperuricaemia in at least 75% of subjects with primary gout, and that it may be the sole cause in up to 25% of these patients.

Overt overproduction — as defined by an increased urinary uric acid level on a low-purine diet — is certainly less common in gout patients in this country than such figures would indicate, and many would agree with Nuki (1976) that they are too high, reflecting an unrepresentative selection of severely affected patients in specialised centres. It has even been suggested that uric acid overproduction as a cause of gout represents less than 1% of the total gouty population (Loffler et al, 1983).

Beyond very rare patients with deficiency of HGPRT or overactivity of PRPP synthetase, no further specific metabolic abnormalities have yet been defined with certainty. Erythrocyte levels of PRPP are normal in idiopathic primary gout although fibroblast cultures from gout overproducers may show increased concentration or generation of this regulatory substrate, sometimes with increased concentration of ribose-5-phosphate (Becker, 1976); the possibility of a defect in glutamine metabolism proposed by Gutman & Yü (1963) has received no support after several lines of further investigation; the possibility of qualitative or quantitative changes in PRPP amidotransferase has not been established (Wyngaarden, 1974); and increased xanthine oxidase activity in gouty overproducers appears to be a secondary phenomenon (Marcolongo et al, 1974). The putative role of abnormal protein binding of urate as a significant factor in gout has yet to be clarified (Klinenberg & Kippen, 1970).

The part played by impaired excretion in primary gout has been controversial. There is considerable overlap of urate clearance between gout patients and normal subjects. Gutman & Yü (1957) found that uric acid clearance averaged 8.7 (s.d.$\pm$2.5) ml/min in normal men and was only slightly less, 7.5 ($\pm$2.4) ml/min, in gout patients. Rather greater differences have been found in other series, for example a mean clearance of 5.8 in normals compared with 3.6 in gout patients in a study in this country (Snaith & Scott, 1971).

A recent study in the New Zealand Maori has demonstrated a reduced clearance of uric acid in young non-gouty non-obese Maoris with normal renal function (4.9 $\pm$ 1.5 ml/min) compared with their Caucasian counterparts, suggesting a genetic component, undoubtedly aggravated by diet and obesity, associated with the high incidence of hyperuricaemia and gout in this race (Gibson et al, 1984).

Excretion of uric acid is increased both in patients and normal subjects if the plasma level is raised by intravenous infusion of urate (Yü et al, 1962), but at equivalent plasma levels the clearance of urate is less in gouty subjects than in normals (Lathem & Rodnan, 1962; Nugent et al, 1964). It is evident that the kidney in many patients with gout does not excrete the load of endogenous uric acid presented to it to the same extent as that of normal subjects, although it remains capable of removing much larger extraneous loads. The studies of Rieselbach et al (1970) indicate that the pattern of urate tubular secretion in gouty overproducers appears to be indistinguishable from normal, whereas normoproducers show diminished secretion, but identification of any specific renal abnormality in gout patients must await more precise methods of examining tubular transport of urate than are currently available.

Diminished uricolysis has never been demonstrated as a cause of hyperuricaemia. Gout patients do not show any diminution of extrarenal disposal of uric acid; indeed, some show an increased extrarenal loss consequent upon hyperuricaemia (Seegmiller et al, 1961; Sorensen, 1962).

It therefore appears likely that while a few patients with primary gout possess a single genetic abnormality, the majority derive their hyperuricaemia from a number of contributory factors, namely quantitative variations in genetically determined metabolic and renal functions, the precise nature of which have yet to be elucidated, to which are added in many instances the effects of external agents, particularly food (with regard to both its purine and calorie content), alcoholic liquors and drugs, especially diuretics. As Acheson & Chan (1969) have said, 'The associates of a high uric acid are the associates of plenty'. Subject to this multifactorial concept, however, the terms 'primary' and 'secondary gout' still serve a useful clinical and descriptive purpose.

FAMILIAL JUVENILE GOUT

In the past decade several studies have highlighted additional rare families with a high incidence of gout clearly of genetic origin but with no as yet defined biochemical basis. It occurs in young subjects (in some affecting both sexes) and generally presents around puberty, but up to the 3rd decade. There appear to be three distinct groups:

1. Uric acid excretion is grossly increased in this group (2 families) and renal function generally reduced at presentation with a concentrating ability disproportionately low for the reduction in GFR. Activity of both HGPRT and PRPP in lysed red cells has been normal in all patients but in one of them HGPRT may not have been fully active in vivo (Westberg et al, 1979).

2. 12 families have been described in the second group following the original report of Duncan & Dixon (1960), also distinguished from the normal gouty population by their young age, associated renal disease — rapidly and progressively fatal in some instances — in the absence of the overt uric acid overproduction seen in the previous group. Concentrating capacity in this group is also disproportionately low for the relatively moderate reduction in GFR in some young family members. Equally unusual is the fact that both males and females are affected and the defect is characterised by a dominant pattern of inheritance (Simmonds et al, 1980a, b). Hypertension has been reported in some but not all families. The basic defect may be primary renal disease (Hollingworth & Scott, 1983). It remains to be established whether these are all the same disorder or possibly different subgroups. Early recognition may be important since it is possible that allopurinol can halt the rapid decline in renal function.

3. In the third group juvenile gout and hyperuricosuria is associated with a chronic compensated haemolytic syndrome of unknown aetiology (Lieberman et al, 1982). 8 patients have been reported. As in the first group, this may be an X-linked recessive disorder strongly expressed in the heterozygous female. However, renal function appears normal.

MANAGEMENT OF GOUT

It is arguable to what extent patients with gout — diagnosed on ground of clinical findings, hyperuricaemia and if possible the demonstration of urate crystals — should be further investigated as to the cause of the underlying elevated concentration of serum uric acid. Certainly a careful clinical history and examination should identify possible contributory factors such as diuretics, obesity, hypertension and renal impairment. In current clinical practice this is often thought to be sufficient, and indeed may be so in the case of the older gout patient with mild hyperuricaemia.

In most patients, however, and certainly in the case of young patients with marked hyperuricaemia, steps should be taken to identify 'overproducers', since among these may be found occasional patients with a specific enzyme deficiency, notably that of HGPRT, a situation which apart from anything else will require a family investigation. Overproducers are also at some risk of developing urate nephrolithiasis.

Uric acid production is most conveniently estimated by measuring the 24-hour urinary uric acid excretion after 5 days' equilibration on a low-purine alcohol-free diet. Measurement of the uric acid to creatinine ratio in spot urine samples is an unreliable method of assessing uric acid production (Wortmann & Fox, 1980). In the absence of renal failure the urinary uric acid is a good index of urate turnover as estimated by isotope techniques such as the rate of decline in excretion of ^{14}C-labelled urate (Scott et al, 1969). A level of urinary acid excretion greater than 600 mg (3.6 mmol) in 24 hours signifies an increase in uric acid production. In the presence of renal failure the urinary uric acid excretion is diminished and urate production can then be estimated only by isotope methods. An increased rate of de novo purine biosynthesis is distinguishable from a raised turnover of preformed purines (as occurs in myeloproliferative disorders) by measuring the rate of incorporation of isotopes such as glycine-1-^{14}C into urinary uric acid (Seegmiller et al, 1963a), but such investigations are not necessary in normal clinical practice.

Patients identified as overproducers should be screened for the presence of a possible enzyme abnormality by methods such as the estimation of HGPRT activity on red cell haemolysates (Seegmiller et al, 1967), preferably in a laboratory where purine enzymatic pathways are customarily studied. For details of methodology see Hoffee & Jones (1978) and Kelley & Weiner (1978).

Apart from consideration of these possible underlying or complicating factors, the treatment of primary gout falls into two parts — the acute attack and long-term management.

Acute gout

Treatment of acute gout is directed solely towards relief of inflammation as rapidly as possible. A common error is to begin immediate treatment with a uricosuric drug or allopurinol. It must be emphasised that control of uric acid plays no part in the treatment of acute gout, and attempts to lower the blood level at this stage may well prolong the episode.

With a severe attack the patient will find it helpful to rest in bed or a chair with protection and elevation of the affected limb. Three drugs are commonly used. Colchicine is the time-honoured remedy: phenylbutazone and indomethacin are equally effective and usually less toxic (Smyth & Percy, 1973).

Colchicine. This drug is best given as the 0.5 mg tablet. The usual dose is 1.0 mg followed by 0.5 mg every 2 hours until the attack subsides. The most frequent toxic effect is diarrhoea, but this does not usually occur until a total dose of 5–6 mg has been taken. There is considerable variation in individual sensitivity however, and sometimes diarrhoea, nausea, or vomiting preclude the effective use of colchicine.

Phenylbutazone should be prescribed in a dose of 200 mg 4 times daily until the attack is relieved. Such a dose is rather too high for the long-term treatment of other disorders such as rheumatoid arthritis, but may be safely given for a few days. However, because of the risk of marrow suppression, this drug has been withdrawn from prescription in the United Kingdom (except for patients with ankylosing spondylitis), although some patients with gout express an individual preference for it.

Indomethacin. This is also useful in acute gout in a dose of 50 mg 4 times daily.

Others of the newer non-steroidal anti-inflammatory drugs, e.g. naproxen 250 mg 3 times daily (Sturge et al, 1977a), are also effective in treating acute gouty arthritis.

These drugs can be used either alone or in combination. They should be administered as early as possible and a gouty patient should always keep a small supply of whichever preparation is most effective for his own particular case, so that he can abort an attack directly he notices the first symptoms.

Salicylate is less effective than these drugs and is therefore rarely indicated. It should be noted that colchicine and indomethacin do not alter the serum uric acid, whereas phenylbutazone and salicylate do (phenylbutazone is weakly uricosuric; salicylate, as noted above, causes urate retention in low dosages and is strongly uricosuric in high dosages). If there is any doubt about the diagnosis it is therefore advisable to draw blood for a uric acid estimation before any drugs are given.

Acute gout sometimes causes a sizeable joint effusion, particularly in the knee. Immediate relief is then given by aspiration of the fluid (which should be examined for the presence of crystals) followed by intra-articular injection of hydrocortisone or prednisolone. Systemic corticosteroids or ACTH are also effective in the treatment of acute gouty arthritis, but are rarely necessary in view of the other medication available.

Considerable interest has recently been taken in drugs which possess combined anti-inflammatory and uricosuric properties, notably azapropazone. These are discussed in Chapter 22. Although such a combination of features might at first sight appear desirable, it has already been pointed out that treatment of the acute attack and long-term control of hyperuricaemia are two very different problems and it remains to be seen if drugs of this type represent a significant therapeutic advance.

Long-term management

When an acute attack has been terminated the question of long-term management is considered, with particular reference to lowering the serum uric acid. This is a decision of some importance, because once started such treatment must be continued regularly and indefinitely. It is therefore necessary for both doctor and patient to be convinced of its necessity.

It is well-recognised that regular prophylactic colchicine, given in a dose of 0.5–1.0 mg daily, can to a greater or lesser degree prevent recurrences of acute articular gout (Yü, 1982), but the drug does not change the serum uric acid or affect the development of tophi. If regular medication is to be given, antihyperuricaemic agents are surely more satisfactory, though the prophylactic use of colchicine is useful during the early stages of urate-lowering drugs.

Indications for lowering the serum urate vary to some extent with individual cases, but treatment should usually be commenced in one of the following situations:

1. Gout with chronic joint changes or tophi
2. Frequent acute attacks
3. Evidence of renal damage
4. Gout accompanied by a considerably elevated serum uric acid — 8.0 mg/100 ml or over — because the disease is then usually progressive, in terms of both frequency of attacks and the development of chronic joint damage.

In the absence of these criteria — for example, following one or two attacks with only a moderately elevated uric acid — there is nothing lost by awaiting the course of events for a while. In particular, long-term treatment should not be started when there is any doubt about the diagnosis. A rare exception is the patient who presents with atypical joint symptoms in the presence of hyperuricaemia and in whom it has not been possible to demonstrate urate crystals, when it may be justifiable to lower the uric acid for some months as a form of therapeutic trial. Such situations are very unsatisfactory, however, and the step should not be taken before the fullest possible investigation has been carried out. The condition of 'non-gout' has been mentioned above (p. 899).

If it is decided to lower the serum uric acid this may be done with either allopurinol or uricosuric drugs. The clinical pharmacology of antihyperuricaemic drugs is reviewed in Chapter 22.

Allopurinol

The drug used most commonly in Britain to lower serum concentrations of uric acid is allopurinol. Currie (1978), conducting a survey in general practice, found that 55.3% of gout patients were receiving no regular urate-lowering medication, 37.9% were receiving allopurinol and 6.8% were taking a uricosuric drug, usually probenecid.

Allopurinol (4-hydroxy-pyrazolo-(3,4-d) pyrimidine) is an inhibitor of xanthine oxidase and is rapidly converted in vivo to its active metabolite, oxipurinol. Its original use was directed towards the degradation of 6-mercaptopurine (6MP) in the chemotherapy of cancer (Rundles et al, 1963). For this reason it is important to reduce dosage of the immunosuppressive drug azathioprine (which is degraded to 6MP in vivo) when given with allopurinol (Shapiro, 1974).

The final maintenance dose depends upon estimations of plasma uric acid, usually lying in the region of 300 or 400 mg daily. Smaller doses may be indicated where there is renal impairment. Allopurinol produces a very rapid fall in serum and urinary uric acid; the effect is sustained and, provided administration is continued regularly, attacks of gout become less frequent and eventually terminate, while tophi become smaller. In the early stages of treatment, however, while 'uric acid is on the move', acute attacks of gout may be frequent and severe; it is a good plan to prescribe concurrent treatment with an anti-inflammatory drug for a few months, such as colchicine 0.5 mg twice daily, and the patient should be warned of the possibility of further gout attacks, continuing allopurinol in the prescribed dosage. There is something to be said for starting with a daily dose of 100 mg, increasing it gradually. Single daily dosage produces a sustained fall in serum urate (Brewis et al, 1975).

Side-effects are extremely rare and allopurinol has now become firmly established in the treatment of gout (Scott et al, 1966). Apart from occasional skin rashes, particularly in patients with renal failure, gastrointestinal symptoms, usually minor, and very rare hypersensitivity reactions (Mills, 1971; Young et al, 1974) allopurinol appears to be a remarkably safe drug. The development of xanthine or oxipurinol stones has been described when the drug is administered to patients with the Lesch–Nyhan syndrome (Seegmiller, 1968; Greene et al, 1969). Oxipurinol stones have also been reported in a patient with uric acid nephrolithiasis treated with high dose allopurinol (Stote et al, 1980). Careful titration of the dose, in children (between 5 and 10 mg/kg depending on renal function) as well as adults, will avoid such complications (Dillon et al, 1984). Xanthine nephropathy or stone has also been documented in patients with malignant disorders, e.g.

lymphosarcoma (Band et al, 1970), treated concomitantly with allopurinol to reduce uric acid levels and it is possible that this complication could likewise be avoided with lower allopurinol doses. This is important because xanthine has a low solubility (not much in excess of 1 mmol/l at any pH) whereas the solubility of uric acid, which is similar to that of xanthine at pH 5.0, can be increased 12-fold by alkalinisation of the urine (12 mmol/l at pH 7.0). An adequate diuresis with alkali might thus be more effective at a lower allopurinol dosage. Allopurinol toxicity in renal failure, and guidelines for its use in this situation, are fully reviewed by Hande et al (1984).

Possible effects of allopurinol on iron metabolism have not been confirmed (Emmerson, 1966; Boyett et al, 1968), but it appears that the drug increases the risk of bone marrow damage in patients with neoplastic diseases who are receiving chemotherapy, particularly cyclophosphamide, probably because of an interaction between allopurinol and cytotoxic drugs (Boston Collaborative Drug Surveillance Program, 1974). Another possible drug interaction is with ampicillin, with which skin reactions appear to be over twice as common in patients who are also taking allopurinol (Jick & Porter, 1981). Crystals of hypoxanthine, xanthine, and oxipurinol have been found in skeletal muscle biopsies from patients with gout who were being treated with allopurinol (Watts et al, 1971), but this finding does not appear to have any clinical significance. A theoretical possibility has been the incorporation of allopurinol ribonucleotide into nucleic acids, but experimental support for this is lacking (Nelson et al, 1973; Nelson & Elion, 1974; Stevenson et al, 1976). Recent suggestions that allopurinol may be associated with the formation of cataract (Lerman et al, 1984) await confirmation and further study is required. Allopurinol hepatoxicity is extremely rare (Al-Kawas et al, 1981).

In the treatment of early uncomplicated gout there is little to choose between the use of allopurinol and uricosuric agents, both of which are effective in lowering the serum uric acid. Allopurinol is rather more potent than uricosuric drugs, but it has been in use for a shorter time, so that caution and prolonged observation for late effects are still necessary. Recent reports have indicated that allopurinol together with the uricosuric agent benzbromarone are more effective than either alone, whilst the metabolism and excretion of metabolites are unaltered (Mertz & Borner, 1983). Isolated reports of patients non-responsive to either form of therapy have appeared (Loffler et al, 1983) and much higher doses may be needed. However, it remains to be established through the finding of other such cases whether compliance was or was not a complicating factor.

It has recently been suggested that overproducers of uric acid are more 'appropriately' treated with allopurinol and under-excretors with uricosuric drugs (Boss & Seegmiller, 1979). Such an argument is superficially attractive but may be specious: most patients with gout show evidence of impaired clearance of uric acid but may nevertheless be managed perfectly well with allopurinol.

There are a number of situations where allopurinol is clearly indicated, either alone or occasionally in combination with uricosuric therapy (Fig. 36.28):

1. Extensive tophaceous gout
2. Gout where there is known to be gross overproduction of uric acid with high urinary excretion
3. Failure of uricosuric agents to control plasma uric acid effectively (bearing in mind, however, that the most common cause of this is failure to take tablets regularly)
4. Intolerance to uricosuric agents
5. Gout associated with severe renal failure, where uricosuric drugs become ineffective (Fig. 36.29)
6. Uric acid stone formation
7. Acute uric acid nephropathy, in which treatment of leukaemia or reticuloses by cytotoxic drugs leads to nucleoprotein breakdown and excretion of massive amounts of uric acid (Watts et al, 1966).

If allopurinol is discontinued, serum levels of uric rise rapidly to pretreatment levels (Loebl & Scott, 1974). Recurrence of gouty arthritis may not occur even over a prolonged period; but once a decision has been made to start the drug allopurinol should probably be continued indefinitely.

It is still questioned whether or not progressive deterioration of renal function occurs in association with gout and if so whether this is prevented by long-term treatment with allopurinol. A

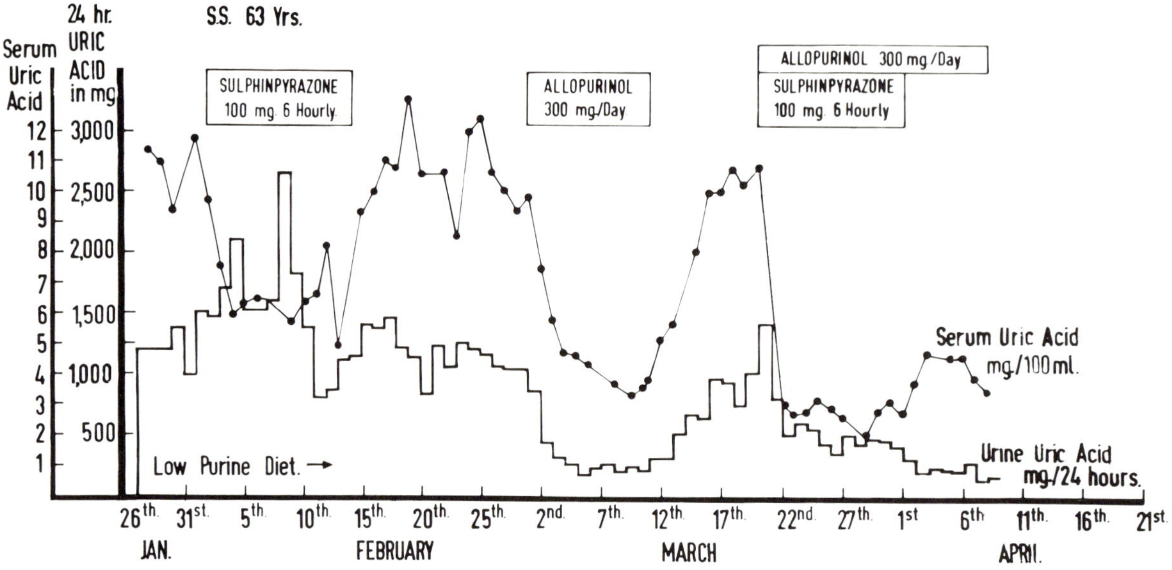

Fig. 36.28 Effects of the uricosuric agent sulphinpyrazone and the xanthine oxidase inhibitor allopurinol, given separately and in combination, upon levels of serum and urinary urate in a patient with gout. (Reproduced by courtesy of the Editor of the *British Medical Journal*.)

controlled study by Gibson et al (1982) indicates that this may indeed be so, but as pointed out earlier in the chapter (p. 893) the conclusions of this study are to some extent vitiated by differences in initial renal function in the two groups studies, so that the question is perhaps still open.

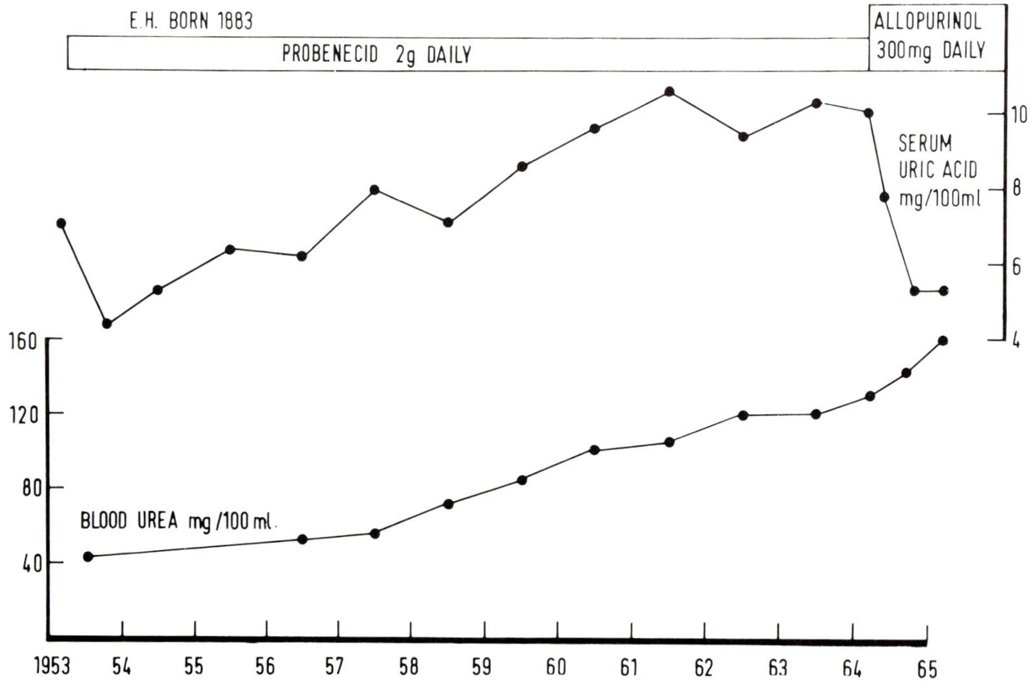

Fig. 36.29 Levels of serum uric acid and blood urea in a patient with gout and progressive renal failure. With increasing azotaemia the uricosuric agent probenecid became ineffective, but the urate level was easily controlled with allopurinol. (Reproduced by courtesy of the Editor of the *British Medical Journal*.)

Uricosuric drugs

Because of the efficiency and acceptability of allopurinol, uricosuric agents are now used much less frequently than previously. These drugs lower the serum uric acid by inhibiting renal tubular reabsorption, thus increasing urinary output. Those used therapeutically in Britain are probenecid and ethebenecid (0.5–1.0 g twice daily) and sulphinpyrazone (100 mg 3 or 4 times daily), the individual maintenance dose, as with allopurinol, being determined by serial concentrations of uric acid, which should be kept at normal levels.

The benzofuran compounds benziodarone and benzbromarone (Delbarre et al, 1973) are very potent uricosuric drugs, acting even when the glomerular filtration rate is reduced to 25–50% of normal. They may possess an additional uricostatic effect, inhibiting purine synthesis. They are widely used on the continent of Europe but are not available in the United Kingdom.

Tienilic acid is a drug of great potential interest, with the unique combination of powerful uricosuric and diuretic properties (Reardon & Scott, 1980; New Zealand Hypertension Study Group, 1983). Following reports of hepatoxicity, marketing permission was withdrawn in the USA, the UK and elsewhere, but the drug is used to good effect in France and other countries.

Sulphinpyrazone is not widely used as a uricosuric agent, but its additional apparent property of reducing morbidity after myocardial infarction is one which should perhaps be taken into consideration in some individual cases (Sherry, 1978).

As with allopurinol, though not to such a great extent, acute attacks of gout may remain troublesome during the early stages of uricosuric treatment, and it is wise to prescribe concurrent treatment with an anti-inflammatory drug for a few months. Uricosuric agents are usually well tolerated; dyspepsia and rashes are uncommon complications. The development of the nephrotic syndrome has been noted with probenecid (Scott & O'Brien, 1968), but this is extremely rare.

As noted above salicylates are uricosuric, but the high dosage necessary makes them generally unacceptable for this purpose. With low plasma levels they actually raise the plasma urate and they also antagonise the action of probenecid and sulphinpyrazone.

Other measures

Severe dietary restriction is generally unnecessary, though moderation should be recommended with regard to high-purine foods, which include sweetbreads, paté, liver, kidney, fish-roe, herrings, shellfish and tinned fish (sardines, etc.) and also alcoholic beverages, particularly beer. Current trends in the consumption of health foods (yeast, etc.) in quantity may also precipitate gouty attacks or alternatively kidney stones. Similar problems can present in subjects consuming high quantities of vitamins (ascorbic acid or nicotinic acid). Gouty subjects tend to be overweight and this may require attention, since reduction in weight itself lowers the serum uric acid (Nicholls & Scott, 1972) and thus corrects mild degrees of hyperuricaemia. Indeed, the patient with gout should receive advice about his whole life-style insofar as he will accept it: for example, a moderate amount of exercise is almost certainly beneficial. The disappearance of gouty symptoms after a patient takes such measures, without recourse to regular drug treatment, is a most rewarding therapeutic exercise.

Hypertension, if present, should be treated as necessary. The question sometimes arises of prescribing thiazide or other diuretics for patients with gout who may have incidental hypertension. These diuretics raise plasma uric acid by their action on the renal tubule and thiazide diuretics may account for an increasing proportion of new patients presenting with gout, especially, it seems, among elderly women. The effect on uric acid can be overcome by uricosuric drugs or allopurinol, the latter in reduced doses to compensate for the oxipurinol-retaining effect of thiazide diuretics, particularly in patients with poor renal function.

Of considerable interest is a recent account describing the abolition of uric acid in the blood of patients with advanced haematological malignancies following the intravenous injection of uricase covalently attached to polyethyleneglycol (David et al, 1981).

ASYMPTOMATIC HYPERURICAEMIA

In these days of health screening and multichannel biochemical investigation, raised serum concentrations of uric acid may be found in persons with no history of gout. The risks, such as they are, of asymptomatic hyperuricaemia have probably been exaggerated.

As pointed out above, prolonged hyperuricaemia certainly carries a proportionate risk of gouty arthritis, but the widely quoted data from the Framingham study (Hall et al, 1967), giving an incidence of 90% of persons with a serum uric acid above 9.0 mg/100 ml developing gout, are based on very small numbers with this degree of hyperuricaemia. Other studies have not confirmed such a high risk: for example, the investigation of Fessel (1972), also already quoted, found that only 3 out of 66 men with such high concentrations (in whom pre-existent gout, cardiovascular and renal disease, and diabetes had been excluded) developed gout after 4 years. In any case, gouty arthritis can be dealt with if and when it occurs.

Rather more concern may be felt about the possible development of kidney disease, with the argument that raised serum concentrations of uric acid should be reduced because of the possibility of progressive renal failure and renal calculi. Evidence is hard to come by, discussed earlier. The findings of a recent American survey (Fessel, 1979), in which a large number of hyperuricaemic individuals and normouricaemic controls were followed over a period of years, indicated that azotaemia attributable to hyperuricaemia is generally mild and develops no more frequently than azotaemia in normouricaemic people. The theoretical risk is probably of no clinical importance, at least unless serum concentrations of uric acid are very high. Similarly, the risks of urolithiasis seem small and no higher in those with hyperuricaemia than in those without: in the American study (Fessel, 1979) the risk was so low, indeed, that it was considered justifiable to await the occurrence of the first stone before starting drug treatment. Nephrologists commonly treat the raised serum uric acid accompanying renal failure with allopurinol; such treatment is justifiable on the grounds that it is harmless (provided that the dose is properly adjusted) and possibly beneficial, but in our present state of knowledge no more can be said than that.

The third problem of asymptomatic hyperuricaemia lies in its possible relation to cardiovascular disease, again discussed above (p. 916). In the absence of associations such as obesity, hypertension and medication hyperuricaemia does not appear to be a coronary risk factor, and there are no grounds whatever for believing that, by itself, lowering the serum concentrations of uric acid will have any effect in reducing the risk of cardiovascular disease.

How, then, should the person with asymptomatic hyperuricaemia be managed? He should certainly receive a full clinical assessment, outlined in the early part of this chapter, as for a patient with overt gout. Very rarely indeed, however, will it be found necessary to prescribe urate-lowering drugs. One such example from our experience was a boy of 12 whose elder brother, presenting with gouty arthritis, was found to have a partial deficiency of hypoxanthine-guanine phosphoribosyltransferase (Bunn et al, 1975). The younger boy was found on investigation to show a similar deficiency with gross elevations of serum and urinary concentrations of uric acid: though free of symptoms and with normal renal function, he was thought to have a considerable risk of developing gout and renal calculi, so that prophylactic treatment with allopurinol was thought to be justified. Uric acid concentrations have remained normal in the subsequent 10 years, and he has remained well, which might not otherwise have been the case.

Mild degrees of hyperuricaemia, at any rate, may, therefore, be observed judiciously but left untreated. Opinions differ with regard to higher concentrations of uric acid — say, above 9.0 mg/100 ml. This degree of sustained asymptomatic hyperuricaemia is extremely rare in the absence of some readily apparent underlying cause; many would hold that such people, particularly if hyperuricosuric, should be treated with allopurinol.

REFERENCES

Abrahamson S, Hoffstein S T, Weissman G 1982 Superoxide anion generation by human neutrophils exposed to monosodium urate. Arthritis and Rheumatism 26: 775–783

Acheson R M, O'Brien W M 1966 Dependence of serum uric acid on haemoglobin and other factors in the general population. Lancet 2: 777–778

Acheson R M, Chan Y K 1969 New Haven survey of joint diseases. The prediction of serum uric acid in a general population. Journal of Chronic Diseases 21: 543–553

Acheson R M, Chan Y K, Payne M 1969 New Haven survey of joint diseases. The interrelationship between morning stiffness, nocturnal pain and swelling of the joints. Journal of Chronic Diseases 21: 533–542

Afzel Mir M, Delamore I W 1974 Hypouricaemia in Hodgkin's disease. Cancer 32: 1508–1511

Agudelo C A, Schumacher H R, Phelps P 1972 Effect of exercise on urate crystal-induced inflammation in canine joints. Arthritis and Rheumatism 15: 609–616

Al-Kawas F H, Seeff L B, Berendson R A, Zimmeerman H J, Ishak K G 1981 Allopurinol hepatoxicity. Annals of Internal Medicine 95: 588–590

Allison A C, Hovi T, Watts R W E, Webster A D B 1975 Immunological observations on patients with Lesch–Nyhan syndrome, and on the role of de novo purine synthesis in lymphocyte transformation. Lancet 2: 1179–1182

Alvsaker J O 1966 Uric acid in human plasma. V. Isolation and identification of plasma proteins interacting with urate. Scandinavian Journal of Clinical and Laboratory Investigation 18: 227–239

Atsmon A, De Vries A, Frank M 1963 Uric acid lithiasis. Elsevier, Amsterdam

Bagnara A S, Letter A, Henderson J F 1974 Multiple mechanisms of regulation of purine biosynthesis de novo in intact tumour cells. Biochimica et Biophysica Acta 374: 259–270

Ball G V, Sorenson L B 1970 The pathogenesis of hyperuricemia and gout in sickle cell anemia. Arthritis and Rheumatism 13: 846–848

Band P R, Silverberg D S, Henderson J F, Ulan R A, Wensel R H, Banerjee T K, Little A S 1970 Xanthine nephropathy in a patient with lymphosarcoma treated with allopurinol. New England Journal of Medicine 283: 354–357

Barcello P 1976 Personal communication

Barlow K A, Beilin L J 1968 Renal disease in primary gout. Quarterly Journal of Medicine 37NS: 79–98

Baron D N, Dent D E, Harris H, Hart E W, Jepson J B 1956 Hereditary pellagra-like skin rash with temporary cerebellar ataxia, constant renal aminoaciduria and other bizarre biochemical features. Lancet 2: 421–428

Batumen V, Maesaka J K, Haddad B, Tepper E, Landy E, Wedeen R P 1981 The role of lead in gout nephropathy. New England Journal of Medicine 304: 520–523

Bearn A G, Yü T-F, Gutman A B 1957 Renal function in Wilson's disease. Journal of Clinical Investigation 36: 1107–1114

Becker M A 1976 Patterns of phosphoribosylphosphate and ribose-5-phosphate concentration and generation in fibroblasts from patients with gout and purine overproduction. Journal of Clinical Investigation 57: 308–318

Becker M A 1984 Phosphoribosylpyrophosphate synthetase superactivity: detection, characterisation of underlying defects and treatment. In: De Bruyn CHMM, Simmonds H A, Müller M M (eds) Purine metabolism in man: IV. Plenum Press, New York, 165A: 327–331

Becker M A, Seegmiller J E 1975 Recent advances in the identification of enzyme abnormalities underlying excessive purine synthesis in man. Arthritis and Rheumatism 18: 687–694

Becker M A, Meyler L J, Seegmiller J E 1973 Gout with purine overproduction due to increased phosphoribosylpyrophosphate synthetase activity. American Journal of Medicine 55: 232–242

Becker M A, Yen R C K, Itkin P 1979 Regional localization of the gene for human phosphoribosylpyrophosphate synthetase on the X-chromosome. Science 203: 1016–1019

Beckett A, Lewis J G 1960 Gout and the serum uric acid in diabetes mellitus. Quarterly Journal of Medicine 29: 443–458

Beighton P, Solomon L, Soskolone C L, Sweet B, Robin G 1974 Serum uric acid concentrations in an urbanized South African Negro population. Annals of the Rheumatic Diseases 33: 442–445

Beighton P, Solomon L, Soskolone C L, Sweet M B E 1977 Rheumatic disorders in the South African Negro. Part IV: Gout and hyperuricaemia. South African Medical Journal 51: 969–972

Bengtsson C, Tibblin E 1974 Serum uric acid levels in women. An epidemiological survey with special reference to women with high serum uric acid values. Acta Medica Scandinavica 196: 93–102

Bennett J S, et al 1972 Hypouricemia in Hodgkin's disease. Annals of Internal Medicine 76: 751–756

Bennett P H, Wood P H N 1966 Population studies of the rheumatic diseases. Proceedings of the Third International Symposium, New York, June 5th–10th, 1966. Excerpta Medica Foundation, Amsterdam

Berkowitz D 1966 Gout, hyperlipidemia, and diabetes interrelationships. Journal of the American Medical Association 197: 77–80

Bluestone R, Kippen I, Klinenberg J R, Whitehouse M W 1970 Effects of some uricosuric and anti-inflammatory drugs on the binding of uric acid to human serum albumin in vitro. Journal of Laboratory and Clinical Medicine 76: 85–91

Bluestone R, Waisman J, Klinenberg J R 1977 The gouty kidney. Seminars in Arthritis and Rheumatism 10: 1–9

Bode C, Schumacher H, Goebell H, Zelder O, Pelzel H 1971 Fructose induced depletion of live adenine nucleotides in man. Hormone and Metabolic Research 3:289

Boogaerts M A, Hammerschmidt D E, Roelant C, Verwilghen R L, Jacob H S 1983 Mechanisms of vascular damage in gout and oxalosis: Crystal-induced, granulocyte mediated, endothelial injury. Thrombosis and Haemostatis 50: 576–580

Boss G R, Seegmiller J E 1979 Hyperuricemia and gout: classification, complications and management. New England Journal of Medicine 300: 1459–1468

Boston Collaborative Drug Surveillance Program 1974 Allopurinol and cytotoxic drugs. Journal of the American Medical Association 227: 1036–1040

Boyett J D, Vogler W R, De Paula Furtado V, Schmidt F H 1968 Allopurinol and iron metabolism in man. Blood 32: 460–468

Boyle J A, Campbell S, Duncan A M, Greig W R, Buchanan W W 1966a Serum uric acid levels is normal pregnancy with observations on the renal excretion of urate in pregnancy. Journal of Clinical Pathology 19: 501–503

Boyle J A, Greig W R, Duncan A M Boyle I T, Buchanan W W 1966b Serum uric acid values in various states of thyroid function. Acta Rheumatologica Scandinavica 12: 204–209

Boyle J A, Greig W R, Jasani M K, Duncan A, Diver M, Buchanan W W 1967 Relative roles of genetic and environmental factors in the control of serum uric acid levels in normouricaemic subjects. Annals of the Rheumatic Diseases 26: 234–238

Boyle J A, McKiddie M, Buchanan K D, Jasani M K, Gray H W, Jackson I M D, Buchanan W W 1969 Diabetes mellitus and gout. Blood and plasma insulin responses to oral glucose in normal weight, overweight and gouty patients. Annals of the Rheumatic Diseases 28: 374–378

Brauer G W, Prior I A M 1978 Prospective study of gout in New Zealand Maoris. Annals of the Rheumatic Diseases 37: 466–472

Breckenridge A 1966 Hyperuricaemia and hypertension. Lancet 1: 15–18

Brewis I, Ellis R M, Scott J T 1975 Single daily dose of allopurinol. Annals of the Rheumatic Diseases 34: 256–259

Brøchner-Mortensen K 1941 100 gouty patients. Acta Medica Scandinavica 106: 81–107

Brooks G W, Mueller E 1966 Serum urate concentrations among university professors. Journal of the American Medical Association 195: 415–418

Brown J, Mallory G K 1950 Renal changes in gout. New England Journal of Medicine 243: 325–329

Bunch T W, et al 1974 Synovial fluid complement determination as a diagnostic aid in inflammatory joint disease. Mayo Clinic Proceedings 49: 715–20

Bunn D N, Moss I K, Nicholls A, Scott J T, Snaith M L, Watson M R 1975 Clinical and biochemical observations on three cases of hypoxanthine-guanine phosphoribosyltransferase deficiency. Annals of the Rheumatic Diseases 34: 249–255

Burch T A, O'Brien W M, Need R, Kurland L T 1966 Hyperuricaemia and gout in the Mariana Islands. Annals of the Rheumatic Diseases 25: 114–116

Bywaters E G L, Holloway V P 1964 Measurement of serum uric acid in Great Britain in 1963. Annals of the Rheumatic Diseases 23: 236–239

Campion D S, Olsen R, Bluestone R, Klinenberg J R 1975 Binding of urate by serum proteins. Arthritis and Rheumatism 18 (Suppl): 747–749

Canoso J J, Yood R A 1979 Acute gouty bursitis: report of 15 cases. Annals of the Rheumatic Diseases 43: 394–397

Castrillo J M, Diaz-Curiel, Rapado A 1984 Hyperuricaemia in primary hyperparathyroidism: incidence and evolution after surgery. Advances in Experimental Medicine and Biology 165A: 151–157

Chait A, Mancini M, February A W, Lewis B 1972 Clinical and metabolic study of hyperlipidaemia. Lancet 2: 62–64

Chalmers R A, Krömer H, Scott J T, Watts R W E 1968 A comparative study of the xanthine oxidase inhibitors allopurinol and oxipurinol in man. Clinical Science 35: 353–362

Chang Y-H, Gralla E J 1968 Suppression of urate crystal-induced canine joint inflammation by heterologous anti-polymorphonuclear leukocyte serum. Arthritis and Rheumatism 11: 145–50

Clarke A M, McKenzie R G 1969 Ileostomy and the risk of urinary uric acid stones. Lancet 2: 395–397

Coe F L 1978 Hyperuricosuric calcium oxalate nephrolithiasis. Kidney International 13: 418–426

Conley C L, Kowal J, D'Antonio J 1957 Polycythaemia associated with renal tumours. Bulletin Johns Hopkins Hospital 101:63

Cowdrey S C 1966 Hyperuricaemia in infectious mononucleosis. Journal of the American Medical Association 196: 319–321

Currie W J C 1978 The gout patient in general practice. Rheumatology and Rehabilitation 17: 205–218

Currie W J C 1979 Prevalence and incidence of the diagnosis of gout in Great Britain. Annals of the Rheumatic Diseases 38: 101–106

Darlington L G 1984 Lean dry gout patients. Advances in Experimental Medicine and Biology 165A: 129–132

Darlington L C, Scott J T 1972 Plasma lipid levels in gout. Annals of the Rheumatic Diseases 31: 487–489

Darlington L G, Slack J, Scott J T 1982 Family study of lipid and purine levels in gout patients. Annals of the Rheumatic Diseases 41: 253–256

Darlington L G, Slack J, Scott J T 1983 Vascular mortality in patients with gout and their families. Annals of the Rheumatic Diseases 42: 270–273

David S, Park Y K, Abuchowski A, Davis F F 1981 Hypouricaemic effect of polyethyleneglycol modified urate oxidase. Lancet 2: 281–283

Davies D F, Shock N W 1950 Age changes in glomerular filtration rate, effective renal plasma flow and tubular excretory capacity in adult males. Journal of Clinical Investigation 29: 496–507

Decker J L, Healey J A, Skeith K D 1968 In: Bennett P H, Wood P H N (eds) Population studies in rheumatic diseases. Excerpta Medica, Amsterdam, p. 66

De Galantha E 1935 Technic for preservation and microscopic demonstration of nodules in gout. American Journal of Clinical Pathology 5: 165–166

Delbarre F, Auscher C, Brouilhet H, De Gery A 1967 Action de l'ethanol dans la goutte et sur le metabolisme de l'acide urique. Semaine des Hopitaux de Paris 43: 659–664

Delbarre F, Auscher C, Saporta L, De Gery A, Danchot J 1973 Treatment of gout with a dibrom derivative of benzofuranes. Revue du Rhumatisme et des Maladies Osteo-Articularies 40: 275–277

DeMars R, Sarto G, Felix J S, Benke P 1969 Lesch–Nyhan mutation: prenatal detection with amniotic fluid cells. Science 164: 1303–1305

Demartini F E, Wheaton E A, Healey L A, Laragh J H 1962 Effect of chlorthiazide on the renal excretion of uric acid. American Journal of Medicine 32: 572–577

Denis G, Launay M P 1969 Carbohydrate intolerance in gout. Metabolism 18: 770–775

Denman A M, Szur L, Ansell B M 1966 Joint complaints in polycythaemia vera. Annals of the Rheumatic Diseases 23: 139–144

De Seze, Phankim-Koupernik M 1964 Syndrome du canal carpien d'origine goutteuse. Revue du Rhumatisme et des Maladies Osteo-Articularies 31: 9–12

Desnick R H, Fiddler M B, Douglas S D, Hudson L D S 1978 Enzyme therapy. II: Immunologic considerations for replacement therapy with unentrapped, erythrocyte- and liposome-entrapped enzymes. In: Gatt S, Freysz, Mandel P (eds) Enzymes of lipid metabolism. Plenum Press, New York, p. 753

Diamond H S 1982 Gout and the kidney. In: Bacon P A, Hadler N M (eds) The kidney and rheumatic disease. Butterworths, London, ch. 19, p. 323

Diamond H S, Paolino J S 1973 Evidence for a postsecretory reabsorptive site for uric acid in man. Journal of Clinical Investigation 42: 1491–1499

Diamond H S, Lazarus R, Kaplan D, Halberstrom D 1972 Effect of urine flow rate on uric acid excretion in man. Arthritis and Rheumatism 15: 338–346

Diamond H S, Carter A C, Feldman E B 1974 Abnormal regulation of carbohydrate metabolism in primary gout.

Annals of the Rheumatic Diseases 34: 554–562
Dieppe P A, Calvert P 1983 Crystals and joint disease. Chapman & Hall, London
Dillon M J, Simmonds H A, Barratt T M, Fairbanks L D, Holland P C 1984 Problems of diagnosis and treatment of adenine (APRT) and hypoxanthine–guanine (HGPRT) phosphoribosyltransferase deficiency in childhood. In: De Bruyn CHMM, Simmonds H A, Müller M M (eds) Purine metabolism in man. IV. Plenum Press, New York, 165A:1.6
Doherty M, Whicher J T, Dieppe P A 1983 Activation of the alternative pathway of complement by monosodium urate monohydrate crystals and other inflammatory particles. Annals of the Rheumatic Diseases 42: 285–291
Dorhout Mees E J, Blom van Assendelft P, Nieuwenhuis M G 1971 Elevation of uric acid clearance caused by inappropriate antidiuretic hormone secretion. Acta Medica Scandinavica 189: 69–72
Dosman J A, Crawhall J C, Klassen G A 1974 Uric acid metabolism following acute myocardial infarction. Advances in Experimental Medicine and Biology 41: 423–427
Dreyfuss F 1960 The role of hyperuricaemia in coronary heart disease. Diseases of the Chest 38: 332–334
Duncan H, Dixon A St J 1960 Gout, familial hyperuricaemia, and renal disease. Quarterly Journal of Medicine 29NS: 127–135
Dunn J P, Brooks G W, Mausner J, Rodnan G P, Cobb S 1960 Social class gradient of serum uric acid levels in males. Journal of the American Medical Association 185: 431–436
Eidlitz M 1961 Uric acid and arteriosclerosis. Lancet 2: 1046–1047
Eisen A Z, Seegmiller J E 1961 Uric acid metabolism in psoriasis. Journal of Clinical Investigation 40: 1486–1494
Emmerson B T 1966 Effects of allopurinol on iron metabolism in man. Annals of the Rheumatic Diseases 25: 700–703
Emmerson B T 1973 Alteration in urate metabolism by weight reduction. Australia and New Zealand Journal of Medicine 3: 410–437
Emmerson B T 1980 The kidney and gout. In: Hamburger, Crosnier, Grunfeld (eds) Nephrology. Wiley-Flammation, New York & Paris, ch. 59, p. 747–756
Emmerson B T 1983 Hyperuricaemia and gout in clinical practice. ADIS Health Science Press, Sydney
Emmerson B T, Knowles B R 1971 Triglyceride concentrations in primary gout and gout of chronic lead nephropathy. Metabolism 20: 721–729
Emmerson B T, Mirosch W, Douglas J B 1971 The relative contributions of tubular reabsorption and secretion to urate excretion in lead nephropathy. Australia and New Zealand Journal of Medicine 1: 353–362
Emmerson B T, Thompson L 1973 The spectrum of hypoxanthine-guanine phosphoribosyltransferase deficiency. Quarterly Journal of Medicine 62: 423–437
Emmerson B T, Row P G 1975 An evaluation of the gouty kidney. Kidney International 8: 65–71
Emmerson B T, Gordon R B, Johnson L A 1976 Urate kinetics in hypoxanthine-guanine phosphoribosyltransferase deficiency: their significance for the understanding of gout. Quarterly Journal of Medicine 45: 49–61
Evans J G, Prior I A M, Harvey H P B 1968 Relation of serum uric acid to body bulk, haemoglobin and alcohol intake in two South Pacific Polynesian populations. Annals of the Rheumatic Diseases 27: 319–325
Faires J S, McCarty D P Jr 1962 Acute synovitis in normal joints of man and dog produced by injections of microcrystalline sodium urate, calcium oxalate and corticosteroid esters. Arthritis and Rheumatism 5: 295–296
Faller J, Fox I H 1982 Ethanol-induced hyperuricemia. Evidence for increased urate production by activation of adenine nucleotide turnover. New England Journal of Medicine 307: 1598–1602
Ferris T F, Gorden P 1968 Effect of angiotensin and norepinephrine upon urate clearance in man. American Journal of Medicine 44: 359–365
Fessel W J 1972 Hyperuricemia in health and disease. Seminars in Arthritis and Rheumatism 1: 275–299
Fessel W J 1979 Renal outcomes of gout and hyperuricemia. American Journal of Medicine 67: 74–82
Fiddis R W, Vlachos N, Calvert P D 1983 Studies of urate crystallisation in relation to gout. Annals of the Rheumatic Diseases 42 (Suppl): 12–15
Fox I H, Wyngaarden J B, Kelley W N 1970 Depletion of erythrocyte phosphoribosylpyrophosphate in man: a newly observed effect of allopurinol. New England Journal of Medicine 283: 1177–1182
Fox I H, Halperin M L, Goldstein M B, Marliss E B 1976 Renal excretion of uric acid during prolonged fasting. Metabolism 25: 551–559
Fredrickson D S, Levy R K, Lees R S 1967 Fat transport in lipoproteins — an integrated approach to mechanisms and disorders. New England Journal of Medicine 276: 273–281
Garrod A B 1876 A treatise on gout and rheumatic gout (rheumatoid arthritis), 3rd Edn. Longman, London
Gartler S M, Scott R C, Goldstein J L, Campbell B, Sparkes R 1971 Lesch–Nyhan syndrome: rapid detection of heterozygotes by use of hair follicles. Science 172: 572–574
Gatter R A 1977 Use of the compensated polarizing microscope. Clinics in Rheumatic Diseases 3: 91–103
Gibbs D, McFadyean I R, Crawford M d'A, de Muinck Keizer E E et al 1984 First trimester diagnosis of Lesch-Nyham syndrome. Lancet ii: 1180–1183
Giblett E R, Anderson J E, Cohen F, Pollara B, Meuwissen H J 1972 Adenosine-deaminase deficiency in two patients with severely impaired cellular immunity. Lancet 2: 1067–1069
Gibson T, Grahame R 1974 Gout and hyperlipidaemia. Annals of the Rheumatic Diseases 33: 298–303
Gibson T, Kilbourn K, Horner I, Simmonds H A 1979 Mechanism and treatment of hypertriglyceridaemia in gout. Annals of the Rheumatic Diseases 38: 31–35
Gibson T, Highton C, Potter C, Simmonds H A 1980 Renal impairment and gout. Annals of the Rheumatic Diseases 39: 417–423
Gibson T, Rodgers V, Potter C, Simmonds H A 1982 Allopurinol treatment and its effect on renal function: a controlled study. Annals of the Rheumatic Diseases 41: 59–65
Gibson T, Rodgers A V, Simmonds H A, Court-Brown F, Todd E, Meilton V 1983 A controlled study of diet in patients with gout. Annals of the Rheumatic Diseases 42: 123–127
Gibson T, Waterworth R, Hatfield P J, Robinson G, Brember K 1984 Hyperuricaemia in young New Zealand Maori men. In: De Bruyn CHMM, Simmonds H A, Müller M M (eds) Purine metabolism in man. IV. Plenum Press, New York, 165A: 123–129
Glynn R J, Campion E W, Silbert J E 1983 Trends in serum

uric acid levels 1961–1980. Arthritis and Rheumatism 26: 87–93

Golding D N 1970 Hypothyroidism presenting with musculoskeletal symptoms. Annals of the Rheumatic Diseases 29: 10–14

Goldstein R A, Becker K L, Moore C F 1972 Serum urate in healthy men — intermittent elevations and seasonal effect. New England Journal of Medicine 287: 649–650

Gorden P, Robertson G L, Seegmiller J E 1971 Hyperuricemia, a concomitant of congenital vasopressin-resistant diabetes insipidus in the adult. New England Journal of Medicine 284: 1057–1060

Gordon T P, Bertouch J V, Walsh B R, Brooks P M 1982 Monosodium urate crystals in asymptomatic knee joints. Journal of Rheumatology 9: 967–969

Goss S J, Harris H 1975 New method for mapping genes in human chromosomes. Nature 255: 680–684

Grahame R, Scott J T 1970 Clinical survey of 354 patients with gout. Annals of the Rheumatic Diseases 29: 461–468

Grahame R, Haslam R M, Scott J T 1968 Sulphobromophthalein retention in gout and asymptomatic hyperuricaemia. Annals of the Rheumatic Diseases 27: 19–26

Greene M L, Fujimoto W Y, Seegmiller J E 1969 Urinary xanthine stones — a rare complication of allopurinol therapy. New England Journal of Medicine 280: 426–427

Greene M L, Marcus R, Aurbach G D, Kazem E S, Seegmiller J E 1972 Hypouricemia due to isolated renal tubular defect. American Journal of Medicine 53: 361–367

Gross J M 1963 Fanconi syndrome developing secondary to the ingestion of outdated tetracycline. Annals of Internal Medicine 58: 523–528

Gutman A B, Yü T-F 1957 Renal function in gout, with a commentary on the renal regulation of urate excretion, and the role of the kidney in the pathogenesis of gout. American Journal of Medicine 23: 600–622

Gutman A B, Yü T-F 1962 Secondary gout. Annals of Internal Medicine 56:675

Gutman A B, Yü T-F 1963 An abnormality of glutamine metabolism in primary gout. American Journal of Medicine 35: 820–831

Gutman A B, Yü T-F 1968 Uric acid nephrolithiasis. American Journal of Medicine 45: 756–779

Gutman A B, Yü T-F, Berger L 1959 Tubular secretion of urate in man. Journal of Clinical Investigation 38: 1178–1781

Hadler N M, Franck W A, Bress N H, Robinson D R 1974 Acute polyarticular gout. American Journal of Medicine 56: 715–719

Hall A P 1965 Correlations among hyperuricemia, hypercholesterolemia, coronary disease and hypertension. Arthritis and Rheumatism 8: 846–852

Hall A P, Barry P E, Dawber T, McNamara P M 1967 Epidemiology of gout and hyperuricemia. American Journal of Medicine 42: 27–37

Hall M C, Selin G 1960 Spinal involvement in gout. A case report with autopsy. Journal of Bone and Joint Surgery 42A: 341–343

Halla J T, Ball G V 1982 Saturnine gout: a review of 42 patients. Seminars in Arthritis and Rheumatism 11: 307–314

Hande K R, Noone R M, Stone W J 1984 Severe allopurinol toxicity. American Journal of Medicine 76: 47–56

Handler J S 1960 The role of lactic acid in the excretion of uric acid in toxaemia of pregnancy. Journal of Clinical Investigation 39: 1526–1532

Hansen O E 1966 Hyperuricemia, gout and atherosclerosis. American Heart Journal 72: 570–573

Harkness R A, Nicol A D 1969 Plasma uric acid levels in children. Archives of Disease in Childhood 44: 773–778

Hauge M, Harvald B 1955 Heredity in gout and hyperuricaemia. Acta Medica Scandinavica 152: 247–257

Hawkins C F, Ellis H A, Rawson A 1965 Malignant gout with tophaceous deposits in small intestine and megaloblastic anaemia. Annals of the Rheumatic Diseases 24: 224–233

Healey L A 1975 Port wine and the gout. Arthritis and Rheumatism 18 (Suppl): 659–662

Healey L A, Wheaton E A, Cutler R E, Demartini F E 1966 Uric acid excretion in diabetic ketoacidosis. Diabetes 15: 357–359

Healey L A, Skeith M D, Simkin P A 1974 Hypouricemia. Archives of Internal Medicine 134: 46–47

Hench P S 1935 A clinic on some diseases of joints. Medical Clinics of North America 19: 551–583

Henderson J F, Paterson A R P 1973 Nucleotide metabolism: an introduction. Academic Press, New York

Herman J, Goldbourt V 1982 Uric acid and diabetes: observations in a population study. Lancet 1: 240–243

Hoffee P A, Jones M E (eds) 1978 Methods of enzymology, Vol II. Purine and nucleotide metabolism. Academic Press, New York, p. 654

Hollingworth P, Scott J T 1983 Familial gout, hyperuricaemia and renal impairment. Annals of the Rheumatic Diseases 42 (Suppl): 87–88

Hollingworth P, Scott J T, Burry H C 1983 Nonarticular gout: hyperuricaemia and tophus formation without gouty arthritis. Arthritis and Rheumatism 26: 98–101

Holmes E W, Kelley W N 1974 Re-evaluation of the pyrazinamide suppression test. Advances in Experimental Medicine and Biology 41B: 739–744

Holmes E W, Wyngaarden J B, Kelley W N 1973 Human phosphoribosylpyrophosphate amidotransferase: two molecular forms interconvertible by purine ribonucleotides and phosphoribosylpyrophosphate. The Journal of Biological Chemistry 248: 6035–6040

Howell R R, Seegmiller J E 1962 Uricolysis by human leucocytes. Nature 196: 482–483

Howell R R, Eanes R D, Seegmiller J E 1963 X-ray diffraction studies of the tophaceous deposits in gout. Arthritis and Rheumatism 6: 97–103

Isömaki H, v Essen R, Ruutsalo H M 1977 Gout, particularly diuretics-induced, is on the increase in Finland. Scandinavian Journal of Rheumatology 6: 213–216

Jain A K, Ryan J R, McMahon F G, Noveck R J 1974 Effect of single oral doses of benzbromarone on serum and urinary uric acid. Arthritis and Rheumatism 17: 146–157

Jaques B C, Ginsberg M H 1982 The role of cell surface proteins in platelet stimulation by monosodium urate crystals. Arthritis and Rheumatism 25: 508–521

Jick H, Porter J B 1981 Potentiation of ampicillin skin reaction by allopurinol or hyperuricaemia. Journal of Clinical Pharmacology 21: 457–458

Jolly D J et al 1983 Isolation of characterization of a full-length expressible cDNA for human hypoxanthine phosphoribosyltransferase. Proceedings of the National Academy of Sciences USA 80: 477–481

Kahn M F 1976 Goutte, obesité et plaisirs de la table.

Comparaison entre 40 goutteux et 40 témoins. Nouvelle Presse Medicale 5: 1897–1898
Katz W A 1975 Deposition of urate crystals in gout: altered connective tissue metabolism. Arthritis and Rheumatism 17: 751–756
Katz W A, Schubert M 1970 The interaction of monosodium urate with connective tissue components. Journal of Clinical Investigation 49: 1783–1789
Katz J L, Weiner H, Yü T-F 1975 Psychobiological variables in the onset and recurrence of gouty arthritis. Journal of Chronic Diseases 28: 51–62
Kaufman J M, O'Brien W M 1976 Hyperuricaemia in mongolism. New England Journal of Medicine 276: 953–956
Kaufman J M, Greene M L, Seegmiller J E 1968 Urine uric acid to creatinine ratio — a screening test for inherited disorders of purine metabolism. Journal of Paediatrics 73: 583–592
Kay N E, Gottleib A J 1973 Hypouricemia in Hodgkin's disease. Cancer 32: 1508–1511
Kellermeyer R W 1968 Hageman factor and acute gouty arthritis. Arthritis and Rheumatism 11: 452–459
Kelley W N 1972 Biochemistry of the X-linked uric aciduria-enzyme defect and its genetic variants. Archives of Internal Medicine 130: 199–206
Kelley W N 1975a Hypouricemia. Arthritis and Rheumatism 18 (Suppl): 731–737
Kelley W N 1975b Disorders of purine metabolism in man. Biochemical Society Transactions 3: 1202–1205
Kelley W N, Meade J C 1971 Studies on hypoxanthine-guanine phosphoribosyltransferase in fibroblasts from patients with the Lesch-Nyhan syndrome. Evidence for genetic heterogeneity. The Journal of Biological Chemistry 246: 2953–2958
Kelley W N, Weiner I M 1978 Uric acid. Handbook of experimental pharmacology 51
Kelley W N, Wyngaarden J B 1983 In: Stanbury J B, Wyngaarden J B, Fredrickson D S, Goldstein J L, Brown M S (eds) The metabolic basis of inherited disease, 5th Edn. McGraw-Hill, New York, ch. 51
Kelley W N, Rosenbloom F M, Seegmiller J E, Howell R R 1968 Excessive production of uric acid in type I glycogen storage disease. Journal of Paediatrics 72: 488–496
Kelley W N, Goldfinger S E, Hardy H L 1969 Hyperuricaemia in chronic beryllium disease. Annals of Internal Medicine 70: 977–983
Kelley W N, Fox I H, Wyngaarden J B 1970 Essential role of phosphoribosylpyrophosphate (PRPP) in regulation of purine biosynthesis in cultural human fibroblasts. Clinical Research 18:457
Kennedy T D, Higgens C S, Woodrow D F, Scott J T 1984 Crystal deposition in the knee and great toe joints of asymptomatic gout patients. Journal of the Royal Society of Medicine 77: 747–750
Kippen I, Klinenberg J R, Weinberger A, Wilcox W 1974 Factors affecting urate solubility in vitro. Annals of the Rheumatic Diseases 33: 313–317
Klein R, Klein B E, Cornono J C, Maready J, Cassel J C, Tyroler H A 1973 Serum uric acid. Its relation to coronary heart disease risk factors and cardiovascular disease. Archives of Internal Medicine 132: 401–410
Klinenberg J R, Kippen I 1970 The binding of urate to plasma proteins determined by means of equilibrium dialysis. Journal of Laboratory and Clinical Medicine 75: 503–510
Kohn P M, Prozan G B 1959 Hyperuricemia — relationship to hypercholesterolemia and acute myocardial infarction. Journal of the American Medical Association 170: 1909–1912
Kosoff Y D, Morris L E, Lublic L 1953 Paraplegia as a complication of gout. Journal of the American Medical Association 152: 37–38
Kozin F, McCarty D J 1976 Protein adsorption to monosodium urate, calcium pyrophosphate dihydrate and silica crystals: relationship to the pathogenesis of crystal-induced inflammation. Arthritis and Rheumatism 19: 433–438
Kuster G et al 1972 Uric acid metabolism in Dalmatian and other dogs. Archives of Internal Medicine 129: 492–496
Kuzell W C, Schaffarzick R W, Naugler W E, Koets P, Mankle E A, Brown B, Champlain B 1955 Some observations on 520 gouty patients. Journal of Chronic Diseases 2: 645–669
Lagier R, MacGee W 1983 Spondylodiscal erosions due to gout: anatomico-radiological study of a case. Annals of the Rheumatic Diseases 42: 350–353
Lalanne M, Henderson J F 1975 Effects of hormones and drugs on phosphoribosylpyrophosphate concentrations in mouse liver. Canadian Journal of Biochemistry 53: 394–399
Lambert J R, Wright V 1977 Serum uric acid levels in psoriatic arthritis. Annals of the Rheumatic Diseases 36: 264–267
Lathem W, Rodnan G P 1962 Impairment of uric acid excretion in gout. Journal of Clinical Investigation 41: 1955–1963
Leathes J B 1906 On diurnal and nocturnal variations in the excretion of uric acid. Journal of Physiology 35: 125–130
Leeper R D, Benua R S, Brener J L, Rawson R W 1960 Hyperuricaemia in myxoedema. Journal of Clinical Endocrinology 20: 1457–1466
Lefkovits A M 1965 Gouty involvement of the larynx. Arthritis and Rheumatism 8: 1019–1026
Lerman S, Megaw J, Frauenfelder F T 1984 Further studies on allopurinol therapy and human cataractogenesis. American Journal of Ophthalmology 97: 205–209
Lester S C, LeVan S K, Steglich C, DeMars R 1980 Expression of human genes for adenine phosphoribosyltransferase and hypoxanthine-guanine phosphoribosyltransferase after genetic transformation of mouse cells with purified human DNA. Somatic Cell Genetics 6: 241–259
Lewis J C 1961 Gout and the haemoglobin level in patients with cardiac and respiratory disease. British Medical Journal 1: 24–26
Liddle L, Seegmiller J E, Laster L 1959 The enzymatic spectrophotometric method for determination of uric acid. Journal of Laboratory and Clinical Medicine 54: 903–913
Lieber C S, Jones D P, Lasowsky M S, Davidson C S 1962 Inter-relation of uric acid and ethanol metabolism in man. Journal of Clinical Investigation 41:1380
Lieberman U A, Samuel R, Halabe A, Joshua H, Lubin E, Zoref-Shani E, Sperling O 1982 Juvenile metabolic gout caused by chronic compensated hemolytic syndrome. Arthritis and Rheumatism 25: 1264–1266
Loeb J N 1972 The influence of temperature on the solubility of monosodium urate. Arthritis and Rheumatism 15: 189–192

Loebl W Y, Scott J T 1974 Withdrawal of allopurinol in patients with gout. Annals of the Rheumatic Diseases 304–307

Löffler W, Gröbner W, Medina R, Zöllner N 1982 Influence of dietary purines on pool size, turnover and excretion of uric acid during balance conditions. Research in Experimental Medicine 181: 113–123

Löffler W, Simmonds H A, Gröbner W 1983 Gout and uric acid nephropathy: some new aspects in diagnosis and treatment. Klinische Wochenschrift 61: 1233–1239

Long W K 1967 Glutathione reductase in red blood cells: variant associated with gout. Science 155: 712–713

Lowenthal M N, Dymond I D 1977 Gout and hyperuricaemia in blacks. South African Medical Journal 52:524

McCarty D J, Hollander J L 1961 Identification of urate crystals in gouty synovial fluid. Annals of Internal Medicine 54: 452–460

MacLachlan M J, Rodnan G P 1967 Effects of food, fast and alcohol on serum uric acid and acute attacks of gout. American Journal of Medicine 42: 38–57

Magid S K, Gray G E, Anand A 1981 Spinal cord compression by tophi in a patient with chronic polyarthritis. Arthritis and Rheumatism 24: 1431–1434

Malawista S E, Seegmiller J E, Hathaway B E, Sokoloff L 1965 Sacroiliac gout. Journal of the American Medical Association 194: 954–956

Malawista S E, Van Blaricom G, Cretella S B, Schwartz M L 1979 The phlogistic potential of urate in solution. Studies of the phagocytic process in human leukocytes. Arthritis and Rheumatism 22: 728–736

Mandel N S 1976 The structural basis of membranolysis. Arthritis and Rheumatism 19:439–445

Mandel N S, Mandel G S 1982 Structures of crystals that provoke inflammation. In: Weissman G(ed) Advances in inflammation research, Vol 4. Raven Press, New York, p. 73–94

Manuel M A, Steele T H 1974 Changes in renal urate handling after prolonged thiazide treatment. American Journal of Medicine 57: 741–746

Marcolongo R, Marinello E, Riario-Sforza G, Pagani R 1972 The inhibition of xanthine oxidase activity by benzodiarne. Clinica Chimica Acta 41: 91–94

Mariani G, et al 1984 Turnover and distribution of ^{14}C-uric acid in psoriatic patients. In: De Bruyn CHHM, Simmonds H A, Müller M M (eds) Purine metabolism in man, IV. Plenum Press, New York 165A– 277–281

Matzkies F, Berg G, Mädl H 1980 The uricosuric action of protein in man. Advances in Experimental Medicine and Biology 122A: 227–231

Medalie J H, Snyder M, Groen J J, Newfeld H N, Goldbourt U, Riss E 1973 Angina pectoris among 10 000 men, 5 years incidence and univariate analysis. American Journal of Medicine 55: 583–594

Melmon K L, Webster M E, Goldfinger S E, Seegmiller J E 1967 The presence of a kinin in inflammatory synovial effusion from arthritides of varying etiologies. Arthritis and Rheumatism 10: 13–20

Mertz D P, Babucke G 1971 Epidemiology and clinical findings in primary gout. Observations between 1948 and 1968. Munchener Medizinische Wochenschrift 113: 617–624

Mertz D P, Borner K 1983 Ausschiedung und Serumkonzentrationen von Allopurinol, Oxipurinol und Oxipurinen under kombinierter behandlung mit Allopurinol/Benzbromaron in steigender Dosierung. Medizinische Welt 34: 974–979

Messerli F H, Frölich E D, Dreslinski G R, Suarez D H, Aristimuno G G 1980 Serum uric acid in essential hypertension: an indication of renal vascular involvement. Annals of Internal Medicine 93: 817–821

Metcalfe-Gibson A, McCallum F M, Morrison R B I, Wrong O 1965 Urinary excretion of hydrogen ion in patients with uric acid calculi. Clinical Science 28: 325–342

Michelis M F, Warms P C, Fusco R D, Davis B B 1974 Hypouricemia and hyperuricosuria in Laennec cirrhosis. Archives of Internal Medicine 134: 681–683

Mielants H, Veys E M, De Weerdt A 1973 Gout and its relation to lipid metabolism. I. Serum uric acid, lipid and lipoprotein levels in gout. Annals of the Rheumatic Diseases 32: 501–505

Migeon B R 1970 X-linked hypoxanthine-guanine phosphoribosyltransferase deficiency: detection of heterozygotes by selective medium. Biochemical Genetics 4: 377–383

Mikklesen W M, Dodge J H, Valkenburg H 1965 The distribution of serum uric acid values in a population unselected as to gout or hyperuricemia. American Journal of Medicine 39: 242–251

Mills R M Jr 1971 Severe hypersensitivity reactions associated with allopurinol. Journal of the American Medical Association 216: 799–802

Milne M D 1966 Urate excretion. Proceedings of the Royal Society of Medicine 77: 308–310

Mody G M, Naidoo D 1984 Gout in South African blacks. Annals of the Rheumatic Diseases 43: 394–397

Moidel R A, Good A E 1981 Coexistent gout and systemic lupus erythematosus. Arthritis and Rheumatism 24: 969–971

Moskowitz R W, Vertes V, Schwartz A, Marshall G, Friedman B 1969 Crystal-induced inflammation associated with chronic renal failure treated with periodic haemodialysis. American Journal of Medicine 57: 450–460

Mudge G H 1971 Uricosuric action of cholecystographic agents. New England Journal of Medicine 284: 929–933

Myers A R, Epstein F H, Dodge H J, Mikklesen W M 1968 The relationship of serum uric acid to risk factors in coronary heart disease. American Journal of Medicine 45: 520–528

Naff G B, Byers P H 1973 Complement as a mediator of inflammation in acute gouty arthritis. I. Studies on the reaction between human serum complement and sodium urate crystals. Journal of Laboratory and Clinical Medicine 81: 747–760

Narins R G, Weisberg J S, Myers A R 1974 Effect of carbohydrates on uric acid metabolism. Metabolism 23: 455–465

Nelson D J, Elion G B 1974 Personal communication

Nelson D J, Bugge C J L, Krasny H C, Elion G B 1973 Formation of nucleotides of (6–^{14}C) allopurinol and (6–^{14}C) oxipurinol in rat tissues and effects on uridine nucleotide pools. Biochemical Pharmacology 22: 2003–2022

New Zealand Hypertension Study Group 1983 Multicentre controlled trial of tienilic acid in hyperuricaemic, hypertensive subjects, with intensive monitoring of liver function. British Journal of Clinical Pharmacology 15: 513–518

Nicholls A, Scott J T 1972 Effect of weight loss on plasma and urinary levels of uric acid. Lancet 2: 1223–1224

Nicholls A, Snaith M L, Scott J T 1973 Effect of oestrogen

therapy on plasma and urinary levels of uric acid. British Medical Journal 1: 449–451
Nishioka K, Mikanagi K 1981 A retrospective study on the cause of death, in Japan, of patients with gout. The Ryumachi 21 (Suppl): 29–33
Nugent C A, MacDiarmid W D, Tyler F H 1964 Renal excretion of urate in patients with gout. Archives of Internal Medicine 113: 115–121
Nuki G 1976 Some aspects of gout and purine metabolism In: Hughes G R V (ed) Modern topics in rheumatology. Heinemann, London, p. 163
Nuki G, Astrin K, Brenton D, Avishank M, Lever J, Seegmiller J E 1973 Purine and pyrimidine nucleotide pools in azaguanine resistant human lymphoblasts deficient in hypoxanthine-guanine phosphoribosyltransferase. American Journal of Human Genetics 25:56A
Nyhan W L, Sweetman L, Carpenter D G, Carter C H, Hoefnagel D 1968 Effects of azathioprine in a disorder of uric acid metabolism and cerebral function. Journal of pediatrics 72: 111–118
Orowan E 1955 The origin of man. Nature 175: 683–684
Ortel R W, Newcombe D S 1974 Acute gouty arthritis and response to colchicine in the virtual absence of synovial-fluid leukocytes. New England Journal of Medicine 290: 1363–1364
Owen-Smith B D 1983 Significance of circadian variations of uric acid elimination. Annals of the Rheumatic Diseases 42 (Suppl):87
Page T, Bakay B, Nissinen E, Nyhan W L 1981 Hypoxanthine-guanine phosphoribosyltransferase variants: correlation of clinical phenotype with enzyme activity. Journal of Inherited Metabolic Diseases 4: 203–206
Pak C Y C, Barilla D E, Holt K, Brinkley L, Tolentino R, Zermekh J R 1978 Effect of oral purine load and allopurinol on the crystallization of calcium salts in urine of patients with hyperuricosuric calcium urolithiasis. American Journal of Medicine 65: 593–599
Pant S S, Moser H W, Krane S M 1968 Hyperuricemia in Down's syndrome. Journal of Clinical Endocrinology 28: 472–478
Perricone E, Brandt K D 1978 Enhancement of urate solubility by connective tissue. Arthritis and Rheumatism 21: 453–460
Peterson J L, McBride O W 1980 Co-transfer of linked eukaryotic genes and efficient transfer of hypoxanthine phosphoribosyltransferase by DNA-mediated gene transfer. Proceedings of the National Academy of Sciences USA 77: 1583–1587
Phelps P 1970 Polymorphonuclear leukocyte motility in vitro. IV. Colchicine inhibition of chemotactic activity formation after phagocytosis of urate crystals. Arthritis and Rheumatism 13: 1–9
Phelps P, McCarty D J Jr 1966 Crystal induced inflammation in canine joints. II. Importance of polymorphonuclear leukocytes. Journal of Experimental Medicine 124: 115–125
Platt P, Dick W C 1983 Crystals and inflammation. Annals of the Rheumatic Diseases 42 (Supple): 4–7
Popert A J, Hewitt J V 1962 Gout and hyperuricaemia in rural and urban populations. Annals of the Rheumatic Diseases 21: 154–163
Postlethwaite A E, Ramsdell C M, Kelley W N 1974 Uricosuric effect of an anticholinergic agent in hyperuricemic subjects. Archives of Internal Medicine 134: 270–275
Praetorius E, Kirk J E 1950 Hypouricaemia: with evidence for tubular elimination of uric acid. Journal of Laboratory and Clinical Medicine 35: 865–868
Pund E E, Hawley R L, McGee H J, Blount S G 1960 Gouty heart. New England Journal of Medicine 263: 835–838
Raddatz D A, Mahowald M L, Bilka P J 1983 Acute polyarticular gout. Annals of the Rheumatic Diseases 31: 162–165
Rae S A, Davidson E M, Smith M J H 1982 Leukotriene B4, an inflammatory mediator of gout. Lancet 2: 1122–1124
Rajan K T 1975 Observations on phagocytosis of urate crystals by polymorphonuclear leucocytes. Annals of the Rheumatic Diseases 34: 54–61
Ramsdell C M, Kelley W N 1973 The clinical significance of hypouricemia. Annals of Internal Medicine 78: 239–242
Rapado A 1969 Gout and saturnism. New England Journal of Medicine 281:851
Rassin D K, Lloyd K G, Kelley W N, Fox L 1982 Decreased amino acids in various brain areas of patients with the Lesch–Nyhan syndrome. Neuropaediatrics 13: 130–134
Ravenscroft P J, Sands J M, Emmerson B T 1973 Studies on the uricosuric action of the hypolipidemic drug halofenate. Archives of Internal Medicine 134: 547–551
Reardon J A, Scott J T 1980 Controlled in-patient study of tienilic acid in treatment of gout and hypertension. Annals of the Rheumatic Diseases 39: 367–372
Reynolds P R, Knapp M K, Baraf H S B, Holmes E W 1983 Moonshine and lead: relationship to the pathogenesis of hyperuricaemia in gout. Arthritis and Rheumatism 26: 1057–1064
Richet G, Mignon F, Ardaillou R 1965 Goutte secondaire des nephropathies chroniques. Presse Medicale 73: 633–638
Rieselbach R E, Sorensen L B, Shelp W D, Steele T H 1970 Diminished renal urate secretion per nephron as a basis for primary gout. Annals of Internal Medicine 73: 359–366
Roch-Ramel F, Wiener I M 1980 Renal excretion of urate: factors determining the action of drugs. Kidney International 18: 665–676
Rockson S, Stone R, van der Weyden M, Kelley W N 1974 The Lesch–Nyhan syndrome: evidence for abnormal adrenergic function. Science 186: 934–935
Rodgers A V, Gibson T, Simmonds H A, Toseland P 1984 The effect of beer ingestion on plasma and urine uric acid in gout and normouricaemic subjects. In: De Bruyn CHMM, Simmonds H A, Müller M M (eds) Purine Metabolism in Man, IV. Plenum Press, New York, 165A: 327–331
Rodnan G P 1982 Treatment of the gout and other forms of crystal-induced arthritis. Bulletin on the Rheumatic Diseases 32: 43–53
Rosenbloom F M, Henderson J F, Caldwell I C, Kelley W N, Seegmiller J E 1968 Biochemical bases of accelerated purine biosynthesis de novo in human fibroblasts lacking hypoxanthine-guanine phosphoribosyltransferase. Journal of Biological Chemistry 243: 1166–1173
Rosenfeld J B 1974 Effect of long-term allopurinol administration on serial GFR in normotensive and hypertensive hyperuricaemic subjects. Advances in Experimental Medicine and Biology 41B: 581–596
Rosenthale M E, Dervinis A, Kassarich J, Sinler S 1972 Prostaglandins and anti-inflammatory drugs in the dog knee joint. Journal of Pharmacy and Pharmacology 24: 149–150

Rouault T, Caldwell D A, Holmes E W 1982 Aspiration of the asymptomatic metatarsophalangeal joint in gout patients and hyperuricemic controls. Arthritis and Rheumatism 25 209–212
Rubin T T, Plag J A, Ranson J A, Clark B R, Rahe R 1969 Serum uric acid levels. Journal of the American Association 208: 1184–1186
Rubinow A, Sennenblick M 1981 Amyloidosis secondary to polyarticular gout. Arthritis and Rheumatism 24: 1425–1427
Rundles R W, Wyngaarden J B, Hirchings G H, Elion B G, Silberman H R 1963 Effects of a xanthine oxidase inhibitor on thiopurine metabolism, hyperuricemia and gout. Transactions of the Association of American Physicians 76: 126–140
Russell I J, Papaioannou C, McDuffie F C, Macintyre S, Kusher I 1983 Effect of IgG and C-reactive protein on complement depletion by monosodium urate crystals. Journal of Rheumatology 10: 425–433
San Miguel J C 1964 Goa y mixedema. Medicina Clinica (Barcelona) 42: 295
Schlosstein L, Kippen I, Bluestone R, Whitehouse M W, Klinenberg J R 1974 Association between hypouricaemia and jaundice. Annals of the Rheumatic Diseases 33: 308–312
Schumacher H R 1977 Pathogenesis of crystal-induced synovitis. Clinics in Rheumatic Diseases 3: 105–131
Scott J T 1969 Causes of hyperuricaemia. Proceedings of the Royal Society of Medicine 62: 851–853
Scott J T 1977a In: Purine and pyrimide metabolism. Ciba Foundation Symposium No. 48. Elsevier/Excerpta Medica, Amsterdam p. 217
Scott J T 1977b Obesity and hyperuricaemia. In: Crystal-induced arthropathies. Clinics in Rheumatic Diseases. Kelley W N ed. London: W B Saunders Co Ltd. 3: 25–35
Scott J T 1978 New knowledge of the pathogenesis of gout. Journal of Clinical Pathology 12 (Suppl): 205–213
Scott J T 1983 Uric acid and the interpretation of hyperuricaemia. Clinics in Rheumatic Diseases 9: 241–255
Scott J T, O'Brien P K 1968 Probenecid, nephrotic syndrome and renal failure. Annals of the Rheumatic Diseases 27: 249–252
Scott J T, Pollard A C 1970 Uric acid excretion in the relatives of patients with gout. Annals of the Rheumatic Diseases 29: 397–400
Scott J T, Sturge R A 1976 The effect of weight loss on plasma and urinary uric acid and lipid levels. Journal of Clinical Chemistry and Clinical Biochemistry 14: 319
Scott J T, Stodell M A 1984 Serum uric acid levels in psoriasis. In: De Bruyn C H M M, Simmonds H A, Müller M M (eds) Purine metabolism in man. IV. Plenum Press, New York, 165A: 283–285
Scott J T, Dixon A St J, Bywaters E G L 1964a Association of hyperuricaemia and gout with hyperparathyroidism. British Medical Journal 1: 1070–1073
Scott J T, McCallum F M, Holloway V P 1964b Starvation, ketosis and uric acid excretion. Clinical Science 27: 209–221
Scott J T, Hall A P, Grahame R 1966 Allopurinol in the treatment of gout. British Medical Journal 2: 321–327
Scott J T, Holloway V P, Glass H I, Arnot R N 1969 Studies of uric acid pool size and turnover rate. Annals of the Rheumatic Diseases 28: 366–373
Seegmiller J E 1968 Seminars on the Lesch–Nyhan syndrome: management and treatment, discussion. Federation Proceedings 27: 1097–1104
Seegmiller J E 1980 Heberden Oration 1979: Human aberrations of purine metabolism and their significance for rheumatology. Annals of the Rheumatic Diseases 39: 103–117
Seegmiller J E, Grayzel A I, Laster L, Liddle L 1961 Uric acid production in gout. Journal of Clinical Investigation 40: 1304–1314
Seegmiller J E, Howell R R, Malawista S E 1962 The inflammatory reaction to sodium urate. Its possible relationship to the genesis of acute gouty arthritis. Journal of the American Medical Association 180: 469–475
Seegmiller J E, Laster L, Howell R R 1963a Biochemistry of uric acid and its relation to gout. New England Journal of Medicine 268: 712–716, 821–827
Seegmiller J E, Grayzel A I, Liddle L, Wyngaarden J B 1963b The effect of 2-ethylamino-1,3,4-thiadiazole on the incorporation of glycine into urinary purines and uric acid in man. Metabolism 12: 507–515
Seegmiller J E, Rosenbloom F M, Kelley W N 1967 Enzyme defect associated with a sex-linked human neurological disorder and excessive purine synthesis. Science (New York) 155: 1682–1684
Sequeira W, et al 1981 Quadriparesis in tophaceous gout. Arthritis and Rheumatism 24: 1428–1430
Shapiro S 1974 Allopurinol and bone marrow depression. Lancet 2:412
Sheikh M I, Møller J V 1968 Binding of urate to proteins of human and rabbit plasma. Biochemica et Biophysica Acta 158:456
Shelp W D, Steele T H, Rieselbach R E 1969 Comparison of urinary phosphate, urate and magnesium excretion following parathyroid hormone administration to normal man. Metabolism 18: 63–70
Sherry S & Committee: The Anturane Reinfarction Trial Research Group (Kane S H, Chairman) 1978 Sulphinpyrazone in the prevention of cardiac death after myocardial infarction. New England Journal of Medicine 298: 289–295
Simkin S A 1973 Local concentration of urate in the pathogenesis of gout. Lancet 2: 1295–1298
Simkin P A, Campbell P M, Larson E B 1983 Gout in Heberden's nodes. Arthritis and Rheumatism 26: 94–97
Simmonds H A, Van Acker K J 1983 Adenine phosphoribosyltransferase deficiency 2,8-dihydroxyadenine lithiasis. In: Stanbury J B, Wyngaarden J B, Fredrickson D A, Goldstein J L, Brown M S (eds) The metabolic basis of inherited disease, 5th Edn, McGraw-Hill, New York. ch. 52, p. 1144–1156
Simmonds H A, Cameron J S, Potter C F, Warren D, Gibson T, Farebrother D 1980a Renal failure in young subjects with familial gout. In: Rapado A, Watts R W E, Bruyn C H M M (eds) Purine metabolism in man. III. Plenum Press, New York, 122:15–21
Simmonds H A, Warren D J, Cameron J S, Potter C F, Farebrother D A 1980b Familial gout and renal failure in young women. Clinical Nephrology 14: 176–182
Simmonds H A, Goday A, Morris G S, Brolsma M F J 1984a Metabolism of deoxynucleosides by lymphocytes in long-term culture deficient in different purine enzymes. Biochemical Pharmacology 33: 763–770
Simmonds H A, Webster D R, Wilson J, Fairbanks L D, Potter D F 1984b Evidence for a new syndrome involving

acute arthritis (Atkins et al, 1970; Dieppe et al, 1982). The male : female ratio was 1.5 : 1 in the large series reported by McCarty but most series have shown a slight female predominance. Asymptomatic chondrocalcinosis is a common finding and there have been many surveys in which the incidence of calcification of the menisci in the knee joints varies with the mean age of the sample. In one large series of 12 268 films it was found 0.42% (Weaver, 1942) but Ellman & Levin (1975) found it in 27.6% of patients in a home for elderly Jews whose mean age was 84.3 years. This increased incidence with age has been confirmed by other workers (Delauche et al, 1977; Wilkins et al, 1983) and it probably affects 5% of the adult population at the time of death. An autopsy study of 840 menisci taken from the knees of 215 cadavers in the dissecting rooms at Philadelphia showed CPPD in all four menisci from 7 cadavers (McCarty et al, 1966). Multiple deposits of dicalcium phosphate dihydrate, a diamorphic form of brushite were found in 5 cadavers. Hydroxyapatite crystals were found as solitary calcifications in one meniscus in 3 cadavers, and were thought to be secondary to trauma. A fourth pattern of calcification involved the vessels supplying the outer third of the meniscus and was also hydroxyapatite. Lagier & Baud (1968) in a study of 320 cadavers found an incidence of CPPD crystal deposits of 6.8%. There are limited data available on the overall clinical prevalence of pyrophosphate arthropathy and hospital figures can be selective. At the Mayo Clinic in 1970/71 the frequency of admission for pseudogout was 0.9 per 1000 (O'Duffy, 1976) and McCarty found hospital cases to occur half as frequently as gout.

Clinical features

In pseudogout the affected joint becomes suddenly painful, warm, swollen and tender and, as with gout, redness of the overlying skin frequently occurs. The attacks on the whole are slightly less severe than in urate gout, but fever, leucocytosis and a rise in the sedimentation rate can occur. The knee is by far the commonest site for an attack and accounts for more than half the reported cases. Other large joints such as the wrist, elbow, shoulder, hip and ankle are the next commonest joints to be involved. It is rare for the big toe joints to be involved in the acute attacks and in a series of 238 cases reported by McCarty (1972) there were only 8 cases involving the first metacarpophalangeal joints and in these the crystals of CPPD were found in the aspirated joint fluid.

The attacks last for a few days up to as long as 4 weeks. Subacute and petite attacks and clustering of attacks can be found with several joints being involved at the same time. There is also a tendency for them to recur in joints previously affected. The attacks of pseudogout are commoner in men than in women (McCarty, 1981: Dieppe et al, 1982) and after trauma, surgery or an acute illness (O'Duffy, 1976).

In most cases there are no abnormalities in serum biochemistry or in haematological findings. The serum calcium, phosphate and alkaline phosphatase levels are within the normal range. Pyrophosphate when measured has been normal, but can be raised in the joint fluid due to crystal shedding from cartilage. Examination of joint fluid by polarised light microscopy is the essential diagnostic investigation, when crystals will be found phagacytosed by leucocytes (Fig. 37.1).

Calcium pyrophosphate crystals are weakly positively birefringent. When a first-order red compensator is used they show a faint blue colour against a red background if the axis of the crystal is parallel to the compensator. X-ray diffraction crystallography is needed for more accurate identification but it is not a routine procedure. The morphology of the crystals can be studied further by electron microscopy (Fig. 37.2), transmission

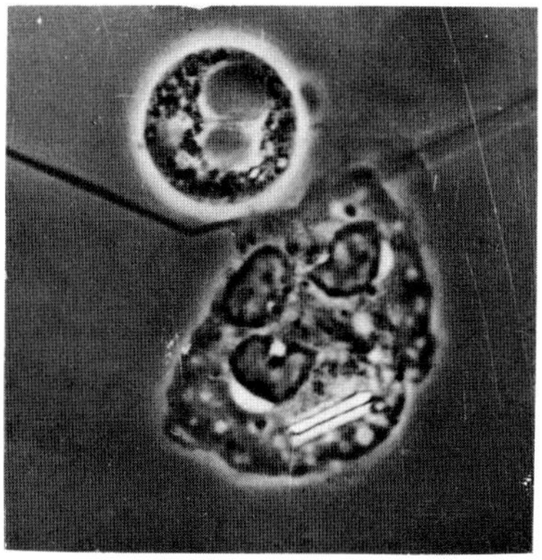

Fig. 37.1 Ingestion of crystals of calcium pyrophosphate by polymorphonuclear leucocyte.

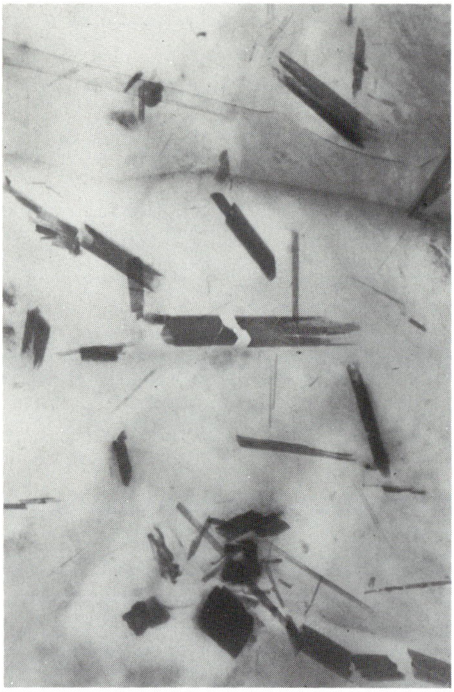

Fig. 37.2 Electron microscopy of pyrophosphate crystals (by courtesy of Dr P. A. Dieppe).

electron microscopy (Fig. 37.3) and scanning electron microscopy (Fig. 37.4).

Radiographs in pyrophosphate arthropathy show characteristic calcifications in both fibro and hyaline cartilage and although the calcifications are not invariably present, they are often of diagnostic value (Figs 37.5–37.8). The knee meniscus is the commonest site of involvement but the triangular ligament at the wrist, distal to the lower end of the ulna and the symphysis pubis also frequently show punctate calcification. When pyrophosphate arthropathy is suspected initial radiographs need only to be taken of the knees, pelvis and wrists, as if calcification is not found here it is unlikely to be seen elsewhere. Hyaline cartilage calcification appears as a dense line parallel to the joint surface and is due to deposits of CPPD in the mid-zone layer. It is seen more often in the large joints such as the knee, wrist, hip, shoulder, elbow and ankle. Smaller joints can be involved but the calcification here is more difficult to detect. Deposits can be

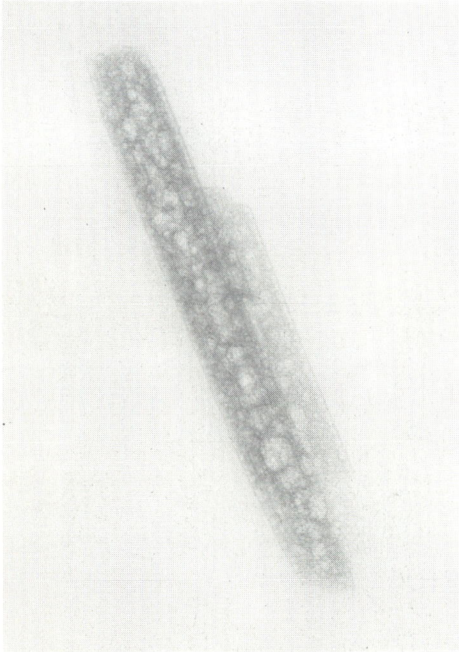

Fig. 37.3 Transmission electron microscopy of CPPD crystal (× 20 000) (by courtesy of Dr P. A. Dieppe)

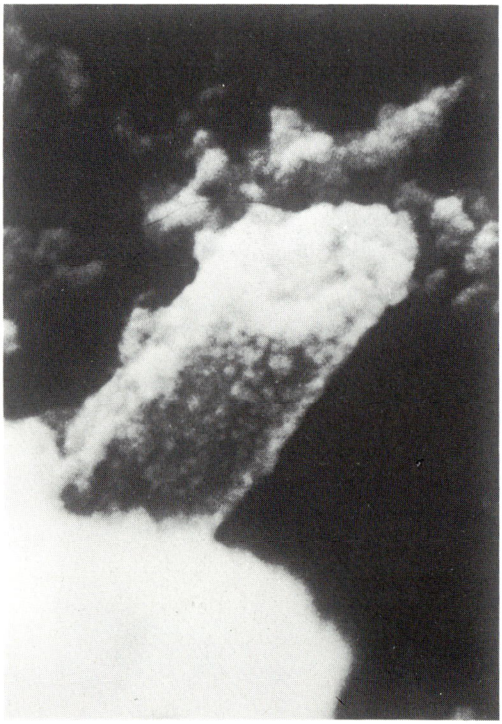

Fig. 37.4 Scanning electron microscopy of CPPD crystal phagocytosed by synovial fluid cell, showing granular appearance of crystal surface (× 120 000) (by courtesy of Dr P. A. Dieppe).

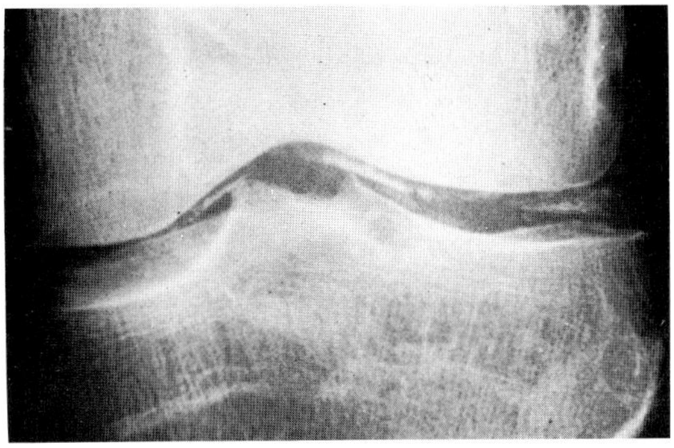

Fig. 37.5 Chondrocalcinosis in the hyaline cartilage and the fibrocartilage meniscus of the knee joint.

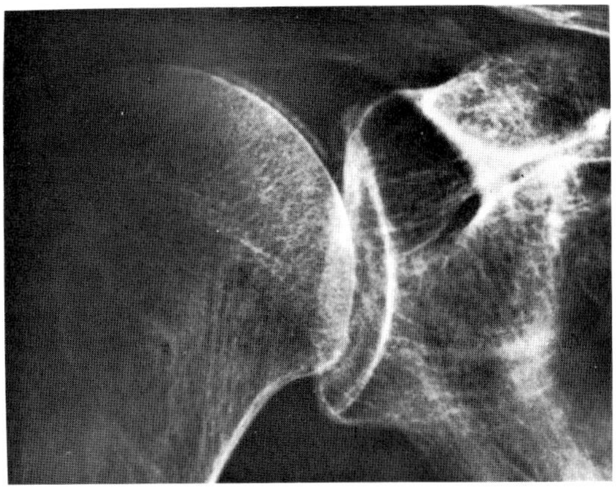

Fig. 37.6 Chondrocalcinosis in the shoulder joint.

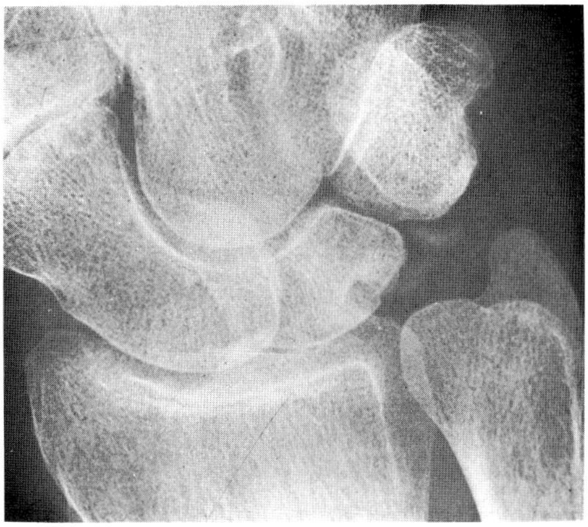

Fig. 37.7 Calcification in the triangular ligament of the wrist joint.

seen in the synovium (Fig. 37.9) and in the tendons close to the joints such as the achilles tendon (Gerster et al, 1977) and the plantar fascia. They can also be seen in the ligamentum flavum as well as in the intervertebral discs (Bywaters et al, 1971; Richards & Hamilton, 1976). Cartilage calcification can lead to degenerative and destructive change in the joints and Resnick (1977) has stressed the characteristic joint distribution in pyrophosphate arthropathy. Sites not normally prone

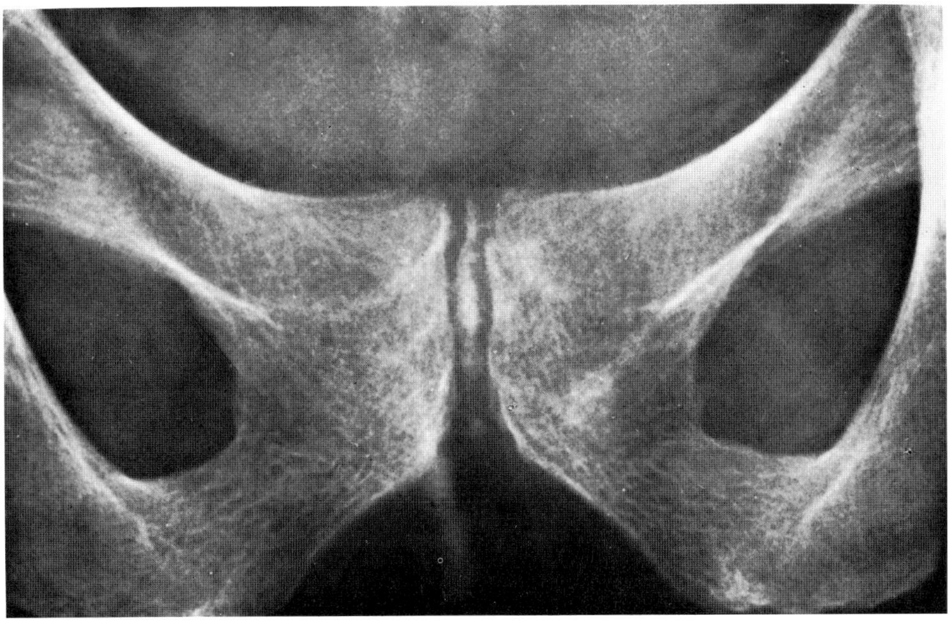

Fig. 37.8 Chondrocalcinosis in the symphysis pubis.

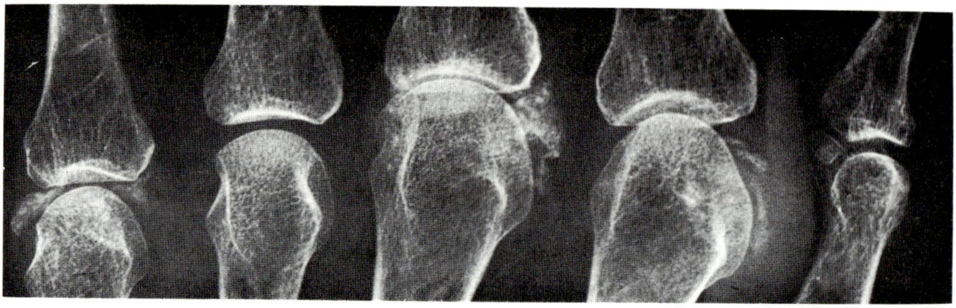

Fig. 37.9 Calcification in the synovial membrane of the metacarpophalangeal joints in hyperparathyroidism.

to osteoarthritis such as the wrists (Resnick & Utsinger, 1974), metacarpophalangeal joints (Martel et al, 1970), elbows and shoulders are commonly affected, and patellofemoral joint space narrowing with the patella wrapped round the femur is a characteristic feature. Flexion contractures and varus deformities of the knee can occur with collapse of the medial tibial plateau or necrosis of the medial femoral condyle.

Patterns of joint involvement

The acute attack of pseudogout is only one of a number of different ways in which pyrophosphate arthropathy can present and McCarty (1975) has distinguished six different clinical patterns.

1. Pseudogout
2. Pseudo-rheumatoid arthritis
3. Pseudo-osteoarthritis
4. Pseudo-osteoarthritis with superimposed acute attacks
5. Lanthantic (asymptomatic CPPD deposits)
6. Destructive or pseudoneurotrophic joints.

The cases with polyarthritis that mimic rheumatoid arthritis are not common (5%) and morning stiffness, swelling and tenderness of the involved joints with a raised sedimentation rate may lead to the wrong diagnosis. Calcium pyrophosphate crystals can also be deposited in the joints of rheumatoid patients (Bywaters, 1972; Dieppe et al, 1982), but this may relate to the cartilage being previously damaged.

The largest group of patients with pyrophosphate arthropathy, approximately 50%, have osteoarthritis (Hamilton, 1981), which can occur with and without attacks of pseudogout. It occurs most commonly in women, and the knee joint is most frequently involved, but it can also be seen in the hips, wrists and shoulders. In the long-term follow-up studies of the Czechoslovak patients, severe osteoarthritis undoubtedly supervened in the majority of cases (Zitnan & Sit'aj, 1976). Mitrovic (1983) stained the cartilage of 250 knees with Indian ink and correlated the fibrillation in the hyaline cartilage with deposition of CPPD crystals in the menisci. He confirmed a definite correlation between osteoarthritis and crystal deposition.

Lanthantic or asymptomatic chondrocalcinosis due to CPPD crystal deposition is not uncommon as the various surveys of elderly populations have shown, but its presence should always alert one to the possibility of associated endocrine or metabolic disease. Calcification of intervertebral discs can also occur and was found by us in 21 of the 67 lumbar spines of patients with pyrophosphate arthropathy. It was not associated with spinal stiffness and was more frequent in the older patients and in those with more widespread peripheral joint involvement (Richards & Hamilton, 1976).

Pyrophosphate arthropathy can also lead to severe destructive arthritis, which is most commonly seen in the knee, hip and shoulder joints (Menkes et al, 1973, 1976; Richards & Hamilton, 1974, Villiaumey et al, 1975). Gerster (1975) found such changes to occur more frequently than in a sex- and age-matched control population of osteoarthritis. Dicalcium phosphate dihydrate crystals have also been reported in association with a destructive arthropathy (Faure et al, 1977). In all these patients there was no evidence of neurological abnormalities but CPPD deposits have been found in 4 consecutively seen patients with Charcot's arthritis (Jacobelli et al, 1973). Some of these patients with tabes dorsalis had symptomless chondrocalcinosis in undamaged joints. While there is undoubtedly evidence that CPPD deposits can lead to destructive changes, there are also many instances where previously damaged joints may be the site of crystal deposition.

Treatment

Treatment of an acute attack of pseudogout can be by aspiration of the joint fluid and an injection of a corticosteroid together with the administration of a non-steroidal antirheumatic drug. Colchicine is effective, but less so than with urate gout. This clinical observation is supported by experimental work which shows that colchicine is less effective in blocking the release of chemotactic factor when CPPD crystals are phagocytosed by leucocytes, compared to the blocking action when urate crystals are engulfed (Phelps, 1969, 1970; Tse & Phelps, 1970). Intravenous colchicine has been used successfully when there have been contraindications for giving non-steroidal antirheumatics, but it is rarely necessary. There is no specific treatment for the chronic joint disease, but intra-articular yttrium-90 can be effective and magnesium carbonate, which exerts a stabilising growth inhibitory effect on CPPD crystals, has also been shown to improve symptoms (Doherty & Dieppe, 1981, 1983).

ASSOCIATIONS WITH METABOLIC AND OTHER DISEASES

Since pyrophosphate arthropathy was recognised there has been a large and increasing number of diseases reported in association with it (Hamilton, 1976, 1981), and there is difficulty deciding which are true associations and which provide clues to pathogenesis. There is a definite relationship with age and with osteoarthritis, but it seems likely that a previously damaged joint or one where there is already pre-existing arthritis may become the site of CPPD deposition. This would explain the occurrence in the hypermobile joint (Bird et al, 1978), after meniscectomy (Doherty et al, 1982) and in the neuropathic joint. Controlled studies have been made which have helped (McCarty et al, 1974: Alexander et al, 1982), but owing to the infrequency of some of the diseases in which deposition occurs, they do not always provide the answer. Hypophosphatasia is one of these rare diseases which are important and another is hypomagnesaemia. Some of the more highly probable associations also include hyperparathyroidism, haemochromatosis, hypothyroidism, amyloidosis and gout, and the isolated reports in Wilson's disease and ochronosis cannot be dismissed. Controlled studies have not confirmed the frequent reports in diabetes mellitus and in Paget's disease.

Hyperparathyroidism

Hyperparathyroidism was one of the first reported, commonest and most important associations (Bywaters, 1959: Zvaifler et al, 1962: Bywaters et al, 1963) and the incidence in the different sexes of patients with pyrophosphate arthropathy varies between 5 and 15%. The relationship may be with sustained hypercalcaemia which is supported by the association with familial hypocalciuric hypercalcaemia (Marx et al, 1982), but there are also reports of elevated parathormone levels in normocalcaemic patients (Phelps & Hawker, 1973: Dunham et al, 1982). When we look at series of patients with proven parathyroid adenomas we find an incidence of chondrocalcinosis between 18 and 41% (Rickewaert et al, 1966: Dodds & Steinbach, 1968: Pritchard & Jessop, 1977) and this has been shown to be due to CPPD deposition. Crystal deposition is proportional to the duration of the disease and its severity and there is a definite relationship with age. The mean age of those with chondrocalcinosis was significantly higher than those without chondrocalcinosis, which is a finding similar to that which we have reported in haemochromatosis. Once present the chondrocalcinosis does not get less or disappear after parathyroidectomy, and there may be an increased incidence of pseudogout immediately following surgery (Bilezikian et al, 1973). This may be due to a fall in intrasynovial ionised calcium levels postoperatively, which results in crystal shedding from cartilage.

Haemochromatosis

In idopathic haemochromatosis acute crystal synovitis and chronic arthritis due to CPPD deposition are found in approximately half the patients.

It has a characteristic distribution and varies from mild involvement of metacarpophalangeal joints to severe disabling arthritis and is described in Chapter 38. It is directly related to iron overload and has also been found in secondary haemochromatosis due to hereditary spherocytosis (Dymock et al, 1970; Berry & Miller, 1973).

Hypothyroidism

Dorwart & Schumacher (1975) reported 12 patients with severe hypothyroidism 7 of whom had pyrophosphate arthropathy, and acute attacks of pseudogout started after thyroid replacement was begun. In a larger series of 48 patients with hypothyroidism the incidence of chondrocalcinosis was 15.9% (Menkes et al, 1979). 40 of these patients were female with a mean age of 59.9 years and 8 male with a mean age of 53 years. Alexander et al (1982) found hypothyroidism in 10.5% of 105 consecutive patients with pyrophosphate arthropathy. It was one of their commonest findings and this suggests that it may produce changes in connective tissue that allows CPPD crystals to be deposited.

Gout

In six different reports up to 8% of patients with pyrophosphate arthropathy have a history of gout, suggesting that urate crystals may act as nucleation sites for calcium pyrophoshate. Stockman et al (1980) in a controlled study reviewed 138 patients with gout, who had a mean age of 55.2 years and found 8 or 5.8% with chondrocalcinosis compared with none in their controls, and this was in agreement with earlier series (Hamilton, 1976).

Hypophosphatasia

This rare disease is an intriguing and important association, as inorganic pyrophosphate is a natural substrate for alkaline phosphatase. These patients have very low levels of alkaline phosphatase, and increased excretion of phosphoethanolamine in the urine. O'Duffy (1970) described a 51-year-old woman with a 27 year history of attacks of pseudogout and widespread chondrocalcinosis, and an X-ray diffraction pattern of CPPD was obtained from material from a symphysis pubis biopsy. Eade et al (1980) reported two further cases, one with severe hypophosphatasia presenting in infancy. She had acute attacks of pseudogout and died in renal failure. At autopsy there was calcification of cartilage and CPPD deposits were seen in the synovial membrane of the knee joint.

Hypomagnesaemia

Another important clue may be the finding of CPPD deposits in some patients with very low serum magnesium levels (Milazzo, 1981), as magnesium will complex with inorganic pyrophosphate to form highly soluble complexes and is an important cofactor for alkaline phosphatase.

Amyloidosis

The calcium binding ability of some amyloids may explain the possible association with amyloid arthropathy (Ryan et al, 1982).

PATHOGENESIS

Pyrophosphate consists of two molecules of orthophosphate joined together with the loss of one molecule of water and is produced in large amounts during the synthesis of all major cell constituents. It is rapidly hydrolysed to orthophosphate by pyrophosphatases, so that intracellular concentrations are low. In contrast, the rate of turnover is high and it has been estimated that several kilograms are produced daily in an adult man. In dogs studied with ^{32}P-labelled pyrophosphate it can be shown that the entire plasma content of pyrophosphate is replaced every 2–10 minutes (Jung et al, 1970). It is a common metabolite, but what are the factors leading to the formation of extracellular deposits of crystals of calcium pyrophosphate? Which are the common sites for crystals to appear and why are they chosen? Do such deposits always lead to symptomatic arthritis or can they sometimes be a natural accompaniment of ageing or occur in already damaged cartilage?

The crystals first appear in the intermediate or mid-zone layer of hyaline cartilage around chondrocytes. There is a calcium concentration gradient from the synovial fluid down to the calcification front with the highest concentration products of calcium and pyrophosphate in the mid-zone. The free calcium concentration may be low in the deeper cartilage due to the strong binding by the matrix vesicles. The pyrophosphate in cartilage could be liberated from the subchondral bone surface and meet raised calcium concentrations coming down through the cartilage from the joint surface. Crystals in joint fluid are probably shed from cartilage and CPPD is also commonly found in fibrocartilage such the knee joint menisci, the symphysis pubis, the intervertebral discs, and some ligaments such as the achilles tendon, plantar fascia and ligamentum flavum. There has also been one case report in which it was deposited in the dura mater (Grahame et al, 1971).

The concentration product of calcium and pyrophosphate is critical to the site of crystal formation, but the chemistry of the cartilage matrix and the presence of absence of nucleating or inhibitory factors may also be important. The matrix has been studied by Bjelle (1972, 1981) in six cartilage biopsies from hereditary cases, where he found different staining characteristics from controls and changes in the composition of the glycosoaminoglycans.

The associated diseases provide useful clues to some of the nucleating and inhibitory factors that may influence crystal formation and emphasise the different pathways and mechanisms that may be involved. Hearn et al (1978) have been able to grow pyrophosphate crystals in vitro and show that crystal growth is increased by iron and inhibited by magnesium, which increases the solubility of calcium pyrophosphate. It is also possible that hydroxyapatite may nucleate the growth of CPPD crystals.

Plasma and urinary levels of inorganic pyrophosphate are normal in patients with pyrophosphate arthropathy, and red cell pyrophosphatase activity is normal, suggesting a local rather than a general metabolic abnormality. The exception is hypophosphatasia, an inherited disorder in which there are low levels of alkaline phosphatase, an enzyme having pyrophosphatase activity. This results in raised levels of plasma pyrophosphate. McGuire et al (1981) have found it 4 times higher than normal and this can result in impaired bone formation.

Lust et al (1976) have shown that chondrocytes in culture from a patient with pyrophosphate arthropathy produced increased amounts of pyrophosphate compared with chondrocytes from osteoarthritic cartilage. Seegmiller et al (1981) have also found increased pyrophosphate in fibroblasts and lymphoblasts cultured from patients with hereditary pyrophosphate arthropathy. The experiments of Howell (1981) support the view that as well as increased production, there is a failure of adequate hydrolysis of pyrophosphate in the environment of the matrix vesicles. He found that neutral pyrophosphatase was present in substantial amounts in growth plate incubates, but not in chondrocalcinotic ones.

It will be seen that many mechanisms play a part in crystal production, and once formed, Dieppe & Calvert (1983) have stressed that an 'amplification loop' may arise, leading to further joint damage and crystal deposition. There is also mounting evidence that crystals will arise in cartilage already damaged from a variety of different causes.

If much remains to be discovered about the local deposition of calcium pyrophosphate in cartilage, more is known about the mechanism of acute crystal-induced inflammation by urate and CPPD crystals. Both are ingested by leucocytes with the formation of phagolysozomes and the release of a non-dialysable chemotactic factor, which in the case of CPPD is only partially blocked by colchicine (Phelps, 1969, 1970). The membranolytic effects of urate and CPPD crystals, and the effect of blocking by hydrogen bonding agents such as polyvinyl pyridine N-oxide, have also been studied by Wallingford & McCarty (1971) and by Weissman et al (1971). Urate crystals rapidly break down the membranes with the release of the lyzozomal enzymes and are effectively blocked by PVPNO. CPPD crystals are less reactive against membranes and their action is not blocked by PVPNO.

APATITE ARTHRITIS

Periarthritic deposits of calcium apatite have been well recognised for some years (McCarty & Gatter, 1966) as has the association with chronic renal failure and haemodialysis (Moskowitz et al, 1967; Caner & Decker, 1964) and interest now centres on the significance of intra-articular calcium apatite crystals and what role they play in the pathogenesis of osteoarthritis (Schumacher, 1975,

1977; Dieppe et al 1976, 1979; Doyle et al, 1977).

Alizarin red staining is proving a useful screening technique for apatite (Paul et al, 1983), and increased specificity has been obtained using scanning electron microscopy, electron probe analysis, and transmission electron microscopy. Dieppe et al (1979) found apatite crystals in 9 of 34 unselected patients with osteoarthritis using scanning electron microscopy, and while using transmission electron microscopy, Schumacher (1983) found apatite in the joint effusions in 44 of 100 patients in a selected population. Crystals have also been demonstrated close to matrix vesicles in hyaline cartilage by Ali (1977) and in the knee joint menisci (McCarty et al, 1966).

Apatite crystals can cause acute inflammatory arthritis when injected into the knees of dogs using the same model as has been used in experiments with urate and calcium pyrophosphate crystals (Schumacher et al, 1977) but not all human joint effusions in which crystals are found show active inflammation; can they sometimes be incidental findings? However, crystals could be phagocytosed by the synovium and lead to the release of proteases and collagenase, which then cause increasing damage and destruction to the joint. This is seen in 'Milkwaukee shoulder', in which there is progressive erosion and destruction of the glenohumeral joint with loss of the rotator cuff and upward subluxation of the femoral head (Fig. 37.10). This type of severe destructive arthritis described by McCarty (1981, 1983) is not confined to the shoulder (Schumacher et al, 1981) and can be very disabling, but fortunately is rare.

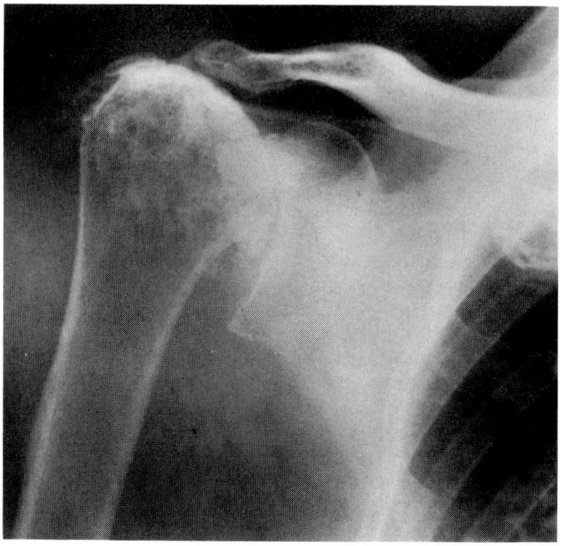

Fig. 37.10 Milwaukee shoulder.

REFERENCES

Alexander G J M, Dieppe P A, Doherty M, Scott D G I 1982 Pyrophosphate arthropathy: a study of metabolic associations and laboratory parameters. Annals of the Rheumatic Diseases 41: 371–376

Ali S Y 1977 Matrix vesicles and apatite nodules in arthritis cartilage. In Willoughby D A, Giroud J P, Velo G P (Eds) Perspectives in inflammation. University Park Press, Baltimore, p 211–224

Atkins C J, McIvor J, Smith P M, Hamilton E, Williams R 1970 Chondrocalcinosis and arthropathy: Studies in haemochromatosis and in idiopathic chondrocalcinosis. Quarterly Journal of Medicine 34: 71–82

Berry E M, Miller J P 1973 Hereditary spherocytosis, haemochromatosis, diabetes mellitus and chondrocalcinosis. Proceedings of the Royal Society of Medicine 66: 9–10

Bilezikian J P, Aurbach G D, Connor T B, Pachas W N, Aptekar R, Wells S A et al 1973 Pseudogout after parathroidectomy. Lancet 1: 445–446

Bird H A, Tribe C R, Bacon P A 1978 Joint hypermobility leading to osteoarthritis and chondrocalcinosis. Annals of the Rheumatic Diseases 37: 203–211

Bjelle A 1972 A morphological study of articular cartilage in pyrophosphate arthropathy. Annals of the Rheumatic Diseases 31: 449–459

Bjelle A 1981 Cartilage matrix in hereditary pyrophosphate arthropathy. Journal of Rheumatology 8: 959–964

Bjelle A, Edvinsson U, Hagstam A 1982 Pyrophosphate arthropathy in two Swedish families. Arthritis and Rheumatism 25: 66–74

Bywaters E G L 1959 Annals of the Rheumatic Diseases 18:64 (discussion)

Bywaters E G L 1972 Calcium pyrophosphate deposits in synovial membrane. Annals of the Rheumatic Diseases 31: 219–221

Bywaters E G L, Dixon A St J, Scott J T 1963 Joint lesions in hyperparathyroidism. Annals of the Rheumatic Diseases 22: 171–187

Bywaters E G L, Hamilton E B D, Williams R 1971 The spine in idiopathic haemochromatosis. Annals of the Rheumatic Diseases 30: 453–465

Caner J E Z, Decker J L 1964 Recurrent acute (? gouty) arthritis in chronic renal failure treated with periodic haemodialysis. American Journal Medicine 36: 57–582

Delaunche M-C, Stehle B, Casson B, Verret J M, Khan M-F 1977 Frequence de la chondrocalcinose radiologique apres 80 ans. Revue du Rhumatisme et des Maladies Osteo-articulaires 44: 555–557

Dieppe P, Calvert P 1983 Crystals and joint disease. Chapman & Hall, London

Dieppe P A, Crocker P, Huskisson E C, Willoughby D A

1976 Apatite deposition disease. A new arthropathy. Lancet 1: 226–269
Dieppe P A, Crocker P R, Corke C F, Doyle D V, Huskisson E C C, Willoughby D A 1979 Synovial fluid crystals. Quarterly Journal of Medicine 48: 533–553
Dieppe P A et al 1982 Pyrophosphate arthropathy: a clinical and radiological study of 105 cases. Annals of the Rheumatic Diseases 41: 371–376
Dodds W J, Steinbach H L 1968 Primary hyperparathyroidism and articular cartilage calcification. American Journal of Roentgenology 104: 884–892
Doherty M, Dieppe P A 1981 The effect of intra-articular yttrium 90 on chronic pyrophosphate arthropathy of the knee. Lancet 1243–1246
Doherty M, Watt I, Dieppe P A Localised chondrocalcinosis in post-meniscectomy knees. Lancet 1982: 1207–1210
Doherty M, Dieppe P A 1983 Double blind, placebo-controlled, trial of magnesium carbonate in chronic pyrophosphate arthropathy. Annals of Rheumatic Diseases 42 (Suppl): 106–107
Dorwart B B, Schumacher H R 1975 Joint effusions, chondrocalcinosis and other rheumatic manifestation in hypothyroidism. A clinico-pathologic study. American Journal of Medicine 59: 780–790
Doyle D V, Dieppe P A, Crocker P R, Ibe K, Willoughby D A 1977 Mixed crystal deposition in an osteoarthritic joint. Journal Pathology 123: 1–4
Dunham J, Bourke B E, Bitensky L E, Chayen J, Loveridge N, Scott J T 1982 Circulating levels of biologically active parathyroid hormone in rheumatic diseases. Annals of the Rheumatic Diseases 41: 569–573
Dymock I W, Hamilton E B D, Laws J W, Williams R 1970 Arthropathy of haemochromatosis. Clinical and radiological analysis of 63 patients with iron overload. Annals of the Rheumatic Diseases 29: 469–476
Eade A W T, Swannell A J, Williamson N 1981 Pyrophosphate arthropathy in hypophosphatasia. Annals of the Rheumatic Diseases 40: 164–170
Ellman M H, Levin B 1975 Chondrocalcinosis in elderly persons. Arthritis and Rheumatism 18: 43–47
Faire G, Netter P, Malanan B, Steinmetz J 1977 Monocrystalline calcium hydrogen phosphate dihydrate in destructive arthropathies of chondrocalcinosis. Lancet 2: 142–143
Faires J S, McCarty D J 1962 Acute arthritis in man and dog after intrasynovial injection of sodium urate crystals. Lancet 2: 682–684
Gaucher A et al 1977 Hereditary diffuse articular chondrocalcinosis. Scandinavian Journal of Rheumatology 6: 217–221
Gerster J C, Vischer T L, Fallet G H 1975 Destructive arthropathy in generalized osteoarthritis with articular chondrocalcinosis. Journal of Rheumatology 2: 265–269
Gerster J C, Baud C A, Lagier R, Bossina I, Fallet G H 1977 Tendon calcification in chondrocalcinosis. Arthritis and Rheumatism 20: 717–722
Graham R, Sutor D J, Mitchenor M B 1971 Crystal deposition in hyperparathyroidism. Annals of the Rheumatic Diseases 30: 597–604
Hamilton E B D 1976 Diseases associated with CPPD deposition diseases. Arthritis and Rheumatism 19: 353–357
Hamilton E B D 1981 Diseases associated with articular chondrocalcinosis. Rhumatologie 32: 457–462
Hamilton E B D 1981 Chondrocalcinosis and osteoarthritis. Epidemiology of osteoarthritis. Ciba-Geigy, Paris p 109–112
Hearn P R, Russell R G G, Elliott J C 1978 Formation product of calcium pyrophosphate crystals in vitro and the effect of iron salts. Clinical Science and Molecular Medicine 54:29P
Howell D S 1981 Calcium pyrophosphate deposition disease. In: Kelly W N, Harris E D, Ruddy S, Sledge S (eds) Textbook of rheumatology. Saunders, Philadelphia p 1438–1454
Jacobelli S, McCarty D J, Silcox D C et al 1973 Calcium pyrophosphate dihydrate crystal deposition in neuropathic joints. Four cases of polyarticular involvement. Annals of Internal Medicine 79: 340–347
Jung A, Russell R G G, Bisaz S, Morgan D B, Fleisch H 1970 Fate of intravenously injected pyrophosphate-^{32}P in dogs. American Journal of Physiology 218: 1757–1764
Kohn N N, Hughes R E, McCarty D J, Faires J S 1962 The significance of calcium phosphate crystals in the synovial fluid of arthritic patients: the pseudogout syndrome. 11 Identification of crystals. Annals of Internal Medicine 56: 738–745
Lagier R, Baud C A 1968 Pathologic calcifications of the locomotor system. Position of chondrocalcinosis. In: Rapports et Communications. IV Symposium European des Tissues Calcifies, Bordeaux, 1967, p 109–113
Lust G, Nuki G, Seegmiller J E 1976 Inorganic pyrophosphate and proteoglycan metabolism in cultured human articular chondrocytes and fibroblasts. Arthritis and Rheumatism 19:479–487
McCarty D J 1972 Pseudogout, articular chondrocalcinosis. In: Hollander J L, McCarty D J (eds) Arthritis and allied conditions, 8th Edn. Lee & Febiger, p. 1140–1160
McCarty D J 1975 Diagnostic mimicry in arthritis. Patterns of joint involvement associated with calcium pyrophosphate dihydrate crystal deposits. Bulletin on the Rheumatic Diseases 25: 804–808
McCarty D J 1981 Calcium pyrophosphate dihydrate crystal deposition disease. Rheumatologie 18: 43–47
McCarty D J 1983 Crystals, joints and consternation. Annals of Rheumatic Diseases 42: 243–253
McCarty D J, Gatter R A 1964 Pseudogout syndrome (articular chondrocalcinosis). Bulletin on the Rheumatic Diseases 14: 331–334
McCarty D J, Gatter R A 1966 Recurrent acute inflammation associated with focal apatite crystal deposition. Arthritis and Rheumatism 9: 804–819
McCarty D J, Hollander J L 1961 Identification of urate crystals in gouty synovial fluid. Annals of Internal Medicine 54: 452–460
McCarty D J, Kohn N N, Faires J S 1962 The significance of calcium phosphate crystals in the synovial fluid of arthritis patients: the pseudogout syndrome. 1. Clinical aspects. Annals of Internal Medicine 56: 711–737
McCarty D J, Hogan J M, Gatter R A, Grossman M 1966 Studies on pathological calcifications in human cartilage. 1. Prevalence and types of crystal deposits in the menisci of two hundred cadavera. Journal of Bone and Joint Surgery 48A: 309–325
McCarty D J, Silcox D C, Coe F, Jacobelli S, Reiss E, Genart H, Ellman 1974 Diseases associated with calcium pyrophosphate dihydrate crystal deposition. American Journal of Medicine 56: 704–714
McCarty D J, Halverson P B, Carrera G F, Brewer B J, Kozin F 1981 'Milwaukee shoulder': association of

microspheroids containing hydroxyapatite crystals, active collagenase and neutral protease with rotator cuff defects. 1. Clinical aspects. Arthritis and Rheumatism 24: 464–473

McGuire M K B, Hearn P B, Russell R G G 1980 Calcium pyrophosphate crystals (their relevance to calcium pyrophosphate dihydrate crystal deposition disease, pseudogout, chondrocalcinosis and pyrophosphate arthropathy): Biochemical and physicochemical aspects. In: Maroudas, Holborrow (eds) Studies in joint diseases. Pitman, London, p 117–156

Marx S J, Spiegel A M, Levine M A, Lasker R D, Fox M An association between neonatal severe primary hyperparathyroidism and familial, hypocalcuric hypercalcemia in three kindreds. New England Journal of Medicine 1982 306: 257–63

Martel W, Champion C K, Thompson G R, Carter T L 1970 A roentgenologically distinctive arthropathy in some patients with pseudogout syndrome. American Journal of Roentgenology 109: 587–605

Menkes C J, Luton J P, Job C, Chanzy M O, Bricaire H, Delbarre F 1979 Hypothyroidism and chondrocalcinosis. 9th European Congress of Rheumatology, Wiesbaden, Abstract 239

Millazzo S C, Ahern M J, Cleland L G, Henderson D R F 1981 Calcium pyrophosphate dihydrate deposition disease and familial hypomagnesemia. Journal of Rheumatology 8: 767–771

Mitrovic D 1983 Pathology of articular deposition of calcium salts and their relationship to osteoarthrosis. Annals Rheumatic Diseases 42 (Suppl): 19–26

Moskowitz R W, Vertes V, Schwartz A, Marshall G, Friedman B 1969 Crystal induced inflammation associated with chronic renal failure and haemodialysis. American Journal of Medicine 47: 450–460

Nyulassy S, Stefanovic Sitaj S, Zitnan D 1976 HLA system in articular chondrocalcinosis. Arthritis and Rheumatism 19: 391–393

O'Duffy J D 1974 Hypophosphatasia associated with calcium pyrophosphate, dihydrate deposits in cartilage. Arthritis and Rheumatism 13: 381–388

O'Duffy J D 1976 Clinical studies of acute pseudogout attacks: comments on prevalence, predispositions and treatment. Arthritis and Rheumatism 19: 349–352

Paul H, Reginato A J, Schumacher H R 1983 Alizarin red S-staining as a screening test to detect calcium compounds in synovial fluid. Arthritis and Rheumatism 26: 191–200

Phelps P 1969 Polymorphonuclear leucocyte motility in vitro. III. Possible release of a chemotactic substance after phagocytosis of urate crystals by polymorphonuclear leucocytes. Arthritis and Rheumatism 12: 197–204

Phelps P 1970 Polymorphonuclear leucocyte, motility in vitro. IV. Colchicine inhibition of chemotactic activity formation after phagocytosis of urate crystals. Arthritis and Rheumatism 13: 1–9

Phelps P, Hawker C D 1973 Serum parathyroid hormone levels in patients with calcium pyrophosphate crystal deposition disease (chondrocalcinosis, pseudogout). Arthritis and Rheumatism 6: 590–596

Pritchard M H, Jessop J D 1977 Chondrocalcinosis in primary hyperparathyroidism. Influence of age, matabolic bone disease and parathyroidectomy. Annals of the Rheumatic Diseases 36: 146–151

Reginato A J 1976 Articular chondrocalcinosis in the Chiloe islanders. Arthritis and Rheumatis19: 395–404

Reginato A J, Valenzuela F, Martinez V 1970 Polyarticular and familial chondrocalcinosis. Arthritis and Rheumatism 13: 197–213

Resnick D, Utsinger P D 1974 The wrist arthropathy of pseudogout occurring with and without chondrocalcinosis. Radiology 113: 633–641

Resnick D et al 1977 Clinical, radiographic and pathological abnormalities in calcium pyrophosphate dihydrate deposition disease (CPPD): Pseudogout. Radiology 122: 1–16

Richards A J, Hamilton E B D 1974 Destructive arthropathy in chondrocalcinosis articularis. Annals of Rheumatic Diseases 33: 196–203

Richards A J, Hamilton E B D 1976 Spinal changes in idiopathic chondrocalcinosis articularis. Rheumatology and Rehabilitation 15: 138–142

Rickewaert A, Solnica J, Lanham C, deSe'ze S 1966 Manifestations articulaires de l'hyperparathyroidie. Presse medicale 74: 2599–2603

Ryan L M, Liang G, Kozin F 1982 Amyloid arthropathy: absence of a paraprotein and possible association with chondrocalcinosis. Journal of Rheumatology 9: 273–278

Schumacher H R 1975 Pathology of the synovial membrane in gout. Light and electron microscopy studies. Interpretation of crystals in electron micrographs. Arthritis and Rheumatism 18: 771–782

Schumacher H R, Somlyo A P, Tse R L, Mairer L 1977 Arthritis associated with apatite crystals. Annals Internal Medicine 87: 411–416

Schumacher H R, Miller J L, Ludivico C, Jessar R A 1981 Erosive arthritis associated with apatite crystal deposition. Arthritis and Rheumatism 24: 31–37

Schumacher H R, Cherian P V, Reginato A J, Bardin T, Rothfuss S 1983 Intra articular apatite deposition. Annals Rheumatic Disease 42 (Suppl): 54–59

Seegmiller J E, Faure G, Netter P, Galcher A, Lust G 1981 Elevated intracellular inorganic pyrophosphate in fibroblasts and lymphoblasts cultured from patients with dominantly inherited chondrocalcinosis. 15th International Congress Rheumatology, Paris, Abstract

Sitaj S, Zitnan D 1967 Spinal changes in chondrocalcinosis. Proceedings VI Congresses Europ en de Reumatologia 547–555

Stockman A, Darlington L G, Scott J T 1980 Frequency of chondrocalcinosis of the knees and avascular necrosis of the femoral heads in gout: a controlled study. Annals of the Rheumatic Diseases 35: 521–525

Tse R L, Phelps P 1970 Polymorphonuclear leucocyte motility in vitro. V. Release of chemotactic activity following phagocytosis of calcium pyrophosphate crystals diamond dust and urate crystals. Journal of Laboratory and Clinical Medicine 76: 403–415

Van Der Korst J L, Geerards J, Driessens F C M 1974 A hereditary type of idiopathic articular chondrocalcinosis. Survey of a pedigree. American Journal of Medicine 56: 307–314

Villiaumey J, Larget-Piet C, Di Menza C, Rotterdam M 1975 Caracteres, symptomatiques et evolutifs des destructions articulaires observees an cours de la chondrocalcinose. Revue du Rheumatisme 42: 263–273

Wallingford W R, McCarty D J 1971 Differential membranolytic effects of microcrystalline sodium urate and calcium pyrophosphate dihydrate. Journal of Experimental Medicine 133: 100–112

Weaver J B 1942 Calcification and ossification of the menisci. Journal of Bone and Joint Surgery 24: 873–882

Weissman G, Zurier R B, Spieler P J, Goldstein I M 1971 Mechanisms of lysosomal enzyme release from leucocytes exposed to immune complexes and other particles. Journal of Experimental Medicine 134: 149s–165s

Wilkins W E, Dieppe P A, Maddison P, Evison G 1982 Osteoarthritis and articular chondrocalcinosis in the elderly. Annals of the Rheumatic Diseases 40:516

Wilkins E, Dieppe P, Maddison P, Evison G 1983 Osteoarthritis and articular chondrocalcinosis in the elderly. Annals Rheumatic Diseases 42: 280–284

Zitnan D, Sit'aj S 1958 Muohopocetna familiarha kalcifikaaz artikularynch chrupick. Bratislavske lekarskelisty 38: 217–228

Zitnan D, Sit'aj S 1963 Chondrocalcinosis articularis. Annals of the Rheumatic Diseases 22: 142–170

Zitnan D, Sit'aj S 1976 Natural course of articular chondrocalcinosis. Arthritis and Rheumatism 19: 363–390

Zvaifler N J, Reefe W E, Black R L 1962 Articular manifestations in primary hyperparathyroidism. Arthritis and Rheumatism 5: 237–249

Arthritis in ochronosis, haemochromatosis and Wilson's disease

OCHRONOSIS

Ochronosis was the name given by Virchow in 1866 to describe the microscopic appearance of the pigment deposited in connective tissue in patients with alkaptonuria. These patients pass urine which turns brownish-black when alkali is added owing to the polymerisation of homogentisic acid. The urine also turns black on standing owing to oxidation taking place; staining of the nappies may be the first clue to the diagnosis. Bodeker (1859) isolated homogentisic acid from urine and Wolkow & Bauman in 1891 identified it as 2,5-dihydroxyphenylactic acid, which is an intermediate metabolite in the synthesis of the amino acids phenylalanine and tyrosine. Garrod (1908) in his classic paper on inborn errors of metabolism cited ochronosis as an example, and La Du et al (1958) were able to show that it was due to a specific enzyme defect. These patients have an absence of the enzyme homogentisic acid oxidase in the liver and kidney, the defect being transmitted by a single autosomal gene. Ochronosis and arthropathy used to occur in patients treated for long periods with dressings soaked in carbolic acid (Beddard, 1910) and have also been seen following the prolonged administration of quinacrine (Ludwig et al, 1963).

The deposits of the brownish-black ochronotic pigment are widespread (Lichenstein & Kaplan, 1954). They are found in the hyaline cartilage of joints and in the annulus fibrosus and nucleus pulposus of intervertebral discs. The tracheal cartilage and the cartilage of the nose and ears are also affected. Deposits are seen in the walls of medium-sized arteries, in the aorta and sometimes in the aortic and mitral valves. Symptomless deposits occur in the renal parenchyma, in the islets of the pancreas and there may be renal and prostatic calculi. The tympanic membrane may be discoloured and the cerumen black. Deafness may result from middle ear involvement. Scleral pigmentation is characteristic and there can be small deposits in the cornea. Deposits occur in the dermis, especially around the sweat glands in the axilla and groin. The sweat may contain homogentisic acid and results in staining of under-clothes.

Ochronosis is of worldwide distribution but large series have been reported from Czechoslovakia (Cervansky et al, 1959; Huttle, 1970). The literature was extensively reviewed by O'Brien et al (1963). The two most important manifestations are ochronotic spondylosis and ochronotic arthropathy affecting the large joints, especially the knee, hip and shoulder. They are commoner and more severe in males than in females and occur at an earlier age. Symptoms are rare before the 4th decade, when stiffness and low back pain may develop. At this stage symptoms are minimal but later on obliteration of the normal lumbar curve occurs, together with kyphosis of the dorsal spine. This leads to obvious deformity, the patient being bent forwards as in severe cases of ankylosing spondylitis. Tell-tale pigmentation of the ears, which become calcified and rigid, discolouration of the nasal cartilage or scleral pigmentation may suggest the diagnosis, but radiology is needed to show the characteristic spinal changes (Fig. 38.1). In a few cases rupture of an intervertebral disc may be a presenting feature (O'Brien et al, 1963; McCollum & Odum, 1965).

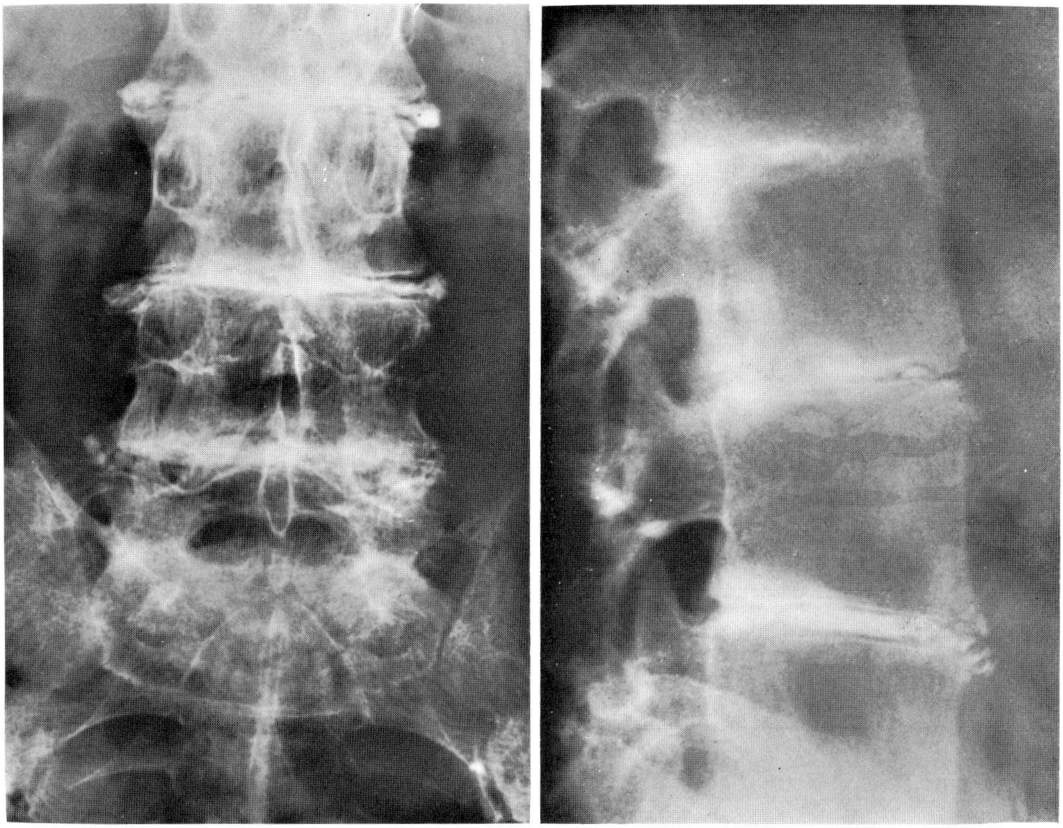

Fig. 38.1 Disc narrowing and calcification in ochronosis (case: Dr W. G. Wenley).

The radiological features of ochronotic spondylosis include calcification of multiple intervertebral discs, which has been shown by Bywaters et al (1970) to be hydroxyapatite. There have been isolated reports of calcium pyrophosphate crystal deposition in ochronosis (Bywaters et al, 1970; Steiger & Lagier, 1972; Rynes et al, 1975) but whether the association is fortuitous or directly related to the ochronosis is uncertain. The apatite deposits in the intervertebral discs affect both the annulus and the nucleus, contrasting with the calcification seen in pyrophosphate arthropathy, hyperparathyroidism and haemochromatosis, which is only in the annulus and is due to calcium pyrophosphate (Bywaters et al, 1971). The disc spaces in ochronotic spondylosis become uniformly narrowed and there is sclerosis of the vertebral plates adjacent to the disc spaces. Osteophytes occur but are not large and in late cases fusion of vertebral bodies is associated with obliteration of the disc spaces. Unlike ankylosing spondylitis the sacroiliac joints do not become fused.

The knee is the commonest peripheral joint to develop arthritis; symptoms develop at a later age then those of ochronotic spondylosis. Joint effusions are common and may contain mononuclear cells with pigment inclusions (Huttle, 1970). Hunter et al (1974) have described the 'ground pepper' sign, stressing that particles of pigmented cartilage can give a characteristic appearance to the joint fluid. Osteochondral loose bodies are sometimes found and are thought to be formed from particles of cartilage which break off into the joint fluid. Ossification in ligments adjacent to joints have also been reported. The symptoms, signs and radiological features are those of severe osteoarthritis. Pain and stiffness are later accompanied by limitation of movement and flexion contracture. Radiologically there is loss of joint space and

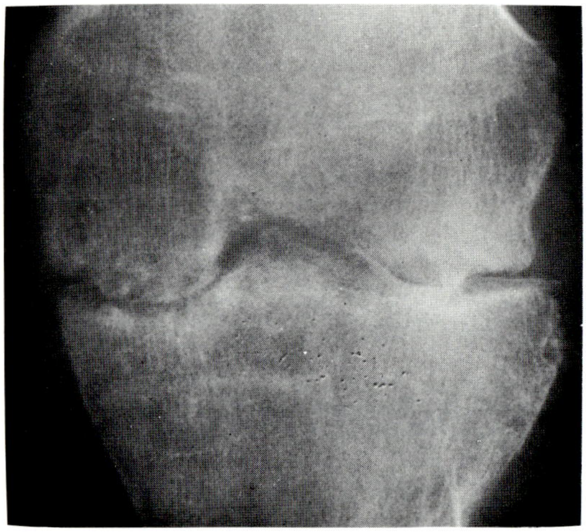

Fig. 38.2 Destructive arthritis of the knee joint in ochronosis (case: Dr W. G. Wenley).

prominent osteophyte formation. Destructive joint changes can occur but are unusual (Fig. 38.2). Shoulder and hip involvement is less frequent, but can be severe and disabling. The small joints of the hands and feet are not affected.

HAEMOCHROMATOSIS

Idiopathic haemochromatosis is an hereditary disorder of iron metabolism in which there is greatly increased absorption and deposition of iron, which leads to the characteristic pattern of tissue damage and clinical signs. The disease does not usually become manifest until after the age of 40, and is 10 times commoner in men than women. There is hepatic fibrosis, and later cirrhosis, cutaneous pigmentation, diabetes, testicular atrophy, cardiomyopathy and arthropathy. HLA typing of these patients has shown that the condition is determined by a locus closely linked with the A locus of the HLA complex on chromosome 6 (Bomford et al, 1977). HLA-A3 is significantly increased and the presence of this allele may be used to assign the putative haemochromatosis susceptibility allele in family studies. Serum iron levels are characteristically raised with a reduced and fully saturated total iron binding capacity. Serum ferritin levels which accurately reflect total body iron stores in idiopathic haemochromatosis are also markedly increased. Ferritin is the most readily available iron storage protein in which ferric oxide is combined with apoferritin, a large molecular weight protein. Iron stores may also be estimated by a chelating agent such as desferrioxamine. The diagnosis is confirmed by the finding of massive siderosis on liver biopsy. Haemochromatosis can also follow repeated blood transfusion and in some severe anaemias ineffective erythropoiesis leads to increased absorption and iron overload even in the absence of transfusion.

Clinical features of arthropathy

In 1964 Schumacher first suggested that a specific arthropathy might be associated with haemochromatosis, and since then many case reports and surveys confirm his initial observation (de Seze et al, 1964; Hamilton et al, 1968; Wardle & Patton 1969; Dymock et al, 1970). In our studies we found it in 31 of 54 male patients, which was similar to the incidence of 44% of 54 patients reported by Dorfman et al (1969). We have since followed up the progression of the disease over 10 years (Hamilton et al 1981).

The arthropathy presents as a degenerative non-inflammatory process, affecting first the small joints of the hands, but later large joints such as the hips, knees and shoulders can be involved, causing considerable disability.

The first symptoms of arthritis usually occur in the 2nd and 3rd metacarpophalangeal joints and are often more severe in the right hand than in the left. At first all that the patient complains of is that he gets minor twinges of pain when he flexes his fingers. He may notice bony swelling of the involved joints and on examining the metacarpophalangeal joints there is limitation of full flexion. Other finger joints may then be affected with resulting bony swelling and deformity, but ulnar deviation does not occur. The distribution of the joints involved resemble rheumatoid arthritis but the superficial clinical appearance of the individual joints is that of osteoarthritis. In the early stages the arthritis causes surprisingly little in the way of symptoms and one may only detect it on careful clinical examination. Gordon & Little (1973) have stressed that it can be the presenting feature of haemochromatosis. In our series 5 patients had symptoms of arthritis, occurring before other symptoms of haemochromatosis, in 5 the initial symptoms occurred together and in the remaining

21 patients they occurred from 1–24 years afterwards (Dymock et al, 1970). In one-third of those patients with arthritis, large joints are involved and the hip has been the joint that has caused most pain and disability. In a recent retrospective survey of 96 patients we found that 7 of them had severe hip disease and 5 had required surgery.

Superimposed on the relatively benign and slowly progressive degenerative joint disease there may be attacks of acute synovitis due to crystals of calcium pyrophosphate. These attacks of pseudogout are usually in the knees, but if a number of joints are involved at the same time the clinical picture may resemble active rheumatoid arthritis, and a number of patients have been mistakenly treated with gold or corticosteroids.

Radiology

The earliest radiographic change to occur in the metacarpal heads is the appearance of small cysts 1–3 mm in diameter. Roughening, irregularity and apparent crumbling or destruction of the metacarpal heads then occurs, which is possibly due to infraction of the cysts (Fig. 38.3). There may also be sclerosis of the metacarpal heads, and narrowing of the joint space is a frequent finding. Prominent cyst formation is sometimes seen in the carpal bones, and in the shoulder subchondral sclerosis and irregularity of the articular surfaces of the humerus can occur. In the hips there are subarticular cystic changes with loss of cartilage, and occasionally dense calcification of the fibrocartilage of the acetabular labrum with deepening of the acetabular cup. In the knee cystic changes are not seen and sclerosis is rare, but loss of cartilage and lipping of the margins of the knee joints are common.

In addition to these features of a degenerative and destructive arthritis, chondrocalcinosis is a striking radiological feature. We found it in over two-thirds of the patients with arthritis and in 6 without other evidence of joint disease. It was seen in the fibrocartilage meniscus in 39 of 108 knees and in the hyaline cartilage of the knee in 17 joints. The next commonest site was in 21 wrists. It was present in 12 hip joints and was in the symphysis pubis 9 times. 7 of 47 patients had calcification in one or more intervertebral discs (Fig. 38.4) and all of these 7 patients had arthropathy and chondro-

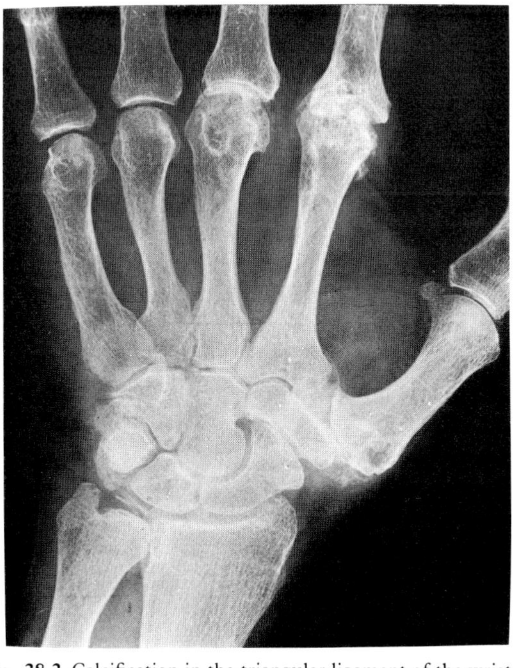

Fig. 38.3 Calcification in the triangular ligament of the wrist and arthritis of the 2nd and 3rd metacarpophalangeal joints in haemochromatosis.

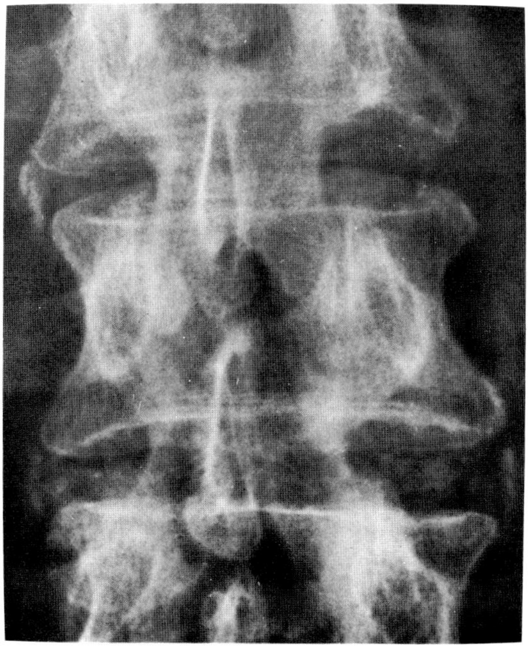

Fig. 38.4 Disc calcification in the annulus fibrosus in idiopathic haemochromatosis.

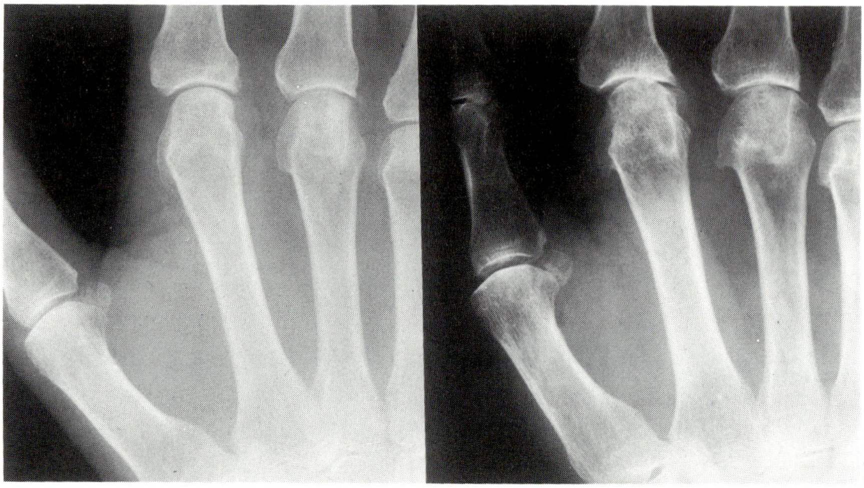

a b

Fig. 38.5 Serial radiographs of metacarpophalangeal joints in haemochromatosis. (a) 1973. (b) 1978.

calcinosis in peripheral joints. The lumbar spine has been examined in detail in 6 patients who came to autopsy (Bywaters et al, 1971) and in 4 calcification was present in the fibres of the annulus fibrosus. Crystals of calcium pyrophosphate dihydrate identified by their shape and their positive birefringence, and in one case by X-ray diffraction, were laid down along the lines of the outer annular fibres. Extra-articular sites of calcification included the Achilles tendon, plantar fascia and ligamentum flavum.

The incidence, severity and radiological progression of the arthritis, and chondrocalcinosis has been recorded over ten years in 18 patients, and it did not get less or disappear, despite adequate venesection therapy (Figs 38.5, 38.6). The chondrocalcinosis spread to involve other joints and became more severe, being found in 7 patients initially and in 13 subsequently. The knees and wrists were the joints most frequently involved (Hamilton et al, 1981).

Pathogenesis

The presence of iron in the synovium was first recorded by Sheldon (1935). We have examined synovium obtained by needle biopsy in 22 patients

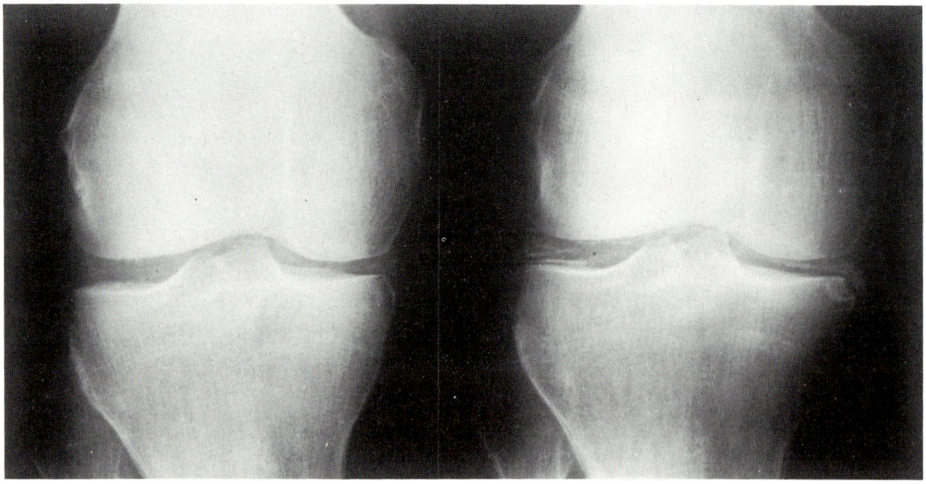

a b

Fig. 38.6 Serial radiographs of right knee in haemochromatosis. (a) 1967. (b) 1978.

and at autopsy in 5 patients and have related the findings to the clinical and radiological evidence of arthropathy and to the measurement of liver and total body iron stores (Walker et al, 1972). Iron deposits were shown on histological examination in 11 patients and when present were always within synovial lining cells as well as sometimes being within phagocytic cells in the stroma. Intimal cell hyperplasia was found in 8, villus formation in 7 and an inflammatory cell infiltrate in 2 cases. No correlation was found between the iron deposits and histological abnormalities and the radiological evidence of an arthropathy. Iron was found in 8 of 19 patients with an arthropathy compared with 3 of 8 patients without an arthropathy. A definite relationship did exist between the presence of synovial iron and the stage of treatment. Four of 18 patients who had completed venesection had synovial iron present, whereas it was found in 7 of 9 untreated patients. The mean chelatable iron store (Smith et al, 1969) in those patients with synovial iron was considerably higher at 1198 μg/kg than the corresponding value of 470 μg/kg for patients in whom there was no synovial iron. In 17 patients in whom the comparison could be made there was also a significant direct relationship between the grading of liver iron and the presence of synovial iron. Using electron microscope Schumacher (1972) has shown that the iron is deposited in the synthetic type B synovial cell to a greater extent than in the phagocytic or type A cell. We have not found iron in cartilage but it has been reported by Sheldon (1935) and Muirden & Senator (1968). De Seze et al (1966) demonstrated the presence of haemosiderin in the chondrocytes of articular cartilage, and Schumacher (1982) using electron microscopy found particles typical of ferritin in both intact and degenerating chondrocytes in 3 or 4 patients who had cartilage biopsies. Both apatite and CPPD crystals were detected in some of the samples, but not in any direct morphologic relationship to the iron deposits.

In our patients with arthritis the mean age at which the joint symptoms presented was 56 years. This age of onset was not related to the duration of time other symptoms of haemochromatosis had been present, but the age of the patient when the first symptom of haemochromatosis appeared was an important factor determining the onset of arthritis. In the arthritic patients the mean age at which the first symptoms of haemochromatosis were noted was 51.9 years compared with 43.4 years in the non-arthritic. The incidence of chondrocalcinosis due to CPPD deposition in hyperparathyroidism is also age-related (Dodds & Steinbach, 1968; Pritchard & Jessop, 1977). There is no evidence that treatment of haemochromatosis improves the joint disease, and 16 of our patients first developed their symptoms after the completion of venesection therapy (Dymock et al, 1970).

It seems likely that the joint damage in haemochromatosis is related to iron overload, especially as we have seen identical joint lesions in secondary haemochromatosis in a man with hereditary spherocytosis who developed characteristic changes in the 2nd and 3rd metacarpophalangeal joints as well as chondrocalcinosis in the hips and knee joint. Berry & Miller (1973) have also reported a similar case of haemochromatosis and chondrocalcinosis in hereditary spherocytosis.

The role of iron salts acting as nucleating agents for crystal formation has been tested in crystal growth in vitro by Hearn et al (1978) and Hearn & Russell (1980). They found that low concentrations of ferric salts promoted crystal growth. The amount of pyrophosphate needed for crystal formation was reduced to one-quarter of that required in the absence of iron. In haemochromatosis there is also evidence to suggest that once present the removal of such crystals may be inhibited by iron. McCarty et al (1981) induced synovial haemosiderosis in rabbits knees by repeated injections of autologous blood. Synthetic triclinic CPPD crystals, radiolabelled with ^{85}Sr and ^{45}Ca were then injected into these joints and the clearance rate of these crystals was compared with that in normal joints. It was significantly reduced by the synovial haemosiderosis suggesting inhibition of intracellular pyrophosphatases by iron, and confirming their earlier work that pyrophosphatase in erythrocytes was inhibited by ferrous ions (McCarty et al, 1970, 1972).

Having described the clinical features and pathology of the arthritis found in patients with idiopathic haemochromatosis, we must continue to ask if these findings are specific for iron overload. I am sure this is not so as the characteristic changes seen in the metacarpophalangeal joints, especially the 2nd and 3rd, have been described in some patients with uncomplicated pyrophosphate arthropathy by Martel et al (1970) and by Resnick & Utsinger (1974). However, they do appear to be seen in much increased frequency in patients with haemochromatosis (Adamason et al, 1983) although the explanation for this is not readily apparent. We also did not find them (1975) when the hands of 50 patients with idiopathic chondrocalcinosis were matched with 100 control subjects.

WILSON'S DISEASE

This is a rare disorder of copper metabolism which is inherited as an autosomal recessive, and the clinical features present during childhood or early adult life. It is characterised by low ceruloplasmin and serum copper levels and increased absorption and retention of copper. Copper is deposited in the basal ganglia and in the liver. This results in neurological symptoms such as tremor, rigidity, dysarthria and inco-ordination, and in cirrhosis of the liver. Renal tubular lesions also occur and a diagnostic feature is the well-known Kayser-Fleisher ring of brown pigment at the corneal margin. Lesions of bones and joints are less well recognised than are the other manifestations of the disease as they are not often the cause of symptoms and are often only detected on radiological examination.

Osteoporosis is a prominent feature and is accompanied by an increased incidence of fractures. Some patients show features of rickets and osteomalacia, thought to be secondary to the renal tubular lesions (Finby & Bearn, 1958). Small bony fragments adjacent to joint margins have been described by Rosenoer & Mitchell (1959) and Mindelzun et al (1970). The suggestion that they may be related to the tremor remains unproven. Feller & Schumacher (1972) describe 4 adult patients with similar ossified bodies adjacent to the wrist joint and suggested that they might be accessory skeletal elements or calcifications in bursae or tendons. There are several case reports of osteochondritis dissecans affecting the femoral condyles or the medial aspect of the talus, and chondromalacia patellae is another frequent finding. Some joints show subchondral or subcortical sclerosis as well as bone irregularity. Premature osteoarthritic changes are often seen, especially in the wrists, the metacarpophalangeal joints and in the knees. Golding & Walsh (1977) found radiological evidence of mild or moderate premature osteoarthritis in a survey of 32 patients aged 7–45 years.

Chondrocalcinosis is rare. It was first described by Boudin et al (1963) and was seen in the knee joints of two patients by Feller & Schumacher (1972). In haemochromatosis and hyperparathyroidism the incidence of chondrocalcinosis is age-related and its relative infrequency in Wilson's disease may be explained by manifestations of the disease presenting in children or early adult life, and until the advent of penicillamine treatment there have been few long-term survivors.

Synovial biopsies were taken from the knees of 7 patients by Kaklamanis & Spengos (1973) who found microvilli formation and intimal cell hyperplasia, as well as chronic inflammatory cell infiltrate in 6 patients. No copper was demonstrated, nor were crystals of calcium pryophosphate found. They did not find any correlation between such synovial changes and the various radiographic abnormalities they detected.

The mechanism of the various joint changes remains unexplained although the tremor has been implicated and, of course, some patients have associated osteoporosis or osteomalacia. A possible explanation remains the direct action of copper on bone or cartilage, although short-term copper over-loading experiments in the rate have not been shown to produce any damage (Wolff, 1960).

REFERENCES

Adamson T C, Resnick C S, Guerra J, Vint V C, Weisman M H, Resnick D 1983 Hand and wrist arthropathies of haemachromatosis and calcium pyrophosphate deposition disease: distinct radiographic features. Radiology 147: 377–381

Atkins C J, McIvor J, Smith P M, Hamilton E, Williams R (1970) Chondrocalcinosis and arthropathy; Studies in haemochromatosis and in idiopathic chondrocalcinosis. Quarterly Journal of Medicine 34: 71–82

Beddard A P 1910 Ochronosis associated with carboluria.

Quarterly Journal of Medicine 3: 329–336
Bensasson M, Dorfman H, Parez-Busquier M, Solnica J, Mery C, Kahn M F, de Seze S 1975 Etude radiographique de la main dans 50 cas de chondrocalcinose articulaire primative. Comparison avec une serie de 100 termoins. Revue du Rheumatisme et des Maladies Osteo-Articulaires 42: 3–11
Berry E M, Miller J P 1973 Hereditary spherocytosis, haemochromatosis, diabetes mellitus and chondro calcinosis. Proceedings of the Royal Society of Medicine, 66: 9–10.
Boedeker C W 1859 Ueber das Alcapton; ein neuer Beitrag zur Frage: welche Staffe des Harus koennen Kupferreduction bewirken? Zeitschrifg fur Rationelle Medizin 7: 130–145
Bomford A, Eddleston A L W F, Kennedy L, Batchelor H R, Williams R 1977 Histocompatibility antigens as markers of abnormal iron metabolism in patients with idiopathic haemochromatosis and their relatives. Lancet, 327–329
Boudin G, Pepin B, Hubault A 1963 Les arthropathies de la maladie de Wilson. Bulletin et Memoires de la Societe Medicale des hopitaux de Paris 114: 617–622.
Bywaters E G L, Dorling J, Sutor J 1970 Ochronotic densification. Annals of the Rheumatic Diseases 29:563
Bywaters E G L, Hamilton E B D, Williams R 1971 The spine in idiopathic haemochromatosis. Annals of the Rheumatic Diseases 30: 453–465
Cervansky J, Sit'aj S, Urbanek T 1959 Alkaptonuria and ochronosis. Journal of Bone and Joint Surgery 41A: 1169–1182
Dodd W J, Steinbach H L 1968 Primary hyperparathyroidism and articular cartilage calcification. American Journal of Roentogenology 104: 884–892
Dorfmann H, Solnica J, Di Menza C L, Seze S de 1969 Les arthropathies des haemochromatoses. Semaine des Hopitaux de Paris, 45: 516–523
Dymock I W, Hamilton E B D, Laws J W, Williams R 1970 Arthropathy of haemochromatosis. Clinical and radiological analysis of 63 patients with iron overload. Annals of the Rheumatic Diseases, 29: 469–476
Feller E R, Schumacher H R 1972 Osteoarticular changes in Wilson's disease. Arthritis and Rheumatism, 15: 259–266
Fielding J 1965 Differential ferrioxamine test for measuring chelatable body iron. Journal of Clinical Pathology 18: 88–97
Finby N, Bearn A G 1958 Roentgenographic abnormalities of the skeletal system in Wilson's disease (hepatolenticular degeneration). American Journal of Roentgenology 79: 603–611
Garrod A E 1908 The Croonian lectures of inborn errors of metabolism, Lecture 11. Alkaptonuria. Lancet 2: 73–79
Golding D N, Walshe J M, Arthropathy of Wilson's disease. Study of clinical and radiological features in 32 patients. Annals of the Rheumatic Diseases 36: 99–111
Gordon D A, Little H A 1973 The arthropathy of haemochromatosis without haemochromatosis. Arthritis and Rheumatism 16: 305–512
Hamilton E, Williams R, Barlow K A, Smith P M 1968 The arthropathy of idiopathic haemochromatosis. Quarterly Journal of Medicine 37: 171–182
Hamilton E B D, Bomford A B, Laws J W, Williams R 1981 The natural history of arthritis in idiopathic haemochromatosis Quarterly Journal of Medicine 50: 321–329
Hearn P R, Russell R G G, 1980 Formation of calcium pyrophosphate crystals in vitro. Implications for calcium pyrophosphate crystal deposition disease (pseudogout). Annals of the Rheumatic Diseases 38: 222–227
Hearn P R, Russell R G G, Elliott J C, 1978 Formation product of calcium pyrophosphate crystals in vitro and the effect of iron salts. Clinical Science Molecular Medicine 54:29
Hunter T, Gordon D A, Ogryzlo M A 1974 The ground pepper sign of synovial fluid: a new diagnostic finding in ochronosis. Journal of Rheumatology 1: 45–53
Huttle S 1970 Synovial effusion: Part 1. Acta Rheumatologica et Balneologica Pistiniana 5
Kaklamanis P, Spengos M, 1973 Osteoarticular changes and synovial biopsy findings in Wilson's Disease. Annals of the Rheumatic Disease 32: 422–427
La Du B N, Zannoni V G, Laster L, Seegmiller J E, 1958 The nature of the defect in tyrosine metabolism in alcaptonuria Journal of Biological Chemistry 230: 251–260
Lichtenstein L, Kaplan L, 1954 Hereditary ochronosis: patholgic changes observed in two necropsied cases. American Journal of Pathology 30: 99–125
Ludwig G D, Tools J F, Wood J C 1963 Ochronosis from quinacrine (Atabrine). Annals of Internal Medicine 59: 378–384
Martel W, Champion C K, Thompson G R, Carter T L, 1970 A roentgenologically distinctive arthropathy in some patients with pseudogout syndrome. American Journal of Roentgenology 109: 587–605
McCarty D J, Pepe P F 1972 Erythrocyte neutral inorganic pyrophosphatase in pseudogout. Journal of Laboratory and Clinical Medicine 79: 277–284
McCarty D J, Pepe P F, Solomon S D, Cobb J 1970 Inhibition of human erythrocyte pyrophosphatase activity by calcium, cupric and ferrous ions. Arthritis and Rheumatism 13:336
McCarty D J, Palmer D W, Garancis J C, 1981 Clearance of calcium pyrophosphatase dihydrate crystals in vivo. 111 Effects of synovial haemosiderosis. Arthritis and Rheumatism 24: 706–710
McCollum D E, Odom G L, 1965 Alkaptonuria, ochronosis and low-back pain. Journal of Bone and Joint Surgery 47A: 1389–1392
Mindelzun R, Elkin M, Scheinberg I H, Sternlieb I, 1970 Skeletal changes in Wilson's disease: A radiological study. Radiology 94: 127–132
Muirden K D, Senator G B, 1968 Iron in the synovial membrane in rheumatoid arthritis and other joint disease. Annals of the Rheumatic Diseases 27: 38–48
O'Brien W M, La Du B N, Bunim J L, 1963 Biochemical, pathologic and clinical aspects of alcaptonuria, ochronosis and ochronotic arthropathy. American Journal of Medicine 34: 813–838
Pritchard M H, Jessop J D, 1977 Chondrocalcinosis in primary hyperparathyroidism. Influence of age, metabolic bone disease and parathyroidectomy. Annals Rheumatic Diseases 36: 146–151
Resnick D, Utsinger P D, 1974 The wrist arthropathy of 'pseudogout' occurring with and without chondrocalcinosis. Radiology 113: 633–641
Rosenoer V M, Mitchell R C, 1959 Skeletal changes in Wilson's disease (hepatolenticular degeneration). British Journal of Radiology 32: 805–809
Schumacher H R 1964 Haemochromatosis and arthritis. Arthritis and Rheumatism 7: 41–50

Schumacher H R 1972 Ultrastructural characteristics of the synovial membrane in idiopathic haemochromatoses. Annals of the Rheumatic Diseases, 31: 465–473

Schumacher H R 1982 Articular cartilage in the degenerative arthropathy of haemochromatosis. Arthritis and Rheumatism 25: 1460–1468

Seze S, de Hubault A, Welfling J, Kahn M F, Solnica J, 1964 Les arthropathies des Haemochromatoses. Revue du Rhumatisme 31: 2472–2481

Seze S, de Hubault A, Kahn M F, Welfling J, Jaffres R, Mitrovic D, Solnica J, 1966 Les arthropathies des haemochromatoses. Semaine des hopitaux de Paris 42: 2472–2482

Sheldon J H, 1935 Haemochromatosis. Oxford University Press, London

Smith P M, Lester A J, Miller J P G, Dymock I W, Pitcher C S, Williams R, 1969 The differential ferrioxamine test in the management of idiopathic haemochromatosis. Lancet 2: 402–405

Walker R J, Dymock I W, Ansell I D, Hamilton E B D, Williams R, 1972 Synovial biopsy in haemochromatosis arthropathy. Annals of the Rheumatic Diseases 31: 98–102

Wardle E N, Patton J T, 1969 Bone and joint changes in haemochromatosis. Annals of the Rheumatic Diseases 28: 15–23

Wolff S M, 1960 Copper deposition in the rat. Archives of Pathology 69: 217–223

P.J.L. Holt

Endocrine disorders

The endocrine hormones permeate the body and regulate the function of many organs and tissues often widely dispersed. It is to be expected that both increased or decreased function of the endocrine glands may result in symptoms within the locomotor system or may be associated with locomotor symptoms as part of a common disease process. Conversely, hormones are used as replacement therapy, pharmacologically to suppress inflammatory processes, or to regulate bone and connective tissue activity. The pathophysiology of these endocrine dependent syndromes described is ill-understood and in many cases more than one process (or at different times, different processes) are involved. However, two main areas may be considered — inflammation and its associated processes, and connective tissue metabolism.

Throughout life normal endocrine gland function alters and the effects of hormone dysfunction vary with the age of onset. Pregnancy is a special example of a reversible physiological state, in which the hormone changes are predictable, but where the physical results vary. Alteration of hormone production may be influenced in many ways — stress, sleep, nutrition. Rovensky et al (1981) have shown growth hormone production to increase and cortisol to decrease after raising the core temperature in thermal baths.

The rarity and ill defined symptomatology of these disorders often lead to misdiagnosis. Hence the importance of clearly defining the clinical features since the symptoms often arise from extra-articular structures, though the patient and often the doctor may misinterpret these as of articular origin. Stiffness after rest is characteristic of inflammatory synovitis; it is also found in the thighs and calf muscles in hypothyroidism. Muscular weakness and fatigue as found in inflammatory arthritis occur in several of the endocrine syndromes to be described.

No attempt will be made to discuss the metabolic pathways involved nor to enter into the more specialised controversies of cause and effect since the basic facts on which these are based are rapidly changing and an intimate knowledge is not necessary for the diagnosis and supervision of these syndromes.

THE ADENOHYPOPHYSIS

Growth hormone (somatotrophin) has a marked and rapid anabolic effect resulting in protein synthesis principally in the form of collagen. Associated with this is a cellular proliferation, particularly of fibroblasts, and an increase in body nitrogen, calcium and phosphorus but no obvious alteration in alkaline phosphatase activity. Growth hormone does not appear to act directly on the cartilage cells but via a plasma component, somatomedin (sulphation factor) (Salmon & Du Vall, 1970; Sledge, 1973) which is a large polypeptide probably produced by the liver in response to growth hormone (Hall, 1971). Since somatomedin has a longer plasma half-life than growth hormone, it has a more prolonged action than the intermittently secreted growth factor (Van Wyk & Underwood, 1978).

Secretion of growth hormone is under the control of the hypothalamus which is itself innervated from the mid brain when a variety of impulses influence secretion. Thus emotional and metabolic pathways are different and sleep induced growth hormone release is produced by a different pathway from hypoglycaemia induced growth hormone release. Recently it has been established that endorphins, which are usually associated with elevation of the pain threshold, may release growth hormone and other pituitary hormones such as ACTH. It has been suggested that this may be part of the general adaption reaction to stress.

Fluctuations of serum growth hormone occur during the day in response to many stimuli, the main secretion occurring during the early phases of sleeping. After adolescence these bursts of secretion become less frequent and thus the total amount secreted daily falls, although the basal levels of growth hormone production remain relatively unchanged and the pituitary can easily be stimulated to produce additional growth hormone until late in life (Cartilidge et al, 1970).

The growth of skeleton and connective tissue is symmetrical even when excessive.

In gigantism and acromegaly the diurnal rhythm is lost with a raised and more continuous secretion throughout the 24 hours, amounting either to a modest increase in basal levels or very gross elevation of production. Occasionally the hypersecretion continues to occur in pulses. Serum from these patients will stimulate human fetal cartilage chondrocytes to grow (Ashton & Francis, 1978).

Before epiphyses close the syndrome of pituitary gigantism is produced, due principally to increased longitudinal growth which may be associated with aches and pains and postural defects but no clear-cut rheumatic syndromes. After closure of the epiphyses, longitudinal growth is no longer possible and a completely different picture — acromegaly — results.

No evidence of autoimmunity exists in this disease nor is there any association with other rheumatic diseases. No significant rheumatic complications of hypopituitism are known.

ACROMEGALIC ARTHROPATHY

The first clinical descriptions are those of Fritzsche & Klebs (1884), and Marie (1886) who gave the name (acral = distal parts); Minkowski (1887) and Broca (1888) described pituitary adenosis, the usual underlying cause of the syndrome. However, pathological descriptions of the skeletal features have been scarce until the work of Kellgren et al (1952), Bluestone et al (1971) and Deterbeck et al (1973).

The physiological functions of the pituitary gland were demonstrated by Aschner (1909) who produced growth arrest in young dogs by hypophysectomy and later Evans & Long (1921) demonstrated that pituitary extracts would restore normal growth to hypophysectomised animals and in excess gigantism.

Clinical features

The only significant (and uncommon) rheumatological complication of gigantism is slipped femoral epiphyses. The rheumatic manifestations of acromegaly always occur during the course of established systemic disease. Both sexes are affected in about equal degree and symptoms start from the age of 20 years onwards, many in the 3rd and 4th decades. The history of acromegaly is usually long since the features are insidious in onset and missed. In Davidoff's series (1926) of 100 cases the diagnosis was not made until some ten years after symptoms could be retrospectively recognised, and arthropathy was not mentioned in this series. Thus there may be the typical facies, thick loose skin, large extremities, general massive build with dorsal kyphosis and hypertension, though none of these may be prominent. An element of depression is often present leading to difficulty in evaluating the severity of the symptomatology. Rheumatic symptoms may occur at both early or late stages of the disease and may persist after the hyperpituitarism has been successfully treated. In many cases the signs of an arthropathy are only detected when specifically looked for and the signs, particularly crepitus, may be out of proportion to the symptoms. The retention and indeed excessive range of joint movement may be misleading. The characteristic tendency to hypermobility, in spite of articular cartilage increase which should produce tighter joints, implies that it is probably mainly due to laxity of para-articular structures.

Five types of rheumatic complaints occur, symptoms of carpal tunnel compression being the commonest, followed by lower backache, peripheral joint pain and Raynaud's phenomenon either singularly or in combination.

Rheumatic complaints in acromegaly
Low backache
Limb arthropathy
Compression neuropathies
Neuromuscular symptoms
Raynaud's phenomenon.

Pain in the jaw associated with a clicking tempero-mandibular joint occurs and is presumably due to the hypermobility and thickened articular cartilages.

Backache

About half the patients with acromegaly suffer from backache, mainly affecting the lumbosacral spine but occasionally involving the rest of the spine (Bluestone et al, 1971). It is usually non-traumatic in origin, of insidious onset and can occur from adolescence on. The range of spinal and hip movements of the acromegalic are maintained into later life and even increased, compared to the normal population where they tend to decrease, patients in the 6th decade often touching their toes with ease (Fig. 39.1). Lateral movement of the spine is also good. This increased spinal movement is found even in the presence of severe backache and local tenderness and is a highly suggestive and characteristic feature. Rigidity and splinting of the spine are not found. Pain in the kyphotic dorsal region is rare and in this part of the spine movement is not increased. Straight leg raising is normal or increased unless hip disease is present. Nerve root compression symptoms or signs referred to the limbs are unusual, tendon reflexes and sensation being intact and muscle weakness difficult to assess.

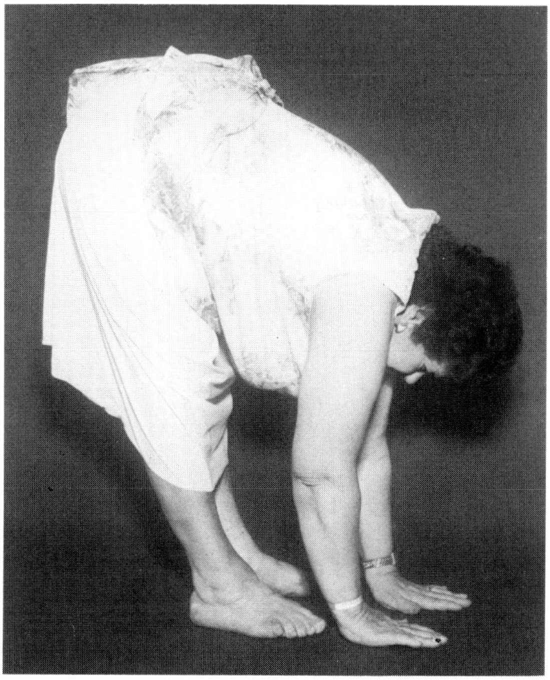

Fig. 39.1 Acromegalic woman aged 70 with back and knee pain. Note mobility of hips, spine and wrists.

Neck movements are usually normal and neck pain is not prominent, though supraclavicular pain may occur.

The pathogenesis of the backache is unknown, but it may be related to the retention of disc height and turgor allowing at least normal, and perhaps excessive, back movement for this age-group, associated with irregular cartilage growth of the end-plate as found elsewhere. Degenerative changes, osteophytosis and ossification of cartilage and ligaments may also contribute. To what extend the back muscles share in the generalised weakness leading to instability, is unknown.

Limb arthropathy

Articular changes are found principally in the larger joints, the knees, shoulders and hips — in that order. The ankle is surprisingly infrequently a problem. Crepitation occurs in the knees and shoulders in the majority of patients with a long history of acromegaly. Typically it is coarse in nature and continuous throughout the range of movement. The association of crepitation throughout movement of the shoulder or knee with little or no pain or other evidence of arthritis is very suggestive of acromegaly. Occasionally a pronounced catch may be felt in the arc of movement of a joint; some of these symptoms may be due to soft tissues rubbing over osteophytes. Some enlargement of the knee due to both fluid, synovial and periarticular thickenning is common. Occasionally osteophytes may be felt. Localised tenderness over the menisci may occur but tests of meniscal integrity (e.g. McMurray's test) are usually negative. The patella is often well clear of the femoral condyle in contradistinction to osteoarthrosis and may be placed more cephalically, suggesting patella alta. A prepatellar bursa is not uncommon.

Symptoms are surprisingly mild and rare, probably due to the relatively thick cartilage present. The initial episodes are usually acute, isolated and temporary, primarily affecting the knee and associated with the appearance of a marked increase in the size of the synovial effusion. These episodes, often attributed to trauma, are sometimes associated with transient locking of the joint. Conversely these patients may complain that their knees 'give way'. Later weakness of the thighs, together with the weight of the upper body, leads to difficulty in rising from a chair. Occasionally mild, more continuous, but ill-defined symptoms are found in the hands though whether these represent a true acromegalic arthropathy or an exacerbation of an underlying osteoarthrosis is uncertain. Full mobility and stability of the joints are maintained unless effusions are large or degenerative joint disease has supervened, when gross joint destruction associated with continuous and severe pain, indistinguishable from osteoarthrosis, occurs. This is most marked in the hip joint which is therefore most likely to present a serious problem. Fisher (1978) has described 'capping' i.e. a layer of bone around the humoral and femoral heads; a preceding slipped epiphysis may contribute to the joint destruction. When degeneration of the knee cartilage occurs, loss of joint space results in angulation and usually a varus deformity, though, as distinct from osteoarthrosis, extension of the knee is not usually lost.

Foot problems seldom arise. Laxity of the forefoot tissue can result in splaying and pressure pain but seldom arthritis.

Compression neuropathies

Connective tissue and bony overgrowth may produce ill-defined paraesthesiae in the limbs. The most characteristic expression of these compression neuropathies is the carpal tunnel syndrome, found in about 50% of cases and usually bilateral. Nocturnal exacerbation is not so prominent as in other forms of this syndrome. Moreover muscle wasting in the hand or gross neurological loss is uncommon. The symptoms characteristically are not relieved by splinting or local injections of hydrocortisone but rapidly disappear after successful hypophysectomy, the latter suggesting that fluid retention probably plays a part.

Spinal cord compression with long tract signs has been reported in acromegaly (Horenstein et al, 1971). Fluctuation of the symptoms and signs with treatment of the pituitary adenoma occurred. Myelograms and histological examination of the specimens removed suggest that the narrowing of the vertebral canal is a combination of vertebral body remodelling and exuberant soft tissue overgrowth within the vertebral canal. In a single case removal of soft tissue and adequate control of pituitary function appeared to prevent recurrence of spinal compression (Longson & Isherwood, 1975) (Fig. 39.2).

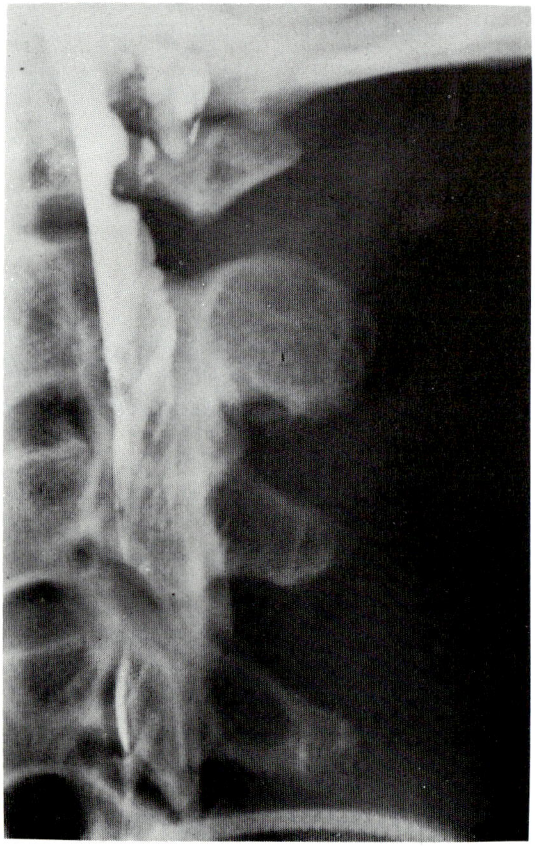

Fig. 39.2 Acromegaly. Cervical myelogram. Note irregularity of the radio-opaque column and its separation from the posterior vertebral body and neural arch by soft tissue thickening. (By courtesy of Drs Longson and Isherwood.)

Neuromuscular manifestations
Many patients with acromegaly complain of fatigue and lethargy, thought to be due largely to their disease process, though fatigue and a depressive element may also contribute, especially with the onset of hypopituitarism. Muscle wasting is not normally found, the clinical impression being of enlarged, but weak, muscles, most marked proximally. However, a myopathy with mild proximal muscle weakness has been demonstrated in 6 out of 11 patients with acromegaly. 5 patients had a raised creatinine phosphokinase; the average mean action potential duration was shorter and in 5 cases hypertrophy of type I and II muscle fibres and in some cases segmental necrosis was found (Mastalgia et al, 1970; Nagulesparen et al, 1976). The significance of this is uncertain.

Kellgren et al (1952) demonstrated increased connective tissue formation between nerve fibres in acromegaly. More recently Lewis (1972) has shown a peripheral neuropathy in two cases of pituitary gigantism and suggested that endoneural fibroblasts, like other fibroblasts, may be affected by growth hormone and that the consequent connective tissue overgrowth may produce the neuropathy. The peripheral nerves may be palpable (Low et al, 1974), but this is rare in the author's experience and paraesthesia has not resulted from compression of thickened nerve. There is no evidence of a direct hormonal effect on nerves and it is unlikely that the impaired glucose tolerance is important (Jadresic et al, 1982).

Raynaud's phenomenon
This is a surprisingly frequent complaint — about 21% of patients — but is rarely observed under hospital conditions. It usually involves the hands and its causation is unknown, there being no evidence of vascular disease in acromegaly.

Pathology
Synovial fluid from these patients is of non-inflammatory type analogous to that of osteoarthrosis, viscid, clear and with few white cells are predominantly of the mononuclear form. Occasionally small cartilage particles are seen and a crystal-induced arthritis is possible since crystals have been found (Lamotte et al, 1966), chondrocalcinosis can occur (Bluestone et al, 1971), and raised levels of plasma inorganic pyrophosphate have been found (Silcox & McCarty, 1973). Rheumatoid factor and other autoantibodies are not raised and evidence of inflammation such as an elevated erythrocyte sedimentation rate is absent.

Morbid anatomical descriptions are limited. Histologically the synovium may show a mild non-specific synovitis. However, the dominant features are the chondrocytic hypertrophy and the remodelling of bone.

Chondrocytic hypertrophy is most characteristically seen as increased chondrocytic activity irregularly distributed in the deeper layers of the cartilage, producing a thickened disorganised cartilage (Fig. 39.3), (Silberberg & Hasler, 1971; Bluestone et al, 1971; Mankin et al, 1978). The overlying cartilage is ulcerated in a patchy manner starting as a fissuring of the surface and eventually resulting in the deep, sharply demarcated ulcers with undermined edges characteristic of acromegalic cartilage degeneration (Erdheim, 1931) (Fig. 39.4). In spite of the relatively thick articular cartilage, cysts may be found in the subchondral bone ends similar to those of osteoarthrosis and presumably forming along the line of the deep cartilage fissures present. Progressive loss of cartilage occurs, resulting in denuded subchondral bone which becomes eburnated and pitted over the articular aspects. This area is surrounded by thinned cartilage and osteophytes. The overall appearance of the articular cartilage can most readily be described as a mixture of degeneration and regeneration, the regenerative process being exuberant and disorganised, occurring at an age when cartilage cellularity is normally diminishing. The degeneration of the articular cartilage probably results mainly from the uneven collagen and proteoglycan production of the basal layers and the resulting stress and strain in the cartilage. Other forms of cartilage may also be involved, for example at the costochondral junction, resulting in enlargement ('beading') of these joints and contributing to the increased anterior posterior diameter of the chest (Waine et al, 1945), and of the larynx, which partly explains the voice changes.

Similarly bone formation in hyaline cartilage

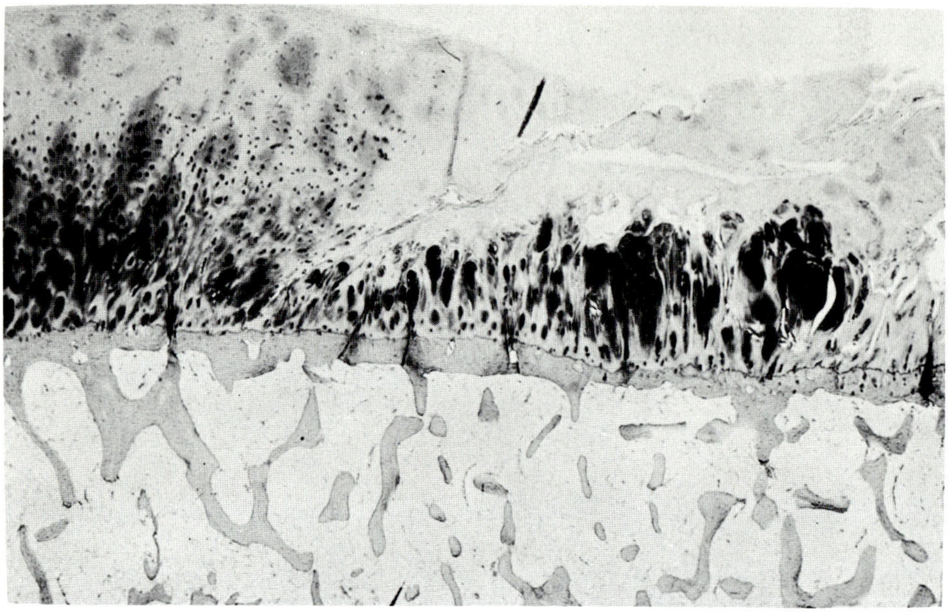

Fig. 39.3 Acromegaly. Femoral head. The uneven and excessive chrondrocytic proliferation is well seen. The cartilage over part of this area is fissured and degenerating. Elsewhere it is hypertrophied. (H & E ×10)

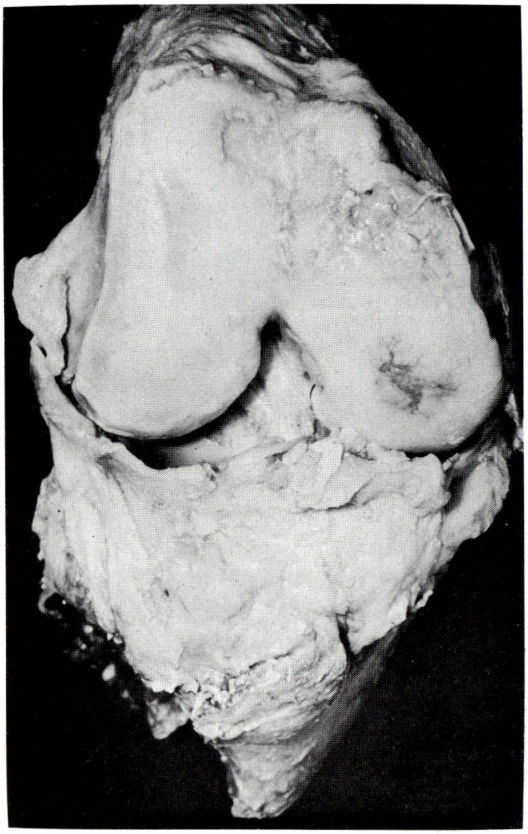

matrix is excessive and the fibrocartilaginous attachments are hypertrophied and later become ossified, thus producing the widespread osteophytic outgrowths. Tissue laxity is a feature of acromegaly, most readily seen in the hyperextensibility of the fingers and skin, but possibly also affecting ligaments. Whether this plays a part in the production of the arthropathy is unknown. Some of the features are similar to those of osteoarthritis and a role for growth hormone in idiopathic osteoarthrosis has been suggested (Dequeker et al, 1975). However, other explanations for these raised hormone levels in osteoarthrosis, such as the stress produced by the painful joints, may explain these differences. The pathology of the joint changes differs from that found in osteoarthrosis in its patchy distribution, its marked regenerative appearance, its occurrence on a background of hypertrophied cartilage with retention of joint space and the relatively late appearance of subchondral sclerosis.

Fig. 39.4 Acromegaly knee. Characteristic condylar and retropatellar ulcers. Note the clearly defined edges of the ulcers and the relatively thick cartilage elsewhere.

Independently of the excessive cartilage growth, bone remodelling occurs at two sites. Periosteal new bone is formed in certain areas such as the shafts of the metacarpal, metatarsal and phalangeal bones, and anterior surfaces of the vertebral bodies. Resorption may be found at other sites such as the posterior surfaces of the vertebral bodies. Endosteal bone remodelling is found in the form of a reduction in the number but an increase in the diameter of bone trabeculae within long bones, the overall result being to maintain bone mass (Delling & Schulz, 1977) although radiologically the appearance may be of osteopenia. Some of these changes may be influenced by the hyperparathyroidism occasionally found (Hartog, 1967).

Radiology

All radiological changes tend to be symmetrical though they may be more severe on one side, especially in the hip or shoulder.

Dorsal kyphosis is a prominent feature but vertebral collapse is not found. Intervertebral disc spaces are increased in height, but without alteration in the vertebral end-plates. These changes are most readily seen in the lumber spine. Although osteophytosis around the disc margin, particularly in the thoracic region, may give the impression of narrowing of the disc, this does not occur. Osteophytosis is most marked on the anterior aspect of the thoracic and lumbar vertebrae and usually affects many segments. When severe it may form bridges, particularly anteriorly, where associated ossification of the anterior parts of the disc is often present as discrete islands of bone.

The vertebral bodies are altered in shape; in particular the anterior/posterior diameter tends to be increased by irregular new bone formation on the anterior aspect of the vertebral bodies which in the cervical region has a caudal prolongation. Posteriorly the vertebral bodies have an increased concavity in the lateral view; this is most readily seen in the lumbar spine (Bluestone et al, 1971; Stuber & Palanio, 1971) (Fig. 39.5). The aetiology of this is unknown but may be due to the soft tissue overgrowth within the canal already referred to.

Radiological changes in the peripheral joints have two stages. The initial feature is widening of the joint space due to thickening of the cartilage,

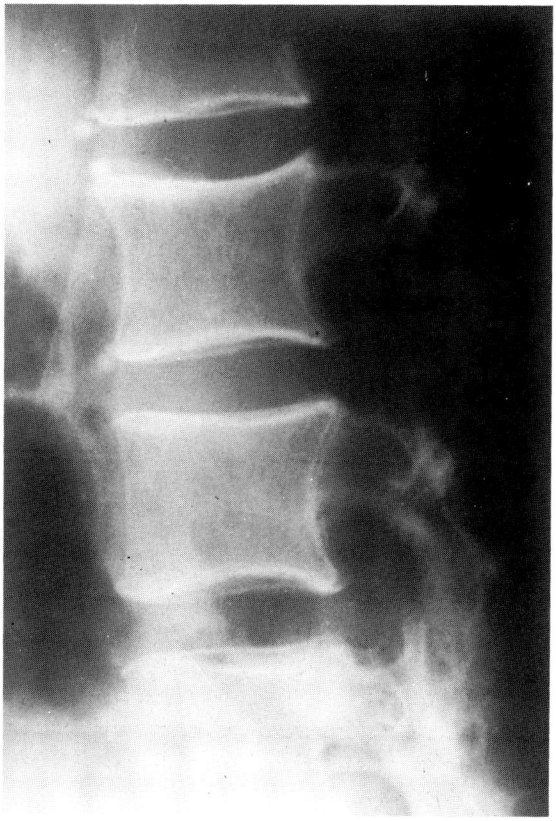

Fig. 39.5 Lumbar spine: increased concavity of anterior and posterior vertebral surfaces with calcification at anterior margins of discs. (Reproduced with permission from Bluestone et al (1971) with kind permission of the Editor, *Annals of the Rheumatic Diseases*.)

occasionally associated with increased soft tissue and, less frequently, synovial fluid shadows. Erosion, marginal sclerosis and malalignment are not features. At a later stage as the cartilage degenerates the changes of secondary degenerative joint disease appear with marginal sclerosis as a late feature (Fig. 39.6). However, certain features remain distinctive. In the hands there is well-marked ungual tufting to give a spade-like terminal phalanx and an osteophytic extension of the joint margins most marked at the bases of the terminal phalanges, produce sclerotic hook-like projections (Fig. 39.7). Small areas of joint capsule calcification or ossification may also be seen. Widening of the ends of the metacarpal bones is another feature and this is associated with remodelling of the phalangeal shafts leading to a uniform thickening of the phalangeal shaft and loss of the normal

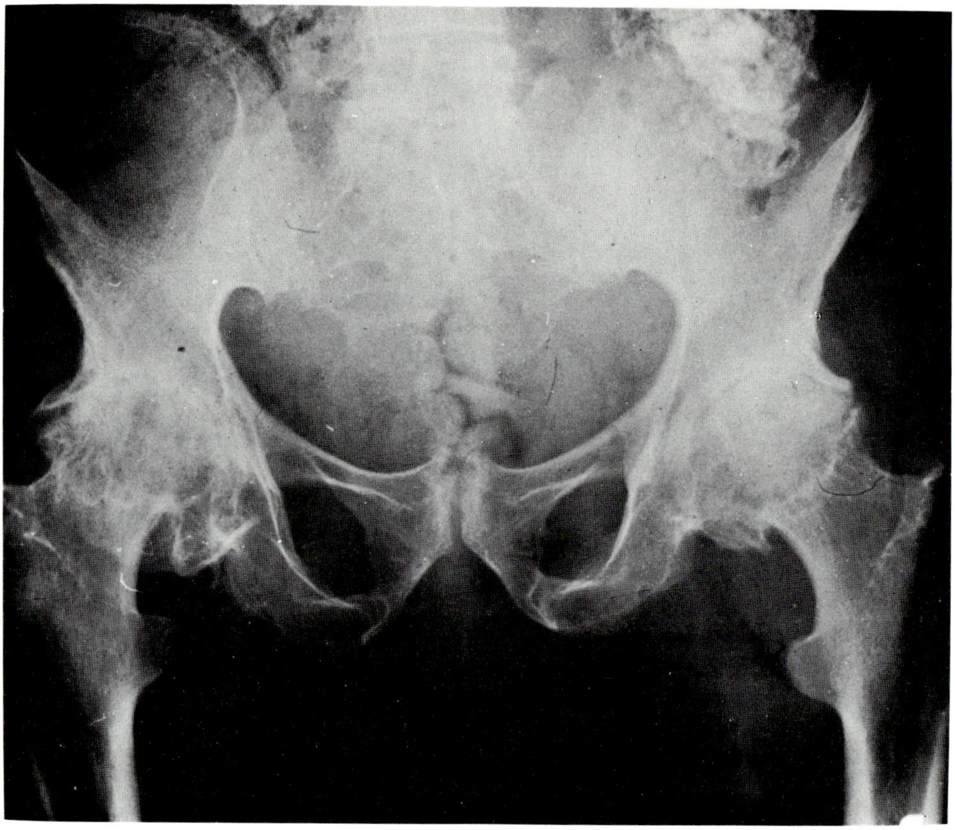

Fig. 39.6 Acromegaly. Osteoarthrosis of the hip occurring in long-standing acromegaly. Note the bony overgrowth and whiskering of the joint margin.

waisted appearance. The sesamoid bone of the thumb may be enlarged (Kleinberg et al, 1966). Occasionally chondrocalcinosis may be seen, most prominently in the knees. The rare association of hyperparathyroidism may produce a picture superficially resembling osteoporosis, but with thick trabeculae.

Diagnosis

The appearance of the patient is usually sufficient to suggest the diagnosis. This can be aided by serial photographs, radiology of the sella turcica or estimation of soft tissue thickness, e.g. of the heel pad (Steinbach & Russell, 1964). Clinical impressions of pituitary activity are of little value since elevated growth hormone levels may not be reflected in clinical symptoms or signs. Of more importance in the assessment of activity is direct measurement of fasting and resting growth hormone levels and its limited suppression during a glucose tolerance test. Single random growth hormone level assays are of little value since the growth hormone is continually varying, often widely, and in response to many stimuli; nor can 24 hour urinary excretion be accurately measured. Urinary calcium excretion is often increased and the serum inorganic phosphate level may be elevated. The increased collagen output as hydroxyproline during active disease and a fall in the excretion is a useful means of following successful therapy. Bone biopsy is unhelpful. Recently Fogelman et al (1980) have demonstrated that bone scans with technetium-99 diphosphonate correlate well with growth hormone and bone turnover but not with alkaline phosphatase levels.

Treatment

Rapid cure of the carpal tunnel syndrome and some regression of spinal nerve compression symptoms follow a successful hypophysectomy. Apart

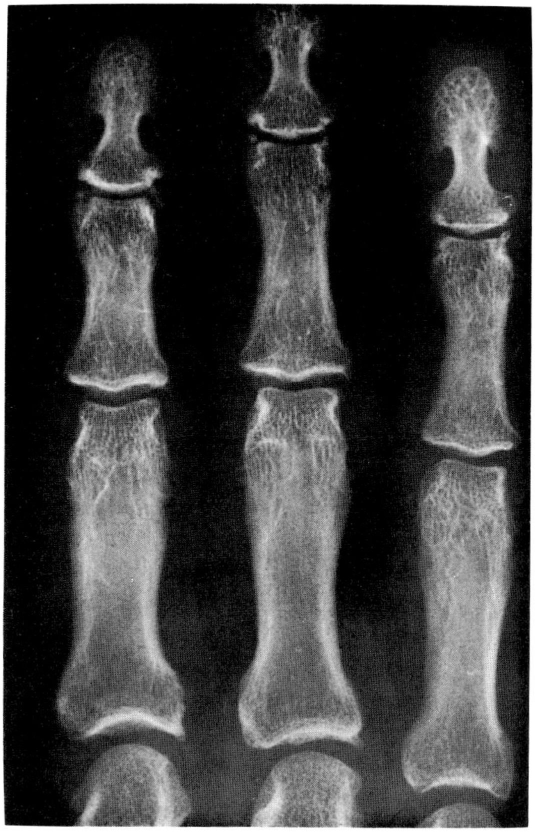

Fig. 39.7 Acromegaly hand. Note spade-like terminal phalanx and capsular ossicles in terminal interphalangeal joints, thickening of phalangeal shafts and retention of joint spaces. (Reproduced with permission from Bluestone et al, 1971).

from this, the rheumatic symptoms are not improved by reduction in growth hormone levels and once osteoarthrosis supervenes it is progressive. Corticosteroid injections either into a joint or into the carpal tunnel are not helpful. Analgesics may be necessary for the peripheral arthritis and backache but at a later stage irreversible degenerative joint disease, particularly in the hips and knees, occurs and surgery is necessary. The bone is strong and takes the implant well, the only problem being that of laxity of the periarticular tissues found in this condition. Postoperative care is necessary in hip arthroplasty to avoid the femoral component jumping out of the socket. Postoperative nursing with the leg in slight abduction may help to prevent this. The long-term results of knee replacement, which may be needed in these patients, have not so far been reported.

THYROID

The active thyroid hormones, thyroxine and triiodothyronine, circulate largely bound to serum proteins, very small amounts being in the active free form. They increase the turnover of protein, carbohydrate, fat and minerals and are thus essential for the normal growth, development and maturation of tissues. In vitro studies have shown thyroid hormone to increase synovial cell function, but to decrease glycosaminoglycan and collagen production by these cells. In physiological concentrations this is reflected in an accumulation of protein; in excess, catabolism particularly of protein results in, among other things, loss of connective tissue; in deficiency bone formation and modelling is defective and mucoid material formed of glycosaminoglycan and protein is laid down extracellularly. The histological picture is varied; osteomalacia or osteoporosis may be present. Drugs such as phenylbutazone and corticosteroids have an antithyroid action; however, other drugs such as aspirin and clofibrate increase thyroid hormone activity.

Support for an autoimmune causation of thyroid disease is strong. Organ-specific and non-specific antibodies together with abnormal cell mediated responses, raised gamma-globulins and other autoimmune disease such as vitiligo, have been found in both hypo- and hyperthyroidism (Beardwell, 1975). Hyperthyroidism is the commonest thyroid disorder followed by hypothyroidism, most of which is iatrogenic and thus usually detected. It is important in assessing surveys of thyroid and rheumatic diseases to differentiate between the different types of thyroid disease, since the type of autoimmunity involved may also differ. It is difficult to assess the true statistics even from large series. Becker et al (1963) surveyed 506 patients with Hashimoto's thyroiditis; only 20 cases of rheumatoid arthritis were found in spite of a 23.5% incidence of symptoms suggestive of connective tissue disease. Most of these had non-specific 'fibrositis' or thoracic shoulder girdle symptoms. Mulhern et al (1966), again in 170 cases of Hashimoto's disease, found a doubtful relationship with rheumatoid arthritis but no 'fibrositis'. Delamere et al (1982) studied 150 patients mainly with thyrotoxicosis, and found no increased incidence of either rheumatoid arthritis or systemic lupus erythematosus. Morning stiffness and weakness of the shoulders were the only significant associations to emerge and they, like other authors, point to the clinical similarity to polymyalgia rheumatica (Thomas & Croft, 1974; How et al, 1977; Dent & Edward, 1978). It should be noted that these associations were mainly found in the older patients.

Many of the autoimmune diseases overlap and serological studies suggest an increased incidence of autoimmune thyroiditis in Sjögren's syndrome (Bloch & Bunin, 1963; Whaley et al, 1973). Clinical thyroid disease occurs in 10–14% of patients with Sjögren's syndrome (Whaley et al, 1973) but no increase of clinical Sjögren's syndrome was found in autoimmune thyroid disease (Williamson et al, 1967). Recently interest has been aroused by the finding of microsomal and thyroglobin antibodies in the synovial fluid of patients with a variety of arthritides not matched by serum antibodies. These synovial fluid antibodies fell with decrease in disease activity suggesting that they were produced in the joint.

Gardner (1969) found that 12% of patients with rheumatoid arthritis dying in hospital, and thus presumably with a preponderance of elderly subjects, had thyroiditis and thyroid fibrosis.

In other cases a syndrome resembling systemic lupus erythematosus has been induced by the use of anti-thyroid drugs of the thiouracil (Amrhein et al, 1970) and thionamide type (Librik et al, 1970).

An association between hypothyroidism and raised serum uric acid levels has been suggested (Leeper et al, 1960), but not wholly confirmed (Boyle et al, 1966). The issue remains controversial (see Ch. 36).

HYPOTHYROIDISM

Sir William Gull (1874) described 5 women with a 'cretinoid state' who had muscle stiffness, joint swelling and thickening of the skin. A further 5 cases were described four years later (Ord, 1878). Since then several rheumatic syndromes have been found in hypothyroidism although the presence of more than one may result in a spectrum of clinical presentations. Moreover, the insidious onset of the vague musculoskeletal symptoms allows their presence to go unnoticed in many cases. Because of intellectual slowing, only a proportion of hypothyroid patients complain of rheumatic symptoms or signs, though direct questioning may increase the frequency. Many of these patients have a mild depressive illness, associated with feelings of tiredness and weakness which, in turn, influences their reaction to the symptoms.

Conversely, rheumatic symptoms may occur in hypothyroid patients who clinically appear euthyroid and may lead to the diagnosis of the underlying thyroid disease. This is particularly true when the carpal tunnel syndrome is the main feature. The clinical picture is further complicated by the patient's reaction to the ambient temperature, usually being exacerbated by cold and alleviated by warmth, such as hospital admission. The effect of temperature is particularly marked in patients with muscle cramps and stiffness.

Rheumatological manifestations of hypothyroidism
Carpal tunnel syndrome
Muscle cramps and stiffness
Myopathy
Arthropathy
Epiphyseal dysplasia

Carpal tunnel syndrome
Median nerve compression at the wrist or, rarely, the median plantar nerve in the foot, is found in about 6–7% of all cases of hypothyroidism (Frymoyer & Bland, 1973). Usually due to compression of the nerve from outside by the myxoedematous tissue and accompanying tenosynovitis, a true neuropathy with myxoedematous infiltration of perineurium and endoneurium also occurs in hypothyroidism (Fincham & Cape, 1968). It differs little from other types of carpal tunnel syndrome except that the symptoms tend to be more persistent and less related to exercise and that local hydrocortisone injections are less effective. Fortunately thyroid replacement produces prompt relief. A rare symmetrical peripheral sensory neuropathy with marked symptoms, but few objective signs, has been described (Nickel et al, 1961).

Muscle cramp, stiffness

Muscle cramps, stiffness and ill-defined skeletal pain in varying degree are common (Collins et al, 1964; Golding, 1970), and may be especially prominent where the onset is acute following iatrogenic hypothyroidism (Donniak et al, 1979). Localisation is poor though the thighs, calves and shoulder regions are most commonly affected and, less frequently, the hands and feet. The symptoms are worse after exercise, especially climbing or descending stairs, when quite severe muscle cramp in thighs and calves may be felt. Movements are slow and deliberate, often out of proportion to cerebration which may appear superficially normal; stiffness, unlike that associated with inflammatory arthritis, is not significantly relieved by exercise. The clinical picture often mimics polymyalgia rheumatica very closely and 'fibrositis' of the shoulder girdle is not uncommonly diagnosed especially in cases of Hashimoto's thyroiditis, where ill-defined pains particularly in the shoulders and chest are frequent, and in these latter cases the response of the limb girdle symptoms to thyroxine may be poor in contradistinction to the response in other forms of hypothyroidism.

Tendon reflexes often show characteristic delayed relaxation and muscles are enlarged and firm but seldom tender or weak (Spiro et al, 1970). This enlargement is mainly due to myxoedematous infiltrations; however, a true myopahty may be present (see below). Tenosynovitis over the wrist, finger flexors and dorsi flexors of the feet is not uncommon and responds poorly to thyroid hormone replacement (Dorwart & Schumacher, 1975).

Myopathy

Features of a myopathy are found, especially in severe hypothyroidism, their true incidence being difficult to define (Lahey, 1926). Proximal muscle pain and weakness with, in some cases, hypertrophy of proximal and distal (calf) muscles, occurs (Hoffman's syndrome in adults and Hercules' syndrome in a cretinous child). Hypotonia, pseudomyotonia or increased muscle enzymes in the serum are found in some patients (Salick et al, 1968; Goldman et al, 1977). Histologically focal necrosis and regeneration, mucinous deposits around the muscle fibres, loss of fibre striations and wide variations in fibre size are the most characteristic findings although the changes are often minimal. Recovery may not always follow treatment (Fessel, 1968) and this complication of hypothyroidism is even less responsive to thyroid replacement therapy than the more common muscle weakness found in the 'rheumatoid–fibrositic' syndrome described earlier. In other cases muscular atrophy or cerebellar lesions have been described which respond poorly to replacement therapy. The true incidence of neuromyopathies in hypothyroidism is unknown. However, Nickel et al (1961) biopsied 12 hypothyroid patients and found myopathic changes in all. No autoimmune defect has been found and although Fessel (1968) felt that the changes were directly due to a lack of action of the thyroid hormone on the muscle cell, the site of defect is unknown; neuromuscular transmission defects, primary neuropathy and primary myopathy/myositis have been proposed (Nickel et al, 1961; Chokroverty, 1976; Mohr & Reid, 1977).

Arthropathy

Usually articular pains are mild and indefinite and overshadowed by the symptoms of the myopathy and sensory neuropathies. Rarely non-tender synovial and periarticular thickening with synovial effusion is found usually affecting knees, hands and feet. The joints may be stiff, but without diurnal variation: signs of inflammation are not present and the synovial fluid has a normal protein content, and is of low cellularity and high viscosity (with a positive string test, i.e. dripping in an unbroken column from a syringe); calcium pyrophosphate crystals may be found (Dorwart & Schumacher, 1975), and pyrophosphate arthropathy occurs (Alexander et al, 1982). Response to treatment is excellent (Bland & Frymoyer, 1970; Frymoyer & Bland, 1973). In these cases only periarticular osteoporosis and soft tissue swelling occur. Various forms of bone collapse have been described. Seedat & Randered (1975) have documented avascular necrosis of the hip, suggesting that it might be due to hypercholesterolaemia. Collapse of the tibial plateau gives a radiological picture similar to that of bone necrosis (Bland & Frymoyer, 1970), and a single case suggestive of osteochondritis of the knee responsive to therapy has been described (Bywaters, 1969). These may, in part, represent epiphyseal dysgenesis which develops in the growing period (Wilkins, 1941); later in life osteolytic lesions, sometimes painful, occur (Weissbein et al, 1959). Recently chondrocalcinosis, with both intra- and extracellular crystals but without attacks of pseudogout, has been documented (Dorwart & Schumacher, 1975). Response of the arthropathy to treatment of the hypothyroidism is good

Congenital hypothyroidism

The delay or absence of epiphyseal development leads to failure of enchondral bone growth and irregular joint surfaces. The late appearance of multiple small centres of ossification produces the fragmented irregular 'stippled' appearance of the epiphysis and 'beaking' of the vertebral body being virtually diagnostic of this disorder and of value in dating its onset (Wilkins, 1941; Fig. 39.8). In cases of juvenile onset failure of linear growth is more prominent with delayed epiphyseal union and growth arrest lines seen in the diaphysis, the dysplasia being most easily seen in larger centres of ossification — femoral and humeral heads and navicular bones.

Replacement therapy leads to bone growth and eventual epiphyseal union. However, delayed growth spurts may result in mechanical deformity and the slipping of epiphyses, especially that of the femoral head (Epps & Martin, 1963; Hirano et al, 1978).

HYPERTHYROIDISM

A degree of myopathy is common and occasionally may be mistaken for arthritis. It usually affects the

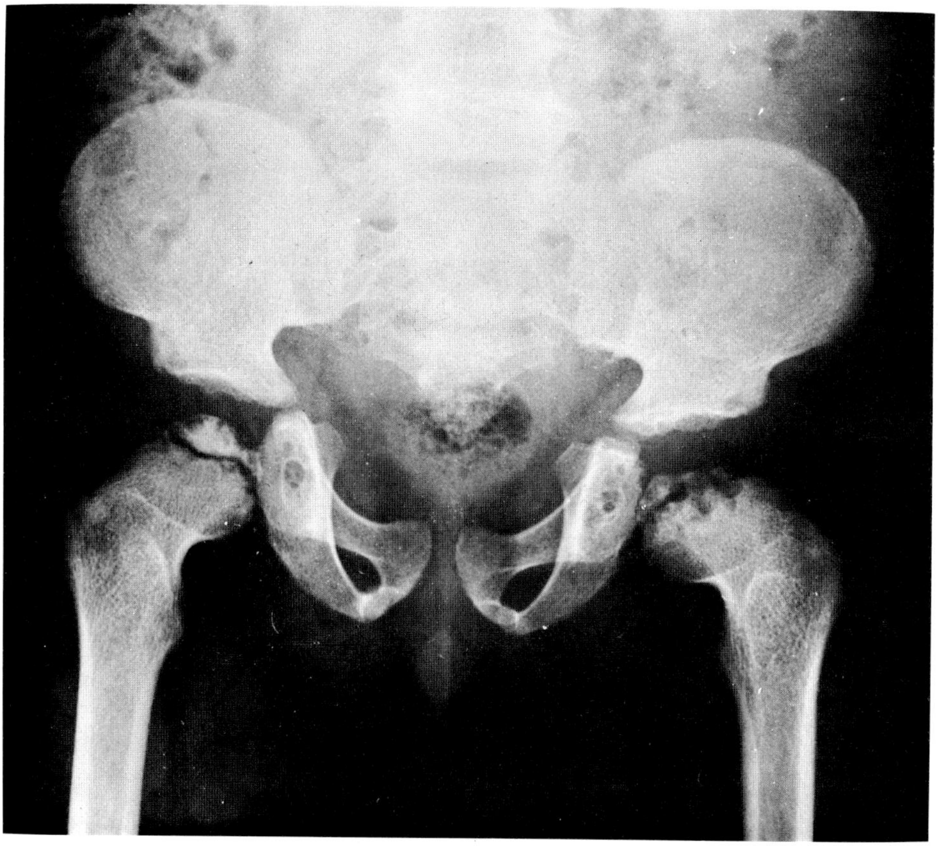

Fig. 39.8 Congenital hypothyroidism. Epiphyseal dysgenesis affecting the femoral heads in an 8-year-old boy (bone age $2\frac{1}{2}$ years). Note the different stages on the two sides and the presence of bone cysts. (By courtesy of Dr J.B. Fawcitt.)

proximal limb muscles and it is associated with weakness and cramp. In severe hyperthyroidism the peripheral muscles may be involved. The symptoms rapidly disappear following treatment of the thyroid overactivity (Ramsay, 1966).

Periarthritis is said to be more frequent in these patients, especially of the shoulder (Skillern, 1943; Meulengracht & Schwartz, 1951). A spectrum of changes have been described in the peripheral joints. The author has not been impressed by either the presence of periarthritis or of peripheral joint fractures in hyperthyroidism.

Osteoporosis is an accepted accompaniment of thyrotoxicosis but rarely leads to problems.

The above probably represent implications of simple thyroid oversecretion as distinct from thyroid acropachy.

THYROID ACROPACHY

This is a distinct syndrome complicating less than 1% of hyperthyroid patients (Gimlette, 1960) and usually follows treatment when the patient may be either euthyroid or hypothyroid. In 1968 only 317 cases had been reported (Kinsella & Beck, 1968). It can occur at any age, the youngest reported case being 14 years old (Thomas et al, 1973). The sexes are equally affected and up to 28 years may separate the onset of thyrotoxicosis and the onset of acropachy (Freeman, 1958).

The fingers and toes only are affected. In its mildest form a fluffy, irregular, lace-like periosteal new bone formation involving metacarpals, metatrrsals and phalanges is found (Fig. 39.9). This is symptomless. Involvement of the rest of the skeleton, e.g. long bones, does not occur and this and the painless periostitis help to differentiate thyroid acropachy from hypertrophic osteoarthropathy. In addition soft tissue swelling of fingers and toes which may be asymmetrical, erythematous and fluctuant, but painless and non-tender and without evidence of inflammation, can be present (Fig. 39.10). Pretibial myxoedema and finger clubbing are found in most, but not all, cases (Nixon & Samol, 1970).

The cause of this syndrome is completely unknown. Long acting thyroid stimulator (LATS), which is an immunoglobulin, has been implicated,

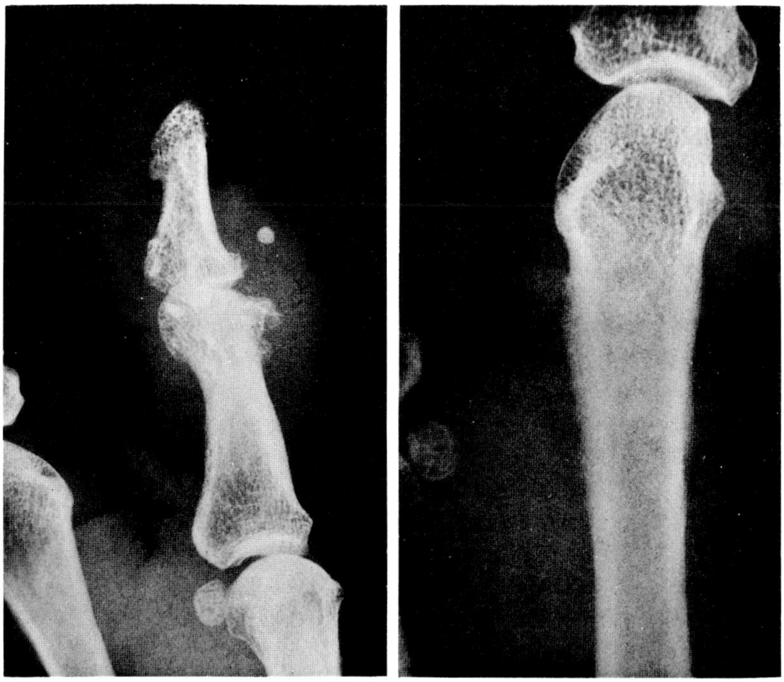

a b

Fig. 39.9 Thyroid acropachy. Typical changes with 'egg-shell' new bone formation around joint and periosteal new bone formation along shape of 2nd metacarpal bone.

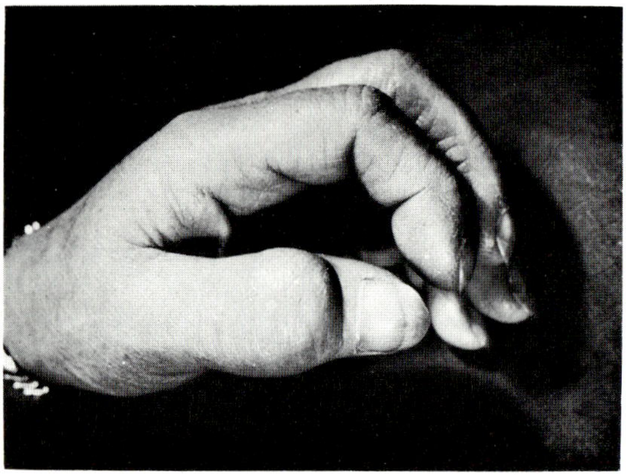

Fig. 39.10 Thyroid acropachy. Diffuse fluctuant non-tender swelling which may be erythematous.

but the evidence is unconvincing, although Lynch et al (1973) have reviewed 10 cases of acropachy and in all cases where it was sought LATS was found. The role of the more recently described human thyroid stimulator (HTS, previously known as 'LATS-protector' — LATS-P) may be more relevant. Investigations other than those of thyroid function are unhelpful. The ESR is normal. Treatment is directed at seeking out other causes of clubbing and correcting the thyroid function, but this has no effect on the acropachy. Reassurance can be given that a crippling arthritis will not develop and the symptoms will diminish, though this may take several years.

ENDOCRINE PANCREAS

Several rheumatic syndromes have been described in association with diabetes mellitus. In some the relationship is not clear nor even completely confirmed. Other factors may be important such as the obesity sometimes present, or even a common immunological mechanism underlying the diabetes and the arthritis. Immune mechanisms may play a part in the pathogenesis of the rheumatic disease. Thus circulating complexes of insulin and anti-insulin antibodies have been found in the sera of patients with insulin-requiring diabetes (Lev-Ran et al, 1971; Kilpatrick & Varella, 1980). These may be partly responsible for the vasculitis together with the increased aggregatability of the platelets, increased capillary permeability and the altered lipid metabolism.

Much of the epidemiological work in diabetes has ignored factors such as obesity, decreasing glucose tolerance normally found with increasing age, racial variations in glucose tolerance, and variations in criteria used (e.g. O'Sullivan & Williams, 1966). There may be a long prediabetic period in type I diabetes mellitus, the main cause of the rheumatic features described, before clinical diabetes appears (Gorsuch et al, 1981) and presumably although the diathesis is present in some people diabetes never appears.

Insulin is rapidly cleared from the circulation and is normally delivered in response to food. Inefficient metabolism leads to loss of bone matrix which is more marked in insulin-requiring diabetics (Levin et al, 1976; McNair et al, 1981). Bone loss appears to be entirely metabolic and not due to microangiopathy, as evidenced by retinal lesions.

In tissue culture, fibroblasts from diabetics show early senescence and if this also occurs with chondrocytes then poor bone formation might result (Goldstein et al, 1969). In similar experiments insulin has been shown to stimulate collagen synthesis and amino acid uptake into bone (Wettenhall et al, 1969; Canalis et al, 1977). In rats made diabetic, the enzymes responsible for degradation and synthesis of cartilage glycosaminoglycan were increased (Silberberg et al, 1977). One of the results of this altered collagen metabolism seems to be an increase in collagen cross-linking resulting in more stable and permanent collagen which thus accumulates (Hamlin et al, 1975; Chang et al, 1980; Buckingham et al, 1981). This accumulation could explain some of the soft tissue lesions discussed later and perhaps enhance the internal sclerosis of arteries. Thus connective tissue metabolism is affected and may account for the periarticular features of the disease. Except for the neuropathic lesions found in diabetes, the association between diabetes and the pathogenesis of all the conditions to be described still needs clarification.

Hyperuricaemia and gout are found in diabetic patients but this may be due to the associated obesity found in both hyperuricaemia and diabetes and in particular Boyle et al (1969) could not find any difference in glucose metabolism between gouty and diabetic patients. Ketoacidosis and dehydration are an uncommon cause of gout in diabetic patients. McCarty et al (1962) in their original description found that 4 of their 7 patients with pseudogout (calcium pyrophosphate crystal deposition disease), had evidence of mild diabetes. Later work (McCarty, 1974; Hamilton, 1976) has failed to confirm this association.

VERTEBRAL ANKYLOSING HYPEROSTOSIS (see also Chs. 28, 29, 34 and 57)

The first description of this syndrome was probably in 1938 by Meyer & Forster. An increased incidence of vertebral ankylosing hyperostosis (Forestier's disease — Forestier & Lagier, 1971a, b) has been found in both diabetes and obesity though the relative importance of these two independent factors is not clear (Julkunen et al, 1971; Julkunen et al, 1975, 1981). An alternative view has been put by Harris et al (1974), who found only 5 diabetics in 54 patients with ankylosing hyperostosis.

The diabetes is usually mild and may be unsuspected or latent. This syndrome is more frequent in older patients and is thought to be uncommon before 40 years of age. However, examples are being found increasingly in younger people and partial forms described with relatively minor spinal and peripheral joint changes in which the borderline with normal ageing may be obscure. There is a slight male preponderance but no association with occupation. Predominantly affecting the dorsal spine, the symptoms are usually minor and the hyperostosis is usually an incidental finding, although when extensive ankylosis occurs minimal spinal restriction without dorsal kyphosis is found. Backache and intermittent root pain, particularly around the chest and shoulders, sometimes following unaccustomed exercise, is the main feature and is usually asymmetrical, rather ill-defined and without the severity or duration found in ankylosing spondylitis. Occasionally hyperostosis of the cervical spine may cause dysphagia. Radiological examination varies from minor ossification in the paravertebral structures to large bony overgrowths forming a flowing continuous layer, mainly on the anterior and right lateral vertebral borders and accentuated at the disc margins to form bony bridges across the vertebral discs (Fig. 39.11). Not all the intervertebral spaces are involved. The changes are most marked in the dorsal region and are more readily seen on lateral views of the spine. All stages of bone overgrowth are found and growth of new bone may extend downwards or upwards along the vertebral body, the changes being asymmetrical. Thus the changes are not uniform throughout the spine. The ossification is only in the anterior fibres of the anterior longitudinal ligament, which is not destroyed or replaced, and to a lesser extent in other adjacent ligaments and intervertebral discs. There are clear areas between the ossified anterior fibres of the anterior longitudinal ligament and the underlying vertebral body since the periosteal bone in this area is not affected (Fig. 39.12). Thus the radio-

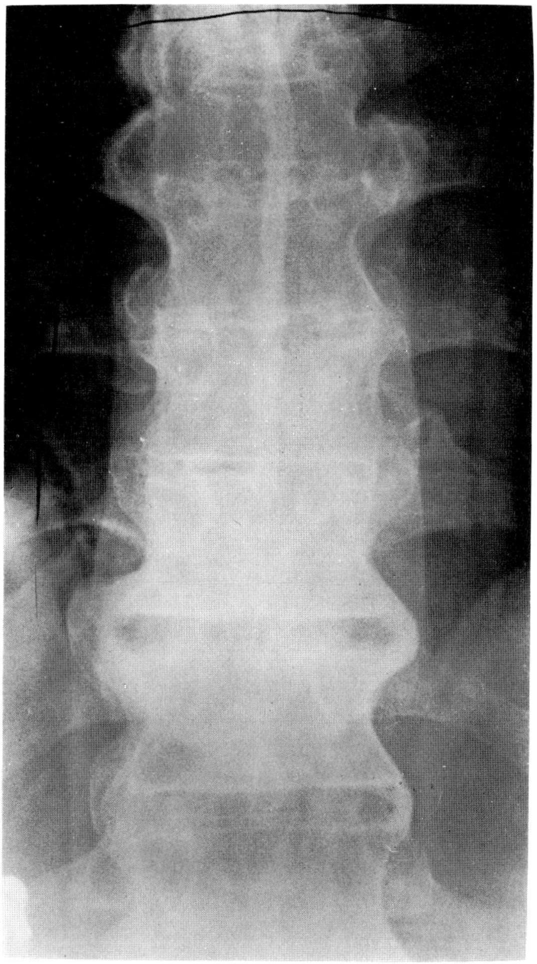

Fig. 39.11 Vertebral ankylosing hyperostosis. Thoracic spine showing complete bridging across vertebral space. (70-year-old obese male with latent diabetes.)

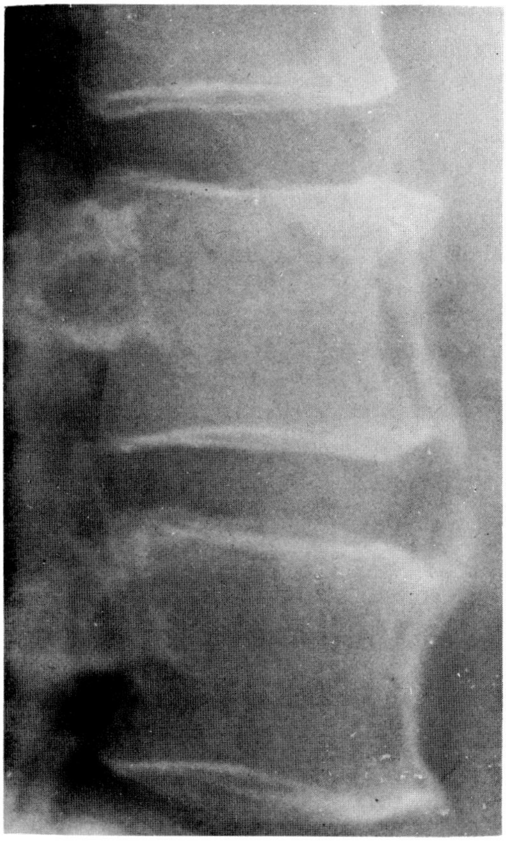

Fig. 39.12 Vertebral ankylosing hyperostosis. Lumbar vertebrae. Note calcification of arterior layers of longitudinal ligaments and radiotranslucent zone between calcification and anterior borders of vertebrae. Bridging of intervertebral spaces incomplete. Intervertebral disc spaces normal. (Obese male age 60 years with latent diabetes. HLA-B27-negative.)

logical picture presents a more undulating appearance than in ankylosing spondylitis. Vernon-Roberts et al (1974) have suggested that fibrous extension from the annulus fibrosus over the surface of the vertebrae lifts the periosteum off and leads to new bone formation, this fibrous extension being impeded by the pressure of the aorta on the left. The elevation of the periosteum over the lateral vertebral surfaces leads to new bone formation on these surfaces. The intervertebral disc spaces are retained and the apophyseal joints not significantly affected, nor are the syndesmophytes completely fused, probably explaining the retained spinal mobility. However, irregularities of the apophyseal joints and in the spinal canal may cause root pressure (Vernon-Roberts et al, 1974). Schmorl's nodes, which are apparently symptomless, are frequently found at post-mortem examination. Radiological progression has been demonstrated (Julkunen et al, 1981).

'Whiskery' bony outgrowths around joints and from bones particularly of the knee, shoulder, hip and sacroiliac joints may occur and non-erosive and non-sclerotic calcaneal spurs are common (Resnick et al, 1975; Resnick et al, 1978) (Fig. 39.13). To this syndrome the term 'diffuse idiopathic skeletal hyperostosis' (DISH) is sometimes given. These peripheral joint changes may cause mild symptoms with effusions. Progression is slow so that the bone changes often appear to be maximal when first observed. Several cases of degenerative hip disease have been seen but this may be a fortuitous association in this predominantly elderly age-group. Differentiation from ankylosing spondylitis is usually possible in particular by the lack of pain, ankylosis of sacroiliac joints or posterior interspinal joints, inflammatory peripheral joint involvement, impairment of chest movements or raised ESR found in ankylosing spondylitis which also tends to occur in a younger age-group.

The pathogenesis is unknown; an association with histocompatability antigen HLA-B27 has been suggested (Shapiro et al, 1976) but not confirmed and genetic or environmental factors are suggested by the increased incidence in Pima indians. Accentuated growth at the edge of the vertebrae suggests that mechanical factors may be important, but previous trauma is not a feature (Julkunen et al, 1975). Although the spinal changes bear superficial resemblance to those found in acromegaly, growth hormone levels are normal (Harris et al, 1974; Littlejohn et al, 1981). Higher levels of insulin, without diabetes, have been found following glucose challenge suggesting abnormal glucose tolerance (Littlejohn et al, 1981). Treatment of this benign condition is purely symptomatic.

OSTEOARTHROSIS

This common rheumatic disease has been said to be more common in the diabetic probably due to

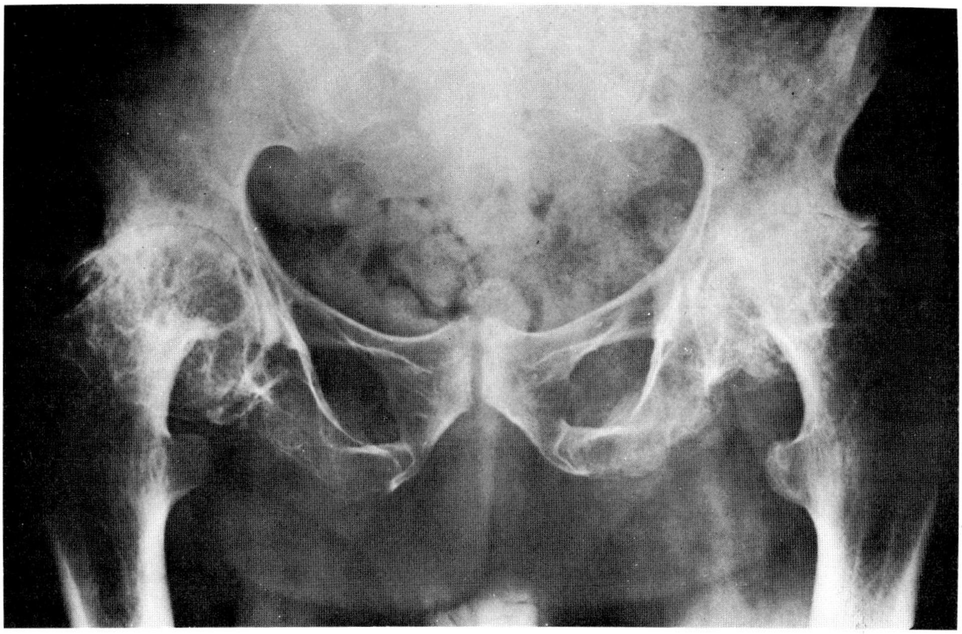

Fig. 39.13 Vertebral ankylosing hyperostosis. Associated changes in hips showing typical 'whiskering' effect on right and changes of secondary osteoarthrosis in both hips.

obesity. However, Silberberg et al (1959) examined 200 sternoclavicular joints at autopsy, thus avoiding the problem of weight-bearing, and found an increased incidence of degenerative changes. Campbell & Feldman (1975) showed an increased incidence of subchondral and periosteal cysts of a degenerative nature mainly in the hands, shoulders and feet of 100 diabetics. However, there was no evidence of bone hypertrophy.

NEUROPATHY

Six forms can be distinguished, though overlap and confusion occur:

Peripheral neuropathy
Neuro-arthropathy — large joints — Charcot
Trophic ulceration — osteomyelitis
Osteolysis
Spinal neuropathy
Carpal tunnel compression syndrome.

Peripheral neuropathy occurs to some extent in about 60% of diabetics and is usually of stocking and glove type with paraesthesiae which may be very painful. The skin, especially of the soles of the feet, is tender and the patients often have a continual urge to move their legs. As the sensory loss progresses, the pain often lessens and weakness becomes more prominent.

Other forms of neuropathy occur: mononeuritis multiplex with radicular or more peripheral involvement (Childs & Yates, 1978); amyotrophy with end-plate involvement and shoulder and thigh involvement which usually resolves. The autonomic nervous system is frequently affected and could play a part in such syndromes as the frozen shoulder syndrome, though this is unproven. Neuroarthropathy affects the large joints which eventually become hypermobile and then flail with gross disorganisation. The ankle, tarsal and metatarsophalangeal joints are primarily affected, not the knee or upper arm as in other forms of Charcot joints (Brunckner & Howell, 1972). The onset may be acute with swelling, oedema and erythema, not unlike gout, but the relative lack of pain, systemic upset, leucocytosis or raised ESR suggest the alternative diagnosis which is aided by the presence of sensory loss. Progressive destruction occurs although function is well maintained (Lippman et al, 1976). The pathogenic mechanisms are not clear. Trauma is important. Vascular defects may occur although angiography can be normal (Lippman et al, 1976). Whitehouse & Wechstein (1978) have suggested that the osteopathy in fact represents the healing stage of a local osteomyelitis. Simple treatment with protection of pressure areas and good diabetic control are probably all that can be given. Sympathectomy has been disappointing. Attempts at surgical fusion are likely to fail.

Predominantly peripheral sensory loss, particularly if associated with plantar callus and underlying fore-foot arthritis, may result in perforating plantar ulcers with secondary infection and osteomyelitis (Fig. 39.14). The clinical features are mild oedema, with web-space swelling but little pain, although the patient tends to walk on the outer side of his foot. Apart from the neuropathy there is usually bone destruction and vascular calcification and the latter is the single most important variable determining prognosis. Surgical treatment is usually necessary.

Forefoot osteolysis is a distinct and very characteristic syndrome in which there is gradual disappearance of bone with few clinical features and it is often a chance finding. The distal metatarsal and proximal phalanges are affected with initial spotty osteoporosis of the periarticular region followed by bone loss (Pogonowska et al, 1967; Schwartz et al, 1969; Clouse et al, 1974). The joint margins tend to be well maintained but juxta-articular cysts appear and may be mistaken for inflammatory erosions (Fig. 39.15). Whittling away of the diaphysis leads to tapered (atrophic) bone with clear outlines (Fig. 39.16). Secondary splintering and fragmentation of the bone may confuse the picture. Pain is variable since obvious neuropathy is not a feature. The vascular supply is good (otherwise bone resorption would not occur) and the bone tends to reform without treatment.

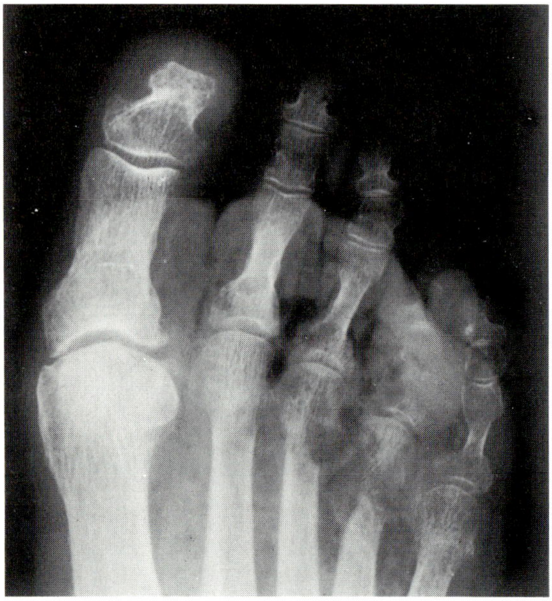

Fig. 39.14 Osteomyelitis. Diabetic of 9 years duration. The main changes are interstitial gas and soft tissue swelling of the web spaces of the toes. Early cortical changes of the heads of 3rd and 4th metatarsals. Bone elsewhere good with no evidence of osteoporosis, vascular calcification or periostitis.

The absence of gross neurological defect, plantar callus or infection, lack of systemic ill-health and eventual healing, tend to point to osteolysis and it is very important to distinguish this condition from osteomyelitis. The treatments are completely different. The diabetic foot is well reviewed by Levin & O'Neal (1977).

Spinal neuropathy is characterised by gross irregular new bone formation often with disorganisation of the intervertebral discs at one or more level. Osteoporosis is not present. The main features are the relatively mild pain and the need to distinguish from secondary infection which may be present. Carpal tunnel compression syndrome is a common form of nerve entrapment syndrome and was associated with diabetes mellitus in 63 of 379 patients (16.6%) of Phelen's (1970) series of carpal tunnel syndrome. Some of these cases may be associated with a peripheral neuropathy, the carpal compression serving to complete the syndrome. This concept is illustrated by Jung et al (1971) who described a 'diabetes hand syndrome' in which there is a diabetic peripheral neuropathy of the upper extremity associated with evidence of median nerve conduction delay at the wrist. In half the patients similar delay was found in the ulnar nerves — which were not compressed. The result was a partial contracture of all the fingers not associated with Dupuytren's contracture (Fig. 39.17). Since median nerve compression is only part of the problem, carpal tunnel decompression may have little effect on the clinical picture.

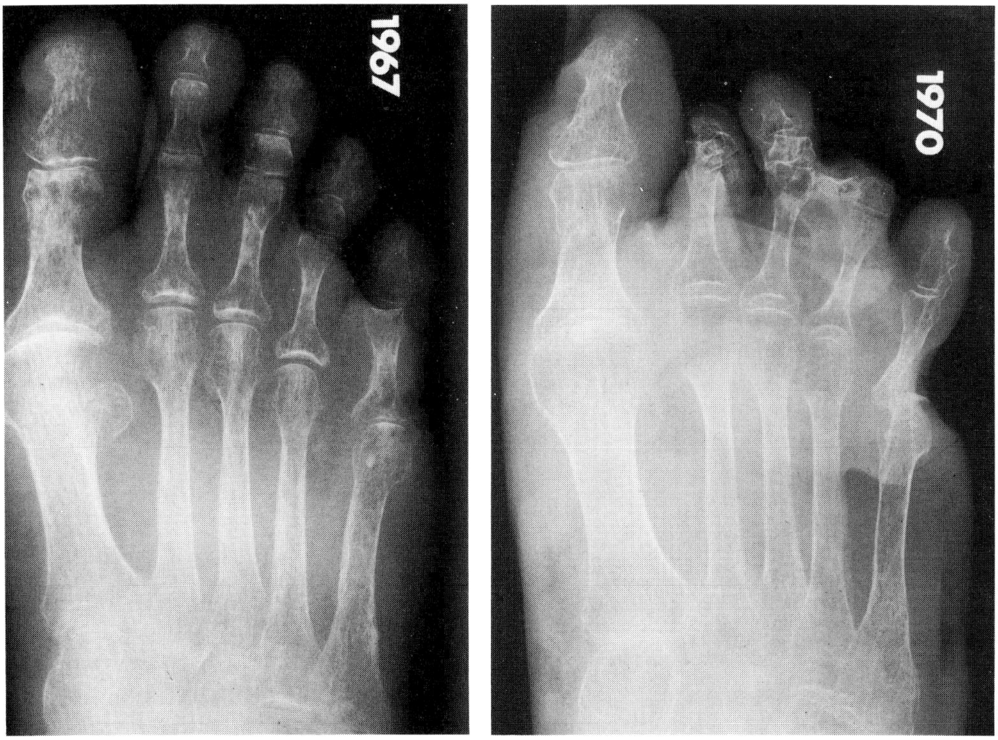

a b

Fig. 39.15 59-year-old female with claudication, developing (a) widespread spotty osteoporosis but without loss of bone cortex or joint space (1967) and later (b) dry gangrene and ulcer crater on lateral side 5th metatarsophalangeal joint (1970). No evidence vascular calcification.

SOFT TISSUE CONTRACTURE

This can take three forms:

Dupuytren's contracture
Diabetic cheiroarthropathy
Periarthritis of the shoulder.

The increased production of stable collagen has already been referred to; both this and microvasculitis with ischaemia and fibrosis probably play a part in the following essentially soft tissue syndromes. A susceptibility to fibrosis may underlie these cases since bilateral symmetrical Dupuytren's contracture, often associated with knuckle pads (Garrod) and plantar nodules, is found in

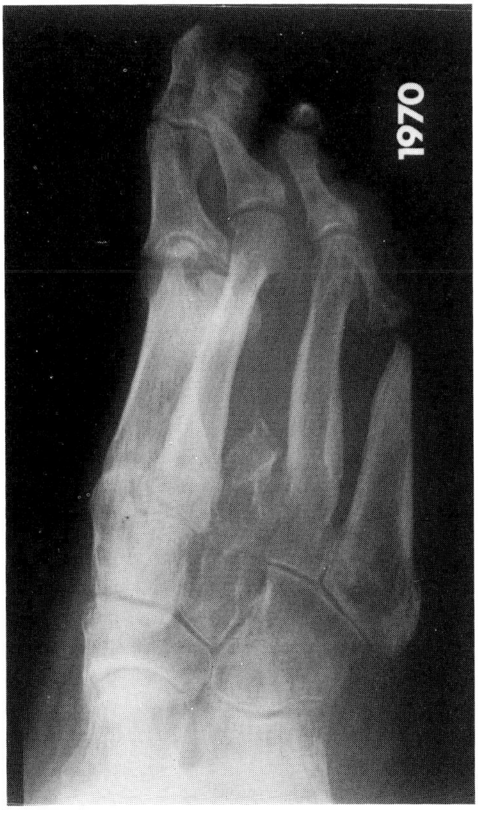

Fig. 39.16 Forefoot osteolysis. 87-year-old female diabetic with osteolysis affecting 3rd and 5th digits. The typical tapered (atrophic) appearance is seen but the bone cortex is well maintained. Widespread osteophorosis and evidence of vascular calcification.

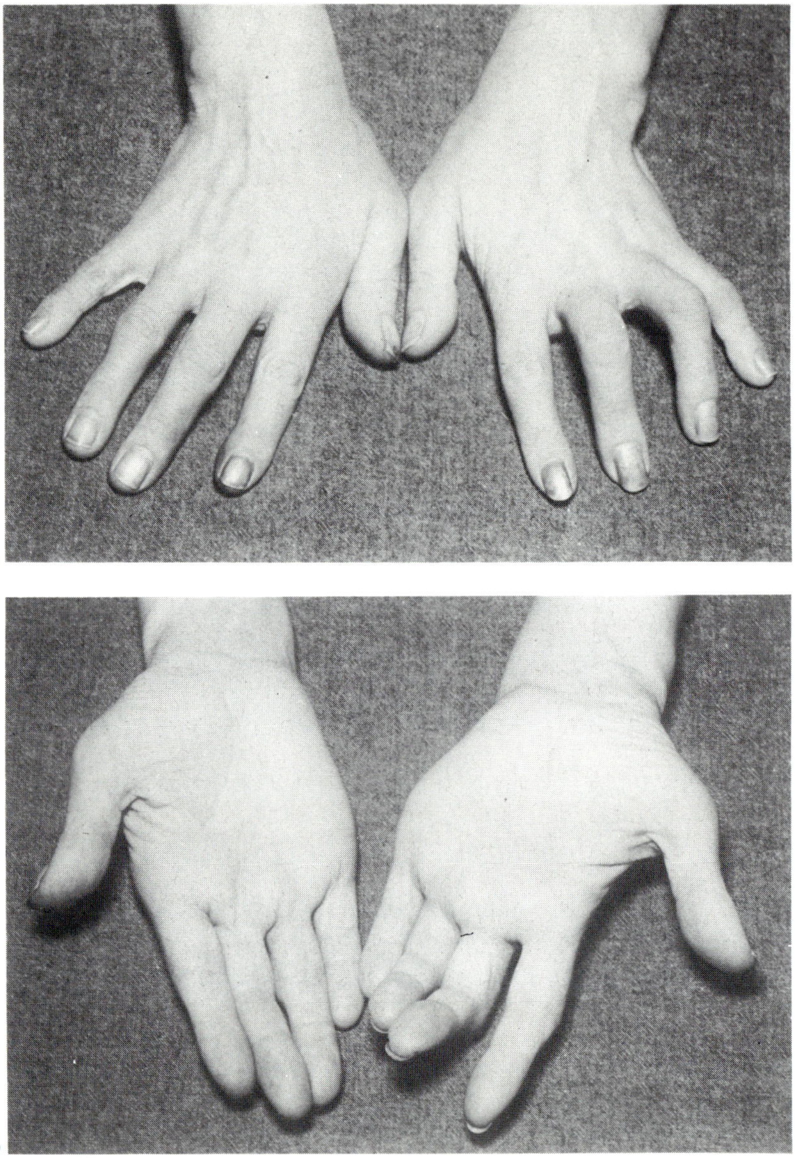

a

b

Fig. 39.17 Diabetic hand. Flexion of fingers (mainly 3rd and 4th) without evidence of Dupuytren's contracture. Minimal evidence of peripheral neuropathy.

epileptics on prolonged administration of anticonvulsants (Critchley et al, 1976).

Dupuytren's contracture

An association between diabetes mellitus and Dupuytren's contracture has long been suspected. Viljanto (1973) found that 25% of patients with Dupuytren's contracture, apparently not due to a neuropathic cause, had diabetes. Other series have given an incidence in diabetes of 21–63%. Although the incidence is obviously raised, it is difficult to interpret since the incidence of Dupuytren's contracture in the controls varied from 5–22%!

The low grade inflammatory reaction produces a nodular thickening in the palmar fascia usually of the ring and middle finger more frequently than the more usual ring and little finger found in idiopathic Dupuytren's contracture (Vitny et al, 1979). Some of these cases may be confused with diabetes cheiroarthropathy (see below).

Other fibrous reactions are found in diabetic patients such as Garrod's pads, firm swellings in the dorsum of the proximal interphalangeal joints and heel pad nodules where the incidence is the same as that in rheumatoid arthritis (unpublished observation). The aetiology is unknown; trauma, vasculitis and the possibility of a genetic factor have been suggested since some cases are familial and Bowser-Riley et al (1975) in a preliminary report have shown chromosomal abnormalities in Dupuytren's contracture. The severity of the contracture does not relate to the length or severity of the diabetes mellitus (Revach & Cabilli, 1972). The prognosis and treatment do not differ from Dupuytren's contracture unrelated to diabetes.

Diabetic cheiroarthropathy (limited joint mobility syndrome)

This is a relatively recently recognised syndrome, though first described in 1957 by Lundbaek in adults with long-standing diabetes. More recently the main interest has been in young insulin requiring diabetics who are said to have a surprisingly high frequency — up to 40%, though to confuse the picture, Jackson et al (1978) did not find any cases among 252 young diabetics. The minimal changes found may explain why it has been previously undetected and, conversely, make the differentiation from the normal difficult.

The cardinal features are a mild to moderate contraction deformity of the fingers in which passive and active extension of the metatarsophalangeal and interphalangeal joints is lost, principally at the proximal interphalangeal joints, the 4th and 5th fingers being most frequently involved (Fig. 39.18). A sensation of stiffness is usually the first complaint, but is unlike inflammatory stiffness in not being relieved by exercise. This is unassociated with any evidence of neuromuscular disease or inflammation, the joints not being tender, though they may be thickened, nor is there evidence of joint destruction. Thickening of the skin of the digits may be present but there is no evidence of Dupuytren's contracture. In the cases seen personally it was impossible to determine convincingly what structure was impairing extension which was limited by some 20 degrees from the horizontal line. In one case flexor tendon nodules not of obvious inflammatory nature and not helped by hydrocortisone injections, have developed. Less frequently other joints are affected, such as toes, wrists, elbows, knees and hips (Grigic et al, 1975). In all cases it seems that it is the soft tissues around the joint, rather than the joint itself, that are involved. Although more frequently described in children (Rosenbloom & Frias, 1974; Benedetti et al, 1975; Grgic et al, 1975), cases are seen in the adult (Jung et al, 1971; Dorwart & Schumacher, 1974). The syndrome usually develops slowly after five or more years of insulin therapy. Progression is unusual and some improvement can occur.

Other rheumatic symptoms, Raynaud's phenomenon and haematological and biochemical evidence of inflammation, are not found. As the number of cases increase strong associations with microvascular disease (Rosenbloom et al, 1981) are found but less so with neurological changes or the

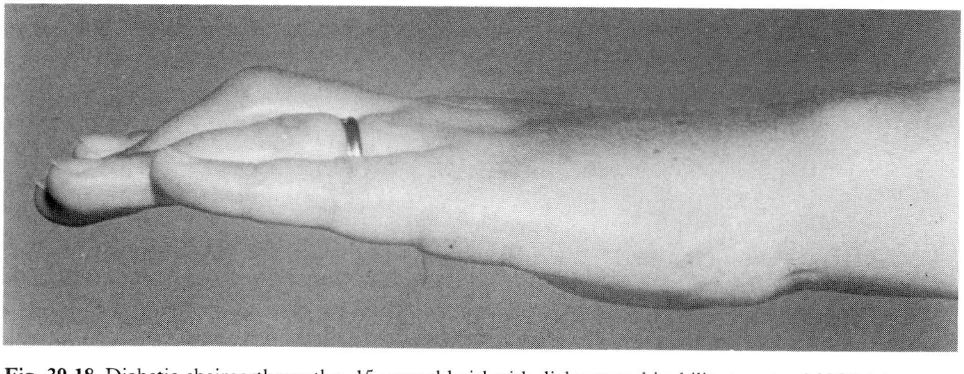

Fig. 39.18 Diabetic cheiroarthropathy. 15-year-old girl with diabetes and inability to extend MCP joints or straighten 3rd and 4th fingers fully. A little thickening in palmar tendon sheaths. No evidence of Dupuytren's contracture.

quality of diabetic control, although these are both important, as is the insulin dependence. Traisman et al (1978) found an equally high incidence of this condition in non-diabetic siblings of patients, suggesting an hereditary factor. Thus at present the clinical picture still requires confirmation and definition and the pathogenesis is confused.

Periarthritis of the shoulder

This is about 4–6 times as frequent in diabetics as in the normal population but does not differ in its characteristics or prognosis (Bridgeman, 1972; Lequesne et al, 1977). Although both shoulders are commonly involved there is no evidence of a polyneuropathy to account for the symmetry. This syndrome is more common in the insulin-dependent diabetic and in those of longer duration. Dupuytren's contracture was not particularly frequent is these series of patients and no laboratory features other than the diabetes mellitus distinguish these patients from the controls. Calcification in the shoulder has been documented (Kaklamanis et al, 1975). The demonstration of changes in the acromioclavicular joints by Campbell & Feldman (1975), has already been referred to. They also found calcific tenosynovitis and vascular and non-vascular calcification, all features that could give rise to the shoulder symptoms. The shoulder–hand syndrome may complicate some of these cases.

EXOCRINE PANCREAS FAILURE

Exocrine pancreas failure is one of the causes of malabsorption and of secondary bone disease. The sometimes associated chronic cystic fibrosis is complicated by two distinct syndromes. The first is a transient migrating polyarthralgia with low grade activity but definite synovial hypertrophy; the exacerbation can be very painful but little deformity results, although the arthritis may eventually persist in a single joint. The second is a form of hypertrophic pulmonary osteoarthropathy (Matthey et al, 1976). No evidence of neuritis or vasculitis is found and the circulating immune complexes associated with recurrent chest infection may be responsible.

Both acute and chronic pancreatic disease can be associated with fat necrosis, the arthritic manifestation of which may be delayed for 2–3 weeks (Potts et al, 1975; Shackleford, 1977; Goluboff et al, 1978). There is fever, tender red subcutaneous nodular swelling of fingers and tender joint effusions. The ESR is raised and during the acute phase so are the serum lipase and amylase. In children post-traumatic pancreatitis may occur and osteolytic lesions may be found without a prior history (Boswell & Baylin, 1973). Radiologically subcutaneous calcification is sometimes found. Treatment is that of pain, shock and the underlying pancreatis.

Over-zealous replacement therapy with pancreatic extracts of high purine content may produce a symptomless hyperuricaemia (Stapleton et al, 1976).

CORTISOL (see also Ch. 20)

Cortisol, the principle active glucocorticoid, is normally secreted continuously, the highest levels being found between 6 and 8 a.m. and the lowest at midnight. In between there is a gradual change with little fluctuation, unless physical or psychological stress occurs, when very high levels may be found. Pathological endogenous secretion is marked by a sustained high level of secretion and loss of the normal circadian rhythm. From the 2nd decade on there is a slow continuous fall in the total daily production of cortisol. No deficiency of cortisol production has been found in rheumatoid patients unless previously treated with corticosteroids or ACTH (reviewed by Jasani et al, 1974). Thus cortisol deficiency as presently measured is not the cause of rheumatoid disease or presumably of other inflammatory arthritides. The clinical impression that during active phases of the disease higher doses of cortisol are needed and tolerated without side-effects is probably due to the increased cortisol metabolism of the hypertrophied inflammatory tissue (Wynne-Roberts & Castor, 1972) and the different metabolic pathways in the inflamed synovium resulting in a reduced effective cortisol concentration locally (Murphy & West, 1969). Further liver enzyme induction, which can be produced by many antirheumatic drugs, is known to increase corticosteroid catabolism though the clinical significance of this is unknown. Cortisol circulates bound to albumin and an α-

globulin (cortisol binding globulin (CBG) or transcortin) and the hypoalbuminaemia often found in severe rheumatic disorders may increase the severity of adverse reactions to administered cortisol (Lewis et al, 1971).

The important functions of the corticosteroids in rheumatological practise can be summarised as follows:

Metabolic

Increased gluconeogenesis impairs collagen (skin, cartilage and bone) and muscle formation and, in large doses, wound healing. Whole body calcium is reduced, partly due to an antagonism of vitamin D activity and thus reduced calcium absorption from the gut, and partly due to increased urinary calcium excretion. Raised cortisol levels reduce growth hormone secretion and impair its action, further reducing longitudinal growth in childhood and bone and cartilage formation at all ages.

Anti-inflammatory

Glucocorticosteroids inhibit inflammatory responses at many levels and in particular reduce the ensuing connective tissue growth. The reaction to infection can be seriously impaired leading to failure to localise infection and, of equal importance, delay in its recognition and treatment. Conversely, increased cortisol may be required to combat the stress of infection in patients on long-term corticosteroid supplements.

Immunological

Many immunological reactions are reduced although large doses of corticosteroids are necessary to do this. As the dose given increases, cell-mediated and, relatively late and only with very large doses, humoral immunity are affected.

Cardiovascular

In conjunction with noradrenaline and angiotensin cortisol maintains arteriolar tone and blood pressure. Failure of maintentenance of blood pressure is one of the features of shock, the diagnosis of which may be delayed in patients on corticosteroid treatment.

The clinical effects of excess corticosteroid follow from this wide spectrum of physiological and pharmacological actions. Both the level and duration of corticosteroid excess are important, temporary elevation of corticosteroid being of little significance. The halogenated corticosteroid compounds, triamcinolone and dexamethasone, are thought to produce a myopathy most readily. Detection is difficult since weakness and fatigue precede wasting, there is no muscle necrosis, nor signs of inflammation such as tenderness and stiffness (Afifi et al, 1968), hence the muscle enzymes are not usually increased nor is electromyography abnormal although prolonged action potentials have been reported (Muller & Kugelberg, 1959). Atrophy of the type II fibres with preservation of type I fibres has been described (Engel, 1966). Improvement may be slow after withdrawal of treatment due to the underlying disease being partly responsible for the myopathy, and in many of the conditions for which corticosteroids are given, there can be difficulty in differentiating weakness due to the disease and due to the corticosteroid given.

Osteoporosis induced by cortisol does not differ significantly from that in other forms of osteoporosis. The part played by administered corticosteroids in the production or acceleration of osteoporosis, particularly when an underlying disease associated with a catabolic state such as rheumatoid arthritis is present, is still not clear. Nor is the pathogenesis of the local form of bone collapse known as aseptic bone necrosis, although it is probably multifactorial. Some of these patients are on corticosteroids which may predispose to the development of the condition possibly by a combination of osteoporosis and fat embolism (Fischer & Bickel, 1971).

Rapid reduction of corticosteroid or following the removal of an adrenal gland may result in a transient painful polyarthritis which has no diagnostic features other than the time of onset and the response to slightly larger than normal maintenance dose of corticosteroids.

Rotstein & Good (1957) described steroid pseudorheumatism in which there was thickening of the skin of the legs, which was tender. There was also tenderness of bones and muscle. Some patients with skin atrophy on corticosteroid, without the full picture, are tender over the soles and heels and find walking painful. No neurological or vascular association has been found and unfortunately there are no investigations of pain tolerance.

IATROGENIC PITUITARY–ADRENAL INSUFFICIENCY

The practical problem of the corticosteroid-treated patient's inability to respond to stress, usually in the form of infections or operations, is a common one. There is usually a history of prior treatment with corticosteroids but to formally assess the status of the pituitary adrenal axis the following tests can be performed. Plasma cortisol taken at 8–9 a.m. or 24 hour urinary 17-oxogenic corticosteroid excretion estimations are relatively easy to perform but do not test the ability to respond to stress. Two tests are used to assess this response. ACTH as a 6 hour infusion or tetracosactrin depot 1 mg followed by a single blood sample 5–6 hours later; or, more conveniently, the synthetic tetracosactrin is given in the early morning and the plasma cortisol measured 30 and 60 minutes later. An incremental increase of 300 nmol/l or a maximal value greater than 550 nmol/l (both measured fluorometrically or by radio-immunoassay) should be obtained. If these results are abnormal the test should be repeated after giving tetracosactrin daily for three days. This test does not exclude ACTH deficiency which is most satisfactorily done by means of an insulin tolerance test in which the blood glucose concentration must fall below 2.2 nmol/l and be associated with symptoms or signs of hypoglycaemia. During the test the plasma cortisol should rise at least 170 nmol/l and to a maximum of over 550 nmol/l.

The practical answer to the problem in most cases is to give cortisone or hydrocortisone just before, during and after the period of stress, subsequently reducing the dose over several days.

PREGNANCY

The physiological state of pregnancy imposes biochemical, immunological, biomechanical and above all psychological stresses of variable degree on the mother. These are acutely reversed following delivery. The importance of these changes on parturition are well known and accepted as part of normal pregnancy; relatively little attention is paid to the immediate musculoskeletal symptoms produced, nor to the later sequelae.

Biochemical changes

Principle among the biochemical changes are increased secretion of hormones, especially oestrogens, progesterone and relaxin. The placenta is a major source of prostaglandins which appear in large quantities at parturition and although clinical improvement of rheumatoid arthritis occurs during pregnancy, no clear benefit has followed administration of oestrogens, progesterone, pregnant blood or placental extracts to patients with inflammatory arthritis. In 1938 Hench noted the suppression of rheumatoid arthritis in 20 of 22 young pregnant women and in 1949 suggested that cortisone was the antirheumatic compound concerned. This increased cortisol effect is due to several factors, the loss of diurnal rhythm, increased production, increased free cortisol and reduced clearance of cortisol. Other biochemical changes such as rises in serum cholestrol, acute phase reactants, e.g. fibrinogen, and altered albumin and globulin ratios seem to be of relatively little importance other than confusing the picture by increasing the erythrocyte sedimentation rate. No difference in the biochemical changes induced by pregnancy has been found between the normal and arthritic patient except in cortisol metabolism, where the rheumatoid process may produce alteration in cortisol breakdown.

Apart from these biochemical alterations, human pregnant serum has been shown to have other effects on the inflammatory response. Thus McArthur et al (1971) found higher free tryptophan levels in both pregnant and jaundiced sera and also following treatment with anti-inflammatory agents. Hempel et al (1970) have demonstrated that pregnant serum contains a factor which will increase the stability of lysosomes; this serum factor is not found in the serum from rats with adjuvant-induced arthritis.

Immunological changes

Alterations of the immune response presumably of a physiological nature but with potential pathogenic consequences, are found during pregnancy and menstruation and have been extensively investigated (reviewed by Persellin, 1981). The most consistent changes in immune and inflammatory responses occur in the second half of pregnancy. Oestrogens, progesterone, testroterone, cortisol, pregnancy-specific glycoprotein (B_1-glycoprotein) and pregnancy associated α_2-glycoprotein (PAG) all increase during pregnancy and fall sharply after parturition. Of these cortisol and α_2-glycoprotein have the main claim to immunoregulation which is designed specifically to retain the fetus but also has non-specific anti-inflammatory effects. Several forms of polymorphonuclear cell and lymphocyte function are reduced, but some of these functions can be restored by washing the cells, implying an acquired reversible defect of the cell from the surrounding serum rather than an inherent defect. This impaired immune/inflammatory response has been demonstrated with infections such as the tuberculin response.

Holt & Popovic (1976) have shown that pregnant serum may have immunoregulatory effects on normal lymphocytes and Oka & Vainio (1966) found that there was a tendency for the antiglobulin to fall during pregnancy although other features affecting the prognosis of rheumatoid arthritis are unchanged. These physiological alterations probably underlie the fluctuating activity of rheumatic diseases during pregnancy. Most of these inhibitory effects demonstrated in vitro disappear within hours of delivery.

During the menstrual cycle, changes, probably of a lesser degree, occur in immune reactions and inflammatory responses and Rudge co-workers (Rudge et al, 1983) have demonstrated the importance of this when assessing the responses of menstruating women to therapy such as in drug trials.

Trials of rubella vaccination suggest that women are most likely to develop joint symptoms if vaccinated within 7 days of menstruation — the safest period being in the last 7 days of the cycle (Best et al, 1974).

Biomechanical changes

The normal female pelvis is more obliquely placed than in the male and this is associated with a greater lumbar lordosis and lumbosacral angulation, and weaker muscles and ligaments. Upon these joints pregnancy imposes obvious mechanical changes of increased weight, an altered centre of gravity, increased lumbar lordosis, increased laxity of both spinal and pelvic ligaments and increased pressure on the pelvic brim. Movement of the lower part of the sacrum occurs backwards and there is also a sliding movement of the sacroiliac joints, although the actual distance between the bones in unchanged. Diastasis of the symphysis pubis is present and gas may be found in both sacroiliac and symphysis pubis during normal pregnancy (Russell, 1969). There is an increase in the angle made by the lumbosacral vertebrae, an area that is already predisposed to cause trouble. Calguneri et al (1982) have shown increased mobility laxity of peripheral joints during pregnancy.

Morphological examination of these joints in normal pregnancy has shown vascular hypertrophy and fissuring of the cartilage, periosteal resorption and bone sclerosis. These features were described by Luschka (1854) and Loeschke (1912) who found reversible changes as early as the 2nd month of pregnancy. These progress with pregnancy and reach a maximum at the 8th–9th month. Following delivery the centre of gravity reverts to normal and there is a period when the abdominal muscles remain lax and indeed may never regain their antepartum strength, an inability to raise the extended legs from the horizontal being not uncommon.

It would be surprising of these various changes did not have an effect on co-existing rheumatic disease.

The interaction of pregnancy and the rheumatic diseases is reviewed by Cecere & Persellin (1981). In general 75% of rheumatoid patients will improve during pregnancy but will invariably relapse after delivery or abortion. This benefit is repeated in subsequent pregnancies. There is no clear evidence that rheumatoid disease is prone to start during pregnancy. Kay & Bach (1965) suggested that women with rheumatoid arthritis are subfertile and have fewer pregnancies, even before they develop their arthritis, and have an earlier menopause. This work has not been confirmed.

The effect of pregnancy on systemic lupus erythematosus is generally felt to be less predictable and less favourable than with rheumatoid arthritis, more cases tending to exacerbate. The main problem has been in differentiating progressive renal disease due to SLE and deteriorating renal function associated with toxaemia. Undoubtedly there has been an improvement due to better management. In the inactive stages of SLE, fertility is probably not superficially impaired, although in active phases and when large doses of corticosteroid are used, amenorrhea is common.

Although most cases of rheumatoid arthritis remit during pregnancy, exacerbation of systemic lupus erythematosus tends to occur and the rare cases of ankylosing spondylitis where both mechanical and inflammatory problems may be present, may get better or worse during pregnancy and delivery, though without permanent deterioration.

Mention of the effect of abnormal pregnancy on skeletal deformities in the newborn should be made. Although not proven, oligohydramnios is thought to lead to such skeletal abnormalities as talipes, scolosis and dislocation of the hip; the evidence has been discussed by Dunn (1976) including his own epidemiological results and, in particular, he finds that affected babies often have more than one deformity. Fetal wastage is quite markedly increased is SLE, particularly if there is renal impairment.

Rheumatic complications of pregnancy

A minor, though troublesome, carpal tunnel compression syndrome is frequent, difficult to treat, but always regresses after delivery. Fluid retention and increased fatty tissue are probably responsible for the compression. An interesting syndrome of recurrent finger clubbing and hypertrophic osteodystrophy occurring during pregnancy has been described by Cullen & Maskery (1966). Osteopenia is found in some pregnant women and depends largely on the previous bone status which is itself subject to geographical variation (Salzberger et al, 1960; Nordin & Roper, 1955). A more clearly defined syndrome (of unknown aetiology) is the transient osteoporosis of the hip.

Transient osteoporosis of the hip in pregnancy

Longstreth et al (1973) have reviewed the literature of transient osteoporosis of the hip and added one case of their own. They found that of the 31 cases, eight were females and six of these were pregnant at the time of onset. In these six cases the onset was in the later stages of pregnancy. Both unilateral and bilateral involvement occurred, the main symptom being pain. In spite of the dramatic radiological appearances, recovery was rapid and usually complete. In the case reported by Longstreth et al (1973) the newborn infant also had radiotranslucent areas and growth arrest lines in the long bones at the age of 2 months.

Two major syndromes occur during pregnancy or following delivery — low back pain with or without symptoms referred to the legs and the pelvic relaxation syndrome. Occasionally both may occur in the same patient, most frequently in the first pregnancy. Recurrence in future pregnancies is very common.

Low back pain

Low back pain in pregnancy is similar in symptomatology to other forms of non-specific low back pain (Mantle et al, 1977). It is frequent (48%); when the symptoms persist after delivery, care should be taken before operating to evaluate whether the symptoms are psychoneurotic in origin. It may result from a combination of the mechanical factors mentioned above, ligamentatous laxity and an underlying predisposition or premorbid change already present in the patient. Walde (1962) has reported that 13 out of 137 patients with pelvic relaxation also had disc herniation and Hagen (1974) discussed five out of 23 patients who developed symptoms of disc herniation in relationship to pregnancy and delivery. Recurrence later in life may escape association with the prior pregnancy and the prognosis of pregnancy induced low back ache in terms of recurrence unassociated with pregnancy is completely unknown. Schmorl (1927) suggested that the lithotomy position used for gynaecological operations might produce tears of the intervertebral discs; at present there is no evidence to support or refute this claim.

Pelvic relaxation syndrome

Interpretation of the origin of pelvic pain is difficult; it often arises in pelvic viscera, being referred to the peripheral segments supplied by the lower lumbar and sacral nerves, that is the anterior abdominal wall, thighs, groins and legs. Although occurring to some degree in many normal pregnancies, the term 'pelvic relaxation' has been applied when excessive symptoms are produced. Thus the borderline between physiological and pathological is indistinct. Local tenderness over the affected joint is a very useful and frequent sign and may be easily elicited in the symphysis pubis by a finger placed over the pubis or in the vagina when the wide separation and local tenderness can be easily appreciated; sacroiliac tenderness is more difficult to determine. Tenderness over the origin of the thigh adductors is frequent and occasional tenderness of the costochondral and costosternal junctions may be found. Characteristically pain occurs during walking, particularly upstairs or turning over in bed. Pain arising in either sacroiliac or symphysis pubis joint will cause a positive Trendelberg's sign with a waddling, hesitant gait. Radiologically laxity of the pelvic joints can sometimes be seen with widening of the symphysis pubis and occasionally unequal height of the pubic bones on weight-bearing on one leg (Fig. 39.19). This may be associated with a clicking sound on movement. However, none of these changes are necessary for the diagnosis. In relaxation of the sacroiliac joints lumbar sacral disc disease may be mimicked with a stiff back and even a positive Lasègue sign (Genell, 1948).

A periarticular sclerosis of the sacroiliac joint affecting the iliac bone only in the middle and lower part of the joint is a symptomless radiological finding (osteitis condensens ilii). It is more frequent in multipara.

Treatment. Prophylactic treatment mainly consisting of practical assessment and routine antenatal classes started before the second half of pregnancy helped to reduce the incidence of backache (Mantle et al, 1981).

During pregnancy treatment is mainly symptomatic with analgesia, rest and sacroiliac belt. Following delivery, spontaneous recovery is usual, although recurrence in subsequent pregnancies is frequent and again conservative treatment suffices in the majority of cases. Prophylactic exercises to strengthen the abdominal muscles should be started after the first post-partum month.

Although the degrees of pubic symphyseal separation, while weight-bearing, either horizontally or vertically, are not decisive, if the width exceeds

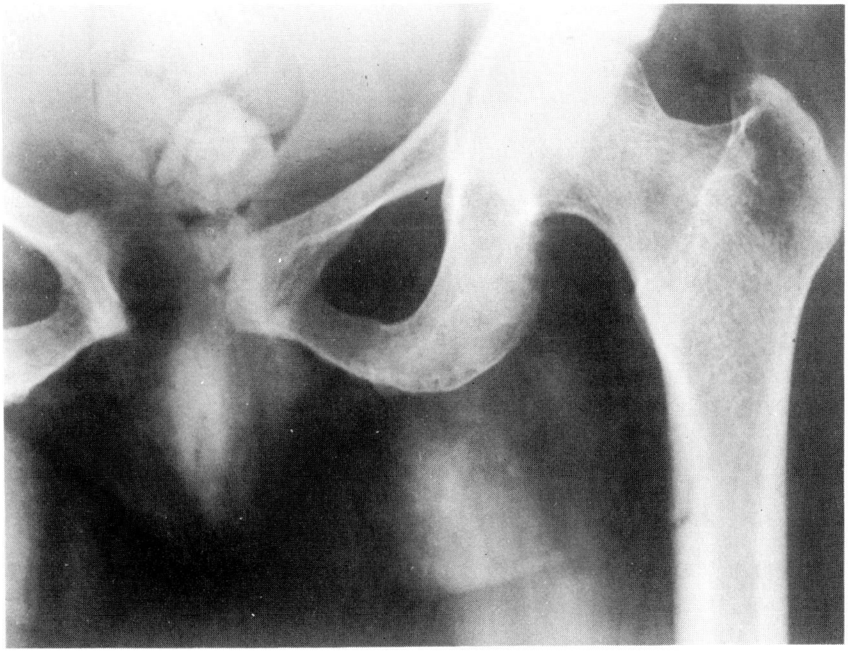

Fig. 39.19 Pelvic relaxation syndrome. Excessive widening of the symphysis pubis has occurred. Patient non-weight-bearing so that there is no inequality of height. (Note also Looser zone of the left femoral shaft — associated with osteomalacia in Asian women). (By permission of Butterworth, London. Dr J. G. B. Russell).

10 mm and the vertical shift is more than 5 mm and if combined with widening and sclerosis of the sacroiliac joints, there is a tendency to a delayed convalescence (Hagen, 1974). It is in these cases that operation may be indicated. Although patients may go through natural childbirth after fusion of the symphysis pubis and sacroiliac joints, whether produced by either surgery or ankylosing spondylitis, it is probably better to delay this operation until after child bearing has ceased.

Osteitis pubis

This painful condition arises usually within 2 months of delivery or other pelvic operation, when it can occur in the male, for example, following prostatectomy (Barnes & Malament, 1963). Pain is felt in the pubic area, groins and inner aspects of thighs and is present when sitting but aggravated by movements such as walking or sneezing. There is spasm of the thigh adductors and abdominal muscles. The gait is waddling and there is tenderness, often severe, of the symphysis pubis. The most comfortable position is lying in bed with the hips slightly flexed. The white cell count and ESR may be normal and radiographs, although also initially normal, later show irregular porosis and 'moth-eaten' erosions which are later replaced by sclerosis as the condition settles. Eventually ankylosis of the symphysis may occur. Local aspiration of an abscess cavity may reveal an infective organism, but the aetiology of the condition is usually obscure and the many treatments which have been advocated probably reflect the variety of theories about the aetiology and the rather poor response often found is usually due to delay in the initial diagnosis. Prolonged treatment with antibiotic and anti-inflammatory drugs is often successful. Occasionally surgical drainage or arthrodesis of the joint are necessary.

MENOPAUSAL ARTHRALGIA

Ill-defined aches and pains without objective finding are not uncommon at the menopause. Although usually mild and of minor consequence, in some patients they can assume major degree and require treatment. Other features of the menopause are not necessarily excessive and serum biochemistry and serology are normal. The cause of these symptoms is unknown, a combination of emotional lability, hormone imbalance, tissue fluid changes and other more subtle biochemical alteration is most probable. The presence of coexisting osteoarthrosis, usually of the generalised type, may account for some of the symptoms. The prognosis is good unless generalised osteoarthrosis develops.

Treatment, where necessary, with small doses of oestrogens rapidly clears the symptoms which seldom last two years.

THE CONTRACEPTIVE PILL

Although rheumatic symptoms do occur in a minority of patients taking oral contraceptive preparations, they are usually mild and do not lead to disability (Ramcharen, 1981). Erythema nodosum and arthralgia occur either in isolation or together. The arthralgia is characteristically migratory, affecting the small and large joints with minimal synovitis and no bone change. Systemic upset is rare and the symptoms usually settle after stopping the drug or, occasionally, after altering the preparation used, but recur with reintroduction of the drug. The appearance of anti-nuclear factors (ANF) in the serum after taking the contraceptive pill is not uncommon, (Bole et al, 1969; Kay et al, 1971), and LE cells are common but DNA antibodies are not raised. Immunoglobin levels may be increased. Withdrawal of the pill results in both a disappearance of LE cells and a marked reduction in positive ANF titres. Depression, which can be severe, was found in 11.8% of patients on contraceptive drugs (Herzberg et al, 1971), and the clinical picture may then closely resemble systemic lupus erythematosus.

The pathogenesis of this syndrome and of the immunological changes is unknown. Oestrogens and hormonal contraceptive therapy have been shown to reduce in vitro lymphocyte reactivity (Hagen & Froland, 1972; Barnes et al, 1974; Alblin, 1974), but increased skin cell-mediated immunity has also been found (Gerretson et al, 1975). Auto-antibodies in general are found more frequently and in higher titre in women.

Whether these patients are examples of drug-induced SLE or patients with an underlying SLE diathesis, is uncertain; however, with the lower doses of contraceptive now being used, this syndrome appears to be becoming much less frequent.

The effect of contraceptive pills on rheumatoid arthritis has been debated, but recent large surveys suggest that the use of oral contraceptives may halve the incidence of rheumatoid arthritis (Wingrave & Kay 1978; Vandenbrouche et al, 1982) However, this work is retrospective and the part played by various components of the contraceptive pill is not clear. There is evidence that the protective effect may be equally strong for ex-users and current users.

REFERENCES

Ablin R J, Bruns G R, Guinan P, Bush J M 1974 The effect of estrogen on the incorporation of H-thymidine by PHA stimulated human peripheral blood lymphocytes. Journal of Immunology 113:705

Afifi A K, Bergman R A, Harvey M C 1968 Steroid myopathy clinical, histological and cytological observations. John Hopkins Medical Journal 123:158

Alexander G M, Dieppe P A, Doherty M, Scott D G I 1982 Pyrophosphate arthropathy: a study of metabolic association and laboratory data. Annals of the Rheumatic Diseases 41; 4:377

Amrhein J A, Kenny F M, Ross D 1970 Granulocytopenia, lupus like syndrome and other complications of propylthiouracil therapy. Journal of Pathology 76:54

Aschner B 1909 Demonstration von Hunden nach Exstirpation der Hypophyse. Munch Med Wochschr 56:2668

Ashton I K, Francis M J D 1978 Response of chondrocytes isolated from human foetal cartilage to plasma somatomedin activity. Journal of Endocrinology 76:473

Barnes E W, MacCuish A C, Loudon N B, Jordan J, Irvine W J 1974 Phytohaemagglutinin-induced lymphocyte transformation and circulating auto-antibodies in women taking oral contraceptives. Lancet 1:898

Barnes W C, Malament M 1963 Osteitis pubus. Surgery Gynaecology and Obstetrics 117:277

Beardwell C G 1975 Immunology of endocrine disease. In: Taylor G (ed) Immunology in medical practice. Saunders, London

Becker K L, Ferguson R H, McConahey W M 1963 The connective tissue diseases and symptoms associated with Hasgimoto's thyroiditis. New England Journal of Medicine 268:277

Benedetti A, Noacco C, Cattano G, Macor S 1975 Juvenile diabetes cheiroarthropathy. VIII European Rheumatology Congress, Helsinki

Best J M, Banatvala J E, Bowen J M 1974 New japanese rubella vaccine. Comparative trials. British Medical Journal 3:221

Bland J H, Frymoyer J W 1970 Rheumatic syndromes of myxedema. New England Journal of Medicine, 282:1171

Bloch K J, Bunim J J 1963 Sjögren's syndrome and its relationship to connective tissue disease. Journal of Chronic Disease 16:915

Bluestone R, Bywaters E G L, Hartog M, Holt P J L, Hyde S 1971 Acromegalic Arthropathy. Annals of the Rheumatic Diseases 30:243

Bole G C, Friedlander M H, Smith C K 1969 Rheumatic symptoms and serological abnormalities induced by oral contraception. Lancet 1:323

Boswell S H, Baylin C J 1973 Metastatic fat necrosis and lytic bone lesions in a patient with painless acute pancreatis. Radiology 106:85

Bowser-Riley S, Bain A D, Nobel J, Lamb D W 1975 Chromosome abnormalities in Dupuytren's disease. Lancet 2: 1282–83

Boyle J A, Greig W R, Duncan A M, Boyle I J, Buchanan W W 1966 Serum uric acid values in various states of thyroid function. Acta Rheumatica Scandinavica 12:204

Boyle J A, McKiddie M, Buchanan K D, Jasani M K, Gray H W, Jackson I M D, Buchanan W W 1969 Diabetes mellitus and gout. Blood sugar and plasma insulin response to oral glucose in normal weight, overweight and gouty patients. Annals of the Rheumatic Diseases 28:374

Bridgeman J F 1972 Periarthritis of the shoulder and diabetes mellitus. Annals of the Rheumatic Diseases 31:69

Broca A 1888 Un squelette d'acromegalie. Archives Generale de Medicine (Paris) 2:656

Bruckner F E, Howell A 1972 Neuropathic Joints Seminar. Arthritis and Rheumatism 2:47

Buckingham B A, Uitto J, Sandborg C, Keens T, Kaufman F, Landing B 1981 Scleroderma-like syndrome and non-enzymatic glycosylation of collagen in children in poorly controlled insulin dependent diabetes. Paediatric Research 15:626 (abstract)

Bywaters E G L 1969 Gout and other metabolic diseases. In: Copeman W S C (ed) Copeman's textbook of the rheumatic diseases, 4th Edn. Churchill Livingstone, Edinburgh

Calguneri M, Bird H A, Wright V 1981 Changes in joint laxity occurring during pregnancy. Annals of the Rheumatic Diseases 41:126

Campbell W L, Feldman F 1975 Bone and soft tissue abnormalities of the upper extremity in diabetes mellitus. American Journal of Roentgenology Radium Therapy Nuclear Medicine 124:7

Canalis M, Dietrich J W, Maini D M, Raisz L G 1977 Hormonal control of bone collagen synthesis in vitro. Effects of insulin and glucagon. Endocrinology 100:668

Cartlidge N E, Black M M, Hall M R 1970 Pituitary function in the elderly. Gerontologia Clinica (Basel) 12:65

Cecere F A, Persellin R H 1981 The interaction of pregnancy and the rheumatic diseases. In: Holt P J L (ed) Clinics of the rheumatic diseases 7:747

Chang K, Witto J, Rowold R A, Grant G A, Kilo C, Williamson J R 1980 Increased collagen cross linkages in experimental diabetes: reversal by beta-aminopropionitrile and D-penicillamine. Diabetes 29 (10):778

Child D L, Yates D A H 1978 Radicular pain in diabetes. Rheumatology and Rehabilitation 17:195

Chokroverty S 1976 Myxedema, myopathy and myasthenia. Transactions of the American Neurological Association 101:226

Clouse M E, Gramn H F, Legg M, Flood T 1974 Diabetic osteoarthropathy. Clinical and roentgenographic observations in 90 cases. American Journal of Roentgenology Radium Therapy Nuclear Medicine 121:22

Collins J A Jr, Zimer F E, Johnson W J, Hough R H 1964 The many faces of hypothyroidism. Postgraduate Medicine 36:371

Critchley E M, Vakil S D, Haywood H W, et al 1976 Dupuytren's disease in epileptics: result of prolonged administration of anticonvulsants. Journal of Neurology, Neurosurgery, Psychiatry 39:498

Cullen D R, Maskery P J 1966 Clubbing of the fingers and hypertrophic osteoarthropathy in pregnancy. Lancet 2:473

Davidoff L M 1926 Studies in Acromegaly III. The anamnesis and symptomatology in one hundred cases. Endocrinology 3:461

Delamere J P, Scott D L, Felix-Davies D D 1982 Thyroid dysfunction and rheumatic diseases. Journal of the Royal Society of Medicine 75:102

Delling G R, Schulz A 1977 Bone cells and remodelling surfaces in acromegaly. Calcified Tissue Research 22 (Suppl):255

Dent G R, Edward O M 1978 Auto-immune thyroid disease and the polymyalgia rheumatica — giant cell arteritis syndrome. Clinical Endocrinology 9:215

Dequeker J, Burssens A, Creytens G, Bouillon R 1975 Ageing of bone: its relation to osteoporosis and osteoarthritis in post-menopausal women. In: Von Keep P A, Lauritzen C (eds) Frontiers of hormone research, Vol 3. Karger, Basel, p. 166

Deterbeck L C, Tressler H A, O'Duffy J A, Randall R V 1973 Peripheral joint manifestations of acromegaly. Clinical, Orthopaedic and Related Research 91:119

Donniak D, Botazzi G F, Russell R G G 1978 Goitrous thyroiditis (Hashimoto's disease). Clinics in Endocrinology and Metabolism 8:63

Dorwart B B, Schumacher H R 1974 Hand deformities resembling rheumatoid arthritis. Seminars in Arthritis and Rheumatism 4:53

Dorwart B B, Schumacher H R 1975 Joint effusions, chondrocalcinosis and other rheumatic manifestations in hypothyroidism. American Journal of Medicine 59:780

Dunn P M 1976 Congenital postural deformities. British Medical Bulletin 32:71

Engel A C 1966 Electron microscopic observations in thyrotoxic and corticosteroid induced myopathies. Mayo Clinic Proceedings 41: 985–986

Epps C H, Martin E D 1963 Slipped capital femoral epiphysis in a sexually mature myxedematous female. Journal of the American Medical Association 183:287

Erdheim J 1931 Pathologie und Klinik in Einzeldarsteilungen, Vol 3. Aschoff, Elias H (eds). Eppinger H, Steinberic & Wenckebach W F, Berlin

Evans H M, Long J A 1922 Characteristic effects upon growth, arteries and ovulation induced by the intraperitoneal administration of fresh anterior hypophysical substance. Proceedings of the National Academy of Science 8:38

Fessel W J 1968 Myopathy of hypothyroidism. Annals of the Rheumatic Diseases 27:590

Fincham R W, Cape C A 1968 Neuropathy in myxedema. A study of sensory nerve conduction in the upper extremities. Archives of Neurology (Chicago) 19:464

Fischer D E, Bickel W H 1971 Corticosteroid induced avascular necrosis — a clinical study of seventy-seven patients. Journal of Bone and Joint Surgery 53A: 859–873

Fisher M S 1978 An unusual bone change in acromegaly. Skeletal Radiology 3:177

Fogelman I, Hay I D, Citron D L, Brastal C H, Turner J G, Bessant M A 1981 Semi-quantitative analysis of the bone scan in acromegaly correlation with human growth hormone values. British Journal of Radiology 53:874

Forestier J, Lagier R 1971A Vertebral ankylosing hyperostosis. In: Hill A C S (ed) Modern trends in rheumatology 2. Butterworth, London

Forestier J, Lagier R 1971B Ankylosing hyperostosis of the spine. Clinical Orthopaedics and Related Research 74:65

Francis M J O, Ellis J P, Hockadry T D R 1974 Skin collagen in diabetes melittus in relation to treatment. Proceedings of the Royal Society of Medicine 67:35

Freeman A G 1958 Gross digital clubbing and exophthalmoplegia in thyroid disease. Lancet 1:57

Fritzsche G, Klebs E 1884 Eine Beitrag zue Pathologie des Reisenwuchses. In: Klinische und Pathologisch-Anatom Untersuchnger. Vogel F C W, Leipzig

Frymoyer J W, Bland J 1973 Carpal tunnel syndrome in patients with myxedematous arthropathy. Journal of Bone and Joint Surgery (AM) 55:78

Gardner D L 1969 Pathology of the Rheumatic Diseases. In: Copeman W S C (ed) Copeman's textbook of the rheumatic diseases, 4th Edn. Churchill Livingstone, Edinburgh

Genell S 1948 Studies on insufficient pelvis (gravidarum et puerperarum). Acta Obstetricia et Gynecologica Scandinavica 28:1

Gerretsen G, Kremer J, Bleumink E, Nâter J P 1975 Dinitrochlorobenzene sensitivation test on women on hormonal contraceptives. Lancet 3:347

Gimlette T M D 1960 Thyroid acropachy. Lancet 1:22

Golding D N 1970 Hypothyroidism presenting with musculoskeletal symptoms. Annals of the Rheumatic Diseases 29:10

Goldman J, Matz R, Mortimer R, Freeman R 1977 High elevations of creatine phosphokinase in hypothyroidism. Journal of the American Medical Association 238:325

Goldstein S, Littlefield J W, Sochdner J S 1969 Diabetes mellitus and ageing: diminished plating efficiency of cultured human platelets. Proceedings of the National Academy of Science 64:155

Goluboff N, Cram R, Ramgotra B, Singh A, Wilkinson S W 1978 Polyarthritis and bone lesions complicating traumatic pancreatitis in two children. Canadian Medical Association Journal 118:924

Gorsuch A W, Spencer K M, Lister J, McNally J M, Dean B M, Bottazzi G F, Cudworth A G 1981 Evidence for a long prediabetic period in type I (insulin dependent) diabetes mellitus. Lancet 2:1363

Grgic A, Rosenbloom A L, Weber F T, Giordano B, Malone J I 1975 Joint contracture in childhood diabetes. New England Journal of Medicine 292:372

Gull W W 1874 On a cretinoid state supervening in adult life in women. Transactions of the Clinical Society London 7:180

Hagen C, Froland A 1972 Depressed lymphocyte response to PHA in women taking oral contraceptives. Lancet 1:1185

Hagen R 1974 Pelvic girdle relaxation from an orthopaedic point of view. Acta Orthopaedica Scandinavica 45:550

Hall K 1971 Effect of intravenous administration of human growth hormone on sulphation factor activity in serum of hypopituitary subjects. Acta Endocrinologica 66:491

Hamilton E D 1976 Diseases associated with CPPD deposition disease. Arthritis and Rheumatism 19:353

Hamlin C R, Kohn R R, Luschin J H 1975 Apparent accelerated ageing of human collagen in diabetes mellitus. Diabetes 24:902

Harris J, Carter A R, Glick E N, Story G O 1974 Ankylosing hyperostosis. Clinical and radiological features. Annals of the Rheumatic Diseases 33:210

Hartog M 1967 Acromegaly and hyperparathyroidism. Proceedings of the Royal Society of Medicine 60:477

Hempel K H, Fernandez L A, Persellin R H 1970 Effect of pregnancy sera on isolated lysosomes. Nature 225:955

Hench P S 1938 Ameliorating effect of pregnancy on chronic atrophic (infectious) rheumatoid arthritis, fibrositis and intermittent hydroarthrosis. Proceedings of staff meeting, Mayo Clinic 13:161

Hench P S, Kendall E C, Slocomb C H, Polley H F 1949 Effect of hormone cortex (17-hydroxy 11-dehydrocorticosterone compound) and of pituitary adrenocorticotrophic hormone on rheumatoid arthritis preliminary report. Proceedings of the Mayo Clinic 14:181

Herzberg B N, Draper K C, Johnson A L, Nicol G C 1971 Oral contraceptives, depression and libido. British Medical Journal 3:495

Hirano T, Stamelos S, Harris V, Dumboric N 1978 Association of primary hypothyroidism and slipped capital femoral epiphysis. Journal of Paediatrics 93:262

Holt P J L, Popovic M 1976 Alterations of T cell function by serum factors in rheumatoid arthritis and systemic lupus erythematosus. In: Dumonde D C (ed) Infections and immunology in the rheumatic diseases. Blackwell, London, p. 467

Horenstein S, Hambrook G, Eyerman E 1971 Spinal cord compression by vertebral acromegaly. Transactions of the American Neurology Association 96:254

How J, Bruscher P D, Walker W 1977 Giant cell arteritis and hypothyroidism. British Medical Journal 2:99

Jackson R L, Holland E, Chatman I D, Guthrie D, Hewitt J E 1978 Growth and maturation of children with insulin dependent diabetes mellitus. Diabetes Care 1:96

Jadresic A, Banks L M, Child D F, Diamant L, Doyle F H, Fraser R T, Joplin G F 1982 The acromegalic syndrome. Relation between clinical features, growth hormone values and radiological characteristics of the pituitary tumours. Quarterly Journal of Medicine 51:189

Jasani M K, Diver M J, Bell A M, Dalakos T G K, Buchanan W W 1974 Some clinical observations on the diurnal rhythm of plasma cortisol (11 — OHCS) in patients with rheumatoid arthritis treated with oral corticosteroid drugs. Current Medical Research and Opinion 2:373

Julkunen H, Heinonen O P, Pyoralav 1971 Hyperostosis of the spine in an adult population. Annals of the Rheumatic Diseases 30:605

Julkunen K, Heinonen O P, Knekt P, Maatela J 1975 The epidemiology of hyperostosis of the spine together with its symptoms and related mortality in a general population. Scandinavian Journal of Rheumatology 4:23

Julkunen H, Knekt P, Aromaa S 1981 Spondylitic deformans and diffuse idiopathic skeletal hyperostosis (DISH) in Finland. Scandinavian Journal of Rheumatology 10:193

Jung Y, Hohmann T C, Gerneth J A, et al 1971 Diabetic hand syndrome. Metabolism 20:1008

Kaklamanis P, Rigas A, Gianatos J, et al 1975 Calcification of the shoulder and diabetes mellitus. New England Journal of Medicine 293:1266

Kay A, Bach F 1965 Subfertility before and after the development of rheumatoid arthritis in women. Annals of the Rheumatic Diseases 24:169

Kay D R, Bole G C, Ledger W J 1971 Antinuclear antibodies, rheumatoid factor and C-reactive protein in serum of normal women using oral contraceptives. Arthritis and Rheumatism 14:239

Kellgren J H, Ball J, Tutton G K 1952 Articular and other limb changes in acromegaly; a clinical and pathological study of 25 cases. Quarterly Journal of Medicine 21:405

Kilpatrick J M, Virella G 1980 Isolation and characterisation of soluble insulin — anti-insulin immune complexes found in vitro and in vivo in sera from patient with diabetes mellitus. Clinical and Experimental Immunology 40:445

Kinsella R A, Beck D F 1968 Thyroid acropachy. Medical Clinics of North America 52:395

Kleinberg D L, et al 1964 The sesamoid index: an aid in the diagnosis of acromegaly. Annals of Internal Medicine 64:1075

Lahey F H 1926 Quadricep test for myasthenia of thyroidism. Journal of the American Medical Association 87:754

Lamotte M, Segrestaa J M, Krassinine C 1966 Arthrite microcristalline calique (pseudogoutte) chez un acromegale. Semaine des Hopitaux de Paris 42:2420

Leeper R D, Bencau R A, Brener J L, Rawson R W 1960 Hyperuricaemia in myxoedema. Journal of Clinical Endocrinology and Metabolism 20:1457

Lequesne M, Dang W, Benasson M, Mery C 1977 Increased association of diabetes mellitus with capsulitis of the shoulder and shoulder hand syndrome. Scandinavian Journal of Rheumatology 6:53

Levin M E, O'Neal L W 1977 The diabetic foot, 2nd Edn. Mosbey, St Louis

Levin M E, Boisseau V C, Avioli L V 1976 Diabetes mellitus and bone mass in juvenile and adult onset diabetes. New England Journal of Medicine 294:241

Lev-Ran A, Joshua H, Mannheimer S 1971 Insulin antibodies in diabetes. Israeli Journal of Medical Science 7:1035

Lewis G P, Jick H, Slone D 1971 The role of genetic factors and serum protein binding in determining drug response as revealed by comprehensive drug surveillance. Annals of the New York Academy of Sciences 179:729

Lewis P D 1972 Neuromuscular involvement in pituitary gigantism. British Medical Journal 2:499

Librik L, Sussman L, Bejar R, Clayton G W 1970 Thyrotoxicosis and collagen-like diseases in three sisters of American Indian extraction. Journal of Paediatrics 76:64

Lippman H I, Perotto A, Farrar R 1976 The neuropathic foot of the diabetic. Bulletin, New York Academy of Medicine 52:1159

Littlejohn G O, Smyth H A 1981 Marked hyperinsulinaemia after glucose challenge in patients with diffuse idiopathic skeletal hyperostosis. Journal of Rheumatology 8:965

Loeschke H 1912 Untersuchungen uber Entstechung und Bedentung der Spaltbildungen in der Symphyse, sowie uber physiologische Erweiterungsvorgange am Becken Schwangerer and Geberander. Archives fur Gynakologie 96:525

Longson D, Isherwood I 1975 Personal communication

Longstreth P L, Malinak L R, Hill C S Jr 1973 Transient osteoporosis of the hip in pregnancy. Obstetrics and Gynaecology 41 4:563

Low P A, McLeod J G, Tutte J R, et al 1974 Peripheral neuropathy in acromegaly. Brain 97:139

Lundback K 1957 Stiff hands in long-term diabetes. Acta Medica Scandinavia 158:447

Luschka H 1854 Die Krenzdermbeinfuge und die

Schambeinfuge des Menschen. Archiv fur pathologische Anatomie and Physiologie (Virchow) 7:299
Lynch P J, Maize J C, Sisson J C 1973 Pretibial myxedema and nonthyrotoxic thyroid disease. Archives of Dermatology 107:107
McArthur J N, Dawkins P D, Smith M J H 1971 Mode of action of antirheumatic drugs. British Medical Journal 2:677
McCarty D J, Kohn N N, Faires J S 1962 The significance of calcium pyrophosphate crystals in the synovial fluid of the arthritic patient: 'The pseudogout syndrome'. Annals of Internal Medicine 56:711
McCarty D J, Silcox D C, Coe F 1974 Diseases associated with calcium pyrophosphate dehydrate crystal deposition. American Journal of Medicine 56:704
McNair P, Christiansen C, Christiansen M S, Madebad S, Faber O K, Binder C, Translol I 1981 Development of bone mineral loss in insulin treated diabetes. A $1\frac{1}{2}$ year follow up study in sixty patients. European Journal of Clinical Investigation 11:55
Mankin H J, Zavin S, Thrasher A, Weinberg E H, Harris W H 1978 Dissociation of the effect of bovine growth hormone in articular acromegaly and in bone of the adult dog. Journal of Bone and Joint Surgery Series A, 60A:1071
Mantle M J, Greenwood R M, Currey H L F 1977 Backache in pregnancy. Rheumatology and Rehabilitation 16:95
Mantle M J, Hremes J, Currey H L F 1981 Backache in pregnancy. Prophylactic influence of Back Care classes. Rheumatology and Rehabilitation 20:227
Marie P 1886 Sur deux cas d'acromégalie. Hypertrophie singulière non congénitale des extrémitiés superieures, inférieures et cephalique. Revue de Medécine 6:297
Masson 1975 Personal communication
Mastalgia F L, Barwick D D, Hall R 1970 Myopathy in acromegaly. Lancet 2:907
Matthay M A, Matthay R A, Mills D M, Lakshminarayan S, Cotton E 1976 Hypertrophic osteoarthropathy in adults with cystic fibrosis. Thorax 31:572
Meulengracht E, Schwartz M 1951 Course and prognosis of humerocapsular periarthritis especially in cases with general symptoms. Nordisk Medicin 46:1629
Meyer M J, Forster E 1938 Consideration pathogeniques sur l'hyperstose moniliforme due flanc droit de la columne dorsale. Revue du Rheumatisme 5:286
Minkowski O 1887 Verber einen Fall von Akromegalie. Berliner Kliniske Wockenschrift 29:371
Mohr P D, Reid H 1977 Myeloneuropathy associated with hypothyroidism. British Medical Journal 1:1005
Mulhern L M, Masi A T, Shulman L E 1966 Hashimoto's disease. A search for associated disorders in 170 clinically detected cases. Lancet 2:508
Muller R, Kugelberg E 1959 Myopathy in Cushing's syndrome. Journal of Neurology and Psychiatry 22: 314–319
Murphy D, West H F 1969 Catabolism and interconversion of cortisol and cortisone in human synovial tissue in vitro. Annals of the Rheumatic Diseases 28:637
Nagulesparen M, Trickey R, Davies M T, Jenkins J S 1976 Muscle changes in acromegaly. British Medical Journal 2:914
Nickel S N, Frame B, Bekin J, Tourtellot E W W, Parker J A, Hughes B R 1961 Myxoedema neuropathy and myopathy: a clinical and pathological study. Neurology 11:125
Nixon D W, Samol E 1970 Acral changes associated with thyroid disease. Journal of American Medical Association 212: 1175–1187
Nordin B E C, Roper A 1955 Post-pregnancy osteoporosis. Lancet 1:431
Oka M, Vainio U 1966 Effect of pregnancy on the prognosis and serology of rheumatoid arthritis. Acta Rheumatologica Scandinavica 12:47
Ord W 1878 On myxoedema: a term proposed to be applied to an essential condition in the 'cretinoid' affection occasionally observed in middle aged women. Medical Chirurgical Transactions, London 61:57
O'Sullivan J B, Williams R F 1966 Early diabetes mellitus in perspective. American Medical Association 198:579
Persellin R H 1981 Inhibitors of inflammatory and immune responses in pregnancy serum. In: Holt P J L (ed) Clinics in rheumatic diseases. Saunders, London, p. 769
Phelan G A 1970 Reflections on 21 years' experience with the carpal tunnel syndrome. Journal of the American Medical Association 212:1365
Pogonowska M J, Collins L C, Dobson H L 1967 Diabetic osteopathy. Radiology 89:265
Potts D E, Mass M F, Iseman M D 1975 Syndrome of pancreatic disease, subcutaneous fat necrosis and polyserosis, case report and review of the literature. American Journal of Medicine 58:417
Ramcharen S (ed) 1981 The Walnut Creek contraceptive drug study: a prospective study of the side effects of oral contraception, Vol III. US Government Printing Office, Washington
Ramsey I D 1966 Muscle dysfunction in hyperthyroidism. Lancet 2:931
Resnick D, Shaul S R, Robins J M 1975 Diffuse idiopathic skeletal hyperostosis (DISH): Forestier's disease with extraspinal manifestations. Radiology 115: 513–524
Resnick D, Shapiro R F, Wiesner K E, Niwayama G, Utsinger P O, Shaell S R 1978 Diffuse idiopathic skeletal hyperostosis (DISH). Ankylosing hyperostosis of Forestier and Rotes-Querol. Seminars in Arthritis and Rheumatism 7:153
Revach M, Cabilli C 1972 Dupuytren's contracture and diabetes mellitus. Israel Journal of Medical Science 774
Rosenbloom A L, Frias J L 1974 Diabetes, short status and joint stiffness: a new syndrome. Clinical Research 22:92
Rosenbloom A L, Silverstein J H, Leyotte D C, Rickardown K, McCallum M 1981 Limited joint mobility in childhood diabetes mellitus indicates increased risk for microvascular disease. New England Journal of Medicine 305:191
Rotstein J, Good B A 1957 Steroid pseudorheumatism. Annals of Internal Medicine 99:545
Rovensky J, Palkovic M, Vilas M, Smondrk J, Jezova D 1981 Plasma concentrations of hormones and lipoprotein after hyperthermia bath in man. In: Palkovic M (ed) Adar Physiol Science, Vol 35. Hormones, lipoprotein and atherosclerosis, p. 155
Rudge S R, Kowanko I C, Drury P L 1983 Menstrual cyclicity of finger joint size and grip strength in patients with rheumatoid arthritis. Annals of the Rheumatic Disease 42:425
Russell J G 1969 Moulding of the pelvic outlet. Journal of Obstetrics and Gynaecology (Brit Comm) 76:817
Salick A I, Colachis S C, Pearson C M 1968 Myxoedema myopathy: clinical electrodiagnostic and pathologic findings in advanced case. Archives of Physical Medicine and Rehabilitation 49:230
Salmon W D Jr, Du Vall M R 1970 In vitro stimulation of

leucine incorporation into muscle and cartilage protein by a serum fraction with sulphation factor activity: differentiation effects from those of growth hormone and insulin. Endocrinology 87:1168
Salzberger M, Ariad I, Serr D M 1960 Osteomalacia in pregnancy. Gynaecologia 150:113
Schmorl G 1927 Veber die an den Wirbelbandsch eiben Vorkommenden Ausuelhnungs und Zerreissungesvorgange und die cladurch an ihnen und der Wirbelspongiosa hervorgerufench Verandenungen. Verhandlung der Deutschen Gesellschaft fur Pathologie 22:250
Schwartz C S, Berenyi M R, Siegal M W 1969 Atrophic arthropathy and diabetic neuritis. American Journal of Roentgenology 106:523
Seedat Y K, Randere M 1975 Avascular necrosis of the hip joints in hypothyroidism. South African Medical Journal 49:2071
Shackleford P C 1977 Osseous lesions and pancreatitis. American Journal of disease of children 131:731
Shapiro R F, Utsinger P D, Wiesner K B, Resnick D, Bryan B L, Castles J J 1976 HLA-B27 and modified bone formation. Lancet 1:230
Silberberg R, Hasler M 1971 Submicroscopic effect of hormones on articular cartilage of adult mice. Archives of Pathology 91:242
Silberberg M, Frank E L, Jarrett S O L, et al 1959 Ageing and osteoarthrosis of the human sternoclavicular joint. American Journal of Pathology 35:851
Silberberg R, Hirschberg C E, Lesker P 1977 Enzyme studies in the articular cartilage of diabetic rats and of rats bearing transplanted pancreatic islets. Diabetes 26:732
Silcox D C, McCarty D J 1973 Measurement of inorganic pyrophosphate in biological fluid. Elevated levels in some patients with osteoarthritis, pseudogout, acromegaly and uraemia. Journal of Clinical Investigation 52:1863
Skillern P C 1943 The association of periarthritis of the shoulder with hyperthyroidism. In: Thomas C C (ed) Transactions of the American Goiter Association, Springfield, Illinois, p. 100
Sledge C B 1973 Growth hormone and articular cartilage. Federation Proceedings 32:1503
Spiro A J, Hirano A, Bellin R L, Finkelstein J W 1970 Cretinism with muscular hypertrophy. Archives of Neurology 23:340
Stapleton F B, Kennedy J, Nousin-Arvanitakis S, Linshaw M A 1976 Hyperuricaemia due to high dose pancreatic extract therapy in cystic fibrosis. New England Journal of Medicine 295:246
Steinbach H L, Russell W 1964 Measurement of the heel pad as an aid to diagnosis of acromegaly. Radiology 82:418
Stuber J L, Palanio E 1971 Vertebral scalloping in acromegaly. American Journal of Roentgenology, Radium Therapy and Nuclear Medicine 112:397
Thomas J, Collipp P J, Sharma R K 1973 Thyroid acropachy. American Journal of Diseases of Children 125:745
Thomas R D, Croft D N 1974 Thyrotoxicosis and giant cell arteritis. British Medical Journal 2:408
Traisman H J, Traisman E S, Maw T J, Wise J 1978 Joint contractions in patients with juvenile diabetes and their siblings. Diabetes Care 1:360
Vandenbrouche J P, Valkenburg H A, Boersma J W, Cats A, Festen J J M, Huber-Bruning O, Rasker J J 1982 Oral contraceptives and rheumatoid arthritis: Further evidence for a preventative effect. Lancet 2:839
Van Wyk J J, Underwood L E 1978 The somatomedins and their activity. In: Litwack J (ed) Biochemical actions of hormones. Academic Press, London
Vernon-Roberts B, Pirie C J, Trenwith V 1974 Pathology of dorsal spine in ankylosing hyperostosis. Annals of the Rheumatic Diseases 33:281
Viljanto J A 1973 Dupuytren's contracture — a review. Seminars in Arthritis and Rheumatism 3:155
Vitny G, Alland A, Galindo A, Galindo F 1979 Maladie de Dupuytren's et diabeti sucre. Revue Francaise d'Endocrinologie Clinique Nutrition et Metabolisme 20:91
Walde J 1962 Obstetrical and gynaecological back and pelvic pain, especially those contracted during pregnancy. Acta obstetrica et gynecologica Scandinavica 4 (Suppl 2): 11
Waine H, Bennett G A, Bauer W 1945 Joint disease associated with acromegaly. American Journal of Medical Science 209: 671
Weissbein A S, Darby J P, Lawson J D 1959 An unusual bone lesion in an adult with mydoedema. Report of a case and review of the literature. Archives of Internal Medicine 104:643
Wettenhall R E H, Schwartz P J, Bernstein J 1969 Actions of insulin and growth hormone on collagen and chondroitin sulphate synthesis in bone organ culture. Diabetes 18:280
Whaley K, Webb J, McAvoy B A, Hughes G R, Lee P, MacSween R N M, Buchanan W W 1973 Sjögren's syndrome: 2 clinical associations and immunological phenomena. Quarterly Journal of Medicine 42:513
Whitehouse F W, Wechstein M 1978 On diabetic osteopathy; a radiographic study of 21 patients. Diabetic Care 1:303
Wilkins L 1941 Epiphyseal dysgenesis associated with hypothyroidism. American Journal of Diseases of Children 61:13
Williamson J, Cant S, Mason D K, Greig W R, Borge J A 1967 Sjögren's syndrome anothyroid diseases. British Journal of Ophthalmology 51:721
Wingrave S J, Kay C R 1978 Reduction in incidence of rheumatoid arthritis associated with oral contraceptives. Lancet 1:569
Wynne-Roberts C R, Castor C W 1972 Uptake of cortisol by rheumatoid and non-rheumatoid fibroblasts in tissue culture. Laboratory Investigation 26:384

Metabolic bone disease

Metabolic bone disease is frequently associated with locomotor symptoms. Bone pains are the most common but joint disturbances including pain, stiffness, or laxity may be an important feature. Symptoms may be acute or chronic. In bone acute pain results from pathological fractures, for example in osteoporosis or hyperparathyroidism, while chronic pain is encountered in Paget's disease, osteomalacia and may also feature in hyperparathyroidism. In joints, acute pain occurs in chondrocalcinosis secondary to parathyroid tumours; chronic pain of osteoarthritis is a common complication of Paget's disease while degenerative spondylosis is a frequent aftermath of spinal crush fractures in osteoporosis. Joint laxity is a common finding in the osteogeneses imperfecta, laxity or stiffness occurs among the mucopolysaccharidoses and limitation of movement without degenerative changes in articular cartilage is a distinctive finding in adults with X-linked hypophosphataemia. Finally soft tissue pain may be associated with ectopic calcification or ossification encountered in pseudohypoparathyroidism and in myositis ossificans.

Knowledge of bone growth, remodelling and ageing, and of their cellular and hormonal control, is still limited but strides have been made since the last edition of this textbook. Some understanding of embryological development is an aid to grasping the complexity of bone dysplasias (Rubin, 1964). An outline of these aspects of bone metabolism is given below.

BONE GROWTH, AGEING AND TURNOVER

Bones are recognisable as anatomical units by 7 weeks' conceptual age, long before they assume the attributes of tissue bone. The primitive long bones and short bones are at first condensations of mesenchymal cells which then differentiate into chondrocytes; a cellular collar develops at the middle of each bone and differentiates into periosteum where tissue bone is first formed by periosteal apposition. The chondrocytes undergo hypertrophy, maturation, and then degeneration at which time they are invaded by capillary vessels from the periosteal collar (Maroteaux, 1979; Garn, 1981) and the process of resorption and true new bone formation is initiated, which continues throughout life. At the bone ends separate centres of ossification, the epiphyses, develop within cartilage beginning in fetal life and appearing at regular intervals throughout childhood to the end of adolescence. While the bone-forming cells, chondrocytes and osteoblasts, are derived from stroma in situ it is now clear that the bone resorbing cell, the osteoclast, is a marrow cell derived from the circulating mononuclear series (Owen, 1978). Growth in length of long bones is accomplished by the cartilage of the epiphyseal growth plate (Fig. 40.1) and ceases in adolescence at the time of epiphyseal fusion. Growth in flat, membrane bones — skull, ilium, ribs — occurs by periosteal apposition, a process which also occurs in long bones where it continues to produce steady widening throughout life (Garn, 1970).

The marrow cavity is first produced, and then maintained, by endosteal resorption which also continues through life except for a brief period in puberty when there is net endosteal new bone formation. The normal newborn skeleton may appear very dense radiologically. Throughout growth periosteal apposition outstrips endosteal resorption except when overtaken by disease such as leukae-

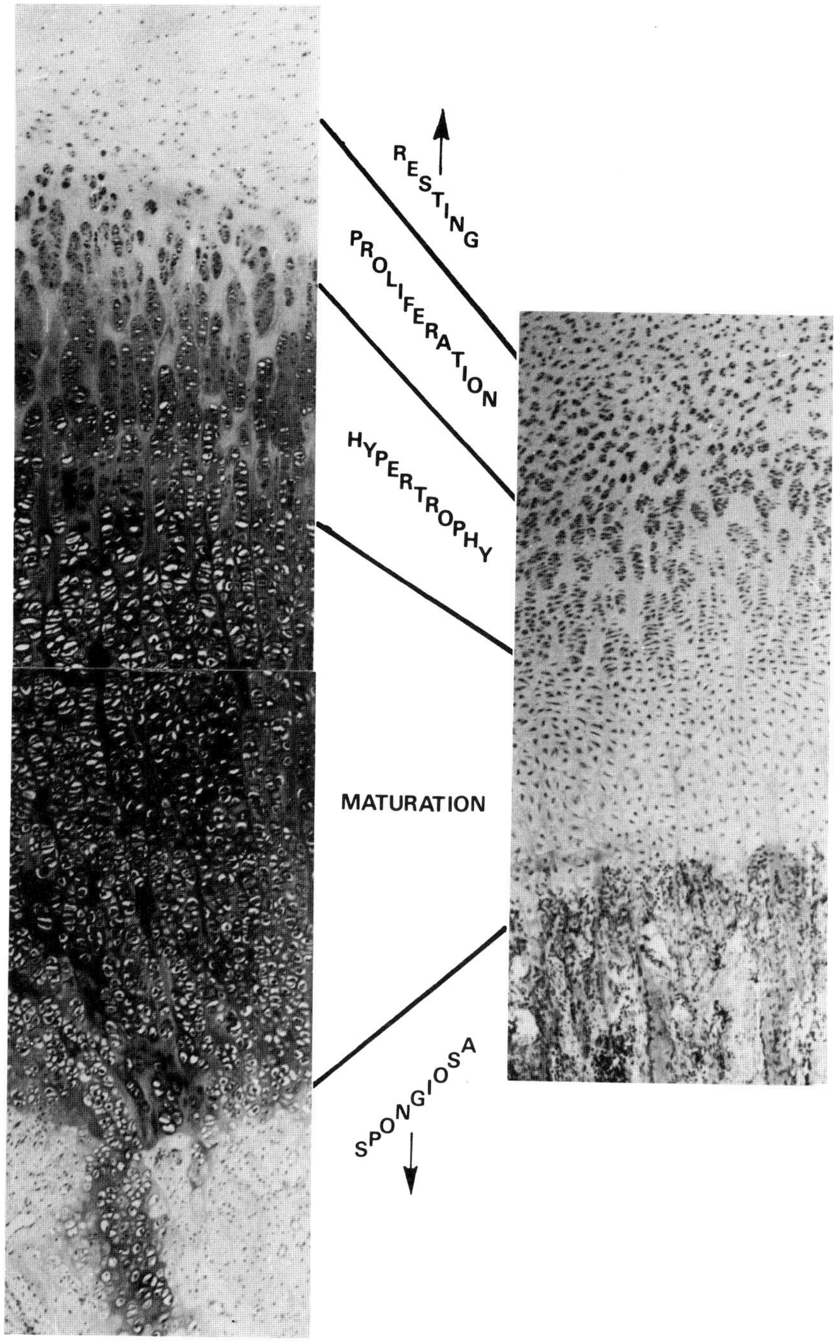

Fig. 40.1 Ricketic (left) and normal (right) growth plates in two 1½-year-old children, one dying from complications of the rickets and the other in an accident. The growth plate is subdivided for descriptive purposes into 5 zones. In the abnormal growth plate the resting and proliferative zones show reduced cellularity; the zones of hypertrophy and maturation are greatly lengthened and the ordered columnar appearance is lost; the zones of maturation and primary spongy bone are minimally vascularised and mineralised. Decalcified sections (H & E × 100) courtesy of Dr P.D. Byers, Institute of Orthopaedics.

mia or juvenile osteoporosis, so that cross-sectional cortical area, and therefore total bone mass, gradually increases. From the end of adolescence to the approximate age of 40 the skeleton is maintained in equilibrium after which time the inexorable changes of involution develop and endosteal resorption predominates during the remainder of life (Garn, 1970). These changes are considered further in the section on osteoporosis.

The skeleton at birth contains about 25–30 g (625–750 mmol) calcium almost all of which is laid down in the last trimester. This is a fairly trivial demand on maternal dietary calcium although lactation requires more, approximately 70 g (1750 mmol). Calcium retention during growth reaches a maximum positive balance of 7.5 mmol daily at the puberty growth spurt, at the time of peak height velocity, and the adult skeleton contains approximately 1 kg calcium. Longitudinal growth is most rapid in the first year of life, about 20 cm, falls to 10 cm in the second year and then halves again during later childhood to 4–5 cm/year until it doubles to a maximum of 10 cm/year at puberty. Ultimately, with involutional changes, height lessens again by a mean of 0.15 cm/year (Cohn et al, 1976; Taylor, 1981).

Compact bone is seen microscopically, under polarised light, in two forms, woven bone and lamellar bone. Woven bone, in which collagen bundles are laid down in many different directions, in seemingly random fashion, is immature bone. It is characteristic of rapid turnover and is thus normal in childhood, occurs with excessive stimulation by parathyroid hormone, and is also a feature of adult Paget's disease. Mature, adult, compact bone exists as concentric lamellar bone. Understanding of the processes involved in its turnover has increased greatly in the last two decades largely due to dynamic studies involving single or double labelling of active mineralisation sites with tetracycline or with toluidine blue (Frost, 1973). The old static histological picture of Haversian systems has thus been replaced by the dynamic concept of bone remodelling units lying parallel to the long axis of the Haversian systems (Fig. 40.2; Parfitt, 1976). Osteoclastic resorption creates a cavity approximately 250 μm in diameter, longitudinally advancing at the rate of about 20 μm daily and taking about 4 mo to complete the cycle of resorption, osteoid neosynthesis and remineralisation (although it is likely that the full life cycle of each remodelling unit is appreciably longer). In the open network of trabecular bone the process is essentially the same but here the processes of initial osteoclastic resorption and subsequent new bone formation take place along the trabecular surfaces where they build up a similar lamellar pattern. The development of simple techniques of bone biopsy from the iliac crest and the processing of undecalcified sections has permitted detailed study, both qualitative and quantitative, of the mineralisation defects which characterise the osteomalacic states.

HORMONAL CONTROL OF BONE METABOLISM

The crucial importance of supply and maintenance of precise ionic calcium concentration in extracellular fluid (ECF), in the presence of a vast skeletal reservoir containing 99% of body calcium has ensured the development of a highly tuned regulatory mechanism for calcium (and phosphorus) homeostasis both in bone and in ECF. This is chiefly accomplished by the parathyroid hormone–vitamin D endocrine system.

Parathyroid hormone (PTH), a polypeptide containing 84 amino acid residues is secreted in direct response to falling calcium concentration in the blood supply to the parathyroid glands (Mayer, 1975). Its synthesis involves 2 precursors, PreProPTH which has an additional sequence of 31 amino acids at the N-terminal end which represents all the structural information encoded in the gene for PTH (Habener & Jacobs, 1982), and ProPTH in which the additional N-terminal sequence is reduced to 6. Biological activity is chiefly contained within the N 1–34 sequence. The actions of PTH, insofar as they affect ECF concentrations of calcium and phosphorus, are well known (Parsons, 1976); they all serve to raise ionic calcium concentration in the ECF. Thus PTH governs intestinal calcium absorption on a day-to-day basis by stimulating 1a-hydroxylation, in renal tubules, of 25-hydroxyvitamin D to form the vitamin D hormone that provides the direct stimulus to intestinal calcium transport (Fraser, 1980). In kidney it promotes renal tubular calcium reab-

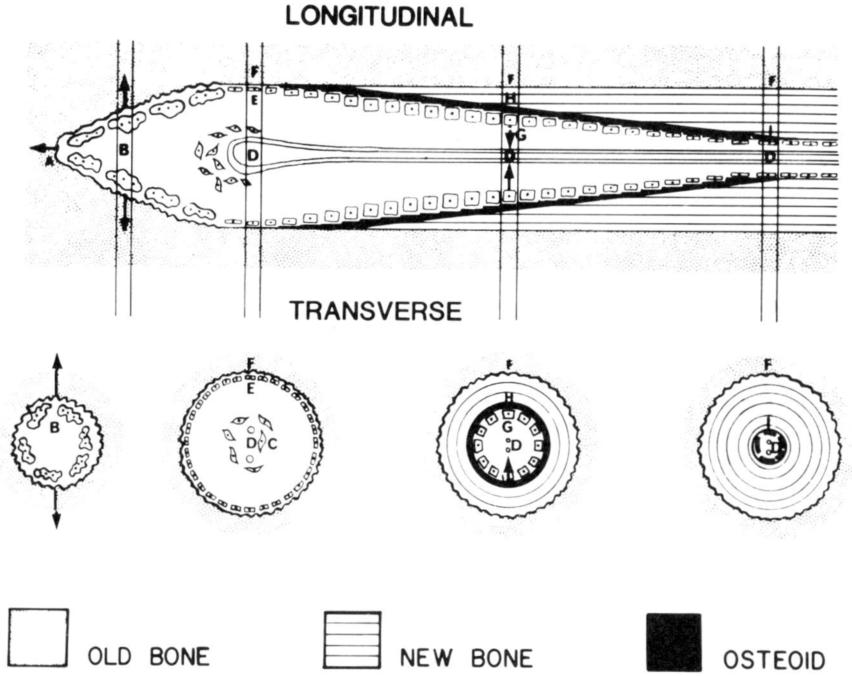

Fig. 40.2 Diagrammatic representation of a cortical remodelling unit; longitudinal and cross-sections. A. Apex and direction of advance. B. Multinucleated osteoclasts enlarging the resorption cavity. C. Mitotically active spindle-shaped cells. D. Capillary loop. E. Mononuclear cells (?post-osteoclasts) lining quiescent zone. F. Cement line separating new bone from old. G. Osteoblasts advancing inwards during radial closure. H. Osteoid seam. I. Flattened cells lining canal of completed Haversian system. (From Parfitt, 1976, with permission of author and publishers.)

sorption (Nordin & Peacock, 1969) and inhibits renal tubular phosphate (and bicarbonate) reabsorption. In bone it constitutes the primary stimulus to osteoclastic resorption and a secondary stimulus to osteoblastic activity. The most obvious physiological results of resorption are seen during growth, in the conversion of the cartilaginous zone of provisional calcification to the metaphyseal zone of primary spongiosa (true bone) and in external (subperiosteal) metaphyseal remodelling as long bones grow in length. A disease model which results from lack of this PTH-stimulated osteoclastic activity is osteopetrosis, or marble bones disease (see below.).

In functional terms, 'vitamin D' may be thought of as a generic name applied to a family of antiricketic compounds (chemically designated as secosteroids). These include the parent vitamins D_2 and D_3, ergo- and cholecalciferol, their 25-hydroxylated derivatives which are the chief circulating forms, and the 1,25-dihydroxylated forms which function as true hormones, together with synthetic compounds such as dihydrotachysterol and alfacalcidol. Vitamin D_2 is synthesised by yeasts. Vitamin D_3 is the true animal pro-hormone whose functional metabolism is shown in Figure 40.3. Among the vitamins it is unique in requiring for its de novo synthesis the ultraviolet portion of the sun's spectrum (290–320 nm) which, in the epidermis, cleaves the B-ring of the precursor sterol 7-dehydrocholesterol to form pre-vitamin D which is then isomerised to cholecalciferol under thermal influence (Holick et al, 1979). It is the alternative availability of the complete prohormone in certain animal foods which gave the 'calciferols' their original designation as a vitamin. Minute concentrations (10^{-10}M) of the ultimate hormone stimulate active transport of calcium and phosphorus across the intestinal mucosal epithelium to provide adequate concentrations for normal mineralisation within cartilage and collagenous osteoid (Fraser, 1980). 1,25-dihydroxyvitamin D is also, paradoxically, an extremely potent stimulus to bone resorption (Raisz et al, 1972). The physiological significance of this, and of a possible but still obscure direct role in mineralisation, remain highly uncertain. But without adequate vitamin D activity a characteristic mineralisation defect results in the appearance of rickets and/or osteomalacia. Figure 40.3 gives an indication of the number of sites where interruption in the functional metabolism of vitamin D may produce this disease. Experimentally 1,25-dihydroxyvitamin D has been observed to stimulate calcium reabsorption in the distal renal tubule (Sutton & Dirks, 1978). Specific receptors for the vitamin D hormones are widespread in cells throughout the body, including fibroblasts and gonads and a possible wider functional role associated with their membranophilic properties is still subject to speculation (Norman & Ross, 1979).

Calcitonin, a 32 amino acid peptide, is secreted by the C-cells of the thyroid gland in response to circumstances opposite to that which stimulate PTH secretion, namely rising plasma calcium (Copp et al, 1962). Experimentally, but not in adult humans, it produces hypocalcaemia by inhibiting PTH-stimulated osteoclastic activity, an effect which is visible cytologically within minutes. In aquatic forms of life it may have osmoregulatory activity (Orimo et al, 1972). In man it has transient natriuretic, calciuric and phosphaturic activity. Immunoassays for calcitonin are still relatively crude, inasmuch as changes within the physiological range cannot be accurately determined, but levels rise in pregnancy and lactation and fall in females after the menopause. These circumstances, together with experimental data, have led some to emphasise a likely physiological, protective role against skeletal mineral loss (MacIntyre et al, 1980). However no tendency to osteoporosis has yet been detected among patients following total or subtotal thyroidectomy who have presumably been rendered calcitonin deficient (but who might be protected by simultaneous hypoparathyroidism). Similarly no disorder of mineral metabolism has been found in patients with medullary thyroid carcinoma in whom calcitonin levels may be many hundreds of time higher than normal. Calcitonin may be employed in treatment of malignant hypercalcaemia, it may eventually find a place in (combined) treatment of osteoporosis, and is of proven value in treatment of Paget's disease (see below).

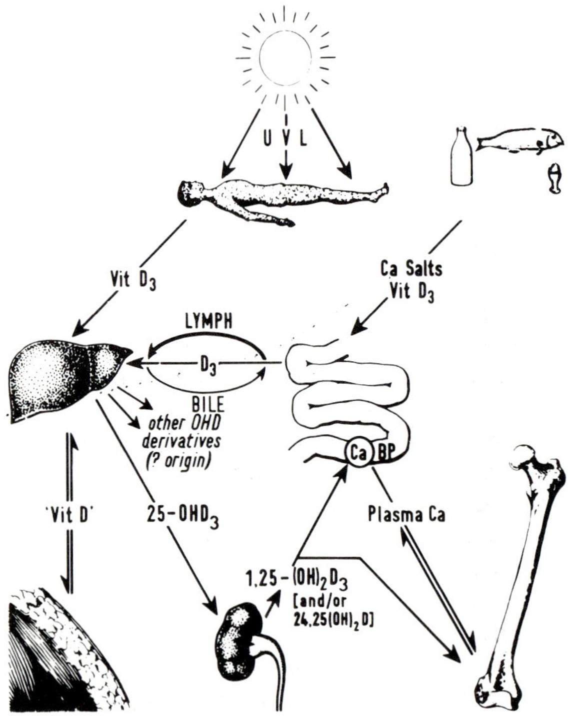

Fig. 40.3 Vitamin D metabolism. Pathways are shown through skin and gut, liver kidney and bone. Interruptions at any sites may produce rickets and osteomalacia. UVL = ultraviolet light; 25-OHD = 25-hydroxyvitamin D; 1,25(OH)$_2$D = 1,25-dihydroxyvitamin D; CaBP = calcium-binding protein(s).

Development and maintenance of skeletal integrity requires additional hormonal effects of growth hormone, somatomedin(s), insulin, thyroid hormone, androgens and oestrogens. Their detailed effects are considered elsewhere (see Ch. 39) and only an outline is required here for adequate balance. Pituitary growth hormone exerts its effects through stimulation of hepatic synthesis of a family of growth factors, somatomedin(s). Somatomedin(s) are stimulated additionally by insulin and are inhibited by cortisol and oestrogens. They stimulate cartilage proliferation and bone growth directly. Bone mass is diminished in insulin-deficient diabetics in whom 1,25-dihydroxyvitamin D levels are also low (without associated rickets). Thyroid hormone plays a vital part in skeletal maturation and stimulates the whole cycle of cartilage proliferation, enchondral growth and ossification (Avioli, 1981). Hypothyroid dwarfs retain infantile (short-limbed) body proportions, in contrast to the proportionate dwarfism encountered in growth-hormone and somatomedin deficiency (Maroteaux, 1979). The rare condition of juvenile hyperthyroidism is, like growth hormone excess, characterised by relative gigantism. Both oestrogens and androgens accelerate skeletal ageing, inhibit cartilage growth and decrease height in rapidly growing adolescents. Testosterone, when it was given as experimental treatment in idiopathic juvenile osteoporosis, produced premature epiphyseal closure and resultant dwarfism. The effects of physiological oestrogen withdrawal after the menopause are considered further in the section on osteoporosis; suffice it to say here that, regardless of the beneficial effects of oestrogen therapy in the group as a whole, measured circulating levels in untreated patients bear little relationship to rates of post-menopausal bone loss (Johnston et al 1979). Oestrogen receptors have never been detected in bone cells, which by contrast contain progestogen receptors. And progestogen treatment may selectively block the association of glucocorticoids with their respective bone cell receptors. The manner in which all these hormonal influences are ultimately coordinated at the cellular level for skeletal development and homeostasis remains uncertain.

BONE DYSPLASIAS

Bone dysplasias constitute a wide field and only a brief outline is possible here. Nevertheless the practical clinical problems they pose can tax combined efforts of rheumatologists, orthotists and orthopaedic surgeons. Several major works are devoted to the subject (Rubin, 1964; Murray & Jacobsen, 1977; Spranger et al, 1974; Bergsma, 1969; Maroteaux, 1979; McKusik, 1972). Most classifications include both known disorders of intermediary metabolism and unknown constitutional or hereditary defects of skeletal development. Known primary metabolic abnormalities are fully described in specialist works (Stanbury et al, 1978) and are summarised in Table 40.1. Only those under heading 'A' are considered further in this chapter.

Other constitutional diseases of bone are briefly summarised in Table 40.2. This is necessarily selective; the original classification lists 82 disorders under 'osteochondrodysplasias' and 40 under 'dysostoses', several subheadings referring simply to 'other forms'. Certain of these conditions, particularly those listed under IC, have themselves revealed a metabolic basis which warrants fuller discussion. While detailed classification has also been attempted on the basis of more unified concepts of developmental disturbance (Rubin, 1964) a large number of diseases clearly remain too difficult to pigeon-hole in this way. A more purely descriptive sequence, based on relative radiological involvement throughout the skeleton, was adopted by Spranger et al (1974) and is shown in Table 40.3; known metabolic abnormalities figure throughout these sections among the total of 82 conditions listed. While this emphasises the major diagnostic role of radiological scrutiny aided by relevant atlases (see above), careful clinical exam-

Table 40.1 Summary of known primary metabolic abnormalities affecting bone (adapted from *International nomenclature of constitutional diseases of bone*: Maroteaux, 1979)

A. Disorders of the parathyroid hormone/vitamin D endocrine system and other defects of calcium and phosphorus metabolism
   1. Metabolic rickets, including X-linked hypophosphataemia and other inherited disorders of renal tubular function (see section on rickets and osteomalacia)
   2. Disorders of parathyroid function, including pseudohypoparathyroidism, hypo-hyperparathyroidism (see section on parathyroid disease)
   3. Hypophosphatasia

B. Complex carbohydrate (e.g. glycosoaminoglycan) disorders
   1. Mucopolysaccharidoses, types I–VII (see Ch. 46)
   2. Mannosidosis, fucosidosis, etc.
   3. Neuraminidase deficiency, mucolipidoses types II & III

C. Lipid disorders
   Niemann–Pick, Gaucher's disease

D. Nucleic acids
   Adenosine-deaminase deficiency, etc.

E. Aminoacid disorders
   Homocystinuria, etc.

F. Metal disorders
   Menke's kinky hair syndrome, etc.

Table 40.2 International nomenclature of constitutional diseases of bone (abbreviated and adapted from Maroteaux, 1979)

I. Osteo-chondrodysplasias: abnormalities of cartilage and/or bone growth and development
- A. Defects of growth of tubular bones and/or spine
  - a. Identifiable at birth
  - b. Identifiable in later life
    - (i) Metaphyseal chondrodysplasia (types Schmid, Janssen, etc.)
    - (ii) Multiple epiphyseal dysplasias
    - (iii) Spondyloepiphyseal dysplasias
    - (iv) Others, e.g. Dyggve–Melchior–Clausen dysplasia, trichorhinophalangeal dysplasia
- B. Disorganised cartilage and fibrous tissue development
  - (i) Enchondromatosis (Ollier)
  - (ii) Polyostotic fibrous dysplasia
  - (iii) Neurofibromatosis
- C. Abnormalities of cortical density and/or remodelling
  - (i) Osteogenesis imperfecta
  - (ii) Osteopetrosis
  - (iii) Melorheostosis
  - (iv) Progressive diaphyseal dysplasis (Camurati–Engelmann)
  - (v) Others, including pyknodysostosis, osteopoikilosis, sclerosteosis

II. Dysostoses: malformation of individual bones singly or in combination
- A. With cranial and facial involvement
- B. With predominant axial involvement
- C. With predominant involvement of extremities

III. Idiopathic osteolyses

IV. Chromosomal aberrations

V. Metabolic abnormalities (see Table 40.1)

Table 40.3 Bone dysplasias (adapted from Spranger et al, 1974)

1. Skeletal dysplasias with predominantly epiphyseal involvement
2. Skeletal dysplasias with predominantly metaphyseal involvement
3. Skeletal dysplasias with major involvement of the spine
4. Mucopolysaccharidoses and mucolipidoses
5. Skeletal dysplasias due to anarchic development of bone constituents (e.g. fibrous dysplasia, enchondromatosis)
6. Osteolyses
7. Skeletal dysplasias with predominant involvement of single sites or segments
8. Skeletal dysplasias with abnormalities of bone density and/or modelling defects

ination for associated soft tissue changes (joints, skin pigmentation, nose, ears, eyes, etc.) is scarcely less important. For example the 'stippled epiphyses' of chondrodysplasia punctata may become almost inapparent as childhood progresses, leaving only radiological long bone asymmetry, but changes including alopecia, cataracts and icthyosiform skin may ensure correct diagnosis. While too few of these conditions are amenable to cure, prognosis regarding disability, both physical and mental, and genetic counselling, are obviously of great importance.

Many of the severe disturbances recognisable at birth are incompatible with life and for present purposes are of academic interest only. Of those identifiable in later life (see Table 40.2 IAb), metaphyseal chondrodysplasia (or 'metaphyseal dysostosis'), type Schmid, poses a diagnostic problem since the metaphyses are wide and flared, the growth plate also widened and very ragged, and appearances are very similar to severe rickets. The dense outline of the abnormal region is of some differential value; deformity and dwarfism result, treatment with vitamin D is of no value and osteotomy when required heals normally.

The multiple epiphyseal dysplasias are not uncommon and there is considerable overlap between the mild (Ribbing) and severe (Fairbank) forms, both inherited as autosomal dominant characteristics. The epiphyses are small and flattened or otherwise distorted (Fig. 40.4) and the condition leads to osteoarthritis early in adult life. It may also result in relative dwarfism. The chief diagnostic problem is differentiation from hypothyroidism. Progress of bony disturbance (but not the joint disturbance) arrests when growth ceases. It may therefore be important to minimise damage during childhood and adolescence by avoiding undue weight-bearing and instead encouraging activity such as cycling and swimming. Mild vertebral abnormalities are not uncommon and the point at which the degree of platyspondyly, for example, warrants classification as 'spondyloepiphyseal' dysplasia is partly a matter of radiological experience. Severe degrees of spondyloepiphyseal dysplasia, possibly with additional metaphyseal abnormalities, causing dwarfism, limb deformities and kyphoscoliosis are too often

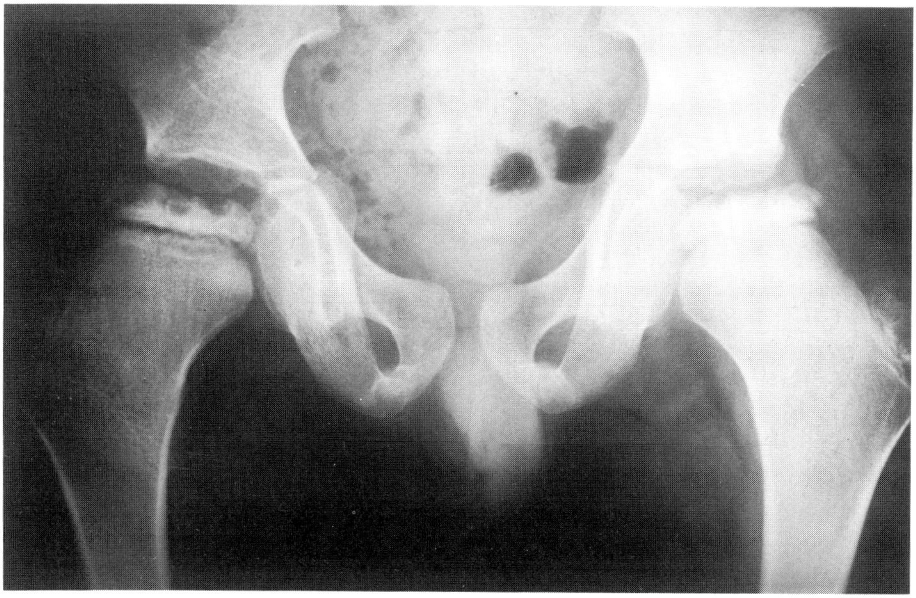

Fig. 40.4 X-ray of pelvis and hips in a child with multiple epiphyseal dysplasia. Note the small, flattened femoral heads. Other epiphyses show similar distortion. Appearances are very similar to hypothyroidism, which needs excluding, but do not respond to treatment.

casually but mistakenly labelled as Morquio–Brailsford syndrome (mucopolysaccharidosis IV, see Ch. 46).

Fibrous dysplasia is a sporadic condition which may involve one or many bones, the polyostotic variety being the original Von Recklinghausen's disease. In association with shaggy ('coast-of-Maine') skin pigmentation and, in females only, precocious puberty, it constitutes the McCune–Albright syndrome (Albright & Reifenstein, 1948). Bizarre, cystic bone lesions develop during childhood with external expansion, narrowed cortices subject to pain and pathological fractures or painless, progressive deformity which may be especially obvious in the region of the femoral neck as extensive coxa vara ('shepherds crook' deformity). Prophylactic surgical pinning and plating of the femoral neck may be required. The skull base may show sclerotic changes and expansion may distort orbital geometry and even lead to blindness. Both polyostotic fibrous dysplasia and neurofibromatosis (inherited as an autosomal dominant characteristic) share an occasional association with hypophosphataemia; rickets and osteomalacia may develop, and spontaneously regress, at any time of life (Dent & Gertner, 1976) as shown in Figure 40.5. Pharmacological vitamin D treatment is necessary.

Osteopetrosis (marble bones disease, Albers-Schoenberg disease) is characterised by an inherited functional defect of the osteoclasts, which lack an ultramicroscopic brush border. In the severe, infantile autosomal recessively inherited form widespread failure of resorption prevents development of marrow cavities; gross hepatosplenomegaly and leucoerythroblastic anaemia result. There is also failure of metaphyseal remodelling in the grossly dense, but brittle, long bones. Skull overgrowth leads to early blindness. Until recently the only available, but poorly effective, therapy was with corticosteroids and dietary calcium deprivation. Strenuous calcium deprivation, undertaken in the hope of providing space for marrow development, is followed by growth of less dense but still unremodelled bone, a ragged appearance at the growth plate reminiscent of rickets, and hypocalcaemia with hypophosphataemia due to the 'hungry bones'. Following both experimental transmission of the disease and its cure by appropriate spleen cell and bone marrow

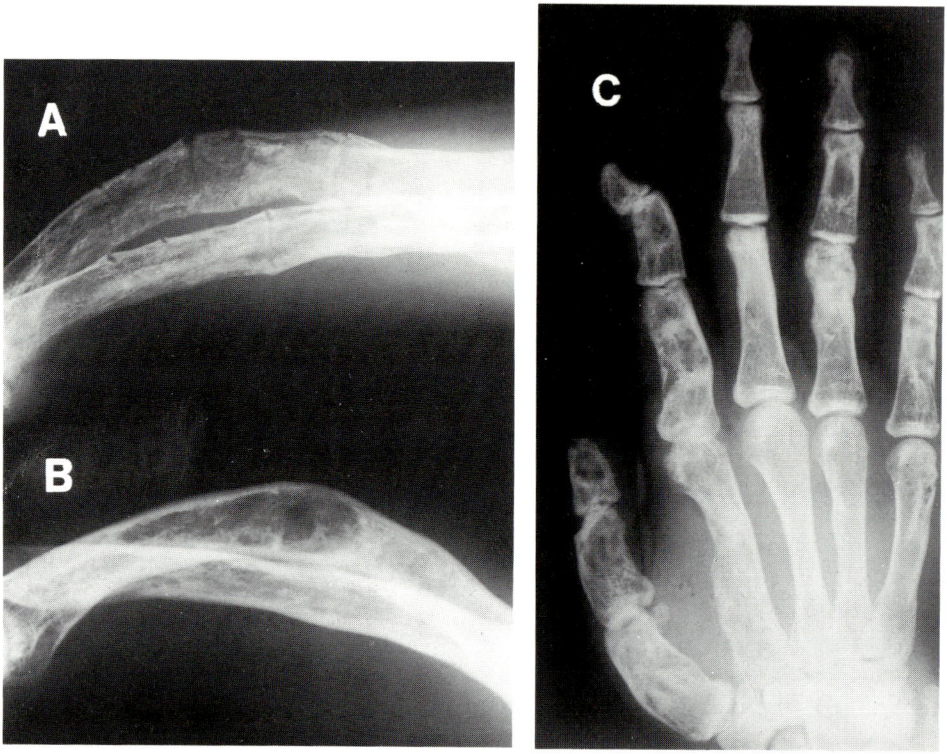

Fig. 40.5 Radiological appearances in polyostotic fibrous dysplasia. (A) Forearm of an 18-year-old male. Note first the bizarre bone deformities and second the profuse osteomalacic, pseudofractures associated with hypophosphataemia (plasma phosphorus 0.51–0.65 mmol/l, 1.5–2.0 mg/dl). (B) The same forearm 5 years later. Vitamin D was only given during the first $2\frac{1}{2}$ years but normal plasma phosphorus was thereafter maintained at levels of 1.03–1.32 mmol/l (3.1–4.2 mg/dl). (C) Later X-ray of the same patient's wrists and hands. Note the random polyostotic distribution of abnormal and completely normal bones.

transplantation in grey lethal osteopetrotic mice (Walker, 1975a, b) two groups have had preliminary success in the human disease following marrow irradiation and histocompatible marrow homotransplantation (Ballet et al, 1977; Coccia et al, 1980). The successful 'osteoclast grafts' have shown early evidence of producing normal bone resorption, subsequently isolated cells in one male infant showing the female chromosomal characteristics of the donor. A milder form of osteopetrosis, with autosomal dominant inheritance and onset later in childhood has also been described, and may be asymptomatic.

Melorheostosis ($\mu\epsilon\lambda o\varsigma$ = limb and $\rho\epsilon\omega$ = I flow) is a curious localised condition characterised by a heaped-up appearance of cortical bone, on either endosteal or periosteal surfaces, which appears like candle-guttering as if flowing down either bone surface. It may present in young adult life with localised bone pain or it may be an asymptomatic, chance finding. There is no specific therapy.

Progressive diaphyseal dysplasia (Camurati–Engelmann disease) was first described by Cockayne (1920) and later by the eponymous authors (Camurati, 1922; Engelmann, 1924). It is inherited as an autosomal dominant characteristic but often appears sporadically. It presents at different ages between childhood and mid-adult life with pain in the shafts and joints of long bones in upper and lower limbs. Cranial overgrowth may lead to neurological compression. The course of the disease is variable; it may appear to regress in adult life, remain static or show steady progression. Delayed sexual and skeletal maturation may be a striking feature but the incidence is not easy to gauge from the literature.

Radiological changes in long bones include ragged cortical thickening on both surfaces, mainly in mid-shaft, irregular medullary cavity and mild abnormality of metaphyseal remodelling (Fig. 40.6). Some patients show raised alkaline phosphatase indicative of increased osteoblastic activity. Recent reports of interest suggest a systemic inflammatory element (Smith et al, 1977; Crisp & Brenton, 1982) with findings of raised ESR, mild normochromic anaemia, autoimmune phenomena in more than one generation, and response to corticosteroid therapy. The condition poses some problems of differential diagnosis from other causes of either more or less regular diaphyseal thickening and bone pain including 'juvenile Paget's disease' (osteoectasia with hyperphosphataemia), craniodiaphyseal dysplasia, generalised cortical hyperostosis with both dominant and recessive (Van Buchem's disease) forms, sclerosteosis and others (Beighton, 1978; Maroteaux, 1979).

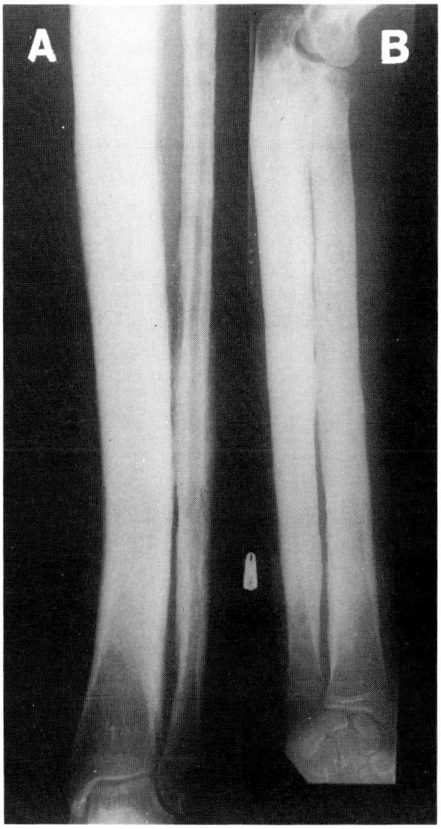

Fig. 40.6 Radiological appearances in progressive diaphyseal dysplasia in a 23-year-old female weighing 35 kg with primary amenorrhoea. Appearances may resemble Paget's disease and the alkaline phosphatase level was raised. (A) Tibia and fibula. (B) Radius and ulna.

Hypophosphatasia is inherited either as an autosomal recessive, lethal form in infancy or as a milder dominant variety in older patients (Rasmussen & Bartter, 1978). It is characterised by absent or low plasma alkaline phosphatase activity, involving the bone isoenzyme, although occasionally total enzyme activity is within normal limits. The infantile disease is characterised by grossly defective mineralisation, radiologically apparent as severe rickets. The normal role of alkaline phosphatase, produced by osteoblasts, in mineralisation is uncertain but one substrate, pyrophosphate, is an inhibitor of mineralisation; in hypophosphatasia pyrophosphate levels are increased in blood and urine (Russell et al, 1971). The disease is also characterised by increased urinary excretion of phosphoethanolamine, a finding of uncertain significance. Hypercalcaemia and hypercalciuria are common and may be considered to result from normal intestinal absorption (Jowsey, 1977) coupled with gross failure of skeletal calcium uptake. Hypercalcaemia may improve during intravenous infusion of alkaline phosphatase-rich plasma from patients with Paget's disease (Whyte et al, 1982). The adult disease is crippling but not fatal and is characterised by bone pain and pathological fractures which suffer non-union. Chondrocalcinosis and arthropathy have been observed (Whyte et al, 1982).

Steady progress continues in the slow clarification of bone dysplasias in terms of metabolic abnormalities involving hereditary enzyme deficiencies, specific defects of cell function and disturbances of gene coding for structural protein synthesis.

OSTEOGENESIS IMPERFECTA

Recent clinical and genetic surveys of osteogenesis imperfecta (fragilitas ossium, the 'brittle bones syndrome') have added to older radiological descriptions and confirmed that the disease(s) occur as several distinct genetic entities (Sillence, 1981; Wynne-Davies & Gormley, 1981) whose number may be expected to grow with simultaneous advances in the chemistry of disordered collagen (Eyre, 1981; Smith & Francis, 1982). While the most superficially recognisable forms of the disease fall into one of two clinical categories it has become increasingly obvious that its older, simple distinction into corresponding *congenita* and *tarda* forms is no longer tenable (Sillence, 1981; Wynne-Davies & Gormley, 1981).

Collagen is the structural protein of bone and provides the organic framework within which all mineralisation occurs; it is therefore vital for skeletal integrity. It is also present in other supporting tissues throughout the body. Five types of collagen have been distinguished to date of which type I is the constituent of bone, dentine, tendon, skin and cornea. All types share the same basic structure of a rod-like triple polypeptide helix, each of the 3 polypeptide chains containing about 1000 amino acid residues particularly rich in glycine and proline (Prockop et al, 1979; Smith & Francis, 1982). Molecular synthesis and elaboration of the ultimate collagen fibres is complex. Each polypeptide chain has its own DNA and mRNA and the sequence of post-translational modification is still uncertain. Steps include hydroxylation, glycosylation, disulphide bondings, helix formation, removal of molecular extensions, aldehyde formation and cross-linking. Biopsy and necropsy studies of skin collagen in osteogenesis imperfecta (OI) indicate possible abnormalities at many stages including increased lysyl hydroxylation, increased solubility of polymeric collagen, increased ratios of type III to type I collagen, ultramicroscopic changes in cross-linkage, fibre thickness and aggregation, chromatographic changes after collagen hydrolysis and altered gel filtration patterns in collagen following fibroblast culture in isotopically labelled media; there is also promise in sophisticated techniques of recombinant DNA. Some work is conflicting, few final answers are yet forthcoming with respect to individual OI syndromes and the reader is referred beyond the present over-simplification for more detailed analysis (Eyre, 1981; Smith & Francis, 1982).

The incidence of OI is 1 in 25 000–50 000, about the same as haemophilia. The most currently accepted classification based on work in Australia is shown in Table 40.4. The lethal form II, the 'thick-bone' type of Fairbank (1951), also shows swollen (beaded) ribs and multiple Wormian bones in the skull, such skull changes not being confined to type II. Very similar conclusions were reached in an Edinburgh-based survey, Wynne-Davies & Gormley (1981) recognising two main groups among the non-lethal forms (corre-

Table 40.4 Proposed nomenclature of osteogenesis imperfecta (adapted from Sillence, 1981)

Type	Suffix	Inheritance	Clinical features	Earlier nomenclature
I*	Congenita (tarda)	Autosomal dominant	Bone fragility, blue sclerae ± presenile hearing loss	Dominant OI with blue sclerae Van der Hoeve's triad OI tarda levis OI tarda type II Eddowe's syndrome
II	Congenita (always)	Autosomal recessive	Extreme bone fragility, crumpled bones, perinatal death	Lethal perinatal OI Lethal congenital OI OI letalis of Vrolik
III	Congenita (tarda)	Autosomal recessive	Severe bone fragility, normal sclerae, severe growth retardation and skeletal deformity	OI congenita of Vrolik Progressively deforming OI with normal sclerae OI tarda gravis Lobstein's disease
IV*	Congenita (tarda)	Autosomal dominant	As in III but all features of variable lesser severity	Lobstein's disease Dominantly inherited OI with normal sclerae

* Types I & IV have been divided in subgroups A & B on the basis of negative or positive dental abnormalities (dentinogenesis imperfecta) which also breed true in family studies.

sponding with types I and III/IV in Table 40.4); their second group was almost entirely sporadic and both were attributed to 'probably separate autosomal dominant genes'. The same 2 groups are implied in the simpler distinction by Bauze et al (1975) into 'mild' and 'severe' forms. The synonyms and eponyms under which OI has been historically discussed have been catalogued (Weil 1981). The best known group (type 1, 'mild') contains Van der Hoeve's triad of fragile bones, blue sclerae and deafness. However presenile hearing loss, when it occurs, is not confined to this group and, contrary to some traditional views, does not consist solely of otosclerosis, which if present is coincidental, but may be conductive, sensorineural and mixed (Bergstrom, 1981). Since all infants tend to have bluish sclerae this ultimately valuable distinction may be least useful at a time when it may be most desirable. The other most generally useful distinguishing feature is patients' stature, dwarfism often being *progressive* in the 'severe'-congenital-sporadic-white sclerae group; in the Edinburgh series the most severely dwarfed patients (height −6 to −14 standard deviations below normal) invariably belonged to this group.

As stated earlier, congenita/tarda distinction is invalid: almost all dominantly inherited conditions show a wide range of severity and perinatal fractures are not rare among type I patients. In severely affected patients of types III and IV X-rays may show a characteristic expanded, cystic appearance at the ends of the long bones which look like the outlines of small marbles within a bag. OI may show additional clinical features which are not confined to any special group. They include kyphoscoliosis, protrusio acetabuli, basilar invagination, frontal bossing, ligamentous laxity, a history of hernia and premature corneal arcus. Discovery of one or more of these features among children or young adults with 'osteoporosis' of uncertain origin may permit, with variable confidence, alternative diagnosis of a form of OI (unspecified). Kyphoscoliosis may lead to pulmonary heart disease. In fatal cases death often results from chest infection among patients with grossly reduced vital capacity and sudden death from cervical cord compression has been recorded among patients with basilar invagination.

Genetic counselling and antenatal diagnosis can be important. The recurrence rate among families with clear dominant or recessive forms is plainly 50% and 25% respectively. The frequency of gene carriers for type II is 1 in 125 and the chance of a normal sibling in this group having an affected child is therefore 1/750 (2/3 × 1/125 × 1/4). The type III *phenotype* may show mixed inheritance; parental consanguinity, or more than one affected sibling, warrants assigning a 25% recurrence risk. On the other hand the risk of a subsequent new dominant mutation is essentially zero. Combining both possibilities, and assuming the actual recessive incidence to be between 10% (Sillence, 1981) and 20% (by analogy with other seemingly sporadic cases that are actually inherited as autosomal recessives), then a 10–20% frequency × 25% risk gives an 'educated guess' of a 2.5–5% recurrence risk once the obvious recessive cases have been eliminated (Lubs & Travers, 1981). Attempts at antenatal diagnosis are indicated particularly when types II–IV are suspected and may be undertaken by abdominal ultrasound at 16 and 20 weeks and by oblique abdominal X-ray at 20 weeks (Lubs & Travers, 1981).

Management of OI involves encouragement and maintenance of physical mobility, orthotics, specialised techniques of orthopaedic surgery and continuing efforts to determine effective systemic therapy. Patients with OI are especially susceptible to the osteoporotic effects of immobilisation. This may partly explain the downhill course that sometimes seems to be reserved until after the patients' first lower limb fracture. Orthotic management is continuously developing (Bleck, 1981); general advice in Britain can be obtained from The Brittle Bones Society.* Systemic therapy remains empirical and its effectiveness is unconfirmed. Most of the therapeutic regimes adopted on theoretical grounds for osteoporosis (see below) have been widely used in OI (Albright, 1981) including heavy dietary mineral supplements, with or without calcitonin, vitamin D and/or fluoride, vitamin D and flavonoids (Catechin). Some of these may be considered potentially valuable and the need for placebo effects among both patients and their doctors will ensure that efforts continue.

* 112 City Road, Dundee DD2 2PW

OSTEOPOROSIS

'Osteoporosis' is defined as the presence of too little, *qualitatively normal*, bone per unit volume (Fig. 40.7). The term has been used by some in a physiological sense to describe the gradual bone loss that occurs with normal ageing, its application is restricted by others to bone mass below any given normal range for age and sex however measured (see below); and some have further reserved it for the development of clinical disease, namely pathological fractures, usage that was implied in the original description by Albright et al, (1941). A first-stage label of 'osteopenia' has also been used, prior to definitive diagnosis, to describe radiological or histological appearances of undermineralisation.

Major recent reviews are available (Barzel, 1979; De Luca et al, 1981; Dixon et al, 1983). Clinical osteoporosis may ultimately follow either normal rates of bone loss from skeletons that are undermineralised at maturity or accelerated bone loss (whether idiopathic or secondary) at any age. Trabecular (spongy) bone is more susceptible than cortical bone to increased resorption. Pathological fractures, the chief clinical effects of osteoporosis, are therefore encountered in those areas where trabecular bone predominates, particularly when also liable to trauma, namely the vertebral bodies (80–95% trabecular bone), proximal femur (45–75% trabecular) and distal radius (27% trabecular); these proportions need to be appreciated in the global context of 4 times more cortical than trabecular bone.

Numerous studies in the past few years have established normal rates of involutional bone loss in males and in females before and after the menopause (Nagant de Deuxchaisnes, 1983). Numerous methods have been used, results from different sampling sites reflecting relative proportions of trabecular and cortical bone. They include:

1. Caliper measurements of cortical thickness or area in metacarpal and phalangeal bones (Barnett & Nordin, 1960; Meema, 1962; Vose & Engel, 1973)
2. Single photon absorptiometry, using I^{125} according to the Cameron & Sorensen (1963) principle, at midshaft radius (90% cortical bone) and distal radius (Wahner et al, 1977).

Vertebral trabecular bone mass may be more selectively evaluated by

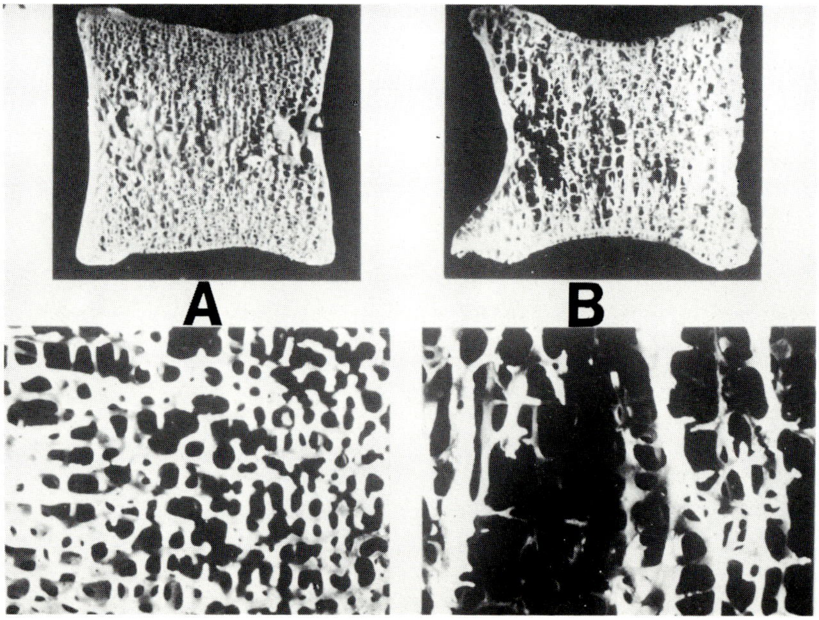

Fig. 40.7 Cross-section through (A) young normal and (B) osteoporotic vertebral bodies. Trabecular bone volume can be quantitated in iliac crest biopsies (see p. 1005).

3. Dual photon absorptiometry (Wilson & Madsen, 1977)
4. Total body neutron activation analysis (TBNAA) (McNeill et al, 1973; Harrison et al, 1981)
5. Computed transverse axial tomography (Ruegsegger et al, 1974; Cann et al, 1980).

Quantitation of trabecular bone volume may be made directly from

6. Iliac crest bone biopsy (Meunier et al, 1973; Courpron et al, 1980).

Less quantitative methods include radiological indices of

7. Femoral trabecular pattern
8. Measurement of vertebral body heights and/or crush fractures.

Fortunately for the understanding of involutional bone loss, and for evaluation of numerous published therapeutic trials, reasonable uniformity of results has emerged. Most measurements indicate that from the age of 40 (or less), males during the remainder of life and females before the menopause lose bone at an approximate rate of 0.1–0.2% per year. This statement needs dual qualification in that on the one hand not all measurements reach statistical significance and, on the other, TBNAA suggests a higher rate in premenopausal females of 0.37%, corresponding to negative calcium balance of 0.2 mmol/day (Cohn et al, 1976). After the menopause mean annual bone loss in females approximates 1.0%. Estimates of total bone loss depend somewhat on the relative amounts of cortical and trabecular bone in the sites sampled. Thus during approximately half a century of life (from the 30s to the 80s) females may lose 47% of trabecular bone as measured by iliac crest biopsy or dual photon absorptiometry of the spine (Riggs et al, 1981) and 28% of total body skeleton by TBNAA. Males lose about a quarter as much bone during the same period.

The incidence of vertebral crush fractures is related to trabecular bone volume (TBV) as a percentage of total volume in iliac crest biopsies from affected patients. Mean TBV in females aged 60–69 is 15.3 ± 4.6% and crush fractures may become the rule when TBV falls to 11% (Meunier et al, 1979; Courpron et al, 1980). Other surveys have reported a vertebral crush fracture prevalence in white females of 19% by age 60 and 45% by age 80, not more than 25% of the white male population being affected at any age (Boukhris & Becker, 1973). Crush fractures may however be asymptomatic in as many as 20–29% of affected subjects (Gershon-Cohen et al, 1953).

The incidence of proximal femoral (subcapital and pertrochanteric) and distal radial (Colles') fractures is shown in Figure 40.8. The morbidity and resulting economic considerations are obvious. The incidence of hip fracture is 70–80 per 100 000 inhabitants per year, an annual total for England and Wales of 40 000 which permanently fills 18% of all orthopaedic beds and claims a mortality of 12–15% (Lewis, 1981). 8% of females and 2.5% of males break their hip but if life were prolonged to 90, 32% of females would suffer these fractures. Below the age of 40 the sex incidence of Colles' fracture is equal; after the age of 60 it is 7 times more common in females. There are, plainly, additional aetiological factors in these fractures besides osteoporosis; they are likely to include neuroleptic and alcohol intake, vertebrobasilar in-

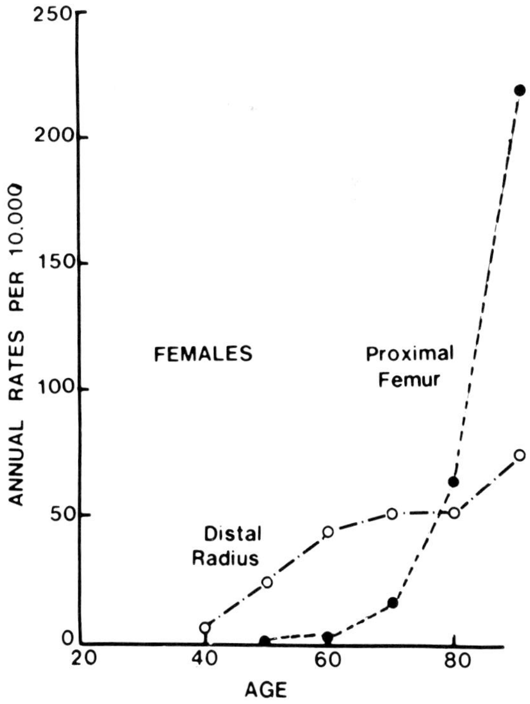

Fig. 40.8 Variation of proximal femoral and distal radial fracture rate with age in British females.

sufficiency, other forms of cerebrovascular and neurological disease, cardiac irregularities, poor eyesight and muscle weakness.

Primary (idiopathic) and secondary forms of osteoporosis are listed in Table 40.5. The aetiology of idiopathic (including postmenopausal) osteoporosis remains uncertain as do pathogenetic mechanisms in many secondary forms. Albright et al (1941) attributed the disease to primary hypoplasia of the osteoblasts. However even the most exhaustive histomorphometric analyses have failed to establish beyond doubt whether the pathogenetic sequence is initiated by a decrease in osteoblastic activity or an increase in bone resorption. Absolute trabecular bone volume is diminished by definition. Most workers have found a decrease in osteoid seam width, a decrease in mineralisation rate using double tetracycline labelling and no significant changes in bone forming surfaces, bone resorbing surfaces and indices of osteoclastic activity (Nagant de Deuxchaisnes, 1983). Others still interpret their data as indicating a primary increase in bone resorption (Nordin et al, 1981).

Whatever the true sequence of events, its cause is likely to be multifactorial in the population as a whole, as discussed further below in relation to treatment. The most widely implicated factors are physical activity, dietary habits (particularly calcium intake) and oestrogen loss in postmenopausal females. Nevertheless there are numerous patients with osteoporosis, females who have undergone normal or late menopause and males without detectable endocrine disturbance, all of whom clearly relate in addition a lifetime of athletic physical activity and optimum mineral and vitamin nutrition. Bone cells contain no oestrogen receptors and despite the relative benefits of oestrogen therapy in therapeutic trials among the postmenopausal osteoporotic population not all individuals appear to respond. There are conflicting data on peripheral levels of oestrone and androstenedione in postmenopausal osteoporosis (Riggs et al, 1973b; Nordin et al, 1980). Dividing women into rapid and slow bone losers, the only hormonal difference found by Johnston et al (1979) was lower progesterone levels among the rapid losers. These data conflict slightly with those of Christiansen et al (1981) who found in addition lowered oestrone levels in fast bone losers; the latter additionally had reduced fat mass. Osteoporosis is more common in slender women and two weight-related factors may protect against

Table 40.5 Forms of primary and secondary osteoporosis

1. Idiopathic
   a. Juvenile
   b. Young adults (both sexes)
   c. ?Following pregnancy
   d. Involutional: males
   e. Involutional (postmenopausal): females
2. Endocrine
   a. Adrenocortical excess
      (i) Cushing's disease
      (ii) Corticosteroid therapy
      (iii) Corticotrophin therapy
   b. Hypogonadiam
   c. Hypopituitarism
   d. Hyperthyroidism
3. Gastrointestinal disease
   a. Postgastrectomy
   b. Malabsorption syndromes (any)
   c. Hepatobiliary disease, especially chronic obstructive jaundice (especially biliary cirrhosis)
4. Nutritional deficiency
   a. Calcium deficiency
   b. Alcoholism (multifactorial)
   c. Protein malnutrition
   d. Scurvy
5. Immobilisation, including localised forms, and neurogenic disturbance
   a. Fractures
   b. Chronic localised arthritis
   c. Arthrodesis
   d. Poliomyelitis, etc.
6. Arthritis
   a. Rheumatoid arthritis
   b. Ankylosing spondylitis
   c. Seronegative polyarthritis
7. Miscellaneous
   a. Chronic renal failure (rare)
   b. Epilepsy
   c. Chronic heparin administration e.g. thromboembolism prophylaxis in pregnancy
   d. Systemic mastocytosis
   e. ?Chronic pulmonary disease
8. Neoplastic disease, e.g. myelomatosis, leukaemia (included for differential diagnosis)

postmenopausal osteoporosis. First, if residual oestrogen levels are important, the major and perhaps exclusive means of achieving this is the peripheral conversion in fat and muscle of androstenedione, secreted by the adrenal glands, to oestrone and thence to oestradiol (Longcope et al, 1968; MacDonald et al, 1978; Frumar et al, 1980). Second is the steady, strengthening effect of weight load (that is, unavoidable 'exercise') on the skeleton.

Other biochemical changes which normally follow the menopause may be either enhanced or diminished in osteoporosis. After much conflicting data it appears that immunoreactive parathyroid hormone levels rise with age but are lower in crush fracture patients (Arnaud et al, 1981). Some have found low 1,25-dihydroxyvitamin D levels in osteoporosis (Gallagher et al, 1979) while others have reported them normal (Nordin et al, 1980; Nagant de Deuxchaisnes, 1983). Plasma phosphorus, plasma and urinary calcium and urinary hydroxyproline rise after the menopause and the calcium and hydroxyproline changes are heightened in osteoporosis. Lastly, urinary free cortisol is raised in patients with rapid postmenopausal bone loss (Manolagas et al, 1979). Many of these observations need to be additionally interpreted in the knowledge that too few reported control groups were weight-matched as well as age-matched, and that illness adds the effects of both physical and emotional stress.

The diagnosis of osteoporotic crush fracture in patients presenting with acute back pain associated with vertebral collapse is made by exclusion. In uncomplicated osteoporosis, plasma and urinary calcium, phosphorus and hydroxyproline are within normal limits; although 24-hour urinary calcium excretion may be elevated if bone loss is acute. Hypercalcaemia never occurs and if present strongly indicates alternative, or dual, aetiology (malignancy, thyrotoxicosis, excessive vitamin D and/or thiazide therapy). Plasma alkaline phosphatase is rarely more than minimally elevated in response to simple fracture. Full blood count and ESR are normal in the absence of alternative, or dual, pathology. Serum protein electrophoresis should be undertaken routinely to exclude myelomatosis. Sternal marrow examination and iliac crest biopsy are warranted if any doubt exists. Rarely, diagnostic and therapeutic difficulties may result from the possible association of coincident benign paraproteinaemia (Hobbs, 1969; Kyle, 1978) and idiopathic osteoporosis. Idiopathic juvenile osteoporosis (Brenton & Dent, 1976) also needs to be distinguished from childhood aleukaemic leukaemia or lymphosarcoma. Isotopic bone scans are non-specific at the crush fracture site but may reveal fractures, or metastastic deposits, elsewhere. Needle biopsy of affected lowest thoracic or lumbar vertebrae may be required if the clinical picture is bizarre or if doubt remains. All secondary causes of osteoporosis should be excluded (Table 40.5) since they may be amenable to therapy.

Results of therapeutic trials have paralleled the clarification of aetiological factors. The deleterious effects in the skeleton of weightlessness in Skylab astronauts, and immobilisation by bed-rest, contrast with the higher than average bone mass of athletes, cross-country runners, marathon runners, swimmers, ballet dancers and weight-lifters, as variably determined by photon absorptiometry or total body calcium (Nagant de Deuxchaisnes, 1983). However when physical activity is determined by questionnaire, conflicting results have been obtained (Zanzi et al, 1981). Animal studies have confirmed the importance of regular stress in determining skeletal strength (Lanyon & Rubin, 1983). Exercise programmes among the elderly have produced good evidence for relative skeletal improvement whether measured by limb-bone photon absorptiometry (Smith et al, 1981), dual photon absorptiometry in the lumbar spine (Krolner et al, 1983) or TBNAA (Aloia et al, 1978). These findings emphasise the importance of active physiotherapy in patients recovering from crush fractures, followed by a permanent programme of daily muscle-strengthening exercises involving both spinal flexion and extension. By the same token, spinal corsets and braces should be discouraged once they are no longer essential to control pain.

Calcium intake may be important in achieving a strong skeleton, in protecting against osteoporotic fractures and in the treatment of established disease. Epidemiological studies of calcium intakes in Finland, Puerto Rico, Yugoslavia and Japan have supported the first two concepts (Nagant de

Deuxchaisnes, 1983). A protective role of calcium supplementation against mineral loss was also supported by metabolic balance data in the 1960s. Subsequent observations did not sustain this belief however until Heaney & Recker (1981) established from longitudinal studies that whereas calcium equilibrium was provided, statistically, by intakes of 800 mg daily before the menopause, after the menopause the same required intake was 1400 mg daily. There is also evidence that calcium supplementation protects against mineral loss judged by photon absorptiometry and against vertebral crush fracture measured by 'spine score'. There is no compelling evidence in favour of any particular form of supplementation, calcium carbonate having been given in some studies and pharmaceutic preparations including effervescent calcium gluconate and microcrystalline hydroxyapatite compound being effective in others.

The benefits of oestrogen replacement therapy have been established in the last few years by studies too numerous to detail (Nagant de Deuxchaisnes, 1983). They include protection against bone mineral loss and height loss; and, after 6 years' treatment, the risk of hip fracture may be reduced by 50–60%. The beneficial effects of oestrogen replacement may be lost after 4 years' discontinuation but by contrast it appears never to be too late to start. While oestrogen therapy reverses most of the biochemical changes discussed above, its precise mode of action remains obscure. Effective regimes include conjugated oestrogens 0.625 mg daily, ethinyl oestradiol and mestranol 25 μg daily and oestradiol valerate 2 mg daily. Dosage must be cyclical (in women who have not undergone hysterectomy) but treatment is not without risk chiefly from endometrial hyperplasia although this can largely be abolished by inclusion of progestational agents. If oestrogen therapy is contraindicated, or not tolerated, progestogen therapy alone (norethisterone or lynestrenol 5 mg daily) may provide similar benefit.

The use of anabolic steroids has long been in disrepute (Riggs et al, 1972; Gordan et al, 1973). Recent studies however have shown that stanozolol may significantly increase total body calcium. Calcitonin therapy by itself may induce secondary hyperparathyroid bone changes which ultimately nullify its initial effect; in combination with high calcium supplementation however there is evidence of benefit albeit expensive and painstaking. Fluoride alone produces osteomalacic histology with defective mineralisation and increased resorption. These deleterious effects are blocked by massive calcium supplementation; trabecular bone volume may increase by 60% in two years (Briançon & Meunier, 1981) and long-term studies have shown highly significant reduction in vertebral crush fracture rate, a benefit even more striking in combination with oestrogen therapy (Riggs et al, 1982). Side-effects are common, particularly gastrointestinal disturbance, and a proportion of patients show no radiological or histological response.

Borderline or defective vitamin D nutrition among the elderly may contribute to the incidence of hip and other fractures. Physiological replacement to ensure optimal nutrition is therefore fully justifiable, and inexpensive. Most studies of pharmacologic therapy, with any vitamin D derivative, have on the other hand been disappointing. Groups so treated, whether alone or in combination with other agents, have tended to show poorer results and danger of intoxication is constant (Nagant de Deuxchaisnes, 1983)

Lastly, patients with osteoporosis require reassurance. Dent & Watson (1966) emphasised the *spontaneous* tendency for crush fractures to lessen or cease with time particularly in younger patients. Residual pain, associated with degenerative spondylosis, may be relieved by non-steroidal anti-inflammatory agents and by a period of lying horizontal during the day. At the same time the disease is not without its rare fatality, mocking efforts to define the responsible agent. Newer approaches to research involve attempts to uncouple the dynamic sequence within the bone remodelling unit, first activating the process, then depressing subsequent osteoclastic activity, freeing the cycle to permit new bone formation and ultimately repeating the phases. Further analysis is premature.

RICKETS AND OSTEOMALACIA

Rickets and osteomalacia are conditions of defective mineralisation in cartilage and bone respectively. They are associated, in historical descriptive sequence, with characteristic clinical (Glisson,

1650), histological (Pommer, 1885; recently reviewed by Aaron, 1978), radiological (Looser, 1920; Chick et al, 1923) and biochemical (Howland & Kramer, 1921) abnormalities which by 1948 (Albright & Reifenstein, 1948) had become fully delineated. The disease may be further defined by reference to its specific aetiological factor, namely inadequate activity of vitamin D. This description embraces both the classical vitamin deficiency disease and the myriad forms of vitamin D resistance (Table 40.6). Others prefer looser terminology based on specific histomorphometric criteria thereby including conditions with similar biopsy appearances such as hypophosphatasia, fluorosis and diphosphonate ingestion in which vitamin D deficiency or resistance play no part. In addition, routine histological methods may not distinguish osteomalacia from Paget's disease or hyperparathyroidism.

In growth cartilage (see Fig. 40.1) defective

Table 40.6 Classification of rickets and osteomalacia, nutritional and metabolic (from Stamp, 1982). Forms which need considering in the differential diagnosis of locomotor symptoms presenting in adolescence or adult life are indicated (*).

A. Privational
- Classic deficiency*
- Asian immigrant children: infants, puberty late rickets*
- Asian immigrant adults*
- Indigenous elderly*, institutionalised groups*
- 'Food faddists'*

B. Gastrointestinal

Partial gastrectomy*

Small bowel malabsorption syndromes*
- Gluten-sensitive enteropathy (coeliac disease)
- Purgative addiction
- Visceral scleroderma
- Regional enteritis
- Surgical resection or bypass
- Mesenteric tuberculosis
- Amyloidosis (primary or secondary)

Chronic pancreatic insufficiency

Hepatobiliary disturbance
- Prematurity
- Biliary atresia
- Neonatal hepatitis
- Primary biliary cirrhosis
- Ascending cholangitis
- Chronic active hepatitis
- Anticonvulsant drugs (?multifactorial)*

C. Hereditary renal disease (usually renal phosphate 'leak' with high phosphate clearance)

Hypophosphataemia*
- X-linked dominant: also rarely autosomal dominant, autosomal recessive

Vitamin D-dependency rickets
- Type I, type II

Fanconi syndromes:
- Cystinosis: infantile form, late childhood form

Fanconi syndrome without cystinosis:
- Childhood form
- Adult form with and without diabetes mellitus*
- Oculocerebrorenal (Lowe's) syndrome
- Wilson's disease (hepatolenticular degeneration)
- Tyrosinaemia
- Glycogenosis with abnormal galactose metabolism
- Familial nephrosis
- (Fanconi tubule without rickets: hereditary fructose intolerance, galactosaemia)

C. Hereditary renal disease (contd)

Bartter's syndrome

Distal renal tubular acidosis ('renal rickets with nephrocalcinosis . . .')*

24,25$(OH)_2$D-dependency rickets

D. Acquired renal disease

1. Mainly glomerular
- Azotaemic renal osteodystrophy (any form)*

2. Mainly tubular
- Hypophosphataemic syndromes*
  - Idiopathic
  - Mesenchymal tumours
    - Benign
    - Malignant
  - Neurofibromatosis
  - Polyostotic fibrous dysplasia

Fanconi syndromes*
- Obstructive uropathy
- Gammopathies: Idiopathic
  - Paraproteinaemia
  - Myelomatosis
- Primary amyloidosis
- Sjögren's syndrome
- Heavy metal poisoning, e.g. cadmium
- Idiopathic Fanconi syndrome: adult forms, with and without diabetes mellitus pancreatic carcinoma.
- ?Association with chronic pancreatic insufficiency

Ureterosigmostomy and ileal bladder

Renal homotransplantation

E. Miscellaneous forms

Phosphate depletion (antacid ingestion)*

Calcium depletion

?Magnesium depletion

Primary hyperparathyroidism*

Diphosphonate ingestion

?Axial osteomalacia*

provisional calcification is associated with a lengthened zone of hypertrophy, with distortion or obliteration of longitudinal cell columns in the zones of hypertrophy and maturation, with resulting lack of normal vascularisation channels, and with excessive osteoclastic resorption in the primary spongiosa (Mankin, 1974; Aaron, 1978). X-ray appearance of the resulting expanded, widened and ragged growth plate is shown in Fig. 40.9. In iliac crest biopsy surface coverage with osteoid and/or osteoid seam width is excessive, defective mineralisation front is revealed by low uptake of tetracycline or toluidine blue and there may be evidence of increased osteoclastic resorption. Total bone volume may be reduced, normal or increased (Frame & Parfitt, 1978). X-rays may show a characteristic Looser's zone, a ribbon-like zone of rarefaction (Fig. 40.10), and signs of secondary hyperparathyroidism (subperiosteal resorption in phalanges) may be evident. In severe forms, vertebral softening leads to symmetrical biconcavity of vertebral bodies ('codfish' vertebrae) with ballooning of the intervertebral discs and loss of upper segment (crown-to-pubis) height.

Signs and symptoms of rickets include swollen epiphyses, 'beading' at the costochondral junctions (the 'ricketty rosary'), Harrison's sulcus in the thorax from the inward pull of the diaphragm at its site of attachment and bowing deformities in the femora and tibiae with loss of lower segment (pubis-to-sole) height. Older children may show genu varum instead and combinations occur as 'windswept legs' (Fig. 40.11); the disease may be manifest in later childhood only as hobbling or inability to run. Symptoms of hypocalcaemia, tetany or paraesthesiae, may occur at any age but are less common; Chvostek's and Trousseau's signs should be looked for but their significance is limited (Stamp et al, 1980). The former is elicited as a brief contraction of one or more superficial facial muscles following light finger percussion of branches of the facial nerve: the latter is production of tetanic carpal spasm (the 'main d'accoucheur') by inflation of a sphygmomanometer cuff to systolic blood pressure for 3 minutes. Proximal myopathy is a characteristic feature of rickets and osteomalacia but may be difficult to distinguish separately from bone pain and tender-

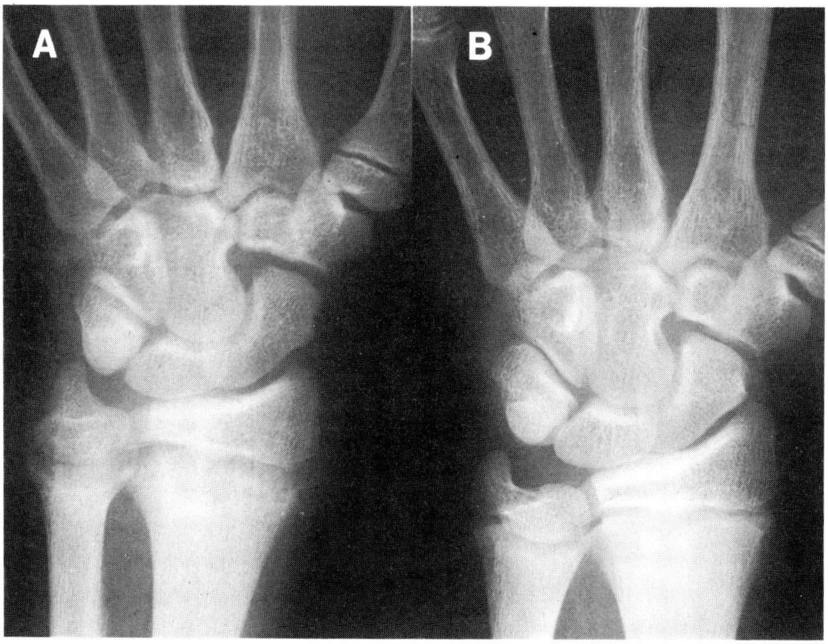

Fig. 40.9 Radiological appearances of rickets (A) in the wrist of a 14-year-old boy and (B) after healing with vitamin D. Appearances may be identical in all forms of rickets regardless of cause. Compare with normal and abnormal histological appearances shown in Figure 40.1.

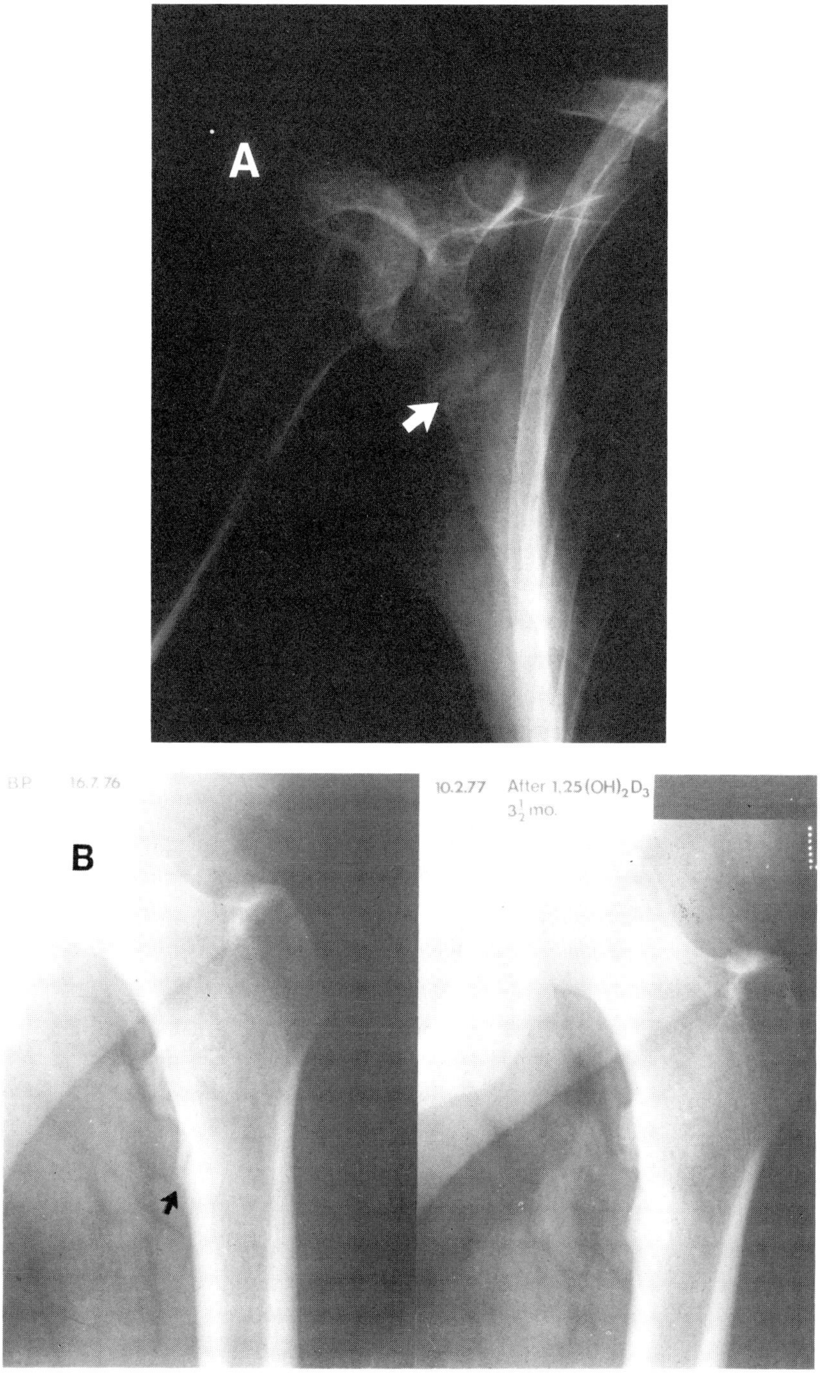

Fig. 40.10 Radiological appearance of Looser's zones (pseudofractures) arrowed in (A) scapula and (B) femur before and after treatment with calcitriol. This is the only diagnostic feature of osteomalacia although signs of secondary hyperparathyroidism (Fig. 40.12) may be present without Looser's zones.

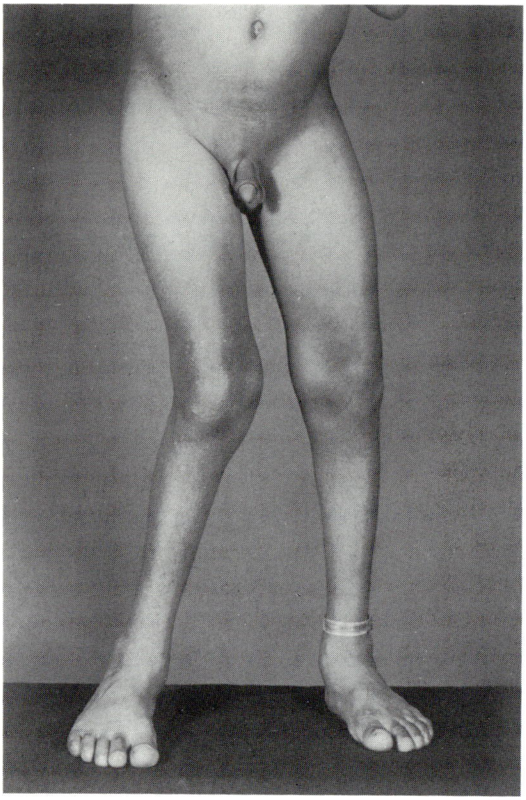

Fig. 40.11 'Windswept' legs in an 8-year-old boy with rickets due to an idiopathic Fanconi syndrome without cystinosis. Renal glomerular function has remained normal during 9 years' treatment and follow-up although well-marked aminoaciduria, renal glycosuria and nephrogenic diabetes insipidus persist.

ness; electromyographic changes, when present, are non-specific; its cause is still uncertain (Frame & Parfitt, 1978).

Symptoms of osteomalacia in the adult are often vague and even when severe may appear non-specific. Bone pain and tenderness result from the pull of tendons on softened bone, the most painful bones (ribs, sternum, hips, vertebrae) having the thinnest cortices. Many patients with osteomalacia have spent years labelled with 'lumbago' or 'neurosis'. Therapeutic disasters have resulted from misdiagnosis of 'polymyositis' and subsequent corticosteroid therapy. Pathological fractures may occur in the severest forms.

The disease may result from any disturbance of the functional metabolism of vitamin D (Fig. 40.3). The gradual elucidation of the many forms covers over five decades of medical history (Dent, 1969). The causes have been recently reviewed in detail (Stamp, 1982); Table 40.6 gives special reference to those forms most likely to involve the differential diagnosis of uncertain locomotor symptoms in adolescence and adult life.

Appropriate clinical and laboratory studies will reveal precise aetiology in every case, and the reader is referred to standard or specialist textbooks for investigation and treatment of associated conditions. Of all these forms, X-linked hereditary hypophosphataemia has unique features the reasons for which are obscure. There is no myopathy unless the patient is immobilised; bones develop thick cortices without evidence of hyperparathyroidism; extraskeletal ossification develops in tendons, ligaments and periarticular tissues and the radiological appearance may ultimately resemble ankylosing spondylitis or fluorosis (Stamp, 1982). Patients are negative for the histocompatibility antigen HLA-B27.

The greater or lesser tendency of all forms to show laboratory features of hypocalcaemia, hypophosphataemia and raised alkaline phosphatase (of bony origin) are well known. However there are frequent exceptions to these findings. Table 40.7 shows main laboratory findings in the major forms of the disease.

Plasma calcium, corrected for albumen concentration, may be within the lower limit of normal in 50% of patients with classical deficiency disease (Stamp et al 1980). Plasma calcium is almost invariably normal in the hypophosphataemic syndromes whether hereditary or acquired. Osteoblastic activity often diminishes in chronic osteomalacia and alkaline phosphatase levels may be minimally raised, or rarely normal, even in severe disease. Plasma phosphorus levels may be elevated in severe untreated childhood rickets ('functional hypoparathyroidism') or in the early healing stages of the disease (Stamp et al, 1980). The frequency of rickets in renal tubular disease is associated with the renal tubular site of 1,25-dihydroxyvitamin D synthesis. In addition to hypophosphataemia, renal tubular defects may include renal glycosuria, amino aciduria and bicarbonate wastage (type II renal tubular acidosis). These four defects constitute Fanconi's syndrome, the chief surviving eponym among the original descriptions in the 1930s by Lignac, Fanconi, De Toni and Debré

Table 40.7 Main biochemical changes in some forms of rickets and osteomalacia and in some superficially similar bone diseases (Dent & Stamp, 1977)

Diagnosis	Plasma Ca* (mmol/l)	Plasma P (mmol/l)	Plasma HCO_3 (mmol/l)	Plasma urea (mmol/l)	Plasma alkaline phosphatase	Urine Ca (mmol/24 h)
Normal adult	2.25–2.62 2.25–2.55 (fasting)	0.82–1.35	24–28	3–7		3–7.5 (♂) 3–6.5 (♀)
Normal children (1–16 years old)	2.25–2.62	1.29–1.94	20–26	3–5		1–5
Chondrodystrophies	Normal	Normal	Normal	Normal	Normal	Normal (high if in an active phase)
Idiopathic osteoporosis	Normal	Normal	Normal	Normal	Normal	Normal
Hypophosphataemic rickets	Normal	0.32–0.81**		Normal	Elevated	Low normal
Classic and other forms of non-acidotic rickets	1.5–2.25	0.32–1.29	20–26	Normal	Elevated	0.5–2.5
Acidotic forms of rickets	1.75–2.37	0.32–0.97	10–22	3–10	Elevated	3.5–9
Renal-glomerular osteodystrophy	1.25–2.25	1.29–>3	10–20	15–>80	Elevated	0.5–2.5
Primary hyperparathyroidism	2.55–>4 (fasting)	0.32–0.97	20–26	Normal or elevated	Normal or elevated	4–15
Hypophosphatasia	2.25–3.5	0.97–1.61	20–28	3–20		High or high normal
Hypohyperparathyroidism	1.25–1.75	1.29–2.26	22–26	Normal	Elevated	0.5–2.5

* All plasma Ca must be corrected for the protein content of the same specimen, albumen concentration being the most important. Many laboratories use a normal reference albumen level of 41 g/l. For each 6 g/l above this, subtract 0.10 mmol/l calcium and vice versa, correcting intermediate values proportionally. Use of a second decimal place for calcium and phosphorus levels was necessitated by the introduction of SI (Système International) units but the laboratory accuracy it implies is unattainable.

** Levels up to 1.02 are compatible with the diagnosis in infancy and early childhood.

(Dent, 1969). Additional defects may involve renal loss of sodium, potassium and water leading to hypokalaemia and nephrogenic diabetes insipidus. The precise relationship of all these forms to possible defects of 1,25-dihydroxyvitamin D synthesis awaits full clarification.

All privational and almost all gastrointestinal forms of osteomalacia are associated with deficiency of the parent vitamin and low circulating levels of 25-hydroxyvitamin D (Stamp, 1982). Treatment of classic deficiency requires only vitamin D_2 or D_3 in doses of 1 000–10 000 iu daily; even lower doses produce supranormal, healing levels of 1,25$(OH)_2$D (Mawer, 1980). In situations of doubt a therapy trial of 1800 iu daily, provided by Caps A & D (*BNF*) two twice daily, is a perfectly valid approach: simple deficiency disease will show clinical and biochemical improvement within 3 weeks while few metabolic (i.e. 'vitamin D-resistant') forms respond to less than 10 000 iu (0.25 mg) daily. Malabsorption syndromes, particularly gluten-sensitive enteropathy, may show considerable resistance to treatment and, even after instituting a gluten-free diet, may benefit from vitamin D dosage as high as 5 mg daily in the first 1–2 months (Dent & Stamp, 1977). Transient worsening of bone pain, a 'stirring-up phenomenon', is frequent in the first 1–2 weeks of successful treatment and patients should if possible be warned in advance of this possibility.

Pharmacological vitamin D treatment may take many months to achieve therapeutic (but unpredictable) plateau levels of 25-OHD (Stamp et al, 1977), the parent vitamin being inactive. Although guidelines for maintenance vitamin D dosage have been established for all metabolic forms of the disease (Dent & Stamp, 1977), therapeutic availability of the potent derivatives 1,25-

dihydroxycholecalciferol (calcitriol) and 1a-hydroxycholecalciferol (alfacalcidol) has improved the outlook for treatment in all renal forms of the disease. Alfacalcidol requires prior 25-hydroxylation in liver before it is effective; animal and human studies indicate that its potency is approximately half that of calcitriol. In most renal forms of rickets and osteomalacia calcitriol in *maintenance* dosage of 0.25–1.5 μg daily approximates the effects of vitamin D in dosage of 0.25–2.0 mg daily. The very high peripheral $1,25(OH)_2D$ concentrations that rapidly follow small doses of vitamin D in classical deficiency (Mawer, 1980), coupled with (limited) study of high dose calcitriol or alfacalcidol in metabolic rickets, suggest that as with vitamin D high dosage of these derivatives (5–10 μg daily, respectively) may be required for optimum therapeutic response in early healing stages. The need for careful follow up to minimise risk of intoxication, even with maintenance dosage, remains.

Phosphate supplements are required in addition for treatment in acquired hypophosphataemic syndromes, provided for example by Phosphate-Sandoz tabs 2–3 times daily. More frequent (5-hourly) phosphate administration has been recommended in X-linked hypophosphataemia (Glorieux et al, 1972) but not all workers find phosphate supplements necessary in this condition (Dent & Stamp, 1977). Bicarbonate supplements are needed in acidotic forms.

PARATHYROID DISORDERS

Primary hyperparathyroidism

Primary hyperparathyroidism is a 'common and polymorphic condition' (Albright et al, 1934) with an overall, current incidence of 1–2 per thousand as revealed by contemporary screening programmes. In many it remains asymptomatic. Surgical results show solitary adenomata in 85–90% of cases, 10–15% have hyperplasia of all four glands, while parathyroid carcinoma is rare (about 1%). Apart from a small subgroup with (often familial) multiple endocrine adenomatosis in childhood or early adult life the incidence increases with advancing age. It is about 4 times more common in females than in males, the overall sex difference being almost entirely due to the predominance of females in the postmenopausal age-group.

Bone and joint manifestations are uncommon. While historically the first diagnoses followed successful parathyroidectomy in patients with severe hyperparathyroid bone disease (osteitis fibrosa cystica), including pathological fractures through 'brown tumours' (Albright & Reifenstein, 1948), and until a decade or more ago bone disease still accounted for 20% of presenting cases, the last few years have shown a striking reduction in the clinical incidence of primary osteitis fibrosa. This change is apparent both in Britain, among the University College Hospital, London, series of over 700 cases covering the years 1952–1982 (L.C.A. Watson, unpublished), and in the USA (Reiss & Canterbury, 1982).

Symptoms of osteitis fibrosa include both pain and pathological fractures in localised brown tumours and more vague, general pains in knees and ankles associated with more diffuse signs of subperiosteal resorption (Fig. 40.12). Erosive bone lesions occasionally resemble rheumatoid arthritis.

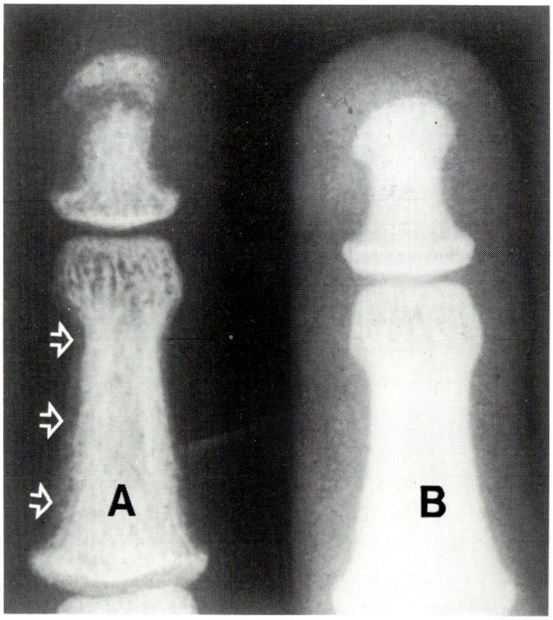

Fig. 40.12 (A) Gross subperiosteal erosions in the phalanges (magnified) of a patient with hyperparathyroidism and osteitis fibrosa. The tips of the arrowheads lie along the periosteum as can be seen by comparison with (B) showing restoration of normal contour after healing; this is a less penetrated X-ray.

Articular symptoms may be still more difficult to interpret. Chondrocalcinosis (pseudogout, see Ch. 37) is 6 times more common in hyperparathyroidism than in age- and sex-matched controls (Dent, unpublished data). However occasional patients, with *or without* radiologically visible calcification in menisci or articular cartilage, present with joint symptoms which range from mild, subacute, remitting polyarthritis in the small joints of the hand and wrist to more clear-cut symptoms and signs of degenerative joint disease. In the past, demonstration of hypercalcaemia was a chance finding and subsequent confirmation of hyperparathyroidism was classified among the 'accidental' diagnoses. Ease of biochemical screening has increased the diagnostic frequency of arthritis and coexistent hyperparathyroidism. In such patients associated symptoms of long-standing hypercalcaemia including a history of urolithiasis, dyspepsia or constipation should be sought as they may strengthen the indications for recommending parathyroid surgery. Parathyroidectomy may well be offered as desirable in any case although both clinician and patient should understand that the chance of rheumatological improvement may be small. Published follow-up of joint symptoms after successful parathyroidectomy is lacking. Despite these reservations the author has occasionally observed gratifying long-term improvement.

Diagnosis of hyperparathyroidism is made by standard means, highly accurate laboratory verification of non-fluctuating hypercalcaemia, with due correction for serum albumen concentration, being paramount. Other typical laboratory features including low or low–normal phosphorus ($<$ 1 mmol/l), high or high–normal chloride ($\leq$ 104 mmol/1), normal renal glomerular function (in patients without osteitis fibrosa) and normal haematological indices including ESR, form the basis of multivariate statistical analysis as a diagnostic aid (Watson et al, 1980). A standard hydrocortisone test, giving 40 mg by mouth 8-hourly for 10 days and measuring fasting calcium on the 6th, 9th and 11th days, is particularly indicated if presentation is unusual; hypercalcaemia persists or even increases slightly in hyperparathyroidism, by contrast with its improvement in hypercalcaemic sarcoidosis. Joint symptoms not surprisingly often improve during the test. All routine radioimmunoassays for circulatory parathyroid hormone frequently show normal levels in subsequently proven hyperparathyroidism.

Hypoparathyroid disorders

The hypoparathyroid disorders include idiopathic hypoparathyroidism, surgical (secondary) hypoparathyroidism, pseudohypoparathyroidism and hypo-hyperparathyroidism; extensive reviews are available (Nusynowitz et al, 1976; Parfitt, 1979; Nagant de Deuxchaisnes & Krane, 1978). Idiopathic hypoparathyroidism may be associated with embryological maldevelopment involving the thymus and aortic arch (Di George's syndrome) and with immune disturbances which may predispose to frequent monilial infection. The disease presents from early childhood to adult life, occasionally after parturition, with variable symptoms including epilepsy, hypocalcaemic tetany or paraesthesiae (carpopedal spasm, laryngeal stridor) and cataract. Surgical hypoparathyroidism may follow thyroidectomy or parathyroidectomy at variable intervals. Both forms may show papilloedema for uncertain reasons. Pseudohypoparathyroidism is characterised by target organ resistance to parathyroid hormone in bone and kidney and by clinical features including short stature, rounded facies, variable brachydactyly (particularly congenital shortening of the 4th metacarpal — McKusick, 1983) and ectopic subcutaneous calcification (with which patients may present, Fig. 40.13). It is twice as common in females as in males and is possibly inherited as an X-linked dominant characteristic (McKusick, 1983). Both idiopathic hypoparathyroidism and pseudohypoparath roidism may show variable mental retardation. Immunoreactive PTH levels are undetectable or low in hypoparathyroidism and raised in pseudohypoparathyroidism and hypo-hyperparathyroidism. In hypo-hyperparathyroidism bone sensitivity to increased PTH secretion results in clinical osteitis fibrosa associated with hypoparathyroid biochemistry. Alkaline phosphatase is raised and radiological bone resorption particularly in the metaphyses resembles rickets. Patients with idiopathic hypoparathyroidism tend to have dense bones; rarely hyperostotic changes may be clinically significant (Jimenea et al, 1971). Pseudohypoparathyroidism also shows hyperostosis but

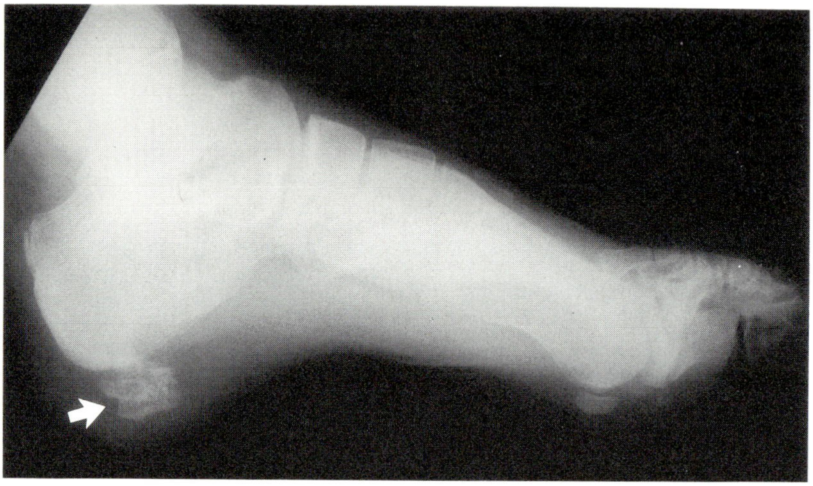

Fig. 40.13 Subcutaneous calcification (arrowed) in the heel of a 9-year-old boy with pseudohypoparathyroidism who presented with pain in the heel on walking.

occasional evidence of subperiosteal resorption indicates variable sensitivity to parathyroid activity in bone. Hypo-hyperparathyroidism may show either clinical features of pseudohypoparathyroidism or patients may be tall and above average in intelligence. Whether this represents a clinical spectrum or discrete varieties of the disease has yet to be established (Nusynowitz et al, 1976).

Diagnosis may be facilitated by intravenous parathyroid hormone infusion. Patients with idiopathic hypoparathyroidism respond by a rise in plasma calcium and in urinary excretion of phosphorus and cyclic adenosine monophosphate (cAMP). Results in pseudohypoparathyroidism suggest different forms of the disease some showing no response in either urinary phosphorus or cAMP and some showing increase in cAMP only (Parfitt, 1979; Nagant de Deuxchaisnes & Krane, 1978; Lewin et al, 1978).

1,25-dihydroxyvitamin D concentrations appear low in all forms (Haussler & McCain, 1979) and intestinal calcium absorption is markedly reduced. Successful treatment entails maintenance with vitamin D or one of its derivatives in similar dosages to those indicated for renal forms of rickets and osteomalacia (see above). Sensitivity to the 'vitamins D' varies considerably. Lastly the designation 'pseudo-pseudohypoparathyroidism' may be used for the phenotype of pseudohypoparathyroidism in the absence of biochemical disturbance. Whether some patients with pseudohypoparathyroidism grow out of their biochemical abnormalities is still uncertain (McKusick, 1983).

PAGET'S DISEASE

Paget's disease is a common condition originally described by Sir James Paget (1877) as 'osteitis deformans'. It is characterised by increased bone turnover, increased production rate of bone remodelling units and overgrowth of immature woven bone (Meunier et al, 1980). New 'cutting cones' of osteoclastic resorption (see Fig. 40.2) are frequently seen invading incompleted bone remodelling units with resulting irregularity of cement lines which form the outer tidemark of each unit. Increased osteoclastic activity also leads to varying degrees of marrow fibrosis. Radiological appearances are of expanded bone with irregularly thickened cortices and coarse distorted trabecular pattern (Fig. 40.14). The bones become softened, may bend and show cortical fractures. There is a recent extensive review (Hamdy, 1981).

The aetiology is unknown. Ultrastructural studies of Pagetic osteoclasts suggest the presence of viral microcylindrical intranuclear inclusion bodies which with immunological techniques variably appear to be either measles virus (Rebel et al, 1980) or respiratory syncytial virus (Mills et al, 1980). Circulating antibody levels to these or related viruses are not elevated and viral disease has not been transmitted in tissue culture.

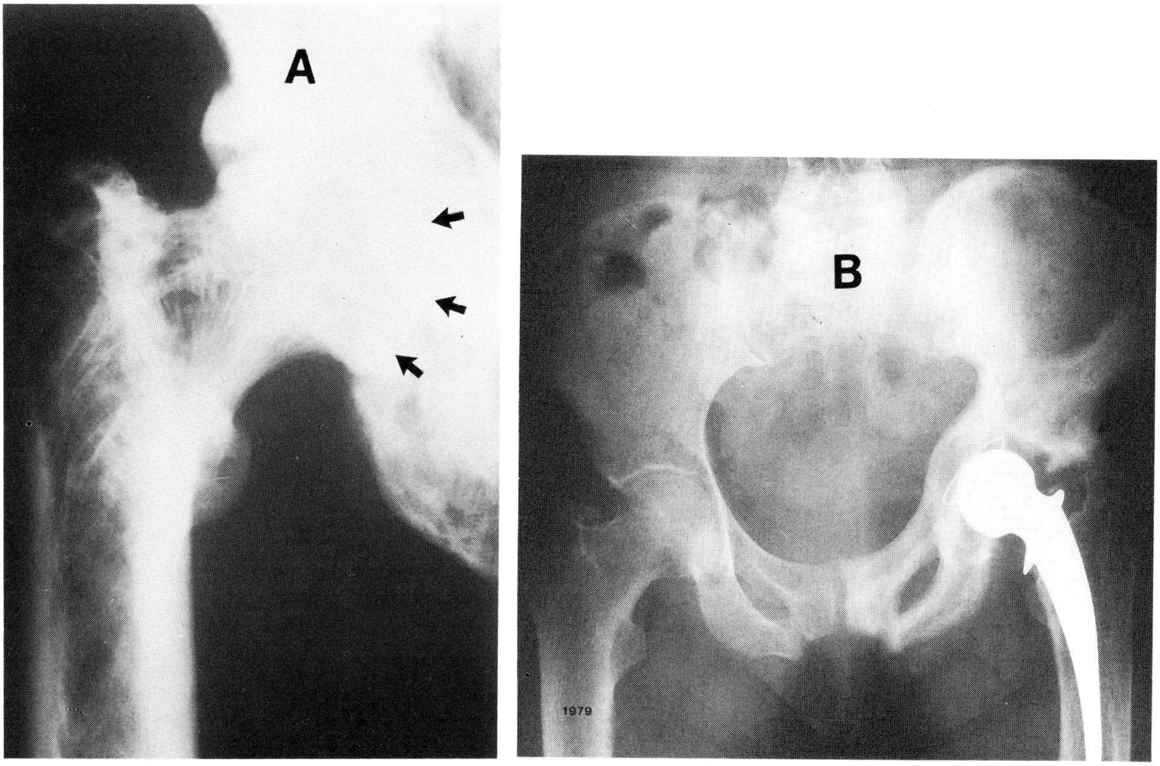

Fig. 40.14 (A) Paget's disease affecting both pelvis and proximal right femur; there is coxa vara. In this situation secondary osteoarthritis may show the unusual distribution of medial, rather than superior, joint space loss (arrowed). (B) Paget's disease affecting the whole left hemipelvis. Despite the generalised increase in density the bone is soft; note the resulting acetabular protrusion. Secondary osteoarthritis has lead to total hip replacement.

Radiological Paget's disease is seen in at least 3.5% of the population over the age of 45 (Pygott, 1957) but varies geographically both within the United Kingdom and throughout the world. It increases with advancing age. The disease is polyostotic although individuals may show involvement of only one bone. No part of the skeleton is immune. The disease typically advances very slowly over years and may even appear static. Only 5% of patients with Paget's disease are probably symptomatic (Collins, 1956), a number which nevertheless totals 30 000–40 000 (Woodhouse, 1977). Females are affected more than males in a ratio of 4 : 3 and occasional dominant inheritance is seen (McKusick, 1983).

Symptoms and complications of Paget's disease include bone pain, bone deformity with or without pain, pathological fractures, secondary osteoarthritis (OA), neurological compression syndromes involving cranial nerves, brainstem (from basilar invagination), spinal cord and spinal root symptoms (Fig. 40.15). Osseous hyperaemia may increase demands on cardiac output, occasionally contributing to cardiac failure. It is postulated that some neurological symptoms may also represent a vascular 'steal'. Malignant change in the form of chondrosarcoma, osteogenic sarcoma or fibrosarcoma is described but is uncommon. Pain is a presenting feature in over 80% of patients (Franck et al, 1974; Altman & Collins, 1980; Winfield & Stamp, 1984). It is important from a therapeutic standpoint to distinguish carefully the source of pain. Over 50% of patients have bone pain described as constant, dull or burning. Over 30% present with clinical osteoarthritis. Lumbar spondylosis and OA of the hip are frequent, the latter occurring at some stage in up to 50% of patients; both types may occur in the absence of adjacent Paget's disease. OA is usually associated with deformity; affected joints are stable, dry and

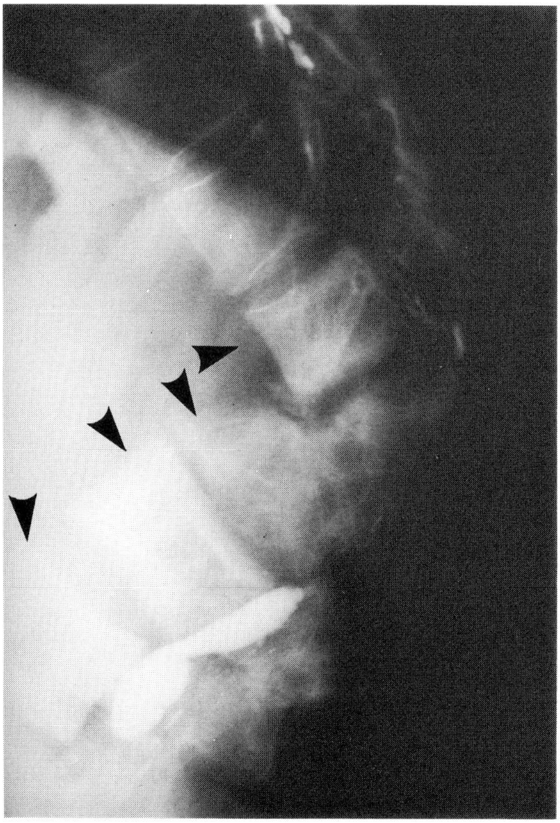

Fig. 40.15 Unusual 'knuckle' kyphosis from severe vertebral collapse in Paget's disease. Note the overall enlargement of certain of the affected bones (all arrowed).

subarticular sclerosis and cyst formation are characteristically absent. Acetabular Paget's disease is more important in the genesis of OA hip than femoral disease (Winfield & Stamp, 1984). When both are present, with coxa vara, more medial joint space loss is seen; advanced disease produces protrusio acetabuli with implications for surgical hip replacement. Sacroiliac Paget's may produce obliteration of that joint. Pathological fractures generally heal well with internal fixation but non-union may occur in approximately 10% (Barry, 1980). Total hip replacement is often satisfactory but complications include increased intraoperative blood loss, later loosening of either component and heterotopic ossification.

Chief biochemical findings reflect the increased bone turnover, with raised plasma alkaline phosphatase and increased liberation and urinary excretion of hydroxyproline-containing peptides. Plasma calcium is normal but hypercalcaemia occurs more readily than normal after immobilisation from fracture (Albright & Reifenstein, 1948). Raised immunoreactive PTH levels have been reported in 12% (Meunier et al, 1980) the reason for which is uncertain. Coexistent hyperparathyroidism appears adversely to affect Paget's disease, and *vice versa* (Albright & Reifenstein, 1948), 5 out of 6 patients studied with both conditions having shown a 'hungry bones' stage following parathyroidectomy (Stamp, 1972).

Simple analgesics, non-steroidal anti-inflammatory agents and physiotherapy control many symptoms. Regular injection of porcine, salmon or human calcitonin appears highly specific for Pagetic bone pain (Bijvoet et al, 1968; Singer et al, 1980; MacIntyre et al, 1980). Side-effects are facial flushing and occasional gastrointestinal disturbance. Oral diphosphonate therapy with sodium etidronate may be effective (Smith et al, 1973; Johnston et al, 1980); its use is somewhat complicated by a dose-related mineralisation defect leading to histological appearance of osteomalacia. Both forms of therapy regularly lower plasma alkaline phosphatase and urinary hydroxyproline. Occasional escape from control occurs as immunological resistance to calcitonin may develop (Singer et al, 1980). The cytotoxic antibiotic mithramycin may also have a small place in therapy (Ryan & Schwartz, 1980; Martin, 1980).

MISCELLANEOUS DISORDERS

Three other conditions justify inclusion for completeness. Fibrogenesis imperfecta ossium is an acquired disorder of collagen metabolism (Swan et al, 1976). It shows a superficial histological appearance of severe osteomalacia but examination under polarised light reveals a pathognomonic loss of normal osteoid birefringence. Ultramicroscopic studies show amorphous collagen. The disease presents in middle or later life with increasing bone pains and tenderness. X-rays show osteopenia and very coarse trabeculation but there is no bony expansion. Alkaline phosphatase levels of bone origin are raised. Effective therapy has not been established; active metabolities of vitamin D and calcium supplements may produce partial response. More complete remission has recently followed melphalan therapy for coexistant monoclonal gammopathy (Stamp et al, 1985).

'Axial osteomalacia' describes a syndrome associated with excessive osteoid and radiologically coarsened trabeculae in spine, ribs and pelvis (Condon & Nassim, 1971). The entity has not universally been accepted (Jowsey, 1977).

Local heterotopic ossification in muscle connective tissue occasionally follows trauma. A rare, generalised disease exists as myositis (or fibrodysplasia) ossificans progressiva (McKusick, 1983). It may be inherited as an autosomal dominant characteristic. Odd phalangeal abnormalities, particularly monophalangy and hallux valgus, are present at birth. The condition then presents in early childhood (rarely up to late adolescence) with repeated brawny soft tissue swellings which have been initially mistaken for fibrosarcoma. Bars of histologically true bone gradually form within muscle connective tissue. The disease runs a progressive, disabling course, with increasing immobility, but may become more static in adult life. The cause of the apparent conversion of fibroblasts to osteoblasts is unknown, and treatment is palliatory. Disorders of heterotopic ossification are the subject of a recent monograph (Connor, 1983).

REFERENCES

Aaron J E 1978 Histological aspects of vitamin D and bone. In: Lawson D E M (ed) Vitamin D. Academic Press, London, p 201–265

Albright F, Reifenstein E C 1948 The parathyroid glands and metabolic bone disease. Williams & Wilkins, Baltimore

Albright F, Aub J C, Bauer W 1934 Hyperparathyroidism. A common and polymorphic condition as illustrated by seventeen proved cases from one clinic. Journal of the American Medical Association 102: 1276–1287

Albright F, Smith P H, Richardson A M 1941 Postmenopausal osteoporosis: its clinical features. Journal of the American Medical Association 116: 2465–2474

Albright J 1981 Systemic treatment of osteogenesis imperfecta. Clinical Orthopaedics and Related Research 159: 88–96

Aloia J F, Cohn S H, Ostuni J A, Cane R, Ellis K 1978 Prevention of involutional bone loss by exercise. Annals of Internal Medicine 89: 356–358

Altman R D, Collins B 1980 Musculoskeletal manifestations of Paget's disease of bone. Arthritis and Rheumatism 23: 1121–1127

Arnaud C D, Gallagher J C, Jerpbak C M, Riggs B L 1981 On the role of parathyroid hormone in the osteoporosis of aging. In: De Luca H F, Frost H M, Jee W S S, Johnston C C Jr, Parfitt A M (eds) Osteoporosis: Recent advances in pathogenesis and treatment. University Park Press, Baltimore, p. 215–225

Avioli L V 1981 The endocrinology of involutional osteoporosis. In: De Luca H F, Frost H M, Jee W S S, Johnston C C Jr, Parfitt A M (eds) Osteoporosis: Recent advances in pathogenesis and treatment. University Park Press, Baltimore, p. 343–351

Ballet J J, Griscelli C, Coutris C, Milhaud G, Maroteaux P 1977 Bone-marrow transplantation in osteopetrosis. Lancet 2:1137

Barnett E, Nordin B E C 1960 The radiological diagnosis of osteoporosis: a new approach. Clinical Radiology 11: 166–174

Barry H C 1980 Orthopaedic aspects of Paget's disease of bone. Arthritis and Rheumatism 23: 1128–1130

Barzel U S (ed) 1979 Osteoporosis II. Grune & Stratton, New York

Bauze R J, Smith R, Francis M J O 1975 A new look at osteogenesis imperfecta. A clinical, radiological and biochemical study of 42 patients. Journal of Bone and Joint Surgery 57I3: 2–12

Beighton P 1978 Inherited disorders of the skeleton. Churchill Livingstone, London

Bergsma D (ed) 1969 Skeletal dysplasias. Birth Defects 5 (4)

Bergstrom L 1981 Fragile bones and fragile ears. Clinical Orthopaedics and Related Research 159: 58–63

Bijvoet O L M, van der Sluys Veer J, Jansen A P 1968 Effects of calcitonin on patients with Paget's disease, thyrotoxicosis, or hypercalcaemia. Lancet i: 876–881

Bleck E E 1981 Nonoperative treatment of osteogenesis imperfecta: orthotic and mobility management. Clinical Orthopaedics and Related Research 159: 111–122

Boukhris R, Becker K L 1973 The inter-relationship between vertebral fractures and osteoporosis. Clinical Orthopaedics and Related Research 90: 209–216

Brenton D P, Dent C E 1976 Idiopathic juvenile osteoporosis. In: Bickel H, Stern J (eds) Inborn errors of calcium and bone metabolism. MTP Press, Lancaster, p. 222–238

Briancon D, Meunier P J 1981 Treatment of osteoporosis with fluoride, calcium and vitamin D. Orthopaedic Clinics of North America 12: 629–648

Cameron J R, Sorenson J 1963 Measurement of bone mineral in vivo: an improved method. Science 142: 230–232

Camurati M 1922 D'un raro caso di osteite simmetrica creditaria degli arti inferiori. Chirurgia degli Organi di Movimento 6: 662–655

Cann C E, Genant H K, Ettinger B, Gordan G S 1980 Spinal mineral loss in oophorectomized women. Determination by quantitative computed tomography. Journal of the American Medical Association 244: 2056–2059

Chick H, Dalyell E J, Hume E M, Mackay H M M, Henderson-Smith H, Wimburger H 1923 Studies of rickets in Vienna 1919–22. Medical Research Committee Special Reports Series 77

Christiansen C, Christiansen M S, Transbol I 1981 Bone mass in postmenopausal women after withdrawal of oestrogen/gestagen replacement therapy. Lancet 1: 459–461

Coccia P F, Krivit W, Cervenka J, Clawson C, Kersey J H, Kim T H, et al 1980 Successful bone-marrow transplantation for infantile malignant osteopetrosis. New England Journal of Medicine 302: 701–708

Cockayne E A 1920 Case for diagnosis. Proceedings of the Royal Society of Medicine 13: 132–136
Cohn S H. Vaswani A, Zanzi I, Ellis K J 1976 Effect of aging on bone mass in adult women. American Journal of Physiology 230: 143–148
Collins D H 1956 Paget's disease of bone-incidence and subclinical forms. Lancet 2: 51–57
Condon J R, Nassim J R 1971 Axial osteomalacia. Postgraduate Medical Journal 47: 817–820
Connor J M 1983 Soft tissue ossification. Springer-Berlag, Berlin
Copp D H, Cameron E C, Cheney B A, Davidson A G F, Henze K G 1962 Evidence for calcitonin — a new hormone from the parathyroid that lowers blood calcium. Endocrinology 70: 638–649
Courpron P, Meunier P J, Edouard C, Giroux J M, Bressot C 1980 Histomorphometrie du tissu osseux spongieux iliaque normal. In: Rasmussen H, Eisenger J, Paecht A (eds) L'Osteoporose. Symposium International, Armour Montagu, Paris, p. 117–139
Crisp A J, Brenton D P 1982 Engelmann's disease of bone — a systemic disorder? Annals of the Rheumatic Diseases 41: 183–188
De Luca H F, Frost H M, Jee W S S, Johnston C C Jr, Parfitt A M (eds) 1981 Osteoporosis: Recent advances in pathogenesis and treatment. University Park Press, Baltimore
Dent C E 1969 Rickets (and osteomalacia), nutritional and metabolic (1919–69). Proceedings of the Royal Society of Medicine 63: 401–408
Dent C E, Gertner J M 1976 Hypophosphataemic osteomalacia in fibrous dysplasia. Quarterly Journal of Medicine 45: 411–420
Dent C E, Stamp T C B 1977 Vitamin D, rickets and osteomalacia. In: Avioli L V, Krane S M (eds) Metabolic bone disease, Vol 1. Academic Press, New York, p. 237–304
Dent C E, Watson L 1966 Osteoporosis. Postgraduate Medical Journal (October Supplement) 42: 583–608
Dixon A St J, Russell R G G, Stamp T C B (eds)1983 Osteoporosis: A multidisciplinary problem. Royal Society of Medicine International Congress and Symposium Series, No. 55, Academic Press, London
Engelmann G 1924 Ein fall von osteopathica Hyperostotica multiplex infantilis. ROEFO: Fortschritte auf dem Gebiete der Roentgenstrahlen und der Nuklearmedizin 39: 1101–1106
Eyre D R 1981 Concepts in collagen biochemistry: evidence that collagenopathies underlie osteogenesis imperfecta. Clinical Orthopaedics and Related Research 159: 97–107
Fairbank H A T 1951 An atlas of general affections of the skeleton. E & S Livingstone, Edinburgh
Frame B, Parfitt A M 1978 Osteomalacia: current concepts. Annals of Internal Medicine 89: 966–982
Franck W A, Bress N M, Singer F R, Krane S M 1974 Rheumatic manifestations of Paget's disease of bone. American Journal of Medicine 56: 592–603
Fraser D R 1980 Regulation of the metabolism of vitamin D. Physiological Reviews 60: 551–613
Frost H M 1973 Bone remodelling and its relationship to metabolic bone disease. Charles C Thomas, Springfield
Frumar A M, Meldrum D R, Geola F, Shamonki I M, Tataryn I V, Deftos L J, Judd H L 1980 Relationship of fasting urinary calcium to circulating oestrogen and body weight in postmenopausal women. Journal of Clinical Endocrinology and Metabolism 50: 70–75
Gallagher J C, Riggs B L, Eisman J, Hamstra A, Arnaud S B, De Luca H F 1979 Intestinal calcium absorption and serum vitamin D metabolites in normal subjects and osteoporotic patients: effects of age and dietary calcium. Journal of Clinical Investigation 64: 729–736
Garn S M 1970 The earlier gain and the later loss of cortical bone. Charles C Thomas, Springfield, Illinois
Garn S M 1981 The phenomenon of bone formation and bone loss. In: De Luca H F, Frost H M, Jee W S S, Johnston C C Jr, Parfitt A M (eds) Osteoporosis: Recent advances in pathogenesis and treatment. University Park Press, Baltimore, p. 3–18
Gershon-Cohen J, Rechtman A M, Schraer H, Blumberg N 1953 Asymptomatic fractures in osteoporotic spines of aged. Journal of the American Medical Association 153: 625–627
Glisson F 1650 De rachitide sive morbo puerili quo vulgo the rickets dicitur tractatus. Adscitis in operis societatum Georgio Bate et abasuero regemortero. Du-Gardi, London
Glorieux F H, Scriver C R, Reade T M, Goldman H, Roseborough A 1972 Use of phosphate and vitamin D to prevent dwarfism and rickets in X-linked hypophosphataemia. New England Journal of Medicine 287: 481–487
Gordan G S, Picchi J, Roof B S 1973 Antifracture efficacy of long-term estrogens for osteoporosis. Transactions of the Association of American Physicians 86: 326–332
Habener J F, Jacobs J W 1982 Biosynthesis and control of secretion of the calcium-regulating peptides. In: Parsons J A (ed) Endocrinology of calcium metabolism. Raven Press, New York, p. 143–181
Hamdy R C 1981 Paget's disease of bone. Praeger Publishers, Eastbourne, New York
Harrison J E, McNeill K G, Sturtridge W C, Bayley T A, Murray T M, Williams C, et al 1981 Three-year changes in bone mineral mass of postmenopausal osteoporotic patients based on neutron activation analysis of the central third of the skeleton. Journal of Clinical Endocrinology and Metabolism 52: 751–758
Haussler M R, McCain T A 1977 Basic and clinical concepts related to vitamin D metabolism and action. New England Journal of Medicine 297: 974–983, 1041–1050
Heaney R P, Recker R R 1981 Osteoporosis-related nutritional influences on bone: calcium. In: De Luca H F, Frost H M, Jee W S S, Johnston C C Jr, Parfitt A M (eds) Osteoporosis: Recent advances in pathogenesis and treatment. University Park Press, Baltimore, p. 253–256
Hobbs J R 1969 Paraproteinaemia. Proceedings of the Royal Society of Medicine 62: 733–736
Holick M F, Holick S A, McNeill S M, Richtand N, Clark M B, Potts J T Jr 1979 The photo-biochemistry of vitamin D_3 in vivo in the skin. In: Norman A W, Schaefer K, v Herrath D, Grigoleit H G, Coburn J W, De Luca H F, Mawer E B, Suda T (eds) Vitamin D: Basic research and clinical application. Walter de Gruyter, Berlin, p. 173–176
Howland J, Kramer B 1921 Calcium and phosphorus in the serum in relation to rickets. American Journal of Diseases in Childhood 22: 105–119
Jimenea C V, Frame B, Chaykin L B, Sigler J W 1971 Spondylitis of hypoparathyroidism. Clinical Orthopaedics and Related Research 74: 84–89
Johnston C C Jr, Norton J A Jr, Khairi R A, Longcope C

1979 Age-related bone loss. In: Barzel U S (ed) Osteoporosis II. Grune & Stratton, New York, p. 91–100
Johnston C C Jr, Khairi M R A, Meunier P J 1980 Use of etidronate (EHDP) in Paget's disease of bone. Arthritis and Rheumatism 23: 1172–1176
Jowsey J J 1977 Metabolic diseases of bone. Saunders, Philadelphia
Krolner B, Toft B, Nielsen S P, Tondevold E 1983 Physical exercise as prophyllaxis against involutional vertebral bone loss: a controlled trial. Clinical Science 64: 541–546
Kyle R A 1978 Monoclonal gammopathy of undetermined significance: natural history in 241 cases. American Journal of Medicine 64: 814–826
Lanyon L E, Rubin C T 1983 Regulation of bone mass in response to physical activity. In: Dixon A St J, Russell R G G, Stamp T C B (eds) Osteoporosis a multidisciplinary problem. Royal Society of Medicine International Congress and Symposium Series. Academic Press, London, p. 51–61
Lewin I G, Papapoulos S E, Tomlinson S, Hendy G N, O'Riordan J L H 1978 Studies of hypoparathyroidism and pseudohypoparathyroidism. Quarterly Journal of Medicine 47: 533–548
Lewis A F 1981 Fracture of neck of the femur: changing incidence. British Medical Journal 283: 1217–1220
Longcope C D, Layne D S, Tait J F 1968 Metabolic clearance rates of and interconversions of estrone and 17-beta-estradiol in normal males and females. Journal of Clinical Investigation 47: 93–106
Looser E 1920 Über Spätrachitis und Osteomalacia: Klinische, röntgenologische und pathologischanatomische Untersuchungen. Deutsche Zeitschrift für Chirurgie 152: 210–357
Lubs H A, Travers H 1981 Genetic counselling in osteogenesis imperfecta. Clinical Orthopaedics and Related Research 159: 36–41
MacDonald P C, Edman C D, Hemsell D L, Porter J C, Siiteri P K 1978 Effect of obesity on conversion of plasma androstenedione to estrone in postmenopausal women with and without endometrial cancer. American Journal of Obstetrics and Gynaecology 130: 448–455
MacIntyre I, Evans I M A, Hobitz H H G, Joplin G F, Stevenson J C 1980 Chemistry, physiology and therapeutic applications of calcitonin. Arthritis and Rheumatism 23: 1139–1147
McKusick V A 1972 Heritable disorders of connective tissue, 4th Edn. Mosby, St Louis
McKusick V A 1983 Mendelian inheritance in man: catalogs of autosomal dominant, autosomal recessive and X-linked phenotypes, 6th Edn. Johns Hopkins University Press, Baltimore
McNeill K G, Thomas B J, Sturtridge W C, Harrison J E 1973 In vivo neutron activation analysis for calcium in man. Journal of Nuclear Medicine 14: 502–506
Mankin H J 1974 Rickets, osteomalacia and renal osteodystrophy. Journal of Bone and Joint Surgery 56A: 101–128, 352–386
Manolagas S C, Anderson D C, Lindsay R 1979 Adrenal steroids and the development of osteoporosis in oophorectomised women. Lancet 2: 597–600
Maroteaux P 1979 Bone diseases of children. Lippincott, Philadelphia
Martin T J 1980 Actions of calcitonin and mithramycin. Arthritis and Rheumatism 23: 1131–1138
Mawer E B 1980 Clinical implications of measurements of circulating vitamin D metabolites. Clinics in Endocrinology and Metabolism 9: 63–79
Mayer G P 1975 Effect of calcium and magnesium on parathyroid hormone secretion in calves. In: Talmage R V, Owen M, Parsons J A (eds) Calcium-regulating hormones. Excerpta Medica, Amsterdam, p. 122–124
Meema H E 1962 The occurrence of cortical bone atrophy in old age and in osteoporosis. Journal of the Canadian Association of Radiologists 13: 27–32
Meunier P, Courpron P, Edouard C, Bernard J, Bringuier J, Vignon G 1973 Physiological senile involution and pathological rarefaction of bone. Clinics in Endocrinology and Metabolism 2: 239–256
Meunier P J, Courpron P, Edouard C, Alexandre C, Bressot C, Lips P, Boyce B F 1979 Bone histomorphometry in osteoporotic states. In: Barzel U S (ed) Osteoporosis II. Grune & Stratton, New York, p. 27–47
Meunier P J, Coindre J M, Edouard C M, Arlot M E 1980 Bone histomorphometry in Paget's disease. Arthritis and Rheumatism 23: 1095–1103
Mills B G, Singer F R, Weiner L P, Holst P A 1980 Cell cultures from bones affected by Paget's disease. Arthritis and Rheumatism 23: 1115–1120
Murray R O, Jacobsen H G 1977 The radiology of skeletal disorders, 2nd Edn. Churchill Livingstone, Edinburgh
Nagant de Deuxchaisnes C 1983 The pathogenesis and treatment of involutional osteoporosis: In: Dixon A St J, Russell R G G, Stamp T C B (eds) Osteoporosis. A multi-disciplinary problem. Royal Society of Medicine International Congress and Symposium Series, No. 55. Academic Press, London, p. 291–323
Nagant de Deuxchaisnes C, Krane S M 1978 Hypoparathyroidism. In: Avioli L V, Krane S M (eds) Metabolic bone disease, Vol 2. Academic Press, New York, p. 218–445
Nordin B E C, Peacock M 1969 Role of kidney in regulation of plasma-calcium. Lancet 2: 1280–1283
Nordin B E C, Peacock M, Aaron J, Crilly R G, Heyburn P J, Horsman A, Marshall D 1980 Osteoporosis and osteomalacia. Clinics in Endocrinology and Metabolism. Saunders, Philadelphia, p. 177–205
Nordin B E C, Aaron J, Speed R, Crilly R G 1981 Bone formation and resorption as the determinants of trabecular bone volume in postmenopausal osteoporosis. Lancet 2: 277–279
Norman A W, Ross F P 1979 Vitamin D seco-steroids: unique molecules with both hormone and possible membranophilic properties. Life Science 24: 759–769
Nusynowitz M L, Frame B, Kolb F O 1976 The spectrum of hypoparathyroid states. Medicine (Baltimore)55: 105–119
Orimo H, Ohata M, Fujita T, Yoshikawa M, Higashi T, Abe J, Watanabe S, Otani K 1972 Ultimobranchial calcitonin of Anguilla japonica. In: Taylor S (ed) Endocrinology 1971. Heinemann, London, p. 48–54
Owen M 1978 Histogenesis of bone cells. Calcified Tissue Research 25: 205–207
Paget J 1877 On a form of chronic inflammation of bones. Medico-Chirurgical Transactions, London 60: 37–63
Parfitt A M 1976 The actions of parathyroid hormone on bone. Relation to bone remodelling and turnover, calcium homeostasis and metabolic bone disease. III. PTH and osteoblasts, the relation between bone turnover and bone loss, and the state of the bones in primary hyperparathyroidism. Metabolism 25: 1033–1069

Parfitt A M 1979 Surgical, idiopathic, and other varieties of parathyroid hormone-deficient hypoparathyroidism. In: Groot L J (ed) Endocrinology, Vol 2. Grune & Stratton, New York, p. 755–768

Parsons J A 1976 Parathyroid physiology and the skeleton. In: Bourne G H (ed) The biochemistry and physiology of bone, Vol 4, 2nd Edn. Academic Press, New York, p. 159–225

Pommer G A 1885 Untersuchungen uber Osteomalacie and Rachitis. Vogel, Leipzig

Prockop D J, Kivirikko K I, Tuderman L, Guzman N A 1979 The biosynthesis of collagen and its disorders. New England Journal of Medicine 301: 13–23, 77–85

Pygott F 1957 Paget's disease of bone, the radiological incidence. Lancet 1: 1170–1171

Raisz L G, Trummel C L, Holick M F, De Luca H F 1972 Dihydroxycholecalciferol, a potent stimulator of bone resorption in tissue culture. Science 175: 768–769

Rasmussen H, Bartter F C 1978 Hypophosphatasia. In: Stanbury J B, Wyngarden J B, Fredrickson J S (eds) Metabolic basis of inherited disease, 4th Edn. McGraw-Hill, New York, p. 1340–1349

Rebel A, Basle M, Pouplard A, Malkani K, Filmon R, Lepatezour A 1980 Bone tissue in Paget's disease of bone. Arthritis and Rheumatism 23: 1104–1114

Reiss E, Canterbury J M 1982 Clinical endocrinology of the parathyroids. In: Parsons J A (ed) Endocrinology of calcium metabolism. Raven Press, New York, p. 183–209

Riggs B L, Jowsey J, Goldsmith R S, Kelly P J, Hoffman D L, Arnaud C D 1972 Short- and long-term effects of estrogen and synthetic anabolic hormone in postmenopausal osteoporosis. Journal of Clinical Investigation 51: 1659–1663

Riggs B L, Arnaud C D, Jowsey J, Goldsmith R S, Kelly P J 1973a Parathyroid function in primary osteoporosis. Journal of Clinical Investigation 52: 181–184

Riggs B L, Ryan R J, Wahner H W, Jiane N S, Maddox V R 1973b Serum concentrations of estrogen, testosterone, and gonadotropins in osteoporotic and nonosteoporotic postmenopausal women. Journal of Clinical Endocrinology 36: 1097–1099

Riggs B L, Wahner H W, Dunn W L, Mazess R B, Offord K P, Melton L J III 1981 Differential changes in bone mineral density of the appendicular and the axial skeleton with aging. Relationship to spinal osteoporosis. Journal of Clinical Investigation 67: 328–355

Riggs B L, Seeman F, Hodgson S F, Taves D, O'Fallon W M 1982 Effect of the fluoride-calcium regimen on vertebral fracture occurrence in postmenopausal osteoporosis; comparison with conventional therapy. New England Journal of Medicine 306: 446–450

Rubin P 1964 Dynamic classification of bone dysplasias. Year Book Medical Publications, Chicago

Ruegsegger P, Niederer P, Anliker M 1974 An extension of classical bone mineral measurements. Annals of Biomedical Engineering 2: 194–205

Russell R G G, Bisaz S, Donath A, Morgan D B, Fleisch H 1971 Inorganic pyrophosphate in plasma in normal persons and in patients with hypophosphatasia, osteogenesis imperfecta and other disorders of bone. Journal of Clinical Investigation 50: 961–969

Ryan W G, Schwartz T B 1980 Mithramycin treatment of Paget's disease of bone. Arthritis and Rheumatism 23: 1155–1161

Sillence D 1981 Osteogenesis imperfecta: an expanding panorama of variants. Clinical Orthopaedics and Related Research 159: 11–25

Singer F R, Fredericks R S, Minkin C 1980 Salmon calcitonin therapy for Paget's disease of bone. Arthritis and Rheumatism 23: 1148–1154

Smith E L, Reddan W, Smith P E 1981 Physical activity and calcium modalities for bone mineral increase in aged women. Medicine and Science in Sports and Exercise 13: 60–64

Smith R, Francis M J O 1982 Disorders of collagen biosynthesis. In: O'Riordan J L H (ed) Recent advances in endocrinology and metabolism. Churchill Livingstone, Edinburgh, London, p. 211–238

Smith R, Russell R G G, Bishop M C, Woods C G, Bishop M 1973 Paget's disease of bone. Experience with a diphosphonate (disodium etidronate) in treatment. Quarterly Journal of Medicine 42: 235–256

Smith R, Walton R J, Corner B D, Gordon I R S 1977 Clinical and biochemical studies in Engelmann's disease. Quarterly Journal of Medicine 182: 273–294

Spranger J W, Langer L O, Wiedemann H-R 1974 Bone dysplasias. Saunders, Philadelphia

Stamp T C B 1972 Phosphorus metabolism in humans. MD Thesis, University of Cambridge

Stamp T C B 1982 The clinical endocrinology of vitamin D. In: Parsons J A (ed) Endocrinology of calcium metabolism. Raven Press, New York, p. 363–422

Stamp T C B, Haddad J G, Twigg C A 1977 Comparison of oral 25-hydroxycholecalciferol, vitamin D, and ultraviolet light as determinants of circulating 25-hydroxyvitamin D. Lancet 1: 1341–1343

Stamp T C B, Walker P G, Perry W, Jenkins M V 1980 Nutritional osteomalacia (and late rickets) in Greater London, 1974–79. Clinical and metabolic studies in 45 patients. Clinics in Endocrinology and Metabolism 9: 81–105

Stamp T C B, Byers P D, Ali S Y, Jenkins M V, Willoughby J M T 1985 Fibrogenesis imperfecta ossium: remission with melphalan. Lancet 1: 582–583

Stanbury J B, Wyngarden J B, Fredrickson J S (eds) Metabolic basis of inherited disease, 4th Edn. McGraw-Hill, New York

Sutton R A L, Dirks J H 1978 Renal handling of calcium. Federation Proceedings 37: 2112–2119

Swan C H J, Shah K, Brewer D B, Cooke W T 1976 Fibrogenesis imperfecta ossium. Quarterly Journal of Medicine 45: 233–253

Taylor W H 1981 In: Persistent pain: Modern methods of treatment. Lipton S, Miles J (eds) Academic Press, London, p. 69–86

Vose G P, Engel A 1973 Relationship of radiographic cortical thickness vs. age in thirteen bones of the hand. Journal of Gerontology 28: 46–49

Wahner H W, Riggs B L, Beabout J W 1977 Diagnosis of osteoporosis: usefulness of photon absorptiometry at the radius. Journal of Nuclear Medicine 18: 432–437

Walker D G 1975a Bone resorption restored in osteopetrotic mice by transplantation of normal bone marrow and spleen cells. Science 190: 784–785

Walker D G 1975b Spleen cells transmit osteopetrosis in mice. Science 190: 785–789

Watson L, Moxham J, Fraser P 1980 Hydrocortisone suppression test and discriminant analysis in differential diagnosis of hypercalcaemia. Lancet 1: 1320–1325

Weil U H 1981 Osteogenesis imperfecta: historical

background. Clinical Orthopaedics and Related Research 159: 6–10

Whyte M P, Murphy W A, Fallon M D 1982 Adult hypophosphatasia with chondrocalcinosis and arthropathy. Variable penetrance of hypophosphatasemia in a large Oklahoma kindred. American Journal of Medicine 72: 631–641

Whyte M P, Valdes R Jr, Ryan L M, McAlister W H 1982 Infantile hypophosphatasia: enzyme replacement therapy by intravenous infusion of alkaline phosphatase-rich plasma from patients with Paget's disease. Journal of Pediatrics 101: 379–386

Wilson C R, Madsen M 1977 Dichromatic absorptiometry of vertebral bone mineral content. Investigative Radiology 12: 180–184

Winfield J, Stamp T C B 1984 Joint complications of Paget's disease. Annals of Rheumatic Diseases 43: 769–773

Woodhouse N J Y 1977 Historical and epidemiological aspects of Paget's disease. In: MacIntyre I (ed) Human calcitonin and Paget's disease. Hans Huber, Bern p. 50–65

Wynne-Davies R, Gormley J 1981 Clinical and genetic patterns in osteogenesis imperfecta. Clinical Orthopaedics and Related Research 159: 26–35

Zanzi I, Ellis K J, Aloia J, Cohn S H 1981 Effect of physical activity on body composition. In: De Luca H F, Frost H M, Jee W S S, Johnston C C Jr, Parfitt A M (eds) Osteoporosis: Recent advances in pathogenesis and treatment. University Park Press, Baltimore, p. 139–146

M.B. Pepys M.L. Baltz

Amyloidosis

Definition and constituents of amyloid

Amyloid is an abnormal protein material which, under a wide variety of different circumstances, may be deposited intercellularly in the tissues and organs of the body. Amyloid deposits may be focal, localised or distributed throughout the body. They may have no apparent clinical effects, being merely an incidental pathological finding, or they may cause serious morbidity and mortality by disrupting the structure and function of vital organs. The name 'amyloid' was introduced by Virchow in 1854 when he observed similarities between the staining properties of the tissue deposits and of starch and cellulose; however as early as 1859 Schmidt and Friedereich & Kekulé demonstrated the protein nature of the deposits.

Amyloid is identified histologically by its binding of the dye Congo red and the pathognomonic apple-green birefringence which it then displays when viewed in polarised light (Fig. 41.1). This tinctorial property is a function of the fact that amyloid deposits are largely composed of protein fibrils which bind the molecules of Congo red in a linear orientation. Amyloid fibrils are rigid, twisting, non-branching, of indeterminate length and 10–15 nm in diameter (Fig. 41.2). They are composed of non-glycosylated polypeptide chains which lie with their long axes perpendicular to the long axis of the fibril and are arrayed in an anti-parallel β-pleated sheet conformation (Fig. 41.3).

Various different polypeptides form amyloid fibrils in the different clinicopathological entities

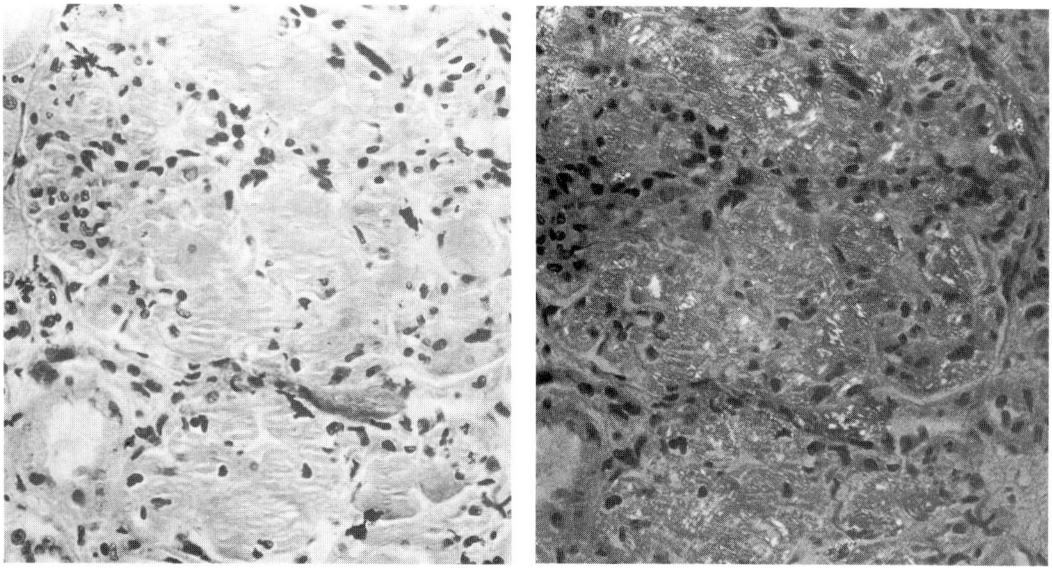

a b

Fig. 41.1 Glomerular amyloid deposits stained with Congo red. (a) Normal illumination. (b) Polarised light showing characteristic birefringence. (× 320)

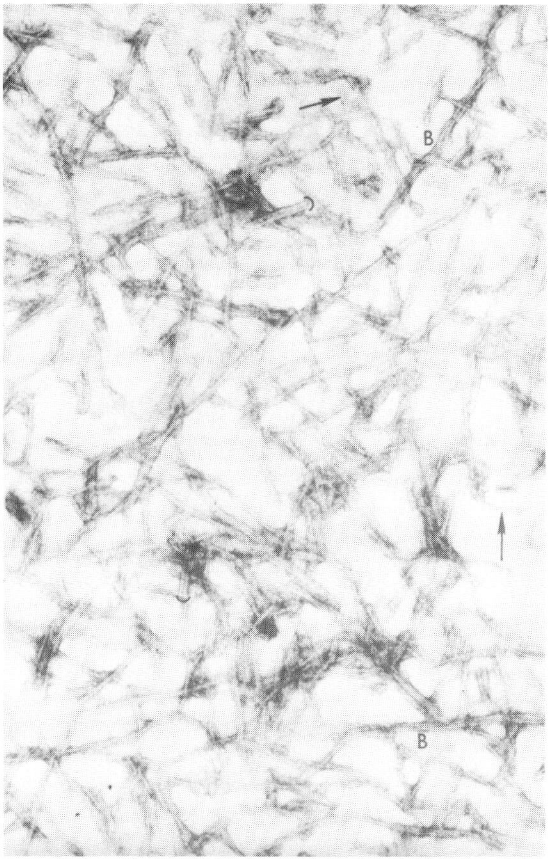

Fig. 41.2 Electron micrograph of negatively stained isolated purified amyloid fibrils. Arrows point to single filaments; most filaments are paired and end together (half circles); thicker bundles (B) comprise filaments twisting around each other (× 65 000). (Reproduced with permission from Franklin & Zucker-Franklin, 1972).

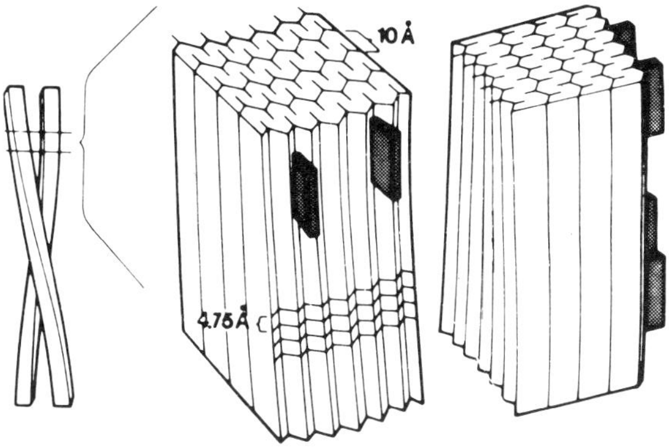

Fig. 41.3 Twisted β-pleated sheet antiparallel configuration of paired filaments of an amyloid fibril. The planar molecular of Congo red binding to the fibril are shown as stippled blocks. (Reproduced with permission from Glenner, 1980a.)

caused by or associated with amyloidosis. The commonest are amyloid A protein (AA) in reactive systemic amyloidosis and fragments of immunoglobulin light chains (AL) in amyloidosis associated with immunocyte dyscrasia (nomenclature of amyloid proteins according to Cohen & Wegelius, 1980). However regardless of the subunit chemistry the β-pleated sheet configuration is always present and is likely to be responsible not only for the typical morphology of the fibrils and their staining characteristics but also for their pathophysiological properties and consequences which are not related merely to the anatomical sites of deposition. Glenner (1980a, b) has therefore recently proposed the more precisely descriptive term 'β-fibrilloses' to include all the different forms of amyloidosis.

A non-fibrillar glycoprotein known as 'amyloid P component' (AP) (reviewed by Pepys et al, 1982; Pepys & Baltz, 1983) is present as a minor constituent of amyloid deposits comprising 6–14% of the weight of the fibrils. It has been demonstrated in all forms of amyloidosis in which it has been sought, with the possible exception of the intracerebral amyloid plaques associated with Alzheimer's disease and senile dementia. AP is intimately associated with the amyloid fibrils and is apparently bound to them in a calcium-dependent fashion, but it is not an integral part of the fibrillar structure. AP is identical to a normal circulating plasma protein, serum amyloid P component (SAP) and an immunochemically cross-reactive protein is a normal integral constituent of the glomerular basement membrane and of elastic fibre microfibrils throughout the body.

Although other materials including mucopolysaccharides, absorbed plasma proteins and reticulin-like tissue proteins have been identified in or associated with amyloid deposits either in situ or after extraction from tissues there is no evidence that any of these is specifically related to the deposition, structure or effects of amyloid.

Importance of amyloid

Amyloid is of considerable interest from the viewpoint of fundamental biochemistry, in particular the mechanisms of formation from a number of completely distinct proteins of the peculiar anti-parallel β-pleated sheet conformation of polypeptide chains which constitute the amyloid fibrils. Proteins composed entirely of this configuration are not normally found in vertebrate proteins though they do occur among invertebrates, an example being silk fibroin (Walton & Blackwell, 1973). Of great physiological interest is the fact that some of the amyloid proteins are derived from precursors which have been stably conserved in evolution and therefore presumably have important functions whether these are known, as in the case of immunoglobulins, or as yet unknown, as in the case of AA or AP. However the clinical importance of amyloidosis, particularly to rheumatologists, lies primarily in the fact that systemic amyloidosis associated with rheumatic diseases is usually a fatal complication of non-fatal primary disorders. Arthropathic manifestations of forms of amyloid unrelated to underlying rheumatic disease may also involve rheumatologists. Hereditary forms of amyloidosis, although rare, are important because of the possible light they may shed on pathogenetic mechanisms in general. Finally of relevance to all physicians is the ubiquitous association of increasing age with amyloid deposition, in the heart, blood vessels, joints and most notably the brain. Amyloid in the walls of cerebral blood vessels, in the intracerebral plaques and in the neurofibrillary tangles is an integral part of the pathology of Alzheimer's disease and senile dementia. These conditions are presently estimated to affect 1.5 million adults in the USA and to be the fourth most common cause of death in that country (Glenner, 1981a).

In the 23 years since Cohen & Calkins (1959) first demonstrated the fibrillar nature of amyloid and especially in the past decade there have been major advances in understanding of the chemistry of amyloid. A number of fibril proteins and their precursors as well as AP have been identified and characterised in detail and there has been some progress in detection and differential diagnosis of amyloid deposits. Understanding of possible pathogenetic mechanisms of amyloid deposition has also advanced but not, unfortunately, to the point where it is able to contribute to therapy. Amyloid deposits only very rarely show spontaneous regression and no generally effective treatment exists for systemic amyloidoisis. There are many recent reviews of different aspects of amyloidosis (Glenner 1980a, b; Glenner et al, 1980; Ignaczak, 1981; Franklin, 1982; Cohen et al, 1982, 1983a; Tribe & Mackenzie, 1982) and the present chapter will therefore deal in detail only with the latest findings, which represent the significant advances of the past few years. (See also the addendum at the end of the chapter.)

CLINICAL AMYLOIDOSIS SYNDROMES

Systemic amyloidosis

Systemic amyloidosis, in which the deposits are widely distributed throughout the body, can arise

1. As a complication of chronic infection, chronic inflammation or malignant neoplasia (reactive systemic amyloidosis, AA fibrils)
2. As a complication of various forms of immunocyte dyscrasia (immunocyte dyscrasia-associated or monoclonal protein amyloidosis, AL fibrils)
3. As a heredofamilial disorder.

The hereditary forms are rare and for obvious reasons tend to be focal in geographical distribution but they are of considerable theoretical importance as natural models of amyloidogenesis as well as having a very high rate of morbidity and mortality. The frequency of the other two main types of systemic amyloid is very much greater and together they contribute the great majority of all cases of amyloidosis which present clinically and/or are diagnosed in life. Their incidence relative to one another varies in different parts of the world and is difficult to determine precisely because the patients at risk are almost always segregated into different specialist clinics on the basis of their primary disease. However the relative incidence of chronic systemic infections such as tuberculosis and leprosy, of chronic rheumatic conditions and of immunocyte dyscrasia is one crucial factor. Other important factors exist but are poorly understood. Apparently identical primary diseases in different ethnic groups or in groups of similar ethnic background living in different geographical areas may have quite different rates of complication by amyloidosis.

The amount and distribution of the deposits both at the macroscopic and at the microscopic level varies greatly both within and between the different forms of systemic amyloidosis, as does the clinical presentation. A comprehensive account of these clinical and pathological features is not included here and interested readers are referred to the many excellent existing reviews, cited above, of these topics.

Reactive systemic (AA) amyloidosis

Causes. AA amyloidosis is the form most commonly encountered by the rheumatologist since one of its most frequent predisposing causes, at least in Western Europe and the USA, is chronic rheumatic disease (see for example Dictor & Hasserius, 1981) especially rheumatoid arthritis, juvenile chronic arthritis and ankylosing spondylitis (Jayson et al, 1971). Cases have also been reported complicating Reiter's syndrome (Miller et al, 1979), dermatomyositis (Galdenman et al, 1962), psoriasis and psoriatic arthritis (Qureshi et al, 1977; David et al, 1982; Sharma et al, 1983), adult Still's disease (Harrington et al, 1981), Behçet's syndrome (Bėroniade, 1975; Rosenthal et al, 1978; Rubies-Prat et al, 1982) and, very rarely, systemic lupus erythematosus (see below). It is very difficult to obtain precise estimates of the incidence of amyloidosis in these different diseases but values in the range of 5–20% have been reported for rheumatoid athritis (Arapakis & Tribe, 1963; Tribe, 1966; Lender & Wolf, 1972; Bywaters, 1978; Wegelius et al, 1980) and around 5% for juvenile chronic arthritis (Schnitzer & Ansell, 1977). There is no doubt that systemic amyloidosis is an important cause of death in young adults who have had juvenile chronic arthritis even when the disease has 'burnt out' some years before. Despite the difficulty in obtaining estimates of incidence it is clear that, in marked contrast to rheumatoid arthritis, systemic lupus erythematosus is only exceptionally complicated by amyloidosis. There are just 7 cases in the English literature and some of these had other conditions predisposing to amyloidosis (Carstens et al, 1980; Huston et al, 1981; Sweat et al, 1981). A similar contrast exists between Crohn's disease, in which amyloid has been reported at a rate of between 1 and 8% (Rashid et al, 1980), and ulcerative colitis in which it is extremely rare (Shorvon, 1977). Possible reasons for this difference, which is of both practical and theoretical importance, are discussed below.

Systemic infections are a very important cause of reactive systemic amyloidosis in many parts of the world. For example, tuberculosis, which is still a significant cause in the United Kingdom (Brandt et al, 1968; Kennedy et al, 1974), is by far the most frequent in India (Rizvi et al, 1974) and leprosy is involved in the areas in which it is endemic (Williams et al, 1965; McAdam et al, 1975). Chronic osteomyelitis is recognised historically as being an important cause and in countries where adequate management is not available it still is. Other forms of localised chronic infection, including bronchiectasis, chronically infected burns and the decubitus ulcers and chronic pyelonephritis of patients with paraplegia also cause AA amyloidosis.

Renal carcinoma and Hodgkin's disease are the malignant neoplasms most commonly associated with the development of reactive systemic amyloidosis; less frequent causes include carcinomas of the gut, lung and urogenital tract (Kimball, 1961; Azzopardi & Lehner, 1966; Sommer & Teppo, 1976; Dictor & Hasserius, 1981; Pras et al, 1982b; Vanatta et al, 1983; Hind et al, 1983b). Cases associated with other neoplasms as diverse as basal cell carcinoma (Lichtenstein & Lee, 1980) and hairy cell leukaemia (Linder et al, 1982) have recently been described.

Clinical features. AA amyloidosis usually involves the main parenchymal organs and commonly presents with proteinuria due to deposition in the renal glomeruli (Jones, 1981). Macroscopic haematuria is very rare and even microscopic haematuria is unusual. The proteinuria is usually nonselective though a selective pattern may occur. In association with the proteinuria, which is often sufficient to cause the nephrotic syndrome, there is a progressive decline in glomerular filtration rate which may cause remission of nephrotic syndrome before terminating in end-stage renal failure. Renal amyloidosis may also present with isolated tubular defects and when, rarely, the medulla rather than the cortex is the main site of amyloid deposition the patient may develop nephrogenic diabetes insipidus.

AA amyloid deposition can affect almost any organ and tissue in the body and may present for example with organomegaly (liver, spleen, thyroid, etc.) in the presence or absence of renal abnormality. In earlier literature the predominantly parenchymal pattern of amyloid deposition occuring as a complication of chronic infection and inflammation was called 'secondary amyloidosis' in contrast to the predominantly mesenchymal distribution of amyloid which usually occurs in association with either overt or occult immunocyte dyscrasia, so-called 'primary amyloidosis'. Although the clinical associations of these patterns are broadly correct there is a great deal of overlap and in view of the present capacity to characterise amyloid fibrils chemically the designations 'primary' and 'secondary' are no longer appropriate.

AA amyloidosis may become clinically evident quite early in the course of predisposing rheumatic disease but the incidence rises with the duration of the primary condition. The mean duration of underlying diseases such as rheumatoid arthritis, juvenile chronic arthritis and ankylosing spondylitis before amyloid is diagnosed is about 12–14 years. For most patients the diagnosis of amyloidosis carries a grave prognosis which is closely related to the presence of renal involvement (Wegelius et al, 1980; Tribe & MacKenzie, 1982). 70% or more have progressive renal disease and around 50% of individuals with reactive systemic amyloid complicating rheumatic disease die within 5 years of the amyloid being diagnosed. By 15 years a further 25% will be dead but the remainder, including those in whom significant renal involvement is absent and some in whom the renal lesion seems to be static or even to regress, clearly have a better prognosis. The advent of chronic haemodialysis and renal transplantation has meant that early deaths from uraemia per se may be avoidable but the extensive deposition of amyloid in other organs and tissues is usually associated with a less favourable prognosis in these patients than in others with end-stage renal failure.

Amyloidosis associated with immunocyte dyscrasia, monoclonal protein (MP) (AL) amyloidosis

Causes. Systemic amyloidosis may be associated with almost any form of dyscrasia of cells of the B lymphocyte lineage, ranging from frank malignancy in the form of multiple myeloma through malignant lymphomas, macroglobulinaemia, heavy chain disease and 'benign' monoclonal gammopathy to occult conditions in which the deposition of amyloid is the only demonstrable evidence of the disorder. Up to 15% of patients with myeloma develop amyloidosis whilst the incidence in the other malignant forms of B cell or plasma cell dyscrasia is lower. The incidence in benign nonoclonal gammopathy is not known but may be around 5–10%. A high proportion of patients with amyloidosis associated with immunocyte dyscrasia have Bence-Jones proteinuria. Since the fibrils in this form of amyloid are composed of monoclonal immunoglobulin light (L) chains it is likely that a monoclonal paraprotein or free light chains should be detected in all patients provided sufficiently sensitive techniques are used. With standard methods this is, however, not always the case and individuals may present with amyloid in the absence of any readily demonstrable serum or urine protein abnormality. In the absence of any previous predisposing inflammatory condition or a family history of amyloidosis it is almost certain that such apparently 'primary amyloidosis' is associated with immunocyte dyscrasia and that analysis of the fibrils will reveal their identity as AL protein. Sometimes Bence-Jones proteinuria or paraproteinaemia manifests itself after presentation and diagnosis of the amyloid.

Clinical features. AL amyloid is often deposited principally in mesenchymal tissues producing clinical effects such as peripheral sensorimotor and autonomic neuropathy, macroglossia, carpal tunnel syndrome, restrictive cardiomyopathy often with low voltage ECG and conduction disturbances, non-thrombocytopaenic purpura sometimes with cutaneous induration, and arthropathy of large joints with little inflammation. Organs less commonly involved include the gut, lung and urogenital tract but, as with AA systemic amyloid, any tissue may be affected. Gastrointestinal symptoms are more common with AL than AA amyloid and may be due to vascular and neuropathic effects as well as to actual deposition within the gut itself. Hyposplenism is occasionally seen and may occur also in AA amyloidosis (Boyko et al, 1981; Gertz et al, 1983). A rare but serious manifestation of AL amyloid is an acquired haemorrhagic diathesis. This may be associated with deficiency of factor X and occasionally also of factor IX or with increased fibrinolysis (Greipp et al, 1981; Liebman et al, 1983). Bleeding may occur in the absence of any identifiable coagulation defect and this is true also in AA amyloidosis in no case of which has any specific factor deficiency been described.

Renal involvement with AL amyloid is not unusual and has the same clinical manifestations as renal disease caused by AA amyloid, but the prognosis is even worse. Patients with myeloma complicated by amyloid have a significantly worse prognosis than those with myeloma alone. Most individuals with renal AL amyloid, even in the absence of myeloma, die of uraemia, heart failure or some other effect of the amyloid within a year of diagnosis (Ogg et al, 1981). It may be that in the absence of any other cause of symptoms, amyloid deposition is more advanced at the time of diagnosis than in cases of AL amyloid with myeloma or AA amyloid with a primary disease already under medical supervision. Alternatively this particular form of AL amyloid may just be more damaging. Although it may occur rarely in young adults, AL amyloid without myeloma is usually seen over the age of 50 years and is more common in men than in women and in Caucasians than in non-Caucasians.

Heredofamilial systemic amyloidosis

These disorders have been extensively reviewed elsewhere (Glenner et al, 1978; Ignaczak, 1981). A large number of different forms exist varying in mode of inheritance, the anatomical distribution of the deposits, the clinical manifestations, and probably the chemical nature of the fibrils. The only fibril protein identified so far is related to prealbumin (AFp) in the Portuguese type (type I) of familial amyloid neuropathy (see below). Predominantly neuropathic, nephropathic and cardiopathic types exist but the amyloid is always distributed more widely than the major clinically affected organ system. New families and new forms of the disease are quite frequently reported.

Familial Mediterranean fever (FMF) is a disease with autosomal recessive inheritance, the pathogenesis of which is not known (Sohar et al, 1967; Eliakim et al, 1981). It is characterised by recurrent attacks of fever which may be associated with polyserositis, arthritis and skin rashes. It occurs amongst most ethnic groups around the Mediterranean and also in Armenians, Arabs and Jews. FMF may be complicated at a relatively early age by systemic AA amyloidosis in a significant proportion of cases. Although it is likely that the AA amyloid occuring in FMF is a typical example of reactive systemic amyloidosis complicating a long-standing inflammatory process, there are some curious features. For example, whilst in some-patients the amyloid follows recurrent severe attacks, in others it may be a very early or even the presenting feature of the disease. Also, Armenian patients and Ashkenazi Jews whose clinical manifestations of FMF are indistinguishable from those of the other ethnic groups, almost never develop amyloidosis (Schwabe & Peters, 1974; Pras et al, 1982a). The reasons are not known but these observations illustrate clearly the multifactorial pathogenesis of amyloidosis.

Localised amyloidosis

Deposits of amyloid localised to particular organs or tissues or distributed focally within one or more tissues occur in a wide variety of different forms. Amyloid of AL type is often found, in amounts ranging from microscopic to massive, in close association with extramedullary plasmacytomas. In some cases the amyloid predominates and the presumptive source of the fibril precursor protein is represented by a more or less intense plasma cell infiltrate. Such lesions have been described in the lung, urogenital tract, skin and elsewhere. Their clinical effects are those to be expected from mass lesions at the sites in which they are found.

Primary localised cutaneous amyloidosis is a distinct condition which may present in macular, papular and a rare nodular form with lesions caused by dermal amyloid deposits (Brownstein & Helwig, 1970; Black, 1976; MacDonald et al, 1980). The nodular form is an example of local AL amyloid, whereas morphological observations suggest that in the macular and papular forms the fibrils are derived from epidermal cell proteins. There have been reports of immunohistochemical staining of the deposits with anti-keratin antibodies (Masu et al, 1980; Kobayashi & Hashimoto, 1981) but other workers have failed to confirm these observations (Noren et al, 1983a). The aetiology of this type of amyloid is not known. The skin is also a common site for deposition of AL amyloid in systemic immunocytic amyloidosis.

Amyloid deposition in the myocardium of the ventricles and the atria and within the heart valves is common with increasing age, the incidence over 60 years of age being around 50% (Cornwell & Westermark, 1980). It may be just an incidental finding at autopsy but in some cases it is associated with significant functional cardiac impairment. The commonest form of senile cardiac amyloid, the fibril protein of which has been designated AS_{C1}, seems to be related to prealbumin (Cornwell et al, 1981). There may be associated deposits of this same type of amyloid in the lungs and in extracardiac vessels but there is no correlation with the presence or extent of the other common forms of senile amyloid affecting the brain or pancreas. A distinct form of cardiac amyloid affecting only the atria apparently has a different chemical origin, as has microfocal amyloid found in the aortic wall of most individuals over the age of 50 years.

Amyloid deposition in the brain and cerebral vasculature is also a common concomitant of ageing and, although more pronounced and seen at an earlier age in patients with Alzheimer's disease (presenile dementia), essentially the same pathology is found in senile brains (Cornwell & Westermark, 1980; Glenner, 1981a). Amyloid is present in vessel walls, in the cortical plaques and in the neurofibrillary tangles. Its origin and protein nature are not known, nor whether the amyloid itself plays a pathogenetic role or is merely an epiphenomenon of ageing and dementia (Vanley et al 1981; Mountjoy et al, 1982; Okoye & Watanabe, 1982). Amyloid in the brain is also a notable feature of the pathology of spongiform encephalopathy of kuru and Jakob–Creutzfeldt type (Masters et al, 1981).

Amyloid is frequently demonstrable in the islets of Langerhans in the ageing pancreas and also in the pancreas of patients with diabetes mellitus at any age (Cornwell & Westermark, 1980). The fibrils may be derived from proinsulin or other peptide products of the islet cells but this has not yet been formally established. Amyloid localised to other endocrine organs, especially in neoplasms thereof (APUDomas), is well recognised (Westermark et al, 1977) and in the case of the deposits found in medullary carcinoma of the thyroid it has been proved by amino acid sequencing that the fibril protein (AE_t) is derived from procalcitonin (Sletten et al, 1976).

Amyloid deposits are present in most osteoarthritic joints at surgery or autopsy, usually in close association with calcium pyrophosphate deposits (chondrocalcinosis) affecting the joint capsule and articular cartilage (Goffin et al, 1981; Sorensen et al, 1981; Ladefoged, 1982; Egan et al, 1982). The clinical significance and the biochemical nature of amyloid in this situation are not known. Rarely systemic AL amyloid may present with, or have as one major manifestation, a serious amyloid arthropathy which can superficially mimic acute polyarticular rheumatoid arthritis affecting large joints (Hickling et al, 1981).

AMYLOID FIBRIL PROTEINS AND THEIR PRECURSORS

The chemical nature of the polypeptide subunits which constitute the fibrils in the major forms of systemic amyloidosis, in some of the hereditary syndromes and in some of the localised forms of amyloid is known from amino acid sequencing of isolated fibril preparations. Related or identical proteins in the plasma or formed locally are also known in some cases and are established as the precursors of the fibril protein. In other cases this precursor–product relationship seems probable but has not yet been confirmed. Biochemical analysis of denatured, dissociated, solubilised preparations of even the purest isolates of amyloid fibrils always reveals material additional to the well recognised AL or AA subunit proteins. This material, most of which has a greater apparent molecular weight than that of the fibril subunit protein (i.e. greater than 5–25 000), is difficult to study and has been very poorly characterised hitherto. It may be related to 'reticulin', representing normal connective tissue matrix material. Similar products can be obtained from extracts of non-amyloid tissue. However it may conceivably be important in contributing to the formation and deposition of amyloid fibrils and, as such, its further study could give valuable information regarding the mechanisms of amyloidogenesis.

AL

AL proteins in each individual case of MP amyloidosis are either whole intact immunoglobulin light chains or fragments thereof or a mixture of the two. The fragments are derived from the N-terminal of the L chain and usually comprise whole or part of the variable (V_L) domain. The molecular weight of AL proteins varies between about 8 and 30 000. Only rarely is the AL from a given subject composed exclusively of intact L chains, V_L or fragments thereof almost always being present. In patients with AL amyloid in whom the monoclonal immunoglobulin has been characterised the L chain of the paraprotein is always identical with or at least clearly the precursor of the AL subunits (Wille et al, 1980; Glenner, 1980a,b).

It is thought that proteolytic cleavage of the paraprotein L chain yields fragment(s) with a propensity for polymerising into anti-parallel β-pleated sheets as amyloid fibrils. Rarely some L chains seem able to do this even without cleavage and the capacity for the whole polypeptide or its fragments to form amyloid must be related, at least in part to their own intrinsic biophysical properties (Glenner, 1980a,b). This concept is supported by the observation that AL protein is more commonly derived from λ chains than from κ chains (Pick et al, 1981; Natvig et al, 1981) despite the fact that among normal immunoglobulin and the paraprotein products of immunocyte dyscrasias, κ chains predominate. Furthermore a new λ subgroup, designated λ_{VI}, was identified on the basis of its isolation as AL protein from two cases of MP amyloidosis before it had been recognised in any other form (Natvig et al, 1981; Sletten et al, 1981; Solomon et al, 1982). On the other hand immunochemical studies have not revealed any antigenic determinant specific for all or even subsets of AL proteins except insofar as they may possess C_L region sequences which are recognised by broad spectrum conventional polyclonal anti-L chain antisera.

AA, SAA and the acute phase response

AA

AA protein was discovered when the subunit protein of amyloid fibrils from patients with reactive systemic amyloidosis was first identified (Benditt & Eriksen, 1972). It is usually of molecular weight about 8000 and consists of 76 amino acid residues. AA subunits of smaller and occasionally of larger size have been characterised (Husby & Sletten, 1980; Isobe et al, 1980) but in all cases the peptides are not glycosylated. The amino acid sequence of AA is not related to any known protein other than its serum counterpart which is called 'serum amyloid A' (SAA) (Benditt et al, 1971; Levin et al, 1972; Ein et al, 1972; Sletten & Husby, 1974). Proteins homologous with human AA/SAA have been identified in the monkey (Hermodson et al, 1972), mouse (Eriksen et al, 1976), rabbit (Anders et al, 1977), mink (Anders et al, 1976; Waalen et al, 1980), guinea-pig (Skinner et al, 1974) and duck (Gorevic et al, 1977). Antisera raised against denatured AA protein cross-react with SAA, and anti-SAA sera react with isolated AA and with AA-type amyloid fibrils. In its native state in serum SAA has an apparent molecular weight of 180 000 (Anders et al, 1975; Levin et al, 1973; Linke et al, 1975) but denaturation with acids, alkalis, chaotropic agents or detergents yields a peptide of approximately 12 000 daltons, the N-terminal portion of which is almost completely homologous with AA (Marhaug et al, 1980). Proteolytic enzymes of leukocyte and serum origin can cleave SAA to yield AA-size or smaller fragments and it is generally believed that this mechanism is involved in the generation of AA during the pathogenesis of amyloidosis (Lavie et al, 1978, 1980; Zucker-Franklin et al, 1980; Silverman et al, 1980; Skogen & Natvig, 1981), although there is no direct evidence of the precursor–product relationship between SAA and AA in vivo.

SAA as an acute phase protein

SAA is a notable acute phase protein, that is its circulating concentration increases rapidly and extensively in response to most forms of tissue injury, infection and inflammation (Rosenthal & Franklin, 1975; Gorevic et al, 1976; McAdam et al, 1978; Hijmans & Sipe, 1979; Benson & Cohen, 1979; de Beer et al, 1982a,b). Macrophages apparently play a central role in induction of the acute phase response of SAA and other acute phase proteins. When stimulated directly by microbial products or other biological toxins, or by the products of immunospecifically or non-specifically activated lymphocytes, macrophages synthesise and secrete a family of closely related, potent, low molecular weight peptide mediators (Sipe et al, 1979; Selinger et al, 1980a,b; McAdam & Dinarello, 1980; Sztein et al, 1981; McAdam et al, 1982; Kampschmidt et al, 1982; Bornstein, 1982). These cause fever (endogenous pyrogen), promote lymphocyte activation (lymphocyte activating factor) and initiate acute phase protein synthesis by hepatocytes (leukocyte endogenous mediator). These diverse mediator activities copurify with each other and have been designated as interleukin 1 (IL1) (Oppenheim & Gery, 1982). It is of some fundamental interest and of possible practical relevance to the pathogenesis of amyloidosis that very low doses of some potent biological toxins, such as abrin, can induce an acute phase response at dose levels which cause no other clinical evidence of toxicity (M. L. Baltz, K. Gomer, A. J. S. Davies & M. B. Pepys, unpublished observations).

In most diseases, including chronic active or remittent inflammation, whether associated with an infective cause or not, SAA levels tend to be raised to an extent which generally reflects disease activity. The non-specific nature of the acute phase response, whether of SAA or of other acute phase proteins, means that measurement of the serum levels of SAA or other proteins cannot be diagnostic for reactive systemic amyloidosis in individual cases (Pepys, 1982; Pepys & Baltz, 1983). However AA amyloidosis is associated with chronic active inflammatory or infectious conditions such as rheumatoid arthritis, Still's disease, ankylosing spondylitis, Crohn's disease, bronchiectasis, chronic osteomyelitis and leprosy in which sustained high levels of SAA are seen. In some of these disorders the risk is definitely greater in particular forms or subsets of the disease in which systemic manifestations such as fever, leukocytosis and the acute phase response are more pronounced, for example: lepromatous rather than tuberculoid leprosy, polyarticular and systemic forms of Still's disease rather than the pauciarticular form, renal carcinoma and Hodgkin's disease among malignant neoplasms. In addition the highly significant differences in incidence of AA amyloidosis between various chronic idiopathic inflammatory diseases have been noted above. It is interesting that these differences correlate precisely with the relative magnitude in the different conditions of the acute phase response in general and of SAA in particular. Systemic lupus erythematosus and ulcerative colitis are remarkable both for the very low rate at which they are complicated by AA amyloidosis and for the modest nature of the acute phase response which is induced even by severe disease activity (de Beer et al, 1982b). This is in marked contrast to the situation in rheumatoid arthritis and Crohn's disease (de Beer et al, 1982b). The overall cumulative rate of production of SAA may thus be one important factor contributing to the pathogenesis of AA amyloidosis and there is evidence in rheumatoid arthritis for a close correlation between persistently high SAA levels and the rapid progression of AA amyloidosis (Falck et al, 1983).

Of interest in this context are those cases of FMF which present with amyloidosis without a previous clinical history of overt attacks of fever and polyserositis. FMF attacks are known to be associated with a major acute phase response but, it is conceivable, on the basis of the experimental work noted above, that in some individuals a sufficient acute phase response may be triggered by a level of the unknown biochemical events underlying FMF which is too low to cause clinical symptoms. Gout represents another intriguing situation because it seems very rarely to be associated with AA amyloidosis. Among 5 earlier cases in the literature most had alternative possible causes, especially chronic infection, for their amyloid, whilst 4 recently reported cases have all been in Israelis suggesting a possible contribution of ethnic factors (Levo et al, 1980; Rubinow & Sonnenblick, 1981). SAA levels have not been measured in any well characterised group of gouty patients with active and quiescent disease and, although it is likely that acute attacks would induce a major acute phase response it is possible that the intermittent nature of the disease is such that cumulative SAA production fails to achieve the level required for amyloidogenesis. Alternatively the colchicine commonly used to treat gout may have protected against amyloidosis (see below).

ApoSAA

In its native form, in undenatured serum, SAA (molecular weight 180 000) is associated with high density lipoprotein (HDL), d = 1.12–1.21 g/ml. This is the case in rabbits (Skogen et al, 1979; Tobias et al, 1982) and mice (Benditt et al, 1979) as well as man (Benditt & Erikson, 1977). It therefore seems to be an apolipoprotein and has been designated as 'apoSAA' (Benditt & Erikson, 1977). This is compatible with its primary structure which contains sequences capable of forming amphipathic helical domains similar to those characteristic of apolipoproteins such as apoA–I (Segrest et al, 1976; Segrest & Feldman, 1977). It has recently been claimed that some apoSAA in man may also be associated with low density (LDL), intermediate density (IDL) and very low density lipoprotein (VLDL) fractions (Marhaug et al, 1982). Earlier reports that albumin is the 'carrier-protein' for SAA in serum (Rosenthal & Franklin, 1977) and of the presence of complexes of SAA with albumin fragments, prealbumin and β_2 microglobulin (Marhaug & Husby, 1981; Marhaug et al, 1983), are probably attributable to in vitro artefacts produced during denaturation of serum and subsequent chromatography under denaturing conditions. However a small portion of material with SAA immunoreactivity and large molecular weight does sediment in the ultracentrifuge with a density greater than that of lipoprotein (Marhaug et al, 1982).

At the peak of the acute phase response apoSAA comprises up to 50% of the total apoproteins of HDL (Hoffman & Benditt, 1982a; Marhaug et al, 1982). SAA-rich HDL isolated from acute phase murine or human serum also contains the 'normal' HDL apoproteins apoA–I and apoC (Benditt et al, 1982; Hoffman & Benditt, 1982a). The other apoproteins of apoSAA-containing human LDL, IDL and VLDL are also the same as in non-apoSAA-containing controls (Marhaug et al, 1982). Furthermore, the proportions and absolute amounts of these 'normal', non-acute phase apoproteins is the same within each class of lipoproteins whether isolated from normal or acute phase serum (Benditt et al, 1982; Hoffman & Benditt, 1982a; Marhaug et al, 1982). However in mice the HDL from acute phase serum includes a particular subset of apoSAA-bearing particles in which there are 2 moles of apoSAA for each mole of apoA-I. These particles also contain about 10% more protein and 10% less phospholipid than non-apoSAA-HDL but in other respects their lipid composition and phospholipid profile are the same as control HDL (Hoffman & Benditt, 1982a). It is not clear yet whether the binding of apoSAA to HDL involves displacement of some phospholipid or whether these changes occurring with the acute phase response take place independently.

Normal levels of apoSAA are very low indeed and this probably explains why it has not previously been widely remarked upon in studies of lipoprotein structure. There are however reports of HDL apoproteins which clearly correspond to apoSAA although they were not identified as such or indeed as acute phase proteins (Shore et al, 1978; Malmendier et al, 1979).

Polymorphism of AA and SAA

AA extracted from amyloid deposits shows microheterogeneity of amino acid sequence and variation in chain length, predominantly at the C-terminal end (Gorevic et al, 1978; Husby & Sletten, 1980; Westermark, 1982; Skogen et al, 1983). Polymorphism of apoSAA isolated from lipoprotein fractions of acute phase serum is also evident. In man 6 isotypes of apoSAA have been demonstrated on the basis of differences in pI (Bausserman et al, 1980; Marhaug et al, 1982), whilst in the rabbit (Tobias et al, 1982) and mouse (Hoffman & Benditt, 1982a) two forms have been identified. None of these proteins is glycosylated and the differences between forms within each species seem to be due to differences in amino acid composition and sequence. There is only one report so far of the complete amino acid sequence of apoSAA. This human protein, designated $apoSAA_1$, consists of 104 residues of which the first 76 from the N-terminal are identical with AA from tissue amyloid deposits, though two variants with a curious double substitution of alanine and valine at residues of 52 and 57 were detected (Parmelee et al, 1982). Each of the two forms of rabbit apoSAA contains 103 residues but no sequence data has yet been reported (Tobias et al, 1982).

Conventional polyclonal antisera to AA react with all the polymorphic forms of apoSAA in a given species but monoclonal antibodies which can differentiate between some of the forms in man have been prepared (McAdam et al, 1982). Further sequence information and the exchange between laboratories of proteins and antibodies will be required in the future to correlate the different nomenclatures and to establish the identities of the different polymorphic forms of apoSAA. An alternative approach to elucidation of the structure and genetic basis of this polymorphism is the application of recombinant DNA technology. There is already evidence at the DNA level for the existence in mice of a series of related but distinct apoSAA sequences (Stearman et al, 1982).

Synthesis of SAA

Although claims have been made for synthesis of SAA by other cell types (Rosenthal & Sullivan, 1978; Linder et al, 1977), the only unequivocal evidence is for production by hepatocytes (Selinger et al, 1980a,b; Benson & Kleiner, 1980; Benson, 1982; McAdam et al, 1982; Tatsuta et al, 1982, 1983). These cells respond to IL1 by increasing their rate of SAA synthesis in vivo or in vitro and this is associated with an increased rate of transcription of mRNA for SAA (Stearman et al, 1982). Murine apoSAA is secreted on its own by hepatocytes and not as a part of an already constituted lipoprotein particle (Hoffman & Benditt, 1982b). If HDL is provided in vitro the newly secreted SAA rapidly binds to it and presumably the same thing happens in vivo in the plasma or intercellular fluid. Production of free apoSAA may explain the small amounts of apoSSA detected in human LDL, IDL, VLDL and free of lipid (Marhaug et al, 1982).

The transcription of mRNA for SAA in liver cell nuclei of mice which have received lipopolysaccharide is increased from 3–12 hours afterwards with a peak at 6.5–9 hours and a subsequent decline (Stearman et al, 1982). Similarly the synthesis of SAA protein and the increase in serum levels of SAA follows very rapidly after an acute stimulus. The rate of rise in circulating SAA concentration is rapid and the increment attained is enormous, reaching as much as 10 000 times normal values in some patients with active inflammatory disease (de Beer et al, 1982b).

The absolute amounts of SAA in terms of weight or molarity which are present in the plasma are difficult to determine in view of the problems of obtaining a suitable calibration standard for assays. ApoSAA concentrations can be measured after denaturation and dissociation from lipoprotein but, where this has been done AA has generally been used for standardisation and it differs from SAA in terms of size and antigenicity (Rosenthal & Franklin, 1975; Sipe et al, 1976; Ignaczak et al, 1977; Benditt & Eriksen, 1977; McAdam et al, 1978; Hijmans & Sipe, 1979). ApoSAA can also be measured in its native form (Benson & Cohen, 1979; de Beer et al, 1982a; Chambers & Whicher, 1983) but a standard native lipoprotein calibrator which is both physicochemically and immunochemically stable is not available, quite apart from the heterogeneity of size and molar apoprotein content of lipoprotein particles. Despite these difficulties, it seems likely that peak acute phase levels of SAA in man and the mouse may be in the range of 1–5 mg/ml.

Functions of SAA

The functions of apoSAA and of the apoSAA-rich HDL particles are not known but the latter are obviously quite different from normal 'non-acute phase' HDL. Benditt et al (1980) and Hoffman & Benditt (1983) have reported that apoSAA-rich HDL is cleared from the plasma very rapidly, with T1/2 of 75–80 minutes in mice. This is much more rapid than the clearance of apoA-I or any other apoproteins for which information is available. They have therefore suggested that the function of apoSAA may be to confer a rapid clearance rate on HDL particles, possibly as a means of eliminating complexes of toxic or unwanted materials with HDL (Ulevitch et al, 1979; 1981). Evidence in support of this hypothesis is provided by the observation that lipopolysaccharide added to rabbit serum forms a complex with HDL and that with acute phase rabbit serum the HDL in the complex contains apoSAA (Tobias et al, 1982). However, ^{125}I-lipopolysaccharide was cleared at the same rate by normal and acute phase rabbits (Tobias et al, 1982).

Further work in this area will be of considerable interest, particularly with respect to possible differences in function of the different polymorphic forms of apoSAA. The limited data available so far indicate that individuals, either animals or men, are capable of making all the different forms in response to various different stimuli although they may not do so to an equal extent on different occasions (Gorevic et al, 1978; Tobias et al, 1982; Bausserman et al, 1982). This may be of particular interest with regard to the pathogenesis of amyloidosis, if, for example, there was an association between certain of the SAA types and the deposition of AA-fibrils (Gorevic et al, 1982). However, no evidence for the existence of any such amyloid-prone form of SAA has yet been obtained (Westermark, 1982; Marhaug et al, 1982).

It has been reported that murine and human SAA, isolated by formic acid denaturation of acute phase serum and subsequent gel filtration chromatography in formic acid, can suppress the T cell-dependent in vitro antibody response to sheep erythrocytes of both murine and human lymphocytes (Benson et al, 1975; Benson & Aldo-Benson, 1979; Aldo-Benson & Benson, 1982). No effect on T cell-independent B cell activation was demonstrated. This interesting observation is difficult to interpret in terms of a physiological role in vivo since the conformation of SAA isolated in formic acid may bear little relation to that of apoSAA in its native state in lipoprotein particles. Furthermore SAA prepared in this way is known to contain other proteins, including albumin fragments, prealbumin and β_2-microglobulin which may be covalently linked to the SAA itself (Marhaug & Husby, 1981; Marhaug et al, 1983). In view of the extreme potency of lymphokines and monokines it is also not possible by conventional biochemical techniques to exclude the possibility of the presence of this type of biologically active peptide in the SAA preparations. In this regard it is of some interest that there are many reports of in vitro immunosuppressive or other cellular effects of a number of putatively pure acute phase proteins (Sipe & Rosenstreich, 1981). Some of these observations have subsequently been shown not to be reproducible with more highly purified proteins or to have been due to low molecular weight contaminants. Interpretation of this type of study should therefore be approached with considerable caution.

Prealbumin

The subunits of amyloid fibrils in type I (Portuguese) familial amyloid polyneuropathy occuring in families of Portuguese (AFp), Swedish (AFs), Japanese (AFj) and Jewish origin are composed of prealbumin (Costa et al, 1978; Skinner & Cohen, 1981; Tawara et al, 1981; Shoji et al, 1981; Pras et al, 1981). Both intact prealbumin subunits and various, presumably proteolytic, cleavage fragments have been identified. There is some evidence for minor heterogeneity of amino acid sequence as well as characteristic differences in amino acid composition between plasma prealbumin and the amyloid fibril protein (Pras et al, 1981). The fibril protein (AS_{C1}) in the commonest form of senile cardiac amyloid is also related to or derived from prealbumin as shown by amino acid sequencing, although the isolated subunits do not react immunochemically with antibody to prealbumin (Sletten et al, 1980). It has recently been reported that amyloid in the neuritic plaques, neurofibrillary tangles and microangiopathic lesions of Alzheimer's disease and senile dementia stain immunohistochemically with anti-prealbumin (Shirahama et al, 1982). These observations have yet to be confirmed by other laboratories or the protein decisively identified by isolation of fibrils and sequencing of their subunit protein.

Hormone proteins

The subunit protein (AE_t) of amyloid fibrils derived from the deposits associated with medullary carcinoma of the thyroid shows amino acid sequence homology with calcitonin and seems to be related to or derived from a procalcitonin molecule or calcitonin precursor (Sletten et al, 1976). Local amyloid deposits associated with other endocrine tumours are thought to be related to their specific hormone products but this has not yet been established.

γ-Trace protein

Fibrils have recently been isolated (Cohen et al, 1983b) from tissue of patients with the rare condition of hereditary cerebral haemorrhage with amyloidosis (Gudmundsson et al, 1972; Wattendorf et al, 1982). The amyloid is confined to the cerebral blood vessels and seems to be responsible for the cerebrovascular catastrophes which occur in these individuals. Amino acid sequencing of the isolated fibril protein has shown homology with γ-trace protein (Cohen et al, 1983b), a peptide of unknown function which is present in blood and CSF and which is itself structurally related to corticotrophin.

AMYLOID P COMPONENT

AP is composed of 10 identical glycosylated polypeptide subunits which are non-covalently associated in two disc-like pentameric rings interacting face-to-face (Pinteric et al, 1976; Osmand et al, 1977; Pepys et al, 1977) (Fig. 41.4). It is apparently identical to the normal serum protein, SAP (Skinner et al, 1980; Pepys & Baltz, 1983), and is distinct in its structure and amino acid sequence from all other proteins with the exception of C-reactive protein (CRP), the classical acute phase protein. CRP and SAP share 50% strict residue for residue identity and when conservative substitutions are taken into account the overall homology is of the order of 70% (Anderson & Mole, 1982). The sequence of SAP isolated from a pool of normal plasma shows microheterogeneity at three different positions (Anderson & Mole, 1982). This is the only evidence so far for polymorphic forms or possible allotypes of SAP but if such variants exist they might be of considerable interest with respect to amyloidogenesis (see below)

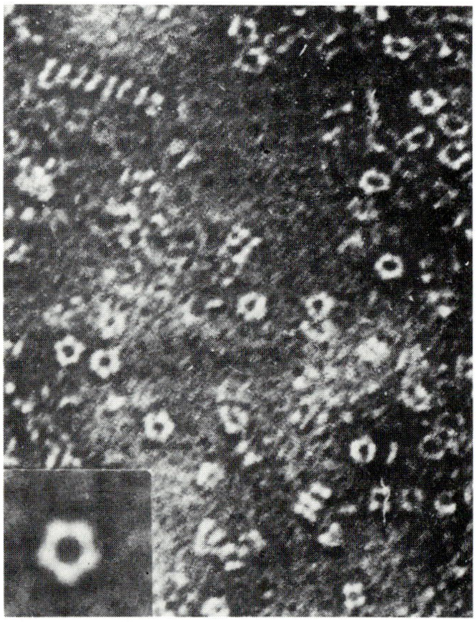

Fig. 41.4 Electron micrograph of negatively stained preparation of human SAP showing pairs of discs side on and face on, and small stacks of molecules (× 570 000). Inset: face view of molecule produced by rotational integration. (Reproduced with permission from Pepys et al, 1977.)

SAP and CRP are clearly members of the same, unique protein 'superfamily' and have presumably been derived during evolution by a process of gene duplication. This duplication must have occurred at a very early stage in vetebrate evolution, if not before, since proteins homologous with and corresponding in functional properties to human SAP and CRP respectively are present in all vertebrates in which they have been sought (Pepys et al, 1978a; Baltz et al, 1982a; Robey et al, 1983). A protein homologous with CRP is even present in an invertebrate, *Limulus polyphemus*, the horseshoe crab (Robey & Liu, 1981; Liu et al, 1982). Such stable conservation during evolution suggests that these proteins have important physiological functions but these have not yet been identified.

Ligand binding by SAP/AP

SAP and AP bind calcium ions and also display specific calcium-dependent ligand binding properties. This was first described in the case of human SAP with respect to agarose (Pepys et al, 1977) and SAP of other species has been isolated and identified on the basis of this same binding specificity. Subsequently SAP was shown to undergo calcium-dependent binding to AA and AL-type amyloid fibrils in vitro (Pepys et al, 1979) and the occurrence of this interaction in vivo probably accounts for the almost universal presence of AP in amyloid deposits.

More recently it has been shown that aggregated human SAP expresses new reactivites which are not expressed by native, non-aggregated SAP (de Beer et al, 1981). These reactivites are directed towards two normal plasma proteins, fibronectin and C4-binding protein. When suitably immobilised SAP is exposed to whole normal human serum it selectively binds these two proteins in a strictly calcium-dependent reaction. A pair of SAP molecules, for example bound by an immobilised IgG anti-SAP molecule, binds a single molecule of fibronectin. SAP within the plasma or in serum is not bound to either fibronectin or C4-binding protein and apparently exists freely as single, uncomplexed molecules (Baltz et al, 1982b).

When isolated, pure human SAP is exposed to free ionised calcium it rapidly aggregates and, if the protein concentration is sufficient, it precipitates out (Baltz et al, 1982b). The mechanism of this phenomenon is not known but it does not seem to depend on the charge or sialation of the SAP since desialated SAP behaves in the same way. Mouse SAP does not aggregate in this fashion.

The chemical identity of the physiological ligand(s) for SAP is not known. SAP does not bind just to any deposit in vivo containing calcium or to any polyanion capable of binding calcium. In the case of agarose the pyruvate moiety, a variable trace constituent, seems to be essential, and the pyruvate acetal of galactose inhibits all the binding reactions of SAP (Hind et al, 1983a). With regard to physiological or pathophysiological ligands recent observations suggest that SAP may be binding to a particular folded conformation of polypeptide chains known as the β-turn. This forms when there are many glycine residues appropriately distributed among bulky and hydrophobic L-amino acids. It consists of a ten atom hydrogen-bounded ring inserted into the polypeptide backbone such that the end peptide moiety has its peptide acyl oxygen directed nearly perpendicular to the plane of the other atoms. This is an exposed position in which it is capable of binding cations and in fact sequences which form β-turns bind Ca^{++} with a high selectivity over Na^{+}, K^{+} or Mg^{++}.

Elastin was the first protein in which β-turns were described and it has a known affinity for binding calcium (Urry, 1974). Amyloid fibrils with their anti-parallel β-pleated sheet structure of polypeptide chains also contain β-turns (Cooper, 1983) and bind calcium (Kula et al, 1977). It has lately been shown that normal elastic fibres throughout the body bear SAP on their surface (Breathnach et al, 1981b) and it is therefore possible that SAP is specifically equipped to recognise peptide sequences which include calcium-binding carbonyl groups in appropriate spatial orientation. The presence of these groups may be the feature in common between such apparently diverse protein ligands of SAP as amyloid fibres, elastic fibres, fibronectin and C4-binding protein.

Serum levels of SAP

SAP is synthesised by hepatocytes (Baltz et al, 1980a; Tatsuta, 1983) and its serum concentration is relatively stable in man, females (mean ± s.d., 33 ± 10 mg/l) having slightly but significantly lower values than males (43 ± 14 mg/l) (Pepys et al, 1978b). The levels in cord sera are much lower (4 ± 2 mg/l) (Pepys et al, 1978b) but rise rapidly during the first weeks of life to reach the lower part of the adult range, around 10–20 mg/l. In chronic inflammatory or neoplastic diseases in which CRP and SAA levels tend to be raised, the SAP concentration also rises but generally remains within the normal range and does not exceed 100 mg/l (Pepys et al, 1978b). Patients with macroglobulinaemia may be exceptional in having higher SAP values than this even with modest rises in acute phase proteins (Jensson et al, 1982;Strachan & Johnson, 1982). In our experience acute stimuli such as major surgery are not followed by any significant or consistent change in SAP levels; however, Hashimoto & Migita (1979) have reported a doubling of SAP levels by the third postoperative day in Japanese subjects undergoing surgery.

Amongst the other species in which SAP levels have been measured, mice are exceptional in two respects: firstly, there are marked genetically determined differences in normal levels between different inbred strains and secondly, SAP is a major acute phase reactant in all strains (Pepys et al, 1979). Acute phase levels of mouse SAP are derived largely by de novo synthesis of the protein, in the liver, rather than from release of preformed stocks (Baltz et al, 1980c). The T1/2 of ^{125}I-SAP measured both by whole body counting and by plasma sampling is about 7.5–9.5 hours in all strains studied (C57Bl, CBA, BALB/c, DBA/2) regardless of whether the animals are normal and healthy or are mounting acute phase responses to acute or chronic stimuli, or have established amyloidosis (Baltz et al, 1980c). Changes in the plasma level are therefore apparently due to alteration in the rate of synthesis of SAP or of its secretion into the circulation. The turnover and synthesis rates of SAP in man have not been measured directly but observations in individuals undergoing plasma exchange suggest that they are very rapid. It is therefore possible that alterations in overall production and availability of SAP in man could take place in the absence of rises in the plasma level.

SAP and amyloidosis

AP has been detected immunochemically using antisera to AP or SAP in deposits or extracts of all forms of amyloid in which it has been sought (Pepys et al, 1982; Pitkanen et al, 1983; Breathnach et al, 1981a, 1983b; Wheeler & Eiferman, 1983), regardless of the chemical nature of the fibril protein, with the possible exception of intracerabral amyloid plaques (Shirahama et al, 1982). Immunohistochemical staining with anti-SAP therefore provides a valuable aid in the tissue diagnosis of all except the latter form of amyloid. Deposits of experimentally induced amyloid in mice (Baltz et al, 1980a) and guinea-pigs (Skinner & Cohen, 1976) also contain AP, as do naturally occurring amyloid deposits in cattle (F. C. de Beer, I. F. Rowe, E. Gruys & M. B. Pepys, unpublished observations).

The significance of this universal association is not known but a possible explanation may simply be that regardless of the chemistry of the subunit proteins, the formed amyloid fibrils all share a common structural feature which happens to be a ligand for SAP. The possible nature of this ligand has been discussed above. Alternatively, there may be a more intimate association between AP and the pathogenesis of amyloidosis. For example in man AP is a normal tissue protein located at sites where early amyloid deposition often occurs (see below), whilst in the mouse SAP is an acute phase reactant, levels of which are raised during experimental induction of amyloidosis and correlate more closely with amyloidogenesis than do those of SAA (Baltz et al, 1980b). It has been suggested that the calcium-dependent aggregation manifested by isolated human SAP may in some way contribute to amyloid fibril deposition (Pinteric & Painter, 1979; Painter et al, 1982), but it cannot be an essential feature of the pathogenesis since mouse SAP, which is also found in amyloid deposits, does not aggregate in the same way (Baltz et al, 1982b). The possible existence of polymorphism in the primary structure of SAP (Anderson & Mole, 1982) raises the question of whether some form of SAP/AP is particularly associated with the development of amyloidosis but there is no evidence on this point as yet.

SAP-related material in normal human tissues

Normal human renal glomerular basement membrane (GBM) and the peripheral microfibrillar mantle of elastic fibres in blood vessels and tissues throughout the body contain a protein which binds anti-SAP antibodies immunospecifically (Fig. 41.5) (Dyck et al, 1980b; Breathnach et al, 1981a,b; 1983a; Houser et al, 1982). It is also present in some other, but not all, vascular basement membranes but is not detectable in renal tubular, dermo-epidermal or other basement membranes (Breathnach et al, 1983a).

The normal tissue AP (TAP) is not eluted from tissue sections except by denaturing solvents which completely destroy tissue architecture, but it can be released in soluble form from isolated GBM by digestion with collagenase. Solubilised TAP from GBM gives reactions of complete identity in gel double immunodiffusion analysis with SAP and anti-SAP. However it is heterogeneous in pI, in molecular size and in polypeptide chain composition. Some of the native material and of the subunits are the same size as SAP but the ma-

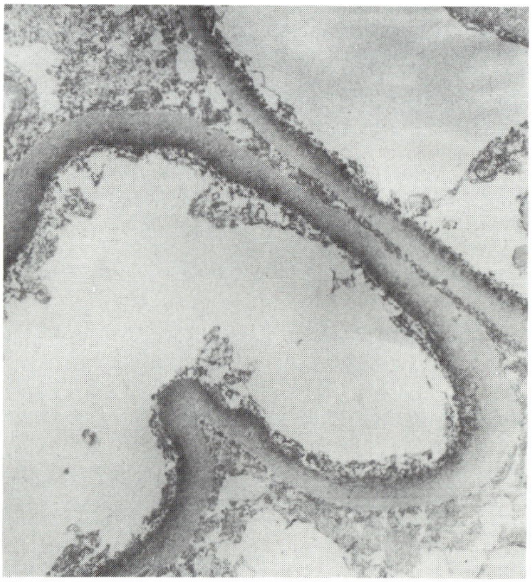

Fig. 41.5 Electron micrograph of normal human glomerular basement membrane stained by immunoperoxidase with anti-SAP antibodies. There is a continuous layer of staining in the lamina rara interna. (× 1600)

jority are heavier, suggesting that the TAP is covalently linked to collagen and/or other matrix proteins in the GBM (Dyck et al, 1980b). SAP itself has no biochemical similarity or immunochemical cross-reactivity with either collagen or the elastic fibre microfibrillar proteins which have been characterised hitherto (Sear et al, 1981). The biological significance of TAP in normal tissues is not known but it is possible that the interaction between aggregated AP and fibronectin (see above) may be relevant.

Immunohistochemical studies with anti-SAP of renal biopsies in various forms of renal disease show distinctive abnormal staining patterns in the GBM and such staining is a simple and sensitive marker for glomerular pathology (Dyck et al, 1980a; Orfila et al, 1982). When used routinely for examination of renal biopsies it also has the advantage of detecting small amounts of amyloid which may otherwise be missed unless Congo red staining is included. Anti-SAP is also a useful reagent for the demonstration of abnormalities in the structure and distribution of elastic fibres in skin biopsies (Breathnach et al, 1982).

PATHOGENESIS OF AMYLOID FIBRIL DEPOSITION

Fibril formation and deposition

A general concept of the likely mechanisms of deposition of amyloid fibrils, involving partial proteolytic cleavage of an abnormal precursor protein into subunits capable of polymerisation into β-pleated sheet fibrils, is now widely accepted (Glenner, 1980a, b) but many areas of ignorance and uncertainty remain. In the great majority of cases there is clear evidence for the presence of a fibril subunit precursor protein which is abnormal either quantitatively, qualitatively or both. The monoclonal immunoglobulin light chains in immunocytic amyloidosis seem certain to be the precursors of AL fibrils, but the precursor product relationship between SAA and AA is less clear. Nonetheless it is very likely indeed that such a relationship exists in AA amyloidosis as it presumably also does between a normal or variant form of plasma prealbumin and the prealbumin subunit of the fibrils in type I familial amyloid polyneuropathy, senile cardiac amyloidosis and possibly Alzheimer's disease and senile dementia.

Proteolytic cleavage of L chains to yield V_L fragments capable of polymerising into Congophilic amyloid-like fibrils has been demonstrated in vitro using pepsin, trypsin, renal tubular or leucocyte lysosomal enzymes to digest isolated Bence-Jones proteins (Glenner et al, 1971; Shirahama et al, 1973; Linke et al, 1973; Epstein et al, 1974). Formation of amyloid fibrils in vitro has also been demonstrated in human myeloma stem cell culture with an apparently close relationship between the newly formed fibrils and macrophages (Durie et al, 1982). Analogous processes probably underlie AL fibril formation in vivo and the presence of intact, undergraded L chains together with V_L fragments in some cases may result from copolymerisation or coacervation.

L chains of λ isotype, for some reason related to their intrinsic properties or to their capacity to interact with other structures in vivo, have a greater tendency to yield β-pleated sheet-forming fragments than κ chains. In other words some precursors are more amyloidogenic than others (Glenner, 1980a, b).

SAA is very susceptible to proteolytic cleavage and is readily degraded by proteinases from monocytes and polymorphs, as well as a number of other serine proteinases, into fragments of a size similar to AA or even smaller (Lavie et al, 1978, 1980; Skogen & Natvig, 1981; Silverman et al, 1982). Although some claims have been made there is as yet no convincing evidence for the existence of a particular specific enzyme or enzymes responsible for the production of AA from SAA in patients with amyloidosis. Also, despite the existence of polymorphic forms of SAA and heterogeneity of AA extracted from fibrils no evidence has yet been forthcoming in favour of a particular amyloidogenic subset of SAA molecules. However this possibility should not be excluded. The recent work on identification and sequencing of prealbumin in some hereditary and senile forms of amyloidosis (see above) suggests that particular amyloidogenic polymorphic forms of this protein may be of pathogenic significance. Further studies of the polymorphism of SAP, AP and TAP would also be of interest in this regard.

The reasons why only some patients with predisposing causes, such as plasma cell dyscrasia or chronic inflammatory disease, develop amyloidosis are still unclear and many different areas for speculation exist in addition to those outlined above. The role of environmental or genetic influences unrelated to the primary amyloidogenic process are apparently very important. For example, the failure of FMF-affected individuals of Armenian, and probably also Ashkenazi, origin to develop amyloidosis (see above), and the remarkable variation observed in the incidence of experimentally-induced AA-amyloid in syngeneic mice at different times and in different laboratories are cases in point. The role of tissue proteins and other matrix elements as possible foci for fibril formation and deposition is quite obscure and there are no clues about the mechanisms underlying the different anatomical distribution of deposits in AA, AL and familial amyloidosis syndromes or even in different individuals with the same type of amyloidosis.

Fibril degradation

Even less is known of the fate of amyloid fibrils than of their initial deposition. Regression of amyloidosis has been documented (Lowenstein & Gallo, 1970; Paraf et al, 1970; Dikman et al, 1977; Cohen et al, 1975; Buxbaum et al, 1979; Cusano et al, 1982), albeit rarely, but since the diagnosis of amyloid depends on histopathology alone it is very difficult to avoid the problems inherent in sampling. Thus even when clinical manifestations attributable to amyloid remit, proof of diminution in the amount of amyloid requires adequate tissue samples before and afterwards to permit precise quantitation. This is rarely possible in a clinical situation but nonetheless deposits both in man and experimental animals (Williams, 1967) can regress or in some cases apparently 'relocate' from one organ or tissue to another (Shirahama & Cohen, 1980). Amyloid does not apparently evoke a significant foreign body or inflammatory reaction but the close association of fibrils with reticuloendothelial cells has been observed in the electron microscope (Shirahama & Cohen, 1967). These may represent 'attempts' at phagocytosis and degradation (Shirahama et al, 1971).

There has been increasing interest lately in the degradation of amyloid fibrils by whole human serum or fractions thereof. These studies are based on the work of Kedar et al (1980) who showed that when serum is placed in wells within an agar gel incorporating AA fibrils, zones of clarification develop around the wells and the fibrils therein lose their capacity to bind Congo red. The precise effects of this 'amyloid degrading factor' (ADF) on the fibrils is not clear but other workers have shown that incubation of AA fibrils in suspension with commercial preparations of elastin, plasmin and kallikrein is associated with cleavage of the AA subunits (Skogen & Natvig, 1981). It has been claimed that the serum ADF activity detected in the gel diffusion assay is a serine proteinase, distinct from elastase or cathepsin G, which is bound to or closely associated with plasma albumin and which is inhibitable by α_1-proteinase inhibitor (Teppo et al, 1982). Indeed preparations of isolated albumin exhibit ADF activity (Maury & Teppo, 1982). AL fibrils seem not to be affected by serum so if this mechanism is involved in systemic amyloidosis it probably concerns the AA type only.

Kedar et al (1980) originally reported that sera of patients with AA amyloidosis had significantly less ADF activity than control sera of either healthy subjects or individuals with predisposing diseases in the absence of amyloid. This observation has been confirmed by several other groups (Wegelius et al, 1982; Maddison et al, 1983; Caspi et al, 1983) but some divergences exist in subsequent findings. Wegelius's group in Finland find that ADF activity in rheumatoid arthritis correlates positively with serum albumin levels and negatively with α_1-proteinase inhibitor levels. They therefore propose that ADF levels are inversely related to the extent of the acute phase response and to external albumin/ADF losses. Albumin is a 'negative' acute phase reactant the synthesis of which by the liver is reduced pari passu with increased production of acute phase proteins including α_1-proteinase inhibitor. Patients with amyloid are usually those with long-standing active disease. Similarly these patients are likely to have proteinuria with loss of albumin and associated ADF. In confirmation of this concept the Finnish group report that in patients with hereditary or immunocyte amyloid, in patients with cirrhosis, or in patients undergoing surgery there is a close correlation between plasma albumin levels and ADF activity (Maury & Teppo, 1982). On the other hand Kedar et al (1982) claim that hypoalbuminaemic sera and effusion fluids may have entirely normal levels of ADF and that the low level of ADF in serum in amyloidotic subjects is due to the concomitant presence of a low molecular weight inhibitor (I^{ADF}). They report that the effect of this inhibitor can be reversed in vitro by addition to the serum of EDTA, citric acid or ascorbic acid (Kedar et al, 1982). However it has not proved possible to confirm either the enzymatic nature of ADF nor enhancement of ADF in amyloidotic patient sera by any of the above chemicals (Caspi et al, 1983, 1984).

Further work is necessary to clarify these observations and to characterise more precisely the factors involved. All work on ADF so far has been done in vitro and it is not know whether the existing observations have any counterpart in vivo. That they may have is suggested by work in experimental animal models of AA amyloidosis in which amyloid deposition, induced by administration of an extrinsic acute phase stimulus, can be greatly accelerated by the simultaneous injection of an extract of amyloidotic tissue. Such tissue extracts contain so-called 'amyloid enhancing factor' (AEF) (Axelrad et al, 1982) and Kedar claims that there is some similarity between AEF and his postulated I^{ADF} (Kedar et al, 1982).

PATHOGENESIS OF THE EFFECTS OF AMYLOID

Amyloid deposits seem to exert their pathological effects largely by their physical presence which distorts the normal architecture of tissues and organs and disrupts their functions. Despite the recent in vitro evidence for factors capable of degrading isolated amyloid fibrils the natural history of amyloid deposits in vivo is to persist and increase leading inexorably in most cases to clinically significant failure of organ or tissue function or to the consequences of a space-occupying mass lesion. Occasionally the amount of amyloid seems to decrease but usually, in that small proportion of patients in which the clinical manifestations remain static or even improve with time, repeat biopsy or eventual autopsy may show little change in the quantity of amyloid present (Tribe & MacKenzie, 1982; Kyle et al, 1982). These findings suggest that some secondary effect of the presence of amyloid may be contributing to organ dysfunction and that this can ameliorate, spontaneously or with therapy, despite persistence of the amyloid per se. The nature of such secondary effects, if any, is not known though van Rijswijk (1981) has suggested that in the kidney interstitial fibrosis may be involved and that when this is rapidly progressive its retardation by treatment with anti-inflammatory and anti-fibrotic agents such as dimethyl sulphoxide (DMSO) or prednisolone may be beneficial (van Rijswijk et al, 1983).

Rare but serious complications of amyloidosis which are not simply a result of the physical bulk of the deposits include clotting factor deficiency and sensitivity to digitalis. Acquired deficiency of factor X and sometimes also other factors occurs only in AL amyloidosis and is probably due to adsorption of the clotting proteins by the fibrils (Furie et al, 1977; McPherson et al, 1977; Griepp et al, 1981). Resection of the amyloid-laden spleen led to an improvement in one case (Rosenstein et al, 1983). However it should be noted that bleeding complications are common in all forms of amyloidosis, occurring in around 40% of cases, in most of which there is no abnormality in the coagulation tests (Yood et al, 1983). Haemorrhage in amyloidosis is therefore usually probably due to direct amyloid infiltration of the blood vessels. Patients with systemic amyloidosis affecting the heart are often exquisitely sensitive to digitalis toxicity, once again because the fibrils seem able to adsorb and therefore concentrate the drug locally (Rubinow et al, 1981).

DIAGNOSIS

Biopsy

Amyloidosis can only be diagnosed positively by histological examination of tissue obtained by biopsy or resection. A high index of suspicion is therefore necessary so that the possibility of amyloid comes to mind during investigation of any case in which it could be involved. If feasible the tissue or organ mainly affected, such as kidney or heart (endomyocardial biopsy, Schroeder et al, 1975), should be biopsied but care must be taken lest this cause complications. It may be preferable to attempt biopsy of a more accessible tissue in the first place. Rectal biopsy including adequate submucosal tissue contains diagnostic amounts of amyloid in over 90% of cases of systemic amyloidosis (Tribe & MacKenzie, 1982). Aspiration of subcutaneous fat from the anterior abdominal wall has been suggested as an alternative source of material (Westermark & Stenkuist, 1973). Skin biopsy is often positive in patients with familial amyloidotic polyneuropathy (Shirahama et al, 1980) and, if it is, spares the patient a direct biopsy of nerve. Splenic aspiration has been used to provide material but rectal or gingival biopsy is probably preferable.

It is essential to undertake a full coagulation screen before subjecting a patient with possible amyloid to any sort of biopsy procedure. Although relatively rare, acquired factor X-deficiency occurring in AL amyloidosis is often associated with severe bleeding usually of a greater extent than can be accounted for by deficiency of factor X alone. This haemorrhagic diathesis may be very difficult to correct and severe enough to preclude biopsy. Bleeding may also occur in the absence of any abnormality in the coagulation tests (Yood et al, 1983).

A variety of stains have been used to identify amyloid histologically (Tribe & Perry, 1979; Glenner, 1981b) but the pathognomonic stain is alkaline Congo red (Puchtler et al, 1962) which yields the classical green birefringence when viewed in polarised light. It is essential that all aspects of the staining procedure, and of tissue inspection thereafter, be performed properly or the diagnosis may be missed. In skilled hands the Congo red stain is undoubtedly excellent but immunohistochemical staining with antisera specific for amyloid proteins (see below) may well prove to be easier and more specific, though this approach also requires detailed attention to technique. When tissue sections are treated with potassium permanganate under specific conditions AA amyloid loses its capacity to bind Congo red whereas this does not occur with AL or prealbumin fibrils (Wright et al, 1977; van Rijswijk & van Heusden, 1979). This method therefore provides for differential diagnosis of the major causes of systemic amyloidosis, but once again it is essential to include both positive and negative control tissues, containing known amyloid fibril types, in each staining run. One of the nephropathic forms of familial amyloidosis (Ostertag type) has recently been shown to have permanganate-sensitive non-AA fibrils (Lanham et al, 1982) so the permanganate test alone cannot diagnose AA amyloidosis.

Amyloid fibrils have a characteristic appearance in the electron microscope and standard transmission electron microscopy of properly fixed tissue specimens can therefore establish the diagnosis alone, or preferably confirm it in association with Congo red and/or immunohistochemical staining.

All forms of amyloid, with the possible exception of senile and presenile cortical plaques, contain AP and immunohistochemical staining with anti-AP serum is therefore a valuable aid to the histopathological diagnosis of amyloid (Breathnach et al, 1981a, 1983b; Shirahama et al, 1981; Pepys et al, 1982; Lanham et al, 1982; Tribe & MacKenzie, 1982) (Fig. 41.6). AA amyloid can also be stained in all cases using anti-AA serum (Fig. 41.7) but AL amyloid presents more of a problem (Livni et al, 1980; Fujihara et al, 1980; Fujihara & Glenner, 1981; Linke & Nathrath, 1982; Hind et al, 1983b). Since the AL subunits are predominantly derived from the V_L region of the L chain they usually lack the common isotypic

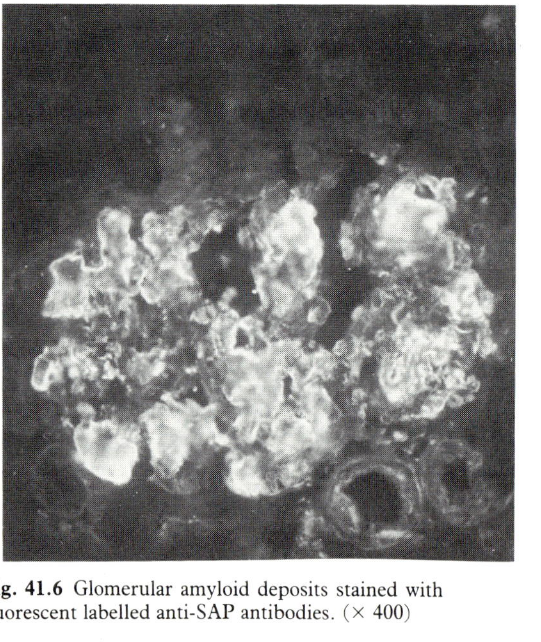

Fig. 41.6 Glomerular amyloid deposits stained with fluorescent labelled anti-SAP antibodies. (× 400)

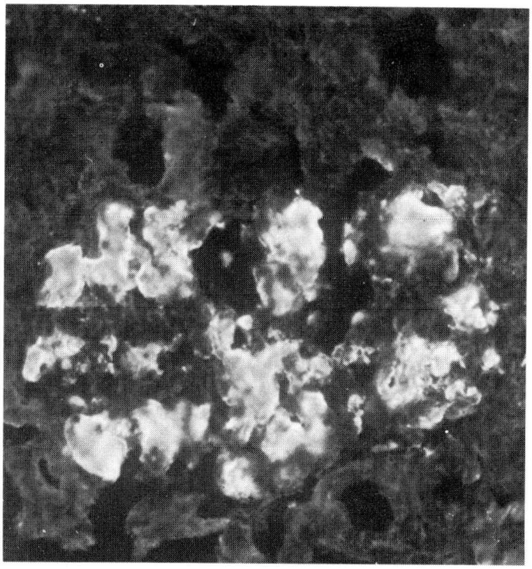

Fig. 41.7 Glomerular amyloid deposits stained with fluorescent labelled anti-AA antibodies. (× 400)

epitopes characteristic of κ and λ chains. It is frequently necessary to use antisera specific for the particular L chain subgroup or individual anti-idiotype antiserum raised against the patients own monoclonal paraprotein to obtain positive staining. However if suitable reagents are available good results are obtained. Staining with anti-prealbumin serum is effective in type I familial amyloid polyneuropathy but is not consistently reproducible with senile amyloid deposits in heart or brain. It is not unlikely that different configurations of the subunit protein in the β-pleated sheet fibrils, or perhaps variant forms of the subunit itself or its cleavage products, may lack the epitopes against which anti-plasma prealbumin antisera are directed. Negative immunohistochemical staining of amyloid deposits in situ in tissues should therefore not be taken as unequivocal evidence of the absence of a particular protein.

Non-invasive techniques

Amyloid deposits always contain calcium, and soft tissue scanning after injection of calcium-seeking isotopes such as [^{99m}Tc]pyrophosphate or diphosphonate, particularly the former, may aid in diagnosis (Yood et al, 1981; Rao et al, 1981; Johnston et al, 1982; Wizenberg et al, 1982; Schiff et al, 1982; Sobol et al, 1982; Falk et al, 1983). This approach has proved particularly useful for cardiac amyloidosis but has also picked up deposits in liver and skeletal muscle. Uptake and prolonged retention of [^{67}Ga]-citrate occurs with amyloidosis in the kidneys and heart but is so non-specific that biopsy confirmation is always required (Banzo-Marraco et al, 1981). Echocardiography is a useful diagnostic tool for cardiac amyloid (Sutton et al, 1982), whereas electrocardiography is notably less so. Most patients with acquired systemic amyloid affecting the heart have abnormal ECGs (Carroll et al, 1982) but this seems not usually to be the case with senile cardiac amyloidosis even when it is very extensive (Cattin et al, 1981).

MANAGEMENT

There is no effective treatment for any form of amyloidosis other than surgical resection of localised masses and replacement therapy for end-stage renal failure. Based on current views of the pathogenesis of amyloid deposition a rational aim is to reduce as far as possible the production and level of the fibril precursor in the hope, at least, that the damage already caused will progress more slowly or, at best, that some resorption of the amyloid may occur (Schnitzer & Ansell, 1977). This aim is very difficult to achieve in most conditions. The only possible exception is FMF in which colchicine seems to be effective in controlling the clinical manifestations in most patients (Goldfinger, 1972; Zemer et al, 1976, 1980). Even in those individuals whose FMF is not completely controlled, colchicine apparently prevents the development of amyloidosis if treatment is started before it occurs. This may be because colchicine is suppressing the secretion of SAA and other acute phase proteins, as it is known to do in experimental animals. Colchicine also prevents the experimental induction by repeated casein injection of AA amyloid in mice (Kedar et al, 1974; Shirahama & Cohen, 1974). Unfortunately in neither mice nor men does colchicine given after the appearance of amyloid cause the amyloid to regress, although some patients with FMF have shown an improvement (Ravid et al, 1977; Walker & Bear, 1982). However if colchicine has a potent anti-inflammatory effect on the primary disease, as in FMF, or can be shown to suppress the acute phase response of SAA to other inflammatory stimuli, then it may be worth trying. Divided doses of up to 2.0 mg/day may be tolerated without ill effect.

In other inflammatory or infective diseases complicated by amyloidosis aggressive treatment of the primary condition is indicated and in a few cases complete control or eradication, for example of localised sepsis, had been associated with regression of the amyloid. Such complete control is however rarely achieved and the use, for example, of sufficient corticosteroids to even approach it in most active rheumatic conditions carries its own hazards. The use of alternative, albeit potentially toxic agents, such as chlorambucil or cyclophosphamide may be justified and in general the best results are likely to be obtained by so closely controlling the primary disorder that amyloid does not ever develop (Schnitzer & Ansell, 1977).

In AL amyloidosis complicating myeloma or other malignant forms of immunocyte dyscrasia the treatment is aimed at reduction or elimination of paraprotein in any case but is unlikely to have much beneficial effect on the amyloid. In otherwise 'benign' immunocyte dyscrasia a choice must be made whether to give steroid and cytotoxic drugs or not. Theoretical arguments in favour exist, as mentioned above, and there have been reports of apparent benefit in some cases but the overall prognosis remains very poor (Kyle & Griepp, 1978; Ogg et al, 1981) and even when there has been some clinical improvement the quantity of amyloid present has not diminished (Kyle et al, 1982).

Dimethyl sulphoxide (DMSO) is a polar aprotic solvent which has been given orally, by infusion and by topical administration to patients with amyloidosis. There have been some reports of benefit (Osserman et al, 1976, 1980; van Rijswijk et al, 1980; Ravid & Kedar, 1980; Ravid et al, 1982) and some experimental work in which resolution of amyloid deposits was observed (Isobe & Osserman, 1976; Hanai et al, 1979; Greenwald et al, 1980). The mode of action is unknown. There is some evidence that DMSO may solubilise amyloid fibrils and it may facilitate their extraction from tissues in vitro (van Rijswijk, 1981). DMSO seems to have a significant anti-inflammatory effect in rheumatoid arthritis, as evidenced by decreases in CRP and SAA levels during treatment with it and this may explain some of its apparent benefit in AA amyloid (van Rijswijk et al, 1980; Kisilevsky et al, 1983). Unfortunately DMSO has a foul pervasive odour, as have its metabolites, and it is therefore extremely unpleasant therapy both for the patient and his relatives and attendants. The evidence of clinical benefit from DMSO is probably insufficient at present to warrant further trials of its use (van Rijswijk et al, 1983).

What is required for treatment of amyloidosis is an agent either which itself disrupts the β-pleated sheet structure of the fibrils or which permits existing mechanisms in the body to do so. It should then be possible for the deposits to be resorbed permitting maximal restoration of function of the affected tissues or organs. Unfortunately no such agent is known or in prospect.

Although many individuals with systemic amyloidosis die within months of diagnosis others survive for considerable periods and vigorous supportive and palliative treatment is necessary. Care must be taken to avoid digitalis toxicity when cardiac amyloid is present and also to avoid salt and water depletion through injudicious use of diuretics. A new approach to treatment of patients with orthostatic hypotension due to autonomic neuropathy is to replete their depleted noradrenaline stores by administration of the precursor substance DL-threo-3,4-dihydroxyphenylserine. This has been tried with some success in patients with familial amyloid polyneuropathy (Suzuki et al, 1981, 1982) and would greatly improve the quality of life in those patients with AL amyloid who may be crippled by this problem. End-stage renal failure should be treated by the usual means of support and amyloid per se is no contraindication to transplantation. However the prognosis of amyloid patients is generally below average as a result of the systemic nature of their disease and effects of their primary condition, if any (Jones 1976; 1981; Jacob et al, 1979; Dorman et al, 1981).

ADDENDUM

There has been significant progress in several different areas of work on amyloidosis since this chapter was first drafted in 1983. Important points include: the cloning of genes for human and mouse SAA; indications that only one of the two polymorphic forms of mouse SAA is laid down as AA fibrils; establishment of immunoassays and DNA probe assays for the genetic variant of prealbumin (Met for Val at position 30) which is associated with familial amyloid polyneuropathy, making presymptomatic diagnosis possible; presymptomatic diagnosis of patients with the hereditary cerebral haemorrhage with amyloidosis syndrome by assays of γ-trace levels in cerebrospinal fluid; isolation and characterisation of a novel protein as the fibril subunit in the cerebral amyloid angiopathy of senile dementia and Alzheimer's disease; preliminary characterisation of the amyloid fibrils for cortical plaques indicating that they are structurally and chemically distinct from all other types of local and systemic amyloid; new X-ray scattering studies of solutions and wet gels of AA amyloid fibrils which, together with secondary structure predictions of SAA, suggest that the AA fibril probably does not consist of the hitherto generally accepted stack of anti-parallel β-pleated sheets. All these topics are dealt with in the proceedings of the Fourth International Symposium on Amyloidosis which was held in November 1984 and are published as *Amyloidosis — The Disease Complex*, G. G. Glenner (ed) Excerpta Medica, Amsterdam, in press.

REFERENCES

Aldo-Benson M A, Benson M D 1982 SAA suppression of immune response in vitro: evidence for an effect on T cell-macrophage interaction. Journal of Immunology 128: 2390–2392

Anders R F, Natvig J, Michaelsen T E, Husby G 1975 Isolation and characterisation of amyloid related SAA as a small molecular weight protein. Scandinavian Journal of Immunology 4: 397–401

Anders R F, Nordstoga K, Natvig J B, Husby G 1976 Amyloid-related serum protein SAA in endotoxin-induced amyloidosis of the mink. Journal of Experimental Medicine 143: 678–683

Anders R F, Natvig J B, Sletten K, Husby G, Nordstoga K 1977 Amyloid-related serum protein SAA from three animal species: comparison with human SAA. Journal of Immunology 118: 229–234

Anderson J K, Mole J E 1982 Large scale isolation and partial primary structure of human plasma amyloid P-component. Annals of the New York Academy of Science 389: 216–234

Arapakis G, Tribe C R 1963 Amyloidosis in rheumatoid arthritis investigated by means of rectal biopsy. Annals of Rheumatic Diseases 22: 256–262

Axelrad M A, Kisilevsky R, Willmer J, Chen S J, Skinner M 1982 Further characterisation of amyloid-enhancing factor. Laboratory Investigation 47: 139–146

Azzopardi J G, Lehner T 1966 Systemic amyloidosis and malignant disease. Journal of Clinical Pathology 19: 539–548

Baltz M L, Dyck R F, Pepys M B 1980a Amyloid P-component in mice injected with casein: identification in amyloid deposits and in the cytoplasm of hepatocytes. Immunology 41: 59–66

Baltz M L, Gomer K, Davies A J S, Evans D J, Klaus G G B, Pepys M B 1980b Differences in the acute phase responses of serum amyloid P-component (SAP) and C3 to injections of casein or bovine serum albumin in amyloid-susceptible and resistant mouse strains. Clinical and Experimental Immunology 39: 355–360

Baltz M L et al 1980c Studies of serum amyloid P component (SAP) as an acute phase reactant in mice. In: Glenner G G, Pinho e Costa P, Falcao de Freitas A (eds) Amyloid and amyloidosis. Excerpta Medica, Amsterdam, p 534–542

Baltz M L et al 1982a Phylogenetic aspects of C-reactive protein and related proteins. Annals of the New York Academy of Science 389: 49–75

Baltz M L, de Beer F C, Feinstein A, Pepys M B 1982b Calcium-dependent aggregation of human serum amyloid P component. Biochimica Biophysica Acta 701: 229–236

Banzo-Marraco J et al 1981 Renal uptake of ^{67}Ga-citrate in renal amyloidosis due to familial mediterranean fever. European Journal of Nuclear Medicine 6: 277–280

Bausserman L L, Herbert P N, McAdam K P W J 1980 Heterogeneity of human serum amyloid A proteins. Journal of Experimental Medicine 152: 641–656

Bausserman L L, Herbert P B, McAdam K P W J 1982 Serum amyloid A polymorphism in a subject with a naturally occurring inflammatory response. Clinica Chimica Acta 118: 201–207

Benditt E P, Eriksen N 1972 Chemical classes of amyloid substance. American Journal of Pathology 65: 231–249

Benditt E P, Eriksen N 1977 Amyloid protein SAA is associated with high density lipoprotein from human serum. Proceedings of the National Academy of Science USA 74: 4025–4028

Benditt E P, Eriksen N, Hermodson M A, Ericsson L H 1971 The major proteins of human and monkey amyloid substances: common properties including unusual N-terminal amino acid sequences. FEBS Letters 19: 169–173

Benditt E P, Eriksen N, Hanson R H 1979 Amyloid protein SAA is an apoprotein of mouse plasma high density lipoprotein. Proceedings of the National Academy of Science USA 76: 4092–4096

Benditt E P, Eriksen N, Hoffman J S 1980 Origin of protein AA. In: Glenner G G, Pinho e Costa P, Falcao de Freitas A (eds) Amyloid and amyloidosis. Excerpta Medica, Amsterdam, p 397–405

Benditt E P, Hoffman J S, Eriksen N, Parmelee D C, Walsh K A 1982 SAA, an apoprotein of HDL: its structure and function. Annals of the New York Academy of Science 389: 183–189

Benson M D 1982 In vitro synthesis of the acute phase

reactant SAA by hepatocytes. Annals of the New York Academy of Science 389: 116–119
Benson M D, Aldo-Benson M 1979 Effect of purified protein SAA on immune response in-vitro: mechanisms and suppression. Journal of Immunology 122: 2077–2082
Benson M D, Cohen A S 1979 Serum amyloid A protein in amyloidosis, rheumatic and neoplasitc diseases. Arthritis and Rheumatism 22: 36–42
Benson M D, Kleiner E 1980 Synthesis and secretion of serum amyloid protein A (SAA) by hepatocytes in mice treated with casein. Journal of Immunology 124: 495–499
Benson M D, Aldo-Benson M A, Shirahama T, Borel Y, Cohen A S 1975 Suppression of in-vitro antibody response by a serum factor (SAA) in experimentally induced amyloidosis. Journal of Experimental Medicine 142: 236–241
Beroniade V 1975 Amyloidosis and Behçet's disease. Annals of Internal Medicine 83: 904–905
Black M M 1976 Primary localised amyloidosis of the skin: clinical variants, histochemistry and ultrastructure. In: Wegelius O, Pasternack A (eds) Amyloidosis. Academic Press, London p 479
Bornstein D L 1982 Leukocyte pyrogen: a major mediator of the acute phase reaction. Annals of the New York Academy of Science 389: 323–337
Boyko W J, Pratt R, Wass H 1981 Functional hyposplensim, a diagnostic clue in amyloidosis. American Journal of Clinical Pathology 77: 745–748
Brandt K, Cathcart E J, Cohen A S 1968 A clinical analysis of the course and prognosis of 42 patients with amyloidosis. American Journal of Medicine 44: 955–969
Breathnach S M, Bhogal B, Dyck R F, de Beer F C, Black M M, Pepys M B 1981a Immunohistochemical demonstration of amyloid P component in skin of normal subjects and patients with cutaneous amyloidosis. British Journal of Dermatology 105: 115–124
Breathnach S M et al 1981b Amyloid P component is located on elastic fibre microfibrils of normal human tissues. Nature 293: 652–654
Breathnach S M, Melrose S M, Bhogal B, de Beer F C, Black M M, Pepys M B 1982 Immunohistochemical studies of amyloid P component in disorders of cutaneous elastic tissue. British Journal of Dermatology 107: 443–452
Breathnach S M, Melrose S M, Bhogal B, de Beer F C, Black M M, Pepys M B 1983a Immunohistochemical studies of amyloid P component distribution in normal skin. Journal of Investigative Dermatology 80: 86–90
Breathnach S M, Melrose S M, Bhogal B, de Beer F C, Black M M, Pepys M B 1983b Ultrastructural localisation of amyloid P component in primary localised cutaneous amyloidosis. Clinical and Experimental Dermatology 8: 355–362
Brownstein M H, Helwig E B 1970 The cutaneous amyloidoses. I. Localised forms. Archives of Dermatology 102:8
Buxbaum J N, Hurley M E, Chuba J, Spiro T 1979 Amyloidosis of the AL type. Clinical, morphologic and biochemical aspects of the response to therapy with alkylating agents and prednisone. American Journal of Medicine 67: 867–878
Bywaters E G L 1978 Amyloidosis. In: Scott J T (ed) Copeman's textbook of the rheumatic diseases, 5th Edn. Churchill Livingstone, Edinburgh, p 746–760
Carroll J D, Gaasch W H, McAdam K P W J 1982 Amyloid cardiomyopathy: characterisation by a distinctive voltage/mass relation. American Journal of Cardiology 49: 9–13
Carstens P H B, Ogden L L, Peak W P 1980 Renal amyloidosis associated with systemic lupus erythematosus. American Journal of Clinical Pathology 74: 835–838
Caspi D, Baltz M L, Pepys M B 1983 Serum amyloid degrading activity. Clinical Science 65:16P
Caspi D, Baltz Marilyn L, Feinstein A, Munn E A, Pepys M B 1984 'Amyloid degrading activity' of human serum: an in-vitro clearing effect which does not involve degradation of amyloid fibrils. Clinical and Experimental Immunology 57: 647–656
Cattin L, Melato M, Antonutto G, Mlaoc M, da Col P G 1981 ECG findings in elderly patients with and without senile cardiac amyloidosis. Journal of Chronic Diseases 34: 503–509
Chambers R E, Whicher J T 1983 Quantitative radial immunodiffusion assay for SAA. Journal of Immunological Methods 59: 95–103
Cohen A S, Calkins E 1959 Electron microscopic observations on a fibrous component in amyloid of diverse origins. Nature 183: 1202–1203
Cohen A S, Wegelius O 1980 Classification of amyloid: 1979–1980. Arthritis and Rheumatism 23: 644–645
Cohen A S, Shirahama T, Skinner M 1982 Electron microscopy of amyloid. In: Harris J S (ed) Electron microscopy of proteins, Vol 3. Academic Press, London, p 165–205
Cohen A S, Sirahama T, Sipe J D, Skinner M 1983a Amyloid proteins, precursors, mediator and enhancer. Laboratory Investigation 48: 1–4
Cohen D H, Jensson O, Feiner H, Frangione B 1983b Amyloid deposits of the Icelandic form of hereditary cerebral haemorrhage are composed of fragments derived from CSF and serum basic protein (gamma) trace. Clinical Research 31:489A
Colien H J, Lessin L S, Hallal J, Burkholder P 1975 Resolution of primary amyloidosis during chemotherapy. Annals of Internal Medicine 82: 466–473
Cooper J H 1974 Selective amyloid staining as a function of amyloid composition and structure: histochemical analysis of the alkaline Congo red, standardised toluidine blue and iodine methods. Laboratory Investigation 31: 232–238
Cooper J H 1983 A histochemical construct of the amyloid fibril. In: Tribe C R, Bacon P A (eds) Amyloidosis EARS. John Wright, Bristol p 31–35
Cornwell G G, Westermark P 1980 Senile amyloidosis: a protein manifestation of the aging process. Journal of Clinical Pathology 33: 1146–1152
Cornwell G C, Westermark P, Natvig J B, Murdoch W 1981 Senile cardiac amyloid: evidence that fibrils contain a protein immunologically related to prealbumin. Immunology 44: 447–452
Costa P P, Figueira A S, Bravo F R 1978 Amyloid fibril protein related to prealbumin in familial amyloidotic polyneuropathy. Proceedings of the National Academy of Science USA 75: 4499–4503
Cusano A J, Bland J H, Lapenas D J, Cohen A S, Libbey C 1982 Juvenile rheumatoid arthritis with renal amyloidosis: a 23-year old survival. Journal of Rheumatology 9: 921–925
David M, Abraham D, Weinberger A, Feuerman E J 1982 Generalised pustular psoriasis, psoriatic arthritis and nephrotic syndrome associated with systemic amyloidosis. Dermatologica 165: 168–171

de Beer F C, Baltz M, Holford S, Feinstein A, Pepys M B 1981 Fibronectin and C4-binding protein are selectively bound by aggregated amyloid P component. Journal of Experimental Medicine 154: 1134–1149

de Beer F C, Dyck R F, Pepys M B 1982a Solid phase immunoradiometric assay for serum amyloid A protein using magnetisable cellulose particles. Journal of Immunological Methods 54: 213–222

de Beer F C, Mallya R K, Fagan E A, Lanham J G, Hughes G R V, Pepys M B 1982b Serum amyloid A protein concentration in inflammatory disease and its relationship to the incidence of reactive systemic amyloidosis. Lancet 2: 231–234

Dictor M, Hasserius R 1981 Systemic amyloidosis and non-haematologica malignancy in a large autopsy series. Acta Pathologica Microbiologica Scandinavia Section A 89: 411–416

Dikman S H, Katin T, Gribetz D, Churg J 1977 Resolution of renal amyloidosis. American Journal of Medicine 63: 430–433

Dorman S A, Gamelli R L, Benziger J R, Trainer T D, Foster R S 1981 Systemic amyloidosis involving two renal transplants. Human Pathology 12: 735–738

Durie B G M, Persky B, Soehnlen B J, Grogan T M, Salmon S E 1982 Amyloid production in human myeloma stem-cell culture, with morphologic evidence of amyloid secretion by associated macrophages. New England Journal of Medicine 307: 1689–1692

Dyck R F, Evans D J, Lockwood C M, Rees A J, Turner D, Pepys M B 1980a Amyloid P-component in human glomerular basement membrane: abnormal patterns of immunofluorescent staining in glomerular disease. Lancet 2: 606–609

Dyck R F et al 1980b Amyloid P-component is a constitutent of normal human glomerular basement membrane. Journal of Experimental Medicine 152: 1162–1174

Egan M S, Goldenberg D L, Cohen A S, Segal D 1982 The association of amyloid deposits and osteoarthritis. Arthritis and Rheumatism 25: 204–208

Ein D, Kimura S, Terry W D, Magnotta T, Glenner G G 1972 Amino acid sequence of an amyloid fibril protein of unknown origin. Journal of Biological Chemistry 247: 5653–5655

Eliakim M, Levy M, Ehrenfeld M 1981 Recurrent polyserositus. Familial Mediterranean fever, periodic disease. Elsevier/North Holland, Amsterdam

Epstein M V, Tan M, Wood I S 1974 Formation of 'amyloid' fibrils in vitro by action of human kidney lysosomal enzymes on Bence-Jones proteins. Journal of Laboratory and Clinical Medicine 84: 107–110

Eriksen N, Ericsson L H, Pearsall N, Lagunoff D, Benditt E P 1976 Mouse amyloid protein A: Homology with non-immunoglobulin protein of monkey amyloid. Proceedings of the National Academy of Science USA 73: 964–967

Falck H M, Maury C P J, Teppo A M, Wegelius O 1983 Correlation of persistently high serum amyloid A protein and C-reactive protein concentrations with rapid progression of secondary amyloidosis. British Medical Journal 286: 1391–1393

Falk R H, Lee V W, Rubinow A, Hood W B, Cohen A S 1983 Sensitivity of technetium-99m-pyrophosphate scintigraphy in diagnosing cardiac amyloidosis. American Journal of Cardiology 51: 826–830

Franklin E C 1982 The amyloid diseases. In: Lachmann P J, Peters D K (eds) Clinical aspects of immunology, 4th Edn. Blackwell, Oxford, Ch 41 p 1231

Franklin E C, Zucker-Franklin D 1972 Current concepts of amyloid. Advances in Immunology 15: 249–304

Friedereich N, Kekulé A 1859 Zur Amyloidfrage. Archiv fur Pathologische Anatomie und Physiologie und fur Klinische Medizin 16: 50–65

Fujihara S, Glenner G G 1981 Primary localised amyloidosis of the genitourinary tract. Immunohistochemical study on eleven cases. Laboratory Investigation 44: 55–60

Fujihara S, Balow J E, Costa J C, Glenner G G 1980 Identification and classification of amyloid in formalin-fixed, paraffin-embedded tissue sections by the unlabelled immunoperoxidase method. Laboratory Investigation 43: 358–365

Furie B, Greene E, Furie B C 1977 Syndrome of acquired factor X deficiency and systemic amyloidosis: in-vivo studies of the metabolic fate of factor X. New England Journal of Medicine 297: 81–85

Galdenman A H, Levine R A, Aundt K A 1962 Dermatomyositus complicated by generalised amyloidosis. New England Journal of Medicine 267: 858–861

Gertz M A, Kyle R A, Greipp P R 1983 Hyposplenism in primary systemic amyloidosis. Annals of Internal Medicine 98: 475–477

Glenner G G 1980a Amyloid deposits and amyloidosis — the β-fibrilloses I. New England Journal of Medicine 302: 1283–1292

Glenner G G 1980b Amyloid deposits and amyloidosis — the β-fibrilloses II. New England Journal of Medicine 302: 1333–1343

Glenner G G 1981a Amyloidosis: the hereditary disorders, including Alzheimer's disease. Journal of Laboratory and Clinical Medicine 98: 807–810

Glenner G G 1981b The bases of the staining of amyloid fibers: their physico-chemical nature and the mechanisms of their dye-substrate interaction. Progress in Histochemistry and Cytochemistry 13: 1–37

Glenner G G, Ein D, Eanes E D, Bladen H A, Terry W, Page D L 1971 Creation of 'amyloid' fibrils from Bence–Jones proteins in-vitro. Science 184: 712–714

Glenner G G, Ignaczak T F, Page D L 1978 The inherited systemic amyloidoses and localised amyloid deposits. In: Stanbury J B, Wyngaarden J B, Frederickson D F (eds) Metabolic basis of inherited disease, 4th Edn. McGraw-Hill, New York, p 1308–1339

Glenner G G, Pinho e Costa P, Falcao de Freitas F (eds) 1980 Amyloid and amyloidosis. Excerpta Medica, Amsterdam

Goffin Y A, Thona Y, Potvliege P R 1981 Microdeposition of amyloid in the joints. Annals of the Rheumatic Diseases 40: 27–33

Goldfinger W E 1972 Colchicine for familial Mediterranean fever. New England Journal of Medicine 287:1302

Gorevic P D, Rosenthal C J, Franklin E C 1976 Amyloid related serum component (SAA). Studies in acute infections, medullary thyroid carcinoma and post surgery. Behaviour as an acute phase reactant. Clinical Immunology and Immunopathology 6: 83–93

Gorevic P D, Greenwald M, Frangione M, Pras M, Franklin E C 1977 The amino acid sequence of duck amyloid A (AA) protein. Journal of Immunology 118: 1113–1118

Gorevic P D, Levo Y, Frangione B, Franklin E C 1978 Polymorphism of tissue and serum amyloid A (AA and

SAA) protein in the mouse. Journal of Immunology 121: 138–140
Gorevic P D, Cleveland A B, Franklin E C 1982 The biological significance of amyloid. Annals of the New York Academy of Science 389: 380–393
Greenwald M, Kedar I, Sohar E 1980 The effect of colchicine and dimethylsulfoxide (DMSO) on the genetic amyloidosis of the white Pekin duck. In: Glenner G G, Pinho e Costa P, Falcao de Freitas A (eds) Amyloid and amyloidosis. Excerpta Medica, Amsterdam, p 584–586
Greipp P R, Kyle R A, Bowie E J W 1981 Factor X deficiency in amyloidosis: a critical review. American Journal of Haematology 11: 443–450
Gudmundsson G, Hallgrimsson J, Jonasson T A, Bjarnason O 1972 Hereditary cerebral haemorrhage with amyloidosis. Brain 95: 387–404
Hanai N, Ishihara T, Uchino F, Imada N, Fujihara S, Ikegami J 1979 Effects of dimethyl sulfoxide and colchicine on the resorption of experimental amyloid. Virchows Archiv Abteilung A, Pathologische Anatomie 384: 45–52
Harrington T M, Moran J J, Davis D E 1981 Amyloidosis in adult onset Still's disease. Journal of Rheumatology 8: 833–836
Hashimoto S, Migita S 1979 Changes of thirty-nine serum protein components following surgical stress. Nippon Ketsucki Gakkai Zasshi 42: 667–677
Hermodson M A, Kuhn R W, Walsh K A, Neurath H, Eriksen N, Benditt E P 1972 Amino acid sequence of monkey amyloid protein A. Biochemistry 11: 2934–2938
Hickling P et al 1981 A study of amyloid arthropathy in multiple myeloma. Quarterly Journal of Medicine 50: 417–433
Hijmans W, Sipe J D 1979 Levels of the serum amyloid A protein (SAA) in normal persons of different age groups. Clinical and Experimental Immunology 35: 96–100
Hind C R K, Collins P M, Pepys M B 1983a Ligand specificity of serum amyloid P component. Clinical Science 65:17P
Hind C R K, Tennent G A, Evans D J, Pepys M B 1983b Demonstration of amyloid A (AA) protein and amyloid P component (AP) in deposits of systemic amyloidosis associated with renal adenocarcinoma. Journal of Pathology 139: 159–166
Hoffman J S, Benditt E P 1982a Changes in high density lipoprotein content following endotoxin administration in the mouse. Journal of Biological Chemistry 257: 10 510–10 517
Hoffman J S, Benditt E P 1982b Secretion of serum amyloid protein and assembly of serum amyloid protein-rich high density lipoprotein in primary mouse hepatocyte culture. Journal of Biological Chemistry 257: 10518–10522
Hoffman J S, Benditt E P 1983 Plasma clearance kinetics of the amyloid-related high density lipoprotein apoprotein, serum amyloid protein (apoSAA), in the mouse. Evidence for rapid apoSAA clearance. Journal of Clinical Investigation 71: 926–934
Houser M T, Scheinman J I, Basgen J, Steffes M W, Michael A F 1982 Preservation of mesangium and immunohistochemically defined antigens in glomerular basement membrane isolated by detergent extraction. Journal of Clinical Investigation 69: 1169–1175
Husby G, Sletten K 1980 The structure of amyloid proteins. In: Glenner G G, Pinho e Costa P, Falcao de Freitas A (eds) Amyloid and amyloidosis. Excerpta Medica, Amsterdam, p 266–273
Huston D P, McAdam K P W J, Balow J E, Bass R, de Lellis R A 1981 Amyloidosis in systemic lupus erythematosus. American Journal of Medicine 70: 320–323
Ignaczak T F 1981 Amyloidosis. In: Kelley W N, Harris E D, Ruddy S, Sledge C B (eds) Textbook of rheumatology. Saunders, Philadelphia, Ch 92 p 1511–1530
Ignaczak T F, Sipe J D, Linke R P, Glenner G G 1977 Immunochemical studies on the nature of the serum component (SAA) related to secondary amyloidosis. Journal of Laboratory and Clinical Medicine 89: 1092–1104
Isobe T, Osserman E F 1976 Effects of dimethyl sulfoxide (DMSO) on Bence-Jones proteins, amyloid fibrils and casein-induced amyloidosis. In: Wegelius O, Pasternack A (eds) Amyloidosis. Academic Press, London p 247–257
Isobe T, Husby G, Sletten K 1980 Characterisation of amyloid protein AA similar to SAA. In: Glenner G G, Pinho e Costa P, Falcao de Freitas A (eds) Amyloid and amyloidosis. Excerpta Medica, Amsterdam, p 331–336
Jacob E T, Bar-Nathan N, Shapira Z, Gafni J 1979 Renal transplanation in the amyloidosis of familial Mediterranean fever. Experience of ten cases. Archives of Internal Medicine 139: 1135–1138
Jayson M I V, Salmon P R, Harrison W 1971 Amyloidosis in ankylosing spondylitis. Rheumatology and Physical Medicine 11: 78–82
Jensson O, Bjornsson O G, Arnason A, Birgisdottir B, Pepys M B 1982 Serum amyloid P-component and C-reactive protein in serum of healthy Icelanders and members of an Icelandic family with macroglobulinaemia. Acta Medica Scandinavica 211: 341–345
Johnston J B, Rayner H L, Travenen L, Greenberg D 1982 Skeletal muscle uptake of Tc 99m pyrophosphate in amyloidosis. American Journal of Haematology 13: 247–251
Jones N F 1976 Renal amyloidosis: pathogenesis and therapy. Clinical Nephrology 6: 459–464
Jones N F 1981 Renal amyloidosis. Journal of Clinical Pathology 34: 1228–1232
Kampschmidt R F, Upchurch H F, Pulliam L A 1982 Characterisation of a leukocyte-derived endogenous mediator responsible for increased plasma fibrinogen. Annals of New York Academy of Science 389: 338–351
Kedar (Keizman) I, Ravid M, Sohar E, Gafni J 1974 Colchicine inhibition of casein-induced amyloidosis in mice. Israel Journal of Medical Science 10: 787–789
Kedar I, Ravid M, Sohar E 1980 Amyloid degrading activity of human serum. In: Glenner G G, Pinho e Costa P, Falcao de Freitas A (eds) Amyloid and amyloidosis. Excerpta Medica, Amsterdam, p 60–62
Kedar I, Sohar E, Ravid M 1982 Degradation of amyloid by a serum component and inhibition of degradation. A dynamic concept of amyloid deposition. Journal of Laboratory and Clinical Medicine 99: 693–700
Kennedy A L, Burton J A, Allison M E M 1974 Tuberculosis as a continuing cause of renal amyloidosis. British Medical Journal 3: 795–797
Kimball K G 1961 Amyloidosis in association with neoplastic disease: report of an unusual case and clinicopathological experience at Memorial Center for Cancer and Allied Diseases during eleven years (1948–1959). Annals of Internal Medicine 55: 958–974

Kisilevsky R, Bondreau L, Foster D 1983 Kinetics of amyloid deposition. II. The effects of dimethylsufoxide and colchicine therapy. Laboratory Investigation 48: 60–67
Kobayashi H, Hashimoto K 1981 Antigenic identity of amyloid in localised cutaneous amyloidosis with keratin. Journal of Investigative Dermatology 76:320
Kula R W, Engel W K, Line B R 1977 Scanning for soft-tissue amyloid. Lancet 1: 92–93
Kyle R A, Greipp R R 1978 Primary systemic amyloidosis: comparison of melphelan and prednisone versus placebo. Blood 52: 818–827
Kyle R A, Wagoner R D, Holley K E 1982 Primary systemic amyloidosis. Resolution of the nephrotic syndrome with melphelan and prednisolone. Archives of Internal Medicine 142: 1445–1447
Ladefoged C 1982 Amyloid deposits in human hip joints. Acta Pathologica et Microbiologica et Immunologica Scandinavica, Section A, 90: 5–10
Lanham J G, Meltzer M L, de Beer F C, Hughes G R V, Pepys M B 1982 Familial amyloidosis of Ostertag. Quarterly Journal of Medicine 51: 25–32
Lavie G, Zucker-Franklin D, Franklin E C 1978 Degradation of serum amyloid A protein by surface-associated enzymes of human blood monocytes. Journal of Experimental Medicine 148: 1020–1031
Lavie G, Franklin E C, Zucher-Franklin D 1980 Characterisation of a series of elastase-like serine proteases of human peripheral blood monocytes that degrade SAA. In: Glenner G G, Pinho e Costa P, Falcao de Freitas A (eds) Amyloid and amyloidosis. Excerpta Medica, Amsterdam, p 448–455
Lavie G, Zucker-Franklin D, Franklin E C 1980 Elastase-type proteases on the surface of human blood monocytes: possible role in amyloid formation. Journal of Immunology 125:175–180
Lender M, Wolf E 1972 Incidence of amyloidosis in rheumatoid arthritis. Scandinavian Journal of Rheumatology 1: 109–112
Levin M, Franklin E C, Frangione B, Pras M 1972 The amino acid sequence of a major non-immunoglobulin component of some amyloid fibrils. Journal of Clinical Investigation 51: 2773–2776
Levin M, Pras M, Franklin E C 1973 Immunologic studies of the major non-immunoglobulin protein of amyloid. I. Identification and partial characterisation of a related serum component. Journal of Experimental Medicine 138: 373–380
Levo Y, Shalev O, Rosenmann E, Eliakim M 1980 Gout and amyloidosis. Annals of the Rheumatic Diseases 39: 589–591
Lichtenstein H L, Lee J C K 1980 Amyloidosis associated with metastasizing basal cell carcinoma. Cancer 46: 2693–2696
Liebman H, Chinowsky M, Valdin J, Kenoyer G, Feinstein D 1983 Increased fibrinolysis and amyloidosis. Archives of Internal Medicine 143: 678–682
Linder E, Lehto V P, Virtanen I, Stenman S, Natvig J B 1977 Localisation of amyloid-related serum protein SAA-like material to intermediate (10 nm) filaments of cultured human embryonal fibroblasts. Journal of Experimental Medicine 146: 1158–1163
Linder J, Silberman H R, Croher B P 1982 Amyloidosis complicating hairy cell leukaemia. American Journal of Clinical Pathology 78: 864–867
Linke R P, Nathrath W B J 1982 Immunochemical typing of amyloid from tissue biopsies. Acta Histochemica, Suppl Band XXV, S: 89–93
Linke R P, Zucker-Franklin D, Franklin E C 1973 Morphologic, chemical and immunologic studies of amyloid-like fibrils formed from Bence-Jones proteins by proteolysis. Journal of Immunology 111: 10–23
Linke R P, Sipe J D, Pollack P S, Ignaczak T F, Glenner G G 1975 Isolation of a low molecular weight serum component antigenetically related to an amyloid fibril protein of unknown origin. Proceedings of the National Academy of Science USA 72: 1473–1476
Livni N, Laufer A, Levo Y 1980 Demonstration of amyloid in murine and human secondary amyloidosis by the immunoperoxidase technique. Journal of Pathology 132: 343–348
Liu T-Y, Robey F A, Wang C M 1982 Structural studies on C-reactive protein. Annals of the New York Academy of Science 389: 151–161
Lowenstein J, Gallo G 1970 Remission of the nephrotic syndrome in renal amyloidosis. New England Journal of Medicine 282: 128–132
McAdam K P W J, Dinarello C A 1980 Induction of serum amyloid A synthesis by human leukocyte pyrogen. In: Agarwal M K (ed) Bacterial endotoxin and host response. Elseiver, Amsterdam, p 167–178
McAdam K P W J, Anders R F, Smith S R, Russell D A, Price M A 1975 Association of amyloidosis with erythema nodosum leprosum reactions and recurrent neutrophil leucocytosis in leprosy. Lancet 2: 572–576
McAdam K P W J, Elin R J, Sipe J D, Wolff S M 1978 Changes in human serum amyloid A and C-reactive protein following etiocholanolone inflammation. Journal of Clinical Investigation 61: 390–394
McAdam K P W J et al 1982 The biology of SAA: identification of the inducer, in vitro synthesis and heterogeneity demonstrated with monoclonal antibodies. Annals of the New York Academy of Science 389: 126–136
MacDonald D M, Fergin P E, Black M M 1980 Localised cutaneous amyloidosis. A clinical review of 100 cases including immunofluorescent studies. In: Glenner G G, Pinho e Costa P, Falcao de Freitas A (eds) Amyloid and amyloidosis. Excerpta Medica, Amsterdam, p 239
McPherson R A et al 1977 Coagulopathy in amyloidosis: combined deficiency of factors IX and X. American Journal of Haematology 3: 225–235
Maddison P J, Bacon P A, Strachan A F, Tribe C R 1983 A marked deficiency of amyloid degrading factor is associated with a poor prognosis in secondary amyloidosis. In: Tribe C R, Bacon P A (eds) Amyloidosis EARS. Wright, Bristol, p. 124–127
Malmendier C L, Christophe J, Ameryckx J P 1979 Separation and partial characterisation of new apoproteins from human plasma high density lipoproteins. Clinica Chimica Acta 99: 167–176
Marhaug C, Husby G 1981 Characterisation of human amyloid-related protein SAA as a polymorphic protein: association with albumin and prealbumin in serum. Clinical and Experimental Immunology 45: 97–106
Marhaug G, Sletten K, Husby G 1980 Primary structure of human amyloid-related serum protein SAA. In: Glenner G G, Pinho e Costa P, Falcao de Freitas A (eds) Amyloid and amyloidosis. Excerpta Medica, Amsterdam, p 337–342
Marhaug G, Sletten K, Husby G 1982 Characterisation of

amyloid-related protein SAA complexed with serum lipoprotein (apoSAA). Clinical and Experimental Immunology 50: 382–389

Marhaug G, Sletten K, Husby G 1983 Studies of SAA and AA-like protein fragment in serum. In: Tribe C R, Bacon P A (eds) Amyloidosis EARS. Wright, Bristol, p. 15–18

Masters C L, Gajdusek D C, Gibbs C J Jr 1981 Creutzfeldt–Jacob disease virus isolations from the Gerstmann–Strausler syndrome with an analysis of the various forms of amyloid plaque deposition in the virus-induced spongiform encephalopathies. Brain 104: 559–588

Masu S, Hosokawa M, Seiji M 1980 Immunofluorescence studies on cutaneous amyloidosis with anti-keratin antibody. Tohoku Journal of Experimental Medicine 132: 121–122

Maury C P J, Teppo A M 1982 Mechanism of reduced amyloid A-degrading activity in serum of patients with secondary amyloidosis. Lancet 2: 234–237

Miller L D, Brown E C, Arnett F C 1979 Amyloidosis in Reiter's syndrome. Journal of Rheumatology 6: 225–231

Mountjoy C Q, Tomlinson B E, Gibson P H 1982 Amyloid and senile plaques and cerebral blood vessels. A semi-quantitative investigation of a possible relationship. Journal of Neurological Science 57: 89–103

Natvig J B, Westermark P, Sletten K, Husby G, Michnelsen T 1981 Further structural and antigenic studies of light chain amyloid patients. Scandinavian Journal of Immunology 14: 89–94

Noren P, Westermark P, Cornwell G G, Murdoch W 1983 Immunofluorescence and histochemical studies of localised cutaneous amyloidosis. British Journal of Dermatology 108: 277–285

Ogg C S, Cameron J S, Williams D G, Turner D R 1981 Presentation and course of primary amyloidosis of the kidney. Clinical Nephrology 15: 9–13

Okoye M I, Watanabe I 1982 Ultrastructural features of cerebral amyloid angiopathy. Human Pathology 13: 1127–1132

Oppenheim J J, Gery I 1982 Interleukin 1 is more than an interleukin. Immunology Today 3: 113–119

Orfila C, Rakotarivony J, Segonds A, Suc J M 1982 Immunofluorescence study of amyloid P-component patterns in human nephropathies. Histochemistry 74: 347–354

Osmand A P, Friedenson B, Gewurz H, Painter R H, Hofmann T, Shelton E 1977 Characterisation of C-reactive protein and the complement subcomponent Clt as homologous proteins displaying cyclic pentameric symmetry (pentraxins). Proceedings of the National of the National Academy of Science USA 74: 739–743

Osserman E F, Isobe T, Farhangi M 1976 Effect of dimethyl sulfoxide (DMSO) in the treatment of amyloidosis. In: Wegelius O, Pasternack A (eds) Amyloidosis. Academic Press, London, p 553–564

Osserman E F, Sherman W H, Kyle R A 1980 Further studies of therapy of amyloidosis with dimethyl sulfoxide (DMSO). In: Glenner G G, Pinho e Costa P, Falcao de Freitas A (eds) Amyloid and amyloidosis. Excerpta Medica, Amsterdam, p 563–569

Painter R H, de Escallon I, Massey A, Pinteric L, Stern S B 1982 The structure and binding characteristics of serum amyloid protein (9.5S α 1-glycoprotein). Annals of New York Academy of Science 389: 199–213

Paraf A, Caste T, Rautureau J 1970 La regression de l'amylose. Disparition d'une amylose hepatique massive apres nephrectomie pour cancer. Presse Medicale 78: 547–548

Parmelee D C, Titani K, Ericsson L H, Eriksen N, Benditt E P, Walsh K A 1982 Amino acid sequence of amyloid-related apoprotein ($apoSAA_1$) from human high density lipoprotein. Biochemistry 21: 3298–3303

Pepys M B 1982 C-reactive protein, amyloidosis and the cute phase response. The Goulstonian Lecture. In: Sarner M (ed) Advanced Medicine 18. Pitman, Tunbridge Wells, p 208–230

Pepys M B, Baltz M L 1983 Acute phase proteins with special reference to C-reactive protein and related proteins (pentaxins) and serum amyloid A protein. Advances in Immunology 34: 141–212

Pepys M B et al 1977 Isolation of amyloid P-component (protein AP) from normal serum as a calcium-dependent binding protein. Lancet 1: 1029–1031

Pepys M B, Dash A C, Markham P E, Thomas H C, Williams B D, Petrie A 1978b Comparative clinical study of protein SAP (amploid P-component) and C-reactive protein in serum. Clinical and Experimental Immunology 32: 119–124

Pepys M B, Dash A C, Fletcher T C, Richardson N, Munn E A, Feinstein A 1978a Analogues in other mammals and in fish of human plasma proteins C-reactive protein and amyloid P-component. Nature 273: 168–170

Pepys M B, Baltz M, Gomer K, Davies A J S, Doenhoff M 1979 Serum amyloid P-component is an acute phase reactant in the mouse. Nature 278: 259–261

Pepys M B, Dyck R F, de Beer F C, Skinner M, Cohen A S 1979 Binding of serum amyloid P-component (SAP) by amyloid fibrils. Clinical and Experimental Immunology 38: 284–293

Pepys M B et al 1982 Biology of serum amyloid. P component. Annals of the New York Academy of Science 389: 286–297

Pick A I, Frohlichmann R, Lavie G, Duczyminer M, Skvaril F 1981 Clinical and haematological studies of 20 patients with amyloidosis and plasma cell dyscrasia. Acta Haematologica 66: 154–167

Pinteric L, Painter R H 1979 Electron microscopy of serum amyloid protein in the presence of calcium: alternative forms of assembly of pentagonal molecules in two-dimensional lattices. Canadian Journal of Biochemistry 57: 727–736

Pinteric L, Assimeh S N, Kells D I C, Painter R H 1976 The utrastructure of Clt, a subcomponent of the first component of complement: an EM and ultracentrifuge study. Journal of Immunology 117: 79–83

Pitkanen P, Westermark P, Cornwell G G, Murdoch W 1983 Amyloid of the seminal vesicles. A distinctive and common localised form of senile amyloidosis. American Journal of Pathology 110: 64–69

Pras M, Franklin E C, Shibolet S, Frangione B 1982 Amyloidosis associated with renal cell carcinoma of the AA type. American Journal of Medicine 73: 426–428

Pras M, Franklin E C, Prelli F, Frangione B 1981 A variant of prealbumin from amyloid fibrils in familial polyneuropathy of Jewish origin. Journal of Experimental Medicine 154: 989–993

Pras M, Bronshpigel N, Zemer D, Gafni J 1982a Variable incidence of amyloidosis in familial Mediterranean fever among different ethnic groups. Johns Hopkins Medical Journal 150: 22–26

Puchtler H, Sweat F, Levine M 1962 On the binding of Congo red by amyloid. Journal of Histochemistry and Cytochemistry 10: 355–364
Qureshi M S A, Sandle G I, Kelly J K, Fox H 1977 Amyloidosis complicating psoriatic arthritis. British Medical Journal 2:302
Rao B K, Padmalatha C, Buchon J A, Lieberman L M 1981 Hepatic and splenic scintigraphy in idiopathic systemic amyloidosis. European Journal of Nuclear Medicine 6: 143–165
Rashid H, Blake D, Gokal R, Gooptu D, Kerr D N S 1980 The association of renal amyloidosis with regional enteritis (Crohn's disease) — report of two cases and review of the literature. Clinical Nephrology 14: 154–157
Ravid M, Kedar I 1980 Prolonged dimethylsulfoxide treatment of systemic amyloidosis in man. In: Glenner G G, Pinho e Costa P, Falcao de Freitas A (eds) Amyloid and amyloidosis. Excerpta Medica, Amsterdam, p 578–579
Ravid M, Robson M, Kedar I 1977 Prolonged colchicine treatment in four patients with amyloidosis. Annals of Internal Medicine 87: 568–570
Ravid M, Shapira J, Lang R, Kedar I 1982 Prolonged dimethylsulfoxide treatment in 13 patients with systemic amyloidosis. Annals of the Rheumatic Diseases 41: 587–592
Rizvi S N A, Gulati P D, Vaishnava H 1974 Tuberculosis and renal amyloidosis. British Medical Journal 4:657
Robey F A, Liu T-Y 1981 Limulin: a C-reactive protein from *Limulus polyphemus*. Journal of Biological Chemistry 256: 969–975
Robey F A, Tanaha T, Liu T-Y 1983 Isolation and characterisation of two major serum proteins from the dogfish, *Mustelus canis*, C-reactive protein and amyloid P-component. Journal of Biological Chemistry 258: 3889–3894
Rosenstein E D, Itzkowitz S H, Penziner A S, Cohen J I, Mornaghi R A 1983 Resolution of factor X deficiency in primary amyloidosis following splenectomy. Archives of Internal Medicine 143: 597–599
Rosenthal C J, Franklin E C 1975 Variation with age and disease of an amyloid A protein-related serum component. Journal of Clinical Investigation 55: 746–753
Rosenthal C J, Franklin E C 1977 Serum amyloid A (SAA) protein — interaction with itself and serum albumin. Journal of Immunology 119: 630–634
Rosenthal C J, Sullivan L 1978 Serum amyloid A. Evidence for its origin in polymorphonuclear leukocytes. Journal of Clinical Investigation 62: 1181–1186
Rosenthal T, Weiss P, Gafni J 1978 Renal involvement in Behcet's syndrome. Archives of Internal Medicine 138: 1122–1124
Rubies-Prat J, de la Figuera M, Obiols G, Guardia J 1982 Amyloidose systemique compliquant un syndrome de Behcet. La Nouvelle Presse Medicale 11:2636
Rubinow A, Sonnenblick M 1981 Amyloidosis secondary to polyarticular gout. Arthritis and Rheumatism 24: 1425–1427
Rubinow A, Skinner M, Cohen A S 1981 Digoxin sensitivity in amyloid cardiomyopathy. Circulation 63: 1285–1288
Schiff S, Bateman T, Moffatt R, Davidson R, Berman D 1982 Diagnostic considerations in cardiomyopathy: unique scintigraphic pattern of diffuse biventricular technetium-99 m-pyrophosphate uptake in amyloid heart disease. American Heart Journal 103: 562–563
Schmidt M B 1859 Ueber das sogenannte 'thierische amyloid' (Substanz der corpuscula amylacea). Annalen der Chemie und Pharmacie 110: 250–255
Schnitzer T J, Ansell B M 1977 Amyloidosis in juvenile chronic polyarthritis. Arthritis and Rheumatism 20: 245–252
Schroeder J S, Billingham M E, Rider A K 1975 Cardiac amyloidosis: diagnosis by transvenous endomyocardial biopsy. American Journal of Medicine 59: 269–273
Schwabe A D, Peters R S 1974 Familial Mediterranean fever in Armenians. Analysis of 200 cases. Medicine 53: 453–462
Sear H J, Grant M E, Jackson D S 1981 The nature of the microfibrillar glycoproteins of elastic fibres. A biosynthetic study. Biochemistry Journal 194: 587–598
Segrest J P, Feldman R J 1977 Amphipathic helixes and plasma lipoproteins: a computer study. Biopolymers 16: 2053–2065
Segrest J P, Pownall H J, Jackson R L, Glenner G G, Pollock P S 1976 Amyloid A: amphipathic helices and lipid binding. Biochemistry 15: 3187–3191
Selinger M J, McAdam K P W J, Kaplan M M, Sipe J D, Rosenstreich D, Vogel S N 1980a In-vitro production of SAA by mouse hepatocytes. In: Glenner G G, Pinho e Costa P, Falcao de Freitas A (eds) Amyloid and amyloidosis. Excerpta Medica, Amsterdam p 486–490
Selinger M J, McAdam K W P J, Kaplan M M, Sipe J D, Vogel S N, Rosenstreich D L 1980b Monokine induced synthesis of serum amyloid A protein by heptocytes. Nature (Lond) 285: 498–500
Sharma S C, Mortimer G, Kennedy S, Thomson J 1983 Secondary amyloidosis affecting the skin in arthropathic psoriasis. British Journal of Dermatology 108: 205–210
Shirahama T, Cohen A S 1967 Fine structure of the glomerulus in human and experimental renal amyloidosis. American Journal of Pathology 51: 869–911
Shirahama T, Cohen A S 1974 Blockage of amyloid induction by colchicine in an animal model. Journal of Experimental Medicine 14: 1102–1107
Shirahama T, Cohen A S 1980 Redistribution of amyloid deposits. American Journal of Pathology 99: 539–550
Shirahama T, Cohen A S, Rodgers O G 1971 Phagocytosis of amyloid: in-vitro interaction of mouse peritoneal macrophages with human amyloid fibrils and their accelerated uptake after dye binding. Experimental and Molecular Pathology 14: 110–123
Shirahama T, Benson M D, Cohen A S, Tanaka A 1973 Fibrillar assemblage of variable segments of immunoglobulin light chains: an electron microscopic study. Journal of Immunology 110: 21–30
Shirahama T, Cohen A S, Rubinow A, Rodgers O G 1980 Ultrastructure of skin biopsies from patients with heredofamilial amyloid polyneuropathy. In: Glenner G G, Pinho e Costa P, Falcao de Freitas A (eds) Amyloid and amyloidosis. Excerpta Medica, Amsterdam p 132–138
Shirahama T, Skinner M, Cohen A S 1981 Immunocytochemical identification of amyloid in formalin-fixed paraffin sections. Histochemistry 72: 161–171
Shirahama T, et al 1982 Senile cerebral amyloid. Prealbumin as a common constituent in the neuritic plaque, in the neurofibrillary tangle, and in the microangiopathic lesion. American Journal of Pathology 107: 41–50
Shoji S, Kameko M, Tsukada N, Kato M 1981 Immunologic and immunohistochemical study of familial amyloid polyneuropathy. Neurology 31: 1493–1496

Shore V G, Shore B, Lewis S B 1978 Isolation and characterisation of two threonine-poor apoliproteins of human plasma high density lipoproteins. Biochemistry 17: 2174–2179
Shorvon P J 1977 Amyloidosis and inflammatory bowel disease. Digestive Diseases 22: 209–213
Silverman S L, Cathcart E S, Skinner M, Cohen A S, Burnett L 1980 A pathogenetic role for polymorphonuclear leukocytes in the synthesis and degradation of SAA protein. In: Glenner G G, Pinho e Costa P, Falcao de Freitas A (eds) Amyloid and amyloidosis. Excerpta Medica, Amsterdam, p 420–425
Silverman S L, Cathcart E S, Skinner M, Cohen A S 1982 The degradation of serum amyloid A protein by activated polymorphonuclear leucoytes: participation of granulocyte elastase. Immunology 46: 737–744
Sipe J D, Rosenstreich D L 1981 Serum factors associated with inflammation. In: Oppenheim J J, Rosenstreich D L, Potter M (eds) Cellular functions in immunity and inflammation. Elsevier/North Holland, New York, p 411–329
Sipe J D, Ignaczak T F, Pollock P S, Glenner G G 1976 Amyloid fibril protein AA: purification and properties of the antigenically related serum component as determined by solid phase radioimmunoassy. Journal of Immunology 116: 1151–1156
Sipe J D, Vogel S N, Ryan J L, McAdam K P W J, Rosenstreich D L 1979 Detection of a mediator derived from endotoxin-stimulated macrophages that induces the acute phase serum amyloid A response in mice. Journal of Experimental Medicine 150: 597–606
Skinner M, Cohen A S 1976 Aspects of the amyloid P component. In: Wegelius O, Pasternack O (eds) Amyloidosis. Academic Press, London, p 339–352
Skinner M, Cohen A S 1981 The prealbumin nature of the amyloid protein in familial amyloid polyneuropathy (FAP) — Swedish variety. Biochemical and Biophysical Research Communications 99: 1326–1332
Skinner M, Cathcart E S, Cohen A S, Benson M D 1974 Isolation and identification by sequence analysis of experimental induced guinea pig amyloid fibrils. Journal of Experimental Medicine 140: 871–876
Skinner M, Pepys M B, Cohen A S, Heller L M, Lian J B 1980 Studies of amyloid protein AP. In: Glenner G G, Pinho e Costa P, de Freitas F (eds) Amyloid and amyloidosis. Excerpta Medica, Amsterdam, p 384–391
Skogen B, Natvig J B 1981 Degradation of amyloid proteins by different serine proteases. Scandinavian Journal of Immunology 14: 389–396
Skogen B, Borresen A L, Natvig J B, Berg K, Michaelsen T E 1979 High density lipoprotein as a carrier for amyloid related SAA in rabbit serum. Scandinavian Journal of Immunology 10: 39–45
Skogen B, Sletten K, Lea T, Natvig J B 1983 Heterogeneity of human amyloid protein AA and its related serum protein SAA. Scandinavian Journal of Immunology 17: 83–88
Sletten K, Husby G 1974 The complete amino acid sequence of non-immuoglobulin amyloid fibril protein AS in rheumatoid arthritis. European Journal of Biochemistry 41: 117–125
Sletten K, Westermark P, Natvig J B 1976 Characterisation of amyloid fibril proteins from medullary carcinoma of the thyroid. Journal of Experimental Medicine 143: 993–998
Sletten K, Westermark P, Natvig J B 1980 Senile cardiac amyloid is related to prealbumin. Scandinavian Journal of Immunology 12: 503–506
Sletten K, Natvig J B, Husby G, Juul J 1981 The complete amino acid sequence of a prototype immunoglobulin-λ light-chain-type amyloid fibril protein AR. Biochemistry Journal 195: 561–572
Sobol S M, Brown J M, Bunker S R, Patel J, Lull R J 1982 Non-invasive diagnosis of cardiac amyloidosis by technetium-99m-pyrophosphate myocardial scintigraphy. American Heart Journal 103: 563–566
Sohar E, Gafni J, Pras M, Heller H 1967 Familial Mediterranean fever. A survey of 470 cases and review of the literature. American Journal of Medicine 43: 227–253
Solomon A, Frangione B, Franklin E C 1982 Bence Jones proteins and light chains of immunoglobulins. Preferential association of Vλ VI subgroup of human light chains with amyloidosis AL λ. Journal of Clinical Investigation 70: 453–460
Sommer T, Teppo L 1976 Hypernephroma and amyloidosis. In: Wegelius O, Pasternack A (eds) Amyloidosis. Academic Press, New York, p 455–470
Sorensen K H, Teglbjaerg P S, Ladefoged C, Christensen H E 1981 Pyrophosphate arthritis with local amyloid deposition. Acta Orthopaedica Scandinavica 52: 129–133
Stearman R S, Lowell C A, Pearson W R, Morrow J F 1982 Regulation of synthesis of amyloid A-related protein. Annals of the New York Academy of Science 389: 106–115
Strachan A F, Johnson P M 1982 Protein SAP (serum amyloid P component) in Waldenstrom's macroglobulineamia, multiple myeloma and rheumatic disease. Journal of Clinical and Laboratory Immunology 8: 153–156
Sutton M G St J, Reichek N, Kastor J A, Giuliani E R 1982 Computerised M-mode echocardiographic anaylsis of left ventricular dysfunction in cardiac amyloid. Circulation 66: 790–799
Suzuki T et al 1981 Orthostatic hypotension in familial amyloid polyneuropathy: treatment with DL-Threo-3, 4-dihydroxyphenylserine. Neurology 31: 1323–1326
Suzuki T et al 1982 Pharmacohiretic studies of oral L-Threo-3, 4-dihydroxy phenylserine in normal subjects and patients with familial amyloid polyneuropathy. European Journal of Clinical Pharmacology 23: 463–468
Sweet J, Bear R A, Lang A P 1981 Amyloidosis and systemic lupus erythematosus. Human Pathology 12: 853–856
Sztein M B et al 1981 The role of macrophages in the acute phase response: SAA inducer is closely related to lymphocyte activating factor and endogenous pyrogen. Cellular Immunology 63: 164–171
Tatsuta E, Shirahama T, Sipe J D, Skinner M, Cohen A S 1982 Kinetics of SAP and SAA production by cultured mouse liver cells. Annals of the New York Academy of Science 389: 467–470
Tatsuta E, Sipe J D, Shirahama T, Skinner M, Cohen A S 1983 Different regulatory mechanisms for serum amyloid A and serum amyloid P synthesis by cultured mouse hepatocytes. Journal of Biological Chemistry 258: 5414–5418
Tawara S, Araki S, Toshimori K, Nakagawa H, Ohtaki S 1981 Amyloid fibril protein in type I familial amyloidotic polyneuropathy in Japanese. Journal of Laboratory and Clinical Medicine 98: 811–822
Teppo A M, Maury C P J, Wegelius O 1982 Characteristics of the amyloid A fibril-degrading activity of human serum. Scandinanvian Journal of Immunology 16: 309–314

Tobias P S, McAdam K P W J, Ulevitch R J 1982 Interactions of bacterial lipopolysaccharide with acute phase rabbit serum and isolation of two forms of rabbit serum amyloid A. Journal of Immunology 128: 1420–1427
Tribe C R 1966 Amyloidosis in rheumatoid arthritis. In: Hill A G S (ed) Modern trends in rheumatology. Butterworths, London, p 121–138
Tribe C R, MacKenzie J C 1982 Amyloidosis. In: Bacon P A, Hadlen N M (eds) The kidney and rheumatic disease. Butterworths, London, p 297–322
Tribe C R, Perry V A 1979 Diagnosis of amyloidosis. Association of Clinical Pathologists (London), Broadsheet 92
Ulevitch R J, Johnston A R, Weinstein D B 1979 New function for high density lipoproteins. Their participation in intravascular reactions of bacterial lipopolysaccharides. Journal of Clinical Investigation 64: 1516–1524
Ulevitch R J, Johnston A R, Weinstein D B 1981 New function for high density lipoproteins. Isolation and characterisation of a bacterial lipopolysaccharide-high density lipoprotein complex formed in rabbit plasma. Journal of Clinical Investigation 67: 827–837
Urry D W 1974 Studies on the conformation and interaction of elastin. In: Wagner W D, Clarkson T B (eds) Arterial mesenchyme and arteriosclerosis. Advances in Experimental and Medical Biology 43: 211–243
van Rijswijk M H 1981 Amyloidosis. Drukkerig van Denderen B V, Groningen
van Rijswijk M H, van Heusden C W G J 1979 The potassium permanganate method. American Journal of Pathology 97: 43–54
van Rijswijk M H, et al 1980 Successful treatment with dimethylsulphoxide of human amyloidosis secondary to rheumatoid arthritis. In: Glenner G G, Pinho e Costa P, Falcao de Freitas A (eds) Amyloid and amyloidosis. Excerpta Medica, Amsterdam, p 570–577
van Rijswijk M H, et al 1983 DMSO and prednisolone in the treatment of systemic AA amyloidosis. In: Tribe C R, Bacon P A (eds) Amyloidosis EARS. Wright, Bristol, p. 108–115
Vanatta P R, Silva F G, Taylor W E, Costa J C 1983 Renal cell carcinoma and systemic amyloidosis: demonstration of AA protein and review of the literature. Human Pathology 14: 195–201
Vanley C T, Aguilar M J, Kleinherz R J, Lagios M D 1981 Cerebral amyloid angiopathy. Human Pathology 12: 609–616
Virchow R 1854 Uber eine im Gehirn und Ruckenmark des Menschen aufgefundene Substanz mit der chemischen Reaction der Cellulose. Vichows Archives Pathologische Anatomie 6: 135–138
Waalen K, Sletten K, Husby G, Nordstoga K 1980 The primary structure of amyloid fibril protein AA in endotoxin-induced amyloidosis of the mink. European Journal of Biochemistry 104: 407–412
Walker F, Bear R A 1982 Long term colchicine therapy for renal amyloidosis in familial Mediterranean fever. Canadian Medical Assoication Journal 127: 1163–1164
Walton A G, Blackwell J 1973 Biopolymers. Academic Press, New York
Wattendorf A R, Bots G T A M, Went L N, Erdtz L J 1982 Familial cerebral amyloid angiopathy presenting as recurrent cerebral haemorrhage. Journal of Neurological Science 55: 121–135
Wegelius O, Teppo A M, Maury C P J 1982 Reduced amyloid A-degrading activity in serum in amyloidosis associated with rheumatoid arthritis. British Medical Journal 1: 617–619
Wegelius O, Wafin F, Falck H M, Tornroth T 1980 Follow-up study of amyloidosis secondary to rheumatic disease. In: Glenner G G, Pinho e Costa P, Falcao de Freitas A (eds) Amyloid and amyloidosis. Excerpta Medica, Amsterdam, p 183–190
Westermark P 1982 The heterogeneity of protein AA in secondary (reactive) systemic amyloidosis. Biochimica Biophysica Acta 701: 19–23
Westermark P, Stenkuist B 1973 A new method for the diagnosis of systemic amyloidosis. Archives of Internal Medicine 132: 522–523
Westermark P, et al 1977 Amyloid in polypeptide hormone-producing tumours. Laboratory Investigation 37: 212–215
Wheeler G E, Eiferman R A 1983 Immuno histochemical identification of the AA protein in lattice dystrophy. Experimental Eye Research 36: 181–186
Wille L E, Olsen E, Forre O, Sletten K, Jentoft H 1980 Demonstration and partial characterisation of an atypical protein in the urine of a patient with primary amyloidosis. Acta Medica Scandinavica 208: 177–182
Williams G 1967 Histological studies in resorption of experimental amyloid. Journal of Pathology and Bacteriology 94: 331–336
Williams R C Jr, Cathcart E S, Calkins E, Fite G L, Rubio J B, Cohen A S 1965 Secondary amyloidosis in lepromatosis leprosy. Possible relationship of diet and environment. Annals of Internal Medicine 62: 1000–1007
Wizenberg T A, Muz J, Sohn Y H, Samtowski W, Weissler A M 1982 Value of positive myocardial technetium-99m-pyrophosphate scintigraphy in the non-invasive diagnosis of cardiac amyloidosis. American Heart Journal 107: 468–473
Wright J R, Calkins E, Humphrey R L 1977 Potassium permanganate reaction in amyloidosis. A histologic method to assist in differentiating forms of this disease. Laboratory Investigation 36: 274–281
Yood R A. Skinner M, Cohen A S, Lee V W 1981 Soft tissue uptake of bone seeking radionuclide in amyloidosis. Journal of Rheumatology 8: 760–766
Yood R A, Skinner M, Rubinow A, Talarico L, Cohen A S 1983 Bleeding manifestations in 100 patients with amyloidosis. Journal of the American Medical Association 249: 1322–1324
Zemer D, Pras M, Sohar E, Gafni J 1976 Colchicine in familial Mediterranean fever. New England Journal of Medicine 294: 170–171
Zemer D, Pras M, Shenner Y, Sohar E, Gafni J 1980 Daily prophylactic colchicine in familial Mediterranean fever. In: Glenner G G, Pinho e Costa P, de Freitas F (eds) Amyloid and amyloidosis. Excerpta Medica, Amsterdam, p 580–583
Zucker-Franklin D, Lavie G, Franklin E C 1980 Evidence for the degradation of serum amyloid A (SAA) on the surface of mononuclear leukocytes. In: Glenner G G, Pinho e Costa P, Falcao de Freitas A (eds) Amyloid and amyloidosis. Excerpta Medica, Amsterdam, p 456–458

SECTION IX

Arthritis in Children

Rheumatic fever

Definition and criteria

Rheumatic fever is characterised clinically by fever, polyarthritis and carditis, histologically by specific granulomata, and bacteriologically by preceding group A beta-haemolytic streptococcal infection. It is surprising, now that rheumatic fever has disappeared from all except the poorest areas of the world, that its significance and relevance have never been higher: it is the only rheumatic disease where we know for certain the exogenous factor.

Prevalence

A century ago acute rheumatism was one of the commonest of the diseases of childhood and adolescence; as late as 1928, according to Sheldon (1948), 20–25% of the beds at the leading London children's hospital were occupied by rheumatic fever cases. It was frequent also in adults: Osler (1882) notes that of 456 cases of rheumatic fever admitted to Montreal General Hospital, 4.4% were cases under 15, 49% aged 15–25, and 26% aged 25–35. By 1926 rheumatic fever cases had fallen to 1.1% of the admissions at Guy's Hospital compared with 5% in 1914 (Osman, 1926); by 1952 they had fallen to 0.23%. At Taplow, admissions for rheumatic fever had fallen from 146 in 1952 to 4 in 1973 (Fig. 42.1), predominantly in the first decade. In the notification areas of England and Wales the incidence of verified rheumatic fever has fallen from 0.05% of the child population in 1948 to 0.014% in 1961 (Fig. 42.2). Between 1961 and 1968 the primary attack rate fell from 0.026% to 0.01% in Czechoslovakia (Sitaj et al, 1970), whereas in Manhattan (1963–1965) it stayed at 0.05% of the child population (Brownell & Baylen-Rose, 1973).

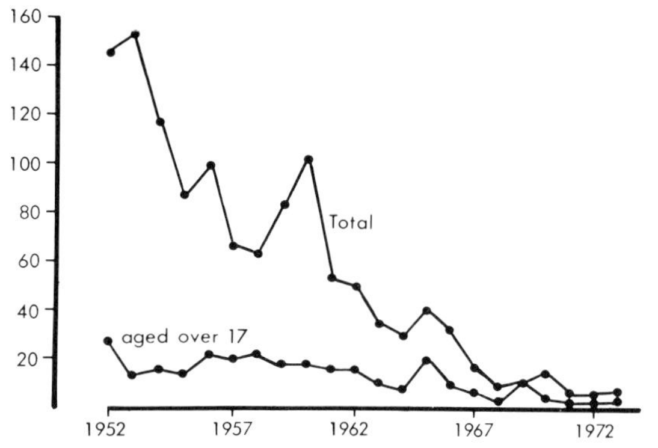

Fig. 42.1 Annual admissions to Taplow of rheumatic fever cases 1952–1973.

The prevalence of rheumatic fever and rheumatic heart disease in a population is a better index of its social importance than is the number of cases affected per year. A survey of 1000 families in Baltimore, USA (Collins et al, 1950), showed that on any particular day 12.8 out of 1000 persons were affected, as compared with 3.5 with tuberculosis. In the Framingham study, 2.7% of adults between 30 and 59 years of age had rheumatic heart disease (Stokes & Dawber, 1956). The annual disability was 758 days per 1000 population compared with 813 for tuberculosis.

A more striking decrease in the severity of the disease has been seen in recent years, well reflected in the mortality rate for rheumatic fever (Fig. 42.3). It will be noted that this fluctuates and decreases with the mortality rate of scarlatina, although the decrease in the latter since 1910 has not been accompanied by any decrease in incidence. The 10 persons per million dying of rheumatic fever, however, are only a small part of the relevant mortality. If we include deaths from rheu-

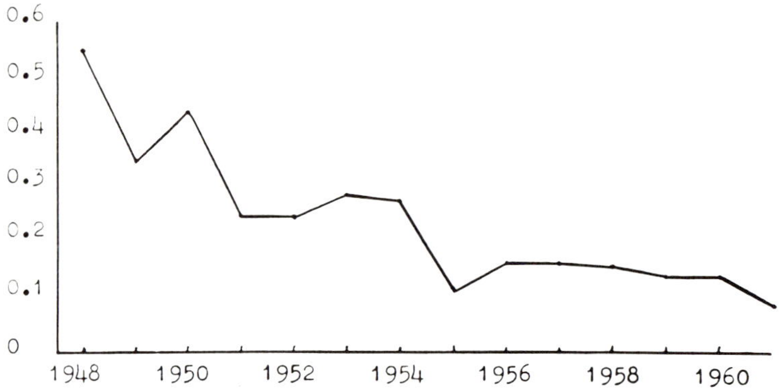

Fig. 42.2 Annual notification of acute rheumatic fever (verified 1948–1960 per thousand children (Ministry of Health).

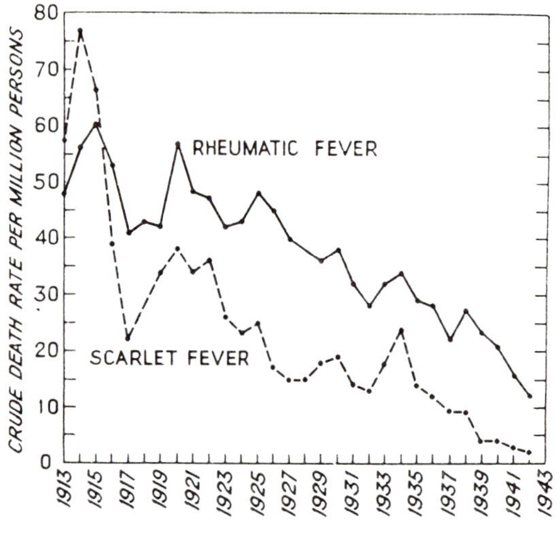

Fig. 42.3 Crude death rates per million persons from scarlet and rheumatic fevers, showing over 30 years the close correspondence between their trends and yearly oscillation. (Glover, 1943. By courtesy of the Editor of *The Lancet*.)

matic heart disease it may be seen (Fig. 42.4) that deaths in England and Wales have fallen only very little in the 12-year period 1948–1960. Most of these deaths are in the young: indeed from the age of 5 up to 20, rheumatic fever and heart disease together is still one of the leading causes of death. In Portugal, with the highest death rate in Europe from rheumatic fever and rheumatic heart disease, 0.73% of school children were said to be affected (Teixeira et al, 1973).

The above figures are based on the 'cause of death' as given in the death certificate. The incidence of gross valvular disease has been found (Hallgrimsson, 1975) to be between 1 and 5% of all autopsies (6% in a large series aged 41–60 at the Royal Postgraduate Medical School of London). Indeed, considering how common streptococcal infection is, minor degrees of heart involvement probably occur in many people without reaching

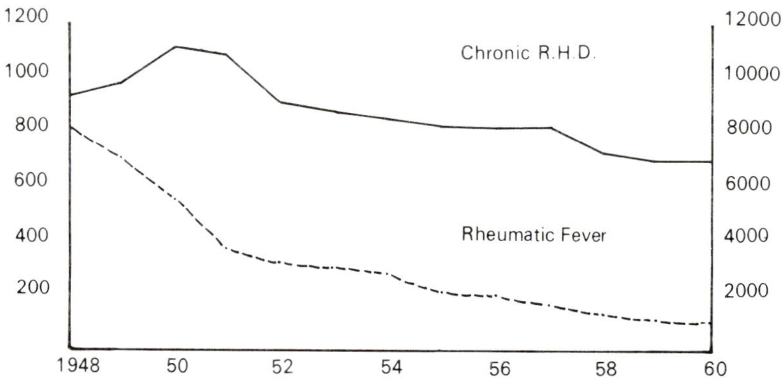

Fig. 42.4 Actual deaths from chronic rheumatic heart disease (top right scale) and from rheumatic fever (lower left scale). England and Wales, all ages, 1948–1960.

the threshold of clinical consciousness and are manifest only perhaps as minor and transient electrocardiographic abnormalities (Rantz et al, 1947). Thus, it seems possible to view the great decline in rheumatic fever in the last century as due primarily to a decrease in severity. It preceded the use of penicillin or sulphonamide.

In less developed countries, rheumatic fever and rheumatic heart disease are still a very big problem, e.g. in India (Agarwal, 1981) or in Egypt, where Abdin & Eissa (1965) in 1000 cases found not only a high proportion of severe carditis but also involvement of children at an earlier age than usually seen in Great Britain (see p. 1063; 'Geographical and seasonal factors'). A similar picture was seen in Jamaica where 21 deaths occurred in 100 cases (Back & De Pass, 1964), and surprisingly in Mississippi, (Pilapil, 1971) where 34% of those with carditis died.

Aetiological factors

Rheumatic fever is one of the sequelae of group A beta-haemolytic streptococcal infection. The very close relationship of streptococcal infection to rheumatic fever is well shown by Coburn & Young's study (1949) of the monthly occurrence of rheumatic fever and scarlet fever over four years at a training establishment. The rheumatic fever peak always accompanies, and in fact occurs slightly after, the peak period of streptococcal infection in February and March of each year (Fig. 42.5). This correspondence and slight lag is shown also in the milk-borne group A haemolytic streptococcal epidemic recorded by Madsen & Kalbak (1940). Although only a very few develop rheumatic fever, everyone from time to time suffers group A streptococcal infection as shown by the level of streptococcal antibody in the blood serum, which after a drop from the maternal level soon after birth to zero, rises steadily with increasing age to reach the normal adult level at the age of 10 (Fig. 42.6; Quinn, 1949). Hence there is certainly more than one factor responsible for the development of rheumatic fever. These will be discussed under the headings of infection, age and sex, geographical and seasonal factors, nutrition and housing, and heredity. It may be possible that 'miniature' rheumatic fever occurs in many people following a series of streptococcal infections but only reaches the threshold of clinical illness when such additional conditioning factors coincide as well.

Infection

While group A haemolytic streptococcal infection always precedes the attack of rheumatic fever, there is no evidence that this organism itself is present in the lesions of the disease or is immedi-

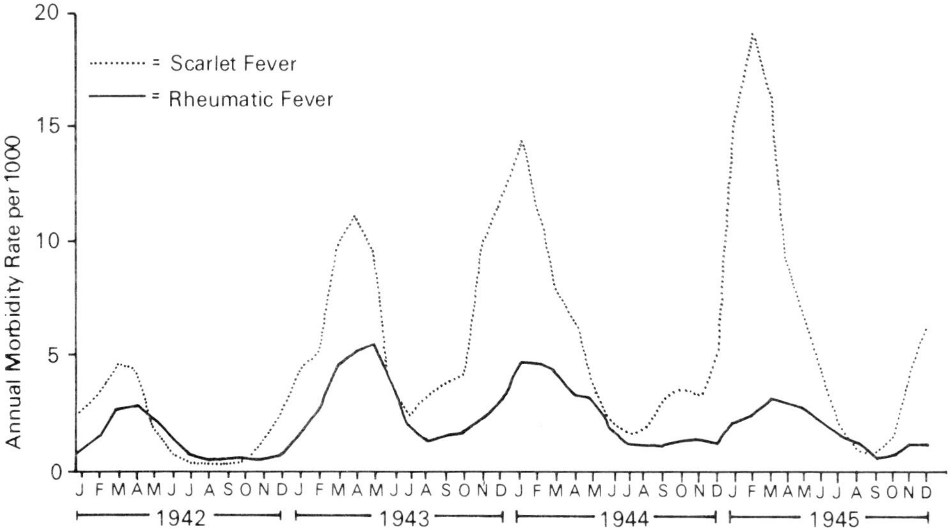

Fig. 42.5 Seasonal trend of scarlet fever and rheumatic fever among Navy personnel. (Coburn & Young, 1949. By courtesy of Williams & Wilkins, Baltimore.)

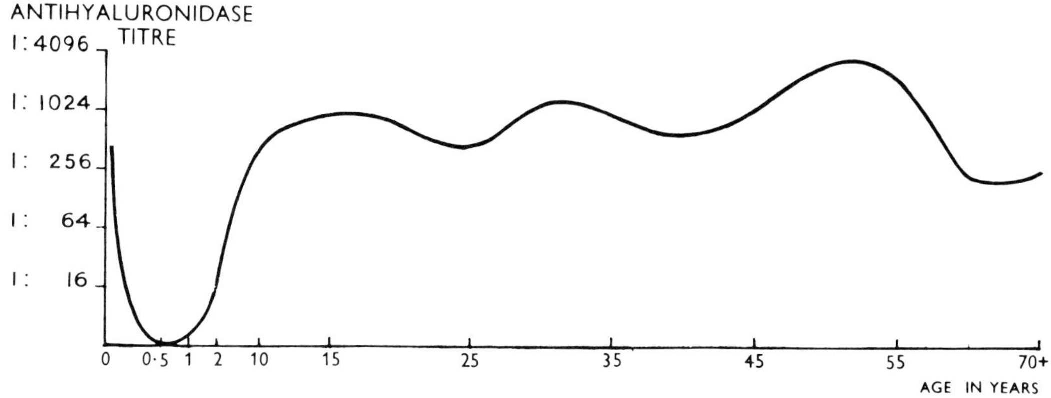

Fig. 42.6 Level of antistreptococcal antibody at various ages. Note rapid fall from maternal blood level after birth and attainment of adult level at about the age of 10 years. (Redrawn from Quinn, 1949. By courtesy of the *Journal of Immunology*.)

ately responsible for its manifestations. Culture of acutely involved valves grew various organisms, including group A beta-haemolytic streptococci, in only 2 out of 44 valves from 11 patients; all those taken with aseptic precautions were sterile (Watson et al, 1961). This did not, however, exclude L organisms (forms of streptococci devoid of cell wall). These are found to produce M-antigen (Sharp et al, 1957) and a specific complement-fixing antigen (Crawford, 1960). However, despite much research, no evidence for L-form participation in rheumatic fever has been found (Quinn & Lowry, 1974). In some cases there may be confusion with rubella virus infection, where synovitis is sometimes seen. Kuttner (1958) was unable to find virus in auricular appendages obtained at commissurotomy. Burch et al (1970) have speculated whether some cases of mitral stenosis could have originated in Coxsackie infection. Some cases of 'rheumatic heart disease' without a history of rheumatic fever may well from their antibody pattern be congenital (non-rheumatic) in origin (Shulman et al, 1974). Others have postulated that streptococci produce myocardial damage by release of extracellular cytotoxic materials such as streptolysin O and streptococcal proteinase, but Aschoff bodies have not been reproduced (Kellner & Robertson, 1954).

Another possibility is that the mucopeptide of the cell wall may exert a direct toxic action in the tissues, after dissociation from the group-specific polysaccharides (Ohanian & Schwab, 1967). Streptococcal bacteriophage and lysogenic strains have received consideration; the latter are found to be more common in children (Kjems, 1960) and associated with high carrier rates and infection with non-typeable group A organisms (Quinn & Lowry, 1974). The fact that bactericidal penicillin will not cut short an attack of rheumatic fever argues against the continued presence of living streptococci, and ASO levels persist equally long in cases given six weeks penicillin in bactericidal dosage as in controls (Carter et al, 1962). We have also found that tetracycline (active against L-forms) is similarly ineffective (Smith & Bywaters, 1966).

If antigenic material were deposited in the heart, a continued reaction against it is a very real possibility. There are many distinct streptococcal cellular products (Fig. 47.7) and Halbert & Keatinge (1961) have shown the presence of 20 distinct extracellular antigens. The cell wall and cell membrane constituents are particularly interesting, since there appear to be antigens therein, eliciting antibodies which are cross-reactive not only with myocardial sarcolemma (Kaplan, 1965) but, as Kingston & Glynn have shown (1971), with fibroblasts, endothelial cells, synoviocytes and astrocytes (Fig. 42.8). While Kaplan found only a few strains capable of producing this antigen, others have found a similar one present in most of the types of group A streptococci, both those producing M protein and those not (Nakhla & Glynn, 1967). It may possibly be localised in the cell (protoplast) membrane itself (Zabriskie & Freimer, 1966) which seems to be difficult to exclude from cell wall preparations. The membrane can, how-

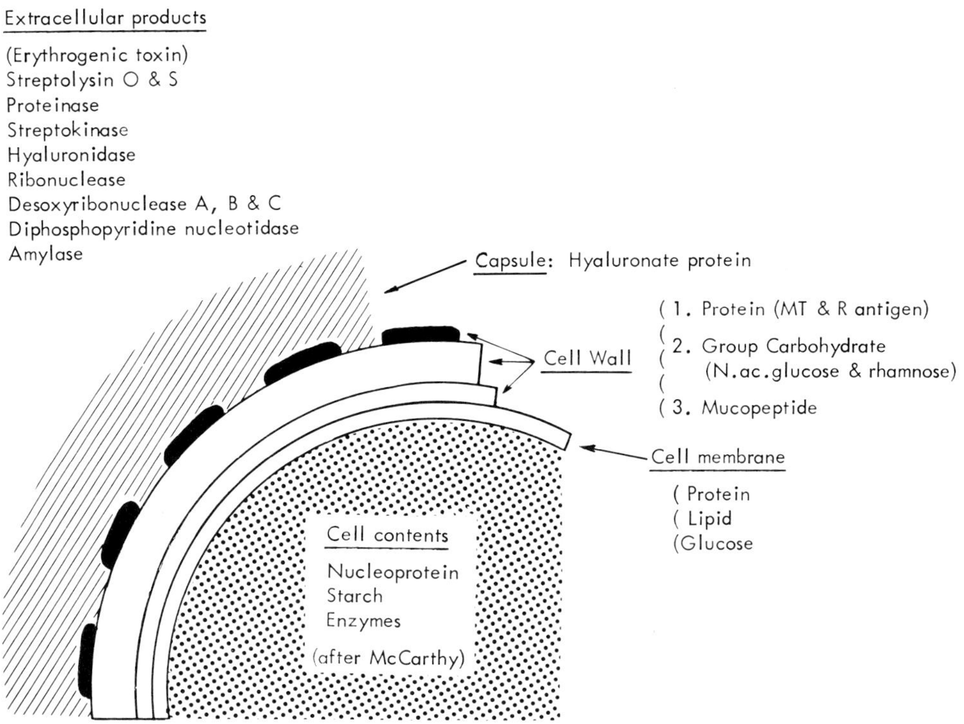

Fig. 42.7 Antigenic and other constituents of group A beta-haemolytic streptococcus.

ever, be isolated by phage lysin breakdown of cell wall components (i.e. protein, mucopeptide and group-specific polysaccharide) and has been shown by the latter authors to be cross-reactive with a similar cell membrane from heart muscle and arterial smooth muscle cells. The cross-reactive antiheart antibody titre is four times as high in rheumatic fever as in uncomplicated streptococcal infection: it lasts for 1–2 years before disappearing and reappears with infections and before recurrences of rheumatic fever. It differs from postcardiotomy antibody since it is absorbed not only by the heart but also by streptococcal membrane (Zabriskie et al, 1970b, 1971). Cell-mediated immune response to streptococcal membrane occurs in nephritis (Zabriskie et al, 1970a) and rheumatic fever (McLaughlin et al, 1972) but leucocytes from the latter were not inhibited by heart muscle antigen. There are many cardiac antigens (Halbert et al, 1973), some organ-specific, others reacting with skeletal muscle.

Of the 60 or so Lancefield serotypes of group A streptococci, no particular type or types have been found particularly associated with rheumatic fever, unlike the well-attested role of certain nephritogenic types in glomerular nephritis. There seems, however, to be a clear distinction between, on the one hand, the tonsillar and upper respiratory tract infections (leading to rheumatic fever in about 0.1% of cases during epidemic and in 0.03% of sporadic sore throats) and, on the other hand, the pyoderma infections, leading, also infrequently, to glomerulonephritis, but not, apparently, to rheumatic fever (Stollerman, 1971). The seasonal peak (in the same place) is different (Bisno et al, 1970), and the organisms associated with high virulence (M antigen) and typeability. There is also a different antibody response, the nephritogenic infections showing less ASO and ADPNase than in rheumatogenic infection (Wannamaker 1970a, b) but equal antidornase B. Surprisingly, severe streptococcal infections, e.g. with bacteriaemia (Duma et al, 1969; Hable et al, 1973) do not develop rheumatic fever. If it is not one particular variety of streptococcus, it may be a particular succession of infections. Murphy (1945) and Murphy & Swift (1949) have shown in rabbits that infection with a particular type leads to suf-

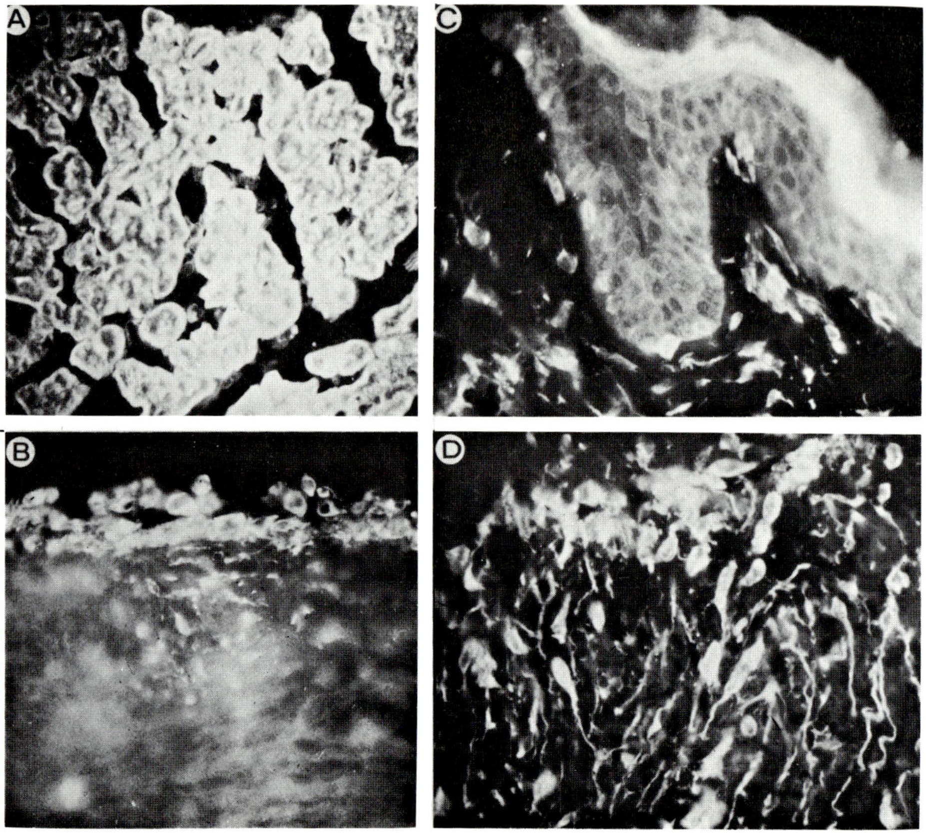

Fig. 42.8 Immunofluorescent localisation of cross-reactive antibody raised in rabbits immunised with group A streptococci on human tissues. (A) Myocardium (×270). Showing subsarcolemmal staining. (Kasp-Grokowska et al, 1972.) (B) Synovial membrane (×480). Showing staining of synoviocytes and fibroblasts. (Kingston & Glynn, 1971.) (C) Skin (×490). Showing staining of fibroblasts, blood vessels and epidermis. (Kingston & Glynn, 1971.) (D) Tricuspid valve (×480). Showing staining of endothelium and fibroblasts. (Kingston & Glynn, 1971.)

ficient M-antibody to protect against subsequent infections with that type, but if rabbits are infected with a series of different types a rheumatic fever-like illness occurs with mycocardial and valvular lesions somewhat resembling the human disease, a high sedimentation rate and even heart failure. Against this hypothesis is the finding of Holborow & Isdale (1956) that patients with rheumatic fever aged below 5 years showed significantly less ASO response than those in older age-groups, confirmed by Wasz-Hockert & Widholen (1956) and contrary to previous claims by Coburn & Pauli (1935). If rheumatic fever depended upon repeated streptococcal infection, the ASO response in young children with rheumatic fever should be higher, instead of lower as in uncomplicated infections (Rantz et al, 1951).

While most workers will agree that in the rheumatic fever group as a whole, antibody titres are higher and last longer than in uncomplicated streptococcal infections, this may not help in any individual case, and these levels are equalled by those with purulent complications such as quinsy or otitis media. There seems to be little difference in immunological reactivity of rheumatic fever subjects to non-streptococcal antigens compared with subjects without rheumatic fever or rheumatic heart disease (Rantz, 1962). Serum complement levels may be raised initially in some patients, returning to normal levels but with a later secondary rise perhaps due to termination of increased complement consumption during rheumatic fever (Schubart et al, 1963), and circulating immune complexes especially in HLA-B5 subjects

(Yoshinoya & Pope, 1979). High and long-maintained levels of antibody to group A-specific carbohydrate have been described by Dudding & Ayoub (1968) as characteristic of rheumatic valvular disease as compared with cases of rheumatic fever or chorea without carditis, although this has been denied (Zimmerman et al, 1971). They have also described low affinity antibody as characteristic of rheumatic fever (Shulman & Ayoub, 1974) and group-specific antibody rise after heart surgery (Ayoub et al, 1974) speculating on its cross-reaction (described by Goldstein et al, 1968) with heart valve extract. The latter reaction could not be confirmed at Taplow by Kasp-Grochowska et al (1972) but the latter authors have identified the cross-reacting component from heart muscle as a plasmalogen-like substance, presumably from cell membrane (Kasp-Grochowska & Glynn, 1977).

The appearance in the serum of rheumatic fever subjects of antibodies reacting both with streptococci and with myocardial sarcolemma (Kaplan et al, 1961), and therefore 'autoimmune' in character, is strong evidence that the streptococcus is concerned in the development of heart damage: this has been confirmed both by Hess et al (1962), by Zitnan & Bosmansky (1966) and by Nakhla & Glynn (1967), although Christensen et al (1979) have expressed doubts about this interpretation of the data. These cross-reacting antibodies do not appear, however, by themselves to be the active agents since they may be found in a high proportion of patients after cardiac surgery and in a number of patients after uncomplicated sore throats. Others using haemagglutination, immunofluorescent and other methods have found anti-heart antibody in 15% of post-cardiotomy patients (Robinson & Brigden, 1963), after myocardial infarction (Van der Geld, 1964; Strausz & Dobias, 1967; Faivre et al, 1967), in endomyocardial fibrosis (Shaper et al, 1967; Van der Geld et al, 1966), in systemic lupus (Das & Cassidy, 1973), chagasic cardiopathy (Cossio, 1974), in heart transplantation (Ellis et al, 1970) as expected, and, perhaps unexpectedly, in congenital heart disease (Nora et al, 1974). Delayed hypersensitivity to streptococcus is also present to high degree (Rajapakse, unpublished observations and also Read et al, 1974). Indeed tolerance to heart grafts involving both humoral and delayed hypersensitivity can be induced by pre-treatment with cross-reactive streptococcal cell membrane (Ellis et al, 1974). Such antibodies may only injure the heart and the brain as in chorea (Husby et al, 1976) if the cell barrier is broken by non-specific damage (Gazenfeld et al, 1966). It seems possible, therefore, that the streptococcus may induce carditis in some individuals because of a cross-reacting antigen, and it would seem that the comparatively rare occurrence of rheumatic fever is therefore associated as much with human individual peculiarity, whether congenital or acquired later, as with streptococcal specificity.

Age and sex

Rheumatic fever is rare before the age of 4, and acute migratory polyarthritis in small children is due usually to Henoch–Schönlein purpura (with or without purpura), to Still's disease or to leukaemia. Niemann et al (1960) cite 0.5% of rheumatic fever with onset before the age of 5, Rosenthal et al (1968) cite 0.5% below the age of 3. Chorea, nodules and rash are rare. One fatal case is recorded at 9 months of age (Powell & Miller, 1969). The peak age for rheumatic fever is about 7 or 8. Sex incidence is about equal except that chorea tends to affect adolescent girls more frequently. Adults nowadays seldom develop rheumatic fever except under epidemic conditions, e.g. in aircraft carriers (Dully, 1973) or army barracks. In such epidemics the disease tends to be mild (Malpas & Landon, 1960). 31% of such attacks occur within 6 months of enlistment. Persistent murmurs developed in those with a previous history of rheumatic fever and it seems doubtful whether such subjects should be exposed to these conditions of potential epidemic infection (Slater & Rosenbaum, 1959). In the aged, rheumatic fever is rarer, atypical (Kjorstad, 1957) and difficult to diagnose (Wee & Goodwin, 1966), being often mistaken for rheumatoid arthritis.

Geographical and seasonal factors

While it is untrue that rheumatic fever is not seen in the tropics, e.g. Honolulu (Yim, 1962), Ceylon (de Silva, 1959), Jamaica (Back & DePass, 1957), Philippines (Alimuriung et al, 1955), Puerto Rico (Palmieri et al, 1962) and India (Webb, 1961), there is a marked decrease in incidence of rheumatic heart disease admitted to hospital, in the incidence of autopsy material in hospitals and in mortality rates from rheumatic fever from north to south in the northern hemisphere. This is well shown in Mills' map of North American mortality distribution (Mills, 1939) and in data from the Metropolitan Life Assurance Co. (1944). Whether this is associated with different streptococcal infection rates is not known. Increased incidence in the cooler months of the year (see Fig. 42.5) might be due to the easier spread of streptococcal infection in the home or barracks. In support of this is the seasonal variation for rheumatic fever admissions, which runs parallel with those of scarlet fever, tonsillitis and erysipelas. It seems probable that most of these differences will prove not to be racial or climatic but due to differing social conditions and streptococcal infection. Thus, Kirschner et al (1959) have shown marked differences in streptolysin O titres between Maoris living in civilised areas and those living in Rara Tonga (Fig. 42.9). The microclimate in the home may be more important than the weather outside.

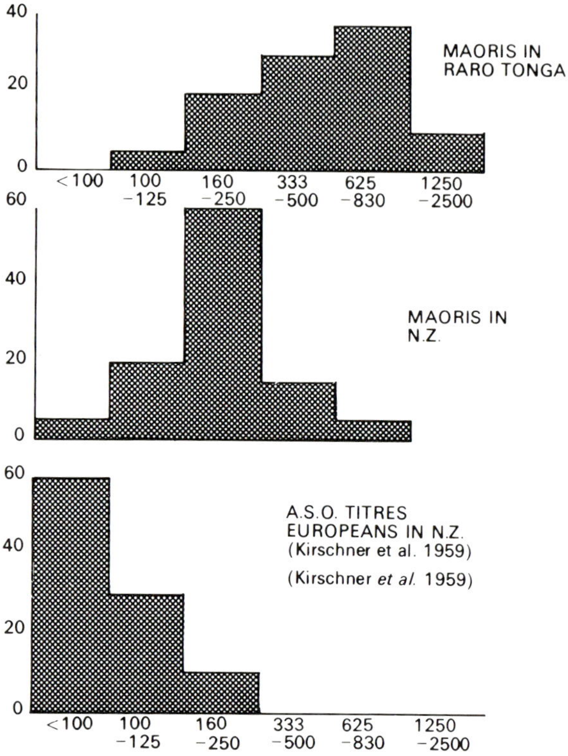

Fig. 42.9 Antistreptolysin O titre in Maoris is higher in Raro Tonga (more primitive) than in New Zealand, and both are higher than in non-Maori New Zealanders. (Kirschner et al, 1959).

Poverty, nutrition and housing

Rheumatic fever is 'essentially a working class disease' said Robert Hutchinson in 1922, commenting on the rarity of rheumatic fever in his private practice and its great frequency in hospital practice. Again, this may be an effect, not of presence or absence, but of severity. In this country the highest mortality from rheumatic heart disease (Morris & Titmuss, 1942) occurred in the five main areas of industrial urbanisation where, side by side with great wealth, there have always been great poverty and appalling slums. Thus, in 1920 the rejection rate for valvular disease of the heart was 22/1000 from industrial Cardiff and 2/1000 from rural Carmarthen (Miller, 1926). If the towns of England and Wales are arranged according to the proportion of inhabitants within the two lowest social grades, a direct correlation of poverty with the rheumatic heart disease death rate is seen (Morris & Titmuss, 1942). A similar result is obtained for various occupational groups, the mortality from valvular disease in males aged 20–45 being for the professions and employing classes 28% under the mean rate and 21% over the mean rate for semi- and unskilled workers. Similar trends are seen in the USA (Collins, 1947). The close correlation with overcrowding (Thomson, 1928; Fig. 42.10) is also seen with the family net income, i.e. money spent per head on food,

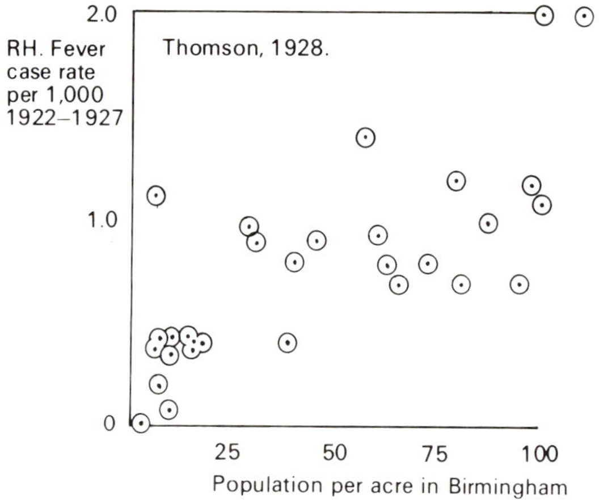

Fig. 42.10 Rheumatic fever case rate per 1000, 1922–1927. Correlation between overcrowding and incidence of rheumatic fever in Birmingham 1922–1927. (Thomson, 1928.)

clothes, fuel and excluding fares, rent and rates (Daniel, 1942).

It seems possible that overcrowding may be important because of the increased liability to infection. Epidemics were not uncommon during the war in camps with a rapid turnover of recruits, but could be controlled with prophylactic sulphadiazine until a resistant strain developed, when the epidemic reached alarming proportions (Coburn & Young, 1949). In families of low compared with those of high social standards, the amount of streptococcal infection is very much higher judged by the antistreptolysin O titre: between 2 and 3 times the number of children up to the age of 9 show high antibody levels in the low social standard group as compared with the high, and these develop earlier. This is dependent on the size of the family in the low standard group but not in the high standard group (Hammon et al, 1950). In a study of umbilical cord blood as an index of family streptococcal infections (Bywaters et al, 1957a), the major difference was between social classes rather than between town and country, primiparae or multiparae, summer or winter, or whether there were children of school age. The importance of increased infection risks in schools and in large families has also been noticed by Hewitt & Stewart (1952).

Genetic factors

Mitral stenosis has been seen in 3 identical twin pairs of a family (Chang, 1961). May Wilson believes on the basis of a series of 112 families she has studied that there is a hereditary susceptibility based on a single autosomal recessive gene with a penetrance of 86% (Wilson & Lubschez, 1944). In Belfast it has been shown (Stevenson & Cheeseman, 1953) that the risk of a sibling developing rheumatic fever is more than doubled if one parent has been affected. The blue-eyed appear less prone by half to rheumatic fever (Hewitt & Stewart, 1952). Certainly it is general experience that rheumatic fever occurs in families although not as frequently as 50 years ago, when Cheadle (1889) could cite families where 5 out of 6 and 11 out of 12 developed rheumatic fever. It is difficult, however, to dissociate the family genes from the familial environment. Kaufmann & Scheerer (1938) showed that in 27 pairs of identical twins affected with rheumatic fever 4 or 5 pairs were both affected, whereas in 43 pairs of non-identical twins 1 or 2 pairs only were both affected. Somewhat similar figures have been published by Taranta et al (1961) and a slightly higher proportion by Claussen (1955). However, in a disease like tuberculosis, Kallmann & Reisner (1943) found concordance in identical twins in 87% and in non-identical twins in 25.6% similar to that in other siblings. Furthermore, there is marked bias in hospital-based series in favour of concordance which is not seen in more randomly or completely collected twin registrations (Moesman, 1959). In our own hospital-selected series of rheumatic fever cases we have 20 twin pairs: only 3 are concordant and these are all non-identical. This favours environmental rather than hereditary mechanisms.

If there is a familial or heritable tendency to develop rheumatic fever we have even less idea of its mechanism. Glynn et al (1959) drew attention to the high proportion of non-secretors of the ABO blood group substances, confirmed by Clarke et al (1960). There was also noted a relative deficiency of group O individuals (Macaffee, 1965) in all series. The explanation may lie in the findings of Van Rijsewijk & Goslings (1963) that non-secretors seem to be more susceptible to infection by streptococcus pyogenes. Falk et al (1973), Faughey et al (1975), Murray et al (1978) and Greenberg et al (1975) report conflicting HLA observations but in general no overall significant association between rheumatic fever and the HLA-A or B series.

A monoclonal antibody identifies mononuclear cells from 75% of rheumatic fever cases, compared with 15% control cases (Zabriskie, 1983, personal communication) and is similar to the original reagent described in 1979 by Patarroyo et al. The remaining 25% are identified by another clonal antibody.

In summary, therefore, rheumatic fever is due to group A beta-haemolytic streptococcal infection, but is conditioned by other factors, possibly hereditarily determined, possibly environmentally determined, of which we know little yet. It seems possible that the actual mechanism is one of immunologically mediated muscle damage.

Epidemiology

The epidemiology of rheumatic fever (Acheson, 1965) is therefore that of the group A haemolytic streptococcus, although cases have been recorded in significant numbers in an outbreak of non-haemolytic group A type-18 infection (James & McFarland, 1971). While the usual spread is by hand contact, and hence is associated with overcrowding, epidemics have been recorded due to milk-borne infection (Madsen & Kalbak, 1940), food infection (Otte & Ritzerfeld, 1961), wound infection (Quinn & Hillman, 1965) and anal carriage (McKee et al, 1966). Both perianal cellulitis (Amren et al, 1966) and impetigo (Markovitz et al, 1965) are responsible in some areas for much streptococcal disease: the latter, endemic in some tropical areas, may occasionally lead to glomerulonephritis but seldom to rheumatic fever. Streptococcal puerperal sepsis is now seldom seen (Ledger & Headington, 1972). The recent decline in incidence of rheumatic fever in highly developed countries is probably due both to better hygiene and to less overcrowding and contact: with less rapid passage, the organism is tending to become less virulent and many strains, except in epidemics, are non-typeable (Stollerman et al, 1965). Detection of the M-associated protein antigen described by Widdowson et al (1971) may be useful in such circumstances.

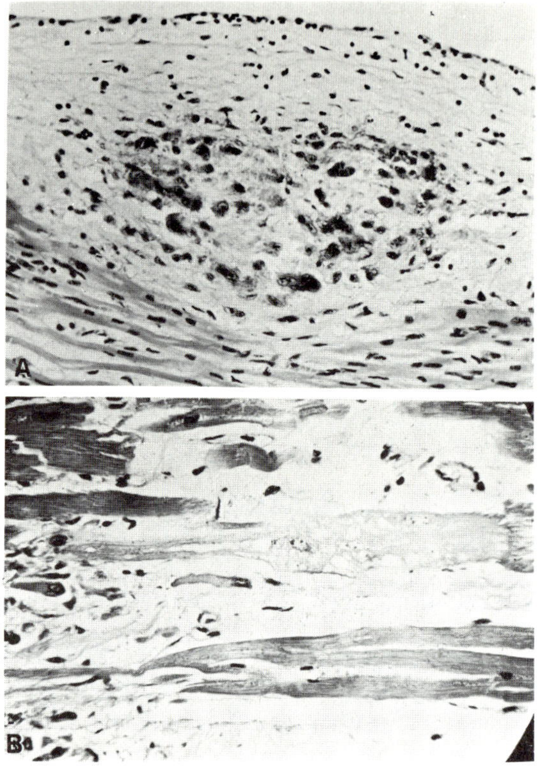

Fig. 42.11 (A) Fully developed Aschoff nodule in subendocardial region superficial to muscle. (B) Myocardium in rheumatic fever showing damaged muscle fibres in various stages of disintegration.

Pathology

The characteristic structural change of rheumatic fever is a peculiar inflammatory reaction in the connective tissue of the moving parts of the body, partly proliferative, partly exudative and ending in fibrosis.

In the heart these granulomata are called after Ludwig Aschoff, who first (1904) emphasised their importance. The node — usually perivascular in position — is composed of large 'owl-eyed' cells, sometimes multinucleated (Fig. 42.11); the large nucleus contains a prominent nucleolus and the cytoplasm is basophil. These are set in an oedematous base with altered connective tissue fibres, plasma cells and lymphocytes. The Anitschkow cell, a characteristic feature of the Aschoff node, is thought to be of myogenic origin (Fenoglio & Wagner, 1973) but is not specific for rheumatic fever (Murphy & Becker, 1966; Serck-Hanssen, 1966). 'Fibrinoid' change in the connective tissue may occur alone, without or before a cellular reaction. This material, for long a subject of enquiry (Geiler, 1960) may be of variable composition, deriving from fibrinogen (Gitlin et al, 1957) gammaglobulin and perhaps in certain situations from smooth muscle (Muirhead et al, 1957; Movat, 1958). Such cardiac granulomata are present in between 80% (Wilson, 1940) and 90% (Gross, 1935) of active cases. Similar granulomata differing in some respects from the cardiac nodes (e.g. by the absence of Anitschkow myocytes; Clawson, 1941) occur in the connective tissue planes of other moving parts such as joint capsules, bursae, tendon sheaths and insertions, aorta, larynx, pharynx and oesophagus (Klinge, 1932). Endocarditis is manifest in the earliest stages as a palisade formation (Fig. 42.12) with adherent platelet thrombus, ultimately forming the well-known warty vegetations along the line of closure of the valve cusps and particularly those on the mitral valve (Fig. 42.13). Fibrinous serositis less often affects

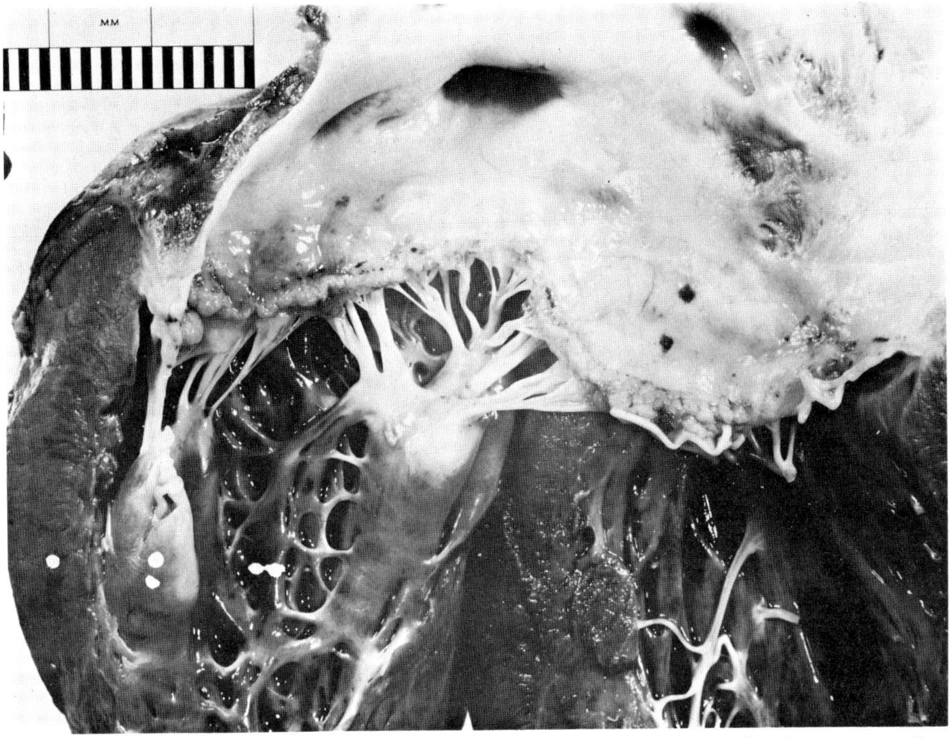

Fig. 42.12 Fresh rheumatic verrucae on the mitral valve in female aet. 17 dying in first known attack of chorea and pancarditis.

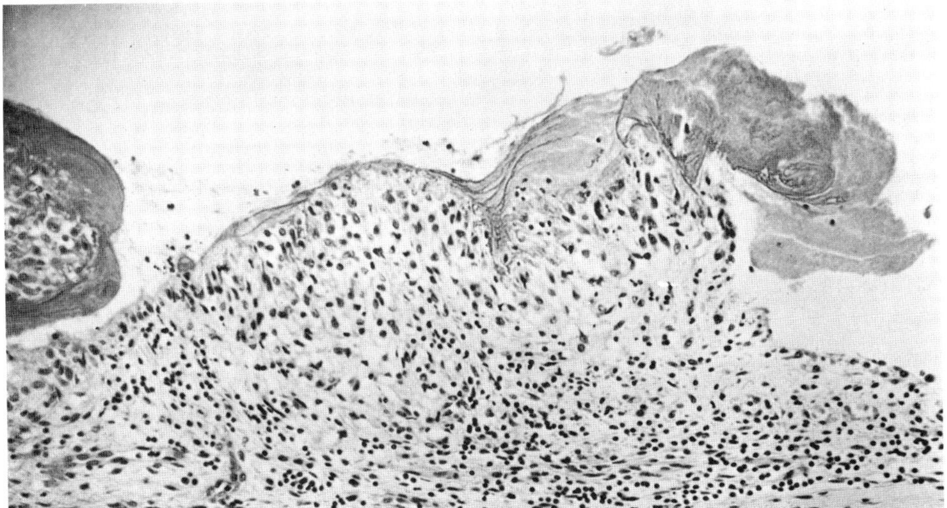

Fig. 42.13 Mitral valve showing early rheumatic lesion. (H & E ×100)

the pericardium, and still less often the pleurae and synovial cavities. Proliferative changes may occur in the vessels. Rarely more marked obliteration occurs and coronary involvement was responsible for 3 sudden deaths out of a series of 13 deaths recorded in young adults with rheumatic fever by Griffith & Huntington (1946). Biopsy of the left auricular appendage during operations for valuvlar disease has revealed a high proportion showing Aschoff nodes in the absence of clinical rheumatic activity and often many years after the last attack of rheumatic fever (Pinniger, 1951) and in all series this proportion has been relatively high (about 20–50%). There is correspondence between their appearance in the left auricle and the remainder of the heart (Ruebner & Boitnott, 1961; Dalldorf & Murphy, 1960; Lannigan, 1961). Kuepper et al (1961) have shown complement fixation in Aschoff nodes as well as in endocardium from rheumatic and congenital cases. Murphy (1960) has pointed out the close relationship between the experimental heart disease produced in rabbits by repeated streptococcal infection leading to muscle fibre degeneration and the appearances of rheumatic carditis, and is of the opinion that the Aschoff cells both in the heart and in the media of arteries are derived from muscle fibres. Certainly some of them appear to derive thus (McDonald, 1975) (Fig. 42.11B) and perhaps all, since Murphy has shown muscle fibres to occur even in the valve cusps (Murphy, 1963). Aschoff node cells in the proximal part of the atrioventricular valves contain actomyosin B characteristic of striated muscle, whereas elsewhere they are characterised by actomyosin A of smooth muscle origin (Becker & Murphy, 1969). Lannigan & Zaki (1965) have described submicroscopic particles in the lesions, possibly L-forms. It has been claimed that pretreatment of patients with steroids before commissurotomy decreases somewhat the extent of Aschoff nodes (Gil et al, 1955; Decourt et al, 1962) but in both series some florid examples were found who had been on long-term and high dosage of steroid. Rheumatic phlebitis of the coronary vessels has been described (Von Glahn & Kuschner, 1961). Aortitis not due to syphilis or ankylosing spondylitis and presumably rheumatic has been seen in a number of patients, particularly in the older literature. An example of our own with gross subintimal aortic thickening has shown widespread amyloid disease, and this has been noted previously (Symmers, 1956).

The *rheumatic nodules* formed over bony prominences and tendon pressure sites consist of a similar granulomatous tissue intimately mixed with fibrinoid (Fig. 42.14): they are distinguishable in the majority of cases from the nodules of rheumatoid arthritis, where there are often large areas of necrosis, a definite palisade layer and less fibrinoid lattice (Bennet et al, 1940; Collins, 1937). However, in juvenile chronic polyarthritis (including Still's disease) the nodules (seen in 5% of patients) resemble closely those of rheumatic fever rather than those of adult rheumatoid arthritis (Bywaters et al, 1958). Nodules in children resembling those of rheumatoid arthritis are usually the subcutaneous nodule of granuloma annulare. Nodules of intermediate type are seen in systemic lupus erythematosus (Bywaters, 1975).

'Rheumatic pneumonia' (Fig. 42.15) consisting

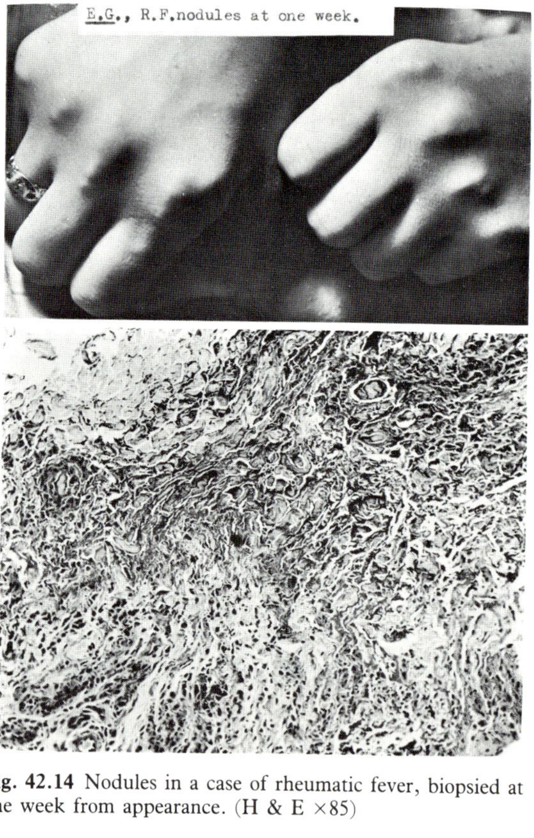

Fig. 42.14 Nodules in a case of rheumatic fever, biopsied at one week from appearance. (H & E ×85)

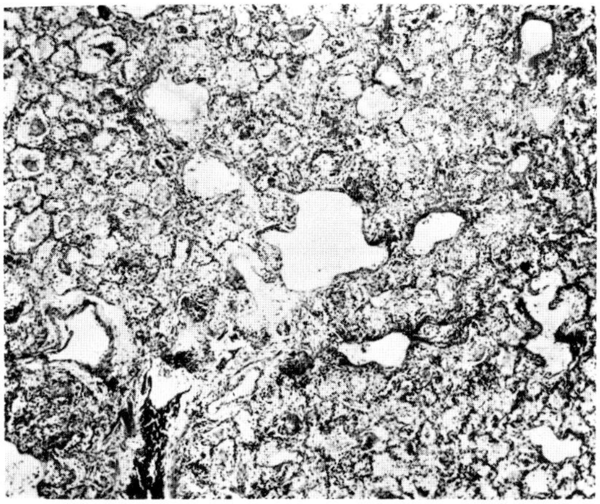

Fig. 42.15 Section of lung in 'rheumatic pneumonia'. Note dilated alveolar ducts lined with fibrin leading from the terminal broncheoli, lower left. (H & E ×30) (From *Modern Practice in Infectious Fevers*, Butterworth, London.)

of a fibrinous exudate lining the terminal bronchioles and their ducts (Hadfield, 1938) is similar to that seen in uraemia or with hexamethonium and is probably due to acute left heart failure often associated with salicylate poisoning (see p. 1077). The non-specific Masson body is left (Herbut & Manges, 1945) and may progress to ossification within the alveoli.

With the subsidence of the active process, complete resolution may occur, or, if the process has been severe and long continued, fibrosis and scarring will appear. This produces valvular deformities in the heart and, in rare instances, deformities of the hands due to fibrosis of joint capsules (Jaccoud's syndrome). Scarring may be the response to low-grade subclinical activity such as that demonstrated histologically in the left auricular appendage by Kuschner et al (1952). Fibrosis in the pericardial surfaces is never as intense as after tuberculosis; while obliteration of the sac is frequent, constriction does not occur although it may do so in rheumatoid patients. Calcification may ultimately occur in some of the fibrotic areas and has been demonstrated radiologically (Epstein, 1940) in the left auricle in the position of MacCallum's patch (1924).

Symptomatology and clinical aspects

The child with rheumatic fever presents a vary variable picture: this may range from the acute and florid attack to minimal comlaints of tiredness, pallor, loss of appetite or vague muscle and limb pains. The classical attack of rheumatic fever follows a sore throat after a so-called 'silent interval' of several days to several weeks: there may still be exudate on the tonsils, or lymph gland enlargement and a scarlatinal rash may have occurred. Postscarlatinal arthritis is rheumatic fever (Watson et al, 1945). The 'silence' of this latent period refers to clinical observations only: it is known that the sedimentation rate remains raised throughout (Rantz et al, 1945).

The onset may be acute, with fever and headache, night sweats, perhaps epistaxis and pain with or without swelling of one or more joints. In many children, however, the onset is more insidious: the child fails to recover after a cold or sore throat, is listless and lacking in energy, may be pallid or is found to be sweating in bed at night.

In adolescents and in adults the presenting picture is more usually that of an acute polyarthritis (q.v.). The course of the disease is less severe and serious heart involvement is much less common if cases are excluded in which old-standing rheumatic heart disease already exists as a residue from a previous childhood attack. Marginate erythema is rare and nodules are seldom seen. The occasional adult will be seen showing the full-blown picture with nodules, carditis and lung changes; more usually they have had previous attacks.

Temperature, pulse and respiration

Fever is usually marked at the onset: it is almost always controlled by adequate dosage of salicylates, prednisolone or ACTH (as also are other fevers, including that of Still's disease). An increase in temperature often means a fresh complication such as endocarditis or pericarditis. In contradistinction to the fever of Still's disease, the morning temperature of rheumatic fever is seldom in the normal range during epidoses of fever; i.e. this is not a remittent fever (McMinn & Bywaters, 1959).

Hyperpyrexia, with attendant delirium and coma ending more often than not in death, seems to have disappeared since 1882, when it was such a problem that a special committee was set up by the Clinical Society of London. We have seen it only once in about 1000 patient years, developing during salicylate therapy; recovery occurred after tepid sponging. A typical case is recorded by Cruickshank (1951) also on salicylate, with residual cerebellar signs. It may well have been due to salicylate.

The sleeping pulse rate rises with temperature and frequently remains high (above 100/minute) when the fever has disappeared, returning only gradually to normal. This sustained sleeping pulse rate increase was previously thought to indicate carditis, but bradycardia is occasionally seen in the presence of active rheumatism (Fig. 42.16).

Breathing becomes rapid and out of proportion to the febrile increase in metabolism when pericarditis, pleurisy or failure develops: not infrequently a rise in nocturnal respiration rate heralds pericardial involvement.

Arthritis

The rheumatic process affects predominantly the joint capsule, with a secondary and subsidiary synovitis (Fig. 42.17). This explains the 'intolerable pain upon moving the affected joint which likewise swells and acquires a faint blush of redness' Heberden, 1802), differing both from the pale, swollen and warm joints of rheumatoid arthritis and the hot, red and dry joints of gout. The larger joints are commonly affected, although any joint or joints may become involved: the affection is classically migratory, lasting a day or so in one joint and then disappearing while already another joint has become involved. The effusion is seldom large in amount, clots and contains 60–90% polymorphs in a total of between 30 000–40 000 cells/mm^3, it is viscous with a total protein between 3–5 g/100 ml. This migratory involvement may continue for days or weeks: salicylates appear to suppress pain and inflammation rapidly in most patients but in a few severe cases we have seen continued and indeed fresh joint symptoms and signs with a salicylate blood level in the region of 30 mg/100 ml (Fig. 42.18). A rather different type of joint involvement is seen in a few patients with

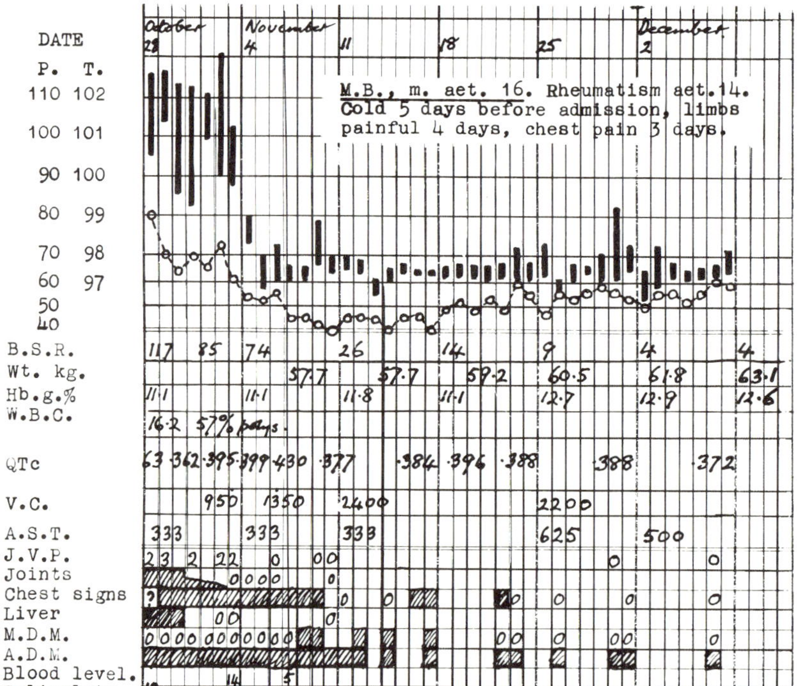

Fig. 42.16 Chart of rheumatic fever case showing bradycardia (sleeping pulse rate per minute = circles beneath temperature maximum and minimum). Note also rapid subsidence after 4 days' salicylate dosage.

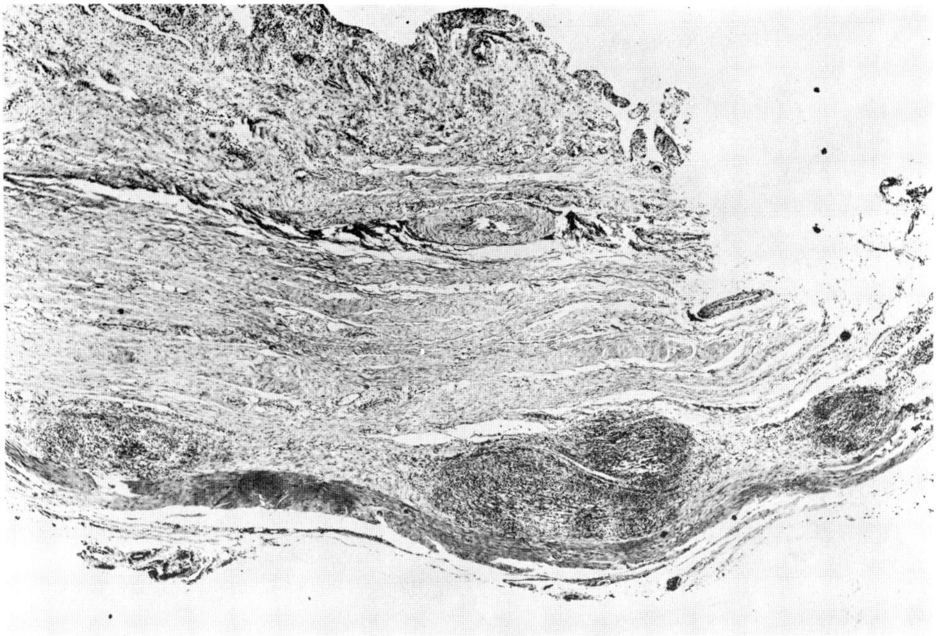

Fig. 42.17 Synovial membrane and capsule from the knee from a case of rheumatic fever showing relatively normal synovial membrane (upper portion) with focal fibrinoid necrosis and granulomata in the deeper part of the joint capsule. (H & E ×15)

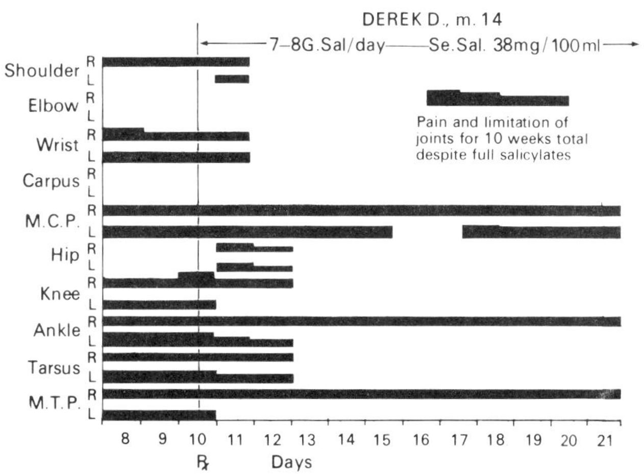

Fig. 42.18 Chart showing prolonged arthritis in boy aet. 14 despite adequate salicylate therapy. Note fresh involvement of elbow. Eventual complete recovery but with residual heart lesions.

chronic swelling and stiffness of the metacarpophalangeal and proximal interphalangeal joints lasting up to 6 months or more from onset, not responding to salicylate; this may closely mimic rheumatoid arthritis or Still's disease but may be distinguished not only because of a typical history and the cardiac signs of rheumatic fever, but also because it subsides completely. This type of lesion is probably due to capsular inflammation: biopsy shows mild synovitis only (Fig. 42.19). There is no serologic evidence of rheumatoid arthritis or lupus erythematosus. Rarefaction is seen radiologically (and can be demonstrated quantitatively — Bywaters, 1949) and interosseous wasting

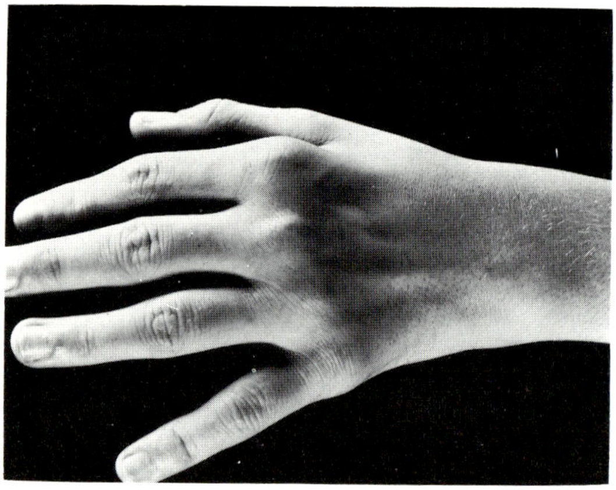

Fig. 42.19 LL male aet. 14. Second attack of rheumatic fever with polyarthritis, pancarditis and chorea. Chronic joint involvement — spindling, thickening and limitation of wrists, proximal and metacarpophalanged joints with ulnar deviation at four months from onset. ESR 1/2 mm/h. ASO 500 units. Rheumatoid factor negative. Follow-up aet. 22 years: normal hands and heart.

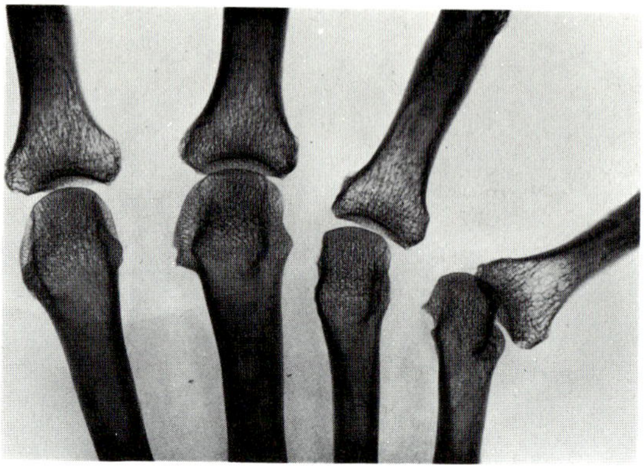

Fig. 42.20 X-ray of right hand showing ulnar deviation, subluxation at metacarpal joints with small lateral erosions of metacarpal heads. This occurred in a woman of 25 years who had had two previous rheumatic attacks with chorea and polyarthritis. No present complaint of joints, but evidence of mitral stenosis, aortic incompetence, normal sedimentation rate and a biopsy showing synovial membrane without evidence of active inflammation. (By courtesy of the *British Heart Journal*.)

heightens the similarity to rheumatoid arthritis. Sometimes dorsal sheath effusions are seen and on occasion the peripheral signs of rheumatic fever consist of a painful pitting oedema of the hand and elbow, similar but more painful than that seen in Henoch–Schönlein purpura. Complete subsidence of the arthritis occurs in almost every case without residual lesions.

Rarely, in cases in which there have been repeated attacks of arthritis, with prolonged pain and disability of the hands, a residual, non-progressive correctable ulnar deviation of the fingers occurs after one of the later attacks. This was described first by Jaccoud in 1869 and is of importance because of its resemblance to rheumatoid arthritis. Similar deformities may also affect the feet. Confusion is particularly easy in the very rare case where subluxation and bony 'erosions' occur (Fig. 42.20) (Bywaters, 1950, 1975). Useful distinguishing points are the history of repeated rheumatic fever attacks, residual heart lesion, normal sedimentation rate, biopsy findings and the lack of symptoms or progression (Grahame et al, 1970). This complication is well recognised in France (e.g. Ravault et al, 1961) and more recently in the USA (Zvaifler, 1962; Ruderman & Abruzzo, 1966). As described recently (Bywaters, 1975), somewhat similar lesions occur in systemic lupus erythematosus. Rather more emphasis has been placed on these chronic joint manifestations in a description designed for the specialist than would have been made in an exposition for undergraduates or general medical education where the dictum is still true that rheumatic fever 'licks the joints but bites the heart' (Lasègue, 1884). The status of streptococcal 'reactive arthritis', lasting a year in B27-positive individuals (Hubbard & Hughes, 1982; Gerstar et al, 1982) remains still unsolved.

Rheumatic torticollis has been described (Rehm, 1878) but apart from temporary migratory involvement of the neck joints it seems probable that such a torticollis is related to the antecedent throat infection, i.e. is the *maladie de Grisel*, a fixed torticollis occurring after any acute pharyngeal infection and thought variously to be due to dislocation (Berkheiser & Seidler, 1931), vertebral osteitis (Swynghedauw et al, 1946), subluxation due to muscle spasm (Grisel, 1930) or spondylarthritis (Odelberg-Johnson, 1932). It is not to be confused with ankylosing spondylitis or the cervical apophyseal involvement seen in Still's disease and some cases of adult rheumatoid arthritis. It is treated with manipulation and extension (Zimmermann, 1967).

'Growing pains' are, in general, not due to rheumatic fever, agreeing with Hawksley (1938). Distinguishing features from the limb pain of rheumatic fever are these: occurrence in lower limbs rather than upper, between joints rather than at joints and towards the end of the day. Such pains are usually due to posture, exertion or fatigue or are of psychological origin (Naish & Apley, 1951).

Skin manifestations

These are by no means common. The typical and characteristic rash is erythema annulare, often called erythema circinatum or erythema marginatum (Fig. 42.21; Bywaters, 1979). It is a fleeting ringed eruption seen in about 10–20% of active cases, usually on the trunk, usually flat, growing in size by annular accretion and leaving slight staining in the centre. A similar ringed rash has been reported in serum sickness and trypanosomiasis (Keil, 1937). The fixed drug rashes and ringed syphilides are not likely to cause confusion but seven other types of annular erythema are to be differentiated (Beare et al, 1966). The characteristic feature of erythema marginatum is its rate of spread, which averages 2–4 mm/12 hours and differentiates it from the rash of Still's disease, which does not spread (Isdale & Bywaters, 1956). The histological appearance (Fig. 42.22) is somewhat similar to that of Henoch-Schönlein purpura

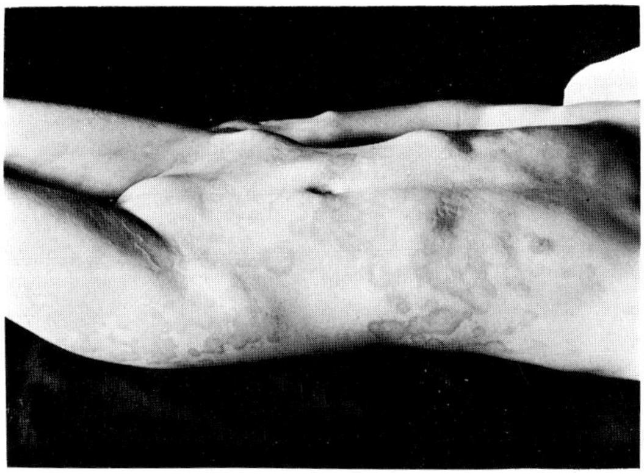

Fig. 42.21 V.S. female aet. 9 in first attack with polyarthritis, carditis, multiple nodules and recurrent rash, later pericardial effusion. Subacute bacterial endocarditis aet. 14 and 17 years. Well at follow-up, aet. 28 years.

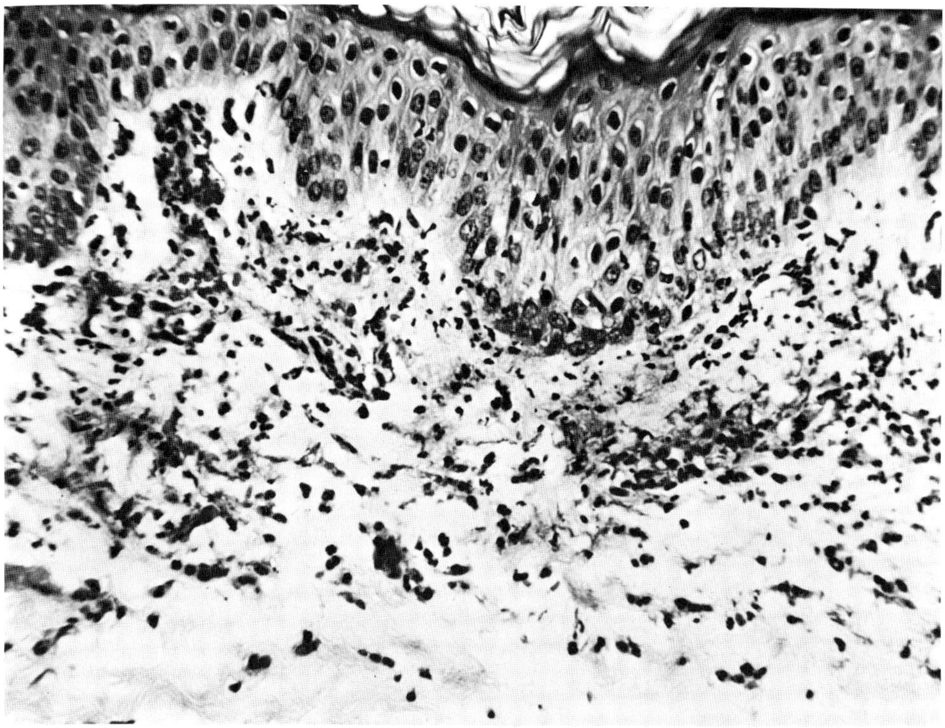

Fig. 42.22 Erythema marginatum. Note polymorphonuclear leucocytes and their debris. (H & E ×280)

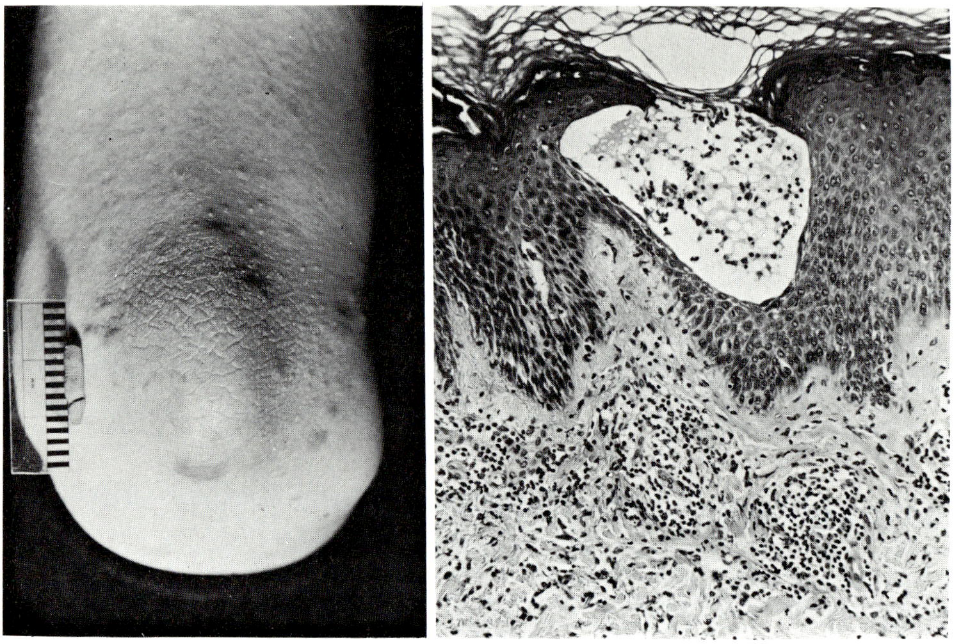

Fig. 42.23 Erythema papulatum on elbow, in A.B. male aet. 13; acute rheumatic fever with aortic and mitral disease. ESR 110 mm/h. Histology on right: H & E × 170.

without the erythrocyte diapedesis (Bywaters et al, 1957b). It may sometimes be raised. Urticaria occurs uncommonly as well as an irregular macular papular rash somewhat resembling that of Still's disease except in its distribution. Erythema papulatum is rare, appearing on the extensor surfaces, particularly hands, knees, and elbows (Fig. 42.23; Bywaters, 1971). Erythema nodosum and Henoch–Schönlein purpura are not rheumatic manifestations: in each of these diseases synovitis may occur and is often mistaken for rheumatic fever (see Ch. 49). Like nephritis, erythema nodosum may occur together with rheumatic fever as a coincidence, but other nodose lesions, such as those due to sulphathiazole, should be excluded.

Nodules

Nodules occur not infrequently (about 30% at Taplow) in juvenile rheumatic fever at the sites of repeated mild traumata over bony prominences such as the spinous processes (Fig. 42.24), knuckles, olecranon and occiput, and where tendons exert pressure on their sheaths (Fig. 42.25), such as in the palm, at the wrist and at the ankle. Over the finger tendons they may cause a mechanical contracture lasting a few days or a week but never, as with rheumatoid tendon nodules, becoming permanent. At the elbow they are preceded by a slight thickening of the subcutaneous tissue, more visible than palpable, which histologically is indistinguishable from the fully developed nodule (see Fig. 42.14).

While they occur usually during the later part of the active stage this is not always so, some occurring with a normal sedimentation rate. They seldom occur in cases without cardiac involvement. The number of nodules seems to bear some relation to the severity of the disease and in one ultimately fatal case they were so numerous as to be uncountable. They may be distinguished clinically (as well as histologically, q.v.) from the nodules of rheumatoid arthritis by their smaller size, usually several millimetres in diameter, their more rapid appearance and disappearance and their tendency to occur in groups of two or three. Biopsy of nodules is occasionally useful in cases, usually adults, where there is difficulty in differentiating rheumatoid arthritis. Unfortunately, in such cases (proved subsequently to be due to rheumatic fever) not only is the nodule clinically larger and more durable than usual but histologically it may show some degree of palisading and necrosis,

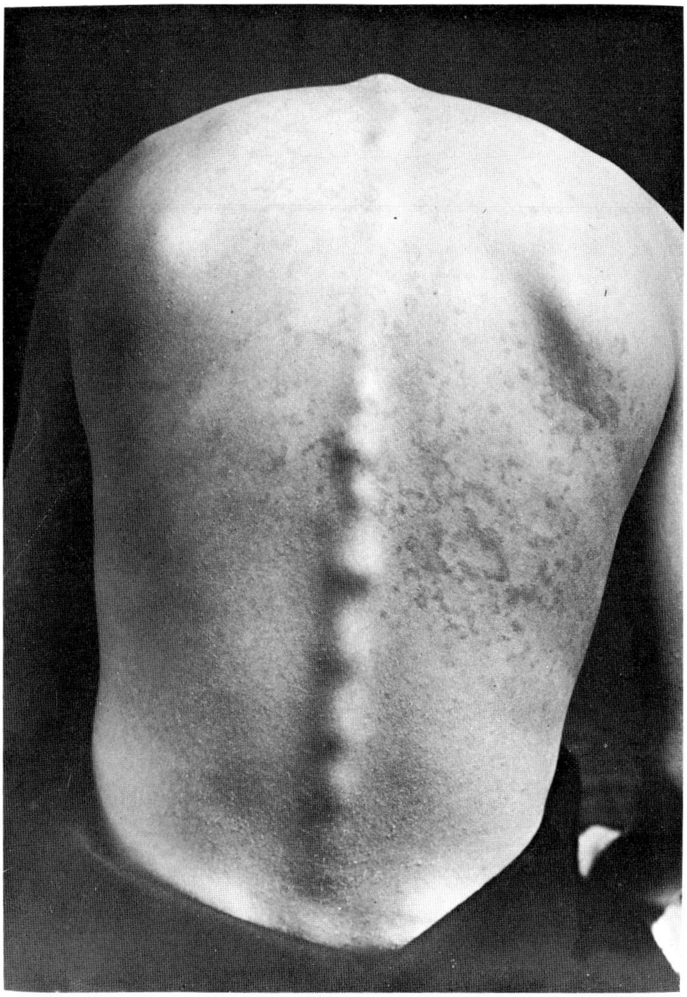

Fig. 42.24 R.R. aet. 12 at 6 weeks from onset, showing nodules over spine and scapula lasting 2 months, with erythema marginatum lasting 4 months.

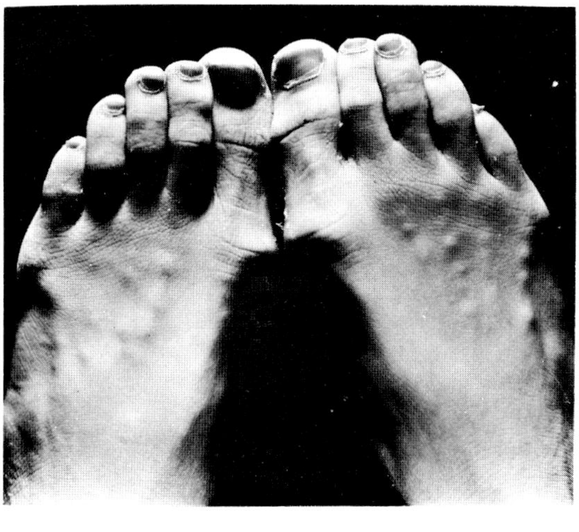

simulating thereby the more acute type of rheumatoid nodule.

Heart

Heart involvement, without which rheumatic fever would be no more important than mumps, was not suspected in rheumatic fever until 1788 (see Ch. 1). Its incidence depends upon the frequency and care with which it is looked and listened for and upon its definition, ranging from the minor and transient increases in conduction time de-

Fig. 42.25 R.G. aet. 18 with polyarthritis and carditis. ESR 80 mm/h. ASO titre 2500. Multiple nodules on elbows, feet, fingers developing 3 weeks after admission

scribed by Rantz et al (1947), occurring in recovery from haemolytic sore throat, to the full-blown carditis of rheumatic fever. A detailed account is given by Cary Coombs (1924) and more recently by Wood (1968). In the early stages a soft apical pansystolic murmur is heard, often with a short, soft inconstant mid-diastolic murmur in the mitral area internal to the apex or an early diastolic murmur in the aortic area (heard best in expiration at the left border of the sternum). In many patients these signs are transient but they may progress to the characteristic murmurs of established valvular disease. They must be distinguished from the innocent systolic murmurs heard in 90% of normal children (Lessof & Brigden, 1957). The characteristics of the pathological murmur are that it lasts throughout systole, is conducted towards and is usually maximal just internal to the apex beat. In the child known to have had a past attack of rheumatic fever, active heart involvement is difficult to diagnose unless fresh murmurs are heard or changes in quality occur.

The electrocardiogram may give some help, particularly in the early stages where the PR interval may be increased above an arbitrary upper limit of 0.20 seconds in adults or 0.18 seconds below the age of 15; minor increases above the Ashman & Hull (1945) standards for the rate and age must be interpreted in the light of subsequent changes, since such increases have been seen in 10% of cases presenting as chorea in the absence of clinical or laboratory signs of cardiac involvement (Heffer, 1941) and indeed in normal children occasionally (Mirowski et al, 1964). These authors reaffirm the well known fact that first degree heart block unusually occurs without other evidence of carditis and that residual cardiac lesions seldom ensue. The length of the QT interval corrected for varying heart rate is of little value.

Rhythm change. Heart block, usually incomplete, and nodal rhythm are complications occasionally seen (Clarke & Keith, 1972). Fibrillation seldom occurs except in the older age-groups or in those with established mitral disease.

Pericarditis. In the early stages of rheumatic fever pericarditis is not of great prognostic significance. It is usually 'dry', manifest by rub and sometimes by electrocardiographic changes. Sometimes an effusion occurs. Later than 4 weeks from onset, pericarditis produces an effusion and has a considerably worse prognosis, lasting very much longer and being accompanied by more pain, by tachypnoea and electrocardiographic change (Thomas et al, 1953). Such an effusion is almost always accompanied by valvular disease and causes a rapid increase in cardiac size, and straightening or bulging of the left border (Besterman & Thomas, 1953). Carditis alone does not cause a rapid increase in size. The onset is often insidious, the child being less lively and looking off colour, or it may be dramatic with increase in fever, and sleeping pulse rate, with precordial pain, orthopnoea, vomiting and an increased jugular venous filling; the signs at the lung bases are probably due to an accompanying pleural effusion (Thomas et al, 1953): there may be signs of collapse. Pressure symptoms due to the effusion are not a marked feature of rheumatic pericarditis (and aspiration is seledom indicated); nor does the scarring except in exceptional cases (McMurray et al, 1951) lead as in tuberculosis to obstruction or constrictive symptoms.

Heart failure. The most useful sign of heart failure is an increase in the jugular venous pressure (measured clinically in the neck at an angle of 45°) although this occurs also early in the development of a pericardial effusion. In children failure is often seen unaccompanied by peripheral oedema or ascites. The vital capacity, however, is markedly decreased. Dyspnoea and orthopnoea are not as striking symptoms of failure as they are in adults. An increased respiratory rate in sleep with periodic variations may be seen in severe relapses accompanied by pericarditis. An increase in bodyweight is the best clinical index over short periods of water and chloride retention and hence, unless the patients are on a low salt diet, of the severity of failure. Intake and output charts are of lesser value but useful when diuretics are being used. Any rapid increase in size of the heart is usually due to pericardial effusion, but more gradual increase occurs with failure and may be accompanied radiologically by lung congestion. Liver damage due to 'central necrosis' is common in severe long-lasting failure: in some of these, actual cardiac cirrhosis may be present with an increase in centrilobular connective tissue. Clubbing of the fingers occasionally occurs in severe long-standing failure and subsides as the heart recovers (Bywaters, 1950); it is important that this is not by itself taken to mean bacterial endocarditis.

Lungs

Lung changes in rheumatic fever are almost invariably secondary to heart involvement. Pleural effusions and basal rales indicative of congestion are common. Rarely massive collapse occurs and usually as rapidly expands (Fig. 42.26). Occasionally in long-standing failure haemosiderosis may occur, consisting of fine soft aggregates 1–3 mm in diameter throughout the lung field (Ellman & Gee, 1951). These may be due to haemorrhage (Taylor & Strong, 1955). A more discreet aggregate about the same size may be due to ossification of the fibrinous products within the alveoli (Elkeles & Glynn, 1946) as a sequel to rheumatic pneumonia. They are found mainly in the lower zones, particularly in men with mitral stenosis, occurring, according to Galloway et al (1961), in 25% of men as against only 9% of women. They should be distinguished from the calcific lesions of pulmonary microlithiasis (Kent et al, 1955).

Rheumatic 'pneumonia' occurs in patients with heart failure and pancarditis (Grunow & Esterly, 1972). It is usually manifest as dyspnoea, orthopnoea and cyanosis, and not infrequently in accompanied by dry cough and a small amount of blood-stained sputum. Radiologically this diffuse opacity spreading out from one or both lung roots (Fig. 42.27) closely resembles uraemic oedema, as

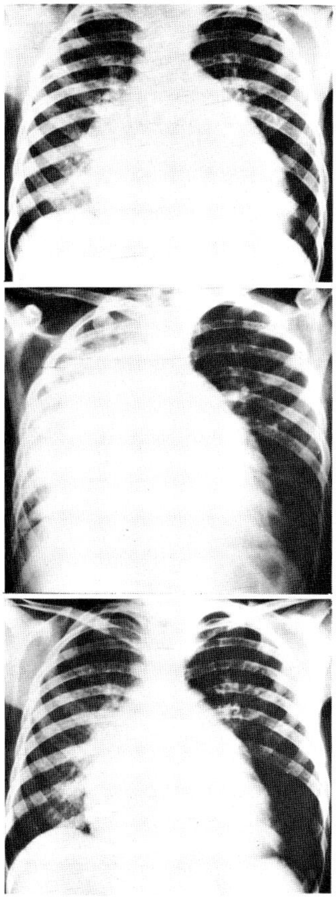

Fig. 42.26 X-rays of heart in male aet. 14 with rapid development of pericardial effusion and collapse of right lung, 2 days after, re-expanding 4 days later. (From *Modern Practice in Infectious Fevers*, Butterworth, London.)

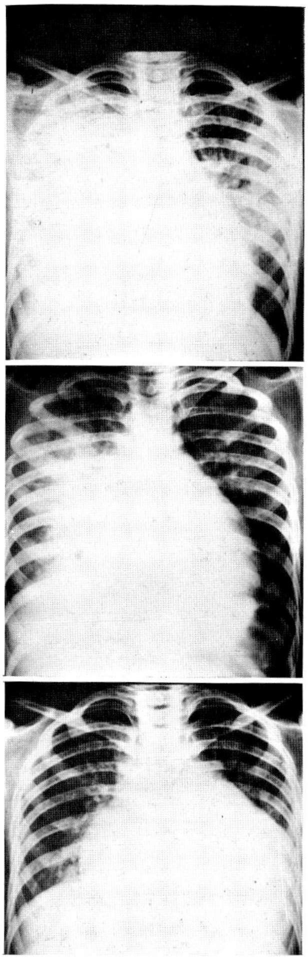

Fig. 42.27 N.O'F. female aet. 8 'Rheumatic pneumonia' clearing before death from cardiac failure. X-ray dated 7, 17, 25 August 1948.

it does also pathologically (Doniach, 1947). This rheumatic 'pneumonia' is often associated with high salicylate blood levels. The increased vascular permeability seen also in acute salicylate poisoning (Hormaechaea et al, 1979; Broderick et al, 1976; Heffner & Sahn, 1981) and outpouring of oedema fluid with or without fibrin is probably a manifestation of acute cardiac insufficiency brought about by failure of the damaged heart to respond to the increase in metabolism due to salicylate. When it occurs, salicylates must be stopped, and prednisone given, together with digitalis, diuretics and a low salt diet (see p. 1089). Penicillin is of no value. Some interstitial fibrosis may occur after repeated episodes (Moolten, 1962) as after iatrogenic pulmonary oedema (Heard, 1962).

Serositis

Abdominal pain may sometimes occur and in a number of cases is the main reason for admission to hospital; appendicectomy in such cases is followed by the development of rheumatic fever (Lin & Rodriquez-Torros, 1969). However, since in some cases of rheumatic fever true appendicitis may develop, it is probably always wise to err on the side of the surgeons, although in most of the cases the appendix which has been removed proves to be normal. The pain may be due to rheumatic peritonitis (Rhea, 1933; Wilson, 1940). It may be referred from the pleurae or the pericardium or it may be due to myositis involving the rectus sheath (Reitman, 1945). In one case it was associated with rheumatic arteritis of the abdominal vessels (Freiberg & Gross, 1934). Cases of segmental ileitis and colitis have been recorded (Felsen, 1940; Herschfield & Marks, 1949). The orchitis occasionally seen in rheumatic fever (Trasoff & Goodman, 1944) may be of a similar nature or may be due to mumps with synovitis mimicking that of rheumatic fever. Yersinial reactive arthritis needs differentiation (Laitinen et al, 1975).

Renal involvement

Renal involvement in the patient with rheumatic fever is usually acute glomerulonephritis (although variable histologic changes may be found; Mendoza et al, 1975; Gibney et al, 1981). In 4 out of 6 cases recorded by Brod (1949) the nephritis followed the rheumatic fever after 2 weeks; in one case it preceded rheumatic fever by 2 weeks; and occurred simultaneously in the last. In a large series of cases in Boston, 4% of nephritis patients had rheumatic heart disease, and 5% of the rheumatic children had glomerulonephritis (Hartman & Bland, 1951). The association is thus less common than the increased Addis count seen with or without cardiac failure (Goldring & Wyckoff, 1930). As both these diseases are due to streptococcal infection, it is odd that they do not more often occur together (Chandrasekhara & Cornfield, 1969). Goldsmith et al (1958) have recorded a family outbreak including cases with glomerulonephritis and rheumatic fever due to a Griffith type 1 streptococcus; rheumatic fever may follow acute glomerulonephritis, i.e. they are not mutually exclusive (Hartman & Bland, 1951). Acute nephritis (with nitrogen retention in half of the cases only) occurred in 0.9% of 1111 cases at Taplow (Ansel & Hill, unpublished). Both Henoch–Schönlein purpura and lupus erythematosus with renal damage, of course, need exclusion.

Chorea minor

Sydenham's chorea was first fully related to rheumatism and heart disease by Sée in 1850 although a few previous authors including Bright (1838) had noted an association. It has only superficial connection with St Vitus, the patron saint of actors and dancers, a Sicilian martyred under Diocletian in AD 303, after whom the dancing manias of the Middle Ages were named. Chorea may occur during the course of an attack of rheumatic fever or without acute rheumatism or a history thereof ('lone chorea'). About half the cases in this latter category have evidence of rheumatic heart disease.

Chorea minor is characterised by spontaneous movements, by ataxia and incoordination and by weakness, which may at times be severe enough to amount to paralysis. Emotional expression may be exaggerated or altered. It is almost always one of the *late* complications of rheumatic fever (Taranta, 1959), although the preceding attack may have been so mild as to pass unnoticed. Evidence for this is: (1) the increased ASO titre seen early, even in 'lone' chorea; (2) its association in the vast majority of cases with present or past rheumatic fever or rheumatic heart disease; (3) the seasonal peak which occurs about 1–2 months later than that of rheumatic fever, and (4) the appearance in later life of mitral stenosis despite absence of carditis in the acute attack (Bland, 1961). Even cases due apparently to other diseases such as diphtheria (Haber, 1937) might well be due to concomitant streptococcal infection.

The only exceptions appear to be hypoparathyroidism, systemic lupus erythematosus and possibly Henoch–Schönlein purpura. More than 27 cases associated with systemic lupus erythematosus have been published (Donaldson and Espiner, 1971). The ASO titre is normal. Hypoparathyroidism may be associated with choreic movements due to a 'functional irritability of the nerve fiber' (McKinney, 1962; Tabaee-Zadeh et al, 1972) as may primary hyperparathyroidism (Lloyd et al, 1965) possibly due to magnesium deficiency (Fisherman, 1965).

Girls are more often affected than boys, particularly in the age-group 11–15 and in pregnancy. In chorea gravidarum one-third of cases have heart disease, one-quarter a previous history of rheumatic fever, and one-half have had previous chorea (Beresford & Graham, 1950) but it may occur in the absence of any preceding infection judged by three antibody levels (Jonas et al, 1972). It appears to be getting less frequent (Gatenby 1956).

Anatomically, changes in the brain may be either absent, indistinguishable from those found in rheumatic fever without chorea, or those of a meningoencephalitis (reviewed by Lessof, 1958). Antistreptococcal antibody binding to astrocytes (Kingston & Glynn, 1976; Darlington et al, 1976), and similar antibodies binding to basal nuclei (Husby et al, 1976) from choreic patients have been described. Although chorea may be due to release of motor activity from higher control by damage to corticostriate pathways, functionally it a appears to be completely reversible, perhaps due to 're-education'.

Symptoms. All degrees of chorea exist, from the very mild to severe and even fatal cases. The onset is generally insidious, the child seeming to be merely restless, inattentive, nervous or emotionally disturbed. Sometimes she is thought by her parents to be naughty or careless, since she tends to drop things, cry without reason, grimace, or stumble. Soon, however, the inco-ordinate nature of the child's movements tends to become manifest. The limbs cannot be held still, and the face twitches, often breaking into the aimless choreic smile. These movements commence often in the upper limbs, and more frequently on the right side. In about a third of cases they remain limited to one side (hemichorea), although in other cases they soon spread equally to all limbs. The movements, unlike those of encephalitis, tend to cease during sleep, but are much increased by any attempt at voluntary movement. Evidence of muscular inco-ordination is provided by asking the child to put out her tongue. This can be done, but it is then suddenly jerked back into the mouth as though the child were playing the trumpet. Weakness and hypotonia of all the muscles are present, and may sometimes progress to the stage of a mild paresis on one or both sides. 'Pendulum' knee jerks may be present. When the arms are stretched out in front, the wrists tend to be drawn into flexion and the metacarpophalangeal joints into extension — the 'choreic hand' (Fig. 42.28). An unsteady hand grip affords a useful graphic assessment — 'milking' grip. Respiration is often jerky and irregular.

Some degree of psychic disturbance is always present, and may show itself by fretfulness, attacks of causeless laughing or crying, or sometimes by violent attacks of rage. Sleep is usually affected, being restless, broken, and accompanied by bad dreams. Severe cases, seldom seen today, need beds with padded protecting rails. The patient is usually afebrile (hyperpyrexia may rarely be seen, associated with salicylate medication) and evidence of associated or previous rheumatic activity may or may not be present (e.g. raised ESR). Thus in the Taplow series (Lessof, 1958) two-thirds had rheumatic fever as well, and half of the remainder had rheumatic heart disease. The attacks last a few days to several months, the child recovering completely.

In some children transient residual movement may be seen and needs to be distinguished from multiple tics (Healy, 1970). The essential difference is the unco-ordinated and purposeless nature of the choreic movements as against the repetitive progressive and limited nature of the tic. Rare hereditary types of chorea or choreoathetosis, either Huntingdon's or the autosomal dominant types of early onset (Haerer et al, 1967), or that associated with hyperuricaemia, need differentiation, as do

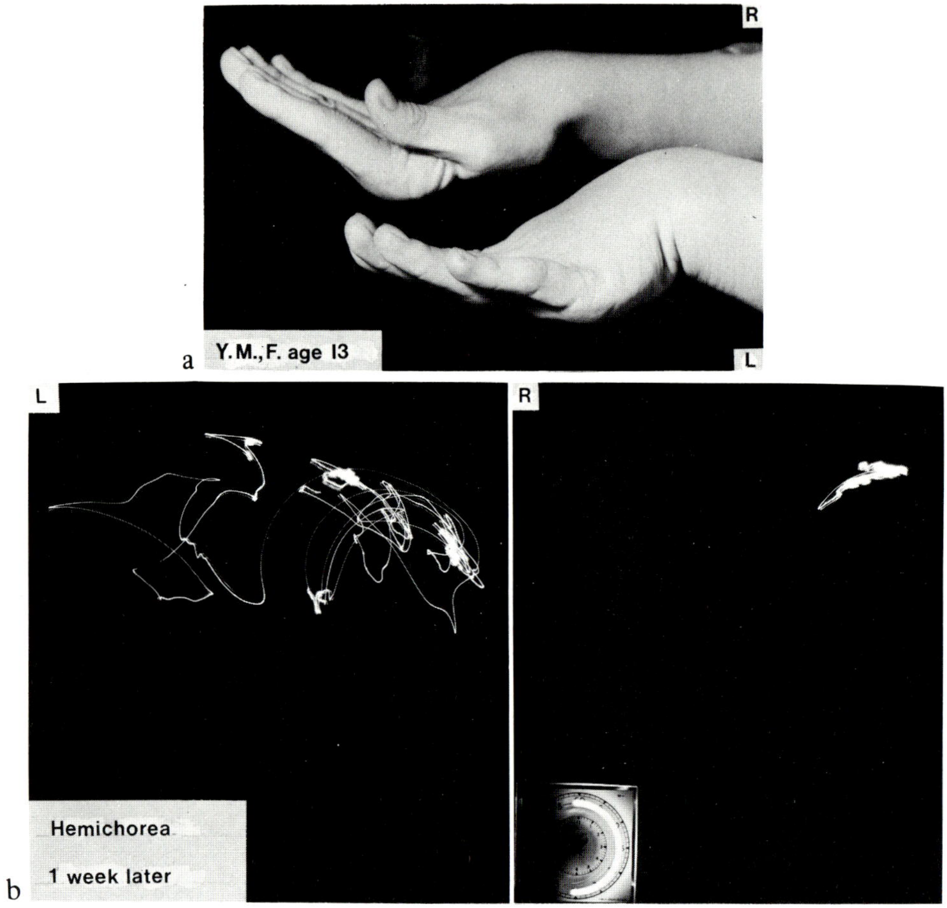

Fig. 42.28 Severe chorea (Y.M. female aet. 13) showing (a) pronator sign and (b) one week later, subsidence of chorea on one side as shown by light tracings over a 30-second exposure.

the abnormal acquired movements in encephalitis, vascular disease, brain tumour, particularly in the region of the aqueduct, or those following perinatal brain injury or phenothiazone administration (Singer & Wong, 1970). The contraceptive pill may precipitate a relapse of chorea (Lewis & Harrison, 1969) or apparently produce such dysfunction de novo (Riddoch et al, 1971), perhaps by facilitating thrombosis. Hereditary tremor and paramyoclonus multiplex are easily distinguished. The rare association with hypo- or hyperparathyroidism, with lupus and with the 'Gilles de la Tourette' syndrome (Melvin et al, 1977) should be considered and the appropriate examination made. Electroencephalography may show abnormal slow waves (Diamond & Tentler, 1962) but these may also be seen in uncomplicated rheumatic fever (Lavy et al, 1964) and are not pathognomonic (Johnson et al, 1964).

Relapses may occur without fresh infection for up to 2 years, but after this period recurrences are usually due to a fresh streptococcal stimulus (Taranta, 1957). Recurrences in a patient who has had 'lone' chorea tend also to be free from other rheumatic manifestations, but as Bland has suggested (1961) and as we have shown in our 10-year follow-up (Thomas, unpublished data), mitral stenosis is particularly prone to occur insidiously in patients with chorea and very transient minimal carditis in hospital. Complications other than this are few; hyperpyrexia has been mentioned. Myositis ossificans has been seen due to muscle damage from forcible restraint (Coste et al, 1950). Transient or permanent blindness may result from optic atrophy due to obstruction of the central retinal artery even in cases of pure chorea without carditis (Hearn & Roper Hall, 1961; Ling et al, 1969). Its pathogenesis is uncertain but minor degrees of obscuration may occur in rheumatic heart disease without chorea (Swash & Earl, 1970). Transient papilloedema with benign intracranial hypertension has also been recorded (Chun et al, 1961).

No treatment is known that shortens the duration of chorea. Bed-rest is the best form of therapy and parents must be warned not to scold or punish the child for clumsiness or grimacing. Hospital lessons are valuable not only as diversional therapy but because failure to keep up with contemporaries due to lack of schooling can cause psychological difficulties. A controlled study (Sacks et al, 1962) has indicated that this is perhaps the major factor in the residual difficulties which these children often display. Even in 'lone' chorea it is best to keep the child in bed until choreic movements have ceased. Severe cases may need full doses of sedatives such as phenobarbitone or chloral, and in the worst cases (chorea gravis and insaniens) paraldehyde is necessary. Many other drugs have been tried but are mostly more dangerous and no more effective (e.g. chlorpromazine or haloperidol — Siegal & Mones, 1971).

In the late stages of the disease reeducation should be undertaken to help the child to regain the finer movements and muscular co-ordination. This may take the form of 'play therapy' with bricks, card-house building, sewing etc. and must be carefully supervised to see that accuracy and neatness are restored — and thus the child's confidence in herself.

Laboratory aids

These are of the greatest value in the management of rheumatic fever by graded rest.

Erythrocyte sedimentation rate. This we have found the most useful single criterion for determining when it is safe to allow increased physical activity without the danger of relapse (Fig. 42.29). The Westergren method is best, using a 200 mm tube and a dilution of 4 parts of blood (fresh or sequestrened) to one of 3.8% sodium citrate, reading the fall at one hour. Correction for anaemia is unnecessary and unwise (Sinton, 1948). The Wintrobe method will sometimes give anomalous results because with undiluted blood the tube diameter is too small to allow free fall, particularly if the haemocrit is over 40% (Shannon & Bywaters, 1957). Thus, values of 5 mm/h may be obtained by the Wintrobe method in a case of severe active rheumatic fever or Still's disease where a simultaneous Westergren method will give values of 60–80 mm/h. The same objection applies to the Rourke–Ernstene method of measuring the maximum fall per minute. It is important to remember that errors due to change of temperature (Fourke & Plass, 1929) or contamination with alcohol (Sykes, 1948) may occur unless due care is observed.

The sedimentation rate runs parallel with plasma viscosity (Lawrence, 1961) which is more easily automated, and increased values are usually due to an increase in plasma fibrinogen. Low results may occur in congestive failure (Payne & Schlesinger, 1935; Wood, 1936) due to impaired liver function and resultant low fibrinogen (Sanghvi & Bohra, 1962) but this is comparatively uncommon (Spagnuolo & Feinstein, 1964). With these exceptions we have not found a normal sedimentation rate in the presence of clinically active rheumatism, provided that the patient is untreated. The converse, however, is not true, since we can confirm Harris's (1945) observation that in adolescent girls a high ESR of about 20 to 30 mm/h may be maintained for several months in the absence of any clinical signs and without any apparent harm despite increased physical activity (Bywaters, 1950).

C-reactive protein. A similar indicator of 'rheumatic' activity is the appearance of C-reactive protein in the plasma. Again this is a non-specific indicator of inflammation but is not affected by congestive heart failure (Rosansky & Davis, 1958). C-reactive protein decreases in serum before the sedimentation rate has reached normal.

Haemoglobin. The hypochromic anaemia of the acute stages of rheumatic fever is not affected by iron therapy but improves spontaneously with recovery. It is similar to the anaemia of sepsis and may be due in part to haemolysis (Reinhold, 1951).

White count. A moderate leucocytosis is generally present.

Immunoglobulins. There is an increase in IgG

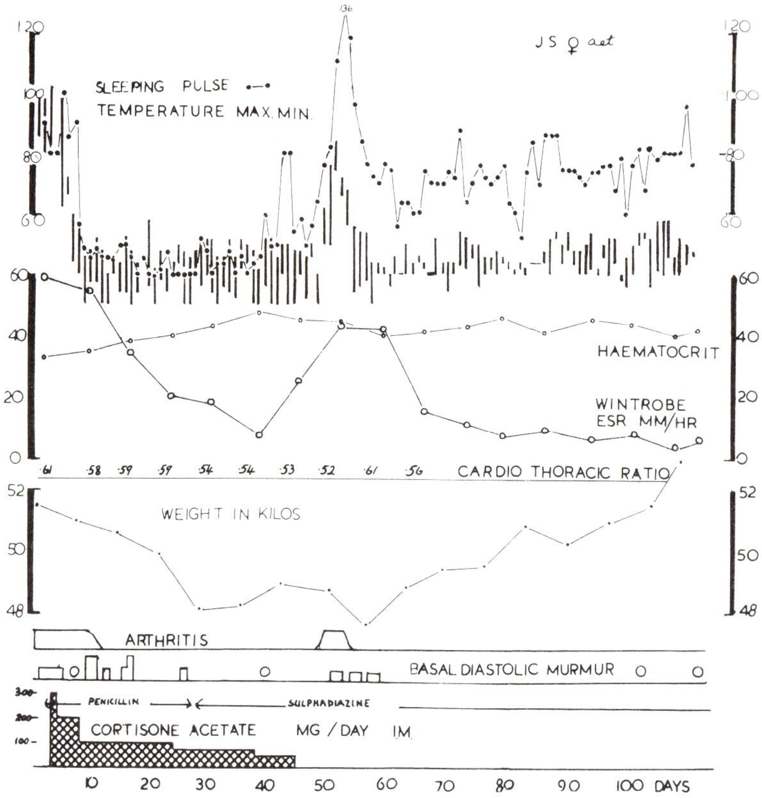

Fig. 42.29 Course of rheumatic fever in child treated with cortisone acetate for 6 weeks. Note rebound following discontinuance, affecting pulse temperature, haematocrit, sedimentation rate, cardiothoracic ratio, body weight, arthritis and basal diastolic murmur from above down, with eventual improvement and recovery.

or IgA in the first two weeks (Schoenfield et al, 1968). IgA increases significantly more in those with heart-reactive antibody rise (Vaccaro et al, 1970).

Serum antistreptolysin O titre. A rise in this titre above the normal level (0–200 units after the age of 8) is useful indicator of preceding streptococcal infection, and as such is of some values where diagnostic doubt exists. A standardised method has been described (Johnson, 1955) and standard sera are available from commercial sources. It is important to distinguish high non-specific titres of 'ASO' due to the inhibitory action of increased lipoproteins in jaundice (Winblad, 1966) and also the rare association of ASO activity with myeloma protein (Zettervall et al, 1966). A significant rise fails to occur after some 20% of streptococcal infections, but other antibodies to extracellular products will increase in these circumstances. Antidesoxyribonuclease B and anti-diphosphopyridine nucleotidase are thought by some to be a better indicator than ASO titre (Wannamaker & Ayoub, 1960) for this purpose. For full discussion and details of methods see Stollerman (1960).

The 'Streptozyme' test has recently been recommended (see footnote, Table 42.2), and the Bacitracin disc, specifically discouraging group A streptococci on blood agar plates.

Complications

The only complication, apart from the inherent manifestations of the disease dealt with above and the accidental effects of treatment dealt with below, is subacute bacterial endocarditis. McIlwayne (1947) claims that the rheumatic process is usually active in cases with acquired heart lesions, basing this view on the presence of active

Aschoff nodes in the heart at post-mortem in 78%: the majority of previous workers, however, agree on half this amount, i.e. 36% in the 262 previous cases cited by McIlwayne. It is, however, rare for active rheumatic fever to be complicated by the development of subacute bacterial endocarditis, although this does occasionally occur in the older age-groups and is a possibility always to be entertained, particularly in view of the efficacy of modern treatment.

Course and prognosis

An attack of rheumatic fever may last a week or a year: in general the more severe the attack the longer it lasts. The average attack lasts about 6 weeks, if the criterion of duration be adopted of the fall to 'normal' levels of the sedimentation rate: shorter, if other criteria are adopted (Taran, 1946). In children a more reliable index of cure is the resumption of normal weight-accretion (taking care to exclude oedematous episodes) (Fig. 42.29).

In some cases a polycyclic course is seen with one or more relapses, lasting in all several months; this must be distinguished from a recurrence or second attack (due to streptococcal reinfection).

In many recovered cases second attacks, and in some multiple attacks, occur. In the pre-prophylactic era, a series studied by May Wilson showed one or more recurrences in 85% of children (Wilson & Lubschez, 1944). They found the risk of recurrences to diminish after the age of 13 and after one year from the attack, but in the Taplow series of pre-prophylaxis cases admitted between 1949 and 1950 there were about 5% recurrences per year for each of the first five years following the initial attack, compared with 1% recurrences per year in a similar number of children given prophylaxis (Bywaters & Thomas, 1958). No decrease of recurrences after puberty was found. In cases treated (1948–1950) with bed-rest alone (compared with others treated with cortisone, aspirin or ACTH) acute signs subsided rather more slowly, but by the 8th week there was little difference between the series (Bywaters & Thomas, 1961).

Residual heart damage was found at 5 years in half the cases who had had no recurrences, and the state of the heart at 5 years was determined almost entirely by its condition on or soon after admission to hospital rather than by the treatment used (Thomas, 1961). This was also the 5-year and the 10-year conclusion of the US./UK. Co-operative Clinical Trial (1960, 1965). Those without carditis in hospital are normal at follow-up and those with carditis tend to have residual damage depending on the severity of the carditis observed during hospital admission. The severity of the residual damage is greater in those cases with prolonged and severe attacks, and the risk of this is increased with the number of recurrences. Enlargement of the heart is usually at its maximum during the attack, and if the patient is adequately rested may ultimately attain a normal ratio to chest diameter since the chest will continue to grow in a child and the heart size remains stationary (Taussig & Goldenberg, 1941). The valvular lesions may become static or they may progress, quite apart from rheumatic activity, as a result of fibrosis and in the absence of any obvious intervening rheumatic activity. On the other hand, if slight in degree, the physical signs indicating valvular disease during the acute attack may completely disappear.

The prognosis may be reviewed in the light of the careful 20-year study of 1000 patients in Boston by Bland & Duckett Jones (1952) whose observations merit detailed attention (Table 42.1). It is worst in those cases with carditis (especially if severe, or associated with progressive enlargement of the heart), in those with prolonged attacks or recurrences and in those with numerous nodules. Our own 10-year follow-up (Thomas, unpublished data) shows similar results but slightly better, perhaps due to the lessening severity of rheumatic fever of recent years. We can also confirm a suggestion of Bland's (1961) that mitral stenosis is particularly liable to follow chorea, even when there has been only minimal carditis during intitial hospitalisation.

The management of pregnancy in a woman with

Table 42.1 After Bland & Duckett Jones (1952)

	Mean age		
	8 years	18 years	28 years
No detectable heart disease	347	323	319 (3 lost)
Rheumatic heart disease	653	475	380 (2 lost)
Dead	0	202	310

rheumatic heart disease is a difficult problem, well reviewed by Bunim & Appel (1950). The chief danger is congestive failure at term due to the increase in output associated with pregnancy (+ 50%) and the extra load due to labour. Embolism may also be fatal. In a number of fatal cases proceeding to term in apparently good health, active Aschoff nodules have been found at post-mortem (McKeown, 1948). The outlook is bad only for those with rheumatic heart disease of some severity. Apart from active rheumatism, and in patients not severely affected, pregnancy does not seem to affect adversely mild established valcular lesions.

While many patients with rheumatic heart disease survive to the usual 60–70 years, the majority die earlier, with the highest rate in the first few years from onset. Death occurs usually from congestive failure in a recurrent attack but rarely now in the initial attack. Before antibiotics subacute bacterial endocarditis accounted for 18% of 100 fatal adult cases in rheumatic heart disease according to Juca & White (1944). Today we can treat those cases successfully both medically and surgically.

Table 42.2 Summary of Duckett Jones Criteria (modified). For guidance in the diagnosis of rheumatic fever. Detailed definitions of the above criteria are given and discussed in *WHO Technical Report Series*, No. 342, Geneva, 1966, and in *Circulation* 13:617.

Major criteria	Minor criteria
I. Carditis	I. Fever
II. Polyarthritis	II. Arthralgia
III. Chorea	III. Prolonged PR interval
IV. Subcutaneous nodules	IV. Increased sedimentation rate, leucocytosis or C-reactive protein
V. Erythema marginatum	V. Evidence of preceding haemolytic streptococcal infection[a]
	VI. History of rheumatic fever or presence of old rheumatic heart disease.

Rheumatic fever is indicated if two major or two minor criteria are met; other diseases need to be excluded.

[a] Bisno & Ofek (1974) commend the Streptozyme test, a two-minute slide agglutination using red cells coated with streptococcal extracellular products, as more sensitive than any single serological test such as antistreptolysin, antikinase, etc.

Differential diagnosis

The criteria for diagnosis put foward by Duckett Jones have been almost universally accepted for the purpose of comparisons and for clinical trials. They are briefly listed here (Table 42.2) and more fully in the WHO Technical Report Series 342 (1966) quoting the modified criteria adopted by the American Heart Association (1956). During a period when 959 bona fide cases of rheumatic fever were admitted to Taplow, there were in addition 196 admissions diagnosed wrongly as rheumatic fever (Hallidie-Smith & Bywaters, 1958). These simulating conditions may be grouped under headings of: functional disease (tachycardia, neuroses, etc.), traumatic and postural disease, infections (the largest category), connective tissue disorders, rheumatic and congenital heart disease, blood dyscrasias, and a few miscellaneous and often unclassified complaints (Table 42.3).

In childhood *appendicitis* is the most common erroneous diagnosis with which in the USA a child with rheumatic fever enters hospital: 19 out of 271 cases according to Hansen (1943). This has already been discussed. In the youngest children it may be necessary to exclude *scurvy*.

Osteomyelitis (Harris, 1960) is perhaps the next most important differential diagnosis particularly in younger children with acute lesions deeply seated, such as the hip. The white blood count affords little help and diagnostic aspiration should be performed: even if negative and with no history of injury or boils it is better to diagnose infection and treat it rapidly with penicillin, since delay may cause irremediable damage. X-rays are of little or no value in the early stage. Staphylococci may cause a scarlet fever-like illness with joint involvement (Dunnett & Schallibaum, 1960). Measurement of staphylococcal alpha haemolysin may be a useful diagnostic aid (Lack & Towers, 1962).

Poliomyelitis is occasionally diagnosed as rheumatic fever since in the initial stages fever, pain, tenderness and even swelling (Poynton, 1943) are prominent features (Brainerd & Sokolow, 1949). *Rubella*, particularly in young women, causes synovitis like that of rheumatic fever (Bennett & Copeman, 1940). Synovial fluid cells are, however, monocytes (Chambers & Bywaters, 1963) not polymorphonuclear as in acute rheumatism. *Mumps*

Table 42.3 Differential diagnosis. (Modified from Hallidie-Smith & Bywaters, 1958)

Final diagnosis of 196 cases referred as rheumatic fever in whom this diagnosis was not confirmed	
Functional (8)	
Physiological tachycardia	3
Hysteria	3
Neurosis and depression	2
Traumatic and postural (11):	
Sprains	5
Slipped femoral epiphysis	2
Torn cartilage, osteochondritis dissecans, chest deformity and backache — one each	4
Infections (91):	
Upper respiratory tract	45
Lower respiratory tract	10
Bone and joint	10
Blood stream	4
Urinary tract	4
Pericarditis	2
'Flu, mononucleosis, measles, polio, hepatitis, erysipelas, paratyphoid and meningitis	16
Connective tissue disorders (42):	
Still's and rheumatoid arthritis	24
Henoch–Schönlein purpura	8
Erythema nodosum	5
Visceral lupus erythematosus	2
Periarteritis nodosum	1
Penicillin sensitivity	1
Granuloma annulare	1
Rheumatic and congenital heart disease (9):	
Rheumatic	7
Congenital	2
Blood dyscrasias (2):	
Iron deficiency anaemia	1
Aleukaemia stem-cell leukaemia	1
Others (33):	
Limb pains	15
Arthralgia	9
Arthritis	5
Fever	3
Gout and syphilis	1
Total	196

arthritis (Lass & Shephard, 1961) and *transient hip syndrome* or 'irritable hips' (Hardinge, 1970) may both need consideration.

Other infections simulating acute rheumatic polyarthritis are *miliary tuberculosis* (Freud et al, 1950) and *meningococcal bacteraemia* (Daniels, 1948); blood cultures or cerebrospinal fluid examination should be made if necessary. Polyarthritis is also seen in the early stage of *hepatitis* and three of the cases recorded by Martini (1950) were diagnosed as rheumatic fever. *Yersinia enterocolitica* arthritis (Winblad, 1973) especially in B-27-positive cases (Sheldon et al, 1982) is a more recent contender.

Another condition to be borne in mind is *acute lymphatic leukaemia* associated with fever, migratory pain and swelling of joints due to periosteal reaction (Fink et al, 1972); other blood diseases such as *sickle cell anaemia* (Diggs, 1965), *myelosclerosis* (Wood and Andrews, 1949) and infective *reticuloendotheliosis* (Knopf, 1947; Diamond & Clark, 1965) may simulate closely rheumatic fever, as also have rarities like *neuroblastoma* (de Lorimer et al, 1969) diagnosed with vanillyl-mandelic acid excretion and curable, and *primary sarcoma of the heart* (Shelburne, 1948), *right atrial myxoma* with fever, effusions in knees, presystolic and diastolic murmurs and a raised ESR (Currey et al, 1967), *type 2 hyperlipoproteinaemia* with migratory polyarthritis (Khachadurian, 1968), *histiocyte reticulosis* (Henderson, 1969) or *rhabdomyosarcoma* (Calabro & Castleman, 1972). *Henoch-Schönlein purpura* is differentiated by the characteristic rash but may coexist (Gairdner, 1948). Other collagen diseases such as *polyarteritis nodosa* and *systemic lupus erythematosus* should also be differentiated. As noted previously, chorea may sometimes complicate systemic lupus erythematosus. *Familial Mediterranean fever* and *Sweet's syndrome* (Krauser & Schumacher, 1975) need differentiation.

Still's disease is frequently mistaken for rheumatic fever and the converse also holds but is less common. In adult seronegative rheumatoid arthritis the confusion is less likely to occur, since fever and rash are comparatively rare (Bywaters, 1971b). Important differential points are the absence in rheumatic fever of enlarged glands and the characteristically *marginate* character of the rash, the less remittent fever and the more migratory joint involvement. The differential sheep cell agglutination test for rheumatoid factor is seldom of value, since it is usually negative in juvenile chronic arthritis. Occasionally, chronic joint swelling with spindling and disability may persist for many months in rheumatic fever; if, in addition, pericarditis is heard, biopsy of the joint may be the only certain method of diagnosis. Amongst heart conditions endomyocardial fibrosis, especially in Africans, needs differentiation since it may also show antiheart antibody (Van der Geld et al, 1966).

In adults, *gout, Reiter's syndrome* and *gonorrhoea* may need to be considered at all ages: the history and the results of serum uric acid estimations and prostatic or cervical secretion examinations respectively constitute the main criteria for differentiation.

Rheumatoid arthritis in adults is perhaps the most important of all simulating diseases, especially in its first few months before X-ray change develops and especially if the latex test is negative. Biopsy of synovial membrane may need to be done if the clinical features are not helpful. A more common mistake seems in our own experience to be the diagnosis of the prolonged chronic afebrile stage of adult rheumatic fever with stationary painful and swollen joints as 'rheumatoid arthritis'; such cases are judged ultimately to be rheumatic fever because of the gradual appearance of a heart lesion or because of the complete subsidence of all joint signs and symptoms. The recurrent type of palindromic rheumatism of Hench which we believe to be a variant of rheumatoid arthritis (Ansell & Bywaters, 1959) may be particularly confusing, especially as heart involvement is much less frequent in adult rheumatic fever (McDanald & Weisman, 1978).

Treatment

Prevention

As in medicine generally, prevention reaps a better harvest than cure. Apart from general measures to improve the health of the nation which are perhaps responsible for the century's decline in rheumatic fever severity and are beyond the scope of this discussion, specific preventative measures can only be applied to a population known to be at risk, such as large groups of institutionalised young people or children who have had rheumatic fever or who come from a rheumatic family. These specific measures are primarily directed against streptococcal infection and are discussed in the section on after-care since they are particularly applicable to the convalescent case. It is obviously both undesirable and impossible to give penicillin to everyone with a sore throat.

The care of the acute attack

The most important of all general therapeutic measures is to limit the work of the damaged heart, since it appears probable that over-exercise of a diseased organ is itself damaging: some interesting evidence has been adduced for poliomyelitis by Ritchie Russell (1949) in this respect. Although cardiac work is greater lying flat than in the sitting position, it is muscular effort which primarily increases metabolic rate and hence cardiac work. Especially in children, the only practical way of limiting muscular activity other than anaesthesia is to lay them flat in bed. Some (Robertson et al, 1946) have felt that prolonged rest is part of the mythology of medicine and indeed there are only two pieces of evidence for it: the first data published were those of Sibson (1877) who showed that 3 out of 24 of the rested patients developed residual heart disease as against 43 out of 127 who were not rested. More recently Taussig & Goldenberg (1941) showed that of a group of children who showed progressive enlargement of the heart following an acute attack, only 50% had been rested and then only for a short time, as against 67 treated with adequate rest out of a group of 68 children with normal cardiac growth.

Increasing physical activity is allowed as soon as the disease shows signs of subsidence, conventionally according to eight grades. One of the best criteria for this is the fall of the sedimentation rate to normal but neither this nor any other single criterion is infallible. In children increasing bodyweight is also very useful as an indicator. In any case, more caution should be exercised if the heart has been seriously damaged: in adults, where cardiac damage is much less common, prolonged rest is sometimes omitted in mild cases.

For many children such prolonged physical inactivity is best enforced away from home in a convalescent home or hospital. The hospital school established in many such institutions does a great deal to reduce the educational gap left by the acute state and to lessen the psychological handicaps of the disease. Parental visits should be encouraged. Care must be taken to guard against intercurrent infection (q.v.) and tooth extractions, etc. should be covered with penicillin.

Salicylates

Today, more than a century after the introduction of salicylates, there is still considerable controversy on their value, their mode of action and the best way of using them (Gross & Greenberg, 1948). The majority view is that they suppress the less important manifestations of the disease if given in adequate dosage; it has still to be shown that cardiac sequelae are less frequent or less severe in salicylate-treated cases. In the large dosage advocated by Coburn (10–15 g/day in adults) with blood levels between 35 and 40 mg/100 ml, fever and pain disappear and the sedimentation rate may sometimes fall, but each of these effects will occur also in non-rheumatic patients (Harris, 1947). Pericarditis, nodules, rash, chorea and pneumonia have been found occasionally to occur at such blood levels (Murphy, 1945). That author and others (Keith & Ross, 1945; Wegria & Smull, 1945) have not found the course shortened (judged by the sedimentation rate) and residual heart disease seem to be the same in the treated and untreated groups. Watkinson (1949) in a careful study has found in adults that the duration of the rise in the sedimentation rate was materially decreased on high salicylate dosage. We have not found any considerable difference between patients treated with salicylate, cortisone and bed-rest alone if recurrences are avoided, apart from the special danger of salicylates (Bywaters & Thomas, 1961) in potential heart failure (Fig. 42.30). Sutcliffe (1955) showed that salicylates could precipitate pulmonary oedema in congestive failure in a patient with active carditis and rheumatic heart disease. With this drug there may be an increase in metabolic rate and in cardiac output (Alexander & Smith, 1962) which the damaged heart can ill sustain. Pulmonary oedema has also sometimes been seen in cases without heart disease due to sodium

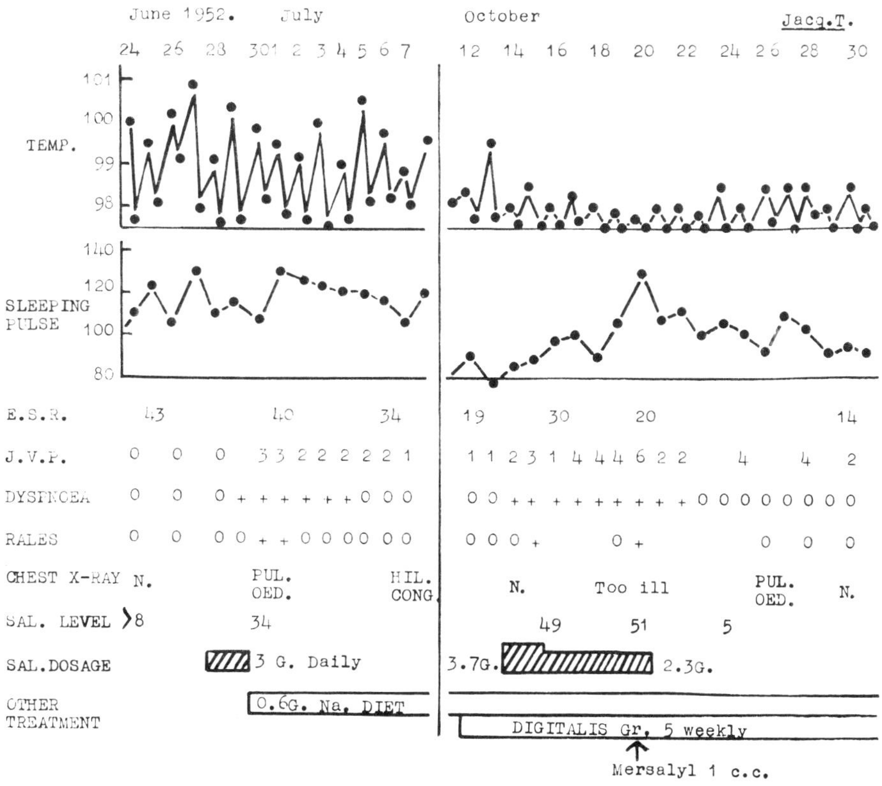

Fig. 42.30 Two episodes of pulmonary oedema with dyspnoea following aspirin administration, in JT with severe active rheumatic heart disease.

retention (Granville-Grossman & Sergeant, 1960).

Tinnitus and deafness, nausea, hallucinations, delirium and a respiratory alkalosis with hyperaemia are reversible and not infrequent toxic effects. The last complication is accompanied by a raised blood pH and a secondary decreased CO_2-combining power due to respiratory loss of CO_2. The only severe effect is bleeding, said to be correctable with vitamin K (Hoffman et al, 1947), but this is rare. If sodium salicylate or acetyl salicylic acid causes gastric discomfort an enteric-coated preparation should be given. The intravenous route has no added advantage. There seems to be no good reason for giving sodium bicarbonate as well as the salicylate. Methyl salicylate used externally on the limbs is a counter-irritant and is seldom necessary if salicylates are given internally to abolish the pain. It must be remembered that this is absorbed and has given rise to severe toxic effects. Salicylates have been shown to have an anti-inflammatory effect (Spector & Willoughby, 1959), but this is apparently not dependent upon their characteristic uncoupling of oxidative phosphorylation (Marks & Smith, 1960).

Gentisate (Meyer & Ragan, 1948), gamma resorcylate (Reid et al, 1951) and 3-OH-2 phenyl cinchoninic acid (Blanchard et al, 1950) appear to have in general a salicylate-like action, but none has any advantage over aspirin. There is no reason to suppose that other newer NSAIDs would not be as useful as aspirin.

Steroid compounds and ACTH

The beneficial effect of these substances in rheumatic fever (Hench et al, 1949) is due to their anti-inflammatory action, which appears in general to be more powerful than that of salicylates, abolishing fever and joint pains rapidly and, if in large enough dosage, raising the haemoglobin and reducing the sedimentation rate towards normal. When hormone treatment is reduced or stopped, the manifestations or disease may reappear (see Fig. 42.29) in a proportion of children, the so-called 'rebound phenomenon' (Elster & Pader, 1959). While fever and joint symptoms subside rapidly, other manifestations are not affected — chorea (Dixon & Bywaters, 1952) nodules, rash. The large-scale controlled trial run jointly in the USA, Canada, and Great Britain showed no significant difference between groups treated for 6 weeks respectively by cortisone, ACTH and aspirin at the 1-, 5- and 10-year follow-up (US/UK Co-operative Clinical Trial, 1965). The major factor in determining the incidence of rheumatic heart disease at the end of five years was the status of the heart at the beginning of treatment. 96% of cases without carditis initially showed no residual heart disease. Cases with initial carditis but without pre-existing heart disease showed no residual heart disease in 82% if mild or in 30% if severe. Taplow experience with controlled trials of 6 or 12 weeks' aspirin, ACTH and bed-rest alone, has shown little difference in cardiac residual in the long-term follow-up, an opinion held also following a controlled trial by Freidman et al (1962). Some other controlled trials have produced data which showed that steroids were beneficial (Dorfman et al, 1961). We feel that steroids without salt-retaining action (e.g. prednisolone) should be given to patients with carditis or marked rheumatic activity: by suppressing activity they lessen the risk of heart failure, or, if failure is already present, allow a satisfactory response to digitalis and diuretics. Salicylates do not adequately control disease activity, and are potentially dangerous in the patient with severe carditis (Fig. 42.30). Continuous prophylaxis is an essential background measure. Complications of steroid treatment, e.g. prednisolone, are comparatively few for the period of 1–3 months usually necessary in rheumatic fever. With high dosage, infections have occurred and suppression of the inflammatory response to such infections may not only facilitate infection but may also abolish the clinical signs by which such infection is normally detected. In recent immigrants tuberculosis is always a possibility. Pancreatitis has been seen only with the massive dosage tried (and abandoned) by Smith and his colleagues (1957).

Penicillin

While it may be of value to institute a 10-day bactericidal course of penicillin at the onset of the rheumatic fever attack, this is of certain value only to prevent spread of streptococcal infection in the ward. There is yet (1975) no evidence that penicillin given after the onset of rheumatic fever even in large dosage for 6 weeks has any effect upon the residual cardiac lesions (Carter et al, 1962; Vaisman et al, 1965).

Treatment of heart failure and other complications

Heart failure must be treated with digitalis, diuretics and restriction of salt intake. If the rheumatic process is active and there is heart failure as well, prednisolone should be used in addition to the above measures in a dosage of 25–50 mg/day (Bywaters & Thomas, 1960).

After-care

The cardiac sequelae of rheumatic fever tend to be more severe in cases with second or later attacks and it is most important to prevent such recurrences. The return of a susceptible child to the very home environment which was one of the factors leading to the disease needs careful watching and in this the general practitioner has been greatly assisted by liaison with the hospital service. To confirm or exclude rheumatic heart disease picked up at school medical examinations or by the practitioner may need specialist advice: a firm diagnosis is essential to obviate cardiac neurosis based on the misinterpretation of innocent systolic murmurs or growing pains. Thus in one study (Bergman & Stamm, 1967) only 18% of 93 schoolchildren with reported rheumatic heart disease were confirmed. It is seldom that the environment can be greatly improved — with the present rate of housebuilding — but useful advice can often be given on diet, allowances, exercise, schooling and chemoprophylaxis. In general, unless the heart is badly affected, moderate indulgence in noncompetitive games should be allowed. Education of the parents on the early signs of a relapse is also valuable.

Prophylaxis

Streptococcal infection is usually spread by direct manual contact rather than by airborne dust or droplets (Rubbo & Benjamin, 1953). The avoidance of streptococcal infection, of overcrowding at home and in the cinema, etc., is important, but a more effective way of avoiding reinfection is by penicillin or sulphonamide pretreatment, introduced originally in 1939 by Thomas & France and by Coburn & Moore. The usual dosage of the latter for children below the age of 10 is 0.5 g of sulphadiazine b.d. or above 10, 0.5 g t.d.s. Undesirable reactions sufficient to require stopping the drug at this dose level are uncommon, and develop usually within the first month of treatment: they include urticaria, drug fever, nausea and vomiting and leucopenia (Fig. 42.31). These are seldom severe and usually reversible although one death from agranulocytosis has been recorded (Stowell & Button, 1941). It is probably wise to do a white blood count weekly for the first month. Another drawback within a large institution is the development of sulphonamide-resistant strains of streptococcus (Stokes, 1947) and epidemics. Most authors who have tried this method of prophylaxis in hospital are convinced of its value. The incidence of recurrences has been reduced from 5.6% per patient year in the unprotected to 1.2% per patient year in those protected with sulphonamide or penicillin (Bywaters & Thomas, 1958). Much greater reduction has been shown in various American series, where the incidence of recurrences in the control unprotected population has been much higher. In patients living at home and looked after by their family doctor, prophylaxis has often been inadequate for various reasons, including parental apathy and lack of supervision (Bywaters et al, 1957b).

Penicillin has certain advantages. Toxic reactions are comparatively rare, consisting mainly of

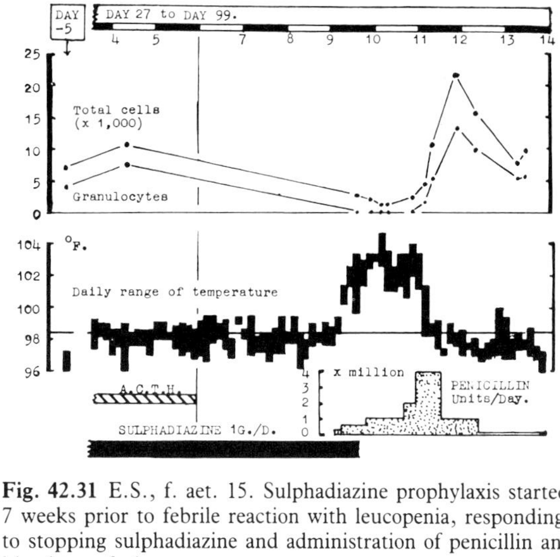

Fig. 42.31 E.S., f. aet. 15. Sulphadiazine prophylaxis started 7 weeks prior to febrile reaction with leucopenia, responding to stopping sulphadiazine and administration of penicillin and blood transfusion.

urticaria and serum sickness-like effects with angioneurotic oedema (Mirabel, 1951). A useful review of untoward penicillin reactions is given by Guthe et al (1959). Penicillin should be given orally twice daily. We have not felt that it matters a great deal whether penicillin V or penicillin G is given. The dosage recommended by the Royal College of Physicians (1957) is 200 000 units crystalline penicillin G tablets twice daily, or alternatively penicillin G 120 mg twice daily. Effective prophylactic levels may be maintained by 1.2 million units long-acting benzathine penicillin G (dibenzyl penicillin) intramuscularly once a month, but the drawbacks of a painful injection have limited the use of this method in Great Britain. Allergic reactions to it are also common — 1.3% according to McFarland (1958). Regular routine prophylaxis should be maintained for at least 5 years from the acute attack or until the child leaves school or any environment of increased streptococcal risk, although patients without evidence of carditis in the acute attack seldom develop carditis later: although recurrences are less frequent in those without rheumatic heart disease, it is wise to use prophylactic measures in such patients since often (as for instance in those sent into hospital with late manifestations such as chorea) it is impossible to say whether transient carditis had originally been present or not.

If prophylaxis has not been instituted or a streptococcal sore throat has developed due to a lapse in prophylaxis, rheumatic fever may be prevented by bactericidal treatment of the sore throat, using 1 million units of penicillin by mouth each day or perhaps better, an initial injection of 1.2 million units composed of crystalline penicillin G, 300 000 units, procaine penicillin, 300 000 units and benzathine penicillin, 600 000 units, to be followed by 300 000 units crystalline penicillin G three times a day by mouth for a total period of 10 days. Massell et al (1951) and Denny et al (1950) showed dramatic reduction of rheumatic fever by this means, even with a 5 day delay in treatment the number of patients protected, as judged by subsequent antibody rise, is considerable (Brock & Siegal, 1953). However, there is some evidence (Hahn et al, 1952) that electrocardiographic changes are reduced much less by antibiotic treatment of sore throat than is overt rheumatic fever. This may not matter.

It seems probable that sulphadiazine and penicillin are both useful in preventing further recurrences of rheumatic fever and that a decision to use one or other of them should depend primarily upon individual circumstances. Tonsillectomy should be performed only on account of recurrent tonsillitis. Steroid treatment of acute and haemolytic streptococcal sore throat does not modify signs or symptoms, the incidence of PR changes or of overt rheumatic (Hahn et al, 1951).

Penicillin-resistant strains of streptococci (Garrod & Waterworth, 1962) and of resistant staphylococci (Harris et al, 1962) may develop in patients on oral penicillin prophylaxis, but endocarditis has been recorded (Parillo et al, 1979). Antibiotic cover for dental extraction, tonsillectomy and gastrointestinal or genitourinary surgery needs special consideration in patients with rheumatic heart disease who are prone to develop subacute bacterial endocarditis. The recommendations of the American Heart Association (1972) appended as Table 42.4 include dosage for maximal blood levels at the time of surgery when bacteraemia is almost universal, and provision for both the type of bacteria to be expected and penicillin allergy. Sound teeth should not be extracted prophylactically since subacute bacterial endocar-

Table 42.4 Prevention of subacute bacterial endocarditis. (After American Heart Association, 1972.)

Dental procedures

1. Intramuscular procain penicillin 600 000 U and penicillin G 200 000 U, 1 hour before and daily for 2 days.
b. Orally 500 mg penicillin V or phenethicillin 1 hour before; 250 mg 6-hourly for 2 days after
   or
   1.2 million U penicillin G 1 hour before and 600 000 U 6-hourly for 2 days after
c. If penicillin allergy or prior oral penicillin prophylaxis:erythromycin 500 mg p.o. at 2 and 1 hours before and 250 mg 6-hourly for 2 days.

Gastrointestinal and genitourinary surgery

a. Penicillin as above+streptomycin 1–2 g intramuscularly 1 hour before and daily for 2 days after
b. Ampicillin 3 g 1 hour before and 1.5 g 6-hourly for 2 days+streptomycin as above
c. Erythromycin p.o. as above or vancomycin 1 g i.v.+streptomycin as above.

ditis can develop in the edentulous (Simon & Goodwin, 1971).

Another potentially useful measure is vaccination with polyvalent M protein, the cell wall substance which engenders type specific immunity. This has been worked at for long by many, but is only recently that technical advances in purification methods have rendered such an approach feasible in man. While rheumatic fever has occurred in immunised patients (Massell et al, 1970), the reasons for this are not clear and it now seems certain that an alum-precipitated polyvalent M protein or peptide fragments thereof (Stollerman, 1980) vaccine afford a measurable degree of protection against upper respiratory streptococcal infection and do not induce heart-reactive antibodies (Beachey et al, 1979).

At the moment, in this as in other fields, preventive methods seem to be more important than curative and specifically antistreptococcal measures. It is unfortunate, however, that it would appear necessary that a child must have one attack of rheumatic fever before it is known that he is susceptible and in need of protection. A great deal more work needs to be done on this, as on all aspects of rheumatic fever, before we can control this form of heart disease, still widely prevalent throughout the world.

REFERENCES

Abdin Z H, Eissa A 1965 Rheumatic fever and rheumatic heart disease in children below the age of 5 years in the tropics. Annals of the rheumatic Diseases 24:389

Acheson R M 1965 The epidemiology of acute rheumatic fever. Journal of Chronic Diseases 18:723

Agarwal B L 1981 Rheumatic heart disease unabated in developing countries. Lancet 2: 910–911

Alexander W D, Smith G 1962 Disadvantageous circulatory effects of salicylate in rheumatic fever. Lancet 1:768

Alimurung M M, Herrera F, Guytingco A, Cruz P M 1955 Heart disease in the Philippines. American Heart Journal 50:293

American Heart Association 1956 Circulation 13:617

American Heart Association 1972 Prevention of rheumatic fever. Report of a WHO Expert Committee. WHO, Geneva

Amren D P, Anderson A S, Wannamaker L W 1966 Perianal cellulitis associated with group A streptococci. American Journal of Diseases of Children 112:546

Ansell B M, Bywaters E G L 1959 Palindromic rheumatism. Annals of the Rheumatic Diseases 18: 331–332

Aschoff L 1904 Zur myocarditisfrage. Verhandlungen der Deutschen Gesellschaft für Urolgie, 8:46.

Ashman R, Hull E 1945 Essentials of Electrocardiography 2nd Edn Macmillan, London

Ayoub E M, Taranta A, Bartley T D 1974 Effect of valvular surgery on antibody to the group A streptococcal carbohydrate. Circulation 50:144

Back E H, de Pass E E 1957 Acute rheumatic fever in Jamaican children. West Indian Medical Journal 6:98

Back E H, de Pass E E 1964 Acute rheumatism in Jamaican children: review of 100 cases. West Indian Medical Journal 13:173

Beachey E M, Stollerman G, Johnson R H, Ofek I, Bisno A L 1979 Human immune response to immunisation with a structurally defined polypeptide fragment of streptococcal M protein. Journal of Experimental Medicine 150: 862–877

Beare J M, Froggart P, Jones J H, Neill D W 1966 Familial annular erythema. An apparently new dominant mutation. British Journal of Dermatology 78: 59–68

Becker C G, Murphy G E 1969 Demonstration of contractile protein in endothelium and cells of the heart valves, endocardium, intima, arteriosclerotic plaques, and aschoff bodies of rheumatic heart disease. American Journal of Pathology 55:1

Bennett G A, Zeller J W, Bauer W 1940 Subcutaneous nodules of rheumatoid arthritis and rheumatic fever; pathologic study. Archives of Pathology 30:70

Bennett R A, Copeman W S C 1940 Notes on rubella with special reference to certain rheumatic sequelae. British Medical Journal 1:924.

Beresford O D, Graham A M 1950 Chorea gravidarum. Journal of Obstetrics and Gynaecology of the British Empire 57:616

Bergman A B, Stamm S J 1967 The morbidity of cardiac nondisease in school children. New England Journal of Medicine 276:1008

Berkheiser E J, Seidler F 1931 Nontraumatic dislocations of atlanto-axial joint. Journal of the American Medical Association 96:517

Besterman E M M, Thomas G T 1953 Radiological diagnosis of rheumatic pericardial effusion. British Heart Journal 15:113

Bisno A L, Ofek I 1974 Serologic diagnosis of streptococcal infection. American Journal of Diseases of Children 127: 676–681

Bisno A L, Pearce I A, Wall H P, Moody M D, Stollerman G H 1970 Contrasting epidemiology of acute rheumatic fever and acute glomerulonephritis. New England Journal of Medicine 283:561

Blanchard K C, Harvey A M, Howard J E, Kattus A, Marshall E J, Newman E V, Zubrod C G 1950 Effect of 3-hydroxy-2-phenylcinchonimic acid upon rheumatic fever. Bulletin of Johns Hopkins Hospital 87:50

Bland E F 1961 In: Proceedings of the 10th Congress of the International League against Rheumatism Rome, 1961, Vol 2. Minerva Medica, Turin, p. 79

Bland E F, Duckett Jones T 1952 The natural history of rheumatic fever: a 20 year perspective. Annals of Internal Medicine 37:1006.

Brainerd H D, Sokolow M 1949 The differential diagnosis of rheumatic fever and infections of the central nervous

system. Journal of Pediatrics 34:204
Bright R 1838 Cases of spasmodic disease accompanying affections of the pericardium. Medico-chirurgical Transactions 22:1
Brock L L, Seigal A C 1953 Studies of the prevention of rheumatic fever: the effect of time of initiation of treatment of streptococcal infections on the immune response of the host. Journal of Clinical Investigation 32:630
Brod J 1949 Acute diffuse glomerulonephritis. American Journal of Medicine 7:317
Broderick T W, Reinke R T, Goldman E 1976 Salicylate induced pulmonary oedema. American Journal of Roentgenology, Radium Therapy and Nuclear Medicine 127: 865–866
Brownell K D, Bailen-Rose F 1973 Acute rheumatic fever in children. Journal of the American Medical Association 224:1593
Bunim J J, Appel S B 1950 A principle for determining prognosis pregnancy in rheumatic heart disease. Journal of the American Medical Association, 142:90
Burch G E, Giles T D, Colcolough H L 1970 Pathogenesis of 'rheumatic' heart disease: critique and theory. American Heart Journal 80:556
Bywaters E G L 1950 The relation between heart and joint disease including 'rheumatoid heart disease' and chronic post-rheumatic arthritis (type Jaccoud). British Heart Journal 12:101
Bywaters E G L 1971b Still's disease in the adult. Annals of the Rheumatic Diseases 30:121
Bywaters E G L 1975 Jaccoud's syndrome. A sequel to the joint involvement of systemic lupus erythematosus. Clinics in Rheumatic Diseases 1:125
Bywaters E G L 1979 Skin manifestations of rheumatic disease. In: Dermatology in general medicine, Fitzpatrick T B ed 2nd Edn. McGraw-Hill, New York
Bywaters E G L, Thomas G T 1958 Prevention of rheumatic fever recurrences. British Medical Journal 2:350
Bywaters E G L, Thomas G T 1960 In: Jones A M (ed) Modern trends in cardiology. Butterworth, London
Bywaters E G L, Thomas G T 1961 Bed rest, salicylates, and steroid in rheumatic fever. British Medical Journal 1:1528
Bywaters E G L, Holborow E J, Johnson G D, Kelley R J 1957a Cord-blood antistreptolysin-O level according to parity and social class as a possible index of familial streptococcal experience. Journal of Hygiene 55:276
Bywaters E G L, Hallidie-Smith K, Thomas G T 1957b Prevention of recurrences of rheumatic fever. British Medical Journal 1:1234
Bywaters E G L, Glynn L E, Zeldis A 1958 Subcutaneous nodules of Still's disease. Annals of the Rheumatic Diseases 17:278
Calabro J J, Castleman B 1972 Case records of the Massachusetts General Hospital. New England Journal of Medicine 286, 205
Carter M E, Bywaters E G L, Thomas G T 1962 Rheumatic fever treated with penicillin in bactericidal dosage for six weeks. British Medical Journal 1:965
Caughey D E, Douglas R, Wilson W, Hassall I B, 1975 HL-A antigens in Europeans and Maoris with rheumatic fever and rheumatic heart disease. Journal of Rheumatology 2:319–322
Chambers R J, Bywaters E G L 1963 Rubella synovitis. Annals of the Rheumatic Diseases 22:263
Chandrasekhara M K, Cornfeld D 1969 Concomitant rheumatic fever and acute glomerulonephritis. Clinical Pediatrics 8:110
Chang F C 1961 Mitral stemosis in identical twins. Report of a family. New England Journal of Medicine 264:923
Chaturvedi U C, Davies J W, Flewett T H 1973 Separation and characterization of cardiac antigen proteins. Clinical and Experimental Immunology 15:613
Cheadle W B 1889 The various manifestations of the rheumatic state. Smith Elder, London
Christensen P, Schalen C, Holm H E 1979 Re-evaluation of experiments intended to demonstrate immunological cross reactions between mammalian tissues and streptococci. Progress in Allergy 26: 1–41
Chun R W, Smith N J, Forster F M 1961 Papilledema in Sydenham's's chorea. American Journal of Diseases of Children 101:641
Clarke C A, McConnell R B, Sheppard P M 1960 ABO blood groups and secretor character in rheumatic carditis. British Medical Journal 1:21
Clarke M, Keith J D 1972 Atrioventricular conduction in acute rheumatic fever. British Heart Journal 34:472
Claussen F 1955 Beiträge der zwillings-forschung zum rheuma-problem. Zeitschrift für Rheumaforschung 14:145
Clawson B J 1941 Relation of 'anitschkow myocyte' to rheumatic inflammation. Archives of Pathology 32:760
Coburn A F, Moore L V 1939 The prophylactic use of sulfanilamide in streptococcal respiratory infections with especial reference to rheumatic fever. Journal of Clinical Investigation 18:147
Coburn A F, Pauli R H 1935 Studies on the immune response of the rheumatic subject and its relationship to activity of the rheumatic process. VI. Antistreptolysin levels. Journal of Clinical Investigation 14:769
Coburn A F, Young D C 1949 Epidemiology of haemolytic streptococcus. Williams & Wilkins, Baltimore
Collins D H 1937 Subcutaneous nodule of rheumatoid arthritis. Journal of Pathology and Bacteriology 45:97
Collins S D 1947 The incidence of rheumatic fever as recorded in general morbidity surveys of families. Public Health Reports Washington, (Suppl) 198:1
Collins S D, Phillips F R, Oliver D S 1950 Specific causes of illness found in monthly canvasses of families; sample of eastern Health District of Baltimore 1938–43. Public Health Reports (Washington) 65:1235
Coombs C F 1924 Rheumatic heart disease Wright, Bristol
Cossio P 1974 Chagasic cardiopathy: antibodies reacting with plasma membrane of striated muscle and endothelial cells. Circulation 50:1252
Coste F, Galmiche P, Brion S 1950 A propos d'un cas curieux de myosite ossifiante bloquant les hanches; reflexions sur les ossifications ectopiques. Revue du Rheumatisme 17:180
Crawford Y E 1960 Studies of a complement-fixing antigen from group A streptococcal L forms. Journal of Immunology 84:86
Cruickshank E K 1951 Hyperpyrexia with cerebellar damage in acute rheumatism. Lancet 1:1052
Currey H L, Mathews J A, Robinson J 1967 Right atrial myxoma mimicking a rheumatic disorder. British Medical Journal 1:547
Dalldorf F G, Murphy G E 1960 Relationship of aschoff bodies in cardiac atrial appendages to the natural history of rheumatic heart disease. American Journal of Pathology 37:507
DeCourt L V, Montenegro M R, Castiglioni R, Sawaya J,

Tranchesi B 1967 Steroid therapy and histologic evidence of subclinical rheumatic carditis. Archives of Interamerican Rheumatology 4:495
DeLorimier A A, Bragg K U, Linden G 1969 Neuroblastoma in childhood. American Journal of Diseases of Children 118:441
Denny F W, Wannamaker L W, Brink W F, Rammelkamp C H, Custer E A 1950 Prevention of rheumatic fever. Journal of the American Medical Association 143:151
Diamond E F, Tentler R 1962 The electroencephalogram in rheumatic fever. Journal of the American Medical Association 182:685
Diamond L K, Clark W H 1965 Case records of the Massachusetts General Hospital. New England Journal of Medicine 272:477
Diggs L W 1965 Sickle cell crises. American Journal of Clinical Pathology 44:1
Dixon A. St. J, Bywaters E G L 1952 Methods of assessing therapy in chorea with special reference to the use of A.C.T.H. Archives of Diseases in Childhood 27:161
Donaldson I, MacG, Espiner E A 1971 Disseminated lupus erythematosus presentive as chorea gravidarum. Archives of Neurology (Chicago) 25, 240
Doniach I 1947 Uremic edema of lungs. American Journal of Roentgenology 58:620
Dorfman A, Gross J I, Lorincz A E 1961 The treatment of acute rheumatic fever. Pediatrics 27:692
Dorling J, Kingston D, Webb J A 1976 Streptococcal antibodies reacting with brain tissue. II. Ultra structural studies. British Journal of Experimental Pathology 57: 255–265
Dudding B A, Ayoub E M 1968 Persistence of streptococcal group A antibody in patients with rheumatic valvular disease. Journal of Experimental Medicine 128:1081
Dully F E 1973 Streptococcal epidemic in an aircraft carrier. Aerospace Medicine 44:1181
Duma R J, Weinberg A M, Medrek T F, Kunz L J 1969 Streptococcal infections: a bacteriologic and clinical study of streptococcal bacteremia. Medicine 48:87
Dunnett W N. Schallibaum E M 1960 Scarlet-fever-like illness due to staphylococcal infection. Lancet 1:1227
Elkeles G, Glynn L E 1946 Disseminated parenchymatous ossification in lungs in association with mitral stenosis. Journal of Pathology and Bacteriology 58:517
Ellis R J, Lillehei C W, Zabriskie J D 1970 Journal of the American Medical Association 211:1505
Ellis R J, Zabriskie J B, Ebert P A 1974 Tolerance to myocardial tissue allografts by pretreatment with cross-reactive streptococcal membrane antigen. Surgery 76:142
Ellman P, Gee A 1951 Pulmonary haemosiderosis. British Medical Journal 2:384
Elster S K, Pader E 1959 Studies on acute rheumatic fever in the adult. II. The rebound phenomenon. Annals of Internal Medicine 51:339
Epstein B S 1940 Roentgenologic differentiation of rheumatic from non-rheumatic mitral valve calcifications. American Journal of Roentgenology 44, 704
Faivre G, Gilgenkrantz J M, Duheille J, Petitier H 1967 Immunofluorescence et syndromes post-commisurotomie ou post-infarctus. Archives des maladies de Coeur et des vaisseaux 60, 484
Falk J A, Fleischman J L, Zabriskie J B et al 1973 A study of HL-A antigen phenotype in rheumatic fever and rheumatic heart disease patients. Tissue Antigens 3:173
Felsen J 1940 Rheumatic intestinal necrosis. Review of Gastroenterology 7:339
Fenoglio J J, Wagner B M 1973 Studies in rheumatic fever. VI. Ultrastructure of chronic rheumatic heart disease. American Journal of Pathology 73:623
Fink C W, Windmiller J, Sartain P 1972 Arthritis as the presenting feature of childhood leukemia. Arthritis and Rheumatism 15:347
Fisherman R A 1965 Neurological aspects of magnesium metabolism. Archives of Neurology 12:562
Freidberg C K, Gross L 1934 Periarteritis nodosa (necrotising arteritis) associated with rheumatic heart disease, with a note on abdominal rheumatism. Archives of Internal Medicine 54.170
Freidman S, Harris T N, Caddell J L 1962 Long-term effects of ACTH and cortisone therapy in rheumatic fever. Journal of Pediatrics 60:55
Freud P, Weisz A, Brunhofer A 1950 Miliary tuberculosis simulating acute rheumatic fever. American Journal of Diseases of Children 79:676
Gairdner D 1948 The Schönlein–Henoch syndrome (anaphylactoid purpura). Quarterly Journal of Medicine 17:95
Galloway R W, Epstein E J, Coulshed N 1961 Pulmonary ossific nodules in mitral valve disease. British Heart Journal 23:297
Garrod L P, Waterworth P M 1962 The risks of dental extraction during penicillin treatment. British Heart Journal 24:39
Gatenby P B B 1956 Chorea gravidarum. Lancet 2:997
Gazenfeld E, Rosenmann E, Davies A M, Laufer A 1966 Isoproterenol induced myocardial lesions in the immunized and non-immunized rat. II. Histopathological lesions after specific immunization. Immunology 10:193
Geiler G 1960 Morphology and pathogenesis of rheumatic lesions. German Medical Monthly 5:208
Gerstar J C, Payot M, Rappoport G 1982 Streptococci and reactive arthritis. Annals of the Rheumatic Diseases 41:646
Gibney R, Reineck J, Bannayan G A 1981 Renal lesions in acute rheumatic fever. Annals of Internal Medicine 94: 322–6
Gil R J, Rodriguez H, Ibarra J J 1955 Incidence of asymptomatic, active rheumatic cardiac lesions in patients submitted to mitral commissurotomy and the effect of cortisone on these lesions. American Heart Journal 59:912
Gitlin D, Craig J M, Janeway J A 1957 Studies on the nature of fibrinoid in the collagen diseases. American Journal of Pathology 33:55
Glynn A A, Glynn L E, Holborow E J 1959 Secretion of blood-group substances in rheumatic fever. British Medical Journal 2:266
Goldring W, Wyckoff J 1930 Studies of kidney in acute infection; observations with urine sediment count (Addis) in acute rheumatic infection. Journal of Clinical Investigations 8:569
Goldsmith J H, Cowan M A, Gooder E 1958 Familial outbreak of acute glomerulonephritis due to Griffith type-1 streptococcus. Lancet 2:674
Goldstein I, Rebeyrotte P, Parlebas J, Halpern B 1968 Isolation from heart valves of glycopeptides which share immunological properties with streptococcus haemolyticus group A polysaccharides. Nature 219:866
Grahame R, Mitchell A B S, Scott J T 1970 Chronic post-rheumatic fever (Jaccoud's) arthropathy. Annals of the Rheumatic Diseases 29:622
Granville-Grossman K L, Sergeant H G S, 1960 Pulmonary

oedema due to salicylate intoxication. Lancet 1:575
Greenberg L J, Gray E D, Yunis E J 1975 Association of HL-A5 and immune responsiveness in vitro to streptococcal antigens. Journal of Experimental Medicine 141: 935–943
Griffith G C, Huntington R W 1946 Sudden death in rheumatic fever. Annals of Internal Medicine 25:283
Grisel P 1930 Enucléation de l'atlas et torticollis nasopharyngien. Presse medicale 38:50
Gross L 1935 Lesions in roots of pulmonary artery and aorta in rheumatic fever. American Journal of Pathology 11:631
Gross M, Greenberg L A 1948 The salicylates. Hillhouse Press, New Haven, Connecticut
Grunow W A, Esterly J R 1972 Rheumatic pneumonitis. Chest 61:298
Guthe T, Idsoe O, Willcox R R 1959 Untoward penicillin reactions. Bulletin of the World Health Organization 19:427
Haber H G 1937 Entzündliche gelenkerscheinungen und chorea minor bei diphtherie im kindesalter. Monatsschrift für Kinderheilkunde 70:332
Hable K A, Horstmeier C, Wold A D, Washington J A 1973 Group A β-hemolytic streptococcemia. Bacteriologic and clinical study of 44 cases. Proceedings, Mayo Clinic 48:336
Hadfield G 1938 The rheumatic lung. Lancet 2, 710
Haerer A F, Currier R D, Jackson J F 1967 Hereditary nonprogressive chorea of early onset. New England Journal of Medicine 276:1220
Hahn E O, Houser H B, Rammelkamp C H, Denny F W, Wannamaker L W 1951 Effect of cortisone on acute streptococcal infections and post-streptococcal complications. Journal of Clinical Investigation 30:274
Halbert S P, Keatinge S L 1961 The analysis of streptococcal infections. VI Immunoelectrophoretic observations on extracellular antigens detectable with human antibodies. Journal of Experimental Medicine 113:1013
Halbert S P, Lin T M, Smith S 1973 The cardiac auto-immune system IX. Auto-immune myocarditis in rabbits immunized with rabbit heart. International Archives of Allergy and Applied Immunology 44, 783
Hallgrimsson J 1975 Chronic rheumatic valvular heart disease: an autopsy study. Acta Pathologica et Microbiologica Scandinavica 83: 633–638
Hallidie-Smith K A, Bywaters E G L 1958 The differential diagnosis of rheumatic fever. Archives of the Diseases of Childhood 33:350
Hammon W M, Sather G E, Hollinger N 1950 Preliminary report of epidemiological studies on poliomyelitis and streptococcal infections; Lansing neutralizing antibody and antistreptolysin 'O' surveys of California cities, Texas, North Carolina, Mexico, Pacific Island, and Japan. American Journal of Public Health and the Nation's Health 40:293
Hansen A E 1943 Conditions causing confusion in diagnosis of rheumatic fever in children; analysis of diagnosis made by practicing physicians in 271 rheumatic subjects. Journal of the American Medical Association 121:987
Hardinge K 1970 The etiology of transient synovitis of the hip in childhood. Journal of Bone and Joint Surgery 52B:100
Harris N H 1960 Some problems in the diagnosis and treatment of acute osteomyelitis. Journal of Bone and Joint Surgery 42B:535
Harris T N 1945 The erythrocyte sedimentation rate in rheumatic fever. Its significance in adolescent and overweight children. American Journal of the Medical Sciences 210:173
Harris T N 1947 Failure of massive salicylate therapy to suppress inflammatory reaction in rheumatic fever. American Journal of the Medical Sciences 213:482
Harris T N, Friedman S, Hallidie-Smith K, Coriell L L, Fabrizio D 1962 Occurrence of penicillin-resistant staphylococci in patients receiving penicillin orally for prophylaxis of recurrences of rheumatic fever. American Journal of Medicine 32:545
Hartman S A, Bland E F 1951 Rheumatic fever and glomerulonephritis. American Journal of Medicine 10:47
Hawksley J C 1938 Incidence and significance of 'growing pains' in children and adolescents. Journal of the Royal Institute of Public Health and Hygiene 1:798
Healey C E 1970 Gilles de la Tourette's syndrome (maladie des tics). Successful treatment with haloperidol. American Journal of Diseases of Childhood 120:62
Heard B E 1962 Fibrous healing of old iatrogenic pulmonary edema ('hexamethonium lung'). Journal of Pathology and Bacteriology 83:59
Hearn G W, Roper Hall M J 1961 Obstruction of central retinal artery associated with chorea. British Medical Journal ii:684
Heberden W 1802 Commentaries on the History and Cure of Diseases, 3rd edn Payne, London
Heffer E T 1941 Electrocardiogram in rheumatic fever; study of sydenham's chorea. Journal of Pediatrics 18:363
Heffner J E, Sahn S A 1981 Salicylate-induced pulmonary oedema. Annals of Internal Medicine 95: 405–409
Hench P S, Slocumb C H, Barnes A R, Smith H L, Polley H F, Kendall E C 1949 Effects of adrenal cortical hormone 17-hydroxy-11-dehydrocorticosterone (compound E) on acute phase of rheumatic fever. Proceedings, Mayo Clinic 24:277
Henderson J I 1969 Histiocytic reticulosis. A review of 20 patients in the paediatric age range. Medical Journal of Australia 2:485
Herbut P A, Manges W E 1945 The 'Masson body' in rheumatic pneumonia. American Journal of Pathology 21:741
Herschfield B M, Marks D N 1949 Segmental colitis associated with rheumatic fever. New York State Journal of Medicine 49:1702
Hess E V, Fink C W, Taranta A, Ziff M 1962 Circulating heart antibodies in rheumatic fever: a clinical study. Arthritis and Rheumatism 5:301
Hewitt D, Stewart A 1952 Some epidemiological aspects of acute rheumatism. British Journal of Social Medicine 6:161
Hoffman W S, Volini I F, Pomaranc M, Nobe C 1947 Biochemical findings in acetylsalicylate therapy of acute rheumatic fever. Journal of Laboratory and Clinical Medicine 32:1528
Holborow E J, Isdale I C 1956 Antistreptolysin response in acute rheumatic fever in children. Lancet 1:649
Hormaechea E, Carlson R W, Rogove H et al 1979 Hypovolaemia, pulmonary edema and protein changes in severe salicylate poisoning. American Journal of Medicine 66: 1046–1050
Hubbard W N, Hughes G R U 1982 Streptococci and reactive arthritis. Annals of the Rheumatic Diseases 41:435
Husby I, Zabriskie J B, Abdin Z H, Williams R C 1976 Antibodies reacting with cytoplasm of subthalamic and caudate nucleus neurons in chorea and acute rheumatic fever. Journal of Experimental Medicine 144: 1094–1110

Hutchinson R 1922 The value of pulse charts in acute carditis in childhood. Lancet 1:1086
Isdale I C, Bywaters E G L 1956 The rash of rbeumatoid arthritis and Still's disease. Quarterly Journal of Medicine 25:377
Jaccoud F S 1869 Lecons de clinique medicale faites a l'Hospital de la Charite, 2nd Edn. Delahave, Paris
James L, McFarland R B 1971 An epidemic of pharyngitis due to a nonhemolytic group A streptococcus at Lowry Air Force base. New England Journal of Medicine 284:750
Johnson D A, Klass D W, Millichap J G 1964 Electroencephalogram in Sydenham's chorea. Archives of Neurology 10:21
Johnson G D 1955 Determination of antistreptolysin. Journal of Clinical Pathology 8:296
Jonas S, Spagnuolo M, Kloth H H 1972 Chorea gravidarum and streptococcal infection. Obstetrics and Gynaecology 39:77
Juca A, White P D 1944 Cause of death in rheumatic heart disease in adults. Journal of the American Medical Association 125:767
Kallmann F J, Reisner D 1943 The future of medical research. Cited by Burnett M, Lancet 1953 1:103
Kaplan M H 1965 Induction of autoimmunity to heart in rheumatic fever by streptococcal antigen(s) cross-reactive with heart. Federation Proceedings 24:108
Kaplan M H, Meyerserian M, Kushner I 1961 Immunologic studies of heart tissue. IV. Serologic reactions with human heart tissue as revealed by immunofluorescent methods: isoimmune, Wassermann, and autoimmune reactions. Journal of Experimental Medicine 113:17
Kasp-Grochowska E, Kingston D, Glynn L E 1972a Immunology of bovine heart valves. I. Cross-reaction with the C-polysaccharide of streptococcus pyogenes. Annals of the Rheumatic Diseases 31:282
Kasp-Grochowska E, Kingston D, Glynn L E 1972b Immunology of bovine heart valves. II. Reaction with connective tissue components. Annals of the Rheumatic Diseases 31:290
Kasp-Grochowska E, Glynn L E 1977 The role of the plasmalogen in the cross reaction between group A Streptococci and human myocardium. British Journal of Experimental Pathology (in press)
Kaufmann O, Scheerer E 1938 Uber die erblichkeit des akuten gelenkrheumatismus. Zeitschrift für Konstitutiouslehre 21:687
Keil H 1937 Rheumatic erythemas: a critical survey. Annals of Internal Medicine 11:2223
Keith J D, Ross A 1945 Observations on salicylate therapy in rheumatic fever. Canadian Medical Association Journal 52:554
Kellner A, Robertson T 1954 Selective necrosis of cardiac and skeletal muscle induced experimentally by means of proteolytic enzyme solutions given intravenously. Journal of Experimental Medicine 99:387
Kent G, Gilbert E S, Meyer H H 1955 Pulmonary microlithiasis. Archives of Pathology 60:556
Khachadurian A K 1968 Migratory polyarthritis in familial hypercholesterolemia (type II hyperlipoproteinemia). Arthritis and Rheumatism 11:385
Kingston D, Glynn L E 1971 A cross-reaction between Str. pyogenes and human fibroblasts, endothelial cells and astrocytes. Immunology, 31, 1003
Kingston D, Glynn L E 1976 Antistreptococcal antibodies reacting with brain tissue: I. Immunofluorescent studies. British Journal of Experimental Pathology 57: 114–128
Kirschner L, Markham N P, Watters P A 1959 Streptococcal infections in tropical regions. New Zealand Medical Journal 58:491
Kjems E 1960 Studies on streptococcal bacteriophages. 4. The occurrence of lysogenic strains among group A haemolytic streptococci. Acta Pathologica et Microbiologica Scandinavica 49:199
Kjorstad H 1957 Rheumatic fever in the aged. Acta Medica Scandinavica 158:337
Klinge F 1932 Das gewebsbild des fieberhaften rheumatismus; zusammenfassende Kritische betrachtung zur trage der geweblichen sonderstellung des rheumatischen gewebsschades. Virchows Archiv für pathologische Anatomie und Physiologie und für klinische Medizin 286:344
Knopf E 1947 Beitrag zur klinik und differentialdiagnose der infektiosen retikulo-endotheliose. Archiv für Kinderheilkunde 134:129
Krauser R E, Schumacher H R 1975 The arthritis of Sweet's syndrome. Arthritis and Rheumatism 18: 35–41
Kuepper K, Langer E, Klein P 1961 Demonstration of complement-binding structures in Aschoff's nodes of surgically removed heart auricles. Virchows Archiv für pathologische Anatomie und Physiologie und für klinische Medizin 334:342
Kuschner M, Ferrer M I, Harvey R M, Wylie R H 1952 Rheumatic carditis in surgically removed auricular appendages. American Heart Journal 43:286
Kuttner A G 1958 Tissue culture studies of auricular appendages obtained at mitral commissurotomy. Proceedings of the Society for Experimental Biology and Medicine 98:392
Lack C H, Towers A G 1962 Serological tests for staphylococcal infection. British Medical Journal 2:1227.
Laitinen O, Leirisalo M, Allander E 1975 Rheumatic fever and yersinia arthritis criteria and diagnostic problems in a changing disease pattern. Scandinavian Journal of Rheumatology 4:145
Lannigan R 1961 Sub-clinical rbeumatic carditis. British Heart Journal 23:35
Lanningan R, Zaki S A 1965 Submicroscopic particles in the lesions of rheumatic carditis. Lancet 1:1098
Lasègue C 1884 Etudes medicales. Tonce 2, Paris
Lass R, Shephard E 1961 Mumps arthritis. British Medical Journal 2:1613
Lavy S, Lavy R, Brand A 1964 Neurological and electroencephalographic abnormalities in rheumatic fever. Acta Neurologica Scandinavica 40:76
Lawrence J S 1961 Assessment of the activity of disease. Lewis, London
Ledger W J, Headington J T 1972 Group A β-hemolytic streptococcus. Obstetrics and Gynecology 39:474
Lessof M, Brigden W 1957 Systolic murmurs in healthy children and in children with rheumatic fever. Lancet 2:673
Lessof M H 1958 Sydenham's chorea. Guy's Hospital Reports 107:185
Lewis P D, Harrison M J G 1969 Involuntary movements in patients taking oral contraceptives. British Medical Journal 4:404
Lin J S, Rodriguez-Torres R 1969 Appendectomy in children with acute rheumatic fever. Pediatrics 43:573
Ling W, Oftedal G, Simon T 1969 Central retinal artery occlusion in Sydenham's chorea. American Journal of

Diseases of Children 118:525
Lloyd H M, Aitken R E, Ferrier T M 1965 Primary hyperparathyroidism resembling rickets of late onset. British Medical Journal 2:853
Macaffee A L 1965 ABO blood groups and rheumatic heart disease. Annals of the Rheumatic Diseases 24:392
MacCallum W G 1924 Rheumatic lesions of the left auricle of the heart. Bulletin of the Johns Hopkins Hospital 35:329
McDanald E, Weisman M H 1978 Articular manifestations of rheumatic fever in adults. Annals of Internal Medicine 89: 917–920
McDonald H G 1975 Myocardial lysis in acute rheumatic fever followed by regeneration of cardiac muscle and origin of Aschoff's bodies. Journal of Clinical Pathology 28:568
McFarland R B 1958 Reactions to benzathine penicillin. New England Journal of Medicine 259:62
MacIlwaine Y 1947 Relationship between rheumatic carditis and subacute bacterial endocarditis. Journal of Pathology and Bacteriology 59:557
McKee W M, Di Caprio J M, Roberts C E, Sherris J C 1966 Anal carriage as the probable source of a streptococcal epidemic. Lancet 2:1107
McKeown E F 1948 Acute rheumatism in pregnancy. Journal of Obstetrics and Gynaecology of the British Empire 55:50
McKinney A S 1962 Idiopathic hypoparathyroidism presenting as chorea. Neurology 12:485
McLaughlin J F, Paterson P Y, Hartz R S, Embiny S H 1972 Rheumatic carditis: In vitro responses of peripheral blood leukocytes to heart and streptococcal antigens. Arthritis and Rheumatism 15:600
McMinn F J, Bywaters E G L 1959 Differences between the fever of Still's disease and that of rheumatic fever. Annals of the Rheumatic Diseases 18:293
McMurray C, Cayer D, Cornatzer W E 1951 Chronic adhesive pericarditis due to rheumatic state, associated with liver damage, serious effusions, and pigmentation; beneficial effect of pericardectomy on phospholipide turnover and other liver functions after failure of medical management. Gastroenterology 17:294
Madsen T, Kalbak K 1940 Investigations on rheumatic fever subsequent to some epidemics of septic sore throat (especially milk epidemics). Acta Pathologica et Microbiologica Scandinavica 17:305
Malpas J S, Landon J 1960 Rheumatic fever in the young adult. Annals of the Rheumatic Diseases 19:262
Markowitz M, Bruton H D, Kuttner A G 1965 The bacteriologic findings, streptococcal immune response, and renal complications in children and impetigo. Pediatrics 35:393
Marks V, Smith M J H 1960 Anti-inflammatory activity of salicylate. Nature 187:610
Martini G A 1950 Uber polyarthritis im vorstadium der inokulationshepatitis. Deutsche medizinische Wochenschrift 75:1464
Massell B F, Sturgis G P, Knobloch J D, Streeper R B, Hall T N, Norcross P 1951 Prevention of rheumatic fever by prompt penicillin therapy of hemolytic streptococcic respiratory infections. Journal of the American Medical Association 146:1469
Massell B F, Honikman L H, Amezcua J 1970 Rheumatic fever following streptococcal vaccination. Journal of the American Medical Association 207, 1115
Melvin H, Van Woert, Yip L C, Balis M E 1977 Purine phosphoribosyltransferase in Gilles de la Tourette syndrome. New England Journal of Medicine 296: 210–212
Mendoza M, Mandalenkis N, Kaner A, Pirani C, Pollak V 1975 Chronic membranoproliferative glomerulonephritis. A patient with recurrent episodes simulating rheumatic fever and acute nephritis. American Journal of Medicine 59:251
Metropolitan Life Assurance Company 1944 Studies in rheumatic fever. New York
Meyer K, Ragan C 1948 Antirheumatic effect of sodium gentisate. Science 108:281
Miller R 1926 Report on environmental and other predisposing causes of rheumatic infections. British Medical Journal (Suppl) 2:5
Mills C A 1939 Medical climatology. Springfield, Illinois
Mirabel L 1951 Penicillin hypersensitivity reaction with purpura of Schonlein–Henoch type, acute nephritis and angioneurotic oedema. Proceedings of the Royal Society of Medicine 44:150
Mirowski M, Rosenstein B J, Markowitz M 1964 A comparison of atrio-ventricular conduction in normal children and in patients with rheumatic fever, glomerulonephritis, and acute febrile illnesses. A quantitative study with determination of the P–R index. Pediatrics 33:334
Moesman G 1959 Factors precipitating and predisposing to RA as illustrated by studies on monozygotic twins. Acta Rheumatologica Scandinavica 5:291
Moolten S E 1962 Pulmonary fibrosis in rheumatic heart disease. American Journal of Medicine 33:431
Morris J N, Titmuss R M 1942 Epidemiology of juvenile rheumatism. Lancet 2:59
Movat H Z 1958 The concept of fibrinoid. American Journal of the Medical Sciences 236:373
Muirhead E E, Booth E, Montgotnery P O'B 1957 Derivation of certain forms of 'fibrinoid' from smooth muscle. Archives of Pathology 63:213
Murphy G E 1945 Salicylate and rheumatic activity; objective clinical-histologic study of effect of salicylate on rheumatic lesions, those of joints and tendon sheaths in particular. Bulletin of the Johns Hopkins Hospital 77:1
Murphy G E 1960 Nature of rheumatic heart disease. Medicine 39:269
Murphy G E 1963 The characteristic rheumatic lesions of striated and of non-striated or smooth muscle cells of the heart. Genesis of the lesions known as Aschoff bodies and those myogenic components known as Aschoff cell or as Anitschkow cells or myocytes. Medicine 42:73
Murphy G E, Becker C G 1966 Occurrence of caterpillar nuclei within normal immature and normal appearing and altered mature heart muscle cells and the evolution of Anitschkow cells from the latter. American Journal of Pathology 48:931
Murphy G E, Swift H F 1949 Induction of cardiac lesions, closely resembling those of rheumatic fever, in rabbits following repeated skin infections with group A streptococci. Journal of Experimental Medicine 89:687
Murray G C, Montiel M, Persellin R H 1978 A study of HLA antigens in adults with acute rheumatic fever. Arthritis and Rheumatism 21: 652–656
Naish J M, Apley J 1951 'Growing pains': clinical study of non-arthritic limb pains in children. Archives of the Diseases in Childhood 26:134
Nakhla L S, Glynn L E 1967 Studies on the antigen in β-haemolytic streptococci that cross-reacts with an antigen in human myocardium. Immunology 13:209
Neimann N. Pierson M, Lascombes G, Petit J, Viver F 1960 Bouillaud's disease in children less than 5-years old.

Archives Francaises de Pediatrie 17:1024
Nora J J, Weishuhn E J, Bourland B J Fluorescent anti-heart IgM and raised levels of serum IgMin newborns with congenital heart diseases. British Heart Journal 36:167
Odelberg-Johnson G 1932 Case of cervical spondyl-arthritis after tonsillectomy. Acta Orthopaedica Scandinavica 2:302
Ohanion S H, Schwab J H 1967 Persistence of group A streptococcal cell walls related to chronic inflammation of rabbit dermal connective tissue. Journal of Experimental Medicine 125:1137
Osler W 1892 Textbook of Medicine. New York: Appleton
Osman A A 1926 Cited by Glover J A. In Lancet 1930 i:499
Otte H J, Ritzerfeld W 1961 An epidemic of streptococcal tonsillitis due to the eating of contaminated food. German Medical Monthly 6:13
Palmieri M R G, Costas R, Rivers R S D 1962 Rheumatic fever in the tropics. American Heart Journal 63:18
Parillo J, Borst G, Mazur M, et al 1979 Endocarditis due to resistant viridans on oral penicillin prophylaxis. New England Journal of Medicine 300: 296–300
Patarroy M E, Winchester R J, Vejerano A, et al 1979 Association of a B-cell alloantigen with susceptibility to rheumatic fever. Nature 278: 173–174
Payne W W, Schlesinger B 1935 Study of sedimentation rate in juvenile rheumatism. Archives of Diseases in Childhood 10:403
Pilapil V R 1971 Rheumatic fever in Mississippi. 104 cases seen over a decade. Journal of the American Medical Association 215:1626
Pinniger J L 1951 The left auricular appendage in mitral stenosis; a study of fifteen cases submitted to valvulotomy. St Thomas's Hospital Report 7:54
Powell O, Miller R E 1969 Rheumatic myocarditis in an infant nine months of age. Journal of Pediatrics 74:123
Poynton F J 1943 Arthritis in poliomyelitis. Lancet 2:433
Quinn R W 1949 Antihyaluronidase content of human blood serum; study in age differences. Journal of Immunology 61:185
Quinn R W, Hillman J W 1965 An epidemic of streptococcal wound infections.
Quinn R W, Lowry P N 1974 Streptococcal L forms and phage. A clinical-epidemiologic study. Yale Journal of Biology & Medicine 47:86
Rantz L A 1962 Hemolytic streptococcal infection and rheumatic fever. Progress in Cardiovascular Disease 4:483
Rantz L A, Boisvert P J, Spink W W 1947 Hemolytic streptococcus sore throat: the post-streptococcic state. Archives of Internal Medicine 79:401
Rantz L A, Moraney M, DiCaprio J M 1951 Antistreptolysin O response following hemolytic streptococcus infection in early childhood. Archives of Internal Medicine 87:360
Rantz L A, Rantz H H, Boisvert P J, Spink W W 1945 Etiology and pathogenesis of rheumatic fever. Archives of Internal Medicine 76:131
Ravault P P, Maitrepierre J, Lejeune E, Normand J, Cretin-Matenaz R 1961 Dislocating rheumatism, articular sequel of Bouillaud's disease. Journal de Medecine Lyon 42:101
Read S E, Fischetti V A, Utermohlen V, Falk R E, Zabriskie J B 1974 Cellular reactivity studies to streptococcal antigens. Migration inhibition studies in patients with streptococcal infections and rheumatic fever. Journal of Clinical Investigation 54:439
Rehm H 1878 In: Gerhard's Handbuch der Kinderkrankheit, Vol 3. p 21
Reid J, Watson R D, Cochran J B, Sprouli D H 1951 Sodium γ-resorcylate in rheumatic fever. British Medical Journal ii:321
Reinhold J 1951 Anaemia of rheumatic fever. British Medical Journal 2:1093
Reitman N 1945 Abdominal manifestations of rheumatic fever; description of right rectus syndrome. Annals of Internal Medicine 22:671
Rhea L J 1933 Rheumatic peritonitis. American Journal of Pathology 9:719
Riddoch D, Jefferson M, Bickerstaff E R 1971 Chorea and the oral contraceptives. British Medical Journal 4:217
Robertson H F, Schmidt R E, Feiring W 1946 Therapeutic value of early physical activity in rheumatic fever; preliminary report. American Journal of Medical Science 211:67
Robinson J, Brigden W 1963 Immunological studies in the post-cardiotomy syndrome. British Medical Journal ii:706
Rosansky R, Davis E 1958 Relation between C-reactive protein and erythrocyte sedimentation rate in rheumatic fever. American Journal of Clinical Pathology 29:331
Rosenthal A, Czoniczer G, Massell B F 1968 Rheumatic fever under 3 years of age Pediatrics 41:612
Rourke M D & Plass E D 1929 Investigation of various factors which effect sedimentation rate of red blood cells. Journal of Clinical Investigation 7:365
Royal College of Physicians of London 1957 Rheumatic fever committee report.
Rubbo S D, Benjamin M 1953 Transmission of haemolytic streptococci. Journal Hygiene 51:278
Ruderman J E, Abruzzo J L 1966 Chronic postrheumatic fever arthritis (Jaccoud's): Report of a case with subcutaneous nodules. Arthritis and Rheumatism 9:640
Ruebner B H, Boitnott J K 1961 The frequency of Aschoff bodies in atrial appendages of patients with mitral stenosis. relationsbip to age, atrial thrombosis, and season. Circulation 23:550
Russell W R 1949 Paralytic poliomyelitis. The early symptoms and the effect of physical activity on the course of the disease. British Medical Journal 1:465
Sacks L, Fenstein A R, Taranta A 1962 A controlled psychologic study of Sydenham's chorea. Journal of Pediatrics 61:714
Sanghvi L M, Bohra B M 1962 The retardation of erythrocyte sedimentation in congestive heart failure. British Heart Journal 24:180
Schoenfeld A E, Rubinstein A, Raviv U 1968 Immunoglobulins in rheumatic fever. Israel Journal of Medical Sciences 4:815
Schubart A F, Rothschild H J, Schroeder W C, Ewald R W, Tuerk J D 1963 Effect of penicillin treatment on serum complement levels in acute rheumatic fever. Annals of the Rheumatic Diseases 22:319
See G 1850 De la Choree; Rapports du rhumatisme et des maladies du coeur. Bailliere, Paris
Serck-Hanssen A 1966 The Anitschkow myocyte. Further evidence of its myogenic origin and non-rheumatic genesis. Acta Pathologica et Microbiologica Scandinavica 66:471
Shannon F T, Bywaters E G L 1957 Cause of anomalous results in the erythrocyte sedimentation rate using Wintrobe's method. British Medical Journal 2:1405
Shaper A G, Kaplan M H, Foster W D, MacIntosh D M, Wilks N E 1967 Immunological studies in the endomyocardial fibrosis and other forms of heart disease in the tropics. Lancet 1:598
Sharp J T, Hijmans W, Dienes L 1957 Examination of the L

forms of group A streptococci for the group-specific polysaccharride and M protein. Journal of Experimental Medicine 105:153
Shelbourne P A 1948 Primary sarcoma of the heart with report of a case. Annals of Internal medicine 29:1139
Sheldon P J H S, Mair N S, Fox E 1982 Yersinia arthritis: a clinical, immunological, and family study of 2 cases. Annals of the Rheumatic Diseases 41: 153–158
Sheldon W 1948 Rheumatic fever. Acta Paediatrica 36: 383
Shulman S T, Ayoub E M 1974 Qualitative and quantitative aspects of the human antibody response to streptococci group A carbohydrate. Journal of Clinical Investigation 54:990
Shulman S T, Ayoub E M, Victorica B E, Gessner I H, Tanner D F, Hernandez F A 1974 Differences in antibody response to streptococcal antigens in children with rheumatic and non-rheumatic mitral valve disease. Circulation 50:1244
Sibson F 1877 In: Reynold's system of medicine, Vol 4. MacMillan, London, p. 526
Siegel G J, Mones R J 1971 Modification of choreiform activity by haloperidol. Journal of the American Medical Association 216:675
Silva S de 1959 Incidence of rheumatic fever in Ceylon. Archives of Disease in Childhood 34:347
Simon D S, Goodwin J F 1971 Should good teeth be extracted to prevent streptococcus viridans endocarditis? Lancet 1:1207
Singer K, Wong M 1970 Severe persistent chorea with phenothiazine therapy. Report of a case. Postgraduate Medical Journal 46:633
Sinton J R 1948 Clinical value of some methods of estimating erythrocyte sedimentation rate
Sitaj S, Urbanek T, Bosmansky K 1970 Some aspects of epidemiology and surveillance of rheumatic fever. Acta Rheumatologica Scandinavica 16:30
Slater J D, Rosenbaum S 1959 Acute rheumatic fever in young men. A clinical and epidemiological study Annals of the Rheumatic Diseases 18:285
Smith M E, Bywaters E G L 1966 Effect of tetracycline on the duration of raised antistreptolysin-O titre in rheumatic fever. Annals of the Rheumatic Diseases 25:332
Smith R T, Good R A, Zak S J 1957 Sequelae of prednisone treatment of acute rheumatic fever. American Journal of Diseases of Children 93:77
Spagnuolo M, Feinstein A R 1964 Congestive heart failure and rheumatic activity in young patients with rheumatic heart disease. Pediatrics 33:653
Spector W G, Willoughby D A 1959 Experimental suppression of the acute inflammatory changes of thermal injury. Journal of pathology and Bacteriology 78:121
Stevenson A C, Cheeseman E A 1953 Heredity and rheumatic fever: study of 462 families ascertained by affected child and 51 families ascertained by affected mother. Annals of Eugenics 17:177
Stokes H L 1947 Prophylactic sulphanilamide in rheumatic fever; preliminary report. Proceedings of the Royal Australian College of Physicians 2:16
Stokes J, Dawber T R 1956 Rheumatic heart disease in the Framingham study. New England Journal of Medicine 255:1228
Stollerman G H 1960 In: Cohen A (ed) Laboratory diagnostic procedures in the rheumatic diseases.
Stollerman G 1971 Rheumatogenic and nephritogenic streptococci. Circulation 43:915
Stollerman G 1980 Streptococcal vaccines and global strategies for prevention of rheumatic fever. American Journal of Medicine 68: 636–638
Stollerman G H, Siegel A C, Johnson E E 1965 Variable epidemiology of streptococcal disease and the changing pattern of rheumatic fever. Medical Concepts in Cardiovascular Disease 34:45
Stowell D D, Button W H 1941 Observations on the prophylactic use of sulfanilamide on rheumatic patients. Journal of the American Medical Association 117:2164
Strausz I, Dobias G 1967 Autoantibodies reacting with heart muscle tissue in coronary heart disease. Journal of Clinical Pathology 20:161
Sutcliffe J 1955 Pulmonary oedema due to salicylates with report of a case. British Journal of Radiology 28:314
Swash M, Earl C J 1970 Transient visual observations in chronic rheumatic heart disease. Lancet 2:323
Swynghedauw P, Bonte G, Laine E 1946 Oséites subceiguës de l'atlas consécutives à des suppinatious mastoidiennes ou latéro-cervicales; contribution à l'étude de la pathogénie de la maladie de Grisel. Revue d'orthopédie et de Chirurgie de l'Appareil Moteur 32:43
Sykes W O 1948 Erythrocyte sedimentation rate. The effect of alcohol as contaminant. British Medical Journal 1:393
Symmers W. St. C 1956 Amyloidosis; 5 cases of primary generalized amyloidosis and some other unusual cases. Journal of Clinical Pathology 9:212
Tabaee-Zadeh M, Frame B, Kapphahn K 1972 Kinesiogenic choreoathetosis and idiopathic hypoparathyroidism. New England Journal of Medicine 286:762
Taran L M 1946 Laboratory and clinical criteria of rheumatic carditis in children. Journal of Pediatrics 29:77
Taranta A 1959 Relation of isolated recurrences of Sydenham's chorea to preceding streptococcal infections. New England Journal of Medicine 260:1204
Taranta A, Stollerman G H The relationship of Sydenham's chorea to infection in group A streptococci. Journal of Diseases in Children 93:37
Taranta A, Torosdag J, Ketrakos J, Jegier W, Ochida I 1961 Proceedings of the 10th International Congress on Rheumatology, Rome
Taussig H B, Goldenberg M 1941 Roentgenologic studies of size of heart in childhood: 3 different types of teleroentgenographic changes which occur in acute rheumatic fever. American Heart Journal 21:440
Taylor H E, Strong G F 1955 Pulmonary hemosiderosis in mitral stenosis. Annals of Internal Medicine 42:26
Teixeira M A, Relvas P M, Milheiro J 1973 A radiofotografia osteo-articular e a prevencao das artroses. Acta Rheumatologica Portuguesa 1:7
Thomas C B, France R 1939 A preliminary report of the prophylactic use of sulfonamide in patients susceptible to rheumatic fever. Bulletin of the Johns Hopkins Hospital 64:67
Thomas G T 1961 Five-year follow-up on patients with rheumatic fever treated by bed rest, steroidsm or salicylate British Medical Journal i:1635
Thomas G T, Besterman E M M, Hollman A 1953 Rheumatic pericarditis. British Heart Journal 15:29
Trasoff A, Goodman D H 1944 Rheumatic orchitis associated with rheumatic pericarditis and effusion; report of case. Medical Annual DC 13:149
U.S./U.K. Co-operative Clinical Trial 1960 Evolution of rheumatic heart disease in children. British Medical Journal 2:1033

U.S./U.K. Co-operative Clinical Trial 1965 Natural history of rheumatic fever and rheumatic heart disease. British Medical Journal 2:607, Circulation 32:457
Vaccaro R, Severi F, Burgio C R 1970 IgA and autoimmunity. Lancet 1:369
Vaisman B S, Guasch L J, Vignan I A, Correa T E, Schuster C A, Mortimer E A, Rammelkamp C H 1965 The failure of penicillin to alter acute rheumatic valvulitis. Journal of the American Medical Association 194:1284
Van der Geld H 1964 Anti-heart antibodies in the postpericardiotomy and the postmyocardial-infarction syndromes. Lancet 2:617
Van der Geld H, Somers K, Peetoom F 1966 Endomyocardial fibrosis. Lancet 1:48
Van Rijsewijk M J, Goslings W R O 1963 Secretor status of streptococcus pyogenes group A carriers and patients with rheumatic heart disease or acute glomerulonephritis. British Medical Journal 2:542
Von Glahn W C, Kuschner M 1961 Rheumatic phlebitis of the coronary veins. American Journal of pathology 6:251
Wannamaker L W 1970a Differences between streptococcal infections of the throat and of the skin. New England Journal of Medicine 282:23
Wannamaker L W 1970b Streptococcal infections of the throat and skin. New England Journal of Medicine 282:78
Wannamaker L W, Ayoub E M 1960 Antibody titers in acute rheumatic fever. Circulation 21:598
Wasz-Hockert O, Widholen O 1956 Etiological role of β-haemolytic streptococci in rheumatic fever and rheumatic cardiac affections. Annals Paediatrial Fenniae 2:284
Watkinson G 1949 Massive salicylate therapy in rheumatic fever. Annals of the Rheumatic Diseases 8:120
Watson R, Frand Rothbard S, Swift H F 1945 Relationship of postscarlatinal arthritis and carditis to rheumatic fever. Journal of the American Medical Association 128:1145
Watson R F, Hirst G K, Lancefield R C 1961 Bacteriological studies of cardiac tissues obtained at autopsy from eleven patients dying with rheumatic fever. Arthritis and Rheumatism 4:74
Webb J K G 1961 The pattern of disease in South Indian children. Postgraduate Medical Journal 37:149
Wee A S T, Goodwin J F 1966 Acute rheumatic fever and carditis in older adults. Lancet 2:239
Wegria R, Smull K 1945 Salicylate therapy in acute rheumatic fever. Journal of the American Medical Association 129, 485
WHO Technical Report Series 342 on Prevention of Rheumatic Fever 1966
Widdowson J P, Maxted W R, Pinney A M 1971 M-associated protein antigen of Group A streptococci. Journal of Hygiene 69: 553–64
Wilson M G 1940 Rheumatic fever. Oxford University Press, London
Wilson M G, Lubschez R 1944 Recurrence rates in rheumatic fever. The evaluation of etiologic concepts and consequent preventive therapy. Journal of the American Medical Association 124:188 and 126:1188
Winblad S 1966 Studies on non-specific antistreptolysin O titre. I. The influence of serum-beta-lipoproteins on the non-specific antistreptolysin O titre. Acta Pathologica et Microbiologica Scandinavica 66:93
Winblad S 1973 Acute joint symptoms in yersiniosis enterocolitica (abstract). Scandinavian Journal of Rheumatism 2:3
Wood E E, Andrews C T 1949 Subacute myelosclerosis. Lancet 2:739
Wood P 1936 Erythrocyte sedimentation rate in diseases of heart. Quarterly Journal of Medicine 5:1
Wood P 1968 Diseases of the heart and circulation, 3rd Edn. Eyre & Spottiswoode, London
Yim H 1962 Rheumatic fever in Hawaii. American Journal of Diseases of Children 103:715
Yoshinoya S, Pope R M 1980 Detection of immune complexes in acute rheumatic fever and their relationship to HLA B5. Journal of Clinical Investigation 65: 136–145
Zabriskie J B, Freimer E H 1966 An immunological relationship between the group A streptococcus and mammalian muscle. Journal of Experimental Medicine 124:661
Zabriskie J B, Hsu K C, Siegal B C 1970b Heart-reactive antibody associated with rheumatic fever: Characterization and diagnostic significance. Clinical and Experimental Immunology 7:147
Zabriskie J B, Read S E, Eillis R J 1971 Cellular and humoral studies in diseases with heart-reactive antibodies. In: Amos B (ed) Progress in Immunology. Academic Press, London, p. 213
Zabriskie J B, Lewshenia R, Moller G, Wehle B, Falk R E 1970a Lymphocytic responses to streptococcal antigens in glomerulonephritis patients. Science 168:1105
Zettervall O, Sjoquist J, Waldenstrom J, Winblad S 1966 Serological activity in myeloma type globulins. Clinical and Experimental Immunology 1:213
Zimmermann H 1967 Maladie du Grisel (Torticollis naso-pharyngien). Helvetica Paediatrica Acta 22:76
Zimmerman R A, Auernheimer A H, Taranta A 1971 Precipitating antibody to group A streptococcal polysaccharide in humans. Journal of Immunology 107:832
Zitnan D, Bosmansky K 1966 Antimyocardial serum factors in rheumatic fever detected by the immunofluorescence method. Acta Rheumatologica Scandinavica 12:267
Zvaifler N J 1962 Chronic post rheumatic fever (Jaccoud's) arthritis. New England Journal of Medicine 267:10

B.M. Ansell E.G.L. Bywaters

Juvenile chronic arthritis

HISTORICAL

In 1897 George Frederic Still described 22 cases of juvenile chronic arthritis. He emphasised 12 florid cases of lymphadenopathy and fever but thought that other cases were similar to those of adult rheumatoid arthritis. A number of individual cases had been recorded previously, (e.g. Cornil, 1864), but Still brought together almost all the distinctive features of the childhood disease, except the rash, and young patients with chronic arthritis were often referred to as having 'Still's disease'. Long-term follow-up confirms Still's view that several different entities are concerned: we feel therefore that it is better to use the general term 'juvenile chronic arthritis' (JCA) for arthritis commencing in childhood. The syndrome originally emphasised by Still consisting of fever, arthritis, lymphadenopathy and splenomegaly, with the addition of rash (Boldero, 1933), may be a specific one, and can occur for the first time in adult life (Bywaters, 1971). The Wissler (1967) or Wissler–Fanconi syndrome ('subsepsis allergica') is a variant of the latter.

DEFINITION

A number of 'diagnostic' or classificatory criteria have been introduced both for clinical and survey purposes (Bywaters, 1968; Kviem et al, 1982). Those introduced by the American Rheumatism Association (Brewer et al, 1977) are complicated for clinical use. The Taplow criteria (Ansell & Bywaters, 1959) had the virtue of simplicity: 'arthritis starting before the age of 16 manifest by two of the following: pain, swelling and limitation in four or more joints reliably observed over a period of at least 3 months, or in one joint for a similar period with biopsy confirmation; other diseases being excluded as far as possible up to 1 year from the onset of the symptoms'. The working criteria put forward from the workshop on the care of rheumatic children (Wood, 1978) and outlined in Table 43.1 form a basis for initial diagnosis but do not indicate the further subgroups which are emerging and indeed may not be obvious by 3 months of illness.

Table 43.1 Criteria for juvenile chronic arthritis (Wood, 1978)

Onset under 16 years
Arthritis of 1 or more joints for 3 months
Exclusion of other defined entities, e.g. psoriatic arthritis, infection, hypogammaglobulinaemia, systemic lupus erythematosus, dermatomyositis, familial Mediterranean fever, etc.
Classification by mode of onset in first 3 months:
Systemic
Polyarthritic (5 or more joints)
Pauciarticular (less than 5 joints)

PREVALENCE AND INCIDENCE

This is a comparatively rare disease: Lawrence (personal communication) estimated that 0.2% of the adult population have a history consistent with polyarthritis during childhood. Looking at four regions adjacent to Taplow over a 10 year period, Bywaters (1968) found 0.06% of the school population in each area affected; this is a minimum prevalence. It agrees well with the point prevalence in 1966 found in the Bristol Child Development Study (personal communication, Butler, 1975). In Finland, Laaksonen (personal communication) in 1977 found a prevalence rate of 1 : 1200 children under the age of 16.

The peak age of incidence, as most authorities agree, is between 1 and 3 years of age and this peak is particularly a female one and is accounted for by the large number of young girls presenting with pauciarticular arthritis (Fig. 43.1). The incidence in males tends to rise around puberty, owing to the onset of seronegative HLA-B27 linked disease. In early teens, girls with seropositive disease tend to predominate.

PATHOLOGY

Joint changes may be similar to those of adult rheumatoid disease (Fig. 43.2a) or may show mild synovitis only (Fig. 43.2b). Because of the greater thickness of juvenile cartilage, bone is eroded only very much later and therefore the reversible stage lasts longer. This phenomenon and its consequence, the absence of X-ray change early, led to the earlier mistaken views that the lesion was periarthritic. Nodules are also uncommon; they occur mainly, but not solely, in the seropositive group (Fig. 43.3a). In the latter they resemble usually the adult nodule but when seen in the seronegative patient resemble more closely that seen in rheumatic fever (Fig. 43.3b) (Bywaters et al, 1958). Arteritis is seen rarely and only in older seropositive children.

AETIOLOGY

Infection and trauma have both been suggested as playing a provocative role. Trauma perhaps may be important in a few cases as a localising factor, and infection as a precipitating one. There are a large number of non-specific immunological abnormalities, which include changes in serum proteins and increased serum concentrations of immunoglobulins (Table 43.2) while particularly those with systemic illness have circulating immune complexes relating to all classes of immunoglobulins (Rossen et al, 1977; Moran et al, 1979). Between 25 and 30% of children carry antinuclear antibodies. Selective IgA deficiency is seen in varying proportions from 2–4% of children with juvenile chronic arthritis and is most common in those children with a pauci-articular onset. It does not appear to alter the manifestations or course (Barkley et al, 1979; Cassidy, 1977). The low complement in the synovial fluid detected by Hedberg (1971) and the demonstration of complexes of IgG and IgG rheumatoid factor in the

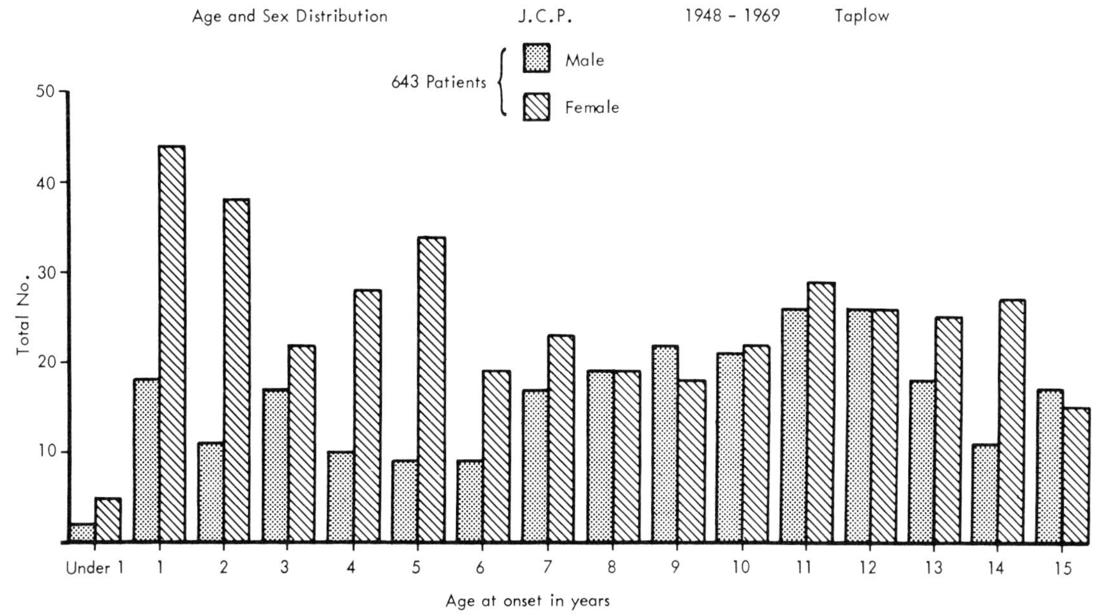

Fig. 43.1 Age and sex distribution of 643 patients with juvenile chronic arthritis.

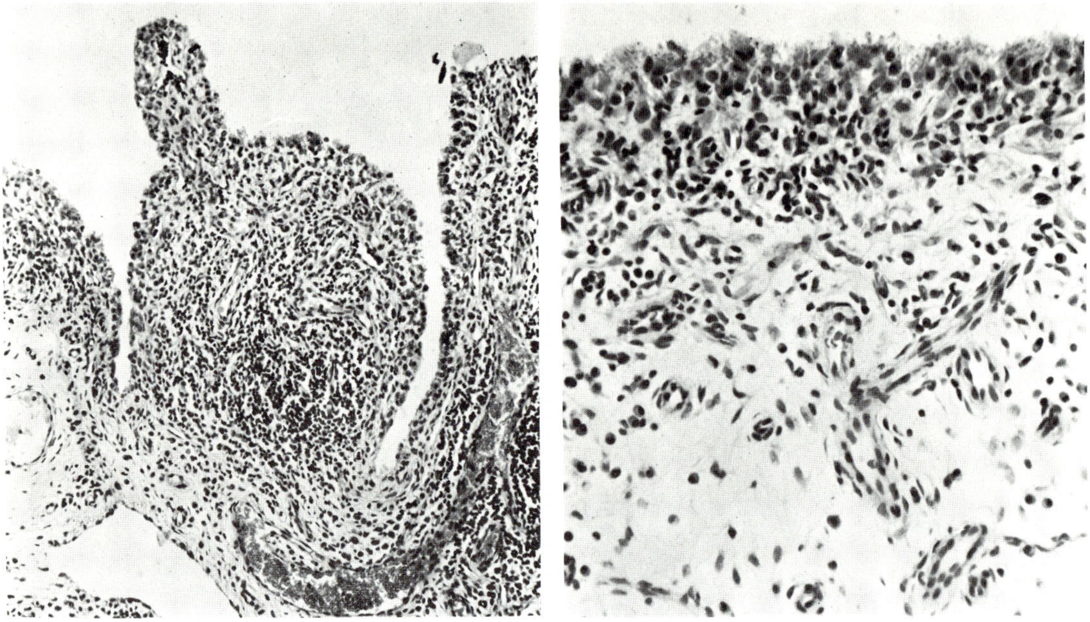

a b

Fig. 43.2 (a) Synovium from knee of a 2-year-old girl at 8 months. No other joints are involved and she went into remission aged 5. 15 years later she is still well. The picture is typical of rheumatoid arthritis with marked infiltration by lymphocytes and plasma cells. (H & E × 130) (b) Synovium from the knee of a 4-year-old girl with seronegative monarthritis for 11 months. Later other joints become involved. Note the relative lack of lymphocytes or plasma cell accumulation. (H & E × 200)

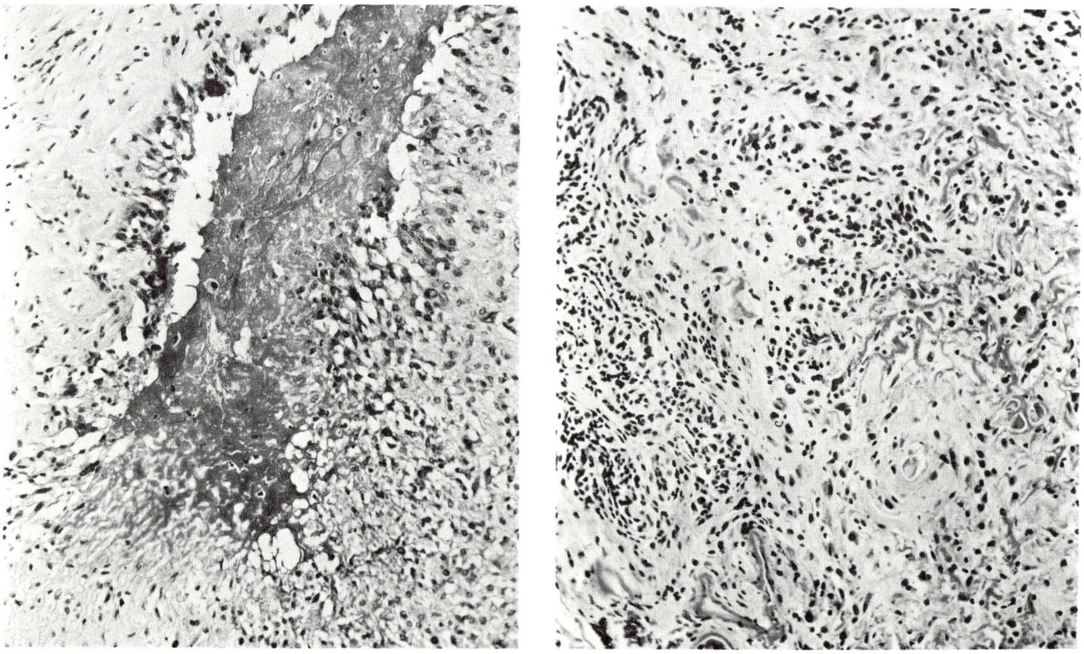

a b

Fig. 43.3 Rheumatoid-type nodule from a female aged 11 with seropositive polyarthritis for 5 years. Note the central necrosis and well-developed palisading. (H & E × 120) Compare with (b) Nodule from a female aged 8 years with seronegative arthritis for 16 months. Note the lattice-like fibrinoid change towards the right margin. (H & E × 110)

Table 43.2 Serum immunoglobin levels, mg/100 ml

	Controls		Juvenile chronic arthritis			
		s.d.	Active	s.d.	Inactive	s.d.
n	136		293		97	
IgG	1123	270	2018	853	1394	371
IgA	199	103	345	218	254	141
IgM	73	34	127	67	95	52
IgD	4.4	4	3.8	3.5	2.7	3

synovial tissues of juvenile patients by Munthe (1972) further suggest an immunological basis.

Høyeraal & Mellbye (1974a) found that 34 patients with juvenile rheumatoid arthritis had significantly higher serum levels of CH50, C4, C3 and C3A than their matched control group, but no difference for Clq, suggesting there may have been increased consumption and therefore increased synthesis. Cell-mediated immunity in juvenile rheumatoid arthritis may be impaired (Høyeraal & Mellbye, 1974b). On the basis of finding an antibody in sera from juvenile patients which was specific for a regulatory subset of T cells, thereby causing its loss, Morimoto et al (1981) suggested that aberrations in suppressor function may be important in the pathogenesis of active JCA, but this has not been confirmed by Williams and his colleagues (1981). Peripheral lymphocytes from patients with systemic disease and possibly also polyarthritis, but not pauciarticular arthritis, have altered responsiveness to mitogens. However, the mechanism and meaning have not been established (Gershwin et al, 1979; Tyndall et al, 1982).

Relapses of systemic illness sometimes occur after intercurrent infection by various organisms (Tyndall et al, 1984). An increased incidence of antibodies to EB virus relative to age has been found in our patients with systemic illness, but these children were all hospitalised and, therefore, at greater risk from becoming infected. The increase in alpha-interferon production demonstrated in relapses of systemic illness (Bacon et al, 1983) further supports the possibility of preceding infection.

Genetic data are also difficult to interpret. Stastny & Fink (1979) noted that the prevalence of HLA-DW4 was considerably lower in children with arthritis than in control subjects or in adults with rheumatoid arthritis, and that there was an increased incidence of DW5 and DW8. Subsequent work has confirmed that in early onset pauciarticular disease, HLA-DW5 and HLA-DR5 are increased, particularly in young children with positive tests for anti-nuclear antibodies. Also increased in the young pauciarticular patients are HLA-DW8 and HLA-DR8, but these appear to have wider clinical associations than HLA-DR5. Cross reactivity between HLA-DR5 and DR8 complicates the interpretation of data relating to these two antigens (Miller & Glass, 1981). In addition to these findings, HLA-DR7 appears reduced in our group of pauciarticular patients. The majority of patients with HLA-B27 are males, with a pauciarticular onset at an older age — usually 9 years or more. Schaller et al (1976) have suggested that these really belong to the spondylitic class. HLA-DR4 is increased in patients with persistently positive IgM rheumatoid factor disease in the same frequency as seen in adult rheumatoid arthritis (Clemens et al, 1983; Førve et al, 1982). It is also suggested that HLA-DR4 may be increased in older onset (8+) seronegative polyarthritis (Morling et al, 1981). It is rare to get more than one member of a family affected by JCA and in those few families reported the disease was similar in the two sibs. HLA studies of 10 sib pairs, in whom all except one pair were pauciarticular at onset, showed haplotype identity of the affected sibs, but no common haplotype to all the families. The interval between the two sibs becoming affected has varied from 5 months to 11 years (Ansell & Clemens, 1982). Among the 7 pairs of identical twins, apart from the spondylitic and psoriatic groups, 4 have become concordant with a mean follow-up of 16 years.

Thus, the most likely cause is a non-specific stimulus in a genetically prone host; further work utilising new technologies in infectious diseases and the rapidly expanding information on host defence mechanisms is essential.

CLINICAL ASPECTS

While the presenting symptoms are usually pain or swelling of joints, or impaired use of a limb, the disease may start systemically in nearly one-third with fever and malaise, joint symptoms being absent and only developing some months later.

Features of systemic onset disease

This mode is particularly common under the age of 5 when boys are affected as frequently as girls. The fever is usually high and remittent, reaching 38.8°C to 39.9°C at night and often subnormal by morning. While this characteristic feature is not always present, such fever is of considerable diagnostic importance since it differs from that found in rheumatic fever, where the temperature seldom swings as much and is more sustained (McMinn & Bywaters, 1959). This fever does not respond to antibiotics but does respond to adequate salicylate dosage (Fig. 43.4) as does also that of rheumatic fever. A rash is seen in the majority, consisting of small red morbilliform macules, usually 2–5 mm in diameter, on arms, legs, face and sometimes trunk, surrounded by a zone of pallor. This is quite characteristic (Fig. 43.5) and is associated with the fever, often being seen, therefore, only towards evening. Rarely in the larger patches central pallor is seen, but unlike the extensive circinate or marginate erythemata in rheumatic fever, these lesions do not spread but appear and disappear only to recur next evening elsewhere (Isdale & Bywaters, 1956).

Very occasionally there is a minor urticarial element to the rash (Schaller & Wedgewood, 1970). This combination of swinging fever and rash is diagnostic of juvenile chronic arthritis even in the absence of joint lesions. It is occasionally seen in patients with an onset in adult life (Elkon et al, 1982), both female and male (Fabricant et al, 1973), even up to the forties, accompanied by other classical features of the juvenile disease such as C2–3 fusion (Bywaters, 1971).

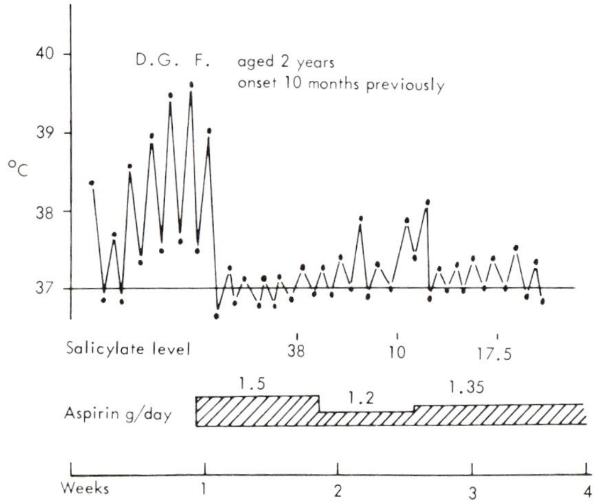

Fig. 43.4 Characteristic fever chart with response to adequate dosage of salicylate, but relapse on inadequate dosage.

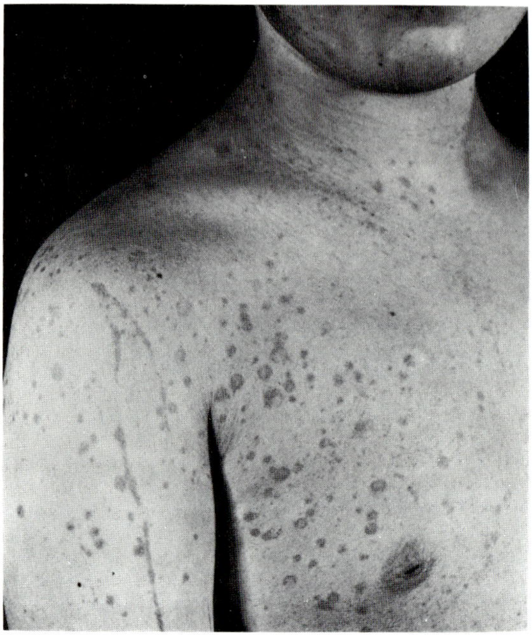

Fig. 43.5 Typical macular rash in a young girl.

Lymphadenopathy and splenomegaly

These classical manifestations are found only in the more severe and active stages of the disease, and in younger patients (Fig. 43.6). Pathologically the lymph nodes show non-specific follicular hyperplasia and often relate topographically to inflamed joints.

The liver may be enlarged, usually associated with splenomegaly. Raised levels of SGOT, SGPT and lactic dehydrogenases are usually due to concomitant drug medication. An occasional patient will have hepatomegaly with grossly abnormal liver function tests when mild periportal round cell infiltration has been seen but its relation to the basic disease process is still uncertain (Schaller et al, 1970). Very occasionally an enlarged liver may be due to fatty changes associated with steroid administration and later in the disease course to amyloidosis.

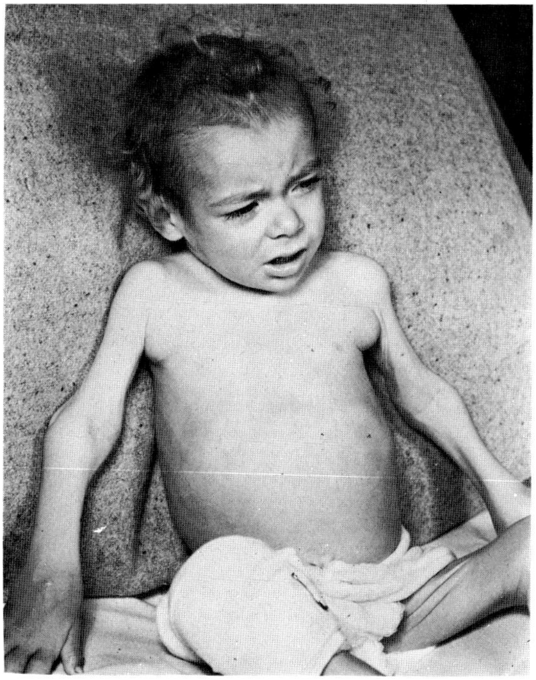

Fig. 43.6 Wasting of muscles, arthritis and marked axillary lymphadenopathy in a 3-year-old boy with disease of 2 years' duration.

Serositis

Pericarditis as an isolated cardiac manifestation is most common with systemic onset disease. It is unusual for the pericarditis to precede the arthritis but may occur with acute exacerbations (Fig. 43.7) and with other manifestations such as rash, lymphadenopathy and splenomegaly. Its duration has ranged from 1–15 weeks; in one-quarter of patients there are recurrent episodes (Lietman & Bywaters, 1963). While the child may have obvious symptoms such as precordial pain or friction, many cases develop insidiously; therefore the frequency with which it is documented depends on the care with which it is sought by echocardiograph (Bernstein et al, 1974). There is no reason to suspect that children who have pericarditis fare worse than others. As yet, none of our patients have proceeded to constriction although one case has been recorded by Keith et al (1958). Cardiac tamponade is occasionally seen (Scharf et al, 1976) and indeed one of our cases has died from tamponade, owing to the parents' unwillingness to send the child back to hospital.

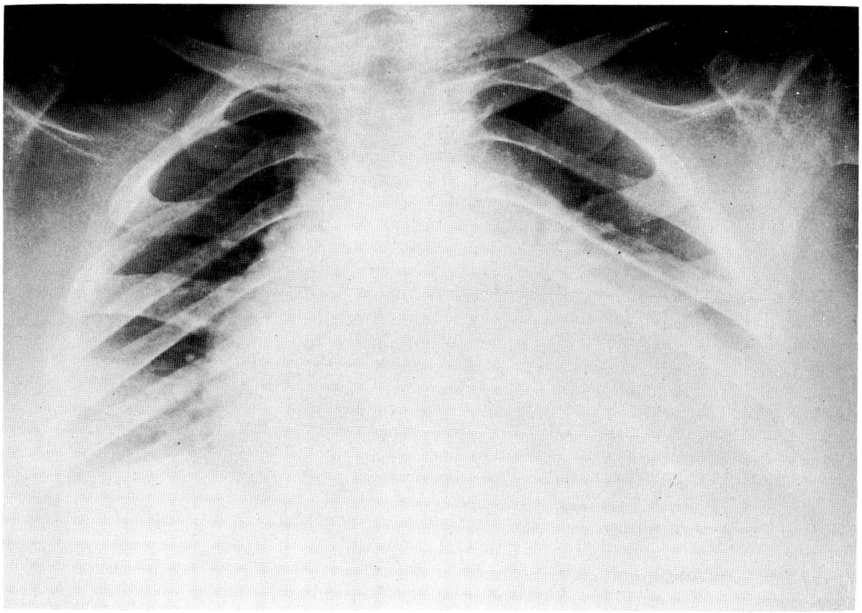

Fig. 43.7 Acute pericardial effusion occurs with an exacerbation of arthritis and rash in a boy aged 10 whose systemic juvenile chronic arthritis had commenced 6 years earlier.

Pleurisy
This is usually seen only with pericarditis.

Other clinical aspects
Myocarditis is rare but may result in cardiomegaly, cardiac failure and even death (Miller & French, 1977; Brewer, 1977). Pulmonary disease is also rare in children (Athreya et al, 1980). Pulmonary fibrosis has been reported in seropositive cases (Brinkman & Chaikof, 1959; Jordan & Snyder, 1964), and we have seen an example in seronegative disease. Encephalitis has been described in 'Still's' disease (Schlesinger, 1949). In our experience cerebral symptoms are usually a complication due not to the disease itself, but to unsuspected fat embolism, to coincidental viral infection, salicylate overdosage or pseudotumour cerebri due to corticosteroids, as drawn attention to by Jan et al (1972).

The kidneys may be involved by amyloid disease, or by gold, penicillamine or renal papillary necrosis (Wortmann et al, 1980). If intrinsic kidney disease is seen, lupus should be excluded, but associated glomerulitis may rarely occur (Antilla, 1972).

Polyarticular onset
This tends to affect girls more frequently than boys and is usually persistently seronegative for IgM rheumatoid factor. Those few older girls who do carry IgM rheumatoid factor do so from within a few months of onset (Ansell, 1980). There is no peak age of incidence, it can be seen within the first year but also occurs at any time throughout childhood. Those first affected in adolescence tend to have a more destructive course possibly because the epiphyseal cartilage is no longer thick. In addition to the polyarthritis there may be lethargy, weight loss, unwillingness to use limbs, morning slowness and low grade fever. Symmetrical involvement of wrists and carpi, proximal interphalangeal joints and flexor tenosynovitis, knees and ankles are the usual presenting joints. Other early involvement includes the neck, while later hind feet, elbows, shoulders, hips and temperomandibular joints may be affected.

Pauciarticular onset
This is the most usual mode of presentation accounting for about 50% of patients seen. Large joints, particularly those of the lower limbs, are most frequently affected and involvement is often asymmetrical. Eventually up to 40% may spread to involve more joints usually as asymmetrical polyarthritis which is severe in about half. If would appear to encompass several entities; the most frequent is that in young children, particularly girls, with a positive ANA, who are at risk for iridocyclitis. Older boys who carry B27 and therefore best grouped as 'juvenile spondylitis' are next, while other children, again particularly girls, remain with only a few joints and without complications; these are often referred to as 'persistent pauciarticular': some pauciarticular onset may ultimately develop psoriasis.

Pattern of joint involvement
Of all joints, the knees are most frequently involved (60%) followed closely by the wrists and carpi. Peculiar to seronegative childhood disease is a relatively high frequency of terminal interphalangeal joint involvement without nail changes or other overt signs of psoriasis. The swelling of the terminal interphalangeal joints looks superficially like Heberden's nodes and later the X-rays show bony overgrowth. This is due to enlargement of the basal epiphyses and not to ossification in the capsular tendinous insertion. Proximal interphalangeal joints are much more commonly affected than metacarpophalangeal joints although the latter may be splinted by severe flexor tenosynovitis. Neck involvement is characteristic, usually affecting the upper part; only rarely is this the first site affected (2%). The neck is held stiffly with loss of extension and rotation: occasionally the patient presents with a torticollis, particularly in the systemic group. Radiological involvement of apophyseal joints is followed by fusion and later the bodies which fuse at the level of the fused apophyseal joints (Fig. 43.8). The resultant ankylosis needs to be differentiated from congenital fusion and it is quite different from the abnormal mobility and subluxation of the elderly rheumatoid, where oncovertebral disease invades the degenerate disc space. Noticeable also is the infrequency of atlantoaxial subluxation in the seronegative group, although it has occasionally been recorded as a presenting feature (Nathan & Bickel, 1968).

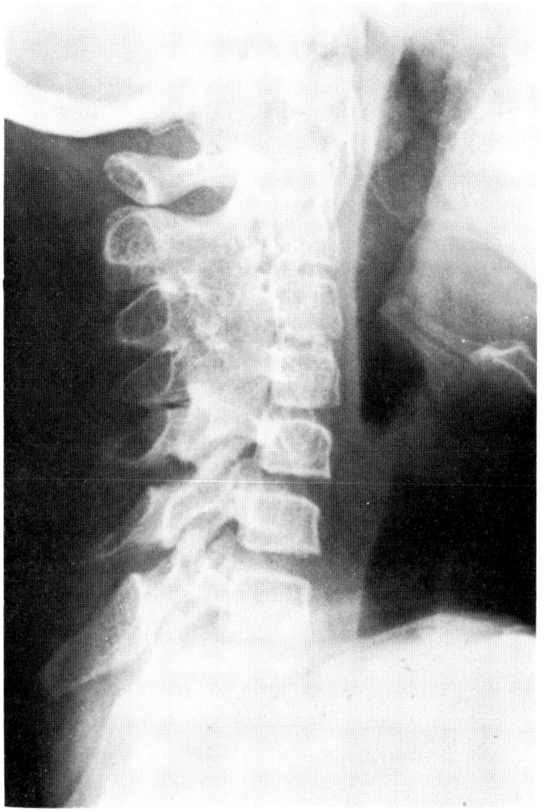

Fig. 43.8 Bony apophyseal fusion between C2/3 and C4 with narrowing at 5/6 and poorly developed cervical vertebrae in a child who has suffered from juvenile chronic arthritis for 10 years.

Hip involvement after systemic illness and in the polyarthritic group is common, while loss of mobility due to knee disease is associated with poor development of the hip in the absence of clinical involvement (Gallino et al, 1984). Hip disease is rarely a presenting feature, but tends to occur with persistent disease activity. The younger the patient the more likely it is to be associated with poor development of the whole joint (Rombouts & Rombouts-Lindemans, 1971), while in older patients protrusio or even fusion of the joint can occur (Gallino et al, 1984). Unilateral involvement is rare, usually in extended particular disease, and is often associated with scoliosis. Scoliosis in juvenile chronic arthritis is not uncommon, affecting about 15%; it is of varying aetiology, including torticollis, hip involvement, unequal leg length as well as idiopathic scoliosis (Rombouts & Rombouts-Lindemans, 1974). Involvement of the temperomandibular joints may lead to limitation of bite and to underdevelopment of the jaw due to premature fusion of the epiphyses; micrognathia may however, be present, without limitation of either temperomandibular joint, but it is associated with loss of neck movement (Ronning et al, 1974).

An interesting characteristic is the relative absence of pain on palpation or active movement of the joints seen in a few children, due perhaps to the lack of the psychic element of pain sense characteristic of the adult (Laaksonen & Laine, 1961). Children above the age of 5 years are able to do visual analogue scores and showed an extremely low awareness of pain (Scott et al, 1977); this helps to maintain function.

Tenosynovitis is seen in numerous sites, particularly the dorsal sheaths of the wrists and around the ankles. Flexor tendon synovitis may be a serious problem in children, frequently causing loss of extension of the fingers; if adhesions develop, serious claw hand deformity may result (Ansell & Bywaters, 1953).

Nodules. Subcutaneous nodules are seen in 4% of seronegative cases, usually on the olecranon. As detailed under 'pathology' the histological appearances resembled more closely those of rheumatic fever than of adult rheumatoid arthritis, showing in most instances no central necrotic area, little fibrosis and no palisading, but instead (see Fig. 43.3b) some fibrinoid lattice, groups of blood vessels and sparse cells with plump nuclei. While those few older children with classical rheumatoid nodules are always seropositive, younger ones are usually seronegative (Bywaters et al, 1958).

Iridocyclitis. 10% of our patients with juvenile chronic arthritis showed evidence of iridocyclitis; two distinct types were seen — acute and chronic (Kanski, 1977). In the majority it was a chronic insidious process, involving both eyes in two-thirds, the second eye being affected within a year or not at all. The first overt sign is a punctate precipitate on the posterior surface of the cornea (Fig. 43.9); partial or complete band keratopathy commonly develops, and later cataract; these together form the ocular triad of Still's disease (Smiley et al, 1957). Chronic iridocylitis is usually symptomless: there is little or no injection of the eye and little pain, so that it is frequently missed

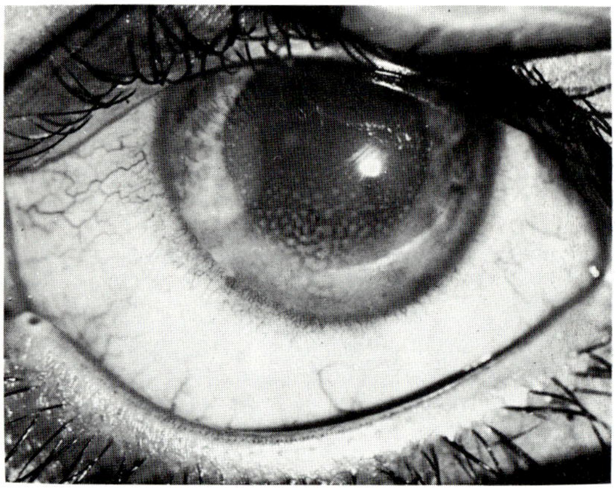

Fig. 43.9 Keratitis punctata in a 9-year-old boy showing also circumcorneal vascularisation and early band keratopathy.

unless routine slit lamp examination is undertaken; a cloudy aqueous fluid cannot be recognised just on clinical examination. The eyes should be checked at least annually, unless the patient is thought to be a special risk because of few joints involved and/or a positive anti-nuclear antibody test, when it is desirable to check at 3–6 monthly intervals. At any time irregularity of the pupil or pigmentary deposits calls for immediate consultation. Patients with chronic iridocyclitis have an early age of onset, are predominantly female, and tend to have a pauciarticular arthritis at onset, which persists in more than half the patients. A particular feature is the high incidence — 88% — of anti-nuclear antibodies in these children (Schaller et al, 1974). Negative correlations include the absence of rheumatoid factor and sacroiliac changes.

This chronic type of uveitis can grumble on for months or years with occasional remissions and exacerbations. A few children run a relatively benign course (Smiley & Kanski, 1978) but in general this is a very serious complication, and unheeded, will often lead to glaucoma or blindness. Prompt treatment with local corticosteroids and mydriatics will usually control the inflammation (Kanski, 1981) but it may not be possible to control the inflammation in every case in this way and the very high daily dosage of corticosteroids previously used to do this is not acceptable. Because of this, cytotoxic drugs have been under study. Azathioprine appears to be of little value. Cyclophosphamide is encouraging (Witmer, 1974), while our experience indicates that chlorambucil is also effective (Mehra et al, 1981).

Mainly boys have acute uveitis with redness, photophobia and pain; this is transitory and usually settles readily on local treatment leaving minimal changes; these tend to develop sacroiliitis or spondylitis. Of those so far tested, all have carried tissue type HLA-B27.

Other features

Growth defects. These may be general or local: as in other chronic diseases of childhood, general growth may be affected by the metabolic changes of severe disease, continuing for many years (Fig. 43.10). A more common cause of failure to grow is the prolonged daily administration of corticosteroids even in dosage as low as

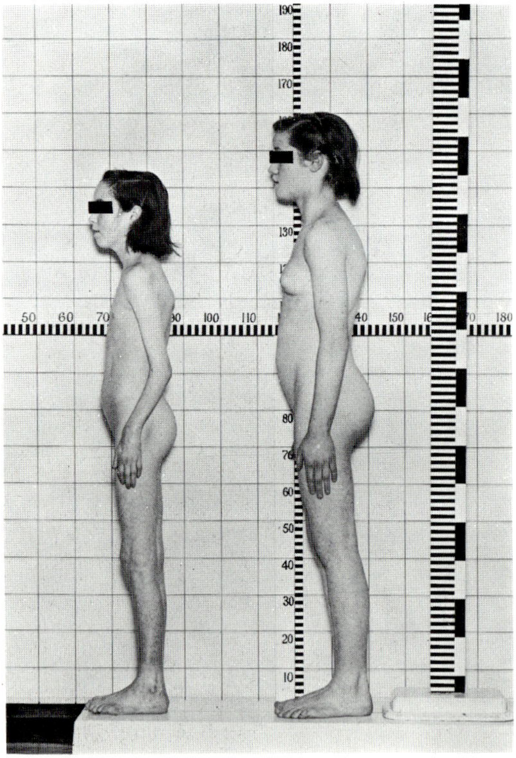

Fig. 43.10 Retarded growth in a 14-year-old girl as compared to her twin. She had juvenile chronic arthritis of 5 years' duration and had never received corticosteroid therapy.

3–5 mg/day of prednisone. Local disturbances of growth arise from slowing or more rarely, acceleration in the region of affected joints which sometimes affects the whole limb. Involvement of joints in younger patients may give rise to the premature appearance of ossification centres or to enlargement of epiphyses; this is easily appreciated if only one side is involved. The knee is frequently involved when temporary increased metaphyseal growth may occur giving rise to overgrowth of the whole leg on the affected side (Ansell & Bywaters, 1956). Conversely, and often in older patients, one whole limb or a foot is shorter as a result of fusion of epiphyses in one site. In young children subperiosteal bone accretion may cause characteristic widening of the phalanges. In older children premature epiphyseal fusion is most striking in the metatarsals or metacarpals with resulting short fingers or toes (Fig. 43.11). Very occasionally there is a destruction of epiphyses by rheumatoid granulation tissue preventing further growth of such epiphyses. Failure of development of cervical vertebrae is seen particularly in children with neck involvement at an early age (Fig. 43.8), while, as previously indicated, failure of mandibular growth is not uncommon in young children.

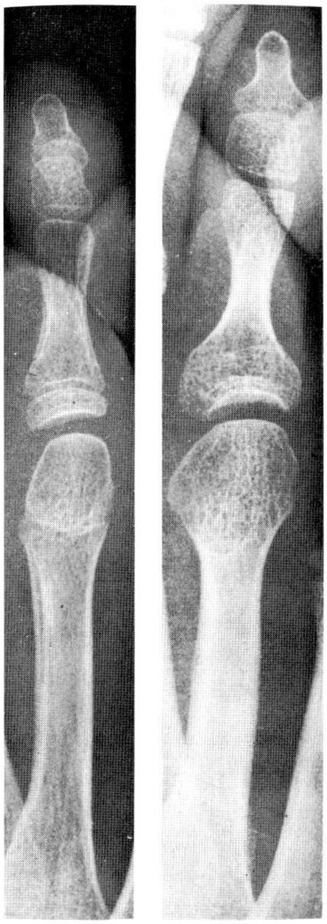

Fig. 43.11 Periostitis in 1963 followed by premature epiphyseal fusion and growth anomaly of basal phalanx and metatarsal.

Fractures. These are most frequent in children whose onset of disease is below 5 years and particularly if they have been treated by immobilisation and corticosteroids (Badley & Ansell, 1960). Vertebral collapse is almost entirely confined to patients with osteoporosis from prolonged oral corticosteroid therapy. Children with pauciarticular disease are also at risk from supracondylar fracture of the femur on the same side as an involved knee.

Amyloidosis. Amyloidosis is the most serious complication because it is nearly always fatal. It occurs mainly in the more severe cases whose disease remains active for prolonged periods, but it has been seen as early as 1 year and as late as 23 years from onset. It is usually detected by the development of proteinuria, but occasionally of diarrhoea, or of unexplained anaemia; ultimately it leads to a nephrotic syndrome with oedema and finally uraemia and death (Fig. 43.12); it is particularly common following persistent activity in the systemic group. The longer the follow-up of the more difficult referral cases the higher the incidence. Once the diagnosis of amyloidosis has been established, the mean duration of life has been 8 years. Therapy should aim at decreasing the overall activity of the disease process and to this end cytotoxic drugs are currently under study (Schnitzer & Ansell, 1977).

Death. The two most important causes of death are infection and amyloidosis. Of 2144 patients seen between 1947 and 1982, 60 died, almost half of these from renal failure (Table 43.3). In the early 1950s this was usually due to infection in the systemic phase. Systemic disease also appears to be at particular risk from amyloidosis later. Other causes of death among those studied include trauma, carcinoma of colon following colitic arthritis, atlantoaxial subluxation, fat embolus from trauma (1) and crush fracture of vertebrae after corticosteroid therapy, and apparently unre-

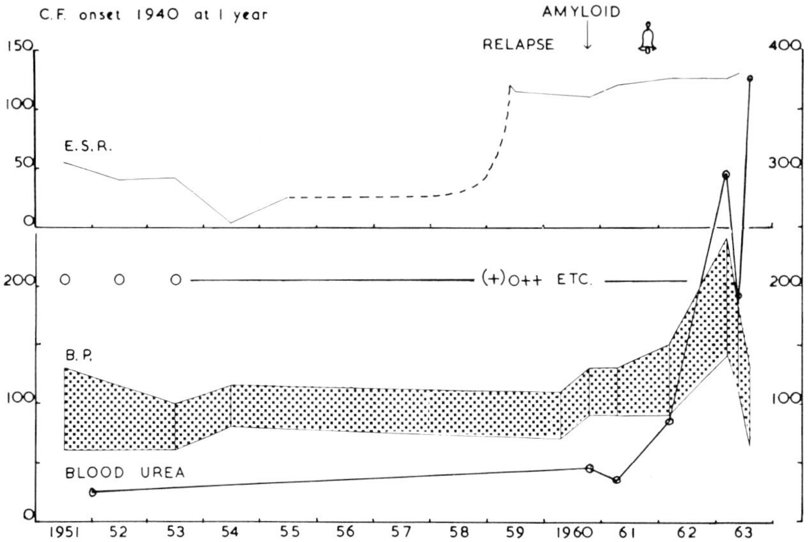

Fig. 43.12 Chart showing proteinuria developing in a relapse 19 years from onset: amyloidosis was diagnosed on renal biopsy and she died from renal failure 3 years later.

Table 43.3 Cause of death in juvenile chronic arthritis (2144 total referrals, Taplow 1947–1982)

Renal failure	26
Infections	22
Heart failure	6
Blood dyscrasia	2
Traumatic	5
Neoplasm	1
Unrelated	1

lated causes such as subarachnoid haemorrhage (1).

DIAGNOSTIC AIDS

Acute phase reactants. The erythrocyte sedimentation rate (ESR) as well as the plasma fibrinogen, C-reactive protein (Gwyther et al, 1982) plasma viscosity, etc., are each of considerable value in estimating the activity of the disease and the effect of treatment, and in the initial differentiation of non-inflammatory conditions, such as chondrodystrophy, osteitis dissecans or parental anxiety syndrome. It must be borne in mind, however, that the ESR can be within normal limits with few joints involved, in inactive disease and, exceptionally, in the older child with active disease in several joints. We prefer the Westergren method for the ESR, since the Wintrobe tube is too narrow for free fall to occur in high haematocrit bloods (Shannon & Bywaters, 1957).

Blood count. There is usually a mild anaemia in active disease but is rare for the haemoglobin to be below 10 g% without some other cause. Particularly in systemic disease the white count may be considerably elevated, e.g. up to 30 000/mm^3, with a high percentage of polymorphs. The platelet count may also be increased up to 900 000/mm^3 in severe disease (Endresen et al, 1977).

Serological. IgM rheumatoid factor tests are negative and remain so. Those children with positive sheep cell agglutination or latex tests tend to have an older age of onset, are frequently girls and have a pattern of illness resembling adult rheumatoid arthritis. Anti-nuclear antibodies are present in 30% of patients with juvenile chronic arthritis, many of whom have chronic iridocyclitis; one-third of those with positive anti-nuclear antibodies have no other specific features. Antibodies to double-stranded DNA are generally absent (Johnson et al, 1975). Serum complement levels show little change. However, immune complexes can be detected by a variety of techniques, particularly in systemic disease (Moran et al, 1979; Rossen et al, 1977). Anti-IgG antibodies are present in the sera of patients, particularly with active disease (Wernick et al, 1981; Schlumpf et al, 1985). What their relevance is to the disease process requires further elucidation. Moore and his colleagues continue to search for hidden rheumatoid factors (Moore et al, 1978).

Immunoglobulins. In general, immunoglobulin levels, with the exception of IgD, are raised (Goel et al, 1974) in active disease as compared to healthy children (see Table 43.2). IgM was particularly high in the seropositive females. A few patients had extremely high levels of serum IgG; the majority of these subsequently developed amyloidosis. Whether high IgA early in systemic disease is associated with poor prognosis is under study. IgA deficiency is occasionally seen, usually in those with a pauciarticular onset (Cassidy, 1977).

Radiological. Soft tissue swelling and osteoporosis are non-specific signs of inflammation and disuse. Juxtra-articular periostitis indicates synovitis; it is probably commoner in children than adults; particularly along phalanges and due to flexor tenosynovitis. Erosions are less frequent and usually occur later than in the adult: they denote the irreversible stage, although occasionally carpal and other erosions have been noted to heal (Bywaters, 1963). A most useful diagnostic sign is growth change — either under or overdevelopment (Martel et al 1962; Ansell & Kent, 1977). As well as X-rays of the involved area, neck and sacroiliac views are of particular value, although lesions in the neck are not usually found without clinical limitation. Sacroiliac changes may be helpful in distinguishing the type of disease present.

Biopsy of synovial membrane. This is of value, particularly in monarticular cases, for exclusion of other disorders such as infections (tuberculosis, fungal, etc.) and pigmented villonodular synovitis or angioma of the synovial membrane (Bywaters & Edmonds, 1976).

DIFFERENTIAL DIAGNOSIS (Table 43.4)

In infants and very young children, disinclination to walk or to use an arm may be due to many different causes besides arthritis, for example, poliomyelitis, Henoch-Schönlein purpura, scurvy, rickets or osteomyelitis. In the older child monarticular disease needs differentiation from tuberculosis, pigmented villonodular synovitis and traumatic lesions. Prolonged fever is the presenting sign of many different conditions; rheumatic fever, although now very much less common, is still an important disease to differentiate. Pericarditis may be the presenting feature and innocent basal systolic murmurs can be thought to indicate rheumatic endocarditis; antistreptolysin O rise is only indicative of previous streptococcal infection and by itself is in no way diagnostic of rheumatic fever. It is useful to remember that rheumatic fever seldom occurs in developed countries, below the age of 4, although in countries where it is still a common scourge it can occur earlier. Fever and polysynovitis below 4 years of age, if not due to juvenile arthritis, are usually due to viral infections or Henoch–Schönlein purpura, while in the first months of life diffuse lipogranulomatosis mimics Still's disease closely. Ultimately, it may be useful to differentiate the arthritis associated with ulcerative colitis, psoriasis, or ankylosing spondylitis; initially it is much more urgent to exclude infective conditions such as osteomyelitis, or staphylococcal or salmonella arthritis (Borella et al, 1963), which can be effectively treated, as well as Kawasaki syndrome (Melish, 1980) and conditions which carry a grave prognosis such as leukaemia, neuroblastoma and lymphosarcoma (Emkey et al, 1973). The clue to these last is the presence of bone pain, i.e. pain on weight-bearing, undue anaemia (Hb below 10 g), or widespread periostitis or motheaten bones on X-ray; confirmation is by bone marrow or lymph node examination. Other types

Table 43.4 Differential diagnosis of juvenile chronic arthritis

Trauma (abuse, thorn synovitis, meniscal tears, slipped epiphysis, osteochondritis dissecans)
Infections (virus, bacteria, fungus, tick borne)
'Reactive' arthritis (rheumatic fever, postdysenteric, Reiter's)
Other autoimmune disorders (systemic lupus erythematosus, dermatomyositis, systemic sclerosis, 'mixed connective tissue disease', sicca syndrome, arteritis)
Inherited and metabolic abnormalities (structural and biochemical abnormalities, e.g. familial Mediterranean fever, Marfan's syndrome, Ehler–Danlos syndrome, haemoglobinopathies, Morquio's disease, Hunter-Scheie's syndrome, Fabry's disease)
Deficiency states (rickets, scurvy)
Neoplastic disease (leukaemia, neuroblastoma)
Miscellaneous, e.g. sarcoidosis, pigmented villonodular synovitis, irritable hip syndrome

of connective tissue disease may need differentiation, including dermatomyositis, systemic sclerosis, systemic lupus erythematosus, mixed connective tissue syndrome, and polyarteritis nodosa, all of which may occur during childhood years. Similarly, polyarthritis identical to juvenile chronic polyarthritis, even with nodule formation, can occur in hypogammaglobulinaemia (Barnett et al, 1970). Chondrodystrophy should also be borne in mind since it is occasionally misdiagnosed as juvenile arthritis, as is Ehlers–Danlos syndrome (Osborn et al, 1981). In the initial attack drug allergy, e.g. to penicillin, with synovitis needs to be excluded; the latter is usually accompanied by an urticarial rash and joint involvement is migratory. Viral infections, particularly rubella, affecting teenage girls (Chambers & Bywaters, 1963), but also mononucleosis and mumps, may be associated with transitory polysynovitis. In children other than of British stock, sickle cell anaemia and Mediterranean fever can mimic Still's disease, as rarely can sarcoidosis (Hetherington, 1982). Finally, hysterical manifestations in the older child may masquerade as rather atypical rheumatoid disease.

PROGNOSIS

While it is impossible to give an exact prognosis for an individual case, the overall picture is the reverse of the gloomy picture depicted from orthopaedic hospitals (Barkin, 1952). Edström in 1958 noted that 62% of 85 patients had recovered without defects; 19% were healed and only 19% crippled or dead. Our own follow up would entirely support his view (Table 43.5). As already indicated, the one potentially fatal complication is amyloidosis and the next most serious complication is infection. Seronegative cases have higher remission rates and maintain function better, compared with seropositive cases, who have more persistent activity and more radiological destruction. Some seronegative cases develop ankylosing spondylitis or gut disease. In all except those with chronic iridocyclitis and pauciarticular arthritis, hip involvement was common (40%) and the state of the hips often determined the ultimate functional status.

Those with seropositive disease and a few with a systemic onset fared badly as regards function and capacity to work (Table 43.5; Fig. 43.13).

Table 43.5 15-year follow-up of 161 JCA patients seen originally within 1 year of onset up to 1962 (Ansell, 1978)

			Life-style	
Final diagnosis	Number	Dead	Normal	Impaired
JCA	107	10	90	7
Mode of onset:				
Systemic	32	8		4
Polyarticular	23	2		2
Pauciarticular	52	0		1
Juvenile ankylosing spondylitis	27	0	27	0
Juvenile rheumatoid arthritis	23	3	14	6
Psoriatic arthritis	4	1	2	1
Total	161	14	133	14

GENERAL MANAGEMENT

The management of these children is not easy and depends throughout on parental co-operation. During the whole period of activity of the disease regular supervision is necessary, and close liaison with the family physician and the school medical authorities is essential to maintain physiotherapy, adequate splintage, suitable drug therapy, adequate schooling and subsequent training for employment. Only such close co-operation between family, medical and social services can give these children a fair chance of growing up with limbs that will enable them to lead a reasonable normal life, and with the outlook and training adequate to secure worthwhile employment. This is the aim of all treatment: the immediate and easy satisfaction obtained by complete rest or steroid therapy with the temporary abolition of pain and inflammation does not, in the long run, merit jeopardising these ends.

Thus, although this is a chronic disease, the ultimate outlook for the majority of children is good, compared with that for adults (Calabro & Marchesano, 1968). It is important to educate the family on the nature of the disease and what can be achieved by intelligent handling and treatment. Our aim is to control the disease so that the child can live at home with occasional supervision, attending either an ordinary or special school, pre-

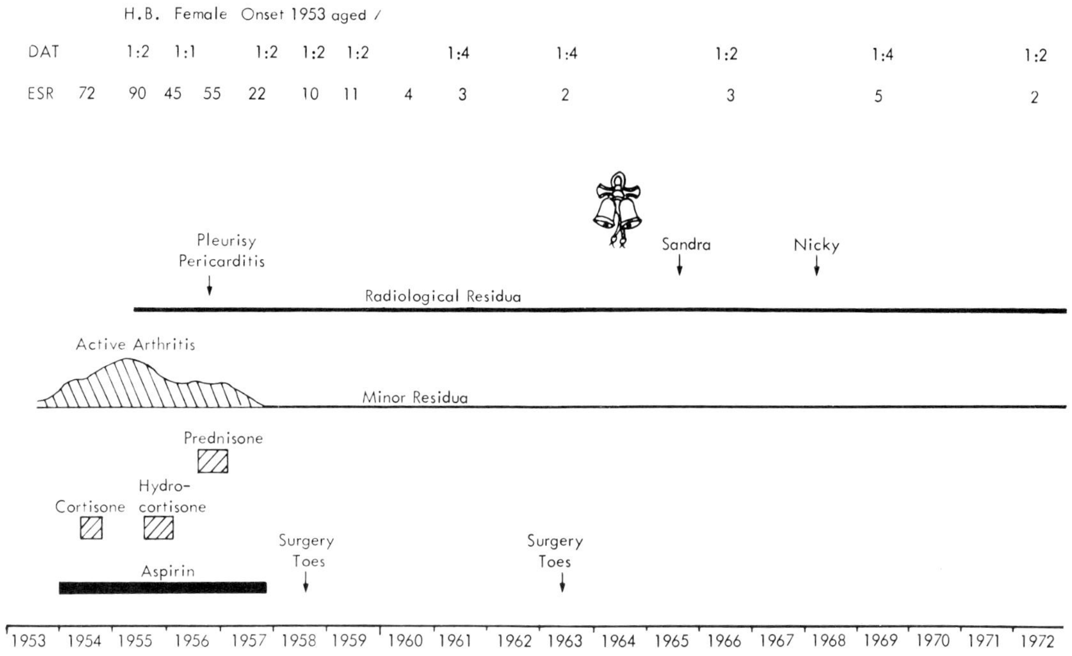

Fig. 43.13 Course of a girl with seronegative arthritis, who had an episode of systemic illness and then recovered with only minor joint residua; note the lack of post-pregnancy exacerbation.

venting as best we can contractures and growth deformities, and maintaining adequate growth of body, mind and spirit (Ansell, 1980). Vigilance has to be maintained throughout the period of activity of the disease process, which may last for many years. The outlook depends, therefore, to a great extent on the courage and resources of the parents; this factor and the pattern of the disease presentation are the most important aspects of the physicians's assessment. It is essential to realise that drug treatment is only one of many measures: of equal or perhaps greater importance are adequate rest and exercise, splinting, surgery, social measures and, above all, the maintainance of psychological support (McAnarney et al, 1974; Wilkinson, 1981).

While the disease is active the child often needs increased rest both at night and during the day. Every effort should be made to get the child up and walking every day; only with severe systemic illness or pain in weight-bearing joints, particularly the hip, or when flexion deformities of the hip and knee need correction, should the child be treated in bed. Too much irreversible damage has been done by prolonged bed-rest to think that it has any major role in the management of juvenile arthritis; muscles and bones waste, joints ankylose, contractures, renal calculi and bed sores develop and, above all, time is lost, and time is a commodity of the highest value during childhood. Deformities can be prevented, especially those affecting the hands and wrists, by wearing splints at night. Should flexion contractures of the knees already be present, correction by serial splinting should be undertaken at the earliest opportunity. Knee contractures are frequently dependent on hip flexion and both require correction at the same time. To prevent and correct hip flexion prone lying is of great value, and this can be done during the daily rest period and for a period each evening. Neck involvement requires special attention in view of the tendency to bony fusion of apophyseal joints; while we cannot prevent fusion we can prevent flexion deformity by use of a plastic neck collar, worn particularly when sitting at a desk or table. Because of the tendency to dropped wrists, this is another site where work splints, e.g. for writing, are useful. Apart from these two sites, work splints are rarely required in children. In the prevention of permanent deformities of the feet, particular attention should be paid to adequate shoes and suitably moulded in-soles. Interesting exercise is the most valuable form of physiotherapy. The exercise programme should begin assisted, followed by active and going on to resisted exercises. When undertaken in the hydrotherapy pool, walking can be instituted, even when weight-bearing on dry land is impossible on account of acute spasm in the hip, or flexion contractures of the hip or knee. The exercise programme must be continued at home under parental supervision and to this end the parents must be both motivated and taught to carry this out.

Drug therapy

Aspirin is one of the most satisfactory agents. The suggested dosage is in the order of 80 mg/kg body weight per day or 2 g/m^2. Most children can be maintained on this for prolonged periods, but as children frequently do not complain of tinnitus it is advisable to control dosage by occasional blood level estimations, aiming at 2.0 mmol/l midway between doses. Salicylates have a marked effect on fever when given in adequate dosage (see Fig. 43.4) as well as on joint swelling and pain. Although many children do not complain of pain, there is frequently a high degree of protective reflex muscle spasm, and this is decreased by the administration of salicylate. Long-acting preparations, such as enteric-coated aspirin or aloxiprin are of particular value when given late at night, in helping to overcome the early morning stiffness. Similarly, the preparation benorylate which, by virtue of its being able to be given twice a day, may be useful. Occasionally salicylates will cause occult gastrointestinal bleeding, dyspepsia or a rash (Rich & Johnson, 1973). Abnormal transaminase levels are not uncommon, although serious liver impairment has not been recorded (Athreya et al, 1975); however, hepatotoxicity can be associated with encephalopathy (Usher et al, 1978; Starko & Mullick, 1983). For such patients control of joint symptoms may be achieved by the use of other non-steroidal anti-inflammatory drugs. Ibuprofen is given three times a day in a daily dosage of 20–30 mg/kg body weight. Naproxen at 10–15 mg/kg per day given in two doses is a useful analgesic and anti-inflammatory agent for controlling joint symptoms. Tolectin at 15–30 mg/kg in 3 doses is also effective and may control fever, which the preceeding two do not. Indomethacin at 2.5 mg/kg can also control fever and joint symptoms but tolerance is poor in children under 5 with frequent nausea and vomiting. 1.5 mg/kg as a single evening dose is useful in older polyarthritic children in overcoming morning stiffness (Ansell, 1982). As yet, the role of other non-steroidal anti-inflammatory drugs accepted in adults including piroxicam and diclofenac are still under study. The process of investigating the safety and place of such drugs in children is time-consuming and tedious (Brewer et al, 1982).

Corticosteroid therapy in high dosage does not appear to cut short the duration of the activity of the disease, to prevent complications, or to alter the long-term prognosis (Lindbjerg, 1964). The indications for such treatment are: severe systemic illness; or severe joint involvement not responding to an adequate conservative regime and, very occasionally, severe iridocyclitis which has not responded to local steroid drops. If the corticosteroid preparation is given in daily divided doses as low as 5 mg prednisone per day, most children will show some degree of hypercortisonism with a moon-face and obesity and almost all fail to grow. Below the age of 5 years, even 3 mg/day causes impairment of growth, while older children may be able to tolerate slightly higher dosage (Blodgett et al, 1956). Prolonged medication is often complicated by osteoporosis and crush fractures of vertebrae and there is the overall suppression of the hypothalamic–pituitary–adrenal axis (Byron et al, 1983) which may produce serious illness with minor infections, such as diarrhoea or tonsillitis. Inhibition of growth cannot be overcome by anabolic steroids nor by human growth hormone (Ward et al, 1966), but growth is resumed and often made up when the child is taken off daily steroid (Fig. 43.14). Because of this serious effect on growth, the use of ACTH (Zutshi et al, 1971), or alternate-day corticosteroid should always be considered (Ansell & Bywaters, 1974).

Once a child has been put on daily divided dosage corticosteroid therapy, it is extremely difficult to return to once daily administration, let alone an alternate-day regime. Because of this, prednisone should never be given more than once daily and whenever possible, even in systemic illness, an

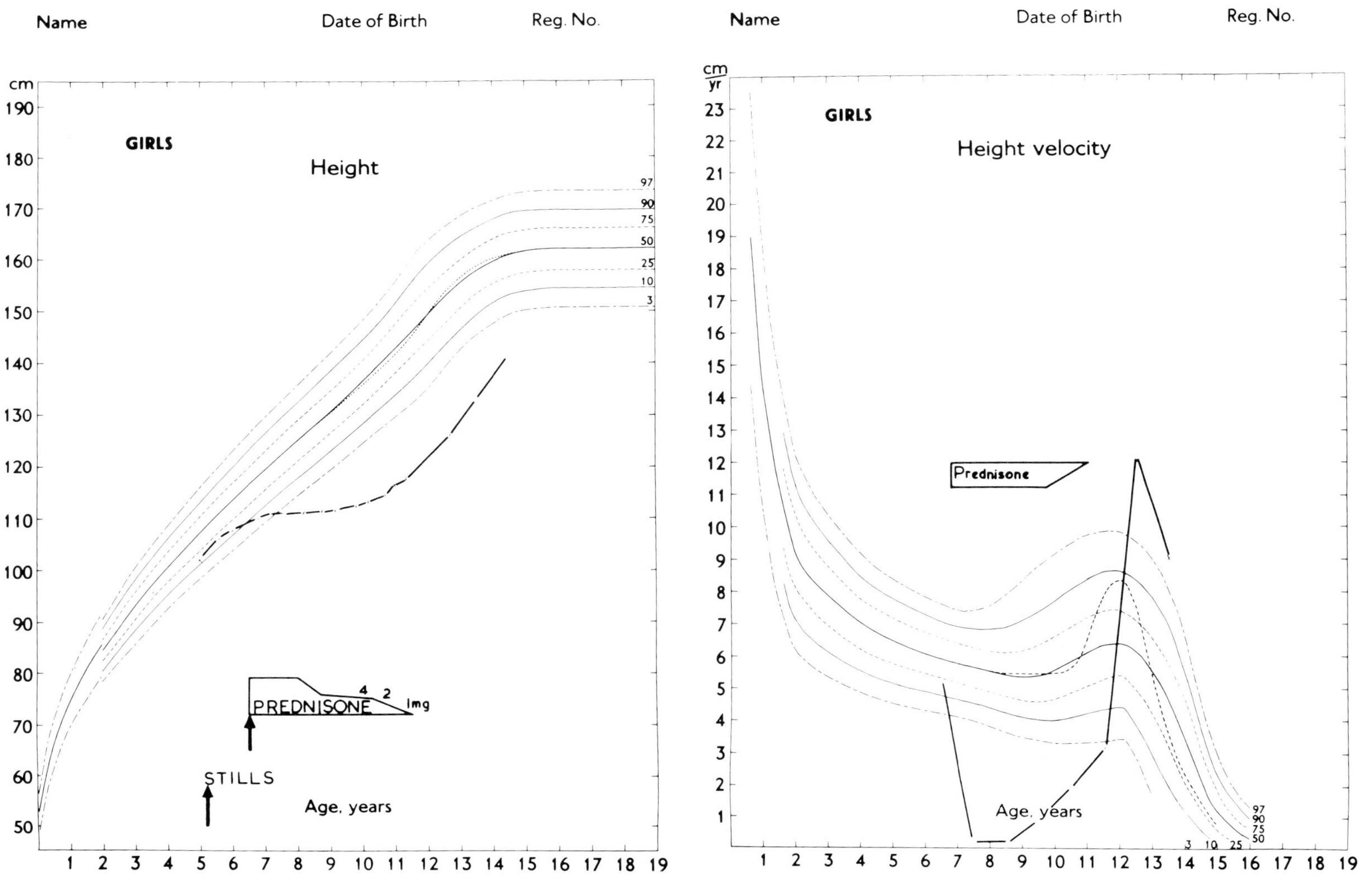

a b

Fig. 43.14 Height (a) and height velocity (b) charts (Tanner) from a girl with severe systemic juvenile chronic arthritis who was being treated with daily prednisone. Note the impaired rate of growth during drug therapy with resumption after cessation and her delayed puberty growth spurt.

alternate-day regime used. Pulsing with methylprednisone at 30 mg/kg on 3 consecutive days has only a very transient effect and may be followed by a rebound in disease activity (Miller, 1980). Thus in serious systemic illness it is sometimes wiser to use corticotrophin in the form of Acthar Gel. The duration of action of this allows rapid alteration in dosage when necessary. If treatment has to be continued this does not cause serious impairment of growth provided the child is not rendered cushingoid. The disadvantage of Acthar Gel is alternate-day injections at home, but children will adapt to this well, and usually give their own: with disposable syringes there is little danger of infection. Hypertension, hypokalaemia and obesity, however, have occurred. There is no advantage in adding corticotrophin to daily prednisone, but once the latter is removed growth proceeds normally (Fig. 43.15). In general, both alternate-day prednisone and alternate-day Acthar Gel have proved satisafactory in controlling severe manifestations without serious interference with, or suppression of, the hypothalamic–pituitary–adrenal axis (Byron et al, 1983). Anabolic steroids are sometimes employed with good effect to increase muscle bulk (Fig. 43.16). Once the active stage of

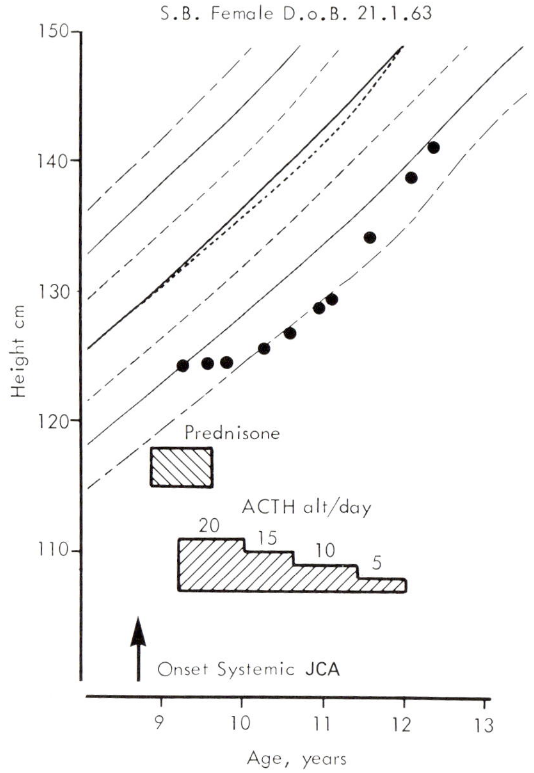

Fig. 43.15 Resumption of growth during therapy with Acthar Gel once daily prednisone was stopped.

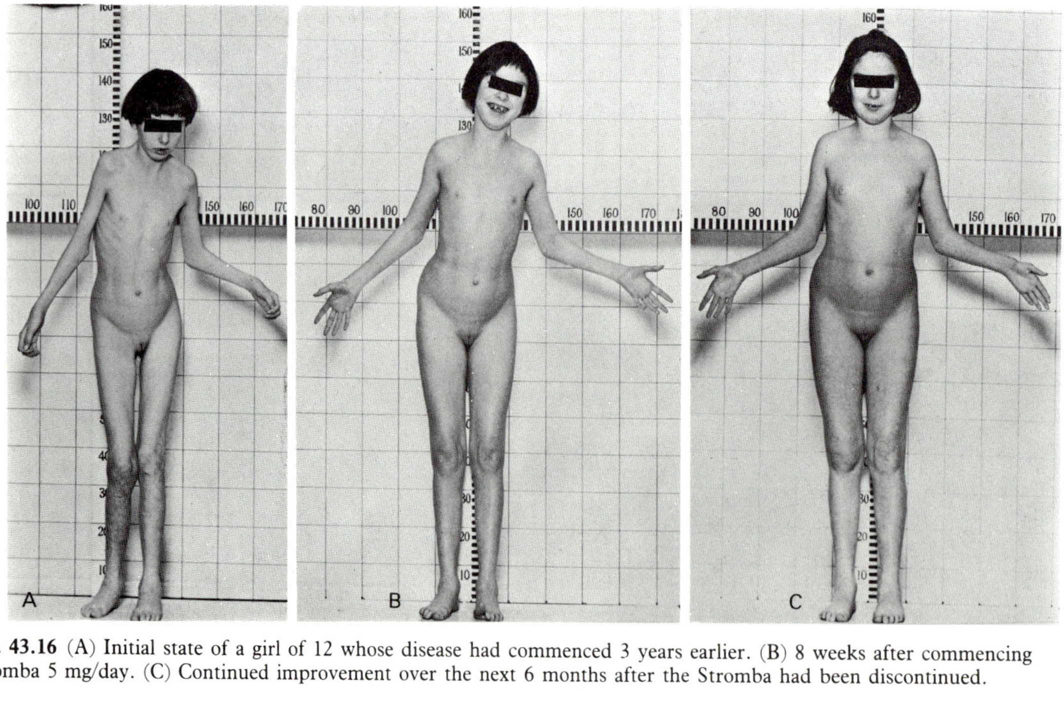

Fig. 43.16 (A) Initial state of a girl of 12 whose disease had commenced 3 years earlier. (B) 8 weeks after commencing Stromba 5 mg/day. (C) Continued improvement over the next 6 months after the Stromba had been discontinued.

the disease has passed, unwanted virilising side-effects or jaundice can occur, so control is required.

Gold salts do not appear to be more toxic than in adults (Levinson et al, 1977) and require the same monitoring. In patients with continuing active polyarthritic joint disease, their use should be seriously considered, as well as in patients on corticosteroids, where dosage reduction is desirable, either because of complications or because the disease remains active (Fig. 43.17). Dosage should be approximately 1 mg of gold per kilo body weight per week, and maintained for a minimum of 6 months provided side-effects do not occur; it is wise to continue with maintenance therapy thereafter, either fortnightly or monthly, according to the severity of the disease, for several years. Some 60% of children can be expected to respond satisfactorily over a 1–3-year period (Ansell & Hall, 1981). Studies with auranofin suggest that this will be similarly effective (Giannini et al, 1983).

The indications for penicillamine administration would appear to be the same as for gold, i.e. severe active disease, or in those cases where it is desirable to reduce corticosteroid therapy (Fig. 43.18). Schairer et al (1975), using a dosage for children of 30 mg/kg body weight, found this to be an effective drug. Dosage of 10–15 mg/kg increasing to 30 mg/kg if there is no effect in 1 year has shown this to be similar in effect to myocrisin over a 3-year comparison (Ansell & Hall, 1981). Autoimmune side-effects appear to be rare, but meticulous monitoring of of blood and urine are essential. Persistent proteinuria with either gold or penicillamine calls for a rectal biopsy because of the risk of amyloidosis with continuing active disease.

Failure on either myocrisin or penicillamine does not necessarily mean the child will not respond to the alternative therapy.

Antimalarials are considered by some to be valu-

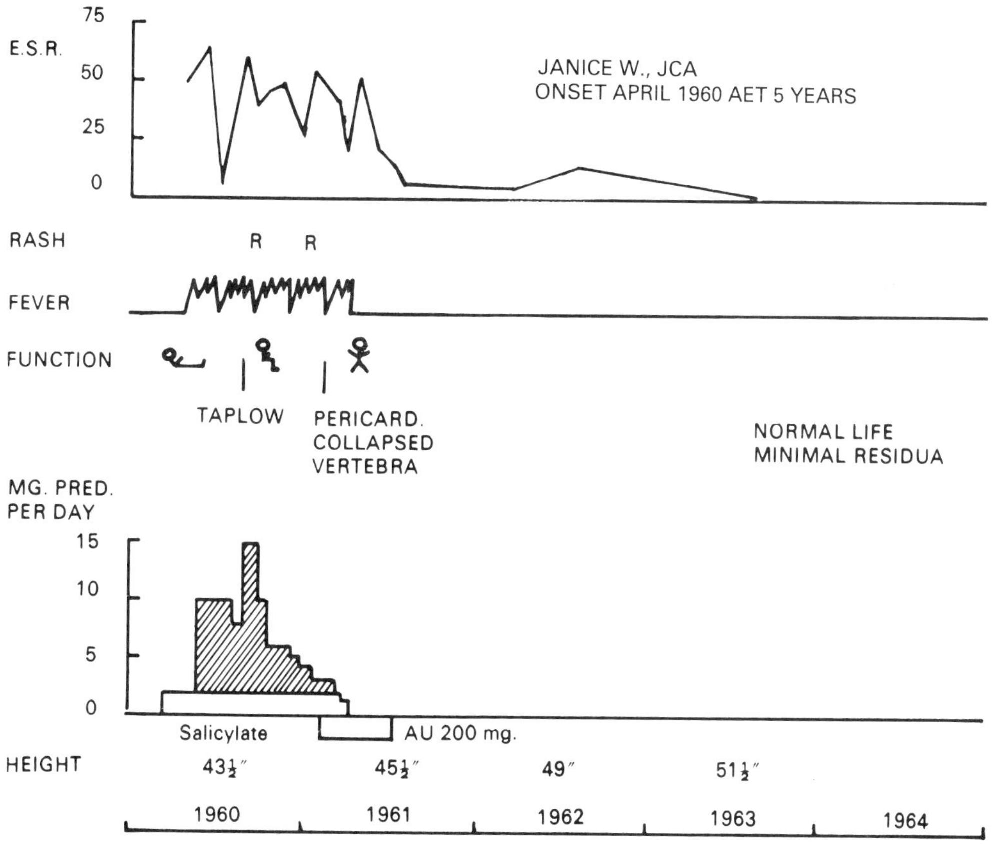

Fig. 43.17 Myocrisin used to help withdrawal of corticosteroids.

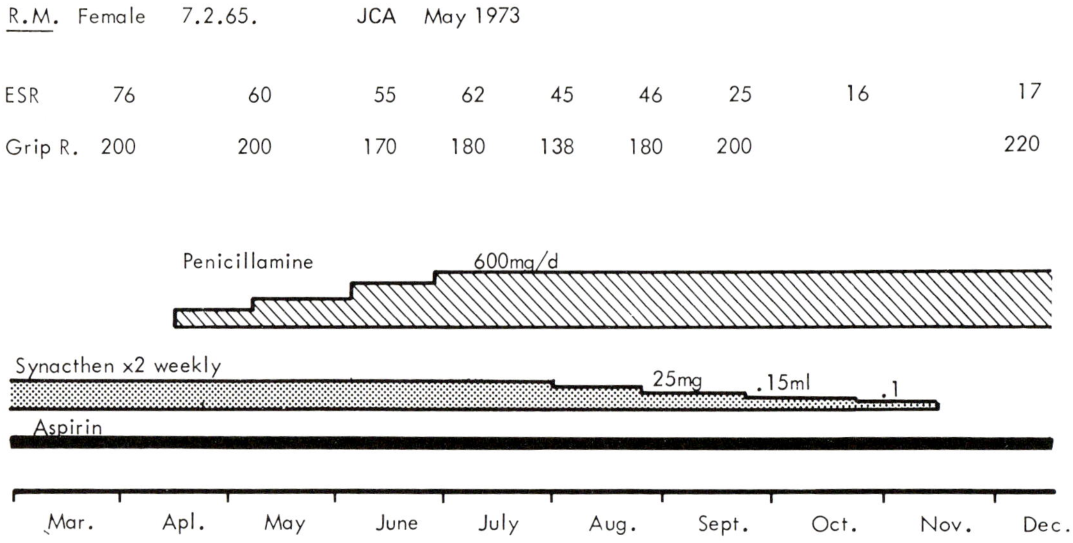

Fig. 43.18 Penicillamine used to help in withdrawal of synacthen.

able in controlling severe disease activity both in the systemic and joint phase. To avoid toxicity, Laaksonen et al (1974) suggest a dosage of 4 mg/kg per day of chloroquine and 5–7 mg/kg per day of hydrochloroquine. As with adults a regular check should be kept on vision; therapy should not be continued for longer than 2 years without a break.

Immunosuppressive therapy

Because of the possible mutagenic and oncogenic effects of these drugs, they should be reserved for cases with amyloidosis, the one potentially fatal complication, or when serious side-effects occur on other forms of therapy and standard methods of management have proved ineffective. Azathioprine in a daily dosage of 2.5 mg/kg body weight has been used, but it is necessary to monitor this carefully with weekly blood counts because of the risk of bone marrow damage (Kolle, 1969). Because it is less mutagenic than the alkylating agents, it is particularly useful for those patients whose standard therapy has engendered serious side-effects (Dale, 1972). Munthe and his colleagues (1975) have also reported favourably on the response of patients whose disease is complicated by amyloidosis. There have been encouraging reports with cyclophosphamide (Skogland et al, 1971), but in view of the very serious danger of bladder damage, as well as the distressing effect of hair loss, it is probably wiser to use chlorambucil. To date this has proved the most potent drug in controlling disease activity and it is acceptable to patients, but from the haematological point of view it is the most difficult to handle and carries, of course, the usual risk of infection. Using it in cases complicated by amyloidosis, at a dosage of 0.15 mg/kg body weight tailored by regular blood monitoring, it has only been possible to maintain continuous therapy over a prolonged period in under one-half of the patients; in addition to the haematological effects, viral infections, particularly chickenpox and herpes zoster, have been a problem in one-quarter (Fig. 43.19) while 1 of 70 of our patients so treated has developed leukaemia after 4 years (Buriot et al, 1979). In those in which it has been possible to maintain adequate dosage, satisfactory amelioration of their joint state and maintenance of renal function have been achieved (Fig. 43.20).

Plasmapharesis may be helpful but is not without danger (Brewer et al, 1981).

SURGERY

In the early case the orthopaedic surgeon may be consulted for advice on splinting and appliances, and for diagnostic biopsy; in the later stages for improvement of function or the management of fracture. It is essential to prevent immobilisation of an involved joint because of its tendency to

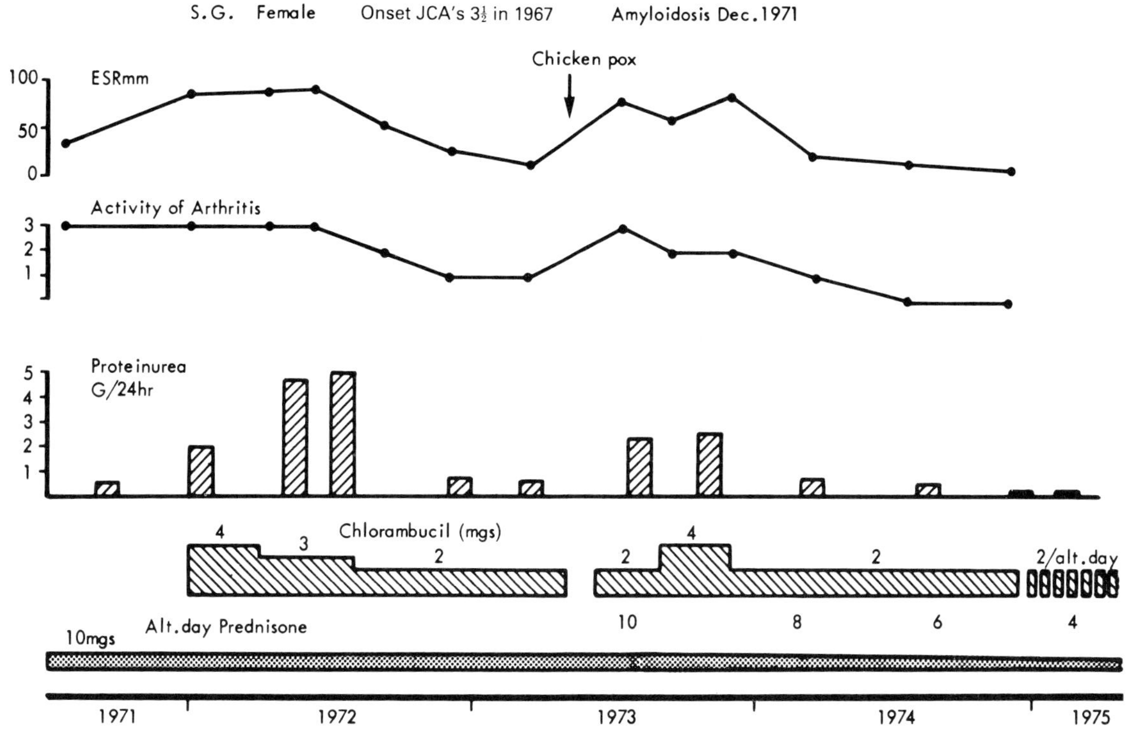

Fig. 43.19 Exacerbation of disease and proteinuria on stopping chlorambucil because of severe chickenpox.

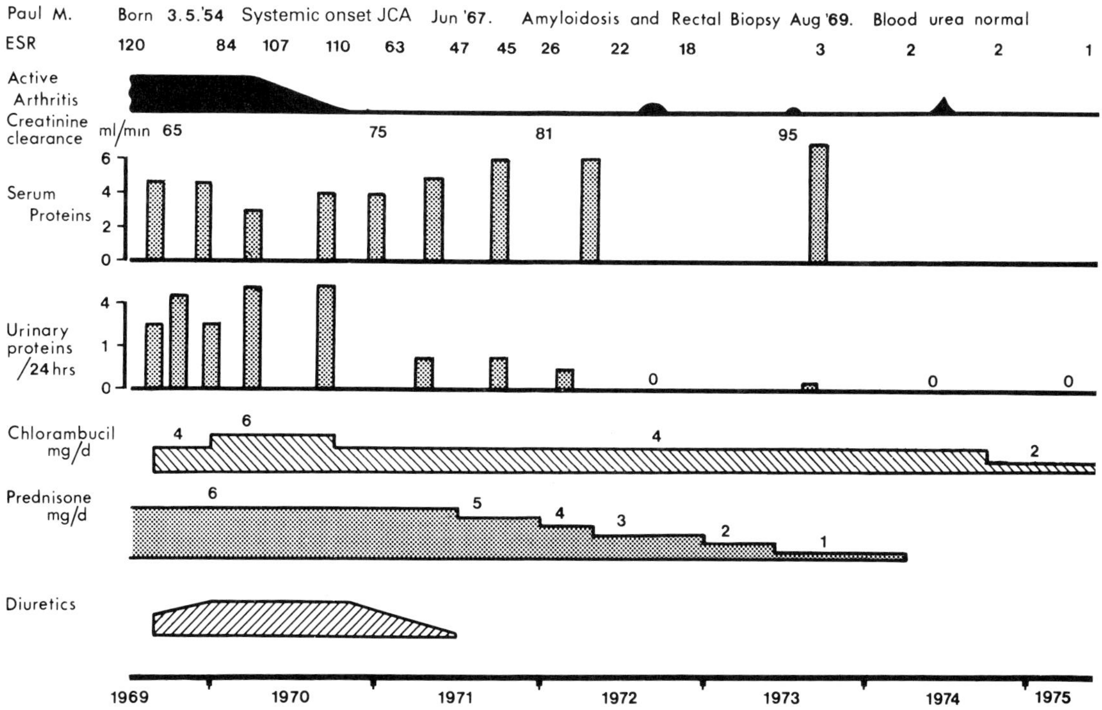

Fig. 43.20 Course of a boy whose disease became complicated by amyloidosis; apparent remission on chlorambucil.

stiffen, so that fractures may need to be treated by pinning or splinting to allow maintenance of joint function (Badley & Ansell, 1960).

Multiple synovectomies are not advocated for children. However, there may well be a place for surgical synovectomy of of a knee, or an elbow, particularly if this is the only severely involved joint and there is evidence of overgrowth and loss of function (Fink et al, 1969). Following synovectomy, remobilisation appears more difficult than in adults, and particularly the knee may require manipulation (Roles, 1978). Because of this it is vital to defer operation until the children are old enough to co-operate in an active physiotherapeutic regime. Prior to this, time may be gained and surgery rendered unnecessary by the occasional injection of long-acting steroid into a knee.

Non-surgical 'synovectomy' of the knee has also been carried out using intra-articular osmic acid. Martio and his colleagues (1972) suggested that at 1 year 46% of patients had improved and that the earlier cases did best; in view of possible radiation problems, we do not use 'isotope' synovectomy. Surgical synovectomy should also be considered when there is a single flexor tendon lesion which is causing severe impairment of flexion of the finger, or when 'triggering' is occurring and it has not responded to a local hydrocortisone injection. Valgus deformities of the knee which are not improving on a conservative regime, including Mermaid splints and wedging of the shoes, in the younger child may warrant supracondylar osteotomy. In the child approaching puberty, provided growth is occurring, stapling of epiphyses is an extremely useful procedure (Ansell et al, 1970) (Fig. 43.21). Soft tissue procedures may be of value in correcting deformities of hips and knees (Swann, 1978).

In adolescence and early adult life severe established deformities may require more extensive orthopaedic measures. Osteotomy of the fused carpi or tarsi may be required while for a severely damaged painful single knee, without hip limitation, arthrodesis is probably still the treatment of choice, although with the better design of prostheses, reconstruction of the knees should become a practical procedure. Total hip replacement can be considered in the severely affected joint, as soon as growth has ceased. Best results are obtained in those patients who have only just lost their ability to walk, not in those who have been confined to bed or a wheelchair for some years. With small femoral heads and shafts as well as persistent anteversion, specially made prostheses may be required. To date, the overall results are better than in adults (Arden, 1978). Other procedures that may need to be considered include orthodontic treatment and plastic reconstruction of micrognathia. Thus, with these as well as the measures previously discussed, the outlook for children with juvenile chronic arthritis has improved still further, although the psychological aspects require careful appraisal throughout the whole course and management (Wilkinson, 1981).

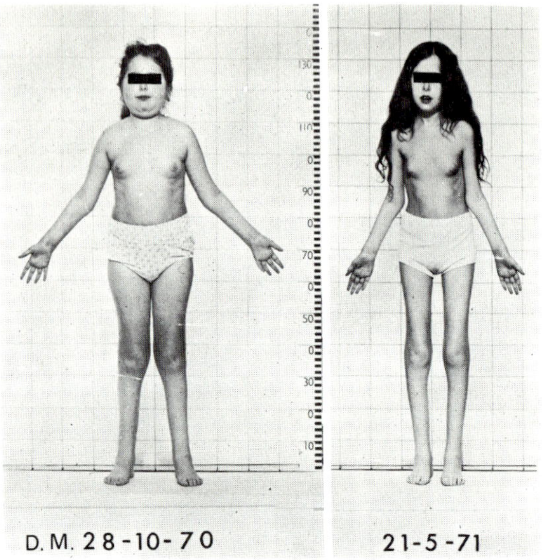

Fig. 43.21 Gross valgus deformity of knees in a patient at puberty rendered Cushingoid by daily corticosteroid. Note improvement in position of knees after stapling, even prior to resumption of growth in height after daily corticosteroids were reduced.

REFERENCES

Ansell M 1978 Chronic arthritis in childhood. Annals of the Rheumatic Diseases 37: 107–120
Ansell M 1980 Rheumatic disorders in childhood. Butterworth, London
Ansell M 1981 Rehabilitation in juvenile chronic arthritis. Clinics in Rheumatic Diseases 7: 469–484
Ansell M 1982 Juvenile chronic arthritis. In: Hart F Dudley (ed) Drug treatment of the rheumatic diseases,

2nd Edn. Adis, London
Ansell B M Bywaters E G L 1953 Finger contractures due to tendon lesions as a mode of presentation of rheumatoid arthritis. Annals of Rheumatic Diseases 12: 283–289
Ansell B M, Bywaters E G L 1956 Growth in Still's disease. Annals of Rheumatic Diseases 15: 295–319
Ansell B M, Bywaters E G L 1962 Diagnosis of probable Still's disease and its outcome. Annals of Rheumatic Diseases 21: 253–262
Ansell B M, Bywaters E G L 1974 Alternate-day corticosteroid therapy in juvenile chronic polyarthritis. Journal of Rheumatology 1: 176–186
Ansell B M, Clemens L E 1982 HLA in chronic arthritis in childhood. In: Dawkins R L, Christiansen F T, Zilko P J (ed) Immunogenetics in rheumatology; Musculoskeletal disease and D-penicillamine. International Congress Series 602. Excerpta Medica, Amsterdam, p 164–166
Ansell B M, Hall M A 1981 Penicillamine in chronic arthritis of childhood. Journal of Rheumatology 8 (Suppl 7):112–115
Ansell B M, Kent P A 1977 Radiological changes in juvenile chronic polyarthritis. Skeletal Radiology 1: 129–144
Ansell B M, Arden G P, MacLennan I C M 1970 Valgus knee deformities in children with juvenile chronic polyarthritis treated by epiphyseal stapling. Archives of Diseases of Childhood 45: 388–392
Antilla Raimo 1972 Renal involvement in juvenile rheumatoid arthritis. Acta Paediatrica Scandinavica (Suppl) 227: 1–73
Arden G P 1978 Total joint replacement. In: Arden G P, Ansell B M (ed) Surgical management of juvenile chronic polyarthritis. Academic Press, London, Ch 10, p 125–160
Arden G P, Ansell B M, Hunter M J 1972 Total hip replacement in juvenile chronic polyarthritis and ankylosing spondylitis. Clinical Orthopaedics and Related Research 84: 130–136
Athreya B H, Moser G, Cecil H S, Myers A R 1975 Aspirin induced hepatotoxicity in juvenile rheumatoid arthritis. Arthritis and Rheumatism 18: 347–352
Athreya B H, Doughty R A, Bookspan M, Schumacher H R, Sewell E M, Chatten J 1980 Pulmonary manifestations of juvenile rheumatoid arthritis. A report of 8 cases and review. Clinics in Chest Medicine 1: 361–374
Bacon T, Tyndall de Vere A, Tyrrell D A J, Denman A M, Ansell B M 1983 Interferon system in patients with systemic juvenile chronic arthritis; in vivo and in vitro studies. Clinical and Experimental Immunology 54: 23–30
Badley B W D, Ansell B M 1960 Fractures in Still's disease. Annals of Rheumatic Diseases 19: 135–142
Barkin R E 1952 Clinical course of juvenile rheumatoid arthritis. Bulletin of the Rheumatic Diseases 3: 19–20
Barkley D O, Hohermuth H J, Howard A 1979 IgA deficiency in juvenile chronic polyarthritis. Journal of Rheumatology 6: 219–224
Barnett E V, Winklestein A, Weinberger H J 1970 Agammaglobulinemia with polyarthritis and subcutaneous nodules. American Journal of Medicine 48: 40–47
Baum J, Fink C 1968 Juvenile rheumatoid arthritis in monozygotic twins. A case report and review of the literature. Arthritis and Rheumatism 11: 33–37
Bernstein B, Takahashi M, Hanson V 1974 Cardiac involvement in juvenile rheumatoid arthritis. Journal of Pediatrics 85: 313–317
Blodgett F M, Burgin L, Iezzoni D, Gribetz D, Talbot N B 1956 Effects of prolonged cortisone therapy on statural growth, skeletal maturation and metabolic status of children. New England Journal of Medicine 254: 636–641
Boldero M E A 1933 A case of Still's disease. Medical Society Transactions (London) 16:55
Borella L, Goobar J E, Summitt R L, Clark G M 1963 Septic arthritis in childhood. Journal of Pediatrics 62: 742–747
Brewer E 1977 Juvenile rheumatoid arthritis — cardiac involvement. Arthritis and Rheumatism 20: 231–236
Brewer E 1982 Methodology and studies of children with juvenile rheumatoid arthritis. Pediatric Rheumatic Collaborative Study Group (PRCSG). Journal of Rheumatology 9: 107–155
Brewer E J, Bass J C, Baum J et al 1977 Current proposed revision of JRA criteria. Arthritis and Rheumatism 20 (Suppl 2): 195–199
Brewer E J, Nickeson R W, Rosen R D, et al 1981 Plasma exchange in selected patients with juvenile rheumatoid arthritis. Journal of Pediatrics 98: 194–200
Brinkam G L, Chaikof L 1959 Rheumatoid lung disease. Report of a case which developed in childhood. American Review of Respiratory Diseases 80: 732–737
Buriot D, Prieur A M, Lebranchu Y, Messerschmitt J, Griscelli C 1979 Acute leukaemia in 3 children with juvenile arthritis treated with Chlorambucil. Archives of French Pediatrics 36: 592–598
Byron M A, Jackson J, Ansell B M 1983 Effect of different corticosteroid regimens on hypothalamic–pituitary–adrenal axis (HPA) and linear growth in juvenile chronic arthritis. Journal of the Royal Society of Medicine 76: 452–457
Bywaters E G L 1963 The hand. In: Carter M (ed) Radiological aspects of rheumatoid arthritis. Excerpta Medica, Amsterdam, p 43
Bywaters E G L 1968 Diagnostic criteria for Still's disease (Juvenile RA). In: Bennett P H, Wood P H N (ed) Population studies of the rheumatic diseases. Excerpta Medica, Amsterdam, Ch 33, p 235
Bywaters E G L 1971 Still's disease in the adult. Annals of Rheumatic Diseases 30: 121–133
Bywaters E G L, Ansell B M 1965 Monarticular arthritis in children. Annals of the Rheumatic Diseases 24: 116–122
Bywaters E G L, Edmonds J 1976 Biopsies and tissue diagnosis in the rheumatic diseases. Clinics in Rheumatic Diseases 2: 179–210
Bywaters E G L, Glynn L E, Zeldis A 1958 Subcutaneous nodules of Still's disease. Annals of Rheumatic Diseases 17: 278–285
Calabro J J, Marchesano J M 1968 The early natural history of juvenile rheumatoid arthritis. Medical Clinics of North America 52: 567–591
Cassidy J T, Petty R E, Sullivan D B 1977 Occurrence of selective IgA deficiency in children with juvenile rheumatoid arthritis. Arthritis and Rheumatism 20: 181–183
Chambers R J, Bywaters E G L 1963 Rubella synovitis. Annals of Rheumatic Diseases 22: 263–268
Clemens L E, Albert E, Ansell B M 1983 HLA studies in IgM rheumatoid factor positive childhood arthritis. Annals of Rheumatic Diseases 42: 431–434
Cornil M V 1864 Memoires lus a la Societe de Biologie. Societe de Biologie: Series 4, 3, 3
Dale I 1972 The treatment of juvenile rheumatoid arthritis with Azathioprine. Scandinavian Journal of Rheumatology 1: 125–127
Edmonds J, Morris R I, Metzger A L, Bluestone R, Terasaki P I, Ansell B M, Bywaters E G L 1974 Follow-up study of

juvenile chronic polyarthritis with particular reference to histocompatibility antigen W27. Annals of Rheumatic Diseases 33: 289–292
Edström G 1958 Rheumatoid arthritis in Still's disease in children. A survey of 161 cases. Arthritis and Rheumatism 1: 497–504
Elkon K B, Hughes G R V, Bywaters E G L et al. Adult onset Still's disease. 20 year follow-up and further studies of patients with active disease. Arthritis and Rheumatism 25: 647–654
Emkey R D, Ragsdale B D, Ropes M W, Miller W 1973 A case of lymphoproliferat ve disease presenting as juvenile rheumatoid arthritis. American Journal of Medicine 54: 825–828
Endresen G K, Høyeraal H M, Kass E 1977 Platelet count and disease activity in juvenile rheumatoid arthritis. Scandinavian Journal of Rheumatology 6: 237–240
Fabricant M S, Stebbins B C, Friou G F 1973 Still's disease in adults. Journal of the American Medical Association 225:273
Fink C W, Baum J, Paradies L H, Carrell B C 1969 Synovectomy in juvenile rheumatoid arthritis. Annals of Rheumatic Diseases 28: 612–616
Fletcher M R, Scott J T 1975 Chronic monarticular synovitis. Diagnostic and prognostic features. Annals of the Rheumatic Diseases 34: 171–176
Florin-Christensen A, Arana R M, Morteo O G, Roux M E B, Hubscher O 1974 IgG, IgA, IgM and IgD antiglobulins in juvenile rheumatoid arthritis. Annals of the Rheumatic Diseases 33: 32–34
Førve O, Doblong J H, Høyeraal H M, Thorsby K 1982 HLA antigens in juvenile arthritis — genetic basis for the different sub-types. Arthritis and Rheumatism 26: 35–38
Friedman M, Greenwood F C 1968 The effect of prolonged ACTH or corticosteroid therapy in children on growth and on pituitary–adrenal and pituitary function. Memoirs of the Soceity for Endocrinology 17: 249–270
Gaisford W 1962 Fatality after Oxyphenbutazone in Still's disease. British Medical Journal 2:1517
Gallino L, Pountain G, Mitchell N, Ansell B M 1984 Developmental aspects of the hip in juvenile chronic arthritis. A radiological assessment. Scandinavian Journal of Rheumatology 13: 310–318
Gershwin M E, Haselwood D, Dorskind K et al 1979 Altered responsiveness to mutogens in sub-group of patients with juvenile rheumatoid arthritis. Journal of Clinical and Laboratory Immunology 1: 293–297
Giannini E H, et al 1983 Auranofin in the treatment of juvenile rheumatoid arthritis. Journal of Pediatrics 102: 138–141
Goel K M, Logan R W, Barnard W P, Shanks R A 1974 Serum immunoglobulins and beta 1C–beta IA globulin concentraions in juvenile rheumatoid arthritis. Annals of the Rheumatic Diseases 33: 35–38
Gwyther M, Schwarz H, Howard A, Ansell B M 1982 C-Reactive protein in juvenile chronic arthritis an indicator of disease activity and possibly amyloidosis. Annals of Rheumatic Diseases 41: 259–262
Hall A, Ansell B M, James D C O, Zylinski P 1975 HL-A antigens in juvenile chronic polyarthritis (Still's disease). Annals of Rheumatic Diseases 36 (Suppl 1): 36–38
Hedberg H 1971 The total complement activity of synovial fluid in juvenile forms of arthritis. Acta Rheumatologica Scandinavica 17: 279–285
Hetherington S 1982 Sarcoidosis in young children. American Journal of Diseases of Childhood 136: 13–15
Hollingworth P, De Vere Tyndall A, Ansell B M et al 1982 Intensive immunosuppression versus prednisolone in the treatment of connective tissue diseases. Annals of the Rheumatic Diseases 41: 557–562
Høyeraal H M, Mellbye O J 1974a High levels in serum complement factors in juvenile rheumatoid arthritis. Annals of the Rheumatic Diseases 33: 243–247
Høyerral H M, Mellbye O J 1974b Humoral immunity in juvenile rheumatoid arthritis. Annals of the Rheumatic Diseases 33: 248–254
Isdale I C, Bywaters E G L 1956 The rash of rheumatoid arthritis and Still's disease. Quarterly Journal of Medicine 25:377
Jan J E, Hill R H, Low M D 1972 Cerebral complications in juvenile rheumatoid arthritis. Canadian Medical Association Journal 107: 623–625
Johnson G D, Konice M, Holborow E J 1975 Comparison of methods employed for the detection of antibodies to ds-DNA. VIII European Rheumatology Congress, Helskinki. Abstract No 42.05
Jordan J D, Snyder C H 1964 Rheumatoid disease of the lung and cor pulmonale. Observations in a child. American Journal of Diseases of Children 108: 174–180
Kanksi J J 1977 Acute anterior uveitis in juvenile rheumatoid arthritis. Archives of Ophthalmology 95: 1784–1797
Kanski J J 1981 Care of children with anterior uveitis. Trans Ophthalmic Surgery (UK) 101: 387–390
Keith J D, Rowe R D, Vlad P 1958 Heart disease in infancy and childhood. Macmillan, New York
Kolle G 1969 'Schaden bei immunsupressiver therapie'. Deutsche Medizinische Wochenschrift 94:2568
Kviem T K, Høyerral H M, Kass E 1982 Diagnostic criteria of rheumatoid arthritis. Scandinavian Journal of Rheumatology 11: 187–192
Laaksonen A L, Laine V 1961 A comparative study of joint pain in adult and juvenile rheumatoid arthritis. Annals of the Rheumatic Diseases 20: 386–387
Laaksonen A-L, Koskiahde V, Juva K 1974 Dosage of antimalarial drugs for children with juvenile rheumatoid arthritis and systemic lupus erythematosus. Scandinavian Journal of Rheumatoloty 3: 103–108
Levinson J E, Balz G P, Bondi S 1977 Gold therapy. Arthritis and Rheumatism 20: 531–535
Lietman P S, Bywaters E G L 1963 Pericarditis in juvenile rheumatoid arthritis. Pediatrics 32: 855–860
Lindbjerg I F 1964 Juvenile rheumatoid arthritis. A follow-up of 75 cases. Archives of Disease in Childhood 39: 576–583
McAnarney E R, Pless I B, Satterwhite B, Friedman S B 1974 Psychological problems of children with chronic juvenile arthritis. Pediatrics 53: 523–528
McMinn F J, Bywaters E G L 1959 Differences between the fever of Still's disease and that of rheumatic fever. Annals of the Rheumatic Diseases 18: 293–297
Martel W, Holt J F, Cassidy J T 1962 Roentgenologic manifestations of juvenile rheumatoid arthritis. American Journal of Roentgenology 88: 400–423
Martio J, Isomaki H, Heikkola T, Laine V 1972 The effect of intra-articular osmic acid in juvenile rheumatoid arthritis. Scandinavian Journal of Rheumatology 1: 5–8
Mehra R, Moore T L, Catalano J D, Neuks S H, Zuckner J 1981 Chlorambucil in the treatment of juvenile rheumatoid arthritis. Journal of Rheumatology 8: 141–144
Melish M C 1980 Kawasaki syndrome; a new infectious

disease. Journal of Infectious Diseases 143: 317–324
Miller J J III 1980 Prolonged use of large intravenous steroid pulses in the rheumatic diseases of children. Pediatrics 65: 989–994
Miller J J III, French J W 1977 Myocarditis in juvenile rheumatoid arthritis. American Journal of Diseases of Childhood 131: 205–209
Miller M L, Glass D N 1981 The major histocompatibility complex antigens in rheumatoid arthritis and juvenile arthritis. Bulletin of the Rheumatic Diseases 31: 21–25
Moller P W, Ansell B M, Bywaters E G L 1969 Myocrisin therapy in Still's disease. Proceedings of the 12th International Congress of Rheumatic Diseases, Prague. Abstract No 675
Moore T L, Zuckner J, Baldassare A R, Weiss T D, Dorner R W 1978 Complement-fixing hidden rheumatoid factor in juvenile rheumatoid arthritis. Arthritis and Rheumatism 21: 935–941
Moran H, Ansell Barbara M, Mowbray J F, Levinsky R J, Soothill J F 1979 Antigen antibody complexes in the serum of patients with juvenile chronic arthritis. Archives of Diseases in Childhood 54: 120–122
Morimoto C, Reinherz E L, Borel Y, Mantzouranis E, Steinberg A D, Schlossman S F 1981 Auto-antibody to an immunoregulatory inducer population in patients with juvenile rheumatoid arthritis. Journal of Clinical Investigation 67: 753–761
Morling N, Hellensen C, Jacobsen B K et al 1981 HLA-A, B, C, D, DR antigens and primed lymphocyte typing (PLT) defined DP antigen in juvenile chronic arthritis. Tissue Antigens 17: 434–441
Munthe E 1972 Complexes of IgG and IgG rheumatoid factor in synovial tissues of juvenile rheumatoid arthritis. Scandinavian Journal of Rheumatology 1: 153–160
Munthe E 1975 In: Jennings J, Jayson M (eds) Proceedings of a symposium on the clinical and immunological aspects of Still's disease. Academic Press, Bristol
Nathan F F, Bickel W H 1968 Spontaneous axial subluxation in a child as the first sign of juvenile rheumatoid arthritis. Journal of Bone and Joint Surgery 50-A: 1675–1678
Osborn T G, Lichtenstein J R, Moore T L, Weiss T, Zuckner J 1981 Ehlers–Danlos syndrome presenting as rheumatic manifestations in the child. Journal of Rheumatology 8: 79–85
Powell R H, Ansell B M 1974 Benorylate in management of Still's disease. British Medical Journal 1:145
Rich R R, Johnson J S 1973 Salicylate hepatotoxicity in patients with juvenile rheumatoid arthritis. Arthritis and Rheumatism 16: 1–9
Roles N 1978 Synovectomy of the knee and elbow. In: Arden G P, Ansell B M (eds) Surgical management of juvenile chronic polyarthritis. Academic Press, London, Ch 4, p 75–95
Rombouts J J, Rombouts-Lindemans C 1971 Involvement of the hip in juvenile rheumatoid arthritis. Acta Rheumatologica Scandinavia 17: 248–267
Rombouts J J, Rombouts-Lindemans C 1974 Scoliosis in juvenile rheumatoid arthritis. The Journal of Bone and Joint Surgery 56B: 478–483
Ronning O, Valiaho M J, Laaksonen A-L 1974 The involvement of the temperomandibular joint in juvenile rheumatoid arthritis. Scandinavian Journal of Rheumatology 3: 89–96
Rossen R D, Brewer E J, Person D A, Templeton J W, Lidsky M D 1977 Circulating immune complexes and antinuclear antibodies in juvenile rheumatoid arthritis. Arthritis and Rheumatism 20: 1485–1490
Sairanen E, Laaksonen A-L 1962 The toxicity of gold therapy in children suffering from rheumatoid arthritis. Annals de Pediatriae Fenniae 8: 105–109
Schairer H, Stoeber E, Kolle G 1975 Results of a controlled trial of gold or D-penicillamine in juvenile rheumatoid arthritis. VII European Rheumatology Congress, Helsinki. Abstract No 11.09
Schaller J, Wedgewood R J 1970 Pruritus associated with the rash of juvenile rheumatoid arthritis. Paediatrics 45: 296–298
Schaller J, Beckwith B, Wedgewood R J 1970 Hepatic involvement in juvenile rheumatoid arthritis. Journal of Pediatrics 77: 203–210
Schaller J, Johnson G D, Holborow E J, Ansell B M, Smiley W K 1974 The association of antinuclear antibodies with chronic iridocyclitis of juvenile rheumatoid arthritis (Still's disease). Arthritis and Rheumatism 17: 409–416
Schaller J G, Ochs H D, Thomas E G 1976 Histocompatibility antigens in childhood onset arthritis. Journal of Pediatrics 88: 926–930
Scharf J, Levy J, Benderly A, Nahir M 1976 Pericardial tamponade in juvenile rheumatoid arthritis. Arthritis and Rheumatism 19: 760–762
Schlesinger B E 1949 Rheumatoid arthritis in the young. British Medical Journal 2: 197–201
Schlumpf U, Howard A, Ansell B M 1985 IgG-anti-IgG antibodies in juvenile chronic arthritis. Scandinavian Journal of Rheumatology (in press)
Schnitzer T J, Ansell B M 1977 Amyloidosis in juvenile chronic polyarthritis. Arthritis and Rheumatism 20 (Suppl 2): 245–252
Scott P J, Ansell B M, Huskisson E C 1977 Measurement of pain in juvenile chronic polyarthritis. Annals of Rheumatic Diseases 36: 186–187
Shannon F T, Bywaters E G L 1957 Cause of anomalous results in the erythrocyte sedimentation rate using Wintrobe's method. British Medical Journal 2:1405
Skoglund R R, Schanberger J E, Kaplan J M 1971 Cyclophosphamide therapy for severe juvenile rheumatoid arthritis. American Journal of Diseases of Children 121: 531–533
Smiley W K, Kanski J J 1978 Eye surgery. In: Arden G P, Ansell B M (eds) Surgical management of juvenile chronic polyarthritis. Academic Press, London, Ch 16, p 235–252
Smiley W K, May E, Bywaters E G L 1957 Ocular presentations of Still's disease and their treatment. Annals of the Rheumatic Diseases 16: 371–383
Starko K M, Mullick F G 1983 Hepatic and cerebral pathology findings in children with fatal salicylate intoxication. Further evidence for a causal relation between salicylate and Reye's syndrome. Lancet 1: 326–329
Stastny P, Fink C W 1979 Different HLA-D associations in adult and juvenile rheumatoid arthritis. Journal of Clinical Investigation 63: 124–130
Still G F 1897 On a form of chronic joint disease in children. Medico-Chirurgical Transactions 80: 47–59
Sturrock R D, Goel G K, Lee P, et al 1974 Associate of HLA-17 and AJ in juvenile rheumatoid arthritis and ankylosing spondylitis. Journal of Rheumatology 1: 269–273
Swann M 1978 Management of lower limb deformities. In: Arden G P, Ansell B M (eds) Surgical management of

juvenile chronic polyarthritis. Academic Press, London Ch 8 p 97–116

Turner M W, Okafor G, Ansell B M 1975 Studies on the isolubilized immunosorbent procedure for the measurement of antiglobulins. In: Jennings J, Jayson M (eds) Proceedings of a symposium on the clinical and immunological aspects of Still's disease. Academic Press, London

Tyndall de Vere A, Bacon T, Parry R, Tyrrell D A J, Denman A M, Ansell B M 1984 Infections and interferon production in systemic juvenile chronic arthritis: a prospective study. Annals of the Rheumatic Diseases 43: 1–7

Usher M H, Grand R J, Gair J D, Gelfand E W 1978 Hepato-toxicity and encephalopathy association with aspirin therapy in rheumatoid arthritis. Journal of Pediatrics 93: 1034–1037

Ward D J, Hartog M, Ansell B M 1966 Corticosteroid-induced dwarfism in Still's disease treated with human growth hormone. Annals of Rheumatic Diseases 25: 416–421

Wernick R, Lospalluto J J, Fink C W, Ziff M 1981 IgG and IgM rheumatoid factors by solid phase radio-immunoassay. A comparison between adult and juvenile rheumatoid arthritis. Arthritis and Rheumatism 24: 1501–1511

Wilkinson A 1981 Juvenile chronic arthritis in adolescence: facing the reality. Rehabilitation Medicine 3: 11–17

Williams R C Jr, Froelich C J, Kilpatrick K, Crowe W E, Levinson J E 1981 Tγ cell subset specificity of lymphocyte reactive factors in juvenile rheumatoid arthritis and systemic lupus erythematosus sera. Arthritis and Rheumatism 24: 585–591

Wissler H 1967 In: Delbane et Paylan (ed) Morceaux choisis sur les rheumatismes inflammatoires chronique de l'Enfant. L'Expansion, Paris, No 2 p 203

Witmer R 1974 Augenkomplikationen bei Kindlicher rheumatoider arthritis. 16 Tagung der Deutschen Gesellschaft fur Rheumatologie, Mainz

Wood P H N 1978 Special meeting on nomenclature and classification of arthritis. In: Munthe E (ed) The care of rheumatic children. Eular, Basel, p 47

Wortmann D W, Kelsch R C, Kuhns L, Sullivan D B, Cassidy J T 1980 Renal papillary necrosis in juvenile rheumatoid arthritis. Journal of Pediatrics 97: 35–40

Zutshi D W, Friedman M, Ansell B M 1971 Corticotrophin therapy in juvenile chronic polyarthritis (Still's disease) and effect on growth. Archives of Disease in Childhood 46: 584–593

Other forms of arthritis in childhood

Although it has become customary to classify juvenile chronic arthritis by mode of onset, long-term follow-up has demonstrated that a number of distinct entities emerge (Table 44.1). These are being defined clinically and supported by appropriate markers. The purpose of this chapter is to highlight these conditions.

Table 44.1 Other forms of arthritis in childhood

Seropositive (IgM rheumatoid factor) juvenile arthritis
Juvenile spondylitis
Arthritis associated with ulcerative colitis or regional enteritis (as in adults)
Reactive arthritis — usually postdysenteric (as in adults)
Psoriatic arthropathy
Polyarthropathy associated with other disorders such as systemic lupus erythematosus, overlap syndrome, familial Mediterranean fever, hypogammaglobulinaemia, sarcoidosis, etc.

Seropositive (IgM rheumatoid factor) juvenile arthritis

Chronic arthritis in childhood associated with persistent IgM rheumatoid factor accounts for some 8% of all arthritis commencing under the age of 16 years. Girls are particularly affected; the age of onset is usually in the region of 10 or 11 years upwards. The most usual presentation is with a polyarthritis affecting the small joints of the hand and feet, often of insidious onset. The characteristic joint distribution is the wrist, with swelling over the ulnar styloid, metacarpophalangeal joints, especially 2 and 3, together with interphalangeal joints and metatarsophalangeal joints. The younger the patient the more likely there is to be hindfoot involvement early. Knee involvement is also seen relatively early and is the most common joint involved in all forms of childhood arthropathy. There is frequently some loss of weight, general malaise and lassitude, but major systemic manifestations are not seen; occasionally there is a slight fever and lymphadenopathy, usually axillary. Initially, the ESR is moderately raised and continues to rise over the first few weeks or months of illness. The haemoglobin tends to fall, the white count is usually normal and the platelets tend to rise. IgM rheumatoid factor tests are positive within weeks and only very rarely do they convert after about 3 months of illness (Ansell, 1983).

The value of seropositivity as a discriminant has been emphasised by Hanson et al (1969), who, in their prospective study, noted that it was the older children who largely accounted for seropositivity and that there was a close correlation with the presence of nodules. Erosions often with periostitis develop early in the hands and feet, so that in our recent prospective study, by 6 months from onset, all except one of the seropositive patients had erosions in either hands or feet (Fink & Ansell, 1980). Immunogenetically, these patients resemble adult rheumatoid arthritis in that 62% carry DR4 (Clemens et al, 1983). A family history of seropositive rheumatoid arthritis was found in 25%, with grandparents being more commonly affected than the parents.

The pattern tends to be one of a progressive joint involvement with stiffness of the shoulders, involvement of the neck, hips, elbows and hindfeet. Flexor tenosynovitis can develop, which is often nodular and gives rise to triggering of fingers. Carpal tunnel syndrome is occasionally seen, and as in adult rheumatoid arthritis, rupture of extensor tendons of the 4th and 5th finger and the thumb is not uncommon. Nodules similar in distribution to that of adult disease and with typical rheumatoid histology are seen in some 30% within the first year of disease. Vasculitis has been extremely uncommon, as has rheumatoid peripheral neuropathy. Entrapment is, however, occasionally seen at elbows and knees and atlanto-axial subluxation can give rise to cord compression relatively early in the disease. Other complications include aortic incompetence (Leak et al, 1981) and pulmonary fibrosis.

The disease tends to remain active with relatively rapid joint destruction (Fig. 44.1) (Williams & Ansell, 1981), so that after 5 years of disease, severe erosive changes were present at many sites with further progression occurring between 5 and 10 years, and this despite the use of gold and penicillamine, albeit somewhat later than one would now prescribe.

Management

Because of the tendency to rapid joint damage, it is essential that joints are protected by appropriate splinting from very early in the course. An acute exacerbation of arthritis, particularly in the lower limbs, may call for a short period of bed-rest, during which time joints must be maintained in good position and muscles allowed to function by appropriate exercises. While non-steroidal anti-inflammatory drugs are valuable in reducing pain, and particularly early morning stiffness, it would seem desirable to treat with gold or penicillamine early — dosages of 1 mg/kg body weight of intramuscular gold weekly or penicillamine up to 15 mg/kg per day, preferably given on an empty stomach. Although some 70% appear to improve during the first year of treatment, breakthrough is not uncommon so that by our 3-year follow-up only 50% were satisfactorily controlled (Ansell et al, 1981). The 30% who do not respond to either of these drugs tend to be those who go on to multiple surgical procedures. Although constituting a small proportion of patients with juvenile chronic arthritis, they account for nearly half the surgical procedures undertaken in our unit.

Because of this high failure rate with usual long-acting drugs, corticosteroids are frequently introduced relatively early. It is desirable that the dosage should be kept to a minimum, and particularly in those children who still have potential growth, an alternate day regime is preferable. As yet, it is not possible to distinguish which child is un-

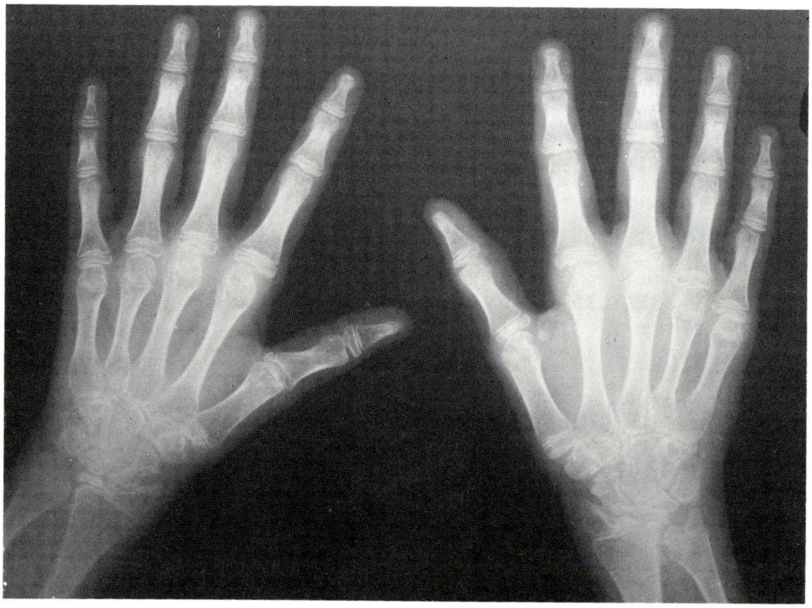

Fig. 44.1 14 months from onset, this 12-year-old girl shows a symmetrical erosive arthritis affecting MCP 1, 2 and 3, with severe wrist involvement including the radioulnar joint with an ulnar growth defect on the right.

likely to respond to long-acting drugs; if this were possible, azathioprine might be considered earlier; because of its possible mutagenic effect this is usually reserved for later in the course.

THE SPONDYLOARTHROPATHIES

Juvenile spondylitis

Although classic ankylosing spondylitis has been described in childhood (Edstrom et al, 1960), children frequently present as a peripheral arthropathy and only later develop sacroiliitis and/or ankylosing spondylitis (Ansell, 1980; Schaller, 1977). The onset is usually from the age of 9 and upwards; boys are affected 6 times more frequently than girls. The peripheral arthritis affects the lower limbs, in particular the knees, ankles and hips, often presenting as a monarticular arthritis, to be followed by other large joints associated with enthesopathy (Jacobs, 1982) (Fig. 44.2). The heel, either due to plantar fasciitis or bursitis around the tendo Achillis, is the commonest site but others include the tibial tubercle and greater trochanter. It has been suggested (Schaller, 1979) that younger children present with arthritis of the knee and/or ankle and teenagers with pain in the hip, either acute or subacute, sometimes associated with discomfort in the low back; this distinction is not, however, clear-cut; very occasionally there is fever, weight loss and myalgia. The arthritis tends to spread in an asymmetric fashion; involvement of interphalangeal and metatarsophalangeal joints of the toes is not uncommon (Fig. 44.3), being seen in 25% of our follow-up group (Ansell, 1980). In the first year of disease, upper limb involvement is seen in less than 10%; when it does occur, it tends to affect the metacarpophalangeal joint of the thumb, occasionally the elbow and wrist. Back pain, discomfort or loss of movement is not common at presentation; very occasionally the child will, however, have atlantoaxial subluxation early in the illness.

At presentation, radiological evidence of sacroiliitis is unusual; the mean duration to definite sacroiliac changes being 6.5 years (Fig. 44.4). However, sacroiliac joint interpretation is extremely difficult in the teenage period. Similarly,

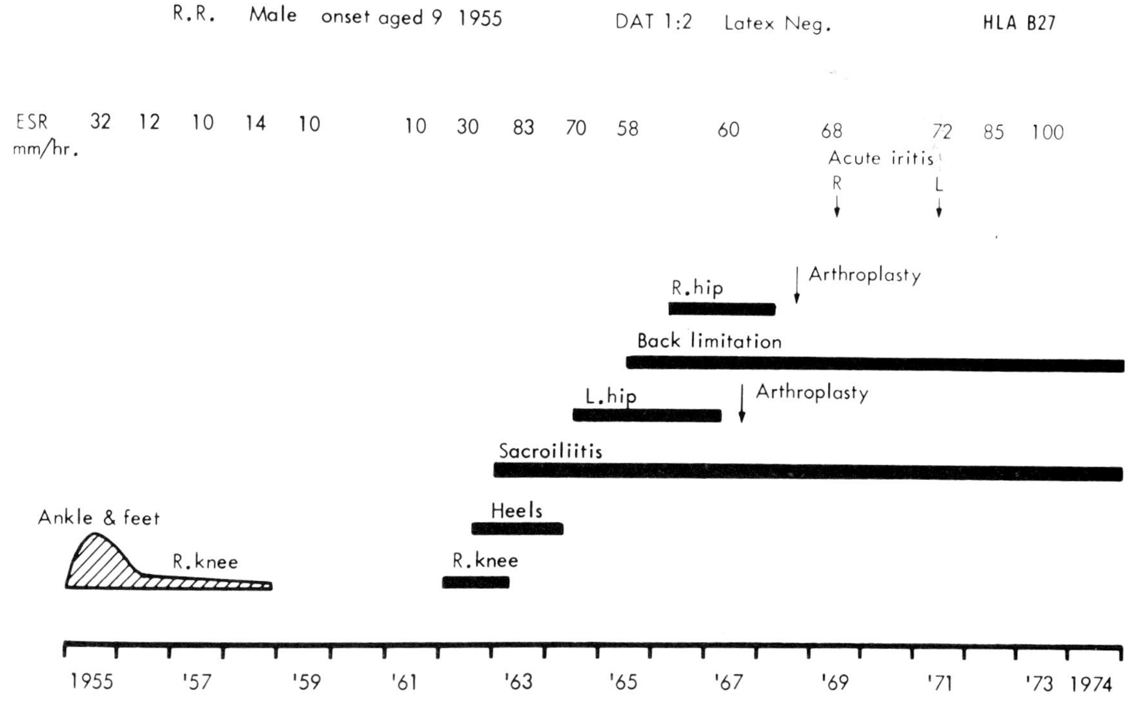

Fig. 44.2 Course of a boy who developed lower limb arthropathy, initially remitted but ultimately had severe ankylosing spondylitis with attacks of acute iritis.

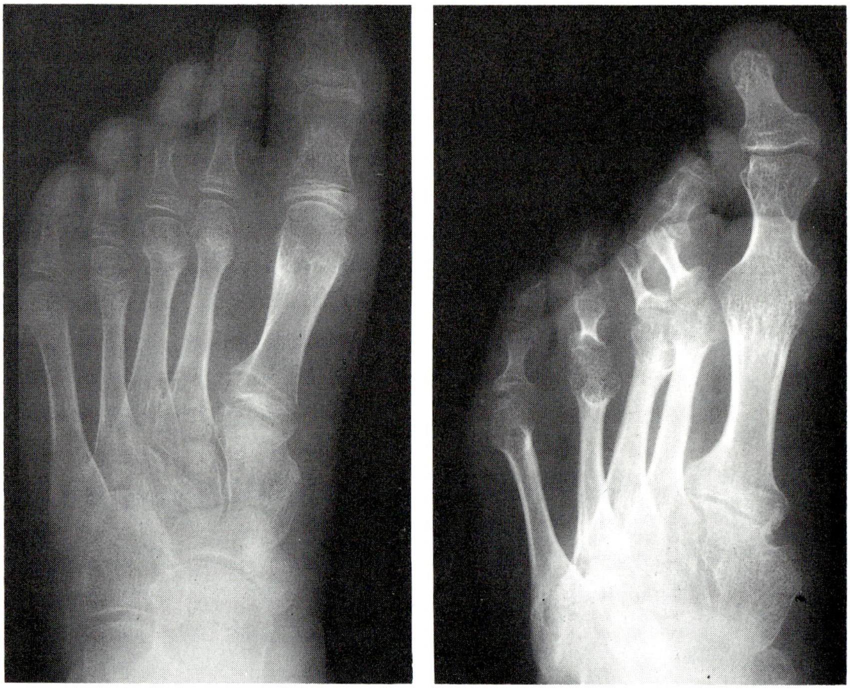

a b

Fig. 44.3 (a) Osteoporosis of foot 6 months after the development of the 2nd toe followed by involvement of MTP 2, 3 and 5 which severely interfered with walking in a 13-year-old boy. (b) Progressive changes after 5 years which caused bony fusion of MTP 1 and an erosive destructive arthritis of MTPs and PIP 2; tarsometatarsal fusion is also occurring.

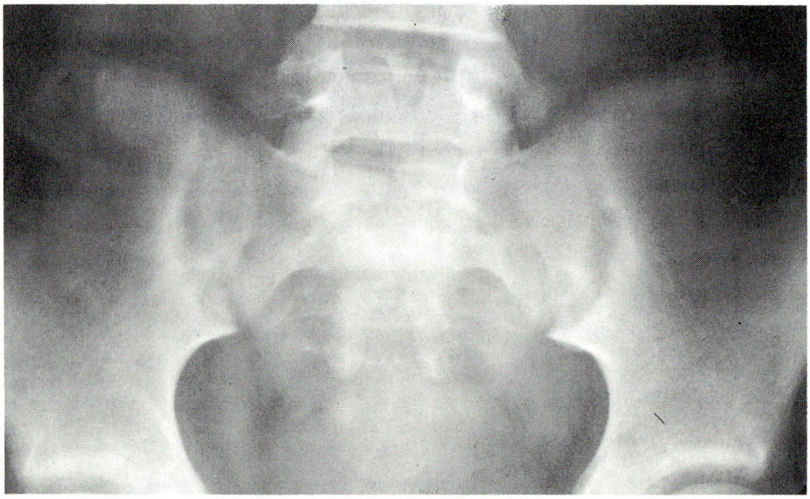

Fig. 44.4 Early sacroiliitis 4 years after an onset of acute arthritis in a hip followed by a knee in a 9-year-old boy.

scanning of sacroiliac joints is difficult as the epiphyseal development interferes with simple scanning techniques; newer methods with computerised tomography may become more helpful. Typical radiological changes of ankylosing spondylitis can develop but these may be delayed for years (Riley et al, 1971). Diagnosis is, therefore, difficult; a family history of ankylosing spondylitis or acute uveitis is helpful; the ESR is usually raised except when there is persistent monoarthritis; the haemoglobin tends to be normal, but can fall with persisting widespread peripheral arthropathy. The IgG tends to be raised; IgM rheumatoid factor and anti-nuclear antibodies are absent; HLA-B27 is present in over 90%.

The course is somewhat variable. In one-half, the peripheral arthropathy will remit, but sacroiliitis develops with or without minor back symptoms and radiological change; about one-tenth will go on to classic ankylosing spondylitis with residual problems in their peripheral joints (Fig. 44.2). Approximately one-third of patients slowly develop further incapacity due to recurrent episodes of peripheral arthropathy, increasing hip problems or progressive changes throughout the spine. The most serious functional disability results from limitation of hip movement, particularly if there is also stiffening of the lumbar spine. Radiologically, a number of different hip changes have been seen (Ansell & Kent, 1977). Complete bony fusion is rare; the most common type is of a gradual elongation of the femoral head with bony overgrowth at the edges (Fig. 44.5), while a few patients develop a progressive erosive change indistinguishable from rheumatoid arthritis. Acute iridocyclitis punctuates the course; in our 15-year follow-up study group this has occurred in 27%. About 5% develop ulcerative colitis or regional enteritis after many years of follow-up. Very occasionally, the late development of amyloidosis has been noted, particularly in those who have had a persistence of their peripheral arthropathy, associated with a high sedimentation rate. Another complication seen occasionally is aortic incompetence; this may be present before obvious spinal changes have occurred (Keans et al, 1980).

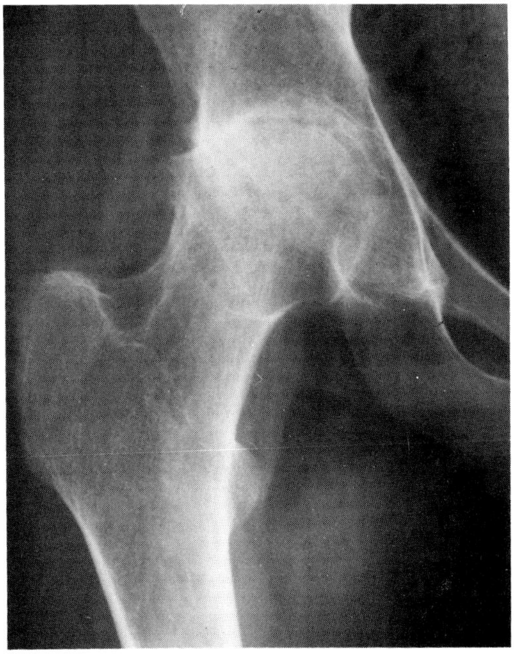

Fig. 44.5 11 years after initial presentation, this 22-year-old is showing elongation of the femoral head, with erosions and narrowing of joint space, and degenerative changes at the base of the femoral head.

Management

In general, joint function should be maintained by exercise; however, occasionally acute spasm around the hip will warrant a period of bed-rest with skin traction. Spasm at the foot is best treated by a period in a walking plaster followed by a T-strap and iron. For plantar fasciitis, local hydrocortisone injections into the most tender site followed by an insole — sorbo rubber or one of the newer plastics — to reduce impact on the painful site.

Non-steroidal anti-inflammatory agents, particularly naproxen, flurbiprofen and indomethacin, are helpful in relieving pain and allowing maintenance of function. Because of its possible side-effects, phenylbutazone, although effective, is best avoided. Very occasionally for those young people who have a period of general ill-health, ACTH is useful. A single troublesome joint or enthesopathy can often be helped by a local corticosteroid injection. Despite the problem of ossification around the prosthesis, hip arthroplasty will need to be considered in those who are becoming unable to walk because of progressive hip damage. Temporomandibular arthroplasty may also need consideration for progressive loss of movement. Atlantoaxial fusion is also occasionally required.

For these few patients who continue to add on peripheral joints over years, azathioprine appears the most useful drug; these patients do not respond to gold or penicillamine.

Inflammatory bowel disease

As in adults, two types of athritis occur, 'intestinal arthritis' and spondylitis. The former is characterised by episodes of synovitis, usually affecting the large joints particularly the knees which are not necessarily associated with exacerbations of the bowel disease. There is no apparent correlation between the arthritis and the severity or type of bowel disease (Lindsley, 1977). Other manifestations, particularly skin lesions such as erythema nodosum, pyoderma gangrenosum, and mucous membrane ulceration, are not uncommon. Spondylitis also presents as a peripheral arthropathy affecting the lower limbs, and can be very difficult to differentiate. The incidence of hip involvement, however, is much higher than in intestinal synovitis and the joint involvement in the spondylitic subgroup does not seem to have the same episodic course. Thus, an adolescent presenting with a lower limb arthropathy, perhaps associated with anaemia, persistently positive occult bloods, growth failure, or vague abdominal pain, should immediately be investigated for underlying bowel disorder, particularly regional enteritis. This is one of the few occasions when it may be justified to consider performing tissue typing to try to establish which pattern of arthritis is present, as intestinal synovitis will improve as the bowel state does, but the same is not true of the spondylitic variety. At times, the arthropathy can antedate the bowel disorder by many years.

Reactive arthritis

During childhood, infective diarrhoea, which can be from any organism — *Salmonella, Shigella, Yersinia* (Leino et al, 1980), *Campylobacter* — is the commonest cause of Reiter's syndrome, although with sexual activity beginning earlier, some sexually acquired cases occur in the early teens. The typical triad of urethritis, conjunctivitis and arthritis, tends to develop within about 10 days, but it can be anything from 3–20 days after the initial incident. As the episode of diarrhoea may have been minimal, a careful enquiry should be made in all cases of acute arthritis. In small children, it is often difficult to spot a urethral discharge, but a history of dysuria may be obtained. Mucocutaneous lesions are not uncommon. They are mild and have to be searched for; they include erythematous ulceration on the hard palate, scattered pustules on the glans penis, and ulceration of the penis. A high fever mimicking that of systemic juvenile chronic arthritis has been recorded, but the typical maculopapular rash does not occur. The term 'incomplete Reiter's syndrome' has been suggested for children who present with polyarthritis and a history of diarrhoea, or feature such as conjunctivitis or mucocutaneous lesions, has been suggested, but these are probably better called 'reactive arthritis' (Jacobs, 1982). HLA-B27 is present in 90% of these patients.

Juvenile psoriatic arthritis

Although the onset of psoriasis occurs before the age of 15 years in about one-third of patients, juvenile psoriatic arthritis is probably underdiagnosed. This may reflect the variety of disease patterns that typify this condition in the adult, as well as the absence of a satisfactory definition for childhood disease. Using the definition of a seronegative inflammatory arthritis with an onset before 16 years and with psoriasis either preceding, coincident with, or following the arthritis and the active exclusion of other defined conditions, it was found to constitute 4% of referrals in our long-term follow-up group (Ansell & Wood, 1976) and the more recent review of early cases (Fink & Ansell, 1980). Girls are more frequently affected that boys in a ratio of 3 : 2, and they tend to be younger than boys, with a mean age of onset of 8.2 years compared with 9.5 years for boys. The mean age of skin involvement was 8.8 years (Shore & Ansell, 1982). The psoriasis may antedate the joint involvement or arthritis may be followed by psoriasis. Relatively uncommonly (9%) the two occur simultaneously. A family history of psoriasis, with or without arthritis, was found in 40% and is a helpful clue when a child presents with an asymmetrical arthropathy.

The most usual presentation is that of pauciarticular arthritis with the knee the commonest joint; approximately half present in this way. Other common sites include a single finger or toe with involvement of metacarpophalangeal, proximal interphalangeal and terminal phalangeal joints, and the flexor tendon, which is usually associated with a marked periosteal reaction. Despite a pauciarticular onset, the majority of children go on to develop an asymmetrical polyarthritis with frequently intermittent episodes of synovitis. The major differences between juvenile chronic arthritis and psoriatic arthritis is the relative lack of systemic manifestations, the intermittent course with variable periods between exacerbations which continue into and through adult life, and very occasionally, a severe destructive, often asymmetric, disease. The gradual development of sacroiliitis, particularly in boys, is seen in something under half. On tissue-typing, there is an increased incidence of HLA-B17 which tends to go with milder disease and HLA-B27 which tends to be in the group later developing sacroiliitis; in contrast to pauciarticular onset juvenile arthritis, HLA-DW5 is unusual (Shore et al, 1981). Anti-nuclear antibody is seen in something under 10% and while iridocyclitis has been seen in young girls, ANA associates with destructive disease rather than iridocyclitis.

In the management of these patients, as in juvenile arthritis, it is important to maintain position and function of joints. For both acute flexor tenosynovitis and persistent swelling of a single joint, a local injection of hydrocortisone in the flexor tendons and a longer acting steroid into a knee or elbow may be extremely helpful. The majority will require only non-steroidal anti-inflammatory drugs. The severity of the peripheral arthritis may occasionally warrant gold, but response is uncertain and in the severe destructive type, cytotoxic therapy may need to be considered. Azathioprine has been found to be effective in controlling both skin and joints. In our follow-up group of 60 (Shore & Ansell, 1982), one patient developed Crohn's disease and one ulcerative colitis, supporting the concept of juvenile psoriatic arthritis as a distinct member of the family of seronegative arthropathies.

The rarer connective tissue disorders

Systemic lupus erythematosus is most common in girls (80%) usually around the age of puberty — it is rare before the age of 5. The overall clinical features are similar to those found in adults (Caero et al, 1981), but it is perhaps noteworthy that fever and lymphadenopathy are more marked. Arthralgia and arthritis are common presenting symptoms, but it is usual to find multisystem involvement at the first consultation. Ragsdale et al (1980), however, have drawn attention to a small group of patients initially diagnosed as juvenile arthritis who were ultimately considered to have SLE as late as $2\frac{1}{2}$–20 years from presentation. There is still disagreement over the significance of renal involvement. King et al (1977) felt that particularly children with a membranous lesion on renal biopsy are likely to become azotaemic and hypertensive and die early from renal failure while Fish et al (1977) have suggested that in general, children and adolescents have a better renal prognosis than adults. It is, however, generally accepted that significant renal disease tends to develop in the first 2 years of the illness in nearly half and that this is one of the most important long-term prognostic factors.

Central nervous system involvement ranks second to nephritis in causing morbidity and mortality. It is unusual as a presenting feature but occasionally chorea or convulsions are the initial manifestations. Overall, it occurs in about one-third, with headache and psychosis the most common later manifestations, while involvement of cranial and peripheral nerves can occur. Sequelae include cerebellar ataxia, focal loss of function, as well as a syndrome of disorientation, loss of memory, and even progressive intellectual deterioration

Mixed connective tissue disease (Ch. 50) can be seen in childhood with features overlapping between juvenile chronic arthritis, polymyositis, systemic sclerosis and systemic lupus erythematosus. The development of acute Raynaud's phenomenon in a child presenting with arthritis should alert one to this possibility (Peskett et al, 1978). Flexor tenosynovitis and myositis appear particularly troublesome while the presence of pulmonary hypertension and cardiac involvement are bad prognostic features (Rosenberg et al, 1979). Follow-up of our patients has indicated that some may pass through an acute synovitis and myositis to end with features suggestive of scleroderma including difficulty in swallowing; a few will develop overt systemic lupus erythematosus, while in others, the synovitis, myositis and flexor tenosynovitis remit, leaving just the Raynaud's phenomenon. At the initial appraisal, it was impossible to assess the ultimate course.

Arthritis may occur in up to one-third of children suffering from dermatomyositis and can be the presenting feature. The presence of Raynaud's phenomenon, together with the rash, particularly over the metacarpophalangeal joints, as well as a relatively low ESR, will help differentiate this (Ch. 54). In childhood, generalised scleroderma and systemic sclerosis are rare; when they do occur the clinical features are indistinguishable and prognosis is similar to that seen in adults (Cassidy et al, 1977; Ch. 55). However, localised disease, both morphea and linear, are relatively more common. Linear scleroderma can also affect the deeper structures, such as muscle and bone, and can cause local contracture and deformity, as well as loss of function. Joint symptoms and diffuse nodule formation in tendons may occur at a distance from the sites of local lesions; these cases need differentiation from synovitis. In general, the symptoms tend to be of stiffness with signs of loss of movement rather than synovitis (Ansell et al, 1976). Limb pain, both myalgia and arthralgia, can be seen in childhood polyarteritis, but with the exception of the so-called 'cutaneous form' (which is characterised by a variety of skin lesions and painful subcutaneous nodules which suggest erythema nodosum, but are smaller, more widespread and considerably more indurated, as well as occurring throughout the body) arthritis is uncommon.

Whether or not the mucocutaneous lymph node syndrome (Kawasaki et al, 1974) is the same as infantile polyarteritis is still not certain. This affects young children, initially mimicking an infection with fever associated with conjunctival infection, erythema of the oropharynx, a variety of rashes and the later development of cardiac abnormalities; some 20% have arthralgia or arthritis and a somewhat higher porportion aseptic meningitis.

Other conditions

In infants and young children, sarcoidosis can cause boggy tendon sheath effusions, marked synovial thickening (often painless), uveitis and cutaneous lesions (Hetherington, 1982). It is unusual to have hilar lymphadenopathy or lung lesions. Familial Mediterranean fever occurs in children of Mediterranean stock and is characterised by recurring attacks of fever, peritonitis, pleurisy, occasionally pericarditis; synovitis occurs in about half (Heller et al, 1966). The episodes of arthritis usually last about a week, but a few persist for months (Sneh et al, 1977). Recurrent attacks in hips and knees may lead to narrowing of joint space and loss of cartilage; neck involvement can cause changes in the apophyseal joint C2/3. They may also be associated with failure of overall growth, thus closely mimicking juvenile chronic arthritis.

REFERENCES

Ansell B M 1980 Juvenile spondylitis and related disorders. In: Moll J M H (ed) Ankylosing spondylitis. Churchill Livingstone, Edinburgh, p. 120–136

Ansell B M 1983 Juvenile chronic arthritis with persistently positive tests for rheumatoid factor. (Sero-positive juvenile rheumatoid arthritis). Annales de Pediatrie 30: 545–550

Ansell B M, Kent P A 1977 Radiological changes in juvenile chronic polyarthritis. Skeletal Radiology 1: 129–144

Ansell B M, Wood P H N 1976 Prognosis in juvenile chronic polyarthritis. Clinics in Rheumatic Diseases, 2, 397–412

Ansell B M, Nasseh G A, Bywaters E G L 1976 Scleroderma in childhood. Annals of the Rheumatic Diseases 35, 189

Ansell B M, Hall M A, Ribeiro S 1981 A comparative study of gold and penicillamine in sero-positive juvenile chronic arthritis. (Juvenile rheumatoid arthritis.) Annals of the Rheumatic Diseases 40:522

Caeiro F, Michaelson F M C, Bernstein R, Hughes G Y R, Ansell B M 1981 Systemic lupus erythematosis in childhood. Annals of the Rheumatic Diseases 40, 325–331

Cassidy J T, Sullivan D B, Dabich L, Pelty R E 1977 Scleroderma in childhood. Arthritis and Rheumatism 20: 351–354

Clemens L E, Albert E, Ansell B M 1983 HLA studies in IgM rheumatoid factor disease. Annals of the Rheumatic Diseases 42: 431–434

Edstrom G, Thune S, Wittbom-Cigen G 1960 Juvenile ankylosing spondylitis. Acta Rheumatologica Scandinavica 6, 161–173

Feinglass E J, Arnett F C, Dorsch C A 1976 Neuro-psychiatric manifestations of systemic lupus erythematosus; diagnosis, clinical spectrum and relationship to other features of disease. 55, 323

Fink C W, Ansell B M, Wood P H N 1980 Juvenile arthritis in England; a long term follow-up. Arthritis and Rheumatism 23, 673

Fish A J, Blau E B, Westberg N G, et al 1977 Systemic lupus erythematosus within the first two decades. Am J Med 62, 99–117

Hanson V, Drexter E, Kornreich H 1969 The relationship of rheumatoid factor to age of onset in juvenile rheumatoid arthritis. Arthritis and Rheumatism 12, 82–86

Heller H, Gafini J, Michaeli D, et al 1966 The arthritis of familial mediterranean fever. Arthritis and Rheumatism 9, 1–17

Hetherington S 1982 Sarcoidosis in young children. American Journal of Diseases in Childhood 130: 13–5

Jacobs J C, Berdon W E, Johnston A D 1982 HLA B27 associated spondylo-arthritis and enthesopathy in childhood; clinical, pathologic and radiographic observations in 58 patients. Journal of Pediatrics 100, 521–528

Kawasaki T, Kpsaki F, Okawa S, Shigematusi I, Yanagawa H 1974 A new infantile acute febrile muco-cutaneous lymph node syndrome (MLNS) prevailing in Japan. Pediatrics 54:271

Kean W F, Anastassiades T P, Ford P M 1980 Aortic incompetence in HLA B27 positive juvenile arthritis. Annals of the Rheumatic Diseases 39: 294–295

King K K, Kornreich H K, Bernstein B H, et al 1977 The clinical spectrum of systemic lupus erythematosus in childhood. Arthritis and Rheumatism 20: 287–294

Leak A M, Millar-Craig M W, Ansell B M 1981 Aortic regurgitation in sero-positive juvenile arthritis. Annals of the Rheumatic Diseases 40, 229–234

Leino R, Makela A, Tillikainen A, Toivanen A 1980 Yersinia arthritis in children. Scandinavian Journal of Rheumatology 9: 245–249

Lindsley C B 1977 Arthritis in inflammatory bowel disease in children. Arthritis and Rheumatism 20 (Suppl 2): 411–413

Peskett S A, Ansell B M, Fiszman P, Howard A 1978 Mixed connective tissue disease in children. Rheumatism and Rehabilitation 17: 245–2

Petty R E, Cummin G R, Curler B E 1979 Pulmonary hypertension in a child with mixed connective tissue disease. Journal of Rheumatism 6:700

Ragsdale C G, Petty R E, Cassidy J T, et al 1980 The clinical progression of apparent juvenile rheumatoid arthritis to systemic lupus erythematosus. Journal of Rheumatology 7, 50–55

Riley M J, Ansell B M, Bywaters E G L 1971 Radiological manifestations of ankylosing spondylitis to age at onset. Annals of the Rheumatic Diseases 30: 138–148

Schaller J G 1977 Ankylosing spondylitis of childhood onset. Arthritis and Rheumatism 20: 398–401

Schaller J G 1979 The sero-negative spondylo-arthropathies of childhood. Clinical Orthopaedics and Related Research 143, 76–83

Shore A, Ansell B M 1982 Juvenile psoriatic arthritis: an analysis of 60 cases. Journal of Pediatrics 100, 529–535

Shore A, Gladman D, Keystone E, Clemens L, Ansell B M 1981 HLA-defined sub-groups of juvenile psoriatic arthritis. Abstract 666. XVth International Congress of Rheumatology. Revue de Rheumatism

Sneh E, Pras M, Michaeli D, Shahn H, Gafini J 1977 Protracted arthritis in familial mediterranean fever. Rheumatism and Rehabilitation 16: 102–106

Williams R, Ansell B M 1981 Radiological assessment in sero-positive juvenile chronic arthritis (juvenile rheumatoid arthritis). Annals of the Rheumatic Diseases 40:526

SECTION X

Other forms of Arthritis

Infective arthritis

Arthritis may result from direct infection of joints by micro-organisms, or as a reaction to a preceding infection. Dumonde & Steward (Ch. 14) have proposed the classification shown in Table 45.1.

Table 45.1 Association between microbial infection and arthritis (Dumonde & Steward)

	Infection known	Microbes in joints	Antigen in joints	Syndrome
Type I	+	+	+	Infective
Type II	+	—	+	Postinfective
Type III	+	—	—	Reactive
Type IV	—	—	—	Inflammatory

This chapter will deal predominantly with type I and type II infections; in suppurative arthritis it is usually possible to find the organism in the joint, although meningococcal infection tends to belong to type II; infections with *Salmonella* can be type I or type III, i.e. arthritis occurring after the infection in the bowel has cleared: it is then termed 'reactive'.

Arthropathy due to syphilis belongs to type II while those associated with viral infections probably also belong in this group. The situation is more complicated in diseases such as Behçet's syndrome where there may be a combination of infection and altered immunity. This chapter is concerned primarily with clinical descriptions and the immediate management of type I and II infections.

BACTERIAL INFECTIONS

Acute suppurative arthritis

The incidence of acute suppurative arthritis has declined since antibiotics have been widely used for the treatment of systemic infections, but it does still occur (Argen et al, 1966; Russell & Ansell, 1972). Clinically it can be mistaken for gout, pseudogout, psoriatic arthropathy or rheumatic fever, or, when it occurs in a joint already the seat of rheumatoid arthritis or crystal deposition, for an exacerbation of the disease (Kellgren et al, 1958; Myers et al, 1969). Predisposing factors include intra-articular injection, debilitating illnesses such as diabetes, rheumatoid arthritis, systemic lupus erythematosus (Quismoro & Dubois, 1975), regional enteritis (London & Fitton, 1970), neuropathic joint disease (Martin et al, 1965), leukaemia (Douglas et al, 1964), abdominal surgery (Smith & Ward, 1966) and injury (Willkens et al, 1960), as well as treatment with corticosteroids or immunosuppressive drugs. If a satisfactory outcome is to be obtained, prompt diagnosis and treatment are required. The administration of an antibiotic before diagnosis may make cultural diagnostic confirmation impossible and can also mask the underlying problem, as can the administration of corticosteroids.

Primary septic arthritis affects either sex and all ages but tends to be more frequent in the young (Borrella et al, 1963; Patterson, 1970; Nade, 1983a). The importance of immunodeficiency in infantile bone and joint infections has been stressed (Kuo et al, 1975). While usually monarticular, multiple joints are involved initially in some 10%; after an initial monarticular onset only very rarely does it spread to other joints. Any joint can be affected but the most common site is the knee, except in infants, particularly premature, when it is the hip (Samilson et al, 1958). Infection reaches the joint by extension from a pre-existing infection in the adjacent soft tissue or bone, by haematogenous spread from a focus of infection elsewhere in the body or rarely by direct introduction into the joint through a puncture wound; very occasionally it appears to be idiopathic. The onset is acute, often with rigors and associated with a high fever, but prodromal symptoms of malaise, arthralgia and low grade fever, persisting for several days before the appearance of obvious arthritis, are not uncommon; this occurred in 25% of the cases reported by Ward et al (1960), while in our experience it was more likely if infections complicated underlying disease (Russell & Ansell, 1972). The affected joint is usually exquisitely painful and tender with limitation of movement; it may be hot and red. The most important diagnostic procedures are blood and synovial fluid cultures, which in a young child may require a general anaesthetic. Blood cultures are positive in about a quarter of cases, while if antibiotics have not been given the synovial fluid will usually give a positive culture. In addition the synovial fluid tends to have a high white cell count, often about 50 000/mm^3 with more than 90% of polymorphonuclear leucocytes; the sugar content tends to be low compared to that of the blood, particularly when a positive culture from the synovial fluid is obtained (Ward et al, 1960). As cultures take time new methods are being introduced, notably detection of products of microbial metabolism or microbe host interaction by gas chromatography (Borenstein et al, 1983) or detection of microbial antigens by counter immunoelectrophoresis (Rytel, 1975). If superficial infection is present, e.g. a bed sore, this too should be cultured as it is likely to grow the same organisms as the joint (Russell & Ansell, 1972). The organism most commonly cultured is *Staphylococcus aureus*; many others have been implicated including alpha and beta haemolytic streptococci, *E. coli*, *Pseudomonas aerogenes*, *pneumococcus* (Argen et al, 1966; Torres et al, 1973) and *Haemophilus influenzae* (Ho et al, 1983). This last is the commonest organism under the age of 2, but can occur in adults, particularly the immunosuppressed; it can then mimic gonococcal disseminated disease including tenosynovitis.

The ESR may be raised, but this is not particularly helpful diagnostically and while there can be a polymorphonuclear leucocytosis in the blood, this is not necessarily present. Initially, unless there is extension from a bone focus, X-rays merely reveal periarticular swelling and a joint effusion. Scanning with ^{99m}Tc phosphate is useful in identifying bone lesions as well as joint inflammation; if this scan is equivocal, ^{67}Ga imaging should be undertaken (Namey & Halla, 1978). After about 2 weeks there will be a uniform osteoporosis spreading out from the joint surface; this is followed by destruction of cartilage and loss of detail in the subchondral bone. When infection is not recognised and treated early, serious damage to the joint can occur (Fig. 45.1). In those with no underlying disorder the hip appears at particular risk.

In management the limb should be splinted in the optimal position or, if severe muscle spasm is present, skin traction may be used. Once blood and synovial fluid have been obtained for culture, appropriate antibiotics should be administered (Nade, 1983a, b). It is advisable to commence with erythromycin and fucidin, which should be given intravenously if the patient is obviously septicaemic, and then change as required when the organism has been cultured and sensitivities known. Methicillin-resistant staphylococci are slowly emerging; these are usually insensitive to cephalosparins but respond to the more toxic vancomycin (Watanakunakorn, 1982). Antibiotics enter the synovial cavity freely, but the synovial fluid should be aspirated when it reaccumulates, as the presence of purulent material may inhibit their action; should reaccumulation occur rapidly, the joint should continue to be aspirated both to relieve intra-articular pressure and remove debris (Goldenberg et al, 1975); intra-articular antibiotics may be valuable. If there is no response to therapy within 72 hours, or destruction of the joint is already present either from the infection itself or it being superimposed on a previously damaged joint, surgical drainage is indicated (Chartier et al, 1959). Once the acute inflammation has subsided, and this usually takes a few days, muscle-setting exercises can begin, followed by active exercises. Resumption of weight-bearing is allowed once all signs of inflammation have subsided. The duration of antibiotic therapy will vary according to the speed with which the initial therapy is commenced, the type of infection and the presence of any underlying disease: in general antibiotics

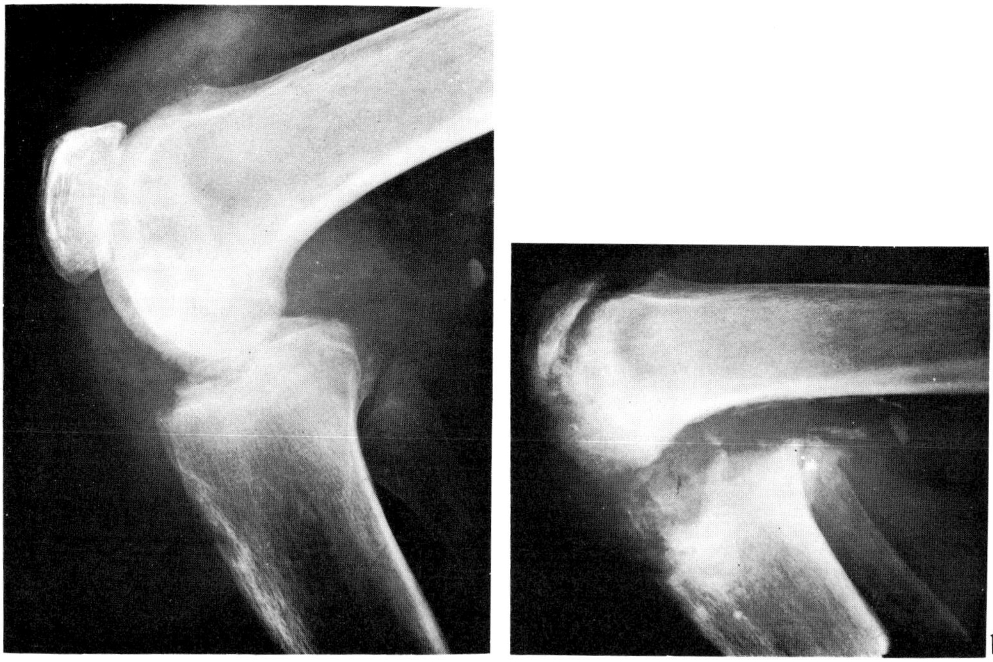

a b

Fig. 45.1 (a) Infection with *Staphylococcus aureaus* in a joint already the seat of rheumatoid arthritis. (b) Gross destruction accrued over 4 months.

should be continued for a minimum of 6 weeks; if infection has complicated pre-existing disease or caused joint destruction prior to diagnosis, 12 or more weeks' therapy is required; they must be continued until there is no clinical evidence of inflammation. The ESR repeated at weekly intervals is a useful guide but it should be realised that if there is pre-existing rheumatoid arthritis or systemic lupus erythematosus the ESR will only fall to its pre-infection level. The prognosis depends on the underlying state of the joint and the speed with which the infection is controlled; provided specific therapy commences quickly and at this time there is a normal or only mildly damaged joint, it is good; if the infection has caused joint destruction this will cause problems, usually later in life; very occasionally amputation may be required as it was in the patient in Figure 45.1. Although *Staphylococcus aureus* is still the most usual organism in rheumatoid arthritis, other organisms are being reported increasingly frequently in the immunocompromised host. These include *Pneumococcus*, *Streptococcus*, particularly C and G, *E. coli*, *Pseudomonas aeruginosa*, *Klebsiella* and *Aerobacter* species, *Serratia marcescens* and *Proteus* species.

In drug abusers, the habitual use of intravenous drugs is associated with *Pseudomonas* and *Serratia* as well as *Staphylococcus*; the last mentioned is usually carried on the skin or in the nose.

SPECIAL PROBLEMS

Gonococcal arthritis

Prompt and adequate treatment of gonorrhoea with antibiotics appears to prevent arthritis; despite this, there is a steadily rising incidence so that it is the commonest cause of infectious arthritis in the USA (Handsfield, 1975). It is particularly common in females (Graber et al, 1960) and the disease is also seen in homosexual males, following gonococcal vulvovaginitis in children and in the neonate (Sponzilli & Calabro, 1961). It is now relatively rare in males as their gonococcal urethritis is usually obvious and therefore promptly treated.

Two clinical forms have been described. The disseminated one is characterised by fever and rigors within 3 weeks of the infection; in women this is not infrequently related to menstruation and pregnancy (Goobar & Clark, 1964; Taylor et al, 1966).

Such patients will have a positive blood culture. At this point there may be polyarthralgia or polyarthritis, often migratory mimicking rheumatic fever although ultimately the infection tends to localise in one or two joints. Skin lesions consisting of small erythematous macules which may become petechial are seen before or with the arthritis; these indicate the septicaemic phase of the illness. The vesicles may become pustular and a dark necrotic centre develop in the pustule. At presentation these skin lesions may differ in size and appearance due to the age of each lesion (Ackerman et al, 1965). Myocarditis, endocarditis, meningitis and pericarditis can also occur in the acute stage (Holmes, 1971) while infrequently suppurative myositis is seen. The other group is predominantly arthritic. 6 of the 28 cases reported by Montgomery et al (1962) were monarticular from the onset as were some of the cases described by Gelfand et al (1975); even so, the arthritis is usually accompanied by fever. The joints most commonly affected are the knees and the ankles, wrists, tarsi and metatarsophalangeal joints. Tenosynovitis of the dorsal sheath or fingers occurs fairly frequently. Gelfand and his colleagues, (1975) compared those patients with a positive blood culture with those in whom the joint culture only was positive and suggest there is evidence for the two clinical forms. However, these probably represent a spectrum of the same disease (Brandt et al, 1974). Diagnosis rests on culture of the gonococcus. This can be from the synovial fluid or tissue, blood, cervix, throat, rectum or skin. The cultures need special care with a proper course of media of paramount importance. Thayer Martin plates are appropriate for cervical, rectal and throat cultures but for blood, skin lesions or synovial fluid the medium should be chocolate agar, TSV broth or a semisolid overlay L-form medium. The value of gonococcal serology is still a matter of controversy (Dans et al, 1977).

Penicillin remains the drug of choice; for disseminated disease therapy is given intravenously for at least 5–7 days; for a septic arthritis it can be either intravenous or high dose oral or intramuscular. There is an increasing incidence of penicillinase-producing gonococci in Great Britain (McCutchan et al, 1982), which strains have usually arisen elsewhere as a result of self-prescribed penicillin prophylaxis for gonorrhoea; thus patients failing to respond to penicillin, or contacts of known cases or travellers from endemic areas should immediately have their gonococcal isolates screened for penicillinase production. For such patients spectinomycin is the treatment of choice, or alternatively, cephoxitin after the oral administration of probenecid. During the acute stage the affected joint or joints should be rested in a splint, aspiration may be required to relieve pain. If therapy has not been initiated satisfactorily it could be, as with any other septic arthritis, that surgical drainage may be required. Inadequate therapy is associated with joint destruction which can be followed by bony fusion. Disseminated infection has been shown to be associated with complement deficiency, particularly C5, C6, C7 and C8 (Peterson et al, 1979).

Meningococcal arthritis

Prior to chemotheraphy, three types of arthritis occurred in acute meningococcal infections (Schein, 1938). The first, developing at the same time as the petechial rash, was an acute transient polyarthritis associated with marked pain and tenderness, thought to be due to haemorrhage into articular structures. The second — the usual one — occurred from the 5th day of the illness onwards and consisted of a purulent arthritis involving a single joint, often the knee; in only one-third could meningococci be isolated from the joint. The third form, that following serum therapy, is not seen nowadays, while the other forms are also less frequent (Pinals & Ropes, 1964; Russell & Ansell, 1972). This second type of arthritis usually develops as the disease comes under control with chemotherapy (Eichner & Deller, 1970), but occasionally arthritis is the presenting feature with only mild systemic illness. Usually two or three large joints are involved but it can be monarticular (Whittle et al, 1973). In a series of 717 cases of meningococcal infection the incidence of arthritis was 6.6% often associated with other allergic complications, cutaneous vasculitis and episcleritis. Histological and bacteriological studies suggested these lesions were not due to persisting infection but to immune complex disease, with a fall in serum C3 and deposition of IgG, IgM, complement and meningococcal antigen in the synovial membrane, and joint fluid leucocytosis (Greenwood et al, 1973); counter-current immunoelectrophoresis can identify meningococcal antigen in the synovial fluid.

Chronic meningococcaemia still occasionally causes difficulty in diagnosis (Gore, 1956); it usually affects young adults and is characterised by rigors, fevers, headache and joint pain, the latter often flitting, and rash. C7 deficiency has been associated with the chronic disease (Adams et al, 1983). The treatment of choice in meningococcal infection is still penicillin, with chloramphenicol and sulphonamides as alternatives.

Brucellosis

Brucellosis results from human infection with one of the brucella organisms. The goat is the natural host of *Brucella melitensis* which is the most invasive of these organisms and accounts for the majority of human infections. The cow is the natural host for *Brucella abortus* which is the most common infection in Great Britain and the United States of America. *Brucella suis* from the hog is the least common infection, but the one thought most likely to cause suppurative lesions. Infection in man is by the gastrointestinal tract through the ingestion of raw milk, or more commonly by direct contact with infected animals, when the organism gains access through minute abrasions in the skin or nasopharynx. The incubation period is usually 21 days, but the interval can be longer. The brucella organisms localise where there is an abundance of reticuloendothelial tissue and by invading the cells are protected from the action of antibiotics. Infection produces recurrent fever with sweating, sickness, myalgia and arthralgia; this last has been said to occur in as many as 32% of patients, while a few patients may have transitory polyarthritis (Hardy, 1937). Involvement of joints, bursae and bones is relatively uncommon, but can cause severe destructive lesions (Kelly et al, 1960). The arthritis is usually monarticular, with the hips and knees being the most frequently involved joints. The presenting feature usually suggests a septic arthritis in the hip, but the knee may cause problems in differential diagnosis as it can cause a recurrent or persistent effusion with little generalised disturbance (Makin et al, 1957). Bursitis was originally recorded in the subdeltoid bursa (Kennedy, 1904), but the most common site is the prepatella where it gives rise to marked enlargement and thickening (Johnson & Weed, 1954). Osteomyelitis in the long bones due to brucellar infections shows no specific features except that it tends to be chronic and may be aggravated by secondary infection with staphylococci (Kelly et al, 1960). In the spine a characteristic spondylitis results, which may develop weeks or months after the initial infection; any site can be affected, but most commonly the lumbar region. The onset is usually acute with severe back pain which may extend down the legs. Radiologically there is involvement of one or more contiguous vertebrae by a destructive lesion with narrowing of the disc space or spaces (Fig. 45.2), a proliferative marginal reaction leading to exostoses and relatively

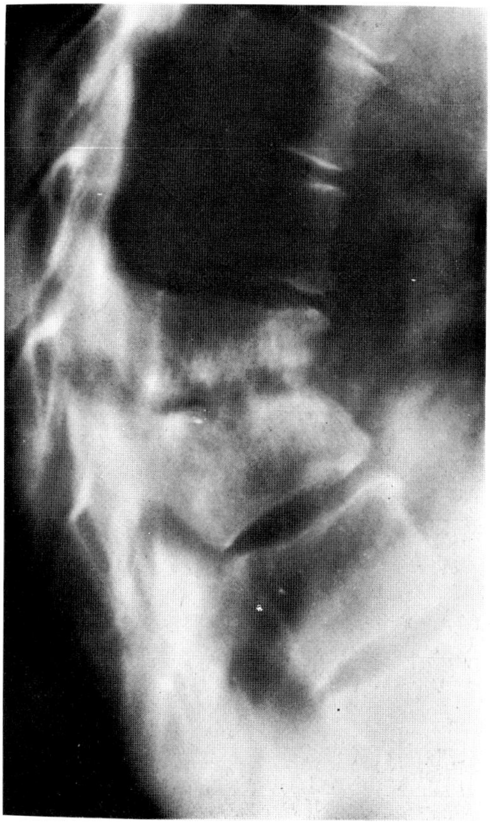

Fig. 45.2 Tomogram of lower thoracic spine showing destruction of contiguous vertebrae and disc space with some proliferation anteriorly as a result of infection with *Brucella melitensis* in a man of 70 who complained of persistent back pain after a holiday in Malta.

early bony fusion between the vertebrae. Occasionally paravertebral abscesses arise (Zammit, 1958; Papathanassiou et al, 1972).

It is often difficult to establish a diagnosis of brucellosis. The only absolute diagnosis is by culture of the organism from joints or bursae, when culture of the synovial tissue is often more valuable than synovial fluid (Coventry et al, 1949). The method of culture is important as it should be in an atmosphere containing approximately 10% of added CO_2 and should be on human blood agar or a specially prepared medium of fresh meat extract agar with added blood and glucose (Weed, 1957). An agglutination titre in the serum of 1 : 80 or greater indicates infection has occurred, but does not necessarily mean that this is the cause of the bone or joint symptoms. The presence of a rising titre and the development of typical spine changes radiologically, however, allows a reasonably confident diagnosis to be made; skin tests are of no diagnostic value. Histologically the synovial membrane shows granulation tissue with interstitial oedema, infiltration with large or small mononuclear cells which can coalesce to cause granuloma (Rotes-Querol, 1957), but the most valuable examination of synovial membrane is that of culture.

Once a diagnosis of brucellosis has been established, a combination of chemotherapy should be employed; currently tetracyclin and streptomycin, given in adequate doses for a minimum of 4 weeks, appears to be useful, as does erythromycin. The use of corticosteroids as an aid to releasing bacteria bound within the reticuloendothelial system may be valuable; for peripheral arthritis it is usually sufficient to treat by splinting and chemotherapy, though if frank suppuration is present, drainage is occasionally required. Grossly thickened bursae are best treated by chemotherapy and excision, while peripheral osteomyelitis may well require local drainage as well as chemotherapy. Brucellar spondylitis calls for some form of immobilisation by case or brace, as well as chemotherapy; occasionally surgery is necessary (Kemp et al, 1974).

MYCOPLASMA

Mycoplasma pneumoniae can cause fever, rashes of many types and transient arthropathy (Jones, 1970). This may also go on to cause the Stevens-Johnson syndrome in which there is systemic pustular as well as extensive vascular lesions in skin and mucous membrane (Sontheimer et al, 1978). In hypogammaglobulinaemia *Mycoplasma* can cause serious problems.

Tuberculosis

The incidence, pattern, and outlook of tuberculosis involving bones, joints and tendons have changed remarkably, owing to preventive measures as well as to the advent of chemotherapy, although it must be remembered that tuberculous arthritis has been recorded following apparently satisfactory vaccination with BCG (Backman & Wallgren, 1954). Not only has there been a change in incidence, but the type of tuberculous involvement appearing now in the clinics is somewhat different (Newton et al, 1982). From being a disease primarily of children and young people, it is now seen at any age, while joints previously damaged by disorders such as rheumatoid arthritis, or degenerative change, can present with a secondary tuberculous infection. In addition it appears to be particularly common and somewhat different in manifestation among some of the immigrant population in this country. This includes the occurrence of multiple sites, tendon sheath involvement and dactylitis, as well as involvement of more than one site in the spine. Although involvement is always thought to be secondary to tuberculosis elsewhere, occasionally there is no obvious primary lesion (Griffiths, 1975).

The most common bony site is the spine; infection begins as a single focus in a vertebral body, usually thoracic, where it gives rise to a central cavity containing caseous material surrounded by fibrous tissue and atrophic bone; more than one vertebra may be involved (Fig. 45.3) (Bailey et al, 1972). This is followed by the development of a cold abscess under the anterior communicating ligament and as this extends other vertebrae can be affected. Clinically it can present as back pain, kyphos due to a collapsed vertebra, a cold abscess, or pain from pressure on surrounding structures (Wilkinson, 1959). Bone lesions in other sites also tend to be silent until there is collapse of bone around the focus, approach of an abscess to the surface or involvement of a neighbouring joint. Vary rarely, disseminated bone lesions, in the ab-

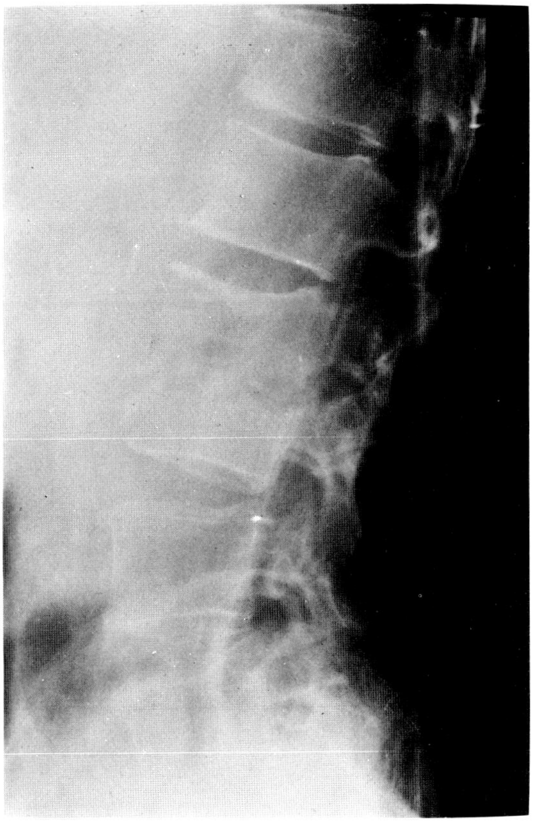

Fig. 45.3 Involvement of two adjacent vertebrae by tuberculosis: note the marked destruction of vertebral bodies with collapse and involvement of disc space.

sence of pulmonary involvement, may be mistaken for metastatic carcinoma (O'Malley & Zelt, 1965).

The majority of joint lesions are secondary to involvement of bone, but primary involvement of the synovial membrane does occur, particularly in the knee (Murray, 1940; Rose, 1959). Any large joint can be involved, but the knee or hip is the most common and usually only singly. Symptoms consist of a gradual loss of movement together with pain, particularly on jarring movements, swelling and marked muscle wasting. Radiologically, the earliest signs are osteoporosis and haziness of the bones. This is followed by erosions with marked irregularity of contours of joint surfaces (Fig. 45.4). Occasionally there are cystic lesions in the metaphysis with involvement of the epiphyseal plate and epiphysis (Hayes, 1961), while involvement of the greater trochanter has a specific radiological appearance with extensive erosive change and a large irregular shadow outside due to calcification of the caseous material in the subgluteal bursa. At times the bony lesions may be atypical and difficult to distinguish from other destructive lesions (Hunt, 1964). Sacroiliitis, which occurs in about 7% of skeletal tuberculosis, tends to be unilateral but can be bilateral (Wallace & Cohen, 1976).

Tuberculous tenosynovitis usually affects the ulnar and radial bursae giving rise to complicated palmar ganglion. Less commonly the extensor tendon sheath of the hand, isolated flexor tendon sheaths of the fingers or toes may be involved; these two are usually secondary to tuberculosis elsewhere (Pimm & Waugh, 1957). Tuberculous dactylitis presents as a painless swelling around a metatarsal or metacarpal (Fig. 45.5); other bones can also be involved; reported in African children (Cremin et al, 1970) these are similar to the cases seen among our immigrant population.

In the diagnosis of tuberculosis a positive Mantoux test is of no value but a negative reaction usually excludes the disease. Biopsy of a lymph node is unrealiable, and an absolute diagnosis of tuberculosis can be established only by the demonstration of tubercle bacilli in smear, culture or guinea-pig inoculation of the synovial fluid or synovial membrane. Histologically the synovial membrane shows evidence of caseation with giant cell formation, but proof of its aetiology rests on demonstration of tubercle bacilli. This is essential as infection with mycobacteria other than tuberculosis is becoming recognised more frequently, particularly after local injury or infection (Kelly et al, 1963; Godwin, 1965; Molony & Connolly, 1973) (see below).

In the management of tuberculosis of the skeletal system a combination of drug therapy with surgery gives the best results (Wilkinson, 1965). The majority of cases can be cured by chemotherapy provided it is taken properly. As with other forms of tuberculosis, rifampicin or ethambutol should be administered together with isoniazid for an adequate period of time, usually at least a year and preferably 18–20 months; occasionally it will still be necessary to use streptomycin. If significant bone destruction has occurred, surgery for removal of caseous and necrotic tissue will probably be required. The exact method and type

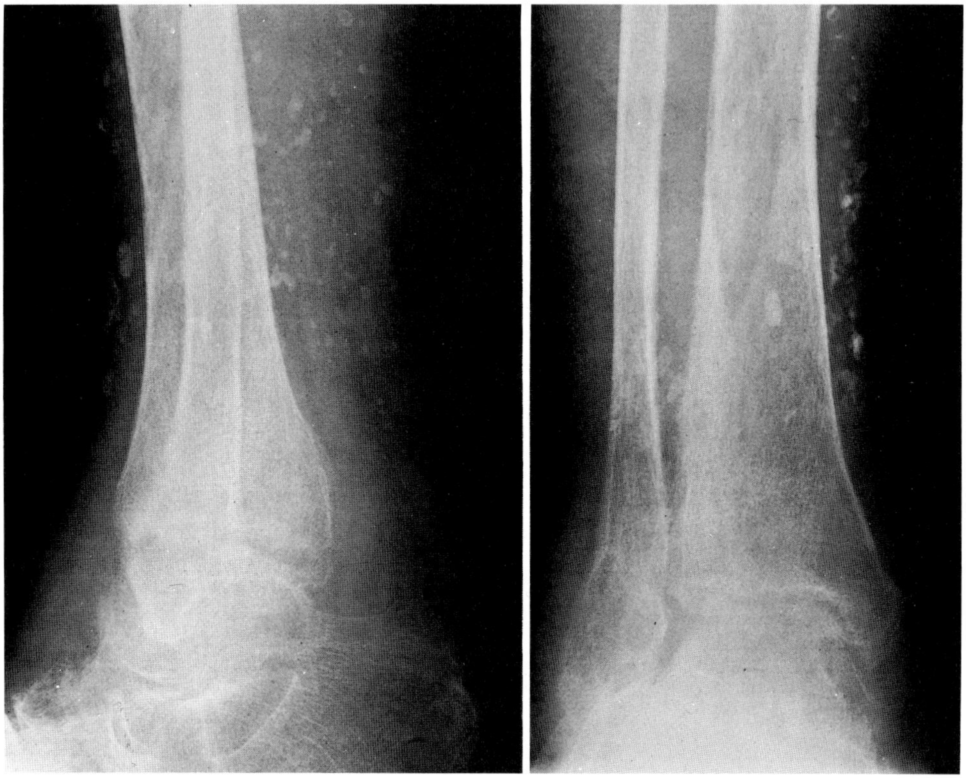

Fig. 45.4 Radiological appearance (a) lateral and (b) anteroposterior, of the ankle and subtalar joint in a patient of 65 who presented with a painful swollen ankle and foot. This was shown on biopsy to be due to tuberculosis.

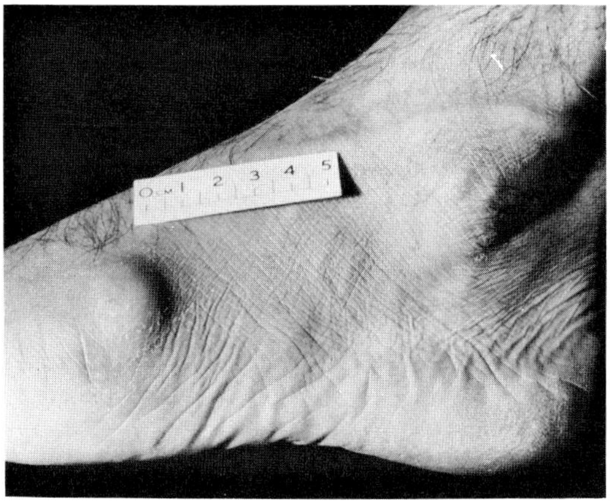

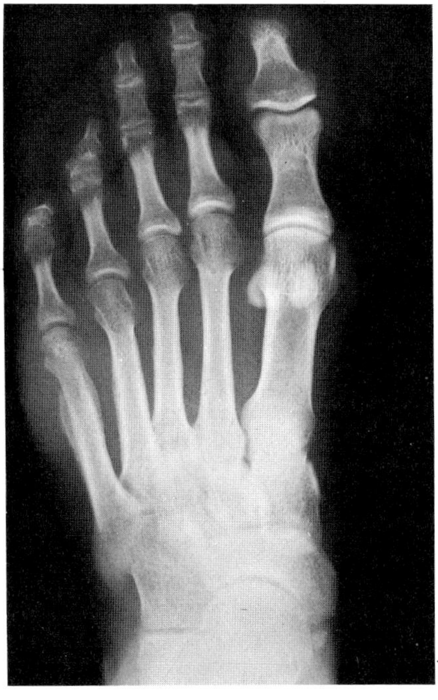

Fig. 45.5 (a) This 27-year-old Kenyan Indian presented with a cystic swelling on the side of his foot: this was aspirated and contained *M. tuberculosis*. (b) This shows the extent of the periostitis in this case of tuberculous dactylitis.

of surgery will depend on the site of the lesion and type of involvement (Griffith, 1975); encouraging results in spiral tuberculosis using a simplified regime (Tuli, 1975) have been reported.

Atypical mycobacteria

These are ubiquitous generally saprophytic organisms that have a low pathogenicity for man: however, they can inject joints, tendons and bursae. Originally this was thought to arise from direct implantation but it is now considered that haematogenous spread is more likely, particularly in the compromised host or with pre-existing joint problems (Girard et al, 1973; Cheatum et al, 1976). In contrast to *Mycobacteria tuberculosis*, atypical mycobacteria not uncommonly cause polyarthritis.

Since many organisms are resistant, or partially so, to the major anti-tuberculous drugs, multiple medications must be tested and often used in combination to obtain a therapeutic response and debridement may be required.

Leprosy

In lepromatous leprosy when there are crops of subacute and inflamed nodules, there may be fever, arthralgia or transient arthritis; the organisms are not usually detected in the joints.

In tuberculoid disease the frequency of bone and joint changes increases with the duration. These changes may be specific, owing to the invasion of the bone by the *Mycobacterium*, or non-specific when they arise from a combination of disturbance of circulation, anaesthesia and pressure, with trauma and secondary infection hastening the destructive process (Paterson, 1955). The specific changes consist of pseudocyst formation in the metaphysis, which can be multiple, and periostitis followed sometimes by bone expansion with decrease in density, thinning of the cortex and rarefaction. The most characteristic non-specific changes are absorption of bones of the bands and feet, probably the result of nerve injury (Riordan, 1960). In the hands it begins in the tufts spreading to the rest of the terminal phalanges, and then other phalanges, while in the feet it often begins in the metatarsal bones and may spread to the tarsal joints leaving the phalanges intact. The patterns of disintegration of the tarsus are well reviewed by Harris & Brand (1966). Charcot joints may also develop in elbows, knees and ankles, secondary to involvement of the central nervous system.

ENTERIC INFECTIONS (see also Ch. 32)

Salmonella

Septic arthritis is a rare complication of salmonella infections although with certain organisms, notably *Cholera suis*, an incidence as great as 2.4% has been reported (Saphra & Wassermann, 1954). Salmonella arthritis tends to occur in infants and young children, and, while it may follow systemic infection, not uncommonly it is the first manifestation of the disease (Carroll et al, 1981). Usually monarticular, any joint can be involved, but particularly the knees, shoulders and hips. The clinical picture is of swelling, often with periarticular oedema, tenderness, pain and limitation of movement, while warmth and redness are not uncommon (David & Black, 1960). It is much rarer in adults. Dual infections have been recorded (Gordon et al, 1949). Both arthritis and osteomyelitis are particularly common in children suffering from sickle cell anaemia (Talbot & Hunt, 1957). The reduction in complement-mediated serum opsonising activity for salmonella may be responsible (Hand & King, 1978). Involvement of vertebrae may cause the so-called 'typhoid spine' (Miller et al, 1963) or cause collapse of vertebrae (Fig. 45.6).

The diagnosis can only be definitely established by culture, although there is usually a high agglutination titre in the blood, and radiologically there may be juxta-articular osteomyelitis. Therapy with systemic antibiotics, of which chloramphenicol is one of the most valuable, may have to be supplemented by intra-articular therapy.

In addition to suppurative arthritis and osteomyelitis, a non-bacterial polyarthritis occurring 5–14 days after infection was reported by Berglof (1963). Among 426 cases of salmonella infection, seen between 1961 and 1962, 12 similar cases were observed (Vartiainen & Hurri, 1964). All these episodes of polyarthritis were in association with *Salmonella typhimurium*, giving an incidence of 2.4% in this type of infection. The arthritis developed some 12 days after the initial illness and frequently resembled rheumatic fever; its duration varied from days to months; conjunctivitis and iridocy-

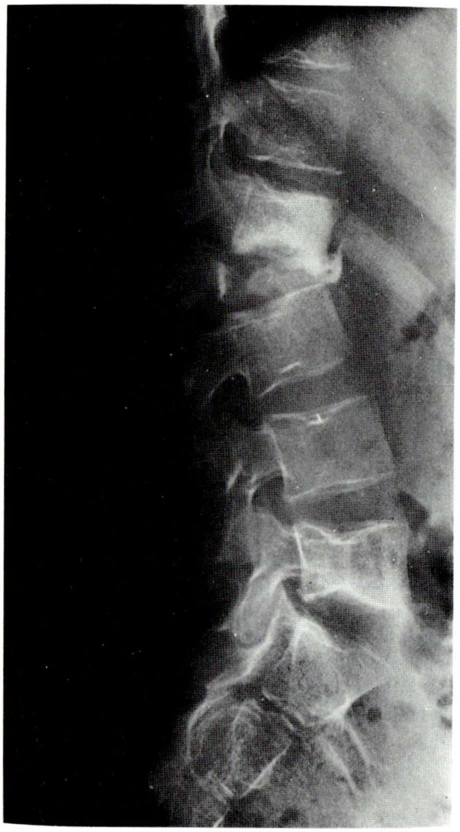

Fig. 45.6 *Salmonella* osteomyelitis of the spine in a boy with sickle cell disease: severe destruction occurred in the spine, already the site of sickle cell changes.

clitis as well as urethritis can occur causing a typical Reiter's syndrome (Ch. 31).

Bacillary dysentery

As with salmonella infections, polyarthritis may develop 2–3 weeks after acute bacillary dysentery. The joints affected are usually knees, elbows, wrists or fingers, the whole picture mimicking rheumatic fever or occasionally a typical Reiter's syndrome develops. These patients also belong to the tissue type HLA-B27 (Aho et al, 1975).

***Yersinia enterocolitica* infection**

The arthritis which follows this mild gastrointestinal illness occurs at an interval 1–21 days after the infection. It can be monarticular but is usually a polyarthritis with knees and ankles being the most commonly involved joints, and is self-limiting; an occasional case is complicated by sacroiliitis (Ahvonen et al, 1969). Although usually reactive, a suppurative oligoarthritis has been seen (Spira & Kabins, 1976). In these cases the organism is detected, but for the others diagnosis is based on rising agglutination titres and occasionally a positive stool culture (Sheldon et al, 1982). Aho et al (1974) noted that 43 of 49 patients with reactive yersinia arthritis belonged to tissue type HLA-B27 while none of those without arthritis carried this tissue type.

***Campylobacter jejuni* enteritis**

This too can cause a reactive arthritis, usually within 2–3 weeks of the diarrhoea (Berden et al, 1979).

Clostridium difficile colitis

Acute arthritis has now been associated with colitis due to *Clostridium difficile* continuing for several weeks after the onset of the diarrhoea (Bolton et al, 1981).

Amoebic dysentery

Numerous extraintestinal symptoms have been attributed to amoebiasis and these include arthralgia, neuralgia, backache and urticaria (Spellberg & Zivin, 1948). 4 cases of polyarthritis with relatively mild gastroinstinal symptoms, but amoebae in the stools and showing regression of their arthritis on the treatment of the amoebiasis, have been reported (Rappaport et al, 1951).

SPIROCHAETAL INFECTIONS

Syphilis

In both congenital and acquired syphilis bone and joint involvement may occur.

Congenital. A number of skeletal manifestations have been described in syphilitic infants. Osteochondritis is is the commonest; this usually presents between the ages of 3 weeks and 3 months with pseudoparalysis of a limb associated with considerable swelling; it may lead to complete epiphyseal separation or fracture of the epiphysis. Much less common lesions consist of metaphysitis, periostitis or osteitis and very rarely dactylitis. In these last types the bone changes are widespread (Caffey, 1939). Other syphilitic stigmata are often mild and the child may be well nourished.

In older children painless effusions in the knees, originally described by Clutton (1886) and subsequently named after him, may occur. These usually arise between the ages of 8 and 16 years and are characterised by symmetrical hydrarthroses of the knees and occasionally elbows. There is little pain or tenderness, and function is not impaired. The condition mimics pyogenic or rheumatoid arthritis and the presence of a raised ESR may make diagnosis difficult (Borrella et al, 1962). Histologically the synovium is vascular, infiltrated with plasma cells and shows lesions suggestive of microgummata (Argen & Dixon, 1963). Other stigmata can usually be found although these may be mild.

Acquired. In the secondary stage, hydrarthrosis of the knee, resembling Clutton's joints, may occur; polyarthritis has been described (Chesney et al, 1924), while the presence of tenosynovitis and periostitis adjacent to a bone may mimic arthritis. In the tertiary stage, bone involvement is not uncommon and the two sites frequently involved are the tibia and the clavicle. The most common lesion is periostitis and this is followed by ossification leading to a characteristic lacey pattern of the bone. Gummatous periostitis may also arise when there is infiltration of the inner layers of the periosteum and subperiosteal connective tissue by small gummata and these cause erosion of the bone. Osteitis diffusa is much less common but can cause marked sclerosis of bone. Gummata arising in the cortex or medullary cavity may spread to cartilage, causing erosion and subsequent joint involvement. This is particularly common in the clavicle where it may cause sternoclavicular involvement (Ehrenpreis, 1957). Joint involvement also results from gummata arising in the soft tissue and infiltrating into the joint or in the synovial membrane itself. Although there may be marked swelling and bone destruction, the local symptoms are slight. As biologically false Wassermann reactions occur not infrequently in diseases such as lupus erythematosus and yaws, it is essential to obtain a positive *Treponema pallidum* complement fixation test (Wilkinson & Sequeira, 1955) before concluding that a lesion is due to syphilis. Neuropathic joint disease (Charcot joints) as a result of syphilis is rare these days. Usually presenting as a monarticular arthritis, in tabes dorsalis the joints most commonly affected are the knee, hip and ankle (Storey, 1964) (Figs 45.7, 45.8); the lumbar and lower dorsal spine can also be involved

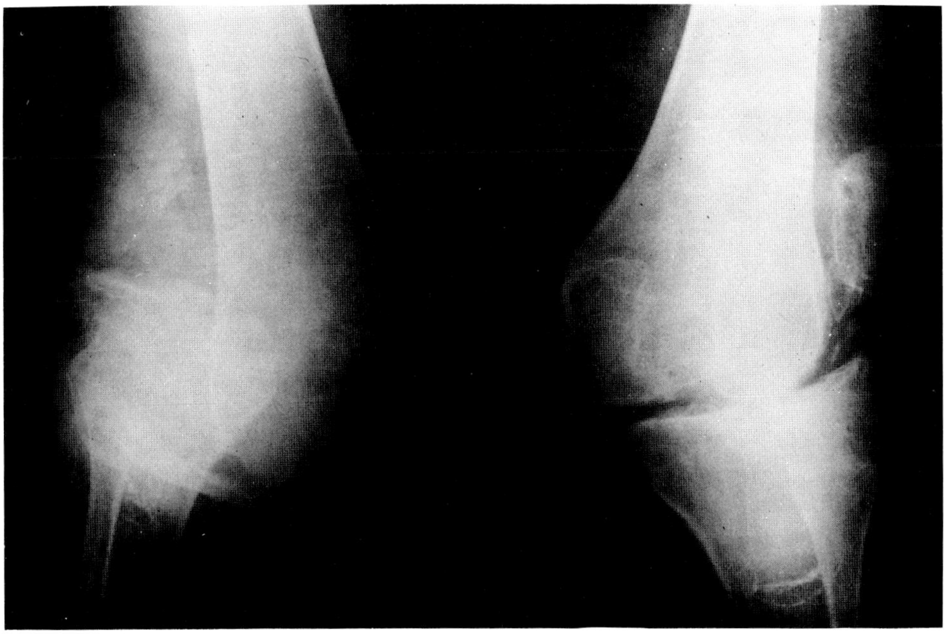

Fig. 45.7 Bilateral Charcot's knee joints in a middle-aged woman, who was unusual in the number of joints involved. Note complete dislocation.

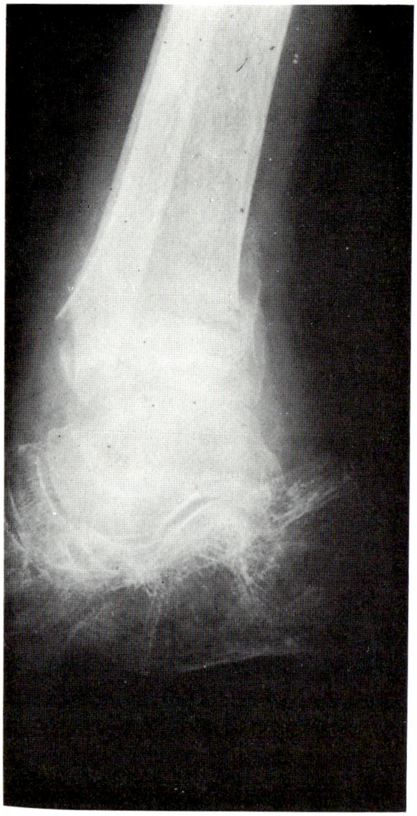

Fig. 45.8 Lateral view of ankle and tarsus in same patient as in Figure 45.7. Note the periostitis of the long bones in addition to the bony proliferation and destruction.

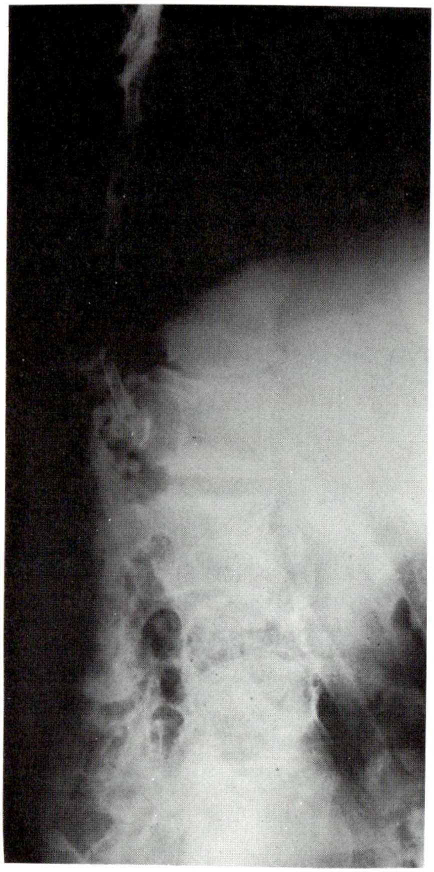

Fig. 45.9 'Charcot's spine'; this is the same patient as illustrated in Figures 45.7 and 45.8.

(Campbell & Doyle, 1954) (Fig. 45.9). The onset of symptoms is insidious with progressive enlargement, effusion and instability, together with coarse crepitus. Other joints can later become involved. Histologically the synovial membrane shows fibrosis with focal calcification (Rodnan et al, 1960). Neuropathic joints are discussed further in Chapter 49.

Yaws

This highly contagious disease, which is restricted to the tropics, is characterised by sores usually on the lower limbs due to infection with *Spirochaeta pertenuis* through a skin break. These are followed by fever, 'rheumatic' pains and the appearance of papules and later bone changes. In the secondary stage there is diffuse subperiosteal new bone fcrmation involving the long bones, particularly the tibia, and this may also give rise to polydactylitis and focal rarefaction of bone (Hackett, 1951). During the growing period involvement of joints and epiphyses may occur while fibrotic nodules in the region of joints can mimic arthritis. In the tertiary stage, which takes from 20–30 years to develop, the most characteristic change is in the lower limbs with 'boomerang' deformity of the the tibia (Goldman & Smith, 1943), which results from the gradual thickening due to periosteal reaction. This tends to be localised and nodular but occasionally there is diffuse osteoperiostitis. Localised cortical destruction and a slow spread of the necrotic process in the cancellous bone and skin leading to ulceration may occur and can give rise to lesions resembling gummata. The distinction between yaws and syphilis is not possible radiologically and as both diseases give a positive Wasserman reaction, a negative *Treponema palli-*

dum immobilisation test is necessary to exclude syphilis. Effective therapy with penicillin, chlortetracycline, oxytetracycline and chloramphenicol in the early stages can prevent mutilating and incapacitating deformities (Furtado, 1957), but seems to have little effect on the gummatous lesions (Cockshott & Davies, 1960).

Rat bite fever

This usually follows a bite from a wild or laboratory rat but has occurred after a bite or minor injury from mouse, cat, dog, weasel or squirrel or following consumption of contaminated food. For many years, there was confusion over the aetiology of this disease, as different workers were able to demonstrate different organisms. There seems no doubt that it may result from infection with *Spirillum minus* or *Actinomyces muris*, the latter being the more frequent (Wilson & Miles, 1955). The disease due to *Actinomyces muris* is also known as 'Haverhill fever'. This is characterised by an incubation period of from 3–10 days followed by the development of a febrile illness with a morbilliform rash, which is occasionally purpuric, and a non-suppurative flitting arthritis. Diagnosis is based on blood culture or agglutination of 1 : 80 or more. The disease tends to be self-limiting, but paroxysms may recur at irregular intervals for weeks or months (Burke et al, 1959). With *Spirillum minus*, the incubation period is longer, varying from 7–21 or more days. Around the site of the wound there is usually redness and swelling while regional lymphadenopathy is marked. The rash may be pustular; joint pains are widespread but the arthritis tends to be monarticular. The illness is more severe than that of Haverhill fever and fatalities have been reported. Diagnosis is again based on culture from blood, pustule or joint. Penicillin is often valuable when a pustular rash is present (Waterson & Wedgewood, 1953).

Leptospirosis

In the group of diseases caused by infection with various leptospira, which are immunologically distinct, the initial manifestations are due to leptospiraemia and characterised by fever and severe myalgia, while arthralgia may occur (Edwards, 1959). Reports of actual arthritis are rare, but one associated with myocarditis due to the *Leptospira pomona* which mimicked rheumatic fever has been recorded (Sutliff et al, 1953).

Lyme arthritis

This is usually a mono- or pauciarticular arthritis affecting particularly children and young adults. It is named after the small community of Lyme, Connecticut where it was first recognised in the 1970s because of the geographical clustering of cases with a peak onset of new cases in the summer and early autumn. The arthritis is often preceded by a characteristic expanding skin lesion known as 'erythema chronicum migrans' which arises from the bite of *Ixodes dammini* (Steere & Malawista, 1979). A spirochete has now been recovered from the leading edge of the skin lesion and from the blood in some early cases; it has not, however, been recovered from the joints (Steere et al, 1983b). Similar spirochetes have been recovered from *I. ticinus*. Malaise, fatigue, chills, fever and headache sometimes associated with a stiff neck, are common symptoms associated with the onset of the skin lesions. Backache, myalgia, nausea and vomiting are also not uncommon. These symptoms, however, usually only last for a few days. In the absence of a skin lesion, which is only seen in three-quarters, or systemic features, diagnosis can be difficult, as the disorder closely mimics pauciarticular onset juvenile arthritis or seronegative asymmetric arthritis of adults. The knee is the most commonly affected joint followed by other large joints and occasionally by small joints of the hands and feet. In the majority the arthritis remains monarticular or pauciarticular but some patients do have migratory joint symptoms. Characteristically the joint swelling can last for a week or so but it may persist for many months and most patients have recurrent acute attacks usually separated by longer periods of remission. In addition to arthritis some patients have developed neurological abnormalities which consisted of meningoencephalitis, cranial nerve palsies and motor or sensory radiculopathy within several months of the skin lesions (Steere et al, 1977). Similarly myocardial conduction abnormalities have also been noted in a few patients months after the original skin lesions. Those patients with severe and prolonged illness appear to have genetic differences from the overall population with DR2 increased and DR7 decreased (Steere et al, 1983c). During the acute phase of arthritis the ESR is usually high; cryoprecipitates have been detected in the serum of some patients while immune complexes are common. Tests for rheumatoid factor and anti-nuclear factor are negative. Synovial biopsies have shown synovial hyperplasia, vascular proliferation and a heavy infiltration of mononuclear cells, the whole picture looking like that of rheumatoid arthritis (Steere et al, 1977). Treatment with tetracycline, then penicillin, then erythromycin, in this order of efficacy seems to be curative and, given early, prevents late complications (Steere et al, 1983a).

Rocky mountain spotted fever

This presents with fever, arthralgia, myalgia, swelling of the hands and feet and rash which appears first on the extremities. It is a rickettsial vasculitis carried by a tick *Dermacentor andersoni*. Athough originally reported from the Rocky Mountain area in the United States, it now appears all over that country. Diagnosis depends on recognition of the clinical pattern of illness and subsequent demonstration of rising serum titres against *Proteus* OX-19 antigen. Treatment with tetracycline needs to be instituted promptly as this is a serious illness (Brown, 1981).

VIRAL INFECTIONS

The occurrence of polyarthritis has been recognised with the increasing frequency in diseases known to be viral in origin as well as in those in which a viral aetiology is suspected. Thus articular pain and swelling occasionally precedes infectious hepatitis (Onion et al, 1971; Fernandez & McCarty, 1971). Upper respiratory infections including influenza (Price et al, 1963) may occasionally have arthritic manifestations. In one of our cases where there was a rise in titre to parainfluenza A, the synovial fluid contained large mononuclear cells such as those described in rubella by Chambers & Bywaters (1963). Other cases with arthropathy accompanied by a mild respiratory infection, an absolute lymphocytosis and cold agglutinins in the blood have been shown to have rising titres to syncitial virus. In rubella, rheumatic symptoms were present in some 15% of 300 patients reviewed by Bennet & Copeman (1940). These varied from transient muscle pain lasting about 48 hours through an illness suggesting rheumatic fever to more persistent polyarthritis. Since then there have been a number of cases reported so that an illness pattern has gradually emerged (Lee et al, 1960; Yanez et al, 1966).

Rubella arthritis usually occurs in the young adult female but has been recorded as early as 14 months; although characteristically developing within a few days after the rash, it can precede the rash or occur without obvious rash. The joints most commonly affected are those of the hands, knees and ankles but any may be involved; occasionally the arthritis can be migratory. Carpal tunnel compression is not infrequent and tendon lesions of the hands may cause stiffness and difficulty in bending the fingers (Lee et al, 1960). The arthritis is usually self-limiting, lasting from 2–28 days but, particularly in older patients, symptoms such as stiffness may persist for considerably longer. Diagnosis is based on a history of contact, rash, post-auricular and occipital lymphadenopathy, typical blood changes, which consist of 'turk' and 'plasma' cells which are present in most cases for about 10 days and may persist for up to 6 weeks (Hillenbrand, 1956), and rising titre of rubella antibodies. Rubella virus may be detected in peripheral blood lymphocytes and synovial fluid if appropriately looked for. Vaccination against rubella may be associated with a polyarthritis; the incidence of this may well depend on the type of vaccine used (Spruance & Smith, 1971). Recurrent episodes of arthritis or arthralgia are not uncommon after vaccination and it has been possible to isolate the rubella virus from the peripheral lymphocytes of a patient two years after vaccination (Chantler et al, 1981).

The synovial fluid protein content is low and the characteristic feature is the sparsity of polymorphs and predominance of mononuclear cells (Chambers & Bywaters, 1963). Histologically this is a non-specific synovitis. The virus has been isolated from an involved joint (Hildebrandt & Maassab, 1966; Denman, 1974). Less specific findings are a moderate rise in erythrocyte sedimentation rate and neutropenia. As with other viral infections, a transiently positive latex test may occur (Johnson & Hall, 1958) but the sheep cell agglutination test is negative while a rise in antibody titre to smooth muscle is common. There is no increase in incidence of HLA-B27 in rubella arthropathy (Robintaille et al, 1976). As the disorder is self-limiting, symptomatic therapy with salicylate is usually all that is necessary, but in cases with severe tendon involvement or carpal tunnel compression steroids may be valuable (Chambers & Bywaters, 1963).

The occurrence of arthritis with *mumps* is well recognised; thus Masondieu (1924) recorded an incidence of 0.44% in 1334 cases. As with other complications in mumps this usually affects young adult males. Occurring some 10–14 days after the parotitis, it is characteristically a migratory polyarthralgia or polyarthritis affecting particularly large joints, but the hands and feet can be involved. It mimics rheumatic fever as it can be associated with serositis, particularly pericarditis or systemic 'Still's' disease in both child and adult (Gordon & Lanter, 1983). Myalgia is also well documented (Gold et al, 1968; Ghosh & Reddy, 1973). While it is self-limiting, lasting from a few days to several weeks and resolving without residua, during the acute phase there may be a rise in the erythrocyte sedimentation rate to more than 100 mm/h (Appelbaum et al, 1952), and a polymorph leucocytosis in blood and synovial fluid. Positive complement fixation tests in the serum are recorded in definite cases (Lass & Shephard, 1961; Caranasos & Felker, 1967). Treatment is symptomatic. In 1970 Ward & Bishop drew attention to a transient synovitis of the knee thought to be due to *chickenpox*, although the virus was not isolated from the joint. Rarely polyarthritis of a migratory type has also been noted (Friedman & Naveh, 1971; Mulhern et al, 1971).

In *adenoviral arthritis*, several days after the onset of fever, coryza and pharyngitis, there is the development of a maculopapular rash and arthritis. These last can be confused with rheumatic fever and systemic onset juvenile arthritis. The disease tends to be self-limiting, remitting over 2–12 weeks. Adenovirus 7 is the most common type; serum cryoprecipitates containing IgA, IgM, IgG_1, IgG_2, C3, C4 and intact adenovirus virion can be detected, as can similar complexes in the synovial fluid (Utsinger, 1977).

A transient, often migratory arthritis affecting particularly the PIP and MCP joints can occur as part of the prodrome of *acute hepatitis* in adults (Inman, 1982). Its incidence has varied from 4–25% in various series (Alarcon & Townes, 1973; Schumacher & Gall, 1974). It is frequently associated with urticaria, and various other erythematous rashes. It tends to persist for some 2–3 weeks, usually subsiding as the jaundice appears but if jaundice remains absent the joint symptoms may persist throughout the illness. About 80% of the patients have hepatitis B antigen at the time of arthritis. A small proportion have positive tests for rheumatoid factor and anti-nuclear antibodies may be present. It has been suggested that it represents a form of serum sickness, with the Australian antigen providing the necessary antigen for stimulation of antibody production, complex formation, complement fixation and tissue damage (Onion et al, 1971).

The *arboviruses*, which have a vertebrate host, usually a mammal, are transmitted to man by a mosquito, tick or sandfly. A variety of clinical disease patterns are recognised, with the most common manifestations fever, arthritis or arthralgia and rash; the three most commonly associated with arthritis are the Ross River virus, Chikungunya and O'Nyong (Haddow et al, 1960).

Since Nimmo (1928) first reported an epidemic of polyarthritis in Narrangera, New South Wales, outbreaks of similar character have been reported from other parts of Australia (Halliday & Horan, 1943). The term 'epidemic polyarthritis' was coined by Dowling (1946), to describe those outbreaks where the clinical and epidemiological features suggested these were a single disease entity, and it is now usually referred to as Ross River virus which has been shown to be an alpha virus of the togaviridae family (Doherty, 1972). Ross River virus antigen has been detected by specific immunofluorescence in monocytes and macrophages from synovial fluid early in the disease (Fraser et al, 1981). It affects young adults and the incubation period appears to be 10 days. The characteristic features are malaise, fever and myalgia followed 12–24 hours later by a maculopapular or urticarial rash, lymphadenopathy and arthritis. This is usually polyarticular with periarticular thickening and tenderness and occasionally effusions in the joints, while swelling of flexor tendon sheaths has been observed. It is transient, settling in about 2 weeks, but persistent pain and some stiffness may remain for up to 2–3 months.

The name 'Chikungunya' has been given to a dengue-like illness observed in Tansania and Asia in which there was such severe joint pain that patients were completely immobilised. In the acute stage, fever and an itchy maculopapular eruption are common. Actual joint inflammation was only found in a small proportion of patients but joint pain might persist for some months (Robinson, 1955; Carey et al, 1969). The causative virus has been isolated from man and mosquitoes (Ross, 1956) and belongs to the arbovirus group.

'O'Nyong-Nyong' is the name given to an epidemic disease in East Africa, characterised by a sudden onset of fever associated with severe joint pain, headache, conjunctivitis, rash and lymphadenopathy; here also there is a tendency for the patients to suffer from protracted joint pain (Shore, 1961). A group 'A' arbovirus, similar but distinct from the one described in Chikungunya, has been isolated from the serum of patients in acute stages and also from mosquitoes (Haddow et al, 1960).

Three types of bone and joint lesions have been described in *smallpox* (Cockshott & MacGregor, 1958). The first is a necrotic non-suppurative osteomyelitis probably due to the smallpox virus. This usually involves the diaphysial ends of long bones destroying the epiphyseal lines and causing deformities by destruction or premature fusion of epiphyses. The second is a suppurative arthritis which is thought to be due to secondary infection of a pustule. The third is a non-suppurative arthritis occurring some 10–28 days after the initial infection. This last tends to affect children of both sexes under 10 years of age; the severity of the smallpox appears to be unimportant but the child is usually malnourished. Not infrequently more than one joint is involved, and when this is so involvement is usually symmetrical, the elbows being the commonest site, then the wrists, hands, ankles, feet and knees. There may be an interval of one or two days between successive joint involvement. The first sign is swelling and this is followed by pain, difficulty in movement and local tenderness; the swelling is primarily soft tissue but there may be an effusion. It is usual to get a low-grade fever and slight leucocytosis but no real toxaemia. Secondary infection is not uncommon, which leads to further joint damage. In the absence of secondary infection the lesions tend to recover in a few months but leave behind limitation of movement and growth abnormalities. The joint fluid is sterile but elementary bodies may be found in it (Cockshott & MacGregor, 1958). Vaccination against smallpox has been recorded as being complicated by bone involvement (Cochran et al, 1963) and by arthritis (Silby et al, 1965). This was a 65-year-old woman who 10 days after vaccination developed an acute arthritis of the right knee from which the vaccinia virus was isolated.

Infectious mononucleosis is due to infection with Epstein–Barr virus (Henle & Henle, 1972) and occurs predominantly in late teenage and early adolescent life; it is characterised by irregular fever with a sore throat, a blotchy rash, lymphadenopathy and splenomegaly. Numerous complications have been recorded including arthralgia, arthritis (Ray et al, 1982) and cardiovascular involvement (Bernstein, 1940). In acute cases the sedimentation rate is frequently raised so that rheumatic fever, systemic juvenile chronic arthritis or rheumatoid arthritis may be simulated. In two of our cases in whom biopsies of affected joints were performed the synovial membrane showed a subacute synovitis with no specific features. The arthritis affected the knees in both, an ankle in one and a wrist in the other. This resolved completely over a few weeks. However, we have also had a case with recurrent episodes of fever and synovitis.

Atypical mononuclear cells are found early in the peripheral blood, the Paul Bunnell test is usually positive and rise in titres against EB virus allows a confident diagnosis to be made. The differential agglutination test shows agglutination of the non-sensitised as well as the sensitised cells and the latex test is negative, so there should be no confusion with rheumatoid arthritis. Particularly in childhood, *cytomegalic virus* infection closely mimicks the clinical features of Epstein–Barr viral infections, including arthritis. A transient arthritis with *Echo virus type 6* has been reported (Sanford & Sulkin, 1959) and it is likely that enteroviral infections may induce arthritis more commonly than has been reported. A febrile systemic illness with seronegative arthritis may be caused by *Coxsackie B* infection (Hurst et al, 1983).

Erythema infectiosum. Epidemics of this mild exanthematous illness are not uncommon in children usually in the winter months and may be associated with a transient arthritis of large joints at the time of the fever and rash (Ager et al, 1966). Erythema infectiosum has now been shown to be due to a parvovirus, an organism of considerable current interest in rheumatology. It is thought to cause transient or more persistent arthritis in adults, the relationship of which to rheumatoid arthritis is under scrutiny.

Cat-scratch fever develops 1 or 2 weeks after a scratch by a cat, regional lymphadenitis persisting for a few weeks or months. Complications include erythema nodosum (Greer & Keefer, 1951), sterile osteolytic bone lesions (Collipp & Koch, 1959), and soft tissue masses (Laskin & Potenza, 1971).

Behçet's syndrome is described in Chapter 49.

FUNGAL INFECTIONS

Infections with fungi may be primary, secondary in illnesses such as lymphoma or SLE (Sieving et al, 1975) or in any other disorder requiring immunosuppression, or as complications during the treatment of bacterial infections with broad spectrum antibiotics. The majority of fungi are acquired from soil or organic dust; some have a worldwide distribution while others occur only in specific geographic areas. However, with the increase in travel in recent years it is no longer sufficient to consider these disorders only in endemic areas. Arthritis may arise directly from haematogenous spread or be secondary to infection in the bone adjacent to the joint. Radiologically this can be confused with tuberculosis, syphilis, osteomyelitis or malignant metastases. The diagnosis of any particular infection is based on the culture of the fungus from the infected bone, synovial fluid or membrane. Skin tests and serological complement fixation tests may be useful as a guide, but considerable cross-reactivity occurs. In the treatment of fungal infections, despite its toxicity, amphotericin B is extremely valuable. It should be given in a dosage of 50 mg intravenously in saline over 6 hours twice weekly for a minimum of 1 month. The possibility of amphotericin B intra-articularly as well as local surgery will also need consideration (Aidem, 1968). The use of oral 5 fluorocytosine in some cases is helpful (Harder & Hermans, 1975). The place of ketaconazole is still under study (Lancet Editorial, 1982; Dismukes et al, 1983).

Aspergillosis is found primarily in the lungs; bone and joint involvement have been recorded in the disseminated type (Tobler & Minder, 1954; Cawley, 1947) and this can lead to serious bone destruction.

Bone involvement with *Actinomyces bovis* is secondary to spread from a soft tissue focus. The bone most frequently involved is the mandible, while ribs, ilium, phalanges and humeri can be affected. Vertebral involvement is due to extension from mediastinal or retroperitoneal infection, and while several vertebrae are usually involved, the discs are spared (Cope, 1951). Radiologically there is dense bony sclerosis extending into the bodies and surrounding many small abscess cavities, producing a honeycomb appearance (Baylin & Wear, 1953). Occasionally long dense spurs may be seen to arise from the vertebral bodies, the whole process being one of sclerosis.

Therapy consists of penicillin in high dosage for a long period of time (Brett, 1951); treatment with tetracycline and neomycin have also been reported as successful but penicillin is still the drug of choice. Removal of damaged tissue may be required. Amphotericin B is usually reserved for those patients who do not respond to antibiotics.

The causative organism of North American blastomycosis, *Blastomyces dermatitidis*, lives primarily in the Ohio and Mississippi river valleys and in the middle Atlantic states. It gains entrance through the lungs or abraded skin and spreads by lymphatic or haematogenous routes. It may be either a localised cutaneous or a systemic disorder involving lungs, skin, bone and joints. With lung infection, erythema nodosum may be a presenting feature (Smith et al, 1955). Bone involvement can be seen in up to 50% (Cherniss & Waisbren, 1956). This is characteristically an osteolytic lesion which is sharply delineated from the adjacent normal bone. Any bone may be involved, especially vertebrae, ribs, tibia and tarsi; extensive vertebral destruction with collapse of vertebral bodies mimics tuberculosis (Baylin & Wear, 1953). Involvement of joints may be due to direct extension when the knees are commonly affected or due to haematogenous spread (Bayer et al, 1979a). Sanders (1967) noted arthritis was a prominent component of the illness in 9 of 74 patients, 6 of these presenting as a monarticular arthritis without evidence of bone change. Diagnosis is established by the finding of the organisms in the synovial fluid but a positive immunodiffusion test present in 80% suggests current infection. Amphotericin B is probably the drug of choice in treatment still (Fountain, 1973).

Coccidiomycosis results from infection with *Coccidioides immitis* and arises only in people who have visited or resided in an endemic area such as the south-western United States, Mexico and South America. Following the inhalation of the fungus there is an acute but benign illness which is characterised by the development of fever, malaise, generalised aching and sometimes conjunctivitis. In about one third of cases, after 8–15 days an acute arthritis develops which can persist for a month before resolving without residua (Dickson & Gifford, 1938). Erythema nodosum may also develop but not necessarily in association with arthritis.

A proportion of patients go on to a chronic disseminated form when arthritis may occur secondary to bone infection or alone. Bone involvement is seen in up to 20% — usually affecting the ends of long bones, particularly the tibial tubercle and ankle malleoli. In the majority only a single site is involved; if there are multiple bone lesions this suggests rapid dissemination and a poor prognosis. The most commonly affected joint is the knee, then the ankle and less commonly the foot, elbow and wrist. Usually, but not always it is monarticular (Bayer & Guze, 1979). The characteristic picture is of swollen red joints with nodular lesions which break down to form discharging sinuses; it can present as a non-specific chronic synovitis (Greenman & Campbell, 1975). Distinction from tuberculosis can be difficult as both processes cause a destructive lesion in bone and may have pulmonary involvement; in coccidiomycosis the lesion tends to be more rapidly destructive; it has also been reported as mimicking sarcoidosis (Shields, 1959). Diagnosis is made by identification of the organism; the characteristic spherules are best seen after digestion with 20% potassium hydroxide. A positive coccidioidin skin test may occur from past as well as present infection. A complement fixation test and an immunodiffusion test may also be helpful. Treatment consists of antifungal agents of which amphotericin B, systemically with or without local intra-articular therapy together with suitable debridgment has proved valuable (Gehlback et al, 1973).

Cryptococcosis (torulosis) results from infection by *Cryptococcus neoformans*, which has a worldwide distribution and shows a predilection for the central nervous system, skin and lungs. Bone involvement is unusual except when there is haematogenous dissemination but occasionally it may be implanted directly into the bone as in dactylitis following injury (Littman & Zimmerman, 1956). No bone is immune but there appears to be particular predilection for bony prominences, skull and vertebrae. The lesion is a destructive one which progresses slowly and insidiously with much soft tissue swelling. Secondary joint involvement is rare. Amphotericin B alone or with oral 5 fluorocytosine are valuable in treatment (Bayer et al, 1980).

Infection with *Histoplasma capsulatum*, *histoplasmosis*, is relatively common and usually benign, with the pulmonary system frequently involved. The acute pulmonary manifestations may be complicated by erythema nodosum (Little & Steigman, 1960). In the chronic stage bone and joint involvement is rare, but Key & Large (1942) reported involvement of a knee joint which clinically closely resembled tuberculosis; the diagnosis was not made until after amputation when it was found that the synovial membrane was a mass of granulation tissue with many phagocytic cells which contained *Histoplasma capsulatum*. In contrast, infection with *Histoplasma duboisin*, found in West Africa and characterised by granulomatous lesions in the skin causing papules and ulcers, is not infrequently associated with arthritis (Cockshott & Lucas, 1964).

Madura foot (Mycetoma pedis) results from invasion of the foot and much less commonly the hand (Linscheid & Dobyns, 1975) by filamentous fungi and occurs widely in the tropics and subtropics. It presents as a painless swelling of the affected part which may be ill-defined or nodular, but eventually pale nodules develop which break down to form sinuses. The causative fungus can be found in the discharge from the sinus (Abbot, 1956). Radiologically the characteristic picture is of involvement of the second row of the tarsal bones and bases of the adjacent metatarsals. Initially there is loss of definition followed by erosion of the cortex and associated with a ragged periosteal reaction which may resemble the bristles of a brush or palisade: in addition there is sclerosis of the affected spongiosa, osteoporosis distal to the involved bones and in contrast to bacterial infection an absence of true sequestra (Davies, 1958). Therapy with an appropriate antibiotic over a prolonged period is desirable together with appropriate surgical management. Recently the culture of *Petriellidium boydis* from joints and its successful treatment by amphotericin B and also ketaconazole has been reported (Haapasaari et al, 1982).

The first case of hydrarthrosis of the knee due to infection with *Cephalosporium* was recorded by Ward et al (1961), while arthritis due to *nocardia* is now being documented (Rao et al, 1981).

Although numerous types of *Sporotrichii* have been recognised it is thought that only *schenckii* is pathogenic for man. *Sporotrichosis* is a subacute infection, usually limited to the skin and subcutaneous tissues but extracutaneous dissemination can occur. Multifocal disease tends to occur only in patients who are immunocompromised. Involvement of bones and joints is usually due to blood-borne dissemination, but may arise by direct extension from cutaneous or subcutaneous lesions (Mikkelsen et al, 1957). Arthritis is uncommon (Bayer et al, 1979) and when it occurs the lesions tend to be destructive, and histologically reveal granulomatous formation. Occasionally there is no obvious primary source as in the case of chronic synovitis of the knee reported by Webster & Willander (1957). The condition must be differentiated from villonodular synovitis and tuberculosis, as well as more common forms of chronic synovitis. Diagnosis is based on a culture of *Sporothrix schenckii* — which is often easier from synovial tissue than fluid. Treatment is with amphotericin B and local debridement if necessary.

Candida infections tend to occur when the host response is depressed as in prolonged antibiotic, corticosteroid and immunosuppressive therapy (Bayer & Guze, 1978). It is tending to increase as more severely ill patients are maintained (Toala et al, 1970): thus Noyes et al (1973) reported a patient who had undergone prolonged intravenous feeding after partial gastrectomy, who developed pain, swelling and loss of movement of one knee followed by pain in the hip; *Candida albicans* was isolated from the knee. While *Candida albicans* is the most frequent offender, *C. tropicalis* and *C. guillermondi* have also been isolated from infected joints. Clinical arthritis has followed documented fungal septicaemia by as long as 12 weeks (Murray et al, 1976). It has also been recognised in a patient following intra-articular corticosteroid (Koga et al, 1968). Amphotericin B or 5 fluorocytosine are the drugs of choice; synovectomy may be required if drug therapy and repeated aspirations fail.

Lymphogranuloma venereum which affects both sexes and all races may be complicated by arthritis (Wright & Logan, 1939). This is polyarticular, showing a predilection for the knees, ankles and wrists. Occasionally it is acute and migratory mimicking rheumatic fever, but more commonly it pursues a chronic course with a tendency to recurrent effusions in the joints which may persist for weeks or months with little or no destruction of cartilage or bone. The synovial fluid is sterile: the Frei cutaneous test is always positive (Dawson & Boots, 1939). The infective agent is now classified with psittacosis as a distinct biological group (Horsfall & Tamm, 1968).

Infection after total joint replacement

The increased use of total prosthetic joint replacement in rheumatoid arthritis particularly, but also in osteoarthrosis, ankylosing spondylitis and systemic lupus erythematosus, carries with it the potential risk of infection. This has varied in different series from negligible (0.4%) (Charnley, 1972) to serious (11%).

It appears to be of three types. The first is the immediate postoperative, which is obvious from the early days. This is minimised by scrupulous aseptic theatre techniques and by an antibiotic cover commencing with premedication and continuing for 2–14 days (Pollard et al, 1979). The second is when the patient heals, albeit slowly, and has no or only minimal discomfort at the site of surgery; months or years later an abscess develops in the neighbourhood of the joint or the prosthesis loosens and infection is found at reoperation. The third is that which occurs at varying intervals from months to (in our experience) eight years after successful surgery. There may be a clear-cut story of preceding infection elsewhere in the body, but this is not always the case. The recognition of this type is very important as immediate prompt treatment with antibiotics and continuation for 6–12 months may allow retention of the prosthesis. For the other two types, although irrigation, drainage and prolonged antibiotic therapy are employed, the vast majority will require removal of the prosthesis.

REFERENCES

Abbott P 1956 Mycetoma in Sudan. Transactions of the Royal Society of Tropical Medicine and Hygiene 50: 11–30

Ackerman A B, Miller R C, Shapiro L 1965 Gonococcemia and its cutaneous manifestations. Archives of Dermatology 91: 227–232

Adams E M, Hustead S, Rubin P, Wagner R, Gewurz A, Graziano F M 1983 Absence of the seventh component of Complement in a patient with chronic meningococcaemia presenting as vasculitis. Annals of Internal Medicine 99: 35–38

Ager E A, Chin T D Y, Poland J D 1966 Epidemic erythema infectiosum. New England Journal of Medicine 275: 1326–1331

Aho K, Ahvonen P, Lassus A, Sievers K, Tiilikainen A 1974 HL-A 27 in reactive arthritis: A study of Yersinia arthritis and Reiter's disease. Arthritis and Rheumatism 17: 521–526

Ahvonen P, Sievers K, Aho K 1969 Arthritis associated with Yersinia enterocolitica infection. Acta Rheumatologica Scandinavica 15: 232–253

Aidem H P 1968 Intra-articular amphotericin B in the treatment of coccidioidal synovitis of the knee. Journal of Bone and Joint Surgery 50A: 1663–1668

Alarcon G S, Townes A S 1973 Arthritis in viral hepatitis: report of two cases and review of the literature. Johns Hopkins Medical Journal 132: 1–15

Appelbaum E, Kohn J, Steinman R E,Shearn M A 1952 Mumps arthritis. Archives of Internal Medicine 90: 217–223

Argen R J, Dixon A St J 1963 Clutton's joints with keratitis and periostitis. Arthritis and Rheumatism 6: 341–348

Argen R J, Wilson C H, Wood P 1966 Suppurative arthritis. Archives of Internal Medicine 117: 661–666

Backman A, Wallgren E I 1954 On tuberculosis of bones and joints of B C G vaccinated children. Acta Paediatrica 43: 252–258

Bailey H L, Gabriel M D, Hodgson A R 1972 TB of the spine in children Operative findings and results in 100 consecutive patients treated by removal of the lesion and anterior grafting. Journal of Bone and Joint Surgery 54A: 1633–1657

Bayer A S, Guze L B 1978 Fungal arthritis I. Candida arthritis. Seminars in Arthritis and Rheumatism 8: 142–150

Bayer A S, Guze L B 1979 Fungal arthritis II. Coccydial synovitis. Seminars in Arthritis and Rheumatism 8: 200–211

Bayer A S, Choi C, Tillman V B, Guze L B 1980 Fungal arthritis V. Cryptococcal and histoplasma arthritis. Seminars in Arthritis and Rheumatism 9: 218–227

Bayers A S, Scott V J, Guze L B 1979a Fungal arthritis III. Sporotrichal arthritis. Seminars in Arthritis and Rheumatism 9: 66–79

Bayer A S, Scott V J, Guze L B 1979b Fungal arthritis IV. Blastomycotic arthritis. Seminars in Arthritis and Rheumatism 9: 145–151

Baylin G J, Wear J M 1953 Blastomycosis and actinomycosis of spine. American Journal of Roentgenology 69:395

Bennet R A, Copeman W S C 1940 Notes on rubella, with special reference to certain rheumatic sequelae. British Medical Journal 1: 924–926

Berden J H, Muytjens H L, van de Putte L B 1979 Reactive arthritis associated with Campylobacter jejuni enteritis. British Medical Journal 1: 380–381

Berglof F E 1963 Arthritis and intestinal infection. Acta Rheumatologica Scandinavica 9: 141–149

Bernstein A 1940 Infectious mononucleosis. Medicine 19: 85–159

Bolton R P, Wood G M, Losowsky M A 1981 Acute arthritis associated with Clostridium difficile colitis. British Medical Journal 283: 1023–1024

Borella L, Goobar J E, Clark G M 1962 Synovitis of the knee joints in late congenital syphillis. Journal of the American Medical Association 180: 190–192

Borella L, Goobar J E, Summit R L, Clark G M 1963 Septic arthritis in childhood. Journal of Pediatrics 62: 742–747

Borenstein D G, Gibbs C A, Jacobs R P 1983 Gas liquid chromatographic analysis of synovial fluid; volatile short chain fatty acids in septic arthritis. Annals of Rheumatic Diseases 42: 362–367

Brandt K D, Cathcart E S, Cohen A S 1974 Gonococcal arthritis: clinical features correlated with blood, synovial fluid and genitourinary cultures. Arthritis and Rheumatism 17: 503–510

Brett M S 1951 Advanced actinomycosis of the spine treated with pencillin and streptomycin. Journal of Bone and Joint Surgery 33B: 215–220

Brown R T 1981 Rocky Mountain Spotted fever. Journal of Current Adolescent Medicine 3: 17–21

Burke W A, Kwong O, Halpern R 1959 Rat bite fever due to Streptobacillus moniliformis: a report of two cases. California Medicine 91: 356–358

Caffey J 1939 Syphilis of skeleton in early infancy; non-specificity of many of the roentgenographic changes. American Journal of Roentgenology 42:637

Campbell D J, Doyle J O 1954 Tabetic Charcot's spine: report of 8 cases. British Medical Journal 1: 1018–1020

Caranasos G J, Felker J R 1967 Mumps arthritis. Archives of Internal Medicine 119: 394–398

Carey D E, Myers R M, de Ranitz C M, Jadva M, Reuden R 1969 The 1964 Chikungunya epidemic at Vallore, South India. Transactions of the Royal Society of Tropical Medicine and Hygiene 64: 434–445

Carroll W L et al 1981 Spectrum of salmonella associated arthritis. Pediatrics 68: 717–720
Cawley E P 1947 Aspergillosis and aspergilli; report of unique case of the disease. Archives of Internal Medicine 80: 423–434
Chambers R J, Bywaters E G L 1963 Rubella synovitis. Annals of the Rheumatic Diseases 22: 263–268
Chantler J K, Ford D K, Tingle A J 1981 Rubella associated arthritis. Rescue or rubella virus from peripheral blood lymphocytes two years post vaccination. Infection and Immununity 32: 1274–1280
Charnley J 1972 Post-operarive infection after total hip replacement with special reference to air contamination in the operative room. Clinical Orthopaedics and Related Research 87: 167–187
Chartier Y, Martin W J, Kelly P J, 1959 Bacterial arthritis: experience in the treatment of 77 patients. Annals of Internal Medicine 50: 1462–147
Cheatum D E, Hudman Y, Jones S R 1976 Chronic arthritis due to Mycobacterium intracellular. Arthritis and Rheumatism 19: 777–778
Cherniss E I, Waisbren B A 1956 North American blastomycosis: A clinical study of 40 cases. Annals of Internal Medicine 44: 105–123
Chesney A M, Kemp J E, Resnik W H 1924 Syphilitic arthritis with oseinophilia; recovery of T pallidum from the synovial fluid. Bulletin of the Johns Hopkins Hospital 35: 235–239
Clutton H H 1886 Symmetrical synovitis of the knee in hereditary syphilis. Lancet 1: 391–393
Cochran W, Connolly J H, Thompson J D 1963 Bone involvement after vaccination against smallpox. British Medical Journal 2: 285–287
Cockshott W P, Davies A G M 1960 Tumoural gummatous yaws. Journal of Bone and Joint Surgery 42B: 785–787
Cockshott W P, Lucas A O 1964 Histoplasmosis duboisii. Quarterly Journal of Medicine 33: 223–238
Cockshott W P, MacGregnor M 1958 Osteomyelitis variolosa. Quarterly Journal of Medicine 27: 369–387
Collipp P J, Koch R 1959 Cat-scratch fever associated with an osteolytic lesion. New England Journal of Medicine 260: 278–280
Cope V Z 1951 Actinomycosis of bone with special reference to infection of the vertebral column. Journal of Bone and Joint Surgery 33B: 205–214
Coventry M B, Ivins J C, Nichols D R, Weed L A 1949 Infection of hip by Brucella suis. Journal of the American Medical Association 141: 320–325
Cremin B J, Fisher R M, Levinsohn M W 1970 Multiple bone tuberculosis in the young. British Journal of Radiology 43: 638–645
Dans P E, Rothenberg R, Holmes K K 1977 Gonoccal serology; how soon how useful and how much. Journal of Infectious Diseases 135: 330–334
David J R, Black R L 1960 Salmonella arthritis. Medicine 39: 385–403
Davies A G 1958 The bone changes of Madura foot; observations on Uganda Africans. Radiology 70: 841–847
Dawson M H, Boots R L 1939 Arthritis associated with lymphogranuloma venereum. Journal of the American Medical Association 113: 1162–1163
Denman A M 1974 Report of Symposium on Viruses, Arthritis and Connective tissue Disorders. Annals of the Rheumatic Diseases 33: 489–492
Dickson E C, Gifford M A 1938 Coccidioides infection (coccidioidomycosis) primary type of infection. Archives of Internal Medicine 62: 853–871
Dismukes W E, Stam A M, Graybill J R et al 1983 Treatment of systemic mycoses with Ketoconazole: Emphasis on toxicity and clinical response in 52 patients. Annals of Internal Medicine 98: 13–20
Doherty R L, Carley J G, Best J C 1972 Isolation of Ross River virus from man. Medical Journal of Australia 1: 1083–1084
Douglas G W, Levin R H, Sokoloff L 1964 Infectious arthritis complicating neoplastic disease. New England Journal of Medicine 270: 299–302
Dowling P G 1946 Epidemic polyarthritis. Medical Journal of Australia 1: 245–246
Edwards G A 1959 Clinical characteristics of leptospirosis. American Journal of Medicine 27: 4–17
Ehrenpreis B 1957 Syphilis of bone in the adult. New York State Journal of Medicine 2: 3486–3488
Eichner H L, Deller J J 1970 Meningococcal arthritis. Arthritis and Rheumatism 13: 272–275
Fernandez R, McCarty D J 1971 The arthritis of viral hepatitis. Annals of Internal Medicine 74: 207–211
Fountain F F 1973 Acute blastomycotic arthritis. Archives of Internal Medicine 132: 684–688
Fraser J R E, Cunningham A L, Clarris B J, Aaskov J G, Leach R 1981 Cytology of synovial effusion in epidemic polyarthritis. Australian and New Zealand Journal of Medicine 11: 168–173
Friedman A, Naveh Y 1971 Polyarthritis associated with chickenpox. American Journal of Diseases in Children 122: 179–180
Furtado T A 1957 Late manifestations of yaws. Archives of Dermatology 76: 446–451
Gehlback S H, Hamilton J D, Conant N F 1973 Coccidioidomycosis. Archives of Internal Medicine 131: 254–255
Gelfand S G, Alfonse T M, Garcia-Kutzbach A 1975 Spectrum of gonococcal arthritis. Evidence for sequential stages and clinical subgroups. Journal of Rheumatology 2: 83–90
Ghosh S K, Reddy T A 1973 Arthralgis and myalgia in mumps. Rheumatology and Rehabilitation 12: 97–99
Girard D E, Bagby G C, Walsh J R 1973 Destructive polyarthritis secondary to mycobacterium Kansassii. Arthritis and Rheumatism 16: 665–669
Godwin M C 1965 Infection of knee joint by Mycobacterium kansasii. Journal of the American Medical Association 194: 88–89
Gold H E, Boxerbaum B, Leslie H J 1968 Mumps arthritis. American Journal of Diseases in Children 116: 547–548
Goldenberg D L, Brandt K D, Cohen A S, Cathcart E S 1975 Treatment of septic arthritis: comparison of needle aspiration and surgery as initial modes of joint drainage. Arthritis and Rheumatism 18: 83–90
Goldmann C H, Smith S J 1943 X-ray appearance of bone in yaws. British Journal of Radiology 16: 234–238
Goobar J E, Clark G M 1964 Rheumatological manifestations of gonorrhea. Archives of Interamerican Rheumatology 7: 1–24
Gordan H S, Hoffman S J, Schultz A, Lomberg F 1949 Serous arthritis of the knee joint. Report of a case caused by Salmonella typhosa and Salmonella montevideo in a child. Journal of the American Medical Association 141: 460–461
Gordon S C, Lanter C B 1982 Mumps arthritis: unusual

presentations as adult Still's. Annals of Internal Medicine 97: 45–47
Gore M 1956 Chronic meningococcemia. Annals of Internal Medicine 45: 142–145
Graber W J, Sanford J P, Ziff M 1960 Sex incidence of gonococcal arthritis. Arthritis and Rheumatism 3: 309–313
Greenman R, Campbell G 1975 Coccidioidal synovitis of the knee. Archives of Internal Medicine 135: 526–530
Greenwood B M, Whittle H C, Bryceson A D M 1973 Allergic complications of meningococcal disease. II. Immunological investigations. British Medical Journal ii: 737–740
Greer W E R, Keefer C S 1951 Cat-scratch fever; disease entity. New England Journal of Medicine 244: 545–548
Griffiths D H 1975 Orthopaedic tuberculosis. British Journal of Hospital Medicine 14: 146–157
Haapasaari J, Essen R V, Kahanpää A, Kostiala A A I, Holmberg K, Ahlquist J 1982 Fungal arthritis simulating juvenile rheumatoid arthritis. British Medical Journal 285: 923–924
Hackett C J 1951 Bone lesions of Yaws in Uganda. Blackwell, Oxford
Haddow A J, Davies C W, Walker A J 1960 O'nyong-nyong fever: and epidemic virus disease in East Africa. I. Introduction. Transactions of the Royal Society of Tropical Medicine and Hygiene 54: 517–522
Halliday J H, Horan J P 1943 Epidemic of polyarthritis in Northern Territory. Medical Journal of Australia 2: 293–295
Hand W L, King N L 1978 Serum opsonisation of salmonella in sickle cell anaemia. American Journal of Medicine 64: 388–395
Handsfield H H 1975 Disseminated gonococcal infection. Clinical Gynaecology and Obstetrics 18: 131–142
Harder E J, Hermans P E 1975 Treatment of fungal infections with Flucytosine. Archives of Internal Medicine 135: 231–237
Hardy A V 1937 Arthritis in brucella melitensis infections. Medical Clinics of North America 21:1747
Harris J R, Brand P W 1966 Patterns of disintegration of the tarsus in the anaesthetic foot. Journal of Bone and Joint Surgery 48B: 4–16
Hayes J T 1961 Cystic tuberculosis of the proximal tibial metaphysis with associated involvement of the epiphysis and epiphyseal plate. Journal of Bone and Joint Surgery 43A: 560–567
Henle W, Henle G 1972 Epstein–Barr virus. The cause of infectious mononucleosis. Oncogenesis and herpesviruses. In: Biggs P M, de-The G, Payne L N (eds) WHO International Agency for Research on Cancer, Lyon, p 269
Hilderbrandt H M, Maassab H F 1966 Rubella synovitis in a one-year-old patient. New England Journal of Medicine 274: 1428–1430
Hillenbrand F K M 1956 The blood picture in rubella. Its place in diagnosis. Lancet 2: 66–68
Ho G Jr, Gadbow J J Jr, Glickstein S L 1983 Haemophilus influenzae septic arthritis in the adult. Seminars in Arthritis and Rheumatism 12: 314–321
Holmes K K, Courts G W, Beatty H N 1971 Disseminated gonococcal infection. Annals of Internal Medicine 74: 979–993
Horsfall F L, Tamm I 1968 Viral and rickettsial infections of man, 4th Edn. Lillincot, Philadelphia
Hunt D D 1964 Problems in diagnosing osteoarticular tuberculosis. Journal of American Medical Association 190: 95–98
Hurst N P, Martynoga A G, Nuke G 1983 Coxsackie B infection and arthritis. British Medical Journal 286:605
Inman R D 1982 Rheumatic manifestations of hepatitis B virus infection. Seminars in Arthritis and Rheumatism 11: 406–420
Johnson E W, Weed L A 1954 Brucellar bursitis. Journal of Bone and Joint Surgery 36A: 133–139
Johnson R E, Hall A P 1958 Rubella arthritis, report of cases studied by latex tests. New England Journal of Medicine 258: 743–745
Jones M C 1970 Arthritis and arthralgia in infection with mycoplasma pneumoniae. Thorax 25: 748–750
Kellgren J H, Ball J, Fairbrother R W, Barnes K L 1958 Suppurative arthritis complicating rheumatoid arthritis. British Medical Journal 1: 1193–1200
Kelly P J, Martin W J, Schirger A, Weed L A 1960 Brucellosis of the bones and joints. Journal of the American Medical Association 174: 347–353
Kelly P J, Weed L A, Lipscombe P R 1963 Infection of tendon sheaths, bursae, joints and soft tissues by acid-fast bacilli other than tubercle bacilli. Journal of Bone and Joint Surgery 45A: 327–336
Kemp H B S, Jackson J W, Keremiah J D, Cook J 1973 Anterior fusion of the spine for infective lesions in adults. Journal of Bone and Joint Surgery 55B: 715–734
Kennedy J C 1904 Notes on case of chronic synovitis, or bursitis, due to organism of Mediterranean fever. Journal of the Royal Army Medical Corps 2: 178–180
Key A J, Large A M 1942 Histoplasmosis of the knee. Journal of Bone and Joint Surgery 24: 281–290
Koga J, Iwabuchi A, Saito Y, Nadamitsu Y 1968 A case of acute arthritis of the knee due to Candida. Orthopaedic Surgery 19: 523–528
Kuo K N, Lloyd-Roberts G C, Orme I M, Soothill J F 1975 Immunodeficiency and infantile bone and joint infection. Archives of Disease in Childhood 50: 51–56
Lancet Editorial 1982 Ketoconazole. 1: 319–320
Laskin R S, Potenza A 1971 Cat-scratch fever — a confusing diagnosis for the orthopaedic surgeon. Journal of Bone and Joint Surgery 53A:1211–1214
Lass R and Shephard E 1961 Mumps arthritis. British Medical Journal 2: 1613–1614
Lee P R, Barnett A F, Scholer J F, Bryner S, Clark W H 1960 Rubella arthritis. A study of twenty cases. California Medicine 93: 125–128
Linscheid R L, Dobyns J H 1975 Common and uncommon infections of the hand. Orthopaedic Clinics in North America 6: 1063–1104
Little J A, Steigman A J 1960 Erythema nodosum in primary histoplasmosis. Journal of the American Medical Association 173:875
Littman M L, Zimmerman L E 1956 Crytococcsis. Grune & Stratton, New York
London D, Fitton J M 1970 Acute septic arthritis complicating Crohn's disease. British Journal of Surgery 57: 536–537
McCutchan J A, Adler M W, Berrie J R H 1982 Penicillinase producing Neisseria gonorrhoeae in Great Britain 1977–81: alarming increase in incidence and recent development of endemic transmission. British Medical Journal 285: 337–340
Makin M, Alkalaj I, Rosansky R 1957 Mono-articular

brucellar arthritis. Journal of Bone and Joint Surgery 39A: 1183–1186
Martin J R, Root H S, Kim S O, Johnson L G 1965 Staphylococcus suppurative arthritis occurring in neuropathic knee joints. Arthritis and Rheumatism 8: 389–402
Masondieu P 1924 Thesis for Doctor of Medicine. Faculty of Paris, No 519
Medical Research Council Working Party on Tuberculosis of the Spine 1982 A ten year assessment of a controlled trial comparing debridement and anterior spinal fusion in the management of tuberculosis of the spine in patients on standard chemotherapy in Hong Kong. Journal of Bone and Joint Surgery 64B: 393–398
Mikkelsen W M, Brandt R L, Harrell E R 1957 Sporotrichosis: a report of 12 cases, including two with skeletal involvement. Annals of Internal Medicine 47: 435–459
Miller G A H, Ridley M, Medd W E 1963 Typhoid osteomyelitis of the spine. British Medical Journal 1: 1068–1069
Molony J, Connolly K 1973 Knee arthropathy secondary to Mycobacterium scrofulaceum. Annals of the Rheumatic Diseases 32: 69–71
Montgomery M M, Poske R M, Pilz C G, Libnoch J A 1962 Acute gonococcal arthritis: clinical findings presenting by 28 patients observed in recent years. Annals of Internal Medicine 56: 688–689
Mulhern L M, Friday G A, Perri J A 1971 Arthritis complicating varicella infection. Pediatrics 48: 827–829
Murray H W, Fialk M A, Roberts R B 1976 Candida. American Journal of Medicine 60: 587–595
Murray R C 1940 Tuberculosis of knee: follow-up investigation of old cases. British Medical Journal 2: 10–12
Myers A R, Millers L M, Pinals R S 1969 Pyarthrosis complicating rheumatoid arthritis. Lancet 2: 714–716
Nade S 1983a Acute haematogeneous osteomyelitis in infancy and childhood. Journal of Bone and Joint Surgery 65B: 109–119
Nade S 1983b Acute septic arthritis in infancy and childhood. Journal of Bone and Joint Surgery 65B: 234–241
Namey T C, Halla J T 1978 Radiographic and videographic techniques. Clinics in Rheumatic Diseases 4: 95–132
Newton P, Sharp J, Barnes K L 1982 Bone and joint tuberculosis in Greater Manchester 1969–79. Annals of the Rheumatic Diseases 41: 1–6
Nimmo J R 1928 Unusual epidemic. Medical Journal of Australia 1:549
Noyes F R, McCabe J D, Fekety F R 1973 Acute candida arthritis. Journal of Bone and Joint Surgery 55A: 169–176
O'Malley B W, Zelt H D 1965 Disseminated bone tuberculosis without pulmonary manifestations. American Journal of Medicine 38: 932–936
Onion D K, Crumpacker C S, Gilliland B C 1971 Arthritis of hepatitis associated with Australian antigen. Annals of Internal Medicine. 75: 29–33
Papathanassiou B T, Papachristou G, Hartofilakidis-Garofalidis G 1972 Brucellar spondylitis. Report of six cases. Acta Orthopaedics Scandinavica 43: 384–391
Paterson D C 1970 Acute suppurative arthritis in infancy and childhood. Journal of Bone and Joint Surgery 52B: 474–482
Paterson D E 1955 Radiological bone changes and angiographic findings in leprosy, with special reference to pathogenesis of 'atrophic' conditions of digits. Journal of the Faculty of Radiologists 7: 35–56
Peterson B H, Lee T J, Synderman R, Brooks G F 1979 Neisseria meningitides and Neisseria gonorrhoea bacteremia associated with C_6, C_7 or C_8 deficiency. Annals of Internal Medicine 90: 917–920
Pimm L H, Waugh W 1957 Tuberculosis tenosynovitis. Journal of Bone and Joint Surgery 39B: 91–101
Pinals R S, Ropes M W 1964 Meningococcal arthritis. Arthritis and Rheumatism 7: 241–258
Pollard J P, Hughes S P F, Scott J E, Evans M J, Benson M K D 1979 Prophylactic antibiotics following total hip replacement — a controlled trial. Journal of Bone and Joint Surgery 61B: 118–119
Price G E, Ford D K, Gofton J P, Robinson H S 1963 An outbreak of 'infectious' polyarthritis in a Haida Indian family. Arthritis and Rheumatism 6: 633–638
Quismorio F P, Dubois E L 1975 Septic arthritis in systemic lupus erythematosus. Journal of Rheumatology 2: 73–82
Rao K V, O'Brien T J, Anderson R C 1981 Septic arthritis due to nocardia steroids after successful kidney transplantation. Arthritis and Rheumatism 24: 99–101
Rappaport E M, Rossian A X, Rosenblum L A 1951 Arthritis due to intestinal amebiasis. Annals of Internal Medicine 34: 1224–1231
Ray C G, Gall E P, Minnich L L, Roediger J, de Benedeth C, Corrigan J L 1982 Acute polyarthritis associated with active Epstein-Barr Virus infection. Journal of the American Medical Association 248: 2991–2993
Riordan D C 1960 The hand in leprosy. Journal of Bone and Joint Surgery 42A: 683–690
Robinson M C 1955 Epidemic of virus disease in southern province, Tanganyika Territory in 1952–53; clinical features. Transactions of the Royal Society of Tropical Medicine and Hygiene 49: 28–32
Robitaille A, Cockburn C, James D C O, Ansell B M 1976 HLA frequencies in less common arthropathies. Annals of the Rheumatic Diseases 35: 271–273
Rodnan G P, Yunis E J, Totten R S 1960 Experience with punch biopsy of synovium in the study of joint disease. Annals of Internal Medicine, 53: 319–331
Rose G K 1959 Tuberculosis of the knee joint. British Journal of Clinical Practice 13:241
Ross R W 1956 Newala epidemic; virus isolation, pathogenic properties and relationship to epidemic. Journal of Hygiene 54: 177–191
Rotes-Querol J 1957 Osteo-articular sites of brucellosis. Annals of the Rheumatic Diseases 16: 63–68
Russell A S, Ansell B M 1972 Septic arthritis. Annals of the Rheumatic Diseases 31: 40–44
Rytel M W 1975 Counter immunoelectrophoresis in diagnosis of infectious disease. Hospital Practice 10: 75–82
Samilson R L, Bersani F A, Watkins M B 1958 Acute suppurative arthritis in infants and children: the importance of early diagnosis and surgical drainage. Pediatrics 21: 798–804
Sanders L L 1967 Blastomycosis arthritis. Arthritis and Rheumatism 10: 91–98
Sanford J P, Sulkin S E 1959 The clinical spectrum of ECHO-virus infection New England Journal of Medicine 261: 1113–1122
Saphra I, Wassermann M 1954 Salmonella cholerac suis; clinical and epidemiological evaluation of 329 infections

identified between 1940 and 1954 in New York Salmonella Center. American Journal of Medical Sciences 228: 525–533
Schein A J 1938 Articular manifestations of meningococcic infection. Archives of Internal Medicine 62:963
Schumacher H R, Gall E P 1974 Arthritis in acute hepatitis and chronic active hepatitis. American Journal of Medicine 57: 655–664
Sheldon P J H S, Main N S, Fox E 1982 Yersinia arthritis; a clinical immunological and family study of two cases. Annals of Rheumatic Diseases 41: 153–158
Shields L H 1959 Disseminated cryptococcosis producing a sarcoid type reaction. Archives of Internal Medicine 104: 763–770
Shore H 1961 O'nyong-nyong fever: an epidemic virus disease in East Africa. III. Some clinical and epidemiological observations in the northern province of Uganda. Transactions of the Royal Society of Tropical Medicine and Hygiene 55: 361–373
Sieving R R, Kaufman C A, Watanakunakorn C 1975 Deep fungal infection in systemic lupus erythematosus. Report of three cases and review of the literature. Journal of Rheumatology 2: 61–72
Silby H M, Farber R, O'Connell C J, Ascher J, Marine E J 1965 Acute monarticular arthritis after vaccination. Report of a case with isolation of vaccina virus from synovial fluid. Annals of Internal Medicine 62: 347–350
Smith J G, Harris J S, Conant N F, Smith D T 1955 An epidemic of North American blastomycosis. Journal of the American Medical Association 158: 641–646
Smith W S, Ward R M 1966 Septic arthritis of the hip complicating perforation of abdominal organs. Journal of the American Medical Association 195: 1148–1150
Sontheimer R D, Garibaldi R A, Krueger G G 1978 Stevens Johnson syndrome associated with mycoplasma pneumoniae infections. Archives of Dermatology 114: 241–244
Spellberg M A, Zivin S 1948 Amebiasis in veterans of World War II with special emphasis on extraintestinal complications, including case of amebic cerebellar abscess. Gastroenterology 10: 452–473
Spira T J, Kabins S A 1976 Yersinia eulercolifiea septicaemia with septic arthritis. Archives of Internal Medicine 136: 1305–1306
Sponzilli E E, Calabro J J 1961 Gonococcal arthritis in the newborn. Journal of the American Medical Association 177: 919–921
Spruance S L, Smith C B 1971 Joint complications associated with derivatives of HPV-77 rubella virus vaccine. American Journal of Diseases of Children 122: 105–111
Steere A C, Malawista S E 1979 Cases of Lyme disease in the United States: locations correlated with distribution of Ixodes dammini. Annals of Internal Medicine 91: 730–734
Steere A C, Malawista S E, Harding S R, Askenase P W, Andiman W A 1977 Erythema Chronicum migrans and Lyme arthritis; the enlarging clinical spectrum. Annals of Internal Medicine 86: 685–698
Steere A C, Hutchinson G J, Rahn D W et al 1983a Treatment of the early manifestations of Lyme disease. Annals of Internal Medicine 99: 22–26
Steere A C, Grodzicki R L, Klornblatt 1983b The spirochaetal etiology of Lyme disease. New England Journal of Medicine 308: 733–740
Steere A C, Bartenhagen N H, Craft J E et al 1983c The early clinical manifestations of Lyme disease. Annals of Internal Medicine 99: 76–82
Storey G 1964 Charcot joints. British Journal of Venereal Disease 40: 109–117
Sutliff W D, Shepard R, Dunham W B 1952 Acute leptospira pomona arthritis and myocarditis. Annals of Internal Medicine 39:134
Talbot J M, Hunt J A 1957 Infection of bone and joint by Salmonellae. British Medical Journal 2: 1095–1096
Taylor H A, Bradford S A, Patterson S P 1966 Gonococcal arthritis in pregnancy. Obstetrics and Gynecology 27: 776–782
Toala P, Schroeder S A, Daly A K, Finland M 1970 Candida at Boston City Hospital. Clinical and epidemiological characteristics and susceptibility to eight antimicrobial agents. Archives of Internal Medicine 126: 983–989
Tobler W, Minder W 1954 Generalistierte chronische aspergillose beim kind und ihre beziehung zur antibiotischen therapie. Helvetica Paediatrica Acta 9: 209–230
Torres J, Rathburn H K, Greenough W B 1973 Pneumococcal arthritis: report of a case and review of the literature. Johns Hopkins Medical Journal 132: 234–241
Tuli S M 1975 Results of treatment of spinal tuberculosis by 'middle-path' regime. Journal of Bone and Joint Surgery 57B: 13–23
Utsinger P D 1977 Immunological study of arthritis associated with adenovirus infection. Arthritis and Rheumatism 20:138
Vartiainen J, Hurri L 1964 Arthritis due to salmonella typhimurium. Acta Medica Scandinavica 175: 771–776
Wallace R, Cohen A S 1976 Tuberculous arthritis. American Journal of Medicine 61: 277–282
Ward J R, Bishop B 1970 Varicella arthritis. Journal of the American Medical Association 212: 1954–1956
Ward J, Cohen A S, Bauer W 1960 The diagnosis and therapy of acute suppurative arthritis. Arthritis and Rheumatism 3: 522–535
Ward H P, Martin W J, Ivins J C, Weed L A 1961 Cephalosporium arthritis. Proceedings of the Mayo Clinic 36: 337–343
Watanakunakorn C 1982 Treatment of infections due to methicillin resistant staphylococcus aureus. Annals of Internal Medicine 97: 376–378
Waterson A P, Wedgewood J 1953 Rat-bite fever. Report of a case due to actinomyces muris. Lancet 1: 472–473
Webster F S, Willander D 1957 Chronic sporotrichal synovitis of the knee. Journal of Bone and Joint Surgery 39A: 207–215
Weed L A 1957 Use of selective medium for isolation of brucella from contaminated surgical specimens. American Journal of Clinical Pathology 27: 482–485
Whittle H C, Abdullahi M T, Fakunle F A et al 1973 Allergic complications of memingococcal disease. I. Clinical aspects. British Medical Journal 2: 733–737
Wilkinson A E, Sequeira P J L 1955 Studies on treponemal immobilization test; use of TPI as verification test in suspected latent syphilis. British Journal of Venereal Diseases 31: 143–154
Wilkinson M C 1959 Treatment of tuberculosis of the spine. British Medical Journal 2: 280–282
Wilkinson M C 1965 The treatment of bone and joint tuberculosis. Annals of the Royal College of Surgeons of England 37: 19–39
Willkens R F, Healey L A, Decker J L 1960 Acute infectious arthritis in the aged and chronically ill. Archives

of Internal Medicine 106: 354–364
Wilson G S, Miles A A 1955 In: Topley and Wilson (eds) Principles of bacteriology and immunology, Vol 2. p 1473
Wright L T, Logan M 1939 Osseous changes associated with lymphogranuloma venereum. Archives of Surgery 39:108
Yanez J E, Thompson G R, Mikkelsen W M, Bartholomew L E 1966 Rubella arthritis. Annals of Internal Medicine 64: 772–777
Zammit F 1958 Undulant fever spondylitis. British Journal of Radiology 31: 683–690

Heritable disorders

DISORDERS OF THE FIBROUS PROTEINS — COLLAGEN AND ELASTIN

This group of hereditary diseases presents a wide variety of clinical features affecting many organs of the body. The one feature that is common to most is a generalised laxity of ligaments, resulting in hypermobility of joints. It is for this reason that they may present to the rheumatologist or orthopaedic surgeon with articular problems. With the exception of those conditions that are due to a known inborn error of metabolism, e.g. homocystinuria, which are transmitted by a recessive mode of inheritance, most of these conditions exhibit a Mendelian dominant pattern of inheritance. They include Marfan's syndrome, osteogenesis imperfecta and the Ehlers–Danlos syndrome, together with pseudo-xanthoma elasticum (PXE) and cutis laxa which generally do not manifest hypermobility of joints. For the sake of convenience, the 'hypermobility syndrome', in which generalised joint laxity occurs in otherwise healthy subjects but which may present similar clinical problems, will also be discussed in this section. For a detailed account of these disorders the reader is referred to the works of McKusick (1972, 1975).

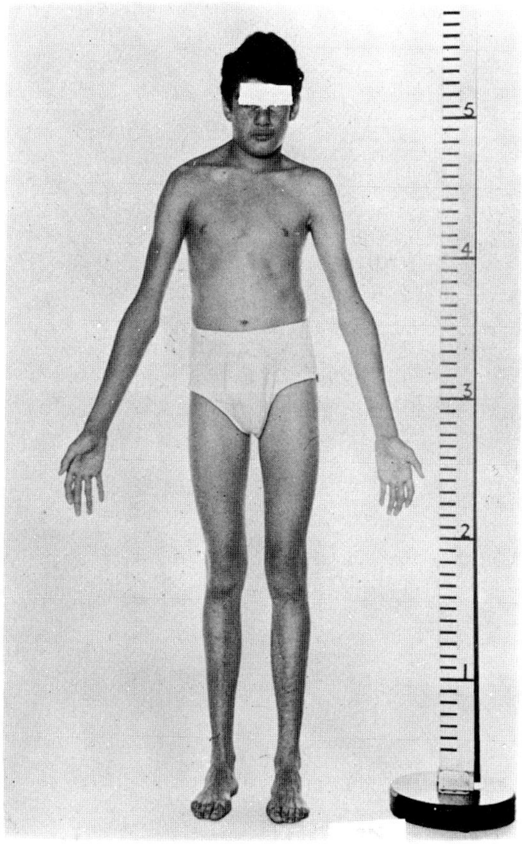

Fig. 46.1 Marfan's syndrome: note the long slender arms and legs with reduced upper segment : lower segment ratio. The patient also has a scoliosis.

Marfan's syndrome

A characteristic feature of Marfan's syndrome is the distortion of the body shape, resulting in long slender extremities (Fig. 46.1); thus the arm-span exceeds the height and the fingers are long and tapered (arachnodactily) (Fig. 46.2). This results in a height : hand-length ratio in excess of 9 and a height : foot-length ratio in excess of 7. Furthermore, the upper segment (crown-to-pubis) : lower segment (pubis-to-floor) ratio is reduced below the normal value of 0.93. The 'metacarpal index' is a useful diagnostic indicator of arachnodactily. It is the average ratio of length : mid-point width of the 2nd, 3rd, 4th and 5th metacarpals as seen on the plain X-ray of the hand (Sinclair et al, 1960). A value of 8.5 or more

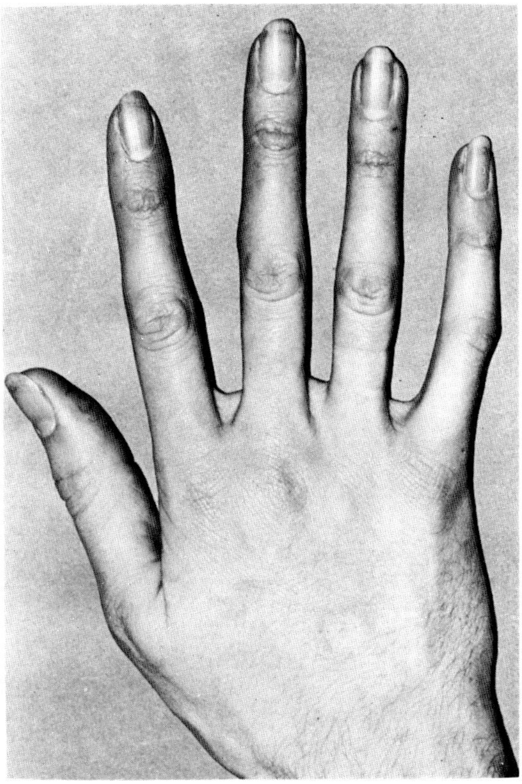

Fig. 46.2 Arachnodactily. The long 'spidery' digits are characteristic of Marfan's syndrome.

indicates arachnodactily. Other skeletal abnormalities include kyphoscoliosis, pectus excavatum, dolichocephaly, a long narrow face, a high arched palate and prognathism. Skeletal symptoms are common and arise as a result of kyphoscoliosis, e.g. backache and dorsal pain, or from the sequellae of the laxity of joints (see below). Other clinical features include dislocation of the lens (ectopia lentis) which is usually bilateral and is caused by an abnormality in the suspensory ligaments of the lens which can be seen on slit-lamp examination. Dilatation of the pupil is necessary to visualise the abnormality in some 30% of cases. Dilatation of the ascending aorta or pulmonary artery may occur, sometimes with dissecting aneurism formation, and the effect is similar to that seen in luetic aortitis. The patient may present with anginal pain, aortic incompetence or rupture of the aorta. Although survival to old age has been reported, few patients with the complete syndrome survive beyond middle age. 'Formes frustes' of the syndrome are common and may be associated with a normal life span. The condition is seen worldwide and it does not favour one or other of the sexes. The mode of inheritance is that of the autosomal dominant but cases also develop by mutation. It seems likely that the basic defect in this condition is in the collagen rather than the elastin, since the turnover rate of collagen is shown to be increased (Laitenen et al, 1968) and this is in keeping with the earlier finding of Prokop & Sjoerdsma (1961) that urinary hydroxyproline excretion is excessive.

Studies of collagen of aortic origin have revealed increased solubility and a decreased cross-linking. Aortic explants obtained at operation for a repair of a dissecting aneurism revealed an increase in the amount of type I collagen synthesis (Krieg & Müller, 1977). This biosynthetic defect of type I collagen appears to be the result of a qualitative and quantitative abnormality affecting the alpha 2 chain (Scheck et al, 1979; Boucek et al, 1981). These observations have led to speculation of a primary gene-determined defect in the alpha 2 (1) peptide. A mutation in one of the alpha 2 (1) genes would be sufficient to cause disruption of fibrillogenesis and result in the molecular phenotype. The lack of support normally provided by type I collagen fibres results in disintegration of the elastic fibres of the ascending aorta which consequently dilates under the continuous stress mediated by the arterial blood pressure. Attempts at repair by hypertrophy of smooth muscle cells are to no avail and the ascending aorta become progressively weaker and may eventually rupture. This disastrous complication may be forestalled by surgical replacement of the aorta.

Fibroblasts from patients with Marfan's syndrome when grown in tissue culture have been shown to accumulate excessive amounts of hyaluronic acid (Metalon & Dorfman, 1968) and this is in keeping with the finding of increased urinary excretion of mucopolysaccharides in these patients (Berenson & Dalferes, 1965).It is clear that the abnormality is a complex one which involves both the collagen and the glycosaminoglycans of the connective tissue matrix.

Homocystinuria

Homocystinuria is a metabolic defect caused by a

deficiency of the enzyme cystathionine synthetase (Uhlendorf & Mudd, 1968) that mimics Marfan's syndrome in that ectopia lentis, pectum excavatum and arachnodactyly are commonly present. Additional features include thrombosis in medium-sized arteries (e.g. coronary arteries), osteoporosis with pathological fractures and mental retardation which are all absent in Marfan's syndrome.

Analysis of the collagen cross-links in skin biopsy samples obtained from three patients with documented homocystinuria showed that the formation of stable intermolecular cross-link formation was reduced as compared with age-matched control subjects (Kang & Trelstad, 1973).

The condition may be confirmed by the detection of homocystine in the urine of affected patients by the nitropruside method of Spaeth & Barbour (1967). Studies of the pedigrees in 20 families containing 38 patients confirmed that the pattern of inheritance is that of an autosomal recessive as is generally the case in Garrodian inborn errors of metabolism. Urinary-stone and tissue deposits are not found as are the case in cystinuria, and cystinosis (Schimke et al, 1965). Treatment with a low methionine diet has been advocated in a number of reports and in some cases a significant reduction in plasma methionine levels has been recorded in the neonatal period (Perry et al, 1966).

Hyperlysinaemia

Gross hypermobility of joints and hypotonicity of muscles associated with marked mental retardation has been shown to be associated with an excess of lysine in blood, urine and cerebrospinal fluid. It is believed that the condition is due to a disturbance of the incorporation of lysine into certain proteins due to an, as yet, unidentified enzymatic defect (Ghadimi et al, 1965).

Pseudo-xanthoma elasticum

In this condition, an elastic-staining material is seen in aggregations in the skin, which becomes coarsened, thickened and grooved, with a yellowish appearance. It is seen particularly on the neck, face and in the folds of the axillae and groins. Angioid streaks are seen in the ocular fundi and a degenerative chorioretinitis may cause serious loss of vision. Thickening of the media of arteries may cause occlusion and result in ischaemic symptoms such as intermittent claudication or angina pectoris. Calcification of peripheral arteries commonly occurs. Gastrointestinal bleeding is another well-recognised complication. Originally, the basic defect was thought to reside in collagen (Hall et al, 1955) but more recently elastin has been implicated (Moran & Lansing, 1958). On the basis of a clinical study of 140 affected individuals, Pope has recognised four distinct groups, two of which are inherited as an autosomal dominant (1974a) and two as an autosomal recessive (1974b). Loose-jointedness was found to occur mainly in the dominant type II group. Harvey et al (1975) have reported that in both dominant types I and II there is a reduction in the in vivo elastic modulus of the skin, whereas in recessive type I the modulus is significantly increased. These findings would suggest that not only is it the collagen that is abnormal in pseudo-xanthoma elasticum but that in the different genetic groups the abnormality in collagen differs.

Ehlers–Danlos syndrome

In this condition, generalised laxity of ligaments often of the more gross variety is combined with hyperextensibility of the skin and a haemorrhagic diathesis. The skin is soft and velvety in texture and when picked up it can be stretched to a much greater extent than normal skin (Fig. 46.3). On releasing the skin, it recoils back to its original position immediately. The skin is thinner than normal and this is at least partly responsible for its greater fragility. Relatively minor trauma may result in breakage of the skin and healing is poor, leading to unsightly scars. These are commonly seen over the bony prominences such as the knees or on the face and often represent minor traumatic incidents in childhood (Fig. 46.4).

The Ehlers–Danlos syndrome is in fact not a homogeneous enity but a clinically and genetically diverse group of connective tissue disorders (Beighton, 1970). At the time of writing, nine types have been delineated (Table 46.1). It should be pointed out that more than 80% of EDS patients have type I and II of the condition and that a further 10% have type III (Beighton, 1983). Many patients, however, showing stigmata of the EDS are not classifiable within the above-mentioned classification.

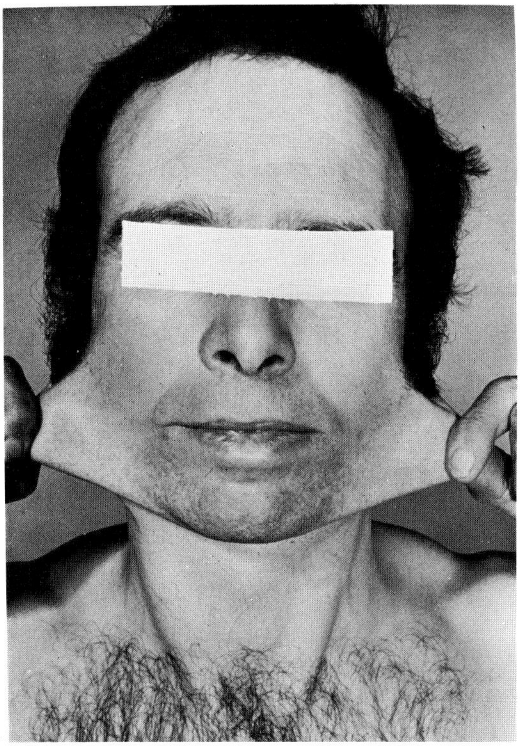

a

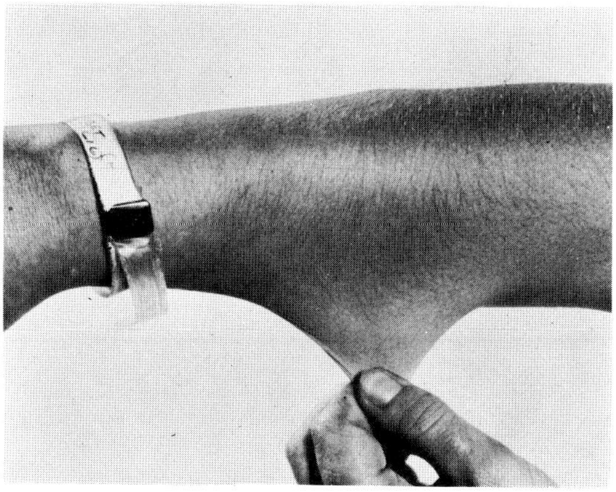

b

Fig. 46.3 Ehlers–Danlos syndrome showing the characteristic cutaneous hyperextensibility.

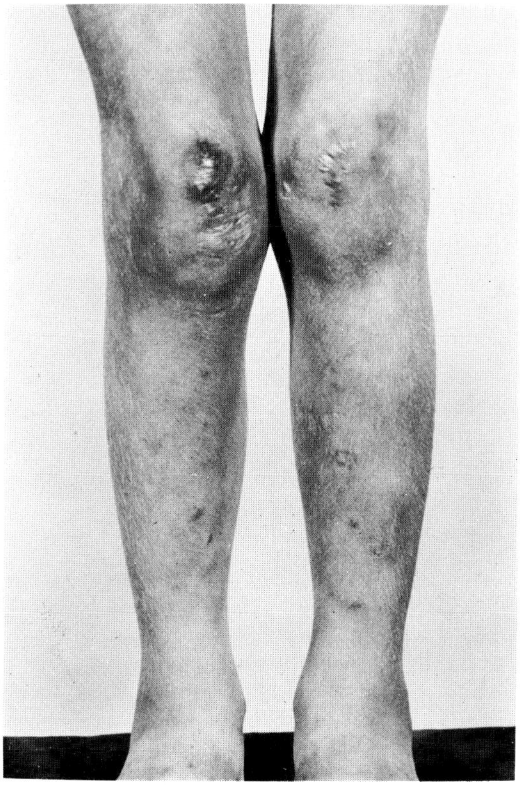

Although the major triad of stretchy skin, lax joints and fragile tissues are constant features to a greater or lesser degree, the variety of clinical manifestations is very wide. In a small number of patients sudden death may occur from rupture of a large vessel or viscus or from major haemorrhage. These complications are seen virtually only in the very rare type IV.

The articular complications of the EDS are identical with those seen in other hypermobility syndromes and are considered below.

Other non-articular sequelae include mitral valve prolapse, hiatus hernia, gastric, duodenal and colonic diverticula, rectal prolapse and inguinal, femoral or umbilical herniae. There is a tendency towards spontaneous bleeding but it is not clear whether this is due to a coagulation defect or abnormalities in the vessel wall or in the perivascular supporting connective tissues.

In the eye as a result of involvement of the sclera ocular distortion occurs and results in myopia. Squints are also common as a result of

Fig. 46.4 Ehlers–Danlos syndrome — unsightly thin gaping scars, the result of previous trauma.

Table 46.1 Clinical features of the various types of Ehlers–Danlos syndrome

Type	Form, frequency	Main features	Mode of inheritance	Metabolic defect
I	Gravis — severe 1 : 625 000	Skin — very stretchable bruisable, fragile Hyperextensible joints — Generalised, severe, varicose veins Premature rupture membranes frequent	Autosomal dominant	Unknown
II	Mitis — mild 1 : 444 444	Mild cutaneous and joint manifestations. Joint hypermobility may be limited to hands and feet. No prematurity.	Autosomal dominant	Unknown
III	Benign hypermobility syndrome 1 : 5 000 000	Joint hypermobility generalised, marked, cutaneous manifestations minimal. Joint complications frequent.	Autosomal dominant	Unknown
IV	Ecchymotic, arterial Sack–Barabas type 1 : 5 000 000	Thin skin, excessive bruising, vessel rupture, bowel rupture Joint hypermobility — fingers only; skin hyperextensibility minimal or absent	Autosomal recessive (severe) Autosomal dominant (variable)	Absent or deficient collagen type III
V	X-linked form 1 : 2 000 000	Skin stretchability striking. Moderate fragility, bruising. Joint hypermobility limited. Floppy mitral valves.	X-linked recessive	Lysyloxidase deficiency.
VI	Ocular-scoliotic form	Fragility of eye globes Severe scoliosis Vascular abnormalities	Autosomal recessive	Hydroxylysine deficiency
VII	Procollagen peptidase deficiency	Severe loose-jointedness, with joint dislocations, short stature, epicanthic folds. Skin soft, slightly stretchable.	Autosomal recessive	Procollagen peptidase deficiency
VIII	New variant (Stewart et al, 1977)	Marked skin fragility, moderate joint hypermobility, minimal bruising and skin hyperextensibility. Advanced generalised periodontitis.	Autosomal dominant	Unknown
IX	Fibronectin deficiency (Arneson et al, 1980)	Joint hyperextensibility, easy bruising, deficient platelet function	Probably autosomal recessive	Fibronectin deficiency

laxity in the tendons of the extrinsic muscles of the eye. The facial appearance may be marred by redundant skin on the upper eyelids.

The skin generally is subject to splitting on minor trauma and surgical repair of incisions or lacerations is hazardous, often resulting in gaping or unsightly scars.

In pregnancy premature rupture of the membranes and resultant premature labour is not uncommon. Other obstetric complications including ante- and post-partum haemorrhage, severe laceration, and uterine prolapse may occur.

Cutis laxa

This is a distinct entity in which the disorder is believed to reside in the dermal elastin, resulting in loosely hanging folds of skin and a characteristic appearance of premature ageing, giving the so-called 'blood-hound facies'. Unlike the Ehlers–Danlos syndrome, with which it is frequently confused, joint mobility is not excessive (Beighton, 1970; Grahame & Beighton, 1971).

Osteogenesis imperfecta (fragilitas ossium)

This is discussed in Chapter 40.

HYPERMOBILITY IN HEALTHY SUBJECTS

Normal subjects exhibit a wide range of joint mobility, even after taking into consideration the influence of age, sex and ethnic factors. Clinically, hypermobility is recognised by the ability of the patients to perform certain passive manoeuvres, including passive dorsiflexion of the 5th metacarpophalangeal joint to 90° (Fig. 46.5a) apposition of the thumb to the volar aspect of the forearm

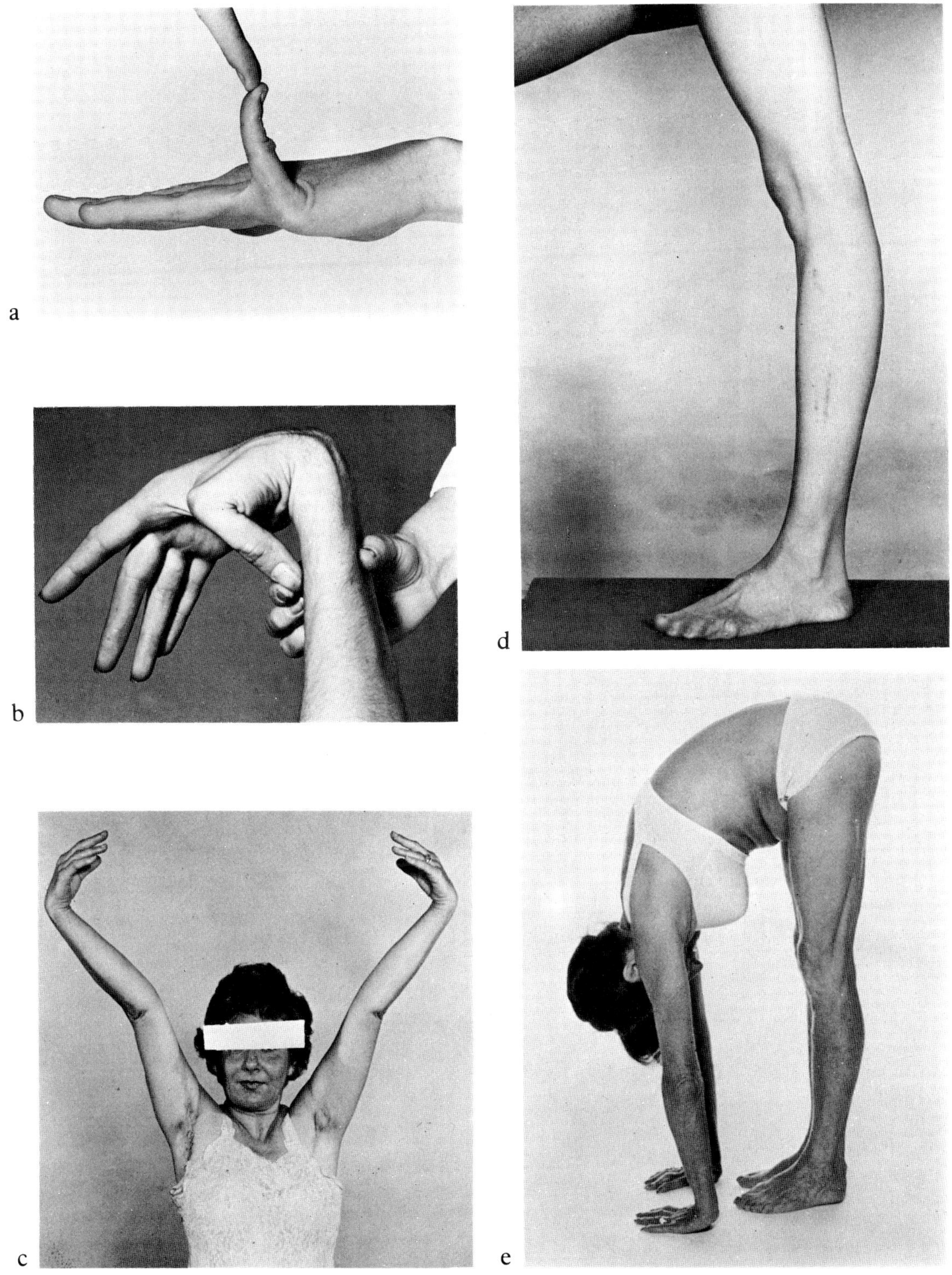

Fig. 46.5 Clinical stigmata of hypermobility. (a) Passive dorsiflexion of 5th metacarpophalangeal joint to 90°. (b) Passive apposition of the thumb to the volar aspect of the forearm. (c) Hyperextension of elbows to more than 10°. (d) Hyperextension of the knee to more than 10°. (e) Forward flexion of the trunk placing hands flat on the floor and with knees extended.

(Fig. 46.5b), hyperextension of the elbow (Fig. 46.5c) and knee (Fig. 46.5d) to beyond 10° and placing the hands flat on the floor by flexing the trunk with the knees fully extended (Fig. 46.5e). Patients suffering from the hereditary diseases referred to earlier in this section have little difficulty in performing these movements; however, it should be noted that approximately 10% of healthy subjects can also be classified as showing generalised hypermobility by these criteria (Carter & Wilkinson, 1964; Beighton et al, 1973). A more refined method of detecting minor differences in joint mobility has been introduced for the 5th metacarpophalangeal joint, by measuring the angle of dorsiflexion that occurs in response to a fixed predetermined force applied to the palmar aspect of the distal interphalangeal crease (Grahame & Jenkins, 1972). With this method it was possible to detect the year by year decline in joint mobility that occurs in children between the ages of 5 and 11 years, which was not revealed by the conventional tests (Silverman et al, 1975). There is very little further reduction in joint mobility during the adolescent years. During adult life there is a further gradual decline in joint mobility (Beighton et al, 1963; Sweetman et al, 1974).

A more sophisticated device for quantitating hyperextension of the metacarpalphalangeal joint of the index finger has been constructed by the Leeds group (Jobbins et al, 1979). With this hyperextensometer it was possible to confirm the relative hyperlaxity of females and the progressive decline in joint range with age in a healthy population (Bird, 1979).

In a survey comparing the different methods of assessing joint mobility currently available (Bird et al, 1979), it was concluded that the original Carter and Wilkinson system, as described above, remains the method of choice for assessing generalised joint laxity.

Negroes and Indians are more mobile than Caucasians (Harris & Joseph, 1949; Schweitzer, 1970) and adult females tend to be more mobile than males at any particular age. This sex difference has also been shown by Loebl (1972) using alternative methods of assessing metacarpophalangeal joint mobility, namely abduction and axial traction. The term 'hypermobility syndrome' (Kirk et al, 1967) has been used to describe articular complaints that arise in hypermobile subjects who are otherwise healthy. Studies on patterns of inheritance have revealed both dominant (Beighton & Horan, 1970) and recessive forms (Horan & Beighton, 1973).

The clinical effects of hypermobility

The clinical effects of hypermobility depend on its degree and are irrespective of its cause. It is not surprising, therefore, that they are more pronounced in the hereditary diseases referred to above, where hypermobility tends to the grosser than in normal subjects with hypermobility, in whom the defect is often less pronounced. Hypermobile joints, because of the ligamentous laxity, are more vulnerable to the effects of trauma and damage to the ligaments is more likely to occur (Nicholas, 1970). For the same reason, dislocation of joints is more likely to occur (Fig. 46.6) and some patients are able to dislocate and reduce their joints at will. Both congenital dislocation of the hip and recurrent acquired dislocation of the patella and shoulder have been shown to be associated with generalised hypermobility (Carter & Wilkinson, 1964; Carter & Sweetman, 1960). Joint effusions, particularly of the knee and ankle have been reported to occur in hypermobile subjects (Sutro, 1947); and as a result of this Baker's cyst formation may occur (Grahame, 1971). Hypermobility has been shown to be associated with chronic back pain, unexplicable on other grounds, and for this disorder the term 'loose back syndrome' has been suggested (Howes & Isdale, 1971). It seems quite likely that the hypermobile spine is predisposed to a number of sequellae including ligamentous trauma, disc prolapse and spondylolisthesis. It should be stated that this represents the author's clinical impression and is not based on controlled studies.

There is good presumptive evidence to suggest that premature osteoarthrosis may be a direct consequence of joint hypermobility, though this is difficult to prove (Fig. 46.7). Arthralgia occurs in hypermobile subjects ('the hypermobility syndrome') in direct relationship to the degree of hypermobility in a population sample (Beighton et al, 1973). The reason for this arthralgia is obscure and requires further elucidation. Symptoms tend to improve as the years go by and the joints lose some of their hypermobility (Kirk et al, 1967).

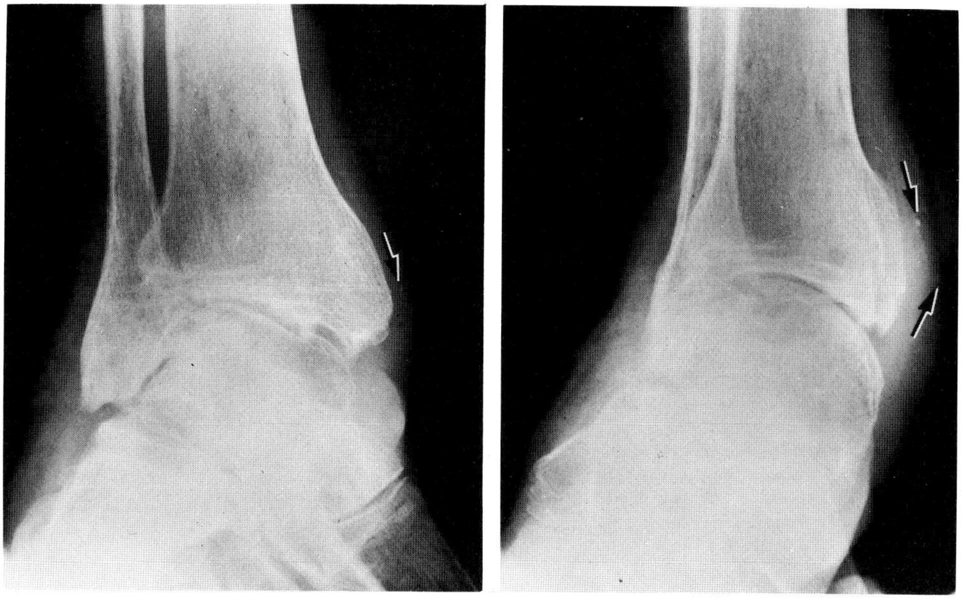

Fig. 46.6 Chronic subluxation and secondary osteoarthrosis of the ankle joints in a subject with Ehlers–Danlos syndrome. Note the calcified subcutaneous spheroids (marked by an arrow).

More recently evidence has been accumulating that suggests the possibility that patients with so-called 'hypermobility syndrome' might be suffering from a generalised disorder (albeit mild) of connective tissue. An increased prevalence of mitral valve prolapse ('floppy mitral valve syndrome'), a reduced upper segment : lower segment ratio, a reduced skin thickness, spinal anomalies and a history of fracture has been found in a group of patients with hypermobility syndrome as compared with control subjects (Grahame et al, 1981). The association between mitral valve prolapse and hypermobility is strengthened by a further investigation which found an increased prevalence of hypermobility in a group of 21 patients with mitral valve prolapse compared with matched controls suffering from other cardiac diseases (Pitcher & Grahame, 1982). It is of interest that studies on valve tissue removed at operation from patients with idiopathic mitral valve prolapse have shown accumulation of procollagen and reduced the collagen content suggesting a deficiency of the enzyme procollagen peptidase as the underlying mechanism (Bonella et al, 1980). Further studies are required to elucidate whether the hypermobility syndrome as we know it is part of a generalised collagen disorder.

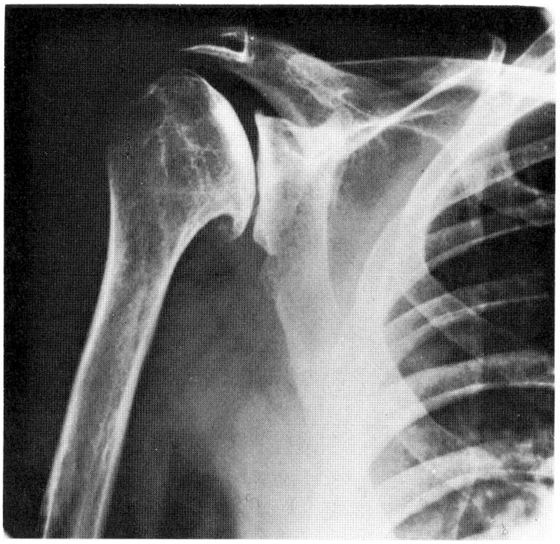

Fig. 46.7 Osteoarthritis of the shoulder joint in a patient suffering from the Ehlers–Danlos syndrome.

A recent review of nearly 200 patients seen in a hypermobility clinic over a 10-year period demonstrated the female preponderance (85%) in this syndrome. This, no doubt, reflects the increased joint laxity that female subjects in general display compared with males. Another striking finding was the numerous lesions and varied pattern of locomotor disorders seen in individual patients. By and large hypermobile subjects do not present with different rheumatological problems from other patients. They merely have more of them and in greater variety (Grahame, 1983a).

Hypermobility in healthy subjects should not be considered solely as a liability. It seems very likely that it is an important selection factor enabling them to compete successfully in many athletic pursuits, e.g. sport (Nicholas, 1970) and ballet dancing (Grahame & Jenkins, 1972).

Management

Joint hypermobility is often overlooked with the result that the patient's symptoms are wrongly ascribed to other conditions. Much unnecessary suffering results from an inappropriate diagnosis of adult (or juvenile) rheumatoid arthritis. Many of the complications of hypermobility, e.g. osteoarthrosis, ligamentous or muscle tear, are amenable to treatment along conventional lines. More difficult to manage however, is the arthralgia, often quite severe, experienced by many hypermobile subjects. Patients can often identify aggravating and relieving factors. Careful note should be made of these in an attempt to achieve relief by their avoidance wherever possible. Symptoms arising in unstable lax weight-bearing joints may be relieved by instituting appropriate exercise programmes, thereby utilising muscle tone to compensate for ligamentous laxity (Grahame, 1983b).

DISORDERS OF THE GROUND SUBSTANCE — THE MUCOPOLYSACCHARIDOSES (Table 46.2)

In this group of conditions there is an inherited disturbance of the mucopolysaccharides (glycosaminoglycans). The widespread and severe abnormalities include gross skeletal deformities and dwarfing due to bone involvement, clouding of the cornea, mental retardation, enlargement of the liver and spleen and cardiac failure. The joints are characteristically hypomobile. Herniae are common. There is widespread deposit of mucopolysaccharide throughout the organs of the body and excessive amounts of mucopolysaccharides are detected in the urine. Another characteristic is the finding of metachromatic granules in the circulating lymphocytes, bone marrow cells, or cultured fibroblasts (Danes et al, 1972). Many clinical variants have been described as follows; type IH (Hurler's syndrome) (Fig. 46.8); type IS (Scheie's syndrome); type IH/S (Hurler–Scheie compound); type IIA (Hunter's syndrome, severe); type IIB (Hunter's syndrome, mild); type III (Sanfillippo's syndrome — types A and B); type IV (Morquio's syndrome); type VI (Maroteaux-Lamy syndrome — types A and B) and type VII (β-glucuronidase deficiency). An autosomal recessive pattern of inheritance is seen in all syndromes except type II which is an X-linked recessive and thus affects males only.

With the exceptions of types IS and III, patients succumb in childhood or adolescence to respiratory infection, cardiac valve thickening or coronary arterial stenosis. The mucopolysaccharide excreted in the urine is dermatan sulphate in types I, II, VI and VII. Heparan sulphate is found in types I, II and III whereas keratan sulphate is seen exclusively in type IV. New possibilities for a rational therapy in these conditions are raised by the observations that administration of normal human plasma to patients with types I and II results in decreased urine excretion of polysaccharides and increased excretion of their degradation products (DiFeranti *et al*, 1971). A report of a beneficial clinical response to the transfusion of leucocytes in a child with type II (Hunter's syndrome) resulted in considerable clinical and biochemical improvement (Knudson et al, 1968). More recently biochemical improvement was temporarily induced in a child with Hunter's syndrome following the transplantation of parental skin (Dean et al, 1975). Leucocyte transfusion was found to be superior to plasma infusion in a comparative study carried out in two patients with Hurler's syndrome (type IH) and Scheie's (type IS) syndrome (Nishioka et al, 1979).

Current work using transplanted human amniochorionic membrane is likely to prove even more successful. This is because the amniotic epithelial cells, though rich in the enzymes deficient in the mucopolysaccaridoses, do not contain HLA-A,B, C, and DR antigens and beta-2-microglobulin are thus unlikely to induce a graft-versus-host reaction (Adinolfi et al, 1982).

Table 46.2 Mucopolysaccharidoses (after McKusick, 1975).

	Designation	Clinical features	Genetics	Excessive urinary MPS	Enzyme deficient
MPS IH	Hurler's syndrome	Early clouding of cornea, grave manifestations, death usually before age 10	Homozygous for MPS IH gene	Dermatan sulphate Heparan sulphate	
MPS IS	Scheie's syndrome	Stiff joints, cloudy cornea, aortic regurgitation, normal intelligence? normal life span	Homozygous for MPS IS gene	Dermatan sulphate Heparan sulphate	α-L-iduronidase Bach et al (1972)
MPS IH/S	Hurler–Scheie compound	Phenotype intermediate between Hurler and Scheie	Genetic compound MPS IH and IS genes	Dermatan sulphate Heparan sulphate	
MPS IIA	Hunter's syndrome, severe	No clouding of cornea, milder course than in MPS IH, but death usually before age 15	Hemizygous for X-linked gene	Dermatan sulphate Heparan sulphate	Sulpho-iduronide sulphatase Bach et al (1973)
MPS IIB	Hunter's syndrome, mild	Survival to 30s–50s, fair intelligence	Hemizygous for X-linked allecle for mild form	Dermatan sulphate Heparan sulphate	
MPS IIIA	Sanfilippo's syndrome A	Identical phenotype	Homozygous for Sanfilippo A gene	Heparan sulphate	Heparan sulphate sulphatase Krease & Neufeld (1972)
MPS IIIB	Sanfilippo's syndrome B	Mild somatic, severe central nervous system effects	Homozygous for Sanfilippo B (at different locus)	Heparan sulphate	*N*-acetyl-α-D-glucosaminidase O'Brien (1972)
MPS IV	Morquio's syndrome (probably more than one allelic form)	Severe bone changes of distinctive type, cloudy cornea, aortic regurgitation	Homozygous for Morquio gene	Keratan sulphate	? Chondroitin sulphate sulphatase Matalon et al (1974)
MPS V	(Vacant (now MPS IS))				
MPS VIA	Maroteaux-Lamy syndrome, severe form	Severe osseous and corneal change normal intellect	Homozygous for M-L gene	Dermatan sulphate	Arylsulphatase B Barton & Neufeld (1972) (MPS VIA and VIB)
MPS VIB	Maroteaux-Lamy, mild form	Mild osseous and corneal change, normal intellect	Homozygous for allele at M-L locus	Dermatan sulphate	
MPS VII	β-glucuronidase deficiency (more than one allelic form?)	Hepatosplenomegaly, dysostosis multiplex, white cell inclusions, mental retardation	Homozygous for mutant gene at β-glucuronidase locus	Dermatan sulphate	β-gluconidase Sly et al (1973)

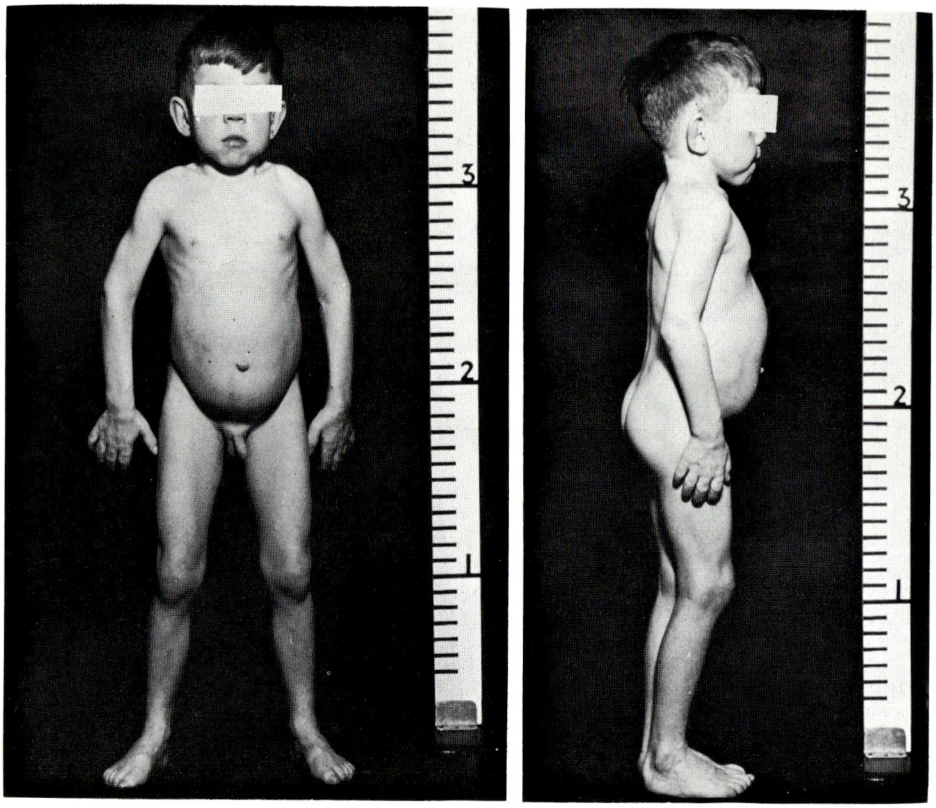

Fig. 46.8 Type I mucopolysaccharidosis (Hurler's syndrome). Note the short stature, coarse features, stubby hands, umbilical hernia and abdominal distension due to hepatosplenomegaly. Age 11½ years.

MISCELLANEOUS HEREDITARY SKELETAL DISORDERS

Over 200 hereditary diseases affecting the skeleton have been described. Many are extremely rare and space permits a description of only a small selection of these in this chapter. For a comprehensive review the reader is recommended to consult the excellent monographs by Wynne-Davies (1973) and Horan & Beighton (1982).

Myositis ossificans progressiva (fibrodysplasia ossificans progressiva) makes its appearance known during childhood. Soft tissues including muscles, ligaments and tendons become replaced by bone. Microdactyly, particularly of the thumb and hallux, is a common finding. It is believed that the primary lesion is a dystrophy of connective tissue which secondarily undergoes calcification. The relationship between the microdactyly and myositis ossificans is unknown. The pattern of inheritance is that of Mendelian dominant.

Osteopoikilosis is characterised by round, circumscribed areas of dense bone of 1 cm or more in diameter. They are found particularly at the ends of long bones and in the small bones of the hands and feet. In addition, skin lesions which are usually oval, white and slightly elevated occur in streaks along the posterior thighs and buttocks. A Mendelian autosomal dominant inheritance is encountered. The basic defect is thought to be a so-called 'hyperplasia' of collagen in the skin and bone matrix (Fig. 46.9).

In *achondroplasia* the trunk is of normal length and the limbs are short, whilst the cranium is bulging and the bridge of the nose is depressed (Fig. 46.10). The condition is inherited as an autosomal dominant but since reproductive capacity is impaired the majority of cases arise by mutation. Four types of neurological deficit have been recently described (Lutter & Langer, 1977). In type

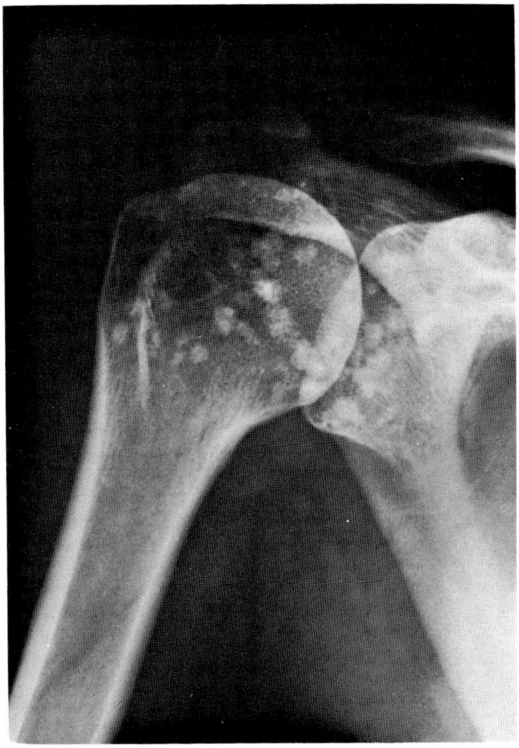

Fig. 46.9 Osteopoikilosis affecting the humerus and scapula.

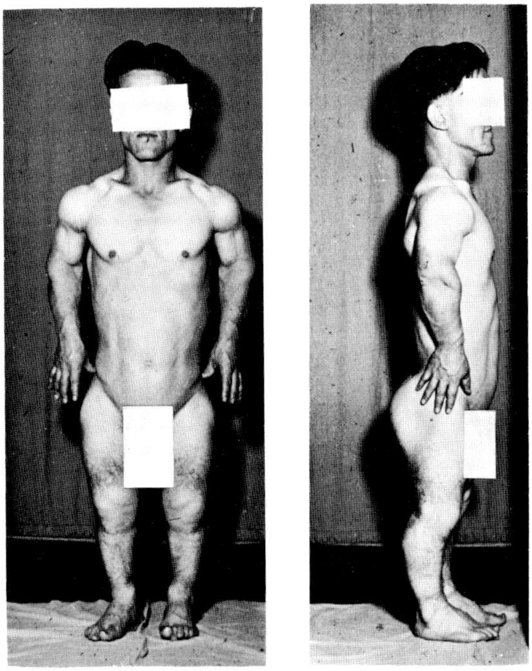

Fig. 46.10 Achondroplasia. The limbs are short while the trunk is normally proportioned. The cranium is bulging.

1 thoracolumbar kyphosis was associated with cord compression, slowly progressive sensory followed by motor and reflex changes dominating the clinical picture. Laminectomy gave variable results. Type 2 presented with intermittent claudication thought to be due to vascular insufficiency. Laminectomy brought good results. Type 2 presented with intermittent claudication thought to be due to vascular insufficiency. Laminectomy brought good results in these patients. Type 3 was characterised by true nerve root compression found at operation to be the result of disc prolapse. In type 4 an acute severe back or neck pain associated with trauma gave rise to paraparesis or paraplegia. Results of operation here were poor due to severe neurological damage. In another study (Morgan & Young, 1980) of spinal stenosis in achondroplasia, surgical decompression was found to give excellent results when compression was localised but long-term results were less satisfactory where the stenosis was generalised throughout the vertebral column. Intelligence is usually not impaired and many patients live a normal life span (Murdoch et al, 1970).

Epiphysial dysplasia. (*1*) *Spondyloepiphysial dysplasia.* This form of short-trunk dwarfism makes its presence felt in childhood and the changes felt in childhood and the changes become more pronounced during adolescence. The major abnormality is seen in the lumbar vertebrae and is revealed on X-ray as humping of bone in the central portions of the vertebral plates, with lack of bone in the region of the ring apophyses (Fig. 46.11). Precocious degenerative changes occur in large joints, notably hips, knees and shoulders. A dominant and an X-linked recessive form have been described.

(2) *Multiple epiphysial dysplasia.* This is another common form of precocious osteoarthrosis of the hip (Fig. 46.12) accompanied by dwarfing. Involvement of the lower tibial epiphysis causes sloping of the tibial surface of the ankle.

In *pycnodysostosis* the stature is short and the bones show increased density but despite this they are fragile and fractures are common. The condition is inherited as an autosomal recessive.

In *osteopetrosis* the bones are also sclerotic, yet fragile. There is a congenital form and one which develops during childhood or adolescence. In the

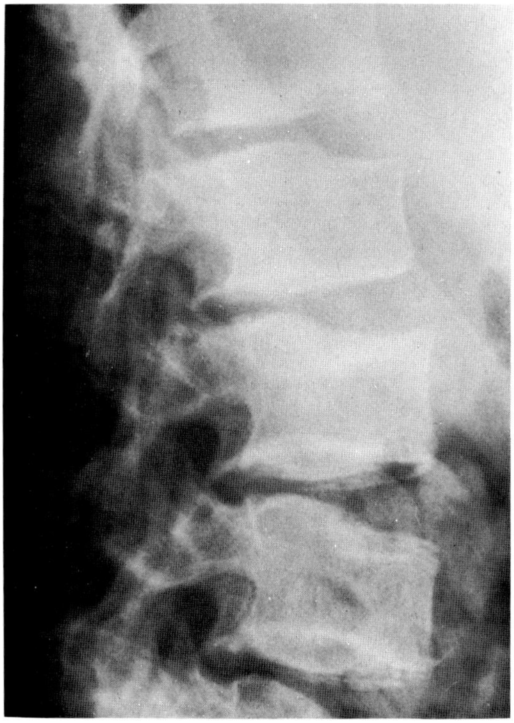

former variety, severe anaemia may develop from replacement of bone marrow by dense bone and affected infants do not survive long. The tarda variety carries a better prognosis but fractures occur as well as stenosis of the cranial nerve foramina.

In the *nail-patella syndrome* (hereditary onycho-osteodysplasia) the finger nails are hypoplastic or absent, as may be the patellae. The gene for this condition is believed to be located on the same chromosome as the ABO blood group. It is inherited as an autosomal dominant trait. Renal failure may occur although the lesion responsible for this has not been elucidated.

In *cleidocranial dysostosis* there is defective development of membrane bones. It is inherited as an autosomal dominant trait but many cases result from mutation. There is often bulging of the frontal parts of the skull with hypoplasia or absence of the clavicles as well as the muscles normally

Fig. 46.11 Involvement of the vertebral body in spondyloepiphysial dysplasia. The heaping up of the posterior portion of the superior vertebral plate is characteristic.

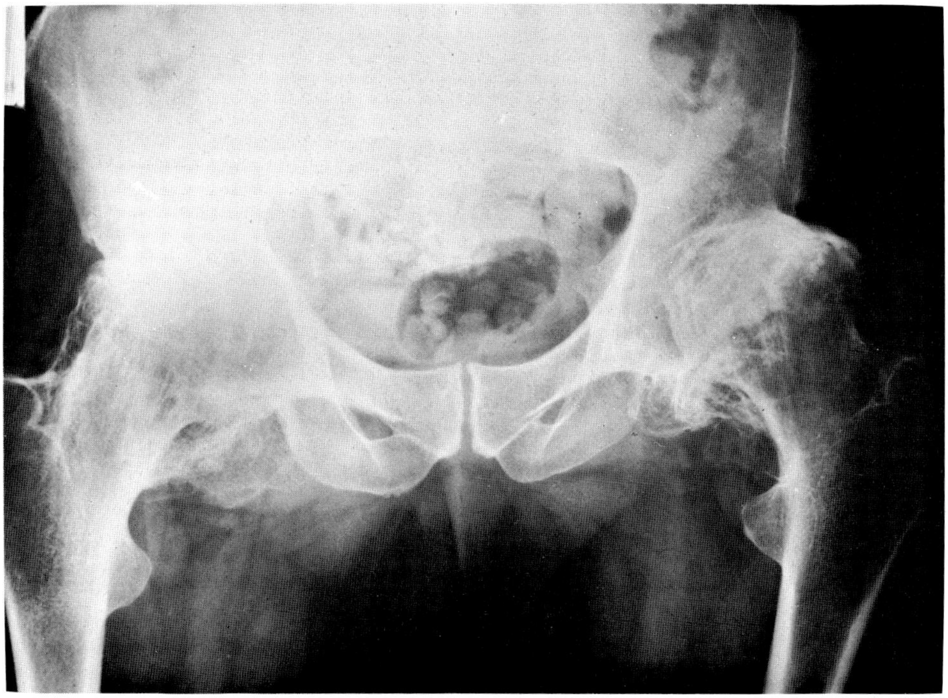

Fig. 46.12 Premature osteoarthrosis of the hips in a patient suffering from multiple epiphysial dysplasia.

attached to the clavicles. The life span is not shortened. Hypoplasia of the acetabulum may lead to dislocation of the hip.

In *diaphyseal aclasis* multiple exostoses occur near the ends of the long bones. The axial skeleton is usually not affected. Symptoms arise from pressure on other structures such as peripheral nerves. The pattern of inheritance is that of autosomal dominance.

REFERENCES

Adinolfi M, Akle C A, McColl I et al 1982 Expression of HLA Antigens, beta 2 microglobulin and enzymes by human amniotic epithelial cells. Nature, 295: 325–327

Arneson M A, Hammerschmidt D E, Furcht I T, King R A 1980 A new form of Ehlers–Danlos syndrome: fibronection corrects defective platelet function. Journal of the American Medical Association 224: 144–147

Bach G, Eisenberg F Jr, Cantz M, Neufeld E F 1973 The defect in the Hunter syndrome deficiency of sulphoiduronide sulphatase. Proceedings of the National Academy of Science 70:2134

Bach G, Friedman R, Weisman B, Neufeld E F 1972 The defect in the Hurtler and Scheie syndrome deficiency of L-iduronidase. Proceedings of the National Academy of Sciences 69:2048

Barton R W, Neufeld E F 1972 A distinct biochemical deficit in the Maroteaux-Lamy syndrome (mucopolysacchariodosis VI) Journal of Pediatrics 80:114

Beighton P 1970 The Ehlers–Danlos syndrome. Heinemann, London

Beighton P 1983 The Ehlers–Danlos syndrome. In: Beighton P, Grahame R, Bird H (eds) Hypermobility of joints. Springer-Verlag, Berlin, Ch 12

Beighton P, Horan F 1970 Dominant inheritance in generalised articular hypermobility. Journal of Bone and Joint Surgery 52B:145

Beighton P, Solomon L, Soskole C L 1973 Articular mobility in an African population. Annals of the Rheumatic Diseases 32:413

Berenson G S, Delferes E R Jr 1963 Urinary excretion in mucopolysaccharides in normal individuals and in the Marfan syndrome. Biochimica et Biophysica Acta 101:183

Bird H A 1979 Joint hypermobility: A dissertation for the degree of Doctor of Medicine, University of Cambridge. p 103

Bird H A, Brodie D A, Wright V 1979 Quantification of joint laxity. Rheumatology and Rehabilitation 18: 161–166

Bonella D, Parker D J, Davies M J 1980. Accumulation of procollagen in human floppy mitral valves. Lancet 1: 880–881

Boucek R J, Noble N L, Gunja-Smith Z, Butler W T 1981. The Marfan syndrome: a deficiency in chemically stable cross-links. New England Journal of Medicine 305: 988–91

Carter C S, Sweetman R 1960 Recurrent dislocation of the patella and of the shoulder; their association with familial joint laxity. Journal of Bone and Joint Surgery 42B:183

Carter C S, Wilkinson J 1964 Persistence of joint laxity and congenital dislocation of the hip. Journal of Bone and Joint Surgery 46B:40

Child A H, Dorrance D E, Jay B, Pope F M, Jones R B, Gosling R G 1981 Ophthalmic Paediatrics and Genetics 1: 59–76

Danes B S, Hutteroth T H, Crewe H 1972 The Hurler syndrome: a study of cultured lymphoid cells lines. Journal of Experimental Medicine 136:644

Dean M F, Muir H, Benson P F, Button L R, Bachelor J R, Bewick M 1975 Increased breakdown of glycosaminoglycans and appearance of corrective enzyme after skin transplants in Hunter syndrome. Nature 257:609

DiFerrante N, Nichols B L, Donnoly P V, Nevi G, Hrgovcic R, Bergland R K 1971 Induced degradation of glycosaminoglycans of Hurler's and Hunter's syndromes by plasma infusion. Proceedings of the National Academy of Science 68:303

Ghadimi H, Billington I, Pecova P 1965 Hyperlysinaemia associated with retardation. New England Journal of Medicine 273:723

Grahame R 1971 Joint-mobility — clinical aspects. Proceedings of the Royal Society of Medicine 64:693

Grahame R 1983a Illustrative case histories. In: Beighton P, Grahame R, Bird H A (eds) Hypermobility of joints. Springer-Verlag, Berlin, Ch 7

Grahame R 1983b Management of articular complications in the hypermobility syndrome. In: Beighton P, Grahame R, Bird H W (eds) Hypermobility of joints. Springer-Verlag, Berlin, Ch 7

Grahame R, Beighton P 1971 Physical properties of the skin in cutis laxa. British Journal of Dermatology 84:326

Grahame R, Jenkins J M 1972 Joint hypermobility, asset or liability. A study of joint mobility in ballet dancers. Annals of the Rheumatic Diseases 31:109

Grahame R, Edwards J C, Pitcher D, Gabell A, Harvey W 1981 A clinical and echocardiographic study of patients with a hypermobility syndrome. Annals of the Rheumatic Disease 40: 541–546

Hall D A, Reed R, Tunbridge R E 1955 Electron microscope studies of elastic tissue. Experimental Cell Research 8:35

Harris H, Joseph J 1949 Variation in extension of metacarpal phalangeal and interphalangeal joints of the thumb. Journal of Bone and Joint Surgery 31B:547

Harvey W, Pope F M, Grahame R 1975 Cutaneous extensibility in Pseudo-xanthoma elasticum. British Journal of Dermatology 97:679

Horan F, Beighton P 1971 Recessive inheritance of generalised joint hypermobility. Rheumatology and Rehabilitation 12:47

Horan F, Beighton P 1982 Orthopaedic problems in inherited skletal disorders. Springer-Verlag, Berlin

Howes R C, Isdale I C 1971 The loose back, an unrecognised syndrome. Rheumatology and Physical Medicine 11:72

Jobbins B, Bird H A, Wright V 1979. A joint hyperextensometer for the quatification of joint laxity. Engineering in Medicine 8: 103–104

Kang A H, Trelstad R L 1973 A collagen defect in homocystinuria Journal of Clinical Investigation 52: 2571–2578

Kirk J A, Ansell B M, Bywaters E G L 1967 The hypermobility syndrome. Annals of the Rheumatic Diseases, 26:419

Knudson A G, DiFerrante N, Curtis G E 1971 The effect of leucocyte transfusion in a child with type II mucopolysaccharidosis. Proceedings of the National Academy of Science USA 68:173

Kresse H, Neufeld E F 1972 The Sanfilippo a corrective factor: purification and mode of action. Journal of Biological Chemistry 247:2164

Krieg T, Müller P K 1977 The Marfan syndrome. Experimental and Cellular Biology 45: 207–221

Laitenin O, Uitto J, Iivanan M 1968 Collagen metabolism of the skin in Marfan's syndrome. Clinica Chimica Acta 21:321

Loebl W 1972 Assessment of mobility of metacarpophalangeal joints. Rheumatology and Physical Medicine 11:356

Lutter L P, Langer L O 1977 Neurological complications in achondroplastic dwarfs — Surgical treatment. Journal of Bone Joint Surgery (AM) 59:87

McKusick V A 1972 Heritable disorders, in concective tissue, 4th Edn. Mosby St Louis

McKusick V A 1975 Mendelian inheritance in man, 4th Edn. Johns Hopkins University Press, London

Matalon R, Arbogast B, Dorfman A 1974 Morquio's syndrome a deficiency of chondroitin sulfate N-acetylhexosamine sulfate sulfatase (Abstract). Pediatric Research 8:436

Metalon D, Dorfman A 1968 The accumulation of hyaluronic acid in the culture of fibroblasts of the Marfan syndrome. Biochimica et biophysica Acta 32:150

Moran T J, Lansang A 1958 Studies on the nature of the abnormal fibres in pseudo xanthoma elasticum. Archives of Pathology 65:688

Morgan D, Young R F 1980 Spinal neurological complications of achondroplasia: results of surgical treatment. Neurosurgery 52:463

Murdoch J L, Walker B A, Hall J G, Abbey H, Smith K K, McKusick V A 1970 Achondroplasia, a genetic and statistical survey. Annals of Human Genetics 33:227

Nicholas J A 1970 Injuries to the knee ligaments. Relationship to looseness and tightness in football players. Journal of American Medical Association 212:2236

Nishioka J, Mizushima T Ono K 1979 Treatment of mucopolysaccharidosis. Clinical and Biochemical aspect of leucocyte transfusion as compared with plasma infusion in patients with Hurler and Scheie's syndrome 140: 194–203

O'Brien J S 1972 Sanfilippo syndrome profound deficiency of alpha acetyglucosaminidase activity in organs and skin fibroblasts from type B patients. Proceedings of the National Academy of Science 69:1720

Perry T L, Dunn H G, Harrison S, Macdougal L, Waddington P D 1966 Early diagnosis and treatment of homocystinuria. Paediatrics 37:502

Pitcher D, Grahame R 1982 Mitral valve prolapse and joint hypermobility: Evidence for a systemic tissue abnormality. Annals of the Rheumatic Diseases 41: 352–354

Pope F M 1974a Autosomal dominant forms of pseudo-xanthoma elasticum. Journal of Medical Genetics 11:152

Pope F M 1974b Two types of autosomal recessive pseudo xanthoma elasticum. Archives of Dermatology 110:209

Prokop D J, Sjoerdsma A 1961 The significance of urinary hydroxyproline in man. Journal of Clinical Investigations 40:843

Scheck M, Siegel R C, Parker J, Chang Y-H, Fu J C 1979 Aortic aneurism in Marfan's syndrome: changes in the ultra structure and composition of collagen. Journal of Anatomy 129, 3: 645–657

Schweitzer G 1970 Laxity of metacarpal phalangeal joints of the finger and interphalangeal joints of the thumb. A comparative interacial study. South African Medical Journal 44:246

Schimke R N, McKusick V A, Huang T, Pollack A D 1965 Homocystinuria studies of 20 families with 38 affected members. Journal of American Medical Association 193:87

Silverman S, Constine L, Harvey W, Grahame R 1975 A survey of joint mobility and in vivo skin elasticity in London school children. Annals of the Rheumatic Diseases 34:177

Sinclair R J G, Kitchin A H, Turner R W D 1960 The Marfan syndrome. Quarterly Journal of Medicine 29:19

Sly W S, Quinton B A, McAlistair W H, Rimoin D L 1973 Beta glucuronidase deficiency report of clinical radiological and biochemical features of new mucopolysacchariodsis. Journal of Pediatrics 82:249

Spaeth G L, Barber G W 1967 Prevalence of homocytinuria amongst the mentally retarded. Evaluation of specific screening test. Paediatrics 40:586

Stuart R E, Hollister D W, Rimoin D L 1977 A new variant of Ehlers–Danlos syndrome: an autosomal dominant disorder of fragile skin, abnormal scarring and generalised periodontitis. Birth defects 13: 85–93

Sutro C J 1947 Hypermobility of knees due to over lengthened capsular and ligamentous tissues. Surgery 21:67

Sweetman B J, Anderson J A D, Dalton E R 1974 Relationships between little finger mobility, lumbar mobility, straight leg raising and low back pain. Rheumatology and Rehabilitation 13:61

Uhlendorf B W, Mudd S H 1968 Cystathionine synthase in tissue culture derived from human skin enzyme defect in homocystinuria. Science 160:1007

Wynne-Davies R 1973 Heritable Disorders in Orthopaedic Practice. Oxford

Arthritis and blood disease

Rheumatic complications, which are predominantly articular, of haematological disease can have an obvious pathogenesis due to bleeding (haemophilia), localised ischaemia (sickle cell disease) or possibly immune complex formation (cryoglobulinaemia). However, in others the pathogenesis is less clear, e.g. immune deficiencies and leukaemia. The rheumatic complications may be the main feature (haemophilia) or be a comparatively minor feature (leukaemia).

The rheumatologist may be faced with the rheumatic features as the presenting aspect of the disease or be an adviser in part management of the prime haematological problem. In either case few practising rheumatologists will acquire a wide experience of this group of disorders and the experience may well be uneven due to epidemiological factors, e.g. sickle cell disease, and the availability of the required facilities to investigate patients.

In the following account no attempt has been made to catalogue every condition and some of the data are based on single case reports or small series of patients; nor will the pathogenetic mechanism of haematologic disease be dealt with in detail. However, it is hoped that the chapter will provide help with the more common problems encountered, with mention only of the interesting rarities. Further reading will be found in the chapter references.

HAEMOPHILIA AND OTHER BLEEDING DISORDERS

Factor VIII is probably manufactured in two stages, both being necessary to produce a fully functional molecule. Functional tests are necessary to identify defects in these two stages since antihaemophilic factor can be physically present but in a non-functional form. Haemophilia A is an X-linked recessive disease while Von Willebrand's disease is an autosomally inherited defect (Table 47.1). These diseases result from abnormalities of complementary parts of the antihaemophilic factor (VIII) molecule. Haemophilia B (Christmas disease) is a similar X-linked recessive disease in which factor IX is functionally defective. Minor variations in the basic defects outlined are found and in some patients multiple errors occur. About a quarter or one-third of patients give no family history of bleeding. The resulting failure of coagulation affects the intrinsic pathway, coagulation

Table 47.1 Haemophilia and other bleeding disorders

Disorder	Occurrence	Defect	Test	Treatment	
Haemophilia A	M	X-linked Factor VIII ↓	Ristocetin-induced platelet aggregation normal Bleeding time normal	Factor VIII	Cryoprecipitate Single donor Concentrate pool
Haemophilia B	M	X-linked Factor IX ↓	Bleeding time normal	Factor IX	Concentrate pool
Von Willebrand's disease	M & F	Autosomal Factor VIII defective	Prolonged bleeding time Ristocetin-induced platelet aggregation ↓	Factor VIII	Concentrate pool

thus depending on the extrinsic pathway which is said to be deficient in synovial tissue; this may partly explain the propensity for joint haemorrhage and destruction (Astrup & Sjolin, 1958).

Haemophilia can be defined as a functional factor VIII level of less than 50% of the average value in the population. Using this definition, a prevalence of 6–8 cases/100 000 is appropriate. A factor VIII level of < 1% will usually give rise to severe disease and a level of > 10% very few problems.

The clinical severity of the disorder approximates to the functional level of factor VIII or IX in plasma although these levels tend to fluctuate (Table 47.2) and the bleeding tendency varies thoughout the year. The disease severity tends to be constant in families though this is probably less so in Von Willebrand's disease. Mild deficiencies rarely lead to persisting musculoskeletal problems and will not be considered further.

Table 47.2 Clinical severity of haemophilia

Factor VIII (IX) level	Clinical severity	Bleeding tendency
< 1%	Severe	Severe bleeds
1–5%	Moderate	Variable
> 5%	Mild	Rarely bleeds

Children are usually detected in one of two ways, either as a family contact or following bruising or prolonged bleeding, sometimes in association with minor operations, or following bleeds into joints or muscles.

The large joints and muscle groups, especially of the lower limb, are most frequently involved (Table 47.3). The hand or foot is rarely involved. The initial bleeds start at the time of mobility, usually walking, but are mainly unrelated to obvious trauma. In the young interpretation is difficult but the muscle or joint is painful and the child dislikes examination. The affected joint is flexed and the surrounding muscles are kept in the relaxed position. Although blood may be aspirated from some joints, especially the more persistently swollen, this is not invariable and undoubtedly some of the bleeding, often with less swelling, occurs into the capsule. The origin of bleeding is uncertain and is one of the less well understood features of this condition.

It is useful to consider the clinical course of the arthropathy in three stages: acute haemarthrosis, subacute and chronic arthropathy.

Acute haemarthrosis

This is often the first manifestation of haemophilia and occurs in about 25–30% of cases. Initially in sporadic cases the child will be thought to have knocked or twisted the joint. In the very young the child can only demonstrate the site of the pain by resisting movement of the joint and initially swelling will be limited. The pain in the joint rapidly increases and is later associated in most cases with swelling, usually globally, of the joint. The joint is painful at rest but becomes exquisitely painful on movement and may be very tender, but it is the pain that always predominates. The effusion is tense and warm and the joint flexed. Skin discolouration of the joint *does not occur*, but bruising elsewhere may be seen. The most commonly affected joints are knee, ankle, elbow, hip and shoulder, in that order. The back and neck are rarely affected. Mild constitutional features such as a fever and leucocytosis can occur, presumably due to the extravasated blood, and the principle differential diagnosis in the initial episode is from a traumatic or septic arthritis, the joint becoming too painful for juvenile arthritis.

Table 47.3 135 patients followed up for more than 4 years with principal joints affected

Disorder	NAR	AR	K	A	E	S	Mono	T	C	Arm
Haemophilia	50	41	35	29	23	6	6	17	13	11
Von Willebrand's disease	17	3	1	3	1	—	2	—	—	—
Christmas disease	7	7	5	4	3	2	1	2	3	—
	74	51	41	36	27	8	9	19	16	11

NAR = No arthritis; AR = recurrent joint bleeds; K = knee; A = ankle; E = elbow; S = shoulder; T = thigh; C = calf; Arm = upper & lower arm muscle; Mono = recurrent bleeds in single joint only.

Subacute arthropathy
Progression to subacute arthropathy is probably determined by the severity of the bleeding defect. the frequency of bleeds and the adequacy of management.

Progression of arthropathy is dependent on recurrent bleeds at fairly frequent intervals, i.e. before the damage from the previous bleeds has fully recovered. This is an important principle because recurrent bleeds lead to synovial hypertrophy, cartilage irregularities, capsular fibrosis and bone overgrowth and eventually to a self-perpetuating chronic arthropathy. It is at this stage that it is noticed that one or more joints are the sites of recurrent bleeds, that the swelling does not settle between bleeds and the doughy synovial thickening persists (Fig. 47.1). The joint is now persistently flexed and muscles wasted. Pain with later bleeds tends to be less than in the initial episodes.

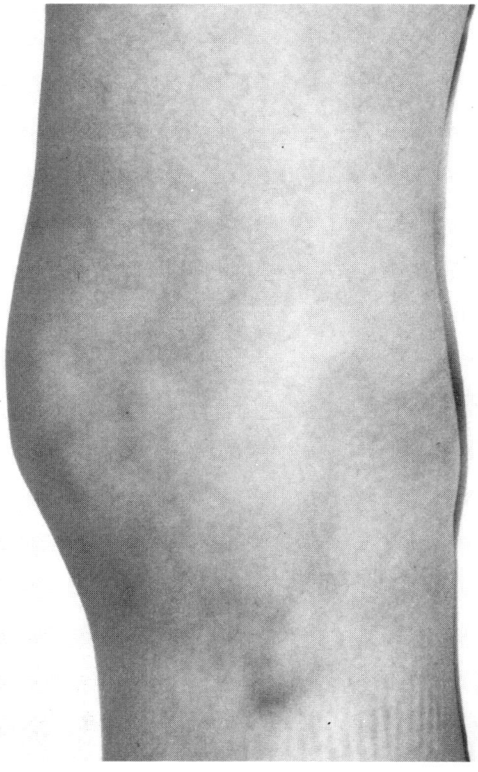

Fig. 47.1 Haemophilia arthropathy, becoming chronic with effusion and periarticular thickening and small popliteal cyst (unusual) on right. Early flexion of knee.

Chronic haemophilic arthropathy
The acute episodes of bleeding are often less at this stage but pain of mild degree tends to persist between bleeding episodes and the joint is persistently flexed often with limitation of the full range of flexion. Between bleeds the joints are usually not tender. The muscles are wasted, especially the quadriceps, but the knee remains relatively stable. Bones may be enlarged; this is most easily felt in the patella which may also be deflected laterally — this is most easily felt in the flexed position — and difficulty may be experienced in inserting the finger between the patella and the lateral femoral condyle. The patient's ability to make kicking movements is severely limited. Elongation of the affected limb may be found due to epiphyseal overgrowth, this in itself encouraging the patient to walk with a flexed knee.

The ankle early loses its range of movement with chronic involvement, the main change being in limitation of lateral movement but also in dorsiflexion (see below).

Soft tissue bleeding
The most important form of this is bleeding into muscle which can lead to more problems than joint involvement. The muscle is painful on movement and later at rest, tender and often in spasm; later a firm thickening can be felt (Aronstam et al, 1983). Obvious discolouration is rare and late and usually dependent. Initially no residua may be apparent and complete recovery occurs, but with further bleeds or inadequate treatment it will be noticed that the joint controlled by the muscle does not reach the limit of its range. Later still the muscle, or part of it, becomes firm and hard and cannot be felt to relax normally or it is band-like. The muscle, or part of it, atrophies and is felt and seen to be small. As the limb, *but not the muscle* which is fibrosed, elongates with normal growth, the inequality between limb and muscle becomes increasingly apparent and joint range is progressively reduced by the muscular contraction. This is most clearly seen at the ankle with the shortening of the calf muscles, leading to a tip-toe gait which in itself adds further stress to the calf muscles and flexing of the knee (Fig. 47.2).

Other sites of bleeding are the biceps muscles with flexion of the elbow and the flexor muscles

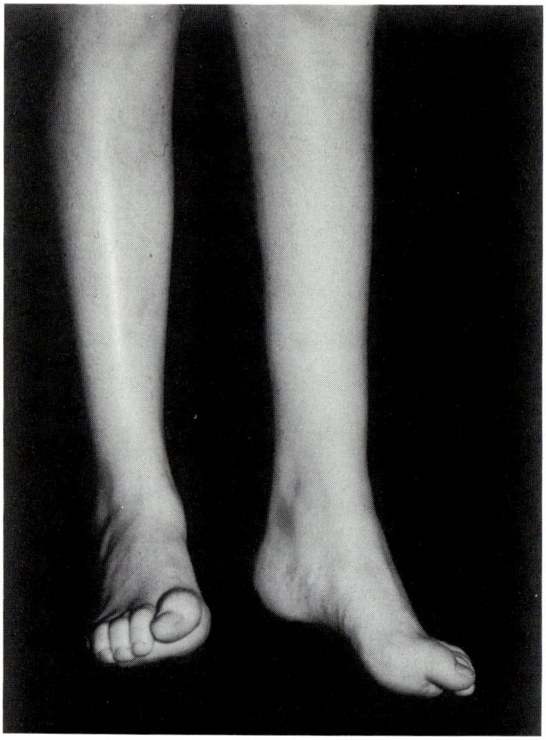

Fig. 47.2 Haemophilia. Contracture and wasting of upper left calf with plantagrade flexion of foot.

Involvement of the palmar and thenar eminences is rare but very painful. It usually follows direct trauma and heals completely.

Pressure involvement of nerves occurs with bleeds into the ilio-psoas muscle (femoral nerve), which is the common site, and in the forearm and palm when the median nerve may be involved. A more subtle neuromyopathy has been suggested by Defaria et al (1979) who have demonstrated EMG abnormalities, elevated creatine phosphokinase levels and type II fibre atrophy. These changes were not directly related to obvious bleeding.

Rarely, a haemophilic pseudotumour may develop at the site of a poorly treated haematoma which, due to persistence and recurrent bleeds, becomes organised and highly vascularised. Progressive enlargement may occur. Two main forms have been described, an adult form usually in the pelvis or femur, and a childhood form distal to the knee. Initial prolonged treatment of the coagulation defect is recommended but surgical removal is usually necessary. Aspiration should not be undertaken (Ahlberg, 1975).

Epilepsy, mental deficiency and limb paresis are found in these patients, presumably due to intracerebral bleeds early in life.

of the forearm, with a flexion deformity of the wrist and fingers, the picture being similar to that of Volkmann's ischaemic contracture (Fig. 47.3).

Aetiopathogenesis

The various theories of causation of joint changes are well described by Arnold & Hilgartner (1977)

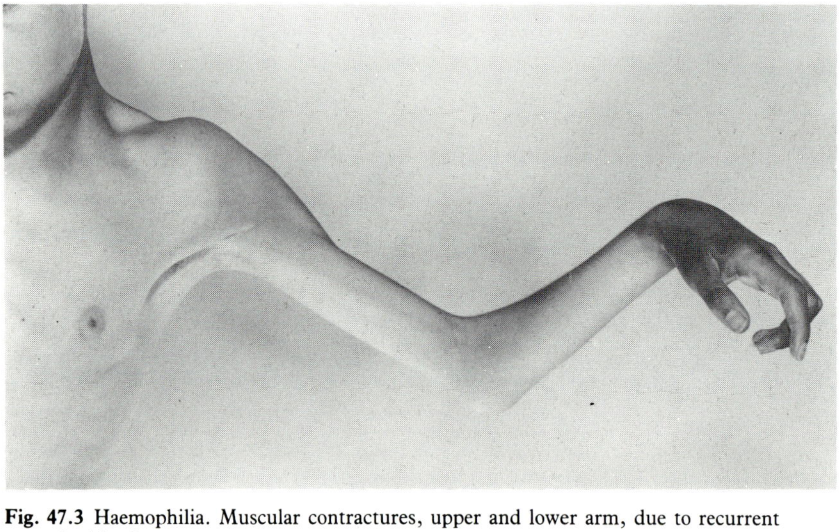

Fig. 47.3 Haemophilia. Muscular contractures, upper and lower arm, due to recurrent muscular bleeding.

and Stein & Duthie (1981). As intimated above, the sites of articular bleeding are not clear. Probably capsular, synovial and subchondral bleeding occur. Anticoagulant antibodies have been demonstrated in the synovial membrane of haemophilia and rheumatoid arthritis which are different from factor VIII antibodies (Rainsford et al, 1982). Relatively little is known about the fate of intra-articular blood. Small intra-articular bleeds may be a frequent occurrence in rheumatoid arthritis but apparently cause few problems (Bennett et al, 1972), and occur in anticoagulated patients (Wild & Zvaifler, 1976) without sequelae. Repeated clinical and, presumably, also subclinical bleeds in thromboasthenia (Klofhorn, 1979) have been associated with haemophilia-like changes. Attempts to reproduce the changes of haemophilia by injecting blood into joints were unsuccessful until Hoaglund (1967) gave repeated injections for 18 weeks into the knees of puppies. This produced the full range of changes found in human haemophilia. Brighton et al (1970) have produced a degenerative arthritis by parenteral iron injections but only if high doses and immature rabbits were used. Iron was deposited in chondrocytes and cartilage. Similar work does not appear to have been done in the adult animal. Research with dogs suffering from haemophilia A has helped to determine the serial changes (Swanton & Wysocki, 1975). A synovial reaction with polymorphonuclear leucocytes, lymphocytes and monocytes occurs early as the synovial membrane hypertrophies. Platelets may be important in increasing the synovial permeability (Bignold, 1980). Iron pigment is deposited. The synovium continues to hypertrophy and form itself into a pannus with undermining and erosion of cartilage; that the proliferating synovium can produce latent collagenase and neutral proteinases similar to those found in rheumatoid arthritis synovium, was shown by Mainardi et al (1978). Later the central cartilage starts to degenerate and fibrillation much like that of osteoarthrosis appears. This is followed by subchondral bone cyst formation (Van Creveld et al, 1971; Hoedemaker & Wagenvoort, 1975).

X-ray features

The range of features is wide (Pettersen et al, 1980). The initial feature is an increase in soft tissue haziness and loss of fat and translucency within the synovial cavity. This is initially transient with each bleeding but later becomes permanent with recurrent bleeds (Figs 47.4, 47.5). Occasional calcification within this soft tissue is seen and similar calcification can be seen in chronic haematomas (Fig. 47.6). The epiphyses lying adjacent to joints may undergo precocious development and enlarge, sometimes asymmetrically; thus they are deeper and wider than might be expected (most easily demonstrated by comparison with the opposite side) (Figs 47.4, 47.5, 47.7). The changes are most characteristically seen at the knee and elbow. The patella is wider in all directions and its lower end is often squared, but

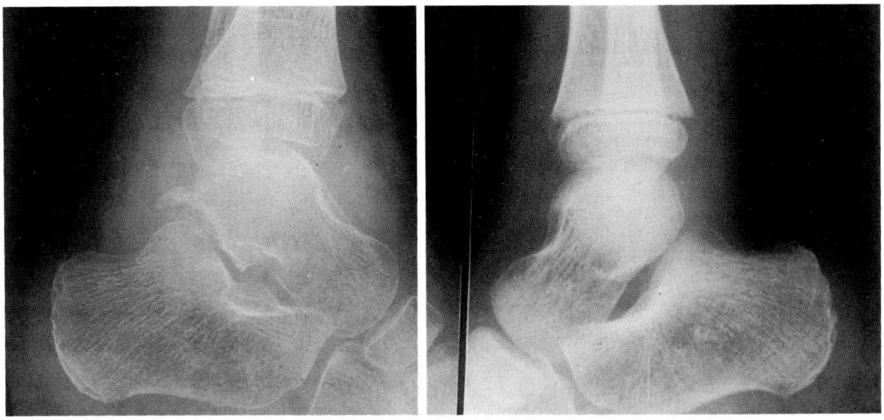

Fig. 47.4 Haemophilia. Ankles. Left shows bone hypertropy, especially of epiphysis, ossicle formation and characteristic thickening of periarticular soft tissue.

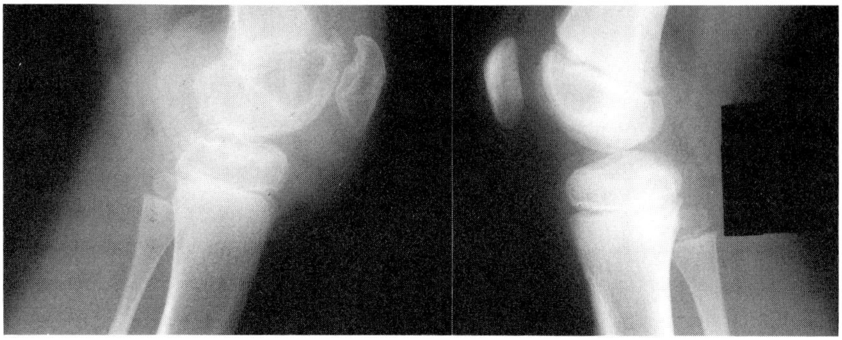

Fig. 47.5 Haemophilia. Knees. Relatively late changes on left of soft tissue thickening, increased epyphiseal growth, loss of patella–femoral cartilage and characteristic 'beaking' of upper pole of patella.

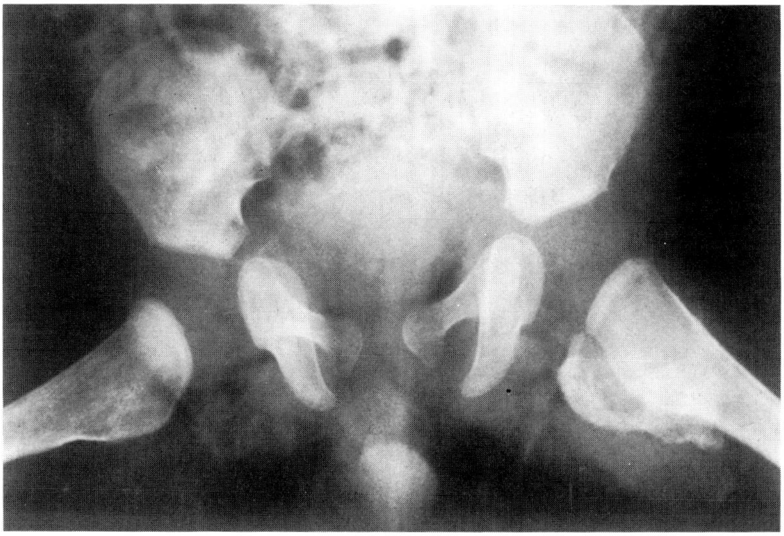

Fig. 47.6 Haemophilia. Left hip, new bone formation at site of haemorrhage medial to upper end of femur.

more characteristically its upper pole has a beaked appearance (Fig. 47.5). The tibial plateaux are often irregular and the femoral condyles, as well as being enlarged, have an enlarged and excavated intercondylar notch (Fig. 47.8), and asymmetrical patella groove with migration of the patella laterally on flexion of the knee (Fig. 47.9). Lateral erosion of tibial and femoral cortices may be seen, especially at ankle level. Periostitis, especially of the lower humerus, is a frequent finding (Fig. 47.7). Juxta-articular bone cysts in the later stages are very characteristic. Cartilage loss is a relatively late finding.

Management

The management of the locomotor problems of haemophilia is only one (although the major one) of several problems the patient may have. It is important to realise that there may be psychological problems within the family and that owing to intracerebral bleeds epilepsy and reduced intelligence are not uncommon. Many of the children have to attend special schools with limitation of their educational potential and, to a lesser extent, limitation of social contact (about 20% of our own series). Fortunately the type of clinical course usually becomes apparent at an early stage

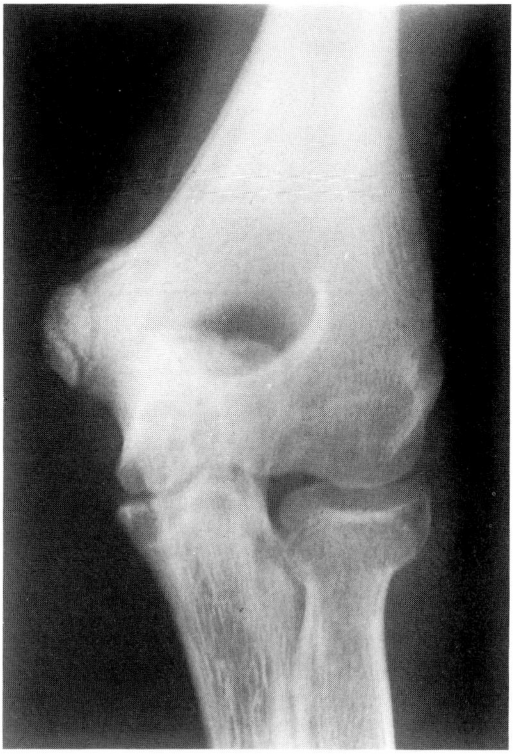

Fig. 47.7 Haemophilia. Elbow. Periostitis of lower end humerus, rarefaction of olecranon fossa. Some widening of upper radial head. Loss of cartilage in humeroulnar joint with periarticular cyst formation.

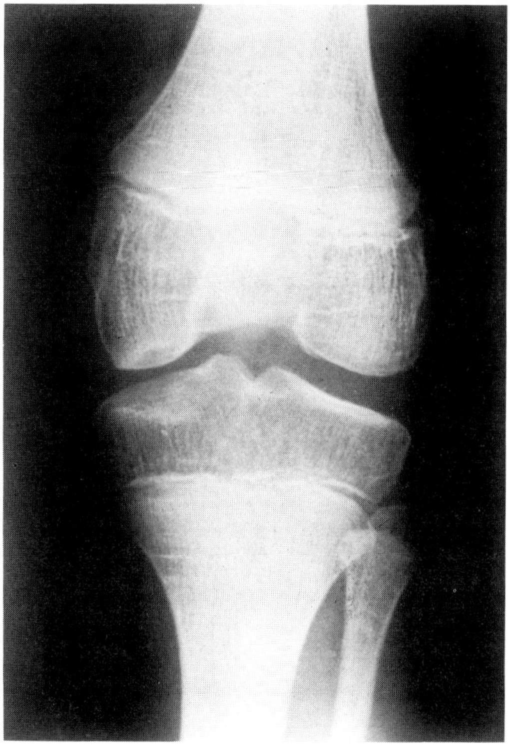

Fig. 47.8 Haemophilia. Early squaring of intercondylar notch. Multiple growth arrest lines.

and allows for forward planning of treatment.

For the acute bleeding episode early and adequate factor VIII and IX replacement, as appropriate, are necessary. Several forms are available but the differences are of little practical importance (see Table 47.1). (The recent description of acquired immune deficiency syndrome (AIDS) will result in greater screening of replacement sources and the use of smaller pools or single donors.) Initially injections of replacement factor will be given

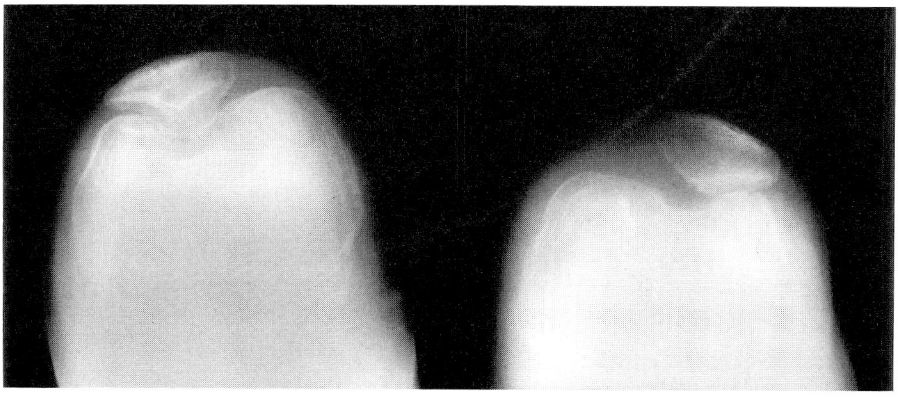

Fig. 47.9 Haemophilia. Knees 'skyline' view to show lateral migration of the patella with narrowing of lateral patella-femoral cartilage.

at hospital; later the relatives or a close friend and eventually the child will learn to give the injections. The increasing trend towards self-administration at home has increased the rapidity of intervention and the independence of the child with less loss of schooling time, etc. While awaiting his injection and for it to become effective, support for the limb is necessary. Often a splint will be available from previous bleeds. Early stabilisation of painful joints and muscles is essential. The effects of the bleed take a variable time to settle, usually varying from 1–3 days. However, if the bleed was large and treated late and particularly if it occurs into muscle, then the relief may take much longer and bleeds into previously affected sites are slower to settle. Presumably due to reduction of non-specific inflammation, much of the pain and some of the swelling of soft tissue bleeds can be removed by corticosteroid, e.g. 30 mg prednisolone initially and reducing over 3 days, given orally. This form of therapy may be indicated where intense pain and severe swelling are present causing nerve pressure or potential muscle fibrosis and shortening. The importance of rapid and adequate treatment of muscle bleeds has been emphasised by Aronstam et al (1983). Large tense synovial effusions often need aspiration but only under cover of replacement therapy. The use of intra-articular corticosteroids is controversial and rarely used. They might inhibit synovial anticoagulant antibodies (Rainsford et al, 1982).

As the pain and tenderness decrease, physiotherapy to obtain slow progressive increases in joint movement and muscle power are commenced. Initially physiotherapy must be supervised but later it can usually be managed by patient and family. Recovery from initial joint bleeds is usually complete. Recovery from intramuscular bleeds is more variable.

If the patient is developing subacute arthritis this is usually indicated by recurrent bleeds in a single joint at decreasing intervals and with incomplete recovery between attacks. In these circumstances it may become necessary to embark on a course of prophylactic injections, i.e. twice and three times a week for 1–3 months to allow the joint function to improve and, in particular, to facilitate physiotherapy. The increasing availability of replacement factor has greatly facilitated this technique. Emergency supplies can often be kept at the patient's home. With increasing practise patients learn to recognise the early symptoms and signs of bleeding and can thus take prophylactic therapy earlier. Care must be taken to ensure that only genuine bleeds are treated as the temptation to overtreat and prevent painful episodes is great. However, prophylactic injections are justified for such events as examinations, weddings, etc. The induction of antibodies to factor VIII is well recognised and is preceded by increasing requirements for replacement factor. Treatment is still controversial but in these patients factor VIII should be given with care.

The question of analgesic and anti-inflammatory therapy is contentious. Paracetamol has no known effect on bleeding and in spite of evidence that non-steroidal anti-inflammatory drugs may diminish haemostasis, we have found that ibuprofen and indomethacin seem relatively safe for short periods; the latter can be taken as a suppository. Addictive drugs must be avoided.

Often small physical adaptations may help. Thus if the ankle joints are affected and are hypermobile, then help is often obtained by using boots instead of shoes. An element of valgus and pes planus which would normally be ignored at this age may be corrected by a wedge through sole and small instep supports.

Soft elasticated protective supports are readily obtained for the knees and elbows.

Calipers and such mechanised supports are probably outdated and should not be necessary if the child is adequately treated early enough.

Van Pad et al (1981) have made the interesting suggestion of using radiosynoviorthesis. This has seemed a worthwhile technique, being simple and resulting in less pain and bleeding but with no evidence of reduced joint destruction. Chromosomal damage was not found.

Surgery has three major functions. Soft tissue may be released, usually by a lengthening of the Achilles tendon or of fibrosed or shortened muscle tissue. Synovectomy is seldom indicated in these patients, though some centres claim goods results (Mannucci et al, 1977; McCollough et al, 1979). Synovectomy is usually used in younger patients; in the older patient the problems are more those of degenerative disease (McCollough et al, 1979).

Surgery is also of use in replacing or arthrodesing certain destroyed joints, typically the hip and knee (Small et al, 1983). This is a rare, but occasional, necessity and like all surgery should be done in a centre with specialised knowledge and facilities.

It should be reiterated that these problems start in young children and thus with aggressive treatment, often over a long time, surprising remodelling and recovery of the joint can occur often obviating proposed surgery. It also follows that these children are growing; thus prophylaxis is necessary in preventing potential problems, such as fibrosis and shortening of muscles which may not be apparent until the bones elongate with growth, i.e. too late. Fortunately the frequency of bleeding episodes seems to decrease as the child gets older and the state of the musculoskeletal system is often dependent on earlier management.

Most patients will be independent and employable; this is primarily dependent on their cerebral status and the development of antibodies to factor VIII or IX which prevents further use of these factors. An increased incidence of liver function abnormality has been found, presumably due to viral infection from replacement therapy, but is seldom a major problem.

Since the child may be physically handicapped, the best possible education should be provided. This involves liaison with the school to explain the circumstances, a joint clinic at which haematological, locomotor and dental problems can be reviewed, usually by different experts, thus saving duplicate clinic attendances which would waste school time, and a nurse home visitor who is able to identify unsuspected problems. This approach also allows incidental problems to be identified and discussed; thus we have seen tuberculosis, dactylitis, juvenile arthritis, epiphyseal dysplasia and osteoma occurring in these children as well as a number of problems such as upper respiratory tract allergy and eneuresis requiring advice — all available instantly.

THROMBOCYTOSIS

Thrombocytosis is a common finding in acute and chronic inflammatory conditions including malignancies. Some correlation with the severity and complications of rheumatoid disease is also found (Hutchinson et al, 1976). Occasionally this may result in thrombosis and ischaemic changes (Ehrenfeld et al, 1977) (Fig. 47.10) or bleeding into the joint (Harris & Ross, 1974). Treatment is with anticoagulants and prednisolone and in the long-term second line antirheumatic therapy to reduce the inflammation and associated thrombocytosis.

HAEMOGLOBINOPATHIES

Haemoglobin forms approximately 95% of the dry weight of the red blood cell. The haemoglobin molecule is made up of polypeptide chains of globin (97%) and the haem group (3%). Thus the principle constituents of the red blood cell are the globin moieties of the haemoglobin molecule. Each haemoglobin molecule contains two pairs of identical polypeptide chains, each chain having a heme group attached to it. Haemoglobin variants may arise from abnormalities of either globin or haem synthesis. Not all these variants produce clinical disease and it is only abnormalities of the α and β globin chain that are associated with locomotor problems and will be considered here.

The predominant haemoglobin (F) of the fetus and newborn is made up of two α and two γ chains. From late in pregnancy β chain synthesis replaces most of the γ chains to produce adult (A) haemoglobin, a process normally complete by 6 months of age. Balanced α and β chain synthesis must be maintained to produce a soluble haemoglobin molecule. For the purposes of this discussion there are two main haemoglobinopathies.

The first is that in which an amino acid substitution occurs in the sequence (usually of a single amino acid) of the β globin chain. Thus this is a qualitative change in haemoglobin production and sickle cell disease is the most important result. Haemoglobins with abnormal amino acid sequences in their globin chains have been given a series of names. The most frequent varieties of pathological significance, for our purpose, are haemoglobin SS (homozygous), haemoglobin C and haemoglobin SC (in which the amino acid chain sequence is altered at two sites).

Thus HbS, when deoxygenated, becomes aligned in insoluble fibres which deform the erythrocyte to produce the sickle-shaped deformity and make the erythrocyte more rigid. The deformed

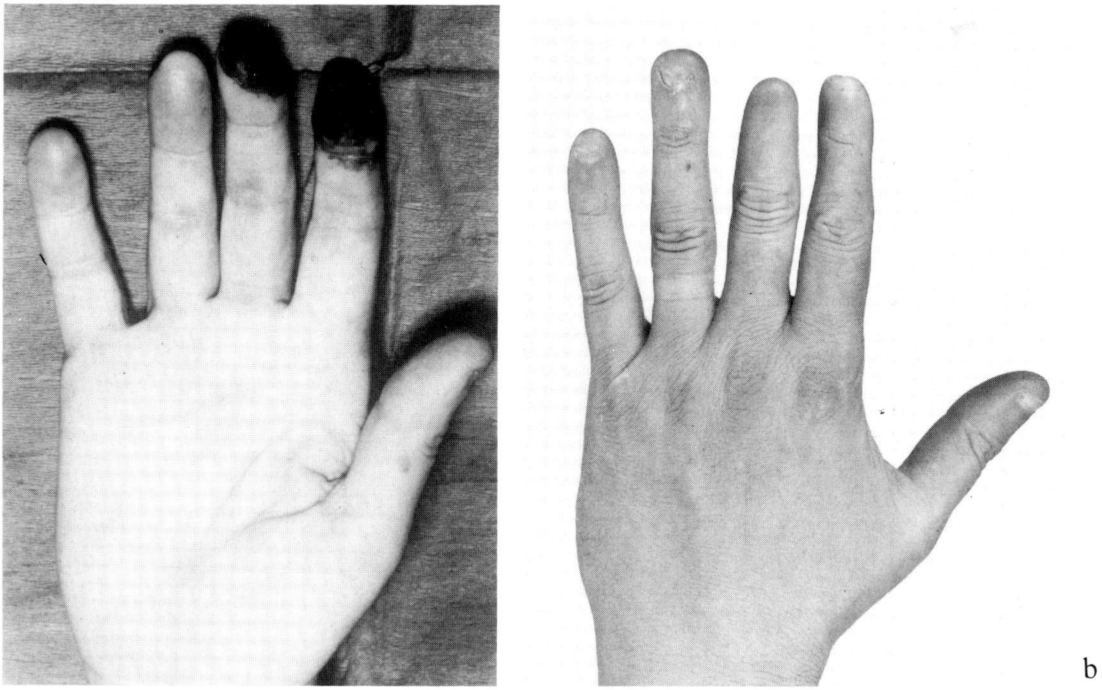

a b

Fig. 47.10 Thrombocytosis during penicillamine treatment of rheumatoid arthritis with gangrene of finger tips (a). No recurrence after 5 years (b).

and inelastic erythrocytes are trapped and block small blood vessels. The extent to which this change occurs is dependent on the concentration of the abnormal haemoglobin, the oxygen tension, the period of oxygen desaturation, pH and the blood flow. These factors often produce local rather than general symptoms. The disease is limited to blacks (African and American) and to a lesser extent people of the Mediterranean littoral and Middle East and requires both parents to carry the gene. In the sickle cell trait a heterozygous state occurs in which normal haemoglobin (HbA) and abnormal haemoglobin (e.g. HbS) occurs in the same erythrocyte, the resulting concentration of abnormal haemoglobin usually being too low to cause sickling of the erythrocyte. It is increasingly recognised that the patient with the homozygous state may survive into adult life, presumably depending, in part, on such factors as environmental health, availability of treatment and the severity of the disease.

The second abnormality is a quantitative change in production of either α or β globin chains, the resulting inbalance between the two chains causing the predominant globin chain produced to precipitate with destruction of immature pro-erythrocytes within the bone marrow (thalassaemia). This results in chronic anaemia and compensatory overactivity and enlargement of the bone marrow in an attempt, usually not realised, to maintain the haemoglobin level. Originally described as 'Mediterranean anaemia', thalassaemia is still most commonly found in people of Mediterranean ancestry.

In both conditions, sickle cell disease and thalassaemia, the resulting increased haemolysis leads to an average erythrocyte half-life of 10–15 days instead of the usual 120 days.

The two defects — an abnormal haemoglobin of sickle cell disease or an abnormal rate of α and β globin production of thalassaemia – are coded on different chromosomes but occur in overlapping racial distribution and may both be present in an individual.

Arthritis (Dorwart & Schumacher, 1981) and aseptic necrosis (Schlumf, 1978) probably due to thalassaemia trait, have been described, but are rare. Arthritis has not been described in sickle cell trait (Dorwart et al, 1977). However, Keeling et al (1974) have described aseptic necrosis in sickle cell trait and it may be blamed for vague skeletal aches and pains.

Sickle cell disease

Expansion of the bone marrow from an early age results in the marrow being found progressively more peripherally. The marrow cavity is widened with fewer, but coarser, trabeculae. Endosteal resorption and persistent new bone formation lead to thinning of the cortex and widening of the bone, the normal wasted appearance of the digits being replaced by a biconvex expanded pattern (Fig. 47.11). These changes, although helpful from the diagnostic point of view, are symptomless. For practical purposes, symptoms only occur in homozygous HbSS disease (Sennara & Gorry, 1978). Bone infarction is the commonest feature to cause symptoms, the result of which depends on the site of the infarction (Fig. 47.12). It is usually multiple and involves the diaphysis (Sennara & Gorry, 1978) (Figs 47.13, 47.14). Thus infarction of the epiphyseal plate may lead to reduced or abnormal growth (Fig. 47.15). Within the bone marrow, fibrosis and dense, sometimes calcified, areas may be found. Cortical lesions and periosteal elevation also occur (Fig. 47.16). In the vertebrae coarsening of the vertical trabeculae occurs. Collapse and

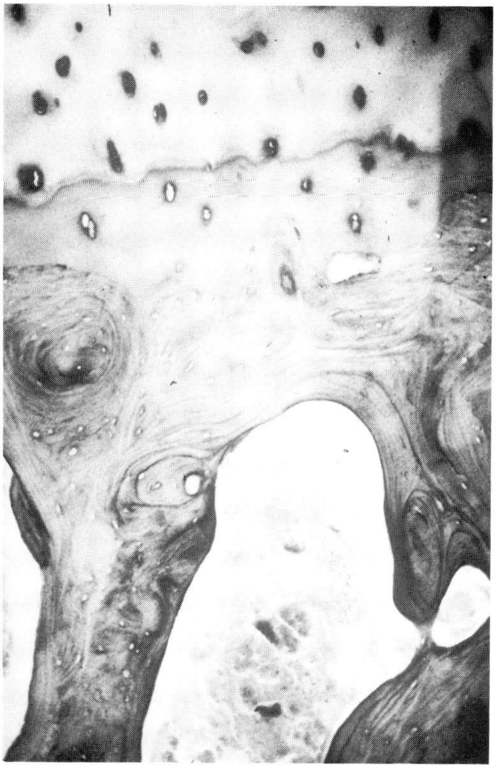

Fig. 47.12 Sickle cell disease. Femoral head. Above — viable articular cartilage. Below — necrotic bone marrow and dead bone with empty ostocyte lacunae. (Courtesy of Dr A. Freemont.)

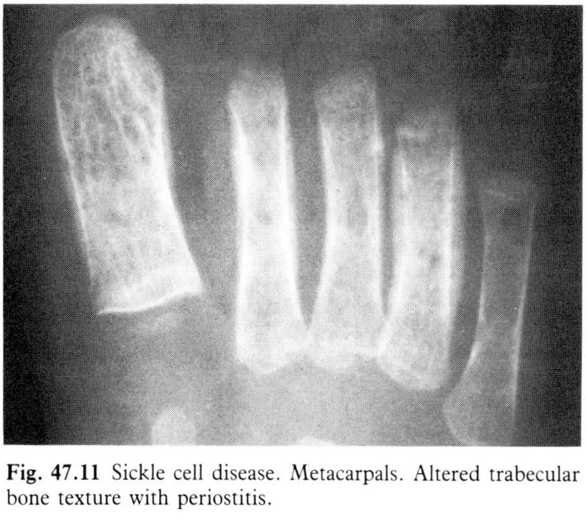

Fig. 47.11 Sickle cell disease. Metacarpals. Altered trabecular bone texture with periostitis.

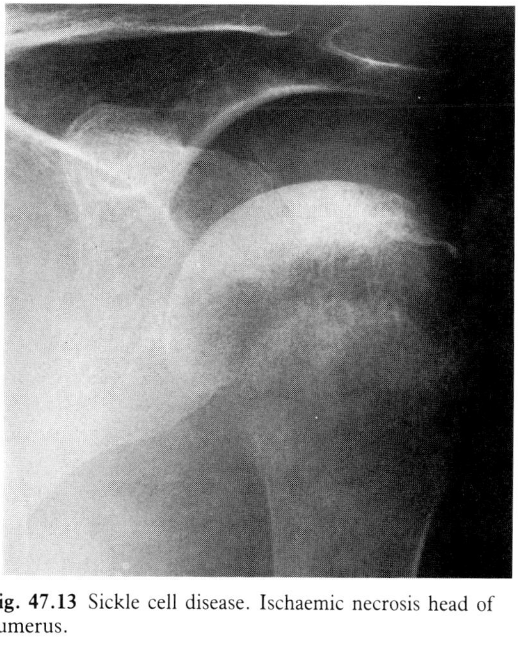

Fig. 47.13 Sickle cell disease. Ischaemic necrosis head of humerus.

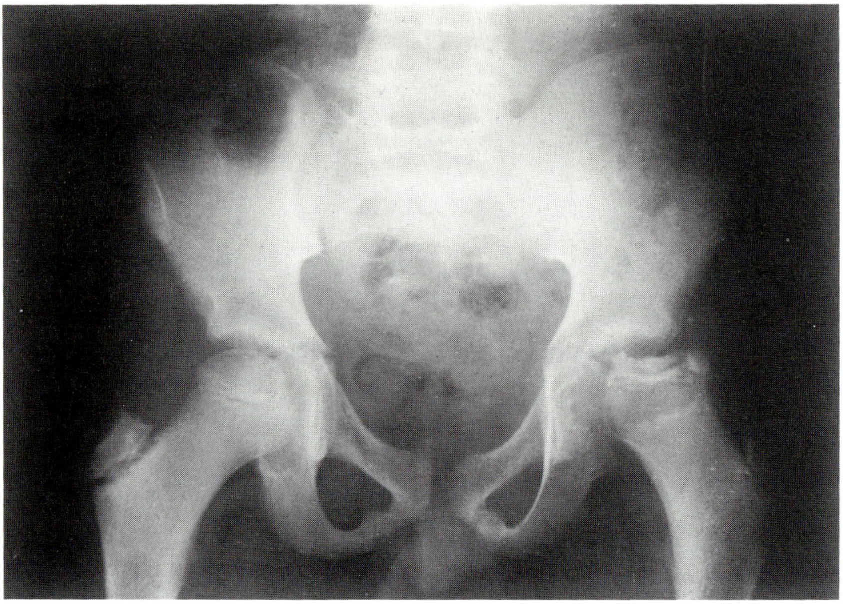

Fig. 47.14 Sickle cell disease. Ischaemia necrosis of head of left femur.

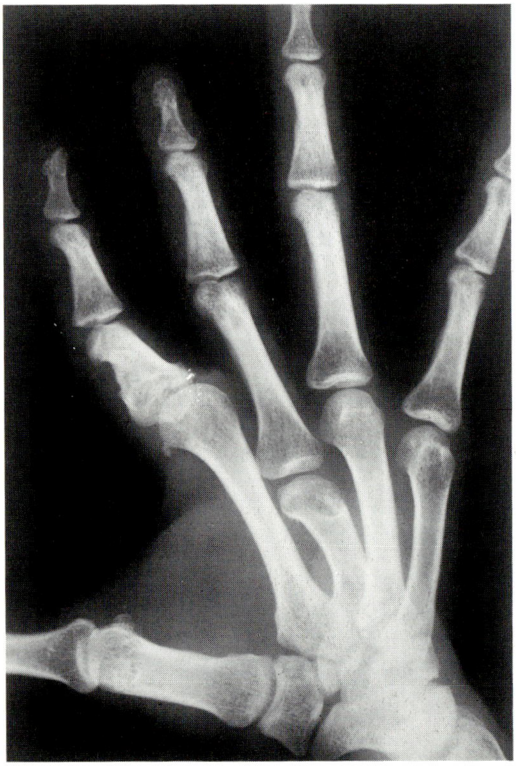

Fig. 47.15 Sickle cell disease. Bone infarction. 2nd proximal phalanx and 3rd metacarpal. Changes may be present in the carpal bones.

end-plate abnormalities may all be seen (Figs 47.17, 47.18). End artery blockage may occur in all the usual sites and at any age but usually between 10 and 30 years with perhaps an increased frequency of infarction of the head of femur (Fig. 47.14). The head of humerus, tibial plateau and femoral condyle are also affected. The pain in long bones and back is often of rapid onset and great severity to be followed later by aches in the same areas. The arthritic symptoms often take a migratory pattern and this, associated with the paucity of physical findings in the joints and the features of anaemia with hyperdynamic circulation, may simulate rheumatic fever, particularly as the two conditions often occur in the same populations. The radiological features of avascular necrosis of the femoral head in this conditions have been well described (Lee et al, 1981). Both hips are involved in half the cases and in two-thirds of these the acetabulum also shows radiological change. The outcome varies with age. In the immature head there is flattening and migration of the head with mushrooming, but little subsequent disability. In the mature head segmental destruction is followed by continuing destruction, pain and osteoarthrosis; thus the outlook is worse in the older patient. Many of the infarctions are probably

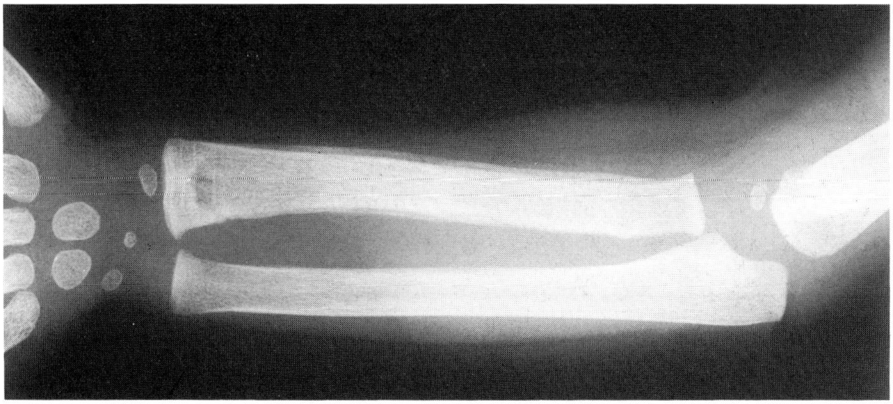

Fig. 47.16 Sickle cell disease. Periostitis shaft of radius.

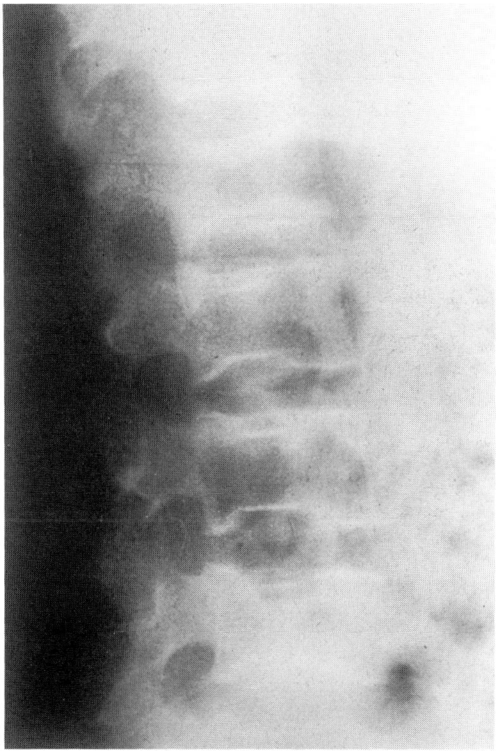

Fig. 47.17 Sickle cell disease. Depression of vertebral end-plates. The depressed areas are dense and may result from infarction. The relative porosity of the vertebral bodies is due to the increased vascularity. Each episode may be intensely painful.

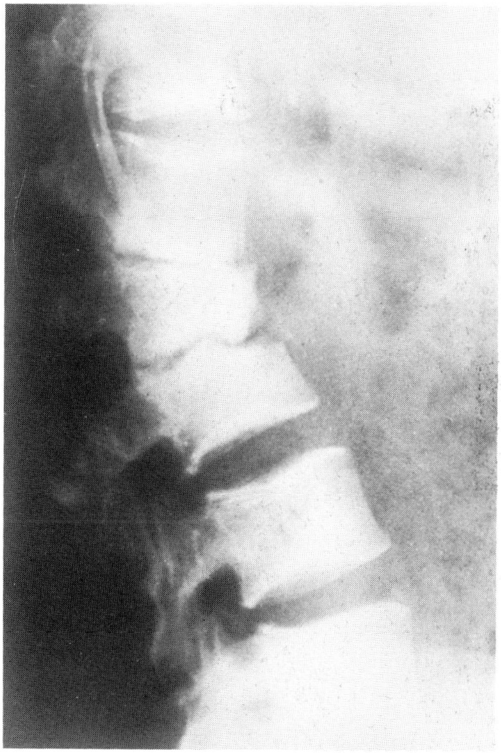

Fig. 47.18 Sickle cell disease. Collapse of the intervertebral discs.

painless but where pain occurs, although immediate radiographs are normal, bone scans may show poor perfusion of the painful area and bone turnover may be increased (Hammell et al, 1973; Alavi et al, 1976). Previous evidence of bone infarction can, of course be present on the initial radiograph and confuse the issue. There may be fever and other constitutional factors such as abdominal pain, renal, cardiac or cerebral disease. Attacks are spontaneous or may follow relative anoxia due to lung infection, flying or at night during sleep. Leg ulcers are common. Longitudinal studies have shown reduced physical and sexual development with retarded bone age (Lubom et al, 1982).

The blood film shows a chronic anaemia with Howell–Jolly bodies, reticulocytosis and sickled erythrocytes.

There is thrombocytosis and leucocytosis during crises and circulating immune complexes have been demonstrated (Hernandez et al, 1981). Jaundice may be apparent. The bone marrow is hyperplastic. Occasionally aplastic crises arise in which the peripheral reticulocytosis does not occur.

The diagnosis is suspected from the history and confirmed by electrophoresis of the haemoglobin.

Synovial effusions

These are more common in sickle cell disease then destructive arthropathy and have the characteristics of non-inflammatory effusions though inflammatory cell counts have been found (Espinoza et al, 1974). They are usually short-lived, affecting one or two joints, mainly the knee, and usually not recurrent. The pathogenesis is obscure but thrombosis of the synovial vessels may be found (Schumacher et al, 1973). Urate crystals occur in these fluids but their significance is not clear (see infra). Sickled red cells can be found in the fluid even in the heterozygous state when they probably result from the low Po_2 and pH of the inflammatory fluid (Casey & Cathcart, 1970; Hasselbacher, 1980). They do not indicate sickle cell arthropathy. Destructive chronic synovitis is rare (Schumacher et al, 1977) and its pathogenesis multiple. Previous damage from aseptic necrosis or infection are the more usual causes of progressive joint destruction. The synovium in these cases has demonstrated marked inflammatory cell infiltration but of quite different form from that found in rheumatoid arthritis and with evidence of microvascular thrombosis.

Osteomyelitis

The frequency of osteomyelitis is increased in sickle cell disease and is predominantly due to *Salmonella* in contradistinction to staphylococcal infection in non-sickle cell patients. The propensity to develop osteomyelitis may be based on bone infarction, reduced bacterial phagocytosis due initially to inability of the spleen to remove particles, this defect being reversible by plasma transfusion (Pearson et al, 1970), and later to splenic fibrosis and to the low oxygen tension present. Wilson et al (1976) and more recently Hind & Kind (1978) have suggested that defects in the alternate complement pathway may lead to defective opsonisation and lysis of micro-organisms, a specific deficiency being in factor B (Wilson et al, 1976). The marrow cavity is usually involved and, although several sites can be affected, the lesions often escape notice for long periods; otherwise the features are those of other types of osteomyelitis. Radiologically distinction from bone infarction can be very difficult and the two conditions may coincide. The bone infection seldom breaks through into the joint and the infrequent septic arthritides probably arise as independent episodes.

Hyperuricaemia

Serum uric acid levels are raised in over one-third of adults with sickle cell disease. Hyperuricaemia is partly due to overproduction of uric acid which can initially be contained by increased renal elimination, but as renal function deteriorates so the hyperuricaemia becomes manifest (Diamond et al, 1979). Occasionally gout, sometimes tophaceous, supervenes (Balloo et al, 1977; Rothschild et al, 1980).

Hand-foot syndrome

This occurs in the young child up to 2 years of age; failure to affect older children is probably due to the bone marrow having been replaced by fibrous tissue. These is a sudden development of global tender warm swellings of the fingers and feet. Fever and leucocytosis may occur and the whole episode lasts about 2 weeks, the features often simulating infection. In the convalescent stage, as the swelling diminishes, the skin tends to scale. Although marked and dramatic radiological changes of infarction, lysis and marked periosteal new bone formation are seen, eventually the bone architecture returns to normal apart from the coarse trabeculae and shortened phalanges or metacarpals.

The cause of this syndrome is unknown but is

usually thought to be due to infarction. Cold, which can cause swelling of the infant fingers, is not a cause.

Thalassaemia

In thalassaemia, due to ineffective haemopoiesis, the bone marrow expands with resultant osseous changes. However, blood vessel blockage and bone infarction are not found (unless sickle cell disease is also present). Again the changes occur from an early age and the ankles seem to be particularly severely involved. Thus 25 of 50 thalassaemic patients had painful ankles especially when weight-bearing. Tenderness and joint effusions occurred in some patients (Gratwick et al, 1978). Similar changes have been noted at the wrists and elbows (Schlumf, 1978). Gratwick et al (1978) have shown widespread iron deposition in synovial tissue and in bone, particularly at the sites of growth and have suggested that this may have an effect on the tissues. Haemosiderosis is probably multifactorial, repeated transfusions, haemolysis and increased intestinal iron absorption playing a part. The serum iron is high with saturation of the iron binding proteins. The pathogenesis of the synovitis is often not clear but probably results in most cases from an extension of the marrow cavity into the joint. Iron deposition in the synovium and urate crystals have also been described.

Radiologically there is osteopenia with widened medullary spaces, thin cortices and coarse trabeculae and evidence of microfractures.

Expansion of the bone marrow of the vertebral bodies and eruption through the thinned periosteum into the epidural space with spinal cord compression has been recorded (Issargarisil et al, 1981). This extramedullary enlargement may readily respond to radiotherapy. Less severe forms of thalassaemia may allow greater bone and extra medullary deformities to develop.

Treatment

This consists of trying to redress the ineffective haemoglobin production by use of repeated over-transfusions of normal blood to maintain a haematocrit above 35%. This reduces the total blood that has to be transfused by resulting in a decrease in whole blood volume and is an attempt to reduce bone marrow expansion. The resulting excess tissue iron is removed with desferrioxamine (Propper et al, 1980). The value of using young erythrocytes is apparent.

Radiotherapy may reduce local extramedullary masses and help to reduce pressure effects.

IRON OVERLOAD ARTHROPATHY

An arthropathy associated with iron overload but without haemochromatosis has been described in a variety of conditions. Transfusional siderosis (Abbot & Gresham, 1972; Sella & Goodman 1973), hereditary spherocytosis (Berry & Miller, 1973) and sideroblastic anaemia (Fitzcharles et al, 1982) have all been associated with arthropathy. The symptoms usually start as an intermittent small joint polyarthropathy which may progress to a polyarthritis initially of small but later of large joints with stiffness, swelling and a raised ESR but rarely radiological changes. The features are not unlike rheumatoid arthritis but back pain seems to be more frequent and the rheumatoid factor is not elevated. The bone marrow is packed with iron and the serum ferritin may be high and out of keeping with the relatively modest elevation of the ESR. Most patients are anaemic.

The pathogenesis of this arthropathy is not clear. Brighton et al (1970) produced a degenerative arthritis in immature but not adult rabbits by parental iron injections in high doses. Choi Ye-Chin et al (1981) have shown iron uptake by chondrocytes without evidence of cytotoxicity. This uptake was reversed by desferroxamine.

Treatment is symptomatic only.

LEUKAEMIA

The question of malignancy developing in patients with rheumatoid arthritis remains unanswered. To date the evidence would suggest that only lymphomas, leukaemia and myeloma are increased and that this is in part related to cytotoxic therapy, (Isomaki et al, 1978; Kirsner et al, 1981; Boyle et al, 1981; Baltus et al, 1983).

Lymphoblastic leukaemia is a relatively common malignancy in children where it is a frequent cause of musculoskeletal pain (Schaller, 1972;

Fink et al, 1972). Joint pain has been said to occur in 60% of these children, the overall incidence is probably less (10–20%), though it is often difficult to ascertain in a sick, miserable child. The pain is most commonly around the metaphysial ends of limb bones, i.e. the growing and most vascular part of the bone. Thus the knee and wrist regions are frequent sites of pain; the ankles, shoulders fingers and other small joints are less frequently involved. Childhood leukaemia may be a cause of the irritable hip syndrome (Ansell, 1978); pain is thought to originate from infiltration of the capsule, periosteum, bone and muscle. Although there may be effusions into the joints, the pain and, in particular, the tenderness, are usually clearly in the bone ends; warmth is unusual and colour changes do not occur. Ill-defined pain and isolated areas of tenderness elsewhere in the skeleton occur and are sometimes of a migrating nature. Tenderness without pain may be present over the sternum, particularly in myelogenous leukaemia. Muscle pain may be severe. The severity of the pain, the sites of tenderness and the general appearance of the child — ill-health, fever, purpura, lymphodenopathy and hepatosplenopathy — together with radiographs showing generalised osteopenia (especially of the vertebrae or metaphysis) or osteolytic lesions or periosteal elevation, are all suggestive. A blood film is usually diagnostic, but bone marrow or lymph node biopsy may be necessary for diagnosis. Willken et al (1980) have discussed the difficulties in differentiating the lymph node changes found in rheumatoid diseases and lymphoma. Immunological methods, in particular the recent development of monoclonal antibodies, may aid this. Sedimentation rate and other acute phase reactants may be raised and are of no help in differentiation from juvenile arthritis. The synovium usually has non-specific changes only but the blastic change in the lymphocytes may suggest the diagnosis.

In the adult the pain is usually less intense and with fewer objective musculoskeletal signs which tend to be less migratory in pattern. Both acute and chronic leukaemia occur and the joints affected — knees, ankle, shoulders, hip and elbow — are much the same in both (Spilberg & Meyer, 1972) (Figs 47 19, 47.20). Back pain and radicular signs may occur from infiltration of the meninges.

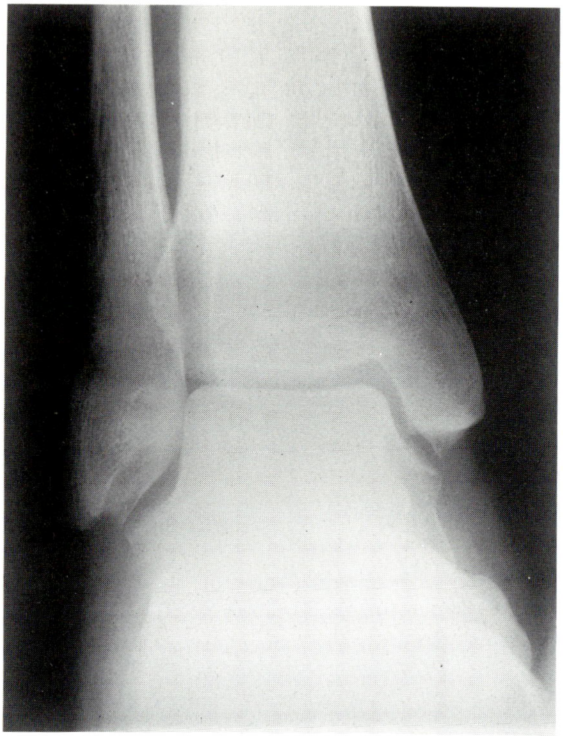

Fig. 47.19 Acute myeloid leukaemia. Periarticular osteoporosis, endosteal resorption, possible erosion of tip of fibula. Joint spaces still well preserved. It is sometimes difficult to differentiate secondary infection.

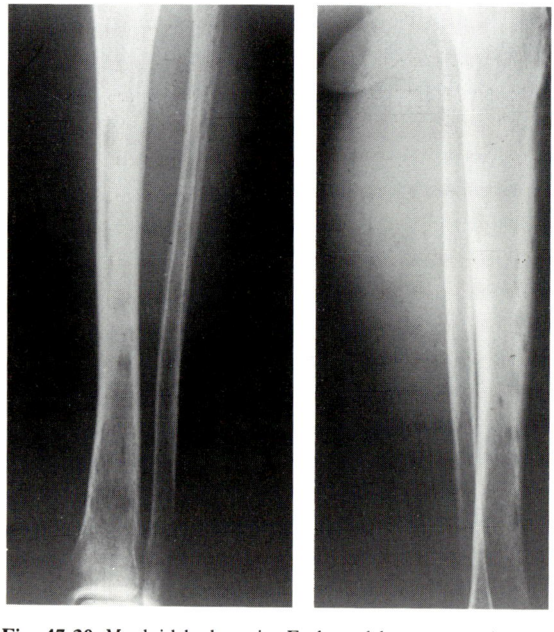

Fig. 47.20 Myeloid leukaemia. Endosteal bone resorption and generalised osteopenia, most marked at metaphysis.

These patients are increasingly susceptible to infection and the resulting sepsis is often less florid and more persistent than other forms of infection.

Response of the musculoskeletal symptoms to treatment parallels that of other features of the leukaemia and both relief and repair of tissue damage can be rapid. Bone pain may often be relieved by non-steroidal anti-inflammatory drugs such as indomethacin. Locomotor symptoms may fluctuate with disease activity and herald both improvement or relapse.

Hyperuricaemia may occur both in the treated and untreated state. Occasionally gout supervenes. The potentiating effect of allopurinol on azathioprine therapy should be remembered (see Ch. 36).

Hairy cell leukaemia (leukaemic reticuloendotheliosis)

This rare type of B cell leukaemia is of interest because of its association with a particular and rare form of vasculitis — polyarteritis nodosa. Although this type of leukaemia was first described in 1958 (Bouroncle et al, 1958) and the clinical features in 71 cases described in 1978 (Golomb et al, 1978), the association with polyarteritis nodosa was not appreciated until 1979 (Elkon et al, 1979). Further cases have been described (Goedert et al, 1981; Le Pogam et al, 1982). The reasons for this association are not clear. Polyarteritis nodosa may appear late, up to 11 years after the initial diagnosis of the leukaemia (Behn & Sykes, 1982). Prior infection, blood transfusions and splenectomy may all play a part perhaps through increasing immune complex formation, although polyarteritis nodosa is not usually associated with circulating immune complexes. Hepatitis B antibody has been rarely detected (Pope et al, 1980).

Rheumatoid arthritis has been reported after (Crofts et al, 1979) and before (Facchini et al, 1981) the onset of hairy cell leukaemia. Sattar & Cawley (1982) describe a man with intermittent non-erosive polyarthritis of large joints who benefitted from treatment with corticosteroids. Hairy cells were found in the synovial fluid which was otherwise unremarkable.

T cell leukaemia

This is another rare form of chronic leukaemia. A single case of symmetrical polyarthropathy with cutaneous nodule formation (Soesbergen et al, 1983) has been described. A marked peripheral lymphocytosis of T cell type was accompanied by lymphocytic infiltration in the synovium of T cell type. Tenosynovitis was a marked feature. Rapid improvement, including clearance of the nodules, followed chlorambucil treatment. With relapse of the leukaemia the arthritis and tenosynovitis returned.

Lymphoma

Classification of the different types of lymphoma is difficult and not essential for this discussion. Lymphomata frequently involve the skeletal system and bone pain is the commonest musculoskeletal feature (Reiner et al, 1977). Periarticular osseous involvement (Fig. 47.21) which sometimes breaks through to the joint space may produce joint pain and swelling with tenderness (Hench et al, 1962; Hustu & Pinkel, 1967). The usual presentation is as a monoarthritis of large joints, although an acute symmetrical polyarthritis of small joints has been described (Martin et al, 1973). The latter case has added interest, demonstrating rapid bone healing with successful treatment (Fig. 47.22). Direct involvement of the synovium by lymphoma and malignant deposits has been suggested (Newton et al, 1984). The synovial fluid is unremarkable and thus of no positive diagnostic help. The diagnosis is usually apparent from the localisation of pain and sometimes tenderness. A radiograph may show osseous changes and a radionuclide scan inflammation or vascularity in the bone rather than the joint. When fever is associated with a monoarthritis or polyarthritis, confusion with joint or bone infection may occur, but, in this age-group, seldom with chronic inflammatory arthritis.

Treatment is symptomatic for the bone or joint pain and specific for the lymphoma.

Myelomatosis

Myelomatosis (multiple myeloma) is a neoplastic proliferation of plasma cells (B lymphocytes) resulting in expansion either locally or in more widespread fashion. Since it usually occurs in the bone marrow there is replacement of the bone marrow locally with destruction of bone trabeculae and later thinning (with or without expansion) of the

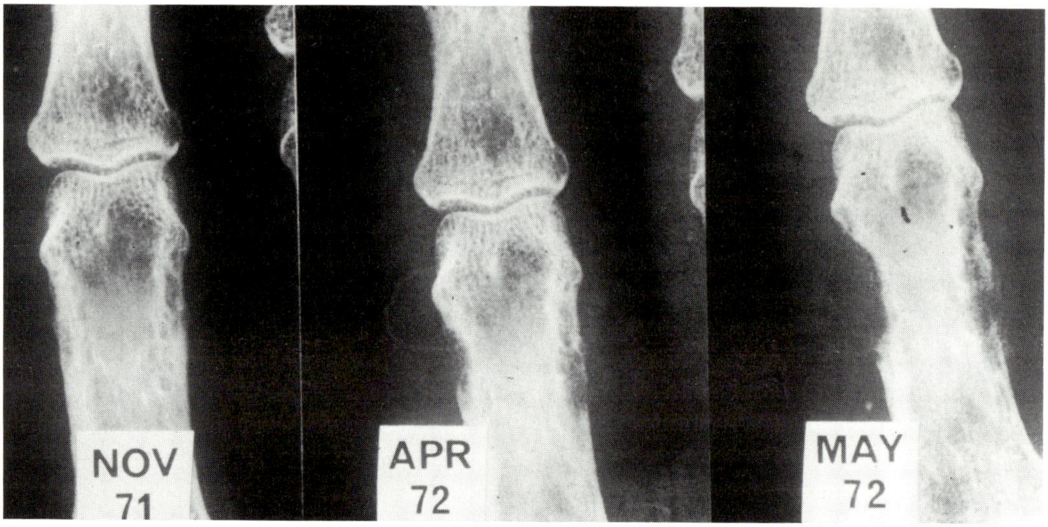

Fig. 47.21 Lymphosarcomatosis leukaemia. Widespread medullary and endosteal porosis.

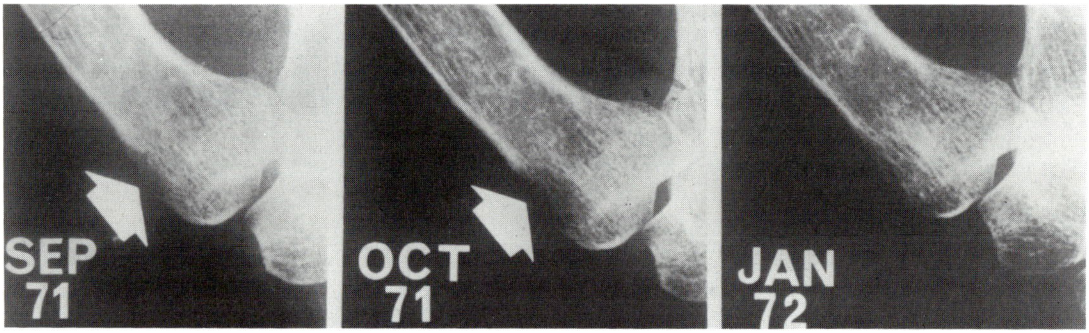

Fig. 47.22 Lymphosarcomatosis leukaemia. 1st metacarpal, subperiosteal erosion with repair due to chemotherapy-induced remission.

cortex. The bone weakens and collapses (vertebrae) or fractures (long bones). The tumour may break through the bone end and invade the joint (Mintz et al, 1978). Extraosseous deposits occur. The result is aches and pains, often of ill-defined character, or the unheralded acute pain and tenderness associated with localised bone fracture. Background ill-health, anaemia, infections, hypercalcaemia and renal failure may all occur.

Radiological changes include osteopenia, sometimes with a frosted glass appearance, localised 'punched-out' radiotranslucent areas or alternatively osteosclerosis, bone fractures and collapse. Rarely a localised mass (plasmacytoma) may be found. See also Chapter 49.

Amyloidosis

Joint involvement is a recognised complication occurring at any time during the course of the disease. Deposits are found in the periarticular tissue, particularly the joint capsule (Gordon et al, 1973b). This characteristically gives rise to a hard, smooth, global, non-fluctuant swelling of the joint capsule which can be felt around the joint, characteristically the shoulder, hip and finger joints. This is not usually tender but movement is markedly diminished by the severe pain provoked, such that the slightest movement may cause severe pain. The patient may assume an immobile hunched posture with marked muscle wasting and osteopenia. Carpal tunnel syndrome symptoms are characteristic features and other neuropathies may occur. Amyloid may be found in idiopathic carpal tunnel syndrome when the postoperative results are less satisfactory (Short & Palmer, 1981). Effusions in joints occur due to periarticular amyloid deposits or deposits within the synovium. The fluid is of high viscosity and contains few cells. Amyloid may be detected in the villous fragments aspirated (Gordon et al, 1973a). See also Chapter 41.

Waldenström's macroglobulinaemia

The lymphocyte proliferation appears to be primarily in lymphoid organs, lymph nodes, spleen and liver where a pattern of follicular hyperplasia may be found. The picture may resemble a malignant lymphoma or lymphatic leukaemia.

The protein production is practically confined to M immunoglobin.This tends to coat red cells due to the presence of anti-I or i antigen producing rouleau formation (Feizi & Kabat, 1972). Waldenström's macroglobulinaemia has similar osseous features to myelomatosis but joint involvement is rare. The hyperviscosity may cause ischaemic changes peripherally with Raynaud's phenomena. Purpura is common. Amyloidosis is rare and seldom affects joints. Neuropathy and myelopathy have been observed.

Diagnosis will rest on suspicion, the presence of anaemia but not leucopenia or thrombocytopenia, a very high ESR and abnormal serum immunoglobins. Monoclonal gammaglobinopathy is rare in rheumatoid disease (Youinou et al, 1983). Rheumatoid factors are not uncommon but anti-nuclear factor and other autoantibodies are rare.

In the urine of about one-quarter of cases of myelomatosis Bence Jones proteins (light chains) are found. They are less frequent in Waldenström's macroglobulinaemia.

Treatment

Myelomatosis tissue is very radiosensitive and local deposits may be treated this way. However, for the more usual generalised form chemotherapy is necessary. To rapidly reduce abnormal protein levels, particularly in macroglobulinaemia, plasmaphoresis may be necessary until chemotherapy becomes effective. Chemotherapy is usually with multiple drugs and the different protocols for both diseases are still being evaluated. Cortisone on its own is of relatively little use though it may reduce the capillary bleeding of macroglobulinaemia.

It is essential to maintain hydration and a moderate diureses to prevent calcium or myeloma protein being deposited in the kidney. Prednisolone may reduce hypercalcaemia. Bone pain can be exceptional and may necessitate local amputation. Occasionally a local tumour may be removable.

Analgesia is important together with appropriate splinting especially of the spine, but overall mobility must be maintained.

Angioimmunoblastic lymphadenopathy

Angioimmunoblastic lymphadenopathy is a recently described, but increasingly diagnosed, disorder (Lukes & Tindle, 1975). It appears to be a relatively benign lymphoproliferative disorder in which fever, sweats, weight loss, rashes, generalised lymphadenopathy, hepatosplenomegaly, anaemia, often haemolysis and a polyclonal hypergammaglobulinaemia occur to a varying degree. Conversion to lymphoma occurs and in some cases may coexist.

The lymph node histology is characteristic showing a pleomorphic cellular infiltrate, primarily of plasma cells and immunoblasts and a marked proliferation and arborisation of blood vessels, thus giving the condition its descriptive title. The aetiopathogenesis is unknown (Lukes & Tindle, 1975; Frizzeri et al, 1975).

A variety of rheumatic features have been described since the association was first noted in 1976 (Bensa et al). In a review of 200 cases of angioimmunoblastic lymphadenopathy to 1977, 7% had arthritis and arthralgia (Cullen et al, 1979). Other reports have dealt with individual cases (Rothwell et al, 1980; Raskin et al, 1982; Davies & Fordham, 1983). The arthritis is acute in onset and symmetrical of small and large joints but not apparently erosive. It is often treated as a seronegative arthritis before the true diagnosis of the lymphadenopathy becomes apparent. A wide age range from 20 years onwards and both sexes are affected. Synovial thickening with warmth and tenderness have been described. The synovial fluid findings are non-specific. The ESR is often normal in spite of the mild inflammation. Although non-specific autoantibodies are found in most cases, antiglobulins are not found. Response, often temporary, of the arthritic manifestation follows non-steroidal anti-inflammatory drugs. More prolonged, and often dramatic, response follows treatment with corticosteroids and cytotoxic agents which may be necessary for treatment of the lymphoma.

Pierce et al (1979) have described the development of Sjögren's syndrome and systemic lupus erthematosus in the course of angioimmunoblastic lymphadenopathy. Moore et al (1976) have described angioimmunoblastic lymphadenopathy developing in a patient with Sjögren's syndrome of 6 years standing and a single case of systemic lupus erythematosus developing following angioimmunoblastic lymphadenopathy has been reported (Popa et al, 1982).

Myeloid metaplasia (myelofibrosis with myeloid metaplasia or myelofibrosis with extramedullary haematopoiesis)

This condition usually follows progressive replacement of the haemopoietic marrow by fibrous tissue and the consequent reactivation of dormant haemopoietic tissue in extramedullary sites. It is of unknown aetiology and is progressively more frequent with advancing age. Occasional extramedullary haemopoiesis may develop without significant bone marrow fibrosis.

The musculoskeletal symptoms are usually a late feature.

Hyperuricaemia is frequent and may lead to classical attacks of gout. Migratory bone and, less frequently, joint pain occur, but persistent arthritis in a joint is rare. The synovium has been shown to be a site of potential haemopoiesis (Heinicke et al, 1983). The initial radiological appearances are of diffuse osteopenia and then either a 'ground glass' appearance of bones or osteosclerosis of several bones. Most frequently the axial skeleton is involved. Periostitis is possibly due to subperiosteal haemorrhages from platelet deficiency or extramedullary haemopoietic tissue. Invariably the spleen is enlarged and this may be seen on radiographs. Increasing anaemia and abnormalities are found in white and red cells and in the platelets on blood film examination. Later immune deficiency and abnormal serum globulin patterns may develop. Bone marrow taps are often 'dry' and a bone trephine biopsy is more useful.

Treatment is limited. Androgens may be given in courses to try to increase the erythropoiesis. Thrombocytosis can be reduced by busulphan and irradiation or removal of the spleen to reduce haemolysis and improve thrombocytopenia but it is often followed by complications.

MULTICENTRIC RETICULOHISTIOCYTOSIS (LIPID DERMATOARTHRITIS)

This is a systemic disease of unknown aetiology in which the histiocytes become filled with lipid and giant cells form. Recent work has shown collagen phagocytosis in this condition (Caputo et al, 1981). Any age can be affected and females slightly more frequently than males (Barrow & Holubar, 1969). The course is long and variable. Polyarthritis is the most frequent presenting feature and then multiple skin nodules, but many systems are involved.

The arthritis is symmetrical affecting all the joints of the fingers and feet together with large joints and spine. Morning stiffness, swollen and sometimes tender joints mimic other forms of inflammatory arthritis. The nodules of fingers, skin and elbows may enhance the similarity. However, their more widespread distribution, including the face, should arouse suspicion. The arthritis is destructive producing 'opera glass' hand deformities. Radiologically, in addition to the destructive joint lesions — often with late preservation of joint space — there are isolated bone translucences and nodules to be seen in the soft tissue (Gold et al, 1975; Malek & Brodkin, 1973).

The skin nodules, which are reddish brown in colour and often widespread, are suggestive of the diagnosis. The ESR is seldom markedly raised. Autoantibodies are not found. Although mild hypercholesterolaemia may be present other lipids are normal. Synovial fluid examination may show foamy cells, though these are more easily seen together with giant cells in synovial biopsies. Similar changes are found in biopsies of the nodules. The foamy appearance is due to a PAS-positive substance (Krey et al, 1974).

Treatment

Although many treatments have been tried there is no evidence of other than symptomatic benefit for which simple non-steroidal anti-inflammatory drugs should be tried.

The course tends to be progressive and up to 30% of cases are complicated by a wide variety of malignancies (Barrow & Holubar, 1969).

CRYOGLOBULINAEMIA

On cooling serum to 4°C for several (usually up to 3) days, precipitates may form. Within these precipitates are globulins — cryoglobulins or cold insoluble globulins. Resolution of part of these precipitates with warming to 37°C identifies the cryoprecipitates. Not all precipitate may redissolve. A major cryoprotein is cryofibrinogen hence the value of clotting the blood sample at 37°C and using the resulting serum, minus cryofibrinogen, for the investigation of cryoglobulins. The cryoprecipitates are not pure immunoglobulins; lipid and other proteins — especially fibronectin — are often present. Indeed fibronectin may have a role in the formation of immune complexes, especially when raised as in inflammatory disease (Beaulieu et al, 1981).

Although cryoglobulins belong to all classes of immunoglobulin those of the 'rheumatoid factors' are the predominant type usually discussed in association with rheumatoid diseases. Immune complexes form a large proportion of the cryoprecipitate and both the classical and alternative pathways of complement activation may be initiated by cryoprecipitation even to the extent of producing hypocomplementaemia. The important point is to establish what the complement level is in vivo, i.e. at 37°C, since cryoprecipitation may lead to falsely low in vitro values. Tarantino et al (1978) have suggested that reduced C4 levels in essential mixed cryoglobulinaemia may be partly due to reduced biosynthesis. The cryoglobulins belong to all classes of immunoglobulin, but the tendency for antiglobulins to form immune complexes results in these antiglobulins being concentrated in these cryprecipitates. Immune complexes are the most frequent cause of cryoprecipitation and their quantity bears some relationship to disease activity. The cryoprecipitates have been shown to contain antiglobulins of different classes (Meltzer et al, 1966A) and anti-DNA and IgM lymphocytoxic antibodies (Winfield et al, 1975a, b). There are both qualitative and quantitative differences between the small amounts of mixed IgM and IgG cryoglobulins found in rheumatic and other inflammatory conditions as diverse as sarcoidosis, chronic inflammation of the liver, bacterial and viral infections and the much larger quantities of monoclonal cryglobulins found in lymphoproliferation disease. The presence of cryoglobulins does not necessarily indicate they are producing disease and symptoms are less frequent in conditions involving the monoclonal cryoglobulins.

Several different classifications of cryoglobulinaemia have been used. A simplified one is given.

Unmixed (monoclonal). This type is usually associated with lymphoproliferative disorders. Only one class of immunoglobulin is found in the cryoprecipitate. Self-association of immunoglobulins is rare and little complement activation occurs.

Mixed (polyclonal). More than one immunoglobulin class is present and almost invariably a 'rheumatoid factor' antiglobulin is involved. The 'rheumatoid factor' (which can be of any class) may be limited to a single immunoglobulin in lymphoproliferative diseases or of several classes in infection or inflammation.

Essential. These cryoglobulins can be either monoclonal or polyclonal. Usually no underlying cause for the gammaglobulinopathy is found. Hepatitis B antibody has been found in 12–85% of cases (Weinberger et al, 1981; Levo et al, 1977).

Symptoms of cryoglobulinaemia are probably produced in two principal ways, as follows.

Hyperviscosity

This may be a prominent feature of 'pure' monoclonal cryoglobulinaemia especially if of the IgM type rather than with the smaller molecules of IgG and IgA types. The formation of cryoprecipitates is due to weak self-association not of immunological nature and thus complement activation is minimal. In addition to the increased viscosity due to large aggregates, deposition of protein on vessel walls occurs; the consequences of this in functional terms are not clear. The features found are Raynaud's phenomenon, cold-induced urticaria, digital gangrene, arterial thrombosis, cutaneous ulcers, congestive cardiac failure and paradoxically spontaneous haemorrhage. Central nervous system features, both transient and permanent, may occur.

Immune complex disease

This is typical of the polyclonal 'mixed' cryoglobulinaemia in which complexes of rheumatoid factor, antigen and complement are found and produce a vasculitis usually of small and, less frequently, of medium arteries.

A variety of skin manifestations is the commonest finding in these patients (Brouet, 1974). This is not surprising since dermal temperatures are usually lower (30°C compared to 37°C) than core temperatures. Purpura — small polymorphic lesions, often with a dark centre especially over the extermities — urticaria and reticulate livido (Fig. 47.23) may be found.

Mixed neuropathies of the periphery are common but central nervous system features are uncommon. Initial paraesthesia may be followed by numbness and motor loss usually of mononeuritic type (Fig. 47.23). Joint involvement is common but mild being a transient arthralgia, mainly of large joints without signs and not usually leading to joint destruction.

Several histological types of glomerulonephritis and intestinal vasculitis occur. The prognosis depends largely on the progress of renal involvement. Hepatosplenomegaly, lymphadenopathy, Sjögren's syndrome and other features of inflammatory connective tissue or lymphoproliferative disease may be found (Gorevic et al, 1980).

Treatment

This is difficult (Gettner et al, 1981). A direct approach by removing abnormal protein with plasmaphoresis is often temporarily but rapidly successful, particularly in hyperviscosity syndromes, but needs repeating frequently. Immune complex disease may also be helped by plasmaphoresis but perhaps less so than in other more typical immune complex diseases such as systemic lupus erythematosus and this probably represents a different ability of plasmaphoresis to alter the underlying immune defects. Attempts to control the inflammatory aspects of immune complex disease with relatively high doses of corticosteroids and cytotoxic drugs are only partially successful.

When there is a clear underlying disease especially of lymphoproliferative nature, this should be treated and the response of the cryoglobulinaemia will mirror the effect of treatment on the un-

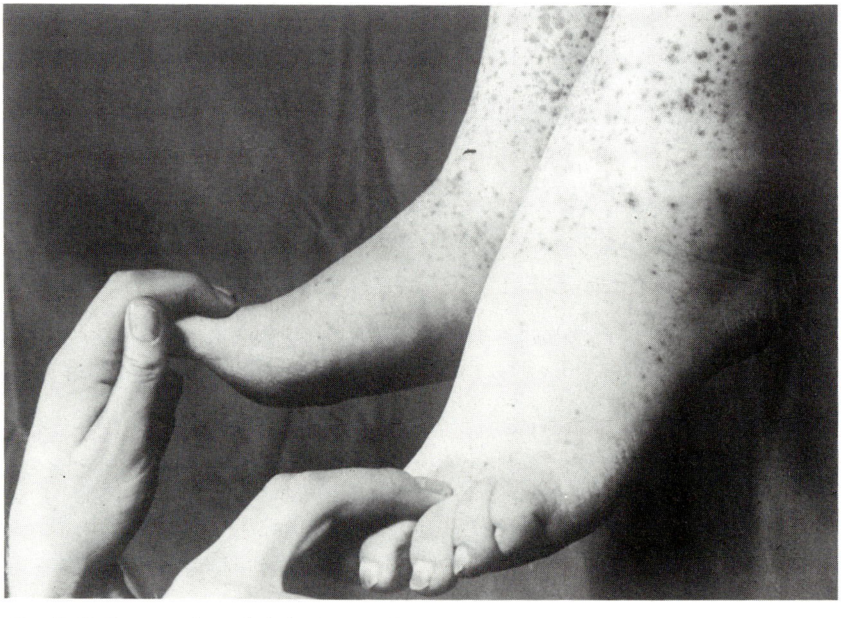

Fig. 47.23 Cryoproteinaemia (mixed type). Typical purpura. Foot drop is present on left due to mononeuritis of lateral poplital nerve.

derlying condition. While severe cooling should be avoided, relatively little benefit follows from the use of warm clothing.

HYPERGAMMAGLOBULINAEMIC PURPURA

This is a condition found as a complication of inflammatory connective tissue disease such as rheumatoid disease, Sjögren's syndrome and SLE. It also occurs in chronic lymphocytic lymphoma. Intermediate-sized immune complexes are found. Purpura and vasculitic lesions of the skin are characteristic. Cutaneous vasculitis also occurs in other conditions such as intestinal disease and lymphoproliferative disorders where the underlying cause, hypergammaglobulinaemia, is probably similar.

HYPERVISCOSITY SYNDROME

Features of hyperviscosity syndrome have been described in rheumatoid arthritis in association with intermediate size complexes (Popa et al, 1975). The spectrum of clinical events is similar to that in cryoglobulinaemia.

IMMUNE DEFICIENCY

The recognition of these defects is relatively recent, Bruton (1952) giving the first clear discussion. They are clinically rare conditions which can be broadly classified into those due to abnormal T lymphocyte cell function which roughly correlates with 'cell-mediated immunity', those due primarily to deficient immunoglobulin production (B cells) and a combination of these two extremes. Loss of a single antibody class, e.g. IgA, is called a 'selective deficiency' (or 'dysgammaglobulinaemia'). The primary division into T and B lymphocyte defects is an oversimplification since regulatory systems exist between these cell types by which they alter each other's immune expression and the defect often involves only some of the cell types present. In patients with severe combined immunodeficiency there is both a T and B cell defect and these children are usually dead by 2 years. The latter form of immunodeficiency will not be considered further. Further subdivision of these dysfunctions is possible into primary (either of early or late onset) immune deficiency and those secondary to malignancy, usually of lymphoreticular type or following immunosuppressive treatment.

In addition immunodeficiency may arise from abnormalities of neutrophil phagocyte and monocytic function or complement deficits. The constant feature of all these deficits is a susceptibility to infection either recurrent or persistent, especially of paranasal sinus and lungs and in the adult gastrointestinal infections.

Associated with some of these abnormalities, autoimmune disease, including synovitis, may be present without detectable evidence of infection. The literature contains many isolated reports in which a variety of immune defects have been associated with arthritis or connective tissue disease and it is difficult to know if these are chance associations or whether the conditions are pathologi cally related. However, certain associations appear to occur more frequently than by pure chance. The recently described acquired immune deficiency syndrome (AIDS) in homosexuals, haemophiliacs and transfused patients, could present with bone or joint sepsis, though at the time of writing this has not been reported.

Hypogammaglobulinaemia (see also Ch. 11)

'Hypogammaglobulinaemia' is a better term than 'agammaglobulinaemia' since these patients are rarely completely devoid of gammaglobulin. All classes of immunoglobulin can be affected but especially the IgG classes are depressed. For practical purposes two types of hypogammaglobulinaemia will be discussed, the sex-linked (Bruton) form of childhood and the (relatively) late onset 'acquired' form. The divide is mainly by time of onset and taken at 2–4 years. Although the acquired form is usually thought to be non-hereditary, the occurrence of other autoimmune diseases and immune abnormalities in some of these families suggests that a familial factor may sometimes be present (Friedmann et al, 1977). A suggested incidence is of about 1/50 000 but this is probably an underestimate and, in particular, ethnic differences are not documented.

The main pathological difference between the sex-linked and acquired forms of hypoglobulinaemia is the reduced lymphoid mass and absence, or markedly reduced number, of surface immunoglobulin-bearing lymphocytes (without total lymphopenia) in the circulation in X-linked hypogammaglobulinaemia. There are normal or increased quantities of lymphoid tissue and normal numbers of surface immunoglobulin-bearing lymphocytes which do not mature into functioning immunoglobulin-producing plasma cells.

There is usually a background of chronic or recurrent sepsis involving nasal sinuses, ears and lungs, and diarrhoea occurs, particularly in the late onset forms. The common form of arthritis is infective, especially in children. One or more joints may be involved with tenderness and swelling. Systemic features are variable and the patient may remain ambulant. The susceptibility is primarily to bacterial infection, resistance to viral and fungal infection being practically normal. The common bacterial organisms are involved but atypical organisms such as *Mycoplasma pneumonia* and T strains now called '*Ureaplasma urealyticum*,' may be implicated. Both these organisms need careful culture conditions for identification and it is essential to obtain joint fluid for examination before treatment. Treatment is with gammaglobulin replacement and appropriate antibodies. Gammaglobulin alone is ineffective.

In 1956 Janeway et al noted the association between 'collagen diseases' and congenital hypogammaglobulinaemia. Shortly afterwards Good et al (1957) reported the association between hypogammaglobulinaemia and rheumatoid arthritis in the adult and with arthritis in children. Arthritis is found in about 30% of children with hypogammaglobulinaemia (Petty et al, 1977). There are important differences in the clinical pictures between the arthritis of hypogammaglobulinaemia and rheumatoid arthritis; nodules, erosions and rheumatoid factors are not found in the hypogammaglobulinaemia patients (Grayzel et al, 1977), who usually obtain some benefit from gammaglobulin injections.

The non-infective arthritis can vary from recurrent painless hydroarthrosis to a more persistent oligoarthritis commonly affecting the knee (in 30% of cases). Pain, swelling, mild ill-health with fever and leucocytosis may occur but the patient usually remains ambulant. Synovial thickening varies in degree and rarely leads to erosions or joint destruction. Interestingly 'rice bodies' may be found (Taborn, 1981). The synovial fluid does not contain large numbers of neutrophils, polymorphs or rheumatoid factor, nor is synovial infiltration prominent, consisting of inflammatory cells but without plasma cells. The lack of neutrophils may reflect the lack of complement activation and consequent chemotaxis. In the adult the non-infective arthritis is more often symmetrical and affects both large and small joints. Tenosynovitis is an important feature.

Dermatomyositis

A dermatomyositis-like picture has been described in association with **hypogammaglobulinaemia** (Wilfert et al, 1977; Webster et al, 1978), apparently due to echovirus or adenovirus infections to which these children are susceptible. There may be arthritis, myalgia with an inflammatory myositis leading to flexion deformities of knees and elbows, and subcutaneous oedema. A variety of rashes and neurological features, including convulsions, have been described, but the question of the relationship of this syndrome to the more usual forms of dermatomyositis is debatable. The creatine phosphokinase and other muscle enzyme levels are usually normal. The central nervous system involvement is the most serious aspect and the usual cause of death. Widespread cortical and cerebellar changes are found and the cerebrospinal fluid culture may yield the virus which is by other techniques difficult to detect.

Selective IgA deficiency

This is the commonest form of immune deficiency and is found in about 1 in 300 of the population, when it is often associated with normal health.

Lone (selective) IgA deficiency is more frequent (about 2–4%) in children with juvenile arthritis (Cassidy et al, 1973), but there is no evidence that it plays a part in the disease process. It has also been linked with a wide variety of autoimmune processes including connective tissue diseases. The lack of secretory IgA may explain the increased absorption of antigens, e.g. cow's milk (Cunningham-Rundles et al, 1978), and collagens

(Wells et al, 1973), in these patients. Moreover there is a high incidence of autoantibodies in these patients, which may represent cross-reactivity with absorbed antigen. The association of atopy with IgA deficiency could have a similar basis, i.e. sensitisation to absorbed allergens.

Iatrogenic IgA deficiency may occur with D-penicillamine treatment of rheumatoid arthritis (Stanworth et al, 1977), but apparently has no clinical significance.

In some of these patients anti-IgA antibodies may be present and treatment of the immune deficiency by blood products may produce severe, even fatal, anaphylactoid reactions. Preliminary injection of a small amount of the blood product as a test dose should be tried.

Pathogenesis of non-infective arthritis in immune deficiency

This is unknown and may well vary in different types of immune deficiency. The absence of benefit from immunoglobulin replacement in IgA deficiency suggests that this is not the prime defect, but that both immune deficiency and autoimmune connective tissue disease represent facets of altered autoimmunity in the patient. The widespread nature of the associated autoimmunities would follow from this. The increased incidence of antibodies to food allergens found in IgA deficiency would support the concept of cross-reactive autoimmunity sometimes resulting in arthritis, though this is probably a rare cause of arthritis. The high incidence of diarrhoea and persistence of enteral infections could result in a reactive type of arthritis.

The presence of autoimmune disease in patients with hypogammaglobulinaemia and of their normal relatives suggests an hereditary defect and it is interesting that metabolic abnormalities (Giblett et al, 1972, 1975) have been described as a cause of immune deficiency.

The possibility of, at present, unrecognised infections in these cases remains.

In contrast to the incidence of arthritis with humoral deficiencies, there is no clear association with lone T cell (cell-mediated) immune deficiencies. Transient arthritis has been described in the Wiskott–Aldrich syndrome (Cooper et al, 1968).

Diagnosis

Apart from the clinical history of recurrent infections, the low levels of IgG, IgA and usually IgM immunoglobulins are suggestive. T lymphocytes appear in normal numbers but there may be a deficiency of Ig-bearing (B) lymphocytes (X-linked agammaglobulinaemia), absence of immunoglobulin or its production by Ig-bearing lymphocytes on stimulation (late onset agammaglobulinaemia). Obvious problems are encountered with young children where up to 3 months of age the maternal immunoglobulins may persist or there may be delay in the maturation of the child's immune system with transient hypogammaglobulinaemia. Tests of the ability to develop immunity after immunisation or lymph node biopsy are only necessary to further define the type of immune deficiency. In the late onset types of hypogammaglobulinaemia underlying causes of immune deficiency such as myeloma and lymphoma should be searched for.

Treatment

Joint aspiration is essential to establish the presence of any infection. It is important to sample as many joints as possible, the early diagnosis of infection bearing on the ultimate diagnosis. The laboratory should be asked to look for *Mycoplasma* and other unusual infections.

The response of the synovitis to intramuscular gammaglobulin is good if bacterial infection (pneumococci and *H. influenza*) is present but has little effect on mycoplasma infection which requires erythromycin and tetracycline.

Adequate replacement immunoglobulin should be given (25 g/kg weekly), intramuscularly or intravenously according to the preparation. However, if the replacement immunoglobulin does not contain specific antibodies, resident infection (e.g. echovirus) may be unaffected. In isolated IgA deficiency replacement is of little use since injection immunoglobulin will not reach mucosal surfaces in adequate quantities. The occasional reactions to IgA infusions have been mentioned.

In rare cases of cellular immunodeficiency grafting of lymphoid tissue has been used with success. The use of 'immune stimulation' such as transfer factor, thymosin or levamisole has been of little use except, apparently, in occasional cases.

Table 47.4 Complement component deficiency and rheumatic disease (after Agnello, 1978; Boyer et al, 1975; Day et al, 1972; Glass et al, 1976; Hauptmann et al, 1974; Jasin, 1977; Rosenfield, 1976; Schaller et al, 1977).

Complement Component		
C1 r	LE	Vasculitis, nephritis, infection
C1 s	LE	
C1 INH	LE	Angioneurotic oedema
C4	LE	Vasculitis
C2	LE	Juvenile arthritis, vasculitis, nephritis, bacterial infection
C3	LE	Bacterial infection
C5	LE	Bacterial infection
C6		Bacterial infection
C7		Bacterial infection
C8	LE	Bacterial infection

LE = Lupus erythematosus.

COMPLEMENT (see also Ch. 13)

A variety of complement component deficiencies have been associated with rheumatic syndromes (Agnello, 1978) (Table 47.4). Primary complement deficiency is not common and is a rare cause of rheumatoid syndromes. However, the true incidence of component deficiencies is not known, nor is it always clear whether the deficiency is primary or secondary to the disease. Many examples have been ascertained because of routine testing in disease and this will tend to bias the result towards an association between disease and deficiency. Complement deficiency, usually of the early components of the cascade, is more frequently a result of the disease than a cause. Deficiency of C2 is probably the most frequent and most investigated deficiency. Biochemical complement deficiency is compatible with good health.

Arthritic symptoms secondary to complement deficiency are of two main types — immune complex disease and pyogenic infection. Poor viral neutralisation and genetic disease associated with HLA regions which are also close to the chromosomal regions coding for some of the complement components, are other factors in the predisposition of these patients to autoimmune disease.

The early stages of the complement cascade play a role in regulating the size and solubility of immune complexes (Casali & Lambert, 1979; Schifferli & Peters, 1982). It is therefore not surprising that deficiencies will lead to abnormalities of immune complex function. Thus immune complex disease is not an unusual feature of these deficiencies. The main features of the resulting syndromes simulate lupus erythematosus with fever, rashes, alopecia, arthralgia, hepatosplenomegaly. These features may be severe; however central nervous system and renal problems are probably less pronounced than in conventional lupus erythematosus. The serological findings are of interest. Antinuclear factor, antibody to double stranded DNA and band immunoglobulin deposits in the skin may be absent. The single most effective screening test is a serum haemolytic complement estimation which is usually at a very low level. There is a tendency for these deficiencies to be familial and thus when atypical cases of lupus erythematosus appear in more than one member of a family, complement defects should be sought.

An increased susceptibility to bacterial infection is found particularly with deficiencies of C3 and the later components. The most frequent infection is neissarial presumably due to defective opsonisation. Where complement deficiency occurs *secondarily* to the disease state a similar increased susceptibility to infection arises. Features suggestive of dermatomyositis and scleroderma occur but are rarely as marked as in these conditions when unassociated with complement deficiency.

C1 inhibitor of various degrees is perhaps more common than true complement deficiency and as well as causing angioneurotic oedema, causes abdominal pain, arthralgia and lupus-like syndromes.

Treatment

The treatment of the above conditions are, on the whole, unsatisfactory except for acute episodes such as with angioneurotic oedema and gonococcal septicaemia when fresh frozen plasma may be lifesaving.

In some cases an absolute deficiency of complement protein exists and in these cases, as in many other examples of absolute selective protein deficiency, replacement therapy may result in autoantibodies being induced.

CONCLUSION

In many of the situations discussed there is an interplay between the disease process and the haematological/immunological system so that the progenitive process is often obscured. These are rare conditions in everyday practice; however failure to recognise them may result in failed treatment. Recognition and investigation is a valuable way to a better understanding of the common autoimmune processes.

Most of the illustrations were obtained from patients seen with my colleagues Dr I. Delamore and Dr D. Evans, to whom I am most grateful.

REFERENCES

Abbot D F, Gresham G A 1972 Arthropathy in transfusional siderosis. British Medical Journal 1: 418–419

Agnello V 1978 The complement deficiency states. Medicine (Baltimore) 57: 1–21

Ahlberg A 1975 On the natural history of haemophilic pseudo-tumour. Journal of Bone and Joint Surgery 57A: 1133–1136

Alavi A, Schumacher H R, Dorwart B B, Kukl D E 1976 Bone marrow scan evaluation of arthropathy in sickle cell disorders. Archives of Internal Medicine 136:436

Ansell B M 1980 Rheumatic disorders in childhood. Butterworth, London

Arnold W D, Hilgarner M W 1977 Haemophilic arthropathy, current concepts of pathogenesis and management. Journal of Bone and Joint Surgery 59A: 287–305

Aronstam A, Browne R A, Wassef M, Hamad Z 1983 The clinical features of early bleeding into the muscle of the lower limb in severe haemophiliacs. Journal of Bone and Joint Surgery 65B: 19–23

Astrup T, Sjolin K E 1958 Thromboplastic and fibrinolytic activity of the synovial membrane and fibrous capsular tissue. Proceedings of the Society of Experimental Medical Biology 97: 852–854

Balloo S P, Khan M A, Kushner I, Harris J W 1977 Secondary gout in haemoglobinopathies: report of two cases and review of the literature. American Journal of Haematology 2: 397–402

Baltus J A M, Boersma J W, Hartman A P, Vandenbroucke J P 1983 The occurrence of malignancies in patients with rheumatoid arthritis treated with cyclophosphanide: a controlled restrospective follow up. Annals of the Rheumatic Diseases 42: 268–373

Barrow M V, Holubar K 1969 Multicentric reticulohistiocytosis, a review of 33 patients. Medicine 48: 287–305

Beaulieu A D, Valet J P, Strevey J 1981 The influence of fibronectin on cryoprecipitate formation in rheumatoid arthritis and systemic lupus erythematosus. Arthritis and Rheumatism 24: 1383–1388

Behn A, Sykes H 1982 Polyarteritis nodosa and hairy cell leukaemia. Rheumatism and Rehabilitation 21: 164–166

Bennett R M, Williams E D, Lewis S M, Holt P J L 1972 Studies of a popliteal synovial fistula. Annals of the Rheumatic Diseases 31: 482–486

Bensa J L, Faure J, Martin H, Solto T J, Shaerer R 1976 Levamisole in angioimmunoblastic lymphadenopathy. Lancet 1:1081

Berry E M, Miller J P 1973 Hereditary spherocytosis, haemochromatosis, diabetes mellitus and chondrocalcinosis. Proceedings of the Royal Society of Medicine 66: 9–10

Bignold L P 1980 The importance of platelets in increased vascular permeability evoked by experimental haemarthrosis in synovium or the rat. Pathology 12: 169–179

Bouroncle B A, Wiseman B K, Doan C A 1958 Leukaemia reticuloendotheliosis Blood 13: 609–630

Boyer J T, Gall E P, Norman M E, Wilson V R, Zimmerman T S 1975 Hereditary deficiency of the seventh component of complement. Journal of Clinical Investigation 56: 905–913

Boyle D J, Day J F, Kassan S S, Thomas M R, Robinson W A, Steigerwald J C 1981 Incidence of malignancy 10 years following cyclophosphamide use for rheumatoid arthritis. Arthritis and Rheumatism 24 (Suppl): P71 Abstract 81

Brighton C T, Bigley E C, Smolenaski B I 1970 Iron induced arthritis in immature rabbits. Arthritis and Rheumatism 13: 848–857

Brouet J C, Clauvel J P, Danor F, Klein M, Selingmann M 1974 Biological and clinical significance of cryoglobins. A report of 86 cases. American Journal of Medicine 57: 775–788

Bruton O C 1952 Agammaglobinaemia. Paediatrics 9:722

Caputo R, Aleasi E, Berti E 1981 Collagen phagocytosis in multicentric reticulohistiocytosis. Journal of Investigative Dermatology 76: 342–346

Casali P, Lambert P H 1979 Purification of soluble immune complexes from serum using polymethyl metacrylate beads coated with conglutinin or C_1q. Clinical and Experimental Immunology 37: 295–309

Casey D F, Cathcart E S 1970 Haemarthrosis and sickle cell trait. Arthritis and Rheumatism 13: 882–88

Cassidy J T, Petty R E, Sullivan D B 1973 Abnormalities in the distribution of serum immunoglobulin concentrations in juvenile rheumatoid arthritis. Journal of Clinical Investigation 52: 1931–1936

Choi Ye-chin, Hough A J, Morris G M, Sokoloff L 1981 Experimental siderosis in vitro. Arthritis and Rheumatism 24: 809–823

Cooper M D, Chase H P, Lowman J T et al 1968 Wiskott-Aldrich syndrome An immunologic deficiency disease involving the afferent limb of immunity. American Journal of Medicine 44: 499–513

Crofts M A, Sharp J C, Joyner M W 1979 Rheumatoid arthritis and hairy cell leukaemia. Lancet 2: 203–204

Cullen M H, Stansfield A C, Oliver R T D, Lister T A, Malpas J S 1979 Angio immunoblastic lymphadenopathy. Report of ten cases and review of literature. Quarterly Journal of Medicine 48: 151–177

Cunningham-Rundles C, Brandies W E, Good R A, Day N K 1978 Milk precipitins, circulating immune complexes and IgA deficiency. Proceedings of the National Academy of Science 75: 3387–3389

Davies P G, Fordham J N 1983 Arthritis and

angioimmunoblastic lymphadenopathy. Annals of the Rheumatic Diseases 42: 516–518
Day N K, Geiger H, Stroud R, Debracco E W, Mancado B 1972 C_1 deficiency: an inborn error associated with cutaneous and renal disease. Journal of Clinical Investigation 51: 1102–1108
Defaria C R, de Mezo-Souza S E, Pinheiro E D 1979 Haemophilic neuromyopathy 42: 600–605
Diamond H S, Meisel A D, Holden D 1979 The natural history of urate overproduction in sickle cell anaemia. Annals of Internal Medicine 90: 752–757
Dorwart B B, Schumacher H R 1981 Arthritis in B thalassaemia trait: clinical and pathological features. Annals of the Rheumatic Diseases 40: 185–189
Dorwart B B, Goldberg M A, Schumacher H R, Alavi A 1977 Absence of increased frequency of bone and joint disease with haemoglobin AS and AC. Annals of Internal Medicine 86: 66–67
Ehrenfeld M, Penchas S, Eliakim M 1977 Thrombocytosis in rheumatoid Arthritis. Annals of the Rheumatic Diseases 36: 571–581
Elkon K B, Hughes G R V, Catovsky D et al 1979 Hairy cell leukaemia with polyarteritis nodosa. Lancet 2: 280–282
Espinoza I R, Spilberg I, Osterland C K 1974 Joint manifestation of sickle cell disease. Medicine 53:295
Facchini A, Mariani E, Ferrolli A et al 1981 Hairy cell leukaemia and rheumatoid arthritis; cause or effect. Arthritis and Rheumatism 24:1587
Felzi T, Kabat E A 1972 Immunochemical studies on blood groups. Journal of Experimental Medicine 135: 1247–1258
Fink C W, Windmiller J, Sartain P 1972 Arthritis as a presenting feature of childhood leukaemia. Arthritis and Rheumatism 15: 347–349
Fitzcharles M A, Kirwen J R, Calvin B J, Currey H L F 1982 Sideroblastic anaemia with iron overload presenting as an arthropathy. Annals of the Rheumatis Diseases 41: 97–99
Friedman J M, Failkow P J, Davies S D, Ocks H D, Wedgwood R J 1977 Auto-immunity in relative of patients with immunodeficiency diseases. Clinical Experimental Immunology 28: 375–388
Frizzeri A G, Moran E M, Rappaport H 1975 Angioimmunoblastic lymphadenopathy. American Journal of Medicine 59: 803–818
Gettner D, Kohn R W, Gorevic P, Franklyn E C 1981 The effect of combination therapy (steroids, immunosuppressive and plasmophoresis) on 5 mixed cryoglobionaemia patients with renal, neurologic and vascular involvement. Arthritis and Rheumatism 24: 1121–1127
Giblett E R, Anderson J E, Cohen F, Pollova B, Meinwissen H J 1972 Adenosine-deaminose deficiency in two patients with severely impaired cellular immunity. Lancet 2: 1067–1069
Giblett E R, Ammann A J, Wara D W, Sandman R, Diamond L K 1975 Nucleoside phosphoglucose deficiency in a child with severely defective T cell immunity and normal B cell immunity. Lancet 2: 1010–1013
Glass D, Raum D, Gilson D 1976 Inherited deficiency of the second component of complement. Rheumatis disease associations. Journal of Clinical Investigation 58: 853–861
Goedert J J, Nupe J R, Smith F S, Stahl N I, Jaffe E S, Fauci A S 1981 Polyarteritis nodosa, hairy cell leukaemia and splenosis. American Journal of Medicine 71: 323–326
Gold R H, Metzger A L, Mirra J M 1975 Multicentric reticulohistiocytosis, an erosive polyarthritis with distinctive clinical, roentgenographic and pathologic features. American Journal of Roentgenology, Radium Therapy and Nuclear Medicine 124: 610–624
Golomb H M, Catovsky D, Golde D W 1978 Hairy cell leukaemia. Annals of Internal Medicine 89: 677–683
Good R A, Rotstein J, Mazzitelo W F 1957 The simultaneous occurrence of rheumatoid arthritis and agammaglobinaemia. Journal of Laboratory and Clinical Medicine 49: 343–357
Gordon D A, Pruzanski W, Ogryzlo M 1973a Synovial fluid examination for the diagnosis of amyloidosis. Annals of the Rheumatic Diseases 32: 428–430
Gordon D A, Pruzanski W, Ogryzle M A, Little H 1973b Amyloid arthritis simulating rheumatoid disease in five patients with multiple myeloma. American Journal of Medicine 55: 142–154
Gorevic P D, Kasab H J, Levo Y et al 1980 Mixed cryoglobinaemia: clinical aspects and long term follow up of forty patients. American Journal of Medicine 69: 287–308
Gratwick G M, Bullough P F, Bohne W H I, Markinson A I, Peterson C M 1978 Thalassaemia osteoarthropathy. American Internal Medicine 88: 494–501
Grazyel A I, Marcus R, Stern R, Winchester R J 1977 Chronic polyarthritis associated with hypergammaglobinaemia: study of two patients. Arthritis and Rheumatism 20: 887–894
Hammell C F, De Nardo S J, De Nardo G L, Lewis J P 1973 Bone marrow and bone mineral scintographic studies in sickle cell disease. British Journal of Haematology 25: 593–598
Harris B K, Ross H A 1974 Haemarthrosis as the presenting manifestation of myeloproliferative disease. Arthritis and Rheumatism 17: 969–970
Hasselbacher P 1980 Sickled erythrocytes in synovial fluid. Arthritis and Rheumatism 23: 127–128
Hauptmann C, Grosshaus E, Heid E 1974 Lupus erythemateuse aigus et deficits hereditaire en complement. A propos d'un cas par deficit complet en C_4. Annales de Dermatologie et de Syphiligraphie 101:479
Heinicke M H, Zarrabi M H, Gorevic P D 1983 Arthritis due to synovial involvement by extramedullary haemopoeisis in myelofibrosis with myeloid metaplasia. Annals of the Rheumatic Disease 42: 196–200
Hench P K, Mayne T G, Kiely J M, Dockerty M B 1962 Clinical study of rheumatic manifestations of lymphoma. Arthritis and Rheumatism 5:301
Hernandez P et al 1981 Circulating immune complexes in sickle cell hepatic crises. Acta Haematologie 65: 15–20
Hind W L, Kind N L 1978 Serum opsonization of salmonella in sickle cell anaemia. American Journal of Medicine 64: 388–394
Hoaglund F T 1967 Experimental haemarthrosis. Journal of Bone and Joint Surgery 49A: 285–298
Hoedemaker K M, Wagenvoort C A 1975 Pathological changes in patients suffering from haemophilia. In: Brinkhouse K M, Hember H C (eds) Handbook of haemophilia, Part 1. American Elsevier, New York
Hustu H O, Pinkel D 1967 Lymphosarcoma, Hodgkins disease and leukaemia in bone. Clinical Orthopaedics 52: 83–93
Hutchinson R M, Davis P, Jayson M I V 1976 Thrombocytosis in rheumatoid arthritis. Annals of the Rheumatic Diseases 35: 138–142
Isomaki H A, Hakulinen T, Joutsenlahti V 1978 Excess risk

of lymphomas, leukaemia and myeloma in patients with rheumatoid arthritis. Journal of Chronic Diseases 31: 691–696
Issargarisil S, Piankijagum A, Wasi P 1981 Spinal Cord Compression in thalassaemia. Archives of Internal Medicine 141: 1033–1036
Janeway C A, Gitlin D, Craig J M, Grice D S 1956 'Collagen diseases' in patients with congenital agammaglobinaemia. Transactions of the Association of American Phyicians 69:93
Jasin H E 1977 Absence of the eighth component of complement in association with systemic lupus erythematosus-like disease. Journal of Clinical Investigation 60: 709–715
Keeling M M, Lockwood W B, Harris E A 1974 Avascular necrosis and erythrocytosis in sickle cell trait. New England Journal of Medicine 190: 442–444
Kirsner A B, Farber S J, Sheon R P, Finker R I 1981 Incidence of malignant disease in patients receiving cytotoxic therapy for rheumatoid arthritis. Arthritis and Rheumatism 41 (Suppl): 32–33
Klofhorn R W, Lightsey A L 1979 Haemarthrosis associated with Glanzmann's thromboasthenia. Arthritis and Rheumatism 22: 1390–1393
Krey P R, Comerford F R, Cohen A S 1974 Multicentric reticulohistoicytosis. Fine structural analysis of the synovium and synovial fluid cells. Arthritis and Rheumatism 17: 615–633
Lee R E J, Golding J S R, Serjeant G R 1981 The radiological features of avascular necrosis of the femoral head in homozygous sickle cell disease. Clinical Radiology 32: 205–214
LePogam P P, Ghandour C, Leprise P Y 1982 Hairy cell leukaemia and polyarteritis nodosa. Journal of Rheumatology 8: 441–442
Levo Y, Gorevic P D, Wassaf H J, Zucker-Franklin D, Franklin E C 1977 The association between hepatis B virus and essential mixed cryoglobulinaemia. New England Journal of Medicine 296: 1501–1504
Luban N L C, Leikin S L, August G A 1982 Growth and development in sickle cell anaemia. Preliminary Report. American Journal of Paediatrics, Haematology, Oncology 4: 61–65
Lukes R J, Tindle B H 1975 Immunoblastic lymphadenopathy: a hyperimmune entity resembling Hodgkin's disease. New England Journal of Medicine 292: 1–7
McCollough N C, Enio J E, Lovett J, Liam E C Y, Niemann K N W, Loughlin E C 1979 Synovectomy or total replacement of the knee in haemophilia. Journal of Bone and Joint Surgery 61A: 69–75
Mainardi C L, Levine P J H, Wibl Z, Harris E D M 1978 Proliferative synovitis in haemophilia: biochemical and morphological observation. Arthritis and Rheumatism 21: 137–144
Malek J, Brodkin R 1973 Multicentric reticulohistiocytosis with extensive bone and joint destruction. New York State Journal of Medicine 73: 2482–2491
Mannucci P M, de Franchis R, Torri G, Pietrograndi V 1977 Role of synovectomy in haemophiliac arthropathy. Israeli Journal of Medical Science 13: 983–987
Martin V M, Bennett R M, Hughes G R V, Holt P J L 1974 Lymphosarcomatous arthropathy. Annals of the Rheumatic Diseases 32: 162–166
Meltzer M, Franklyn E C 1966 Cryoglobinaemia — a study of twenty nine patients. I. IgG and IgM cryoglobulin and factors affecting cryoprecipitability. American Journal of Medicine 40: 828–836
Meltzer M, Franklin E C, Elias K, McCullough R T, Cooper N 1966 Cryoglobulinaemia — a clinical and laboratory study. II. Cryoglobulin with rheumatoid factor activity. American Journal of Medicine 40: 837–856
Mintz G, Robles-Suavedra R J, Enriquiz R D, Jimeney R T, Juan M A 1978 Haemarthrosis as the presenting manifestation of true myeloma joint disease. Arthritis and Rheumatism 21: 148–151
Moore S B, Harrison E C, Weiland L H 1976 Angioimmunoblastic lymphadenopathy. Mayo Clinica Proceedings 51: 273–280
Newton P, Freemont A J, Noble J, Scott N, Grennan D M, Hilton R C 1984 Secondary malignant synovitis. Quarterly Journal of Medicine 53:135
Pearson H A, Cornelius F A, Schwarz A D, Zilson J H, Wolfson S L, Spencer R P 1970 Transfusion — reversible functional asplenia in young children with sickle cell anaemia. New England Journal of Medicine 283: 334–337
Pettersen H, Ahlberg A, Nilsom I M 1980 A radiologic classification of haemophilic arthropathy. Clinics of Orthopaedic Related Research 149: 153–159
Petty R E, Cassidy J T, Tubergen D C 1977 Association of arthritis with hypogammaglobulinaemia. Arthritis and Rheumatism 20: 441–443
Pierce D A, Stern R, Jaffer R, Zubman J, Talal N 1979 Immunoblastic sarcoma with Sjögren's syndrome and systemic lupus erythematosus in a patient with immunoblastic lymphadenopathy. Arthritis and Rheumatism 22: 911–916
Popa G, Nastase V, Hanganu E 1982 Angioimmunoblastic lymphadenopathy associated with systemic lupus erythematosus. Folia Haematology 109: 430–434
Pope R M, Mannik M, Gilliband B C, Tiller D C 1975 The hyperviscosity syndrome in rheumatoid arthritis due to intermediate complexes formed by self association of IgG-rheumatoid factor. Arthritis and Rheumatism 18: 97–106
Propper R D, Button L N, Nathan D G 1980 New approaches to the transfusion management of thalassaemia. Blood 55: 55–60
Rainsford S G, Aronstam A Holborow E J, McLellan L 1982 Anticoagulant antibodies in the synovial membranes of patients suffering from haemophilia, rheumatoid arthritis and other rheumatic disorders. Journal of Clinical Pathology 35: 673–80
Raskin R J, Tesar J T, Lawless O J 1982 Polyarthritis in immunoblastic lymphadenopathy. Arthritis and Rheumatism 25: 1481–1485
Reiner R R, Chalner B A, Young R C, Reddick R, Johnson R E 1977 Lymphoma presenting in bone: Results of histopathology: stageing and therapy. Annals of Internal Medicine 87: 50–55
Rosenfield S I, Bacon J, Sleigbigel R T, Liddey J P 1976 Hereditary deficiency of the fifth component of complement in man. II. Biological properties of C5 deficiency in human serum. Journal of Clinical Investigation 57: 1635–1643
Rothschild B M, Sienkneckt C W, Kaplan S B, Spindler J S 1980 Sickle cell disease associated with uric acid deposition disease. Annals of the Rheumatic Diseases 39: 392–395
Rothwell R S, Mant M J, Davies P 1980 Angioimmunoblastic lymphadenopathy associated with polyarthritis. Annals of the Rheumatic Diseases 39: 406–409

Satter M A, Cawley M I D 1982 Arthritis associated with hairy cell leukaemia. Annals of the Rheumatic Diseases 41: 289–291

Schaller J 1972 Arthritis as a presenting manifestation of malignancy in children. Journal of Paediatrics 81: 793–797

Schaller J G, Gillibrand B C, Ochs H D, Liddey J P, Agodoa L C Y, Rosenfield S I 1977 Severe systemic lupus erythematosus with nephritis in a boy with deficiency of the fourth component of complement. Arthritis and Rheumatism 20: 1519–1525

Schifferli J A, Peters D K 1982 Complement-mediated inhibition of immune precipitation. II. Analysis by sucrose density gradient ultracentrifugation. Clinical and Experimental Immunology 47: 563–569

Schlumf U 1978 Thalassaemia minor and aseptic necrosis, a coincidence? Arthritis and Rheumatism 21:280

Schumacher H R, Andrews R, McLoughlin G 1973 Arthropathy in sickle cell disease. Annals of Internal Medicine 78: 203–211

Schumacher H R, Dorwart B B, Bond J, Alavi A, Miller W 1977 Chronic synovitis with early cartilage destruction in sickle cell disease. Annals of the Rheumatic Diseases 36: 413–419

Sella E J, Goodman A G 1973 Arthropathy secondary to transfusional haemochromatosus. Journal of Bone and Joint Surgery 55A: 1077–81

Sennara H, Gorry F 1978 Orthopaedic aspects of sickle cell anaemia allied to haemaglobinopathies. Clinics in Orthopaedics 130: 154–57

Short W H, Palmer A K 1981 Amyloidosis and the carpal tunnel syndrome. Orthopaedic Review 10: 89–94

Small M, Steven M M, Freeman P A 1983 Total bone arthroplasty in haemophilic arthritis. Journal of Bone and Joint Surgery 65B: 163–5

Soesbergen R M Van, Feltkamp-Vroom T M, Feltkamp C A, Somers R, Van Beck W P 1983 T cell leukaemia presenting as chronic polyarthritis. Arthritis and Rheumatism 25: 87–91

Spilberg I, Meyer G J 1972 The arthritis of leukaemia. Arthritis and Rheumatism 15: 630–635

Stanworth D R, Williamson J P, Shadforth M, Feli-Davies D, Thompson R 1977 Drug induced IgA deficiency in rheumatoid arthritis. Lancet 1: 1001–1002

Stein H, Duthie R B 1981 The pathogenesis of chronic haemophilic arthropathy. Journal of Bone and Joint Surgery 63B: 601–609

Swanton M C, Wysocki G P 1975 Pathology of the joint in canine haemophilia A. In: Brinkhous K M, Hemker H C (ed) Handbook of haemophilia, Part 1. American Elsevier, New York

Taborn J D, 1981 Rice bodies in hypogammaglobulinaemic arthritis. Journal of Rheumatology 8: 165–8

Tarantion A, Anelli A, Constantino A, De Vuchi A, Monti G, Massaro L 1978 Serum complement pattern in essential mixed cryoglobinaemia. Clinical Experimental Immunology 32: 77–85

Van Creveld S, Hoedemaker P J, Kingman M J et al 1971 Degeneration of joints in haemophiliacs under treatment by modern methods. Journal of Bone and Joint Surgery 53B: 296–302

Van Pad T, Bosch P J I, Van de Putti L B A, Boerbooms A M Th, Geerdink P J 1981 Radiosynoviorthesis in haemophilic joint disease. Rheumatology 40: 237–239

Webster A D B, Tripp J H, Hayward A R et al 1978 Echovirus encephalitis and myositis in primary immunoglobulin deficiency. Archives of Diseases in Children 53: 33–37

Weinberger A, Berliner S, Prinklas J 1981 Articular manifestation of essential cryoglobinaemia. Seminars in Arthritis and Rheumatism 13: 224–229

Wells J V, Michaeli D, Fudenberg H H 1973 Antibodies to human collagen in subjects with selective IgA deficiency. Clinical and Experimental Immunology 13: 203–208

Wild J H, Zvaifler N J 1976 Haemarthrosis associated with sodium warfarin therapy. Arthritis and Rheumatism 19: 98–102

Wilfert C M, Buckley R H, Mohanakumer T et al 1977 Persistent and fatal central nervous system echovirus infections in patients with agammaglobulinaemia. New England Journal of Medicine 296: 1485–1489

Willkens R F, Roth G F, Husby G, Williams R C 1980 Immunocytological studies of lymph nodes in rheumatoid arthritis and malignant lymphoma. Annals of the Rheumatic Diseases 39: 147–157

Wilson W A, Hughes G R V, Lachman P J 1976 Deficiency of factor B of the complement system in sickle cell anaemia. British Medical Journal 1: 367–369

Winfield J B, Koffler D, Kunkel H G 1975a Specific concentration of polynucleotide immune complexes in the cryoprecipitates of patients with systemic lupus erythematosus. Journal of Clinical Investigation 56: 563–570

Winfield J B, Winchester R J, Wernet P, Kunkel H G 1975b Specific concentration of anti-lymphocyte antibodies in the serum cryoprecipitates of patients with systemic lupus erythematosus. Clinical and Experimental Immunology 19: 399–408

Youinou P, Le Goff P, Renier J C, Hurey D, Mossec P, Morrow W J W 1983 Relationship between rheumatoid arthritis and nonoclonal gammapathy. Journal of Rheumatology 10: 210–215

Osteonecrosis

Bone in the living animal is a dynamic structure, comprised of an inorganic extracellular matrix and viable cells, including osteocytes, osteoclasts and osteoblasts. The term *osteonecrosis* applies primarily to the death of osteocytes, but radiological features do not become apparent until subsequent alteration in the extracellular matrix occurs, and this usually results from attempted biological repair. It is therefore important to appreciate that, while the diagnosis of osteonecrosis is often based upon typical radiological features, there may be a long latent period between the primary event (osteocyte death) and secondary structural changes in the extracellular matrix.

Varying terminologies have been used to describe this condition. The recognition in the late 19th century that bone necrosis could occur in the absence of underlying sepsis prompted the term *aseptic necrosis*. Later studies revealed the importance of disruption of blood supply following fractures (Phemister, 1940) and *avascular necrosis of bone* became accepted terminology. However, occlusion of blood vessels cannot be demonstrated in all cases, and the term *osteonecrosis* is now most commonly used.

Osteonecrosis is of importance to both rheumatologists and orthopaedic surgeons. Joint pain may occur before radiological changes are present, although the mechanism whereby this occurs is ill-understood. When structural collapse of articulating surfaces occurs, secondary osteoarthritis develops. Osteonecrosis is also a well-recognised and disabling complication of systemic lupus erythematosus and a potential complication of any therapeutic regime employing high dose corticosteroids. In children, these disorders may mimic juvenile chronic polyarthritis, particularly if several epiphyseal centres are involved. Although histological and radiological progression of osteonecrosis may follow similar patterns regardless of aetiology, it is apparent that a wide range of disorders, varying from genetically determined conditions to trauma, may cause bone necrosis and, therefore, in all cases an attempt should be made to identify the causative factor.

CLASSIFICATION

Osteonecrosis may be broadly divided into two subgroups. Firstly, the process may occur in developing bone. In this situation, cartilage development is also affected and the term *osteochondrosis* is applied. Secondly, necrosis may occur in adult bone. In the osteochondroses, although genetic and environmental factors may play some role in the aetiology, these are not as clearly definable as in the adult group, where an inciting factor can usually be identified.

Inevitably, exceptions to this classification occur, and osteonecrosis of bone occurring in children with systemic lupus erythematosus or complicating slipped femoral epiphysis is well recognised. Conversely, an obvious precipitating factor may not be apparent in cases of osteonecrosis of the lunate (Keinböck's disease) occurring in the adult.

OSTEOCHONDROSES

Although the precise pathological mechanisms underlying the development of osteochondroses are not fully understood, it seems probable that alteration in the blood supply to developing bone has an important role. Approximately 50 different anatomical sites have been identified and many of these bear eponymous titles of the authors of the initial descriptions, coinciding with the development of radiology in the early part of this century which allowed the differentiation of these disorders from chronic joint infections, in particular tuberculosis. Osteochondrosis is not, however, restricted to man, and has been described in both pigs and bull calves when fed on regimes which produce rapid weight gain. The occurence of osteochondritis dissecans in the knee and hock joints of young thoroughbred race horses is well recognised and often has disastrous effects upon subsequent racing ability (Olsson & Reiland, 1978). In man, these disorders can be divided into those where a single centre is involved and those where multiple centres are affected (Thiemann's disease, multiple epiphyseal dysplasias, etc.). In the former group, further subdivision based upon the anatomical location in relationship to developing long bone is shown in Figure 48.1. If the physis (epiphyseal cartilage) is involved then growth of the bone is affected. In epiphysoid bones, i.e. non-long bones, no diaphysis is present but growth disturbance may still occur, i.e. in Scheuermann's

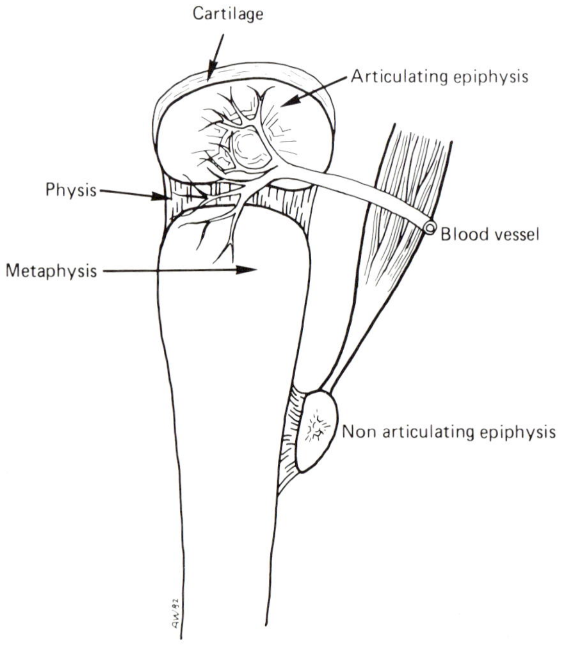

Fig. 48.1 Schematic representation of anatomical localisation of the osteochondroses (after Siffert, 1981).

Table 48.1 Classification of osteochondroses

Site	Eponym
Single epiphyseal nucleus	
Femoral head	Legg–Calve–Perthe
Navicular	Kohler
Metatarsal head	Freiberg
Capitellum	Panner
Vertebral body*	Calve
Non-articulating epiphysis	
Tibial tubercle	Osgood–Schlatter
Inferior pole patella	Sindig Larsen
Os calcis	Sever
Physis	
Tibia	Blount
Vertebral	Scheuermann
Multiple	
Proximal phalanx	Thiemann
Multiple epiphyseal dysplasia	
Spondyloepiphyseal dysplasia	

* Often due to underlying granuloma

disease. A nosological classification of the osteochondroses, based upon the patterns of localisation shown in Figure 48.1 is given in Table 48.1.

The precise mechanisms operating in the aetiology of osteochondritis dissecans are less clear, as this may represent the end result of a subchondral fracture, partial segmented loss of vascularity, or only partial revascularisation of an initially larger necrotic segment (Siffert, 1981).

Aetiological factors

Most of the osteochondroses tend to develop shortly after the appearance of the bony epiphyseal nucleus and any condition which delays ossification of this nucleus is associated with an increased risk of osteochondroses which may explain why, with the exception of Freiberg's disease, boys with their delayed skeletal maturity predominate.

In Perthes' disease, there appears to be a constitutional predisposition to the disorder, in that it develops bilaterally in up to 20% of children, and may be related to familial factors, as 10% of affected children have a family history of the disorder. Environmental factors also influence the disease, as there are regional variations in incidence, and an association with poorer socioeconomic groups.

Racial factors are of relevance in certain disorders, as Perthes' disease is predominantly seen in whites, whereas Blount's disease occurs more commonly in blacks.

Trauma and stress can also be implicated, as reflected by the observation that both Scheuermann's and Perthes' diseases occur more commonly in children with limb dysplasias following thalidomide, where excessive mechanical forces have been applied to the unaffected skeleton. The wide range of apparent factors predisposing to osteochondroses led Duthie & Houghton (1981) to propose a model for the development of osteochondroses in which the same clinical and radiological pattern may emerge from the spectrum of grossly abnormal stresses on normally developing bone and cartilage to normal stresses applied to congenitally abnormal bone and cartilage.

CLINICAL AND RADIOLOGICAL FEATURES OF SOME OF THE OSTEOCHONDROSES

Disorders of the articular epiphysis

Femoral head (Perthes' disease)

Originally described independently by Perthe, Legg and Calvé in 1910, this remains the most common and most disabling of the osteochondroses, with an incidence of approximately 0.01% in the white population. Boys are more commonly affected, but the disease, when present in girls, tends to be more severe.

The disorder usually presents as either hip pain, occasionally with radiation to the knee, or limp, in a child typically between the ages of 1 and 6 years. Clinical features which tend to indicate a poor prognosis are delay between onset of disease and diagnosis, children over the age of 6, obesity and adduction deformities. The most objective assessment of disease severity remains radiological (Fig. 48.2) and because of the tendency to affect only portions of the femoral head in the early stages, lateral views of the hip, as well as anterior posterior projections, are required. Catterall (1971) graded the radiological appearances on a I–IV scale, with I representing changes in only the anterior portion of the epiphysis and IV entire femoral head involvement, with flattening and marked metaphyseal reaction. The prognosis progressively worsens with radiological severity and other radiological changes which indicate a poor prognosis include premature fusion of the epiphysis and lateral subluxation (Catterall, 1981).

Conservative treatment with avoidance of weight-bearing and abduction splinting is usually favoured for the milder groups (I and II), whereas surgical treatment, with an abduction femoral osteotomy, appears to offer the greatest success in the more severe grades (III and IV), with a satisfactory outcome being obtained in 51% of such patients (Canario et al, 1980). However, a central problem to the evaluation of treatment programmes lies in the poor inter-observer correlation

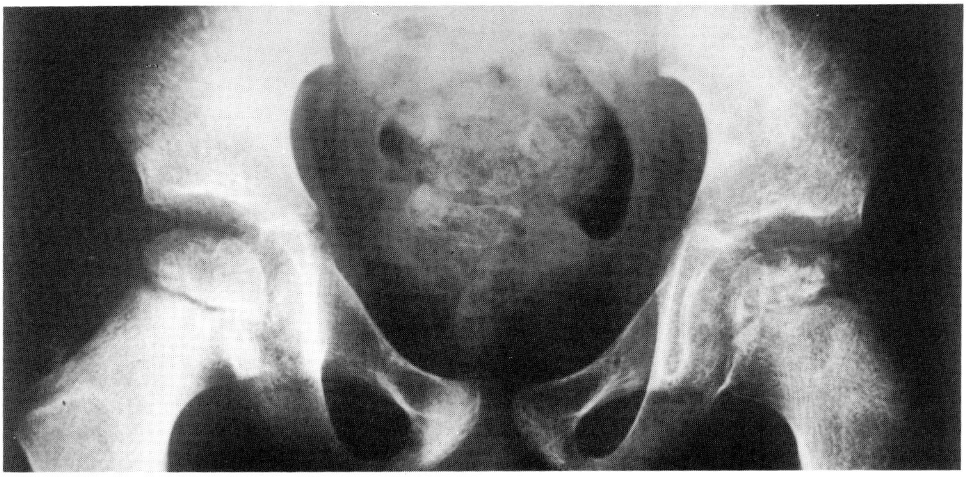

Fig. 48.2 Perthes' disease of the left femoral head. (Courtesy of Dr P. Hacking, Department of Radiology, Royal Victoria Infirmary, Newcastle upon Tyne.)

of the Catterall grading of hip radiographs (Hardcastle et al, 1980).

A radiological appearance identical to Perthes' disease may be seen following a variety of other conditions, including hip dislocation, cretinism, multiple epiphyseal dysplasias, Gaucher's disease, sickle cell disorders, and slipped femoral epiphysis. However, in these groups the capacity to regenerate a normal femoral head is reduced and the prognosis is worse.

Navicular (Köhler's disease)
Initially described in 1908, this condition is the next most common of the osteochondroses (Fig. 48.3). It usually presents in boys, between the ages of 2 and 9 years, with a mean of 5 years. Foot pain with 'point' tenderness are the most reliable clinical features. The prognosis is excellent, with the condition clinically and radiologically resolving usually within 18 months. The resolution may be more rapid if a short leg cast is used. Non-weight-bearing does not dramatically improve the prognosis (Williams & Cowell, 1981).

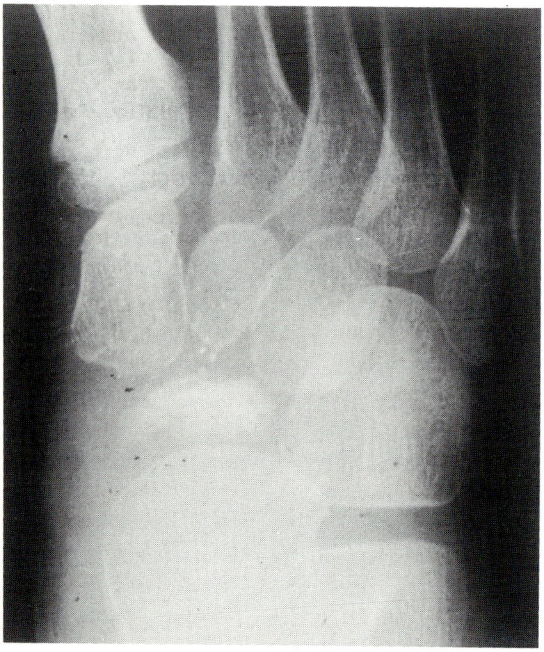

Fig. 48.3 Köhler's disease of tarsal navicular. (Courtesy of Dr P. Hacking, Department of Radiology, Royal Victoria Infirmary, Newcastle upon Tyne.)

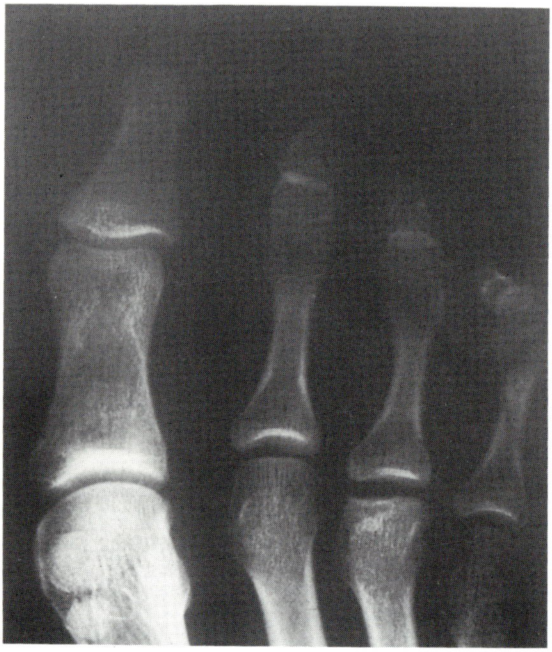

Fig. 48.4 Freiberg's disease affecting the 3rd metatarsal head.

Metatarsal head (Freiberg's disease)
First described in 1914, this condition usually affects the 2nd metatarsal head, but is occasionally seen in the 3rd and 4th metatarsals (Fig. 48.4). It usually presents as metatarsalgia in a girl between the ages of 12 and 15 years, and understandably is frequently referred with a diagnosis of juvenile rheumatoid arthritis. The aetiology of the condition is not known, but changes in female footwear fashions do not appear to be the main factor. Treatment with a metatarsal arch support may afford relief of symptoms but the radiological appearance often does not return to normal and some persistent metatarsalgia may remain. Symptoms may precede radiological changes (Omer, 1981).

Capitellum (Panner's disease)
Described originally in 1927, this appears to be an 'over-use' disorder affecting the dominant arm of boys between the ages of 8 and 14 years and presenting as elbow pain (Fig. 48.5). Frequently, the medial epicondyle is also involved, and this type of lesion is commonly seen in young baseball pitchers and appropriately called 'little leaguer's elbow'. The lesion resolves with rest.

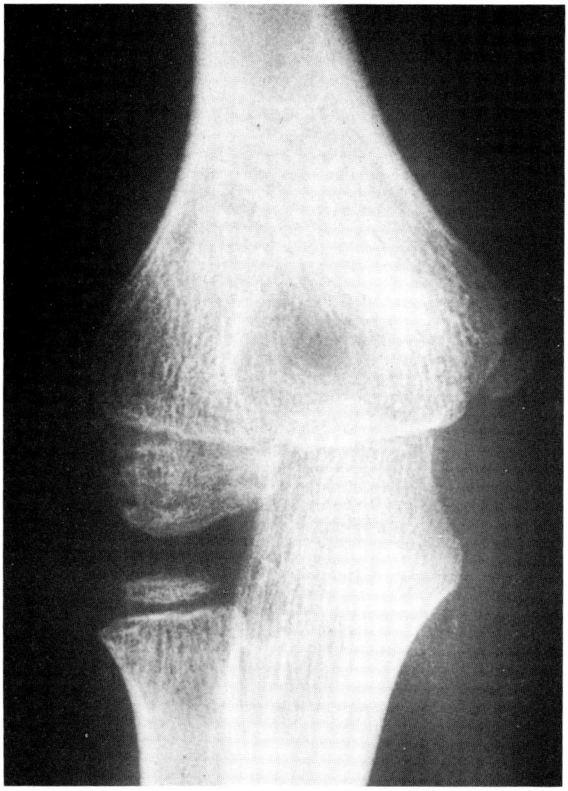

Fig. 48.5 Panner's disease of capitellum. (Courtesy of Dr P. Hacking, Department of Radiology, Royal Victoria Infirmary, Newcastle upon Type.)

Osteochondritis dissecans

Although differing in some ways from the previously described osteochondroses, it is included in this section as part of the articulating epiphysis is involved, although the pathogenic mechanisms may be fundamentally different.

Most commonly, the condition affects the knee, when typically the medial femoral condyle is involved (Fig. 48.6). Occasionally, it is seen in the ankle, when the talus is involved, and in the hip after Perthes' disease.

When the knee is affected, the patient is usually male, in his 2nd decade, and often gives a history of predisposing trauma. Recurrent patellar subluxation and associated hypermobility are present in 10% of cases (Mubarak & Carroll, 1981). Pain and swelling are the most characteristic features and true locking may be present if a cartilaginous or bony-cartilaginous fragment has become detached. The diagnosis can usually be made on radiological appearances, although intercondylar (tangential) views are frequently required to demonstrate the lesion. Arthroscopy may allow confirmation of the diagnosis and removal of a small loose body if present.

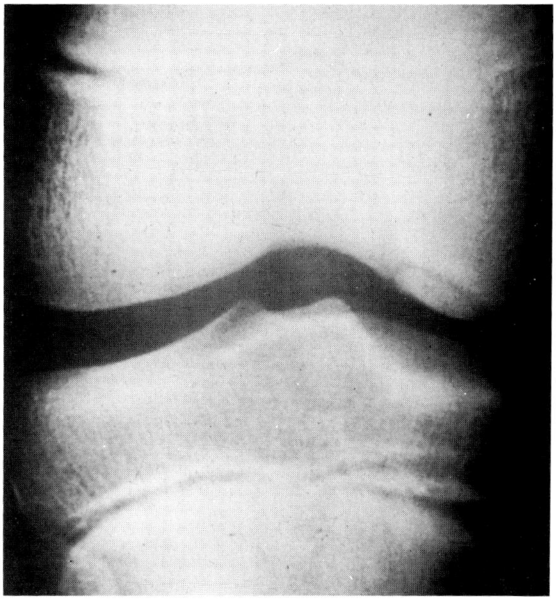

Fig. 48.6 Osteochondritis dissecans of the medial femoral condyle. (Courtesy of Dr P. Hacking, Department of Radiology, Royal Victoria Infirmary, Newcastle upon Tyne.)

The prognosis depends upon the age of the patient, being better in younger subjects. Loose bodies require removal; partially detached fragments may be reattached to the underlying bone which is usually 'drilled' in an attempt to induce new cancellous bone formation (Pappas, 1981).

Disorders of non-articular epiphyses

Tibial tuberosity (Osgood–Schlatter disease)

This disorder was described independently by Osgood and Schlatter in 1903. Males around the age of 15 years are most commonly affected, and athletes seem particularly prone to the condition. Typically, a history is obtained of pain, swelling and tenderness over the tibial tubercle, worse on activity. The diagnosis is supported by the radiological demonstration of fragmentation of the tibial tubercle with occasional new bone formation. The interpretation of the X-ray appearance may, however, be difficult because of the marked variation in patterns of ossification of the tibial tubercle. The condition usually remits over several months with cessation of athletic activities. Occasionally, painful ossicles may form in the patellar tendon which require excision (Katz, 1981) (see also Ch. 60).

Inferior pole of patella (Sindig-Larsen syndrome)
Described independently by Sindig in 1921 and Larsen in 1922, this also represents a traction epiphysitis of the patellar tendon, affecting its insertion into the inferior pole of the patella. Teenage boys are usually affected, with local patellar pain on activity. The condition needs to be differentiated from chondromalacia patellae. X-rays show fragmentation of the inferior patella epiphysis, but again considerable variation in the normal ossification of this centre may make radiological confirmation difficult. The condition resolves with restriction of activities.

Os calcis (Sever's disease)
This disorder, originally described in 1912, presents as pain on the inferior or posterior aspect of the heel in children between the ages of 10 and 15 years. Radiographs show fragmentation of the epiphysis, which even in normals may be much more sclerotic than adjacent bone. It is, therefore, advisable to obtain views of the contralateral heel for comparison, assuming the disease is unilateral (Edeiken, 1981). A heel cup or heel lift may alleviate symptoms. The condition spontaneously resolves.

Disorders of physeal epiphysis

Spinal osteochondroses (Scheuermann's disease)
First described in 1921, this condition must be distinguished from the so-called 'osteochondrosis of the primary vertebral center' (Calvé's disease). In Scheuermann's disease, several vertebrae are affected, usually in mid-thoracic to upper lumbar regions, with irregularity of the epiphyseal plate, anterior wedging, and disc herniation (Schmorl's nodes). Complete vertebral collapse is uncommon. Calvé's disease, in contrast, affects only one vertebral body, with collapse of that vertebra and with the occasional radiological presence of an associated intravertebral vacuum cleft. Although Calvé's disease was initially thought to represent ischaemic necrosis, it is now recognised that the underlying lesion is often an eosinophilic granuloma and vertebral biopsy is mandatory.

Scheuermann's disease usually presents between the ages of 13 and 17 years, and is uncommon under 10. Pain in the mid-thoracic region or deformity with kyphosis and scoliosis are the most common clinical features, but radiological surveys suggest that the disease may be much more prevalent than clinically suspected (Resnick, 1981). A histological review of 100 post-mortems on individuals between the ages of 8 and 20 years revealed classical changes in 5 and transitional changes in 17 (Aufdermaur, 1981). Herniation of the disc, to produce Schmorl's nodes, may occur in either the mid or anterior vertebral body and be associated with loss of disc height. Schmorl's nodes do not appear to develop in young people in the absence of spinal osteochondrosis (Edeiken, 1981). Stoddard & Osborn (1979) found radiological evidence of previous Scheuermann' disease more commonly in patients presenting later in life with back pain and spondylosis, than in a matched population without back pain, and postulate that Scheuermann's disease, as well as producing pain in adolescence, may also predispose to the development of spondylosis.

Osteochondrosis deformans tibiae (Blount's disease)
Originally described in 1937, this disorder appears to affect the medial tibial physis and is most commonly seen in blacks. It can occur on early walking, between 1 and 2 years, when it usually presents as relatively asymptomatic varus angulation of the tibia with associated internal tibial rotation. The treatment of choice at present is tibial osteotomy performed before the age of 8 (Larigerskiold, 1981).

A variant of this disorder is occasionally seen in adolescents, when acute, painful, varus angulation of the tibia occurs. This is frequently the result of underlying osteomyelitis.

The multiple epiphyseal dysplasias
These groups of disorders are uncommon and classification frequently confusing. However, as they may present either mimicking juvenile polyarthritis or ankylosing spondylitis if spinal in-

volvement is present, and appear to predispose the development of osteoarthrosis, they are of importance of rheumatologists.

Involvement of multiple epiphyses may occur in several apparent systemic diseases, including Gaucher's diseases, congenital hypothyroidism, and the mucopolysaccharidoses.

In other multiple epiphyseal dysplasias, an underlying systemic illness appears to be present and these often follow familial patterns of inheritance, but the precise biochemical defects have not been identified (Ansell et al, 1975; Beighton, 1978).

This section concentrates on those disorders where the primary pathology resides in the developing epiphysis and where no associated constitutional factors are present.

Thiemann's disease

This uncommon disease, which may arise sporadically or follow either recessive or autosomal dominant patterns of inheritance, affects the distal epiphysis of the proximal phalanx of the hand, but spares the thumb. Females between the ages of 10 and 13 are most commonly affected and because of the accompanying swelling and stiffness of the proximal interphalangeal joints the disease mimics juvenile chronic polyarthritis. However, serological and haematological abnormalities are not present and the radiological appearance is characteristic (Fig. 48.7) (Molloy & Hamilton, 1978; Melo-Gomes et al, 1981).

Multiple epiphyseal dysplasias

These are a heterogeneous group of disorders, occasionally showing either autosomal dominant or recessive modes of inheritance. By definition, several sites are usually involved and symptoms appear in early childhood. Hip disease may give rise to premature osteoarthritis and early fusion of the epiphysis in the fingers produces a short, stubby appearance of the hands. Severe dwarfing does not occur (Wynn-Davies, 1973).

Spondyloepiphyseal dysplasia

The distal and proximal joint involvement resembles multiple epiphyseal dysplasia, but involvement of the physeal epiphysis of the vertebral bodies is also present. Some restriction of growth results and severe, premature, degenerative, spinal disease occurs. This appearance, in a young patient, may clinically resemble ankylosing spondy-

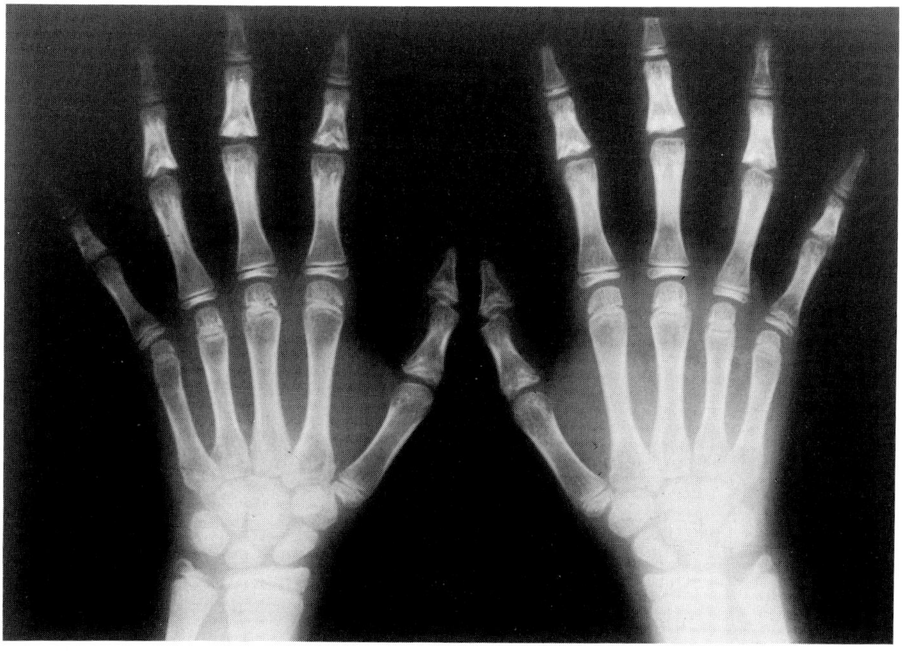

Fig. 48.7 Thiemann's disease, affecting proximal interphalangeal epiphyses.

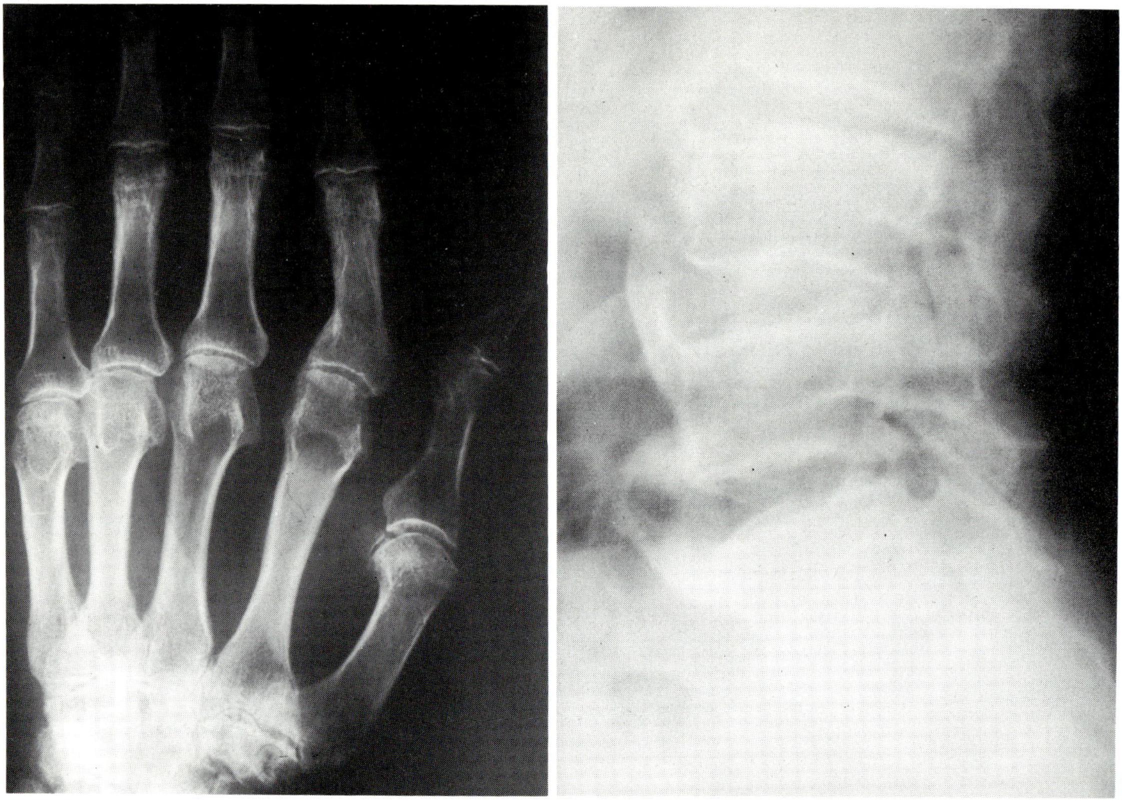

Fig. 48.8 Remodelling of epiphysis and premature degenerative arthritis in a 28-year-old male with previous spondyloepiphyseal dysplasia. (a) Hand radiograph. (b) Lumbar spine.

litis but the radiographic features are diagnostic and sacroiliac involvement is not seen (Fig. 48.8).

OSTEONECROSIS

This section concentrates upon the clinical and pathological features of osteonecrosis occurring in adult bone and the various aetiological factors. Many of the underlying disorders can, however, produce osteonecrosis in developing bone and in that situation the appearance, both histologically and radiologically, is identical to osteochondroses. The prognosis in children, although still guarded, tends to be better than in the adult. A schematic representation of the aetiological factors inducing bone necrosis in both adult and developing bone, is shown in Figure 48.9.

A list of the many recognised disorders causing osteonecrosis is given in Table 48.2.

Pathology

Osteonecrosis is the result of death of osteocytes (histologically recognisable as empty lacunae), osteoblasts and osteoclasts. A variety of pathological changes result from such an event, ranging from complete reconstitution of necrotic bone in children to prolonged mechanical and structural integrity of infarcted bone, as may occur after intracapsular fracture of the femoral neck, or to rapid collapse and destruction of affected bone, as is seen in steroid-associated osteonecrosis.

Following bone necrosis, a process of repair occurs; the rate at which this proceeds is probably affected by both the age of the patient and concomitant therapy (e.g. corticosteroids.). It must also be appreciated that varying stages of the reparative process are observed in different areas of bone at any moment in time and isolated bone biopsies may not reflect the changes present

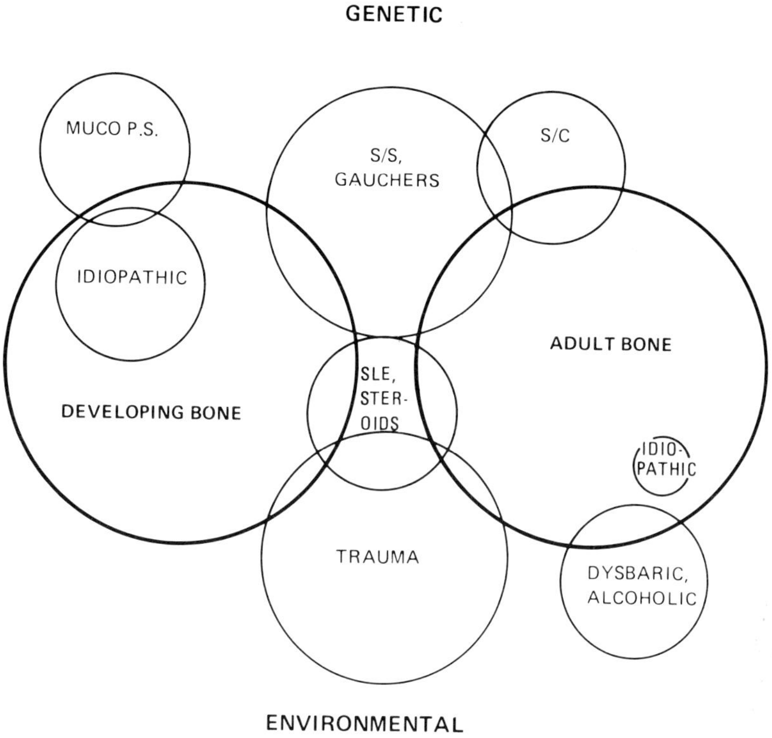

Fig. 48.9 Venn diagram illustrating factors capable of inducing necrosis in developing and adult bone.

Table 48.2 Classification of causes of osteonecrosis

1. **Idiopathic**
   Osteonecrosis of the lunate (Kienbock's disease)
   Medial tibial plateau
2. **Traumatic**
   Fractures
   Dislocation
   Slipped femoral epiphysis
3. **Genetically-determined**
   Haemoglobinopathies (S/S, S/C and S/thal)
   Gauchers disease
   Mucopolysaccharidoses
4. **Treatment-related**
   Corticosteroids
   Chemotherapy
   Organ transplantation
   Radiotherapy
5. **Miscellaneous**
   Systemic lupus erythematosus
   Dysbaric osteonecrosis
   Alcoholism, hyperlipidaemia and hyperuricaemia
   Pregnancy
   Hypothyroidism
   Pancreatitis

throughout the infarcted area. Typically, the earliest changes after bone necrosis are those of revascularisation extending from viable marrow adjacent to necrotic trabeculae, producing the radiological appearance of increased radiolucency around necrotic bone. From the vascular tissue mesenchymal cells differentiate into osteoblasts, which migrate and lay down unwoven bone on the framework of dead trabeculae. The net effect is of increased bone density and, radiologically, the infarcted area appears sclerotic. Simultaneous osteoclastic absorption of the necrotic bone also occurs. If osteoclastic activity exceeds osteoblastic, as often appears to be the case in subchondral bone, then weakened subchondral lines appear (radiologically equivalent to the crescentic line) (Fig. 48.10). This may result in collapse of the articular surface (Fig. 48.11). The cartilage and chondrocytes remain viable throughout this process, receiving nutrition from the synovial fluid, but when collapse of the articular surface has oc-

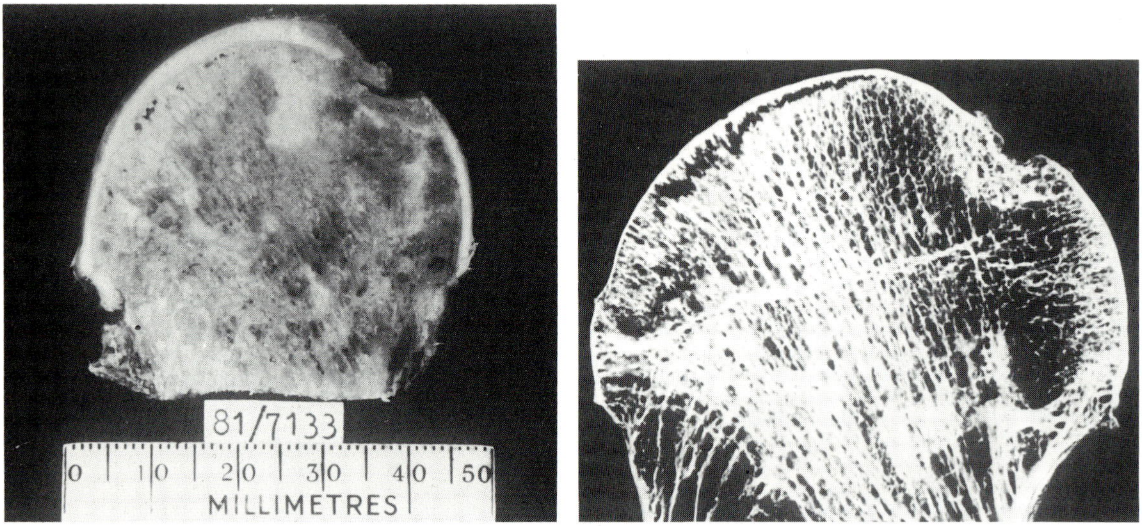

Fig. 48.10 Macroscopic appearance (a) and slab radiograph (b) of an osteonecrotic femoral head showing subchondral fracture but intact articulating surface. (Courtesy of Dr A. Malcolm, Department of Pathology, Royal Victoria Infirmary, Newcastle upon Tyne.)

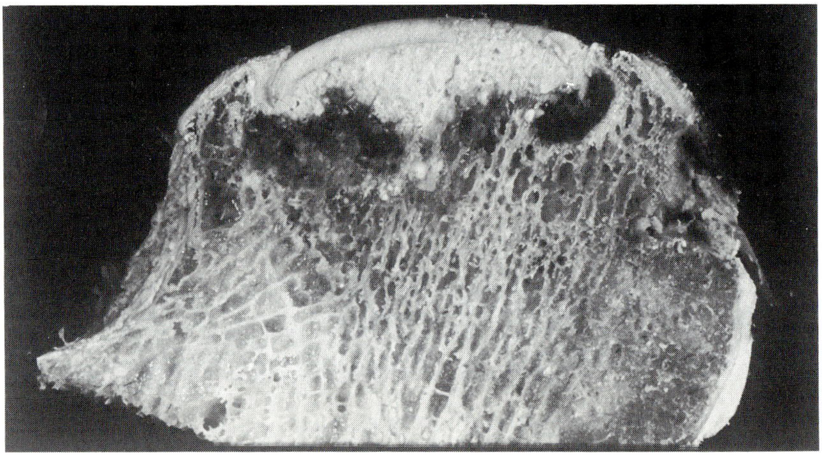

Fig. 48.11 Macroscopic appearance of an osteonecrotic femoral head showing collapse of articulating surface overlying a subchondral fracture. (Courtesy of Dr A. Malcolm, Department of Pathology, Royal Victoria Infirmary, Newcastle upon Tyne.)

curred, secondary osteoarthrosis, with cartilage loss, results. Detailed reviews of the histological features and factors influencing them are given by Catto (1976) and Glimcher & Kenzora (1979).

Experimental models

Kenzora et al (1978) were able to demonstrate a sequence of pathological and radiological events in the femoral heads of rabbits which had undergone osteotomy of the femoral head and division of the ligamentum teres. This pattern reflected the changes seen in man, and demonstrated the dynamic process of attempted repair by osteoblasts and simultaneous reabsorption of necrotic bone by osteoclasts. The mechanism whereby corticosteroids induce osteonecrosis is less clear. Rabbits treated with corticosteroids develop hypercholesterolaemia and an increase in marrow fat cell diameter. These changes may, in part, be reversed by clofibrate (Wang et al, 1978). Earlier studies had demonstrated localisation of intra-arterially injected fat emboli in subchondral vessels, in rabbits, but these had usually disappeared within 10 weeks of injection.

Miniature swine have been used to study dysbaric osteonecrosis because of their susceptibility to developing bone necrosis after exposure to compressed air. Thomas et al (1982) showed that presently used decompression tables do not allow adequate equilibration of marrow fat nitrogen in these animals and may explain why dysbaric osteonecrosis has not lessened in frequency in the past six years.

Idiopathic osteonecrosis

Idiopathic osteonecrosis of adult bone occurring in the absence of either underlying bone disease or extraneous factors is uncommon. Two conditions that approach this description are described.

Osteonecrosis of lunate (Kienböck's disease)

This usually presents in the young adult with wrist pain and occasionally gives rise to a carpal tunnel syndrome. It occurs more commonly in people with heavy manual occupations, but has been described in association with systemic diseases (Fig. 48.12). Undisplaced fractures which compromise the vasculature of the lunate, akin to scaphoid fractures, have been demonstrated in many of the so-called 'idiopathic' group (Beckenbaugh et al, 1980).

The natural history of the condition is extremely variable and, although revascularisation of the lunate is uncommon, many achieve good functional and symptomatic results with conservative treatment, including splinting, and do not require surgical intervention.

Osteonecrosis of the medial tibial plateau

This is a disorder of the elderly, and presents as acute onset knee pain, often with an associated non-inflammatory synovial effusion. Classical radiological findings may not be present initially but isotopic bone scanning often demonstrates an area of increased uptake in the medial tibial plateau. In the absence of pre-existing osteoarthrosis, the prognosis is good, with symptoms resolving over one year (Houpt et al, 1982).

Trauma

Osteonecrosis after trauma has been recognised for many years. In this situation, interruption of the vascular supply can usually be clearly identified, and the term 'avascular necrosis' is appropriate.

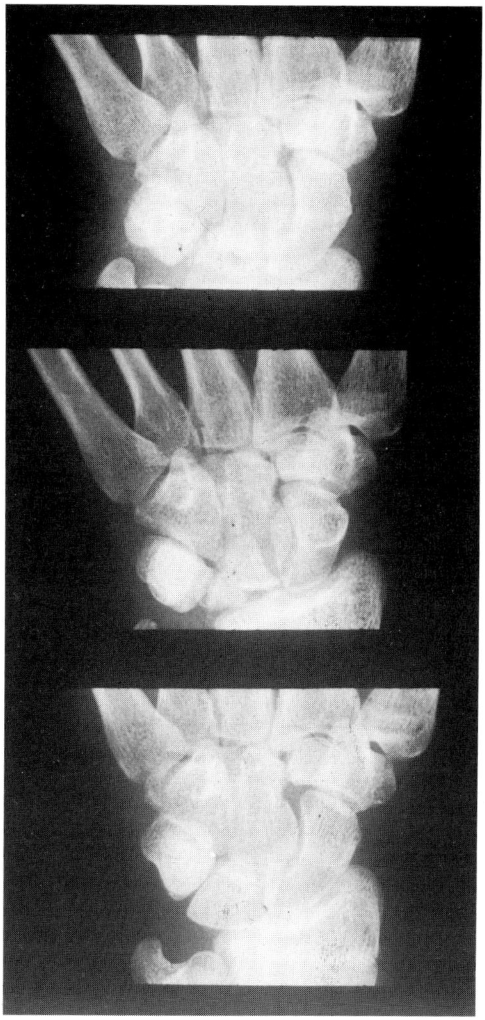

Fig. 48.12 Kienbock's disease of lunate developing in a young girl with SLE (progression is shown from bottom to top). Courtesy of the Editor, *Annals of Rheumatic Diseases*.

Fractures

Radiological evidence of osteonecrosis develops in up to 50% of patients following fracture of the neck of the femur, with distribution of the retinacular vessels. The vascularity obtained through the ligamentum teres is usually inadequate to maintain viability of the femoral head (Fig. 48.13). Radiological changes, however, do not usually become apparent within the first 6 months. The incidence is increased if displacement or delayed union occurs (Jacobs, 1978). Osteonecrosis of the proximal part of the scaphoid following fracture is well recognised, and less frequently seen in the

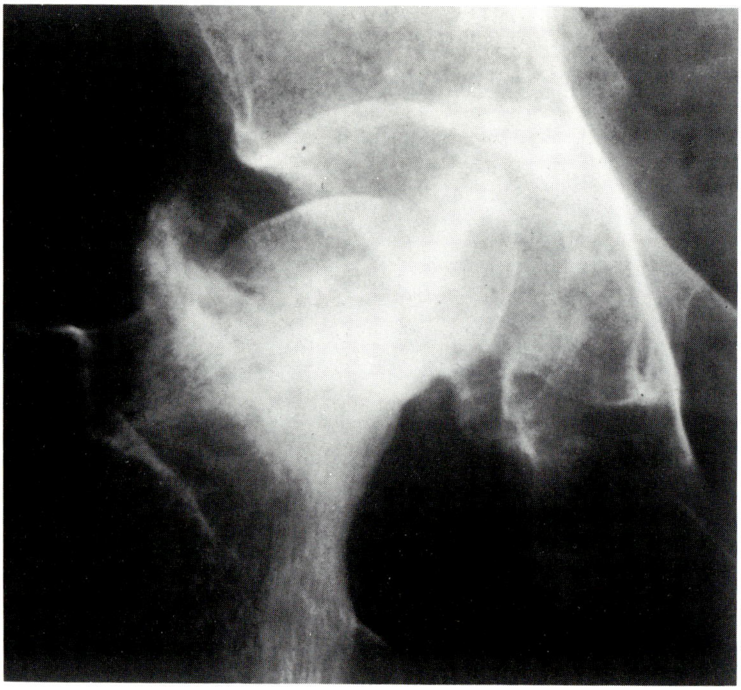

Fig. 48.13 Osteonecrosis of the femoral head following previous fractured neck of femur.

humeral head after fracture of the surgical neck of the humerus.

Dislocation
Femoral head necrosis after hip dislocation is well recognised, the incidence being greater with posterior dislocations (14%), compared to anterior dislocation (3.2%); and this reflects the severity of the damage to retinacular blood supply (Jacobs, 1978).

Slipped femoral epiphysis
Although not strictly traumatic, disruption of femoral head vascularity is probably the major factor inducing osteonecrosis in this condition. The incidence is approximately 16% following slipped femoral epiphysis, and the outcome is poor, with permanent destruction and remodelling of the head (Hall, 1957).

Genetically determined osteonecrosis

Haemoglobinopathies
Sickle cell disease and its variants predominate in the causation of bone infarction. The site, age, and presentation vary depending on the haemoglobinopathy but radiological evidence of bone infarction is present in 30% of subjects with either S/S, S/C or S/thal disease. Bone infarction does not appear to be more common in patients with the sickle trait (S/A).

In sickle cell disease (S/S), medullary infarction occurs more commonly than juxta-articular osteonecrosis, and presents frequently in children between the age of 6 months and 2 years. At this stage, haemopoietic marrow is still present in the distal tubular bones, and infarction in these sites gives rise to symmetrical pain and swelling of the hands and feet, sometimes with associated features of fever and leucocytosis. Radiological changes showing marked periosteal reaction around the shaft ('bone within bone' appearance) may develop. When bone crises arise in the older patient, usually at more proximal sites or in the spine, the differential diagnosis from osteomyelitis becomes more difficult, and as well as standard microbiological techniques, bone scanning with Tc polyphosphonates may prove helpful, as this has been shown to demonstrate isotopically 'cold' areas in the early stages of infarction, compared to increased uptake in osteomyelitis (Chung et al, 1978).

Sickle cell S/C haemoglobinopathies are a milder form of disease, without the severe anaemia of S/S disease. These patients usually survive into adult life but are more prone to developing osteonecrosis of the femoral and humeral heads (Golding et al, 1959) (Fig. 48.14). Frequently, in these patients there is a delay between the onset of symptoms and the characteristic radiological changes of osteonecrosis (Chung & Ralston, 1969). Although total joint replacement has been successfully undertaken in many of these patients, they do present anaesthetic challenges regarding the avoidance of hypoxia and the minimisation of tourniquet times if surgery is being performed on distal joints (Schumacher, 1975).

Bone infarction is rarely seen in thalassaemia, in either the heterozygote (minor) or homozygote (major) states unless the thalassaemia gene is present in association with the sickle cell gene (S/thal), where osteonecrosis of bone, usually the femoral head, tends to occur, often in adult life (Golding et al, 1959).

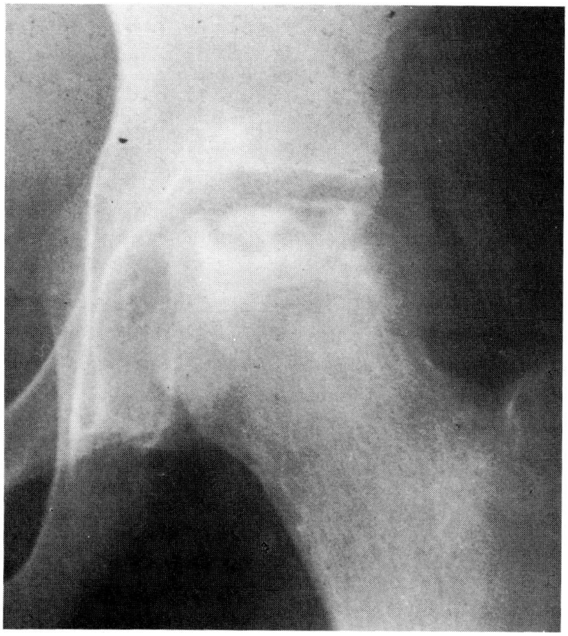

Fig. 48.14 Osteonecrosis of the femoral head with collapse of articulating surface in a patient with S/S sickle cell disease. (Courtesty of Dr R. Lee, Department of Radiology, Royal Victoria Infirmary, Newcastle upon Tyne.)

Gaucher's disease

Osteonecrosis of the femoral head was detected in 75% of patients with Gaucher's disease who had musculoskeletal symptoms (Amstutz & Carey, 1966). The age of onset was variable, but when it occurred in children the appearance resembled Perthes' disease and recovery was occasionally observed. Osteonecrosis of other sites, usually the humeral head, may also be present.

Mucopolysaccharidoses

The mucopolysaccharidoses (MPS) are a biochemically defined group of conditions characterised by enzymatic deficiences of glycosaminoglycan degradation. In many of these, the associated intellectual impairment dominates the clinical picture but in Morquio's syndrome (MPS type IV) and the Marateaux–Lamy syndrome (MPS type VI) intellectual function is normal and the musculoskeletal problems associated with epiphyseal dysplasia may be the presenting feature. Clouding of the cornea may occur in both conditions but definitive diagnosis depends upon the demonstration of selective enzymatic defects and excess of keratan sulphate (MPS IV) and dermatan sulphate (MPS VI) in the urine (Khan & De Seze, 1975; Beighton, 1978).

Treatment related

Corticosteroids

In many conditions in which corticosteroids are thought to play an important aetiological role in the development of osteonecrosis, other pathological states already exist, such as systemic lupus erythematosus and metabolic bone disease in renal transplantation patients. In these conditions, it is often difficult to apportion responsibility for the production of osteonecrosis.

However, there is considerable evidence that corticosteroids per se may induce aseptic bone necrosis in animals (Fisher et al, 1972). In man, osteonecrosis of the femoral head has been described as a clinical feature of Cushing's syndrome and Cushing's disease (Madell & Freeman, 1964; Sharon et al, 1977). Similarly, osteonecrosis following steroid therapy has occurred in a variety of conditions, such as pemphigus, erythema multiforme, multiple sclerosis, and thrombocytopenic purpura, where no underlying bone pathology is suspected (Heinmann & Freiberger, 1960).

Cases of osteonecrosis involving both femoral and both humeral heads have been reported following short courses of high dose dexamethasone therapy for neurosurgical conditions. In these situations there were intervals, varying from 7–22 months, between the administration of dexamethasone and the development of symptomatic osteonecrosis (McCluskey & Gutteridge, 1982). These observations are supported by the observed incidence of osteonecrosis following combination chemotherapy for lymphoma. Following these regimes, 1.3% of patients developed osteonecrosis but the interval between onset of symptoms and cessation of chemotherapy was often over 1 year (Lancet editorial, 1982). Prednisolone in total dosage ranging from 2.1–26 g was present in the chemotherapeutic regimes. Two patients developed osteonecrosis after cytotoxic drugs alone.

Gregg and co-workers (Gregg et al, 1980), questioned the importance of corticosteroids alone in inducing aseptic bone necrosis in children. They were unable to detect any radiological evidence of bone necrosis in children under the age of 11 with the nephrotic syndrome who had received prednisolone in total dosage ranging from 2–64 g.

Organ transplantation

Osteonecrosis remains a major complication of renal transplantation, with an incidence of 13 and 21% in two large recent series (Ibels et al, 1978; Elsmtedt, 1981). Although femoral head involvement is the most common and troublesome site, multiple bone involvement is frequently present. The interval between transplantation and development of osteonecrotic symptoms is usually 1 year or less. These series failed to detect an association between total steroid dosage or the number of rejection crises and the development of osteonecrosis, but an earlier study (Murray, 1973) noted a fall in incidence from 34% to 10%, when the mean total prednisolone dosage in the first 3 post-operative weeks was reduced from 2.9 g to 1.2 g. A relationship with the number of rejection crises, and hence total steroid dosage, was found by Hartington et al (1971). Osteonecrosis in renal transplant children under the age of 10 years appears to be less common (Stern & Watts, 1979), and when present affects the distal femoral condyle more frequently than the femoral head.

The suggestion that pre-existing renal osteodystrophy may also predispose to osteonecrosis is supported by findings of an increased incidence in renal transplant patients with hyperparathyroidism (Ibels et al, 1978), and hypophosphataemia (Elsmtedt, 1981). Although abnormalities in serum lipids are present in post-transplant patients, these are the same in the groups with and without osteonecrosis. However, the central importance of corticosteroids is evidenced by the description of bilateral femoral head osteonecrosis occurring in two patients who had received cardiac transplants. In these cases, the interval between transplantation and development of osteonecrosis was longer than in the renal group, being 2 years and 4 years. Both patients underwent successful bilateral total hip replacements (Burton et al, 1978).

Radiotherapy

Bone necrosis following radiotherapy is rarely seen nowadays with more carefully controlled dosage regimes (Looney, 1956). The most likely sites of involvement are the mandible after radiotherapy for head and neck cancer. Morrish et al (1981) observed an incidence of 21%, and found the complication to be dose-related, all patients with osteonecrosis having received more than 75 Gy. It also occurred more commonly in dentulous patients who subsequently required tooth extraction.

Miscellaneous

Systemic lupus erythematosus

As life expectancy improves in systemic lupus erythematosus (SLE), so non-fatal complications of the disease or its treatment become more apparent. Osteonecrosis occurring in SLE was initially described by Dubois & Cozens (1960). The relative importance of the underlying disease, compared to its therapy, is difficult to establish, but cases of osteonecrosis occurring in patients with both SLE and discoid LE who have not received corticosteroids are reported (Dubois & Cozens, 1960; Leventhal & Dorfmann, 1974).

The incidence appears to be approximately 10%,

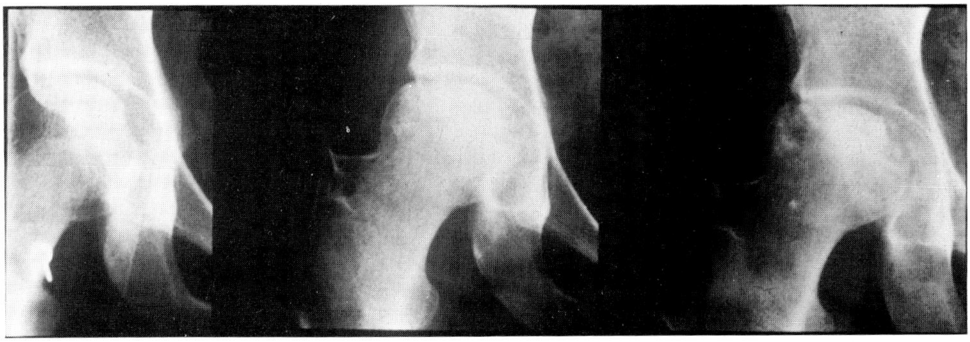

Fig. 48.15 Progressive changes of femoral head osteonecrosis in patient with SLE.

though considerable variation occurs depending upon duration of follow-up and severity of SLE, and hence, treatment regimes. A 40% incidence of radiological osteonecrosis was observed in children with steroid-treated SLE, although only one-third of the radiologically involved sites were symptomatic (Bergstein et al, 1974). Although a variety of clinical factors have been implicated in the various series, including Raynaud's phenomenon and polymyositis (Zizic et al, 1980) and leucopenia (Smith et al, 1976), these are not consistent findings. Several studies have suggested that symptomatic osteonecrosis tends to occur relatively early in the disease, usually within 3 years of onset (Klippel et al, 1979; Abeles et al, 1978; Griffiths et al, 1979).

Femoral head involvement occurs most commonly (Fig. 48.15), and symptoms may precede classical radiological changes by up to 6 months. Multiple joint disease may be present in 80% of affected individuals (Figs 48.16, 48.17) and in one case a total of 6 joints were involved. The aetiology has not been clearly defined, but evidence of active or previous vasculitis in nutrient vessels has not been detected histologically (Leventhal & Dorfmann, 1974). Although corticosteroids are not a prerequisite, osteonecrosis is observed more commonly in patients receiving steroid therapy, par-

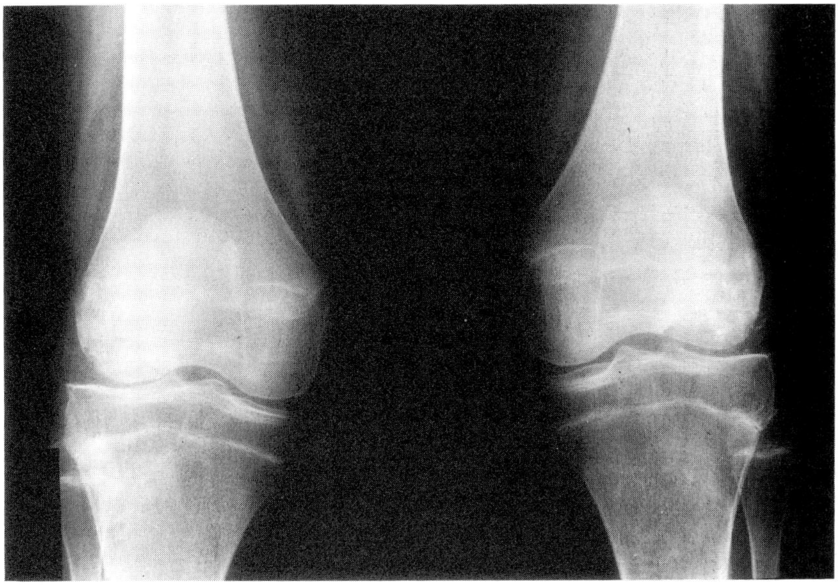

Fig. 48.16 Bilateral lateral femoral condyle osteonecrosis in a 19-year-old female with SLE.

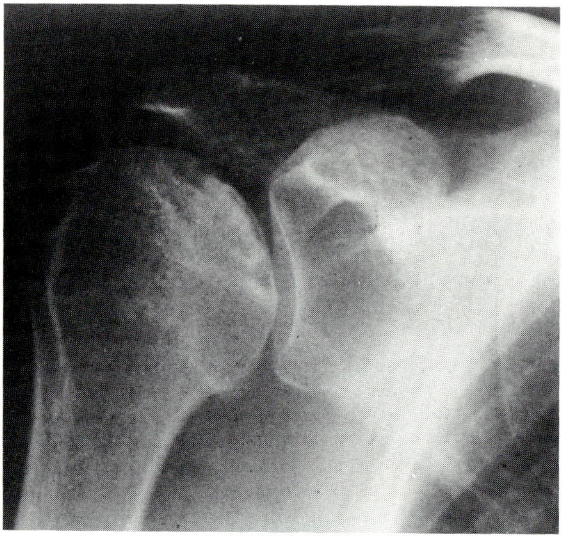

Fig. 48.17 Osteonecrosis of the humeral head with crescentic line in a young female with SLE.

ticularly when high dose steroid treatment has been given in the early stages of the disease (Abeles et al, 1978; Griffiths et al, 1979). The use of cytotoxic drugs in either oral or intravenous form does not appear to either enhance the incidence or lessen it by virtue of their steroid-sparing effects (Dinant et al, 1982).

As radiological changes develop late in the evolution of the disorder and represent irreversible destruction, early diagnosis is of considerable importance. Using a variety of diagnostic procedures, including isotopic scanning, intraosseous manometry, and intraosseous venography, Zizic et al (1980) were able to detect histological bone necrosis in SLE patients before radiological changes had become apparent.

Dysbaric osteonecrosis

Although compressed air had been used in tunnelling to prevent water seepage since 1841, it was not until 1911 that reports of aseptic bone necrosis appeared, and it was in 1936 that similar pathology was described in divers using compressed air. Bone necrosis is a potentially late hazard to any subject breathing air at greater than 2 atmospheres absolute. It initially presented much greater problems in tunnelling workers than divers, for although the pressures under which tunnellers operated was less than in diving, the exposure periods were much longer (Davidson, 1976).

Nitrogen solubility in fatty tissue is 5 times that of non-fatty tissue, and it has been suggested that nitrogen gas exchange occurs more slowly in marrow fat than other tissues (Chryssanthou, 1978). It is, therefore, postulated that osteonecrosis may be induced by nitrogen release within bone marrow on decompression. The nitrogen bubbles so formed may occur within vessels, causing occlusion, or raise intraosseous pressure, so that extravascular occlusion occurs. In the acute situation, post-mortem examination of divers dying of decompression sickness has shown generalised nitrogen bubble formation, and platelet microthrombi in intraosseous blood vessels (Kawashima et al, 1978).

The incidence of both acute decompression sickness and osteonecrosis has fallen since the introduction of strict decompression schedules, but osteonecrosis was still detectable in half the Japanese diving fishermen of one village, where decompression programmes were not adhered to (Ohta & Matsunage, 1974). This compares with an incidence of 4% in Royal Navy divers.

In a detailed review of nearly 5000 divers, the Decompression Sickness Central Registry (1981) found that the incidence of osteonecrosis was related to the number of episodes of acute decompression sickness, depth dived — being 22% in divers who had descended below 300 m (30 atmospheres absolute), duration of diving experience, and both weight and skinfold thickness of divers.

Radiologically, the most commonly observed lesions are infarctions of the shaft, particularly in the distal femur. These may present as either lytic or sclerotic lesions, are asymptomatic and rarely progress to involve articulating surfaces. Although less common, the juxta-articular lesions are clinically more damaging, as they may progress to involve the articular surface, with collapse of subchondral bone (Fig. 48.18). In contrast to other forms of induced osteonecrosis, the humeral head is the site most commonly involved (McCullum & Walder, 1966; Decompression Sickness Central Registry, 1981).

Rarely, decompression illnesses and osteonecrosis may effect aviators in unpressurised craft above 18 000 feet, and they represent a potential

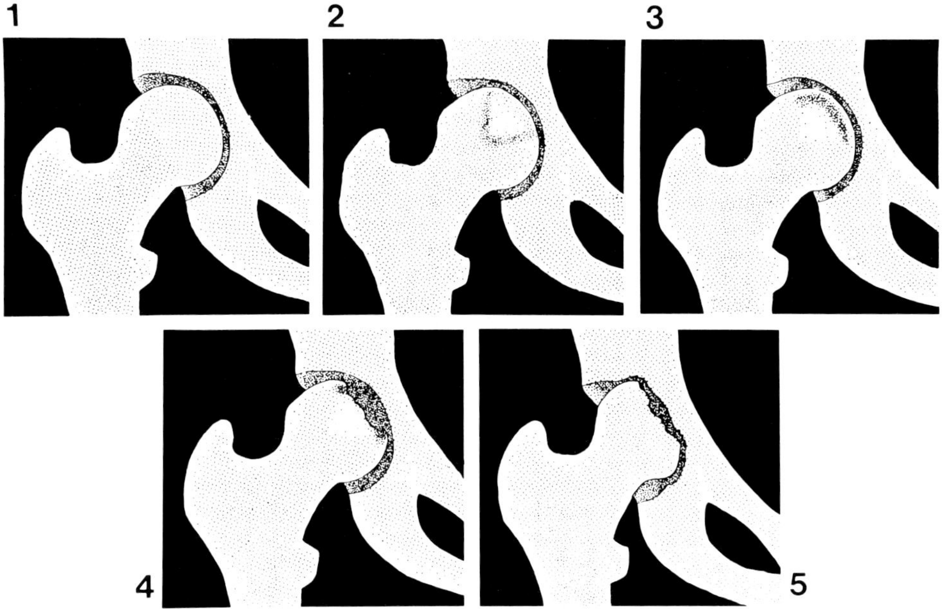

Fig. 48.18 Schematic representation of the radiological progression of osteonecrosis. 1. Normal. 2. Wedge-shaped sclerotic necrotic segment with adjacent radiolucent area of revascularisation. 3. Development of subchondral fracture (crescentic line). 4. Collapse of articulating surface. 5. Secondary osteoarthrosis.

hazard following the use of hyperbaric oxygen for medical purposes (Davidson, 1976).

Alcoholism, hyperlipidaemia and hyperuricaemia
Patterson et al (1964) reported that heavy alcohol consumption was the cause of osteonecrosis in 17% of their unselected series; the usual site of involvement being the femoral head. Radiological involvement of the clinically uninvolved hip was often present but, although the radiological changes were never seen to regress, many of these hips remained asymptomatic for periods of up to 5 years (Lee et al, 1980). Abnormalities of liver biochemistry or histology are usually present in these patients (Jones & Engleman, 1967). The mechanism of osteonecrosis in these patients is not clear, and may be related to the associated abnormalities of serum lipids. Hungerford & Zizic (1978) detected increased intraosseous pressure with an abnormal stress test in many patients before radiological changes were apparent, but this finding is not confined to alcohol-induced osteonecrosis.

The described association of hyperuricaemia and osteonecrosis probably reflects the abnormalities of purine metabolism seen in alcoholics; Stockman et al (1980) were unable to detect any cases of bone necrosis in a radiological survey of 138 gouty patients. Osteonecrosis occurring in association with familial hypercholesterolaemia or hypertriglyceridaemia is extremely uncommon, and suggests that factors other than pure hyperlipidaemia must be operating before bone necrosis occurs (Palmer et al, 1981).

Pregnancy
The development of femoral head necrosis during pregnancy is extremely uncommon. In several of the recorded cases other possible contributing factors, such as corticosteroid therapy, have been present (Kay et al, 1972). In the cases where no precipitating factor has been found the symptoms have usually developed after the 30th week of pregnancy and, although unequivocal radiological changes have developed, these resolved with conservative management after delivery (Zolla-Pazner et al, 1980).

Hypothyroidism
A condition clinically and radiologically resembling Perthes' disease may develop in children

with congenital hypothyroidism. Five cases of osteonecrosis affecting either the femoral head or the lunate have been described in adult hypothyroidism (Rubinstein & Brooks, 1977).

Pancreatitis

Rarely, osteonecrosis appears to complicate chronic relapsing pancreatitis, but as alcohol abuse may frequently be found in such patients it is difficult to establish the aetiological factor.

DIAGNOSTIC PROCEDURES

Strictly, the diagnosis of osteonecrosis rests upon pathological findings. However, as the process does not inevitably lead to surgical intervention, it is commonly accepted that a diagnosis of osteonecrosis can be made on clinical and radiological grounds. Unfortunately, by the time radiologically overt changes are apparent in adult bone, the pathological processes have often reached an irreversible state, and eventual collapse of the articulating surface occurs. There is, therefore, the need for more sensitive diagnostic procedures which can detect osteonecrosis in 'at risk' individuals before irreversible pathological changes are pesent. This section discusses both the radiological features and some of the other diagnostic methods currently employed. These techniques are reviewed in greater detail by Nixon (1984).

Radiological

Conventional plain radiography

Although there are congent reasons for not extrapolating radiological features into pathological states (Glimcher & Kenzora, 1979), there does appear in many patients to be a radiological progression of changes closely akin to those seen in experimentally induced osteonecrosis when juxta-articular lesions are present. These are illustrated in Figure 48.18. Variations in radiological positioning may make certain of the changes more apparent, for example, tangential or intercondylar views for osteochondritis dissecans, and the 'frog leg' view for the crescentic line in femoral head osteonecrosis (Sweet & Madewell, 1981). Tomography may also demonstrate changes not obvious in standard radiographs.

Intraosseous venography

This has been most clearly defined for the femoral head. Injected contrast in normal bone shows complete clearance within 5 minutes through 3 extraosseous veins with no diaphyseal reflux into the shaft. Disturbance of this pattern may be seen early in osteonecrosis before classical, standard, radiological changes are apparent (Zizic et al, 1980).

Radioisotopic imaging

The bone-seeking isotope, [^{99m}Tc]methylene diphosphonate, has routinely been employed. In post-renal transplantation patients, decrease in activity has been observed in femoral heads prior to the radiological onset of osteonecrosis. Once X-ray changes are present, with attempted repair and new bone formation, increased radioactivity is seen (D'Ambrosia et al, 1978).

Decreased activity has not, however, been found in patients with suspected osteonecrosis of the medial femoral condyle. In this group, increased activity was always noted but preceded radiological changes (Greyson et al, 1982). A similar pattern has been observed in experimentally induced osteonecrosis in rabbits, where increased uptake of [^{99m}Tc]diphosphonate was detectable 3 weeks after induction and preceded radiological changes by 4 months (Gregg, 1977).

Intraosseous manometry

Increased intraosseous pressure above the normal of 30 mmHg was noted in both early and late osteonecrosis of the femoral head (Arlet et al, 1968). It is, however, not a reliable prediction of early disease and the technique has been extended to measure intraosseous compliance by the injection of normal saline. Exaggerated increases in pressure, with delay in returning to baseline, were found by Hungerford & Zizic (1978) in patients prior to the development of radiological changes.

TREATMENT

The overriding principles of therapy depend upon knowledge of the natural history of the untreated disease.

Children often have the capacity to reconstitute anatomically normal bone after episodes of osteonecrosis or osteochondroses and therefore the emphasis is on conservative management. The main exceptions to this rule are Perthes' disease, where surgical intervention offers the best chance of avoiding residual deformity of the femoral head if radiologically severe changes are detected and Blount's disease, where tibial osteotomy is required to prevent residual tibia vara.

Adult bone, unfortunately, lacks the reparative potential of growing bone, and conservative treatment is normally ineffective in preventing the progression of destructive changes, particularly in weight-bearing joints, when radiological evidence of osteonecrosis is present. The exception to this rule is spontaneous osteonecrosis of the tibial plateau in the elderly which usually resolves spontaneously.

The rate at which destruction and collapse of the affected bone occurs is, however, extremely variable, even in the femoral head. This variability is even more apparent in the humeral head, where only 14% of the juxta-articular lesions observed in divers were shown to affect the articulating surface.

Symptomatically, lesions of the femoral head give rise to the greatest degree of disability, and studies of surgical management have therefore concentrated on this problem.

If radiological subchondral fractures are present, total hip replacement is usually deemed the treatment of choice when symptoms demand. Similarly, techniques other than total hip replacement have been unsatisfactory in steroid-induced osteonecrosis when radiological features are present (Springfield & Enneking, 1978).

A variety of alternative surgical procedures have been employed in patients with post-traumatic femoral head osteonecrosis before the development of subchondral fractures; these include cortical bone grafting using the fibula to provide a strut akin to the trochanteric pin, muscle pedicle grafts, and rotational osteotomies. All are claimed by various groups to be effective and do not preclude total hip replacement if later required (Nixon, 1984).

Hungerford & Zizic (1978, 1980) have concentrated upon early treatment of osteonecrosis, basing their diagnosis on increased intraosseous pressure and histological appearance on biopsy. They employ a technique of surgical core decompression, which is claimed to arrest, reverse, or delay the progression of changes, depending upon the degree of radiological involvement. Their comparative study of this technique and medical treatment, in patients with SLE osteonecrosis, appears promising in that only 13% of surgically decompressed patients eventually required total hip replacement, compared to 68% of the medically treated group. However, the follow-up was shorter in the decompressed group and further studies will be required to fully evaluate the techniques. Although osteonecrosis of the humeral head is usually less disabling, 25% of patients in one series required surgical intervention in the form of a hemiarthroplasty (Cruess, 1978).

Once osteonecrosis has developed at one site, reduction of corticosteroid dosage does not prevent the subsequent development of osteonecrosis at other sites, and no doubt reflects the long latency between osteocyte death and the development of clinical and radiological features (Griffiths et al, 1979).

ALLIED CONDITIONS

Osteolysis appears most commonly in distal phalanges, is frequently asymptomatic, and appears to be related to changes in vascular supply producing chronic ischaemia. A wide variety of clinical disorders may produce this appearance, including diabetes mellitus, frostbite, and scleroderma. An adjacent periosteal reaction may also be present, and in diabetics this may mimic osteomyelitis. The differentiation is important, as osteolysis in this condition often heals completely (Pastan & Cohen, 1978).

Painful but transient osteolysis has also been described in adult bone adjacent to more proximal joints. Here, there may be a non-inflammatory joint effusion and systemic disturbance with a raised ESR; radiological features are those of subchondral osteopenia, and isotopic scans show increased uptake of methylene diphosphonate. The condition appears to resolve slowly and spontaneously (Jacox et al, 1982). This condition is probably allied to *regional migratory osteoporosis*, which again is a self-limiting condition, usually affecting the lower limb joints of middle-aged females. A raised ESR is often present, and electromyographic studies have shown denervation changes during the acute episodes. Steroids do not appear to influence the natural history (McCoid et al, 1978). Bone biopsies have shown only osteoporotic changes (Pantazopougous et al, 1973). Clinically and radiologically, there are similarities to the reflex sympathetic dystrophies seen in the shoulder–hand and hip–foot syndromes.

These disorders should not be confused with *diffuse childhood osteoporosis* which usually presents as pathological fractures without an inflammatory component. Calcitonin deficiency has been demonstrated in one case and the abnormalities corrected by calcitonin replacement (Stevenson et al, 1982).

REFERENCES

Abeles M, Urman J D, Rothfield N F 1978 Aseptic necrosis of bone in SLE. Relationship to corticosteroid therapy. Archives of Internal Medicine 138: 750–754

Amstutz H C, Carey E J 1966 Skeletal manifestations and treatment of Gaucher's disease. Journal of Bone and Joint Surgery 48A: 679–701

Ansell B M, Bywaters E G L, Elderkin F M 1975 Familial arthropathy with rash, uveitis and mental retardation. Proceedings of the Royal Society of Medicine 68: 584–585

Arlet J, Ficat P, Sebbag D 1968 Interet de la mesure de la pression intra-medullaire dans le massif trochanterier dez le homme en particulier pour le diagnotic de l'osteonecrose femoro-capitale. Review of Rheumatology 35: 250–253

Aufdermaur M 1981 Juvenile kyphosis (Scheuermann's disease): radiography, histology and pathogenesis. Clinical Orthopaedics and Related Research 154: 166–174

Beckenbaugh R D, Shives T C, Dobyns J H, Linscheid R L 1980 Kienbock's disease. Clinical Orthopaedics and Related Research 149: 98–106

Beighton P 1978 Inherited disorders of the skeleton. Churchill Livingstone, Edinburgh

Bergstein J M, Wiens C, Fish A J, Vemier R L, Michael A 1974 Avascular necrosis of bone in SLE. Journal of Paediatrics 85: 31–35

Burton D S, Mochizuki R M, Halpern A A 1978 Total hip arthroplasty in the cardiac transplant patient. Clinical Orthopaedics and Related Research 130: 186–190

Canario A T, Williams L, Wientroub S, Catterall A, Lloyd-Roberts G C 1980 A controlled study of the results of femoral osteotomy in severe Perthes' disease. Journal of Bone and Joint Surgery 62B: 438–440

Catterall A 1971 The natural history of Perthes' disease. Journal of Bone and Joint Surgery 53B: 37–53

Catterall A 1981 Legg-Calvé–Perthes' syndrome. Clinical Orthopaedics and Related Research 158: 41–52

Catto M 1976 Pathology of aseptic necrosis. In: Davidson J K (ed) Aseptic necrosis of bone. Excerpta Medica, Amsterdam, p. 3–100.

Chryssanthou C P 1978 Dysbaric osteonecrosis. Etiological and pathogenetic concepts. Clinical Orthopaedics and Related Research 130: 94–106

Chung S M K, Ralston E L 1969 Necrosis of the femoral head associated with sickle cell anaemia and its genetic variants. Journal of bone and Joint Surgery 51A: 33–58

Chung S M K, Alavi A, Russell M O 1978 Management of osteonecrosis in sickle cell anaemia and its genetic variant. Clinical Orthopaedics and Related Research 130: 158–174

Cruess R L 1978 Experience with steroid-induced avascular necrosis of the shoulder and etiologic considerations regarding osteonecrosis of the hip. Clinical Orthopaedics and Related Research 130: 86–93

D'Ambrosia R D, Shoji H, Riggins R S, Stadalnik R C, De Nardo G L 1978 Scintigraphy in the diagnosis of osteonecrosis. Clinical Orthopaedics and Related Research 130: 139–143

Davidson J K 1976 Dysbaric osteonecrosis. In: Aseptic necrosis of bone. Excerpta Medica, Amsterdam, Ch. 4, p. 145–212

Decompression Sickness Central Registry 1981 Aseptic bone necrosis in commercial divers. Lancet 2: 384–388

Dinant H J, Decker J L, Klippel J H, Balow J E, Plotz P H, Steinberg A D 1982 Alternative modes of cyclophosphamide and azathioprine therapy in lupus nephritis. Annals of Internal Medicine 96: 728–736

Dubois E L, Cozens L 1960 Avascular bone necrosis associated with SLE. Journal of the American Medical Association 174: 971–996

Duthie R B, Houghton G R 1981 Constitutional aspects of osteochondroses. Clinical Orthopaedics and Related Research 158: 19–27

Edeiken J 1981 Roentgen diagnosis of diseases of bone, 3rd edn. Bone ischaemia and osteochondroses. ch 6, p 679. Williams & Wilkins, Baltimore

Elsmedt E 1981 Avascular bone necrosis in the renal transplant patient. Clinical Orthopaedics and Related Research 158: 149–157

Fisher D E, Bickel W H, Holley K E, Ellefson R D 1972 Corticosteroid-induced aseptic necrosis. Clinical Orthopaedics 84: 200–206

Glimcher M J, Kenzora J E 1979 The biology of osteonecrosis of the human femoral head and its clinical implications. 1. Tissue biology. Clinical Orthopaedics and Related Research 138: 284–309

Golding J S R MacIver J E, Went L N 1959 The bone changes in sickle cell anaemia and its genetic variants. Journal of Bone and Joint Surgery 41B: 711–718

Gregg P J 1977 The use of radio-isotopes in aseptic bone necrosis. In: Evans A, Walden D N (eds) Aseptic bone necrosis, London CIRIA Underwater Engineering Group, p. 77–83

Gregg P J, Barsoum M K, Soppit D, Jackson R H 1980 Avascular necrosis of bone in children receiving high dose steroid treatment. British Medical Journal 281:116

Greyson N D, Lotern M M, Gross A E 1982 Radionuclide evaluation of spontaneous femoral osteonecrosis. Radiology 142: 729–735

Griffiths I D, Maini R N, Scott J T 1979 Clinical and radiological features of osteonecrosis in SLE. Annals of the Rheumatic Diseases 38: 413–422

Hall J E 1957 The results of slipped femoral epiphysis. Journal of Bone and Joint Surgery 39B: 659–673

Hardcastle P H, Ross R, Hamalainen M, Mata A 1980

Catterall grouping Hardcastle P H, Ross R, Hamalainen M, Mata A 1980 Catteral grouping of Perthes' disease. Journal of Bone and Joint Surgery 62B: 428–431
Hartington K D, Murray W R, Kountz S L, Belzer F O 1971 Avascular necrosis of bone after renal transplantation. Journal of Bone and Joint Surgery 53A: 203–215
Heinmann W G, Freiberger R A 1960 Avascular necrosis of femoral and humeral heads after high dose corticosteroids. New England Journal of Medicine 263: 672–675
Houpt J B, Alpert B, Lotern M 1982 Spontaneous osteonecrosis of the medial tibial plateau. Journal of Rheumatology 9: 81–90
Hungerford D S, Zizic T M 1978 Alcoholism associated ischaemic necrosis of the femoral head. Early diagnosis and treatment. Clinical Orthopaedics and Related Research 130: 144–152
Hungerford D S, Zizic T M 1980 The treatment of ischaemic necrosis of bone in SLE. Medicine (Baltimore) 59: 143–148
Jacobs B 1978 Epidemiology of traumatic and non-traumatic osteonecrosis. Clinical Orthopaedics and Related Research 130: 51–67
Jacox R F, Waterhouse C, Taves D R 1982 Transient painful osteolysis — A metabolic study. Journal of Rheumatology 9: 279–283
Jones J P, Engleman E P 1967 Avascular necrosis of bone in alcoholism. Arthritis and Rheumatism 10: 287–288
Jones J P Jnr, Sakovich L 1966 Fat embolism of bone: A roentgenographic and histological investigation, with the use of intra-arterial Lipiodol, in rabbits. Journal of Bone and Joint Surgery 48A: 149–164
Ibels S L, Allen C A, Huffer W E, Weil R 1978 Aseptic necrosis of bone following renal transplantation: experience in 194 transplant recipients and review of the literature. Medicine (Baltimore) 57: 25–45
Kahn M F, De Seze S 1975 Rheumatic manifestations of heritable disorders of connective tissue. Clinics in Rheumatic Diseases 1: 3–36
Katz J F 1981 Nonarticular osteochondroses. Clinical Orthopaedics and Related Research 158: 70–76
Kawashima M, Torisu T, Hayashi K, Kitano M 1978 Pathological review of osteonecrosis in divers. Clinical Orthopaedics and Related Research 130: 107–117
Kay N R M, Park W M, Bark M 1972 The relationship between pregnancy and femoral head necrosis. British Journal of Radiology 45: 828–831
Kenzora J E, Steele R E, Yosipovitch Z H, Glimcher M J 1978 Experimental osteonecrosis of the femoral head in adult rabbits. Clinical Orthopaedics and Related Research 130: 8–50
Klipper A R, Stevens M B, Zizic T M, Hungerford D S 1976 Ischaemic necrosis of bone in systemic lupus erythematosus. Medicine (Baltimore) 55:251
Klippel J H, Gerber L H, Pollak L, Decker J L 1979 Avascular necrosis in SLE. Silent symmetric osteonecrosis. American Journal of Medicine 67: 83–87
Lancet editorial 1982 Osteonecrosis caused by combination chemotherapy. Lancet 1: 433–434
Larigerskiold A 1981 Tibia vera: osteochondrosis deformans tibiae. Blount's disease. Clinical Orthopaedics and Related Research 158: 77–82
Lee C K, Hansen H T, Weiss A B 1980 The 'silent hip' of idiopathic ischaemic necrosis of the femoral head in adults. Journal of Bone and Joint Surgery 62A: 795–800
Leventhal G H, Dorfmann H D 1974 Aseptic necrosis of bone in SLE. Seminar in Arthritis and Rheumatism 4: 73–93
Looney W B 1956 Late effects of early medical and industrial use of radioactive materials. Their relation to the more accurate establishments of maximum permissible amounts of radioactive elements in the body. Journal of Bone and Joint Surgery 38A: 175–218
McCluskey J, Gutteridge D H 1982 Avascular necrosis of bone after high doses of dexamethasone during neurosurgery. British Medical Journal 284: 333–334
McCoid W C, Nies K M, Campion D S, Louie J S 1978 Regional migratory osteoporosis. Arthritis and Rheumatism 21: 834–838
McCullum R I, Walder D N 1966 Bone lesions in compressed air workers. Journal of Bone and Joint Surgery 48B: 207–235
Madell S H, Freeman L M 1964 Avascular necrosis of bone in Cushing's syndrome. Radiology 83: 1068–1070
Melo-Gomes J A, Melo-Gomes E, Viana-Queiros M 1981 Thiemann's disease. Journal of Rheumatology 8: 462–467
Molloy M G, Hamilton E B D 1978 Thiemann's disease. Rheumatology and Rehabilitation 17: 179–180
Morrish R B, Chan E, Silverman S, Meyer J, Fu K K, Greenspan D 1981 Osteonecrosis in patients irradiated for head and neck carcinoma. Cancer 47: 1980–1983
Mubarak S J, Carroll N C 1981 Juvenile osteochondritis dessicans of the knee: etiology. Clinical Orthopaedics and Related Research 157: 200–211
Murray W R 1973 Hip problems associated with organ transplants. Clinical Orthopaedics and Related Research 90: 57–69
Nixon J E 1984 Early diagnosis and treatment of steroid induced avascular necrosis of bone. British Medical Journal 288: 741–744
Ohta Y, Matsunage H 1974 Bone lesions in divers. Journal of Bone and Joint Surgery 56B: 3–16
Olsson S E, Reiland S 1978 The nature of osteochondrosis in animals. Acta Radiologica Supplementa 358: 299–306
Omer G E 1981 Primary articular osteochondroses. Clinical Orthopaedics and Related Research 158: 33–40
Palmer A K, Hensinger R N, Costenbader J M, Basset D R 1981 Osteonecrosis of the femoral head in a family with hyperlipoproteinaemia. Clinical Orthopaedics and Related Research 155: 166–171
Pantazopoulos T, Exarchon E, Hantofilakidis G 1973 Idiopathic transient osteoporosis of the hip. Journal of Bone and Joint Surgery 55A: 315–321
Pappas A M 1981 Osteochondrosis dissecans. Clinical Orthopaedics and Related Research 158: 59–69
Pastan R S, Cohen A S 1978 The rheumatologic manifestations of diabetes mellitus. Medical Clinics of North America 62: 829–839
Patterson R J, Bickel W H, Dahlem D C 1964 Idiopathic avascular necrosis of the head of the femur. Journal of Bone and Joint Surgery 46A: 269–282
Phemister D B 1940 Changes in bones and joints resulting from interruption of circulation: non-traumatic lesion in adults with bone infarction. Archives of Surgery 41: 1455–1482
Resnick D 1981 The osteochondroses. In: Resnick D, Niwayama G (eds) Diagnosis of bone and joint disorders, Vol III. Saunders, Philadelphia Ch. 78
Rubinstein H M, Brooks M H 1977 Aseptic necrosis of bone in myxoedema. Annals of Internal Medicine 87: 580–581
Ruderman M, McCarty D J 1964 Aseptic necrosis in systemic

lupus erythematosus. A report of a case involving six joints. Arthritis and Rheumatism 7: 709–717
Schumacher H R 1975 Rheumatological manifestations of sickle cell disease and other hereditary haemoglobinopathies. Clinics in Rheumatic Diseases 1: 37–52
Sharon P, Kaplinsky N, Leiba S, Frankl O 1977 Aseptic necrosis of head of femur: presenting manifestation in Cushing's disease. Journal of Rheumatology 4: 73–75
Siffert R 1981 Classification of the osteochondroses. Clinical Orthopaedics and Related Research 158: 10–18
Smith F E, Sweet D E, Brunner C M, Davis J S 1976 Avascular necrosis in SLE, an apparent predileciton for young patients. Annals of the Rheumatic Diseases 35: 227–232
Springfield D S, Enneking W J 1978 Surgery for aseptic necrosis of the femoral head. Clinical Orthopaedics and Related Research 130: 175–185
Stern P J. Watts H G 1979 Osteonecrosis after renal transplantation in children. Journal of Bone and Joint Surgery 61A: 851–856
Stevenson J C, White M C, Jopling F, McIntyre I 1982 Osteoporosis and Calcitonin deficiency. British Medical Journal 285: 1010–1011
Stockman A, Darlington L G, Scott J T 1980 Frequency of chondrocalcinosis of the knees and avascular necrosis of the femoral heads in gout: a controlled study. Annals of the Rheumatic Diseases 39: 7–11
Stoddard A, Osborn J F 1979 Scheuermann's disease or spinal osteochondrosis: its frequency and relationship with spondylosis. Journal of Bone and Joint Surgery 61B: 56–58
Sweet D E, Madewell J E 1981 Pathogenesis of osteonecrosis. In: Resnick D, Niwayama G (eds) Diagnosis of bone and joint disorders, Saunders, Philadelphia, Ch. 76.
Thomas I H, Evans A, Walder D N 1982 Saturation of mini pig marrow with nitrogen during exposure to compressed air. Lancet 2: 127–129
Wang G J, Moga D B, Richemer W G, Sweet D E, Reger S I, Thompson R C 1978 Cortisone-induced bone changes and its response to lipid clearing agents. Clinical Orthopaedics and Related Research 130: 81–85
Williams G A, Cowell H R 1981 Kohler's disease of the tarsal navicular. Clinical Orthopaedics and Related Research 158: 53–58
Wynn-Davies R 1973 Heritable disorders in orthopaedic practice. Blackwell, Oxford
Zizic T M, Hungerford D S, Stevens M B 1980 Ischaemic bone necrosis in SLE. The early diagnosis of ischaemic necrosis of bone. Medicine (Baltimore) 59: 134–142
Zolla-Pazner S, Pazner S S, Lanyi V, Meltzer M 1980 Osteonecrosis of the femoral head during pregnancy. Journal of the Americal Medical Association 244: 689–690

49

C.G. Barnes

Miscellaneous

Included in this chapter are those miscellaneous conditions not described elsewhere since they are not conveniently classified with the more major rheumatic diseases. Although miscellaneous arthritis is the subject, many conditions described are not considered to be primarily rheumatological but may present with, or include, rheumatic manifestations. These may be a true inflammatory synovitis, or lesions of bone, tendons and other tissues which may mimic joint disease. An attempt is made to group some of these conditions according to pathogenesis or presentation without implying a classification of disease.

INFLAMMATORY ARTHROPATHIES

The conditions described in this section may all include inflammatory arthritis but with features which distinguish them from other forms of synovitis. They may, therefore, be erroneously diagnosed as 'atypical rheumatoid arthritis'; they must be included in the differential diagnosis of rheumatoid arthritis which remains the most common form of inflammatory arthritis. Similarly those conditions occurring principally in childhood, e.g. the arthritis of Henoch–Schönlein purpura and Clutton's joints, contribute to the differential diagnosis of juvenile chronic arthritis (see Ch. 43).

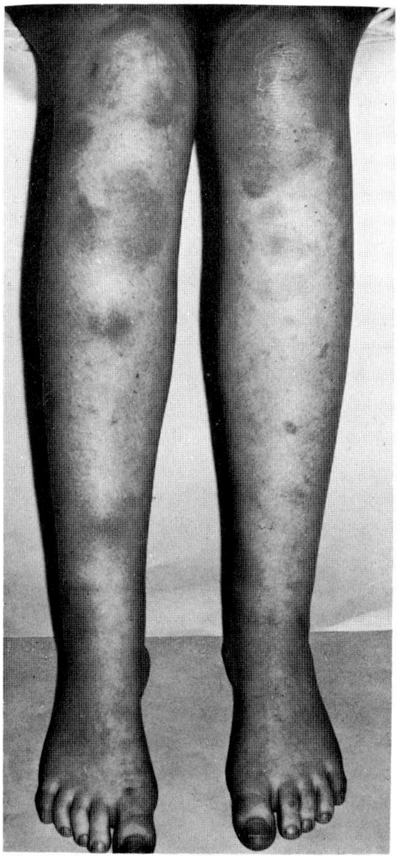

Fig. 49.1 Erythema nodosum lesions on the lower legs.

Erythema nodosum

Erythema nodosum — nodular cutaneous eruptions which are red, tender and warm, which never ulcerate and which resolve leaving a bruised discolouration — of any cause may be associated with arthralgia or a true synovitis. The lesions are normally situated on the lower legs (Fig. 49.1) but they may occur on the thighs, forearms, hands and face. The histological appearance is one of non-specific cutaneous vasculitis without thrombosis, with an infiltrate of lymphocytes, granulocytes, eosinophils and histocytes in the subcutaneous tissue (Gardner, 1965; Blomgren, 1974). Erythema nodosum is considered to be an allergic cutaneous vasculitis (Fine & Meltzer, 1968), or a hypersensitivity response to a number of possible infections — streptococcal, tuberculous, meningococcal or fungal — but also occurs in association with sarcoidosis (q.v.), Behçet's syndrome (q.v.), leprosy, ulcerative colitis (Sams & Winkelmann, 1968), Crohn's disease, and occasionally as a drug-induced eruption, for example following the ingestion of sulphonamides or oral contraceptives (Blomgren, 1974).

Joint manifestations occur in about 75% of patients with erythema nodosum. Arthralgia is a prominent feature, often preceding the appearance of skin lesions, and may be followed by a symmetrical arthritis of the knees, ankles, wrists, elbows, small joints of the hands and shoulders. The affected joints are painful, tender and stiff with synovial swelling and effusion, and the ESR is raised. Destructive changes within the joints are not seen radiologically and spontaneous remission without residua is usual within 3–6 months (Truelove, 1960). Recurrences may occur, usually associated with the development of more cutaneous lesions.

Treatment of the arthritis is symptomatic, salicylates producing relief in most cases although corticosteroid treatment is sometimes necessary in persistent severe cases. Detection of the underlying cause, where possible, is the main consideration.

Sarcoidosis

Two patterns of joint disease are associated with sarcoidosis, and may be the presenting feature of the disease. An incidence of joint complaints of between 12 and 70% in patients with sarcoidosis has been reported. Women are more frequently affected than men.

Erythema nodosum (see above) occurring in one-third of patients with sarcoidosis may be associated with a peripheral polyarthritis affecting small and medium-sized joints, which may develop early in the disease, and pulmonary lesions, usually hilar lymph node enlargement (Lofgren, 1953; Neville et al, 1983). The distinction made between hilar adenopathy and pulmonary parenchymal infiltration in sarcoidosis is not as clear-cut as previously thought (Neville et al, 1983). Thus erythema nodosum and arthritis may also be associated with the more infiltrative form of the disease.

In one series it is recorded that only two-thirds of these patients produced typical skin lesions (Gumpel et al, 1967). In patients diagnosed by mediastinal adenopathy and biopsy there is no difference in the characteristics of the arthropathy between those with and without erythema nodosum (Pennec et al, 1982). The arthritis is indistinguishable from that associated with erythema nodosum of any cause and is self-limiting, but while present may produce severe joint pain, limitation, stiffness and synovial swelling. Peripheral joints are symmetrically involved, most commonly the ankles, knees, proximal interphalangeal and metacarpophalangeal joints, wrists and elbows. In these cases histological examination of the synovium reveals non-specific inflammatory changes. Remission of sarcoidosis occurs in 80% of patients within 2 years (Neville et al, 1983).

In the other pattern, seen most commonly in Negroes, sarcoid infiltration is present in various organs, bones and joints being involved either as an early or late feature (Spilberg et al, 1969; Neville et al, 1977). Sarcoid infiltration of synovium produces pain and swelling of one or both knees, but the small joints of the hands, ankles and shoulders are also frequently involved. Effusions are common (Gumpel et al, 1967). The synovium of tendon sheaths may be similarly involved. Bone involvement is seen radiologically as cystic 'punched-out' lesions, cortical 'erosions', osteoporosis or mottled rarefaction usually of the metacarpals, metatarsals and phalanges. The cortical 'erosions' may be associated with tender overlying nodules detectable clinically, which may also develop on extensor surfaces of the forearms leading to confusion with rheumatoid nodules (Boyd & Andrews, 1981). Destruction of a terminal phalanx may occur, associated with lupus pernio of the affected fingers. The disease runs a chronic course of exacerbations and remissions. Although little destructive joint change usually occurs (Spilberg et al, 1969), joint deformity and radiological erosive changes have been recorded (Menkes et al, 1982). Bone involvement implies chronicity of the sarcoidosis and a poor prognosis (Neville et al, 1983).

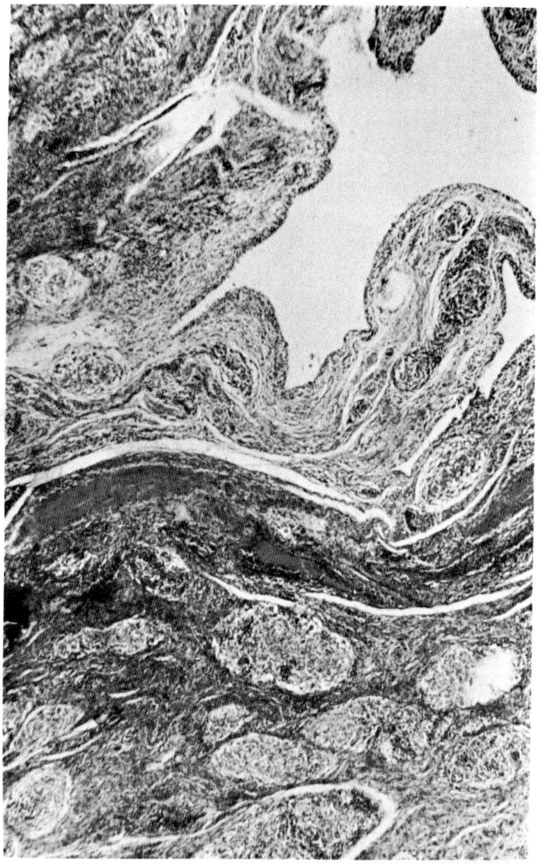

Fig. 49.2 Synovial sarcoid. Numerous non-caseating granulomata in the subsynovial connective tissue with little evidence of hyperplasia of surface synovial cells.

Diagnosis depends ultimately on biopsy of an affected organ; and the synovium (Fig. 49.2) may be seen to contain the typical non-caseating giant cell granulomata of sarcoidosis (Siltzbach & Duberstein, 1968).

The sedimentation rate is elevated, and a raised plasma gamma-globulin is frequently present; the Mantoux test usually remains negative. Hypercalcaemia is present in a minority of patients and the Kveim test will also give histological proof of the diagnosis. Tests for rheumatoid factor are usually negative. Examination of the joint fluid reveals an inflammatory effusion with numerous leucocytes which may be predominantly neutrophils or lymphocytes (Menkes et al, 1982).

A true sarcoid myopathy has also been reported as a rare manifestation of the disease (Talbot, 1967) which responds favourably to systemic corticosteroid treatment.

Behçet's syndrome

The original description of this syndrome consisted of a triad of painful oral and genital ulceration and iritis (Fig. 49.3a, b, c) (Behçet, 1940). Since then it has been recognised that many other systems may be involved including the skin and joints, and the cardiovascular, central nervous and gastrointestinal systems, together with venous thrombosis and vasculitis. A positive family history is now a well recognised association both of Behçet's syndrome itself (Lehner & Barnes, 1979a) and of isolated buccal ulceration (Mason & Barnes, 1969; Ben Ayed & Hamza, 1976).

The aetiology remains unknown. A viral aetiology was suggested by Behçet himself and later by other workers (Behçet, 1940; Sezer, 1953, 1956; Evans et al, 1957). Although later studies did not confirm a viral aetiology (Dudgeon, 1961; Yamanouchi et al, 1981) a possible association with herpes simplex virus type 1 has been suggested (Eglin et al, 1982). There does not seem to be evidence of infectivity in the various published surveys. Alternative hypotheses include tuberculous infection and an immunological disturbance manifested by the detection of antibodies against buccal mucosa (Oshima et al, 1963; Shimizu et al, 1965; Lehner, 1967; Cooper & Penny, 1974). Both popliteal and aortic aneurysms have been reported (Hills, 1967; Enoch et al, 1968) in which cases histological examination showed the vessel wall to be infiltrated with acute and chronic inflammatory cells together with an endarteritis of the vasa vasorum, without giant cell formation. Fibrinoid necrosis and panarteritis have also been reported (Hills, 1967; O'Duffy et al, 1971).

A number of immunological disturbances have been detected including the formation of immune complexes, increased leucocyte chemotaxis, reduced leucocyte phagocytic activity, increased serum IgA and reduced parotid secretion IgA levels and elevated serum complement level. Demyelinating antibodies have been detected in patients with neurological manifestations. These disturbances have been reviewed by Lehner & Barnes (1979b) and Shimizu et al (1979).

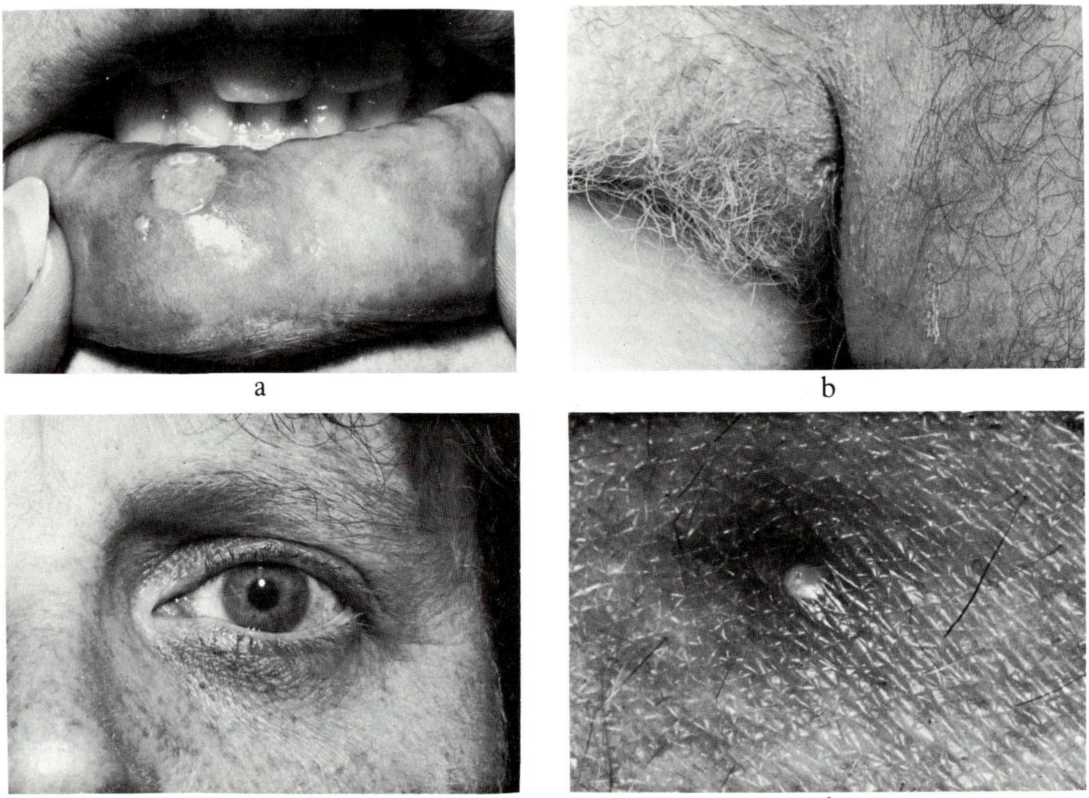

a b c d

Fig. 49.3 Behçet's syndrome. (a) Buccal ulceration. (b) Genital ulceration. (c) Uveitis. (d) Skin 'pustule'.

The diagnosis rests on the grouping together of the various features into a symptom complex in that no absolutely specific diagnostic test exists. Thus it has been suggested that a 'definite' diagnosis may be made when 3 of the 4 principal symptoms of orogenital ulceration, eye and skin lesions, are present, or 2 of these with 2 less common manifestations (Mason & Barnes, 1969).

Similar criteria are suggested by O'Duffy (1974) and by the Behçet's Disease Research Committee of Japan (1974). 'Incomplete' and 'complete' forms are diagnosed dependent on the occurrence of only 2, or more than 2, of the major features but the suggestion that a 'possible' diagnosis may be made in the presence of only 1 major feature (Behçet's Disease Research Committee of Japan, 1974) does not seem to be acceptable since almost all of the features individually may occur in isolation or as part of other diseases. Further classifications which serve to describe the predominant manifestations in an individual patient are:

1. Buccal aphthosis
   Mucocutaneous aphthosis
   General aphthosis

   (Touraine, 1955)
2. Mucocutaneous
   Arthritic, Neurological, Ocular } type

   (Lehner & Batchelor, 1979)
3. Oculo-Behçet
   Neuro-Behçet
   Vasculo-Behçet
   Entero-Behçet

   (Shimizu et al, 1979)

The possible manifestations are as follows.

Major features

Buccal ulceration (Fig. 49.3a)

Genital ulceration (and bladder ulceration) (Fig. 49.3b)

Skin lesions:
- Sterile pustules (sometimes following venepuncture or intradermal injection of sterile saline (Fig. 44.3d))
- Erythema nodosum
- Erythema multiforme
- Ulceration with residual scarring

Eye lesions:
- Uveitis (Fig. 49.3c) with or without hypopyon
- Corneal ulceration
- Retinitis/chorioretinitis
- Retrobulbar neuritis

Minor (or less common) features

Arthritis

Gastrointestinal lesions:
- Duodenal ulceration
- Ulcerative colitis

Cardiac lesions:
- Pericarditis
- Myocarditis (Higashihara et al, 1982)
- Endocarditis and valve lesions

Vascular lesions:
- Vasculitis
- Aneurysm formation
- Thrombophlebitis including the venae cavae (Mounsey, 1966; Kansu et al, 1972)

Central nervous system lesions:
- Brainstem syndrome
- Meningomyelitis syndrome
- Confusional states (Evans et al, 1957)
- Papilloedema
- Hemiplegia

Renal lesions:
- Proteinuria/microscopic haematuria

Glomerulonephritis (Beaufils et al, 1980; Williams & Lehner, 1979)

Pleuropulmonary lesions: various

Epididymitis

Amenorrhoea

Family history of a complete or incomplete syndrome.

Other reported possible associations include lyphoblastic lymphoma, pancreatitis, peripheral neuropathy, subungual infection (O'Duffy et al, 1971), cystitis, cryoproteinaemia, bullous skin eruption (Fiddes, 1971; Cooper & Penny, 1974), benign intracranial hypertension (Kalbian & Challis, 1970), and amyloidosis (Rosenthal et al, 1975; Dilsen et al, 1981).

There is an association with the possession of the HLA-B5 antigen (Bw51 split) especially in Japanese and Turkish populations (Ohno et al, 1975; Lehner & Batchelor, 1979; Yazici et al, 1980). Skin hypersensitivity to an intradermal needle prick, with or without the injection of 0.1 ml physiological saline, with the production of a sterile pustule within 48 hours (a positive 'pathergy' test) is present in a majority of Japanese (Suzuki & Mizuno, 1981) and Turkish patients (Yazici et al, 1980, 1984), but not in Europeans (Davies et al, 1984). Yazici et al (1980) consider the presence of both the HLA-B5 antigen and a positive pathergy test to be virtually diagnostic of Behçet's syndrome in Turkish patients.

There is a wide variation in the prevalence of the disease, and of its manifestations, in different parts of the world. The prevalence in Japan is estimated as 1: 10 000 (Yamamoto et al, 1974; Shimizu, 1977) maximal in the northern island of Hokkaido, compared with 0.064 : 10 000 in Yorkshire (Chamberlain, 1977) and 1 : 800 000 in Minnesota (O'Duffy, 1978). There is known to be a high prevalence of the disease in the Eastern Mediterranean area, and increasing numbers of cases are being reported from North Africa and China. Gastrointestinal lesions are reported in 50% of Japanese patients but rarely in Europeans whereas pleuropulmonary lesions have only been reported from Turkey.

Arthritis is listed as a 'minor feature' although it occurs in approximately 45% of patients (Barnes, 1979). The arthritis presents as a monarticular or symmetrical polyarticular synovitis with pain, swelling and stiffness of the involved joints affecting the knee most frequently (Fig. 49.4) and is usually subacute or chronic, occasionally episodic, rarely leads to permanent deformity and in many cases is self-limiting (Fig. 49.5) (Mason & Barnes, 1969; Ben-Dov & Zimmerman, 1982; Yurdakul et al, 1983). Synovial rupture of the knee has been recorded in Behçets syndrome as in other arthropathies which may therefore mimic venous thrombosis (Dawes et al, 1983). Arthralgia is common. Dilsen et al (1979) recorded involvement of the sacroiliac joints but this is not the experience of other investigators (Mason & Barnes, 1969; Cham-

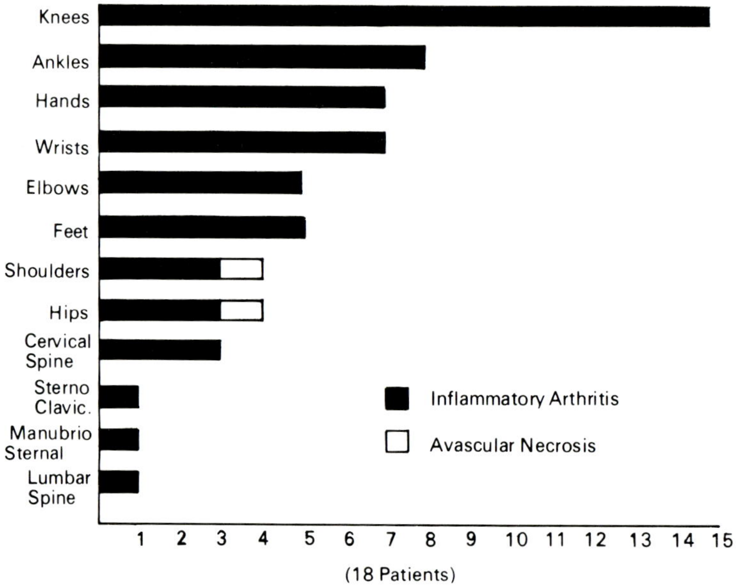

Fig. 49.4 Behçet's syndrome. Joints affected (from Mason & Barnes, 1969, with permission of the Editor of the *Annals of the Rheumatic Diseases*)

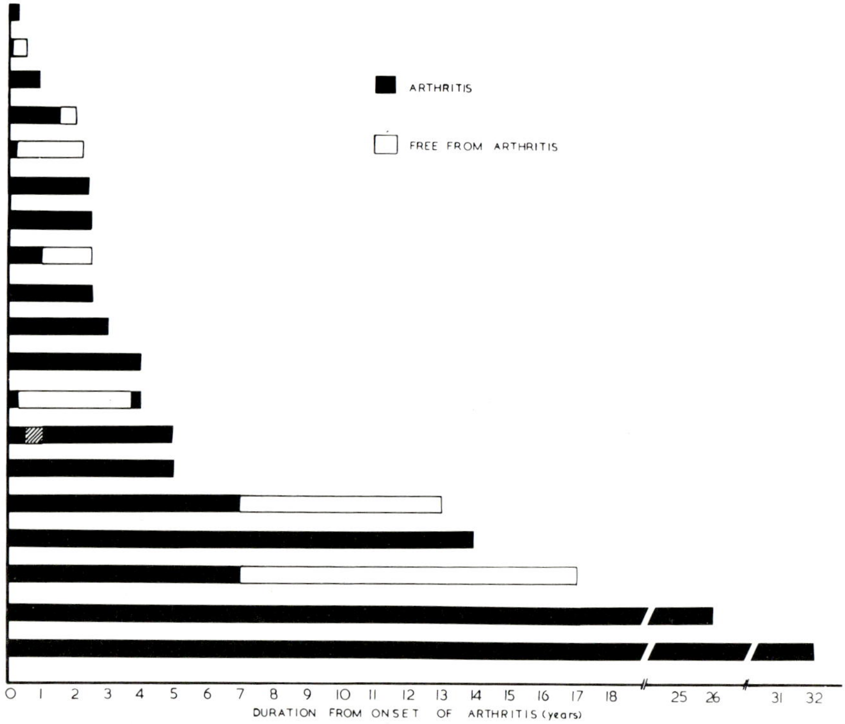

Fig. 49.5 Behçet's syndrome. Course of the arthritis (from Mason & Barnes, 1969, with permission of the Editor of the *Annals of the Rheumatic Diseases*).

berlain, 1977; Yazici et al, 1981), and it is, therefore, probably inappropriate to include Behçet's syndrome in the group of seronegative spondarthritides. A raised ESR indicates the inflammatory nature of the disease and α_2 and γ-globulin levels may be raised. Tests for rheumatoid factor are negative. Although the arthritis is usually non-destructive, both joint deformity and erosive changes, radiologically and histologically, have been reported (Vernon-Roberts et al, 1978; Ben-Dov & Zimmerman, 1982; Yurdakul et al, 1983). Histological examination of the synovium usually shows involvement of the superficial zones which are replaced by dense inflamed granulation tissue composed of lymphocytes mingled with macrophages, vascular elements, fibroblasts and neutrophils, without evidence of infection. Pannus formation may also be present. However there are also reports of a less specific synovitis including the formation of lymphoid follicles (Vernon-Roberts et al, 1978; Gibson et al, 1981; Yurdakul et al, 1983). The histological changes however are usually different from those seen in other inflammatory arthropathies and may be added to the list of diagnostic criteria.

No specific treatment is known. Corticosteroids are not considered to influence the disease but may be required to treat sight-threatening uveitis. Venous thrombosis may be treated with anticoagulants and the use of fibrinolytic agents has been recommended (Cunliffe & Menon, 1969). Sporadic reports of the use of antiproliferative agents, for example azathioprine or cyclophosphamide, alone or in combination with steroids, have appeared suggesting their beneficial effect, but there has not been a controlled trial of these agents (Rosselet et al, 1968; Buckley & Gibbs, 1969; Mamo & Azzam, 1970; Cooper & Penny, 1974; Kansu et al, 1972; Lessof et al, 1979). Controlled trials of the use of transfer factor (Denman et al, 1979) of levamisole (Lehner & Wilton, 1979) and of colchicine (Aktulga et al, 1980) have been performed without significant effect although the latter may improve erythema nodosum and arthralgia.

Symptomatic treatment of arthritis with non-steroidal anti-inflammatory analgesics is required, and oral and genital ulcers may be relived by local corticosteroid preparations.

Anaphylactoid (Henoch–Schönlein) purpura (see also Ch. 52)

The combination of purpura, arthritis, gastrointestinal and renal lesions bears the eponymous title of Henoch–Schönlein purpura, following the descriptions of the joint manifestation by Schönlein and gastrointestinal manifestations by Henoch. The basic pathology consists of a widespread vasculitis involving arterioles and small capillaries. Increased vascular permeability leads to the development of oedema and extravasation of blood. In skin biopsies a perivascular accumulation of inflammatory cells may be seen with an associated necrotising arteriolitis (Gairdner, 1948). This has been variously attributed to an allergy to a number of possible agents including streptococci (Bywaters et al, 1957), assorted foods (including various meats, eggs, etc.), insect bites, and drugs — notably penicillin (Spring, 1951; Casser, 1956).

Circulating immune complexes and IgA incorporation in these complexes and deposition in the skin, have been detected (Levinsky & Barratt, 1979).

The development of Henoch–Schönlein purpura in patients with familial Mediterranean fever (q.v.), also a disease in which immune complexes may be present, has been reported, several episodes developing after penicillin injections (Flateau et al, 1982).

Children of both sexes are affected, but boys more frequently than girls, with a peak incidence at 3 years. The disease is occasionally seen in adults. A rapid onset is usual with mild pyrexia, raised sedimentation rate, and polymorphonuclear leucocytosis.

The purpura is non-thrombocytopenic and characteristically affects the buttocks, legs and soles of the feet, although it may occasionally affect the trunk, head and arms. The lesions develop as red macules or papules which subsequently become purpuric, the purpuric lesions being papular and sometimes proceeding to vesiculation and coalescence, with ecchymoses and necrosis. Urticaria, especially of the face and legs, may be the presenting feature.

Abdominal pain, usually colicky, heralds the gastrointestinal lesions, which may precede other manifestations. This is due to haemorrhage and oedema of the gut wall, sometimes producing intestinal haemorrhage or intussusception (Allen et al, 1960).

Joint involvement consists of a transient, nonmigratory arthritis with synovial swelling, pain and stiffness, usually affecting more than one joint. The ankles, knees, hips, wrists and elbows are usually affected, with a preponderance of lower limb joint involvement. Effusions into affected joints show the characteristics of an inflammatory fluid with a high white cell count, mainly of polymorphonuclear leucocytes. Joint destruction does not occur and complete resolution is the rule.

Acute proliferative or focal glomerulonephritis, presenting as proteinuria and haematuria, and occasionally leading to chronic glomerulonephritis and hypertension, is recorded in 50% of patients (Bywaters et al, 1957), renal failure being the cause of death in 4% (Derham & Rogerson, 1956). Histologically a focal glomerulitis is present with proliferation of endothelial cells and fibrinoid deposition (Vernier et al, 1961).

Haemorrhage at other sites, e.g. intracranial and ocular, has been reported, as have headache, hypertensive encephalopathy and convulsions (Lewis & Philpott, 1956).

Treatment is mainly symptomatic. Corticosteroids have not been shown to affect the renal lesion favourably, but they may be of value in treating arthritis and gastrointestinal haemorrhage (Allen et al, 1960). Surgical intervention for intussusception may be required. The prognosis however is generally good, the exceptions being the uncommon cases of intestinal perforation and intussusception, progression of the renal disease to chronic glomerulonephritis and renal failure, and intracranial haemorrhage.

Familial Mediterranean fever (familial recurrent polyserositis)

This disease, inherited as an autosomal recessive trait, affects Sephardic (non-Askanazi) Jews and occasionally Armenians and Arabs. It is characterised by episodes of fever with abdominal and thoracic pain due to a non-specific serositis affecting the peritoneum and pleura (Sohar et al, 1967). Synovitis may also develop (Heller et al, 1966), characterised by transient monarticular, or occasionally polyarticular, episodes of pain, synovial swelling and effusion, either in isolation or together with abdominal and thoracic pain. The joints most commonly affected are the knees, ankles and hips. Fluid from the peritoneum, pleural cavity or a joint shows a high, predominantly polymorphonuclear, cell content and is sterile.

Although the episodes of arthritis are short-lived and resolve spontaneously a more chronic destructive arthritis may develop in joints subjected to repeated attacks (Jessop, 1969; Herness & Makin, 1975). The affected joint then develops into a condition indistinguishable from secondary osteoarthrosis.

The radiological changes within affected joints are localised osteoporosis in the early stages, the development of early destructive changes which may be mistaken for rheumatoid erosions, and lastly those of degenerative joint disease.

The development of secondary amyloidosis is a well-recognised complication of the disease leading to death from renal failure (see Ch. 41).

The cause of familial Mediterranean fever remains unknown although evidence is accumulating that it is an immunologically mediated disease. Circulating immune complexes, complement consumption and raised levels of plasma cyclic nucleotides during attacks and serum lymphocytotoxins have been detected (Zlotnick et al, 1979; Savi et al, 1978; Reimann et al, 1970; Levo et al, 1980; Paykoc et al, 1979). Episodes of Henoch — Schönlein purpura (q.v.), thought to be an immune complex disease, have been reported as occuring in patients with familial Mediterranean fever (Flateau et al, 1982).

The only treatment considered to alleviate frequency and severity of attacks of the disease is colchicine, which may may be used as a long-term prophylactic in a dose of 1.0–2.0 mg daily. It has been reported that some patients with familial Mediterranean fever on long-term prophylaxis with colchicine may develop mild steatorrhoea (Ehrenfeld et al, 1982).

Hyperlipoproteinaemias

A group of disorders has been described which involve elevation of one or more of the fractions of plasma lipoproteins — chylomicrons consisting

Table 49.1 The hyperlipoproteinaemias (N = normal)

Type	Plasma appearance	Plasma lipids: Cholesterol	Plasma lipids: Triglycerides	Lipoprotein abnormality	Primary form	Secondary to
I	Milky	N or +	+ + + +	Chylomicrons	Autosomal recessive	Diabetes mellitus Pancreatitis Alcoholism
II Familial hypercholesterolaemia	Clear	+ + +	N or +	β + + + Pre-β N or +	Autosomal dominant	Hypothyroidism Hypoproteinaemia Obstructive hepatic disease Myeloma Macroglobulinaemia Hypercalcaemia
III	Turbid/milky	+ +	+ +	Abnormal β/pre-β lipoprotein	?Autosomal recessive	–
IV	Turbid/milky	N or +	+ +	Pre-β + + +	Autosomal recessive	Diabetes mellitus Pancreatitis Alcoholism Glycogen storage disease Hypercalcaemia Hypothyroidism Dysglobulinaemias Progestogens Gout Gaucher's disease
V	Turbid or milky	+ +	+ + +	Chylomicrons + Pre-β + +	?Autosomal dominant	–

Table 49.2 Rheumatic syndromes associated with the hyperlipoproteinaemias

Type	Skin	Tendon	Joints	Plasma uric acid
I	Xanthomata			
II	Xanthomatosis	Xanthomata	Migratory polyarthritis	
III	Xanthomata + palmar crease deposits	Xanthomata		Elevated
IV	Xanthomata (rare)		Arthralgia Arthritis	Elevated
V	Xanthomata			Elevated

largely of alimentary triglycerides; β-lipoprotein of which approximately half is cholesterol and half protein (apoprotein B); pre-β-lipoprotein consisting of triglycerides and cholesterol in a ratio of approximately 5 : 1; and α-lipoproteins containing approximately 50% protein and 18% cholesterol. The designation of these fractions depends on their mobility on paper electrophoresis — for example β-lipoprotein has the mobility of β-globulins.

Five groups have been described (Fredrickson et al, 1967; Rifkind, 1970) which are summarised in Table 49.1 and various rheumatic disorders may be associated with these lipoprotein abnormalities (Table 49.2).

Xanthomata are present in all the five patterns of abnormality and have been classified as:

1. *Eruptive*: yellow papules containing triglycerides with surrounding erythema on the knees, buttocks, back and shoulders. These may be present in types I, III, IV and V.

2. *Involving tendons*: localised xanthomatous

deposits occur in the tendons of the palm and dorsum of the hand, the patella tendon, around the elbow and in the Achilles tendon (Glueck et al, 1968). These are present in types II and III.

3. *Lytic lesions in bone*: these have been recorded in type V leading to pathological fractures (Siegelman et al, 1972). Replacement of trabecular cancellous bone and endosteal erosion of the cortex accompany hypertrophy of the marrow which contains excessive lipid deposits. Aseptic necrosis of bone also occurs, possibly due to vascular occlusion by lipid-containing cells or fat droplets.

Type II hyperlipoproteinaemic (hypercholesterolaemic) arthritis

A migratory polyarthritis may develop in patients with type II hyperlipoproteinaemia otherwise characterised by the presence of xanthelasma, premature arcus senilis, eruptive xanthomatosis, and premature atherosclerosis (Khachadurian, 1968; Rooney et al, 1975). While tendon xanthomata may produce mechanical defects or apparent tendinitis (e.g. Achilles tendinitis) the polyarthritis is a distinct entity. Large peripheral joints are affected by pain, varying from a mild arthralgia to severe disablement, accompanied by swelling, redness and tenderness. The swelling of joints has been attributed to synovitis on the basis of raised joint fluid white cell counts (Glueck et al, 1968). Conversely, on the basis of a normal joint fluid white cell count and radio-isotope studies, it has been suggested that this is a periarthritis rather than true synovitis (Rooney et al, 1978). The duration of involvement of any particular joint lasts from a few days to a month, with migration from one joint to another, which may lead to an erroneous diagnosis of rheumatic fever. The arthritis may involve the knees, ankles, hips, elbows, wrists and also the smaller joints of the hands. Although hyperuricaemia may be associated with types III, IV and V hyperlipoproteinaemia, there is no evidence to suggest that the polyarthritis of type II hyperlipoproteinaemia is due to a uric acid crystal synovitis.

Treatment is entirely symptomatic with anti-inflammatory analgesics together with treatment aimed at lowering the hypercholesterolaemia.

Type IV hyperlipoproteinaemic arthralgia and arthritis

A series of middle-aged patients has been described by Goldman et al (1972) with type IV hyperlipoproteinaemia who presented with joint pain and morning stiffness. Women were affected twice as frequently as men and the onset was variably acute or insidious. In this series recurrent joint swelling was reported by the patients but, despite joint pain and tenderness, no objective synovitis was detected.

More recently the development of a mild, but persistent, synovitis affecting both large and small peripheral joints in association with type IV hyperlipoproteinaemia has been reported (Buckingham et al, 1975). In this series metaphyseal and epiphyseal cysts were seen radiologically, and joint fluid contained an increased number of white cells of which 90% were mononuclear. Histology revealed synovial cell hyperplasia with villus formation but infiltrated with only a few mononuclear cells. Of their 12 patients, 2 were hyperuricaemic and 6 had positive tests for rheumatoid factor.

Hyperuricaemia and the hyperlipoproteinaemias

Hyperuricaemia is reported in association with hypertriglyceridaemia (type III, IV, V but not type I) and there is an increased incidence of gout in these patients, who are also obese and show impaired glucose tolerance tests (Berkowitz, 1964, 1966).

Clutton's joints

Congenital syphilis may be associated with a painful symmetrical arthritis of the knees, or occasionally of the elbows and ankles (Gray & Philp, 1963). Since it develops in childhood or in young adults it can present a problem in the differential diagnosis of juvenile chronic polyarthritis.

The knees become painful and swollen with an acute or insidious onset, and with definite synovial thickening and effusion. Biopsy reveals a non-specific synovitis: there is a multiplication of surface synovial cells, increased vascularity, infiltration with plasma and round cells with fibrinoid changes, and sometimes suggestion of gummatous formation (Argen & Dixon, 1963). Radiologically periostitis of the tibiae may be seen.

The arthritis is however self-limiting without permanent damage, treatment as far as the joints are concerned therefore being entirely symptomatic. The diagnosis depends on the detection of other stigmata of congenital syphilis together with positive serological tests for syphilis.

Traumatic synovitis

Injury to a normal joint can produce a transient synovitis. Hypermobile joints are especially susceptible to trauma (see Ch. 46), as are joints affected by degenerative arthropathy. Injury to a joint at the time of the onset of rheumatoid or psoriatic arthritis can lead to severe involvement of that joint by the inflammatory disease (Williams & Scott, 1967).

Direct injury in the form of a blow or fall and indirect twisting or jarring accidents, e.g. while skiing, will produce synovitis in otherwise fit, usually young, patients. The joint becomes painful and limited, with swelling due to effusion and mild synovial thickening and is both tender and warm.

X-rays and laboratory tests remain normal and spontaneous full recovery within 4–6 weeks is usual. During this time treatment is entirely symptomatic, the majority of cases requiring mild analgesia, or anti-inflammatory analgesic drugs only.

Occasionally very severe pain and tenderness develops with local muscle spasm and gross limitation. This tends to occur in the knees, and occasionally elbows, and may indicate the presence of an associated haemarthrosis. In this case, temporary splinting, aspiration of the effusion and subsequent physiotherapy to regain full joint range and strengthen wasted muscles (e.g. quadriceps) may be necessary.

Bony injury related to the trauma, either a fracture adjacent to, or into, a joint, or a torn knee meniscus, provide the principal problems in differential diagnosis.

Acne arthritis

Severe acne (acne fulminans: acne conglobata) may occasionally be associated with arthralgia and arthritis. This was first described by Burns & Coleville (1959) since when only about a score of case reports have been published (Davis et al, 1981; Clement et al, 1982).

There is a strong male predominance and arthralgia and arthritis accompany a severe exacerbation of acne, usually affecting the trunk, with fever and weight loss. Arthralgia usually affects the hips, knees and shoulders, and occasionally ankles, wrists and hands, whereas the arthritis described almost always affects lower limb joints and may be of acute polyarticular or oligoarticular onset. Synovitis of the knees has been reported, associated with elevation of the ESR, leucocytosis and negative rheumatoid factor and anti-nuclear antibody tests. Sacroiliac joint involvement clinically and radiologically has been reported in two male patients, one with radiological total spinal fusion, neither of whom possessed the HLA–B27 antigen. In one series of 4 patients 3 possessed the HLA-B27, and all DRw4 antigens.

Microbiological examination of joint fluid has not revealed an infective organism and blood cultures have also been sterile. It has been suggested that an immunological mechanism may be the pathogenesis of the arthralgias and arthritis following the reporting of reduced delayed hypersensitivity reactions (Rajka, 1977; Palatsi, 1977), reduced serum complement levels (Lane et al, 1976) and the presence of circulating immune complexes (Clement et al, 1982). It has, therefore, been suggested that this may represent another form of 'reactive' arthritis associated with an exacerbation of acne involving an infective agent in the skin (Davis et al, 1981; Clement et al, 1982).

Arthralgia and arthritis are reported to resolve with treatment with anti-inflammatory analgesics, coincident with treatment of the acne topically and with antibiotics. Corticosteroids have occasionally been necessary to treat both the skin and joint manifestations.

Pustulotic arthro-osteitis (see also Ch. 28, p. 733)

The description of the rheumatic manifestations associated with a pustular rash on the palms and soles of the feet (pustulosis palmaris et plantaris), distinct from psoriasis although an overlap is reported (Ashurst, 1964), has recently led to the proposal, from Japan, of use of the diagnostic term 'pustulotic arthro-osteitis' (Sonozaki, 1981a, b).

Symptoms arising from the anterior chest wall

are common to all cases with musculoskeletal involvement including pain and swelling of the sternoclavicular and manubriosternal joints, and of the costoclavicular region, which may simulate Tietze's syndrome. Radiologically costoclavicular ossification, hypertrophy of the clavicle, and erosions or sclerosis of the manubriosternal joint have been reported. This was recorded in 9.4% of 128 patients with pustulosis palmaris et plantaris (Sonozaki, 1981b).

Additionally spondylitis, spondylodiscitis, sacroiliitis and peripheral inflammatory arthritis have been reported. Peripheral arthritis involves the metacarpophalangeal and proximal interphalangeal joints, elbows, knees, hips, ankles and wrists in order of frequency. In contrast to psoriatic arthritis distal interphalangeal joints were involved in only 1 of 53 patients. Mono- or oligoarticular involvement was usual and was non-erosive and seronegative for rheumatoid factor; the arthritis lasted for only 1–2 months and radiology of peripheral joints did not show erosive changes. No other systemic features were present and there was no specific association with a particular histocompatibility antigen. No definite familial aggregation of cases has been detected with the exception of one report of a family in which four brothers and two sisters were affected (Kumagaya et al, 1973). In the majority of cases the skin eruption coincided with the development of musculoskeletal symptoms, but in some cases developed either before or after the onset of arthritis, usually within 2 years. Exacerbations or remissions of skin disease were usually associated with increase or decrease of arthritis.

Histologically a non-speicific synovitis or an enthesopathy was detected without evidence of infection.

Treatment remains entirely symptomatic with anti-inflammatory analgesics.

It has been suggested, therefore, that pustulotic arthro-osteitis may be a specific condition, distinct from other inflammatory arthritides, which should be classified in the group of seronegative spondarthritides.

Pyoderma gangrenosum

Pyoderma gangrenosum is a non-bacterial, ulcerating, destructive skin lesion (Fig. 49.6) of unknown aetiology which may be associated with ulcerative colitis (Perry & Brunsting, 1957), paraproteinaemias (Thompson et al, 1973), or paroxysmal nocturnal haemoglobinuria (Holt et al, 1980). Arthritis or arthralgia have been reported in association with pyoderma gangrenosum, including sporadic cases of typical rheumatoid arthritis (Stolman et al, 1975).

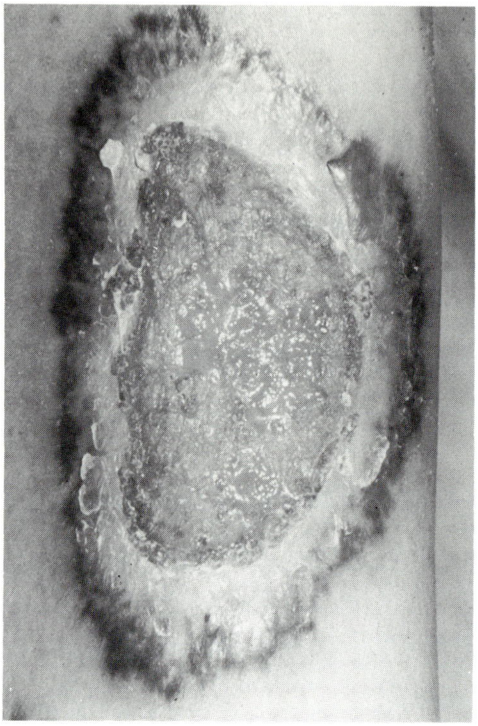

Fig. 49.6 Pyoderma gangrenosum.

Three forms of polyarthritis have been recorded in patients with pyoderma gangrenosum — typical rheumatoid arthritis, colitic arthropathy in those patients with ulcerative colitis (q.v.) and a progressive erosive seronegative polyarthritis (Holt et al, 1980). The latter may occur without associated ulcerative colitis, paraproteinaemia or psoriasis. The arthritis may develop before, and is unrelated to, the activity of the skin lesions. It is unlike rheumatoid arthritis in that the joints involved include the 1st carpometacarpal and terminal interphalangeal joints and sacroiliac joints in addition to the elbows, temporomandibular joints and cervical spine. Progressive joint destruction occurs leading to joint deformity and disability. Although the pyoderma itself usually responds rapidly to systemic corticosteroid therapy joint disease progresses despite this treatment and is equally unresponsive to pencillamine and anti-inflammatory analgesics (Holt et al, 1980).

Synovial fluid is sterile and contains a high neutrophil count. Serum complement levels are normal and no confirmed evidence of cryoprecipitate or immune complex deposition is available. Skin histology does not reveal arteritis and no association with any specific histocompatibility antigen has been discovered.

Arthritis associated with intestinal bypass surgery (see also Ch. 28, p. 734, Ch. 32, p. 814)

Intestinal (jejunocolic and jejunoileal) bypass surgery is performed as treatment of gross obesity. The proximal jejunum is divided and anastomosed to the ascending colon or ileum, the majority of the small intestine thus being left as a blindloop.

This procedure may lead to a number of complications including renal and hepatic damage, cholecystitis, electrolyte disturbances, thrombocytopenia, malabsorption syndromes and osteomalacia (Franck et al, 1979). The latter has also been reported in congenital megaoesophagus and megaduodenum (Manicourt & Orloff, 1979).

Arthralgia and arthritis may develop rapidly post-operatively, within one month, or after several years. Pain, swelling, warmth, redness and stiffness of affected joints develop acutely, most commonly affecting the knees but also frequently of small and medium-sized joints symmetrically. The arthritis is frequently episodic with remissions and acute exacerbations although effusions are uncommon. Radiological erosions and permanent joint damage has not been reported, tests for serum rheumatoid and anti-nuclear factors are negative (Delamere et al, 1983, Clegg et al, 1980).

Infection of joints has not been detected but circulating immune complexes are present in some patients and it is postulated that some of the complications of this procedure may be immune-complex-mediated, possibly related to absorbed bacterial antigens from the intestinal blind loop (Clegg et al, 1980; Moake et al, 1977; Rose et al, 1977). Patients undertaking rapid weight reduction by other means do not develop similar problems (Delamere et al, 1983).

Treatment is entirely symptomatic but surgical reversal of the bypass results in resolution of the arthropathy.

ARTICULAR OR PARA-ARTICULAR TUMOURS

The conditions discussed under this heading fall into the differential diagnosis of a monarticular arthropathy. One may classify these tumours pathologically, although there is considerable doubt whether many of them should be considered as true neoplams, as follows:

1. Arising within synovium
   a. By metaplasia:
      Synovial chondromatosis (osteochondromatosis)
   b. Unknown aetiology:
      Pigmented villondular synovitis
   c. Benign neoplasms:
      Haemangioma
      Lipoma
   d. Malignant neoplasms:
      Secondary neoplastic deposits
      Primary synovioma (synovial sarcoma)
      Melanotic sarcoma
      Synovial chondrosarcoma
2. Arising from bone/cartilage
   a. Development defect:
      Enchondromatosis (Ollier's disease)
      Diaphyseal aclasis
   b. Malignant neoplasms:
      Chondrosarcoma
      Giant cell tumour (osteoclastoma)
      Osteosarcoma (osteogenic sarcoma)
   c. Myelomatosis
   d. Osteoid osteoma
3. Arthropathies associated with non-articular neoplastic disease
   a. Lymphosarcomatous arthritis
   b. Carcinoma arthritis
   c. Secondary neoplastic deposits

Arising within synovium

Synovial chondromatosis and osteochondromatosis

There has been considerable confusion over the terminology of this condition arising from the use of the term 'osteochondromatosis' for other unrelated conditions. The situation is clarified in Table 49.3.

Table 49.3 Terminology of synovial chondromatosis and osteochondromatosis

Present terminology	Terms used previously
Synovial chondromatosis	
Synovial osteochondromatosis	
Diaphyseal aclasis	Osteochondromatosis Hereditary multiple exostosis
Enchondromatosis (Ollier's disease)	Osteochondromatosis Maffuci's syndrome (when associated with haemangiomata)

Cartilaginous plaques form within the synovium of joints, and occasionally in the synovium of tendon sheaths, by metaplasia (Murphy et al, 1962; Jeffreys, 1967); these may subsequently ossify (osteochondromatosis). The condition is regarded as benign and is not thought to lead to the even rarer condition of synovial chondrosarcoma (King et al, 1967). Men are affected more frequently than women, usually in youth and middle-age, with monarticular involvement of the knee or hip, or less commonly the elbow or shoulder. The involved joint becomes episodically painful and swollen with limitation of movement, or 'locking', due to the mechanical presence of the cartilaginous plaques which may separate and form loose bodies within the joint. An associated effusion is frequently present.

Radiographs of the affected joint may be normal, since cartilaginous deposits are radiolucent, or may reveal multiple opacities when ossification has occurred (Fig. 49.7 a–d) seen also histologically (Fig. 49.7e). Secondary degenerative changes may develop prematurely. Treatment is surgical, involving the removal of loose bodies or synovectomy, when symptoms are severe enough to justify surgery.

Pigmented villonodular synovitis

The correct classification of this condition remains in doubt. Although it has been included with other intra-articular tumours, and has formerly been classified as a low grade malignant tumour of synovium, some authorities suggest that it represents a benign haemangioma or is of inflammatory origin (Byers et al, 1968: Bobechko & Kostvik, 1968; Granowitz et al, 1976). The finding of virus-like structures has also been reported (Molnar et al, 1971). It should probably be regarded as an inflammatory granulomatous condition, and true malignant change does not occur.

The term 'pigmented villonodular synovitis' was introduced by Jaffe et al (1941); as implied by the title there is a chronic proliferation of synovial tissue, which is dark brown in colour, owing to the presence of excessive amounts of haemosiderin. The synovium proliferates forming villi which clump together, sometimes diffusely, sometimes being entirely localised or nodular.

Histologically the villi have a coating of synovial lining cells. In the connective tissues of the stroma there are sheets of compact round and polyhedral cells, many of which may be multinucleate. Haemosiderin is present in the lining cells and in the cells of the stroma. In some, but not all, cases an excessive number of mitoses is seen which in the past has led to the classification of this disease as a neoplasm and caused diagnostic confusion with synovial sarcoma (Nilsonne & Moberger, 1969). Histiocytes containing foamy, lipoid material and haemosiderin, plasma cells and lymphocytes are also present within the stroma. Clefts lined by pigment-containing synovial cells are frequently observed in this disease (Fig. 49.8) (Clark, 1958).

Pigmented villonodular synovitis may develop in intra-articular synovium or in the synovial lining of tendon sheaths or bursae. The diffuse form is usually present in joints, whereas the nodular form is found more frequently within tendon sheaths. Both sexes are equally affected at any age (Bobechko & Kostvik, 1968; Clark, 1958). Localised bone involvement may occur (Kindblom & Gunterberg, 1978) and may resemble a primary bone neoplasm (Jergesen et al, 1978).

Diffuse pigmented villonodular synovitis presents as a painless swelling of one joint, most commonly the knee (Granowitz & Mankin, 1967), but hip, shoulder, elbow or wrist involvement is not unusual. Initially the swelling is intermittent but it eventually becomes chronic and painful, with clinical signs of both synovial hypertrophy and ef-

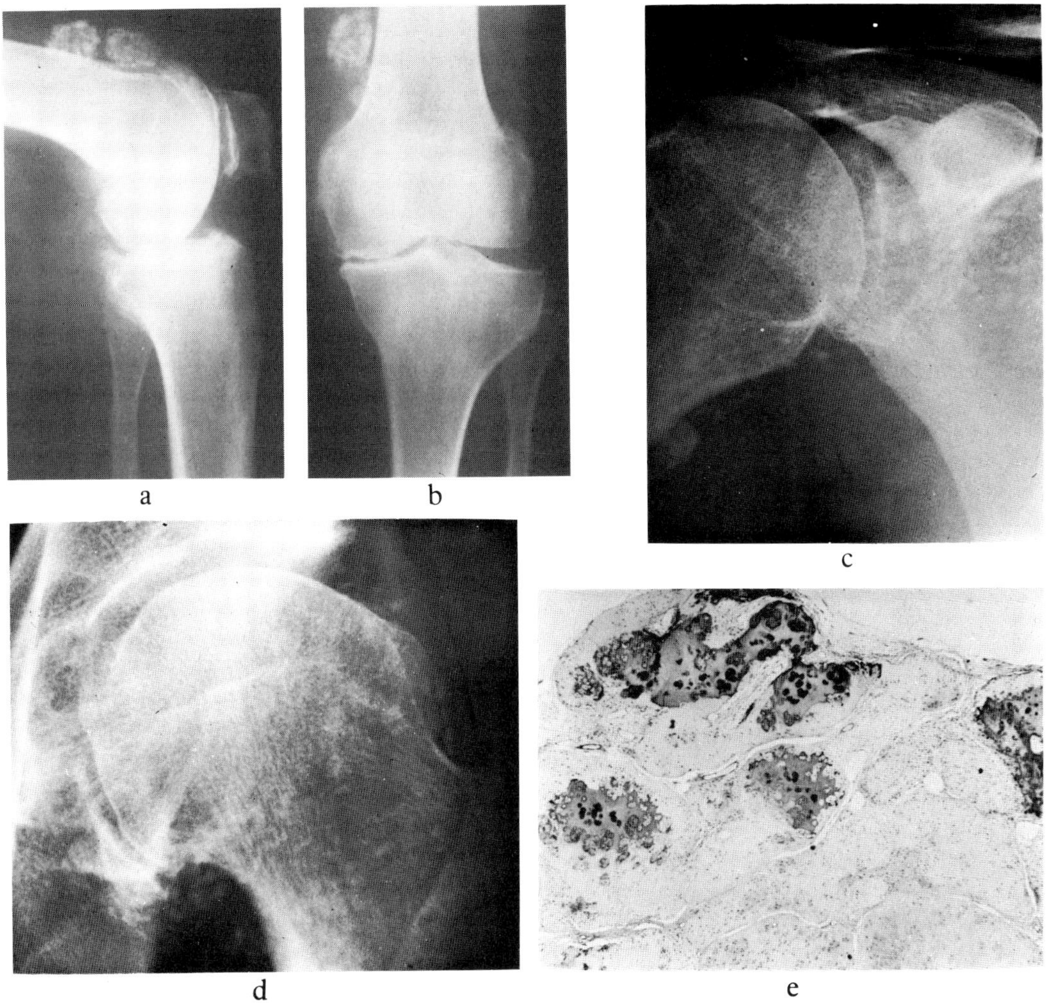

Fig. 49.7 Synovial osteochondromatosis. (a & b) Radiograph of the knee. (c) Radiograph of the shoulder. (d) Radiograph of the hip. (e) Histology of synovium showing numerous nodules of hyaline-type cartilage, some undergoing calcification.

fusion. It has been suggested that this may develop after local trauma (Vilppula et al, 1982).

Radiologically there is initially normal preservation of the cartilaginous joint space and mineralisation of bone, but marginal erosion of juxta-articular bone, cystic changes, localised osteoporosis and narrowing of the joint space occur as late features (Breimer & Freiberger, 1958; Smith & Pugh, 1962; Schajowicz & Blumenfeld, 1968; Pantazopoulos et al, 1975).

Aspiration of the joint produces a heavily blood-stained fluid, the differential diagnosis therefore being the other causes of haemarthrosis, including synovial haemangioma, coagulation disorders, trauma and malignant tumours. Thus the involvement of a single joint with a blood-stained fluid, radiological bone destruction and histological evidence of excessive mitoses may lead to a diagnosis of synovial sarcoma, the correct diagnosis being indicated by the presence of multinucleate giant cells, and lipid and haemosiderin deposits within histiocytes. Treatment by synovectomy is advised in progressive cases although recurrences are common, and radiotherapy may be used for treatment for postoperative recurrences (Granowitz et al, 1976).

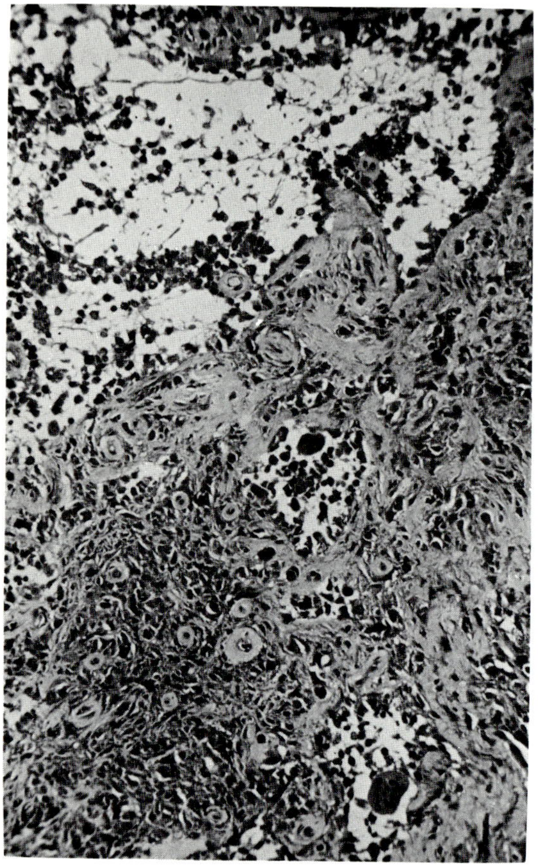

Fig. 49.8 Pigmented villonodular synovitis — part of lesion showing fibrous tissue stroma with aggregates of rounded and polyhedral cells and spaces lined with synovial-type cells and with some multinucleate giant cells.

Localised nodular lesions may occur within joints when they lead to symptoms suggesting a mechanical derangement. Thus in the knee episodic pain with locking and a sensation of instability develops, similar to that experienced with a torn meniscus (Granowitz & Mankin, 1967; Fechner & Fraire, 1972).

Localised nodular involvement of tendon sheaths with palpable swelling is difficult to differentiate both clinically and histologically from a fibrous xanthoma (Jones et al, 1969). Response to surgical excision of the affected synovium is good.

Benign tumours

Benign tumours of joints are uncommon but must be considered in the differential diagnosis of any monarticular swelling. This includes xanthomata, haemangiomata and lipomata (Coventry et al, 1966). Diagnosis can only be confirmed by biopsy. Synovial haemangiomata are uncommon; they may be sessile or pedunculated, the latter sometimes producing symptoms attributed to the mechanical presence of the tumour. The knee is the usual joint affected (Reeves, 1966; Stevens et al, 1969), although involvement of the elbow has also been reported (Larsen & Landry, 1969). Joint swelling is painless and aspiration reveals a heavily bloodstained fluid.

Malignant tumours

Secondary neoplastic deposits. The most common malignancies found within joints are secondary deposits from common extra-articular primary neoplasms, for example those arising in the breast and lung, when they simulate a monarticular arthritis (Goldenberg et al, 1975).

Synovioma (synovial sarcoma). Synovial sarcoma characteristically develops adjacent to, and very rarely within, a joint or from the synovium of tendon sheaths or bursae. The origin of this sarcoma, adjacent to joints, is thought to be due to neoplastic change within mesenchymal cells which differentiate into the appearance of synovium (Cadman et al, 1965; Hajdu et al, 1977).

Histologically the tumour consists of two components which have been confirmed by electron microscopy (Gabbiani et al, 1971). A fibrosarcomatous component of malignant spindle cells is usually present in at least some areas of the tumour. The synovial component consists of malignant round or clear cells arranged in sheets, cords or nests and lining numerous clefts or spaces. The latter are an important diagnostic feature histologically. The lining cells of these clefts may contain a mucin-like secretion (Fig. 49.9). Characteristically the tumour is heterogeneous although the biphasic features listed above are usually to be found in different areas of the tumour. Some monophasic types occur, consisting of malignant spindle cells only which are, therefore, difficult to distinguish from other spindle cell sarcomata.

Synovial sarcomata are highly malignant, metastasising rapidly usually to the lungs, but also to bone, regional lymph nodes, skin and medias-

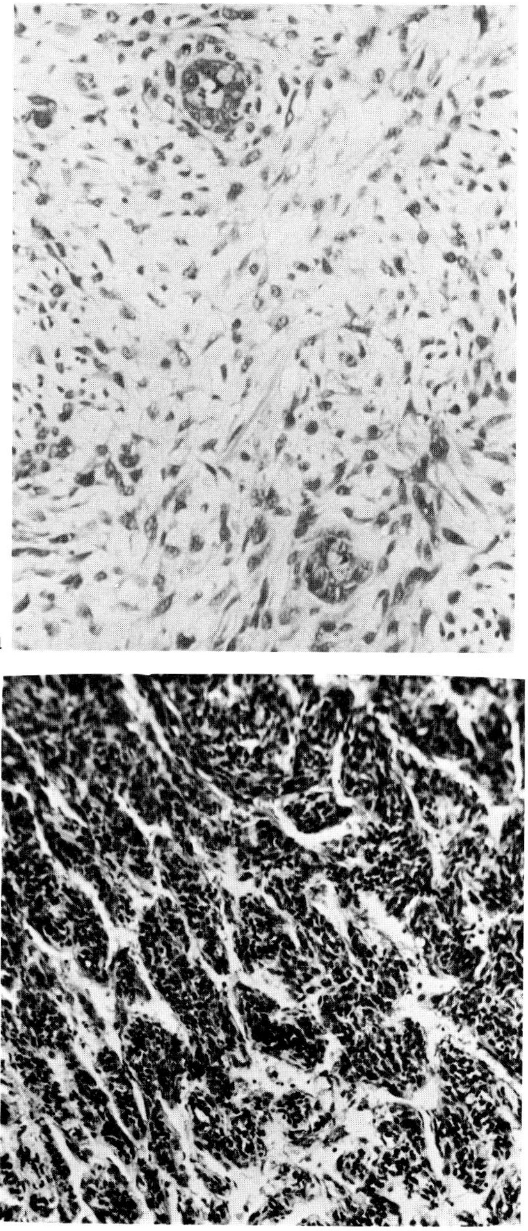

a

b

Fig. 49.9 Synovial sarcoma. (a) Biphasic pattern comprising predominantly spindle cell element but with two islands of cells resembling epithelial cells. (b) Mixed solid fibrosarcomatous area with clefts lined by synovial type cells. (H & E × 400)

tinum (Ryan et al, 1982). Bone deposits are osteolytic.

This is a rare tumour but affects both sexes equally, usually in the 20–60 year age group, although cases presenting in children have been reported (Lee et al, 1974). Lower limbs are more commonly affected than the upper limbs, and the tumour may present in the hand or foot, or adjacent to the knee, elbow or shoulder (Kogstad, 1970). While it is usually accepted that synoviomata develop in the extremities they may rarely arise from the spine, particularly the neck (Batsakis et al, 1967), temporomandibular region or pleura (Ryan et al, 1982). Monarticular involvement is the rule, the differential diagnosis being from an inflammatory synovitis especially when the hand or foot is involved.

Synoviomata present as slowly growing swellings which are only painful and tender in approximately half the cases, diagnosis being made by biopsy. Effusions also occur; they are usually heavily blood-stained. Radiological examination reveals a soft tissue mass sometimes with speckled calcification, adjacent bony erosion occurring as a late feature (Fig. 49.10).

Treatment is by radical excision, involving amputation when the tumour develops peripherally, postoperative radiotherapy or cytotoxic therapy usually being advised. Alternatively complete disappearance of metastatic tumour in patients treated

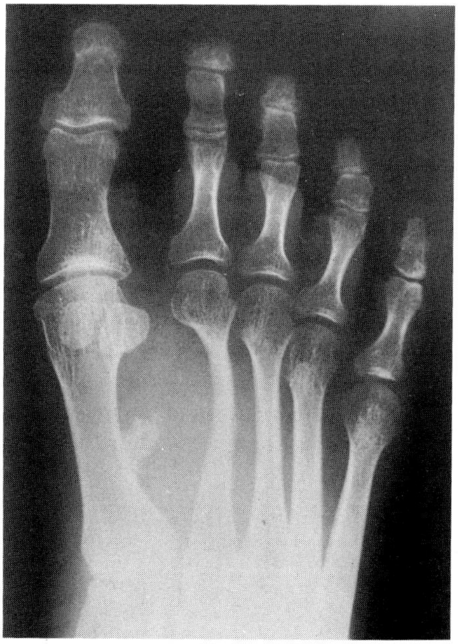

Fig. 49.10 Synovial sarcoma. Radiograph of foot showing thinning and bowing of metatarsals and calcification in the tumour.

with cytotoxic drugs alone has been reported although with subsequent recurrence (Ryan et al, 1982).

Recurrences after local excision are common. While the long-term prognosis is poor, 50–60% 5-year survival rates have been reported after radical surgery and irradiation (Raben et al, 1965; Rissanen & Holsti, 1970), and the average life expectancy from the onset of symptoms has been assessed at 6.5 years (Cadman et al, 1965). The median survival with cytotoxic agents has been recorded as 10 months (Ryan et al, 1982) with a group of patients surviving for longer.

Melanotic sarcoma. A rare form of tumour arising from tendons or aponeurosis may develop in the extremities, usually in the foot or around the ankle, and sometimes in the palm of the hand. This tends to recur after excision and may eventually metastasise.

Histologically it consists of nests of clear cells with prominent nucleoli, separated by fibrous septa, which contain melanin pigment. The condition may therefore be confused with synovial sarcoma (Mackenzie, 1974).

Synovial chondrosarcoma. Even more rarely sarcomatous change has been diagnosed histologi cally in cartilaginous deposits within joint synovium, usually from the knee and hip. It remains doubtful whether this develops in the synovium involved by the benign condition of synovial chondromatosis (King et al, 1967).

Arising from bone/cartilage

Developmental defects

Enchondromatosis (Ollier's disease). This is a rare developmental disease in which cartilage islands remain in the metaphyses and diaphyses of the long bones and of the digits. Since these islands persist, adjacent epiphyseal plate growth is disturbed producing both shortening and deformities. An associated haemangiomatous malformation may also be present, then known as Maffuci's syndrome (Richardson & Diddams, 1962; Anderson, 1965). Such haemangiomata are superficial, appearing as blue cutaneous swellings on one or both hands or feet, and sometimes in internal viscera.

The cartilage islands enlarge and produce nodular tumours on the surface of the bone, which may become chondrosarcomatous.

The affected hands and feet thus become deformed with swellings adjacent to joints, which may be mistaken for arthritis. The swellings are however hard and bony and the diagnosis is confirmed radiologically. Lucent chondromata are then seen expanding the shafts of the affected bones, occasionally with associated exostoses, with distortion of the normal contour (Fig. 49.11).

Diaphyseal aclasis (hereditary multiple exostosis). This rare inherited condition consists of the presence of multiple, cartilage-capped, bony exostoses arising from long bones and from the shoulder girdle. Since these arise alongside the epiphyseal plate, their presence may produce bony swellings adjacent to joints and affect normal growth of the involved bone (Solomon, 1961, 1963). Thus, they may lead to local deformity of bone, for example valgus deformity of the lower leg, bowing or deviation of the forearm, shortening of the bone or limb, or premature degenerative change within joints adjacent to areas of disturbed bone growth. The diagnosis is made radiologically (Fig. 49.12).

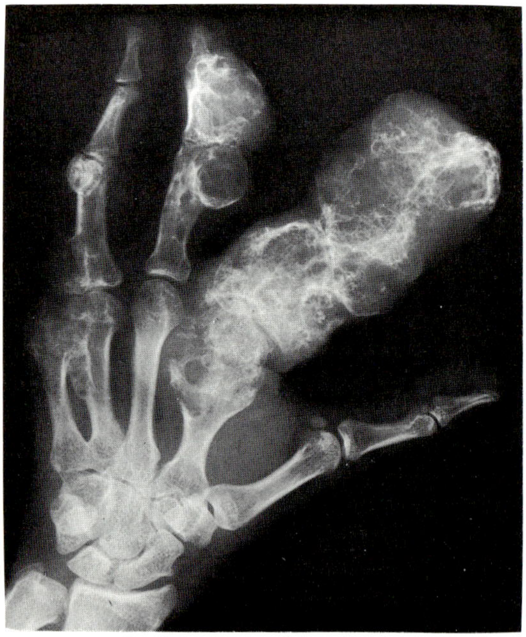

Fig. 49.11 Enchondromatosis.

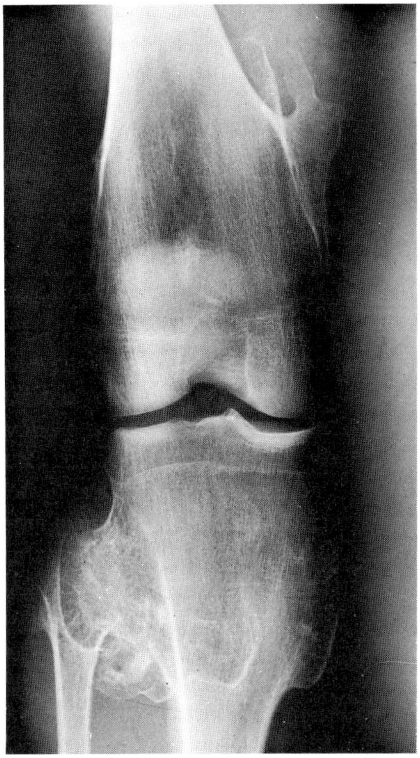

Fig. 49.12 Diaphyseal aclasis. Radiograph showing multiple exostoses of the femur, tibia and fibula with a normal knee joint.

Malignant change has been reported in the cartilage of the exostosis.

Malignant neoplasms

Chondrosarcoma, fibrosarcoma and reticulum-cell sarcoma (histiocytic lymphoma) of bone. Chondrosarcomata and fibrosarcomata may arise as solitary tumours from bones of the spine, limb girdles or limbs themselves, or as periosteal chondrosarcoma (Bertoni et al, 1982), with a variable risk of metastasising. Surgical ablation where possible and radiotherapy, although many of these tumours prove to be radioresistant, are the usual methods of treatment (Bertoni et al, 1982; Gitelis et al, 1981).

Reticulum-cell sarcoma (histocytic lymphoma) may present as an isolated swelling arising from bone despite the diffuse nature of the neoplasm which derives from lymphocytes. This is well reviewed by Sweet et al (1981).

Giant cell tumours (osteoclastoma) and osteosarcomata (osteogenic sarcomata). Sweetnam (1982) has reviewed the terminology of primary tumours arising in bone. 'Osteogenic sarcoma' is a term implying all primary bone tumours, thus including chondrosarcoma and fibrosarcoma but if these are excluded one is left with the more accurate term 'osteosarcoma'. Osteosarcoma may be recognised and defined histologically by the formation of osteoid by malignant osteoblasts whereas osteoclastomata is a giant cell tumour.

Both these tumours may occasionally arise as a swelling adjacent to a joint which may be painful and thus may be confused with either a monarticular arthropathy or synovioma. The differentiation lies in the radiological appearance of the tumour with bone expansion and destruction indicating its bony origin (Fig. 49.13), and in histological exmination of biopsy material.

Osteosarcomata usually arise from the metaphyseal region of long bone most commonly around the knee, but have also been reported as developing in a bone affected by fibrous dysplasia (Bloch, 1962; Húvos et al, 1972), from periosteum (Bertoni et al, 1982) and following irradiation (Sweetnam, 1982). Osteosarcoma developing in bone affected by Paget's disease is the most malignant form. Osteosarcoma metastasises to the lungs, and rarely to a distant bone.

Amputation of the affected limb has always been the principal form of treatment for osteosarcoma, even if only for palliation to prevent local painful recurrence after conservative treatment. The traditional treatment was radiotherapy followed by amputation 6 months later if pulmonary metastases were not detected. However an improved prognosis is achieved by radical ablative surgery, although prosthetic replacement of some long bones is now possible, followed by one of a number of schemes of treatment with combinations of cytotoxic drugs (Bleyer et al, 1982; Sweetnam, 1982). Embolisation of a giant cell tumour with subsequent resection is also described (Channon & Williams, 1982).

Myeloma

This is one of the most common neoplastic causes of backache, and of vertebral collapse which may

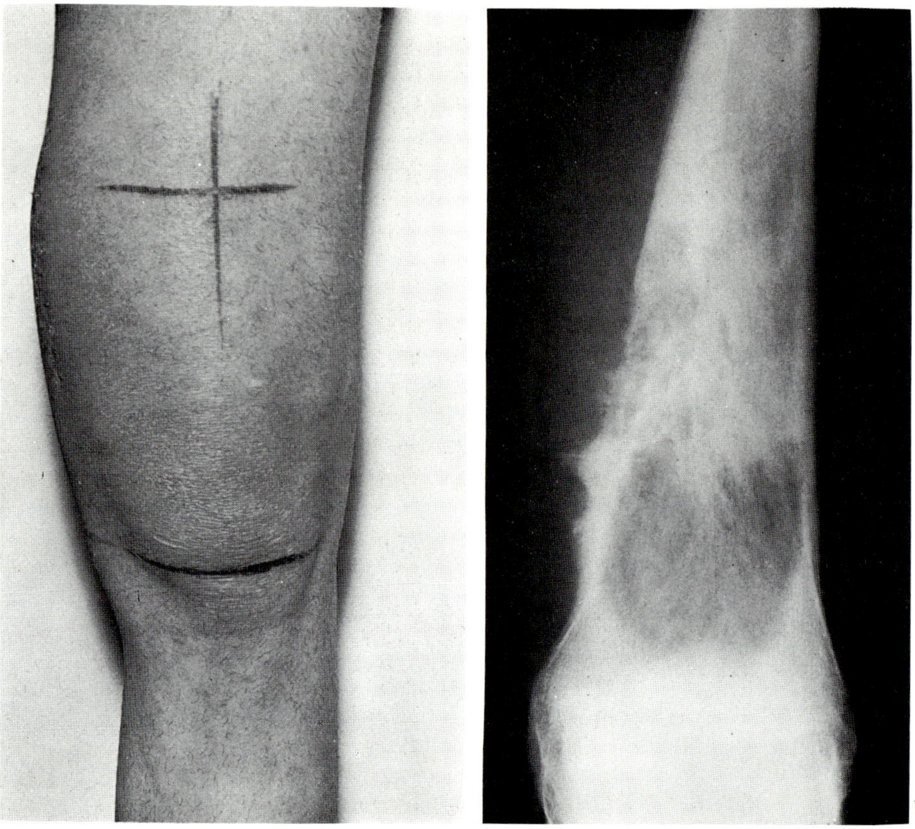

Fig. 49.13 Osteosarcoma. (a) Swelling adjacent to the knee arising from the lower femur. (b) Radiograph of the femoral neoplasm.

produce long tract or nerve root pressure. The diagnosis is initially suspected by the finding of a high ESR and confirmed by detecting characteristic X-ray changes, plasma and urinary protein abnormalities, and excessive numbers of, often abnormal, plasma cells in the bone marrow.

Radiologically myeloma may appear as:

1. Generalised radiolucency (Fig. 49.14A)
2. Discrete multiple osteolytic lesions characteristically in the calvarium, mandible (Fig. 49.14B), and clavicles (Fig. 49.14C); sclerotic deposits have been recorded but these are rare
3. A solitary large radiolucent area (plasmacytoma)
4. Pathological fracture including vertebral collapse (Fig. 49.14A)

Myeloma is a cause of para-amyloid which itself, together with other causes of amyloidosis, may produce a polyarthritis arising from amyloid infiltration of synovium and articular cartilage, often with an associated carpal tunnel syndrome (Hickling et al, 1981). Secondary gout may also accompany myelomatosis.

Osteoid osteoma

Osteoid osteoma (Sherman, 1947; Lichtenstein, 1965) is a benign bone tumour consisting of vascular fibrous tissue, fibroblastic proliferation and the presence of spicules of newly formed osteoid tissue (Fig. 49.15a). These typically develop in young adults, males being more frequently affected than females, as single lesions in the long bones, especially the femur, tibia and fibula.

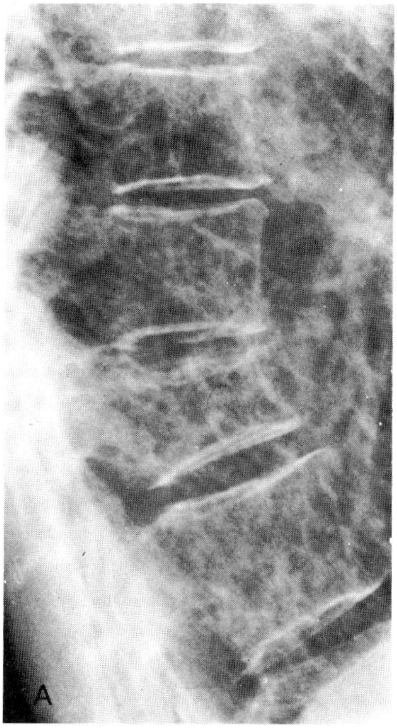

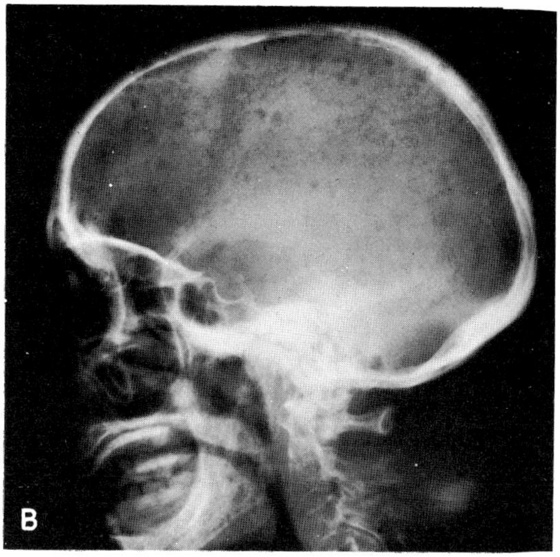

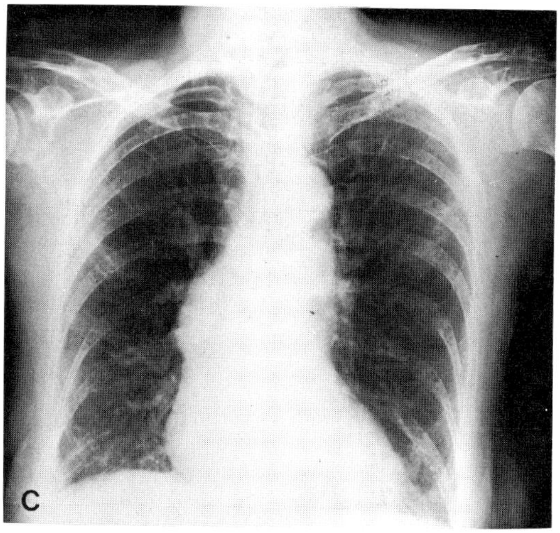

Fig. 49.14 Multiple myeloma. (A) Generalised translucency of vertebrae with collapse. (B) Radiograph of skull showing discrete osteolytic lesions in calvarium and mandible. (C) Radiograph of chest showing discrete osteolytic lesions in ribs, clavicles and scapulae.

Upper limb and spinal involvement also occur. The tumour may become sufficiently large to produce clinical swelling of bone.

Pain is the presenting symptom which is localised, continuous and often severe. Many patients experience complete but temporary relief from small doses of aspirin (Cohen et al, 1982).

Diagnosis depends on radiography and radio-isotope bone scans. Radiographically the lesions appear as a rarefied area of bone surrounded by sclerosis, often with a central nidus of dense bone (Fig. 49.15b). Radio-isotopic bone scan reveals a localised increased uptake of the isotope by the tumour (Winter et al, 1977) in most cases.

Osteoid osteomata developing in bone within a joint capsule may be associated with a non-specific or lymphofollicular synovitis with joint effusion which has been reported as occurring at the hip or elbow (Snarr et al, 1973; Cronemeyer et al, 1981). This, together with an elevated ESR, may therefore mimic primary inflammatory monarticular joint disease.

Treatment is by localisation and complete surgical excision of the lesion which may be assisted by intraoperative radio-isotopic uptake techniques

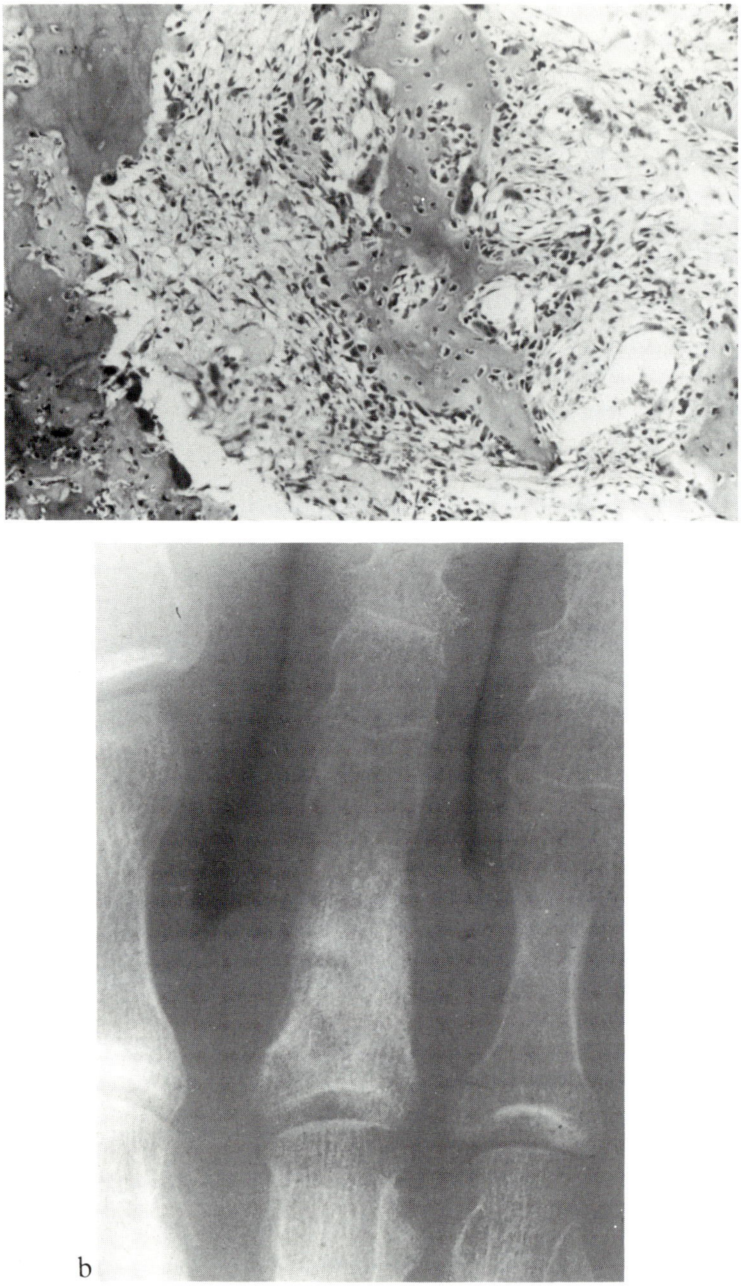

a

b

Fig. 49.15 Osteoid osteoma. (a) Osteoid osteoma, high power view showing part of the nidus of the tumour (centre) and the sclerotic surrounding bone (left). (b) Radiograph showing osteoid osteoma of a proximal phalanx of the toe with overlying periosteal reaction. (H & E × 600)

(Ghelman et al, 1981). In excised specimens a greatly increased rate of prostaglandin synthesis has been demonstrated (Makley & Dunn, 1982).

Arthropathies associated with non-articular neoplastic disease

Neoplasms arising from organs not related to the locomotor system (e.g. lung), or arising as a multifocal process (e.g. reticulosis), may present as a rheumatic disease with joint involvement, or with bone infiltration. Arthritis has been reported as a presenting feature of distant malignancies other than as hypertrophic (pulmonary) osteoarthropathy (q.v.).

Lymphosarcomatous arthritis
Lymphosarcoma has been described as producing multiple joint pain with local tenderness and clinical evidence of synovitis. Biopsy of the synovium reveals lymphosarcomatous change, and radiologically multiple radiolucent areas adjacent to joints are seen (Martin et al, 1973).

Carcinoma arthritis
Carcinomas of the pancreas, prostate, breast, bladder, ovary and lung, and also a rhabdomyosarcoma and a melanoma, have all been reported as being associated with arthritis. In the case of the acinar cell carcinoma of the pancreas this may also produce areas of fat necrosis with tender subcutaneous nodules.

Monarticular, or asymmetrical polyarticular, involvement of larger joints, sparing the wrists and hands, is usual with signs of active synovial inflammation. This polyarthritis, like the neoplasm with which it is associated, is predominantly a disease of later life and usually precedes the presentation of the neoplasm. The sedimentation rate is raised, tests for rheumatoid factor are negative, and biopsy reveals a non-specific synovitis (Calabro, 1967; Virshup & Sliwinski, 1977; Bennett et al, 1976; Murray & Persellin, 1980; Weinblatt & Karp, 1981; Shenberger & Morgan, 1982).

Malignant cells have been detected in the synovial fluid of patients with 'metastatic carcinomatous arthritis' in patients with bronchogenic carcinoma (Fam et al, 1980).

Secondary neoplastic deposits
In bone these present as local pain, or pathological fractures including collapse of vertebrae. Characteristically the pain is of 'boring' constant nature both at rest and on exertion, although often exacerbated by the latter. Diagnosis depends on radiological evidence of the secondary deposit although many cases present with pain before radiological abnormality is apparent. In these cases a radio-isotope bone scan will often reveal areas of increased uptake of the isotope.

Secondary malignant deposits occuring in bone adjacent to a joint may simulate an arthritis by the development of joint effusion (Gall et al, 1974).

HYPERTROPHIC OSTEOARTHROPATHY

The combination of finger-clubbing, painful tender swelling of bones and joints, commonly the ankles and wrists, and radiological periostitis form the characteristic presentation of this disease. In addition a recurrent mild synovitis with effusion in large joints, especially knees, may occur, possibly secondary to adjacent periosteal pathology. The overlying skin is usually red, warm and frequently oedematous, and tenderness may be elicited from the long bones adjacent to affected joints. The sedimentation rate is raised, although synovial fluid contains a low white cell count and therefore does not have the characteristics of an inflammatory effusion. The progress of the disease is typically one of remissions and relapses.

Radiologically a narrow band of irregular periosteal new bone is seen at the distal ends of the long bones (Fig. 49.16) — especially of the radius, ulna, tibia and fibula — which progressively extends proximally. The periosteal new bone may be separated from the cortex by a translucent zone, or appear as cortical thickening (Greenfield et al,

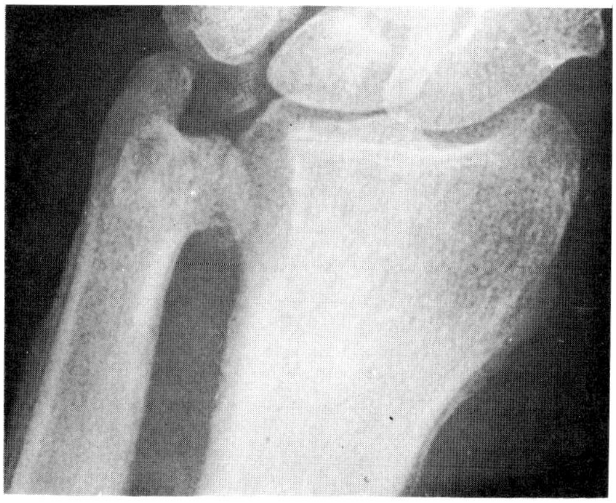

Fig. 49.16 Hypertrophic osteoarthropathy showing periosteal new bone. (Reproduced with permission from Currey H L F (ed) *An Introduction to Clinical Rheumatology*, 3rd Edn. Pitman, London.)

1967). In advanced cases similar appearances are seen in widely separated parts of the skeleton including the bones of the hands and feet, the diaphyses of other long bones, vertebrae and clavicles (Yacoub & Simon, 1966; Greenfield et al, 1967). Tufting of the distal phalanges also occurs.

The pathogenesis of this condition remains uncertain but hypertrophy of periosteal tissue dependent on vagal stimulation has been suggested (Dixon, 1963), a concept supported by the observation that symptoms and signs of hypertrophic (pulmonary) osteoarthropathy may regress after vagotomy without excision of the primary lesion (Flavell, 1956; Yacoub, 1965; le Roux, 1968). Parasympathetic blockade with propantheline has also been reported to alleviate the disease (Lopez-Enriquez, 1980; Schwartz, 1981). Similarly eradication of the cause (see below) leads to resolution of all manifestations of hypertrophic osteoarthropathy, and treatment of a neoplasm with chemotherapy may also be effective in relieving the rheumatic symptoms (Evans, 1980).

Histologically the radiological appearances are confirmed by the finding of layers of subperiosteal cancellous new bone formation surrounding the cortex of the diaphysis of the affected long bones.

The terminology of this condition may produce difficulties. The formerly accepted name of 'hypertrophic pulmonary osteoarthropathy' (HPOA) implied an aetiology secondary to a pulmonary pathology and this is the most common cause. Of the pulmonary causes bronchial carcinoma is the most frequent, the incidence of HPOA being variously assessed as between 1.2% (le Roux, 1968) and 10% (Flavell, 1956). All other forms of primary lung neoplasm, except the cylindromic form of bronchial adenoma, and also pulmonary metastases from extrathoracic tumours, have been recorded as leading to HPOA (Stenseth et al, 1967; Yacoub et al, 1967), as have 25% of pleural fibrosarcomata (le Roux, 1968). The coincidence of both HPOA and metastatic synovial and bony deposits from bronchogenic carcinoma has been reported (Fam & Cross, 1979) which coincidence, as the authors state, has therapeutic implications. Other non-neoplastic pulmonary conditions associated with HPOA are suppurative lung diseases including bronchiectasis and empyema, tuberculosis and aspergillosis (Yacoub & Simon, 1966).

There are, however, many causes of hypertrophic osteoarthropathy in which pulmonary pathology is not the primary disease, and thus the disease should be known as 'hypertrophic osteoarthropathy'. Among the very large number of described causes of this are congenital cyanotic heart disease (McLaughlin et al, 1967), biliary atresia (Cavanaugh & Holman, 1965), biliary cirrhosis (Mendlowitz, 1942), portal cirrhosis (Buchan & Mitchell, 1967; Han & Colins, 1968; Epstein et al, 1979), intestinal lymphoma (Bakhshandeh et al, 1971), Hodgkin's disease (Mullins & Lenhard, 1971), ulcerative colitis (Honska et al, 1957; Farman et al, 1976), Crohn's disease (Neale et al, 1968; Fielding & Cooke, 1971), gastrointestinal neoplasms (Hollis, 1967), and pseudomembranous enterocolitis (Ueno et al, 1981a).

Thus secondary hypertrophic oesteoarthropathy may be associated with many varied diseases although most relate to the respiratory or gastrointestinal systems, a recent report of the association with cystic fibrosis (Wasser et al, 1982) also demonstrating this. A rare primary form does, however, exist and is then known as 'pachydermoperiostosis'.

Pachydermoperiostosis (Touraine–Solente–Gole syndrome)

Males are affected almost exclusively by this condition which may be inherited as a Mendelian dominant trait, either autosomal or sometimes sex-linked (Fischer et al, 1964; Rimoin, 1965). Chromosome studies have been found to be normal (Susmano et al, 1967).

The characteristic features, in the absence of other underlying disease, are clubbing, periostosis leading to enlargement of the extremities, thickening of the skin and scalp (pachydermia) and an arthropathy. Profuse sweating is often prominent. Bone marrow failure has also been reported in association with this condition (Metz & Dowell, 1965). The onset is usually during or soon after puberty and the process becomes inactive within 5 years (Calabro et al, 1966; Salfeld & Spalckhaver, 1966).

The 'arthropathy', however, consists of painful swelling due to periostitits adjacent to joints, usually the knees, wrists and ankles (Fig. 49.17). There is no actual inflammatory synovitis (Calabro

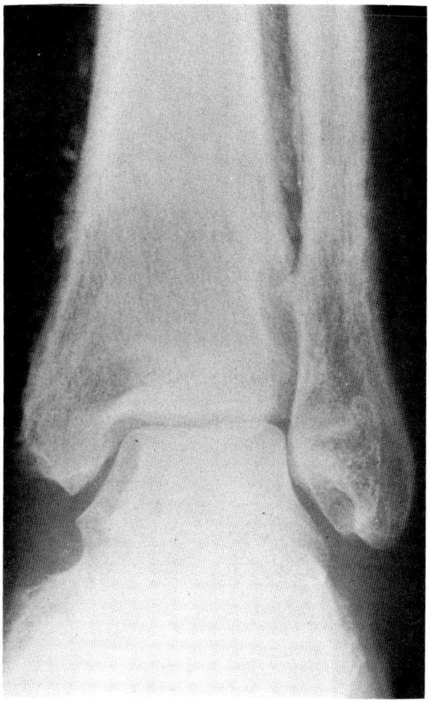

Fig. 49.17 Pachydermoperiostosis showing prolific periosteal new bone of the lower tibia and fibula.

et al, 1966). This, however, may lead to an erroneous diagnosis of juvenile polyarthritis, clubbing being the hall-mark of pachydermoperiostosis.

Thyroid acropachy

Thyroid acropachy is a similar rare condition of digital clubbing and periostosis seen in a small minority of patients with longstanding hyperthyroidism often with exophthalmos and pretibial myxoedema (Scanlon & Clemett, 1964; Williams, 1967; Ford, 1970; Bland et al, 1979). Swelling of the hands and feet may occur, and the skin may develop an indurated fissured texture which, it has been suggested, may be due to lymphatic obstruction (Rothschild & Yoon, 1982).

MISCELLANEOUS CONDITIONS

One could argue that some of the conditions included in this section could be classified with other diseases, but most have sufficiently distinctive features to warrant discussion in their own right. The importance of these conditions depends on the fact that they may be associated with systemic disease (e.g. neuropathic joints and atrial myxoma) or erroneously may be diagnosed as a progressive disabling joint disease (e.g. Dupuytren's contracture).

Neuropathic (Charcot's) joints

The disorganisation of joints due to neurological disease, either peripheral neuropathy or cord lesions, has been attributed to loss of pain sensation. However, in some cases pain sensation may be present and the exact cause for this type of joint disease is therefore uncertain.

In all cases, however, there appears to be a combination of some diminution of pain sensation, impairment of position sense and trauma leading to disorganisation of the joint, which sometimes develops very rapidly.

Many conditions have therefore been identified as associated with the development of neuropathic joint disease:

1. Tabes dorsalis (the original Charcot's joints)
2. Diabetes mellitus with peripheral neuropathy
3. Syringomyelia
4. Leprosy
5. Congenital indifference to pain
6. Charcot–Marie–Tooth disease
7. Paraplegia
8. Myelomeningocoele
9. Subacute combined degeneration of the cord
10. Familial amyloid polyneuropathy (Pruzanski et al, 1981).

The affected joint progressively undergoes destructive changes with profuse new bone formation and resultant bony deformity. Effusions are common, crepitus is prominent and painless instability usual. Although pain may become a prominent feature late in the disease the presenting symptoms are usually swelling, deformity, weakness or instability. Acute episodes of pain, swelling, redness, and tenderness with effusion may also occur subsiding spontaneously over a period of weeks or months (Storey, 1964).

Radiologically (Figs 49.18, 49.19) there is a combination of:

1. Loss of cartilage joint space
2. Roughening of subchondral bone

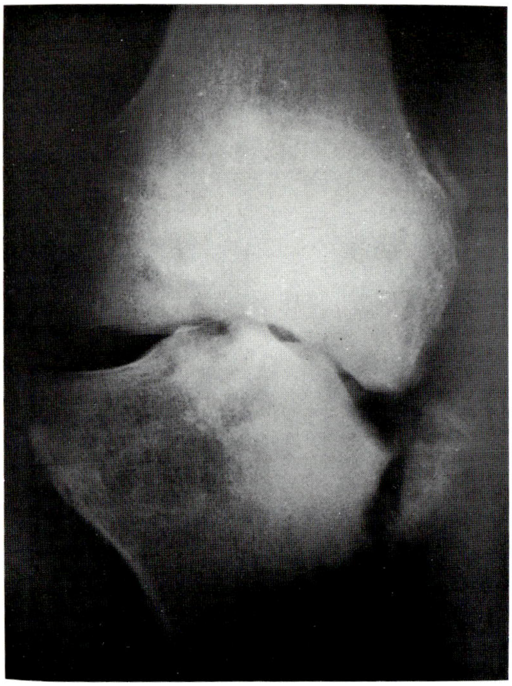

Fig. 49.18 Neuropathic arthropathy of the knee showing narrowing of the joint space, sclerosis, subluxation, fragmentation of the tibial plateau and new bone formation.

3. Sclerosis of bone ends
4. Massive new bone formation with resultant deformity
5. Loose bodies within the joint.

In tabes dorsalis the knees, feet and spine are characteristically affected. Similary the lower limb involvement is more common in diabetes mellitus (Sinha et al, 1972) when painful involvement of the tarsus is characteristic although wrist involvement has also been reported (Feldman et al, 1969). Congenital indifference to pain also leads to lower limb joint destruction (Fizgerald, 1968). In those conditions affecting only the lower limbs, for example, paraplegia and Charcot–Marie–Tooth disease (Bruckner & Kendall, 1969), weakness may contribute to the pathogenesis. By contrast upper limb joint involvement is more common in syringomyelia.

Infection, haemarthrosis, dislocation and fracture adjacent to the affected joint may complicate the condition, and spinal involvement may lead to compression of the spinal cord.

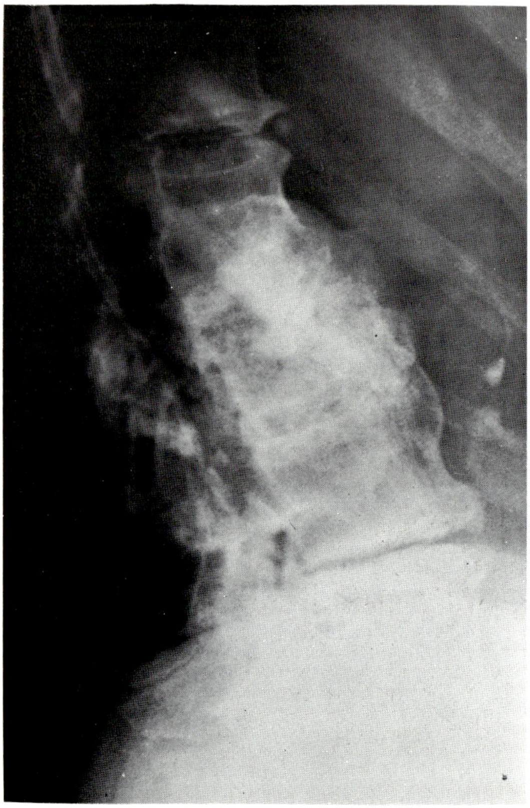

Fig. 49.19 Neuropathic arthropathy of the spine showing loss of disc spaces, sclerosis and prolific new bone formation.

Treatment consists of the relief of pain, where present, and stabilisation of the unstable joint using splints, or calipers, or occasionally by surgical arthrodesis.

Although hypertrophic change is the usual description of neuropathic joints a destructive and resorptive arthropathy has been described in association with diabetes mellitus with neuropathy. An atrophic arthritis mutilans pattern of joint involvement of peripheral joints, affecting the upper limb 5 times more frequently than the lower limb was recorded in these patients (Schwarz et al, 1969).

Dupuytren's contracture and diathesis

Contracture of the palmar fascia leading to flexion deformity of the fingers at the metacarpophalangeal joints occurs 6–10 times more often in men than in women (Viljanto, 1973), and may produced variable degrees of disability from an in-

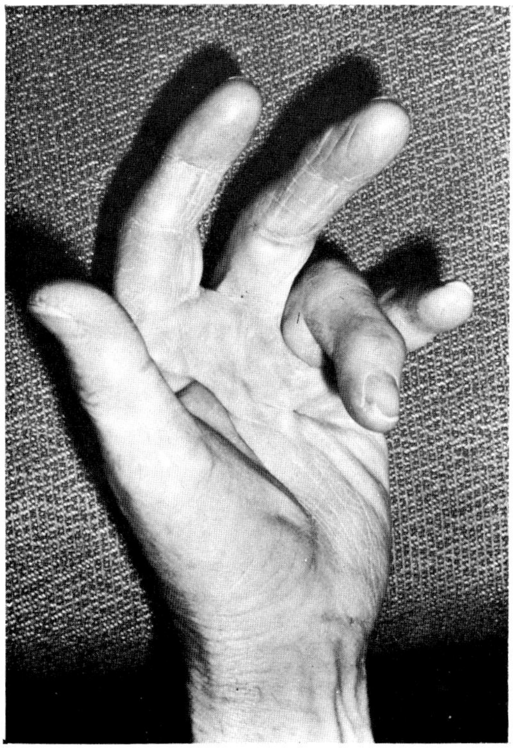

Fig. 49.20 Dupuytren's contracture showing thickening and contraction of the palmar fascia with inability to extend the ring metacarpophalangeal joint (by courtesy of Mr B. Helal).

ability to extend the ring MCP joint (Fig. 49.20) to a completely closed hand. Surveys have shown an incidence of 1–3% of the population (Viljanto, 1973) being most common in Northern Europe and rare in coloured races (Hueston, 1962). It is probably inherited as a Mendelian dominant trait (James, 1974) and may occur solely as a mild isolated contracture of the palmar fascia without deformity of the hand. A strong association is also present with epilepsy and alcoholism (Wolfe et al, 1956). Study of histocompatibility antigens has not revealed any association of a particular antigen with Dupuytren's contracture (Hunter et al, 1981).

A distinction can therefore be drawn between Dupuytren's contracture affecting the palmar fascia alone, and Dupuytren's diathesis. The latter may present as a spectrum of manifestations ranging from nodule formation in the palmar fascia alone to the complete syndrome of palmar contracture, fibrous plantar nodules, Peyronie's disease (pain and curvature of the penis on erection), epilepsy, gum hypertrophy (possibly due to anticonvulsant therapy), stiff shoulders and Garrod's pads, the fleshy swellings over the dorsum of the proximal interphalangeal joints arising from the extensor paratenon (Lettin, 1964; Hueston, 1975). Synovitis does not occur in this syndrome.

The pathology consists of a proliferation and thickening of the connective tissue of the palmar and plantar fasciae with the formation of fibrous nodules. This does not affect adjacent tendon sheaths, muscles, blood vessels or nerves. The nodules are formed of fibroblasts with an irregular pattern, or arranged in bundles, with a prominent network of reticulin. Contraction of the proliferative fascia leads to the deformity of the hand (Gabbiani & Manjo, 1972; Viljanto, 1973).

It has been suggested that contracture may occur primarily in the palmar aponeurosis, and that repeated ruptures occur with the formation of scar tissue which contracts ('intrinsic theory'). An alternative theory is that there is some change in adjacent tissues provoking contracture of the palmar aponeurosis ('extrinsic theory'). The relationship to trauma is debateable but it has been suggested that repeated occupational trauma does not contribute to the condition, whereas a specific local injury such as a burn, penetrating wound or an ulnar nerve lesion may do so (Hueston, 1968; Viljanto, 1973).

Treatment depends entirely on the extent of the disability. However, the only satisfactory means of correcting the palmar contracture is by surgical incision of the palmar fascia (fasciotomy) as a palliative procedure, or excision of the affected fascia (fasciectomy), occasionally with associated skin grafting. Amputation of the little finger at the metacarpophalangeal joint, or through the 5th metacarpal, has also been advocated where the contracture is entirely confined to this finger.

Relapsing polychondritis

As the name suggests this condition is characterised by episodes of inflammation around hyaline and fibrocartilagenous structures leading to their dissolution (Pearson et al, 1960).

Cartilaginous structures commonly affected are the external ear, nasal cartilage, and those of the respiratory tract including the larynx and tracheal and bronchial rings.

Additional features include polyarthritis, inflammatory eye disease (scleritis, episcleritis, keratitis, conjunctivitis, uveitis), cochlear and vestibular damage, and cardiovascular lesions (aortic or mitral regurgitation, pericarditis, aortic aneurysm) (McAdam et al, 1976). A wide variety of conditions with which relapsing polychondritis may be associated has been reported; McAdam et al (1976) noted that 30% of their patients had another preceding or coexistent condition. The conditions listed in the literature include rheumatoid arthritis, Sjögren's syndrome, systemic lupus erythematosus, progressive systemic sclerosis, Raynaud's phenomenon, thyroid disorders, ulcerative colitis, pernicious anaemia, malignancy, tuberculosis, psoriasis, syphilis, alopecia universalis, diabetes insipidus, diabetes mellitus, renal tubular acidosis, herpes zoster and simplex, Hodgkin's disease and glomerulonephritis (Donlan et al, 1966; Odkuist, 1970; Miller et al, 1974; McAdam et al, 1976; Meyer et al, 1981; Ueno et al, 1981b; Kronberg, 1981; Piette et al, 1982).

The cause of relapsing polychondritis remains unknown. An abnormality of cellular immune mechanisms has been postulated (Herman & Dennis, 1973) with disturbance of cell-mediated immunity to proteoglycan (Rajapkse & Bywaters, 1974). Circulating antibodies to native type II collagen have been detected but these are also found in rheumatoid arthritis. However antibodies to cartilage have been demonstrated also as have circulating immune complexes (Ebringer et al, 1981; Kronberg, 1981; Meyer et al, 1981; Ueno et al, 1981b). Elevation of the sedimentation rate and of gamma-globulin levels, and anaemia, are present. These immunological abnormalities and the association with the diseases listed indicate the immunological mediation of the disease.

Histologically there is a loss of basophilic staining of cartilage matrix due to loss of acid mucopolysaccharide, perichondral inflammation with fibrocytic reaction and perivascular cellular infiltration of plasma cells and lymphocytes, and cartilage destruction with replacement by fibrous tissue (Verity et al, 1963; Kaye & Jones, 1964; McAdam et al, 1976) (Fig. 49.21).

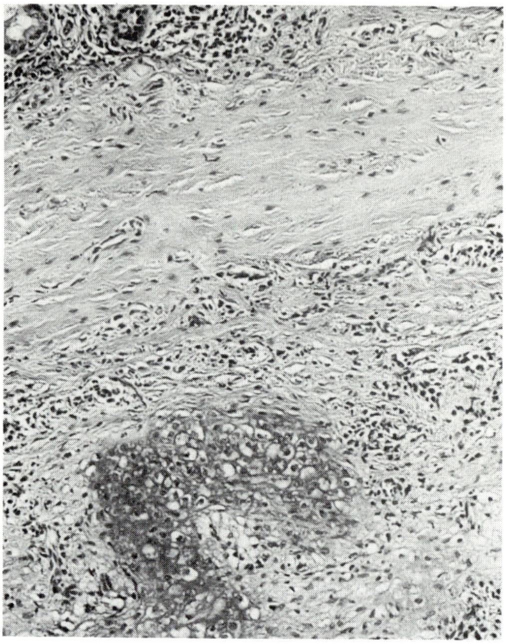

Fig. 49.21 Relapsing polychondritis. Biopsy of trachea, showing heavy lymphocytic infiltrate and destruction of cartilage, replacement fibrosis (top) and markedly abnormal residual cartilage (bottom). (H & E ×400)

The maximum age of onset is in the 5th decade, males being more frequently affected than females. 50% of patients present with ear and joint involvement. Swelling, redness, pain, warmth and tenderness of the external ear or nose develop with subsequent collapse of the cartilage and deformity, that of the nose (Fig. 49.22) being associated with rhinorrhoea which may be confused with sinusitis or chronic rhinitis. Respiratory tract involvement presents as hoarseness, dyspnoea and inspiratory stridor (Verity et al, 1963; McAdam et al, 1976). Severe large airways obstruction may be demonstrated by pulmonary function tests (Gibson & Davis, 1974).

Involved joints become swollen and tender, with effusions in peripheral joints, although non-synovial cartilaginous joints (e.g. symphysis pubis) and costochondral junctions are also affected. Joint involvement is oligoarticular or polyarticular most commonly affecting the large and small joints of the upper limbs (Fig. 49.23), and also the hips and knees (McAdam et al, 1976). Although migratory

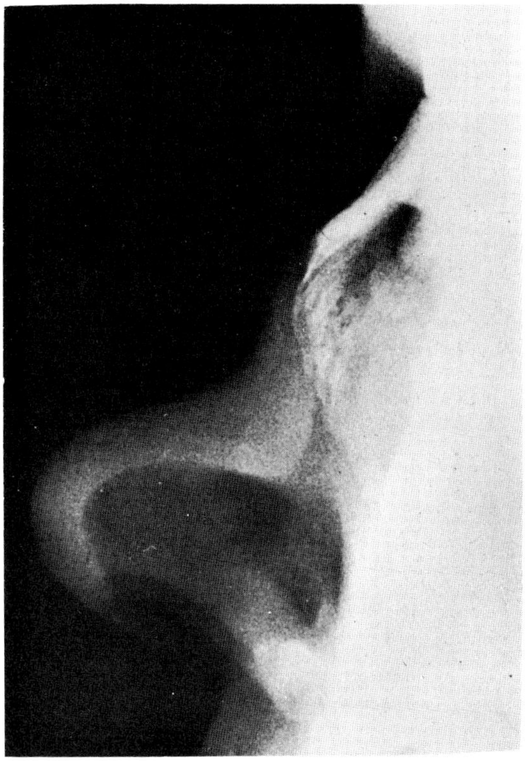

Fig. 49.22 Relapsing polychondritis. Radiograph showing collapse of the nasal cartilage. (Reproduced with permission from Currey H L F (ed) *An Introduction to Clinical Rheumatology*, 3rd Edn. Pitman, London.)

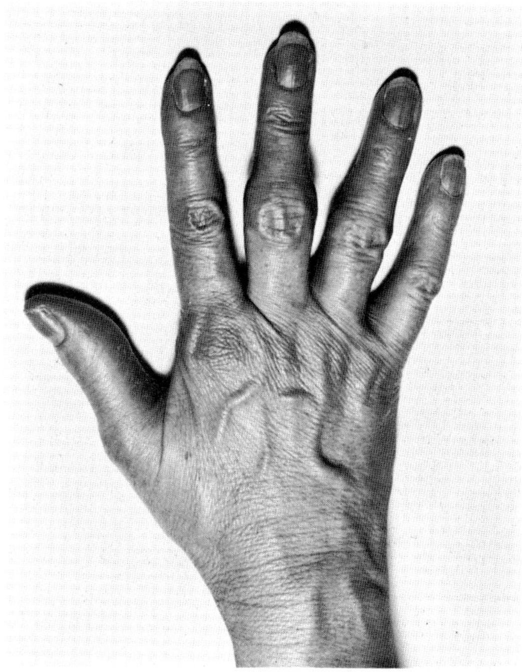

Fig. 49.23 Relapsing polychondritis showing swelling of the proximal interphalangeal joints.

joint manifestations occur continuous inflammation is more common. Cartilage inflammation is the characteristic pathology although articular involvement is usually recognised as a polyarthritis, with negative tests for rheumatoid factor usually without erosive radiological change. However radiological 'erosions' may develop (Fig. 49.24), presumably due to cartilage destruction and inflammatory reaction, leading to erroneous diagnosis of rheumatoid arthritis, especially if hoarseness is attributed to cricoarytenoid joint involvement, the correct diagnosis being revealed by the detection of involvement of other cartilagenous structures which may require laryngoscopy.

Treatment remains symptomatic with analgesics unless serious and potentially life-threatening manifestations develop, especially of the larynx and trachea, when corticosteroids and immunosuppressives may suppress the inflammatory process. Tracheostomy may be required.

McAdam et al (1976) reported that 30% of their patients died on average 4.2 years after diagnosis, from respiratory or cardiovascular manifestations of the disease or from malignancy.

Eosinophilic fasciitis

This conditions was first described by Shulman (1974) as a diffuse fasciitis with hypergammaglobulinaemia and an eosinophilic leucocytosis. The more concise term of 'eosinophilic fasciitis' may be misleading as eosinophils are not always present in the fasciitis itself.

The disease, which affects young and middle-aged men and women, is usually of rapid onset, apparently often after unusual strenuous exertion and in the autumn or winter (Moutsopoulos et al, 1980). Tightness and thickening of the skin and subcutis of the limb and trunk develop with loss of surface features, restriction of movement and contractures for example of the shoulders and elbows. The disease is usually symmetrical and

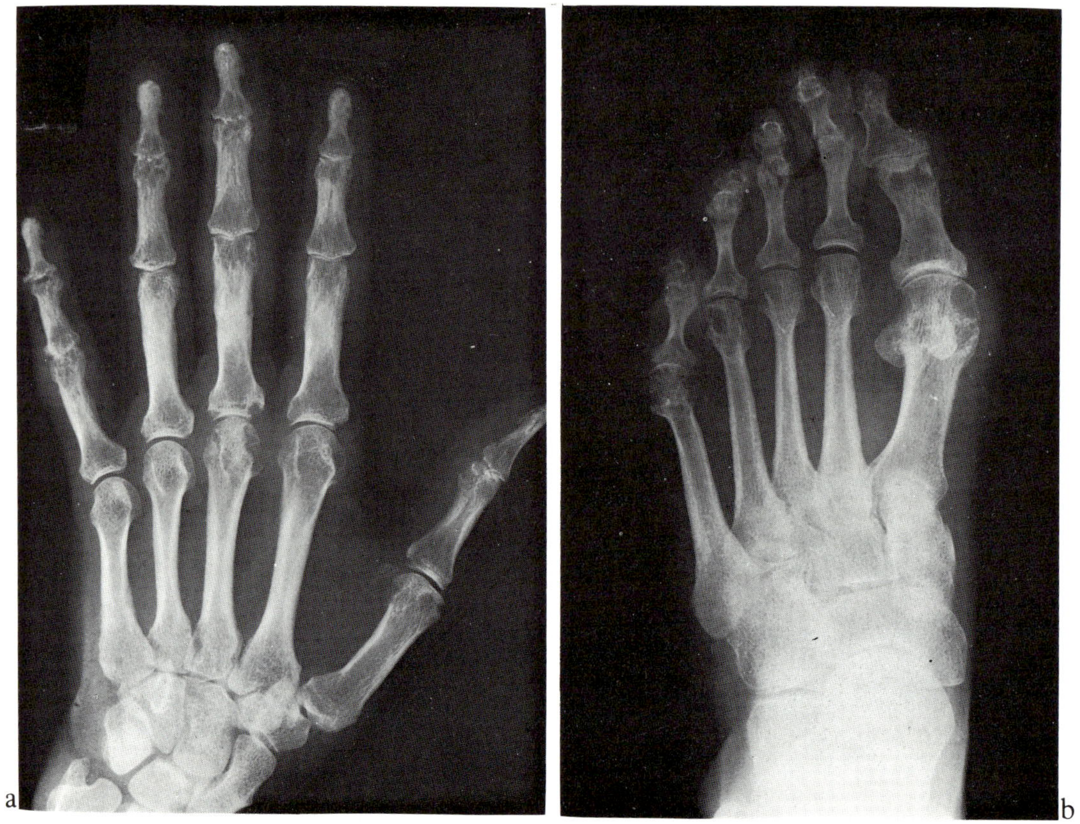

Fig. 49.24 Relapsing polychondritis. Radiographs of (a) hand and (b) foot, showing 'erosions'.

generalised, sparing the face although localised fasciitis in a child has been reported (Kaplinsky et al, 1980a). Raynaud's phenomenon very rarely occurs (Kaplinsky et al, 1980b). Polymyositis may occur and superficial inflammatory changes may be present at the surface of muscles adjacent to active fasciitis (Schumacher, 1976). Telangiectasia, oesophageal involvement and calcinosis have not been recorded. Proteinuria, splenomegaly and pulmonary involvement rarely occur (Caspi et al, 1982). Other clinical features include polyarticular synovitis (Rosenthal & Benson, 1980; Kent et al, 1981) affecting small and medium-sized joints of upper and lower limbs, and peripheral nerve entrapment syndromes (carpal tunnel syndrome, ulnar and lateral popliteal nerves) (Barnes et al, 1979; Kaplinsky et al, 1980b; Wollheim et al, 1981). Association has been reported with Hashimoto's thyroiditis and Grave's disease (Smiley et al, 1980), Hodgkin's disease (Michaels, 1982), aplastic anaemia and thrombocytopenia. Peripheral blood eosinophilia is recorded in the majority of, but not all, patients (Moore & Zuckner, 1980; Moutsopoulos et al, 1980) as is hypergammaglobulinaemia, but rheumatoid factor and anti-nuclear antibody tests are usually negative and circulating immune complexes have not been detected (Moutsopoulos et al, 1980).

Diagnosis is made by a full thickness biopsy through skin and subcutaneous tissue to muscle. The deep fascia is greatly thickened with fibrosis and infiltration with inflammatory cells (lymphocytes, plasma cells and histiocytes), which may spread into the superficial zone of muscle (Fig. 49.25). Eosinophils are only occasionally seen histologically. In contrast to scleroderma, skin and skin appendages are rarely affected.

Treatment with corticosteroids results in resolution of the disease in the majority of patients, usually within 2–4 years. However there are case

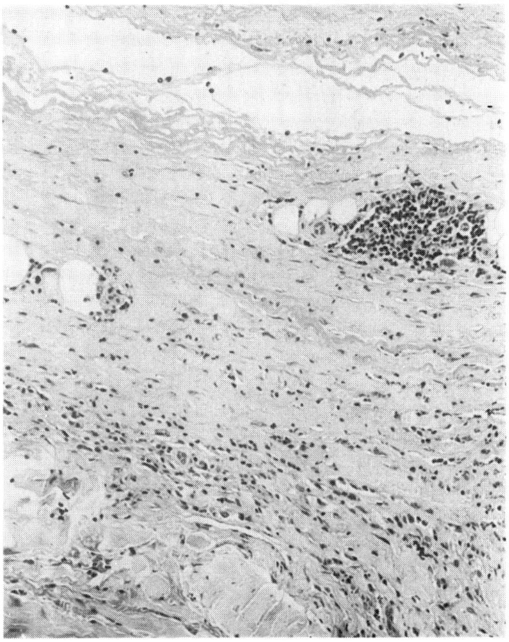

Fig. 49.25 Fasciitis with eosinophilia, showing fibrin deposition and chronic inflammation in the fibrous tissue of the fascia and extension of the inflammatory process into the superficial part of the underlying skeletal muscle (at bottom of illustration). (H & E ×400)

reports appearing of chronic skin and subcutaneous thickening and contracture which are not, or only partly, responsive to steroid treatment (Bertken & Shaller, 1983).

The place of eosinophilic fasciitis in the classification of the rheumatic disease is uncertain as is its cause. The condition has been considered by some as a variant of progressive systemic sclerosis (scleroderma). However others consider that the usual lack of visceral involvement, eosinophilia and the histological changes distinguish eosinophilic fasciitis from other conditions and that it should be categorised separately (Moutsopoulos et al, 1980).

No definite or consistent immunological disturbances have been detected. The presence of eosinophilia raises the possibility of hypersensitivity to an unknown allergen, and one case following treatment with phenytoin, which resolved on cessation of the drug, has been reported (Buchanan et al, 1980). Granulomatous vasculitis has been detected histologically in two cases (Lewkonia et al, 1982).

Atrial myxoma

Arthralgia with Raynaud's phenomenon, weight loss and fever may accompany an atrial myxoma. Although the arthralgia is located in both the limb girdles and peripheries no true clinical synovitis is present. Multiple systemic manifestations have also been recorded simulating polyarteritis nodosa (Thomas, 1981). The ESR is raised, normochromic anaemia and elevation of α_2 and γ-globulins are present, tests for serum rheumatoid factors remain negative.

Although the myxoma may produce embolisation the rheumatic manifestations are widespread and not likely to be embolic phenomenona. Surgical removal of the tumour produces relief of symptoms (Currey et al, 1967; Thomas, 1981).

REFERENCES

Aktulga E, et al 1980 A double-blind study of colchicine in Behçet's disease. Haematologica 65: 399–402

Allen D M, Diamond L H, Howell D A 1960 Anaphylactoid purpura in children (Henoch-Schönlein syndrome). American Journal of Diseases of Children 99: 833–854

Anderson I F 1965 Mafucci's syndrome — report of a case with review of the literature. South African Medical Journal 39: 1066–1070

Argen R J, Dixon A S 1963 Clutton's joints with keratitis and periostitis. A case report with histology of synovium. Arthritis and Rheumatism 6: 341–348

Ashurst P J C 1964 Relapsing pustular eruptions of the hands and feet. British Journal of Dermatology 76: 169–180

Bakhshandeh K, Nasr K, Haghighi P, Haghshenas M 1971 Clubbing and osteoarthropathy associated with primary upper small intestinal lymphoma. Journal of Tropical Medicine and Hygiene 74: 117–119

Barnes C G 1979 Behçet's syndrome — joint manifestations and synovial pathology. In: Lehner T, Barnes C G (eds) Behçet's syndrome: clinical and immunological features. Academic Press, London, Ch. 17, p. 199

Barnes L, Rodnan G P, Medsger T A, Short D 1979 Eosinophilic fasciitis — a pathologic study of 20 cases. American Journal of Pathology 96: 493–518

Batsakis J G, Nishiyama R H, Sullinger G D 1967 Synovial sarcoma of the neck. Archives of Otolaryngology 85: 327–331

Beaufils H et al 1980 Kidney involvement in Behçet's syndrome. Virchows Archives A of Pathology, Anatomy and Histology 388: 187–198

Behçet H 1940 Some observations on the clinical picture of the so-called triple symptom complex. Dermatologica (Basel) 81: 73–83

Behçet's Disease Research Committee of Japan 1974 Behçet's disease: guide to diagnosis of Behçet's disease. Japanese Journal of Ophthalmology 18: 291–294
Ben Ayed H, Hamza M 1976 La maladie de Behçet. Imprimerie Officielle, Tunis
Ben-Dov I, Zimmerman J 1982 Deforming arthritis of the hands in Behçet's disease. Journal of Rheumatology 9: 617–618
Bennett R M, Ginsberg M H, Thomsen S 1976 Carcinomatous polyarthritis: the presenting symptom of an ovarian tumour and association with a platelet activating factor. Arthritis and Rheumatism 19: 953–959
Berkowitz D 1964 Blood lipid and uric acid interrelationships. Journal of the American Medical Association 190: 856–858
Berkowitz D 1966 Gout, hyperlipaemia and diabetes. Journal of the American Medical Association 197: 77–80
Bertken R, Shalter D, 1983 Chronic progressive eosinophilic fasciitis: report of a 20 year failure to attain remission Annals of the Rheumatic Diseases 42: 103–105
Bertoni F, Boriani S, Laus M, Campanacci M 1982 Periosteal chondrosarcoma and periosteal osteosarcoma. Journal of Bone and Joint Surgery 64B: 370–376
Bland J H, Frymayer J W, Newberg A H, Revers R, Normal R J 1979 Rheumatic syndrome in endocrine disease. Seminars in Arthritis and Rheumatism 9: 23–64
Bleyer W A et al 1982 Improved three-year disease-free survival in osteogenic sarcoma. Journal of Bone and Joint Surgery 64B: 233–238
Bloch C 1962 Post radiation osteogenic sarcoma. American Journal of Roentgenology 87, 1157–1162
Blomgren S E 1974 Erythema nodosum. Seminars in Arthritis and Rheumatism 4: 1–24
Bobechko W P, Kostvik J P 1968 Childhood villonodular synovitis. Canadian Journal of Surgery 11, 480–486
Boyd R E, Andrews B S 1981 Sarcoidosis presenting as cutaneous ulceration, subcutaneous nodules and chronic arthritis. Journal of Rheumatology 8: 311–316
Breimer C W, Freiberger R H 1958 Bone lesions associated with villonodular synovitis. American Journal of Roentgenology 79: 618–629
Bruckner F E, Kendall B E 1969 Neuroarthropathy in Charcot–Marie–Tooth disease. Annals of the Rheumatic Diseases 28: 577–583
Buchan D J, Mitchell D M 1967 Hypertrophic osteoarthropathy in portal cirrhosis. Annals of Internal Medicine 66: 130–135
Buchanan R C, Gordon D A, Muckle T J, McKenna F, Kraag G 1980 The eosinophilic fasciitis syndrome after phenytoin (Dilantin) therapy. Journal of Rheumatology 7: 733–736
Buckingham R B, Bole G G, Bassett D R 1975 Polyarthritis associated with type IV hyperlipoproteinaemia. Archives of Internal Medicine 135: 286–290
Buckley C E, Gibbs J P 1969 Cyclophosphamide therapy of Behçet's disease. Journal of Allergy 43: 273–283
Burns R E, Coleville J M 1959 Acne conglobata with septicemia. Archives of Dermatology 79: 361–362
Byers P D, Cotton R E, Deacon O W, Lowy M, Newman P H, Sissons H A, Thomson A D 1968 The diagnosis and treatment of pigmented villonodular synovitis. Journal of Bone and Joint Surgery 50B: 290–309
Bywaters E G, Isdale I, Kempton J J 1957 Schönlein — Henoch purpura. Quarterly Journal of Medicine 50: (NS26) 161–175
Cadman N L, Soule E H, Kelly P J 1965 Synovial sarcoma. Cancer 18: 613–627
Calabro J J 1967 Cancer and arthritis. Arthritis and Rheumatism 10: 553–567
Calabro J J, Marchesano J M, Abruzzo J L 1966 Idiopathic hypertrophic osteoarthropathy (pachydermoperiostosis): onset before puberty. Arthritis and Rheumatism 9:496
Caspi D, Fishel R, Varon M, Yona E, Baratz M, Yaron M 1982 Multisystem presentation of eosinophilic fasciitis. Rheumatology and Rehabilitation 21: 218–221
Casser L 1956 Anaphylactoid purpura following penicillin therapy. Journal of the Medical Society of New Jersey 53: 133–134
Cavanaugh J J A, Holman G H 1965 Hypertrophic osteoarthropathy in childhood. Journal of Paediatrics 66: 27–40
Chamberlain M A 1977 Behçet's syndrome in 32 patients in Yorkshire. Annals of the Rheumatic Diseases 36: 491–499
Channon G M, Williams L A 1982 Giant-cell tumour of the ischium treated by embolisation and resection. Journal of Bone and Joint Surgery 64B: 164–165
Clark W S 1958 Pigmented villonodular synovitis. Bulletin of the Rheumatic Diseases 8: 161–162
Clegg D O, Samuelson C O, Williams H J, Ward J R 1980 Articular complications of jejunoileal bypass surgery. Journal of Rheumatology 7: 65–70
Clement G B, Vasey F B, Fenske N A, Bridgeford P, Germain B F, Espinoza L R 1982 Acne arthritis: clinical manifestations, human leukocyte antigens, and circulating immune complexes. Arthritis and Rheumatism 25 (Suppl):S12 Abstract 58
Cohen M D, Harrington T M, Ginsberg W W 1982 Osteoid osteoma: a review of 95 patients. Arthritis and Rheumatism 25 (Suppl):S154 Abstract E93
Cooper D A, Penny R 1974 Behçet's syndrome: clinical immunological and therapeutic evaluation of 17 patients. Australian and New Zealand Journal of Medicine 4: 585–596
Coventry M B, Harrison E G, Martin J D 1966 Benign synovial tumours of the knee: a diagnostic problem. Journal of Bone and Joint Surgery 48A: 1350–1358
Cronemeyer R L, Kirchmer N A, Smet A A de, Neff J R 1981 Intra-articular osteoidosteoma of the humerus simulating synovitis of the elbow. Journal of Bone and Joint Surgery 63A: 1172–1174
Cunliffe W J, Menon I S 1969 Treatment of Behçet's syndrome with phenformin and ethyloestrenol. Lancet 1: 1239–1240
Currey H L F, Mathews J A, Robinson J 1967 Right atrial myxoma mimicking a rheumatic disorder. British Medical Journal 1: 547–548
Davies P G, Fordham J N, Kirwan J R, Barnes C G, Dinning W J 1984 The Pathergy test and Behçet's syndrome in Britain. Annals of the Rheumatic Diseases 43: 70–73
Davis D E, Viozzi F J, Miller F, Blodgett R 1981 The musculoskeletal manifestation of acne fulminans. Journal of Rheumatology 8: 317–320
Dawes P T, Raman D, Haslock I 1983 Acute synovial rupture in Behçet's syndrome. Annals of the Rheumatic Diseases 42: 591–592
Delamere J P, Baddeley R M, Walton K W 1983 Jejuno-ileal bypass arthropathy: its clinical features and associations Annals of the Rheumatic Diseases 42: 553–557
Denman A M, Hollingworth P, Webster A D B, Pelton B K,

Rhodes E L 1979 Failure of transfer factor in the treatment of Behçet's syndrome: a double-blind trial. In: Lehner T, Barnes C G (eds) Behçet's syndrome; clinical and immunological features. Academic Press, London, Ch. 23, p. 277
Derham R J, Rogerson M M 1956 The Schönlein–Henoch syndrome with particular reference to renal sequelae. Archives of Diseases in Childhood 31: 364–368
Dilsen N, Konice M, Ovul C 1979 Arthritic patterns in Behçet's disease. In: Dilsen N, Konice M, Ovul C (eds) Behçet's disease. Excerpta Medical International Congress, Series 467. Excerpta Medica, Amsterdam, p. 145
Dilsen N, Konice M, Ovul C, Erbengi T, Gursoy E 1981. Three cases of renal amyloidosis with Behçet's disease. In: International Conference on Behçet's Disease. Japan Medical Research Foundation, p. 56
Dixon A St J 1963 Unusual effects of bronchial carcinoma and other lung tumours. Thorax 18:197
Donlan D G, Lemmon G B, Teitelbaum S L 1966 Relapsing polychondritis: analytical literature review and studies on pathogenesis. American Journal of Medicine 41: 285–299
Dudgeon J A 1961 Virological aspects of Behçet's disease. Proceedings of the Royal Society of Medicine 54: 104–106
Ebringer R, Rook G, Swana G T, Bottazzo G F, Doniach D 1981 Autoantibodies to cartilage and type II collagen in relapsing polychondritis and other rheumatic diseases. Annals of the Rheumatic Diseases 40: 473–479
Eglin R P, Lehner T, Subak-Sharpe J H 1982 Detection of RNA complementary to Herpes-Simplex virus in mononuclear cells from patients with Behçet's syndrome and recurrent oral ulcers. Lancet 1: 1356–1356
Ehrenfeld M, Levy M, Sharon P, Rachmilewitz D, Eliakim M 1982 Malabsorption of long-term colchicine therapy in recurrent polyserositis (familial Mediterranean fever). Arthritis and Rheumatism 25 (Suppl):S141, Abstract E17
Enoch B A, Castillo-Olivares J L, Khoo T C L, Grainger R G, Henry L 1968 Major vascular complications in Behçet's syndrome. Postgraduate Medical Journal 44: 453–459
Epstein O, Ajdukiewicz A B, Dick R, Sherlock S 1979 Hypertrophic hepatic osteoarthropathy. Clinical roentgenologic, biochemical, hormonal and cardiorespiratory studies, and review of the literature. American Journal of Medicine 67: 88–97
Evans A D, Pallis C A, Spillane J D 1957 Involvement of the nervous system in Behçet's syndrome. Lancet 2: 349–353
Evans W K 1980 Reversal of hypertrophic osteoarthropathy after chemotherapy for bronchogenic carcinoma. Journal of Rheumatology 7: 93–97
Fam A G, Cross E G 1979 Hypertrophic osteoarthropathy, phalangeal and synovial metastases associated with bronchogenic carcinoma. Journal of Rheumatology 6: 680–686
Fam A G, Kolin A, Lewis A J 1980 Metastatic carcinomatous arthritis and carcinoma of the lung: a report of two cases diagnosed by synovial fluid cytology. Journal of Rheumatology 7: 98–104
Farman J, Twersky J, Fierst S 1976 Ulcerative colitis associated with hypertrophic osteoarthropathy. Digestive Diseases 21: 130–135
Fechner R E, Fraire A E 1972 Intra-articular localised nodular synovitis of the knee. Archives of Pathology 93: 473–476
Feldman M J, Becker K L, Reefe W E, Longo A 1969 Multiple neuropathic joints including cases in patients with diabetes mellitus. Journal of the American Medical Association 209: 1690–1692
Fiddes P H 1971 Behçet's syndrome with a cryoparaprotein. Medical Journal of Australia 1: 1275–1277
Fielding J F, Cooke W T 1971 Finger clubbing and regional enteritis. Gut 12: 442–444
Fine R M, Meltzer H D 1968 Erythema nodosum — a form of allergic cutaneous vasculitis. Southern Medical Journal 61: 680–686
Fischer D S, Singer D H, Feldman S M 1964 Clubbing: a review, with emphasis on hereditary acropachy. Medicine (Baltimore) 43: 459–479
Fitzgerald J A W 1968 Neuropathic arthropathy secondary to atypical congenital indifference to pain. Proceedings of the Royal Society of Medicine 61: 663–664
Flateau E, Kohn D, Schiller D, Lurie M, Levy E 1982 Schönlein–Henoch syndrome in patients with familial Mediterranean fever. Arthritis and Rheumatism 25: 42–47
Flavell G 1956 Reversal of pulmonary hypertrophic osteoarthropathy by vagotomy. Lancet 1: 260–262
Ford P M 1970 Thyroid acropachy. Proceedings of the Royal Society of Medicine 63: 284–285
Franck W A, Hoffman G S, Davis J S, Alpern H D, Olson J E 1979 Osteomalacia and weakness complicating jejunoileal bypass. Journal of Rheumatology 6: 51–56
Fredrickson D S, Levy R I, Lees R S 1967 Fat transport in lipoproteins — an integrated approach to mechanism and disorders. New England Journal of Medicine 276: 34–44, 94–103, 148–156, 215–225, 273–281
Gabbiani G, Manjo G 1972 Dupuytren's contracture: fibroblast contraction? An ultrastructual study. American Journal of Pathology 66: 131–147
Gabbiani G, Kaye G I, Lattes R, Manjo G 1971 Synovial sarcoma. Electron microscopic study of a typical case. Cancer 28: 1031–1039
Gairdner D 1948 The Schönlein–Henoch syndrome (anaphylactoid purpura). Quarterly Journal of Medicine NS17: 95– : 95–122
Gall E P, Didizian N A, Park Y 1974 Acute monoarticular arthritis following patella metastasis, a manifestation of carcinoma of the lung. Journal of the American Medical Association 229: 188–189
Gardner D L 1965 Pathology of the connective tissue diseases. Edward Arnold, London
Ghelman B, Thompson F M, Arnold W D 1981 Intraoperative radioactive localisation of an osteoid-osteoma. Journal of Bone and Joint Surgery 63A: 826–827
Gibson G J, Davis P 1974 Resp? Respiratory complications of relapsing polychondritis. Thorax 29: 726–731
Gibson T, Laurent R, Highton J, Wilton M, Dyson M, Millie R 1981 Synovial histopathology of Behçet's syndrome. Annals of the Rheumatic Diseases 40: 376–381
Gitelis S, Bertoni F, Picci P, Campanacci M 1981 Chondrosarcoma of bone. Journal of Bone and Joint Surgery 63A: 1248–1256
Glueck C J, Levy R I, Fredrickson D S 1968 Acute tendinitis and arthritis. Journal of the American Medical Association 206: 2895–2897
Goldenberg D L, Kelley W, Gibbons R B 1975 Metastatic adenocarcinoma of synovium presenting as an acute arthritis, diagnosis by closed synovial biopsy. Arthritis and Rheumatism 18: 107–110
Goldman J A, Glueck C J, Abrams N R, Steiner P, Herman J H 1972 Musculoskeletal disorders associated with type IV hyperlipoproteinaemia. Lancet 2: 449–452

Granowitz S P, Mankin H J 1967 Localised pigmented villonodular synovitis of the knee. Journal of Bone and Joint Surgery 49A: 122–128

Granowitz S P, D'Antonio J, Mankin H L 1976 The pathogenesis and long-term results of pigmented villonodular synovitis. Clinical Orthopaedics and Related Research 114: 335–351

Gray M S, Philp T 1963 Syphilitic arthritis. Annals of the Rheumatic Diseases 22: 19–25

Greenfield G B, Schorasch H A, Shkolnik A 1967 The various roentgen appearances of pulmonary hypertrophic osteoarthropathy. American Journal of Roentgenology 101: 927–931

Gumpel J M, Johns C J, Shulman L E 1967 The joint disease of sarcoidosis. Annals of the Rheumatic Diseases 26: 194–205

Hajdu S I, Shiu H, Fortner J G 1977 Tendosynovial sarcoma. A clinicopathological study of 136 cases. Cancer 39: 1201–1217

Han S Y, Colins L C 1968 Hypertrophic osteoarthropathy in cirrhosis of the liver. Radiology 91: 795–796

Heller H, et al 1966 The arthritis of familial Mediterranean fever. Arthritis and Rheumatism 9: 1–17

Herman J H, Dennis M V 1973 Immunopathologic studies in relapsing polychondritis. Journal of Clinical Investigation 52: 549–558

Herness D, Makin M 1975 Articular damage in familial Mediterranean fever. Journal of Bone and Joint surgery 57A: 265–267

Hickling P, et al 1981 A study of amyloid arthropathy in multiple myeloma. Quarterly Journal of Medicine NS 200: 417–433

Higashihara M, Mori M, Takeuchi A, Ogita T, Miyamoto T, Okimoto T 1982 Myocarditis in Behçet's disease — a case report and review of the literature. Journal of Rheumatology 9: 630–633

Hills E A 1967 Behçet's syndrome with aortic aneurysm. British Medical Journal 4: 152–154

Hollis W C 1967 Hypertrophic osteoarthropathy secondary to upper gastrointestinal tract neoplasm. Annals of Internal Medicine 66: 125–130

Holt P J A, Davies M G, Saunders K C, Nuki G 1980 Pyoderma gangrenosum. Clinical and laboratory findings in 15 patients with special reference to polyarthritis. Medicine (Baltimore) 59: 114–133

Honska W L, Strenge J, Hammarsten J F 1957 Hypertrophic osteoarthropathy and chronic ulcerative colitis. Gastroenterology 33: 489–492

Hueston J T 1962 Digital Wolfe grafts in recurrent Dupuytren's contracture. Plastic and Reconstructive Surgery 29: 342–344

Hueston J T 1968 Dupuytren's contacture and specific injury. Medical Journal of Australia 1: 1084–1085

Hueston J T 1975 Dupuytren's contracture selection for surgery. British Journal of Hospital Medicine 13: 361–370

Hunter T, Shanahan W R, Robertson G A, Stranc M F, Schroeder M L 1981 The distribution of histocompatibility antigens in patients with Dupuytren's contracture. Arthritis and Rheumatism 24: 1218–1219

Huvos A G, Higinbotham N L, Miller T R 1972 Bone sarcoma arising in fibrous dysplasia. Journal of Bone and Joint Surgery 54A: 1047–1956

Jaffe H L, Lichtenstein L, Sutro G J 1941 Pigmented villonodular synovitis, bursitis and tenosynovitis. Archives of Pathology 31: 731–765

James J I P 1974 In: Hueston J T, Tubiana R (eds) Dupuytren's disease, 1st English Edn. Churchill Livingstone, Edinburgh

Jeffreys T E 1967 Synovial chondromatosis. Journal of Bone and Joint Surgery 49B: 530–534

Jergesen H E, Mankin H J, Schiller A L 1978 Diffuse pigmented villonodullar synovitis of the knee mimicking primary bone neoplasm. Journal of Bone and Joint Surgery 60A: 825–829

Jessop J D 1969 Familial Mediterranean fever. Proceedings of the Royal Society of Medicine 62: 199–200

Jones F E, Soule E H, Coventry M B 1969 Fibrous xanthoma of synovium (giant cell tumour of tendon sheath, pigmented nodular synovitis). Journal of Bone and Joint Surgery 51A: 76–86

Kalbian V V, Challis M T 1970 Behçet's disease: a report of 12 cases with 3 manifesting as papilledema. American Journal of Medicine 49: 823–828

Kansu E, et al 1972 Behçet's syndrome with obstruction of the venae cavae. Quarterly Journal of Medicine NS41: 151–168

Kaplinsky N, Bubis J T, Pras M 1980a Localised eosinophilic fasciitis in a child. Journal of Rheumatology 7: 541–543

Kaplinsky N, Revach M, Katz W A 1980b Eosinophilic fasciitis. Report of a case with features of connective tissue disease. Journal of Rheumatology 7: 536–540

Kaye R L, Jones D A 1964 Relapsing polychondritis. Annals of Internal Medicine 60: 653–664

Kent L T, Cramer S F, Moskowitz R W 1981 Eosinophilic fasciitis. Clinical, laboratory and microscopic considerations. Arthritis and Rheumatism 24: 677–683

Khachadurian A K 1968 Migratory polyarthritis in familial hypercholesterolaemia (type II hyperlipoproteinaemia). Arthritis and Rheumatism 11: 385–393

Kindblom L G, Gunterberg B 1978 Pigmented villonodular synovitis involving bone. Journal of Bone and Joint Surgery 60A: 830–832

King J W, Spjut H J, Fechner R E, Vanderpool D W 1967 Synovial chondrosarcoma of the knee joint. Journal of Bone and Joint Surgery 49A: 1389–1396

Kogstad O 1970 Malignant synovioma. Acta Rheumatologica Scandinavica 16: 81–90

Kronberg I J 1981 Autoimmune disturbances in relapsing polychondritis and primary alopecia. Arthritis and Rheumatism 24:862

Kumagaya H et al 1973 Two brothers with pustulosis palmaris et plantaris associated with lesions of the bilateral clavicles. Orthopaedic Surgery and Traumatology 22: 522–523

Lane A M, Leyden J I, Spiegel R J 1976 Acne arthralgia. Journal of Bone and Joint Surgery 58A: 673–675

Larsen I J, Landry R M 1969 Haemangioma of the synovial membrane. Journal of Bone and Joint Surgery 51A: 1210–1212

Lee S M, Hajdu S I, Exelby P R 1974 Synovial sarcoma in children. Surgery, Gynaecology and Obstetrics 138: 701–704

Lehner T 1967 Behçet's syndrome and autoimmunity. British Medical Journal 1: 465–466

Lehner T, Barnes C G 1979a Criteria for diagnosis and classification of Behçet's syndrome. In: Lehner T, Barnes C G (eds) Behçet's syndrome: clinical and immunological features. Academic Press, London, Ch. 1, p. 1

Lehner T, Barnes C G 1979b Behçet's syndrome: clinical and

immunological features. Academic Press, London
Lehner T, Batchelor R 1979 Classification and an immunogenetic basis of Behçet's syndrome. In: Lehner T, Barnes C G (eds) Behçet's syndrome: clinical and immunological features. Academic Press, London, Ch.2, p.13
Lehner T, Wilton J M A 1979 The therapeutic and immunological effects of levamisole in recurrent oral ulceration and Behçet's syndrome. In: Lehner T, Barnes C G (eds) Behçet's syndrome; clinical and immunological features. Academic Press, London, Ch. 24, p. 291
Lessof M H, Jefferys D B, Lehner T, Mattock M, Sanders M D 1979 Corticosteroids and azathioprine; their use in Behçet's syndrome. In: Lehner T, Barnes C G (eds) Behçet's syndrome; clinical and immunological features. Academic Press, London, Ch. 22, p. 267
Lettin A W F 1964 Dupuytren's diathesis: a case report. Journal of Bone and Joint Surgery 46B: 220–225
Levinsky R J, Barratt T M 1979 IgA immune complexes in Henoch-Schönlein purpura. Lancet 2: 1100–1103
Levo Y, Waisman Y, Ehrenfeld M, Levy M, Eliakim M 1980 Lymphocytotoxins in recurrent polyserositis. Israel Journal of Medical Sciences 16: 203–205
Lewis I C, Philpott M G 1956 Neurological complications of the Schönlein-Henoch syndrome. Archives of Diseases in Childhood 31: 369–371
Lewkonia R M, Marx L H, Atkinson M H 1982 Granulomatous vasculitis in the syndrome of diffuse fasciitis with eosinophilia. Archives of Internal Medicine 142: 73–75
Lichtenstein L 1965 Osteoid osteoma. In: Bone tumours, 3rd Edn. Mosby, St Louis, Ch. IX, p. 90
Lofgren S 1953 Primary pulmonary sarcoidosis. II. Clinical course and prognosis. Acta Medica Scandinavica 145: 424–431
Lopez-Enriquez E, Morales A R, Robert F 1980 Effect of atropine sulfate in pulmonary hypertrophic osteoarthropathy. Arthritis and Rheumatism 23: 822–824
McAdam L P, O'Hanlan M A, Bluestone R, Pearson C M 1976 Relapsing polychondritis: prospective study of 23 patients and a review of the literature. Medicine (Baltimore) 55: 193–215
Mackenzie D H 1974 Clear cell sarcoma. Journal of Pathology 114: 231–232
McLaughlin G E, McCarty D J Jr, Downing D F 1967 Hypertrophic osteoarthropathy associated with cyanotic congenital heart disease. Annals of Internal Medicine 67: 579–587
Makley J T, Dunn M J 1982 Prostaglandin synthesis by osteoid osteoma. Lancet 2:42
Mamo J G, Azzam S A 1970 Treatment of Behçet's disease with chlorambucil. Archives of Ophthalmology 84: 446–450
Manicourt D H, Orloff S 1979 Osteomalacia complicating a blind loop from congenital megaoesophagus — megaduodenum. Journal of Rheumatology 6: 57–64
Martin V M, Bennett R M, Hughes G R V, Holt P J L 1973 Lymphosarcomatous arthropathy. Annals of the Rheumatic Diseases 32: 162–166
Mason R M, Barnes C G 1969 Behçet's syndrome with arthritis. Annals of the Rheumatic Diseases 28: 95–103
Mendlowitz M 1942 Clubbing and hypertrophic osteoarthropathy. Medicine (Baltimore) 21: 296–306
Menkes C J, Feldman J-L, Job-Deslandre C 1982 Chronic sarcoid arthritis Arthritis and Rheumatism 25 (Suppl): S154, Abstract E96
Metz E N, Dowell A 1965 Bone marrow failure in hypertrophic osteoarthropathy. Archives of Internal Medicine 116: 759–764
Meyer O, Cyna J, Dryll A, Cywinder-Golenzer C, Wassef M, Ryckewaert A 1981 Relapsing polychondritis — pathogenic role of anti-native collagen type II antibodies. Journal of Rheumatology 8: 820–824
Michaels R M 1982 Eosinophilic fasciitis complicated by Hodgkin's disease. Journal of Rheumatology 9: 473–476
Miller S B, Donlan C J, Roth S B 1974 Hodgkin's disease presenting as relapsing polychondritis. Arthritis and Rheumatism 17: 598–602
Moake J L, Kageler M V, Cimo P L 1977 Intravascular hemolysis, thrombocytopenia, leukopenia and circulating immune complexes after jejunoileal bypass surgery. Annals of Internal Medicine 86: 576–578
Molnar Z, Stein W H, Stoltzner G H 1971 Cytoplasmic tubular structures in pigmented villonodular synovitis. Arthritis and Rheumatism 14: 784–787
Moore T L, Zuckner J 1980 Eosinophilic fasciitis. Seminars in Arthritis and Rheumatism 9: 228–235
Mounsey J P D 1966 Behçet's syndrome — a spectrum. Transactions of the St John's Hospital Dermatological Society 52: 197–200
Moutsopoulos H M, Webber B L, Pavlidis N A, Fostiropoulos G, Goules D, Shulman L E 1980 Diffuse fasciitis with eosinophilia: a clinicopathologic study. American Journal of Medicine 68: 701–709
Mullins G M, Lenhard R E 1971 Digital clubbing in Hodgkin's disease. Johns Hopkins Medical Journal 128: 153–157
Murphy F B, Dahlin D C, Sullivan C R 1962 Articular synovial chondromatosis. Journal of Bone and Joint Surgery 44A 77–86
Murray G L, Persillin R H 1980 Metastatic carcinoma presenting as monarticular arthritis: a case report and review of the literature. Arthritis and Rheumatism 23: 95–100
Neale G, Kelsall A R, Doyle F H 1968 Crohn's disease and diffuse symmetrical periostitis. Gut 9: 383–387
Neville E, Carstairs L S, James D G 1977 Sarcoidosis of Bone. Quarterly Journal of Medicine (NS46) 182: 215–227
Neville E, Walker A N, James D G 1983 Prognostic factors predicting the outcome of sarcoidosis: an analysis of 818 patients. Quarterly Journal of Medicine (NS 52) 208: 525–533
Nilsonne U, Moberger G 1969 Pigmented villonodular synovitis of joints. Histological and clinical problems in diagnosis. Acta Orthopaedica Scandinavica 40: 448–460
Odkuist L 1970 Relapsing polychondritis. Acta Otolaryngologica 70: 448–454
O'Duffy J D 1974 Suggested criteria for diagnosis of Behçet's disease. Journal of Rheumatology 1 (Suppl 1): 18(abstract)
O'Duffy J D 1978 Summary of international symposium on Behçet's syndrome. Journal of Rheumatology 5: 229–233
O'Duffy J D, Carney J A, Deodhar S 1971 Behçet's disease. Report of 10 cases, 3 with new manifestations. Annals of Internal Medicine 75: 561–570
Ohno S, Nakayama E, Sugiura S, Itakura K, Aoki K, Aizawa M 1975 Specific histocompatibility antigens associated with Behçet's disease. American Journal of Ophthalmology 80: 636–641
Oshima Y, et al 1963 Clinical studies on Behçet's syndrome. Annals of the Rheumatic Diseases 22: 36–45
Palatsi R 1977 Delayed hypersensitivity and febrile acne

conglobata. Acta Dermatovener (Stockholm) 57: 51–53
Pantazopoulos Th, Stavrou S, Stamos C, Kehayas G, Hartofilakidis-Gerofalidis G 1975 Bone lesions in pigmented villonodular synovitis. Acta Orthopaedica Scandinavica 46: 579–592
Paykoc S, Sumer N, Ertan A, Akit A 1979 Cyclic nucleotides in familial Mediterranean fever. New England Journal of Medicine 300: 1160–1161
Pearson C M, Kline H M, Newcomer V D 1960 Relapsing polychondritis. New England Journal of Medicine 263: 51–58
Pennec Y, Youinou P, Goff P le, Boles J M, Menn G le 1982 Comparison of the manifestations of acute sarcoid arthritis with and without erythema nodosum. Scandinavian Journal of Rheumatology 11: 13–16
Perry H O, Brunsting L A 1957 Pyoderma gangrenosum: a clinical study of 19 cases. Archives of Dermatology 75: 380–386
Piette J C, Beaufils H, Wechsler B, Herson S, Godeau P 1982 Relapsing polychondritis with glomerulonephritis. Arthritis and Rheumatism 25 (Suppl):S149, abstract E67
Prusanski W, Baron M, Shupak R 1981 Neuroarthropathy (Charcot joints) in familial amyloid polyneuropathy. Journal of Rheumatology 8: 477–481
Raben M, Calabrese A, Higinbotham N L, Phillips R 1965 Malignant synovioma. American Journal of Roentgenology 93: 145–153
Rajapakse D A, Bywaters E G L 1974 Cell mediated immunity to cartilage proteoglycan in relapsing polychondritis. Clinical and Experimental Immunology 16: 497–502
Rajka G 1977 Cell mediated immunity and acne conglobata. Acta Dermatovener (Stockholm) 57: 141–143
Reeves B 1966 Haemangioma of the knee joint. Proceedings of the Royal Society of Medicine 59: 705–706
Reimann H A, Coppola E D, Villegas G R 1970 Serum complement defects in periodic diseases. Annals of Internal Medicine 73: 737–740
Richardson J A, Diddams A C 1962 Maffuci's syndrome. Archives of Internal Medicine 109: 186–191
Rifkind B M 1970 The hyperlipoproteinaemias. British Journal of Hospital Medicine 4: 683–692
Rimoin D L 1965 Pachydermoperiostosis (idiopathic clubbing and periostosis). Genetic and physiological considerations. New England Journal of Medicine 272: 923–931
Rissanen P M, Holsti 1970 Synovial sarcoma and its treatment. Oncology 24: 108–117
Rooney P J, Dallantype D, Buchanan W W 1975 Disorders of the locomotor system associated with lipid metabolism and the lipoidoses. Clinics in Rheumatic Diseases 1: 163–194
Rooney P J, Thind J, Madkour M M, Spencer D, Dick W C 1978 Transient polyarthritis associated with familial hyperbeta-lipoproteinaemia. Quarterly Journal of Medicine (NS 47) 187: 249–259
Rose E, Espinoza L R, Osterland C K 1977 Intestinal bypass arthritis: association with circulating immune complexes and HLA B27. Journal of Rheumatology 4: 129–134
Rosenthal J, Benson M D 1980 Diffuse fasciitis and eosinophilia with symmetric polyarthritis. Annals of Internal Medicine 92: 507–509
Rosenthal T, Bank H, Aladjem M, David R, Gafni J 1975 Systemic amyloidosis in Behçet's disease. Annals of Internal Medicine 83: 220–223
Rosselet E, Saudan Y, Zenklusen G 1968 L'effect de l'azathioprine (Imuran) dans la maladie de Behçet. Schweizerische Medizinische Wochenschrift 98: 627
Rothschild B M, Yoon B H 1982 Thyroid acropachy complicated by lymphatic obstruction. Arthritis and Rheumatism 25: 588–590
Roux B T 1968 Bronchial carcinoma with hypertrophic pulmonary osteoarthropathy. South African Medical Journal 42: 1074–1075
Ryan J R, Baker L H, Benjamin R S 1982 The natural history of metastatic synovial sarcoma. Clinical Orthopaedics and Related Research 164: 257–260
Salfeld K, Spalckhaver I 1966 Zur Kenntnis der Pachydermoperiostosis. Dermatologische Wochenschrift 152: 497–511
Sams W M Jr, Winkelmann R K 1968 The association of erythema nodosum and ulcerative colitis. Southern Medical Journal 61: 676–679
Savi M, Asinari G, Gaudiano V, Olivetti G, Neri T M 1978 Unusual immunologic findings in familial Mediterranean fever. Archives of Internal Medicine 138: 644–645
Scanlon G T, Clemett A R 1964 Thyroid acropachy. Radiology 83: 1039–1042
Schajowicz F, Blumenfeld I 1968 Pigmented villonodular synovitis of the wrist with penetration into bone. Journal of Bone and Joint Surgery 508: 312–317
Schwarz G S, Berenyi M R, Siegel N W 1969 Atrophic arthritis and diabetic neuritis. American Journal of Roentgenology 106: 523–529
Schwartz J A 1981 Pro-Banthine for hypertrophic osteoarthropathy. Arthritis and Rheumatism 24:1588 (letter)
Sezer F N 1953 The isolation of a virus as the cause of Behçet's disease. American Journal of Ophthalmology 36: 301–315
Sezer N 1956 Further investigations on the virus of Behçet's disease. American Journal of Ophthalmology 41: 41–55
Shenberger K N, Morgan G J 1982 Recurrent malignant melanoma presenting as monarthritis. Journal of Rheumatology 9: 328–330
Sherman M S 1947 Osteoid osteoma. Journal of Bone and Joint Surgery 29: 918–930
Shimizu T 1977 Behçet's disease: a systemic inflammatory disease. In: Vascular lesions of collagen diseases and related conditions. University of Tokyo Press, Tokyo, Ch. VI–1, p. 201
Shimizu T, Katsuka Y, Oshima Y 1965 Immunological studies on Behçet's syndrome. Annals of the Rheumatic Diseases 24: 494–500
Shimizu T, Ehrlich G E, Inaba G, Hayashi K 1979 Behçet disease (Behçet syndrome). Seminars in Arthritis and Rheumatism 8: 223–260
Shulman L E 1974 Diffuse fasciitis with hypergamma-globulinaemia and eosinophilia: a new syndrome. Journal of Rheumatology 1 (Suppl 1): 82
Schumacher H R 1976 A scleroderma-like syndrome with fasciitis, myositis and eosinophilia. Annals of Internal Medicine 84: 49–50
Siegelman S S, Schlossberg I, Becker N H, Sachs B A 1972 Hyperlipoproteinaemia with skeletal lesions. Clinical Orthopaedics 87: 229–232
Siltzbach L E, Duberstein J L 1968 Arthritis in sarcoidosis. Clinical Orthopaedics 57: 31–50
Sinha S, Munichoodappa C S, Kozak G P 1972 Neuro-arthropathy (Charcot joints) in diabetes mellitus. Medicine 51: 191–210

Smiley A M, Husain M, Indenbaum S 1980 Eosinophilic fasciitis in association with thyroid disease. Journal of Rheumatology 7: 871–876

Smith J H, Pugh D J 1962 Roentgenographic aspects of articular pigmented villonodular synovitis. American Journal of Roentgenology 87: 1146–1156

Snarr J W, Abell M R, Martel W 1973 Lymphofollicular synovitis with osteoid osteoma. Radiology 106: 557–560

Sohar E, Gafni J, Pras M, Heller J 1967 Familial Mediterranean fever, a survey of 470 cases and review of the literature. American Journal of Medicine 43: 227–253

Soloman L 1961 Bone growth in diaphysial aclasis. Journal of Bone and Joint Surgery 43B: 700–716

Soloman L 1963 Hereditary multiple exostosis. Journal of Bone and Joint Surgery 45B: 292–304

Sonozaki H, et al 1981a Clinical features of 53 cases with pustulotic arthro-osteitis. Annals of the Rheumatic Diseases 40: 547–553

Sonozaki H, et al 1981b Incidence of arthro-osteitis in patients with pustulosis palmaris and plantaris. Annals of the Rheumatic Diseases 40: 554–557

Spilberg I, Silzback L E, McEwan C 1969 The arthritis of sarcoidosis. Arthritis and Rheumatism 12: 126–137

Spring M 1951 Purpura and nephritis after administration of procaine penicillin. Journal of the Americal Medical Association 147: 1139–1141

Stenseth J H, Clagett O T, Woolner L B 1967 Hypertrophic pulmonary osteoarthropathy. Diseases of the Chest 52: 62–68

Stevens J, Katz P L, Archer F L, McCarty D J 1969 Synovial haemangioma of the knee. Arthritis and Rheumatism 12:647

Stolman L P, Rosenthal D, Yaworsky R, Horan F 1975 Pyoderma gangrenosum and rheumatoid arthritis. Archives of Dermatology 111: 1020–1023

Storey G O 1964 Charcot's joints. British Journal of Venereal Disease 40: 109–117

Susmano A, Shah P, Krompotic E 1967 Normal sex-chromosomal complement in a case of familial osteoarthropathy. Lancet 2: 131–133

Suzuki K, Mizuno N 1981 Intracutaneous test with physiological saline in Behçet's disease. In: International Conference on Behçet's Disease. Japan Medical Research Foundation. p 44

Sweet D L, Mass D P, Simon M A, Shapiro C M 1981 Histiocytic lymphoma (reticulum-cell sarcoma) of bone. Journal of Bone and Joint Surgery 63A: 79–84

Sweetnam R 1982 Osteosarcoma. British Journal of Hospital Medicine 28: 112–121

Talbot P S 1967 Sarcoid myopathy. British Medical Journal 4: 465–466

Thomas M H 1981 Myxoma masquerading as polyarteritis nodosa. Journal of Rheumatology 8: 133–137

Thompson D M, Main R A, Beck J S, Albert-Recht F 1973 Studies on a patient with leucocytoplastic vasculitis, pyoderma gangrenosum and paraproteinaemia. British Journal of Dermatology 88: 117–125

Touraine A 1955 L'aphtose: données récentes et synthese. Presse Medicale 63: 1493–1495

Truelove L H 1960 Articular manifestations of erythema nodosum. Annals of the Rheumatic Diseases 19: 174–180

Ueno Y, Cassell S, Barnett E V 1981a Hypertrophic osteoarthropathy and pseudomembranous enterocolitis. Journal of Rheumatology 8: 825–828

Ueno Y, Chia D, Barnett E V 1981b Relapsing polychondritis associated with ulcerative colitis. Journal of Rheumatology 8: 456–461

Verity M A, Larson W M, Madden S C 1963 Relapsing polychondritis. American Journal of Pathology 42: 251–269

Vernier R L, Worthen H G, Patersen R D, Colle E, Good R A 1961 Anaphylactoid purpura. Pediatrics 27: 181–193

Vernon-Roberts B, Barnes C G, Revell P A 1978 Synovial pathology in Behçet's syndrome. Annals of the Rheumatic Diseases 37: 139–145

Viljanto J A 1973 Dupuytren's contracture: a review. Seminars in Arthritis and Rheumatism 3: 155–176

Vilppula A H, Yli-Kerttula U I, Aine R A T, Ojala A T 1982 Pigmented villonodular synovitis. Scandinavian Journal of Rheumatology 11: 145–149

Virshup A M, Sliwinski A J 1973 Polyarthritis and subcutaneous nodules associated with carcinoma of the pancreas. Arthritis and Rheumatism 16: 388–392

Wasser K B, et al 1982 Pulmonary hypertrophic osteoarthropathy in cystic fibrosis: a survey of 375 patients. Arthritis and Rheumatism 25 (Suppl): S154 Abstract E94

Weinblatt M E, Karp G I 1981 Monarticular arthritis: early manifestation of a rhabdomyosarcoma. Journal of Rheumatology 8: 685–688

Williams B L 1967 Acropachy in a case of thyrotoxicosis. Proceedings of the Royal Society of Medicine 60: 899–900

Williams D G, Lehner T 1979 Renal manifestations of Behçet's syndrome. In: Lehner T, Barnes C G (eds) Behçet's syndrome: clinical and immunological features. Academic Press, London. Ch. 21, p. 259

Williams K, Scott J T 1967 Influence of trauma on the development of chronic inflammatory polyarthritis. Annals of the Rheumatic Diseases 26: 532–537

Winter P F, Johnson P M, Hilal S K, Feldman F 1977 Scintigraphic detection of osteoid osteoma. Radiology 122: 177–178

Wolfe S J, Summerskill W H J, Davidson C S 1956 Thickening and contraction of the palmar fascia (Dupuytren's contracture) associated with alcoholism and hepatic cirrhosis. New England Journal of Medicine 255: 559–563

Wollheim F A, Lindstrom C G, Eiken O 1981 Eosinophilic fasciitis complicated by carpal tunnel syndrome. Journal of Rheumatology 8: 856–860

Yacoub M H 1965 Cervical vagotomy for pulmonary osteoarthropathy. British Journal of Diseases of the Chest 59: 28–31

Yacoub M H, Simon G 1966 Hypertrophic pulmonary osteoarthropathy and intrathoracic inflammatory conditions. British Journal of Diseases of the Chest 60: 81–86

Yacoub M H, Simon G, Ohnsorge J 1967 Hypertrophic pulmonary osteoarthropathy in association with pulmonary metastases from extrathoracic tumours. Thorax 22: 226–231

Yamamoto S et at 1974 A nation-wide survey of Behçet's disease in Japan: I. epidermiological survey. Japanese Journal of Ophthalmology 18: 282–290

Yamanouchi K, Shishido A, Kobune F, Sakata H, Inaba G 1981 Virological approaches on Behçet's disease in Japan. In: International Conference on Behçet's Disease, Japan Medical Research Foundation, p. 15

Yazici H, Tuzlaci M, Yurdakul S 1981 A controlled survey of sacroiliitis in Behçet's disease. Annals of the Rheumatic Diseases 40: 558–559

Yazici H, Tuzun Y, Pazarli H, Yalcin B, Yurdakul S, Muftoglu A 1980 The combined use of HLA-B5 and the pathergy test as diagnostic markers of Behçet's disease in

Turkey. Journal of Rheumatology 7: 206–210
Yazici H, Chamberlain M A, Tuzun Y, Yurdakul S, Muftuoglu A 1984 A comparative study of the pathergy reaction among Turkish and British patients with Behçet's disease. Annals of the Rheumatic Diseases 43: 74–75
Yurdakul S, et al 1983 The arthritis of Behçet's disease: a prospective study. Annals of the Rheumatic Diseases 42: 505–515
Zlotnick A et al 1979 Circulating immune complexes in familial Mediterranean fever, systemic lupus erythematosus and HBs AG carriers. Harefuah 97: 55–57

SECTION XI

Inflammatory Disorders of Connective Tissue

Overlap syndromes and mixed connective tissue disease

Diagnosis of a disease depends on (1) knowledge of its aetiology or pathogenesis or (2) recognition of a clinical feature or combination of features unique to that disease. Neither of these criteria are fulfilled in the diagnosis of the autoimmune connective tissue diseases — rheumatoid arthritis (RA), systemic lupus erythematosus (SLE), polymyositis and scleroderma. The aetiology of all these diseases is unknown and they all have clinical or serological features in common, e.g. arthritis, Raynaud's phenomenon and rheumatoid factors. Where a feature is relatively disease-specific, e.g. articular erosions in RA, the association is not exclusive and is not necessarily present in all patients with the disease. This has led to the development of scoring systems used for the criteria in the diagnosis of RA (Ropes et al, 1958), SLE (Cohen et al, 1971) and polymyositis (Bohan et al, 1977). Although these criteria do not provide rigid diagnostic boundaries they have helped in the standardisation of disease groups for research purposes. When patients fulfil criteria for more than one disease they are commonly referred to as 'overlap syndromes'. See also Chapter 12 and the following chapters in Section XI.

OVERLAP SYNDROMES

Overlap between RA and SLE has been recognised for at least 25 years (Haserick, 1955). It has been suggested that RA patients with clinical features of SLE also have serological features in common, such as LE cells (Kievits et al, 1956; Wilkens & Decker, 1963). An important question which has not been resolved by a controlled epidemiological survey is whether these overlap syndromes represent more than a chance association. Since approximately 1% of the population have rheumatoid arthritis it would not be surprising to find 1% of an SLE series who also had RA. Given that most published series arise from referral centres, selection for relatively severe or complicated disease could lead to a relatively high proportion of patients with features of both diseases.

It is unlikely that chance association would account for the frequent reports of overlaps between scleroderma and polymyositis, both relatively rare diseases. Polymyositis, i.e. a destructive inflammatory myopathy, has been described in 12% of scleroderma patients (Clements et al, 1978) and scleroderma in 8–10% of patients presenting with polymyositis (Bohan et al, 1977; Venables et al, 1981). Similarly polymyositis occurs in approximately 10% of SLE patients (Borenstein et al, 1978) and SLE in 4–6% of patients presenting with polymyositis (Bohan et al, 1977; Venables et al, 1981). The overlap between SLE and scleroderma is more difficult to evaluate because of the lack of universally accepted criteria for the diagnosis of scleroderma, though both diseases have a number of clinical features in common, including Raynaud's phenomenon, dactylitis, oesophageal involvement and arthritis (Sharp, 1981).

MIXED CONNECTIVE TISSUE DISEASE (MCTD)

Antibodies to nuclear ribonuclear protein

A high proportion of patients with overlapping features of SLE, scleroderma and polymyositis have antibodies to nuclear ribonuclear protein (nRNP). The antigen was described as a ribonuclease (RNase) sensitive component of a saline extract of thymus called extractable nuclear antigen (ENA)

Table 50.1 Major precipitating antigen systems present in thymus extracts

Antigen (other names)	Clinical associations
nRNP (Mo)	MCTD, SLE, scleroderma
SS-B (La, Ha)	Sicca syndrome, SLE
SS-A (Ro)	Sicca syndrome, SLE
Sm	SLE
Scl-70	Scleroderma
Jo-1	Polymyositis

More than 15 other antigens have been described. The above list represents those that have been reproducibly identified in a number of different centres and occur in at least 20% of patients within the above disease groups.

(Sharp et al, 1971), and later shown to be immunologically identical to the Mo antigen (Mattioli & Reichlin, 1971). Because thymus extracts contain a number of antigens (Table 50.1), determination of antibodies to nRNP requires not only a detection system but also a means of distinguishing nRNP from other antigens in the substrate. Anti-nRNP antibodies can be demonstrated by immunofluorescence, haemagglutination (Sharp et al, 1971) and as precipitating antibodies by counter-immunoelectropheresis (CIE) (Kurata & Tan, 1966) and immunodiffusion (Mattioli & Reichlin, 1971). On indirect immunofluorescence, anti-nRNP containing sera give a fine speckled nuclear staining pattern with a characteristic sparing of the nucleoli (Fig. 50.1). Because other antibody systems, particularly anti-Sm and anti-SS-B, give very similar patterns on immunofluorescence this technique is best used as a screening test only. Haemagglutination is sensitive and quantitative but relies on the demonstration of RNase sensitivity of the antigen and it is possible that other RNase-sensitive antigens could give a false positive reaction with some sera. CIE and immunodiffusion can define the reacting antigen by lines of immunological identity as well as by enzyme sensitivity (Fig. 50.2). Because of the 'double check' available in the precipitating antibody assays these tend to be more commonly used in most laboratories.

Clinical features

Mixed connective tissue disease was originally described as 'An apparently distinct rheumatic disease syndrome associated with a specific antibody to an extractable nuclear antigen' (i.e. anti-nRNP) (Sharp et al, 1972). The clinical features found in patients with this antibody are shown in Table 50.2. The remarkable diversity of clinical features and the prominence of arthritis, Raynaud's

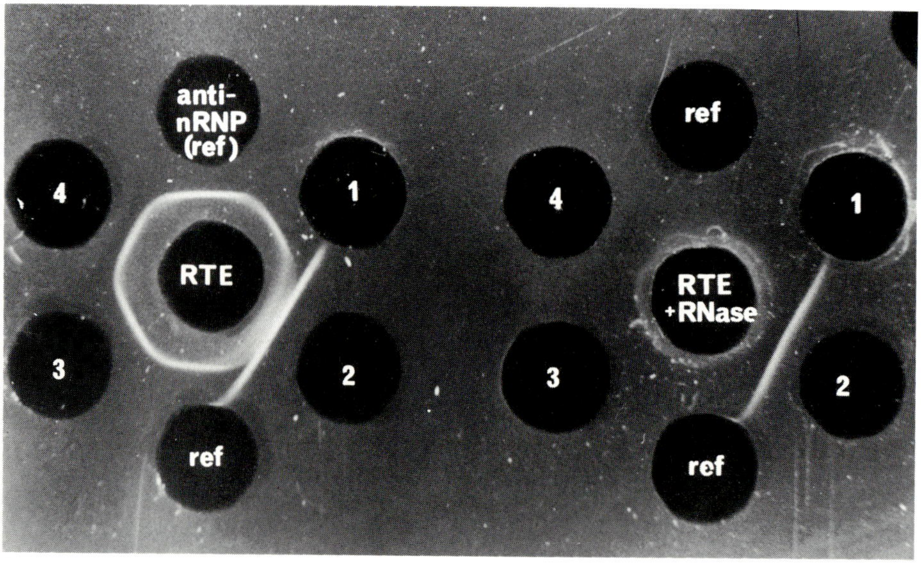

Fig. 50.1 Speckled nuclear staining pattern of an anti-nRNP serum by indirect immunofluorescence on Hep_2 cells.

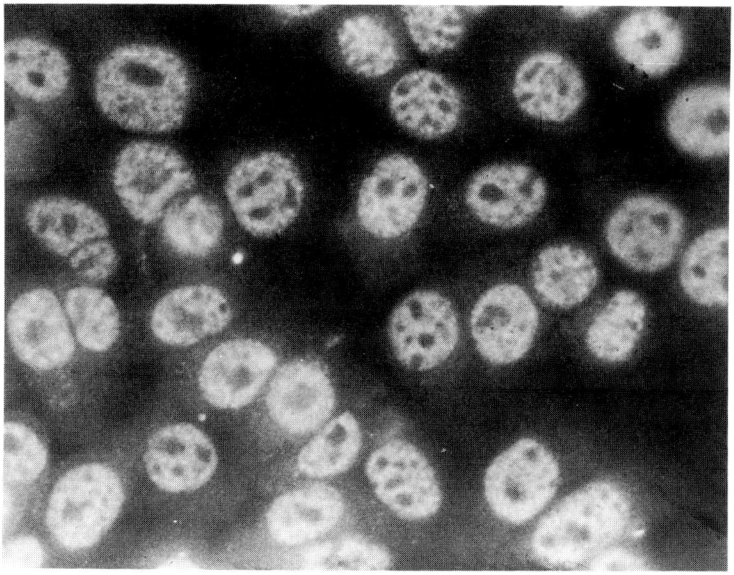

Fig. 50.2 Demonstration of precipitating antibodies to nRNP by immunodiffusion. The centre well of each hexagon contains rabbit thymus extract (RTE) as a source of soluble antigens. An anti-nRNP serum is placed in the top and bottom wells and four test sera (1–4) in the remaining wells. All four sera have produced a precipitin which gives a line of identity with that of the anti-nRNP reference serum and disappears after the extract is digested with RNase. Serum 2 has formed a second precipitin with an RNase-resistant antigen which was subsequently identified as Sm.

phenomenon, myositis and scleroderma-like features have been confirmed by most authors. The disease occurs predominantly in middle-aged females (F : M 4 : 1, mean age 37 years). However, the important claim of a 'good prognosis' associated with a relatively low frequency of renal and neurological disease has been challenged by other studies (see below).

Arthritis

Arthralgia occurs in over 90% of most series of MCTD patients and clinical evidence of synovitis in over two-thirds. In most cases the arthritis is peripheral and symmetrical affecting PIPs, MCPs and wrists (Bennett & O'Connell, 1978; Halla & Hardin, 1978), large joints such as knee and elbow being involved in 25–80% of patients. The axial skeleton is almost invariably spared. In Sharp et al's report (1976) 68% had arthritis, which in the majority was non-deforming, though 3 out of the 25 (12%) also had rheumatoid-like features with ulnar deviation in 2 and subcutaneous nodules in 1. A more recent study (Halla & Hardin, 1978) suggests that destructive changes may be more common. 8 out of 19 patients were described as presenting with 'RA-like disease'. X-rays showed osteoporosis in 8 and erosions, predominantly of the ulnar styloid and MCPs in 5. In a series reported by Bennett & O'Connell (1978) arthritis was present on 100% of 20 patients, marginal erosions were detected in 60% and ARA criteria for classical RA fulfilled in 60%. With the exception of one patient, who also had typical arthritis mutilans resembling psoriatic arthritis, the erosions were small, punched out and asymmetrical and did not lead to joint deformity.

The majority of MCTD patients have rheumatoid factors and in view of the high frequency of erosions, some authors have stressed the importance of distinguishing between MCTD and RA by examining the serum for antibodies for nRNP (Sharp et al, 1972). Whether such a differential diagnosis is of practical importance is questionable though it may have therapeutic implications, particularly as adverse reactions to gold have been noted in MCTD patients treated as RA (Halla & Hardin, 1978).

Raynaud's phenomenon

A striking association between antibodies to nRNP and Raynaud's phenomenon is undisputed in most studies. It is often a presenting symptom of MCTD and may be severe, leading to gangrene of digits though rarely calcinosis (Sharp et al, 1976). It is often associated with signs of digital vasculitis such as periungual infarcts or pulp lesions. Antibodies to nRNP have been reported to occur in up to 30% of patients with 'idiopathic' Raynaud's. Whether these represent a subset of 'early MCTD' remains to be established.

Fibrosing alveolitis

Although abnormalities in lung function testing occur in 67–84% of patients with MCTD, symptoms of lung disease occur in under 50% (Harman et al, 1977). The majority of the symptomatic patients had infiltrates on X-ray though loss of volume was reported to be less frequent. Initially, like other manifestations of MCTD, the lung lesions were thought to be mild and responsive to steroid therapy, though more recently (Esther et al, 1981) attention has been drawn to the development of pulmonary hypertension as a serious late complication.

Table 50.2 Clinical characteristics of patients with antibodies to nuclear ribonuclear protein. (After Sharp et al, 1976; based on 100 patients.)

	% patients with anti-nRNP
Arthritis/arthralgia	95
Raynaud's phenomenon	85
Decreased oesophageal motility	67
Impaired pulmonary diffusing capacity	67
Swollen hands	66
Myositis	63
Lymphadenopathy	39
Skin rash	38
Sclerodermatous changes	33
Fever	33
Serositis	27
Splenomegaly	19
Hepatomegaly	15
Renal disease	10
Neurological abnormalities	10

Other features

The other clinical findings in MCTD listed in Table 50.2 are covered by the overlap features (see below) of this disease. However, other authors have highlighted certain features in their studies. These include Sjögren's syndrome, infrequent in Sharp's series but found in 12 out of 25 patients by Alarcon-Segovia (1976). Trigeminal neuralgia, originally reported as clinically unimportant (Sharp et al, 1976), was found in 4 out of 21 patients by Cohen et al (1979). Hepatosplenomegaly, malabsorption syndrome and Hashimoto's thyroiditis have also been noted (Wolfe et al, 1977) but these are relatively rare.

OVERLAP FEATURES OF MCTD

Polymyositis, dermatomyositis and myocarditis

Inflammatory muscle disease, with proximal muscle weakness and tenderness, raised muscle enzymes and electromyographic changes characteristic of polymyositis are reported to occur in 50–63% of patients with MCTD. Muscle biopsy changes, with interstitial inflammatory infiltrates, fibre necrosis and regeneration, are indistinguishable from those of polymyositis and dermatomyositis described by Walton & Adams (1958). The characteristic skin changes of dermatomyositis, with a violaceous rash over the eyelids, was described in 3 out of 25 patients in Sharp's original study (Sharp et al, 1972), and 'several' others had erythematous changes over the knuckles and interphalangeal joints. Myocarditis, though apparently uncommon in adults with MCTD (about 10%) is reported to occur 3 times more frequently in children with MCTD (Signsen et al, 1977). Some investigators have highlighted the frequency of subclinical cardiac involvement in both adults and children and have suggested that it may be an important cause of death (Oetgen et al, 1981).

Cardiac abnormalities detected on ECG were also present in approximately one-fifth of patients with primary polymyositis (Bohan et al, 1977) and the same study described other features of MCTD, particularly Raynaud's phenomenon in 20% and arthralgia in 26%. Despite the clinical similarities between some patients with polymyositis and those with MCTD many early studies have had no apparent difficulty in distinguishing between the two 'entities' on the basis of the presence of anti-nRNP. In a recent study we have shown that the quantitation of antibodies to nRNP in patients with myositis does not provide a cut-off point which divides them into two distinct diseases though, like previous reports, there was a striking correlation between the titre of anti-nRNP and the number of systemic features (Venables et al, 1981).

Scleroderma-like features

Apart from Raynaud's phenomenon, other features common to scleroderma also occur in about 25% of patients (Wolfe et al, 1977). Oesophageal involvement, indistinguishable from that of scleroderma, occurs in the majority (Sharp et al, 1972) but is usually asymptomatic (Winn et al, 1976). The 'sausage-like' swelling of the fingers, noted as a relatively characteristic feature of MCTD is similar to that seen in early scleroderma. The oedema is non-pitting and is due to an inflammatory exudate within the dermis and subcutaneous tissues. Sclerodactly, where skin thickening and tightening is associated with dermal collagen deposition is also present in about 60% of MCTD patients and may represent the end result of the oedematous phase and is histologically identical to scleroderma (Sharp, 1976). Whether scleroderma proximal to the digits is a feature of MCTD remains a subject of debate and confusion. Such patients probably represent the diagnostic boundary between MCTD and scleroderma and might well comprise the 30% of scleroderma patients reported to have anti-nRNP (Kurata & Tan, 1966) or the 3 MCTD patients from Sharp's original series who subsequently developed classical scleroderma (Brody et al, 1977).

SLE-like features and renal disease

Features of SLE were reported to occur in nearly 90% of patients with anti-nRNP by Reichlin & Mattioli (1974) and in 65% of 308 patients described by Wolfe et al (1977). SLE-like rashes occurred in approximately one-third of the 100 patients described by Sharp in 1976. Like SLE, lymphadenopathy (occasionally mimicking lymphoma), fever and serositis also occurred, but it was suggested that the MCTD population differed in the much higher frequency of Raynaud's phenomenon and myositis (Sharp, 1981), and the lower prevalence (around 10%) of renal disease and central nervous system involvement. This difference was reflected in the relatively low prevalence in MCTD of the serological 'markers' of SLE: namely anti-DNA antibodies (12%), antibodies to the Sm antigen (Tan & Kunkle, 1966) (0%), LE cells (14%) and hypocomplementaemia (4%). Other studies have described a higher prevalence of renal disease in association with anti-nRNP ranging from around 20% of patients whose sera contained anti-nRNP alone (Bennett & Spargo, 1977; Lemmer et al, 1982) to 57% when anti-nRNP was present with antibodies to other nuclear antigens (Hochberg et al, 1981). In addition to the low prevalence of renal disease in MCTD it is frequently claimed that when it occurs it is relatively 'mild' (Sharp et al, 1972). However, there have been reports of patients who died of progressive renal failure (Sharp et al, 1976; Hochberg et al, 1981; Venables et al, 1981). The renal biopsy findings most frequently reported in association with anti-nRNP are mesangial proliferative changes or membranoproliferative nephritis (Wolfe et al, 1977; Bennett & Spargo, 1977; Venables et al, 1983).

Bennett & Spargo (1977) have suggested that the membranous nephropathy may account for the apparently good prognosis associated with MCTD in earlier studies. In SLE, membranous nephritis tends to follow a slowly progressive course over many years (Hayslett et al, 1973). If MCTD nephritis is similar it will probably take many more years of follow-up before the true renal prognosis is established.

DIAGNOSIS OF MCTD

When first described, MCTD was unique in that it appeared to be the only rheumatic disease entity which could be defined by a single antibody system (Sharp, 1972). Not only was the antibody almost invariably present in high titre but it was absent in all but 2 of over 400 control sera. SLE sera giving similar serological reactions could be distinguished by either their relatively low titre (less than 1 : 1000) or by the presence of antibodies to RNase-resistant antigens (including Sm). The initial optimism of this early report has not been supported by subsequent studies. Amongst the 100 patients with high titre anti-RNP reported in 1976 only 74 were thought to have MCTD (Sharp et al, 1976); the remaining 26 included 12 with SLE and 8 with scleroderma. Since then anti-nRNP has been described in a variety of conditions including rheumatoid arthritis (8–13%), scleroderma (17–31%), SLE (26–56%), Sjögren's syndrome (3–17%) and in the occasional normal serum (Notman et al, 1975; Kurata & Tan, 1976; Venables et al, 1981). Because of the frequent occurrence of the antibody in well-defined rheumatic diseases, attempts have been made to redefine diagnostic criteria for MCTD. Alarcon-Segovia (1976) and Bennett & O'Connell (1978) have suggested, in addition to overlapping clinical features, the presence of high titre anti-nRNP (greater than 1 : 6400) and the absence of antibodies to DNA and Sm. The serological criteria, presumably designed to differentiate between patients with SLE and MCTD would also exclude some patients with typical clinical features of MCTD. The presence of DNA antibodies would have excluded 3 (12%) of Sharp's original series and 50% of those described by Notman et al (1975). In a study of patients with polymyositis and overlap syndromes, many of whom had clinical features of MCTD, we have shown that they could all be excluded from the diagnosis by the rigid application of these serological criteria (Venables et al, 1981).

In addition to difficulties with serological diagnosis some authors have questioned whether MCTD is a useful concept in clinical diagnosis. It has been mentioned that most patients with MCTD have features of SLE, polymyositis, scleroderma or RA. Reichlin & Mattioli (1974) have stated that in their experience with anti-Mo (nRNP)-positive patients, the ratio of patients with a clinical picture of SLE to those with the features of MCTD was about 8 : 1. Similarly, Gaudreau et al (1978) found that only 22% of patients with anti-nRNP had 'overlap' syndromes mainly between SLE, scleroderma and polymyositis and the remainder could be fitted into straightforward clinical subgroups of which SLE was the most frequent. In a more recent study Munves & Sehur (1983) found that MCTD as a diagnosis accounted for only 3% of patients in whom anti-RNP was detected, while over 50% were thought to have SLE.

Although disappointing as an aid in clinical diagnosis it is generally agreed that anti-nRNP antibodies are associated with certain clinical features, myositis and lung disease being particularly important as both are potentially life-threatening or lead to severe disability. The detection and measurement of antibodies to nRNP may be a useful addition to the armamentarium of the clinical immunology laboratory even if its role is restricted to advising the clinician to look for these lesions before they become clinically apparent. Whether the presence of anti-nRNP is helpful in treatment or prognosis will be discussed below.

PROGNOSIS AND RESPONSE TO TREATMENT

MCTD and anti-nRNP antibodies were reported to be associated with an 'excellent' response to corticosteroid therapy (Sharp et al, 1972). In a series of over 300 patients (Wolfe et al, 1977) the same conclusion was reached after observing a mortality of 7% with a mean disease duration of 7 years. Reichlin & Mattioli (1974) regarded anti-nRNP as a marker of one end of the spectrum of SLE whose favourable prognosis was due to the relative lack of antibodies to DNA. In assessing the prognosis of MCTD it is important to recognise that much of the data in the early series was retrospective and interpretation could be biased in that only surviving patients would be available for study. A true assessment of survival should therefore be made in relation to time of follow-up rather than to disease duration at the time of presentation.

There is little information concerning comparative studies with diseases which resemble MCTD. It has been suggested that, although the early sclerodermatous skin changes may respond to corticosteroid therapy, over the long-term the scleroderma-like features may be the least steroid-reponsive of the various manifestations of MCTD (Sharp, 1981; LeRoy Maricq & Buhalen, 1980). Polymyositis in MCTD shows improvement with high dose corticosteroids (Sharp et al, 1976). However, there is no evidence that such treatment is more effective than in primary polymyositis which is also responsive to corticosteroid therapy providing the dose is adequate (Bradley, 1977). In a retrospective study published by Bohan et al (1977) the survival statistics in patients with myositis were favourable for 87–91% of all groups except those with malignancy. Their 'overlap group' which included patients with features of MCTD did not appear to fare any better than the remaining patients.

The 'favourable' prognosis of MCTD is often stated to be due to the relatively low frequency of renal disease when compared to groups of patients with SLE. Whether such a comparison is valid is open to question as a substantial proportion of MCTD patients have clinical features which resemble polymyositis or scleroderma rather than SLE. Reichlin & Mattioli (1972) partially resolved this problem when they compared the frequency of renal disease in a group of patients with anti-RNP, presenting with SLE-like features. Like Sharp they found that the frequency of renal disease in patients with anti-nRNP was less than 10% compared to over 70% in patients with antibodies to double-stranded (ds) DNA. However, this study is subject to two major criticisms: first, the period of follow-up is not stated and secondly, the 'control' group with antibodies to ds DNA appeared to have a particularly bad prognosis in that 30% had died. Comparison of the prognosis of MCTD and SLE requires the rigorous application of epidemiological techniques particularly as the prognosis of SLE is apparently improving (Gordon et al, 1980). A recent study which attempted to apply such criteria has indicated that the presence of anti-nRNP in SLE is not associated with a better prognosis (Hochberg et al, 1981) though the association of this antibody with Raynaud's phenomenon and myositis was again confirmed.

TREATMENT

Treatment of MCTD is with non-steroidal anti-inflammatory drugs, corticosteroids or, in a few patients, cytotoxic drugs such as azathioprine or cyclophosphamide. Treatment is based on the extent of organ involvement determined by standard clinical and laboratory evaluation. Raynaud's phenomenon, sclerodactly and proximal scleroderma are largely unresponsive though painful oedematous fingers may respond to treatment with corticosteroids. The arthritis may be treated with non-steroidal anti-inflammatory drugs or a small dose of prednisolone. Unfortunately there are no published data concerning the effect of gold therapy in a controlled trial though isolated reports would suggest that it is liable to lead to toxicity. The treatment of major organ involvement is the same whether or not anti-nRNP is detected in the serum. Polymyositis requires treatment with high dose steroids (40–60 mg/day prednisolone) and the dose maintained until a clinical response is observed, usually around 6 weeks (Walton & Adams, 1968). The necessity for a large dose is stressed, because many clinicians who have read the early reports of an 'excellent' or 'favourable' prognosis assume that a low starting dose of steroids is adequate for myositis in MCTD. There is no evidence to support this view: indeed Sharp et al (1972) used 1 mg/kg prednisolone for the initial treatment of 15 out of 25 of his patients. The ability to tail off the steroids to a maintenance dose of around 10 mg/day is completely in accordance with experience with primary polymyositis (Bradley, 1977; Bohan et al, 1977). Fibrosing alveolitis, because it can progress to pulmonary hypertension, also requires aggressive early treatment, sometimes in combination with cytotoxic drugs (Sharp et al, 1976). If, as has been suggested, such intervention improves the long-term prognosis, the finding of anti-nRNP in the serum represents an important 'pointer' for the possibility of lung disease. When renal disease occurs it has been suggested that it is no different from that of SLE and 'should be treated as such' (Sharp, 1981).

MCTD AS A 'DISTINCT CLINICAL ENTITY'

Over the last ten years the weight of opinion has swung against the concept of MCTD as a distinct entity. Patients with anti-nRNP may be asymptomatic individuals, suffer from mild Raynaud's phenomenon associated with arthritis (Peltier et al, 1978), have typical scleroderma and/or polymyositis or, particularly in children, suffer from severe SLE with renal involvement. Such patients would appear to be too heterogeneous to constitute a single diagnostic entity. The presence of anti-nRNP as a 'marker' antibody is disappointing. Not only is the antibody found in relatively well-defined diseases but some patients with typical clinical features of MCTD are anti-nRNP negative or, in our experience, may even have the 'wrong' antibody such as anti-SS-B(La).

The good prognosis of MCTD and responsiveness to treatment has not stood the test of time. There is no evidence that scleroderma with anti-nRNP has a better outlook than scleroderma without the antibody. Nor has it been shown that the finding of anti-nRNP in patients with polymyositis makes any difference in the necessity for, and the responsiveness to, high dose steroids. Even the long held belief that anti-nRNP in SLE confers a favourable prognosis is being challenged by recent studies. One attempt to resolve this confusion was the proposal that the patients with MCTD-like features should either be assigned to the group that they resemble most closely, e.g. SLE or scleroderma, or described as 'undifferentiated connective tissue disease' (UCTD) (Leroy et al, 1980). This term has the advantage that it circumvents the fallacy of diagnosing a disease by a single serological test and takes account of the patients who subsequently develop a classical rheumatic disease syndrome. A disadvantage is the assumption that the clinical features of these patients will 'differentiate' into a recognisable disease. Experience has shown that a number of patients continue to suffer from multisystem syndromes for years and may die without developing typical scleroderma, polymyositis or SLE. For this reason the author favours the term 'overlap syndrome'. Although not a diagnosis, it conveys information, particularly if the overlapping features are incorporated in the description, e.g. 'scleroderma/polymyositis overlap' or 'SLE/scleroderma overlap'. The term 'UCTD' could then be used for patients whose clinical features are insufficient to fulfil diagnostic criteria for any of the above diseases, if there is evidence that it is early and showing signs of progression.

REFERENCES

Alarcon-Segovia D 1976 Symptomatic Sjögren's syndrome in mixed connective tissue disease. Journal of Rheumatology 3: 191–200

Bennett R M, Spargo B M 1977 Immune complex nephropathy in mixed connective tissue disease. The American Journal of Medicine 63: 534–541

Bennett R M, O'Connel J 1978 The arthritis of mixed connective tissue disease. Annals of the Rheumatic Diseases 37: 397–403

Bohan A, Peter J B, Bohan R L, Pearson C M 1977 A computer- assisted analysis of 153 patients with polymyositis and dermatomyositis. Medicine (Baltimore) 65: 255–286

Borenstein D G, Fye W B, Arnett F C, Stevens M B 1978 The myocarditis of systemic lupus erythematosus. Annals of Internal Medicine 89: 619–624

Bradley W G 1977 Polymyositis. British Journal of Hospital Medicine (April): 351–355

Brody S, Nimelstein S, McShane D and Holman H 1977 Mixed connective tissue disease (MCTD): A follow-up of the original 25 cases. XIV. International Congress of Rheumatology, San Francisco, USA, June 26 (Abstract 68)

Clements P J, Furst D E, Campion D S, Bohan A, Harris R, Levy J, Paulus H E 1978 Muscle disease in progressive systemic sclerosis: Diagnostic and therapeutic considerations. Arthritis and Rheumatism 21: 62–71

Cohen A S, Reynolds W E, Franklin E C 1971 Preliminary criteria for the classification of systemic lupus erythematosus. Bulletin on the Rheumatic Diseases 21: 643–648

Cohen M L, Dawkins B, Dawkins R L, Owen E T 1979 Clinical significance of antibodies to ribonucleoprotein. Annals of the Rheumatic Diseases 39: 74–78

Esther J M, Sharp G C, Agia G, Hurst D J, Maricq H R 1981 Pulmonary hypertension in patients with mixed connective tissue disease and antibody to nuclear ribonucleo protein. Arthritis and Rheumatism 24: Supplement 104 (Abstract)

Gaudreau A, Amor B, Kahn M F, Rychewaert A, Sany J, Peltier A P 1978 Clinical significance of antibodies to soluble extractable nuclear antigens (anti-ENA). Annals of the Rheumatic Diseases 37: 321–327

Gordon M F, Stolley P D, Schinnar 1981 Trends in recent systemic lupus erythematosus mortality rates Arthritis and Rheumatism 24: 762–773

Halla J T, Hardin J G 1978 Clinical features of the arthritis of mixed connective tissue disease. Arthritis and Rheumatism 21: 497–503

Harman C, Wolfe J F, Lillard S, Held C, Cordon R and Sharp G C 1976 Pulmonary involvement in mixed connective tissue disease (MCTD). Arthritis and Rheumatism 19: Supplement 105 (Abstract)

Haserick J R 1955 Modern concepts of systemic lupus erythematosus. A review of 126 cases. Journal of Chronic Diseases 1: 317–326

Hayslet J P, Kashgarian M, Bensch K G, Spargo B M, Freedman L R, Epstein F H 1973 Clinical pathological correlations in the nephrotic syndrome due to primary renal disease. Medicine (Baltimore) 52: 93–120

Hochberg M C, Dorsh C A, Feinglass E J, Stevens M B

1981 Survivorship in systemic lupus erythematosus: Effect of antibody to extractable nuclear antigen. Arthritis and Rheumatism 24: 54–59

Kievits J M, Goslings J, Schuit H R E, Hijmans W 1956 Rheumatoid arthritis and the positive LE cell phenomenon. Annals of the Rheumatic Diseases 15: 211–216

Kurata N and Tan E M 1976 Identification of antibodies to nuclear acidic antigens by counterimmunoelectropheresis. Arthritis and Rheumatism 19: 574–579

Lemmer J P, Curry N H, Mallory J H, Waller M V 1981 Clinical course in patients with high titre antibodies to ribonucleoprotein (RNP). Arthritis and Rheumatism (Suppl 25: S108 (Abstract)

Le Roy E C, Maricq H R, Kaleh M B 1980 Undifferentiated connective tissue disease syndromes. Arthritis and Rheumatism 23: 341–343

Mattioli M, Reichlin M 1971 Characterisation of a soluble nuclear ribonucleoprotein antigen reactive with SLE sera. The Journal of Immunology 107: 1281–1290

Munves E F, Sehur P H 1983 Antibodies to Sm and RNP. Prognosticators of disease involvement. Arthritis and Rheumatism 26: 848–853

Notman D D, Kurata M D, Tan E M 1975 Profiles of antinuclear antibodies in systemic rheumatic diseases. Annals of Internal Medicine 83: 464–469

Oetgen W J, Mutter M L, Davis J E, Lawless O J 1981 Cardiac abnormalities in mixed connective tissue disease. Arthritis and Rheumatism 44: Supplement 104 (Abstract)

Reichlin M, Mattioli M 1972 Correlation of a precipitin reaction to an RNA protein antigen and a low prevalence of nephritis in patients with systemic lupus erythematosus. The New England Journal of Medicine 286; 769–775

Reichlin M, Mattioli M 1974 Antigens and antibodies characteristic of systemic lupus erythematosus. Bulletin on the Rheumatic Diseases 24: 756–760

Ropes N W, Bennet G A, Cobb S 1958. Revision of diagnostic criteria for rheumatoid arthritis. Bulletin on the Rheumatic diseases 9: 175–180

Sharp G C 1981 Mixed connective tissue disease and overlap syndromes. In: Textbook of Rheumatology Eds. Kelley, Harris, Ruddy & Sledge. 1151–1161

Sharp G C, Irvin W S, LaRoque R L, Velez C, Daly V, Kaiser A D, Holman H R 1971 Association of autoantibodies to different nuclear antigens with clinical patterns of rheumatic disease and responsiveness to therapy. The Journal of Clinical Investigation 50: 350–359

Sharp G C, Irvin W S, Tan E M, Gould R G, Holman H R 1972. Mixed connective tissue disease — an apparently distinct rheumatic disease syndrome associated with a specific antibody to extractable nuclear antigen (ENA). The Americal Journal of Medicine 52: 148–159

Sharp G C, Irvin W S, May C M, Holman H R, McDuffie F C, Hess E V, Schmid F R 1976 Association of antibodies to ribonucleoprotein and Sm antigens with mixed connective tissue disease, systemic lupus erythematosus and other rheumatic diseases. The New England Journal of Medicine 295: 1149–1154

Singsen B M, Bernstein H H, Kornreich H K, King K K, Hansen V, Tan E M 1977 Mixed connective tissue disease in childhood. Journal of Pediatrics 90:893

Tan E M, Kunkle H G 1966 Characteristics of a soluble nuclear antigen precipitating with sera of patients with systemic lupus erythematosus. Journal of Immunology 96: 464–471

Venables P J W, Mumford P A, Maini R N 1981 Antibodies to nuclear antigens in polymyositis: relationship to autoimmune 'overlap syndromes' and carcinoma. Annals of the Rheumatic Diseases 40: 217–233

Venables P J W, Tung Yi, Woodrow D F, Moss J, Maini R N 1983 Relationship of precipitating antibodies to soluble cellular antigens and histologically defined renal lesions in systemic lupus erythematosus. Annals of the Rheumatic Diseases 42: 17–22

Walton J H, Adams R D. 1958 Polymyositis. Williams and Wilkins, Baltimore

Wilkens R D, Decker J L 1963 Rheumatoid arthritis with serologic evidence suggesting systemic lupus erythematosis: Clinical serologic and chromatographic studies. Arthritis and Rheumatism 6: 720–735

Winn D, Gerhardt D, Winship D and Sharp G C 1976 Esophageal function in steroid treated patients with mixed connective dissue disease (MCTD) Clinical Research 24:545 (Abstract)

Wolfe J R, Kingsland J, Lindberg D, Sharp G C 1977 Disease pattern in patients with antibodies only to nuclear ribonucleoprotein (RNP). Clinical Research 25:488 (Abstract)

Polymyalgia rheumatica and giant cell arteritis

In recent years there has been an increasing tendency to consider giant cell arteritis and polymyalgia rheumatica as closely related conditions. The precise nature of the association is not known, but the two conditions affect the same patient population and frequently occur together in the same individual; for this reason they are discussed together in this chapter.

There is often considerable delay in making the diagnosis, partly because of the frequent absence of physical signs and lack of specific laboratory tests, but also because the systemic features of the disease are not recognised as being due to underlying arteritis. There is still a need to increase awareness that giant cell arteritis is a systemic disease, that it is fairly common in older patients and that it may present in a wide variety of ways.

HISTORICAL BACKGROUND

Horton and his colleagues are usually credited with the first description of giant cell arteritis. In 1932 they published a paper entitled 'An undescribed form of arteritis of the temporal vessels'; and they suggested the name 'temporal arteritis'. However, in 1890 Jonathan Hutchinson, a surgeon at the London Hospital, had described 'A peculiar form of thrombotic arteritis of the aged, which is sometimes productive of gangrene'. An elderly porter at the hospital is described as having 'red streaks' on his head, which prevented him from wearing his hat. These proved to lie over his temporal arteries, which were inflamed and swollen on both sides. At first, feeble pulsation could be detected, but this ceased and the redness subsided. The old man lived for several years without any other manifestation of arterial disease. Giant cell arteritis may have been recognised in the 10th century — *The Tadkivat* of Ali Ibn Isa (940–1010 AD) suggests excision of the temporal artery to treat, among other complaints, headache in patients subject to chronic eye disease, including conditions where the temporal muscles become hot and inflamed, with loss of sight in some cases.

Dequeker (1981) describes two paintings — Jan Van Eyek's work in the municipal museum of Bruges depicting the Holy Virgin with Canon Van der Paele (1436) and Pieri di Cosimo's 1505 portrait of Francesco Gamberti, now in the Rijks museum, Amsterdam. Both show signs of temporal arteritis, and the recorded health data support the clinical diagnosis. Perhaps the main reason why temporal arteritis was not noted historically is that the mean life span was too short for a sufficient number of cases to develop and be recognised as examples of a specific diagnosis.

Horton et al (1932) described the typical histological appearances at temporal artery biopsy. The arteritis was at first thought to be a benign condition, limited to the temporal arteries, but later reports emphasised its widespread nature (Gilmour, 1941).

Polymyalgia rheumatica was probably first described by Bruce in 1888. He was a physician practising at Strathpeffer Spa in Scotland, and described 5 patients aged from 60–70 years who suffered from widespread muscular and joint pains. He introduced the term 'senile rheumatic gout'. In the early 1950s several authors (Kersley, 1951; Meulengracht & Schwartz, 1952; Forestier & Certonciny, 1953) used a variety of names to describe a similar condition adding constitutional symptoms and an elevated sedimentation rate to the symptom complex but it was Barber (1957) who suggested the present name.

Several authors mentioned myalgic symptoms in early reports of temporal arteritis but Porsman (1951) first pointed out the similarity between temporal arteritis and 'arthritis of the aged'. In 1960 Paulley & Hughes reported on 67 patients, emphasising the occurrence of 'an arthritic rheumatism' in giant cell arteritis, providing more solid clinical evidence for the relationship between polymyalgia rheumatica and giant cell arteritis. Histological support came from the work of Alestig & Barr (1963) who reported arteritis in temporal artery biopsies in 7 out of 9 patients with polymyalgia rheumatica. Further reports, in particular Hamrin and colleagues' (1965) findings of temporal arteritis in 51 of 93 patients with polymyalgia, have confirmed the coexistence of the two conditions, although the nature of the relationship remains unclear. Those wishing to preserve the identity of the two diseases point out that arteritis is not found in many patients with polymyalgia, and that in some central arthritis and ligamentous disease can explain the pattern of myalgia (Coomes & Sharp, 1961; Bruk, 1967).

EPIDEMIOLOGY

The incidence of polymyalgia rheumatica and temporal arteritis has been difficult to establish, partly because firm diagnostic criteria do not exist, particularly for polymyalgia, and because symptoms in both diseases are wide ranging; patients may present to many different departments. The incidence of the disease is based on hospital populations. Huston et al (1978) reported an increased incidence during the years 1970–1974 compared to 1950–1959, probably reflecting increased diagnostic awareness. The 1970–1974 incidence rate of biopsy-positive cases found at Olmsted County, Minnesota amounted to 17.4 per 100 000 in the population aged 50 years or more, a figure not very different from Bengtsson & Malmvall's (1981) finding of 16.8 per 100 000 in the same age-group in Göteborg, Sweden. The age-specific rate in Olmsted County increased from 1.4 per 100 000 in the age-group 50–59 years to 29.6 per 100 000 in the age-group 70–79.

The temporal arteries and aorta of all adults who died in Malmö throughout one year were examined by Östberg (1973), and although active temporal arteritis was not found, evidence of previous arteritis was found in 1.7% of the 889 cases. It was found that in 75% of these subjects there had been either biopsy evidence or a clinical history suggestive of temporal arteritis. This study certainly suggests that giant cell arteritis may be underdiagnosed, but further studies are required. The variety of symptoms and lack of specificity of signs and symptoms contribute to make such studies difficult, and indeed the epidemiology of polymyalgia rheumatica has been less well defined. Silman & Currey (1982) found 3 cases of polymyalgia in 247 residents over 65 years in old peoples' homes and day centres. Only one case had been previously diagnosed.

Polymyalgia has been found to account for 1.3–4.5% of the patients attending rheumatic disease clinics but clearly these figures are influenced by the type of clinical load (Dixon et al, 1966; Mowat & Hazleman, 1974). It is probably half as frequent as rheumatoid arthritis in patients over 70 years of age.

Familial aggregation of polymyalgia rheumatica and giant cell arteritis has been reported by several workers. Liang et al in 1974b again emphasised this intriguing relationship. In addition to their own 4 pairs of first degree relatives, they noted a further 6 pairs in the world literature occurring in a patient population of less than 500. Clustering of cases in time and space was seen in Liang's and another study (Kvernebo & Brath, 1980), and suggests that in addition to a genetic predisposition environmental factors may be important. Kyle et al (1983) described a husband who developed polymyalgia rheumatica within 1 month of his wife's relapse; and Rhodes (1976) noted that 9 of 11 cases seen over 6 years in a practice of 3000 lived in one small part of the same village, and of these 2 lived in the same house, 2 were neighbours and 2 others close friends.

Polymyalgia rheumatica and giant cell arteritis are well recognised in England and Scandinavian countries, and in the USA. Most reports of these conditions derive from Northern States, especially where there is a large population of Scandinavian extraction. However, the diseases are recognisable worldwide and there have been several recent reports of their occurrence in American Negros. Sandford & Berney (1977) described 5 cases of polymyalgia and 1 of temporal arteritis to which they added 3 and 4 additional case reports respectively from the literature. They noted no difference in clinical findings or in the response to corticosteroids from those described in Caucasians.

Tissue typing has produced conflicting reports. Hazleman et al (1977) found that HLA-B8 was significantly more common in polymyalgia (59%) and temporal arteritis (50%) than in controls (27%). Another study reported an increase in HLA-D3 and DR4 (Lowenstein et al) but others have found no significant increase in the frequency of any antigen (Terasaki et al, 1976; Hunder et al, 1977; Mattingley et al, 1978). It seems unlikely that there is a significant increase in any HLA antigen in either disease but Mattingley et al (1978) point out that as there does seem to be a tendency for the disease to be common in those of Scandinavian stock, an appropriate control group should be tested. Also the controls for all these series are perhaps inappropriate since all investigators have used blood donors who are not age-matched and not always sex-matched with the patients with polymyalgia who tend to be over 60 with a female preponderance. Although Bender et al (1976) found no indication of postnatal selection at the HLA loci, Smith & Walford (1977) have reported that the frequency of HLA-B8 is decreased in cohorts of elderly women, suggesting the possibility of an increased mortality rate in such patients.

AETIOLOGY AND PATHOGENESIS

At present it is impossible to define the underlying pathological abnormality in polymyalgia and, indeed, it may well be that there are several different mechanisms responsible for a largely similar pattern of pain. The relative homogeneity of groups of patients and the apparent rapid clinical response to corticosteroids does not exclude this possibility. Although the increasing incidence of giant cell arteritis and polymyalgia rheumatica after the age of 50 implies a relationship to ageing the meaning of this observation is not understood.

A distinct prodromal event is often noted by patients, the association of an illness resembling influenza or viral pneumonia often being striking (Bell & Klinefelter, 1967). However, these viral infections are probably coincidental and viral studies have produced negative results (Mowat & Hazleman, 1974).

The known association of hepatitis B with polyarteritis nodosa led Bacon et al (1975) to seek a similar association in polymyalgia. Although hepatitis antigen was not found in any of the 12 patients tested before the commencement of corticosteroid therapy, hepatitis B surface antibody was found in 9 cases. This finding has not been confirmed (Liang et al, 1976).

Fessel (1969) suggested that contact with pet birds, especially parakeets, might be a factor in aetiology, representing some immunological reaction to psittacosis or constituent of their food. Others (Ornilla et al, 1970; White & Innes 1972) have been unable to support this suggestion.

Both the humoral and cellular immune systems have been implicated in pathogenesis. Giant cell arteritis is limited to vessels with an internal elastic lamina, and an electron microscopic study (Parker et al, 1975) showed fragmentation of the elastic lamina with mononuclear cell accumulation compatible with cell-mediated injury. Fragments of elastic tissue can be demonstrated within giant cells and Smith (1969) showed that giant cells engulf fibrillar material thought to be altered internal elastic membrane. Immunoglobulins and complement have also been detected in the vessel wall of patients with arteritis by immunofluorescence. Deposits have been noted both intra- and extracellularly of all immunoglobulin classes plus C_3, adjacent to the internal elastic lamina in many cases (Liang et al, 1974a; Park & Hazleman, 1978). The presence of immunoglobulin or complement within a lesion does not prove that it has been caused by hypersensitivity. Such a finding may be due to non-specific immune complex deposition at the site of vascular injury of different cause. Using an immunoperoxidase method, Gallagher & Jones (1982) found only intracellular deposits and did not detect extracellular complement. This pattern of intracytoplasmic staining for immunoglobulins would be anticipated in any chronic inflammatory reaction.

Eghtedari and colleagues (1976) demonstrated increased numbers of circulating lymphoblasts in patients with active polymyalgia rheumatica and Malmvall & Bengsson (1976) found immunoglobulins to be elevated in similar patients. These observations have led to the suggestion that these diseases may have an immunological basis, perhaps an age-related autoimmune process directed against arterial wall constituents. Hazleman et al (1975) reported that lymphocytes of patients showed transformation responses to arterial antigen higher than in other related diseases, but other workers were unable to repeat their findings (Jones et al, 1980). Park et al (1981c) have also failed to find any difference in in vitro lymphocytotoxicity to arterial smooth muscle between the cells from patients with active untreated GCA/PMR and normal controls.

Park et al (1981a) measured immune complexes in patients by three different methods. Although complexes of undetermined composition were found in 44% of patients with active, untreated disease using one system, in general there was poor correlation between the results of the three assays and no clear correlation between the presence of immune complexes and the ESR, graded disease activity and the presence of arteritis. However, the incidence was higher than in normal controls. Using the Raji cell immunoassay, immune complex concentrations showed a positive correlation with the erythrocyte sedimentation rate and gamma-globulin levels (Papaioannou et al, 1982). However, Malmvall et al (1981) found no increase in immune complexes; varying results may be due to different methods of detection and of case selection. However, the proximity of inflammatory cells and immune deposits to the elastic tissue may well be significant. The fragmentation and destruction of the internal elastic membrane suggests that an autoimmune reaction is directed against the elastic tissue, but the possibility that an extraneous antigen alone, or one closely associated with the elastic tissue, is the cause cannot be disregarded. Elastin was initially thought to be non-immunogenic; however, antibodies have been raised to elastins (Darnule, 1980) and both inter- and intraspecific cross-reactivity are reported. It has been proposed that a serum cytotoxic factor leads to endothelial breakdown and then to disruption of the internal elastic lamina.

PATHOLOGY

The arteritis is histologically a panarteritis with giant cell granuloma formation, often in close relationship to a disrupted internal elastic lamina. Large and medium-sized arteries are affected and the involvement is patchy and 'skip lesions' are often found. They were identified in 28% of patients by Klein et al (1976), and were as short as 330 μm, but long portions of arteries may be involved. More patients with 'skip lesions' had normal arteries to palpation but they did not have a more benign disease. The gross features are not characteristic; the vessels are enlarged and nodular and have little or no lumen. Thrombosis often develops at sites of active inflammation; later, these areas may recanalise. The lumen is narrowed by intimal proliferation (Fig. 51.1) This is a common finding in arteries and may result from advancing age or nearby chronic inflammation or low blood flow.

The adventitia is usually invaded by mononuclear and occasionally polymorphonuclear inflammatory cells, often cuffing the vasa vasorum, and here fibrous proliferation is frequent. The medial changes are dominated by the giant cells, which vary from small cells with 2–3 nuclei up to masses of 100 μm containing many nuclei. Here there is invasion by mononuclear cells resembling histiocytes. Fibrinoid necrosis is infrequent. Giant cells are not seen in all sections and therefore are not required for the diagnosis if other features are compatible. The more sections that are examined in the area of arteritis, the more likely it is that giant cells will be found (Huston et al 1978). A progression of changes can be demonstrated from the active infiltrative phase to the scarred artery with little cellular infiltrate. At first the most severe changes are centred on the internal elastic lamina, which becomes swollen and fragmented (Parker et al 1975), and portions of this can be demonstrated within giant cells with surrounding plasma cell and lymphocytic infiltration. Corticosteroids reduce the inflammatory cell infiltrate so temporal artery biopsy should, if poss-

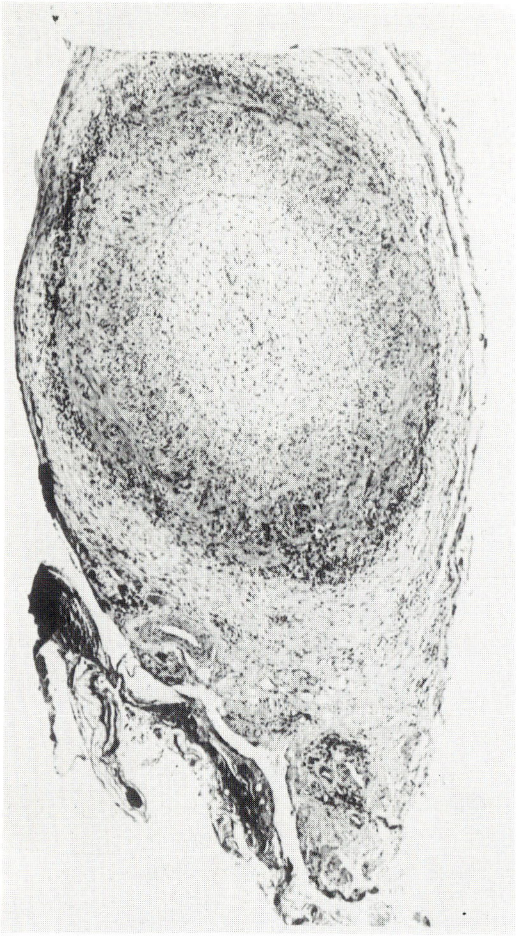

Fig. 51.1 Section of temporal artery showing occlusion of lumen due to intimal thickening with inflammatory changes in media. (H & E × 28)

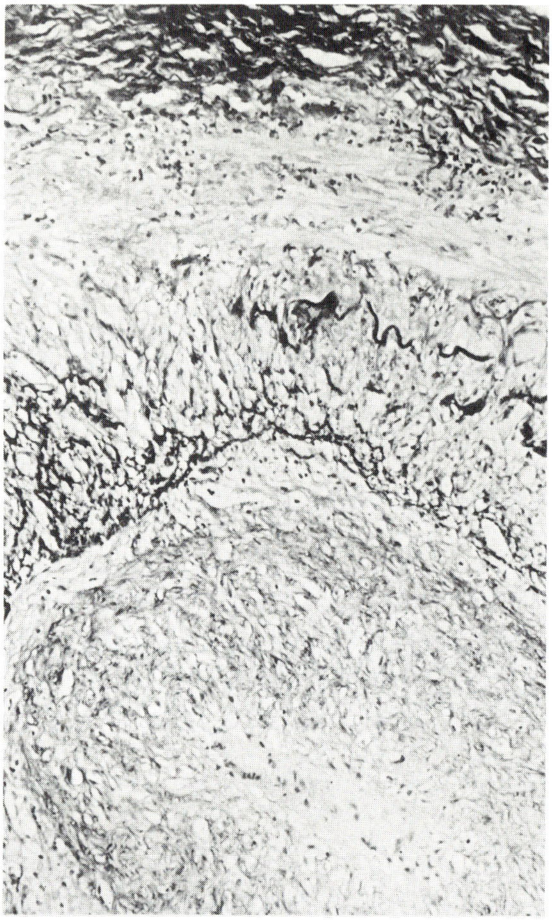

Fig. 51.2 Section of temporal artery showing disruption of the internal elastic lamina with collagenous replacement. (× 140)

ible, be carried out before treatment is started.

Histological changes also occur in temporal arteries with advancing age; they differ only in degree with those encountered in giant cell arteritis and it can sometimes be difficult to distinguish between them (Ainsworth et al, 1961). However, an inflammatory cell infiltrate does not occur except in relationship to large plaques of atherosclerosis. The degree of intimal thickening in arteritis is usually greater, a well-developed smooth muscle layer is seen by the lumen, loss of the internal elastic lamina is considerable. Healed arteritis has collagenous replacement of the media extending between the breaks in the internal elastic lamella (Fig. 51.2) and this is the most important change. The biopsy finding of healed vasculitis by no means excludes the possibility of active lesions elsewhere. Not infrequently episodes of vasculitis are recurrent. The widespread nature of the vasculitis has been well documented, and occasionally veins are affected.

Involvement of the aorta (Fig. 51.3) and its branches, the abdominal vessels and the heart have all been described (Klein et al, 1975). Although there is a high incidence of involvement of the head and neck vessels in giant cell arteritis, it is interesting that the intracranial vessels are seldom involved. Wilkinson & Russell (1972) studied the head and neck vessels and they demonstrated a

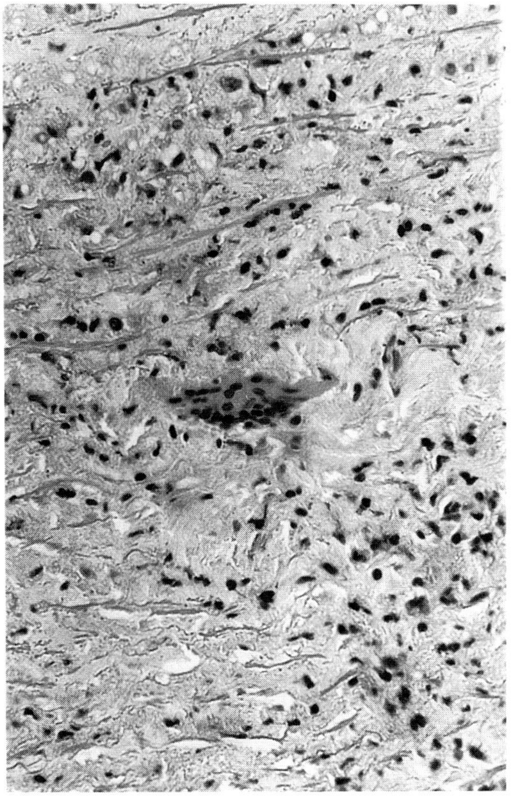

Fig. 51.3 Section of ascending aorta showing an area of giant cell infiltration. (H & E × 270)

close correlation between the susceptibility to arteritis and the amount of elastic tissue present in the arterial wall. The highest incidence of severe involvement was noted in the superficial temporal arteries, vertebral arteries and ophthalmic and posterior ciliary arteries. The internal carotid, external carotid, and central retinal arteries were affected less frequently. In some instances follow-up biopsy or autopsy surveys have shown persistence of mild chronic inflammation even though symptoms have resolved (Fauchald et al, 1972).

There is little to support a concept of primary muscle disease in polymyalgia rheumatica. Serum aldolase and creatine phosphokinase are normal and there is no abnormality on electromyography (Bruk, 1967). Muscle biopsy has shown type II atrophy and there is no evidence of inflammatory changes (Brooke & Kaplan, 1972). Histochemical examination of muscle has demonstrated some abnormalities of the motor nerve terminals and end-plates, which have been interpreted as consistent with a neuropathy (Isaacs et al, 1973). However, it has been suggested by other workers that these changes are non-specific.

Liver biopsy can show non-specific inflammatory change or focal liver cell necrosis. There are occasional reports of granulomata and hepatic arteritis (McCormack et al, 1978).

Synovial biopsy has shown non-specific inflammatory changes (Henderson et al, 1975), with lymphocytic infiltration of knees, sternoclavicular joints, and shoulders.

CLINICAL FEATURES

Age, sex and onset

The mean age at onset of giant cell arteritis and polymyalgia rheumatica is approximately 70 years, with a range of about 50 to more than 90 years of age. Younger patients have been reported but these are atypical. Women are affected about twice as often as men.

The onset of the disease can be dramatic and some patients can give the date and hour of their first symptom. Equally, the onset can be insiduous and in most instances the symptoms have been present for weeks or months before the diagnosis is established, a mean of 6.2 months in one series (Mowat & Hazleman, 1974). Constitutional symptoms, including fatigue, anorexia and weight loss and depression, are present in the majority of patients and may be an early or even an initial finding and can lead to delay in diagnosis (Jones & Hazleman, 1981). They may be striking and suggest neoplasia. Mowat & Hazleman (1974) noted a weight loss of 3–23 kg (mean 6 kg) in 32 of 59 patients. A hidden malignancy can mimic the symptoms of polymyalgia rheumatica but these patients do not usually respond to corticosteroids. Knorring & Somer (1974) emphasised that the possibility of an underlying tumour must be considered even in long-standing cases of polymyalgia rheumatica, although at present there is no evidence to suggest that malignancy is more common in patients with polymyalgia than in other people. Deterioration in health or a poor initial response to steroids must always be taken seriously and a search for an occult neoplasm made. Patients may present with a pyrexia. In some cases the onset is associated with recent bereavement.

Polymyalgia rheumatica

Patients usually locate the source of their pain and stiffness to the muscles. The onset is commonest in the shoulder region and neck with eventual involvement of the shoulder and pelvic girdles and the corresponding proximal muscle groups.

Involvement of distal limb muscles is unusual. The symptoms are usually bilateral and symmetrical. Stiffness is usually the predominant feature, is particularly severe after rest, and may prevent the patient getting out of bed in the morning. If the symptoms are severe, aching is more persistent. The muscular pain is often diffuse and movement accentuates the pain; pain at night is common. Muscle strength is usually unimpaired, although the pain makes interpretation of muscle testing difficult. There is tenderness of involved structures including periarticular structures such as bursae, tendons and joint capsules, although the muscle tenderness is generally not as severe as that in myositis. In late stages muscle atrophy may develop, with restriction of shoulder movement. An improvement of shoulder range is rapid with corticosteroid therapy, unlike that seen in frozen shoulder. Occasionally the painful arc sign of subacromial bursitis is present; this is important to recognise as a local injection of corticosteroid will give relief and save the patient from an increase in systemic corticosteroid dosage.

Inflammatory synovitis and effusions have been noted by several authors (Bruk, 1967; Mowat & Hazleman, 1974), the reported incidence varying from 0–100% in various series (Henderson et al, 1975). Synovitis of the knees, wrists and sternoclavicular joints is most common, but involvement is transient and mild. Bruk (1967) found erosive changes in joints and/or sclerosis of the sacro iliac joints in 17 of 80 patients although they were difficult to demonstrate in the sternoclavicular joints except by tomography. Such changes have not been reported by others although Andrews (1965) found a significant increase in both unilateral and bilateral radiographic sacroiliac joint disease compared with control populations. O'Duffy and colleagues (1976) found abnormal technetium pertechnetate scintigrams in 24 of 25 patients and showed widespread uptake over several joints, particularly shoulders, knees, wrists and hands. Isotope scans in the author's unit have not confirmed this finding.

The arthroscopic appearances are indistinguishable from rheumatoid arthritis (Henderson et al, 1975); the synovial tissue shows non-specific inflammatory changes (O'Duffy et al, 1976) and the synovial fluid has the appearances of a mild inflammatory exudate. The synovitis of polymyalgia differs from that of rheumatoid arthritis in that it does not cause typical juxta-articular osteoporosis and erosions, and reports of more pronounced joint changes may be partly explained by the variable diagnostic criteria used. An association between carpal tunnel syndrome and polymyalgia has been noted by several authors (Richards, 1978); local steroid injection and/or surgical decompression are sometimes necessary.

Giant cell arteritis

Headache is the most common symptom and is present in two-thirds or more of patients (Hamilton et al, 1971). It usually begins early in the course of the disease and may be the presenting symptom. The pain is severe and localised to the temple but it may be occipital or be less defined and precipitated by brushing the hair. It can be severe even when the arteries are clinically normal and conversely may subside even though the disease remains active. The nature of the pain varies; some patients describe it as shooting and others as a more steady ache. Scalp tenderness is common, particularly around the temporal and occipital arteries, and may disturb sleep. Tender spots or nodules or even small skin infarcts may be present for several days. The vessels are thickened, tender and nodular with absent or reduced pulsation (Fig. 51.4). Occasionally they are red and clearly visible.

Visual disturbances have been described in 25–50% of cases (Hamilton et al 1971), although the incidence of visual loss is now regarded as much lower, about 6–10% in most series (Jones & Hazleman, 1981b). This is probably because of earlier recognition and treatment. Visual symptoms include diplopia, ptosis and transient or permanent, partial or complete blindness. Visual loss

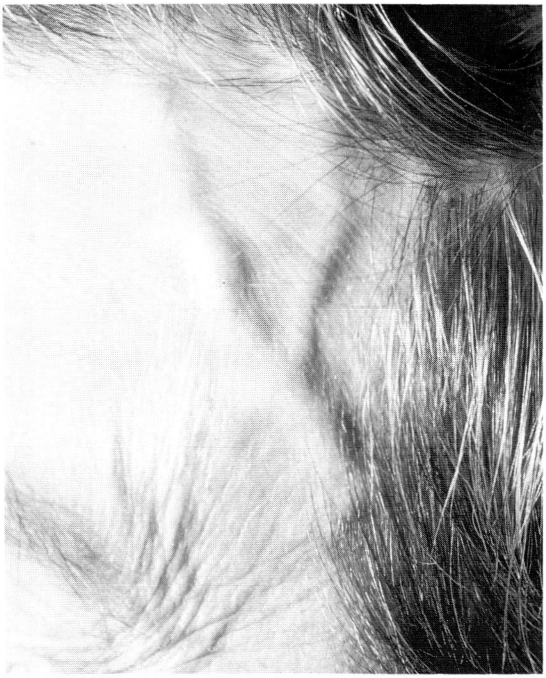

Fig. 51.4 Photograph showing enlarged thickened temporal artery.

is caused by ischaemia of the optic nerve secondary to arteritis of the posterior ciliary or ophthalmic artery and less commonly occlusion of the retinal arterioles. Rarely arterial lesions cause infarction of the occipital cortex with visual loss. The ophthalmoscopic findings are variable and depend on the vessels affected, but the most common pattern is ischaemic optic neuropathy due to posterior ciliary arteritis. In addition to narrowed vessels and a few circumpapillary haemorrhages, there may be oedema of the disc due to blocking of axoplasmic flow at the nerve head. This interference with axoplasmal transport is responsible for the transient cotton wool spots seen later on.

Occlusion or inflammation of the anterior ciliary vessels gives rise to either anterior segment necrosis with uveitis or scleritis. The latter takes the form of a necrotising anterior scleritis which remains localised to one area of the globe, usually adjacent to or underlying one of the rectus muscles, and may prove difficult to control. Blindness may be the initial symptom but tends to follow other symptoms by several weeks or months, being frequently preceded by transient visual symptoms. Once established, the visual deficit is usually permanent.

Pain on chewing, due to claudication of the muscles of mastication, occurs in up to two-thirds of patients. Tingling in the tongue, loss of taste, and pain in the mouth and throat can also occur, presumably due to vascular insufficiency.

The widespread nature of the vasculitis has been previously mentioned. Clinical evidence of large artery involvement is present in 10–15% of cases, and in some instances aortic dissection and rupture occur (Salisbury & Hazleman, 1981). Tenderness in areas distant from arteries may be present even when the vessels are clinically normal. Bruits are often hear over large arteries and there may be tenderness, particularly over the subclavian artery (these bruits are presumably due to arteritis, as they disappear with treatment). An early sign of arteritis is increased sensitivity of the carotid sinus. Light pressure will often lead to transient asystole for two or more beats, and it is therefore advisable for the patient to be lying down.

Less common features of giant cell arteritis include hemiparesis, peripheral neuropathy, deafness, depression and confusion. Involvement of the coronary arteries has led to myocardial infarction; and aortic regurgitation and congestive cardiac failure may occur. Abnormalities of thyroid and liver function are well described and will be detailed later in the chapter.

RELATIONSHIP BETWEEN POLYMYALGIA RHEUMATICA AND GIANT CELL ARTERITIS

Paulley & Hughes (1960) were the first to link the two conditions, suggesting that polymyalgia was a prodromal manifestation of temporal arteritis. Alestig & Barr (1963) supported this observation when they found temporal arteritis in patients with polymyalgia rheumatica who had no symptoms or signs of arteritis. Certainly it is difficult to maintain a practical distinction between them by clinical or histological criteria. Patients originally suffering from polymyalgia rheumatica have later had symptoms of cranial arteritis and in a number of patients with typical myalgia and no symptoms from the temporal region, biopsies have shown arteritic changes. Fauchald et al in 1972 studied 94 patients and found histological evidence of giant cell arteritis in 61. Systemic involvement was similar in the groups with or without clinical and/or biopsy evidence of arteritis. Of those with myalgia alone 40% had a positive biopsy and of those with a proven arteritis only 11 did not have myalgia.

In patients with polymyalgia rheumatica who have no symptoms or signs of arteritis, positive temporal biopsies are found in 10–15%. Those wishing to preserve the identity of the two diseases base their argument on the latter figure and of the failure to find evidence of arteritis in many patients with polymyalgia followed up for many years. Conversely there are many similarities between the two conditions. The age and sex distribution is similar; the biopsy findings show an identical pattern; the laboratory features are similar even though many are non-specific inflammatory changes. In addition there is similarity in the myalgia and the associated systemic features, and in the response to corticosteroid therapy.

The onset of myalgic symptoms may precede, coincide with, or follow that of the arteritic symptoms. No difference has been found between the characteristics of those myalgic patients with a positive biopsy and those with no histological evidence of arteritis (Fauchald et al, 1972). Mild aching and stiffness may persist for months after other features of giant cell arteritis have remitted. There is little evidence to suggest that the musculoskeletal symptoms are related to vasculitis. Many patients with giant cell arteritis do not have polymyalgia rheumatica, even when large vessels are involved. In addition the finding of joint swelling in some patients and the production of pain by the injection of 5% saline solution into the acromioclavicular, sternoclavicular and manubriosternal joints (Coomes & Sharp, 1961) suggests that polymyalgia rheumatica may in some patients be a particular form of proximal synovitis.

LABORATORY FINDINGS

The erythrocyte sedimentation rate is usually greatly elevated and provides a useful means of monitoring treatment, although it must be appreciated that some elevation of the ESR may occur in otherwise healthy elderly people. Establishing a raised ESR is the key investigation although a normal ESR is occasionally found in patients with active biopsy-proven disease (Hazleman & Mowat, 1974).

Anaemia, usually of a mild hypochromic type, is common and resolves without specific treatment but a more marked normochromic anaemia occasionally occurs and may be a presenting symptom (Jones & Hazleman, 1981a). Leucocyte and differential counts are generally normal; platelet counts are also usually normal but may be increased. Protein electrophoresis may show a non-specific rise in α_2-globulin with less frequent elevation of α_1-and γ-globulins. Quantification of acute phase proteins and α_1-antitrypsin, orosomucoid, haptoglobin and C-reactive protein are no more helpful than the ESR in the assessment of disease activity (Park et al, 1981b).

Abnormalities of thyroid and liver function have also been well described. Thomas & Croft (1974), in a retrospective survey of 59 cases of giant cell arteritis, found 5 patients with hyperthyroidism. The arteritis followed the thyrotoxicosis by intervals of 4–15 years in three cases, and in two occurred simultaneously. Individual cases of hypothyroidism have also been reported. Dent & Edwards (1978) found 7 cases of PMR or GCA in 250 patients with autoimmune thyroid disease. All cases occurred in women over 60, giving a prevalence of 9.3% in this age-group. Raised serum values for alkaline phosphatase were found in up to 70% of patients with polymyalgia rheumatica (Mowat & Hazleman, 1974). Bromsulphthalein retention is also often abnormal and transaminases may be mildly elevated. Long & James (1974) report on a liver biopsy which showed portal and intralobular inflammation with focal liver cell necrosis and a small epithelioid cell granuloma. The pathological significance of these abnormalities is unclear. Abnormal liver scans may also occur (Kyle et al, 1982).

DIAGNOSIS

The diagnosis of polymyalgia rheumatica is initially one of exclusion. The differential diagnosis (Table 51.1) in an elderly patient with muscle pain, stiffness and a raised ESR is wide because

Table 51.1 Differential diagnosis in polymyalgia rheumatica

1. Neoplastic disease
2. Joint disease
   a. Osteoarthrosis, particular of the cervical spine
   b. Rheumatoid arthritis
   c. Connective tissue disease
3. Multiple myeloma
4. Leukaemia
5. Lymphoma
6. Muscle disease
   a. Polymyositis
   b. Myopathy
7. Infections, e.g. brucellosis, bacterial endocarditis
8. Bone disease, particularly osteomalacia
9. Hypothyroidism
10. Parkinsonism
11. Functional

the prodromal phases of several serious conditions can mimic it. In practice non-specific clinical features and the frequent absence of physical signs makes diagnosis difficult.

Polymyalgia rheumatica can usually be differentiated from late onset rheumatoid arthritis by the absence of prominent peripheral joint pain and swelling. In patients with polymyositis, the muscular weakness is the predominant factor limiting movement, whereas in polymyalgia rheumatica pain causes limited function.

The diagnosis of giant cell arteritis should be considered in any patient over the age of 50 years who has recent onset of headache, transient of sudden loss of vision, myalgia, unexplained fever or anaemia or high erythrocyte sedimentation rate. Because the symptoms and signs may vary in severity and be transient, patients suspected of having this disease must be questioned carefully about recent as well as current symptoms. The arteries of the head, neck and limbs should be examined for tenderness, enlargement, thrombosis and bruits. A previous history of headaches, scalp tenderness, jaw claudication and other symptoms may not at first be mentioned by the patient. If a temporal artery biopsy is performed, and as the involvement may be focal, a symptomatic or clinically abnormal segment of the artery should be chosen. Klein et al (1976) emphasised the need for long arterial specimens if blind biopsy is to be undertaken. Angiography of the temporal arteries is not usually helpful — there is no characteristic abnormality and false positives (usually due to atheroma) are not uncommon. An angiographic examination of the aortic arch and its branches may prove helpful in patients with symptoms of large artery involvement.

Temporal artery biopsies need not be carried out in all patients with polymyalgia rheumatica. If clinical evidence for giant cell arteritis is absent and if symptoms are mild and of recent onset or conversely stable and of long duration then the patient can be followed closely without biopsy. Blindness is uncommon in such patients.

There is usually little difficulty in separating giant cell arteritis from other forms of arteritis, because of the different distribution of lesions, histopathology, and organ involvement. However, occasionally necrotising arteritis can involve the temporal artery (Morgan & Harris, 1978).

Delay in diagnosis

The systemic features of the disease can be vague and easily overlooked: they include fever, anorexia and weight loss. Conversely they can be striking and may suggest neoplasia. Despite a typical pattern of musculoskeletal symptoms and the presence in many of significant systemic features, there is often considerable delay of several months before diagnosis (Mowat & Hazleman, 1974, Jones & Hazleman, 1981a). This delay is partly because of the frequent absence of physical signs and lack of specific laboratory tests. Patients and doctors also tend to ascribe the symptoms to degenerative joint disease expected in an older population, or even to psychological illness; and the patient herself may attribute her aches and pains to family tensions and other problems. In others the systemic features of the disease and laboratory abnormalities can lead to diagnostic confusion and often extensive investigation.

TREATMENT

Although anti-inflammatory drugs will lessen the painful symptoms they are not as effective as corticosteroids, and only corticosteroids will prevent the complications of arteritis. Initially the steroids should be given in a sufficient dosage to control the disease and then maintained at the lowest dose which will control the symptoms and lower the erythrocyte sedimentation rate. In giant cell arteritis corticosteroids should be given, preferably after the diagnosis has been confirmed histologically. However, where GCA is strongly suspected there should be no delay in starting therapy as the temporal artery biopsy will still show inflammatory changes for several days after corticosteroids have been started and the result is unlikely to alter therapeutic decisions. If the temporal (or other) artery biopsy shows no arteritis but the clinical suspicion of the disease is strong, corticosteroid treatment should be started. The great danger is in delaying therapy as blindness may occur at any time. There are no clinical trials to help decide on the correct initial dose; prednisolone 60 mg/day is commonly prescribed. Some ophthalmologists suggest an initial dose of at least 60 mg as they have seen blindness occur at a lower dose, but this has to be balanced against the potential complication of high dosage in this age-group. It is suggested that reduction in dosage is made by 5 mg at weekly intervals when the symptoms are fully controlled and the sedimentation rate has fallen. The reduction is more gradual when dosage falls below 20 mg daily (1 mg every 1–2 weeks) and when 10 mg is reached, by 1 mg every 2–4 weeks. These dosage levels are suggestions only and not to be interpreted rigidly as individual cases vary greatly. Clinical relapse may occur without a rise in sedimentation rate and the sedimentation rate may rise without corresponding symptoms.

In general most patients with polymyalgia rheumatica can be controlled on 10 mg prednisolone daily, but the severity of symptoms dictates the choice of dosage. Again dosage is gradually lowered when symptoms are fully controlled and the sedimentation rate is normal (1 mg reductions every 3 or 4 weeks). Patients with polymyalgia rheumatica are usually elderly, almost all have arthritis of neck and back. It is therefore of importance to try to distinguish between the aches and pains of osteoarthritis and the very different symptoms of polymyalgia.

The author believes that there is no justification for treating polymyalgia with non-steroidal anti-inflammatory agents. All patients should receive corticosteroid and indeed this may be used to confirm the diagnosis, since failure to show a significant response within 3–4 days to an adequate dose virtually excludes the diagnosis. Whilst non-steroidal anti-inflammatory agents will often improve the symptoms they do not control the underlying arteritis and vascular complications may develop. Hunder (1974), however, considers that non-steroidal anti-inflammatory drugs may be tried in patients with polymyalgia rheumatica if there are no symptoms or signs of vascular involvement and especially in those with normal temporal artery biopsies. They suggest that if patients do not respond adequately in the first few weeks, prednisolone should then be started.

Jones & Hazleman (1981b) emphasise that there is no method of identifying those patients who will develop complications of their disease. Temporal artery biopsy was of no value in predicting which patients would be likely to develop signs of giant cell arteritis. Indeed in this series of 85 patients the 6 patients who developed prominent loss of vision had no clinical evidence of giant cell arteritis in the early stages of the disease. Fauchald et al (1972) and Hamilton et al (1971) considered that all patients with polymyalgia should be treated with high doses of corticosteroids as if they had giant cell arteritis. However, it should be emphasised that high dose corticosteroids in this elderly group of patients will produce a morbidity and mortality of their own, and this must be weighed against the severity of the disease. For this reason lower doses of steroids are used in this group. Alternate day regimes appear less effective (Hunder et al, 1975) though side-effects are reduced, and there is less suppression of the hypothalamic–pituitary–adrenal axis. The suppressive effects of cytotoxic drugs have not been studied in a systematic fashion.

There is controversy over the length of time for which treatment is required but at least 18 months is likely. Recurrence of symptoms is common on reducing the dose of steroid and reduction of 1 mg in the late stages may be associated with increase of symptoms. Recrudescence of disease may also occur in an unpredictable fashion and has been noted several years after presentation. In many patients, resolution occurs over 2–3 years. Jones & Hazleman (1981b) found that a third of their patients required 10 mg of prednisone or more after 1 year's treatment, and Coomes et al (1976) found that treatment was necessary for 5 years or longer in 84% of their patients with polymyalgia. Jones & Hazleman (1981b) found that arteritis and complications developed up to 9 years after the onset of polymyalgia (mean 1 year). Patients require regular follow-up and should be instructed to report to their doctor if there is any exacerbation of their myalgia or if there are visual symptoms. The clinician should be alert to the development of signs of giant cell arteritis at any time in the long course of this disease and not become complacent in the management of the apparently fit corticosteroid-treated patient.

Treatment schedules will improve when we better understand the natural history of the disease. We are currently unable to identify those at risk from exacerbation and we do not know how long or frequently to follow-up the patient. However, we are dealing with an elderly population and attention to detail over prescribing with clear instructions, and supervision if necessary, will do much to avoid problems with compliance. Polymyalgia is a very satisfying condition to treat but full patient-cooperation and careful follow-up is necessary.

REFERENCES

Ainsworth R W, Gresham G A, Balmforth G V 1961 Pathological changes in temporal arteries removed from unselected cadavers. Journal of Clinical Pathology 14: 115–119

Alestig K, Barr J 1963 Giant cell arteritis: biopsy study of polymyalgia rheumatica, including one case of Takayasu's disease. Lancet 1: 1228–1230

Ali Ibn Isa, Woods C A (trans) 1936 Memorandum book of a 10th century oculist. Northwestern University, Chicago

Andrews F M 1965 Polymyalgia rheumatica. Practitioner 205: 635–640

Bacon P A, Doherty S M, Zuckerman A J 1975 Hepatitis-B antibody in polymyalgia rheumatica. Lancet 2: 476–478

Barber H S 1957 Myalgic syndrome with constitutional effects. Polymyalgia rheumatica. Annals of the Rheumatic Diseases 16: 230–237

Bell W R, Klinefelter H F 1967 Polymyalgia rheumatica. John Hopkin's Medical Journal 121: 175–187

Bender K, Mayerova A, Klotzbucher B, Burckhardt K, Miller C 1976 No indication of postnatal selection at the HLA loci. Tissue Antigens 7: 118–121

Bengtsson B E, Malmvall B A 1981 The epidemiology of giant cell arteritis including temporal arteritis and polymyalgia rheumatica. Arthritis and Rheumatism 24: 899–904

Brooke M H, Kaplan H 1972 Muscle pathology in rheumatoid arthritis, polymyalgia rheumatica, and polymyositis: A histochemical study. Archives of Pathology 94: 101–106

Bruce W 1888 Senile rheumatic gout. British Medical Journal 2: 811–813

Bruk M I 1967 Articular and vascular manifestations of polymyalgia rheumatica. Annals of the Rheumatic Diseases 26: 103–113

Coomes E N, Sharp J 1961 Polymyalgia rheumatica. A misnomer? Lancet 2: 1328–1331

Coomes E N, Ellis R M, Kay A G 1976 A prospective study of 102 patients with polymyalgia rheumatica syndrome. Rheumatology and Rehabilitation 15: 270–276

Darnule T V, Likhite V, Darnule A T 1980 Enhancement of humoral immune response against human lung elastin peptides. Experientia 36: 606–607

Dent G R, Edwards O M 1978 Autoimmune thyroid disease and the polymyalgia rheumatica–giant cell arteritis syndrome. Clinical Endocrinology 9: 215–219

Dequeker J V 1981 Polymyalgia rheumatica with temporal arteritis, as painted by Jan Van Eyck in 1436. Canadian Medical Association Journal 124: 1597–1598

Dixon A St. J, Beardwell C, Kay A, Wanka J, Wong Y T 1966 Polymyalgia rheumatica and temporal arteritis. Annals of the Rheumatic Diseases 25: 203–208

Eghtedari A A, Esselinckx W, Bacon P A 1976 Circulating immunoblasts in polymyalgia rheumatica. Annals of the Rheumatic Diseases 35: 158–162

Fauchald R, Rygvold O, Oystese B 1972 Temporal arteritis and polymyalgia rheumatica. Clinical and biopsy findings. Annals of Internal Medicine 77: 845–52

Fessel W J 1969 Polymyalgia rheumatica, temporal arteritis and contact with birds. Lancet 2: 1249–1250

Forestier J, Certonciny A 1953 Pseudopolyarthritis rhizomelique. Revue du Rheumatisme et des Maladies Osteo-Articulaires 20:854

Gallagher P, Jones K 1982 Immunohistochemical findings in cranial arteritis. Arthritis and Rheumatism 25: 75–79

Gilmour J R 1941 Giant cell chronic arteritis. Journal of Pathology 53: 263–268

Hamilton C R J R, Shelley W M, Tumulty P A 1971 Giant cell arteritis: Including temporal arteritis and polymyalgia rheumatica. Medicine (Baltimore) 50: 1–25

Hamrin B, Jonsson N, Landberg T 1965 Involvement of large vessels in polymyalgia arteritica. Lancet 1: 1193–1196

Hazleman B L, Maclennan I C M, Esiri M M 1975 Lymphocyte proliferation to artery antigen as a positive diagnostic test in polymyalgia rheumatica. Annals of the Rheumatic Diseases 34: 122–127

Hazleman B L, Goldstone A, Voak D 1977 Association of polymyalgia rheumatica and giant cell arteritis with HLA-B8. British Medical Journal 3: 989–991

Henderson D R F, Tribe C R, Dixon A St J 1975 Synovitis in polymyalgia rheumatica. Rheumatology and Rehabilitation 14: 244–249

Horton B T, Magath T B, Brown G E 1932 An undescribed form of arteritis of the temporal vessels. Mayo Clinic Proceedings 7: 700–701

Hunder C G 1974 Polymyalgia rheumatica. Journal of Rheumatology 1:140

Hunder G G, Sheps S G, Allen G L, Joyce J W 1975 Daily and alternate day corticosteroid regimes in treatment of giant cell arteritis: Comparison in a prospective study. Annals of Internal Medicine 82: 613–617

Hunder G G, Taswell H F, Pineda A A, Elveback L R 1977 HLA antigens in patients with giant cell arteritis and polymyalgia rheumatica. Journal of Rheumatology 4: 321–323

Huston K A, Hunder G G, Lie J T, Kennedy R H, Elveback L R 1978 Temporal Arteritis. A 25 year epidemiologic, clinical and pathologic study. Annals of Internal Medicine 88: 162–167

Hutchinson J 1890 On a peculiar form of thrombotic arteritis of the aged which is sometimes productive of gangrene. Archives of Surgery 1: 323–327

Isaacs H, Frere G 1973 Non-specific arthralgia and myalgia with subclinical neuropathy. South African Medical Journal 2: 1581–1584

Jones J G, Hazleman B L 1981a Polymyalgia rheumatica and giant cell arteritis — a difficult diagnosis. Journal of the Royal College of General Practitioners 31: 283–289

Jones J G, Hazleman B L 1981b Prognosis and management of polymyalgia rheumatica. Annals of the Rheumatic Diseases 1: 1–5

Jones J G, Park J R, Hazleman B L 1980 Lack of consistent peripheral blood lymphocyte transformation responses in polymyalgia rheumatica and giant cell arteritis. Journal of Rheumatology 7: (6) 891–894

Kersley G D 1951 A myalgic syndrome of the elderly. Proceedings II Congress of European Rheumatology, Barcelona. Revista Espanola de Rheumatismo, p 388

Klein R G, Hunder G G, Stenson A W, Sheps S G 1975 Large artery involvement in giant cell (temporal) arteritis. Annals of Internal Medicine 83: 806–809

Klein R G, Campbell R J, Hunder G G, Carney J A 1976 skip lesions is temporal arteritis. Mayo Clinic Proceedings 51: 504–508

Knorring J Von, Somer T 1974 Malignancy in association with polymyalgia rheumatica and giant cell arteritis. Scandinavian Journal of Rheumatology 3: 129–133

Kvernebo K, Brath H K 1980 Polymyalgia arteritica. A report on 5 cases within a family. Scandinavian Journal of Rheumatology 9: 187–189

Kyle V, Jones J, Hazleman B 1982 Abnormal liver scans in PMR/GCA. Annals of the Rheumatic Diseases 41:636

Kyle V, Hazleman B L, King R H 1983 Polymyalgia rheumatica/giant cell arteritis in husband and wife. Clinical Rheumatology (in press)

Liang G C, Simkin P A, Mannick M 1974a Immunoglobulins in temporal arteries. Annals of Internal Medicine 81: 19–24

Liang G C, Simkin P A, Hunder G G, Wilske K R, Healey L A 1974b Familial aggregation of polymyalgia rheumatica and giant cell arteritis. Arthritis and Rheumatism 17: 19–24

Liang M, Greenberg H, Pincus T, Robinson W S 1976 Hepatitis B antibodies in polymyalgia rheumatica. Lancet 1:43

Long R, James O 1974 Polymyalgia rheumatica and liver disease. Lancet 1:77

Lowenstein M B, Bridgeford P H, Vasey F B, Germain B F, Espinoza L R 1982 Increased frequency of HLA-DR3 and DR4 in polymyalgia rheumatica-giant cell arteritis. Arthritis and Rheumatism 25 (No. 4 Suppl):S31

McCormack L R, Astanta R W, Foroozar P 1978 Liver involvement in giant cell arteritis. Digestive Diseases 23 (Suppl): 725–745

Malmvall B E, Bengtsson B A, Kaijser B, Nilsson L A, Alestig K 1976 Serum levels of immunoglobulin and complement in giant cell arteritis. Journal of the American Medical Association 236: 1876–1878

Malmvall B E, Bengtsson B A, Nilsson L A, Bjursten L M 1981 Immune complexes, rheumatoid factors and cellular immunological parameters in patients with giant cell arteritis. Annals of the Rheumatic Diseases 40: 276–280

Mattingley P C, Mowat A G, Gunson H H, Jackman C 1978 HLA antigens in polymyalgia rheumatica. British Medical Journal 2: 989–990

Meulengracht E, Schwartz M 1952 The cause and prognosis of periarthrosis humeroscapularis with special regard to cases and general symptoms. Acta Medica Scandinavica 143:350

Morgan G J Jr, Harris E D Jr 1978 Non-giant cell temporal arteritis: Three cases and a review of the literature. Arthritis and Rheumatism 21: 362–363

Mowat A G, Hazleman B L 1974 Polymyalgia rheumatica: A clinical study with particular reference to arterial disease. Journal of Rheumatology 1: 190–202

O'Duffy D J, Wahner H W, Hunder G G 1976 Joint imaging in polymyalgia rheumatica. Mayo Clinic Proceedings 51: 519–524

Ornilla E, Swannell A S, Dixon A St J 1970 Myalgia and bird-keeping. Lancet 2: 96–98

Ostberg G 1973 On arteritis with special reference to polymyalgia arteritica. Acta Pathologica Microbiologica Scandinavia 237 (Suppl): 1–59

Papaioannoau C C, Gupta R C, Hunder G G, McDuffie F C 1980 Circulating immune complexes in giant cell arteritis and polymyalgia rheumatica. Arthritis and Rheumatism 23:1021

Park J R, Hazleman B L 1978 Immunological and histological study of temporal arteries. Annals of the Rheumatic Diseases 37: 238–243

Park J R, Jones J G, Harkiss G D, Hazleman B L 1981a Circulating immune complexes in polymyalgia and giant cell arteritis. Annals of the Rheumatic Diseases 40: 360–365

Park J R, Jones J G, Hazleman B L 1981b Relationship of the erythrocyte sedimentation rate to acute phase proteins in polymyalgia rheumatica and giant cell arteritis. Annals of the Rheumatic Diseases 40: 493–495

Park J, Jones J G, Hazleman B L 1981c In vitro lymphocytotoxicity to cultured human arterial smooth muscle cells in patients with giant cell arteritis and polymyalgia rheumatica. Journal of Rheumatology 8: 125–128

Parker F, Healey L A, Wilske K R, Odland G F 1975 Light and electron microscopic studies on human temporal arteritis with special reference to alterations related to senescence atherosclerosis and giant cell arteritis. American Journal of Pathology 79: 57–70.

Paulley J W, Hughes J P 1960 Giant cell arteritis or arteritis of aged. British Medical Journal 2: 1562–1567

Porsman V A 1951 Proceedings II Congress European Rheumatology. Editorial Scienta, Barcelona, p 479

Rhodes D J 1976 Giant cell arteritis in general practice. Journal of the Royal College of Practitioners 26: 337–346

Richards A J 1978 Carpal tunnel syndrome and polymyalgia rheumatica in the elderly. Arthritis and Rheumatism 21: 865–868

Salisbury R S, Hazleman B L 1981 Successful treatment of dissecting aortic aneurysm due to giant cell arteritis. Annals of the Rheumatic Diseases 40: 507–508

Sandford R G, Berney S N 1977 Polymyalgia rheumatica and temporal arteritis in blacks — clinical features and HLA-

typing. Journal of Rheumatology 4:435
Silman A J, Currey H L F 1982 Polymyalgia rheumatica in a defined elderly community. Rheumatology and Rehabilitation 21: 235–237
Smith G S, Walford K L 1977 Influence of the main histocompatability complex on ageing in mice. Nature 270: 727–729
Smith K R 1969 Electron microscopy of giant cell (temporal) arteritis. Journal of Neurology, Neurosurgery and Psychiatry 32: 348–352
Terasaki P J, Healey L A, Wilske K R 1976 Distribution of HLA haplotypes in polymyalgia rheumatica. New England Journal of Medicine 295:905
Thomas R D, Croft D N 1974 Thyrotoxicosis and giant cell arteritis. British Medical Journal 2: 408–409
White A G, Innes E H 1972 Polymyalgia rheumatica and contact with melopsittacus undulatus. Rheumatology and Physical Medicine 11: 380–384
Wilkinson I M S, Russell R W R 1972 Arteries of the head and neck in giant cell arteritis. A pathological study to show the pattern of arterial involvement. Archives of Neurology 27: 378–382

52

D.G.I. Scott

Vasculitis

Definition

'Vasculitis' literally means 'inflammation of blood vessels'. Although many clinical syndromes are characterised by vascular inflammation, vasculitis implies histopathological change. Within this framework there is a spectrum of disease dependent upon the size of vessels involved (artery, arteriole, capillary, venule) and the type of inflammatory infiltrate (acute leucocytoclastic, eosinophilic, lymphocytic, granulomatous, etc.). Difficulties in understanding vasculitic diseases arise because the size of blood vessel and the inflammatory infiltrate may vary within patients with a specific clinical disease, the inflammatory response changes with time, and different clinical patterns of disease may be associated with identical histopathological changes. For example rheumatoid arthritis may be complicated by acute necrotising arteritis, leucocytoclastic and lymphocytic small vessel vasculitis and granulomatous lesions (rheumatoid nodules); these vascular lesions may all be detected in one patient at the same time or sequentially. A similar spectrum of vascular involvement may occur in Wegener's granulomatosis and allergic granulomatous angiitis.

The term 'systemic' indicates multiple organ involvement in diseases such as polyarteritis nodosa, but localised forms of polyarteritis, Wegener's granulomatosis and allergic granulomatous angiitis have been described. Similarly small vessel vasculitis may be widespread or restricted to the retina or the skin.

Vasculitis is thus best described as a clinicopathological process characterised by inflammation and necrosis of blood vessels. This recognises the diverse clinical and pathological nature of vascular inflammation and the problems that exist in combining clinical and histological patterns of disease.

Classification

Many different classification systems have been described based on clinical features, histopathology and aetiology. Most are based on the classic review by Zeek who in 1952 subdivided vasculitis into hypersensitivity angiitis, allergic granulomatous angiitis, rheumatic arteritis, periarteritis nodosa and temporal arteritis. More recent classifications use the term polyarteritis nodosa *group* to indicate that polyarteritis is not a distinct disease entity.

A simple classification is shown in Table 52.1; this uses the term 'systemic necrotising arteritis' to indicate that arterial involvement is essential for inclusion in this group. This classification is based on the *largest* vessel involved as this may have an

Table 52.1 Classification of vasculitis

1. Systemic necrotising arteritis
   a. Polyarteritis nodosa group
      e.g. Classical, hepatitis B associated polyarteritis nodosa (PAN)
      Infantile PAN, Kawasaki's disease
      Arteritis of RA, SLE, other connective tissue diseases
   b. With granulomatosis
      e.g. Allergic granulomatous angiitis
      Wegener's granulomatosis
2. Small vessel or hypersensitivity vasculitis
   e.g. Henoch–Schönlein purpura
   Essential mixed cryoglobulinaemia
   Vasculitis of RA, SLE, other connective tissue diseases
3. Large vessel, giant cell arteritis
   e.g. Temporal arteritis
   Takayasu's arteritis

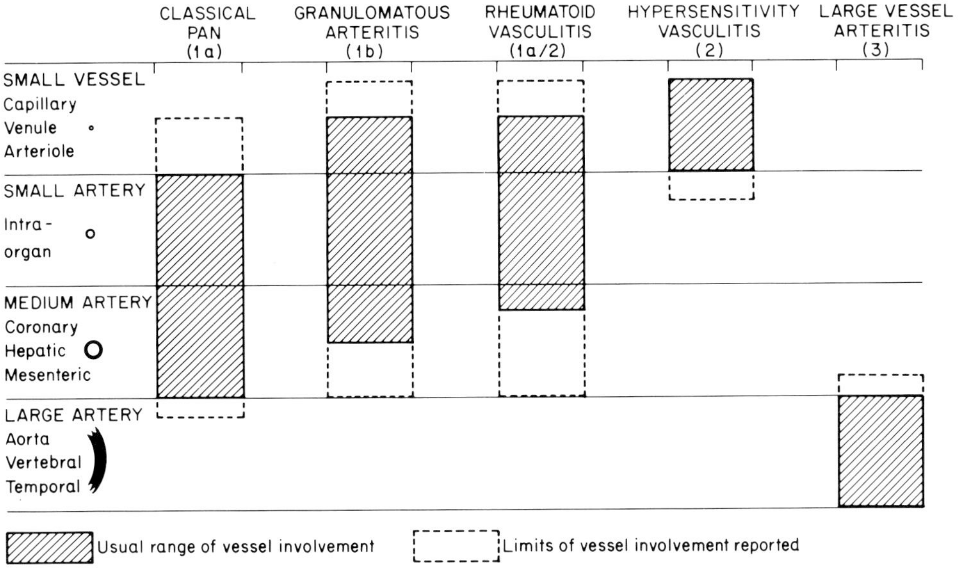

Fig. 52.1 Relationship between vessel size and classification groups (shown in parenthesis).

important bearing on prognosis and treatment. By depicting the range of vessel size (Fig. 52.1), the overlap between granulomatous vasculitis, rheumatoid vasculitis and classical polyarteritis nodosa is clearly shown and justifies the use of a broad systemic necrotising arteritis group.

Granulomatous vasculitis is sometimes classified separately from polyarteritis nodosa. However, some patients show features of both and may be classified as overlap syndromes (Fauci et al, 1978). It is more useful to consider the relationship between vasculitis and granulomatosis as a spectrum ranging from pure arteritis at one end to pure granulomatosis at the other with many diseases showing some features of both (Fig. 52.2). Patients with pulmonary involvement may have distinctive clinical features, a different aetiology and a higher incidence of granulomatosis, but the extrapulmonary vascular lesions are often identical to those seen in classical polyarteritis nodosa with

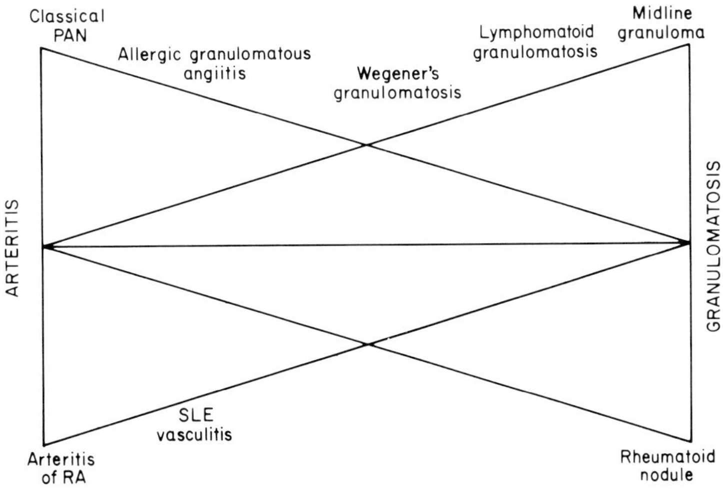

Fig. 52.2 Relationship between arteritis and granulomatosis (based on Alarcon-Segovia, 1980).

the same potentially serious consequences.

It may seem more appropriate to base classification on aetiological factors. The problems created by such an approach are most clearly seen when the role of hepatitis B surface antigen is examined. Immune complexes containing hepatitis BsAg have been implicated in the aetiology of classical polyarteritis nodosa (Gocke et al, 1970), small vessel vasculitis (Gower et al, 1978), urticarial vasculitis (Neumann et al, 1981), cryoglobulinaemic vasculitis (Levo et al, 1977), as well as glomerulonephritis (Combes et al, 1971), arthritis (Onion et al, 1971) and temporal arteritis (Bacon et al, 1975). Hepatitis BsAg and antibody have even been demonstrated in vessel walls in patients with chronic aggressive hepatitis in the absence of active vasculitis (Nowoslawski et al, 1972).

The lack of complete understanding of aetiology and pathogenesis and the wide spectrum of clinical and histological patterns of disease explain the difficulties in formulating useful classification systems. Patients with systemic necrotising arteritis have severe life-threatening disease which may respond to aggressive cytotoxic therapy. By contrast, patients with small vessel vasculitis or temporal arteritis have more benign disease usually responsive to corticosteroids. This suggests that whatever the clinical pattern of disease, or the aetiology, prognosis is dependent on the size and type of vessel involved and a simple histological classification is at present the most appropriate.

PATHOGENETIC MECHANISMS

The most frequently postulated mechanism for the production of vasculitis is the deposition of circulating immune complexes. This may depend on local factors which make blood vessels susceptible to injury as well as the role of the individual immune response of the host to antigenic challenge.

Circulating immune complexes and vasculitis

Experimental studies in animals have established that exposure to antigen results in the production of soluble immune complexes in the circulation, their deposition in blood vessel walls and vascular damage (Cochrane & Dixon, 1976). Lesions can be induced locally by an Arthus reaction and parenterally as in experimental serum sickness or by the intravenous administration of preformed immune complexes.

Circulating immune complexes may activate the complement system generating anaphylotoxins capable of degranulating mast cells and chemotactic factors for neutrophils, the dominant cell in early vasculitic lesions. The complement system is critical as depletion of complement components beyond C_2 blocks the development of vascular inflammation despite immune complex deposition (Henson & Cochrane, 1971). Complement may also be protective by neutralising viral antigen (Notkins, 1971) and by the solubilisation of immune complexes (Miller & Nussenzweig, 1975). In rheumatic diseases and infection an antibody to activated complement components (immunoconglutinin) may be produced resulting in increased clumping of immune complexes. The balance between complement solubilisation and immunoconglutinin-induced clumping may be critical to the deposition of circulating immune complexes.

Polymorphonuclear leucocytes are also critical as their depletion abolishes the vasculitis of the Arthus reaction or serum sickness (Kniker & Cochrane, 1965). Polymorphs phagocytose immune complexes and release lysosomal enzymes which may destroy the basement membrane and internal elastic lamina of the vessel wall.

The endothelial cell interaction with immune complexes and polymorphs is also important. Fc receptors for human IgG (Johnson et al, 1975; Matre, 1977) and C1q receptors (Andrews et al, 1981) on endothelial cells provide a binding site for circulating immune complexes. Polymorphs adhere avidly to endothelial cells and may be cytotoxic in the presence of complement mediated by the release of oxygen free radicals (Sacks et al, 1978; Weiss et al, 1981).

The endothelial cell is an important early site of ultrastructural change in vascular inflammation (Dobrescu et al, 1983). Reactions between circulating blood cells and serum with endothelial cells are therefore potentially important in the pathogenesis of vasculitis. In addition to immune complex interactions with endothelial cells, nonimmune factors (probably oxidised lipoproteins) in sera from patients with systemic necrotising arteritis, and peripheral blood mononuclear cells from patients with Takayasu's arteritis have been shown to be cytotoxic to cultured human umbilical cord endothelial cells (Scott et al, 1984).

Endothelial cells secrete a variety of factors involved in the coagulation process and prostacyclin (Jaffe & Weksler, 1979). Activated platelets secrete vasoactive mediators including thromboxane A2 and Cupps & Fauci (1981) suggest that the balance between thromboxane A2 (promotes platelet aggregation) and prostacycline (inhibits platelet aggregation) may be important in the induction of local vasculitic lesions.

Mechanical factors may be involved in the localisation of immune complexes. Serum sickness lesions predominate at vessel branching points (Kniker & Cochrane, 1968), hypertension increases the severity of vascular lesions (Fisher & Bark, 1961) and hydrostatic pressure may explain the frequent localisation of cutaneous vasculitis to lower limbs.

Experimentally induced reticulo-endothelial blockade results in delayed clearance of immune complexes (Haakenstad & Mannik, 1974) and an increased risk of their tissue deposition. Such blockade may in part explain the association between vasculitis and lymphoproliferative disorders such as hairy cell leukaemia (reviewed by Elkon et al, 1979). Delayed reticuloendothelial clearance of sensitised erythrocytes has been described in other diseases associated with vasculitis including systemic lupus erythematosus and rheumatoid arthritis (Lockwood et al, 1979; Williams et al, 1979) and impaired complement-mediated phagocytosis by monocytes has been reported in patients with cutaneous vasculitis and rheumatoid arthritis (Hurst & Nuki, 1981).

Immune complexes in clinical vasculitic diseases

Circulating immune complexes have been described in the majority of vasculitic diseases by a variety of methods. Two diseases extensively studied for the role of immune complexes in their pathogenesis are rheumatoid vasculitis and hepatitis B associated polyarteritis nodosa.

Circulating immune complexes have been detected in patients with rheumatoid vasculitis by a wide variety of techniques. The presence of cryoglobulinaemia (Weisman & Zvaifler, 1975; Erhardt et al, 1979) and anticomplementary activity (Scott et al, 1981a) is associated with vasculitis as opposed to synovitis. Complement activation is common, detected by serum hypocomplementaemia and raised levels of the complement breakdown product C3d (Scott et al, 1982b). Serial studies have shown a close relationship between active vasculitis and anti-complementary activity, IgG rheumatoid factor and hypocomplementaemia (especially C4) suggesting that complement activating immune complexes may have an important pathogenetic role (Scott et al, 1981a). These complexes are large (greater than 19s) and contain IgM and IgG rheumatoid factors and C3 (Jones et al, 1980; Elson et al, 1983). Other autoantibodies may also be involved including 7s IgM rheumatoid factor (Roberts-Thompson et al, 1981) and precipitating antibodies to extractable nuclear antigens (Venables et al, 1980; Quismorio et al, 1983).

Immunoglobulin and complement are detected in the walls of affected blood vessels (Conn et al, 1972; Rapoport et al, 1980) and immune complex deposition can be induced by the intradermal injection of histamine (MacFarlane et al, 1981). In susceptible (seropositive) patients, intradermal histamine can induce various degrees of leucocytoclastic vasculitis in dermal vessels as well as IgM and C3 deposition. Seronegative patients have neither immune nor histological changes (Jorizzo et al, 1983). There is therefore considerable evidence to implicate immune complex deposition in the pathogenesis of rheumatoid vasculitis.

Circulating immune complexes are commonly detected in patients with the polyarteritis nodosa group of systemic necrotising arteritides. Hypocomplementaemia and complement activation are usually restricted to patients with hepatitis B associated disease (see below). Immunoglobulin and complement may be detected in the walls of affected blood vessels but rarely in affected glomeruli in patients with renal involvement (Ronco et al, 1983). The correlation between levels of circulating immune complexes and disease activity is often poor suggesting that other mechanisms may be involved.

Non-infective exogenous agents including foods, drugs and immunisation procedures have also been implicated in the aetiology of systemic vasculitis (Mullick et al, 1979; Blumberg et al, 1980; Phanuphak & Kohler, 1980).

Viral infection

Animal models demonstrate that vasculitis may occur in response to direct viral replication within blood vessel walls (e.g. equine viral arteritis) as well as through the deposition of immune complexes (Aleutian disease of mink) (reviewed by Sergent, 1980). Viral replication has been demonstrated in cultured human endothelial cells (Friedman et al, 1981) and viral infection of human endothelial cells increases granulocyte adherence (MacGregor et al, 1980). However, the importance of such direct viral infection in human vasculitic disease is unknown.

Immune mechanisms are strongly implicated in hepatitis B-associated polyarteritis nodosa — the best recognised viral-associated systemic vasculitis in man. Hepatitis BsAg has been detected in circulating immune complexes (Gocke et al, 1970; Trepo et al, 1974; Sergent et al, 1976), in cryoglobulins (Levo et al, 1977), in affected blood vessel walls (Gocke et al, 1970; Michalak, 1978), and has been eluted from the kidneys together with immunoglobulin by treatment known to dissociate antigen–antibody bonds (Michalak, 1978). Higher levels of hepatitis BsAg containing immune complexes (analysed by precipitation techniques) are seen in patients with hepatitis B-associated cutaneous *venulitis* than those with hepatitis B-associated polyarteritis nodosa, but levels of hepatitis BsAg in the antigen fraction of the complex are greater in polyarteritis and correlate with clinical improvement (Gupta & Kohler, 1984). However, the association between disease activity and levels of other immune complex assays, or circulating free hepatitis BsAg and Ab, is often poor, stressing that antigen identification does not explain the entire pathogenetic mechanism.

A variety of other viral antigens have been reported in patients with vasculitis. These include cytomegalovirus (Bamji &Salisbury, 1978; Doherty & Bradfield, 1981), herpes zoster (Mackenzie et al, 1981), herpes simplex (Phinney et al, 1982), and Epstein–Barr virus (Hoffman & Frank, 1979). These associations do not always implicate immune complex-mediated disease but stress the importance of searching for viral antigens in vasculitis.

Other mechanisms

Atopy is a feature of allergic granulomatous vasculitis and Wegener's granulomatosis. Elevated IgE levels are described in both diseases (Conn et al, 1976) and may suggest a fundamental defect in T cell control. Basophils in the presence of IgE and an appropriate antigen degranulate releasing histamine and platelet activating factor, leading to platelet clumping and release of more vasoactive amines.

Cell-mediated mechanisms may be important in the production of granulomatous vasculitis (reviewed by Cupps & Fauci, 1981). Animal studies have demonstrated vasculitis in vivo following intravenous injection of activated splenic lymphocytes (cocultured with an endothelial cell line) suggesting direct lymphocyte-mediated vascular inflammation (Hart et al, 1983). We have recently described increased numbers of circulating activated lymphocytes and lymphocyte-mediated cytotoxicity on cultured human endothelial cells in vitro in patients with Takayasu's arteritis and temporal arteritis (Scott et al, 1984). Immunohistological studies show that the inflammatory lymphoid vascular infiltrates comprise predominantly T lymphocytes in the granulomatous vasculitides and large vessel giant cell arteritis. The majority of these T lymphocytes stain with specific monoclonal antibody markers for T helper cells in Churg–Strauss vasculitis (Winkelmann et al, 1983) and temporal arteritis (Banks et al, 1983). One patient with Takayasu's arteritis studied in our own laboratory showed a vascular infiltrate comprising 90% T lymphocytes, nearly all staining with the marker for T suppressor/cytotoxic cells. Studies of circulating lymphocytes using monoclonal antibody markers in these different vasculitic diseases have given conflicting results. Few functional assays have been reported but in small numbers of patients we found impaired T suppressor cell activity in rheumatoid vasculitis but not polyarteritis nodosa (Scott, 1981).

Some patients with cutaneous vasculitis have strong delayed hypersensitivity reactions to streptococcal and mycobacterial antigens despite the absence of the antigen in the lesions (Miescher et al, 1967). It is possible that certain subjects develop such a high degree of cell-mediated immunity to microbial antigens that minute amounts of antigen in the vasculature will lead to protracted reactions of type IV hypersensitivity. This mechanism may be important in some post-infective or allergic vasculitides (Dumonde & Richards, 1981).

Immunogenetic studies have revealed important associations between HLA markers and a variety of diseases. The numbers of patients with vasculitis included in such studies are often small but the following associations have been reported — Wegener's granulomatosis with HLA-DR2 (Elkon et al, 1983), polyarteritis nodosa with HLA-DR7 (Scott et al, 1982b), rheumatoid vasculitis with HLA-DR4 (Scott et al, 1981c) and with HLA-B8, DR3 (Cunningham et al, 1982) and temporal arteritis with HLA-DR4 and DR3 (Lowenstein et al, 1983), HLA-DR4 and Cw6 (Armstrong et al, 1983), and also with the immunoglobulin allotype Gm2 (Demaine et al, 1983). These genetic markers may be important for the different clinical and histological expression of vasculitic diseases.

Vasculitis may be seen as the result of various aetiological agents acting through different (mainly immunological) mechanisms in a susceptible host. Immune complex deposition is the most extensively studied pathogenetic mechanism but the regulation of the immune response, genetic susceptibility and other immunological mechanisms require further study.

CLINICAL SYNDROMES — SYSTEMIC NECROTISING ARTERITIS

Classical polyarteritis nodosa

The initial description of this disease was by Rokitansky (1852) although Kussmaul & Maier (1866) first used the term 'periarteritis nodosa' to describe a disease characterised by intimal inflammation in medium-sized arteries leading to nodular aneurysms in a 27-year-old man. The term 'polyarteritis' is now used to indicate that many vessels are involved and that histology reveals a panarteritis with acute inflammatory cell infiltration and fibrinoid necrosis of the media, adventitia and endothelium (Fig. 52.3). Nuclear debris from degenerating neutrophils (leucocytoclasis) is common in early lesions but mononuclear cells are also involved in later stages. Giant cells are rarely seen. Lesions may be segmental (involving small sections of the artery) and focal (involving part of the artery wall). Segmental lesions lead to occlusion whereas focal lesions may give rise to aneurysm formation. Infarction due to arterial occlusion and haemorrhage due to aneurysmal rupture are the two most important features of this disease. The evolution of the vascular lesions closely parallel those of serum sickness (Arkin, 1930). Chronic or 'burnt out' arteritis is characterised by a lack of inflammatory infiltrate, fibrous replacement of the subendothelial layer and destruction of the internal elastic lamina (Fig. 52.4). All stages of evolution may be present at any given time.

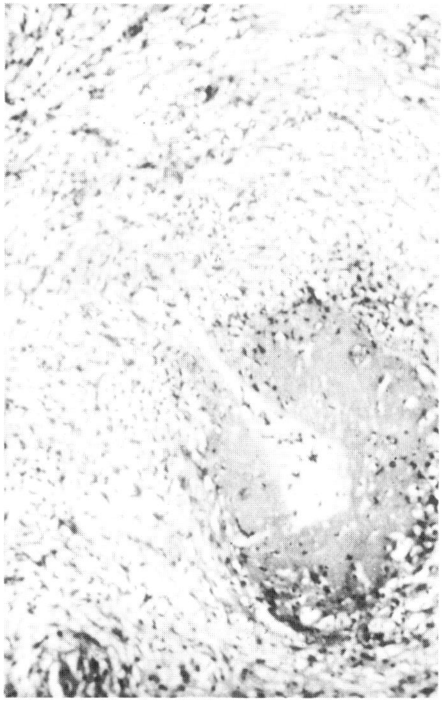

Fig. 52.3 Polyarteritis nodosa; acute necrotising arteritis with fibrinoid necrosis and aneurysm formation in a small testicular artery (reproduced by courtesy of Dr C. R. Tribe.). (H & E × 200)

Polyarteritis nodosa has been described in all age-groups including the elderly as well as infants and children when it may be associated with a febrile illness, characteristic mucocutaneous lesions and lymphadenopathy (Kawasaki et al, 1974). The mean age at onset is 45 but may be higher in a District General Hospital population (Scott et al,

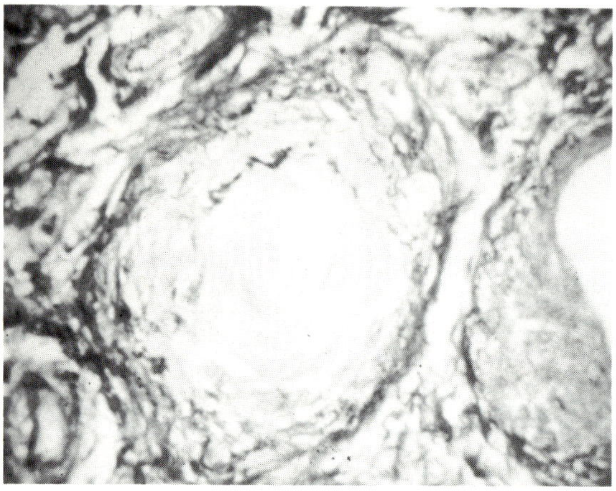

Fig. 52.4 Polyarteritis nodosa; chronic arteritis. Elastic stain showing complete disruption of the internal elastic lamina in a renal artery with almost complete occlusion of the lumen. (Reproduced by courtesy of Dr C. R. Tribe.) (van Geison × 200)

1982a). It is slightly commoner in males (male to female ratios range from 4 : 1 to 1.3 : 1) and its incidence is approximately 5/million/year.

Diagnosis

Classical polyarteritis nodosa can involve any organ system and may be confused with a variety of diseases. Polyarteritis nodosa should be considered in the differential diagnosis of

a. Pyrexia of unknown origin
b. Acute abdominal pain with features suggesting more than one organ involvement
c. Neuropathy or myopathy
d. Glomerulonephritis, unexplained haematuria or hypertension
e. Cutaneous rashes, especially ulcers, livedo reticularis or nodules
f. Myocardial ischaemia in young patients
g. Unexplained neurological disease especially if associated with systemic symptoms and a raised erythrocyte sedimentation rate.

The two 'diagnostic' procedures commonly used are tissue biopsy and visceral angiography. The demonstration of aneurysms at visceral angiography merely reflects the intensity of the arteritis but is not specific to classical polyarteritis nodosa. Aneurysms have been reported in Wegener's granulomatosis (Baker & Robinson, 1978; Moutsopoulos et al, 1983), allergic granulomatous angiitis (Travers et al, 1979), rheumatoid arthritis (Webb and Payne, 1970; Paci et al, 1983), thrombotic thrombocytopenic purpura (Straer et al, 1973), systemic lupus erythematosus (Longstreth et al, 1974), Behçet's syndrome (Durieux et al, 1981), bacterial endocarditis (Clark et al, 1972), and atrial myxoma (Leonhardt & Kullenberg, 1977), as well as in non-vasculitic diseases (reviewed by Travers et al, 1979). Angiography is still a useful investigation demonstrating the widespread nature of arterial involvement and confirming that there is arterial as opposed to small vessel disease (Fig. 52.5). Visceral angiography should include coeliac as well as renal arteries and aneurysms are detected in up to 70% of cases of polyarteritis nodosa (Chatel et al, 1979; Travers et al, 1979). Serial studies may reflect the episodic nature of vascular inflammation (Fisher, 1981) and healing with successful treatment (Fauci et al, 1978).

Renal biopsy is the most useful site for tissue diagnosis. Where possible renal biopsy should follow visceral angiography because of the potential danger of aneurysmal rupture. However, angiography itself is not without risk and has been reported to precipitate renal failure in polyarteritis nodosa (Kaur et al, 1982). Renal biopsy may help differentiate classical polyarteritis nodosa from Wegener's granulomatosis or small vessel vasculitis. Arteritis is characteristic of polyarteritis nodosa, crescentic glomerulonephritis suggests Wegener's granulomatosis and focal necrotising glomerulonephritis or glomerulitis suggests small vessel vasculitis (Mills & McCroskery, 1981). There may be considerable overlap between these histological features and necrotising glomerulitis and arteritis often coexist in patients with Wegener's granulomatosis or polyarteritis nodosa. Other patients have aneurysms demonstrated angiographically but only necrotising glomerulitis at renal biopsy (Fig. 52.6) suggesting that the term 'microscopic polyarteritis' which is used to describe focal necrotising glomerulonephritis is often inappropriate. Immunofluorescence and electron-microscopy help differentiate focal glomerulonephritis due to small vessel vasculitis in diseases such as systemic lupus erythematosus, Henoch–Schönlein purpura and essential mixed cryoglobulinaemia (positive glomerular immunofluorescence for immunoglobulin and complement, electron-

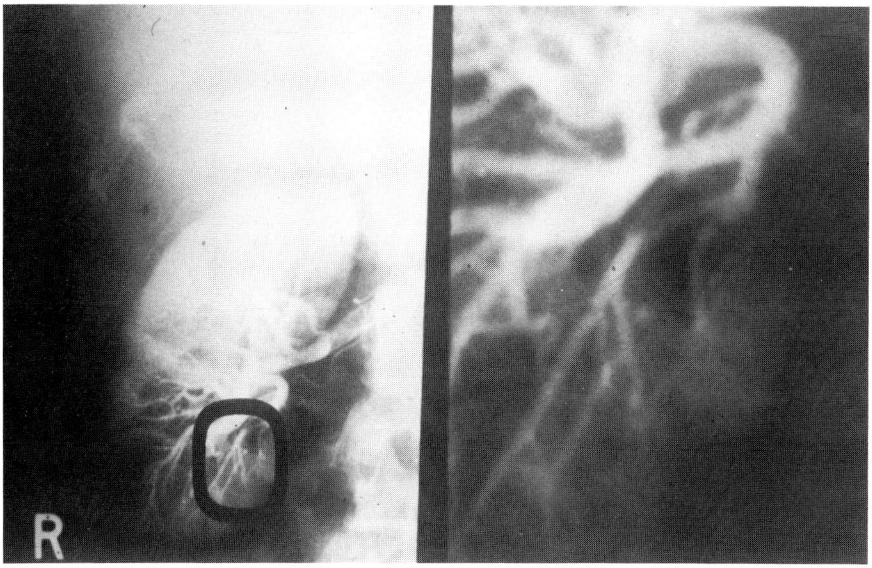

Fig. 52.5 Polyarteritis nodosa; right renal angiogram. Enlarged view shows small microaneurysm.

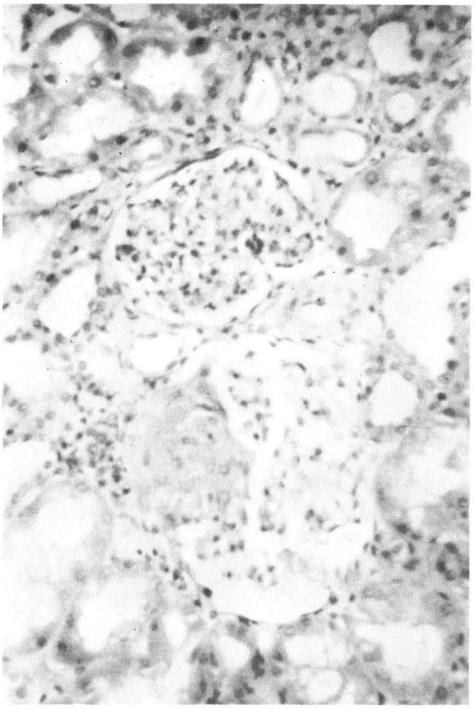

Fig. 52.6 Polyarteritis nodosa; renal biopsy showing focal necrotising glomerulonephritis. Note the small area of fibrinoid material in the affected glomerulus with a normal glomerulus above. This patient also had microaneurysms detected at visceral angiography. (Reproduced by courtesy of Dr C. R. Tribe.) (H & E × 770)

dense deposits) from focal glomerulonephritis associated with polyarteritis nodosa or granulomatous vasculitis (negative glomerular immunofluorescence, no electron dense deposits) (Scott et al, 1982a; Ronco et al, 1983).

Other biopsy sites may be helpful in difficult cases. These include skeletal muscle (Maxeiner et al, 1952) especially if painful lower limb muscle is biopsied (Verztman, 1980), testis (Dahl et al, 1960), rectum (Tribe et al, 1981), and sural nerve, especially in patients with neuropathy (Wees et al, 1981). Vasculitis is a peculiarly focal phenomenon and sections of the entire biopsy should be examined in order to include affected vessels.

Biopsies of cutaneous lesions give the highest frequency of positive results. Interpretation may be difficult as only small vessels are usually obtained and the correlation between results of skin biopsy and systemic disease is often poor. Classification is based on the size of the *largest* vessel involved, so a combined approach using angiography and multiple tissue biopsies may be necessary.

Clinical features (*Table 52.2*)

General systemic symptoms are common early features of classical polyarteritis nodosa, particularly fever and weight loss which are present in over

Table 52.2 Major clinical features in classical polyarteritis nodosa

Age (years)	45/60*
Sex ratio (M : F)	2 : 1
Systemic symptoms	80%
Fever	*70%*
Weight loss	*70%*
Kidney	75%
Hypertension	50%
Arthralgia/myalgia	65%
Arthritis	*50%*
Skin	50%
Neuropathy	50%
CNS	*25%*
Heart	50%
Abdominal pain	45%

* Older age-group seen in a District General Hospital

two-thirds of patients. Fever and myalgia may be the most useful clinical features for differentiating polyarteritis nodosa from rheumatoid vasculitis or small vessel vasculitis.

Kidney. Renal disease is common and prognosis is largely dependent on the extent of renal damage. Haematuria, proteinuria and impaired creatinine clearance are the most frequent clinical findings and require urgent investigation (e.g. biopsy). Although renal insufficiency is usually mild or moderate, severe renal impairment and oligoanuria are associated with a particularly poor prognosis and require early aggressive treatment (Verztman, 1980). However the incidence of acute renal failure may depend on the referral pattern. 6 of the last 25 patients presenting to a Regional Nephrology Unit with acute renal failure due to primary glomerular disease had polyarteritis nodosa. 4 of these patients died despite aggressive cytotoxic therapy, stressing the severity of prognosis in acute renal failure (Turney, Adu & Michael, personal communication).

The nephrotic syndrome is rare and suggests renal vein thrombosis rather than glomerulonephritis (Miller et al, 1954). Tubular damage, papillary necrosis and aneurysmal rupture giving rise to perirenal or retroperitoneal haematoma are infrequent but important manifestations of renal disease.

Hypertension may develop in 50% of patients but is considerably rarer at presentation. Hyperreninaemia and hyperaldosteronism have been described (White & Schambelan, 1980; Pickering et al, 1981) suggesting that hypertension is a secondary phenomenon. Chronic hypertension may persist and contribute to deteriorating renal function despite inactive or treated arteritis.

Musculoskeletal. Diffuse arthralgias and myalgias are common. A transient non-deforming, non-erosive large joint arthritis is much commoner than is generally recognised occurring in up to 50% of patients. Synovial biopsy may show vascular lesions identical to those seen in other organs (Smukler & Schumacher, 1977). Synovial fluid shows inflammatory changes with a moderate leucocytosis, predominantly neutrophils with intracellular inclusions (Kritridou, 1977). Synovial fluid hypocomplementaemia has been described in patients with hepatitis B-associated disease (Duffy et al, 1976). Myalgia commonly affects lower limbs and may be associated with arteritis or neuropathy.

Heart. Cardiac involvement is present in over two-thirds of patients at necropsy and is second only to renal disease as a cause of death (Holsinger et al, 1962; Kitridou, 1977). The most common clinical manifestation is congestive cardiac failure which may result from coronary arteritis, hypertension or both. Acute pericarditis occurs in up to 30% of patients (Holsinger et al, 1962). Arhythmias, usually supraventricular, develop in 20% of patients and tachycardia is often disproportionate to any fever and may be of serious prognostic significance (Hughes, 1979). These rhythm disturbances may be related to the involvement of the highly vascular sinoatrial node (James & Birk, 1966). Cardiac disease is very common in children with infantile polyarteritis or Kawasaki's disease. Coronary artery aneurysms are detected in over 20% of children with Kawasaki's disease and coronary artery aneurysmal rupture is the commonest cause of death.

Gut. Abdominal pain, major abdominal bleeding and intestinal infarction or perforation are serious problems occurring in approximately 15% of cases and have a high mortality (Lopez et al, 1980). Small bowel and mesenteric arteries are the commonest site of infarction and rupture but the complications of polyarteritis nodosa embrace almost the entire diagnostic spectrum of the acute abdomen. These patients most frequently present as surgical emergencies (Colton & Butler, 1967). Angiography reveals the widespread nature of intra-abdominal disease. Aneurysms are detected in coeliac vessels in 50% of cases (Chatel et al, 1979) and in superior mestenteric arteries in 39% (D'Izarn et al, 1976; Chatel et al, 1979). Hepatic angiography may detect aneurysms more frequently than intestinal or renal angiography (Travers et al, 1979).

Abdominal pain is common in the absence of overt intra-abdominal disease and may represent ischaemia or microinfarction of the liver, spleen or mesentery; the overall incidence of gastrointestinal involvement may be as high as 50% (Camilleri et al, 1983). Abnormal liver function is also common and may be due to hepatitis, hepatic infarction or intrahepatic aneurysm formation. Other rare forms of gastrointestinal involvement include peptic ulceration and bleeding (Camilleri et al 1983; Shepherd et al, 1983), intestinal angina (Bircher et al, 1965), ischaemic colitis (Wood et al, 1979), and pancreatitis (French, 1953).

Nervous system. Neurological dysfunction occurs in 80% of patients with polyarteritis nodosa (Moore & Cupps, 1983). Peripheral nerve abnormalities occur in over 50% of patients and vasculitis may be demonstrated in 76% of peripheral nerves examined at necropsy (Lovshin & Kernohan, 1948). Mononeuritis multiplex is the most characteristic manifestation of polyarteritis nodosa; nerves most commonly affected are the lateral popliteal, sural, radial, ulnar and median. Nerve damage occurs in response to ischaemia from vasculitis affecting the vasa nervorum (Lovshin & Kernohan, 1948) and may be detected at sural nerve biopsy. A mixed peripheral neuropathy is also common but sensory signs are usually less pronounced than motor disturbance such as distal paralysis, muscle wasting and loss of reflexes. Mixed peripheral neuropathy may be due to the spread of distal mononeuritis leading to diffuse symmetrical changes (Fig. 52.7). Cranial nerves are rarely affected but involvement of the ocular, facial and acoustic nerves has been reported (Dudley & Goodman, 1969; Lake-Bakaar, 1978).

Central nervous system disease includes organic psychosis, confusional states, convulsions, hemiplegia, cerebellar dysfunction and subarachnoid haemorrhage in up to 40% of patients (Ford & Siekert, 1965; Kitridou, 1977). Hypertensive or uraemic encephalopathy should be excluded. Rarer manifestations are necrotising or transverse myelopathy (Castaigre et al, 1970), spinal subarachnoid haemorrhage (Henson & Croft, 1956), and features resembling multiple sclerosis (Verztman et al, 1972).

Ocular disease affects 20% of patients and may be due to vasculitis (choroiditis, central retinal artery occlusion, scleritis, intraocular haemorrhage, optic neuropathy) or secondary to hypertension. Patients may present with sudden unilateral loss

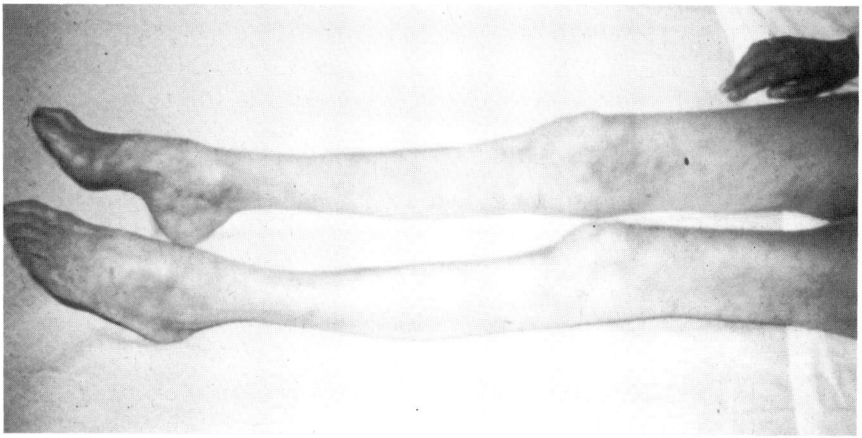

Fig. 52.7 Polyarteritis nodosa; mononeuritis multiplex. Bilateral foot drop with marked muscle wasting.

of vision, transient or permanent field defects and amaurosis fugax.

Lung. Pulmonary disease is characteristic of allergic granulomatous angiitis and Wegener's granulomatosis but relatively infrequent in classical polyarteritis nodosa. It is important to recognise that patients may not fit these strict clinical classifications and necrotising arteritis with pulmonary involvement carries the same severe prognosis as those with no lung disease (Rose & Spencer, 1957). Rarer but important pulmonary lesions in classical polyarteritis nodosa include pulmonary artery thrombosis, haemoptysis and diffuse intrapulmonary haemorrhage (Bocanegra et al, 1981; Leatherman et al, 1982).

Testes. Testicular symptoms are rare in systemic diseases. In classical polyarteritis nodosa, orchitis and epididymitis may affect 18% of patients (Dahl et al, 1960; Frohnert & Sheps, 1967) and arteritis may be seen at necropsy in up to 80% (Kitridou, 1977).

Skin. The incidence of cutaneous lesions varies considerably between different series and ranges from 5–65% (Gilliam & Smiley, 1976; Travers et al, 1979; Cohen et al, 1980; Scott et al, 1982a). A variety of rashes have been described including urticaria, non-specific maculopapular rashes, livedo reticularis, necrotic lesions (Fig. 52.8) and purpura (Lyell & Church, 1954; Hughes, 1979), but the nodules described by Kussmaul & Maier (1866) are rare. Other less common cutaneous lesions include nailfold and nail-edge infarcts, splinter haemorrhages and erythema multiforme. More serious lesions such as peripheral gangrene due to major vessel occlusion can occur (Fig. 52.9) but are relatively uncommon (Lyell & Church, 1954; Travers et al, 1979).

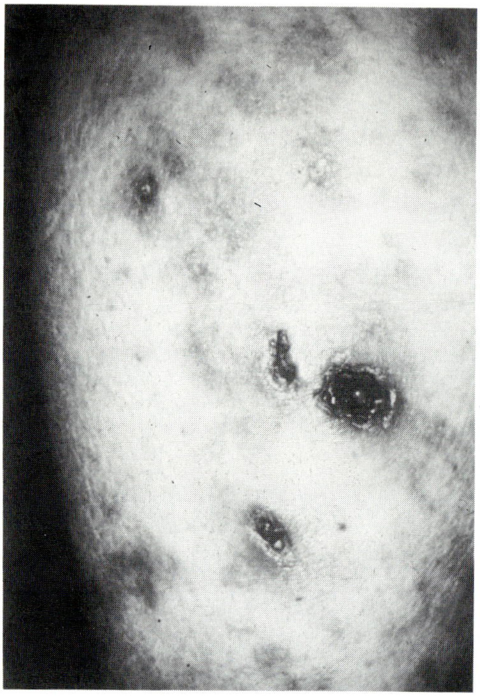

Fig. 52.8 Polyarteritis nodosa; small cutaneous infarcts on the thigh.

Localised polyarteritis nodosa

Cutaneous lesions with histological appearances identical to those of polyarteritis nodosa may occur in the absence of systemic disease (Borrie, 1972). Nodules, livedo reticularis and ulcers are the commonest lesions; they may be associated with muscle and nerve lesions but only in the limb affected by cutaneous disease. Complement levels are normal, immune complexes and cryoglobulins are rarely detected and tests for hepatitis B surface antigen are negative. Lesions tend to run a chronic course but the overall prognosis is good. This form of localised polyarteritis nodosa may be associated with inflammatory bowel disease (Dyer, et al, 1970; Solley et al, 1975).

Necrotising arteritis may also occur locally (without systemic involvement) in the breast (Dega & Hunder, 1974), gastrointestinal tract including appendix, gall bladder and colon (Fayemi et al, 1972; Meyer & Lichtenstein, 1982) uterus and testis (Scott et al, 1982a). The cause of these localised lesions is unknown but stresses the importance of including 'systemic' in the definition of necrotising arteritides.

Laboratory tests in classical polyarteritis nodosa (Table 52.3)

There are no specific laboratory abnormalities in classical polyarteritis nodosa. The incidence of hepatitis B infection is varied, dependent probably on its incidence in the general population from which the patients originate. For example, hepatitis B infection is found in the majority of patients with polyarteritis nodosa from Poland (Michalak, 1978) and Brazil (Verztman, 1980) but is rare (less

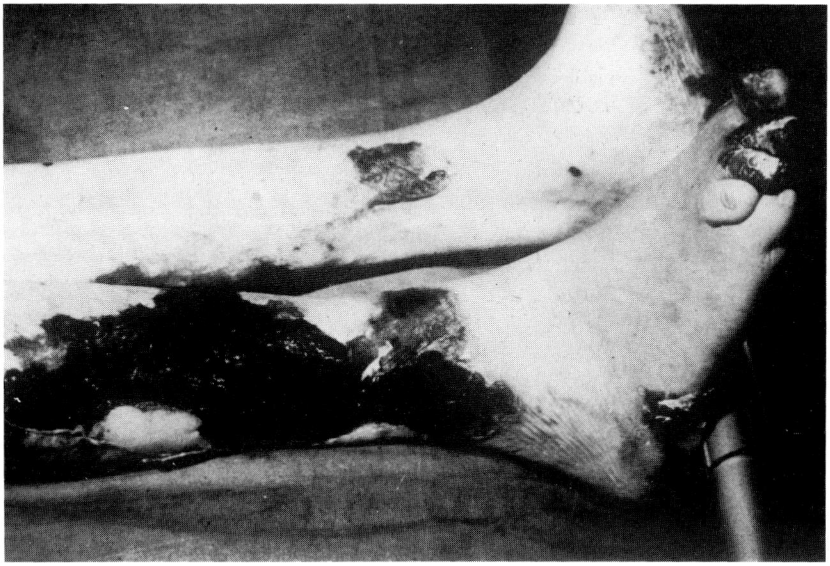

Fig. 52.9 Polyarteritis nodosa; extensive cutaneous infarction and peripheral gangrene.

Table 52.3 Laboratory abnormalities in classical polyarteritis nodosa[1]

ESR > 20 mm/h	94%
Leucocytosis (wbc > 10 × 10^9/1)	85%
Anaemia	66%
Rheumatoid factor	40%
Anti-nuclear antibodies	7%
Immune complexes	85%
Hypocomplementaemia	15%
Renal function abnormality	70%
Proteinuria	65%
Haematuria	60%
Liver function abnormality	60%
Hepatitis BsAg	5–80%[2]

[1] Figures derived from Cupps & Fauci (1981) and Scott et al (1982)

[2] Incidence of hepatitis BsAg varies greatly in different series (see text)

than 15%) in the patients studied at the Mayo Clinic, USA (Cohen et al, 1980), Michigan, USA (Sack et al, 1975) and in South West England (Scott et al, 1982a).

Leucocytosis is common (over 80% of patients) and may help differentiate necrotising arteritides from small vessel vasculitis or rheumatoid vasculitis (Scott et al, 1982a). Eosinophilia is commoner in patients with allergic granulomatous angiitis but occurs in approximately 20% of patients with classical polyarteritis nodosa even in the absence of pulmonary disease. A mild anaemia, raised erythrocyte sedimentation rate, thrombocytosis and raised immunoglobulins are common.

Rheumatoid factor is detected in 40% of patients but anti-nuclear antibodies are rare. Hypocomplementaemia and complement activation is restricted to patients whose disease is associated with hepatitis B infection. Circulating immune complexes are common (up to 90% of cases) but levels often fail to reflect disease activity and are less value in serial studies than the leucocyte count or C-reactive protein (Hind et al, 1984).

Liver function tests are frequently abnormal and levels of alkaline phosphatase may reflect disease activity (Elkon & Hughes, 1980).

An abnormal urinary sediment usually indicates active renal disease, and functional tests such as creatinine clearance are important for monitoring progressive renal damage and response to treatment.

Examination of the cerebrospinal fluid in patients with central nervous system disease may show increased pressure, pleocytosis, raised levels of protein and xanthochromia (Ford & Siekert, 1965).

Prognosis

The 5-year survival rate of untreated polyarteritis nodosa is less than 20%. The commonest causes of death are renal failure and cardiac lesions. Other features associated with a particularly poor prognosis are gastrointestinal infarction and aneurysm rupture especially of cardiac, cerebral and renal vessels. The majority of deaths occur within 3 months as a direct consequence of arteritis. Later deaths may be due to recurrence (rare), secondary phenomena (chronic renal failure, hypertensive complications), or complications of treatment.

Treatment

Corticosteroids improve the 5-year survival to 50% (Frohnert & Sheps, 1967). However, Cupps & Fauci (1981) suggest that such treatment may only induce a partial remission or mask smouldering disease activity. Corticosteroids may aggrevate vascular damage leading to hypertension, and prolonged treatment may be associated with an increased risk of sepsis — an important cause of late mortality.

Cytotoxic drugs, particularly cyclophosphamide, may improve 5-year survival to over 80% (Leib et al, 1979). Oral cyclophosphamide (2 mg/kg.day^{-1}) plus oral prednisolone 60 mg initially but rapidly reduced to alternate day regime after 2 weeks is currently considered the treatment of choice resulting in complete and sometimes dramatic remissions even in advanced disease (Fauci et al, 1979). Slow improvement of neuropathy may occur (Moore & Fauci, 1981) and relapses are rare with this form of therapy. Similar dramatic early responses and improved survival have been reported in small numbers of patients treated with intravenous cyclophosphamide plus methylprednisolone (Scott et al, 1982a). It is important to use cytotoxic therapy as early as possible; Cohen et al (1980) reported no improvement in survival in patients in whom cytotoxic therapy was introduced late for active disease failing to respond to corticosteroids alone. Cyclophosphamide is excreted by the kidneys so smaller doses may be necessary in patients with severe renal impairment especially when the intravenous route is used. Plasma exchange may be a useful adjunct to cytotoxic immunosuppressive therapy in patients with renal disease (Lockwood et al, 1979).

Significant improvement in the use of antihypertensive agents, the management of renal failure and the use of antibiotics are also important to the improved survival reported in recent years.

Polyarteritis nodosa may be a 'curable' disease. If long-term complications of treatment are to be avoided, careful titration of cytotoxic and corticosteroid therapy is necessary to obtain maximum benefit and minimal side-effects. Attempts to withdraw treatment should be considered where remission has seen maintained for more than 6 months.

GRANULOMATOUS VASCULITIS

Allergic granulomatous angiitis

This rare disease may be considered as a subgroup of classical polyarteritis nodosa. The spectrum of clinical disease is similar, vascular lesions may be identical (acute necrotising arteritis of small and medium-sized arteries), and both diseases have a similar overall prognosis. Certain features help differentiate allergic granulomatous angiitis from classical polyarteritis nodosa and suggest that different pathogenetic mechanisms are involved. These are

a. A strong association with asthma and blood eosinophilia
b. Significantly higher incidence of lung disease
c. More frequent involvement of small vessels
d. The presence of intra- and extravascular granulomata.

The characteristic histological changes are vasculitis, eosinophilic infiltration and granulomata with macrophages, giant cells and epithelioid cells. Granulomata are most commonly seen in the skin and epicardium (Churg & Strauss, 1951; Rose & Spencer, 1957).

Allergic granulomatous angiitis was established as a clinical entity by Churg and Strauss in 1951 and is often called Churg–Strauss vasculitis although the first description of the disease was by Ophuls in 1923.

Diagnosis

Diagnosis is based on the characteristic history, blood eosinophilia, and the demonstration of vasculitis using biopsy sites similar to those described for investigating classical polyarteritis. Lung or skin biopsy may be useful for detecting the eosinophilic infiltrate or granulomata. Lanham et al (1984) stress the importance of clinical features in diagnosis as classical (though not pathognomonic) histological changes are found in only a minority of cases. Because of previous dependence on pathological changes for diagnosis, this disease is probably underdiagnosed.

Clinical features (Table 52.4)

The male preponderance is similar to polyarteritis nodosa (3 : 1) but diagnosis is usually made at a younger age (mean 38 years). There is a prodromal phase which consists of allergic disease which often arises unusually late in individuals who may have no family history of atopy. The atopic disease usually consists of asthma, often preceded by allergic rhinitis. The second phase is characterised by peripheral blood eosinophilia, eosinophilic tissue infiltrates especially affecting the lungs with transient pulmonary infiltrates seen on X-ray. This phase may recur over a period of years but is ultimately interrupted by a third life-threatening vasculitic phase with many of the clinical features of classic polyarteritis nodosa (Lanham et al, 1984). Features differing from classical polyarteritis nodosa include

a. Cutaneous lesions which are more common, especially purpura due to leucocytoclastic vasculitis and nodules due to granulomata
b. Life-threatening gastrointestinal bleeding and intestinal infarction which are rarer, reflecting the lower incidence of aneurysms detected at angiography (abdominal pain is still common with an overall incidence almost identical to classical polyarteritis nodosa)
c. Additional cardiac features which include nodular pericarditis, endothelial fibrosis and eosinophilic infiltrates and
d. Less severe renal disease.

Laboratory features are similar to those of classical polyarteritis nodosa. However, hepatitis B infection is not associated with allergic granulomatous angiitis, blood eosinophilia is much more frequent (90%) and raised levels of IgE are common (Conn et al, 1976; Lanham et al, 1984). Complement levels are normal but circulating immune complexes can be detected in some patients. Renal biopsies show features suggesting small vessel vasculitis — focal necrotising glomerulonephritis, sometimes with crescent formation. Arteritis is seen less frequently than in classical polyarteritis nodosa. IgM and C3 have been detected in affected glomeruli in some patients, suggesting a possible role for immune complex deposition in pathogenesis (Lanham et al, 1984).

Table 52.4 Major organ involvement in granulomatous arteritis [1]

	Allergic granulomatous angiitis	Wegener's granulomatosis
Lung	90%	95%
Sinus/nasopharynx	(70%)[2]	95%
Kidney	60%	80%
Skin	70%	50%
Joints	60%	65%
Neuropathy	65%	30%
Eye	rare	50%

[1] Figures derived from Cupps & Fauci (1981), Scott et al (1982), Fauci et al (1983) and Lanham et al (1984)

[2] Allergic rhinitis is common in allergic granulomatous angiitis but the severe, often destructive granulomatous infiltration of the nasopharynx is a feature of Wegener's granulomatosis only.

Prognosis

Without treatment the overall prognosis is similar to that of classical polyarteritis nodosa with a 5-year survival rate of less than 10%. With the introduction of steroids this figure improves to over 60% in some series (Cupps & Fauci, 1981; Lanham et al, 1984). 50% of all reported deaths are cardiac though most were reported in the pre-steroid era. Causes of death include myocardial infarction and intractable cardiac failure. Cardiac granulomata are often detected at necropsy.

Treatment

Chumbley et al (1977), Vertzman (1980) and Lanham et al (1984) suggest that allergic granulomatous angiitis responds better to high dose corticosteroids (40–60 mg/day) than does classical polyarteritis nodosa. However, relapses are not uncommon in corticosteroid-treated patients and Fauci et al (1978) advocate the use of cyclophosphamide in a similar oral regime to that used to treat classical polyarteritis nodosa either in severely ill patients as initial treatment or in those patients who fail to respond to corticosteroids alone. Despite successful treatment the allergic symptoms often return when treatment is discontinued.

Wegener's granulomatosis

Wegener's granulomatosis may also be considered as a variety of polyarteritis nodosa. Clinical features are similar and acute necrotising arteritis is a common histological finding. However the frequent, often severe, involvement of the nasopharynx and lungs by necrotising granulomatous vasculitis may dominate the clinical picture suggesting different pathogenetic mechanisms and Wegener's granulomatosis is more often classified as a distinct clinical syndrome. Nasopharyngeal lesions and the absence of an allergic history or significant eosinophilia help distinguish Wegener's granulomatosis from allergic granulomatous angiitis. Small vessel involvement as well as arteritis is characteristic of both diseases.

The first descriptions of Wegener's granulomatosis were by Klinger (1931) and Wegener (1936). However, Fahey et al (1954) and Goodman & Churg (1954) were responsible for its recognition as a clinical entity.

Immunological mechanisms have been implicated in the aetiology of Wegener's granulomatosis but without any distinctive pattern of abnormality. Circulating immune complexes may be detected (Howell & Epstein, 1976) and immune deposits have been described in the lung (Shasby et al, 1982) and kidney (Horn et al, 1974) in a minority of cases. Cellular mechanisms have also been implicated in some cases (Niinaka et al, 1978; Gephardt et al, 1983). The importance of circulating factors in pathogenesis is suggested by reports of Wegener's granulomatosis recurring in a transplanted kidney (Curtis et al, 1983).

Diagnosis

Systemic multiple organ disease with prominent lung and nasopharyngeal involvement suggests a diagnosis of Wegener's granulomatosis. Open lung biopsy is the most definitive diagnostic procedure, showing characteristic histological changes in most cases (Fauci et al, 1983), followed by renal or gingival biopsy. Endobronchial lung biopsies and nasopharyngeal biopsies are often unhelpful, showing non-specific changes. The characteristic histology shows vasculitis and granulomata with well formed giant cells (Fig. 52.10) and central necrosis. Any combination of granuloma, vasculitis and necrosis may be present at a given site.

Renal biopsy may reveal crescentic glomerulonephritis with or without arteritis (Mills & McCroskery, 1981) or focal glomerulonephritis; granulomata and vasculitis are rarely seen. Immune deposits are only detected in the glomerulus in a minority of patients by immunofluorescence or electron microscopy. Although vasculitis is rarely found at gingival biopsy, the presence of granulomata with acute or chronic inflammation is so unusual in other diseases as to be highly suggestive of Wegener's granulomatosis (Scott & Finch, 1972). Aneurysms have been detected in a few patients but the role of visceral angiography has not been established.

Clinical features (Table 52.4)

Males are slightly more commonly affected and the mean age at diagnosis is 43 years (range 14–75)

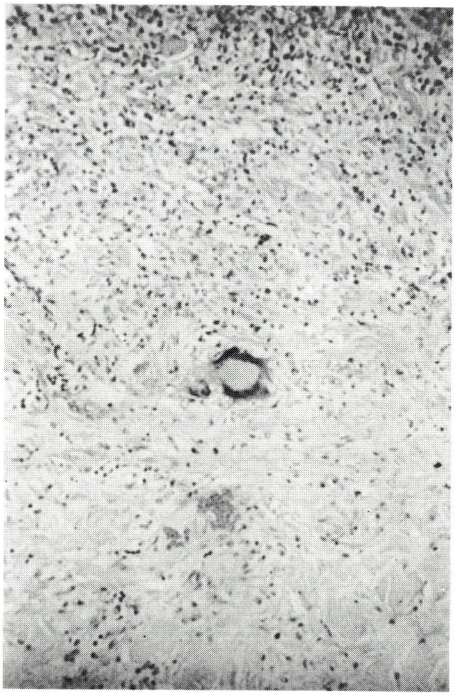

Fig. 52.10 Wegener's granulomatosis; section of a large cutaneous granuloma showing a large multinucleated giant cell. (H & E × 200)

(Fauci et al, 1983). Most patients present with problems relating to the upper respiratory tract. Necrotising granulomata may be found in the nasopharynx, nasal septum, maxillary, ethmoid, frontal and sphenoid sinuses. Symptoms of sinusitis, rhinitis, nasal obstruction, otitis media, pain and hearing loss (due to Eustachian tube obstruction) are commoner than the more dramatic secondary effects of granulomatous invasion and destruction leading to saddle nose deformity (Fig. 52.11), orbital compression, proptosis and intracranial disease. Generalised systemic symptoms usually follow within months but a delay of several years between respiratory tract disease and systemic vasculitis has been described (MacFarlane et al, 1983). Lower respiratory tract symptoms are a presenting feature in one-third of patients.

Lung involvement is associated with cough, dyspnoea, chest pain and haemoptysis. Severe pulmonary haemorrhage is an uncommon but important problem (Leatherman et al, 1982). Chest X-ray may reveal solitary or multiple nodules (Fig. 52.12), infiltrates, cavitation, focal areas of atelectasis or pleural effusions. Hilar lymphadenopathy is extremely rare.

Paranasal sinus involvement may be complicated by secondary bacterial infection, which may simulate reactivation of Wegener's granulomatosis (Pinching et al, 1980). Oral ulceration is common but perforation of the hard or soft palate suggests midline granuloma and not Wegener's granulomatosis.

Renal involvement occurs in up to 80% of cases. Typical biopsy changes may be seen in the absence of any clinical features of renal disease (Fauci & Wolff, 1977). Nephrotic syndrome may occur as a complication of glomerular disease in contrast to its association with renal vein thrombosis in classical polyarteritis nodosa.

Ocular involvement is much commoner in Wegener's granulomatosis than polyarteritis nodosa. Lesions include conjunctivitis, granulomatous episcleritis, sclerouveitis, and scleromalacia

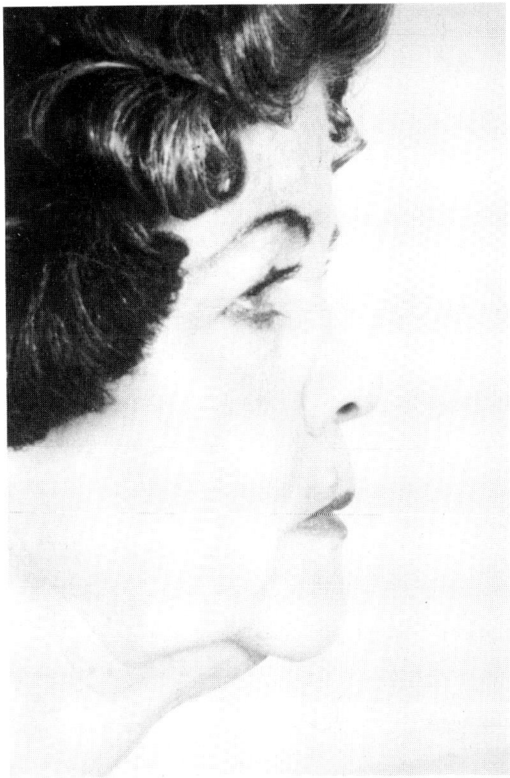

Fig. 52.11 Wegener's granulomatosis; saddle nose deformity due to nasal cartilage destruction. (Courtesy of the Editor of the *Annals of Rheumatic Diseases*.)

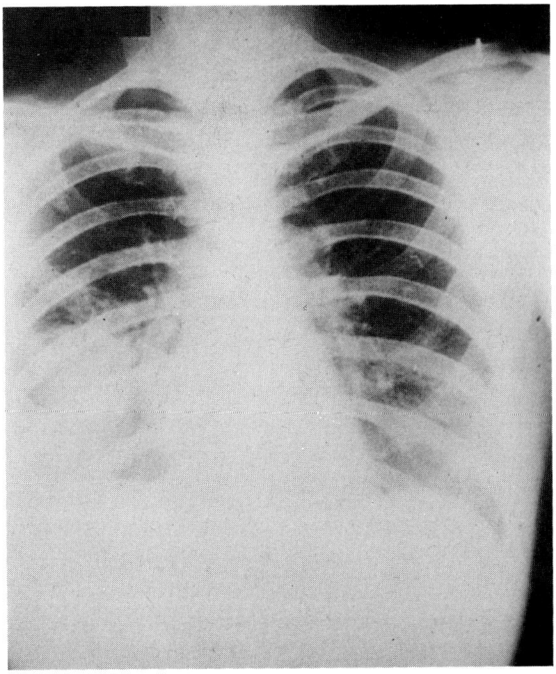

Fig. 52.12 Wegener's granulomatosis; chest X-ray showing large granuloma in the right lower zone.

perforans (Wolff et al, 1974). Other serious but less frequent problems include acute blindness (Haynes et al, 1977) and severe proptosis (Vermees et al, 1978) which is often resistant to treatment.

A transient arthritis similar to that seen in classical polyarteritis nodosa develops in approximately 60% of patients. Occasionally small joints are involved mimicking rheumatoid arthritis (Pritchard & Gow, 1976).

Intracranial spread of granulomatous lesions may involve structures at the base of the brain including the pituitary and cranial nerves (Drachman, 1963), but peripheral neuropathies are identical to those seen in classical polyarteritis nodosa.

Carrington & Liebow (1966) describe a limited form of Wegener's granulomatosis with predominantly lower respiratory tract involvement but without renal disease. The more recent descriptions of indolent Wegener's and the demonstration of renal abnormalities at biopsy in the absence of clinically apparent renal disease suggests that this limited form of Wegener's granulomatosis is rare (Churg, 1983).

Laboratory tests

Laboratory abnormalities such as anaemia, leucocytosis and hyperglobulinaemia are similar to those described in classical polyarteritis nodosa. However, extreme elevations of the erythrocyte sedimentation rate (more than 100 mm/h) are more often seen and high levels of IgE (Conn et al, 1976) suggest Wegener's granulomatosis or allergic granulomatous angiitis rather than polyarteritis nodosa. Rheumatoid factors are detected in approximately 60% but, as in polyarteritis nodosa, anti-nuclear antibodies are very rarely found. Tests for hepatitis B infection are uniformly negative. Sinus and chest X-rays may reveal granuloma, infiltration or bone destruction. Computer-assisted tomography is useful in the assessment of ocular disease (Haynes et al, 1977; Vermees et al, 1978).

Prognosis

Without treatment the mean survival from the onset of renal disease is 5 months (Walton, 1958) and the overall 2-year survival rate is less than 10%. Corticosteroids have very little effect on prognosis but may produce dramatic improvement of serious ocular disease.

Treatment

Cyclophosphamide has revolutionised treatment and Wegener's granulomatosis is now often considered a 'curable' disease (Wolff et al, 1974; Israel et al, 1977; Fauci et al, 1983). Oral cyclophosphamide is the most usual method of treatment but in contrast to polyarteritis nodosa, prolonged therapy may be required as recurrences occur up to 10 years after presentation. Fauci et al (1983) describe complete remission in 79 out of 85 patients (92%) with Wegener's granulomatosis studied over a 21-year period when treated with a combination or oral cyclophosphamide (2 mg/kg. day^{-1}) and prednisolone (1 mg/kg. day^{-1}) changing to alternate days by 1 month and reducing to 20 mg alternate days by 6 months. One-third of their cases are now off all treatment and they suggest tapering the cyclophosphamide after 1 year of complete remission. Relapses do occur (30%) but respond after restarting treatment. Only 10 patients died, 6 with active disease and 4 from other causes confirming the efficacy of this type of cytotoxic regime.

Lymphomatoid granulomatosis

This disease is not a true inflammatory necrotising arteritis. There is direct invasion of vessel walls by atypical lymphoid, plasmacytoid and reticulo-endothelial cells with varying numbers of mitoses. Granulomata tend to be less distinct than in Wegener's granulomatosis and the vasculitis is neither leucocytoclastic nor associated with fibrinoid necrosis. Although cutaneous and cerebral features may occur, this disease is mainly restricted to the lungs. Progressive pulmonary disease often leads to respiratory failure which is the commonest cause of death. Transformation to frank lymphoma is well documented (Liebow et al, 1972).

Overlap syndromes and other necrotising arteritides

Problems exist particularly in differentiating classical polyarteritis nodosa from allergic granulomatous angiitis. Patients who show some features of both diseases (overlap syndromes) include those with 'polyarteritis' following hypersensitisation who frequently have eosinophilia and allergic histories but rarely granulomata (Phanuphak & Kohler, 1980) and also patients with 'polyarteritis' associated with acute serous otitis media (Sergent & Christian, 1974). The problem of classification was highlighted in a recent series of 37 patients with systemic necrotising arteritis (but excluding Wegener's granulomatosis). 10 patients had a preceeding history of asthma, 13 patients pulmonary infiltration on chest X-ray, but only 6 had both asthma and pulmonary infiltrates. Eosinophilia was commoner in, but not restricted to, patients with lung disease. Granulomata were detected at biopsy or necropsy in 4 patients: all had acute necrotising arteritis confirmed histologically but in the absence of clinically apparent lung disease (Scott et al, 1982a).

Other diseases with distinctive clinical features may be associated with acute necrotising arteritis. These include the 'polyarteritis' associated with hairy cell leukaemia (Elkon et al, 1979), with relapsing polychondritis (Somers & Potuleice, 1978) and with angioimmunoblastic lymphadenopathy (Alarcon-Segovia, 1977). Early recognition and treatment of the vasculitis (as described in classical polyarteritis nodosa) is important as early prognosis depends on the vasculitis rather than the underlying disease.

Rheumatoid vasculitis

Vasculitis is an uncommon but important complication of rheumatoid arthritis encompassing almost the entire spectrum of clinical and histological features associated with vascular inflammation.

Vascular lesions complicating rheumatoid arthritis were first described by Bannatyne in 1898 but the direct association between vasculitis and rheumatoid disease was not recognised until the late 1940s and early 1950s. It is now accepted that vasculitis may be responsible for many of the extra-articular lesions of rheumatoid disease. The commonest lesions are small microinfarcts of the nail edge, nailfold or along the course of digital arteries (Fig. 52.13). These may be detected in as many as 30% of hospital in-patients (Dequeker & Rosberg, 1967) but in the absence of systemic symptoms have a benign prognosis (Bywaters & Scott, 1963). Their presence should, however, alert the physician to the possibility of systemic

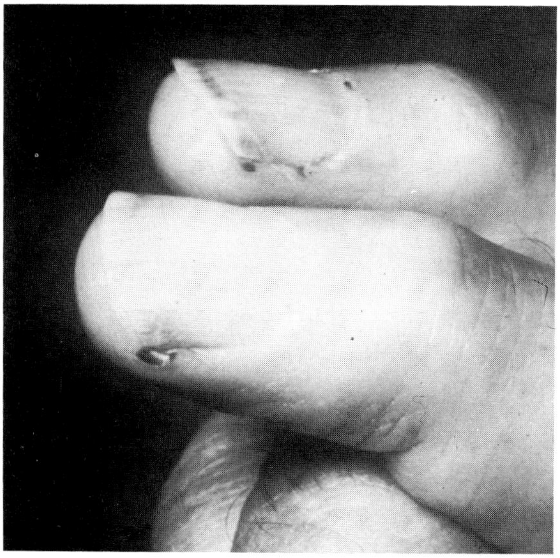

Fig. 52.13 Rheumatoid vasculitis; typical nailfold and nail-edge infarcts.

vasculitis which is much less frequent (8 per million of the population per year) but associated with a more serious prognosis.

Systemic vasculitis is associated with a wide range of clinical features such as skin rashes, ulceration, peripheral gangrene, neuropathy and visceral infarction. There is also a wide range of histological findings, including acute necrotising arteritis (Fig. 52.14), indistinguishable from polyarteritis nodosa (Ball, 1954; Tribe et al, 1981), subacute arteritis with mainly round cell infiltrates with or without fibrinoid necrosis (Sokoloff et al, 1951; Tribe et al, 1981) and acute leucocytoclastic vasculitis (Soter et al, 1974). These different histological changes may coexist in the same patient at the same time or sequentially suggesting that they represent a spectrum of disease. However, the presence of acute necrotising arteritis is associated with a particularly poor prognosis (Scott et al, 1982c). Histology of digital lesions shows a bland intimal proliferation often with obliteration of the lumen but relatively few inflammatory cells.

Diagnosis

The most useful biopsy sites for histological diagnosis are the rectum (Tribe et al, 1981), sural nerve (Conn et al, 1974; Wees et al, 1981) and skin. Skin biopsy often shows an acute leuco-

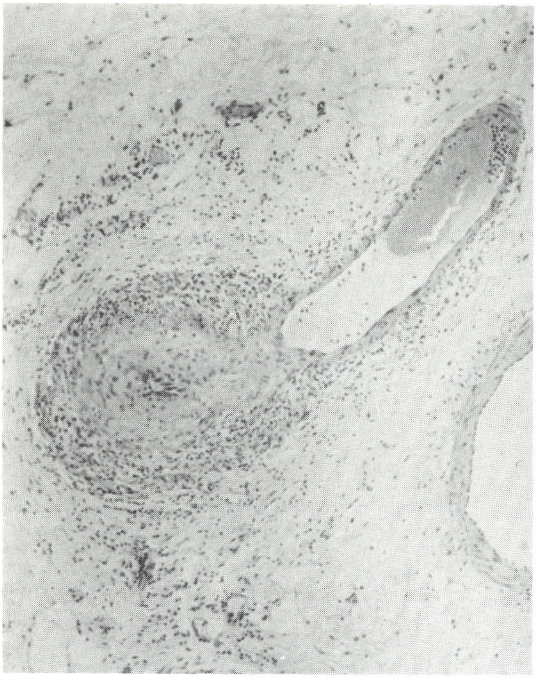

Fig. 52.14 Rheumatoid vasculitis; gastrectomy specimen showing acute necrotising arteritis. (Reproduced by courtesy of Dr C. R. Tribe.) (H & E × 200)

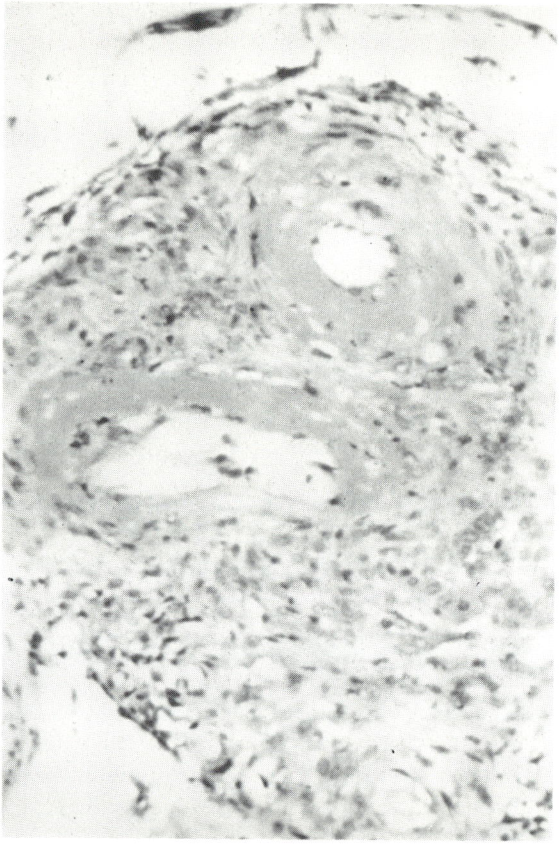

Fig. 52.15 Rheumatoid vasculitis; rectal biopsy showing acute necrotising arteritis. (Reproduced by courtesy of Dr C.R. Tribe.) (H & E × 200)

cytoclastic small vessel vasculitis whereas rectal biopsy may reveal acute necrotising arteritis in the same patient (Fig. 52.15). It is important to take a deep biopsy from the posterior rectal wall to obtain sufficient submucosal arteries for histological examination. This technique reveals necrotising arteritis in over 40% of patients with clinical evidence of systemic rheumatoid vasculitis. Sural nerve biopsy is most useful in patients with peripheral neuropathy. The role of visceral angiography is unknown but it would be surprising if aneurysms were not detected in some patients. Brachial arteriography frequently shows narrowing or occlusion of digital arteries (Fig. 52.16) especially in patients with clinically apparent digital lesions (Scott et al, 1961).

The role of immune complexes in the pathogenesis of rheumatoid vasculitis has previously been discussed. Despite histological and many clinical similarities, immunological mechanisms in necrotising arteritis associated with rheumatoid disease are quite distinct from those in polyarteritis nodosa. Corticosteroids have been implicated in the aetiology of systemic rheumatoid vasculitis and although it is now apparent that necrotising arteritis often occurs in the absence of corticosteroids, many critical observers believe than an explosion of rheumatoid vasculitis occurred during the 1950s coinciding with an era of uncontrolled steroid therapy and that such cases are less frequent today (Scott, 1976).

Clinical features

The clinical features of 60 patients with systemic rheumatoid vasculitis are shown in Table 52.5. This study excluded patients with digital lesions in the absence of systemic disease. Systemic vasculitis was defined by the presence of one or more of the following.

a. Mononeuritis multiplex

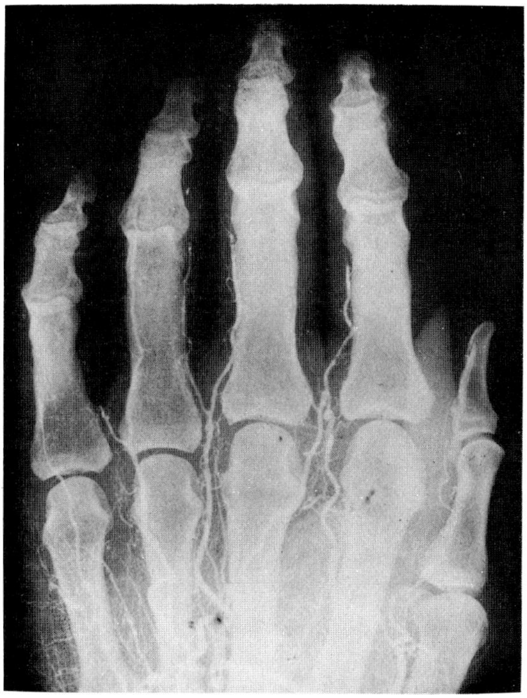

Fig. 52.16 Rheumatoid vasculitis; digital vascular occlusion demonstrated by brachial arteriography. (Reproduced by courtesy of Dr J. T. Scott.)

b. Peripheral gangrene
c. Biopsy evidence of acute necrotising arteritis and
d. Typical digital lesions, or biopsy evidence of small vessel vasculitis only if associated with active systemic extra-articular disease.

It is important to recognise that the clinical features listed in Table 52.5 are not all a direct consequence of vasculitis. Rheumatoid nodules may be responsible for some cutaneous ulcers, nodular scleritis, some cases of pulmonary fibrosis and cardiac lesions such as valvulitis and heart block. Vasculitis is now thought not to play any role in the development of these rheumatoid nodules (Rasker & Kuipers, 1983).

The wide range of clinical disease shows many similarities with polyarteritis nodosa. Cutaneous lesions are the most frequent. These include digital lesions, small finger pulp infarcts (often associated with intracutaneous nodules), cutaneous rashes including purpura, papules, livedo reticularis, bullous eruptions and pustules. The role of vasculitis

Table 52.5 Clinical features in 60 patients with systemic rheumatoid vasculitis

Organ	Number of patients (%)	Details (number of patients)
Skin	54 (90%)	Digital vasculitis (34), ulcers (32), rash (19), gangrene (8)
Nodules	52 (87%)	Rheumatoid nodules (52)
Systemic	50 (83%)	Weight loss (49), hepatosplenomegaly (13)
Neuropathy	26 (43%)	Sensory (20), motor (10), CNS (3)
Lung	24 (40%)	Fibrosing alveolitis (13), pleurisy/effusion (9) nodules (3)
Heart	20 (33%)	Arhythmia (10), pericarditis (8), aortic incompetence (3), myocardial infarct (3)
Kidney	15 (25%)	Active sediment (12), amyloid (4)
Eye	10 (17%)	Scleritis (9), Sjögren's syndrome (4)
Gut	8 (13%)	Abdominal pain (6), colitis (2)

in the development of cutaneous ulcers is varied. Vasculitic ulcers are often deep, have punched out edges and develop suddenly in unusual sites (Fig. 52.17); they are frequently associated with digital lesions or biopsy evidence of vasculitis elsewhere. Chronic leg ulcers may have a different aetiology but also deteriorate in the present of ac-

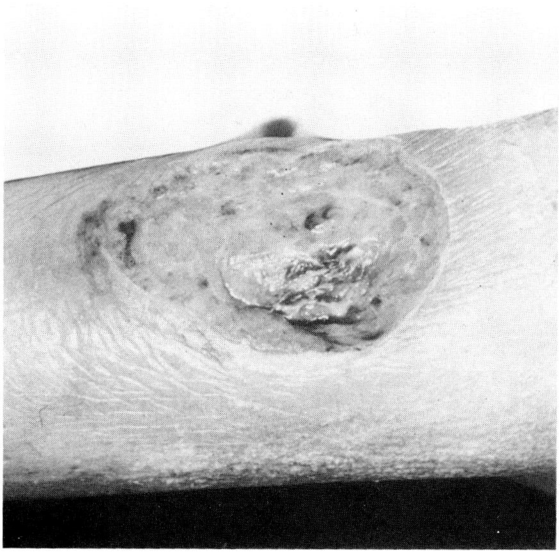

Fig. 52.17 Rheumatoid vasculitis; deep cutaneous ulcer in the calf due to vasculitis.

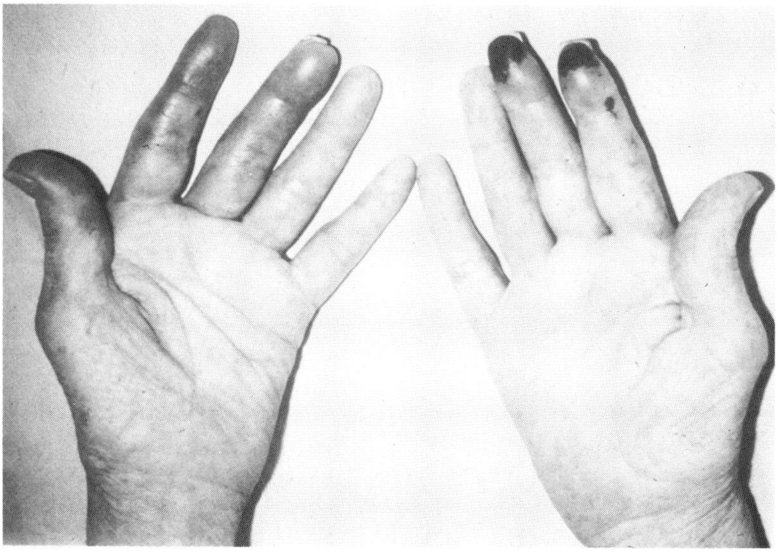

Fig. 52.18 Rheumatoid vasculitis; peripheral gangrene.

tive vasculitis at other sites. Ulceration of fingers or gangrene (Fig. 52.18) may develop in the more severe cases of digital vasculitis (Bywaters, 1957; Scott et al, 1961) and the distinctive cutaneous ulceration known as 'pyoderma gangrenosum' may be due to vasculitis in patients with rheumatoid disease (Stolman et al, 1975).

Neurological lesions may arise from a variety of causes including entrapment and cervical cord compression as well as vasculitis. The most common vasculitic neuropathy is a distal sensory neuropathy which is often benign; mononeuritis multiplex is less common but more serious particularly if extensive (Fig. 52.19). Widespread distal sensory motor neuropathy carries a particularly evil prognosis (Pallis & Scott, 1965).

Generalised systemic symptoms are common, particularly weight loss. In the absence of active synovitis, vasculitis should be considered in the differential diagnosis of severe weight loss in patients with rheumatoid disease.

Renal involvement is less common and less severe than in polyarteritis nodosa. Proteinuria and haematuria may be detected in up to 40% of patients (Schmid et al, 1961) but the urinary sediment usually returns to normal with resolution of

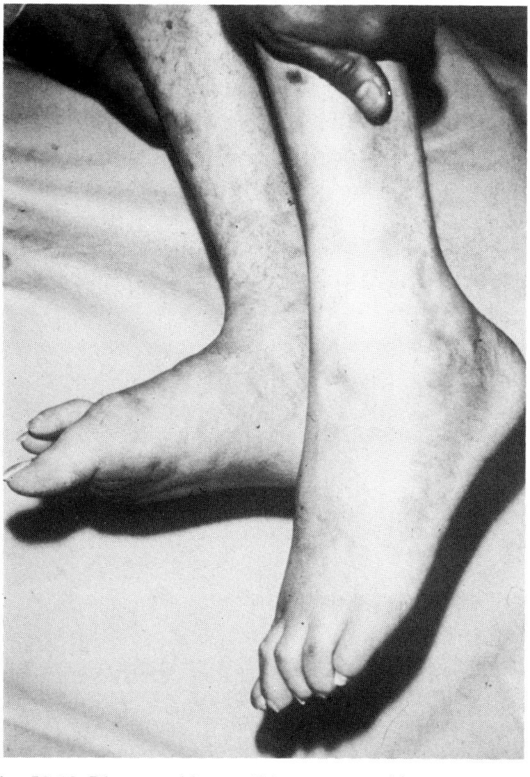

Fig. 52.19 Rheumatoid vasculitis; mononeuritis resulting in left foot drop.

other clinical features of vasculitis. Renal histology is often non-specific but acute necrotising arteritis has been described in some patients (Meriwether et al, 1967; Scott et al, 1981c).

Major organ infarction is uncommon but associated with a particularly poor prognosis. The best documented lesions are coronary arteritis (Voyles et al, 1980), intestinal infarction and perforation due to arteritis (Adler et al, 1962) and cerebral arteritis (Ramos & Mandybur, 1975; Watson et al, 1977) where angiographic abnormalities may be detected (Paci et al, 1983). The ability of rheumatoid vasculitis to mimick almost the entire spectrum of vasculitic disease is highlighted by even rarer reports of pulmonary arteritis (Walker & Wright, 1968), temporal arteritis (Fournie et al, 1976) and aortic arch syndrome (Falicov & Cooney, 1964).

Laboratory tests (Table 52.6)

A mild anaemia is common and usually associated with an elevated erythrocyte sedimentation rate and raised levels of acute phase proteins. Thrombocytosis is not uncommon but leucocytosis is much rarer than in polyarteritis nodosa. These laboratory tests do not help differentiate vasculitis from uncomplicated rheumatoid arthritis. Almost all patients are seropositive, usually with high titres of IgM rheumatoid factor. Anti-nuclear antibodies are also common. The most useful laboratory tests for differentiating rheumatoid vasculitis from uncomplicated rheumatoid synovitis are raised levels of complement-activating immune complexes such as cryoglobulins or anticomplementary activity and hypocomplementaemia, especially low levels of C4. Some radioimmunoassays for IgG rheumatoid factor have shown a very close association between high levels and the presence of vasculitis (Allen et al, 1981; Quismono et al, 1983). The relationship between IgM and IgG rheumatoid factors and vasculitis is shown in Figure 52.20. Anticomplementary activity, C4 and IgG rheumatoid factor levels are also useful for monitoring the activity of rheumatoid vasculitis.

Table 52.6 Laboratory abnormalities in 60 patients with systemic rheumatoid vasculitis

Anaemia	70%
Leucocytosis (> 10 × 10^9/l)	14%
Thrombocytosis (> 400 × 10^9/l)	40%
RA latex-positive	92%
Rose Waaler titre (mean)	1/256
Anti-nuclear antibodies	60%
Low C3	12%
Low C4	62%
Immune complexes	100%
Cryoglobulins	78%
Anticomplementary activity	58%

Prognosis

Vasculitic lesions are frequently recurrent (over 60%) and this may be responsible for the cumulative mortality of 40% within 5 years (Bywaters & Scott, 1963; Wilkinson & Torrance, 1967; Scott et al, 1981c). Major organ infarction, widespread sensory motor neuropathy and histological evidence of necrotising arteritis at rectal biopsy are associated with a particularly poor prognosis.

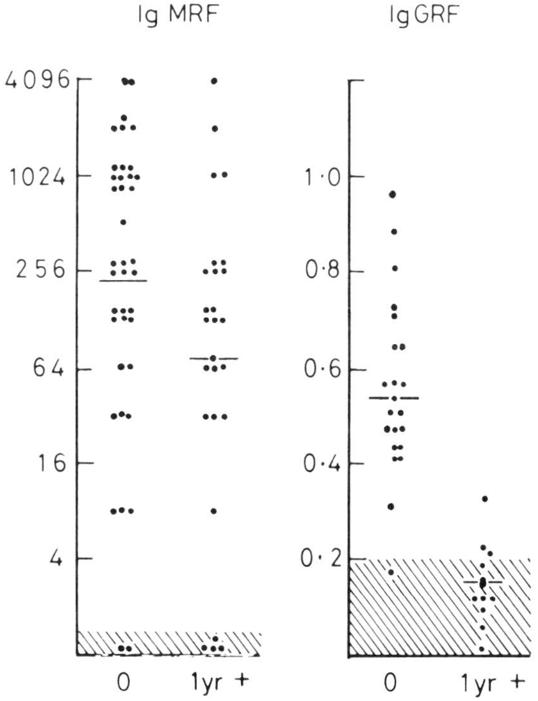

Fig. 52.20 Rheumatoid vasculitis; IgM RF and IgG RF levels at the time of vasculitis (O) and at follow-up at least 1 year from the onset of vasculitis (1 yr+); the normal range is represented by the shaded area and the mean titres by the horizontal bars. (Reproduced by permission from Scott et al, 1981c.)

Treatment

Treatment has been poorly defined due to the small numbers of patients included in therapeutic studies. Benefit has been claimed with D penicillamine (Jaffe, 1970), plasma exchange (Goldman et al, 1979; Scott et al, 1981b) and cyclophosphamide (Weismann & Zvaifler, 1975; Abel et al, 1980). In a small controlled trial Nicholls et al (1973) were unable to demonstrate any improvement attributable to azathioprine.

Therapeutic responses have been studied in 45 of the 60 patients with systemic rheumatoid vasculitis shown in Tables 52.5 and 52.6. 21 were treated with intermittent bolus intravenous injections of cyclophosphamide plus methylprednisolone and 24 with a variety of other more conventional antirheumatic or cytotoxic drugs. The intravenous therapy was associated with more frequent healing of vasculitic lesions, particularly leg ulcers and neuropathy, a lower rate of relapse, fewer serious complications and a lower mortality. One particularly dramatic effect was the rapid healing of motor function in patients with mononeuritis treated early (Scott & Bacon, 1984). Aggressive cytotoxic therapy should be reserved for patients with *systemic* rheumatoid vasculitis, particularly those with evidence of an underlying arteritis as opposed to small vessel vasculitis. A combination of plasma exchange and intravenous cyclophosphamide plus methylprednisolone may be necessary for severely ill patients.

Vasculitis associated with other connective tissue diseases

Vasculitis is a common feature of many connective tissue diseases. In systemic lupus erythematosus lesions of small arterioles and capillaries predominate but large muscular arteries may be involved occasionally with aneurysm formation (Longstreth et al, 1974). Major peripheral arterial occlusion (Dubois & Arterberry, 1962; Gladstein et al, 1979), ileal or colonic perforation due to mesenteric arteritis (Zizac et al, 1975), and severe renal damage due to arteriolar or intralobular artery lesions (Baldwin & Gallo, 1975) have been described. Intra-abdominal arteritis is associated with a very high mortality (90%) similar to polyarteritis nodosa (Ziczac et al, 1983). Over a third of renal biopsies showing diffuse proliferative lupus glomerulonephritis are reported to show an associated arteritis or arteriolitis. The presence of such vasculitis is associated with more severe glomerular injuries and a poorer prognosis (Bhuyan et al, 1983).

Destructive obliterative vascular changes occur in practically every organ in progressive systemic sclerosis but there is still no agreement as to whether these changes are primary or secondary.

Perivascular collections of lymphocytes are commonly seen in muscle biopsies from patients with dermatomyositis, but their significance is unknown. Diffuse arteritis is most commonly detected in children with dermatomyositis (Banker, 1975) and patients with myositis associated with Sjögren's syndrome (Alexander et al, 1982a). In adults the presence of cutaneous vasculitis may be associated with an increased risk of underlying malignant disease (Feldman et al, 1983).

Sjögren's syndrome is also associated with cutaneous vasculitis, systemic vasculitis and cerebral symptoms which may be attributable to vasculitis. An antibody to a cytoplasmic antigen (anti-Ro/anti-SSA) is found more frequently in these patients than in uncomplicated Sjögren's syndrome (Alexander et al, 1982a, b).

Small vessel vasculitis is responsible for many of the clinical manifestations of Behçet's syndrome. Occasionally large arteries are involved but in these cases the primary site of pathology is the vasa vasorum.

Necrotising arteritis has been reported in up to 50% of patients with Cogan's syndrome, a condition characterised by interstitial keratitis and audiovestibular disease (Cheson et al, 1976). However it is likely that some of these cases had either polyarteritis nodosa or Wegener's granulomatosis which are known to be associated with ocular and auditory manifestations leading to an overestimation of the importance of Cogan's syndrome as a primary vasculitic disease (Haynes et al, 1980).

SMALL VESSEL OR HYPERSENSITIVITY VASCULITIS

Inflammation of small blood vessels (arterioles, capillaries and venules) is a feature of many of the diseases described above. As classification is based on the largest vessel involved, the characteristic feature of small vessel vasculitis is the lack of any muscular artery involvement. Although small vessel vasculitis can involve any organ system, it rarely progresses to life-threatening complications and cutaneous lesions dominate the clinical picture.

Histology reveals a characteristic neutrophilic infiltrate, leucocytoclasis, tissue destruction, fibrinoid changes, haemorrhage and secondary healing (Fig. 52.21). Damaged vessels are usually at the same stage of involvement at any given time in contrast to the spectrum of acute, subacute and chronic changes which may coexist in systemic necrotising arteritis. Primary lymphocytic infiltration has been described (Soter et al, 1976) but mixed cellular patterns are more common and different cellular infiltrates probably represent a continuous evolution from acute to chronic vasculitis.

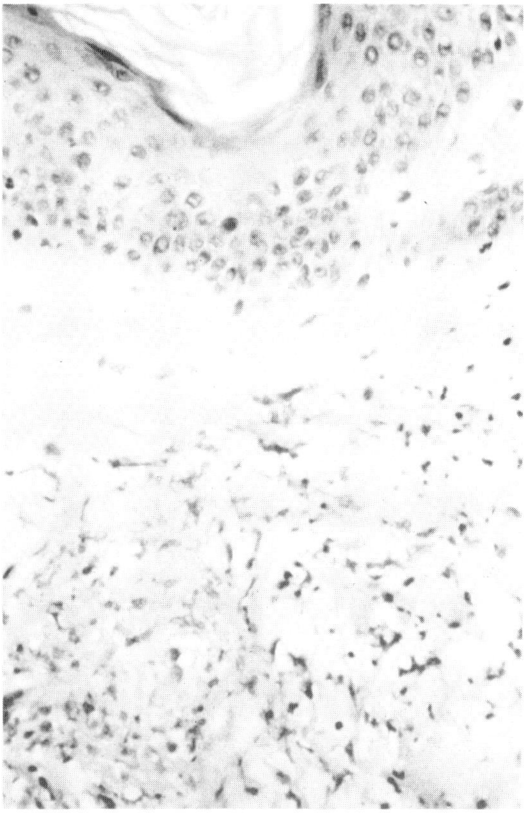

Fig. 52.21 Leucocytoclastic vasculitis affecting small dermal vessels with widespread nuclear debris. (Reproduced by courtesy of Dr C. R. Tribe.) (H & E × 200)

The term 'hypersensitivity' describes the frequent relationship of these diseases to precipitating antigens such as drugs, foreign protein or infection. Large series suggest that females are more commonly affected than males (Winkelmann & Ditto, 1964; Cream, 1976). Immune complexes are usually implicated in aetiology and a variety of antigens (hepatitis B, streptococcal, staphylococcal, microbacterial organisms) as well as immunoglobulin and complement may be demonstrated in cutaneous lesions (Parish, 1971; Sams et al, 1975; Braverman & Yen, 1975). Two distinctive clinical syndromes associated with small vessel vasculitis are Henoch–Schlönlein purpura and essential mixed cryoglobulinaemia.

Henoch–Schönlein purpura (see also Ch. 49)
This disease is characterised by the combination of purpura, arthritis, haemorrhagic gastrointestinal disease and glomerulonephritis. Children are most commonly affected but Henoch–Schönlein purpura has been described in adults (Cream et al, 1970).

Streptococcal infection, drug hypersensitivity and food allergy are commonly implicated although tumour antigens may be important in some adults (Cairns et al, 1978; Kauffman et al, 1980). IgA containing immune complexes are found in the sera in early disease (Levinsky & Barratt, 1979) and immunoglobulins (especially IgA) and complement are detected in cutaneous and renal lesions (Evans et al, 1973; Giangiacomo & Tsai, 1977). Alternative complement pathway activation is suggested by presence of factor B and C3 in affected lesions and by the description of Henoch–Schönlein purpura in patients with congenital absence of C2 (Sussman et al, 1973). These studies suggest that abnormal local IgA-mediated immune responses to an infectious agent in the respiratory tract or to food in the gastrointestinal tract may be important.

Purpura usually affects the lower limbs. Joint involvement (mainly large joints) is commoner and more severe in adults. Gastrointestinal symptoms, thought to result from small vessel vasculitis with haemorrhage into bowel wall, include abdominal pain, intussusception and gastrointestinal haemorrhage. Renal involvement is usually mild although a progressive glomerulonephritis may occur and renal failure is the commonest cause of death (Cream et al, 1970).

Corticosteroids have not been shown to influence the course of renal disease but may improve gastrointestinal symptoms in contrast to their lack of effect in polyarteritis affecting the gut (Lopez et al, 1980). In rare cases with progressive renal disease, a trial of cytotoxic drugs may be justified.

Essential mixed cryoglobulinaemia

In 1966 Meltzer & Franklin described a group of patients with purpura (due to leucocytoclastic small vessel vasculitis), arthralgia, muscle weakness and renal disease. The characteristic laboratory abnormality was the presence of a cryoglobulin made up of IgM rheumatoid factor and IgG. Other diseases associated with cryoglobulinaemia were excluded and this syndrome was therefore called essential mixed cryoglobulinaemia and classified as a small vessel hypersensitivity vasculitis. This classification has persisted but recent studies suggest that the cryoglobulinaemia is often not 'essential'; hepatitis Bs antigen may be detected in some cryoglobulins (Levo et al, 1977); digital gangrene, leg ulcers, intestinal vasculitis (Reza et al, 1974) and peripheral neuropathy (Gorevic, 1980) suggest larger vessel involvement, and necropsy studies have revealed widespread necrotising arteritis affecting the kidneys, heart, gastrointestinal tract, nervous system, muscle and lungs (Gorevic et al, 1980). Many patients with essential mixed cryoglobulinaemia should therefore be reclassified within the systemic necrotising arteritides.

Renal involvement is associated with a poor prognosis (probably due to associated arteritis). Plasma exchange (Lockwood et al, 1979), cytotoxic drugs (Ristow et al, 1976) or combined plasma exchange and immunosuppression (Geltner et al, 1981) may be associated with clinical improvement.

Other small vessel vasculitides

Gilliam & Smiley (1976) reviewed the wide range of diseases associated with small vessel vasculitis. These include subacute bacterial endocarditis, chronic active hepatitis, ulcerative colitis, primary biliary sclerosis, Goodpasture's syndrome and intestinal bypass surgery.

Cutaneous vasculitis

Systemic features including arthralgia and occasional arthritis may occur in patients with distinctive cutaneous vasculitic syndromes. These include erythema elevatum diutinum (reviewed by Katz et al, 1977), and hypocomplementaemic urticarial vasculitic syndrome (reviewed by Zeiss et al, 1980).

LARGE VESSEL ARTERITIS

Temporal arteritis

Temporal arteritis is a systemic granulomatous panarteritis of large elastic arteries. The principal vessels involved are the internal and external carotids, temporal, occipital and ophthalmic arteries. The media becomes thickened by infiltration with mononuclear cells, neutrophils and eosinophils; giant cells are present in varying degrees but may be quite rare. Smooth muscle necrosis and disruption of the internal elastic lamina occurs and intimal proliferation may lead to thrombosis, occlusion and recanalisation.

Temporal (giant cell) arteritis is relatively common and sometimes associated with the syndrome of polymyalgia rheumatica. For a full description see Chapter 51.

Takayasu's arteritis

Like temporal arteritis, Takayasu's arteritis is a granulomatous panarteritis affecting large elastic arteries. Clinical features, the distribution of vascular involvement and histology show important differences between these diseases, and Takayasu's arteritis usually affects young women between the ages of 15 and 25 years at presentation in contrast to the older age-group affected by temporal arteritis.

Takayasu (1908) described a curious fundal appearance in a 21-year-old woman. In the discussion that followed this presentation, the association was made between the ocular lesions and absent radial pulses, and in the ensuing years the widespread nature of the vascular inflammation affecting the aortic arch and its branches was described.

Inflammatory changes predominate in the adventitia consisting of mononuclear cells, reticular cells, neutrophils and an occasional multinucleate giant cell. Later the granulomata become fibrotic, collagen is deposited in the adventitia and intimal thickening leads to narrowing and may proceed to thrombosis.

Infection and direct antibody mediated arterial damage were popular postulated pathogenic mechanisms but have not been substantiated. Recent studies suggest that genetic factors may be important and a variety of HLA antigen associations have been described. The most impressive figures come from a North American series which showed a strong association with HLA-DR4 and a B cell alloantigen MB3 (Volkman et al, 1982). Recent studies in our own laboratory suggest that cytotoxic T lymphocytes may be directly involved in the pathogenesis of Takayasu's arteritis (Scott et al, 1984).

There is a biphasic pattern of diseases. In the acute stage, systemic symptoms including fever, malaise, weight loss and arthralgia predominate. Mono- and polyarticular arthritis have been described occasionally suggesting a diagnosis of rheumatoid arthritis (Serre et al, 1970). Less frequent manifestations include scleritis, skin nodules, pleurisy and pericarditis (reviewed by Strachan, 1964). The chronic phase, characterised by signs and symptoms of vascular occlusion, develops after an interval of months or decades (mean 8 years) but as the systemic phase is often undiagnosed this distinction is not always apparent.

Absence of at least one arterial pulse, especially radial, ulnar and carotid is very common. Bruits are often detected in the supraclavicular area. Involved arteries are tender (especially carotid) and claudication of the arms is an important symptom. Other features include hypertension due to renal artery stenosis, palpitations, cardiac failure, coronary thrombosis and aortic incompetence. Transient visual failure due to ischaemia may be precipitated when the head is extended leading to a characteristic 'face down' posture. Retinal changes are usually due to hypertension. Syncope is common but cerebral infarction rare.

There are no specific laboratory abnormalities. Marked elevations of the erythrocyte sedimentation rate and acute phase proteins, elevated immunoglobulins, a mild anaemia and leucocytosis are common. Rheumatoid factor and anti-nuclear antibodies are rarely detected. Diagnosis is confirmed by arch-aortography and it is important to visualise the whole aorta to define the extent of disease. Narrowing or occlusion are the usual findings but saccular or fusiform aneurysms can occur. The most frequently involved sites are the subclavian, descending aorta, renal, carotid and pulmonary arteries. Echocardiography is a useful non-invasive technique for serial examination of the aortic root (Tanaka et al, 1979).

Corticosteroids provide symptomatic relief in some patients and previously absent pulses may become palpable (Fraga et al, 1972). Vascular surgery may be required in selected cases. Reports on prognosis are conflicting but most modern series show a mortality of less than 15% (Nakeo et al, 1967; Lupi-Heirera et al, 1977), possibly related to corticosteroid therapy. The role of cytotoxic agents in this disease has not been evaluated.

REFERENCES

Abel T, Andrews B S, Cunningham P H, Brunner, C M, Davis J S, Horwitz D A 1980 Rheumatoid vasculitis: effect of cyclophosphamide on the clinical course and levels of circulating immune complexes. Annals of Internal Medicine 93: 407–413

Adler R H, Norcross B M, Lockie L M 1962 Arteritis and infarction of the intestine in rheumatoid arthritis. Journal of the American Medical Association 180: 922–926

Alarcon-Segovia D 1977 The necrotizing vasculitides. A new pathogenetic classification. Medical Clinics of North America 61: 241–260

Alarcon-Segovia D 1980 Classification of the necrotizing vasculitides in man. Clinics in Rheumatic Diseases 6: 223–232

Alexander E L, Josifek L, Provost T T, Alexander G E 1982a Myositis/vasculitis in a primary Sjogren's syndrome. Arthritis and Rheumatism 25(Suppl 4): S15 (Abstract)

Alexander E L, Provost T T, Stevens M B, Alexander G E 1982b Neurologic complications of primary Sjogren's syndrome. Medicine (Baltimore) 61: 247–257

Allen C, Elson C J, Scott D G I, Bacon P A, Bucknall R C 1981 IgG antiglobulins in rheumatoid arthritis and other arthritides: relationship with clinical features and other parameters. Annals of the Rheumatic Diseases 40: 127–131

Andrews B S, Shadforth M, Cunningham P, Davis J S 1981 Demonstration of a Clq receptor on the surface of human endothelial cells. Journal of Immunology 127: 1075–1080

Arkin A 1930 A clinical and pathological study of periarteritis nodosa. Report of five cases, one histologically healed. American Journal of Pathology 6: 401–426

Armstrong R D, Behn A, Myles A, Panayi G S, Welsh K I 1983 Histocompatability antigens in polymalgia rheumatica and giant cell arteritis. Journal of Rheumatology 10: 659–661

Bacon P A, Doherty S M, Zuckerman A J 1975 Hepatitis-B antibody in polymyalgia rheumatica. Lancet 2: 476–478

Baker S B, Robinson D R 1978 Unusual renal manifestations of Wegener's granulomatosis. Report of two cases. American Journal of Medicine 64: 883–889

Baldwin D S, Gallo G R 1975 Lupus nephritis. Clinics in Rheumatic Diseases 1: 639–664

Ball J, 1954 Rheumatoid arthritis and polyarteritis nodosa. Annals of the Rheumatic Diseases 13: 277–290

Bamji A, Salisbury R 1978 Cytomegalovirus and vasculitis. British Medical Journal 1:623

Banker B Q, 1975 Dermatomyositis of childhood. Ultrastructural alteration of muscles and intramuscular blood vessels. Journal of Neuropathology and Experimental Neurology 34: 46–75

Banks P M, Cohen M D, Ginsburg W W, Hunder G G 1983 Immunohistologic and cytochemical studies of temporal arteritis. Arthritis and Rheumatism 26: 1201–1207

Bannatyne G A 1898 Rheumatoid arthritis, 2nd Edn. John Wright, Bristol

Bell W R, Klinefelter H F 1967 Polymyalgia rheumatica. John Hopkins Medical Journal 121: 175–187

Bengtsson B A, Malmvall B E 1981 An alternate-day corticosteroid regimen in the maintenance therapy of giant cell arteritis. Acta Medica Scandinavica 209: 347–350

Bhuyan U N, Malaviya A N, Dash S C, Malhotra K K 1983 Prognostic significance of renal angiitis in systemic lupus erythematosus (SLE). Clinical Nephrology 20: 109–113

Biller J, Asconap'e J, Weinblatt N E, Toole J F 1982 Temporal arteritis associated with a normal sendimentation rate. Journal of the American Medical Association 247: 486–487

Bircher J, Bartholomew G, Cain J C, Adson M A 1966 Syndrome of intestinal arterial insufficiency ('abdominal angina'). Archives of Internal Medicine 117: 632-638

Blumberg S, Bienfang D, Kantrowitz F G 1980 A possible association between influenza vaccination and small-vessel vasculitis. Archives of Internal Medicine 140: 847–848

Bocanegra T S, Espinoza L R, Vasey F B, Germain B F 1981 Pulmonary haemorrhage in the systemic necrotizing vasculitis associated with hepatitis B. Chest 80: 102–103

Borrie P 1972 Cutaneous polyarteritis nodosa. British Journal of Dermatology 87: 87–95

Braverman I M, Yen A 1975 Demonstration of immune complexes in spontaneous and histamine induced lesions and in normal skin of patients with leukocytoclastic angiitis. Journal of Investigative Dermatology 64: 105–112

Brennan M J, Sandyk R 1982 Reversible quadriplegia in a patient with a giant-cell arteritis. South African Medical Journal 62: 81–82

Bywaters E G L 1957 Peripheral vascular obstruction in rheumatoid arthritis and its relationship to other vascular lesions. Annals of the Rheumatic Diseases 16: 84–103

Bywaters E G L, Scott J T 1963 The natural history of vascular lesions in rheumatoid arthritis. Journal of Chronic Diseases 16: 905–914

Cairns S A, Mallick N P, Lawler W, Williams G 1978 Squamous cell carcinoma of the bronchus presenting with Henoch–Schönlein purpura. British Medical Journal 2: 474–475

Camilleri M, Pusey C D, Chadwick V S, Rees A J 1983 Gastrointestinal manifestations of systemic vasculitis. Quarterly Journal of Medicine 52: 141–149

Carrington C B, Liebow A A 1966 Limited forms of angiitis and granulomatosis of Wegener's type. American Journal of Medicine 41: 497–527

Castaigre P, Cambier J, Escowrople R, Brunet P 1970 Les manifestations nerveuses centrales de la periarterite nouese. A propos d'une anatomaclinique. Annals of Internal Medicine 121: 375

Chatel A, Gornier T H, Brigot J M, Toulg C, Helenon C H 1979 L'arteriographie dans la periarterite noueuse. Journal de Radiologie 2: 113–120

Cheson B D, Bluming A Z, Alroy J 1976 Cogan's syndrome: a systemic vasculitis. American Journal of Medicine 60: 549–555

Chumbley D C, Harrison E G, DeRemee R A 1977 Allergic granulomatosis and angiitis (Churg-Strauss syndrome). Report and analysis of 30 cases. Mayo Clinic Proceedings 52: 477–484

Churg 1983 Pulmonary angiitis and granulomatosis revisited. Human Pathology 14: 868–883

Churg J, Strauss L 1951 Allergic granulomatosis, alleric angiitis and periarteritis nodosa. American Journal of Pathology 27: 277–302

Clark R E, McNamara T O, Palubinskas A J 1972 Intrarenal mycotic aneurysm detected angiographically. British Journal of Radiology 45: 66–67

Cochrane C G, Dixon F J 1976 Antigen-antibody complex induced disease. In: Miescher P A, Muller-Eberhard H J (Eds) Textbook of immunopathology, Vol 1, 2nd Edn. Grune & Stratton, New York

Cohen R D, Conn D L, Ilstrup D M 1980 Clinical features, prognosis and response to treatment in polyarteritis. Mayo Clinic Proceedings 55: 146–155

Colton C L, Butler T J 1967 The surgical problem of polyarteritis nodosa. British Journal of Surgery 54: 393–396

Combes B, Stastny P, Shorey J, Eigenbrodt E H, Barrera A, Hull A R et al 1971 Glomerulonephritis with deposition of Australia antigen–antibody complexes in glomerular basement membrane. Lancet 2: 234–237

Conn D L, McDuffie F C, Dyck P J 1972 Immunopathological study of sural nerves in rheumatoid arthritis. Arthritis and Rheumatism 15: 135–143

Conn, D L, McDuffie F C, Holley K E, Schroeter A L 1976 Immunologic mechanisms in systemic vasculitis. Mayo Clinic Proceedings 51: 511–518

Cream J J 1976 Clinical and Immunological aspects of cutaneous vasculitis. Quarterly Journal of Medicine 45: 255–276

Cream J J, Gumpel J M, Peachey R D G 1970 Schönlein–Henoch purpura in the adult. Quarterly Journal of Medicine 39: 461–484

Cunningham TJ, Tait B D, Mathews J D, Muirden K D 1982 Clinical rheumatoid vasculitis associated with the B8 DR3 phenotype. Rheumatology International 2: 137–139

Cupps T R, Fauci A S 1981 The vasculitides, Major problems in internal medicine, Vol XXI. Saunders, Philadelphia

Curtis J J, Diethelm A G, Herrera G A, Crowell W T, Whelchel J D 1983 Recurrence of Wegeners granulomatosis in a cadaver renal allograft.

Transplantation 36: 452–454
Dahl E V, Baggenstoss A H, Deweerd J H 1960 Testicular lesions of periarteritis nodosa with special reference to diagnosis. American Journal of Medicine 28: 222–228
Dega F J, Hunder G G 1974 Vasculitis of the breast: an unusual manifestation of polyarteritis. Arthritis and Rheumatism 17: 973–976
Demaine A G, Vaughan R W, Behn A R, Myles A B, Panayi G S, Welsh K I 1983 Immunoglobulin (Gm) allotype frequencies in patients with giant cell arteritis and polymyalgia rheumatica. Journal of Immunogenetics 10: 343–348
Dequeker J, Rosberg G 1967 Digital capillaritis in rheumatoid arthritis. Acta Rheumatologica Scandinavica 13: 299–307
Dickson E R, Maldonado G E, Sheps S G, Cain J A 1973 Systemic and giant-cell arteritis with polymyalgia rheumatica. Reversible abnormalities of liver function. Journal of the American Medical Association 224: 1496–1498
Dixon A St J 1976 Polymyalgia rheumatica. In: Scott J T (ed) Copeman's textbook of rheumatology, 5th Edn. Churchill Livingstone, Edinburgh
D'Izarn J J, Boulet C P, Couvard J P, Bonnin A, Ledoux-Lebard G 1976 L'arteriographie dans la periarterite noueuse. Journal de Radiologie et Electrologie et de Nucleare 57: 505–509
Dobrescu G, Dobrescu A, Stoica L, 1983 Ultrastructural aspects in skin allergic vasculitis. Morphologie et Embryologie (Bucuresti) 29: 31–34
Doherty M, Bradfield J W 1981 Polyarteritis nodosa associated with acute cytomegalovirus infection. Annals of the Rheumatic Diseases 40: 419–421
Drachman D A, 1963 Neurological complications of Wegener's granulomatosis. Archives of Neurology 8: 145–155
Dubois E L, Arterberry J D 1962 Gangrene with manifestations of systemic lupus erythematosus. Journal of the American Medical Association 181: 366–374
Dudley J P, Goodman M 1969 Periarteritis nodosa and bilateral facial paralysis. Archives of Otolaryngology 90: 139–146
Duffy L, Linsky M, Sharp J T, Davis J S, Person D A, Hollinger B et al 1976 Polyarthritis, polyarteritis and hepatitis B. Medicine (Baltimore) 55: 19–37
Dumonde D R, Richards T J 1981 The significance of immunological investigation in cardiovascular disease. In: Lessof M H (ed) Immunology of cardiovascular disease. Marcel Dekker, New York, Ch. 2, p.75–104
Durieux P, Bletry O, Huchon G, Wechsler B, Cheretien J, Godeau P 1981 Multiple pulmonary arterial aneurysms in Behcet's disease and Hughes–Stovin syndrome. The American Journal of Medicine 71: 736
Dyer H, Verbov J L, Dawson A M Borrie P F, Stansfeld A G 1970 Cutaneous polyarteritis nodosa associated with Crohn's disease. Lancet 1: 648–650
Elkon K B, Hughes G R V 1980 Vasculitis. In: Bellingham J (Ed) Advanced Medicine, No 16. Pitman Medical, Tunbridge Wells
Elkon K B, Hughes G R V, Catovsky D, et al 1979 Hairy cell leukaemia with polyarteritis nodosa. Lancet 2: 280–282
Elkon K B, Sutherland D C, Rees A J, Hughes G R V, Batchelor J R, 1983 HLA-antigen frequencies in systemic vasculitis: Increase in HLA-DR2 in Wegeners granulomatosis. Arthritis and Rheumatism 26: 102–105
Elson C J, Scott D G I, Blake D R, Bacon P A, Holt P D J 1983 Complement-activating rheumatoid-factor-containing complexes in patients with rheumatoid vasculitis. Annals of the Rheumatic Diseases 42: 147–150
Erhardt C C, Mumford P, Maini R N 1979 The association of cryoglobulinaemia with nodules, vasculitis and fibrosing alveolitis in rheumatoid arthritis and their relationship to serum Clq binding activity and rheumatoid factor. Clinical and Experimental Immunology 38: 405–413
Esiri M M, MacLennan I C M, Hazleman B L 1973 Lymohocyte sensitivity to skeletal muscle in patients with polymyositis and other disorders. Clinical and Experimental Immunology 14: 25–35
Evans D J, Gwyn-Williams D, Peters D K, Sissons J G P, Boulton-Jones J M, Ogg C S et al 1973 Glomerular deposition of properdin in Henoch-Schönlein syndrome and idiopathic focal nephritis. British Medical Journal 2: 326–328
Fahey J, Leonard E, Churg J, Goodman G 1954 Wegener's granulomatosis. American Journal of Medicine 17: 168–179
Falicov R E, Cooney D F 1964 Takayasu's arteritis and rheumatoid arthritis. Archives of Internal Medicine 114: 594–600
Fauci A S, Wolff S M 1977 Wegener's granulomatosis and related diseases. In: Dowling H F (ed) Disease-a-month, Vol 23, No. 7
Fauci A S, Haynes B F, Katz P 1978 The spectrum of vasculitis. Clinical, pathologic, immunologic and therapeutic implications. Annals of Internal Medicine 89: 660–676
Fauci A S, Haynes B F, Katz P, Wolff S M 1983 Wegeners granulomatosis: prospective clinical and therapeutic experience with 85 patients for 21 years. Annals of Internal Medicine 98: 76–85
Fauci A S, Katz P, Haynes B F, Wolff S M 1979 Cyclophosphamide therapy of severe systemic necrotizing vasculitis. New England Journal of Medicine 301: 235–238
Fayemi A D, Ali M, Braun E J 1972 Necrotizing vasculitis of the gall bladder and the appendix. American Journal of Gastroenterology 67: 608–612
Feldman D, Hochberg M C, Zizac T M, Stevens M B 1983 Cutaneous vasculitis in adult polymyositis/dermatomyositis. Journal of Rheumatology 10: 85–89
Fisher E R, Bark J 1961 Effect of hypertension on vascular and other lesions of serum sickness. American Journal of Pathology 39: 665–675
Fisher R G 1981 Renal artery aneurysm in polyarteritis nodosa: a multi episodic phenomenon. American Journal of Roentgenology 136: 983–985
Ford R G, Siekert R G 1965 Central nervous system involvement in periarteritis nodosa. Neurology (NY) 15: 114–122
Fournie A, Durroux R, Ayrolles C, Boussigues J Y, Gay R 1976 Maladie de Horton et polyarthrite rheumatoide. Revue du Rhumatisme et des Maladies Osteoarticulaires 43: 309–212
Fraga A, Mintz G, Valle L, Flores-Izquierdo G 1972 Takayasu's arteritis: frequency of systemic manifestations (study of 22 patients) and favourable response to maintenance steroid therapy with adrenocorticosteroids (12 patients). Arthritis and Rheumatism 15: 617–624
French G 1953 Polyarteritis nodosa presenting as acute diabetes mellitus. British Medical Journal 1: 1262
Friedman H M, Macarak E J, MacGregor R R, Wolf E J, Kefalides N A 1981 Virus infection of endothelial cells.

Journal of Infectious Diseases 143: 266–273
Frohnert P P, Sheps S G 1967 Long-term follow up study of periarteritis nodosa. American Journal of Medicine 43: 8–14
Geltner D, Kohn R W, Gorevic P, Franklin E C 1981 The effect of combination therapy (steroids, immunosuppressives, and plasmapheresis) on 5 mixed cryoglobulinaemic patients with renal, neurologic and vascular involvement. Arthritis and Rheumatism 24: 1121–1127
Gephardt G N, Ahmad M, Tubbs R R 1983 Pulmonary vasculitis (Wegener's granulomatosis). Immunohistochemical study of T and B cell markers. American Journal of Medicine 74: 700–704
Giangiacomo J, Tsai C C 1977 Dermal and glomerular deposition of IgA in anaphylactoid purpura. American Journal of Diseases of Children 131: 981–983
Gilliam J N, Smiley J D 1976 Cutaneous necrotizing vasculitis and related disorders. Annals of Allergy 37: 328–339
Gladstein G S, Ruynes R I, Parhami N, Bartholomew L E 1979 Gangrene of the foot secondary to systemic lupus erythematosus with large vessel vasculitis. Journal of Rheumatology 6: 549–553
Gocke D J, Hsu K, Morgan C, Bombardieri S, Lockshin M, Christian C L 1970 Association between polyarteritis and Australia antigen. Lancet 2: 1149–1153
Goldman J A, Casey H L, McIlwain H, Kirby J, Wilson C H, Miller S B 1979 Limited plasmapheresis in rheumatoid arthritis with vasculitis. Arthritis and Rheumatism 22: 1146–1150
Goodman G C, Churg J 1954 Wegener's granulomatosis. Pathology and review of the literature. Archives of Pathology 58: 533–553
Gorevic P D, Kassab H J, Levo Y, et al 1980 Mixed cryoglobulinaemia: clinical aspects and long-term follow up of 40 patients. American Journal of Medicine 69: 287–308
Gower R G, Sausker W F, Kohler P F, Thorne G E, McIntosh R M 1978 Small vessel vasculitis caused by hepatitis B virus immune complexes. Journal of Allergy and Clinical Immunology 62: 222–228
Graham E, Holland A, Avery A, Russell R W R 1981 Prognosis in giant-cell arteritis. British Medical Journal 282: 269–271
Gupta R C, Kohler P F 1984 Identification of HBsAg determinants in immune complexes from hepatitis B virus-associated vasculitis. Journal of Immunology 132: 1223–1228
Haakenstad A O, Mannik M 1974 Saturation of the reticulo-endothelial system with soluble immune complexes. Journal of Immunology 1112: 1939–1948
Hamilton C R, Shelley W M, Tumulty P A 1971 Giant-cell arteritis: including temporal arteritis and polymyalgia rheumatica. Medicine (Baltimore) 50: 1–27
Hart M N, Sadewasser K L, Cancilla P A, DeBault L E 1983 Experimental autoimmune type of vasculitis resulting from activation of mouse lymphocytes to cultured endothelium. Laboratory Investigation 48: 419–427
Hauser W A, Ferguson R H, Holley K E, Kurland L T 1971 Temporal arteritis in Rochester, Minnesota, 1951 to 1967. Mayo Clinic Proceedings 46: 597–602
Haynes B F, Fishman M C, Fauci A S, Wolff S M 1977 The ocular manifestations of Wegener's granulomatosis: fifteen years experience and review of the literature. American Journal of Medicine 63: 131–140
Haynes B F, Kaiser-Kupfer M I, Mason P, Fauci A S 1980 Cogan syndrome: studies in 13 patients, long term follow up and a review of the literature. Medicine (Baltimore) 59: 426–441
Hazleman B, Golstone A, Voak D 1977 Association of polymyalgia rheumatica and giant-cell arteritis with HLA-B8. British Medical Journal 2: 989–991
Healey A, Wilske K R 1980 Presentation of occult giant-cell arteritis. Arthritis and Rheumatism 23: 641–643
Henson P M, Cochran E C G 1971 Acute immune complex disease in rabbits. The role of complement and of a leucocyte dependant release of vaso active amines from platelets. Journal of Experimental Medicine 133: 554–571
Henson R A, Croft P D 1956 Spontaneous spinal subarachnoid haemorrhage. Quarterly Journal of Medicine 25: 53–66
Hind C R K, Savage C O, Winearls C G, Pepys M B 1984 Objective monitoring of disease activity in polyarteritis by measurement of serum C-reactive protein concentration. British Medical Journal 288: 1027–1030
Hoffman G S, Frank W A 1979 Infectious mononucleosis, auto-immunity and vasculitis. Journal of the American Medical Association 242: 2735–2736
Holsinger D R, Osmundson P J, Edwards J E 1962 The heart in periarteritis nodosa. Circulation 25: 610–618
Horn R G, Fauci A S, Rosenthal A S, Wolff S M 1974 Renal biopsy pathology in Wegener's granulomatosis. American Journal of Pathology 74: 4231–433
Howell S B, Epstein W V 1976 Circulating immunoglobulin complexes in Wegener's granulomatosis. American Journal of Medicine 60: 259–268
Hughes G R V 1979 Connective tissue diseases, 2nd Edn. Blackwell, Oxford
Hunder G G, Allen T L 1978–1979 Giant-cell arteritis: a review. Bulletin on the Rheumatic Diseases 29: 980–986
Hurst N P, Nuki G 1981 Evidence for defect of complement mediated phagocytosis by monocytes from patients with rheumatoid arthritis and cutaneous vasculitis. British Medical Journal 1: 2081–2083
Israel H L, Patchefsky A S, Saldana M J 1977 Wegener's granulomatosis and benign lymphocytic angiitis and granulomatosis of the lung: recognition and treatment Annals of Internal Medicine 87: 691–699
Jaffe I A 1970 The treatment of rheumatoid arthritis and necrotizing vasculitis with penicillamine. Arthritis and Rheumatism 13: 436–443
Jaffe E A, Weksler B B 1979 Recovery of endothelial cell prostacycline production after inhibition by low doses of aspirin. Journal of Clinical Investigation 63: 532–533
James T N, Birk R 1966 Pathology of the cardiac conduction system in polyarteritis nodosa. Archives of Internal Medicine 117: 561–567
Johnson P M, Trenchev P, Faulk W P 1975 Immunological studies of human placentae. Binding of complexed immunoglobulin by stromal endothelial cells. Clinical and Experimental Immunology 22: 133–138
Jones V E; Cowley P J, Allen C, Elson C J 1980 The isolation of immune complexes containing IgM rheumatoid factor and recovery of IgG rheumatoid factor from the complexes. Journal of Immunological Methods 37: 1–14
Jorizzo J L, Daniels J C, Apisarnthanarax P, Gonzalez E B, Cavallo T 1983 Histamine-triggered localized vasculitis in patients with seropositive rheumatoid arthritis. Journal of American Academy of Dermatology 9: 845–851
Katz S I, Gallin J I, Hertz K C, Fauci A S, Lawley T J 1977 Erythema elevatum diutinum: skin and systemic

manifestations, immunologic studies and successful treatment with dapsone. Medicine *Baltimore* 56: 443–455
Kauffmann R H, Herrmann W A, Meijer C J L M, Daha M R, Van Es L A 1980 Circulating IgA-immune complexes in Henoch-Schönlein purpura. A longitudinal study of their relationship to disease activity and vascular deposition of IgA. American Journal of Medicine 69: 859–866
Kaur J S, Goldberg J P, Schrier R W 1982 Acute renal failure following arteriography in a patient with polyarteritis nodosa. Journal of the American Association 247: 833–844
Kawasaki T, Kosaki F, Osawa S, Shitematsu I, Yamatawa S 1974 A new infantile acute febrile mucocutaneous lymph node syndrome (MCLS) prevailing in Japan. Pediatrics 54: 271–280
Kitridou R C 1977 Polyarteritis and related disorders. In: Katz W (Ed) Rheumatic diseases — Diagnosis and treatment. Lippincott, Philadelphia
Klein R G, Hunder G G, Stanson A W, Shets S G 1975 Large artery involvement in giant-cell (temporal) arteritis. Annals of Internal Medicine 83: 806–812
Klinger H 1931 Grenzformen der periarteritis nodosa. Frankfurter Zeitschrift fur Pathologie 42: 445–480
Kniker W T, Cochrane C G 1965 Pathogenic factors in vascular lesions of experimental serum sickness. Journal of Experimental Medicine 122: 83–97
Kniker W T, Cochrane C G 1968 The localisation of circulating immune complexes in experimental serum sickness: the role of vasoactive amines and hydrodynamic forces. Journal of Experimental Medicine 127: 119–135
Kussmaul A, Maier R 1866 Ueber eine bisher nicht beschriebene eigenthemliche arteriener-krangung (periarteritis nodosa), die mit Morbus Brightil und reapid fortschreitender allgemeiner Muskellahmung einhergeht. Deutsches Archiv fur Klinische Medizin 1: 484–517
Lake Bakaar 1978 Polyarteritis nodosa presenting with bilateral nerve deafness. Journal of the Royal Society of Medicine 71: 144–147
Lanham J G, Elkon K B, Pusey C D, Hughes G R 1984 Systemic vasculitis with asthma and eosinophilia: a clinical approach to the Churg-Strauss syndrome. Medicine (Baltimore) 63: 65–81
Leatherman J W, Sibley R K, Davies S F 1982 Diffuse intrapulmonary haemorrhage and glomerulonephritis unrelated to anti-glomerular basement membrane antibody. American Journal of Medicine 72: 401–410
Leib E S, Restivo C, Paulus H E 1979 Immunosuppressive corticosteroid therapy of polyarteritis nodosa. American Journal of Medicine 67: 941–947
Leonhardt E T G, Kullenberg K P G 1977 Bilateral atrial myxomas with multiple arterial aneurysm — a syndrome mimicking polyarteritis nodosa. American Journal of Medicine 62: 792–794
Levinsky R J, Barratt T M 1979 IgA immune complexes in Henoch–Schönlein purpura. Lancet 2: 1100–1103
Levo V, Gorevic P D, Kassab H J, Zucker-Franklin D, Franklin E C 1977 Association between hepatitis-B virus and essential mixed cryoglobulinaemia. New England Journal of Medicine 296: 1501–1504
Liebow A A, Carrington C R B, Friedman P J 1972 Lymphomatoid granulomatosis. Human Pathology 3: 457–558
Lockwood C M, Worlledge S, Nicholas A, Cotton C, Peters D K 1979 Reversal of impaired splenic function in patients with nephritis or vasculitis (or both) by plasma exchange. New England Journal of Medicine 300: 525–530
Longstretch P L, Korobin M, Palubinskaa A J 1974 Renal microaneurysms in a patient with SLE. Radiology 113: 63–65
Lopez L R, Schokett A L, Stanford R E, Claman H N, Kohler P F 1980 Gastro-intestinal involvement in leucocytoclastic vasculitis and polyarteritis nodosa. Journal of Rheumatology 7: 677–684
Lovshin L L, Kernoham J W 1948 Peripheral neuritis in periarteritis nodosa: a clinicopathological study. Archives of Internal Medicine 82: 321–338
Lowenstein M B, Bridgeford P H, Vasey F B, Germain B F, Espinoza L R 1983 Increased frequency of HLA DR3 and DR4 in polymyalgia-giant cell arteritis. Arthritis and Rheumatism 26: 925–927
Lupi-Herrera E, Sanchez-Torres G, Marcushamer J, Mispierta J, Harowitz S, Vela J E 1977 Takayasu's arteritis. Clinical study of 107 cases. American Heart Journal 93: 94–103
Lyell A, Church R 1954 The cutaneous manifestations of polyarteritis nodosa. British Journal of Dermatology 66: 335–343
MacFarlane D G, Burton P A, Bacon P A 1981 Histamine skin test in vasculitis. Revue du Rhumatisme et des Malades Osteoarticulaires. Numero special, Juin, Abstract No. 0533
MacFarlane D G, Bourne J, Dieppe P A 1983 Indolent Wegener's granulomatosis. Annals of the Rheumatic Diseases 42: 398–407
MacGregor R R, Friedman H M, Macarak J, Kefalides N A 1980 Virus infection of endothelial cells increases granulocyte adherance. Journal of Clinical Investigation 65: 1469–1477
MacKenzie R A, Forbes G S, Karnes W E 1981 Angiographic findings in herpes zoster arteritis. Annals of Neurology 10: 458–464
Matre R 1977 Similarities of Fc receptors on trophoblasts and placental endothelial cells. Scandinavian Journal of Immunology 6: 935–958
Maxeiner S R, McDonald J R, Kirklin J W 1952 Muscle biopsy in the diagnosis of periarteritis nodosa. Surgical Clinics of North America 32: 1–25–1233
Meltzer M, Franklin E C 1966 Cryoglobulinaemia: a study of 29 patients. American Journal of Medicine 40: 828–836
Meriwether J H, Weinberger H J, Gleason I O 1967 The renal vascular lesion in rheumatoid disease. Arthritis and Rheumatism 10: 298 (Abstract)
Meyer G W, Lichenstein J 1982 Isolated polyarteritis nodosa affecting the caecum. Digestive Diseases Science 27: 467–469
Michalak T 1978 Immune complexes of hepatic B surface antigen in the pathogenesis of periarteritis nodosa. American Journal of Pathology 90: 619–628
Miescher P A, Paronetto F, Koffler D 1967 Immunofluorescent studies in human vasculitis. In: Grabar P, Miescher P A (eds) Immunopathology, 4th International Symposium. Schawabe, Basel
Miller G, Hoyt J C, Pollack B E 1954 Bilateral renal vein thrombosis and the nephrotic syndrome associated with lesions of polyarteritis nodosa. American Journal of Medicine 17: 856–860
Miller G W, Nussenzweig V 1975 A new complement function: Solubilisation of antigen-antibody aggregates. Proceedings of the National Academy of Science

U.S.A. 72: 418–422
Mills J A, McCroskery P A 1981 Periarteritis nodosa, hypersensitivity angiitis and related syndrome: clinical and pathological aspects. In: Bacon P A, Hadler N M (eds) The Kidney and Rheumatic Disease, Butterworth International Medical Reviews, Vol 1, Butterworth, London
Moore P M, Cupps T R 1983 Neurological complications of vasculitis. Annals of Neurology 14: 155–167
Moore P M, Fauci A S 1981 Neurologic manifestations of systemic vasculitis: a retrospective and prospective study of the clinicopathologic features and responses to therapy in 25 patients. The American Journal of Medicine 71: 517–524
Morgan G J, Harris E D 1978 Non-giant cell temporal arteritis. Three cases and a review of the literature. Arthritis and Rheumatism 21: 362–366
Moutsopoulos H M, Avgerinos P C, Tsampoulas C G, Katsiotis P A 1983 Selective renal angiography in Wegeners granulomatosis. Annals of the Rheumatic Diseases 42: 192–195
Mullick F G, McAllister H A, Wagner B M, Fenoglio J J 1979 Drug related vasculitis. Clinicopathologic correlations in 30 patients. Human Pathology 10: 313–325
Nakeo K, Ikeda M, Kimata S, et al 1967 Takayasu's arteritis, clinical report of 84 cases and immunological studies of 7 cases. Circulation 35: 1141–1155
Neumann H A M, Berretty P J M, Reinders-Folmer S C C 1981 Hepatitis-B surface antigen deposition in the blood vessel walls of urticarial lesions in acute hepatitis-B. British Journal of Dermatology 104: 383–388
Nicholls A, Snaith M L, Maini R N, Scott J T 1973 Controlled trial of azathioprine in rheumatoid vasculitis. Annals of the Rheumatic Diseases 32: 589–591 (Abstract)
Niinaka T, Okochi T, Watanabe Y, Sakai S, Takahasi Y, Yamamura Y 1978 Lymphocyte functions in Wegener's granulomatosis. Journal of Medicine 9: 491–501
Notkins A L 1971 Infectious virus–antibody complexes interaction with anti-immunoglobulins, complement and rheumatoid factor. Journal of Experimental Medicine 134: 41S–51S
Nowoslawski A, Krawczynski K, Brozosko W J, Madalinski K 1972 Tissue localisation of Australia antigen immune complexes in acute and chronic hepatitis and liver cirrhosis. American Journal of Pathology 68: 31–48
Onion D H, Crumpacker C S, Gilliband B C 1971 Arthritis of hepatitis associated with Australia antigen. Annals of Internal Medicine 75: 29–33
Ophuls W 1923 Periarteritis acuta nodosa. Archives of Internal Medicine 32: 870–898
Paci R, Guiffrida C M, Marangolo M, Ventura F, Di Paola F 1983 Neuroradiologic picture of cerebral vasculitis in rhematoid arthritis. Neuroradiology 25: 343–345
Pallis C A, Scott J T 1965 Peripheral neuropathy in rheumatoid arthritis. British Medical Journal 1: 1141–1147
Papaioannou C C, Gupta R C, Hunder G G, McDuffie F C 1980 Circulating immune complexes in giant-cell arteritis and polymyalgia rheumatica. Arthritis and Rheumatism 23: 1021–1025
Parish W E 1971 Studies on vasculitis. 1. Immunoglobulins, BIC, C-reactive protein, and bacterial antigens in cutaneous vasculitis lesions. Clinical Allergy 1: 97–109
Park J R, Jones J G, Harkiss D G, Hazleman B L 1981 Circulating immune complexes in polymyalgia rheumatica and giant-cell arteritis. Annals of the Rheumatic Diseases 40: 360–365
Phanuphak P, Kohler P F 1980 Onset of polyarteritis nodosa during allergic hyposensitization treatment. American Journal of Medicine 68: 479–485
Phinney P R, Fligiel S, Bryson Y J, Porter D D 1982 Necrotizing vasculitis in a case of disseminated neonatal herpes simplex infection. Archives of Pathology and Laboratory Medicine 106: 64–67
Pickering T G, Lockshin M D, Eisenmenger W J 1981 Renin-dependent hypertension in polyarteritis nodosa. British Medical Journal 282: 1758
Pinching A J, Rees A J, Pussell B A, Lockwood C M, Mitchison R S, Peters D K 1980 Relapses in Wegener's granulomatosis: the role of infection. British Medical Journal 281: 836–838
Pritchard M H, Gow J 1976 Wegener's granulomatosis presenting as rheumatoid arthritis (2 cases). Proceedings of the Royal Society of Medicine 69: 501–504
Quismorio F P, Beaardmore T, Kaufman R L, Mongan E S 1983 IgG Rheumatoid factors and anti-nuclear antibodies in rheumatoid vasculitis. Clinical and Experimental Immunology 52: 330–340
Ramos M, Mandybur T I 1975 Cerebral vasculitis in rheumatoid arthritis. Archives of Neurology 32: 271–275
Rapoport R J, Kozin F, Mackel S E, Jordon R E 1980 Cutaneous vascular immunofluorescence in rheumatoid arthritis. Correlation with circulating immune complexes and vasculitis. American Journal of Medicine 68: 325–3331
Rasker J J, Kuipers F C 1983 Are Rheumatoid nodules caused by vasculitis? A study of 13 early cases. Annals of the Rheumatic Diseases 42: 384–388
Reza M J, Roth B E, Pops M A, Goldberg L S 1974 Intestinal vasculitis in essential mixed cryoglobulinaemia. Annals of Internal Medicine 81: 632–634
Ristow S C, Griner P F, Abraham G N, Shoulson I 1976 Reversal of systemic manifestations of cryoglobulinaemia. Archives of Internal Medicine 136: 467–470
Roberts-Thomson P J, Wernick W, Ziff M 1981 Low molecular weight IgM in rheumatoid arthritis and other rheumatic diseases. Arthritis and Rheumatism 24: 795–802
Rokitansky K 1852 Ueber einege der wichtigsten krankheiten der arterien. Deukschriften der kais. Akadamie der Wissenschaflen besondess Agbedrucket 4: 49
Ronco P, Verroust P, Mignon F, Kourilsky O, Vanhille P, Meyrier A, Mery J P, Morel-Maroger L 1983 Immunopathological studies of polyarteritis nodosa and Wegeners Granulomatosis: a report of 43 patients with 51 renal biopsies. Quarterly Journal of Medicine 52: 141–149
Rose G A, Spencer H 1957 Polyarteritis nodosa. Quarterly Journal of Medicine 26: 43–81
Sack M, Cassidy J T, Bole G G 1975 Prognostic factors in polyarteritis. Journal of Rheumatology 2: 411–420
Sacks T, Moldow C F, Craddock P R, Bowers T K, Jacob H S 1978 Oxygen radicals mediate endothelial cell damage by complement stimulated granulocytes. Journal of Clinical Investigation 62: 1161–1167
Sams W M, Cloman H N, Kohler P F, McIntosh R M, Small P, Mass M F 1975 Human necrotizing vasculitis, immunoglobulins and complement in vessel walls of cutaneous lesions and normal skin. Journal of Investigative Dermatology 64: 441–445
Schmid F R, Cooper N S, Ziff M, McEwan C 1961 Arteritis in rheumatoid arthritis. American Journal of Medicine 30: 56–83

Scott D G I 1981 Systemic vasculitis in Bath–Bristol area: clinical, pathological and therapeutic studies. MD thesis, Bristol
Scott D G I, Bacon P A 1984 Intravenous cyclophosphamide and methylprednisolone in treatment of systemic rheumatoid vasculitis. American Journal of Medicine 76: 377–384
Scott D G I, Bacon P A, Allen C, Elson C J, Wallington T 1981a IgG rheumatoid factor, complement and immune complexes in rheumatoid synovitis and vasculitis: comparative and serial studies during cytotoxic therapy. Clinical and Experimental Immunology 43: 54–63
Scott D G I, Bacon P A, Bothamley J, Allen C, Elson C J, Wallington T 1981b Plasma exchange in rheumatoid vasculitis. Journal of Rheumatology 8: 433–439
Scott D G I, Bacon P A, Tribe C R 1981c Systemic rheumatoid vasculitis: a clinical and laboratory study of 50 cases. Medicine (Baltimore) 60: 288–297
Scott D G I, Bacon P A, Elliott P J, Tribe C R, Wallington T 1982a Systemic vasculitis in a district general hospital 1972–1980: clinical and laboratory features, classification and prognosis of 80 cases. Quarterly Journal of Medicine 203: 292–311
Scott D G I, Bacon P A, Elson C J, Wallington T 1982b Polyarteritis nodosa and systemic rheumatoid vasculitis have a different immunological mechanism. Arthritis and Rheumatism 25(Suppl 4): S15(Abstract)
Scott D G I, Blake D R, Blann A, Salmon M, Brailsford S, Winyard P, Bacon P A 1984 The role of lymphocytes and serum factors in vasculitic diseases. Annals of the Rheumatic Diseases 43: 116 (abstract)
Scott J T 1976 Clinical aspects of neuropathy in rheumatoid arthritis. In: Feltkamp T E W (Ed) Non-articular forms of rheumatoid arthritis. Proceedings of IVth ISRA symposium. Stafleu, Leyden, P. 46–54
Scott J, Finch L D 1972 Wegener's granulomatosis presenting as gingivitis. Review of the clinical and pathological features and report of a case. Oral Surgery 34: 920–933
Scott J T, Hourihane D O, Doyle F H, Steiner R E, Laws J W, Dixon A St J et al 1961 Digital arteritis in rheumatoid disease. Annals of the Rheumatic Diseases 20: 224–233
Sergent J S, 1980 Vasculitis associated with viral infection. Clinics in Rheumatic diseases 6: 339–350.
Sergent J S, Christian C L 1974 Necrotizing vasculitis after acute serous otitis media. Annals of Internal Medicine 81, 195–199
Sergent J S, Lockshin M D, Christian C L, Gocke D J 1976 Vasculitis with hepatitis B antigenaemia. Medicine (Baltimore) 55: 1–17
Serre H, Simon L, Lamboley C 1970 Les manifestations articulaires de la maladies de Takayasu. Seminars hopital de Paris 46: 1587–1602
Shasby D M, Schwarz M I, Forstot J Z, Theofilopoulos N, Kassan S S 1982 Pulmonary immune complex deposition in Wegener's granulomatosis. Chest 81: 338–340
Shenberger K N, Meharg J G, Lane C D 1981 Temporal arteritis presenting as ataxia and dementia. Postgraduate Medical Journal 69: 246–249
Shepherd H A, Patel C, Bamforth J, Isaacson P 1983 Upper gastrointestinal endoscopy in systemic vasculitis presenting as an acute abdomen. Endoscopy 15: 307–311
Smith C A, Fidler W J, Pinals R S 1983 The epidemiology of giant cell arteritis. Report of a ten year study in Shelby County, Tennessee. Arthritis and Rheumatism 26: 1214–1219
Smukler N M, Schumacher R 1977 Chronic non destructive arthritis associated with cutaneous polyarteritis. Arthritis and Rheumatism 20: 1114–1120
Sokoloff L, Wilens S L, Bunim J J 1951 Arteritis of striated muscle in rheumatoid arthritis. American Journal of Pathology 27: 157–173
Solley G O, Winkelmann R K, Robelstad R A 1975 Correlation between regional enterocolitis and cutaneous polyarteritis nodosa. 2 case reports and review of the literature. Gastroenterology 69: 235–239
Somers G, Poluliece P 1978 Relapsing polychondritis: relationship to periarteritis nodosa. British Medical Journal 2: 603–604
Soter N A, Austen K F, Gigli I 1974 The complement system in necrotizing angiitis of the skin. Analysis of complement component activities in serum of patients with concomitant collagen-vascular disease. Journal of Investigative Dermatology 63: 219–226
Soter N A, Mihm M C, Gigli I, Dvorak H F, Austen K F 1976 Two distinct cellular patterns in cutaneous necrotizing angiitis. Journal of Investigative Dermatology 66: 344–350
Stolman L P, Rosenthal D, Yaworsky R, Horan F 1975 Pyoderma gangrenosum and rheumatoid arthritis. Archives of Dermatology 111: 1020–1023
Strachan R W, 1964 The natural history of Takayasu's arteriopathy. Quarterly Journal of Medicine 33: 57–69
Straer J D, Beaufils P, Morel-Maroger L, Richett G 1973 Vascular nephropathies with acute renal failure. In: Kincaid-Smith P, Mathew T H, Becker E L (eds) Glomerulonephritis, morphology, natural history and treatment, Vol 1. Wiley, New York, p. 1035–1046
Sussman M, Jones J H, Almeida J D, Lachmann P 1973 Deficiency of the second component of complement associated with anaphylactoid purpura and presence of mycoplasma in serum. Clinical and Experimental Immunology 14: 531–539
Takayasu M 1908 Case with unusual changes of the central vessels in the retina. Societatis Ophthalmologicae Japonicae 12: 554
Tanaka H, Mihara K, Ookura H, et al 1979 Echocardiographic findings in patients with aortitis syndrome. Angiology 30: 620–633
Travers R L, Allison D J, Brettle R P, Hughes G R V 1979 Polyarteritis nodosa: a clinical and angiographic analysis of 17 cases. Seminars in Arthritis and Rheumatism 8: 184–199
Trepo C G, Zukerman A J, Bird R C 1974 The role of circulating hepatitis B antigen-antibody immune complexes in the pathogenesis of vascular and hepatic manifestations of polyarteritis nodosa. Journal of Clinical Pathology 27: 863–868
Tribe C R, Scott D G I, Bacon P A 1981 The place of rectal biopsy in the diagnosis of systemic vasculitis. Journal of Clinical Pathology 34: 843–850
Venables P J W, Erhardt C C, Maini R N 1980 Antibodies to extractable nuclear antigens in rheumatoid arthritis: relationship to vasculitis and circulating immune complexes. Clinical and Experimental Immunology 39: 146–153
Vermess M, Haynes B F, Fauci A S, Wolff S M 1978 Computer assisted tomography of orbital lesions in Wegener's granulomatosis. Journal of Computer Assisted

Tomography 2: 45–48
Verztman L 1980 Polyarteritis nodosa. Clinics in Rheumatic Diseases 6: 297–318
Verztman L, Depaola D, Rubinstein J, Lederman R 1972 Angiitis necrosantes In: Verztman L, Depaolo D (Eds) Doencas difusas to tecido conjuntivo. Gernasa, Brazil
Volkman D J, Mann E L, Fauci A S 1982 Association between Takayasu's arteritis and a B-cell alloantigen in North Americans. New England Journal of Medicine 306: 464–465
Voyles W F, Searles R P, Bankhurst A D 1980 Myocardial infarction caused by rheumatoid vasculitis. Arthritis and Rheumatism 23: 860–863
Walker W C, Wright V 1968 Pulmonary lesions and rheumatoid arthritis. Medicine (Baltimore) 47: 501–520
Walton E W 1958 Giant cell granuloma of the respiratory tract (Wegener's granulomatosis). British Medical Journal 2: 265–270
Watson P, Fekete J, Deck J 1977 Central nervous systemic vasculitis in rheumatoid arthritis. Canadian Journal of Neurological Science 4: 269–272
Webb J, Payne W H 1970 Abdominal apoplexy in rheumatoid arthritis. Australian Annals of Medicine 2: 168–170
Wees S J, Sunwoo I N, Ooh S J 1981 Sural nerve biopsy in systemic necrotizing vasculitis. American Journal of Medicine 71: 525–532
Wegener F 1936 Uber generalisierte, septische gefasserkrankungen. Verhandlungen der Deutschen Gesellschaft fur Pathologie 29: 202–209
Weisman M H, Zvaifler N J 1975 Cryoimmunoglobulinaemia in rheumatoid arthritis. Journal of Clinical Investigation 56: 725–739
Weiss S J, Young J, LoBuglio, Slivka A, Nimeh N F 1981 Role of hydrogen peroxide in neutrophil-mediated destruction of cultured endothelial cells. Journal of Clinical Investigation 68: 714–721
White R H, Schambelan M 1980 Hypertension, hyperreninemia, and secondary hyperaldosteronism in systemic necrotizing vasculitis. Annals of Internal Medicine 92: 199
Wilkinson M, Torrance W N 1967 Clinical background of rheumatoid vascular disease. Annals of the Rheumatic Diseases 26: 475–479
Williams B D, Pussell B A, Lockwood C M, Cotton C 1979 Defective reticuloendothelial system function in rheumatoid arthritis. Lancet 1: 1311–1314
Winkelmann R K, Ditto W B 1964 Cutaneous and visceral syndrome of necrotizing or "allergic" angiitis: a study of 38 cases. Medicine (Baltimore) 43: 59–89
Winkelmann R K, Beuchner S A, Powell F C, Banks P M 1983 The T lymphocyte and cutaneous Churg–Strauss granuloma. Acta Dermatologica Venereol (Stockholm) 63: 199–204
Wolff S M, Fauci A S, Horn R G, Dale D C 1974 Wegener's granulomatosis. Annals of Internal Medicine 81: 513–525
Wood M K, Read D R, Kraft A R, Barreta T M 1979 A rare cause of ischemic colitis: polyarteritis nodosa. Diseases of the Colon and Rectum 22:428
Zeek P M 1952 Periarteritis nodosa: A critical review. American Journal of Clinical Pathology 22: 777–790
Zeiss C R, Burch F X, Marder R J, Furey N L, Schmid F R, Gewurz H 1980 A hypocomplementaemic vasculitis urticarial syndrome. Report of four new cases and definition of the disease. American Journal of Medicine 68: 867–875
Zizac T M, Classen J N, Stevens M B 1983 Acute abdominal complications of systemic lupus erythematosus and polyarteritis nodosa. American Journal of Medicine 73: 525–531
Zizac T M, Shulman L E, Stevens M B 1975 Colonic perforations in systemic lupus eruthematosus. Medicine (Baltimore) 54: 411–426

Systemic lupus erythematosus

Although environmental and hormonal factors play a clear part in the pathogenesis of systemic lupus erythematosus (SLE), it is now apparent that there is an important genetic component to the disease. In a recent study (Fielder et al, 1983) some 80% of SLE patients were found to have a null allele at the C4 locus on the 6th chromosome. SLE has, in recent years, emerged from being a rare disease to one which is now commonly seen on general medical and rheumatology wards. It is characterised by widespread organ involvement, a variety of clinical manifestations, and a tendency to exacerbation and remission. There are marked immunological abnormalities, notably the presence in the serum of a wide variety of anti-nuclear antibodies. One group of antibodies, those directed against DNA, are the most constant feature, and thus the diagnostic hallmark of this disease.

HISTORICAL

The term 'lupus' was, for several centuries applied to a variety of facial skin lesions, though by the 19th century it had become apparent that a distinct form existed in young women. In 1872, Hebra & Kaposi noted that 'constitutional' symptoms could be associated. However, the credit for the fullest clinical delineation of the disease goes to William Osler, who in 1904 suggested a vascular basis for SLE and described a 'disease of unknown aetiology, with polymorphic skin lesions — hyperaemia, oedema and haemorrhage — arthritis occasionally, and a variable number of visceral manifestations, of which the most important are gastrointestinal crises, endocarditis, pericarditis, acute nephritis and haemorrhage from the mucous surfaces. Recurrence is a special feature of the disease and attacks may come on month after month or even throughout a long period of years' (Osler, 1904). Over the following half-century pathological descriptions were added, but the next major advance came with the discovery of the LE cell phenomenon by Hargraves et al (1948) and the identification of the LE cell factor as an antinuclear antibody (Miescher et al, 1953).

This led rapidly to the discovery of other antinuclear antibodies, notably, in 1957, to the discovery of antibodies against native DNA (Robbins et al, 1957; Seligmann 1957; Miescher & Strassle 1957; Cepellini et al, 1957) and to the introduction of the clinically useful DNA-binding test (Pincus et al, 1969; Cohen et al, 1971; Hughes, 1971). These discoveries had two clinical consequences — firstly a marked increase in the prevalence of the disease, largely due to the recognition of milder and atypical forms of SLE, and secondly, for the same reason, a steady improvement in the overall prognosis of the disease.

EPIDEMIOLOGY

SLE is rare in males. Most series agree on a female : male ratio of 9 : 1 (Estes & Christian, 1971). The disease is commonest during the child-bearing years; new cases are rare over the age of 40.

The prevalence of SLE appears to be increasing worldwide — in parts of south-east Asia it may exceed that of rheumatoid arthritis. SLE may be more prevalent in Negro populations. Over a 10-year period (1956–1965) the age-adjusted mortality prevalence rates were 3 times greater for black females than white females in New York City, and 4.3 times greater in Jefferson County, Alabama

(Siegel & Lee, 1973). While epidemiological studies have been limited, the disease appears to be less common in the UK than, for example, the USA and the West Indies. The highest reported incidence and prevalence is in black females. In New York, a prevalence figure in black females of 1 in 1000 was noted (Siegel & Lee, 1973). A study in San Francisco (Fessel, 1974) noted that in black women aged 15–64 the prevalence was 1 in 245 — a figure far higher than, for example, pernicious anaemia, and comparable with figures recorded in a West Indian female population (Wilson & Hughes, 1976). Family studies have revealed an increased incidence of SLE, other connective tissue diseases, and serological abnormalities in relatives of SLE patients (Leonhardt, 1964). A few well-documented reports of SLE in monozygotic twins exist, though discordant twin studies have also been reported. HLA and complement allotype studies in SLE families will be discussed later.

PATHOLOGY

The most striking histological feature is the so-called 'fibrinoid necrosis' which affects especially the small arteries, arterioles and capillaries. Fibrinoid, which contains large amounts of gamma-globulin and fibrin, together with complement, is also seen in interstitial collagen and membranes such as pleura and joint capsules. The other feature highly suggestive of SLE is the haematoxylin body, resulting from the in vivo effect of antinuclear factor on damaged tissue cells, leading to pyknosis of nuclei, with resultant phagocytosis.

With the possible exception of the 'onion-skin' thickening of the arterioles of the spleen (see below) no pathological feature is pathognomonic for SLE. For this reason, the pathological changes in each organ will be discussed with the clinical findings.

CLINICAL FEATURES

General

Table 53.1 gives the incidence of major clinical manifestations in 150 SLE patients studied at Columbia Presbyterian Medical Center, New York (Estes & Christian, 1971).

Table 53.1 Major clinical manifestations of SLE in 150 patients. (After Estes & Christian, 1971).

Manifestation	% incidence
Musculoarticular	95
Cutaneous	81
Fever	77
Neuropsychiatric	59
Renal	53
Pulmonary	48
Cardiac	38

General malaise is usual in active SLE and may be the result of a number of contributing factors, including anaemia, fever, arthralgia and myalgia. There may be marked depression or other psychological problems (to be discussed more fully in the section on CNS lupus). A frequent clinical feature in SLE patients is allergy to drugs or chemicals, and SLE patients may give a history of drug allergies long before their SLE becomes apparent. Fever may also be the presenting manifestation of SLE. The fever is most commonly low grade, but can, in some patients, be dramatic. There is no characteristic fever pattern, but patients can sustain temperatures of over 40°C (104°F) for days without swings to normality. In one patient with CNS lupus seen by the author, the temperature swung between 35°C(95°F) and 40°C(104°F), possibly due to hypothalamic involvement. The presence of fever is an important clinical finding in the differential diagnosis of a patient with polyarthritis, and should always lead to a suspicion of SLE as a possible diagnosis.

Anorexia and insidious weight loss occur in up to two-thirds of SLE patients (Harvey et al, 1954), though these are usually features of active disease.

Skin

Table 53.2, from a review by Gilliam & Sontheimer (1982), lists the main clinical spectrum of skin manifestation of SLE.

Almost every type of skin and mucous membrane lesion has been described in SLE. The 'classical' butterfly eruption (Fig. 53.1) is now seen in less than half of SLE patients — again due to the recognition of the wider spectrum of the disease. More common is transient facial erythema. Erythematous rashes may occur on the forehead, neck, eyelids, and, in general, in areas exposed to light. Ultraviolet light sensitivity is a prominent feature in up to 40% of patients, ex-

Table 53.2 Cutaneous manifestations of SLE in 520 patients (From Dubois E L 1974 *Lupus erythematosus*, by kind permission of the author.)

	Number of patients	%
Butterfly rash	191	36.7
Photosensitivity	170	32.7
Chronic discoid lesions	149	28.6
Alopecia, non-scarring	111	21.3
Butterfly eruption	109	20.9
Petechiae, purpura, ecchymoses	103	19.8
Maculopapular lesions, non-specific	99	19.0
Raynaud's phenomenon	96	18.4
Conjunctivitis	52	10.0
Maculopapular lesions, sun-exposed areas	47	9.1
Mucous membrane lesions	47	9.1
Diffuse hyperpigmentation	44	8.4
Urticaria	46	6.9
Erythema, articular	34	6.5
Fractured frontal hair	29	5.6
Leg ulcer	29	5.6
Subcutaneous nodules	26	5.0
Periorbital oedema	25	4.8
Thrombophlebitis	24	4.6
Facial oedema	24	4.6
Jaundice	20	3.8
Alopecia, scarring	19	3.6
Pruritis, marked	15	2.8
Gangrene, digital	7	1.3
Palatal erythema	7	1.3
Periungal erythema	6	1.1
Bullae	2	0.4

posure to sunlight resulting in a flare not only of the skin rash, but also of systemic features. Other prominent manifestations include urticaria, palmar and plantar rashes, digital and elbow vasculitis and subungual erythema. An important clinical feature is livedo reticularis which may be the only clinical manifestation of vasculitis, and vasculitic leg ulcers occur in a few cases. Mouth ulcers of a variety of types are frequent, and were included as one of the original criteria for classification of the disease by the American Rheumatism Association (p. 1342).

Discoid lesions occur in up to 20% of patients with classical SLE (Grigor et al, 1978). An interesting subgroup of patients is characterised by widespread, reversible skin lesions, superficially resembling discoid LE, but not scarring. This syndrome, called 'subacute cutaneous lupus erythematosus' (SCLE) has been found to frequently have anti-Ro antibodies, and preliminary studies have suggested that there is a preponderance of HLA-DR3 (Sontheimer et al, 1981) — though this has yet to be confirmed.

Alopecia is one of the most important manifestations of SLE. In a series of SLE patients studied at the Hammersmith Hospital, alopecia occurred in 64% (Davis et al, 1973). The hair loss is patchy and is often associated with new hair growth on the forehead. Occasionally, total alopecia may occur. The aetiology is obscure but it serves both as a barometer of disease activity in some patients, and an important factor in the differential diagnosis from other connective tissue disorders.

Skin biopsy is of value in the investigation of SLE. Immunofluorescent studies reveal the presence of deposits of gammaglobulin and complement (usually in the dermal–epidermal junction) in up to 90% of SLE cases. These findings are

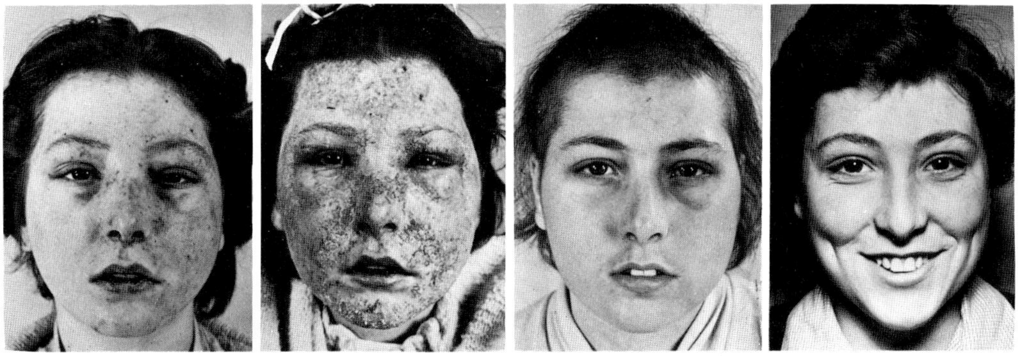

Fig. 53.1 Severe facial rash in SLE, showing serial improvement during 3 months of steroid therapy. (Reproduced by kind permission of Professor E.G.L. Bywaters, Hammersmith Hospital, and the publishers of Gazewood & Lightwood (eds) *Pediatrics for the practitioner* (1953).)

noted in clinically unaffected skin in up to 50% of SLE patients, and in virtually 100% of discoid lesions (Kay & Tuffanelli, 1969). The number of non-SLE skin biopsies with similar deposits is low, though they are very occasionally found in other connective tissue diseases. The gamma-globulin and complement may be deposited as immune complexes (see Ch. 13). In one study the antibody was shown to be complexed with DNA (Tan & Kunkel, 1966). Electron microscopy of SLE skin biopsies has revealed virus-like or cytoplasmic tubular aggregates (CTA) similar to those seen in the kidneys and other organs of SLE patients.

Rheumatoid-like nodules occur in under 5% of SLE patients. Panniculitis is a rare but well-recognised feature of the disease and is occasionally precipitated by a sudden reduction in prednisolone dosage.

Musculoskeletal system

The major musculoskeletal problem in SLE is tendonitis, and not arthritis. Patients with mild to moderate disease activity frequently complain of difficulty in straightening the fingers. Occasionally, flexor tendonitis becomes more severe and, in some unfortunate patients, leads to severe deformities (resembling the 'Jaccoud' arthritis of rheumatic fever) (Fig. 53.2). Although arthritis may occur, erosive disease is rare, and even in those cases where erosions are reported, they are usually minute. Much more common is joint pain. Arthralgia occurs in over 90% of patients. In a few

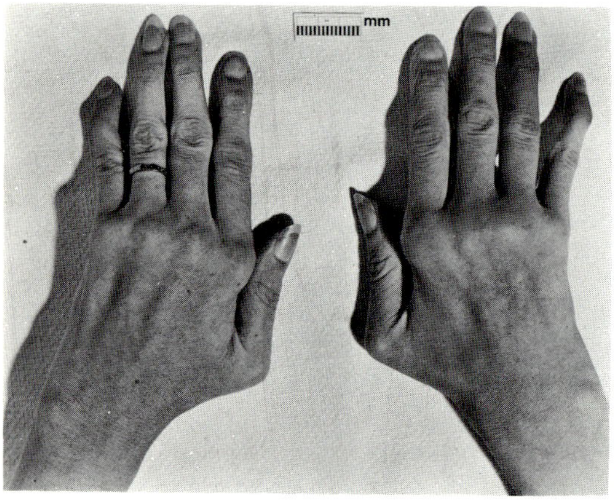

Fig. 53.2 Hands of late deforming ('Jaccoud-like') stage of SLE. (Professor E.G.L. Bywaters, Hammersmith Hospital.)

SLE patients, generalised body pain may be so intense that movement is difficult.

One of the continuing problems in the management of SLE patients in aseptic necrosis, most commonly affecting the hip, but occasionally involving multiple joints including those of the hands and feet (Lightfoot & Lotke, 1972). Although vasculitic ischaemia has occasionally been invoked on a pathogenic factor, in the great majority of patients the lesion is directly associated with excessive steroid usage.

As the use of corticosteroids in SLE becomes more conservative, it is possible that this complication may become less prevalent (Hughes, 1982).

An inflammatory myositis may occur, and should be suspected in patients with periorbital oedema. Myositis tends to be more prominent in mixed connective tissue disease and other 'overlap' syndromes (see Ch. 50).

Myasthenia is occasionally associated with SLE (Wolf & Barrows, 1966; Alarcon-Segovia et al, 1963) as are thymomas.

Cardiovascular system

The incidence of cardiac involvement in SLE depends on definition. Major, clinically significant, cardiac disease probably occurs in the minority of patients (e.g. 18% of the hospital SLE patients studied in our unit — Grigor et al, 1978). While older studies highlighted non-infective endocarditis of Libman and Sacks, more recently, two different cardiac problems — early coronary artery disease and congenital heart block — have come under scrutiny.

Pericarditis remains the commonest problem, with substernal pain on deep breathing. It is almost invariably associated with pleurisy (Estes & Christian, 1971). Echocardiography reveals abnormalities in up to two-thirds of hospital SLE patients routinely studied (Davis et al, 1973) though significant constriction is unusual, and tamponade distinctly rare.

Myocarditis is unusual. Bulkley & Roberts (1975) detected myocardial inflammation in only 8 of 36 autopsied cases of SLE. Statistically more important may be the effects of hypertension or chronic steroid therapy.

Although murmurs are found in up to 70% of SLE patients (Shearn, 1959) these do not signify

Libman–Sacks endocarditis (a diagnosis rarely made and usually only at autopsy) (Fig. 53.3). Aortic and mitral valve insufficiency are rare complications (Shulman & Christian, 1969; Paget et al, 1975).

More recently, significant coronary artery disease has been reported in long-standing SLE. Haider & Roberts (1981) in an autopsy study found that one half of the patients had 76–100% narrowing of at least one major coronary artery. It has been suggested that with the increased survival in SLE, and long-term steroid usage, late myocardial infarction may become an important complication in SLE, though this is as yet unproven.

Pulmonary hypertension

Another relatively recent observation is the possibly frequent complication of pulmonary hypertension. During the past year in my unit, 12 SLE patients have had documented pulmonary hypertension. Whilst once it was thought that the hypertension was associated with Raynaud's phenomenon or 'spasm', this is clearly not the case.

An observation made by members of my unit is, I believe, of significance. Anti-phospholipid antibodies (see below) are now recognised to be important features in SLE, and are associated with thrombosis and abortion. In the study of anticardiolipin antibodies by Harris et al (1983), those with the highest titres included a number of patients with pulmonary hypertension. Furthermore, of 7 patients with SLE and pulmonary hypertension, 6 had the lupus anti-coagulant (Asherson et al, 1983), suggesting that intrapulmonary thrombotic episodes might be a contributing mechanism.

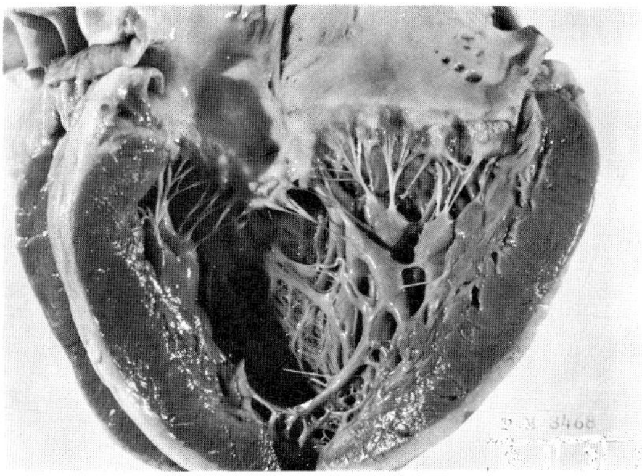

Fig. 53.3 Libman-Sacks endocarditis. Small non-infected vegetations on and below the line of closure of the mitral valve. (Dr Shirley Amin, University Hospital of the West Indies.)

Congenital heart block

Esscher & Scott (1979) estimated that one-third of children born with complete heart block will have mothers who have, or will develop, SLE or a similar connective tissue disease. The mechanism of this naturally transmitted disorder is unknown. Nor is it known whether other cardiac defects in the fetus are a factor in the high spontaneous abortion rate in SLE. Though the condition of the offspring is relatively benign, the extent of the problem of not yet known. We have recently seen SLE and congenital heart block in two successive generations of one family.

Blood vessels

The vasculitis of SLE predominantly affects small arteries, arterioles and capillaries and major organ or limb infarction is rare — a differentiation from polyarteritis nodosa.

The commonest clinical sites of vasculitis are in the skin, where digital and elbow lesions and livedo reticularis predominate. Raynaud's phenomenon occurs in between 5 and 26% of SLE patients; unlike systemic sclerosis this is rarely a prominent feature of the disease. Subgroups of patients with Raynaud's phenomenon and features of SLE, systemic sclerosis and dermatomyositis are described in more detail in Chapter 50. Gangrene of the extremities is a rare complication (Dubois & Arterberry, 1962). Vasculitis of systemic vessels leads, on rare occasions, to a variety of intra-abdominal lesions, but most commonly presents as intermittent abdominal pain. Rarely, cardiac, hepatic and renal infarction may be due to vasculitis. Cerebral vasculitis is discussed on page 1333.

Thrombophlebitis occurs in approximately 10% of SLE patients (Estes & Christian, 1971; Gladman & Urowitz, 1980) and may be a recurring problem in certain patients. Indeed, in some patients, widespread venous thrombosis (including renal and axillary vein thrombosis) is prominent. A small number with pulmonary hypertension in

SLE have, in our patients at the Hammersmith, had a clear past history of multiple venous thrombosis. Recent work has suggested that some of these patients may have a tendency to hypercoagulation (Byron & Hughes, 1982; Boey et al, 1983; Harris et al, 1983; Asherson et al, 1983).

Lungs and pleurisy

Pleurisy occurs in 50–60% of patients and may be the presenting manifestation of the disease. As distinct from rheumatoid arthritis, the pleural fluid sugar is usually normal (Carr et al, 1970). Recurrent pleurisy and adhesions may contribute over the years to a gradual elevation of the diaphragms and 'shrinking lungs'.

A variety of pulmonary manifestations occur including recurrent pneumonia, atelectasis or, more rarely, diffuse florid mottled pulmonary shadowing. In the series of Estes & Christian (1971) 14 of 150 patients had diffuse lung infiltrates and 9 had X-ray evidence of pulmonary fibrosis.

The radiological findings are very variable, pleural changes predominating (Bulgrin et al, 1960).

Pulmonary function tests show a combination of pulmonary restriction, vascular obstruction and airway obstruction (Gold & Jennings, 1966). The earliest sign of lung involvement is usually an impairment of diffusing capacity. In a study of our own SLE patients, 30 consecutive SLE patients underwent full lung function tests. In 24 (80%) the tests were abnormal, although only a minority complained of symptoms referable to the respiratory system. In a number of patients, abnormal diaphragmatic function was observed, possibly accounting for the raised diaphragms seen on chest X-ray in these patients (Gibson et al, 1977) (Fig. 53.4).

Other rarer pulmonary problems (reviewed by Turner-Stokes & Turner-Warwick 1982) include pneumonitis, pulmonary infarction, pulmonary haemorrhage, as well as the far more common secondary problems of infection and congestive failure.

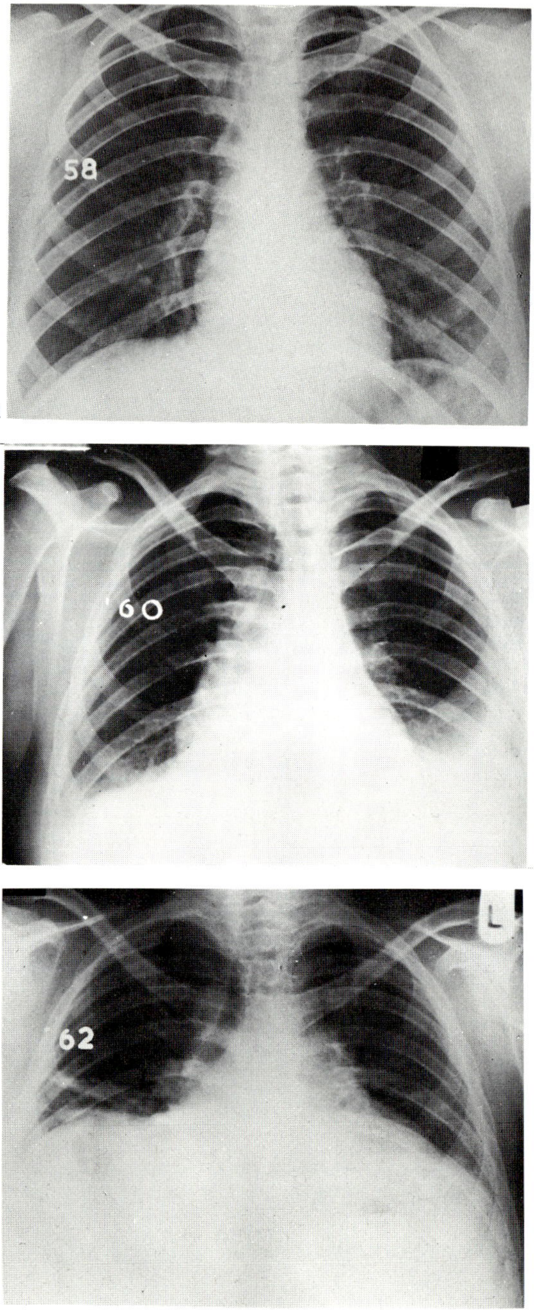

a b c

Fig. 53.4 Pleural adhesions and plate-like atelectases and 'shrinking lungs' in SLE. (Professor E.G.L. Bywaters, Hammersmith Hospital.)

Reticuloendothelial system

Mild to moderate lymphadenopathy occurs in 50% of SLE patients during disease exacerbations. Biopsy of nodes shows non-specific lymphadenitis. Splenomegaly occurs in fewer patients (approximately 15–20%) (Harvey et al, 1954). The histological changes are non-specific, with the exception of fibrinoid necrosis and a characteristic concentric periarterial fibrosis of the smaller arteries in the Malpighian corpuscles of the spleen — the so-called 'onion-skin lesions' (Fig. 53.5). The thymus is small or of normal size (Hare & MacKay, 1969) though thymomas have been reported in SLE patients (Larsson, 1963).

Studies of RES clearance have sent support to the concept that certain patients with SLE may have impaired splenic function (Lovy et al, 1980). It is conceivable, though not proved, that this may turn contribute to the impaired clearance of circulating immune complexes, and possibly to renal disease (Elkon et al, 1980). Another potential sequel of impaired splenic function is infection. Of 4 cases of salmonellosis in SLE reported by Lovy et al (1981), 2 showed clinical evidence of hyposplenism.

Gastrointestinal system

Sjögren's syndrome frequently co-exists with SLE (Bloch et al, 1965). Acute abdominal pain is an occasional feature and may be a presenting symptom of the disease. A variety of mechanisms may cause the pain — peritonism (usually associated with serositis elsewhere), intestinal arteritis, pancreatitis and perforation, particularly in patients on corticosteroid therapy, are the commonest. Diarrhoea is rarely a prominent feature of the disease, although it does occur. Major liver involvement is strikingly rare apart from occasional perihepatitis. Chronic active hepatitis with LE cells — so-called 'lupoid hepatitis' — is unrelated to SLE (Hughes, 1973).

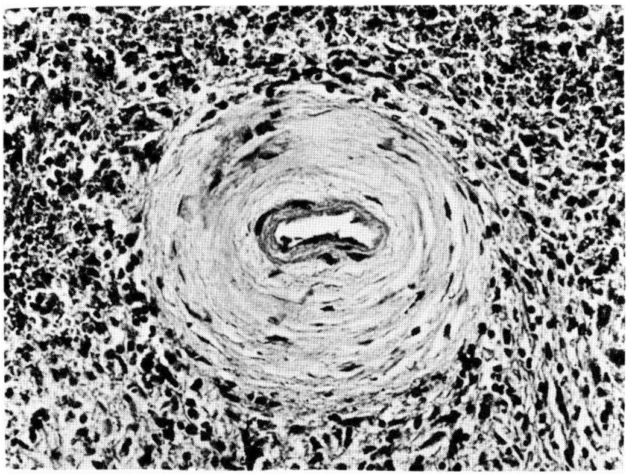

Fig. 53.5 Spleen. Periarterial fibrosis leading to the almost pathognomonic 'onion-skin' thickening.

Kidney

The incidence of clinical renal involvement in SLE is around 50% (Estes & Christian, 1971). Electron-microscopy studies suggest that the majority of SLE patients have subclinical involvement, though most renal lesions are transient and reversible.

The changing patterns of diagnosis of SLE and the recognition of milder disease, suggests that any textbook figures on the incidence of renal involvement in SLE should be treated with circumspection.

It seems likely that transient renal depositon of complexes occurs in *all* patients at some time during their disease (Hughes, 1971). In large clinical series (Estes & Christian, 1971; Grigor et al, 1978) the incidence of significant renal involvement (proteinuria, etc.) is around 50%. The subject has been reviewed extensively by Adu & Cameron (1982).

No histological lesion is pathognomonic for SLE. The changes include thickening of the glomerular basement membrane, proliferative glomerulitis, and fibrinoid change (Fig. 53.6). One 'classical' appearance, the 'wire-loop' thickening of the glomerular basement membrane, again is suggestive but not pathognomonic of SLE.

Traditionally, three major types of renal involvement are described on light microscopy. Table 53.3 shows the comparative incidences of these types of renal lesions taken from three large studies.

Focal nephritis carries the best prognosis and is usually reversible. The diffuse proliferative lesion carries the worst prognosis and is the most resistant to therapy. Membranous nephritis may present with nephrotic syndrome and carries a reasonably good prognosis (Baldwin et al, 1970). These categories are not hard and fast and patients with, for example, focal nephritis may progress into diffuse proliferative disease (Baldwin & Gallo, 1975).

Immunofluorescence is an important tool in the examination of SLE renal biopsies and has contributed significantly to an understanding of the immune complex mechanisms in SLE (Agnello et al, 1973). Marked variations in the deposition of gamma-globulin and complement can occur (Fig. 53.7). At least four patterns of immunofluorescent staining are described (Koffler et al, 1969): linear, mesangial, granular and 'lumpy'. In all but the rare linear pattern, complement and im-

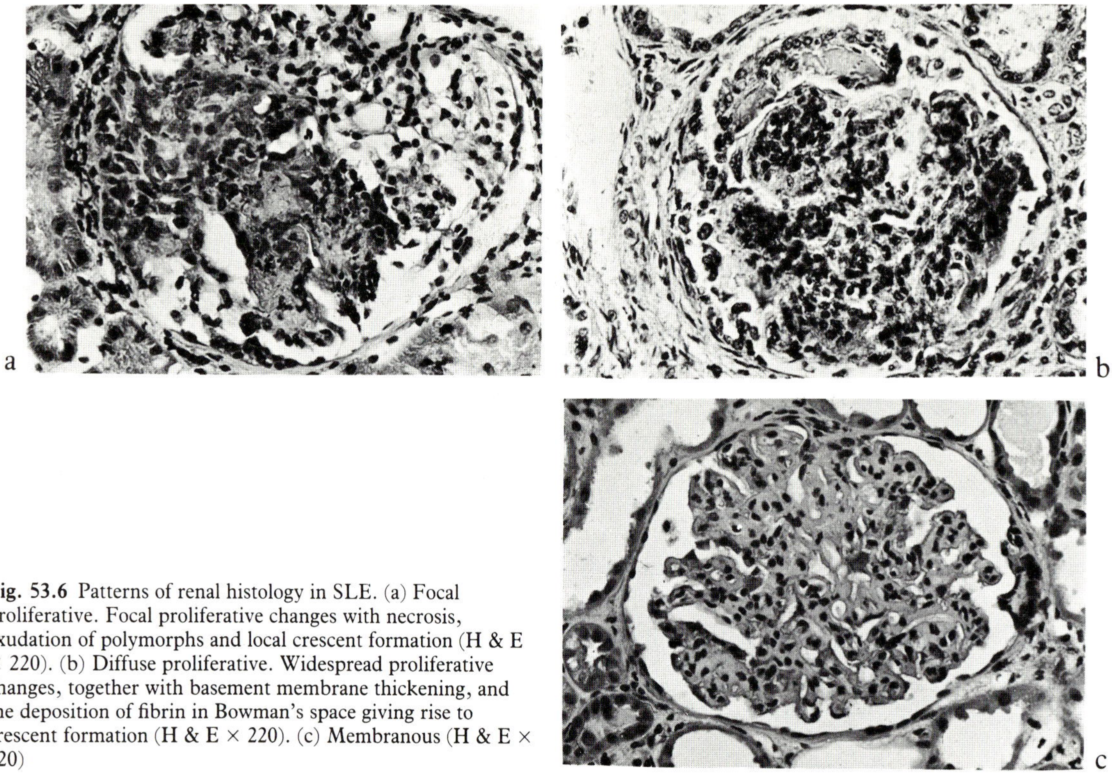

Fig. 53.6 Patterns of renal histology in SLE. (a) Focal proliferative. Focal proliferative changes with necrosis, exudation of polymorphs and local crescent formation (H & E × 220). (b) Diffuse proliferative. Widespread proliferative changes, together with basement membrane thickening, and the deposition of fibrin in Bowman's space giving rise to crescent formation (H & E × 220). (c) Membranous (H & E × 220)

Table 53.3 Classification of SLE nephritis (%)

Source	Focal	Diffuse proliferative	Membranous
Pollak et al (1964)	30	61	9
Baldwin et al (1970)	27	46	27
Estes & Christian (1971)	64	13	13
Adu & Cameron (1982)	23	64	15

munoglobulin are observed in similar distribution, suggesting their deposition together as immune complexes. Glomerular deposits of properdin have also been demonstrated (Rothfield et al, 1972). Granular deposits are associated with active glomerulonephritis, while 'lumpy' deposits occur with more advanced histological and clinical renal

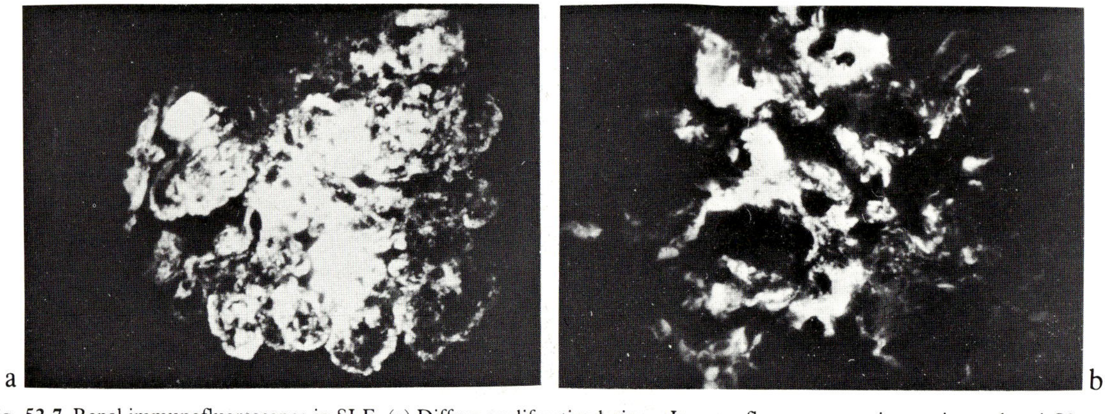

Fig. 53.7 Renal immunofluorescence in SLE. (a) Diffuse proliferative lesions. Immunofluorescence using conjugated anti-C3 antiserum (× 220). Glomerulus shows granular and lumpy deposits along the basement membrane and in the mesangium. A thrombus is seen in one capillary lumen (bottom right). (b) Predominantly mesangial staining. (Dr Shirley Amin, University Hospital of the West Indies.)

disease. Mesangial deposits may be seen in kidneys without histological evidence of glomerular injury. The antigen involved has proved difficult to demonstrate but is known to consist predominantly of native DNA (Koffler et al, 1967).

Although heavy deposits of fibrin are unusual, a study by Kant et al (1981) revealed fibrin deposits or thrombi in a focal and segmental distribution in 34 of 103 biopsies. Intrarenal thrombi were especially associated with necrosis, endothelial hypercellularity and crescents.

Electron microscopy may reveal electron dense deposits, either mesangial or subendothelial, the latter being associated with a poorer prognosis (Grishman et al, 1973) (Fig. 53.8). Virus-like particles are seen in the majority of SLE renal biopsies (Hurd et al, 1971). These interwoven tubular structures were initially thought to be myxovirus in nature, but are currently felt to be due to alteration of the endoplasmic reticulum resulting from cell injury. While they do not occur in normal kidneys, they are not specific for SLE (Fig. 53.9).

Amyloid is remarkably rare in SLE, an observation of interest in view of the poor CRP and SAA acute phase response in SLE (Pepys et al, 1982).

A rare though possibly underdiagnosed feature of SLE is renal vein thrombosis (Appel et al, 1976). In two of our patients, renal vein thrombosis was associated with the presence of the 'lupus anticoagulant', a finding known to predispose to a thrombotic tendency (Asherson et al, 1984).

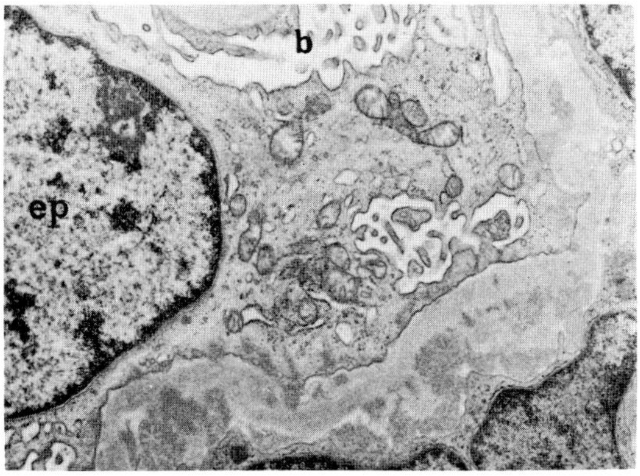

Fig. 53.8 Electron-microscopy of SLE glomerulus, showing dense deposits on subendothelial aspects of the basement membranes. ep = epithelial cell; b = Bowman's capsule. (Mrs J. Audrescht, University Hospital of the West Indies.)

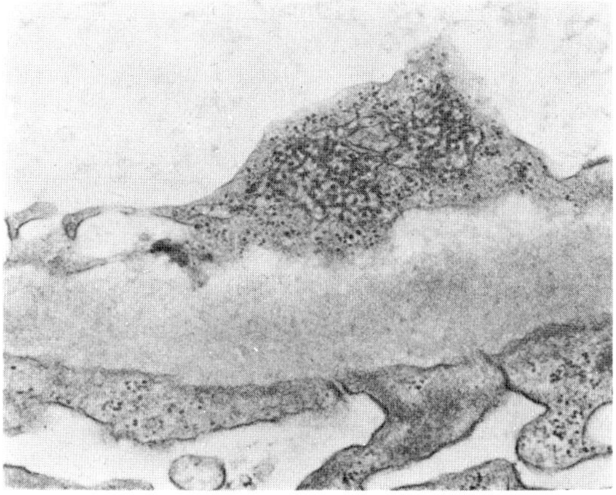

Fig. 53.9 Tubuloreticular structure on basement membrane. (Mrs J. Audrescht, University Hospital of the West Indies.)

The clinical manifestations of renal disease in SLE are those of any nephritis, the commonest, and usually reversible, feature being proteinuria.

Central nervous system disease

It is now recognised that CNS involvement is one of the major problems in SLE both in terms of management and prognosis (Hughes, 1980).

While Kaposi, 100 years ago, noted recurrent delirium in 2 out of 11 patients, CNS involvement has been underemphasised until recently. In the series of Estes & Christian (1971) neuropsychiatric involvement was noted in 59%.

The commonest clinical manifestation is that of a psychiatric illness, ranging from a mild affective disorder to florid psychosis. The spectrum of neurological involvement in CNS lupus is wide, and includes seizures, hemiplegia, cranial nerve lesions, cerebellar ataxia, chorea, aseptic meningitis and (less commonly) peripheral neuropathy (Bennett et al, 1972).

In one group of 6 patients a disease resembling multiple sclerosis was associated with findings suggestive of SLE. The commonest neurological finding was spastic paraplegia. The CSF in all patients showed a paretic Lange curve and the serum gave a biological false-positive test for syphilis (Fulford et al, 1972).

The CSF is normal in the majority of patients, though in those with arachnoiditis, the protein content is raised.

The pathogenesis of cerebral lupus is poorly understood. Cerebral vasculitis alone may not account for the clinical or pathological findings (Johnson & Richardson, 1968). Evidence has accumulated suggesting that CNS deposition of immune complexes may play a role in the pathogenesis. The CSF complement level is reduced in some, though by no means all, cases (Petz et al, 1971) and CSF DNA anti-DNA complexes have been demonstrated (Keefe et al, 1974). However the lack of evidence of vasculitis in many cases and the variety of neuropsychiatric manifestations suggest that to ascribe all the changes to one mechanism — immune complex deposition — is an oversimplistic view. For this reason, the observation that antilymphocyte antibodies may show cross-reactivity with brain tissue has pathogenetic implications, and Bluestein & Zvaifler (1976) have demonstrated a weak association between the presence of lymphocytotoxins and cerebral involvement in SLE.

Our own studies confirmed this finding and suggested that at least one population of anti-lymphocyte antibodies might show cross-reactivity with brain (Bresnihan et al, 1977, 1979).

A further cause of cerebral injury in SLE is cerebral thrombosis. A very strong association was observed between the presence of anti-cardiolipin antibodies and focal or widespread cerebral thrombosis in SLE (Harris et al, 1984).

Investigation of these patients is difficult. The EEG frequently shows diffuse abnormalities and may be useful in a patient with psychosis alone. Arteriography is almost always normal, brain scans are difficult to interpret in this condition and CSF findings, including (as has been mentioned) complement levels, are generally unhelpful.

Ocular lesions

The commoner ocular lesions are exudates ('cytoid bodies') and haemorrhages. Fortunately blindness is extremely rare. Rarely, perivascular sheathing and fibrosis may be seen in the fundus (Bishko, 1972; Spaeth, 1967). Fluorescein retinal angiography may occasionally show leakage of dye but has not been found to be a reliable investigation in our hands (Lanham et al, 1982).

Abnormal Schirmer's tests suggestive of Sjögren's syndrome are detectable in up to a half of all SLE patients (Dubois, 1974).

Blood

The commonest abnormality is a normochromic, normocytic anaemia. Very rarely, the marrow may become severely hypoplastic (Burkhardt, 1965). In one of our patients, progressive leucopenia and anaemia finally ended in marrow failure. In this patient, return of normal marrow function followed 'pulse' cyclophosphamide treatment (Walport et al, 1982). Haemolytic anaemia is described in 6–15% in the series of Dubois (1952), though in more recent series, including as they do milder cases, the number of SLE patients with major haemolytic anaemia is rare.

Leucopenia (usually between 2000 and 4500/mm^3) occurs in nearly one-half of SLE patients. In our patients, an absolute lymphopenia has been a more common finding (Davis et al, 1973). Leucocytosis is rare in the absence of infections or steroid therapy. Thrombocytopenia occurs in 5–10% of patients and may be the presenting manifestation of the disease, though this is rare. The relationship between thrombocytopenia and SLE is complex. Recent studies of anti-nuclear antibodies and their role as markers for 'subsets' of SLE patients have led to suggestions that one group of patients with anti-Ro (anti-SSA) antibodies might have a propensity for thrombocytopenia (Morley & Hughes, 1981). Also, antibodies directed against phospholipid antigens in platelet membranes have recently been shown to be associated with thrombocytopenia in SLE (Harris et al, 1984). If proved to be true, these findings might provide markers for those patients with idiopathic thrombocytopaenic purpura who subsequently develop SLE. Coagulation defects are discussed elsewhere.

INFECTIONS IN SLE

A tendency to infection is a recognised feature of SLE, over and above that relating to uraemia, immunosuppression and other iatrogenic causes (Staples et al, 1974). A variety of explanations for this tendency is possible, including lower complement levels, defective phagocytosis and impaired RES activity. Whether mild untreated SLE predisposes to infection remains to be seen.

SLE AND PREGNANCY

Pregnancy is not contraindicated in SLE provided that renal and cardiac function are good (Zurier, 1975; Grigor et al, 1977). The fetal death rate is somewhat higher than normal (Estes & Larson, 1965). There is a slight tendency to clinical exacerbation during the first trimester and during the puerperium. The major obstetric feature in SLE is the high incidence of spontaneous abortions, not only in established SLE but dating back to before the diagnosis of SLE was established (Grigor et al, 1977).

The reasons for the higher spontaneous abortion rate at around 12 weeks in unclear, though a number of factors may contribute. The finding of heart block in the offspring of SLE mothers (Chang, 1982) might suggest that more serious congenital cardiac defects may lead to abortion. An alternative explanation might implicate the clotting defect, where the lupus anticoagulant impairs placental function (Byron, 1982; Boey et al, 1983). A third finding is that in certain SLE patients with spontaneous abortions, circulating antibodies were detected which were absorbable in vitro by placental trophoblast antigens (Bresnihan et al, 1977b). A syndrome has been proposed consisting of thrombosis, spontaneous abortion and neurological disease (Hughes, 1983; Hughes, 1984; Derue et al, 1985).

SLE VARIANTS

Discoid lupus

Discoid LE is a chronic skin disease characterised by erythema, scaling, follicular plugging and scarring. The lesions often have a characteristic 'butterfly' distribution on the nose and cheeks and may be chronic and disfiguring. Alopecia is common and mucocutaneous ulcers may occur.

Manifestations suggestive of systemic involvement are rare and occur in 5% only (Beck & Rowell, 1963) though synovitis occurs in up to 50% (Dubois & Martel, 1956). Abnormal serological findings such as positive ANF tests and leucopenia occur in up to one-third of patients (Shrank & Doniach, 1963). Raised titres of anti-DNA antibodies were detected in 7 out of 25 patients with discoid LE. None of these patients has as yet developed systemic features (Davis et al, 1974).

Abortion, thrombosis and neurological disease

The syndrome of reported abortions, repeated thrombotic episodes and neurological disease has recently been described in detail (Hughes, 1983; Hughes, 1984). These patients are frequently ANA-negative, and usually have high titres of anticardiolipin antibodies. Other features of the syndrome are livedo reticulosis and labile hypertension (Hughes, 1984). Preliminary evidence suggests that steroid and/or immunosuppressive therapy might, by reducing the titre of anti-phospholipid antibodies, allow successful pregnancy to occur (Lubbe et al, 1983; Derue et al 1985).

ANA-negative lupus

Anti-Ro (anti-SSA) antibodies are predominently cytoplasmic. It has long been recognised, especially by dermatologists, that patients with otherwise typical lupus may be ANA-negative. One such group, those with subacute cutaneous LE (SCLE) may or may not be ANA-positive. Even in those patients who are ANA-negative, anti-Ro antibodies are occasionally described (see below).

Drug-induced lupus

Lupus-like syndromes have been recognised as an occasional complication of therapy with certain drugs for over 30 years (Table 53.4). More frequent by far is the finding of positive anti-nuclear antibodies in asymptomatic patients taking these drugs.

The clinical features depend largely on the speed of diagnosis. In the majority of patients with 'drug-induced lupus', the syndrome consists of arthralgias together with the finding of circulating anti-nuclear antibodies. Continuation of the drug may result in progression to pleurisy, fever, myalgias, rashes, etc. Renal involvement is rare. The sex ratio is more even than in idiopathic SLE, though in our studies of hydralazine lupus, a female predominance remained (Batchelor et al, 1980).

There appear to be minor differences in clinical emphasis between the syndromes produced by various drugs (reviewed by Harmon & Portanova, 1982). In the vast majority of patients however,

Table 53.4 Drugs implicated in the induction of a lupus-like syndrome

Cardiovascular	Procainamide Quinidine Practolol
Antimicrobial	Isoniazid Penicillin Sulphonamides Griseofulvin Streptomycin Tetracycline Nitofurantoin
Anticonvulsant	Phenytoin (diphenylhydantoin) Methoin (mephentoin) Ethosuximide Troxidone (trimethadione) Primidone
Antihypertensive	Hydralazine Methyldopa Reserpine
Antithyroid	Propylthiouracil Methylthiouracil
Psychotropic	Chlorpromazine Lithium carbonate
Miscellaneous	D-penicillamine Oral contraceptives Methysergide Phenylbutazone Allopurinol Gold salts Aminoglutethimide

the syndrome subsides on stopping the drug (Hughes, 1982b).

Serologically, drug-induced lupus differs fundamentally from idiopathic SLE in that ani-DNA antibodies are almost invariably absent (Hughes 1971; Hughes et al, 1981). Sera from certain procainamide-induced lupus patients contain antibodies against histones, and more recently, certain hydralazine lupus sera were shown to have antibodies against a different group of histones (reviewed by Harmon & Portanova, 1982). To date we have been unable to demonstrate antibodies against saline-soluble non-histone antigens (Hughes et al, 1981).

The aetiology of the syndrome may reflect host factors as well as the offending drug. Alarcon-Segovia (1975) suggested that a 'lupus diathesis' might exist in those individuals developing the syndrome. Recently, we demonstrated a striking association between the development of hydralazine lupus and HLA-DR3; indeed, if confirmed, the figures suggest that the combination of female sex, slow acetylator status and HLA-DR3 almost guarantees the development of symptoms in those taking sufficient drug (Batchelor et al, 1980).

MIXED CONNECTIVE TISSUE DISEASE

Sharp et al (1972) proposed this term for a small group of patients in whom a disease resembling systemic sclerosis also contains 'overlap' features of SLE and dermatomyositis. The disease has three points worthy of distinction from SLE: First, Raynaud's phenomenon is prominent and almost universal; secondly, renal disease is rare and the long-term prognosis is good; thirdly, the sera of these patients have three distinguishing immunological features — the absence of DNA antibodies, strongly positive 'speckled' pattern ANF tests, and antibodies in high titre to 'extractable nuclear antigen' (ENA). ENA is a mixture of antigens of which one ribonucleoprotein (RNP) is RNase-sensitive. Anti-RNP antibodies are found in all cases of mixed connective tissue disease, often in high titre. A small percentage of SLE patients demonstrate anti-RNP antibodies, though in lower titre (Bresnihan et al, 1977). The subject is discussed in Chapter 50.

IMMUNOLOGICAL FEATURES OF SLE

SLE is characterised by the heterogeneity of its abnormal serological findings. At its simplest, the picture is one of impaired suppressor T cell function with the production of diverse humoral antibodies. More detailed descriptions of the common immunological abnormalities occurring in many of the rheumatic diseases are given elsewhere in this volume, and the following is a summary.

Suppressor T cell function

Although earlier work gave conflicting data on the ratio of helper to suppressor cells in SLE, most of the recent assays have shown evidence of impaired suppressor T cell function during active disease. Miller & Schwartz (1979) demonstrated impaired suppressor cell function not only in 11 out of 15

SLE patients, but in 13 of 50 healthy first-degree relatives.

Anti-nuclear antibodies

Anti-nuclear antibodies (ANA) exist in all known immunolobulin classes. Most, if not all, can be detected by fluorescent antibody techniques (Beck, 1961). The interpretation of 'patterns' of immunofluorescence has, to a large extent, been superceded by more precise identification of nuclear antigens. Whilst these antigen–antibody systems are discussed in Chapter 12, a short revision seems appropriate.

Table 53.5 lists the more widely measured anti-nuclear and anti-cytoplasmic antigen–antibody systems. The use of counter-immunoelectrophoresis, 'Western blotting' and other analyses have resulted in the recognition of at least a dozen other systems (reviewed by Bernstein & Hughes, 1983).

In clinical practice, the demonstration of ANFs by immunofluorescence provides the most widely used screening test in SLE. The test lacks diagnostic specificity for SLE, but a negative ANA test is extremely rare in active disease: two possible 'explanations' for occasional ANA-negative SLE are the occasional example of slow conversion to ANA and DNA positivity, and 'Ro-positive' lupus.

Table 53.5 Major anti-nuclear and anti-cytoplasmic antibodies

Antigen	Biological properties	Clinical comments
DNA	Anti-double stranded DNA antibodies highly specific for DNA. A number of antigen sites on DNA molecule identified	The most specific test for DNA. Most commercial DNA test preparations contain single stranded DNA, contributing to 'borderline' values
RNA	Antibodies against a variety of natural and synthetic ribonucleosides and nucleotides.	Found in a small percentage of SLE patients
RNP	A complex antigen of protein and RNA	MCTD (high titre) 100% SLE (low titer) 20%
Ro (SSA)	Predominantly cytoplasmic	'ANA-negative lupus' Sjögrens syndrome Thrombocytopenia Mothers of babies with congenital heart block
La (SSB)	Usually associated with anti-Ro	Sjögrens syndrome
Sm	Usually associated with anti-RNP	SLE (predominantly in blacks)
Jo-1	Antigen probably histidyl tRNA	Polymyositis (Approx 25%) associated with 'overlap' features
Anti-histones	Against single or multiple nuclear histones	Found in certain cases of drug-induced lupus

LE cells

The LE cell test detects IgG antibody against DNA-histone. It has been largely superceded by the simpler ANA and more specific anti-DNA antibody tests.

Anti-DNA antibodies

The discovery in 1957 that SLE sera contain antibodies against native (double stranded) DNA was important for two reasons: first, because DNA antibodies have come to be regarded as the single most specific marker of this disease, and secondly because the DNA–anti-DNA complex system is the predominant immune complex involved in the nephritis of SLE.

In the 14 years since the introduction of the DNA-binding (Farr) test by Pincus et al (1969), this test system has provéd the most widely acceptable (Hughes et al, 1971; Hughes, 1975). Attention to details such as the physicochemical conditions of the assay (Pincus, 1971; Lewkonia et al, 1977) is a relatively straightforward matter but standardisation of the substrate remains a major problem, despite the plethora of workshops and symposia on the subject.

Despite the high diagnostic value of anti-DNA antibodies, fluctuations do not necessarily closely parallel clinical activity. In particular, some patients appear to do well for long periods of time with persistently high anti-DNA antibody titres. The recognition that high DNA-binding values do not per se indicate more serious disease has contributed to a more conservative approach to the treatment of serological abnormalities in otherwise clinically well SLE patients (Hughes, 1982) (Figs 53.10, 53.11).

Anti-ENA (extractable nuclear antigens)

a. Anti-RNP antibodies are found in up to one-quarter of SLE patients, usually in lower titre than that seem in mixed connective tissue disease. It does not seem that the presence of anti-RNP is associated with any particular disease pattern in SLE (Bresnihan et al, 1977a).

b. Anti-Ro (subsequently also called 'anti-SSA') antibodies are found in one-quarter of SLE patieents (Bernstein & Hughes, 1981). In our studies, it was found to be associated with thrombocytopenia, and indeed was found in 25% of our patients with ITP (Morley & Hughes, 1981).

It has also been associated with sicca syndrome (see Ch. 56), with 'ANA-negative lupus' and 'subacute cutaneous LE', and, interestingly, is found in the serum of 60% of mothers of infants with congenital heart block.

c. Anti-Sm. Although claims have been made for the association of anti-Sm with CNS involvement in SLE, this has not been our experience. The interesting racial differences in the frequency of Sm suggests that it may have HLA associations (Bernstein & Hughes, 1983).

d. Anti-histones. These antibodies were noted by Tan and colleagues to be present in procainamide-induced lupus. Studies are in progress to assess that possibility that other drug-induced lupus syndromes may have distinguishable antihistone antibody profiles.

Antiviral antibodies

A number of raised viral antibody titres have been found in SLE — notably raised anti-measles antibody titres (Phillips & Christian, 1970). The aetiological significance of these findings is uncertain though they may simply reflect the hyperactive state in SLE, broadly paralleling as they do the elevated immunoglobulin levels seen in this disease.

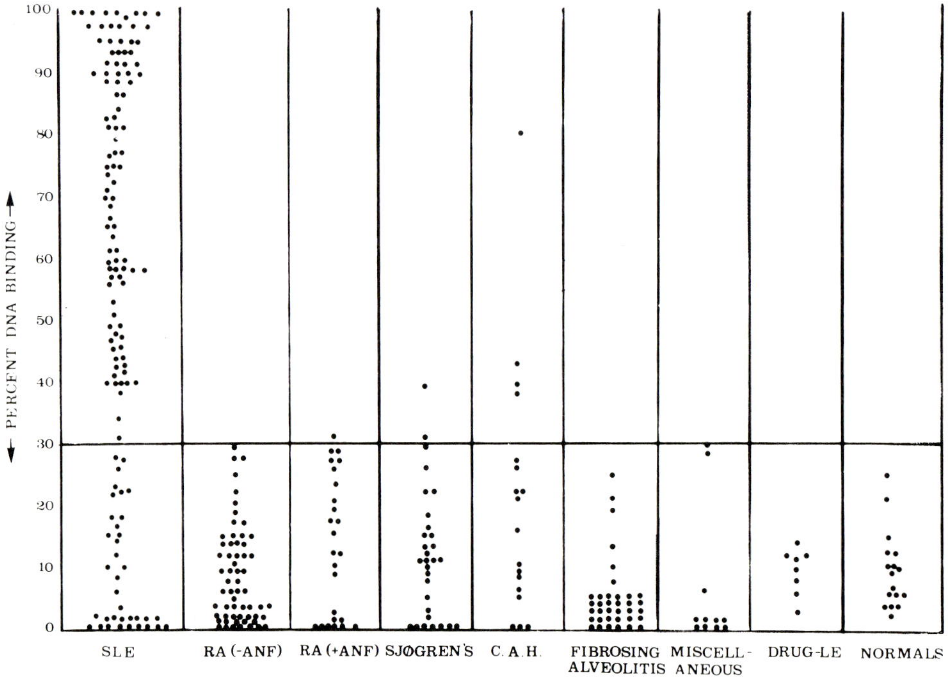

Fig. 53.10 DNA-binding in 262 ANF-positive sera. A control group of ANF-negative rheumatoid arthritis patients is shown. CAH = chronic active hepatitis. (From Hughes, G.R.V. *Ninth symposium of advanced medicine*. Pitman Medical (1973). By permission of the Editors.)

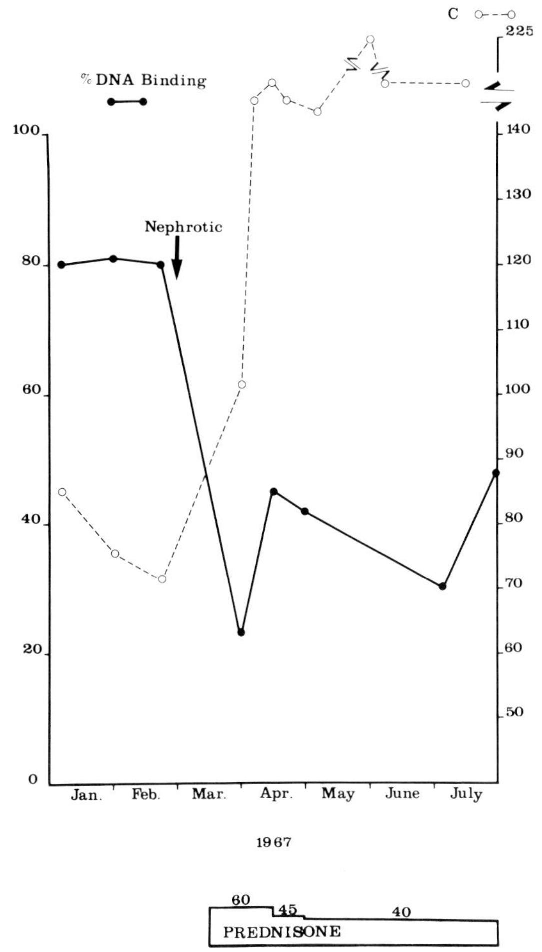

Fig. 53.11 Serial study of DNA binding and complement in SLE.

Rheumatoid factors

Both IgG and IgM rheumatoid factors are found in up to a third of SLE patients. It is not clear whether they play any pathogenetic or protective role.

Biological false-positive (BFP) tests for syphilis

Up to 30% of SLE patients demonstrate BFP reactions (Harvey & Shulman, 1974). A small percentage of patients also give 'true positive' tests, though the reaction can be distinguished by its 'beaded' appearance, presumably due to action of anti-DNA antibody on the spirochaetal DNA (Kraus et al, 1970).

Circulating anticoagulants

The so-called 'lupus anticoagulant' — an anti-lipid antibody — is, paradoxically, associated with a marked tendency to venous thrombosis (reviewed by Byron, 1982). In a recent study from our unit, careful measurement revealed the presence of the lupus anticoagulant in the plasma of 31 of 60 patients with SLE. Of these 31, thromboses (DVT, renal, cerebral or axillary vein) were seen in 19. There was also a clear association with the presence of abortions, thrombocytopenia and biological false-positive tests for syphilis (Boey et al, 1983). More recent reports from our group have suggested associations between anti-phospholipids such as the lupus anticoagulant with cerebral thrombosis (Harris et al, 1983), thrombocytopenia (Harris et al, 1984), multiple abortions (Derue et al, 1985), renal vein thrombosis (Asherson et al, 1984), Budd–Chiari syndrome (Hughes, 1984) and pulmonary hypertension (Asherson et al, 1983).

Serum complement levels

Measurements of serum complement (most usually C3, C4 and total haemolytic complement levels) provide the single most important investigation in SLE. In the great majority of SLE patients a lowered complement level is indicative of renal involvement (Schuer & Sandson, 1968; Cohen et al, 1971), and usually precedes other clinical evidence of such involvement. The classical pathway is predominantly involved, with recruitment of properdin (alternate) pathway (Schuer, 1975).

Cryoglobulins

Cryoglobulins may be detected in up to 80% of SLE sera (Christian et al, 1968) being associated with disease activity, in particular renal disease, and with reduced serum C3 and C1q complement levels (Hanauer & Christian, 1967; Stastny & Ziff, 1969). They contain IgG, IgM and C1q. Some, if not the majority, of SLE cryoglobulins are immune complexes, with the IgG or IgM component possessing rheumatoid factor, anti-DNA, anti-lymphocyte or anti-RNP activity (Winfield et al, 1975; Zvaifler & Bluestone, 1976).

Recently, a modification of the standard cryoprecipitation technique has made it more sensitive (Mola et al, 1983).

Anti-erythrocyte antibodies

Positive direct antiglobulin (Coombs) tests are found in up to 65% of SLE patients (Mongan et al, 1967) though haemolytic anaemia occurs in only 6–15%. The use of different antisera has established that in SLE the red cells are coated with either complement and IgG or complement along (Worlledge, 1967).

Anti-leucocyte antibodies

The variety of techniques used for detection of leucocyte antibodies makes figures difficult to compare, though an incidence of positive direct antiglobulin consumption tests for leucocytes has been reported (Dausset et al, 1961).

Lymphocytotoxic antibodies (LCAs)

Antibodies directed against lymphocyte surface determininants are found in the serum of patients with SLE as well as in a variety of other diseases, particularly viral infections. The antibody groups most frequently recognised are the cold-reactive lymphocytotoxic antibodies — IgM, and reacting preferentially at 4°C in the standard laboratory (Terasaki) microtoxicity method.

In addition to being found in 80% of SLE patients, they have also been reported in up to 50% of unrelated household contacts of SLE patients. Their role, if any, in the T cell disturbance in SLE is uncertain. However, evidence has been presented that certain LCAs may cross-react with antigenic sites on placental trophoblast, possibly contributing to spontaneous abortion in SLE, and with sites on brain (Bresnihan et al, 1979).

Anti-neuronal antibodies

One group of LCAs was found to be cross-reactive both with fetal erythrocytes (Goldberg et al, 1978) and with neurones. The neuronal activity was greater with cortical neurones than with cerebellar and caudate neurones, and was found predominantly in SLE patients with neuropsychiatric disease (Bresnihan et al, 1979; Hughes, 1980).

Organ-specific antibodies

One of the interesting paradoxes of SLE is that in this disease, characterised as it is by the proliferation and variety of circulating antibodies, organ-specific antibodies are surprisingly uncommon.

AETIOLOGY

Evidence exists for genetic, hormonal and environmental factors all contributing to the gross immunological and clinical abnormalities in SLE.

Genetic factors

Epidemiological studies have shown an increase in the prevalence of hypergammaglobulinaemia, antinuclear antibodies, BFP tests for syphilis and clinical SLE and other connective tissue diseases in family members of patients with SLE (Siegel &Lee, 1973).

There are also a number of well-documented reports of SLE occurring in monozygotic twins.

Further evidence that a genetic predisposition to develop SLE or 'lupus diathesis' exists comes from the frequent development of SLE in patients with chronic BFP reactions and those with previous histories of thrombocytopenic purpura (Rabinowitz & Dameshek, 1960; Catterall, 1973). Increasing numbers of cases of SLE have been reported in persons with isolated complement component deficiencies, particularly C2 and C4 (Day et al, 1973; Schur, 1975). No definite relationship between any particular HLA group and SLE has yet been confirmed, though possible HLA relationships with isolated complement deficiencies and BFP reactors have yet to be reported.

The major evidence suggesting a genetic aetiology for SLE is summarised by Walport et al (1982). In a family study of SLE recently completed in the UK, we found that 83% of patients with SLE had a null allele for C4A, C4B, compared with 43% of normal controls. There was strong linkage disequilibrium between DR3 and the null alleles for C4A and C4B (Fielder et al, 1983). It remains to be seen whether this subtle inherited complement deficiency is directly involved in the pathogenesis of SLE.

Hormonal factors

In almost all series studied, the female to male ratio in SLE is 9 : 1. Indeed in the main child bearing years, the ratio may be as high as 20 : 1 (Inman, 1978). Further evidence from animal studies, studies of sex hormones in SLE patients, twin studies, and frequent case reports of Klinefelter's syndrome and SLE has underlined the major role of sex hormones, not only in the modulation of the immune response but in the pathogenesis of SLE (reviewed by Talal, 1982).

Viral agents

Most of the data implicating a virus aetiology for the SLE comes from the study of animal models of disease. In the dogs studied by Lewis, Schwartz and colleagues (see below), cell-free filtrates were shown to transmit the disease. In humans, no direct evidence for a universal aetiological agent exists at present. Nonetheless, it is intriguing that lymphocytotoxic antibodies, often associated with viral infection, are demonstrable in up to 50% of unrelated household contacts of SLE patients (DeHoratius & Messner, 1975). Direct observations of human tissue suggesting the presence of C-type virus particles still remain unconfirmed (reviewed by Pincus, 1976).

UV light

The provocative effect of sunlight on SLE disease activity has been mentioned earlier. Interesting observations have been made regarding the immunogenecity of DNA after UV irradiation. Such irradiation alters native DNA in vivo and in vitro to form thymine dimers which are antigenic. While immunisation of animals with DNA fails to result in antibody production, UV-DNA is a strong immunogen, producing high titre UV-DNA antibodies. Tan and his colleagues have, in a series of elegant experiments, demonstrated immune complex deposition in the kidney of animals, UV-irradiated and subsequently given UV-DNA antigen, and in the skin in animals immunised and then exposed to UV light (Tan 1976; Natali and Tan 1972, 1973).

Animal models

Speculation concerning infective and genetic aetiologies for SLE has been enhanced by the findings in New Zealand mice, and in a group of dogs developing a lupuslike syndrome.

The New Zealand mouse

The New Zealand black (NZB) mouse develops a spontaneous haemolytic anaemia. When, however, the animal is crossed with the clinically well white (NZW) mouse, the F_1 hybrid, particularly the female, develops a lupus-like disease, with ANF, DNA and RNA antibodies, hypergammaglobulinaemia, haemolytic anaemia and immune complex nephritis.

While the severity of the disease can be modified by cross-breeding experiments, transmission is not simply autosomal. The sex differences in disease incidence and severity in these animals, as in human SLE, cannot be accounted for simply by hormonal factors (Steinberg et al, 1971).

In addition to DNA–anti-DNA complexes, these animals are also known to have circulating virus–antivirus complexes, the virus being predominantly C-type gross leukaemia virus, to which the animal appears to break tolerance. The relative roles of infection, genetic and immunological factors in the genesis of SLE in these animals has been reviewed elsewhere (Whaley et al, 1975).

Canine SLE

Lewis et al (1965) reported a group of dogs in which SLE, characterised by haemolytic anaemia, thrombocytopenia, nephritis, arthritis, lymphadenopathy, LE cells and DNA antibodies spontaneously developed.

In a series of interesting experiments, these workers were able to transmit the disease by cell-free extracts of canine spleens. In addition they were able to induce serological abnormalities (including positive ANF rests) in mice, using the canine filtrate. Serial passage of spleen cells from these serologically positive mice resulted in the early appearance of positive ANF tests in murine recipients.

These early results were taken to indicate the presence in canine SLE of a virus, capable of spreading by both horizontal and vertical routes (reviewed by Hughes, 1982a).

DIFFERENTIAL DIAGNOSIS

The differential diagnosis of SLE is wide. The criteria laid down by the ARA (Table 53.6) are for

Table 53.6 ARA criteria for classification of SLE

	Percentage incidence		
	ARA Series	Hammersmith Hospital Davies et al (1974)	Memphis Trimble et al (1974)
1. Facial erythema	64	64	40
2. Discoid lupus	17	31	32
3. Raynaud's phenomenon	20	19	44
4. Alopecia	43	64	40
5. Photosensitivity	37	17	28
6. Oral and nasal ulceration	15	22	16
7. Arthritis without deformity	90	89	100
8. LE cells (2 or more)	92	75	48
9. Chronic false positive serological tests for syphilis (longer than six months)	12	8	12
10. Proteinuria (>3.5 g/day)	20	25	16
11. Cellular casts	48	17	16
12. Pleuritis	60	30	
Pericarditis	19	19	60
13 Psychosis or convulsions	19	19	20
14. Haemolytic anaemia	16	14	
Leucopenia	40	47	52
Thrombocytopenia	11	14	

classification purposes only and are of little value in diagnosis of individual cases — indeed it is probable that the vast majority of mild SLE patients do not meet the minimum 4 criteria.

This author suggests, in Table 53.7, a number of other features which have frequently been found helpful in reaching a diagnosis.

This list is somewhat arbitrary, but serves to emphasise the importance of history taking in diagnosis. If it is believed that lupus is a genetically determined disease, it follows that the disease, or at least the diathesis, has been present since birth.

It is not uncommon for SLE patients presenting clinically at the age of 25 following their first pregnancy to have recalled an attack of 'rheumatic fever' at the age of 15, or epilepsy dating back to the early teens. A past history of migraine (often premenstrual) is frequent, and some women give a history of recurrent abortions. In laboratory testing, the finding of anti-DNA antibodies is of paramount importance. However, of use in our experience is the finding of *lymphopenia*, its extent often mirroring disease activity. So persistent is the finding of a low CRP level in SLE (it is not uncommon to see SLE patients with an ESR of over 100 mm/h and a zero CRP level) that we have suggested it be considered as a classification criterion (Lanham et al, 1980).

Table 53.7 SLE — additional features in diagnosis

Female sex
Age under 40
Migraine
Recurrent abortions
Alopecia
Livedo
Tendonitis
EEG abnormalities
Epilepsy (often for many years)
Anti-DNA antibodies
High ESR with low CRP
Hypocomplementaemia
Lymphopenia
Lupus anticoagulant

In the older patient, the diagnosis can be difficult. Sjögren's syndrome with anti-nuclear antibodies is a common differential diagnosis, and may, in some patients, be the residuum of previous mild SLE.

MANAGEMENT

The case for a more conservative management of SLE has been published elsewhere (Hughes, 1982). The asymptomatic patient with no renal disease requires no therapy. A rapidly rising anti-DNA antibody level, or (perhaps even more significantly) a rapidly falling complement level suggests closer patient monitoring, though even here, insititution of therapy may not be required. Even in the more ill hospital patients reported from our unit by Grigor et al (1978), the *mean* prednisolone dose was 7.5 mg daily.

General measures

The patient with mild SLE can, and normally

does, lead a normal lifestyle. Pregnancy is not contraindicated, provided that renal function if adequate. Despite the theoretical dangers of the contraceptive pill in SLE, problems and disease flares are surprisingly rare (Travers & Hughes, 1978). It seems advisable to use low-oestrogen preparations. The development of anticardiolipin assays (Harris et al, 1983) may help predict those at risk of thrombosis.

Photosensitivity to UV light is well known in SLE, though it may be a variable phenomenon, some patients being photosensitive only during flares of disease. Approximately one-half of patients give a definite history of UV sensitivity (Tan 1976). While UV-barrier creams are widely recommended, their efficacy is somewhat variable.

Present evidence suggests that drugs known to cause drug-induced lupus, such as hydralazine, anti-tuberculous agents do *not* exacerbate idiopathic SLE and are thus not contraindicated in this disease.

Two drugs which require caution in SLE are sulphonamides (including Septrin) and penicillin, both of which may cause a flare of disease.

Aspirin

Small dose salicylates are widely used in mild SLE. High doses of aspirin frequently produce hepatotocity. Seaman & Plotz (1976) noted moderate to marked elevation of serum transaminases within two weeks of full dose aspirin therapy. A notable finding was the association of hepatotoxicity with active disease. In our own studies (Travers & Hughes, 1978), the return to normal levels following the stopping of aspirin therapy was rapid. Initial data suggested that aspirin derivatives without the orthoacetyl group did not produce this side-effect.

Aspirin and the kidney

It has been noted that a number of SLE patients on aspirin developed mild reduction in glomerular filtration rates (Kimberley & Plotz, 1977; Travers & Hughes, 1978). It has been suggested that this effect is through a deterioration in renal circulation produced by the anti-prostaglandin mechanism of aspirin. The same effect has been noted with indomethacin, naproxen, ibuprofen and fenoprofen (Kimberley et al, 1978).

In the majority of patients in our clinics this effect is hardly discernible.

Non-steroidal anti-inflammatory drugs

These are the first-line drugs in the mild rheumatic complaints of SLE. Side-effects are rare though idiosyncratic reactions have been ascribed to ibuprofen in a small number of patients (Sonnenblick & Abraham, 1978).

Antimalarials

These drugs are now regarded as a major part of therapy in SLE, especially as fears of retinal toxicity have lessened with the use of smaller doses. They have been used in the treatment of discoid LE since 1894 though it is clear that their effect extends far beyond the skin and joints. The mechanism of action of these drugs remains unknown (reviewed by Lanham & Hughes 1982). The most commonly used drug is hydroxychloroquine (200 mg daily). Some advocate a loading dose of 400 mg daily though many patients are unable to tolerate this dose. Retinopathy appears now to be related to the higher doses previously used. McKenzie (1981) reviewed 84 patients who had consumed in excess of 1 kg of antimalarials in low daily dosage. None of these individuals had retinopathy, whereas a second group of patients with chloroquine retinopathy had all taken lower total doses but higher daily doses. Other antimalarials used are chloroquine (250 mg daily) and mepacrine (50–100 mg daily). Despite the improved safety with recurrently used antimalarial regimes, 6-monthly ophthalmological checking is required.

Corticosteroids

The majority of patients with SLE require corticosteroids at some time during the course of their disease. Steroid dosage is an individualistic clinical decision (Wasner & Fries, 1978). For acute and severe disease 60 mg daily is recommended. We rarely resort to higher dosage of steroids in our practice. Prolonged higher dosage of corticosteroids, especially in CNS disease, leads to a greater morbidity from treatment than from the underlying disease (Sargent et al 1975). A major problem with high dose steroid therapy is aseptic bone necrosis. There is an almost linear relationship between the magnitude and duration of corticosteroid dosage and the incidence of aseptic necrosis (Dimante, 1978). A second major problem is infection. Although the list of immunologial and other defects that may lead to increased susceptibility to infection in SLE is long (Staples et al, 1974), it is almost certain that treatment may be the culprit in the majority of cases (Quismorio & Dubois, 1975).

It is our practice therefore as soon as clinical improvement is seen to reduce steroid therapy below 20 mg and ultimately to alternate day steroid therapy, and if possible, no drugs at all.

Immunosuppressive agents

Controlled trials of these agents have proved almost impossible. Most people with large clinical experience of SLE are convinced that the addition of agents such as azathioprine does have a steroid-sparing effect in the majority of patients. In proliferative nephritis the combination of azathioprine and steroids is now common practice (reviewed by Adu & Cameron, 1982). The choice of immunosuppressive agent is still disputed. The high ratio of toxicity with cyclophosphamide, in particular the haemorrhagic cystitis and ovarian failure make it an unattractive therapeutic choice in the majority of young women with SLE. Ginzler et al (1976) attempted to minimise these side-effects by combining lower doses with both azathioprine and prednisolone.

It is, perhaps, surprising that malignancy of the reticuloendothelial system while occasionally reported in SLE patients receiving immunosuppressive agents (Hehir et al, 1979) is rare.

Pulse steroid therapy

During the past few years attempts have been made to find a rapidly effective form of immunosuppression. These attempts have included the use of intravenous 'bolus' methylprednisolone therapy (e.g. 1 g i.v. on 3 successive days). There is little doubt that in occasional patients there is a dramatic and prolonged period of improvement though repeated attempts this form of therapy have, in our experience, been less than satisfactory. The subject is reviewed by Kimberley (1982). Similar trials are in progress using pulse cyclophosphamide (e.g. 500 mg i.v. of cyclophosphamide). This form of treatment looks very prom-

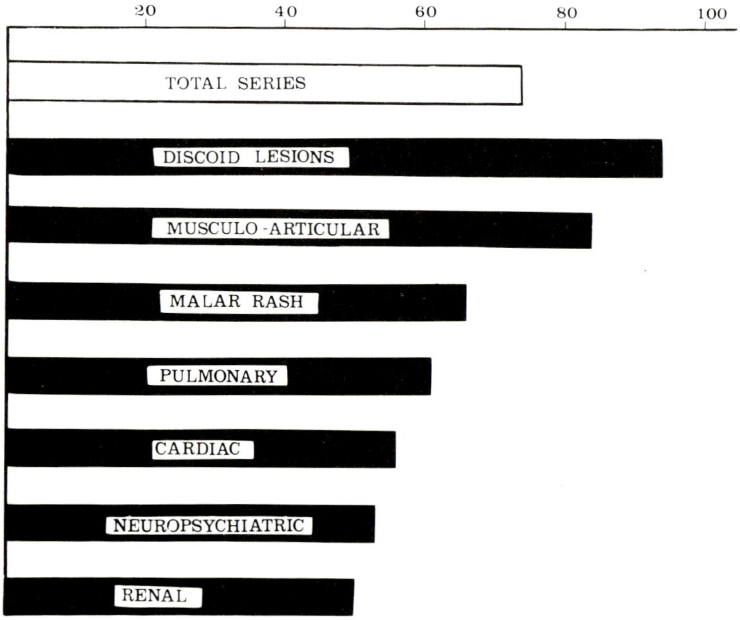

Fig. 53.12 Estimated 5-year survival (%) for seven manifestations of SLE. (From Estes & Christian, 1971.)

ising. In a recent patient with lupus-associated marrow aplasia, the use of intravenous cyclophosphamide reversed severe haematological deficit (Walport et al, 1982).

Plasmapheresis

Over the past decade a number of centres have advocated the use of plasma exchange in SLE (reviewed by Jones, 1982). Although the theoretical attractions of removal of antibody complexes, etc. make this form of therapy appealing, the long-term effects in most patients with SLE have been disappointing (Hughes & Ryan, 1980).

Sex hormone modulation

In view of the marked effect of the female sex hormones in SLE and the occasional premenstrual exacerbations of disease, attempts have been made in experimental animals to modulate the disease with sex hormones. While this is not possible in humans, a recent report demonstrated clinical and serological improvement in two women with marked premenstrual exacerbations of disease who were treated with danazol (Morley & Hughes, 1982).

PROGNOSIS

The prognosis of SLE is improving year by year, owing largely to the recognition of milder forms of the disease. Most centres now show 5- and even 10-year survival figures in the 90% and over range (Fig. 53.12). Higher mortality figures are still published in poorer populations. In a recent study of children with SLE the prognosis appeared to be similar to that in adults (Caeiro et al, 1981). Although aggressive therapy during the acute disease may be life-saving, the trend in recent years has been towards a more conservative approach to the subacute and subclinical SLE patient. While often more demanding both for patient and physician, this approach is beginning to be regarded as superior not only in terms of morbidity but possibly also in reducing mortality in SLE.

REFERENCES

Adu D, Cameron J S 1982 Lupus nephritis. Clinics in Rheumatic Diseases 8:153

Agnello V, Koffler D, Kunkel H G 1973 Immune complex systems in the nephritis of systemic lupus erythematosus. Kidney International 3:390

Alarcon-Segovia D 1975 Drug induced lupus syndromes. Clinics in Rheumatic Diseases 1

Alarcon-Segovia D, Galbraith R F, Maldonado J E, Howard F M Jr 1963 Systemic lupus erythematosus following thymectomy for myasthenia gravis. Report of two cases. Lancet 2:662

Appel G B, Williams G S, Meltzer J I, Pirani C I 1976 Renal vein thrombosis, nephrotic syndrome & SLE. Annals of Internal Medicine 85:310

Asherson R A, Mackworth-Young C G , Boey M L, Hull R G, Saunders A, Gharavi A E, Hughes G R V 1983 Pulmonary hypertension in SLE. British Medical Journal 287: 1024–1025

Asherson R A, Lanham J G, Hull R G, Boey M L, Gharavi A E, Hughes G R V 1984 Renal vein thrombosis in systemic lupus erythematosus. Clinical and experimental Rheumatology 2/1: 75–79

Baldwin D Gallo G R 1975 Lupus nephritis. Clinics in Rheumatic Diseases 1:639

Baldwin D, Lowenstein J, Rothfeild N F, Gallo F, McCluskey R T 1970 The clinical course of proliferative and membranous forms of lupus nephritis. Annals of Internal Medicine 73:929

Batchelor J R, Welsh K I, Tinoco R M, et al 1980 Hydralazine-induced SLE: influence of HLA-DR and sex on susceptibility. Lancet 1:1107

Becker G J, Waldburger M, Hughes G R V, Pepys M B 1980 Value of C-reactive protein measurement in the investigation of fever in SLE. Annals of the Rheumatic Diseases 39:50

Bennett R, Hughes G R V, Bywaters E G L, Holt P J L 1972 Neuropsychiatric problems in SLE. British Medical Journal 4:342

Bernstein R, Hughes G R V 1983 Antinuclear antibodies in lupus-like syndromes. In: 19th Symposium of Advanced Medicine. Pitman, London

Bishko F 1972 Retinopathy in systemic lupus erythematosus. A case report and review of the literature. Arthritis and Rheumatism.15:57

Bloch K J, Buchanan W W, Wohl M J, Bunim J J 1965 Sjögren's syndrome. A clinical, pathological and serological study of sixty-two cases. Medicine 44:187

Bluestein H G, Zvaifler N J 1976 Brain reactive lymphocytotoxic antibodies in the serum of patients with SLE. Arthritis and Rheumatism 19:844

Boey M L, Colaco C B, Gharavi A E, 1983 Thrombosis in SLE: striking association with the presence of the circulating 'lupus anticoagulant.' British Medical Journal 287: 1021–1023

Bresnihan B, Bunn C, Snaith M L, Hughes G R V 1977a Antiribonucleoprotein antibodies in connective tissue diseases: estimation by counterimmunoelectrophoresis. British Medical Journal 1:610

Bresnihan B, Grigor R R, Oliver M, Hughes G R V 1977b Immunological mechanism for spontaneous abortion in systemic lupus erythematosis. Lancet 2:1205

Bresnihan B, Grigor R R, Hughes G R V 1977C A

prospective analysis of anti-RNP antibodies in SLE. Annals of the Rheumatic Diseases 36:55
Bresnihan B, Oliver M, Grigor R, Hughes G R V 1977d Brain reactivity of lymphocytotoxic antibodies in SLE with and without cerebral involvement. Clinical and Experimental Immunology 30:333
Bresnihan B, Hohmeister R, Cutting J, et al 1979 The neuropsychiatric disorder in SLE: evidence for both vascular and immune mechanisms. Annals of the Rheumatic Diseases 38:301
Bulgrin J G, Dubois E L, Jacobson G (1960) Chest roentgenographic changes in systemic lupus erythematosus. Radiology 74:42
Bulkley B H, Roberts W C 1975 The heart in SLE and the changes induced in it by corticosteroid therapy. American Journal of Medicine 58:234
Burkhardt R 1965 The bone marrow in systemic lupus erythematosus. Seminars in Haematology 2:29
Byron M A 1982 The clotting defect in SLE. Clinics in Rheumatic Diseases 8:137
Caeiro F, Michielson F M C, Bernstein R M, Hughes G R V 1981 SLE in childhood. Annals of the Rheumatic Diseases 40:325
Carr D T, Lillington G A, Mayne J G 1970 Pleural fluid in systemic lupus erythematosus. Proceedings of the Mayo Clinic 45:409
Cepellini R, Polli C, Calada F 1957 A DNA-reacting factor in serum of a patient with lupus erythematosus. Proceedings of their Society for Experimental Biology and Medicine 96:572
Chang R W 1982 Cardiac manifestations of SLE. Clinics in Rheumatic Diseases 8:197
Christian C L, Hatfield W B, Chase P H 1963 Systemic lupus erythematosus, cryoprecipitation of sera. Journal of Clinical Investigation 42:823
Cohen S A, Hughes G R V, Noel G L, Christian C L 1971 Character of anti-DNA antibodies in systemic lupus erythematosus. Clinical and Experimental Immunology 8:551
Dausset J, Colombani J, Colombani M 1961 Study of leukopenias and thrombocytopenias by the direct antiglobulin consumption test in leucocytes and/or platelets. Blood 18:672
Davis P, Atkins B C, Josse R G, Hughes G R V 1973 Criteria for the classification of SLE. British Medical Journal 3:88
Davis P, Atkins B, Hughes G R V 1974 Antibodies to native DNA in discoid lupus erythematosus. British Journal of Dermatology 91:175
Day N K, Geiger H, McLean R, Michael A, Good R A 1973 C2 deficiency. Development of lupus erythematosus. Journal of Clinical Investigation 52:1601
De Horatius R J, Messner R P 1975 Lymphocytotoxic antibodies in family members of patients with SLE. Journal of Clinical Investigation 55:1254
Derue G J, Englert H J, Harris E N, Gharavi A E, Morgan S H, Hull R G, Hughes G R V 1985 Abortion in systemic lupus: association with antiphospholipid antibodies. Journal of Obstetrics and Gynaecology 5: 107–109
Dimant J 1978 Computer analysis of factors influencing the appearance of aseptic necrosis in patients with SLE. Journal of Rheumatology 5:136
Donadio J V, Holley K E, Wagoner R D, Ferguson R H, McDuffie F C 1974 Further observations on the treatment of lupus nephritis with prednisone and combined prednisone and azathioprine. Arthritis and Rheumatism 17:573
Dubois E L 1974 Lupus erythematosus. USC Press
Dubois E L, Arterberry J D 1962 Gangrene as a manifestation of systemic lupus erythematosus. Journal of the American Medical Association 181:366
Dubois E L, Martel S 1956 Discoid lupus erythematosus: an analysis of its systemic manifestations. Annals of Internal Medicine 44:482
Elkon K B, Sewell J R, Ryan P F J, Hughes G R V 1980 Splenic function in non-renal systemic lupus erythematosus. American Journal of Medicine 69:80
Esscher E & Scott J S 1979 Congenital heart block and maternal SLE. British Medical Journal 1:1235
Estes D, Christian C L 1971 SLE A prospective analysis. Medicine 50:85
Estes D, Larson D L 1965 Systemic lupus erythematosus and pregnancy. Clinical Obstetrics and Gynaecology 8:307
Fielder A H L, Walport M J, Batchelor J R, et al 1983 British Medical Journal 286:425
Fulford K W M, Catterall R D, Delharty J J, Doniach D, Kremer M 1972 A collagen disorder of the nervous system presenting as multiple sclerosis. Brain 95:373
Gibson G J, Edmonds J P, Hughes G R V 1977 Diaphragm function and lung involvement in systemic lupus erythematosus. American Journal of Medicine 53:926
Gilliam J N, Sontheimer R D 1982 Skin manifestations of SLE. Clinics in Rheumatic Diseases 8:207
Ginzler E, Diamon H, Guttacauria M, Kaplan D 1976 Prednisolone and azathioprine compared to prednisone plus low-dose azathioprine and cyclophosphamide in the treatment of diffuse lupus nephritis. Arthritis and Rheumatism 19:693
Gladman D D, Urowitz M B 1980 Venous syndromes and pulmonary embolism in SLE. Annals of the Rheumatic Diseases 39:340
Gold W M, Jennings D B 1966 Pulmonary function in patients with systemic lupus erythematosus. Annual Review of Respiratory Diseases 93:556
Goldberg L S, Bresnihan B, Hughes G R V 1978 Lymphocytotoxic antibodies in SLE: evidence for reactivity with i antigen. Clinical and Experimental Immunology 31:443
Grigor R R, Lewkonia R M, Hawkins D F, Hughes G R V 1977 Pregnancy in SLE. Proceedings of the Royal Society of Medicine 70:99
Grigor R, Edmonds J, Lewkonia R, Bresnihan B, Hughes G R V 1978 SLE. A prospective analysis. Annals of the Rheumatic Diseases 37:121
Grimley P M, Decker J L, Michelitch H J, Frantz M M 1973 Abnormal structure in circulating lymphocytes from patients with SLE and related disease. Arthritis and Rheumatism 16:313
Grishman E, Purush J C, Lee S L, Chung J 1973 Renal biopsies in lung nephritis: correlation of electron microscopic findings with clinical course. Nephron 10:25
Haider Y S, Roberts W C 1981 Coronary arterial disease in SLE: quantification of degrees of narrowing in 22 necropsy patients (21 women) aged 16–37 years. American Journal of Medicine 70:775
Hanauer L B, Christian C L 1967 Studies of cryoproteins in SLE. Journal of Clinical Investigation 46:400
Hare W, MacKay I 1969 Thymic size in systemic lupus erythematosus. Archives of Internal Medicine 124:60
Hargraves M M, Richmond H, Morton R, 1948 Presentation

of two bone marrow elements: the 'tart' cell and the 'LE' cell. Mayo Clinic Proceedings 23:25
Harmon C E, Portanova J P 1982 Drug-induced lupus. Clinics in Rheumatic Diseases 8:121
Harris E N, Gharavi A E, Boey M L, Patel D M, Mackworth-Young C G, Loizou S, Hughes G R V 1983 Anticardiolipin antibodies: detection by radioimmunoassay and association with thrombosis in SLE. Lancet 2: 1211–1214
Harris E N, Gharavi A E, Asherson R A, Boey M L, Hughes G R V 1984 Cerebral infarction in systemic lupus; association with anticardiolipin antibodies. Clinical and Experimental Rheumatology 2: 47–51
Harvey A M, Shulman L E, Tumulty P A, Conley C L, Schoenrich E H 1954 Systemic lupus erythematosus: review of literature and clinical analysis of 138 cases. Medicine 33:291
Hehir M, Sewell J, Hughes G R V 1979 Lymphoma in a patient with SLE receiving long-term azathioprine. Annals of the Rheumatic Diseases 38:94
Hughes G R V 1971 Significance of anti-DNA antibodies in SLE. Lancet 2:861
Hughes G R V 1973a Immunological factors in systemic lupus erythematosus. In: 9th Symposium of Advanced Medicine 67. Walker J C (ed), Pitman, London
Hughes G R V 1973b Annotation: the diagnosis of systemic lupus erythematosus. British Journal of Haematology 25:409
Hughes G R V 1975 Antinuclear antibodies in SLE — clinical and pathological significance. Clinics in Rheumatic Diseases 1
Hughes G R V (1980) CNS lupus: Diagnosis and treatment. Journal of Rheumatology 7:405
Hughes G R V 1982a The Treatment of SLE: The case for conservative management. Clinics in Rheumatic Diseases 8: 299–313
Hughes G R V 1982b Hypotensive agents, betablockers and drug-induced lupus. British Medical Journal 284:936
Hughes G R V 1983 Thrombosis, abortion, cerebral disease and the lupus anticoagulant. British Medical Journal 287: 1088–1089
Hughes G R V 1984 Autoantibodies and connective tissue diseases. (The 1983 Prosser White Oration). Clinical and Experimental Dermatology 9:535
Hughes G R V, Ryan P F J 1980 Conference report. Plasma exchange. Annals of the Rheumatic Diseases 39:95
Hughes G R V, Cohen S A, Christian C L 1971 Anti-DNA activity in systemic lupus erythematosus. A diagnostic and therapeutic guide. Annals of the Rheumatic Diseases 30:259
Hughes G R V, Rynes R I, Gharavi A, Ryan P F J, Mansilla R 1981 The heterogeneity of serologic findings and predisposing host factors in drug-induced lupus erythematosus. Arthritis and Rheumatism 24:1070
Hurd E R, Gigenbrodt E, Worthen H, Strunk S S, Ziff M 1971 Glomerular cytoplasmic structures in renal biopsies of patients with systemic lupus erythematosus and other diseases. Arthritis and Rheumatism 14:539
Inman R D 1978 Current comment: Immunologic sex differences and the female predominance in SLE. Arthritis and Rheumatism 21:849
Johnson R T, Richardson E P 1968 The neurological manifestations of systemic lupus erythematosus. Medicine 47:337
Jones J V 1982 Plasmapheresis in SLE. Clinics in Rheumatic Diseases 8:243
Kay D M, Tuffanelli D C 1969 Immunofluorescent techniques in clinical diagnosis of cutaneous disease. Annals at Internal Medicine 71:753
Keefe E B, Bardana E J, Harbeck R J, Pirofsky B, Carr R I 1974 Lupus meningitis. Antibody to DNA and DNA: anti DNA complexes in cerebrospinal fluid. Annals of Internal Medicine 80:58
Kimberley R P 1978 Renal prostaglandins in SLE. Lancet 2:553
Kimberley R P 1982 Pulse methylprednisolone in SLE. Clinics in Rheumatic Diseases 8:261
Kimberley R P, Plotz P H 1977 Aspirin-induced depression of renal function. New England Journal of Medicine 296:418
Koffler D, Schur P H, Kunkel H G 1967 Immunological studies concerning the nephritis of systemic lupus erythematosus. Journal of Experimental Medicine 126:607
Koffler D, Schur P H, Kunkel H G 1969 Variable patterns of immunoglobulin and complement deposition in the kidneys of patients with SLE. American Journal of Pathology 56:305
Kraus S J, Haserick J R, Lantz M A 1970 Fluorescent treponemal antibody-absorption test reactions in lupus erythematosus. New England Journal of Medicine 282:1287
Lanham J G, Hughes G R V 1982 Antimalarial therapy in SLE. Clinics in Rheumatic Diseases 8:279
Lanham J G, et al 1980 CRP levels in SLE — a classification criterion? Arthritis and Rheumatism 23:6
Lanham J G, Barrie T, Kohner E M, Hughes G R V 1982 SLE retinopathy: evaluation by fluorescein angiography. Annals of Rheumatic Diseases 41:473
Lanham J, Walport M, Hughes G R V Congenital heart block and connective tissue disease. Journal of Rheumatology 10: 823–825
Larsson D 1963 Thymoma and systemic lupus erythematosus in the same patient. Lancet 2:665
Leonhardt E T G 1964 Family studies in SLE. Acta Medica Scandinavica (Suppl 416) 176:5
Lewis R M, Schwartz R S, Henry W B 1965 Canine systemic lupus erythematosus. Blood 25:143
Lewis R M, Andre-Schwartz, Harris G S, Hirsch M S, Black P H, Schwartz R S 1973 Canine systemic lupus erythematosus. Transmission of serologic abnormalities by cell-free filtrates. Journal of Clinical Investigation 52:1893
Lewkonia R M, Barth P T, Hale G M, Hughes G R V 1977 Specificity and clinical relevance of antibodies to double-stranded DNA. Annals of the Rheumatic Diseases 36 (Suppl):114
Lightfoot R W Jr, Hughes G R V 1976 Significance of persisting serologic abnormalitis in SLE. Arthritis and Rheumatism 19:837
Lightfoot R W Jr, Lotke P A 1972 Osteonecrosis of metacarpal heads in SLE. Value of radiostrontium scintimetry in different diagnosis. Arthritis and Rheumatism 15:486
Lovy M, et al 1980 Hyposplenism in SLE. Journal of Rheumatology 7:760
Lovy M, Ryan P, Hughes G R V 1981 Concurrent SLE & salmonellosis. Journal of Rheumatology 8: 605.
Lubbe W F, Butler W S, Palmers S J, Liggins G C 1983 Fetal survival after prednisolone suppression of maternal lupus-anticoagulant. Lancet 1: 1361–1362
McKenzie A H 1981 Ocular safety of huge cumulative

antimalarial dosage. Arthritis and Rheumatism 24 (Suppl):570
Miescher, P, Strassle R 1957 New serological methods for detection of LE factor. Vox Sang 2:283
Miescher P, Fauconnet M, Berand T 1953 Experimental immunonucleophagocytosis and the LE phenomenon. Experimental Medicine and surgery 11:173
Miller K B, Schwartz R S 1979 Familial abnormalities of suppressor-cell function in SLE. New England Journal of Medicine 301:803
Mola E M, Gharavi A E, Joshi V R, Patel B M, Colaco C B, Hughes G R V 1983 Enhancement of cryoprecipitation from hypotonic serum: a comparative study in normals and in patients with connective tissue diseases. Clinical and Experimental Rheumatology 1:35
Mongan E S, Leddy J P, Atwater E C, Barnett E V 1967 Direct antiglobulin (Coombs) reactions in patients with connective tissue disease. Arthritis and Rheumatism 10:502
Morley K D, Hughes G R V 1981 Thrombocytopenia and anti Ro. Lancet 2:940
Morley K D, Hughes G R V 1982 Systemic lupus erythematosus: two patients treated with Danozol. British Medical Journal 284:1431
Natali P G, Tan E M 1972 Experimental renal disease induced by DNA anti DNA immune complexes. Journal of Clinical Investigation 51:345
Natali P G, Tan E M 1973 Experimental skin lesions in mice resembling systemic lupus erythematosus. Arthritis and Rheumatism 16:579
Osler W 1904 Manifestations of the erythema group of skin diseases. American Journal of Medical Science 127:1
Paget S A, Bukley B N, Brauer L E, Seningen R 1975 Mitral valve disease of SLE: a cause of severe congestive heart failure reversed by valve replacement. American Journal of Medicine 59:134
Pepys M B, Lanham J G, de Beer F C 1982 C-Reactive protein in SLE. Clinics in Rheumatic Diseases 8:91
Petz L D, Sharp G C, Cooper N R, Irwin W S 1971 Serum and cerebrospinal fluid complement and serum autoantibodies in systemic lupus erythematosus. Medicine 50:259
Pincus T 1971 Immunochemical conditions affecting the measurement of DNA antibodies using ammonium sulphate precipitation. Arthritis and Rheumatism 14:623
Pincus T 1976 The role of C-type particles in the pathogenesis of SLE. In: Hughes G R V (ed) Modern topics in rheumatology. Heinemann, London
Pincus T, Schur P H, Rose J A, Decker J L, Talal N 1969 Measurement of serum DNA-binding activity in SLE. New England Journal of Medicine 281:701
Phillips P E, Christian C L 1970 Myxovirus antibody increases in human connective tissue diseases. Science 168:982
Pollak V E, Pirani C L, Schwartz F 1964 Natural history of the renal manifestations of systemic lupus erythematosus. Journal of Laboratory and Clinical Medicine 63:537
Quimby F W Schwartz R S 1982 Systemic lupus erythematosus in mice and dogs. In: Lachmann P, Peters D K (eds) Clinical aspects of immunology, 4th Edn. Blackwell, Oxford, p. 1217–1230
Rabinowitz Y, Dameshek W 1960 SLE after 'idiopathic' thrombocytopenic purpura. Annals of Internal Medicine 52:1
Reichlin M 1976 Mixed connective tissue disease. In: Hughes G R V (ed) Topics in rheumatology. Heinemann, London
Robbins W C, Holman H R, Deicher H, Kunkel H G 1957 Complement fixation with cell nuclei and DNA in lupus erythematosus. Proceedings of the Society of Experimental Biology 96:575
Rothfield N F, Ross H A, Minta J O, Lepow I H 1972 Glomerular and dermal deposition of properdin in systemic lupus erythematosus. New England Journal of Medicine 287: 681
Schur P H 1975 Complement in lupus. Clinics in Rheumatic Diseases 1: 51a
Schur P H, Sandson J 1968 Immunologic factors and clinical activity in systemic lupus erythematosus. New England Journal of Medicine 278:533
Seaman W E, Plotz P H 1976 Effect of aspirin on liver tests in patients with RA or SLE and in normal volunteers. Arthritis and Rheumatism 19:155
Sergent J S, Lochshin M D, Klempner M S, Lipsky B A 1975 Central nervous system disease in SLE. American Journal of Medicine 58:644
Seligmann M 1957 Mise en evidence dans le serum de malades de lupus erythematosus dissemine d'une substance determinant une reaction de precipitation avec l'acide desoxyribonucleique. CR Academy of Sciences (Paris) 245:243
Shearn M A 1959 The heart in SLE. American Heart Journal 58: 452
Sharp G C, Irwin W S, Tan E M, Gould R G, Holman H R 1972 Mixed connective tissue disease. An apparently distinct rheumatic disease syndrome associated with a specific antibody to an extractable nuclear antigen (ENA). American Journal of Medicine 52:148
Shulman H J, Christian C L 1969 Aortic insufficiency in systemic lupus erythematosus. Arthritis and Rheumatism 12:138
Shrank A B, Doniach D 1963 Discoid lupus erythematosus. Correlation of clinical features with serum autoantibody pattern. Archives of Dermatology 87:677
Siegel M, Lee S L 1973 The epidemiology of systemic lupus erythematosus. Seminars in Arthritis and Rheumatism 3:1
Sonnenblick M, Abraham A S 1978 Ibuprofen sensivity in SLE. British Medical Journal 1:619
Sontheimer R D, Stastny P, Gilliam J N 1981 HLA associations in subacute cutaneous lupus erythematosus. Journal of Clinical Investigation 67:312
Spaeth G L 1967 Corneal staining in systemic lupus erythematosus. New England Journal of Medicine 276:1168
Staples P J, Gerding D N, Decker J L, Gordon R S 1974 Incidence of infection in systemic lupus erythematosus. Arthritis and Rheumatism 17:1
Stastny P, Ziff M 1969 Cold-insoluble complexes and complement levels in SLE. New England Journal of Medicine 280:1376
Steinberg A D, Pincus T, Talal N 1971 The pathogenesis of autoimmunity in New Zealand mice 3. Factors influencing the formation of antinucleic acid antibodies. Immunology 20: 523
Talal N 1982 Sex hormones and modulation of immune response in SLE. Clinics in Rheumatic Diseases 8:23
Tan E M 1976 Sunlight as a potential aetiological factor in systemic lupus erythematosus. In: Hughes G R V (ed) Modern topics in rheumatology. Heinemann, London
Tan E M, Kunkel H G 1966 An immunofluorescent study of the skin lesions in SLE. Arthritis and Rheumatism 9:37
Travers R, Hughes G R V 1978a Salicylate hepatotoxicity in

SLE: a common occurrence? British Medical Journal 2:1532
Travers R, Hughes G R V 1978b Oral contraceptive therapy and SLE. Journal of Rheumatology 5:448
Turner-Stokes L, Turner-Warwick M 1982 Intrathoracic manifestations of SLE. In: Clinics in Rheumatic Diseases 8:229
Walport M J, Black C M, Batchelor J R 1982 The immunogenetics of SLE. In: Clinics in Rheumatic Diseases 8:3
Walport M J, Hubbard W N, Hughes G R V 1982 Reversal of aplastic anaemia secondary to SLE by high dose intravenous cyclophosphamide. British Medical Journal 285:769
Wasner C, Fries J F 1978 Treatment decisions in SLE. Arthritis and Rheumatism 21:601
Whaley K, Hughes G R V, Webb J 1976 Systemic lupus erythematosus in man and animals. In: Buchanan W W, Dick W C (ed) Recent advances in rheumatology-2. Churchill Livingstone, Edinburgh
Wilson W, Hughes G R V 1976 Immunosuppressives in the rheumatic diseases. In: Hughes G R V (ed) Modern topics in rheumatology. Heinemann, London
Winfield J B, Koffler, D, Kunkel H G 1975 Specific concentration of polynucleotide immune complexes in the cryoprecipitates of patients with SLE. Journal of Clinical Investigation 56:563
Winfield J B, Winchester R J, Wernet P, Fu S M, Kunkel H B 1976 Nature of cold-reactive antibodies to lymphocyte surface determinants in systemic lupus erythematosus. Arthritis and Rheumatism 18:1
Wolf S M, Barrows H S 1966 Myasthenia gravis and systemic lupus erythematosus. Archives of Neurology 14:253
Worlledge S 1967 Autoimmunity and blood diseases. Practitioner 199:171
Zurier R B 1975 SLE and pregnancy. Clinics in Rheumatology 1:613

B.M. Ansell

Polymyositis and dermatomyositis

Copemans text RH Diseases

J TScott '86

Polymyositis and dermatomyositis comprise a group of disorders in which there is a diffuse non-suppurative inflammation of striated muscle; in dermatomyositis there are, in addition, characteristic skin manifestations. The association with skin manifestations was first described by Univerricht in 1887; it has only been in the last 20 years or so that the frequency of inflammatory lesions of muscle without typical or with atypical dermal lesions has been appreciated. In adult life dermatomyositis, and to a lesser extent polymyositis, can be associated with malignancy.

Classification has been controversial (Pearson & Currie, 1974; Dawkins, 1977) and it is still not entirely satisfactory but much of the recent literature has used that suggested by Bohan & Peter (1975) based on the earlier work of Pearson (1966) (Table 54.1). Myositis may be an important part of other collagen vascular diseases, notably systemic lupus erythematosus (Isenberg et al, 1981; Ch. 53) and overlap or mixed connective tissue disease (Ch. 50) as well as scleroderma (Medsger et al, 1968; Ch. 55); rheumatoid arthritis itself is associated with only a nodular myositis which does not cause symptoms; treatment with penicillamine can induce polymyositis (Doyle et al, 1983; Nishikai et al, 1974). All these conditions are characterised by abnormal electromyograms, raised creatine phosphokinase and typical myositic histological features, although occasionally in systemic lupus erythematosus a vacuolar myositis is seen (Pearson & Yamasaka, 1958). In polyarteritis histological changes may be present in muscles without any symptoms or there may be a diffuse muscle-aching as part of the general disease. Very occasionally giant cell arteritis affecting the muscles is symptomatic.

Table 54.1 Classification of polymyositis (after Bohan & Peter, 1975)

Group	Type
1	Primary idiopathic polymyositis
2	Primary idiopathic dermatomyositis
3	Dermatomyositis/polymyositis in association with neoplasia
4	Childhood dermatomyositis/polymyositis
5	Polymyositis/dermatomyositis associated with collagen vascular disease

In older patients it is also important to exclude polymyalgia rheumatica as although the predominant symptom is stiffness rather than weakness, disuse can lead to muscle wasting. Here investigations such as electromyography, creatine phosphokinase and muscle biopsy which are all normal are helpful (Ch. 51). Other conditions in which myositis itself may present include sarcoidosis; this can only be distinguished by the presence of typical granulomatous changes in the muscle biopsy (Silverstein & Silzbach, 1969; Douglas et al, 1973). Other clinical features will suggest the underlying diagnosis. Rarely, infestations such as trichinosis and infections such as toxoplasmosis cause muscle pain and weakness. Thyrotoxic myopathy can mimic polymyositis; it tends to affect middle-aged men when weakness and wasting is profound with relatively little pain; appropriate tests of thyroid function will differentiate this form of muscle disease. In general, in endocrine disorders such as Addison's disease, Cushing's syndrome and hypopituitarism, muscle weakness is usually a secondary feature and the diagnosis self-evident. The same is also true of hyperparathyroidism and metabolic bone diseases which not infrequently show weakness of proximal limb muscles. Diabetic amyotrophy tends to give anterior thigh pain and quadriceps-wasting rather than a more diffuse syndrome; carcinomatous neuromyopathy produces a proximal motor weakness and neurological signs are present in addition. It is said to occur particularly in carcinoma of the lung or breast (Croft & Wilkinson, 1963).

In childhood, subacute polymyositis has to be differentiated from muscular dystrophy when minor skin changes are helpful, while in dystrophy there is a selective pattern of muscular weakness, slow onset and progressive unremitting course; the muscles involved, and often the family history are helpful. Creatinine phosphokinase is of no help as it can be very high in certain types of muscular dystrophy. Acute polymyositis must be distinguished from paroxysmal myoglobinuria. This occurs particularly in childhood, although it is occasionally seen in adult life, when it is most likely to occur following exercise (McArdle, 1963); in this condition the attacks are recurrent. Another problem in childhood is the rare presentation of dermatomyositis with arthalgia and/or tendon nodules. This then needs differentiating from scleroderma and juvenile chronic arthritis (Ansell & Bywaters, 1962).

AETIOLOGY

Lymphocyte infiltration around and within degenerating muscle fibres suggests an immunological basis. Most patients have normal complement levels, although typical dermatomyositis has been reported in the presence of congenital C2 deficiency (Leddy et al, 1975), a few patients will have a rise in immunoglobulins, while antibodies to nuclear antigens have been reported in variable concentrations but these are without diagnostic specificity. Since Reichlin & Mattioli (1976) first described serological reactions characteristic of polymyositis, considerable work on the heterogeneity of the precipitating antibodies has been performed. Thus Wolfe et al (1977) described an antinuclear antibody with distinct specificity for polymyositis, while Venables and his colleagues (1981) noted that anti-RNP was the main antibody detected, and that neither anti-RNP or anti-DNA antibodies defined a distinct clinical entity or excluded malignant disease. The Jo-1 antibody system seems the most consistently described, occurring in the order of 30% of patients with polymyositis, much less commonly in dermatomyositis and not in controls; it is also found in considerable frequency in the overlap syndrome (MCTD). Irrespective of race or clinical subgroup all anti-Jo-1-positive patients either had HLA-DR3 or HLA-DRw6 or both (Arnett et al, 1981). The relevance of the antibody systems being described remains, as yet, uncertain.

Peripheral blood lymphocytes from active untreated cases of myositis have been shown to have direct cytotoxic effects on muscle cell cultures derived from human fetal and from animal sources (Currie et al, 1971; Dawkins & Mastaglia, 1973), while Johnson et al (1972) have shown that lymphocytes from such patients release lymphotoxins during incubation with autologous muscle tissue. The effector population of lymphocytes in polymyositis has not been identified so that in vitro measurement of myotoxicity has been difficult to perform. A sensitive in vitro muscle cell killing, utilising carnitine which cannot be synthesised by cardiac and skeletal muscle so that it is preferentially taken up from the culture by the myotubes, has been developed by Cambridge & Stern (1981) and provides the first reasonably specific test for myotoxicity. Using monoclonal markers to a variety of human leucocyte antigens Rowe et al (1981) have demonstrated the presence of large numbers of T-lymphocytes in the infiltrates of polymyositis patients: these observations support the importance of cell-mediated mechanisms in the aetiology of this disorder. However, in children with dermatomyositis the possibility that muscle injury is the result of immune complex deposition in the vessel wall has not been excluded. Whitaker & Engle (1972) were able to demonstrate immunoglobulin and complement deposited in the vessel walls of skeletal muscles in 9 of 11 children with dermatomyositis, 3 of 12 adults with dermatomyositis and 2 of 7 adults with polymyositis. A larger number of vessels with positive immunofluorescence was seen in childhood dermatomyositis than in adult.

Precipitating factors

There is no known precipitating factor. Photosensitisation is common in dermatomyositis and exposure to sunlight may initiate an eruption on the face, arms or legs. Drug hypersensitivity can occasionally be incriminated, the most recent reports relating to penicillamine (Doyle et al, 1983) while viral infections have received particular attention (Isaacson, 1967). Severe transient myositis in children has been documented following influenza (Middleton et al, 1970; Dietzman et al, 1974). Electron-microscopic studies have demonstrated nuclear and cytoplasmic structures resembling many different viruses, e.g. Coxsackie (Mastaglia & Walton, 1970), myxovirus (Chou, 1968; Sato et al, 1971), picornavirus (Chou & Gutman, 1970). In the dermatomyositis seen in hypogammaglobulinaemia, with histological findings identical to idiopathic myositis, echovirus has been grown from muscle and CSF (Webster et al, 1978). In adults, malignancy and dermatomyositis, and to a lesser extent polymyositis, have been linked since the 1950s (Williams, 1959). Arundell et al (1960) give an incidence of 34.2% which is higher than is generally quoted (Callen, 1982). The muscle disease often precedes any obvious symptoms of tumour and the courses of the dermatomyositis and the malignancy may not follow each other. In nearly all cases the neoplasm has been a carcinoma, particularly lung, prostate, female genitalia, breast or large intestine, although occasionally a reticulosis, thymoma or myeloma have been recorded (Beck, 1968). The exact nature of the relationship between malignancy and dermatomyositis has escaped elucidation.

INCIDENCE

Polymyositis and dermatomyositis can develop at any age, but most commonly between 30 and 60 years with females being affected twice as commonly as males (Barwick & Walton, 1963); in those over 40 associated with malignancy, the female predominance is less marked. The frequency of these disorders is unknown; Rose & Walton (1966), found 89 new cases over a 12-year span, 1954–1965, from an estimated region of 3.3 million persons. The suggested incidence of 0.5 per 100 000 could well be an underestimate.

MANIFESTATIONS

The most common presenting symptom is muscular weakness affecting particularly the legs and occurs in more than 50%; skin rash accounts for a further 24%, while joint or muscle pain or features such as fever, general fatigue and Raynaud's phenomenon make up the remainder (Walton & Adams, 1958). Not only is the early clinical picture of polymyositis variable in form, but also in its rate of onset and progression of symptoms. Muscle weakness is present in all cases, and in its absence a clinical diagnosis cannot be made with certainty. In the acute case this may come on very rapidly with severe constitutional symptoms, oedematous skin rash and rapid loss of strength, whereas in the subacute or chronic case it comes on slowly, usually affecting the lower limbs first. This causes the gradual development of weakness in the pelvic musculature with increasing difficulty in getting out of a chair. Later it may become difficult for the patient to climb up and down stairs, get up from the floor, or out of a bath; there is also a tendency to fall, with difficulty in rising without assistance. After the onset of weakness in the pelvic girdle, there tends to be loss of strength in the shoulder girdle muscles and ultimately there may be weakness of the anterior neck muscles so that the patient cannot raise his head from the pillow, and weakness of back muscles so that he cannot sit up unaided. Involvement of the posterior pharyngeal muscles gives a picture of partial bulbar palsy with dysphagia and dysphonia and often a marked nasal voice. In rapidly advancing cases, or in severe long-standing cases, progressive involvement of the respiratory muscles can prove fatal (Medsger et al, 1971). Initially in a few cases there is also muscle pain, tenderness and induration; these are most often seen in association with skin lesions. As the disease advances or persists, contractures or shortening of muscles tend to develop. This can involve the biceps brachialis, producing contractures at the elbows; the wrist flexors, preventing full extension of the wrists without flexion of the fingers; and the hamstrings and quadriceps, causing contractures at hips and knees. Atrophy of muscles is a late event.

The typical rash of dermatomyositis is ultimately seen in about 40% of patients, while atypical skin lesions varying from a hide-bound apparent thickening mimicking systemic sclerosis or widespread dermal atrophy, to a transient erythema or a scaling eruption mimicking eczema, occurs in a further 20%. Usually in conjunction with active muscle disease, there are dusky red patches which are slightly elevated, smooth or scaly over the elbows and on the knuckles (Fig. 54.1), knees and medial malleoli. Eventually these areas become shiny, red and somewhat atrophic and the skin tends to flake; these are fequently referred to as 'collodion patches' (Fig. 54.2). The typical facial rash of dermatomyositis consists of a dusky heliotrope eruption in the periorbital region and occasionally on the forehead (Fig. 54.3); involvement of neck, shoulders and front and back of chest may occur. On the upper eyelids a dusky suffusion can be seen, at times accompanied by telangiectasia. In conjunction with the facial ery-

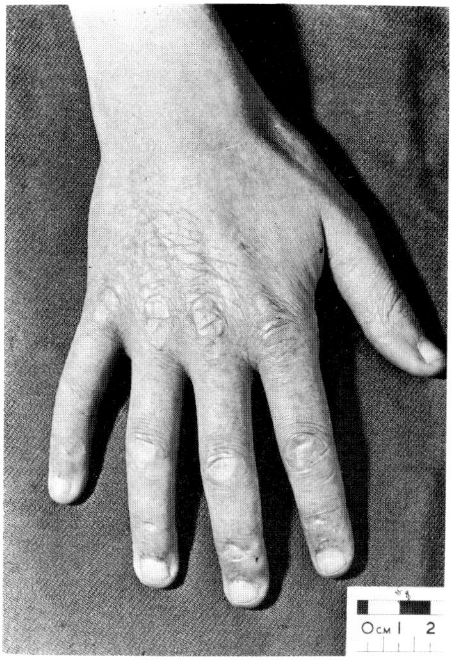

Fig. 54.2 Typical collodion patches over metacarpal and interphalangeal joints.

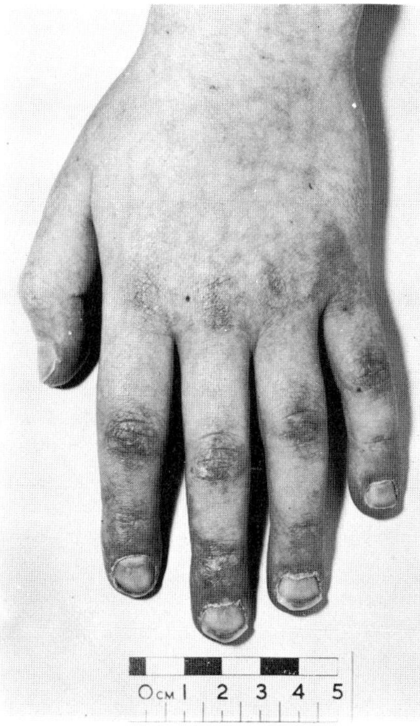

Fig. 54.1 Dusky patches over the proximal interphalangeal joints, and to a lesser extent metacarpophalangeal and terminal interphalangeal joints in acute dermatomyositis.

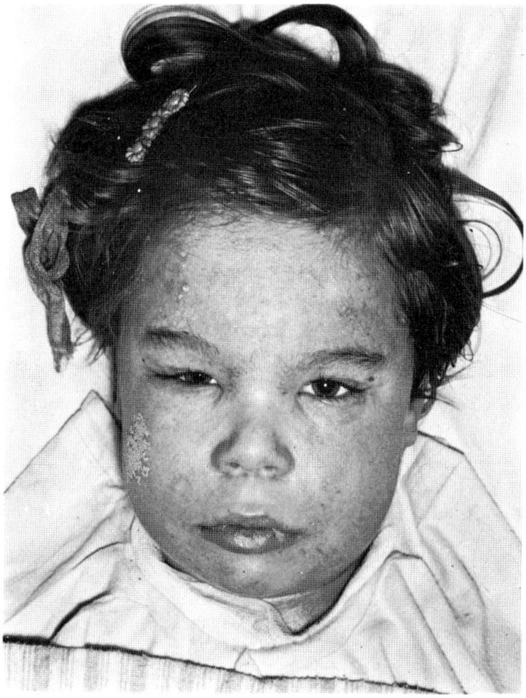

Fig. 54.3 Facial appearance in a child with acute dermatomyositis; note the oedema together with generalised rash.

thema, a scaly rash may occur on the extensor surface of the forearms, and down the front of the legs, again purplish in colour. If the rash is acute there may be intradermal and subcutaneous oedema. Around the nail beds there is characteristic telangiectasia (Fig. 54.4). While usually muscle and joint changes go hand in hand, occasionally one sees maximal skin changes with minimal muscle changes; Pearson & Currie (1974) have recorded typical skin changes in two patients without evidence of muscle involvement.

Other features include Raynaud's phenomenon which occurs in about one-third of patients, and mild or transitory arthritis has been recorded in about one-third of cases. Thus, acute arthralgia or even arthritis may initially make one suspect systemic lupus erythematosus or early rheumatoid arthritis rather than polymyositis. Very rarely the articular symptoms are present for one or more years before muscular weakness appears (Pearson, 1959). Dysphagia is recorded in nearly 30% of cases. There would appear to be two components, weakness of the pharyngeal muscles and hypomotility of the oesophagus (Donoghue et al, 1960); only rarely has oesophageal stricture been recorded. Small bowel disease, identical to that seen in scleroderma, has been recorded in 3 of 200 patients (Pearson & Currie, 1974).

Other visceral manifestations recorded include those involving the cardiac muscle which causes non-specific T-wave changes and even heart block (Schaumburg et al., 1971; Fernandez-Herlihy, 1971), with ultimately typical pathological changes

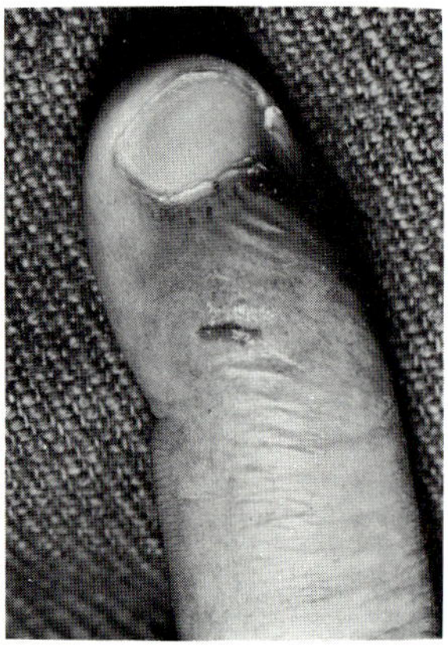

Fig. 54.4 Telangiectasia at the nail edge.

(Walton & Adams, 1958; Askari & Huettner, 1982; Denbow, 1979). Occasionally pericarditis is observed. Pulmonary involvement appears to be of two types, an acute infiltrative lesion occurring in an active phase of the disease and associated with rapid improvement on corticosteroids, and a chronic fibrosing alveolitis (Duncan et al, 1974). Renal involvement is extremely rare, but Kagen (1971) has drawn attention to myoglobin in the serum in active cases, and one patient had renal failure due to myoglobinuria. Ocular and nervous system defects have also been reported, but these are also extremely rare (Susac et al, 1973).

CHILDHOOD DERMATOMYOSITIS

The two specific features which set this type in a separate class are the presence of vasculitis (Banker, 1975) and the late development of calcinosis. Girls are affected more commonly than boys; the onset has been recorded as young as 14 months, although usually it affects slightly older children most commonly between the 4th and 10th birthday (Cook et al, 1963; Wedgewood et al, 1953).

The onset is acute in 50% and those who start slowly can pass into an acute phase; those with an insidious onset may slowly progress to severe contractures, or recover, leaving residua such as calcinosis. In childhood a rash nearly always occurs and, together with weakness, is the usual presenting feature. Pain is much more common than in adults, as is oedema, not just of the face and over muscles, but also of the hands and feet. In acute cases this is associated with fever, loss of weight and general malaise (Cook et al, 1963; Schaller, 1973). Banker & Victor (1966) pointed out the high incidence of vasculitis in these children and this may well account for the very high incidence of serious skin ulceration (Fig. 54.5). The mucous membranes can be involved; dysphagia and ulceration of the oesophagus is relatively common; ulceration in other parts of the intestine as an infarction can give rise to abdominal pain, haematemesis and melaena. Death from perforations of these lesions is still occasionally seen. Retinitis, characterised by extensive exudative deposition mimicking the cytoid bodies of systemic lupus erythematosus with haemorrhages, is well recognised

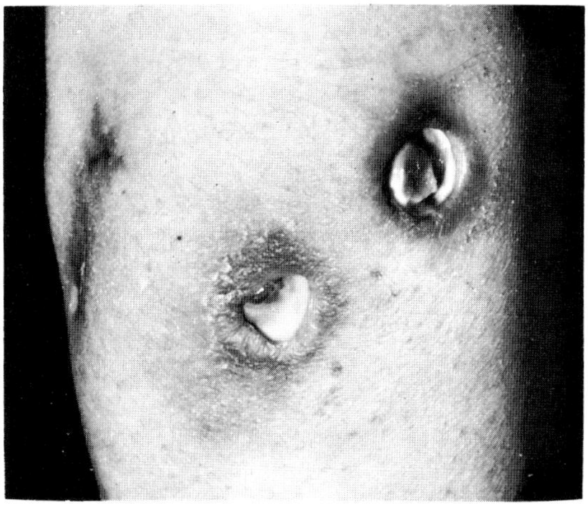

Fig. 54.5 Severe ulceration around the elbows in a boy of 14.

(Fruman et al, 1976). Acute pulmonary manifestations can occur (Dubowitz & Dubowitz, 1964), as can myocardial involvement. Winkelman (1982) has suggested that these constitute a separate group with poor response to corticosteroids. However our more recent experience suggests that such patients often respond to high dose corticosteroid with or without cytotoxic therapy, and that there is overlap with the more chronic form, which closely resembles adult dermatomyositis clinically.

Dermatomyositis in childhood can very occasionally be associated with other disorders; thus it has been recorded in leukaemia (Hanson & Kornreich, 1967) and also in hypogammaglobulinaemia (Gotoff et al, 1972; Webster et al, 1978). In this latter situation there appears to be marked oedema with severe induration of the tissues and relatively little rash; at post-mortem one such patient had extensive round cell infiltration of the liver which was thought to represent a malignant lymphoma (Page et al, 1963). With these exceptions, the prognosis in the childhood disease is better than in the adult form.

The actual duration of the acute phase varies from a few months, with complete reversal of the physical signs and symptoms, through recurrent periods of activity but eventual recovery over 2–3 years, to the very occasional continuation of activity over many years with extensive muscle-wasting, severe contractures and widespread calcinosis. Only very rarely is there a rapid progression to death, usually from respiratory failure, or complications of therapy. The severity of the vasculopathy in the pretreatment muscle biopsy may be of value in identifying those likely to have a prolonged and severe course (Crowe et al, 1982).

Calcinosis has been seen to occur in our childhood cases as early as 6 months after the onset of symptoms and as late as 15 years and has occurred in varying degrees (Sewell et al, 1978). It is a deposition of calcium salts in the connective tissue in the subcutaneous panniculus and fascial planes which can occur anywhere. It may be circumscribed, affecting the subcutaneous tissues predominantly and in only one site (Fig. 54.6), or multiple with small or large lesions which extrude through the skin giving rise to necrosis; this is particularly common on the buttocks (Fig. 54.7). It can also affect the fascial planes of the muscles (Fig. 54.8) and cause such extensive deposition that it has been decribed as calcinosis universalis.

There is usually no demonstrable alteration in serum levels of calcium, phosphate or alkaline phosphatase, although occasionally the last is transiently raised. Recent interest has centred on the increase in excretion of gamma carboxyglutamic

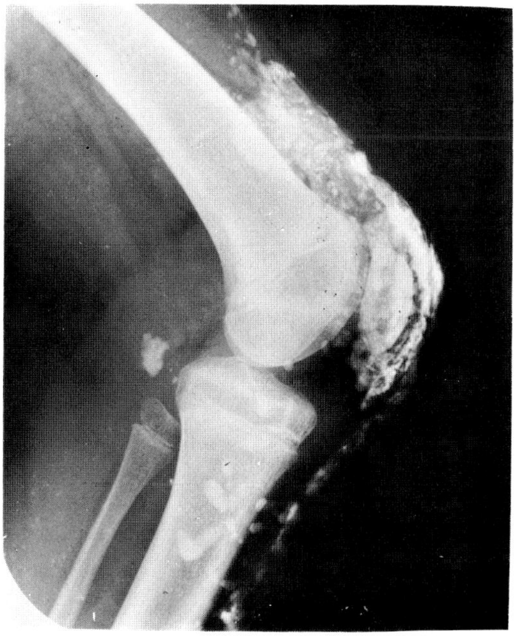

Fig. 54.6 Extensive calcinosis affecting particularly subcutaneous tissue.

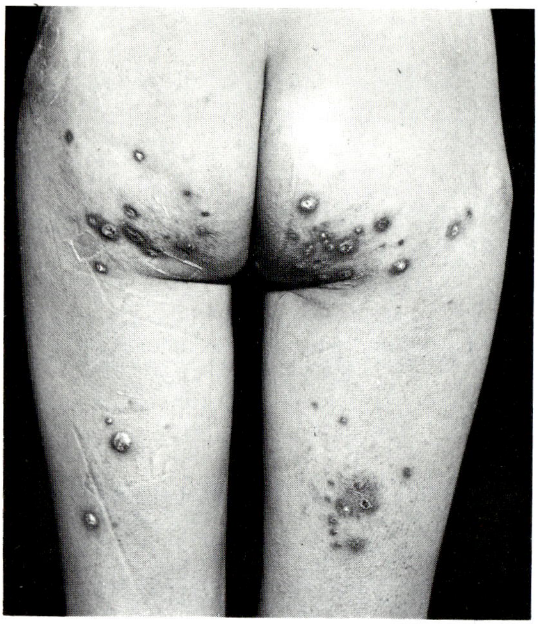

Fig. 54.7 Calcinosis in the subcutaneous tissue of buttocks and thighs, in places ulcerating through the skin.

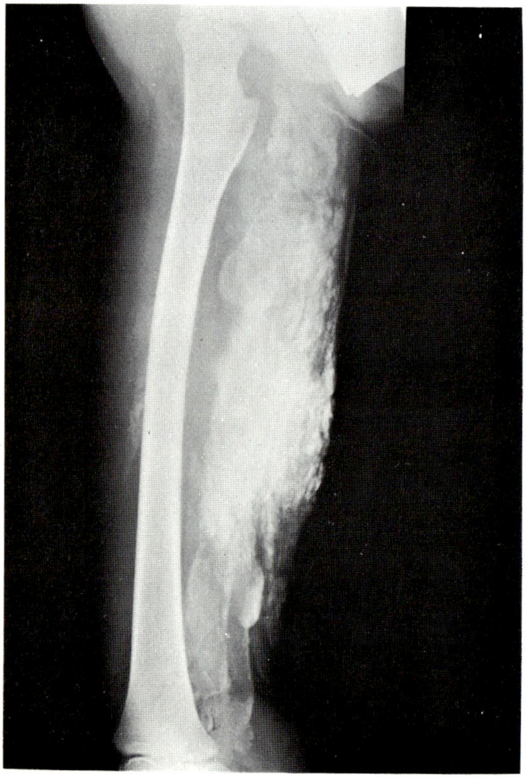

Fig. 54.8 Calinosis in the interfascial planes of the muscles and in subcutaneous tissues.

acid in children with dermatomyositis, which was three-fold that of controls in those with calcinosis (Lian et al, 1982). Histologically there may be fibrosis, some mild round cell infiltration with a few giant cells and fibroblast proliferation, but when the fascial planes of the muscles are severely involved secondary atrophy of muscle occurs (Fig. 54.9). When this calcinosis is extensive it can cause severe disability. Ultimately a patient who has become crippled as a result of muscle-wasting and calcinosis may succumb from inanition or bronchopneumona. In one of such cases the calcinosis was shown to contain 15 mg of calcium per 100 mg of wet weight (Loewi & Dorling, 1964); it has been identified by X-ray defractions as hydroxyapatite (Cochrane & Davis, 1965).

Comparing our patients whose dermatomyositis occurred under the age of 16 with a similar group in which it first developed over that age (Hamilton et al, 1970), the outstanding differences were the florid and severe rash, the high incidence of pain and oedema, as well as the rapid development of contractures in the young patients. Calcinosis, both in the subcutaneous and interfascial planes of the muscles, was seen in only 2 adults aged 21 and 23 at onset, but was extremely common in the juveniles. Anti-nuclear antibodies were detected in nearly half of the juveniles tested. The incidence of dysphagia, Raynaud's phenomenon and arthritis were similar, but radiological changes suggestive of previous erosion were confined to the children (Fig. 54.10). In some patients the late changes, both clinical and radiological, can mimic scleroderma (Fig. 54.10) (Sewell et al, 1978). Another

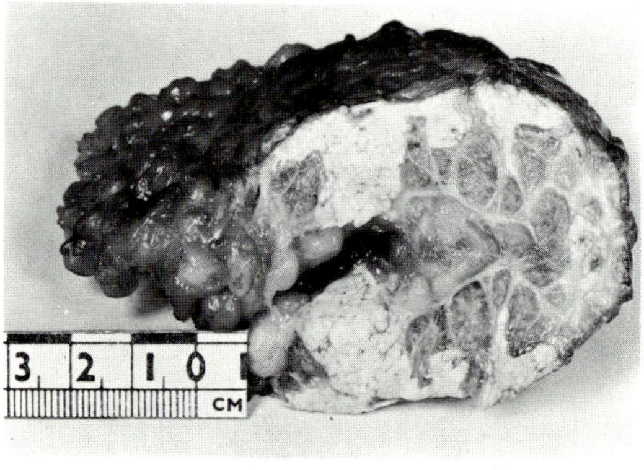

Fig. 54.9 Extensive calcinosis infiltrating the muscle.

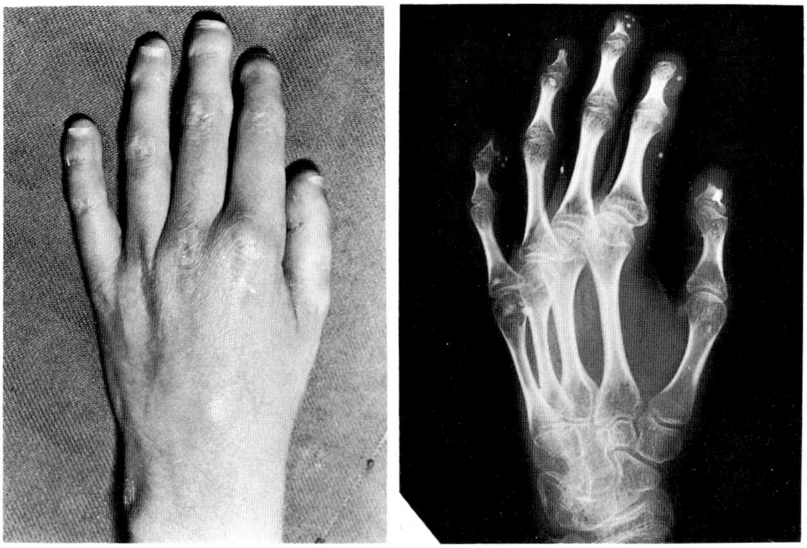

Fig. 54.10 (a) The clinical appearance with collodion patches but also atrophy of finger tips looking like scleroderma. These changes have developed over a 25-year period after a typical attack of dermatomyositis in the pre-corticosteroid era. (b) This shows carpal changes consistent with those seen in juvenile chronic arthritis. Note also changes mimicking scleroderma in that there is loss of terminal phalanges, and calcinosis.

feature of the juvenile group was the presence of tendon nodules. Presentation with tendon nodules and arthralgia or even frank arthritis, closely mimics juvenile arthritis and can be difficult to differentiate until typical rash or calcinosis develops (Ansell & Bywaters, 1962).

Prognosis

The prognosis varies with the age of onset of the symptoms and whether there is associated malignancy or not (Degos et al, 1971). In general the prognosis is worse in the older age-group, not only due to malignancy (Arundell et al, 1960), but also to heart and lung complications (Medsger et al, 1971). Children tend to do well and maintain their function (Sullivan et al, 1972) but there is the occasional child who deteriorates rapidly (Ansell et al, 1971). Of 18 juvenile patients studied for a mean of 18.5 years from diagnosis (Chalmers et al, 1982) 6 had some degree of residual weakness, but only 3 had residual disability and this was from flexion contractures and calcinosis. Recovery from the acute phase in childhood and young adult life may be followed by an appearance resembling scleroderma (Fig. 54.10), while at times calcinosis causes severe impairment of muscle function (Sewell et al, 1978). The alteration which corticosteroids have made in prognosis is borne out by comparison of cases; prior to corticosteroids mortality was in the order of 50%, but following the use of corticosteroids the mortality of those not associated with malignancy is in the order of 14% (Rose & Walton, 1966; Winkelmann et al, 1968).

Laboratory aspects

The ESR is normal in about half the cases; elevation is particularly common in acute cases and in such cases there is frequently a neutrophil leucocytosis. The most important blood investigation is serum creatine phosphokinase, as it is the most sensitive enzyme of muscle damage; in active disease the levels are usually high, falling when the condition responds to corticosteroid therapy, often before improvement is evident clinically; once chronic, with slow progression and much muscle fibrosis, the creatine phosphokinase may return to normal. Other serum enzymes such as aldolase, SGOT and SGPT may also be raised in the acute phase (Vignos & Goldwyn, 1972). Non-specific elevations of acute phase reactants include alpha-2 and gamma-globulins. Anti-nuclear antibodies are seen in a proportion; this is more common in children than adults (Pachman et al, 1980). Relatively rarely the Jo-1 antibodies are positive. Antibodies to DNA are negative and C3 is normal. Immune complexes may be seen in active juvenile dermatomyositis (Pachman et al, 1980). Electromyographically there is a characteristic triad of polymyositis

1. Spontaneous fibrillation and positive or saw-tooth potentials which are indistinguishable from those found in denervation and occur at complete rest
2. Polyphasic or short duration potentials which appear on voluntary contraction, of small amplitude and duration when compared with normal motor unit potentials
3. Salvos of repetitive potentials or 'pseudomotic-myotonic' chains of oscillations of high frequency which are evoked by mechanical stimulation of the nerve or movement of the electrode (Marinacci, 1965).

Histologically the muscle shows degeneration of muscle fibres, regenerative activity, infiltrates of chronic inflammatory cells, especially near blood vessels, phagocytosis of necrotic fibre substance, interstitial fibrosis and variation in cross sectional diameter of the adjacent muscle fibres (Figs 54.11, 54.12); the last two occur particularly in the advanced stages of acute polymyositis (Adams, 1973). Angiitis is a prominent feature of dermatomyositis in childhood (Banker & Victor, 1966; Banker, 1975), so that it is considered that the major abnormality in dermatomyositis in childhood is in the wall of the intramuscular blood vessels. The angiopathy results in multiple thrombus formation and infarction of muscle. The electron-microscopic features of polymyositis are gradually being delineated (Mastalgia & Walton, 1971; Banker, 1975).

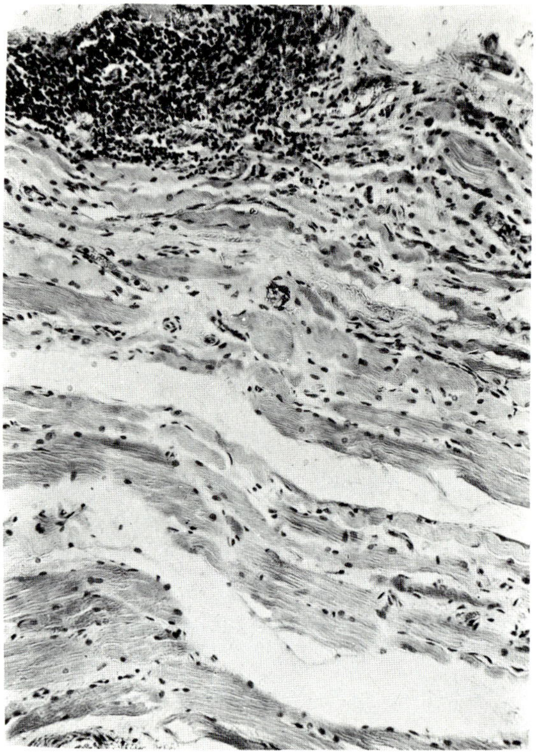

Fig. 54.11 Biopsy of muscle showing marked inflammatory infiltration. The muscle fibres show considerable variation in size with degeneration of fibres, some regeneration and fibrosis.

Management

During the acute phase of the disease bed-rest is imperative and only as strength returns should assisted exercises commence; care should be taken to avoid over-stretching weak and inflamed muscles. During this phase it is important that the limbs are maintained in a good position and the use of Plastazote or similar soft-type splinting is extremely valuable in avoiding the development of contractures. Once inflammation is subsiding a more active physiotherapeutic regime can be introduced. Special problems will require special management, e.g. a semisolid diet for dysphagia or a respirator for intercostal muscle weakness. That a routine malignancy search is of little value in ascertaining whether dermatomyositis is associated with neoplasm is suggested by the review of Callen (1982). However, a suspicious history, or signs on careful routine examination as well as basic laboratory tests are valuable, and if there is any suspicion, appropriate investigations including CAT scanning should be performed.

Corticosteroids proved to be the first effective therapy capable of suppressing disease activity in polymyositis and dermatomyositis and thereby altering the natural course of the disease. The initial

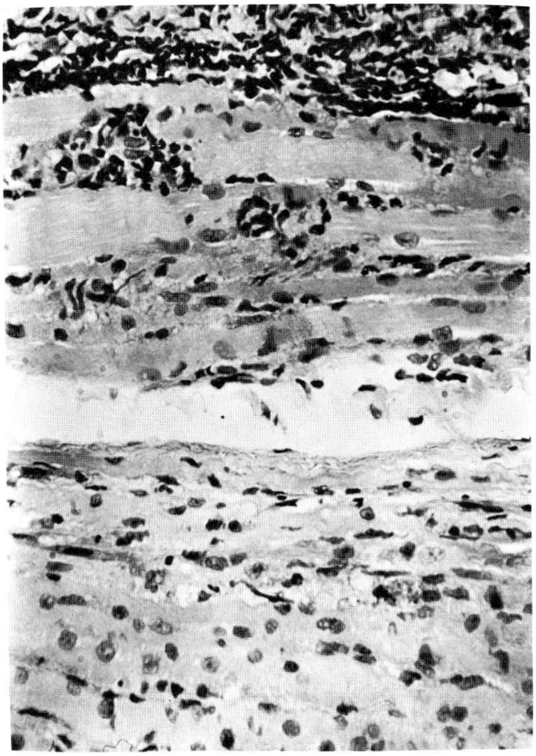

Fig. 54.12 A higher power section of the same muscle showing the perivascular cuffing with inflammatory cells, particularly mononuclears, the extensiveness of the infiltration and the marked variation in nuclear size in the muscles according to their state: note the very large nuclei in the regenerating fibres in the lower part of the section.

dose should be reasonably high, usually about 60 mg of prednisone daily in adults and perhaps 1–2 mg/kg daily in children. At times it may be necessary to go above this dosage level to bring the myositis under control, but as soon as this happens, every effort should be made to reduce the dosage. The place of alternate-day therapy is not yet certain; particularly in children, once the acute phase has been controlled it is desirable to reduce the dose on alternate days initially and finally get onto an alternate-day regime (Engel et al, 1971). Serial analysis of creatine phosphokinase levels is a useful guide, as is maintenance muscle strength and of vital capacity. If the disease does not appear to be responding to high dosage corticosteroid therapy, a search for malignancy should be instituted, even if the original screen was negative.

It has been suggested (Pearson, 1972) that complications of corticosteroid therapy are rare, but this has not been our experience, nor that of Benson & Aldo (1973) who drew attention to hypertension, diabetes and severe osteoporosis causing crush fractures of vertebrae. If these have occurred, or the patient has become unresponsive to corticosteroid therapy, immunosuppressive drugs should be considered irrespective of the presence of malignancy. The first of these drugs to receive particular attention was methotrexate (Malaviya et al, 1968). This can be given alone or in combination with corticosteroids. It was initially suggested as intravenous therapy in the order of 0.8 mg/kg bodyweight at weekly intervals, provided that prior to each weekly injection the blood count was satisfactory and there was no evidence of liver dysfunction. Subsequently oral therapy of 5 mg five days a week has been suggested (Sokolof et al, 1971). However, in addition to its effect on the liver and on the haemopoetic systemic, pruritis and pneumonitis have been recorded; Arnett et al (1973), when treating patients with unresponsive disease, noted that 2 of 5 developed lung problems. It is possible that the oral route does produce more toxicity than the intravenous route. Thus Metzger et al (1974a) treated 22 patients with intravenous methotrexate using from 0.5–0.8 mg/kg bodyweight given intravenously at intervals of 5–7 days and later spaced out at longer intervals; they noted that half the patients showed some minor degree of toxicity including stomatitis, sore throat, skin rash, purpura, fever and some gastrointestinal side-effects, but 75% benefitted.

The maximum effect appears to come in at about 10 weeks and continues; the intravenous route can be maintained for months if not years. Benson & Aldo (1973), using azathioprine in a dosage of 1.5–2 mg/kg body weight and adjusted just to depress the white blood count in patients who were either unresponsive to corticosteroids, or had developed side-effects, reported a favourable effect. This can be given orally with a fair degree of safety, although nausea and dyspepsia may be troublesome. In those young patients unresponsive to corticosteroids, or in those in whom side-effects from corticosteroids may call for their reduction or withdrawal, cyclophosphamide

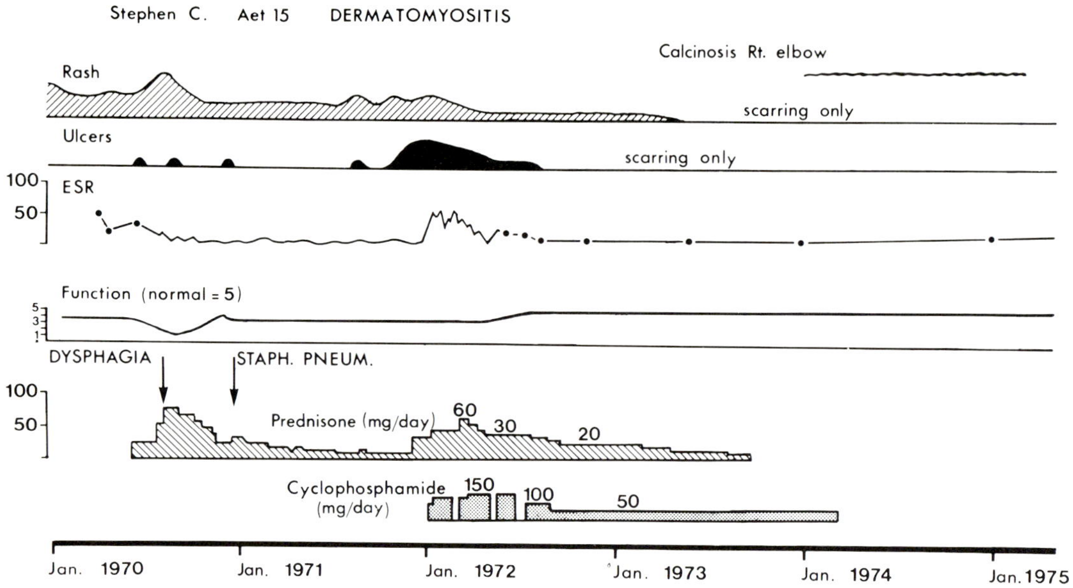

Fig. 54.13 Course of a boy whose illness was complicated initially by dysphagia, and subsequently severe ulcerating lesions and muscle weakness which responded on addition of cyclophosphamide to the basic regime of corticosteroids. He has no residual weakness, extensive skin scarring and some calcinotic lesions at one elbow.

has proved to be effective; a dosage of up to 4 mg/kg bodyweight has been used. In general this has been given orally in continuous therapy, gradually reducing as the patient improved (Fig. 54.13). Of 8 juvenile patients so treated, 2 relapses occurred after stopping cyclophosphamide, but recommencement of therapy led to improvement. Chlorambucil is equally effective. In adults not responding to 60 mg perdnisone over 1 month intensive immunosuppression with antilymphocyte globulin and azathioprine in addition to high dose steroid is valuable (Hollingworth et al, 1982). Total body irradiation has been reported to cause remission in at least 2 single patients with progressive polymyositis who had been unresponsive to other forms of treatment (Hubbard et al, 1982), while Brewer et al (1980) reported beneficial effects from plasmaphoresis in a child with dermatomyositis. In adults a course of plasmaphoresis may be beneficial in unresponsive patients.

In young people the use of corticosteroids and immunosuppression do not appear to have stopped the development of calcinosis; the lesions in the subcutaneous tissues may discharge through the skin and subsequently heal, resolve spontaneously (Sewell et al, 1978), or be accessible to surgical

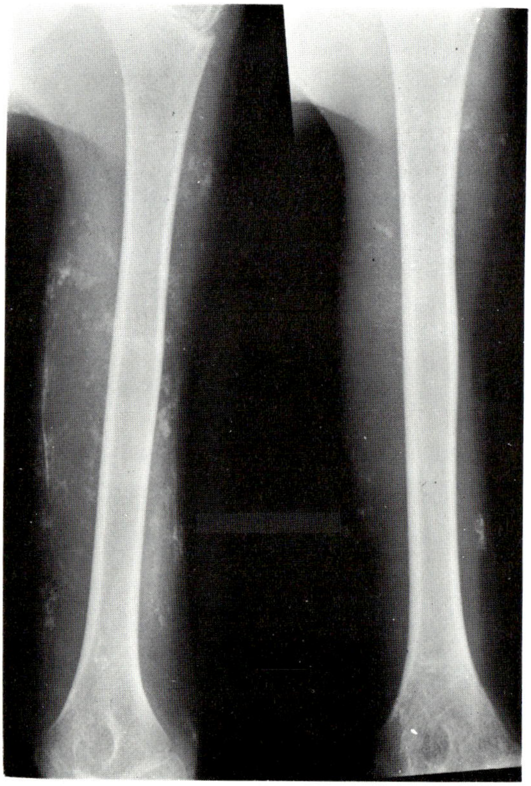

Fig. 54.14 Improvement in the radiological appearance of the thigh muscles, over a year in a girl aged 11, 6 years from the onset of her dermatomyositis.

removal. Those in the interfascial planes, which give rise to more problems, remain as yet an unsolved problem. Intravenous edathanil disodium given over a 3-week period was suggested as useful by Davies & Moe (1959); this has not been our experience in the calcinosis of dermatomyositis, nor that of Metzger et al (1974b). A low calcium diet and disodium hydrogen phosphate in a dose of 4 g at each meal has also proved ineffective. The successful treatment of calcinosis circumscripta with probenecid (Dent & Stamp, 1972) led to our using this. Less than half of our patients completing more than 1 year of therapy have shown any evidence of regression and this could have been spontaneous (Fig. 54.14).

Activity may persist for months or years and it is important that these cases are carefully followed and kept on the lowest dosage of appropriate drugs. Intercurrent infection will require prompt treatment; calcinotic nodules may need removal, and morale will certainly need boosting from time to time.

REFERENCES

Adams R D 1973 The pathologic substratum of polymyositis. In: Pearson CM, Mastofi FK (eds) The striated muscle. Williams & Wilkins, Baltimore, p. 292

Ansell B M, Bywaters E G L 1962 Diagnosis of probable Stills and its outcome. Annals of the Rheumatic Diseases 21: 253–262

Ansell B M, Hamilton E, Bywaters E G L 1971 The course and prognosis in juvenile dermatomyositis. In: Clinical studies in myology. Proceedings of the 2nd International Congress on Muscle Diseases. Excerpta Medica, Amsterdam, p. 560

Arnett F C, Whelton J C, Zizic T M, Stevens M B 1973 Methotrexate therapy in polymyositis. Annals of the Rheumatic Diseases 32: 536–546

Arnett, Frank C, Hush, Thomas J, Bias, Wilmr B, Nishikua M, Reichlin M 1981 The Jo-1 antibody system in myositis — relationship to clinical features and HLA. Journal of Rhematology 8: 925–930

Arundell F D, Wilkinson R D, Haserick J R 1960 Dermatomyositis and malignant neoplasms in adults. Archives of Dermatology 82: 772–775

Askari A D, Huettner T L 1982 Cardiac abnormalities in polymyositis/dermatomyositis. Seminars in Arthritis and Rheumatism 12: 208–219

Banker B O 1975 Dermatomyositis of childhood. Ultrastructural alterations of muscle and intramascular blood vessels. Journal of Neuropathology and Experimental Neurology 34: 46–75

Banker B Q, Victor M 1966 Dermatomyositis (systemic angiopathy) of childhood. Medicine 45: 261–289

Barwick D D, Walton J N 1963 Polymyositis. American Journal of Medicine 35: 646–660

Beck P 1968 Myelomatosis presenting as dermatomyositis. British Medical Journal 1: 747–748

Benson M D, Aldo M A 1973 Azathioprine therapy in polymyositis. Archives of Internal Medicine 132: 547–551

Bohan A, Peter J B 1975 Polymyositis and dermatomyositis. New England Journal of Medicine 292: 344–347; 403–407

Brewer E J, Gianninni E H, Rosser R D, Patten B, Barkley E 1980 Plasma exchange therapy of a child onset dermatomyositis patient. Arthritis and Rheumatism, 23, 509–519

Callen J P 1982a The value of malignancy evaluation in patients with dermatomyositis. Journal of the American Academy of Dermatology 6: 253–259

Callen J P 1982b Dermatomyositis and malignancy. Clinics in Rheumatic Diseases 8: 369–381

Cambridge G, Stern C M 1981 The uptake of tritium labelled carintine by monolayer cultures of human foetal muscles and its potential as a label in cytotoxicity study. Clinical Experimental Immunology 43: 211–219

Chalmers A, Sayson R, Walters K 1982 Juvenile dermatomyositis — medical, social and economic status in adulthood. Canadian Medical Association Journal 126: 31–35

Chou S M 1968 Myxovirus-like structures and accompanying nuclear changes in chronic polymyositis. Archives of Pathology 86: 649–658

Chou S M, Gutmann L 1970 Picornavirus-like crystals in subacute polymyositis. Neurology 20: 205–213

Cochrane W, Davis D V 1965 An electron microscopic study of a case of dermatomyositis. Annals of the Rheumatic Diseases 24: 147–152

Cook C D, Rosen F S, Banker B Q 1963 Dermatomyositis and focal scleroderma. Pediatric Clinics of North America 10: 979–1016

Croft P B, Wilkinson M 1963 In: Brain L, Noris F (eds) The remote effects of cancer on the nervous system. Grune & Stratton, London

Crowe W K, Bove K E, Levinson J E, et al 1982 Clinical and pathogenetic implications of histopathology in childhood poly dermatomyositis. Arthritis and Rheumatism 25: 126–139

Currie S, Saunders M, Knowles M, Brown A E 1971 Immunological aspects of polymyositis. The in vitro activity of lymphocytes on incubation with muscle antigen and with muscle cultures. Quarterly Journal of Medicine 40: 63–84

Davies H, Moe P J 1959 Favorable response of calcinosis universalis to *edathamil* dosodium. Pediatrics 24: 780–785

Dawkins R 1977 In: Holborow E J, Reeves G W (eds) Immunology in medicine. Academic Press, London

Dawkins R, Mastaglia F L 1973 Cell-mediated cytotoxicity to muscle in polymyositis. New England Journal of Medicine 288: 434–438

Degos R, Civatte J, Belaich S 1971 The prognosis of adult dermatomyositis. Transactions of the St John's Hospital Dermatological Society 57: 98–104

Denbow C E 1979 Cardiac involvement of polymyositis. Arthritis and Rheumatism 22: 1088–1092

Dent C E, Stamp T C B 1972 Treatment of calcinosis

circumscripta with Probenecid. British Medical Journal 1: 216–218
Dietzman D E, Schaller J, Ray C G, Reed M E 1974 Myositis associated with influenza and infection. Pediatric Research 8:423.
Donoghue F D, Winkelmann R K, Moersch J H 1960 Esophageal defects in dermatomyositis. Annals of Otology (St Louis) 69: 1139–1145
Douglas A C, Macloed J G, Matthews J D 1973 Symptomatic sarcoidosis of skeletal muscle. Journal of Neurology, Neurosurgery and Psychiatry 36: 1034–1040
Doyle D R, McCurley T L, Sergeant J S 1983 Fatal polymyositis in D-penicillamine treated rheumatoid arthritis. Annals of International Medicine 3: 327–330
Dubowitz L M, Dubowitz V 1964 Acute dermatomyositis presenting with pulmonary manifestations. Archives of Disease in Childhood 39: 293–296
Duncan P E, Griffin J P, Garcia A, Kaplan S B 1974 Fibrosing alveolitis in polymyositis. A review of histologically confirmed cases. American Journal of Medicine 57: 621–626
Engel W K, DeVivo D C, Warmolts J R 1971 High-single-dose alternate-day prednisone (HSAD-PRED) in neuromuscular diseases. Excerpta Medica International Congress Series No. 237, p. 59
Fernandez-Herlihy L 1971 Heart block in polymyositis. New England Journal of Medicine 284: 1101–1101
Fruman L S, Sullivan D B, Petty R T 1976 Retinopathy in juvenile dermatomyositis. Journal of Pediatrics 88: 267–269
Gotoff S P, Smith R D, Sugar O 1972 Dermatomyositis with cerebral vasculitis in a patient with agammaglobulinemia. American Journal of Diseases of Children 123: 53–56
Hanson V, Kornreich H 1967 Systemic rheumatic disorders in childhood: lupus erythematosus, anaphylactoid purpura, dermatomyositis and scleroderma. Parts I & II. Bulletin on Rheumatic Diseases 17: 435–440; 441–446
Hollingworth P, De Vere Tyndall A: Ansell B M et al 1982 Intensive immunosuppression versus prednisolone in the treatment of connective tissue disorders. Annals of Rheumatic Diseases 41: 557–562
Hubbard W N, Walport J J, Halnan K E, Beaver R P, Hughes G R Y 1982 Remission from polymyositis after total radiation. British Medical Journal 284: 1915–1916
Isenberg D A, Snaith M I 1981 Muscle disease in S L E. A study of its nature, frequency and course. Journal of Rheumatology 8: 917–924
Janis J F, Winkelmann R K 1968 Histopathology of the skin in dermatomyositis. Archives of Dermatology 97: 640–650
Johnson R L, Fink C W, Ziff M 1972 Lymphotoxin formation by lymphocytes and muscle in polymyositis. Journal of Clinical Investigation 51: 2435–2449
Kagen L J 1971 Myoglobulinemia and myoglobinuria in patients with myositis. Arthritis and Rheumatism 14: 457–464
Leddy J P, Griggs R C, Klemperer M R, Frank M M 1975 Hereditary complement (C_2) deficiency with dermatomyositis. American Journal of Medicine 58: 83–91
Lian J B, Puchman L M, Gundberg C M, Partridge E H, Maryjowski 1982 Gamma-carboxyglutamatge excretion and calcinosis in juvenile dermatomyositis. Arthritis and Rheumatism 25: 1094–1100
Loewi G, Dorling J 1964 Calcinosis, histological and chemical analysis. Annals of Rheumatic Diseases 23: 272–279
McArdle B 1963 Metabolic myopathies. American Journal of Medicine 35: 661–672
Malaviya H N, Many A, Schwartz R S 1968 Treatment of dermatomyositis with methotrexate. Lancet 2: 485–488
Marinacci A A 1965 Electromyography in the diagnosis of polymyositis. Bulletin of the Los Angeles Neurological Society 30: 191–200
Mastaglia F L, Walton J N 1970 Coxsackie virus-like particles in skeletal muscle from a case of polymyositis. Journal of Neurological Sciences 11: 593–599
Mastaglia F L, Walton J N 1971 An ultrastructural study of skeletal muscle in polymyositis. Journal of Neurological Sciences 12: 473–504
Medsger T A, Rodnan G P, Moossy J, Vester J W 1968 Skeletal muscle involvement in progressive systemic sclerosis (scleroderma). Arthritis and Rheumatism 11: 554–568
Medsger T A, Dawson W N, Masi A T 1970 The epidemiology of polymyositis. American Journal of Medicine 48: 715–723
Medsger T A, Robinson H, Masi A T 1971 Factors affecting survivorship in polymyositis: a life-table study of 124 patients. Arthritis and Rheumatism 14: 249–258
Metzger A L, Bohan A, Goldberg L S, Bluestone R, Pearson C M 1974a Polymyositis and dermatomyositis: combined methotrexate and corticosteroid therapy. Annals of Internal Medicine 81: 182–189
Metzger A L, Singer F R, Bluestone R, Pearson C M 1974b Failure of disodium etidronate in calcinosis due to dermatomyositis and scleroderma. New England Journal of Medicine 291: 1294–1296
Middleton P J, Alexander R M, Szymanski M T 1970 Severe myositis during recovery from influenza. Lancet 2: 533–535
Nishikai M, Reichlin M 1980 Heterogeneity of precipitating antibodies in polymyositis and dermatomyositis. Arthritis and Rheumatism 23: 881–888
Nishikai M, Funatsu Y, Homma M 1974 Monoclonal gammopathy penicillamine-induced polymyositis and systemic sclerosis. Archives of Dermatology 110: 253–255
Pachman L M, Cook N 1980 Juvenile dermatomyositis — a clinical and immunologic study. Journal of Pediatrics 96: 226–234
Page A R, Hansen A E, Good R A 1963 Occurrence of leukemia and lymphoma in patients with agammaglobulinemia. Blood 21: 197–206
Pearson C M 1959 Rheumatic manifestation of polymyositis and dermatomyositis. Arthritis and Rheumatism 2: 127–143
Pearson C M 1966 Polymyositis. Annual Review of Medicine 17: 63–82
Pearson C M, Yamazaki J N 1958 Vacuolar myopathy in systemic lupus erythematosus. American Journal of Clinical Pathology 29: 455–463
Pearson C M, Currie S 1974 Polymyositis and related disorders. In: Walton J N (ed) Disorders of voluntary muscle, 3rd Edn. Churchill Livingstone, Edinburgh, Ch. 16, p. 614
Reichlin M, Mattioli M 1976 Description of a serological reaction characteristic of polymyositis. Clinical Immunological Immunopathology 5: 12–20
Rose A L, Walton J N 1966 Polymyositis: A survey of 89 cases with particular reference to treatment and prognosis. Brain 89: 747–768
Rowe D, Isenberg D A, McDougal J, Beverly P C L 1981

Characterisation of polymyositis infiltrates using monoclonal antibodies to human leucocyte antigens. Experimental Immunology 45: 290–298
Sato T, Walker D L, Peters H A 1971 Chronic polymyositis and myxovirus-like inclusions, electron microscopic and viral studies. Archives of Neurology 24: 409–418
Schaller J 1973 Dermatomyositis. Journal of Pediatrics 83: 699–702
Schaumburg H H, Nielson S L, Yurchak P M 1971 Heart block in polymyositis. New England Journal of Medicine 284: 480–481
Sewell J R, Liyanage B, Ansell B M 1978 Calcinosis in juvenile dermatomyositis. Skeletal Radiology 3: 137–143
Silverstein A, Siltzbach L E 1969 Muscle involvement in sarcoidosis. Archives of Neurology 21: 235–241
Sokoloff M C, Goldberg L S, Pearson C M 1971 Treatment of corticosteroid-resistant polymyositis with methotrexate. Lancet 1: 14–16
Sullivan D B, Cassidy J T, Petty R E 1972 Prognosis in childhood dermatomyositis. Journal of Pediatrics 80: 555–563
Susac J, Garcia-Mullen R, Glaser J S 1973 Ophthalmoplegia in dermatomyositis. Neurology 23: 305–310
Unverricht H 1887 Polymyositis acuta progressiva. Zeitschrift fur Klinische Medizin 12: 533–549
Venables P J W, Mumford P A, Maini R N 1981 Antibodies to nuclear antigens in polymyositis: relationship to autoimmune 'overlap syndromes' and carcinoma. Annals of the Rheumatic Diseases 40: 217–223
Vignos P J, Goldwyn J 1972 Evaluation of laboratory tests in the diagnosis and management of polymyositis. American Journal of the Medical Sciences 263: 291–308
Walton J N, Adams R D 1958 Polymyositis. Livingstone, Edinburgh
Webster A D B, Tripp J H, Hayward A R, et al 1978 Echovirus encephalitis and myositis in primary immunoglobulin deficiency. Archives of Diseases of Childhood 53: 33–37
Wedgewood R J P, Cook C S, Cohen J 1953 Dermatomyositis; report of 26 cases in children with a discussion of endocrine therapy in 13. Pediatrics 12: 447–466
Whitaker J N, Engel W K 1972 Vascular deposits of immunoglobulin and complement in idiopathic inflammatory myopathy. New England Journal of Medicine 286: 333–338
Williams J C Jr 1959 Dermatomyositis and malignancy: a review of the literature. Annals of Internal Medicine 50: 1174–1182
Winkelmann R K, Mulder D W, Lambert E H, Howard F M, Diessner G R 1968 Dermatomyositis-polymyositis: comparison of untreated and cortisone-treated patients. Mayo Clinic Proceedings 43: 545–556
Winkelmann R K 1982 Dermatomyositis in childhood. Clinicals in Rheumatic Diseases 8: 353–368
Wolfe J F, Adelstein E, Sharp G C 1977 Antinuclear antibody with distinct specificity for polymyositis. Journal of Clinical Investigation 59: 176–178

Systemic sclerosis

Systemic sclerosis is a multisystem disorder characterised by collagen proliferation, inflammatory cell infiltration, vascular obstruction and ischaemic atrophy. The term 'scleroderma' refers to the cutaneous features alone. Although scleroderma occurs in the great majority of cases of systemic sclerosis, it is not universally present and the term 'scleroderma' should not be regarded as synonymous with the multisystem disease complex. 'Morphoea' is a form of scleroderma restricted to the skin with well demarcated plaques of fibrosis. In morphoea visceral involvement hardly ever occurs and it is thought unlikely that morphoea is related to systemic sclerosis.

CLASSIFICATION AND EPIDEMIOLOGY

A scheme for classifying various forms of systemic sclerosis is shown in Table 55.1. Although there is considerable overlap in the cutaneous and visceral manifestations between these various forms of the disorder the pattern of disease is usually distinct and helpful in assessing the likely prognosis. In an effort to aid the recognition of this disorder, Masi et al (1980) have established diagnostic criteria for the presence of definite systemic sclerosis (Table 55.2).

The disorder is uncommon with estimates of the annual incidence varying between 2.3 and 12 cases per million population (Medsger & Masi, 1978; Kurland et al, 1969). The disorder may present at any age with a peak incidence in the 4th or 5th decade (Rodnan & Medsger, 1975, Medsger & Masi, 1978). It is recognised but uncommon in children (Cassidy et al, 1977; Kornreich et al, 1977) but in young people there is relatively a much higher incidence in females than males, being 15 : 1 in those under 45 years in contrast with 2 : 1 in those over this age (Medsger & Masi, 1971). There are no racial differences in incidence but the prognosis does seem somewhat worse for Negroes than Caucasians (Masi & D'Angelo, 1967). There may be an association of systemic sclerosis with being married, alcohol intake and performing manual and less skilled work (Medsger & Masi, 1978).

Occupational factors may be relevant with reports of an increased incidence in stonemasons (Bramwell, 1914), coalminers (Rodnan et al, 1967) and goldminers (Erasmus, 1957). Scleroderma-like conditions have developed in workers exposed to

Table 55.1 Classification

Localised cutaneous
Morphea
— Single or multiple plaques
— Generalised
Linear scleroderma
Systemic sclerosis
CREST syndrome
Diffuse
Overlap syndromes
Eosinophilic fasciitis
Drug- and chemical-induced

Table 55.2 Preliminary criteria for the diagnosis of systemic sclerosis (after Masi et al, 1980)

Major criterion
Proximal scleroderma (to MCP^s and MTP^s)
Minor criteria
Sclerodactyly
Digital tip pitting or loss of substance of distal fingerpad
Bibasilar pulmonary fibrosis
At least the major or two or more minor criteria required for the diagnosis of systemic sclerosis

vinyl chloride (Jayson, 1977), other chlorinated hydrocarbons (Jablonska, 1975; Sparrow, 1977) and epoxy resins (Yamakage et al, 1980). Features of systemic sclerosis were amongst long-term follow-up consequences of the widespread connective tissue changes which occurred in an epidemic in Spain and thought to be due to adulterated cooking oil (Toxic Epidemic Study Group, 1982). Certain therapeutic agents have produced scleroderma-like conditions. In particular bleomycin (Finch et al, 1980) and tryptophan and carbidopa (Sternberg et al, 1980) have been identified. The development of peritoneal fibrosis following practalol and retroperitoneal fibrosis with methysergide therapy may be due to comparable mechanisms. Connective tissue disease and in particular systemic sclerosis may develop after cosmetic surgery and injection of a foreign substance. Paraffin has been incriminated as the most likely cause (Kumagai et al, 1984). A scleroderma-like syndrome may occur in association with childhood diabetes mellitus (Rosenbloom et al, 1981) and there is a reported association with malignancy (Talbott & Barrocas, 1979); this is doubtful except possibly with lung cancer as an end-stage event in advanced pulmonary fibrosis.

Although rare, there have been a sufficient number of familial cases reported (Camus et al, 1970; Frayha et al, 1977; Gray & Altman, 1977; Strosberg et al, 1977) to stimulate interest in genetic studies and there are reports of increased prevalences of HLA-DR1, DR3 and DR5 (Black et al, 1984), B8 and DR3 (Kallenberg et al, 1981) and DR5 (Gladman et al, 1981). There may be an increased association of DRw3 will the CREST syndrome (Germain et al, 1981) and B8 may be a marker for rapidly progressive disease with widespread visceral involvement (Hughes et al, 1978).

PATHOLOGY AND CLINICAL FEATURES

The pathological changes and clinical features of systemic sclerosis are due to a variable combination of mild chronic inflammatory cell infiltration, connective tissue proliferation, vascular obstruction and ischaemic atrophy. These features occur in variable combination in the different organ systems and lead to characteristic pathological and clinical changes.

Presenting features. The onset of the disorder is usually between 30 and 50 years of age. The most frequent presenting feature is of Raynaud's phenomenon and, particularly in the CREST syndrome (p. 1375), the true diagnosis may not be recognised for many years (Rodnan & Medsger, 1975). There may be progressive induration and stiffening of the skin with difficulty in using the hands. Less frequently polyarthritis, dysphagia, small bowel problems and other visceral features may be present at the onset. Although the pathological changes are widespread, clinical evidence of involvement may not be obvious in the various body systems. Table 55.3 shows the frequency of clinical and pathological evidence of organ system involvement in series of patients with systemic sclerosis.

Table 55.3 Frequency of organ involvement (%)

	Pathological (D'Angelo et al, 1969)	Clinical (LeRoy, 1976)
Skin	98	90
Oesophagus	74	52
Small intestine	48 }	15
Large intestine	39 }	
Lungs	81 }	43
Pleura	81 }	
Heart	81	40
Pericardium	53	11
Muscle	41	20
Kidney	58	35

Raynaud's phenomenon and peripheral vascular disease

Raynaud's phenomenon is a syndrome of reversible peripheral ischaemia occurring predominantly in the hands but also in the feet and occasionally elsewhere. The syndrome is usually precipitated by exposure to cold and sometimes by emotion or other poorly recognised events. The fingers first turn white and then become cyanosed. During the rewarming phase they may turn bright red due to profound vasodilation. Pain with numbness and paraesthesiae is common. When Raynaud's phenomenon persists for several years without evidence of any underlying disorder it is called 'primary Raynaud's disease'. Frequently Raynaud's phenomenon is the presenting feature of a connective tissue disorder and particularly systemic sclerosis. However, the other features making the diagnosis may only become apparent in subsequent years and only be recognised on careful examination and investigation.

With more severe peripheral ischaemia, the systemic sclerosis patient may develop small areas of infarction at the finger tips. Most common are small areas of ulceration (Fig. 55.1) which heal giving the appearance of pitting and atrophy of the pulp of the fingertip (Fig. 55.2). Radiographs show lysis of the tips of the terminal phalanges (Fig. 55.3). Larger areas of ulceration may develop at the finger tips and elsewhere (Fig. 55.4), particularly over sites exposed to trauma. There is a risk of secondary infection due to poor peripheral vascular supply. Recurrent infection of the fingers with terminal pulp atrophy may eventually require amputation. Some patients may end up losing several digits (Fig. 55.5).

Examination of the skin will show dilated capillaries. These telangiectasiae are particularly prominent on the face (Fig. 55.6) and the palms of the hands but also occur elsewhere. The nailbeds may appear swollen and capillary microscopy (Maricq, 1981) will show a characteristic pattern (Fig. 55.7) of enlarged and deformed capillary loops surrounded by avascular areas (Maricq et al, 1980). There is a correlation between these nailbed changes and multisystem involvement by systemic sclerosis (Maricq et al, 1976).

The vascular lesions in the hands may be demonstrated by arteriography. It is difficult to evaluate transient changes in patients with Raynaud's phenomenon alone but in more advanced disease there may be segmental blocks in the digital vessels with loss of the more distal circulation (Fig. 55.8).

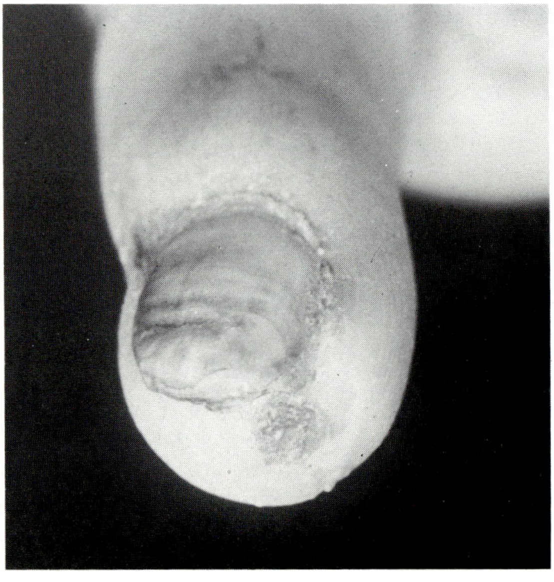

Fig. 55.1 Ulceration and scarring of the fingertips.

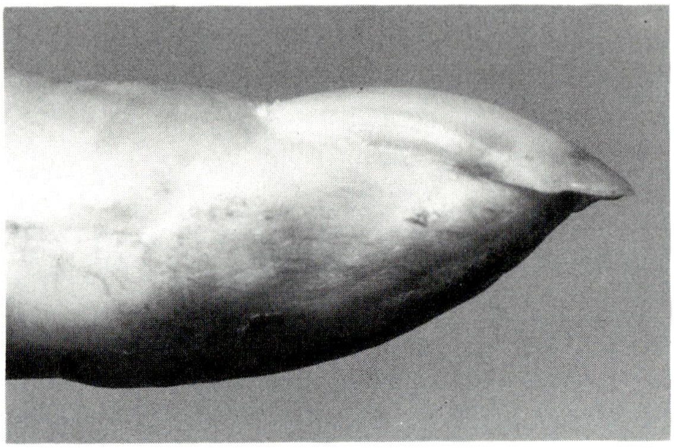

Fig. 55.2 Atrophy of the pulp of the fingertip.

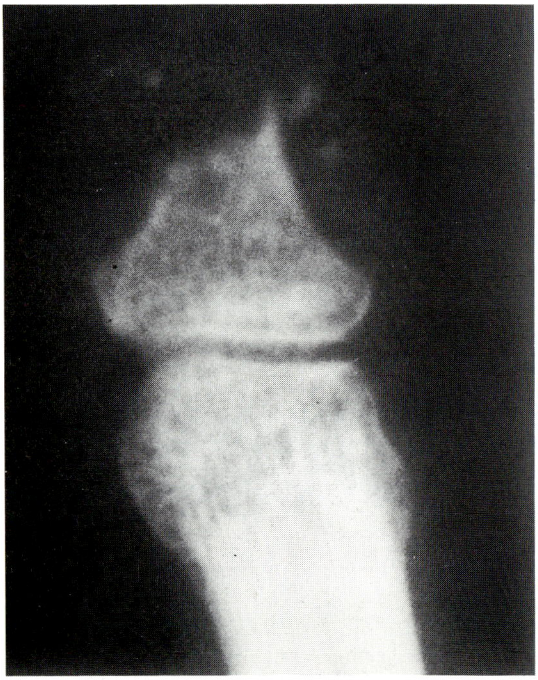

Fig. 55.3 Lysis of the tip of the terminal phalanx with some scattered areas of soft tissue calcification.

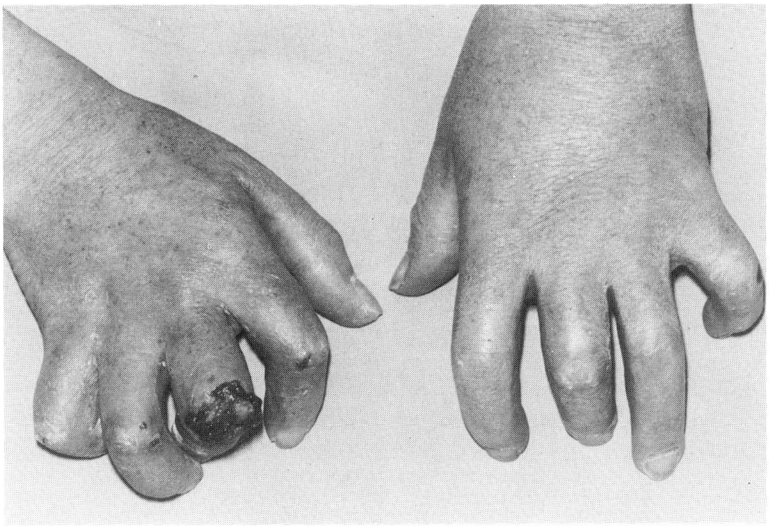

Fig. 55.4 Indolent infection in the skin overlying the proximal interphalangeal joint of the right middle finger.

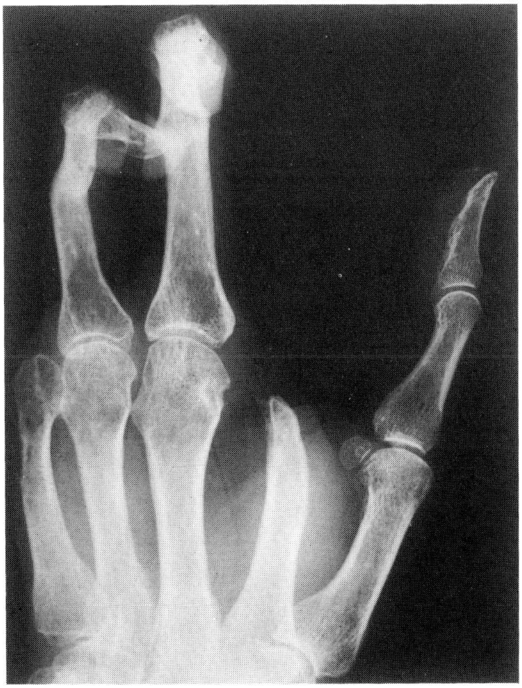

Fig. 55.5 Radiograph to show multiple amputations and fusion of the interphalangeal joints.

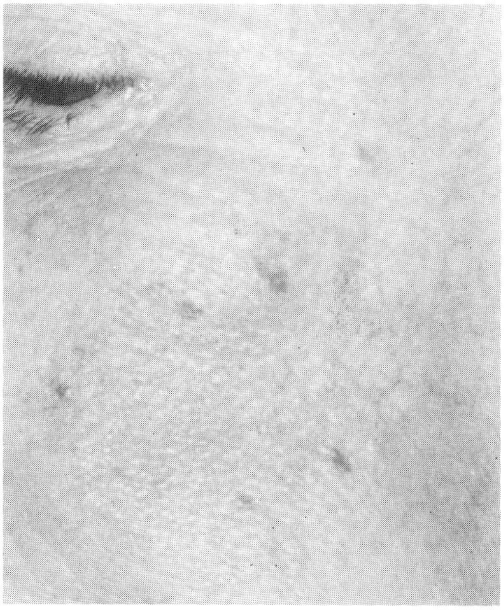

Fig. 55.6 Telangiectasiae in the skin of the face.

Skin changes

These are usually most prominent in the fingers and the face but many patients have a more widespread pattern occasionally sparing the extremities. The term 'sclerodactyly' refers to changes limited to the fingers and not spreading proximal to the metacarpophalangeal joints. 'Acrosclerosis' describes changes predominantly in a peripheral distribution particularly affecting the hands and feet, the distal forearms and legs, and the face predominantly in a circumoral distribution. The term

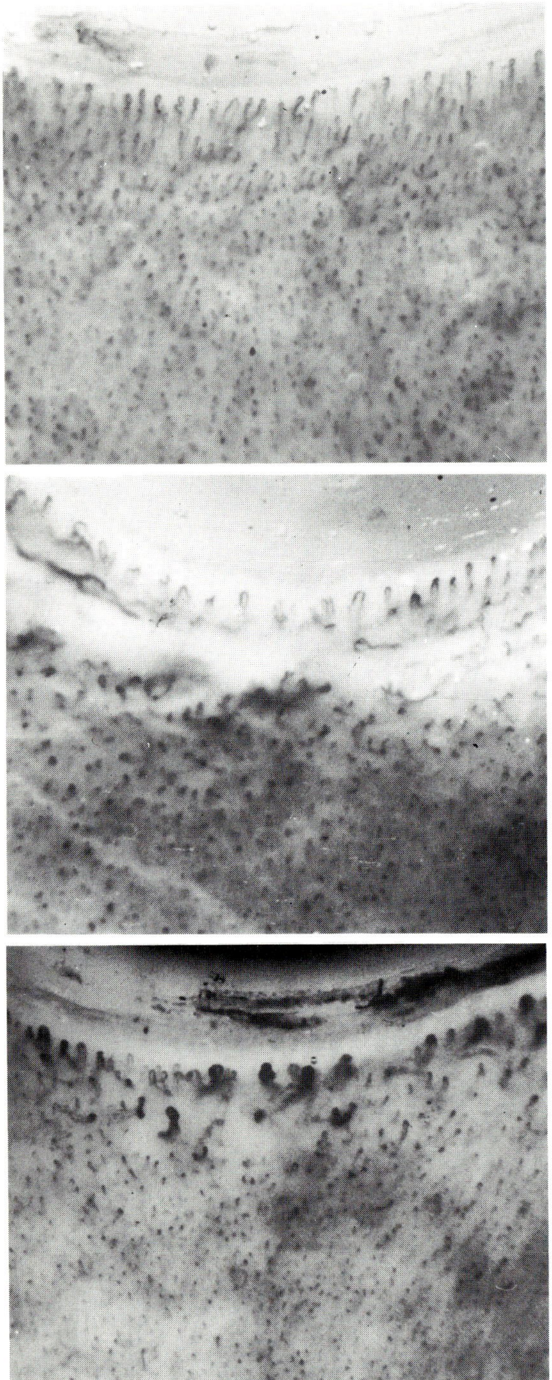

a

b

c

Fig. 55.7 Nail-bed capillaries. (a) Normal subjects. (b) Scleroderma pattern showing moderately enlarged loops and considerable loss of capillaries resulting in a large avascular zone. (c) Scleroderma pattern abnormalities with strikingly enlarged capillaries and also some loss of capillaries (by courtesy of Dr H. Maricq).

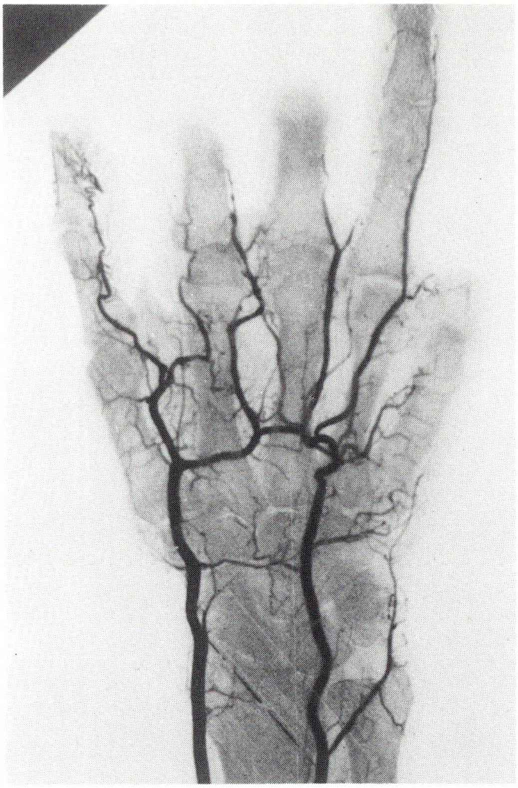

Fig. 55.8 Arteriogram showing multiple vascular occlusions resulting in the loss of several digits.

'proximal scleroderma' means that the disease has involved skin proximal to the metacarpophalangeal joints and generally implies involvement of the trunk.

The typical findings in areas involved by scleroderma are of tightness and induration. It is difficult to pinch the skin and there may be loss of hair in involved sites. There may be patchy areas of depigmentation and hyperpigmentation particularly on the limbs. The tightness of the skin may lead to limitation of joint movement and commonly patients are unable to straighten their fingers, which lie curled with slight flexion deformities (Fig. 55.9). In some patients extensive skin changes involve the whole body which may appear as if encased in a suit of armour.

There may be difficulty in opening the mouth with tightness around the lips and the appearance of radial furrows in the surrounding skin (Fig. 55.10). The tautness of the skin on the nose may produce a 'beak-like' appearance. These

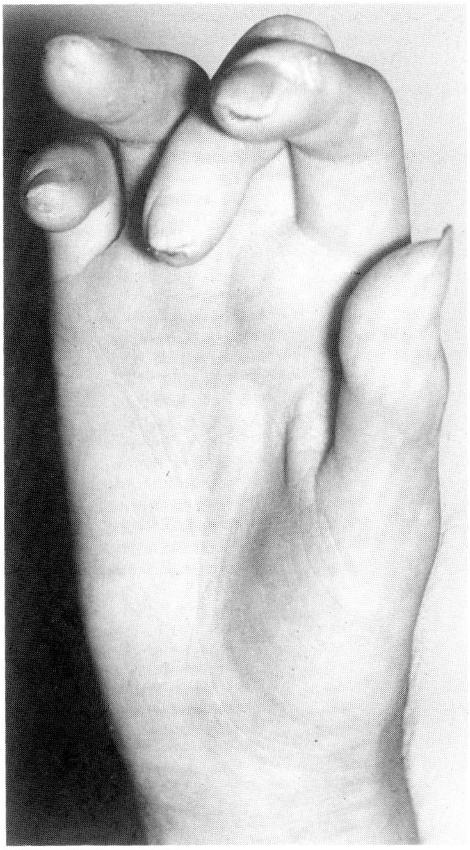

Fig. 55.9 Advanced scleroderma involvement in the hand with flexion deformities of the fingers and digital pitting scars on the fingertips.

changes together with telangiectasia make the facial appearance of scleroderma readily recognisable.

These easily recognised sclerodermatous features are often preceded by a transient oedematous phase which may not be obvious before being replaced by induration. The skin appears swollen and pressure with the thumb may leave a fingerprint on the skin surface.

Long-term follow-up examination may show spontaneous resolution of skin changes particularly in the forearm where on occasion they return almost to normal.

Calcinosis may develop in the skin and subcutaneous tissues, particularly in the fingers (Fig. 55.11) but also elsewhere. The skin may ulcerate and discharge this material. Calcinotic deposits are readily recognised on radiographs (Fig. 55.12).

In the indurative phase (Fig. 55.13), a biopsy of the skin will show atrophy and thinning of the epidermis. There is thickening of the dermis due to gross collagen proliferation. The thickness of the skin on biopsy is used as an index of progress (Rodnan et al, 1979). Electron-microscopy of the collagen shows the fibres to be a mixture of sizes indicating the recent synthesis of new collagen fibrils. There is atrophy and disappearance of the appendages such as the hair follicles and sweat glands. However, in early involvement the skin

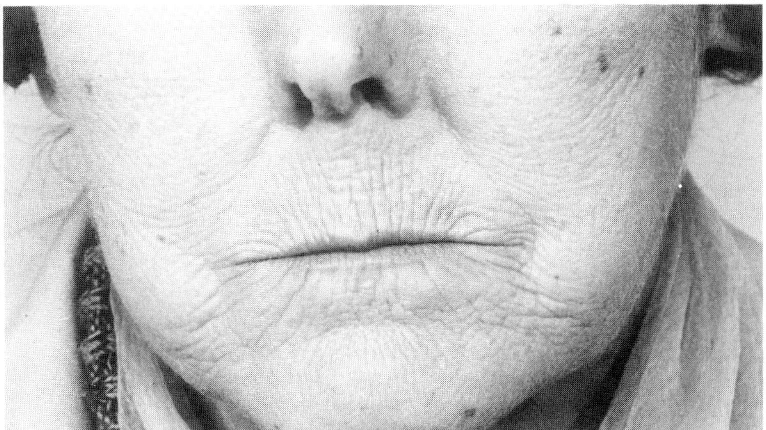

Fig. 55.10 Scleroderma facies with tight pinched lips surrounded by radial furrowing and telangiectasia on the face.

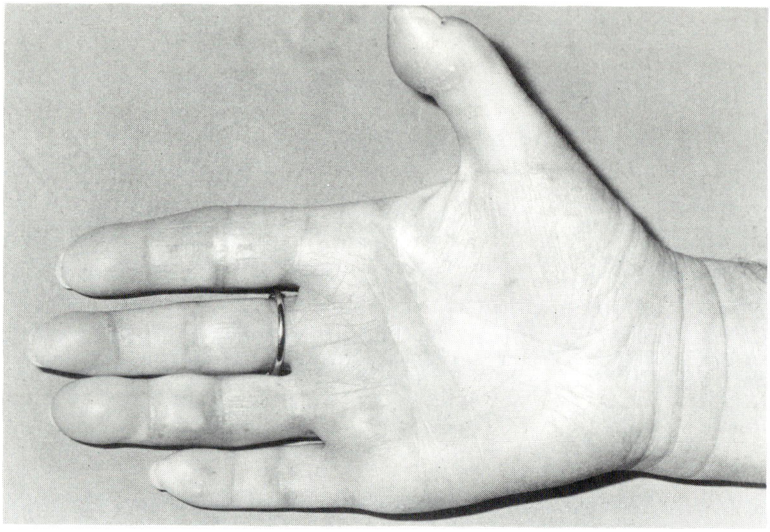

Fig. 55.11 Calcinotic lesions in the skin of the fingers.

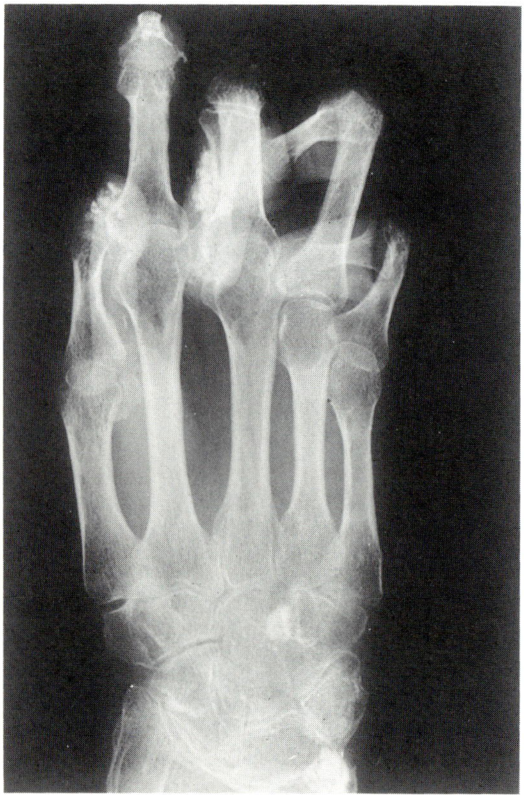

Fig. 55.12 Radiograph to show severe flexion deformities of the fingers with soft tissue calcinosis.

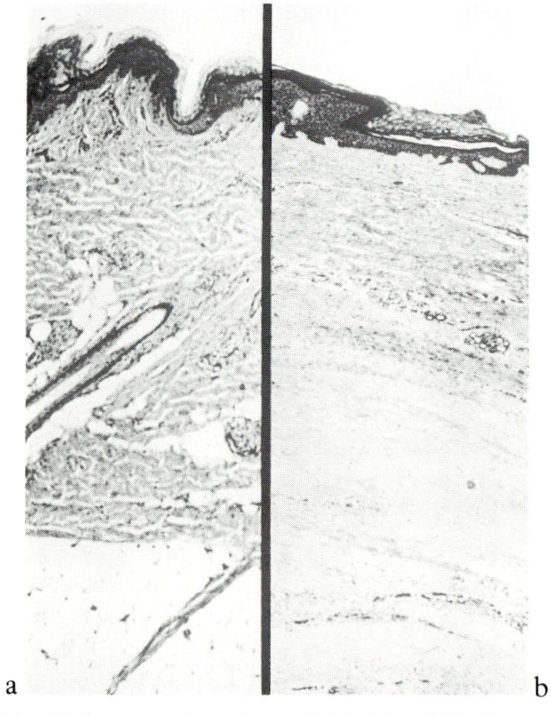

Fig. 55.13 A comparison of normal skin (a) and skin from a patient with scleroderma (b) The epidermis in the latter is atrophied, the dermis thickened and the dermal appendages are lost. (×45)

may appear relatively normal except for the presence of a sparse infiltration of chronic inflammatory cells predominantly deep in the dermis (Fig. 55.14). These cells may be concentrated around small blood vessels (Fleishmajer et al, 1977). If anything these infiltrates are more frequent in morphoea than in systemic sclerosis. Immunofluorescent examination may show deposition of immunoglobulins in the skin in patients with overlap syndromes but not in those with systemic sclerosis with an acrosclerotic distribution (Connolly & Winkelmann, 1977).

Tendons and joints

Although involvement of tendons and joints is common (Lovell & Jayson, 1979), it may be difficult to distinguish from stiffness and joint contractures produced by the skin changes. There can be mild synovitis of the joints and tendon sheaths with deposition of fibrin on the surface of the synovial membrane; in some cases this produces pain, tenderness and loss of function. It may be possible to palpate and hear a coarse leathery crepitus on movement. This usually arises from the patellofemoral joint or the tendons of the distal forearms or legs.

On radiographs (Figs 55.5, 55.12) there may be deformity, loss of joint space, subluxation and rarely fusion of damaged joints. Examination of the synovium usually shows relatively mild inflammatory changes, dense fibrosis and a thick layer of fibrin on the synovial surface (Rodnan & Medsger, 1968; Clark et al, 1971). Joint destruction and fusion are uncommon (Fig. 55.15).

Muscle and neurological involvement

Mild muscle involvement is common (Medsger et al, 1968; Clements et al, 1970) and pathological examination reveals a mild chronic inflammatory cell infiltration usually in a perivascular distribution, muscle fibre atrophy and fibrous replacement. The muscle changes occur predominantly in the limb girdles with weakness but not usually significant pain and seem more common in those with overlap syndromes. However most patients will have electromyographic abnormalities (Hausmanowa-Petrusewicz et al, 1982). Investigation may show mild elevation of the serum creatine

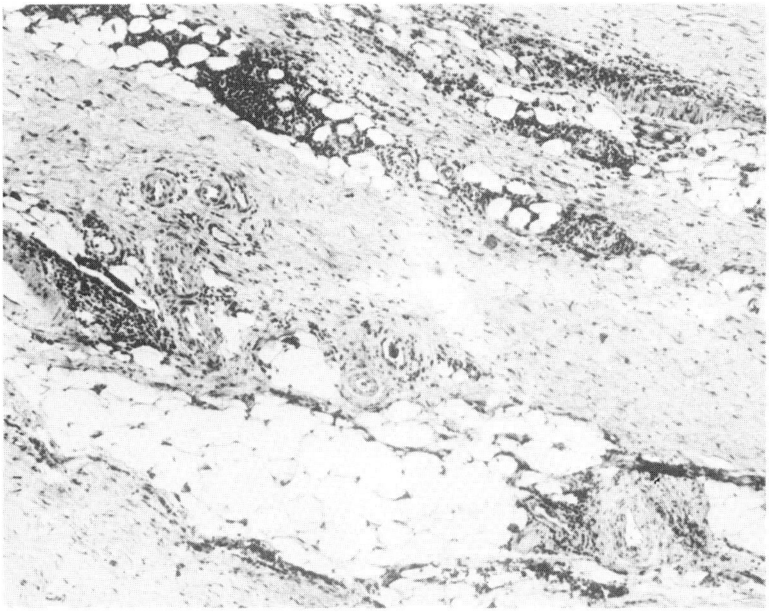

Fig. 55.14 The earliest lesions of scleroderma in which there is a sparse lymphocytic infiltrate. This is most prominent at the dermal, subcutaneous fat junction and around the dermal appendages. (×150)

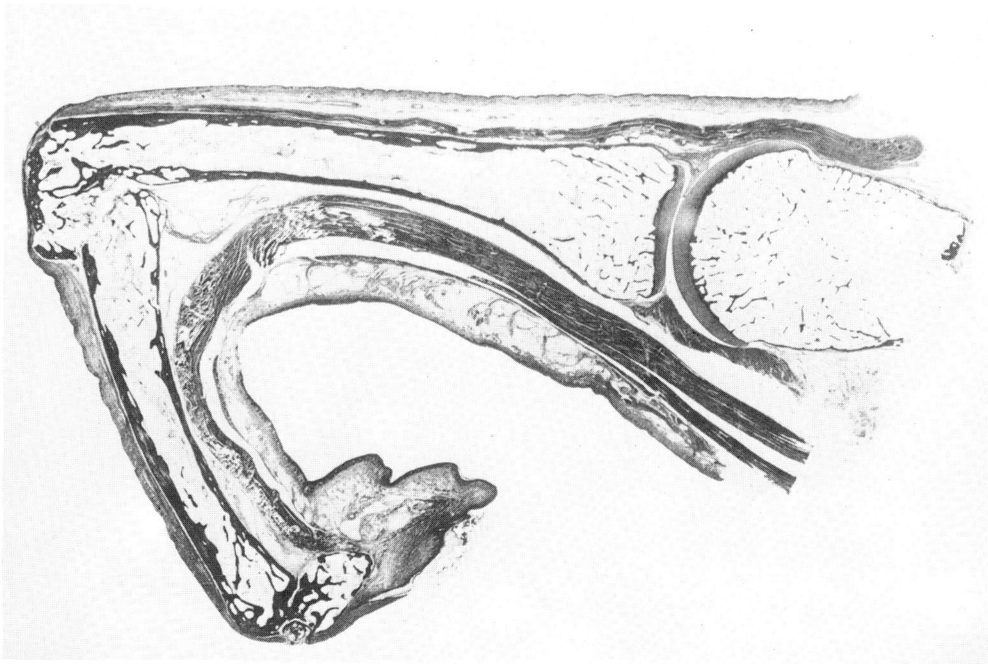

Fig. 55.15 A longitudinal section through the index finger of a patient with scleroderma. There is loss of pulp and bone of the distal phalanx, ankylosis of both interphalangeal joints and fusion of the extensor tendons with the overlying dermis. (×1–8)

phosphokinase and aldolase with an increase in the urinary excretion of creatine and a specific antibody directed against a calf thymus nuclear extract (Wolfe et al, 1977).

Neurological involvement is rare but there is an association with trigeminal neuralgia (Farrell & Medsger, 1982). This symptom may be presenting feature of systemic sclerosis but generally follows its onset by a matter of months.

Gastrointestinal involvement

Oesophageal changes are extremely common and have been found in up to 90% of patients (Orringer et al, 1976). There is atrophy of the muscle coats of the oesophageal wall and dilation of the lumen (Treacy et al, 1963) with interference with neuromuscular co-ordination and loss of tone in the distal oesophageal sphincter. Disordered peristalsis may be recognised radiographically in 55% and manometrically in 73% of subjects (Turner et al, 1973).

The predominant symptoms are of lower oesophageal dysphagia with difficulty in swallowing, particularly if lying flat. Damage to the lower oesophageal sphincter leads to reflux and severe heartburn. In the more advanced case, a stricture may develop making the dysphagia considerably worse. Barium swallow examination may reveal disordered peristalsis, oesophageal reflux, stricture formation and a dilated oesophagus (Fig. 55.16). Upper oesophageal changes fortunately are rare but, when they do occur, lead to incompetence of the cricopharyngeal apparatus and inhalation of food into the trachea (Rajapakse et al, 1981).

Similar pathological changes affect the small intestine (Fig. 55.17). Disordered motility may lead to secondary bacterial overgrowth and a malabsorption syndrome. Small bowel involvement is common (Bluestone et al, 1969) but often symptom-free. Those patients with more severe disease may develop steatorrhoea and weight loss. Barium examination of the small intestine reveals dilated intestinal loops with thickened folds and a 'wire spring' appearance of the small bowel when not distended. The passage of food is delayed and there may be flocculation. Rarely the small bowel becomes grossly distended with loss of onward peristalsis. This is known as intestinal pseudo-

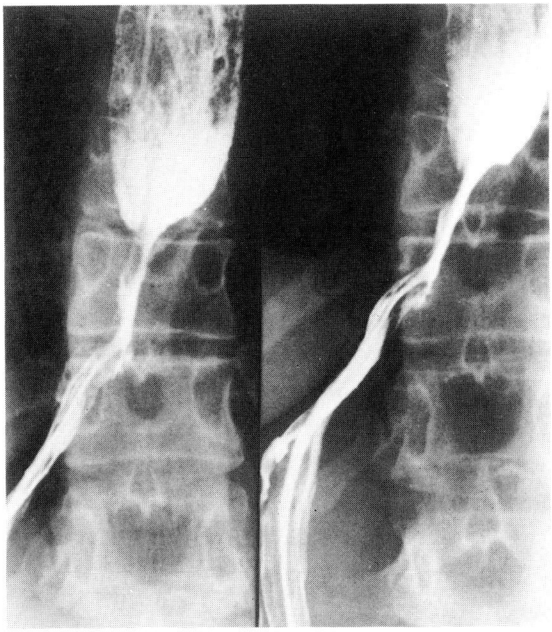

Fig. 55.16 Barium swallow examination showing an oesophageal stricture with a dilated oesophagus above.

obstruction because of the resemblance to organic obstruction of the small bowel. It is frequently a fatal complication.

Involvement of the large intestine leads to ballooning of the intestinal wall and the appearance of pseudodiverticulosis (Fig. 55.18). Occasionally a pseudodiverticulum may perforate (Jayson et al, 1972). Large bowel disease may also present with obstruction (Davis et al, 1976) or infarction of the colon (Edwards & Lennard-Jones, 1960).

Salivary glands

The parotid and submandibular glands may be affected by inflammatory cell infiltration, collagen deposition and glandular atrophy. Although obvious Sjögren's syndrome occurs in only a small proportion of patients, careful testing will show some evidence in almost all subjects (Alarcon-Segovia et al, 1974).

Pulmonary involvement

Involvement of the respiratory system is common.

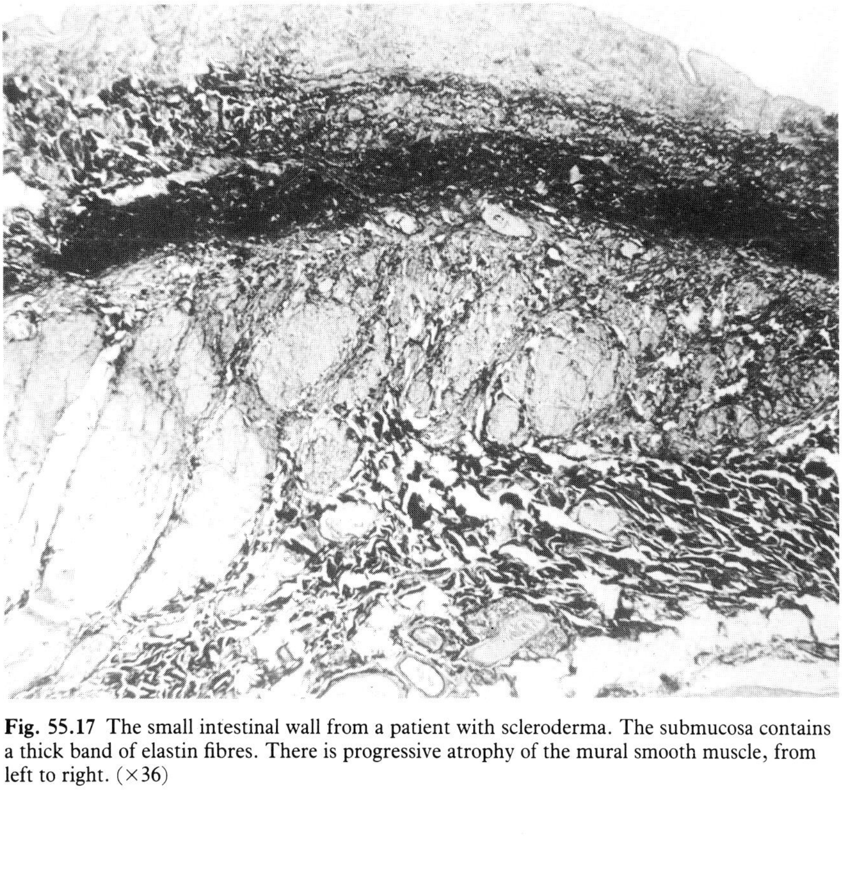

Fig. 55.17 The small intestinal wall from a patient with scleroderma. The submucosa contains a thick band of elastin fibres. There is progressive atrophy of the mural smooth muscle, from left to right. (×36)

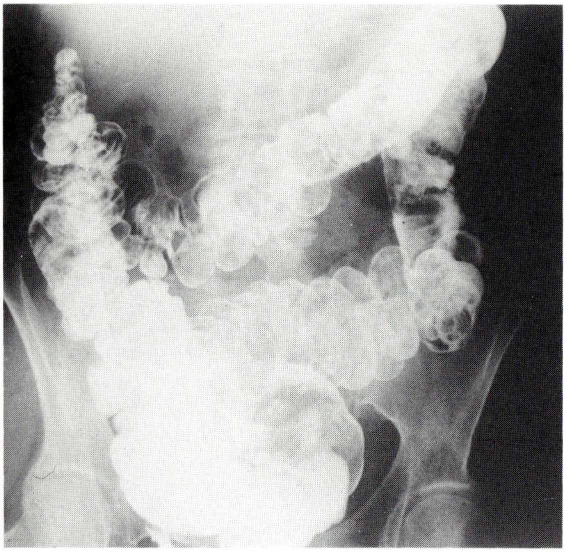

Fig. 55.18 Barium enema showing pseudodiverticulosis affecting the whole colon.

Pulmonary function tests will show a mixture of restrictive, obstructive, and small airway changes in a large proportion of patients frequently with ventilation/perfusion mismatching (Guttadauria et al, 1977). The diffusing capacity decreases in the cold seasons (Emmanuel et al, 1976) and with a cold challenge (Furst et al, 1981) suggesting a form of Raynaud's phenomenon affecting the lungs.

Fibrosing alveolitis usually starts in the lower lobes and spreads slowly upwards. There is progressive development of dyspnoea with fine basal rales. Radiographs show fine reticular changes which give rise to a honeycomb appearance in more severe cases. Rarely an alveolar cell carcinoma develops but this is believed to be the result of hyperplastic changes in advanced pulmonary fibrosis (Zatuchni et al, 1953; Collins et al, 1958).

Hyperplastic changes may develop in the smaller pulmonary arteries and arterioles leading to pulmonary hypertension. Death may result from rapidly progressive respiratory failure (Young & Mark, 1978). This complication is associated with the CREST variant of systemic sclerosis and is not related to pulmonary fibrosis which frequently occurs separately (Salerni et al, 1977).

Cardiac involvement

At autopsy, McWhorter & LeRoy (1974) found pericardial involvement with fibrinous adhesions or effusion in two-thirds of patients in contrast with clinical evidence of pericarditis in only about 7% during life. Cardiac wall fibrosis may lead to a cardiomyopathy with intractable congestive heart failure, rhythm changes, angina pectoris despite normal coronary arteries, and sudden death (Bulkley et al, 1976). The suggestion that there is a form of myocardial Raynaud's phenomenon has been raised. There seems to be an association between sclerodermatous involvement of the cardiac and peripheral muscles (West et al, 1981).

Kidney involvement

Renal disease is responsible for 43% of deaths in systemic sclerosis. Two-thirds of all deaths and three-quarters of renal deaths occur in the autumn and winter. There is a decrease in renal perfusion on cutaneous cooling in contrast with the normal increase. This suggests that there is a form of renal Raynaud's phenomenon which may play a part in the pathogenesis of permanent renal damage (Cannon et al, 1974).

In an extensive study of 210 patients over 20 years of age Cannon et al (1974) used proteinurea, azotaemia and hypertension as markers of renal involvement. One or more of these markers developed in 45% at a median onset of 3 years. Over the follow-up period death occurred in 10% of patients without markers but 60% of those with one or more of these features. Renal deaths occurred due to combination of malignant hypertension and acute renal failure. An elevation in the blood renin levels associated with the development of hypertension (Gavras et al, 1977) provides the basis for treatment with an angiotensin-converting enzyme inhibitor. Acute renal failure with severe hypertension may develop suddenly, particularly in patients with proximal and diffuse scleroderma and rarely in the CREST syndrome. Histological examination of the kidneys shows similar features to those of malignant hypertension with mucoid intimal proliferation and thickening in small arteries (Fig. 55.19) producing vascular obstruction and fibrinoid necrosis of arterioles and glomeruli (Fennell et al, 1961).

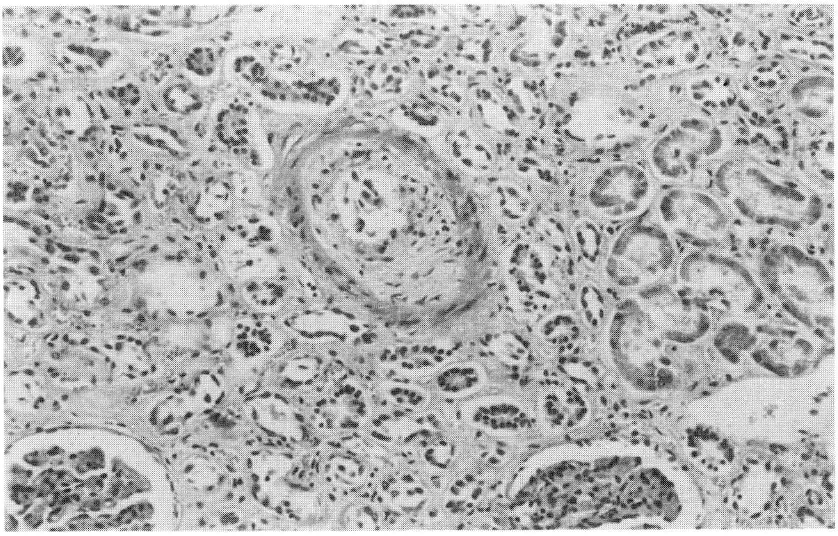

Fig. 55.19 Renal biopsy. There is intimal proliferation and adventitial fibrosis affecting the arteriole.

Disease subtypes and overlap syndromes

Most patients can be classified into one or more subtypes of the disease. This is helpful in determining prognosis although in any individual the disease pattern may extend to include a broader range of features.

The CREST syndrome is a combination of **C**alcinosis, **R**aynaud's phenomenon, o**E**sophageal involvement, **S**clerodactyly and **T**elangiectasia (Winterbauer, 1964). It is the same as the syndrome described by Thibierge & Weissenbach (1911). Most patients present with Raynaud's phenomenon and may develop peripheral ulceration and pitting in the pulps of the fingers and occasionally gangrene. Commonly it is many years before the true diagnosis is recognised (Rodnan & Medsger, 1975). In general the long-term prognosis for life is relatively good but these patients may develop severe and fatal pulmonary hypertension. The association of primary biliary cirrhosis with systemic sclerosis also seems to be with this variant (Reynolds et al, 1971). The CREST syndrome is specifically associated with an antibody directed against the centromere of dividing cells (Fig. 55.21c) (Tan et al, 1980) which provides a useful diagnostic and prognostic test.

In diffuse scleroderma there is early involvement of the skin of the trunk and limbs. These patients are at much greater risk of progressive visceral disease and have a significantly worse life expectancy (Bennett et al, 1971).

Mixed connective tissue disease (Sharp et al, 1972) is an overlap syndrome combining the features of systemic sclerosis, systemic lupus erythematosus, dermatomyositis and other autoimmune diseases. It is unlikely that it is a separate disease. It does seem specifically associated with an antibody to a ribonuclease-sensitive extractable nuclear antigen (Sharp et al, 1976) although it is not present in all cases. Although the prognosis is better than those of systemic sclerosis and systemic lupus erythematosus separately, renal involvement has been recorded (Bennet & Spargo, 1977). A similar syndrome has been observed in children (Singsen et al, 1977) but if anything the prognosis is rather worse than in adults with more frequent involvement of the heart and kidneys and also thrombocytopaenia (see Ch. 50).

Shulman (1974, 1975) described an apparently distinct syndrome known as eosinophilic fasciitis which is doubtfully related to excessive physical exertion. The patient develops sclerodermatous change particularly in the limbs and sometimes the trunk but without Raynaud's syndrome or visceral disease. The blood sedimentation rate is elevated with eosinophilia and hypergammaglobulinaemia. A biopsy shows marked thickening of the deep fascia with collagenous hypertrophy and a perivascular or scattered infiltrate of plasma cells and lymphocytes with occasional lymphoid follicles. Visceral involvement is rare and the skin changes will usually respond to steroid therapy (see Ch. 49).

PATHOGENESIS

Connective tissue changes

The most striking change in the skin is the progressive tethering and induration. Biopsies show a progressive increase in dermal thickness due to collagen proliferation (Rodnan et al, 1979). Biochemical assays indicate that the total collagen content is increased but the various collagen types are present in their normal proportions (Lovell et al, 1979). Chemical analysis shows an excess of readily reducible intermolecular cross-links (Herbert et al, 1974). On electron-microscopy the collagen fibres contain fibrils of a wide range of sizes. Many are thin with incomplete cross-banding and embryonic beaded filaments reminiscent of fetal skin collagen (Hayes & Rodnan, 1971). In vitro cultures of fibroblasts from sclerodermatous skin shows an increased production of collagen (LeRoy, 1974). This increase is more marked in fibroblasts derived from the deeper than the superficial dermis and may be a property of the cell as it continues through subcultures of up to 15 generations (Buckingham et al, 1978). There is some evidence that scleroderma serum selectively potentiates high collagen producing clones of fibroblasts and suppresses low collagen producing clones (Botstein et al, 1982). Mitogenic activity for fibroblasts found in systemic sclerosis serum could stimulate fibroblast replication and fibrosis. A lymphokine derived from stimulation of human mononuclear cells may play a role in stimulating fibroblasts to secrete excess collagen (Johnson & Ziff, 1976). Alternatively the presence of circulating antibodies to types I and IV collagen raise the possibility that immunity to autologous collagen may play a fundamental role in the pathogenesis of the disease (Mackel et al, 1982). Deficiency of collagenase may interfere with the removal of excess collagen in the skin (Brady, 1975).

In the deep dermis there is also an increase in fibronectin (Cooper et al, 1979) but its role is uncertain. The earliest changes in scleroderma may be a massive increase of glycosaminoglycan (Ishikawa & Horiuchi, 1975). Systemic sclerosis fibroblasts in cell culture synthesise excess glycosaminoglycan (Buckingham et al, 1983), and intraperitoneal injections into mice of urinary glycosaminoglycans from systemic sclerosis patients will produce a scleroderma-like disease (Ishikawa et al, 1975). The significance of these changes remains to be determined.

Microcirculatory changes

Measurements of the peripheral microcirculation in the skin confirm the clinical evidence of peripheral ischaemia with an excessive further reduction on exposure to cold (Coffman & Cohen, 1971; LeRoy et al, 1971; Haavik Nilsen & Jayson, 1980).

The principle pathological changes occur in the capillaries, arterioles and small arteries. There is an extreme reduction in the numbers of capillaries to perhaps only 20% of normal and those remaining show endothelial swelling and reduplication of the basement membrane (Norton et al, 1968). In the small arteries (150–500 μ) there is marked intimal thickening due to proliferation and swelling of endothelial cells and the deposition of a mucoid ground substance with fine collagen fibrils (Fig. 55.20). Around the adventitia is a cuff of fibrous tissue and there may be an infiltration of mononuclear cells. In the late stages these features may be replaced by blood vessel fibrosis and atrophy. In the smaller arterioles (50–150 μ) the principle changes are of intimal sclerosis with fibrinoid change and necrosis (Campbell & LeRoy, 1975). Obstruction of the digital vessels can be detected on arteriography in the vast majority of cases (Dabich et al, 1972) but there is a poor correlation between the severity of vascular disease and the sclerodermatous change in the skin. This raises some doubt about whether the vascular damage can be regarded as the cause of the excessive fibrosis.

There is no evidence of sympathetic hyperactivity (Fries, 1969). Sapira et al (1972) failed to confirm the presence of elevated catecholamines (Peacock 1959) although blood vessels from systemic sclerosis patients may show altered responses on exposure to catecholamines (Winkelmann et al, 1977). Abnormalities of serotonin metabolism may be relevant. Serotonin is known to

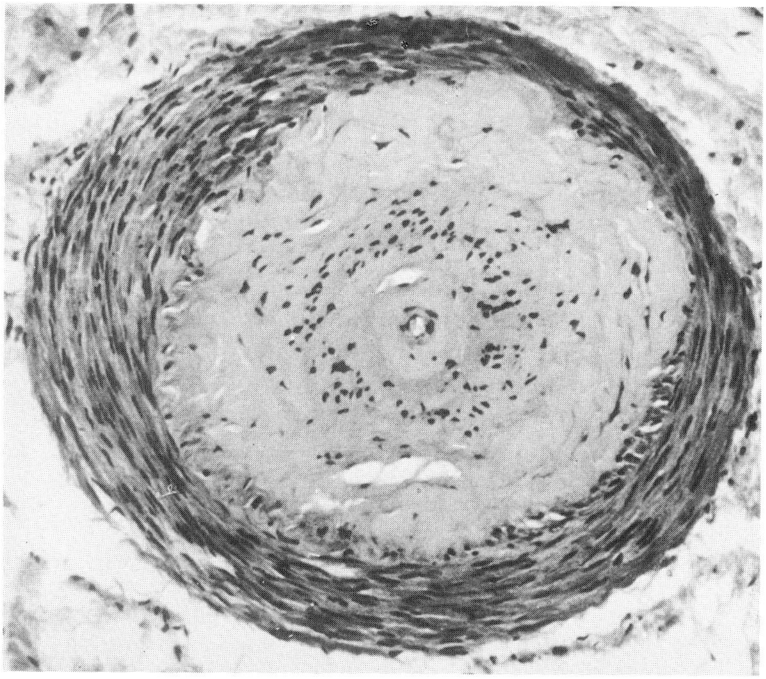

Fig. 55.20 A digital artery from a patient with scleroderma. The intima is thickened by globular, relatively acellular hyaline material. The lumen is narrowed. (×96)

cause Raynaud's phenomenon (Halpern et al, 1960; Scherbel & Harrison, 1959; Winkelmann et al, 1976.) Abnormalities of serotonin metabolism occur in systemic sclerosis (Stachow et al, 1977). Carcinoid tumours may be associated with scleroderma-like lesions (Fries et al, 1973) and a scleroderma-like illness has been reported during treatment with L-5-hydroxytryptophan and carbidoba (Sternberg et al, 1980) and was thought due to high serotonin levels. In vitro testing shows that serotonin can stimulate fibroblast growth (Boucek & Noble, 1973).

Endothelial cell damage is indicated by elevated factor VIII/von Willebrand antigen and von Willebrand factor activity in systemic sclerosis (Kahaleh et al, 1981) with evidence of in vivo platelet activation (Kahaleh et al, 1982). However, the evidence for a circulating endothelial cell cytotoxic factor is controversial (Kahaleh et al, 1979; Summers et al, 1984).

In systemic sclerosis and Raynaud's phenomenon the reduced peripheral circulation may be due to reduced red cell deformability (Dodds et al, 1979) and hyperviscosity of the blood (Goyle & Dormandy, 1976) which is particularly marked at low shear rates (McGrath et al, 1977) as in the smaller blood vessels. There is elevation of the fibrinogen levels which is a result of impaired fibrinolytic activity (Cunliffe & Menon, 1969; Jarrett et al, 1978; Holland & Jayson, 1982) and defective plasminogen plasminogen activator release from vascular endothelia (Holland & Jayson, 1985). This may also be responsible for poor clearance of fibrin deposits in the walls of small blood vessels (Fennell et al, 1961) so exacerbating the vascular problem.

Complement-fixing serological factors may react with blood vessel walls (Tan & Pearson, 1972), and immune complex deposition in the intimal lesions of small arteries within the kidney (Lapenas et al, 1978) may play a pathogenetic role.

Inflammatory and immunological changes

A number of observations suggest that inflammatory and immunological abnormalities play a role in the pathogenesis of the disease. In overlap syndromes, there is a mixture of features of systemic lupus erythematosus and other rheumatic disorders (Sharp et al, 1972) and a systemic sclerosis-like syndrome may follow graft-versus-host disease after bone marrow transplantation (Furst et al, 1979). Biopsies frequently show chronic inflammatory cell infiltration in the skin (Fleischmajer et al, 1977) and immunofluorescent examination of the skin (Winkelmann et al, 1977) and kidney (Lapenas et al, 1978) may show immunoglobulin and complement deposition. A mixed cryoglobulinaemia is often present but shows little correlation with the clinical features and is of uncertain pathogenic significance (Husson et al, 1976).

On detailed testing anti-nuclear antibodies are found in virtually all cases (Tan et al, 1980). The anti-nuclear factor is usually of the speckled or nucleolar patterns (Fig. 55.21) but its presence shows no correlation with disease severity or outcome (Jordan et al, 1971). Alarcon-Segovia & Fishbein (1975) reported the association of uracil-specific antibodies against single-stranded RNA. Douvas et al (1979) found an antibody against a nuclear protein Scl-70 in about 20% of systemic sclerosis patients, which seems specifically restricted to this disorder. Despite the presence of these autoantibodies there is impaired in vitro antibody function possibly due to the presence of suppressor monocytes (Segond et al, 1982).

With respect to cell-mediated immunity there is a reduction of antibody-dependent and phytohaemagglutinin-induced lymphocyte cytotoxicity

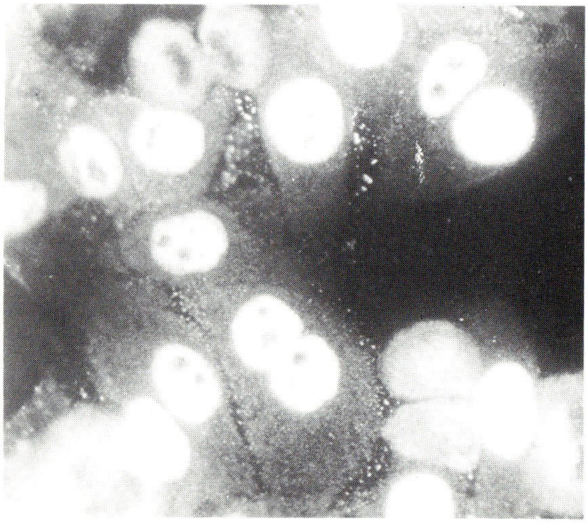
a

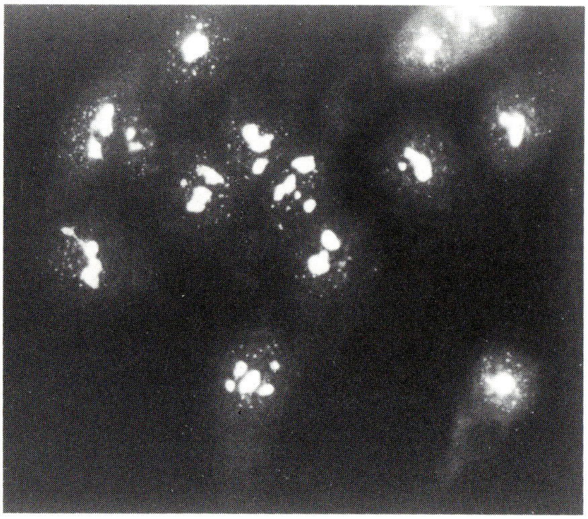
b

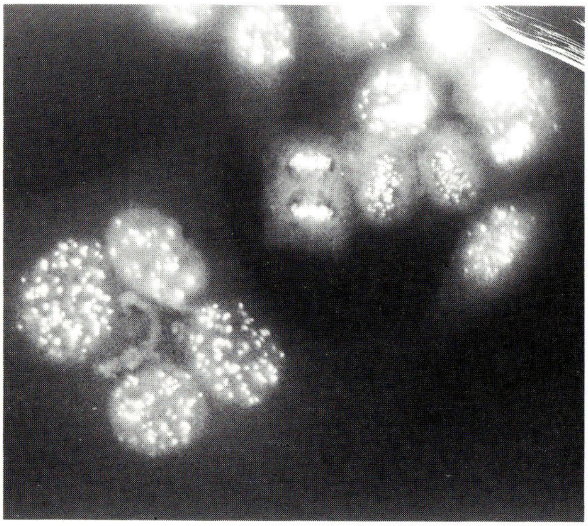
c

Fig. 55.21 (a) Diffuse staining of nucleus by anti-nuclear factor typical of systemic lupus erythematosus. (b) Nucleolar pattern in systemic sclerosis. (c) Anti-centromere antibody and discrete speckled pattern obtained in a patient with the CREST syndrome.

(Horwitz & Garrett, 1977; Wright et al, 1979). There is a reduction in the numbers of circulating T lymphocytes which correlates to a certain degree with the extent of visceral disease (Hughes et al, 1976). In the skin there is an excess of T lymphocytes (Kondo et al, 1976) which may be responsible for lymphokine stimulation of collagen synthesis by fibroblasts (Johnson Ziff, 1976).

There is an increased frequency of chromosomal breaks (Emerit, 1979) and sister chromosomal exchanges (Sherer et al, 1981) in systemic sclerosis patients. However, the significance of these findings is uncertain as there is also an increased chromosomal breakage rate in their non-affected relatives.

PROGNOSIS

Overall the 5-year survival rate is between 70 and 80% (Bennett et al, 1971; Barnett, 1978). The survival time appears better in Caucasians than in negroes (Masi & D'Angelo, 1967). Patients with sclerodactyly or acrosclerosis have a much better prognosis than those with diffuse scleroderma (Barnett, 1978; Tuffanelli & Winkelmann, 1962). The following have been identified as associated with a reduced survival: older age at presentation; trunk involvement; excess alcohol intake; cigarette smoking; elevated ESR; anaemia; evidence of cardiac, pulmonary, or renal disease (Bennett et al, 1971; Medsger & Masi, 1973). The principle cause of death due to systemic sclerosis is renal failure. Cannon et al (1974) used proteinurea, azotaemia and hypertension to indicate renal involvement. In the absence of these markers only 10% of these patients died over 20 years in contrast with 60% of those with one or more of these features. An unexplained increase in plasma renin levels in an otherwise stable patient may herald imminent deterioration of renal function and may be of great prognostic importance (Gavras et al, 1977).

TREATMENT

This should be considered under the following headings:

a. General/symptomatic
b. Improvement of peripheral blood flow
c. Anti-inflammatory drugs
d. Anti-fibrotic drugs
e. Treatment of specific organ involvement

General/symptomatic treatment

Care must be taken to protect the patient and particularly the hands and feet against cold exposure. Warm clothes and gloves with thermal liners or electrically heated by a portable battery pack are important for cold weather. Patients must stop smoking and drugs known to precipitate Raynaud's phenomenon such as β-blockers and ergotamine must be avoided. The patient should avoid trauma to the fingers and any infections must be treated promptly. Lanolin creams may produce some apparent softening of the skin and cosmetic preparations such as 'Covermark' are helpful for unsightly telangiectasiae. Physiotherapy and splinting to prevent and control deformities are of little value.

Improvement of peripheral microcirculation

Peripheral vasodilation with measureable increases in the capillary microcirculation of the skin are provided by the use of oral reserpine (Coffman & Cohen, 1971), guanethidine (LeRoy et al, 1971), methyldopa (Varadi & Lawrence, 1969), nifedipine, intra-arterial reserpine (Haavik Nilsen & Jayson, 1980) and intravenous infusions of prostaglandin E_1 (Martin et al, 1981) and I_2. The latter may also act by improving red cell deformability (Dowd et al, 1981). The benefit from these infusions seems only temporary but they may allow the healing of otherwise intractable skin ulcers. 1% topical glyceryl trinitrite used as an ointment in ischaemic areas may also improve the circulation locally (Franks, 1982). Sympathectomy can provide some symptomatic relief but does not seem to influence the long-term course of the disease (Johnston et al, 1965).

The fibrinolytic abnormalities can be improved by intravenous infusion of low molecular weight dextran (Cunliffe & Menon, 1969) with an increase in the peripheral microcirculation (Tomlinson et al, 1985). Fibrinolytic enhancement using the anabolic steroid stanazolol (Jarrett et al, 1978) and plasmapheresis (O'Reilly et al, 1979) have also been used to reduce fibrinogen levels. Controlled studies indicate their possible values. Plasmapheresis also may act by improving red cell deformability (Dodds et al, 1979).

Anti-inflammatory and immunosuppressive therapy

Although non-steroidal anti-inflammatory drugs may relieve the mild synovitis which frequently occurs in systemic sclerosis, there is no evidence that they affect the development of sclerodermatous skin change or the course of the disease. Studies of the effects of steroids have proved disappointing (Zion, 1955; Medsger & Masi, 1973). However many patients had advanced disease. There does seem some useful benefit particularly in patients with early disease, inflammatory cell infiltration, immunoglobulin and complement deposition on skin biopsies, and with clinical evidence of overlap syndromes (Winkelmann et al, 1977). There is no firm evidence that immunosupressive therapy is of any value (Steigerwald, 1974).

Anti-fibrotic drugs

The lathyritic effect of D-penicillamine on collagen (Nimni, 1968) led to trials of this compound in systemic sclerosis. Particularly in early disease it can prevent disease progress and lead to improved elasticity in the skin (Bluestone et al, 1970; Jayson et al, 1977). However, there is little evidence that it affects the progress of the vascular or visceral features of the disease. Beta-amino propionitrile is an effective lathyritic agent. In treating systemic sclerosis favourable changes were noted in dermal collagen but its use was limited by severe side-effects (Keiser & Sjoerdsma, 1967).

Colchicine is known to depolymerise microtubules and inhibit the excretion of collagen from fibroblasts in vitro. Despite a favourable uncontrolled study (Alarcon-Segovia et al, 1979), a controlled evaluation (Guttadauria et al, 1977) failed to detect any useful benefit. Potasium amino benzoate (POTABA) has not been shown to influence the disease outcome (Medsger & Masi, 1973). Experience with the weak oestrogen cyclofenil which is known to decrease proteoglycan synthesis in connective tissue (Black et al, 1983) suggests that it is of some value.

Management of specific organ involvement

The various complications will require appropriate management. In general it may be possible to provide symptomatic relief but it is doubtful whether the underlying pathological changes are altered.

Metoclopramide significantly improves oesophageal motility (Ramirez-Mata et al, 1977) and will help to control dysphagia. In the presence of stricture, oesophageal dilatation may prove necessary and for reflux there are reconstructive procedures at the oesophageal gastric junction (Orringer et al, 1981). Malabsorption due to secondary bacterial overgrowth will respond to oral antibiotics such as tetracycline or metronidazole. Intestinal pseudo-obstruction is frequently a fatal complication. Some patients respond to conservative management. Occasionally a volvulus is discovered at laparotomy with restoration of bowel function when corrected. There have been cases of total ileal resection subsequently managed by a parenteral nutrition regime (personal observation). With large bowel disease it is important to avoid both diarrhoea and constipation by dietary regulation.

Cardiac failure will often prove resistent to treatment but it is important to exclude pericarditis and to manage arrhythmias and conduction defects in the appropriate ways. Pulmonary involvement is usually due to progressive fibrosing alveolitis or pulmonary hypertension. There is doubtful benefit from penicillamine therapy. Otherwise management depends upon prompt treatment of secondary infection and other symptomatic therapy.

Acute renal failure with malignant hypertension is the principal cause of death due to systemic sclerosis. In the past this complication had a universally fatal outcome. More recently the use of dialysis, nephrectomy and renal transplantation (LeRoy & Fleischmann, 1978) provided only very limited success. With aggressive treatment of hypertension there have been reports of patients surviving (Mitnick & Feig, 1978; Wasner et al, 1978). However, the oral angiotensin-converting enzyme inhibitor Captropil can be dramatically effective in reversing systemic sclerosis renal crises (Lopez-Ovejero et al, 1979). It is important to treat patients promptly at the onset of acute renal failure and hypertension. It seems more effective in the absence of malignant hypertension (Whitman et al, 1982). Improvement in the digital artery circulation has also been found (Miyazaki et al 1982). This benefit does not seem due to inhibited production of angiotensin II but may be a consequence of accumulation of circulating kinins.

CONCLUSION

Oh that this too, too solid flesh would melt
Thaw and resolve itself into a dew.
Hamlet, Act I, Scene ii, 129–130

REFERENCES

Alarcon-Segovia D, Fishbein E 1975 Immunochemical characterisation of the anti-RNA antibodies found in scleroderma and systemic lupus erythematosus. I Differences in reactivity with Poly (U) and Poly (A). Journal of Immunology 115: 28–31

Alarcon-Segovia D, Ibanez G, Hernandez-Ortiz J, Velazquez-Forero F, Gonzalez-Jimenez Y 1974 Sjögren's syndrome in progressive systemic sclerosis (Scleroderma). American Journal of Medicine 57: 78–85

Alarcon-Segovia D, Ramos-Niembro F, Ibanez de Kasep G, Alcocer J, Tamayo R P 1979 Long-term evaluation of colchicine in the treatment of scleroderma. Journal of Rheumatology 6: 705–712

Barnett A J 1978 Scleroderma (progressive systemic sclerosis). Progress and course based on a personal series of 118 cases. Medical Journal of Australia 2: 129–134

Bennett R, Bluestone R, Holt P J L, Bywaters, E G L 1971 Survival in scleroderma. Annals of Rheumatic Diseases 30: 581–588

Bennett R M, Spargo B H 1977 Immune complex nephropathy in mixed connective tissue disease. American Journal of Medicine 63: 534–541

Black C M, Jayson M I V, White A G, Million R M 1983 A double blind comparison of cyclofenil and placebo in systemic sclerosis (SS). Annals of the Rheumatic Diseases 42:229

Black C M, Maddison P J, Welsh K I et al 1984 HLA antigens in scleroderma. British Journal of Rheumatology 23: 267–271

Bluestone R, MacMahon M, Dawson J M 1969 Systemic sclerosis and small bowel involvement. Gut 10: 185–193

Bluestone R, Grahame R, Holloway V, Holt P J L 1970 Treatment of systemic sclerosis with d-Penicillamine. Annals of Rheumatic Diseases 29: 153–158

Botstein G R, Sherer G K, LeRoy E C 1982 Fibroblast selection in scleroderma. Arthritis and Rheumatism 25: 189–195

Boucek R J, Noble N L 1973 Histamine, norepinephrine and bradykinin stimulation of fibroblast growth and modification of the serotonin response (37714). Proceedings of the Society for Experimental Biology and Medicine 144: 929–933

Brady A H 1975 Collagenase in scleroderma. Journal of Clinical Investigation 56: 1175–1180

Bramwell B 1914 Diffuse scleroderma: its frequency; its occurrence in stone-mason's; its treatment by fibrolysin — elevations of temperature due to fibrolysin injections. Edinburgh Medical Journal 12: 387–401

Buckingham R B, Prince R K, Rodnan G P, Taylor R 1978 Increased collagen accumulation in dermal fibroblast cultures from patients with progressive systemic sclerosis (Scleroderma). Journal of Laboratory and Clinical Medicine 92: 5–21

Buckingham R B, Prince R K, Rodnan G P 1983 Progressive systemic sclerosis (PSS, scleroderma) dermal fibroblasts synthesize increased amounts of glycosaminoglycan. Journal of Laboratory and Clinical Medicine 101: 659–669

Buckley B H, Ridolfi R L, Salyer W R, Hutchins G M 1976 Myocardial lesions of progressive systemic sclerosis. Circulation 53: 483–490

Campbell P M, LeRoy E C 1975 Pathogenesis of systemic sclerosis: A vascular hypothesis. Seminars in Arthritis and Rheumatism 4: 351–368

Camus J-P, Emerit I, Reinert Ph, Guillien P, Grouzet J, Fourot J 1970 Sclérodermie familiale avec syndrome de Sjögren. Annalle de Médicine Interne 121: 149–161

Cannon P J, Hassar M, Case D B, Casarella W J, Sommers S C, LeRoy E C 1974 The relationship of hypertension and renal failure in scleroderma (progressive systemic sclerosis) to structural and functional abnormalities of the renal cortical circulation. Medicine 53: 1–46

Cassidy J T, Sullivan D B, Dabich L, Petty R 1977 Scleroderma in children. Arthritis and Rheumatism 20: 351–354

Clark J A, Winkelmann R K, McDuffie F C, Ward L E 1971 Synovial tissue changes and rheumatoid factor in scleroderma. Mayo Clinic Proceedings 46: 97–103

Clements P J, Furst D E, Campion D S, Bohan A, Harris R, Levy J, Paulus H E 1978 Muscle disease in progressive systemic sclerosis. Arthritis and Rheumatism 21: 62–71

Coffman J D, Cohen A S 1971 Total and capillary fingertip blood flow in Raynaud's phenomenon. New England Journal of Medicine 285: 259–263

Collins D H, Darke C S, Dodge D G 1958 Scleroderma with honeycomb lungs and bronchiolar carcinoma. Journal of Pathology and Bacteriology 76: 531–540

Connolly S M, Winkelmann R K 1981 Direct immunofluorescent findings in scleroderma syndromes. Acta Dermatovener (Stockholm) 61: 29–36

Cooper S M, Keyser A J, Beaulieu A D, Ruoslahti E, Nimni M E, Quismorio F P Jr 1979 Increase in fibronectin in the deep dermis of involved skin in progressive systemic sclerosis. Arthritis and Rheumatism 22: 983–987

Connolly S M, Winkelmann R K 1981 Direct immunofluorescent findings in scleroderma syndromes. Acta Dermatovener (Stockholm) 61: 29–36

Cunliffe W J, Menon I S 1969 Blood fibrinolytic activity in diseases of small blood vessels and the effect of low molecular weight dextran. British Journal of Dermatology 81: 220–225

Dabich L, Bookstein J J, Zweifler A, Zarafonetis C J D 1972 Digital arteries in patients with scleroderma. Archives of Internal Medicine 130: 708–714

D'Angelo W A, Fries J F, Masi A T, Shulman L E 1969 Pathologic observations in systemic sclerosis (scleroderma). American Journal of Medicine 46: 428–440

Davis R P, Hines J R, Flinn W R 1976 Scleroderma of the colon with obstruction: Report of a case. Diseases of the Colon and Rectum 19: 256–259

Dodds A J, O'Reilly M J G, Yates C J P, Cotton L T, Flute P E, Dormandy J A 1979 Haemorrheological response to plasma exchange in Raynaud's syndrome. British Medical Journal 2: 1186–1187

Douvas A S, Achten M, Tan E M 1979 Identification of a nuclear protein (Scl-70) as a unique target of human antinuclear antibodies in scleroderma. Journal of Biological Chemistry 254: 10514–10522

Dowd P M, Kovacs I B, Bland C J H, Kirby J D T 1981 Effects of prostaglandins I_2 and E_1 on red cell deformability in patients with Raynaud's phenomenon and systemic sclerosis. British Medical Journal 2:350

Edwards D A W, Lennard-Jones J E 1960 Diffuse systemic sclerosis presenting as infarction of the colon. Proceedings of the Royal Society of Medicine 53: 877–879

Emerit I 1979 Chromosomal abnormalities in progressive systemic sclerosis. Clinics in Rheumatic Diseases 5: 201–214

Emmanuel G, Saroja D, Gopinathan K, Gharpure A, Stuckey J 1976 Environmental factors and the diffusing capacity of the lung in progressive systemic sclerosis. Chest 69 (Suppl): 304–307

Erasmus L D 1975 Scleroderma in gold-mines on the Witwatersrand with particular reference to pulmonary manifestations. South African Journal of Laboratory and Clinical Medicine. 3: 209–231

Farrell D A, Medsger T A Jr 1982 Trigeminal neuropathy in progressive systemic sclerosis. American Journal of Medicine 73: 57–62

Fennell R H Jr, Reddy C R R M, Vazquez J J 1961 Progressive systemic sclerosis and malignant hypertension. Archives of Pathology 72: 209–215

Finch W R, Rodnan G P, Buckingham R B, Prince R K, Winkelstein N A 1980 Bleomycin-induced scleroderma. Journal of Rheumatology 7: 651–659

Fleischmajer R, Perlish J S, Reeves J R T 1977 Cellular infiltrates in scleroderma skin. Arthritis and Rheumatism 20: 975–984

Franks A G Jr 1982 Topical glyceryl trinitrate as adjunctive treatment in Raynaud's disease. Lancet 1: 76–77

Frayha R A, Tabbara K F, Geha R S 1977 Familial CRST Syndrome with sicca complex. Journal of Rheumatology 4: 53–58

Fries J F 1969 Physiologic studies in systemic sclerosis (scleroderma). Archives of Internal Medicine 123: 22–25

Fries J F, Lindgren J A, Bull J M 1973 Scleroderma-like lesions and the carcinoid syndrome. Archives of Internal Medicine 131: 550–553

Furst D E, Clements P J, Graze P, Gale R, Roberts N 1979 A syndrome resembling progressive systemic sclerosis after bone marrow transplantation. Arthritis and Rheumatism 22: 904–910

Furst D E, Davis J A, Clements P J, Chopra S K, Theofilopoulos A N, Chia D 1981 Abnormalities of pulmonary vascular dynamics and inflammation in early progressive systemic sclerosis. Arthritis and Rheumatism 24: 1403–1413

Gavras H, Gavras I, Cannon P J, Brunner H R, Laragh J H 1977 Is elevated renin activity of prognostic importance in progressive systemic sclerosis? Archives of Internal Medicine 137: 1554–1558

Germain B F, Espinoza L R, Bergen L L, Vagesh M, Vasey F B 1981 Increased prevalence of DRw3 in the CREST syndrome. Arthritis and Rheumatism 24: 857–859

Gladman D D, Keystone E C, Baron M, Lee P, Cane D, Mervert H 1981 Increased frequency of HLA-DR5 in scleroderma. Arthritis and Rheumatism 24: 854–856

Goyle K B, Dormandy J A 1976 Abnormal blood viscosity in Raynaud's phenomenon. Lancet 1: 1317–1318

Gray R G, Altman R D 1977 Progressive systemic sclerosis in a family. Arthritis and Rheumatism 20: 35–41

Guttadauria M, Diamond H, Kaplan D 1977 Colchicine in the treatment of scleroderma. Journal of Rheumatology 4: 272–276

Guttadauria M, Ellman H, Emmanuel G, Kaplan D, Diamond H 1977 Pulmonary function in scleroderma. Arthritis and Rheumatism 20: 1071–1079

Haavik Nilsen K, Jayson M I V 1980 Cutaneous microcirculation in systemic sclerosis and response to intra-arterial reserpine. British Medical Journal 1: 1408–1411

Halpern A, Kuhn P H, Shaftel H E, et al 1960 Raynaud's disease, Raynaud's phenomenon and serotonin. Angiology 11: 151–167

Hausmanowa-Petrusewicz I, Jablonska S, Blaszczyk M, Matz B 1982 Electromyographic findings in various forms of progressive systemic sclerosis. Arthritis and Rheumatism 25: 61–65

Hayes R L, Rodnan G P 1971 The ultrastructure of skin in progressive systemic sclerosis (scleroderma). 1. Dermal collagen fibres. American Journal of Pathology 63: 433–442

Herbai G, Blom B, Bostrom H 1977 Treatment of progressive systemic sclerosis (scleroderma, PSS) with a new drug influencing connective tissue. Acta Medica Scandinavica 201: 203–206

Herbert C M, Lindberg K A, Jayson M I V, Bailey A J 1974 Biosynthesis and maturation of skin collagen in scleroderma and effect of D-penicillamine. Lancet 1: 187–192

Holland C D, Jayson M I V 1985 Venous blood fibrinolysis and fibrinolytic potential in primary Raynaud's phenomenon and systemic sclerosis associated Raynaud's phenomenon. Progressive Systemic Sclerosis. Gower, New York

Horwitz D A, Garrett M A 1977 Lymphocyte reactivity to mitogen in subjects with systemic lupus erythematosus, rheumatoid arthritis and scleroderma. Clinical and Experimental Immunology 27: 92–99

Hughes P, Holt S, Rowell N R, Dodd J 1976 Thymus-dependent (T) lymphocyte deficiency in progressive systemic sclerosis. British Journal of Dermatology 95: 469–473

Hughes P, Gelsthorpe K, Doughty R W, Rowell N R, Rosenthal F D, Sneddon I B 1978 The association of HLA-B8 with visceral disease in systemic sclerosis. Clinical and Experimental Immunology 31: 351–356

Husson J M, Druet P, Contet A, Fiessinger J N, Gamilleri J P 1976 Systemic sclerosis and cryoglobulinemia. Clinical Immunology and Immunopathology 6: 77–82

Ishikawa H, Horiuchi I R 1975 Initial change of glycosaminoglycans in systemic scleroderma. Dermatologica 150: 334–345

Ishikawa H, Suzuki S, Horiuchi R, Sato H 1975 An approach to experimental scleroderma using urinary glycosaminoglycans from patients with systemic scleroderma. Acta Dermatovener 55: 97–107

Jablonska S 1975 Scleroderma and pseudo scleroderma. Polish Medical Publishers, Warsaw

Jarrett P E M, Morland M, Browse N L 1978 Treatment of Raynaud's phenomenon by fibrinolytic enhancement. British Medical Journal 2: 523–525

Jayson M I V 1977 Vinyl chloride diseases. Annals of Rheumatic Diseases 36 (Suppl): 39–41

Jayson M I V, Lovell C, Black C M, Wilson R S E 1977 Penicillamine therapy in systemic sclerosis. Proceedings of the Royal Society of Medicine 70 (Suppl 3): 82–88

Jayson M I V, Salmon P R, Gough J, Poliness T, Bishton R L 1972 Spontaneous bowel perforation in intestinal scleroderma. Post-graduate Medical Journal 48: 56–58

Johnson R L, Ziff M 1976 Lymphokine stimulation of collagen acumulation. Journal of Clinical Investigation 58: 240–252

Johnston E N M, Summerly R, Birnstingl M 1965 Prognosis in Raynaud's Phenomenon after Sympathectomy. British Medical Journal 1: 962–964

Jordan R E, Deheer D, Schroeter A, Winkelmann R K 1971 Antinuclear antibodies: their significance in scleroderma. Mayo Clinic Proceedings 46: 111–113

Kahaleh M B, Osborn I, LeRoy E C 1981 Increased factor VIII/von Willebrand factor antigen and von Willebrand factor activity in scleroderma and in Raynaud's phenomenon. Annals of Internal Medicine 94: 482–484

Kahaleh M B, Osborn I, LeRoy E C 1982 Elevated levels of circulating platelet aggregates and betathromboglobulin in scleroderma. Annals of Internal Medicine 96: 610–613

Kahaleh M B, Sherer G K, LeRoy E C 1979 Endothelial injury in scleroderma. Journal of Experimental Medicine 149: 1326–1335

Kallenberg C G M, Van der Voort-Beelen J M, D'Amaro J, The T H 1981 Increased frequency of B8/DR3 in scleroderma and association of the haplotype with impaired cellular immune response. Clinical and Experimental Immunology 43: 478–485

Keiser H R, Sjoerdsma A 1967 Studies on beta-amino proprionitrile in patients with scleroderma. Clinical Pharmacology and Therapeutics 8: 593–602

Kondo H, Rabin B S, Rodnan G P 1976 Cutaneous antigen-stimulating lymphokine production by lymphocytes of patients with progressive systemic sclerosis (scleroderma). Journal of Clinical Investigation 58: 1388–1394

Kornreich H K, Koster-King K, Bernstein B H, Singsen B H, Hanson V 1977 Scleroderma in childhood. Arthritis and Rheumatism 20: 343–350

Kumagai Y, Shiokawa Y, Medsger T A Jr, Rodnan G P 1984 Clinical spectrum of connective tissue disease after cosmetic surgery. Arthritis and Rheumatism 27: 1–12

Kurland L T, Hauser W A, Ferguson R H, Holley K E 1969 Epidemiologic features of diffuse connective tissue disorders in Rochester, Minn. 1951 through 1967, with special reference to systemic lupus erythematosus. Mayo Clinic Proceedings 44: 649–663

Lapenas D, Rodnan G P, Cavallo T 1978 Immunopathology of the renal vascular lesion of progressive systemic sclerosis (scleroderma). American Journal of Pathology 91: 243–258

LeRoy E C 1974 Increased collagen synthesis by scleroderma fibroblasts in vitro. Journal of Clinical Investigation 54: 880–889

LeRoy E C 1976 Scleroderma (systemic sclerosis). In: Modern Topics in Rheumatology. Heinemann, London

LeRoy E C, Downley J A, Cannon P J 1971 Skin capillary blood flow in scleroderma. Journal of Clinical Investigation 50: 930–939

LeRoy E C, Fleischmann R M 1978 The management of renal scleroderma. American Journal of Medicine 64: 974–978

LeRoy E C, Kahaleh M B, Mercurio S 1983 A fibroblast mitogen present in scleroderma but not control sera. Inhibition by proteinase inhibitors. Rheumatology International 3: 35–38

Lopez-Ovejero J A, Saal S D, D'Angelo W A, Cheigh J S, Stenzel K H, Laragh J H 1979 Reversal of vascular and renal crisis of scleroderma by oral angiotensin-converting-enzyme blockade. New England Journal of Medicine 300: 1417–1419

Lovell C R, Jayson M I V 1979 Joint involvement in systemic sclerosis. Scandinavian Journal of Rheumatology 8: 154–160

Lovell C R, Nicholls A C, Duance V C, Bailey A J 1979 Characterisation of dermal collagen in systemic sclerosis. British Journal of Dermatology 100: 359–369

McGrath M A, Peek R, Penny R 1977 Blood hyperviscosity with reduced skin blood flow in scleroderma. Annals of Rheumatic Diseases 36: 569–574

Mackal A M, DeLustro F, Harper F E, LeRoy E C 1982 Antibodies to collagen in scleroderma. Arthritis and Rheumatism 25: 522–531

McWhorter J E, LeRoy E C 1974 Pericardial disease in scleroderma (systemic sclerosis). American Journal of Medicine 57: 566–575

Maricq H R 1981 Widefield capillary microscopy. Arthritis and Rheumatism 24: 1159–1165

Maricq H R, Spencer-Green G, LeRoy E C 1976 Skin capillary abnormalities as indicators of organ involvement in scleroderma (systemic sclerosis), Raynaud's Phenomenon and Dermatomyositis. American Journal of Medicine 61: 862–870

Maricq H R, LeRoy E C, D'Angelo W A et al 1980 Diagnostic potential of in vivo capillary microscopy in scleroderma and related disorders. Arthritis and Rheumatism 23: 183–189

Martin M F R, Dowd P M, Ring E F J et al 1981 Prostaglandin E1 infusions for vascular insufficiency in progressive systemic sclerosis. Annals of Rheumatic Diseases 40: 350–354

Masi A T, D'Angelo W A 1967 Epidemiology of fatal systemic sclerosis (diffuse scleroderma). Annals of Internal Medicine 66: 870–883

Masi A T, Rodnan G P, Medsger T A et al 1980 Subcommittee for scleroderma criteria of the ARA Diagnostic and Therapeutic Criteria Committee Preliminary Criteria for the classification of systemic sclerosis (scleroderma). Arthritis and Rheumatism 23: 581–590

Medsger T A Jr, Masi A T 1971 Epidemiology of systemic sclerosis (scleroderma). Annals of Internal Medicine 74: 714–721

Medsger T A Jr, Masi A T 1973 Survival with scleroderma — II: A life-table analysis of clinical and demographic factors in 358 male US veteran patients. Journal of Chronic Diseases 26: 647–660

Medsger T A Jr, Masi A T 1978 The epidemiology of systemic sclerosis (scleroderma) among male US veterans. Journal of Chronic Diseases 31: 73–85

Medsger T A Jr, Rodnan G P, Moosy J, Vester J W 1968 Skeletal muscle involvement in progressive systemic sclerosis (scleroderma). Arthritis and Rheumatism 11: 554–568

Mitnick P D, Feig P U 1978 Control of hypertension and reversal of renal failure in scleroderma. New England Journal of Medicine 299: 871–872

Miyazaki S, Miura K, Kasai Y, Abe K, Yoshinaga K 1982 Relief from digital vasospasm by treatment with captopril and its complete inhibition by serine proteinase inhibitors in Raynaud's phenomenon. British Medical Journal 1: 311–312

Nimni M E 1968 A defect in the intramolecular and

intermolecular cross-linking of collagen caused by penicillamine. Journal of Biological Chemistry 243: 1457–1466

Norton W L, Hurd E R, Lewis D C, Ziff M 1968 Evidence of microvascular injury in scleroderma and systemic lupus erythematosus: Quantitative study of the microvascular bed. Journal of Laboratory and Clinical Medicine 71: 919–933

O'Reilly M J G, Talpos G, Roberts V C, White J M, Cotton L T 1979 Controlled trial of plasma exchange in treatment of Raynaud's syndrome. British Medical Journal 1:1113

Orringer M B, Dabich L, Zarafonetis C J D, Sloan H 1976 Gastroesophageal reflux in esophageal scleroderma: Diagnosis and implications. Annals of Thoracic Surgery 22: 120–130

Orringer M B, Orringer J S, Dabich L, Zarafonetis C J D 1981 Combined Collis gastroplasty — fundoplication operations for scleroderma reflux esophagitis. Surgery 90: 624–630

Peacock J H 1959 Peripheral venous blood concentrations of epinephrine and norepinephrine in primary Raynaud's disease. Circulation Research 7: 821–827

Rajapakse C N A, Bancewicz J, Jones C J P, Jayson M I V 1981 Pharyngo-oesophageal dysphagia in systemic sclerosis. Annals of Rheumatic Diseases 40: 612–614

Ramirez-Mata M, Ibanez G, Alarcon-Segovia D 1977 Stimulating effect of metroclopramide in oesophagus and lower oesophageal sphincter of patients with PSS. Arthritis and Rheumatism 20: 30–34

Reynolds T B, Denison E K, Frankl H D, Lieberman F L, Peters R L 1971 Primary biliary cirrhosis with scleroderma, Raynaud's phenomenon and telangiectasia. American Journal of Medicine 50: 302–312

Rodnan G P, Medsger T A Jr 1968 The rheumatic manifestations of progressive systemic sclerosis (scleroderma). Clinical Orthopaedics and Related Research 57: 81–93

Rodnan G P, Medsger T A Jr 1975 Progressive systemic sclerosis — CREST syndrome: Observations on natural history and late complications in 90 patients. Arthritis and Rheumatism 18:423

Rodnan G P, Benedek T G, Medsger T A, Cammarata R J 1967 The association of progressive systemic sclerosis (scleroderma) with coal miners' pneumoconiosis and other forms of silicosis. Annals of Internal Medicine 66: 323–334

Rodnan G P, Lipinski E, Luksick J 1979 Skin thickness and collagen content in progressive systemic sclerosis and localized scleroderma. Arthritis and Rheumatism 22: 130–140

Rosenbloom A L, Silverstein J H, Lezotte D C, Richardson K, McCallum M 1981 Limited joint mobility in childhood diabetes mellitus indicates increased risk for microvascular disease. New England Journal of Medicine 305: 191–194

Salerni R, Rodnan G P, Leon D F, Shaver J A 1977 Pulmonary hypertension in the CREST syndrome variant of progressive systemic sclerosis (scleroderma). Annals of Internal Medicine 86: 394–399

Sapira J D, Rodnan G P, Scheib E T, Klaniecki T, Rizf M 1972 Studies of endogenous catecholamines in patients with Raynaud's phenomenon secondary to progressive systemic sclerosis (scleroderma). American Journal of Medicine 52: 330–337

Scherbel A L, Harrison J W 1959 Response to serotonin and its antagonists in patients with rheumatoid arthritis and related diseases. Angiology 10: 29–33

Segond P, Salliere D, Galanaud P, Desmottes R M, Massias P, Fiessinger J N 1981 Impaired primary in vitro antibody response in progressive systemic sclerosis patients: role of suppressor monocytes. Clinical and Experiemental Immunology 47: 147–154

Sharp G C, Irvin W S, May C M et al 1976 Association of antibodies to ribonucleoprotein and Sm antigens with mixed connective-tissue disease, systemic lupus erythematosus and other rheumatic diseases. New England Journal of Medicine 295: 1149–1154

Sharp G C, Irvin W S, Tan E M, Gould R G, Holman H R 1972 Mixed connective tissue disease — An apparently distinct rheumatic disease with a specific antibody to an extractable nuclear antigen (ENA). American Journal of Medicine 52: 148–159

Sherer G K, Jackson B B, LeRoy E C 1981 Chromosome breakage and sister chromatid exchange frequencies in scleroderma. Arthritis and Rheumatism 24: 1409–1413

Shulman L E 1974 Diffuse fasciitis with hypergammaglobulinaemia and eosinophilia: a new syndrome? Journal of Rheumatology 1 (Suppl 1): 46 (Abstract)

Shulman L E 1975 Diffuse fasciitis with eosinophilia: a new syndrome. Transactions of the Association of American Physicians 88: 70–86

Singsen B H, Kornreich H K, Koster-King K et al Mixed connective tissue disease in children. Arthritis and Rheumatism 20: 355–360

Sparrow G P 1977 A connective tissue disorder similar to vinyl chloride disease in a patient exposed to perchlorethylene. Clinical and Experimental Dermatology 2: 17–22

Stachow A, Jablonska S, Skiendzielewska A 1977 5-hydroxytryptamine and tryptamine pathways in scleroderma. British Journal of Dermatology 97: 147–154

Steigerwald J C 1974 Chlorambucil therapy in progressive systemic sclerosis. Journal of Rheumatology 1 (Suppl 1): 74

Sternberg E M, Van Woert M H, Young S N et al 1980 Development of a scleroderma-like illness during therapy with L-5-Hydroxytrytophan and carbidopa. New England Journal of Medicine 303: 782–787

Strosberg J M, Peak B, Harris E D Jr 1977 Scleroderma with intestinal involvement fatal in two of a kindred. Journal of Rheumatology 4: 46–52

Summers G D, Weiss J B, Jayson M I V 1984 Studies of the growth of human endothelial cells in serum from patients with scleroderma and other rheumatic diseases. Rheumatology International 5: 9–13

Talbott J H, Barrocas M 1979 Progressive systemic sclerosis (PSS) and malignancy, pulmonary and non-pulmonary. Medicine 58: 182–207

Tan E M, Pearson C M 1972 Rheumatic disease sera reactive with capillaries in the mouse kidney. Arthritis and Rheumatism 15: 23–28

Tan E M, Rodnan G P, Garcia I, et al 1980 Diversity of antinuclear antibodies in progressive systemic sclerosis. Arthritis and Rheumatism 23: 617–625

Thibierge G, Weissenbach R-J 1911 Concretions calcaires sous-cutanees et sclerodermie. Annals de Dermatologie et de Syphiligraphie 5: 129–155

Tomlinson I, Haavik Nilsen K, Jayson M I V 1985 Effects of peripheral vaso-dilators on cutaneous microcirculation in systemic sclerosis. Progressive Systemic Sclerosis. Gower, New York

Toxic Epidemic Syndrome Study Group 1982 Toxic epidemic syndrome, Spain, 1981. Lancet 2: 697–702
Treacy W L, Baggenstoss A H, Slocumb C H, Code C F 1963 Scleroderma of the esophagus. Annals of Internal Medicine 59: 351–356
Tuffanelli D L, Winkelmann R K 1962 Diffuse systemic scleroderma. A comparison with acrosclerosis. Annals of Internal Medicine 57: 198–203
Turner R, Rittenberg G, Lipshutz W, Schumacher H R, Miller W, Cohen S 1973 Esophageal dysfunction in collagen disease. American Journal of Medical Sciences 265: 191–199
Varadi D P, Lawrence A M 1969 Supression of Raynaud's phenomenon by methyldopa. Archives of Internal Medicine 124: 13–18
Wasner C, Cooke R, Fries J F 1978 Successful medical treatment of scleroderma renal crisis. New England Journal of Medicine 299: 873–857
West S G, Killian P J, Lawless O J 1981 Association of myositis and myocarditis in progressive systemic sclerosis. Arthritis and Rheumatism 24: 662–667
Whitman H H III, Case D B, Laragh J H et al 1982 Variable response to oral angiotensin-coverting-enzyme blockade in hypertensive scleroderma patients. Arthritis and Rheumatism 25: 241–248
Winkelmann R K, Carapeto F J, Jordan R E 1977 Direct immunofluorescence in the diagnosis of scleroderma syndromes. British Journal of Dermatology 96: 231–238
Winkelmann R K, Goldyne M E, Linschied R L 1976 Hypersensitivity of scleroderma cutaneous vascular smooth muscle to 5-hydroxytraptamine. British Journal of Dermatology 95: 51–56
Winkelmann R K, Goldyne M E, Linscheid R L 1977 Influence of cold on catecholamine response of vascular smooth muscle from resistance vessels of scleroderma skin. Angiology 28: 330–339
Winterbauer R H 1964 Multiple telangiectasia, Raynaud's phenomenon, sclerodactyly, and subcutaneous calcinosis: A syndrome mimicking hereditary haemorrhagic telangiectasia. Bulletin of the John Hopkins Hospital 114: 361–383
Wolfe J F, Adelstein E, Sharp G C 1977 Anti-nuclear antibody with distinct specificity for polymyositis. Journal of Clinical Investigation 59: 176–178
Wright J K, Hughes P, Rowell N R, Sneddon I B 1979 Antibody-dependent and phytohaemagglutinin-induced lymphocyte cytotoxicity in systemic sclerosis. Clinical and Experimental Immunology 36: 175–182
Yamakage A, Ishikawa H, Saito Y, Hattori A 1980 Occupational scleroderma-like disorder occurring in men engaged in polymerization of epoxyresins. Dermatologica 161: 33–44
Young R H, Mark G J 1978 Pulmonary vascular changes in scleroderma. American Journal of Medicine 64: 998–1004
Zatuchni J, Campbell W M, Zarafonetis C J D 1953 Pulmonary fibrosis and terminal bronchiolar ('alveolar-cell') carcinoma in scleroderma. Cancer 6: 1147–1158
Zion M M, Goldberg B, Suzman M M 1955 Corticotrophin and cortisone in the treatment of scleroderma. Quarterly Journal of Medicine 24: 215–227

M.L. Snaith

Sjögren's syndrome

DEFINITION

The syndrome has conventionally been the association of pathological dryness of the mouth (xerostomia) and eyes (xerophthalmia) with rheumatoid arthritis or one of the other autoimmune connective tissue diseases such as systemic lupus erythematosus (SLE) or scleroderma. In everyday medical practice doctors are concerned with coping with the clinical problems ad hoc, rather than with the requirement for precise definition for the purposes of clinical research or epidemiology. However, as more specific autoantibodies and autoantigens are demonstrated, as the mechanisms of autoimmunity are discovered and as immunogenetic prognosis indicates the possibility for selecting powerful treatment early in the disease process it becomes important to define disease entities more precisely, at least for the purposes of communication.

A broadly accepted definition of Sjögren's syndrome (SS) now is:

Primary Sjögren's syndrome
a. Keratoconjunctivitis sicca (KCS) plus
b. Xerostomia

as either glandular (localised) or extraglandular (systemic) sicca syndrome.

Secondary Sjögren's syndrome
a. Keratoconjunctivitis sicca and/or
b. Xerostomia
plus
c. A chronic inflammatory connective tissue disease.

Difficulties, perhaps pedantic, may arise over the definitions of the separate manifestations, e.g. whether the associated rheumatoid arthritis is classical or definite, with or without erosions or rheumatoid factor. Symptomatic KCS or xerostomia may appear many years before the 'associated' autoimmune disease, during which time 'primary Sjögren's syndrome' would be correct, following which 'secondary' would be more accurate. These concepts may be shown schematically as in Figure 56.1.

The disadvantage of this representation is that it implies a degree of homogeneity of the sicca syndrome, which is probably untrue. No diagram can reflect accurately the nuances of the situation as it is known at present.

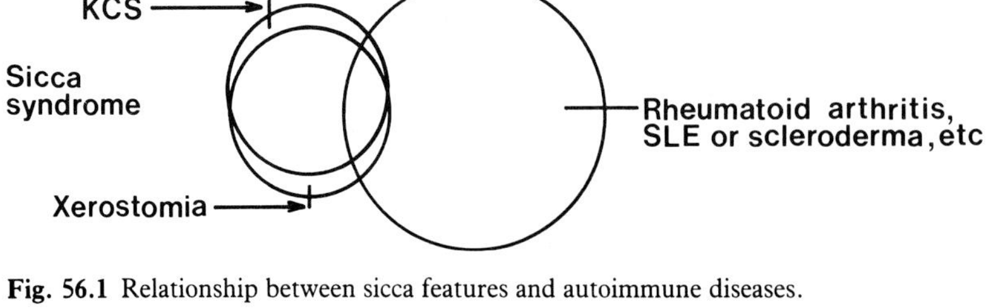

Fig. 56.1 Relationship between sicca features and autoimmune diseases.

THE SPECTRUM OF SJÖGREN'S SYNDROME

We are considering a syndrome of clinical and pathological manifestations. Patients tend to be in their middle age, particularly when the associated condition is rheumatoid arthritis, and tend to be female, as in autoimmune disorders in general. SS has however been reported in children, with a range of manifestations similar to the adult (Bernstein et al, 1977). The central features, KCS and xerostomia, are linked to a number of different connective tissue disorders, each of which may have separate associations. It is difficult therefore to ensure that one is observing direct and not indirect associations and the reader should bear this in mind when disease associations with the sicca syndrome are reported. Likewise, despite the recent demonstrations of characteristic immunogenetic and autoantibody profiles in SS it is not always easy clinically to draw a firm line between extension of primary extraglandular SS and an associated but pathologically unrelated disease. The effects of selection bias because of sub-specialty interests may influence any reported series, even where a multidiscipline clinic exists to overcome it (Berkeson, 1955). With these provisos one can design a scheme for the spectrum of SS, as follows.

Conditions which may be associated with, and in those instances be pathogenetically related to, sicca syndrome in primary Sjögren's syndrome:

Vasculitis (panarteritis, necrotising arteritis)
Hyperglobulinaemic purpura
Lymphoproliferation and related disorders
Hepatosplenomegaly
Parotid enlargement
Fibrosing alveolitis and obstructive airways disease
Raynaud's syndrome
Renal tubular acidosis
Glomerulonephritis
Polyneuritis
Anaemia, leucopenia, thrombocytopenia
Myositis

Disorders known to be complicated by sicca syndrome, i.e. secondary Sjögren's syndrome:

Rheumatoid arthritis
Systemic lupus erythematosus (and subsets, e.g. mixed connective tissue disease)
Scleroderma and progressive systemic sclerosis
Chronic active hepatitis
Primary biliary cirrhosis
? Polymyositis and dermatomyositis

HISTORY

Strict priority would award the eponym to one of the several late 19th and early 20th century authors who described patients, with in some instances histopathological details, who probably had what we perceive as Sjögren's syndrome in one or other of its forms (discussed in detail by Shearn, 1971). In France today Gougerot usually shares with Sjögren the eponym to acknowledge his recognition of the widespread dryness of the mucous membranes of the mouth, eyes, nose larynx and vulva (Escande, 1977). Sometimes Morlock Houwer's name is added since he pointed to the association of dry eyes, dry mouth and arthritis (Shearn, 1971). It is however the name of Henrik Sjögren, a Swedish ophthalmologist, which is most widely used, in recognition of his classic 1933 monograph and the subsequent contribution made over a generation which formed the basis for our present understanding of this disorder (Sjögren, 1933). Mikulicz' syndrome as a separate disease entity lived on until it became clear that in emphasising salivary gland swelling the fact that histologically Mikulicz' syndrome and Sjögren's syndrome are identical had been overlooked (Morgan & Castleman, 1953).

THE CLINICAL PRESENTATION OF SJÖGREN'S SYNDROME

Xerophthalmia

A patient with xerophthalmia due to KCS has an eye that looks so irritable that it should be watering but is not. It feels gritty, uncomfortable and tired and is photophobic; there is accumulated sticky matter at the lid margins, especially overnight. A dry, dusty atmosphere is especially uncomfortable and may influence tests of tear-flow. Interestingly antidepressants and possibly other drugs which affect salivary production do not seem to induce dry eyes. Superimposed infection, due especially to staphylococcus, may occur. Sensation is sometimes actually reduced and conjunctival or corneal scarring is a risk.

Xerostomia

Most people with pathological xerostomia will notice the dryness but do not always complain of it spontaneously. Advancing age, habitual mouth breathing, anxiety and antidepressants can all lead to dryness. Cigarette smoking actually stimulates salivary flow but heavy smokers often seem to have a dry atrophic mouth. The lack of symptomatic dryness does not exclude sub-normal salivary gland function or pathological change revealed by biopsy (see below). None the less if the patient cannot eat a dry biscuit without recourse to water, salivation is probably inadequate. Dental problems occur early: dental pain, gingivitis, mouth odour and severe caries. The distorted canaliculi and inspissated secretions may lead to duct blockage and retrograde infection. Angular stomatitis is common and the tongue is often fissured. Swelling of the parotids or submandibular glands may be bilateral and painless: the so-called 'chipmunk facies'. The risk of glandular lymphoma is increased in SS (see below) and rapid or painful swelling may indicate this complication.

Other results of impaired exocrine functions

In severe forms of the sicca syndrome the abnormal glandular secretions may affect the nasal airways with blockage of the nose, sinusitis, otitis media, deafness due to Eustachian tube involvement, sore throat or a post-cricoid web reminiscent of Plummer–Vinson (Doig et al, 1971). Dyspareunia or discomfort due to vaginal dryness may be a problem. The skin may be dry. It is less easy to determine the extent of specific gastrointestinal manifestations but gastric, pancreatic and gall bladder dysfunction, together with constipation, are all described (Mason et al, 1973).

Symptoms as a result of the associated disorder

The rheumatologist is clearly likely to see patients firstly because of the associated rheumatic condition. Because rheumatoid arthritis is so common this will be a frequent combination though only about half of all patients with KCS are said to have rheumatoid arthritis (Whaley et al, 1973a). The sicca syndrome of SS with rheumatoid arthritis tends to be relatively mild, that of SS with SLE or scleroderma rather more severe. This clinical impression that the sicca syndrome of rheumatoid arthritis is different from primary SS or SS/SLE has been strengthened by the immunological information that has been accumulated in recent years (see below). The awareness of the association between arthritis and sicca syndrome emphasised in the writings of Sjögren and indeed earlier seems likely to result in physicians actively seeking it, with a tendency to exaggerate the SS/RA link compared with others. The frequency of sicca features in patients with SLE is uncertain, but experience indicates that the more one looks for them the more one finds them (e.g. 30–60%; Moutsopoulos et al, 1980). The frequency in polymyositis and scleroderma is also not known. The more uncommon a disorder, the more such surveys have to be based in referral centres, with the risk of association (Berkeson, 1953).

Irrespective therefore of the frequency of the association, patients may present as a result of SLE, scleroderma, autoimmune liver disease, polymyositis or autoimmune thyroid disease. The sicca syndrome in these patients may be sufficiently severe as to bring the patient to specialist attention for its sake rather than the associated disorder: which may indeed not become manifest until months or years later. The patient should not therefore be categorised as primary SS except in retrospect. Perhaps immunogenetic and other data may in future permit earlier categorisation of the type of disease from which the patient is suffering with possibilities for earlier treatment.

THE DIAGNOSIS OF KERATOCONJUNCTIVITIS SICCA

In much of the rheumatological literature on SS an abnormal Schirmer's test is used to define patients with pathologically dry eyes. The standardised filter paper strips that are available provide a quick and easy test instrument for this. Its very availability however may provide a false sense of security, that a low reading on a Schirmer's means a pathologically dry eye and a high reading a normal one. Tear secretion, like any body function, is complex and there is not necessarily a close relationship between dysfunction, pathology and symptoms. There is no major problem in diagnosing a severely dry eye but the investigation of the questionably dry eye (Mackie, 1982) demands more than a five minute Schirmer's test done in a busy clinic. The following are the available means of investigation for possible KCS:

1. Schirmer's test
2. Bengal rose staining of the conjunctiva and cornea
3. Slit lamp examination, revealing abnormal debris in the tear film
4. Tear film break-up time
5. Tear protein profiles
6. Tear film osmolality and fluorescein dilution test.

The normal tear film consists of three main layers: a thin inner mucin layer produced mainly by the goblet cells of the conjunctiva; a major aqueous layer produced by the main and accessory lacrimal glands and a thin superficial lipid layer, from the marginal meibomian glands. It is aqueous tear deficiency which is paramount in KCS. Disturbed tear physiology results in instability of the tear film with rapid drying with an abnormal tear film break-up time and an increased concentration of mucin, demonstrated by Bengal rose staining (Plate 56.1) which also stains dead and dying epithelial cells. Disturbance of the epithelial growth pattern results in adherent epithelial strands, detectable with a slit lamp and microscope (Plate 56.2).

Schirmer's test

The folded end of a 5 × 20 cm filter paper strip (Whatman No. 41) is placed in the lower conjunctival sac. Conventionally the eye is closed but Mackie (1982) argues that this may result in an erroneous reduction in tear diffusion along the strip and recommends the eye be open. He also suggests the strip be moved to another site if there is no wetting after 2 minutes. With this modification a 95% confidence limit gave an abnormal result as less than 6 mm wetting after 5 minutes. If no secretion is observed despite moving the filter paper, an inhalation of 5% ammonium chloride solution held 6 inches away from the patient's face may produce normal tear flow (sometimes referred to as the Schirmer II test).

Tear film break-up time (BUT)

When the aqueous layer is reduced, the hydrophobic lipid layer may come in contact with the mucin, with break-up of the normal thin layer of tears on the conjunctiva. This is observed by the use of a bright beam of light and a lens. Normally the BUT will be anywhere between 10 seconds and 2 minutes and this test has been criticised on this account. However its protagonists (Manthorpe et al, 1981) maintain that it is a useful test and can be made quantitive. It is probably another situation where, when a minor degree of subnormal function is present, the test is unreliable but

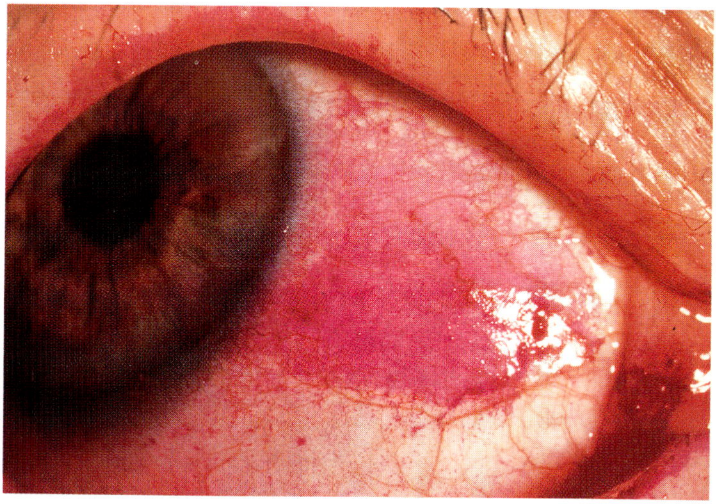

Plate 56.1 Rose Bengal staining of corneal conjunctiva.

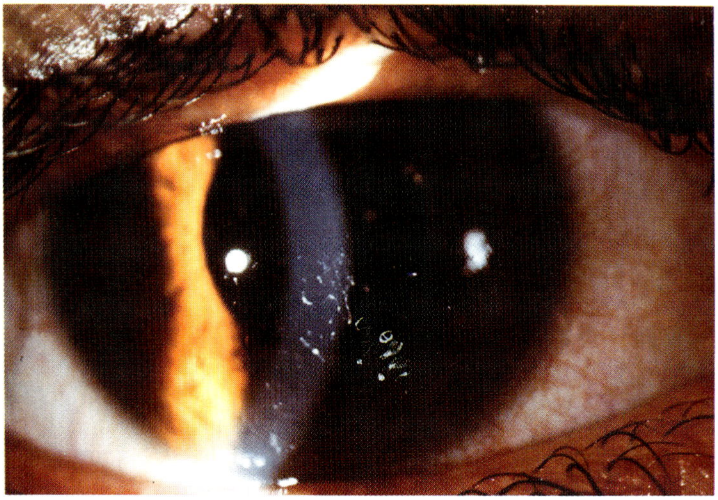

Plate 56.2 Slit lamp photograph showing the epithelial and mucus strands of keratoconjunctivitis sicca.

when there is obvious dryness the test is also unequivocal.

Tear protein profiles

Lysozyme can be measured accurately using a micrococcus agar plate (against suitable standards) and is a more sensitive indicator of early xerophthalmia than Schirmer testing (Mackie & Seal, 1981). Enzyme-linked assays for lactoferrin and cerulopasmin may also prove useful in the diagnosis of patients where the quality rather than the quantity of tears is in doubt.

Osmolality and fluorescein dilution

Osmolality, reflecting tear constituents, and fluorescein dilution, the rate of tear clearance, have been used to detect early ophthalmic sicca and also to provide a measure of severity. However neither has met with widespread acceptance.

INVESTIGATING THE SALIVARY GLANDS

The need for an assessment of salivary gland function is established by the clinical circumstances: dryness may be so obvious as to be not worth measuring, since indices of function do not reveal cause. When doubt exists, or a measure of change is desired, investigations along the following lines are available:

1. Salivary flow rate
2. Sialanalysis
3. Imaging and functional radiology, sialography and scintigraphy
4. Biopsy.

These investigations do not necessarily reveal disease to the same extent, since they reflect different aspects of structure and function. They are also, with the exception of biopsy, physiological studies and standardised techniques must be used if meaningful results are to be obtained, taking into account factors such as age, anxiety, pain. conditioned reflexes and altered taste sensation. A variety of drugs affect salivary flow, including antidepressants, analgesics, antihistamines and antihypertensives (Mandel & Wotman, 1976).

Salivary flow

The secretory rate of each gland may be measured but the sublingual and submaxillary require collecting apparatus individually moulded to the mouth. Total saliva is normally about 1.0–1.5 litres in 24 hours, mostly during the day and largely from the parotid and submaxillary glands. Total unstimulated saliva is easily collected and is preferred by some (Ben-Aryeh, 1982) but forms only 5% of the maximum stimulated flow. Its ease of collection must be weighed against the crudeness of the method. Parotid secretions, about half of the total, are collected either by cannulation (as during sialography) or by using a special suction cup. Maximal stimulation may be by timed application to the edge of the tongue of a specified solution of citric acid or lemon juice or by intravenous pilocarpine (Seward et al, 1966). A concensus gives a lower limit of normal for maximal stimulation of 0.5 ml per gland per minute.

Sialanalysis

The saliva of established xerostomia is distinctly viscid as well as meagre. The concentrations of sodium, potassium and IgA are elevated compared to normal controls. This does not distinguish between primary and secondary SS but there may be alteration in composition before diminution in flow rate (Ben-Aryeh, 1982). If material is to be stored frozen, it may be necessary to add EDTA to prevent precipitation of glycoproteins. Normal ranges should probably be established for each laboratory as differences are reported depending upon the method of collection and between spontaneous and stimulated flow.

Sequential salivary scintigraphy

Briefly the technique involves intravenous administration of 5–10 MCi of sodium pertechnetate (^{99m}technetium) and sequential gamma imaging of the whole head and neck (Daniels et al, 1979). If thyroid function is normal, comparison may be made with the salivary glands. Previous scanning methods using iodine have been superseded by the development of technetium. The test may be made sensitive and semiquantitative by 'blind' interpretation and appropriate normal control experience within the same institution, obtained by taking advantage of scans being performed for diagnostic purposes of other organs. The tracer is not localised in the minor salivary glands (Akker et al, 1976) which are those usually biopsied (see below). It takes over an hour to perform and requires a dose of radiation (albeit moderate, with a short-life isotope).

Sialography

The parotid duct is cannulated and 0.5–2.0 ml of contrast material (preferably water soluble) is injected slowly to avoid pain to the patient. Dikjstra (1980) suggested standard views and reviewed the interpretation of sialograms. In SS there may be either or both sclerosis of the ductuli and dilatation of the acini which may progress to gross destruction. Idiopathic dilatation of the salivary ducts which is found in a significant proportion of the general population may mimic lymphoid infiltration due to SS. Sarcoidosis is the other main pathology to be distinguished from SS. Sialography is of particular relevance where a glandular lymphoma is suspected.

Overall it must be emphasised that sialographic abnormalities can be found in 15% of the normal population, the incidence increasing with age (Dikjstra, 1980).

Salivary gland biopsy

Although scintigraphy and parotid flow rates assess major salivary function, it seems that minor salivary morphology reflects that of the major glands — a fortunate fact as biopsy of the major glands carries too many hazards to be of much use in clinical investigation unless malignant change is suspected. The technique of biopsy is described in detail elsewhere (Chisholm & Mason, 1968). Briefly, the lower lip is grasped and everted, avoiding areas of overlying mucosal damage; after local anaesthesia, a 3–5 cm appropriate incision is made in the lip. The salivary glands bulge and are dissected out. Mucosa is not removed. The incision is closed with absorbable sutures. This is a well tolerated procedure, soreness settling within a few days and healing completely within a week. Chisholm & Mason's scheme (1968) for grading lip biopsy changes is widely used and discriminates well between normal and pathological tissue. A slight lymphocytic infiltration may occur in otherwise normal gland tissue (Fig. 56.2). Normally however no foci of lymphocytes are found (a focus being an aggregate of 50 or more lymphocytes and histiocytes). Unequivocally pathological tissue, grade 4, equals 4 or more foci per 4 mm square of tissue (Fig. 56.3). Other related criteria were suggested by Tarpley et al (1974) who pointed to the importance of the presence of a plasma cell infiltrate, particularly with regard to local immunoglobulin synthesis. Daniels (1984) has recently reviewed the procedure and interpretation.

Other secretory glands

The term 'autoimmune exocrinopathy' has been

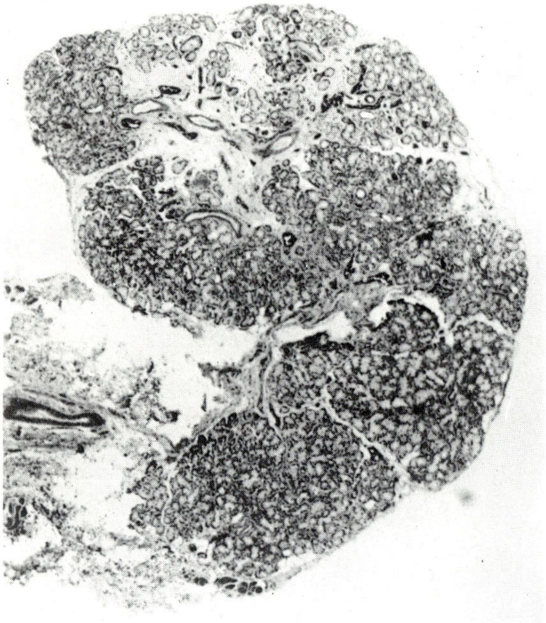

Fig. 56.2 Normal salivary gland biopsy.

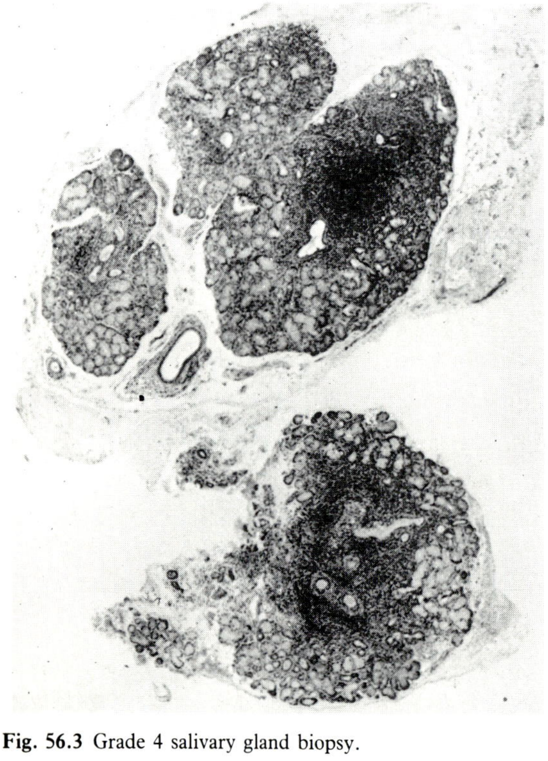

Fig. 56.3 Grade 4 salivary gland biopsy.

coined (Strand & Talal, 1979). This indicates the potential involvement of the glands of the pancreas, oesophagus, stomach, small and large intestines, vagina and skin. Abnormalities, usually involving lymphocytic infiltration and fibrosis, have been reported in biopsy material from several of these organs. The value of performing functional assessments even when possible is more difficult to assess, because of inevitably small series, the lack of control investigations and lack of specificity of the findings. These investigations are not therefore helpful in diagnosis and they will be discussed below in their respective sections.

SYSTEMIC FEATURES

Arthritis

About half of all patients with SS have rheumatoid arthritis. Factors of definition and selection will inevitably provide differences in reported series, even with international criteria. A further 15% or so will have arthralgia or arthritis in the absence of a classifiable form of arthritis. Those patients with systemic lupus erythematosus or scleroderma may well of course have rheumatic symptoms as a result of joint or soft tissue involvement.

The converse situation, the reported frequency of symptomatic SS in patients with rheumatoid arthritis, varies from 20–30% depending upon the patient population surveyed and the methods used. A post-mortem study of salivary gland histology indicated that lymphocytic infiltration may be ubiquitous (Waterhouse & Doniach, 1966). In the majority of patients the rheumatoid arthritis precedes the sicca features by 5–10 years, but they may commence simultaneously or occasionally the sicca features precede the arthritis by up to several years.

The arthritis of patients with SS and RA (SS–RA) is clinically similar to that of rheumatoid patients with no sicca features. The sicca symptoms however are usually much less severe in patients with RA than those with SS alone or associated with SLE, scleroderma or polymyositis (Moutsopoulos et al, 1979b)

Little is known about the influence of medication in those rheumatoid patients with SS but the effect of phenylbutazone on salivary glands (producing swelling) should be recalled. Penicillamine seems to be capable of inducing autoimmune disorders such as SLE or pemphigus and it is prudent to bear in mind the possibility that SS might be inducible in susceptible individuals. An indication of the pivotal position of SS in relation to autoimmune disease is given in the comparison with other forms of chronic inflammatory arthritis: in a survey of patients with psoriatic arthritis, ankylosing spondylitis and Reiter's syndrome, evidence of SS could not be found (Whaley et al, 1971).

Raynaud's phenomenon and disease

Raynaud's is associated with connective tissue diseases in general, particularly scleroderma. Benign Raynaud's phenomenon occurs in the normal population and it may be many years before a systemic connective tissue desease develops in the susceptible individual. The true frequency in SS patients is therefore difficult to give but it may amount to about one-fifth (Mason et al 1973). There seems no doubt that the frequency of Raynaud's phenomenon is relatively increased in patients with sicca syndrome alone compared to those with accompanying rheumatoid arthritis (Moutsopoulos et al, 1979b).

Gastrointestinal disease

SS involves all salivary tissue and associated atrophy of oesophageal mucosa may occur (Doig, 1971). Dysphagia arising from oesophageal dysmotility is likely to be due to associated systemic sclerosis or inflammatory myopathy, either of which may involve the gastrointestinal tract rather selectively. Indeed oesophageal dysmotility like arthralgia may, admittedly rarely, be a common denominator in any connective tissue disease syndrome (Stevens et al, 1964). Appropriate dynamometric or radio-contrast studies should be performed to delineate the underlying mechanism of such dysphagia. Hypochlorhydria, atrophic gastritis and parietal cell antibody have been found quite frequently, but do not, it seems, imply an overall increased risk of pernicious anaemia (Whaley et al, 1973b). Serum pepsinogen levels are reduced, possibly in association with atrophic gastritis (Maury et al, 1982). Scintigraphic studies may offer a simple non-intensive method of studying this (Katona et al, 1982). Pancreatic function may be mildly (and infrequently) distorted (Fenster et al, 1964).

Liver disease

Of 43 patients with primary SS studied retrospectively, Pavlidis (1982) found two with liver involvement. 23 of Bloch's 62 patients (Bloch et al, 1965) had hepatomegaly but the contribution from primary and secondary SS is not given. In the earlier reports, interpretation of the evidence is difficult as tests for liver function such as flocculation tended to reflect hyperglobulinaemia and liver biopsy surveys have understandably not been done. Antibodies to mitochondria, smooth muscle or liver cell membrane were found in up to one-third of patients with primary or secondary SS (Manthorpe et al, 1981). Using antimitochondrial antibody as a marker Whaley and associates found 6% of patients had liver involvement (Whaley et al, 1970). The frequency of sicca features in patients selected by autoimmune liver disease is much higher. Of a combined series of patients with either chronic active hepatitis, primary biliary cirrhosis or cryptogenic cirrhosis Golding et al (1970) found evidence of SS in 52%. All 14 patients with primary biliary cirrhosis investigated by Alarcon-Segovia et al (1973) had evidence of SS.

Muscle disease

Frank polymyositis is a known but infrequent accompaniment of SS (Bloch et al, 1965). A mild inflammatory myositis occurs in rheumatoid arthritis, being more readily identifiable the more severe the RA although only rarely assuming a major role. Likewise, muscle biopsies in patients with SS frequently reveal asymptomatic abnormalities (12 of 23 in the series of Denko & Old, 1969). Immunoglobulin and complement deposits, with ultrastructural changes, have been found (Ringel et al, 1982). Of Pavlidis's retrospective series (Pavlidis et al, 1982) of patients with primary SS, 6 had muscle involvement at diagnosis and 9 at follow up. Presumably this was at a level less than that required to make a diagnosis of polymyositis complicated by sicca features, which would have produced a category of secondary SS. Primary polymyositis patients have not been examined in number for the frequency of SS, but by inference from SLE and scleroderma it would not be surprising if such evidence were found. Dermatomyositis in children and adults has also not been investigated in detail for evidence of KCS or xerostomia. Since this condition is somewhat different in adults from that in children it would be of particular interest to obtain such information. Nor is there any evidence of SS occurring in association with neoplasia in general in the older adult.

Renal disease

Renal disease in a patient with SS may be due to associated lupus nephritis, scleroderma kidney, analgesic nephropathy or amyloidosis — all secondary to or part of the associated connective tissue disease. However, these having been accounted for, there remains a proportion of patients with nephropathy. Whilst there is no unique lesion, tubular disorders are prominent. Nephrogenic diabetes insipidus, Fanconi's syndrome and renal tubular acidosis are all described in patients with primary SS. Such defects may also occur in patients with SLE and primary biliary cirrhosis (Blythe, 1982). Perhaps the denominator is SS? Adult patients with renal tubular acidosis fall into two main groups: familial (equal sex incidence, no autoantibodies), and non-familial (female preponderance, frequent autoantibodies) (Feest & Wrong, 1982). Indeed although the frequency of SS in patients with non-familial renal tubular acidosis is uncertain, it is probably high enough to justify investigating renal tubular acidosis patients along these lines (azotaemia is unusual in SS in the absence of glomerulonephritis, which usually implies lupus nephritis with DNA antibodies). There is an understandable paucity of histological evidence as the degree of renal dysfunction in SS rarely merits needle biopsy and the material thus obtained will usually not include papillary tissue. A mechanism that has been suggested is a direct nephrotoxic effect of the hyperglobulinaemia typical of SS, by analogy with myeloma. However the level of serum globulins seems to bear no correlation with the development of tubular dysfunction. Taken together with the lymphocytic infiltration of the interstitial tissues of the kidneys (Feest et al, 1978), it is rather more likely that the nephritis of SS is due to the disease process (Shioji et al, 1970).

Cutaneous manifestations

Vasculitis of one form or another is an integral part of the connective tissue disease spectrum and an overall association with SS is to be expected and is found. The manifestations range from the benign nailfold infarcts seen in RA to arteritic lesions more typical of polyarteritis nodosa. In patients with primary SS the purpura of hyperglobulinaemia seem prominent. This affects particularly the lower extremities, is often transient and may be made worse by exercise or fatigue. SS should be considered in all patients with non-thrombocytopenic purpura. Lesions are not necessarily benign however, with splanchnic and cerebral involvement being described. Vasculitis may be a presenting symptom or one that develops after years of other features of the sicca complex, a situation characteristic of SS. SS has been described in patients with pemphigus (Wallach et al, 1979) and dermatitis herpetiformis (Fraser et al, 1979). In addition, vasculitis is thought to be the pathology underlying the neuropathy of SS (see below). Histopathological data are lacking with specific regard to the vasculitis of SS, as distinct from that of polyarteritis nodosa or rheumatoid disease. Evidence is accumulating however that autoantibodies to the extractable nuclear antigen Ro (SSA) may be associated with vasculitis (Alexander et al, 1983) (see below). Perhaps complexes of a certain size or stability are required in order for deposits to accumulate in sites appropriate for vasculitis.

Nervous system

Major neurological involvement in SS is relatively uncommon and peripheral sensory neuropathy, probably the commonest non-compressive neuropathy (i.e. aside from carpal tunnel syndrome) is rarely very extensive or severe. An accompanying vasculitis may indicate the pathogenesis with occlusion of the vasa nervorum. Electrophysiological and biopsy studies showed in one instance an axonal neuropathy predominantly of myelinated fibres (Peyronnard et al, 1982). This Sjögren's neuropathy is somewhat similar to that occurring in RA alone, although it may precede the sicca features.

Involvement of the central nervous system is distinctly uncommon. As in connective tissue disorders in general, trigeminal neuropathy seems to be the most frequently described cranial nerve problem: of 109 patients with SS there were 9 with a peripheral neuropathy and 4 with trigeminal involvement (Kaltreider & Talal, 1969).

16 patients with central nervous system complications of primary SS have been reported as a series (Alexander et al, 1982). Most of them also had some peripheral involvement, including one instance of recurrent third nerve palsy (although interestingly no trigeminal problems). 4 patients had spinal cord disorders including subarachnoid haemorrhage. Cerebral involvement ranged from nystagmus through recurrent hemiparesis to aseptic meningoencephalitis. The emphasis was on focal and intermittent involvement rather than the diffuse and often protracted cerebritis of SLE.

The pathogenesis of central nervous system involvement is again inferentially vasculitis (12 of the 16 had peripheral vasculitis) although direct histopathological evidence for this is scanty. Of the 12 with vasculitis, 83% had antibodies to the soluble nuclear antigen Ro (SSA), which is separately found to associate with vasculitis (see above). Evidence for direct cell-mediated neurological damage is meagre (Shearn, 1971).

Pulmonary disease

Whilst pulmonary involvement is common (20–30%) in patients with SS, there is no unique lesion. An array of pulmonary problems have been described affecting airways or pulmonary parenchyma: chronic bronchitis, bronchiectasis, asthma, irreversible airways obstruction, diffuse interstitial pneumonia and fibrosing alveolitis. Conditions such as pleural effusion, linear basal atelectasis and the 'shrinking lung' syndrome, or fibrosing alveolitis, intrapulmonary nodules or pleural effusions may be ascribed to SLE or RA respectively in SS secondary to either of these diseases. Tests for lung function will tend to reflect these disorders, with restrictive defects predominating (Oxholm et al, 1982). Pulmonary problems in SS have been ascribed to the effects of the sicca features, with hyposecretion of viscid mucus and secondary infection. Certainly the dryness of the upper respiratory tract leads to mucosal crusting in the nasal and oropharynx, sore throats and a hoarse voice. The term 'bronchitis sicca' has been used to denote patients in whom inspissated secretions cause a chronic dry cough, with peculiar difficulty in expectoration and attacks of secondary infection. A reduction in mucosal defence because of shortage of IgA has also been postulated (Shearn, 1971). Clear descriptions of this syndrome are however lacking. The mucociliary clearance of radiolabelled polystyrene particles was found to be normal from central airways, with increase in the whole lung clearance rate. This diminished aerosol penetrance is similar to that found in asthmatics and was interpreted as indicating peripheral airways obstruction (Fairfax et al, 1981). This could be due to small mucus plugs as occurs in asthma. Histological examination of the lungs in SS may reveal various degrees of consolidation, lipoid pneumonia or changes typical of fibrosing alveolitis. The features perhaps more specific for SS alone are lymphoproliferative: polyclonal B and T lymphocyte and plasma cell infiltrates of the septa and small airways (Strimlan et al, 1976; Newball & Brahim, 1977). Indeed airways obstruction may be due as much to this diffuse pneumonitis as to mucus plugging. Cardiac disease ascribed to SS alone is rare although pericarditis as part of associated RA or SLE is not.

Haematological disturbances

There is no haematological disorder unique to patients with SS. If the associated condition is SLE for example, any finding of lymphopenia will be ascribed to the lupus. Apart from this instances, leucopenia in general occurs relatively infrequently. A mild anaemia of chronic disease can be expected. Thrombocytosis occurs with associated active RA. Thrombocytopenia has been reported (Berrebi et al, 1982). Pernicious anaemia is probably more common in patients with SS than controls (Whaley et al, 1973b).

MISCELLANEOUS ASSOCIATIONS WITH SJÖGREN'S SYNDROME

Other causes of a sicca syndrome

The most likely reasons for an erroneous impression of SS are those mentioned above, such as old age in general, the post-menopause in women, or drugs. However some other pathological conditions may produce a sicca syndrome. Amyloidosis, itself perhaps complicating RA, may infiltrate the lachrymal and salivary glands and produce a sicca syndrome. Indeed, in a search for amyloid, a minor salivary gland should perhaps be biopsied before the rectal mucosa, which may occasionally bleed profusely (Simon & Moutsopoulos, 1979). A sicca-like condition in type 5 hypolipoproteinaemia has been described (Reinertsen et al, 1980) but the resemblance is somewhat superficial with a normal biopsy. Haemochromatosis involves the salivary glands, producing dryness which appeared to respond to bromhexine (Blandford et al, 1979). Perhaps of more relevance to the pathogenesis of SS, patients following allogeneic bone marrow grafts have been observed to develop a similar clinical picture including lymphoid infiltrates of salivary glands. However autoantibodies are lacking, so one cannot infer too much similarity in pathogenesis (Gratwohl et al, 1977). Thiabendazole (an antihelminthic) has been incriminated as a cause of a sicca syndrome (Fink et al, 1979).

THE IMMUNOPATHOLOGY OF SJÖGREN'S SYNDROME

Humoral immunity (general)

Hyperglobulinaemia is characteristic of SS, but not invariable. Marked elevation of serum globulin is less often a feature of secondary than of primary SS where hyperviscosity syndromes or hyperglobulinaemic purpura may be of major clinical importance. This non-specific B cell activity is presumably related in some way to the high prevalence of autoantibodies and immune complexes in these patients and to the lymphadenopathy, occasionally massive (pseudolymphoma — see below), which is found. Lymphocytes obtained from salivary gland biopsies and cultured in vitro secrete immunoglobulin (Cummings et al, 1974).

Anti-nuclear antibodies

The prevalence of anti-nuclear antibodies detected by immunofluorescence is greater in primary SS than in SS with rheumatoid arthritis (for example, 88% and 56% respectively in the series of Bloch et al, 1965). The staining patterns are variably diffuse, speckled or occasionally nucleolar. Titres of ANA do not bear a clear relationship to activity of disease.

The heterogeneity of SS, initially indicated clinically and by the fluorescent patterns of ANA, was later amplified by the demonstration of diverse antigen–antibody systems, using immunoprecipitation and complement fixation. Because of differences in technique, in sources of antigen and probably in classification of the patients whose sera were used to identify these antigens, it was not always apparent whether or not different workers were describing the same system. As a result of interlaboratory collaboration, the picture has become clearer. The antibodies designated Sjd (Anderson et al, 1961), Ro (Clark et al, 1969), and SSA (Alspaugh & Tan, 1975), all have similar specificities as do La, SSB (Alspaugh & Maddison, 1979), Sjt (Anderson et al, 1961) and Ha (Akizuki et al, 1977). The antibodies concerned may have identical specificities but the macromolecular antigens with which they react, whilst sharing common antigenic determinants, do not necessarily have identical physicochemical properties. For example, SSA (Ro) antigen extracted from human spleen is not digested by trypsin, in contrast to the antigenically similar material obtained from the continuously growing diploid lymphocyte line (originally from a patient with hereditary spherocytosis) known as WIL 2. Likewise, there may be subtle differences between SSB (La, Ha) from different sources (Alexander & Provost, 1981). These differences may become less apparent when the antigens are purified (Venables et al, 1983). Recent work has shown them to be soluble complexes of protein with small RNA nucleotides (Lerner & Steitz, 1981). The molecular weight of SSA (Ro) is of the order of 150 000 Daltons; that of SSB (La) is less than 100 000 (Teppo et al, 1982).

The precise localisation and function of these soluble antigens within the cell remains to be determined. Fluorescence and other evidence indicates that SSA (Ro) is probably cytoplasmic and SSB (La) is both cytoplasmic and nuclear (Maddison and Reichlin, 1979). However differences between substrates and the manner of antigen expression influence the findings. Monoclonal antibodies raised against purified antigens used as specific immunogens are promising experimental tools (Hyams, 1984).

The immunoglobulin class of antibodies to SSB has been examined (Helve et al, 1982) using an ELISA assay. IgG and IgM antibodies were detected mainly in the sera of patients with SS but also in patients with chronic active hepatitis. IgA antibodies were found in the sera from patients with RA, SLe and primary biliary cirrhosis.

Clinical importance of anti-SSA (Ro) and SSB (La) antibodies

SSA (Ro) antibodies possibly occur in as many as half of all patients with SS, the frequency of SSB (La) antibodies being more variously reported (10–80%) (Alexander & Provost, 1981). The specificity for the various types of SS is also under debate but the prevalence seems greatest in those patients with primary SS and SS-SLE although one French group found lower overall prevalences, with no difference between the subgroups (Mayer et al, 1982). An apparently strong clinical correlation is that of SSA (Ro) with vasculitis, whether it be in patients with primary SS or SLE (Alexander et al, 1983). Patients with ANA-negative SLE are also found on closer examination to have a high frequency of SSA and SSB (Maddison, 1982) as do both patients and mothers in the rare neonatal lupus syndrome (Lockshin et al, 1983). The finding of SSB in patients with polyarthralgia may also predict the later development of SS rather than RA (Isenberg et al, 1982). Another clinically rather distinct subgroup of patients with predominantly cutaneous manifestations of SLE (subacute cutaneous lupus erythematosus) tend to carry the SSA-Ro and SSB-La antibodies. Finally there is probably an immunogenetic association between HLA-B8 and DR3 with SSA-Ro antibodies (see below).

Aside from the clinical value of defining subgroups, these antibodies are of great interest to cell biologists as probes in the investigation of the distribution and cellular roles of small nuclear and cytoplasmic ribonuclear proteins (Lerner & Steitz, 1981).

DNA antibodies

Anti-native DNA or DNA protein antibodies, whilst most typical of SLE, are found in about one-quarter of patients with SS or RA. Their specificity may however differ somewhat. In addition some rheumatoid factors may have antinuclear binding specificity (Karsh et al, 1982). Whereas in SLE the finding of DNA antibodies indicates the likelihood of concurrent or impending nephritis, this is not so for SS unless the titre is very high, in which case perhaps the patient actually has SLE and will develop nephritis. Other nuclear antibodies such as anti-golgi complex and anti-polyADP-ribose are described but their place in the clinical assessment of patients is not yet proven.

Rheumatoid factors and immune complexes

Classical rheumatoid factor (by sheep cell agglutination) is found in abundance (approaching 100%) in all varieties of SS, especially and inevitably in SS-RA but also in SS alone (Bloch, 1965). Antiglobulins of subclasses IgG and IgA are found in excess of normal (Dunne et al, 1979) in blood and saliva in patients with RA, with systemic sicca syndrome and with RA complicated by SS (Elkon et al, 1981). Such rheumatoid factors may well contribute to the formation of the circulating immune complexes which are found by several methods in pathological quantities in the majority of patients with SS of all types (Yoshinoya et al, 1982). The pathogenicity of these circulating complexes is not proven, although presumptively lesions such as interstitial nephritis, the unusual glomerulonephritis of primary SS, arthralgia and vasculitis could all involve immune complex deposition. Levels do not usually correlate with disease activity in SS. The handling of immune complexes by the reticuloendothelial system has been studied using clearance of radiolabelled antibody-coated erythrocytes (Moutsopouolos et al, 1980b). Whilst this technique could not be expected to reflect accurately the variety of antigen–antibody interactions which occur in health and disease, clearance was abnormally prolonged in most patients with SS. The clearance rates for immunologically inert microaggregated albumin were normal.

Other autoantibodies

Organ-specific antibodies occur more commonly in SS than in healthy people; specificities include smooth muscle, skeletal muscle, liver cell membrane, parietal cell, pancreas, ovary and thyroid. Although raised (about 30%) the frequency of organ-specific antibodies does not approach that of ANA, anti-SSA/B or antiglobulins. Unfortunately the critical follow-up studies to determine whether the findings of a given antibody predicts for disease in this group of patients are lacking. A possible exception is thyroid disease. Pathological similarities exist between autoimmune thyroiditis and the salivary glands in SS and an increased incidence of antibodies to thyroid microsomes and thyroglobulin has long been apparent (Bloch et al, 1965; Strand & Talal, 1980). However no difference in the prevalence of keratoconjunctivitis sicca could be found in patients with thyroid disease of various kinds (including thyroiditis) and hospital controls (Williamson et al, 1967). Antibodies to salivary duct (SDA) are commonly found in SS, more often (50–70%) in SS–RA than in primary SS (10–20%) or in RA alone (20–30%) (MacSween et al, 1967; Manthorpe et al, 1981), the apparently relevant antibody thus bearing an inverse relationship to the usual severity of end-organ disease. The specificity for salivary duct antigens seems to be high; this together with, if anything, an inverse correlation between SDA and focal lymphocytic sialadenitis in biopsy specimens has prompted suggestions that, variously, SDA is an irrelevant epiphenomenon or a protective blocking antibody (Whaley et al, 1969; Moutsopoulos et al, 1980a).

Cellular immunity

There may be impairment of certain cell-mediated immune reactions such as mitogenic lymphocyte transformation and antigen-stimulated leucocyte migration; cutaneous anergy has also been demonstrated (Michalski et al, 1978). The humoral evidence of hyperglobulinaemia, autoantibodies and immune complexes indicate a B cell hyper-reactivity, which in turn implies disordered immunoregulation. However, this B cell activity is not usually reflected in increased spontaneous polyclonal antibody formation by circulating B cells; lymphopenia is uncommon, and there is no overall depletion in peripheral blood T lymphocytes. These are all in contrast to SLE (Fauci & Moutsopoulos, 1981). In SS, suppressor T cells with an IgG Fc receptor (Ts) are depleted in blood and lip biopsy specimens (Moutsopoulos & Fauci, 1980c; Fox et al, 1982); mitogen-induced plaque formation is reduced in some patients; and the autologous mixed lymphocyte reaction may be reduced (inferentially affecting the generation of suppressor T lymphocytes). As in SLE, serological and cellular factors interact: the apparent reduction in Ts cells was reversed by treatment of total lymphocytes with trypsin. That this was a serum factor (possibly immune complexes) is indicated by the finding that serum from such patients would also block the expression of the Fc receptor on normal lymphocytes. These abnormalities in immunoregulation were found mostly in patients with extraglandular primary SS (Moutsopoulos & Fauci, 1980c).

GENETICS OF SJÖGREN'S SYNDROME

There is no very obvious evidence of a familial tendency in SS, the reported instances being exceptional. However, there is both laboratory and epidemiological evidence for a genetic influence on the expression of RA and SLE, both of which are associated with SS. In patients with primary SS, increased frequencies of DRw3 (or DR3) and, in linkage disequilibrium, HLA-B8, are found and in those with SS secondary to RA only an increase in DRw4. In addition an increased incidence of certain HLA-linked B cell alloantigens was found in both primary and secondary SS (Moutsopoulos et al, 1979a). DW2 and DW3 have also been observed to be associated with higher titres of antibody to the SSB antigen (Manthorpe et al, 1982). It may be that there is a common immune response gene influencing expression of, say, antinuclear antibodies; however the autoimmune diseases remain clinically and probably immunogenetically complex and heterogenous.

LYMPHOPROLIFERATION AND MALIGNANCY IN SJÖGREN'S SYNDROME

B cell hyper-reactivity with hyperglobulinaemia, autoantibody formation and immune complexes are characteristic of SS. That a frankly malignant picture could emerge became apparent in the early 1960s and the concept developed of a spectrum of benign to malignant lymphoproliferation (Anderson & Talal, 1972). Of 136 patients with SS traced retrospectively, 7 cases of non-Hodgkin's lymphoma were found, giving a relative risk of about 44 compared with the general population (Kassan & Grady, 1978). Marked parotid enlargement treated with local radiotherapy was associated with an even greater risk of malignancy. There was also an increased risk of skin cancer. Other surveys have confirmed these findings — that patients with SS are unusually likely to develop neoplasia, particularly lymphoid. There may be an analogy here with the New Zealand mouse (NZB/Wf1) which has features resembling SLE and SS and which tends to develop lymphoma. The MRL/l mouse also develops autoimmune disease and salivary periductal lymphoid infiltrates. The autosomal recessive lpr gene here appears to be responsible for the massive but non-malignant lymphadenopathy, which is of T cell phenotype (Hang et al, 1982).

The spectrum concept implies a potential progression from the benign glandular lymphoid infiltrates of SS, whether or not accompanied by a connective tissue disease. The intermediate stage, termed 'pseudolymphoma' (Anderson & Talal, 1972) involved new or progressive lymphadenopathy, splenomegaly, hyperglobulinaemic purpura and perhaps renal disease with extraglandular but benign lymphoreticular hyperplasia. Steroid treatment can cause regression of this stage. Finally extraglandular malignant lymphoma (which has been shown to be of B cell lineage) (Zulman et al, 1978) develops in a small proportion of patients.

It may be inferred from this concept that pseudolymphoma is a premalignant stage. The histological picture of benign lymphoepithelial lesion (BLEL) probably should not be regarded as benign, at least in its potential, as was originally thought (Godwin, 1952). In one series of 45 biopsy cases, presenting as salivary gland tumours, 40 were malignant or pre-malignant (Schmid et al, 1982). This raises the possibility that some patients with SS actually have an undeclared lymphoid neoplasm, to which perhaps there is an associated hyperplastic reaction. Whether or not this risk of malignancy is further increased by the use of cytotoxic drugs is uncertain. Meanwhile a high index of suspicion should be maintained in patients with SS particularly primary. Although lymphoproliferation may be benign, a policy of early biopsy, especially of enlarging nodes or salivary glands may be advisable. Malignant transformation, detected morphologically or immunohistochemically by, for example, light chain restriction, may also be heralded by reduction in previously high serum globulin levels and perhaps the appearance of a monoclonal band in the plasma.

TREATMENT OF SJÖGREN'S SYNDROME

General management

To a patient with active RA or SLE uncomfortable dryness of the mouth and eyes is an extra burden. Yet it may be that this problem is overlooked in the concern to treat another more obvious one such as nephritis or disabling arthritis. Conversely, the systemic nature of the condition may not be apparent if xerostomia, for example, is the predominant complaint.

There is something to be said for a multidisciplinary approach to multisystem disease, so that the patient is saved from having to present herself to successive subspecialists for advice on the various aspects of her disorder. Therein however lies management by committee, often unsatisfactory for patients.

Treating the problems of reduced secretions

For most patients treatment of the dry eyes is satisfactorily accomplished by using some form of tear substitute. Methylcellulose eyedrops (Hypromellose) are commonly used in the UK. More complicated formulations such as 'Tears Naturale' and 'BJ6' or a 20% solution of the mucolytic acetylcysteine may offer certain advantages. The tears should be dropped in as often as required, usually 2–4 times daily. Surgical obliteration of the nasolacrimal duct to limit drainage is sometimes necessary. Soft contact lenses, to reduce evaporation, have been tried and largely found wanting. Staphylococcal infection may supervene and appropriate measures should be taken (with ophthalmological advice). Various saliva substitutes have been mostly unsatisfactory for the symptomatic relief of xerostomia (Klestov et al, 1981). Sugar-free acid drops or lemon juice are usually suggested as sialogogues, although one would think that the dryness itself would provide maximum stimulus to salivation. Liquid in any form is what is really needed to facilitate mastication and to wash away food remnants. A sensible patient rapidly discovers the optimal quantity and frequency of liquid to enable her to swallow and talk comfortably. Antidepressants and antihistamines are to be avoided if possible because of the additional effect on secretion. Regular dental supervision is advisable, as gingivitis, caries and oral thrush seem commoner than usual and dentures may become ill-fitting. A bland lubricant helps with vaginal dryness. Bromhexine 24–48 mg/day orally has been advocated and in a controlled trial against a placebo appeared to produce improvement in tear secretion, although not in salivation (Frost-Larsen et al, 1978).

Surgical intervention is necessary in those rare instances of acute suppurative parotitis not responding to antibiotics, or duct blockage from calculus. Contrary to all other advice in the literature, a Hungarian report of parotidectomy in 15 patients with SS concluded that it was safe and beneficial, with overall improvement in salivation (Berenyi, 1974).

Systemic treatment

In patients with secondary SS it is most likely that the nature and intensity of systemic treatment will be dictated by the accompanying connective tissue disease (RA, SLE, etc.). The marked variations in sicca symptoms, both real and by comparison with the associated connective tissue disease, make it difficult to know if, for example, treatment of SS/RA with D-penicillamine results in improvement in the sicca features.

Patients with primary glandular SS require symptomatic relief as outlined above. Extraglandular disease manifested by renal tubular acidosis, arthralgia, Raynaud's syndrome, etc., may also be satisfactorily managed symptomatically (with, respectively, alkalis, anti-inflammatory drugs, guanethidine blocks, etc.). Complications such as myositis, lung infiltrations or haemolytic anaemia will usually be regarded as indications for systemic treatment with corticosteroids. The dose will be dictated by the circumstances but one should remember that SS is a chronic disease; one is looking for control, not cure. Dosage should be carefully restricted to the absolute minimum necessary to produce improvement in whichever aspect of the disorder one is concerned with. A claim has been made that the combination of thyroxine with prednisone is especially effective (Denko & Bergenstal, 1960).

The lymphoproliferative and malignant complications (see above) of SS will also merit treatment dictated by their nature. The important step in these circumstances is to achieve a tissue diagnosis. The finding of a lymphoma will necessitate discussion with oncological colleagues and appropriate treatment as for a lymphoma unassociated with connective tissue disease. The programme of treatment for lymphoma often includes short intermittent courses of treatment with corticosteroids and these may result in an acute flare-up of arthritis upon termination of a particular course. The possible oncogenic effects of immunosuppressive agents such as azathioprine or cyclophosphamide must also be remembered if such immunosuppressive treatment of non-malignant SS lymphoproliferative complications are undertaken. Controlled trials of cytotoxic drugs either alone or in combination with steroids are lacking, but clearly if steroid toxicity is becoming unacceptable in the face of continuing disease activity the addition of azathioprine 2–2.5 mg/kg (where renal function is normal) is reasonable. Most physicians would regard cyclophosphamide 1–2 mg/kg or chlorambucil 2–6 mg/day as being the alternatives, albeit carrying greater risk of toxicity.

Drug reactions

Side-reactions to drugs, initially penicillin and sulphonamides, more recently D-penicillamine and gold, have been said to be unduly common in SS (Bloch, 1965). However these findings have been since questioned and to date there is no conclusive evidence to suggest that one's clinical practice should be modified.

AETIOLOGY OF SJÖGREN'S SYNDROME

The foregoing discussions indicate the complexity of Sjögren's syndrome. Indeed it seems quite likely that the sicca syndrome, or 'autoimmune exocrinopathy', is a final common pathology of expression for a number of different pathological entities involving lymphoid hyperplasia and autoaggression. The murine models (NZB/W — Kessler, 1968; MRL/l — Hang et al, 1982) so far confirm the genetic and autoimmune nature of the human disease. A canine model also exists (Quimby et al, 1979). Perhaps the relationship that has been noted between salivary tissue and thymus (Martinez-Hernandez et al, 1973) will help us to understand the expression of autoimmunity in this manner. It does not, however, as yet explain the genesis of the syndrome, nor how to reverse the situation.

REFERENCES

Akizuki M, Boehm-Truitt M J, Kassan S S, Steinberg A D, Chused T M 1977 Purification of an acidic nuclear protein antigen and demonstration of its antibodies in subsets of patients with sicca syndrome. Journal of Immunology 119: 932–938

Akker H P van den, Sokole E B, Schoot J B van der 1976 Origin and location of the oral activity in sequential salivary gland scintigraphy with ^{99m}Tc-pertechnetate. Journal of Nuclear Medicine 17: 959–964

Alarcon-Segovia D, Diaz-Jouanen E, Fishbein E 1973 Features of Sjögren's syndrome in primary biliary cirrhosis. Annals of Internal Medicine 79: 31–36

Alexander E L, Provost T T 1981 Ro (SSA) and La (SSB) antibodies. Seminars in Immunopathology 4: 253–73

Alexander E L, Provost T T, Stevens M B, Alexander G E 1982 Neurological complications of primary Sjögren's syndrome. Medicine (Baltimore) 61: 247–57

Alexander E L, Arnett F C, Provost T T, Stevens M B 1983 Sjögren's syndrome: association of anti-Ro (SS-A) antibodies with vasculitis, haematological abnormalities and serological hyperactivity. Annals of Internal Medicine 98: 155–159

Alspaugh M A, Maddison P J 1979 Resolution of the identity of certain antigen–antibody systems in systemic lupus erythematosus and Sjögren's syndrome: an inter-laboratory collaboration. Arthritis and Rheumatism 22: 796–798

Alspaugh M A, Tan E M 1975 Antibodies to cellular antigens in Sjögren's syndrome. Journal of Clinical Investigation 55: 1067–1073

Anderson J R, Cray K G, Beck J S, Kinnear W F 1961 Precipitating autoantibodies in Sjögren's disease. Lancet 2: 456–60

Anderson L G, Talal N 1972 The spectrum of benign to malignant lymphoproliferation in Sjögren's syndrome. Clinical and Experimental Immunology 10: 199–124

Ben-Aryeh H, Spielman A, Sjargel R et al 1982 Sialochemistry in the diagnosis of salivary gland involvement in Sjögren's syndrome. In: Machtey I (ed) Progress in rheumatology. J Wright, Boston, p. 69–75

Bereny B 1974 Oral surgical approach to the treatment of Sjögren's syndrome. International Journal of Oral Surgery 3: 304–313

Berkeson J 1955 The statistical study of association between smoking and cancer. Mayo Clinic Proceedings 30:319

Bernstein B, Koster-King W, Singsen B, Kornreich H K, Hansen V 1977 Sjögren's syndrome in childhood. Arthritis and Rheumatism 20: 361–362

Berrebi A, Shalind M, Talanor M, Vorst E 1982 Thrombocytopenia in Sjögren's syndrome. Arthritis and Rheumatism 25:1510

Blandford R L, Dowdle J R, Stephens M R, Walker D M 1979 Sjögren's syndrome associated with idiopathic haemochromatosis. British Medical Journal 1:1323

Bloch K J, Buchanan W W, Wohl M J, Bunim J J 1965 Sjögren's syndrome: a clinical pathological and serological study of 62 cases. Medicine (Baltimore) 44: 187–231

Blythe W B 1982 Renal tubular disorders in the rheumatic diseases. In: Bacon P A, Hadler N M (eds). The kidney and rheumatic diseases. Butterworths, London, p. 267–281

Chisholm D M, Mason D K 1968 Labial salivary gland biopsy in Sjögren's disease. Journal of Clinical Pathology 21: 656–660

Clark G, Reichlin M, Tomasi T B 1969 Characterisation of a soluble cytoplasmic antigen reactive with sera from patients with systemic lupus erythematosus. Journal of Immunology 102: 117–122

Cummings N A, Schall G L, Asofsky R, Anderson L G, Talal N 1971 Sjögren's syndrome: newer aspects of research, diagnosis and therapy (NIH Conference). Annals of Internal Medicine 25: 937–950

Daniels T E 1984 Labial salivary gland biopsy in Sjögren's syndrome. Arthritis and Rheumatism 27: 147–156

Daniels T E, Powell M R, Sylvester R A, Talal N 1979 An evaluation of salivary scintigraphy in Sjögren's syndrome. Arthritis and Rheumatism 22: 809–814

Denko C W, Bergenstal D M 1960 The sicca syndrome (Sjögren's syndrome). Archives of Internal Medicine 105: 849–858

Denko C W, Old J W 1969 Myopathy in the sicca syndrome (Sjögren's syndrome); a study of sixteen cases. Archives of Internal Medicine 105: 849–858

Dijkstra P F 1980 Classification and differential diagnosis of sialographic characteristics in Sjögren's syndrome. Seminars in Arthritis and Rheumatism 10: 10–17

Doig J A, Whaley K, Dick W C, Nuki G, Williamson J, Buchanan W W 1971. Otolaryngological aspects of Sjögren's syndrome. British Medical Journal 4: 460–464

Dunne J V, Carson D A, Spiegelberg H L, Alspaugh M A, Vaughan J H 1979 IgA rheumatoid factor in the sera and saliva of patients with rheumatoid arthritis and Sjögren's syndrome. Annals of Rheumatic Diseases 38: 161–165

Elkon K B, Caeiro F, Gharavi A E, Patel B M, Ferjencik P P, Hughes G R V 1981 Radio-immunoassay profile of antiglobulins in connective tissue diseases: elevated levels of IgA antiglobulin in systemic sicca syndrome. Clinical and Experimental Immunology 46: 547–556

Escande J P 1977 Conception actuelle du syndrome de Gougerot Sjögren. Revue Rhumatisme et Maladies Osteoarticulaires 44: 455–459

Fairfax A J, Haslam P L, Pavla D, Sheahan N F, Bateman S R M, Agnew J E, Clarke S W, Turner-Warwick M 1981 Pulmonary disorders associated with Sjögren's syndrome. Quarterly Journal of Medicine 50: 279–295

Fauci A S, Moutsopoulos H M 1981 Polyclonally triggered B cells in the peripheral blood and bone marrow of normal individuals and in patients with systemic lupus erythematosus and primary Sjögren's syndrome. Arthritis and Rheumatism 24: 577–583

Feest T G, Lockwood C M, Morley A R, Uff J S 1978 Renal histology and immunopathology in distal renal tubular acidosis. Clinical Nephrology 10: 187–190

Feest T G, Wrong O M 1982 Renal tubular acidosis. In: Jones N F, Peters D K (eds) Recent advances in renal medicine. Churchill Livingstone, Edinburgh, p. 243–271

Fenster F, Buchanan W W, Lasker, Bunim J J 1964 Studies of pancreatic function in Sjögren's syndrome. Annals of Internal Medicine 61: 498–508

Fink A I, MacKay C Y, Cutler S S 1979 Sicca complex and cholangiostatic jaundice in two members of a family probably caused by Thiabendazole. Ophthalmology (Rochester) 86: 1892–6

Forstot J Z, Forstot S L, Greer R O, Tan E M 1982 The incidence of Sjögren's sicca complex in a population of patients with kerato-conjunctivitis sicca. Arthritis and Rheumatism 25: 156–160

Fox R I, Carstens S A, Fong S, Robinson C A, Howell F, Vaughan J H 1982 Use of monoclonal antibodies to analyse peripheral blood and salivary gland lymphocyte subsets in Sjögren's syndrome. Arthritis and Rheumatism 25: 419–426

Fraser N G, Rennie A G R, Donald D 1979 Dermatitis herpetiformis and Sjögren's syndrome. British Journal of Dermatology 100: 213–215

Frost-Larsen K, Isager H, Manthorpe R 1978 Sjögren's syndrome treated with Bromhexine: a randomised clinical study. British Medical Journal 1: 1579–1581

Gerhardt R E, Loebl D H, Rao R N 1978 Interstitial immunofluorescence in nephritis of Sjögren's syndrome. Clinical Nephrology 10: 201–207

Godwin J T 1952 Benign lymphoepithelial lesion of the parotid gland. Cancer 5: 1089–1103

Golding P L, Bown R, Mason A M S, Taylor E 1970 Sicca complex in liver disease. British Medical Journal 4: 340–342

Gratwohl A A, Moutsopoulos H M, Chused T M 1977 Sjögren-type syndrome after allogeneic bone marrow transplantation. Annals of Internal Medicine 87: 703–706

Hang L, Theofilopoulos A N, Dixon F J 1982 A spontaneous rheumatoid arthritis-like disease in MRL/1 mice. Journal of Experimental Medicine 155: 1690–1701

Helve T, Teppo A M, Kurki P, Wegelius O 1982 Human antibodies to the nuclear SS-B68 antigen: an assay for antibodies of IgG, IgM and IgA classes. In: Machtey I (ed) Progress in Rheumatology. J Wright, Boston, p. 51–55

Hyams J 1984 Rheumatoid sera unravel microtubule organizers. Nature 308: 604–5

Isenberg D A, Hammond L, Fisher C, Griffiths M, Stewart J, Bottazzo G F 1982 Predictive value of SS-B precipitating antibodies in Sjögren's syndrome. British Medical Journal 284: 1738–1740

Kaltreider H B, Talal N 1969 Neuropathy of Sjögren's syndrome. Annals of Internal Medicine 70: 751–762

Karsh J, Halbert S P, Anken M, Kline Z, Steinberg A D 1982 Anti DNA, anti deoxyribonucleoprotein and rheumatoid factor measured by ELISA in patients with systemic lupus erythematosus, Sjögren's syndrome and rheumatoid arthritis. International Archives of Allergy and Applied Immunology 68: 60–69

Kassan S S, Grady M 1978 Sjögren's syndrome: an update and overview. American Journal of Medicine 64: 1037–1046

Katona G, Burgos-Vargas R, Zimbron A 1982 The scintigraphic approach of gastric dysfunction in Sjögren's syndrome with ^{99m}Pertechnetate. In: Machtey I (ed) Progress in rheumatology. J Wright, PSG, Boston, p. 77–83

Kessler H S 1968 A laboratory model for Sjögren's syndrome. American Journal of Pathology 52: 671–685

Klestov A C, Webb J, Latt D et al 1981 Oral Medicine and Oral Surgery 51: 594–599

Lerner M R, Steitz J A 1981 Snurps and scryps. Cell 25: 298–300

Lockshin M D, Gibofsky A, Peebles C L, Gigli I, Fotiano M, Hurwitz S 1983 Neonatal lupus erythematosus with heart block. Arthritis and Rheumatism 26: 210–213

Mackie I A, Seal D V 1981 The questionably dry eye. British Journal of Ophthalmology 65: 2–9

MacSween R N M, Goudie R B, Anderson J R et al 1967 Occurrence of antibody to salivary duct epithelium in Sjögren's disease, rheumatoid arthritis and other arthritides. Annals of Rheumatic Diseases 26: 402–411

Maddison P J Reichlin M 1979 Deposition of antibodies to a soluble cytoplasmic antigen in the kidneys of patients with systemic lupus erythematosus. Arthritis and Rheumatism 22: 858–863

Maddison P J 1982 Seronegative SLE. Clinics in Rheumatic Diseases 8: 105–119

Mandel I D, Wotman S 1976 The salivary secretions in health and disease. Oral Science Review 8: 25–47

Manthorpe R, Frost-Larsen K, Isager H, Prause J U 1981 Sjögren's syndrome: a review with emphasis on immunological features. Allergy 36: 139–153

Manthorpe R, Teppo A M, Bendixen G, Wegelius O 1982 Antibodies to SS-B in chronic inflammatory connective tissue diseases. Arthritis and Rheumatism 25: 662–667

Martinez-Hernandez A, Nakane P K, Pierce G B 1973 The relationship between the submaxillary gland and the thymus. Laboratory Investigation 29: 226–271

Mason A M S, Gumpel J M, Golding P L 1973 Sjögren's syndrome — a clinical review. Seminars in Arthritis and Rheumatism 2: 301–331

Maury P J, Rasanen V, Teppo A M, Helve T, Wegelius O 1982 Serum pepsinogen 1 in rheumatic diseases: reduced level in Sjögren's syndrome. Arthritis and Rheumatism 25: 1059–1063

Meyer O, Chabrand-Ahond L, Kahn M F, Ryckewaert A 1982 Determination of the presence of soluble SS-A, SS-B and RNP anti-nuclear antigen antibodies in pure or associated forms of Sjögren's syndrome. Rhumatisme et Maladies Osteoarticulaires 49/6: 421–425

Michalski Y P, McCombs C, Fye K H, Daniels T E, Terasaki P I, Talal N 1978 Impaired lymphocyte response in Sjögren's syndrome associated with HLA-B8. Journal of Clinical and Laboratory Immunology 1: 25–29

Morgan W S, Castleman B 1953 A clinicopathologic study of 'Mikulicz' disease. American Journal of Pathology 29: 471–503

Moutsopoulos H M, Mann D L, Johnson A H, Chused T M 1979a Genetic differences between primary and secondary sicca syndrome. New England Journal of Medicine 301: 761–763

Moutsopoulos H M, Webber B L, Vlagopoulos T P, Chused T M, Decker J L 1979b Differences in clinical manifestations of sicca syndrome in the presence and absence of rheumatoid arthritis. American Journal of Medicine 66: 733–736

Moutsopoulos H M, Fauci A S 1980 Immunoregulation in Sjögren's syndrome: influence of serum factors on T cell subpopulations. Journal of Clinical Investigation 65: 519–528

Moutsopoulos H M, Klippel J H, Pavlidis N et al 1980a Correlative histologic and serologic findings of sicca syndrome in patients with systemic lupus erythematosus. Arthritis and Rheumatism 23: 36–40

Moutsopoulos H M, Chused T M, Mann D L et al 1980b Sjögren's syndrome (sicca syndrome). Annals of Internal Medicine 92: 212–226

Newhall H H, Brahim S A 1977 Chronic obstructive airways disease in patients with Sjögren's syndrome. American Review of Respiratory Diseases 115: 295–304

Oxholm P, Bundgaard A, Madsen E B, Manthorpe R, Rasmussen F V 1982 Pulmonary function in patients with primary Sjögren's syndrome. Rheumatology International 2: 179–181

Pavlidis N A, Karsh J, Moutsopoulos H M 1982 The clinical picture of primary Sjögren's syndrome: a retrospective study. Journal of Rheumatology 9: 685–90

Peyronnard J M, Charron L, Beaudet F, Couture F 1982 Vasculitic neuropathy in rheumatoid disease and Sjögren's syndrome. Neurology (NY) 32: 839–845

Quimby F W, Schwartz R S, Poskitt T, Lewis R M 1979 A disorder of dogs resembling Sjögren's syndrome. Clinical Immunology and Immunopathology 12: 471–476

Reinertsen J L, Schaefer E J, Brewer H B, Moutsopoulos H M 1980 Sicca-like syndrome in type V hyperlipoproteinaemia. Arthritis and Rheumatism 23: 114–8

Ringel S P, Forstot J Z, Tan E M, Wehling C, Griggs R C, Butcher D 1980 Sjögren's syndrome and polymyositis or dermatomyositis. Archives of Neurology 39: 157–163

Schmid U, Helbron D, Lennert K 1982 Development of malignant lymphoma in myoepithelial sialadenitis (Sjögren's syndrome). Virchow Archiv 395: 11–43

Seward H F G, Hamilton D I, Patey D H 1966 An investigation of the value in clinical practice of the Curry Test for parotid function. British Journal of Surgery 53: 190–193

Shearn M 1971 Sjögren's syndrome. Lloyd H Smith Jnr (ed) Major problems in internal medicine, Vol 2. Saunders, Philadelphia, p. 617–71

Shioji R, Furayama T, Onedera S, Saito H, Ito H, Sasaki Y 1980 Sjögren's syndrome and renal tubular acidosis. American Journal of Medicine 48: 456–463

Simon B G, Moutsopoulos H M 1979 Primary amyloidosis resembling sicca syndrome. Arthritis and Rheumatism 22: 932–934

Sjögren H 1933 Zur Kenntnis der keratoconjunctivitis sicca. Acta Ophthalmologie (Suppl 2) 10: 1–151

Stevens M B, Hookman P, Siegel C I 1964 Aperistalsis of the oesophagus in patients with connective tissue disorders and Raynaud's phenomenon. New England Journal of Medicine 270: 1218–1222

Strand V, Talal N 1980 Advances in the diagnosis and concept of Sjögren's syndrome (autoimmune exocrinopathy). Bulletin on the Rheumatic Diseases 30: 1046–1052

Strimlan C V, Rosenow E C, Divertie H B, Harrison E G 1976 Pulmonary manifestations of Sjögren's syndrome. Chest 70: 354–361

Tarpley T M, Anderson L G, White G L 1974 Minor salivary gland involvement in Sjögren's syndrome. Oral Surgery 37: 64–74

Teppo A M, Gripenberg M, Kuki P, Bahlieu K, Helve T, Wegelius O 1980 Purification and characterization of a nuclear SS-B antigen. Scandinavian Journal of Immunology 15: 1–7

Venables P J W, Russell P J, Buchanan R R C et al 1983 Quantitation and detection of isotopes of anti-SS-B antibodies by ELISA and Farr assays using affinity purified antigens. Arthritis and Rheumatism 26: 146–155

Wallach D, Pecking A, Delvincourt C, Cottenot F, Najean Y 1979 Gougerot–Sjögren syndrome and pemphigus. Parallel development of the dryness syndrome and autoimmune dermatosis. Annals of Dermatology and Venereology 106: 181–186

Waterhouse J P, Doniach I 1966 Postmortem prevalence of focal lymphocytic adenitis of the submandibular gland. Journal of Pathology and Bacteriology 91: 53–64

Whaley K, Chisholm D M, Goudie R B et al 1969 Salivary duct autoantibody in Sjögren's syndrome: correlation with focal sialadenitis in the labial mucosa. Clinical and Experimental Immunology 4: 273–82

Whaley K, Goudie R B, Williamson J, Nuki G, Dick W C, Buchanan W W 1970 Liver disease in Sjögren's syndrome and rheumatoid arthritis. Lancet: 861–863

Whaley K, Chisholm D M, Williamson J, Dick W C, Nuki G, Buchanan W W 1971 Sjögren's syndrome in psoriatic arthritis, ankylosing spondyliitis and Reiter's syndrome. Acta Rheumatologica Scandinavica 17: 105–114

Whaley K, Williamson J, Chisholm D W, Webb J, Mason D K, Buchanan W W 1973a Sjögren's syndrome 1: sicca components. Quarterly Journal of Medicine 42: 279–304

Whaley K, Webb J, McAvoy B A et al 1973b Sjögren's syndrome 2: Clinical associations and immunologic phenomena. Quarterly Journal of Medicine 42: 513–548

Williamson J, Cant J S, Mason D K, Greig W R, Boyle J A 1967 Sjögren's syndrome and thyroid disease. British Journal of Ophthalmology 51: 721–726

Yoshinoya S, McDuffy S, Alarcon-Segovia D, Pope R M 1982 Detection and partial characterization of immune complexes in patients with rheumatoid arthritis plus Sjögren's syndrome and with Sjögren's syndrome alone. Clinical and Experimental Immunology 48: 339–347

Zulman J, Jaffe R, Talal N 1978 Evidence that malignant lymphoma of Sjögren's syndrome is a monoclonal B-cell neoplasm. New England Journal of Medicine 289: 1215–220

SECTION XII

Topographical Rheumatology (Regional Disorders)

M.I.V. Jayson

Back pain, spondylosis and disc disorders

The back extends from the neck to the coccyx, and back pain includes pain felt in the cervical, dorsal, lumbosacral and coccygeal areas and may spread into the shoulder and pelvic girdles and radiate to the limbs. Despite the frequency of back symptoms, understanding of their underlying causes is often unsatisfactory. This is partly due to the difficulties of precise definition. Pain is a subjective sensation; without conscious appreciation, pain does not exist, only neurological impulses. In the present context, back pain must be of sufficient degree for the patient to seek medical advice. The looseness of this definition makes epidemiological and statistical surveys difficult to interpret and much information relates to figures of sickness absence from work, obtained in the knowledge that factors other than the severity of the pain might be relevant.

The magnitude of the problem

Back pains, including symptoms felt in both the cervical and lumbar regions present some of the commonest causes of disability (Table 57.1). About 2% of the adult population seek medical advice for back pain each year. Wood & Badley (1982) estimated that in Britain back troubles cause 26.9 spells and 949 days of incapacity per 1000 male workers with a total of 14 million working days lost per annum. This underestimates the total problem in that female workers and those not in employment were not included. Amongst rheumatic complaints as a whole, back pain accounts for about 31% of spells of loss of work and 29% of the total time lost through ill-health by male industrial workers. However, as a cause for permanent disability, back pain is of lesser significance. Harris et al (1971) reported approximately 65 000 people in Great Britain identified as impaired by 'slipped disc' or 'lumbago' in contrast to about 1 000 000 from rheumatic diseases as a whole.

Radiological evidence of disc degeneration is common (Table 57.2). The prevalences of both back pain and disc degeneration increase with age. (Lawrence et al, 1963; Lawrence, 1969). However, the correlation between radiological evidence of lumbar spondylosis and back pain is poor (Lawrence, 1977). When age-related factors are taken into account there is no correlation between back pain and the development of osteophytes in the spine although there is a residual correlation with disc degeneration (Torgerson & Dotter, 1976). Comparable degrees of radiological change occur in most countries, but in less developed countries symptoms of back pain are less frequent (Bremner et al, 1968).

Table 57.1 Frequency of spinal symptoms in adults. (From Lawrence, 1969.)

Sex	Pain (%)			
	Neck/Shoulder/Brachial		Back/Hip/Sciatic	
	Present	Past	Present	Past
Male	9	28	11	40
Female	12	34	19	33

Table 57.2 Radiological evidence of disc degeneration in adults. (From Lawrence et al, 1963)

Sex	Disc degeneration (%)	
	Cervical	Lumbar
Male	40	60
Female	37	44

There is an increased prevalence of back pain in those who perform heavy manual labour (Lawrence, 1969; Anderson, 1980) and particularly if the work involves bending or twisting the spine or if there is a risk of sudden unexpected movements (Buckle et al, 1980). Car and truck drivers, especially if required to travel long distances, have an increased frequency of back pain and prolapsed intervertebral disc (Buckle et al, 1980; Kelsey, 1975). The use of vibrating tools or vibrations transmitted from vehicle seats may lead to spinal problems particularly if the vibration is at the natural resonant frequency of the body (Frymoyer et al, 1980; Wilder et al, 1982).

There is an increased incidence of radiological evidence of lumbar spondylosis in subjects with osteoarthritis of the hips (Saunders et al, 1979). It is not clear whether this association is the result of a generalised degenerative process affecting both the hip and spine or whether the mechanical consequences of osteoarthritis of the hips lead to spinal problems and vice versa.

THE STRUCTURE AND FUNCTION OF THE SPINE

The 7 cervical, 12 dorsal and 5 lumbar vertebrae, together with the sacrum and coccyx, have a common underlying structure with differences reflecting the functions of the various sites. In the lumbar spine, the vertebrae are heavily built (Fig. 57.1) reflecting the stresses which they transmit and are in contrast with the lightly built cervical vertebrae which carry much less load but are more mobile. The total ranges of movement of the neck and the relative contributions of its different parts have been reviewed by Penning (1968). The vertebrae are linked principally by the intervertebral discs and apophyseal joints. Also there are the uncovertebral joints in the neck and the costotransverse joints in the thoracic region.

Posterior and posterolateral protrusion of the intervertebral disc can impinge upon the posterior longitudinal ligament, nerve root, and other sensitive structures, producing local and referred pain. The structure and properties of the disc are therefore of special interest.

Each disc consists of a central nucleus pulposus surrounded by the annulus fibrosus. The nucleus is normally a gel-like structure with randomly orientated collagen fibres embedded in a matrix largely consisting of water and protein polysaccarides (Rosenberg et al, 1967). Stevens et al (1979) compared the proteoglycans of the intervertebral disc with those in hyaline cartilage. The fundamental structure is similar but disc proteoglycans contain a greater proportion of keratan sulphate, a lesser proportion of chondroitin sulphate and are shorter in length principally due to a shorter region of core protein carrying the chondroitin sulphate side chains. There are some subtle differences between the proteoglycans of the nu-

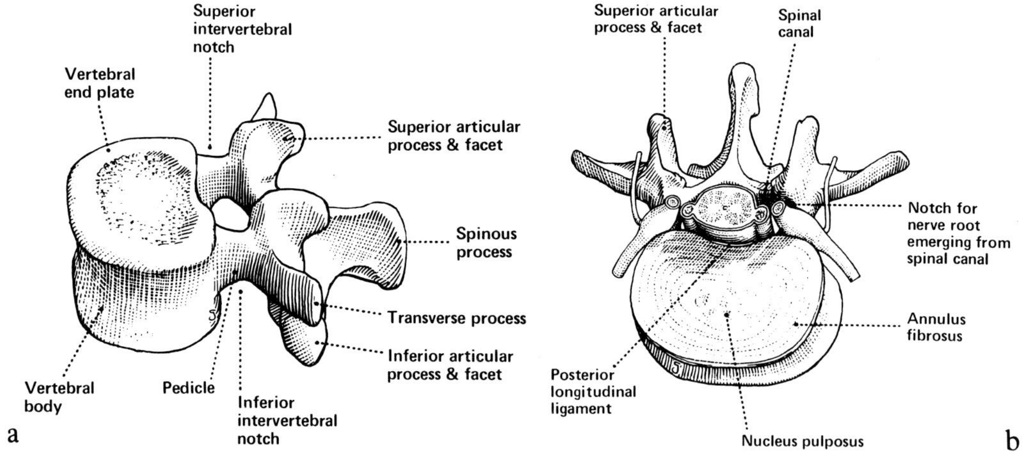

Fig. 57.1 A typical lumbar vertebrae in (a) lateral view; (b) axial view — showing the close relationship of the nerves of the cauda equina to the posterior and posterolateral surfaces of the intervertebral disc.

cleus pulposus and the annulus fibrosus, the latter showing a greater capability of aggregating with hyaluronic acid. The proteoglycan concentration normally increases to a maximum in about the 3rd decade of life and then decreases (Murayama, 1972). With ageing (Hirsch et al, 1953) the water content of the disc decreases and there is an increase in collagen so that it becomes more fibrous. With disc degeneration, prolapse and spondylolisthesis (Hirsch et al, 1953; Davidson & Woodhall, 1959; Roberts et al, 1982) there is a decrease in the proteoglycan content. Lipson & Muir (1981) followed the changes in proteoglycan in an animal model of intervertebral disc degeneration. Incision of the disc leads to prolapse and a fall in water and proteoglycan content. This is followed by a transient increase of both, which represents an attempt at repair and then further loss with scar formation until a pattern of disc degeneration results which is similar to that found in human disease (Adams & Muir, 1976).

The annulus fibrosus consists principally of extremely strong collagen fibres arranged in laminae running concentrically to encircle the nucleus pulposus but also spiralling obliquely from one vertebral body to the other and intertwining with one another so as to form a complex finger trap arrangement (Fig. 57.2). It is this arrangement which enables the annulus fibrosus to resist the enormous pressures that may develop with the intervertebral disc. The alternate laminae lie at about 30° to the spinal axis first one way and then the other (Happey, 1976). This arrangement of the

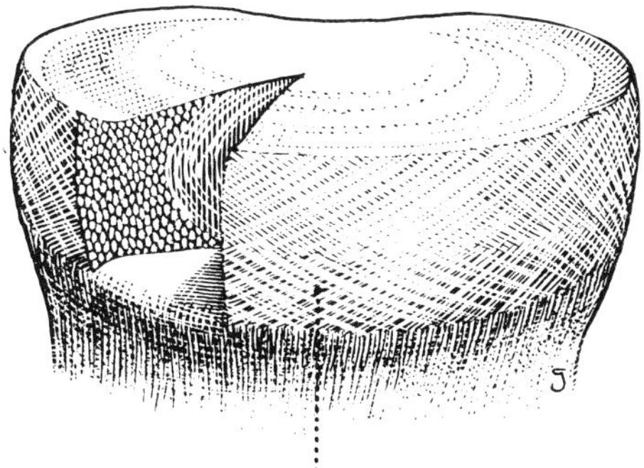

Fig. 57.2 The collagen bundles in the annulus fibrosis interlace to form a strong network which can resist increases in nuclear pressures.

annulus fibrosus affords little resistance to flexion and extension movements of the spine but provides high resistance to horizontal subluxation and rotation (Galante, 1967; Hirsch & Sonnerup, 1968). The gel-like structure of the normal nucleus redistributes pressures upon it in an isotropic fashion, i.e. equally in all directions. Increases in pressure are accommodated by a slight increase of girth of the annulus which is accomplished by a small alteration in the angle of crossing fibres (Horton, 1958). When disc degeneration occurs, the nucleus becomes more fibrous and its gel-like properties are lost. Loads are then redistributed in an anisotropic fashion, i.e. not equally in all directions, so that localised high pressure points develop at the inner annulus wall and may potentiate annular failure. Theoretical analysis (Hickey & Hukins, 1980) together with experimental observations (Brown et al, 1957; Jayson et al, 1973) indicate that under compressive load the vertebral end-plates will usually give way rather than the annulus fibrosus. It is only when there is already severe disorganisation of the disc that increases in intranuclear pressure can cause posterior or posterolateral prolapse. During ageing of the annulus, electron-microscopic examination shows the appearance of large collagen fibres which may be associated with an increase of strain and perhaps be associated with the risk of annular tears (Hickey & Hukins, 1982).

However, during flexion of the spine, stresses are concentrated at the areas of maximal curvature of the disc, which are usually at its posterolateral borders (Hickey & Hukins, 1980). Compression combined with excessive flexion of a disc that perhaps shows some minor degeneration may be sufficient to cause posterior or posterolateral prolapse (Adams & Hutton, 1982).

Analysis of the collagen of the disc shows that of the nucleus to be predominantly type II as found in normal cartilage. The annulus fibrosus contains both types I and II. The outer margin is almost entirely type I with a smooth transition to become almost entirely type II at its inner margin and junction with the nucleus pulposus (Eyre & Muir, 1977). This structural change correlates with function in that the nuclear collagen predominantly withstands compressive loads in the same way as cartilage but the outer annulus meets tensile stresses similar to those experienced by tendon. There is little change in the proportions of types I and II with age but in degenerative spondylosis there is excess synthesis of type I collagen in both the annulus and nucleus (Herbert et al, 1975). These fibres are relatively coarse and may interfere with the optimum mechanical and biochemical efficiency of the disc. This change could play a part in the genesis of spondylosis but more likely occurs as a response to disc damage. Biochemical examination indicates the presence of degradative enzymes within the disc (Sedowofia et al, 1982). These include collagenases, gelatinases and elastases. In particular collagenases are present in higher concentration in the nucleus than the annulus and are found in both active and latent forms. At the L5 disc, the concentrations of these proteolytic enzymes correlate with disc degeneration. It seems that the disc contains enzymes capable of degrading its own matrix and which may well play a part in the pathogenesis of disc degeneration.

Nachemson & Morris (1964) and Nachemson (1965) measured the pressures within the nuclei of the lumbar discs of both volunteers and patients with degenerative spondylosis. Vertical load is normally carried by the nucleus but when the disc is degenerate an increasing amount is borne by the annulus. The least stress on the normal disc is with the body reclining, with higher levels for standing, unsupported sitting, leaning forward and weight-lifting (Fig. 57.3). A poor posture, lifting heavy objects in an incorrect fashion and sitting without a lumbar support produces increased levels of intradisc pressure and may be responsible for back pain (Nachemson, 1980). The lowest lumbar discs bear the greatest body weight. They also transmit the greatest torque when the body is flexed forwards as they are nearest to the hips. It is hardly surprising that disc prolapse is most frequent in the lower lumbar discs (Armstrong, 1965) and is associated with heavy manual work (Anderson, 1971).

The apophyseal joints are true synovial joints with fibrous capsules lined by synovium. Degenerative arthritis frequently involves these joints with production of osteophytes which may impinge upon nerve roots emerging through the intervertebral foramina (see Fig. 57.1). In addition,

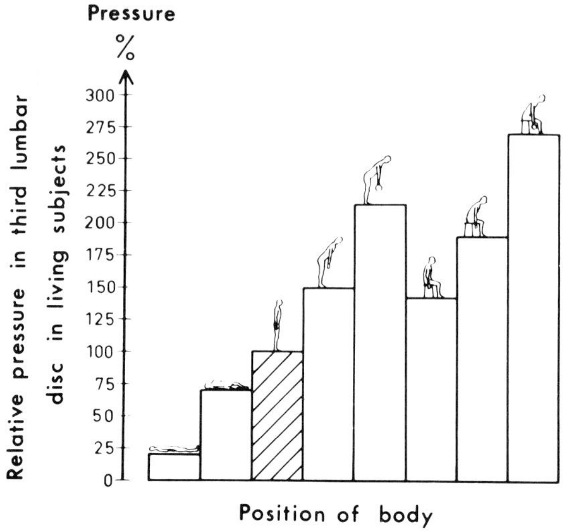

Fig. 57.3 The variations of pressure within the nucleus pulposus of the third lumbar disc in a variety of postures related to that in the upright position (by courtesy of Professor A. Nachemson).

in the neck, the vertebral arteries pass through the transverse foramina of the transverse processes of the vertebrae. They too may be affected, producing transient vertebrobasilar arterial insufficiency related to neck movements.

Each cervical and dorsal apophyseal joint is orientated so that its centre of rotation lies within the intervertebral disc. In contrast the lumbar apophyseal joints are much more anteroposteriorly inclined with their centres of rotation behind the discs. They stabilise the lumbar intervertebral joints against torsion and attempts at this movement will produced shear stresses in the disc and may account for the association of disc damage with load-bearing while the spine is twisted (Farfan et al, 1970).

From practical observations and theoretical analyses, Farfan et al (1972) and Hickey & Hukins (1980) demonstrated the influence of geometric factors on the patterns of disc degeneration. In the upper lumbar spine the round shape of the discs and the more vertically orientated joint surfaces provide maximum protection against torsion. In the lower lumbar spine increased ovality of the lumbar discs and greater inclination of the apophyseal joint surfaces diminish the effectiveness in resisting torsion and could account for the higher incidence of annular ruptures. Discs with flattened or re-entrant posterior surfaces have posterolateral margins of maximal curvature where torsional stress is concentrated and tend to develop posterolateral ruptures. On the other hand discs with rounded posterior surfaces develop midline ruptures. Anterior annular tears occur in both the upper and lower lumbar spine (Hilton et al, 1980) and may be the result of degeneration and mechanical damage respectively. Asymmetric articular processes lead to asymmetric disc degeneration whereas symmetric disc degeneration is more common when the processes are symmetrical. It is not uncommon to find the same pattern of disc degeneration at several levels in any individual spine (Jayson & Barks, 1973).

Back pain may arise due to stimulation of the nerve roots or sensory nerve endings in the back. Sensory nerve endings are present in fetal intervertebral discs but they degenerate and are not found in the adult nucleus pulposus or inner annulus (Jackson et al, 1966). Wyke (1980) and Yoshizawa et al (1980) identified nociceptive receptors in adults in the sites listed in Table 57.3. There is no alteration in disc degeneration and in particular no ingrowth of nerve fibres into degenerate areas. In particular, nerve endings in the outer annulus are found adjacent to the posterior longitudinal ligament which could well be a source of back pain in disc degeneration or prolapse (Hirsch et al, 1963; Jayson & Barks, 1973). The central pathways from these pain receptors pass through dense anastomotic plexuses involving the nerves from several spinal segments. Stimulation of any of these nerve endings can lead to diffuse pain and makes localisation of the source of symptoms difficult (Pedersen et al, 1956). The central perception of pain is modulated by the release of endorphins and enkephalins in the hypothalmic system. Preliminary evidence suggests that some back pain sufferers release less endorphins and enkephalins than normal (Dodds et al, 1983). This may in part explain the gross variation in severity of symptoms between patients with apparently similar pathologies.

Table 57.3 Sites of nociceptive receptors in relation to the back

1. In the skin and subcutaneous tissues
2. In the fibrous capsules of the apophyseal and sacroiliac joints
3. In the outer layers of the annulus fibrosus
4. In the longitudinal ligaments of the spine, and particularly the posterior longitudinal ligament
5. In the periosteum and attached fasciae, aponeuroses and tendons
6. In the walls of blood vessels in and around the spine
7. In the dura mater and epidural adipose tissues.

CLASSIFICATION OF BACK PAIN

Table 57.4 provides a classification for the more common causes back pain. Although shown separately, many of these problems are inter-related. In particular, spondylosis and apophyseal osteoarthrosis are often secondary to other spinal disease.

Table 57.4 Causes of back pain

Structural	Prolapsed intervertebral disc Spondylosis and apophyseal osteoarthrosis Senile ankylosing hyperostosis Spinal stenosis Spondylolisthesis Other congenital anomalies Scheuermann's osteochondritis Fractures Non-specific
Inflammatory	Ankylosing spondylitis and related inflammatory spondylopathies Rheumatoid arthritis Infection
Neoplastic	Primary tumours Metastases, reticuloses and myelomatosis
Paget's disease Metabolic	Osteoporosis, osteomalacia, hyperparathyroidism Chondrocalcinosis Ochronosis
Referred pain	

LUMBOSACRAL PAIN

Mechanical disorders of the spine, arising perhaps as inherited abnormalities or following injury or repeated heavy use, are responsible for most low back pains. However, it is always important to exclude other possible causes as many of the structural abnormalities can be found in symptom-free individuals.

Prolapsed intervertebral disc

Despite being first described relatively recently (Mixter & Barr, 1934), the clinical syndrome of prolapse of an intervertebral disc is now diagnosed very commonly. Indeed, of all rheumatic complaints in adult working males, disc disease is the most frequent single diagnosis (Anderson, 1971). It is those who undertake the heaviest work who appear at the greatest risk. Andrae (1929) found pathological evidence of posterior prolapse in 15.2% of routine autopsies. The L4–5 and L5–S1 discs are the most commonly affected (Armstrong, 1965) but prolapse of any of the lumbar discs can occur (Aronson & Dunsmore, 1963). More than one disc can be affected in any subject and evidence of past disc prolapse is often found at autopsy without any previous relevant history.

Nuclear material bursts through the annulus fibrosus (Fig. 57.4) and can displace and damage ligaments, periosteum, blood vessels and the dura in addition to nerve roots. The displaced nuclear and annular material heals by fibrosis and shrinking so that eventually symptoms will remit. As the annulus is weak there is considerable risk of recurrence and later secondary degenerative changes may occur. Local scarring can involve the nerve sheath leading to persistent pain. The lumbar nerve roots pass behind the discs (see Fig. 57.1) to emerge through the intervertebral foramen, each of which is bounded by the posterolateral part of the disc, the pedicles and the articular processes. Disc prolapse is usually to one side of the midline and sometimes into the intervertebral foramina producing local and referred pain. An L4–5 prolapse most often damages the L5 root and an L5–S1 prolapse the S1 root. However, a single extensive posterolateral prolapse can damage more than one nerve root.

A central posterior fissure and prolapse can damage the posterior longitudinal ligament which is innervated by the sinuvertebral nerve, producing central back pain. These fissures are difficult to recognise except by discography (Park et al, 1979). It is rare but possible for a large central posterior prolapse to compress the cauda equina. In general this only happens if the spinal canal is already narrowed by congenital stenosis (see below) or some space-occupying lesion.

Intervertebral disc tissue can also prolapse vertically up or down into the adjacent vertebral bodies (Fig. 57.5). In autopsy examinations, Schmorl & Junghanns (1971) found these 'Schmorl's nodes' in about 38% of spines, but radiographically (Fig. 57.6) in only 13.5%. Although vertical prolapse may occur through an area of weakness of vertebral end-plate, most arise due to acute or recurrent stress. Under load the vertebral end-plate

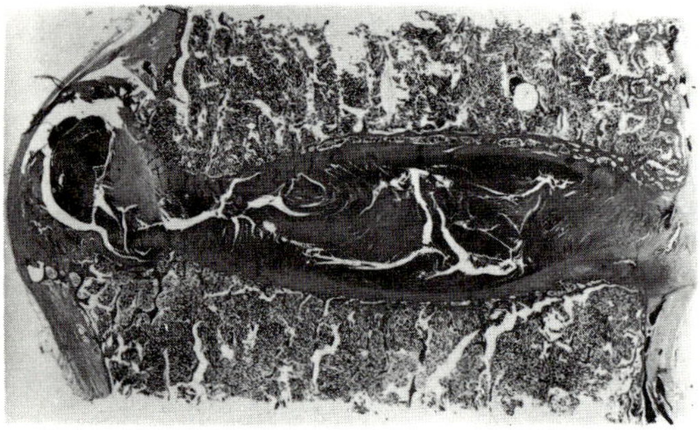

Fig. 57.4 Section through a lumbar disc showing a herniation of the nucleus pulposus surrounded by fibrous tissue and osteophytic new bone formation. The remaining nucleus shows extensive fissuring. (H & E × 50) (By courtesy of Dr B. Vernon-Roberts and the Editor of *The lumbar spine and back pain.*)

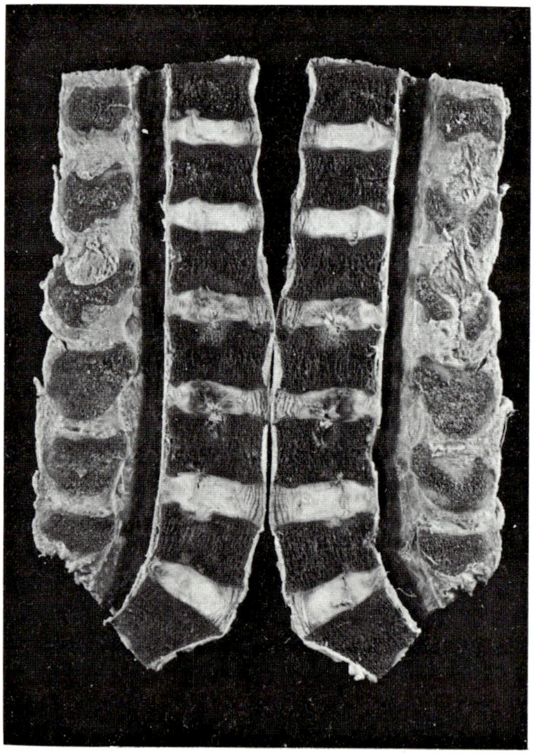

Fig. 57.5 Sagittal section of the lumbar spine showing multiple Schmorl's nodes with and without disc degeneration (By courtesy of Dr B. Vernon-Roberts.)

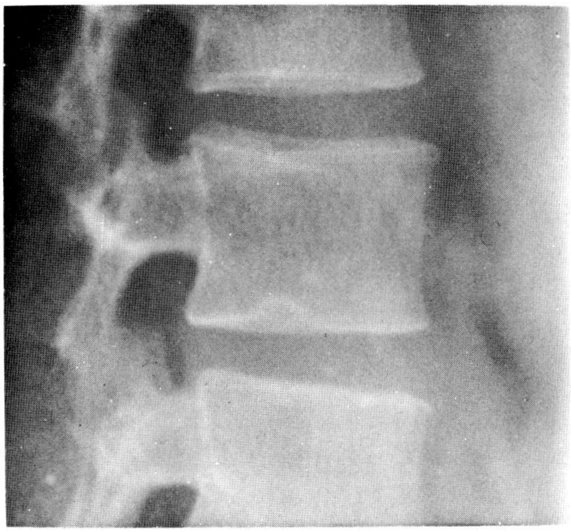

Fig. 57.6 Radiograph to show Schmorl's nodes.

is more likely to give way than the healthy annulus fibrosus (Brown et al, 1957; Jayson et al, 1973). The mineral content of the vertebral bone influences the type of fracture of the vertebral end-plate. When the bone has a normal or high mineral content and the disc is normal, a central fracture of the vertebral end-plant develops in contrast with spines with a low mineral content and a degenerate disc when wedge fractures of the vertebral bodies occur (Hansson & Roos, 1981).

Prolapse of a lumbar intervertebral disc produces pain both in the back and referred into one or other lower limb. The distribution and nature of the pain vary widely. It may develop suddenly particularly during some stress involving bending, twisting and lifting and be so sudden and severe that the patient becomes stuck and unable to straighten up. Sometimes it appears gradually several hours after the event or there may be no obvious precipitating factors. There are two types of referred pain. Pressure on the ligaments and other tissues of the spine produces pain that is dull, poorly defined and felt in the muscles of the same embryonic level. The distribution of this pain is of little help in determining the level of the prolapse. Nerve root damage produces cutaneous symptoms that are much better localised, with the distribution of numbness and paraesthesiae being rather more helpful than pain. Most cases of 'sciatica' are thought to be due to such root damage by lumbar disc lesions. Table 57.5 shows the principal effects of nerve root damage that are used in identifying the level of the lesion but there may be considerable overlap between adjacent roots and more than one root may be compressed by prolapse of a single disc. Symptoms are made worse by spinal movements and particularly flexion, and also by manoeuvers that may raise the cerebrospinal fluid pressure, such as coughing, sneezing, micturition and defaecation. The symptoms pursue a variable course. They may remit rapidly and completely, or, at the other extreme, they may become worse with gradual extension of the pain and the neurological signs. Sometimes the condition becomes chronic and always the patient who has had one episode of a prolapsed intervertebral

Table 57.5 Principal changes used for identifying the sites of lumbar nerve root lesions. (Note that this table does not list the total distribution of each root.)

Root	Superficial paraesthesiae and sensory change	Muscle weakness	Tendon reflex change
L2	Upper thigh, anterior, medial and lateral surfaces	Flexion and adduction of hip	None
L3	Anterior surface of lower thigh. Anterior and medial surfaces of knee	Adduction of hip. Extension of knee	Knee jerk possibly descreased
L4	Antero-medial surface of leg	Extension of knee. Dorsiflexion and inversion of foot	Knee jerk decreased
L5	Antero-lateral surface of leg, dorsum and medial surface of foot especially dorsal surface of hallux	Extension and abduction of hip. Flexion of knee. Dorsiflexion of foot and toes, especially hallux	None
S1	Lateral border and sole of foot, back of heel and lower calf	Flexion of knee. Plantar flexion and eversion of foot	Ankle jerk decreased

disc is at risk of further acute episodes of pain.

The patient stands with a rigid spine avoiding forward flexion, but usually allowing lateral flexion and rotation in one or both directions. Moll & Wright (1980) have described techniques for measuring spinal movements. There may be a sciatic scoliosis (Fig. 57.7). due to spasm of the paraspinal muscles, which can be appreciated by palpation. This scoliosis is an automatic reflex to protect damaged nerve roots. There may be local tenderness on palpation or percussion which help to indicate the level of the prolapse. Normally the extended lower limb can be elevated to nearly 90° by flexing the hip. This movement can be severely limited by a lower lumbar disc prolapse as the movement pulls on the dura and nerve roots that are already damaged. With the hip flexed just short of producing pain dorsiflexion of the ankle produces similar symptoms. A further variant is Lasègue's test in which the hip and knee are flexed. Knee straightening then produces pain. Sensory loss, motor weakness and reflex changes may be detected in the lower limbs and may indicate the particular nerve root involve (Table 57.5).

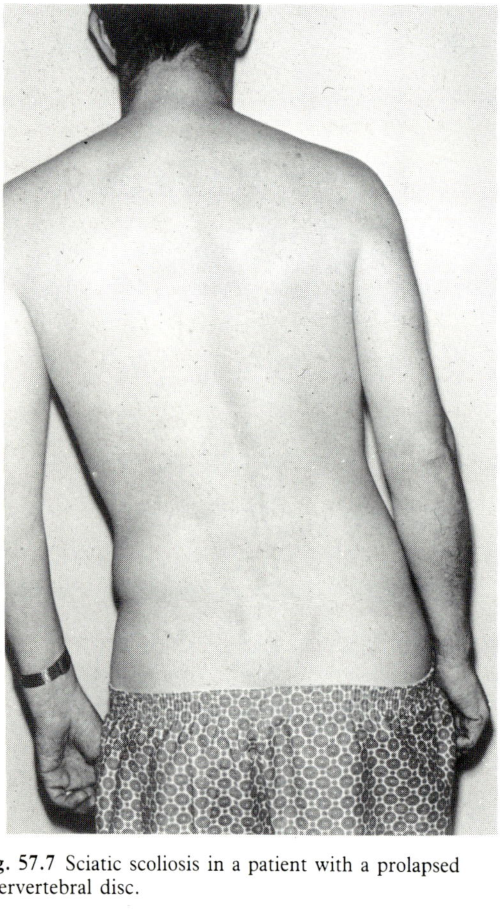

Fig. 57.7 Sciatic scoliosis in a patient with a prolapsed intervertebral disc.

Central posterior prolapse of the lumbar disc is rare and problems most often arise if there is previous narrowing of the spinal canal — spinal stenosis. The prolapse may damage the cauda equina with pain, paraesthesiae and sensory loss in the low back, buttocks, perineum and lower limbs and may interfere with micturition, defaecation, erection and ejaculation. Urinary retention can even occur with an otherwise symptomless prolapse (Love & Emmett, 1967). In some patients with spinal stenosis (see below) the blood supply to the damaged cauda equina is only just adequate. Exercise, such as walking a certain distance, leads to pain and paraesthesiae which are relieved by rest (Blau & Logue, 1961).

Investigations

The blood sedimentation rate and plasma viscosity are normal and no abnormalities are found in other haematological or biochemical tests. At lumbar puncture, the cerebrospinal fluid is usually normal but the protein may be raised if there is a large prolapse with a spinal block. The following radiological procedures may be used in the investigation of patients with a suspected disc prolapse:

1. Conventional radiography. With an acute prolapse there may be no abnormality except perhaps for the scoliosis. Disc narrowing may subsequently develop and later secondary spondylitic changes appear.

2. Myelography. This investigation is only indicated is spinal surgery is contemplated. Iodised oil is introduced into the subarachnoid space and can be removed at the end of the examination. The outline of the subarachnoid space can be seen and diagnosis depends upon finding localised deformities in relation to the disc spaces (Fig.57.8). It is therefore of great value for the diagnosis of a central disc prolapse or of a large eccentric lesion, but it may not identify a posterolateral prolapse if the nerve root is not sufficiently filled with contrast of if the lesion is very lateral. Unfortunately myelography using iodised oil may be followed by ar-

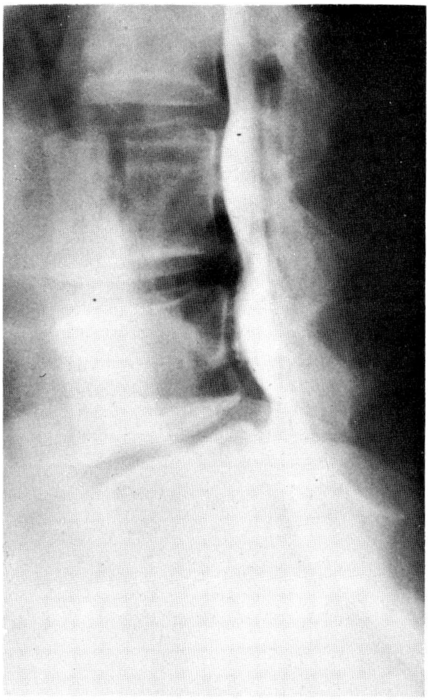

Fig. 57.8 Myelogram lateral view showing marked indentation of the myodil column at L4–5 with lesser indentation at L3–4 and 2–3. This indicates a large prolapse at L4–5 and possible lesser prolapses at the higher levels.

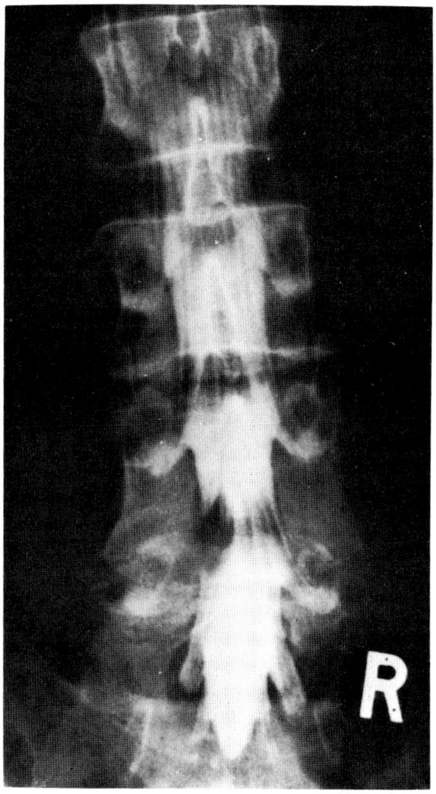

Fig. 57.9 Radiculogram. There is a large protrusion at the L4–5 level which is central and to the left-hand side with distortion and displacement of the L5 root sheath.

achnoiditis (Lilequist, 1974). This technique is now used less often than formerly for the investigation of lumbar nerve root lesions.

3. Radiculography. A water-soluble radio-opaque dye is introduced into the subarachnoid space. The dye penetrates along the nerve root sheath allowing the roots to be seen clearly (Fig. 57.9). As the dye is very irritant to the spinal cord and brain the technique is restricted to examination of the lower lumbar and lumbosacral nerve roots and the patient is kept upright during introduction of the dye, throughout the examination and for about 6 hours afterwards. This technique has largely replaced myelography in investigating lumbar disc disorders.

4. Epidural myelography. Water-soluble contrast medium is injected into the extradural space through the sacral hiatus. As a disc protrusion will impinge upon the extradural space before the dural sac itself, it should allow improved diagnosis of minor lesions. Indeed, Mathews & Yates (1969) thought the technique sufficiently accurate to demonstrate the reduction of size of lumbar disc prolapse following treatment. However, the contrast medium may flow poorly through the epidural space, producing difficulties in interpretation.

5 Vertebral venography. The ascending lumbar vein is catheterised via the femoral vein under local anaesthetic. Injection of water-soluble contrast medium allows examination of the vertebral venous system and disc protrusion may be recognised as obstructed veins (Mace, 1976).

6. Discography. This technique was first described by Lindblom (1948) and involves direct injection of low-toxicity water-soluble dye directly into the intervertebral disc under fluoroscopic control. Interpretation depends upon:

a. Injection, volume and pressure. The normal disc will only accept about 0.5 ml of contrast medium and will resist further injection. Much larger volumes can be injected easily into degenerate discs.

b. Pain production.

Injection into the diseased disc may reproduce the patient's symptoms. This can help identify the disc which is at fault.

c. Local anaesthetic and steroid. Injection into a disc responsible for a patient's symptoms should relieve the pain sometimes for several weeks. Again this relief would indicate the source of the problem.

d. Appearance. The normal nucleus is round or oval and may be uni- or bilocular. Disorganisation of disc structure and prolapse can be readily seen (Fig. 57.10).

7. Computerised axial tomography. CAT scanning can demonstrate prolapse of a disc into the vertebral canal when combined with radiculography and, with the latest generation of machines, without the need for contrast medium (Williams et al, 1980). This non-invasive method for detecting prolapse may well become the most effective investigation technique in the future.

8. Nuclear magnetic resonance. NMR appears to offer enormous potential advantages for imaging the spine. Its use for examining changes in hydration and chemical composition of the disc has yet to be exploited.

Lumbar spondylosis and apophyseal osteoarthrosis

Although spondylosis strictly refers to degeneration of the intervertebral disc and the latter term to the disease of the apophyseal joints, the two usually coexist and are considered together as degenerative spondylosis. Schmorl & Junghanns (1971) found these changes in 80% of male and 60% of female spines at 50 years and in virtually all subjects by 70 years. Despite well-marked spondylosis, many subjects deny major back symptoms so that when present their clinical significance may be in doubt. Lawrence (1977) found only a 12% difference in the frequency of back problems between those with the least and those with the grossest radiographic changes. Torgeson & Dotter (1976) were able to find some relation between back pain and radiographic evidence of disc space narrowing but not with the development of osteophytes.

The pathological appearances include disorganisation of the internal structure of the disc with loss of the clear distinction between the nucleus pulposus and the annulus fibrosus. The disc becomes narrowed and, if several are involved, the spine may become shorter (Fig. 57.11). Osteophytes develop around the vertebral rims (Fig. 57.12) and when gross they can meet and even fuse. Osteoarthritic changes in the apophyseal joints are similar to those in osteoarthrosis of any other synovial joint (see Ch. 33). There is erosion of cartilage, sclerosis of the articular bone and production of osteophytes which

a 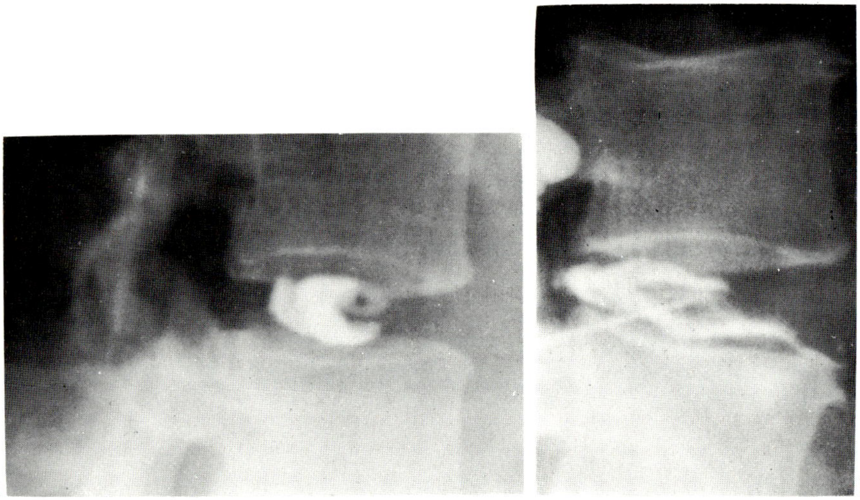 b

Fig. 57.10 Discograms. (a) Normal showing a central nucleus. (b) A degenerate disc with posterior prolapse of the nucleus substance.

If the LSR is 0.2 or more then the job should be altered in order to make it easier.

Posture and manual handling techniques

The risk of back problems can be minimised by careful attention to posture. Appropriate advice should be given not only to back sufferers but also to all those involved in occupations for which there is a risk of back problems. For those required to stand for most of the day it is important to be able to move about, to work with the head up and not in a slouched position, to work at a bench at the appropriate height, and for women to avoid wearing high heels. Lifting heavy objects requires the kinetic handling technique in which the subject crouches down with the knees apart and the object between the feet and close to the body. Heavy objects should always be carried close to the body in a comfortable position and never lifted above shoulder height. Torsion of the spine combined with heavy load carrying appears particularly hazardous and should be avoided. A careful choice of chairs with appropriate lumbar support and the design of tables and desks to suit the individual all help to minimise back problems. Mantle et al (1981) have demonstrated the benefit of a back care programme in preventing back pain in pregnant patients.

Pre-employment screening

Many industries undertake medical examinations prior to employing workers in order to minimise the risk of health problems. In general pre-employment screening has not been of great value in this field as physical characteristics and radiological changes correlate poorly with the development of back pain. However, Kosiak et al (1968) excluded workers if any radiological changes was found in the spine, with a significant fall in incidence of back problems; but this was at a cost of rejecting over a quarter of all job applicants. Such a screening programme involves considerable X-radiation and many who would never develop back pain would be excluded from employment. Ultrasonic measurements of vertebral canal diameters may provide some indication of those at risk (Macdonald et al, 1984). At the present time, however, the only reliable guide seems to be that subjects who have suffered severe back pain in the past are likely to develop further problems in the future.

Early treatment

Many larger factories have physiotherapy departments available for treating their workforce. There is a very high remission rate in workers treated in this way but it is not clear whether this is a specific benefit of early treatment or due to many trivial problems resolving spontaneously. Bergquist-Ullmann & Larsson (1977) found that a programme of advice on back care in a factory environment produced at least as good if not better results than more formal physiotherapy treatment.

COCCYGEAL PAIN

Occasionally coccygeal pains arise from congential deformities, injuries and fractures, infections, neoplasms and arthritis of the sacrococcygeal joint. However, such symptoms are usually of unknown cause and therefore should be called 'non-specific coccygeal pain' or 'coccydynia'. In many instances this syndrome is associated with chronic anxiety states.

Treatment is often unsatisfactory but involves cushioning to prevent pressure on the coccyx while sitting, local heat applied by shortwave diathermy, injection of local anaesthetic with or without steroids and, extremely rarely, surgical excision of the coccyx.

DORSAL PAIN

Pain in the thoracic region is less common than in the low back and neck. It is important to exclude inflammatory, neoplastic, metabolic and referred causes. Prolapse of a thoracic intervertebral disc is extremely rare. Many patients show evidence of degenerative changes and these are often secondary to Scheuermann's osteochondritis. Sometimes the symptoms are of uncertain aetiology and should therefore be termed 'non-specific dorsal pain'.

Scheuermann's osteochondritis

This is a condition of unknown cause in which there is irregular ossification of the vertebral epiphyseal end-plates principally in the lower dorsal but also in the upper lumbar spine (Butler, 1955). The condition is analogous to osteochondritis elsewhere and may represent a form of avascular necrosis. It predominantly affects adolescent males who develop a smooth dorsal kyphosis with round shoulders and a flat chest. There may be aching pain which becomes more marked in later years with the development of secondary degenerative spondylosis.

The radiological appearances are characteristic. There is fragmentation of the epiphyseal plate with increased density and irregularity of the vertebral surfaces. The disc spaces become narrowed and the vertebrae become wedged, being narrower anteriorly (Fig. 57.26). There may be multiple herniations of the nuclei into the vertebral bodies (Schmorl's nodes) due to weakness of the vertebral end-plates.

Treatment is unsatisfactory but involves physiotherapy exercises predominantly aimed at preservation of posture.

Diffuse idiopathic skeletal hyperostosis (DISH)

Forestier & Rotes-Querol (1950) drew attention to a syndrome of exuberant new bone formation occurring around the spine and principally affecting the dorsal and dorsolumbar regions. It leads to stiffening of the spine but many patients are symptom-free. Bony spurs are found at multiple levels and often fuse to form bridges (Fig. 57.27) and are more marked on the right-hand side of the spine than the left. The appearances are quite different from those of ankylosing spondylitis and there is no association with HLA-B27. In contrast with spondylosis, the disc spaces may remain intact (Vernon-Roberts et al, 1974). The earliest changes occur in the 'waist' of the vertebral body away from the intervertebral disc and new bone is formed along the insertion of fibrous tissue into the anterior cortical surface. It progresses along the fibres at an angle to the cortical surface and distinct from it until the condition is advanced (Fornasier et al, 1983).

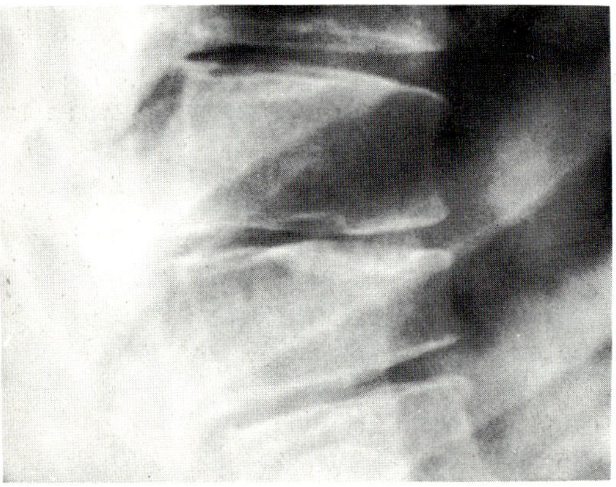

Fig. 57.26 Scheuermann's osteochondritis of the dorsal spine. Note the anterior wedging of the vertebral body and irregularity of the vertebral end-plates.

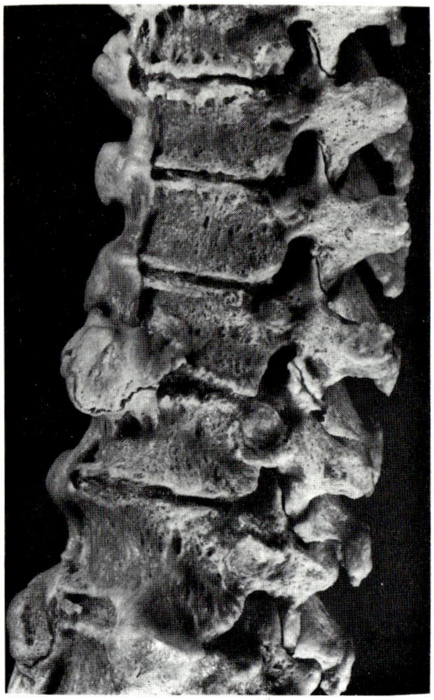

Fig. 57.27 Anklyosing hyperostosis. Left side of the macerated dorsal spine. The bone added on the right side of each vertebral body has a distinct left margin with, in places, an underlying space where it has extended over the anterior longitudinal ligament. Note also the addition of bone around the articular margins of the apophyseal and costovertebral joints. (By courtesy of Dr B. Vernon-Roberts and the Editor of the *Annals of Rheumatic Diseases.*)

This condition may form part of a generalised disease process as similar subperiosteal new bone formation may occur around the pelvis (Harris et al, 1974) and elsewhere.

The aetiology of this condition is unknown, but it may have a hormonal or metabolic basis (Dwosh, 1983). There seems to be an association with impaired glucose tolerance, frank diabetes and obesity (Julkunen et al, 1971); see also Chs 34 and 39.

OTHER CAUSES OF BACK PAIN

Inflammatory

Seronegative spondylopathies

Ankylosing spondylitis and the related inflammatory seronegative spondylopathies are described in Section VI. Advanced ankylosing spondylitis with a dorsal kyphosis, loss of lumbar lordosis and loss of spinal movement in all directions, is easily recognised. However, mild ankylosing spondylitis with back pain in the absence of deformity and radiological changes is not an uncommon cause of back pain and may affect 1–1.5% of the population (Calin & Fries, 1975). Helpful points in recognising ankylosing spondylitis include a young age of onset, insidious development of back pain, the persistence of back pain for over 3 months, the aggravation of back pain by rest and relief by exercise. Tissue typing will show the subjects to be of type HLA-B27 but the absence of this tissue type is more helpful in excluding this diagnosis than is its presence for making it — many HLA-B27-positive individuals do not develop this disorder.

Rheumatoid arthritis

The clinical features and pathology of rheumatoid involvement of the spine are described in Section V. The disease most often involves the neck but rarely the lumbar spine. In advanced cases destructive changes with the development of a scoliosis may be found. The presence of back pain in association with typical clinical and laboratory features of rheumatoid arthritis should prompt a detailed examination of the spine.

Polymyalgia rheumatica

This condition is common in the elderly and often presents with pain and stiffness in the shoulder and limb girdles and with aching in the cervical and lumbar regions (Ch. 51). It is often confused with cervical and lumbar spondylosis particularly as appropriate radiological changes are usually found in this age-group. Useful points in the differential diagnosis are that in polymyalgia the symptoms are aggravated by rest and relieved by exercise, the blood sedimentation rate is high and there is a dramatic therapeutic response to oral corticosteroids.

Infection

Infection of the spine may follow surgery to the spine or elsewhere, and particularly urological procedures (Garcia & Grantham, 1960). There is an association with diabetes and cutaneous sepsis. It can produce osteomyelitis of the vertebral body, infection of the disc or an epidural abcess. The most common organism is *Staphyloccus aureus*, but *E. coli*, *Proteus* and *Pseudomonas pyocyanea* may be found. In this country infections of the spine due to brucellosis and typhoid are rare, but spinal tuberculosis is still occasionally seen, particularly among immigrant communities.

The presenting features vary widely. At one extreme there is constant pain, limited movements and spasm of the paraspinal muscles around the affected area and the patient becomes ill with pyexia and a raised sedimentation rate. At the other, chronic backache develops insidiously with minimal systemic signs (Griffiths & Jones, 1971).

It is important to identify the causative organism to allow appropriate chemotherapy, and culture of the blood and material obtained by needle aspiration or open biopsy may be needed.

Tuberculous infection of the vertebrae, described by Percival Pott in 1779, starts predominantly in the anterior metaphyseal regions of the vertebra with bone destruction. Caseating abscesses may spread to the spinal canal with meningeal irritation and cord or nerve root compression, and may present in the neck, the posterior mediastinum or as an iliopsoas abscess. Both tuberculosis and brucellosis may involve one or other sacroiliac joint. Radiographs show destruction of bone perhaps with new bone formation in the healing stage. In contrast with metastases, the infection can spread into and destroy the intervertebral disc, and involve the adjacent vertebra.

When herpes zoster affects the cervical or lumbar nerve roots the prodromal symptoms can be confused with other causes of spine and root pain. After a few days the characteristic cutaneous vesicles appear and give the correct diagnosis.

Neoplasms

Tumours involving the spine are extremely important causes of back pain. Most frequent are malignant metastases. Osteolytic lesions most often arise from carcinomas of the breast, bronchus, kidney, thyroid, prostate and other organs; osteosclerotic metastases (Fig. 57.28) usually arise from the prostate. Reticuloses and leukaemia may produce deposits in the spine. Multiple myeloma can present as a solitary plasmacytoma or as multiple lytic lesions of bone. Primary growths are rare but include benign tumours such as haemangioma of the vertebral body which appears as vertical striations on X-ray, meningioma and neurofibroma and malignant tumours such as osteosarcoma, chordoma and others.

In malignancy the patient may show general features of ill-health with loss of weight, pyrexia and a raised blood sedimentation rate. However, these changes do not always occur and sometimes the patient appears well. This stresses the need for a complete general examination in all patients with back pain including, when indicated, a rectal examination. Back pain develops insidiously. It is persistent and slowly increases, perhaps with an acute exacerbation if a fracture occurs. When the neoplasm involves the nerve roots or the spinal cord, neurological changes appear. They progress steadily but, especially if haemorrhage occurs into the tumour, they can advance dramatically.

Treatment of malignant tumours may involve surgery or radiotherapy. Hall & MacKay (1973) obtained worthwhile improvement in 35% of patients following laminectomy and decompression for incomplete paraplegia.

Paget's disease

The bones of the spine can be involved by Paget's disease and recognised on X-ray as sclerosis of the bone with thickening and coarsening of the trabecular pattern (Fig. 57.29.) Sometimes there are no symptoms and these changes are discovered by chance radiological findings. Paget's disease can nevertheless produce severe persistent pain or, by encroachment into the vertebral canal, the clinical pattern of spinal stenosis. Rarely malignant transformation takes place.

Metabolic bone disease

The spine may be involved by a variety of disorders of bone metabolism. These include osteoporosis, osteomalacia and hyperparathyroidism (Ch. 40), chondrocalcinosis (Ch. 37) and och-

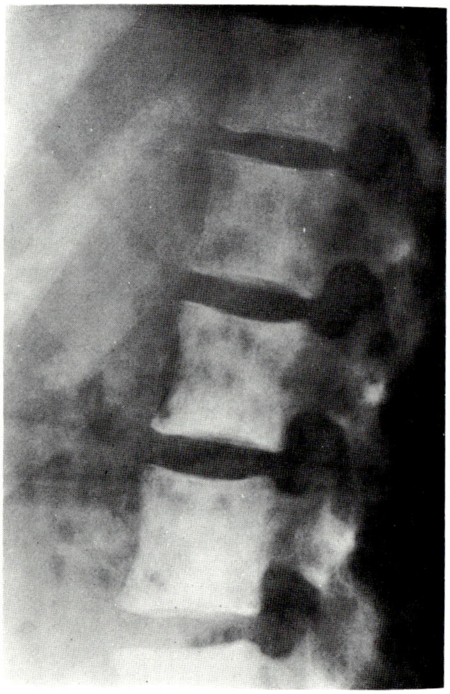

Fig. 57.28 Osteosclerotic metastases in the lumbar spine from carcinoma of the prostate.

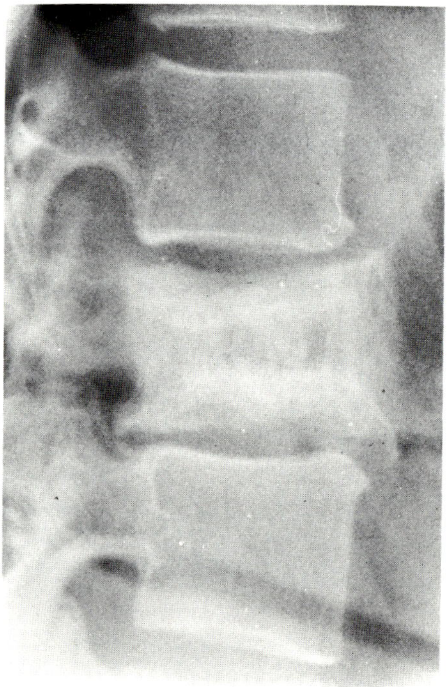

Fig. 57.29 Paget's disease of the 3rd lumbar vertebra.

mentioned, the commonest root to be affected is the 7th cervical which produces moderate weakness of triceps, sometimes weakness of the extensors and flexors of the wrists and fingers, depression of the triceps reflex and sensory impairment mainly over the index finger. It is much less common to see involvement of C6 or C8.

The signs that may be elicited in less common syndromes will be outlined as they are discussed. Standard anteroposterior and lateral X-ray films of the neck and the sedimentation rate (ESR) are useful screening tests for the exclusion of serious underlying disease.

Table 58.2 outlines a scheme for the discussion of the diagnosis and treatment of the commoner conditions affecting this area.

Table 58.2 Sites of origin of neck pain.

1. Synovial joints
   Apophyseal
   Atlanto axial
2. Intervertebral discs
3. Nerve roots, spinal cord
4. Vertebral bodies
   Developmental
   Anomalies
5. Muscles, ligaments
6. Arteries
   Vertebral
   Cranial
   Polymyalgic
7. Deep lymphatic glands:
   retropharyngeal space
8. Thoracic viscera

Synovial joints

Several forms of inflammatory arthritis show a predilection for involvement of the facet joints of the cervical spine. These include: rheumatoid disease, psoriatic arthritis, ankylosing spondylitis, Reiter's disease and colitic arthritis. Usually evidence of the disease will be manifest elsewhere by the time symptoms in the neck arise, but rarely rheumatoid disease can first present as pain and stiffness in the neck. Examination reveals symmetrical restriction of head movement, particularly of lateral flexion.

The drug treatment of inflammatory spondylitis should follow the regimen for the underlying disease. Partial rest and support of the neck can be provided by a felt or plastic collar, but prolonged immobilisation should be avoided, particularly in ankylosing spondylitis, since permanent restriction of movement may result.

Some patients with progressive rheumatoid spondylitis may develop excessive mobility at the joint between the odontoid peg of the axis and the anterior arch of the atlas. When the neck is flexed the odontoid peg subluxes backwards towards the spinal cord. In a survey of outpatients with rheumatoid arthritis significant atlantoaxial subluxation was found in 25% of 76 patients (Mathews, 1969), but only 5 showed evidence of minor spinal cord lesions. Treatment by cervical brace or spinal fusion is unnecessary unless there are symptoms or signs of progressive cord damage. Particular care must be exercised when these patients are anaesthetised, indeed it is a sound policy for all rheumatoid patients undergoing surgery to leave the Ward wearing a collar as a reminder to all staff. They are well advised to wear a collar when driving, against the risk of a whip-lash injury. Similarly, the patients should either be exempted from the compulsory wearing of seat-belts, or use a high supporting neck rest.

Due to erosion of the lateral masses of the atlas, vertical (Swinson et al, 1972) or lateral subluxation can occur. Subaxial luxation can occur particularly at the levels of C4, 5, 6. As with cervical spondylosis at this level, vascular involvement is particularly likely to occur, leading to ischaemic myelopathy.

Cervical spondylosis

The cervical apophyseal joints, particularly the lower ones, are a common site for degenerative spondylosis. Along with changes in the facet joints, degenerative changes in the discs give rise to narrowing and osteophytic outgrowths. In the majority of the elderly no symptoms, other than the restriction of range, are noticed. Some patients experience persistent aching in the neck and shoulders, though the signs and radiographs are not qualitatively different from those of symptomless patients. Sensitivity to pain and nervous tension seem to be factors producing symptoms. Forcible treatments are best avoided, but many patients obtain great relief from gentle stretching mobilisation by a physiotherapist, aimed at restoring movement. The restrictive effects of a collar are unlikely to be beneficial and more likely to lead to increased stiffness and discomfort.

The anterior part of the spinal cord receives most of its blood supply through the anterior spinal artery augmented at intervals by segmental feeders: at cord level C4–5 there tends to be a relative watershed. Arteriosclerotic obstruction and osteophytic outgrowths associated with relative narrowing of the cervical canal can all contribute to an ischaemic myelopathy (Wilkinson, 1971). Most often this affects the C5 spinal segment producing a well recognised syndrome. There is weakness of shoulder abduction (deltoid) and external rotation (infraspinatus) associated with suppression of the supinator reflex (C5 lower motor neurone lesion) and a brisk finger jerk (C7, 8 upper motor neurone lesion). The lower limbs are spastic with extensor plantar responses. The condition often remains relatively static for many years. Evidence of vascular impairment precludes active mechanical treatment. If there is evident deterioration, myelography may indicate mechanical block, in which case decompressive laminectomy may help. If no block is evident anterior tethering may be the cause, in which case best relief may be obtained by anterior decompression and fusion (Magnaes & Hauge, 1980).

Intervertebral discs

Opinion is still divided on the basic cause of acute cervical torticollis. There is circumstantial evidence that in adults a fragment of the annulus impinges against the sensitive dura mater or the nerve root sheath, producing asymmetrical restriction of cervical movements, deformity and secondary muscle spasm. Rest in a makeshift collar is a safe first aid measure for severe pain. Lying prone or supine with the head dependent is a simple domestic way of applying traction. The physiotherapists may produce dramatic relief of pain and restoration of movement by gentle traction or mobilisation of the neck (Cyriax, 1978). However, these neck lesions are usually self-limiting, and if there is any clinical doubt that complications may exist it is preferable to await spontaneous resolution.

Nerve roots and spinal cord

Some cases of cervical torticollis are accompanied by pain radiating down the limb, either from the outset or after a phase of pain confined to the neck. This pain may become very severe and be continuous at rest. Often in such cases nerve root interruption occurs shown by the appearance of uniradicular neurological signs, commonly C7 root, and the spontaneous resolution of pain. A firm collar and strong analgesics will afford some relief when the pain is at its height. Occasionally cervical traction performed either reclining or sitting, may help intractable pain. A multicentre trial (British Association of Physical Medicine, 1966) showed that the majority of patients lost their symptoms within 3 months whatever treatment was given. Minor weakness recovers spontaneously in 3–6 months, but sensory symptoms may persist, analagous to cases with root lesions in the leg (Yates, 1964). It follows that prolonged administration of placebo treatment, such as electrotherapy, on such patients is a waste of time and resources. Only rarely does lateral root entrapment give rise to chronic persistent pain. Electrodiagnosis (EMG) can be most helpful in giving objective evidence of root compromise, either in the presence of denervation potentials (fibrillation) within the distribution of a single nerve root, or a difference in the cortical evoked responses compared with the normal side. Foraminal decompression, with or without intervertebral fusion, is only very occasionally justified.

Compression of the 1st thoracic root at the thoracic outlet and of the median nerve in the carpal tunnel may produce aching in the arm associated with paraesthesiae in the hand. Typically the paraesthesiae are worse at night and are not exacerbated by neck movements. However, either of these conditions may occur in association with cervical spondylosis, and it may be impossible to determine clinically which is the predominant factor. Electrodiagnosis can be of great help, particularly in detecting carpal tunnel compression.

The thoracic outlet syndrome results from pressure upon the emerging neurovascular bundle in that situation. Contributory factors include the presence of a cervical rib or other bony abnormality, a fascial band behind the scalenus anterior muscle, trauma and vascular disease. Ischaemic features due to intermittent compression of the subclavian artery (coldness and discolouration of the hand) are present in addition to neurological symptoms (pain and paraesthesiae, usually in the C8T1 area of distribution). In addition to electrodiagnosis, arteriography and venography may be necessary to establish this sometimes difficult diagnosis (Urschell & Razzuck, 1972).

If the weakness in the arm is severe or progressive and extends beyond the territory of one nerve root it is unlikely to be due to a simple disc protrusion. Multiradicular involvement can be confirmed by EMG and causes, such as malignant infiltration of the brachial plexus or spinal tumour, should be sought. Significant spinal cord compression may present with spastic weakness of the legs and paraesthesiae in the limbs. The important signs are sustained knee of ankle clonus and extensor plantar responses, and these preclude any attempts at mechanical treatment. A neurological opinion, myelography or CT scan should be arranged urgently (Fig. 58.2).

Vertebrae

Developmental abnormalities

Several varieties of vertebral dysostosis may affect the cervical spine (Beighton, 1978), some of them being genetically determined. In the Klippel–Feil anomaly congenital fusion of cervical vertebrae may coexist with a low hairline, webbing of the neck and scapular elevation.

Unilateral underdevelopment of one side of a cervical vertebra, hemivertebra, is normally painless until later life when secondary degenerative changes arise from unequal wear. Associated with this anomaly one shoulder may be fixed higher than the other ('Sprengel's shoulder'). There may be a diffuse congenital stenosis of the spinal canal, particularly in association with a chondrodysplasia such as achondroplasia. Spondylotic encroachment can give rise to cervical cord and cauda equina compression. In cases where both lumbar and cervical stenoses coexist, personal experience in several cases has shown that cervical decompression

a

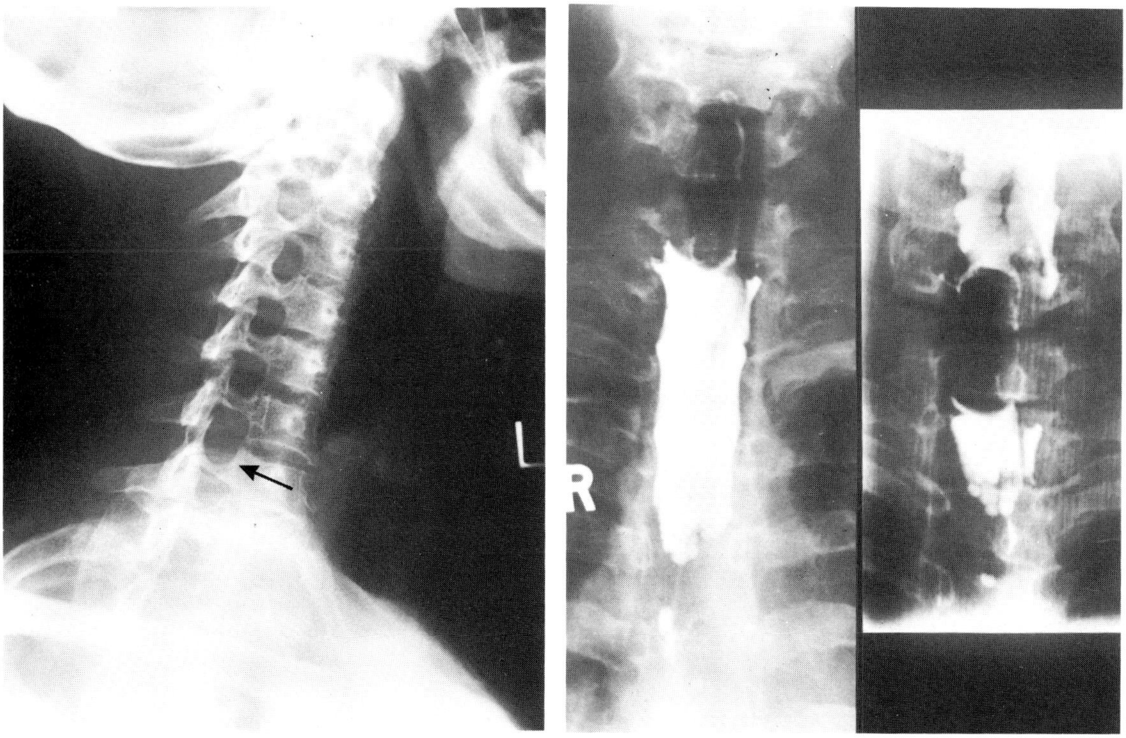

b

Fig. 58.2 Neurofibroma (a) Oblique X-rays. The C6–7 foramen is enlarged by 'dumb-bell' tumour pressure. (b) Myelogram shows an almost complete block. Full recovery occurred after excision.

should be performed first as this may give rise to sufficient clinical improvement without further action. If not, then lumbar decompression should follow.

Vertebral disease

Neoplastic deposits or sepsis in bone give rise to a constant pain, which often persists at rest. The neck is usually held completely rigid and a period of rest and support in a collar produces no amelioration, such as is seen with mechanical torticollis. X-ray films may show localised osteolysis or collapse, the earliest detectable change being asymmetrical disappearance of pedicles. However, a complete reliance should not be placed on a negative report since X-ray changes may not be evident for several months after the onset of symptoms. The ESR will usually be elevated so that in practice either this or the radiograph will be abnormal. These are essential screening investigations in such cases.

Muscles and ligaments

Chronic neck pain without the localising signs of organic disease already described is extremely common. Patients who are depressed or emotionally disturbed seem to complain disproportionately of neck pain. Poor 'hang-dog' cervical posture, with secondary stretching of cervical muscles and ligaments, may be a factor. Strong reassurance after careful examination, coupled with postural instruction, helps. It is preferable to avoid the use of medicaments if possible, but intermittent use of a mild sedative or antidepressant benefits some patients.

Persistent neck pain after injury, particularly traffic collisions producing a 'whip-lash' effect, is common. Once again the symptoms are usually quite disproportionate to the signs, and it is hard to avoid the conclusion that emotional instability and compensation wrangles are major factors. X-ray films of the cervical spine, with a lateral view in full flexion and extension should always be taken. Having thus excluded traumatic subluxation, it is possible that partial tears of the interspinous ligaments may be responsible. On this supposition the injection of hydrocortisone and local anaesthetic sometimes produces relief. After prolonged medicolegal wrangling patients tend to lose confidence, and if a collar has been recommended they feel dependent on it and unsteady without it. Rehabilitation to normal life and employment requires a firm positive approach. The patient must be strongly reassured that there is no real instability or danger while being weaned from the collar. Gentle manual mobilisation, augmented by postural exercises helps to restore normal function.

Arteries

The vertebral arteries run up the cervical spine in foramina just anterior to the facet joints and then join to form the basilar artery, which is the main arterial supply to the hind brain. In elderly patients one vertebral artery, or both, may be largely occluded by atheromatous changes. If an osteophyte from a degenerative facet joint further obstructs the flow, transient ischaemia of the hind brain may occur on neck movements. This may be manifested by drop attacks, transient paraesthesiae, positional vertigo, or visual disturbances. Such symptoms are an absolute contraindication to any mobilising treatment of the neck and immobilisation in a collar or brace should be advised.

Polymyalgia rheumatica

As indicated in Chapter 51, polymyalgia is a syndrome reflecting several underlying diseases, including arteritis of the aged, temporal arteritis, neoplasia and infection. The pains in the neck and periscapular muscles are often associated with a central arthritis producing moderate restriction of movement in the cervical spine, shoulders and hips. Response to modest steroid therapy is usually dramatic, but some milder cases run a benign self-limiting course and can be relieved by non-steroid anti-inflammatory drugs, but careful supervision is advisable.

Temporal arteritis

The temporal and occipital arteries may be involved in temporal arteritis causing severe head pain and occasionally a torticollis. Usually the patient is elderly and may notice severe malaise, fever and night sweats. The temporal arteries are thickened and the pulses impaired. The ESR is usually markedly raised (more than 50 mm/h). An arterial biopsy confirms the diagnosis. Since the arterial supply to the retina may be obstructed at any time, producing permanent blindness, there should be no delay in starting vigorous corticosteroid therapy which may need to be continued for a considerable time.

Cervical glands

Infection in the deep cervical glands in the retropharyngeal space may cause a painful torticollis, particularly in children. Though an acute disc lesion can rarely produce dysphagia, in adults this symptom may indicate an inflammatory process. On the lateral X-ray film of the cervical spine the thin soft-tissue shadow behind the pharyngeal air space may be thickened and distorted by retropharyngeal sepsis (Fig. 58.3). Through the mouth distortion of the posterior pharyngeal wall may be apparent. The responsible organism is often *Mycobacterium tuberculosis* but occasionally *Streptococcus* is responsible. Following identification of the responsible organism by aspiration or open drainage, the appropriate antibiotic produces resolution.

Thoracic viscera

Apical lung disease can present with a painful torticollis, particularly pneumonia in children. Cardiac or mediastinal pain can be referred into the jaw and neck but a careful history and examination will show that the cervical spine is not the source.

SHOULDER

The shoulder joint mechanism is unique because of its great mobility. This is derived from four separate mechanisms:

1. The glenohumeral joint which provides 90° abduction (half the range of elevation) and approximately 180° of internal and external rotation
2. The sternoclavicular and
3. The acromioclavicular joints allow the clavicle to act as a mobile stabilising strut during the remaining 90° of full elevation
4. The scapula rotates against the chest wall, stabilised by various muscles including trapezius, rhomboids, levator scapulae and serratus anterior.

Such a mechanism is complex and a number of painful structures lie in close proximity. The di-

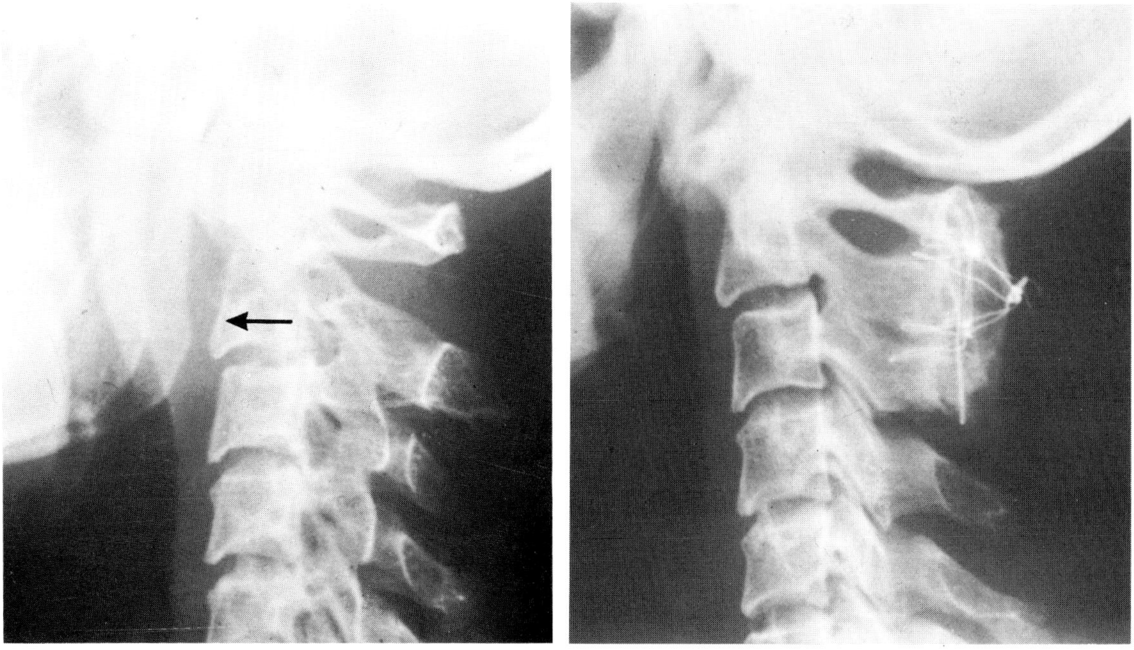

a b

Fig. 58.3 Tuberculous caries of odontoid. (a) Retropharyngeal swelling indicated by arrow. (b) Swelling resolved after antituberculous therapy and fusion. (Courtesy of Dr J.A. Mathews.)

agnosis of shoulder pain is therefore dependent on a systemic examination based on a sound knowledge of applied anatomy.

Terminology

Exchange of ideas and comparison of research data are often impossible owing to confusion over terminology. No perfect system exists but the following terms can be defined:

1. 'Arthritis', 'capsulitis' and 'synovitis' are synonymous and indicate an inflammatory lesion of the glenohumeral synovial joint lining within the capsule.
2. Rotator cuff lesions are outside the capsule — extracapsular — and where possible the structure involved should be specified, e.g. supraspinatus, infraspinatus, subscapularis tendinitis or subacromial bursitis. There is no agreement on the meaning of the term 'pericapsulitis' and it is better avoided.

History

Careful history-taking can give useful clues as to the nature of the lesion. A spontaneous onset characterises chronic subdeltoid bursitis. Minor trauma, such as lifting or athletic overuse, often produces a supraspinatus tendinitis. Significant injury is required to produce a post-traumatic arthritis.

Tendon lesions cause pain on certain movements, whereas an early frozen shoulder and bursitis are characterised by continuous pain at rest. Knowledge of the patient's occupation and passtimes are essential and these may need to be modified to obtain relief.

Examination

On inspection the outline of the shoulder can provide useful clues. The normal rounding of the shoulder is disturbed by swelling in chronic bursitis or an inflammatory arthritis. A step is visible following traumatic subluxation of the acromioclavicular joint. Dislocation produces a sharp angulation, while a lesion of the circumflex nerve produces marked wasting of the deltoid.

Diffuse muscle wasting appears rapidly with sepsis and malignant deposits but more slowly as a rheumatoid shoulder undergoes ankylosis. Marked wasting is not usually seen with a frozen shoulder because some joint movement is preserved.Associated with the shoulder–hand syndrome there may be marked puffiness and stiffness of the hand.

The patient is asked to elevate the arm noting whether it is (1) full and painless; (2) full with the presence of a painful arc; (3) restricted. The same observations are then made when the arm is elevated passively. Finally the range of glenohumeral movement is tested with the scapula firmly fixed, gripped by one hand.

From these observations it can be deduced whether:

1. Full elevation is prevented by muscular weakness or accompained by pain as in an extracapsular lesion
2. Glenohumeral movement is restricted, indicating an intracapsular lesion or arthritis.

Extracapsular lesions

Full painless elevation is possible. If a painful arc is present this indicates inflammation of either the subacromial bursa or the supraspinatus or infraspinatus tendon, or the acromioclavicular joint, as these structures are either moved or squeezed during elevation.

Subacromial bursa. Chronic bursitis is characterised by the gradual onset of persistent pain most often referred to the deltoid insertion. There may have been trauma, particularly from a repetitive rotatory action such as in decorating. Occasionally psoriatic arthritis or gout may first present in this fashion. Characteristically the pain persists at rest for many months or years leading to many sleepless nights. There is a painful arc on passive elevation and particularly pain on passive rotation of the abducted humerus. Resisted isometric contractions are all moderately uncomfortable.

Acute calcific bursitis is rare and produces severe pain from the outset. The bursa may be swollen and hot, so that sepsis is suspected, and there may be a mild pyrexia and leucocytosis. No passive or active movements can be tolerated. Aspiration is often fruitless but should be attempted in case pus can be reported to contain calcium apatite microcrystals (McCarty & Gatter,

1966). X-rays sometimes show a fluffy calcific deposit within the bursa which subsequently disappears (Fig. 58.4), and it has been postulated that this is a form of pseudogout (Pinals & Short, 1960).

Both acute and chronic bursitis can often be relieved by subacromial injection of an insoluble steroid mixed with a dilute anaesthetic for comfort. Subsequent gout-like exacerbation can be suppressed by indomethacin or colchicine. Rest in a sling for a few days may help.

Tendinitis. The common lesions involve the supraspinatus and infraspinatus tendons which blend into the capsule of the glenohumeral joint and are inserted into the greater tuberosity. Both give rise to a painful arc on passive elevation. When the muscles are tested in static contraction a supraspinatus lesion causes sharp discomfort on resisted abduction and an infraspinatus lesion on resisted external rotation. Steroid injections either into the relevant tenoperiosteal junction (Cyriax, 1978) or subacromial space (Richardson, 1975) may have a beneficial effect. In older patients degenerative changes are widespread and small tears of the capsule are common so that the joint frequently connects with the subacromial bursa. The history and clinical picture is less clear-cut but a subacromial steroid injection (Steinbrocker, 1972) is often effective. Ligamentous calcification is of little diagnostic value, being sometimes present on the painless side.

Particularly in the elderly, trauma may lead to extensive rupture of the musculotendinous cuff. Passive movements are relatively painless but voluntary abduction and external rotation are grossly weakened. An arthrogram reveals an extensive tear and electrodiagnosis excludes a lower motor neurone lesion such as in neuralgic amyotrophy (see below).

In younger patients the capsule can be resutured but the shoulder must be kept in an abduction plaster for several months. This procedure is not justified in older patients who will certainly end up with a stiff shoulder which is of less use than a weak one.

Acromioclavicular joint. Subluxation of the joint by falling on to the point of the shoulder is common. Degenerative arthrosis can also be complicated by persistent pain. By careful palpation the joint can be easily and effectively injected.

a

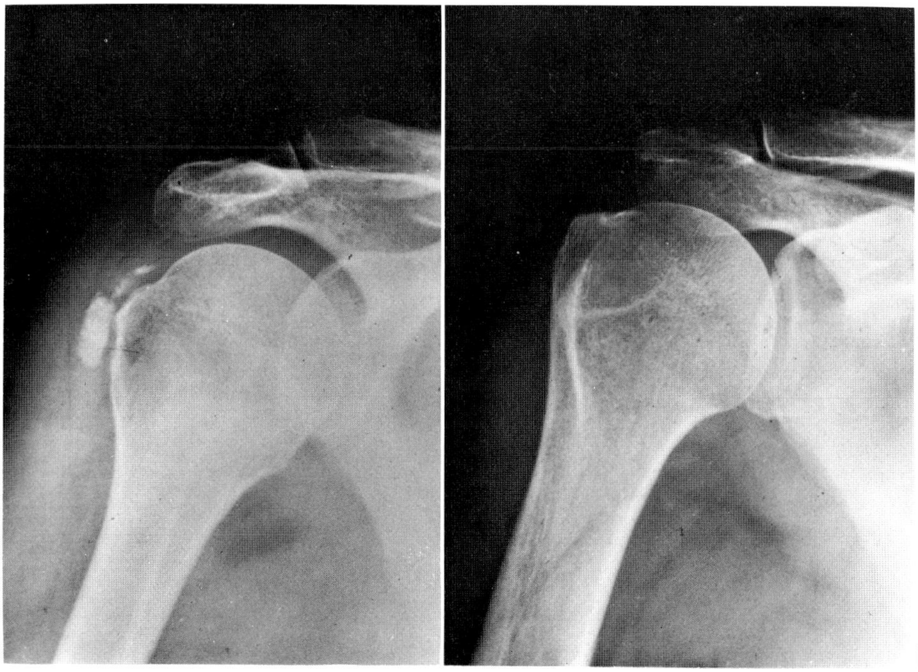

b

Fig. 58.4 Acute calcific bursitis. (a) Fluffy deposit within bursa. (b) Disappearance after 1 month.

Intracapsular lesions

Arthritis of the shoulder may be an isolated lesion (monoarthritis) or part of a generalised arthropathy. Whatever the underlying cause the pattern of joint restriction is similar: when tested, with the humerus by the side, external rotation is more restricted than abduction and internal rotation. Mild bilateral involvement as seen in polymyalgia rheumatica may be missed unless the range of external rotation is carefully tested.

Trauma. Increasing pain and stiffness follow an injury. Intra-articular steroid will often diminish the pain. There is a tendency for the stiffness to lessen slowly with normal use, but sometimes it persists, presumably owing to dense adhesions. If there is still significant deficiency of glenohumeral range 12 months from the injury, manipulation under anaesthetic is justified. The tearing sound produced is due to rupture of the capsule and adhesions which will quickly reconstrict unless the procedure is covered by an intra-articular steroid injection. It is best to admit the patient so that the shoulder can be stretched several times a day for 3 days, and intravenous analgesia can be given for each session. If this elaborate regime is followed excellent results are achieved.

Inflammatory arthritis. The shoulder is commonly affected in rheumatoid arthritis and occasionally in psoriasis and ankylosing spondylitis. In the early stages the changes are mainly inflammatory and intra-articular steroid injection can be most beneficial.

The joint can be stretched gently to preserve range, but if too vigorously stretched a flare is induced. Later cartilage erosion and capsular scarring produce irreversible stiffness and finally a fibrous ankylosis.

In polymyalgia rheumatica there are usually stiffness and tenderness of both shoulders accompanied by stiffness of the cervical spine. Pain and stiffness are often marked but the response to systemic steroid treatment is so dramatic that other treatment is not usually necessary.

If a fibrous ankylosis is painful, arthrodesis of the shoulder eases the pain without loss of function. Some good results from prosthetic replacement have been reported.

Frozen shoulder. There is further discrepancy about nomenclature in this condition. Most apply the term to the development of a painful stiff shoulder without significant trauma. Many cases seem to occur spontaneously but several general conditions leading to immobilisation of the arm may predispose, such as hemiplegia, chest wall surgery, coronary thrombosis, diabetes and herpes zoster of cervical nerve roots. The possibility of bronchial carcinoma must also be considered.

For 3–6 months there is increasing pain which persists at night. This is followed by a second static phase for a similar period. In the third phase movement gradually returns as the joint 'unfreezes' spontaneously. Characteristically, glenohumeral movement, although fairly restricted, is not totally lost and thus muscle wasting is not a marked feature.

Shoulder–hand syndrome. In some cases, pari passu with first phase of the frozen shoulder syndrome, there is in addition to capsulitis of the shoulder evidence of sympathetic over-activity in the arm with increased deep limb flow and sweating (Steinbrocker, 1972). The whole hand is swollen and there is pain on movement of all joints, save the distal interphalangeal joints. In the second phase the hand becomes cold with atrophic skin and contractures of the finger joints and long flexor tendons. Superficially the condition resembles rheumatoid arthritis but it is usually unilateral, and X-rays show marked disuse osteoporosis (Sudeck), which is characteristically patchy, but never erosions.

In some patients there appears to be a constitutional and sometimes familial predisposition to produce this phenomenon. Van der Korst et al (1960) pointed out the tendency for epileptic patients on suppressive treatment to develop the shoulder–hand syndrome. Lettin (1964) used the term 'Dupuytren's diathesis' in describing an epileptic patient with marked nodular fibrous thickening of the palmar and plantar fascia, fibrous pads on the knuckles and excessive hypertrophy of the gums who developed the shoulder–hand syndrome. Other underlying conditions, as mentioned above in association with frozen shoulder, must be borne in mind.

Treatment. Prophylaxis involves the assiduous attention to all patients at risk who are exhorted to keep the hand and shoulder mobile with exercises repeated several times a day. Once the condition is established the treatment at the shoulder depends on the phase.

First phase. Active stretching of the shoulder cannot be tolerated. Various forms of heat treatment usually increase the pain but ice can be comforting to both the shoulder and hand. Some mobility may be preserved by pendulum exercises. Radiotherapy, intra-articular or systemic steroids and stellate ganglion block (Williams et al, 1975) have been stated to ease the pain, but satisfactory control data are scanty. A nocturnal suppository of indomethacin helps the patient to sleep. In the hand the first priority must be to prevent joint and flexor tendon contractures, which can be intractable. In contrast to the shoulder the hand can be actively stretched after ice application. The patient must continue regular active exercise with a rubber 'squeegee'.

Second phase. Once rest pain has eased the shoulder can usually be actively stretched without producing a flare. This can be started by a physiotherapist, but the main onus must be on the patient to follow a routine several times a day. Experience suggests that full function usually returns more quickly with an active regime rather than awaiting spontaneous resolution.

Other arthropathies are as follows:

1. Sepsis within the joint usually produces severe pain and rigidity. Any of the pyogenic organisms may be involved. Tuberculous involvement is less dramatic and is usually accompanied by marked muscle wasting.

2. Neuropathic involvement is virtually pathognomonic of syringomyelia (Fig. 58.5). Marked radiological changes are evident in a relatively painless joint.

3. Aseptic necrosis of the subchondral bone occurs in sickle cell disease (Fig. 58.6) and caisson disease. Destruction of the overlying articular cartilage leads to progressive degenerative change. Prolonged systemic steroid therapy as in systemic

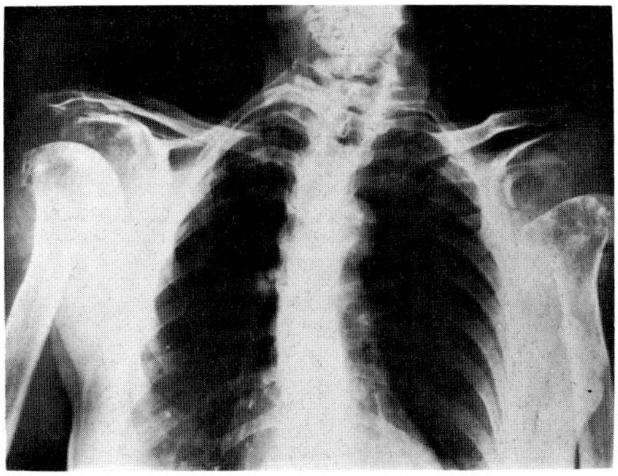

Fig. 58.5 Bilateral arthropathy of shoulders in syringomyelia.

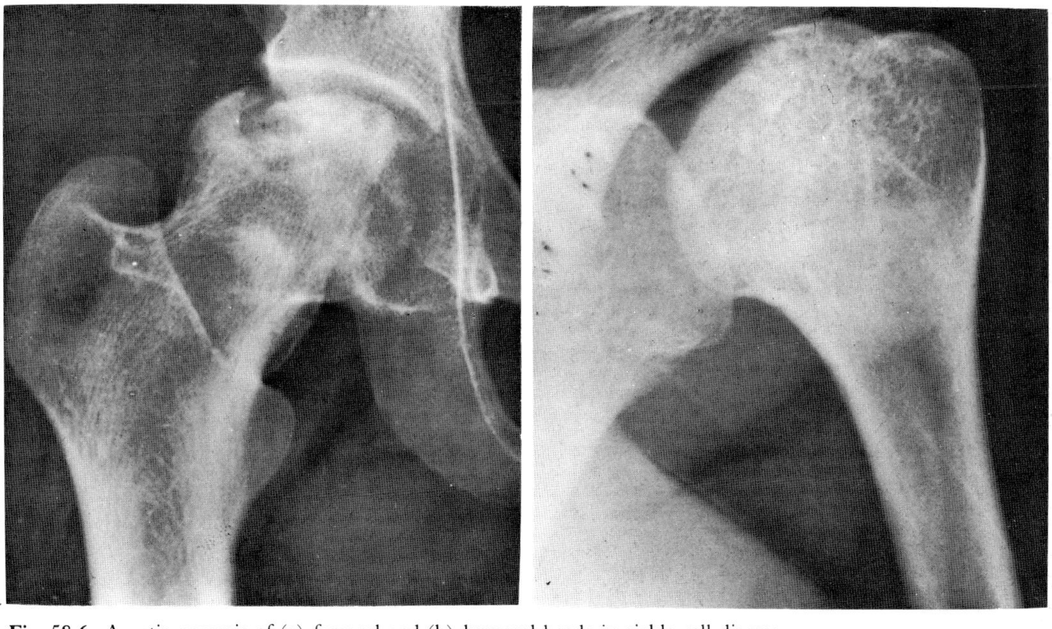

a b

Fig. 58.6 Aseptic necrosis of (a) femoral and (b) humeral heads in sickle cell disease.

lupus or renal transplant has a similar effect: the mechanism is not known but fat microembolisation has been postulated. In haemophilia multiple subchondral bleeds have the same effect but recurrent haemarthroses seem to produce little joint damage.

4. 'Milwaukee' shoulder is a term coined by McCarty and others (1980) to describe a progressive destructive arthropathy associated with extensive intracapsular calcium apatite deposition. They postulated that microapatite crystals are liberated into the joint by repetitive trauma. These activate collagenases and proteinases, which cause further damage of the joint. One such patient, paraplegic and chairbound from poliomyelitis, had severe changes in both shoulders (Fig. 58.7); presumably due to wear from overuse.

Periscapular myalgia

This condition could be called 'housewives shoulder' but the term 'fibrositis' is better avoided. The complaint is of aching in the periscapular muscles (levator scapulae and rhomboids) after light use. The patient is usually tense and anxious and somewhat depressed. Apart from a kyphotic posture and drooping of the shoulders no abnormality can be detected in the spine or shoulders. Tender 'trigger spots' can be found along the medial border of the scapula. Persistent postural tension in muscles may be the cause and temporary relief can be given by a muscle relaxant, such as diazepam, and massage of the tender spots. Long-term management consists of reassurance after complete assessment and instruction in basic posture.

Neuralgic amyotrophy

It has been postulated that a latent or slow virus may be the cause of this radiculitis which presents with severe pain in the neck and shoulder girdle. Any surgical procedure, inoculation in the arm or minor trauma can act as the trigger, but often it appears spontaneously. Weakness usually develops rapidly and this can variously be in the territory of one or several roots, a nerve trunk or even individual muscles — the 'mosaic' form — while sensory loss is usually minimal. A unilateral lesion

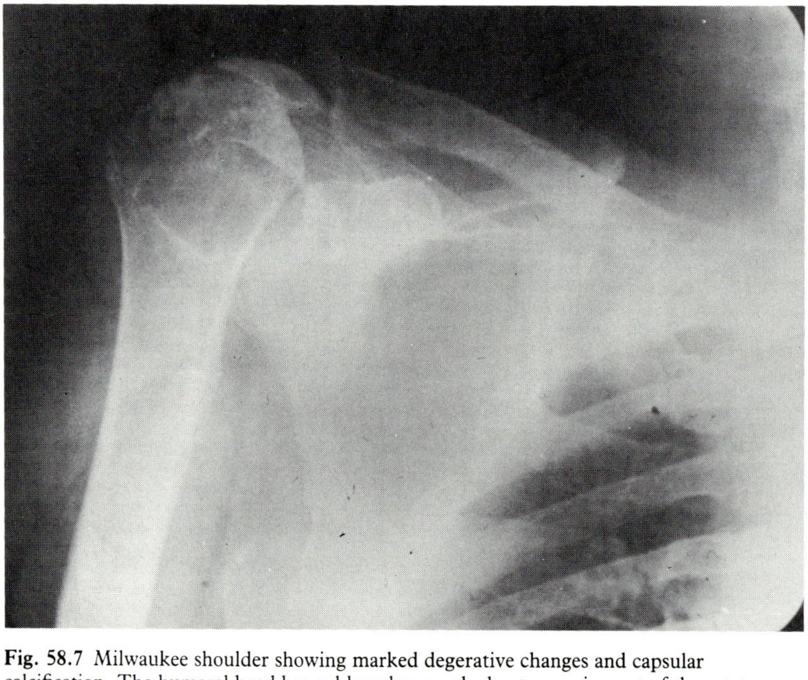

Fig. 58.7 Milwaukee shoulder showing marked degerative changes and capsular calcification. The humeral head has subluxed upwards due to wearing out of the rotator cuff.

of supraspinatus and infraspinatus innervated by the suprascapular nerve is seen occasionally while another is a lesion of the nerve to serratus anterior producing winging of the scapulae. A few motor fibres often survive and full or partial recovery usually occurs. Electromyography is invaluable in delineating the lesion and assessing prognosis.

REFERENCES

Beighton P 1978 Vertebral dysostoses. In: Inherited disorders of the skeleton. Churchill, London

British Association of Physical Medicine 1966 Pain in the neck and arm: a multi-centre trial of the effects of physiotherapy. British Medical Journal 1: 253–258

Corrigan B, Maitland G D 1983 Practical orthopaedic medicine. Butterworths, London

Cyriax J 1978 Diagnosis of soft tissue lesions. In: Textbook of orthopaedic medicine, 7th Edn. Bailliere Tindall & Cassell, London

Hilton J 1863 Rest and pain. Bell & Daldy, London.

Lettin A W F 1964 Dupuytren's diathesis: a case report. Journal of Bone and Joint Surgery 46D: 220–225

McCarty D J, Gatter R A 1966 Recurrent acute inflammation associated with focal apatite crystal deposition. Arthritis and Rheumatism 9: 804–819

McCarty D J, Halverson P B, Guillormo F C, Brewer B J Kozin F 1981 Milwaukee shoulder. Arthritis and Rheumatism 24: 464–484

Pinals R S, Short C L 1966 Calcific periarthritis involving multiple sites. Arthritis and Rheumatism 9: 566–574

Richardson A T 1975 The painful shoulder. Proceedings Royal Society of Medicine 68:731

Steinbrocker O 1972 The painful shoulder in arthritis and allied conditions. In: Hollander and McCarty 8th Edn. Lea & Fibige, Philadelphia

Steinbrocker O. Spitzer, N. Friedman H H 1948 The Shoulder-hand syndrome in reflex dystrophy. Annals of Internal Medicine 29: 22–52

Swinson D R, Hamilton E D B, Mathews J A. Yates D A H 1972 Vertical subluxation of the axis in rheumatoid arthritis. Annals of the Rheumatic Diseases 31: 359–363

Urschell H C, Razzuk M A 1972 Management of the thoracic outlet syndrome. New England Journal of Medicine 286: 1140–1143

Van der Kost J K, Colenbrander H, Cats A 1960 Phenobarbital and the shoulder-hand syndrome. Annals of the Rheumatic Diseases 25: 553–555

Wilkinson M 1971 Cervical spondylosis. Heinemann, London

Williams N E, Seifert M H, Cuddigan J H P, Wise R A 1975 Treatment of capsulitis of the shoulder. Rheumatology and Rehabilitation 14: 237–239

Yates D A H 1964 Unilateral lumbo-sacral root compression. Annals of Physical Medicine 7: 169–179

59

H.L.F. Currey

The upper limb

Rheumatological disorders involving the cervical spine and shoulder are discussed in Chapter 58. This section deals with conditions arising distal to the shoulder joint.

Clinical separation of the various causes of pain in the arm can be difficult. Accurate localisation of the pain, analysis of provoking factors, and meticulous physical examination are the sheet anchors of diagnosis. Investigations seldom prove helpful, and may be misinterpreted: for example, accepting minor radiological changes as evidence that arm pain arises in the cervical spine. Investigations are of value mainly in screening for underlying causes of arm pain. The ESR or chest X-ray — like examination of the breasts — may provide the clue to an unexpected cause of skeletal pain. In the shoulder–hand syndrome (p. 1444) for example, the chest radiograph may reveal an underlying bronchial carcinoma.

Two important causes of diagnostic confusion are the frequently poor localisation and wide radiation of arm pains, and the apparent tendency for different types of arm pain to occur together in one arm of the same patient. Pain arising in the glenohumeral joint is usually felt at about the insertion of the deltoid muscle and, unlike nerve root pain arising in the cervical spine, it seldom radiates below the elbow. Pain localised to the tip of the shoulder is likely to arise from the acromioclavicular joint or from the diaphragm. There is also a tendency for pain arising from localised arm conditions such as tennis elbow or carpal tunnel syndrome to disseminate more widely the longer the condition persists. Thus longstanding pain from median nerve compression at the wrist may be described as a diffuse ache reaching up the forearm.

Primary neurological conditions may mimic rheumatic disorders in the arm, particularly in the early stages. *Pre-eruptive herpes zoster* is a well known trap. Before the appearance of the tell-tale clusters of vesicles on an erythematous base, the pain may appear to be of skeletal origin. A superficial, smarting quality of the pain, or a history of contact with varicella, may be useful pointers to the true diagnosis. The initial events in *neuralgic amyotrophy* (Parsonage & Turner, 1948) may be similarly misleading. The premonitory pain in the neck, shoulder and upper arm is likely to be mistaken for mechanical nerve root pressure in the cervical spine. The true situation may be suspected from a history of antecedent trauma, inoculation or viral infection, and is revealed by the sudden appearance within a week or two of lower motor neurone weakness and wasting in one or more shoulder girdle muscles, for example deltoid or serratus anterior. Occasionally there is some sensory loss too.

BICIPITAL TENDINITIS

Subacute and chronic inflammatory lesions are common at both the upper and lower ends of the biceps muscle. *Tendinitis of the long head of biceps* presents as shoulder pain which is exacerbated by both shoulder flexion and forearm supination. There is also tenderness anteriorly along the course of the bicipital groove. A local corticosteroid injection into this tender site is often curative. *Biceptal tendinitis at the elbow* presents as antecubital fossa pain which is aggravated by resisted elbow flexion and forearm supination. There is local tenderness over the tendon at the elbow. Treatment by local corticosteroid injection must take account of the nearby large blood vessels. *Rupture of the long head of biceps* usually, but not always, results from an excessive strain. The clinical picture is dramatic: resisted elbow flexion produces a prominent bulbous enlargement distal and lateral to the usual biceps muscle belly bulge. Early surgical repair is effective.

HUMERAL EPICONDYLITIS (TENNIS AND GOLFER'S ELBOW)

The lateral and medial humeral epicondyles at the elbow provide the common origins for the wrist and finger extensor and flexor muscles respectively. These fibro-osseous attachments are the sites of the inflammatory changes which underlie the extremely frequent minor, but troublesome, condition known as 'tennis elbow' (lateral epicondylitis) and the less common 'golfer's elbow' (medial epicondylitis). The exact pathogenesis of these lesions is not known, but it is likely that minor mechanical tears at the bony attachments of these muscle groups produce an 'enthesopathy' similar to that which occurs in the 'painful heel' (plantar fasciitis).

Young and middle-aged adults are mainly affected, and there may be an occupational factor, particularly a combined forearm/wrist movement against resistance which provokes pain and may be causally related. In 'tennis elbow' the patient complains of the (usually) gradual onset of an unpleasant dull ache over the lateral aspect of one elbow. This is aggravated by activity and, characteristically, sharp exacerbations of pain may be triggered by manoeuvres which involve supination of the forearm with the wrist dorsiflexed and against resistance. Occasionally, the pain is felt diffusely and is poorly localised.

On examination the elbow joint itself is clinically normal. Except in very severe cases the range of passive elbow and forearm joint movements are full and painless, and there is no swelling. A positive diagnosis depends on eliciting two physical signs: active wrist dorsiflexion against resistance provokes a sharp exacerbation of pain, and firm pressure with a fingertip over the lateral humeral epicondyle locates a tender point. This tenderness is sharply localised and may require careful probing to locate.

In 'golfer's elbow' pain and tenderness are located over the medial humeral epicondyle, and it is resisted palmar flexion of the wrist which provokes discomfort.

Untreated, epicondylitis waxes and wanes over a period of months. It can settle spontaneously, possibly because a provoking activity is avoided, or it may occasionally become severe enough to interfere seriously with an occupational or sporting activity. (Playing tennis is not a particular association.)

The standard treatment is a local injection of corticosteroid. A popular technique is to inject a mixture of corticosteroid and local anaesthetic. However, it probably causes the patient less discomfort if the site is first infiltrated down to periosteum with a small volume of lignocaine. Without withdrawing the needle, the syringe is then replaced by one containing a corticosteroid, and 50 mg of hydrocortisone (or equivalent) is infiltrated into and around the site of maximum tenderness. Following the injection it appears sensible to restrict forceful activities of the arm, particularly any which have previously provoked the pain, for a period of 2 or 3 weeks. An alternative injection technique which avoids the use of a needle is to employ a 'hypospray' gun. Both techniques are liable to be followed by a period of increased pain 6–12 hours later, and both are effective in about 75% of cases (Hughes & Currey, 1969). Repeat injections have the same success rate. Thus a small proportion of cases fail to respond despite repeated injections. The fate of these is uncertain. Some may eventually recover spontaneously. Others come to surgery, but this is rarely necessary. A variety of minor local operative procedures (e.g. repositioning the muscle origin) appear to be effective. It has been suggested that some cases of 'unresponsive' tennis elbow may actually represent local entrapment of a small branch of the radial nerve: 'radial tunnel syndrome' (Roles & Maudsley, 1972). The treatment of golfer's elbow is exactly comparable, but injection techniques must take account of the presence of the ulnar nerve running behind the medial epicondyle.

Recently claims have been made for the effectiveness of treating 'tennis elbow' by applying a tight band or elastic bandage round the proximal forearm (or even the wrist) during periods of activity. This simple method appears worth testing, especially in mild cases.

OLECRANON BURSITIS

The olecranon bursa, lying over the proximal subcutaneous surface of the ulna at the elbow, is the bursa most commonly recognised as being involved in rheumatic disorders. These range from chronic or subacute effusions believed to be due to repetitive trauma in leaning on the elbow ('student's elbow') to acute pyogenic infective bursitis. Effusions may also occur in rheumatoid arthritis, and typical rheumatoid nodules may develop in the walls of such bursae. In chronic tophaceous gout it is not uncommon for the bursa to be distended with fluid (containing crystals) but without evidence of inflammation. Rarely acute gouty attacks may involve the bursa.

Differentiation from solid lesions lying over or near the olecranon process is usually not difficult. In addition to rheumatoid nodules and gouty tophi, these include calcinotic deposits (as found in scleroderma and dermatomyositis), xanthomata, the now very rare nodules of rheumatic fever, and tumours such as lipomata and neurofibromata.

Clinically effusions into the olecranon bursa are obvious ('water on the elbow') and aspiration of fluid is very simple. Any inflamed bursa requires aspiration in order to exclude crystals (by polarised light microscopy) or infection.

Infected bursae require appropriate antibiotic treatment, while an inflamed (non-infected) olecranon bursitis can be managed by aspiration followed by local injection of a corticosteroid preparation. Non-inflamed bursae required no treatment. Occasionally they are excised if effusions are chronic or recurrent.

ENTRAPMENT NEUROPATHY

The two common obstructive neuropathies in the arm — median nerve compression at the wrist and ulnar nerve compression at the elbow — may both either mimic, or result from, a rheumatic complaint. Occasionally the radial nerve may be involved.

Carpal tunnel syndrome

On the volar surface of the wrist the carpal bones form a concavity which is bridged over by the flexor retinaculum to create the carpal tunnel. In their passage through this tunnel the long flexor tendons in their sheaths occupy most of the available space. Any increase in the bulk of the contents of the canal is thus liable to compress the median nerve as it runs amongst the tendons. The ulnar nerve lies in a separate compartment and is very rarely involved.

Median nerve compression without any obvious precipitating cause is most common in middle-aged women. There are, however, a very large number of recognised causes, all of which operate by increasing bulk within the canal. These conditions include general factors such as fluid retention from any cause, pregnancy, obesity, myxoedema, acromegaly and amyloidosis, and local lesions such as ganglia, callus resulting from a wrist fracture, or a gouty tophus. A common and important cause is rheumatoid arthritis, in which carpal tunnel symptoms may occur early (due to flexor tenosynovitis) or late (due to wrist subluxation or other destructive changes). Other forms of inflammatory arthritis and pyrophosphate deposition can occasionally produce the carpal tunnel syndrome.

In a mixed peripheral nerve, pressure interferes with conduction in sensory fibres before affecting motor fibres. Hence it is that median nerve compression at the wrists can often be diagnosed with confidence on the characteristic sensory symptoms before any neurological deficit can be found on examination, and sometimes before electrical conduction studies reveal any abnormality. The typical complaint is of being woken at night by an unpleasant numb tingling sensation affecting the palmar aspect of the radial side of the hand. Although localisation of these sensory symptoms may be vague (see above) the patient will almost invariably volunteer that relief is obtained by hanging the arm down over the side of the bed and wringing the hand. Increased activity by day (e.g. housework or gardening) will often provoke or worsen the complaint that night. If the condition progresses the patient may notice more constant sensory changes, for example inability to feel a pin when picking it up between forefinger and thumb, awkwardness in executing fine movements with the fingers, and thenar muscle wasting.

In mild cases there may be no abnormal physical signs and, even in patients with typical sensory symptoms, it may be difficult to demonstrate any sensory loss. The median nerve transmits sensation from the palmar aspect of the radial $3\frac{1}{2}$ digits, but this is somewhat variable. More severe cases show impaired sensation in this distribution. Motor weakness is also a marker of severity. Power is conveniently tested in the abductor pollicis brevis muscle by asking the patient to place the back of the hand flat on a table top, then to raise the thumb vertically upwards against resistance from a starting position beside the palm. Power in the opponens muscle is tested by getting the patient to pinch together the tips of the thumb and little finger while the examiner attempts to force them apart with his own index finger. Muscle wasting may be apparent as a characteristic loss in bulk of the thenar eminence. Tapping or pressing with the tip of a finger over the point where the median nerve traverses the carpal tunnel may provoke a sensation like an electric shock in the distribution of the median nerve (Tinel's sign). Symptoms may also be reproduced by sustained passive wrist flexion (Phalen's sign) or extension (prayer sign).

Electrical testing can be valuable in difficult cases (see Ch. 68). It may, however, reveal no abnormality in the mildest cases (the patients symptoms being more sensitive than the test). A characteristic finding is delay in median nerve motor conduction from just above the wrist to the abductor pollicis brevis muscle. In severe cases there may be electrical signs of denervation in this muscle. Retrograde sensory conduction from the index finger to above the wrist may be slowed or impaired. Electrical testing can also be of value in excluding a more generalised peripheral neuropathy (indicated by slowing of motor conduction in other limb nerves), as well as in the differential diagnosis from cervical nerve root lesions.

Management is eminently satisfactory. Dramatic relief of symptoms (and confirmation of the diagnosis) is usually readily obtained either by providing a night wrist splint which holds the joint in the neutral position, or by injecting about 0.1 ml of a soluble corticosteroid preparation (e.g. betamethasone) into the carpal tunnel. The median nerve lies approximately in the centre of the wrist under the tendon of palmaris longus (when this is present). These measures usually suffice for mild cases. Resistant cases, and those in whom a motor deficit is present, require surgical division of the flexor retinaculum. This is curative. Underlying causes must of course be sought.

It is particularly important for clinicians to be aware of the high frequency of carpal tunnel syndrome in rheumatoid arthritis (Barnes & Currey, 1967). The condition is easily overlooked, both pain and muscle-wasting being ascribed to the rheumatoid disease. This is a serious error, for a superadded neurological deficit has a disproportionately severe effect on hand function already compromised by joint and tendon damage. The error is avoided if patients are routinely questioned about paraesthesia. The peripheral sensory (digital) neuropathy occasionally found in rheumatoid arthritis can be another source of difficulty. In these circumstances, electrical testing can provide useful confirmation.

Ulnar neuropathy

Ulnar nerve compression at the elbow is often due to disease of the nearby joint. Lying in a groove behind the medial humeral epicondyle it is vulnerable to pressure from osteophytic outgrowths, from synovial hyperplasia, and from cystic extensions of the synovial cavity. The patient notices paraesthesia in the ulnar $1\frac{1}{2}$ fingers and awkwardness in executing fine finger movements. Motor power is conveniently tested as abduction (ulnar deviation) of the little finger (abductor digiti minimi). Severe involvement may produce a partial 'claw hand'. Electrical testing pinpoints the lesion to the level of the elbow. All but the mildest cases require surgical transposition of the nerve to the front of the elbow. This is highly effective, although recovery of established neurological defects may take many months.

Radial neuropathy

Synovial cysts extending from the elbow joint can occasionally compress the posterior interosseous branch of the radial nerve to produce wrist and finger drop. This has to be differentiated from extensor tendon rupture. Sensation is not affected. Surgical correction is curative.

Mention has been made above about the theory that some cases of resistant 'tennis elbow' may represent entrapment of a small branch of the radial nerve.

DE QUERVAIN'S SYNDROME (TENOVAGINITIS OF ABDUCTOR POLLICIS LONGUS)

A number of painful conditions about the wrist may be mistaken for arthritis of that joint. The differentiation is important: primary osteoarthritis of the carpus is rare, so the diagnosis of arthritis of the wrist usually implies a serious inflammatory condition such as rheumatoid arthritis.

Three painful conditions at the wrist arise in the anatomical snuff box (Fig. 59.1). They are ununited fractures of the scaphoid, primary osteoarthritis of the 1st carpometacarpal joint, and tenovaginitis of the tendon of abductor pollicis longus. Inflammatory changes can arise in any of the long tendons where they cross the distal ends of the forearm bones, presumably resulting from mechanical factors operating at the point where the tendon is angulated over the edge of the bone. Much the most commonly involved tendon is abductor pollicis longus. The resulting clinical picture (De Quervain's syndrome) is characteristic.

The condition usually presents in young or middle-aged adults, and there may be an occupational factor such as the use of heavy shears in the clothing industry. The patient complains of an unpleasant dull ache on the radial side of the wrist, which is precipitated or aggravated by use of the thumb. On examination the wrist and thumb joints are normal, but pressure by the examiner's finger over the point where the extensor pollicis longus tendon crosses the radial styloid process (Fig. 59.1) produces a sharp pain when the patient extends and abducts the thumb. Occasionally, there may be crepitus or a sausage-like swelling in the line of the tendon indicating an effusion in the sheath. Treatment by injection into the tendon sheath of 0.2 ml of a corticosteroid preparation through a fine needle is usually successful. Failing that, the first carpometacarpal joint may be immobilised in a splint for a few weeks, or the tendon sheath can be released surgically. Predisposing occupational factors may require attention.

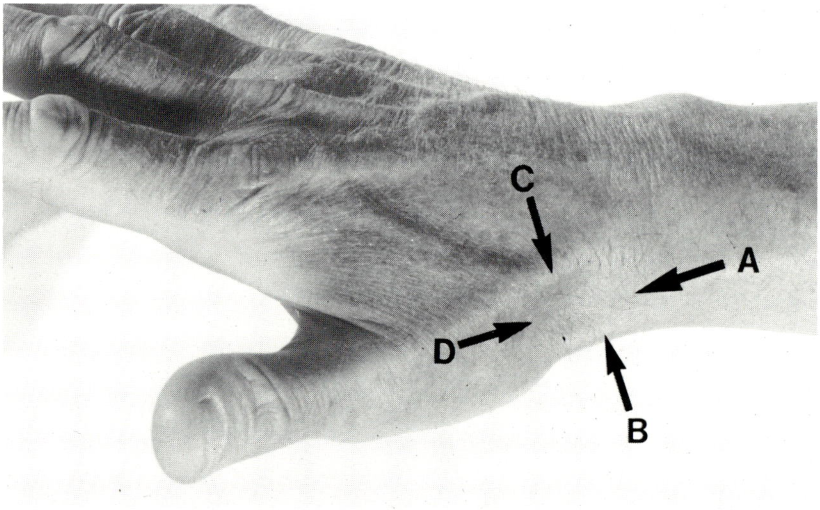

Fig. 59.1 The anatomical snuff box. The borders of the snuff box are: A — Tip of the radial styloid process; B — Tendon of abductor pollicis longus; C — Tendon of extensor pollicis longus; D — First carpometacarpal joint. The scaphoid bone occupies the middle of the snuff box.

STENOSING TENOVAGINITIS ('TRIGGER FINGER')

This common minor condition results from an incomplete obstruction to the movement of a finger flexor tendon in its sheath. It most commonly affects the middle finger in the dominant hand of middle-aged women. Rheumatoid arthritis is an important predisposing cause.

The patient complains that flexion and/or extension of the finger proceeds to a certain point, then 'sticks'. A forced effort is required to overcome the resistance, and the movement is then completed with a sometimes audible snap. Passive force may be required to overcome the obstruction. Any discomfort is usually only mild.

The site of obstruction is easily located by the examiner palpating the flexor tendon during flexion and extension of the digit. The lesion is almost invariably opposite the metacarpophalangeal joint.

The first line of treatment is an injection of 0.25 ml of a corticosteroid preparation through a fine needle into the tendon sheath. If that fails, surgical release of the obstructed segment of sheath is a relatively simple matter. At operation a thickening of the tendon is found where it passes beneath the pulley opposite the metacarpophalangeal joint, and the sheath is narrowed at this point. Apart from rheumatoid arthritis, the cause of trigger finger is usually uncertain. However, local chronic trauma (e.g. occupational) is sometimes an important factor. Rare systemic causes include gout, systemic sclerosis, chronic infections, and type II hyperlipoproteinaemia.

WRITER'S CRAMP (OCCUPATIONAL CRAMP)

When a patient presents with loss of function in a hand, this is usually clearly due either to an articular or to a neurological problem. Occasionally, however, the patient describes progressive difficulty in executing some frequently performed manoeuvre which previously presented no difficulty, and for which no neurological or articular cause is apparent. Typically the movements involved are repetitive and rapid, need precision, and are required by the patient to earn a living. An example is the left hand fingering movements of a musician who plays a stringed instrument. The condition has been best studied amongst clerks who, in the days before automation, used to spend their working days making entries in ledgers. The initial complaint is of some loss of precision in handwriting, soon followed by slowing. Attempts to continue writing produce increasing awkwardness, with spasm and pain in the muscles involved. Eventually, writing becomes impossible. Clinical examination of the limb reveals no abnormality.

The mechanism of these occupational cramps is unknown. By the time that the patient is seen, there is usually good evidence that anxiety about his ability to carry on his occupation has become a major factor in perpetuating the disability. At this stage it is likely to be difficult to unravel the relative contributions of a pre-existing personality defect, doubts on the patient's part about his ability to manage his occupation anyhow, and the role of stress from other causes. Management starts with the careful exclusion of organic causes such as early Parkinsonism or dystonia. Psychological and personality assessment are likely to indicate the interplay of factors mentioned above — without opening up any obvious directions for effective intervention. Traditionally writer's cramp is treated by avoiding the occupation in question for a period of weeks and by changing the activity, for example by switching from a 'fountain' to a 'dip-in' pen. However, neither these measures nor formal psychological treatment are reliably effective, and the prognosis for complete recovery from an established disability is not good (Hudgson, 1983).

RAYNAUD'S PHENOMENON

Raynaud's phenomenon is a common accompaniment of inflammatory rheumatic diseases. It is due to transient functional spasm of digital arteries, sometimes superimposed on varying degrees of organic occlusion, triggered usually by exposure to cold, occasionally by vibration or even warmth. Rarely the toes may be affected as well as the fingers. In the typical cycle cold exposure causes some or all of the fingers to turn white, and this is accompanied by an unpleasant, numb, tingling sensation. After 15 or 30 minutes, occasionally longer, capillary dilatation produces a purple and white marbled effect. This then gives way to an erythematous flush before the cycle is completed by the fingers returning to normal.

Raynaud's phenomenon may result from a very wide variety of causes. It is common in schoolgirls, in whom the condition is usually benign, although it can produce trophic changes. The appearance of Raynaud's phenomenon for the first time in adult life is much more sinister. It can result from mechanical pressure in the thoracic outlet or from the use of vibrating tools, but much more commonly it heralds the appearance of a systemic connective tissue disease such as rheumatoid arthritis, systemic sclerosis, polymyositis, polyarteritis or SLE. The closest link is with systemic sclerosis (Ch. 55) in which Raynaud's phenomenon may precede other features of the disease by months or even years, and trophic changes may be severe.

The first line of treatment is avoidance of smoking and of cold exposure. Recent interest has centred on pharmacological control of digital spasm by either slow calcium channel antagonists (Smith & Kendry, 1982) or prostaglandin E_1 infusions (Martin & Tooke, 1982) or by plasmapheresis (Talpos et al, 1978). Cervical sympathectomy remains of limited and usually transient value. It is usually employed when skin viability is critically threatened.

DUPUYTREN'S CONTRACTURE

Dupuytren's contracture is a fibrotic process involving the palmar fascia which may superficially mimic a rheumatic disorder. It is discussed on page 1254.

REFERENCES

Barnes C G, Currey H L F 1967 Carpal tunnel syndrome in rheumatoid arthritis. A clinical and electrodiagnostic survey. Annals of the Rheumatic Diseases 26: 226–233

Hudgson P 1983 Writer's cramp (leading article). British Medical Journal 286:585

Hughes G R V, Currey H L F 1969 Hypospray treatment of tennis elbow. Annals of the Rheumatic Diseases 28: 58–62

Martin M F R, Tooke J E 1982 Effects of prostaglandin E_1 on microvascular haemodynamics in progressive systemic sclerosis. British Medical Journal 285: 1688–1690

Parsonage M J, Turner W A 1948 Neuralgic amyotrophy. The shoulder girdle syndrome. Lancet 1: 973–978

Roles N C, Maudsley R H 1972 Radial tunnel syndrome: Resistant tennis elbow as a nerve entrapment. Journal of Bone and Joint Surgery 54B: 499–508

Smith C Douglas, McKendry R J R 1982 Controlled trial of nifedipine in the treatment of Raynaud's phenomenon. Lancet: 2: 1299–1301

Talpos G, Horrocks M, White J M, Cotton L T 1978 Plasmapheresis in Raynaud's disease. Lancet: 1: 416–417

teomalacia. Overuse fractures (stress fractures) of the pubic rami occur in military recruits (Meurman, 1980) and in joggers and distance runners (Pavlov et al, 1982). Treatment is by rest and analgesics, with isometric exercises or hydrotherapy to maintain muscle tone until healing has occurred.

The pubic rami are a common site for metastatic carcinomatous deposits which may result in a pathological fracture.

Both pyogenic and tuberculous osteomyelitis of the pubic rami occur and are treated appropriately.

Intrapelvic lesions

It has already been noted that much pain experienced in or around the region of the hip joint may be referred from lesions of the spine. Lesions of the intrapelvic viscera may also cause pain felt in and around the hip joint, often accompanied by protective spasm of the hip flexors and obturator internus. This is particularly so if there is peritonitis, or a local inflammatory lesion such as an appendix abscess or pyosalpinx, lying close to the obturator foramen.

Iliopsoas bursitis and cysts of the hip

Iliopsoas bursitis in rheumatoid arthritis may cause oedema of the leg due to compression of the femoral vein (Ford et al, 1981). Synovial cysts may also arise from the hip joint and have been reported as penetrating into the pelvis where they may cause compression symptoms (Watson & Ochsner, 1967; Coventry et al, 1959).

PATTERN OF PAIN REFERRAL FROM THE HIP JOINT

Abnormalities of the hip joint or structures closely related to it may cause pain felt deep in the hip, in the groin, in the buttock, over the greater trochanter, in the front or the back of the thigh, or in the knee. Pain may be experienced in one or several of these sites in a given subject: but pain arising from the hip is often most severe either deep in the groin or in the lower part of the front of the thigh and the knee joint.

It is well recognised that disease of the hip in children, for instance epiphysiolysis (slipping upper femoral epiphysis) or Perthes' disease, may cause pain which is experienced only in the knee. It is less well recognised that adults suffering from hip disease may also complain only of pain felt in and around the knee joint. This occurs at any age but seems especially common in the elderly. Many elderly subjects also have radiological changes of symptomless osteoarthritis in the knee, to which their pain may be wrongly ascribed unless movements of the hip have been tested. It is often difficult to persuade such a patient to accept treatment to the hip once they have been told that radiological examination has confirmed the presence of 'arthritis' in the knee. Careful clinical examination of the hip joint is mandatory in all patients who complain of pain in the knee; and while testing movements of the knee joint it is important to support the thigh so as to prevent concomitant movement of the hip, especially rotation, which may cause pain apparently arising from the knee. The Trendelenburg test will usually be abnormal when hip disease is the source of the pain.

Avascular necrosis

Avascular necrosis in the femoral head may arise as a primary event, secondary to a number of predisposing causes, or during the course of established osteoarthritis or inflammatory joint disease (see Ch. 48). The initial pain may be severe, but the typical X-ray appearances are thought to coincide with the period of revascularisation, and may not be seen until some months have elapsed. If this sequence is not appreciated confusion may be caused by the apparently normal initial radiograph.

OTHER CAUSES OF PAIN IN FRONT OF THE THIGH

Referred spinal pain

Lesions of the lower dorsal or lumbar spine, particularly those involving the segments L1, L2 and L3, may result in pain referred down the front of the thigh (Kellgren, 1939). Such pain is usually made worse by movements of the spine. When there is nerve root irritation, the femoral nerve stretch test (hyperextension of the hip with the knee flexed) will result in accentuation of the pain.

Lesions of the femoral neck and upper femur

Just as pain arising within the hip joint may be experienced only in the knee, so may pain arising from lesions in the femoral neck or in the upper femur. Bone tumours and osteomyelitis may occur in the femur. The femoral neck and upper femoral shaft are a common site for insufficiency fractures in metabolic bone disease.

Osteoid osteoma

Osteoid osteoma is probably a very slow-growing benign neoplasm, though some believe that it is infective in origin or due to a vascular lesion. The condition presents with pain, often of a deep boring character, which is seldom aggravated by exercise or by position, and which may be troublesome at night. Pain is often relieved to a greater extent by salicylate than by other analgesic or anti-inflammatory drugs. The natural history of the condition is not known; but it is commonly diagnosed between the ages of 10 and 30 years and occurs equally in males and females. If the lesion occurs in a superficial bone there may be a tender swelling; usually there are no abnormal physical findings. It may occur in any bone, including the vertebrae, but is most common in the bones of the lower limb, and particularly around the hip and in the femur (Murray & Jacobson, 1971). Histologically the lesion shows three characteristic zones: an inner zone of vascular granulation tissue containing active osteoblasts is separated by a zone of calcification and osteoid from a surrounding zone of trabecular bone formation. Radiologically the lesion appears as an area of increased radiolucency surrounded by a zone of bone sclerosis, sometimes with an overlying periosteal reaction. In the centre of the radiolucent area there may be a radiodense nidus, though this cannot always be demonstrated even by tomography. The lesion may be small, and in trabecular bone the sclerosis may not be marked, so that osteoid osteoma may not always be demonstrable by conventional radiography (Fig. 60.2). However the lesion usually shows increased activity on radionucleotide bone scanning.

Treatment is by resection of the lesion. Complete removal is preferable, but partial removal of sclerotic bone and the nidus often provides symptomatic improvement.

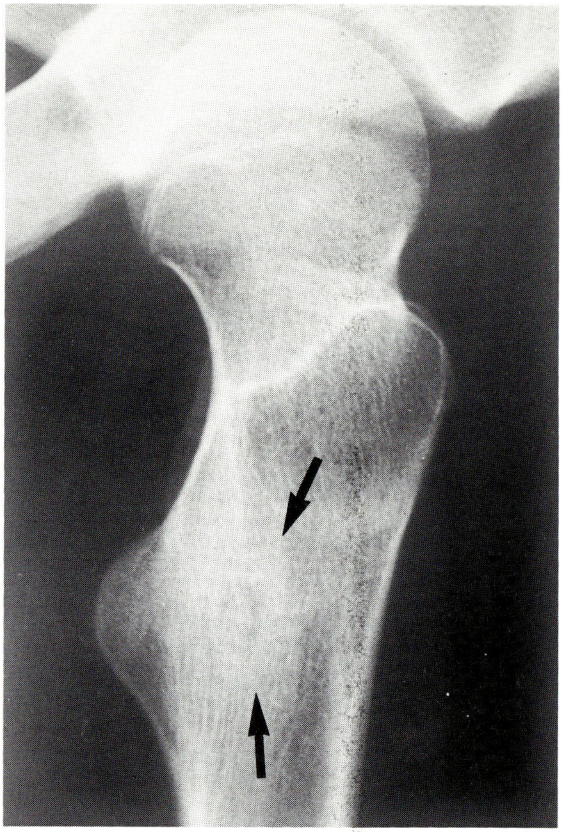

Fig. 60.2 Osteoid osteoma in the right femur of a 15-year-old girl who had complained for nearly 2 years of pain in the right knee. The abnormality was shown only on the lateral view and was confirmed by a scintiscan. Her pain was relieved when the lesion was excised.

Paget's disease (osteitis deformans)

Paget's disease is described in Chapter 40. The disease usually begins between the ages of 40 and 60 and the initial symptom is often pain in the leg, in the thigh or around the hip. When juxta-articular bone is involved in the acetabulum, femur, or tibia, arthritis often develops in the corresponding joint.

Affected long bones are thickened but brittle and are liable to pathological fractures. These often develop as horizontal cracks across the upper femur. Although often incomplete at first, such transverse fractures may be the cause of an increase of pain in Paget's disease, and, if not treated by rest or preventative surgical stabilisation, usually progress to a complete transverse pathological fracture (Grundy, 1970).

Rarely, osteogenic sarcoma may develop in bone affected by Paget's disease: this may be accompanied by an increase in pain and swelling.

Herpes zoster

Herpes zoster results from infection of one or more posterior root ganglia with the varicella virus, causing pain in the distribution of the affected root. This is followed after an interval by a vesicular rash in the same distribution which often heals with scab formation and scarring. The interval between the onset of pain and the appearance of the rash varies from a few days to two weeks or more, and until the rash appears the cause of the pain may defy diagnosis. It is thought that early treatment of the skin lesions with idoxuridine solution will reduce the frequency and severity of post-herpetic neuralgia. The condition is unusual below the age of 50 unless there is some impairment of immune mechanisms. Lumbar or sciatic nerve roots are not infrequently affected.

NERVE ENTRAPMENT SYNDROMES

Compression or entrapment syndromes of nerves usually cause pain, and sometimes sensory impairment or weakness, in the distribution of the nerve. Nerve pain is frequently mistaken for pain due to arthritis: where peripheral nerves run in confined spaces close to joints or synovial tissue they may themselves be affected by pressure damage as a result of synovial swelling, causing additional symptoms which it is important to recognise and treat (Kopell & Thompson, 1960; Nakano, 1975).

Sciatic nerve compression

This is commonly experienced temporarily from sitting too long in one position causing the leg to 'go to sleep'. A complete lesion of the sciatic nerve causes paralysis of all muscles below the knee and, in a high lesion, of the hamstring muscles, with sensory loss in the outer part of the foot and calf. Such lesions are usually due to deep penetrating wounds but have been reported in patients suffering from haemophilia or who are treated with anticoagulants (Lange, 1966), due possibly to intramuscular or intraneural bleeding.

Femoral nerve compression

Compression lesions of the femoral nerve result in weakness of extension of the knee with an absent knee jerk, slight weakness of hip flexion, and impaired sensation over the dorsum and inner side of the foot (Biemond, 1970). Damage to the nerve may follow intrapelvic tumour or injury, pressure from a psoas abscess, or haemorrhage into the iliacus muscle due to haemophilia (Goodfellow & Fearn, 1965) or to anticoagulant therapy (Lange, 1966; Fearn, 1968). The haematoma compresses the nerve within the iliopsoas sheath (Simeone et al, 1977), but bleeding into the psoas muscle is rare. Femoral nerve compression has also been recorded due to pressure from an enlarged psoas bursa in rheumatoid arthritis.

Meralgia paraesthetica

The lateral cutaneous nerve of the thigh is derived from the 2nd and 3rd lumbar roots. As it enters the thigh the nerve is wedged between the origin of the sartorius muscle, the bony margin of the pelvis and the attachment to the anterior superior iliac spine of the inguinal ligament. Compression of the nerve at this site leads to a sharp, burning pain, hyperalgesia, paraesthesiae and numbness over the lateral aspect of the thigh. Symptoms are often present at rest but are made worse by extending the hip and by exercise such as walking. When the pain is brought on by walking it may be mistaken for ischaemic pain due to arterial insufficiency. The problem may be precipitated by an acute blow, by repetitive minor trauma or by pressure from a tight belt or corset (Kitchen & Simpson, 1972; Sunderland, 1978), and is aggravated by rapid gain in weight or by pregnancy. Rarely, the nerve may be compressed by a lesion within the pelvis or where it pierces the deep fascia laterally in the thigh.

Mild cases require no treatment. In more severe cases weight reduction, avoidance of local pressure and local steroid injections may be tried. Uncommonly, surgical decompression may be needed.

Lateral popliteal nerve palsy

The lateral popliteal (common peroneal) nerve is particularly liable to injury by pressure as it winds round the lateral side of the neck of the fibula deep to the fibres of origin of the peroneus longus muscle, which form a bridge with attachments to bone both proximal and distal to the nerve. Arteriosclerotic or diabetic subjects and patients with vasculitis are at greatest risk. Damage may be caused by a direct blow, by pressure during sleep or during operation, by a tight bandage or plaster cast, by synovitis of the superior tibiofibular joint (Stack et al, 1965), or by traction during an inversion injury to the ankle. Synovial effusion in the knee joint may rarely cause pressure on the lateral popliteal nerve: this is more likely to occur when the superior tibiofibular joint communicates with the knee. There is often pain in the outer side of the leg with weakness of dorsiflexion and eversion of the foot, with an area of impaired sensation on the front and outer side of the calf and the dorsum of the foot. Subsequent instability of the ankle due to residual weakness causes considerable disability (Sidey, 1969). Nerve conduction velocity studies may help to confirm the diagnosis.

Slow recovery usually occurs over a period up to 12 months. Weak muscles should be supported by splinting, and prolonged physiotherapy may be needed to restore muscle coordination. If recovery is delayed, surgical exploration and decompression may be successful.

Tarsal tunnel syndrome

The medial and lateral plantar nerves arise as terminal branches of the posterior tibial nerve usually within, or just distal to, the 'tarsal tunnel' which is formed by the flat, fibrous flexor retinaculum bridging across from the medial malleolus of the tibia to the medial margins of the calcaneum. The nerve and its branches are sometimes bound down by fibrous bands within the tunnel, which is traversed also by the tendons of the posterior tibial muscle and of the long flexors of the toes and their accompanying synovial sheaths, and by the posterior tibial artery and veins. Narrowing of the tunnel due to injury or arthritic deformity, synovial swelling or thickening of the other tunnel contents (Macfarlane & DuToit, 1974) may result in compression of the posterior tibial nerve or its branches. This causes burning pain, with paraesthesiae, in the sole of the foot, particularly the medial side, which is often worse at night. As with carpal tunnel syndrome, the pain often spreads proximally from the site of compression and may radiate up the leg and thigh in a sciatic nerve distribution. Pressure applied locally over the tarsal tunnel may accentuate the symptoms. There may be sensory impairment in the territory of either the medial or the lateral planter nerve but not involving the dorsum of the foot (Lam, 1967; DiStefano et al, 1972). It is usually not possible to show weakness of the short flexor muscles in the foot. The differential diagnosis includes other local causes of pain in the foot, such as interdigital neuroma, inflammatory arthritis, peripheral neuritis, sciatic nerve pain and peripheral vascular disease. Conduction velocity studies in the posterior tibial nerve across the flexor retinaculum may help to confirm the diagnosis (Baylan et al, 1981).

Local steroid injection into the tarsal tunnel is sometimes helpful. Definitive treatment is by surgical decompression, with careful dissection to ensure that the posterior tibial nerve and its branches are free of all encircling fibrous bands.

Sural nerve compression

The sural nerve is a sensory branch of the medial popliteal nerve. Cases have been described in which pain in the ankle and foot, sometimes with paraesthesiae or numbness on the outer side of the foot, has been relieved by decompression of the sural nerve where it lies close to the peroneal tendons behind the lateral malleolus (Pringle et al, 1974).

Interdigital neuroma and compression of the digital nerves (Morton's metatarsalgia) are discussed later in the chapter.

LESIONS AROUND THE KNEE JOINT

The knee is commonly involved by osteoarthritis, and by rheumatoid arthritis and other inflammatory joint diseases. It is also the joint most commonly affected by monarticular synovitis, both in the adult (Fletcher & Scott, 1975) and in children (Bywaters & Ansell, 1965). The differential diagnosis of synovitis of the knee is discussed in Chapter 5.

Internal derangements

Internal derangements of the knee, including meniscal tears, ligamentous injuries and loose bodies, cause pain and swelling which may be intermittent and which are frequently aggravated by exercise. There may be locking of the knee, usually in some degree of flexion, and the knee may give way on weight-bearing, due to sudden pain causing inhibition of the quadriceps muscle. These problems and their management are discussed in textbooks of orthopaedic surgery and in specialist monographs on the knee (Smillie, 1980; Jackson & Waugh, 1984). Chronic irritation due to an internal derangement may cause persisting effusion and thickening of the synovium, the histology of which may show inflammatory changes similar to those found in early, mild rheumatoid arthritis (Soren, 1978).

Osteochondritis dissecans in the knee may cause symptoms similar to those of internal derangements and is discussed in Chapter 48.

Synovial shelf syndrome

The anatomy of the synovial folds within the knee has been known for many years. Appreciation of their functional significance has increased during the past decade, consequent upon greater use of the arthroscope in seeking the precise diagnosis in patients with symptoms of internal derangement of the knee. The medial synovial shelf, known also as the 'plica synovialis mediopatellaris', crosses the medial suprapatellar plica in the coronal plane to be inserted into the infrapatellar fat-pad. The medial shelf is of variable width and is present in nearly 50% of subjects. When the knee is flexed beyond 30 degrees it lies in contact with the medial femoral condyle. Irritation of this synovial fold gives rise to the 'synovial shelf syndrome' or 'plica syndrome'. This is aggravated when the knee is kept flexed for long periods and is characterised by tenderness over the medial side of the knee in the line of the synovial shelf, with pain in the front of the knee after prolonged sitting or when climbing or descending stairs, and in the absence of patellofemoral joint disease. The presence of the shelf is confirmed by arthroscopy and treatment is by arthroscopic excision (Vaughan-Lane & Dandy, 1982). The long-term effects of this treatment are awaited, but excellent or good results are reported in 83% of knees reviewed 1–2 years after the operation.

Lesions of the patella

Chondromalacia patellae

This name has been applied to a syndrome, mainly encountered in adolescents and young adults, with females predominating, which is poorly understood and difficult to diagnose with certainty (British Medical Journal, 1981). Deep-seated aching is felt towards the front of the knee behind the patella, with pain, and sometimes instability, during active movements with the knee flexed. There may be recurrent effusion and sometimes retropatellar crepitus. There is often tenderness of the posterior surface of the patella, or pain when the patella is compressed against the femur: but there may be no abnormal physical signs. The patients are frequently athletic and may suffer considerable disability. Arthroscopy can be helpful by excluding other causes of the symptoms and may demonstrate softening, swelling, fibrillation or erosion of the retropatellar cartilage. When present, these changes are most commonly found on the medial facet (Goodfellow et al, 1976). In a series of patients examined arthroscopically the retropatellar cartilage appeared normal in 49% (Leslie & Bentley, 1978). It is not clear whether or not such patients should be regarded as having chondromalacia without overt changes in the cartilage: nor is it clear how often demonstrable abnormalities in the cartilage are the cause of the symptoms (Goodfellow, 1984).

Many authors in the past regarded the changes in the cartilage in chondromalacia patellae as being indistinguishable from those of early osteoarthritis (Collins, 1949), although clinically there is no evidence that chondromalacia predisposes to the later development of retropatellar osteoarthritis. Reported changes in the bone of the patella, however, are unlike those of osteoarthritis, with thinning of the subchondral bone plate and both focal and diffuse osteoporosis of the underlying trabecular bone (Darracott & Vernon-Roberts, 1971). In 4 out of 11 patellae showing these changes there was no microscopic abnormality in the superficial zone of the articular cartilage.

Spontaneous improvement usually occurs during a period of months or years. It is important to reassure the patient that there is no abnormality present likely to cause permanent damage. A reduction in the level of physical activity is helpful. Physiotherapy and isometric quadriceps exercises often help, but sometimes make the symptoms worse. Non-steroid anti-inflammatory drugs (aloxiprin) are disappointing (Bentley et al, 1981). A variety of surgical procedures have been advocated, including realignment of the patellar tendon, release of the lateral quadriceps, and patellectomy (Bentley, 1978; Osborne & Fulford, 1982). Resurfacing of the patella has also been attempted (Insall et al, 1980). There is no general agreement that any particular operation is universally helpful.

Dislocation of the patella

Medial dislocation is usually the result of injury, but may occur in cases of severe genu varum. Recurrent dislocation of the patella nearly always occurs towards the lateral side. Predisposing features are injury, congenital hypoplasia of the patella or of the lateral femoral condyle, hypermobility syndromes, muscle weakness, genu valgum and an abnormally high patella or patella alta (Ficat & Hungerford, 1977; Aichroth, 1984). Trouble usually begins in adolescence or in early adult life, and girls are more commonly affected than boys. Recurrent subluxation implies similar displacement, but with the patella riding on the lateral femoral condyle without complete dislocation.

In mild cases the patient complains of the knee giving way as the patella slips momentarily over the femoral condyle. When subluxation is less frequent each episode is usually precipitated by a sudden contraction of the quadriceps with the knee partly flexed and with the foot everted. There is considerable pain and often subsequent disability and swelling of the knee. Rarely a general anaesthetic may be needed to reduce the dislocation. A useful physical sign is the patient's 'apprehension', aroused by any manipulation of the knee which is likely to induce lateral displacement of the patella.

Treatment initially should be conservative with intensive physiotherapy designed to strengthen the quadriceps muscle, and especially vastus medialis (Heywood, 1961; Crosby & Insall, 1976). If the dislocations recur with such frequency as to seriously disable the patient, operation will be necessary. A variety of procedures have been described (Ficat & Hungerford, 1977; Aichroth, 1984) designed to realign the extensor apparatus of the knee and to reposition and stabilise the patella. Late patellofemoral osteoarthritis may develop (Hampson & Hill, 1975). When there is severe degeneration of the articular surface, patellectomy may be indicated, combined with stabilisation to prevent subsequent dislocation of the patellar tendon.

Habitual dislocation implies dislocation at every flexion and extension movement of the knee.

Osteoarthritis of the patellofemoral joint

This is covered in Section VII.

Nail–Patella syndrome

Hereditary onycho-osteodysplasia or 'the nail–patella syndrome' is a rare condition inherited as an autosomal dominant, but showing considerable clinical variation, and affecting both ectodermal and mesodermal structures (Wynn-Davies & Fairbank, 1976). In the hand the nails are hypoplastic, split or absent on one or several digits, especially the thumb. The patellae are hypoplastic or absent, and there may be hypoplasia of the lateral femoral condyle and of the head of the fibula. There is sometimes hypoplasia of the capitellum at the elbow with posterior subluxation of the radial head, and occasionally an abnormal scapula. Iliac horns, when present, are diagnostic.

There may be loss of extension and limitation of supination at the elbow, but musculoskeletal symptoms usually relate to recurrent dislocation of the patella. In about one-third of cases the syndrome is associated with proteinuria and renal dysfunction, which may ultimately result in renal failure (Hawkins & Smith, 1950). Microscopy shows changes in the glomerular basement membrane.

Patellar tendinitis

Otherwise known as 'jumper's knee' or Sinding–Larsen–Johansson disease, this condition presents in otherwise healthy children or adolescents with pain, swelling and tenderness localised usually to the inferior pole of the patella, but occasionally affecting the upper pole (Sinding-Larsen, 1921; Johansson, 1922). Radiographs may show irregular calcification at the upper or lower pole of the patella and the condition is thought to be due to chronic traction strain analogous to Osgood-Schlatter disease of the tibial tubercle. A similar condition occurs in athletic young adults.

Treatment is by avoidance of the precipitating activity. Rarely a period of rest in a plaster of Paris cylinder may be needed. Local injections of prednisolone have also been advocated, but these should not be given into the substance of the patellar tendon because of the risk of subsequent rupture.

Bursitis around the knee

Numerous bursae occur near the knee in relation to the attachments of the various muscles and ligaments (Bywaters, 1979). Many of these bursae communicate constantly or occasionally with the knee joint and are affected by diseases of that joint. Among recognised syndromes are the following.

Prepatellar bursitis

This subcutaneous bursa is present in 90% of people and covers the lower half of the patella and the upper part of the patellar tendon. There may be synovitis in the bursa, with effusion, as part of rheumatoid arthritis or it may be affected by acute gout. Friction due to prolonged kneeling results in fibrous thickening of the bursal wall with effusion ('housemaid's knee'). Treatment is by rest, aspiration and steroid injection. Complete excision of the bursal sac may be needed if there is chronic or recurrent inflammation.

Rarely the bursa is the site of pyogenic or tuberculous infection, which may be associated with osteomyelitis of the patella. The knee joint itself seldom becomes infected. Treatment is by incision and drainage with appropriate chemotherapy. The prepatellar bursa is said to be a common site for gummatous infiltration.

Coalminer's 'beat knee' is a combination of chronic frictional inflammation of the bursa with haemorrhage, and often with secondary pyogenic infection (Sharrard, 1963) and is still a prescribed industrial disease in the UK. It has become rare now that the use of knee-pads is universal in the coal mines.

Infrapatellar bursitis

There are two infrapatellar bursae. The deep infrapatellar bursa lies between the front of the tibia and the back of the lower part of the patellar tendon. It is separated from the synovial cavity of the knee joint by the infrapatellar fat pad. There is occasionally a small, superficial infrapatellar bursa lying subcutaneously in front of the insertion of the patellar tendon. Priests and nuns are said not to get prepatellar bursitis because they kneel in an upright posture, but they are afflicted by infrapatellar bursitis ('clergyman's knee'). Inflamed or infected deep infrapatellar bursitis presents as a tender, fluctuant swelling on either side of the patellar ligament with tenderness on pressure over the ligament itself and pain on movements of the knee, especially on active extension.

Anserine bursitis

The tibial intertendinous bursa lies deep to the combined insertions of the sartorius, gracilis and semitendinosus muscles (the 'pes anserinus') separating them from the medial ligament of the knee and from the upper part of the tibia. It may become inflamed, enlarged and painful (Moschowitz, 1937). Treatment is as for prepatellar bursitis.

Semimembranosus bursitis and popliteal cysts

Of the numerous bursae which have been described behind the knee the most constant is the semimembranosus bursa lying between the medial head of the gastrocnemius and the semimembranosus tendon. It may communicate with other bursae and frequently is in communication with the cavity of the knee joint (Wilson et al, 1938). The bursa may be inflamed and enlarged as a result of frictional irritation, especially in children, in whom communication with the knee joint is uncommon: in adults with osteoarthritis or rheumatoid arthritis involvement of this bursa is usual. Baker (1877) was one of the first to draw attention to the formation of popliteal cysts in association with disease of the knee joint. Baker's cysts, or popliteal cysts, may be formed either by enlargement of the semimembranosus or gastrocnemius bursae, or by direct herniation of synovium from the back of the knee joint. The differential diagnosis includes lipoma, xanthoma, fibrosarcoma, haemangioma and other vascular tumours, varicose veins and lymphadenopathy (Mayerding & Van Demark, 1943).

In children good results are obtained by aspiration and steroid injection or by simple excision. In adults treatment should usually be directed to the accompanying intra-articular pathology (see below in paragraphs on synovial rupture and calf cysts).

Other lesions around the knee

Hoffa's disease
The infrapatellar fat-pad syndrome was described by Hoffa (1904), although other authors have disputed its existence as a separate entity in the absence of traumatic or inflammatory synovitis in the knee joint. The condition often occurs in young people, sometimes after a mild injury. There is tender swelling of the infrapatellar fat-pad with hypertrophy of its intra-articular fringes which are then caught between the articular surfaces of the knee. Laxity of the quadriceps may contribute by failing to draw up the fat-pad during extension. Pain is felt behind the patellar tendon and there may be stiffness and episodes of effusion. True 'locking' does not occur but the knee may give way. Bleeding into the fat-pad can lead to calcification visible on X-ray. The swollen fat-pad results in a fullness on each side of the patellar tendon at the front of the knee with local tenderness.

Treatment is usually conservative with exercises to strengthen the quadriceps muscle. A raise to the heel of the shoe to prevent full extension of the knee while walking may also be helpful. Rarely excision of the prominent, intra-articular fatty folds, or even excision of the whole fat-pad may be necessary.

Torsion, or volvulus, of part of the infrapatellar fat-pad may occur following injury, possibly on the basis of pre-existing hypertrophy and thickening, and can simulate an acute meniscus lesion (Bulmer, 1966). Treatment is by excision of the infarcted tissue.

Osgood–Schlatter disease
Osgood, in 1903, described epiphysitis of the upper end of the tibia in boys, and Schlatter described a similar condition some months later. Also known as 'apophysitis of the tibial tubercle', this condition presents usually in a child aged 10–15 years with pain in the front of the knee after exertion, often with swelling and local tenderness over the tibial tubercle. The pain is accentuated by strong quadriceps contraction. Boys are more frequently affected than girls. Radiographs may show enlargement and fragmentation of the epiphysis of the tibial tubercle (Fig. 60.3). In the past the condition was regarded as an example of juvenile osteochondritis: it is now usually regarded as a simple traction epiphysitis associated with overuse (Smillie, 1980).

In many cases treatment is not required: others may need a reduction in the level of physical activity. If pain is severe the leg should be rested in a plaster of Paris cylinder.

Osgood–Schlatter disease should not be confused with the similar clinical picture which may occur in teenagers and young adults as a result of enthesopathy of the insertion of the patellar tendon due to ankylosing spondylitis (Fig. 60.4) (see also Ch. 29).

Synovitis of superior tibiofibular joint
This synovial joint so seldom causes clinical problems that when it does so the cause of the symptoms tends to be overlooked. It may be involved early in ankylosing spondylitis or other seronegative spondarthritides. Synovial cysts arising from the joint may be a cause of lateral popliteal nerve palsy (Stack et al, 1965). Treatment is with anti-inflammatory drugs and, perhaps, intra-articular steroid injection.

Pellegrini–Stieda disease
Although first described by Köhler in 1903 this condition is usually known by the names of the authors who wrote about it some two years later. It is thought to represent calcification and ossification in a haematoma resulting from partial avulsion of the medial ligament of the knee from the femoral condyle. The alternative name is 'post-traumatic para-articular osteoma'.

Clinically, a period of temporary improvement after an injury is followed by increasing pain and tenderness. The characteristic finding is the ap-

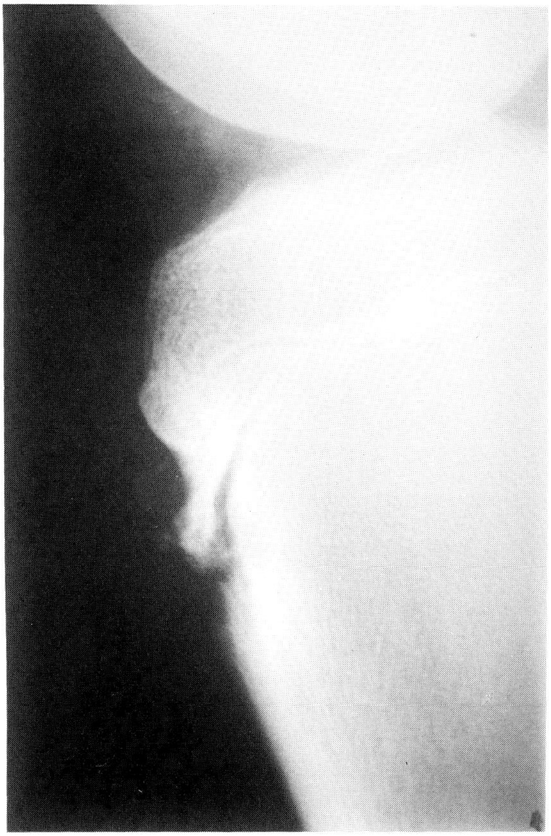

Fig. 60.3 Osgood–Schlatter disease of the tibial tubercle in a 12-year-old boy.

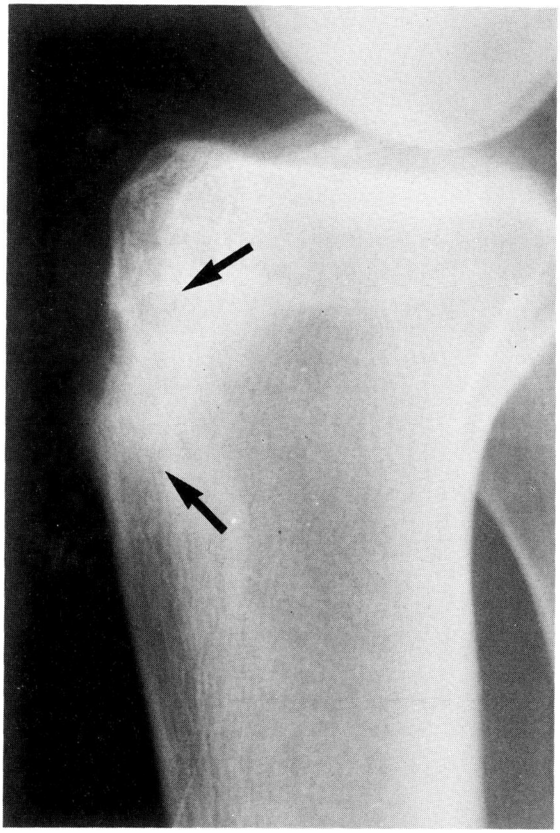

Fig. 60.4 Enthesopathy of the insertion of the patellar tendon in an 18-year-old woman who has ankylosing spondylitis.

pearance on the radiographs of an area of new bone formation, usually semilunar in outline, near the attachment of the medial ligament to the condyle.

Local steroid injections may be helpful if the condition is recognised before ectopic bone has appeared. Otherwise treatment is by muscle strengthening exercises and gradual mobilisation within the limits of pain.

Acute calcification

Acute, painful ligamentous calcification is most commonly seen around the shoulder joint, but it can occur in any ligament and is not uncommon around the knee (Fig. 60.5).

Tendinitis

The tendon of origin of the popliteus muscle arises from the lateral condyle of the femur, and for the first 2.5 cm is intracapsular, being covered on its deep surface by the synovial membrane of the knee joint. Inflammation causes lateral knee pain, and sometimes tenderness.

The tendon of insertion of the biceps muscle is attached to the head of the fibula. It occasionally becomes inflamed, causing pain which is most severe when the knee is actively flexed against resistance.

The tendons of insertion of the other hamstring muscles and their associated bursae may become inflamed, causing pain in the back of the knee. This is said to happen especially as a result of sudden activity without an adequate period of warming up.

LONG LEG SYNDROME

Inequality of leg length from whatever cause, true or apparent, alters the mechanisms of gait and pos-

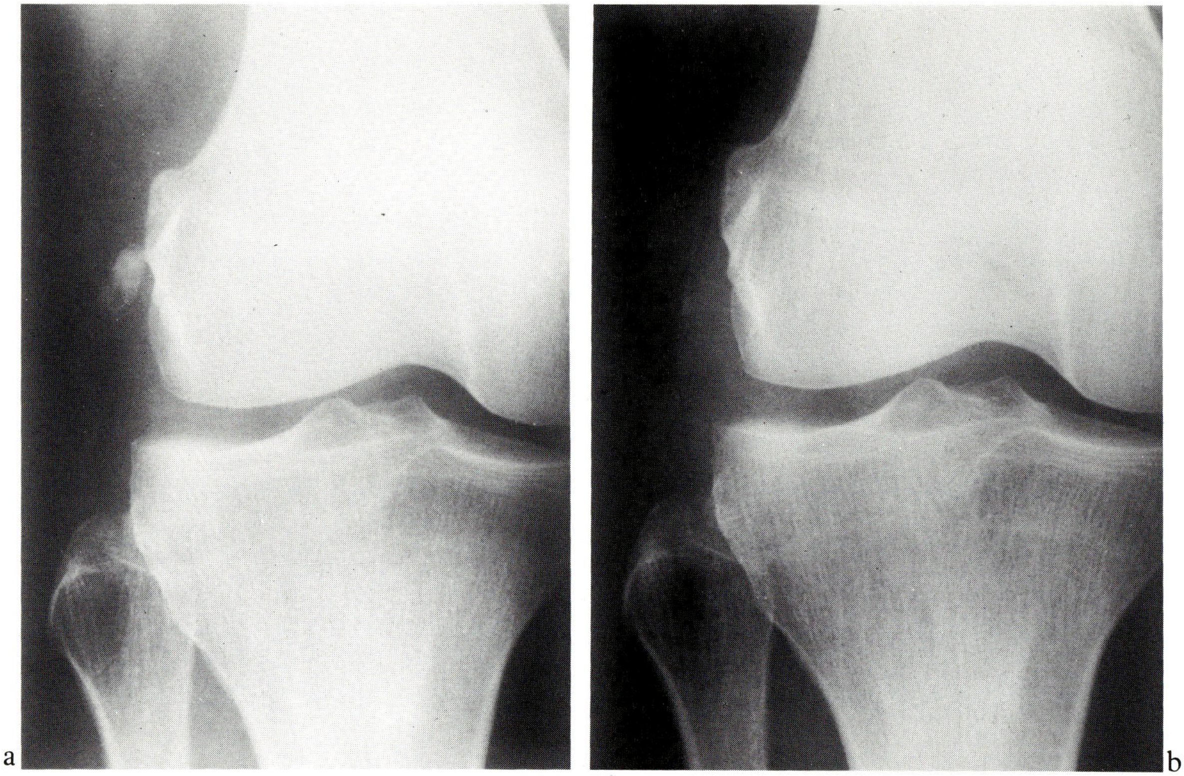

Fig. 60.5 Acute calcification of the lateral ligament of the knee in a 57-year-old woman (a) at presentation with an extremely painful knee (b) 3 weeks later by which time the calcium had resorbed and she was free of pain.

ture. The inequality may arise from congenital deformities or following disease or injury. Synovial inflammation in juvenile chronic arthritis may lead to overgrowth and true lengthening of the more severely affected limb: severe inflammation however is more likely to lead to premature epiphyseal closure and shortening. Disease of the hip with adduction or abduction deformities will lead respectively to apparent shortening or lengthening of the affected leg relative to the other side. Persistent uncorrected leg inequality with compensatory pelvic tilt and lumbar scoliosis may lead to backache and ultimately to premature degenerative changes in the spine resulting from the abnormal stresses.

The knee of the longer leg tends to be held in flexion, even during the stance phase of walking, with consequent abnormal stresses on the lateral compartment. In a knee affected by rheumatoid arthritis this leads to premature collapse of the lateral tibial and femoral condyles. In the previously normal knee, lateral compartment osteoarthritis may be induced (Dixon & Campbell-Smith, 1969; British Medical Journal, 1971).

Uncorrected leg length inequality is similarly associated with increased stress and premature degenerative change in the hip of the longer leg (Gofton & Trueman, 1971).

It is important, therefore, that leg length inequality from whatever cause should be detected and a correction should be applied by building up the shoe of the shorter leg whenever the discrepancy is 1.5 cm or greater. This should be done whether or not the inequality in length is causing symptoms at the time when it is first recognised.

SYNOVIAL RUPTURE AND CALF CYSTS

Deep venous thrombosis in the calf is a potentially dangerous condition, which, when untreated, carries a risk of pulmonary embolism and of chronic swelling of the leg. Unnecessary anticoagulation is also hazardous: this is particularly so if anticoagulants are given to patients who, at the same time, need to take non-steroid anti-inflammatory drugs or oral corticosteroids, who may be anaemic, and who are prone to peptic ulceration. Synovial rupture, with leakage of inflammatory synovial fluid from the knee into the tissues of the calf may result in symptoms and physical signs which are indistinguishable from those of deep venous thrombosis (Katz et al, 1977).

Intra-articular pressure

In a normal subject lying horizontally, at rest, with the leg extended and the muscles relaxed, the intra-articular pressure in the knee joint is similar to or slightly below atmospheric pressure (Jayson & Dixon, 1970a; Levick, 1979). Strong isometric contraction of the quadriceps may result in a negative intra-articular pressure as great as −100 mmHg (Jayson & Dixon, 1970b). If an effusion is present, however, or if the joint is artificially distended with saline or with plasma, there is a slight positive pressure at rest, and a similar contraction of the quadriceps will raise intra-articular pressure to greater than 300 mmHg (Caughey & Bywaters, 1963). A large effusion will inhibit quadriceps contraction. Flexion of the knee in the presence of an effusion may result in even higher intra-articular pressures, up to 1000 mmHg. The mean pressures induced are higher in rheumatoid patients than in healthy control subjects (Jayson & Dixon, 1970b). Pressures of these levels have resulted in rupture of the knee joint, both in cadaver experiments (Dixon & Grant, 1964) and in healthy and rheumatoid volunteers. Rupture usually occurs posteriorly where the capsule is weak between the attachments medially of the semimembranosus and semitendinosus muscles and the medial head of gastrocnemius. Occasionally a pre-existing popliteal cyst may rupture. Rupture of the suprapatellar pouch is uncommon.

Synovial rupture

Rupture of the knee joint presents with pain and stiffness in the muscles of the calf, followed by swelling and tenderness with pitting oedema around the ankle (Dixon, 1964; Good, 1964). An acute onset is usual, but occasionally the symptoms develop gradually. The patient is sometimes aware of an episode of sudden pain in the back of the knee, or of a sensation of something having 'given way' in the popliteal fossa. More commonly the initial symptoms start in the calf. Homan's sign is usually positive. By the time the patient seeks medical advice there is seldom a tense effusion in the knee joint; but there may be a history of swelling of the knee, or of a popliteal swelling, which has diminished as the calf has become painful.

Synovial rupture is a common complication of inflammatory joint disease; but it occurs in osteoarthritis and has been recorded in subjects who had no history of preceeding abnormality in the knee (Kilcoyne et al, 1978; Macfarlane & Bacon, 1980). In such patients confusion with venous thrombosis is even more likely. Synovial rupture may occur late in the course of rheumatoid arthritis and there may be more than one episode in the same patient. Rupture is more likely to occur, however, when the joint has only recently been affected by the disease, and before significant fibrosis of the capsule has occurred. Patients with rheumatoid arthritis may first present for medical advice because of synovial rupture.

The escaping synovial fluid in inflammatory arthritis is rich in leucocytes, enzymes and inflammatory mediators. This fluid tracking through the tissues of the calf results in pain, tenderness and oedema extending to the ankle. The overlying skin may be warm, and sometimes redness and pitting oedema extend anteriorly to the subcutaneous surface of the tibia. Synovial rupture occurring in septic arthritis has even more serious consequences (Hall & Healy, 1968; Richards, 1981). Bleeding at the time of rupture may also contribute to inflammation in the calf.

Haemorrhage into the calf muscles, due to a torn muscle, or a bleeding disorder, may cause symptoms and signs similar to those of synovial rupture. In such a case as blood tracks down through the calf, bruising may appear around the ankle: this sign is not always present, and its absence cannot be relied on as excluding haemorrhage (Fig. 60.6).

Calf cysts

Cysts in the calf often lie in the intermuscular planes, usually between gastrocnemius and soleus,

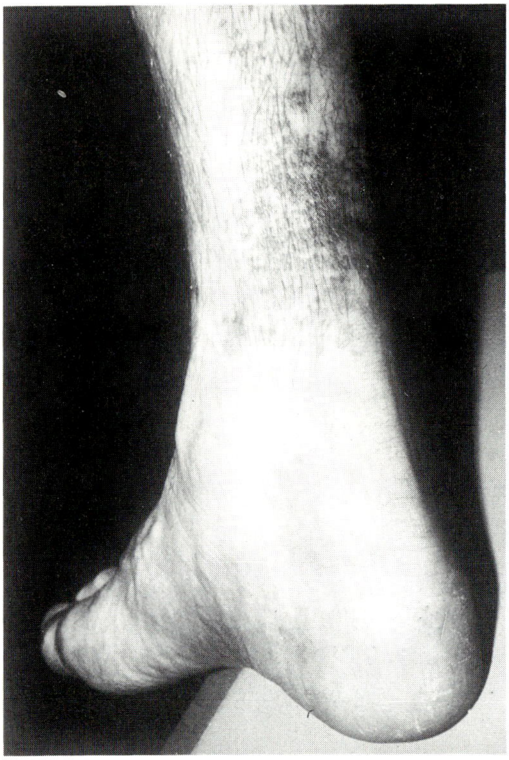

Fig. 60.6 Subcutaneous bruising above the ankle in a middle-aged man who had complained of sudden pain and swelling in the calf.

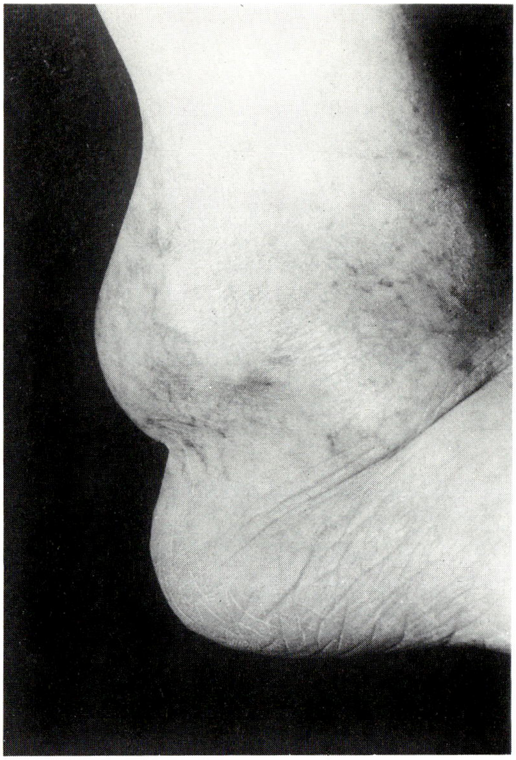

Fig. 60.7 Cystic swelling presenting at the back of the ankle in a 53-year-old woman with rheumatoid arthritis for 11 years. Investigation showed this to be the continuation of a calf cyst in communication with the knee joint.

but occasionally deep to soleus. They most commonly present as a tender swelling in the mid-calf (Beatty, 1959). Occasionally the cyst extends down to the level of the Achilles tendon and may present as a fluctuant cystic swelling at the ankle (Fig. 60.7). Rarely a cyst may extend proximally between the muscles of the thigh (Hench et al, 1966). Cysts may arise by enlargement and extension of a pre-existing popliteal cyst and be lined by synovium. Alternatively, recurrent or chronic synovial leakage may result in loculation of fluid with formation of a pseudocyst lined by nonspecific fibrous and inflammatory tissue (Harvey & Corcos, 1960). Occasionally such a cyst forms after a single episode of synovial rupture. These collections of fluid may seal off and form an isolated cyst in the calf. More commonly the cyst remains in continuity with the synovial cavity of the knee joint. The cyst is filled with fluid which resembles synovial fluid and frequently contains large masses of fibrin clot (Taylor, 1969).

If the intra-articular pressure in the knee increases, so does the pressure within the cyst. In contrast, when the knee is aspirated pressure within the cyst remains unaltered. Arthrography shows that fluid under pressure will usually pass from the knee joint into the cyst; but it is rarely possible to demonstrate the passage into the knee of contrast medium injected into the cyst. Jayson & Dixon (1970c) have postulated the presence of a valvular mechanism which allows fluid to be pumped from the knee to the cyst, but not to return. Such an arrangement may act as a safety-valve, preventing the development of very high intra-articular pressures (Genovese et al, 1972).

Investigation of calf cysts and synovial rupture

It is sometimes possible to establish the diagnosis of synovial rupture on the history and physical examination alone. When there is doubt, arthrography is a simple procedure which will usually confirm synovial leakage or the presence of a cyst (Hall & Scott, 1966); though if arthrography is delayed for some days after an acute rupture, then healing may prevent demonstration of the leak. A water-soluble radio-opaque dye is injected into the knee joint and it is usually necessary for the patient to exercise after injection of the contrast medium either by quadriceps contractions, walking or gentle knee flexion. Facilities for screening are helpful but are not essential, for plain X-ray films before and after exercise can give all the necessary information. Contrast medium outlining a cyst has a well-defined margin and usually shows filling defects due to fibrin clot. The shadow of fluid leaking along tissue planes typically has an ill-defined, feathery margin.

Ultrasonic scanning is helpful in showing the presence of a cyst in the popliteal fossa or calf (Meire et al, 1974); but it does not reliably demonstrate synovial rupture and leakage when there is no loculation of fluid or cyst formation.

Coexisting thrombosis and synovial rupture

Unfortunately, positive findings on arthrography or ultrasonic scanning do not entirely exclude coexisting deep vein thrombosis (Prescott et al, 1978; Gordon et al, 1979; Simpson et al, 1980; Belch et al, 1981). For this reason venography may be preferred to arthrography as the initial investigation. In the absence of thrombophlebitis the venogram may show distortion of the peroneal or popliteal veins due to extrinsic pressure exerted by fluid or by a cyst in the calf. This pressure on the veins often causes a reduced venous blood flow, which may be wrongly interpreted as indicating thrombosis, if ultrasonic scanning using the Doppler technique is relied on to support the diagnosis. Radio-iodine-labelled fibrinogen studies may also give false positive results (Gibbons et al, 1975), due probably to the presence of clot and fibrin in the calf, which wrongly suggest thrombosis.

Management of synovial rupture and synovial cysts

Usually all that is required to control acute or recurrent synovial leakage is conservative treatment to reduce the volume and pressure of fluid in the knee joint.

Following an episode of synovial rupture, or following an increase in pain and tension within a cyst in the calf, the limb should be rested, on a splint if necessary, together with the administration of simple analgesics. Residual effusion in the knee should be aspirated; and if there is active synovitis then an intra-articular injection of steroid should be given. Aspiration of the cyst alone is usually unhelpful, and if there is still an effusion in the knee the cyst will refill within a few hours or days. Steroid injected directly into the knee will pass into the cyst but not in the opposite direction.

If conservative treatment fails then anterior synovectomy of the knee joint may be needed. Operation on the cyst, or on the back of the knee joint, is rarely indicated. If the synovitis is controlled, or after anterior synovectomy, most popliteal and calf cysts will regress (Jayson et al, 1972; Pinder, 1973). Excision of the cyst alone without treatment directed against the synovitis in the knee joint is unsatisfactory and leads to recurrence of the cyst (Harvey & Corcos, 1960) or even to failure to heal with fistula formation (Bennett et al, 1972).

ANTERIOR TIBIAL COMPARTMENT SYNDROME

The anterior tibial compartment syndrome has been well documented since it was first described by P R Vogt in 1943 in an unpublished communication to the Oregon State Medical Society. Its main feature is pain in the muscles of the anterior compartment of the leg due to ischaemic necrosis (Leach et al, 1967).

Pain in the anterior tibial muscles, sometimes accompanied by local crepitus, is not uncommon during or after unaccustomed exercise, but is relieved quickly by resting. The anterior tibial syndrome occurs usually in healthy but physically untrained young men in association with strenuous exercise of the leg muscles, such as marching or running. Pain starts during or shortly after exertion, but may be delayed for several hours. It is dull and aching at first but increases in severity until there is intense pain in the front of the leg. The pain is accentuated by any movement, active or passive, of the leg or foot, and is not relieved by rest or elevation. The pretibial muscles become tender and swollen with increased local temperature and redness of the overlying skin. The dorsiflexors of the foot and toes become paralysed, starting usually with the tibialis anterior and extensor hallucis muscles, but sometimes sparing extensor digitorum longus. Contracture of the affected muscles often prevents foot drop. The anterior tibial nerve may be damaged, resulting in weakness of extensor digitorum brevis and sensory loss on the dorsum of the foot in the region of the first interdigital cleft. Circulation in the anterior tibial artery is usually intact and preservation of the dorsalis pedis pulse does not exclude the syndrome. The patient may be febrile and frequently the blood neutrophil count is raised, features which may suggest an erroneous diagnosis of cellulitis.

The syndrome may develop with rapidity. If effective treatment is to be undertaken before irreversible muscle necrosis has occurred, then early clinical diagnosis is essential without awaiting the results of laboratory investigations. As soon as muscle weakness has developed, surgical decompression of the anterior tibial compartment by a wide fasciotomy becomes urgent. The deep fascia should be incised from just below the level of the tibial tubercle down to the level of the extensor retinaculum at the ankle. As the fascia is opened the swollen muscles bulge through. If these muscles are pinkish-white and flush when decompressed, then recovery is likely: but grey and obviously necrotic muscle should be excised. The sooner that operation is carried out after the onset of symptoms the greater is the expectation of recovery.

The aetiology of this syndrome is obscure. It is assumed that swelling of muscles results from the stress of unaccustomed exercise, and that the subsequent rise in pressure in the closed anterior compartment leads to obstruction of capillary circulation. Consequent ischaemic damage institutes a vicious cycle of increasing swelling and tension which can only be relieved by decompression. Recent observations regarding the greater severity of microscopic damage to untrained muscle used in extrinsic contraction may be relevant. A similar syndrome may also occur in cases in which there is a demonstrable arterial lesion due to embolism, thrombosis or injury.

STRESS FRACTURES OF THE TIBIA AND FIBULA

Stress fractures, particularly near the junction of the upper and middle thirds, are a not uncommon cause of 'shin splints' in athletes (especially distance runners and joggers) and in military recruits. Local bone tenderness may give a clue to the diagnosis. Radionucleotide bone scanning may identify the lesion at a time before the conventional radiographs show abnormality (Fig. 60.8).

Patients who have longstanding rheumatoid arthritis are likely to be osteoporotic; if systemic steroids have been given the severity of the osteoporosis is increased. Such patients are liable to insufficiency fractures, not only in the spine, pubic rami and femur, but also in the tibia and fibula. The typical late deformities in the rheumatoid knee, of fixed flexion, valgus and external rotation, pose abnormal stresses on the leg during weight-bearing, and these stresses are increased if, as is so often the case, there is an accompanying valgus deformity of the ankle and hind-foot. Stress/insufficiency fractures are common in such patients and repeated fractures are the rule

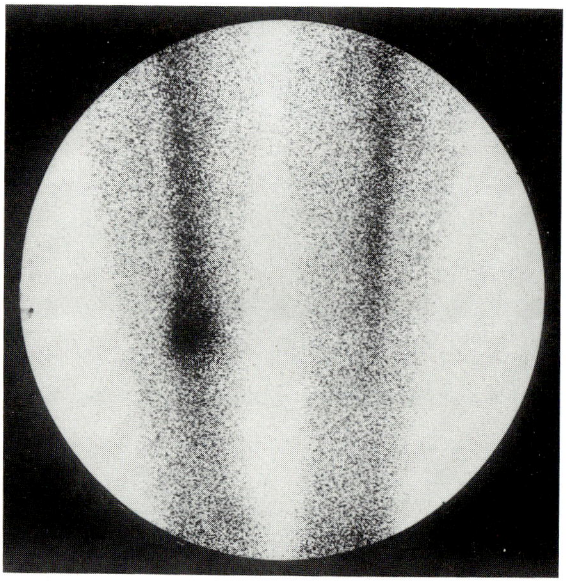

Fig. 60.8 Stress fracture of the tibia of a professional football player demonstrated by scintiscan at a time when the conventional X-ray showed no abnormality (by courtesy of Mr J. P. Jackson).

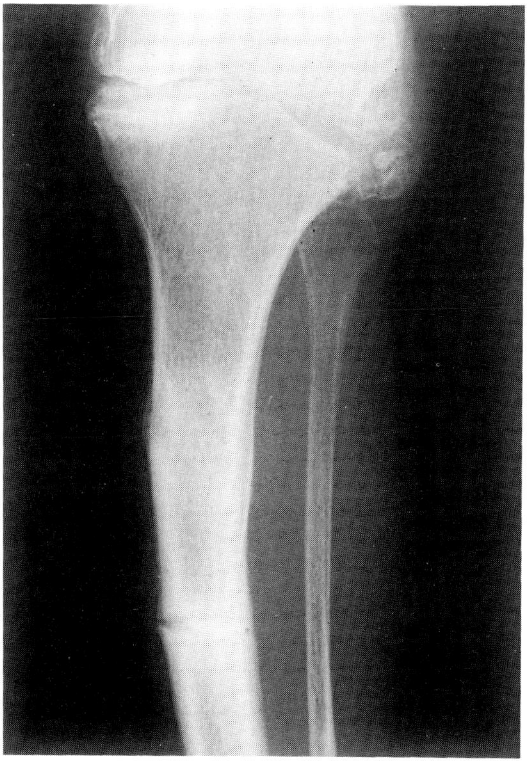

Fig. 60.9 Multiple stress fractures of the tibia of a 48-year-old woman with longstanding rheumatoid arthritis. She had never been treated with corticosteroids.

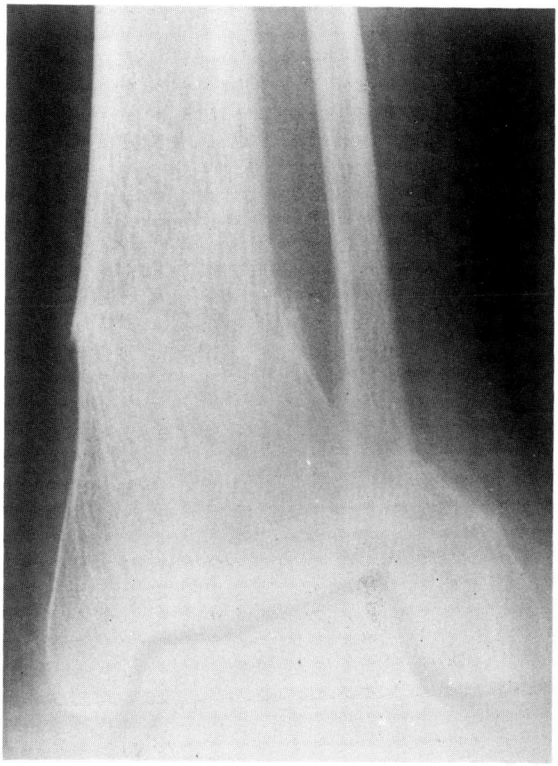

Fig. 60.10 Insufficiency fracture of the tibia and fibula above the ankle in a 52-year-old woman with longstanding rheumatoid arthritis and osteoporosis. She complained of increasing pain in her ankle for 3 weeks so that she had become barely able to stand.

(Fig. 60.9). A series of unrecognised and uncorrected incomplete fractures may readily result in a gradually increasing valgus bowing within the tibia itself, thus increasing the abnormal stresses and increasing the difficulty of subsequent reconstructive surgery. These fractures often develop insidiously, and if situated near the ankle or knee the pain which they engender may readily be mistaken for an exacerbation of pain arising from the nearby joint (Fig. 60.10).

INTERMITTENT CLAUDICATION

Arterial insufficiency as a result of peripheral vascular disease characteristically causes cramp-like pain in the leg muscles, induced by walking. After a certain distance the patient, usually a man, is forced to stop by pain; but after a few minutes rest he is able to walk on again for a similar distance. Although the calf is the most common site for the pain, the precise location of pain depends on the vessels involved. Ischaemic pain in the buttocks and Leriche's syndrome are discussed earlier in this chapter. The patient may complain of 'arthritis', but there will usually be objective evidence of impaired arterial circulation.

Neurogenic intermittent claudication results from ischaemia of the cauda equina on exercise, associated usually with spinal stenosis (see Ch. 57.). Aching pain in the legs on exertion is accompanied usually by numbness and tingling, and sometimes by overt muscle weakness. The symptoms are eased by rest and relief is usually increased by flexing the lumbar spine: the patient may therefore stop and pretend to retie his shoelace.

PAINFUL ANKLE AND HEEL

Lesions of the Achilles tendon

Complete and incomplete rupture
Rupture of the Achilles tendon is usually complete and occurs predominantly in middle-age following a sudden plantar-flexion force of the foot. At the moment of rupture the patient feels a sharp pain, as if he were struck from behind. Indeed, patients not infrequently complain of being kicked. Immediately, there is a visible defect as the ends of the tendon retract; but after 24 hours or so the intact tendon sheath may be distended by haematoma and the lesion presents as a tender swelling of the tendon. The diagnosis is often missed, but palpation will usually reveal the defect, and despite continuity of the tendon sheath there will be weakness of plantar-flexion of the foot.

In younger patients there is more likely to be an incomplete rupture near the musculotendinous junction. It is likely that pains in the calf attributed to rupture of the plantaris tendon are in fact due to incomplete rupture of the Achilles tendon.

A recent rupture should be repaired surgically. Conservative treatment with the foot immobilised in plantar flexion also gives reasonable results, but there is a risk of re-rupture (Gilles & Chalmers, 1970).

Heterotopic calcification and osseous metaplasia have both been described in the Achilles tendon. Opinions differ as to whether such changes are the cause or the effect of rupture (Fisher & Woods, 1970).

Peritendinitis
This is a common cause of chronic pain in the back of the heel occurring primarily, but not exclusively, in athletes. There may be diffuse swelling and tenderness on both sides of the tendon. Often there is crepitus.

Treatment is by rest and by steroid infiltration into the paratenon — but *not* into the tendon itself, because of the risk of inducing rupture. In chronic cases operation has been suggested with stripping of the paratenon.

Bursitis

Retrocalcaneal bursitis
The Achilles tendon is inserted into the middle of the posterior surface of the calcaneum. The retrocalcaneal (subachilles) bursa is interposed and may become inflamed as a result of overuse or injury, or as part of a generalised synovitis. Pain is accentuated by dorsiflexion of the foot, and the bulging, tender bursa can be palpated on each side of the tendon. Treatment is as for prepatellar bursitis.

Postcalcaneal bursitis
Inflammation of this small subcutaneous, and probably adventitious, bursa results from friction as a result of poorly fitting footwear, and when there is a prominence of underlying bone is one cause of 'pump bumps'. The swelling is lower down on the heel over the insertion of the tendon and there is often chafing or inflammation of the overlying skin.

Calcaneal epiphysitis

The insertion of the Achilles tendon into the calcaneal epiphysis may become inflamed, usually in boys aged between 9 and 15, causing pain and tenderness behind the heel. Most of these cases are related to trauma or repeated strain and the occurrence of an avascular necrosis of the epiphysis (Sever's disease) is now doubted. Radiographs of the normal calcaneum frequently show several dense ossification centres in the epiphysis.

Enthesopathy in ankylosing spondylitis causes similar symptoms, occasionally with an erosion of the calcaneum.

Tenosynovitis

Tenosynovitis may occur in any of the dorsal or flexor tendon sheaths around the ankle, particularly in rheumatoid arthritis. Idiopathic tenosynovitis may also occur (Parvin & Ford, 1956). These lesions usually respond well to steroid injection into the tendon sheath.

Ligamentous injuries

Sprains of the ankle result usually from a forced inversion injury causing damage to one or several of the components of the lateral ligament. Injury to the medial ligament is less common. Acute sprains are treated by immobilisation, or if severe in a young subject, by open repair. Chronic strain of the lateral ligament is seen in middle-aged women who complain that the ankle is weak and gives way under them. If radiographs with varus and valgus stress fail to demonstrate a major ligamentous defect with instability, then treatment is by intensive muscle re-education, including exercises on the wobble-board (Leach et al, 1981).

Occasionally a 'weak ankle' may be the consequence of a peroneal entrapment neuropathy (Sidey, 1969).

Pain under the heel

Tender heel pad
Though there is seldom a history of trauma this may be the result of a simple contusion. Pain is felt on weight-bearing and may persist for weeks or months. There is usually a local tender spot, often not in the midline. The wearing of a sponge rubber insole, excavated so as to avoid pressure at the point of maximum tenderness, may help. Local infiltration with steroid is painful but is sometimes effective.

Plantar fasciitis and calcaneal spur
The pain and point of maximum tenderness are more anterior and in the midline over the attachment of the plantar fascia to the calcaneum. Pain may arise as an isolated feature or as part of a generalised disease. In seronegative spondarthritis, and occasionally in rheumatoid arthritis, there may be erosion of bone at the fascial attachment. The presence of a plantar spur is of little significance, unless serial radiographs show that it has arisen by healing of such an erosion. Irregular periostitis is a feature of Reiter's disease.

Treatment is by rest, sponge rubber insoles and non-steroid anti-inflammatory drugs.

Painful os calcis
The calcaneum itself may be painful on weight-bearing in osteoporotic patients, especially in active young patients with metabolic bone disease or in older patients with conditions such as myelomatosis. Stress fractures of the calcaneum result from overuse (Leabhart, 1959). The calcaneum is composed almost entirely of trabecular bone, and stress fractures may be difficult to detect: a bone scan may reveal lesions which are not apparent on conventional radiographs. Fractures of the normal os calcis as a result of a fall from a height may not cause obvious deformity and may also be overlooked. Such undetected fractures may later provoke painful subtalar arthritis.

Hypertrophic osteoarthropathy
Hypertrophic pulmonary osteoarthropathy is the combination of finger clubbing, painful tender swelling of joints and periosteal new bone formation which sometimes accompanies intrapulmonary or inflammatory bowel disease. The wrists and ankles are particularly affected; but in severe cases there may be diffuse tarsal and metatarsal involvement. There may be synovitis with effusion which is often intermittent and the overlying skin may be red and warm. In addition to finger clubbing and signs of constitutional illness, there is usually tenderness of the long bones adjacent to the joints (Holling, 1967).

Thyroid acropachy is a rare condition which may present a similar picture, though affecting primarily the digits (Gimlette 1960) and often accompanied by pretibial myxoedema. Children may be affected (Thomas et al, 1973) (see Ch. 39).

THE PAINFUL FOOT

The human foot has become greatly specialised to provide balance and a stable support for body weight while standing: in addition it provides a spring or lever by which the body is propelled forwards. These objectives are fulfilled by the grouping together of a number of small, spongy, elastic bones, supported in a series of resilient arches by muscular function and the plantar fascia. Rose (1979) has described the foot as being functionally like a six-legged stool (that is, a three-legged stool with additional support from the toes between two of its legs) in which one leg, the calcaneum, is posterior with the other five legs, the metatarsal rays, being anterior. The talus is balanced on this stool and transmits body weight through the subtalar joint. Pronation or supination at the subtalar joint are accompanied respectively by flattening or increasing height of the medial longitudinal arch.

Clinical examination of the painful foot should include examination of the shoes for abnormal wear. The joints of the foot and ankle complex should be tested individually for tenderness and passive range of movement. The posture of the foot should be noted at rest, on weight-bearing and during walking, as should the ability of the patient to walk on tip-toe and on the heel with the toes off the ground. Careful neurological examination and inspection of the blood supply and skin may be needed.

Lesions of the mid-foot

Midtarsal arthritis

The midtarsal joint may be involved as part of a generalised inflammatory arthropathy or by osteoarthritis. Osteoarthritis in middle-age may result from previous injury to the ankle. The development of midtarsal osteoarthritis in a young adult should raise suspicion of a developmental abnormality such as a calcaneal bar (calcaneonavicular bar).

If the foot falls into a valgus position during prolonged standing, as a result of poor muscle control and obesity, midtarsal pain will result. If not corrected this may, over a number of years, lead to midtarsal osteoarthritis. Postural exercises usually lead to improvement and long-arch supports are usually indicated only when there is weakness.

An exostosis or osteophyte at the joint between the navicular and the cuneiform may become painful due to excessive friction with the formation of a bursa. The prominent bone may need to be excised.

Köhler's disease

Köhler's disease is a form of osteochondritis affecting the tarsal navicular in young children. There is pain and swelling in the midtarsal region with tenderness over the navicular. Radiographs show increased density of the navicular which is compressed from before backwards. Sometimes the bone has a fragmented appearance. Evolution continues for 2 years or so before there is gradual resolution. It is not possible to protect the foot from weight-bearing for the whole of this period, but immobilisation in a walking cast for 2 or 3 months usually relieves the pain. A few patients develop talonavicular osteoarthritis in later years.

Stress fractures

Stress fractures of the tarsal navicular occur, predominantly in male athletes (Torg et al, 1982).

Flat foot

Mobile flat foot

Many children and many athletes stand at rest with an apparent flat foot. A flat foot which is mobile, strong and painless, and which has good toe action is a normal foot.

Rigid flat foot

A rigid flat foot is one in which the long arch cannot be restored by muscle action. There is often loss of alignment between the tarsal bones and secondary osteoarthritis may develop. Many patients can be relieved by active foot exercises and the use of a valgus support in well-fitting shoes. In severe cases talonavicular, naviculocuneiform or talocalcaneal arthrodesis may be necessary.

Spasmodic flat foot

Peroneal or spasmodic flat foot is one in which there is spasm of the peroneal muscles resulting in an eversion deformity of the foot. The onset is often after starting work which involves much standing so that the condition is sometimes known as 'apprentice's foot'. It may be associated either with developmental abnormalities and intertarsal bridges (e.g. calcaneonavicular bar) or with acquired inflammatory states and occupational strains (Outland & Murphy, 1960). Oblique tarsal radiographs may reveal a bony bridge — but occasionally the bar is a synchondrosis, when the appearance is of incomplete bony bridging.

Treatment of intertarsal bridging is surgical. Even in children, however, excision of the bar alone may not be sufficient and localised arthrodesis may also be necessary.

Pes cavus

Pes cavus, or claw-foot, may be familial or idiopathic and does not always signify an underlying neurological abnormality. Nevertheless two-thirds have some degree of neurological involvement (Brewerton et al, 1962) and claw-foot is the typical deformity in minimal poliomyelitis, peroneal muscular atrophy and Friedreich's ataxia. The development of a cavus foot for the first time in a teenager, during the growth spurt, indicates the need for a careful search for evidence of diastematomyelia or other spinal abnormality.

The intrinsic muscles of the foot normally flex the metatarsophalangeal joint and extend the interphalangeal joints. When they are paralysed or weak the forefoot drops and the unopposed action of the extrinsic muscles results in increased arching of the foot, with clawing of the toes and contracture of the plantar fascia. There may be also some adduction and inversion of the forefoot with a tendency to secondary contracture of the Achilles tendon.

Many cases required no treatment. Surgical correction of the claw-toes reduces disability arising from corns and callouses and makes the choice of footwear easier. Severe cases may merit more radical bone and tendon surgery.

Metatarsal pain

Hallux valgus and hallux rigidus
Faulty shoes are the biggest single cause of problems with the forefoot. Congenital abnormalities (metatarsus primus varus and metatarsus brevis) may account for some cases of hallux valgus, but the majority result from deformities induced by compression of the toes during childhood and adolescence. Hallux valgus is rare among peoples who habitually walk barefoot (Wilson, 1980).

In middle-age flattening of the anterior arch and splaying of the forefoot is common and the pull of the tendons tends to inrease the valgus deformity of the big toe. An inflamed bunion may add to the discomfort. The first metatarsophalangeal joint is especially prone to minor trauma with the development of secondary osteoarthritis. When this leads to a stiff and painful joint the condition is called 'hallux rigidus'.

In minor cases removal of an exostosis underlying the bunion may be all that is needed. Temporary relief in hallux rigidus may be obtained by the fitting of a metatarsal-bar on the outside of the sole of the shoe. Numerous reconstructive operations have been advocated for hallux valgus (Wilson, 1980).

March fracture
This is a stress fracture of one of the metatarsal necks, usually the 2nd, causing local pain and tenderness. It is suggested that there is an underlying abnormality in that the affected metatarsal may be abnormally long. The typical callus around the fracture site may not be apparent on the radiographs at first. The condition often develops after prolonged walking or marching.

Treatment is by immobilisation in a walking plaster until pain has been relieved.

Freiberg's disease
Also known as 'Köhler's disease of the metatarsal head', and as 'Freiberg's Infraction', this condition presents with pain in the forefoot, often severe, followed by flattening and broadening of the affected metatarsal head. Again the 2nd metatarsal is most commonly affected, less often the 3rd. The condition usually occurs in children but is seen in adults. It is usually regarded as being a form of osteochondritis.

During the acute phase, support in a walking plaster may be needed.

Morton's metatarsalgia
This is usually caused by a plantar digital neuroma arising in the cleft between the 3rd and 4th, or sometimes the 2nd and 3rd, toes. There may be intense local pain on weight-bearing with paraesthesiae and sensory disturbance in the affected toes. Similar symptoms arise from pressure on the digital nerve by a synovial cyst or bursa (Bossley & Cairney, 1980).

Rheumatoid arthritis
It should be remembered that metatarsal pain may be a presenting feature in rheumatoid arthritis. If pain is confined to the forefoot, diagnosis of the underlying inflammatory disease may be delayed.

Other causes of foot pain

Chilblains (lupus pernio) have become relatively uncommon now that central heating in cars and buildings is almost universal. Nevertheless they may still present as a cause of painful red swollen digits.

Peripheral neuritis, due to diabetes, alcoholism, or other causes, may present with pain in the foot. Patients with diabetes may develop neuropathic arthritis, often in the midtarsal joints. Ischaemia may also cause intractable pain in the foot. This is commonly due to atheromatous peripheral vascular disease, but iliac artery occlusion due to rheumatoid vasculitis has been reported (Rudge et al, 1981). More commonly vasculitis presents with local cutaneous or digital infarcts.

Sudeck's atrophy

This is an ill-understood vascular disturbance, possibly due to an abnormality of autonomic nerve function. In the foot it causes burning pain at rest associated with a sequence of dystrophic skin changes and the development of marked osteoporosis in the bones of the foot. During the acute phase the foot may be warm and swollen, later it is cold and contracted. This chronic painful condition may be triggered by minor trauma.

An apparently similar condition affecting the knee or ankle is known as transient osteoporosis and may recover over a period of months.

REFERENCES

Aichroth P M 1984 Dislocation of the patella. In: Jackson J P, Waugh W (eds) Surgery of the knee joint. Chapman & Hall, London, Ch. 8, p. 192–209

Baker W M 1877 On the Formation of synovial cysts in the leg in connection with disease of the knee joint. St Bartholomew's Hospital Reports 13: 245–261

Baylan S P, Paik S W, Barnert A L, Ko K H, Yu J, Persellin R H 1981 Prevalence of the tarsal tunnel syndrome in rheumatoid arthritis. Rheumatology and Rehabilitation 20: 148–150

Beatty D C 1959 Rheumatoid cysts in the calf. Proceedings of the Royal Society of Medicine 52: 1106–1108

Belch J J F, McMillan N C, Fogelman I, Capell H, Forbes C D 1981 Combined phlebography and arthrography in patients with painful swollen calf. British Medical Journal 282:949

Bennett R M, Hughes G V R, Bywaters E G L, Holt P J L 1972 Studies of a popliteal synovial fistula. Annals of the Rheumatic Diseases 31: 482–486

Bentley G 1978 The Surgical treatment of chondromalacia patellae. Journal of Bone and Joint Surgery 60B: 74–81

Bentley G, Leslie I J, Fischer D 1981 Effect of aspirin treatment on chondromalacia patellae. Annals of the Rheumatic Diseases 40: 37–41

Biemond A 1970 Femoral neuropathy. In: Vinken P J, Bruyn G W (eds) Handbook of clinical neurology, Vol 8. Diseases of Nerves, Part II. American Elsevier, New York

Bossley C J, Cairney P C 1980 The intermetatarsophalangeal Bursa — Its significance in Morton's metatarsalgia. Journal of Bone and Joint Surgery 62B: 184–187

Brewerton D A, Sandifer P, Sweetnam R 1962 Pes cavus. Journal of Bone and Joint Surgery 44B:741

British Medical Journal 1971 Leading article — Short leg syndrome. British Medical Journal 1:245

British Medical Journal 1981 Leading article — Chondromalacia patellae. British Medical Journal 282:1014

Bulmer J H 1966 Torsion of the infrapatellar fat pad. British Medical Journal 2:628

Bywaters E G L 1979 Lesions of bursae, tendons and tendon sheaths. Clinics in Rheumatic Diseases 5: 893–926

Bywaters E G L, Ansell B M 1965 Monoarticular arthritis in children. Annals of the Rheumatic Diseases 24: 116–122

Caughey D E, Bywaters E G L 1963 Joint fluid pressure in chronic knee effusions. Annals of the Rheumatic Diseases 22: 106–109

Cochrane G M 1971 Osteitis pubis in athletes. British Journal of Sports Medicine 5: 233–235

Collins D H 1949 The pathology of articular and spinal disorders. Arnold, London

Coventry M B, Mitchell W C 1961 Osteitis pubis. Observations based on a study of 45 patients. Journal of the American Medical Association 178: 898–905

Coventry M B, Polley H F, Weiner A D 1959 Rheumatoid cysts of the hip: Report of three cases. Journal of Bone and Joint Surgery 41A: 721–730

Crosby E B, Insall J 1976 Recurrent dislocation of the patella. Relation of treatment to osteoarthritis. Journal of Bone and Joint Surgery 58A: 9–13

Darracott J, Vernon-Roberts B 1971 The bony changes in chondromalacia patellae. Rheumatology and Physical Medicine 11: 175–179

DiStefano V, Sack J T, Whittaker R, Nixon J E 1972 Tarsal-tunnel syndrome. Review of the literature and two case reports. Clinical Orthopaedics and Related Research 88: 76–79

Dixon A St J 1964 Acute rupture of the knee in rheumatoid arthritis. Proceedings of the Royal Society of Medicine 57: 1129–1130

Dixon A St J, Campbell-Smith S 1969 Long leg arthropathy. Annals of the Rheumatic Diseases 28: 359–364

Dixon A St J, Grant C 1964 Acute synovial rupture in rheumatoid arthritis. Clinical and experimental observations. Lancet 1: 742–745

Donovan M S, Sosman M C 1942 Tuberculosis of the greater trochanter and its bursa. American Journal of Roentgenology 48: 719–725

Fearn C B d'A 1968 Iliacus haematoma syndrome as a complication of anticoagulant therapy. British Medical Journal 2: 97–98

Ficat R P, Hungerford D S 1977 Disorders of the patello-femoral joint. Williams & Wilkins: Baltimore.

Fisher T R, Woods C G 1970 Partial rupture of the tendo calcaneus with heterotopic ossification. Journal of Bone and Joint Surgery 52B: 334–336

Fletcher M R, Scott J T 1975 Chronic monarticular synovitis. Diagnostic and prognostic features. Annals of the Rheumatic Diseases 34: 171–176

Ford M J, Martynoga A G, Nuki G 1981 Iliopsoas bursitis in rheumatoid arthritis: An unusual cause of leg oedema. British Medical Journal 282: 947–948

Fraser I 1932 A very large bursa. Lancet 1: 290–291

Genovese G R, Jayson M I V, Dixon A St J 1972 Protective value of synovial cysts in rheumatoid knees. Annals of the Rheumatic Diseases 31: 179–182

Gibbons D, Phillips M, Prossor I M 1975 Ruptured popliteal cyst simulating deep vein thrombosis with false positive radiofibrinogen uptake. Postgraduate Medical Journal 51: 735–736

Gillies H, Chalmers J 1970 The management of fresh ruptures of the tendo achillis. Journal of Bone and Joint Surgery 52A: 337–343
Gimlette T M D 1960 Thyroid acropachy. Lancet 1: 22–24
Gofton J P, Trueman G E 1971 Studies in osteoarthritis of the hip, Part II. Osteoarthritis of the hip and leg-length disparity. Canadian Medical Association Journal 104: 791–799
Good A E 1964 Rheumatoid arthritis, Baker's cyst and 'thrombophlebitis'. Arthritis and Rheumatism 7: 56–64
Goodfellow J 1984 Chondromalacia patellae. In: Jackson J P, Waugh W (eds) Surgery of the knee joint. Chapman & Hall, London, Ch. 9, p 210–233
Goodfellow J W, Fearn C B d'A 1965 Iliopsoas haematoma. Journal of Bone and Joint Surgery 47B:184
Goodfellow J, Hungerford D S, Woods C 1976 Patello-femoral joint mechanics and pathology. 2. Chondromalacia patellae. Journal of Bone and Joint Surgery 58B: 291–299
Gordon G V, Edell S, Brogadir S P, Schumacher H R, Schimmer B M, Dalinka M 1979 Baker's cysts and true thrombophlebitis. Report of two cases and review of the literature. Archives of Internal Medicine 139: 40–42
Grundy M 1970 Fractures of the femur in Paget's disease of bone. Journal of Bone and Joint Surgery 52B: 252–263
Hall A P, Healey L A 1968 Infected synovial cysts arising as a complication of septic arthritis in a patient with rheumatoid arthritis. Arthritis and Rheumatism 11: 579–584
Hall A P, Scott J T 1966 Synovial cysts and rupture of the knee joint in rheumatoid arthritis. Annals of the Rheumatic Diseases 25: 32–40
Hampson W G J, Hill P 1975 Late results of transfer of the tibial tubercle for recurrent dislocation of the patella. Journal of Bone and Joint Surgery 57B: 209–213
Harris N H, Murray R O 1974 Lesions of the symphysis in athletes. British Medical Journal 4: 211–214
Harvey J P, Corcos J 1960 Large cysts in lower leg originating in the knee occurring in patients with rheumatoid arthritis. Arthritis and Rheumatism 3: 218–228
Hawkins C F, Smith O E 1950 Renal dysplasia in a family with multiple hereditary abnormalities including iliac horns. Lancet 1: 803–808
Hench P K, Reid R T, Reames P M 1966 Dissecting popliteal cyst simulating thrombophlebitis. Annals of Internal Medicine 64: 1259–1264
Heywood A W B 1961 Recurrent dislocation of the patella. Journal of Bone and Joint Surgery 43B: 508–517
Hoffa A 1904 The influence of adipose tissue with regard to the pathology of the knee joint. Journal of the American Medical Association 43: 795–796
Holling M E 1967 Pulmonary hypertrophic osteoarthropathy. Annals of Internal Medicine 66: 232–234
Insall J, Tria A J, Aglietti P 1980 Resurfacing of the patella. Journal of Bone and Joint Surgery 62A: 933–936
Jackson J P, Waugh W (eds) 1984 Surgery of the knee joint. Chapman & Hall, London
Jayson M I V, Dixon A St J 1970a Intra-articular pressure in rheumatoid arthritis of the knee. I. Pressure changes during passive joint distension. Annals of the Rheumatic Diseases 29: 261-265
Jayson M I V, Dixon A St J 1970b Intra-articular pressure in rheumatoid arthritis of the knee. III. Pressure changes during joint use. Annals of the Rheumatic Diseases 29: 401–408
Jayson M I V, Dixon A St J 1970c Valvular mechanisms in juxta-articular cysts. Annals of the Rheumatic Diseases 29: 415–420
Jayson M I V, Dixon A St J, Kates A, Pinder I, Coomes E N 1972 Popliteal and calf cysts in rheumatoid arthritis. Treatment by anterior synovectomy. Annals of the Rheumatic Diseases 31: 9–15
Johansson S 1922 A previously undescribed lesion of the patella. Hygiea 84: 161–166
Katz R S, Zisic T M, Arnold M D 1977 The pseudothrombopblebitis syndrome. Medicine 56: 151–164
Kellgren J H 1939 On the distribution of pain arising from deep somatic structures with charts of segmental pain areas. Clinical Science 4: 35–46
Kilcoyne R F, Imray T J, Stewart E T 1978 Ruptured Baker's cyst simulating acute thrombophlebitis. Journal of the American Medical Association 240: 1517–1518
Kitchen C, Simpson J 1972 Meralgia paresthetica. A review of 67 patients. Acta Neurologica Scandinavica 48: 547–555
Kopell H P, Thompson W A L 1960 Peripheral entrapment neuropathies of the lower extremity. New England Journal of Medicine 262: 56–60
Lam S J S 1967 Tarsal tunnel syndrome. Journal of Bone and Joint Surgery 49B: 87–92
Lange L S 1966 Lower limb palsies with hypoprothrombinaemia. British Medical Journal 2: 93–94
Leabhart J W 1959 Stress fractures of the calcaneus. Journal of Bone and Joint Surgery 41A: 1285–1290
Leach R E, Hammond G, Stryker W S 1967 Anterior tibial compartment syndrome. Journal of Bone and Joint Surgery 49A: 451–462
Leach R E, Osamu N, Richard P G, Stockel J 1981 Secondary reconstruction of the lateral ligaments of the ankle. Clinical Orthopaedics and Related Research 160: 201–211
Leslie I J, Bentley G 1978 Arthroscopy in the diagnosis of chondromalacia patellae. Annals of the Rheumatic Diseases 37: 540–547
Levick J R 1979 An investigation into the validity of subatmospheric recordings from synovial fluid and their dependence on joint angle. Journal of Physiology 289: 55–67
Macfarlane D G, Bacon P A 1980 Popliteal cyst rupture in normal knees. British Medical Journal 281: 1203–1204
Macfarlane I J A, DuToit S N 1974 A ganglion causing tarsal tunnel syndrome. South Africa Medical Journal 48: 2568
Mayerding H W, Van Demark R E 1943 Posterior hernia of the knee. Journal of the American Medical Association 122: 858–861
Meire H B, Lindsay D J, Swinson D R, Hamilton E B D 1974 Comparison of ultrasound and positive contrast arthrography in the diagnosis of popliteal and calf swellings. Annals of the Rheumatic Diseases 33: 221–224
Meurman K O A 1980 Stress fracture of the pubic arch in military recruits. British Journal of Radiology 53: 521–524
Moschowitz E 1937 Bursitis of the sartorius bursa: An undescribed malady simulating chronic arthritis. Journal of the American Medical Association 109:1362
Murray R O, Jacobson H G 1971 Osteoid osteoma. In: The radiology of the skeletal disorders. Churchill Livingstone, Edinburgh & London, p. 388
Nakano K K 1975 The entrapment neuropathies of rheumatoid arthritis. Orthopaedic Clinics of North America 6: 837–860
Osborne A H, Fulford P C 1982 Lateral release for

chondromalacia patellae. Journal of Bone and Joint Surgery 64B: 202–205
Outland T, Murphy I D 1960 Peroneal flat foot. Clinical Orthopaedics 16: 64–73
Parvin R W, Ford L T 1956 Stenosing tenosynovitis of the common peroneal tendon sheath. Journal of Bone and Joint Surgery 38A: 1352–1357
Pavlov H, Nelson T L, Warren R F, Torg J S, Burstein A H 1982 Stress fractures of the pubic ramus. A report of twelve cases. Journal of Bone and Joint Surgery 64A: 1020–1025
Pinder I M 1973 Treatment of the popliteal cyst in the rheumatoid knee. Journal of Bone and Joint Surgery 55B: 119–125
Prescott S M, Pearl J E, Tikoff G 1978 Pseudo-pseudothrombophlebitis: Ruptured popliteal cyst with deep venous thrombosis. New England Journal of Medicine 299: 1192–1193
Pringle R M, Protheroe K, Mukherjee S K 1974 Entrapment neuropathy of the sural nerve. Journal of Bone and Joint Surgery 56B: 465–468
Richards A J 1981 Ruptured popliteal cyst and pyogenic arthritis. British Medical Journal 282: 1120–1121
Rose G K 1979 Soft tissue and bony operations for pes cavus and planus. In: Rob C, Smith R (eds). Operative surgery, 3rd Edn. Orthopaedics. Butterworths, London & Boston, p. 894–900
Rudge S R, Macfarlane A, Lloyd Jones J K 1981 Coronary and peripheral vascular occlusion due to rheumatoid arteritis. Postgraduate Medical Journal 57: 196–198
Sharrard W J W 1963 Aetiology and pathology of beat knee. British Journal of Industrial Medicine 20: 24–31
Sidey J D 1969 Weak Ankles. A study of common peroneal entrapment neuropathy. British Medical Journal 3: 623–626
Simeone J F, Robinson F, Rothman S L G, Jaffe C C 1977 Computerised tomographic demonstration of a retroperitoneal haematoma causing femoral neuropathy. Report of two cases. Journal of Neurosurgery 47: 946–948
Simpson F G, Robinson P J, Bark M Losowsky M S 1980 Prospective study of thrombophlebitis and 'pseudothrombophlebitis'. Lancet 1: 331–333
Sinding-Larsen M F 1921 A hitherto unknown affection of the patella. Acta Radiologica 1: 171–173
Smillie I S 1980 Diseases of the knee joint, 2nd Edn. Churchill Livingstone, Edinburgh
Soren A 1978 Histodiagnosis and clinical correlation of rheumatoid and other synovitis. Georg Thieme, Stuttgart. J B Lippincott, Philadelphia, Toronto
Stack R E, Bianco A J, MacCarty C S 1965 Compression of the common peroneal nerve by ganglion cysts. Report of 9 cases. Journal of Bone and Joint Surgery 47A: 773–778
Sunderland S 1978 In: Nerves and nerve injuries, 2nd Edn. Churchill Livingstone, Edinburgh, Ch. 72, p. 1007–1010
Swartout R, Compere E 1974 Ischiogluteal bursitis — The pain in the arse. Journal of the American Medical Association 227: 551–552
Taylor A R 1969 Arthrography of the knee in rheumatoid arthritis. British Journal of Radiology 42: 493–497
Thomas J, Collip P J, Sharma R K 1973 Thyroid acropachy. American Journal of Diseases of Children 125: 745–746
Torg J S, Pavlov H, Cooley L H et al 1982 Stress fracture of the tarsal navicular. Journal of Bone and Joint Surgery 64A: 700–712
Vaughan-Lane T, Dandy D J 1982 The synovial shelf syndrome. Journal of Bone and Joint Surgery 46B: 475–476
Watson J D, Ochsner S F 1967 Compression of the bladder due to 'rheumatoid' cyst of the hip joint. American Journal of Roentgenology 99: 695–696
Wilson D W 1980 Treatment of hallux valgus and bunions. British Journal of Hospital Medicine 24: 548–558
Wilson P D, Eyre-Brook A L, Francis J D 1938 A clinical and anatomical study of the semimembranosus bursa in relation to popliteal cyst. The Journal of Bone and Joint Surgery 20: 963–984
Wynne-Davis R, Fairbank T J 1976 Nail–patella syndrome. In: Fairbank's atlas of general affections of the skeleton, 2nd Edn. Churchill Livingstone, Edinburgh, Ch. 45, p. 158–159

SECTION XIII

Physical Treatment, Rehabilitation and Surgical Treatment

Physical treatment of the rheumatic diseases

The local features of rheumatic diseases result from mixtures of inflammation and degeneration, and in some patients systemic features are also present. Where an obvious and remediable cause exists the approach is self-explanatory. This section deals with aspects of management which are not dramatic or curative but can provide support in both the general and local sense. The methods used require a logical approach and skilled help from therapists and can provide useful relief at all stages of the disease processes. Scientific studies are scarce but there can be little doubt that a range of supportive measures is available for rheumatic sufferers whose benefit can be obtained at lesser risk than many of the much discussed drug regimes. At the same time the addictive properties of the undoubted soothing effect of such treatments should be resisted.

As the techniques available are not specific, and the processes of inflammation and degeneration so frequently occur together, the principles of treatment will be emphasised leaving the details of application to be decided by a clinical judgement of the balance between these two main pathological components. Thus the application of physical treatments can be considered conveniently under the headings

1. Systemic — applicable mainly to generalised inflammatory disease
2. Local — applicable to local effects of inflammatory or degenerative joint disease.

When inflammation is the main feature most relief is obtained by a regime of rest; when degeneration is dominant there is much to be said in favour of movement.

SYSTEMIC ASPECTS OF TREATMENT

By tradition the most important single factor in the treatment of inflammation is 'rest'. On the other hand most clinicians believe that to maintain function in damaged joints some 'physical activity' must be maintained. This section is concerned with the means of administering and reconciling these two apparently conflicting principles of treatment together with the techniques available to implement them satisfactorily. Definitive decisions about treatment can seldom be made early in diseases whose course is unpredictable, such as rheumatoid arthritis and other inflammatory disorders. Variability in the natural history of disease and difficulties in quantifying physical treatments add to the difficulty in organising properly controlled clinical trials.

Rest

Hilton (1863) advocated rest for the relief of pain resulting from inflammation and this remains a fundamental approach. However, with the availability of potent anti-inflammatory drugs it becomes particularly important to assess the benefit of rest both in terms of cost and time so that individual judgements for patients can be made. In general terms it can be said that when the whole patient is 'inflamed' the whole patient should be rested. By contrast when individual joints are inflamed only these particular joints need rest. To express this in terms of a generalised inflammatory joint disease is to say that the systemic features such as fever, anaemia, tachycardia, malaise and loss of weight require rest in bed whilst inflammation of joints in the absence of generalised features requires only local supportive measures. The evidence that treatment according to this hypothesis produces worthwhile long- or medium-term results is still lacking but some studies show benefit in the short-term.

The multiple medical dangers of going to bed have been eloquently described by Asher (1947). Despite the risks to a wide range of body systems a period of bedrest may be very helpful in the treatment of active rheumatoid arthritis especially when systemic features are evident. It is usually necessary to admit a patient to hospital to achieve adequate bedrest, as only rarely can adequate domiciliary medical, nursing and physiotherapeutic facilities be provided. Before recommending moving an elderly patient from home to hospital the psychological trauma of separating such a patient from the usual environment must be weighed against the undoubted risks of unsupervised domestic bedrest. Ideally bedrest should be continuous and it is particularly difficult to justify admission to hospital unless this optimum use of time is made. Duthie et al (1964) felt that patients who were admitted early in the course of their rheumatoid arthritis and whose disease was of acute onset fared better than those with less active and more chronic forms. They argue that this may be partly due to early exposure to physical methods of treatment. However this study does not establish whether admission, recumbency, or the treatment received, rather than the nature of the disease process, accounted for the differences between the groups or that admission confers long-term advantages. In practice it is the aim to admit patients whenever there is a significant acute attack which does not settle within a week or so of home bedrest.

A counsel of perfection is to maintain absolute bedrest until all evidence of disease activity has subsided. This could often involve a period of several months, so a compromise is usually necessary. Guidelines are needed to determine the period of immobilisation and it is necessary to set criteria by which changes in disease activity can be measured. A wide range of techniques is used, e.g. observation of body temperature and pulse rate, or estimation of the duration of morning stiffness, haemoglobin or erythrocyte sedimentation rate. In addition measurements of local disease activity such as temperature, range of movement or grip strength may be helpful. Again we lack the evidence that bedrest favourably influences the long-term course of the disease and as a matter of expedience it is not customary to insist on a period of more that 2 or 3 weeks, to be followed by mobilisation. Reactivation of disease is taken as an indication to intensify anti-inflammatory drug treatment or to accept long-term limitations of mobility.

During the period of bedrest the physiotherapist and nursing staff should ensure that an optimum posture is adopted (Figs 61.1, 61.2). Actively inflamed joints are more than usually susceptible to stretching of the joint capsule setting the scene for subsequent contracture and deformities which are

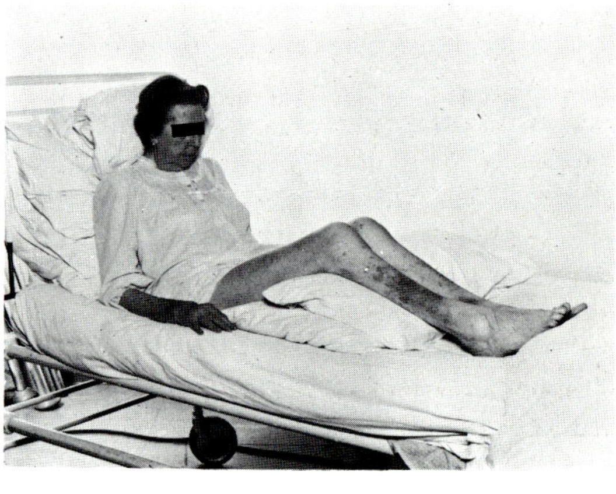

Fig. 61.1 Poor posture in bed encourages contractures of the hips and knees and may lead to neck and ankle problems.

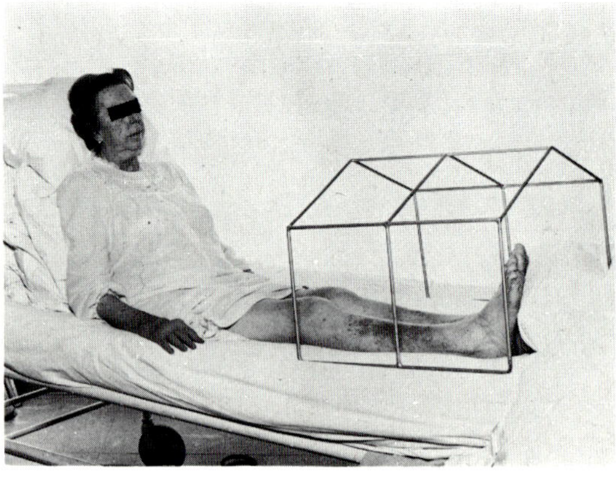

Fig. 61.2 Attention to pillows enables the neck, knees and ankles to be correctly supported. A bed cradle relieves pressure from the feet.

difficult or impossible to correct. Particular attention should be given to maintaining an orthodox neck posture and full extensibility of hips and knees. A bed cradle should be inserted to relieve inflamed ankles and feet of the weight of bed clothes.

Several trials have been conducted in attempts to clarify the relative importance of admission to hospital, rest in bed and immobilisation of joints. Mills et al (1971) set out to investigate the value of bedrest for patients admitted with rheumatoid arthritis. One group of 20 patients was confined to bed for 22 hours a day for 4 weeks, 18 hours a day for a further 6 weeks, allowing walks to the bathroom in the first period and longer walks in the second. Another group of 22 patients was admitted but no restriction imposed on physical activity. Assessments were made fortnightly for 10 weeks. They found that over half the patients improved and there was no overall difference between the two groups except that the more active cases benefited from the more severe restriction. It could perhaps be concluded from this study that admission to hospital care itself was so helpful that differences in the amount of rest were no longer apparent. Lee et al (1974) have made another attempt to assess the value of admission to hospital for bedrest. 16 patients were admitted and confined to bed for at least 13 hours daily; 14 further patients were managed without admission and their physical activity was unsupervised. At the end of 1 month, half of the in-patient group had improved by several objective criteria whereas the out-patients were unchanged. No evidence of longterm benefit is provided nor are criteria available to help select patients most likely to benefit.

The reasons for admission to hospital are both varied and to some extent empirical and can be medical or social. Most patients benefit from rest itself, the availability of medical and paramedical services and from familiarisation with their disease. They are also made aware of the variety of treatments available. Bedrest is usually continued until the evidence of disease activity has substantially diminished and a basic regime has been established which is likely to maintain this improvement.

In the absence of clear evidence that bedrest has any longterm beneficial effect on rheumatoid disease the decision to admit to hospital should also be the indication to review and improve basic drug treatment.

Movement

Although many clinicians have long suspected the value of movement for patients whose active polyarthritis has largely gone into remission only recently has there been evidence supporting this. Nordemar et al (1981) compared 23 patients with moderate disease activity who participated in regular physical training with 23 who did not. Over a period of 4–8 years the group in training showed significant improvements in activity index, sick-leave requirements, number of joints involved and a diminished rate of progress of radiological erosion. The authors argue that this effect tallies with the known effects of exercise on articular cartilage nutrition, and strength of cartilage, ligaments and tendons.

A case can thus be made for regular group training under the guidance of a physiotherapist, concentrating on non weight-bearing exercises. These could be applicable to many patients with low grade generalised arthritis who could not otherwise be obtaining exercise.

LOCAL ASPECTS OF TREATMENT

The indications for local as opposed to general treatment are not always clear-cut, nor are the two needs mutually exclusive.

Rest

It seems unnecessarily restrictive to impose a regime of bedrest on a patient with a small number of active joints and relatively little systemic disturbance; yet where joints are spontaneously painful despite recumbency and especially if sleep is disturbed, local splintage can be at least comforting. In many instances individual joints can be rested while the patient remains ambulant. It is most frequently helpful to splint wrists, knees and ankles. The splints must be readily available and can be made from plaster of Paris, polyethylene 'Polythene' or a malleable or other thermoplastic material. Supporting the policy of immobilising inflamed joints is the study of Kindersley (1936) who noted that inflammation lessened if joints were splinted in unpadded plaster for periods of 1–3 weeks. He found that after an initial period of discomfort lasting 48 hours there was symptomatic relief both locally and reflected by improvement in general health and appetite. He also postulated that the relief of pain was associated with lessening of muscle-wasting. Duthie (1951) and Swanson (1956) as well as other observers comment that under similar conditions there can be a reduction in systemic disease and increase in well-being. Harris & Copp (1962) studied the effect of immobilisation on local disease activity. They compared 18 pairs of active rheumatoid knees; one of the pair was totally immobilised in plaster of Paris for 4 weeks; its fellow was splinted for only 3 days when the plaster was split and the knee then treated with daily assisted exercises. They found that there was no difference in the reduction of the disease activity between the two groups nor any marked patient preference. There was not surprisingly some extra stiffness in the knees which had just been subjected to 4 weeks of immobilisation but this was not apparent by the 8-week stage. They could find no evidence to recommend the longer period of immobilisation. On the other hand Partridge & Duthie (1963) demonstrated that reduction of disease activity is more rapid when immobilisation is more complete. 34 patients had their limbs immobilised in unpadded plastic splints for 4 weeks; a control group was similarly splinted but the splints were removed twice daily for exercises. Both groups improved and in no case did ankylosis occur.

It is generally worth immobilising joints until evidence of local activity has diminished, during which time arrangements can be made for improved supportive therapy.

Modified rest

Attempts to protect joints from some of the stresses to which they are normally subjected are frequently made and can be of great value. By using splints and supports a form of partial rest may be achieved which permits a certain amount of physical activity whilst preventing painful stresses. The principles entailed are immobilisation, support and relief of weight while allowing modified but useful functional activity. In general a position of comfort and rest which prevents restricting deformity must be found. A great many rival materials and techniques are available, all of whose exponents rightly extol their virtues. In practice it is advisable to familiarise oneself with those most readily available and to build up an expertise in conjunction with the physiotherapists, occupational therapists and surgical appliance manufacturers who are directly responsible for supply and fitting. In this way the best use can be made of available expertise and enthusiasm; it is more useful to discuss the principles involved rather than details.

Splint materials vary in their convenience and relative merits and no one is ideal in all respects. The properties needed are *strength*, *lightness*, *comfort* and *speed of supply*. Materials frequently used include plaster of Paris, which needs little equipment, 'Polythene', which is light and strong, and 'Plastazote', a brand of thermoplastic polyethylene which is quickly made, is rather soft but can be easily reinforced. A supporting splint should reach approximately two-thirds the length of the limb on each side of the joint to be really effective.

For arm splints lightness is very important. An elbow splint can be made to support the joint at the right angle and mid-pronation, so that feeding and toilet activities can be managed. A wrist splint (Fig. 61.3) should hold the joint in approximately 10° of dorsiflexion and stop short of the metacarpophalangeal joints. This position allows good use of finger and thumb flexors. The fingers can be stabilised but allowed to function by a variety of lively, i.e. moveable, splints. Splints to restrict movement of the thumb carpometacarpal joint are also useful, particularly in osteoarthritis (Fig. 61.4).

The legs often need relief from weight-bearing. Unfortunately this may require the transfer of this function to the arms, which may not be capable of the extra effort involved. The simplest means of achieving this is with a single walking stick used on the less affected side. Care must be taken that the pressure of a handle does not lead to median nerve damage at the wrist or ulnar nerve damage in the palm and attention must be given to providing a large and comfortable handle. A pair of sticks spreads the load very much better. If the finger grip is poor or the wrists painful or

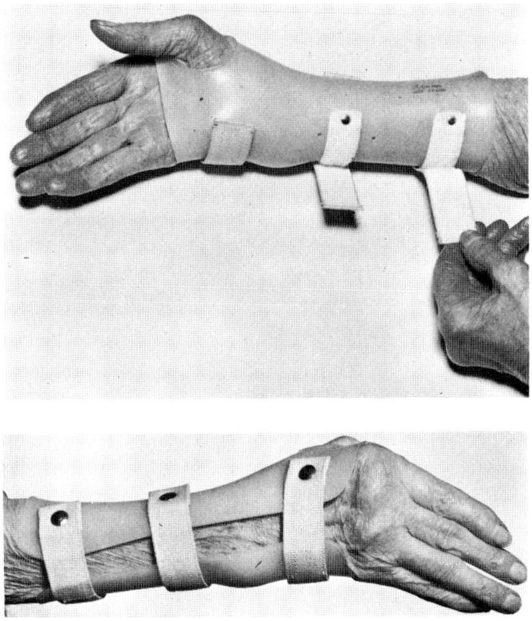

Fig. 61.3 A wrist splint should support the joint in a functional position. 'Velcro' fastenings make it easier for the crippled hand to adjust.

unstable, the demand must be moved proximally and a forearm crutch substituted. A wide variety of tripods, tetrapods and walking frames is available and the most practical approach to selection is by trial assessment in a physiotherapy gymnasium. Weight can be transferred directly from shoe to pelvis by means of ischial-bearing weight-relieving calipers and these can have locking hinges at the knees; however these are seldom used by patients with rheumatoid arthritis owing to their weight and complexity. A small measure of weight can be transferred from calf to thigh with a knee cylinder (Fig. 61.5) and this also helps stabilise the knee. However this too is a little cumbersome and stiffening the knee can be inconvenient. Hinged knee splints are available, though not entirely satisfactory. Ankle and subtaloid joints can be encased in strong light-weight splint casts (Fig. 61.6) with good results but here the difficulty in fitting shoes can be a serious problem. The painful stress of a valgus hind-foot can be self-perpetuating because the fall of weight medial to the ankle tends to aggravate the deformity. This situation can be helped by an inner raise on the heel or a floated-out, i.e. medially, sole to the shoe. More severe varieties of valgus ankle with a flat longitudinal arch of the foot can be helped by fitting a lower leg iron with a T-strap to draw the foot inwards (Fig. 61.7). Support can also be obtained from moulded heel caps which help maintain on orthodox and mechanically sound position for the ankle and subtaloid joints. Metarsophalangeal joints frequently sublux leaving the patient to bear weight on painful prominent metatarsal heads — a crip-

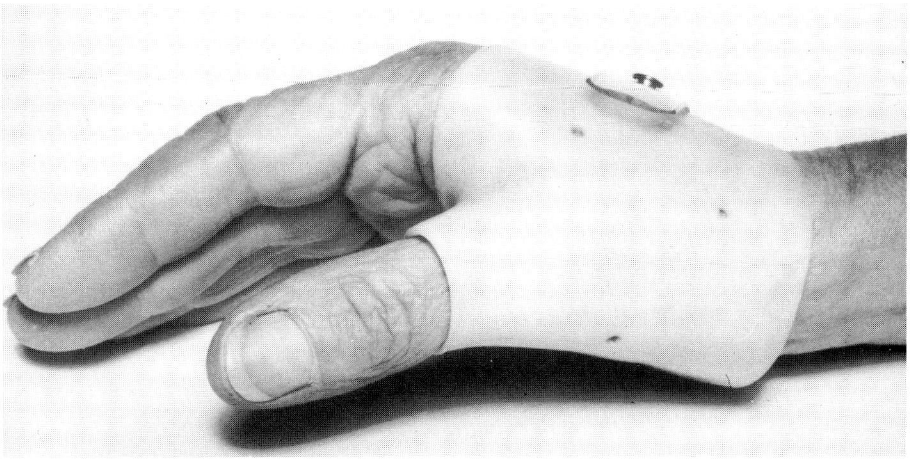

Fig. 61.4 This splint immobilises the thumb carpometacarpal joint, commonly affected by trauma or osteoarthrosis.

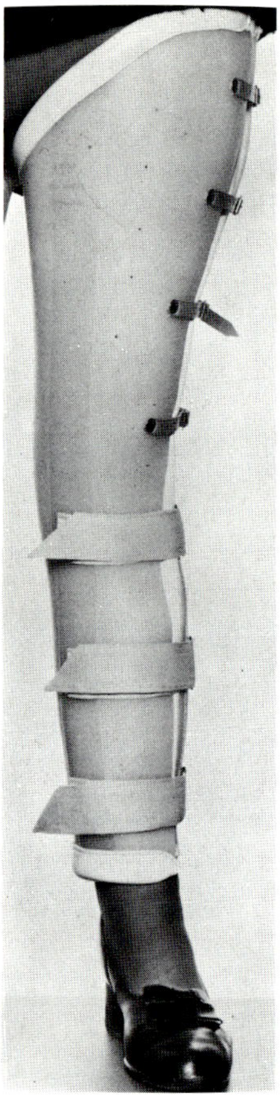

Fig. 61.5 A knee cylinder can help with stability. Where firm fixing is needed conventional strap and buckle are preferable.

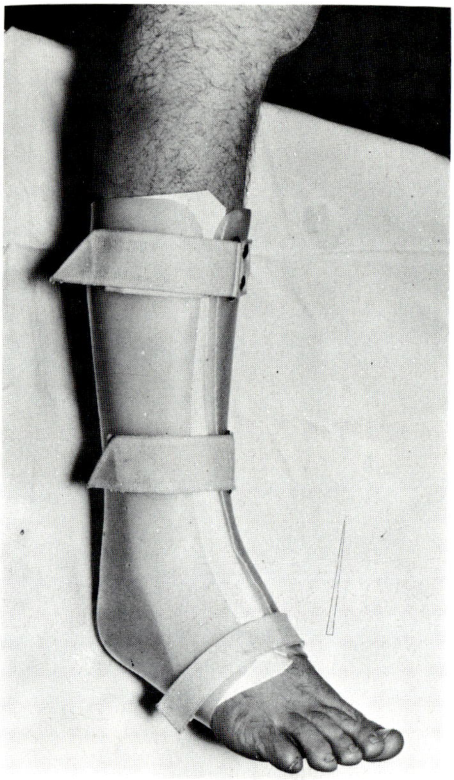

Fig. 61.6 A lightweight splint may stabilise the ankle and subtaloid joints but makes shoe fitting difficult.

pling problem. In most patients some relief can be obtained by supplying and fitting metatarsal supports (Fig. 61.8) whose object is to transfer weight back from the prominent painful heads to the non-painful metatarsal shafts. Longitudinal arch supports help to correct a valgus foot deformity. Like all devices which occupy space in shoes they will seldom be acceptable unless the necessary shoes to accommodate them are purchased. A rocker sole (Fig. 61.9) effectively helps by resting the hallux metatarsophalangeal joint.

Not infrequently the complexity of the problem arising from pain and deformity at ankle, subtaloid, mid-tarsal and metatarsophalangeal joints is such that specially designed and fitted boots or shoes will prove more satisfactory. These are usually made from conventional leather or one of the newer moulded plastic materials. Boots give greater support, particularly at the ankle and subtaloid level, whereas shoes will suffice if the problem lies more distally in the foot. Conventional leather is longer lasting and has more satisfactory potential for support, whereas moulded plastic can be made quickly and is lighter weight. In general leather is necessary for outdoor use but plastic is satisfactory indoors.

Movement (Table 61.1)

The apparent conflict between rest and movement has been mentioned in the opening paragraph of this section. An understanding of the various types of exercise and their respective places in management avoids any conflict of interests. It is crucial within the use of the term 'exercise' to recognise the principles and place of each variety in the course of recurrent arthritis activity. Exercises may be given with either of two main objectives: to maintain or improve the range of joint move-

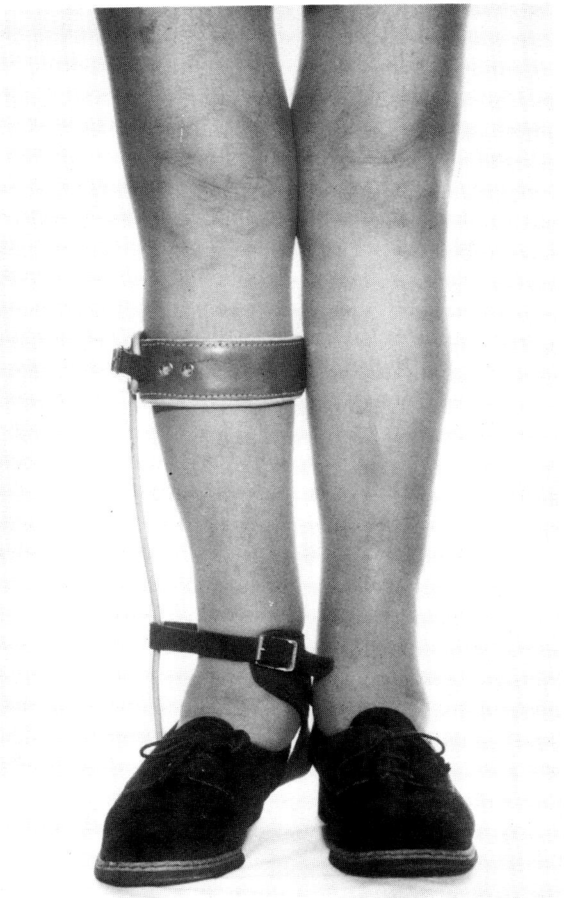

Fig. 61.7 A lower leg caliper and T-strap needs careful fitting to correct the valgus.

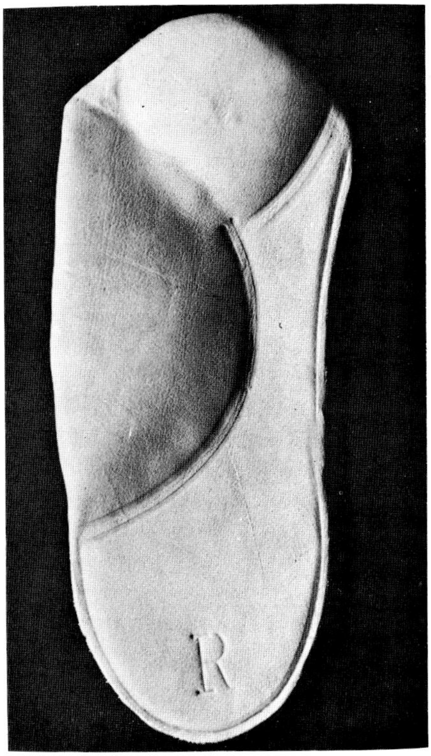

Fig. 61.8 This insole helps to reduce pain by taking weight behind painful metatarsal heads and helping to correct a valgus flat foot.

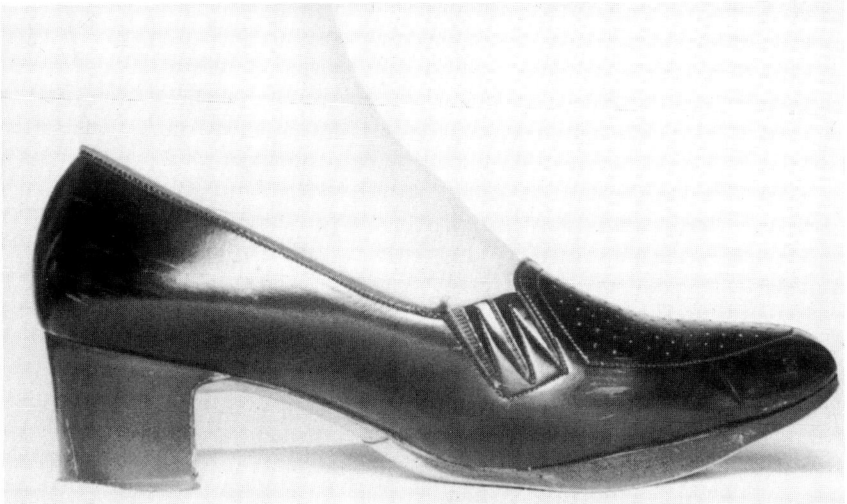

Fig. 61.9 A rocker sole effectively rests the metatarsophalangeal joint of the great toe, often affected by osteoarthrosis or gout.

Table 61.1 Indications for various types of exercise or movement

Type	Purpose
Passive exercise (movement)	To prevent stiffening of an otherwise immobilised joint (extreme form 'manipulation'). Possibly promotion of healing.
Active exercise — assisted	To encourage return of movement as joint activity settles.
Active exercise — resisted	To build up muscle power when joint activity has settled (extreme form 'isometric or 'static').

ment; to increase muscle strength and improve joint stability. A further benefit claimed for movement is that healing of cartilaginous defects is promoted. Salter et al (1980) drilled holes in the hyaline knee cartilage of 120 adolescent and 27 adult rabbits. They showed that whereas only 8% of defects healed in the immobilised joints, 52% healed in 3 weeks in joints subjected to continuous passive movement.

Passive exercises (movement)

This term indicates that the joint movement is performed entirely without active patient co-operation. During a phase of rest and splintage it is common practice to remove an immobilised joint from its support once or twice daily and for a therapist to take it gently through a full range. This may lessen the amount of stiffness remaining to be overcome when the period of rest ends, without prejudicing resolution of activity. It is important to have skilled therapists to undertake this form of passive movement as the patient may be unable to move a joint whose muscles are inhibited by pain, and unskilled over-zealous forcing of movement carries with it the danger of damage to weakened ligaments. Relatives may be taught to continue with these techniques at home.

By contrast the extreme form of passive movement 'manipulation' is indicated in the situation where a joint has no clinically evident inflammation but has deformity and restriction of movement due to fibrotic contracture of its capsule. Choosing joints for such treatment requires care. Joints in which there is residual activity will usually react by becoming more inflamed and these more vigorous passive movements should not be attempted. If the bony components of a joint have subluxed it may be impossible to increase the range passively without actually increasing the subluxation. This situation may be detected clinically or radiologically and in such instances alternatives to passive treatment must be sought. Gentle manipulations are often given by physiotherapists and require skill and judgement. The 'feel' of the joint, particularly the 'end feel' of a range of movement will indicate whether any increase in range is likely to be achieved. As with many forms of physical treatment the effect is more rapid when given frequently but gently. Often better relaxation can be obtained by administering preliminary heat. When a joint range has been increased it is necessary to maintain the benefit and it is usually helpful to make serial splints where applicable, e.g. the knee. With some joints, for example the shoulder, it is feasible to instruct the patient to continue the passive stretching at home by domestic methods utilising walls or roller towels. By these means a contracted joint capsule may be 'stretched' — a euphemism for tearing the non-extensible fibrous tissue which is limiting movement.

When the 'end feel' of a joint range suggests that tough fibrous restriction tissue exists, the combination of heat and passive movement is unlikely to achieve worthwhile progress. Here it may be worth trying a manipulation under general anaesthetic as full movement can then be achieved without heed to discomfort. It may be possible to break adhesions and again to stretch or tear the fibrotic capsule to improve the joint range. With the relaxed and unconscious patient it is easier to cause damage and joint bleeds and occasionally bony fractures have been produced. In any event it is probably worth injecting a corticosteroid to lessen the risk of a post-manipulation flare of activity and where applicable the improvement should always be maintained by splintage.

It will be evident from this discussion that passive movements have a very limited part to play in the treatment of rheumatoid arthritis and may often be harmful.

Active exercises — assisted

After a period of acute joint inflammation or enforced rest in splints it may be difficult for a patient to regain joint movement spontaneously. Attempts to move such joints unaided may be so feeble or painful as to lead to demoralisation. Assistance can be provided in overcoming weakness or weight transmission.

Many physiotherapeutic methods are available to assist movement of a joint manually. In principle the patient is asked to initiate a gentle movement and the therapist will then help by continuing it. A wide range of gadgets is also available for achieving the same end. Pulleys, ropes and wheels can be used to help with shoulder, arm, hip and leg movements, the assistance being provided by the momentum of the device, the contralateral limb, or weights. As a patient progresses through series of treatments and the joint tolerance is seen to increase, the amount of assistance can be reduced to such a level that virtually unaided movement is taking place.

The use of a hydrotherapy pool (Fig. 61.10) is a very effective way of assisting movement to which all rheumatology units should have access. The buoyancy effect of the water relieves weight, reducing the effort needed for movement and leaving the therapist free and uncluttered to assist. In addition the warmth of the water seems to provide added relief of pain and consequent muscle spasm making for easier co-operation. The optimum size of a pool is determined by the number of patients to be treated in it at a time. A convenient depth for a useful buoyancy effect is 1.3 m (4 ft) and a gently sloping floor is helpful to accommodate patients of different heights. Shallow steps, a rail and hoist are essential. The temperature is usually maintained at a little over

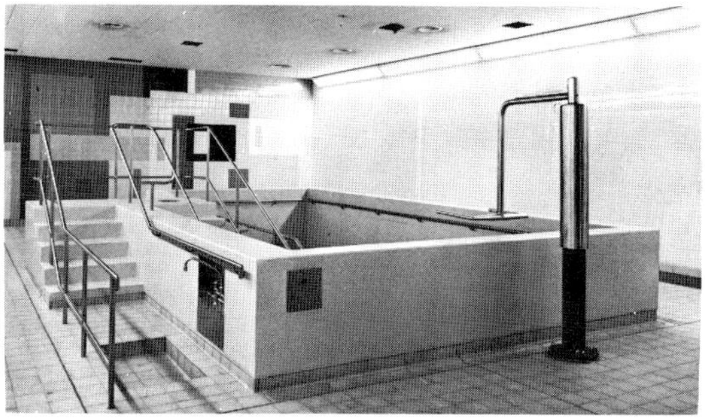

Fig. 61.10 (Courtesy John Laing & Son Ltd.) A modern hydrotherapy pool. Shallow steps with a rail and a hoist help patient in and out.

35°C (95°F). Although hydrotherapy is specially useful for treating weight-bearing joints, shoulder movements are also enhanced. In some rehabilitation centres small individual tanks are available in which a limited range of hydrotherapy treatments can be given.

Active exercises — resisted

When the pain and activity have settled sufficiently an arthritic patient should be encouraged in active joint movement. As bearing surfaces may be damaged, stress should be avoided. In particular leg exercises should be non-weight-bearing. When active movement is easily accomplished the muscle strength can be more rapidly regained by resisting movement. In their extreme form these exercises are 'static' or 'isometric'. The principle is to obtain the maximum amount of muscle exercise with the minimum approximation of its points of attachment and thus the minimum of joint movement. In this way the muscle can be increased in bulk, strength and the minimum of trauma imparted to the relevant joint. This type of exercise is most used for weight-bearing joints whose stability depends partly on muscle strength — the prime example of this being the knee. Wasting of the quadriceps muscle is a regular sequel to knee inflammation; the muscle rapidly loses strength and the accompanying instability with increased side-to-side and anteroposterior movement leads to a loss of confidence in walking. In particular vastus medialis, which is responsible for the last few degrees of extension, wastes early, delaying restoration of function. Resisted knee exercises may be started even when a patient is confined to bed with the joint splinted. The therapist will instruct the patient to 'set' the quadriceps muscle or attempt to force the back of the knee into the bed. In general the best effect is obtained by teaching a suitable regime and advising the patient to spend a few minutes on the exercise each hour of the waking day.

Delorme (1945) has studied exercise techniques for restoring quadriceps muscle power after knee surgery and injuries. He found that low repetition rate high resistance exercises were better for restoring muscle power than high repetition low resistance exercises which produced better endurance. He found it important to restore power first, and this should certainly be the case for the rheumatoid knee, but unfortunately his technique included full knee extension which might cause pain and patellofemoral damage in the arthritic joint. Cuddigan (1973) also studied the effects of quadriceps exercises on muscle strength. An important finding was that in rheumatoid patients improvement was very slow and he concluded that 'patients should be made aware of the need for a continuing long-term dedicated physiotherapeutic routine if they are to achieve and maintain quadriceps strength'.

Unfortunately quadriceps exercises are not easily dissociated from movement of the patellofemoral joint but in an unsplinted knee the tibiofemoral joint can be flexed to 30°, the patella thus being immobilised by its ligament. A severely wasted quadriceps muscle may be outside the patient's voluntary control and in this situation treatment is best initiated with the help of faradic stimulation, the tangible and visible effects of which help in re-education.

In no other situation in the body is a joint so dependent upon muscle for stability but it is feasible to devise analagous techniques for trunk and other limb muscle groups and these also can be applied during a phase of rest.

ACCESSORY TREATMENTS

Thermal methods of treatment are in widespread use for the treatment of rheumatic conditions including rheumatoid arthritis. They are often requested by patients and ordered by their physicians and surgeons. Most techniques are very demanding of therapists' time and great care must be taken that they are not used to the exclusion of other more important methods of treatment. In general it should be said that application of heat or cold in isolation can have no more than a temporary soothing effect and when used in this way must be self-administered by the patient. However these techniques can be used to provide analgesia and relaxation prior to physical methods of treatment, thus enabling them to be applied more effectively. In these circumstances they will need to be given by the therapist involved.

Although numerous hypotheses have been advanced there has been no convincing evidence produced to establish that alteration of temperature in any way influences rheumatological pathological processes. However the possibility should not be totally discounted at least in the case of ultrasound. Dyson et al (1968) have shown that ultrasound improves the healing of surgically inflicted wounds of rabbits' ears by a mechanism which is independent of healing and Harvey et al (1975) have claimed that ultrasound stimulates fibroblast activity in tissue culture. Despite the observed local physiological effects of heating such as hyperaemia and vasodilatation, only recently has evidence been published claiming efficacy (Binder et al, 1985). Evidence does exist of the relationship between intra-articular temperature changes and those occuring in superficial layers. Hollander & Horvath (1949) showed by simultaneous skin and intra-articular thermometry that microwaves elevated the intra-articular temperature slightly more than the surface temperature, shortwave diathermy elevated both equally, whereas infra-red, paraffin and hot water mainly affected the skin. They also demonstrated a slight temperature rise on joint movement. Harris & Millard (1956) also showed that heating by shortwave elevated the intra-articular temperature and that radioactive sodium was then cleared more quickly from the synovial cavity of the normal knee. Later studies by Harris (1963) showed enhanced clearance in osteoarthrosis and reduction in rheumatoid arthritis, as well as increased clearance with exercise in both conditions.

Discussion amongst therapists frequently revolves around the rival benefits of heat and cold. Here some comparative evidence is available. Kirk & Kersley (1968) studied 20 rheumatoid knees belong to 14 patients. Using a crossover technique, knees received 5 days of ice packs or 5 days of hot packs followed after a 9-day interval by the alternative; both treatments were accompanied by exercises. Objective assessment did not show any difference between the two treatments both groups showing some improvement although cold was preferred by more patients and more knees. There is a clinical impression that active rheumatoid arthritis is made more uncomfortable by heating and their trial lends weight to this idea.

62

M.A. Chamberlain

Rehabilitation in the rheumatic diseases

Modern rehabilitation, particularly in relation to rheumatology, owes a great debt to the previous author of this chapter, the late Dr. Philip Nichols, who referred to the tradition of spa treatment of rheumatic disorders. Spas continue to flourish in continental Europe, providing physical therapy (hydrotherapy, mud therapy, 'straight' physiotherapy and a variety of more exotic treatments) but in Britain, Scandinavia and the USA, they have largely disappeared, and rehabilitation centres are becoming more commonplace, functioning increasingly on a base of scientific knowledge. The techniques and treatment regimes now used derive largely from times of great need, such as the Second World War (especially the Battle of Britain) and from the time of poliomyelitis epidemics in Scandinavia. In the former, the Royal Air Force ran some seven rehabilitation centres, and patients, who numbered amongst them highly motivated pilots, undertook intensive, highly structured and carefully progressed programmes of physiotherapy, exercise and occupational therapy. These treatment patterns, which produced such excellent results, were carried over into civilian rehabilitation centres by doctors such as Philip Nichols (Wynn Parry, 1982).

Following the Scandinavian poliomyelitis epidemic of the late 1950s Sweden has been in the forefront of rehabilitation and most district hospitals have large and excellent departments devoted to it. Similarly their welfare services for the disabled are comprehensive and generous. In the UK the most significant advances have come, perhaps, with the passing of the Chronic Sick and Disabled Persons' Act (1970), with the founding of rehabilitation demonstration centres, and with the establishment of the Society for Research into Rehabilitation, which draws its members from a wide range of professions. Developments on the medical side of rehabilitation have been somewhat different from North American experience, in that it is becoming generally agreed that physicians in each of the major specialties will remain concerned with the long-term management of their patients, i.e. with their rehabilitation. Since the rheumatic conditions represent some 20% of chronic disability in an industrialised society, it is clear that their correct and sympathetic management will contribute a great deal to the proper functioning of that society.

DEFINITION

The World Health Organisation defines rehabilitation as 'the combined and co-ordinated use of medical, social, educational and vocational measures for training and retraining the individual to the highest possible level of functional ability'. Such a definition is useful but fails to involve the patient: it would be more appropriate to envisage an *enabling* process designed to restore the patient to as much autonomy as possible, incorporating his aims and wishes and using his resources: a cynical colleague was heard to define the process as one converting the consumer of welfare benefits to a taxpayer. Many rheumatic patients would indeed wish it were so.

To the rheumatologist concerned with the total management of his patient, it is worth looking at the WHO classifications of Wood & Baddeley (1979), for although the terminology is at first sight difficult to grasp, it has the merit of precision previously lacking in discussions on handicap and disability, particularly in the social sciences literature. In brief, it is a method of extending our horizons from the diagnostic label, through its functional implications, towards its interaction with the environment. Thus the patient has a primary *impairment* (say a traumatic hand amputation), which leads to a functional *disability* (loss of a whole range of bimanual function), which in turn confers a *handicap* (less for a solicitor perhaps than for a violinist or an acrobat, and less for the retired violinist or a retired acrobat).

We can thus see that until problem-orientated medical recording was widely adopted, traditional clinical practice largely concerned itself with impairment, whereas medical rehabilitation is directed at minimising disability and handicap. The doctor who begins to consider the patient's disease in relation to life-style and environment quickly finds himself having to pay regard to social service provision, to social, economic and political policy.

It is the task of the rheumatologist to maintain the patient's ability to participate as fully as possible in life around him. To this end he will need first to assess the patient as accurately as possible and, second, to call up numerous resources. He will need to plan both shortand long-term aims and make use of outpatient, inpatient and domiciliary services.

ASSESSMENT OF THE RHEUMATIC PATIENT

Assessment of the disease by the physician or metrologist

One may use methods such as the duration of morning stiffness, the joint score or Ritchie articular index, the visual analogue scale for pain (see Ch. 65), the presence of anaemia, weight loss, fever, the ESR and C-reactive protein as the clinician or metrologist feels appropriate. For research, particularly if the results are to be useful to social services departments, it may be more appropriate to use the Amelia Harris classification (1971) of disability (Table 62.1) rather than Steinbrocker's functional grading (1949) which is more dependent on cultural and economic factors. The recently introduced Stanford Health Assessment (Fries et al, 1980) of disability is quick to administer and promises to be useful.

Table 62.1 Classification of Handicap (after Harris, 1971)

Category 1	Contains people who need help going to or using the WC practically every night. In addition, most of those in this group need to be fed and dressed or, if they can feed and/or dress themselves, they need a lot of help during the day with washing and WC, or are incontinent.
Category 2	Contains people who need help with the WC during the night but not quite so much help with feeding, washing, dressing, or, while not needing night-time help with the WC, need a great deal of day-time help with feeding and/or washing and the WC.
Category 3	Contains those who are permanently bedfast or confined to a chair and need help to get in and out, or are senile or mentally impaired, or are not able to care for themselves as far as normal everyday functions are concerned, but who do not need as much help as categories 1 and 2.
Category 4	Contains people who either have difficulty doing everything, or find most things difficult and some impossible.
Category 5	Contains people who find most things difficult, or three or four items difficult and some impossible.
Category 6	Contains people who can do a fair amount for themselves but have difficulty with some items, or have to have help with one or two minor items.
Category 7	Contains people who can do everything themselves, but have difficulty with one or two items.
Category 8a	Contains people to whom physical impairment presents no difficulty in taking care of themselves, but whose main impairment is mental, endocrinal, sensory, etc
Category 8b	Contains people to whom impairment presents no difficulty in taking care of themselves.

The patient's ability to respond to therapeutic measures depends much on the *nature* of the disease: the patient with an inflammatory arthropathy is unwell and many joints are inflamed. If inflamed knees are spared by the use of crutches the shoulders may then flare up. The patient with isolated osteoarthrosis is relatively fortunate: he is usually well, if obese, and can learn to compensate for the damaged joint by the use of another part of the body. Patients with complications of the disease (e.g. uveitis in ankylosing spondylitis) are less fortunate.

Those who are blind or deaf or very elderly may have difficulty following the physiotherapist's instructions and those who have other diseases may be too unwell to do so.

Assessment by the physiotherapist

The physiotherapist is able to provide information on the patient's physical performance and such assessment before and after therapy and surgery is valuable. Physiotherapists may be asked to chart joint range. This is, for example, very useful at the shoulder, as it can be correlated to some extent with functional difficulties (Fig. 62.1), assuming elbow function is unimpaired. On occasion, where one is looking for recovering muscle power, e.g. in polymyositis, Oxford gradings of muscle function (Table 62.2) are appropriate. More often, one needs to know whether a patient can roll from side to side (i.e. can turn himself unaided in bed at night, thus preventing the development of pressure sores), can rise from the horizontal to sitting, and can *transfer* from bed to chair (or wheelchair), and from chair (or wheelchair) to commode or toilet, or can rise (aided, or with one or two helpers) from sitting to standing. This is a great demand on damaged knee and hip joints, some 3–7 times body weight being transferred through them. Assessment is also made of posture, of walking (aided or unaided) and of performance up and down stairs.

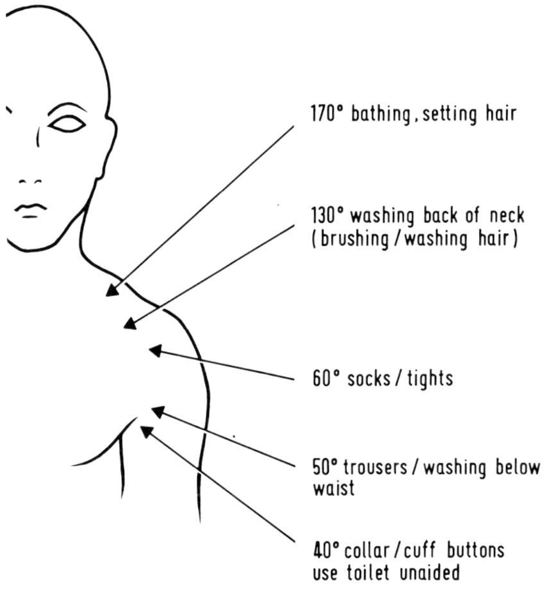

Fig. 62.1 Angles of abduction at the shoulder, related to functional activities.

Table 62.2 Oxford grading of muscle contraction of power and function (MRC grading memorandum No. 45, HMSO, 1976)

0	No contraction
1	Flicker or trace of contraction
2	Active movement, with gravity eliminated
3	Active movement against gravity
4	Active movement against gravity and resistance
5	Normal power

Grades 4-, 4 and 4+ may be used to indicate movement against slight, moderate and strong resistance respectively.

Assessment by the occupational therapist

Those treating the patient with rheumatic diseases need to know how the disease is affecting the patient's life-style. The occupational therapist is able to provide much information on the activities of daily living (ADL), often under the following general headings: personal care (washing, toilet, dressing); feeding and food preparation; household duties (care of clothes, house cleaning and maintenance); care of children and other family members; vocational (paid and voluntary) work; hobbies and recreation, including outdoor activities. The first few categories are largely related to *dexterity* and to reach, lifting, handling, carrying; one also needs to consider *mobility*, both inside and outside the house, and on foot, and by both private and public transport.

There are over 200 ADL forms, and the process of simplifying these and grouping functional difficulties has only just begun (Smith, 1976). A suggested simple form is illustrated (Table 62.3). There is also merit in ADL forms incorporating numerical scores: although crude, these give some semi-objective data indicating where change is (or is not) occurring, and allowing pre- and postoperative comparisons (Table 62.4).

It is also useful to gain some idea of the patient's *dependence* on others for various tasks. A complementary social assessment to this is given in Table 62.5; the critical period during which a patient may be left unattended will govern the patient's need for help and the freedom of the caring relative to engage in employment or hobbies. Table 62.6 (after Kushlick) puts in perspective the involvement of the carer vis-à-vis the advising professionals.

Table 62.3 Activities of daily living: a simple assessment form

Activity	Dependent	With help	Independent
Feeding			
Dressing			
Bed			
Chair			
Toilet			
Bath			
Kitchen			
Housework			
Washing			
Shopping			
Mobility			

Table 62.5 Priority of personal needs (after Bernard Isaacs)

Critical interval	Arise at short and unpredictable intervals (requiring continuous availability of means of being met)
Short interval	Arise every few hours by day (circadian)
Long interval	Arise once every day or less frequently

Assessment by the disablement resettlement officer

Educational and vocational histories are valuable in assessing a patient's further ability to work. A practical trial of the relevant skills should perhaps first be undertaken in the occupational therapy department before sending most patients for assessment at an employment rehabilitation centre. The Manpower Services Commission has the services of a vocational psychologist who should be able to help the referring physician by document-

Table 62.4 A semi-objective assessment form for activities of daily living

Diagnosis	Dates						Comments	Goal
ADL A. Dressing								
B. Feeding								
C. Washing								
D. Lavatory								
E. Bathing with aids								
F. Bathing without aids								
G. Cooking snacks								
H. Cooking meals								
MOBILITY I. Non-ambulatory transfer bed to wheelchair								
J. Non-ambulatory transfer wheelchair to toilet/commode								
K. Non-ambulatory using wheelchair								
L. Ambulatory with Zimmer								
M. Ambulatory with elbow crutch								
N. Ambulatory with stick								
O. Ambulatory no aids								
P. Pressure areas								

Codes

A–O
4. Independent
3. Supervision
2. Assistance
1. Dependent

P
4. None
3. Single superficial sore
2. Single deep sore
1. Multiple sores

Table 62.6 Ambiguity of direct care, showing the involvement of carers in the life of a disabled person (after Albert Kushlick)

DC 24 (24 hours)	Members of client's family (often parent or spouse) — interactions mainly in single location every day of week
DC 12 (12 hours)	e.g. Nurses, houseparents, residential assistants — interactions mainly in single location on a shift basis
DC 2–6 (2–6 hours)	e.g. Teachers and occupational therapists — interactions usually in same location, and consisting of programmes during morning or afternoon of 5-day working week.
DC 10 (10 minutes)	e.g. Physicians, social workers, and educational psychologists — interact with clients in many different locations throughout day; ('hit-and-runners' — often interact mainly with other DCs)

ing not only the patient's current skills but also his potiential for retraining or employment.

Assessment by the clinical psychologist

He is rarely involved in the treatment of rheumatoid patients although in Germany, for instance, clinical psychologists work in association with self-help groups, and certainly there are occasions when modification of mal-adaptive behaviour is desirable. The author is referred to further discussion in texts of rehabilitation such as that by Nichols (1976).

Assessment by the nurse

Nursing the rheumatic patient is a highly skilled undertaking: patients can easily lose the ability to undertake tasks which they do at home daily, albeit with great difficulty, if these are done for them in hospital: it may not be the fault of the nurse, merely perhaps of the ward environment where, for example, the toilet may lack a high seat or rails which would allow the patient to manage unaided.

The nursing assessment should thus take note of not only the patient's physical state (e.g. is the skin intact, are the nails cut?) but also of dynamic features (can the patient turn herself at night, how does she get herself to the lavatory, how are rest and activity alternated, how is comfort maintained?). Aids used should be documented and used in hospital (do the nurses know that the patient with cervical spine involvement wears a collar when the hair is washed?); all nurses should know why such aids are used, and be familiar with details of drug administration. Long- and short-term nursing aims are stated in similar terms to those employed by occupational therapists.

The nurse should ensure that patients learn self-medication and relatives know what part they have to play in helping the patient to lead as normal an existence as possible. Both patients and relatives should be helped to an understanding of the disease and its effects.

Assessment by the health visitor

It is a great help to have health visitors in one's team as their approach is orientated to home problems. Because of the practical help they bring their advice to the patient is often heeded, and they will help interpret the doctor's instructions on management and explain the nature of the illness in appropriate language. They can also bring back to the physician much information on the family, the physical features of the home, and the formal and informal supports used by the family. Information in the following areas is sought:

1. Aids and adaptations (requested and in situ)
2. Finances (benefits and allowances)
3. Level of function, e.g. mobility (including use of public transport); speech; hearing; vision
4. Self care skills, e.g. dressing, feeding, washing, toilet, continence, bathing, hair care, foot care, smoking
5. Drug regime (understood?)
6. Domestic care: cooking, housework, laundry, diet, shopping heating
7. Professional visitors
8. Outings and outpatient appointments
9. Hobbies
10. Health visitor action and advice.

Assessment by the social worker

The medical social worker's assessment will contain information on the patient and his family and the strengths of their relationships (particularly marital). The educational, vocational and family histories are relevant. It is helpful to know how leisure time is spent and how the family interacts with the neighbourhood. What neighbourhood support is used? What formal support is provided?

What are the *financial* obligations of the patient? Patients may be eligible for several of the following: sickness benefit (short-term capacity up to 28 weeks); injury benefit (incapacity due to industrial accident or prescribed occupational disease, up to 26 weeks); invalidity benefit or allowance (incapacity lasting beyond 28 weeks); unemployment supplement; mobility allowance (beginning 6 months after onset of illness, the patient being unable or virtually unable to walk); attendance allowance, level of benefit depending on amount of help required by day and by night; and the non-contributory invalidity pension for married women.

The social worker needs to know the general nature of treatment being undertaken; conversely she will have assessed the areas of stress and change and the possibility of providing help and counselling. She does not see herself as solely the provider of benefits or as the point of liason with social services provision, though these are obviously part of her work.

In summary, the **assessment** of the patient takes due regard of:

The disease process (general and local effects)

Other diseases or disabilities

The patient and his intellectual, emotional, financial and other resources

The family situation and interactions and their emotional resources

The local milieu including informal support network

The local environment (inside and outside the home) and the patient's mobility within this environment.

Planning is undertaken for both short-term and long-term needs, with documentation of change in the areas under study or treatment. Patients with temporary disability will require intensive therapy, those with chronic disease need continued support and help to maintain their level of function.

RESOURCES AND THERAPY AVAILABLE TO THE RHEUMATIC PATIENT

Most rheumatic sufferers are rarely admitted to hospital and most rheumatologists do substantially more outpatient than inpatient work. Much of the responsibility for *co-ordinating* professionals and resources will therefore lie also with the patient's general practitioner, who will use the local rheumatological service as appropriate, and accessible. Nevertheless, where the disorder is complex and ever-changing, the doctor with the most appropriate clinical experience should assume overall responsibility for the pattern, pace and direction of the patient's rehabilitation and the provision of services. Some of the numerous services available are illustrated in Table 62.7, from which it can be seen that they are provided from a great variety of statutory and voluntary sources. Resources available include the following.

Physiotherapy

Physiotherapy is frequently required by the arthritic subject and may be given in hospital, or by domiciliary physiotherapists at a local health centre or the patient's home. A course of treatment may consist of something like 12 sessions, given 2–3 times per week, lasting some 40 minutes (20 minutes of heat, ice or short-wave diathermy, followed by 20 minutes of specific exercises). Patients travelling by ambulance may have to endure several hours' travel, arriving home too exhausted to have benefited from the treatment. Also, to be effective, exercises must be repeated at least daily: it is thus probable that many exercises should be *taught* in the physiotherapy department (in one or two sessions) and then done by the patient at home daily. There is evidence that such exercises will only be done regularly if a follow-up assessment appointment is made (Chamberlain, 1982) at which progress is measured. There is little place for passive treatments except perhaps in conjunction with early treatment using strict bed rest and joint splintage in hospital. Active assisted exercises will gradually be replaced by resisted exercises; hydrotherapy will be used where appropriate and available. Group therapy not only utilises physiotherapists' time well but is enjoyable to patients as many exercises can be disguised as games, encouraging cooperation and competition. Physiotherapy is a scarce resource, undoubtedly of great value where appropriate, yet largely unevaluated and it should not be used as placebo.

Table 62.7 Requirements of, and services for rheumatic patients

Referring and Providing } Agencies	Requirements
Hospital (loans service)	**Walking and mobility aids**
General practitioner	Wheelchairs
	Vehicles
Medical social worker	Transport
Social worker in community	Aids to daily living
Health visitor	**Home adaptations**
District nurse	Home equipment — beds
Occupational therapist } Hospital	— hoists
Physiotherapist } Community	— incontinence
Local authority social services	— alarm equipment
Local authority housing	— rails
Local authority education	— ramps
Environmental health	— stairlifts
Red Cross	**Housing**
Womens' Royal Voluntary Service	Rehousing
Aids centres	Sheltered housing
Societies for disabled	Part III accommodation
	Housing to mobility standards
Artificial Limb and Appliance Centre	Wheelchair housing
Manpower Services Commission	
Gas board	**Support at home**
	Home help
	Meals on Wheels
	Recreational needs
	Sports for disabled
	Access to normal facilities
	Holidays
	Hobbies and clubs — disabled
	— non-disabled

Only a few of the connections from the individuals and organisations in the first column to the facilities in the second have been drawn in. Perhaps the reader would like to complete them, when the complexity of the situation will become apparent!

Occupational therapy

Formal physiotherapy can be complemented by similar exercises in occupational therapy — one can encourage an increased range of shoulder function, for instance, by using games on a wall-mounted magnetic board; quadriceps exercises can be provided by fretwork or the rehabilitation bicycle.

Indeed the occupational therapy department has a great deal to offer the arthritic, as it deals with the interaction between the person, his disease and the environment: it is sad that there are still parts of the world without occupational therapists, where such help for arthritics is correspondingly limited. Some of the help this department can give is discussed below, although space precludes detailed discussion.

Personal care

Dressing. This should be simplified as far as possible by the use of light-weight, easy-care fabrics of suitable design (e.g. front opening bra, or blouses with raglan sleeves). A dressing stick may be necessary (Fig. 62.2). Fastening should be easily managed, using velcro (Fig. 62.3), large buttons and large handles on zips. Those confined to wheelchairs outside may get very cold unless dressed in thermal underwear, warm trousers and perhaps a travel sack and kagoule (Fig. 62.4). Thin tights are cold and difficult to put on even with an aid.

Washing and grooming. This is best performed with the patient seated, with sponges, combs and lipsticks mounted on angulated, long

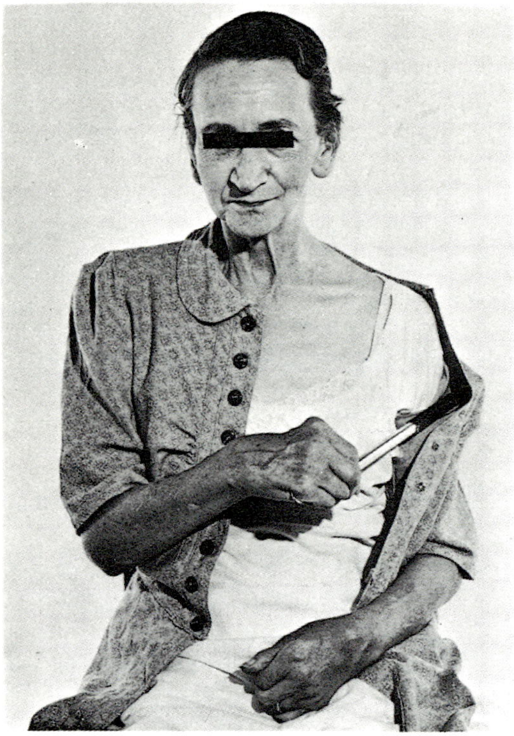

Fig. 62.2 Using a simple 'dressing-stick' made of perspex with one end covered with pimpled rubber.

handles. Hair is probably best kept in a short simple style; where atlantoaxial dislocation is present, a soft collar is worn when the hair is washed.

Bathing. Bathing is often abandoned because of the difficulty of climbing over the bath edge and the patient's fear of falling. A shower (with seat) is ideal but rarely available, but the provision of simple aids (bath board, seat and non-slip mat, toegther with a rail on the adjacent wall) helps many (Fig. 62.5). Adequate quadriceps function is especially important here.

Toilet and perineal hygiene. The problems here are of access, of low seating and of poor hand function: the latter makes it difficult for the patient to clean the perineum, and to insert tampons, pessaries and suppositories.

Wherever possible there should be a toilet or commode on the same level as the living area. Access rails on stairs should be provided and firmly fixed rails around the toilet are usually necessary.

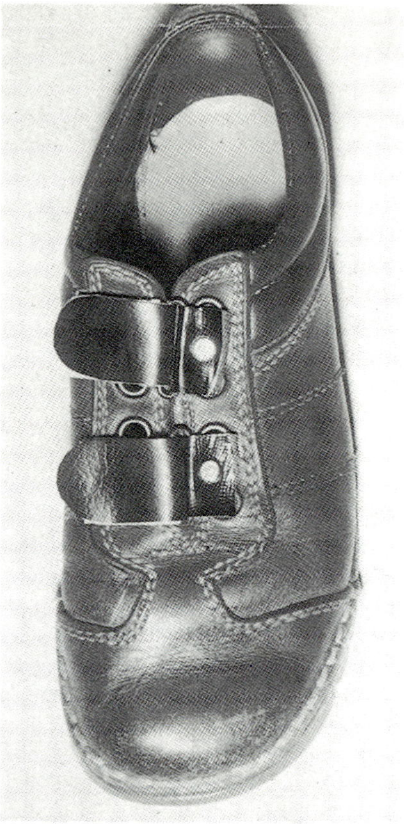

Fig. 62.3 Velcro fastening modifying patients' shoes so they can be more easily fastened by the rheumatic hand.

A raised toilet seat is helpful to those in whom arthritis involves the hip (Fig. 62.6).

Seating. Ellis (1982) showed that forces of the order of 3–7 times body weight are transmitted through the knee on rising. It is easy to understand therefore that poor quadriceps function may result in a patient rarely leaving her chair, with the result that function is further depressed and the patient's activities decline. The single most important feature which arthritics require of their easy chair (Fig. 62.7) is that they are able to get out of it (Munton et al, 1981). It should have a high seat, sufficient back support, comfortable arm rests and adequate support for the thighs. It should be possible for the patient to get the feet under the chair to bring the centre of gravity forward to aid rising. Spring seats and power rise chairs are occasionally useful.

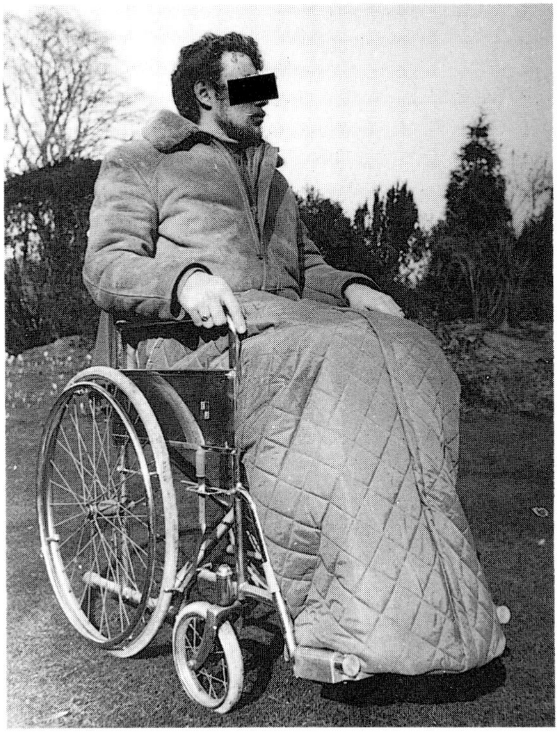

Fig. 62.4 A wheelchair user is immobile and needs to use a travel sack to keep warm.

Aids. There are now around 7000 commercially available aids to daily living and it is quite impossible for every occupational therapy department to stock all of them. Thus, recourse may be had by therapists, patients, their relatives and, indeed, doctors, to aids centres and aids exhibitions. These centres usually have a permanent collection of aids (including larger ones such as hoists, chairs and wheelchairs), and an information bank. Certain commercial aids may require adaptation by the occupational therapy technician, a member of the hospital medical physics department or a volunteer for REMAP (Rehabilitation Engineering Movement Advisory Panel), all of whom may help with aids specially made for an individual patient's particular requirements.

When *prescribing aids* certain principles must be clear. It goes without saying that the patient's diagnosis, prognosis, and functional implications are known. Staff must understand what functional problems are currently of greatest importance to the patient. Wherever possible a problem should be overcome by the use of normal equipment (freezer, washing machine, tumble dryer). If an aid is prescribed it should be the sim-

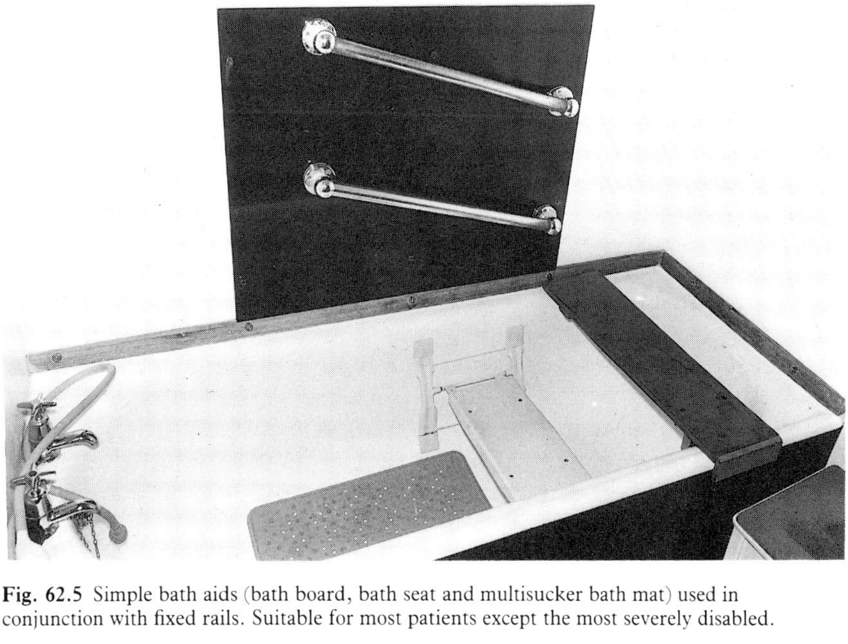

Fig. 62.5 Simple bath aids (bath board, bath seat and multisucker bath mat) used in conjunction with fixed rails. Suitable for most patients except the most severely disabled.

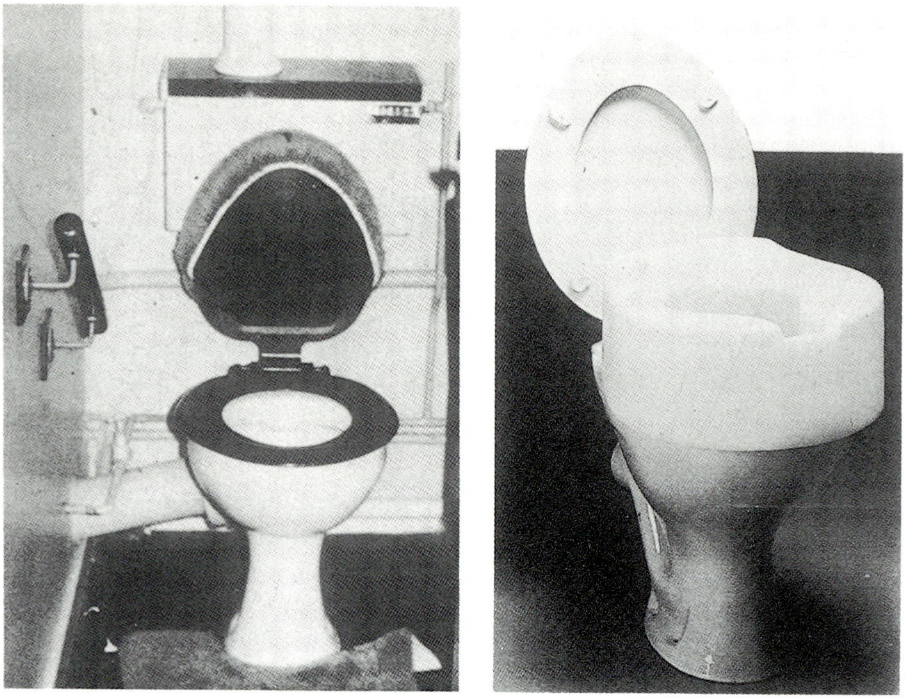

a b

Fig. 62.6 (a) Lavatory with fixed rails. (b) Lavatory with removable raised seat.

plest, sturdiest and least expensive one that does the job properly. It should be tried out by the patient before purchase. Some of the commonest and simplest home aids include: a large grip for a key, tap turners, (Fig. 62.8), trolleys which can be used also as a walking aid (Fig. 62.9) and long-handled equipment (Fig. 62.10).

Only the most severely incapacitated patient requires environmental controls such as the POSSUM (Patient Operated Selector Mechanism) system, whereby switches will operate lights, television, the opening of front doors and so on.

Food preparation and domestic duties

Arthritics rarely need a specialised diet, although they may find it difficult to get out to get fresh vegetables, and become folate deficient; they may also have little money for expensive meats requiring little preparation, or for fridges and freezers. Nevertheless, they should be helped to learn to prepare food safely in a way which conserves their energy. Thus, convenience food can be used where available and patients can be taught to prepare sufficient for several days' meals.

Patients should sit to prepare foods when possible; the kitchen should be designed or redesigned to allow its ergonomically efficient use, with surfaces along which pans can be slid, and with equipment accessible and light-weight (Fig. 62.11). Gas and electricity boards are frequently helpful in providing adaptations to equipment. A trolley is a splendid means of carrying articles (Fig. 62.9) and doubles as a walking frame. Frequently such modifications are best made as a result of a domiciliary visit by the therapist.

Cutlery, like other tools, needs comfortable, large handles and should wherever possible, look acceptable (Figs 62.12–62.14). Many women with arthritis continue to attempt their household tasks unmodified. Merete Brattstrom (1973) has pointed out that many customary ways of cutting bread and lifting vacuum cleaners, for example, may damage joints such as the metacarpophalangeals. The principles of *joint protection* can be of help in sparing joints at risk. In the department, women newly afflicted with arthritis meet in groups with occupational therapists to discuss these matters. In the same way, rheumatoid mothers of young chil-

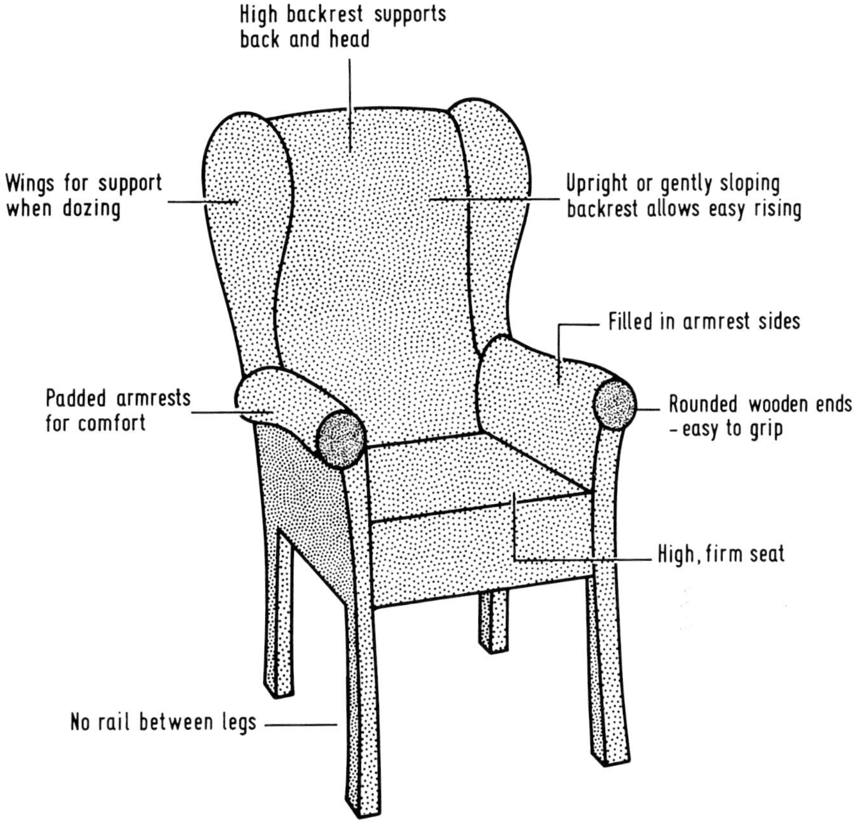

Fig. 62.7 A good easy chair for a patient with arthritis.

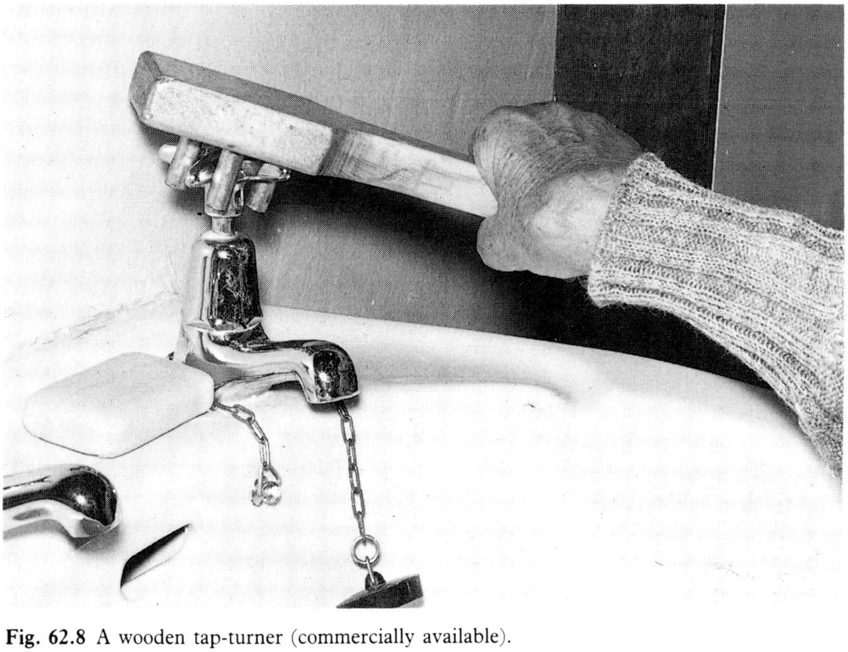

Fig. 62.8 A wooden tap-turner (commercially available).

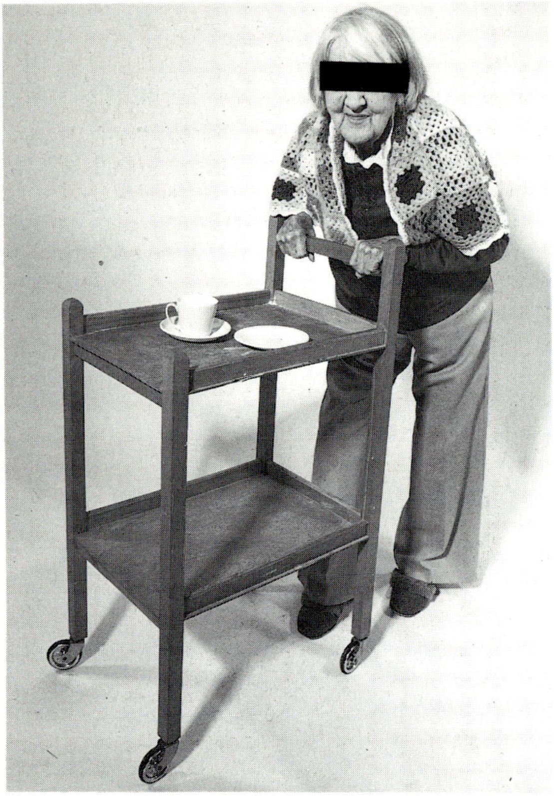

Fig. 62.9 An arthritic person with poor mobility may prefer to use a trolley inside the house. It is impossible to carry a cup of tea and use a conventional walking frame.

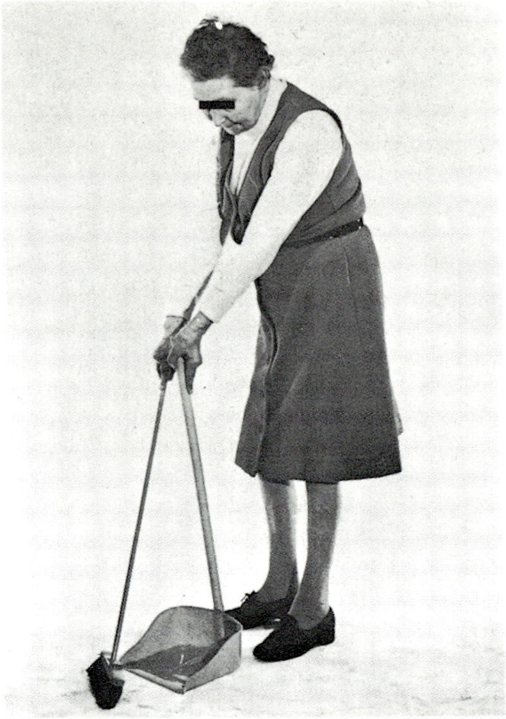

Fig. 62.10 Using a long-handled dustpan and brush.

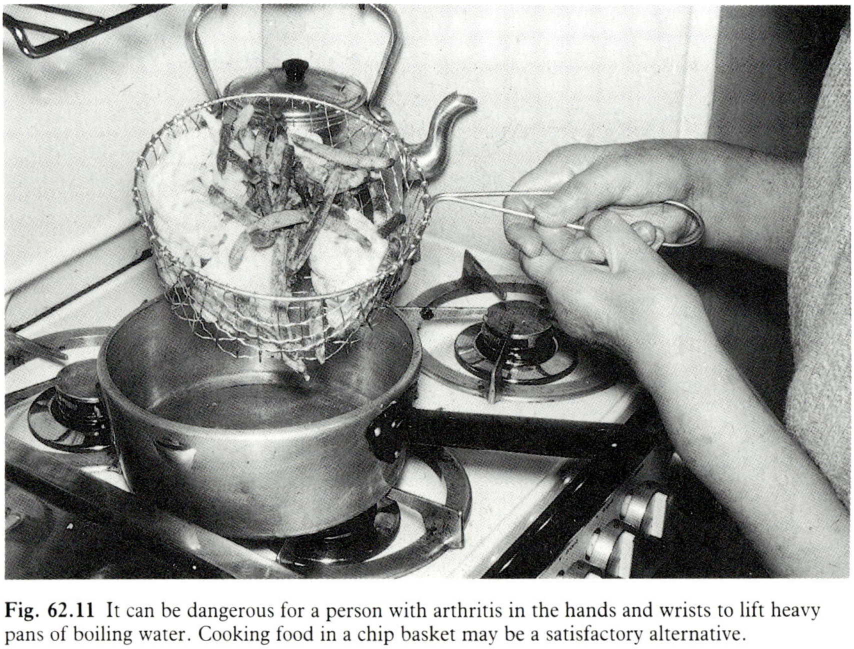

Fig. 62.11 It can be dangerous for a person with arthritis in the hands and wrists to lift heavy pans of boiling water. Cooking food in a chip basket may be a satisfactory alternative.

Advice is often best taken not only from professionals but from those similarly afflicted: the National Ankylosing Spondylitis Society offers a lively forum and good written information to its members; Arthritis Care has many local groups meeting regularly, a successful newsletter, hotels and caravans available. Younger sufferers do not necessarily welcome meetings based on a common disability but may prefer a telephone or written network: the under 35 group is available to them. We are experimenting with a parents group for those who have arthritic children. Patient education groups (based on rheumatology departments) are also found. Many countries have self-help groups doing similar work; in many cases sufferers enjoy fundraising for research or for the welfare of arthritics.

All subjects need written information in simple, attractive forms. The Arthritis and Rheumatism Council publishes a series of such booklets; SPOD produces leaflets; organisations such as the Disabled Living Foundation have a vast range of information, and source books such as the *Directory for the disabled* (Darnborough) are most helpful. Local access guides and social services literature may be available.

KEY SITUATIONS

Certain constellations of problems occur with sufficient frequency to warrant discussion in detail.

Management of early, severe inflammatory polyarthritis

In some patients the disease has an acute onset which renders them generally ill with weight loss, anaemia and fever. In others the diagnosis is not obvious, or complications necessitate inpatient admission for investigation and diagnosis; in yet others the domestic situations (toddlers or elderly relatives to look after, or poor resources) make it imperative to admit the patient for rest. In these cases it is probably most appropriate to admit patients to rheumatology units and wards where skills are concentrated. Further, close collaboration between rheumatologists and orthopaedic surgeons and with remedial therapists responsible for the assessments and treatments referred to, yields good results.

In the early stages, generalised rest in bed (with the limbs correctly positioned, on a firm mattress), local rest in splints (for inflamed joints), graded physiotherapy and adequate pain relief may be most helpful. Duthie (1967) showed that in this way, the patient and family could be educated and over 60% could be kept at work until retirement. The figures may differ now, as unemployment hits the disabled hard; on the other hand, selective, early surgery should have helped others to remain employed.

Prophylaxis; prevention of deformity; advice to the adolescent arthritic

The correct management of ankylosing spondylitis, for example, over many years contributes substantially to the patient's well-being, and the minimising of handicap. The matter is dealt with in detail in Chapter 29. It suffices perhaps to say that it devolves most heavily on the physiotherapist. She gives advice on posture in bed, at work and at leisure, and on daily exercise and sport. Such a young patient will also need to consider other factors including work (the disablement resettlement officer should be consulted more than he usually is) and the acquisition of vocational skills (the specialist careers officer located at the local education department can be a great help for the 16–18 age-group), mortgages and insurance (with persistence, disadvantages can often be reduced and the National Ankylosing Spondylitis Society has much information).

Arthritis in a single, weight-bearing joint

Here we are frequently talking of osteoarthrosis, which though perhaps less severe and less complex than rheumatoid arthritis is responsible for much more disability in total. If considering osteoarthrosis of the hip, for example, we find that surgeons rarely contemplate prosthetic replacement unless the hip disease is advanced and the patient requests surgery. Further, mild arthritis will not necessarily progress rapidly and inexorably to the advanced stage that necessitates surgery. Thus, in early or mild arthritis one aims to:

1. Reduce the load on the joint
2. Increase joint range and prevent deformity
3. Increase muscle power around the joint

4. Decrease pain
5. Alter patients' demands of the joint
6. Decrease environmental adversities.

Let us consider the help various staff may give the patient:

Physiotherapy
To reduce the load on a weight-bearing joint the patient should use a stick in the opposite hand (with the stick handle level with the stick handle level with the wrist when the arm is hanging by the side). The Fisher stick has a comfortable handle for the rheumatic hand.

The patient should also reduce weight to the ideal weight. Even though this will not necessarily prevent further deterioration in the radiological appearance of the joint, the ensuing mechanical advantage can be substantial.

Most people do not require a full range of joint function. But a minimum 90° is necessary at the knee to ascend and descend stairs (and more to kneel); at the hip the mid-range must be conserved, and it must be remembered that a small intermalleolar separation means that high kerbs and steps cannot be negotiated; restricted hip abduction may preclude sexual intercourse and be an indication for surgery.

Flexion deformity tends to occur at the hip with loss of extension and abduction, and with contracture of the joint capsule. Repeated daily exercises (active assisted with sling suspension, then active), particularly of extension and abduction, are necessary and should be combined with periods of prone lying to reduce hip flexion. Fixed flexion of the *knee* is exacerbated by remaining seated (e.g. in a wheelchair) for long periods. It must be combatted energetically or reversed by splintage (serial if necessary) in increasing extension or by reversed sling suspension (Dickson), and by vigorous repeated quadriceps exercise followed by supervised ambulation on crutches.

The improvement of muscle power round the joint may be associated with decreased pain. Conversely, it may be necessary to gain the patients' co-operation in such active therapy programmes by ensuring that maximum pain relief is given at these times by proper timing of analgesics, by giving physical modalities (heat, ice, hydrotherapy) and also by intra-articular steroid injections.

Occupational therapy
It is the occupational therapist's province to carry out (or initiate) home and work adaptations to decrease the demands on the involved joint. Ground floor accommodation (or at least a ground floor toilet) is often helpful. Firmly fixed rails on the stairs and in the toilet, high seating (and high lavatory seat) are appreciated.

Entering and leaving the bath can be hazardous and should be undertaken from the seated position. A bath board, seat and non-slip mat are helpful; ambulifts and hoists are only required for more severely disabled subjects and it should be remembered that most bathrooms and lavatories have little space for such impedimenta. A shower separate from the bath is a boon.

Putting on socks and tights, lacing shoes and cutting toenails are a difficulty and a little help from a relative is probably preferable to the stocking aid, or elastic shoe laces which have to be used by those who live alone.

The patient may be willing and able to alter his life-style, to walk less over uneven terrain, to use a car (a bus step is often too high), to change his style of carrying out various activities. Other remedial staff should be consulted as outlined earlier.

Chronic polyarthritis in the adult
Here we have to consider (a) the impingement of pain and loss of function in one joint on another and (b) interaction between the disease, the environment and the patient's role in society. Again, we would call up resources as outlined above, aiming to maintain or hopefully improve, the patient's independence. A few points (as follow) are worth remembering.

No assessment of domestic activities or function at work is realistic until pain and stiffness are brought under control by non-steroidal anti-inflammatory drugs or by long-term antirheumatic agents. One sees anaemia, fever and the complications of disease taking their toll: the patient has neither the will nor energy to enter a rehabilitation programme or to plan a change in life-style. Further, attempts to spare one joint such as the knee place undue stresses on another such as the shoulder.

The wage-earner is threatened by loss of work and hence of status within and without the family; the mother is threatened by loss of her function; the sexual role of the arthritic may diminish — loss of energy and libido may result from disease and drugs, joints may be painful and have restricted movement, which interferes with intercourse; the patient and partner may no longer view the sufferer as sexually attractive and the relationship may decline to that of parent–child. Loss of money and of mobility may compound the problems. In all these situations it is important that the doctor acts in such a way as to support the patient's key role in the family, giving advice on support services that enhance this role, and also offering approval of whatever sexual demonstration of affection is appropriate, giving counselling on contraception, and considering the role of drug therapy during pregnancy and lactation.

ADDRESSES

Arthritis Care, 6 Grosvenor Crescent, London SWX 7 ER.

Arthritis and Rheumatism Council, 41 Eagle Street, London WCAR 41R.

RADAR, 25 Mortimer Street, London W1N 8AB.

Joint Aids Centres Committee, Leicester Aids Centre, 76 Clarendon Park Road, Leicester L2 3AD.

Mobility Information Service, Copthorne Community Hall, Shelton Road, Shrewsbury, Shrops.

National Ankylosing Spondylitis Society, c/o The Royal National Hospital for Rheumatic Diseases, Bath, BA1 1RL.

Sexual Problems of the Disabled, c/o RADAR, 25 Mortimer Street, London.

Disabled Living Foundation, 346 Kensington High Street, London W14 8NS.

REFERENCES

Badley E, Lee J, Wood P H N 1979 Patterns of disability related to joint involvement in rheumatoid arthritis. Rheumatology and Rehabilitation 18: 105–109

Brattstrom M 1973 Principles of joint protection in rheumatoid disease. Lund, Sweden: Student Literatur

Chamberlain M A, Buchanan J, Hanks H 1979 The arthritic in an urban environment. Annals of the Rheumatic Diseases 381: 51–56

Chamberlain M A, Care G, Harfield B 1982 Physiotherapy in osteoarthrosis of the knees: a controlled trial of hospital versus home exercises. International Rehabilitation Medicine 4:101

Cornwell M 1975 Early years. Disabled Living Foundation Publication

Darnborough A, Kinrade D 1985 Directory for the Disabled, 5th Edn. Woodhead-Faulker, Cambridge

Davis P R, Troup J D G 1964 Pressures in the trunk cavities when pulling pushing and lifting. Ergonomics 7: 465–474

Dixon A St J 1981 Footwear in arthritic feet. Clinics in Rheumatic Diseases 8: 4–377

Ellis M 1982 Forces in the human knee during rising from a chair. PhD Thesis, University of Leeds

Fligg H, Wright V 1981 The community and hospital nurse in relation to arthritis. Clinics in Rheumatic Diseases 7:321

Fries J F, Spitz R, Kraines G, Holman H R 1980 Measurement of patient outcome in arthritis. Arthritis and Rheumatism 23: 137–145

Goldsmith S 1976 Designing for the disabled, 3rd Edn. RIBA

Harris: A: 1971 Handicapped and impaired in Great Britain, Part I. HMSO, London

Kushlika A 1980 How much do we care? International Rehabilitation Medicine 2:103

Multicentre Trial (1966) Pain in the neck and arm: a multicentre trial on the effects of physiotherapy. British Medical Journal 1: 253–258

Munton J S, Ellis M I, Chamberlain M A, Wright: V: 1981 An investigation into the problems of easy chairs used by the arthritic and the elderly. Rheumatology and Rehabilitation 20: 164–173

Manpower Services Commission. Aids and adaptations for disabled employees. Leaflet No. EPL71 (revised)

Nichols P J R 1976 Rehabilitation medicine. Butterworth, London, Oxford Regional Health Authority. Equipment for the disabled

Smith D 1976 The Northwick Park stroke rehabilitation study. Rheumatology and Rehabilitation 15: 163–166

Steinbrocker O, Traeger: C H, Batterman R C 1949 Functional grading. Journal of the American Medical Association 140:659

Williams: E, Hill, Crewe R, Cochrane G 1982 Wheelcharis: A guide to clinical prescription. DHSS Appliance Service, Warbreck Hill, Blackpool, HMSO

Wynn Parry C B 1982 The 1981 Philip Nichols Memorial Lecture. International Rehabilitation 4: 59–64

Surgical treatment of arthritis

Most rheumatologists would find it impossible to provide adequate care for their patients without ready access to the services of an orthopaedic surgical department. In many units up to 10% of patients attending the outpatient clinic will undergo an orthopaedic surgical procedure each year. The need for surgical treatment may be even higher. Allander (1974) in a survey of 293 patients with rheumatoid arthritis found that 8% would benefit from a major reconstructive procedure while the function of 30% would be improved by a minor procedure. However, 60% of those requiring major surgery and 30% of those requiring minor surgery refuse such procedures, while further active and passive selection procedures reduce the final operative load to 10% of the total. However, such surgical treatment cannot be considered or undertaken in isolation.

Rheumatoid arthritis is a complex disease and simple descriptions of the pathological processes fail to provide any explanation of the impact of the disease upon an individual patient. The wide spectrum of the disease means that a single description is quite inadequate as an explanation of the likely future disability for all patients, while the very variable progress of the disease means equally that a carefully chosen description cannot be used to explain the likely future disability in an individual patient. Other forms of inflammatory arthritis can follow a similar variable and unpredictable path.

It follows, therefore, that clinical decisions must be based upon continual assessment. Further, the impact of the disease upon the domestic, social, economic, employment and sexual lives of the patient means that a single doctor cannot undertake such an assessment or determine which are the best therapeutic alternatives to follow. At the same time, although the more predictable nature of osteoarthritis and its usual monarticular damage may make continual assessment less necessary, many of these patients are elderly and have other diseases which may impair their ability to withstand major joint surgery. The valuable part that the rheumatologist/general physician can play in the pre- and postoperative assessment and management of these patients has been described (Bossingham et al, 1980). It is important, if unnecessary medical problems are to be prevented and precious operating theatre time is not to be wasted due to late cancellation of medically unfit patients, that better preoperative surveillance must be undertaken, probably by the general practitioner, and likely difficulties communicated to the hospital team, bearing in mind that there may be considerable delay on a waiting list between reaching a decision to operate and undertaking such surgery.

As in many branches of medicine and as emphasised elsewhere in this book various forms of treatment cannot be considered or undertaken in isolation. A team approach is essential. The orthopaedic surgeon has become a member of such a team, so that together with the general practitioner, rheumatologist, physiotherapist and occupational therapists, nurses, social workers and disablement resettlement officers, he can play his part in the delivery of total patient care. All members of the arthritis team should be involved at all stages in the patient's management, for it is only in this way that all available forms of treatment can be considered for every patient. However, it is important that a single doctor undertakes overall responsibility for the patient's management and for patients with rheumatoid arthritis and other forms of inflammatory arthritis this is best done by a rheumatologist, since surgical treatment is but an item in their continuing lifetime management. Medical and surgical services should be available in the same hospital and ideally in a combined unit and not, as is sometimes the case, many miles apart.

It is clearly incumbent upon the rheumatologist to be aware of the range of operative procedures currently available, the likely results and the optimum time at which they should be considered. There is now a bewildering number of total joint replacements available, particularly for the hip, knee and finger joints. This chapter will not attempt to list, let alone describe, all these prostheses because in many cases their longer term value has not been proven. However, a selection of commonly used procedures and prostheses will be described and the future trends indicated. If advances are to be made, combined clinics must exist at which patients who present a wide range of functional problems are discussed as well as those who clearly fulfil current operative indications. Since orthopaedic surgeons will always have individual preferences and skills with the often unpredictable ability to achieve better results with some procedures than others, this chapter will examine some of the factors responsible for success or failure of these orthopaedic procedures and will discuss some of the problems, real or imaginary, that can arise when patients with arthritis undergo such surgical treatment. Finally, it will become clear that it is often impossible to answer the often asked question, 'When should a patient be referred for surgical treatment?', since the moment will vary greatly depending upon the nature and severity of the patient's disease and the arthritis team's interpretation of that patient's needs.

AIMS OF SURGICAL TREATMENT

The aims of surgical treatment are threefold:

An improvement in function

Such improvement may relate to the domestic, social, economic, employment or sexual implications of the patient's deformity and disability. In essence almost all treatment in arthritis is directed towards an improvement in function, since it is functional difficulties of which the patients either directly or indirectly complain.

Relief of pain

Many surgeons will argue that relief of pain is the prime and often the only reason for operating. Such an approach may imply some lack of confidence in the ability of the operation or prosthesis to improve function, but more usually reflects greater difficulty in demonstrating improved postoperative function than pain relief. In most cases pain relief leads to a functional improvement. However, in some instances surgical treatment may not improve function, particularly when a joint is arthrodesed, but may simply allow the patient to sit or sleep without pain.

Improvement in appearance

In most patients the deterioration in function and appearance will have taken place gradually and they are much more concerned about function than appearance. Thus it is uncommon, except in young women and some patients with juvenile rheumatoid arthritis, to operate for cosmetic reasons alone. However, it must be admitted that an improvement in appearance can be a great morale booster.

PATIENT ASSESSMENT

Although exact numbers are hard to determine it has been calculated that 80 000 total hip and 40 000 total knee arthroplasties were performed in the USA in 1976 with the annual numbers continuing to grow (Hori et al, 1978). In some parts of the world and certainly in the UK the success of surgical treatment for arthritis has created new problems. Quite simply the demand for such surgery, particularly total hip replacement but increasingly total knee replacement, has not been paralleled by an expansion in surgical staff and operating facilities (Office of Health Economics, 1982) Waiting lists have grown longer and indeed continue to grow as patients with less severe disease are added now that it is recognised they would benefit from what was previously an unproved technique. Problems will be compounded if the revision rate for total joint prostheses, currently running at 25% of the patient load in some North

American Centres (Cracchiolo, 1982), is reflected in British and other National practices.

Solutions have varied from the calculated need for new hospitals with more surgeons (Morris, 1978) to a simpler solution in the face of increasing financial stringency of using existing facilities and staff more efficiently (HMSO, 1981). The use of limited resources must therefore be considered during the assessment of patients. It is no longer possible simply to select patients who would benefit from surgery but rather some sort of priority listing must be achieved if the most good is to be done for the most patients. While all clinical medicine is to some extent an expression of a doctor's and a patient's choice, pragmatic decisions based upon shortage are much less acceptable.

Surgical decisions of whether to operate and if so upon which joint are often difficult to make. This is partly due to the complex disabilities arising from multiple joint disease and partly because almost all orthopaedic surgery, in contradistinction to most other surgical treatment, is both elective and demanding upon the patient. Thus, except in the case of stabilisation of the upper cervical spine, surgery has little or no effect upon the patient's general health or life expectancy. Further, many procedures place considerable demands upon the patient, particularly in co-operating fully with the physiotherapists and occupational therapists, if a satisfactory result is to be achieved. Although, theoretically, similar considerations apply to patients with osteoarthritis, the older average age of such patients, the usual involvement of but a single joint, the absence of significant systemic features of the disease and the shorter postoperative recovery period mean that surgical decisions are usually reached more easily.

A correct surgical decision will usually be made in patients with rheumatoid arthritis and related diseases if all members of the arthritis team can independently assess the patient's difficulties and likely response to treatment and then arrive at a conference decision, on whether to operate and upon which joint. The final decisions on the type of operation must then be made by the surgeon and physician in the light of various technical and medical considerations discussed later. Such assessments should concentrate upon the following factors.

The patient's requirements

The patient's requirements must be clearly identified. These will, as suggested above, usually be centred upon an improvement in function. To this end the paramedical and nursing staff should undertake, as far as possible, a practical measurement of the patient's domestic, social, employment and sexual difficulties. For example, it is easy to accept as reasonable a patient's wish to be able to walk to the shops, when a home visit will quickly show that none of the therapeutic alternatives could possibly provide the required functional improvement. Similarly, although hip disease has been identified as an important cause of sexual difficulties, particularly in women, hip surgery while relieving some problems may expose other (Baldursson & Brattstrom, 1979).

An attempt has been made to develop a scoring system that not only identifies those in need but also, by the use of questions based upon functionally important aspects of motion which were shown to be sensitive measures of postoperative change, identifies those most likely to benefit from a procedure, in this case total hip replacement (McDowell et al, 1978). Certainly not all patients are pleased with their surgical results. In some their expectations may have been set too high (Howarth et al, 1981). Thus it is important that both patient and surgeon be realistic in their aims.

Local joint disease

Measurement of existing muscle strength, joint movement and stability together with radiographic analysis, will allow an assessment of how these might be influenced by exercises and surgery. Increasing use of biomechanical measurements has allowed greater insight into abnormal patterns of joint and muscle usage. Gait analysis and functional testing have suggested that the results of hip and knee surgery are more dependent upon patient than prosthetic characteristics (Murray et al, 1976; Andriacchi et al, 1982). Changes in foot loading before and after surgery can be measured (Simkin, 1981), quadriceps bulk and activity can be accurately measured using ultrasonography (Young et al, 1980) and exercise test methods of walking speed, cadence, stride length and oxygen consumption can be employed to show notable postoperative improvements (MacNicol et al, 1980).

These latter findings are important considerations when faced with the prospect of major joint replacement in the patient with ischaemic heart disease. It is clear that provided that his heart disease allows him to undergo the initial surgical stress, his future activities will impose less strain upon his heart; the calculated mean oxygen consumption required to walk 1 kilometre comes down from 19.27 to 9.35 litres six months after hip replacement.

Extent and severity of polyarthritis

An evaluation of the polyarthritis is essential, since the response to surgery will be influenced by involvement of other joints. Thus the results of a knee operation may be affected not only by foot and hip involvement but also by the patient's ability to use carefully selected walking aids with their upper limbs in the immediate postoperative period. Further, experience shows that in patients requiring both hip and knee surgery, the hip operation should be undertaken first as this facilitates subsequent mobilisation of the knees; and stabilisation and relief of pain at the wrist may make subsequent hand surgery unnecessary. On the other hand the apparently ambitious project of replacing both knees during a single operation or within a very short time of each other has been advocated as it leads to better results and the restoration of a more normal gait than when the joints are replaced several months apart (Hardaker et al, 1978).

Therefore, it may be necessary to plan a programme of surgical therapy. This inevitably raises unanswerable questions, for although the outcome of one or two sequential procedures can be predicted, both from the patient's and surgeon's viewpoint, further procedures introduce less predictable factors relating to the cumulative chance of surgical success and the effect upon the patient of an extended stay in hospital. Thus one should be wary of accepting the challenge of terminating a patient's wheelchair life by submitting her to four joint replacements (both hips and both knees) during a single lengthy admission. On the other hand, the replacement of these four joints, because of slowly progressive disease, over a period of years is an entirely different proposition commonly undertaken and frequently successful. For example the replacement of 104 joints in 26 patients by this creeping substitution followed for a mean of 51 months was accompanied by good results, a preference for hip surgery and only 5 revision procedures (McDonald, 1982).

It is implicit in these first three stages of assessment that the patient may not have the ability to identify her difficulties clearly or to be the best judge of her own requirements. The customer is frequently wrong and she may require a sympathetic explanation of the aims of the measures that are being undertaken.

The patient's mental response

Formal preoperative psychological assessment has not been used as a predictor of the postoperative result and is probably unnecessary in most cases since the patient will have been in contact with the therapeutic team over a period of years. However, the patient's mental response to her disease and disability must be assessed and hence a judgement made upon her likely co-operation in achieving satisfactory postoperative progress and the optimum result. Patients are naturally anxious to appear to conform to normal patterns of behaviour and can be expected to claim that a return towards previous functional levels is their major wish. Nevertheless, detailed and unhurried assessment and examination of the response to earlier therapeutic efforts and hospitalisation may show that they really do not wish or require a major change in function or that depression or a poor tolerance of pain may mean that they cannot co-operate in extended and physically and mentally demanding periods of treatment away from home.

Family response

An assessment must be made — after interview and ideally a home visit — of the patient's family's reaction to her disease, deformity and disability. This important item is often neglected. In many families patterns of activity and responsibility will have evolved over the years and will have become both convenient and fixed, so that improved function in the patient may not be utilised. Thus a husband may never allow his arthritic wife to resume domestic responsibilities because her shortcomings and often slow tempo of work interferes with the routine which he now finds both satisfactory and satisfying. Further, a first-hand view of the domestic architecture may show that despite its capacity for simple adaptation by the provision of extra rails, convenient toilets, elimination of steps, etc , that the demands placed upon the patient will remain too great and that the results of the contemplated surgery will never be utilised.

It is fashionable to talk of patient motivation and to ascribe therapeutic success or failure to the patient's 'good' or 'bad' motivation. It should now be clear that if some time is spent in a detailed preoperative assessment of the patient (time which can also be used to increase muscle strength and reduce joint inflammation and contracture), little should be left to chance in arriving at the correct surgical decision, and the arthritis team must carry most of the responsibility for failure.

GENERAL SURGICAL CONSIDERATIONS

The final decision to operate and as to which procedure to employ can only be made by the surgeon, after all aspects of total patient care have been considered and the patient's needs have been accurately assessed. However, there are several other considerations which can influence surgical decisions or the outcome of the procedure.

The patient's general health

As with any elective operation the patient's cardiorespiratory reserve must be adequate. Although systemic features of rheumatoid and related disease, particularly those affecting the heart, lung and kidney, may influence the patient's suitability for major surgery, the extent and severity of the arthritis usually have little effect upon the immediate surgical results. However, in patients with severe long-standing disease the possibility of amyloidosis, with a very low serum albumin, and marked osteoporosis must be remembered as factors which may affect postoperative recovery.

Evidence of capillary vasculitic lesions has been stated to be a contraindication to hand surgery (Holt, 1969). Although commonsense suggests that widespread lesions will impair skin nutrition and wound healing, there are no satisfactory comparative studies and personal experience has shown that it is usually unnecessary to impose such restrictions.

Although many patients are anaemic, the anaemia being proportional to the activity of the disease, there is no evidence to show there is an increased risk in operating upon patients who have adapted to haemoglobin values as low as 10.5 g/dl (Garner et al, 1973). Those with lower values are best transfused a few days preoperatively. Many patients are underweight and this often gives them an advantage over osteoarthritic patients, since obesity undoubtedly reduces the benefits of surgical treatment and should be treated.

Finally, the life expectancy of patients with rheumatoid arthritis is reduced (Uddin et al, 1970; Rasker & Cosh, 1981; Allebeck, 1982). This is a reflection of the duration and severity of the disease, death in some cases being directly related to the effects of the disease while in others it is related to drug therapy including corticosteroids, surgery and infection. However, the mean reduction of some 4–8 years is less than many imagine and will affect surgical decisions in only a few cases.

The patient's local disease

Although it is implicit in the concept of total care that the patient should be receiving any necessary drugs or physical therapy in an attempt to reduce the inflammatory reaction, it is unnecessary to control the activity of the local joint disease before operating. Procedures involving synovectomy may be simpler if the synovial inflammation, which frequently spreads to surrounding ligaments and muscles, is controlled and the vascularity of the tissue reduced by a short period of rest. In particular, it is an advantage to correct deformities secondary to inflammation, such as flexion of the knee, since such correction will simplify the surgical procedure and the resultant improvement in muscle control and development will speed postoperative recovery. The operation may have more than a local effect, since the removal of an inflamed synovial membrane may not only control local disease but also improve the general disease, as if the involved joint was acting as a 'trigger' to the inflammatory process (Fink et al, 1969).

Wound healing

It is often supposed that surgical wounds are more liable to become infected and to heal poorly in rheumatoid patients compared with osteoarthritic patients and it is further supposed that treatment with corticosteroids is likely to exaggerate these tendencies. Certainly there are various factors which, alone or in combination, might be expected to influence wound healing.

1. An increased incidence of bacterial infection in the chest and joints of patients with rheumatoid arthritis has been reported (Baum, 1971)
2. The skin of rheumatoid arthritic patients is significantly thinner than in healthy controls, but this bears no relation to the duration or activity of the disease. This skin thinning is slightly exaggerated by corticosteroid therapy (Grahame, 1969; Schorn & Mowat, 1977)
3. Many patients have a reduced white cell count and in those with Felty's syndrome there will be neutropenia (less than 2.5×10^9 cells/l)
4. Anaemia (Mowat, 1976)
5. Low serum albumin values are common, being proportional to the activity of the disease and are not necessarily a manifestation of nephrosis secondary to amyloidosis or drug therapy
6. Peripheral oedema, usually in the legs, may be associated with low serum albumin values (less than 25 g/l) or increased capilliary diffusion (Jayson et al, 1971), but is more usually due to dependence and immobility or venous and lymphatic occlusion by a posterior knee cyst
7. Wound haematomas secondary to aspirin and related drug therapy
8. Vasculitis with skin ischaemia
9. Reduced neutrophil leucocyte chemotactic activity; a vital activity if the cell is to reach the wound to remove bacterial and other debris and take part in wound healing (Mowat, 1976)
10. The known impairment of wound healing in experimental animals given massive doses of corticosteroids (Garner et al, 1973).

However, in a study of wound healing in 100 matched rheumatoid and osteoarthritic patients, only minor differences were noted (Garner et al, 1973). There was no difference between wound healing in seropositive and seronegative patients, and the rate of healing was unrelated to the duration and severity of the disease, or the degree of anaemia. Corticosteroid therapy was associated with a modest increase in wound infections, but, perhaps more importantly, produced a significant increase in the mean number of days to wound healing if it had been given, irrespective of dose, for more than 3 years. The actual dosage of corticosteroids, which was within the usual range of 2.5–10 mg of prednisolone per day, seemed less important.

Mowat (1976) has found that although the impairment in neutrophil chemotaxis is chiefly related to the prior ingestion of immune complexes, metabolic factors, possibly endogenous corticosteroid production, are also important since elective orthopaedic surgical treatment is associated with an improvement to almost normal values with a subsequent, gradual return to preoperative values over a 14-day period. Further, patients receiving corticosteroid therapy in low dosage showed a higher initial but lower final chemotactic index compared with those patients who had never been treated with these drugs. These findings accord with the wound healing results described above and suggest extra care should be taken over the wounds in those who have received corticosteroids for more than 3 years.

Finally, there has been some concern over wound healing in the increasing number of patients being treated with D-penicillamine. This drug alters the normal metabolism of collagen by inhibiting cross-linking and reducing protein synthesis, and this is associated with an increase in skin thinning (Schorn & Mowat, 1977). These authors found that although D-penicillamine therapy was associated with a modest increase in the mean time to wound healing this was comparable with the delay produced by corticosteroid therapy and was not associated with any special problems. Once again special care is required but it is unnecessary to stop the drug during the operative period.

Although most surgeons and physicians will have seen occasional instances of serious delay in wound healing and troublesome wound infection in patients with rheumatoid arthritis, these are the exception, and even when they occur are not necessarily more frequent or more severe than in comparable osteoarthritic controls (Garner et al, 1973). It is hardly ever necessary to restrict postoperative mobilisation or delay stitch removal beyond the limits set for the patients with degenerative arthritis.

Similar considerations probably apply to other forms of inflammatory arthritis but have been little studied. However, the potential risk of wound infection when operating through psoriatic skin has been examined. Lambert & Wright (1979) noted only 2 infections in 54 operations on 41 patients and commented that evidence of the Köbner phenomenon elsewhere on the patient's skin did not necessarily mean the development of incisional psoriasis.

Patient handling and intubation

The anaesthetist and all who handle the cervical spine of the unconscious rheumatoid patient must remember that many have an unstable neck, usually with atlantoaxial subluxation. Since the majority of patients are symptomless and radiographs are unhelpful in predicting those that are likely to have trouble, all must be handled carefully. We currently send every patient to the operating theatre in a soft collar, which although it is removed, nevertheless serves as a useful reminder to the theatre staff.

Occasionally involvement of the temporomandibular joints will limit mouth opening, while in a few patients, usually those with juvenile rheumatoid arthritis which has extended into adult life, the cervical spine may have ankylosed, adding to the problems with intubation caused by failure of growth of the mandible, temporomandibular joint changes and malocclusion of the teeth (Larheim et al, 1981). Patients with ankylosing spondylitis with cervical spinal fusion in flexion may present special difficulties.

Perversely the early loss of teeth and their replacement by dentures in many patients with inflammatory joint disease reduces the problems with intubation. Teeth are lost partly because dental hygiene is inadequate with poor upper limb function, partly due to direct disease effects upon the gums and partly due to the lack of saliva and accelerated dental caries with Sjögren's syndrome (Malmstrom & Calonius, 1975).

Drug therapy

All drug therapy should be continued over the operative period lest there be an increase in general disease symptoms. It is common practice to perhaps double the dose of any corticosteroid drug for 24–48 hours using intramuscular injections of hydrocortisone in equivalent dose. This is probably both unnecessary and unwise. The plasma cortisol value rises rapidly during surgical procedures, usually reaching a peak at 6 hours, and although an exaggerated adrenal response may be maintained for up to 3 days, the normal circadian rhythm is usually restored the following day (Myles & Daly, 1974). Although corticosteroid-treated patients may have a reduced response due to suppression of the hypothalmic–pituitary–adrenal axis this is often less than expected, and the insulin–hypoglycaemia test correlates well with the surgical stimulus. Additional corticosteroid therapy may be associated with an increased risk of wound or intercurrent infection and may impair initial wound healing by reducing fibroblast activity (Myles & Daly, 1974). See also Chapter 20.

The possibility that intercurrent drug therapy such as gold, D-penicillamine and immunosuppressive agents may cause reduced white cell and platelet counts must be remembered; there is also a possible risk of sensitivity to halothane leading to liver damage, following repeated exposure to the drug during a programme of surgical therapy (Lancet Editorial, 1980; Williams et al, 1977).

Aspirin produces modest hypoprothrombinaemia and, in common with other non-steroidal anti-inflammatory agents which inhibit prostaglandin synthetase, will reduce platelet adhesion. Aspirin has an irreversible inhibitory effect upon the enzyme and the alteration in platelet adhesion persists for the rest of the platelet's life. In general, the other drugs have a reversible competitive inhibitory effect and the platelets recover after drug withdrawal. Although these changes rarely lead to the formation of a wound haematoma, they must be considered in relation to deep venous thrombosis. Aspirin and some of the newer non-steroidal anti-inflammatory drugs compete with warfarin for the same binding protein in the serum. Formal studies of the extent of this interaction in patients is only available for a few drugs and in some cases the expected interference has hypersensitivity to various metals can occur, the relationship between such skin sensitivity and prosthesis loosening is not established. Some authors (Benson et al, 1975) feel that metal sensitivity, particularly to chrome cobalt prostheses, is an important factor in their loosening while others (Evarts, 1978; Lancet Editorial, 1980) consider that the case has not been proved. Prospective skin testing, while recognising the high incidence (10% or more) of sensitivity to the metals in the normal population and the potential for an individual to show changing sensitivity with time, suggests that the use of metal on plastic prostheses produces no change in skin sensitivity while the use of metal on metal prostheses, now largely abandoned, may be accompanied by an increase (Benson et al, 1975; Deutman et al, 1977; Rooker & Wilkinson, 1980). It is perhaps unrealistic to suppose that skin reactivity should mimic reactivity in deeper tissues and the argument would be more persuasive if there was clear immunological evidence of such hypersensitivity with raised serum or local levels of IgE and clear changes in leucocyte reactivity to metal ion solutions. Although trivalent chromium–albumin complexes have been shown to inhibit leucocyte migration and that this correlates with skin reactivity to chromium (Tio, 1976), preliminary studies on synovial fluid from around loose prostheses have failed to demonstrate significant formation of leucocyte migration inhibition factor or induce lymphocyte transformation (Brown et al, 1977).

Although in some patients there is no doubt from the history and the clinical findings that a prosthesis is loose, in many it can be extremely difficult to determine whether persistent pain in a joint is due to minor degrees of loosening or settling of one or other components of the prosthesis. Standard radiographs including stress views often fail to provide the necessary information and direct examination under an image intensifier is notoriously difficult to interpret since the smallest amount of limb rotation gives a false appearance of prosthesis movement. The use of radio-opaque cement allows accurate evaluation of its location, bulk and structure, while cement fractures, cementophytes and fragments can be detected. The addition of barium sulphate to the cement does not significantly alter its biomechanical properties. Bone scanning, often combining the information from ^{99m}Tc-diphosphonates and ^{67}Ga-citrate, can provide valuable information since reversion to a normal pattern occurs in most patients 5 months after hip replacement, although heterotopic ossification may extend the interval to 9 months (Salvati et al, 1976; Schneider et al 1982). There is an urgent need for developments in this field and agreement upon standard methods of investigation.

TYPES OF OPERATION

There are four major types of operation currently used on the joints of patients with arthritis — synovectomy, arthroplasty, osteotomy and arthrodesis.

Synovectomy

Removal of part or whole of the synovial lining of a joint was first used in rheumatoid arthritis in 1887 by Schüller following its beneficial effect in tuberculosis. However, synovectomy was only undertaken in significant numbers of patients from the mid-1950s onwards following promising results when tried in a variety of joints. At present the operation is only considered of value when performed on finger joints, the wrist, elbow and knee joints. Taylor & Hill (1978) have reviewed the subject.

The chief indications for synovectomy are pain and swelling of a joint unresponsive to medical therapy. Although encouraging results of syno vectomy have been reported in damaged joints (Geens, 1969; Gschwend, 1980), most authors stress that the operation must be performed early — usually after 3–6 months of persistent disease and before significant cartilage and bone damage have occurred — to obtain the best results (Goldie, 1974). Follow-up studies indicate a steady deterioration in the percentage of good results from up to 80% at 1 year to 50% or less at 5 years. Earlier uncontrolled studies tended to support the hope that the operation, by removing the disease tissue, would have a prophylactic effect and that the rate of joint damage would be at least retarded if not halted. However, it has become clear to most surgeons, supported by the results of the prospective trial of knee synovectomy undertaken by the Arthritis and Rheumatism Council and British Orthopaedic Association that this was a forlorn hope.

Since at best only 85% of the synovial tissue is excised and similar results may follow generous synovial biopsy, the mechanism by which synovectomy produces relief of pain and swelling is not entirely clear. Certainly the excised subsynovial tissue is well supplied with pain fibres. Further, a reduction in intra-articular inflammation will produce a parallel reduction in inflammation in joint capsule and periarticular structures which are also well supplied with pain fibres. However, sequential studies of joint fluid and synovium and arthrography (Taylor & Ansell, 1972) following synovectomy have shown that a synovial lining regrows within 2–3 months from existing mesenchymal elements in the joint and in most cases is of a similar pathological type, with similar chemical and immunological activity, to that excised at operation. However, such recurrence of proliferative synovial tissue may take several months longer to become clinically detectable (Goldie, 1974). It has been suggested that the thickness of the connective tissue base to the new synovial membrane is vital in determining whether the patient will have a recurrence of symptoms; only occurring in those with a thin connective tissue base (Mitchell & Shepard, 1972).

It must be emphasised that synovectomy produces reasonably predictable results in terms of relief of pain and swelling for periods of 3–5 years. More detailed results are discussed in the relevant surgical sections, particularly those on the hand and knee. However, since the operation is associated with all the usual surgical risks, may lead to significant loss of movement, particularly in finger joints, requires inpatient treatment for approximately 3 weeks in the case of the knee joint, and has now been shown not to have a prophylactic value, its place in management is being questioned.

Growing experience with radioisotope synoviorthesis in rheumatoid arthritis suggests that the initial attempt at reducing persistent synovitis should be by this method, the result appearing comparable with surgical synovectomy with low morbidity (Gumpel, 1978; Boussina et al, 1979). There may still be a place for chemical synovectomy (Menkes, 1979). Further, increasing use of the arthroscope has suggested that joint lavage may be almost as beneficial as synovectomy.

Arthroplasty

Any operation which reconstitutes a joint is described as an arthroplasty. In a few cases the operation consists simply of excision of the damaged joint surfaces and synovial tissues, e.g. metacarpophalangeal joints, metatarsophalangeal joints and hip. With other joints, particularly the knee, elbow and metacarpophalangeal joints, some biological material of human or animal source is inserted following excision of joint surfaces in an attempt to keep the raw surfaces apart and to encourage the formation of a fibrous arthroplasty. Such material as chromatised pig's bladder, fascia lata and skin have had their protagonists, but are now rarely used, surgeons preferring to use metal or plastic to separate joint surfaces and increasingly, following the success of total hip replacement, to replace the joint completely. Various forms of joint replacement, particularly for the hips, have been available for 40 years, but all of the earlier devices proved entirely unsatisfactory as they failed to fulfil the criteria for success which have been clearly established over the past 15 years, particularly by Charnley. In general, a total joint replacement should fulfil the following criteria:

Clinical criteria

1. Relieve pain
2. Restore movement and stability
3. Correct deformity.

Technical and design criteria

1. Be chemically and physically inert in the biological environment
2. Should not generate electrolytic current between the components
3. Be long-wearing
4. Produce minimal wear particles. Such particles should not cause cell damage and should be self-cleared by the device so as to minimise their progressive destructive effect
5. Have low friction characteristics
6. Be firmly fixed to bone
7. Have inherent stability
8. Should mimic normal joint function.

do not always show advantages over those achieved with discarded prostheses. Some 80% of patients have good results, pain relief being more certain than functional gain. The results are better in rheumatoid arthritis compared with osteoarthritis perhaps because these patients expect less and are more appreciative of modest functional gain.

It has become clear that young patients with a single damaged joint and with no other physical impairment are not suitable for total replacement — the failure rate is too high. Previous joint sepsis seriously prejudices success. Refinements in technique, for example, questioning the need for patella replacement or resurfacing, continue. Failure, almost always loosening, results from a combination of poor bone, unbalanced soft tissues, malignment, poor cementing, overuse or abuse, bone or prosthetic fracture and infection. The failure rate accelerates 2 years after surgery so that by 5 years as little as half the patients may be painfree with the original prosthesis in situ (Tew & Waugh, 1982). Revision using the same or another prosthesis can be associated with the same 80% success rate despite the problems of infection, skin coverage and scar tissue (Rand and Bryan, 1982) and in many cases is worth trying since the results of salvage arthrodesis are very variable. The need for significant bone resection, the presence of infection and the uncertainty over the merits of external, internal or intramedullary fixation has led to successful arthrodesis in 25–100% of cases in various series (Stalberg, 1982). Many of the new nonlinked arthroplasties allow the replacement of a single compartment. Although this may be appropriate with any from of arthritis it has particular application with osteonecrosis at the knee which usually affects the femoral condyle. There are many disease associations including rheumatoid arthritis, systemic lupus erythematosus, hyperuricaemia and high dose corticosteroid therapy (Jones, 1978) and in some older patients no clear cause (Bauer, 1978). The sudden onset of pain, perhaps with local bone tenderness, the normal early radiographs, the diagnostic value of bone scintigraphy and the characteristic late radiographic features are now readily recognised (Griffiths et al, 1979; Smith et al, 1981).

As with other knee operations a tourniquet is applied and a compression bandage is required in the immediate postoperative phase. Gentle flexion and ambulation with support are usually allowed from the 5th day, this being a compromise time between the conflicting needs of wound healing and movement. Prophylactic antibiotics are given at the time of surgery and for a few days postoperatively. Most patients will require a 2–3 unit transfusion and osteoarthritic patients some form of anticoagulation.

Osteotomy

High tibial osteotomy if accurately carried out will relieve pain in three-quarters of patients with early osteoarthritis of the knee, particularly those with a varus deformity (Harding, 1976; Tjornstrand et al, 1981). The operation is particularly suitable for the younger, physically active patient, so serving a group for whom total replacement is not recommended (Brueckmann & Kettlekamp, 1982). Patients with rheumatoid arthritis usually have some involvement of both medial and lateral joint compartments and since they more commonly have a valgus than a varus angular deformity the results are rather disappointing.

Benjamin (1969) has described a double osteotomy with division of both tibia and femur a few centimetres from the joint line, the femoral division being within the joint capsule. The operation might be expected to produce changes in venous blood flow in bone (Marmor, 1972), but is probably less useful in correcting angular deformities. In consequence the results, particularly in the hands of those inexperienced in the technique, are rather disappointing and Benjamin describes significant pain relief in only two-thirds of cases, many of whom lose significant movement (Benjamin & Helal, 1980). Thus, in rheumatoid arthritis the operation should only be used in those with good knee flexion (Angel et al, 1974). Indeed, the results of this procedure may be no better than an equivalent time spent in a plaster of Paris cylinder (Huskisson & Phillips, 1973). Any osteotomy of the knee requires up to 6 or 8 weeks of support. Modern, light-weight calf bracing not only avoids the discomfort and vascular complications of several weeks in plaster of Paris but also allows early movement (Brueckmann & Kettlekamp, 1982).

Arthrodesis

Primary arthrodesis of the knee joint usually performed by the Charnley compression technique (Charnley & Lowe 1958) is a very reliable operation. However, up to 3 months rigid immobilisation is required, one of them non-weight bearing, and this may cause difficulties in patients with poor skin and venous congestion in the leg. Arthrodesis should be used with caution in patients with rheumatoid arthritis, particularly in younger patients in whom the operation may accentuate the rate of damage in the other major lower limb joints and eventually become a functional handicap. The great advantage of the operation is the production of a pain-free, stable limb, while the osteoporotic bone in these patients does not alter the technique or lead to a higher rate of non-union (2–4%). Thus many surgeons tend to combine arthroplasty of one knee with arthrodesis of the contraletral, more severely damaged joint. Such an approach has considerable merit, provided that the patient has been shown capable of coping with a stiff, straight limb in the home by the use of some form of knew splint or brace. Others consider that movement should be retained if at all possible and thus recommend arthroplasty as the primary operation. However, since, as indicated earlier, it may be difficult to convert an arthroplasty to an arthrodesis, careful planning of the order of operations may be required.

Arthrodesis of the knee undoubtedly imposes considerable additional strains upon the ipsilateral hip and if the shoe raise is too great upon both hips, as the leg cannot be swung through easily. In the presence of a fused or very stiff ankle the stress upon the hip is even greater. Prevention of damage to the contralateral knee depends upon the development and maintenance of strong quadriceps muscles around this knee and a correct raise to the shoe on the arthrodesed side (Fig. 63.7) (Brattström & Brattström, 1971).

In summary, the range of surgical alternatives at the knee is considerably greater than at other joints, reflecting both the complexity of the joint mechanics and the uncertainties of the surgical solutions. While it is impossible to lay down firm rules, useful guidelines in the choice of procedure are listed in Table 63.3.

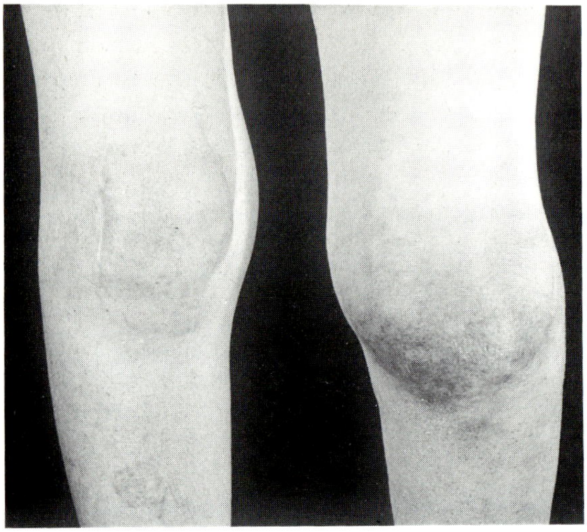

Fig. 63.7 Arthrodesis of the right knee has not been accompanied by correction of the resulting inequality in leg length, with the consequent development of active synovitis and flexion deformity in the left knee. This joint settled completely with conservative therapy.

Table 63.3

Extent of Joint Damage	Treatment
1. Synovial proliferation (RA) Loose bodies (OA)	Synovectomy Arthroscopic debridement
2. Minimal cartilage damage	MacIntosh (RA) Osteotomy (OA)
3. Moderate damage including osteonecrosis	1, 2 or 3 compartment, non-linked hinge arthroplasty
4. Severe damage ± instability	Linked hinge arthroplasty or arthrodesis

RA = rheumatoid arthritis; OA = osteoarthritis

HIP JOINT

Probably more has been written about total hip replacement than any other orthopaedic operation. Recent clinical experience in a variety of diseases, including rheumatoid arthritis, has been summarised by Jayson (1971) and Stinchfield (1973), the latter detailing in various papers the results of 18 154 operations using many different devices. The historical development of these devices has been described elsewhere (Newman, 1971), but credit for the current designs is due to the work of Charnley and of McKee and Watson Farrar. A very large range of devices incorporating modest alterations are available and as might be expected none has been shown to be definitely superior to any other (Stinchfield, 1973). Some of the modifications allow an easier operative technique, a lower incidence of prosthesis dislocation, a reduced incidence of cement reaching the pelvis with the use of the 'Mexican hat' and a theoretical reduction in the risk of infection by incorporating antibiotic into the bone cement.

A variety of surgical approaches to the hip joint are employed (Fig. 63.8), some of which allow replacement of both hips at a single operation though this is demanding on the cardiovascular system with the need for a larger transfusion and means that subsequent ambulation is difficult. There is considerable debate over the advantages and disadvantages of removal of the greater trochanter and its subsequent refixation with wires, screws or bolts. Charnley (1972) has claimed that its removal simplifies the operation and allows an adequate correction of the common adduction deformity. Many surgeons confirm these findings and emphasise that a more accurate siting of the prosthesis, often only possible with trochanteric removal, ensures for it a longer life. The incidence of trochanteric slip following wire breakage (Fig. 63.9) varies from series to series with a mean of 4%. Wire breakage after 6 weeks is unlikely to affect union of the trochanter but wire fragments may migrate subcutaneously and require removal. Despite this surgeons do not suggest that removal requires a slower rate of postoperative mobilisation, although in a few rheumatoid patients with particularly osteoporotic bone there may be a significant incidence of wire slipping, allowing upward displacement of the trochanter. This may occasionally require rewiring if there is pain or a tendency towards a Trendelenburg gait.

The requirements for blood transfusion (3–4 units), anticoagulation and prophylactic antibiotics are similar to those in total knee replacement. The patients are encouraged to move their hips immediately with some form of sling or pillow keeping the limb in abduction. Ambulation is allowed from the 3rd to 7th day and the return of a normal gait with or without the use of one stick can be expected at 1 month, although there is likely to be further improvement up to 1 year after operation.

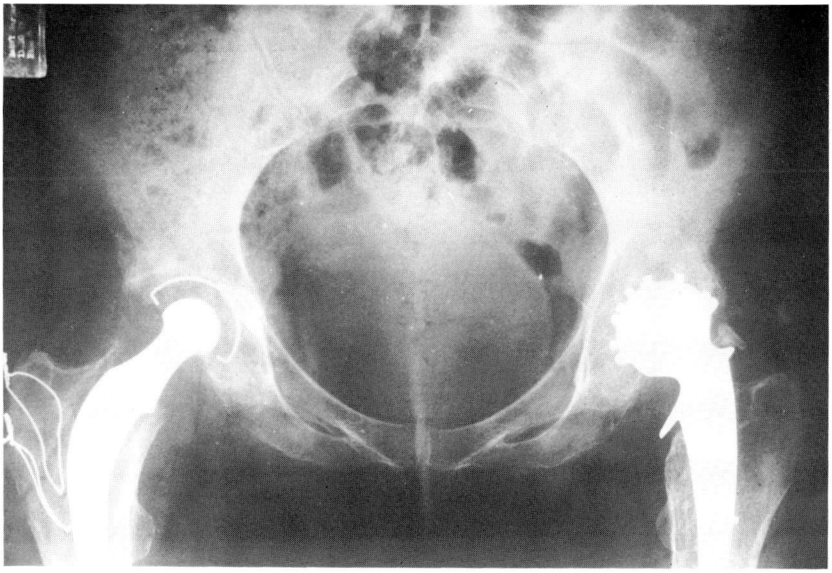

Fig. 63.8 Bilateral total hip replacement. McKee-Farrar prosthesis in the left hip and Charnley prosthesis in the right. The greater trochanter on the right has been reattached with wires. Also on the right the marker wire in the high-density polyethylene acetabular cup and the cement retaining 'Mexican hat' are clearly shown.

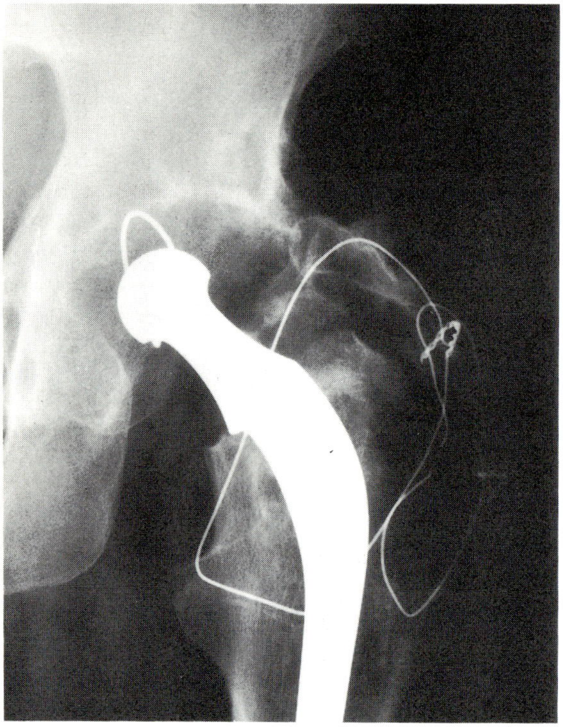

Fig. 63.9 Charnley total hip replacement with early breakage of the trochanteric wires and upward movement of the trochanter associated with pain and haematoma but eventually satisfactory hip abduction.

The success rate, regardless of the underlying disease, is similar, with over 90% of patients having a good or excellent result on the basis of relief of pain, the ability to walk without a stick and the overall functional gain (Evart, 1978; Stinchfield, 1973). Nevertheless there is a risk that in the face of these exciting and largely predictable results that the operation is oversold, that patients in speaking to their surgeon, talking to satisfied recipients and reading articles in the lay and possibly medical press, may believe that all pain is removed, that the gain in function is almost limitless and that there are no complications. The influence of changes in general health, of often irreversible changes in the pattern of daily living in the face of arthritis and of arthritis in other joints, usually the contralateral hip and the knees, is largely ignored by patients anxiously awaiting hip surgery and only partly listening to the cautionary advice of surgeons, therapists and nurses (Haworth et al, 1981).

The results in ankylosing spondylitis are perhaps not quite so good, 73% of 86 hips being graded good or excellent after 10 years (Williams et al, 1977). This is partly because there is an increased risk of heterotopic ossification around the arthroplasty with some 10% becoming ankylosed (Resnick et al, 1976; Williams et al, 1977) and partly because the replacement of an ankylosed joint produces a much less satisfactory total range of movement (96°) than a merely stiff joint (150°) (Bisla et al 1976).

A number of complications may be encountered:

Superficial infection

Some 4 or 5% of cases will have a superficial wound infection, the incidence being no higher in patients with rheumatoid arthritis, whether they are receiving corticosteroids or not.

Deep infection

Although infection may involve the prosthesis at an early stage, the greatest long-term concern is over late infection. The incidence of early infection in osteoarthrosis is low (1%) but rises with time perhaps to 5% after 10 years (Charnley, 1973), although more recent studies suggest 2% (Andrews et al, 1981). The rate of infection is increased in patients with rheumatoid arthritis, reaching 0.5% in the series of Andrews et al (1981), although a ratio to that in osteoarthritis of 1.75 : 1 is more usual. There is growing evidence that late infection is due to haematogenous spread rather than being a manifestation of infection at the time of surgery (BMJ Editorial, 1977). Although unproven, this carries important implications for the treatment and eradication of any intercurrent infection, whether it be in the urinary tract, chest, teeth or feet during the lifetime of a patient who has a prosthetic joint. In patients with rheumatoid arthritis the traditional indicators of sepsis, elevated ESR and white cell count, may be unhelpful. Periostitis along the femoral shaft and resorption of bone around the prosthesis with the development of a denser 'rattle' line are the important radiographic signs (Mendes, 1973). The problems of identifying prosthesis loosening have been discussed earlier. In only a few patients will a discharging sinus develop. In some cases it may be difficult to distinguish between loosening of the prosthesis with an associated tissue reaction producing turbid fluid and infection. Although *Staphylococcus aureus* is the usual organism, others, including anaerobic organisms, may be implicated. Irradication of the infection with the prosthesis in situ is very difficult (Roles, 1971), while removal of the prosthesis and conversion to an excision arthroplasty is often a considerable surgical undertaking. Because of this problem and despite the foregoing comments about blood-borne infection, an expensive and largely untested programme of antibiotic therapy is used at the time of surgery, for example oral cloxacillin for a week, wound lavage with neomycin and polymixin, the addition of fusidic acid or gentamycin to the cement and chloramphenicol powder in the wound at the end of the operations (Andrews et al, 1981).

Wound haematoma

The incidence varies considerably from 1–10% in different series reflecting the quality of surgical technique and anticoagulant control. As indicated earlier, aspirin and related drugs may provide sufficient anticoagulation for rheumatoid arthritics and their usage is associated with a lower incidence of wound haematoma, a complication which delays wound healing and encourages infection.

Fatal complications

Inevitably, because many of the patients are elderly, particularly those with osteoarthritis, some patients will die of cardiorespiratory complications. Pulmonary embolism occurs in some 2% of patients and is often fatal. Fat embolism probably occurs frequently but only rarely produces clinical features, including occasional deaths (Sevitt, 1972). Alterations to the technique of insertion of the cement into the femoral shaft have probably reduced the risk of fat embolism.

Heterotopic ossification

New bone formation in the remnants of the joint capsule and surrounding muscles is common. The incidence and its clinical importance is dependent upon standard methods of classification (Brooker et al, 1973), and although detectable radiographically in up to 30% of patients (Evarts, 1978), it is in only 1–2% that it is sufficient to limit movement and cause discomfort. The much higher incidence in ankylosing spondylitis leading to ankylosis in up to 10% of hips (Bisla et al, 1976) suggests a possible relationship to the carriage of the tissue antigen HLA-B27 but this has not been confirmed (Mattingly et al, 1978). In those with this tendency, attempts have been made to control the process either when the joint is reoperated upon or when the contralateral hip is replaced, by the use of diphosphonates or radiation (Evarts, 1978).

Prosthesis dislocation

The incidence of prosthesis dislocation whether early or late is closely related to its design. The deep McKee-Farrar cup rarely allowed dislocation but the small head of the Charnley prosthesis dislocates in 0–4% of cases both shortly after the operation and in subsequent longer follow-up. Avoidance by the patient of full flexion — particularly combined with rotation as when rolling in bed and sitting on low chairs or toilets — for 1–2 months has reduced the incidence of early dislocation; changes to the device, particularly the acetabular component, and improved techniques have reduced the incidence of both early and late dislocation to a reported 0.4% over 4706 operations (Etienne et al, 1978).

Prosthesis loosening

Loosening of one or other component remains an occasional problem and its cause is not clearly defined. The various causes have been discussed earlier, although in many cases it may reflect a technical failure at the time of surgery (Evarts, 1978). The incidence of prosthesis loosening increases with time and is greater with the higher friction metal-on-metal devices such as the the McKee-Farrar and Ring prostheses that are now rarely used. It is interesting in an aging population, many of whom will die from unrelated causes with an entirely satisfactory arthroplasty, to employ actuarial techniques to the survival of the prosthesis rather than the patient. Thus with a metal-on-metal prosthesis 53% survive 11 years, with an annual probability of removal of 5.5%, while with metal-on-plastic prostheses survival is 88% after 8 years with an annual removal rate of 1.5%. If these trends continue, the 20-year survival chance would be 33% and 74% respectively (Dobbs, 1980).

Prosthesis wear

Despite extensive laboratory testing the ultimate life-span of these prostheses is unknown. Charnley (1973) found that the average wear of the high-density polyethylene acetabular cup was 1.2 mm in 10 years and no cup had to be replaced because of wear. Fracture of the femoral stem is not uncommonly due to either trauma or overuse, but more usually it stems from inadequate support in bone (Evarts, 1978). A wide range of femoral stems are now available so that their length, strength and angulation can be chosen to suit the weight and potential demands of the patient.

Cement

Concern over the possible danger of using methylmethacrylate bone cement has largely disappeared. More than 20 years experience in man and extensive animal experiments have shown it to be safe (Charnley, 1970). Fears that some component of freshly prepared and implanted cement was responsible for dramatic and occasionally fatal changes in the blood pressure also seem to have been allayed (Phillips et al, 1971).

The unpredictable results of subtrochanteric osteotomy (Fig. 63.10) and the only moderate success of cup arthroplasty except in expert hands (Collins & Johnston, 1972) mean that there is now no case for any operation but total hip replacement as the primary procedure in the treatment of the severely damaged hip joint of patients of any age. Nevertheless the problems associated with current hip arthroplasties have led to studies with surface arthroplasties. A variety of still evolving techniques are available, the aims being the preservation of femoral bone stock and the ease of revision. Indications may come to include those younger

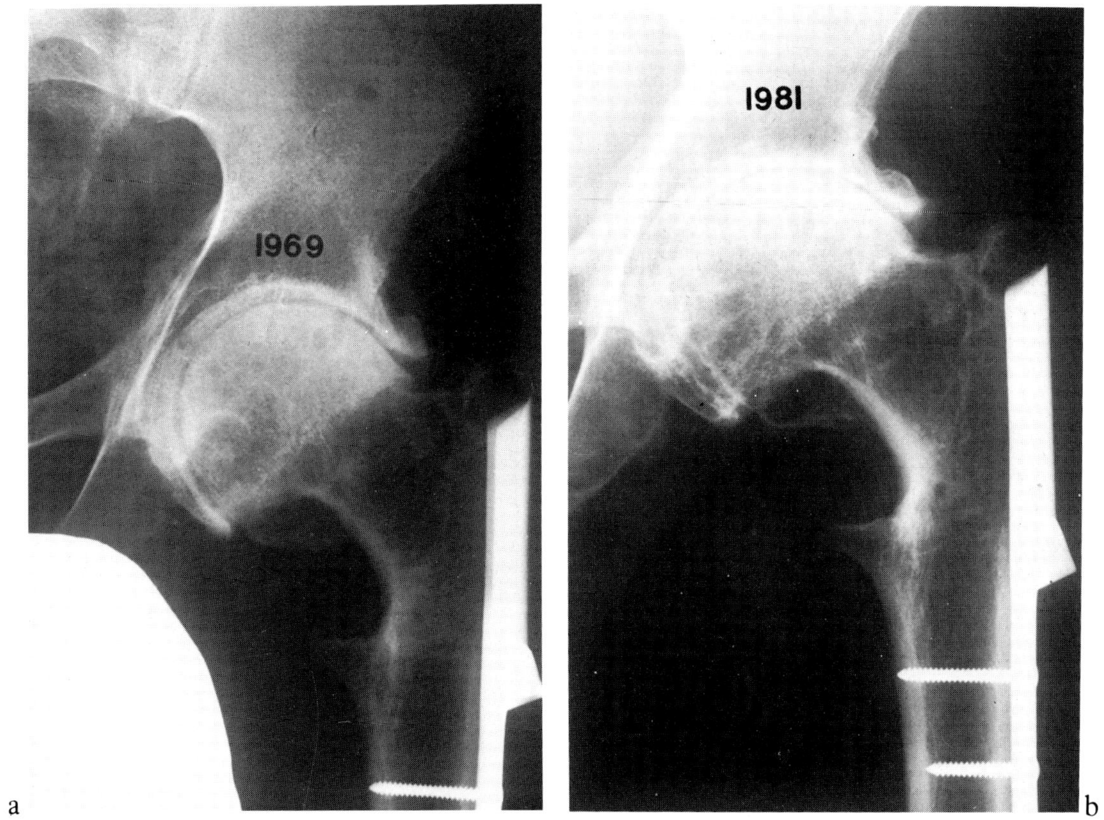

Fig. 63.10 Radiographs 12 years apart of a hip that has undergone trochanteric osteotomy showing the limited disease progression and cartilage preservation that made the operation popular before the widespread use of hip replacement.

osteoarthritic patients who have a high loosening rate, heavier patients, those with inactive inflammatory arthritis with persistent osteoporosis and those with limited avascular necrosis from whatever cause when assessed by bone scanning and more sensitive intraosseous venography (Steinberg, 1982).

In occasional patients in whom the device has become infected, or in whom loosening has been associated with marked bone necrosis, excision arthroplasty, achieved by removing both components may be required. The results of this procedure are generally satisfactory in terms of movement and pain relief (Girdlestone, 1943). If undertaken as a primary procedure the operation is associated with considerable instability and almost inevitably 5 cm of leg shortening. However, as a second procedure in the presence of considerable fibrosis these problems are less marked. Patients will require some 6 weeks of bedrest with traction of the leg in abducted position and the gradual introduction of full weight-bearing over a period of 6–12 months.

THE SPINE

Much of spinal surgery is a specialised field with the work being done both by orthopaedic surgeons and neurosurgeons, depending upon the site and nature of the lesion and the interest and expertise of the two departments. However, the spinal involvement in rheumatoid arthritis and ankylosing spondylitis is well known to rheumatologists and may occasionally require surgical treatment.

Cervical spinal disease in rheumatoid arthritis

Changes in the cervical spine in rheumatoid arthritis are common; several studies describe their development and frequency. Hancock (1978) has reviewed much of the earlier work and described the three common lesions, there sometimes being combinations of one or more in the same patient. Atlantoaxial subluxation (AAS), with an increase in the distance between the anterior surface of the odontoid process and the posterior surface of the anterior arch of the atlas shown on the lateral radiograph of the fully flexed neck (upper limit of normal: 2.5 mm in females, 3.0 mm in males), is found in up to one-quarter of patients. Subaxial subluxation (SAS), usually in the midcervical spine, occurs in up to 20% of cases depending upon the strictness of the criteria using lateral radiographs in flexion and extension. Upward translocation of the odontoid (UT), or more accurately downward movement of the skull onto the odontoid due to the collapse of the lateral masses of the atlas, occurs in 4–8% of cases. The height of the odontoid projecting above MacGregor's line is measured; this line joining the posterior edge of the hard palate and the most caudal point on the occipital curve. The upper limit of normal on the lateral radiograph is 4.5 mm.

More recent series have confirmed these figures, although the incidence, severity and need for surgical treatment clearly depends upon the starting point of the prospective study, these factors reflecting disease duration, disease severity and the need for steroid therapy. 100 patients followed from disease onset for a mean of 7.2 years showed 10 cases of AAS, 20 of SAS, 1 of UT and 2 of combined AAS and UT. 80% of the lesions appeared within 2 years of disease onset and were commoner in women but in no case was there significant neurological abnormality and no surgery was required (Winfield et al, 1981). In contrast, in a prospective 5-year study of 163 patients with later disease, 21 of whom died from problems unrelated to the neck, and with only 106 being available for evaluation, the incidence of neck lesions increased from 43% (46) to 70% (74). There was evidence of radiographic deterioration in 80% of these involved patients and neurological progression in 36%, the combination of SAS and UT carrying the worst prognosis. Surgery was required in 7 patients (Pellicci et al, 1981).

Detailed and sequential clinical and radiographic assessment of these patients is important. Neck pain should always be investigated while some patients will present with neurological features or sometimes simply difficulty in walking without any neck pain. Evaluation can be difficult since the presence of extensive joint disease makes normal neurological examination unreliable while some patients will have a peripheral neuropathy as part of their disease. Further, changes in the neck, the osteoporosis and the difficulty of positioning the neck mean that adequate radiographs may be difficult to obtain. Tomographs and computerised axial tomography may be helpful (Kaufman & Glenn, 1983).

The large majority of patients can be managed conservatively using some form of cervical collar, usually by day and night, and by being given appropriate advice about how to protect their necks from sudden movement. A small number of patients require surgical treatment, rarely for intractable pain alone but more usually for pain combined with significant progression of neurological lesions. While the use of a collar or sometimes carefully controlled inpatient traction or the application of a halopelvic brace may allow neurological signs to stabilise or improve, these methods should not be used for long if neurological signs deteriorate since the degree of recovery is a function of the severity at the time of surgery (Conaty & Morgan, 1981).

Several different surgical approaches to the upper cervical spine have been described (Newman & Sweetman, 1969; Hancock, 1978; Conaty & Morgan, 1981), but a posterior midline one is the most popular. Reducible AAS can be stabilised by preparing the bone surfaces and packing bone chips from the iliac crest between the spines of the first two vertebrae which are also wired together (Fig. 63.11). Irreducible AAS with or without UT requires incorporation of the occiput into the fused area using additional cancellous bone strips, while SAS requires laminectomy and fusion (Fig. 63.12). The results are generally good although bone graft in irreducible AAS has a tendency to be resorbed and for some instability to remain. Postoperatively a variety of methods of fixation are employed from fairly simple collars, through halopelvic bracing to skull traction on a stryker frame (Hancock, 1978; Benjamin & Helal, 1980). The results can be followed both radiographically and neurologically.

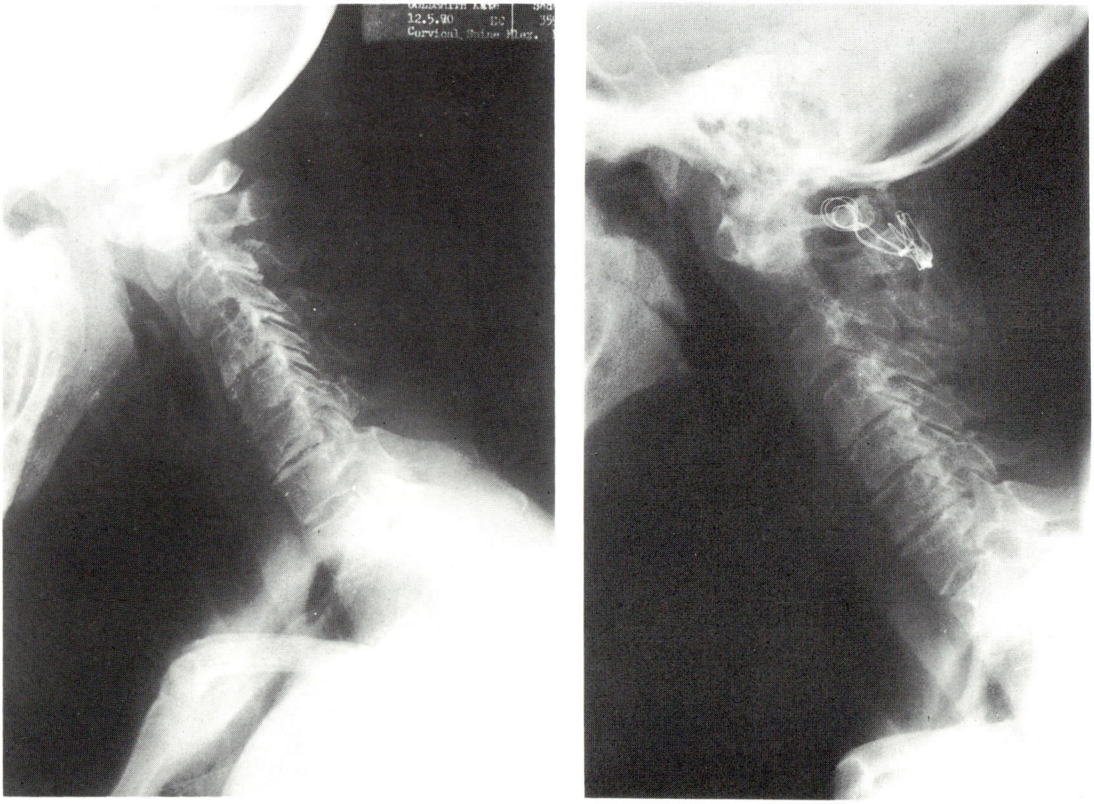

a b

Fig. 63.11 Pre- and postoperative lateral radiographs of the cervical spine in flexion showing reduction in the degree of atlantoaxial subluxation following the insertion of bone chips between the occiput and the upper 3 cervical vertebrae and the wiring of the 1st and 2nd vertebrae.

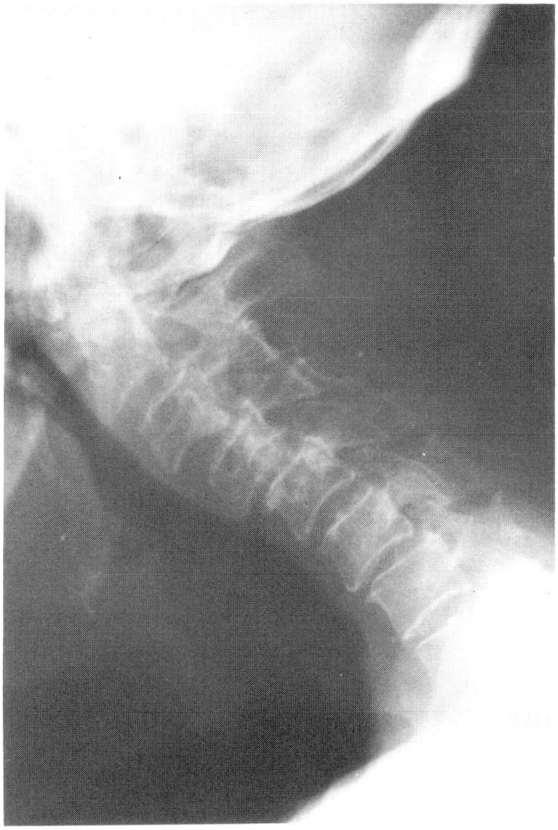

Fig. 63.12 Subaxial subluxation at several levels in a patient with rheumatoid arthritis.

The spine in ankylosing spondylitis

The spinal rigidity combined with kyphosis and an extended neck in late ankylosing spondylitis can give rise to a number of mechanical and function problems. Although the overall posture and ability of the patient to look forward may be improved by replacement of hips which are almost always fused in such cases there remain indications for spinal osteotomy (Law, 1976). In the lumbar spine the indications for osteotomy are:

1. To enable the patient to stand erect
2. To improve the almost exclusively diaphragmatic respiration
3. To eliminate compression of the rib margin
4. To improve the operative field in the abdomen remembering the increased incidence of peptic ulceration and inflammatory bowel disease in these patients.

The posterior excision osteotomy, best done at the lumbar 3–4 level, remains in use. It can achieve 50° of correction and the extent of postoperative immobilisation depends upon the use of any internal fixation (Smith-Petersen et al, 1945; McMaster & Coventry, 1973; Law, 1976). A wide range of complications including death are recorded and there is certainly a risk of both nerve root and cauda equina damage.

In the cervical spine the indications for osteotomy are:

1. To enable the patient to see ahead
2. To prevent atlantoaxial subluxation. This can occur in this disease exactly as in rheumatoid arthritis due to direct inflammatory effects, rather than to simple mechanical effects from the kyphosis
3. To relieve tracheal and oesophageal obstruction
4. To relieve nerve root and cord compression.

A similar posterior approach is adopted usually at the cervical 6–7 or cervical 7 thoracic 1 levels (Law, 1976; Simmons, 1972), although some favour a two-stage procedure involving both anterior and posterior approaches (Yeoman, 1981). Undoubtedly the risks, particularly to the cord and the vertebral arteries are greater than in the lumbar spine and some surgeons prefer that the patient remains conscious so that neurological and vascular assessments can be maintained. Such techniques also eliminate the difficulties of intubation for general anaesthesia. A correction of 40° is possible. Internal fixation is used and the need for postoperative immobilisation minimised.

SHOULDER

The need for surgical treatment of the arthritic shoulder is poorly documented. Osteoarthritis may follow trauma or overuse but the diagnosis of moderate involvement can be overlooked in the face of periarthritic soft tissue lesions and referred pain from the neck. Further, it is often suggested that severe rheumatoid involvement is uncommon but a recent survey which recorded the damage in five clinical and radiographic grades noted that 38 of 100 patients had grade 4 or 5 disease with complete cartilage loss, sometimes with subluxation. The authors concluded that there was a need for earlier surgery (Crossan & Vallance, 1980). Reluctance to provide a surgical solution is enhanced by the knowledge that any operative procedure on the shoulder joint is liable to induce capsulitis (frozen shoulder) with persisting postoperative pain and considerable difficulty in encouraging the return of movement.

Synovectomy is rarely undertaken for the relief of pain in rheumatoid arthritis, although occasionally performed in conjunction with the removal of a cyst whether in relation to the shoulder joint or subacromial bursa (Fig. 63.13). However, Cruess (1980) has advocated wider use of synovectomy and has emphasised the need for a full clearance since 20% of patients have invasion of the deltoid bursa and disruption of the rotator cuff and one-third of patients have acromioclavicular joint involvement that might benefit from concomitant synovectomy.

A number of simple procedures have been tried for the relief of pain associated with cartilage and bone damage. These include excision of the distal 3 cm of the acromion which eliminates pain arising from compression of the subacromial bursa or due to direct contact from the upward subluxing humerus. This operation may be followed by some increase in instability and weakness of the shoulder and almost certainly further upward subluxation of the humerus. Excision of the humeral head also produces a weak and unstable shoulder. Wainwright (1974) reported promising results with glenoidectomy, a procedure which does not preclude future use of some form of joint replacement. These types of arthroplasty may reduce pain but it is unusual to find the range of movement increased; indeed the patient is unlikely to regain even as much as half the normal range.

For many years Neer's prosthesis, which only replaced the humeral head, was available for the treatment of more severe arthritis. This device was quite effective in reducing pain and had a good record in terms of loosening and infection, but since it only replaced part of the joint, the chance of a gain in movement was limited. This prosthesis may still be useful in those patients with avascular necrosis of the humeral head whether due to frac-

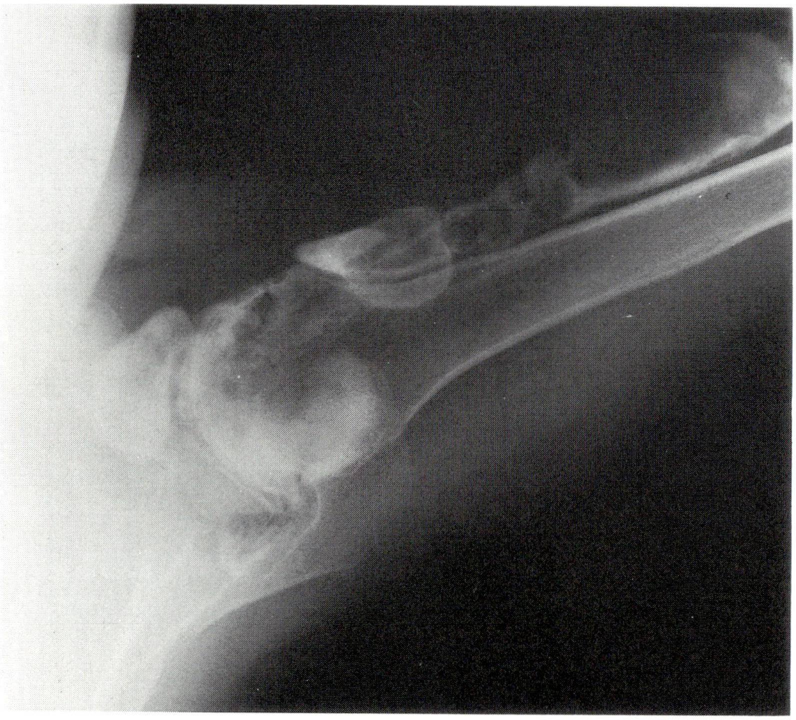

Fig. 63.13 An axilla view of a shoulder arthrogram showing the connection with the subdeltoid bursa which has produced a painful cystic extension down the arm.

ture or the more usual causes including SLE. Over recent years a variety of total replacements have become available. Neer et al (1982) have reviewed the state of the art and have described their encouraging results in 194 cases (50 rheumatoid arthritis) followed from 24–91 months. Only 4 patients failed to achieve any benefit and although there were complications in 24 cases there was only one infection and no case of loosening. In patients with severe shoulder pain, impaired upper limb function and sleep disturbance due to extensive joint damage, arthrodesis in 45° abduction, 25° of flexion and some 20° of internal rotation, usually employing some means of internal fixation, should be considered. The results in both osteoarthritis and rheumatoid arthritis are good, especially when the patient has good elbow and scapula movement (Cofield & Biggs, 1979).

ELBOW

Before discussing the elbow joint itself, it is appropriate to consider the surgical treatment of rheumatoid nodules, bursae and tendinitis, which, although they may occur in a variety of different sites, are particularly common problems in the region of the elbow joint.

Nodules

Surgical removal of rheumatoid nodules may be demanded because they have broken down and are discharging; have become infected and are a potential source of bacteraemia; are cosmetically unacceptable or are an irritation to the patient because of their size. Unfortunately surgical excision of these nodules is not always easy and should not be delegated to the most junior surgeon. Incomplete excision may lead to a persistently discharging wound and a continued risk of bacteraemia. Further, such nodules have a striking tendency to recur unless the mechanical factors and the underlying vasculitis responsible for their development are avoided and controlled respectively. Thus surgery should be accompanied by the use of disease-modifying drugs such as penicillamine.

Bursae

Rheumatoid bursae may require surgical excision because of repeated inflammatory episodes, breakdown, discharge and infection or for cosmetic reasons. As many bursae have one of more connections with the underlying joint, surgical excision may lead to the development of a persistently discharging sinus and such treatment should only be undertaken when local conservative therapy has failed.

Tendinitis

Surgical treatment of common flexor or common extensor tendinitis is rarely more successful than conservative therapy which should include rest, local steroid injections, ultrasound, etc.

Synovectomy of the elbow joint

Although a quarter of rheumatoid arthritics may eventually have elbow involvement, the onset of synovitis is often insidious and destructive changes tend to appear late in the course of the disease (Freyberg, 1969). Synovectomy alone is rarely undertaken although it may be performed in conjunction with cystectomy, the cysts usually appearing anterolaterally where they may cause pressure on blood vessels or on the posterior interosseus nerve, resulting in weakness of the finger extensors. More satisfactory results are achieved by delaying the operation until there is radiographic evidence of joint damage particularly in the radiohumeral compartment when synovectomy can be combined with excision of the radial head (Porter et al, 1974).

The joint is opened through a short lateral incision and approximately 2 cm of the radius is excised. A second medial incision, although it may result in removal of more synovial tissue, does not improve the surgical results. The operation is performed with a tourniquet, so a compression bandage, perhaps combined with a plaster of Paris is applied to hold the elbow in 90° flexion with the forearm in midrotation for 3–5 days. The arm should be elevated in a comfortable sling to reduce postoperative oedema. The operation is associated with few complications and some 80% of patients have relief of pain and a modest improvement (10–15°) in both elbow flexion and forearm rotation. The remaining 20% do less well, but it is unusual for patients to show no improvement or be made worse. The operation is often surprisingly successful even in cases showing severe joint damage (Wilson et al, 1975; Dickson et al, 1976).

Arthroplasty

Progressive damage at the elbow joint — particularly of the ulnar-humeral compartment — from whatever cause, is difficult to treat. A variety of different forms of excision arthroplasty with removal of part of both humeral and ulnar bones, often with the interposition of some biological or chemical material, have been described. Such procedures involve the insertion of silastic sheet or sponge and may produce acceptable results in a few older patients with a good range of shoulder and wrist joint movement. Stability can be improved with the use of removable 'K' wires but movement is sacrificed (Stein et al, 1975).

Replacement arthroplasty of the elbow joint is gradually becoming more reliable. Dee's (1972) early results using a constrained hinge were promising but subsequent follow-up showed that all became loose, usually in the humerus (Fig. 63.14), while a few became infected, both complications demanding prosthetic removal (Souter, 1973). The amount of bone excised meant that arthrodesis was impossible, patients having to endure an unstable, weak joint, often with some form of external bracing. Such results behove others to tread carefully with new prostheses, not only for the elbow joint, and postal results on 400 semiconstrained prostheses, only 10 of which were personally performed by their designer, are not valid in advancing this difficult field (Schlein, 1976).

Measurements of the forces about the elbow suggest that unconstrained surface replacements are likely to be the most successful (Amis et al, 1979). Recent results in patients followed for $3\frac{1}{2}$–4 years seem to support this contention. 80 arthroplasties of a semiconstrained type produced only 60% with good results and a significant number of complications (37), loosenings (11) and infection (7) (Morrey et al, 1981), while 69 unconstrained devices were associated with 87% good results, a lower but still important incidence of complications, but only one case of loosening (Ewald et al, 1980). Occasionally in a badly damaged joint there is compression of the ulna nerve which needs to be transposed to an anterior position.

Arthrodesis

Arthrodesis of the elbow joint is occasionally indicated, particularly if other upper limb joints have a good range of motion. Most patients find that 90° of flexion with the forearm in mid-rotation is the best position although it is important to assess carefully the patient's individual requirements preoperatively.

WRISTS AND TENDON SHEATHS

In inflammatory arthritis wrist surgery is frequently combined with synovectomy of the tendon sheaths, particularly of the extensor tendons.

Synovectomy

Synovectomy of the wrist joint alone is rarely undertaken. However, it may be performed in conjunction with clearance of the flexor tendons and their decompression on the volar aspect of the wrist (Mannerfelt & Norman, 1969). Occasionally, large cysts develop in relation to the flexor tendons and fluid can be balotted backwards and forwards between the palm and the lower forearm under the anterior carpal ligament — a compound palmar ganglion. Synovectomy of the wrist and flexor tendons may also be combined with decompression of the median nerve in the carpal tunnel (see below). Synovectomy of the dorsum of the wrist should always include synovectomy of the related extensor tendon sheaths and vice versa. The main indications for this operation, which is among the most successful undertaken for rheumatoid arthritis, include reduced hand and wrist function due to persistent pain in the distal radioulnar joint and evidence of extensor tendon rupture, stretching or weakness. Several mechanisms are involved in the production of tendon damage or rupture. These include direct mechanical damage by the eroded lower end of the ulna, direct invasion of tendons by rheumatoid synovitis and ischaemic damage due to rheumatoid vasculitis and to mechanical constriction of the tendons under the extensor retinaculum. The commonest tendon to rupture is the extensor digitae minimae followed by the extensor tendons to the little to index fingers in sequence. Rupture of the extensor pollicis longus tendon, usually in the region of

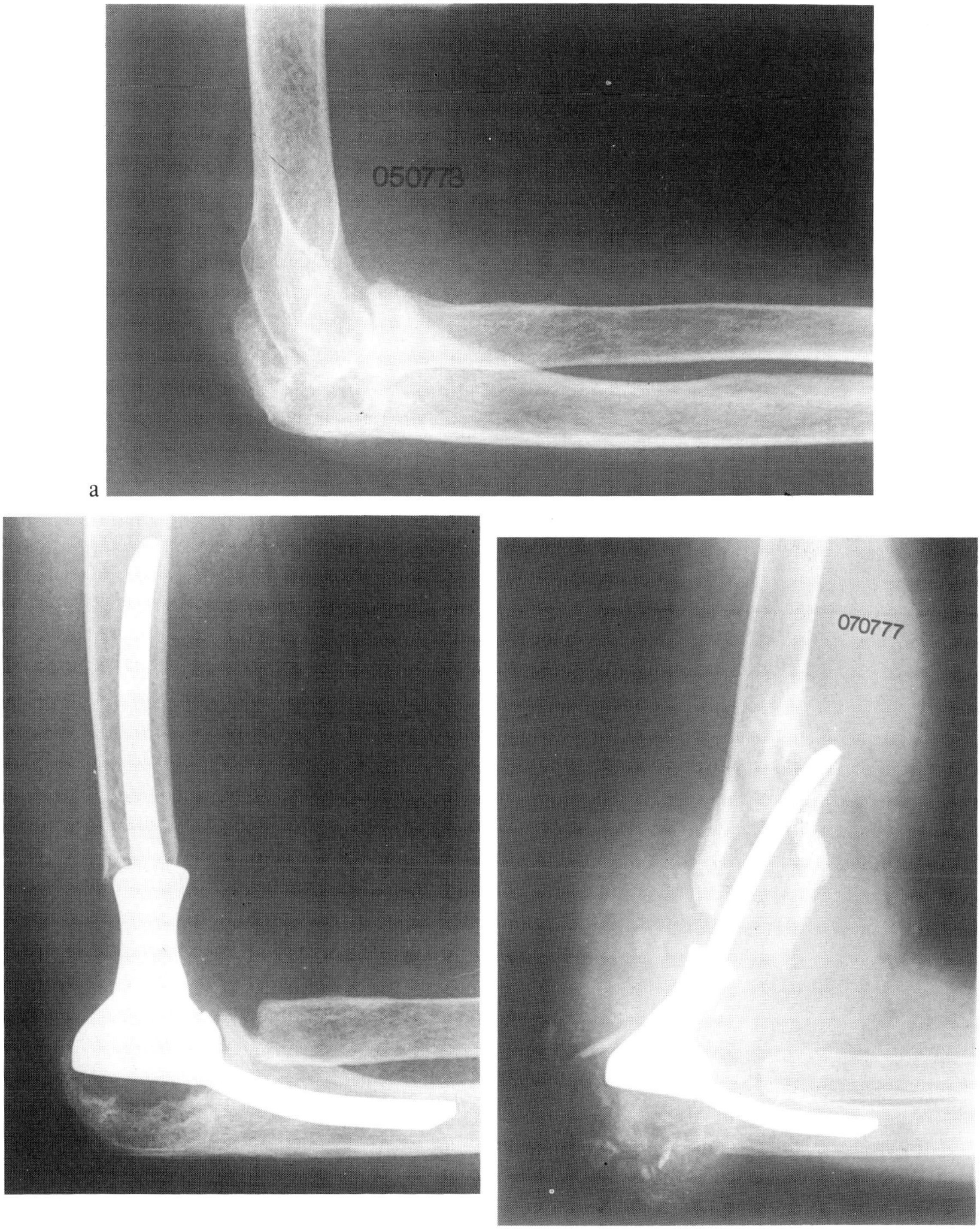

a b c

Fig. 63.14 A series of lateral radiographs, taken over a 4-year period, of the right elbow. The initial extensive cartilage and bone erosion in both the radiohumeral and ulnar humeral compartments led to the excision of the radial head and the insertion of a Dee total replacement. This subsequently loosened, particularly the humeral component, with extensive bone erosion and fracture. There was no infection. Removal produced a pain-free, flail elbow.

Lister's tubercle, also commonly occurs. The various mechanisms involved in tendon damage have persuaded different authors to suggest excision of the lower end of ulna with synovectomy of the distal radioulnar joint (Fig. 63.15), tendon sheath synovectomy or simply decompression of the tendons by division of the extensor retinaculum. However, the best results are achieved by combining all three procedures, resulting in relief of pain and a modest increase in movement at the distal radioulnar joint with consequent improvement in hand function in over 90% of patients. There is no evidence of any loss of stability at the wrist and indeed both the head of the radius and lower end of the ulna can be excised in the same forearm without loss of stability, perhaps due to the limited demands of most rheumatoid arthritics (Cracchiolo & Marmor, 1969; Vaughan-Jackson, 1962).

This very common combined operation is associated with some residual discomfort on the radial side of the wrist and half the patients complain of a clicking sensation due to the movement of the extensor carpi ulnaris tendon over the excised ulnar end during forearm rotation so that some surgeons reroute this tendon. However, the clicking is generally not troublesome and is not clearly related to the amount of bone excised (usually 2 cm) (Rasher et al, 1980). Bowing of the tendons, which might be expected with division of the extensor retinaculum, is only occasionally noted and does not impair hand function (Edwards & Mowat 1973).

Synovectomy of the wrist and extensor tendons has no prophylactic effect on the progress of the disease in the carpus but does appear to prevent subsequent stretching or rupture of tendons. There is a tendency for the small carpal bones to move down into the space created by excision of the lower end of the ulna but this is not generally associated with an increased rate of development of ulnar drift of the fingers and most surgeons do not feel that silastic replacement of the ulna end is necessary (Edwards & Mowat, 1973; Rasher et al, 1980).

Although the problem of extensor tendon involvement in inflammatory arthritis has been acknowledged for many years, the less clinically obvious involvement of the flexor tendons has

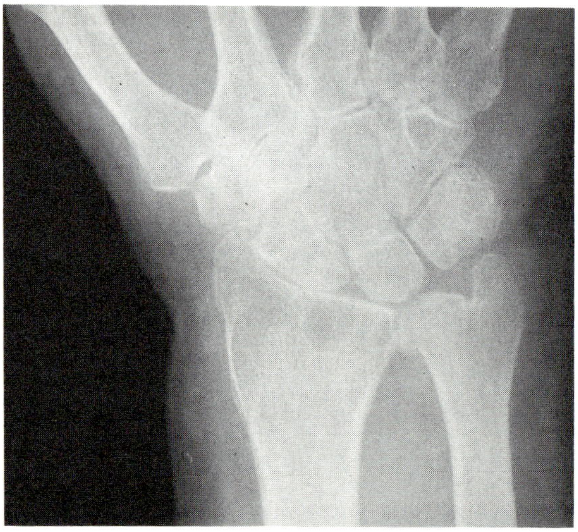
a

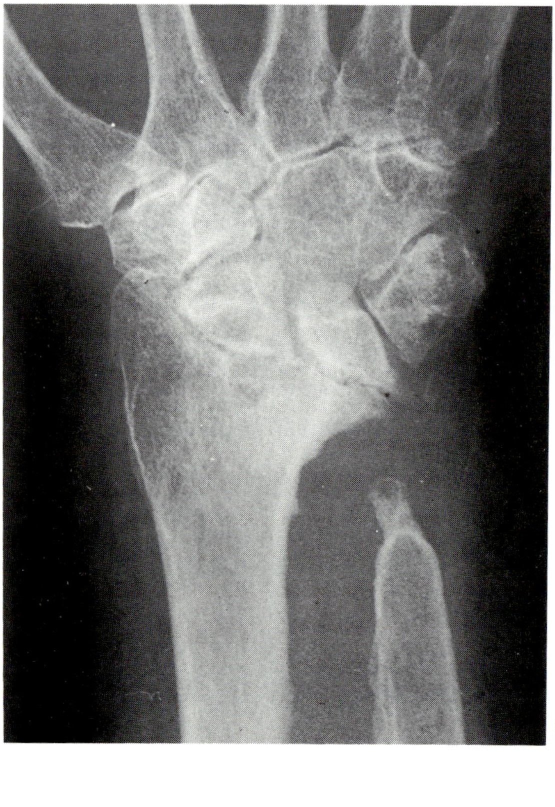
b

Fig. 63.15 (a) Typical preoperative radiograph of the wrist showing soft tissue swelling and involvement of the distal radioulnar joint. (b) Radiograph of the same hand 3 years after synovectomy and excision of the lower end of ulna showing progression of the radiographic changes in the carpus, some regrowth of bone on the lower end of the ulna and the very common broadening of the radius to support the lunate bone.

begun to receive more attention. It may occur in 35–55% of patients, usually early in the disease, and requires careful palpation, checking for the presence of nodules that can cause triggering of the fingers and rarely of the wrist (Carvell et al, 1983) and the use of the Savill pinch test to detect involvement in the fingers (Macauley et al, 1981). In a follow-up of 201 hands (Table 63.4) which underwent flexor tendon synovectomy, good results were noted in 70% of patients with most of the poor results reflecting the progression of the joint disease; an observation of the interrelationship between joints and other structures that can invalidate results, whether pain or function is being measured, and which is often ignored in surgical reports. A recurrence of the synovial proliferation was found in 37% of cases but in very few did this require reoperation. It is interesting to note the low incidence of tendon rupture compared with that of extensor tendons (Dahl et al, 1976).

Table 63.4

Flexor tenosynovitis with pain alone	129
Flexor tenosynovitis with trigger fingers	45
Flexor tenosynovitis with carpal tunnel syndrome	27
Flexor tenosynovitis with tendon rupture	4
Total	201

Tendon repairs

As indicated above, rupture of flexor tendons is uncommon, later onset of disease and greater pain and dysfunction compared with extensor tendon disease leading to better and earlier medical and prophylactic surgical treatment. This is fortunate since satisfactory repair and adequate postoperative tendon excursion is technically difficult to achieve. However, rupture of extensor tendons is not uncommon although adequate prophylactic surgery and the use of disease-modifying drugs should usually prevent rupture. With rupture of the extensor tendons to the index to little fingers, the simplest and most satisfactory results are produced by joining the ruptured tendon to the others. Unless treated very promptly it is rarely possible to repair a rupture of the extensor pollicis longus tendon but satisfactory results are produced by the transfer of extensor indicis proprius (Staub & Ranawat, 1969). Tendon repair is followed by plaster of Paris support for some 3 weeks postoperatively when finger movement can be encouraged with the use of a dorsal dynamic splint.

Other forms of wrist surgery

A variety of arthroplasties requiring bony excision and the interposition of materials such as silicone sheet have been described and although there is a variable relief of pain and gain in stability there is some loss of movement (Jackson & Simpson, 1979). Arthrodesis of the more severely damaged wrist produces very satisfactory results, particularly when patients have only a limited range of painful wrist movement. A variety of techniques for wrist arthrodesis exist, either using plaster of Paris alone to hold wrist position or combined with internal fixation using a long nail inserted either in the 2nd digital cleft or the 3rd metacarpal passing across the carpus into the radius. The operation is usually combined with excision of the lower end of ulna, some surgeons using the excised bone as chips to aid arthrodesis. Most patients find that arthrodesis in a neutral position or in a few degrees of flexion the most satisfactory, particularly for toilet purposes, rather than the usually recommended position of 10° of extension (Dobyns & Linscheid, 1971).

Replacement arthroplasty at the wrist is as yet in an early phase and although it is valuable in some post-traumatic cases it is doubtful whether it will ever have wide usage, particularly in the presence of polyarticular disease, when the simpler existing techniques produce such satisfactory results.

NERVE COMPRESSION SYNDROMES

Median nerve compression symptoms are very common in the early phases of inflammatory arthritis due to proliferative synovitis in the wrist joint and around the flexor tendons in the carpal tunnel. However, such causes only account for some 5% of cases, trauma, osteoarthritis and 'idiopathic' factors being more common (Nicolle & Woolhouse, 1965). The condition is commoner in women, often being related to fluid retention, while in men it is a useful rule not to accept a diagnosis of idiopathic carpal tunnel without a careful search in the arm and neck for an underlying cause.

Diagnosis, particularly in the presence of arthritis, may be difficult since not all patients present with classic features. Some patients respond to local splintage at night, diuretics and local injections of corticosteroid, although the initial 90% benefit associated with the latter is followed by a relapse rate of two-thirds in the following year (Woods, 1980). Any identifiable cause must be treated, disease-modifying drugs being successful in many patients with rheumatoid arthritis. Surgical decompression requires a careful technique to avoid damaging the palmar cutaneous branch of the median nerve and hence unpleasant dysaesthesia (Nicolle & Dickson, 1979). Some one-third of cases will have immediate relief of symptoms, one-third recover within 6 months but the final third may take up to 3 years to recovery fully (Nicolle & Woolhouse, 1965). Poor results reflect delay in diagnosis and treatment and once motor signs are present a full recovery is less likely (Cracchiolo, 1971). Bone density in the hand can be used to confirm returning function (Schorn et al, 1978).

Compression of the ulnar nerve at the wrist — 'syndrome de la loge de Guyon' — is much less common and extremely rare in rheumatoid arthritis (Taylor, 1974).

In most operations on the wrist and hand there can be problems in wound healing due to the development of postoperative oedema, and in rheumatoid patients, due to the thin skin over the dorsum of the wrist. A meticulous technique, wound drainage, the careful application of a compression bandage and the use of a plaster of Paris support for 3–5 days will overcome these problems while not compromising the need for early mobilisation after many procedures.

FINGERS

The types and results of finger surgery in patients with rheumatoid arthritis are the most difficult to describe since they vary so markedly from surgeon to surgeon. Undoubtedly better results are achieved by surgeons experienced in this field who devote much of their time to hand surgery and who are supported by experienced and dedicated therapists whose contribution to initial assessment, splint-making and exercise programmes is critical. It is perhaps more important in the hand than at any other joint to carefully assess preoperative function and to decide whether the planned surgery can produce any functional improvement. Patients often demonstrate surprisingly adequate function in severely damaged and cosmetically unattractive hands. The important functions of the hand are:

1. Pinch
   Pinch movements are of four types:
   a. Power pinch with pulp to pulp opposition
   b. Fine pinch with tip to tip opposition
   c. Tripod pinch with opposition of the thumb to the pulp of the index and middle fingers
   d. Key pinch with opposition of the thumb against the radial side of the index finger.
2. Grip
   There are three types of grip:
   a. Power grip, as in holding a hammer with the thumb locked over the index and middle fingers
   b. Composite grip and pinch for less powerful function with a palm grip combined with pinch of the thumb and index finger
   c. The hook or baggage grip with flexion of the proximal and distal interphalangeal joints.
3. Grasp
4. Flat hand

Assessment of hand function

The number of suggested methods of assessing hand function testify to the absence of any one simple method (Fig. 63.16). Some document so much anatomical and functional information that they are valueless in most busy clinics, while other commonly used functional tests may be too susceptible to learning techniques and of so little practical use to the patient as to be equally valueless to the surgeon (e.g. hammering in nails, picking up paper-clips, etc.). Whenever possible the patient should select individual tests of function that she finds difficult as this then allows sensible and realistic postoperative comparisons (Ansell, 1969). The patient's subjective assessment of pain and cosmetic appearance should also be

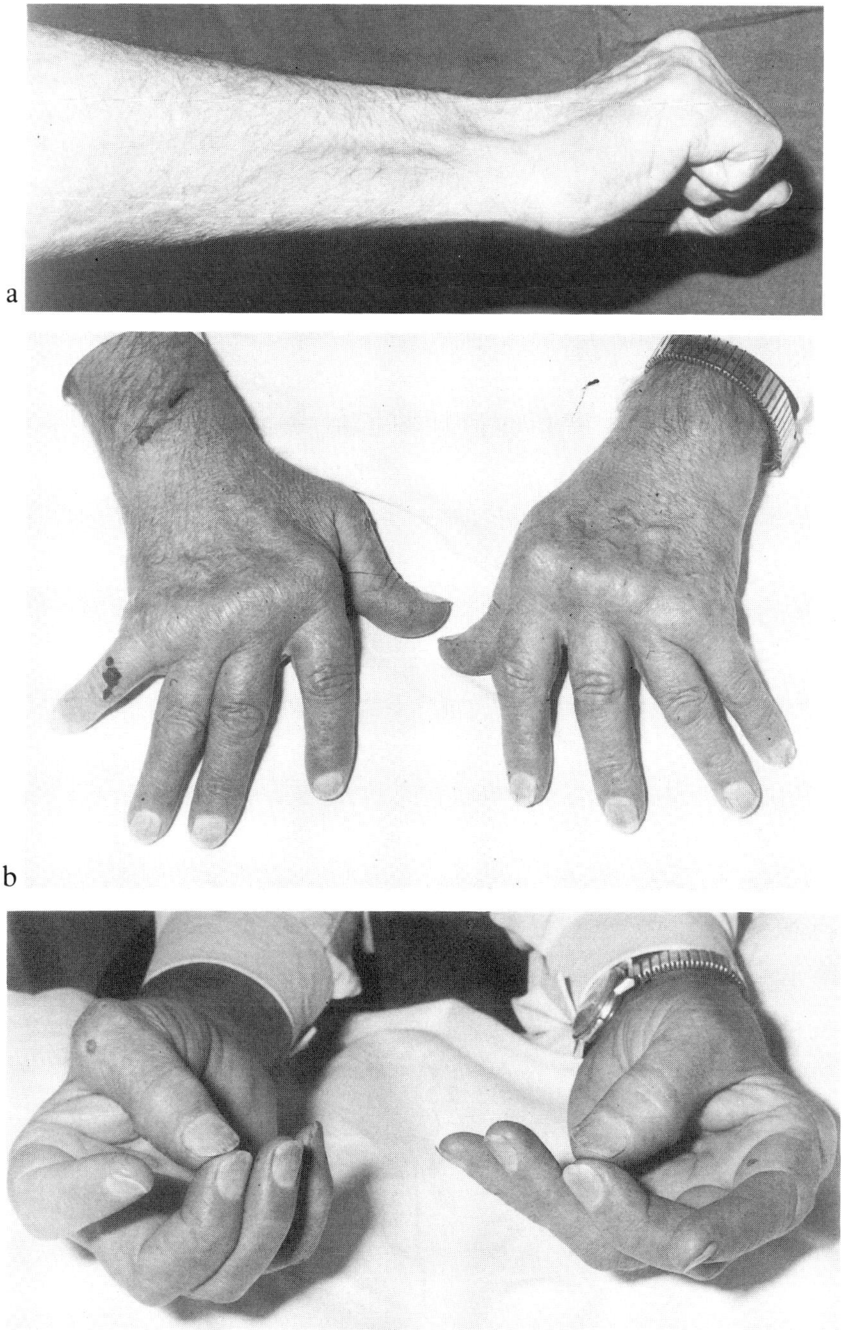

a b c

Fig. 63.16 Hand function may be well preserved despite extensive involvement of the small joints

recorded. A variety of more objective measurements include grip strength, articular index and the measurement of pinch and finger flexion (Nicolle & Dickson, 1979) but it must be remembered that different observers and very mild changes in patient co-operation can make marked changes in such measurements. A valuable objective assessment of the amount a hand or individual digits are used is a radiographic measurement of bone density since this has been correlated with function, improving postoperatively and after drug control of active synovitis (Dickson et al, 1973; Schorn & Mowat, 1977). The technique is also of value in deciding whether patients use their hands when they claim severe pain and dysfunction and refuse to co-operate with functional testing, e.g. in hysteria. With all these tests it must be appreciated that much hand function is dependent upon having a pain-free, stable wrist joint, and that changes in this joint, whether for better or worse, which are almost inevitable in diseases like rheumatoid arthritis, may invalidate sequential measurements.

Once surgical solutions begin to be considered it is essential that the potential gains in terms of pain relief, function, appearance and prophylaxis for future damage are carefully balanced against the risk of a bad result. Souter (1979) has developed a likely score sheet for each operative alternative in the wrist and hand based upon these factors when the maximum potential score for each operation is 20 (Table 63.5).

Table 63.5 A success rating for hand and wrist surgery

	Operation	Credit score
Group 1	Fusion MP thumb	16–18
	Excision lower end ulnar	15–18
	Extensor tendon synovectomy	15–18
Group 2	Flexor tendon synovectomy	12–15
	MP arthroplasty	11–15
Group 3	PIP fusion	12–15
	Wrist stabilisation	11–18
Group 4	Correction swan-neck	12–14
	MP/PIP synovectomy	10–11
	IP thumb fusion	9–18
Group 5	PIP arthroplasty	7–10
	Correction boutonnière	6– 8

Souter (1979) has emphasised the need for careful assessment, remembering that the nature of the underlying disease and the patients ability to learn new functional tricks means that much may be salvaged. Surgical intervention should be used to bolster this tendency. It is useful to start with an operation with a high score and to build upon the rapport so gained with the patient. The postoperative care may be demanding and operations that have mutually exclusive care, e.g. tendon clearance and joint fusion, must not be combined. For the technical satisfaction of the surgeon and to illustrate to potential patients the expected benefits of hand surgery, a range of standard clinical photographs are invaluable.

Synovectomy

Many surgeons feel that synovectomy of the proximal interphalangeal joints is of doubtful value, since although it may relieve pain, loss of movement is usually unacceptable. Certainly some of the reported successful results are in patients with mild and slowly developing disease in whom the prognosis was probably good (Ellison et al, 1971). However, this criticism cannot be levelled at several European groups: Gschwend (1980) reports that in 233 operations in 93 patients (Pahle) and 214 operations in 92 patients (Raunio), 80% had relief of pain and swelling without loss of movement. Similar results, 72% with pain relief and only 18° loss of flexion, have been described for operations on late cases (Edstrom et al, 1976), although no author claims prophylactic benefit for the procedure. Much the same debate rages over synovectomy at the metacarpophalangeal joints, although there is perhaps more willingness to admit that pain is relieved. An attempt to mount a carefully controlled trial was largely defeated by the small number of cases entered and the large number of surgeons undertaking the operations: 41 MCP joints in 13 patients with 28 control joints in 9 patients, and the discouraging results should, perhaps, be interpreted in this light (ARC/BOA Synovectomy Trial, 1975). Individual surgeons, some of whom have included control cases in their series, report pain relief, loss of swelling and no significant loss of movement over 2–5 year periods in 60–90% of cases (Gschwend, 1980). Once again even in late cases 90% may have continuing pain relief after 3 years with only 8° loss of movement (Edstrom et al, 1976). These results must emphasise the specialised nature of this surgery. These synovectomies need to be extensive, clearing all parts of the joint, particularly around the volar plate, the future integrity of which is essential if subluxation at the MCP joint and swan-neck deformity at the PIP joints is to be prevented, and around the related tendons. Soft tissue repair of the extensor expansion and reefing of the radial

With chronic disease, moveover, the joint may become progressively deformed. The surrounding muscles may have wasted, and the tendons may have become inflamed (tenosynovitis), thickened (trigger finger) or ruptured (long extensor tendons of the hand). General examination of any joint therefore must comprise a routine such as:

— look: for swelling and deformity
— feel: for signs of inflammation, swelling and tenderness
— move: to see if the range of movement is limited or abnormal, and measure if necessary with a goniometer
— check: to see the state of the surrounding soft tissues.

Temporomandibular joint
This may be involved in rheumatoid arthritis, and may therefore be swollen, though this is often hard to detect, and may not be symmetrical. However, opening of the mouth may be restricted and painful.

Cervical spine
First this should be inspected to see if there is any increase in the natural lordosis, or whether the neck is held inclined to one side, as this may imply subluxation of the vertebrae. If this is observed, care should be taken in any movement of the cervical spine. The patient should be asked to move the spine to the left, then to the right, and any limitations of rotation noted. Next the patient should flex the neck as far forward as possible, then extend it to the limit backwards. Crepitus may be experienced by the patient on movement and even heard by the examiner. Lateral bending to the left and right should also be attempted. The tendon reflexes in arms should be examined. For example, an inverted supinator reflex would imply a lesion at C5–6 level. If paraesthesiae are complained of then sensation in the upper limbs and occiput should be examined most diligently.

Dorsal spine
Movements can be tested by lateral rotation, flexion and extension preferably with the patient seated so that the buttocks are anchored. The dorsal spine should be observed for evidence of increased kyphosis (as may be seen in osteoporosis), abnormal angulation (abscess or metastatic bone disease) or restriction of movement (ankylosing spondylitis). The vertebrae may be generally tender where an abscess or metastasis is present.

Lumbar spine, sacrum and sacroiliac joints
Movement of the lumbar spine should be tested with the patient standing and with the observer first at the side. With the knees straight the patient is then asked to attempt to touch the toes. The examiner should meanwhile keep an eye on movement of the lumbar spine itself, as the ability to touch the toes may come largely from hip mobility. To check lumbar spine flexion it is best to rely on Shober's method, as refined (Macrae & Wright, 1969). In this method, with the patient erect the sacroiliac dimples are marked and the lumbosacral junction identified in the midline. An ink mark is made on the skin at this point, with another mark 5 cm below and a third 10 cm above, again in the midline. The patient is then asked to bend forward as far as possible with the knees straight and the distraction between the upper and lower marks is measured (Fig. 64.3). The distraction should be between 6 and 7 cm in most adults. This may be severely restricted or even nil in ankylosing spondylitis. Lateral flexion of the spine is obtained by asking the patient to bend to each side in turn without forward flexion, running one hand down the outside of the leg as far as possible. Extension is measured by getting the patient to bend backwards as far as possible. Again tenderness of the vertebrae should be noted, or abnormal angulation. In lower lumbar disc disease there may be flattening of the lumbar lordosis. Straight leg-raising is measured with the patient lying supine. With the knee straight and the sacrum firmly on the couch, the leg is lifted in an arc as high as it will go until further movement is stopped by pain. The lower limb stretch reflexes should be elicited and sensation checked.

The sacrum may be tender, as may the sacroiliac joints, when actively inflamed in sacroiliitis. The sacroiliac joints have their surface markings in the dimples of Venus. Gentle pressure is applied at these points. When upper lumbar disc disease is

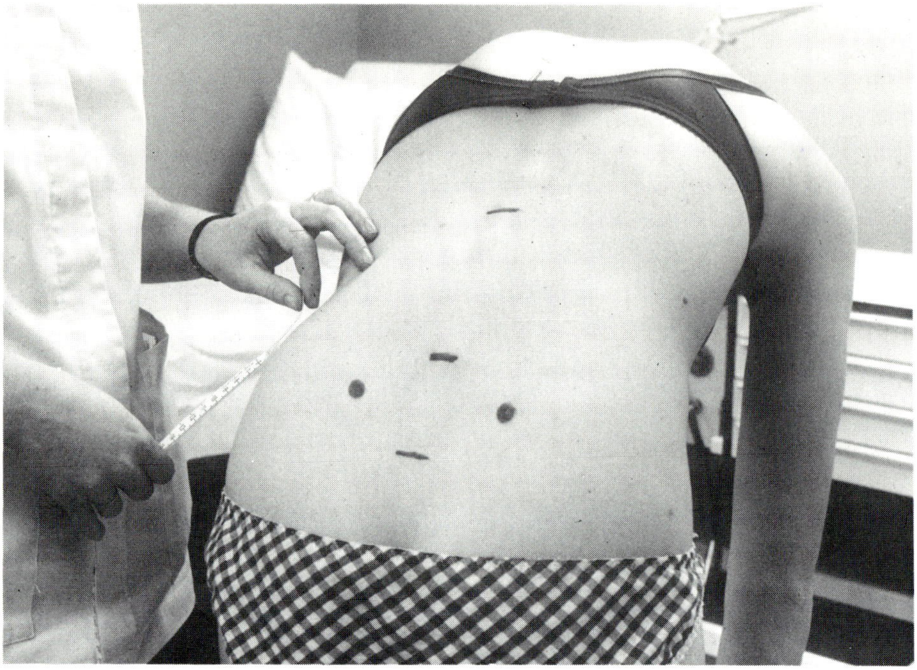

Fig. 64.3 Schober's method for measuring spinal mobility.

suspected, the femoral nerve stretch test is carried out. The patient lies prone, and then each knee in turn is fully flexed — if positive, this will induce discomfort in the anterior thigh.

Sternoclavicular joints and ribs

The sternoclavicular joints may be affected in rheumatoid arthritis, gonococcal arthritis, and degenerative disease, for example. They may be swollen and tender, and movement can be tested by asking the patient to lift up the shoulders. The movement of the ribs may be restricted and painful when the costovertebral joints are affected, as in ankylosing spondylitis. Deep breathing may be painful or there may be limitation in chest expansion.

Shoulder and acromioclavicular joints

First the examiner should look at the scapulae from behind to see if there is any wasting of supra- or infraspinatus muscles. The shoulder should be examined anteriorly for tenderness or effusion. A quick appreciation of shoulder movement can be obtained by asking the patient to attempt to clasp the hands first behind the head and next in the small of the back (Fig. 64.4). This tests most movements of the joint. More carefully, each shoulder should then be actively abducted with the elbow fully extended. Supraspinatus tendinitis will cause a painful arc when abduction reaches about 90°. Adduction can be checked by getting the patient to put the hand anteriorly on the opposite shoulder. Forward flexion and backward extension are elicited by moving the straightened arm fully

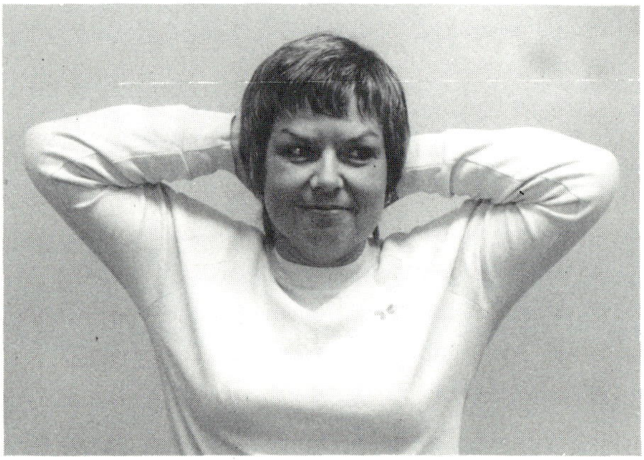

Fig. 64.4 Simple assessment of shoulder movement.

forwards and backwards. Rotator cuff lesions will limit all movements of the shoulder. Biceps tendinitis may be elicited by local tenderness over the biceps groove in the anterior humerus whilst getting the patient to flex the forearm. The acromioclavicular joints may be associated with localised bursitis. There may be local tenderness, and pain on abduction of the shoulder.

Elbow joint

Movements may be checked by asking the patient to fully flex and extend the forearm. Loss of extension particularly may occur in rheumatoid arthritis. Olecranon bursitis and rheumatoid nodules may occur along the subcutaneous (posteromedial) surface of the ulna. If the thumb is placed just anterior to the lateral epicondyle of the joint and the forearm is then pronated and supinated, the radial head may be felt to rotate. If diseased, this may be painful, and crepitus elicited. Tenderness over the lateral epicondyle may be associated with 'tennis elbow' and over the medial epicondyle in 'golfer's elbow'.

Wrist joint

This joint is commonly affected in rheumatoid arthritis and may be subluxed. It may also be swollen with synovitis (mild degrees of swelling must be sought with care), and there may be rupture of the lateral long extensor tendons of the fingers where they run over the dorsum of the joint. Movement may be very painful, and it may be very tender. On the palmar surface of the joint the median nerve may suffer entrapment in the carpal tunnel. The presence of the carpal tunnel syndrome may be checked by placing a sphygmomanometer cuff on the arm in the usual way and inflating it to the mid-point between systolic and diastolic blood pressure. If the test is positive typical numbness and paraesthesiae will develop in the ring, middle and index fingers after a few minutes. Similar symptoms occur on direct digital pressure over the carpal tunnel (Tinel's sign). Less commonly, entrapment of the ulnar nerve in its less vulnerable position may occur. Movements of the wrist are tested by full flexion and extension (Fig. 64.5) and deviation by lateral movement to the ulnar and radial sides.

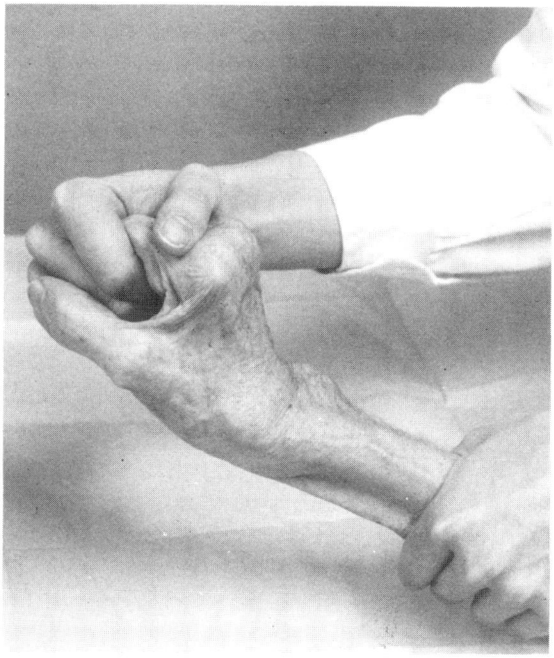

Fig. 64.5 Examination of the wrist joint.

Hand, thumb and fingers

Inspection of the hands and fingers may reveal a wealth of detail. There may be evidence of Raynaud's phenomenon. Vasculitis may be present as palmar erythema or nail-bed lesions in rheumatoid arthritis and SLE. In rheumatoid disease there may be spindling of the fingers. In the sero-negative spondarthritidies the interphalangeal joints are more likely to be involved; rheumatoid arthritis is most likely to cause swelling of the metacarpophalangeal joints. Scleroderma may show thinning and tethering of the skin over the finger tips, with subcutaneous chalky deposits which may ulcerate. The skin may be pigmented. Tenderness of the joints is elicited by firm (not too firm) pressure laterally over the finger joints and knuckles (Fig. 64.6) followed by palpation of individual joints. Heberden's or Bouchard's nodes should be looked for over the distal and proximal interphalangeal joints. There may be subluxation of the metacarpophalangeal joints with ulnar deviation, and swan-neck or boutonnière deformities of the fingers. Hand function may be severely impaired, and grip strength reduced. This can be measured by inflating a rubber bulb attached to a sphygmomanometer to 30 mm Hg and then inviting the

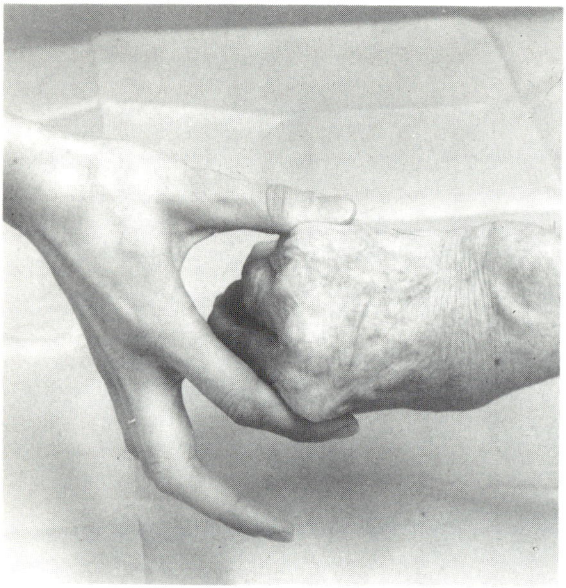

Fig. 64.6 Test to elicit tenderness of the metacarpophalangeal joints by firm lateral pressure.

patient to squeeze the bulb in the palm of the hand as tightly as possible. The average of 3 pressure readings is taken. Movement of each finger in turn should be checked, to see if there is any limitation of flexion or extension. With the thumb over each flexor tendon sheath in the palm, flexion of the appropriate finger will elicit the presence of flexor tendon nodules. At the same time, Dupuytren's contractures in the palms can be looked for. If the patient is a longstanding smoker there will be nicotine staining of the fingers; and if he has developed a lung carcinoma he may have clubbing of the fingers with hypertrophic pulmonary osteoarthropathy.

Hip

The patient is asked to stand, and observed from behind to see if there is any tilting of the pelvis. He is then asked to stand on each hip in turn — if the hip sags on the non-weight-bearing side rather than the normal elevation then this indicates disease of that hip (Trendelenberg test). The patient is then asked to lie down supine. If inflamed or diseased the hip may be held in flexion. This can be checked by making sure the patient's sacrum is flat on the couch. True shortening of the hip can be checked by measuring from the anterior superior iliac spine to the medial malleolus on the same side. Rotation of the hip is measured by first flexing the knee to 90° and then moving the knee laterally then medially (Fig. 64.7). Abduction and adduction with the knee straight should then be checked. Flexion is measured by flexing first the knee and then the hip. Extension is measured by backward movement of the straight leg with the patient lying on one side.

Knee

First this should be inspected for wasting of the quadriceps muscles and the presence of an effusion. Synovial thickening can be felt lateral and superior to the patella. Small effusions can be elicited by patella tap. Very small effusions can be shown by Kellgren's sign. First the joint on the medial side of the patella is emptied by firm pressure with the fingers. The back of the hand is then stroked hard along the lateral side of the patella, and fluid will be seen to bulge across medially under the patella. Extension and flexion of the knee should be elicited, and lateral instability may be checked with the leg straight. The femur is held firmly and the tibia is moved laterally from side to side. Anteroposterior instability can be noted by bending the knee to a right angle with the foot placed firmly down on the couch. An anteroposterior movement if present can then be produced by moving the tibia forwards and backwards (Fig. 64.8). Varus and valgus deformity of the knee and any flexion deformity should be noted. Hyperextension is sometimes seen. Posteriorly, particularly if an effusion is present, a Baker's cyst may be felt in the popliteal fossa. If there is disease of the patellofemoral component of the knee this can sometimes be confirmed by pressing firmly down on the patella with the knee straight and then moving the patella from side to side. Crepitus may be felt, and it may cause pain.

Ankles, subtaloid and mid-tarsal joints

These can best be examined with the knee straight. An effusion should be looked for and any evidence of tenosynovitis of the surrounding tendons. Minor degrees of ankle swelling may be seen from behind, with the patient standing, the two

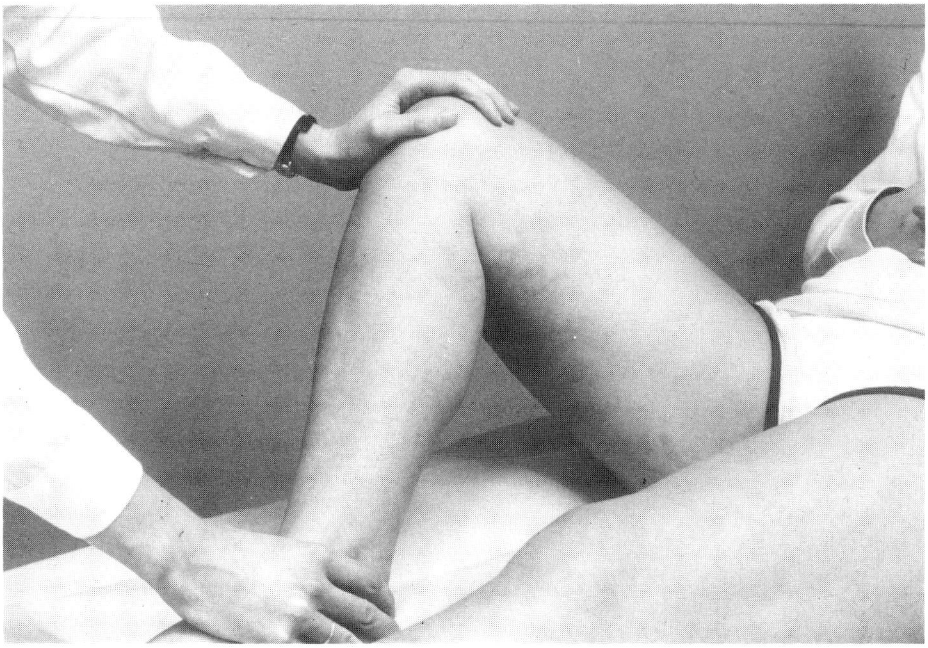

Fig. 64.7 Method of measuring hip rotation.

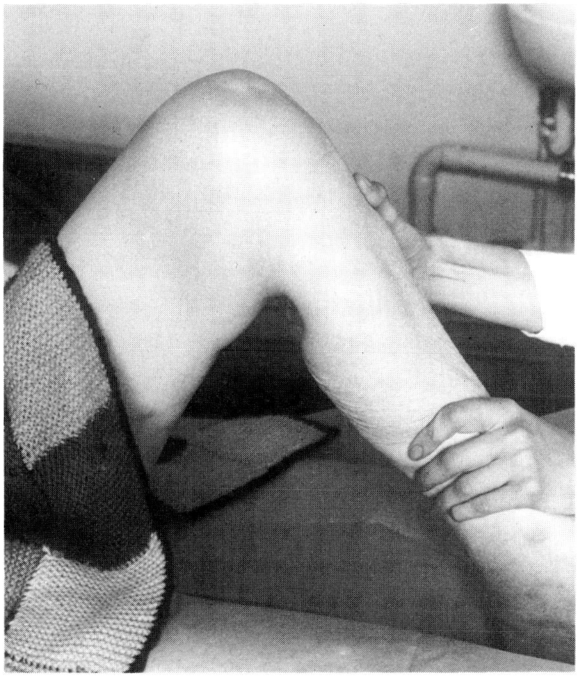

Fig. 64.8 Method for checking anteroposterior instability of the knee.

sides being compared. Extension, plantar flexion and varus and valgus movements should then be tested.

Feet and toes

First the feet should be examined with the patient standing. There may be splaying of the toes with widening of the forefoot in rheumatoid arthritis. Women particularly may have hallux valgus deformity with flattening of the foot, or alternatively the shape of the natural arch may be exaggerated. Tenderness of the metatarsophalangeal joints is looked for by pressure laterally over them followed by individual palpation of the joints: such tenderness is an extremely important sign in early rheumatoid arthritis. The sole of the foot should be carefully inspected for callosities, and no examination of the foot is complete until the shoes have been checked for abnormal wear. In plantar fasciitis there may be tenderness over the plantar surface of the calcaneum and tendinitis of the Achilles tendon may present with tenderness on pressure over its insertion.

REFERENCES

Bernhard G L, Large R L, Hensley G T 1969 Aortic disease with valvular insufficiency as the principal manifestation of SLE. Annals of Internal Medicine 71:81

Bird H A, Wright V 1982 Drugs in surgery. In: Applied drug therapy of the rheumatic disease. Wright, Bristol, Ch. 12, p. 235

Bulkley B H, Robert W E 1973 Ankylosing spondylitis and aortic regurgitation. Description of the characteristic cardiovascular lesion from a study of eight necropsy patients. Circulation 48:1014

Hejmanicik M R, Wright J C, Suirst R, Jennings F L 1964 Cardiovascular manifestations of SLE. American Heart Journal 68:119

Huskisson E C 1974 Measurement of pain. Lancet 2: 1127–31

Macrae I F, Wright V 1969 Measurement of back movement. Annals of Rheumatic Diseases 28:584

Ritchie D M, Boyle J A, McInnes J M, Jasani K, Dalakos G, Grieveson P, Buchanan W 1968 Clinical studies with an articular index for the assessment of joint tenderness in patients with rheumatoid arthritis. Quarterly Journal of Medicine 37: 393–406

Stack B H R, Grant I W B 1965 Rheumatoid interstitial lung disease. British Journal of Diseases of the Chest 59:202

Thould A K, Stansfeld A G, Balme W H 1965 Chronic atrophic perichondritis. Annals of Rheumatic Diseases 24: 563–7

Young R H, Mark G J 1978 Pulmonary vascular change in scleroderma. American Journal of Medicine 64:998

Wilkinson M 1962 Rheumatoid pericarditis. British Medical Journal 2:1723

Clinical trials and therapeutic evaluation

Once upon a time, eminent authorities used experience to advise their colleagues about the use of various treatments. But because judgement proved difficult for the eminent authorities and their experience was sometimes fallacious, a better system was devised. Treatment was given to some patients and withheld from others so that the effects of the treatment could be measured and this exercise was called a clinical trial. Clinical trials became the basis on which eminent authorities advised their colleagues, though it soon became apparent that clinical trials could themselves be both difficult and fallacious. It was then necessary to do clinical trials of clinical trials and the rules and regulations which follow are the result.

DESIGN

Aims of clinical trials in rheumatology

Clinical trials are used to assess the effects of a wide variety of treatments including drugs, operations and physical methods of therapy; the basic principles apply to all of them. Most studies of clinical trial methodology have been carried out with drugs, which will therefore be considered first.

The type of trial required to assess the effectiveness of a drug depends on the nature of the activity of the drug. A classification of antirheumatic drugs is shown in Table 65.1 (Huskisson, 1974a). Simple analgesics relieve pain without any effect on inflammation; their action begins within an hour of administration of the drug and lasts for a few hours. Analgesics with anti-inflammatory effects also relieve pain but have an additional effect on inflammation which can be recognised by changes such as reduction in swelling. Though drugs of this type have the same effect as simple analgesics in single doses, when given regularly their activity increases, reaching a peak usually within a few days of administration. Steroids have a pure anti-inflammatory effect with a time course similar to that of the analgesic–anti-inflammatory drugs. They relieve pain only by reducing inflammation. Drugs with a specific activity in rheumatoid arthritis take months to reach their maximum activity. They also affect joint pain and swelling, but have additional actions on aspects of the disease process itself, for example, reducing the titre of rheumatoid factor and promoting the disappearance of nodules. Various drugs have specific effects in other diseases, for example, colchicine and allopurinol in gout and antibiotics in septic arthritis, and these properties require a different approach for their evaluation.

Table 65.1 Classification of antirheumatic drugs

Type	Example
Simple analgesics	Paracetamol
Analgesics with anti-inflammatory properties	Indomethacin
Pure anti-inflammatory drugs	Prednisolone
Drugs with a specific activity in rheumatoid arthritis	Penicillamine
Drugs with a specific activity in other diseases	Allopurinol

One may require from a trial not evidence of effectiveness but an indication of the incidence of side-effects. A clear statement of the aims of the trial is an essential first step — it is seldom possible to document completely the properties of a compound in one trial and it is a mistake to try to collect too many facts in any one study: by trying to measure two things at once one may measure neither. A programme of trials is normally required and such a programme is shown in Table 65.2. In this programme a compound is screened first for simple analgesic activity, secondly for anti-inflammatory effects, thirdly for toxicity and for a specific action in rheumatoid arthritis. An anti-inflammatory study may fail to detect simple analgesic activity and is inadequate to assess the toxicity of a compound. Each trial serves its own purpose.

Writing a protocol — information required to do it

Having defined the aim of the study it is wise to write a protocol outlining the details of the experiment — at this stage many problems will become apparent. An outline of the protocol and the details which should be included as given in Table 65.3.

It is desirable to have certain information before designing a particular study and this will have been provided from animal studies, studies in volunteers and perhaps from pilot trials in patients.

Table 65.2 Stages in the development of a compound and the information which should be produced at each stage

Study	Information produced
1. Animal tests	Type of activity Efective blood levels Potential toxicity Half-life
2. Volunteer studies	Dose required to produce effective blood levels Optimum formulation
3. Pilot trial and dose-finding	Type of activity Approximate effectiveness Dose Time course Early toxicity
4. Single dose analgesic study	Analgesic potency
5. Three-way crossover trial	Anti-inflammatory effects
6. 6 months group comparative trial	Specific effects in rheumatoid arthritis Toxicity
7. Comparisons with other compounds of similar type	Comparative effectiveness and toxicity
8. Controlled marketing	Incidence of unusual side-effects

Table 65.3 The protocol

Heading	Details to be included
Title; aims	
Basic design	Single or multiple dose (specify duration) Open, double blind or blind observer Crossover or group-comparative (parallel group) Comparative treatment and/or placebo
Patients	How many? In/outpatients Characteristics required Exclusions
Treatments	What treatment is given before the trial Specify for each treatment (unknown, standard, placebo) dose, frequency and time of administration, formulation and duration Method of blinding Allocation of treatment Variations allowed What happens if treatment is not tolerated and at the end of the study Other treatments allowed/not allowed Who gives it — instructions
Measurements	Clinical and laboratory effects; side-effects; patient co-operation Which? How often? Time of day. By whom?
Analysis	Type of analysis Significance levels

Though there is very little correlation between the effectiveness of drugs in animal models and their eventual success in man, animal tests should give an indication of the type of activity to be expected. For example, tests of pain such as the tail flick method in rats are useful for predicting analgesic activity, and tests of inflammation such as carrageenan oedema for predicting anti-inflammatory activity. There are few correlations between toxicity in animals and man but animal tests may at least suggest which organs should be considered as potential sites for toxic effects. Effective blood levels in animals provide the best clue to the dosage which will be required in man and the dose required to produce similar blood levels in volunteers is a good starting point for trials in patients. The plasma half-life of the compound is of great importance since a long half-life may be an indication that the appearance of the peak activity of the drug will be delayed and that the effects may persist after it has been stopped — this is particularly important for crossover trials.

Chronopharmacology

The time course of the action of a treatment is of the greatest importance in designing clinical trials; each type of drug has its own characteristic time course and these are illustrated in Figure 65.1. Measurement of the effect of a treatment must be made at a time when that effect is at its greatest, for simple analgesics after 2 or 3 hours, for most anti-inflammatory drugs after 1 week and, for drugs with a specific effect like that of penicillamine, after 6 months. If a compound takes 1 week to work it is foolish to give it for a shorter time and unnecessary to give it for longer. The effects of simple analgesics must be measured 2 or 3 hours after administration — it is unnecessary to give them for a week and the effect may be missed in this way since the week is composed of many hours of little or no pain-relief as well as a few hours of pain-relief (Huskisson, 1974b). The effects of most anti-inflammatory drugs are apparent after 1 week but the time taken to reach the maximum effect may vary, especially in compounds with a long half-life. All forms of treatment have a characteristic time course; the benefits of an operation for rheumatoid arthritis may be greatest after a few weeks, when the effects of the surgical trauma have subsided. Thereafter there may be a continued slow deterioration as a result of the natural history of the disease. Side-effects also occur at characteristic times. For example most patients who will develop gastrointestinal side-effects while taking full anti-inflammatory doses of aspirin do so within the first month of treatment; loss of taste due to penicillamine usually occurs after about 6 weeks treatment and nephrotic syndrome from the 4th month; measurement must be made after an appropriate period of treatment in all these cases.

Chronopharmacology is also concerned with the relationship of the administration of drugs to the time of day; for example, indomethacin in a large dose is likely to be effective and well tolerated when given at night but less effective and toxic when the same dose is given in the morning (Huskisson, 1976).

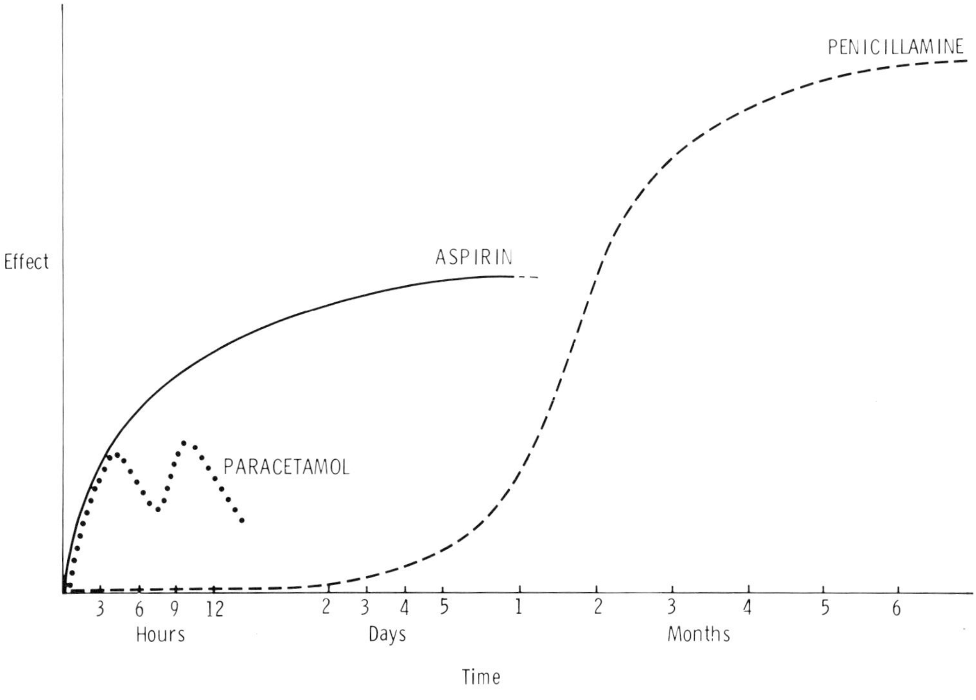

Fig. 65.1 Characteristic time course of various drugs.

Pharmacokinetics

It is highly desirable to know the blood level profile of a compound before starting work, as well as its distribution in the body, metabolism and route of excretion. Absorption may be affected by food. The blood level profile may affect the time course of the action of the drug and may vary considerably from patient to patient so that a subgroup may have higher, lower, more or less prolonged blood levels and consequently more or less effect or toxicity. Accumulation at a particular site may be an advance warning of toxicity and the pathway of excretion may be important if patients with renal or hepatic impairment are to be treated. All too often there is no correlation between blood level changes and effectiveness or toxicity, so that no conclusions can be drawn about clinical effects from the blood levels.

PILOT TRIALS, OPEN TRIALS AND UNCONTROLLED TRIALS

It is a fundamental and immutable principle of clinical trials that the unknown treatment should be compared either with no treatment or with another treatment — there is no place for uncontrolled trials except in diseases whose outcome is completely predictable such as those with a high mortality rate. Established rheumatoid arthritis seldom undergoes spontaneous remission, so that a drug which regularly cured the disease might not need a controlled trial! In rare diseases, there are sometimes insufficient cases to provide controls.

Similarly open trials are to be condemned. A minimum requirement is that the patients should be assessed by an impartial observer who is unaware of the treatments given and has no interest in the outcome. Doctors who give treatment have a special relationship with the recipient which makes it difficult for them to make an unbiased assessment of the treatment.

Pilot trials, which are usually open and uncontrolled, are often useful as a prelude to controlled experiments. They may give an indication of the type of action to be expected, the time course of the action, side-effects and how to overcome them, and optimum dosage. A drug like penicillamine provides a good example of the value of a pilot trial; it takes months to reach its best effects and has unpleasant and dangerous side-effects which can be minimised by an appropriate dosage regime and sometimes overcome in other ways. A pilot trial would enable the investigator to get to know the drug, to learn how to use it, and to plan a trial of the appropriate duration to detect various effects and side-effects. The results of the pilot trial, though useful to the investigator are seldom of value to others because of the unpredictable influence of the placebo effect. Great caution should be exercised before drawing any firm conclusions from such trials.

Design of studies of simple analgesics

It is a general principle of clinical trials that drugs should be tested under conditions as close as possible to those in which they are used. Simple analgesics are usually given in single doses for relief of pain which is otherwise uncontrolled and they should be tested in the same way. There is an additional reason why single dose studies are likely to be successful — maximum activity is seen 1–3 hours after administration and this is therefore the optimum time for measuring pain relief. The appearance of a tablet may have an effect of its own, red being the most effective colour for placebo in the relief of pain (Huskisson, 1974b). It is therefore desirable that treatments which are compared should appear identical. Simple analgesics relieve pain for a few hours and have no effect on the underlying condition so that crossover methodology can safely be used. Ideally, an unknown drug should always be compared with a standard compound such as paracetamol or aspirin as well as placebo, using a three-way crossover design (Fig. 65.2). Comparison of the standard with placebo shows whether the patients were capable of response; comparison of the unknown drug with placebo shows whether the unknown drug was effective; comparison of the unknown drug with the standard provides a measure of the extent of its effectiveness.

In such a study the order of treatment should

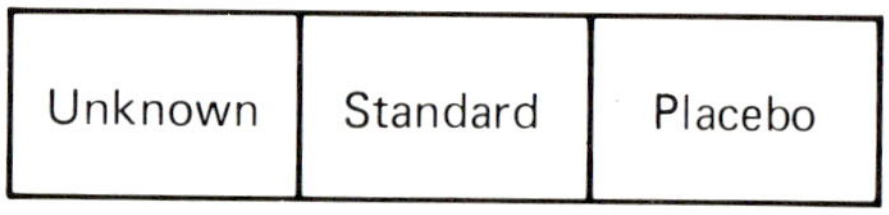

Fig. 65.2 The three-way crossover trial.

be randomised and balanced so that an equal number of patients has each possible order of treatment.

It is difficult to make exact statements about the numbers of patients required for such a study but experience suggests that 24 patients are sufficient to show differences between currently available analgesics and placebo and between more effective and less effective analgesics. Any patient with pain which is of sufficient severity to require the regular use of analgesics may be included, but the nature of the painful condition must be specified. Drugs with anti-inflammatory properties, for example, may have greater analgesic potency in conditions like rheumatoid arthritis in which inflammation is prominent.

No other treatment should be given during the period in which pain or pain relief is being measured. Treatment given at other times during the study must be standardised.

Such a study will document the analgesic potency of a compound without shedding any light on the effects of multiple doses, side-effects, addiction potential or the development of tolerance. If these properties are to be documented it is necessary to design separate longer-term experiments.

Design of studies of anti-inflammatory drugs

Anti-inflammatory drugs usually take a few days to reach their peak effect; fenoprofen, for example, has reached its effect after 1 week and in the next 6 months its effect is neither greater nor less (Huskisson et al, 1974). Naproxen, despite a relatively long plasma half-life, achieves most of its action within 24 hours and even piroxicam, with a much longer half-life is fully effective within 3 days (Huskisson, 1981). It is therefore usually necessary to give an anti-inflammatory drug for 1 week to test its effectiveness; if the drug is stopped its effects soon wear off and it is therefore possible to use a three-way crossover design (Fig. 65.2) as for analgesic trials. The duration of each period of treatment must be based upon the known or predicted time course of the action of the drug. The assumption must be made that patients equilibrate on each treatment and their state at the end of each period of treatment is used in the analysis — changes during periods of treatment cannot be used because the starting point is different depending on the order of treatment. Patients relapse while taking only placebo and may suffer considerable discomfort — it is highly desirable that a trial against placebo should be used early in the course of the investigation of a new compound but the repeated use of trials of placebo is quite unnecessary and does not justify the distress which is caused to the patients. Similarly it is seldom if ever necessary or justifiable to give placebos for longer than 1 week to patients with active inflammatory arthritis; such patients obtain little relief from so-called 'rescue analgesics'. A short-term parallel group study (Fig. 65.3) can be used as an alternative to a crossover for the demonstration of anti-inflammatory activity but requires more patients to achieve the same power. The advantages and disadvantages have been reviewed by Paulus (1981). The standard anti-inflammatory used in such studies has until recently been aspirin though the increasing use of agents such as propionic acid derivatives suggests that one of these should be used as the standard, particularly for the evaluation of similar compounds. The older anti-inflammatory agents such as aspirin are more difficult to use as standards because of their characteristic side-effects which often 'unblind' the observer. Indomethacin causes a further problem because of the additional effects of a large dose at night. If this is omitted, the drug is much less effective — if it is included, side-effects are more

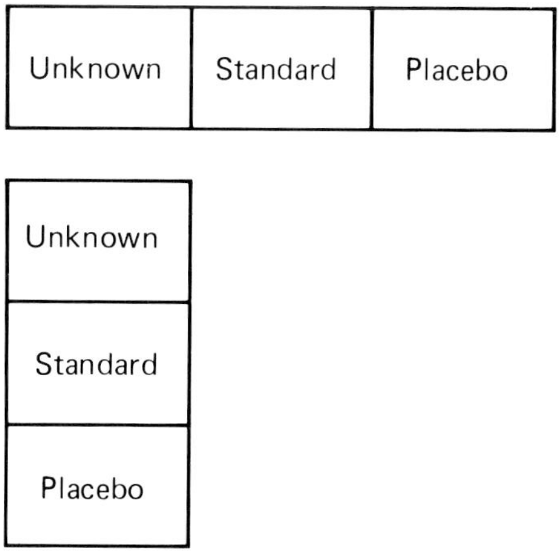

Fig. 65.3 Two designs for studying the efficacy of a non-steroidal anti-inflammatory drug, using crossover or parallel group methodology.

likely and it is necessary to use a complicated pill-taking regime to maintain double blindness.

Rheumatoid arthritis provides an ideal model for testing anti-inflammatory agents because it is common and has obvious inflammatory features. Bed-rest has a beneficial effect on the disease and improvement continues for at least 3 weeks after admission (Lee et al, 1974), so that it is usual to conduct such studies in outpatients. 12–18 patients are sufficient to show differences between existing anti-inflammatory agents and placebo, but much larger numbers are required to show differences between individual drugs. There is an enormous difference between the capacity of individuals to respond to such drugs, which is a further advantage of a three-way crossover design.

Particular problems arise with the provision of tablets for double blind studies. It is is now clear that very minor changes in formulation may cause enormous changes in bioavailability (Garnham, 1974). If a new drug is to be compared with a standard, the standard must be used in the form in which it is known, the generally available marketed product. The formulation should not be changed in any way but if it is, bioavailability studies must be carried out; a comparable blood level profile in man is the minimum acceptable evidence of equivalence.

Sometimes this problem can be overcome by the double placebo method, using placebos for each of the active agents concerned. The disadvantage of this method is that it is necessary for the patient to take two types of tablet, often at different times of day, with an increased risk of errors.

Increasingly one may ask whether double blindness is really necessary (Huskisson & Scott, 1976). It is far more important that the observer should be unaware of the nature of the treatment being assessed and this can be achieved by the use of a blind observer — treatment is given by the doctor in the usual way and assessment carried out by an independent person. Most patients do not need to be blind since they do not have preconcieved ideas about the value of any particular new treatment — it is however important that the standard drug used in a study should not be recognised by the patient as a treatment he has had before and liked or disliked. Single blind trials, using a blind observer have particular advantages for treatments which look different, those which are given by different routes (it is unnecessary as well as unkind to give placebo injections for example), those with characteristic effects or characteristic side-effects which would be recognised by the observer and those with different, unusual or complicated dosage schedules.

Patients must not be allowed to take anti-inflammatory drugs such as aspirin during anti-inflammatory trials though simple analgesics such as paracetamol can be permitted. Small doses of steroids (less than 5 mg daily of prednisolone or equivalent) are usually permitted provided that the dose has been constant for at least 6 months and the patients have active disease. The use of specific drugs such as gold or penicillamine is not permitted unless such treatment has been given for at least 6 months and the patient's condition is stable.

Design of studies for slow-acting drugs and slowly appearing phenomena such as toxicity

Crossover trials are ideal for treatments which take only a short time to work, and for phenomena which take only a short time to develop and which are reversible in an equally short time. It is seldom advisable to use crossover methodology with treatment periods of longer than two weeks. Drugs with a specific action in rheumatoid arthritis take 6 months to produce their maximum effect, and gastric toxicity of anti-inflammatory drugs may take 4 weeks or longer to appear: these phenomena therefore require prolonged trials and it is necessary to use a group comparative or parallel group study (Fig. 65.4). If the study forms part of a comprehensive investigation of a compound, it is often convenient to combine the demonstration of specific activity in rheumatoid arthritis and toxicity. Such trials may be double blind but it is often more convenient to use a blind observer — if side-effects unblind the observer in a double blind trial, the trial becomes open and it may be better to settle for a single blind trial from the beginning. The

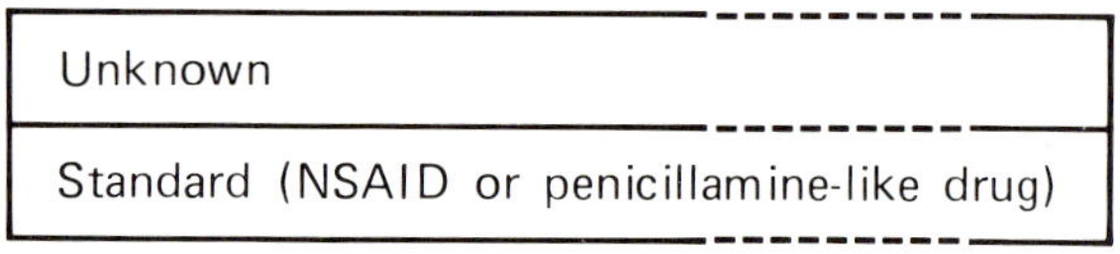

Fig. 65.4 Design for long-term studies to investigate toxicity or long-term effects of drugs like penicillamine.

comparative drug will vary according to the purpose of the study; in toxicity studies, a comparable compound should be used, an anti-inflammatory for an anti-inflammatory, an analgesic for an analgesic. If a penicillamine-like compound is to be tested, penicillamine is ideal as the comparative drug. Placebo can seldom be used for long periods unless full anti-inflammatory therapy is allowed in addition.

2 groups of 12 patients are sufficient to demonstrate the effect of penicillamine with anti-inflammatory drugs compared to anti-inflammatory drugs alone. At least 100 patients in each group are required for a formal toxicity study and this number would show the differences in the incidence of gastrointestinal side-effects between a major anti-inflammatory drug like aspirin and one of the newer propionic acid derivatives like ibuprofen. They should be outpatients throughout the study. In toxicity studies, patients should be excluded if they have other diseases which might interfere with the evaluation of the toxicity of the compound, such as hepatic or renal disease. Patients treated with penicillamine and similar compounds should be those who have not been controlled by or have progressed despite the optimal use of anti-inflammatory drugs. It is unfortunately a matter of chance in most cases whether the two groups are comparable — if the numbers are large enough, they should be comparable in most respects. The chances can be improved by stratification — for example patients with severe pain might be separated from those with moderate or mild pain and separate allocation schedules used for each pain category. The groups might still be unbalanced for another measurement such as articular index. While it is desirable that in terms of age, sex, duration of disease, anatomical and functional status, there is no evidence that any of these factors influences the response to treatment. Where a particular factor is known to influence response, it is essential to ensure that it is the same in both groups. One can stratify for many different factors provided that the subgroups remain of a reasonable size and the number of factors therefore depends on the total number of patients.

In trials of penicillamine-like drugs the patients are usually controlled on optimal anti-inflammatory therapy before the start of the study and maintained if possible on the same dose. Attempts may be made to reduce symptomatic therapy and the reduction used as a measure of the effectiveness of the trial drug. When penicillamine is used as a comparative drug, it is wisest to use a blind observer and to ensure that the patients do not discuss their side-effects with the observer.

Further studies — post-marketing surveillance

The trials outlined above will provide a clear-cut documentation of the type of activity and toxicity to be expected from a compound but will leave many questions unanswered. At this stage, further comparisons with other compounds will usually be required and these will follow the same basic design. When two anti-inflammatory agents are compared a crossover will usually provide the best design but the use of placebo is not necessary if both compounds are known to be effective. Formal controlled toxicity studies will provide only the most frequent side-effects and it will be necessary to accumulate information on large numbers before rare side-effects appear — this is usually best achieved by an early period of controlled marketing as was carried out with ibuprofen (Buckler et al, 1970). Various systems of post-marketing surveillance have been proposed.

MEASUREMENT

There is no perfect measurement for patients with arthritis and current favourites are those which have proved to be of value in demonstrating the effectiveness of drugs in current use. A range of measurements is shown in Table 65.4 which emphasises that the measurement must reflect the aim of the experiment; each trial will therefore require different measurements, depending on its aims. If a drug is being tested for its ability to lower serum uric acid, the uric acid must be measured and if a drug is supposed to be analgesic, pain relief must be measured. While it is quite in order to devise new measurements, they must be validated and their properties defined before they are used as a basis for statements about the effects of treatment. The most important properties of a measurement are its reproducibility, inter- and intraobserver variation, sensitivity, specificity, objectivity and relevance to the condition being measured. It is

Table 65.4 Measurements required for drugs with different types of activity

Type of activity sought	What to measure
Analgesic	Pain relief
Anti-inflammatory	Pain Duration of morning stiffness Analgesic requirements Proximal interphalangeal joint circumference Articular index
Specific action in rheumatoid arthritis	Pain or pain relief Duration of morning stiffness Proximal interphalangeal joint circumference Articular index ESR Rheumatoid factor titre
Side-effects	Response to standard question 'Has the treatment upset you?'

also necessary to consider the safety and acceptability of the method, its requirements in time and apparatus, the effect of external conditions such as time of day and changes in temperature and its applicability to any part of any patient.

Measurement of pain

Pain is the major symptom of rheumatic disease and relief of pain is the object of most treatment. It is not possible to say that a treatment was of benefit to a patient unless his pain was relieved, and no matter how sophisticated measurement of individual disease states become, it will always be necessary to show that the patient felt better.

Pain is a subjective phenomenon, its severity is known only to the sufferer, and the sufferer alone can measure it. A variety of methods has been used to measure pain (Huskisson, 1974c).

The simple descriptive scale

The simple descriptive pain scale described by Keele in 1948 divided pain into agonising, severe, moderate and mild; though definitions were included in the original description, they are seldom used — patients are readily able to categorise their pain in this way (Huskisson, 1974c). The disadvantage of the scale is its lack of sensitivity (Huskisson et al, 1970). A patient with mild pain has only one possible grade of improvement and the changes which are produced by non-steroidal anti-inflammatory drugs are less than one grade of the scale. There are not sufficient descriptions which can be placed in an agreed order of ascending severity to give the scale more divisions (Melzack & Torgerson, 1971).

The visual analogue scale

The visual analogue scale (Fig. 65.5) provides a more sensitive method for measuring pain which is now widely used. It is a line, usually 10 cm in length, which is taken to represent the continuum of the experience of pain. The ends are defined as the extremes of the experience. The patient marks the scale at a point which corresponds to his experience and the distance from the lower end of the scale to that point is taken as the severity of pain.

The performance of a visual analogue scale is profoundly affected by its design. The distribution of results on such a scale is uniform. The uniformity of results is important for the sensitivity of the method. If results are clustered around particular parts of the scale, the sensitivity is lost. The distribution of results on a simple visual analogue scale remains uniform and does not differ whether the scale is vertical or horizontal (Scott & Huskisson, 1979B). The correlation of results on such scales is very high, confirming the good reproducibility of the method. But the situation changes when descriptions are added to the line, making a graphic rating scale (Scott & Huskisson, 1976) (Fig. 65.6). When such a scale is used in the horizontal position, the result are predominantly localised to points corresponding to the descriptions. The scale

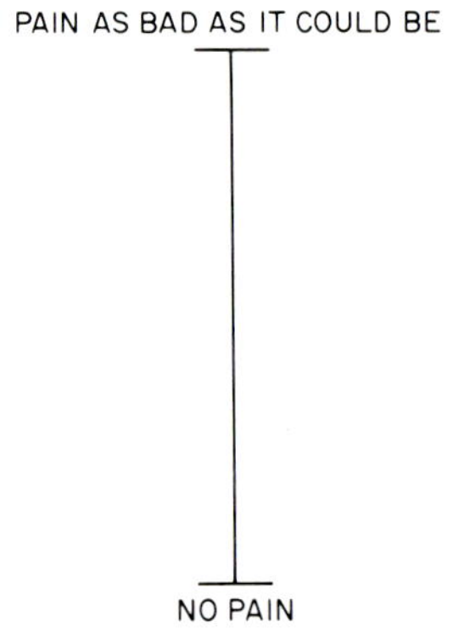

Fig. 65.5 Visual analogue pain scale. It can be vertical or longitudinal.

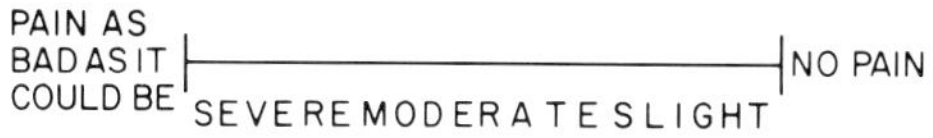

Fig. 65.6 Graphic rating scale. It must be horizontal and the words must be spaced out along the line.

is used by most patients as a simple descriptive scale and the sensitivity is lost. A scale with descriptions produces a uniform distribution of results only when the line is horizontal and the descriptions are spread evenly along its length. It is probably wise to avoid descriptions, except at the ends of the line and also to avoid numbers. Certain numbers like 5 and 10 are likely to be preferred, again causing clustering and loss of sensitivity. Visual analogue scales must have stops at their ends to limit the distribution of results.

It is often said that patients should not be allowed to see the results of previous measurements when assessing pain. The reverse is true (Scott & Huskisson, 1979a). As time passes, patients tend to forget the severity of their pain at a particular point and at later dates will tend to make an overestimate. They should therefore be allowed to see previous scales.

The visual analogue scale provides the patient with a robust, sensitive and reproducible method of measuring pain. Results correlate well with other methods of assessing pain. The method is independent of language and is applicable to most situations.

Other methods

Other methods have been suggested but have not proved attractive. Pain severity can be measured by matching its severity to that of experimental pain which can be measured in terms of the stimulus (Hardy et al, 1952). Objective manifestations of pain are unreliable indicators of pain severity — facial signs and vocal signals are expressed by only a few and irregularly. The concept of the visual analogue scale has been extended to the use of colours, deep red representing severe pain. A series of facial expressions has also been used, similar to that which is available for guests of the Holiday Inn to express their degree of satisfaction.

Measurement of pain relief

There are several advantages to measuring pain relief rather than pain. When pain is measured on two occasions and the second reading subtracted from the first, the difference will always be proportional to the first reading or the initial severity of the pain (Huskisson, 1974c). This is highly undesirable since in a group comparative trial, if initial pain severity is not equal is the two groups, differences may arise not due to treatment but to imbalance of the groups. This relationship is not found if pain is measured directly. All patients start from the same artificial base line on a pain relief scale. When pain scores are subtracted, it is also necessary to assume that differences in different parts of the scale are equal — severe to moderate scores the same as mild to none. Also relief is perhaps a more usual mode of expression by the patient of the effects of treatment.

Methods used to measure pain relief are similar. A simple descriptive scale (slight, moderate and complete pain relief), a visual analogue scale or the graphic rating method are again satisfactory.

Indirect methods — preference, global rating and analgesic requirements

Many of the measurements used in trials of antirheumatic therapy are simply indirect measures of pain. This applies to many functional measurements such as grip strength (Ingpen, 1968). Great caution should be exercised in the interpretation of changes in such measures which cannot be regarded as substitutes for pain measurement. One such measurement is preference which is a useful indication of effectiveness in crossover trials of anti-inflammatory drugs. Preference may moreover reflect the side-effects of a drug as well as its therapeutic effects and a patient may prefer the less effective drug, even placebo, if the more effective has unpleasant side-effects (Huskisson, 1974B). Preference may also be the result of several different effects or effects on several different aspects of the disease (Huskisson & Grayson, 1974). Experience however suggests that the major factor influencing patient preference for drugs is efficacy (Huskisson et al, 1981).

Global scales are another popular measure of the efficacy of a drug. Treatment can be graded both by physician and patient using descriptions like excellent, good, fair, poor and useless. It is doubtful whether the physician can make such assessments since it is difficult to see how he could overrule a patient's decision. The patient's view provides a robust but crude assessment which may have particular value in counting responders and non-responders.

Analgesic requirements measure pain indirectly — patients whose pain is relieved need less analgesic, less anti-inflammatory and less steroid therapy. The reverse does not necessarily apply.

Other measures of disease severity; measurement of inflammation

Apart from the measurement of pain, it is desirable to include some measurement of disease severity and when it is intended to document anti-inflammatory activity as distinct from analgesic activity, to include some measurement of inflammation.

Stiffness

In rheumatoid arthritis, the duration of morning stiffness is a useful guide to the severity of the inflammatory process. It is easily recorded by the patient and is reduced by anti-inflammatory drugs. Stiffness can be measured directly and shown to reflect anti-inflammatory activity (Ingpen, 1968) but since measured stiffness correlates well with the duration of morning stiffness, it seems best to use the simpler measurement.

Swelling

One of the most useful measures of the anti-inflammatory effects of drugs in rheumatoid arthritis is proximal interphalangeal joint circumference (Boardman & Hart, 1967). A small amount of practice is necessary to perfect the technique using the Geigy gauge which was developed from the use of jeweller's rings. A reduction in swelling can be produced by the major anti-inflammatory drugs, aspirin, indomethacin and phenylbutazone but not by the newer anti-inflammatory agents such as ibuprofen (Huskisson et al, 1971), or fenoprofen (Huskisson et al, 1974). Another limitation of the method is the variability of response; it is impossible to predict which patients will show reductions in joint size and it is therefore essential to include an active control and placebo in an experiment in order to show whether or not the patients were capable of response.

The circumference of the knee joint can be measured with a tape measure. This measurement is highly reproducible, even between observers, and much superior to a numerical grading of swelling on a four-point scale (Marks et al, 1978). However the knee is not perfectly cylindrical and it may be difficult to ensure that repeated measurements are made at the same point. There is a good correlation between the volume of fluid aspirated and the change in knee circumference (Kirwan et al, 1979). Intraobserver error in this measurement has been found to be lowest when the circumference is measured as the mid-point of the patella and increased with distance from this point (Nicholas et al, 1976). In the same study, the variation in results from day to day and observer to observer was used to calculate that a significant reduction in circumference would be 1.5 cm at the mid-patella level, 2.7 cm and 3.5 cm at levels 7 and 15 are higher. The removal of 40 ml of fluid from the knee produces a reduction of 1 cm making it clear that very profound changes are required to influence knee joint circumference. Non-steroidal anti-inflammatory drugs are not so potent! The patellar pouch is visible on X-ray and its enlargement enables the radiologist to report an effusion. The size of this structure can best be measured using xeroradiography (Gumpel et al, 1980). These authors showed that, as with knee circumference, the volume of fluid withdrawn from the knee correlated well with reduction in size of the pouch. Gumpel et al (1980) calculated from the reproducibility of the measurement that a significant reduction in the size of the pouch would be achieved by removal of 20 ml of fluid, making this the most sensitive method available to date. Plethysmography has also been used to measure swelling.

One must hope that advances in non-invasive scanning techniques will bring some improvement in the measurement of swelling and a badly needed objective measure of this important aspect of inflammation.

Grip strength, tenderness and articular index

Grip strength and articular index are indirect measures of pain: though they may appear to be objective, they are not, since the pain threshold of the patient influences both the effort he is prepared to expend and the tenderness to which he will admit. They are often used in trials and have some value in confirming the results of pain measurement. Grip is easily measured with a modified sphygmomanometer cuff. Of the variety of articular indices available, that described by Ritchie et al (1968) is most widely used, with the great advantage of simplicity and speed. It is based on the tenderness of a series of joints and can be carried out by an experienced person in less than 2 minutes. There is a large interobserver variation so that the same person must carry out the measurement on all occasions. A similar index has been developed by Doyle et al (1981) for use in osteoarthritis, modified to take account of the different distribution of joint involvement.

Measurement of the tenderness of single joints may be required in conditions other than rheumatoid arthritis where only one or two joints are involved. It may then be useful to use a mechanical method to induce pain and an example is the dolorimeter (McCarty et al, 1965).

Functional measurements

The measurement of functional ability and disability is clearly desirable but present methods leave much to be desired. Measurement of walking time is perhaps the oldest but it depends on effort expended, is improved by repetition and is insensitive to the effects of drugs when compared with other methods. Various scales of functional status have been devised (Steibrocker et al, 1949; Savage, 1958; Empire Rheumatism Council, 1955), but again these are insensitive, requiring a major change in the condition of the patient to show improvement. Each patient has his own functional problems and individualised measurements may provide the only solution to the problem. This was demonstrated in studies comparing various methods of assessing functions such as tying shoe laces and writing (Huskisson et al, 1976). The time taken to complete the tasks was noted, the observer rated them and the patient expressed the subjective degree of difficulty on a visual analogue scale. There were poor correlations between the measures which did not well reflect the effects of treatment with gold and penicillamine, even though patients improved by standard criteria like pain. In a subsequent experiment (Scott & Huskisson, 1977) three visual analogue scales were used in a similar context, measuring global functional ability, a standard task for all patients and a particular task chosen by each patient as being difficult. Measurements of the chosen task showed a greater degree of impairment and responded better than the other functional measures to treatment. This measure in fact responded as well as pain though there was no significant correlation between changes in pain and in function. It is interesting that in the studies discussed above and in a study of grip strength the patients assessment did not correlate well with other measures of the phenomenon. One may ask whether it is more relevant that a patient cannot squeeze a bag or that he feels that he cannot. There is certainly an argument for subjective measurement of disability and the importance of choosing a particular disability for each patient is obvious. Unlike pain, which is universal, disability is a very individual thing.

The alternative to measuring an individual function for each patient is to devise an index which covers a wide range of tasks. Lee et al (1974) devised such a scale in which a series of activities of daily living were graded on a three-point scale of difficulty. The sum of the scores made up an index which has been used to demonstrate the benefits of treatment. Several other attempts have been made to devise such indices including the Nc-Master Health Index Questionnaire which measures physical as well as social and emotional function, the Arthritis Impact Measurement Scale (Meenan, 1981) and the Standard Health Assessment Questionnaire (Fries et al, 1980). One must hope that comparisons of these methods will lead to the emergence of a generally acceptable scale which all centres will use.

Objective measures of inflammation

Two newer methods have been introduced with a view to making objective measurements of inflammation, isotope counting and thermography.

Inflamed joints are warm and this can be demonstrated by radiometry or infra-red thermography. The infra-red thermogram is a temperature map of the surface of the joint and the map has to be changed into a number before it can be analysed. Various attempts have been made to create thermographic indices (Collins et al, 1974, Huskisson et al, 1973). The joint temperature is related to ambient temperature so that this must either be kept constant (Collins et al, 1974) or allowed for by comparing the area of the joint with a control area (Huskisson et al, 1973). Ring et al (1974) used the thermographic index to show reduction in joint temperature in rheumatoid arthritis by intra-articular steroids and oral salicylates but not paracetamol. It remains for this method to be compared with standard clinical measurements in the context of a controlled trial for correlations to be demonstrated with other measures of inflammation. Reduction in joint temperature by anti-inflammatory drugs appears to be slow, taking a great deal longer to achieve than reduction of pain, for example. This may explain the failure of thermography on short-term trials (Huskisson et al, 1973). The method appears to offer the most immediate prospect of an objective measure of the effects of anti-inflammatory drugs.

If an isotope such as technetium-99 is injected intravenously, the counts over inflamed joints are higher than those over normal joints. The measurement is reproducible and is reduced by intra-articular injection of steroids (Dick et al, 1970). It can be applied to small as well as large joints (Dick et al, 1972). Though some authors have shown changes in counts over individual joints, the changes do not correlate with other measures of inflammation and cannot therefore be regarded as showing anti-inflammatory effects (Huskisson et al, 1973).

Greater interest attaches to the technetium index, the sum of counts over a number of joints showing a good correlation with the articular index (Oka et al, 1971; Huskisson et al, 1973). Though this index is not reduced by short-term administration of prednisolone (Berry & Huskisson, 1974), it is reduced by 6 months treatment with penicillamine (Huskisson et al, 1975). It may therefore represent an objective measure of the effects of drugs with a specific activity in rheumatoid arthritis.

The technique of technetium counting is of the greatest importance. Because the isotope has a short half-life, it is impossible to give exact doses and the counts must be corrected for this variable. Joints must be counted at a fixed time interval after injection, usually 20 minutes, when the count rates have reached a plateau. Apparatus and positions of counter and joints must be standardised and external conditions controlled.

Other isotopes have been used for similar purposes. Berry & Huskisson (1974) used indium because it is a better measure of blood flow and though counts were high in rheumatoid arthritis, there was no correlation with articular index and no advantage over technetium. Xenon is inconvenient because it must be given by intra-articular injection with the possible errors of mixing with variable volumes of synovial fluid (Dick et al, 1970). It seems that technetium is the best isotope. Both these methods require expensive apparatus, a controlled environment and skilled operators. On present evidence, their advantages do not justify their inclusion in routine clinical trials.

Laboratory measures

In rheumatoid arthritis, measurement of ESR, rheumatoid factor titre and perhaps immunoglobulin levels are of undoubted value in completing the profile of the action of specific drugs like penicillamine and gold. Some of the more recent non-steroidal anti-inflammatory drugs have been reported to lower the ESR but the significance of this finding is not yet known and the measurement cannot yet therefore be recommended.

Progression and outcome

It is not enough to relieve pain. The aim of drugs like penicillamine is to control symptoms but also to retard or arrest the progression of rheumatoid arthritis. Radiological progression can be measured in a number of ways. The first attempt to grade X-ray changes was the publication of standard grading systems but these are too crude to measure changes over periods of time as short as 1 or 2 years. The most successful method to date has been that of Sharp et al (1971), which was used to show that gold therapy slowed radiological progression (Sigler et al, 1974) and later that penicillamine was more effective than gold (Gibson et al, 1976). Larsen (1981) has devised a simpler system based on an index devised from standard X-rays of a number of joints. His system has not yet been compared with that of Sharp et al (1971) or used to show effects on radiological progression with drugs.

6% of cases where a false-positive result was obtained (Jackson & Abe, 1972). Arthroscopy is a particularly useful tool for the rheumatologist or orthopaedic surgeon in the patient who complains of knee pain in the absence of any abnormality on physical or radiological examination.

Assessment of the extent of synovial or cartilage disease

In chronic diseases such as rheumatoid arthritis where the severity of synovitis has a natural history of great variation, it is often difficult to detect by clinical examination whether the local disease activity is at any one time increasing or decreasing. By arthroscopy it is possible to tell whether a persistently swollen knee joint is swollen as a result of proliferative rheumatoid disease in the synovial membrane or whether the synovitis is relatively mild and the joint is packed with large quantities of intra-articular fibrin. Arthroscopy has an important part to play in assessing the need for surgical synovectomy.

Operative arthroscopy

There is an increasing use amongst orthopaedic surgeons of arthroscopic surgery of the knee. The various procedures performed are operations on menisci — particularly the removal of mobile fragments from a torn meniscus, with normal meniscal tissue being retained — removal of loose bodies and foreign bodies, patellar shaving with a chondrotome and perarthroscopic synovectomy performed with a powered shaver. A survey of 1000 arthroscopic operations (Dandy & O'Carroll, 1982) showed that the indications for operation were internal mechanical derangement in 565 patients, anterior knee pain in 246, disorders of the synovium in 77, ligament injuries in 63 and degenerative joint disease in 49.

Therapeutic benefit and complications

It has been shown (Burman et al, 1934; Jason, 1976) that many patients derive a therapeutic benefit from arthroscopy. The precise reason for this is ill-understood but it is probable that the benefit results from irrigation of the joint and the removal of large quantities of intra-articular fibrin. In a series of patients with rheumatoid arthritis, Sakakibara (1973) showed that 67% of patients noticed an improvement in their symptoms following the procedure. The removal of intra-articular loose bodies from the anterior part of the knee joint with biopsy forceps and the division of intra-articular fibrous bands are simple procedures with obvious clinical benefit. Complications arising from the examination are minimal. Sepsis resulting from arthroscopy is rare; haemarthrosis is also rare though it is not uncommon for patients with a minor inflammatory synovitis to develop a small effusion of the knee 24 hours after the procedure. There is no evidence to suggest that arthroscopy leads to any long-term damage to intra-articular structures and it may therefore be seen to be a valuable technique associated with the most minimal complications.

Arthroscopy as a research tool

Sequential arthroscopic studies in the assessment of systemic and particularly intra-articular therapy has so far little been used, although the potential value of this technique is large. The effect of intra-articular corticosteroids on synovitis has been studied (Robles-Gill, 1973) and improvement has been seen in 80% of cases. One-quarter of these showed complete resolution of inflammatory change. The local effect of radioactive colloids in chronic rheumatoid synovitis has also been studied (Yates, 1973) and again significant changes have been reported in visual and histological appearances. Synovial biopsy material obtained at arthroscopy has been used for immunofluorescent and ultrastructural examination and has also provided specimens for tissue culture research.

TECHNIQUE OF THE EXAMINATION

Arthroscopy of the knee joint may be performed with either local or general anaesthesia. For most rheumatological purposes, local anaesthesia is adequate. If operative procedures are to be performed with the arthroscope or if a thorough examination of the menisci is necessary, then general anaesthesia is required so that a valgus or varus strain may be exerted on the joint. Strict asepsis is required. Arthroscopy is not a procedure to be performed in the outpatient clinic or the hospital ward. An operating theatre or endoscopy suite is required and full sterile precautions with gowned and gloved operators are necessary. The arthroscopic cannulae may be autoclaved though the optical telescopes rapidly deteriorate with repeated autoclaving. These items are commonly sterilised by immersion in 2% aqueous glutaraldehyde (Cidex), though repeated sterilisation does damage light-transmitting fibre bundles and this eventually reduces the intensity and colour temperature of transmitted light.

If the procedure is to be performed under local anaesthesia then it is important that the patient should be calm, relaxed and co-operative. To achieve this a light premedication with intravenous diazepam 10–20 mg is used. The knee is supported in 15–20° of flexion and the skin prepared with an antiseptic solution.

Successful arthroscopy does not require an existing effusion in the joint. Examination may be performed quite adequately if 60–100 ml of normal saline is first injected into the joint space. Where a large effusion is present, instrumentation is made easier, although even in this instance the synovial fluid should be replaced by an equal volume of saline in order to obtain a clear view. It may be necessary for the joint to be flushed several times before the telescope is inserted. After skin preparation, local anaesthetic is injected into the skin and deeply into the joint capsule. Sterile normal saline at room temperature is then injected into the joint space. The trocar and cannula may be inserted into the knee joint medially or laterally and the various positions are shown in Figure 66.3. The most commonly used site for insertion is position C, midway between the head of the fibula and the lower pole of the patella. A small incision (5 mm) is made and with the patient lying horizontal with the knee flexed 20°, the sharp trocar and cannula are advanced with slight pressure through the subcutaneous fat in an upwards and medial direction until the joint capsule is punctured (Fig. 66.4). As soon as the capsule has been punctured the sharp trocar is replaced by a blunt one in order to prevent damage to the articular cartilage and bleeding from the synovial membrane. The trocar is advanced behind the patella so that the tip lies in the medial part of the suprapatellar pouch. The trocar may now be removed and fluid and debris drained from the joint. Surprisingly large quantities of loose fibrin debris may be obtained. The joint is then thoroughly irrigated with saline — either by alternate emptying and refilling of the cavity via the cannula or by the insertion of a separate large-bore needle into the suprapatellar pouch through which saline is introduced. When the effluent saline is clear, the telescope is inserted and the joint examined. If the lateral infrapatellar approach (position C) has been used, approximately 90% of the anterior part of the knee joint may be examined (Fig. 66.5). The suprapatellar pouch is examined fully and changes

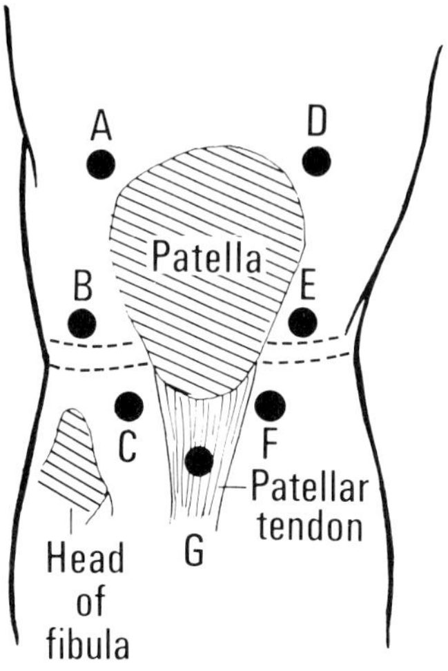

Fig. 66.3 Sites of entry into the knee joint (right). A, Lateral approach via the suprapatellar pouch. B, Lateral mid-patellar approach. C, Lateral infrapatellar approach. D, Medial approach via the suprapatellar pouch. E, Medial mid-patellar approach. F, Medial infrapatellar approach. G, Anterior approach through the patellar tendon.

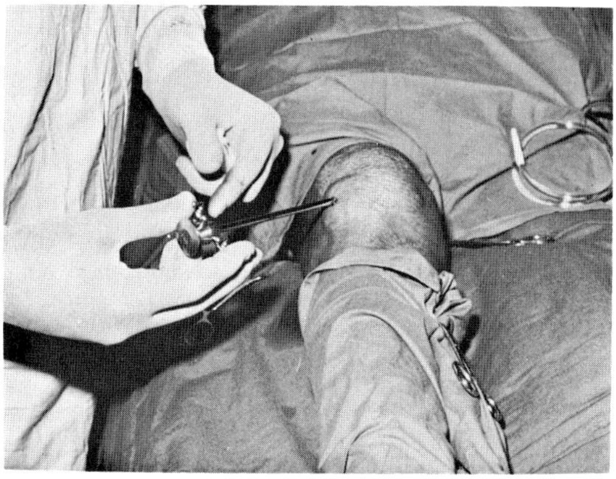

Fig. 66.4 Instrumentation of the right knee by the lateral infrapatellar approach.

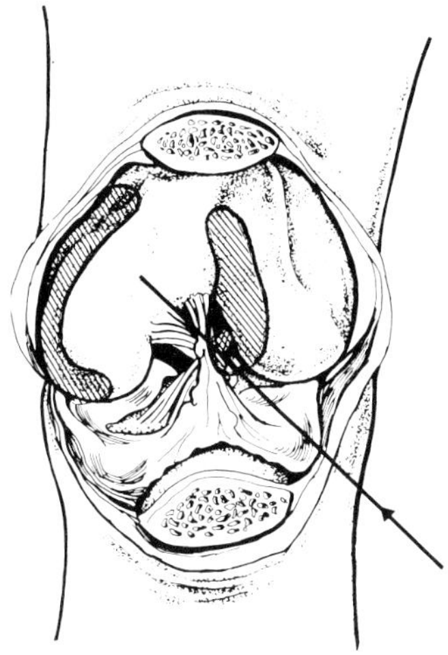

Fig. 66.5 Internal structures of the knee joint visualised by the lateral infrapatellar approach (shaded areas cannot be seen).

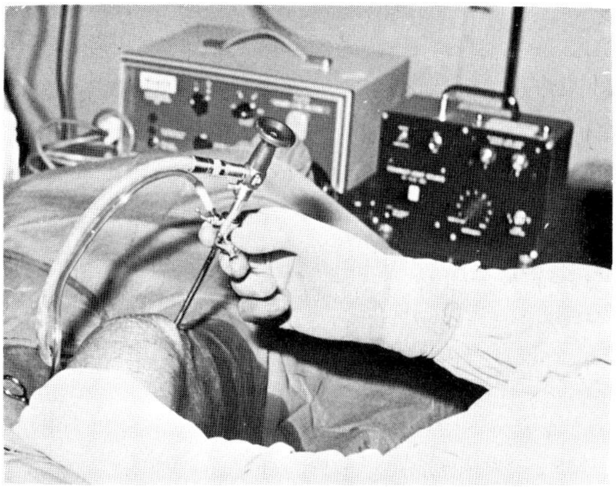

Fig. 66.6 Insertion of the arthroscope in a semi-vertical position for examination of cruciate ligaments and menisci.

are noted. By slowly withdrawing the arthroscope and pivoting the instrument about its point of insertion the medial joint wall may then be examined. The junction of the suprapatellar pouch and the true knee joint is marked by an indentation in the joint capsule, the plica synovialis suprapatellaris (Plate 66.1). This fold does not appear to have any clinical relevance and will be obscured in joints where there is a significant degree of synovial hypertrophy. After the suprapatellar pouch has been examined, the medial joint wall, the medial femoral condyle and the plateau of synovial membrane covering the anterior aspect of the lower end of the femur should be visualised. The arthroscope is then turned 180° about its axis and the back of the patella may clearly be seen. The articular facets of the patella are fully examined if the patella is gently manipulated with the operator's free hand. Normal synovial membrane appears pale pink and through it the fibrous joint capsule is seen (Plate 66.1). Articular cartilage is a pale cream colour and is normally smooth and shiny (Plate 66.1). To examine the medial meniscus and the cruciate ligaments, the arthroscope has to be withdrawn by a further 2–3 cm and pivoted in a semi-vertical position (Fig. 66.6). The patient's knee is then flexed to 90° and the arthroscope carefully advanced under direct vision into the intercondylar notch. The anterior cruciate ligament is now seen (Plate 66.1) fanning out as it passes from femur to tibia. The posterior cruciate ligament is partly obscured by and lies immediately behind the anterior cruciate. In order to see the medial meniscus well it is necessary to apply a valgus strain to widen the medial tibiofemoral space. The lateral margin of the normal medial meniscus (Plate 66.1) appears as a sharp concave edge. The posterior portion of the medial meniscus cannot be seen by anterior approach since the medial femoral condyle intervenes. Furthermore, in patients with a significant proliferative synovitis, examination of the menisci and even the cruciate ligaments is usually obscured by the diseased synovial membrane filling the intercondylar notch. The lateral meniscus may be seen by a lateral infrapatellar approach, although examination of the lateral meniscus is made easier if a medial approach is used.

To complete the inspection, the lateral joint wall and the lateral femoral condyle are visualised. The arthroscope is withdrawn so that the tip of the telescope is only just within the joint space. The telescope is then removed from the cannula and the blunt trocar inserted again. Together these are advanced up the lateral joint space and the telescope reinserted. Examination of the whole of the lateral wall is possible as the arthroscope is slowly withdrawn.

When inspection of the joint is complete, synovial biopsies may be taken under direct vision from specific areas or from a standard site. Since the suprapatellar pouch may often appear normal when gross synovial changes are seen in other areas

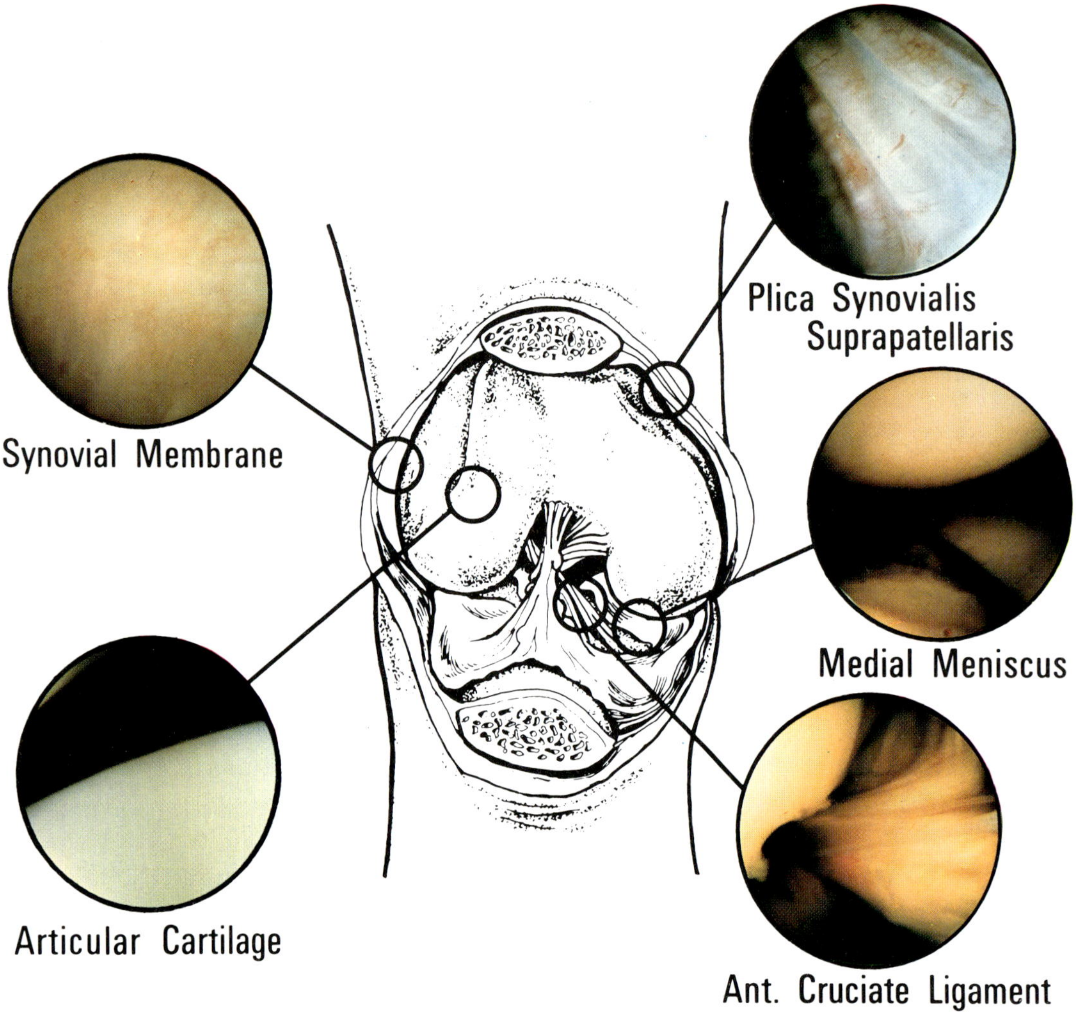

Plate 66.1 Arthroscopic appearances of a normal knee joint.

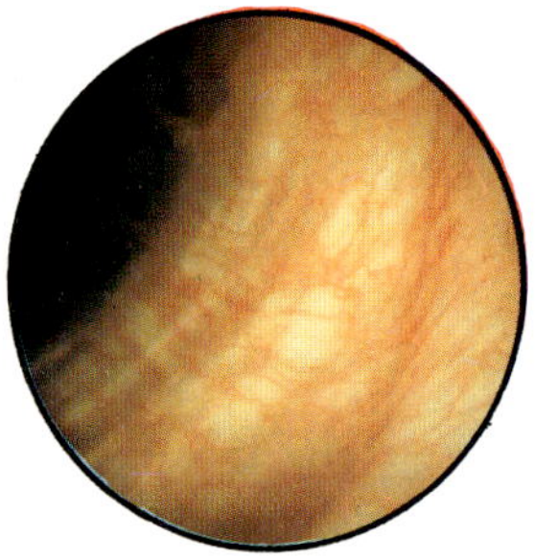

Plate 66.2 Synovial hyperaemia (early rheumatoid synovitis).

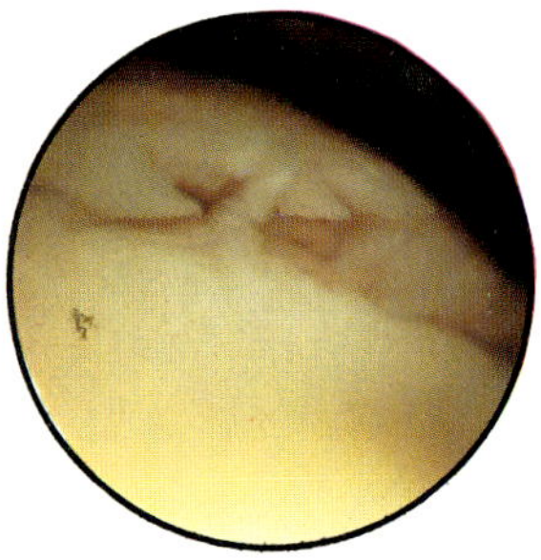

Plate 66.3 Synovial hypertrophy (rheumatoid synovitis) with synovial membrane protruding over the anterior aspect of the medial femoral condyle.

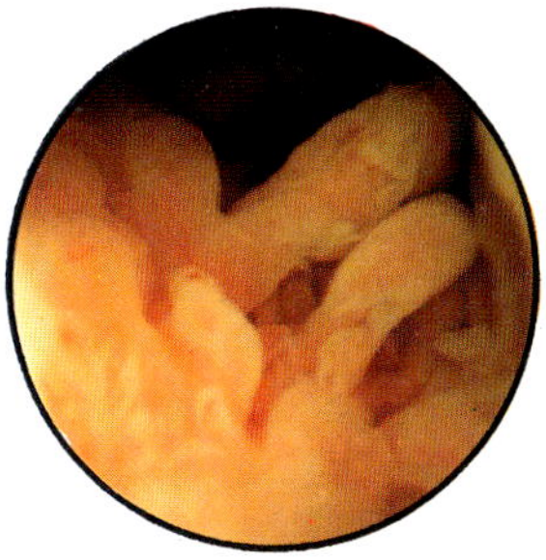

Plate 66.4 Pedunculated 'active' villi of rheumatoid disease.

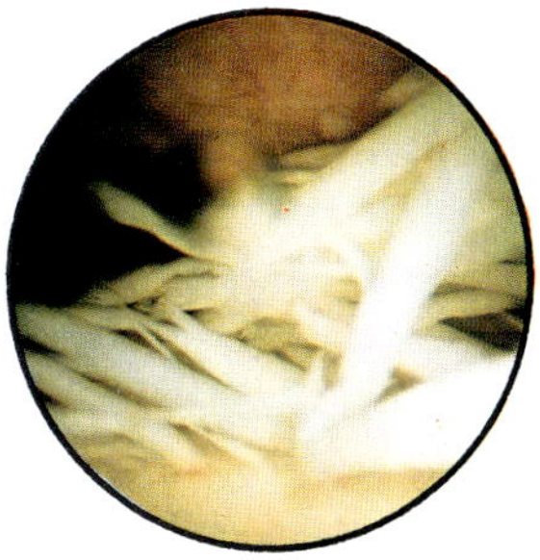

Plate 66.5 Fibrosed villi (late rheumatoid disease).

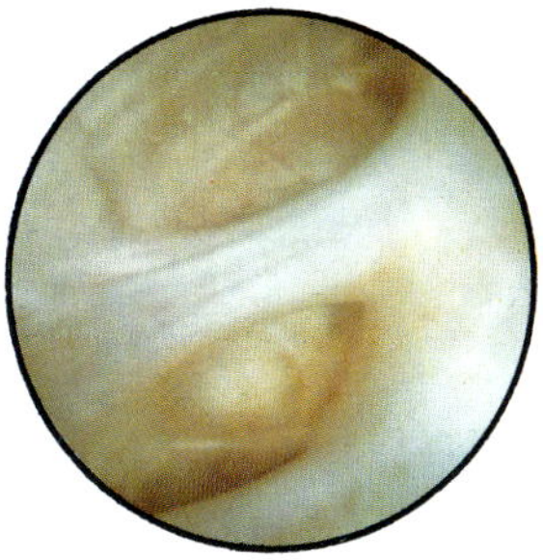

Plate 66.6 Fibrous band adhesion (fibrin bridge) seen high on the lateral knee joint wall in rheumatoid synovitis following yttrium-90 synoviorthesis.

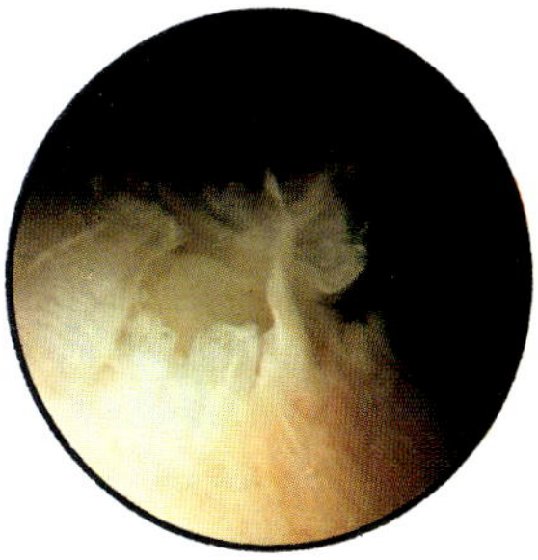

Plate 66.7 Early pannus encroachment onto articular cartilage in rheumatoid synovitis.

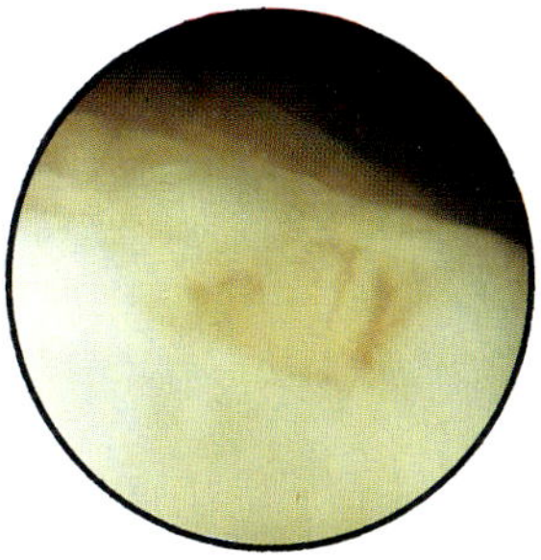

Plate 66.8 Cartilage erosion (centre) containing granulation tissue.

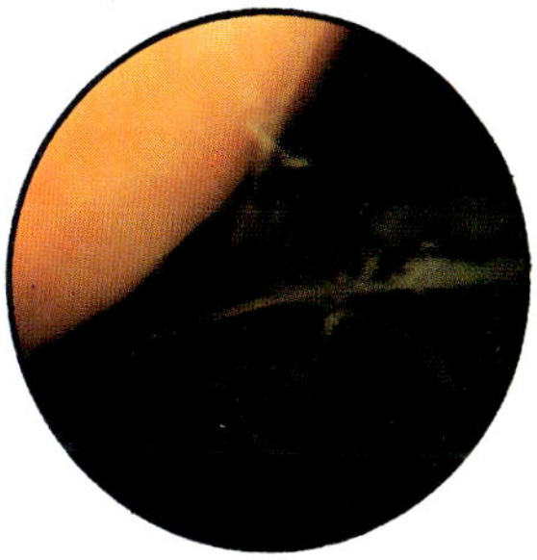

Plate 66.9 Acute non-specific synovitis of Reiter's syndrome with synovial hyperaemia and a fine surface fibrin web.

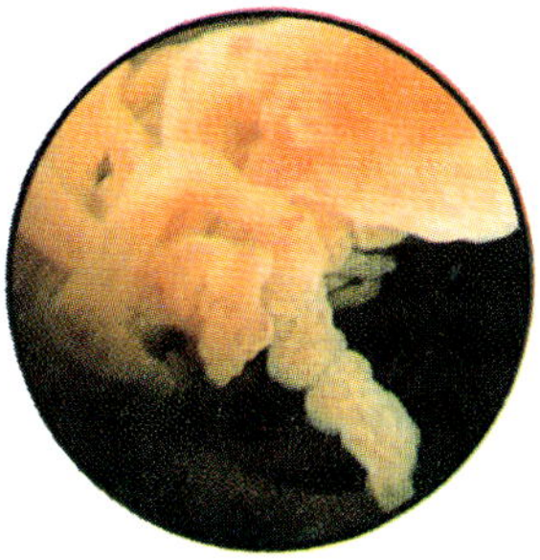

Plate 66.10 Pigmented villonodular synovitis.

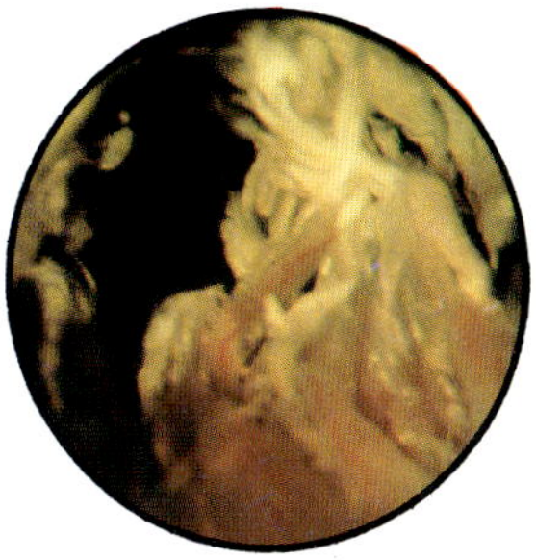

Plate 66.11 Pyrophosphate crystal deposits in the tips of inflammatory synovial villi (chondrocalcinosis).

of the joint, more suitable sites for synovial biopsy are along the medial or lateral joint walls where the disease is usually more pronounced. Photographs may be taken with a single lens reflex camera and to conclude the procedure any remaining saline in the joint space is aspirated, the cannula removed from the knee and the stab incision closed with one stitch.

Whilst arthroscopy of the knee is technically relatively simple and yields a lot of information, that of other joints is a complicated and more difficult procedure. The main reason for this is that other joints are less distensible and there is insufficient room to manoeuvre the arthroscope within the joint. Consequently several approaches are required to inspect a joint adequately, and even then, if there is significant synovitis, articular cartilage is often obscured by inflammatory tissue.

Although a large diameter arthroscope has been used to examine cadaveric shoulder joints (Burman, 1931), smaller 'needle' telescopes are used for patients. These telescopes consist of a single solid rod of special optical glass (Selfoc), around which a layer of fibres transmit light for illumination of the object. A thin metal sheath protects the delicate optical system. As a result of the very small diameter of the instrument, the possible distortion of the image and chromatic aberration are significant factors limiting accuracy of examination. Furthermore, these telescopes are extremely fragile, and arthroscopy of most small joints is more safely performed under general anaesthetic since movement of the joint during the examination may break the instrument inside the patient.

The joints most frequently examined with a needle arthroscope are the elbow, ankle, wrist, metacarpophalangeal joints and the hips, although shoulders, interphalangeal and acromioclavicular joints have also been inspected.

The elbow is placed in a position of 45° flexion, and a needle is inserted through the capsular ligament between the olecranon process of the ulna and the lateral epicondyle of the humerus. Through this needle 10–15 ml of normal saline are injected into the joint cavity and the needle removed. The trocar and cannula may then be inserted into the joint by a posterior approach laterally or medially (Fig. 66.7), the telescope inserted and synovial membrane and part of the articular cartilage examined. Anterior approach to the elbow joint may also be made laterally or medially, but in view of anastomosis of branches of the branchial, ulnar and radial arteries around the anterior aspect of the elbow, a posterior approach is preferable.

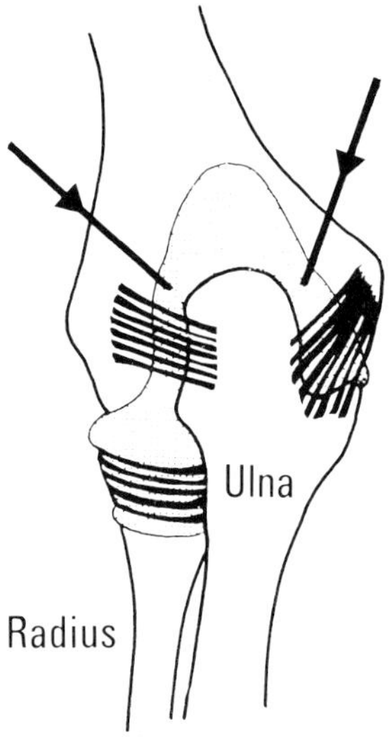

Fig. 66.7 Sites of entry into the posterior aspect of the elbow joint (left).

For the ankle joint, an anteromedial approach is usually employed (Fig. 66.8) and in this way the major part of the anterior tibio-talar articulation is seen. Preliminary distension of the joint with sa-

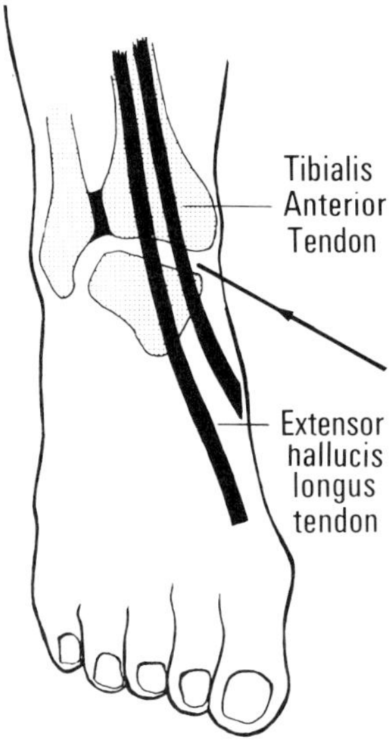

Fig. 66.8 Site of entry into the ankle joint (right).

line makes no appreciable difference in arthroscopy. The arthroscope is inserted between the medial malleolus and the tibiotalar joint line at a point just medial to the tendon of tibialis anterior.

The hip joint is perhaps the most difficult and hazardous joint to arthroscope. It is not possible to introduce the instrument into the acetabulum unless the hip is dislocated. The visible field is limited to the part of the femoral head which lies anteriorly outside the acetabulum and also the junction of the femoral neck with the head. With the patient supine and the hip in extension and internal rotation, an anterior paratrochanteric approach is used. The trocar and cannula are introduced just anterior to the greater trochanter and pointed towards the mid-point of the inguinal ligament. In an adult, the cannula is advanced to a depth of approximately 9 cm before the anterior joint space is punctured, the telescope inserted and part of the joint visualised.

Metacarpophalangeal joints are relatively easy to examine. Traction is applied to the finger and the joint space widened. The trocar and cannula are inserted at a position between the extensor tendon of the finger and the collateral ligament. Saline is injected into the joint through the cannula and the telescope inserted. After inspection, biopsies may be taken through the cannula, although not under direct vision.

ARTHROSCOPIC APPEARANCES IN DISEASE

Physiological variations

Physical factors may influence the macroscopic appearance of synovium. First, by increasing the temperature of the irrigating saline, there is a conspicuous increase in the size of blood vessels (Miki, 1941). The effect is however short-lived since the temperature of the saline equilibrates with that of the synovium within a few minutes, and for practical purposes it is quite satisfactory to use irrigating fluid at room temperature. The effect of increased hydrostatic pressure of the irrigating saline is, however, more important. As pressure rises within the joint, it has been shown that the synovial membrane rapidly blanches. Since intra-articular pressure rises exponentially with the volume of saline injected (Urayama, 1956), a maximum volume of 80 ml of saline should be used for initial distension of the knee joint, and after this a drip set is used with a constant hydrostatic pressure of approximately 30 cm to continue joint irrigation. This system reduces sudden rises in intra-articular pressure if the patient flexes his quadriceps muscles.

Inflammatory synovitis

Just as major variations in histological appearances have been shown to occur in different areas of any one joint (Cruikshank, 1952), so also do major variations in the synovial arthroscopic appearances occur in different areas of an inflamed joint (Robles-Gill, 1973; Yates & Scott, 1975).

There is, however, in rheumatoid synovitis a significant correlation between indices of total synovial disease judged arthroscopically and histologically when synovial biopsies are taken from a standard area on the medial joint wall. The great advantage of arthroscopy in assessing disease activity is therefore that most of the surface synovium may be visualised whereas only a small fraction of the total amount may be examined histologically. The examiner should not only look for individual specific features but also should assess the overall disease activity of the joint and how much of the appearances represent acute or chronic changes.

In rheumatoid arthritis there is a great variability in the appearances of the synovial membrane. In patients with recent onset of disease, there is no gross synovial hypertrophy but the membrane appears hyperaemic. An increased number of vessels which are also dilated are seen in areas of the synovial membrane (Plate 66.2) and a significant pathological feature is that the membrane bleeds easily when touched with the end of the arthroscope. The synovial membrane may also be hypertrophied with vessels no longer clearly seen. The combination of synovial cellular infiltration and oedema, coupled with surface fibrin exudation gives the membrane a dense, evenly coloured appearance like pale pink wax. An indication of the degree of hypertrophy may be obtained by examining the junction of the most anterior part of the femoral condyle (medial or lateral) with the plateau of synovium overlying the lower end of the femur. In the normal joint the articular cartilages seem to be higher than the synovial plateau. When synovial hypertrophy is marked, the synovium is seen above the femoral condyle, and pannus may be seen over part of the articular cartilage (Plate 66.3). In more pronounced cases of synovial hypertrophy the membrane becomes fissured and has the appearance of cobblestones. Further hypertrophy of these cobblestones leads to the development of fat, elongated, pedunculated villi with clubbed ends (Plate 66.4). These villi still have a dense pink/red waxy appearance and correspond with those villi described as characteristic of RA (Palmer, 1967), In histological section they are packed with mononuclear cells and it has been demonstrated (Yates & Scott, 1975) that when present, the intensity of this villous proliferation correlates significantly with the lymphocyte infiltration in the synovium.

Also seen in rheumatoid synovitis are white, avascular villi (Plate 66.5). Occasionally, these fibrous villi form a bridge of fibrin within the joint linking two synovial surfaces. These fibrin bridges may also be seen in the region of the surgical incision in patients who have had a previous surgical arthrotomy and they may be the cause of intermittent localised knee pain. Avascular villi are often found in patients with a clinical remission of inflammatory activity and may represent a stage of tissue repair whereby rheumatoid villi become fibrosed. An intermediate type of villus may be seen; in this case the pink 'active' villus is partly covered with a layer of opaque fibrin. In cases of burnt out RA the only abnormality of the synovium is a smooth layer of opaque fibrin on the synovial surface. No villus proliferation is seen but there is often considerable destruction of the articular cartilage and cruciate ligaments. Similar synovial appearances, together with band-like adhesions (Plate 66.6) have also been seen in knees treated with intra-articular radio-isotopes to obtain a medial synovectomy for chronic inflammatory arthritis.

In any stage of rheumatoid synovitis, a synovial pannus may be seen encroaching on to articular cartilage (Plate 66.7). This in turn leads to bony erosions containing granulation tissue (Plate 66.8) and destruction of articular cartilage.

Loose masses of intra-articular fibrin may be seen in any form of inflammatory synovitis, but particularly in RA owing to its chronicity. These 'rice bodies' are frequently found in the recesses of the suprapatellar pouch, but when present in large quantities may become trapped between the articulating surfaces. It is likely that the removal of these fibrin bodies at arthroscopy accounts for the therapeutic effect of the procedure.

These changes of chronic inflammatory synovitis seen in RA may be differentiated from the more acute changes seen in the arthritides of Reiter's syndrome, ankylosing spondylitis and ulcerative colitis, where the main arthroscopic features are of synovial hyperaemia and formation of a fine opaque web of fibrin on the surface of the membrane. This web (Plate 66.9) is usually less dense and less opaque than the fibrin deposition seen in RA. Villi are often seen arising from the surface of the synovium in these arthritides, but they are thin, almost transparent and blood vessels are conspicuous within them. However, in the few cases of Reiter's syndrome where joint involvement is chronic, and in most cases of psoriatic arthropathy, the villi appear more opaque and histologically they are seen to be oedematous and with moderate cellular infiltration. A useful feature distinguishing these villi from 'active' villi seen in RA is that fine blood vessels may still be seen within the stroma of the former at arthroscopy.

Pigmented villonodular synovitis

This is a rare cause of monarthritis of the knee, though the arthroscopic appearances are particularly characteristic. An evenly blood-stained synovial effusion will alert the arthroscopist to the possibility of pigmented villonodular synovitis. Large villi are seen in the synovial membrane. These have a nodular appearance (Plate 66.10) and areas of brown pigment are seen in these villi. Biopsy reveals the characteristic histological appearance.

Crystal synovitis

The arthroscopic appearances of crystal synovitis are characteristic, and in pyrophosphate arthropathy the synovial changes occur a long time before any radiological signs of intra-articular calcification. Deposits of calcium pyrophosphate are seen not only in the articular cartilage but also in the menisci and in tips of inflammatory villi (Plate 66.11).

In acute gout, similar white urate deposits are also seen in the articular cartilage and in the synovial membrane. In gout however, there is only minimal villus formation, and the deposits tend to occur in smooth synovium over which forms a fine web of fibrin. This reflects the acute nature of the inflammation in a episode of gout.

Degenerative joint disease and internal derangement of the knee

Most of the articular cartilage of a knee joint may easily be examined and abnormalities such as fissuring, pitting or flaking of cartilage and osteophyte formation identified. When the patellofemoral joint is visualised, the free hand may be used to tilt the patella in all directions thus enabling the majority, if not all, of the surface of the patella to be seen.

Tears of the menisci are not always seen directly, due to the femoral condyles obstructing part of each meniscus. If, however, the joint space is widened by applying a valgus or varus strain and manual pressure applied to the peripheral edge of the meniscus, examination is more thorough. Presumptive evidence of meniscus damage may nevertheless be drawn from seeing an irregular, buckled internal margin of the meniscus.

Partial or complete rupture of an anterior cruciate ligament may be detected without difficulty. Small longitudinal tears in the anterior cruciate ligament are occasionally seen but do not appear to be of any clinical significance.

ARTHROGRAPHY

Injection of a contrast medium gives another convenient method of examining radiologically the internal anatomy of synovial joints, bursal sacs and cystic swellings which communicate with joints. Radio-opaque contrast medium is most commonly used, although gas alone, xeroradiography (Raman et al, 1982), or a combination of radio-opaque medium and gas (double contrast arthrography) may be injected. The procedure is most commonly performed on knee, shoulder, hip and wrist joints (Bryan, 1974) and standard injection techniques are used.

Single contrast arthrography of the knee demonstrates well a rupture of the joint capsule and Baker's cysts (Taylor, 1969). Herniation of the joint capsule occurs almost invariably in a posterior direction and is most commonly secondary to chronic inflammatory synovitis of rheumatoid disease. A popliteal cyst may extend upwards into the thigh (Fig. 66.9) or, more often, downwards into the calf (Fig. 66.10). Arthrography has been

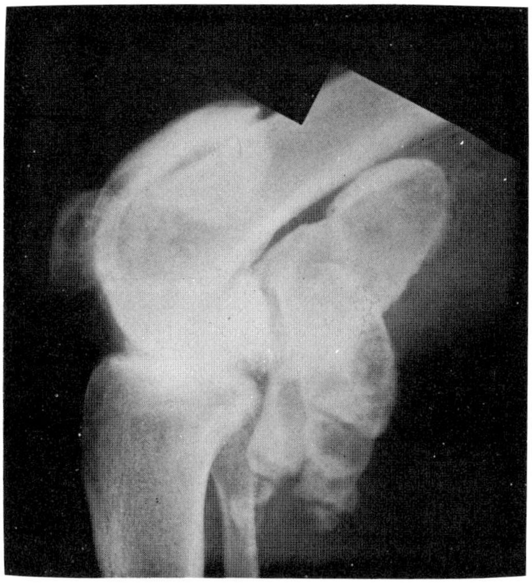

Fig. 66.9 Arthrograph of a multiloculated popliteal cyst extending into the thigh.

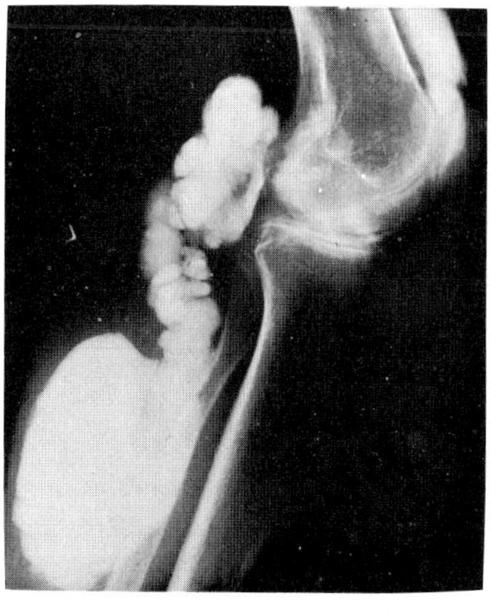

Fig. 66.10 Arthrograph of a large calf cyst communicating with the knee joint. (Reproduced by kind permission of Hall & Scott, 1966.)

shown (Hall & Scott, 1966) to be the most accurate means of determining the full extent of calf cysts which may otherwise be difficult to detect clinically.

Double contrast arthrography of the knee has been shown to be of great value in radiological assessment of the menisci, the articular cartilages, and internal ligaments (Butt & McIntyre, 1969). In this procedure, synovial fluid is aspirated and the knee joint is injected with 80–100 cc of gas (25% air, 75% carbon dioxide) through a serum needle. 5 ml of radio-opaque contrast medium are then injected and the needle withdrawn. After injection, the knee is exercised with weight-bearing and knee flexion. X-ray films may then be taken. In experienced hands, great accuracy may be obtained in the correct diagnosis of meniscus and ligamentous lesions by this method (Thijn, 1979).

Arthrography of the hip joint is of the greatest value in children for the further investigation of congenital dislocation and Perthes' disease. General anaesthetic is required, and since the procedure also demands strict asepsis, the technique is usually performed in an operating theatre. Anterior paratrochanteric approach is most appropriate, and a small lumbar puncture needle may be used to puncture the anterior part of the joint capsule under fluoroscopy and radio-opaque medium injected.

The non-invasive technique of ultrasonic examination of soft tissues has been described and in the diagnosis of popliteal cysts (Fig. 66.11) is shown to be as useful as contrast arthrography. It is probable that continued technical developments in radiology such as CT scanning and NMR scanning will reduce the need for invasive procedures for joint examination.

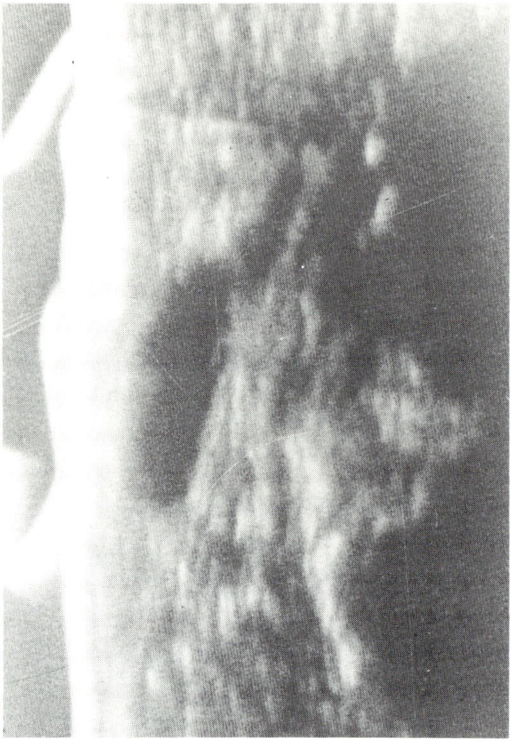

Fig. 66.11 Ultrasound scan of a popliteal cyst. The scan has been taken behind the knee joint and the popliteal cyst is shown as the black elliptical shadow in the centre of the picture with a thin communicating channel coming from the back of the knee joint on the right.

SYNOVIAL BIOPSY

For many years before the introduction of antibiotics, synovial biopsy was considered a dangerous procedure. It is now recognised to be a simple procedure which produces information which may be of great clinical significance. It is obviously a procedure which is reserved for the diagnostic problem rather than for the patient with a straightforward disease. Not only is the histopathological picture important, but synovial biopsy obtains material for immunofluorescence analysis and may be the only means of identifying the organism in patients with a septic arthritis.

Several methods of obtaining a synovial biopsy are possible. In the knee joint, arthroscopy enables a biopsy to be obtained under direct vision. If arthroscopy is not available, a needle biopsy technique may be used. The first punch biopsy needle to be widely used for obtaining synovial tissue was described by Polley & Bickel (1951). This instrument, 5 mm in diameter, was mainly used for biopsies in the knee. Owing to its size, it is impractical for use in other joints. As with arthroscopy, it is preferable to perform the procedure in an operating theatre or purpose-built procedures room. The needle is inserted into the suprapatellar pouch after local analgesia and the formation of a small effusion by the injection of sterile normal saline.

External pressure is applied with a finger to

push the synovium into the hooked lip at the end of the biopsy needle which is then pulled backwards a few centimetres to obtain synovial tissue.

It is important to differentiate between synovial tissue (usually firm and pink) and loose intra-articular debris and fibrin which is thin, soft and white or cream in colour. The biopsy should be repeated until adequate synovial tissue has been obtained.

It is surprising how rarely a haemarthrosis is produced. When the biopsy has been obtained, the needle is withdrawn from the joint space and any remaining fluid aspirated.

A simplified synovial biopsy needle (Parker & Pearson, 1963) was subsequently developed and this needle, being considerably smaller in diameter, has been used extensively for obtaining tissue from the knee, ankle, elbow and wrist joints and from synovial sacs and bursae (Schumacher & Kulka, 1972). The technique of the procedure is similar to that described by Polley & Bickel (1951).

The interpretation of the synovial biopsy may often be difficult for the pathologist. Unusual diseases involving the synovial membrane (amyloidosis, sarcoidosis, tuberculosis, pigmented villonodular synovitis, multicentric retriculohistiocytosis or Whipple's disease) may prove easy diagnoses for the pathologist, whereas common diseases such as osteoarthritis and rheumatoid arthritis may prove difficult to differentiate or to assess the activity of disease. It is well recognised that not only may macroscopic appearances vary from site to site within a joint, but there may also be major variations in histopathological changes in the synovial membrane (Cruikshank, 1952). The histological features may be assessed using the ARA criteria of changes consistent with rheumatoid arthritis. Three or more of the following should be present: marked villous hypertrophy; proliferation of superficial synovial cells often with palisading (Fig. 66.12); marked infiltration of chronic inflammatory cells (lymphocytes or plasma cells predominating) with tendency to form 'lymphoid nodules' (Fig. 66.13); deposition of compact fibrin either on the surface or interstitially; foci of necrosis. Occasionally, multinucleate giant cells may be seen in the rheumatoid synovial membrane (Fig. 66.14).

Although the histopathology may be consistent with RA, there is no single pathological feature which is characteristic, and intense proliferative synovitis may also be seen in osteoarthritis. From a clinical viewpoint, it may often be more valuable

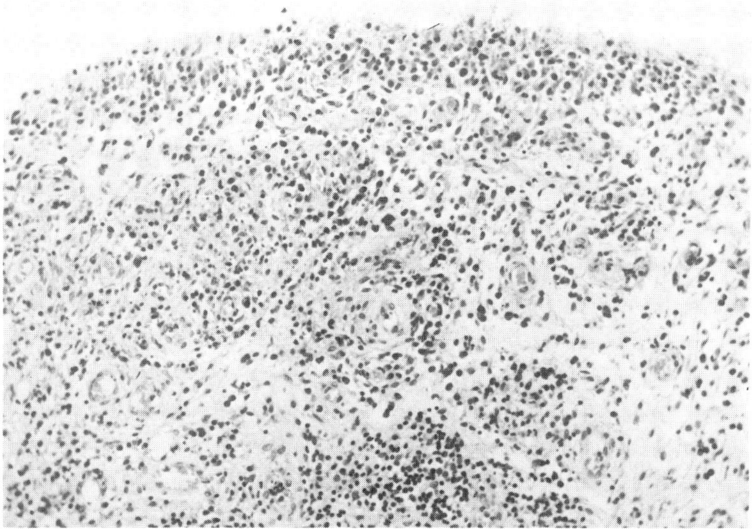

Fig. 66.12 Rheumatoid synovitis × 160. There is palisading of the surface layer of synovium (top). Dark-staining small lymphocytes and plasma cells are seen in groups around the subsynovial blood vessels.

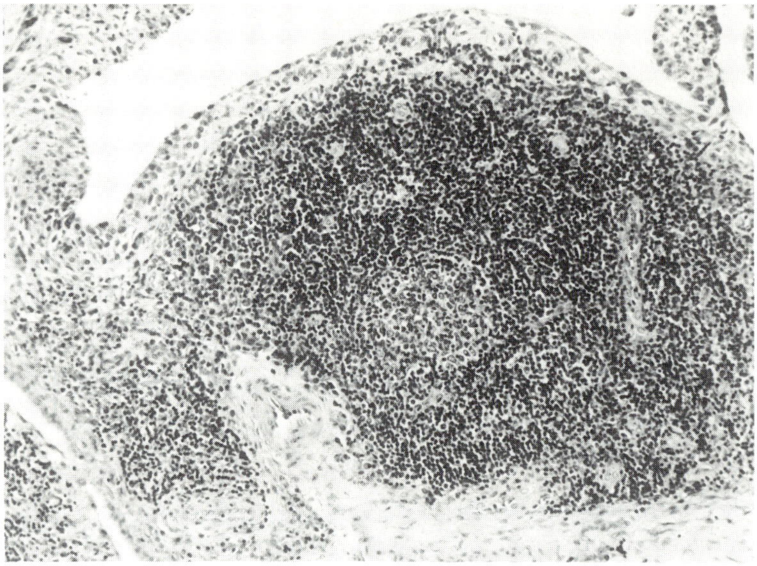

Fig. 66.13 Rheumatoid synovitis × 110. There is a marked infiltrate of lymphocytes and plasma cells with 'lymphoid follicle' formation.

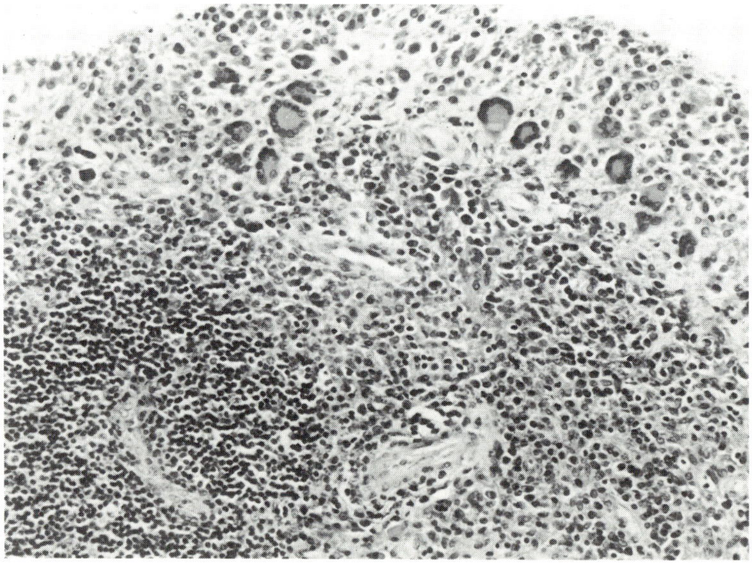

Fig. 66.14 Rheumatoid synovitis × 160. Many multinucleate giant cells are seen between the palisading lining layer (top) and the perivascular aggregates and plasma cells (bottom).

to assess the biopsy for the dominant phase of the four phases of synovitis categorised by Britton et al (1970). These phases are as follows:

1. *Exudative*. Synovial congestion of vessels and oedema with some exudation of neutrophilic leucocytes and fibrin deposition.
2. *Infiltrative and proliferative*. Infiltration by lymphocytes, plasma cells, and histiocytes, proliferation of fibroblasts, synovial cell hy-

perplasia, and conspicuous capillaries.

3. *Necrotic*. Areas of necrosis of lining cells and also in subsynovial connective tissue together with some fibrin deposition.
4. *Fibrotic*. Predominant fibrosis without mononuclear cell infiltration or necrosis.

The histopathological features of the synovitis of ankylosing spondylitis, Reiter's disease and ulcerative colitis are again similar to those of RA, although the inflammatory changes tend to be less marked and proliferation of the synovial lining layer is minimal.

REFERENCES

Alm A, Gillquist J, Liljedahl S-0 1974 The diagnostic value of arthroscopy of the knee joint. Injury 5:319

Bircher E 1922 Beitrog zur Pathologie (Arthritis deformans) und Diagnose der Meniscusverletzungen (Arthroendoskopie). Bruns Beiträge zur Klinischen Chirurgie 127:239

Britton M C, Ruddy S, Corson J M, Sosman J L, Schur P H, Austen K F 1970 The complenent system in rheumatoid synovitis. Immune reactions and experimental models in rheumatic diseases. In: Gordon D (ed) Proceediings of the 4th Canadian Conference on Research in the Rheumatic Diseases, Toronto. p. 40

Bryan G L 1974 Arthrography. In: Diagnostic radiology, 2 Edn. Churchill Livingstone, Edinburgh, p. 327

Burman M S 1931 Arthroscopy or the direct visualisation of joints; an experimental cadaver study. Journal of Bone and Joint Surgery 13:669

Burman M S, Finkelstein H, Mayer L 1934 Arthroscopy of the knee joint. Journal of Bone and Joint Surgery 16:255

Butt W P, McIntyre J L 1969 Double contrast arthrography of the knee. Radiology 92:487

Casscells S W 1971 Arthroscopy of the knee joint — A review of 150 cases. Journal of Bone and Joint Surgery 53A:287

Cruikshank B 1952 Interpretation of multiple biopsies of synovial tissue in rheumatic diseases. Annals of the Rheumatic Diseases 11:137

Dandy D J, O'Carroll P F 1982 Arthroscopic surgery of the knee. British Medical Journal 285: 1256–1258

Edgar M A, Louy M 1973 Arthroscopy of the knee: A preliminary review of fifty cases. Proceedings of the Royal Society of Medicine 66:512

Fletcher M R, Scott J T 1975 Chronic monarticular synovitis; Diagnostic and prognostic features. Annals of the Rheumatic Disease 34:171

Hall A P, Scott J T 1966 Synovial cysts and rupture of the knee joint in rheumatoid arthritis: An arthrographic study. Annals of the Rheumatic Diseases 25:32

Hench P S 1954 In discussion at American Rheumatism Association meeting. Annals of the Rheumatic Diseases 13:353

Hopkins H, Kapany N S 1954 A flexible fibrescope, using static scanning. Nature 173:39

Jackson R W, Abe I 1972 The role of arthroscopy in the management of disorders of the knee. Journal of Bone and Joint Surgery 54B:310

Jayson M I V 1976 Arthroscopy. Clinics in Rheumatic Diseases 2: 77–91

Jayson M I V, Henderson D R F 1973 Arthroscopy in the diagnosis of inflammatory joint disease. Rheumatology and Rehabilitation 12:195

Meire H, Lindsay D J, Swinson D R, Hamilton E B D 1974 Comparison of ultrasound and positive contrast arthrography in the diagnosis of popliteal and calf swellings. Annals of the Rheumatic Diseases 33:221

Miki M 1941 Influences of the temperature and pressure of the medium on the arthroscopic findings of the blood vessels of the synovial membrane. Journal of the Japanese Orthopaedic Association 16:405

Palmer D G 1967 Synovial villi: an examination of these structures within the anterior compartment of the knee and metacarpophalangeal joints. Arthritis and Rheumatism 10:451

Parker R H, Pearson C M 1963 A simplified synovial biopsy needle. Arthritis and Rheumatism 6:172

Polley H F, Bickel W H 1951 Punch biopsy of synovial membrane. Annals of the Rheumatic Diseases 10:277

Raman D, Haslock I, Newton D R L 1982 Air arthrography with xeroradiography. Hospital Update 8: 1323–1327

Robles-Gil J 1973 Arthroscopy: a procedure to research (monograph)

Sakakibara J 1973 Therapeutic value of arthroscopy in the treatment of rheumatoid arthritis. Excerpta Medica International Congress Series No 299:41

Schumacher H R, Kulka J P 1972 Needle biopsy of the synovial membrane — experience with the Parker-Pearson technic. New England Journal of Medicine 286:416

Taylor A R 1969 Arthrography of the knee in rheumatoid arthritis. British Journal of Radiology 42:493

Thijn C J P 1979 Arthrography of the knee joint. Springer Verlag, Berlin

Urayma H 1956 A study on the intra-articular pressure. Journal of the Japanese Orthopaedic Association 30:213

Watnabe M, Takeda S, Ikeuchi H 1969 History of arthroscopy. In: Atlas of arthroscopy, 2nd Edn. Springer Verlag, Berlin

Yates D B 1973 Arthroscopy of the knee after the injection of 90Y. Annals of the Rheumatic Diseases 32 (Suppl):48

Yates D B, Scott J T 1975 Rheumatoid synovitis and joint disease: relationship between arthroscopic and histological changes. Annals of the Rheumatic Diseases 34:1

Injection techniques

The local use of steroids has to a large extent revolutionised the treatment of many soft tissue lesions, and has also proved to be a useful adjunct to the physician's overall management of the inflammatory arthritides, particularly rheumatoid arthritis. It needs to be stressed, however, that in the latter case local steroid injection is not a treatment in itself, for at the best the effect is usually no more than a temporary palliation of symptoms.

INDICATIONS AND CONTRAINDICATIONS

Local steroid injection is indicated if there is clinical evidence of inflammation, i.e. warmth, tenderness and swelling. Apart from the main indication of the active rheumatoid joint, or more rarely in other forms of inflammatory arthritis, such injections are sometimes indicated in painful conditions following trauma, or more occasionally in an acute phase of osteoarthrosis.

Before considering the local use of steroids, it is vital that any suspicion of infection should be excluded. In addition it must be borne in mind that injections repeated with undue frequency have been reported to accelerate destructive changes in weight-bearing joints. Thus Chandler & Wright (1958) noted that 13 out of 25 knees showed significant radiological deterioration after observation for only 2 months, and Chandler et al (1959) later reported a Charcot-type arthropathy after steroid injection into a hip joint. However, Hollander (1970) considers such events to be rare, but stressed that careful radiological supervision should be practised. McCarty & Hogan (1964) have shown that there is a migration of leucocytes into a joint following local steroid injection and suggest that this may be a factor in increasing cartilage destruction. If such a deterioration of joints does indeed occur, another factor may be tendency of the patient to overuse the joint during periods of freedom from pain following injection. This may be particularly so in those suffering from rheumatoid arthritis since the measure of relief obtained is often so great that further injections tend to be demanded by the patient before a suitable interval has elapsed.

Needless to say, absolute sterility of apparatus is essential, particularly with intrasynovial injections. Nevertheless the incidence of infection following this procedure would seem from experience to be extremely low, and the technique does not deserve the censure it has received from some quarters.

The exact mode of action of locally injected steroids is unknown, although it would appear that the primary action is to suppress the local inflammatory process, whether this be in soft tissues or due to synovitis. In the latter case it is known that the synovial cells take up a proportion of the injected material, which may continue to be present therein for as long as 2 weeks. Some absorption into the general circulation does occur, particularly after large doses, but it is probable that this is not significant as regards the production of systemic side-effects. Thus the presence of intercurrent disease such as diabetes mellitus, which might well be influenced by the use of systemic steroids, is not usually a contraindication to their local use.

MATERIALS

Not only hydrocortisone acetate but many of its analogues are recommended for local injection. In selecting the preparation to be used, consideration must be given to: (1) the bulk of material to be injected, and (2) the probable duration of action. In general it may be said that hydrocortisone acetate (HCA) is cheap, effective and proven by many years of experience. Its analogues do not seem to have a proportionately powerful effect when injected locally as they do when used orally, and they are in the main very much more expensive. However, there seems to be good evidence that some of them have the advantage of producing a more prolonged action, although this is usually outweighed by their much increased cost. Among preparations available are hydrocortisone t-butyl acetate, prednisolone t-butyl acetate, methylprednisolone, dexamethasone t-butyl acetate and triamcinolone hexacetonide, .but for routine use HCA is recommended.

Prior to the injection of the steroid, the use of a local anaesthetic is a matter of personal choice. The advantages are an increase of comfort for the patient, while for the operator anaesthetisation of the tissues allows some probing with the needle should a joint cavity be difficult to enter. In addition, in soft tissue lesions the disappearance of local tenderness or increase of function following injection of the anaesthetic may act as a useful guide as to the accuracy of the injection of steroid which is to follow. If a local anaesthetic is used, 1% lignocaine hydrochloride can be recommended, since it is rapidly acting, and in the small doses required, relatively non-toxic.

Presterilised syringes and needles of the disposable type should be used, and thorough skin cleansing practised.

THE SHOULDER

Apart from involvement of the shoulder joint itself in a generalised arthritis, there are some extra-articular lesions which usually respond well to local injection.

Supraspinatus tendinitis

Lesions of the rotator cuff are common in the middle and older age-groups and most frequently affect the supraspinatus tendon. The subacromial bursa is in such close anatomical relationship to the supraspinatus tendon that clinical distinction between tendinitis and bursitis may be impossible; indeed inflammation of one often leads to involvement of the other. It is therefore convenient, and often more effective, if both are injected with a single technique. In obese or very muscular patients it may be necessary to use a long needle, such as a size No. VI serum. The patient should sit with the affected arm hanging loosely to the side. The gap between the humeral head below and the arch of the acromion above is found by palpation at the most lateral point of the shoulder, and the skin marked. The syringe is filled with 1% lignocaine and the needle inserted at the skin mark. The point is then advanced inwards and slightly backwards along the line of the supraspinous fossa, injecting a little local anaesthetic on the way (Fig. 67.1). Resistance will be felt as the point of the needle first enters the substance of the supraspinatus tendon, having passed through the subacromial bursa which lies immediately above the tendon. Having injected more local anaesthetic, it may now be useful to withdraw the needle, and after a suitable interval to re-examine the patient, since an accurately placed injection should now have abolished the typical painful arc of elevation. The syringe is then recharged with 50 mg HCA and the injection repeated as before. Some patients experience pain for a few hours after this injection. Occasionally a second injection may be required for complete control of symptoms.

Bicipital tendinitis

This is less common than supraspinatus tendinitis,

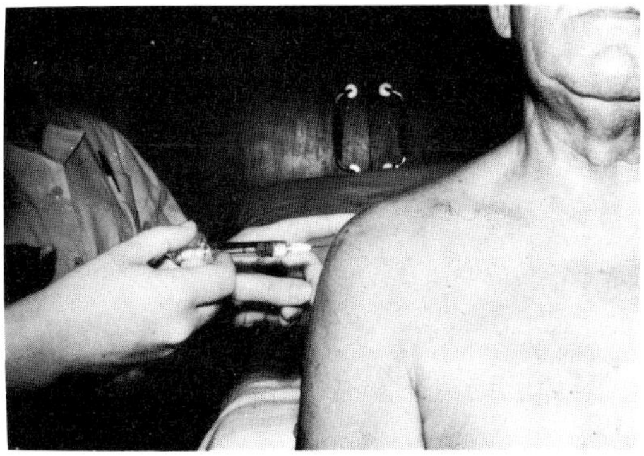

Fig. 67.1 Injection of the supraspinatus tendon. The needle is pointed slightly backwards along the line of the supraspinous fossa.

and is often overlooked as a cause of shoulder pain. The long head of biceps is invested in a synovial sheath, and the condition is therefore one of tenosynovitis. Tenderness is maximal at the bicipital groove in the humeral head. This groove is more readily palpable and the injection more easily given if the arm is held in external rotation. The skin is marked at the point of maximum tenderness. A No. 12 (23G × 13/16 inch) needle is usually adequate and is inserted just below the skin mark. The needle is then directed upwards into the bicipital groove, injecting local anesthetic as the point advances. When the needle enters the substance of the tendon, resistance to injection increases sharply; the point should then be slightly withdrawn until this resistance diminishes, when the needle should be in the synovial sheath. The needle should be left in situ and the syringe recharged with 50 mg HCA, which is then injected. Afterwards pain is less common than with supraspinatus tendinitis (Fig. 67.2).

The acromioclavicular joint

This joint is sometimes affected by trauma, or may be the seat of degenerative change. It is readily accessible to injection since it lies directly beneath the skin. The joint space is small, and a No. 20 (25G × 5/8 inch) needle is normally adequate. The joint space between the outer end of the clavicle and the acromion is usually easily palpable, particularly if the patient is asked to hunch the shoulder up and down. After the skin has been marked, the needle may be directed immediately downwards into the joint cavity. Because the joint cavity itself is small, it is usually not possible to inject more than 12.5 mg of HCA.

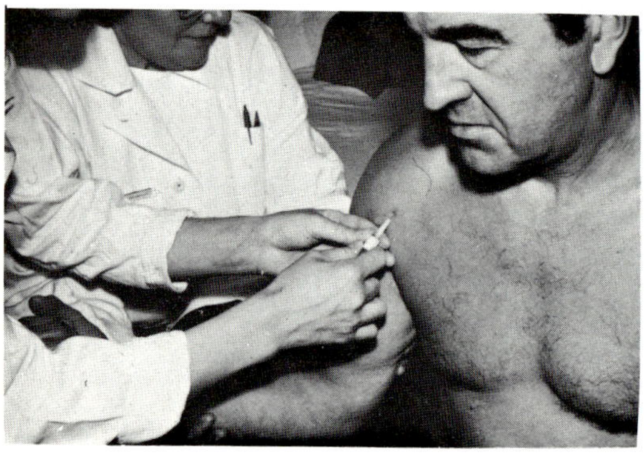

Fig. 67.2 Injection of the tendon of the long head of the biceps.

The shoulder joint

The main indication for injection of this joint is involvement by rheumatoid arthritis; less commonly it may be required in traumatic lesions or osteoarthrosis. Whatever the cause, in the age-group in which injection of the shoulder is required, tears in the rotator cuff have usually occurred, so that the joint cavity communicates directly with the subdeltoid bursa. For this reason the lateral approach is to be preferred, as both may be injected by a single technique.

The positioning of the patient and the skin marking are as for injection of the supraspinatus tendon. A No. VI serum needle is inserted just below the most lateral part of the acromial arch and directed at right angles to the skin with a slight anterior bias. The needle will then pass through the substance of the supraspinatus tendon on its way into the joint cavity, the latter being reached with the needle is almost at full depth. The shoulder joint may also be approached anteriorly at a point just medial to the head of the humerus and 2 cm below the tip of the coracoid process, the needle being directed slightly medially. This approach is useful if a large effusion is present within the joint.

THE ELBOW

The most common lesion at the elbow requiring local injection is the so-called ‘tennis elbow’, less frequently the ‘golfer’s elbow’, and occasionally the elbow joint itself when involved in an inflammatory arthritis.

Tennis elbow

This is a common and disabling lesion which usually responds well to local infiltration with HCA. The most tender point at the external humeral epicondyle is the site of election for the injection. This is found by palpation, and the skin marked. A No. 12 (23G × 3/16 inch) needle is adequate. Although local anaesthetic is not essential, it makes for a more comfortable injection. The needle is inserted at right angles to the skin at the mark, and lignocaine injected as the needle is ad-

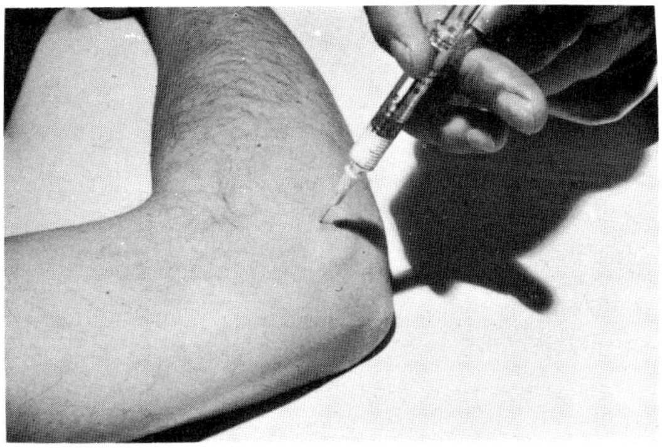

Fig. 67.3 Tennis elbow. The point of the needle should ultimately rest on the periosteum of the external humeral epicondyle.

vanced (Fig. 67.3). For the success of the injection, it appears necessary that the needle point should eventually rest on the periosteum of the humeral epicondyle. 25 mg of HCA is usually sufficient, and considerable resistance is often encountered to the injection owing to the tough fibrous nature of tissues at the common extensor origin. After-pain is common for about 12–24 hours, and the patient should be warned that this may occur.

Golfer's elbow

This condition exactly mirrors tennis elbow, but occurs at the medial humeral epicondyle. The technique of injection is precisely the same as for tennis elbow (Fig. 67.4). The proximity of the ulnar nerve in the humeral groove should be borne in mind.

The elbow joint

Once again, rheumatoid arthritis is the usual indication for injection of this joint. The patient sits with the elbow resting on a table and flexed to 90°, and with the forearm in pronation. A No. 12 (23G × 13/16 inch) needle is adequate. The point of entry is the gap between the lower end of the lateral humeral epicondyle, the head of the radius, and the olecranon. The needle should be directed slightly downwards towards the hand when the joint space will be entered. 50 mg of HCA is an adequate dose (Fig. 67.5).

THE WRIST

Apart from the troublesome tendon lesions which occur around the region of the wrist, compression of the median nerve in the carpal tunnel is common, and may be symptomatic of other conditions, including rheumatoid arthritis, myxoedema, or pregnancy.

The carpal tunnel syndrome

Whatever the cause, prompt and complete relief of symptoms usually follows local steroid injection in this condition. Unfortunately, however, more than 50% of patients suffer a relapse of symptoms after an interval of 1–6 months, and in such cases operative decompression is to be preferred. A No. 20 (25G × 5/8 inch) needle should be used. The patient sits facing the operator with the affected hand resting palm upwards on the table. The patient is then asked to flex the wrist against resist-

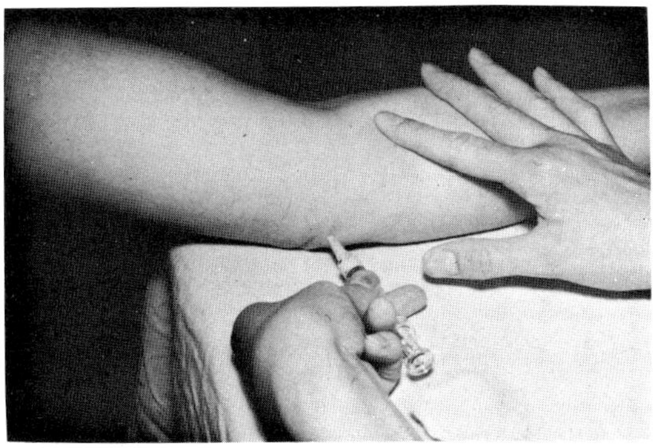

Fig. 67.4 Injection over the medial humeral epicondyle for 'golfer's elbow'.

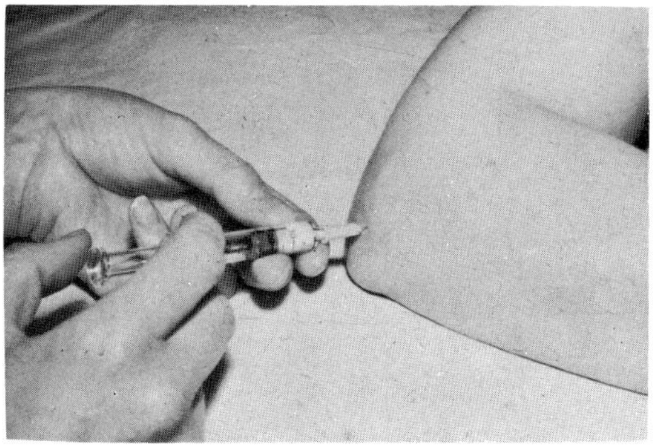

Fig. 67.5 Injection of the elbow joint, the needle entering the gap between the lateral humeral epicondyle, the head of the radius and the olecranon.

ance; if a palmaris longus tendon is present, this is easily seen and palpated. A skin mark is then made just to the radial side of this tendon at the distal crease of the wrist. This is the site of election for the injection. If no palmaris longus is present, the gap between the tendons of flexor digitorum sublimis and flexor carpi radialis is identified. The skin is then marked where the distal crease of the wrist crosses this gap. Numerous small surface veins are usually present around this area, and care should be taken to avoid them.

Local anaesthetic should not be used for this injection, owing to the unpleasant numbness of the median fingers which follows. 1 ml (25 mg) of HCA is used, and the needle inserted at the skin mark at an angle of 45° pointing towards the fingertips. The needle needs to be inserted nearly to its hilt when the tip should be within the carpal tunnel (Fig. 67.6).

Complications of this injection are very rare, and the response rate, albeit sometimes only temporary, is so high that failure should lead to a critical review of the diagnosis.

Tenosynovitis

The wrist is a common site for this condition, usually affecting the tendon and sheath of abductor pollicis longus or extensor pollicis brevis at the radial styloid process. These tendons are easily seen and palpated when the thumb is abducted against resistance. The most tender point of the tendon is located, and this point, and the line of the tendon, marked on the skin. A No. 20 (25G × 5/8 inch) needle should be used. The syringe is loaded with lignocaine, and the needle inserted obliquely along the line of the tendon at the point just distal to the point of maximum tenderness. The operator then places a finger on the tendon proximal to the site of skin puncture. The needle is advanced while the local anaesthetic is slowly injected. When the point of the needle is in the sheath of the tendon, the injected fluid will blow up the sheath; this can be seen and also easily felt by the palpating finger. The needle is then carefully left in situ, while the syringe is recharged with 25 mg of HCA, and the injection completed. A high success rate is usual (Fig. 67.7).

The wrist joint

It is perhaps because this is a complex of many small articulations that injection of this joint does not have the high success rate of simpler articulations such as the knee. The joint may be approached from the dorsal aspect, or from the ulnar side, and in general the latter is usually easier. A No. 12 (23G × 13/16 inch) needle is recommended. The patient's forearm and hand are rested on the table in pronation, with the hand held in ulnar deviation. The lower end of the ulnar styloid process is palpated, and the needle inserted just distal to this. The needle is advanced at right angles to the skin, and sudden loss of resistance to injection indicates penetration of the joint (Fig. 67.8).

THE HAND

Local injection of steroid is occasionally called for in rheumatoid arthritis affecting the metacarpo-

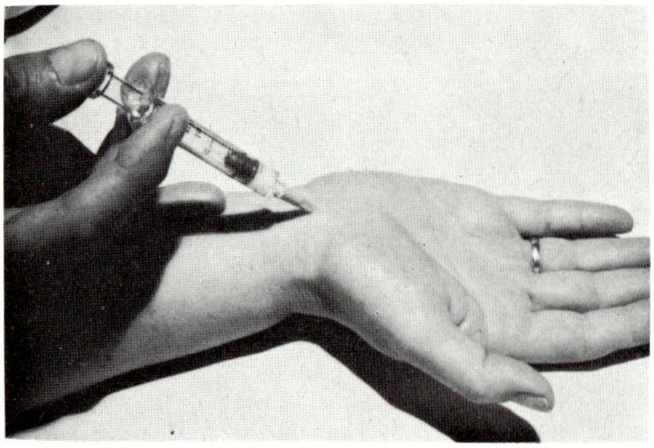

Fig. 67.6 The carpal tunnel. The needle is angled forwards at 45° towards the fingertips.

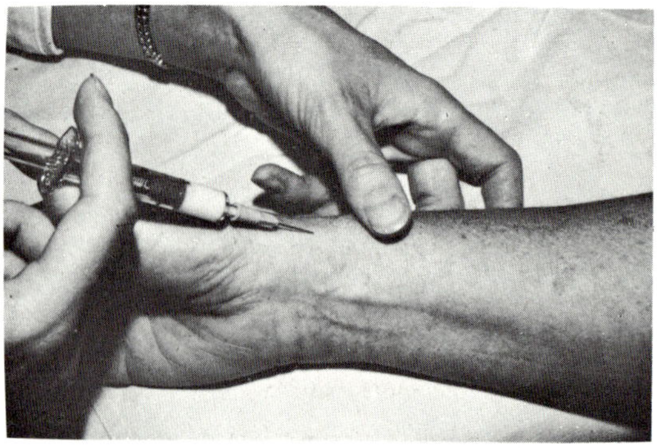

Fig. 67.7 Injection of tenosynovitis at the radial styloid.

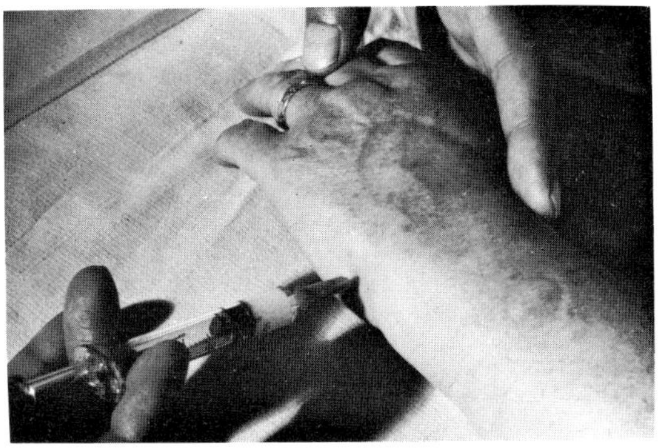

Fig. 67.8 The lateral approach to injection of the wrist joint.

phalangeal or interphalangeal joints of the fingers. In osteoarthrosis it is rarely called for except in involvement of the 1st carpometacarpal joint. Tendinitis or tenosynovitis is also an occasional indication.

The finger joints

The space available for the introduction of a needle into these joints is very small, and accurate palpation of the joint line is essential. Whether it be the metacarpophalangeal or interphalangeal joint, the needle is best inserted on the dorsal surface of the joint to one or other side of the extensor tendon. The joint space will be at its widest if the affected joint is held in a position of mid-flexion, and this will be enhanced if an assistant applies traction meanwhile (Fig. 67.9). A No. 20 (25G × 5/8 inch) needle is the maximum size practical for these injections, and usually no more than 12.5 mg of HCA can be forced into the joint due to its small size.

The 1st carpometacarpal joint

This joint is commonly affected by osteoarthrosis, which, due to the leverage exerted during the pinch grip, can be quite disabling. It is one of the few joints affected by osteoarthrosis where the response is not only satisfactory but also often long-lasting. Once again the joint space is very small and accurate palpation of the joint line needs to be carried out. This is best done, and the joint space widened, if the patient flexes the thumb into the palm and grips it with the flexed fingers. The injection is given dorsally, to one or other side of the extensor tendon, and as with the small finger joints, a No. 20 (25G × 5/8 inch) needle is the maximum size for practical use (Fig. 67.10).

Trigger finger

Catching of the flexor tendons of the fingers within their synovial sheaths is a common symptom in both early and late rheumatoid arthritis, but may also arise as an apparently idiopathic condition. A tender nodule in the palm can usually be palpated over the line of the flexor tendon just proximal to the crease of the metacarpophalangeal joint. Local injection of steroid has a high success rate whatever the cause, but failure will necessitate surgery. The technique of injection is the same as that described for tenosynovitis at the wrist (Fig. 67.11).

THE HIP

Indications for steroid injection in and around the hip joint are rare, the techniques are difficult, and the results less rewarding than in other areas.

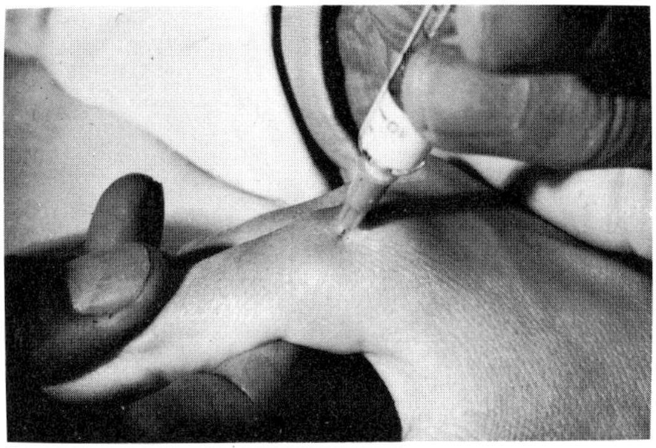

Fig. 67.9 Injection of a finger joint. Traction on the digit helps by widening the joint space.

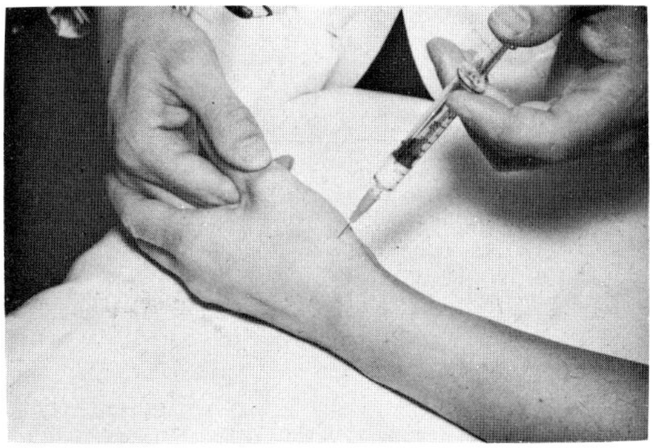

Fig. 67.10 Injection of the 1st carpometacarpal joint.

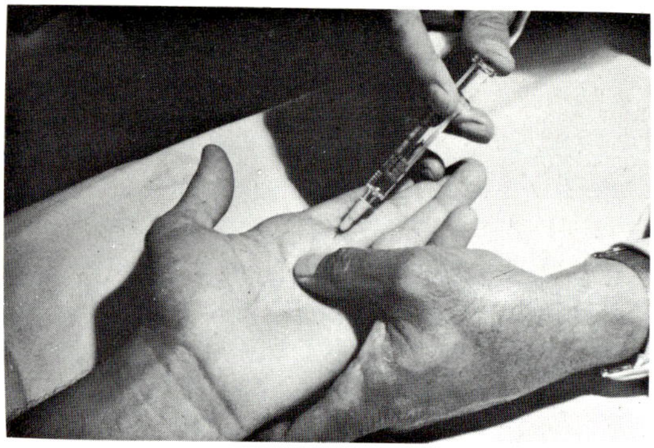

Fig. 67.11 Flexor tendinitis. The operator's index finger palpates for distension of the tendon sheath.

The hip joint

Owing to its depth beneath the surface, this is a joint into which it is difficult to place an accurate injection, and practice under the guidance of an experienced operator is necessary before it should be attempted. The lateral approach to the joint is usually considered to be the most satisfactory. The patient should lie on his side with the affected hip uppermost and flexed to 45°. The outline of the greater trochanter should be palpated, and marked on the skin. A point 1 cm below and 1 cm anterior to the highest point of the trochanter is then marked as the point of entry of the needle (Fig. 67.12). The skin and subcutaneous tissues at this point are then infiltrated with local anaesthetic, and the needle withdrawn. A needle of at least 4 inches in length is then attached to a syringe containing more local anaesthetic, and inserted at the needle mark. This needle is then slowly advanced in the direction of the femoral neck, being slightly withdrawn and given a dorsal bias whenever the bone of the femoral neck is encountered. In this way the needle point is gradually slid up the femoral neck until the thick capsule of the hip joint is encountered. At this point, increased resistance, followed by a sudden 'give' will be felt, when the needle point should be within the joint capsule. It is rarely possible to aspirate fluid from the hip.

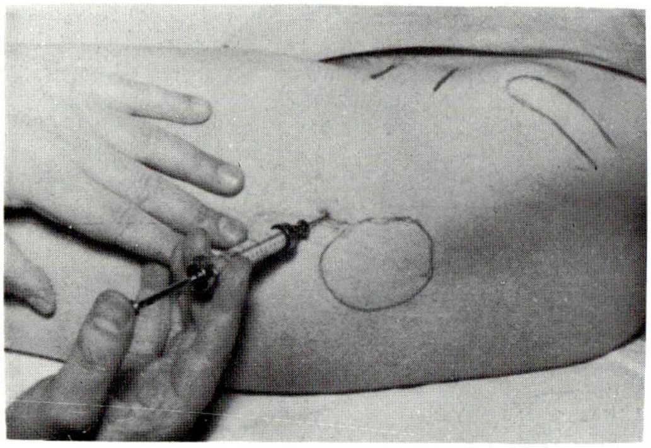

Fig. 67.12 The lateral approach to injection of the hip joint.

The anterior approach is preferred by some. In this case the patient lies supine, with the hip extended and in slight external rotation. The needle is introduced about 3 cm lateral to the femoral pulse and 2 cm below the anterior superior iliac spine. It is directed at an angle of 60° posteriorly and medially through the tough capsular ligaments until bone is reached. The tip of the needle is then slightly withdrawn and the injection given.

Supratrochanteric bursitis

This lesion to some extent mirrors subdeltoid bursitis at the shoulder, although it is very much more rare. Calcification within the bursa may sometimes be seen on radiographs. The bursa lies on the superior surface of the femoral neck, outside the joint capsule. It is difficult to locate with a needle, and its injection is very much a hit and miss affair. The lateral approach to the hip joint is used, but the depth of injection is less.

THE KNEE

The knee joint itself is perhaps the easiest joint in the body to inject, and as it is so often distended by an effusion, and so commonly involved in the inflammatory arthritides, it offers an easy route for such procedures as needle biopsy, or the examination of fluid withdrawn by arthrocentesis. The supra- and infrapatellar bursae may also respond satisfactorily to steroid injection when involved in an inflammatory process.

The knee joint

Provided the patient is able fully to extend the knee, the medial approach is best. The patient sits on the couch with the knee fully extended. The mid-point (widest point) of the patella is palpated, and the gap between this point and the uppermost part of the medial femoral condyle is found and marked. A No. 12 (23G × 13/16 inch) needle is usually adequate unless a large effusion needs to be aspirated; if so a larger bore needle is preferable. The needle is inserted immediately below the mid-point of the patella and advanced at right angles to the skin when the joint should be entered without difficulty (Fig. 67.13). Pressure downwards on the suprapatellar pouch will widen the gap between the patella and femoral condyle if fluid is present within the knee.

Supra- and infrapatellar bursae
These bursae are occasionally involved by inflammation in such conditions as housemaid's or clergyman's knee. In such situations they are usually warm and distended with fluid, being easily palpable. As they lie superficially, aspiration and injection simply involves introducing a suitable needle directly into the distended tissues.

THE ANKLE AND FOOT

Tenosynovitis may occur around the ankle as it does round the wrist joint, and the techniques of injection are the same. The mortice joint of the ankle is often involved in inflammatory arthritis and responds well to local steroids. The small joints of the foot require injection less frequently than the corresponding joints in the hand, but the techniques of injection are identical. Achilles tendinitis, and the painful heel, are other indications for local injection.

The ankle joint
The patient sits on a couch with the foot slightly plantar flexed, and with some eversion. The gap between the lateral side of the medial malleolus and the tendon of tibialis anterior is palpated, and the needle inserted just above the level of the tip of the malleolus. It is directed laterally, posteriorly, and with a slight upward bias, when the joint should be entered. Alternatively, the joint may be entered anteriorly, the joint line between the tibia and talus to be defined by palpation, care being taken to avoid the dorsalis pedis artery (Fig. 67.14). A No. 12 (23G × 13/16 inch) needle is suitable.

Achilles tendinitis
This troublesome condition will usually respond to alteration of footwear or a calcaneal pad. Resistant cases sometimes benefit from local steroid injection, particularly if an adventitious bursa has formed beneath the tendon. Injection simply consists of infiltrating HCA around and beneath the tender portion of the tendon. The needle should not be inserted into the substance of the tendon since complete rupture of the tendon has been reported following steroid injection, and therefore cases showing evidence of tearing of fibres of the tendon are best treated by other means.

The painful heel
This may be ascribed to plantar fasciitis or to the

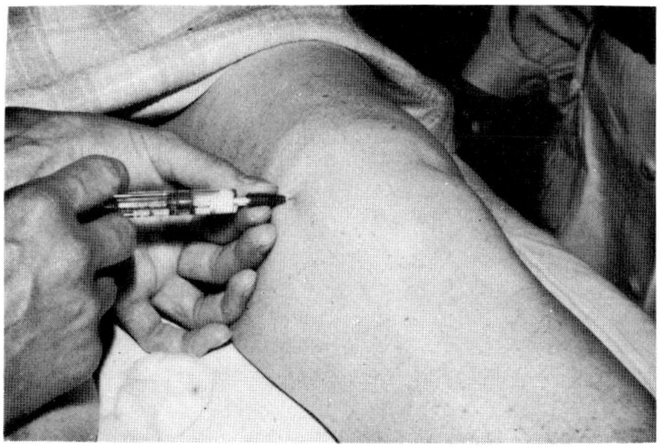

Fig. 67.13 The medial approach to aspiration or injection of the knee joint beneath the lower surface of the patella.

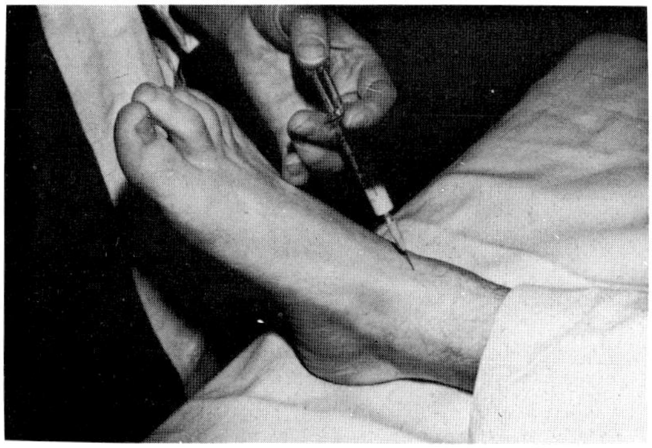

Fig. 67.14 The anterior approach to the ankle joint.

presence of a calcaneal spur, but whatever the cause local steroid injection may be successful in giving relief. There is usually a localised tender spot in the middle of the heel pad, which is the site of election for injection. A No. 12 (23G × 13/16 inch) needle is used and inserted at right angles to the skin at the tender point. For the success of this injection, as with tennis elbow, it seems necessary to advance the tip of the needle until it rests on the periosteum of the os calcis. 25 mg of HCA is adequate.

MISCELLANEOUS

Apart from the common indications described above, many other soft tissue lesions affecting muscles and ligaments, whether traumatic or inflammatory, may respond well to local infiltration of steroid. In such cases, a preliminary infiltration of the suspected site of the lesion with local anaesthetic is often a useful guide as to the accuracy of diagnosis, since in the latter case pain should be abolished, and function restored.

REFERENCES

Chandler G N, Wright V 1958 Lancet 2:661
Chandler G N, Jones D T, Wright V, Hartfall S J 1959 British Medical Journal 1:952
Hollander J L 1970 Maryland State Medical Journal 19:62
McCarty D J, Hogan J M 1964 Arthritis and Rheumatism 7:359

Electrodiagnosis in the rheumatic diseases

Electrodiagnostic techniques may be useful in both the investigation and the management of certain of the rheumatic diseases. Technical details of the methods used are outside the scope of this chapter and if required can be found in the specialised literature (Desmedt, 1973; Licht, 1971). In essence the techniques useful in this group of diseases are:

1. Latency measurements — measurements of time elapsed between electrical stimulation of a peripheral nerve and the detection of its appropriate motor or sensory response
2. Measurement of sensory and motor nerve conduction speed
3. Detection and interpretation of electrical potentials within muscle obtained by needle electrodes (electromyography).

All these techniques, either singly or in combination, can give information about the state of the lower motor neurone system from the anterior horn cell down to the muscle fibre and can localise the level of the lesion to three main sites: the anterior horn cell, the peripheral nerve fibre, and the muscle fibre. Furthermore it is often possible to indicate with reasonable precision the likely level and severity of a peripheral nerve lesion in the entrapment syndromes.

ELECTRODIAGNOSTIC METHODS

Latency measurements

With modern equipment it is easy to determine the time taken between stimulating a peripheral nerve and collecting the appropriate response at a distance. This response may be as a muscle action potential collected by surface electrodes on the muscle belly, in which case motor nerve latency is measured (Fig. 68.1). For sensory nerve latencies two alternative methods may be used: the mixed peripheral nerve can be stimulated at the same site as for motor nerve latencies, and the antidromic sensory nerve potential collected from a pure sensory nerve branch, again by surface electrodes (Fig. 68.1); or the sensory nerve can be stimulated peripherally and the orthodromic nerve action potential collected more proximally. The author much prefers the antidromic technique which allows the simultaneous recording of motor and sensory latencies on different channels of the oscilloscope, thus minimising patient discomfort with no loss of accuracy.

It is not possible to calculate nerve conduction speed from a single latency reading, because although the distance between the point of stimulation and the point of collection can be measured, there is a great variation in the diameter of nerve fibres as they approach their termination. This, together with the uncertainties of delay at the neuromuscular junction, and variability of the speed of propagation of depolarisation of the muscle fibre membrane, makes any such calculation meaningless.

Nerve conduction speed

This can be calculated by stimulating the same peripheral nerve at two points on the limb and collecting from the same position in each case, thus giving two latency measurements. Subtraction of one latency from the other will indicate the time taken by the nerve impulse to pass from one point of stimulation to the other point of stimulation; from this reading and the distance between the two points the speed is easily obtained

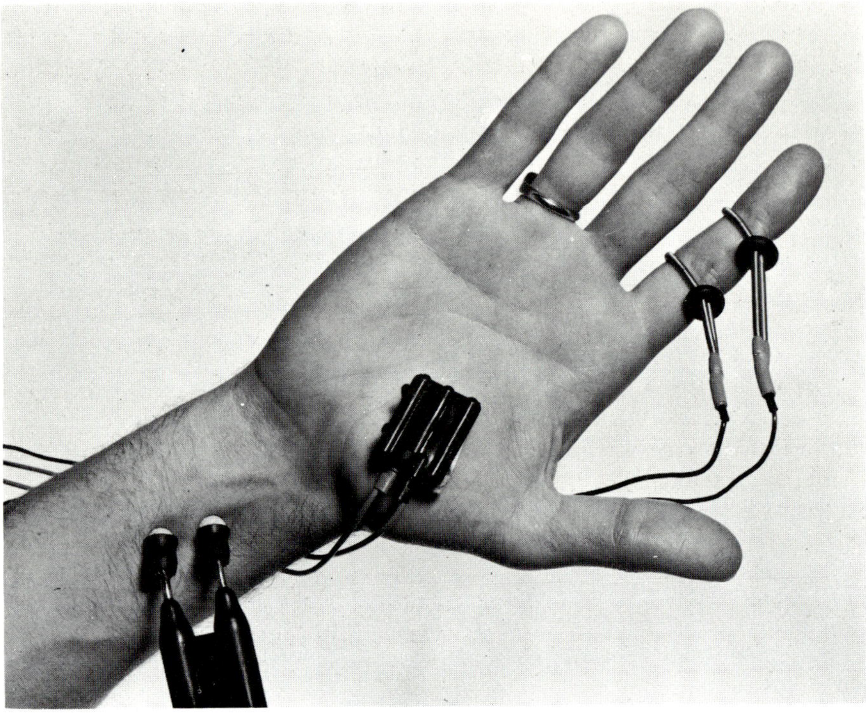

Fig. 68.1 Electrode arrangement for measurement of simultaneous motor and sensory nerve latencies showing stimulating electrodes at the wrist, muscle action potential pick-up over the thenar muscles and digital nerve ring electrodes.

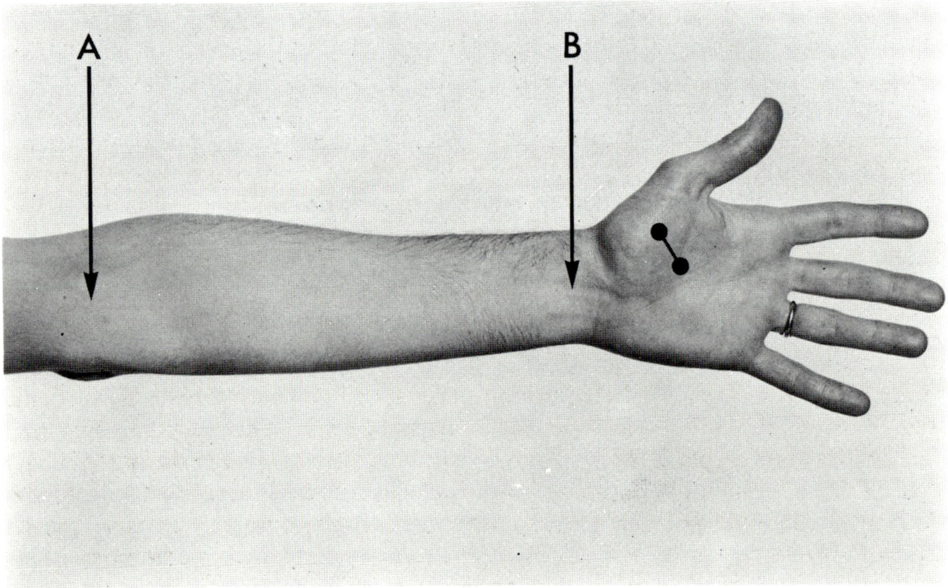

Fig. 68.2 Calculation for obtaining nerve conduction speed:
Distance A to B in millimetres ÷ (latency A − latency from B) ms.
= mm/ms.
= m/s.

(Fig. 68.2). Depending on the readings obtained the answer may appear as a figure comprising one or more decimal places (e.g. 53.42 m/s); such as result gives an entirely spurious impression of accuracy to the clinician receiving the report because the various surface measurements of the distance between the two points of stimulation can contain errors amounting to 10% (Campbell, 1971). It is the author's practice to report nerve conduction speeds to the nearest 5 m/s, so that apparent differences of speed in serial measurements which are due really to measurement error are avoided.

Although this method has only been used as a clinical routine for the past 15 years or so, motor nerve conduction speed was measured by DuBois-Reymond in 1866 with remarkably accurate results considering the limitations of the equipment then available.

Electromyography

This technique consists of sampling appropriate muscles with a coaxial needle electrode about the same size as an ordinary hypodermic needle. The muscle is sampled during relaxation for detection of spontaneous activity, and during voluntary contraction for detection and interpretation of motor unit action potentials.

Denervation is indicated by the detection of fibrillation and/or positive potentials when the voluntary muscle is completely relaxed. Myotonic discharges occur following voluntary contraction or needle movement in myotonia. Diseases involving the anterior horn cells such as progressive muscular atrophy, or the muscle fibres in myopathies are differentiated by characteristic changes in the wave form of the motor unit action potentials.

Peripheral neuropathies may result from two separate pathological processes — segmental demyelination or axonal degeneration. The electrodiagnostic findings vary accordingly: in segmental demyelination, latency measurements are lengthened and nerve conduction speeds diminish; on electromyography no denervation potentials are detected. In axonal degeneration, nerve conduction speeds can be normal if even a single fast-conducting motor nerve fibre is spared, reduced if only slow-conducting fibres are spared, or absent if axonal degeneration is total as in nerve transection; electromyography will reveal denervation potentials at rest with reduction in numbers of motor unit action-potentials on maximal volitional effort, the amount of this reduction being proportional to the numbers of peripheral motor nerve fibres which have degenerated. Conditions producing segmental demyelination if severe or prolonged can progress to axonal degeneration so that mixed electrodiagnostic patterns can occur.

In summary, electrodiagnostic techniques do not give a clinical diagnosis but indicate the site and type of lesions involving the lower motor neurones and muscle fibres.

CLINICAL APPLICATIONS IN THE RHEUMATIC DISEASES

These methods are useful in the diagnosis and assessment of a number of conditions occurring in the rheumatic diseases: the differential diagnosis of muscle wasting, the nerve compression and entrapment syndromes, the diagnosis and assessment of peripheral neuropathy, and the detection and assessment of myopathic disorders.

Nerve compression and entrapment

The clinical aspects of these have been discussed in Chapters 26, 59 and 60. Segmental demyelination is the initial response of the nerve fibre to compression and therefore a lengthening of latency measurement occurs when the nerve is stimulated above and the evoked response collected below the site of the lesion. This test is at its most sensitive when these two points are close together; latency measurements in the carpal tunnel syndrome provide the best example of this, where the median nerve can be stimulated just proximal to the carpal ligament and the evoked motor and antidromic sensory responses collected a short distance peripheral to the ligament. The importance of sensory latency measurement has been stressed for some time and providing this is done the accuracy of the test is in the order of 90% (Campbell, 1962 and subsequent unpublished figures). Normal latency measurements are up to 3.5 ms for sensory nerve and 4.5 ms for motor nerve. In unilateral lesions a difference between the two sides of 1 ms is considered significant.

The ulnar nerve may be compressed at the wrist as a result of synovial proliferation but this is much less common than carpal tunnel compression of the median nerve. Compression or entrapment around the elbow is a more usual site of ulnar nerve involvement and may occur with synovial proliferation or as a result of direct mechanical pressure from elbow crutches, etc. Ulnar nerve involvement may be detected by latency measurements across the elbow or by slowing of nerve conduction speeds from elbow to wrist.

The lateral popliteal nerve is similarly vulnerable as it winds around the head of the fibula and the motor latency from just proximal to the suspected site of the lesion to tibialis anterior, or nerve conduction speed from knee to ankle can confirm this diagnosis.

Peripheral neuropathy

The clinical patterns of peripheral neuropathy seen in rheumatoid arthritis have been described and classified by Pallis & Scott (1965); of these the entrapment neuropathies have already been discussed. Localised digital sensory neuropathy occurs as a result of ischaemia and because of its very localised distribution (for instance only part of the digital nerve on one side of the finger may be involved) electrical tests are of little or no help. In the distal sensory neuropathy of the leg the clinical distribution is usually symmetrical and sensory nerve conduction speeds are slowed, suggesting segmental demyelination. The smallest and most severe group is that caused by arteritis of the vasa nervorum; this will often start as a mononeuritis multiplex proceeding rapidly to a symmetrical mixed polyneuropathy involving arms and legs. Axonal degeneration is the predominant lesion so that conduction speeds on the whole are normal whilst electromyographic evidence of denervation is marked (Weller et al, 1970). Such arteritic lesions occur most commonly in polyarteritis nodosa but may also happen in systemic lupus erythematosus or as a rare accompaniment of any of the connective tissue diseases.

Drug-induced neuropathy has been reported after administration of gold salts (Doyle & Cannon, 1950), indomethacin (Eade et al, 1975), and penicillamine (Meyboom, 1977).

Myopathic disorders

The detection of myopathic changes is not difficult for the trained electromyographer but it remains largely a matter of personal interpretation. Although considerable advances have been made, the quest for an objective measure of myopathic change remains unfulfilled. Nevertheless, electromyographic diagnosis gives a good degree of accuracy, the main problem areas being the assessment of improvement of deterioration in serial investigations, and the detection of minor changes as in unaffected carriers of muscular dystrophy.

In a pure myopathy the degenerative changes are limited to the muscle fibres themselves: as the disease process attacks muscle fibres randomly within the motor unit there is no total loss of motor units as in the neuropathies but instead all affected motor units have a reduced complement of functioning muscle fibres, producing a wave form of either short duration or disintegrated outline. In neuromyopathy the degenerative or inflammatory process involves also the terminal nerve fibres, thereby causing denervation in still viable muscle fibres. These conditions produce signs of denervation electromyographically (fibrillation and positive potentials) as well as the short duration and disintegrated potentials characteristic of a myopathy. This division between pure myopathy and neuromyopathy is not absolute and fibrillation potentials in muscular dystrophy have been reported, though never seen in the author's experience. In particular, signs of denervation cannot always be detected in those conditions which usually produce them and the absence of a particular type of potential should never be regarded as positive evidence excluding such a condition.

Polymyositis and dermatomyositis are the two connective tissue diseases which classically and regularly give the changes of neuromyopathy, although dermatomyositis may on occasion produce skin changes for some considerable time before muscles are involved. Myopathic changes may also be found frequently in systemic sclerosis and scleroderma, in mixed connective tissue disease, and occasionally in systemic lupus erythematosus, rheumatoid arthritis and Sjögren's syndrome. Serial investigations at intervals of about 6 weeks may be used to assess the progress of the disease or the efficacy of treatment, but whatever method of quantifying the degree of myopathy is used a reasonable degree of accuracy can only be achieved if the same observer performs the investigation on each occasion.

Myotonic discharges may also be heard in neuromyopathy, though rarely to the same extent as in myotonia dystrophica or myotonia congenita: they have a very characteristic sound, either high pitched with a rapidly declining frequency ('dive-bomber discharge') or a regular lower frequency sound like a motor car engine missing on one cylinder. They probably arise from areas of increased muscle fibre excitability due to degenerative or inflammatory processes, and diminish or disappear with treatment. Very occasionally small patches of myotonia can be detected in muscular dystrophy and polyneuritis.

The metabolic disorders with which myopathies may be associated do not on the whole come within the scope of this chapter, with the exception of osteomalacia and possibly xanthinuria. In osteomalacia the position is far from clear; some patients have the waddling gait suggestive of pelvic girdle muscle weakness without necessarily showing electromyographic signs of myopathy, whilst others, without clinical evidence of muscle weakness, have the electromyographic characteristics. Henson (1966) and Smith & Stern (1967) could find no relationship between the existence of a myopathy and levels of total serum calcium. Distinction between levels of total calcium and ionised calcium does not appear to have been made and the direct influence of vitamin D on muscle function still has to be determined. Control of the osteomalacia causes resolution of the myopathy.

Myopathy has been described in xanthinuria (Chalmers et al, 1968), the cause of the myopathy apparently being the presence of intramuscular crystals of xanthine and hypoxanthine: it is therefore conceivable that treatment of gross overproduction of uric acid with allopurinol could produce this complication, but if it does occur it does not appear to be of clinical significance.

Drug-induced myopathies can be caused by several substances used in the treatment of the rheumatic diseases: corticosteroids and chloroquine (Whisnant et al, 1963) are the drugs most commonly implicated though colchicine has been reported by Markand & D'Agostino (1971) to produce myopathic changes in rats. The steroid myopathies are an interesting and important group and myopathic changes may be caused by most corticosteroids, either endogenously produced as in the myopathy of Cushing's syndrome, or more usually as a result of steroid medication: rapid reversal of both histological and electromyographic abnormalities occurs on withdrawal of the steroid or on substitution of a different compound. The presence of fluorine in the molecule, as in triamcinolone and dexamethasone, seems to predispose to myopathic change and these two substances produce the most severe effects.

ACTH can also produce myopathic change and cases have been reported where high serum ACTH levels in patients after bilateral adrenalectomy have been associated with clinical and electromyographic signs of myopathy (Prineas et al, 1968).

Finally, although the consensus of opinion is that electrodiagnosis in polymyalgia rheumatica gives normal findings, Buchthal (1970) has reported mild myopathic change in a few patients.

Myasthenia gravis and myasthenic syndrome

Variable weakness affecting proximal muscles and especially muscles of the face and of deglutition is of course the cardinal clinical feature of myasthenia gravis, but it must be stressed that myasthenia gravis is a specific clinical entity, whereas the myasthenic syndrome is simply the association of variable muscular weakness in the symptom complex of disease processes entirely separate from myasthenia gravis. The point needs emphasis because the distinction is sometimes missed and because certain electrodiagnostic techniques can make a clear differentiation.

Myasthenia gravis, though not usually classified as one of the rheumatic diseases, is now accepted as an autoantibody disease. This view was originally propounded by Simpson (1974), and Lindstrom et al (1976) showed the presence of antibody to acetylcholine receptor and its specificity in myasthenia gravis. There is only one electrodiagnostic test truly specific to myasthenia gravis, namely the demonstration of an abnormal resistance to the depolarising neuromuscular blocking agent decamethonium, as described by Churchill-Davidson & Richardson (1952). Diseases producing the myasthenic syndrome give normal findings in this investigation, which is thus of considerable value in the differential diagnosis of variable weakness.

Another useful test, though less specific, is that of increased 'jitter'. When recordings are taken from two single muscle fibres in the same motor unit the time interval between the firing of the two fibres varies at each discharge, and is usually in the order of 20 μs. The figure is markedly increased in cases of myasthenia gravis to around 100 μs and is valuable in the detection of early or mild cases. However, some increase over normal values may also be found in other neuromuscular diseases, though not to the same degree as in myasthenia gravis.

The myasthenic syndrome can occur in polymyositis and dermatomyositis regardless of whether these conditions are associated with a carcinoma: carcinomatous myasthenia is a further separate entity with its own characteristic electrodiagnostic features (the Eaton–Lambert phenomenon).

Finally, penicillamine can induce myasthenia gravis in treatment of both rheumatoid arthritis (Bucknall et al, 1975) and Wilson's disease and such patients produce antibody to acetylcholine receptor (Vincent & Newsom-Davis, 1982). The mechanism of this is not understood and antibodies have been demonstrated in penicillamine-treated patients without myasthenic symptoms (Martin et al, 1980). There is a full return to normality some weeks after withdrawal of penicillamine.

REFERENCES

Buchthal F 1970 Electrophysiological abnormalities in metabolic myopathies and neuropathies. Acta Neurologica Scandinavica (Suppl) 43:129

Bucknall R C, Dixon A St J, Glick E N, Woodland J, Zutshi D W 1975 Myasthenia gravis associated with penicillamine treatment for rheumatoid arthritis. British Medical Journal 1:600

Campbell E D R 1962 Carpal tunnel syndrome: assessment and treatment. Proceedings of the Royal Society of Medicine 55:401

Campbell E D R 1971 Peripheral neuropathy: electrodiagnostic aspects. Proceedings of the Royal Society of Medicine 64:293

Chalmers R A, Johnson M, Pallis C, Watts R W F 1969 Xanthinuria with myopathy. Quarterly Journal of Medicine 38:493

Churchill-Davidson H C, Richardson A T 1952 The action of decamethonium iodide in myasthenia gravis. Journal of Neurology, Neurosurgery and Psychiatry 15:129

Desmedt J E 1973 New developments in electromyography and clinical neurophysiology Karger, Basel

Doyle J B, Cannon E F 1950 Severe polyneuritis following gold therapy for rheumatoid arthritis. Annals of Internal Medicine 33:1468

Eade O E, Acheson E D, Cuthbert M F, Hawkes C H 1975 Peripheral neuropathy and indomethacin. British Medical Journal 2:66

Henson R A 1966 The neurological aspects of hypercalcaemia. Journal of the Royal College of Physicians 1:41

Licht S 1971 Electrodiagnosis and electromyography, 3rd edn. E Licht, New Haven

Lindstrom J M, Seybold M E, Lennon V A, Whittingham S, Duane D D 1976 Antibody to acetylcholine receptor in myasthenia gravis. Neurology 26:1054

Markand O N, D'Agostino A N 1971 Ultrastructural changes in skeletal muscle induced by colchicine. Archives of Neurology Chicago 24:72

Martin V M, Vincent A, Clarke C 1980 Anti-acetylcholine receptor antibodies in penicillamine treated patients without myasthenia gravis. Lancet 2:705

Meyboon R H B 1977 Heavy metal antagonists. Side Effect of Drugs Annual 1:190

Pallis C A, Scott J T 1965 Peripheral neuropathy in rheumatoid arthritis. British Medical Journal 1:1141

Prineas J W, Hall R, Barwick D D, Watson A J 1968 Myopathy associated with pigmentation following adrenalectomy for Cushing's syndrome. Quarterly Journal of Medicine 37:63

Simpson J A 1974 Myasthenia gravis and myasthenic syndromes. In: Walton J N (ed) Disorders of voluntary muscle. Churchill Livingstone, Edinburgh

Smith R, Stern G 1967 Myopathy osteomalacia and hyperparathyroidism. Brain 90:593

Vincent A, Newsom-Davis J 1982 Acetylcholine receptor antibody characteristics in myasthenia gravis. Clinical and Experimental Immunology 49:266

Weller R O, Bruckner F E, Chamberlain M A 1970 Rheumatoid neuropathy: a histological and electrophysiological study. Journal of Neurology, Neurosurgery and Psychiatry 33:592

Whisnant J P, Espinosa R E, Kierland R R, Lambert E H 1963 Chloroquine neuromyopathy. Proceedings of the Staff Meetings of the Mayo Clinic 38:501

Modern imaging techniques

COMPUTERISED TOMOGRAPHY (CT)

Conventional X-rays had until recent years been the physicians' major ally in the imaging or rheumatic disorders. The introduction of computer technology into radiology has greatly increased the sensitivity of modern imaging techniques and allowed the soft tissues to be visualised with similar clarity to that of bones.

The low resolution of CT compared to plain radiographs is compensated for by the increased information in the structure–space relationships and from the knowledge of relative tissue densities (Abrams & McNeil, 1978). The immediate potential for CT in the early diagnosis of the inflammatory and metabolic arthropathies would, with some notable exceptions, seem to be rather limited. There is, however, considerable potential for evaluation of secondary mechanical sequelae of the arthropathies as well as in the assessment of lesions of the spine, trauma, intra-abdominal and paraspinal abscesses, and musculoskeletal tumours.

SACROILIITIS

The complex anatomy of the sacroiliac joints makes conventional radiology and radioisotope evaluation of sacroiliitis difficult, and often unrewarding (Dequecker et al, 1978; Carrera, 1983). Computed tomography, because of its tomographic nature, produces high resolution images which clearly show cortical and subchondral bone as well as surrounding soft tissues.

It is well known that patients may have clinical evidence of sacroiliitis for years prior to the appearance of radiological changes. Current therapeutic methods require a confident diagnosis and several studies show CT to be superior in both detecting and defining early disease of the sacroiliac joints (Carrera et al, 1981; Kozin et al, 1981; Lawson et al, 1982). The expense of CT precludes its routine use for assessment of sacroiliac joints but it can be used when plain film findings are equivocal or when there is a strong suspicion of disease despite normal plain films (Fig. 69.1).

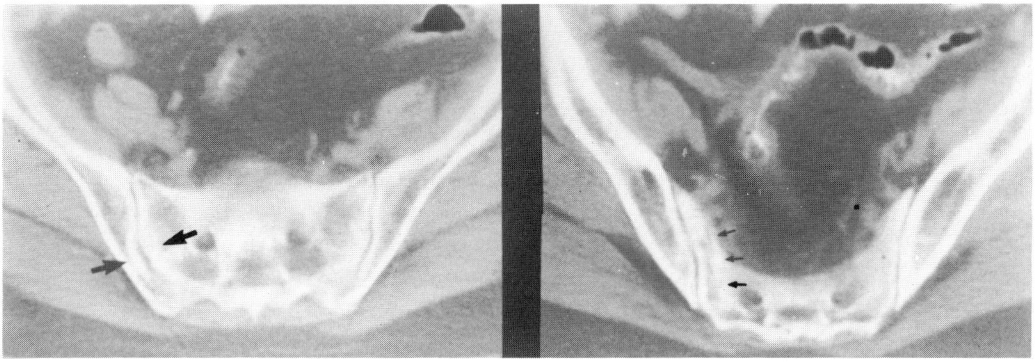
a b

Fig. 69.1 (a) Irregular sclerosis on both sides of the right sacroiliac joint (arrowed) with joint space maintained. (b) Subcortical bone resorption (arrowed) on sacral side of joint. Note the normal left sacroiliac joint on both images.

DISORDERS OF THE SPINE

The development of high resolution scanners has added impetus to the utilisation of CT for spinal studies. Although the technique is a relatively new development it is increasingly becoming the definitive technique for the diagnosis of many spinal disorders.

Disc herniation

CT effectively and efficiently demonstrates disc disease and accurate distinction between a bulging and a herniated disc is usually possible (Fries et al, 1982; Genant et al, 1982; Haughton & Williams, 1982; Teplick & Haskin, 1983). The precise role of CT in clinical management is not yet certain and correlation between CT and clinical findings is still being evaluated.

With increasing age the nucleus pulposus loses its elasticity and shrinks. The surrounding annulus fibrosus weakens with this nuclear retraction, the inner layers buckle inwards and the outer layers bulge outwards to produce a bulging or protruding disc. Trauma may selectively rupture the annulus fibrosus allowing the nucleus to be extruded through successive layers of annulus and when the herniation is beyond the annulus it results in a prolapsed disc. Prolapse is usually in a posterolateral direction. Bulging discs normally demonstrate a bulge of the disc margin beyond the margins of the vertebral body while herniated discs may be recognised as a focal protrusion (Fig. 69.2).

Facet joints

Osteoarthritis in a lower lumbar facet joint may cause pain referred to the lower extremities, which is indistinguishable from a herniated disc (Carrera et al, 1981). Hypertrophic changes in the superior articular facets may also cause pain by compressing a spinal nerve in the neural canal of which the facet joint forms part.

The facet joints are innervated by tiny branches from the adjacent spinal nerves. Stimulation of these nerves results in poorly localised pain in the distribution of the adjacent spinal nerves (Dory, 1981). Degenerative disease of facet joints proceeds from synovitis to joint capsule laxity, articular erosion, osteophytes and subperiosteal new bone formation. CT demonstrates findings from each of these stages of degeneration (Haughton & Williams, 1982).

Facet arthropathy is difficult to demonstrate on plain films but CT readily visualises the joints and can help distinguish facet arthropathy from disc disease as a cause of symptoms and thus save the

a

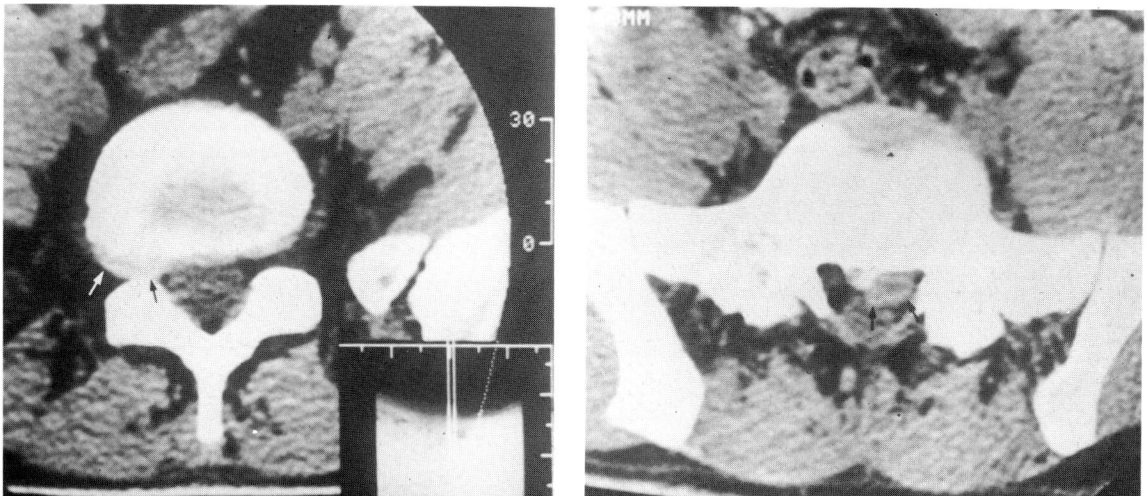

b

Fig. 69.2 (a) Right posterolateral disc protrusion (arrowed) at L4/5 level obstructing lateral recess and intervertebral canal. (b) Large posterior L5/S1 disc protrusion (arrowed) in a patient who has had a laminectomy.

patient from unnecessary radiculography and/or laminectomy.

Facet joint disease may be demonstrated in 5–43% of patients with back pain depending on the indications for CT scanning (Haughton & Williams, 1982) (Fig. 69.3).

Spinal stenosis

Spinal stenosis may be defined as any condition which results in narrowing of the spinal canal, the lateral recesses (subarticular segment of the nerve root canal) or of the intervertebral canals (infrapedicular segment of the nerve root canal and intervertebral foramen).

Causes of spinal stenosis (from Dorwart R.H. et al, 1983)

I. Congenital–developmental stenosis
   1. Idiopathic
   2. Achondroplasia
   3. Hypochondroplasia
   4. Morquio's mucopolysaccharidosis
   5. Dysplasias associated with lax atlantoaxial joints (metatrophic dwarfism), spondyloepiphyseal dysplasia, Kniest's disease, multiple epiphyseal dysplasia, chondrodysplasis punctata
   6. Down's syndrome

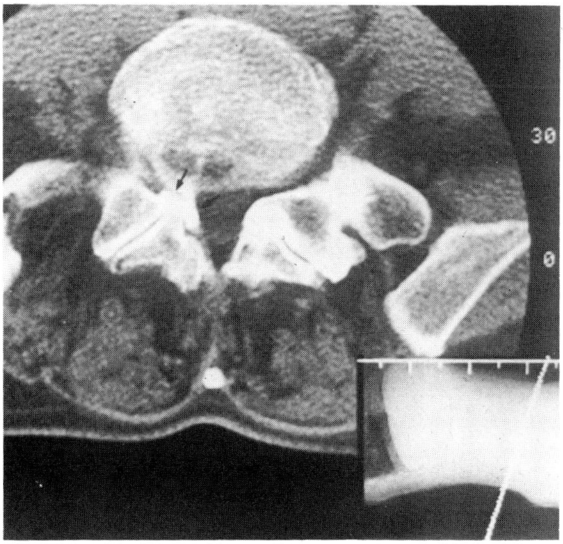

Fig. 69.3 Osteoarthritis of the facet joints with osteophyte (arrowed) on right side causing narrowing of the lateral recess.

   7. Hypophosphatemic vitamin D-resistant rickets

II. Acquired stenosis
   1. Degenerative
      a. Spondylosis and arthrosis
      b. Soft tissue stenosis
      c. Isolated intervertebral disc resorption
      d. Degenerative spondylolisthesis
   2. Combined
      Any possible combinations of congenital or developmental stenosis, degenerative stenosis, and protrusions or intervertebral disc material
   3. Spondylolysis
      a. Without spondylolisthesis
      b. With spondylolisthesis
   4. Iatrogenic
      a. Post-laminectomy
      b. Post-fusion (anterior or posterior)
   5. Post-traumatic, late changes
   6. Miscellaneous
      a. Ankylosing spondylitis
      b. Calcification or ossification of the posterior longitudinal ligament
      c. Diffuse idiopathic skeletal hyperostosis
      d. Calcification or ossification of the ligamentum flavum
      e. Conjoined origin of lumbosacral nerve roots (relative stenosis of neural canal)
   7. Metabolic
      a. Paget's disease of bone
      b. Epidural lipomatosis (Cushing's syndrome or long-term steroid therapy)
      c. Acromegaly
      d. Fluorosis
      e. Calcium pyrophosphate dihydrate deposition disease (pseudogout)

CT criteria for spinal stenosis

The sagittal AP diameter of the central canal should be measured at the superior margin of the lamina with the scanning plane parallel to the vertebral end-plates. An absolute measurement of less than 11.5 mm is pathological (Ullrich et al, 1980).

Measurements must take into account the soft tissue components such as the ligamentum flavum and the discs. Attempts should be made to assess the total cross-sectional area of the canal.

Scarcity or absence of epidural fat is suggestive of stenosis but not conclusive as some normal patients have very little fat in the bony canal. At disc level all patients have fat in the epidural spaces and absence at this level is indicative of disease (Dorwant & Genant, 1983).

CT narrowing of lateral recesses and of the intervertebral canals is similar to central stenosis. Abnormal bony, calcific and soft tissue densities obliterate fat that normally surrounds nerve roots. Absolute measurements of less than 3 mm at the lateral recesses level is pathological (Lee et al, 1978 (Figs 69.4, 69.5).

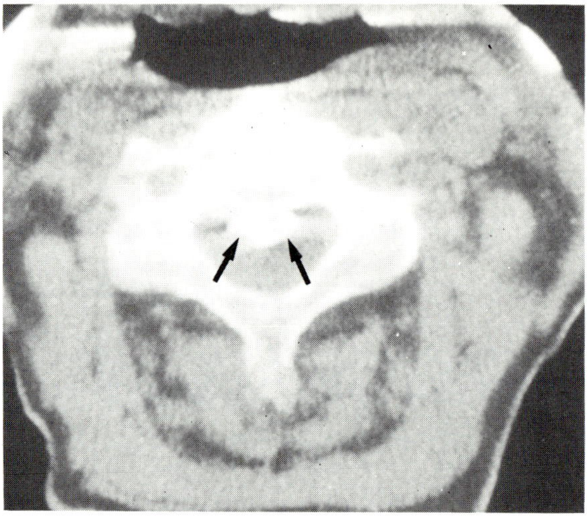

Fig. 69.5 Cervical spinal stenosis secondary to calcification of the posterior longitudinal ligament (arrowed).

TRAUMA

While plain films should still be the first line of investigation in traumatic lesions of the axial skeleton there is often risk in moving patients with unstable spinal lesions. CT causes minimal discomfort and risk to the patient, gives more information on both the bones and the contents of the spinal canal and has a lower radiation dose than conventional tomography (Keene et al, 1982). High resolution scans will show small bone fragments, displaced fragments, foreign bodies and haematoma formation.

CT often provides unique information about pelvic fractures and in particular allows accurate assessment of the acetabular structures which are often difficult to see on plain X-rays. It will show the presence of small intra-articular bone fragments and posterior lip fragments as well as evaluation of the spatial relationships of major fracture fragments (Harley et al, 1982; Boijsen & Ekelung, 1982).

Fractures of long bones are best assessed on

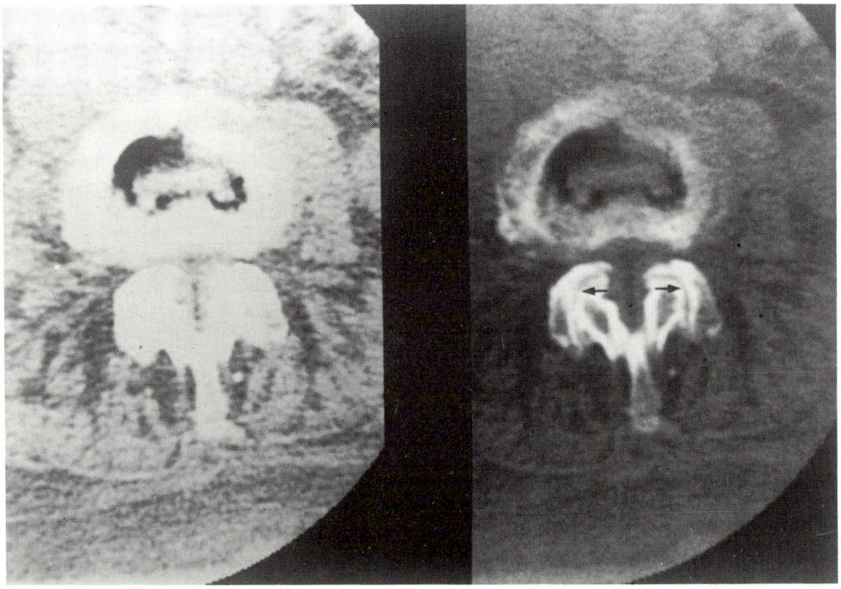

Fig. 69.4 (a) Narrow slit-like spinal canal secondary to degenerative spondylosis. (b) Same image at different settings showing irregular, narrowed, sclerotic facet joints.

plain films but with the leg in plaster it may be difficult to detail postoperative results. CT will allow accurate evaluation of position and condition not effaced by the overlying plaster cast (Reim et al, 1982) (Figs 69.6, 69.7).

SOFT TISSUE LESIONS

A large number of patients present to the general practitioner or rheumatology clinic with painful rheumatic symptoms which do not arise strictly from joint disease but from other connective tissues of the locomotor system. Soft tissue lesions causing anatomical distortion are often easily and accurately localised on CT scans. Qualitative analysis of tissue densities will provide useful information about the nature of many of these lesions such as cysts, abscesses and fatty tumours. The display of the relationship of lesions to the surrounding tissues and the neurovascular bundles provides information which allows accurate preoperative evaluation of extent and accessibility (Fig. 69.8)

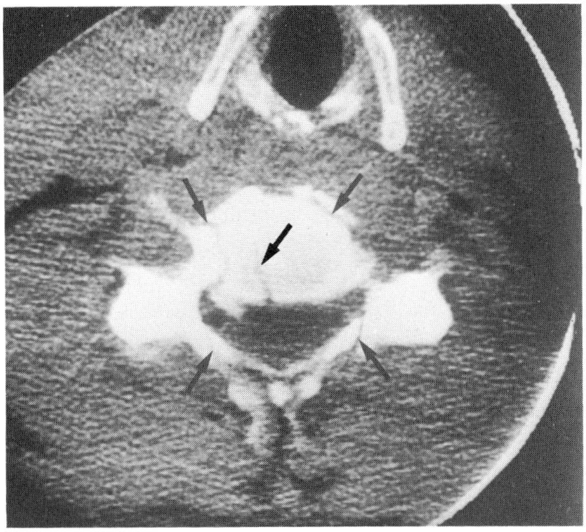

Fig. 69.6 Multiple fractures (arrowed) in cervical vertebra. These fractures are difficult to demonstrate on plain radiographs.

FEMORAL ANTEVERSION

Femoral anteversion is the inclination of the femoral head with reference to the transcondylar plane of the distal femur. The angle of anteversion is increased in CDH, Perthes' disease, neuromuscular disease and in destructive arthritides (Hernandez et al, 1981). Conventional radiology may be difficult to perform in small children and is associated with a high radiation dose. CT offers a simple and direct method of measuring the angle of anteversion. A section taken at the level of the femoral head, neck and trochanteric region is superimposed on a section through the femoral condyles.

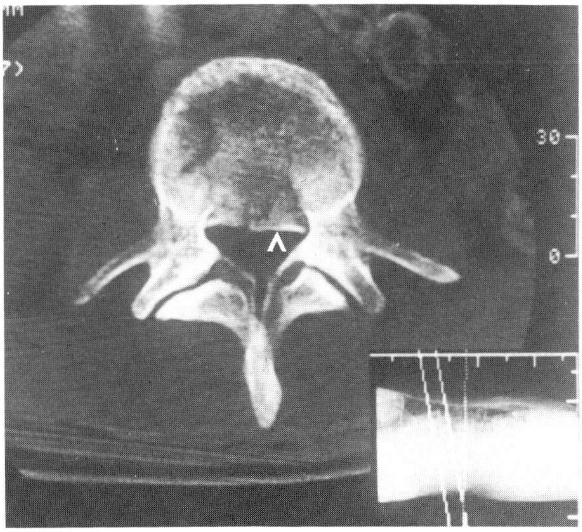

Fig. 69.7 Crush fracture of lumbar vertebra with large fragment (arrowed) protruding into spinal canal.

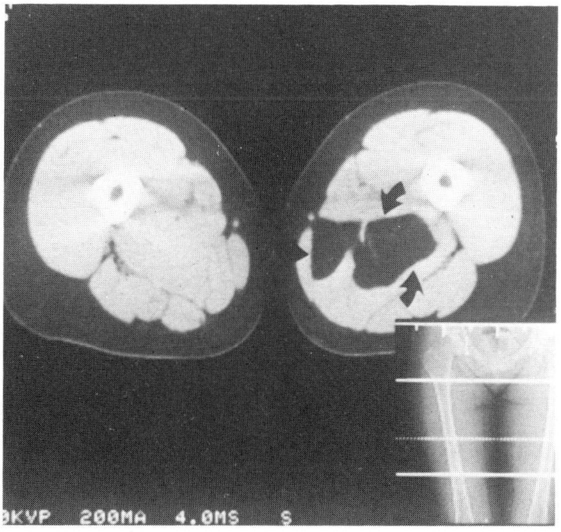

Fig. 69.8 Lipoma (arrowed) in left thigh. The scout view (inset) indicates the level of scan and facilitates accurate delineation of the tumour.

The angle between the femoral neck and the transcondylar axis gives the angle of anteversion (Fig. 69.9).

QUANTITATIVE BONE MINERAL ANALYSIS

A variety of methods exist for quantitative bone mineral analysis, each with its own limitations. CT, because of its unique ability to objectively measure tissue densities, provides an exciting new and potentially highly accurate method for such analysis. CT can clearly define a specific volume of cancellous bone in the axial skeleton, which is the site senstive to many metabolic stimuli, and accurately measure the density. The degree of osteopenia can be measured, response to therapy monitored and likelihood of vertebral collapse assessed from standardised tables (Genant et al, 1983; Cann et al, 1980).

THE USE OF ISOTOPES

Radio-isotope bone scanning has been used for joint activity assessment for about 20 years. Its limited usage reflects the fact that arthritis generally is a clinical diagnosis which, in the majority of cases, is established by other means. It also reflects the low specificity of the procedure. A large number of inflammatory joint diseases have been examined using radionuclide techniques but in none to date has it been widely used. During this period, however, there has been evolution in the range and specificity of bone radiopharmaceuticals and in the sophistication of data analysis. The development of the latter may lead to more objective quantification of the disease process and increased use in assessing therapy.

RADIOPHARMACEUTICALS

Isotopes for potential use in bone/joint imaging

1. ^{99m}Tc pertechnectate
2. ^{99m}Tc phosphonates
3. ^{67}Gallium citrate
4. ^{111}Indium-labelled white cells

The skeletal system has in the past been imaged using such tracers as strontium-85 and 87 and fluorine-18. These had disadvantages of high radiation doses to the patient and long half-lives.

These have been superceded by the ^{99m}Tc compounds, which are easily accessible (molybdenum generator), have an ideal 140 KeV photon emission energy for utilisation with the gamma camera, and a short half-life.

In the patient with arthritis, increased tracer accumulation of plasma protein-bound ^{99m}Tc pertechnetate will reflect:

a. Increased bone blood flow
b. Synovial effusions

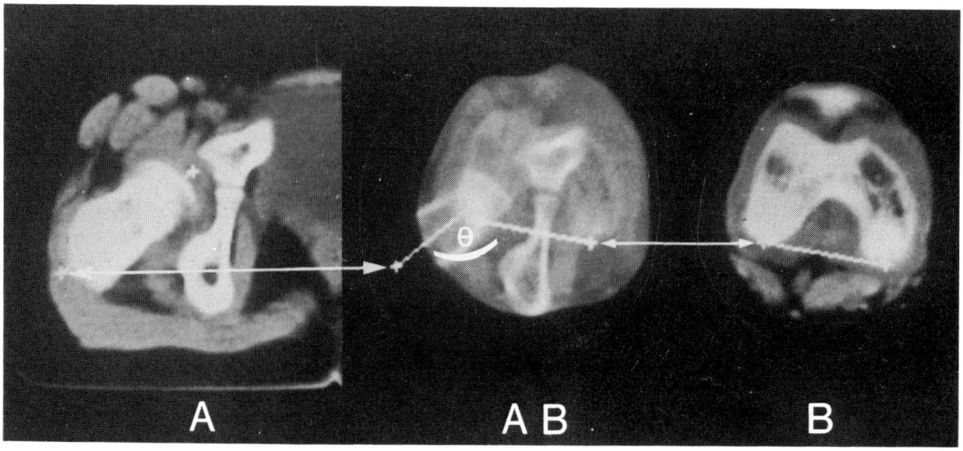

Fig. 69.9 A, Section taken at the level of the hip indicating the line of the femoral neck. B, Section through the distal femur indicating the transcondylar plane. AB, Superimposition of the two images allows the angle of anteversion (θ) to be measured.

c. Increased vascularity of the synovium and its increased transport across a diseased membrane
d. Swelling and soft tissue involvement.

There is however a high soft tissue background with a resultant poor target to background activity ratio: this leads to poor image detail. Its advantage over the ^{99m}Tc phosphate agents however is its specificity for active synovitis.

The ^{99m}Tc phosphates (methylene diphosphate) absorb onto the bone surfaces reacting with hydroxypatite. The resultant scan reflects more the bone activity resultant upon hypervascularity at the subchondral and metaphyseal areas. There is a much improved target to background ratio (resulting in improved images) as the tracer is more readily excreted; 50% of the administered dose is excreted by the kidneys in the first 24 hours. Studies have shown ^{99m}Tc phosphates to be more specific than pertechnetate in the evaluation of the arthropathies.

The most commonly used bone-seeking agent now is ^{99m}Tc methylene diphosphate, incorporating techniques of early- and late-phase imaging with a large field of view gamma camera.

^{67}Ga can also play a role in musculoskeletal assessment, particularly in conjunction with the standard bone scan. It can be advantageously used in:

a. The early diagnosis of osteomyelitis
b. Separating cellulitis and osteomyelitis
c. Identifying pyogenic polyarthritis
d. Detecting infection in a joint either with or without underlying non-infectious arthritis.

^{67}Ga citrate binds to plasma proteins and leucocytes and accumulates at the sites of abscesses and in some tumours. It has a greater affinity for polymorphonuclear leukocytes than lymphocytes — presumably because they have a higher concentration of lactoferrin to which gallium has a high binding affinity.

However, no one explanation can account for gallium accumulation; it has been shown also that it concentrates at areas of tissue damage with no bacterial invasion.

Gallium concentrates mildly in sterile reactive bone; this knowledge is essential for the practical assessment of combined technetium/gallium scans. In the presence of a positive ^{99m}Tc bone scan and a negative gallium scan, active infection is highly unlikely.

^{111}In labelling of white cells, if effective and resulting in viable cells, is an alternative method of detecting infection. The labelled polymorphs accumulate at sites of infection. The use of both gallium and indium as specific differentiators is indicated if the ^{99m}Tc scan is positive.

THE POTENTIAL OF RADIONUCLIDE IMAGING IN JOINT DISEASE

1. Diagnostically to establish the pattern of synovial involvement
2. To follow the effects of therapy
3. To evaluate the complications of joint disease
4. To evaluate the complications of joint replacements.

Pattern of involvement

A large number of studies have shown the value of radionuclide imaging with bone-seeking agents in documenting preradiographic involvement. This has been shown to be the case in ankylosing spondylitis, psoriatic arthritis, gout and other arthropathies. Only if scans are used as X-ray alternatives can one gain any benefit in radiation exposure, however. The marked sensitivity but low specificity of tracer techniques make them highly unlikely to be used alone. Certainly in the initial assessment, correlation with plain X-ray changes are needed. A negative scan however may be particularly useful when synovial involvement is (a) central and inaccessible, (b) involving few joints with little soft tissue involvement, or (c) of doubtful credence (Figs 69.10, 69.11).

Clinicians will have to answer whether earlier demonstrable synovitis would affect clinical management.

For validity of assessment, joint scanning should follow the established protocols of Kontzen et al (1978). Normality/abnormality is established by comparison with the contralateral side. It is normally possible with a large field of view gamma camera to include both areas of interest; if not, joints must be scanned for the same length of time. The normal pattern of joint uptake in hands is described by Hoffer & Genant (1976).

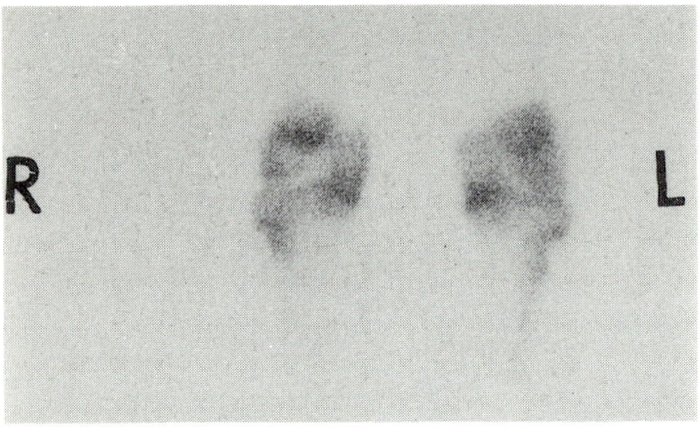

Fig. 69.10 The ^{99m}Tc MDP scan of a young man with seropositive erosive rheumatoid arthritis (feet only) and no clinical evidence of joint effusions. There is evidence of symmetrical synovitis of the knees with no focal accumulation at the sites of erosion.

Quantitative indexation of activity

Several methods of quantitating synovitis have been used but none have received general acceptance. These are as follows (Wallace et al, 1981):

1. Graph of count rates (Alarcon-Segovia et al, 1967)
2. Percentage uptake of isotope dose given (Whaley et al, 1968)
3. Rheumatoid activity index (Oka et al, 1971)
4. Highest number of counts/minute (Park et al, 1977)
5. Time to reach a specific number of counts (Green, 1979)
6. NSAID drug index (Oka et al, 1971)

$$\frac{\text{Count in hottest joint}}{\text{Background counts}}$$

7. Tc index (Cohen & Lorber, 1971)

$$\frac{\text{Count rates}}{\text{Administered dose}}$$

8. Radionuclide arthritis index (Weiss et al, 1965)

$$\frac{\text{Joint counts}}{\text{Bone counts}}$$

9. Sacroiliac (SI) index (Hays & Green, 1972)

$$\frac{\text{SI uptake}}{\text{Sacral uptake}}$$

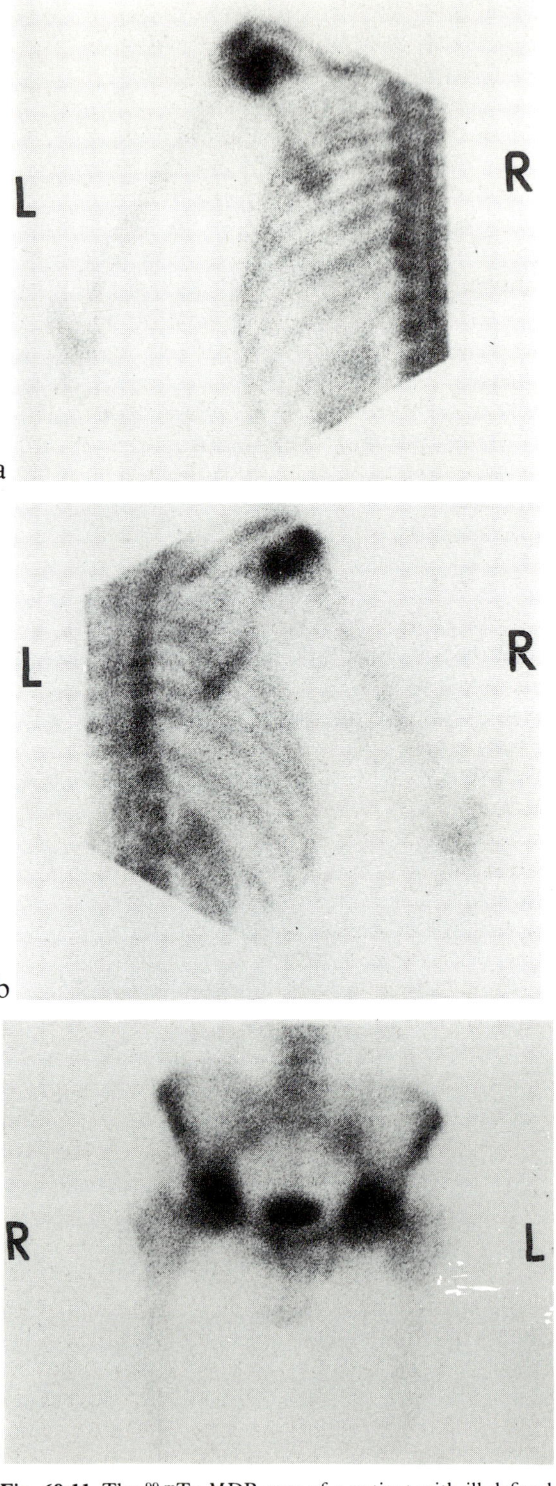

a

b

c

Fig. 69.11 The ^{99m}Tc MDP scan of a patient with ill-defined polyarticular pain, suggestive of large joint distribution, showing focal tracer accumulation in (a & b) both shoulders and (c) hips, confirming an active synovitis at these sites.

10.

$$\frac{\text{Count rate/unit area} \times \text{radiopharmaceutical dose}}{\text{Weight}}$$

(Rosenspire et al, 1980)

Rosenspire et al (1980) compared four methods of quantitating activity using a computer. The most effective measurement was quantitated counts/unit area adjusted. Despite this the conclusion was that joint inflammation could not be reliably evaluated in their rheumatoid arthritis patients.

Greyson (1979–80) has advocated the use of a combined approach to assessment — an early blood pool phase and a delayed standard bone scan for characterising arthritides as hyperaemic or non-hyperaemic.

Isotopes in drug studies

A number of studies have used scintigraphy for peripheral joint assessment progress or regress. They fall into two main groups:

1. Those that compare scanning with other techniques
2. Those that use scanning to evaluate efficacy of therapy.

The results demonstrate that scintigraphy

a. generally shows good correlation with the clinical state
b. Performed serially, compared favourably with knee X-ray examinations and synovial biopsy (Boerbooms & Buys, 1977)
c. Had comparable value to serial radiographic evaluation (Weissberg et al, 1978; Hays & Green, 1972; McCarthy et al, 1970).

The reports on its value in assessing the efficacy of the NSAIDs are confusing, three out of six finding poor correlation — usually with the shorter-acting agents.

The studies that considered the longer-acting agents are more positive. Sturrock et al (1974) showed significant alteration in the ^{99m}Tc 04 count rates in patients treated with gold and penicillamine and, in the study of Huskisson et al (1976), the scanning results were impressive in the penicillamine group.

Sacroiliac joint quantification

The sacroiliac joint remains a difficult joint to assess radiographically, particularly in the young. The possibility of a more quantitative method has been enthusiastically looked at. The value of a quantitative index, however, remains controversial, with conflicting evidence as to its value.

It is impossible to visually assess activity in the sacroiliac joints; computer comparisons are needed. The method usually employed involves comparing the peak uptake of each sacroiliac joint to the mid-sacral peak (equal areas). Background subtraction may be used to decrease the variable effect of body build, renal function, etc. The ratios thus obtained have been looked at in:

a. Normal subjects
b. Patients with known moderate and severe disease involvement
c. Those suspected of having early involvement.

Increased activity ratios have been generally reported in the cases with active erosive changes (grades 2 and 3), and normal or even decreased ratios in relation to end-stage disease (grade 4). The normal range of ratio index lies between 1.0 and 1.5, above 1.7 being considered abnormal. Namey et al (1977) consider that failure to separately analyse the sacroiliac joints and to take into account that sacroiliitis is rarely continuously active has led to the disparity in results as regards the qualitative index diagnosis of sacroiliitis.

Overlap does occur however; in the Spencer et al (1979) study, there was a large overlap with no statistically significant separation between the AS group and the controls. Dequeker et al (1978) and Berghs et al (1978) also found group separation impossible.

However, in a study of 24 patients Szanto & Lindvall (1978) found changes in 23 patients on follow-up radiographic analysis that had, on initial analysis, a normal radiograph but increased SI index. They concluded that quantitative analysis may add to the weight of evidence for an early diagnosis. Agnew et al (1982) reported a high index in 10 out of 13 patients with inflammatory bowel disease that had backache. They postulate an association with X-ray negative sacroiliitis.

Sacroiliac joint imaging is generally agreed to be less useful in the under 20 age-group. Goldberg et al (1978) reported similar indices in normal children to those in the definitely abnormal adult range.

In recent studies Snaith et al (1982) found quantitative scanning of little value in differentiating inflammatory conditions from mechanical problems associated with low back pain. In the experience of Chase et al (1983) its overall sensitivity is no greater than that of a standard radiograph and they felt its role in a clinical situation to be limited.

Spencer et al (1979) concluded that it is unlikely that scintigraphy will be of diagnostic value in the absence of improved methodology.

Role in the complications of arthritis

Joint infection complicating the inflammatory arthropathies may, if joint fluid is available and accessible, be established by simple joint aspiration. A gallium scan may be useful in the absence of direct analysis — a normal to mild local accumulation of uptake resulting from the inflammatory arthritis but an intense concentration in the presence of infection. The concept of concordant/discordant ^{99m}Tc bone scans/^{67}Ga scans is useful in analysis of possible infected or inflamed joints. Cellulitis without pyarthrosis will show a hot ^{99m}Tc blood pool image due to soft tissue hypervascularity, but the bone uptake images will be normal or only mildly increased. If there is complicating synovitis, a gallium scan may be additionally needed for assessment. Out experience with ^{111}indium-labelled white cells also indicates good correlation of focal accumulation at sites of infection.

Bone scanning is generally accepted as being the prime method of investigating osteomyelitis in both adult and child (there is some controversy over the early interpretation in the neonatal period). A hot ^{99m}Tc scan is seen within 1–3 days of the onset of infection — days to weeks before any radiographic changes may become visible. A false-negative cold scan in the acute phase, however, may result from vessel thrombosis or compression of osseous circulation by pus (Fig. 69.12). Detection of abnormality in children and young adults again depends on the comparison of symmetrical metaphyseal activity of the Tc tracer isotope. Gallium citrate sequential scans are

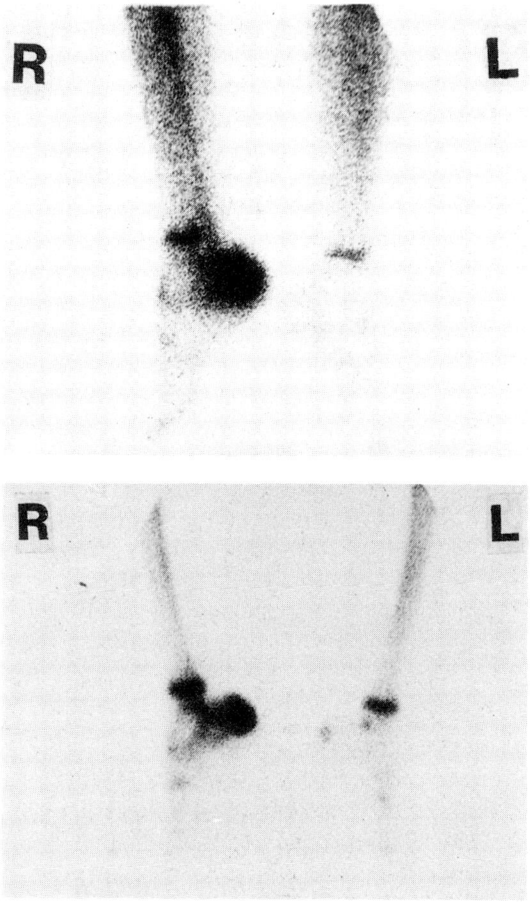

a

b

Fig. 69.12 An 11-year-old with a painful right heel and negative X-rays. (a) The early ^{99m}Tc MDP scan is 'hot', consistent with intense hyperaemia. (b) The delay scan shows focal accumulation of tracer in the calcaneum. These views, in conjunction with the negative X-rays, are those of acute calcaneal osteomyelitis. This was substantiated at surgery.

considered by some investigators to be of value, particularly in children with early blood borne infection. They may also prove to be the best indicator of disease reactivity in the presence of chronic bone changes. Due to some accumulation in reactive bone, the Gallium scan assessment is best made in conjunction with a ^{99m}Tc bone scan.

Bone infarction and aseptic necrosis

The bone infarction changes visible on X-ray represent the revascularisation stage and therefore do not reflect early change. Theoretically, bone trace isotopes should be able to reflect both (a) the early avascular phase and (b) the later hyperaemic revascularisation phase (Fig. 69.13).

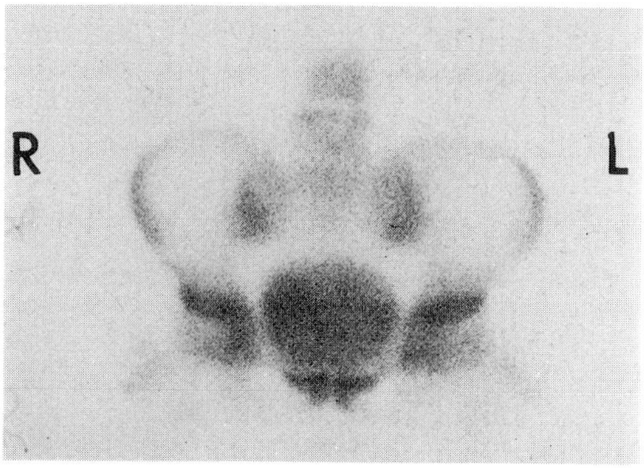

Fig. 69.13 The ^{99m}Tc MDP scan in a 13-year-old girl with seropositive juvenile rheumatoid arthritis being treated with steroids and now complaining of a painful right hip. There is a slightly reduced uptake of tracer in the right femoral head consistent with the early hypovascular phase of ischaemic necrosis. Changes consistent with revascularisation were confirmed on follow-up X-rays.

In conditions such as compromise of femoral neck blood supply by fracture, slipped epiphysis, steroid therapy, and sickle-cell disease, ^{99m}Tc scanning shows increased activity in the hip and aids in the early diagnosis of complications. However, poor specificity does not allow differentiation from coexistent active synovitis. In patients with pre-existing joint disease or in children with 'hot metaphyses' it may not, in the clinical situation, be as useful as expected. The use of high resolution collimators and multiple projection scanning is to be recommended. An alternative to the bone scanning agent technetium phosphate is *technetium sulphur colloid*. This tracer demonstrates the functional state of the marrow and is a reflection of its haemopoietic activity.

Webber et al (1977) have shown a symmetrical decrease of Tc sulphur colloid activity in about one-third of normal patients investigated, so that only asymmetrical decrease in activity can be considered significant.

In patients predisposed to both infection and infarction, e.g. sickle-cell anaemia, combined technetium and gallium scans aid diagnosis.

Back pain and crush fractures (Fig. 69.14)
Radionuclide ^{99m}Tc scanning provides the most accurate diagnosis of early disease/treatment-related osteoporotic spinal crush fractures. Activity in the involved segments will predate X-ray

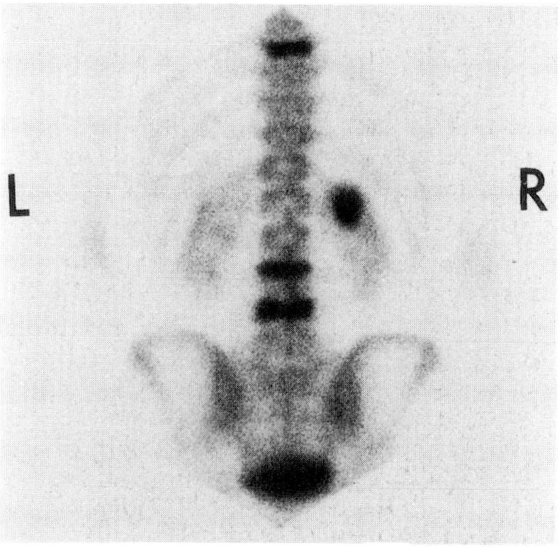

Fig. 69.14 The ^{99m}Tc MDP scan of a middle-aged man on steroids complaining of low lumbar back pain. Avid tracer accumulation at the T8, L3 and L4 levels is consistent with recent crush fractures at these sites.

changes and will aid in determining, in the presence of other accelerated vertebral body changes, what is recent (increased activity = 6/12 or less). Bone mineral analysis can be quantified using either single photon energy absorptiometry from a ^{125}I source (Lanzl & Strandjord, 1964; Cameron et al, 1968) or dual photon energy absorptiometry using a ^{153}gadolinium source (Wilson & Madsen, 1977).

Hypertrophic osteoarthropathy
Hypertrophic osteoartbropathy may present as adjacent joint pain/synovitis. It is a diametaphyseal periostitis of long bones associated with a number of conditions frequently in chest or liver. Terry et al (1975) and Rosenthall & Kirsh (1977) claim that in the early symptomatic but negative radiograph stage bone scintigraphy may be diagnostic. Characteristically a double stripe of activity may be seen, sparing the articular ends.

Reflex dystrophy syndrome
Radiographically, in a typical example (shoulder–hand) there is a spotty osteoporosis in the affected part; blood flow is theoretically increased as is bone turnover. The Tc scan substantiates this theory, showing an increased early pool or hypervascular phase as well as a generalised increase in

bone and joint activity. The history and distribution are usually diagnostic.

Salivary scintigraphy in Sjögren's syndrome and sarcoidosis

Sequential salivary scintigraphy using ^{99m}Tc sodium pertechnetate can be used to evaluate and follow the course of Sjögren's syndrome (Daniels et al, 1979). Abnormal pertechnetate uptake is usually a feature of late disease, and early involvement of the parotid glands in Sjögren's syndrome may be detected using ^{67}Ga citrate (G. Ball, J. Logic: unpublished data).

Miskin et al (1978) found salivary gland uptake of gallium in 75% of their patients with sarcoidosis. Such gallium uptake may be related to increased synthesis and deposition of lactoferrin, which has been shown to occur in parotitis (Tabak et al, 1978; Weiner et al, 1981). In another study, 9 out of 27 patients with sarcoidosis demonstrated bilateral parotid uptake (all 9 had clinically acute sarcoid) — a much higher incidence than in untreated lymphomas, Hodgkin's disease or tuberculosis (Wiener & Potal, 1979).

Lung imaging in fibrosing diseases of the lung

^{67}Gallium scanning may prove to have a useful role in the assessment of patients with inflammatory joint-associated interstitial lung disease. Niden et al (1976) found a close correlation between inflammatory activity detected by gallium and at biopsy. This may be particularly useful due to the limi-

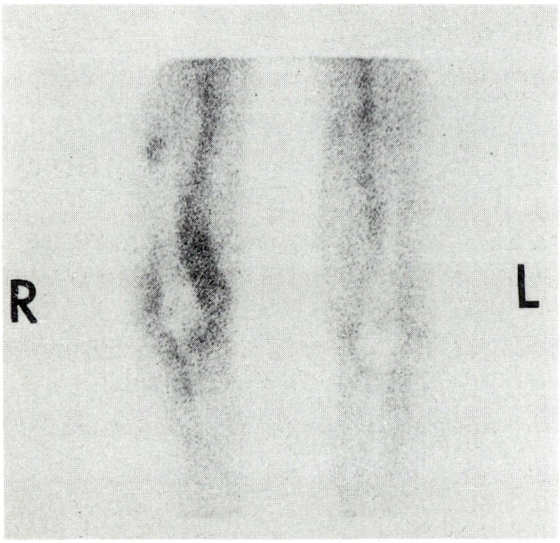

a

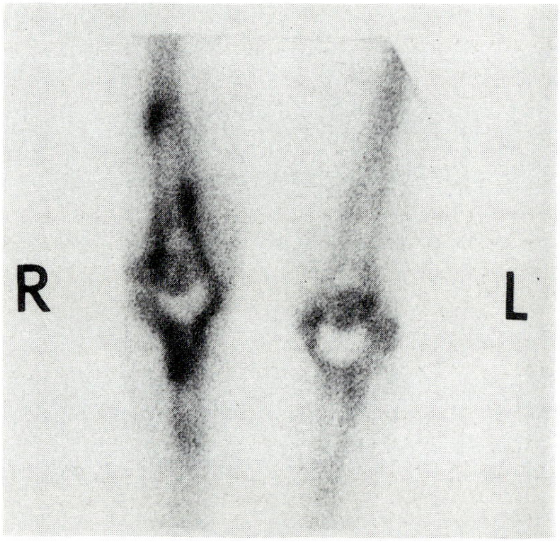

b

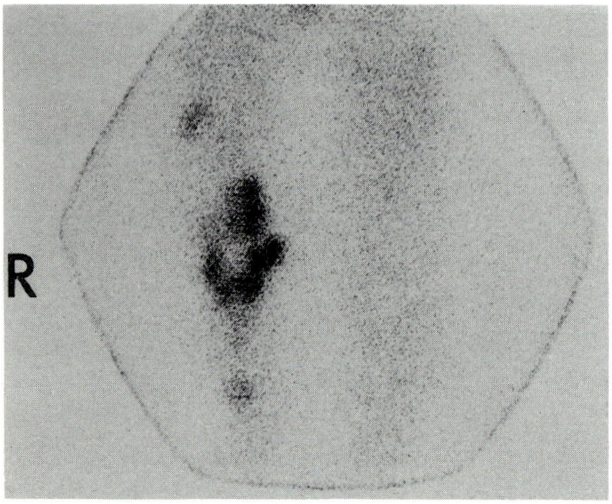

c

Fig. 69.15 (a) Hot immediate ^{99m}Tc MDP scan in patient with a painful total knee replacement (inserted approximately 1 year previously). (b) Delayed (2 hour) ^{99m}Tc MDP scan showing focal accumulation of tracer in relation to both tibial and femoral components. (c) Accumulation (at 22 hours) of ^{111}Indium-labelled white cells, confirming the diagnosis of infection.

tation of standard radiography in these circumstances. Line et al (1978) used gallium scans to evaluate the extent and relative activity of the inflammatory process in patients with idiopathic pulmonary fibrosis. They estimated the size, intensity and texture of the regional pulmonary uptake of ^{67}gallium in order to quantify the amount of pulmonary ^{67}gallium activity in the form of an index.

The index in the review group showed a significant difference from the control group and correlated well with the degree of interstitial cellularity seen on lung biopsy. Gallium scintigraphy may prove to be of value to predict these presumed inflammatory flare-ups and for monitoring the effects of therapy. Pulmonary ^{67}gallium accumulation is considered by a number of observers to be a useful index of disease activity in the follow-up of pulmonary sarcoidosis (Beaumont et al, 1982; van Unnik et al, 1983).

Joint replacement

The role of joint replacement in the management of the patient with arthritis is well established. Despite the success of these procedures, complications associated with both mechanical loosening and deep infection do arise. Radio-isotope bone imaging has been used in an attempt to differentiate between the causes of a 'painful joint'. The ^{99m}Tc scan returns to normal usually within 12 months of surgery (earlier scans would need serial assessment to be of any value). A negative ^{99m}Tc scan can be used as an effective screening method. A positive scan indicates complication — loosening or infection. Discrimination on the basis of pattern distribution has proved unreliable. A number of studies using ^{67}Ga citrate have shown the value of a positive scan in the diagnosis of infection (acceptably low false-negative and false-positive rates) (Fig. 69.15). Early results using ^{111}In-labelled white cells are also promising.

REFERENCES

Abrams H, McNeil R 1978 Medical implications of computed tomography. New England Journal of Medicine 298: 255, 310

Adams F G, Horton P W, Stenhouse G 1980 The clinical comparison of skeletal imaging agents. European Journal of Nuclear Medicine 5: 257–260

Agnew J E, Pocock D G, Jewell D P 1982 Sacroiliac joint uptake ratios in inflammatory bowel disease — relationship to back pain and to the activity of bowel disease. British Journal of Radiology 55: 821–826

Alarcon-Segovia D, Trujeque M, Tovar E, Adame M A 1967 Scintillation scanning of joints with TC^{99m}. Arthritis and Rheumatism 10:262

Alavi A, Bond J P, Kuhl D E, Grech R H 1974 Scan detection of bone marrow infarcts in sickle cell disorder. Journal of Nuclear Medicine 15: 1003–1006

Ash J M, Gilday D L 1980 The futility of bone scanning in neonatal osteomyelitis. Journal of Nuclear Medicine 21: 417–420

Barraclough D, Russell A S, Percy J S 1977 Psoriatic spondylitis: A clinical, radiological and scintiscan survey. Journal of Rheumatology, 4: 282–287

Beaumont D, Herry J Y, Le Cloirec J, Le Jeune J J, de Labarthe B 1982 Sensitivity of ^{67}Ga scanning in sarcoidosis. Detection of biopsy proven pulmonary lesions radiographically undetectable. European Journal of Nuclear Medicine 7: 41–43

Bekerman C, Genant H K, Hoffer P B, Kozin F, Ginsberg M 1975 Radionuclide imaging of the bones and joints of the hand. Radiology 118: 653–659

Berghs H, Remans J, Drieskens L, Kiebooms A, Polderman J 1978 Diagnostic value of sacroiliac joint scintigraphy with ^{99m}technetium pyrophosphate in sacroiliitis. Annals of Rheumatic Diseases 37: 190–194

Boerhooms A, Buys W 1977 Rapid assessment of ^{99m}Tc-pertechnetate uptake in the knee joint as a parameter of inflammatory activity. Arthritis and Rheumatism 20: 348–352

Boijsen E, Ekelund L 1982 Computed tomography in orthopaedic trauma. Computed tomography in orthopaedic radiology. Thieme, Stuttgart

Cameron J R, Mazess R B, Sorenson J A 1968 Precision and accuracy of bone mineral determination by direct photon absorptiometry. Investigative Radiology 3:141

Cann C E, Genant H K 1980 Precise measurement of vertebral mineral content using computed tomography. Journal of Computer Assisted Tomography 4: 493–500

Carrera G 1983 Computed tomography in sacroiliitis. Clinics in Rheumatic Diseases 9: 2 403–415

Carrera G F, Wilkins A L, Haughton V M 1980. Radiology 137: 433–437

Carrera G F, Foley W D, Ryan L M 1981 Computed tomography of sacroiliitis. American Journal of Roentgenology 136:41

Chalmers I M, Lentle B C, Percy J S, Russell A S 1979 Sacroiliitis detected by bone scintiscanning: A clinical, radiological and scintigraphic follow-up study. Annals of Rheumatic Diseases 38: 112–117

Chase W F, Houk R W, Winn R E, Hinzman G W 1983 The clinical usefulness of radionuclide scintigraphy in suspected sacroiliitis — a prospective study. British Journal of Rheumatology 22: 67–72

Cohen M, Lorber A 1971 Avoiding false positive joint scans by the use of labelled albumin. Arthritis and Rheumatism 14: 32–40

D'ambrosia R D, Shoji H, Riggins R S, Stadalnik R C,

DeNardo G L 1978 Scintigraphy in the diagnosis of osteonecrosis. Clinical Orthopaedics and Related Research 130: 139–143

Daniels T E, Powell M R, Sylvester R, Talal N 1979 An evaluation of salivary scintigraphy in Sjögren's syndrome. Arthritis and Rheumatism 22: 809–814

Davis M A, Jones A L 1976 Comparison of ^{99m}Tc-labelled phosphate and phosphonate agents for skeletal imaging. Seminars in Nuclear Medicine 6: 19–31

Davis P, Lentle B C 1978 Evidence of sacroiliac disease as a common cause of low backache in women. Lancet 2: 496–497

Davis P, Thomson A B R, Lentle B C 1978 Quantitative sacroiliac scintigraphy in patients with Crohn's disease. Arthritis and Rheumatism 21: 234–237

Dequeker J, Goddeeris T, Walravens M, DeRoo M 1978 Evaluation of sacroiliitis: Comparison of radiological and radionuclide techniques. Radiology 128: 687–690

Desaulniers M, Fuks A, Hawkins D, Lacourciere Y, Rosenthall L 1974 Radiotechnetium polyphosphate joint imaging. Journal of Nuclear Medicine 15: 417–423

Dick W C, Grennan D M 1976 Radioisotopes in the study of normal and inflamed joints. Clinics in Rheumatic Diseases 2: 67–76

Donnelly B, Johnson P M 1975 Detection of hypertrophic pulmonary osteoarthropathy by skeletal imaging with ^{99m}Tc-labelled diphosphonate. Radiology 114: 389–391

Dorwart R H, Vogler J B, Helms C A 1983 Spinal stenosis. Radiologic Clinics of North America 21: 301–325

Dorwart R H, Genant H K 1983 Anatomy of the lumbosacral spine. Radiologic Clinics of North America 21: 201–220

Dory M 1981 Arthrography of the lumbar facet joints. Radiology 140:23

Dunn E C, Ebringer R W, Ell P J 1980 Quantitative scintigraphy in the early diagnosis of sacro-iliitis. Rheumatology and Rehabilitation 19: 69–75

Duszynski D O, Kuhn J P, Afshani E, Riddlesberger M M 1975 Early radionuclide diagnosis of acute osteomyelitis. Radiology 117: 337–340

Esdaile J, Hawkins D, Rosenthall L 1979 Radionuclide joint imaging in the seronegative spondyloarthropathies. Clinical Orthopaedics and Related Research 143: 46–52

Esdaile J M, Rosenthall L, Terkeltaub R, Kloiber R 1980 Prospective evaluation of sacroiliac scintigraphy in chronic inflammatory back pain. Arthritis and Rheumatism 23: 998–1003

Fries J W, Abodeely D A 1982 Computed tomography of herniated and extruded nucleus pulposus. Journal of Computer Assisted Tomography 65: 874–887

Garcia D A, Tow D E, Kapur K K, et al 1976 Relative accretion of ^{99m}Tc-polyphosphate by forming and resorbing bone systems in rats: its significance in the pathologic basis of bone scanning. Journal of Nuclear Medicine 17: 93–97

Garnett E S, Cockshott W P, Jacobs J 1977 Classical acute osteomyelitis with a negative bone scan. British Journal of Radiology 50: 757–760

Genant H K, Kozin F, Bekerman C, McCarty D, Sims J 1975 The reflex sympathetic dystrophy syndrome. Radiology 117: 21–32

Genant N K, Chafetz N, Helm C A 1982 Computed tomography of the lumbar spine. University of California Press, San Francisco

Genant H K, Cann C E, Boyd D P, et al 1983 Quantitative computed tomography for vertebral mineral determination. Proceedings of Henry Ford Hospital Symposium on Clinical Disorders of Bone and Mineral Metabolism, Detroit

Gilday D L, Paul D J, Paterson J 1975 Diagnosis of osteomyelitis in children by combined blood pool and bone imaging. Radiology 117: 331–335

Goldberg R P, Genant H K, Shimshak R, Shames D 1978 Applications and limitations of quantitative sacroiliac joint scintigraphy. Radiology 128: 683–686

Gomez E, Green F A, Hays M T 1974 New techniques for identification of synovitis and evaluation of joint disease. Bulletin on the Rheumatic Diseases 25: 786–790

Green F A 1979 Joint scintiscans — present status. Journal of Rheumatology 6: 370–373

Greyson N D 1979–80 Radionuclide bone and joint imaging in rheumatology. Bulletin on the Rheumatic Diseases 30: 1034–1038

Handmaker H, Leonards R 1976 The bone scan in inflammatory osseous disease. Seminars in Nuclear Medicine 6: 95–103

Harcke H T 1978 Bone imaging in infants and children. A review. Journal of Nuclear Medicine 19: 324–329

Harley J D, Mack L A, Winquist R A 1982 CT of acetabular fractures: comparison with conventional radiography. Americal Journal of Roentgenology 138: 413–417

Haughton V M, Williams A L 1982 Computed tomography of the spine. Mosby, St Louis

Hayes R L 1978 The medical use of gallium radionuclides. Seminars in Nuclear Medicine 6: 183–190

Hays M T, Green F A 1972 The pertechnetate joint scan. II. Clinical correlations. Annals of Rheumatic Diseases 31: 272–277

Hernandez R J, Tachdijan M O, Poznanski A K, Dias L S 1981 CT determination of femoral torsion. American Journal of Roentgenology 137: 97–101

Ho G, Sadovinikoff N, Malhotra C M, Claunch B C 1979 Quantitative sacroiliac joint scintigraphy — a critical assessment. Arthritis and Rheumatism 22: 837–844

Hoffer P B, Genant H K 1976 Radionuclide joint imaging. Seminars in Nuclear Medicine 6: 121–137

Hoffer P B, Huberty J, Khayam-Bashi H 1977 The association of Ga 67 and lactoferrin. Journal of Nuclear Medicine 18: 713–717

Horoszowski H, Ganel A, Kamhin M, Zaltzman S, Farine I 1980 Sequential use of technetium 99mMDP and gallium 67 citrate imaging in the evaluation of painful total hip replacement. British Journal of Radiology 53: 1169–1173

Hunter J, Hattner R, Murray W, Genant H 1980 Loosening of the total knee arthroplasty — detection by radionuclide bone scanning. American Journal of Roentgenology 135: 131–136

Huskisson E C, Scott J, Balone H W 1976 Objective measurement of rheumatoid arthritis using Tc index. Annals of Rheumatic Diseases 35: 81–82

Jones D C, Cady R B 1981 'Cold' bone scans in acute osteomyelitis. Journal of Bone and Joint Surgery 63B: 376–378

Keene J S, Goletz T H, Lilleas F, et al 1982 Diagnosis of vertebral fractures — a comparison of conventional radiography, conventional tomography and computed axial tomography. Journal of Bone and Joint Surgery 64: 586–594

Kontzen F, Namey T, Tobin M, Dubovsky E, Tauxe W N 1978 Technical aspects of joint imaging. Journal of Nuclear Medicine Tech 6:110

Kozin F, Carrera G F, Ryan L M et al 1981 Computed

tomography in the diagnosis of sacroiliitis. Arthritis and Rheumatism 24:1479.
Lanzl L H, Strandjord N 1964 Radioisotope device for measuring bone mineral. Proceedings of symposium on Low Energy. X — Sources and Applications. Illinois Institute of Technology Research, Chicago
Larson S M 1978 Mechanisms of localization of gallium-67 in tumours. Seminars in Nuclear Medicine 8: 193–203
Lawson T L, Foley W D, Carrera G F, Berland L L 1982 The sacro-iliac joints, anatomic, plain roentgenographic and computed tomography analysis. Journal of Computer Assisted Tomography 6:307
Lee B C P, Kazam E, Newman A D 1978 Computed tomography of spine and spinal cord. Radiology 128: 95–102
Lentle B C, Russell A S, Percy J S, Scott J, Jackson F 1976 Bone scintiscanning updated. Annals of Internal Medicine 84: 297–303
Lentle B C, Russell A S, Percy J S, Jackson F 1977 The scintigraphic findings in ankylosing spondylitis. Journal of Nuclear Medicine 18: 524–528
Lentle B C, Russell A S, Percy J S, Jackson F 1977 The scintigraphic investigation of sacroiliac disease. Journal of Nuclear Medicine 18: 529–533
Line B R, Fulmer J D, Reynolds H Y 1978 Gallium 67 citrate scanning in the staging of idiopathic pulmonary fibrosis — correlation with physiologic and morphological features and bronchoalveolar lavage. American Review of Respiratory Disease 118: 355–365
Lisbona R, Rosenthall L 1977 Observations on the sequential use of ^{99m}Tc-phosphate complex and ^{67}Ga imaging in osteomyelitis, cellulitis and septic arthritis. Radiology 123: 123–129
McCarthy D J, Policyn R E, Collins P A, Gottschalk A 1970 ^{99m}Tc scintiphotography in arthritis. I. Technic and interpretation. Arthritis and Rheumatism 131: 21–31
Miskin F S, Tanaka T T, Niden A H 1978 Abnormal gallium scan patterns of the salivary gland in pulmonary sarcoidosis. Annals of Internal Medicine 89: 933–934
Meyers M H, Downey N T, Moore T M 1977 Determination of the vascularity of the femoral head with Tc 99 m sulphur colloid. Journal of Bone and Joint Surgery 59A: 658–664
Namey T, McIntyre J, Buse M, LeRoy E 1977 Nucleographic studies of axial spondarthritides: I. Quantitative sacroiliac scintigraphy in early HLA-B27-associated sacroiliitis. Arthritis and Rheumatism 20: 1058–1064
Namey T C, Halla J T 1978 Radiographic and nucleographic techniques in the diagnosis and management of septic arthritis and osteomyelitis. Clinics in Rheumatic Diseases 4: 95–132
Newman E F, 1983 Gallium-67 citrate scanning in orthopaedics. Journal of Bone and Joint Surgery, 65B:517
Niden A H, Miskin F S, Khurana M M 1976 Gallium 67 citrate lung scans in interstitial lung disease. *Chest* 69: 266–268
Oka M, Rokonsen A, Rutosi A 1971 Tc^{99m} in the study of systemic inflammatory activity in rheumatoid arthritis. Acta Rheumatologica Scandinavica 17: 27–30
Oren V O, Uszler J M, White J 1978 Diagnosis of uveoparotid fever by 67-Ga citrate imaging. Clinical Nuclear Medicine 3: 127–129
Park H M, Terman S A, Ridolfo A S, Wellman H N 1977 A quantitative evaluation of rheumatoid arthritic activity with Tc 99 m EHDP. Journal of Nuclear Medicine 18: 973–976
Parret J, Peyrin J O 1979 Radioisotopic investigations in salivary pathology. Clinical Nuclear Medicine 4: 250–261
Reis N D, Zinman C, Besser M I B, et al 1982 High resolution computerised tomography in clinical orthopaedics. Journal of Bone and Joint Surgery 64: 20–25
Rosenspire K C, Kennedy A C, Russomanno L, Steinbach J, Blau M, Green F A 1980 Comparison of 4 methods of ^{99m}Tc pyrophosphate uptake in rheumatoid arthritis joints. Journal of Rheumatology 7: 461–468
Rosenthall L, Kirsh J 1977 Observations on radionuclide imaging in hypertrophic pulmonary osteoarthropathy. Radiology 120: 359–362
Rothwell R S, Davis P, Lentle B C 1981 Radionuclide bone scanning in females with chronic low back pain. Annals of the Rheumatic Diseases 40: 79–82
Rushton N, Coakley A J, Tudor J, Wraight E P 1981 The value of bone and gallium scanning in the assessment of painful total hip replacements. Journal of Bone and Joint Surgery 63B: 636–637
Russell A S, Davis P, Percy J S, Lentle B C 1977 The sacroiliitis of acute Reiter's syndrome. Journal of Rheumatology 4: 293–296
Russell A S, Lentle B C, Percy J S 1975 Investigation of sacroiliac disease. Comparative evaluation of radiological and radionuclide techniques. Journal of Rheumatology 2: 45–51
Scott D L, Smith A H, Eastmond C J, Hayter C J, Wright V 1980 An evaluation of the techniques of sacroiliac scintiscanning. Rheumatology and Rehabilitation 19: 76–82
Seltzer S, Weissman B, Finberg H, Markisz J 1982 Improved diagnostic imaging in joint diseases. Seminars in Arthritis and Rheumatism 11: 315–330
Shearman J, Esdaile J, Hawkins D, Rosenthall L 1982 Predictive value of radionuclide joint scintigrams. Arthritis and Rheumatism 25: 83–86
Snaith M L, Galvin S E, Short M D 1982 The value of quantitative radioisotope scanning in the differential diagnosis of low back pain and sacroiliac disease. Journal of Rheumatology 9: 435–440.
Spencer D G, Adams F G, Horton P W, Buchanan W W 1979 Scintiscanning in ankylosing spondylitis: A clinical, radiological and quantitative radioisotope study. Journal of Rheumatology 6: 426–431
Sturrock R D, Nicholson R, Wojtulewski J A 1974 Tc counting in rheumatoid arthritis. Arthritis and Rheumatism 12: 417–420
Sullivan D C, Rosenfield N S, Ogden J, Gottschalk A 1980 Problems in the scintigraphic detection of osteomyelitis in children. Radiology 135: 731–736
Szanto E, Lindvall N 1978 Quantitative ^{99m}Tc pertechnetate scanning of the sacro-iliac joints: A follow-up study of patients with suspected sacroiliitis. Scandinavian Journal of Rheumatology 7: 93–96
Tabak L, Mandel I D, Karlan D, et al 1978 Alterations in lactoferrin in salivary gland disease. Journal of Dental Research 57: 43–47
Teplick J G, Haskin M E 1983 CT and lumbar disc herniation. Radiologic Clinics of North America 21: 259–288
Terry D W, Isitman A T, Holmes R A 1975 Radionuclide bone images in hypertrophic pulmonary osteoarthropathy. American Journal of Roentgenology 124: 571–576
Thomas R H, Resnick D, Alazraki N P, Daniel D, Greenfield R, 1975 Compartmental evaluation of osteoarthritis of the knee: A comparative study of

available modalities. Radiology 116: 585–594

Tsau M, Chen W, Scheffel U, Wagner H N 1978 Studies on gallium accumulation in inflammatory lesions. I. Gallium uptake by human polymorphonuclear leucocytes. Journal of Nuclear Medicine 19: 36–43

Ullrich C G, Binet E F, Sanecki M G, 1980 Quantitative assessment of the lumbar spinal canal by computed tomography. Radiology 134: 137–143

Van Unnik J G, van Royen E A, Alberts C, van der Schoot J B 1983 A method of quantitative ^{67}Ga scintigraphy in the evaluation of pulmonary sarcoidosis. European Journal of Nuclear Medicine 8: 351–353

Wallace D J, Brachman M, Klinenberg J R 1981 Joint scanning in rheumatoid arthritis — a literature review. Seminars in Arthritis and Rheumatism 11: 172–176

Webber M M, Wagner J, Gragin M D 1977 Radionuclide patterns of femoral head disease. International Journal of Nuclear Medicine and Biology 4: 167–177

Weiner R, Hoffer P B, Thakur M R 1981 Lactoferrin: its role as a Ga^{67} protein in polymorphonuclear leukocytes. Journal of Nuclear Medicine 22: 32–37

Weiss T, Maxfield W, Murison P, Hidalgo J 1965 Iodinated human serum albumin (I^{131}) localization studies of rheumatoid arthritis joints by scintillation scanning. Arthritis and Rheumatism 8:976–987

Weiss T E, Shuler S E 1974 Joint imaging as a clinical aid in diagnosis and therapy of arthritic and related diseases. Bulletin on the Rheumatic Diseases 25: 791–793

Weissberg D L, Resnick D, Taylor A, Becker M, Alazraki N 1978 Rheumatoid arthritis and its variants: Analysis of scintiphotographic, radiographic, and clinical examinations. American Journal of Roentgenology 131: 665–673

Whaley K, Pack A I, Boyle J A, et al 1968 The articular scan in patients with rheumatoid arthritis — a possible method of quantitating joint inflammation using radiotechnetium. Clinical Science 35: 547–552

Wiener S N, Patel B P 1979 ^{67}Ga-citrate uptake by the parotid glands in sarcoidosis. Radiology 130: 753–755

Williams F, McCall I W, Park W, O'Connor B, Morris V 1981 Gallium scanning in the painful total hip replacement. Clinical Radiology 32: 431–439

Williamson B R J, McLaughlin R E, Wang C J, Miller C W, Teates C D, Bray S T 1979 Radionuclide bone imaging as a means of differentiating loosening and infection in patients with a painful total hip prosthesis. Radiology 133: 723–726

Wilson C R, Madsen 1977 Dichromatic absorptiometry of vertebral body mineral content. Investigative Radiology 12:180

Index

Entries in italic type denote pages where illustrations appear; entries in bold type indicate a complete chapter on the subject.

Abdomen, physical examination 1574
Achilles tendon
  lesions 1474
  peritendinitis 1474
  rupture 1474
  tendinitis, injection technique 1619
Achondroplasia 1172–1173, *1173*
Acne arthritis 1239
Acquired immune deficiency syndrome (AIDS) 1199
Acromegalic arthropathy
  association with hypertrophic arthropathy 966
  backache 961
  clinical features 960
  compression neuropathies 962
  limb arthropathy 961–962
  neuromuscular manifestations 963
  pathology 963–965
  radiology 966–967
  treatment 966–967
Acromegaly 960
  association with osteoarthrosis 851–852
Acromioclavicular joint, osteoarthrosis 864
Acropachy, thyroid 1253, 1457
Acrosclerosis 1367
ACTH (Corticotrophin) 544–545
  see also Corticosteroids
  in acute gout 921
  in juvenile chronic arthritis 1114
  in rheumatic fever 1088
Acthar Gel, in juvenile chronic arthritis 1116, *1116*
Actinomyces bovis 1153
Acute anterior uveitis 727–728
Addresses, of organisations associated with rehabilitation 1517
Adductor origin, strain 1458
Adenine phosphoribosyltransferase (APRT) 904
Adenohypophysis 959–960
Adenoviral arthritis 1151
AIDS 1199
Aids, rehabilitation 1504–1514
Albers-Schoenberg disease (osteopetrosis) 999–1000
Alcohol, associations with
  gout and hyperuricaemia 915
  hypertriglyceridaemia 196
  osteonecrosis 1223
Alkaptonuria, and osteoarthrosis 853
Allopurinol 569–574
  in gout, long term management 922–924, *924*
Alopecia, in systemic lupus erythematosus 1327
American Rheumatism Association (ARA) 16, 34
Amoebic dysentery, arthritis 1146
Amyloid
  constituents 1024–1025
  definition 1024–1025
  fibril
    degradation 1040–1041
    deposition 1039–1041
    formation 1039–1040
    proteins and their precursors 1031
  importance 1025–1026
  pathogenesis of effects 1041
  P component 1036–1039
  senile 1030
Amyloidosis 691–692, **1024 – 1053**
  addendum (1985) 1044–1045
  in ankylosing spondylitis 752
  association with
    immunocyte dyscrasia, monoclonal protein amyloidosis 1028–1029
    causes 1028
    clinical features 1028–1029
    prevalence 1029
  clinical syndromes 1026–1030
  diagnosis 1041–1043
    biopsy 1041–1043
  familial Mediterranean fever 1029
  heredofamilial systemic 1029
  in juvenile chronic arthritis 1109
  leukaemia 1194–1195
  localised 1029–1030
  management 1043–1044
  in psoriatic arthritis 779
  in pyrophosphate arthropathy 944
  in rheumatoid arthritis 638
  systemic 1029
    associations 1027
    causes 1027
    clinical features 1027–1028
    reactive 1027
Anabolic steroids, in juvenile chronic arthritis 1116
ANA-negative lupus 1335
Anaphylactoid (Henoch-Schönlein) purpura 1235–1236
  abdominal pain 1235–1236
  association with familial Mediterranean fever 1235
  clinical features 1235
  joint involvement 1236
  pathology 1235
  sex incidence 1235
  treatment 1236
Angioimmunoblastic lymphadenopathy 1195–1196
  lymph node histology 1195
  rheumatic features 1195
  treatment 1196
Ankle
  see also Achilles tendon
  arthroscopy 1604–1605
  bursitis 1474
  calcaneal ephphysis 1474
  examination 1578–1579
  injection technique 1619–1620
  ligamentous injuries 1474
  osteoarthrosis 868
  surgery 1534–1535
  'weak ankle' 1474
Ankylosing hyperostosis (Forestier's disease) *764*
  epidemiology 97–98
  osteoarthrosis 859–860
Ankylosing spondylitis 321–322, 429–430, **745 – 774**
  aetiology 760–762
  association with Crohn's disease, ulcerative colitis, Whipple's disease 762
  see also Crohn's disease, ulcerative colitis, Whipple's disease
  axial tomography 757
  back pain 1429
  bone and joint changes, other than spine 756–757
  clinical features 747–750
  complications 751–752

Ankylosing spondylitis *cont*
amyloidosis 752
central nervous system 751–752
heart disease 751
iritis 751
pulmonary 752
treatment 752
course 762–763
Crohn's disease 808–810
definition 745
diagnostic criteria 745–746, *745*
differential diagnosis 764–765
from ankylosing hyperostosis *764*
enthesopathy of insertion of patellar tendon 1466, *1467*
epidemiology 70–72
genetic factors 760–761
genitourinary infection 761–762
hip replacement 1542
historical background 746
intubation 1524
irradiation 767
laboratory findings 759–760
HLA-B27 760
T-cells 760
levamisole therapy 562
management 765–768
appliances 765
patients' handbook 765
physical measures 765
medication 766
nomenclature 745
pathogenesis 760–762
pathology 757–759
apophyseal ankylosis 758
peripheral arthritis 756
physical signs 747–750
chest and spinal rigidity 747–749
extra-articular bony tenderness 749
peripheral joint involvement 749–750
posture 750, *750*
physical treatment 765
exercise 1495
prevalence 746–747
prognosis 762–763
scintigraphy 757
spine 1547
indications for osteotomy 1547
summary 768
surgery 767–768
therapeutic evaluation 1593
ulcerative colitis 811–813
Whipple's disease 814
Annulus fibrosus 1409, *1409*
Anterior tibial compartment 1471–1472
Antibodies 365–70, 394
see also Autoantibodies
Antigens
see also Immune complexes
Anti-malarial drugs **525 – 534**
chloroquine 528–530
in juvenile chronic arthritis 1117–1118
in SLE 1343
Antinuclear antibodies
see also Immune complexes
in SLE 1337, *1337*
Apatite arthritis 945–946
Aponeuroses 219
Apophyseal joint
involvement in ankylosing spondylitis 756, *756*
Apophyseal osteoarthrosis 1416–1418
Appliances
in ankylosing spondylitis 765
rehabilitation 1504–1514
Apprentice's foot 1476
Arachnoiditis 1423
Arborviruses 1151–1152
Arteritis
giant cell 1278–1291
granulomatous *1305*
large vessel 1316
polymyalgia rheumatica 1278–1291
Takayasu's 1316–1317
temporal **1278 – 1291**, 1316, 1440–1441
Arthralgia, menopausal 986
Arthritis
acne 1239
acute
clostridium difficile colitis 1146
suppurative 1137–1139
adenoviral 1151
in adolescents, advice 1515
apatite 945–946
associated microbial infections 443–447
classification *444*, *446*
carcinoma 1251
cervical 622
in childhood 1125–1133, *1125*
see also Juvenile Chronic Arthritis
connective tissue disorders, rarer 1131–1132
dermatomyositis 1131
familial Mediterranean fever 1132
mixed connective tissue disease 1131
Raynaud's phenomenon 1131–1132
sarcoidosis 1132
SLE 1131
juvenile psoriatic arthritis 1130–1131
HLA–B27 1130
incomplete Reiter's syndrome 1130
reactive arthritis 164, 166, 169–170, 322, 428–429, 728
juvenile spondylitis 1127–1130
complications 1129
course 1129
diagnosis 1129
drugs 1129
family history 1129
HLA–B27 1129
inflammatory bowel disease 1130
investigations 1129
iridocyclitis 1128
management 1129
onset 1127
radiology 1127–1129
sex ratio 1127
surgery 1129
seropositive juvenile arthritis 1125–1127
complications 1126
disease progression 1126
management 1126
onset 1125
pattern 1125
sex distribution 1125
spondyloarthropathies 1127–1130
complications, radionuclide imaging 1636
Crohn's disease 806–808
deformans *see* Osteoarthrosis
differential diagnosis 161–164
dysentery, bacillary 1146
enteric infections 1145–1146
enteropathic 808–818
experimental, animal models **468 – 485**, *468*
see also Experimental arthritis
gonococcal 1139–1140
gut infection 815–816
association with arthritis *815*
haemochromatosis 952–956
infective 1137–1161
inflammatory
intestinal bypass surgery 814–815, 1241
aetiology 814–815
treatment 815
shoulder 1444
lepromatous 1145
Lyme 1149–1150
lymphosarcomatous 1251
meningococcal 1140–1141
in mixed connective tissue disease 1271–1272
mumps 1151
in ochronosis 950–952
psoriatic 775–786
juvenile 1130–1131
reactive 164, 166, 169–170, 173, 322, 428–429, 728
campylobacter jejuni 1146
yersinia enterocolitica 1146
rubella 1150–1151
in single weight-bearing joint 1515–1516
in Sjögren's syndrome 1392–1393
smallpox 1152
surgical treatment 1518–1565
see also Surgery
tuberculous 1142–1144
Wilson's disease 956
Arthritis and blood disease **1177 – 1206**
complement 397–404, 1202
cryoglobulinaemia 1197–1198
deficiency 400–401, *1202*
haemoglobinopathies 1185–1191
haemophilia 1177–1185
hyperviscosity syndrome 1199
immune complex disease 1198
see also Immune complexes
immune deficiency 1199–1201
iron overload arthropathy 1191
leukaemia 1191–1196
lipid dermatoarthritis 1196–1197
multicentric reticulohistocytosis 1196–1197
clinical features 1196
course 1197

Arthritis and blood disease *cont*
purpura, hypogammaglobulinaemic 1199
thrombocytosis 1185
Arthritis and Rheumatism Council 15
Arthrocentesis 259
Arthrodesis 1531
elbow 1550
fingers 1559
hand/wrist 1559
in osteoarthrosis 879
Arthrography 1607–1608
double contrast 1607
single contrast 1607
ultrasonic examination 1607, 1608
xeroradiography 1607
Arthropathy
acromegalic 960–976
associated with non-articular neoplastic disease 1250–1251
chronic subluxing (Jaccoud's) 5
hypertrophic 1251–1253, 1475
in hypothyroidism 969–970
inflammatory 1229–1241
iron overload 1191
pyrophosphate 938–949
shoulder 1447
Arthroplasty
criteria 1530–1531
elbow 1550
fingers 1557–1559
hand/wrist 1557–1559
hinge replacement 1537–1538
complications *1538*
non-linked total knee replacement 1538–1539
replacement in osteoarthrosis 878
Arthroscopy 1597–1607
appearances
crystal synovitis 1606–1607
degenerative joint disease of knee internal derangement 1606–1607
inflammatory synovitis 1605–1606
physiological variations 1605
pigmented villonodular synovitis 1606
rheumatoid synovitis 1606
comparison with arthrotomy 1597–1598
examination technique
ankle 1604–1605
elbow 1604
hip 1605
knee joint 1599–1604
metacarpophalangeal joints 1605
fibreoptic arthroscope 1597, *1597, 1598*
historical background 1597
surgery 1535–1604
value and uses
assessment of extent of cartilage or synovial disease 1599
complications 1599
investigation of internal derangement of knee 1598–1599
non-arthritis 1598–1599
operative 1599
as research tool 1599
synovial biopsy 1598
therapeutic benefit 1599
Arthrotomy
comparison with arthroscopy 1597–1598
Articular indices 1591
Articular tumours 1241–1253
(or para-articular)
arising from bone/cartilage 1246
arthropathies associated with non-articular neoplastic disease 1250–1251
carcinoma arthritis 1251
lymphosarcomatous arthritis 1251
secondary neoplastic deposits 1251
benign 1244
developmental defects
diaphyseal aclasis 1246–1247, *1247*
enchondromatosis 1246, *1246*
differential diagnosis 1241
malignant neoplasms 1247–1250
chondrosarcoma 1247
fibrosarcoma 1247
giant cell tumours 1247
osteo-sarcoma 1247, *1248*
reticulum-cell sarcoma 1247
secondary neoplastic deposits 1244
synovioma 1244–1246
melanotic sarcoma 1246
myeloma 1247–1248, *1248*
osteoid osteoma 1248–1250, *1250*
pathological classification 1241
synovial chondromatosis 1241–1242
terminology *1242*
synovial chondrosarcoma 1246
Aschoff 6
Aschoff nodules 1066, *1066*
Aseptic necrosis
see also osteonecrosis 1207–1228
bone 837–838
leading to osteoarthritis 849, *850*
Legg-Perthes disease 851
radionuclide imaging 1636–1637
Aspergillosis 1153
Aspirin
see also Salicylates **500 – 513**
drug interactions 508
intra-articular injection 587
preparations 509
in SLE 1343
Asymptomatic hyperuricaemia 925–926
Atrial myxoma 1259
Attachment proteins 187–190
chondronectin 190
fibronectin 187–189
laminin 189–190
lubricating glycoprotein 190
Auranofin 530
side-effects 532
Auricular ankylosis 622
Autoantibodies 355–371
antibodies against nuclear antigens 362–366, *363*
clinical incidence of positive tests 364–366
specificities *364*
anti-cartilage antibodies 369
anti-collagen antibodies 369
anti-DNA antibodies 366–368
methods of detection 367–368
anti-dsDNA antibodies 368
clinical incidence 368
antiglobulins 356–362
anti-intermediate filament antibodies 370
anti-keratin antibodies 370
anti-perinuclear factor 370
anti-salivary duct antibody 370
assays, comparison *368*
lymphocytotoxic 368–369
rheumatoid factors 356–362
and complement activation 361–362
raised levels, incidence in rheumatoid disease 360–361
Autoimmune reactions 343
Avascular necrosis 1459
see also Osteonecrosis **1207 – 1228**
sickle cell disease 1188
Axial osteomalacia 1019
Azapropazone 521–522
in management of gout 921
Azathioprine 547–554

Bacillary dysentery arthritis 1146
Back pain
arachnoiditis 1423
classification 1411
causes *1411*
coccygeal pain 1427
disc degeneration
influence of geometric factors 1410
radiology 1407, *1407*
disc disorders 1407–1434
DISH 1428
early treatment 1427
epidemiology 99–104
exposure to cold and damp 1425
fibrositic nodules 1424
fibrositis 1424
fractures 1422–1423
frequency *1407*
inflammatory 1429
infection 1429
polymyalgia rheumatica 1429
rheumatoid arthritis 1429
seronegative spondylopathies 1429
local anaesthetic and steroid injection 1416
loose back syndrome 1424
lumbosacral pain 1411–1426
apophyseal osteoarthrosis 1416–1418
congenital abnormalities 1422
investigations 1414–1416
appearance 1416
CAT scanning 1416
conventional radiography 1414
discography 1415–1416
epidural myelography 1415
injection 1415
myelography 1414
nuclear magnetic resonance 1416

Back pain *cont*
pain production 1416
radiculography 1415
vertebral venography 1415
lumbar nerve roots, identification of sites, principal changes used *1413*
lumbar spondylosis 1416–1418
posture 1414
prolapsed intervertebral disc 1411
referred pain 1413–1414
Schmorl's nodes 1412, *1413*
lumbosacral strain 1424
magnitude of problem 1407
management 1425–1426
metabolic bone disease 1430–1431
neoplasms 1429–1430
nerves 1411, *1411*
non-specific low back pain 1423–1425
nucleus pulposus, variations of pressure 1410, *1410*
occupational factors 1408
Paget's disease 1430
posture 1424
pre-employment screening 1427
prevalence 1408
prevention 1426–1427
limitation of load bearing lift/strength rating 1426–1427
manual handling techniques 1427
posture 1427
radionuclide scanning 1637
referred pain 1431
sacroiliac strain 1424
Scheuermann's osteochondritis 1427–1428
Schmorl's nodes 1412, *1413*
sciatica 1413
sciatic scoliosis 1414, *1414*
spinal stenosis 1418–1420
causes *1419*
diagnosis 1420
management 1420
spine, structure and function 1408–1411
spondyolisthesis
association with lumbar spondylosis 1421
degenerative 1421–1422
spondyolysis 1420
spondylolytic spondylolisthesis 1422
spondylosis 1407–1434
'stuck' back 1424
treatment 1425–1426
Bacteria
see also infections, bacterial 1137–1145
Baillou, Guillaume de 4–5, *4*
Baker's cysts 669, 1465–1466, *669*
in hypermobile subjects 1168
Balanitis, of Reiter's disease 791–792, *792*
Bamboo spine 754, *754*
Basement membranes 215–217, *215*
chondronectin 217
fibronectin 216
laminin 216
B-cells 273, 310–313, 336–337
see also immune response, immunogenetics
autoimmune reactions 344
immune deficiency 1199
Sjögren's syndrome 1398–1399
synovial disease 607, 613
Behçet's disease 324, 1231–1235
arthritis 1233, 1234, *1234*
associations 1233
classification 1232–1233, *1232*
possible manifestations 1232–1233
diagnosis 1232
epidemiology 81
family history 1231
forms 1232
histology 1235
HLA 1233
immunological disturbance 1231
joints affected *1234*
levamisole therapy 562
prevalence 1233
treatment 1235
Benign intracranial hypertension 537
Benorylate 509
Biochemistry of conective tissue
see also Connective tissue **177 – 198**
Biomechanics 231
Blastomycosis, North American 1153–1154
Blood
see also Arthritis and blood disease **1177 – 1206**
abnormalities in SLE 1334
AIDS 1199
complement deficiency and rheumatic disease 1202, *1202*
cryoglobulinaemia 1197–1198
haemoglobinopathies 1185–1191
haemophilia 1177–1185, *1177*
hypergammaglobulinaemia purpura 1199
hyperviscosity syndrome 1199
hypogammaglobulinaemia 1199–1200
immune complex disease 1198
immune deficiency 1199–1201
iron overload arthropathy 1191
leukaemia 1191–1196
thrombocytosis 1185, *1186*
Bloodhound facies 1166
Blount's disease 1212
Bone
aseptic necrosis 837–838
Brittle Bones Society 1003
disease 612–622
dysplasias *998*
calcitonin 229
cancellous 227
collagen 227
compact 227
constitutional diseases, international nomenclature *998*
formation 227
hormonal control of metabolism 994–997
infarction, radio nuclide imaging 1636–1637
lamellar 227
metabolic bone disease **992 – 1023**
ageing 992–994
axial osteomalacia 1019
back pain 1130–1131
bone dysplasias 997, *998*
constitutional diseases, international nomenclature *998*
primary metabolic abnormalities *997*
endocrine disorders 987
fibrodysplasia ossificans progressiva 1019
fibrogenesis imperfecta ossium 1018
growth 992–994
heterotopic ossification 1019
hypophosphatasia 1001
infarction, radionuclide imaging 1636–1637
metabolism, hormonal control 994–997, *995*
multiple epiphyseal dysplasia 998–999, *999*
myositis ossificans progressiva 1019
osteogenesis imperfecta 1001–1003
proposed nomenclature *1002*
osteopetrosis 999–1000
osteoporosis 1004–1008, *1006*
oestrogren replacement therapy 1008
Paget's disease 1016–1018
parathyroid disorders 1014–1015
chondrocalcinosis 1015
diagnosis 1015
hypoparathyroidism 1015–1016
osteitis fibrosa 1014
primary hyperparathyroidism 1014–1015
rickets and osteomalacia 1008–1004, *1009*
biochemical changes 1012–1013, *1013*
vitamin D therapy 1013–1014
turnover 992–994
van der Hoeve's triad 1003
osteitis fibrosa 1014
osteocollagen 227
osteogenesis imperfecta 1001–1003
osteomalacia 1008–1014, *1009, 1013*
osteoporosis 1004–1008, *1006*
Paget's disease 1016–1018
parathormone 229
parathyroid disorders 1014–1015
primary metabolic abnormalities *997*
rickets 1008–1014, *1009, 1013*
vitamin D 229
woven bone 227
Bouchard's nodes 861, *863*
Boutonnière finger deformities, surgery 1559–1560, *1559*
British Association of Physical Medicine 16
British Association for Rheumatology and Rehabilitation (BARR) 16
British Council for Rehabilitation of the Disabled 15
British League Against Rheumatism 15
British Rheumatism and Arthritis Association 15
British Society for Rheumatology 16

Brittle Bones Society 1003
Brucellosis 1141–1142
Bunion 1477
Bursae
  injection techniques 1619
    infrapatellar 1619
    suprapatellar 1619
  surgical excision 1549
Bursitis
  acute calcific 1442, *1443*
  chronic 1442
  effusions 1450
  iliopsoas 1459
  infrapatellar 1465
  injection technique, supratrochanteric 1618
  olecranon 1450
  retrocalcaneal 1474
  semimembranous 1465
  student's elbow 1450
  treatment 1450
  trochanteric 1465
  water on the elbow 1450

Calcaneal epiphysitis 1474
Calcaneal spur 1475
Calcific tendonitis 165, *165*
Calcification,
  acute, in knee 1467
Calcitonin 229
Calcium pyrophosphate crystal deposition 857, 859, 938–949
Calcospherites 839–840, *840*
Calve's disease 1212
Campylobacter jejuni arthritis 1146
Candida infections 1155
Caplan's syndrome 681
Carcinoma arthritis 1251
Cardiac disease, in rheumatoid arthritis 627–630
Carpal tunnel syndrome 172, 1125, 1194
  in acromegalic arthropathy 967
  frequency in rheumatoid arthritis 1451
  in hypothyroidism 968
  injection technique 1615–1616, *1616*
    complications 1616
  management 1450–1451
  in myeloma 1248
  in rubella arthritis 1150
Cartilage
  age changes 225
  angiogenesis factors 223
  blood vessels 223
  destruction in rheumatoid arthritis 615–618
  fibrillation
    age factor 824–825
    nature 825–831
    pathology 831–833
  growth 221
  immunity 224
  mechanics 223–224
  neoplastic 222
  proteoglycans
    function 193–194
    structure 190–192
  thickness 225
  transplantation 224–225
CAT scanning in back pain 1416
Catabolin 223, 234, 617
Cat-scratch fever 1153
Cauda equina syndrome, axial tomography 757
Central nervous system disease in SLE 1333–1334
Cephalosporium 1155
Cervical spine 1435–1441
  anatomical relationships *1435*
  disease in rheumatoid arthritis 1545–1546
  examination 1575
  intubation 1524
  surgery 1545–1546
Charcot's joints 975, 1147, *1147*
  associated conditions 1253
  destructive arthropathy 1254
  in leprosy 1145
  radiology 1253–1254
  tabes dorsalis 1254
  treatment 1254
Cheiroarthropathy, diabetic 979–980, *979*
Chest, physical examination 1574
Chickenpox arthritis 1151
Chikungunya virus 1151–1152
Chilblains 1478
Children, therapeutic evaluation, 1593–1594
Chlorambucil 547–554
Chloroquine 528–530
  clinical experience 528–529
  pharmacological properties 528
  side-effects 529–530
  therapeutic usage 529
Choline magnesium trisalicylate 510
Chondrocalcinosis
  see also pyrophosphate arthropathy 938–949, *941*
  acromegalic arthropathy 966
  asymptomatic 942
  epidemiology 79
  gout 944
Chondrocytes 203, *203*
  acromegalic arthropathy 963, *964*
  enzyme activity 205
  growth 205
  respiratory activity 205
Chondromalacia patellae 1463–1464
Chondronectin 190, 217
Chondroprotective compounds, in treatment of osteoarthrosis 877
Chondrosarcoma 1247
Chorea 1078–1081, 1131
  see also rheumatic fever
  complications 1080–1081
  differential diagnosis 1079
  relapse 1080–1081, *1080*
  symptoms 1079
  treatment 1081
Christmas disease 1177, *1177*
Chronic subluxing arthropathy (Jaccoud's) 5
Chronopharmacology, in clinical trials 1583
Class III loci (C4, C2, Factor B) 316–317
Claw-foot 1476–1477
Clergyman's knee 1465
Clinical trials **1581 – 1596**
  analgesics, simple 1584–1585
    design of studies, three-way crossover *1584*
  anti-inflammatory drugs 1585–1586
    design of studies, short-term parallel group *1585*
  articular indices 1591
  chronopharmacology 1583
  design 1581–1584
    aims 1581
    anti-rheumatic drugs, classification *1581*
    programme *1582*
    protocol, how to write 1582
  dolorimeter 1591
  inflammation
    infra-red thermography 1591–1592
    objective measurements 1591
    technetium index 1592
  measurements
    Arthritis Impact Measurement Scale 1591
    articular index 1590–1591
    composite indices 1593
    disease severity 1590–1592
    functional 1591–1592
    grip strength 1590–1591
    indirect methods 1589–1590
    inflammation 1590–1591
    laboratory 1592
    McMaster Health Index Questionnaire 1591
    number 1593
    pain
      graphic rating 1589, *1589*
      other methods 1589
      relief, methods 1589
      simple descriptive scale 1588
      visual analogue scale 1588–1589
    range 1587–1594, *1587*
    side-effects 1594
    Standard Health Assessment Questionnaire 1591
    stiffness 1590
    swelling 1590
    tenderness 1590–1591
    toxicity 1594
  open trials 1584
  outcome 1584
  pharmacokinetics 1584
  pilot trials 1584
  post-marketing surveillance 1587
  progression, radiological 1592–1593
  slow acting drugs, design of studies 1586–1587, *1586*
  slowly appearing phenomena (e.g. toxicity) 1586–1587, *1586*
  statistics 1594
    interpretation 1595
  therapeutic evaluation

Clinical trials *cont*
ankylosing spondylitis 1593
children 1593–1594
gout 1593
osteoarthrosis 1593
treatment other than drugs 1594
uncontrolled trials 1584
Clostridium difficile colitis arthritis 1146
Clutton's joints, 1147, 1238–1239
Coalminer's 'beat knee' 1465
Coccidiomycosis 1154
Coccygeal pain 1427
Colchicine 522–523
in management of acute gout 921
Cold
physical treatment 1494
Colitis
clostridium difficile arthritis 1146
Collagen 178–186, 210–212, *211*
biosynthesis 182, *182*
degradation 185–186
structure 178–182
Complement 397–404
in absence of immunoglobulin 404
activation 397–398
in arthritis and blood disease 1202
binding, of immune complexes 379–380
biological activities 399–400, *399*
C3a, C5 generation 400
deficiency
as acquired abnormality 400–401
genetic determination; predisposition to disease 401
deficiency and rheumatic disease 1202, *1202*
arthritis symptoms 1202
investigations 1202
other diseases 404
polyarteritis nodosa 404
rheumatoid arthritis 403–404
serological findings 1202
SLE 402–403
treatment 1202
vasculitis 404
deposits in tissues in absence of immunoglobulin 404
immune precipitates, solubilisation 400
interaction with receptors 399–400
measurement
hypercatabolism 402
methods 401
in rheumatic diseases 401–402
tissue fixation 402
pathways 397–398, *398*
role in clearance of immune complexes 383
sequence 397–399
Computerised axial tomography (CAT scanning) in back pain 1416
Computerised tomography (CT) 1627–1632
disorders of spine
disc herniation 1627
facet joints 1628–1629
spinal stenosis 1629
femoral anteversion 1631–1632
quantitative bone mineral analysis 1632
sacroiliitis 1627
soft tissue lesions 1631
trauma 1630–1631
Connective tissue
adipose 219
biochemistry 177–197
attachment proteins 187–190
cartilage proteoglycan structure 190
chondronectin 190
collagen 178–186
biosynthesis 182–185, *182*
degradation 185–186
structure 178–182
elastin 186–187
fibronectin 187–189
glycosaminoglycans 190
laminin 189–190
lubricating glycoprotein 190
proteoglycans 190
biosynthesis by chondrocytes 192–193
dermatan sulphate 194–195
function in cartilage 193–194
heparan sulphate 195
hyaluronate 194
compact 219
elastic 219
fibrofatty 219
juxta-articular 620
loose 218–219
Connective tissue diseases in childhood 1131–1132
Connective tissue and joints
structure and function **199 – 250**
aponeuroses, ligaments, tendons 219–220
articular surfaces 235–239
basement membranes 215, *215*
bone 227–229
cartilage 220–227
cells 207–210
chondrocytes 203, *203*
enzyme activity 205
growth 205
osteo blasts 205
osteoclasts 206
osteocytes 207
collagen 210–212, *211*
comparative anatomy 200–201
elastic material 212–215
fibres 210
reticular 215
histiocytes 210
joint capsule fascia 218–219
labra intra-articular discs, menisci 220
lubrication 239–241
non-fibrillar extracellular matrix 217
organised connective tissue 218–219
symphyses 241–244
synovial joints 232
synovial tissue 232
synovium, effect on cartilage catabolin 233–235
units of structure and function 201
Contraceptive pill
rheumatic symptoms 986–987
Corticosteroids 535–545
acute gout, management 921
benign intracranial hypertension 537
corticotrophin (ACTH) 544–545
local treatment 545
drug interaction 537–538
in rheumatic diseases 538
intra-articular injections 584–586
in juvenile chronic arthritis 1114
metabolism 535
osteonecrosis, role in aetiology 1219–1220
physical treatment 1495
potency *536*
side-effects 537–544
gastrointestinal 541–542
growth, impairment 543–544
hypothalamo-pituitary adrenal axis 542–543
osteonecrosis 542
osteoporosis 542
skin atrophy 542
in SLE 1343–1344
synthetic 535–536
treatment
dermatomyositis 540
Felty's syndrome 539
giant cell arteritis 540
other conditions 521
polyarteritis nodosa 539
polymyalgia rheumatica 540
polymyositis 540
rheumatoid arthritis 538–539
SLE vasculitis 539
Wegener's granulomatosis 539–540
withdrawal 537
Corticotrophin (ACTH)
see also corticosteroids 544–545
Cortisol 980–982
anti-inflammatory 981
cardiovascular 981
immunological 981
metabolic 981
CPPD
(calcium pyrophosphate crystal deposition)
association with osteoarthrosis 857, 859
Cramp, occupational (writer's) 1453
C-reactive protein, in rheumatic fever 1081
CREST syndrome 1375
Crohn's disease
association with ankylosing spondylitis 762
enteropathic arthritis
aetiology 807
clinical features 806–807
food allergy 808
investigations 807
pathogenesis *807*
treatment 808
musculoskeletal disorders 809–810
Cryoglobulinaemia 1197–1199
essential 1197
essential mixed in vasculitis 1316
hyperviscosity 1197

Cryoglobulinaemia *cont*
mixed (polyclonal) 1197
unmixed (monoclonal) 1197
Cryoglobulins in SLE 1339
Cryptococcosis (torulosis) 1154
Crystal arthropathies
see also Epidemiology, Gout
epidemiology 75–79
Crystal synovitis
arthroscopic appearance 1607
Crystals in gout
identification by polarising microscope 895, *895, 986*
Cutaneous vasculitis 1316
Cutis laxa 1166
Cysts, calf 1469–1471
Cytomegalic virus 1152
Cytotoxic drugs 547–554
azathioprine 547–554
chlorambucil 547–554
clinical pharmacology 547–549
cyclophosphamide 547–554
mechanisms 548–549
methotrexate 547–554
rationale 547
side-effects 552–554
structure *548*
treatment
dermatomyositis 551–552
juvenile chronic arthritis 551
polyarteritis nodosa 552
polymyositis 551–552
psoriatic arthritis 551
rheumatoid arthritis 549–550
SLE 550–551

Dagger sign 756, *756*
Debridement, in osteoarthrosis 879
Decompression sickness, acute
in aviators 1223
osteonecrosis, incidence 1223
radiology 1222, *1223*
Deformity, prevention 1515
De Quervain's syndrome 1452
Dermatoarthritis, lipid 1196–1197
Dermatomyositis 324, **1350 – 1363**
aetiology 1351–1352
in childhood 1132, 1354–1361
electromyographic triad 1358
laboratory aspects 1357–1358
prognosis 1357
classification 1350–1351
clinical manifestations 1352–1354
cytotoxic drug therapy 551–552
differential diagnosis 1355
epidemiology 87
hypogammaglobulinaemia, association 1200
incidence 1352
management 1358–1361
overlap with mixed connective tissue disease 1272–1273
precipitating factors 1352
Diabetes mellitus
associations
obesity 972
osteoarthrosis 852
carpal tunnel syndrome 978–979
Charcot joints 975
cheiroarthropathy 979–980, *980*
Dupuytren's contracture 978–979
gout 972
hyperuricaemia 917, 972
neuropathy 975–976
osteoarthritis 974–975
osteolysis (forefoot) 976
osteomyelitis 976
periarthritis of shoulder 980
peripheral neuropathy 975
soft tissue contracture 977
spinal neuropathy 976
trophic ulceration 976
vertebral ankylosing hyperostosis 973, 974
Diagnosis
see also Electrodiagnosis
acute phase reactants 1110
aids 1110–1111
blood count 1110
differential **161 – 174**, 1111–1112, *1111*
immunoglobulins 1111
laboratory tests 173–174
radiology 172–173, 1111
serology 1111
synovial membrane biopsy
Diaphyseal aclasis 1246–1247, *1247*
Diaphyseal dysplasia, progressive 1000
Diclofenac 517
Diffuse idiopathic skeletal hyperostosis (DISH) 656, 734–735, 1428
see also ankylosing hyperostosis, Forestier's disease
and osteoarthrosis 859–860
Diflunisal 509
Disc disorders 1407–1434
Discoid lupus 1335
Discs, intervertebral 1438
DISH
see also diffuse idiopathic skeletal hyperostosis, ankylosing hyperostosis, Forestier's disease
Dolorimeter 1591
D-penicillamine 557–558
see also penicillamine
comparison with levamisole *560*
side-effects
after gold therapy 532
in Sjögren's syndrome 1400
Drug-induced lupus 1335–1336, *1336*
Drugs
see also under individual drugs, pharmacokinetics
anti-malarials in SLE 1343
anti-rheumatic in clinical trials, classification 1594, *1581, 1582*
(for details see Clinical Trials)
aspirin in SLE 1343
corticosteroids in SLE 1343
cytotoxic 547–554
hypouricaemic 569–583
immunosuppressive 547–554
immunosuppressive agents in SLE 1344
isotopes in drug studies 1635
NSAIDs in SLE 1343
in osteoarthrosis 875–876
side effects in Sjögren's syndrome 1400
in surgical treatment 1524–1526
uricosuric 574
in long-term management of gout 925
DTC (diethyldithiocarbamate) 557
Dupuytren's contracture 978–979, 1454
epidemiology 110
Dupuytren's contracture and diathesis 1254–1255
Dupuytren's diathesis 1444
Dysentery arthritis
amoebic 1146
bacillary 1146

Echovirus, type 6 1152
Ehlers-Danlos syndrome 1164–1166, *1165, 1166*
articular complications 1165
clinical manifestations 1165
connective tissue disorders, types 1164
eye 1166
non-articular sequelae 1165
pregnancy 1166
skin
appearance 1164
trauma 1166
Elastin 186–187, 213–215
Elbow
arthrodesis 1550
arthroplasty 1550
arthroscopy 1605
effusions 1450
examination 1577
golfer's 1449–1450
humeral epicondylitis 1449–1450
injection techniques 1614–1615, *1615*
olecranon bursitis 1450
radial neuropathy 1452
student's elbow 1450
surgery 1549–1550
synovectomy 1549–1550
tennis 1449–1450
treatment 1449–1450
ulnar neuropathy 1452
water on the elbow 1450
Electrodiagnosis 1621–1626
clinical applications
myasthenia gravis 1625
myasthenic syndrome 1626
myopathic disorders 1624–1625
nerve compression 1623
nerve entrapment 1624
peripheral neuropathy 1624
electromyography 1623
latency measurements 1621
methods 1621
nerve conduction speed 1621–1623, *1622*
techniques 1621

Electromyography 1623
Enchondromatosis 1246, *1246*
Endocarditis 5
Endocrine disorders 959–991
  acromegalic arthropathy 960–967
  adenohypophysis 959–960
  hyperthyroidism 970–971
  hypothyroidism 968–970
  iatrogenic pituitary-adrenal insufficiency 982
  pregnancy 982–986
  in rheumatoid arthritis 638
  thyroid 967–968
  thyroid acropachy 971
Endocrine pancreas 972–980
Enteropathic arthritis 806–818
  ankylosing spondylitis 808–810, *809*
    aetiology 809
    clinical features 808
    HLA-B27 809
    investigations 808–809
    treatment 809
  Crohn's disease 806–808
    aetiology 807
    clinical features 806–807
    investigations 807
    pathogenesis *807*
    treatment 808
  gut infection 815–816, *815*
    aetiology 816
    investigations 816
    treatment 816
  intestinal bypass surgery 814–815
  ulcerative colitis 810–813
    aetiology 810–811
    ankylosing spondylitis 811–812
    clinical features 810
    investigations 810, *811*
    joints involved *811*
    musculoskeletal disorders 813
  Whipple's disease 813–814
    aetiology 814
    clinical features 813
    HLA-B27 814
    investigations 813–814
    treatment 814
Enteropathic reactive arthritis (ERA) 815–816
Enthesis 219
Enthesopathy 219, **723 – 744**, 1449
  see also Seronegative Spondarthritides
  ankylosing spondylitis 757–758, *758*, *759*
  epidemiology 106–107
  insertion of patellar tendon 1467, *1467*
Enzymes, abnormalities in gout 904–906
Eosinophilic fasciitis 1257–1259, *1259*
Epidemiology 59–142
  acute back pain 100–101
  aetiological factors 110
  anatomical abnormalities 98
  ankylosing hyperostosis 97–98
  ankylosing spondylitis 70–72
  applications 124–126
  arthrosis 88–94
  back pain 99–104
  Behcet's disease 81
  biological attributes 114–116
  bone disorders 109–110
  chondrocalcinosis 79
  chronic back pain 101
  congenital dislocation of hip 108
  connective tissue diseases 82–88
  crystal arthropathies 75–79
  dermatomyositis 87
  developmental anomalies 98
  disc prolapse 99
  dorsopathies 88–94
  drug-induced lupus 85
  Dupuytren's contracture 110
  enteropathic arthropathy 73–74
  enthesopathies 106–107
  external influences 111–114
  generalised osteoarthrosis 94–95
  genotype 116–121
  gout 76–79
  HLA-B27 72–73
  hypermobility 107–108
  hypogammaglobulinaemia 81–82
  individual characteristics 114
  inflammatory arthropathies 79–82
  inherited conditions 107
  juvenile chronic arthritis 67–70
  Lyme disease 81
  micro-organisms 79–80
  non-articular rheumatism 106–107
  occupational disorders 105–106
  occurrence of back pain 100
  osteoporosis 110
  other spondylarthropathies 72–75
  Paget's disease 109–110
  peripheral joints, arthrosis 90–94
  polyarteritis nodosa 88
  polyarticular arthrosis 94
  polymyalgia rheumatica 104–105, 1279–1280
  psoriatic arthropathy 75
  reactive arthritis 72–80
  Reiter's disease 74–75, 788–789
  rheumatoid arthritis 63–67
  rheumatic disorders, individual 59–142
  rheumatic fever 108–109, 1066
  septic arthritis 79–80
  Sjögren's syndrome 88
  SLE 82–86, 1325–1326
  soft-tissue syndromes 104–107
  spinal stenosis 98–99
  spondylosis 95–99
  systemic sclerosis 86–87
  techniques 121–124
  transient back pain 100
Epiphyseal dysplasia
  in congenital hypothyroidism 970
  multiple 998–999, *999*
Epstein-Barr virus 438–440, 1152
Erbium (^{169}Er), intra-articular irradiation 589–590
Erosive osteoarthrosis 735, 856–857
Erosive spondylopathy 734
Erythema infectiosum, parvovirus cause 1153
Erythema nodosum 1229–1230, *1229*
  associations 1230
  histology 1229
  joint manifestations 1230
  treatment 1230
Erythrocyte sedimentation rate (ESR)
  in ankylosing spondylitis 799
  in juvenile chronic arthritis 1110
  in osteoarthrosis 869
  in Reiter's disease 798
  in rheumatic fever 1081
European League Against Rheumatism (EULAR) 15
Examination, physical 1573–1580
Exercise 1490–1492
  active
    assisted 1491
    hydrotherapy 1492
    resisted 1491–1492
  passive (movement) 1490
  in spondylitis 1495
Exocrine function, impaired in sicca syndrome 1388
Exocrine pancreas, failure 980
Experimental arthritis, animal models **468 – 485**
  autoimmunisation 478–480
  bacterial products, effect 471–476
  infective arthritis 469–471
  oral 6-sulphanilamidoindazole 480
  osteoarthrosis 480–481
  protein immunisation 476–478
  synovitis, crystal induced 482
Extractable nuclear antigen (ENA)
  see also Immunology
  in SLE 1338
Exudation 283–286
  formation 283–285, *285*
  origin of cells 286–287
Eyes, physical examination 1574

Familial juvenile gout 919–920
Familial Mediterranean fever 1029
  in childhood, mimicking juvenile chronic arthritis 1132
  familial recurrent polyserositis 1236
Fascia 219
Felty's syndrome 689
  association with rheumatoid arthritis 640–641, *641*
  corticosteroid therapy 539
Femoral anteversion, computerised tomography 1631–1632
Femur
  aseptic necrosis of proximal capital epiphysis 851
  slipped epiphysis leading to osteoarthrosis 850–851
Fenbufen 520
Fenclofenac 517–518
Fever
  cat-scratch 1153
  rheumatic 1057–1099
  Rocky Montain spotted 1150
Fibroblasts 201–203

Fibroblasts *cont*
in inflammation 288–290
Fibrodysplasia ossificans progressiva 1019
Fibrogenesis imperfecta ossium 1019
Fibronectin 187–189, 216–217
Fibrosarcoma 1247
Fibrosing alveolitis
in mixed connective tissue disease 1272
in systemic sclerosis 1374
Fibrosis 201
Fibrositic nodules 1424
Fibrositis 14, 20, 150, 1424
of shoulder 1446
Fibula, stress fractures 1472–1473
Fingers
clubbing in ulcerative colitis 813
in hypertrophic osteoarthropathy 1475
deformities
boutonnière 1559, *1559*
swan-neck 1560
injection techniques 1617, *1617*
stenosing tenovaginitis 1453, 1617, *1617*
surgery 1554–1560
trigger finger 1453, 1617, *1617*
Foot
examination 1579
flat 1476
forefoot
hallux rigidus 1533
hallux valgus 1533
osteoarthrosis 868
surgery 1531–1534
Freiberg's disease 1477
Freiberg's infraction 1477
hindfoot
osteoarthrosis 868
injection technique 1619–1620
Köhler's disease of metatarsal head 1477
march fracture 1477
metatarsal pain 1477
Morton's metatarsalgia 1477
painful foot, causes 1475–1478
pes cavus (claw-foot) 1476–1477
rheumatoid arthritis 1477
Foot drop
in rheumatoid vasculitis *1312*
Forestier's disease (ankylosing hyperostosis)
diabetes 973–974
epidemiology 97–98
osteoarthrosis 859–860
Fractures, vertebral
spinal pain 1422–1423
Freiberg's disease 1210, 1477, *1210*
Freiberg's infraction 1477
Frozen shoulder 1444
Fungal infection 1153–1155

Galen 3
Garrod, Sir Alfred 8, *8*
Gastrointestinal tract
in Sjögren's syndrome 1393
in systemic sclerosis 1372–1373
pathology 1372
Gaucher's disease 1219
and osteoarthrosis 853–854
Geigy gauge 1590
Genitourinary infection, causing ankylosing spondylitis 761–762
Geodes 258, 670
Giant cell arteritis 324
clinical features 1284–1285
corticosteroid therapy 540
and polymalgia rheumatica **1278 – 1291**
Giant cell tumours 1247
Gigantism 960
Glucose-6-phosphate, deficiency in gout 910
Glutathione reductase, increased activity in gout 910
Glycosaminoglycans 190
Goerkerman (Ingram) treatment of psoriatic arthritis 782
Gold 559
analysis 532
auranofin 531
comparison with D-penicillamine 532–533
dosage 531
effect on immune response 530–531
formation 530
in juvenile chronic arthritis 1117, *1117*
patient selection 531
rheumatoid arthritis, intra-articular injection 587
side-effects 532
in Sjögren's syndrome 1400
tissue antigens 533
therapeutic recommendation 531–533
Golfer's elbow 1449–1450
injection technique 1616, *1615*
Gonococcal arthritis 1139–1140
Gout **883 – 937**
see also Hyperuricaemia and Uric acid
acute
clinical features 884–886
differential diagnosis 898
long-term management 921–925
pathology 887–888
age of onset 884, *884*
alcohol 915
blood levels of uric acid 899–901
bodyweight, relation to uric acid 914–915, *915*
chronic
clinical features 884–887
differential diagnosis 898–899
pathology 890–891
chronic tophaceous
clinical features 886–887
corticosteroid injection 585
crystal identification 895, *895, 896*
diagnosis 894–899
differential diagnosis 164, 166, 897–899
epidemiology 76–79
familial juvenile 919–920
Heberden's nodes 898
historical background 6–9, 883
hyperlipoproteinaemia 1238
hyperuricaemia 906–917
age range 914
genetic factors 914
race 914
sex ratio 914
hypouricaemia 917–918, *917*
hypouricaemic drugs 569–583
intelligence 915
joints involved 885
lead poisoning 913
Lesch-Nyhan syndrome 906–909, *907*
leukaemia 1193
management 920–925
allopurinol 922–924, *924*
diet 925
hypertension 925
life-style 925
long-term management 921–925
uricosuric drugs 925
monosodium urate monohydrate, crystalline 890
histological demonstration 890
myeloid metaplasia 1196
pathology 887–891
crystal deposition 888–889
inflammatory response 889–890
prevalence 883–884
primary
association with hypertension, renal disease 892–894
hyperuricaemia, causes 918–919
uric acid calculi 892
prodromal symptoms 885
purines 902–905
pyrophosphate arthropathy 944
radiology 897
renal lesions 893–894
saturnine gout 913
secondary
accompanying myelomatosis 1248
serum uric acid 894–895
conversion scale *899*
levels 899, *899*
sex ratio 884, *884*
in sickle cell disease 1190
social class 915
synovial tissue, examination 895–896
therapeutic evaluation 1593
tophi 169
examination 895–86, *896*
urates, sites of deposition 891, *891*
uric acid
calculi 892
formation 892
hyperuricaemia 901
lithiasis 892
metabolism 901
Granulation tissue 202
Graunloma(s), Crohn's disease 810
Granulomatous arteritis
see also granulomatous vasculitis
Granulomatous vasculitis 1293–1294, 1304–1314, *1305*
overlap with polyarteritis nodosa 1293–1294
relationship to arteritis *1293*
Gut infection 815–816
association with arthritis *815*

Haemarthrosis, recurrent in haemophilia
intra-articular radiotherapy 590
Haemochromatosis
chondrocalcinosis 953–954
clinical features 952–953
differential diagnosis 953
HLA 952
osteoarthrosis 853
pathogenesis 954–956
pseudo-gout 953
pyrophosphate arthropathy 943–944, 954
radiology 953–954
sex ratio 952
Haemoglobin
rheumatic fever 1081
uric acid levels 917
Haemoglobinopathies 1185–1191
osteoarthrosis 854
osteonecrosis 1218–1219
sickle cell disease 1186–1190
thalassaemia 1186, 1191
Haemophilia 1177–1185, *1177*
aetiopathogenesis 1180–1181
arthropathy, subacute 1179
chronic arthropathy 1179
clinical severity 1178
corticosteroid therapy 1184
definition 1178, *1177*
factor VIII and IX replacement 1183
haemarthrosis
acute 1178
recurrent, intra-articular radiotherapy 590
management 1182–1185
muscular contractures *1180*
osteoarthrosis 854
patient education 1185
patient independence 1185
physical adaptations 1184
physiotherapy 1184
prophylactic injections 1184
radiology 1181—1185
radiosynoviorthesis 1184
soft-tissue bleeding 1179–1180
splinting 1184
surgery 1184–1185
Hagemann factor 296
Hairy cell leukaemia 1193
Hand
arthroscopy 1605
examination 1577–1578
injection techniques 1616–1617, *1617, 1618*
osteoarthritis, surgery, 1560
success rating *1556*
surgery 1554–1560
Hand-foot syndrome in sickle cell disease 1190
Hallux rigidus 1477
Hallux valgus 1477
Haverhill fever 1149
Headache
giant cell arteritis 1284
temporal arteritis 1440
Heart
mitral valve prolapse associated with hypermobility 1169
physical examination 1574
rheumatic fever 1066
clinical picture 1075–1076
failure 1076–1077
pericarditis 1076
rhythm change 1076
treatment 1089
rheumatic pneumonia 1077–1078
treatment 1089
SLE 1328–1329
subacute bacterial endocarditis
complicating rheumatic fever 1082
prevention *1090*
systemic sclerosis 1374
Heat
physical treatment 1493–1494, *1493*
Heberden, William 5, 16, *5*
Heberden Library 16
Heberden Oration 16
Heberden Round 16
Heberden Society 16
Heberden's nodes 861, *838*
in gout 898
heredity 856
in primary osteoarthrosis 856
Heel, painful 1474–1475
Henoch-Schönlein purpura 1235–1236, 1315–1316
Hepatitis, acute
arthritis 1151
Hepatitis B 435–437
Hereditary multiple aclasis 1246–1247, *1247*
Heritable disorders 1162–1176
bloodhound facies 1166
cutis laxa 1166
Ehlers-Danlos syndrome 1164–1166, *1165, 1166*
of fibrous proteins 1162
homocystinuria 1163–1164
hyperlysinaemia 1164
hypermobility (in healthy subjects) 1166–1170, *1167*
mucopolysaccharidoses 1170–1171, *1171*
osteogenesis imperfecta 1001–1003, *1002*
pseudo-xanthoma elasticum 1164
skeletal
achondroplasia 1172–1173, *1173*
cleiodocranial dyostosis 1174
diaphyseal aclasis 1175
epiphyseal dysplasia 1173
fibrodysplasia ossificans progressiva 1172
microdactyly osteopoikilosis *1173*
multiple epiphyseal dysplasia 1173
myositis ossificans progressiva 1172
osteopetrosis 1173–1174
pycnodyostosis 1173
spondyloepiphyseal dysplasia 1173
Herpes zoster 1461
Heterotopic ossification 1019
Hilton's law 1436
Hip
arthography 1607–1608
arthroscopy 1605
congenital dislocation, epidemiology 108
cysts 1459
examination 1578
injection techniques 1617–1618
joint 1618, *1618*
supratrochanteric bursitis 1618
joint replacement surgery in osteoarthrosis 877–878
osteoarthrosis 866–867
pattern of pain referral from joint 1459
and pelvis 1455–1456
'snapping' 1456
total replacement 1540–1545
see also Surgery
Histiocytic lymphoma 1247
Histoplasma capsulatum, histoplasmosis 1154
Histoplasma duboisin 1154
Historical background of rheumatic diseases **3 – 18**
History-taking 1567–1573
HLA, associations with disease 317–320
with rheumatic diseases 320–326, *320*
HLA-B27 730–733
acne arthritis 1239
ankylosing spondylitis 760
associated disorders 320, *320*
bacillary dysentery 1146
Reiter's disease 791
yersinia arthritis 322, 428–429, 1146
Hoffa's disease 1466
Homocystinuria 1163–1164
Host immunity 337
Housemaid's knee 1465
Housewife's shoulder 1446
HPOA (hypertrophic pulmonary osteoarthropathy) 1251–1253
Human MHC (HLA) system 312–316
Human thyroid stimulator (HTS) 972
Humeral epicondylitis 1449–1450
Hurler's syndrome 1171–1172, *1172*
Hyaluronate 195
Hydroxyapatite crystals
deposition, association with osteoarthrosis 859
detection in synovial fluid 271–272
Hypercalcaemia, in hyperuricaemia 914
Hypergammaglobulinaemic purpura 1199
Hyperlipidaemia, osteonecrosis 1223
Hyperlipoproteinaemia 1236–1238
abnormality patterns 1237, *1237*
eruptive 1237
involving tendons, lytic lesions in bone 1237–1238
hyperuricaemia 1238
Type II (hypercholesterolaemic) arthritis 1238
Type IV arthralgia, arthritis 1238
xanthomata 1237–1238
Hyperlysinaemia 1164
Hypermobility
associations
chronic back pain 1168
loose back syndrome 1168

Hypermobility *cont*
mitral valve prolapse 1169
clinical effects 1168
clinical stigmata *1167*
connective tissue disorder 1169
epidemiology 107–108
management 1170
premature osteoarthrosis 1168
race 1168
sex ratio 1168–1169
syndrome 1168
Hyperparathyroidism
association with acromegalic arthropathy 966
chondrocalcinosis 1015
diagnosis 1015
osteitis fibrosa 1014
primary, bone disease 1014–1015
pyrophosphate arthropathy 943
Hypersensitivity vasculitis 1314–1316
Hypertension 925
essential, in hyperuricaemia 193
Hyperthyroidism 970–971
Hypertriglyceridaemia
alcohol induced 916
in gout 916
Hypertrophic osteoarthropathy 1251–1253, 1475, *1251*
histology 1252
pachydermoperiostosis 1252–1253, *1253*
pathogenesis 1252
primary 1252
pulmonary 1475
pulmonary osteoarthropathy 1252
radiology 1251–1252
radionuclide scanning 1637
secondary, associations 1252
Hypertrophic pulmonary osteoarthropathy (HPOA) 1252
Hyperuricaemia
see also Gout, Uric acid
age range 914
alcohol 915
asymptomatic 925–926
bodyweight, relation to uric acid 914–915, **915**
cardiovascular disease 916–917
diabetes 917
familial juvenile gout 919–920
genetic factors 914
gout 906
causes in primary 918–919
haemoglobin and uric acid levels 917
hypercalcaemia 914
hyperlipoproteinaemia 1238
hyperparathyroidism 914
hypertriglyceridaemia 916
intelligence 915
lead poisoning 913
leukaemia 1193
myeloid metaplasia 1196
myxoedema 914
osteonecrosis 1223
plasma
lipids 916
proteins and uric acid levels 917
race 914
saturnine gout 913
sex ratio 914
in sickle cell disease 1190
social class 915
Hyperviscosity syndrome 689, 1189
Hypogammaglobulinaemia 1199–1200
epidemiology 81–82
Hypo-hyperparathyroidism 1016
Hypomagnesaemia, pyrophosphate arthropathy 944
Hypoparathyroidism 1015–1016
Hypophosphatasia 1001
calcinosis 944
pyrophosphate arthropathy 944
Hyposplenism 1028
Hypothyroidism 968–970
arthropathy 969–970
carpal tunnel syndrome 968
congenital 970
epiphyseal dysplasia 970
muscle 969
myopathy 969
osteonecrosis 1223–1224
pyrophosphate arthropathy 944
rheumatological manifestations 968
Hypouricaemia 917–918, *917*
Hypouricaemic drugs 569–583
allopurinol 569–574, *470*
chemistry 569
dose 572
drug interactions 573–574
historical background 569
kidneys 572
pharmacological properties 570–572
side-effects 573
therapeutic effect 573–574
anti-inflammatory drugs 579–580
benzbromarone 578–579
diuretics 579
lipid-lowering 580
probenecid 575–577
sulphinpyrazone 577–578
thiopurinol 574
uricosuric 574, 579, *575*
Hypoxanthine guanine phosphoribosyl transferase (HGPRT)
decreased activity in Lesch-Nyhan syndrome 906
purine metabolism 901

Iatrogenic pituitary-adrenal insufficiency 982
Ibuprofen 518–519
Iga, selective deficiency 1200–1201
Iliopsoas bursitis 1459
Imaging techniques **1627 – 1642**
computerised tomography 1627–1632
radionuclide scanning 1633–1642
Immune complex disease
concept 386–387
experimental
adjuvant disease 389
aetiology *387*
allergic arthritis 389
arthus reaction 387
prognosis 1198
purpura 1198
serum sickness 387–388, *387*
skin manifestations 1198
spontaneous lupus 389
treatment 1198
Immune complexes 376–397
antigen-antibody interactions 377
assays, use in clinical practice 396–397
biological properties 379
cell interaction 380
circulating immune complexes
clearance 382–383
fate 382–386
tissue deposition 383–385
complement binding 379
composition 377
detection, methods
cryoprecipitation 394–395
gel filtration 394
interaction with complement 395
interaction with rheumatoid factors 396
microscopy 390–392
electronmicroscopy 392–393
other assays 396–397
polyethylene glycol (PEG) precipitation 395
ultracentrifugation 393–394
effect on immune response 380
enhanced antibody production 380
historical background 376
immune reactions, blocking 381
immunoglobulins, structure 377
lattice structure 378, 382–383
nature of antigen 383
pathogenecity 385–386
permeability of vessels 383
physicochemical properties 378
reactions with rheumatoid factors 381–382
regulation of antibody production 380–381
role of complement 395–396
size 378, 382–383
solubility 378–379, *379*
tissue
damage 385–386
deposition 383–385
receptors 385
uptake by reticuloendothelial system 383
Immune deficiency 1199–1201
AIDS 1199
B-cell defects 1199
dermatomyositis associated with hypogammaglobulinaemia 1200
hypogammaglobulinaemia
acquired, late onset 1199
associations 1200
background 1200
bacterial infection 1200
clinical picture,
differences with arthritis of rheumatoid arthritis 1200
familial factor 1199
incidence 1199

Immune deficiency *cont*
non-infective arthritis 1200
onset, time 1199
pathological differences 1200
sex-linked (Bruton) 1199
selective Iga deficiency
diagnosis 1201
frequency in juvenile arthritis 1200
non-infective arthritis, pathogenesis 1201
treatment 1201
T-cell defects 1199
Immune response, autoimmune disease 345–346
Immunodeficiency and arthritis 334
Immunogenetics **309 – 330**
clinical genetics 309
experimental autoimmune disease 312
H-2 complex of mouse 310–312
HLA associations
disease 317–320
rheumatic disease 320–326, *320*
human MHC (HLA) system 312–316
immune response genetics 310–312
other genetic polymorphisms 326
Immunoglobulins
altered, following antigen-binding 379
in rheumatic fever 1081–1082
structure 377–378
Immunological mechanisms 331–354, *331, 332*
Immunology
in SLE 1336–1340
anti-DNA antibodies 1337–1338, *1338, 1339*
anti-ENA 1338
antinuclear antibodies 1337, *1337*
antiviral antibodies 1338
LE cells 1337
rheumatoid factor 1339
T-cell suppressor function 1336
Sjögren's syndrome 1396–1398
synovial fluid 272–273
Immunomodulators 554–563
clinical properties of *560*
D-penicillamine 554–558
DTC 554
gold 559
levamisole 560–561
thymopoietin 559, 561–562
effect on T-cells *558*
immunological abnormalities 555
isoprinosine 554
levamisole 555–557
levamisole therapy in
ankylosing spondylitis 562
Behçet's disease 562
other rheumatic diseases 562
SLE 562
rheumatoid arthritis 562
thymic factors 558–559, *559*
Immunoproliferative disorders 346–349
Immunoregulation, chronic arthritis 341–342, *341*
Immunosuppression, physical therapies 554
Immunosuppressive agents in SLE 1344
Immunosuppressive drugs 547–554
Immunosuppressive therapy in juvenile chronic arthritis 1188
Indomethacin 516–517
in acute gout 921
Infection
see also infective arthritis **1137 – 1161**
acute hepatitis 1151
adenoviral arthritis 1151
after total joint replacement 1155–1156
ankylosing spondylitis 429–430
arboviruses 1151–1152
association with arthritis 443–447
classification *444, 446*
back pain 1429
bacterial 423–430, 1137–1145
candida 1155
chickenpox 1151
clinical considerations 452–457
Coxsackie B 1153
cytomegalic virus mimicking Epstein-Barr viral infections 1152
enteric 1145–1146
fungal 1153–1155
genetic considerations 452–457
genitourinary 427–428
gonococcal 1139–1140
immunity 411–412
inflammatory polyarthritis 427–428
inflammatory rheumatic diseases, involvement 418, *422*
interleukin 455
intestinal, reactive arthritis 428–429
investigation 412–423, *423, 418, 422*
leptospirosis 1149
microbial 411–467
mumps 1151
paramyxoviruses 434–435
parvoviruses 437–438
pathological considerations 452–457
prokaryotic, conclusions 430–431
rat bite fever 1149
reactive immunopathology 447–452
recent progress 423–424
rheumatic diseases, involvement in aetiology and pathogenesis 456–457, *457*
rheumatic fever 424–425
rheumatoid arthritis 424–425
Rocky Mountain spotted fever 1150
in SLE 1334
smallpox 1152
spirochaetal 1146–1150
syphilis 1146–1148
viral 1150–1153
in vasculitis 1296
see also viruses
Infectious mononucleosis 1152
Infective arthritis **1137 – 1161**
actinomyces bovis 1153
acute hepatitis 1151
acute suppurative arthritis 1137–1139
adenoviral 1151
after total joint replacement 1155–1156
amoebic dysentery 1146
arthritis associated with microbial infection *1137*
aspergillosis 1153
atypical mycobacteria 1145
bacillary dysentery 1146
bacterial infections 1137–1145
blastomycosis 1153–1154
North American geography 1153
brucellosis 1141–1142
campylobacter jejuni enteritis 1146
candida infections 1155
cat-scratch fever 1153
complications 1153
cephalosporium 1155
chickenpox 1151
Chikungya virus 1151–1152
clostridium difficile colitis 1146
coccidiomycosis 1154
Coxsackie B infection 1153
Crohn's disease 809
cryptococcosis 1154
cytomegalic virus 1152
Echovirus type 6 1152
enteric infections 1145–1146
erythema infectiosum, parvovirus cause 1153
experimental models 469–471
fungal infections 1153–1155
gonococcal 1139–1140
Haverhill fever 1149
histoplasma capsulatum, histoplasmosis 1154
infectious mononucleosis 1152
leprosy 1145
leptospirosis 1149
Lyme arthritis 1149–1150
lymphogranuloma venereum 1155
madura foot (mycetoma pedis) 1154–1155
meningococcal 1140–1141
mumps 1151
mycoplasma 1142–1145
mycoplasma pneumoniae 1142
nocardia 1155
O'Nyong-Nyong virus 1151–1152
petrullidium boydis 1155
rat-bite fever 1149
Rocky Mountain spotted fever 1150
Ross River virus 1151–1152
rubella 1150–1151
salmonella 1145–1146
smallpox 1152
spirochaetal infections 1146–1150
sporotrichosis 1155
syphilis 1146–1148
tuberculosis 1142–1144
viral infections 1150–1153
yaws 1148–1149
yersinia enterocolitica 1146
Inflammation **281 – 308**
cell types 284
cellular infiltration 286–288
control of inflammatory response 293, *294, 295*
healing process 288–290, *289*
historical background 281, *281*

Inflammation *cont*
inflammatory process 282–290, 303–304
local events *282*
measurement 1590–1592
mediators 296–303
modulators 296–303
objective measurements 1591–1592
in rheumatic diseases 304
systemic response 290–293, *292*
Inflammatory arthritis of shoulder 1444
Inflammatory arthropathy 1229–1241
acne arthritis 1239
anaphylactoid purpura 1235–1236
Behçet's syndrome 1231–1235
Clutton's joints 1238–1239
erythema nodosum 1229–1230, *1229*
Henoch-Schönlein purpura 1235–1236
hyperlipoproteinaemia 1236–1238
intestinal bypass surgery arthritis 1241
pigmented villondular synovitis 1242–1244
pustolotic arthro-osteitis 1239–1240
pyoderma gangrenosum 1240–1241
sarcoidosis 1230–1231
traumatic synovitis 1239
tumours 1241–1253
Inflammatory back pain 1429
Inflammatory bowel disease in children 1130
Inflammatory polyarthritis, early, severe, rehabilitation 1515
Inflammatory synovitis, arthroscopy 1605–1606
Infrapatellar bursitis 1465
Injection techniques **1612 – 1626**
Achilles tendinitis 1619
ankle 1619–1620
elbow 1614–1615, *1615*
fingers 1617, *1617, 1618*
foot 1619–1620
hand 1616–1617
heel, painful 1619–1620
hip 1617–1618, *1618*
knee 1618–1619
miscellaneous 1620
shoulder 1613–1614, *1613*
steroid, local 1612–1620
wrist 1615–1616, *1616, 1617*
Interleukin 1, 234, 291–293, 617, *291*
infection 455
in rheumatoid synovial membrane 601
Intermittent claudication 1473
International Classification of Diseases (ICD) 23, 27, 28, 45
International League Against Rheumatism (ILAR) 15, 16
definition of rheumatology 3–4
Interspinous ossification 756
Intervertebral joints 242–244
age changes 243–244
annulus fibrosus 242
nucleus pulposus 242–244
Intestinal bypass surgery arthritis 814–815, 1241
dermatitis syndrome 734

Intra-articular discs 220
Intra-articular therapy **584 – 591**
aspirin 587
corticosteroid 584–585
gold in rheumatoid arthritis 587
irradiation 588–590
^{169}Er in small joints 589–590
special indications for use 590
^{90}Y in large joints 588–589
orgotein 587
osmic acid 587–588
in osteoarthrosis 876
side-effects 586–587
silicone oil in osteoarthrosis 587
soft-tissue lesions, non-articular 585–586
synoviorthesis 587
Iridocyclitis 1128
in juvenile chronic arthritis 1107–1108
Iron overload arthropathy 1191
Irritable hip syndrome 1192
Ischaemic pain 1457
Ischial tuberosity 1457
Ischial whiskering 757–758, *757*
Isoprinosine 557
Isotopes 1632–1639

Jaccoud's arthropathy 5
Joint capsule 219
Joints
acromioclavicular 1443–1444
antigen persistence 331–334
apophyseal 1410
arthrography 1607–1608
arthroscopic appearances 1605–1607, *1602, 1604*
arthroscopy 1603–1605
articular surfaces 235–239
aspiration 259
Charcot 975, 1147, 1253–1254, *1147*
Clutton 1147
elbow, surgery 1549–1550
examination 1574–1579
function 199–250
gout
acute 885
chronic 886
hip 1459
total replacement 1540–1545
imagine techniques 1627–1642
injection techniques 1612–1620
knee 1462–1467
cysts 1536
surgery 1535–1540
limited joint mobility syndrome 979–980, *979*
lubrication 239–241
neuropathic 975, 1253–1254
osteoarthrosis 861–869
prosthetic
infection 1527–1528
painful 1528–1529
replacement
in osteoarthrosis 877–878

radionuclide scanning 1639
shoulder 1441–1447
frozen 1444
surgery 1547–1549
structure 199–250
superior tibiofibular synovitis 1467
surgery 1534–1535
assessment 1520–1521
symphyses 241–242
synovial 229–232
cervical spine 1437–1438
in systemic sclerosis 1371
wrists, surgery 1550–1553
Jumper's knee 1464
Juvenile chronic arthritis (Still's disease) **1100 – 1124,** *22*
Acthar Gel 1116, *1116*
ACTH therapy 1114
aetiology 1101–1103
age distribution 1101, *1101*
amyloidosis 1109
anabolic steroids 1116
association with rheumatoid arthritis 638
clinical aspects 1103–1106
corticosteroid therapy 1114
growth impairment 1114
criteria 1100
cytotoxic drug therapy 551
death, causes 1109, 1110, *1110*
definition 1100
diagnosis 1111–1112, *1111*
drugs 1114–1118
anti-malarials 1117–1118
gold 1117, *1117*
treatment 1114–1118, *1117, 1118, 1119*
encephalitis 1106
epidemiology 67–70
fever 1104, *1104*
fractures 1109
growth defects 1108, 1114, *1108, 1115, 1116*
heredity 1103
historical background 1100
immunological basis 1101–1103
incidence 1100–1101
iridocyclitis 1107–1108
joint involvement, pattern 1106–1107
keratitis punctata *1108*
kidney involvement 1106
liver enlargement 1104
lone Iga deficiency 1200
lymphadenopathy 1104
management 1112–1114
myocarditis 1106
nodules 1107
NSAIDs 1114
onset
pauciarticular 1106
polyarticular 1106
pericarditis 1105
pleurisy 1106
prevalence 1100–1101
prognosis 1112, *1112, 1113*
pulmonary fibrosis 1106
serositis 1105

Juvenile chronic arthritis (Still's disease) *cont*
sex distribution 1101, *1101*
splenomegaly 1104
surgery 1118–1120
synovial membrane biopsy 1111
systemic features 1104
tenosynovitis 1107
Juvenile psoriatic arthritis 778, 1130–1131
Juvenile rheumatoid arthritis 21

Kashin-Beck disease 855
Keratitis punctata *1108*
Keratoconjunctivitis sicca 683–684, 1386–1390, *684*
diagnosis 1389–1390
fluorescein dilution 1390
osmolality 1390
Schirmer's test 1389
tear film break-up time 1389
tear protein profiles 1390
Ketoprofen 520
Ketosis, effect on uric acid excretion 912, *913*
Kidney, in systemic sclerosis 1374
Kienböck's disease 1217, *1217*
Kinesiology 231
Knee
acute calcification 1467
arthrography 1607–1608
arthroscopy 1598–1604
appearances 1607, *1602, 1603*
bursitis 1465
examination 1578
injection techniques 1618–1619
joint replacement in osteoarthrosis 878
lesions 1462–1467
differential diagnosis 1466
Hoffa's disease 1466
internal derangements 1463
Osgood-Schlatter disease 1466
Pellegrini-Stieda disease 1466–1467
superior tibiofibular joint, synovitis 1466
synovial shelf syndrome 1463
osteoarthrosis 867–868
patella 1463–1465
chondromalacia patellae 1463–1464
dislocation 1464
nail-patella syndrome 1464
popliteal cysts 1465–1466
differential diagnosis 1466
pre-patellar bursitis 1465
surgery 1535–1540
arthroplasty 1536–1539
arthroscopic 1535–1536
choice of procedures *1540*
joint cysts 1536
osteotomy 1539
synovectomy 1536
total knee replacement 1538–1539
synovial biopsy 1608–1611
tendinitis 1467
Kohler's disease 1210, 1476, *1210*

Laboratory tests, differential diagnosis 173–174
Labra 220
Lactic acidaemia 912
Laminin 189–190, 216
Laryngeal arthritis 622
Lateral popliteal nerve palsy 1461–1462
LE cells in SLE 1337
Lead poisoning 913
Leg
long-leg syndrome 1467–1468
Legg-Perthes disease in children, leading to adult osteoarthritis 851
Leprosy arthritis 1145
Leptospirosis 1149
Leriche's syndrome 1457
Lesch-Nyhan syndrome 906–909, *907*
xanthine stone formation 909
Leukaemia 1191–1196
amyloidosis 1194–1195
angioimmunoblastic lymphadenopathy 1195–1196
association with rheumatoid arthritis 1191
hairy cell leukaemia 1193
irritable hip syndrome 1192
leukaemic reticuloendotheliosis 1193
lymphoblastic 1191–1192
lymphoma 1193
myelogenous 1192
differentiation from juvenile arthritis 1192
myeloid 1193, *1192*
myeloid metaplasia 1196
myelomatosis 1193–1194
T-cells 1193
Waldenström's macroglobulinaemia 1195
Leukaemic reticuloendotheliosis 1193
Levamisole 555–557, 560–561
comparison with penicillamine in rheumatoid arthritis *560*
Ligaments 219–220
Limb, lower **1455 – 1480**
ankle, painful 1474–1475
anterior tibial compartment syndrome 1471–1472
bursitis 1465–1466
foot, painful 1475–1478
heel, painful 1474–1475
intermittent claudication 1473
knee joint, lesions 1462–1467
lesions 1455–1480
long leg syndrome 1467–1468
nerve entrapment syndrome 1461–1462
pain 1455–1460
stress fractures 1472–1473
synovial rupture 1468–1471
Limb, upper **1448 – 1454**
Lipid dermatoarthritis 1196–1197
Liver, involvement in Sjögren's syndrome 1393
Liver disease
penicillamine 526–527
Long leg syndrome 1467–1468
Loose back syndrome 1168, 1424
Looser's zone 1010, 1458, *1011*
Lumbar spine flexion check 1575, *1576*
Lumbar spondylosis 1414–1418
Lumbosacral pain 1411–1426
Lumbosacral strain 1424
Lubricating glycoprotein 190
Lungs
changes in rheumatic fever 1077
involvement in SLE 1330
radionuclide scanning in fibrosing diseases 1638–1639
'shrinking' 1330, *1330*
Lupus
ANA-negative 1335
discoid 1335
drug-induced 1335–1336, *1336*
Lyme arthritis 1149–1150
epidemiology 81
Lymphoma 1193
histiocytic 1247
Lymphogranuloma venereum 1155
Lymphosarcomatous arthritis 1251

Madura foot 1154–1155
Manubriosternal joint in osteoarthrosis 864
Marble bones disease 999–1000
March fracture 1477
Marfan's syndrome 1162–1163, *1162, 1163*
McCune-Albright syndrome 999
McGregor's line 658
Measurements 1591
Melanotic sarcoma 1246
Melorheostosis 1000
Menginococcal arthritis 1140–1141
Menisci 220
Menopausal arthralgia 986
Meralgia paraesthetica 1461
Metabolic bone disease **992 – 1023**
see also Bone
Metacarpophalangeal joints, osteoarthrosis 861–863
Methotrexate 547–554
Mexican hat 1541, *1541*
Microbial infection **411 – 467**
see also Infection
Microdactyly 1172
Microscopy
electron 266
stained smears 263–266
wet preparations 266–268
Milwaukee shoulder 863–864, 974, 1446, *946*
Miscellaneous conditions 1229–1266
Mixed connective tissue disease (MCTD) **1269 – 1277**, 1375
antibodies to nuclear ribonuclear protein, 1269–1270, *1270*
arthritis 1271–1272
clinical characteristics 1272, *1271*
clinical features 1270–1271
clinical findings 1272, *1272*
diagnosis 1274–1275
diagnostic criteria 1275

Mixed connective tissue disease (MCTD) *cont*
as 'distinct clinical entity' 1275–1276
epidemiology 88
fibrosing alveolitis 1272
overlap features 1272–1273
overlap with SLE 1336
prognosis 1274–1275
Raynaud's phenomenon 1272
treatment 1275
response 1274–1275
Morton's metatarsalgia 1477
Mouth, physical examination 1574
Mucin clot test 261
Mucopolysaccharidoses 1170–1171, *1171, 1172*
osteonecrosis 1219
Multicentric reticulohistocytosis 1196–1197
Multiple myeloma 1193–1194
Mumps arthritis 1151
Muscle, in systemic sclerosis 1371
Myalgia, pericapsular 1446
Myasthenia gravis, electrodiagnosis 1625–1626
Myasthenic syndrome, electrodiagnosis 1625–1626
Mycetoma pedis 1154–1155
Mycobacteria, atypical arthritis 1145
Mycoplasma pneumoniae arthritis 1142
Myeloid metaplasia 1196
Myeloma 1247–1248, *1248*
Myelomatosis 1193–1194
Myocarditis, overlap with MCTD 1272–1273
Myocrisin 530
Myopathic disorders, electrodiagnosis 1624–1625
Myopathy, in hypothyroidism 969
Myositis ossificans progressive 1019
Myxoedema, hyperuricaemia 914

Necrosis, avascular
see also osteonecrosis **1207 – 1228**
Nail-patella syndrome 1464
Naproxen 519
Natural killer (NK) cells, immune response 337
Neck and shoulder **1435 – 1447**
arteries 1440
cervical spine
examination 1436
functional anatomy 1435–1437
Hilton's law 1436
segmental innervation 1435–1436, *1436*
sites of origin of pain *1437*
torticollis 1436
cervical spondylosis 1437–1438
contra-indications for mobilising treatment 1440
intervertebral discs 1438
ligaments 1440
muscles 1440
nerve roots, spinal cord 1438–1439
polymyalgia rheumatica 1440
posture, poor cervical 1440
shoulder 1441–1447
synovial joints 1437–1438
temporal arteritis 1140–1141
thoracic outlet syndrome 1438–1439
thoracic viscera 1441
vertebrae
developmental abnormalities 1439–1440
disease 1440
Sprengel's shoulder 1439
whip-lash effect 1440
Necrosis, aseptic
see aseptic necrosis 837–838
Neoplasms, back pain 1429–1430
Nerves
back pain 1411, *1411*
carpal tunnel syndrome 1450–1451
central nervous system disease in SLE 1333–1334
compression syndromes 1461–1462
surgery 1553–1554
ulnar nerve 1554
electrodiagnosis 1621–1626
entrapment
neuropathy 1450–1451
syndromes 1461–1462
intermittent claudication 1473
neuralgic amyotrophy 1446–1447
neurologic conditions, primary, mimicking rheumatic disorders 1448
neuropathy 1452
peripheral neuritis causing foot pain 1477–1478
roots 1438–1439
damage 1413
lumbar 1413
pain pathways 155
trunks
pain pathways 155
in systemic sclerosis
Neuralgic amyotrophy 1446–1447
Neuropathic joints 975, 1253–1254
Neuropathy, in diabetes 975–976
Nocardia 1155
Nodules 1126
in juvenile chronic arthritis 759
rheumatoid, in ankylosing spondylitis 759
subcutaneous 169–170, 674–676, *170*
surgical excision, from elbow 1549
tendon 169–170
Nomenclature **19 – 58**
preferred terms 20, *20*
seronegative polyarthritis 26–27
Non-articular rheumatism 13–14
chronic 13–14
indurated nodules 13–14
polymyalgia rheumatica 14
sciatica 13
Non-steroidal anti-inflammatory drugs (NSAIDs) **514 – 524,** *518*
action, mechanisms 514–515
benzotriazines
azapropazone 521–522
colchicine 522–523
oxicams 522
piroxicam 522
indoleacetic acids
indomethacin 516–517
sulindac 517
tolmetin 517
phenylacetic acids
diclofenac 517
fenclofenac 517–518
proprionic acids
fenbufen 520
fenoprofen 519–520
ibuprofen 518–519
ketoprofen 520
naproxen 519
tienilic acid 520–521
pyrazolones
phenylbutazone 521
selection 515
in SLE 1343
use 515
NSAIDs *see above*
Nuclear magnetic resonance, in back pain 1416
Nucleoprotein, increased turnover in gout 910
Nucleus pulposus, pressure variations 1410, *1410*

Occupation, relation to osteoarthrosis 855–856
Occupational cramp 1453
Occupational disorders, epidemiology 105–106
Ochronosis 950–952
Ocular disease, relationship with rheumatoid arthritis 638
Oestrogen replacement therapy in osteoporosis 1008
Olecranon bursitis 1450
Ollier's disease 1246, *1246*
Onycho-osteodysplasia 1464
O'Nyong-Nyong virus 1151–1152
Organ transplantation, complicated by osteonecrosis 1220
Orgotein, intra-articular injection 587
Os calcis 1212
painful 1475
Osgood-Schlatter disease 1211–1212
Osmic acid, in synoviorthesis 587–588
Osteitis deformans 1460
Osteitis fibrosa 1014
Osteitis pubis 986, 1457
Osteoarthritis
see Osteoarthrosis
Osteoarthropathy
hypertrophic 1251–1253, 1475, *1253*
radionuclide scanning 1637
Osteoarthrosis **821 – 880**
aetiology 821–841
alkaptonuria 853
apophyseal 1416–1418

Osteoarthrosis *cont*
articular index 1591
clinical aspects 846–872
clinical categories 847
diabetes 974–975
diarthrodial joints 821–824
differential diagnosis 870
experimental models 853–854
Gaucher's disease 853–854
haemachromatosis 853, 950–958
haematological disorders 1177–1185
haemoglobinopathies 854, 1177–1196
haemophilia 854, 1177–1185
historical background 9–10, 846
individual sites 861–868
intra-articular injection
corticosteroid 585
silicone oil 587
investigations 869–870
Kashin-Beck disease 855
management, medical 874–880
mixed crystal deposition 859
mucopolysaccharidoses 853
neurological disorders 854
occupation, relationship 855–856
ochronosis 950–958
pathology 821–824
premature, result of hypermobility 1168
prevalence 846–847
primary 856–860
secondary 851–856
sex hormones 852–853
signs 860–861
sport 855
storage diseases
see Heritable Disorders and Miscellaneous (Chs 46 & 49)
surgery 877–879
hand 1560
symptoms 860–861
synonyms 821
synovial joints 229–241
classification *231*
therapeutic evaluation 1593
thyroid disease 852
Wilson's disease 853, 950–958
Osteoblasts 205–206
Osteochondritis
dissecans 1211, *1211*
Scheuermann's 1427–1428
Osteochondromatosis 1241–1242
Osteochondrosis 1207
see also Osteonecrosis
Osteoclastoma 1257
Osteoclast grafts 1000
Osteoclasts 205, 207
Osteocytes 205–207
Osteogenic sarcomata 1247
Osteogenesis imperfecta 1001–1003, 1002
Osteoid osteoma 1248–1250, 1460, *1250, 1460*
Osteolysis, differential diagnosis from osteonecrosis 1225
Osteoma, post-traumatic, para-articular 1466–1477
Osteomalacia 1008–1014
axial 1019
hip pain 1456
Osteonecrosis **1207 – 1228**
alcoholism 1223
allied conditions 1225–1226
classification 1207, *1215*
in corticosteroid therapy 524
diagnostic procedures 1224
dysbaric, incidence in
acute decompression sickness 1222
aviators 1222
radiology *1223*
environmental *1215*
experimental models 1216–1217
genetically determined 1218–1219
hyperlipidaemia 1223
hyperuricaemia 1223
hypothyroidism 1223–1224
idiopathic 1217, *1217*
miscellaneous conditions 1220–1222, *1221*
multiple epiphyseal dysplasias 1212–1213
non-articular 1207–1213
osteochondroses 1209–1213
disorders of articular epiphysis 1209–1211
disorders of physeal epiphysis 1212
spinal 1212
pancreatitis 1224
pathology 1214–1216
pregnancy 1223
radiological progression *1223*
terminology 1207
trauma 1217–1218
treatment 1224–1225
corticosteroid 1219–1220
organ transplantation 1220
related 1219–1220
radiotherapy 1220
Osteopetrosis 999–1000, 1173–1174
Osteophytes 622, 833–834, 836–837
in ankylosing hyperostosis 859, *859*
in cervical spondylosis 1437
differentiation from syndesmophytes in osteoarthrosis of spine 754, 865–866, *754, 865*
Osteoporosis
ankylosing spondylitis 755, *755*
corticosteroid therapy 542
differential diagnosis from osteonecrosis 1226
diffuse childhood 1226
regional migratory 1226
epidemiology 110
oestrogen replacement therapy 1008
in surgery 1527
in Wilson's disease 956
Osteosarcomata 1247
Osteotomy 1531
hip 878
knee 879, 1539
indications for in ankylosing spondylitis 1547
Oestrogen replacement therapy, in osteoporosis 1008
Ott's disease 851
Overlap syndromes 1269–1277
Oxford grading of muscle function 1499, *1499*

Pachydermoperiostosis 1252–1253, *1253*
Paget's disease 1016–1018, 1460
back pain 1430
epidemiology 109–110
juvenile 1001
osteosarcoma 1247
Pain **143 – 160**
abnormalities 158
assessment of severity 156
chemical algogens 157
deep 148–153
definition 143–144
distribution 151, *150, 152*
inhibitory controls 147, *145*
localisation 147
measurement 1588–1589
of relief 1589
scales
graphic rating 1588–1589, *1589*
visual analogue 1588–1589, *1588*
mechanisms 156–158
nerve roots 156
nerve trunks 155
pathways 144–147
protective role 143
psychogenic 158
receptors 144–147
referred 148, 150, 153–154
skin 147
reflex tenderness 154
source 143
temperature changes 157–158
threshold 156
transition, focal to segmental 152–153
types 144
visceral 154–155
Paleopathology 3, 4, 11
Palindromic rheumatism 167–168
Pan American League Against Rheumatism (PANLAR) 15
Pancreas, endocrine 972–980
failure 980
Pancreatitis, osteonecrosis 1224
Panner's disease 1210, *1211*
Para-articular tumours 1241–1253
Paramyxoviruses 434–435
Parathormone 229
Parathyroid bone disease 1014–1016
Parvoviruses 437–438
Patella 1463–1465
see also Knee
chondromalacia patellae 1463
dislocations 1464
lesions 1463
nail-patella syndrome 1464
tendinitis 1464
Pellegrini-Stieda disease 1466–1477
Pelvis
see also Hip and pelvis 1455–1456

Pelvis *cont*
intra-pelvic lesions 1459
Penicillamine 525–528, 532–533
Penicillin therapy
gonococcal arthritis 1140
meningococcal arthritis 1141
rat-bite fever 1149
rheumatic fever 1088
side-effects in Sjögren's syndrome 1400
yaws 1149
Periarthritis of shoulder, in diabetes 980
Pericapsular myalgia 1446
Pericarditis in rheumatic fever 1076
Peripheral arthritis and B27 322
Peripheral neuritis causing foot pain 1477–1478
Peripheral neuropathy, electrodiagnosis 1624
Peripheral vascular disease in systemic sclerosis 1365–1366
Peritendinitis 1474
Perths disease 1209–1210
Pes cavus 1476–1477
Petrullidium boydis 1155
Pharmacokinetics **489 – 499,** *493, 494*
in clinical trials 1584
Phenylbutazone 521
in management of acute gout 921
5-phosphoribosyl-l-pyrophosphate (PRPP)
increased activity in gout 909
in purine biosynthesis 902
Physical examination 1573–1580
Physical treatment
see Treatment, physical **1483 – 1496**
Pigmented villonodular synovitis 1242–1244
arthroscopic appearance 1606
intra-articular radiotherapy 590
Piroxicam 522
Pituitary-adrenal insufficiency, iatrogenic 982
Plant-thorn synovitis 166
Plantar fasciitis 1475
Plasma proteins, uric acid levels 917
Polarised light microscopy, crystal identification 268–271
Polyarteritis nodosa **1293 – 1304**
association with hairy cell leukaemia 1193
clinical features 1299–1304
corticosteroid therapy 539
cytotoxic drug therapy 552
diagnosis 1298–1299
epidemiology 88
overlap with granulomatous vasculitis 1293–1294
Polyarthritis, rehabilitation
adult, chronic 1516–1517
early, severe inflammatory 1515
surgery, assessment 1521
Polychondritis, relapsing 1255–1257
Polymyalgia rheumatica 324, **1278 – 1291**
aetiology 1280–1281
back pain 1429
clinical features 1283–1284
corticosteroid therapy 540
diagnosis 1286–1287
differential diagnosis *1287*
epidemiology 104–105, 1279–1280
and giant cell arteritis **1278 – 1291**
historical background 1278–1279
neck involvement 1440
overlap with MCTD 1272–1273
pain in hips and pelvis 1455–1456
pathogenesis 1280–1281
pathology 1281–1283
shoulder involvement 1440
treatment 1287–1288
Polymalgia rheumatica and giant cell arteritis **1278 – 1291**
abnormalities of liver and thyroid function 1286
laboratory findings 1286
relationship 1285–1286
Polymyositis **1350 – 1363**
acute, differential diagnosis 1351
aetiology 1351–1352
classification 1350–1351, *1350*
clinical manifestations 1352–1354
cytotoxic drug therapy 551–552
differential diagnosis 1350
epidemiology 87
incidence 1352
laboratory aspects 1351
management 1358–1361
Polyostotic fibrous dysplasia 999, *1000*
Popliteal cysts 1465–1466
Posture 1424, 1427
in ankylosing spondylitis 750, *750*
in back pain 1410, 1414, *1414*
in bed rest 1484, *1484*
pericapsular myalgia 1446
poor, cervical 1440
physical examination 1573
Pregnancy
Ehlers-Danlos syndrome 1166
osteonecrosis 1223
rheumatic complications 982–986
rheumatic fever 1083–1084
SLE 1335
Prepatellar bursitis 1465
Probenecid 575–577
Progressive systemic sclerosis
penicillamine therapy 526
Proteins, attachment 187–190
chondronectin 190
fibronectin 187–189
laminin 189–190
lubricating glycoprotein 190
Proteoglycans 190–195
Protocol, in clinical trials
instructions on writing 1582, *1582*
Protrusio acetabuli 851
Pseudocysts 618, *619*
Pseudofracture 1010, *1011*
Pseudogout
see pyrophosphate arthropathy 938–949
corticosteroid injection 585
diabetes 973
Pseudohypoparathyroidism 1016, *1016*
Pseudopodagra 165, *165*
Pseudo-pseudohyperparathyroidism 1016
Pseudotumour cerebri 537
Pseudo-xanthoma elasticum 1164
Psoriatic arthritis 322, **775 – 786**
aetiology 776–777
age of onset 778
amyloidosis 779
ancillary investigations 779–780
associations
rheumatoid arthritis 640
spondylitis 778
clinical features 777
cytotoxic drug therapy 551
definition 775, *775*
differential diagnosis 781–782
environmental factors 776–777
epidemiology 75
familial aggregation 776–779
genetic background 776
HLA aetiology 776
juvenile 778, 1130–1131
laboratory findings 779–780
nail changes 777–778, *778*
ocular inflammation 779
pathology 777
prevalence 775–776
prognosis 779
radiology 780–781
sex ratio 776
spondylitic heart disease 779
treatment 782–783
Pubic rami, lesions 1458–1459
Public symphysis, stress lesions 1458
Pulmonary involvement in systemic sclerosis 1373–1374
Pulmonary hypertension in SLE 1329
Pulse steroid therapy in SLE 1344
Purines
biosynthesis 902, *903*
derivation 902
high-purine diet 910
influence of endogenous chemicals 905–911
Purpura
hypergammaglobulinaemic 1199
in immune complex disease 1198
Pustulotic arthro-osteitis 1239–1240
Pyoderma gangrenosum 1240–1241
Pyrophosphate arthropathy **938 – 949**
amyloidosis 944
apatite arthritis 945–946
associations with metabolic disease 943–944
in haemochromatosis 954
hereditary 938
hypomagnesaemia 944
hypophosphatasia 944
hypothyroidism 944
intra-articular therapy 590
Milwaukee shoulder 946, *946*
pathogenesis 944–945
radiology 940–941
sporadic 938–943

Radial neuropathy 1452

Radioisotopic imaging, osteonecrosis 1224
Radiological features 752–757
  sacroiliitis 752–753, *752*
  spinal changes 753–757
Radionuclide imaging 1632–1639
  aseptic necrosis 1636–1637
  back pain 1637
  bone infarction 1636–1637
  crush fractures 1637
  fibrosing diseases of lungs 1638–1639
  joint replacement 1639
  hypertrophic osteoarthropathy 1637
  radiopharmaceuticals 1632
  reflex dystrophy syndrome 1637–1638
  role in arthritis complications 1636
  sacroiliac joint quantification 1635–1636
  salivary scintigraphy 1638
  use of isotopes 1632
  use in joint disease 1533–1635
Radiopharmaceuticals 1632–1633
Radiotherapy, in osteoarthrosis 876
Raynaud's phenomenon 1153–1154
  in acromegaly 963
  atrial myxoma 1259
  childhood 1131
  MCTD 1272
  SJögren's syndrome
  systemic sclerosis 1365–1366
Reactive arthritis 164, 166, 169–170, 173, 322, 428–429, 728
  see also Sexually Acquired Reactive Arthritis
  campylobacter jejuni 1146
  in childhood 1130
  epidemiology 72, 80
  gut infection 815–816
  yersinia enterocolitica 1146
Referred pain 148, 150, 153–154
Reflex dystrophy syndrome, radionuclide scanning 1637–1638
Rehabilitation **1497 – 1517**
  addresses 1517
  adult chronic polyarthritis, management 1517
  aids and adaptations 1503–1514
  assessment of patient 1498–1502
  classification of handicap *1498*
  health visitor 1514
  key situations 1515–1517
  nursing 1514
  occupational therapy 1503
  patient education 1514–1515
  physiotherapy 1502
  resources 1503
  social work 1514–1515
  spa treatment 1497
  WHO definition 1497–1498
Reiter's disease **787 – 805**
  aetiology 790–791
  age of onset 788, *788*
  arthritis 792–794
  bacillary dysentery 1146
  balanitis 791–792
  blood tests 798
  clinical features 791
  complications
    frequency *791*
    neurological 796
  differential diagnosis 799
  epidemiology 74–75, 788–789
  family studies 789–790, *789*
  gut infection 815–816
  heart involvement 796
  historical background 787
  HLA-B27 791
  incidence 788
  incomplete forms 1130
  integumentary lesions 794–795
  joint involvement 792–793, *792, 793*
  management 799–801
  ocular lesions 794
  oral lesions 795–796
  other lesions 790
  pathology 798
  prevalence 787–788
  pulmonary involvement 796
  radiological features 796–798
  recurrence 794
  residual disability 793–794, *793*
  salmonella 1146
  sex ratio 788
  spinal involvement 794
  synovial fluid 798
  triad 787
  urogenital lesions 791–792
  venereal transmission 788
Relapsing polychondritis 1255–1257
Renal disease
  overlap in MCTD 1273
  in Sjögren's syndrome 1394
Respiratory disease 630–633
Rest
  see physical treatment of rheumatic diseases 1483–1496
Resticuloendothelial system in SLE 1330
Reticulohistocytosis, multicentric 1196–1197
Reticulum cell sarcoma 1247
Retrocalcaneal bursitis 1474
Retroviruses 440–442
Rheumatic complications in pregnancy 894–986
Rheumatic diseases
  see also Rheumatological practice
  arrangements for care 52–53
  attitudes 54
  burden on society 49
  classification 24–30, *28*
  community burden 45
  consequences of rheumatic disorders 41–44, *42*
  control of rheumatic disorders 50–52
  International Classification of Diseases 37–30
  knowledge 53–54
  mortality 44
  nomenclature 2–24, *20, 22, 23, 24*
  physical treatment **1483 – 1496**
  rheumatic disorders in hospital 45–46, *46*
    outside hospital 47–49
  rheumatic suffering 39–50
  skills 54
  WHO International Classification of Impairments, Disabilities and Handicaps 41
Rheumatic fever **1057 – 1099**
  acute attack, management 1086
  aetiology 1063–1065
  after-care 1089
  age incidence 1063
  arthritis 1070–1073
  chorea 1087–1081, *1080*
  see chorea for detail
  clinical aspects 1069
  complications 1082–1083
  course 1083
  criteria 1057
  definition 1057
  differential diagnosis
    Duckett-Jones criteria *1084*
    Hallidie-Smith and Bywaters criteria *1085*
    from rheumatoid arthritis 1086
  environmental factors 1064–1065
  epidemiology 108–109, 1066
  erythrocyte sedimentation rate 1081
  genetic factors 1065
  geographical factors 1063–1064
  heart involvement 1075–1076, 1079, 1089
    clinical aspects 1075–1076
    failure 1076
    pericarditis 1076
    rhythm change 1076
    subacute bacterial endocarditis 1082
  historical background 4–6
  hospital admission 1057
  infection 1059–1063
    and streptococci 1059–1063, *1065*
  laboratory aids 1081–1082
  lung changes 1077
  mortality 1064
  nodules 1068, 1074, *1068, 1075*
  pathology 1066
  pneumonia 1069, *1069*
  pregnancy 1083–1084
  prevalence 1057–1059
  prognosis 1083
  prophylaxis 1089–1091
    vaccination 1091
  pulse 1069–1070
  renal involvement 1078
  respiration 1069–1070
  rheumatic pneumonia 1077
    treatment 1078
  seasonal factors 1063–1064, *1058*
  serositis 1078
  sex incidence 1063
  skin manifestations 1073–1074
  streptococci 424–425, 1059–1063, *1065*
  symptomatology 1069
  temperature 1069–1070
  therapy 1086–1091
    ACTH 1088
    penicillin 1088

Rheumatic fever *cont*
salicylates 1087–1088
steroid 1088
Rheumatic heart disease 1057–1058, 1063
mortality 1064
prevalence 1057–1058, *1058*
Rheumatoid arthritis **515 – 719**
aetiology 597–599
aetiopathogenesis 595–602
amyloidosis 691–692
anaemia 685–688, 713–714
ankle 671
articular features 655–674
articular manifestations 653–705
back pain 1429
bacterial infection 425–427
Baker's cysts 669, *669*
bones 691–692
cardiac involvement 682–683
cardiovascular system 712–713
carpal tunnel syndrome 1451
cervical spine 657–660
disease, surgery 1545–1546
clinicopathological spectrum 595–597
corticosteroid therapy 539
course 655
cytotoxic drug therapy 549–550
death statistics 643–644, *643, 644*
definition 595–597
diagnostic criteria 595
differential diagnosis 692–693
drugs 710–712
ear 674
elbow 660
environmental factors 597–598
epidemiology 63–67
explanation 706–707
extra-articular complications 712–714
Felty's syndrome 11, 640–641, 689, *640*
foot 671–673
gastrointestinal tract 678–679
genetic factors 589–599
hand 661–668
historical background, 10–12, 653–654
history-taking 706
hyperviscosity syndrome 689
infection 714
intra-articular corticosteroid 584–585
intra-articular gold 587
juvenile chornic arthritis 638
knee 699–671
lungs 713
lymph nodes 690
management 706–719
medication 709–712
neuropathy 713
ocular complications 713
ocular manifestations 683–684
onset 654
pathology 604–652, *604*
anatomical consequences 618–620
articular diseases 605
associated syndromes 638, 640–642
bone disease 621–622
cartilage destruction 615–618
cell proliferation 611–612
coincidental disease 624–638
consequences of treatment 642–643
medical 642
surgical 642–643
diagnostic biopsy 622–624
fibrosis and repair 614–615, *615*
immunopathology 612, *612, 613*
juxta-articular connective tissues 620–621
synovial disease 605
patients' problems 707–709
penicillamine 527–528
peripheral neuropathy 678
prodromal symptoms 654–655
prognosis 655
psoriatic arthropathy 640
pulmonary involvement 680–682
retroviruses 440–442
septic complications 692
shoulder 660
Sjögren's syndrome 684–685, *685*
skin lesions 690
subcutaneous nodules 674–676
surgery 714–715
systemic manifestations 674–691
vasculitis 676–678, 1309–1314
wrist 661–668
Rheumatoid factor 355–362, *359*
in SLE 1339
Rheumatoid synovitis, arthroscopic appearance 1606
Rheumatoid vasculitis 676–678
clinical features 1310–1313, *1311*
diagnosis 1309–1310
laboratory tests 1313, *1313*
prognosis 1313
treatment 1314
Rheumatological practice **19 – 58**
see also Rheumatic diseases
Rice bodies 261, 1200
Rickets 1008–1014, *1009, 1013*
Rider's bone 1458
Rigid spine syndrome 765
Ritchie index (articular) *1571, 1591*
Rocky Mountain spotted fever 1150
Romanus lesion 755, *755*
Rose-Waaler test 356
Ross River virus 1151–1152
Rubella arthritis 1150–1151

Sacroiliac joint, radionuclide imaging, quantification 1653–1636
Sacroiliac strain 1424
Sacroiliitis
ankylosing spondylitis, radiology 752, *752, 753*
computerised tomography 1627
elicitation of pain 749
pain 1456–1457
Salicylates **500 – 513**
acute gout, management 921
aspirin 508–509, 587, 1343
benorylate 509
chemistry 500
choline magnesium trisalicylate 510
diflunisal 509
historical background 6, 500
pharmacological properties 500–502
in rheumatic fever 1087–1088
salsalate 509
side-effects 503–509
blood, coagulation 506
cardiovascular 505
central nervous system 505
dyspepsia 504
endocrine 505
gastrointestinal bleeding 504
gastrointestinal toxicity 503–504
hypersensitivity 507
kidney 504
liver 505
pregnancy 506
protective 507
pulmonary 506
salicylate intoxication 506–507
therapeutic properties 502–503
therapeutic use in rheumatic diseases 507–508
Salivary glands
in Sjögren's syndrome, investigations 1390–1392
in systemic sclerosis 1364
Salivary scintigraphy 1638
Salmonella
arthritis 1145–1146
infection predominantly causing osteomyelitis in sickle cell disease 1190
Salsalate 509
SARA
see Sexually Acquired Reactive Arthritis
Sarcoidosis 1230–1231
childhood 1132
diagnosis 1230
incidence 1230
joint disease, patterns 1230
in negroes 1230
prognosis 1230
radiology 1230
remission 1230
salivary scintigraphy 1638
sarcoid myopathy 1231
sex ratio 1230
Sarcoma
chondrosarcoma 1247
fibrosarcoma 1247
melanotic 1246
osteosarcoma 1247, *1248*
reticulum-cell 1247
synovial 1244–1246
Scheuermann's disease 1212
Scheuermann's osteochondritis 1427–1428
Schirmer's test 1389
Schmorl's nodes, 1212, 1412, *1413*
Sciatica 1413
Sciatic nerve compression 1461
Sciatic scoliosis 1414, *1414*
Sclerodactyly 1367
Scleroderma
see systemic sclerosis **1364 – 1385**

Scleroderma *cont*
-like features in MCTD 1273
Sclerosis, systemic **1364 – 1385**
Scoliosis, sciatic 1414, *1414*
Septic arthritis, epidemiology 80–81
Seronegative spondarthritides **723 – 744**
see also Ankylosing spondylitis, Enteropathic arthritis, Psoriatic arthritis, Reiter's disease
acute anterior uveitis 727–728
aetiopathogenesis 735–736
associations 736–737
clinical overlap 724–727, *724*
criteria 723–733, *725*
DISH 733–735
disorders showing spondarthritis-like features 733–735
erosive osteoarthritis 735
erosive spondyloarthropathy 734
familial aggregation 728–730
HLA-B27 730–733
intestinal bypass arthritis, dermatitis syndrome 734
irradiation 767
pustulotic arthro-osteitis 733–734
reactive arthritis 728
undifferentiated seronegative peripheral arthritis 733
Seronegative spondylopathies, back pain 1429
Seropositive (Igm rheumatoid factor) juvenile arthritis 1125–1127
Serositis 1078
Serum antistreptolysin O titre in rheumatic fever 1082
Serum complement levels in SLE 1339
Serum urate, indications for lowering in acute gout 922
Serum uric acid
alcohol, effect of 915
in gout 894–895
values 899
hypouricaemia 917–918, *917*
Sever's disease 1212
Sex hormones and osteoarthrosis 852–853
Sexually acquired reactive arthritis (SARA) 320, 423–424, 815–816
see also reactive arthritis
bacterial infection 427–428
Sharpey's fibres 227
Shober's method (lumbar spine flexion check) 1575, *1576*
Shoulder
acromioclavicular joint 1443–1444, 1614
acute calcific bursitis 1442–1443, *1443*
arthrography 1607–1608
arthropathies 1445–1446
aseptic necrosis 1445–1446
chronic bursitis 1442
examination 1442, 1576–1577
extra-capsular lesions 1442
fibrositis 1446
frozen 1444
history-taking 1442
housewife's 1446
inflammatory arthritis 1444
intra-capsular lesion 1444
mechanisms 1442–1442
Milwaukee shoulder 1446
muscle wasting 1442
and neck 1441–1447
see Neck and shoulder **1435 – 1477** for detail
neuralgic amyotraphy, mosaic form 1446–1447
osteoarthrosis 863–864
periarthritis in diabetes 980
pericapsular myalgia 1446
posture 1446
sepsis 1445–1446
shoulder-hand syndrome 1444–1445
subacromial bursa 1442–1443
surgery 1547–1549
syringomelia *1445*
tendinitis 1443
tendinitis, injection techniques
bicipital 1613–1614
supraspinatus 1613, *1613*
terminology 1442
trauma 1444
Shoulder-hand syndrome 1444–1445
Dupuytren's diathesis 1444
predisposition 1444
treatment 1444–1445
'Shrinking' lungs 1330, *1330*
Sicca syndrome 323
Sickle-cell disease 1186–1190
avascular necrosis 1188–1189
diagnosis 1190
gout 1190
hand-foot syndrome 1190
hyperuricaemia 1190
osteomyelitis predominantly caused by *Salmonella* infection 1190
racial factor 1186
radiology *1187, 1189*
synovial effusions 1190
Sindig-Larsen syndrome 1212
Sindig-Larsen-Johansson disease 1464
Sjögren's syndrome 684–685, **1386 – 1403,** *685*
aetiology 1400–1401
arthritis 1392–1393
associated conditions 1387
miscellaneous 1395–1396
other causes of sicca syndrome 1395–1396
rheumatoid arthritis 641–642
symptoms 1388
autoimmune exocrinopathy 1390–1391
clinical manifestations 1394
cutaneous manifestations 1394
definition 1386
differential diagnosis 1386
drug reactions 1400
epidemiology 88
exocrine function, impaired 1388
gastrointestinal disease 1393
genetics 1398
haematological disturbances 1395
historical background 1387
immunopathology 1396–1398
keratoconjunctivitis sicca, diagnosis 1389–1390
liver involvement 1393
lymphoproliferation 1398–1399
malignancy 1398–1399
neurological involvement 1394–1395
pathological manifestations 1387
primary 1386
pulmonary involvement 1395
Raynaud's phenomenon 1393
relationship between autoimmune diseases and sicca features *1386*
Schirmer's test 1389
secondary 1386
SLE 1331
systemic features 1392–1395
treatment 1399–1400
drugs, side effects 1400
general management 1399
problems of reduced secretions 1399–1400
systemic 1400
xeropthalmia 1387
xerostomia 1388
Skin
atrophy in corticosteroid therapy 542
changes in systemic sclerosis 1367–1371
in SLE 1327–1328
Small vessel vasculitis 1314–1316
Smallpox arthritis 1152
Snapping hip 1456
Soft tissue lesions
computerised tomography 1631
non-articular corticosteroid injection 585–586
Solganol 530
South-East Asia and Pacific Area League against Rheumatism (SEAPAL) 15
Spa treatment 10, 14, 1497
Spinal cord 1438–1439
Spinal stenosis 1418–1420
causes 1629, *1419*
computerised tomography 1629
criteria 1629–1630
diagnosis 1420
epidemiology 98–99
management 1420
Spine
cervical intubation 1524
computerised tomography 1628–1630
examination 1575–1576
function 1408–1411
osteoarthrosis 864–866
radionuclide scanning 1637
referred pain 1457, 1459
spinal cord 1438–1439
structure 1408–1411
surgery 1545–1547
in osteoarthrosis 897
Spondarthritides
historical background 12–13
seronegative **723 – 744**
Spondylitis
brucellar 1142
exercise 1495

Spondylitis *cont*
juvenile 1127–1129
physical treatment 1495
Spondyloarthropathies **723 – 744**
see also seronegative spondarthritides
in children 1127–1132, *1127*
Spondylodisciitis 755–756, *755*
Spondylolisthesis 1420–1422
spondylotic 1422
Spondylosis 1420–1422
Spondylosis
back pain **1407 – 1434**
cervical 1437–1438
disc disorders 1407–1434
epidemiology 95–99
lumbar 1416–1418
Spondylotic spondyolisthesis 1422
Sporotrichosis 1155
Sprengel's shoulder 1439
Starvation, predisposing factor in gout 912, *913*
Statistics 1594
Stenosis, spinal 1418–1420
causes 1629, *1419*
computerised tomography, criteria 1629–1630
diagnosis 1420
management 1420
Sternoclavicular joint, osteoarthrosis 864
Steroids in rheumatic fever 1088
Stevens-Johnson syndrome 726, 1142, *726*
Still's disease
see Juvenile chronic arthritis **1100 – 1124**
Stiff man syndrome 765
Stiffness, measurement 1590
'Stuck' back 1424
Student's elbow 1450
Sudek's atrophy 1478
Sulindac 517
Sulphinpyrazone 577–578
Superior tibiofibular joint synovitis 1466
Suppurative arthritis, acute 1137–1139
Sural nerve compression 1462
Surgery **1518 – 1565**
aims 1519
ankle 1534–1535
arthrodesis 1531, 1559
arthroplasty 1530–1531
arthroscopy 1535–1536
drug therapy 1524–1525
elbow 1549–1550
feet 1531–1534
fingers 1554–1559
deformities 1559–1560, *1559*
general considerations 1522
health, local disease
hand 1554–1559
in osteoarthrosis 1560
influencing factors 1523
intestinal bypass surgery arthritis 814–815, 1241
dermatitis syndrome 734
intubation 1524
knee 1535–1536, 1539–1540, *1540*
hip, total replacement 1540–1545
complications 1542–1545
nerve compression syndromes 1553–1554
osteotomy 1531
patient assessment 1519–1522
patient handling 1524
shoulder 1547–1549
spine 1545–1547
synovectomy 1529–1530
technical considerations 1526–1528
thromboembolism 1525–1526, *1526*
wrist 1550–1553, 1554–1559
wound healing 1522–1524
Swelling, measurement, Geigy gauge 1590
Sydenham Thomas 5, 7, 8
Syndesmophyte(s)
in ankylosing spondylitis 754, 757–758, *758, 759*
differentiation from osteophyte(s) 754, *754*
psoriasis 781
Syndrome de la loge de Guyon 1554
Synovectomy 1529–1530, 1536
hand and wrist 1556–1557
elbow joint 1549–1550
wrists and tendon sheaths 1550–1553
Synovial biopsy
arthroscopic methods 1597, 1608–1609
interpretation 1609
histopathology of synovitis 1609–1610
Synovial cells 207–209, 258, 264
Synovial chondromatosis 1241–1242
Synovial chondrosarcoma 1246
Synovial effusions in sickle cell disease 1190
Synovial fluid **251 – 277**, 824
analysis 259–273
arthrocentesis 259
cell counts
differential 266
total 261–263, *261*
composition 251–257
examination 251–277
formation 257–258
gross appearances 260–263, *260*
hydroxyapatite crystals, detection 271–272
immunology 272–273
intra-articular pressure 258
joint aspiration 259
micro-organisms 272
microscopy 263–266
mucin clot test 261
in osteoarthrosis 869–870
pathology 838–839
in Reiter's disease 798
removal 257–258
rice bodies 261
samples 259–260
volume 260
Synovial joints 229–232
classification 229–231, *231*
cervical spine 1437–1438
movement 231–232
structure 229–231
Synovial membrane 334–340, *339*
Synovial rupture 1469–1471
co-existing thrombosis 1471
investigation 1469
management 1470
Synovial sarcoma 1244–1246
Synovial shelf-syndrome 1463
Synovial tissue 232
in gout, examination 895–896
Synovioma 1244–1246
Synovitis
crystal, arthroscopic appearance 1607
histopathology 1610–1611
inflammatory, arthroscopic appearance 1605–1606
methods of quantitation 1634
pigmented villondular 1242–1244
arthroscopic appearance 1606
radionuclide imaging 1633–1634
relationship with osteoarthrosis 840–841
rheumatoid, arthroscopic appearance 1606
superior tibiofibular joint 1466
traumatic 1239
Synovium 824
cartilage-catabolin, effects on 233–235
osteoarthrosis, pathology 839–840
synovial chondromatosis 1241–1242
Syphilis
acquired 1147–1148
congenital 1146–1147
Syringomelia 1445, *1445*
Systemic lupus erythematosus (SLE) 323–324, **1325 – 1349**
aetiology 1330–1341
age of onset 1131
animal models 1341
ANA-negative lupus 1335
blood
abnormalities 1334
vessels 1329–1330
cardiovascular system 1328–1329
central nervous system
disease 1333–1334
involvement 1131
in childhood 1131
clinical features 1131, 1325–1334
clinical manifestations 1326, *1326, 1327*
congenital heart block 1329
corticosteroid therapy 540
cytotoxic drug therapy 550–551
differential diagnosis 1341–1342
additional features *1342*
ARA criteria *1342*
drug-induced lupus 1335–1336, *1336*
epidemiology 85
effect of UV light 1341
epidemiology 82–86, 1325–1326
gastrointestinal system 1331
genetic factors 1340
historical background 1325
hormonal factors 1340–1341
hypercatabolism, tissue fixation and 402–403
immunological features 1336–1340
infection 1334

Systemic lupus erythematosus (SLE) *cont*
levamisole therapy 562
–like features in MCTD 1273
management 1343–1345
anti-malarials 1343
aspirin 1343
corticosteroids 1343–1344
general 1342
immunosuppressive agents 1344
NSAIDs 1343
plasmapheresis 1345
pulse steroid therapy 1344
sex hormone therapy 1345
musculoskeletal system 1328
ocular lesions 1334
organ-specific antibodies 1340
osteonecrosis 1220–1222
radiological changes 1222, *1221*
overlap with MCTD 1336
pathology 1326
pregnancy 1335
prevalence 1325
prognosis 1131, 1345, *1344*
pulmonary hypertension 1329
pulmonary involvement, pleurisy 1330
racial incidence 1326
renal involvement 1331–1333, *1332*
reticuloendothelial system 1330–1331
retroviruses 440–442
sex ratio 1325
'shrinking' lungs 1330, *1330*
thrombophlebitis 1329–1330
tissue fixation and hypercatabolism 402–403
variants 1335–1336
abortion 1335
discoid lupus 1335
neurological disease 1335
thrombosis 1335
vasculitis 1329–1330
viral agents 1341
Systemic sclerosis 324, **1364 – 1385**
age incidence 1364
cardiac involvement 1374
changes
connective tissue 1376
immunological 1377–1379
inflammatory 1377–1379
microcirculatory 1376–1377
classification 1364–1365, *1364*
clinical features 1365–1376
CREST syndrome 1375
diagnostic criteria 1364, *1364*
disease sub-types 1375–1376
electromyographic abnormalities 1371
environmental factors 1365
eosinophilic fasciitis 1375–1376
epidemiology 86–87, 1364–1365
frequency of organ involvement *1365*
gastrointestinal involvement 1372–1373
pathology 1372
genetic factors 1365
incidence 1364
joints 1371
kidney involvement 1364
mixed connective tissue disease 1375
muscle involvement 1371
neurological involvement 1371
occupational factors 1364–1365
overlap syndromes 1375–1376
pathogenesis 1376–1379
pathology 1365–1376
peripheral vascular disease 1365–1366
presenting features 1365
prognosis 1379
pulmonary involvement 1373–1374
fibrosing alveolitis 1374
hyperplastic changes 1374
race factor 1364
Raynaud's phenomenon 1365
salivary glands 1373
sex ratio 1364
skin changes 1367–1371
acrosclerosis 1367
proximal scleroderma 1368
sclerodactyly 1367
typical findings 1368–1371
specific organ involvement, management 1380–1381
tendons 1371
treatment 1379–1381
anti-fibrotic drugs 1380
anti-inflammatory therapy 1380
general 1379
immunosuppressive therapy 1380
improvement of peripheral microcirculation 1379–1380
symptomatic 1379

Takayasu's arteritis 1316–1317
Tarsal tunnel syndrome 1462
T-cells 273
ankylosing spondylitis 760
effect of immunomodulators *558*
immune deficiency 1199
immunogenetics 310–313
leukaemia 1193
in rheumatoid synovial membrane 600–601
suppressor function in SLE 1336
in synovial disease 607, 613–614
Temporal arteritis **1278 – 1291**, 1316, 1440–1441
Temporomandibular arthritis 622, 864
Tendinitis 1443
Achilles 1619
bicipital 1448–1449
knee 1467
patellar 1464
surgery 1549
Tendons 220
repairs 1553
rupture *1553*
in systemic sclerosis 1371
Tennis elbow 1449–1450
injection technique 1614–1615, *1615*
Tenosynovitis, ankle 1474
injection technique 1616, *1616*
Tenovaginitis
of abductor pollicis longus 1452
stenosing 1453
Thalassaemia 1186, 1191
haemosiderosis 1191
pathogenesis of synovitis 1191
race factor 1186
radiology 1191
radiotherapy 1191
treatment 1191
Therapeutic evaluation **1581 – 1596**
see Clinical Trials for detail
Thiemann's disease 851, 1213, *851, 852, 1213*
Thiopurinol 574
Thoracic outlet syndrome 1438–1439
Thoracic pain 1427
Thrombocytosis 1185
correlation with complications and severity of rheumatoid disease *1186*
Thromboembolism, in surgery 1525–1526, *1526*
Thrombosis (deep vein) and synovial rupture 1471
Thymopoietin 559, 561–562
Thyroid 967–968
acropachy 971, 1263, 1475
and osteoarthrosis 852
Tiaprofenic acid 520–521
Tibia, stress fractures 1472–1473
Tienilic acid, in management of gout 925
Tolmetin 517
Tophi 886–887
in gout, examination 895–896, *866*
Torticollis 1436–1438, 1440–1441
Torulosis 1154
Touraine-Solente-Gole syndrome 1252–1253, *1253*
Trapezium excision in osteoarthrosis 878
Trauma
computerised tomography 1630–1631
inflammation 294
traumatic synovitis 1239
Treatment, physical
see Rheumatic diseases, physical treatment **1483 – 1496**
Treatment, surgical
see Surgery **1518 – 1565**
Trigger finger 1453
Trochanteric bursitis 1456
Tuberculosis
arthritis 1142–1143
diagnosis 1143
incidence 1142
management 1143–1144
pattern 1142
sites 1142–1143
Tumours
arising from bone/cartilage 1246–1250
articular 1241–1253
arthropathies associated with non-articular neoplastic disease 1250–1251
back pain 1429–1430
benign 1244
malignant 1244–1250

Ulcerative colitis
aetiology 810–813
association with ankylosing spondylitis 762, 810–812
clinical features 810–812, *811*
enteropathic arthritis 810–813
finger clubbing 813
HLA-B27 813
investigations 810–812
joints involved *811*
musculoskeletal disorders 813
spondylitis 812
treatment 811–812
Ulnar neuropathy 1451
Undifferentiated connective tissue disease (UCTD) 1276
Urate(s)
acute gout 887–890
chronic gout 891
crystals in gout 891, *891*
deposition, sites 891, *891*
identification 895, *895, 896*
histological demonstration 890
increased clearance causing hypouricaemia 917–918
monosodium urate monohydrate, crystalline 890
Uric acid
see also Hyperuricaemia
asymptomatic hyperuricaemia 925–926
calculi 892
formation 892
cardiovascular disease 916–917
decreased excretion
alterations in fluid volume, renal function 911
effects of drugs 911–912
effects of starvation and ketosis 912, *913*
essential hypertension 913
hypercalcaemia 914
hyperparathyroidism 914
lactic acidaemia 912
lead poisoning 913
myxoedema 914
saturnine gout 913
excretion 905–906
gout
see also Gout
serum levels 894–895, 899
conversion scale 899n, *899*
haemoglobin plasma protein 917
hyperuricaemia
age variations 901
from increased formation 906–909
genetic factors 901, 908
non-gouty conditions 899
sex ratio 900–901
increased formation 906–911
lithiasis 892
metabolism 901
formation 901
structural formulae *902*
molecular components 901
origins *902*
Uricosuric drugs in long-term management of gout 925
Uveitis 322

van Breemen, Jan 15, *15*
van der Hoeve's triad 1003
Vascular disease, peripheral in systemic sclerosis 1365–1366
Vasculitis **1292 – 1324**
associated with other connective tissue diseases 1314
classification 1292–1294, *1292, 1293*
clinical syndromes
lymphoid granulomatosis 1308
overlap syndrome with other necrotising arteritides 1308–1309
polyarteritis nodosa
classical 1297–1304
localised 1302
systemic necrotising arteritis 1297–1309
corticosteroid therapy 539
definition 1292
granulomatous 1293–1294, 1304–1306
allergic angiitis 1304–1306
clinical features *1305*
diagnosis 1304–1305
differential diagnosis from polyarteritis nodosa 1304
laboratory features 1305
overlap with polyarteritis nodosa 1293–1294
prognosis 1305
relationship to arteritis 1293
treatment 1305–1306
large vessel arteritis 1316–1317
Takayasu's 1316–1317
temporal 1316
pathogenetic mechanisms 1294–1297
rheumatoid 1309–1314, *1309*
in SLE 1329–1330
small vessel arteritis 1316
viral infection 1296
Vertebrae
cervical,
developmental abnormalities 1439–1440
disease 1440
fracture, spinal pain 1422–1423
intervertebral discs 1438
Vertebral ankylosing hyperostosis, diabetes 973–974
Viral infection in vasculitis 1296
Virus(es) 1152–1153
infection 1150–1153
Visual disturbances in giant cell arteritis 1284–1285
Vitamin D 229
in bone metabolism 995–997, *996*
von Gierke's disease 910
von Recklinghausen's disease 999
von Willebrand's disease 1177–1178, *1177*

Waldenström's macroglobulinaemia 1195
diagnosis 1195
management 1195
Wegener's granulomatosis 539–540, 1306–1308
clinical features 1306–1308
diagnosis 1306
laboratory tests 1308
prognosis 1308
treatment 1308
Whip-lash injury 1440
Whipple's disease 729–730
aetiology 814
association with ankylosing spondylitis 762, 814
clinical features 813–814
enteropathic arthritis 813
HLA-B27 814
investigations 813–814
treatment 814
White cell count in rheumatic fever 1081
WHO International Classification of Impairments, Disabilities and Handicaps 41
Wilson's disease 956
and osteoarthrosis 853
Wrist
arthrography 1607–1608
De Quervain's syndrome 1452
examination 1577
injection techniques 1615–1616, *1616, 1617*
median nerve compression 1450
osteoarthrosis 863
surgery 1550–1560
success rating *1556*
tenovaginitis of abductor pollicis longus 1452
writer's cramp 1453

Xanthine oxidase
inhibitors 905, 915, 922–924, *924*
principal action in man 905
Xanthomata in hyperlipoproteinaemia 1237–1238
Xeropthalmia 1387
Xerostomia 1388
X-rays in differential diagnosis 172–173

Yaws 1148–1149
Yersinia enterocolitica arthritis 322, 428–429, 1146
Yttrium (^{90}Y), intra-articular irradiation 588–589